MW01254896

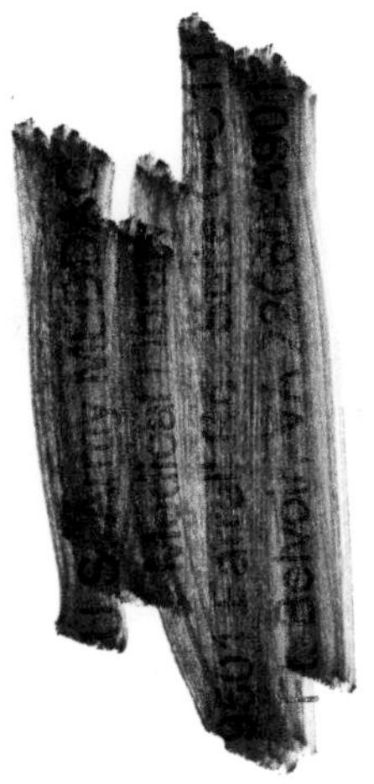

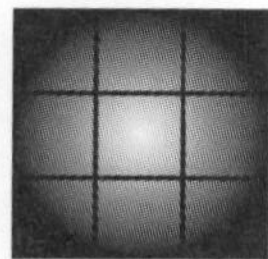

American Academy
of Pediatrics

# Textbook of Adolescent Health Care

**Editor in Chief**

*Martin M. Fisher, MD, FAAP*

**Coeditors**

*Elizabeth M. Alderman, MD, FAAP*

*Richard E. Kreipe, MD, FAAP*

*Walter D. Rosenfeld, MD, FAAP*

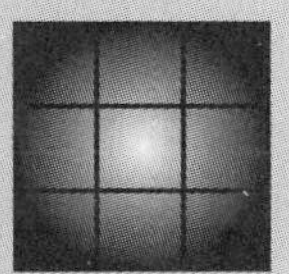

American Academy of Pediatrics

# Textbook of Adolescent Health Care

*Martin M. Fisher, MD, FAAP*

**Editor in Chief**

*Chief, Division of Adolescent Medicine*
*Steven and Alexandra Cohen Children's Medical Center of New York*
*North Shore-Long Island Jewish Health System*
*New Hyde Park, New York*
*Professor of Pediatrics, Hofstra North Shore-LIJ School of Medicine*

**Coeditors**

*Elizabeth M. Alderman, MD, FAAP*
*Professor of Clinical Pediatrics*
*Division of Adolescent Medicine*
*Albert Einstein College of Medicine*
*Children's Hospital at Montefiore*

*Richard E. Kreipe, MD, FAAP*
*Professor of Pediatrics*
*Director, Leadership Education in Adolescent Health (LEAH) Training Program*
*Medical Director, Western New York Comprehensive Care Center for Eating Disorders*
*Division of Adolescent Medicine, Department of Pediatrics*
*Golisano Children's Hospital, University of Rochester Medical Center*

*Walter D. Rosenfeld, MD, FAAP*
*Chairman of Pediatrics*
*Goryeb Children's Hospital*
*Atlantic Health*
*Morristown, New Jersey*

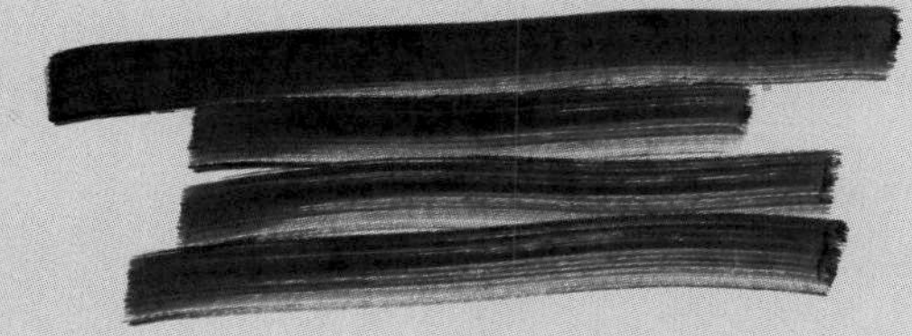



American Academy of Pediatrics

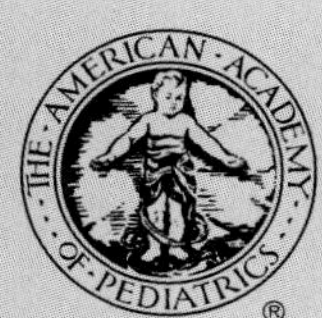


DEDICATED TO THE HEALTH OF ALL CHILDREN™

*Director, Department of Marketing and Publications:* **Maureen DeRosa, MPA**
*Director, Division of Product Development:* **Mark Grimes**
*Senior Developmental Editor:* **Diane Lundquist, MS**
*Editorial Assistant:* **Carrie Peters**
*Director, Division of Publishing and Production Services:* **Sandi King, MS**
*Manager, Publications Production and Manufacturing:* **Theresa Wiener**
*Director, Division of Marketing and Sales:* **Kevin Tuley**
*Manager, Clinical and Professional Publications Marketing:* **Linda Smessaert**
*Cover Design:* **Linda Diamond**

Library of Congress Control Number: 2010915359
ISBN-13: 978-1-58110-269-7
MA0403

The recommendations in this publication do not indicate an exclusive course of treatment or serve as a standard of medical care. Variations, taking into account individual circumstances, may be appropriate.

Every effort has been made to ensure that the drug selection and dosage set forth in this text are in accordance with the current recommendations and practice at the time of publication. It is the responsibility of the health care provider to check the package insert of each drug for any change in indications and dosage and for added warnings and precautions.
The mention of product names in this publication is for informational purposes only and does not imply endorsement by the American Academy of Pediatrics.

The publishers have made every effort to trace the copyright holders for borrowed material. If they have inadvertently overlooked any, they will be pleased to make the necessary arrangements at the first opportunity.



Printed in the United States of America.
Publisher's Cataloging-In-Publication Data
(Prepared by The Donohue Group, Inc.)

American Academy of Pediatrics textbook of adolescent health care / Martin M. Fisher, editor in chief; coeditors: Elizabeth M. Alderman ... [et al.].

p. : ill. ; cm.

Includes bibliographical references and index.
ISBN: 978-1-58110-269-7

1. Adolescent medicine. 2. Adolescent psychology. 3. Teenagers–Health and hygiene. I. Fisher, Martin, 1950- II. Alderman, Elizabeth Meller. III. American Academy of Pediatrics. IV. Title: Textbook of adolescent health care

RJ550 .A64 2011
616.00835 2010915359

9-286/0411
1 2 3 4 5 6 7 8 9 10

# Dedication

We dedicate this textbook to the countless professionals who have contributed to the knowledge contained in it, to health care professionals who will use that knowledge to improve the health of adolescents and young adults, and to the well-being of present and future generations of youth to whom we have dedicated our careers.

To my wife Miriam, for her understanding and respect; my children: Adina and Josh, Jessica, and Robert and Sara, who embody the potential inherent in young people; and my grandchildren Ariella and Alex, who remind me anew of the miracle of human development.

*Martin M Fisher, MD*

To my parents and sisters, to whom I owe my wonderful adolescence, my husband, Eric, with love, for supporting all my work toward bettering the health and lives of adolescents, and our children, Sara and Jeremy, still teenagers, who have been my best teachers.

*Elizabeth M Alderman, MD*

To my family: my parents who tolerated and nurtured my own adolescence; my brother and sister who provided role models as I grew into young adulthood; my wife for her endless patience and unwavering love and support for me; my niece and nephew who are parenting our family's next generation of adolescents; and to our current/future adolescents Elizabeth, Garrett, Nolan, Katelyn, Colin and Katherine who each give us hope for the future. You all inspire me.

*Richard E Kreipe, MD*

To my patients and all of my mentors who have taught me so much; to my parents and my sister Linda who tolerated and loved me as an adolescent; and, to my wife Lynne, and children, Ben and Alexandra, who have provided perspective and steadfast love while ensuring my humility; without them I could never have fully appreciated both the wonders and the struggles of being an adolescent and a parent.

*Walter D Rosenfeld, MD*

# Foreword

The biopsychosocial model defines the intimate relationship among biological, psychological, and social issues in our conceptualization of health and disease.[1] All activities relevant to adolescent health (health care, teaching, and research) should embrace this model to fully understand the profound relationships among biological, psychological, and social factors in the maintenance of health; the prevention of disease; the diagnosis and treatment of both biological and psychological conditions occurring during infancy and childhood; and the understanding of unique conditions that occur during adolescence with potentially profound effects on the development of the adolescent and one's health during adulthood. Adolescent health care providers are in the unique position to practice the biopsychosocial model of disease and to train our young people to understand these complex relationships. Investigators who seek to understand normal adolescent development, the relationship of environment and family to adolescent health and disease, and the complex interplay among biology, psychological factors, and social factors will do well to incorporate the biopsychosocial model into our activities be they at the bedside, the ambulatory setting, or in the community.

One only has to scan the major sections of this new textbook to understand the biopsychosocial model in adolescent health and disease. What is most striking is not only the comprehensive nature of the text, but also the new and contemporary issues that are addressed. The first section, The Foundations of Adolescent Health, includes traditional information on the epidemiology and care of the adolescent in several settings. In addition, the authors provide updated information on brain and cognitive development as our understanding of cognitive development explodes with the use of new technology. These new technologies tell us that beneath the skull there are demonstrable changes in the brain that evolve during adolescence and young adulthood that we have observed clinically for years but for which we did not understand the underlying mechanisms of the cognitive changes. These changes affect all aspects of health and disease. The family and environment, similar to earlier sections, are covered thoroughly.

The second section, Adolescent Sexuality and Reproductive Health, provides information with which most practitioners of adolescent health are familiar, such as adolescent sexual behaviors and reproductive health. There is new information, however, about the sexual health care needs of all adolescents as we learn more about the full expression of adolescent sexuality, through our research and through talking with heterosexual, gay, lesbian, and transgender youth. The third section, Medical and Surgical Conditions, is the most comprehensive section in the book and provides one place in which all medical and surgical conditions are included, which for the practitioner should expedite the availability of information. The fourth section, Psychosocial Issues, includes specific behaviors/conditions, psychiatric and behavioral issues, and educational issues. In these last 2 sections, important emphases are given to medical, surgical, and psychological/social conditions that first present during adolescence.

This text should be available to all practitioners of adolescent health. It provides a comprehensive and complete picture of the complexity of adolescent health care and should be the standard text for training programs and for those wishing to practice outstanding, contemporary adolescent health care delivery. I have known each editor over many years and admire their many years of devotion to the care of adolescents and now to this most comprehensive textbook. They have remarkable accumulated knowledge among them that they share generously through their collective wisdom as well as through their inclusion of outstanding authors to write the specific sections of this text. Each editor has a remarkable ability to grasp and to understand the pressure on youth and their families as a result of major changes in families and in our culture. We thank them for the creation of this text as a cornerstone for adolescent health activities.

Adolescents are the barometers of the health of our nation. Their health and behavior reflect what is occurring within their homes, schools, and the greater culture. We need to nurture our adolescents and allow them to meet their full potential. By assisting adolescents and their families toward optimum health, we shall ensure the health of each young person and ultimately the health of our nation.

1. Engel, G.L. The need for a new model; a challenge for biomedicine. *Science*. 1977; 196: 129–136

*Elizabeth R. McAnarney, MD*
*Professor of Pediatrics*
*Chair Emerita*
*University of Rochester Medical Center*

# Preface

As this textbook goes to publication at the start of the second decade of the 21st century, the field of adolescent health and medicine enters its seventh decade. Perhaps a quick historical overview will serve to map its progress before we delineate today's challenges and how we have tried to address them in this textbook. In 1941 a symposium on adolescence was held under the auspices of the American Academy of Pediatrics (AAP), the publisher of this textbook. That symposium is considered to be the initiating event demonstrating the incorporation of adolescent medicine into pediatric practice. Most of the studies presented at the symposium were by boarding school and college health physicians on topics related to emotional health, physical fitness, and nutrition.[1]

The 1950s and 1960s saw the development of hospital-based adolescent medicine programs in a scattering of cities in the United States and culminated in the establishment of the multidisciplinary Society for Adolescent Medicine in 1968. As the health issues of adolescents became better defined and more widely appreciated, the need for appropriate clinical services, better training, more research, and advocacy became apparent. The AAP formed the Committee on Adolescence in 1976, which guides AAP policy on health issues pertaining to adolescents, and in 1979 the AAP formally organized a Section on Adolescent Health, which provides continuing medical education in the field of adolescent medicine for the practicing pediatrician. The decades of the 1970s and 1080s saw the expansion of existing programs and the addition of new ones. The *Journal of Adolescent Health Care* was established in 1980, and in 1991 its name was changed to the *Journal of Adolescent Health*. The past 2 decades have witnessed the growth of the field internationally, as well as the recognition and expansion of its multidisciplinary nature—hence the name change of its professional organization to the Society for Adolescent Health and Medicine. Other organizations with a focus on adolescent health care were subsequently created, such as the North American Society for Pediatric and Adolescent Gynecology, the Society for Research in Adolescence, and the Academy for Eating Disorders. And to ensure standards, a subspecialty Board and Fellowship certification were established in North America in 1994.

Several textbooks on adolescent health have been published through these years, marking the state of knowledge along the way. This *Textbook of Adolescent Health Care* represents both the accumulation of that knowledge and a concerted effort by our team of experienced and respected professionals to address the rapidly evolving contemporary challenges facing us. Two recent documents (one from the Bureau of Children, Youth and Families at the Institute of Medicine[2] and one written by leaders in interdisciplinary adolescent health training in the United States[3]) suggest ways to address these challenges. Specifically, we need to (1) ensure that high-quality adolescent health care services are accessible, acceptable, appropriate, effective, and equitable; (2) make disease prevention, health promotion, and behavioral health a major component of routine health services, with a focus on the particular needs of specific groups of adolescents who may be especially vulnerable to risky behavior or poor health; (3) engage community health care providers, health organizations, and community agencies to develop coordinated, linked, and interdisciplinary adolescent health services; (4) maintain confidential health services so that adolescents have access to these services when necessary to protect their health; (5) expand professional training in adolescent medicine and adolescent health care to address the emerging needs of both specialists and primary care providers; (6) address the trainee and faculty career development issues specific to women and racial/ethnic minorities to ensure equity and enhance academic success in the field of adolescent health care; (7) demonstrate to all levels of trainees and faculty from a variety of professional disciplines the wide range of opportunities in adolescent medicine and health care, including clinical care, teaching, program development, scholarship, and research; and (8) encourage sharing of and research on best practices in adolescent health care, especially with respect to emerging issues.

We believe that the timing as well as the content and organization of the *Textbook of Adolescent Health Care* make it an invaluable resource for helping adolescent health professionals meet the challenges outlined above. Moreover, to maintain accuracy and relevance, the printed book will be followed by online revisions and updates that will be made available in succeeding years. The information is oriented to meet the needs of the many disciplines (including pediatricians and pediatric subspecialists, internists and family practitioners, nurses and nurse practitioners, social workers, and psychologists) as well as the levels of trainees (students, residents, and fellows) who care for adolescent patients. The multidisciplinary authorship is designed to not only provide the most expert review of the subject matter but to also foster a better integrated approach to adolescent health care so that professionals from disparate areas are more likely to work collaboratively to provide the best thinking, research, and care for this population.

Comprising 196 chapters, the book is organized into 4 sections. The first section, consisting of 48 chapters, and provides comprehensive and contemporary coverage of the foundations of adolescent health. It includes chapters on history and epidemiology; growth and development; approaches to the patient and family; health supervision and prevention; and such management issues as complementary and alternative medicine; assessment and management of acute and chronic pain; death, dying, and palliative care; pharmacology; and health policy and financing. Additional chapters focus on office-based and non–office-based settings (including hospital-based practice, school-based health care, college health, health care of incarcerated youth, and care of adolescents in military settings), and care of special populations (those who live outside of their family homes, adopted adolescents, adolescents with chronic illness and special health care needs). This opening section also addresses multiple family issues (connection between parents and adolescents, parenting issues, divorce and separation, adopted adolescents, adolescents with gay or lesbian parents, and those adolescents facing illness in the family).

Sections 2, 3, and 4 make up the bulk of the textbook. These are devoted to reproductive health and adolescent sexuality, medical and surgical disorders, and the psychosocial challenges faced by adolescents and their families. These chapters correspond to the content specifications for the Board Examination in Adolescent Medicine as developed by the parent American Board of Pediatrics (in conjunction with the Boards of Internal Medicine and of Family Practice), which stipulate that approximately 50% of questions come from the medical/surgical category, 25% reproductive health/adolescent sexuality, and 25% mental health/psychosocial issues. To allow this reference to be used as a study aid, these content specifications partially informed the development of chapters. However, a more important role for this textbook is as a guide for clinical management and psychosocial care.

The editors value the opportunity we have had to work on a project that we believe can help advance the field of adolescent health and medicine, to which we have devoted our careers. We thank the AAP and its staff, especially Diane Lundquist, for their support through the several years it has taken to put this book together. We thank the authors for providing their expertise and collaborating with us in such a highly professional manner. And we thank our families for their love and encouragement throughout.

*Martin M. Fisher, MD, FAAP, FSAHM*
*Elizabeth M. Alderman, MD, FAAP, FSAHM*
*Richard E. Kreipe, MD, FAAP, FSAHM*
*Walter D. Rosenfeld, MD, FAAP, FSAHM*
*Editors,* Textbook of Adolescent Health Care

## REFERENCES

1. Alderman EM, Rieder J, Cohen MI. The history of adolescent medicine. *Pediatr Res.* 2003;54:137–147

2. Committee on Adolescent Health Care Services and Models of Care for Treatment, Prevention, and Healthy Development, National Research Council. *Adolescent Health Services: Missing Opportunities*. Lawrence RS, Gootman JA, Sim LJ, eds. Washington, DC: National Academies Press; 2009

3. Hergenroeder AC, Benson PAS, Britto MT, et al. Adolescent medicine: workforce trends and recommendations. *Arch Pediatr Adolesc Med.* 2010;164(12):1086–1090

# Contributors

**Heather R. Adams, PhD**
University of Rochester Medical Center
Division of Child Neurology
Rochester, New York
192: *Neuropsychologic Testing of Adolescents*
194: *Psychoeducational Assessment of Adolescents*

**William P. Adelman, MD, FAAP**
Adolescent Medicine Consultant to the Army Surgeon General
Chief, Pediatric Primary Care Services
Walter Reed National Military Medical Center
Associate Professor of Pediatrics
Uniformed Services University of the Health Sciences
Bethesda, Maryland
68: *Disorders of Male Genitalia*

**Dale M. Ahrendt, MD, FAAP**
Program Director, Adolescent Medicine Fellowship
San Antonio Uniformed Services Health Education Consortium
Consultant to the Air Force Surgeon General for Adolescent Medicine
San Antonio, Texas
28: *Health Care of Adolescents in Military Settings*

**Harvey Aiges, MD, FAAP**
(deceased)
100: *Disorders of the Liver and Pancreas*

**Lindsey Albrecht, MD**
University of California Davis
Department of Pediatrics
Section of Endocrinology
Sacramento, California
70: *Disorders of Puberty*

**Elizabeth Alderman, MD, FAAP, FSAHM**
Professor of Clinical Pediatrics
Division of Adolescent Medicine
Albert Einstein College of Medicine
Children's Hospital at Montefiore
Bronx, New York
40: *Socioeconomic Status*
61: *The Uterus and Adnexa*
195: *Gifted Adolescents*

**Seth Ammerman, MD, FAAP**
Clinical Professor, Division of Adolescent Medicine
Department of Pediatrics
Stanford University
Lucile Packard Children's Hospital
Palo Alto, California
173: *Tobacco*

**Arash Anoshiravani, MD, MPH**
Division of Adolescent Medicine
Stanford School of Medicine
Medical Director, Santa Clara County Juvenile Custody Institutions
Santa Clara Valley Medical Center
San Jose, California
186: *Disorders of Behavior*

**Richard Antaya, MD, FAAP**
Associate Professor
Department of Pediatrics
Yale University School of Medicine
New Haven, Connecticut
144: *Acne*

**Martha Arden, MD, FAAP**
Private Practice of Adolescent Medicine
Associate Professor of Clinical Pediatrics
Albert Einstein College of Medicine
Bronx, New York
25: *School-based Health Care*

**Arthur Atlas, MD, FAAP**
Director, Respiratory Center for Children
Goryeb Children's Hospital
Morristown, New Jersey
Assistant Professor of Pediatrics
University of Medicine and Dentistry of New Jersey
Newark, New Jersey
89: *Lower Respiratory Infections*

**Mark P. Atlas, MD, FAAP**
Steven and Alexandra Cohen Children's Medical Center of New York
New Hyde Park, New York
Hofstra North Shore-LIJ School of Medicine
110: *Lymphadenopathy and Splenomegaly*

**Beth Auslander, PhD**
Assistant Professor
University of Texas Medical Branch
Galveston, Texas
7: *Adolescent Sexual Development*

**Banu Aygun, MD**
Assistant Member, St Jude Children's Research Hospital
Assistant Professor of Pediatrics, University of Tennessee
Health Science Center
Memphis, Tennessee
107: *Sickle Cell Disease*

**Janice L. Bacon, MD, FAAP**
Professor and Chair
Edward J. Dennis III, MD, Endowed Chair of Obstetrics and Gynecology
University of South Carolina School of Medicine
Columbia, South Carolina
60: *Cervical Findings and Papanicolaou Smear*

**Gloria Balague, PhD**
Clinical Assistant Professor
University of Illinois at Chicago
Chicago, Illinois
167: *Sport Psychology*

**Sophie J. Balk, MD, FAAP**
Attending Pediatrician
Children's Hospital at Montefiore
Professor of Clinical Pediatrics
Albert Einstein College of Medicine
Bronx, New York
46: *Environmental Health*

**Christy Beneri, DO**
Assistant Professor of Clinical Pediatrics
Division of Infectious Diseases
State University of New York-Stony Brook
Stony Brook, New York
136: *Common Viral Infections in Adolescents*

**Molly Curtin Berkoff, MD, MPH, FAAP**
Assistant Clinical Professor
Department of Pediatrics
University of North Carolina at Chapel Hill
Chapel Hill, North Carolina
168: *Physical Abuse*

**Frank M. Biro, MD, FAAP**
Director, Division of Adolescent Medicine
Cincinnati Children's Hospital Medical Center
Rauh Chair of Pediatrics
University of Cincinnati College of Medicine
Cincinnati, Ohio
4: *Normal Pubertal Physical Growth and Development*

**Andrew D. Blaufox, MD**
Chief, Electrophysiology
The Heart Center
Steven and Alexandra Cohen Children's Medical Center of New York
Associate Professor, Clinical Pediatrics
Hofstra North Shore-LIJ School of Medicine
86: *Sudden Cardiac Death*

**Robert Blum, MD, MPH, PhD, FAAP**
William H. Gates Sr Professor and Chair
Johns Hopkins Urban Health Institute, Director
Baltimore, Maryland
3: *International Adolescent Health*

**Margaret J. Blythe, MD, FAAP**
Professor of Pediatrics & Adjunct Professor of Gynecology
Indiana University School of Medicine
Indianapolis, Indiana
23: *Documentation, Coding, and Billing*

**Paula K. Braverman, MD, FAAP**
Professor of Clinical Pediatrics
Division of Adolescent Medicine
Cincinnati Children's Hospital Medical Center
University of Cincinnati College of Medicine
Cincinnati, Ohio
53: *Sexually Transmitted Infections*

**Susan R. Brill, MD, FAAP**
Clinical Associate Professor of Pediatrics
Drexel University College of Medicine
Director of Adolescent Medicine
The Children's Hospital at Saint Peter's University Hospital
New Brunswick, New Jersey
179: *Abuse of Prescription Drugs*

**Claire Brindis, DrPh**
Professor of Pediatrics and Health Policy
PRL-IHPS
San Francisco, California
21: *Health Policy and Financing for Adolescent and Young Adult Health Services*

**Simon Brooker, DPhil**
Reader in Tropical Epidemiology and Disease Control
London School of Hygiene and Tropical Medicine
London, United Kingdom
142: *Parasitic Infections*

**Lauren Bruckner, MD, PhD**
Assistant Professor of Oncology & Pediatrics
Golisano Children's Hospital
University of Rochester Medical Center
Rochester, New York
113: *Hematopoietic Stem Cell (Bone Marrow) Transplantation*

**Donald A.P. Bundy**
Program Leader and APOC Coordinator
Human Development Network
The World Bank
Washington, DC
142: *Parasitic Infections*

**Judith T. Burgis, MD, FAAP**
Associate Professor and Interim Chair
Director, Division of Gynecology
Department of Obstetrics and Gynecology
University of South Carolina School of Medicine
Columbia, South Carolina
60: *Cervical Findings and the Papanicolaou Smear*

**Alexandra Carey, MD, FAAP**
Rockwood Clinic
Spokane, Washington
63: *Menstrual Disorders: Dysmenorrhea and Premenstrual Syndrome*

**Dennis E. Carey, MD**
Division of Pediatric Endocrinology
Hofstra North Shore-LIJ School of Medicine
Steven and Alexandra Cohen Children's Medical Center of New York
New Hyde Park, New York
75: *Bone Health and Disorders*

**Jacqueline Casillas, MD**
David Geffen School of Medicine at UCLA
Los Angeles, California
114: *Cancer Survival Issues*

**Kathryn Castle, PhD**
Associate Professor, Departments of Psychiatry and Pediatrics
Director, General Ambulatory Service
Director, Clinical Psychology Postdoctoral Training Program
University of Rochester Medical Center
Rochester, New York
43: *Cultural Considerations in Adolescent Health Care*

**Marina Catallozzi, MD**
Assistant Professor of Clinical Pediatrics
Section of Adolescent Medicine, Department of Pediatrics
Columbia University College of Physicians & Surgeons
Heilbrunn Department of Population and Family Health
Mailman School of Public Health
New York, New York
2: *Epidemiology of Mortalities and Morbidities in Adolescents*

**Manju Chandra, MD, FAAP**
Director, Division of Pediatric Nephrology
Winthrop University Hospital, Mineola
Professor of Clinical Pediatrics
Stony Brook University School of Medicine
Stony Brook, New York
119: *Voiding Disorders*

**Severine Chavel, MD**
Assistant Clinical Professor of Dermatology
Yale School of Medicine
New Haven, Connecticut
144: *Acne*

**Ashton Chen, DO**
Assistant Professor, Pediatrics
Pediatric Nephrology
Wake Forest University Baptist Medical Center
Winston-Salem, North Carolina
117: *Nephritis and Nephrosis*

**Eulalia R.Y. Cheng, MD**
Division of Pediatric Pulmonology
University of Rochester Medical Center
Rochester, New York
91: *Vocal Cord Dysfunction in Adolescents*

**Joseph N. Chorley, MD, FAAP**
Associate Professor of Pediatrics
Baylor College of Medicine
Primary Care Sports Medicine Specialist
Texas Children's Hospital
Houston, Texas
158: *Disorders of the Upper Extremities*

**Alwyn Cohall, MD, FAAP**
Professor, Clinical Public Health and Pediatrics
Mailman School of Public Health
Columbia University
Director, Harlem Health Promotion Center
New York, New York
40: *Socioeconomic Status*
57: *Sexual Dysfunction*

**W. Andrew Collins, PhD**
Professor of Child Development
University of Minnesota
Minneapolis, Minnesota
6: *Adolescent Psychosocial Development and Behavior*

**Edward E. Conway, Jr, MD, MS, FAAP, FCCM, FCCP, FHM**
Chairman, Milton and Bernice Stern Department of Pediatrics
Chief, Pediatric Critical Care
Beth Israel Medical Center
Professor of Clinical Pediatrics
Albert Einstein College of Medicine
Bronx, New York
95: *Pulmonary Embolism*
134: *Altered States of Consciousness*

**Howard E. Corey, MD**
Director, Children's Kidney Center of New Jersey
Goryeb Children's Hospital
Morristown, New Jersey
115: *Proteinuria and Hematuria*

**Susan M. Coupey, MD, FAAP**
Professor of Pediatrics and Chief, Adolescent Medicine
Albert Einstein College of Medicine
Children's Hospital at Montefiore
Bronx, New York
64: *Abnormal Uterine Bleeding*

**Kanti Craig, MD, MS**
Lieutenant Commander Medical Corps
US Navy
4: *Normal Pubertal Physical Growth and Development*

**Barbara Cromer, MD, FAAP**
Professor of Pediatrics
Case Western Reserve University School of Medicine
Director, Division of Adolescent Medicine
Metro Health Medical Center
Cleveland, Ohio
12: *Adherence Issues*

**Keith R. Cruise, PhD, MLS**
Assistant Professor
Fordham University
Department of Psychology
Bronx, New York
27: *Health Care of Incarcerated Adolescents*

**Anne Davis, MD, MPH**
Associate Professor of Clinical Obstetrics and Gynecology
Columbia University Medical Center
New York, New York
56: *Abortion in Adolescents*

**Peter M.G. Deane, MD, FAAP**
Allergist and Rheumatologist
Allergy, Asthma and Immunology of Rochester, P.C.
Clinical Assistant Professor of Medicine and Pediatrics
University of Rochester School of Medicine and Dentistry
Rochester, New York
151: *Environmental Allergies*

**Kristin Delisi, MSN, CRNP**
Children's Hospital of Pittsburgh of UPMC
Department of Adolescent Medicine
Pittsburgh, Pennsylvania
8: *Medical History*

**Jennifer E. Dietrich, MD, MSC**
Assistant Professor, Department of Obstetrics & Gynecology
Assistant Professor, Department of Pediatrics
Baylor College of Medicine
Houston, Texas
58: *Physiology of Menstruation*

**Joan DiMartino-Nardi, MD**
Clinical Professor of Pediatrics
Albert Einstein College of Medicine
Northern Westchester Hospital
Mount Kisco, New York
71: *Pituitary Disorders*

**Diane di Mauro, PhD**
HIV Center for Clinical and Behavioral Studies
New York State Psychiatric Institute at Columbia University
Sociomedical Sciences Department
Mailman School of Public Health at Columbia University
New York, New York
57: *Sexual Dysfunction*

**Barbara Anne Eberhard, MD**
Associate Professor of Clinical Pediatrics
Hofstra North Shore-LIJ School of Medicine
Steven and Alexandra Cohen Children's Medical Center of New York
New Hyde Park, New York
122: *Vasculitis and Associated Illnesses*

**Laura Edwards-Leeper, PhD**
Assistant in Psychology
Children's Hospital Boston
Instructor in Psychology
Harvard Medical School
Boston, Massachusetts
51: *Medical Treatment of the Transgender Adolescent*

**Abigail English, JD**
Director
Center for Adolescent Health & the Law
Chapel Hill, North Carolina
11: *Legal and Ethical Issues in Adolescent Health Care*

**Michal E. Eisenberg, MD**
Department of Physical Medicine & Rehabilitation
UMDNJ—Kessler Institute for Rehabilitation
West Orange, New Jersey
165: *Rehabilitation and Strength Training*

**Michele J. Fagan, MD**
Assistant Professor of Clinical Pediatrics
Children's Hospital at Montefiore
Bronx, New York
180: *Overdose of Prescription Drugs*

**Michael J. Falk, MD, FRCPC**
Attending Physician
Department of Emergency Medicine
St Luke's/Roosevelt Hospital Center
New York, New York
171: *Adolescents in Gangs*

**Ronald A. Feinstein, MD, FAAP**
Division of Adolescent Medicine
Hofstra North Shore-LIJ School of Medicine
Steven and Alexandra Cohen Children's Medical Center of New York
New Hyde Park, New York
27: *Health Care of Incarcerated Adolescents*

**Leonard G. Feld, MD, PhD, MMM, FAAP**
Sara H. Bissell & Howard C. Bissell Endowed Chair in Pediatrics
Chief Medical officer
Levine Children's Hospital
Carolinas Medical Center
Clinical Professor of Pediatrics
University of North Carolina School of Medicine
Charlotte, North Carolina
116: *Urinary Tract Infections*

**Martin A. Finkel, DO, FAAP**
Professor of Pediatrics
Medical Director
Child Abuse Research Education & Service (CARES) Institute
School of Osteopathic Medicine
University of Medicine & Dentistry of New Jersey
Stratford, New Jersey
169: *Sexual Abuse and Assault*

**Martin M. Fisher, MD, FAAP, FSAHM**
Chief, Division of Adolescent Medicine
Steven and Alexandra Cohen Children's Medical Center of New York
North Shore Long Island Jewish Health System
New Hyde Park, New York
Professor of Pediatrics
Hofstra North Shore-LIJ School of Medicine
9: *Physical Examination and Laboratory Screening*
124: *Chronic Fatigue Syndrome*

**Joseph T. Flynn, MD, MS, FAAP**
Director, Pediatric Hypertension Program
Seattle Children's Hospital
Professor of Pediatrics
University of Washington School of Medicine
Seattle, Washington
118: *Hypertension: Significance, Diagnosis, and Management*

**Chin-To Fong, MD**
Chief, Division of Genetics
Department of Pediatrics, Medicine, Biochemistry & Biophysics, Medical Humanities, and Dentistry
University of Rochester School of Medicine and Dentistry
Rochester, New York
149: *Genetic Predisposition to Common Disorders*
150: *Special Issues of Genetic Testing in Adolescent Patients*

**Michelle Forcier, MD, MPH, FAAP**
Clinical Practice Director Adolescent Medicine
Children's Memorial Hospital, Chicago
Assistant Professor of Pediatrics
Northwestern University's Feinberg School of Medicine
Chicago, Illinois
49: *Adolescent Sexual Behaviors*

**Pavel Fort, MD**
Division of Pediatric Endocrinology
Steven and Alexandra Cohen Children's Medical Center of New York
New Hyde Park, New York
73: *Diabetes Mellitus*

**Graeme Frank, MD, FAAP**
Associate Professor
Hofstra North Shore-LIJ School of Medicine
Steven and Alexandra Cohen Children's Medical Center of New York
North Shore Long Island Jewish Medical Center
New Hyde Park, New York
69: *Growth Disorders*

**Donna Futterman, MD, FAAP**
Associate Professor of Pediatrics
Director, Adolescent AIDS Program
Montefiore Medical Center
Albert Einstein College of Medicine
Bronx, New York
138: *HIV and AIDS in Adolescents*

**Robert Garofalo, MD, MPH**
Associate Professor, Department of Pediatrics
Children's Memorial Hospital/Northwestern University
Howard Brown Health Center
Chicago, Illinois
49: *Adolescent Sexual Behaviors*

**Erica J. Gibson, MD**
Assistant Clinical Professor of Pediatrics
Columbia University Medical Center
Medical Director of School Based Health
New York Presbyterian Hospital
New York, New York
61: *The Uterus and Adnexa*

**Melanie A. Gold, DO, FAAP, FACOP**
Clinical Associate Professor of Pediatrics
Division of Adolescent Medicine
Department of Pediatrics
University of Pittsburgh School of Medicine
Staff Physician
Research Coordinator for Student Health Services
Division of Student Affairs
University of Pittsburgh Student Health Services
Pittsburgh, Pennsylvania
8: *Medical History*

**Neville H. Golden, MD, FAAP**
Chief, Division of Adolescent Medicine
Professor of Pediatrics
Stanford University School of Medicine
Palo Alto, California
75: *Bone Health and Disorders*
76: *Anorexia Nervosa*

**Harris Goldstein, MD**
Dean for Scientific Resources
Director, Einstein/MMC Center for AIDS Research
The Charles Michael Chair in Autoimmune Diseases
Professor of Pediatrics and Microbiology & Immunology
Albert Einstein College of Medicine
New Hyde Park, New York
153: *Immunodeficiencies*

**Mark A. Goldstein, MD, FAAP**
Chief, Division of Adolescent and Young Adult Medicine
Massachusetts General Hospital
Harvard Medical School
Boston, Massachusetts
77: *Bulimia Nervosa*
155: *ENT Disorders*

**John-Paul Gomez, MD**
Medical Director of the Pediatric Psychiatry Liaison Service
Lehigh Valley Hospital and Health Network
Allentown, Pennsylvania
Assistant Professor of Clinical Psychiatry
Penn State College of Medicine
Hershey, Pennsylvania
189: *Psychiatric Emergencies in Adolescents*

**James T. Goodrich, MD, PhD, DSci (Hon)**
Director and Professor
Leo Davidoff Department of Neurological Surgery
Children's Hospital at Montefiore
Albert Einstein College of Medicine
Bronx, New York
131: *CNS Trauma*
132: *Intracranial Vascular Malformations*

**David Gordon, MD**
Assistant Professor of Neurological Surgery
Albert Einstein College of Medicine
Montefiore Medical Center
Bronx, New York
132: *Intracranial Vascular Malformations*

**Richard Gorlick, MD, FAAP**
Associate Professor of Molecular Pharmacology and Pediatrics
Albert Einstein College of Medicine at Yeshiva University
Vice Chairman
Division Chief of Hematology/Oncology
Department of Pediatrics
The Children's Hospital of Montefiore
Bronx, New York
161: *Bone Tumors*

**Beth S. Gottlieb, MD, MS**
Director, Pediatric Rheumatology
Director, Pediatric Rheumatology Fellowship Training Program
Steven and Alexandra Cohen Children's Medical Center of New York
New Hyde Park, New York
Hofstra North Shore-LIJ School of Medicine
120: *Systemic Lupus Erythematosus*

**Melanie K. Greifer, MD**
Attending Physician
Steven and Alexandra Cohen Children's Medical
Center of New York
New Hyde Park, New York
Assistant Professor of Pediatrics
Albert Einstein College of Medicine
Bronx, New York
104: *Inflammatory Bowel Disease*

**Robin H. Gurwitch, PhD**
Professor
Cincinnati Children's Hospital Medical Center
National Center for School Crisis and Bereavement
Cincinnati, Ohio
48: *Disasters*

**J. Nathan Hagstrom, MD, FAAP**
Associate Professor of Pediatrics
University of Connecticut School of Medicine
Division Head, Hematology-Oncology
Connecticut Children's Medical Center
Hartford, Connecticut
108: *Hemostasis and Thrombosis*

**Elena C. Haliasos, MD**
Dermatologist
New Jersey
147: *Miscellaneous Dermatologic Disorders in Adolescence*

**Cindy A. Haller, MD**
Attending Physician, Pediatric Gastroenterology and Nutrition
Steven and Alexandra Cohen Children's Medical Center of New York
New Hyde Park, New York
98: *Disorders of the Esophagus*

**Chad Hamner, MD**
Trauma Medical Director
Attending Pediatric Surgeon
Cook Children's Medical Center
Fort Worth, Texas
163: *Chest Wall Abnormalities*

**Ronald C. Hansen, MD**
Chief, Pediatric Dermatology
Phoenix Children's Hospital
Professor, Dermatology & Pediatrics
University of Arizona College of Medicine
Tucson, Arizona
Consultant, May Clinic Scottsdale
Scottsdale, Arizona
146: *Alopecia*

**Henry Hasson, MD**
Pediatric Neurology
Assistant Professor of Neurology and Pediatrics
SUNY Downstate Medical Center
Maimonides Medical Center
Brooklyn, New York
127: *Seizures in Adolescents*

**Albert C. Hergenroeder, MD, FAAP**
Professor of Pediatrics
Baylor College of Medicine
Chief, Adolescent Medicine and Sports Medicine Section
Texas Children's Hospital
Houston, Texas
159: *Disorders of the Lower Extremities*

**S. Paige Hertweck, MD, FAAP**
Professor, Pediatric Adolescent Gynecology Department
Obstetrics, Gynecology and Women's Health
Chief of Gynecology
Kosair Children's Hospital
Louisville, Kentucky
58: *Physiology of Menstruation*

**David Herzog, MD**
Director, Harris Center for Education and Advocacy in Eating Disorders, Massachusetts General Hospital
Harvard Medical School Endowed Professor in the Field of Eating Disorders
Boston, Massachusetts
77: *Bulimia Nervosa*

**Geri Hewitt, MD, FAAP**
Nationwide Children's Hospital, Columbus
Ohio State University Medical Center, Columbus
Associate Clinical Professor, Department of Obstetrics and Gynecology and Pediatrics
Columbus, Ohio
62: *Amenorrhea*

**Sara Hirschfeld Lee, MD**
Assistant Professor of Pediatrics
Rainbow Babies and Children's Hospital
Case Western Reserve University School of Medicine
Cleveland, Ohio
12: *Adherence Issues*

**Christopher H. Hodgman, MD**
Professor of Psychiatry Emeritus and Clinical Professor of Pediatrics
University of Rochester School of Medicine
Rochester, New York
188: *Psychotic Disorders in Adolescents*

**Andrew R. Hong, MD, FAAP**
Assistant Professor of Surgery & Pediatrics
Albert Einstein College of Medicine
Division of Pediatric Surgery
Steven and Alexandra Cohen Children's Medical Center of New York
New Hyde Park, New York
163: *Chest Wall Abnormalities*

**Peter Hotez, MD, PhD, FAAP**
President, Sabin Vaccine Institute
Walter G. Ross Professor and Chair
Department of Microbiology, Immunology and Tropical Medicine
The George Washington University and Sabin Vaccine Institute
Editor in Chief
PLoS Neglected Tropical Diseases
Washington, DC
142: *Parasitic Infections*

**Denise Hug, MD, FAAP**
Children's Mercy Hospital and Clinics
Assistant Professor, University of Missouri-Kansas City
Kansas City, Missouri
154: *Eye Disorders*

**Elba A. Iglesias, MD, FAAP**
Attending, Adolescent Medicine
Miami Children's Hospital
Division of Adolescent Medicine
Miami, Florida
64: *Abnormal Uterine Bleeding*

**Norman T. Ilowite, MD, FAAP**
Chief, Division of Rheumatology
Children's Hospital at Montefiore
Professor of Pediatrics
Albert Einstein College of Medicine
Bronx, New York
121: *Juvenile Idiopathic Arthritis*

**Elizaveta Iofel, MD**
Assistant Professor of Pediatrics
Division of Pediatric Gastroenterology and Nutrition
Bristol-Myers Squibb Children's Hospital
University of Medicine and Dentistry of New Jersey—Robert Wood Johnson University Hospital
New Brunswick, New Jersey
103: *Diarrhea in the Adolescent*

**Patricia Irigoyen, MD**
Assistant Professor
Pediatric Rheumatology
Children's Hospital at Montefiore
Bronx, New York
121: *Juvenile Idiopathic Arthritis*

**Marc S. Jacobson, MD, FAAP, FAHA**
Professor of Pediatrics and Epidemiology
Albert Einstein College of Medicine
Great Neck, New York
81: *Hyperlipidemia and Atherosclerosis*

**Yasmin Jayasinghe, MBBS, FRANZCOG**
Consultant Gynecologist
Department of Gynecology
Royal Children's Hospital
Melbourne, Australia
Research Collaborator, Mayo Clinic
Rochester, Minnesota
66: *Breast Disorders in the Female*

**Sandra H. Jee, MD, MPH, FAAP**
Assistant Professor of Pediatrics
University of Rochester
Starlight Pediatrics, Research Director
Rochester, New York
29: *Adolescents in Foster Care*

**Poonam Jha, MD, FAAP**
Instructor of Psychiatry and Behavioral Sciences
Feinberg School of Medicine, Northwestern University
Chicago, Illinois
Attending, Child and Adolescent Psychiatry
Children's Memorial Hospital
Chicago, Illinois
185: *Disorders of Anxiety in Adolescents*

**Alain Joffe, MD, MPH, FAAP**
Director, Student Health and Wellness Center
Johns Hopkins University
Associate Professor of Pediatrics
Johns Hopkins Medical Institutions
Baltimore, Maryland
68: *Disorders of Male Genitalia*
175: *Marijuana*

**Jennifer Johnson, MD, FAAP**
Senate Emeritus
Department of Pediatrics
University of California, Irvine
Orange, California
30: *Immigrant Adolescents*

**Margery Johnson, MD**
Medical Director, Outpatient Psychiatry
Children's Memorial Hospital
Northwestern University—Feinberg School of Medicine
Chicago, Illinois
185: *Disorders of Anxiety in Adolescents*

**Karolyn Kabir, MD, FAAP**
Assistant Professor of Pediatrics
Director, Young Mother's Clinic
Division of Adolescent Medicine
The Children's Hospital
Denver, Colorado
55: *Adolescent Parenthood*

**Tsoline Kojaoghlanian, MD**
Assistant Professor
Pediatric Infectious Diseases
Children's Hospital at Montefiore
Albert Einstein College of Medicine
Bronx, New York
88: *Upper Respiratory Tract Infections*

**Bill G. Kapogiannis, MD, FAAP**
Program Director
Adolescent Medicine Trials Network for HIV/AIDS Interventions
Pediatric, Adolescent and Maternal AIDS Branch
Eunice Kennedy Shriver National Institute of Child Health and Human Development
National Institutes of Health
Bethesda, Maryland
20: *Pharmacologic Considerations*

**Sandra Kaplan, MD, FAAP**
(deceased)
35: *Divorce, Separation, and Blended Families*

**Niranjan Karnik, MD, PhD**
Assistant Professor of Psychiatry & Behavioral Neuroscience
University of Chicago Pritzker School of Medicine
Chicago, Illinois
186: *Disorders of Behavior*

**Debra K. Katzman, MD, FRCPC**
Head, Division of Adolescent Medicine
Professor of Paediatrics
Medical Director, The Eating Disorder Program
The Hospital for Sick Children and University of Toronto
Toronto, Ontario
76: *Anorexia Nervosa*

**DenYelle Baete Kenyon, PhD**
Assistant Scientist, Health Disparities Research Center, Sanford Research
Assistant Professor, Pediatrics, Sanford School of Medicine
University of South Dakota
Sioux Falls, South Dakota
39: *Peers*

**Dipak Kholwadwala, MD**
Steven and Alexandra Cohen Children's Medical Center of New York
New Hyde Park, New York
84: *Valvular Heart Diseases*

**Diana King, MD, FAAP**
Assistant Professor of Pediatrics
Albert Einstein College of Medicine
Pediatric Emergency Medicine—Children's Hospital at Montefiore
Bronx, New York
95: *Pulmonary Embolism*

**Jonathan D. Klein, MD, MPH, FAAP**
University of Rochester
Division of Adolescent Medicine
Rochester, New York
13: *Screening in Adolescent Health Care*

**Sylvain Kleinhaus, MD**
Professor Emeritus of Surgery and Pediatrics
Albert Einstein College of Medicine
Director, Pediatric Surgery
Montefiore Medical Center
Bronx, New York
102: *Appendicitis*

**John R. Knight, MD, FAAP**
Associate Professor of Pediatrics
Harvard Medical School
Director, CeASAR
Children's Hospital Boston
Boston, Massachusetts
181: *Office Management and Laboratory Testing*
182: *Treatment Options*

**Cheryl Kodjo, MD, MPH, FAAP**
Associate Professor of Pediatrics
Division of Adolescent Medicine
Associate Dean of Advising
University of Rochester School of Medicine and Dentistry
Rochester, New York
43: *Cultural Considerations in Adolescent Health Care*

**Patricia K. Kokotailo, MD, FAAP**
Professor of Pediatrics
Associate Dean for Faculty Development and Faculty Affairs
University of Wisconsin School of Medicine and Public Health
Madison, Wisconsin
174: *Alcohol*
176: *Stimulants*

**David N. Korones, MD**
Professor of Pediatrics, Oncology, and Neurology
University of Rochester Medical Center
Rochester, New York
19: *Palliative Care and Psychological Aspects of Death and Dying in Adolescence*
111: *Malignant Solid Tumors*
112: *Brain Tumors in Adolescents*

**Beverly Kosmach-Park, HSN, CRNP**
Clinical Nurse Specialist
Department of Transplant Surgery
Children's Hospital of Pittsburgh
Pittsburgh, Pennsylvania
32: *Solid Organ Transplantation*

**Tanya Kowalczyk Mullins, MD, MS, FAAP**
Assistant Professor of Clinical Pediatrics
Division of Adolescent Medicine
Cincinnati Children's Hospital Medical Center
University of Cincinnati College of Medicine
Cincinnati, Ohio
53: *Sexually Transmitted Infections*

**Richard E. Kreipe, MD, FAAP, FSAHM**
Professor of Pediatrics
Division of Adolescent Medicine
Department of Pediatrics
Golisano Children's Hospital
University of Rochester School of Medicine and Dentistry
Rochester, New York
10: *The Approach to Symptoms in the Adolescent Patient*
15: *Anticipatory Guidance*
183: *Somatoform Disorders*

**Paula Kreitzer, MD**
Division of Pediatric Endocrinology
Hofstra North Shore-LIJ School of Medicine
72: *Thyroid Disorders in Adolescents*

**Leonard Kristal, MD, FAAP**
Clinical Assistant Professor of Dermatology
State University of New York-Stony Brook
Stony Brook, New York
147: *Miscellaneous Dermatologic Disorders in Adolescents*

**David Krol, MD, MPH, FAAP**
Team Director, Senior Program Officer
Robert Wood Johnson Foundation
Princeton, New Jersey
157: *Adolescent Oral Health*

**Martha Y. Kubik, PhD, RN**
Associate Professor
School of Nursing
University of Minnesota
Minneapolis, Minnesota
39: *Peers*

**John Kulig, MD, MPH, FAAP**
Director, Adolescent Medicine
Floating Hospital for Children at Tufts Medical Center
Professor of Pediatrics, Public Health and Family Medicine
Tufts University School of Medicine
Boston, Massachusetts
172: *Overview: Substance Abuse*
177: *Opiates*

**Michael LaCorte, MD, FAAP**
Associate Chief of Staff for Brooklyn and Staten Island
Attending Pediatric Cardiologist
Steven and Alexandra Cohen Children's Medical Center of New York
New Hyde Park, New York
82: *Congenital Heart Disease*

**John Langley, MD**
Mental Health Service
St Michael's Hospital
Director, Postgraduate Education
Division of Child Psychiatry
University of Toronto
Toronto, Ontario
187: *Personality Disorders in Adolescents*

**Nicole Larson, PhD, MPH, RD**
Research Associate
Division of Epidemiology and Community Health
School of Public Health
University of Minnesota
Minneapolis, Minnesota
16: *Adolescent Nutrition and Physical Activity*

**Eric Lazar, MD, FAAP**
101: *Diseases of the Gall Bladder*

**Rebecca K. Lehman, MD**
Instructor of Neurology and Pediatrics
University of Rochester Medical Center
Rochester, New York
129: *Movement Disorders and Ataxia*

**Irene W. Leigh, PhD**
Professor of Psychology
Chair, Department of Psychology
Gallaudet University
Washington, DC
156: *Medical and Psychosocial Considerations for Deaf Adolescents*

**Pieter le Roux, MD**
Department of Psychiatry
University of Rochester School of Medicine and Dentistry
Rochester, New York
191: *Mental Health Treatment Modalities for Adolescents*

**Sharon Levy, MD, MPH, FAAP**
Assistant Professor of Pediatrics
Harvard Medical School
Medical Director, Adolescent Substance Abuse Program
Children's Hospital Boston
Boston, Massachusetts
181: *Office Management and Laboratory Testing*
182: *Treatment Options*

**Zhicheng Li, MD**
Chief, Division of Spinal Intervention
Wilmington Health
Wilmington, North Carolina
126: *Headaches*

**Marita E. Lind, MD, FAAP**
Assistant Professor of Pediatrics
CARES Institute
University of Medicine and Dentistry of New Jersey
School of Osteopathic Medicine
Stratford, New Jersey
169: *Sexual Abuse and Assault*

**Paul S. Links, MD, MSc, FRCPC**
Professor of Psychiatry
Department of Psychiatry
Faculty of Medicine
University of Toronto
Toronto, Ontario
187: *Personality Disorders in Adolescents*

**Nathan Litman, MD, FAAP**
Professor of Pediatrics
Albert Einstein College of Medicine
Chief of Service, Pediatrics
Director, Division of Pediatric Infectious Diseases
Children's Hospital at Montefiore
Bronx, New York
160: *Bone and Joint Infections*

**Deborah M. Lopez, MD, FAAP**
Director, Pediatric Intensive Care Unit
Director, Pediatric Sedation Service,
North Naples Hospital
Naples, Florida
94: *Pneumothorax*

**Dionne Louis, MD, FAAP**
University of Oklahoma Health Sciences Center
Department of Dermatology
Oklahoma City, Oklahoma
145: *Dermatitis and Papulosquamous Diseases*

**Kevin K. Makino, MD/PhD Student**
Department of Community and Preventive Medicine
University of Rochester School of Medicine and Dentistry
Rochester, New York
13: *Screening in Adolescent Health Care*

**Husam Mallah, MD**
Pediatric Gastroenterology
University of Rochester
Rochester, New York
105: *Celiac Disease*

**Robert W. Marion, MD**
Professor, Pediatrics & Obstetrics & Gynecology and Women's Health
Chief, Divisions of Genetics & Developmental Medicine
Children's Hospital at Montefiore
Albert Einstein College of Medicine
Bronx, New York
133: *Myelomeningocele*
148: *Genetic Disorders*

**James Markowitz, MD, FAAP**
Attending Physician
Division of Pediatric Gastroenterology
Steven and Alexandra Cohen Children's Medical Center of New York
North Shore—LIJ Health System
New Hyde Park, New York
98: *Disorders of the Esophagus*
104: *Inflammatory Bowel Disease*

**Andrea Marks, MD, FAAP**
Associate Clinical Professor of Pediatrics
Mount Sinai School of Medicine
Associate Attending Pediatrician
Mount Sinai Medical Center
New York, New York
22: *The Adolescent-Friendly Practice*

**Barbara Marshall, MD**
Medical Director, Pediatric Endocrinology
Mary Bridge Children's Hospital and Health Center
Tacoma, Washington
71: *Pituitary Disorders*

**Susan Massengill, MD**
Director, Pediatric Nephrology
Levine Children's Hospital
Associate Professor of Pediatrics
University of North Carolina School of Medicine
Charlotte, North Carolina
116: *Urinary Tract Infections*

**Marguerite M. Mayers, MD, FAAP**
Director, Pediatric Infectious Diseases Clinic
Children's Hospital at Montefiore
Professor of Clinical Pediatrics
Albert Einstein College of Medicine
Bronx, New York
141: *Mycobacterial*

**Amy Mayhew, MD, MPH**
Child and Adolescent Psychiatry Fellow
Cambridge Health Alliance, Harvard Medical School Teaching Affiliate
Cambridge, Massachusetts
150: *Special Issues of Genetic Testing in Adolescent Patients*

**Christina M. McCann, PhD**
Adjunct Staff, Departments of Psychiatry and Pediatrics
Rochester General Hospital
Rochester, New York
191: *Mental Health Treatment Modalities for Adolescents*

**Susan H. McDaniel, PhD**
Dr. Laurie Sands Distinguished Professor of Families & Health
Director, Institute for the Family, Department of Psychiatry
Associate Chair, Department of Family Medicine
University of Rochester Medical Center
Rochester, New York
38: *Family Systems Approaches to Adolescent Health and Illness*

**Ann H. McMullen, RN, MS, CPnP**
Nurse Practitioner (retired)
University of Rochester Cystic Fibrosis Center
University of Rochester Medical Center
Rochester, New York
92: *Cystic Fibrosis*

**Diane F. Merritt, MD, FAAP**
Professor of Obstetrics and Gynecology
Director of Pediatric and Adolescent Gynecology
Washington University School of Medicine
St Louis, Missouri
59: *Perineal and Vaginal Abnormalities*

**Amy B. Middleman, MD, FAAP**
Associate Professor of Pediatrics
Baylor College of Medicine
Houston, Texas
14: *Immunizations*

**Kristin Mmari, DrPh, MA**
Assistant Scientist
Department of Population, Family, and Reproductive Health
Johns Hopkins Bloomberg School of Public Health
Baltimore, Maryland
3: *International Adolescent Health*

**Jonathan W. Mink, MD, PhD, FAAP**
Professor and Chief of Child Neurology
Departments of Neurology, Neurobiology & Anatomy, Brain & Cognitive Sciences, and Pediatrics
University of Rochester
Rochester, New York
129: *Movement Disorders and Ataxia*

**Megan A. Moreno, MD, MS Ed, MPH, FAAP**
Assistant Professor
University of Wisconsin-Madison
Department of Pediatrics
Madison, Wisconsin
174: *Alcohol*

**Libia Moy, MD**
Attending Physician
Division of Pediatric Gastroenterology
Hofstra North Shore-LIJ School of Medicine
Steven and Alexandra Cohen Children's Medical Center of New York
New Hyde Park, New York
100: *Disorders of the Liver and Pancreas*

**Kristi M. Mulchahey, MD**
Private Practice
Atlanta Gyn Associates
Atlanta, Georgia
65: *Hyperandrogenism*

**Gregory J. Mulford, MD, FAAP**
Chairman, Department of Rehabilitation
Morristown Memorial Hospital
Medical Director, Post Acute Services
Atlantic Health
Morristown, New Jersey
Clinical Associate Professor of Physical Medicine and Rehabilitation
University of Medicine and Dentistry of New Jersey
Newark, New Jersey
165: *Rehabilitation and Strength Training*

**Tina Paul Mulye, MPH**
Research and Policy Center Project Associate
University of California
San Francisco, California
21: *Health Policy and Financing for Adolescent and Young Adult Health Services*

**Pamela J. Murray, MD, MPH**
Associate Professor of Pediatrics
University of Pittsburgh School of Medicine
Children's Hospital of Pittsburgh
Pittsburgh, Pennsylvania
32: *Solid Organ Transplantation*
63: *Menstrual Disorders: Dysmenorrhea and Premenstrual Syndrome*

**Joshua P. Needleman, MD**
Associate Professor of Clinical Pediatrics
Weill Cornell Medical College
New York, New York
90: *Asthma*

**Dawn Nero, PsyD**
Supervising Psychologist
New York Presbyterian Hospital
Instructor of Clinical Psychology in Child & Adolescent Psychiatry
Columbia University
New York, New York
184: *Mood Disorders in Adolescents*

**Judith O'Haver, PhD, RN, CPNP-PC**
Assistant Professor
Arizona State University
College of Nursing & Healthcare Innovation
Pediatric Nurse Practitioner
Dermatology Department
Phoenix Children's Hospital
Phoenix, Arizona
146: *Alopecia*

**Scott E. Olitsky, MD, FAAP**
Chief of Ophthalmology
Children's Mercy Hospitals and Clinics
Professor of Ophthalmology
University of Missouri, Kansas City School of Medicine
Kansas City, Missouri
154: *Eye Disorders*

**Ponrat Pakpreo, MD, MPH, FAAP**
Adolescent Medicine Clinic
Sacred Heart Children's Hospital
Spokane, Washington
15: *Anticipatory Guidance*

**David M. Paperny, MD, FAAP**
Assistant Professor of Pediatrics and Adolescent Medicine
University of Hawaii School of Medicine
Director, Kaiser Permanente Adolescent Services
Honolulu, Hawaii
42: *Computers, Technology, and the Internet*

**M. Jane Park, MPH**
Policy Research Coordinator
Division of Adolescent Medicine, Department of Pediatrics
University of California
San Francisco, California
21: *Health Policy and Financing for Adolescent and Young Adult Health Services*

**Doris Pastore, MD, FAAP**
Adolescent Young Adult Medicine Practice
Associate Professor of Pediatrics
Mount Sinai School of Medicine
New York, New York
25: *School-based Health Care*

**Dilip R. Patel, MD, FAAP, FSAHM, FACSM, FAACPDM**
Professor, Department of Pediatrics and Human Development
Michigan State University College of Human Medicine
East Lansing, Michigan
Pediatric Residency Training Program
Michigan State University Kalamazoo Center for Medical Studies
Kalamazoo, Michigan
166: *Hyperthermia*

**Mahesh C. Patel, MD**
Assistant Professor
University of Illinois Medical Center at Chicago
Department of Medicine, Section of Infectious Diseases
Chicago, Illinois
153: *Immunodeficiencies*

**Charlotte J. Patterson, PhD**
Professor of Psychology
Department of Psychology
University of Virginia
Charlottesville, Virginia
37: *Adolescents with Lesbian or Gay Parents*

**Michael J. Pettei, MD, PhD, FAAP**
Associate Professor of Pediatrics
Hofstra North Shore-LIJ School of Medicine
Chief, Pediatric Nutrition
Division of Gastroenterology and Nutrition
Steven and Alexandra Cohen Children's Medical Center of New York
North Shore-Long Island Jewish Health System
New Hyde Park, New York
99: *Peptic Ulcers and Other Disorders of the Stomach and Duodenum*
103: *Diarrhea in the Adolescent*

**Anthony R. Pisani, PhD**
Assistant Professor of Psychiatry and Pediatrics
University of Rochester Medical Center
Wynne Center for Family Research
Center for the Study and Prevention of Suicide
University of Rochester
Rochester, New York
38: *Family Systems Approaches to Adolescent Health and Illness*

**Laura S. Plummer, MD**
Pediatric Ophthalmologist and Adult Strabismus Surgeon
Children's Mercy Hospital and Clinics
Assistant Professor, University of Missouri-Kansas City School of Medicine
Assistant Clinical Professor, Kansas University
Kansas City, Missouri

**Margaret Polaneczky MD, FAAP**
Associate Professor
Weill Medical College of Cornell University
New York, New York
52: *Contraception*

**Heather Munro Prescott, PhD**
Professor of History
Central Connecticut State University
New Britain, Connecticut
1: *History of Adolescent Medicine and Health Care*

**Lisa Albers Prock, MD, MPH, FAAP**
Director, Adoption Program
Developmental Medicine Center
Children's Hospital Boston
Assistant Professor
Harvard Medical School
Boston, Massachusetts
36: *Adoption and Adolescence*

**Sujatha Rajan, MD, FAAP**
Assistant Professor
Division of Pediatric Infectious Diseases
Steven and Alexandra Cohen Children's Medical Center of New York
New Hyde Park, New York
136: *Common Viral Infections in Adolescents*
137: *Infectious Mononucleosis and Mononucleosis-Like Syndromes*

**Dennis N. Ranalli, DDS, MDS**
Expert Consultant, Committee on the Adolescent
American Academy of Pediatric Dentistry
Professor, Department of Pediatric Dentistry
Senior Associate Dean
University of Pittsburgh School of Dental Medicine
Pittsburgh, Pennsylvania
157: *Adolescent Oral Health*

**Cynthia Rand, MD, MPH, FAAP**
Assistant Professor, Pediatrics
University of Rochester School of Medicine and Dentistry
Rochester, New York
15: *Anticipatory Guidance*

**Arlene Redner, MD, FAAP**
Associate Chief, Oncology
Steven and Alexandra Cohen Children's Medical Center of New York
New Hyde Park, New York
111: *Malignant Solid Tumors*

**Gary Remafedi, MD, MPH, FAAP**
Professor, Department of Pediatrics
University of Minnesota
Minneapolis, Minnesota
50: *Issues Affecting Gay, Lesbian, and Bisexual Youth*

**Clement L. Ren, MD, FAAP**
University of Rochester
Department of Pediatrics
Division of Pediatric Pulmonology
Rochester, New York
92: *Cystic Fibrosis*

**Cynthia P. Rickert, PhD**
Assistant Professor, Social Sciences
Ivy Tech Community College
Indianapolis, Indiana
184: *Mood Disorders in Adolescents*

**Vaughn I. Rickert, PsyD**
Donald P. Orr Professor of Pediatrics
Director, Section of Adolescent Medicine
University of Indiana School of Medicine
Riley Hospital for Children
Indianapolis, Indiana
184: *Mood Disorders in Adolescents*

**Jessica Rieder, MD, MS, FAAP**
Department of Pediatrics, Division of Adolescent Medicine
Children's Hospital at Montefiore
Albert Einstein College of Medicine
Bronx, New York
79: *Obesity*

**Rachel G. Riskind, MA**
Doctoral Student
University of Virginia
Charlottesville, Virginia
37: *Adolescents with Lesbian or Gay Parents*

**Arthur Leon Robin, PhD**
Child Psychiatry and Psychology Department
Children's Hospital of Michigan
Detroit, Michigan
33: *Communication Between Parents and Adolescents*
196: *ADHD in Adolescents*

**Deanne Mraz Robinson, MD**
Yale Dermatology Resident
Yale New Haven Hospital
New Haven, Connecticut
149: *Genetic Predisposition to Common Disorders*

**Reuben Rohn, MD, FAAP**
Professor of Pediatrics, Eastern Virginia Medical School
Director, Adolescent Medicine/Endocrinology, Children's Hospital of the King's Daughter
Norfolk, Virginia
67: *Pubertal Gynecomastia*

**Angela Romano, MD, FAAP**
Pediatric Cardiologist
Steven and Alexandra Cohen Children's Medical Center of New York
New Hyde Park, New York
80: *Chest Pain in Adolescents*

**Ellen Rome, MD, MPH, FAAP**
Head, Section of Adolescent Medicine
Cleveland Clinic Children's Hospital
Associate Professor of Pediatrics
Cleveland Clinic Lerner College of Medicine
Cleveland, Ohio
78: *The Female Athlete Triad*

**Marilyn Rosen, MLS**
Reference Librarian
Edward G. Miner Library
University of Rochester School of Medicine and Dentistry
Rochester, New York
17: *Complementary and Alternative Medicine*

**Susan Rosenthal, PhD**
University of Texas Medical Branch
Galveston, Texas
7: *Adolescent Sexual Development*

**Thomas M. Rossi, MD**
Department of Pediatrics
Division of Gastroenterology and Nutrition
University of Rochester School of Medicine and Dentistry
Rochester, New York
105: *Celiac Disease*

**David H. Rothstein, MD, FAAP**
Attending Surgeon
Children's Memorial Hospital
Chicago, Illinois
163: *Chest Wall Abnormalities*

**John D. Rowlett, MD, FAAP**
Professor of Pediatrics
Eastern Kentucky University
Richmond, Kentucky
47: *Adolescents at Work*

**Paul T. Rubery, MD, FAAP**
Associate Professor of Orthopaedic Surgery and Pediatrics
University of Rochester School of Medicine
Rochester, New York
162: *Disorders of the Spine*

**Lorry G. Rubin, MD, FAAP**
Chief, Pediatric Infectious Diseases
Steven and Alexandra Cohen Children's Medical Center of New York
North Shore-Long Island Jewish Health System
New Hyde Park, New York
135: *Fever of Unknown Origin*
139: *Bacterial Infections*

**Desmond K. Runyan, MD, DrPh, FAAP**
Professor of Social Medicine and Pediatrics
University of North Carolina School of Medicine
Chapel Hill, North Carolina
168: *Physical Abuse*

**Olle Jane Z. Sahler, MD, FAAP**
Golisano Children's Hospital at Strong
University of Rochester Medical Center
Rochester, New York
17: *Complementary and Alternative Medicine*
18: *Pain in Adolescents: Pathophysiology and Management*
19: *Palliative Care and Psychological Aspects of Death and Dying in Adolescence*

**Alexandra Salazar, MS, RD, CDE**
New York, New York
79: *Obesity*

**Robert Sammartano, RPA-C**
Senior Surgical Physician Assistant, Pediatric Surgery
Program Director, Postgraduate Residency in Surgery for Physician Assistants
American Association of Surgical Physician Assistants
Chief Delegate for Surgery—House of Delegates
American Academy of Physician Assistants
Bronx, New York
102: *Appendicitis*

**Joseph S. Sanfilippo, MD**
University of Pittsburgh Medical School
Magee Women's Hospital
Pittsburgh, Pennsylvania
58: *Physiology of Menstruation*

**John Santelli, MD, MPH**
Harriet & Robert H. Heilbrunn Professor and Chairman
Heilbrunn Department of Population and Family Health
Mailman School of Public Health
Columbia University
New York, New York
2: *Epidemiology of Mortalities and Morbidities in Adolescents*

**Anju Sawni, MD, FAAP**
Assistant Professor of Pediatrics
Division of Adolescent Medicine
Children's Hospital of Michigan
Wayne State University School of Medicine
Detroit, Michigan
196: *ADHD in Adolescents*

**Michael Scharf, MD, FAAP**
Assistant Professor in Psychiatry and Pediatrics
Director, Child and Adolescent Psychiatry Fellowship
Director, Pediatric Psychiatry Consultation and Liaison Service (Inpatient)
Acting Director of Child and Adolescent Psychiatry
Senior Medical Director for Children and Youth
University of Rochester Medical Center
Rochester, New York
190: *Adolescent Psychopharmacology*

**Marcie Schneider, MD, FAAP, FSAHM**
Associate Clinical Professor of Pediatrics
Albert Einstein College of Medicine
Associate Attending
Greenwich Hospital
Greenwich, Connecticut
9: *Physical Examination and Laboratory Screening*
148: *Genetic Disorders*

**S. Kenneth Schonberg, MD, FAAP**
Professor of Pediatrics
Albert Einstein College of Medicine/Children's Hospital at Montefiore
Bronx, New York
24: *The Adolescent In-Patient Unit*

**David J. Schonfeld, MD, FAAP**
Director, National Center for School Crisis and Bereavement
Director, Division of Developmental and Behavioral Pediatrics
Cincinnati Children's Hospital Medical Center
Cincinnati, Ohio
48: *Disasters*

**Stephanie G. Schuckalo, RN, MSN, APN**
Pediatric Nurse Practitioner
Goryeb Children's Hospital at Atlantic Health
Morristown, New Jersey
97: *Functional GI Disorders*

**Marjorie Kaplan Seidenfeld, MD, FAAP**
Medical Director
Barnard College Primary Care Health Service
New York, New York
26: *College Health*

**C. Wayne Sells, MD, MPH, FAAP**
Director, Division of Adolescent Health
Associate Professor of Pediatrics
Department of Pediatrics
Oregon Health & Science University
Portland, Oregon
50: *Issues Affecting Gay, Lesbian, and Bisexual Youth*

**Ashish R. Shah, MD, FAAP**
Pediatric Pulmonologist
Director, Pediatric Sleep Medicine
Atlantic Health
Morristown, New Jersey
Assistant Professor of Pediatrics
University of Medicine and Dentistry of New Jersey
New Brunswick, New Jersey
93: *Sleep Disorders*

**Jeanelle Sheeder, MSPH, PhD**
Assistant Professor of Obstetrics and Gynecology and Pediatrics
University of Colorado Denver, School of Medicine
Research Director, Colorado Adolescent Maternity Program (CAMP)
Denver, Colorado
54: *Adolescent Pregnancy*

**Ashok Shende, MBBS, FAAP**
Pediatric Hematologist/Oncologist (retired)
Bryside, New York
109: *Disorders of the White Blood Cells*

**Sujit Sheth, MD, FAAP**
Associate Professor of Pediatrics
Columbia University Medical Center
New York, New York
106: *Disorders of the Red Blood Cells*

**Maggie Sifain, MD**
91: *Vocal Cord Dysfunction in Adolescents*

**Shlomo Shinnar, MD, PhD, FAAP**
Professor of Neurology, Pediatrics and Epidemiology and Population Health
Hyman Climenko Professor of Neuroscience Research
Director, Comprehensive Epilepsy Management Center
Montefiore Medical Center
Albert Einstein College of Medicine
Bronx, New York
126: *Headaches*
127: *Seizures in Adolescents*

**Mary Short, PhD**
Associate Professor
University of Houston-Clear Lake
Houston, Texas
7: *Adolescent Sexual Development*

**Scott H. Sicherer, MD, FAAP**
Professor of Pediatrics
Jaffe Food Allergy Institute
Mount Sinai School of Medicine
New York, New York
152: *Food Allergies*

**Alex W. Siegel, PhD**
University of California
Berkeley, California
5: *Adolescent Brain and Cognitive Changes*

**Daniel J. Siegel, MD, FAAP**
Mindsight Institute
Los Angeles, California
5: *Adolescent Brain and Cognitive Changes*

**David M. Siegel, MD, MPH, FAAP**
Professor of Pediatrics and Medicine
University of Rochester School of Medicine and Dentistry
Edward H. Townsend Chief of Pediatrics
Rochester General Hospital
Rochester, New York
123: *Fibromyalgia Syndrome in Adolescents*

**Renee E. Sieving, RN, PhD**
Associate Professor, School of Nursing and Department of Pediatrics
Deputy Director, Healthy Youth Development—Prevention Research Center
University of Minnesota
Minneapolis, Minnesota
39: *Peers*

**Kathy Silverman, DO, FAAP**
Director of Adolescent Medicine Services
Blythedale Children's Hospital
Valhalla, New York
Assistant Professor—Pediatrics
Montefiore Medical Center
Bronx, New York
24: *The Adolescent In-Patient Unit*

**Patricia Simmons, MD, FAAP**
Professor and Chair, Division of Pediatric and Adolescent Gynecology
Departments of Pediatric and Adolescent Medicine and Obstetrics and Gynecology
Mayo Clinic
Rochester, Minnesota
66: *Breast Disorders in the Female*

**Peter J. Simon, MPH**
Heilbrunn Department of Population and Family Health
Mailman School of Public Health at Columbia University
New York, New York
184: *Mood Disorders in Adolescents*

**Eric Small, MD, FAAP**
Assistant Clinical Professor of Pediatrics, Orthopedics, and Rehabilitation Medicine
Mount Sinai School of Medicine
New York, New York
164: *Preparticipation Evaluation*

**Brian Snyder, MD**
North Shore University Hospital
Manhasset, New York
Long Island Jewish Medical Center
New Hyde Park, New York
131: *CNS Trauma*

**Sunil K. Sood, MD, DCH**
Chairman, Department of Pediatrics
Southside Hospital
North Shore-LIJ Health System
Attending Physician, Pediatric Infectious Diseases
Steven and Alexandra Cohen Children's Medical Center of New York
Professor of Clinical Pediatrics
Albert Einstein College of Medicine
Bronx, New York
140: *Tick-Borne Diseases*
143: *Prevention of Travel-Related Infections*

**Norman P. Spack, MD, FAAP**
Endocrine Division
Children's Hospital Boston
Department of Pediatrics
Harvard Medical School
Boston, Massachusetts
51: *Medical Treatment of the Transgender Adolescent*

**Mary Spagnola-Marsh, PhD**
Fellow, Department of Psychiatry
Wynne Center for Family Research
University of Rochester
Rochester, New York
38: *Family Systems Approaches to Adolescent Health and Illness*

**Michael A. Spaulding-Barclay, MD, MS, FAAP**
Medical Director, Eating Disorders Center
Children's Mercy Hospitals and Clinics
Section of Adolescent Medicine
Assistant Professor of Pediatrics
University of Missouri—Kansas City School of Medicine
Kansas City, Missouri
23: *Documentation, Coding, and Billing*

**Phyllis W. Speiser, MD**
Chief, Pediatric Endocrinology
Steven and Alexandra Cohen Children's Medical Center of New York
New Hyde Park, New York
Professor of Pediatrics
Hofstra North Shore-LIJ School of Medicine
74: *Adrenocortical Disorders*

**Alfred J. Spiro, MD, FAAP**
Professor of Neurology and Pediatrics
Albert Einstein College of Medicine
Director, MDA Muscle Disease Clinic
Montefiore Medical Center
Bronx, New York
128: *Motor Unit Disorders*

**Elizabeth R. Sowell, PhD**
Department of Neurology
David Geffen School of Medicine at UCLA
Developmental Cognitive Neuroimaging
Los Angeles, California
5: *Adolescent Brain and Cognitive Changes*

**Elisabeth M. Stafford, MD, FAAP**
Colonel, US Army (retired)
Clinical Professor of Pediatrics
University of Texas Health Science Center at San Antonio
San Antonio Uniformed Services Health Education Consortium Adolescent Medicine Fellowship
San Antonio, Texas
28: *Health Care of Adolescents in Military Settings*

**Laurence Steinberg, PhD**
Department of Psychology
Temple University
Philadelphia, Pennsylvania
6: *Adolescent Psychosocial Development and Behavior*
34: *Parenting the Adolescent*

**Hans Steiner, MD**
Professor Emeritus
Stanford University School of Medicine
Stanford, California
186: *Disorders of Behavior*

**Kenneth J. Steinman, PhD, MPH**
Clinical Assistant Professor
Division of Health Behavior and Health Promotion
The Ohio State University College of Public Health
Columbus, Ohio
44: *Religion and Spirituality*

**Mitchell Steinschneider, MD, PhD**
Professor of Neurology and Neuroscience
Albert Einstein College of Medicine
Bronx, New York
130: *Demyelinating Diseases*

**Catherine Stevens-Simon, MD, FAAP**
(deceased)
54: *Adolescent Pregnancy*
55: *Adolescent Parenthood*

**Mary Story, PhD, RD**
Professor, School of Public Health
University of Minnesota
Minneapolis, Minnesota
16: *Adolescent Nutrition and Physical Activity*

**Victor C. Strasburger, MD, FAAP**
Professor of Pediatrics
Professor of Family & Community Medicine
Chief, Division of Adolescent Medicine
University of New Mexico School of Medicine
Albuquerque, New Mexico
41: *The Media*

**Deborah Studen-Pavlovich, DMD**
Chair, Committee on the Adolescent
American Academy of Pediatric Dentistry
Professor and Chair, Department of Pediatric Dentistry
University of Pittsburgh School of Dental Medicine
Pittsburgh, Pennsylvania
157: *Adolescent Oral Health*

**Dennis M. Styne, MD, FAAP**
Department of Pediatrics
Section of Endocrinology
Sacramento, California
70: *Disorders of Puberty*

**Gina Sucato, MD, MPH, FAAP**
Department of Pediatrics, Division of Adolescent Medicine
University of Pittsburgh School of Medicine
Pittsburgh, Pennsylvania
32: *Solid Organ Transplantation*

**Nanette Sudler, PhD**
Psychologist
Center for Child & Family Development
Morristown, New Jersey
193: *Academic Overachievement and Underachievement*
195: *Gifted Adolescents*

**Young-Jin Sue, MD**
Attending Physician, Pediatric Emergency Services
Children's Hospital at Montefiore
Clinical Associate Professor of Pediatrics
Albert Einstein College of Medicine
Bronx, New York
180: *Overdose of Prescription Drugs*

**Moira Szilagyi, MD, PhD, FAAP**
Associate Professor of Pediatrics, University of Rochester
Medical Director, Starlight Pediatrics
Monroe County Department of Public Health
Rochester, New York
29: *Adolescents in Foster Care*

**Tina Q. Tan, MD, FAAP**
Professor of Pediatrics
Northwestern University Feinberg School of Medicine
Infectious Diseases Attending; Co-Director—Travel Medicine Clinic and International Adoptee Clinic
Clinical Practice Director, Division of Infectious Diseases
Children's Memorial Hospital
Chicago, Illinois
125: *Central Nervous System Infections*

**Pierre-Paul Tellier, MD, FAAP**
Director, McGill Student Health Services
Associate Professor Family Medicine
McGill University
Montreal, Quebec
178: *Hallucinogens, Club Drugs, Inhalants, and Other Substances of Abuse*

**Brook E. Tlougan, MD**
Resident Physician
The Ronald O. Perelman Department of Dermatology
New York University School of Medicine
New York, New York
146: *Alopecia*

**Steven Tobias, PsyD**
Director
Center for Child & Family Development
Morristown, New Jersey
193: *Academic Overachievement and Underachievement*
195: *Gifted Adolescents*

**Sima Shelly Toussi, MD**
Assistant Professor, Division of Pediatric Infectious Diseases
Weill Cornell Medical College
New York, New York
153: *Immunodeficiencies*

**Howard Trachtman, MD, FAAP**
Chief, Division of Nephrology
Steven and Alexandra Cohen Children's Medical Center of New York
New Hyde Park, New York
117: *Nephritis and Nephrosis*

**H. Michael Ushay, MD, PhD, FAAP, FCCM**
Associate Professor of Clinical Pediatrics
Albert Einstein College of Medicine
Medical Director, Pediatric Critical Care Unit
The Children's Hospital at Montefiore
Bronx, New York
87: *Shock in the Adolescent Patient*

**Elise W. van der Jagt, MD, MPH, FAAP**
Professor of Pediatrics and Critical Care
University of Rochester School of Medicine and Dentistry
Chief, Pediatric Hospital Medicine
Golisano Children's Hospital/University of Rochester Medical Center
Rochester, New York
18: *Pain in Adolescents: Pathophysiology and Management*

**Nishka R. Vijay, MD, FRCPC**
Staff Psychiatrist
Pembroke Regional Hospital
Pembroke, Ontario
187: *Personality Disorders in Adolescents*

**Karen Z. Voter, MD, FAAP**
Associate Professor of Pediatrics
University of Rochester School of Medicine and Dentistry
Rochester, New York
92: *Cystic Fibrosis*

**Christine A. Walsh, MD, FAAP**
Professor of Clinical Pediatrics
Divisions of Pediatric Cardiology and Critical Care Medicine
Albert Einstein College of Medicine
Director, Pediatric Dysrhythmia Center
Co-Director, Montefiore/Einstein Cardio-Genetics Center
Children's Hospital at Montefiore
Bronx, New York
85: *Cardiac Dysrhythmias*

**Curren Warf, MD, MS Ed, FAAP, FSAHM**
Head, Division of Adolescent Medicine
Clinical Professor of Pediatrics
Department of Pediatrics
BC Children's Hospital
Department of Pediatrics
University of British Columbia
Vancouver, British Columbia
45: *Cults and Adolescents*
170: *Prostitution and Sex Trafficking*
171: *Adolescents in Gangs*

**Melissa Weddle, MD, MPH, FAAP**
Associate Professor of Pediatrics
Oregon Health and Science University
Portland, Oregon
176: *Stimulants*

**Eric C. Weiselberg, MD, FAAP**
Division of Adolescent Medicine
Director, Deaf Health Services
Steven and Alexandra Cohen Children's Medical Center of New York
North Shore-LIJ Health System
New Hyde Park, New York
156: *Medical and Psychosocial Considerations for the Deaf Adolescent*

**Patience White, MD, FAAP**
Professor of Medicine and Pediatrics
George Washington University School of Medicine and Health Services
Consultant, BMCH Healthy and Ready to Work National Center
Bethesda, Maryland
31: *Transition of Adolescents with Special Health Care Needs to Adulthood*

**Thomas Williams, MD, PhD**
190: *Adolescent Psychopharmacology*

**Albert C. Yan, MD, FAAP**
Associate Professor, Pediatrics & Dermatology
Section Chief, Pediatric Dermatology
Children's Hospital of Philadelphia
University of Pennsylvania School of Medicine
Philadelphia, Pennsylvania
145: *Dermatitis and Papulosquamous Diseases*

**Anji Yetman, MD, FAAP**
Professor, Pediatrics
University of Utah Health Sciences Center
Director, Adult Congenital Cardiac Program
Primary Children's Medical Center
Salt Lake City, Utah
83: *Carditis in the Adolescent*

**Nader Youssef, MD, FAAP**
Senior Medical Director
NPS Pharmaceuticals
Digestive Health Care Center, PA
Hillsborough, New Jersey
96: *The Approach to Abdominal Pain*
97: *Functional GI Disorders*

**Lonnie Zeltzer, MD, FAAP**
UCLA Mattel Children's Hospital
Pediatric Pain Program
Los Angeles, California
114: *Cancer Survival Issues*

**Susan Yussman, MD, MPH, FAAP**
Department of Pediatrics
University of Rochester Medical Center
Rochester, New York
17: *Complimentary and Alternative Medicine*

**Adam J. Zolotor, MD, MPH**
168: *Physical Abuse*

# Table of Contents

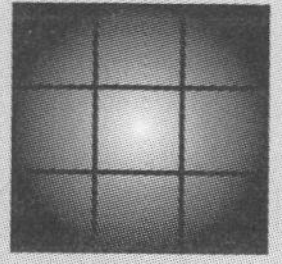

Part 1

# Foundations of Adolescent Health

SECTION 1 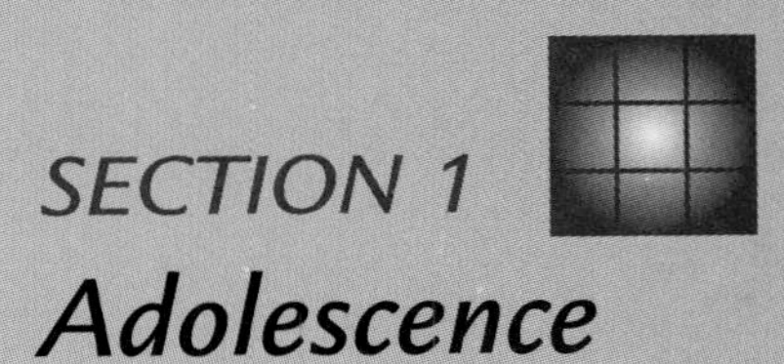

# Adolescence

# CHAPTER 1

## History of Adolescent Medicine and Health Care

HEATHER MUNRO PRESCOTT, PHD

### HISTORY PRECEDING ORGANIZED ADOLESCENT HEALTH CARE

Interest in providing specialized health care to adolescents is a product of ideas about youth that emerged during the early 20th century. The work of developmental psychologist G. Stanley Hall was primarily responsible for establishing adolescence as a distinct developmental category.[1] Hall was also the first to suggest establishing a branch of medicine for adolescents, writing that his book had prompted a deluge of letters from parents and relatives of young people asking for medical advice. "Had I been a physician," Hall wrote, "I might have easily worked up a lucrative practice from such cases."[2]

Yet a new medical field dedicated to this age group did not appear until the 1950s, when adolescent medicine evolved as a subspecialty of pediatrics.[3] This did not mean that adolescents' health care needs were ignored. Rather, the settings in which young people received health care have changed considerably over the course of history.

Prior to the early 20th century, most adolescents, as well as children and adults, received health care from female family members within the home. This was especially true in colonial America, when the number of trained physicians was much lower than in Europe. Advice for caring for sick family members was available in newspapers, almanacs, and domestic medical manuals written by physicians. When an ailment proved to be beyond the healing capabilities of a homemaker, she would rely on a midwife, who typically had training and experience not only in labor and delivery but diagnosis and treatment of illness.[4]

Enslaved African-American youth also received most of their health care within the household or plantation. Typically, slaves received health care from older slave women, who relied on home remedies adapted from West African healing traditions. Owners of large plantations also contracted with local white physicians to provide care for slaves of all ages.[5] After the importation of slaves was outlawed in 1808, slaveholders took special interest in protecting the fertility of young female slaves, because the only legal way to increase the slave population was through reproduction. The estimated mean age of menarche among adolescent female slaves was 15.[6]

### LATE 19TH CENTURY

Prior to the 1920s, a significant percentage of adolescents were compelled to start working for wages at an early age to help support their families. The first national labor data on youth employment, collected in 1880, indicate that 32% of all males and 12% of all females aged 10 to 19 worked for wages. These figures varied considerably according to race and ethnic background; the labor force participation rate of children aged 10 to 19 was considerably higher among black males (66%) and females (44%) than among white males (43%) and females (13%). Likewise, the rate among foreign-born children exceeded that of their counterparts born in the United States—by about 9% and 16% among males and females, respectively. These differences may be largely attributable to the higher earnings levels of white and native-born families. In addition, labor force participation among rural children exceeded urban rates by about 8%.[7]

The poor conditions of many places of employment took a heavy toll on young persons' health. Work in crowded textile mills and sweatshops led to high rates of respiratory illnesses, especially tuberculosis, which was the leading cause of death among adolescents and young adults at the turn of the 20th century. Young workers frequently were injured by heavy machinery too large for them to operate safely. Although some factories, mines, and logging camps contracted with physicians to provide medical service to employees on a fixed per annum basis, most employers did not provide health care or health insurance for their employees.[8] Those who were absent from work because of illness or injury typically lost their jobs.

Larger cities built general hospitals and freestanding dispensaries to provide free health care for growing numbers of poor and immigrant adolescents who needed medical attention. The first children's hospital in the United States opened in Philadelphia in 1855. Several other large cities, such as Boston, Washington, DC, Detroit, and Chicago, created children's hospitals in the late 19th century. In 1909, there were only 25 children's hospitals in the country, compared with 4,359 general hospitals. Children's hospitals seldom treated patients over the age of 12. Administrators of general hospitals recognized that young children needed to be separated from the rest of the hospital population, but they placed adolescents with adult patients. Thus, those who could afford to do so still employed private physicians and nurses to care for them within their homes.[9]

During the 19th century, a variety of public agencies and private philanthropic organizations created institutions for sick and needy adolescents. Although not all of these were designed for health care, the rapid spread of illness among those housed in close quarters necessitated the creation of hospitals and infirmaries as auxiliaries to orphanages, almshouses, and asylums for adolescents with physical, cognitive, or sensory disabilities. Boarding schools for Native American children, started in the late 1870s to separate Native American children from their traditions and make them truly "American," proved to be breeding grounds for contagious diseases, especially tuberculosis and trachoma.[10] White adolescents in private and public schools also were vulnerable to epidemic diseases, such as measles, whooping cough, scarlet fever, diphtheria, and tuberculosis. School boards attempted to control the spread of disease by requiring school children and adolescents to be vaccinated against smallpox, diphtheria, and other diseases prior to attending school. Then as now, a number of parents objected strongly to compulsory vaccination. Some felt that vaccination was dangerous, whereas others resented the intrusion of state officials into private family matters. To prevent the spread of disease and to protect students' health, schools began in the 1890s to hire physicians as medical inspectors. These physicians identified a set of diseases that seemed to be caused and/or exacerbated by the environment of 19th-century schools, many of which lacked adequate light, ventilation, heat, or sanitary facilities. Medical experts noted that American school rooms, especially those in urban areas, were breeding grounds for the spread of disease and called for reforms that would eliminate hazards to student health.[11]

## EARLY 20TH CENTURY

At the same time, child welfare reformers successfully lobbied for legislation to protect the nation's children and youth. Their activism led to the creation of the US Children's Bureau in 1912. This agency led efforts to improve child health and welfare, as well as movements to outlaw child labor and mandate school attendance through the age of 16. As a result of these reforms, school attendance for adolescents grew dramatically. According to US Census figures, in 1890 only 6.7% of 14- to 17-year-olds were enrolled in high school. By 1920, this figure had risen to 32.3% and by 1930 more than 50% of adolescents were enrolled in junior and senior high schools. During the Great Depression, widespread unemployment and New Deal legislation further restricting child labor pushed high school attendance rates to 75% and graduation rates to 50%.

### FIRST ADOLESCENT OUTPATIENT CLINIC

The first mention of an outpatient clinic specifically for adolescents was in a 1918 article from *Archives of Pediatrics*. The article described a separate clinic for girls aged 11 to 16 established by San Francisco physician Amelia E. Gates, MD, as a branch of the children's clinic at the Stanford University Medical School 2 years earlier. Gates observed that malnourishment was a common problem among her patients, with a significant number recorded as underweight for their age, anemic, or having some other dietary deficiency. Postural defects and scoliosis were present in more than one-quarter of her patients. Investigation and treatment of menstrual problems formed a large part of the work of the clinic. Gates wrote it was "surprising how many girls come to us with no knowledge either of the advent or the meaning of the menstrual function," because of erroneous information gathered from other girls or lack of adequate instruction from mothers. Gates believed that one of her main objectives was to make up for this lack of information. Diseases of the teeth and gums were the most common of all, but Gates lacked sufficient facilities for even the most basic dental work.

Gates observed that when the clinic started, she was concerned mainly with medical issues, but she soon found that given her clientele, who came predominantly from working-class families in the Bay area, she and her staff "could hardly confine ourselves to medical work alone," but that the "psychical phenomenon" of the adolescent period was central to their functions as well. A number of the girls in her clinic were referred from associated charities and under the care of foster mothers. The staff also had to deal with other problems in the home, mental overstrain in school, worries about finding employment after graduation, and "the various social maladjustments of our modern life." The clinic "assumed the character of a girls club," providing after-school activities and "wholesome amusement" for the girls' leisure hours. According to Gates, many of the girls looked forward to coming to the clinic, "knowing they can bring their small troubles and worries and feeling sure of a sympathetic understanding and an attempt at effective help." Gates wrote that even after finding jobs, former patients still "hold their allegiance to the clinic and return to us from time to time," usually because of physical disability caused by work-related injuries.[12]

### RELATIONSHIP AMONG HEALTH, ACADEMIC SUCCESS, AND ACCESS TO CARE

During the late 1910s and 1920s, the educational psychologist Lewis Terman argued that public schools also should treat physical illnesses and defects that hindered a student's academic success. He proposed that schools hire nurses, who would not only examine students at school but follow up on cases by visiting the students' homes to ensure that medical treatment was being followed. He also realized that many families, especially immigrant, urban, and rural poor, could not afford medical care on their own. Therefore, he argued that the second essential step in promoting the health of students was to create medical clinics in the nation's schools. These suggestions met with fierce opposition from the American Medical Association (AMA) and other medical organizations, who saw this as the first step toward "socialized medicine." Terman replied that free medical and dental clinics for the nation's children and youth were no different from universal public school education supported by taxpayer dollars. Nevertheless, opposition from the AMA led public schools to abandon school medical clinics as a health care strategy. Instead, they limited their role to providing health education and ensuring that students were properly vaccinated and in sufficiently good health to attend school.[13]

Instead, traditional fee-for-service practice remained the primary model for adolescent health care delivery for decades. Access to these services depended heavily on one's ability to pay. The shortcomings of this system became painfully apparent during the Great Depression of the 1930s, as millions of Americans lost their jobs and could no longer afford physicians' fees. Among the most destitute were the nation's rural farm families, who had the lowest per capita income in the nation and experienced the highest rates of preventable illnesses such as pellagra, hookworm, syphilis, tuberculosis, malaria, and typhoid fever. To address the plight of the nation's farm families, Franklin D. Roosevelt and Congress created the Farm Security Administration (FSA). In addition to providing low-interest loans and other financial benefits to impoverished farmers, the FSA also created a network of prepaid medical cooperative plans that at the agency's peak enrolled more than 650,000 poor rural farmers and their families. Because the FSA targeted those who had few resources to pay for medical care and was a voluntary program that allowed for free choice of physician, the program did not encounter the same attacks from medical organizations about the "socialization of medicine" as did other state-funded health care programs. Although the FSA was disbanded during World War II, the agency's medical program served as a model for the growth of third-party insurance in the postwar period.[14]

## LATE 20TH CENTURY

World War II and its aftermath led to increased attention on the health of adolescents, especially of the nation's young men. Data collected by the Selective Service indicated that 25% of the 18- and 19-year-old registrants who reported for the draft were rejected for military service. Despite the efforts of the FSA, rejection rates were higher for farmers (41%) than for other occupational groups. Racial discrimination and unequal access to health care also led to higher rates of rejection among blacks than among white registrants. These observations led William M. Schmidt, MD, regional medical consultant for the US Children's Bureau, to call once again for the creation of medical clinics in the nation's schools, as well as reforms in medical education that would better equip pediatricians and general practitioners to care for adolescents.[15]

### FIRST HOSPITAL-BASED ADOLESCENT UNIT AND THE SOCIETY FOR ADOLESCENT MEDICINE

The mainstream medical profession continued to oppose school-based medical care, as well as President Truman's efforts to establish national health insurance. However, these calls for increased attention to the health of adolescents led to the emergence of adolescent medicine as a pediatric subspeciality. The first medical unit in the United States devoted exclusively to adolescents was founded by J. Roswell Gallagher, MD, at Boston Children's Hospital in 1951. The Adolescent Unit represented a major shift in approach to the teenage patient: before the 1950s, most physicians who treated adolescents discussed the patient's health problems with the parent and seldom allowed young people to speak for themselves. In contrast, Gallagher and his staff insisted that teenaged patients needed a doctor of their own who would see patients separately from their parents, who would protect their confidentiality, and who would place teenagers' concerns first. The Boston Adolescent Unit served as a model for other hospitals in North America. By the mid-1960s, there were 55 adolescent clinics in hospitals in the United States and Canada, and today more than half of all children's hospitals in the United States have units dedicated to the health care of teenagers. The expansion of adolescent health services led to the creation of a professional organization for adolescent specialists, now called the Society for Adolescent Health and Medicine (SAHM), established in 1968, and the founding of its official professional journal *The Journal of Adolescent Health Care*, first published in 1980 (now the *Journal of Adolescent Health*).[16] In 1991, an application was made by leaders in the field to institute a board-certification examination for physicians interested in becoming subspecialists in adolescent medicine.[17] The American Board of Pediatrics is the parent board for this examination. However, because of a joint agreement with the American Board of Family Practice and the American Board of Internal Medicine, after completing 3-year residencies in pediatrics, family medicine, or internal medicine, physicians become board-eligible following the successful completion of a fellowship program certified by the Accreditation Council on Graduate Medical Education.

### INNOVATIONS IN THE LATE 20TH CENTURY

During the 1960s, adolescents began engaging in behavior that placed them at risk for new health problems. Changing social norms during this period exposed teenagers to new social morbidities such as sexually transmitted diseases, drug addiction, violence, and pregnancy. Although these problems affected the population as a whole, they affected teenagers disproportionately. This may be responsible for the fact that adolescent mortality has risen since 1960, whereas mortality for other age groups has declined.[18] President Lyndon Baines Johnson's War on Poverty included programs to eliminate vast inequities in the distribution of health services in American society. Reforms to Title XIX of the Social Security Act of 1935 authorized the Medicaid program. The US Children's Bureau sponsored a series of special projects grants to train pediatricians in adolescent medicine, which were funded by Title V (Maternal and Child Health Services) of the Social Security Act. Title V funds also were used to create Children and Youth (C & Y) projects, which provided matching funds to state health departments and to medical schools and affiliated hospitals to create new health care services for school-aged children, especially those in underserved areas with high concentrations of low-income families. By 1972, there were 59 C & Y projects in 28 states, the District of Columbia, the US Virgin Islands, and Puerto Rico, serving a total of half a million children and adolescents. The Office of Economic Opportunity (OEO) created by the Economic Opportunity Act of 1964, during Johnson's War on Poverty, funded neighborhood health centers in the nation's cities. The Job Corps and Neighborhood Youth Corps also included health programs for adolescents enlisted in their programs.[17]

Other initiatives to improve access to health care services emerged at this time as well. The American Academy of Pediatrics (AAP), through its Community Access to Child Health (CATCH) program, fostered the development of School-Based Health Centers (SBHC) during the late 1960s and 1970s. The CATCH program had its roots in the work of Philip J. Porter, MD, a faculty member at Harvard who in 1965 became chief of pediatric services at Cambridge Hospital, a municipal hospital affiliating with the Harvard School of Medicine. At the same time, Porter became Director of Maternal and Child Health for the Cambridge City Health Department. After interviewing health care professionals, public health officials, youth clubs and organizations, parents, teachers, and students, Porter developed a program in Cambridge that replaced traditional school nurses with clinical nurses who were directly involved in patient care. These were eventually replaced with pediatric nurse practitioners (PNPs), who created comprehensive school-based clinics, provided visiting nurses for follow-up care in the home, and coordinated care in public health clinics. The success of this program led Porter to look for similar models elsewhere and to persuade the Robert Wood Johnson Foundation (RWJF) to fund the Healthy Children program in 1983. This program dramatically increased the number of SBHCs throughout the country.[19]

## 21ST-CENTURY ADOLESCENT MEDICINE AND HEALTH CARE

Since the early 20th century, experts in adolescent medicine, health, and health care have led the way in working toward ensuring that all adolescents have access to quality medical care, regardless of race, gender, sexual orientation, or socioeconomic status. Adolescent specialists argue that giving teenagers age-appropriate care not only helps reduce the most troubling adolescent health problems, such as pregnancy and substance abuse, but also can prevent adult health problems by educating young people about the importance of lifelong healthy habits.

Despite the growth of services for this age group, gaps in access remain. In America, states have the Medicaid and State Child Health Insurance Programs; more than 8 million or 11% of those under the age of 18 lack health insurance coverage from public or private sources. It remains to be seen whether the United States will follow the lead of other industrialized countries and provide universal coverage for its most vulnerable citizens. The combination of the recent global economic crisis and a new federal administration in the United States presents both an opportunity and challenge to address the health care needs of adolescents in a comprehensive way.

Two major professional groups, the AAP and SAHM, have focused on improving clinical services provided to adolescents and young adults through Web-based materials (www.aap.org/sections/adolescenthealth/strengths.cfm;www.adolescenthealth.org/clinicalcare.htm) to educate physicians, nurses, and other health care professionals caring for this population. Similarly, the European Training in Effective Adolescent Care and Health (EuTEACH) Programme (www.euteach.com) addresses an even broader audience of individuals interested in improving adolescent health and health care. All of these efforts are grounded in initiatives to build on the strengths of adolescents in a developmentally appropriate way to improve their health as they enter adulthood.

## REFERENCES

1. Hall GS. *Adolescence: Its Psychology and Its Relation to Physiology, Anthropology, Sociology, Sex, Crime, Religion, and Education*. New York, NY: D Appleton and Co; 1904

2. Hall GS. Adolescence: the need of a new field of medical practice. *The Monthly Cyclopædia of Practical Medicine.* 1905;8:242

3. Prescott HM. *"A Doctor of Their Own": The History of Adolescent Medicine*. Cambridge, MA: Harvard University Press; 1998

4. Tannenbaum RJ. *The Healer's Calling: Women and Medicine in Early New England*. Ithaca, NY: Cornell University Press; 2002

5. Fett SM. *Working Cures: Healing, Health, and Power on Slave Plantations*. Chapel Hill, NC: University of North Carolina Press; 2002

6. Trussell J, Steckel R. The age of slaves at menarche and their first birth. *J Interdiscip Hist.* 1978;8:477-505

7. Carter S, Sutch R. Fixing the facts: editing of the 1880 US Census of occupations with implications for long-term labor force trends and the sociology of official statistics. *Historical Methods.* 1996;29:5-24

8. Gunn JL. Factory work for doctors: the early years of the section on industrial medicine and public health of the College of Physicians of Philadelphia. *Trans Stud Coll Phys Phil.* 1995;17:61-93

9. Rosenberg CE. *The Care of Strangers: The Rise of America's Hospital System*. New York, NY: Basic Books; 1987

10. Child B. Homesickness, illness, and death: Native American girls in government boarding schools. In: Blair B, Cayliff SE, eds. *Wings of Gauze: Women of Color and the Experience of Health and Illness*. Detroit, MI: Wayne State University Press; 1993:168-179

11. Meckel RA. Going to school, getting sick: the social and medical construction of school diseases in the late nineteenth century. In: Stern AM, Markel H, eds. *Formative Years: Children's Health in the United States*. Ann Arbor, MI: University of Michigan Press;2002: 185-207

12. Gates AE. The work of the adolescent clinic of Stanford University Medical School. *Arch Ped.* 1918;35: 236-243

13. Sedlak MW, Schlossman S. The public school and social services: reassessing the progressive legacy. *Educational Theory.* 1985;35:371-383

14. Grey MR. *New Deal Medicine: The Rural Health Programs of the Farm Security Administration*. Baltimore, MD: Johns Hopkins University Press; 1999

15. Schmidt WM. Physical fitness and health problems of the adolescent: health service in a high school—what it can offer. *Am J Pub Health.* 1945;35:579-583

16. Moore E, Brookman RR. Society for Adolescent Medicine: a capsule history. *J Adolesc Health.* 1998; 23(suppl 6):168-174

17. Gallagher JR. The origins, development, and goals of adolescent medicine. *J Adol Health Care.* 1982;3:57-63

18. Schulenberg J, Maggs JL, Hurrelmann K. *Health Risks and Developmental Transitions During Adolescence*. New York, NY: Cambridge University Press; 1997

19. Hutchins VL, et al. Community Access to Child Health (CATCH) in the historical context of community pediatrics. *Pediatrics.* 1999;103(6):1373-1383

# CHAPTER 2

# Epidemiology of Morbidities and Mortalities in Adolescents

MARINA CATALLOZZI, MD • JOHN SANTELLI, MD, MPH

## INTRODUCTION

This chapter describes the leading causes of death and severe morbidity among adolescents internationally and in the United States. Data sources for this information vary widely, and there are more data available from the United States than from other countries. Data reporting sources also vary in age groupings, with some sources combining childhood and adolescence, others separating in 5-year increments, and still others grouping all adolescents. For example, the Centers for Disease Control and Prevention (CDC) and World Health Organization (WHO) use 10 to 19 years of age as the boundaries of adolescence, but they sometimes include young adults (up to 24 years of age) in reporting causes of morbidity or mortality that span adolescence and young adulthood. Thus, there are no universal standards for adolescent or young adult ages, nor for groupings by developmental phase (ie, early, middle, late adolescents or young adults). We define adolescents as youth 10 to 19 years of age, but some topics include those up to 24 years of age.

## ISSUES WITH DATA SOURCES

Population projections are estimates of future population. They put forth likely population changes based on assumptions about births, and deaths, as well as international migration, and domestic migration over time.[1]

Morbidity and mortality statistics are derived from a variety of sources, each with their own set of limitations. Vital statistics are compiled for the United States by the National Center for Health Statistics (NCHS) using data reported to state health departments. The NCHS publishes data on births, deaths, abortions, fetal deaths, fertility, life expectancy, marriages, and divorces. Registration of births, deaths, and other vital occurrences in the United States is a function of state and local governments; each state requires a continuous and permanent birth and death registration system. Mortality statistics by cause of death are compiled in accordance with WHO regulations according to the *International Classification of Diseases*, 9$^{th}$ edition, Clinical Modification (ICD-9-CM).[2]

Morbidity data are more difficult than mortality data to collect and compile. In general, morbidity data are derived from hospital admission and discharge information, outpatient medical visit data, and regularly performed health and behavior surveys, such as the Youth Risk Behavior Study (YRBS). Many individuals with an illness do not access the medical system, presenting significant limitations to completing morbidity data.

Infectious diseases reporting tends to be more reliable than the reporting of noninfectious diseases because many infectious diseases are verifiable through microbiological identification of an organism, presenting less subjectivity in establishing a diagnosis. There is considerable public health infrastructure on a local, state, and national level to maintain statistics on reportable infectious diseases. Much of this reporting takes place automatically from laboratory to health department. Underascertainment of infectious diseases may occur because a diagnosis is missed, infections are asymptomatic, laboratory testing is not done, or known infections are not reported.

Representative behavioral data are difficult to obtain, and usually gathered through user self-administered surveys. The most widely cited example of this in the United States is the Youth Risk Behavior Surveillance System (YRBSS) conducted by the CDC. The YRBSS surveys a representative sample of 9th through 12th graders. It is conducted every 2 years and includes national, state, and local information. It was developed to monitor health risk behaviors that lead to morbidity and mortality in youth. Although large systems such as these provide prevalence rates of risk behaviors and allow detection of changes in behavior trends, the data are limited by self-report and the youth needing to be in school the day the survey is administered. Adolescents no longer enrolled in school, who are arguably at high risk of unhealthy behaviors, are not surveyed.[3] Despite the limitation with data sources, the United States collects this data in a way in which trends can be followed and interventions made to address problematic issues.

Figure 2-1 depicts an ecological model in which adolescent morbidity and mortality outcomes depend not only on specific behaviors but also on the adolescent's social, biological, cultural, and other contexts. Strong,

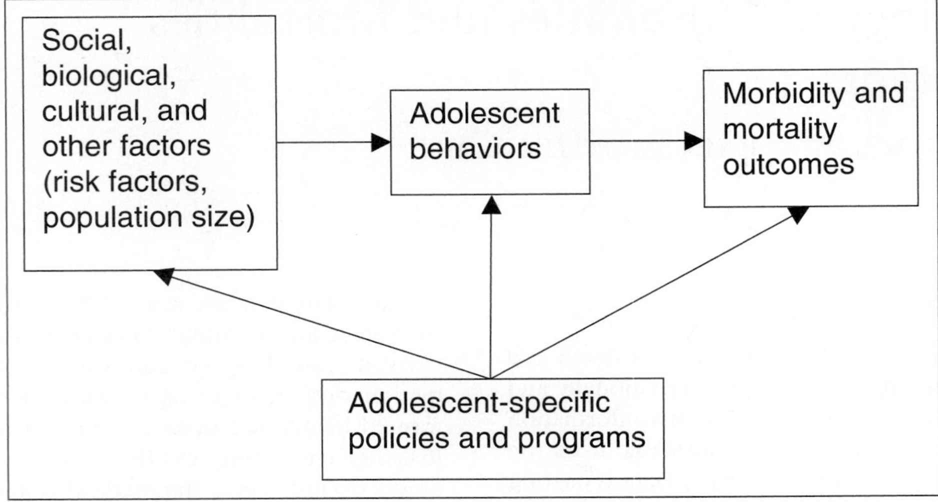


**FIGURE 2-1** Conceptual model showing factors affecting adolescent morbidity and mortality

evidence-based policies and programs that are specific to adolescents and are developmentally appropriate can affect morbidity and mortality and improve the lives of adolescents.

## GLOBAL TRENDS IN ADOLESCENT POPULATION, MORTALITY

Worldwide, the adolescent population is increasing, particularly in developing countries. Blum and Nelson-Mmari[4] have studied morbidity and mortality among young people (see Chapter 3) and have found that adolescent health is affected by improved child survival (resulting in more youth), rural to urban migration (with higher rates of violence and sexually transmitted infections in urban environments), older age at first marriage (which has more effect on girls because it enhances choices for school and work), expanded educational opportunities, and economic and cultural globalization. Globalization has a major effect on adolescent morbidity and mortality by changing the context in which young people live. For example, transnational tobacco company marketing can more openly target youth in developing countries, increasing tobacco-related morbidities. Obesity has emerged as a worldwide problem as calorie-dense diets become available in developing countries. Travel and migration have made AIDS a worldwide epidemic for young people.[4]

Causes of morbidity globally mirror those found in the United States (Table 2-1, Table 2-2). The leading cause of death in adolescents and young adults worldwide is unintentional injury. In the United States, traffic injuries are the main cause of unintentional injury deaths. There are also high rates of sports accidents, burns, poisonings, fire- and burn-related injuries, and drownings (Table 2-3). In developing countries where inroads are being made with regard to treatment and prevention of infectious diseases, unintentional injury is becoming more prominent. In sharp contrast to the United States, however, the second-leading cause of death of adolescents and young adults worldwide is HIV/AIDS and other infectious diseases. In Africa, it is the leading cause of death in persons 15 to 29 years of age. By some estimates, over the last 20 years half of the 60 million persons infected with HIV contracted the infection sometime between 15 and 24 years of age. This so-called invisible epidemic (infection in young people often unaware of their status) has been

**Table 2-1**

**Five Leading Causes of Death, United States, All Races, Both Sexes, 2006**

| *Rank* | *Ages 10–14y* | *Ages 15–19y* |
|---|---|---|
| 1 | Unintentional injury | Unintentional injury |
| 2 | Malignant neoplasms | Homicide |
| 3 | Homicide | Suicide |
| 4 | Suicide | Malignant neoplasms |
| 5 | Heart disease | Heart disease |

Source: Heron M, Tejada-Vera B. Statistics Reports: Deaths: Leading Causes for 2005. National Vital Statistics Reports, 2009;58:8

**Table 2-2**

**Five Leading Causes of Death, Worldwide, Ages 15 to 19y, 2000**

| *Rank* | *Africa* | *Europe* | *North America* | *South America* | *Southeast Asia* | *Worldwide* |
|---|---|---|---|---|---|---|
| 1 | AIDS | Unintentional | Unintentional | Intentional | Unintentional | Unintentional |
| 2 | Infection | Suicide | Suicide | Unintentional | Infection | AIDS |
| 3 | Intentional | Intentional | Intentional | Suicide | AIDS | Infection |
| 4 | Unintentional | Infection | Cancer | Infection | Suicide | Intentional |
| 5 | Suicide | AIDS | Infection | AIDS | Intentional | Suicide |

Adapted from Blum and Nelson-Mmari, The health of young people in a global context. *JAH*. 2004;35(5):402–418.

purported to be the driving force behind the continued epidemic.[4,5] In areas such as sub-Saharan Africa, the disease disproportionately affects young women who are more vulnerable to HIV infection due to social, cultural, and biological factors. Their partners are frequently older men who hold an economic advantage over them—this makes condom negotiation less successful. Additionally, the vaginal surface area and immature cervical tissue of adolescent females makes transmission easier and places the female at increased risk of HIV infection.[4,5]

Although homicide related to interpersonal violence and drug use is an issue in the United States, homicide related to war is the most important form of homicide in developing countries.[4] Suicide is the third most frequent cause of death in industrialized countries such as the United States, but it is only the fifth most frequent cause of death worldwide in the adolescent age group. Rates of suicide are rising (likely secondary to issues such as globalization mentioned previously) and are seen in young men who have access to firearms.[4]

**Table 2-3**

**Five Leading Causes of Unintentional Injury Deaths in the US, 2006, All Races, Both Sexes**

| *Rank* | *Ages 10 to 14y* | *Ages 15 to 19y* |
|---|---|---|
| 1 | Motor vehicle traffic | Motor vehicle traffic |
| 2 | Drowning | Poisoning |
| 3 | Other land transport | Drowning |
| 4 | Fire/burn | Other land transport |
| 5 | Suffocation | Firearm |

Source: Heron M, Tejada-Vera B. Statistics Reports: Deaths: Leading Causes for 2005. National Vital Statistics Reports, 2009;58

Morbidities in developing countries that affect adolescents and young adults include reproductive health issues—particularly early and unwanted pregnancy, unsafe abortions; sexually transmitted infections (other than HIV) that go undiagnosed and untreated; and female genital mutilation. Birth and abortion are significant causes of mortality among young women. Access to safe, confidential, and effective treatment is a priority for adolescents and young adults in the United States and in developing countries.[4]

Violence, in particular sexual coercion and abuse, has been a worldwide issue in particular for young women. Young men also experience high rates of physical and sexual abuse and coercion.[4] The negative consequences of violence are far reaching and include increases in other risk behaviors (sexual risk-taking, substance use) and mental health morbidity. Mental health issues are becoming more recognized and prioritized among youth. In 2003, WHO reported that by the year 2020, psychiatric disorders in adolescents would be one of the leading causes of morbidity.[4,6] Access to psychiatric care remains a problem even in developed countries, and in particular in the United States. Depression is the most common psychiatric condition for adolescents and has been shown to overlap with other morbidities and mortalities. Tobacco, alcohol, and drug use continue to increase globally and are laying important groundwork for unhealthy choices in adolescents. For example, most tobacco users begin use prior to age 18. Alcohol use has been cited as the primary killer of adolescent males in Europe by the Global Burden of Disease because of its association with unintentional and intentional injuries.[4]

Globally, improved adolescent health depends on programs that decrease the risk of motor vehicle accidents (MVAs; eg, safety belts, speed limits, graduated driver's licensing), educate teens regarding reproductive health (particularly safe sex and condom use), reduce the number of teens with access to firearms (or who are involved with combat), and provide accessible mental health services.

## THE GROWING ADOLESCENT POPULATION, UNITED STATES

The adolescent population in the United States has increased markedly over the last 2 decades. In fact, the population of 10- to 19-year-olds in the United States grew by 16.6% (from 34.9 million to 40.7 million) from 1990 to 2000.[7] The steady increase since the 1990s is projected to continue through the year 2030 (Figure 2-2). Although this increase in the adolescent population will continue, it will not increase as sharply as the general population in the United States.[7-10] Until 1990, there were more young adolescents (10–14), but the adolescent population is now older. Older adolescents (15–19) will make up most of the increased population of adolescents. At the same time, the adolescent population is more racially and ethnically diverse than the general population, and projections indicate this trend will continue. Although the current adolescent population, when compared with adults, has greater percentages of black-non-Hispanic, Hispanic, and American Indian/Alaskan native-non-Hispanic individuals, the Hispanic adolescent population is projected to account for most of the increase among racial and ethnic groups within the adolescent population over the next 10 to 20 years.[7,9,10]

With an increase in the adolescent population of color comes an increase in the proportion of adolescents living in poverty, as race and poverty are closely associated in the United States. All of these changes have an effect on services and programs developed for adolescents over the coming years in the United States.[7,9,10]

## ADOLESCENT MORBIDITIES AND MORTALITIES IN THE UNITED STATES

From a historical perspective, the 10 great public health achievements in the 20th century illustrate how concerted public health programs and efforts can prevent morbidity and mortality among teens.[11] These public health achievements include: (1) immunizations, (2) motor vehicle safety, (3) workplace safety, (4) control of infectious diseases, (5) declines in death from

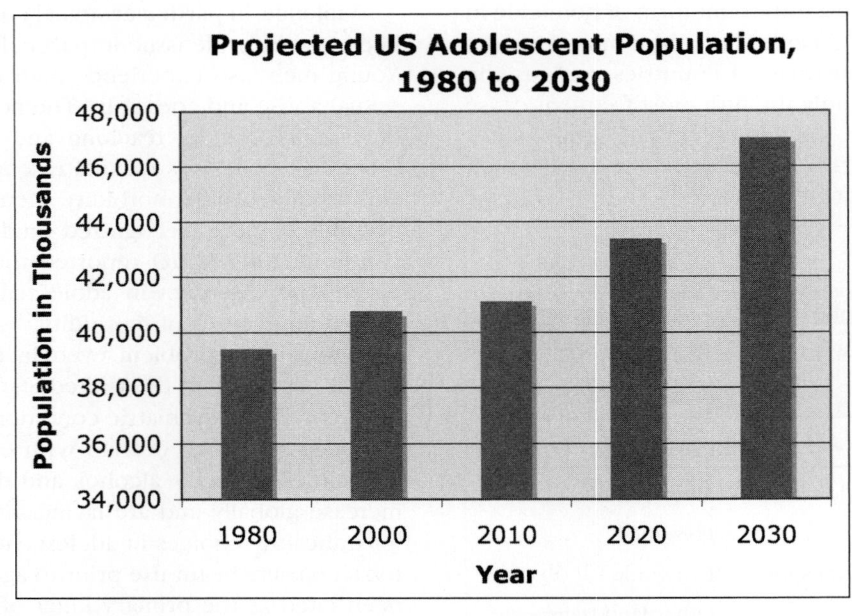


FIGURE 2-2 Projected US Adolescent Population, 1980 to 2030. (Data from National Adolescent Health Information Center (2003). Fact Sheet on Demographics: Adolescents. San Francisco, CA: Author, University of California, San Francisco; and Centers for Disease Control WONDER. Population Projections: United States by State, Age, and Sex, for the Years 2004–2030. Available at: wonder. cdc.gov/wonder/help/PopulationProjections. html#Age%20Group. Accessed April 23, 2009.)

heart disease and stroke, (6) safer and healthier foods, (7) healthier mothers and babies, (8) family planning, (9) fluoridation of drinking water, and (10) tobacco control.

Mortality rates for adolescents and young adults in the United States have decreased from 1980 to 2005.[12] However, continued high rates of preventable death underscore that there is more work to be done in terms of prevention. It is important to understand the causes of morbidity and mortality to be able to direct primary and preventive health care for adolescents. As part of the Healthy People 2010 Initiative, the CDC put forward 21 critical health objectives focused on many of these causes in the hope of guiding future programs and policies for teens (see Box 2-1).

**Box 2-1**

***21 Critical Health Objectives for Adolescents and Young Adults (aged 10–24y)***

- **Reduce mortality of adolescents and young adult**
  1. Reduce deaths of adolescents and young adults
  2. Reduce deaths caused by motor vehicle crashes
  3. Reduce deaths and injuries caused by alcohol and drug-related motor vehicle crashes
- **Unintentional injury**
  4. Increase use of safety belts
  5. Reduce the proportion of adolescents who report they rode with a driver who had been drinking alcohol in the past 30 days
- **Violence**
  6. Reduce homicides
  7. Reduce physical fighting among adolescents
  8. Reduce weapon carrying by adolescents on school property
- **Substance abuse and mental health**
  9. Reduce the proportion of persons engaging in binge drinking of alcoholic beverages
  10. Reduce past month use of illicit substances (marijuana)
  11. Reduce the suicide rate
  12. Reduce the rate of suicide attempts by adolescents that require medical attention
  13. Reduce the proportion of children and adolescents with disabilities who are reported to be sad, unhappy, or depressed
  14. Increase the proportion of children with mental health problems who receive treatment
- **Reproductive health**
  15. Reduce pregnancies among adolescent females
  16. Reduce the number of new cases of HIV/AIDS diagnosed among adolescents and adults
  17. Reduce the proportion of adolescents and young adults with *Chlamydia trachomatis* infections
  18. Increase the proportion of adolescents who have never had sexual intercourse, are not currently sexually active, and if sexually active used a condom the last time they had sexual intercourse
- **Chronic diseases**
  19. Reduce tobacco use by adolescents
  20. Reduce the proportion of children and adolescents who are overweight or obese
  21. Increase the proportion of adolescents who engage in vigorous physical activity

Source: US Department of Health and Human Services. *Healthy People 2010*. Vols 1 and 2. Washington, DC: US Government Printing Office, November 2000. Available at: wonder.cdc.gov/data2010; www.cdc.gov/HealthyYouth/adolescenthealth/NationalInitiative/pdf/21objectives.pdf.

Over the past 3 decades there has been a clear shift from infectious etiologies of morbidity and mortality to those related to intentional and unintentional injuries.[10,11] In fact, the United States CDC reports 4 categories of injuries responsible for 71% of adolescent deaths. These include MVAs (31%), homicide (15%), other unintentional accidents (14%), and suicide (11%).[13-15] This underscores the fact that, although adolescence should be a time of good health with relatively low rates of chronic illness, engagement in risk behaviors not only results in untoward poor health outcomes in adolescents, but it can place these individuals at risk for serious disease as adults. This is particularly important with regard to cardiovascular disease and cancer, accounting for 39% and 23%, respectively, of deaths for adults 25 years of age and older.[14] For example, the 2007 YRBS finds high rates of risk factors for cardiovascular disease and cancer among adolescents. Youth aged 14 to 18 have poor eating habits, with only 21% of youth eating fruits and vegetables at least 5 times/day in the previous 7 days. They also report low rates of physical activity, with only 35% meeting recommended levels of physical activity and 54% attending physical education class. There are high rates of overweight, with 13% classified as obese and 16% as overweight. Eating disorders (anorexia nervosa and bulimia nervosa) generally present during the adolescent years. Additionally, tobacco use is high, with 54% reporting ever trying cigarette smoking and 23% smoking cigarettes in the past month.[15] Hence, adult morbidity and mortality should be affected by health policies and programs that support behavior changes in adolescence.

## UNINTENTIONAL INJURIES

Unintentional injuries are the leading cause of death for persons 10 to 24 years of age in the United States. These preventable deaths increase dramatically for those children 1 to 4 years old to persons 15 to 24 years of age (44% to 79%). Given that injury generally reflects developmental capacity, infants are more likely to sustain injuries from burns, drownings, and falls.[16] As children become mobile they are more likely to have injury from ingestions and poisonings. Thus, while 1- to 4-year-olds are most likely to die of unintentional injury and 10- to 14-year-olds of pedestrian injury, 15- to 24-year-olds are more likely to die of traffic accidents and death secondary to firearms (including homicide, suicide, legal intervention, and unintentional).[16,17] In summary, although mortality rates have decreased since the 1980s, most adolescent and young adult deaths are preventable. Higher mortality rates are seen with increasing age—young adults have 5 times the mortality rate of younger adolescents.[16]

Males are more likely than females to die from each cause of death at every age.[14,16] This seems to be related to differences in behavior and exposure to higher-risk situations. In the United States, the highest mortality rates, particularly with regard to injury, are seen in black and American Indian/Alaskan native males. These racial and ethnic disparities are particularly prominent for homicides. The racial differences in overall mortality rates also appear to be related to socioeconomic factors with impoverished children and adolescents experiencing death rates that are 2 to 5 times higher than individuals who do not live in poverty.[14,16]

Unintentional injuries accounted for 45.5% of all deaths in adolescents and young adults in 2004. Of these, MVAs were responsible for 31.3%, or nearly one-third of mortality. Other unintentional injuries accounted for 14.1% and included poisoning, drowning, fires/burns, and falls.[14] Although this group of unintentional injuries has decreased since 1981, it is still significant.

With respect to MVAs in the United States, American Indian/Alaskan native males have the highest MVA mortality rates.[18] In 2006, youth 16 to 20 years old accounted for about 7% of the overall population, but 14% of fatal crashes involved drivers in that age group.[19] Eighteen percent of all drivers involved in police-reported accidents were 15 to 20 years old. Among drivers involved in fatal MVAs who were 16 to 20 or 21 to 24 years old, 19% and 33%, respectively, had blood alcohol concentration levels at least 0.08 g/dL.[20] Among the 16- to 20-year-olds, the number of fatal crashes increased by 12% over the previous decade. Alcohol-related MVA deaths remain a major public health issue.[19]

Drivers who drink are more than twice as likely to be male and less likely to use restraints.[18] Seventy-four percent of young drunk drivers who were killed in MVAs were not restrained. Apart from not wearing seat belts when driving after drinking, not wearing a seat belt generally is common and more likely to result in a fatality if there is an MVA. Although overall there has been an increase in seat belt use since 1991, seatbelt use increases with age in adolescent females but decreases with age in males.[15,18] There has been an overall reduction in MVA mortality, especially male MVA mortality attributed to increases in minimum age drinking laws. By 1988, states with lower drinking ages were found to have higher alcohol-related car accidents; Congress passed a law upheld by the US Supreme Court to withhold highway funding from any state with a minimum drinking age younger than age 21. This resulted in all states meeting the minimum drinking age of 21 years.[21] The National Highway Traffic Safety Administration (NHTSA) estimates that more than 900 lives were saved by these laws in 2004 alone. Also, although the rates of males and females who drink and drive or ride with a driver who has been drinking have decreased markedly (11.7% to 8.1%, 39.8% to 29.6%, respectively), males are still more likely to drink and drive than females, and both genders are likely to ride with a driver who has been drinking.[15,18] The highest fatality rates in these situations occur in American Indian/Alaskan natives.

Despite improvements, motor vehicle safety is still a substantial issue, and MVAs are still the leading cause of death for adolescents and young adults. Motor vehicle safety for adolescents needs to focus on changing personal behavior (eg, safety belts, helmets, decreased drinking and driving) and changing the physical and social environment. For example, many states have increased the age at which a driver's license can be obtained and lengthened the time in which a new driver needs to be supervised in a graduated process. Other states have laws about the number of teens who can drive in a car together to avoid drinking and driving or other distractions for new teen drivers. Strictly enforced underage drinking laws are also effective.[16]

Other injury-related prevention efforts can include mandatory bike helmets, enforced traffic laws regarding bike riders, early swim lessons, mandated swimming competencies in schools, and proper supervision of athletes by trained individuals (ensuring preparticipation physical examinations, adequate hydration, presence of a medical response system at sporting events).[15] As is true of most preventive efforts, they are best initiated early, before unhealthy risk behaviors have been established.

## HOMICIDE AND VIOLENCE

Homicide is the second-leading cause of death for adolescents and young adults 10 to 24 years old, responsible for 14.2% of all deaths in that age group.[15,22] This is particularly a problem for young men of color. Young men are more likely to die from homicide than their female counterparts, and this difference is more marked as age increases. Males 10 to 14 years old are nearly twice as likely to die from homicide as females, but males 20 to 24 years old are 6.4 times more likely to be homicide victims than female counterparts. This trend has been consistent for more than 25 years. Also, male adolescents are more likely to engage in violent behavior than their female peers. They report higher rates of being in a physical fight, being threatened/injured with a weapon, and carrying a weapon. In contrast, males and females are equally likely to report dating violence.[15,22]

Although homicide rates in adult males in the United States peaked in the early 1990s, there is still a significant problem in young adult black males. Homicide is the leading cause of death for 10- to 24-year-old black, non-Hispanic males, representing 44.5% of all deaths in this group. This is clearly an issue that needs to be addressed because these young men are 2.7 to 15.8 times as likely to die of homicide compared with other racial/ethnic groups.[15,22]

Antiviolence education can take place in the home and the school. Conflict resolution skills, modeling nonviolent resolution of conflict, decreased access to violent images and video games, and decreased access to firearms (particularly in the home) can begin to decrease violence among teens.[16]

## SUICIDE AND DEPRESSION

Suicide is the third-leading cause of death in this age group in the United States, accounting for 12.3% of all deaths in 10- to 24-year-olds in 2004.[15,23] There is a marked increase in suicide rates between early adolescence and young adulthood, with rates 10 times higher in 20- to 24-year-olds compared to 10- to 14-year-olds. In the United States, the highest rates of suicide are among American Indian/Alaskan native male adolescents. Across populations, the trend toward increasing suicide rates with advancing age continues until age 49, then decreases between 50 and 74 years of age, and again increases after age 75. Although female adolescents and young adults are more likely to attempt suicide than their male counterparts, males are 5 times more likely to complete suicide. This higher completion rate is secondary to the method used—males use more lethal methods, such as firearms or hanging, whereas ingestion is more likely in females.[15,23]

Advocacy for suicide prevention includes educating those who work with adolescents to recognize the risk factors for suicide and how to appropriately screen for suicidality. To prevent homicide and suicide, firearms should not be accessible in the home. Access to mental health care should be a major prevention priority for adolescents, because they are one of the highest risk groups for suicide.[16]

## HIV AND SEXUALLY TRANSMITTED INFECTIONS

Among American high school students in 2005, 47% reported ever having sexual intercourse. This is a decrease from 1991 when 54% of students were sexually active.[15] Additionally, more students are reporting condom use at last intercourse (62.8% in 2005 compared to only 46.2% in 1991).[15] Despite these changes, there continues to be a high prevalence of chlamydia infections in young adults (more than 4% of all young adults in the National Longitudinal Study of Adolescent Health [Add Health] data-set) and an overall increase in chlamydia rate for adolescents since 1996.[24,25] This is particularly important for young women because their chlamydia rates are 4.2 times higher than same age males. There also is racial disparity in chlamydia infections, with black young adult infections 6-fold higher than in white young adults. The prevalence of gonococcal infections is low (only 0.43%) because of the increased likelihood of symptoms, detection, and treatment compared to chlamydia. However, there is still a markedly increased prevalence rate of gonorrhea (2.13%) for young black adults compared to other groups. There continues to be a gender and racial disparity, with more girls and more blacks of both genders infected. This is an important public health issue related to screening strategies, access to health care, and long-term morbidity. Higher rates of chlamydia and gonorrhea may be related to the 32% higher risk of ectopic pregnancy in black women compared to white women.[24,25]

Racial disparities also exist with regard to syphilis and HIV. Whereas syphilis is relatively uncommon, there are higher rates among young adults, especially black, non-Hispanic males. Black non-Hispanic youth proportionally represent more cases of HIV and AIDS than their peers, with 13- to 19-year-olds responsible for 69% of all new HIV infections in their age group.[25]

These high rates of sexually transmitted infections in teens underscore not only the need for access to confidential reproductive and sexual health care, but also the importance of prevention. Comprehensive sex education programs are necessary for all adolescents and must include information regarding sexual decision making, safer sex, birth control options, and information regarding sexually transmitted diseases. Only by providing youth with this information can they make healthy decisions regarding sex.

## PREGNANCY/REPRODUCTIVE HEALTH

Despite decreases in the teenage pregnancy rate over time in the United States, the rates remain among the highest in developed countries. There are about 750,000 pregnancies annually in 15- to 19-year-olds in the United States. There was a steady decline in teenage pregnancy rates in the United States to its lowest rate in 30 years, with a 36% decrease between a peak in 1990 to a nadir in 2005. The decline is the result of small increases in abstinence and larger changes in contraceptive practices.[26] However, there have been small increases in pregnancy rates among 15- to 19-year-olds in recent years for reasons that are not fully understood. Racial disparities in pregnancy rates still exist, with black and Hispanic adolescent females having a pregnancy rate twice that of white adolescents.[25-27] These facts highlight the need for comprehensive sexual and reproductive health education to inform adolescents about safer sex and birth control options.

## SUBSTANCE ABUSE

There has been a decline in substance use since the mid-1990s in the United States. Overall, there has been a significant decline in lifetime, past year, and past month use of any illicit drug other than marijuana among 10th grade students in the Monitoring the Future Survey. There also continues to be decreases in cigarette smoking in both Monitoring the Future (www.monitoringthefuture.org) and the YRBS (down from 27.5% in 1991 to 20.0% in 2007). However, daily cigarette smoking is reported by more than 1 in 8 12th graders, and past month cigarette use more than triples between adolescence (ages 10–18) and young adulthood (ages 19–24).[9,28,29]

There have also been decreases in marijuana use (34.2% to 31.8%), steroid use, ecstasy (decreased availability from 30.2% to 27.4%), and methamphetamine use. Modest decreases were also seen for lifetime and past year alcohol use. However, in the YRBS, 43% of students reported drinking alcohol during the past month, with 26% having episodic heavy drinking (ie, binge drinking) during the past month.[9,29-31]

Of great concern is the continued high use of prescription drugs among 12- to 17-year-olds, in particular the high level of Vicodin abuse. In 2006, 1 in 10 12th graders reported past year use of Vicodin. Nonmedical use of over-the-counter cough or cold medications, added to the Monitoring the Future Survey in 2006, was reported by 5.8% of 12th graders in 2007. Younger adolescents continued to report higher rates of current inhalant use (3.9% among 8th graders compared to 2.5% and 1.2% in 10th and 12th graders, respectively).[15,28-31]

Attitudes toward substance abuse, which are thought to predate changes in rates and patterns of abuse (perceptions of low risk, high acceptance, and availability leading to increased abuse), were relatively stable. Decreased perceived risk of harm among 12th graders with respect to LSD is most concerning, along with the decreased perceived risk of harm among 8th graders with respect to marijuana and inhalants. With regard to race and ethnicity, among black, Hispanic, and white 12th graders, whites have the highest rates of past 30-day alcohol abuse, whereas American Indian/Alaskan native-non-Hispanic and white students had the highest rates of past 30-day illicit drug use. Use of any illicit drug is equal for males and females in adolescence, though in young adulthood, males had higher rates of alcohol, cigarette, and illicit drug use than females across all race and ethnic groups.[15,28,29]

In terms of overlapping risk behaviors, there are still high rates (23.3%) of sexually active students who drank alcohol or used drugs before last intercourse.[15] Access to mental health and drug treatment service specific to teenagers is important in the treatment of substance abuse. In terms of preventive measures, strictly enforced underage drinking laws are effective. Additionally, parents and families must be vigilant for signs of substance use and intervene when necessary.

## POLICY IMPLICATIONS: FUTURE DIRECTIONS/AREAS FOR PREVENTION AND INTERVENTION

Although there has been considerable success in decreasing teenage mortality, the hope is that high-risk behaviors and environments can be identified early and that interventions (eg, individual, family, community, etc) can help decrease premature morbidity and mortality, both in adolescence and adulthood. Ecological models that view adolescents and their environments as having a dynamic, bidirectional relationship in which youth both affect and are affected by their environment hold the most promise. The context that adolescents are living in must be examined (biology, environment, social factors) and preventive measures implemented to avoid behaviors that lead to morbidity and mortality—tobacco use, not using seat belts, use of alcohol, weapon carrying—and focus on positive behaviors, protective factors, and resiliency. Maintaining a normal ideal body weight, exercising, delaying sexual initiation, and making good choices should be the emphasis as opposed to a focus on what to avoid. A focus on health and prevention early in adolescence will hopefully result in healthier young adults.

## REFERENCES


1. Hollmann FW, Mulder T, Kallan J. Methodology and assumptions for the population projections for the United States: 1999 to 2100. *Population Division Working Paper No. 38.* Washington, DC: Population Projections Branch, Population Division, Bureau of the Census, US Department of Commerce; 2000

2. US Census Bureau. *Statistical Abstract of the United States: 2009.* Washington, DC: US Census Bureau; 2008

3. Centers for Disease Control and Prevention. Youth risk behavior surveillance—United States, 2007. Surveillance summaries, January 6, 2008. *MMWR.* 2008:57(No SS-4)

4. Blum RW, Nelson-Mmari K, The health of young people in a global context. *J Adoles Health.* 2004;35:402–418

5. Kiragu K. Youth and HIV/AIDS: Can we avoid catastrophe? *Population Reports, Series L, No 12.* Baltimore, MD: The Johns Hopkins University Bloomberg School of Public Health, Population Information Program; 2001

6. World Health Organization. *Caring for Children and Adolescents with Mental Disorders. Setting WHO Directions.* Geneva, Switzerland: WHO; 2003

7. National Adolescent Health Information Center. *Fact Sheet on Demographics: Adolescents.* San Francisco, CA: University of California, San Francisco; 2003

8. Centers for Disease Control WONDER. Population projections: United States by state, age, and sex, for the years 2004–2030. Available at: wonder.cdc.gov/wonder/help/PopulationProjections.html#Age%20Group. Accessed April 23, 2009

9. Kipke MD. *Risks and Opportunities: Synthesis of Studies on Adolescence.* Washington, DC: Forum on Adolescence, National Research Council and Institute of Medicine; 1999

10. Sells CW, Blum RW. Morbidity and mortality among US adolescents: an overview of data and trends. *Am J Pub Health.* 1999;86(4):513–519

11. Centers for Disease Control and Prevention. Ten great public health achievements—United States, 1900–1999. *JAMA.* 1999;281:1481

12. US Department of Health and Human Services, Health Resources and Services Administration, Maternal and Child Health Bureau. *Child Health USA 2007.* Rockville, MD: US Department of Health and Human Services; 2008

13. National Center for Injury Prevention and Control. Fatal injury and leading causes of deaths reports. Atlanta, GA: Centers for Disease Control and Prevention; 2006. Available at: www.cdc.gov/injury/wisqars/index.html. Accessed August 10, 2010

14. National Adolescent Health Information Center. *Fact Sheet on Mortality: Adolescents & Young Adults.* San Francisco, CA: University of California, San Francisco; 2006

15. Centers for Disease Control and Prevention. Youth risk behavior surveillance—United States, 2005. Surveillance summaries, June 9, 2006. *MMWR.* 2006;55(No SS-5)

16. DuRant RH, Smith KS. Vital Statistics and Injuries, In: Neinstein LS, Gordon CM, Katzman DK, Rosen DS, Woods ER, eds. *Handbook of Adolescent Health.* Philadelphia, PA: Lippincott Williams & Wilkins; 2007

17. US Department of Health and Human Services. Trends in the well-being of America's children and youth 2003: HC3.2 Child and youth mortality. Washington, DC: Office of the Assistant Secretary for Planning and Evaluation, Department of Health and Human Services; 2003. Available at: aspe.hhs.gov/hsp/03trends/. Accessed April 23, 2009

18. National Adolescent Health Information Center. *Fact Sheet on Unintentional Injury: Adolescents & Young Adults.* San Francisco, CA: University of California, San Francisco; 2007

19. Chang D. *Traffic Safety Facts Research Note: Comparison of Crash Fatalities by Sex and Age Group.* Washington, DC: National Highway Traffic Safety Administration, National Center for Statistics & Analysis; 2008

20. National Center for Statistics and Analysis, Traffic Safety Facts 2006 Data. *Alcohol Impaired Driving.* Washington, DC: National Highway Traffic Safety Administration; 2008

21. Alcohol Policy Information System. Highlight on underage drinking. Available at: www.alcoholpolicy.niaaa.nih.gov/UnderageDrinking.html. Accessed May 4, 2010

22. National Adolescent Health Information Center. *Fact Sheet on Violence: Adolescents & Young Adults.* San Francisco, CA: University of California, San Francisco; 2007

23. National Adolescent Health Information Center. *Fact Sheet on Suicide: Adolescents & Young Adults.* San Francisco, CA: University of California, San Francisco; 2006

24. Miller WC, Ford CA, Morris M, et al. Prevalence of chlamydial and gonococcal infections among young adults in the United States. *JAMA.* 2004;291:2229–2236

25. National Adolescent Health Information Center. *Fact Sheet on Reproductive Health: Adolescents & Young Adults.* San Francisco, CA: University of California, San Francisco; 2007

26. Santelli JS, Lindberg LD, Finer LB, Singh S. Explaining recent declines in adolescent pregnancy in the United States: the contributions of abstinence and improved contraceptive use. *Am J Public Health.* 2007;97:150–156

27. Guttmacher Institute. *US Teenage Pregnancy Statistics: National and State Trends and Trends by Race and Ethnicity.* New York, NY: Guttmacher Institute; 2006

28. National Adolescent Health Information Center. *Fact Sheet on Substance Use: Adolescents and Young Adults.* San Francisco, CA: National Adolescent Health Information Center, University of California, San Francisco; 2007

29. Johnston LD, O'Malley PM, Bachman JG, Schulenberg JE. *Monitoring the Future National Results on Adolescent Drug Use: Overview of Key Findings, 2008* (NIH Publication No. 09-7401). Bethesda, MD: National Institute on Drug Abuse; 2009

30. NIDA InfoFacts. *High School and Youth Trends. Prescription and Over-the-Counter Medications.* Bethesda, MD: National Institute of Drug Abuse, National Institutes of Health, US Department of Health and Human Services; July 2008

31. NIDA InfoFacts. *High School and Youth Trends. Inhalants.* Bethesda, MD: National Institute of Drug Abuse, National Institutes of Health, US Department of Health and Human Services; June 2008

# CHAPTER 3

# International Adolescent Health

KRISTIN MMARI, MA, DrPH • ROBERT WM. BLUM, MD, MPH, PHD

## INTRODUCTION

Adolescents between 10 and 19 years of age account for 18% of the world's population—representing the largest proportion ever. Behaviors that adolescents adopt during this life stage have critical implications for their future health, morbidity, and mortality. These behaviors are shaped by multiple contexts and external forces—many of which have radically altered the landscape of adolescent health around the world. An ecological approach, in which the environment influences adolescents and adolescents influence their environment, provides the best understanding of adolescent health issues, regardless of geography.

This chapter briefly reviews key social and demographic transitions that affect adolescent and young adult health globally. Subsequently, the leading causes of morbidity and mortality are discussed; and finally, implications for the future of adolescent health and well-being are identified. Because the data rarely discriminate among categories of young people, throughout this chapter the terms "adolescents," "youth," and "young people" are used interchangeably. The World Health Organization (WHO) defines *adolescents* as those between the ages of 10 to 19 years, whereas *youth* are those between the ages of 15 to 24 years, and *young people* include all those between the ages of 10 to 24 years.

## DEMOGRAPHIC AND SOCIAL TRENDS

### GROWING ADOLESCENT POPULATION

As noted previously, today's cohort of adolescents is the largest in history. In the last 25 years, the number of young people in the world has increased by 500 million; and 86% of the world's youth now live in developing countries. The picture is much different in industrialized countries, where the population of youth is declining. In Europe, for example, the number of young people in 2006 totaled 140 million; by 2025, it is projected to decline to 111 million. Conversely, the population of young people in sub-Saharan Africa is anticipated to rise from 305 million in 2006 to 424 million 20 years hence.

### MIGRATION

Beyond population growth, demographic shifts are the result of rural-to-urban and cross-national migration. In 1960, two-thirds of the world population lived in rural areas; by 2030 it will have declined to 40%. Not only is there absolute growth in urban populations, but migratory patterns have shifted as well. Over the past 20 years, large numbers of rural young women, 18 to 24 years old, have come looking for work in major urban areas. The result is that in a number of cities in Latin America and Asia, young adult females outnumber their male counterparts. Elsewhere, the demand (real or perceived) for laborers in cities has resulted in a significant influx of males seeking employment.

In general, large cohorts of young people in urban areas mean that many developing countries can expect a substantial increase in the supply of labor. This can have advantages and disadvantages to local economies. In some Asian settings, the temporarily young age structure of the labor force has been credited as a major factor in enabling sustained economic growth. However, at the same time, a disproportionately high number of young adults in a population can also create new challenges, especially for young men. For example, historical data show that cycles of civil unrest and conflict tend to coincide with periods when young people comprise an unusually large proportion of the population.

### MARRIAGE

Marriage is of particular importance because of the high percentage of young people who marry, with special effect on the quality of adolescent girls' lives. Today young people are marrying at ages older than their parents did; and data suggest that substantially smaller percentages of women marry before the age of 20 years than in previous generations. During the past few decades, the age at marriage has risen most rapidly in Asia, the Middle East, and some part of Latin America. Changes, however, are less striking in sub-Saharan Africa, where early marriage is particularly prevalent. Even in countries where the average age of marriage is relatively high, national figures mask the fact that early marriage may still be prevalent in certain districts. In fact, there is evidence to suggest that in some settings, early marriage may be increasing, especially in societies facing numerous challenges related to poverty and HIV.

### EDUCATION

The other important social trend affecting the health environment of adolescents is the rapid spread of formal education in the developing world. Today, nearly half of all countries mandate education through 14 years of age. Between 1980 and 2005, the percentage of boys enrolled in secondary schools rose from 54% to 63%. For girls, the increase was even more dramatic, rising from 44% to 56%. Comparing girls' education by region from 1980 to 2005: in sub-Saharan Africa girls' education increased from 15% to 33%, in Asia from 34% to 51%, and today in Latin America, there is no gender difference in education of adolescent males and females. The rewards for formal education are especially prominent for adolescent girls, where research has shown positive associations between being in school and protective sexual and reproductive health behaviors, such as delaying first sex, abstaining from sex, and using condoms.

Indeed, the health environment for young people has been dramatically altered by these global societal and epidemiological shifts that have been taking place over the past few decades. Many of these changes have brought great improvements, whereas others have created greater risks for young people, such as the increased risk for HIV among young women in sub-Saharan Africa. As mortality and morbidity trends are examined in the section that follows, it is important to keep in mind that many of these health problems have been shaped by multiple social and economic contexts of young people—all of which are ever-changing.

## ADOLESCENT MORTALITY AND MORBIDITY

### MORTALITY AND PRIMARY CAUSES OF MORTALITY

Considering only mortality rates, adolescence appears to be a relatively healthy period of life. Young people between 10 and 24 years of age are the least likely to die compared with any other age group. In developing countries, the risk of dying between the ages of 10 and 25 years is about 2.5%, compared with about 9% for those between birth and age 10. Although mortality rates among young people in developing countries are low, they are more than double the rates for young people in industrialized countries.

Reliable data on specific causes of adolescent mortality in developing countries are limited, particularly in many of the countries of sub-Saharan Africa. Despite this constraint, the WHO's Global Burden of Disease project calculates mortality estimates based on existing data and various statistical modeling techniques. Although there is regional variation, from a global perspective the major causes of mortality among those ages 15 to 29 years include: (1) unintentional injuries; (2) HIV/AIDS; (3) homicide and war; (4) suicide, and (5) maternal mortality.

#### Unintentional Injuries

For industrialized countries, unintentional injuries represent the leading cause of death for adolescents and young adults. In the United States, injuries kill more adolescents than all diseases combined, with at least 1 adolescent dying of an injury every hour of every day. In developing countries, where industrialization is growing and infectious diseases increasingly are being controlled, unintentional injury will soon become a cause for concern equal to the industrialized world. In a survey of the causes of death among adolescents in South Africa, unintentional injuries were found to account for 57% of all mortality in the 10- to 19-year-old age group, and similar results have been found in Papua New Guinea, Nigeria, Singapore, and a number of South American countries. Within the category of unintentional injuries, traffic-related fatalities are by far the most prevalent in most world regions. For adolescents 15 to 24 years of age, traffic-related injuries are the leading cause of injury deaths among 11 industrialized countries, ranging from a low of 12 to 15 per 100,000 in England, the Netherlands, Norway, and Israel to a high of 49 deaths per 100,000 in New Zealand.

However, traffic accidents are not the only injuries threatening the lives of young people. Recreational and sports accidents in developed countries, burns and poisonings in developing countries, and falls and drowning in every region also represent major risks. In Brazil, drowning is second only to traffic accidents as a cause of death in young people 10 to 14 years of age. Drowning also accounts for 15% of all adolescent deaths in Uruguay, 10% in Paraguay, 8.3% in Costa Rica, and 7% in Argentina and Mexico. In Asia, drowning is the leading cause of mortality due to accidents in children and young adults, and in many countries of the continent, it accounts for up to 30% of accidental deaths, although some of these may be disguised suicides.

#### HIV/AIDS

HIV/AIDS is the second-leading cause of death worldwide among those 15 to 29 years of age, and it is the number 1 cause of mortality in sub-Saharan Africa. Currently there are approximately 12 million young people who are HIV infected around the world, with 75% of those living in sub-Saharan Africa. Additionally, half of all new cases of HIV in sub-Saharan Africa are among youth. Because the majority of HIV infections are sexually transmitted, the vulnerability of young people is strongly influenced by their sexual behaviors, such as early age of sexual initiation, early marriage, multiple sexual partners, and commercial sex work. Most developing regions show substantially higher HIV prevalence among females aged 15 to 24 years compared to males. This is especially true in sub-Saharan Africa, where prevalence rates among females are more than double those of males. Factors that predispose young women to increased risk include: the power differential between genders, genital trauma, cervical immaturity, greater surface area of exposure for females than males, and higher concentration of the HIV virus in semen than in vaginal secretions. In settings where HIV is heterosexually transmitted (and especially in sub-Saharan Africa), the evidence appears strong that circumcision reduces the risk of transmission by as much as 50%. Globally, however, not all HIV is heterosexually transmitted. In Western Europe and North America, two-thirds of all HIV-infected people are males, with anal intercourse a primary mode of transmission. In much of Asia, the primary route of transmission is through IV drug use, so there is little gender variation of HIV in that area.

### Homicide and War

Health data from many parts of the world confirm that injuries due to violence are also among the chief causes of mortality for young people, particularly adolescent males. Available data indicate that the most violent region in the world is the Americas, where homicide rates are highest among young men ages 15 to 24 years. According to the Pan American Health Organization (PAHO), homicide is the second-leading cause of death among young males aged 15 to 24 years in 10 out of 21 countries with populations greater than 1 million, with the highest being in Colombia (267 per 100,000 in 1994), Puerto Rico, Venezuela, and Brazil (72 per 100,000). The United States, at 38 per 100,000, is 4 times higher than the next highest rate among the 21 industrialized countries, and highest when compared to Western European countries, Canada, Australia, and New Zealand.

Mortality as a result of war probably claims more adolescent lives in developing countries than do other forms of homicide, as young people 10 to 24 years old are the majority of soldiers in most developing countries. A 1996 UNICEF report found that adolescents have been used as combatants in many conflicts in countries such as Liberia, Mozambique, Cambodia, Myanmar, and Sierra Leone. In fact, according to WHO (1998), more than 100 million young people have been involved in armed conflict, either as soldiers, civilians, or refugees.

### Juvenile Suicide

Although suicide is the fifth-leading cause of mortality globally, it is the second-leading cause of death for youth in industrialized countries. The highest rates of juvenile suicide occur in Northern Europe, North America, the Pacific Basin, and the Far East, with the lowest rates in Latin America, sub-Saharan Africa, Mediterranean countries, and Muslim countries. In India and China, suicide represents the leading cause of death for youth.

In most regions of the world, suicide is more common for males than females. According to data from the WHO Mortality Database, suicide rates for young people in the 15- to 19-year-old age group were higher among males than females in nearly every country examined. In fact, young males' overall suicide rate among industrialized and developing countries was 2.6 times that of females, with the exceptions of Sri Lanka, El Salvador, Cuba, Ecuador, and China, where female suicide rates exceeded those of their male counterparts.

### Maternal Mortality

Maternal mortality persists among the top 5 leading causes of death globally, and in many countries of the world it is 1 of the 3 leading causes of death among young women. Maternal mortality is defined as death that occurs within 42 days of delivery. About 80% of maternal deaths are due to maternal hemorrhage, sepsis, unsafe abortion, obstruction, and eclampsia, whereas 20% result from complications of diabetes, malaria, and HIV. In many low- and middle-income countries, the lifetime risk of maternal death is 1 in 61, compared with 1 in 2,800 in more industrialized regions of the world.

The risk of maternal mortality among those 10 to 14 years of age is much greater than for older teenagers (15–19 years). A study in Bangladesh showed that girls 10 to 14 years of age had a maternal mortality rate 5 times that of women 20 to 24 years of age, whereas for 15- to 19-year-olds the rate was twice that of the 20- to 24-year-olds. Similarly, in Jamaica and Nigeria, pregnant women under age 15 were 4 to 8 times more likely to die during pregnancy and childbirth than those 15 to 19 years old.

## MORBIDITY TRENDS

### Sexual and Reproductive Health Morbidities

Young people who engage in unprotected sex are at risk for sexually transmitted infections (STIs), including HIV, and pregnancy. According to WHO estimates, 1 in 20 adolescents worldwide acquires an STI each year, and of the estimated 340 million new STIs, at least 111 million occur in young people under the age of 25. Sexually transmitted infections deserve attention not only because of their high prevalence, but also because they frequently go undetected and untreated, and can result in serious reproductive morbidity and mortality.

However, reporting of STIs is often poor, and the actual prevalence among adolescents may be higher than inadequate figures indicate. As a result of the underreporting of STIs, their immediate effects on adolescents may not be apparent.

In addition to STIs, a substantial number of sexually active young women become pregnant, which is often both unplanned and unwanted. National health data for 15- to 19-year-olds usually include rates of births rather than pregnancy rates. The worldwide birth rate for adolescents is 65 per 1,000 girls. However, this average includes a wide range of 37 per 1,000 in Mauritius to 229 per 1,000 in Guinea, and an intemediate birth rate in sub-Saharan Africa of 143 per 1,000 girls for 15- to 19-year-olds. Many of these births occur to adolescents who are not married. In much of sub-Saharan Africa, for example, one-third of births to women 15 to 19 years old are among unmarried adolescents; the proportion is quite low (4%–6%) in Burkina Faso, Mali, Niger, and Nigeria, but exceeds three-quarters in Botswana and Namibia. Typically in Latin America and the Caribbean, 12% to 25% of adolescent births are to unmarried teenagers.

Adolescent birth rates are intertwined with rates of spontaneous and induced abortions. Throughout the world, estimates indicate that 46 million pregnancies are voluntarily terminated every year, 27 million legally and 19 million outside the legal health care system. All but 3% of unsafe abortions occur in developing countries. Importantly, from a public health standpoint, 14% of all unsafe abortions in developing countries (or about 2.5 million abortions) are in women younger than 20 years of age.

### Mental Health Disorders

Until recently, the magnitude of the burden of disease related to adolescent mental disorders has been difficult to quantify. Now, with the global crisis involving adolescents affected by war, orphaned by AIDS, and forced to migrate for economic and political reasons, the dimensions of the burden of compromised mental health are increasingly evident—and alarming. Worldwide, up to 20% of children and adolescents suffer from a disabling mental illness. The WHO indicates by the year 2020 adolescent psychiatric disorders will increase by more than 50% worldwide to become 1 of the 5 leading causes of disability among adolescents.

One of the most common mental disorders affecting adolescents and young people worldwide is depression. When comparing depressive symptoms among adolescents in 28 developed countries, has been shown that adolescents in the United States had the highest levels of depressive symptoms, whereas Austrian teens reported the lowest levels. The primary concern with depression among adolescents is that it is often combined with substance abuse, which puts adolescents at even greater risk for suicide.

### Alcohol

In many countries, overdoses of alcohol and other drugs compete with road accidents as leading causes of death in young people. Psychoactive substance use occurs in all known societies, with heavy episodic or binge drinking especially common among young people. In 2000, the use of alcohol and illicit drugs was estimated to contribute 9.8% of the total global burden of disease for people 15 to 29 years of age. This burden disproportionately affected males and people living in industrialized countries. Although alcohol use seems to have stabilized and binge drinking has declined somewhat in North America recently, adolescent alcohol use in Latin America has increased 400% over the past 25 years. In Australia, 47% of 11th graders indicate that they drink at least weekly. It appears that as income increases, so does alcohol consumption, in industrialized and developing countries.

### Tobacco

Tobacco use is also a major health problem in many countries. According to 1 estimate, between 68,000 and 84,000 people under the age of 20 in low- and middle-income countries begin smoking every day. Smoking usually starts before age 18. Recent trends show an even earlier age of initiation and rising smoking prevalence rates among children and adolescents. For example, according to the Global Youth Tobacco Survey, the highest prevalence of early initiation of cigarette smoking is in China, Poland, and Zimbabwe, where nearly one-third of the students who ever smoked cigarettes started smoking before the age of 10 years. Moreover, nearly 70% of students 13 to 15 years of age have ever smoked cigarettes in the Ukraine, Poland, and the Russian Federation. In surveys across developing countries, 15% of male students and 7% of female students are currently smoking cigarettes. In most countries, boys are more likely than girls to use tobacco. When this tendency is reversed, it usually is due to a successful advertising campaign by the tobacco industry to make cigarettes look fashionable.

## CONCLUSIONS

When examined globally, there are a number of conclusions that can be drawn with significant consequences for the future of young people. First, in both relative terms and absolute numbers there are more young people now than ever before. These numbers will continue to increase over the next 50 years, especially in developing countries, whereas the relative proportion of youth in industrialized countries will decline. In addition, transnational migration means that what was viewed as distant concerns are frequently now relevant to domestic as well as international health.

Trends that have, and will continue to have, a major impact include: (1) the decline of infectious causes of mortality, (2) the rise of urban living, globalization, and education, and (3) the delay in the age of marriage. Emerging issues include: (1) traffic-related mortalities, (2) clandestine abortion, (3) mental health disorders, including suicide, (4) homicide, (5) tobacco and alcohol-related morbidities, and most importantly, (6) HIV/AIDS. Although the HIV/AIDS epidemic has, in large part, helped draw attention of governments worldwide to the reproductive health needs for adolescents, far less attention has been given to addressing the issues of traffic-related mortalities, mental health disorders, suicide, and tobacco and alcohol-related morbidities for adolescents.

To be effective in creating new youth policies and programs for these new morbidities, it is important to pay attention to local and regional variations influenced both by variations in disease prevalence and frequency of related health behaviors, but also by the enormous differences in cultural and social beliefs and practices as well as economic contexts in which these conditions and behaviors occur. In some settings, rapid social changes are destabilizing the traditional paths of youth development, which often results in thrusting youth and society into uncertain confusion regarding how to move forward in the future. In addition, economic decline in developed countries and competition for financial resources in developing countries almost universally affect health care services. Even more lacking are services for mental health disorders, because priority is most often given to those illnesses labeled as physical.

For young people themselves, health may not be a top priority. The views of young people have rarely been studied or taken into consideration for designing policy and programs—particularly in the developing world. Studies on young people's assessments of their health needs in industrialized countries have shown that they tend to focus more on physical concerns, such as acne, menstruation, and weight, and psychosocial concerns, such as relationships with their family and peers. However, few if any of these would feature among the priorities established by government health planners on the basis of quantitative assessments of need. Yet, if interventions that target young people are going to be accepted by, and be salient to them, the viewpoint of young people must be investigated and incorporated into programs. It is uncommon for adults and adolescents to view issues from a similar perspective. Finding common ground between adults and adolescents is essential to finding solutions that will work; positive youth development approaches are being used in a number of areas to good effect in this regard. Youth need to be seen as part of the solution; in doing so, we increase the likelihood that not only will our interventions be accepted, but they will be more effective because they will be more consistent with the health priorities of young people.

## BIBLIOGRAPHY


1. Bearinger L, Sieving R, Ferguson J, Sharma V. Global perspectives on the sexual and reproductive health of adolescents: patterns, prevention, and potential. *Lancet.* 2007;369: 1220–1231

2. Blum R, Rinehart P. *Reducing the Risk: Connections That Make a Difference in the Lives of Youth*. Bethesda, MD: Add Health; 1997

3. Brown P. Choosing to die—a growing epidemic among the young. *Bull World Health Organ.* 2001;29(12):1175–1177

4. Guest P. Mobility transitions within a global system: migration in the ESCAP region. *Asia-Pacific Popul J.* 1999;14(4): 57–72

5. Lammers C, Blum R. International health. In: Friedman SB, Schonberg SK, Fisher MM, Alderman EM, eds. *Comprehensive Adolescent Health Care*. 2nd ed. Philadelphia, PA: Mosby-Year Book, Inc; 1997:17–22

6. Larson RW. Globalization, societal change, and new technologies: what they mean for the future of adolescence. In Larson R, Brown B, Mortimor J, eds. *Adolescents' Preparation for the Future: Perils and Promise*. Ann Arbor, MI: Society for Research on Adolescence; 2002

7. Mathers CD, Stein C, Ma Fat D, et al. *Global Burden of Disease 2000: Version 2 Methods and Results. Global Programme on Evidence for Health Policy Discussion Paper No 50.* World Health Organization; 2002

8. Mensch B, Bruce J, Greene M. *The Uncharted Passage: Girls' Adolescence in the Developing World*. New York, NY: Population Council; 1999

9. National Research Council and Institute of Medicine. *Growing Up Global: The Changing Transitions to Adulthood in Developing Countries. Panel on Transitions to Adulthood in Developing Countries.* Lloyd CB, ed. Committee on Population and Board on Children, Youth, and Families. Division of Behavioral and Social Sciences Education. Washington, DC: The National Academies Press; 2005

10. PAHO. *Health in the Americas*. Washington, DC: PAHO Scientific Publications 569; 1998

11. Patel V, Flisher A, Hetrick S, McGorry P. Mental health of young people: a global public health challenge. *Lancet.* 2007;369:1302–1313

12. Peters L, Tonkin R. Measuring adolescent health status. In: Tonkin RS, ed. *Clinical Paediatrics. International Practice and Research. Vol. 2. Current Issues in the Adolescent Patient.* London: Bailliere Tindal; 1994, 385–407

13. Scheidt P, Overpeck MD, Wyatt W, Aszmann A. Adolescents' general health and well-being. *Health and Health Behaviour among Young People. WHO Policy Series: Health Policy for Children and Adolescents, International Report* 1:24–38. Copenhagen, Denmark: WHO; 2000

14. Toumbouruou JW, Stockwell T, Neighbors C, Marlatt G, Sturge J, Rehm J. Interventions to reduce harm associated with adolescent substance use. *Lancet.* 2007;369:1391-1401

15. UN Department of Economic & Social Affairs. Temporal trends in population, environment, and development. *Population, Environment and Development: The Concise Report*; 2001: 11

16. United Nations Educational, Social, and Cultural Organization (UNESCO). *World Education Report, 1997.* Paris: UNESCO; 1997

17. United Nations. *World Population Prospects, the 2002 Revision, Volume 1: Comprehensive Tables*. New York, NY: United Nations; 2003

18. Van Look P. *On Being an Adolescent in the 21st Century*. Geneva, Switzerland: World Health Organization, Division of Reproductive Health and Research; 2001

19. Warren CW, Riley L, Asma S, et al. Tobacco use by youth: a surveillance report from the Global Youth Tobacco Survey Project. *Bull World Health Organ.* 2000;78:868–876

20. Wasserman D, Cheng Q, Jiang G. Global suicide rates among young people aged 15–19. *World Psychiatry.* 2005;4(2):114–120

21. World Health Organization. *Caring for Children and Adolescents with Mental Disorders. Setting WHO Directions.* Geneva, Switzerland: WHO; 2003

22. World Health Organization. *Global Burden of Disease*. Geneva, Switzerland: WHO; 2000

SECTION 2

# Growth and Development

# CHAPTER 4

## Normal Pubertal Physical Growth and Development

KANTI R. CRAIG, MD • FRANK M. BIRO, MD

### INTRODUCTION

In contrast to the term adolescence, which refers to the psychosocial changes that occur between childhood and adulthood, puberty refers to the physiologic and anatomic changes associated with reproductive capacity. Puberty is a period of development that includes changes in nearly every body system. The onset of puberty is marked by an increase in the amplitude of luteinizing hormone (LH) pulses that reflect an increased amplitude of luteinizing hormone release hormone (LHRH) pulses, most notable during sleep. In this process the hypothalamus is decreasingly sensitive to negative feedback by gonadal sex steroids, and the hypothalamic–pituitary–gonadal (HPG) axis matures with respect to pituitary release of follicular-stimulating hormone (FSH) and LH from an infantile to adult pattern.[1] Prepubertally, central nervous system gamma-aminobutyric acid (GABA) and GABAergic-releasing inhibitory neurons inhibit the LHRH pulse generator.[2] Thus, activation of the LHRH pulse generator and the HPG axis results from a decrease in inhibition and increase in the input of excitatory amino acid neurotransmitters (including glutamate) and possibly astroglial-derived growth factors.[2] In addition, leptin serves as 1 of several permissive factors that does not trigger but allows the onset of puberty.[2]

The past decade has produced several studies investigating factors that influence the onset of puberty, including nutritional status, genetics, and environmental modulators.[3] The body mass index (BMI) of children in the United States has increased dramatically over the past 2 decades, and the overnutrition of youth has accounted for, in part, a younger age at the onset of puberty.[4] Race and ethnicity may also affect the onset of puberty. Analyses from the National Health and Nutrition Examination Survey (NHANES)[5] data suggest that black girls and boys reached the onset of pubertal development (thelarche) one year before their white peers. Additionally, there may be important interactions between these factors, as demonstrated by a greater decrease in age of menarche among black girls, when contrasted with white girls.[6]

Generally occurring with pubertal maturation are changes in cognitive (development of formal operational thought) and social (the process of adolescence) realms. Perhaps the most obvious change associated with puberty is the physical transformation of a girl into a woman and a boy into a man. Although a minor increase in height velocity is an early event for girls and boys, this can only be detected by accurate, longitudinal measurement of height several times a year.[7] The visible, and therefore easily detectable sequence of sexual maturation events in clinical practice was categorized by Reynolds and Wines[8] in the 1940s and modified and disseminated widely by Marshall and Tanner in the 1960s.[9,10] These changes are known popularly as Tanner Stages, and van Wieringen[11] subsequently published descriptive photos representing the changes associated with each stage of sexual maturity rating (SMR).

### PUBERTY IN GIRLS

#### SEXUAL MATURITY RATING OF PUBIC HAIR AND BREAST TISSUE

There are 5 stages of SMR for pubic hair and genital development. Figure 4-1 demonstrates pubic hair staging in girls. Stage 1 SMR is prepubertal; pubic hair is absent. Stage 2 SMR demonstrates fine, sparse, straight hair along the vulva. Darker, coarser, and slightly curly hair that extends over the mid-pubis represents Stage 3. Sexual maturity rating Stage 4 has adult-type hair that covers the external genitalia but does not extend to the

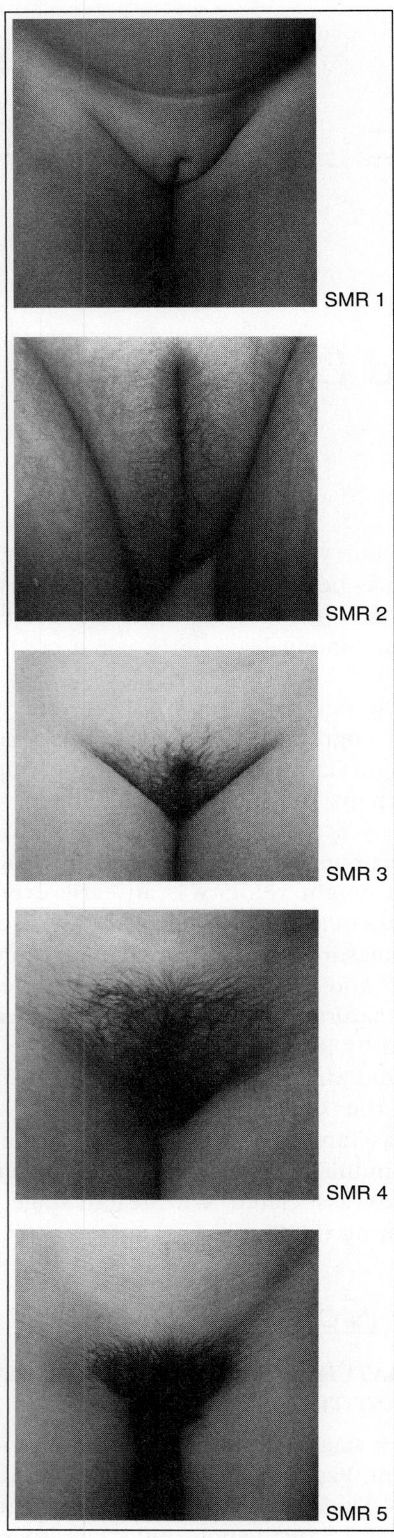


**FIGURE 4-1** Stages of female pubic hair development. Photos courtesy Carlos J. Bourdony, MD, former Director of Pediatric Endocrinology, San Juan City Hospital, San Juan, Puerto Rico.

medial thighs. Finally, Stage 5 SMR has adult-type hair that extends onto the medial thighs. Extension of the adult-type hair up the linea alba or to the anterior thigh is still considered Stage 5 pubic hair development. It is important to consider that the initiation of sexual hair development in the genital and axillary areas is under the influence of the HPA axis, with dihydroepiandrosterone (DHEA) and DHEA-sulfate as the hormones responsible for the first stages of sexual hair development. The HPG and HPA axes are relatively independent of each other, but often coincide.

Figure 4-2 demonstrates breast development. Stage 1 is prepubertal breast, without palpable breast tissue, and a small areola on the same plane as the chest wall skin. Stage 2 reveals the breast "bud" immediately under the enlarging areola. Further enlargement of the breast tissue beyond the margins of the areola, but without separation of the areolar contour from the plane of the chest wall, is Stage 3 (M-3 in photo). Stage 4 has the formation of a secondary mound of the darkening and widening areola above the remainder of the breast tissue, the so-called double-mound effect. Lastly, Stage 5 is defined by recession of the areola to the same level as the skin overlying breast tissue and projection of the papilla beyond the contour of the areola and breast. Some normal adult women do not reach Stage 5 breast development, or only do so during pregnancy. Therefore, SMR Stage 4 can be considered sexually mature; most females at SMR 4 breast development also have menstruated.

In girls, although height velocity predates onset of secondary sex characteristics,[7,12] this is usually not noticeable clinically in adolescent health care, but only detectable with frequent and accurate measurements generally performed in longitudinal growth studies. Utilizing data from the Pediatric Research in Office Settings (PROS) and from NHANES III[4] studies, 50% and 95% of black girls will have attained SMR breast Stage 2 development by ages 9 and 11, respectively, and 50% and 95% of white girls by ages 10 and 12, respectively. Figure 4-3 illustrates the typical sequence of pubertal events in US girls. Globally, there is significant variability in the ages of these developmental changes, as illustrated in Figure 4-4. As seen in Figure 4-3, girls continue to grow after menarche, but at a decreasing rate, usually growing no more than 2 inches following this event. The usual interval between menarche and ovulatory cycles is 14 to 24 months. A later age at menarche is associated with a longer interval before most of the cycles are ovulatory.[13]

Investigations frequently use menarche as the marker of puberty in girls, especially in international studies. For example, the European Prospective Investigation into Cancer (EPIC) showed that the age of menarche

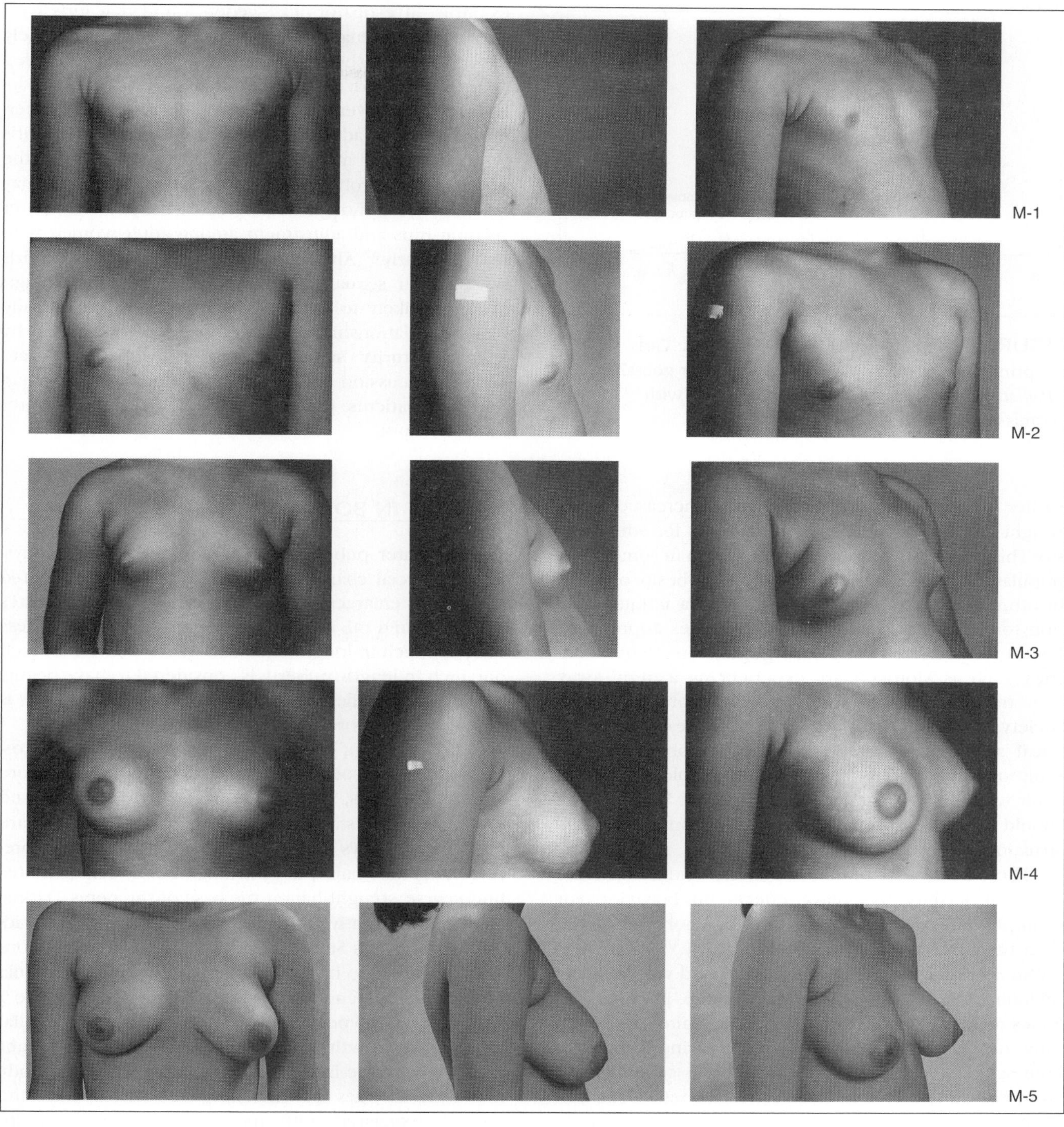


**FIGURE 4-2** Stages of female breast development. Photos courtesy Carlos J. Bourdony, MD, former Director of Pediatric Endocrinology, San Juan City Hospital, San Juan, Puerto Rico.

(their marker for the onset of puberty) has steadily decreased while final adult height has increased.[14] Longitudinal data from Korea confirm a secular trend of increasing adult female height and a younger age of menarche.[15] Repeated studies in Korea show the age of menarche decreasing from 16.8 years to 12.7 years old.[15] In the United States, the age of menarche has declined slightly from age 12.53 to 12.34 from 1999 to 2002.[16]

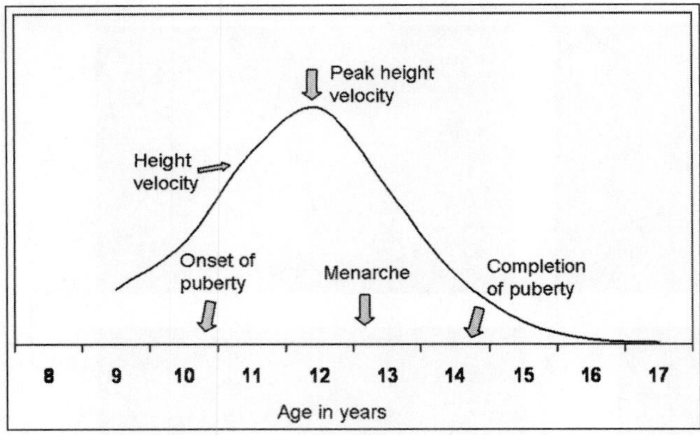


**FIGURE 4-3** Sequence of pubertal events: Girls. (Reprinted from Biro FM. Puberty–Whither goest? *J Pediatr Adolesc Gynecol* 2006;19:163–165, with permission from Elsevier.)

Earlier menarche is associated with increased adult weight and height[6] and an increased risk for adult obesity. This possibility may be more common in some black populations. Given the adverse effects of obesity on adult health, the primary care physician is in a unique position to encourage healthy lifestyle changes appropriate for the preteen and early teen population. Many countries, such as Morocco, are experiencing a trend away from traditional culture toward more "urban" or modern society. Morocco has also observed a decrease in menarcheal age and a higher prevalence of premenarcheal symptoms, previously observed only in older teens or adult women.[17] The global decrease in age of menarche should promote early and open discussion about menstruation and potential complications.

The timing of entry into puberty and indeed the onset of fertility may have effects on behavior. For example, late maturing girls may be more protected than their peers who enter puberty early.[18,19] Different cultures appreciate the changes associated with puberty including menarche in unique ways. Studies in the United States reveal a decreased self-esteem in white girls beginning at age 11 that slowly recovers during the senior high school years (15–18 years).[20] This is coincident to an increased rise in body mass as well as transformation from concrete to formal thought patterns. Black girls, on the other hand, were noted to have overall higher self-esteem when entering mid-adolescence. Such a difference may be due to the observation that black girls may experience pubertal maturation before transfer to middle school; therefore, these girls may have more time to adjust to the physical changes.[20]

The phenomena of a change in self-esteem have been observed in other industrial nations as well. For example, investigators in Sweden found that girls who experienced menarche before age 11 were more likely to exhibit risk behaviors. High-risk activity included delinquency and sexual experiences throughout adolescence. However, by adulthood there were no differences in social adjustment scores compared with girls who had a later menarche. These data suggest that the psychosocial problems observed in adolescence may be limited,[19] although other studies have noted poorer relationships and adjustment among adult women who matured early.[18] Although a complex relationship, girls who appear sexually mature, despite chronologic age, are more likely to be involved with boys romantically. Platonic relationships do not appear to be affected by sexual maturity status.[21] Providers may incorporate such a discussion into anticipatory guidance for parents and patients, particularly as their daughters enter middle school.

## PUBERTY IN BOYS

As boys enter puberty they experience multiple physical and social changes. One of the first changes noted clinically is enlargement of the testes. Prepubertal testes are less than 4 mL in volume, which corresponds to less than one inch in longitudinal axis. Once the testes reach one inch in length, puberty is considered to have begun. For more specific measurement, testicular volume is measured by an orchidometer (Figure 4-5).

The growth of the testes results in increased testosterone that is associated with penile lengthening before widening occurs, as well as the growth of facial and pubic hair. The stages of pubic hair development are the same for boys and girls. That is, Stage 1 SMR is prepubertal; pubic hair is absent. Stage 2 SMR demonstrates fine, sparse, straight hair at the base of the penis. Darker, coarser, and slightly curly hair that extends over the midpubis represents Stage 3. The Stage 4 has thicker, more curled, adult-type hair that covers the external genitalia but does not extend to the medial thighs. Finally, Stage 5 SMR has adult-type hair that extends onto the medial thighs. The growth spurt associated with peak height velocity, decrease in body fat and increase in lean body mass, and changes that include gynecomastia and acne are all associated with increased androgen activity. The presence of such changes in the absence of testicular enlargement (<1 inch) should trigger an investigation of other sources of androgen, such as the adrenal gland with adrenal hyperplasia because the source of androgen is not prepubertal-sized testes. The SMR of boys uses the same criteria as for girls. There are no definitive criteria for penile enlargement as there is for testicular volume. Figure 4-6 shows the classic photos

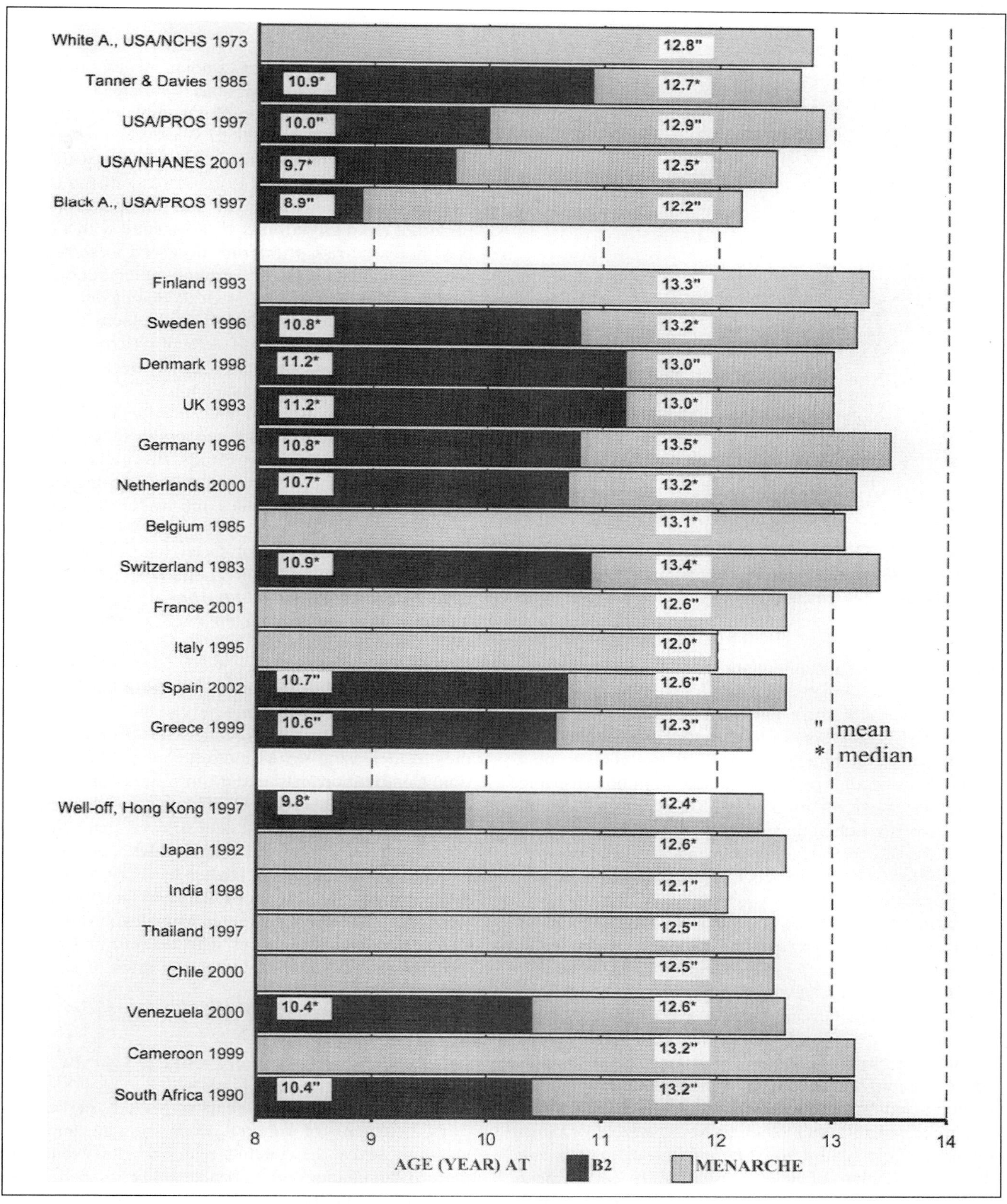


FIGURE 4-4 Average (mean or median) ages at onset of female breast development (B2) or menarche in different well-off populations around the world (From Parent A, Teilmann G, Juul A, Skakkebaek NE, Toppari J, Bourguignon JP. The timing of normal puberty and the age limits of sexual precocity: variations around the world, secular trends, and changes after migration. *Endocr Rev.* 2003;24:668–693. Copyright 2003, The Endocrine Society, with permission.)

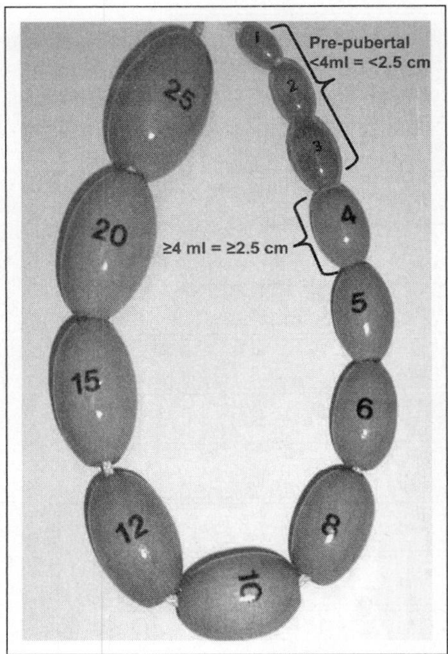


FIGURE 4-5 Orchidometer used for measuring testicular volume in males.

used by Tanner in defining the sexual maturity stages that bear his name.

Boys typically enter puberty later than girls; using the NHANES[5] data, 98% of black and 95% of white boys had genital development by age 13; there seems to be a trend toward earlier pubertal maturation in non-Hispanic white and Mexican-American males.[5] Concurrent with entry into the pubertal growth spurt, testicular enlargement is usually the first external manifestation of puberty in boys. These changes precede Tanner stage 2 pubic hair by approximately 6 months. Palpation of the testes by the primary medical provider allows for assessment of volume as well as screening for masses or varicoceles. It also serves as a forum for the younger teen to be assured that he is "normal." Of note, approximately one-half to one-third of boys develop gynecomastia during early to mid-puberty. This palpable, subareolar breast tissue can be unilateral or bilateral and may persist for 12 to 18 months. These findings are usually physiologic but can be due to decreased androgen production (such as Klinefelter syndrome), medications (such as ketoconazole or cimetidine), and, rarely, testicular tumors. Obesity may imitate the clinical findings of gynecomastia, but the enlargement is due more to fat than glandular breast tissue. Physiologic cases resolve spontaneously; reassurance is helpful. Surgical management and laboratory evaluation for testosterone insufficiency are reserved for prolonged symptoms or significantly increased breast size.[22]

A common complaint among males, and some females, is swelling of the tibial tubercle, a feature of Osgood-Schlatter syndrome. This complaint is observed during the peak height velocity years when osteoblastic alkaline phosphatase activity associated with bone growth is peaking around 12 to 14 years of age in boys. Treatment is mainly supportive and nonoperative.[23] This period of rapid growth may be associated with a temporary increased risk of fracture observed in adolescents. Longitudinal data suggest that bone mineral density may decline prior to the age of peak height velocity and rebounds after the boy's peak height velocity is attained. This may lead to a period of skeletal weakness, because the body draws on cortical bone to meet the mineral demands of the expanding skeleton.[24]

Puberty also heralds the activity of androgens throughout the body in both genders, leading to changes in the skin and sebaceous glands. The higher levels of androgen act on the sebaceous glands to increase the number of sebaceous lobules and overall follicular size in boys and girls and predispose teens to acne. Because of stimulation of terminal facial hair in boys, those with genetic predisposition to tightly spiraled hair may develop *pseudofollicularis barbae*. Primary treatment includes stopping shaving followed by trials of antibiotics and topical steroids.[25]

The effects of androgen (testosterone) extend also into the psychological and social development of the pubertal male. Testosterone levels in males increase 10- to 20-fold during adolescence. Testosterone contributes to increasing sexual interest,[26] as well as competition. Competition may extend into areas of crime and delinquency if there is not effective social constructs and guidance. Longitudinal data showed that boys with higher salivary testosterone levels had a greater likelihood of sexual initiation. Higher levels of testosterone were associated with more frequent coital activity.[27] Generally, self-esteem increases in males during adolescence. However, some boys with delayed or late entry into puberty experience increasing rates of substance abuse and lower self-esteem.[27]

## PUBERTAL SEQUENCING AND TEMPO

Although girls may show signs of puberty earlier than boys, 2 elements of pubertal progression are important for both sexes. Sequencing refers to the predictable pattern of changes in secondary sex characteristics, in which elements proceed in a consistent sequence from individual to individual. For girls, the first clinically important event is the beginning of breast development, also called thelarche, which represents the emergence of SMR 2 with breast budding. The growth of

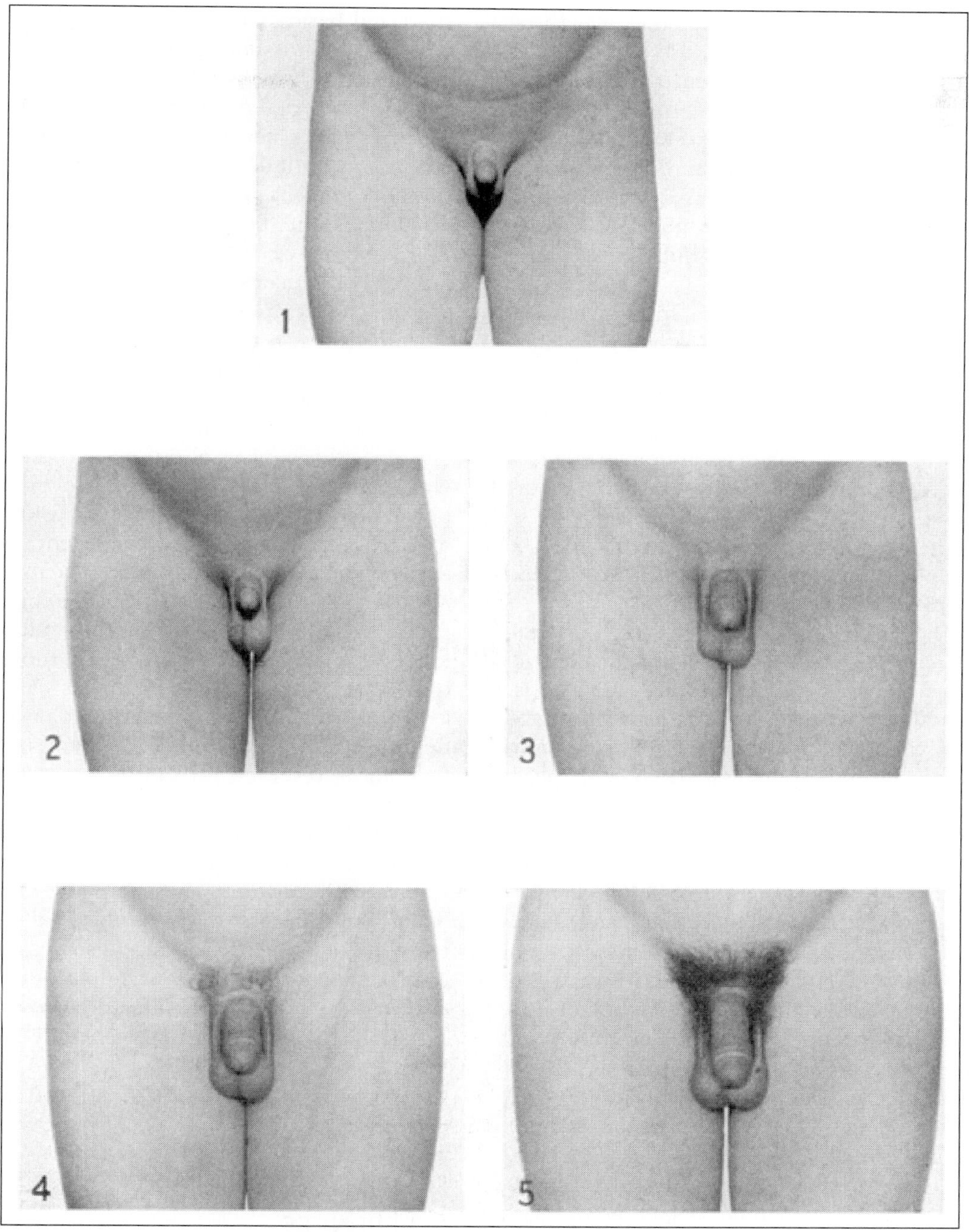


**FIGURE 4-6** Stages of male pubic hair development. (Reprinted with permission from Tanner JM. *Growth at Adolescence*. Oxford, UK: Blackwell Scientific Publications; 1955.)

breast tissue is caused by estrogen being released from the ovaries due to stimulation by gonadotropins, which are secreted from the anterior pituitary in response to hypothalamic gonadotropin-releasing hormone (GnRH). Estrogens also cause skeletal growth and maturation, resulting in the pubertal growth spurt and peak height velocity, which reliably follows the onset of breast development by about 1 year. Finally, menstruation occurs when the ovaries develop an adequate number of mature follicles in response to gonadotropin levels sufficient to stimulate the ovaries to produce enough estrogen to proliferate the endometrium and enough progesterone to cause endometrial secretory changes. Thus, the onset of menses, menarche, is a relatively late pubertal event. Because estrogen causes bone growth as well as closure of the growth plates at the ends of long bones, height usually increases less than 2 inches after menarche. Although the initial development of pubic hair, pubarche, tends to be related temporally with puberty, it is due to adrenal activity producing dehydroepiandrosterone (DHEA and DHEA-S) in response to HPA activation, and not related to gonadal activity. Hence, the onset of pubic hair development is also called adrenarche.

If the events of thelarche-height spurt-menarche occur out of their normal sequence, pathological conditions should be considered. For example, bleeding from the vagina without preceding breast development or growth in height is pathological until proven otherwise. Likewise, the absence of menses after a female has achieved breast development to SMR 4 and has completed her growth spurt, is cause for concern. This is especially true if menarche has not occurred within 2 years of the height spurt, since the interval from peak height velocity to menarche is usually about 1 year.

For boys, the initial clinically relevant pubertal events are not readily visible. Testicular enlargement to 4 mL, which corresponds to 1 inch in longitudinal axis, results in production of testosterone that causes lengthening and then widening of the penis, followed later in puberty by the growth spurt associated with peak height velocity. As noted, if the testes remain small, they cannot be producing enough androgen to cause the various secondary sex characteristics typical of puberty and non-gonadal source must be sought if pubertal changes occur earlier than expected. On the other hand, small testes can be associated with various conditions, such as Klinefelter syndrome. Therefore, familiarity with the normal timing of onset as well as the sequencing of progression and normal volumes of testes is an important part of routine health care of adolescent males.

Tempo refers to the velocity at which puberty proceeds. Unlike the sequencing of pubertal events, the pattern of which is predictable from person to person, tempo can be highly variable. For example, breast development can proceed from thelarche to SMR in less than 2 years, but may also take more than 6 years to completion. Although early developers have a higher peak height velocity than late developers, they also fuse their epiphyses at an earlier age. For males, growth in height can continue into young adulthood.

## HEALTHY BEHAVIORS AND ADOLESCENTS

Common to both genders is the maturation and development of the ocular system. Routine screening during a physical examination should include the Snellen eye chart and basic eye examination. Children who remain nonmyopic into adolescence have a distinctly different lens, and those teens who develop myopia have a lens that is thicker and steeper. Throughout puberty the lens gets flatter and thinner, contributing to increasing myopia.[28] Continued counsel on eye safety during sports and hobbies is critical for this age group.

One of the tasks of a provider for adolescents is to encourage healthy behaviors for the patient's future. For females entering puberty, bone health is of particular importance. Early bone mass density is the most critical factor in preparing strong bones for later life. Research from Ireland concluded that while carbonated soft drinks had no significant effect on bone mineral density in boys, girls were affected. Specifically, the consumption of carbonated beverages was inversely related to bone mineral density in the population of girls 12 to 15 years old.[29] This finding may reflect adolescent girls' preference for low-calorie diet beverages at the expense of calcium-rich foods. Additionally, the timing of peak height velocity is the prime age to begin screening for scoliosis. The prevalence of scoliosis in the American adolescent population is approximately 2%. Scoliosis can be defined as a curve greater than 10 degrees. Curves of 10 to 15 degrees require no formal treatment, only monitoring. Imaging is reserved for curves greater than 20 to 40 degrees.[30]

Other important points to consider in adolescents include smoking behaviors, dietary patterns, and physical activity patterns. These are the 3 areas that are major contributors to preventable disease and mortality in adults (cardiovascular diseases, cerebrovascular disease, and cancer). For example, few people begin regular tobacco smoking after the age of 18, and adult physical activity patterns are generally adopted by that time. These issues should be discussed with parents of children and younger adolescents and with all adolescent patients..

## REFERENCES

1. Biro FM. Puberty. *Adolescent Medicine.* 2007;18:425–433

2. Grumbach MM. The neuroendocrinology of human puberty revisited. *Hormone Research.* 2002;57(suppl):2–14

3. Biro FM. Secular trends in menarche. *J Pediatr.* 2005;147: 725–726

4. Herman-Giddens ME, Kaplowitz PB, Wasserman R. Navigating the recent articles on girls' puberty in Pediatrics: what do we know and where do we go from here? *Pediatrics.* 2004;113:911–917

5. Sun SS, Schubert CM, Liang R, et al. Is sexual maturity occurring earlier among US children? *J Adolesc Health.* 2005;37:345–355

6. Freedman DS, Khan LK, Serdula MK, Dietz WH, Srinivasan SR, Berenson GS. The relation of menarcheal age to obesity in childhood and adulthood: the Bogalusa Heart Study. *BMC Pediatrics.* 2003;3:3

7. Parent A, Teilmann G, Juul A, Skakkebaek NE, Toppari J, Bourguignon JP. The timing of normal puberty and the age limits of sexual precocity: variations around the world, secular trends, and changes after migration. *Endocr Rev.* 2003;24:668-693

8. Reynolds EL, Wines JV. Individual differences in physical changes associated with adolescence in girls. *Am J Dis Child.* 1948;75:329-350

9. Marshall WA, Tanner JM. Variations in pattern of pubertal changes in girls. *Arch Dis Child.* 1969;44:291-303

10. Marshall WA, Tanner JM. Variations in the pattern of pubertal changes in boys. *Arch Dis Child.* 1970;45:13-23

11. Roede MJ, van Wieringen JC. Growth diagrams 1980: Netherlands third nation-wide survey. *Tijdschr Soc Gezondheitszorg.* 1985;63(suppl):1-34

12. Biro FM. Puberty—Whither goest? *J Pediatr Adolesc Gynecol.* 2006;19:163-165

13. Laufer MR. The physiology of puberty. In: Emans SJ, Laufer MR, Goldstein DP, eds. *Pediatric and Adolescent Gynecology,* 5th ed. Philadelphia, PA: Lippincott Williams & Wilkins; 2004:

14. Onland-Moret NC, Peeters PH, van Gils CH, et al. Age at menarche in relation to adult height: the EPIC study. *Am J Epidemiol.* 2005;162:623-632

15. Hwang JY, Shin C, Frongillo EA, Shin KR, Jo I. Secular trend in age at menarche for South Korean women born between 1920 and 1986: the Ansan Study. *Ann Hum Biol.* 2003;30:434-442

16. Irwin CE Jr. Pubertal timing: is there any new news? *J Adolesc Health.* 2005;37:43-44

17. Montero P, Bernis C, Loukid M, Kilali K, Baali A. Characteristics of menstrual cycles in Moroccan girls: prevalence of dysfunctions and associated behaviours. *Ann Hum Biol.* 1999;26:243-249

18. Graber JA, Seeley JR, Brooks-Gunn J, Lewinsohn PM. Is pubertal timing associated with psychopathology in young adulthood. *J Am Acad Child Adolesc Psychiatry.* 2004;43: 718-726

19. Johansson T, Ritzen EM. Very long-term follow-up of girls with early and late menarche. *Endocr Dev.* 2005;8:126-136

20. Biro FM, Striegel-Moore RH, Franko DL, Padgett J, Bean JA. Self-esteem in adolescent females. *J Adolesc Health.* 2006;39: 501-507. Epub 2006 Jul 10

21. Compian L, Gowen LK, Hayward C. Peri-pubertal girls' romantic and platonic involvement with boys: associations with body image and depression symptoms. *J Res Adolescence.* 2004;14(1):23-47

22. Rosen D. Question from the clinician: adolescent gynecomastia. *Pediatr Rev.* 2003;24:317-319

23. DeLee J, Stanitski C. Overuse injuries of the skeletally immature athlete. In: DeLee JC, Drez D Jr. *Orthopedic Sports Medicine.* 2nd ed. Philadelphia, PA:WB Saunders;1993:1834

24. Faulkner RA, Davison KS, Bailey DA, Mirwald RL, Baxter-Jones AD. Size-corrected BMD decreases during peak linear growth: implications for fracture incidence during adolescence. *J Bone Miner Res.* 2006;21:1864-1870

25. Habif TP. Bacterial infections. In: Habif TP, ed. *Clinical Dermatology: A Color Guide to Diagnosis and Therapy*, 4th ed. Philadelphia, PA: Mosby;2003:280-281

26. Halpern CT, Udry JR, Suchindran C. Monthly measures of salivary testosterone predict sexual activity in adolescent males. *Arch Sex Behav.* 1998;27:445-465

27. Biro FM, Dorn LD. Puberty and adolescent sexuality. *Pediatric Ann.* 2005;34:777-784

28. Garner LF, Stewart AW, Owens H, Kinnear RF, Frith MJ. The Nepal Longitudinal Study: biometric characteristics of developing eyes. *Optom Vis Sci.* 2006;83:274-280

29. McGartland C, Robson PJ, Murray L, et al. Carbonated soft drink consumption and bone mineral density in adolescence: The Northern Ireland Young Hearts Project. *J Bone Miner Res.* 2003;18(9):1563-1569

30. Greiner KA. Adolescent idiopathic scoliosis: radiologic decision-making. *Am Fam Physician.* 2002;65(9):1814-1822

# CHAPTER 5

## Adolescent Brain and Cognitive Changes

ELIZABETH R. SOWELL, PHD • ALEX W. SIEGEL • DANIEL J. SIEGEL, MD

### OVERVIEW

Clinicians working with adolescents can benefit greatly from an understanding of the developmental changes in the adolescent brain and cognition. Recent brain imaging studies indicate that significant neural development occurs throughout childhood and adolescence and into young adulthood (approximate ages 7–30).[1-11] These structural changes in the brain coincide with an array of observed cognitive and behavioral shifts in development.[12-21] Current in vivo brain imaging methods do not allow examination of cellular changes, but postmortem studies show that the brain undergoes a synaptic pruning process during childhood and adolescence that appears to increase neural efficiency.[22,23] In this pruning process, unneeded neural connections are eliminated—enhancing the functional efficiency of remaining synaptic circuits. A second process that occurs during the childhood and adolescent years is myelination. Myelin acts as insulation around long axons, increasing the speed of electrical conduction 100-fold and in this way further contributing to the efficiency of the circuit as a whole. Like the pruning process, myelination is not complete until long after the adolescent period, continuing well into adulthood.[24]

Brain imaging studies show that the prefrontal cortex is one of the most rapidly developing brain regions during adolescence.[2,9] The frontal cortex is primarily responsible for integrating differentiated areas of the brain into a functional whole. Integration is the primary force behind the development of executive function, a cognitive capacity that changes significantly during adolescence.[13-16] Executive function includes a range of cognitive processes such as planning, decision making, delayed gratification, attentional resource allocation, and working memory.[20,25,26] In addition to its executive functioning capacities, the prefrontal cortex mediates self-reflection and various aspects of social and emotional function. The prefrontal cortex sends inhibitory signals to the subcortical limbic regions involved in the generation of affective responses. This tonic inhibitory influence supports coordination and balance, which are hallmarks of neural integration.[27] With enhanced prefrontal integrative development, the capacity for self-understanding and empathy may be enhanced following adolescent changes in brain remodeling.

In this chapter, we summarize the exciting new perspectives on the correlation between adolescent brain changes and cognitive, social, and emotional development. Clinicians can benefit from this new knowledge by gleaning insights that will help them care for adolescents and their families during this period of change and challenge.

### BRAIN DEVELOPMENT BEFORE ADOLESCENCE

During the in utero period, driven by genetic information, the nervous system develops its basic architecture with the migration of neurons in the central and peripheral regions. In the brain, the differentiation of major regions follows a caudo-rostral progression from the brainstem upward to the limbic areas and cortex. At birth, these higher cortical regions are the least developed and the most open to continued differentiation. This increase in the complexity of cortical synaptic connections is influenced both by genetics and experience. Experience has been shown to produce structural changes in the brain. Specifically, neural firing patterns in response to internal or external stimuli lead to synaptic growth among those activated neurons. "Neurons which fire together, wire together" is a phrase revealing the fundamental principle by which associated neurons potentially become synaptically linked following an experience.[27]

During the first 3 years of life, genetically driven synapse formation creates a higher density of cortical synapses than will exist in adulthood. Synaptic proliferation continues, with experience shaping neural connections throughout the school years and beyond. Synaptic densities peak at different ages for different brain regions, but most regions evaluated in postmortem studies reach their peak by about 3 to 4 years of age. Synaptic pruning follows with losses continuing into adulthood.[2,19]

The sexual and somatic changes of puberty (described in Chapter 4, Physical Growth and Development) may correspond to some, but not all, neural changes seen in the brain. Brain maturation continues long after puberty, and early sexual maturation may not involve concomitant neurobehavioral changes of the later adolescent years. Clinically this suggests that physicians should be aware that conditions such as precocious puberty do not coincide with early cognitive or brain maturation.

## BRAIN CHANGES IN ADOLESCENCE

Results from recent brain mapping studies show dynamic changes in gray matter that occur throughout childhood and adolescence. Our knowledge of when (and thus where) the changes occur is largely limited by the age groups studied. Thus, it is difficult to know at what exact ages the changes take place. It seems reasonable to conclude from studies of gray matter change across the life span that the curve of gray matter loss during middle and late childhood is steeper in dorsal parietal cortices than it is in frontal cortices.[10] Other studies have also shown more prominent loss in parietal lobes between childhood (7–11 years) and adolescence (12–16 years). Later, from 16 to at least 30 years of age, gray matter loss is more prominent in larger aspects of dorsal prefrontal cortices.[23] Figure 5-1 illustrates these effects. Given studies looking at gray matter changes across the life span it seems that gray matter in the more lateral cortices of the occipital, temporal, and frontal lobes may have been more actively lost earlier in development, and the primary language cortices of the perisylvian region undergo continued gray matter thickening to about age 30, at which point a gradual decline is then observed. Figure 5-2 illustrates these findings. Longitudinal studies have been consistent with this pattern of frontal and parietal gray matter loss and have confirmed cortical thickening in primary language cortices along with thinning of the frontal and parietal lobes.[11]

Gray matter changes during childhood and adolescence are nonlinear as shown in Figure 5-2, and some studies have shown gray matter volume increases during the preadolescent period followed by decreases during the postadolescent period.[2] Some have attributed these gray matter changes, observed with magnetic resonance imaging (MRI), to cellular changes, such as synaptogenesis or synaptic pruning. Synaptic pruning is thought to be instrumental in the fine-tuning of functional regions in the brain (particularly in the prefrontal, parietal, and temporal cortices). The benefit of such a developmental phase of neural "remodeling" may be that such synaptic elimination enables the remaining circuits to process information more efficiently. This enhances the ability of differentiated brain regions to cooperate and support high-level cognitive control. Postmortem studies have shown that synaptic pruning continues throughout

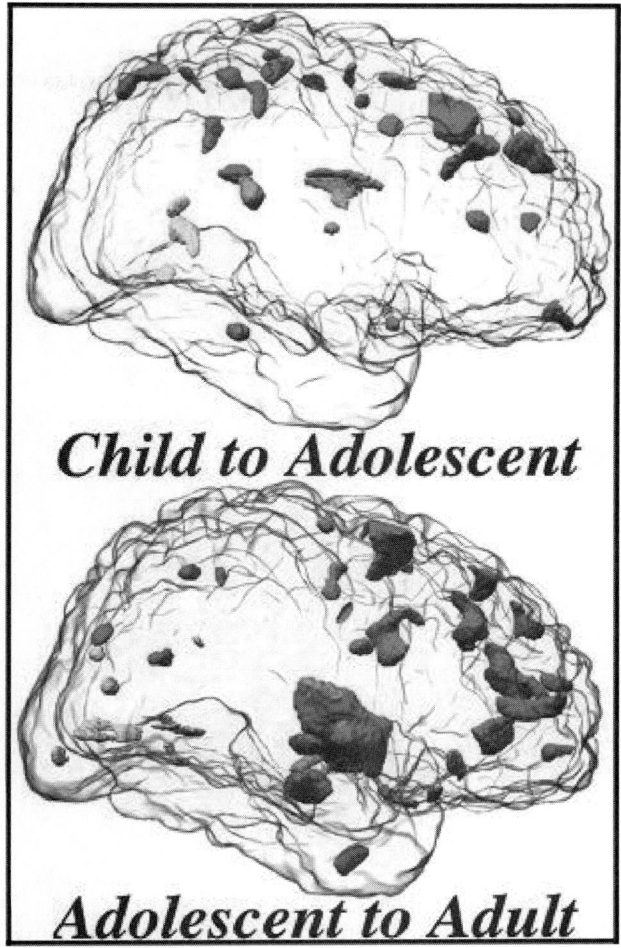


FIGURE 5-1 Top: Child minus adolescent statistical map for the negative age effects representing gray matter density reductions observed between childhood and adolescence and Bottom: adolescence and adulthood. These maps are 3-dimensional renderings of the traditional statistical maps shown inside the transparent cortical surface rendering of one representative subject's brain. Lobes and the subcortical region were defined anatomically on the same subject's brain. Color coding is applied to each cluster based on its location within the representative brain. Clusters are shown in the frontal lobes (purple), parietal lobes (red), occipital lobes (yellow), temporal lobes (blue), and subcortical region (green). Note the increase in maturational changes in the frontal lobes between adolescence and adulthood relative to the same region in the child-to-adolescent map. (Bottom image reprinted from Sowell ER, Thompson PM, Holmes CJ, Jernigan TL, Toga AW. In vivo evidence for post-adolescent brain maturation in frontal and striatal regions. *Nat Neurosci.* 1999;2:859-861, with permission from Macmillan Publishers, Ltd.)

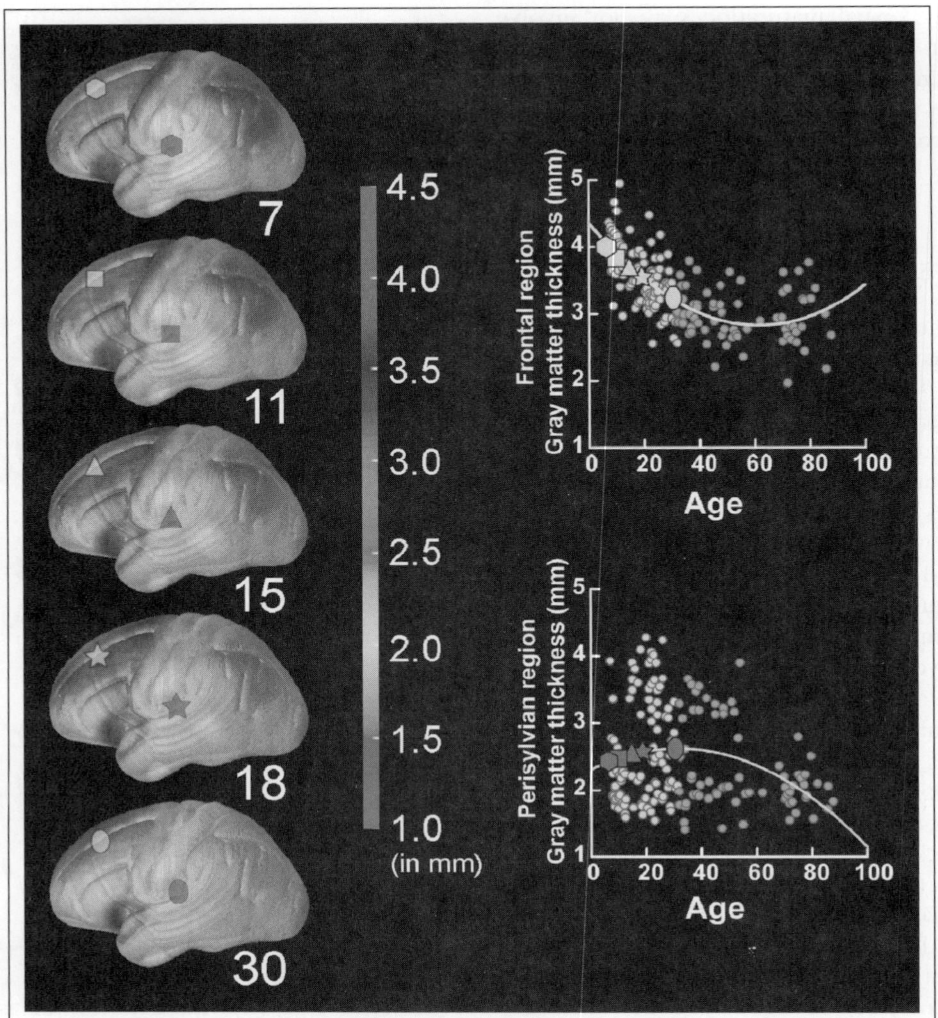


**FIGURE 5-2** Each map represents average cortical thickness in millimeters, color coded according to the color bar, for each of the represented ages between 7 and 30 years. Graphs represent the age function in each of 2 regions, dorsal frontal (top) and posterior perisylvian (bottom). Symbols for each age map shown on the left are placed in the appropriate age location on the regression line for each graph. Perisylvian thickness values are shown in red for each map in the bottom graph, and dorsal frontal thickness values are shown in yellow on the top graph. The data points in the graphs represent each subject (under age 30 represented here in white) and highlight the variability across subjects. Variability in regional patterns is also appreciated, with gray matter thickening between 7 and 30 years in perisylvian cortices and cortical thinning during the same time frame in dorsal frontal regions (based on data presented in Sowell et al, *Nat Neuroscience*. 2003; Sowell et al, *Cereb Cortex*. 2007). (See color insert.)

adolescence,[23] perhaps resulting in a thinning of gray matter. These structural changes are thought to influence the ongoing shift in the adolescent's capacity to process information in an increasingly complex environment.

Synaptic pruning described here is not likely solely responsible for an increase in cognitive efficiency during adolescence; myelination may play a key role as well. One of the most consistent findings of recent MRI studies is that certain brain regions, such as the prefrontal cortex, undergo a steady increase in white matter (thought to reflect continued myelination) during adolescence and well into the adult years.[2,10] The subsequent increase in the speed of neuronal transmission may directly support the rapid linkage of previously disparate circuits. This linking process, called neural integration, may permit more highly refined and regulated processes to emerge.[27] From the behavioral perspective, this integration may ultimately lead to an increase in self-control; indeed, adolescence marks the beginning of adult-level cognitive behavior control. Though the journey to arrive at this level of achievement may be marked by more stormy noncontrolled emotional outbursts and impulsive behaviors in the early adolescent period, further development results in a more mature capacity for self-regulation. Overall, the concurrent processes of synaptic pruning and myelination along with an eventual increase in the speed and capacity of information processing are thought to be related to the increase in the ability to have consistent cognitive behavior control.[28]

## EXECUTIVE FUNCTIONS AND SOCIAL EMOTIONAL DEVELOPMENT

Cognitive control of behavior is better known as "executive function." These skills enable the individual to have selective attention, voluntary inhibition of impulses, more complex decision making, and working memory to hold these in mind. Executive functions overall seem to become more robust,[13,15] perhaps related to the synaptic pruning and myelination of adolescence. The dorsal lateral prefrontal region may play a significant role in these executive domains, as do areas in the more medial prefrontal cortex and anterior cingulate regions.[25]

Social cognition, sometimes referred to as "social intelligence," includes the capacity for self-awareness, perspective taking, and the ability to understand other minds (empathy).[14,29,30] These processes depend on the middle areas of the prefrontal cortex as well as the temporal and parietal regions—all of which undergo significant maturational changes during adolescence. Social cognition seems to undergo a perturbation during puberty followed by a massive development in efficiency and complexity that progresses during adolescence.[14]

Some studies suggest that the coordination and balance of the lower limbic areas, such as the amygdala, by the prefrontal regions may become less efficient during the early part of the adolescent period.[31-35] Though detailed research is not yet available, clinical impressions of adolescent intensity and instability of emotional responses, especially during the early period of these neural changes, may be understood to be more than merely the old notion of rising hormone levels or shifts in self-identity and group identity. Independent studies of the interconnectedness of the prefrontal region with the subcortical affect-generating limbic zones, such as the amygdala, reveal that inhibitory fibers regulate limbic firing (for review, see references 14, 19, 27, 30). With a reorganization of prefrontal architecture, it may be possible for this capacity for higher, "top-down" control to become temporarily disabled. Some research findings, for example, support this view in illuminating the ways the response to facial expressions during early adolescence is governed more by amygdala response than by the prefrontal assessment of these nonverbal signals seen in adults.[32,34] Thus, facial expressions typically interpreted as *fear* by adults may be perceived by early adolescents as showing *anger*.

A comprehensive review of functions subserved by the prefrontal areas, focusing especially on the midline regions including the areas known as the orbitofrontal cortex, the anterior cingulate cortex, and the medial and ventral prefrontal cortices, reveals at least 9 important dimensions:[30]

1. Regulation of the balance and coordination of the autonomic branches of the parasympathetic (brakes) and sympathetic (accelerator) divisions
2. Capacity for attuned, resonant interpersonal communication
3. Emotional balance: enabling limbic arousal to be modulated within a tolerable range
4. Flexible responses that permit a pause for reflection before enacting behaviors
5. Empathy: understanding the point of view of another
6. Insight: connecting awareness of oneself in the past with present experience and anticipated future action
7. Fear modulation: the shifting of the impact of amygdala-based fear responses as they are extinguished by GABA (gamma amino butyric acid) inhibitory input from the prefrontal regions
8. Intuition: being in touch with "gut responses" and utilizing these to inform rational decision making
9. Morality: acting on behalf of the larger good, even when alone

Brain maturation studies of the prefrontal areas during this period support clinical impressions that these 9 functions develop as the individual moves from childhood through adolescence into adulthood. One possible explanation for emotionally "explosive" behaviors sometimes exhibited by adolescents is that the emerging integrative functions of this region may be especially sensitive to excessive input from the lower limbic areas. The outcome of a momentary suspension of the prefrontal inhibitory functions could lead to intensification of such emotional reactions. Alternatively, it is possible that the inhibitory functions of the frontal cortices are not yet mature enough to negotiate the increasingly complex social stimuli of today's teens. Here we see that factors that might lead to the impaired integrative effects of prefrontal fibers might be accompanied by suspension of, or lack of, maturity in any or all of these dimensions. Limbic reactivity or stress can induce such a "low-road state." For clinicians, this perspective can be quite useful in helping adolescents and their parents improve their communication in the face of repeated "irrational" behaviors when the teen—or parent—has become emotionally upset. Explaining these brain functions to families can create the distance necessary for tense situations to be transformed into opportunities to repair disconnections and open the channels of communication again. This view may explain the "tumultuous teen" years characterized by transient shifts in many of these 9 functions during early adolescence. The persistence of such instability for lengthy periods of time or beyond the early adolescent period may warrant further clinical evaluation to rule out emerging psychiatric conditions such as mood or anxiety disorders.

## CLINICAL IMPLICATIONS

Across all cultures studied, scientists have found 2 common features during the adolescent period: (1) Youth during this age prefer to be with their peers, not their parents; and (2) adolescents begin to do things in "new" ways, different from the way their parents and other authorities carried out behaviors.[36] These universal characteristics imply that such behaviors are not learned; rather, they are genetically transmitted. What is the evolutionary advantage offered by such cross-cultural developments in behavior? Through their efforts to align themselves with peers and to create new patterns of behavior, adolescents may prevent society from becoming rigid or stagnant. Thus, the commonly encountered "generation gap" between adolescents and their elders might have a biological foundation.

This drive to create new behavior patterns creates an opportunity for society to change. As the brain undergoes significant alterations during this period, this developmental stage is also a time for the person to acquire new knowledge, skills, and ways of thinking. However, periods of brain growth offer not only opportunity for positive changes but also vulnerability to risk. During adolescence, the drive to carry out behaviors in new ways also pushes adolescents toward high-risk behavior. What creates opportunity also creates vulnerability.

This perspective can help clinicians support parents and teachers during this often challenging developmental period. Though neuroscience is just beginning to illuminate the steps to these universal changes, it is likely that alterations in neurotransmitter release may be at the heart of the high-risk behavior. Although folk psychology suggests that "raging hormones" or some kind of blindness to risk may be at work enabling these impulsive and potentially dangerous behaviors to occur, research suggests in fact that alterations in the brain may reveal the actual source of these shifts. Some studies suggest that the motivational brain circuitry (orbitofrontal cortex, striatum, and amygdala) is activated differently in adolescents than in adults.[36] Such changes in the regions that assess risk-benefit ratios for behaviors and that control impulsivity may help elucidate the changes in the decision-making process during this time period.

For example, studies of sexual behaviors in adolescence reveal that instead of adolescents underestimating risk, they actually overestimated the chances of risky behaviors such as unwanted pregnancy or acquiring a sexually transmitted disease.[37] What seemed to be the cause of these risky behaviors was not unfamiliarity with danger but some assessment that overvalued the meaning of the rewards. Such behavioral decisions seemed to be made more based on sheer computational analysis in which the overvalued benefits outweighed the downside risks, even if they were overestimated. This view would lead the way toward clinical interventions that did not rely on better education about risk (the teens already were overestimating the chances of a negative outcome), but instead supported a more intuitive sense of what might be the "right thing" to do, not so much what, via adolescent logic, appeared to be the right conclusion.

Clinicians helping parents raise adolescents can encourage their active involvement during this period in a way that supports the genetically driven push to differentiate and socialize in new ways. With high-risk elements prominent in modern society, from fast cars to fast drugs and potentially fatal sexually transmitted diseases, more than ever youth need the help of their parents through this period of significant neural change. By the end of adolescence in the mid-20s, the acquisition of more integrated functioning can enable the next generation to survive and hopefully thrive in their new world.

## FUTURE RESEARCH

It is important to note that only a few studies to date have directly evaluated relationships between changing brain function, changing brain structure, and cognitive abilities during childhood and adolescence. Thus, at this point we can really only speculate that the synaptic pruning and myelination characteristics of adolescent brain maturation actually drive changes in cognition and behavior.

For the clinician, research will likely illuminate more fully the specific ways in which neural maturation correlates with the behavioral changes during this period. Working with adolescents and their families can integrate the present knowledge that brain growth—synaptic pruning and myelination—will continue well into the 20s in areas known to be important for emotional and cognitive functions central in the individual's life. Knowing about these changes can help the clinician support families and encourage healthy relationships and communication in the face of the often evocative behaviors and challenges to limits and authority that adolescents have inherited as a genetic legacy of our species. Keeping adolescents safe while at the same time helping them learn to become autonomous and thrive in an ever-changing and fast-paced world is the challenge for clinicians and parents alike.

## REFERENCES


1. Courchesne E, Chisum HJ, Townsend J, et al. Normal brain development and aging: quantitative analysis at in vivo MR imaging in healthy volunteers. *Radiology.* 2000; 216:672-682

2. Giedd JN, Blumenthal J, Jeffries NO, et al. Brain development during childhood and adolescence: a longitudinal MRI study. *Nat Neurosci.* 1999;2:861-863

3. Gogtay N, Giedd JN, Lusk L, et al. Dynamic mapping of human cortical development during childhood through early adulthood. *Proc Natl Acad Sci U S A.* 2004; 101:8174-8179

4. Paus T. Mapping brain maturation and cognitive development during adolescence. *Trends Cogn Sci.* 2005;9:60-68

5. Paus T, Zijdenbos A, Worsley K, et al. Structural maturation of neural pathways in children and adolescents: in vivo study. *Science.* 1999;283:1908-1911

6. Pfefferbaum A, Mathalon DH, Sullivan EV, et al. A quantitative magnetic resonance imaging study of changes in brain morphology from infancy to adulthood. *Arch Neurol.* 1994;51(9):874-887

7. Sowell ER, Delis D, Stiles J, Jernigan TL. Improved memory functioning and frontal lobe maturation between childhood and adolescence: a structural MRI study. *J Int Neuropsychol Soc.* 2001;7:312-322

8. Sowell ER, Thompson PM, Tessner KD, Toga AW. Mapping continued brain growth and gray matter density reduction in dorsal frontal cortex: inverse relationships during postadolescent brain maturation. *J Neurosci.* 2001;21:8819-8829

9. Sowell ER, Thompson PM, Holmes CJ, Jernigan TL, Toga AW. *In vivo* evidence for post-adolescent brain maturation in frontal and striatal regions. *Nat Neurosci.* 1999;2:859-861

10. Sowell ER, Peterson BS, Thompson PM, Welcome SE, Henkenius AL, Toga AW. Mapping cortical change across the human life span. *Nat Neurosci.* 2003;6:309-315

11. Sowell ER, Thompson PM, Leonard CM, Welcome SE, Kan E, Toga AW. Longitudinal mapping of cortical thickness and brain growth in normal children. *J Neurosci.* 2004;24(38): 8223-8231

12. McGivern RF, Andersen J, Byrd D, Mutter KL, Reilly J. Cognitive efficiency on a match to sample task decreases at the onset of puberty in children. *Brain Cogn.* 2002;50:73-89

13. Anderson V, Anderson P, Northam E, Jacobs R, Catroppa C. Development of executive functions through late childhood and adolescence in an Australian sample. *Dev Neuropsychol.* 2001;20:385-406

14. Blakemore SJ, Choudhury S. Development of the adolescent brain: implications for executive function and social cognition. *J Child Psychol Psychiatry.* 2006;47(3/4):296-312

15. Brocki KC, Bohlin G. Executive functions in children aged 6 to 13: a dimensional and developmental study. *Dev Neuropsychol.* 2004;26:571-593

16. Klenberg L, Korkman M, Lahti-Nuuttila P. Differential development of attention and executive functions in 3- to 12-year-old Finnish children. *Dev Neuropsychol.* 2001;20:407-428

17. Leon-Carrion J, Garcia-Orza J, Perez-Santamaria FJ. The development of the inhibitory component of the executive functions in children and adolescents. *Int J Neurosci.* 2004;114:1291-1311

18. Casey BJ, Tottenham N, Liston C, Durston S. Imaging the developing brain: what have we learned about cognitive development? *Trends Cogn Sci.* 2005;9:104-110

19. Dahl RE, Spear LP, eds. *Adolescent brain development: vulnerabilities and opportunities. Annals of the New York Academy of Sciences. Vol 1021* 2004; New York, NY: NYAS; 2004

20. Luciana M, Conklin HM, Cooper CJ, Yarger RS. The development of nonverbal working memory and executive control processes in adolescents. *Child Development.* 2005;76: 697-712

21. Tamm L, Menon V, Reiss AL. Maturation of brain function associated with response inhibition. *J Am Acad Child Adolesc Psychiatry.* 2002;41:1231-1238

22. Rakic P, Bourgeois JP, Goldman-Rakic PS. Synaptic development of the cerebral cortex: implications for learning, memory, and mental illness. *Prog Brain Res.* 1994;102:227-243

23. Huttenlocher PR, Dabholkar AS. Regional differences in synaptogenesis in human cerebral cortex. *J Comp Neurol.* 1997;387:167-178

24. Yaklovlev PI, Lecours AR. The myelogenetic cycles of regional maturation of the brain. In: Minkowski A, ed. *Regional Development of the Brain in Early Life. Oxford: Blackwell Scientific;* 1967;3-70

25. Fuster JM. Frontal lobe and cognitive development. *J Neurocytol.* 2002;31:373-385

26. Hooper CJ, Luciana M, Conklin HM, Yarger RS. Adolescents' performance on the development of decision making and ventromedial prefrontal cortex. *Dev Psy.* 2004;40:1148-1158

27. Siegel DJ. *The Developing Mind: Toward a Neurobiology of Interpersonal Experience*. New York, NY: Guilford; 1999

28. Luna B, Garver KE, Urban TA, Lazar NA, Sweeney JA. Maturation of cognitive processes from late childhood to adulthood. *Child Dev.* 2004a;75:1357-1372

29. Nelson E, Leibenluft E, McClure EB, Pine DS. The social reorientation of adolescence: a neuroscience perspective on the process and its relation to psychopathology. *Psychol Med.* 2005;35:163-174

30. Siegel DJ. *The Mindful Brain: Reflection and Attunement in the Cultivation of Well-Being*. New York, NY: WW Norton; 2007

31. Baird AA, Gruber SA, Fein DA, et al. Functional magnetic resonance imaging of facial affect recognition in children and adolescents. *J Am Acad Child Adolesc Psychiatry.* 1999;38: 195–199

32. Herba C, Phillips M. Annotation: development of facial expression recognition from childhood to adolescence: behavioural and neurological perspectives. *J Child Psychol Psychiatry.* 2004;45:1185–1198

33. Killgore WDS, Oki M, Yurgelun-Todd DA. Sex-specific developmental changes in amygdala responses to affective faces. *Neuroreport.* 2001;12:427–433

34. Monk CS, McClure EB, Nelson EE, et al. Adolescent immaturity in attention-related brain engagement to emotional facial expressions. *NeuroImage.* 2003;20:420–428

35. Thomas KM, Drevets WC, Whalen PJ, et al. Amygdala response to facial expressions in children and adults. *Biol Psychiatry.* 2001;49:309–316

36. Spear LP. The adolescent brain and age-related behavioral manifestations. *Neurosci Biobehav Rev.* 2000;24:417–463

37. Kelley AE, Schochet T, Landry CF. Risk taking and novelty seeking in adolescence: Introduction to Part I. In: Dahl RE, Spear LP, eds. *Adolescent Brain Development: Vulnerabilities and Opportunities. Annals of the New York Academy of Sciences. Vol 1021.* New York, NY: NYAS; 2004:27–32

# CHAPTER 6

# Adolescent Psychosocial Development and Behavior

LAURENCE STEINBERG, PHD • W. ANDREW COLLINS, PHD

## INTRODUCTION

Psychosocial development in adolescence is characterized by 2 interrelated developmental tasks: the development of increasingly mature connections and commitments to individuals and social institutions outside the family (ie, developing a sense of *interdependence*) while simultaneously attaining competence and autonomy from the influence of others (ie, developing a sense of *independence*). Positive psychosocial development in adolescence is the outcome of a long and cumulative process influenced by the individual's prior psychosocial development, the transformative physical and cognitive changes of the adolescent period, and the social and interpersonal contexts in which the adolescent lives.[1] Table 6-1 provides a framework for the boundaries of the various domains related to adolescent psychosocial development.

## DEVELOPING A SENSE OF INDEPENDENCE

Independence is a multifaceted construct that refers to a lengthy list of phenomena that vary in their interrelatedness. This subsection emphasizes research on *emotional autonomy*, which refers to subjective feelings of independence, especially in relation to parents, and *behavioral autonomy*, which refers to the capacity for independent decision-making and self-governance.

### EMOTIONAL AUTONOMY

Development of emotional autonomy involves increases in adolescents' subjective sense of independence, especially in relation to parents or parental figures. At least in the early stages of adolescence, emotional autonomy is achieved in part by separating oneself from and arguing with one's parents; through this process, the relationship is transformed and the adolescent develops both a new behavioral repertoire and a new image of his or her parents.[2] At the end of this process are 3 interrelated outcomes: a changed adolescent, who now views himself or herself in a different light; a changed parent, who now views his or her child (and perhaps himself or herself) in a different light; and a changed parent–child relationship, which is likely to be more egalitarian than it had been before.[3]

The development of emotional autonomy begins with individuation from parents and ends with the achievement of a sense of identity.[1] Theory and research

**Table 6-1**

**Boundaries of Adolescence**

| *Domain* | *Beginning* | *Ending* |
|---|---|---|
| **Biological** | Onset of puberty | Capable of reproduction |
| **Emotional** | Detaching from parents | Separate sense of identity |
| **Cognitive** | Emergence of formal operations | Consolidation of formal operations |
| **Interpersonal** | Shift toward peers | Capacity for intimacy |
| **Social** | Training for adult roles | Adult status |
| **Education** | Junior high school | Completion of schooling |
| **Legal** | Juvenile status | Majority status |
| **Chronologic** | Designated age (eg, 10) | Designated age (eg, 20) |
| **Cultural** | Begin training for ceremonial rite of passage | Completion of ceremonial rite of passage |

Source: Steinberg L. *Adolescence*. 8th ed. New York, NY: McGraw-Hill; 2008. Reprinted with permission from The McGraw-Hill Companies, Inc.

recently has shifted toward the idea that emotional autonomy results from a progressive negotiation between adolescent and parents over issues related to the granting and exercise of adolescent autonomy.[3] Thus, the process of individuation is less about the adolescent's attempt to separate from his or her parents than it is about a transformation in the implicit and explicit assumptions and beliefs that shape interactions among family members. This is not to say that all elements of this negotiation process are conscious or deliberate, that the involved parties are always agreeable participants, or that the day-to-day experience of renegotiating the terms of the parent–adolescent relationship is necessarily pleasant. This new view of emotional autonomy, however, emphasizes the different ways in which adolescents and parents construe their relationship, the different expectations they bring to the kitchen table, the different frames they use to interpret their experiences with each other, and the ways in which these cognitions shape patterns of interaction among family members.[3]

Several conclusions have emerged from studies of emotional autonomy. First, over the course of adolescence individuals' subjective sense of independence increases significantly, as indicated by feelings of separateness from their parents and changes in their perceptions of them, with older adolescents less likely than preadolescents to idealize their parents or believe in their omnipotence.[4] Notably, although this process begins early in adolescence with the deidealization of parents and challenges to parental authority, it unfolds over the entire adolescent period, and fully mature images of one's parents do not begin to appear until late in adolescence.[5]

Second, the development of emotional autonomy is a far more gradual and far less dramatic phenomenon than originally suggested in "storm and stress" perspectives on adolescence.[2,6] Detachment from parental ties is neither the norm nor is it associated with positive adjustment or psychological well-being. No studies suggest that active rebellion or unrelenting oppositionism is necessary for later healthy psychosocial development, and many studies indicate that the overt repudiation of parents by the adolescent likely forecasts problems, not success, in the development of emotional independence.[2]

Third, whereas the process of individuation is significant during early adolescence, identity development is salient in late adolescence and early adulthood. Indeed, research on identity development indicates few age differences in early, or even middle, adolescence; rather, the end of the adolescent decade appears to be the critical time for the development of a coherent sense of identity.[7] Thus, the process of discovering *that* one has a separate identity (the process of individuation) precedes the process of discovering *what* that identity is (the process of identity development). Middle adolescence is important as the time during which the psychosocial concerns of adolescence shift from individuation from parents to the establishment of a sense of identity.[1]

Fourth, the most visible autonomy-related transformations in family relations, such as the widely reported increase in bickering and squabbling over matters of parental authority, occur relatively early in the period.[8] The timing of these changed family patterns suggests that interpersonal changes that reflect the development of emotional autonomy precede improvements in actual self-governance, which may not take place until the middle portion of the period, or the development of a sense of identity, which takes place relatively late in adolescence.

Finally, there are sizable individual differences in the extent to which significant others in the adolescent's life permit or encourage the development of emotional independence, and these differences are meaningfully related to measures of adolescent psychosocial adjustment, especially in the realms of self-reliance, self-perceptions, and mental health. Parents who are warm but not intrusive facilitate the development of healthy emotional independence. The same factors associated with the development of healthy individuation—parental warmth, involvement, and tolerance of expressions of individuality—also appear to contribute to the development of a healthy sense of identity.[1]

## BEHAVIORAL AUTONOMY

Behavioral autonomy encompasses multiple capacities involved with self-reliance, but the construct has appeared in 2 different forms of research on adolescence.[1] In one, behavioral autonomy refers to the capacity for competent self-governance in the absence of external guidance or monitoring, as when, for example, an adolescent functions on his or her own without parents in a new or challenging situation or behaves ethically when outside the purview of adult supervision. In the other, behavioral autonomy refers to the capacity to function independently in the face of excessive external influence, as when, for example, the adolescent must resist peer pressure to behave in a way that goes against his or her better judgment or personal preferences.

Research on the development of behavioral autonomy has for the most part been conducted within the broader framework of socialization research, with a focus on the role of the family. Studies find that parents facilitate the development of behavioral autonomy in 4 chief ways: (1) serving as models of competent decision-makers; (2) encouraging independent decision making in the family context; (3) rewarding independent decision making outside the family context; and (4) instilling in the adolescent a more general sense of self-efficacy through responsive and demanding, or "authoritative," parenting.[1]

The period between early and middle adolescence, from around age 13 until 15, appears to be an important transitional time in the development of behavioral autonomy. Adolescents become increasingly motivated to seek independence from parents during this period while not yet having the psychosocial maturity for mature self-regulation when alone or in the company of their friends. Recent advances in developmental neuroscience have led several writers to link findings from studies of brain maturation to findings from studies of self-governance.[9] Changes in the limbic system may impel the adolescent toward sensation-seeking and risk-taking, both of which require greater independence from parental control and precede maturation of the prefrontal cortex that undergirds various aspects of executive function, affecting self-regulation, impulse control, planning, and foresight (see Chapter 5, Brain and Cognitive Development). This disjunction between biologically driven behaviors fueled by emotions and the ability to modulate those emotions creates a gap that some writers have likened to "starting the engines with an unskilled driver."[10] This gap between the degree of autonomy adolescents seek and are granted on the one hand and their actual capacity for self-governance on the other may leave individuals prone to poor judgment so that they place themselves in difficult or challenging situations before developing the capacity for mature self-regulation.[9] Given the physiologic changes in the brain during the second decade of life, and the variability of adolescents acquiring the skills required in mature decision making, granting privileges such as operating a motor vehicle based solely on chronologic age is open to question. The concept of graduated driver's licenses for adolescents is based on such an understanding; an adolescent must first demonstrate an ability to drive with adult supervision before being able to drive alone during daylight hours; the privilege of being able to drive with other adolescents is a relatively late step in this process because decision making is influenced by the social context of having peers in the vehicle.

## DEVELOPING A SENSE OF INTERDEPENDENCE

Achieving interdependence in adolescence is part of a process begun at birth.[1] With respect to health care, 3 aspects of interdependence develop in important ways during adolescence: *attachment*, *intimacy*, and *sexuality*. Attachment to caregivers forms a substrate upon which other attachments can be built, and the processes of forming and transforming attachments continues throughout and beyond adolescence as a component of interdependence. Same-gender peer relationships during childhood provide initial experiences of intimacy, but intimate relationships with opposite-sex peers typically first develop during adolescence.[11] Though some rudiments of sexuality are present in infancy and childhood, sexual activity itself generally begins during adolescence, bringing with it issues of relationships, social and personal responsibility, health, and safety.[12]

### ATTACHMENT

The construct of attachment in infant–caregiver relationships refers to a unique or distinct connection that supports infants' efforts to feel safe from threatening conditions and to be regulated emotionally. Two largely compatible explanations have been offered for links between attachments in infancy and those in adolescence. One is a carry-forward model, in which functions and representations of caregiver–child attachment relationships (referred to as "internal working models") organize expectations and behaviors in later relationships.[13] A second explanation is that relationships with caregivers prior to adolescence expose individuals to components of effective relating, such as empathy, reciprocity, and self-confidence, which shape interactions in other, later relationships.[14] In turn, childhood and adolescent friendships serve as templates for subsequent close relationships outside of the family, including romantic relationships.[1]

The significance of attachment for individuals and their relationships both before and during adolescence is apparent in findings from longitudinal studies. For example, secure early attachment during infancy predicts the features of relationships with extrafamilial partners during adolescence.[15] Similarly, early attachment security predicts competence with peers both during middle childhood and adolescence, whereas negative early experiences significantly predict hostility in interactions with romantic partners in early adulthood over and above the contributions of proximal relationships with peers and parents.[16] Other things being equal, a foundation of interdependence in early life appears to be a significant forerunner of continued interdependence in one's closest relationships in adolescence and adulthood.

### INTIMACY

As a psychosocial task of adolescence, intimacy refers to mutual openness and responsiveness in at least some relationships with age-mates. In addition, concepts of friendship first incorporate notions of intimacy in early adolescence.[11] The development of intimacy capabilities during adolescence undoubtedly builds on the hallmark physical, cognitive, and social changes of the period. Many scholars speculate that adolescents become increasingly capable of intimate relationships as a more sophisticated understanding of social relations emerges and as adolescents' ability to infer the thoughts and feelings of others sharpens.[1]

As with attachment, there are strong links between the quality of adolescents' friendships and the nature of family relationships in earlier periods, as well as changes in the abilities of relationship partners during adolescence.[16] The degree of flexible control, cohesion, and respect for privacy in families also has been linked positively to intimacy in late-adolescent romantic relationships, with especially strong associations for women. In contrast, negative emotionality in parent–adolescent relationships is correlated with negative emotionality and poor quality interactions with romantic partners in late adolescence.[1]

Spending larger amounts of time with peers and correspondingly less time with adults during adolescence contributes to the development of intimacy by increasing comfort with peers and encouraging self-disclosure as well as openness to others' self-revelations. Shared interest in mastering distinctive contexts and social systems of adolescence also stimulates a desire to communicate with peers, and biological changes associated with puberty also may occasion more frequent discussion with friends, who may offer a more comfortable arena than parent–child relationships for discussing issues of physical changes, sex, and dating. The superficial sharing of activities that sufficed between childhood friends is supplanted during adolescence by the potential for mutual responsiveness, concern, loyalty, trustworthiness, and respect for confidence between adolescent friends. Increases during adolescence in mutuality, self-disclosure, and intimacy with friends have been documented in several studies.[11] Gender differences in both the extent and significance of intimacy are common and widely discussed. During adolescence, girls' friendships consistently involve more knowing and sensitivity, more giving and sharing, and more taking and imposing than boys' friendships do. For males and females, same-sex friendships provide the main arena for the development of intimacy in early and middle adolescence. Intimacy in opposite-sex friendships, whether romantic or platonic, is a relatively late feature.[1] Thus, physical intimacy in sexual relationships, as discussed in the following section, is only one aspect of the broader concept of intimacy in adolescence.

## SEXUALITY

In adolescence, the psychosocial task of sexuality refers to adjusting to a sexually maturing body, managing sexual desires, forming sexual attitudes and values, learning about others' expectations, experimenting with sexual behaviors, and integrating these dimensions into one's sense of self.[12] Because adolescents' sexual behavior is discussed elsewhere (see Chapter 7, Sexual Development), the focus of this subsection is social, attitudinal, and emotional aspects of sexuality rather than sexual activity per se.

It is more difficult to generalize about the development of sexuality in adolescence than about attachment or intimacy because cultural norms surrounding sexual behavior are highly variable and influential.[1] Gender differences in the psychosocial experience of sexuality are especially pronounced due to social (eg, the greater facility girls have in emotional intimacy compared to boys) as well as physical differences (eg, the earlier maturation of girls and the possibility of pregnancy). Girls are judged more harshly than boys for engaging in some types of sexual activities and are consequently more likely than boys to express ambivalence about their sexuality and to fear harsh judgments if viewed as sexually active. Females generally emphasize emotional aspects of sexual relationships, whereas males more often emphasize physical satisfaction and release, though within-gender views are highly variable.[17]

Further sources of individual variation in the development of psychosocial sexuality include significant others, especially relationships and processes involving family members, best friends, and romantic partners. Longitudinal and cross-sectional evidence alike implicate positive parent–adolescent relationships in delayed initiation of intercourse, less frequent intercourse, and fewer sexual partners. Peers, especially best friends, also contribute to individual differences in sexual expectations, attitudes, and behaviors, albeit more among girls than boys.[18]

Timing of sexual initiation is an especially important influence on the psychosocial sequelae of sexual activity. Adolescents who become sexually active at a young age (eg, initiating intercourse before age 16) generally exhibit greater risk for problematic outcomes compared to adolescents who defer sexual activity. As a group, early-active adolescents tend to be less achievement oriented, more alienated from their parents, and more likely to exhibit other problem behaviors, such as drug or alcohol abuse, because of their relative psychosocial immaturity and more general orientation to unconventionality. Moreover, as a general rule the younger the onset of such activity in girls, the more likely it is to be perceived as forced upon them. Individuals who become sexually active at age 16 or older have no more problems than their abstinent peers, however.[18]

One concern about early sexual behavior is that a premature focus on sexual expression may interfere with successful integration of physical sexuality with attitudinal, emotional, and identity components. For example, Maccoby[19] has observed that sexually adventurous female adolescents, unlike their male counterparts, may experience social condemnation, peer derision, and stereotyping that interfere with more positive developmental opportunities. Many adolescents report negative experiences stemming from perceived pressure to engage in sexual activity that they did not desire or for which they felt unready.[17] Accordingly, many observers have advocated that public-school sex-education efforts include more detailed and comprehensive programs that directly address issues of attitudes, values, and responsible sexual decision making (including decisions to abstain from sexual activity) in contrast to the largely ineffective abstinence-based models.[20]

## FACILITATING POSITIVE PSYCHOSOCIAL DEVELOPMENT IN ADOLESCENCE

It is difficult to imagine a period in human development distinguished by psychosocial changes of the same magnitude as those characteristic of adolescence. The individual enters adolescence highly dependent on parents for guidance and governance and engaged in relationships that for the most part lack intimacy and depth. By the end of the adolescent years, however, if all goes well, the individual emerges with a healthy sense of responsible independence, a developing sense of identity, and the capacity to form deep and meaningful relationships with friends and romantic partners.

Although positive psychosocial development in adolescence is built on a strong foundation of healthy independence and interdependence established in infancy and childhood, experiences during the adolescent years matter as well. The main ingredients during adolescence for successful psychosocial development are a family environment in which parents are responsive, demanding, and supportive of the adolescent's need for individuation, involvement in a social network of same- and opposite-sex peers who are on a healthy developmental trajectory of psychosocial maturation, and opportunities to experiment with and explore new responsibilities and relationships.

## REFERENCES


1. Collins WA, Steinberg L. Adolescent development in interpersonal context. In: Eisenberg N, vol. ed. Volume Three: *Social, Emotional, and Personality Development.* Damon W, Lerner RM, eds. *Handbook of Child Psychology.* 6th ed. Hoboken, NJ: John Wiley & Sons, Inc.; 2006:1003–1067

2. Steinberg L. Autonomy, conflict, and harmony in the family relationship. In: Feldman S, Elliot G, eds. *At the Threshold: The Developing Adolescent.* Cambridge, MA: Harvard University Press; 1990:255–276

3. Collins WA. Relationships and development: family adaptation to individual change. In: Shulman S, ed. *Close Relationships and Socioemotional Development.* New York, NY: Ablex; 1995: 128–154

4. Steinberg L, Silverberg S. The vicissitudes of autonomy in early adolescence. *Child Dev.* 1986;57:841–851

5. Youniss J, Smollar J. *Adolescent Relations with Mothers, Fathers, and Friends.* Chicago, IL: University of Chicago Press; 1985

6. Collins WA, Laursen B. Parent–adolescent relationships and influences. In: Lerner R, Steinberg L, eds. *Handbook of Adolescent Psychology.* 2nd ed. New York, NY: Wiley; 2004: 331–361

7. Nurmi JE. Socialization and self-development: channeling, selection, adjustment, and reflection. In: Lerner R, Steinberg L, eds. *Handbook of Adolescent Psychology.* 2nd ed. New York, NY: Wiley; 2004: 85–124

8. Steinberg L. We know some things: adolescent–parent relationships in retrospect and prospect. *J Res Adoles.* 2001;11: 1–19

9. Steinberg L. Risk-taking in adolescence: what changes, and why? *Ann New York Acad of Sci.* 2004;1021:51–58

10. Nelson C, Bloom F, Cameron J, Amaral D, Dahl R, Pine D. An integrative, multidisciplinary approach to the study of brain-behavior relations in the context of typical and atypical development. *Dev Psychopath.* 2002;14: 499–520

11. Savin-Williams RC, Berndt TJ. Friendship and peer relations. In: Feldman SS, Elliott GR, eds. *At the Threshold: The Developing Adolescent.* Cambridge, MA: Harvard University Press; 1990:277–307

12. Brooks-Gunn J, Paikoff R. Sexuality and developmental transitions during adolescence. In: Schulenberg J, Maggs JL, eds. *Health Risks and Developmental Transitions during Adolescence.* New York, NY: Cambridge University Press; 1997:190–219

13. Waters E, Cummings EM. A secure base from which to explore close relationships. *Child Development.* 2000; 71: 164–172

14. Collins WA, Sroufe LA. Capacity for intimate relationships: a developmental construction. In: Furman W, Feiring C, Brown BB, eds. *Contemporary Perspectives on Adolescent Romantic Relationships.* New York, NY: Cambridge University Press; 1999:123–147

15. Sroufe LA, Fleeson J. The coherence of family relationships. In: Hinde RA, Stevenson-Hinde J, eds. *Relationships within Families: Mutual Influences.* Oxford: Oxford University Press; 1988:27–47

16. Collins WA, Van Dulmen M. "The course of true love(s)...": origins and pathways in the development of romantic relationships. In: Booth A, Crouter A, eds. *Romance and Sex in Adolescence and Emerging Adulthood: Risks and Opportunities.* Mahwah, NJ: Erlbaum; 2006:63–86

17. Moore S, Rosenthal D. *Sexuality in Adolescence: Current Trends.* 2nd ed. New York, NY: Routledge; 2006

18. Steinberg L. *Adolescence.* 8th ed. New York, NY: McGraw-Hill; 2008

19. Maccoby EE. *The Two Sexes: Growing Up Apart, Coming Together.* Cambridge, MA: Harvard University Press; 1998

20. Landry D, Kaeser L, Richards C. Abstinence promotion and the provision of information about contraception in public school district sexuality education policies. *Family Planning Perspectives.* 1999;31:280–286

# CHAPTER 7

# Adolescent Sexual Development

MARY B. SHORT, PHD • BETH A. AUSLANDER, PHD • SUSAN L. ROSENTHAL, PHD

## INTRODUCTION

Adolescence typically is defined as the life stage between 10 and 20 years of age. For clinical purposes it may be divided into 3 stages based on approximate chronologic age: early (10–14 years), middle (15–17 years), and late (18–20 years). As adolescents grow and develop across these stages (as described in Chapters 4, 5, and 6), their sexual experiences and romantic relationships may emerge and change over time. In healthy development, adolescents manage their sexual feelings and behaviors so that they feel positively about their bodies and sexuality and do not place themselves at risk for negative psychological or physical consequences. This chapter summarizes the literature on adolescent sexual/romantic relationships, the prevalence of sexual behaviors, influences on the initiation of intercourse, and opportunities for intervention within the health care setting. For an in-depth discussion of issues related to gay, lesbian, and bisexual youth, please refer to Chapter 50.

## SEXUAL/ROMANTIC RELATIONSHIPS

Adolescent sexual/romantic relationships involve sexual attractions and may include sexual behaviors. One component of this dimension is the adolescent's sexual identity. Sexual identity refers to how a person sees him or herself in terms of sexual attractions, behaviors, thoughts and feelings, fantasies, and lifestyle.[1] This includes being attracted to the opposite sex, the same sex, or both sexes. As adolescents explore their sexual attractions, behavior and identity may not coincide. For example, an adolescent may describe herself as attracted to other females but may not have engaged in any sexual behavior with females. Conversely, an adolescent may describe himself as heterosexual in all elements of sexual identity but may also engage in sexual behavior with males. In the former case, she may be following socially normative dating with males, whereas the latter case could represent same-sex-for-pay behavior. Because these can be confusing issues for adolescents and may change over time, it is critical that clinicians not prematurely characterize an adolescent's sexual identity.

Thus, rather than inquire about sexual identity, a health care provider should ask about sexual attractions and behaviors in nonjudgmental, gender-neutral terms and place these questions in the context of routine health concerns. This does not mean that discussion of sexual identity is not important, but the topic may be more easily raised in the context of specific behaviors that may or may not relate to sexual identify. Furthermore, it is important to be sensitive to other health issues that teens may face in relation to sexual behaviors. Compared with heterosexual adolescents, gay, lesbian, bisexual, and transgender youth are more likely to be victims of violence, experience emotional problems, attempt suicide, abuse alcohol and drugs, and engage in risky sexual and delinquent behaviors.[2,3]

Young adolescents begin to develop physical attractions to, and a desire for intimacy with others. Often the initial exploration of these feelings is conducted in groups (eg, a group of boys and girls will go to a movie, with some of the pairs considered to be couples). As adolescents enter middle and late adolescence, the focus becomes less on the peer group and more on a dyad. Although the proportion of adolescents who report being in a steady relationship increases dramatically throughout the high school years,[4] it can be developmentally appropriate for young adolescents to have brief or nonexclusive relationships. However, dating in early adolescence has been associated with other risk factors, including behavioral problems, poor school performance and motivation, and a higher likelihood of engaging in sexual intercourse.[4,5]

Within the context of romantic relationships, adolescents begin to share information, solve problems, make mutual decisions, and compromise with their partners. A satisfactory romantic relationship has been linked to positive self-perception, including social acceptance and attractiveness to others.[4] However, not all dating relationships are healthy or safe. Up to 32% of adolescents have reported experiencing physical violence in a dating relationship, and up to 40% report having an unwanted sexual experience.[6-8] Those who have been victimized have a greater likelihood of engaging in general risk behaviors (eg, attempted suicide, substance use, episodic heavy drinking, and physical fighting) and sexually risky behavior, such as not using a condom.[7,8] Although there are some demographic characteristics (eg, being older, having a baby with the partner, being depressed) associated with the likelihood of being a victim of dating violence, all adolescents are potentially at risk and should be screened regularly in a sensitive and nonjudgmental manner.[6,8,9] Adolescents may be reluctant to share information about unhealthy behaviors in their dating relationships because they may feel responsible for the violence, think they deserved it, or feel they are at risk for violence in the future.

## TALKING WITH ADOLESCENTS ABOUT SEXUAL BEHAVIORS

Talking with adolescents about sexual behaviors in the context of a health care visit can be awkward for patients and professionals if it is not considered part of a complete health history. If inquiries about sexual behaviors are viewed as distinct from the remainder of a health assessment or are addressed only under certain circumstances, then communication about the topic can be difficult. For example, preceding the entire medical history with the introductory statement, "I am going to ask you questions about your health today that I ask all of my patients your age," could be followed at the appropriate time in the visit with, "Now I would like to talk to you about sexual behaviors that can affect young people's health." A modification of the guidelines suggested by the Centers for Disease Control and Prevention appears in Box 7-1.[10]

Given the different permutations of responses given to the questions listed previously, one should be prepared to address issues arising with respect to safety, reducing risks, or emotional distress. An alternative means of introducing the discussion is the use of a screening questionnaire, such as those available in the Guidelines for Adolescent Preventive Services[11] that include trigger items about sexual behaviors and identity.

### Box 7-1

#### *Guidelines for Talking with Adolescents about Sexual Behaviors*

1. Establish normalcy of topic: "I ask these questions of all my patients."
2. Determine if adolescent has ever had sex, using straightforward questions:
   - "Have you ever had sex with males, females, or both?" If yes,
     - "In the past 2 months, how many partners have you had sex with?"
     - "In the past 12 months, how many partners have you had sex with?"
3. Determine behaviors that constitute "having sex": "To understand any health risks, I need to make sure I understand what kind of sex you have had."
   - "Have you had vaginal sex, meaning penis in vagina?" If yes,
     - "Do you use condoms: never, sometimes, or always?"
       - If always, reinforce healthy behavior.
       - If sometimes: "In what situations or with whom do you not use condoms?"
       - If never: "Why don't you use condoms?"
     - "Are you or your partner trying to get pregnant?" If no,
     - "What are you doing to prevent pregnancy?"
   - "Have you had anal sex, meaning penis in rectum/anus?" If yes, ask condom questions.
   - "Have you had oral sex, meaning mouth on penis/vagina?"

Adapted from the CDC: Sexually transmitted diseases treatment guidelines, 2006. *MMWR*. August 4, 2006, Vol 55(RR11). Available at: www.cdc.gov/mmwr/preview/mmwrhtml/rr5511a1.htm.

## PREVALENCE OF SEXUAL BEHAVIORS

Adolescents engage in a variety of sexual behaviors. Understanding this range of sexual behaviors, both noncoital and coital, will help provide necessary health care, education, and counseling to adolescents. Although some adolescents engage in a "typical" progression of sexual behaviors (ie, kissing, to breast touching, to genital touching, and then sexual intercourse), not all adolescents proceed through these behaviors, nor in the same order. Thus, as described previously, a complete medical history includes a sexual history that addresses the full range of behaviors, particularly with respect to oral and anal sex, that can affect health.

### MASTURBATION

Although there are few current data on the masturbation practices of adolescents, masturbation is a frequent behavior in male and female adolescents of various ages. Across studies, boys are more likely to masturbate than girls. Among 11- and 12-year-olds, 27% of boys and 18% of girls report masturbating.[12-14]

### GENITAL TOUCHING

A few studies have investigated adolescents' experiences with masturbation of, or by, a partner. Overall, more adolescents participated in this behavior than sexual intercourse, and among virgins, approximately 16% to 30% have experienced masturbation with a partner compared with 73% to 85% of nonvirgins.[14–16]

### ORAL AND ANAL SEX

Some adolescents engage in oral or anal sex. However, specific data about the prevalence of these behaviors in the adolescent population are limited. Because of the lack of information, it is difficult to determine whether these behaviors have increased in prevalence over the years.

Even though some people have hypothesized that oral sex may be replacement behavior for sexual intercourse so that individuals can maintain their "virgin" status,[17] it appears that nonvirgin adolescents engage in oral sex more frequently than virginal adolescents. Research has found that approximately 9% to 56% of adolescent virgins report engaging in oral sex behavior, as compared to 63% to 93% of nonvirgins.[14–16,18–20] Adolescents may view oral sex as having minimal or no psychological or physical risk, which may be why sexually experienced adolescents have more oral sex partners than vaginal intercourse partners.[21,22]

Some studies have examined the frequency of anal sex in both sexually experienced and inexperienced adolescents. Studies with nonvirgin adolescents have found that approximately 16% to 21% of teens reported having anal sex.[16,18,19] In a study with "virgin" adolescents, approximately 1% of the adolescents reported having anal sex.[15] Further, adolescents who engaged in sexual intercourse at a young age (<15 years of age) are more likely to have engaged in anal sex than adolescents who initiated sexual intercourse at or older than 15 years of age.[18]

### VAGINAL SEXUAL INTERCOURSE

Compared to earlier surveys of 15- to 19-year-olds, data from 2007 suggest that a larger number of adolescents in the United States are delaying the onset of sexual intercourse. For example, in 1991, 54% of adolescents engaged in sexual intercourse; in 2007, these percentages dropped to 48%.[23] Overall, it is estimated that 48% of high school students are sexually experienced[20,23] and about 35% of adolescents are currently sexually active (ie, had sexual intercourse in the past 3 months).[23] Although more adolescents are delaying intercourse and more than half of those having intercourse are using condoms, there is still a number of adolescents engaging in high-risk behaviors. For example, approximately 15% of American high school students report having 4 or more vaginal sex partners,[23] and approximately one-third of adolescents used only withdrawal or no method of protection.[24] Of particular concern is that in the fifth grade—at an average age of 11 years old—5% of girls and 17% of boys report having engaged in sexual intercourse.[25] Compared to adolescents who initiate sexual intercourse later, those who initiate intercourse earlier are more likely to engage in sexually risky behaviors (ie, have more sex partners), have adverse outcomes (ie, unwanted pregnancy and sexually transmitted infections [STIs]), and engage in other health-risk behaviors, such as substance use.[18,26,27]

Intentions to engage in sexual behavior in the near future strongly predict actual behavior. Thus, health care providers should inquire about both intentions and actual behaviors, including oral, vaginal, and anal sex. In addition, very young adolescents have opportunities to engage in sexual behaviors, and some engage in behaviors that place them at risk. Thus, health care providers should begin discussions about sexual health with adolescents at an early age so that adolescents are prepared when they find themselves alone with a romantic partner and as they move through the range of behaviors. During such conversations, it is important to remember that some self-described virgins engage in oral and anal sex, whereas nonvirgins may not.

## INFLUENCES ON SEXUAL INITIATION

Many factors influence the timing of initiation of adolescent sexual behavior. Early pubertal development is a risk factor for engaging in early intercourse.[28] However, regardless of the timing of pubertal development, the family can play a key protective role against early sexual activity, or it can create an environment that does not discourage early initiation. Parents can support healthy decision making and protect the adolescent from negative peer influence in a number of ways. Adolescents tend to delay sexual activity when they have a strong relationship (eg, feeling "connected") with their parents, when their parents monitor their teens' behaviors and whereabouts, when adolescents believe they are being monitored by their parents even if they are not, and when parents communicate openly about sexuality, including their disapproval of early sexual behavior.[25,29,30] In contrast, parenting styles characterized by overcontrol and hostility or permissiveness have been linked with early adolescent sexual behavior and sexually risky behaviors.[28] Furthermore, when girls have older sisters who are teen parents, they are more likely to engage in sexual intercourse at an early age, possibly because it is more acceptable in that family environment.[31]

Peers also can be influential in adolescents' choices to become sexually active, particularly for those adolescents who have strained relationships with their parents.[29,30] When their peers are or are perceived to be sexually active and supportive of early sexual initiation, adolescents are more likely to initiate sex at an early age,[28-30,32] and the likelihood increases further when the adolescents feel they would gain their friends' respect by having sex.[32] With regard to partners, most adolescents initiate sexual intercourse in the context of a steady, committed romantic relationship; however, there are a few adolescents who initiate sexual intercourse with a casual partner.[18] Further, having a "significant other" at an early age or having partners who are 2 or more years older increases the likelihood that adolescents will engage in sexual intercourse at an earlier age.[33]

The cultural context of the adolescent's life also plays a role in the timing of sexual initiation. For example, engaging in other risk behaviors, such as substance abuse, is associated with engaging in sexual intercourse at an early age. But there also are factors that protect against engaging in sexual activity at an early age. For example, individuals who have higher academic performance, religiosity, self-esteem and positive body image tend to delay sexual initiation and continue to make healthier sexual choices.[34-36] "Chastity pledges" are intended to be another protective strategy against early initiation of sexual activity; adolescents who make such private or personal promises do tend to delay sex until later ages than those who do not make pledges.[37] However, compared to adolescents who did not make a pledge, they have a higher likelihood of having oral sex, anal sex, and unprotected intercourse. Furthermore, adolescents who make chastity pledges have STI rates comparable to nonpledgers, even though they tend to be sexually active for less time and with fewer partners.[38] Another concern is the effect of the media on sexual behavior. Overall, research shows that adolescents exposed to sexual content in the mass media have an increased likelihood of initiating sexual intercourse at an early age.[39]

Thus, no single intervention will ensure that all adolescents delay sexual initiation. Interventions need to be culturally and developmentally appropriate, adapting to the adolescent changing in the context of his or her own individual growth and development, but also in the context of his or her environment. Although this section has focused on those factors associated with helping young teenagers wait to have intercourse, it is equally important to help them continue to make wise sexual decisions as they age. Many of the same factors that influence sexual initiation influence other high-risk sexual behaviors.

## OPPORTUNITIES FOR INTERVENTION IN THE HEALTH CARE SETTING

Because sexual development is central to the process of adolescence, health care providers have an opportunity to engage adolescents in discussions about healthy sexual development, including preventive health care related to human papillomavirus (HPV) infection.

### ANTICIPATORY GUIDANCE TO ADOLESCENTS AND PARENTS

Health care providers can support adolescents' healthy sexual development by talking to adolescents and their parents and by encouraging parent–adolescent conversations. Ideally, discussions about sexuality have begun between the parents and the adolescent before the clinician begins those conversations. The third edition of the American Academy of Pediatrics *Bright Futures Guidelines for Health Supervision of Infants, Children, Adolescents, and Their Families*[40] includes materials on the promotion of healthy sexual development across the pediatric age span. By having routine conversations about puberty and sexuality as part of normal development, health care providers can offer anticipatory guidance and identify adolescents who need referrals for specialized medical or behavioral services. Many adolescents want to discuss sexuality with their provider, but many of them do not initiate the conversation and prefer that the clinician initiate the conversation.[41] The American Academy of Pediatrics[42] recommends that these discussions include the following: (1) anticipatory guidance for parents (ie, supervision and communication needs), (2) nonjudgmental/age-appropriate screening methods for risk behaviors (eg, previsit questionnaires), and (3) developmentally appropriate education messages about healthy sexual decision making. Research shows that asking about high-risk sexual behaviors and providing information about risks and prevention can help increase adolescents' knowledge about sexual health and at least temporarily reduce sexual activity and decrease unprotected sex.[43,44]

### NEW OPPORTUNITIES AND CHALLENGES FOR THE HEALTH CARE PROVIDER

Two vaccines have been licensed for the prevention of HPV for girls and boys, and other vaccines for sexually transmitted diseases are in development. The Advisory Committee on Immunization Practices (ACIP)[45] recommends routine vaccination of females age 11 or 12 years with 3 doses of HPV vaccine. The vaccination series in girls can be started beginning at 9 through 25 to 26 years of age. In 2009, the ACIP made a provisional recommendation that the 3-dose series of quadrivalent HPV vaccine may be given to males age 9 through 26 years to reduce their likelihood of acquiring genital warts. Ideally, the vaccine should be administered before potential exposure to HPV through sexual contact in both males and females. Although this vaccine was developed to prevent cervical cancer, the 3-shot series of this vaccine provides an opportunity for health care providers to discuss issues of puberty and sexuality with early adolescents.[46] There was initially concern that parents would resist the concept of a vaccine for an STI; however, data do not support this concern. Parents are more influenced by the efficacy of the vaccine and the seriousness of the disease than by the route of transmission. However, integrating these vaccines into the routine health care of adolescents will provide challenges with regard to affordability and accessibility for all adolescents.

## SUMMARY

Adolescence is an important time for development of sexual health. Health care providers have an opportunity to help adolescents not place themselves at psychological or physical risk while also promoting healthy sexual development. This can be accomplished by establishing trust, respect, and confidentiality with the adolescent and by supporting parents as they supervise and communicate with their teens. In addition, as leaders in the community, health care providers can advocate for a societal context that supports the adolescents' exploration of sexual feelings, identity, and behaviors in a safe and healthy manner.

## REFERENCES


1. Diamond LM. New paradigms for research on heterosexual and sexual-minority development. *J Clin Child Adolesc Psychol.* 2003;32:490–498

2. Friedman MS, Koeske GF, Silvestre AJ, Korr WS, Sites EW. The impact of gender-role nonconforming behavior, bullying, and social support on suicidality among gay male youth. *J Adolesc Health.* 2006;38:621–623

3. Udry JR, Chantala K. Risk assessment of adolescents with same-sex relationships. *J Adolesc Health.* 2002;31:84–92

4. Zimmer-Gembeck MJ, Siebenbruner J, Collins WA. Diverse aspects of dating: associations with psychosocial functioning from early to middle adolescence. *J Adolesc.* 2001;24:313–336

5. Cooksey EC, Mott FL, Neubauer SA. Friendships and early relationships: links to sexual initiation among American adolescents born to young mothers. *Perspect Sex Reprod Health.* 2002;34:118–126

6. Blythe MJ, Fortenberry JD, Temkit M, Tu W, Orr DP. Incidence and correlates of unwanted sex in relationships of middle and late adolescent women. *Arch Pediatr Adolesc Med.* 2006;160:591–595

7. Roberts TA, Auinger P, Klein JD. Intimate partner abuse and the reproductive health of sexually active female adolescents. *J Adolesc Health.* 2005;36:380–385

8. Centers for Disease Control. Physical dating violence among high school students—United States. *MMWR.* 2006. Available at: www.cdc.gov/mmwr/preview/mmwrhtml/mm5519a3.htm. Accessed August 26, 2006

9. Lehrer JA, Buka S, Gortmaker S, Shrier LA. Depressive symptomatology as a predictor of exposure to intimate partner violence among US female adolescents and young adults. *Arch Pediatr Adolesc Med.* 2006;160:270–276

10. Centers for Disease Control. Sexually transmitted diseases treatment guidelines, 2006. *MMWR.* 2006;54(No. RR-4)

11. American Medical Association. Guidelines for adolescent preventive services. Available at: www.ama-assn.org/ama/pub/physician-resources/public-health/promoting-healthy-lifestyles/adolescent-health/guidelines-adolescent-preventive-services.shtml. Accessed August 11, 2010

12. Larsson I, Svedin CG. Sexual experiences in childhood: young adults' recollections. *Arch Sex Behav.* 2002;31:263–273

13. Smith AM, Rosenthal DA, Reichler H. High schoolers' masturbatory practices: their relationship to sexual intercourse and personal characteristics. *Psychol Rep.* 1996;79:499–509

14. Schwartz IM. Sexual activity prior to coital initiation: a comparison between males and females. *Arch Sex Behav.* 1999;28:63–69

15. Schuster MA, Bell RM, Kanouse DE. The sexual practices of adolescent virgins: genital sexual activities of high school students who have never had vaginal intercourse. *Am J Public Health.* 1996;86:1570–1576

16. Feldman L, Holowaty P, Harvey B, Rannie K, Shortt L, Jamal A. A comparison of the demographic, lifestyle, and sexual behaviour characteristics of virgin and non-virgin adolescents. *Can J Hum Sex.* 1997;6:197–209

17. Remez L. Oral sex among adolescents: is it sex or is it abstinence? *Family Planning Perspectives.* 2000;32:298–304

18. Edgardh K. Sexual behaviour and early coitarche in a national sample of 17-year-old Swedish girls. *Sex Transm Infect.* 2000;76:98–102

19. Brewster KL, Tillman KH. Who's doing it? Patterns and predictors of youths' oral sexual experiences. *J Adolesc Health.* 2008;43:73–80

20. Lindberg LD, Jones R, Santelli JS. Noncoital sexual activities among adolescents. *J Adolescent Health.* 2008;43:231–238

21. Halpern-Felsher BL, Cornell JL, Kropp RY, Tschann JM. Oral versus vaginal sex among adolescents: perceptions, attitudes, and behavior. *Pediatrics.* 2005;115:845–851

22. Prinstein MJ, Meade CS, Cohen GL. Adolescent oral sex, peer popularity, and perceptions of best friends' sexual behavior. *J Pediatr Psychol.* 2003;28:243–249

23. Santelli J, Carter M, Orr M, Dittus P. Trends in sexual risk behaviors, by nonsexual risk behavior involvement, US high school students, 1991–2007. *J Adolesc Health.* 2008;e-pub: 1–8

24. Anderson JE, Santelli JS, Morrow B. Trends in adolescent contraceptive use, unprotected and poorly protected sex, 1991-2003. *J Adolesc Health.* 2006;38:734-739

25. Rose A, Koo HP, Bhaskar B, Anderson K, White G, Jenkins RR. The influence of primary caregivers on the sexual behavior of early adolescents. *J Adolesc Health.* 2005;37:135-144

26. Kaestle CE, Halpern CT, Miller WC, Ford CA. Young age at first sexual intercourse and sexually transmitted infections in adolescents and young adults. *Am J Epidemiol.* 2005;161:774-780

27. O'Donnell BL, O'Donnell CR, Stueve A. Early sexual initiation and subsequent sex-related risks among urban minority youth: the reach for health study. *Fam Plann Perspect.* 2001;33:268-275

28. L'Engle KL, Jackson C, Brown JD. Early adolescents' cognitive susceptibility to initiating sexual intercourse. *Perspect Sex Reprod Health.* 2006;38:97-105

29. Donenberg GR, Bryant FB, Emerson E, Wilson HW, Pasch KE. Tracing the roots of early sexual debut among adolescents in psychiatric care. *J Am Acad Child Adolesc Psychiatry.* 2003;42:594-608

30. Fasula AM, Miller KS. African-American and Hispanic adolescents' intentions to delay first intercourse: parental communication as a buffer for sexually active peers. *J Adolesc Health.* 2006;38:193-200

31. East PL, Kiernan EA. Risks among youths who have multiple sisters who were adolescent parents. *Fam Plann Perspect.* 2001;33:75-80

32. Sieving RE, Eisenberg ME, Pettingell S, Skay C. Friends' influence on adolescents' first sexual intercourse. *Perspec Sex Reprod Health.* 2006;38:13-19

33. Marin BV, Kirby DB, Hudes ES, Coyle KK, Gomez CA. Boyfriends, girlfriends, and teenagers' risk of sexual involvement. *Perspect Sex Reprod Health.* 2006;38:76-83

34. Ethier KA, Kershaw TS, Lewis JB, Milan S, Niccolai LM, Ickovics JR. Self-esteem, emotional distress, and sexual behavior among adolescent females: inter-relationships and temporal effects. *J Adolesc Health.* 2006;38:268-274

35. Wingood GM, DiClemente RJ, Harrington K, Davies SL. Body image and African-American females' sexual health. *J Womens Health Gend Based Med.* 2002;11:433-439

36. Lammers C, Ireland M, Resnick M, Blum R. Influences on adolescents' decision to postpone onset of sexual intercourse: a survival analysis of virginity among youths aged 13 to 18 years. *J Adolesc Health.* 2000;26:42-48

37. Bersamin MM, Walker S, Waiters ED, Fisher DA, Grube JW. Promising to wait: virginity pledges and adolescent sexual behavior. *J Adolesc Health.* 2005;36:428-436

38. Bruckner H, Bearman P. After the promise: the STD consequences of adolescent virginity pledges. *J Adolesc Health.* 2005;36:271-278

39. L'Engle KL, Brown JD, Kenneavy K. The mass media are an important context for adolescents' sexual behavior. *J Adolesc Health.* 2006;38:186-192

40. American Academy of Pediatrics. Promoting sexual development and sexuality. Available at: brightfutures.aap.org/pdfs/Guidelines_PDF/9-Promoting-Healthy-Sexual-Development.pdf. Accessed February 9, 2009

41. American Academy of Pediatrics: Committee on Psychosocial Aspects of Child and Family Health and Committee on Adolescence. Sexuality education for children and adolescents. *Pediatrics.* 2001;108:498-502

42. Boekeloo BO, Schamus LA, Simmens SJ, Cheng TL, O'Connor K, D'Angelo LJ. A STD/HIV prevention trial among adolescents in managed care. *Pediatrics.* 1999;103:107-115

43. Mansfield CJ, Conroy ME, Emans SJ, Woods ER. A pilot study of AIDS education and counseling of high-risk adolescents in an office setting. *J Adolesc Health.* 1993;14:115-119

44. Centers for Disease Control. CDC's advisory committee recommends human papillomavirus virus vaccination. June 24, 2006. Available at: www.cdc.gov/media/pressrel/r060629.htm. Accessed May 4, 2010

45. Centers for Disease Control. Quadrivalent human papillomavirus vaccine. Recommendations of the Advisory Committee on Immunization Practices (ACIP). *Morbid Mortal Wkly Rep.* 2007;56(No. RR-02):1-24

46. Short MB, Rupp R, Stanberry LR, Rosenthal SL. Parental acceptance of adolescent vaccines within school-based health centres. *Herpes.* 2005;12:23-27

SECTION 3

# Approach to the Patient and Family

# CHAPTER 8

## Medical History

KRISTIN DELISI, MSN, CRNP • MELANIE A. GOLD, DO

A critical component of the health encounter with any patient is medical history.[1] A thorough medical history can elicit information and provide the adolescent patient with information and advice about health-related behaviors. In addition to the traditional components of medical history (chief complaint, past medical and surgical history, hospitalizations, allergies, and immunizations) obtained from the parent(s) and the adolescent, the adolescent medical history should include an assessment of the adolescent's physical and emotional well-being, biopsychosocial health, strengths, and risk-taking behaviors. Thus, health care professionals define their purview as inclusive rather than exclusive of the most likely disorders and dysfunctions affecting teenagers today.[2] The thorough medical history demonstrates to the adolescent that the health care professional understands the adolescent's world, enhancing the likelihood that useful, or even critical, information will be elicited and that a meaningful therapeutic relationship will ensue.

### ESTABLISHING RAPPORT IN AN ADOLESCENT HEALTH SETTING

When eliciting a history from an adolescent, it helps to focus primarily on style rather than content. A patient-centered interaction style helps build rapport by establishing a partnership with the adolescent. Older views of history-taking held that information flowed unilaterally from the health care professional to the patient. This style is less effective with adolescents because it fails to acknowledge psychosocial influences on health. Patient-centered communication encourages and facilitates discussion of psychosocial issues that can directly and indirectly influence health-related behaviors.

When establishing rapport with the adolescent patient, it is essential to discuss the rules of confidentiality and limits. Confidentiality issues need to be addressed with both the patient and the parent before questions about sensitive topics are asked of the adolescent during the history. It is not reasonable to expect an adolescent to reveal personal information unless confidentiality can be assured. Health care professionals must also determine the limits of confidentiality based on the specific laws of the state they practice in and their own comfort. Common limits of confidentiality include current homicidality, suicidality, and physical or sexual abuse. State-specific guidelines are available from the American Medical Association and the National Center for Adolescent Health and Law. For more in-depth information on confidentiality laws by state, see *State Minor Consent Laws: A Summary*, available from the Center for Adolescent Health and the Law,[3] or visit www.adolescenthealthlaw.org.

In addition to ensuring confidentiality, there are several key opening strategies for establishing rapport and conveying interest and willingness to listen. These include *open-ended questions, affirmations, reflections, and summaries (OARS)*.[4] Open-ended questions invite elaboration and explanation from the adolescent's perspective and cannot be answered by one- or two-word answers like "yes," "no," or "last Wednesday." Open-ended questions encourage the adolescent to express personal thoughts or concerns and avoid feeling interrogated by being asked multiple close-ended questions. For the developmentally younger adolescent, it helps to clarify a potentially vague open-ended question such as "What brings you in today?" by adding response options such as "Are you here for a general physical, a specific concern or problem, or some other reason? Tell me why you are here." *Affirmations* are expressions of appreciation for the adolescent's participation and can greatly enhance rapport. Examples of affirmations are: "I really appreciate your willingness to be so honest with me" and "That's a great idea, you really know how to take care of yourself." *Reflections* indicate to the adolescent that you have an accurate understanding of the teen's perspective and experience. Reflections can restate or paraphrase what the adolescent has said using words that are the same or similar in meaning and content or they can be more complex extensions of meaning or emotion that the adolescent has not yet given voice to. Reflections are most effective when expressed in a warm, nonjudgmental, and empathic tone. *Summaries* are also helpful to establish rapport because they collect several of the adolescent's previously expressed thoughts, feelings, or concerns, and may also include a new perspective of how these pieces of the story fit together. Summaries can also be an effective way to pull together essential components of the discussion when preparing to shift the focus from data gathering (eg, history-taking) to counseling and providing information or advice.

## HISTORY FROM PARENT AND ADOLESCENT

When the adolescent and parent(s) or guardian(s) are both present for the health visit, it can be helpful to include the parent(s) or guardian(s) initially in the history-taking to provide insight to the parent's concerns and the reason for the encounter. When the parent(s) or guardian(s) are present, it helps to introduce yourself to the adolescent first and invite the adolescent to introduce the health care professional to the other people in the room. This sends the message that the adolescent is the primary focus of the visit and will be viewed as the expert regarding the teen's relationships. Early in the interview, the adolescent and parent(s) or guardians(s) should be informed that the adolescent will be interviewed alone for the second part of the medical history, followed by the physical examination. The health care professional should explain that many parents appreciate the opportunity to meet with the health care professional first and that the adolescent will be interviewed second to preserve confidentiality. Most adolescents appreciate such candidness, and this sequence does not alienate them but serves to engender their trust. Some younger adolescents are not ready for a completely independent relationship with their health care professional and are relieved that their parents have a relationship with the health care professional. If the adolescent specifically requests that a parent stay for the entire interview, document this in the medical record and keep in mind that the parent's presence may limit the extent to which the adolescent will provide sensitive information. This also presents a challenge during subsequent visits if exclusion is necessary for more private concerns.

### MEDICAL HISTORY

Medical history obtained from the parent includes the "chief complaint," the adolescent's past medical history, the family medical history, and the social history pertinent to the adolescent's life at home, in school, and with peers. The parent's chief complaint is the problem of greatest concern. The adolescent may report a chief complaint identical to, similar to, or totally different from the primary concerns of the parent. Observing parent–adolescent interactions during the medical history can be both interesting and a significant indicator of family functioning. The parent is usually most familiar with the adolescent's early medical history: the perinatal period, early developmental milestones, serious or chronic illnesses, hospitalizations, operations, significant injuries or accidents, allergies, regular use of medications, and immunizations.

### FAMILY HISTORY

The family history should include the ages and health status of the parents and siblings and note whether any relatives (grandparents, aunts, uncles, first cousins) have genetic or familial medical conditions. These conditions include heart disease, sudden death, hypertension, hypercholesterolemia, coagulation disorders, major organ system disease, or contagious diseases such as tuberculosis or hepatitis. Psychiatric disorders, which may also have a genetic component, including depression, anxiety, schizophrenia, alcoholism, substance abuse, or eating disorders, are also reviewed. A genogram can often be a helpful way to record family medical history. The family medical history provides more than a list of diseases; it also gives a clue to the context of the adolescent's "health environment." The family history may also include information pertaining to the parents' (and siblings') type of work, level of education, and location (if not residing with the adolescent).

### PSYCHOSOCIAL HISTORY

In the psychosocial (developmental) history, the parent is asked to describe the adolescent's personality, strengths, weaknesses, and general adjustment to family life, school, and peer group. If time is limited, the parent may simply be asked what specific concerns exist in any of these areas. Meeting alone with the parent for an initial interview may be a controversial approach to adolescent health care. This initial time with the parent may not be necessary when the adolescent has grown up in a pediatric or family medicine practice.[5] However, in a first visit the health care professional is in a better position to elicit specific data regarding the adolescent's health and to become acquainted with the parent if interviewed alone. Interviewing the parent alone with the full knowledge of the adolescent, rather than a phone conversation behind the adolescent's back, can be helpful and nonproblematic. Health care professionals must develop a style that works best for them and their patients.

## HISTORY FROM ADOLESCENT

Most adults understand the need for confidentiality and the need for teens to communicate privately with their health care professional. The parent or guardian often gladly leaves the room, and it is rare for a parent to persistently object to leaving the adolescent alone with a health care professional. Once alone with the adolescent it helps to restate and review the rules and limitations of confidentiality. It is especially important to discuss confidentiality at the beginning of the psychosocial interview. Explain specifically to adolescents that they will be asked personal questions because the information is important to understanding their health needs.

Components of the medical history obtained from the adolescent interviewed alone include the chief complaint, a detailed review of systems that includes items particularly pertinent to adolescence, the patient's version of the psychosocial history, and the crucial medicosocial history that reviews various health risk behaviors. Talking candidly and openly with the adolescent about numerous important and sensitive areas of the teen's life can be a challenging task. The key to a thorough and meaningful interview is to put the adolescent at ease and to gain trust, even if this requires modifying the professional's typical approach and goals. The "art" of achieving this trust at a first meeting with an adolescent can be cultivated and perfected by the health care professional. Naturally, it is easier to establish a relationship with some adolescents than with others. The initial interview sets the tone for future encounters, and the primary goal is to engender the adolescent's confidence in the health care professional as an adult who understands the adolescent's world, is nonjudgmental, enjoys talking with the adolescent, and is committed to responding to the adolescent's needs.

### CHIEF COMPLAINT

As already noted, the adolescent's chief complaint may be identical to, similar to, or completely different from the parent's. Some adolescents initially appear to have no complaints at all. As the adolescent becomes increasingly comfortable during the course of the initial interview and as "trigger" questions are asked, specific concerns may emerge. Likewise, at a subsequent visit, the adolescent may raise an issue that was not discussed at the first meeting or that was not a problem at that time.

### REVIEW OF SYSTEMS

A review of systems includes questions about each major organ system (head, eyes, ear, nose, and throat, cardiopulmonary, gastrointestinal, dermatologic, genitourinary, gynecologic, endocrinologic, musculoskeletal, neurologic, hematologic, psychiatric) as well as more general complaints such as malaise and fatigue. The adolescent may benefit from discussion regarding menstrual cramps or acne, even if it was not important enough to mention without prompting.

### PSYCHOSOCIAL REVIEW OF SYSTEMS

The psychosocial history is the most important part of the adolescent health encounter. Because adolescence is a time of growth and development, threats to health are likely to arise as adolescents begin to socially explore and experiment. Increased risk-taking behavior can be a normal part of adolescent development. Problems that may accompany exploration, however, are not easily detected on the standard review of systems that health care professionals inquire about. A refined system for organizing the psychosocial history, known by the acronym HEEADSSS, can be successful in an adolescent health setting. The HEEADSSS model was developed in 1972 by Harvey Berman, MD, of Seattle and refined by Eric Cohen, MD, and John M. Goldenring, MD, in 1988.[6]

The HEEADSSS inventory was developed to help health care professionals deal with contemporary causes of adolescent morbidity and mortality including obesity, eating disorders, and unintentional injury and violence. HEEADSSS stands for Home, Education/Employment, Eating, peer-group Activities, Drugs, Depression/Suicide, Sexuality, Safety, and Spirituality. Designed to encourage communication, this method of interviewing can enhance the health care professional's ability to spot potential problems early. The interview is meant to be an adjunct to the formal guidelines for adolescent preventive care used in traditional adolescent practice (Box 8-1). This complementary strategy is practical and time-tested to help health care professionals build on and incorporate the traditional guidelines into their office practice. The HEEADSSS questions should be asked without a parent in the room unless the adolescent specifically gives permission or asks for a parent's presence. If the questions are asked and answered with other people in the room, document this in a chart and note that this was by patient request.

Innovative computerized screening methods for asking HEEADSSS questions have been reported and young people seem to enjoy this mode of recording

**Box 8-1**

***Guidelines for Adolescent Preventive Care***

*Guidelines for Adolescent Preventive Services (GAPS)*
**American Medical Association**
www.ama-assn.org

*Health Supervision III*
**American Academy of Pediatrics**
www.aap.org

*Bright Futures*
**Maternal and Child Health Bureau, Health Resources and Services Administration of the United States Department of Health and Human Services**
www.brightfutures.aap.org

biopsychosocial information.[7] Computerized questionnaires may be useful in some settings, but many adolescents will not answer sensitive questions truthfully when it pertains to information such as drugs or sexual behavior. Rapport and trust are essential when convincing an adolescent that it is safe to reveal personal elements of the history. Questionnaires (by computer or on paper) should not be a substitute for direct, face-to-face communication when eliciting or confirming psychosocial information.

When asking about particularly sensitive topics such as sexuality or substance use, it is critical to reassure the adolescent about confidentiality. Nonjudgmental language is especially important when inquiring about behaviors the adolescent knows are socially undesirable. It is helpful to reassure about confidentiality when initiating discussions about sensitive topics when the adolescent is alone and to explain why you are asking sensitive questions (eg,"I am asking you these questions to help me find out if you might have any health problems from the things that you are doing, to tell me what kind of exam I should do, or what types of tests to order"). When asking about sexual history, it is important to avoid asking vague questions like "Are you currently sexually active?" This question is unclear in terms of the time frame and type of sexual behavior. Ask adolescents to describe specific sexual behaviors and add "second-tier" questions to assess comfort with behaviors. It is also important to use gender-neutral terms and pronouns such as "partner" and avoid "your boyfriend" or "your girlfriend," and "he" or "she," when referring to sexual partners. Gender-biased language dissuades gay, lesbian, bisexual, or questioning youth from discussing same-gendered sexual attractions and behaviors.

Table 8-1 summarizes sample HEEADSSS questions. Questions in **bold** are considered essential. Questions in *italics* are next in importance and should be asked if time permits. The remaining questions are for going into more depth when time allows or the situation demands it. The CRAFFT questions in Chapter 174, Alcohol are used to further assess reports of drug and alcohol use and help identify behavior patterns suggestive of a substance-use disorder or problem that may require referral.[8]

## PROMOTING HEALTHY BEHAVIORS WITH ADOLESCENTS IN THE OFFICE SETTING

The information collected during the medical and psychosocial histories should be used by health care professionals to identify both issues or problems and positive attributes and resiliencies. Positive supports identified in the history suggest the presence of resilience or the ability to adapt and overcome adversity and can be noted with affirmations by the health care professional. When risks are identified with concomitant positive behaviors, productive interventions for behavior change can improve outcomes.

The transtheoretical model of behavior change hypothesizes that individuals have different counseling needs based on their readiness to change.[9] For example, if an adolescent is not ready to or interested in quitting smoking cigarettes, counseling discussions about ways to take action, such as setting a quit date, would be counterproductive and mismatched. Assessing an adolescent's current "readiness for change" is essential when assessing health risk behaviors. Motivational interviewing (MI), which is a counseling style that is respectful, acknowledges choices and ambivalence, and reduces resistance by supporting autonomy, is well-suited for adolescents when promoting healthy behaviors.[4,10] Patient-centered skills such as using active listening with reflections can communicate that the health care professional appreciates the adolescent's fundamental beliefs regarding health and illness, the stage of readiness to change, and his or her confidence in the ability to make a change.

*Agenda setting* can be a helpful initial strategy for establishing a working partnership with an adolescent in a busy office setting.[11] The adolescent is asked to set his or her own agenda by identifying which health behavior he or she wishes to discuss first. For example, in setting the agenda a health care professional can ask: "What would you like to discuss today? We could talk about smoking, exercise, eating, or drinking alcohol, all of which affect your health. You will be the best judge of where to start. I would like to know what is important for you to talk about." Once the adolescent defines his

**Table 8-1**

## Summarizing the HEEADSSS Interview

| *Topic* | *Sample Questions* |
|---|---|
| *Home* | • **Tell me about where you live and who lives with you.**<br>• *Do you live in a house or apartment?*<br>• *Do you share a room or have your own?*<br>• **Are there any new people living in your home?**<br>• **How are your relationships with parents, siblings, other important relatives?**<br>• **What are the rules like at home?**<br>• *Have you ever been homeless or in shelter care?*<br>• *Have you ever been in foster care or residential group home?* |
| *Education* | • **Do you attend school? Which one? What grade are you in?**<br>• **Are you in gifted, regular, or special education classes?**<br>• **What are your favorite and least favorite subjects?**<br>• **How do you do in school in terms of grades?**<br>• **In the past year, how many days of school have you missed? Why?**<br>• **What are your educational goals?**<br>• *Have you ever had to repeat a year of school? Why?*<br>• *Have you ever been suspended? Why?*<br>• Do you feel connected to your school?<br>• Do you feel as if you belong?<br>• Who are the adults at school you feel you could talk to about something important? |
| *Employment* | • **Do you work after school?**<br>• **What type of work do you do?**<br>• **How many hours a week?**<br>• **What are your future career goals?**<br>• **What do you want to do when you grow up in terms of a job?**<br>• *Do you have any home chores? Do you get an allowance?* |
| *Eating* | • **How do you feel about your weight?**<br>• **Do you want to weigh more or less or stay the same?**<br>• **What do you think your ideal or perfect weight should be?**<br>• **How many meals and snacks do you eat per day?**<br>• **Tell me what you would eat in a typical day.**<br>• *Do you ever skip meals? Why? How often?*<br>• *How do you control your weight? With exercise, vomiting, diuretics, laxatives?*<br>• **How often do you have a bowel movement? Do you have any problems with your bowel movements?**<br>• What would it be like if you gained (lost) 10 pounds? |
| *Activities* | • **How do you like to spend your free time? What do you like to do for fun?**<br>• **Do you play any sports?**<br>• **Which ones and how many hours a week?**<br>• *What hobbies, clubs, church, or school activities do you do?*<br>• *How many hours of television per week do you watch? How many hours a week are you on the computer (sedentary)?* |

*(Continued)*

**Table 8-1 (Continued)**

| *Topic* | *Sample Questions* |
|---|---|
| *Drugs* | • **How many of the people who you hang out with smoke cigarettes? How many drink alcohol? And how many use drugs?**<br>• **Do you smoke or chew tobacco?**<br>• **Do you drink alcohol?**<br>• **What kind? Beer, wine, wine coolers, hard liquor?**<br>• **How often do you use tobacco, alcohol, or drugs?**<br>• **How much and how often?**<br>• *Have you ever blacked out or passed out?*<br>• *Did you ever do anything you regretted while drunk or high?*<br>• *When do you most often use alcohol or drugs? Socially? Alone? Time of day? Day of week?*<br>• *How do you feel about cutting back or quitting?*<br>• **What other drugs have you used or tried? Marijuana, inhalants, cocaine or crack, heroin, pills, LSD, ecstasy, crystal meth, or other drugs?**<br>• **Do you use anabolic steroids?**<br>• *Have you ever gotten treatment or counseling for drug use?*<br>• *How do you support your alcohol or drug use? Have you ever had any arrests?* |
| *Depression/ Suicidality* | • **How do you usually feel: happy, sad, or a bit of both?**<br>• **What makes you feel stressed?**<br>• **What do you do to relieve stress? How do you cope?**<br>• **Do you have an adult you can talk to when things are challenging? Who is that?**<br>• **Have you ever thought about trying to hurt or kill yourself?**<br>• *Have you ever tried to hurt or kill yourself?*<br>• *What did you do? Whom did you tell?*<br>• *Have you ever gotten counseling and/or therapy?*<br>• *Have you ever been in a psychiatric hospital? Why? How long did you stay?* |
| *Sexuality* | **For female adolescents:**<br>• **How old were you when you started your menstrual periods?**<br>• **How often do you have a period?**<br>• **How long are your periods? How heavy is your flow?**<br>• **Do you use pads, tampons, or both?**<br>• **Do you have menstrual cramps?**<br>• *What do you use to treat your cramps?*<br>• **How often do you miss school because of cramps?**<br>**For all adolescents:**<br>• **When you think of people to whom you are attracted, are they guys, girls, both, neither, or are you not sure?**<br>• **How comfortable are you with your feelings of attraction?**<br>• *When you think of yourself as a person, do you think of yourself as male, female, neither, or both?*<br>• *How comfortable are you with your feelings?*<br>• **Have you ever had the kind of sex where . . . (add specific type of contact, eg, penis in vagina, mouth on penis, mouth on vagina, penis in rectum, etc.)?**<br>**If above is answered as yes to specific sexual contacts, then ask:**<br>• **How old were you when you first . . . (describe sexual contact)?**<br>• How often do you have pain during sexual intercourse or other sexual activities? |

*(Continued)*

**Table 8-1 (Continued)**

| *Topic* | *Sample Questions* |
|---|---|
| | • Are you satisfied with how often you have sexual relations and with what you do with your sexual partner? |
| | • *Any problems becoming aroused, getting an erection, getting lubricated (wet), or having an orgasm?* |
| | • **Have you ever been pregnant or gotten someone pregnant? What concerns do you have about being able to get pregnant or get someone else pregnant?** |
| | • **What have you used in the past to prevent pregnancy? What are you using now? For methods that you stopped, why did you stop?** |
| | • **How many people have you had sexual relationships with in your lifetime? What about the past 3 months?** |
| | • **Have you ever heard of sexually transmitted infections (STI) like gonorrhea, chlamydia, trichomonas, herpes, or warts? What concerns do you have about STIs?** |
| | • **If ever had sexual contact ask: Have you ever had an STI?** |
| | • *Have you ever exchanged sex for drugs, money, food, or a place to stay?* |
| *Safety* | • **Have you ever been forced to have sex or been touched in a sexual way against your will?** |
| | **If above is answered as yes, then ask:** |
| | • **By whom and is this still going on?** |
| | • **In what ways does that experience affect your day-to-day life?** |
| | • **In what ways does that experience affect your sexual relationships now?** |
| | • **How often do you wear protective sports gear when you play sports?** |
| | • **Have you ever been a victim of violence in your home, neighborhood, or school?** |
| | • **Do you wear a seat belt when riding in a car?** |
| | • **Do you have access to weapons? Is there a gun at home?** |
| | • *Do you ever ride in a stolen car, in a car with a drunk driver, in a car late at night?* |
| | • *Do you use sunscreen when in the sun?* |
| *Spirituality* | • **What role does spirituality play in your life?** |
| | • What do you consider to be your religion? |
| | • How often do you participate in religious activities? |
| | • How important are your spiritual beliefs in your day-to-day life? |
| | • *How do your beliefs influence your health and attitudes about drug and alcohol use, sex, and contraception?* |

**Bold** = essential questions *Italics* = as time permits
Plain text = optional or when situation requires

or her interests or concerns, the health care professional can focus the discussion on these topics. If the adolescent has trouble setting the agenda, the health care professional can encourage the adolescent by showing him or her pictures of behaviors that affect peoples' health. The empty circles are for other issues that might be of concern to the adolescent (see Figure 8-1).

*Readiness rulers* and *importance and confidence rulers* can assess how ready an adolescent is to change a health behavior, how important the change in behavior is, and how confident the adolescent is in his or her ability to make a change. By asking key questions regarding readiness to change, importance of change, and confidence in ability to change, health care professionals help the adolescent weigh the risks and benefits of change. An adolescent may be interested in making a change and feel it is important but may have little confidence in his or her ability to be successful. A visual scale showing highest and lowest readiness, importance, and confidence levels may facilitate this discussion because the adolescent can point to the number that represents how he or she feels about

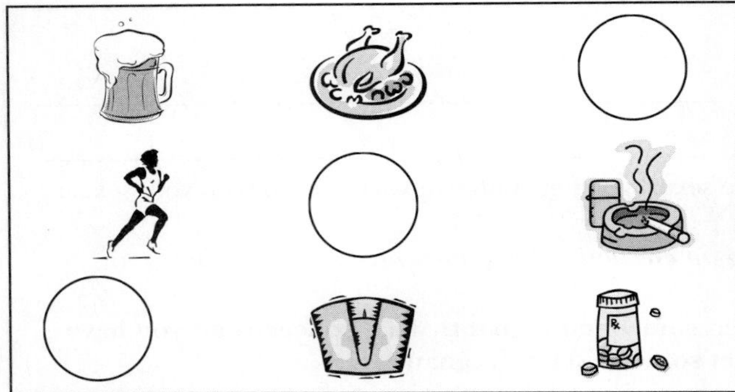

FIGURE 8-1 Agenda-Setting Chart

change (see Figure 8-2). Exploration of importance and confidence of change can help resolve ambivalence and enhance motivation for change. (Box 8-2 provides examples of how to assess importance and confidence for behavior change.)

## MOTIVATING BEHAVIOR CHANGE IN THE ADOLESCENT HEALTH SETTING

Motivational interviewing is a patient-centered yet directive strategy for promoting health behavior change,[4] and can help health care professionals focus on a patient's own perspectives and motivations rather than on his or her deficits. Most of the literature supports the use of MI to address alcohol abuse and dependence.[12] A continually updated bibliography of efficacy studies using MI is available at www.motivationalinterview.org. Motivational interviewing and its adaptations in health care have been described in detail by Miller and Rollnick[4] and by Rollnick, Mason, and Butler.[11] A basic understanding of the general goals and spirit of MI can enhance the health care professional's ability to move an adolescent toward behavior change by selectively eliciting and strengthening the adolescent's own reasons and values for change. Practical applications of MI can be learned and applied effectively to a broad range of health behaviors. Behavior change counseling strategies can be used in a busy clinical practice without full competence and skillfulness in the overall method of MI.

0 1 2 3 4 5 6 7 8 9 10

Least Important — Most Important

0 1 2 3 4 5 6 7 8 9 10

Least Confident — Most Confident

FIGURE 8-2 Example of Importance and Confidence Ruler

### Box 8-2

### *Using Importance and Confidence Rulers*

*Assessing Importance of Behavior Change*

"On a scale from 0 to 10 where 10 is the most important and 0 is the least important, what number would you give for how important it is to you right now to change ______ (insert behavior such as smoking, physical activity, diet, etc.)?" Then ask, "Why is it a ____ (current number) instead of a ________ (1 or 2 points lower)?" Reflect on what the adolescent says and then ask, "What else makes it important?" and repeat asking, "What else?" until the adolescent says, "That's it." Then summarize what was said up to that point and then ask, "What would need to happen to make it just a little bit more important to you to change ________ (insert behavior), say 1 or 2 points higher?" Then summarize.

*Assessing Confidence in Ability to Make Behavior Change*

Confidence can be similarly assessed by asking, "On a scale from 0 to 10, what number would you give for how confident you are right now to ______________ (insert behavior change)? What makes your confidence level a ____ (current number) instead of a __ (1 or 2 points lower)?" Reflect on what the adolescent says and then ask, "What else makes you this confident?" and repeat "What else?" until the adolescent says, "That's it." Then summarize what was said up to that point and then ask, "What would need to happen to make you feel a little bit more confident?" Then summarize.

*Hint:* Another option to save time is to ask what number the adolescent would assign to how important it is to change and how confident he or she is that he or she could change, and then focus the discussion on whichever rating is lower. If both are equally low (≤2), focus on importance first. If both are equally high (≥9), ask "What's keeping you from making this change?"

The spirit of MI includes *collaboration, evocation*, and supporting individual *autonomy*. Motivational interviewing is a *collaborative* approach to behavior change counseling that establishes a partnership between the health care professional and the adolescent by emphasizing a side-by-side companionable style. Health care professionals partner with adolescents about their health care when they evoke, listen to, and reflect the adolescent's perceptions of why changing a health behavior may be beneficial. Motivational interviewing uses reflective listening to help the adolescent hear his or her own arguments for change. "Change talk" occurs when the health care professional helps the adolescent identify and recognize the disadvantages of continuing unhealthy behaviors (maintaining the status quo), why change might be beneficial, and what might help the adolescent make a successful change. *Collaboration* leads directly to the *evocative* element of MI. Instead of the health care professional communicating, "I am the expert and I have what you need," *evocation* communicates, "You have what you need and your perspective is important." Motivational interviewing is an approach that evokes from the adolescent what he or she needs for change. Resisting the natural inclination to argue for change allows health care professionals to elicit from the adolescent his or her own reasons and arguments for change. Behavior change is more likely to occur when the adolescent hears him or herself talk about personal reasons for change. A third essential element of the spirit of MI is supporting *autonomy,* which means stating that the adolescent ultimately decides whether to change, and if change is desired, how to change. Health care professionals need to release the idea that they have to "convince" or "make" an adolescent change and resist the temptation to tell an adolescent "you have to" or "you must" or "should" change. Supporting *autonomy* involves accepting the concept that the adolescent has the choice to exercise change, particularly when it comes to his or her own health behavior, and verbalizing this concept to the adolescent.

Practical applications of the spirit of MI can be learned and applied effectively to a broad range of health behaviors. Behavior change counseling strategies can be applied and used effectively in a busy clinical practice without having full competence and skillfulness in the overall method of MI. *Open-ended questions* are likely to elicit "change talk" by inviting the adolescent to do most of the talking and by encouraging elaboration. *Affirmations* provide support and enhance rapport by expressing appreciation for the adolescent's efforts. They affirm "change talk" and strengthen the adolescent's confidence in the ability to change. *Empathic reflections* give voice to a reasonable guess of what the adolescent is trying to convey. A statement that guesses the adolescent's next thought adds momentum and invites elaboration and exploration. Deeper reflections most likely to add momentum are those that reflect unspoken emotion or meaning. *Summaries* gather and give voice to the adolescent's own perspectives on the advantages and disadvantages of change. Summaries replay the adolescent's previously expressed thoughts, feelings, or concerns related to behavior change to encourage identification of inconsistencies among the adolescent's goals, values, beliefs, and current behavior. A strategic summary can motivate the impulse to resolve these inconsistencies and elicit "change talk." A summary may include the health care professional's understanding of how the adolescent's feelings or concerns fit together. When used effectively, these fundamental MI counseling skills diminish resistance and enhance confidence for change.

Motivational interviewing assumes that readiness to change is not an adolescent trait but a fluctuating product of interpersonal interaction between the adolescent and the health care professional. Health care professionals can facilitate intrinsic motivation to change by eliciting it from the adolescent; motivation is not imposed by the health care professional. Four basic principles of MI include: (1) *expressing empathy;* (2) *developing discrepancy;* (3) *rolling with resistance;* and (4) *supporting self-efficacy. Empathy* communicates acceptance and understanding. Acceptance is effective for facilitating change while pressure to change generally elicits resistance, especially with the adolescent patient. An atmosphere of safety and security promotes self-focus and self-disclosure. Supportive and nonjudgmental communication leads to interpersonal interactions that create an alliance with the adolescent. Helping the adolescent identify *discrepancy* between current status or behavior and important personal goals, values, and beliefs can motivate change. Ambivalence occurs when an adolescent feels two ways about a behavior change, and it is a normal stage of change. An adolescent innately perceives advantages and disadvantages of keeping behavior the same (the status quo) and of making change. Healthy change occurs when an adolescent verbally explores his or her current experience without negative judgment. Health care professionals can elicit and strengthen the adolescent's arguments for change and perceptions of the undesirability of the status quo. Unless the adolescent identifies his or her own reasons for change consistent with personal goals, values, and beliefs, MI will not facilitate change.

*Resistance* is when the adolescent gives voice to one side of the ambivalence (the nonchange side). Responses to resistance should emphasize personal choice and control, reflect the reasons for status quo, convey agreement to disagree, or refocus the discussion. Resistance is a signal to change strategies so that new perspectives are invited but not imposed. One response is to acknowledge what the adolescent has stated as his or her own unique perspective by summarizing the adolescent's own reasons for maintaining status quo before reattempting to elicit "change talk." The health care professional can have a significant positive or negative influence over the amount of resistance an adolescent exhibits during an interaction. Supporting *self-efficacy* helps reduce resistance by empowering the adolescent to find his or her own solutions for change. Motivational interviewing assumes that people have individual reasons and desires to move

**Table 8-2**

**Components of Effective Brief Interventions in Behavior Change Counseling: FRAMES**

| *Component* | *Health Care Professional Role* | *Effect* |
|---|---|---|
| **Feedback** | With permission and in an objective, noncoercive manner, provide personalized information regarding risks and/or consequences associated with current behavior | Raises awareness of negative consequences associated with behavior, increases problem recognition, and develops discrepancy between actual and ideal circumstances while communicating attentiveness and interest |
| **Responsibility** | Communicate that any decision about whether to change is solely the adolescent's and that change will only occur if the adolescent chooses to take steps to change | Minimizes resistance, supports autonomy, paves the way for offering expert perspective |
| **Advice** | With permission and in a concerned and supportive manner, offer a clear recommendation for a particular change | Provides a sense of comfort, direction, or inspiration from expert guidance |
| **Menu of options** | Elicit or offer a range of alternatives for how to accomplish a desired goal, and engage the adolescent to actively weigh options to determine which would fit him or her best | Increases likelihood of keeping commitment to change, enhances sense of freedom and control, provides concrete assistance in changing |
| **Empathy** | Communicates accurate understanding of the adolescent's experience in a warm, nonjudgmental manner | Builds alliance, creates atmosphere of safety, promotes disclosure, and helps clarify adolescent's perceptions |
| **Self-efficacy** | Support adolescent's belief in ability to succeed at change and communicate optimism about the prospects for him or her doing so | Prevents defensive or hopeless reactions to problem recognition, enhances confidence and willingness to attempt behavior change |

in a positive direction and to feel strong, healthy, and in control. The adolescent is the most valuable resource in finding ways to be successful at behavior change. It is the health care professional's job to partner with the adolescent to identify ways to succeed. Hopefulness in the ability to change is found in helping the adolescent identify a range of effective alternatives. Furthermore, when the health care professional is optimistic that the adolescent can be successful, change is more likely to ensue.

The acronym FRAMES has been used by Bien, Miller, and Tonigan[13] to describe the 6 components of effective brief behavior change interventions. The 6 components, the health care professional's role, and the effect they have are illustrated in Table 8-2.

## CONCLUSIONS

The medical history is used by health care professionals to elicit information and to provide the adolescent with information and advice about health-related behaviors. A patient-centered interaction style helps establish a partnership between the professional and the adolescent. When the health care professional conveys interest and a willingness to listen to the adolescent patient, critical information can be elicited and a meaningful therapeutic relationship can be established. The professional has the opportunity to address risks and build upon strengths. Becoming familiar with motivational interviewing allows the professional to help adolescents seek their own change in areas of health.

## INTERNET RESOURCES

- American Medical Association: www.ama-assn.org
- American Academy of Pediatrics: www.aap.org
- Bright Futures: www.brightfutures.aap.org
- Motivational Interviewing: Resources for Clinicians, Researchers, and Trainers: www.motivationalinterview.org
- Center for Adolescent Health and the Law: www.adolescenthealthlaw.org
- Adolescent Health Working Group: ahwg.net/index.htm

## REFERENCES


1. Marks A, Fisher M. Health assessment and screening during adolescence. *Pediatrics.* 1987;80(suppl):135–158

2. Marks A, Malizio J, Hoch J, et al. Assessment of the health needs and willingness to utilize health care resources of adolescents in a suburban population. *J Pediatr.* 1983;102:456–460

3. English A, Kenney KE. *State Minor Consent Laws: A Summary.* 2nd ed. Chapel Hill, NC: Center for Adolescent Health & the Law; 2003

4. Miller WR, Rollnick S. *Motivational Interviewing: Preparing People for Change.* 2nd ed. New York, NY: Guilford Press; 2002

5. Neinstein LS. *Adolescent Health Care: A Practical Guide.* 2nd ed. Baltimore, MD: Williams & Wilkins; 1991

6. Goldenring JM, Rosen DS. Getting into adolescent heads: an essential update. *Contemporary Pediatrics.* 2004;21:64–90

7. Paperny DM, Hedberg VA. Computer-assisted health counselor visits: a low-cost model for comprehensive adolescent preventive services. *Arch Pediatr Adolesc Med.* 1999;153(1):63–67

8. Knight J, Sherritt L, Shrier L, et al. Validity of the CRAFFT Substance Abuse Screening Test among adolescent clinic patients. *Arch Pediatr Adol Med.* 2002;156:607–614

9. Prochaska JO, DiClemente CC, Norcross JC. In search of how people change. *Am Psychol.* 1992;47:1102–1114

10. Rogers CR. *A Way of Being.* Boston, MA: Houghton Mifflin; 1980

11. Rollnick S, Mason P, Butler C. *Health Behavior Change: A Guide for Practitioners.* London: Churchill Livingstone; 1999

12. Miller WR. Motivational interviewing with problem drinkers. *Behavioral Psychotherapy.* 1983;11:147–172

13. Bien TH, Miller WR, Tonigan JS. Brief interventions for alcohol problems: a review. *Addiction.* 1993;88:315–336

# CHAPTER 9

# Physical Examination and Laboratory Screening

MARCIE B. SCHNEIDER, MD • MARTIN FISHER, MD

## INTRODUCTION

Adolescents generally require physical examinations for 3 reasons: routine checkups; medical clearance for school, sports, or employment; and evaluation and treatment of an illness. Evaluation of the health status of adolescents usually also includes laboratory testing. The first part of this chapter focuses on the general checkup, including discussion of the issues of privacy and confidentiality and description of the actual physical examination of the adolescent—how it differs from the examination of children or adults and why it is particularly important in this age group. The second part of the chapter is focused on laboratory testing, including the use of routine laboratory tests, screening laboratory tests that depend upon an adolescent's lifestyle and medical issues, and interpretation of laboratory results in the adolescent age group.

How frequently a physical examination should be performed in well adolescents has been debated. In 1985, the American Academy of Pediatrics (AAP)[1] recommended that adolescents be seen every 2 years for health maintenance. However, given the complex physical and psychological changes occurring during the adolescent years, many clinicians believe that every adolescent should undergo a yearly physical examination to permit close monitoring and to provide preventive care and anticipatory guidance. In 1989, the US Preventive Services Task Force[2] recommended annual comprehensive visits for adolescents, including a physical examination, discussion of behavioral issues, and preventive care.

The Guidelines for Adolescent Preventive Services (GAPS),[3] a health care package developed by the American Medical Association in 1992, attempted to differentiate between the need for preventive services and the need for a physical examination. The GAPS recommendations included an annual routine health visit for persons aged 11 to 21 years (for developmental monitoring, preventive services, and anticipatory guidance), but only 3 complete physical examinations during those years (1 each in early, middle, and late adolescence). This approach was not widely accepted, however, and in 1995, the AAP[4] published new recommendations for preventive pediatric health care that included yearly visits for a complete physical examination, developmental and behavioral assessment, and anticipatory guidance.

*Bright Futures*, a report sponsored by The Maternal and Child Health Bureau of the United States Department of Health and Human Services,[5] which provides guidelines for health supervision of children and adolescents, also recommended yearly health supervision visits for adolescents, including a physical examination, in its first 2 editions, published in 1990 and 1994. Most recently, *Bright Futures*,[6] now under the auspices of the AAP, has published a third edition that incorporates all of the GAPS and AAP recommendations and applies evidence-based approaches to its recommendations. This new edition recommends a yearly health supervision visit for adolescents that includes developmental surveillance, observation of the parent–child interaction, a physical examination, screening tests, immunizations, and anticipatory guidance for the teen and parents. Specific aspects of the most recent *Bright Futures* recommendations for the physical examination and laboratory testing are included in this chapter.

## PREPARATION FOR THE PHYSICAL EXAMINATION

Although the physical examination of adolescents is similar to that of children, patient privacy and confidentiality are especially important. It is the physician's role to ensure that the patient receives comprehensive care in a comfortable manner and that parents' concerns about their teenager are addressed.

Whether to perform the physical examination of the adolescent alone or with a chaperone has received much attention as of late. There have been arguments on both sides. On the one hand, it is desirable to perform the physical examination of the adolescent alone for several reasons. Adolescents have an increased need for privacy once puberty begins and are often uncomfortable with changes in their bodies. Although adolescents may be embarrassed to expose their bodies, they find the examination tolerable because it serves a necessary purpose—the assurance of good health and normalcy. However, revealing their bodies to more than one person during the examination may be embarrassing and unwarranted. In addition, the physical examination may provide the only chance for the physician and patient to be alone; as such, it offers a time for the patient to express confidential concerns. The health care provider can address the patient's concerns and pose any confidential questions not previously asked, such as issues related to sexuality. The physical examination may reveal acne, gynecomastia, or breast asymmetry that may not have been reported to the clinician, possibly because the teenager may have been worried or embarrassed. The clinician can use this opportunity to mention the finding, inquire about the patient's concerns, obtain a history of the problem, and discuss the evaluation and possible treatment approaches. Finally, examining the adolescent alone delivers the message to patient and family that the "child" is growing up. It acknowledges that certain issues are confidential between health care provider and patient and that the adolescent has the right to privacy. This is a first step in shifting the responsibility of health care from the parent to the adolescent.

Despite the sound reasons presented for examining adolescents alone, however, certain conditions warrant examining the patient in the presence of a parent or another chaperone. The decision as to who should be present during the physical examination is based on legal, developmental, and medical considerations, as well as the needs of the patient, parent, and physician. In the currently changing legal climate, the presence of a chaperone while examining adolescent patients, especially for examination of the breasts and genitals, but also for general examinations, is becoming more prevalent. This is certainly so for male examiners with female patients, but also becoming more prevalent for female examiners with male patients and for female examiners with female patients and male examiners with male patients.

Legally, a physician in the United States can perform a pelvic examination with the consent of the patient alone (ie, without parental consent). In most states in the United States, minors may seek evaluation and treatment without parental consent for pregnancy, contraception, sexually transmitted infections (STIs), and abortion (see Chapter 11, Legal and Ethical Framework, for further details).[7] Each state, however, has the right to regulate adolescents' access to such care.[8] Health care providers who plan to perform pelvic examinations must familiarize themselves with their state's regulations regarding the rights of minors with respect to sexuality-related issues. As noted previously, in the current medico-legal climate, it is wise to have a female chaperone present for any pelvic examination performed by a male health care provider. Individual clinicians may also opt to have a chaperone present for breast and testicular examinations.

Developmentally, teenagers in their early adolescent years, or those who are older but developmentally immature, may feel more comfortable with a parent or other staff member present during the physical examination. Data show that many adolescents (especially during the early adolescent years), when given the choice, opt to have a family member accompany them during the genitalia examination.[9] When the patient is severely mentally handicapped, a parent may interpret the patient's needs to the clinician and provide the support necessary to the patient for a successful examination. Family or staff also may be used in situations in which assistance is needed in examining the patient, for example, with a wheelchair-bound patient who needs to be lifted onto a table.

Preparation is necessary for establishing the new routine of examining adolescents without a parent present so that there will be no surprises. The clinician continuing to provide care for a patient can begin preparation for examining the patient alone during late childhood by reminding the patient and parents at each routine visit that the structure of the visit will change at a certain point in time, usually the onset of puberty. If the clinician is seeing a teenager for a first visit, the structure of the visit can be presented at the onset to both patient and parents. Each should be offered the opportunity to express concerns. Examination of the patient alone should not present a difficulty; if it does, psychosocial problems requiring exploration might exist within the family.

## CONDUCTING THE PHYSICAL EXAMINATION

For a complete physical examination, adolescents ideally should wear a hospital gown and underwear. Patients should be reassured that their privacy will be respected and that only the areas being examined at that moment will be revealed under the gown. It is important to assure patients that while wearing the gown they will receive an adequate physical examination and that all areas of the body will be examined.

Adolescents, especially in the early adolescent years, may be more embarrassed about their bodies than children or adults would be; therefore it is logical to begin the physical examination with the least sensitive and least embarrassing areas. The examiner should start with the vital signs, followed by the head and neck examination, working down to the feet in an orderly fashion. Examination of the genitalia may be uncomfortable for the patient (as well as for some health care providers). Talking through the examination and describing various aspects of it as one proceeds may help to delineate the professional boundaries and ease any tension. Breast and testicular examinations may often be performed as part of the general examination of teenagers. The pelvic examination, if necessary, is reserved for the end, because it is the only time that a chaperone may be needed, and a set-up for laboratory tests is required.

The 5 major areas in any complete examination of the adolescent are (1) measurement of vital signs and growth parameters; (2) examination of the head and neck; (3) cardiac, respiratory, abdominal, and neurologic examination; (4) musculoskeletal examination; and (5) examination of the genitalia.

## MEASUREMENT OF VITAL SIGNS AND GROWTH PARAMETERS

Vital signs traditionally include measurement of temperature, blood pressure, pulse, and respiratory rate. Blood pressure and pulse are important parameters to check in the routine examination of the adolescent. Because many adolescents are nervous before their physical examination, an elevated blood pressure or pulse should be checked again at the end of the visit, when the patient feels more comfortable.

Although heart rate significantly decreases in the first few years of life, little change is apparent during the late childhood, adolescent, and adult years. Generally, adolescents have heart rates of less than 80 beats per minute. Routine pulse checks may help identify the occasional adolescent with an irregular heartbeat. The cardiovascular physical examination should emphasize (but not necessarily be limited to: (1) precordial auscultation in both the supine and standing positions to identify, in particular, heart murmurs consistent with dynamic left ventricular outflow obstruction; (2) assessment of the femoral artery pulses to exclude coarctation of the aorta; (3) recognition of the physical stigmata of Marfan syndrome; and (4) brachial blood pressure measurement in the sitting position.

Because 1% to 2% of teenagers in the general population are estimated to have hypertension, it is important that adolescents be screened for elevated blood pressure at each checkup.[10] Hypertension is defined as blood pressure greater than the 95th percentile for gender, age, and height, when repeated on 3 separate occasions. "Prehypertensive" or "high normal" blood pressure is defined as that between the 90th and 95th percentiles and is an indication for lifestyle changes. As with children, blood pressure changes during the adolescent years necessitate the use of standardized curves to determine whether a particular adolescent has elevated blood pressure for his or her age. Updated figures are available based on age, sex, and height for the 50th, 90th, 95th, and 99th percentile blood pressure levels (see Chapter 118, Hypertension).

Blood pressure ideally should be measured in the right arm, with the patient sitting and the arm raised to the level of the heart. The bladder width of the blood pressure cuff should cover 40% of the arm circumference at a midway point between the olecranon and the acromion. The bladder length should cover 80% to 100% of the circumference of the arm. Therefore, the bladder width-to-length should be 1:2. In an adolescent, the Korotkoff sounds recorded are K1 and K5. (K1 is the onset of sound, ie, systolic blood pressure; K5 is the disappearance of sound, ie, diastolic blood pressure.) In a child, K1 and K4 (muffling of sound) are used. The reason for this difference is that K5, often difficult to detect in children, may eventually occur simultaneously with K4 and is easier to detect by adolescence.[10] A patient with elevated blood pressure determined on 3 separate occasions should be evaluated for the cause of the hypertension.

Growth parameters that should be measured regularly during the adolescent years include height and weight, and from this information, body mass index (BMI) should be calculated. Yearly, these should be plotted on the growth charts published by the Centers for Disease Control and Prevention (CDC) in 2000.[11] Changes in height take place most dramatically during the early to middle adolescent years. Boys undergo a growth spurt at an average of 14 years of age, whereas girls undergo their growth spurt approximately 2 years earlier, at an average of 12 years of age. Chronic illnesses (eg, Crohn disease, asthma) may adversely affect growth even before they become apparent, and physiologic delays in growth also affect many youths. Height should be measured at each checkup, with the patient in bare feet and standing straight; ideally a stadiometer attached to the wall should be used, because scale measurements of height are often inaccurate. The patient's height is then plotted on a standardized growth chart (Figure 9-1). Separate growth charts exist for certain disorders, including Down syndrome, Turner syndrome, and achondroplasia. The height at each checkup can then be compared with that at previous visits to monitor the progression of the patient's growth. A major change in percentiles on the growth chart requires further evaluation.

Weight changes that occur during early adolescence may be even more dramatic than changes in height. The average teenager gains 30 to 50 pounds during the early adolescent years. Adolescents should be weighed at each checkup, because the incidence of obesity and eating disorders, including anorexia nervosa and bulimia nervosa, increases during adolescence, and patients with chronic illnesses, such as Crohn disease or diabetes, may present with weight loss. Patients should be weighed in a hospital gown to obtain accurate and comparable weights from visit to visit. As with height, the weight should be plotted on a standardized growth chart (Figure 9-1). The weight at each visit can then be compared with previous measurements to check for a normal progression. A significant change in percentiles

(A)

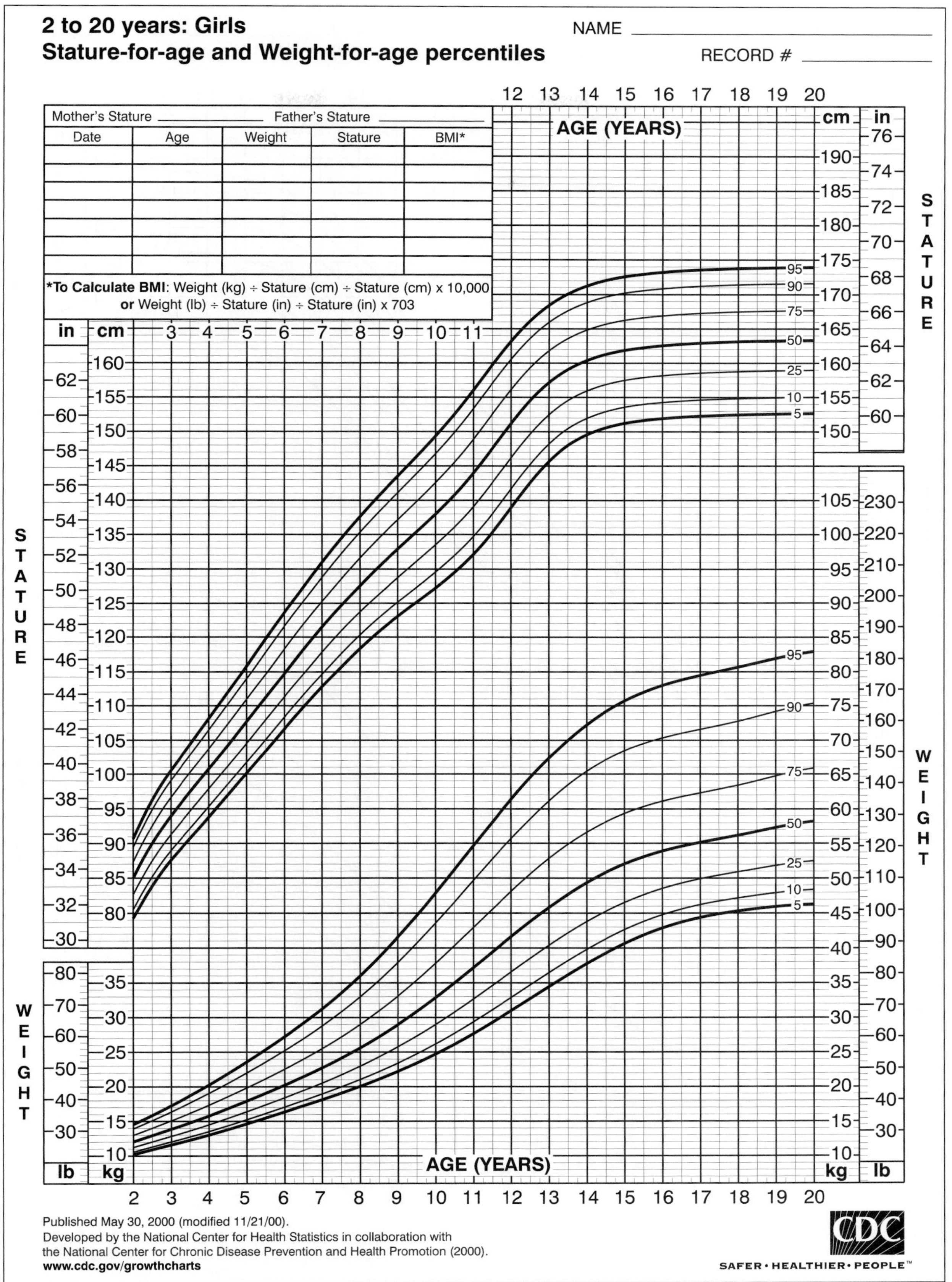


FIGURE 9-1 2000 CDC growth charts for the United States, stature-for-age and weight-for-age percentiles, 2 to 20 years; (A) girls; (B) boys.

(B)

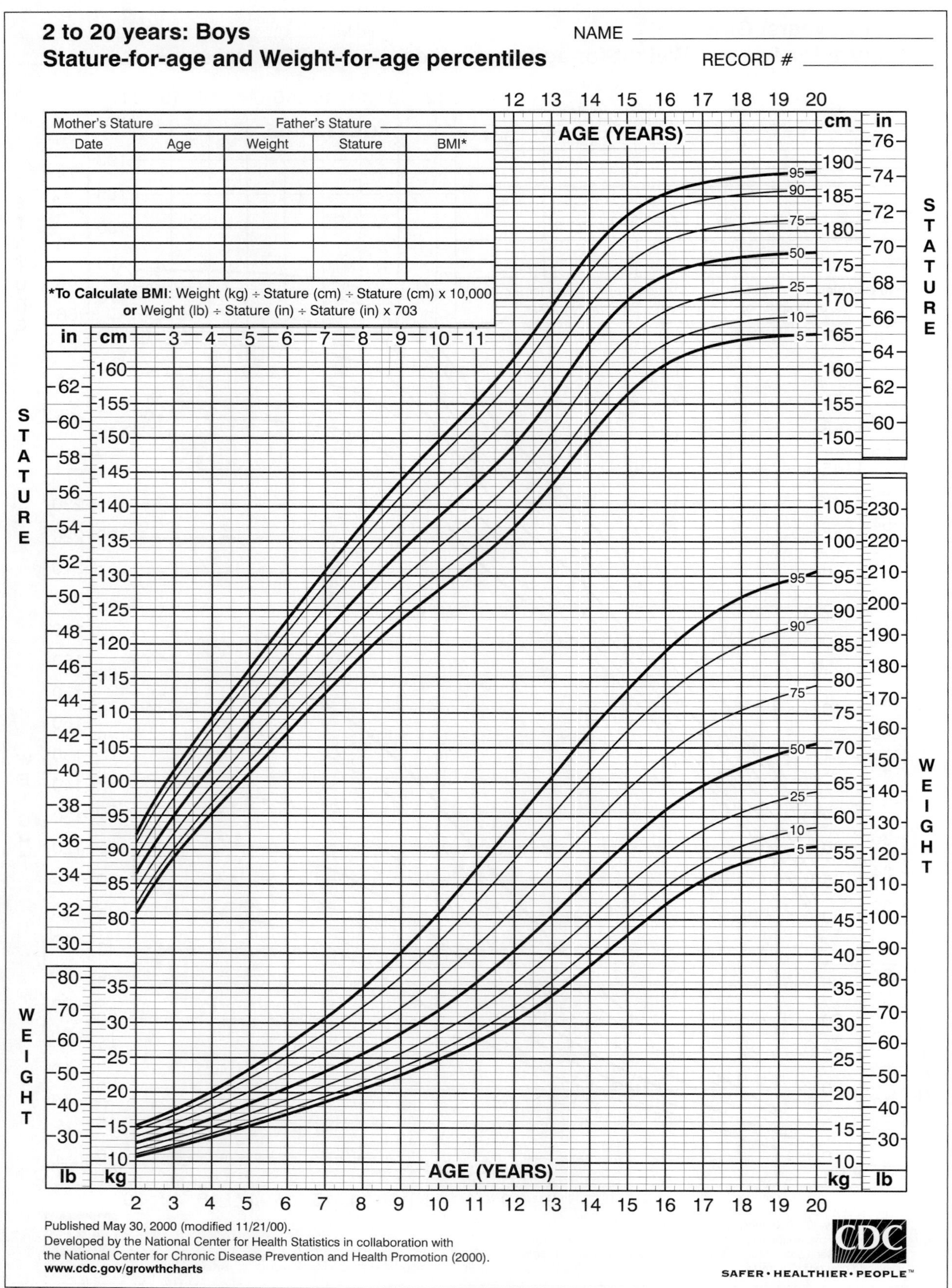


FIGURE 9-1 (Continued)

on the weight curve indicates the need for an evaluation of possibly inappropriate weight loss or gain.

Body mass index, defined as weight in kilograms divided by height in meters squared, should be plotted yearly (Figure 9-2). An adolescent with a BMI between the 85th and 95th percentile for age and sex is considered to be in the "overweight" category, whereas an adolescent with a BMI above the 95th percentile is considered to be in the "obesity" category. Any significant change in BMI from year to year requires further evaluation. In the most recent *Bright Futures* recommendations, measurements of blood pressure, weight, and height, along with calculation and plotting of BMI, are considered to be well-warranted by the evidence for inclusion in the yearly examination of all adolescents.[6]

## EXAMINATION OF THE HEAD AND NECK

Included in this part of the examination are evaluation of the eyes, ears, nose, throat, teeth, skin, neck, and lymph nodes.

The complete eye evaluation includes inspection of the eyes and eyelids, ocular motility, examination of the pupil and red reflex, and an attempt at ophthalmoscopy. Lastly, visual acuity should be assessed. Visual acuity worsens in the teenage years: approximately 1 in every 4 17-year-old has vision of 20/40 or worse, at which level glasses are recommended. Visual acuity is most easily measured by the Snellen chart. Referral to a specialist is recommended if the vision in either eye is worse than 20/40, if strabismus is found, if results of the funduscopic examination are abnormal, or if any other eye abnormalities are detected.[12] The new *Bright Futures*[6] guidelines recommend that vision be checked 3 times during the adolescent years, 1 time each during early, middle, and late adolescence. Additional screening can be done at other times as well, if the primary care provider feels there is an indication to do so.

Evaluation of the ear, nose, and throat differs little for teenagers from that for other age groups. There are no specific evidence-based recommendations for this part of the examination in the new *Bright Futures* guidelines.[6] Many adolescents are routinely tested for hearing problems in school, although the value of auditory screening of adolescents in the school setting has been questioned.[13] Screening for hearing loss in the general medical office, with a high level of ambient noise, is difficult. Patients complaining of hearing loss, with a history of a borderline or abnormal school hearing test or with frequent exposure to loud noise, should be referred for formal audiologic testing.

Adolescents experience changes in dentition (primary teeth change to permanent), facial structures, hormone levels, and personal habits (smoking, snacking)—factors that affect the oral cavity. Decayed, missing, or filled teeth and gingivitis increase with age. From 13% to 50% of teenagers have malocclusion that would benefit from orthodontic treatment. Physical examination of the teeth gives the physician an opportunity to identify any acute problems and to discuss the need for preventive dental care. Every patient should be referred for a dental checkup at least once a year.[14]

Examination of the adolescent should include evaluation of the skin, especially for acne. Although acne may be most common and bothersome on the face, the chest and back should also be evaluated. Adolescents may have other dermatologic findings, including fungal or bacterial infections, café au lait spots, scars, nevi, striae, tattoos, and piercings (see Chapter 147, Miscellaneous Skin Diseases).

The neck should be checked for thyroid size, masses, or tenderness. If an abnormal thyroid gland is present, thyroid function tests should be performed. Lymph nodes should be evaluated at each checkup. The cervical (submandibular, submental, preauricular, postauricular, occipital, anterior, and posterior), supraclavicular, axillary, epitrochlear, and inguinal nodes should be checked. If lymphadenopathy is found, the cause should be investigated (see Chapter 110, Lymphadenopathy and Splenomegaly).

## CARDIAC, RESPIRATORY, ABDOMINAL, AND NEUROLOGIC EXAMINATION

Examination of the cardiac, respiratory, abdominal, and neurologic systems in adolescents does not differ significantly from that in late childhood or early adulthood. It is the rare teenager who is diagnosed with an abnormality in these systems for the first time during adolescence, and it is equally rare for an asymptomatic teenager to be diagnosed with a chronic disease affecting these organs during the adolescent years. However, anecdotal reports and the case report literature abound with cases of just such adolescents, emphasizing the need for vigilance in performance of the cardiac, respiratory, abdominal, and neurologic examinations in "healthy" adolescents. The *Bright Futures*[6] guidelines include this part of the examination in the yearly checkup without specific evidence-based recommendations. Further discussion of the cardiac examination as part of the preparticipation sport examination is found in Chapter 164, Preparticipation Examination.[6]

## MUSCULOSKELETAL EXAMINATION

Musculoskeletal aches and injuries are common during the adolescent years because of increased involvement in competitive sports during a time of rapid growth. In addition, several musculoskeletal disorders may occur during these years, including Osgood-Schlatter disease and slipped capital femoral epiphysis. Generally,

(A)

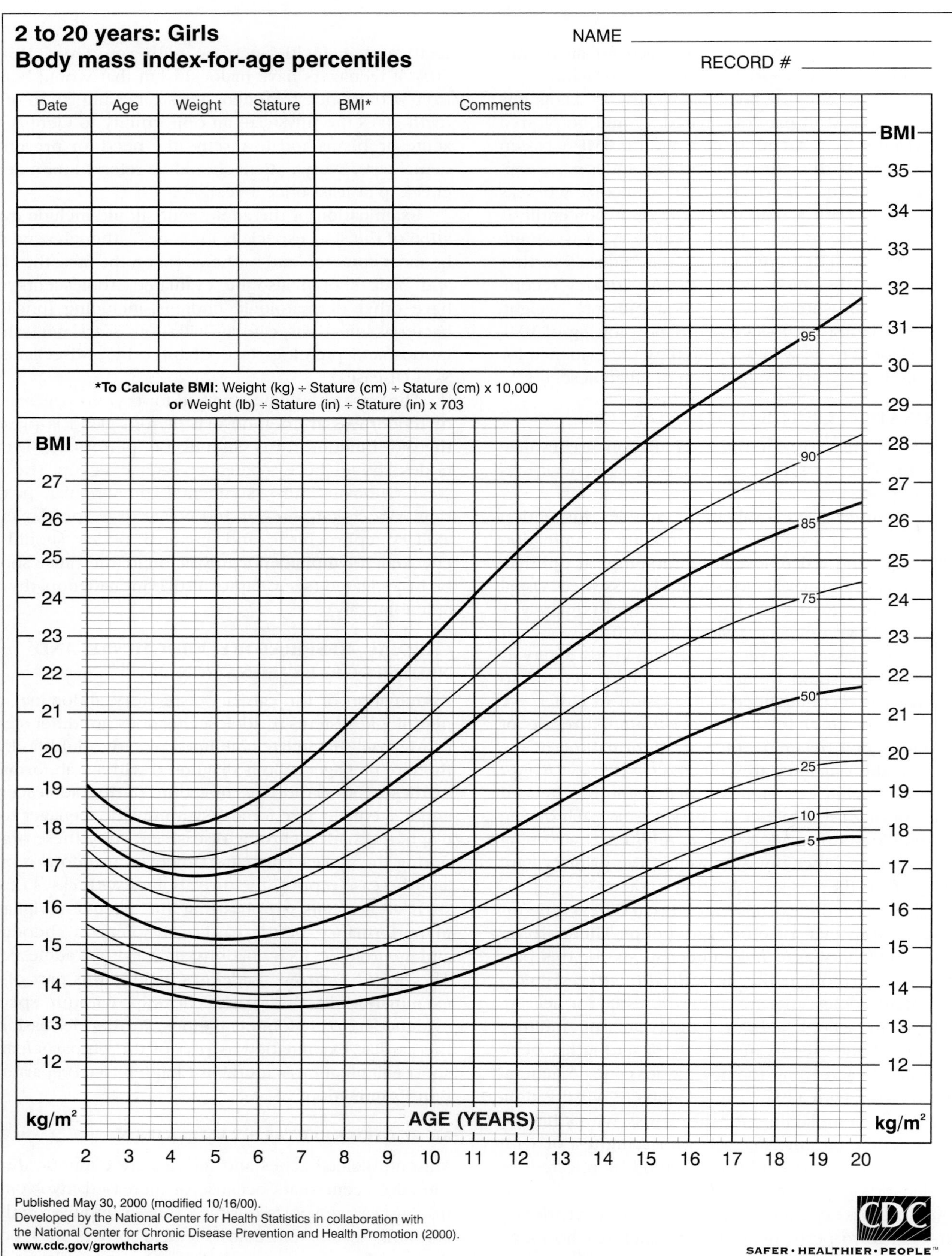


**FIGURE 9-2** 2000 CDC growth charts for the United States, BMI-for-age percentiles, 2 to 20 years; (A) girls; (B) boys.

(B)

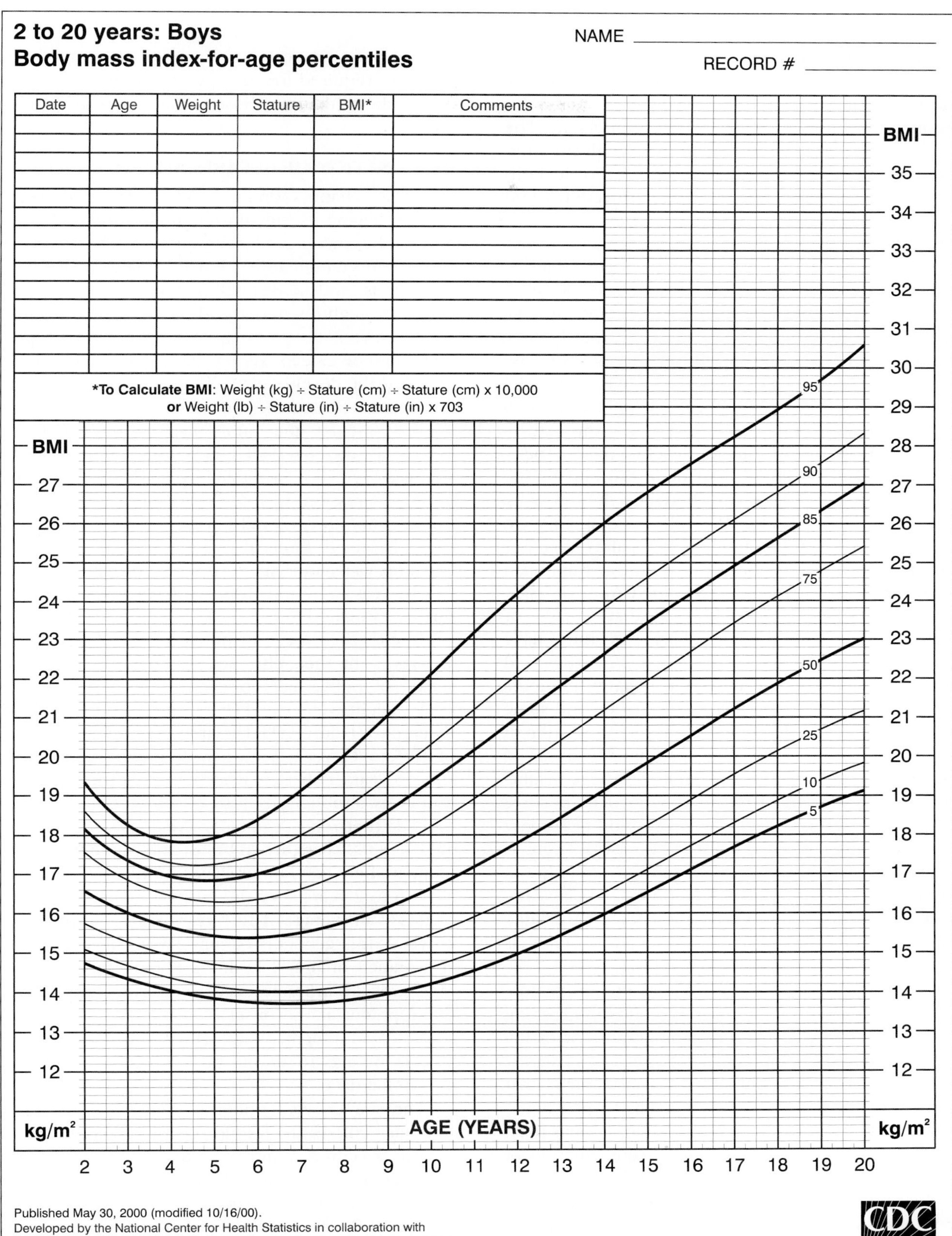


FIGURE 9-2 (Continued)

a complete musculoskeletal evaluation is advised for adolescents involved in competitive athletics, and evaluation of specific areas of the musculoskeletal system is required for those with particular complaints. The general practitioner must be comfortable with the musculoskeletal examination of adolescents to avoid both under- and overreferral for radiologic procedures and specialty evaluations.

Scoliosis is present in 1% to 2% of adolescents, occurring somewhat more frequently in girls than in boys. The scoliosis screening examination includes evaluation of the spine with the patient in 3 standing positions. The patient's back is first examined from behind, with the patient standing upright. In this position the patient can be evaluated for shoulder alignment, scapular prominence, hip prominence, asymmetric arm to body distance, and pelvic asymmetry. A string can be dropped from the occiput to the level of the buttocks; if a curvature of the spine is evident, the end of the string will not fall in the crease between the buttocks. The patient is then examined while bending forward 90 degrees, with arms extended and palms together (Adams test). In this position, a rib or lumbar hump can be seen. Finally, the patient is examined from the side while he or she stands in such a way that thoracic or lumbar lordosis may be noted. Scoliosis screenings have been performed in schools for the past 2 decades, and these have resulted in the detection of large numbers of cases that have required further evaluation and some cases that have resulted in bracing and the prevention of later surgery. More recently, questions have been raised about whether the costs of this approach (ie, consultations and x-rays for the large number of false-positive cases) outweighs the benefits (ie, prevention of surgery for the small number of true positive cases). There is less question, however, about the utility of screening as part of the yearly physical examination by clinicians; the most recent *Bright Futures*[6] recommendations include scoliosis screening in early and middle adolescence as part of the complete physical examination.

Clinical experience has shown that not every adolescent with a positive finding on scoliosis screening needs to be referred for further radiographic or orthopedic evaluation. Development of a specially designed inclinometer called a Scoliometer, an instrument that measures the angle of trunk rotation, has helped determine whom to refer for further evaluation.[15] It has been found that patients with an angle of trunk rotation of less than 5 to 7 degrees are extremely unlikely to have a curve that requires any type of treatment. Patients who have scoliosis determined on physical examination and a small angle of trunk rotation can be followed clinically rather than being referred for radiographic and orthopedic evaluation. The frequency of follow-up is guided by the pubertal stage of the patient; more frequent visits are required for those who are prepubertal or in early puberty than for those at the end of their pubertal growth.

## EXAMINATION OF BREASTS AND GENITALIA

Genitalia change dramatically during adolescence. Tanner staging is the most common method used to follow the pubertal development of the genitalia in adolescents. Tanner and Marshall[16,17] studied 192 English schoolgirls and 228 English schoolboys during the 1960s throughout puberty. They noted that secondary sex characteristics developed in a consistent pattern that could be categorized in stages. These characteristics included the development of breasts and progression of pubic hair in girls, and changes in the genitalia (testes, scrotum, penis) and pubic hair in boys. Other secondary sex characteristics such as axillary and facial hair changes were not included in Tanner's stages, because their progression varies considerably during puberty. Adolescents are generally evaluated for Tanner staging (see Chapter 4, Physical Growth and Development) at checkup visits so that those with normal development can be reassured and those with abnormalities can be further evaluated.[18]

In girls the course of pubertal events generally progresses from thelarche (breast budding) to pubarche (onset of pubic hair appearance) to the time of the peak height velocity (PHV; growth spurt) and, lastly, menarche (Figure 9-3). Thelarche occurs at a mean age of 10.5 to 11 years, with a wide range of normal, from 8 to 13 years. Pubarche usually follows thelarche within 6 months, although in up to 25% of girls, pubarche may precede thelarche. Peak height velocity generally occurs at 12.1 ± 0.8 years, when breast and pubic hair development are between Tanner stages 2 and 3 (which is generally 1.5 to 2 years after the onset of puberty). Menarche begins at an average of 12.7 years, with a range from 9 to 16 years; this generally occurs 2.3 ± 1.1 years from the appearance of breast budding (Tanner breast stage 2). Most girls are in Tanner stage 3 of breast and pubic hair development at the onset of menarche. A girl without breast development by age 13 or without the onset of menses by age 16 should be evaluated for pubertal or menarchal delay.[19]

The sequence of pubertal events in boys includes testicular enlargement, followed by pubarche and PHV (Figure 9-4). In a minority of boys, pubarche precedes testicular enlargement. Genital changes in boys begin at a mean age of 11.6 years, with a range from 9.5 to 13.8 years. Pubarche occurs at a mean of 11.8 years. Peak height velocity occurs on average at 14.1 ± 0.9 years, which is generally during genital stage 4 and pubic hair stage 3 or 4. Boys experience their growth spurt at a

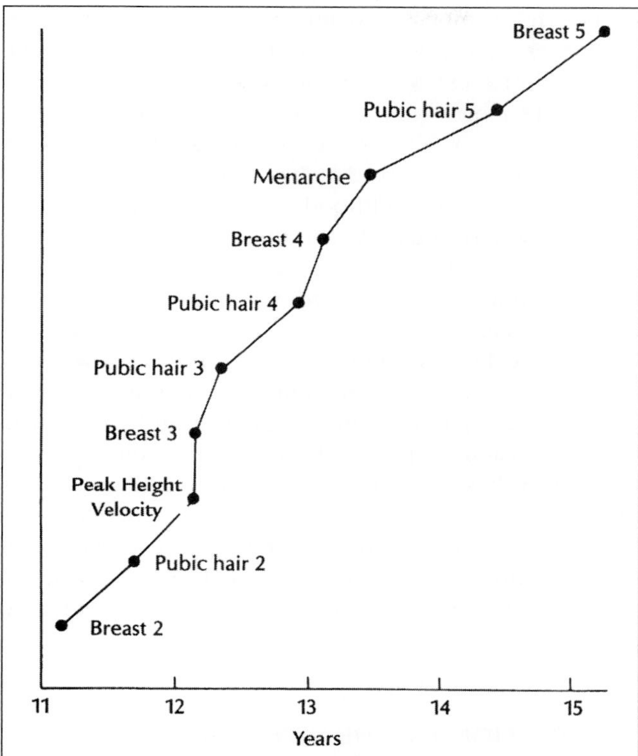


**FIGURE 9-3** Sequence and mean age of pubertal events in females. (Reprinted from Root AW. Endocrinology of puberty. *J Pediatr.* 1973;83:1–19, with permission from Elsevier.)

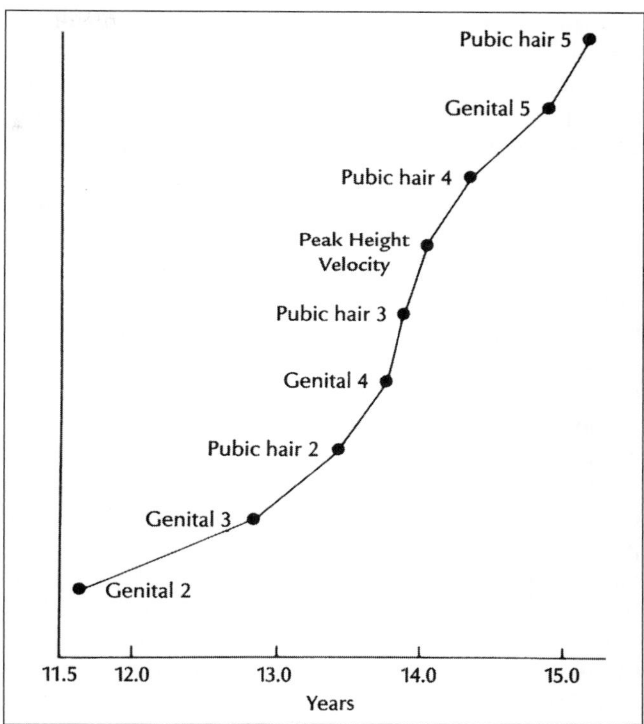


**FIGURE 9-4** Sequence and mean age of pubertal events in males. (Reprinted from Root AW. Endocrinology of puberty. *J Pediatr.* 1973;83:1–19, with permission from Elsevier.)

much later time and in a more advanced sexual maturational stage than girls; this accounts for the height differences of boys and girls in junior high school.[19]

The female breast examination is performed to detect breast masses; most important would be those masses that may become or are already malignant. It has been recommended by some that the breast examination be incorporated into the general checkup of female patients as soon as breast budding appears.[20] However, because breast cancer is extremely rare in the teenage years, and because the examination is often embarrassing, especially to younger adolescents, it seems reasonable to postpone the examination until girls are older and emotionally more mature. *Bright Futures*[6] leaves the breast examination to the discretion of the clinician.

The breast examination may be done with the patient in a sitting and/or lying position. It is important that the arm be above the head during examination of the breast, because the tail of the breast extends into the axilla and may otherwise be missed. Examination of the breast includes inspection for assessment of Tanner stage; detection of any variations or abnormalities in the configuration of breast, areola, or nipple; and palpation for consistency of breast tissue and the presence of any masses. Palpation begins at the external borders of the breast and progresses in concentric circles toward the nipple. Finally, the nipple is gently squeezed to express any discharge. See Chapter 66, Breast Disorders in the Female, for a discussion of abnormalities of the breast examination and variations of normal.

Palpation of the breast will reveal fibrocystic disease in up to 50% of adolescents. Because this condition occurs so frequently, appears to be hormonally modulated, and is not associated with an increased risk of breast cancer, Love et al[21] recommended that fibrocystic disease be renamed "physiologic nodularity" or "lumpy breasts." The finding of physiologic nodularity on breast examination in teenagers is common and cause for reassurance, not alarm.

The clinician can use the time during the breast examination to teach the adolescent how to examine her own breasts. Debate exists over the usefulness of teaching breast self-examination to adolescents. Some believe that it causes more anxiety about breast cancer than necessary in an age group that almost never has the disease, may lead to an increase in surgery, and most adolescents are not likely to follow through on appropriate self-examination. Despite these concerns, others believe that teaching breast self-examination to adolescents is worthwhile, if only to stress an important habit that will take on added significance later in life. The American Cancer Society circulates a pamphlet that teaches women how to examine their breasts in 3 stages: in the shower, standing before a mirror, and in a prone position. *Bright Futures*[6] does not make a recommendation for teaching the breast examination.

Gynecomastia develops in many boys during adolescence; approximately two-thirds of boys are affected, with the peak occurrence at age 14. Gynecomastia occurs bilaterally in approximately three-fourths of patients, with the 2 sides enlarged either sequentially or simultaneously.[22] Embarrassment may prevent many teenage boys from mentioning gynecomastia to their physicians. In examining the male breast, it is essential to differentiate breast tissue from fat tissue. Chapter 67 contains more details about gynecomastia.

Testicular examination is performed to determine the presence of testicular masses, varicoceles, hydroceles, and hernias. The examination includes inspection for size, shape, and Tanner stage; palpation for consistency and masses of the testes, vas deferens, and epididymis; and evaluation for the presence of a hernia by inserting an index finger into the external inguinal ring while the patient coughs. If testicular size is in question, an orchidometer (a string of testicular models marked by size in cubic centimeters) is used to measure testicular volume. Because testicular cancer is the most common cancer in young adult males, the physician may consider teaching patients testicular self-examination. As is the case with breast examination, the value of teaching testicular self-examination remains controversial, because it is argued by some that the anxiety created, combined with the time and money spent to teach the examination, may outweigh the possible benefits.[23] *Bright Futures*[6] does not make a recommendation for teaching testicular examination but does recommend performing an examination to evaluate for the presence of a hydrocele, hernia, varicocele, or mass.

Pelvic examination has been recommended for some females who are sexually active (see the following), have a vaginal discharge and/or suspicion of a sexually transmitted infection, or have primary or secondary amenorrhea, severe dysmenorrhea, or irregular menses. The pelvic examination includes inspection of the external genitalia (for lesions and anatomic abnormalities), vagina (for estrogen effect and discharge), and cervix (for erosion and eversion); and palpation of the cervix (for firmness and tenderness), uterus (for size, tenderness, and position), and adnexa (for size, tenderness, and masses). Many adolescents have an erythematous, nonfriable, symmetric ring around the external os of the cervix. This is referred to as eversion, representing an endocervix that has not yet inverted, as it generally does by adulthood. It is important to recognize eversion of the cervix so that it is not mistaken for an erosion or infection.

Recommendations regarding the performance of a pelvic examination in adolescents who are sexually active have been changing during the past few years. Conceptually, the examination is required to obtain cultures for chlamydia and gonorrhea and to perform a Papanicolaou (Pap) test. With the availability of sensitive urine-based testing for chlamydia and gonorrhea, and a recent recommendation by the American College of Obstetricians and Gynecologists (ACOG)[24] that Pap tests not be routinely performed until 21 years of age, the need for a pelvic examination has decreased dramatically.

## COMPLETION OF THE PHYSICAL EXAMINATION

On completion of the physical examination, patients can change back into their clothes so that they can feel more comfortable when the findings are presented. Findings, evaluation, and treatment of confidential and nonconfidential problems can then be discussed. Anticipatory guidance about health issues enlists the patient as an active participant in his or her health care. Finally, the parents can be invited back into the room to discuss nonconfidential findings and health implications and to review such issues as recommended immunizations and laboratory screening tests.

## LABORATORY TESTING

Findings from the history-taking and physical examination determine whether the adolescent requires routine laboratory screening tests, specialized laboratory tests indicated because of the individual's lifestyle or background, or problem-oriented laboratory testing due to a specific complaint or physical finding. The clinician determines which tests belong in each of these 3 categories; which test results must be interpreted differently in the adolescent compared with patients who are younger or older; and arrangements to be considered in managing special adolescent problems such as the need for confidentiality, limited fees, and fear of needles.

## ROUTINE LABORATORY SCREENING

Laboratory tests considered in routine screening of all adolescents include those that can detect problems that are potentially serious if not discovered, are relatively common in the population, are amenable to treatment, and are acceptable to adolescents and their families. The tests should be simple and convenient, yielding results that are both reliable (ie, similar on repeated measures) and valid (ie, sensitive and specific).[25] According to this definition, few tests should be ordered routinely for adolescent patients, regardless of their apparent health status or health risks. Tests that have been considered during the past 20 years have included hematologic screening, serum chemistries, urinalysis, lipid profile testing, evaluation of immunity to certain infections, and hormonal testing.

Initially, several specialists in adolescent medicine gave their views of which tests to perform, and how often,[25,26] and several national organizations presented their recommendations in official reports. These included the *Guidelines for Health Supervision* by the AAP in 1988; GAPS by the American Medical Association in 1992; and the *Bright Futures Guidelines for Health Supervision of Infants, Children, and Adolescents* in 1990 and 1994.[1,3,5] Because there are no specific right or wrong answers in determining the advisability of laboratory screening tests, the recommendations of the various reports have not always agreed. Accordingly, the most recent *Bright Futures*[6] guidelines, now published by the AAP, have used an evidence-based approach in developing recommendations for laboratory screening in adolescents.

## HEMATOLOGIC SCREENING

An estimated 8% of adolescent girls and 3% of adolescent boys are anemic, usually as a result of iron deficiency.[25,26] Several factors characteristic of the adolescent age group, including rapid growth, poor eating habits, and increased menstrual blood loss in some females, are thought to account for these abnormally low levels. The *Bright Futures*[6] guidelines recommend annual screening in females who have moderate to heavy menses, chronic weight loss, or nutritional deficits. Hemoglobin and hematocrit values remain unchanged in girls but increase significantly in boys during the adolescent years because of the effects of androgen production on hematopoiesis. Possibly because of the presence of the sickle cell gene in the community, mean hemoglobin levels of black adolescents of both sexes are approximately 1 mg/dL lower than those of their white counterparts. Screening for sickle cell trait (using the sickle prep) and thalassemia (using the mean corpuscular volume) in at-risk populations is not currently recommended in any of the national guidelines, with the exception of giving consideration to sickle cell screening in athletes who may be at risk of consequences from high-intensity training in hot climates or high altitudes. Research in recent years has shown that some adolescents, especially those who participate in sports activities, may have subtle degrees of anemia not detectable by hemoglobin or hematocrit determination, but more sophisticated screening (using ferritin levels) is also not generally recommended. There is universal agreement that total and differential leukocyte counts serve no purpose in clinically well children and adolescents.[27]

### SERUM CHEMISTRIES

Some clinicians and many hospitals have a policy of determining electrolyte values and other serum chemistries (including liver function tests, albumin levels, blood urea nitrogen, and creatinine levels) in all adolescent patients. However, there is no evidence that these are useful screening tests for this age group. Although abnormalities may be disclosed in the rare teenager with undetected disease or in the adolescent with surreptitious bulimia nervosa or substance abuse problems, the relatively high cost and large number of false-positive results far outweigh the benefits.

### URINALYSIS

A complete urinalysis that includes either a microscopic or a dipstick evaluation is not currently being recommended by the *Bright Futures*[6] guidelines as part of routine health care for adolescents. Problems for which a urinalysis is advocated in younger or older patients, including urinary tract infection, adult-onset diabetes mellitus, and renal disease, do not appear with the same frequency or implications in the adolescent age group. Some clinicians, however, continue to perform routine dipstick urinalyses on their adolescent patients in the belief that the small expense justifies its use in detecting urethritis or a urinary tract infection (which may be indicated by a positive nitrite or leukocyte esterase test), diabetes mellitus (indicated by glycosuria), or renal disease (proteinuria and/or hematuria). Some have recommended urinalysis to screen for eating disorders. Poor eating habits may be indicated by ketonuria, bulimia may possibly be indicated by an alkaline pH,[28] and water loading may be suspected in those with a low specific gravity.

### LIPID PROFILE

No area of screening has engendered more controversy than the questions of whether children and adolescents should receive routine screening for cholesterol levels. In 1992, an Expert Panel on Blood Cholesterol

Levels in Children and Adolescents of the National Cholesterol Education Program (NCEP) recommended selective, rather than universal, screening in adolescents, and this recommendation was adopted by both the GAPS and *Bright Futures* reports in the 1990s and continues to be endorsed by the most recent *Bright Futures* guidelines.[3,5,6,29] Recommendations of the Expert Panel include the following: (1) measurement of total cholesterol should be performed in all young adults over 19 years of age and in those younger adolescents whose parents have a serum cholesterol level greater than 240 mg/dL; (2) adolescents with an unknown family history or who have multiple risk factors for future cardiovascular disease (eg, smoking, hypertension, obesity, diabetes mellitus, excessive consumption of dietary fats) may be screened for total serum cholesterol at the discretion of the physician; and (3) those with a family history of cardiovascular disease in a parent or grandparent under the age of 55 should be screened with a fasting lipoprotein analysis. Recommendations based on the results of these screening tests are presented in Chapter 81, Hyperlipidemia and Atherosclerosis. Although many physicians have opted for universal screening of all adolescents, the Expert Panel chose not to recommend universal screening because (1) tracking of values into adulthood is not completely consistent, (2) universal screening could lead to unwarranted labeling of many adolescents, (3) for most individuals it is either difficult or unnecessary to begin therapy before adulthood, and (4) there is insufficient evidence of the long-term safety and efficacy of drug therapy for hyperlipidemia in childhood and adolescence.[29]

## SCREENING FOR TUBERCULOSIS

Tuberculin testing remains an important part of tuberculosis control efforts in teenagers. However, which teenagers to test, which test to use, how often to test, and how to interpret the results are all questions that have been re-evaluated in recent years. The most recent *Bright Futures* guidelines, in keeping with the recommendations of other national organizations, do not recommend routine testing but instead recommend that testing be performed in adolescents with specific risk factors (residence in high prevalence area, exposure to tuberculosis, immigrant status, homelessness, history of incarceration, employment in a health care facility).[6] Testing is still recommended using the standard purified protein derivative (PPD) test, although new blood tests have recently been developed to test for exposure to tuberculosis (see Chapter 141, Mycobacterial Infections).

The PPD is performed using an intradermal injection of 5 tuberculin units (eg, the Mantoux test) of PPD.[30] Although induration of 10 mm or more in the Mantoux test at 48 to 72 hours has traditionally been considered a positive reaction, more specific readings, aimed at decreasing both the false-positive and false-negative rate, have come into effect.[31] At this time, the skin tests are considered positive if induration is (1) ≥5 mm in persons with recent close contact with tuberculosis, with a positive chest x-ray finding, or who are immunosuppressed; (2) ≥10 mm in persons with known risk factors such as the foreign-born, the homeless, intravenous drug users, or those with other diseases associated with tuberculosis; and (3) ≥15 mm in those without other risk factors. Adolescents who have received bacilli Calmette-Guérin (BCG) vaccine should also be tested, because BCG vaccination causes an inconsistent tuberculin response that decreases with time, and these individuals should be treated no differently from those who never received the vaccine.

## SCREENING IN SPECIAL CIRCUMSTANCES

Certain adolescents, by virtue of their activities or background, may be considered for additional laboratory screening tests despite the lack of any overt physical findings or complaints. This group includes teenagers, both straight and gay, who are sexually active or involved with drug or alcohol use; those from foreign countries; and those being seen specifically for a presports or preoperative examination. Controversy exists over the specific tests warranted, with a tendency to include more testing in each of these circumstances than for the general population because of the greater risks and smaller numbers of involved adolescents.

### Sexually Active Adolescents

All teens who are sexually active are at risk of acquiring several STIs, and females are at risk for the development of cellular changes, which may be precursors of cervical neoplastic disease. Screening for the presence of infection in both sexes is recommended, but as noted previously, Pap test recommendations in adolescents have changed to age 21 for all adolescent females.[24] The reasons for the decreased emphasis on Pap tests in adolescents are a result of the findings that more than 90% of cellular changes in adolescents revert to normal with no intervention and that cervical cancer takes several years to develop. Although there is no policy, many advocate for screening immunocompromised sexually active adolescent females with pap smears earlier and more frequently. This issue is discussed in greater detail in Chapter 60, Cervical Findings and the Pap Smear.

Testing for chlamydia and gonorrhea remain important components of screening for sexually active adolescents. Chlamydial infection has been found in 5% to 25% of sexually active adolescents in multiple settings, is frequently asymptomatic in both sexes, and may lead to future fertility problems in females. Gonorrhea is seen less frequently, but is most common in the adolescent and young adult age groups, can be asymptomatic in both sexes, and can cause severe clinical infection. Testing is recommended annually in all sexually active adolescents for both chlamydia and gonorrhea with good evidence for chlamydia screening per the US Preventive Services Task Force. DNA probes and nucleic acid antigen tests (NAATs) are commercially available for both gonorrhea and chlamydia testing from genital or urine specimens.

Other STIs for which laboratory screening methods are available include trichomoniasis, bacterial vaginosis, and candidiasis; each may be detected on a saline wet mount of vaginal secretions. There is no screening test for asymptomatic genital herpes, nor is there a readily acceptable screening test for human papillomavirus (HPV), different types of which are associated with venereal warts and cervical neoplastic disease. Pap tests that reveal abnormalities may be tested for HPV. Cervical cancer is caused, in most cases, by HPV types 16 and 18. The HPV vaccines developed in the past few years should help to decrease the risks of cervical cancer worldwide, although general Pap smear recommendations for the foreseeable future will not change.

Some authorities are beginning to suggest recommending offering HIV testing for all adolescents and adults as a general public health measure. However, screening for HIV and syphilis are both recommended in all national guidelines for adolescents who are considered to be at a high risk for infection. This includes those adolescents who are living in a high prevalence area, who have another STI, males having sex with other males, and males or females who have had sex with multiple partners, who have a history of past or present injection drug use, have exchanged sex for money or drugs, or have had a sex partner who has done so, or who have had a past or present partner with HIV infection.[32]

### Alcohol and Drug Use

Laboratory screening may be considered in 2 distinct ways when treating adolescents involved with drug and alcohol use. Screening for alcohol or drugs may be useful in monitoring some teenagers suspected of substance abuse, and screening for certain sequelae of substance abuse may be useful in others. Sophisticated laboratory techniques have made the analysis of serum or urine for illicit substances readily available.[33] Few advocate these tests in mass screenings of adolescents, except perhaps for those participating in high-level sports or high-risk jobs. Although parents or a school may sometimes request that an adolescent be screened for substance use, many clinicians prefer to offer the test to the patient, using acceptance or refusal as a basis for further decision making and counseling. Urine screening for illicit drugs may be useful for evaluation in the emergency department setting or for ongoing care of an adolescent known to be a substance abuser. These patients, especially if there is a history of intravenous drug use, may also benefit from screening for liver function abnormalities, hepatitis B and C, and HIV screening, provided that appropriate counseling is available.

### Adolescents from Foreign Countries

Adolescents from Asia, Africa, and South America are routinely screened for ova and parasites. Because BCG vaccination is used widely in these continents for prevention of tuberculosis, interpretation of tuberculin testing may be more difficult for foreign-born adolescents. It is recommended, however, that tuberculin testing be interpreted no differently in these adolescents, because the duration of BCG immunity is so variable and unpredictable from country to country.

### Presports Evaluation

The adolescent who plans to join in organized sports activities generally undergoes a specialized evaluation before being allowed to participate. Chapter 164 provides more details about the preparticipation examination.

### Preoperative Screening

Screening for a surgical procedure had traditionally involved a series of blood tests (blood counts, clotting studies, blood bank specimen), a urinalysis, a chest radiograph, and an electrocardiogram (ECG). Studies have raised questions about the value of the blood tests and the urinalysis in children and adolescents, but these tests generally continue to be performed. Several large-scale studies have shown that neither the chest radiograph nor the ECG need be performed in the "healthy" adolescent with no previous evidence of pulmonary or cardiac disease; most institutions no longer include these tests in the preoperative procedures for children and adolescents.

## SPECIAL CONSIDERATIONS IN INTERPRETATION AND PERFORMANCE OF TESTS

Several factors in the interpretation and performance of laboratory tests in adolescents are different from the considerations ordinarily applied to either children or adults. The physical changes of adolescence have an impact on the results expected for certain tests, and several psychosocial issues affecting teenagers require special accommodations in the procedures needed in order to perform testing adequately in this age group.

### Laboratory Values

In most laboratory tests the range of the normal standard is no different for adolescents than for children and adults; however, specific biochemical, hematologic, and hormonal tests have significant differences, often with major clinical implications. These differences may be due solely to the effects of growth, they may vary with the Tanner stage, or they may represent a normal progression from childhood values to ultimate adult levels. Specific tests with clinical implications are discussed in the following.

***Serum Alkaline Phosphatase*** Because of skeletal growth, significantly elevated alkaline phosphatase levels are characteristic of early adolescence, especially at Tanner stages 2 to 4. In a laboratory test with normal childhood or adult values in the low to mid-100s, a value in the mid-300s would be perfectly acceptable in growing adolescents. Such values would not call for an evaluation for renal, bone, or liver disease, as might be the case for other age groups.

***Cholesterol and Triglyceride Levels*** Progression in cholesterol and triglyceride levels from childhood to adulthood is reflected in the 95th percentile values for total cholesterol and triglycerides of 200 and 150 mg/dL, respectively, in adolescents. These values would be considered at the lower levels of borderline in the adult. Further work-up and dietary counseling in adolescents must be based on age-appropriate levels.

***Hemoglobin or Hematocrit Levels*** Because of the hematopoietic effects of testosterone, hemoglobin and hematocrit levels increase significantly in boys, from a mean hematocrit of 39% at Tanner stage 1 to 44% at Tanner stage 5. Similar differences do not occur in girls, who may experience a decrease in hemoglobin or hematocrit levels during adolescence if the onset of menstruation includes prolonged or heavy periods. Research reveals that black adolescents have hematocrit values 1% to 3% lower than those of their white counterparts.

### OFFICE LABORATORY TESTS

Specific psychological and social issues must be considered when providing health care to adolescent patients, and laboratory testing is no exception. Because many adolescents are afraid of needles and may not understand the need for them, and because physical or psychological coercion is generally not appropriate, it often is necessary to employ a gentle but firm approach when drawing blood from teenagers. Confidential health care issues often necessitate arrangements of alternative payment options for the teenagers who need a Pap test, a pregnancy test, or testing for STIs. Many routine laboratory tests are available as rapid, office-based tests. Testing for pregnancy, mononucleosis, strep throat, and anemia may be offered in the office setting without involving an outside laboratory. Advantages include rapidity of diagnosis, which fits well with the "do-it-now" time frame within which many adolescents function, and avoiding large bills often generated by outside laboratories. However, interpretation of these tests and further decision-making must be handled with great care, because the sensitivity and specificity of these tests may not be as satisfactory as desired in all cases. The ability to perform and interpret some of these tests may be regulated by the federal Clinical Laboratory Improvement Amendments (CLIA) regulations. Rapid testing for HIV, which has become available during the past few years, requires specific attention as to how posttest counseling will be handled, especially for those with a positive result. Attention to details such as these often distinguishes the successful management of medical concerns in the teenage patient.

## REFERENCES


1. Green M, ed. *Guidelines for Health Supervision*. Elk Grove Village, IL: American Academy of Pediatrics; 1985

2. Fisher M, ed. *Guide to Clinical Preventive Services: An Assessment of the Effectiveness of 169 Interventions. Report of the US Preventive Services Task Force.* Baltimore, MD: Williams & Wilkins; 1989

3. Elster AB, Kuznets NJ, eds. *AMA Guidelines for Adolescent Preventive Services—Recommendations and Rationale*. Baltimore, MD: Williams & Wilkins; 1994

4. American Academy of Pediatrics Committee on Practice and Ambulatory Medicine. Recommendations for preventive pediatric health care. *Pediatrics.* 1995;96:373–374

5. Green M, ed. *Bright Futures: Guidelines for Health Supervision of Infants, Children, and Adolescents*. Arlington, VA: National Center for Education in Maternal and Child Health; 1994

6. Hagan JF, Jr, Shaw JS, Duncan PM, eds. *Bright Futures: Guidelines for Health Supervision of Infants, Children, and Adolescents.* 3rd ed. Elk Grove Village, IL: AAP; 2008

7. English A, Kenney KE. *State Minor Consent Laws: A Summary.* 2nd Ed. Chapel Hill, NC: Center for Adolescent Health and the Law; 2003

8. Boonstra H, Nash E. Minors and the right to consent to health care. *The Guttmacher Report.* 2000;3(4)

9. American Academy of Pediatrics Committee on Practice and Ambulatory Medicine. The use of chaperones during the physical examination of the pediatric patient. AAP Policy Statement. *Pediatrics.* 2005;115(5):1438. (doi:10.1542/Peds.2005-0464)

10. National High Blood Pressure Education Program Working Group on High Blood Pressure in Children and Adolescents. The fourth report on the diagnosis, evaluation, and treatment of high blood pressure in children and adolescents. *Pediatrics.* 2004;114(2 suppl 4th report):555–676

11. Ogden CL, Kuczmarski RJ, Flegal KM, et al. Centers for Disease Control and Prevention. 2000 growth charts for the United States: Improvements to the 1977 National Center for Health Statistics version. *Pediatrics.* 2002;109(1):45-60

12. Committee on Practice and Ambulatory Medicine of American Academy of Pediatrics, Section on Ophthalmology of American Academy of Pediatrics, American Association of Certified Orthoptists, American Association for Pediatric Ophthalmology and Strabismus, and American Academy of Ophthalmology. Eye examination in infants, children, and young adults by pediatricians. *Pediatrics.* 2003;111(4): 902-907

13. Nietupska O, Harding N. Auditory screening of school children: fact or fallacy? *Br Med J.* 1982;284:717-720

14. American Academy of Pediatric Dentistry 2010-2011 Oral Health Policies and Clinical Guidelines, Dietary Recommendations for Infants, Children, and Adolescents, Clinical Guidelines Revised, Oral and Dental Aspects of Child Abuse and Neglect, Infant Oral Health Care Revised, Adolescent Oral Health Care. Available at: www.aapd.org/media/policies.asp. Accessed August 24, 2010

15. US Preventive Services Task Force. Screening for idiopathic scoliosis in adolescents: recommendation statement. Rockville, MD: Agency for Healthcare Research and Quality; 2004 June 4

16. Marshall WA, Tanner JM. Variations in pattern of pubertal changes in girls. *Arch Dis Child.* 1969;44:291-303

17. Marshall WA, Tanner JM. Variations in pattern of pubertal changes in boys. *Arch Dis Child.* 1990;45:13-23

18. Tanner JM. *Growth at Adolescence.* 2nd ed. Oxford: Blackwell Scientific; 1962

19. Root AW. Endocrinology of puberty. *J Pediatr.* 1973;83:1-19

20. Beach RK. Routine breast exams: a chance to reassure, guide, and protect. *Contemp Pediatr.* 1987;70:100

21. Love SM, Gelman RS, Silen W. Fibrocystic "disease" of the breast—a nondisease? *N Engl J Med.* 1982;307:1010-1014

22. Nydick M, Bustos J, Dale JH, Rawson RW. Gynecomastia in adolescent boys. *JAMA.* 1961;178:449-454

23. Brenner JS, Hergenroeder AC, Kozinetz CA, Kelder SH. Teaching testicular self-examination: education and practices in pediatric residents. *Pediatrics.* 2003;111(3):e239

24. Cervical cytology screening. ACOG Practical Bulletin No. 109. American College of Obstetricians and Gynecologists; December 2009

25. Marks A, Fisher M. Health assessment and screening during adolescence. *Pediatrics.* 1987;80:133-158

26. Cromer BA, McLean CS, Heald FP. A critical review of comprehensive health screening in adolescents. *J Adolesc Health.* 1992;13:1S-65S

27. Moyer VA, Grimes RM. Total and differential leukocyte counts in clinically well children. *Am J Dis Child.* 1990;144: 1200-1203

28. Arden MR, Budow L, Bunnell DW, et al. Alkaline urine is associated with eating disorders (letter). *Am J Dis Child.* 1991;145:28-30

29. National Cholesterol Education Program. Highlights of the Report of the Expert Panel on Blood Cholesterol Levels in Children and Adolescents. *Pediatrics.* 1992;89:495-501

30. Starke JR. The tuberculin skin test. *Pediatr Ann.* 1993;22:612-620

31. American Thoracic Society. Diagnostic standards and classification of tuberculosis. *Am Rev Respit Dis.* 1990;142:725-735

32. United States Preventive Services Task Force. Screening for HIV: recommendation statement. *Ann Int Med.* 2005;143:32-37

33. Gray KM, Upadhyaya HP, Deas D, Brady KT. Advances in the diagnosis of adolescent substance abuse. *Ann Int Med.* 2005;143:32-37

# CHAPTER 10

# The Approach to Symptoms in the Adolescent Patient

RICHARD E. KREIPE, MD

*Partially supported by HRSA/MCHB Grant 5 T71MC00012-09-00.*

## INTRODUCTION

The best approach for a professional to take in caring for an adolescent is determined by a number of factors. For the adolescent who is not feeling well, there is an additional layer of complexity. This chapter addresses some of the factors to consider when evaluating and treating adolescents with symptoms.

## CONTEXTS OF INTERACTIONS WITH SYMPTOMATIC ADOLESCENTS

The multiple factors that determine the approach to an adolescent patient by a health care professional include the setting and nature of the encounter, the reason for the encounter (chief complaint in medical parlance), the developmental level of the adolescent, the training and comfort of the provider in working with adolescent patients, and the individual styles and personalities of the patient and the professional. In addition, parents can either facilitate or hinder a productive health care encounter with an adolescent. Several of these factors may be beyond the control of the provider, but being aware of them can improve communication and connection with an adolescent. A number of these issues are addressed in the chapters on performing the medical history and physical examination (Chapters 8 and 9) as well as those on the adolescent-friendly practice and practices in hospital, school-based, college, incarceration, and military settings (Chapters 22 and 24 through 28). Each of these chapters provides valuable practical information related to the approach to the adolescent patient participating in health care. Symptoms that cause an adolescent to feel ill or not well add a layer of complexity to these other variables, especially when they are considered in the context of an adolescent's psychological status and coping skills.

### CASE SCENARIOS

#### Case #1

A 14-year-old female who had been evaluated for severe, unrelenting headaches by specialists in ophthalmology, allergy, and otolaryngology was hospitalized by a neurologist because the headaches had made it impossible for her to attend school regularly. She had a history of abdominal pain, vomiting, and diarrhea attributed to "food allergies," chronic fatigue and rheumatic symptoms attributed to "fibromyalgia," recurrent chest pain attributed to "costochondritis," and "staring spells." Suspecting that the magnetic resonance imaging (MRI) of the head and other planned testing would be normal, the neurologist requested an adolescent medicine consultation on admission. As the patient was being transported from her hospital room to have her MRI, her mother turned to the adolescent medicine specialist and said, "I hope they find something."

With respect to symptoms, there was a clear implication that only a test like an MRI would provide the mother with the answer to the adolescent's headaches. The sequence of moving from 1 specialist to another, as exemplified by this case, is often seen in patients with pain symptoms such as headaches. The primary care provider's role in addressing symptoms that can have a variety of etiologies is to obtain a thorough history and physical examination to guide any testing or referral for consultations that might be considered. As noted in the discussion of somatoform disorders (Chapter 183), normal findings should be interpreted as reassuring because they indicate the absence of infection, tumor, displacement, or destruction of normal tissues, or other pathological processes about which the patient, parents, or physician might be concerned.

Moreover, the physical examination often provides clues regarding the source of the pain. Because this adolescent's headache was localized to the area overlying the masseter and temporalis muscles, and palpation elicited tenderness, the cause of the pain was reliably interpreted as muscle contraction. The triggers for muscle tension leading to chronic headache include a variety of factors. Frequently, it is helpful to note that different triggers (lack of sleep, not eating breakfast, bright lights, allergies, worry) can each result in muscle spasm.

Therefore, an approach to headache that only focuses on one potential trigger, or focuses only on analgesic medication is less likely to succeed than an approach that addresses each of the possible triggers in a comprehensive evaluation and treatment plan. This patient responded well to a program that focused on being more proactive in her recovery, which included the mom not repeatedly asking her daughter about what symptoms she was experiencing. The program also included a well-balanced meal plan with regular meals and snacks, mind–body techniques to lessen her gastrointestinal symptoms of a functional bowel disorder, regular but not excessive exercise, and cognitive behavioral sessions to build coping skills related to depression about her numerous symptoms.

**Case #2**

A 12-year-old male had what seemed like seizures while playing soccer. Treatment for asthma had been initiated 8 months earlier, but without improvement in his wheezing. An electroencephalogram (EEG) with video monitoring was normal during repetitive movement of his right arm and legs, and pulmonary function tests revealed flow-volume loops with inspiratory flattening, characteristic of vocal cord dysfunction. The patient was worried that he would not be able to play for his school soccer team that had won the state championship the previous 2 years.

Whereas the first case involved a situation in which symptoms would not be explained by diagnostic testing, the second case unexpectedly revealed tests that effectively "ruled out" diagnoses that had been linked with the adolescent's symptoms. Thus, the dilemma facing the clinician treating this patient was how to address the presumed diagnosis of seizures and the more longstanding diagnosis of asthma—when the patient had neither. First, the seriousness of the symptoms could be noted, because seizures and asthma can be life-threatening if not properly treated. Then, a reassuring comment such as, "The good news is that on further testing you don't have seizures or asthma, although it previously seemed as if you might have both," could be followed by an explanation of how wheezing just like asthma can occur "when the muscles of the vocal cords contract when you don't want them to so airflow is restricted and makes noise."

This description also would lay the groundwork for a physiologic explanation for his involuntary muscle movements. "Messages carried by nerves coming from the brain tell muscles what to do—either relax or contract. The problem is that the muscles on the right side of your body are contracting and relaxing really fast when you don't want them to. That can be pretty upsetting. Again, the good news is that your EEG is normal, which means that these are not seizures, but they are also not under your control. Maybe we can call them 'episodes' because they start and stop on their own and we expect them to get better over time. Lots of different things can cause these episodes, and stress definitely can make them worse, just like it can cause your vocal cords to close up when you don't want them to. I know that you are worried about not being able to play soccer and don't want to have to take medicines all the time. I believe that you will be able to come off the asthma medicines, but I want you to start a physical therapy program to re-train your nerves and muscles to be working together the way you want them to. It will also be good to have someone to talk to about your other worries. You've been through a lot and you need to get back on track."

**Case #3**

A 15-year-old female presented to the emergency department of a university hospital with incapacitating, chronic mid-epigastric pain not relieved with narcotics after a 5-day hospitalization at a community hospital. She was admitted to the gastroenterology service. After an exhaustive evaluation, no organic cause for her pain was found and she was transferred to the adolescent medicine service because the patient and her mother refused discharge until "something was done about" her pain. The history obtained by the adolescent medicine specialist revealed that her estranged father was recently remarried, taught at her high school, and had a stepson with lymphoma. Her father had not visited her during either hospitalization, but had shown much attention to his stepdaughter when she was initially ill with abdominal pain. A combat veteran, he interpreted the negative testing as meaning that there was nothing really wrong with her. Her mother was in the process of separating from her third husband. The patient described herself as "much more mature than my classmates" and as a "drama queen" considering an acting career. Regular outpatient visits with the adolescent medicine specialist, using a somatically oriented, cognitive behavioral approach to symptomatic relief and resolution of ongoing family conflicts resulted in gradual symptom improvement.

Two years later, at age 17, the patient presented to her primary care provider with acute lower abdominal pain. Due to her history, the visit focused on stressors and she still had not resolved conflicts with her family members, but was planning to move to New York City to become an actress. Brief palpation of her abdomen revealed tenderness, but she seemed to overreact to the physical examination. She was prescribed antacids and it was recommended that she work on her family relationships. Five days later she presented to her gynecologist because of worsening pain. During the pelvic examination, 75 cc of pus from a ruptured pyosalpinx spontaneously drained from her posterior vaginal vault.

This case illustrates the challenge to an adolescent health care provider regarding symptoms that change over time but are assumed to be due to the same mechanism. Although there appeared to be competition with her stepsister for attention and she had conflicted relationships with her parents, as well as with her peers—displaying histrionic and narcissistic features—an interim history for other causes of her symptoms and an appropriate physical examination did not occur at her encounter with her primary care provider. At that time an interim history would have revealed that she was sexually active with her 21-year-old boyfriend but was not using condoms, a pelvic examination likely would have revealed cervical motion tenderness, and a culture might have revealed gonorrheal cervicitis. In addition, the location and quality of the pain from her pelvic inflammatory disease was different than her other chronic pain symptoms. Thus, when adolescent patients have chronic symptoms, it is important to repeatedly update the history to determine any changes between encounters and it is also critical to perform a physical examination if symptoms have changed over time.

### Case #4

An 18-year-old male was evaluated for recurrent, localized back pain that was worse at night, but responded quickly to ibuprofen. He was a well-known scholar-athlete from a small rural town who was feeling "overwhelmed" because he also needed to work part time to help supplement a low family income. The best player on a winless football team, he joked to his physician that it would be good to have an "excuse" to not be on the team. He reported trouble sleeping because of the pain and "all the things on my mind." Because a physical examination and standard x-rays of the spine were both unremarkable, fluoxetine was added to the ibuprofen because of symptoms of depression and anxiety. When the pain did not improve, he was referred to an adolescent medicine specialist for counseling. However, due to the history, a computed tomographic (CT) scan was obtained first and it revealed a suspected, small vertebral osteoid osteoma. Once this benign tumor was removed, his pain did not return, but he continued to work on coping with stress, expressing relief that his pain was not "all in his head," as he had presumed when prescribed fluoxetine.

A common mistake in addressing an adolescent's physical symptoms is to ascribe them to psychological factors. This patient's symptoms were serious enough to warrant a physical examination and standard x-rays. However, when these were negative and the patient reported several sources of stress, anxiety, and possibly depression, a psychiatric diagnosis was made. Although he may have been depressed and anxious, there were clues to suggest an unrecognized anatomic cause of his back pain. First, the pain was localized, whereas psychosomatic pain tends to be more generalized. Second, the pain kept him from getting to sleep at night, and on further questioning he was sometimes awakened by pain, but it was quickly relieved by nonsteroidal anti-inflammatory medications. This history is characteristic of osteoid osteoma, a benign tumor that has no findings on physical examination and frequently goes undetected on routine x-rays, occurring most commonly in the femur and tibia. A CT or MRI scan of the site of pain reveals a small "donut" (central clearing around a rim of sclerosis) lesion, sometimes only 1 cm in diameter. Although these tumors can regress spontaneously over time, surgery is indicated for persistent pain (see Chapter 161, Bone Tumors).

## BIOPSYCHOSOCIAL MODEL

As detailed in Chapter 183, the biopsychosocial model facilitates the approach to complex conditions such as somatoform disorders. However, it is equally applicable and appropriate in routine adolescent health care, especially when addressing the adolescent who has symptoms, whether biological, psychological, or social in origin. Proposed in the literature by Engel[1] at the University of Rochester in a landmark 1977 article, the biopsychosocial approach offers a means of incorporating existing as well as emerging and new areas such as psychoneuroimmunology that better explain the cause and treatment of all symptoms that might present in health care settings than does the traditional dualistic approach in which illness is dichotomized into 2 domains: the body or the mind. It "supplements and enriches the discoveries of biomedicine, rather than undermining them."[2]

Central to the biopsychosocial model is viewing hierarchical natural systems as an interactive continuum in a patient's experience of symptoms. Engel[2] noted that "each level of hierarchy represents an organized dynamic whole... (with) qualities and relationships distinctive for that level of organization... In no way can the methods and rules appropriate for the study and understanding of the cell as cell be applied to the study of the person as person or the family as family." Furthermore, "each system as a whole has its own unique characteristics and dynamics; as a part it is a component of a higher-level system."[3] However, "neither the cell nor the person can be fully characterized as a dynamic system without characterizing the larger system(s) (environment) of which it is a part."[3] Therefore, "with the systems hierarchy as a guide, the physician from the outset considers all information in terms of systems levels and the possible relevance and usefulness of data from each level for the patient's further study and care."[3] In practice with respect to symptoms, Frankel and colleagues[4] note that "a comprehensive understanding of every aspect of care from diagnosis to treatment depends upon an appreciation of both linear and nonlinear processes associated with disease and illness." In practice, all aspects of care related to symptoms, from diagnosis to effective treatment, depend on an understanding of both linear and nonlinear processes associated with illness.

Although an adolescent's report of symptoms is sometimes considered "subjective," Cassell[5] has noted that patients, including adolescent patients, do not have either the option nor the interest to be objective about their own illness. He also notes that although the phrase "taking a history" is sometimes used by health care professionals, a history is unavoidably and actually an *exchange* of information.[5]

## COMMUNICATION REGARDING SYMPTOMS

The word communication is derived from the Latin *communicare*, meaning to share, or to have in common. Adolescents may not see themselves as having much in common with their health care providers, and sometimes may seem reluctant to share information. However, reducing or eliminating symptoms are common goals in a health care encounter when an adolescent does not feel well. The best way to establish shared goals is through language, most commonly spoken language. For patients who do not speak the same language as the provider or who do not have spoken language because of hearing impairment or other conditions, the use of a translator or interpreter becomes necessary.

### LANGUAGE

Spoken language in clinical interactions has 2 dimensions, each relevant to the patient and the provider regarding symptoms: receptive and expressive. Although adolescent patients are rarely aware of these issues, clinicians treating adolescents must attend to both receptive and expressive language for the patient and the provider. To emphasize the importance of this concept, Cassell[5] has noted that "spoken language is our most important diagnostic and therapeutic tool, and we must be as precise in its use as is a surgeon with a scalpel."

Unfortunately, language can be an impediment in working with adolescents with symptoms. First, patients may use the same words to describe different symptoms or may use different words to describe the same symptoms. Second, there is an intrinsic degree of ambiguity regarding what a patient means when describing symptoms. Third, misinterpretation of symptoms can lead to a limited or overly expansive differential diagnosis that may not include the actual condition causing the symptoms. Fourth, beliefs about the symptoms on the part of the adolescent, parents, grandparents, or other important individuals are often more important than what is spoken about the symptoms. As a basic principle, Cassell[5] suggests that providers "accept that physical symptoms always have a physical basis no matter what the underlying cause." Understanding the significance and meaning of symptoms is important in the diagnosis and in planning treatment. Because using descriptive words to describe the symptoms of pain (sharp, dull, burning, throbbing) may limit the expression of the significance and meaning of pain, it is often helpful to have patients "tell their story" and use the words they apply to describe their experience.

In addition to spoken or interpreted language, the astute diagnostician will not only interpret the body language of the adolescent patient as part of the evaluation but will also make use of body language and other techniques to facilitate the adolescent's expressive language. These techniques include (1) giving the patient undivided attention (writing as little as possible and making direct eye contact), (2) using reflective language to clarify traditional elements of the history (eg, timing, location, radiation, quality, severity, precipitants and relievers of pain, as well as any associated symptoms), (3) using a conversational style to identify things that the patient is unable to do as a result of the symptoms, and (4) developing a differential diagnosis that includes specific diagnoses or diseases that the patient (and parents) might be worried about. All of these elements are directed at helping the clinician understand the *story* and *meaning* of the illness, as well as the *suffering* caused by it. Cassell[5] notes, "Thinking about symptoms, attaching meaning to them, searching for explanations, are as much a part of the illness as are its physical expressions. These thoughts are not *caused* by the illness, they are *part* of the illness."

Symptoms cause suffering when the cause is unknown or when there is uncertainty regarding the future. Cassell[6] has noted that "suffering is experienced by persons, not merely by bodies, and has its source in challenges that threaten the intactness of the person as a complex social and psychological entity." Interestingly, clinicians also suffer when they are unable to provide relief of an adolescent's suffering due to symptoms. Cassell[7] notes that "physicians are less skilled at what were once thought to be the basic skills of doctors—discovering the history of an illness though questioning and physical examination, and working toward healing the whole person." These are skills that may be more necessary in adolescent health care than for any other age group.

**REFLECTIVE LISTENING**

Reflective listening is not the same as not talking, but it requires being attentive to subtle nuances of verbal and body language in the adolescent. Often, the provider should not expect to get "facts," but an "understanding of what it is like for the patient to be sick"—for the patient and sometimes the parents. Central to this process should be an exploration of the fears, worries, or concerns that might be evoked by the symptoms—for either the adolescent or the parents. However, because what may be stressful to one adolescent may be inconsequential to another, it is important not to make assumptions. There are 2 major fears that adolescents with symptoms often have: (1) an unrecognized physical illness, and/or (2) unrelenting symptoms. As Epstein and colleagues[8] note, in determining any prior assessment procedures or treatment experiences, the emphasis needs to be on the "experience of the illness."

**NONVERBAL COMMUNICATION**

Communicating with adolescents who have symptoms need not occur only through spoken or body language. Specifically, asking the patient to keep a detailed daily journal that includes all activities and symptoms can provide written documentation of daily patterns that are impossible to capture in conversation. This also emphasizes to the adolescent that the symptoms are being taken seriously. Alternatively, patients may find it easier to communicate about their illness through poems or drawings. All of these nonverbal formats serve the dual purpose of aiding in the diagnostic process by adding dimensions not usually included in traditional medicine, as well as being therapeutic because they give patients an opportunity to express themselves by a means other than through somatic symptoms.

## PHYSICAL EXAMINATION FOCUSED ON SYMPTOMS

Although a routine physical examination in the absence of symptoms is a relatively low-yield diagnostic activity, for symptomatic adolescents the "laying on of hands" provides an important validation of their concerns, even though those symptoms may be considered by the provider to be relatively minor. Even if they are unlikely to provide any new information regarding the diagnosis, procedures such as indirect ophthalmoscopy, deep tendon reflex testing, cranial nerve evaluation, and evaluation of cerebellar function for patients with headaches, or a thorough examination of the lungs for patients with chronic cough, or 4-quadrant inspection, palpation, percussion, and auscultation of the abdomen for patients with recurrent abdominal pain, indicate that the symptoms are being taken seriously.

## SUMMARY

Given the unique developmental features of adolescents and the wide range of settings in which those adolescents who have symptoms of illness are seen by health care professionals, it is important for providers to have a means of interacting with adolescents who may have symptoms that range from inconsequential to life-threatening. This chapter uses case scenarios to highlight the challenges providers face and also details the features of the biopsychosocial model that will minimize problems that arise in relation to the evaluation and treatment of symptoms in adolescents. Communication is a key feature of connecting with adolescents; language, reflective listening, nonverbal communication, and the physical examination are all elements of communicating a caring and thoughtful approach to an adolescent's symptoms that emphasizes the essential feature of caring for adolescents. As noted by Peabody[9] more than 80 years ago, "The secret of patient care is in caring for the patient."

## REFERENCES

1. Engel GL. The need for a new medical model: a challenge for biomedicine. *Science.* 1977;196:129–136

2. Frankel RM, Quill RE, McDaniel SH. The future of the biopsychosocial approach. In: Frankel RM, Quill TE, McDaniel SH, eds. *The Biopsychosocial Approach: Past, Present, Future.* Rochester, NY: The University of Rochester Press; 2003

3. Engel GL. The application of the biopsychosocial model. In: Frankel RM, Quill TE, McDaniel SH, eds. *The Biopsychosocial Approach: Past, Present, Future.* Rochester, NY: The University of Rochester Press; 2003

4. Frankel RM, Quill RE, McDaniel SH. Introduction to the biopsychosocial approach. In: Frankel RM, Quill TE, McDaniel SH, eds. *The Biopsychosocial Approach: Past, Present, Future.* Rochester, NY: The University of Rochester Press; 2003

5. Cassell EJ. *Talking with Patients.* Cambridge, MA: MIT Press; 1985

6. Cassell EJ. The nature of suffering and the goals of medicine. *N Engl J Med.* 1982;306:639–645

7. Cassell EJ. *The Nature of Suffering and the Goals of Medicine.* 2nd ed. Oxford, UK: Oxford University Press; 2003

8. Epstein RM, Quill TE, McWhinney IR. Somatization reconsidered: incorporating the patient's experience of illness. *Arch Intern Med.* 1999;159(3):215–222

9. Peabody FW. The care of the patient. *JAMA.* 1927;88: 877–882

# CHAPTER 11

# Legal and Ethical Issues in Adolescent Health Care

ABIGAIL ENGLISH, JD

## INTRODUCTION

Health care professionals who take care of adolescents 12 to 21 years old must become familiar with a broad range of laws and ethical principles to navigate their way appropriately through the myriad legal questions and ethical concerns that arise in caring for this age group. In the United States, the laws encompass a complex patchwork of state and federal statutes, regulations, and court decisions that concern the legal status of children and the roles and responsibilities of parents. Many of the laws deal with reproductive health and rights, as well as other health issues common in adolescence, such as mental health and substance use. The ethical principles are grounded in concepts of autonomy, beneficence, nonmaleficence, and justice. Human rights principles also merit consideration in relation to the ethical obligations of health care professionals. Key questions arise with respect to consent for health care, confidentiality protection for health care information, and financial access to health care services. In considering these questions, it is important to note that for adolescents, particularly those who are under the age of majority—18 years old—and are considered minors, finding the most appropriate ways to include parents or other trusted adults while honoring the adolescents' need for privacy is an important task for health care professionals.

## CONSENT FOR HEALTH CARE

When minor children need health care, the consent of a parent is usually required. There are many exceptions to this requirement that either allow other adults, or courts, to give consent or that allow minors to consent for their own care. Understanding these options is essential.

### PARENTAL CONSENT

Historically, the requirement of parental consent for children's health care is based in principles of common law and in many states is not found in specific statutes.[1] Nevertheless, consent of a parent or other legally authorized adult is required in most situations in which a minor child or adolescent needs health care. Alternatives to parental consent may include consent by legal guardians, other adult relatives, caretakers, and custodians, sometimes including foster parents. Courts may also give consent and may authorize others such as social workers or probation officers to do so for young people in state custody.[1,2]

Major exceptions exist to the requirement of parental consent. One that applies to children and adolescents of all ages is the exception for emergencies in which prior consent is not required, in large measure because it is implied.[1] Life-saving treatment should be initiated while consent is being sought. Another exception of particular significance for adolescents who are minors is the requirement of parental consent that arises when minors are legally authorized to give consent for their own care.[2]

### MINOR CONSENT

Every state in the US has laws that expressly allow minors to give their own consent for health care in a variety of circumstances. These laws can be broadly grouped into those that allow minors to give their own consent based on the *services* that the minor is seeking, and those that are related to having attained a particular *status*. Each state has some laws in both categories.

#### Minor Consent Based on Services

Every state has one or more laws that authorize minors to consent to certain services.[2,3] These services most frequently include contraceptive services; pregnancy-related care; diagnosis and treatment of sexually transmitted infections (often referred to in the statutes as venereal disease), human immunodeficiency virus (HIV), or acquired immunodeficiency syndrome (AIDS), and reportable or contagious diseases; examination and treatment related to sexual assault; counseling and treatment for drug or alcohol problems; and mental health treatment, particularly outpatient care.[2,3] Not all states have statutes covering all of these services. Among those that do, some of the statutes contain age limits, which most frequently fall between the ages of 12 and 15 years.[2]

The issue of abortion has been the subject of extensive legislation and litigation in many states. Currently most states require some form of parental involvement—either consent or notice—for a minor to obtain an abortion.[2,4] Some states have enacted statutes that have been enjoined by the courts and are not being enforced.[2,4] However, even in those states in which a parental involvement law (or a law requiring the involvement of another adult, such as a grandmother or adult sibling) is being enforced, there also exist provisions for a "judicial bypass" allowing a minor to demonstrate to a court that she is sufficiently mature to give her own consent without parental involvement or, if she is not sufficiently mature, that it would be in her best interest to have the abortion without parental consent or notification.[2,4]

#### Minor Consent Based on Status

Every state also has one or more laws that authorize minors who have attained a specific status to give consent for their own health care.[2] These laws typically authorize one or more of the following groups of minors to do so: emancipated minors; those who are living apart from their parents, including runaways or homeless youth; minors serving in the armed forces; married minors; minors who are the parents of a child; high school graduates; and minors who have attained a certain age, such as 15 or 16.[2] Moreover, in a few states, explicit statutes authorize minors who are "mature minors" to consent for care, although the laws do not generally use that term, but rather contain criteria related to capacity to give informed consent.[2]

## EMANCIPATED MINORS

The legal concept of the emancipated minor has a long history in common law dating to colonial times. Traditionally, minors who were married, serving in the military, or living apart from their parents with parental consent or acquiescence were considered to be "emancipated" from the custody and control of their parents, enabling them to keep their own wages and enter into binding contracts.[1] More recently, a number of states have enacted specific statutes allowing minors who meet similar criteria to seek a court order of emancipation.[5] Some of these statutes mention consent for health care as a consequence of emancipation; others do not.[2,5] However, a strong argument can be made that minors who meet traditional criteria for emancipation should be able to consent for their own health care, even without a statute.

## MATURE MINORS

Another important legal doctrine in the care of adolescents is the "mature minor" doctrine.[1,6] Even in the absence of a specific statute, "mature minors" may have the legal capacity to give consent for their own care.[1,2,6] Unless a state has explicitly rejected the mature minor doctrine, in most states it means that there is little likelihood a health care professional will incur liability for failure to obtain parental consent provided that the minor is an older adolescent (typically at least 15 years) who is capable of giving, and has given, an informed consent and the care is not high risk, is for the minor's benefit, and is within the mainstream of established medical opinion.[1,2,6] The basic criteria for determining whether a patient is capable of giving an informed consent are that the patient must be able to understand the risks and benefits of any proposed treatment or procedure and its alternatives and must be able to make a voluntary choice among the alternatives.[1,2,6] These criteria apply to minors as well as adults.

### ADOLESCENT AUTONOMY AND PARENTAL INVOLVEMENT

When caring for an adolescent, some tension may arise between honoring the adolescent's developing need for autonomy and finding ways to involve parents in the adolescent's care. Ultimately, all parties—the adolescent, the parents, and the health care professional—share a common interest in protecting the adolescent's health and making sure the adolescent gets the necessary care. At times, however, the adolescent may want increased autonomy and the parent may seek greater involvement. These situations challenge the skill of the clinician to mediate the situation, avoid confrontation, honor ethical principles, and act consistent with legal requirements.

## CONFIDENTIALITY OF HEALTH CARE INFORMATION

Maintaining confidentiality in the delivery of health care services to adolescents serves important purposes. Among the most compelling is encouraging adolescents to seek timely care and to provide a candid and complete health history.[7] Additional reasons include supporting adolescents' growing sense of autonomy and protecting them from the discrimination and humiliation that could result from disclosure of confidential information.

Findings from decades of research demonstrate the importance of confidentiality in adolescent health care.[7] Numerous studies have shown that without assurances of privacy, adolescents will sometimes avoid seeking care entirely, refuse specific services, alter their choice of provider, or withhold significant information.[7] Research has also shown that even young adults in their late teens or early 20s remain concerned about the privacy of their health care information and whether it will be disclosed to their parents.[7]

Confidentiality protections are rarely, if ever, absolute, so health care professionals must be able to answer 3 key questions: What *may* be disclosed based on their discretion and professional judgment? What *must* be disclosed? What *may not* be disclosed? In answering these questions, the following considerations are relevant:

- What information *is* confidential (because it is considered private and is protected against disclosure)?
- What information *is not* confidential (because such information is not protected)?
- What *exceptions* are there in the confidentiality requirements?
- What information can be released *with consent*?
- What other mechanisms allow for *discretionary* disclosure without consent?
- What *mandates* exist for reporting or disclosing confidential information?[8]

Even confidential information usually may be disclosed with the permission of the patient or another appropriate person. Often, when minors can legally consent to their own care, they also have the right to control disclosure of confidential information about that care. However, there are a number of circumstances in which disclosure over the objection of the minor might be required even if the minor had consented to the care. For example, if a specific law requires disclosure to parents; if a legal obligation to report suspected physical or sexual abuse applies; or if the minor poses a severe danger to him or herself or to others.[9]

When the minor does not have the legal right to consent to care or to control disclosure, the release of confidential information must generally be authorized by the minor's parent or the person (or entity) with legal custody or guardianship.[9] However, it is still advisable—from an ethical perspective—for the health care professional to seek the agreement (assent) of the minor to disclose confidential information or, at minimum, to advise the minor at the outset of treatment of any limits to confidentiality.[9] Fortunately, issues of confidentiality and disclosure generally can be resolved by discussion and informal agreement between a health care professional, the adolescent patient, and the parents without reference to legal requirements.

## CONFIDENTIALITY LAWS

The confidentiality obligation has numerous sources in law and policy. They include the federal and state constitutions; federal statutes and regulations related to funding programs; state statutes and regulations (such as medical confidentiality and medical records laws, physician-patient and psychotherapist-patient privilege statutes, professional licensing laws, and funding programs); court decisions; and professional ethical standards. Extensive federal medical privacy regulations, known as the "Health Insurance Privacy and Accountability (HIPAA) Privacy Rule," (see below) affect the care of adolescents and adults and are of critical importance.

### Confidentiality in State Minor Consent Laws

Many—but not all—of the state laws that allow minors to consent for their own health care also contain provisions addressing the confidentiality and disclosure of information about that care.[2] In many instances, the laws specify that the information may not be disclosed without the permission of the minor patient.[2] Sometimes, however, the laws grant discretion to the physician or treating health care professional to disclose information to a minor's parent, even over the objection of the minor; usually such laws contain criteria for when this may be done, such as if it is necessary to protect the health of the minor.[2] Conversely, some of the minor consent laws require that parents be involved or informed, but contain exceptions if, in the judgment of the treating professional, it would not be in the minor's interest to do so.[2]

### Federal Laws Protecting Confidentiality

Several federal laws provide confidentiality protection for health care services received by adolescent minors based on their own consent.[2,10] These include the Title X Family Planning Program, the federal drug and alcohol confidentiality regulations, Medicaid, and the HIPAA Privacy Rule.[2,10] The Title X Family Planning Program, which has been in existence for nearly 4 decades, is of particular importance because it contains very strong confidentiality protections and allows minors in every state to receive confidential family planning services in Title X-funded sites without parental consent, regardless of whether their state has an explicit law authorizing minors to give their own consent for contraception or family planning services.[11] The HIPAA Privacy Rule, although of more recent vintage, also contains provisions that are essential for health care professionals to be aware of when treating adolescent patients.

### HIPAA Privacy Rule

The HIPAA Privacy Rule, issued in final form in 2002, built on the framework of consent and confidentiality laws that had been developed over the past several decades.[12] Specifically, when minors are authorized to consent for their own health care and do so, the rule treats them as "individuals" who are able to exercise rights over their own protected health information.[12] Also, when parents have acceded to a confidentiality agreement between a minor and a health professional, the minor is considered an "individual" under the rule.[12]

Generally, the HIPAA Privacy Rule gives parents access to the health information of their unemancipated minor children, including adolescents.[12] However, on the issue of when parents may have access to protected health information for minors who are considered "individuals" under the rule and who have consented to their own care, it defers to "state and other applicable law."[12]

Thus, the laws that allow minors to consent for their own health care have acquired increased significance with the advent of the HIPAA Privacy Rule. The rule must also be understood in the broader context of other laws that affect disclosure of adolescents' confidential health information to their parents. Specifically, if state or other law explicitly *requires* information to be disclosed to a parent, the regulations allow a health care provider to comply with that law and disclose the information.[12] If state or other law explicitly *permits*, but does not require, information to be disclosed to a parent, the regulations allow a health care provider to exercise discretion to disclose or not.[12] If state or other law *prohibits* the disclosure of information to a parent without the consent of the minor, the regulations do not allow a health care provider to disclose it without the minor's consent.[12] If state or other law is *silent* or unclear on the question, an entity covered by the rule has discretion to determine whether or not to grant access to a parent to the protected health information, as long as the determination is made by a health care professional exercising professional judgment.[12]

### Mandatory Disclosure

Varied legal requirements may result in mandatory disclosure of health care information that is otherwise protected as confidential. Particularly significant among such requirements are the child abuse reporting laws that exist in every state and require health care professionals to make reports to child welfare or law enforcement authorities when they know or suspect that a child has been the victim of physical or sexual abuse or neglect.[13] Significant confusion for health care professionals has resulted from the inclusion, in some state laws and by some law enforcement officers, of voluntary sexual activity of minors within the scope of mandatory reporting of child abuse.[13] The laws and their interpretation and application vary widely among the states, and health care professionals must learn about local requirements.

Other important situations in which health care professionals may be *required* to disclose adolescents' confidential health information include those in which an adolescent presents a serious risk of doing harm to self or others,[10] or an adolescent is seeking an abortion and state law requires parental consent or notification or a judicial bypass proceeding,[4] or (in 1 or 2 states) parental consent or notification is required for minors to receive contraception or family planning services paid for by state funds.[14]

## FINANCIAL ACCESS TO HEALTH CARE

Laws that pertain to consent, confidentiality, and payment in health care for adolescents are inextricably intertwined.[15] Financial obstacles can impede access to essential services. The issue is particularly critical for adolescents from low-income families or those, such as homeless youth, who have no family support, and even more critical when a young person needs confidential care.[15–18]

Legal provisions that allow adolescents to give consent for care and protect their confidentiality do not ensure access to care. Financing care is also an essential element of confidentiality. Some of the state minor consent laws specify that if a minor is authorized to consent to care, it is the minor, rather than the parent, who is responsible for payment.[2] In reality, however, few, if any, adolescents are able to pay for health care out of pocket unless there is a sliding fee scale with very minimal payments required. Although most adolescents have private health insurance coverage, they can rarely use that coverage without information reaching the policyholder, who usually is a parent.[16] The potential is greater for them to receive confidential care through Medicaid, but policies and practices in this regard are varied and uneven among the states.

There are some federal and state health care funding programs that enable minors to obtain confidential care with little or no cost to them. Most important is the previously noted federal Family Planning Program funded under Title X of the Public Health Services Act.[11] As significant a role as these programs play, they do not ensure access to comprehensive health services for teens. The financing available through insurance is thus all the more important.

Adolescents are uninsured and underinsured at higher rates than other groups in the population, although young adults are uninsured at the very highest rates.[16,19] Those adolescents and young adults living below the poverty level are at the greatest risk for lacking health insurance. Private employer-based coverage for adolescents has declined, but coverage through public insurance programs such as Medicaid and the State Children's Health Insurance Program has increased.[16,19] Enrollment of all adolescents and young adults who are eligible for these programs would significantly decrease the number of uninsured in this age group and have great potential for improving their access to care. At the time of this writing, health care reform legislation that also could reduce the number of uninsured adolescents and young adults is being debated in the United States.[20]

## ETHICS, HUMAN RIGHTS, AND HEALTH CARE ACCESS

Access to health care for adolescents and young adults and the provision of care to this age group by health care professionals are significantly affected by myriad laws. However, the laws merely establish broad parameters within which health care professionals act. The laws do not answer many critically important questions within those parameters. With respect to the creation of the laws and to actions taken within their framework, principles of ethics and human rights are highly relevant and should be strongly considered.

Ethical principles that are relevant to the care of adolescents and young adults include respect for *autonomy*—supporting the patient's own wishes, ideas, and choices; *nonmaleficence*—avoiding harm to the patient; *beneficence*—doing good for the patient or taking action to further the patient's welfare; and *justice*—giving all patients a fair opportunity to receive health care on the same basis as other groups.[9] The application of these principles can and should guide the development of laws affecting health care as well as the actions of health care professionals in delivering care.

Although the United States has not fully embraced all international agreements embodying principles of human rights, those principles are gaining increased attention as important for guiding health policy and the development of laws.[21] Notably, a document of great significance that articulates key health care rights—the UN Convention on the Rights of the Child—has not been signed by the United States.[21] Nevertheless, the health-related principles articulated in that convention and in documents elaborating on its meaning are important ones for the health care of young people.[21] The right to health is recognized in the convention, and governments are obligated to provide access to health care services.[21] The special status and specific rights of adolescents are also recognized by the United Nations Committee on the Rights of the Child, which interprets the convention. Adolescents are "active rights holders," that is, persons with their own human rights, including the right to nondiscrimination, the right to express views freely, the right to legal protections about health care, the right to information, the right to privacy and confidentiality, and right to protection from abuse, neglect, violence, and exploitation.[21]

## CONCLUSION

Providing high-quality, age-appropriate health care to adolescents and young adults requires an understanding of myriad laws related to consent, confidentiality, and financial access. When informed by strong principles of ethics and human rights, those laws are more likely to meet the needs of this age group, and the care they receive is likely to be of higher quality.

## INTERNET RESOURCES

- American Academy of Pediatrics: Policy Statements: aappolicy.aappublications.org/policy_statement/index.dtl
- Center for Adolescent Health and the Law: www.cahl.org
- Guttmacher Institute State Center: www.guttmacher.org/statecenter/adolescents.html
- National Center for Youth Law: www.youthlaw.org/health
- Society for Adolescent Medicine: Position Papers and Position Statements: www.adolescent-health.org/advocacy.htm

## REFERENCES


1. Holder AR. *Legal Issues in Pediatrics and Adolescent Medicine*. 2nd ed. New Haven, CT: Yale University Press; 1985

2. English A, Kenney KE. *State Minor Consent Laws: A Summary*. 3rd ed. Chapel Hill, NC: Center for Adolescent Health and the Law; 2009

3. Boonstra H, Nash E. Minors and the right to consent to health care. *Guttmacher Report on Public Policy.* 2000;3:4–8

4. Dennis A, Henshaw SK, Joyce TJ, Finer LB, Blanchard K. *The Impact of Laws Requiring Parental Involvement in Minors' Abortions: A Literature Review*. New York, NY: Guttmacher Institute; 2009. Available at: www.guttmacher.org/pubs/ParentalInvolvementLaws.pdf. Accessed September 28, 2009

5. Juvenile Law Center. Emancipation in the United States, 2007. Available at: jlc.org/factsheets/4/. Accessed September 28, 2009

6. Sigman GS, O'Connor C. Exploration for physicians of the mature minor doctrine. *J Pediatrics.* 1991;119:520–525

7. Ford CA, English A. Limiting confidentiality of adolescent health services: what are the risks? *JAMA.* 2002;288(6):252–253

8. English A. Understanding legal aspects of care. In: Neinstein LS, et al, eds. *Adolescent Health Care: A Practical Guide*. 5th ed. Philadelphia, PA: Lippincott Williams & Wilkins; 2008;124–132

9. Ford CA, English A, Sigman G. Confidential health care for adolescents: a position paper of the Society for Adolescent Medicine. *J Adolesc Health.* 2004;35:160-167

10. Morreale MC, Stinnett AJ, Dowling EC. *Policy Compendium on Confidential Health Services for Adolescents.* Chapel Hill, NC: Center for Adolescent Health and the Law; 2005. Available at: www.cahl.org/PDFs/PolicyCompendium/PolicyCompendium.pdf. Accessed April 22, 2010

11. Gold RB. Title X: three decades of accomplishment. *The Guttmacher Report on Public Policy.* 2001;4:5-8. Available at: www.guttmacher.org/pubs/tgr/04/1/gr040105.pdf. Accessed September 28, 2009

12. English A, Ford CA. The HIPAA privacy rule and adolescents: legal questions and clinical challenges. *Perspect Sex Reprod Health.* 2004;36:80-86

13. Protecting adolescents: Ensuring access to care and reporting sexual activity and abuse: position paper of the American Academy of Family Physicians, American Academy of Pediatrics, American College of Obstetricians and Gynecologists, Society for Adolescent Medicine. *J Adolesc Health.* 2004;35:420-423

14. Brindis CD, English A. Measuring public costs associated with loss of confidentiality for adolescents seeking confidential reproductive health care: how high the costs? How heavy the burden? *Arch Pediatr Adolesc Med.* 2004;158:1182-1184

15. Brindis C, Morreale M, English A. The unique health care needs of adolescents. *Future of Children.* 2003;13:117-135

16. Adams S, Newacheck P, Park MJ, Irwin CE Jr. Health insurance across vulnerable ages: patterns and disparities from adolescence to the early 30s. *Pediatrics.* 2007;119:e1033-1039

17. Halley M, English A. *Health Care for Homeless Youth: Policy Options for Improving Access.* Chapel Hill, NC: Center for Adolescent Health and the Law; 2008. Available at: www.cahl.org/PDFs/HealthCareForHomelessYouth.pdf. Accessed April 22, 2010

18. English A, Stinnett AJ, Dunn-Georgiou E. *Health Care for Adolescents and Young Adults Leaving Foster Care: Policy Options for Improving Access.* Chapel Hill, NC: Center for Adolescent Health and the Law; 2006. Available at: www.cahl.org/PDFs/FCIssueBrief.pdf. Accessed September 28, 2009

19. Morreale MC, English A. Eligibility and enrollment of adolescents in Medicaid and SCHIP: recent progress, current challenges. *J Adolesc Health.* 2003;32(suppl):25-39

20. English A, Park MJ, Shafer MA, et al. Health care reform and adolescents—an agenda for the lifespan: position paper of the Society for Adolescent Medicine. *J Adolesc Health.* 2009;456:310-315

21. English A, Santelli J, Rogers AS. Legal and ethical issues in adolescent health care and research. In: DiClemente RJ, Santelli J, Crosby RA, eds. *Adolescent Health: Understanding and Preventing Risk Behaviors.* San Francisco, CA: Jossey-Bass; 2009;531-548

# CHAPTER 12

## Adherence Issues

BARBARA A. CROMER, MD • SARA LEE, MD

### INTRODUCTION

Adherence to therapeutic and preventive regimens is central to adolescent health care and well-being. Compliance has been defined as the "extent to which a patient's behavior coincides with the clinical prescription."[1] In this passive definition, a person is either compliant or noncompliant. In the context of health care, a "noncompliant" adolescent is often construed to be intentionally ignoring recommendations or passively disobedient. Therefore, the term "adherence" is favored over the term "compliance" because it is less pejorative. That is, in the context of a therapeutic relationship in which adolescents work with their health care providers in a partnership to maintain or improve their health, they are considered to be adherent to the plan. However, nonadherence may indicate a need to change the strategy, rather than blame the adolescent for not "following orders," as might occur when an adolescent is judged to be "noncompliant." Therapeutic interventions are best developed with a goal of facilitating and supporting compliance by reducing barriers and encouraging autonomy. The consequences of not following therapeutic suggestions can be significant. Nonadherence may result in unnecessary medication changes or inappropriate dosage increases that are potentially toxic. Failure to adhere to a treatment regimen can lead to increased complications and hospitalizations. Adherence becomes particularly important and challenging during adolescence. As adolescents change and mature, unique therapeutic management issues develop. This chapter addresses the adherence issues facing adolescents and those involved in their care.

### ASSESSING ADHERENCE

Adherence is low in all populations, and it may be lowest in adolescents. A number of studies[1] have demonstrated that approximately 50% of adolescents with chronic conditions do not comply with care recommendations. Adherence to treatment recommendations tends to be higher in certain clinical situations—as in the treatment of acute, symptomatic illnesses versus the practice of preventive health measures such as diet modifications. Complex personal and environmental influences create unique considerations in each case.

Clinicians' predictions of adolescent patient adherence often do not match more objective measures, such as pill counts.[2] This inability to predict adherence may in part reflect the wide variety of factors related to nonadherence. Studies have failed to demonstrate any consistent findings with respect to race, socioeconomic status, or gender. Thus, there is no typical "picture" of an adherent (or nonadherent) patient.

Nonadherence should be suspected in any patient who is not responding to therapy as expected. However, because biological responses vary, adherence of every adolescent patient should be frequently assessed. There are multiple methods of assessing adherence. Direct measures include bioassays and electronic monitoring. Bioassays of certain drugs can aid both in the assessment of adherence and in medication adjustment. They are most helpful for a drug that must be taken regularly, has a long half-life, and reaches a steady state. However, such assays are costly and may require invasive measures such as venipuncture. Also, given variations in metabolism among adolescents, they may not be a reliable indicator of adherence. A notable exception to this is hemoglobin A1c measurement in diabetes mellitus because it indicates the average blood glucose level over a 3-month period. Electronic monitoring devices include glucometers and electronic microprocessors in the lid of pill bottles that record the opening of bottles for the removal of tablets. Direct observation of medication taking is another method of ensuring adherence, but it is time consuming and costly. Even direct observation of oral medication is unreliable for patients who are adept at hiding their medications in their cheeks or palms while appearing to swallow them. Such "cheeking" or "palming" is most commonly associated with psychiatric medications.

Indirect measures of adherence include pill counts, refill tallies, therapeutic outcomes, and patient or parent reports. The simplest method of assessing adherence is to ask the patient. This should be done in an open, empathetic, and nonjudgmental manner. Ask "How many times this week were you able to take your medication?" or "How many times do you think you missed your medication this week?" rather than "Did you take your medication?" However, self-reports of adherence may be unreliable. A study[3] examining self-reported adherence to oral contraceptives showed agreement between self-report and electronic monitoring less than half of the time.

In assessing potential adherence, patients can be asked about their intentions. Patients who report no intention of following recommendations are unlikely to be adherent. In addition, patients who have been adherent in the past are likely to be adherent in the future; in 1 study 4 of young women starting oral contraceptives, 81% of those who were taking their birth control pills rated their past adherence as good.

## DETERMINANTS OF ADHERENCE

Despite efforts to identify psychosocial factors, such as demographic background or personality characteristics associated with adherence, research findings vary from study to study. Although, as stated previously, no definitive profile of the compliant patient has been drawn, many factors have been identified as contributing to adherence.

### DEVELOPMENTAL ISSUES

Nonadherence during adolescent development is, in some respects, expected. Adolescence is a time of cognitive development as most teenagers progress from concrete to abstract thought and formal operations. As a result of cognitive immaturity, younger adolescents may have difficulty understanding abstract concepts related to illness or appreciating the long-term benefits of preventive health practice. Adolescents may also lack problem-solving skills and be unable to grasp the long-term consequences of their behaviors. Those who can perceive the consequences of their behaviors may cope with a difficult situation through denial or by "acting out" in the form of nonadherence. Adolescents' beliefs that they are invulnerable and not susceptible to illness may lead to risky health behaviors. Impulsivity also may be a factor in nonadherence.[5]

Along with cognitive changes, adolescence is a time of physical changes (see Chapter 4, Physical Growth and Development). Pubertal changes lead adolescents to focus on their bodies; chronic illness may complicate their developing body image. Adherence to therapy decreases if the treatment has cosmetic side effects, such as systemic corticosteroids causing acne, weight gain, or a "Cushingoid" appearance. Adolescents who seek an idealized body, but who require body-changing medication(s), may encounter a daily (possibly several times a day) reminder that this goal is unattainable.[6]

As body image forms, so does an adolescent's sense of identity. Adolescence is a time of individuation and separation from the family as the adolescent moves toward independent adulthood. When an illness forces a return to dependency, nonadherence may be a means of asserting control. Illness may also contribute to self-worth, which in turn can influence adherence. The presence of a psychological problem, particularly depression, is a major predictor of poor adherence.[7]

### HEALTH BELIEF MODEL

In the Health Belief Model,[8] adherence depends on (1) perceived susceptibility to disease; (2) subjective estimation of disease severity; (3) estimation of the effectiveness of the prescribed regimen; and (4) perceived physical, psychological, and financial costs of adherence to the prescribed regimen.[1] Perceived susceptibility to disease is an important determinant of adherence to both preventive and therapeutic health advice; however, as previously stated, adolescents may have difficulty assessing their susceptibility to disease because of their cognitive level and their own sense of invulnerability.

Adolescents may also have difficulty understanding the severity of their illness. Severity of disease contributes variably to adherence. Although several studies have shown an association between increased disease severity and increased adherence, others have failed to show a connection, particularly in patients with a chronic illness such as cystic fibrosis or juvenile rheumatoid arthritis.[9] The third facet of the model involves the patient's perceived benefit of treatment. For example, adolescents with HIV have been shown to be more compliant with therapies that they believe improve their quality of life.[10] In the fourth part of the model, patients must weigh the possible benefits of treatment against the "cost" or barriers to adherence, including expense, physical discomfort, and psychological stress.

### ENVIRONMENTAL FACTORS

In attempting to adhere to a treatment regimen, adolescents function in an environment with unique challenges. Compared to adult patients, adolescents have less privacy, mobility, and financial independence, and are subject to school regulations, as well as family and peer pressure. Family support and structure are important components of adherence. Smaller, 2-parent families with stable housing have been associated with improved adherence.[9] Improved adherence has also been associated with parents who are supportive, flexible, and able to problem solve.[11] Too much parental control may decrease adherence by provoking autonomy struggles and rebellion, but some parental involvement is essential. A study of family teamwork in adolescents with diabetes found that parents and teens working together to manage the illness could improve outcomes.[12]

Peer influence can be difficult to differentiate from parental influence. Peers are overwhelmingly important to adolescents, and their influence on adherence can be either negative or positive. When the course of a disease or its treatment affects an adolescent's ability to conform to the peer group, nonadherence may result. Conversely, in selected circumstances, interventions focusing on maintaining a normal appearance and level of activity (eg, medication to improve acne or control asthma) may be helpful in improving adherence. However, if high-dose oral corticosteroids are required to control a disease, the resulting Cushingoid appearance may hinder adherence. Peer counseling also is effective in increasing adherence through positive peer modeling.[13]

### PROVIDER–PATIENT RELATIONSHIP

The relationship between the health care provider and an adolescent can affect adherence. Adolescents who are happy with their clinician and the care provided are more likely to be compliant.[14] In 1 study, the adolescent's belief that the provider would be honest predicted adherence with appointments for repeat Papanicolaou smears.[5] Adolescents need ample time during their visits for questions and answers. They also need to be treated with respect and assured of at least some measure of confidentiality.

### TREATMENT REGIMEN

Many aspects of the treatment regimen itself can influence adherence. Adolescents, like adults, are less compliant with more complex regimens. Unexpected or undesirable side effects also decrease the likelihood of adherence, as does a longer duration of therapy. Palatability of medications can also be problematic; for example, many patients with asthma do not like the taste of inhalers.

### EFFECT OF CHRONIC DISEASE

Chronic illness, defined as an illness that "requires at least 6 months of continuous medical care, permanent lifestyle changes, and continuous behavioral adaptation to the unpredictable course of the illness,"[15] is a major determinant of adherence. Chronic illness tends to intensify the determinants of nonadherence as they become intertwined with the disease process, and adolescents with chronic illnesses may have decreased adherence compared to both adults and younger children. The physiological effects of the illness itself may interfere with normal pubertal growth and development, resulting in altered body image and poor self-esteem. Caring for the illness may result in family and autonomy conflicts, as well as disturbed peer relationships. In addition, adolescents with chronic diseases can have increased likelihood for depression and anxiety.

### PREVENTIVE TREATMENTS

Preventive treatment, particularly that involving asymptomatic disease and lifestyle changes, is associated with nonadherence. Overweight and obesity in adolescents is rapidly increasing in prevalence and may be viewed as a form of nonadherence to dietary and activity recommendations. The promotion of overeating and sedentary lifestyle behaviors contributes to the problem.

## INTERVENTION STRATEGIES FOR IMPROVING ADHERENCE

As our understanding of the determinants of adherence increases, it is clear that there is no single intervention for nonadherence. Indeed, there are many interventions from which to choose. Providers must assess an adolescent's reasons for nonadherence, such as whether (1) the patient does not know what is expected of him or her; (2) the patient lacks the skills or resources needed to implement treatment; (3) the patient lacks confidence in his or her ability to implement treatment; (4) the patient does not believe that implementing the treatment will affect outcome; (5) the patient considers the demands of treatment to be excessive, with a poor cost–benefit ratio; (6) the patient associates negative or nonreinforcing consequences with treatment follow-through; (7) the provider–patient relationship is poor; (8) the patient lacks continuity of care; and (9) characteristics of the clinical setting do not facilitate continuity of care. After these factors are examined, an intervention strategy may be devised (see Box 12-1).

In devising intervention strategies, the clinician should be aware that there are few rigorous research trials of adherence interventions. A recent Cochrane review of adherence to medications indicated that although a variety of simple interventions—including counseling, written information, and phone calls to patients—improved short-term adherence, interventions for longer-term adherence were complex and relatively ineffective with respect to clinical outcomes.[16]

### EDUCATIONAL STRATEGIES

Educational strategies designed to increase an adolescent's knowledge about the illness and its therapy can improve adherence. Taking into account the developmental stage and cognitive level of an adolescent, the practitioner must be aware of his or her ability to identify, explain, and solve complex problems. When teaching

## Box 12-1

### *Interventions to Improve Adherence*

*Educational Interventions*

- Detail correct procedures both verbally and in writing.
- Emphasize the benefits of the treatment regimen.
- Counsel regarding expected side effects and their management.
- Describe prognosis with and without adherence.
- Inform of conceptual basis of disease.

*Behavioral Interventions*

- Consider formal goal setting.
- Contract with patient for adherence.
- Establish behavioral cues for medication taking.
- Institute self-monitoring gradually.

*Enlisting Family Support*

- Involve parent in direct supervision of treatment.
- Enlist parent in providing general support for adherence.
- Enlist peers in providing support to the adolescent.

*Tailoring of Treatment Regimen*

- Minimize number of drugs and dosage frequency.
- Choose regimens with minimal side effects.
- Listen to the patient and negotiate possible treatment options.
- Increase number and duration of visits with continuity of providers.

adolescents about the skills needed to carry out the treatment protocol, that information should be presented both in verbal and reader-appropriate written form, and should be brief, organized, and personalized. Providers should also describe the natural history of the disease with and without adherence, but avoid "scare tactics" or overestimating risk. In accordance with the Health Belief Model, adherence among teens with type 1 diabetes improved when providers emphasized the benefits of treatment rather than the risks of nontreatment.[17] However, in clinical practice it is not unusual for an adolescent male with type 1 diabetes to become interested in better adherence to his treatment when he learns that erectile dysfunction is one of the complications of poorly controlled diabetes. Finally, although increased knowledge does not reliably correlate with increased adherence, adolescents should be provided with instruction as to the conceptual basis of the disease and its pathophysiology.

Adolescents also need education about the side effects and goals of treatment so that they may begin therapy with realistic expectations. Patients should be taught techniques to limit the discomfort of procedures, as well as ways to minimize unwanted side effects. The goals of the patient may not match those of the practitioner and need to be recognized as a potential barrier to therapy. This is another reason for the provider and the patient to work toward common goals.

#### BEHAVIORAL STRATEGIES

Education is most effective when combined with behavioral strategies. With self-monitoring, such as readings from outpatient glucometers in diabetes or peak flow meters in asthma, patients can learn to recognize symptoms, anticipate problems, and make adjustments to prevent those problems from occurring. Such feedback loops are reinforcing because they provide adolescents with a sense of control over their symptoms and enhance a sense of autonomy in managing their illness. For adolescents with type 1 diabetes who are able to use an insulin pump, there is a closed electronic feedback loop that provides more precise control of blood glucose levels. Adolescents with diabetes who are able to use an insulin pump effectively are not required to measure blood glucose or have insulin injections several times a day, further enhancing their sense of autonomy. Other behavioral strategies include formalized goal setting and behavioral contracts. Patients can use other health habits, such as tooth brushing in the evening or in the morning, to cue their medication and can devise charts to monitor their progress. Self-administered reminders, such as cell phone alarms, are also effective for some adolescents. As the adolescent learns self-regulatory skills, a slowly graduated assumption of self-care is advised.

#### INVOLVEMENT OF THE FAMILY

Although adolescents gradually assume responsibility for their own health as they develop, family support and involvement are important to their success in becoming and remaining adherent. Ideally, the health care provider should meet with the adolescent and his or her parent(s) and the adolescent alone. Cohesive families with good communication skills enhance adherence. To maximize the positive contribution of the family, parents can help adolescents with their self-monitoring plan and provide regular positive feedback. For instance, family-based behavioral treatments are successful in helping overweight pediatric patients adhere to weight loss regimens.[18] For adolescents who require increased supervision, parents must strike a balance between enhancing and interfering with developing autonomy. If the family interactions are dysfunctional, they can impede adherence, and such families may benefit from mental health services, such as medical family therapy. Parents of adolescents with chronic illnesses may also find parent support groups helpful for the development of coping skills.

**TAILORING THE TREATMENT REGIMEN**

In devising an intervention strategy to facilitate adherence, the adolescent must be considered as a developing individual with unique needs. When confronted with a nonadherent teen, the health care provider should refrain from showing anger or disappointment and instead examine the reasons for nonadherence, allowing the patient to ask questions and express frustrations. The health care provider should empower the adolescent to be an active participant in his or her treatment plan. For example, written action plans for asthma help patients both manage and prevent exacerbations.[19] Providers can negotiate with patients to adjust the regimen in a way that will improve adherence. The fewest number of daily doses and the fewest number of drugs possible should be used. Providers should consider the intrusiveness of the treatment into the patient's life; adolescents are reluctant to take medications at school because it may indicate that they are different from their peers. Allowing the teen to take the medication in the evening—to avoid the schedule fluctuations associated with rushing to school or sleeping late on the weekend—increases adherence.[20] Side effects should be minimized or treated with secondary medications.

Organizational strategies also can be applied to refining the treatment regimen. Increased duration and frequency of visits, particularly a minimal delay between the first and second appointment, may increase adherence. Improving the clinical experience by ensuring continuity of providers also is important and may include visits with the nurse. Clerks may be used to help patients with logistical problems such as transportation and to aid in data collection to reduce appointment waiting times in clinical settings.

**PUBLIC HEALTH INTERVENTIONS**

Public health interventions are essential to promoting adherence to healthy lifestyles. School-based interventions, such as limiting vending machines and offering fruits and vegetables, can potentially decrease obesity by facilitating healthy food choices. Physical activity can be increased with such interventions as enhanced access to outdoor parks and decreased sedentary behaviors.[21]

## CONCLUSION

Adherence issues are shared by the individual adolescent and the provider. Although potentially frustrating for both participants, adherence can be seen as an opportunity to enhance the relationship between the health care provider and the adolescent, as well as to improve the overall health and well-being of the adolescent.

## REFERENCES


1. Kyngäs HA, Kroll T, Duffy ME. Compliance in adolescents with chronic illness: a review. *J Adolesc Health.* 2000;26:379–388

2. Riekert KA, Drotar D. Adherence to medical treatment in pediatric chronic illness: critical issues and answered questions. In: Drotar D, ed. *Promoting Adherence to Medical Treatment in Chronic Childhood Illness: Concepts, Methods, and Interventions.* Mahwah, NJ: Lawrence Erlbaum; 2000:3–32

3. Potter L, Oakley D, de Leon-Wong E, Canamar R. Measuring compliance among oral contraceptive users. *Fam Plann Perspect.* 1996;28(4):154–158

4. Litt IF. Know thyself: adolescents' self-assessment of compliance behavior. *Pediatrics.* 1985;75(4):693–696

5. Kahn JA, Goodman E, Huang B, Slap GB, Emans SJ. Predictors of Papanicolaou smear return in a hospital-based adolescent and young adult clinic. *Obstet Gynecol.* 2003;101:490–499

6. Chigier E. Compliance in adolescents with epilepsy or diabetes. *J Adolesc Health.* 1992;13(5):375–379

7. Osterberg L, Blaschke T. Adherence to medication. *N Engl J Med.* 2005;352:487–497

8. Rosenstock IM. Why people use health services. *Milbank Mem Fund Q.* 1966;44:94–124

9. Staples B, Bravender T. Drug compliance in adolescents: assessing and managing modifiable risk factors. *Pediatr Drugs.* 2002;4(8):503–513

10. Belzer ME, Fuchs DN, Luftman GS, et al. Antiretroviral adherence issues among HIV-positive adolescents and young adults, *J Adolesc Health.* 1999;25(5):316–319

11. Fielding D, Duff A. Compliance with treatment protocols: interventions for children with chronic illness. *Arch Dis Child.* 1999;80:196–200

12. Anderson BJ, Brackett J, Ho J, Laffel LMB. An intervention to promote family teamwork in diabetes management tasks. In: Drotar D, ed. *Promoting Adherence to Medical Treatment in Chronic Childhood Illness: Concepts, Methods, and Interventions.* Mahwah, NJ: Lawrence Erlbaum; 2000:347–365

13. Friedman IM, Litt IF. Adolescents' compliance with therapeutic regimens: psychological and social aspects and intervention. *J Adolesc Health Care.* 1987;8:52–56

14. Kyngäs H, Hentimen M, Barlow JH. Adolescents' perceptions of physicians, nurses, parents, and friends: help or hindrance in compliance with diabetes self-care. *J Adv Nurs.* 1998;27(4):760–769

15. LeBlanc LA, Goldsmith T, Patel DR. Behavioral aspects of chronic illness in children and adolescents. *Pediatr Clin North Am.* 2003;50:859–878

16. Haynes RB, Yao X, Degani A, Kripalani S, Garg A, McDonald HP. Interventions for enhancing medication adherence. *Cochrane Database Syst Rev.* 2008 Apr 16;(2):CD000011

17. Palardy N, Greening L, Ott J, et al. Adolescents' health attitudes and adherence to treatment for IDDM. *J Dev Behav Pediatr.* 1998;19(1):31–37

18. Epstein LH, Paluch RA, Gordy CC, Dorn J. Decreasing sedentary behaviors in treating pediatric obesity. *Arch Pediatr Adolesc Med.* 2000;154:220–226

19. Bhogal S, Zemek R, Ducharme FM. Written action plans for asthma in children. *Cochrane Database Syst Rev.* 2006 Jul 19;(3):CD005306

20. Jonasson G, Carlsen KH, Mowinkel P. Asthma drug adherence in a long-term clinical trial. *Arch Dis Child.* 2000;83(4):330–333

21. Epstein LH, Raja S, Gold SS, Paluch RA, Roemmich JN. Reducing sedentary behavior: the relationship between park area and the physical activity of youth. *Psychol Sci.* 2006;17(8):654–659

SECTION 4

# Health Supervision and Preventive Care

# CHAPTER 13

## Screening in Adolescent Health Care

Jonathan D. Klein, MD, MPH • Kevin K. Makino, BA

### INTRODUCTION

In adolescent health care, screening is a process in which the likelihood that an adolescent has a condition, or has the propensity to develop a condition, is assessed. The goal of screening is to reduce or eliminate morbidity and mortality of preventable or treatable health problems. Because it entails the use of specific measures or tools to determine risk, screening is different from anticipatory guidance. Anticipatory guidance involves communication, generally on an individual level, about common concerns or problems that may be associated with a specific health risk behavior (such as substance use), or an event that may be associated with heightened risk of health problems (such as transition from high school to college). Depending on the goal of a screening activity, it can range from obtaining clinical history using a screening questionnaire, to conducting a specific aspect of a physical examination, to performing laboratory testing.

For example, in some large school districts, high school sports preparticipation evaluations are sometimes conducted on a number of student athletes at a given time in 1 setting, using "stations" staffed by a group of health professionals, each focused on a specific element of the evaluation (history, cardiac examination, musculoskeletal examination). The purpose of this activity is to screen for conditions in which participating in a given sport might put the adolescent or other athletes at risk of illness, injury, or death. Those who "pass" the screening usually are permitted to participate in the sport(s) for which they were screened, whereas those who "fail" the screening procedure require further evaluation, rehabilitation, or some other intervention, before a final decision about participation is made. In this context, key historical data typically are collected on a sports-focused screening questionnaire, including items about injuries, and syncope with exertion. A screening history of fainting with activity suggests aortic stenosis or hypertrophic cardiomyopathy; this would generally result in the adolescent "failing" the screening and referral for further evaluation. If the screening cardiac auscultation were to reveal a murmur suggestive of either of these conditions, high-intensity exercise should be avoided until the adolescent has had a definitive diagnostic evaluation. Some schools include screening for iron deficiency in female athletes because of the relatively high prevalence of anemia in that population.

Used properly, screening is a powerful tool in primary care and can increase the efficiency of a preventive care visit and quickly organize important information, facilitating prioritizing the agenda for a visit. In addition, many screening tests and questionnaires have been validated in clinical trials, ensuring that the information collected is accurate. Unfortunately, recommendations regarding the conditions for which one should screen and the timing of screening can be confusing. Adolescents often are not screened for many of the conditions for which they should be screened.[1] This chapter reviews the elements of appropriate screening for adolescents, discusses current recommendations for adolescent screening, and provides practical tips for implementing screening recommendations into practice. It provides an overview of current recommendations. However, because guidelines are undergoing constant change as evidence-based practice suggests modifications, they focus more on developing the skills needed to interpret and apply recommendations as they emerge.

### THE "APPROPRIATENESS" OF SCREENING

Screening is an invaluable asset in the primary care visit, but like all tools it has limitations. Even noninvasive screening tests can be associated with unforeseen risks and are associated with costs. Thus, the decision regarding when a screening test is considered "appropriate" should be based on a consideration of the condition or disease for which the screen is designed, the test(s) used for the screening, and the population or individual being screened.

Although screening is a clinical construct, an understanding of the underlying epidemiologic concepts and mathematical equations is required to fully appreciate the appropriate use and application of screening tests. More detailed explanations (including the equations underlying these principles) are available in epidemiology texts.[2]

## DISEASE CHARACTERISTICS

Because the courses of disease follow different trajectories, some conditions are more suitable targets for screening than others. For screening to be justified in a given population, the condition being screened for should possess certain characteristics. First, it should be a health problem with significant morbidity or mortality, or a large burden of suffering. Screening for relatively minor conditions is not cost-effective, especially if applied to the entire population. Second, the condition should have an asymptomatic period in its course, during which periodic screening could identify cases before individuals present with symptoms. If symptoms arise with the onset of illness, screening is less valuable because the symptoms would likely lead to presentation and diagnosis. Third, early intervention or treatment, initiated before the adolescent would have presented with symptoms, must be able to alter the course and clinical outcome. If there is no treatment able to alter the course of illness, or if there is no effective treatment, then screening is difficult to justify.

## TEST CHARACTERISTICS: SENSITIVITY AND SPECIFICITY

Assuming that a condition is a suitable target for screening based on the 3 disease characteristics listed previously, it is necessary to identify a screening tool with appropriate test characteristics. Important test characteristics include sensitivity and specificity. A screening test with 100% *sensitivity* is positive in *all* individuals who have the condition being tested for. A screening test with 100% *specificity* is positive *only* in individuals who have the condition being tested for. An optimal screening test would have 100% sensitivity and 100% specificity, meaning that *every* individual having a positive test would actually have the condition (true positive), and *no* individual with a negative test would actually have the condition (true negative).

Many screening tests are characterized by an inverse relationship between sensitivity and specificity. For example, if the nature of a condition dictates the need for a screening test that identifies affected individuals with a positive test, it would be appropriate to use a test with very high sensitivity. This could be accomplished by setting a very low cutoff threshold for a "positive" result. However, setting a low threshold for a positive test to achieve extremely high sensitivity tends to be associated with more false-positive tests, in which individuals who do not have the condition have a positive screening test. Whether the screening measure is the level of human chorionic gonadotropin (hCG) in a urine pregnancy test, or systolic blood pressure in hypertension screening, for many tests the upper and/or lower thresholds are set at the "normal physiologic range." In addition, the ability of a test to measure a biologic marker, such as urine hCG or substances of abuse, is related to its sensitivity and specificity. These same considerations apply to the physical examination and to history-based screens. For example, asking an adolescent "Do you ever feel extremely sad?" is a more sensitive but less specific screen for depression than asking "Have you ever been so depressed that you thought about taking your own life?" In general, screening tests are designed to have a higher sensitivity than specificity, because the goal is to identify those patients at a high enough risk to justify further evaluation—often requiring additional measures or diagnostic tests to identify those who do or do not have the condition for further testing or treatment. By comparison, diagnostic tests tend to have much higher specificity, but are often more expensive, invasive, and/or time-consuming than screening tests, as their major intent is to identify those with a specific condition.

## POPULATION CHARACTERISTICS

Sensitivity and specificity are core concepts for understanding the performance of any test, and are usually the first (sometimes the only) information available about a particular screening tool. However, they provide limited information regarding the interpretation of a positive or negative test result for a specific patient. In clinical settings, it is important to know the likelihood that an adolescent truly has a condition if a test is positive (positive predictive value, PPV) or does not have a condition if the test is negative (negative predictive value, NPV). Thus, to interpret a test result, one needs to know not only the sensitivity and specificity of the screening test, but also the pretest probability of the specific condition under consideration. This is usually estimated using the prevalence of the condition or disease in a representative population of which the adolescent is a member.

A screening test will either be positive (the adolescent seems to have the condition) or negative (the adolescent does not seem to have the condition). In addition,

**Table 13-1**

**Two-by-Two Table of Screening Test Results and Condition Status**

| | *Adolescent Patient Status* | |
|---|---|---|
| *Screening Test Result* | *Condition Present* | *Condition Absent* |
| Positive test: Appears to have the condition | a true positive (TP) | b false positive (FP) |
| Negative test: Appears to not have the condition | c false negative (FN) | d true negative (TN) |
| | Sensitivity of test = a ÷ (a + c) | Specificity of test = d ÷ (b + d) |

the adolescent being screened either has the condition under consideration or does not have it. Thus, there are 4 possible combinations, based on the screening test result and the patient's status, that can be sorted into a 2-by-2 table (Table 13-1). The common notation of the 4 cells in this classification is: a = true positive (TP) in which the test positive and the condition is present; b = false positive (FP) in which the test is positive but the adolescent does not have the condition; c = false negative (FN) in which the test is negative, but the adolescent actually has the condition being screened for; and d = true negative (TN) in which the test is negative and the adolescent does not have the condition.

The PPV of a screening test is the probability that an adolescent who has a positive test result actually has the condition being screened for. It is the ratio of TP results to the total number of positive results in a population (TP ÷ [TP + FP]). Similarly, the NPV is the probability that an adolescent who has a negative test result actually does not have the condition (TN ÷ [TN + FN]). The PPV and NPV provide information about the usefulness of the test based on the test result, shown as the row a patient is assigned to in Table 13-1. In contrast, sensitivity and specificity provide information on the value of the test based on the adolescent's actual health status, as depicted by their column in Table 13-1.

Screening test performance is affected by disease prevalence. For example, if a test with a sensitivity of 0.93 and specificity of 0.89 were used to screen a population of 1,000 patients, its PPV and NPV would change dramatically depending on whether the population carried a low (1%) or higher (40%) chance of having the condition being tested, as shown in Table 13-2.

The determination of the need for a screening test for an adolescent patient from a low-risk population depends on the severity of the condition and the sensitivity and specificity of the test. However, if an adolescent population has only a 1% pretest likelihood of having a condition, and the performance characteristics of the screening test include 93% sensitivity and 89% specificity, fewer than 8% of patients with a positive test will have the condition being screened for. Therefore, a screening

**Table 13-2**

**Variability of Pretest Positive Predictive Value (PPV) Relative to Low- vs High-Prevalence Adolescent Population Characteristics**

| | *Low-Risk (Prevalence = 0.01)* | | | *High-Risk (Prevalence = 0.40)* | | |
|---|---|---|---|---|---|---|
| *Screening Test Result* | *Condition Present* | *Condition Absent* | *Total* | *Condition Present* | *Condition Absent* | *Total* |
| Positive | 9 (TP) | 109 (FP) | 118 positive | 372 (TP) | 66 (FP) | 438 positive |
| Negative | 1 (FN) | 881 (TN) | 882 negative | 28 (FN) | 534 (TN) | 562 negative |
| Total | 10 | 990 | 1,000 | 400 | 600 | 1,000 |
| PPV = TP ÷ (TP + FP) | | 9 ÷ (9 + 109) = 7.9% | | | 372 ÷ (372 + 66) = 84.9% | |
| NPV = TN ÷ (TN + FN) | | 881 ÷ (881 + 1) = 99.9% | | | 534 ÷ (534 + 28) = 95.0% | |

Test characteristics: Sensitivity of test = 0.93; specificity of test = 0.89.

test with these characteristics would probably not be recommended for general use in a low-risk population. In contrast, the same test might be very useful in screening a high-risk population in which the prevalence is 40%, because its predictive power for both positive and negative results would both be in the 85% to 95% range.

### RISKS OF INAPPROPRIATE SCREENING

The importance of determining the appropriateness of screening extends beyond the need for useful test results. False-positive results may cause harm to an adolescent due to the emotional stress that can occur when a healthy adolescent believes that she or he has a condition based on a positive screening test result. There can also be significant stigmatization from inappropriate labeling with FP results. Physical harm can also result from unnecessary invasive follow-up testing or presumptive treatment. Unnecessary costs can also be incurred with a FP test that requires diagnostic work-up and follow-up. False-negative screening tests may also cause harm by providing false reassurance to those who actually have a condition. This could result in delayed diagnosis, increased likelihood of disease transmission in the case of contagious diseases, and increased morbidity or mortality.

If the previous requirements (for the condition, the screening test, and the population) are satisfied, screening allows clinicians to identify patients at higher risk for developing serious conditions, and to take action to minimize those risks. Many screening tests meet these criteria. A variety of groups review the scientific literature and make up-to-date screening recommendations (see Useful Web Sites for specific links to guidelines for screening for priority health risks of youth). Clinicians tend to adapt guidelines and recommendations to their specific patient population and the available resources.

## SCREENING RECOMMENDATIONS

This section summarizes current recommendations for adolescent screening by various professional and scientific organizations in the context of a well-adolescent preventive care visit. It focuses on the most commonly recommended and widely available screens, including a chart of screens and the recommended follow-ups for each (Table 13-3). These recommendations have a strong evidence base; however, guidelines tend to change over time as new technology and new information becomes available. Therefore,

**Table 13-3**

**Recommended Screenings**

| *Screening Recommendation* | *Suggested Follow-Up for Positive Result* | *Strength of Recommendation* |
|---|---|---|
| **Demographic Information/Before the Visit** | | |
| Special settings (Chs. 24–28) and populations (Chs. 29–31) | | |
| Patient is homeless | Screen for TB, HIV | *** |
| Patient is incarcerated (Ch. 27) | Screen for TB, HIV, syphilis | *** |
| Treatment setting is high-risk for HIV | Screen for HIV infection | *** |
| Patient lived in an area with high TB prevalence | Screen for TB | *** |
| Patient's population prevalence for infectious diseases | | |
| ≥1% prevalence of HIV infection | Screen for HIV | *** |
| High prevalence of syphilis (on the basis of geography and ethnicity) | Screen for syphilis | ** |
| **Family History** | | |
| Elevated cardiovascular risk | Screen fasting lipid levels | *** |
| **Past Medical and Surgical History** | | |
| Hearing loss | Objective hearing test | ** |
| Vision loss | Objective vision test | ** |
| History of sexually transmitted infection (STI) | Consider screening for other STIs | *** |
| **Social History** | | |
| Home environment and family relationships | | |

*(Continued)*

**Table 13-3 (Continued)**

| *Screening Recommendation* | *Suggested Follow-Up for Positive Result* | *Strength of Recommendation* |
|---|---|---|
| Exposure to abuse and/or neglect | Refer to appropriate agency and to a mental health professional | ** |
| School and peers | | |
| Academic performance | GAPS: "Adolescents with a history of truancy, repeated absences, or poor or declining performance should be assessed for the presence of conditions that could interfere with school success. These include learning disability, attention-deficit/hyperactivity disorder, medical problems, abuse, family dysfunction, mental disorder, or alcohol or other drug use" | *** |
| Exposure to violence (bullying/gangs/intimate partner violence) | | * |
| Sexuality | | |
| Sexual identity | GLBTQ patients may be at higher risk for exposure to violence or threatening behavior, depression, and high-risk behavior | ** |
| Sexual history | All sexually active adolescents should be screened for HIV infection, unless the prevalence of undiagnosed HIV infection among their population has been documented as $< 0.1\%$. Sexually active females should have an annual pelvic exam and annual screening for gonorrhea and chlamydia. Adolescents engaging in high-risk behaviors (men who have sex with men, trading sex for drugs and money, having multiple sex partners, or having a partner who is high-risk) should also be screened for syphilis | *** |
| Mental and emotional health | | |
| Depression and suicidal ideation | Refer to a mental health professional | ** |
| Body image | Refer to a mental health professional | ** |
| **Health Behaviors** | | |
| Substance use (general screen) (Also see Chapter 15) | | |
| Any substance (alcohol, tobacco, prescription or OTC medications, illicit substances) | Advise on cessation, refer to a mental health professional | *** |
| Intravenous drug user | Vaccinate against HAV, HBV; screen for HIV, HCV, syphilis | *** |
| **Physical Exam** | | |
| Vital signs | | |
| Height and weight/BMI | Overweight: Conduct dietary and health assessment to determine cardiovascular risk and design potential intervention strategy if BMI $\geq$ 95th percentile for age, or if BMI $\geq$ 85th percentile for age and has increased by at least 2 units in the past year or the patient is otherwise at high risk for cardiovascular disease | *** |

*(Continued)*

**Table 13-3 (Continued)**

| *Screening Recommendation* | *Suggested Follow-Up for Positive Result* | *Strength of Recommendation* |
|---|---|---|
| Blood pressure | Evaluate for essential versus secondary hypertension, and follow up as appropriate | ** |
| Genitourinary | | |
| Pelvic examination (sexually active females) | Follow up as appropriate | *** |
| Ranking System: | | |
| *** = universally recommended, strong evidence | | |
| ** = generally recommended, fair evidence | | |
| * = recommended by some; inconsistent evidence | | |
| GLBTQ, gay/lesbian/bisexual/transgender/questioning; HIV, human immunodeficiency virus; TB, tuberculosis | | |

Web site addresses for professional societies and scientific bodies that generate high-quality screening guidelines have been provided at the end of this chapter to help readers in using the most current guidelines.

Most of the following screening recommendations pertain to the patient history component of the visit, although some are tied to the physical examination; laboratory screenings are addressed separately in Chapter 9. It is important to note that if certain topics are not covered in this section, it does not mean that these topics should not be discussed with patients. Many important issues (eg, seat belt and helmet usage) are better addressed by anticipatory guidance than by screening, as discussed in Chapter 15 of this textbook.

## BEFORE THE VISIT

In establishing the agenda for adolescent well visits, providers should take into account demographic considerations based on their knowledge of the patient to be seen. For new patients, this information is collected during the visit. As discussed in the previous section, population disease prevalence is a critical factor in determining the conditions for which a screening test might be appropriate. For example, it is recommended that patients in high-prevalence settings and geographic areas be screened for sexually transmitted infections (STIs) regardless of individual risk factors. In particular, providers may consider screening some patients for syphilis on the basis of population risk, the prevalence of which varies both by region (higher in the South and in certain metropolitan regions) and ethnicity (higher among Hispanics and blacks than in whites). Readers can access information online about their specific area's STI prevalence rates, as well as available programs and services, at the National Center for HIV/AIDS, Viral Hepatitis, STI, and tuberculosis (TB) prevention Web sites, the addresses for which are provided at the conclusion of this chapter. In addition to geographic and demographic considerations, adolescents seen in non-office-based settings (such as at a school-based health clinic, detention facility, or military setting) or who belong to special populations (including immigrant children or children with special health care needs) may also be at exceptionally high risk for certain conditions and should be screened accordingly.

## MEDICAL AND SURGICAL HISTORY

Certain elements in the medical and surgical history are particularly useful for screening. For example, asking adolescents if they have noticed any loss of hearing or vision in the past year can be helpful in determining which patients may need objective testing. Another high-yield question is to ask about a history of STI. Patients who have had an STI in the past are at significantly higher risk for subsequent infections and should be screened thoroughly.

## SOCIAL HISTORY

The confidential social history provides a critical opportunity to ask high-yield screening questions. Because many health risk behaviors covary, although not necessarily being causally related to each other, the identification of 1 such behavior should lead to an exploration of commonly associated behaviors. For example, adolescents who have academic difficulty are more likely to have mental health concerns and engage in risky behaviors. Gay/lesbian/bisexual/transgender/questioning (GLBTQ) adolescents are more likely to suffer from depression. When patients screen positive for one such factor, providers should recognize that their pretest likelihood for the associated concern—the patient's baseline risk—goes up, and thus they should prioritize screening for associated conditions as well.

Important topics to ask all adolescents about include exposure to violence (at home, with peers, or in relationships) and the adolescent's perceptions of school and academic performance, which may be related to unrecognized learning disabilities, medical problems, abuse, substance use, or depression. When discussing sexuality, patients should be asked about their sexual identity and feelings, as well as their sexual behaviors. Finally, clinicians should specifically ask whether a patient has experienced depressive symptoms or suicidal ideation.

### HEALTH BEHAVIORS

Providers should ask all adolescents about their substance use history, including alcohol, tobacco, illicit substances, and recreational use of prescription and over-the-counter medications. If the patient reports having used illicit substances, it is important to inquire about intravenous drug use as well.

### PHYSICAL EXAMINATION

The physical examination in a preventive care visit is designed primarily to establish baseline measurements for the adolescent and to monitor for physical abnormalities of potential concern. These features make it a nonspecific screening maneuver because, in the absence of symptoms or history, the likelihood of identifying a new abnormality on physical examination is small. Because this textbook contains a separate chapter devoted to the physical examination and laboratory screening (see Chapter 9), only 2 components of the examination specifically thought of as screening will be addressed in this section. The patient's height and weight should be used to calculate body mass index (BMI) percentile, which in turn allows the clinician to determine over- or underweight, and therefore risk of cardiovascular disease, eating disorders, or metabolic disease. In late 2009, the American College of Obstetricians and Gynecologists recommended that females, regardless of sexual activity history, should not have a Pap test before age 21, after which routine Pap is only needed every other year. See Chapter 60, Cervical Findings and the Pap Smear for more comprehensive information.

### THE EVOLUTION OF SCREENING GUIDELINES

The screening tests described previously are supported by research and are expected to remain stable well into the future. However, recommendations change over time as new evidence enters the literature. For example, although scoliosis screening has historically been a cornerstone of adolescent physical examination screening, recent concerns over potential risks due to treatment of nonclinically significant disease have led to its removal from many guidelines.[3] Similar concerns have led to the removal of recommendations for teaching patients to perform breast self-examinations.[4] Other research has led to stronger recommendations—better treatment options and changing population risks have led to broader HIV screening guidelines that support the screening of all sexually active adolescents.[5] To stay abreast of future changes in the evidence base for screenings, readers are advised to take advantage of the resources offered by primary care societies (eg, the American Academy of Pediatrics) and by the US Preventive Services Task Force (USPSTF), the Web addresses for both of which are provided at the conclusion of this chapter.

## PRACTICAL TIPS FOR IMPLEMENTATION

As discussed previously, numerous clinical studies have shown that adolescent screening tests are underperformed, often to a greater degree than providers realize. This final section presents proven strategies to help readers avoid some of the pitfalls responsible for this trend[6–10] and includes tips that pertain to practice structure and organization as well as for individual providers.

One of the most important requirements for consistently performing screening is making the time to do so. Computerized scheduling systems can help plan annual preventive service visits for patients; similarly, prompting or decision-support systems can remind providers when scheduled screens are overdue so that they can be incorporated into the patient's clinical encounter. Other tools can help ensure that all opportunities for screening within each visit are taken advantage of. The most common of these are written patient questionnaires or trigger questionnaires, such as those available from Bright Futures, adapted from earlier efforts by the Guidelines for Adolescent Preventive Services (GAPS) forms.

In screening for healthy and risk behaviors, it is also important for a practice to identify resources to help clinicians, adolescents, and families respond to problems or issues identified. Preparation to respond to issues that are identified in screening includes making use of counseling and health promotion adjuncts, both delivered in the office and/or linked to community resources. Use of clinical staff other than physicians in the care setting can not only facilitate these interactions but can also be a more efficient and cost-effective use of clinical resources. Large practices may consider having health educators, nutritionists, or mental health professionals on-site for easy referral and treatment of patients. Providers may also choose to pursue opportunities to learn skills in communicating information to patients, assessing patients' readiness to change behaviors, and negotiating action plans.

## INTERNET RESOURCES

- Bright Futures: brightfutures.aap.org/index.html. "A national health promotion and disease prevention initiative that addresses children's health needs in the context of family and community." Materials include the *Bright Futures Guidelines for Health Supervision of Infants, Children, and Adolescents*, a downloadable chart of the Bright Futures/American Academy of Pediatrics *Recommendations for Preventive Pediatric Health Care*, and numerous other resources.
- US Preventive Services Task Force (USPSTF): www.ahrq.gov/clinic/USpstfix.htm. "An independent panel of experts in primary care and prevention that systematically reviews the evidence of effectiveness and develops recommendations for clinical preventive services." The Web site includes links to topic-specific recommendations and documentation (including e-mail updates for new or revised recommendations), a downloadable *Pocket Guide to Clinical Preventive Services*, and the free Electronic Preventive Services Selector (ePSS) software for PDAs.
- The American Medical Association (AMA) Guidelines for Adolescent Preventive Services (GAPS): www.ama-assn.org/ama/pub/physician-resources/public-health/promoting-healthy-lifestyles/adolescent-health/guidelines-adolescent-preventive-services.shtml. "A comprehensive set of recommendations that provides a framework for the organization and content of preventive health services... designed to be delivered ideally as a preventive services package during a series of annual health visits between the ages of 11–21." The Web site includes links to the *GAPS Recommendations Monograph* and downloadable screening questionnaires in English and Spanish for use with younger adolescents, middle/older adolescents, and parents/guardians.
- The Society for Adolescent Health and Medicine (SAHM): www.adolescenthealth.org/. "A multidisciplinary organization of health professionals who are committed to advancing the health and well-being of adolescents." The Web site includes links to the organization's position papers and position statements on a wide range of topics, including *Clinical Preventive Services for Adolescents*.
- The Centers for Disease Control and Prevention (CDC) Guide to Community Preventive Services (www.thecommunityguide.org/index.html) is a free resource to help choose programs and policies to improve health and prevent disease in a community. Systematic reviews are used to address which program and policy interventions have been proven effective, and what effective interventions cost. Additionally, CDC's National Center for HIV/AIDS, Viral Hepatitis, STD, and TB Prevention: www.cdc.gov/nchhstp/stateprofiles/usmap.htm. "State Profiles include statistical and other information on HIV/AIDS, Viral Hepatitis, STD, and TB for all 50 states and Washington, District of Columbia, as of September 2007. They also include descriptions of prevention and control programs supported by CDC and state public health officials."

## REFERENCES


1. Halpern-Felsher BL, Ozer EM, Millstein SG, et al. Preventive services in a health maintenance organization: how well do pediatricians screen and educate adolescent patients? *Arch Pediatr Adolesc Med.* 2000;154:173–179

2. Gordis L. *Epidemiology.* 3rd ed. Philadelphia, PA: Saunders; 2004

3. US Preventive Services Task Force. *Screening for idiopathic scoliosis in adolescents: a brief evidence update for the US Preventive Services Task Force*; 2004

4. Kosters JP, Gotzsche PC. Regular self-examination or clinical examination for early detection of breast cancer. *Cochrane Database of Systematic Reviews.* 2007;2

5. Branson BM, Handsfield HH, Lampe MA, et al. Centers for Disease Control and Prevention (CDC). Revised recommendations for HIV testing of adults, adolescents, and pregnant women in health-care settings. *MMWR Recomm Rep.* 2006;55:1–17

6. Klein JD, Allan MJ, Elster AB, et al. Improving adolescent preventive care in community health centers. *Pediatrics.* 2001;107:318–327

7. Bordley WC, Margolis PA, Stuart J, Lannon C, Keyes L. Improving preventive service delivery through office systems. *Pediatrics.* 2001;108:E41

8. Lustig JL, Ozer EM, Adams SH, et al. Improving the delivery of adolescent clinical preventive services through skills-based training. *Pediatrics.* 2001;107:1100–1107

9. Ozer EM, Adams SH, Lustig JL, et al. Can it be done? Implementing adolescent clinical preventive services. *Health Serv Res.* 2001;36:150–165

10. Klein JD, Sesselberg TS, Gawronski B, Handwerker L, Gesten F, Schettine A. Improving adolescent preventive services through state, managed care, and community partnerships. *J Adolesc Health.* 2003;32:91–97

# CHAPTER 14

# Immunizations

AMY B. MIDDLEMAN, MD, MSED, MPH

Immunizations have long been a pillar of infant and childhood preventive care. For many years, adolescents were considered to have outgrown the need for vaccines with the exception of the tetanus/diphtheria (Td) booster needed to enter either middle or high school, depending on state regulations. However, in recent years, several new vaccines have been developed that specifically target the adolescent age group, and more vaccines appropriate for adolescents are in development. The concept of vaccinating throughout the adolescent and adult years to prevent disease is becoming an important public health activity.

## RECENT EVOLUTION OF VACCINES FOR ADOLESCENTS IN THE UNITED STATES

Prior to 1995, the Advisory Committee on Immunization Practices (ACIP), the advisory group to the Centers for Disease Control and Prevention (CDC) on national immunization recommendations, published the recommended immunization schedule only periodically.The first schedule was published in 1983 and included 3 vaccination series: diphtheria/pertussis/tetanus, oral polio virus, and measles/mumps/rubella (DPT, OPV, MMR), plus the Td booster for 14- to 16-year-old adolescents. The second schedule, published in 1989 included the *H influenza* vaccine recommendation, and the third schedule in 1994 included the hepatitis B virus (HBV) vaccination recommendations (www.cdc.gov/vaccines/recs/acip/default.htm). Of particular interest, there were no adolescent recommendations in the 1994 immunization schedule, illustrating the lack of emphasis from a national perspective on vaccination of the adolescent age group.

More recently, the CDC has been working to develop a standard immunization platform for the 11- to 12-year age group. Beginning in 1995, the immunization schedule was endorsed by the CDC, the American Academy of Pediatrics (AAP), and the American Academy of Family Physicians (AAFP). This was the first schedule that specifically indicated that the Td booster could be given at an 11- to 12-year medical visit (www.cdc.gov/vaccines/recs/acip/default.htm). The CDC, AAP, AAFP, and the American Medical Association (AMA) anticipated the need for further focus on adolescent immunization as early as 1996 when they published the first recommendation for improving vaccination coverage among adolescents.[1] By this time, the Td was not the only adolescent vaccine recommended for adolescents. In 1995, the ACIP recommended HBV vaccination for all 11- to 12-year-olds who had not previously received the vaccination series; in 1996, the immunization schedule included the first universal vaccination recommendation for adolescents since the first recommendation of the Td booster at age 14 to 16 years old in 1983. Construction of the 11- to 12-year-old immunization platform had begun.

### SPECIFIC VACCINATION RECOMMENDATIONS FOR ADOLESCENTS

There are multiple new recommendations that utilize the 11- to 12-year immunization platform as well as several older vaccination recommendations that require attention during the adolescent years. Adolescent recommendations are addressed now on the second page of the ever-expanding Immunization Schedule. This schedule is updated and reformatted annually, and the most updated schedule is always easily available on the CDC Web site (www.cdc.gov).

There are several standing vaccination recommendations for adolescents. The HBV has been recommended universally for neonates since 1991; since 1997 ACIP has recommended HBV vaccine for unvaccinated 0- to 18-year-olds.[2] Up to the 19th birthday any adolescent who has not previously received or completed the vaccination series should receive needed doses.[3] Recommendations are currently primarily risk-based for adolescents 19 years of age and older, although all adults requesting vaccination against HBV should receive the vaccination without having to acknowledge a specific risk factor.[4] Hepatitis A vaccination recommendations were recently updated in 2006.[5] Again, although universal vaccination recommendations exist for those 12 to 23 months of age, children older than age 2 years can be vaccinated at subsequent visits. "Catch-up" vaccination is recommended for adolescents with specific risk factors (eg, chronic liver disease, clotting disorders, men having sex with men, use of injection and noninjection illicit drugs, plans to travel to an endemic area) or for those who live in states, counties, or communities that currently maintain hepatitis A immunization programs; "catch-up" can be considered for all other adolescents. Efficacy data for these and all adolescent vaccines are listed in Table 14-1.

Other consistent recommendations include appropriate catch-up for any missed inactivated polio vaccine (IPV), MMR, or varicella (2 doses are currently recommended for all vaccine recipients)[6] vaccines for all adolescents. Adolescents in specific high-risk categories also require catch-up using the polysaccharide pneumococcal vaccine (www.cdc.gov/vaccines/recs/schedules).

## INFLUENZA VACCINE

Influenza disease symptoms include fever, sore throat, dry cough, gastrointestinal symptoms, headache, extreme fatigue, and muscle aches. It is transmitted primarily through respiratory droplets. Approximately 36,000 Americans die each year from seasonal flu. Recently, an increasing number of pediatric deaths have been associated with coinfection with methicillin-resistant *Staphylococcus aureus*. Vaccination against influenza represents a unique challenge as recommendations now include annual universal immunization of all those 6 months of age and older with influenza vaccine.

Healthy adolescents can receive the live attenuated influenza vaccine (LAIV). It is especially important to assure vaccination of chronically ill youth and those in specific risk categories (most of whom should receive the inactivated vaccine) including: (1) those receiving long-term aspirin therapy; (2) females who will be pregnant during the flu season; and (3) those with chronic disorders of the pulmonary or cardiovascular system, chronic metabolic disease, hemoglobinopathies, immunodeficiency, and other disorders.[7] Coverage rates are historically low for this vulnerable population; data from the Behavior Risk Factor Surveillance System collected in February 2005 demonstrated 35% coverage among those aged 2 to 17 years who had 1 or more high-risk medical conditions during 2004–2005.[7]

High coverage rates are desirable to prevent epidemic spread of seasonal flu, but immunization against seasonal flu also serves a potential role in the prevention of pandemic influenza. As more people are immunized against seasonal flu and less virus circulates, there is theoretically less opportunity for recombination of human influenza A strains with viruses of animal origin—the first step in creating potentially deadly new virus strains with pandemic potential. The likelihood of adherence among adolescents for this and other vaccines may be enhanced by newer technologies for vaccine administration such as live attenuated intranasal vaccine and more concentrated delivery efforts to the adolescent population (see the section following, entitled "Policy Improvements to Enhance Adolescent Immunization Rates").

## TDAP VACCINE

Pertussis, caused by *Bordetella pertussis* bacterium, is referred to as the "100-day cough"; it often starts with symptoms similar to the common cold, yet it causes disease symptoms that include paroxysmal coughing, difficulty sleeping, post-tussive vomiting, apnea, cyanosis, and pneumonia. Treatment for the disease is symptomatic only. Vaccination against pertussis has been a mainstay of childhood vaccination since the DPT vaccine was developed in the 1940s. More recently the vaccine incorporated an acellular pertussis component that has been available since 1991 (DTaP). Until the tetanus, diphtheria, and acellular pertussis (Tdap) vaccine was developed, there was no pertussis vaccine indicated for use in those 7 years of age and older because of the risk profile of the vaccine. Data indicate that the incidence of pertussis in the late 1990s was significant in the United States and that the incidence among adolescents was the highest of the age groups between 10 and 49 years of age. Immunity to pertussis wanes 5 to 8 years after natural disease and vaccination.[8] Teens have therefore been left particularly vulnerable to disease outbreaks and serve as potential conduits of disease to vulnerable infants, children, and adults. Studies suggested that approximately 1 million cases of pertussis occur annually in the United States among those older than 15 years of age.[9] Reported cases of pertussis often occurred in the context of middle and high school outbreaks, with increased spread of disease resulting from delay in diagnosis.[9]

In 2005, 2 formulations of Tdap vaccines were approved for single-dose use by the Food and Drug Administration (FDA), 1 for 10- to 18-year-olds (the indication has subsequently been expanded to include 10- through 64-year-olds), the other for 11- to 64-year-olds. The tetanus and diphtheria components are similar to those found in the Td booster. The ACIP/AAP-approved recommendations for use of Tdap among adolescents 11 to 18 years of age are to receive Tdap in place of Td for booster immunization at 11 to 12 years of age. Originally a 5-year interval was encouraged between Td and Tdap to decrease the risk of local/systemic reactions. To simplify recommendations, and due to lack of data supporting intervals, language regarding intervals was removed from the Tdap recommendations in October 2010. It is ideal to administer Tdap and the MCV4 vaccine simultaneously. (Both vaccines contain diphtheria toxoid, and serial administration may increase the risk of reactions.)[9]

**Table 14-1**

## Adolescent Vaccines and Their Efficacy

| *Vaccine* | *Trade Name* | *Manufacturer* | *Dose* | *Recommended Schedule (for Multiple Dose Regimens)* | *Reported Efficacy/Seroprotection* |
|---|---|---|---|---|---|
| Hepatitis A vaccine (HAV) | **Havrix** | GlaxoSmithKline | 12 months through 18 years: 0.5 ml ≥19 years: 1.0 ml Intramuscularly (IM) | 0, 6–12 months | Approximately 100% seroconversion with 2 doses in all age groups[10] |
| | **Vaqta** | Merck | 12 months through 18 years: 0.5 ml IM ≥19 yrs: 1.0 ml IM | 0, 6–18 months | Approximately 100% seroconversion with 2 doses in all age groups[11] |
| Hepatitis A/Hepatitis B vaccine | **Twinrix** | GlaxoSmithKline | ≥18 years: 1.0 ml IM | 0, 1, 6 months | Similar seroconversion rates as hep A and hep B components alone[12] |
| Hepatitis B vaccine (HBV) | **Engerix-B** | GlaxoSmithKline | 0 through 19 years: 0.5 ml IM >19 yrs: 1.0 ml IM | 0, 1, 6 months (See Product Information for alternative schedules) | Seroprotection rate for healthy adults and adolescents: 96% at month 7[13] |
| | **Recombivax HB** | Merck | 11 through 15 years: 1.0 ml IM | 0, 4–6 months | Seroprotection rate for healthy young adults (20–39 years) and adolescents: 98%, 99%, respectively[14] |
| | | | 0 through 19 years: 0.5 ml IM >19 yrs: 1.0 ml IM | 0, 1, 6 months | |
| Bivalent human papillomavirus (HPV2) vaccine | **Cervarix** | GlaxoSmithKline | 9 through 26-year-old females: 0.5 ml IM | 0, 1, 6 months | Approximately 99% effective against CIN2/CIN3 caused by HPV 16, 18[15] |
| Quadrivalent human papillomavirus (HPV4) vaccine | **Gardasil** | Merck | 9 through 26-year-old males and females: 0.5 ml IM | 0, 2, 6 months | Approximately 100% effective against CIN2/CIN3 or AIS caused by HPV 16, 18 Approximately 99% against genital warts caused by HPV 6,11[16] |
| Polysaccharide meningococcal (MPSV4) vaccine | **Menomune** | Sanofi Pasteur | 2 through 55 years: 0.5 ml SC | | Four-fold increase in bacteriocidal antibodies to all serogroups in greater than 90-95% of subjects among those aged 11–18 yrs[17] |
| Conjugate meningococcal (MCV4) vaccine | **Menactra** | Sanofi Pasteur | 2 through 55 years: 0.5 ml IM | | Four-fold increase in bacteriocidal antibodies to all serogroups in greater than 82–97% of subjects in those aged 11–18 yrs[18] |
| | **Menveo** | Novartis | 11 through 55 years: 0.5 ml | | |

(*Continued*)

**Table 14-1 (Continued)**

| *Vaccine* | *Trade Name* | *Manufacturer* | *Dose* | *Recommended Schedule (for Multiple Dose Regimens)* | *Reported Efficacy/Seroprotection* |
|---|---|---|---|---|---|
| Measles, mumps, and rubella (MMR) vaccine | **MMR II** | Sanofi Pasteur | ≥12 months of age: 0.5 ml SC | | 99% clinical efficacy reported for each component |
| Measles, mumps, rubella, and varicella (MMRV) vaccine | **ProQuad** | Merck | 12 months through 12 years: 0.5 ml SC | | Similar to individual components alone (MMR II and varicella) |
| Polysaccharide pneumonococcal (PPSV23) vaccine | **Pneumovax 23** | Merck | ≥2 years: 0.5 ml IM or SC | | Variable based on age and disease status[19] |
| Tetanus, diphtheria, acellular pertussis (Tdap) vaccine | **Adacel** | Sanofi Pasteur | 11 through 64 years: 0.5 ml IM | | Pertussis: approximately 85% efficacy inferred against WHO-defined pertussis[20] |
| | **Boostrix** | GlaxoSmithKline | 10 through 64 years: 0.5 ml IM | | Pertussis: approximately 89% efficacy inferred against WHO-defined pertussis[21] |
| Varicella | **Varivax** | Merck | ≥12 years: 0.5 ml SC | 12–13 years: 0, 4–8 weeks ≥13 years: 0, at least 3 months | Approximately 70–90% efficacy for prevention of varicella[22] |

Influenza vaccine data vary and are not included in this table.

The recommendations for use of Tdap among those 19 to 64 years of age are fourfold: (1) to replace a single dose of Td with Tdap for patients who received their last dose more than 10 years earlier; (2) to protect against pertussis with a single dose of Tdap in settings of increased risk as soon as feasible; (3) to replace Td with Tdap for adults requiring wound prophylaxis if they have not previously received Tdap; and (4) to immunize all adults who anticipate having close contact with an infant ≤12 months of age, all women who anticipate becoming pregnant, and health care personnel who have direct patient contact.[23] For those older than 10 years of age with no record of the primary DTaP series, at least 1 (preferably the first) of the "catch-up" series of 3 Td vaccinations should include a Tdap.

Td has long been recommended for use in pregnant women who received their last Td more than 10 years earlier to prevent maternal and neonatal tetanus. If pregnant women use Tdap, antibodies transferred passively to the infant might interfere with the response to DTaP immunization during infancy. Tdap is not currently recommended during pregnancy, although pregnancy is not a contraindication for use of the vaccine. Use of the vaccine is contraindicated for those who have had a severe allergic reaction to any component of the vaccine and for those with a history of encephalopathy not attributable to an identifiable cause within 7 days of administration of a vaccine containing pertussis components.[9] For a full list of contraindications and precautions as well as the most updated recommendations, consult www.cdc.gov.

## CONJUGATE MENINGOCOCCAL VACCINE

*Neisseria meningitidis*, a gram-negative bacterium, causes meningitis and meningococcemia with potentially devastating sequelae including death. The onset of disease can be misleading and appears similar to any viral illness including the flu, making early diagnosis difficult. The CDC data indicate that the incidence of cases of meningococcal disease in the United States in 2004 was 0.5 to 1.1 per 100,000 population. The disease incidence is highest among infants and children younger than 4 years of age; however, there is an important incidence peak again from age 15 through early adulthood.[24] In addition, adolescents and young adults with meningococcal disease are more likely than younger children to die from the disease. The 5 most common serogroups of *N meningitidis* that cause disease are serogroups A, B, C, Y, and W-135. Serogroup A is common in Africa and China but rare in the United States, serogroup B is common among infants and younger children, serogroup C is more common among older children and adults, and serogroup Y is becoming increasingly common in the United States. Serogroup W-135 is relatively uncommon but has been implicated in outbreaks of meningitis among the hajj pilgrims.[25] Although vaccines targeting serogroup B, which accounts for approximately 20% of adolescent meningococcal disease, do exist and are in use in New Zealand and Cuba, these vaccines are not appropriate for use in the United States. The United States harbors multiple strains of serogroup B bacteria, making meningococcal B vaccine development for this country challenging.

A quadrivalent polysaccharide vaccine addressing serogroups A, C, Y, and W-135 was introduced in the US military in 1982.[26] In 2000, the CDC encouraged the use of the vaccine for those going to college in response to data that an increased risk of disease was associated with "behaviors associated with dormitory and college life."[26] Many states supported the use of vaccine by passing mandates for either education regarding the disease and vaccination or actual immunization prior to college entry.

The conjugate vaccine, an intramuscular vaccine approved in 2005 for use among those 11 to 55 years old, offers significant health benefits. The presence of a carrier protein in the conjugate vaccine confers a more vigorous T-cell response to vaccination. This T-cell response likely provides a strong anamnestic response and may eliminate the carrier state of the targeted disease, representing significant advantages over polysaccharide vaccine. It is also assumed that, like other conjugate vaccines, the duration of protection will be longer than that achieved after vaccination with the polysaccharide vaccine; confirmation of this assumption will require follow-up study.

Use of the conjugate vaccine is contraindicated for those who have had a severe allergic reaction to any component of the vaccine. The safety of vaccination with MCV4 during pregnancy has not yet been established; use of the polysaccharide vaccine is indicated for vaccination during pregnancy.

The recommendations of the ACIP and the AAP regarding the use of MCV4 have evolved since FDA approval of the vaccine. This is due to increasing capacity to produce adequate supply of vaccine and the emergence of additional. The initial 2005 recommendations for use of the vaccine included routine vaccination in 5 categories, including those who (1) are 11 to 12 years of age, (2) are entering high school (approximately 15 years of age), (3) have special circumstances, including college freshmen living in dormitories, military recruits, or travelers to specific geographic areas, (4) have functional asplenia or terminal complement deficiencies, and (5) are working with *N meningitidis* isolates in the laboratory setting.[24] Vaccination was later recommended for all 11–12-year-olds and 13–18-

year-olds not previously vaccinated. In October 2010, due to concerns about waning titers after 1 dose, ACIP voted to recommend a dose of vaccine at 11 to 12 years of age, with a second dose to be given at age 16 years. In addition, a 2-dose primary series is recommended for those at high risk for medical indications; booster doses are recommended every 5 years for those older than age 7 who remain at increased risk of disease.[27] Updated dosing schedules can be found at www.cdc.gov.

Concerns regarding vaccination safety have been raised in conjunction with this vaccine. As of January 2007, 19 cases of Guillain-Barré syndrome (GBS) occurring ≤ 6 weeks after vaccination had been reported to the Vaccine Adverse Events Reporting System (VAERS); 17 of these cases were among 11–19 year olds. The VAERS system is a passive reporting system and is not designed to determine definitive causal relationships. Large, hypothesis-driven studies have since revealed no evidence of increased risk of GBS associated with MCV4 (www.cdc.gov/vaccines/recs/acip/downloads/mtg-slides-jun10/07-3-menin.pdf).

### HUMAN PAPILLOMAVIRUS VACCINE

Human papillomavirus (HPV) is a class of nonenveloped, double-stranded DNA viruses of which there are more than 100 genotypes, approximately 40 of which affect the anogenital region. Genital HPV infection is transmitted primarily through sexual contact, most notably sexual intercourse. Modeling estimates that more than 80% of sexually active women will have acquired genital HPV by 50 years of age.[28] Most HPV infections are cleared by the host immune system and are self-limited. The genital types of HPV are categorized into 1 of 2 groups: *low-risk* types (eg, types 6 and 11), which are associated with recurrent respiratory papillomatosis and genital warts; and *high-risk* types (eg, types 16 and 18), which are more likely to be associated with persistent infection leading to cellular changes associated with the development of cervical cancer as well as vulvar, vaginal, anal, and penile cancers.

Acquisition of HPV has been found to occur soon after sexual debut; in 1 prospective study, the cumulative incidence of HPV infection among US college women was 38.9% by 24 months after sexual debut, with 10.4% having acquired HPV 16.[29] It is estimated that each year, 3.5 to 5.0 million Pap tests among the approximately 50 million performed in the United States will require follow-up due to an abnormality; approximately 11,000 cases of cervical cancer are diagnosed annually (in 2003, 8.1 per 100,000 women were diagnosed). The median age of cervical cancer diagnosis is 47 years.[28]

Each HPV genotype has a unique L1 capsid protein. The L1 protein is capable of self-assembling to form empty shells that are called virus-like particles (VLPs). Current vaccines against HPV that are FDA approved or under FDA consideration are comprised of these VLPs that induce an immune response in the host receiving the vaccine. A quadrivalent vaccine (HPV4) addressing HPV types 6, 11, 16, and 18 was FDA approved in 2006, and a bivalent vaccine (HPV2) addressing types 16 and 18 has been available in the United States since 2009. Both vaccines are administered intramuscularly in a series of 3 0.5-mL doses (0, 1–2, 6 months). Efficacy studies for both vaccines indicate efficacy of between 99% and 100% against the HPV 16 and 18 related cervical intraepithelial neoplasia (CIN) 2/3 and cervical adenocarcinoma *in situ* among those naïve to the vaccine genotypes for at least 5 years postvaccination. Safety and immunogenicity for the quadrivalent vaccine have been established for males 9 to 15 years of age;[28] data among males 16 to 26 years of age indicate 90.4% vaccine efficacy against all external genital lesions (defined as external genital warts and penile intraepithelial neoplasia 1/2/3) and 85.6% against persistent infection.[15] The FDA approved the HPV vaccine for adolescent males in 2009 and the vaccine may be administered to males ages 9 to 26 years.[30] The most updated recommendations can be found at www.cdc.gov.

Because the vaccine uses the L1 antigen, and L1 antigen expression is diminished once the virus genome is incorporated into the host genome (late in infection), this vaccine is a prophylactic vaccine and is effective against HPV types with which the host has not yet been infected. For this reason, the vaccine is recommended for younger adolescents, with catch-up for older adolescents. The ACIP has recommended use of the quadrivalent vaccine, FDA approved for use among females age 9 to 26 years, for all females age 11 to 12 years. In 1 of its most sweeping recommendations, ACIP has also recommended vaccination for all females age 13 to 26 years who have not previously received the vaccine. Previous abnormal Pap test results are not a contraindication for immunization. Patients must be informed that vaccination will not be therapeutic for lesions already acquired but will provide protection against HPV types to which they have not yet been exposed. The vaccine is not recommended for use during pregnancy, although data indicate no causal association of vaccine with adverse events in pregnancy; the vaccine is in pregnancy category B. If a patient becomes pregnant during the vaccination series, the remainder of the series can be completed postpartum.

Current HPV vaccines do not address all oncogenic strains, and everyone may not respond to vaccination. Therefore, no changes in cervical cancer screening guidelines are recommended at this time.

## SAFETY

Safety is always a consideration with immunization practices. There are risks and benefits associated with using all vaccines. For the adolescent vaccinations, there have been some specific issues as well as some general issues to consider.

There have been general recommendations published regarding immunization administration, including recommendations for adolescents.[31] The spacing of vaccination often sparks provider inquiry. Current CDC recommendations reiterate that for multiple-dose series, doses should not be given at intervals less than the minimum intervals recommended or earlier than the minimum age recommended. Doses given 4 days or fewer before the minimum interval are still considered valid; doses given with a shorter interval are considered suboptimal and need to be repeated when appropriate with the minimal interval respected between the invalid and subsequent dose. When vaccine doses are late, although protection may not be optimized until the series is completed, there is no need to restart the vaccination series (with the only exception being oral typhoid vaccine).[31]

Simultaneous administration of vaccines (during the same office visit, delivered in separate syringes at different sites) is ideal for vaccination adherence, and extensive experience supports the safety of this strategy. When not administered simultaneously, inactivated vaccines and live oral vaccines (typhoid and rotavirus vaccines) can be administered any time before or after a different inactivated or live vaccine. Data conflict regarding nonsimultaneous administration of various live vaccines. To minimize risk of interference, injectable and nasally administered live vaccines should be administered at least 4 weeks apart whenever possible.[31] Although combination vaccines for adolescents are rare, combination vaccines are generally preferred over separate component injections. The decision should be based on available scientific data.

Despite the relative safety of nonsimultaneous administration of inactivated vaccines, due to the relatively large amount of diphtheria toxoid in the MCV4 vaccine (estimated to be approximately 6 times that contained in the Tdap vaccine), some experts recommend a 1-month interval between Tdap and MCV4 vaccines. This precaution may decrease the risk of local reactions, including the deposition of immune complexes at the site of injection known as Arthus reactions.

Whenever feasible, use of vaccines from the same manufacturer is recommended for multiple-dose series; however, vaccination should not be deferred because the brand used for previous doses is not available or known. This issue is more complex with the advent of the 2 HPV vaccines that address different numbers of HPV genotypes, and no data are currently available. Although interchangeability may not affect overall efficacy against HPV types 16 and 18, the differences between the valency as well as the adjuvants now employed for the vaccines may limit interchangeability.

Severe adverse reactions to vaccinations are rare. Syncope can occur after vaccination; this reaction is more common among adolescent and young adults.[31] For this reason, as well as to monitor severe allergic reaction, a minimum of 15 minutes of observation post-vaccination is recommended by the CDC for all patients. Specific recommendations for vaccination during pregnancy are available on the CDC Web site. Data regarding adverse outcomes for the fetus exist for smallpox vaccine only; the risk to fetuses from vaccination with live vaccines is currently theoretical. Vaccination during pregnancy is actively recommended for influenza and HBV vaccines only at this time.

The safety of the specific immunizations targeting adolescents has been described briefly above. The CDC Web site maintains safety data as well as the most updated immunization schedule recommendations for all indicated vaccines (www.cdc.gov).

Through the Immunization Safety Office at the CDC, adverse event data are collected by multiple entities: the VAERS is a national passive surveillance system monitored by the CDC and the FDA; the Vaccine Safety Datalink links data from multiple large health maintenance organizations; and the Clinical Immunization Safety Assessment Centers network represents cooperation between academic centers and the CDC to study data and create management protocols. In addition, pharmaceutical companies are required to monitor the safety of their vaccines during phase IV protocols monitored by the FDA. Each modality may have limitations; data points collected through passive reporting via VAERS, for example, require further study to determine true associations; however, such data can effectively and quickly note a potential relationship between vaccine administration and a specific outcome. Based on an Institute of Medicine (IOM) report released in 2005, the Immunization Safety Office is initiating a comprehensive and scientifically robust research agenda that includes extensive internal and external input.[32] This mission will expand the assessment of the safety of vaccines received by children, adolescents, and adults.

Many vaccines are in various stages of development, including vaccines against pandemic flu, HIV, meningococcal disease caused by serogroup B, and malaria. A tuberculosis nasal subunit vaccine is being tested, and West Nile, hepatitis C vaccine, herpes simplex, Cytomegalovirus (CMV), Ebola virus, and leishmaniasis vaccines, among others, are all in various stages of development and target various populations. The technology associated with vaccine development, including the development of new adjuvants and diverse modes of administration, is burgeoning. As the field of vaccine development expands, vaccine safety monitoring will continue to be an important component of maintaining public health.

## WHAT WILL ENHANCE ADOLESCENT IMMUNIZATION RATES?

There are significant concerns regarding adolescent adherence to the new immunization recommendations. Increased cost of the newer vaccines has strained the public health system and has introduced new challenges to private health care providers. In addition, the experiences over the past few years with supply and demand within the adolescent population of MCV4 and the safety concerns inherent with any new vaccination recommendation have sparked national debate about implementation and vaccine safety. There are several policy strategies that might enhance the success of adolescent immunization. These strategies include: (1) development of stable immunization platforms for teens; (2) use of alternative sites for immunization; (3) state vaccination mandates; and (4) state and national funding for vaccine administration and infrastructure in the public and private sectors. Providers caring for adolescents can play an important role as well by implementing practice changes such as the use of standing orders, recall systems, and immunization information systems (IIS); avoiding missed opportunities to immunize, simultaneous administration of multiple immunizations, the use of screening tools, and education for themselves and the patients. The specifics of all these strategies are being debated at a national level among multiple stakeholders.[33] Policy and provider practice changes to improve immunization rates are imminent.

## POLICY IMPROVEMENTS TO ENHANCE ADOLESCENT IMMUNIZATION RATES

### Immunization Platforms

In 2006, the Society for Adolescent Health and Medicine (SAHM) published a position statement regarding adolescent immunization. One of the cornerstones of this statement includes a recommendation for 3 distinct immunization platforms throughout adolescence to encourage immunization while being cognizant of health care utilization patterns and insurance coverage issues that play a role in adherence.[34] The Infectious Diseases Society of America also supports well visits in early, middle, and late adolescence to increase vaccine delivery.[35] This idea supports the already existing adolescent preventive health care schema of annual preventive health visits recommended by the AAP, AMA, Maternal and Child Health Bureau, and SAHM. The first platform, already in place, is the 11- to 12-year-old immunization platform. Data support that 11- to 12-year-olds access health care more frequently than older adolescents, allowing for greater potential success with immunization. The second platform, at 14 to 15 years of age, would allow teens to catch up with immunization recommendations made since their 11- to 12-year preventive health visit and to complete any vaccination series not yet completed. The third, final, adolescent platform is recommended for those 17 to 18 years of age. This platform would serve the same role as the 14- to 15-year-old platform yet would also allow all catch-up to occur prior to a potential shift in insurance coverage that might impede vaccination adherence. Vaccination platforms have helped establish immunization and preventive care standards for infants and children, with the intention that an extension of these platforms into adolescence will enhance the same standards for adolescents. Immunization is shifting from a solely infant and child issue to a much more inclusive strategy to prevent disease across the life span. Creative strategies to encourage adherence among adolescents, young adults, and older adults will be needed to protect as many individuals as possible, both through individual immunization and through the herd immunity that can create a dome of protection over our most vulnerable community members.

### Alternative Immunization Sites

Data indicate that although most adolescents seek care at physician offices,[36] more than a quarter (27%) use multiple sources of care, depending on the desired services, including family planning and community clinics.[37] National Ambulatory Medical Survey data from 2002 indicate that 32% of visits for 17- to 21-year-old females were to obstetricians/gynecologists,[38] and gynecologists are already becoming involved in HPV vaccination, hopefully with the capacity to expand their immunization delivery to include other needed vaccines. Emergency departments (ED) are an unlikely site for multiple or catch-up immunizations; however, the ED is an excellent source of vaccination for wound management (Tdap). Pharmacies are convenient and community-based; pharmacy vaccination clinics have been successful and safe among adult populations, with influenza vaccination in particular,[39] and many states continue to lower the minimum age of immunization allowed in commercial pharmacies as they become more comfortable immunizing in the stores. Study regarding the feasibility of using alternative immunization sites for adolescent vaccination is ongoing.

One alternative immunization site in particular may be most appropriate for adolescents. The most likely site to capture the greatest number of adolescent vaccine recipients is the school. School immunization strategies were highly successful for increasing rates of hepatitis B immunization among adolescents in the 1990s,[40-44] with immunization rates as high as 94% among those participating. School immunization programs also help eliminate disparities in access to immunizations, an important goal in the administration of public health services, and many schools have the capacity to link to local/state registries.

Obtaining parental consent is cited as a significant barrier to school-based immunization initiatives. Federal law requires that health care providers provide a copy of the relevant vaccination information materials produced by the CDC to either the parent/legal representative of any child or to the adult vaccine recipient prior to administering each dose of a vaccine.[45] The relative laxity of this law considers that immunization is critically important to the public's health. Additional laws pertaining to parental consent or signature for immunization differ per state. For example, some states allow adolescents to consent to immunizations associated with reproductive health, such as HBV vaccine, citing the relevant protections of adolescents' ability to consent for care on such issues. To further the goal of increased vaccination rates among adolescents, states must develop immunization strategies that are as inclusive as possible or practical of parental involvement yet do not hinder immunization of a relatively difficult-to-reach population, a challenge for any decision-making organization. Consistency of such policies among states would also be beneficial.

### State Mandates

State mandates for immunization are not new. Every state in America has vaccine mandates.[46] Mandates have been particularly effective among the adolescent population, which currently has no other standard or expectation of vaccination adherence.[47] In a study of the effect of school mandates on adherence to the hepatitis B vaccination series,[48] adolescents were significantly more likely to have completed the series in states with mandates (75%) than in states without mandates (39%). Many argue that mandates for a disease such as HPV, which is not "casually transmitted," are inappropriate. Obviously, hepatitis B infection among adolescents is not transmitted via casual contact, although there is a large percentage of cases for which the etiology is not known. In the end, "the mode of transmission is thought to be a distinction without meaningful difference, and the result is the same."[46] Many people become infected with disease each year, and the threat to public health is preventable with vaccination.

Mandates need to be implemented with care and with awareness of the highly political nature of the mandating process. Several public health organizations have published "checklists" of factors that should be in place prior to attempting to carefully implement a state vaccination mandate. These include adequate funding for vaccination purchase and administration—particularly important with some of the new, more expensive vaccines; public acceptance of the vaccine; resolution of any safety concerns regarding the vaccine; and an opt-out plan for parents that is not so lenient that it weakens mandates in general and allows for the development of pockets of youth vulnerable to vaccine-preventable disease.[49-51] Until such time that mandates for adolescent vaccines have been strengthened, providers can capitalize on existing mandates for the Td/Tdap vaccine and immunize simultaneously for other recommended vaccines. It would also be helpful to attempt to diminish variation in policies among states by creating policies consistent with ACIP and professional organization guidelines.

### State and Federal Funding

There are 2 major federal funding sources for immunization in the United States. The Vaccine for Children Program (VFC), operational since 1994, is an entitlement program that provides vaccine to all eligible individuals from birth until their 19th birthday and funds approximately 40% of all of the doses of childhood vaccines distributed in the United States. Eligible children include those who are eligible for Medicaid, uninsured, American Indian or Alaska Native children, and those who are underinsured (their insurance does not cover vaccines) and receive vaccination through federally qualified health centers (FQHCs) or rural health clinics (RHCd) (www.cdc.gov/vaccines/programs/vfc/default.htm).

Federal dollars via the Vaccination Assistance Act (VAA) are distributed to states to fund vaccination infrastructure and any needed vaccines. Each state utilizes those funds at its own discretion, and with ever-increasing vaccination costs, these funds are often used to immunize constituents who are underinsured children or those 19 years of age and older who are ineligible for VFC coverage and cannot afford vaccination. The VFC funding has increased dramatically over the past several years to keep pace with the increased number of vaccine recommendations for children; VAA funding has remained relatively stagnant over the same time period.[52] Many states have attempted to maintain or increase coverage of the underinsured segment of the population using either state funds or VAA funds. The new vaccine recommendations for adolescents have necessitated a flux in vaccine policy (eg, changing the designation of FQHCs or RHCs) and funding coverage.

Support has been provided by the CDC with the goal of identifying, recruiting, enrolling, and training providers of adolescents interested in becoming VFC providers, and many states now have a State Adolescent Immunization Coordinator. Further funding is clearly required to improve vaccine delivery of the increasing number and increasingly expensive recommended vaccines for adolescents.

Financial concerns also plague vaccination administration in the private sector. Pediatricians, family physicians, and other providers who immunize regularly are facing financial barriers to reimbursement as the cost of the newer vaccines increases. Recent data reveal that the cost of supplying vaccine alone, exclusive of administration costs such as nursing time, can be 17% to 28% higher than the cost of the vaccine itself. These costs include depreciation of refrigerators needed for storage, wastage of product, accidental loss, nonpayment for product, and ordering and tracking vaccinations.[53] In addition, providers pay for vaccine supply prior to administering it, increasing the "up-front" costs for providers and increasing the financial burden on a medical practice. In some states, these vaccine stores are taxable as practice capital. Literature supports that physician reimbursement for varicella vaccine, for example, significantly affects immunization practices.[54] Reimbursement for the actual administration of vaccines also differs with various insurance plans and within different states for administration of vaccine through VFC. Clearly, private providers of vaccines need a financial reprieve that could ultimately increase immunization rates among youth. The summary of an AAP/AMA Immunization Congress that took place in the spring of 2007 supports the consensus that coverage for vaccine provision and administration requires significant attention.[33]

Further funding is required to support the implementation of other important vaccination infrastructure including immunization information systems (IIS). Because adolescents access care at multiple sites for multiple and varied health care needs, use of an IIS allows providers to track adolescent vaccination needs and completion regardless of site of care. Despite the initial effort required to establish and maintain such a system, the benefits of such a system can be dramatic. By linking the IIS from Houston and Harris County (HHCIR) to the Louisiana state IIS (LINKS) after Hurricane Katrina hit the Gulf Coast in 2004, the government saved millions of dollars in health care resources by averting unnecessary vaccine administration among those displaced by the storm.[55]

Shifts are also occurring in the collection of immunization completion data. The Health Employer Data and Information Set (HEDIS) eliminated its adolescent immunization completion measures for 2008 and is updating them for future use. However, the CDC has expanded its data collection on completion rates to include adolescents across all 50 states (CDC, personal communication). The key to this collection will, of course, be the continuation of adequate funds. Because successful adolescent immunization is a priority for the CDC at this time, these data will likely be available for many years.

Funding for vaccination in the public and private sectors is an important element in eliminating socioeconomic disparities in immunization rates. In 1993, the IOM recommended the use of a new insurance mandate for private and public health plans combined with a government subsidy and voucher plan for vaccines recommended by ACIP.[56] The IOM report also suggested increased rigor regarding societal benefits and costs within ACIP when deliberating vaccine recommendations. As noted earlier, multiple professional and governmental organizations are aware of the enlarging financial burden resulting from the influx of new vaccines. A shift in the financial structure that currently supports immunization in this country—1 of the most valuable and cost-effective primary prevention strategies in public health—is eagerly anticipated.

## PROVIDERS' STRATEGIES TO ENHANCE ADOLESCENT IMMUNIZATION RATES

Although there has been little time to accrue data regarding the efficacy of provider strategies in implementing adolescent vaccine recommendations, some strategies used among children and adults have been shown to be effective and are appropriate for use for the adolescent population. The Task Force on Community Preventive Services recommends the following provider strategies with strong evidence to support them:

- provider reminder/recall systems (often available as part of an IIS)
- assessment and feedback for providers
- standing orders (strong evidence for adults, insufficient evidence for children)

Other strategies include scheduling time slots for immunizations only, use of an IIS to improve vaccination efficiency, and the use of screening tools. Examples of all these strategies are available at the Immunization Action Coalition Web site (www.immunize.org). Professional organization literature often updates providers regarding new recommendations, and provider continuing medical education is a critical component for vaccination adherence among adolescents. Research supports the critical role that providers play in parental and adolescent decision making for immunizations.[57] Provider education is critical for parent and adolescent education. Despite a fear of shots, adolescents often consult parents, and parents often consult providers for guidance regarding immunization decisions.

## SUMMARY

Vaccines are one of the most cost-efficient and effective public health strategies developed. Vaccination has traditionally targeted young infants and children and, more recently, senior adults. Yet primary prevention of disease is a concept that applies across the life span. The effective immunization of the adolescent population is the first step to expanding this primary prevention strategy up the ladder of age. New and exciting vaccines for disease prevention now exist for adolescents, and the responsibility is ours to effectively deliver these products to our youth. By working on both policy and individual provider levels, success will become a more imminent reality.

## REFERENCES


1. Centers for Disease Control. Immunization of adolescent recommendations: Advisory Committee on Immunization Practices, Academy of Pediatrics, The American Academy of Physicians, and the American Medical Association. *MMWR Morb Mortal Wkly Rep.* 1996;45(RR-13)1-16

2. Centers for Disease Control. Update: Recommendation to prevent hepatitis B virus transmission—United States. *MMWR Morb Mortal Wkly Rep.* 1999;48(2):33-34

3. Centers for Disease Control. A comprehensive immunization strategy to eliminate transmission of hepatitis B virus infection in the United States. *MMWR Morb Mortal Wkly Rep.* 2005;54 (RR16):1-23

4. Centers for Disease Control. A comprehensive immunization strategy to eliminate transmission of hepatitis B virus infection in the United States. *MMWR Morb Mortal Wkly Rep.* 2006;55 (RR16):1-25

5. Centers for Disease Control. Prevention and control of influenza: Recommendations of the Advisory Committee on Immunization Practices (ACIP). *MMWR Morb Mortal Wkly Rep.* 2007;56(Early Release):1-54

6. Centers for Disease Control. Notice to readers: update on supply of vaccines containing varicella-zoster virus. *MMWR Morb Mortal Wkly Rep.* 2007;56(18):453

7. Centers for Disease Control. Prevention and control of influenza: recommendations of the Advisory Committee on Immunization Practices (ACIP). *MMWR Morb Mortal Wkly Rep.* 2006;55(RR-10):1-42

8. Tan T, Trindade E, Skowronski D. Epidemiology of pertussis. *Pediatr Infect Dis J.* 2005;24:S10-S18

9. Centers for Disease Control. Preventing tetanus, diphtheria, and pertussis among adolescents: use of tetanus toxoid, reduced diphtheria toxoid, and acellular pertussis vaccines. *MMWR Morb Mortal Wkly Rep.* 2006;55:1-34

10. Product information: Havrix. Rixensart, Belgium: GlaxoSmithKline Biologicals; 2006

11. Product information: Vaqta. Whitehouse Station, NJ: Merck & Co, Inc; 2006

12. Product information: Twinrix. Rixensart, Belgium: GlaxoSmithKline Biologicals; 2006

13. Product information: Engerix-B (hepatitis vaccine [recombinant]). Rixensart, Belgium: GlaxoSmithKline Biologicals; 2006

14. Product information: Recombinant HB (hepatitis B vaccine [recombinant]). Whitehouse Station, NJ: Merck & Co, Inc; 2006

15. Dubin G. HPV-008: phase III study of the efficacy of GSK's cervical cancer candidate vaccine in 15- to 25-year-old women. Presented at: ACIP meeting; June 2007; Atlanta, GA

16. Product information: Gardasil. Whitehouse Station, NJ: Merck & Co, Inc; 2006

17. Product information: Menomune. Swiftwater, PA: Sanofi Pasteur, Inc; 2007

18. Product information: Menactra. Swiftwater, PA: Sanofi Pasteur, Inc; 2007

19. Product information: Pneumovax. Whitehouse Station, NJ: Merck & Co, Inc; 2006

20. Product information: Tetanus toxoid, reduced diphtheria toxoid, and acellular pertussis vaccine absorbed ADACEL. Swiftwater, PA: Sanofi Pasteur, Inc; 2005

21. Product information: Tetanus toxoid, reduced diphtheria toxoid, and acellular pertussis vaccine absorbed Boostrix. Rixensart, Belgium: GlaxoSmithKline Biologicals; 2005

22. Centers for Disease Control. Prevention of varicella: recommendations of the Advisory Committee on Immunization Practices (ACIP). *MMWR Morb Mortal Wkly Rep.* 2007;56(RR-4):1-40

23. Centers for Disease Control. Preventing tetanus, diphtheria, and pertussis among adults: use of tetanus toxoid, reduced diphtheria toxoid, and acellular pertussis vaccine. *MMWR Morb Mortal Wkly Rep.* 2006;55(RR17):1-33

24. Centers for Disease Control. Prevention and control of meningococcal disease: recommendations of the Advisory Committee on Immunization Practices (ACIP). *MMWR Morb Mortal Wkly Rep.* 2005;54(RR-7):1-21

25. Granoff D, Harris S. Protective activity of group C anticapsular antibodies elicited in two-year-olds by an investigational quadrivalent *Neisseria meningitidis*-diphtheria toxoid conjugate vaccine. *J Pediatr Infect Dis.* 2004;23(6):490-497

26. Centers for Disease Control. Meningococcal disease and college students. *MMWR Morb Mortal Wkly Rep.* 2000;49 (RR07):11-20

27. Centers for Disease Control. Recommended immunization schedules for persons aged 0 through 18 years—United States, 2010. *MMWR Morb Mortal Wkly Rep QuickGuide.* 2010 Jan 8; 58(51&52):1-4

28. Centers for Disease Control. Quadrivalent human papillomavirus vaccine: recommendations of the Advisory Committee

on Immunization Practices (ACIP). *MMWR Morb Mortal Wkly Rep.* 2007; **56**(RR02):1-24

29. Winer RL, Lee S-K, Hughes JP, Adam DE, Kiviat NB, Koutsky LA. Genital human papillomavirus infection: incidence and risk factors in a cohort of female university students. *Am J Epidemiol.* 2003;157(3):218-226

30. Centers for Disease Control. FDA licensure of quadrivalent human papillomavirus vaccine (HPV4, Gardasil) for use in males and guidance from the Advisory Committee on Immunization Practices (ACIP). *MMWR Morb Mortal Wkly Rep.* May 28, 2010; 59(20):630-632

31. Centers for Disease Control. General recommendations on immunization: recommendations of the Advisory Committee on Immunization Practices (ACIP). *MMWR Morb Mortal Wkly Rep.* 2006;55(RR-15):1-47

32. Broder K, Iskander J. CDC's Immunization Safety Office development of a research agenda: update. Presented at ACIP meeting; June 2007; Atlanta, GA

33. American Medical Association. 2007 National Immunization Congress: Adult and Adolescent Immunization Summary; 2007

34. Middleman A, Rosenthal S, Rickert V, et al. Adolescent immunizations: a position paper of the Society for Adolescent Medicine. *J Adolesc Health.* 2006;38(3):321-327

35. Infectious Diseases Society of America. Actions to strengthen adult and adolescent immunization coverage in the United States: policy principles of the Infectious Diseases Society of America. *CID.* 2007;44(44):e104-e108

36. Ziv A, Boulet J, Slap G. Utilization of physician offices by adolescents in the United States. *Pediatr Ann.* 1999;104(1): 35-42

37. Klein J, McNulty M, Flatau C. Adolescents' access to care: teenagers' self-reported use of services and perceived access to confidential care. *Arch Pediatr Adolesc Med.* 1998;152(7): 676-682

38. Gonik B, Jones T, Contreras D, Fasano N, Roberts C. The obstetrician-gynecologist's role in vaccine-preventable diseases and immunization. *Obstetr Gynecol.* 2000;96(1):81-84

39. D'Heilly S, Blade M, Nichol K. Safety of influenza vaccinations administered in nontraditional settings. *Vaccine.* 2006;24 (18):4024-4027

40. Centers for Disease Control. Hepatitis B vaccination of adolescents—California, Louisiana, and Oregon, 1992-1994. *MMWR Morb Mortal Wkly Rep.* 1994;43:605-624

41. Middleman A. Race/ethnicity and gender disparities in the utilization of a school-based hepatitis B immunization initiative. *J Adolesc Health.* 2004;34(5):414-419

42. Cassidy W. School-based adolescent hepatitis B immunization programs in the United States: strategies and successes. *Pediatr Infect Dis J.* 1998;17(7) (suppl):S43-S46

43. Wilson T. Economic evaluation of a metropolitan-wide, school-based hepatitis B vaccination program. *Public Health Nursing.* 2000;17(3):222-227

44. Boyer-Chuanroong L, Woodruff B, Unti L, Sumida Y. Immunizations from ground zero: lessons learned in urban middle schools. *J Sch Health.* 1997;67(7):269-272

45. Atkinson W, Pickering L, Schwartz B, Weniger B, Iskander J, Watson J. General recommendations on immunization: Recommendations of the Advisory Committee on Immunization Practices (ACIP) and the American Academy of Family Physicians (AAFP). *MMWR Recommendation Report.* 2002;51(RR02):1-36

46. Stewart A. Mandating HPV vaccination—private rights, public good. *N Engl J Med.* 2007;356(19):1998-1999

47. Averhoff F, Linton L, Peddecord K, Edwards C, Wang W, Fishbein D. A middle school immunization law rapidly and substantially increases immunization coverage among adolescents. *Amer J Publ Health.* 2004;94(6):978-984

48. Jacobs RJ, Meyerhoff AS. Effect of middle school entry requirements on hepatitis B vaccination coverage. *J Adolesc Health.* 2004;34(5):420-423

49. Omer S, William K, Halsey N, et al. Nonmedical exemptions to school immunization requirements: secular trends and association of state policies with pertussis incidence. *JAMA.* 2006; 296(14):1757-1763

50. Thompson JW, Tyson S, Card-Higginson P, et al. Impact of addition of philosophical exemptions on childhood immunization rates. *Amer J Prev Med.* 2007;32(3):194-201

51. Salmon DA, Teret SP, MacIntyre CR, Salisbury D, Burgess MA, Halsey NA. Compulsory vaccination and conscientious or philosophical exemptions: past, present, and future. *Lancet.* 2006;367(9508):436-442

52. Lee G. Emerging gaps in vaccine financing for underinsured children in the US. Presented at: ACIP meeting; June 2007; Atlanta, GA

53. Cain K, Reuben M. Take steps to ensure contracts include fair vaccine payments. *AAP News.* 2007;28 (3):1

54. McInerny TK, Cull WL, Yudkowsky BK. Physician reimbursement levels and adherence to American Academy of Pediatrics well-visit and immunization recommendations. *Pediatr.* 2005; 115(4):833-838

55. Boom J, Dragsbaek A, Nelson C. The success of an immunization information system in the wake of Hurricane Katrina. *Pediatr.* 2007;119(6):1213-1217

56. Hinman AR. Financing vaccines in the 21st century: recommendations from the National Vaccine Advisory Committee. *Amer J Prevent Med.* 2005;29(1):71-75

57. Rosenthal S. Protecting their adolescents from harm: parental views on STI vaccination. *J Adolesc Health.* 2005;37(3): 177-178

# CHAPTER 15

# Anticipatory Guidance

PONRAT PAKPREO, MD, MPH • CYNTHIA RAND, MD, MPH

Adolescence is a developmental period of physical, social, and emotional transition. During this time, health care providers offer guidance to parents and adolescents about anticipated physical, psychosocial, and emotional development at well-adolescent office visits. Anticipatory guidance offers adolescents the opportunity to talk about common concerns and guide adolescent decision making with appropriate and accurate health information. It also provides an opportunity to answer questions or concerns from adolescents wondering, "Am I normal?" For parents, it is an opportunity to address the ways they can help their teenagers make healthy and safe decisions. Discussions like these promote personal responsibility and participation in health care, increase patient comfort, and can reduce major causes of adolescent morbidity and mortality.

To be effective, anticipatory guidance should be timely, developmentally appropriate, and relevant to the adolescent, the family, and the community to which the adolescent is connected. Variability in the tempo of physical and emotional maturation during adolescence broadens the spectrum of adolescent health behaviors and beliefs encountered by providers. Such variation warrants taking sufficient time during the well-adolescent visit to provide comprehensive services. Because adolescents see their health care provider less often than younger children, acute visits may also provide opportunities to provide anticipatory guidance or answer adolescent concerns. Although many adolescents are relatively healthy, there is a significant amount of change and transition that occurs during this developmental period warranting periodic surveillance and anticipatory guidance. As such, several professional organizations recommend that adolescents have an annual well-adolescent visit.[1–4] Despite these recommendations, adolescents, particularly those who are uninsured, have low rates of preventive visits. In one study, only half (49%) of all adolescents and 24% of uninsured adolescents had a well-adolescent visit in the previous year.[5] Factors associated with adolescents not receiving anticipatory guidance in the United States include (1) lack of insurance, (2) lack of a medical home, (3) not being a citizen of the United States, and (4) English not being the primary language at home.[5] Barriers to the provision of anticipatory guidance from the clinician perspective include (1) poor reimbursement, (2) insufficient training and self-efficacy, (3) reluctance to discuss sensitive issues, (4) ineffective communication skills, (5) insufficient time to cover anticipatory guidance topics, (6) perceived ineffectiveness of counseling, and (7) few adolescent encounters for health supervision visits.[6–8]

Although anticipatory guidance remains the backbone of prevention in pediatrics, there has been a paucity of evidence to show the efficacy of brief counseling in changing patient behavior.[9,10] In one study, fewer than 25% of parents who received anticipatory guidance reported that they planned to change their behavior.[11] Evidence for preventive counseling effectiveness is variable. Several well-designed reviews have evaluated the effect of counseling on injury prevention; counseling regarding seat belt and bike helmet use has been shown to be effective.[9] However, evidence is lacking on the effectiveness of brief, office-based counseling for secondary smoke exposure, drinking and drug use, violent behavior, or increasing physical activity. More intensive, multifaceted programs have been shown to be effective, particularly for smoking cessation, pregnancy prevention, sexually transmitted infection (STI) prevention, and increasing physical activity. For many issues it is difficult to study the effectiveness of a brief intervention; therefore, lack of evidence does not imply that providing advice is unimportant.

The American Academy of Pediatrics (AAP) describes its guidelines for the health supervision of children, *Bright Futures*, as "evidence-informed" rather than "evidence-based" due to the lack of well-done studies on the efficacy of anticipatory guidance. Randomized controlled trials, the standard for best evidence, are generally not feasible in the study of effective well-child care, as withholding the standard of care would be unethical.[12] Despite limited availability of evidence, anticipatory guidance serves an important role in letting the adolescent and parent know that the provider feels comfortable discussing a broad variety of issues and serves as a resource either for counseling or referral if an individual needs more intensive intervention. In addition, providing information that predicts an adolescent's future physical, cognitive, social, and emotional development prepares parents and adolescents for changes and potential challenges to come.

## SOURCES OF GUIDELINES FOR ANTICIPATORY GUIDANCE

Several national organizations have developed guidelines for the provision of anticipatory guidance to adolescents, among other preventive services offered. A recent review of these guidelines[6] showed that although multiple national organizations recommend general anticipatory guidance, specific recommendations vary, based partly on how the recommendations were developed. For example, the United States Preventive Services Task Force (USPSTF)[13] guidelines are based on the existence of published evidence for each service, whereas the American Medical Association's Guidelines for Adolescent Preventive Services (GAPS)[3] rely on expert opinion and consensus. A comparison of these recommendations is shown in Table 15-1.[6] The American Academy of Family Physicians (AAFP)[14] guidelines are similar to those recommended by the AAP. To ease some of this inconsistency, the newest edition of *Bright Futures*[1] includes the most comprehensive list of anticipatory guidance topics.

**Table 15-1**

**Comparison of Professional Organization's Recommendations for Adolescent Anticipatory Guidance**

| | *EPSDT* | *AAP* | *BF* | *GAPS* | *USPSTF* | *AAFP* | *HEDIS* |
|---|---|---|---|---|---|---|---|
| General anticipatory guidance | ■ | ■ | ■ | ■ | ☑ | ☑ | ■ |
| Violence prevention—general | □ | ■ | ■ | ■ | ?[a] | □ | □ |
| Injury prevention—general | ☑ | ■ | ■ | ■ | ■ | ■ | □ |
| Encourage use of lap/shoulder belt | □ | ■ | ■ | ■ | ■ | ■ | □ |
| Encourage adolescent drivers to minimize risk of automobile accident | □ | □ | ■ | ■ | □ | ■ | □ |
| Encourage use of bicycle/motorcycle/ATV helmets | □ | ■ | ■ | ■ | ■ | ■ | □ |
| Encourage use of protective gear for work or sports | □ | ■ | ■ | ■ | □ | □ | □ |
| Encourage use of smoke detector and development of fire emergency plan | □ | □ | ■ | □ | ■ | ■ | □ |
| Encourage safe storage/removal of firearms | □ | ■ | ■ | ■ | ■ | □ | □ |
| Avoid high noise levels | □ | □ | ■ | □ | □ | □ | □ |
| Avoid tobacco use | □ | □ | ■ | ■ | ■ | ?[b] | ■ |
| Avoid underage drinking and illicit drug use | □ | ■ | ■ | ■ | ■ | □ | □ |
| Avoid alcohol/drug use while driving, swimming, boating, etc | □ | ■ | ■ | ■ | ■ | ■ | □ |
| STI prevention including abstinence, condom use, and avoiding high-risk behavior | □ | □ | ■ | ■ | ■ | ■ | □ |
| Counsel how to avoid unintended pregnancy/encourage contraception use | □ | □ | ■ | ■ | ■ | □ | □ |
| Counsel regarding healthy diet | ■ | ■ | ■ | ■ | ■ | ■ | □ |
| Encourage adequate calcium intake | □ | □ | ■ | □ | ■ | ■ | □ |
| Encourage regular physical activity | □ | □ | ■ | ■ | ■ | ?[b] | □ |
| Limit TV/computer time | □ | □ | ■ | □ | □ | □ | □ |

*(Continued)*

**Table 15-1 (Continued)**

| | *EPSDT* | *AAP* | *BF* | *GAPS* | *USPSTF* | *AAFP* | *HEDIS* |
|---|---|---|---|---|---|---|---|
| Encourage to learn how to swim | ☐ | ☐ | ■ | ☐ | ☐ | ☐ | ☐ |
| Avoid excess midday sun and use protective clothing for at-risk patients | ☐ | ☐ | ■ | ☐ | ■ | ☐ | ☐ |
| Try to get 8 hours of sleep per night | ☐ | ☐ | ■ | ☐ | ☐ | ☐ | ☐ |
| Practice time management skills | ☐ | ☐ | ■ | ☐ | ☐ | ☐ | ☐ |
| Continue to build sense of identity | ☐ | ☐ | ■ | ☐ | ☐ | ☐ | ☐ |
| Develop community involvement | ☐ | ☐ | ■ | ☐ | ☐ | ☐ | ☐ |
| Follow family rules | ☐ | ☐ | ■ | ☐ | ☐ | ☐ | ☐ |
| Understand the importance of your spiritual needs and try to fill them | ☐ | ☐ | ■ | ☐ | ☐ | ☐ | ☐ |

■ yes; ☑ implied; ☐ not mentioned; ? not clear

EPSDT (Early and Periodic Screening, Diagnosis, and Treatment); AAP (American Academy of Pediatrics); BF (Bright Futures); GAPS (Guidelines for Adolescent Preventive Services); USPSTF (United States Preventive Services Task Force); AAFP (American Academy of Family Physicians); HEDIS (Health Plan Employer Data Information Set).

[a]The USPSTF reports insufficient evidence to recommend for or against counseling for violence prevention.

[b]The AAFP reports insufficient evidence to support the effectiveness of counseling adolescents regarding tobacco use or regular physical activity.

Reprinted from Richmond TK, Freed GL, Clark SJ, Cabana MD. Guidelines for adolescent well care: is there a consensus? *Curr Opin Pediatr.* 2006;18:365-370, with permission from Wolters Kluwer Health.

In *Bright Futures*,[1] recommended anticipatory guidance topics covered at each age visit are prioritized. Due to the longitudinal perspective in delivery of this guidance, all topics need not be addressed at every visit.[18] The GAPS were developed by the American Medical Association[3] in the 1990s as a screening (not diagnostic) tool and a framework to provide comprehensive adolescent health care. In addition to training and educational materials, the GAPS include questionnaires for adolescents and their parents to fill out during the adolescents' annual visit (see Chapter 13, Screening) so that providers can target risk behaviors most relevant for the adolescent. Studies have shown that incorporating the GAPS into adolescent visits increases documented discussion of risk behaviors,[19] as well as delivery of educational materials, and can improve access to and quality of care.[20] The GAPS screening forms provide an opportunity to discuss sensitive topics, as well as general health topics that adolescents may be hesitant to bring up directly.

Medicaid mandates coverage of clinical preventive services for adolescents younger than 21 years of age under the Early and Periodic Screening, Diagnosis, and Treatment (EPSDT) program.[21] States have autonomy in deciding the periodicity of visits and screening tools, but they must include health education and anticipatory guidance. However, data show that many adolescents do not receive EPSDT services for which they are eligible (education, counseling, and visits).[22] The Healthcare Effectiveness Data and Information Set (HEDIS)[23] is a tool used by most health insurers in the United States to measure performance on care provided. The HEDIS measures, updated annually, now include a specific measurement of physical activity and nutrition counseling in addition to measuring the rate of annual well visits for adolescents. Adherence to HEDIS measures is low for both adolescent immunization and well visits and is linked to physician reimbursement for those services.[24]

## APPROACH TO THE VISIT

Ensuring that adolescents feel comfortable in the office setting is essential to providing useful anticipatory guidance. An adolescent-friendly office may include an adolescent area in the waiting room, age-neutral décor, adolescent-focused policies (confidentiality), and age-appropriate reading material. Adolescents are more likely to disclose risky behaviors and pay greater attention to anticipatory guidance if confidential care is emphasized,[25] the physician is known to the patient,[26] the provider's full attention is given to each adolescent, and interruptions are avoided as much as possible during a visit. Often it helps to interview the parent and adolescent together at the beginning of the visit to elicit any parental or shared concerns. A discussion with the adolescent and the parent about confidentiality (and its few limitations, such as when the adolescent is at serious risk of self- or other harm) should be done early in adolescence. Confidentiality is discussed further in Chapter 11, Legal and Ethical Issues. During adolescence, anticipatory guidance changes from information directed at parents to risk reduction and health education for the adolescent. To be successful, the adolescent must be engaged in the discussion rather than be the target of a lecture. Rapport with the adolescent can be achieved by supporting the adolescent's emerging autonomy, respecting individual differences by being nonjudgmental, and focusing on the adolescent's strengths.

Anticipatory guidance can be incorporated into the visit as it progresses. For instance, tooth-brushing and the breast or testicular self-examination can be discussed during the physical examination. More sensitive issues are better discussed after the exam is complete and the patient is dressed. Rather than providing open-ended advice, anticipatory guidance should be relevant to the needs of the adolescent. By breaking up information provided over several visits if possible, patients are less likely to be overwhelmed by excessive information. According to the 2005 National Medical Ambulatory Care Survey,[12] the average length of well-child visits for adolescents was 19.8 minutes. Because time is limited, providing handouts, Web sites, book references, and other multimedia resources such as DVDs may be effective ways to provide information to parents and adolescents. Families may review these topics later, and the provider can then focus on more targeted anticipatory guidance during the visit. When concerns arise that require more in-depth counseling, it is best to schedule a follow-up visit. For parents of younger children, recall of topics diminishes as the number of topics increases (≥9 topics), and the same is likely true for adolescents.[27] Finally, it is important to leave sufficient time at the end of the visit to allow the adolescent one more opportunity to ask questions.

## COUNSELING TECHNIQUES

Many approaches can be used to provide prevention education to adolescents, and providers develop their own style over time, but several methods have been shown to be more effective than others.[9] In general, patient-centered approaches and those reinforced over time are associated with better adherence to counseling provided, and several techniques can be incorporated into a busy practice. A strengths-based approach applies concepts from positive youth development to the medical office setting—rather than focusing on what is wrong, this method focuses on what is right.[28,29] Demonstration of an adolescent's specific strengths is associated with increased healthy behaviors and fewer risk behaviors. By assessing and encouraging an adolescent's strengths and assets, providers can promote healthy choices and convey confidence in the adolescent's ability to change a behavior or continue making positive choices.[28]

When risky behaviors are identified, it is important to assess the adolescent's interest in changing that behavior. The Stages of Change model[30] describes the way in which individuals progress through behavior changes. Counseling approaches that incorporate elements of this model have shown promise in changing adolescent behavior, including decreasing tobacco use among adolescents.[31] In the *precontemplative* stage, a patient is not yet willing to acknowledge that there is a problem with a behavior. In this case, brief advice should be given, because patients can become defensive when urged to make a change in something they do not consider a problem. In the *contemplative* stage, patients are ambivalent about changing behavior but are willing to consider one. In this stage, individuals are more open to receiving information about their habit, and health education may be appropriate at this stage because it allows patients to reflect on their behavior. During the *preparation stage*, individuals have made a commitment to change and gather information about how to do so, and *action* is the stage in which patients modify their behavior. This is followed by *maintenance*, when individuals work to prevent relapse.

Motivational interviewing is a patient-centered counseling approach shown to help patients change behavior, and it is consistent with the stages of change.[32] It has been effective for decreasing alcohol use,[33] controlling tobacco and marijuana addiction,[34] and increasing treatment adherence to medications.[35] In addition to assessing motivation for change and building a patient's intrinsic motivation, this technique uses reflective listening to help patients resolve their ambivalence about a behavior change. Reflective listening shows an adolescent that the provider has heard what he or she has to say by paraphrasing key points made, with a wording that signals the provider is unsure of their interpretation. Using phrases such as "So you're saying," or "It sounds like" encourage the adolescent to continue talking (see Chapter 8, Medical History, for more in-depth discussion of motivational interviewing).

## ANTICIPATORY GUIDANCE AND STAGES OF ADOLESCENT DEVELOPMENT

Because adolescents transition through various stages of development, anticipatory guidance can be given based upon differences in identity formation, risk-taking behaviors, autonomy development, and physical maturation at each stage. Early (10–14 years of age), middle (15–17 years), and late adolescent (18–21 years) stages of development are discussed in greater detail in Chapter 10, (Approach to Symptoms in Adolescents). A brief summary of each stage is given here to help the clinician determine where in the spectrum of adolescence a particular adolescent's behavior and cognitive thinking falls with respect to the provision of developmentally appropriate anticipatory guidance.

**Early adolescence** is a developmental stage in which early pubertal development takes place; thinking is "concrete"; youth are preoccupied with physical changes to their bodies and may be self-conscious or uncertain about their appearance and attractiveness to others.

- Physical development: development of secondary sexual characteristics; early adolescents frequently compare their own bodies to those of peers.
- Identity formation: developing sense of self as unique with testing of authority and limits; need for greater privacy; developing their own value system influenced by family and peer values; learning to control impulses.
- Sexual identity: increasing interest in sexual development and self-exploration.
- Parental relationships: seeking increased independence from parents, yet still ambivalent about taking increased responsibility in many aspects of their lives.
- Peer relationships: peer relationships often consist of same-sex groups; intense relationships with peers; conformity to peer group is important.
- Cognition: cognition is "concrete operational," focused on the here-and-now; lacking well-developed abstract thinking.

**Middle adolescence** features continued physical maturation; more intense testing of limits with "experimental" behaviors that may be considered "high-risk" (eg, sexual behaviors or drugs) and considered by adolescents as part of approaching adulthood; being concerned about personal attractiveness; becoming more introspective, with movement toward "formal operational" thinking; continued development of judgment and desire for greater autonomy.

- Physical development: continued linear growth; continued development of secondary sexual characteristics, often completed in females; body image important.
- Identity formation: increasing empathy toward others (less emphasis on self); increased intellectual ability and creativity; increasing feelings of omnipotence and invincibility ("personal fable") that may be associated with risk-taking behaviors.
- Sexual identity: growing interest in dating and sexual intimacy; experimentation with sexual behaviors; continued development of sexual identity.
- Parental relationships: growing desire for autonomy and separation and individuation from parents.
- Peer relationships: peers have a strong influence on the adolescent.
- Cognition: increasing ability for abstract thinking and idealism; decision making and behaviors influenced by psychosocial factors and influence of peers and media.

**Late adolescence** is when final physical maturation typically occurs (although many girls complete external pubertal changes in middle adolescence) and appearance approaches that of mature adults; sexual identity is consolidated; more idealistic; body image more stable; greater independence and interdependence; importance of family is realized; relationships are more intimate; future (career, family, goals, etc) explored in more depth.

- Physical development: physical maturation is generally complete for most older adolescents (although males may continue to grow into adulthood).
- Identity formation: most adolescents have developed a sense of self; a "rational and realistic conscience"; sense of perspective; practical vocational goals; for some, the beginning of financial independence; further refinement of moral, religious, and sexual values.
- Sexual identity: generally accepted; adolescents who are gay, lesbian, bisexual, or transgender may have questions or concerns that emerged in middle adolescence.
- Parental relationships: many adolescents become closer to their parents; preparation for future changes in living situation; less dependent upon parents.

- Peer relationships: adolescents are less concerned with group conformity and more interested in intimate and romantic relationships.
- Cognition: older adolescents are capable of more abstract thinking and demonstrate more problem-solving ability and ability to delay gratification; less impulsivity.

Although this is a generalized description based upon age ranges, some adolescents display behaviors that may reflect an earlier or later stage of development. The format of this chapter is based on the fluidity of development; the provider can determine if topics presented are relevant for a particular adolescent and a given visit.

## SUGGESTED TOPICS FOR ANTICIPATORY GUIDANCE IN ADOLESCENCE

Due to time constraints, it is often difficult to address all recommended preventive and health promotion topics during a well-adolescent visit. The context of each adolescent's life experiences and the relevancy of anticipatory guidance topics need to be considered. Described in the following are a general grouping of topics that fall under the categories of physical development, cognitive development, and social-emotional development. Anticipatory guidance for parents may be found in Chapter 34 (Parenting the Adolescent). In general, asking parents if they have concerns about their adolescent, growth and development or behaviors, either directly or through questionnaires such as GAPS forms for parents, provide opportunities to engage in relevant anticipatory guidance.

### PHYSICAL DEVELOPMENT

#### Puberty and Sexuality

One of the hallmarks of adolescence is pubertal development. By offering anticipatory guidance, the provider can serve a vital role in reviewing anticipated physical changes before they occur; discussions about growth, breast and genitalia development, body hair, menstruation, sweating, voice changes, and body fat distribution can help the adolescent be emotionally prepared for these changes. Indeed, many early adolescents worry about whether or not they are normal. Adolescents who mature earlier or later than their peers may also be concerned. Reassurance about the variability in timing and tempo of puberty may allay some fears. For adolescents who express body image dissatisfaction, consideration of a possible eating disorder and careful assessment is essential.

As adolescents begin to develop secondary sex characteristics, they become more interested and anxious about the changes occurring in their own bodies and those of their friends. Early adolescents are reassured to know that sexual feelings and masturbation are normal behaviors, and the health care provider can serve as a resource for questions about sexual feelings and development. Clinicians should discuss abstinence from sexual activity as developmentally appropriate, particularly for early adolescents, and provide appropriate risk-reduction guidance regarding sexual behaviors.[36] Providers should balance this with a discussion about preventing STIs, including human immunodeficiency virus (HIV), contraceptive methods, and sexual identity, ideally before patients become sexually active. Having this discussion early in the course of adolescent development lets patients know that the health care provider is a resource for these services when they do decide to engage in sexual activity. Questions should be asked in an open-ended manner so that adolescents who are lesbian, gay, bisexual, transgender, or questioning feel comfortable with this discussion. In middle and late adolescence, the issues previously mentioned can be reiterated and become more focused to the specific needs of the adolescent. A discussion about avoiding forced sex, being in a monogamous relationship, and the elements that comprise a healthy relationship (consensual, honest) can be beneficial.[37] In addition to the previous discussion about preventing unwanted pregnancy and STIs by using contraceptives and condoms correctly and consistently, adolescents should be aware of how to get and use emergency contraception.[38]

#### Health Promotion

Promoting physical health, positive body image, and healthy eating are important aspects of anticipatory guidance. Oral health is also an important component to health promotion and disease prevention. It is recommended that providers review the adolescent's daily oral health routine and encourage fluoride supplements, if indicated, up to age 16 years.[39] This recommendation is based on fluoride levels of local water sources. Adolescents should have twice yearly dental visits to prevent significant caries, monitor malocclusion and growth of second and third molars, and provide education.

With respect to nutrition, physical activity, and weight, it is crucial to assess the parents' and adolescent's concerns, tailor the discussion to the adolescent's needs, and include the parents as active participants in any lifestyle changes.[40] With the growing epidemic of childhood and adolescent obesity, recent expert recommendations[41] suggest counseling patients to (1) limit consumption of sugar-sweetened beverages, (2) increase intake of fruits and vegetables, (3) eat breakfast daily,

(4) limit eating in fast-food restaurants, (5) have family meals, (6) limit portion sizes, (7) limit screen time to no more than 2 hours a day, (8) remove television and computers from adolescent's bedrooms, and (9) participate in 60 minutes/day of moderate-to-vigorous activity to help adolescents maintain a healthy weight. Because most bone mineral accretion occurs during the second decade of life (peak rate 12.5 years of age in girls, 14 in boys), it is essential to optimize calcium intake during this time.[42] Encouraging sufficient calcium intake to achieve 1,300 mg/day can help maintain bone health for adolescents. Daily vitamin D supplementation, 400 IU per day, is also recommended. Menstruating females, and males going through the peak growth period are at risk for iron deficiency; iron-rich foods and iron supplementation may be appropriate. Folic acid-containing foods or supplementation for women of childbearing age, including adolescents, is warranted to help prevent neural tube defects.[43]

Skin cancer is clearly linked to cumulative and early exposure to ultraviolet radiation, yet adolescents are using natural and artificial radiation at increasing rates and often associate tanned skin with physical attractiveness.[44] To prevent sun damage, providers should discuss the application of sunscreen during outdoor activity, as well as the risks of indoor tanning.

Many adolescents suffer from excessive sleepiness, most often due to poor sleep hygiene. Providers should ask about sleep patterns, total quantity of sleep obtained, and any other sleep-related symptoms.[45] Awakening and going to bed at the same time every day and having a consistent morning and bedtime routine are important components of good sleep hygiene. Poor sleep may be a sign of depression, sleep apnea, or excessive caffeine intake. Lack of sleep can contribute to an adolescent's moodiness, physical symptoms such as tiredness, poor school performance, or increased attention-deficit/hyperactivity disorder (ADHD) symptoms.

## COGNITIVE DEVELOPMENT

As most adolescents progress from concrete operational thinking during early adolescence to more logical and abstract thinking in late adolescence, their judgment continues to develop. The prefrontal cortex, the area of the brain involved in decision making, planning, and impulse control, does not fully mature until individuals are in their 20s (see Chapter 5, Brain and Cognitive Development).[46] Opportunities for progressively increasing responsibilities, independent decision making, and trying again when an adolescent makes a mistake all contribute to the development of judgment. Along with this development, the desire for independence affects risk-taking behaviors. Early and middle adolescents often lack insight into the consequences of their actions. Emotional issues, such as yearning for peer acceptance, often interfere with an adolescent's ability to think in more complex ways. Parental monitoring is important to maintain adolescents' safety as their cognitive abilities expand.

### Injury Prevention

As they mature, adolescents spend more time with their friends and less time with their parents, making them more susceptible to the attraction of taking chances, which places them at risk for injuries. Indeed, focusing on risk-taking behavior is developmentally appropriate as the leading causes of mortality and morbidity in this age group (10–18 years old) are due to accidents (45%), homicide (12%), and suicide (10.3%).[47]

Inexperience behind the wheel of a motor vehicle and risk-taking behaviors while being a driver or passenger contribute to motor vehicle accidents.[48] Many states have graduated driver licensing laws to promote time to acquire and demonstrate proficiency in driving skills (and judgment) before gaining additional driving privileges. These laws have been shown to lower the rate of motor vehicle accidents among adolescents. A discussion of safe driving habits is appropriate for the middle and older adolescent, and may include: avoiding distractions while driving (texting, talking on a cell phone, eating), always wearing a lap-shoulder belt, limiting nighttime driving among inexperienced drivers, limiting the number of passengers, and making sure passengers wear a seat belt. In 2006, alcohol was associated with 25% of fatal accidents involving drivers 15 to 20 years old; 58% of adolescents riding as passengers in motor vehicles who died in motor vehicle accidents were not wearing seat belts.[49] The Insurance Institute for Highway Safety estimates that in fatal motor vehicle accidents, alcohol was involved in 18% of 16- to 17-year-old and 31% of 18- to 20-year-old drivers, respectively.[50] It is crucial to discuss the risk of cognitive impairment due to drinking alcohol or smoking marijuana and driving and to ensure that adolescents who are under the influence (or who are passengers in a vehicle with a driver under the influence) have a "designated driver" or someone to call to provide a ride home. This is an excellent opportunity for parents and adolescents to agree to a "no-questions-asked" policy for a parent to provide a safe ride home any time an adolescent needs one; the day following such an occurrence provides parents and the adolescent an opportunity to discuss how to avoid such situations in the future.

Homicide and suicide follow vehicular injury as the second and third most common causes of death for adolescents. Adolescents who use drugs are more prone to violence-related injury, including gang violence. Anticipatory guidance should include a discussion about weapon carrying, keeping guns out of the home or, at a minimum, keeping them stored unloaded and locked in the home.[51] Offering suggestions for managing conflict nonviolently and avoiding risky situations can potentially protect the adolescent from injury. Asking about dating violence may open the door for the adolescent to discuss a common but often ignored issue. Mood disorders, particularly depression and anxiety, are common during adolescence. It is important to ask directly about suicidal thoughts or attempts and to let the adolescent know the provider can serve as a resource for mood or emotional issues. Providing adolescents strategies for coping with stress can contribute to their emotional well-being.

Because alcohol and tobacco use often begin in adolescence, health care providers should make substance use/abuse an ongoing part of anticipatory guidance throughout adolescence. Three-quarters of mortality in the 15- to 19-year-old age group is due to unintentional injury, homicide, and suicide, and alcohol is involved in one-third of these cases.[52] Almost one-quarter of 12th graders consider themselves current smokers, and half of them have tried an illicit drug. Understanding the prevalence, patterns, cultural differences, and health consequences of substance abuse in the community can help the physician provide appropriate anticipatory guidance at regular office visits. This includes encouraging adolescents not to smoke or use smokeless tobacco, drugs, alcohol, inhalants, steroids, or diet pills. If a patient does smoke, assess his or her interest in quitting (see Chapter 173, Tobacco). To reduce their exposure, encourage adolescents to choose friends who do not use alcohol or smoke and to avoid settings in which alcohol and tobacco are readily available. In some adolescent populations, tattooing and body piercing are associated with other high-risk behaviors and should be discussed.[53] By serving as a confidential resource, providers can help adolescents quit or cut down on their use of tobacco, alcohol, and illicit drugs and refer to appropriate prevention services in the community.

To prevent head injuries while riding a bicycle, providers should inform parents and patients of the importance of wearing a bicycle helmet when riding and discuss the dangers of riding without one.[54] Off-road vehicles (eg, all-terrain vehicles, mopeds, minibikes) are particularly dangerous for adolescents under age 16 and should not be used by those without a driver's license.[55] Adolescents and parents should be aware of the necessity of wearing a helmet, using eye protection, and wearing reflective clothing to reduce injuries while riding one. To prevent injuries during sports participation, health care providers should advise adolescents to use appropriate protective gear during sports (eg, helmets, eye protection, mouth and wrist guards, athletic supporters, and knee/elbow pads). For athletes, providers should engage in an open discussion about the risks of performance- or growth-enhancing, or ergogenic aids, such as anabolic steroids, to determine a healthy way to meet their athletic goals without using drugs.[56]

### School

During adolescence, youth typically experience 2 to 3 changes in their school environment, moving from elementary to middle school/junior high and again to high school. Differences in academic expectations and social structure can be challenging for some students. Connectedness to school is associated with fewer risk-taking behaviors and better health outcomes.[57] Poor academic performance may be an indicator of learning disorders, stress, or emotional disturbances, such as depression and/or anxiety, and peer and/or family problems. In 2005, an estimated 9.4% of high school students dropped out of school.[58] A high school dropout is defined as an individual 16 to 24 years old who is not enrolled in, or has not completed, high school (in a civilian and noninstitutionalized setting). Racial and ethnic disparities exist: 23% of Hispanic, 11% of black, and 6% of non-Hispanic white students dropped out of high school in 2005.[58] Adolescents spend a significant portion of their day at school. Parents are encouraged to stay connected with teachers so that they are able to keep current with their adolescent's academic performance, behavior, and overall well-being. This allows parents to help their adolescent before problems occur or progress too far. Parental monitoring of school performance is related to increased likelihood of staying in school. Many teachers are able to answer common parental questions about normal social development and academic concerns.

In addition to the previous safety issues, adolescents may also become victims of bullying and cyberbullying. Safe and appropriate use of cell phones, other texting devices, and Internet safety are important topics for parents and health care providers to discuss. Adolescents make healthier choices if they stay connected with their family, if parents maintain a clear presence and appropriate level of supervision, and if clear limits and expectations are set. Discussing school performance and peer relationships, as well as an adolescent's goals, can give the provider insight into an adolescent's daily life and level of connectedness with his or her family, school, and community.

## SOCIAL AND EMOTIONAL DEVELOPMENT

### Connectedness

Adolescence is a period of identity formation and development of autonomy and individuality. This formative period is influenced by the people and community that surround the adolescent. Connectedness is a sense of belonging within different settings of a community and the different people associated in those settings. Adolescents who feel connected to their families, schools, and communities are healthier and engage in fewer risk-taking behaviors. Assessment of adolescents' connectedness in various areas may be helpful. These areas include: positive supports (eg, trusted, caring adults with whom they can confide in; older peers or relatives; friends), family relationships (eg, what role do they play in the family, do they feel they are a valuable member of the family), peer relationships (eg, do they have a number of friends), school (eg, they participate in school activities, are able to identify talents they may want to pursue, future goals related to education/vocation/leisure activities, feel as if they fit in to the school community or that they have their own niche in their school community), and community (eg, work, access to safe recreation, volunteerism, service activities, spiritual and cultural opportunities). When adolescents are involved in community activities, they also feel they have a place in the larger community. Changes in peers, moves to different cities or towns, changes within the family (eg, loss of a parent's job, divorce, illness, and death), and changes in schools may disrupt established connections that provide a sense of belonging and security to many youth.

### Families

During adolescence relationships with parents change, shifting from the primary influence of parents to that of peers who may have different values and beliefs. This is especially true during early and middle adolescence. This shift of influence can be challenging if these new values and beliefs contrast with family-held values. It is particularly challenging for immigrant families in which there may be significant differences between the culture and values of parents and those of adolescents. In many ways, parents may feel they or their values are rejected. It is important for parents to continue to communicate with their adolescents and have discussions about these differences. An adolescent's perception of being able to have an open discussion about differences supports healthy discussion as adolescents develop their value and belief systems. Also, parents should continue to model the behavior and values they want to impart to their adolescents. Indeed, connectedness with parents has been shown to be a protective factor from development of risky behaviors.[59] Most young adults express values that often mirror family values.

Parents need to continue to be involved with their adolescents by appropriately participating in shared activities, monitoring, and supervising activities and peers. As adolescents develop a sense of self, they may voice the need for more privacy or "space." It may seem to parents that they have to expend more effort to be involved as adolescents naturally seek more privacy. This "space" represents the opportunity to have new experiences and to test judgment and decision-making abilities. "Space" also is an opportunity for adolescents to assume more responsibility, become more independent, and develop confidence. Ultimately, "space" reflects the gradual process of individuation, separation, and identity development. However, most adolescents want their parents to be involved ("at a distance"). Adolescents continue to need limits and boundaries as they develop judgment, explore their external world, and discover themselves. A clear discussion about family rules and expectations for appropriate behavior and activities is important in establishing a base from which an adolescent can reference, especially during early and middle adolescence. Adolescents make healthier choices if they stay connected with their family, if parents maintain a clear presence and appropriate level of supervision, and if clear limitations and expectations are set. From all of these changes in values and relationships within the family grow independence and autonomy, self-confidence, and self-efficacy.

### Peers

During adolescence, peer relationships change from interest in same-sex peer group activities in early adolescence, to a smaller network of friends with similar interests and activities during middle adolescence, and to increasingly intimate and intense relationships during older adolescence. Early adolescent friendships are often intense (ie, "BFFL: Best Friends for Life"). From early to late adolescence there is a shift from a desire for conformity and looking and acting like peers (through dress, activities, interests, and behaviors) to individual expression.

As with school, potential changes in groups of friends or significant others should be anticipated. Friendships often change, and it is important for the adolescent to have a number of different friends upon which they can rely. Adolescents who have a difficult time forging new friendships may struggle and become socially isolated when they get into an argument with their one friend. Emotional trauma may occur if adolescents become victims of bullying or cyberbullying. As adolescents try to fit in with each other, peer pressure may influence risk-taking behaviors (eg, sexual activity, alcohol, and other drug use) as well as healthy activities (eg, sports, nutrition, and hobbies). The leading causes of death and morbidity (unintentional accidents, suicide, and homicide) may be preventable with timely and appropriate intervention. Also, safe and appropriate use of cell phones, other text-messaging devices, and Internet safety are important topics for parents and health care providers to discuss. Discussions about friendships, peer pressure, and dangers of high-risk behaviors, providing local resources for safe adolescent activities, and helping adolescents and parents recognize the symptoms of anxiety and depression are all an important part of anticipatory guidance.

### Competency Building

Competency is the ability to handle situations effectively.[60] Competency is believed to be an important component of many resiliency models; resiliency is the ability to "spring back" from adversity. Examples of competency include Kim's[57] description of 5 key youth attributes: a positive sense of self, self-control, decision-making skills, moral system of belief, and social connectedness. Ginsburg[60] describes 7 key components to resiliency: competence, confidence, connection, character, contribution, coping, and control. An assessment of youth competency is in step with a strengths-based approach to anticipatory guidance.

Adolescents develop increasing self-efficacy and less dependence upon adults for self-care (eg, personal hygiene, feeding oneself, homework, school attendance, and driving) by taking on progressive responsibility and developing judgment (eg, driving, safety, and peer pressure). As adolescents mature, they take on increasing responsibility such as chores at home, group activities such as sports or the school newspaper, leadership positions, and jobs. Developmentally appropriate assumption of responsibility teaches adolescents to understand the limits parents (or others) have set and their consequences. Increasing responsibility and independence provide adolescents with the opportunities to practice and demonstrate judgment and earn trust. School is one situation in which increasing individual responsibility is inherent as adolescents become more responsible for independent homework, attendance, and course selection. Successful participation in school demonstrates appropriate time management, decision making, and organizational skills.

Adolescents with chronic illnesses or special health care needs may be expected to assume responsibility for their own medication. Many health care practitioners encourage adolescents to become responsible for their own health care; however, they often do not provide explicit recommendations on how to do so. It is not uncommon for parents to have difficulty letting go of responsibility or shifting complete responsibility to an adolescent. Over time, a gradual shift in responsibility with parental oversight ("double-checking") can be helpful. For example, a pillbox for oral medications allows an adolescent to assume responsibility for taking medications, yet it provides parents a way to check the pillbox at the end of the day without directly "nagging" their adolescent. Participation in health care responsibility in early adolescence may promote better medical adherence and readiness to assume greater responsibility later in adolescence.

### Coping Skills and Conflict Resolution

Positive coping skills and the ability to handle conflict are important life skills. Assessing an adolescent's ability to handle commonly occurring change and stress (eg, change in schools, parental divorce, or household moves) may help identify areas of need and whether or not they can be addressed through office interventions or need referral to mental health resources. The art of negotiation, having a large repertoire of positive stress-reducing skills, dealing with anger, and conflict resolution are important skills. Encouraging parents to converse with their children about these and other topics will facilitate communication when they become adolescents. Also, parents should be supported in modeling appropriate coping strategies. If adolescents or their families need more assistance, providers should refer them to appropriate resources.

### Transitioning Care

Not only does adolescence encompass physical, cognitive, and social-emotional changes, the adolescent may experience other life changes. For example, changes in health insurance coverage due to age, parental employment, moving, and parental divorce may require a change in providers and access to medical and mental health care. Although it may be difficult to anticipate those changes, providers should be prepared to discuss those changes with families and offer resources when available. One predictable change is the natural aging out of pediatric practices. Anticipatory guidance should be given regarding the transition from a pediatric practice to adult primary care and/or adult subspecialists. Transitioning health care should be introduced early in adolescence and revisited periodically to facilitate a smoother transition. During early or middle adolescence it may entail making sure the teen knows his or her medical history, becomes comfortable talking with the physician separately, and is aware of confidentiality issues. During middle adolescence it may be about taking more responsibility in personal health promotion. During middle to late adolescence it may include discussions about health insurance and access to health care, particularly finding an adult provider, when an adolescent moves out of the house and begins working or going to college.

## CONCLUSION

Adolescence is a complex period of development in which there is tremendous physical, cognitive, and social-emotional growth. Staying connected to adolescents by seeing them regularly, providing appropriate anticipatory guidance, and serving as a resource if the adolescent and parent have concerns or questions can improve adolescent health and well-being, as well as satisfy the health care provider. Health care providers have an opportunity to influence adolescent development in many ways, and it is a privilege to be part of that growth.

## INTERNET AND PRINT RESOURCES FOR PARENTS AND ADOLESCENTS

- Adolescent Health Transition Project. Washington Department of Health: depts.washington.edu/healthtr/.
- Greydanus DE, Bashe P, American Academy of Pediatrics. *Caring for your teenager: the complete and authoritative guide*. New York: Bantam Books; 2003.
- Resources for Adolescents, Patients, and Parents. American Academy of Pediatrics: www.aap.org/moc/AdolHandouts_AAPMbrs/Resources.htm.

## REFERENCES


1. Hagan JF, Shaw JS, Duncan P. *Bright Futures Guidelines for Health Supervision of Infants, Children, and Adolescents*. 3rd ed. Elk Grove Village, IL: American Academy of Pediatrics; 2008

2. Gerend MA, Magloire ZF. Awareness, knowledge, and beliefs about human papillomavirus in a racially diverse sample of young adults. *J Adolesc Health.* 2008;42:237–242

3. American Medical Association Department of Adolescent Health. *Guidelines for Adolescent Preventive Services (GAPS): Recommendations Monograph*. 2nd ed. Chicago, IL: American Medical Association, Department of Adolescent Health; 1995

4. Blaschke GS, Lopreiato JO, Bedingfield B, et al. Choosing the Bright Futures Guidelines: lessons from leaders and early adopters. *Pediatr Ann.* 2008;37:262–272

5. Selden TM. Compliance with well-child visit recommendations: evidence from the Medical Expenditure Panel Survey, 2000–2002. *Pediatrics.* 2006;118:e1766–1778

6. Richmond TK, Freed GL, Clark SJ, Cabana MD. Guidelines for adolescent well care: is there consensus? *Curr Opin Pediatr.* 2006;18:365–370

7. Norkin-Goldstein E, Dworkin P, Bernstein B. Time devoted to anticipatory guidance during child health supervision visits: how are we doing? *Ambul Child Health.* 1999;5:113–120

8. Galuska DA, Fulton JE, Powell KE, et al. Pediatrician counseling about preventive health topics: results from the Physicians' Practices Survey, 1998–1999. *Pediatrics.* 2002;109:E83–103

9. Moyer VA, Butler M. Gaps in the evidence for well-child care: a challenge to our profession. *Pediatrics.* 2004;114:1511–1521

10. Munro J, Coleman P, Nicholl J, Harper R, Kent G, Wild D. Can we prevent accidental injury to adolescents? A systematic review of the evidence. *Inj Prev.* 1995;1:249–255

11. Magar NA, Dabova-Missova S, Gjerdingen DK. Effectiveness of targeted anticipatory guidance during well-child visits: a pilot trial. *J Am Board Fam Med.* 2006;19:450–458

12. Olson LM, Tanner JL, Stein MT, Radecki L. Well-child care: looking back, looking forward. *Pediatr Ann.* 2008;37:143–151

13. US Preventive Services Task Force. AHRQ. The guide to clinical preventive services. 2008. Available at: www.ahrq.gov/clinic/pocketgd09/pocketgd09.pdf. Accessed May 4, 2010

14. Summary of Recommendations for Clinical Preventive Services. Revision 6.8. Leawood, KS: American Academy of Family Physicians; 2008

15. US Preventive Services Task Force. The guide to clinical preventive services 2005: recommendations of the US Preventive Services Task Force. Available at: www.ahrq.gov/clinic/pocketgd.pdf. Accessed January 9, 2006

16. Elster A, Kuznets N. *AMA Guidelines for Adolescent Preventive Services (GAPS).* Baltimore, MD: Williams & Wilkins; 1994

17. Elster A. Comparison of recommendations for adolescent clinical preventive services developed by national organizations. *Arch Pediatr Adolesc Med.* 1998;152:193–198

18. Hagan JH, Jr. Discerning bright futures of electronic health records. *Pediatr Ann.* 2008;37:173–179

19. Gadomski A, Bennett S, Young M, Wissow LS. Guidelines for Adolescent Preventive Services: the GAPS in practice. *Arch Pediatr Adolesc Med.* 2003;157:426–432

20. Klein JD, Allan MJ, Elster AB, et al. Improving adolescent preventive care in community health centers. *Pediatrics.* 2001;107:318–327

21. EPSDT and Title V Collaboration to Improve Child Health Resources and Services Administration. 2008. Available at: www.hrsa.gov/epsdt/. Accessed January 6, 2009

22. Hull PC, Husaini BA, Tropez-Sims S, Reece M, Emerson J, Levine R. EPSDT preventive services in a low-income pediatric population: impact of a nursing protocol. *Clin Pediatr (Phila).* 2008;47:137–142

23. National Committee for Quality Assurance. HEDIS 2009 summary table of measures, product lines and changes. Available at: www.ncqa.org/Portals/0/HEDISQM/HEDIS2009/2009_Measures.pdf. Accessed January 10, 2009

24. McInerny TK, Cull WL, Yudkowsky BK. Physician reimbursement levels and adherence to American Academy of Pediatrics well-visit and immunization recommendations. *Pediatrics.* 2005;115:833–838

25. Fairbrother G, Scheinmann R, Osthimer B, et al. Factors that influence adolescent reports of counseling by physicians on risky behavior. *J Adolesc Health.* 2005;37:467–476

26. O'Malley AS. Current evidence on the impact of continuity of care. *Curr Opin Pediatr.* 2004;16:693–699

27. Barkin SL, Scheindlin B, Brown C, Ip E, Finch S, Wasserman RC. Anticipatory guidance topics: are more better? *Ambul Pediatr.* 2005;5:372-376

28. Duncan PM, Garcia AC, Frankowski BL, et al. Inspiring healthy adolescent choices: a rationale for and guide to strength promotion in primary care. *J Adolesc Health.* 2007;41:525-535

29. Ozer EM. The adolescent primary care visit: time to build on strengths. *J Adolesc Health.* 2007;41:519-520

30. Prochaska JO. *Systems of Psychotherapy: A Transtheoretical Analysis*. Homewood, IL: Dorsey Press; 1979

31. Grimshaw GM, Stanton A. Tobacco cessation interventions for young people. *Cochrane Database Syst Rev.* 2006:CD003289

32. Miller WR, Rollnick S. *Motivational Interviewing: Preparing People for Change*. 2nd ed. New York, NY: Guilford Press; 2002

33. Marlatt GA, Baer JS, Kivlahan DR, et al. Screening and brief intervention for high-risk college student drinkers: results from a 2-year follow-up assessment. *J Consult Clin Psychol.* 1998;66:604-615

34. McCambridge J, Strang J. The efficacy of single-session motivational interviewing in reducing drug consumption and perceptions of drug-related risk and harm among young people: results from a multi-site cluster randomized trial. *Addiction.* 2004;99:39-52

35. Borrelli B, Riekert KA, Weinstein A, Rathier L. Brief motivational interviewing as a clinical strategy to promote asthma medication adherence. *J Allergy Clin Immunol.* 2007;120:1023-1030

36. Blythe MJ, Diaz A. Contraception and adolescents. *Pediatrics.* 2007;120:1135-1148

37. Feldman E. Contraceptive care for the adolescent. *Prim Care.* 2006;33:405-431

38. American Academy of Pediatrics Committee on Adolescence. Emergency contraception. *Pediatrics.* 2005;116:1026-1035

39. American Academy of Pediatrics Section on Pediatric Dentistry and Oral Health. Preventive oral health intervention for pediatricians. *Pediatrics.* 2008;122:1387-1394

40. Johnson G, Kent G, Leather J. Strengthening the parent-child relationship: a review of family interventions and their use in medical settings. *Child Care Health Dev.* 2005;31:25-32

41. Davis MM, Gance-Cleveland B, Hassink S, Johnson R, Paradis G, Resnicow K. Recommendations for prevention of childhood obesity. *Pediatrics.* 2007;120(suppl 4):S229-253

42. Greer FR, Krebs NF. Optimizing bone health and calcium intakes of infants, children, and adolescents. *Pediatrics.* 2006;117:578-585

43. American Academy of Pediatrics Committee on Genetics. Folic acid for the prevention of neural tube defects. *Pediatrics.* 1999;104:325-327

44. MacNeal RJ, Dinulos JG. Update on sun protection and tanning in children. *Curr Opin Pediatr.* 2007;19:425-429

45. Millman RP. Excessive sleepiness in adolescents and young adults: causes, consequences, and treatment strategies. *Pediatrics.* 2005;115:1774-1786

46. Giedd JN. Structural magnetic resonance imaging of the adolescent brain. *Ann N Y Acad Sci.* 2004;1021:77-85

47. National Center for Injury Prevention and Control. Centers for Disease Control and Prevention. Web-based injury statistics query and reporting system (WISQARS). Available at: www.cdc.gov/ncipc/wisqars. Accessed January 18, 2009

48. Weiss JC. The teen driver. *Pediatrics.* 2006;118:2570-2581

49. National Highway Traffic Safety Administration. Youth traffic safety statistics (adolescent safety statistics). Available at: nhtsa.gov. Accessed January 18, 2009

50. Insurance Institute for Highway Safety. Fatality facts 2006: teenagers. Available at: www.iihs.org/research/fatality_facts_2006/teenagers.html. Accessed January 18, 2009

51. American Academy of Pediatrics Committee on Injury and Poison Prevention. Firearm-related injuries affecting the pediatric population. *Pediatrics.* 2000;105:888-895

52. Kulig JW. Tobacco, alcohol, and other drugs: the role of the pediatrician in prevention, identification, and management of substance abuse. *Pediatrics.* 2005;115:816-821

53. Carroll ST, Riffenburgh RH, Roberts TA, Myhre EB. Tattoos and body piercings as indicators of adolescent risk-taking behaviors. *Pediatrics.* 2002;109:1021-1027

54. Finnoff JT, Laskowski ER, Altman KL, Diehl NN. Barriers to bicycle helmet use. *Pediatrics.* 2001;108:E4

55. American Academy of Pediatrics. Committee on Injury and Poison Prevention. All-terrain vehicle injury prevention: two-, three-, and four-wheeled unlicensed motor vehicles. *Pediatrics.* 2000;105: 1352-1354

56. American Academy of Pediatrics Committee on Sports Medicine and Fitness. Adolescents and anabolic steroids: a subject review. *Pediatrics.* 1997;99:904-908

57. Kim TE, Guerra NG, Williams KR. Preventing youth problem behaviors and enhancing physical health by promoting core competencies. *J Adolesc Health.* 2008;43:401-407

58. High school dropout rates. Child trends. Available at: www.childtrendsdatabank.org. Accessed January 18, 2009

59. DeVore ER, Ginsburg KR. The protective effects of good parenting on adolescents. *Curr Opin Pediatr.* 2005;17:460-465

60. Ginsburg KR. *A Parent's Guide to Building Resilience in Children and Teens: Giving Your Child Roots and Wings*. Elk Grove Village, IL: American Academy of Pediatrics; 2006

# CHAPTER 16

# Adolescent Nutrition and Physical Activity

NICOLE LARSON, PhD, MPH, RD • MARY STORY, PhD, RD

## IMPORTANCE OF HEALTHY EATING AND PHYSICAL ACTIVITY FOR ADOLESCENTS

Adolescence is characterized by dramatic changes in physical, cognitive, social, and emotional development that affect nutrition and physical activity. It is a nutritionally vulnerable period of life because rapid physical growth creates a high demand for energy and nutrients.[1] During the second decade of life, young people attain the final 15% to 20% of their adult height, gain 50% of their ideal adult body weight, and accumulate 45% of their peak skeletal mass.[2] If energy intake is inadequate, linear growth may be compromised and sexual maturation delayed. Poor diet during adolescence also increases the risk for problems such as iron deficiency, dental caries, and poor school performance. On the other hand, physical inactivity and excessive consumption of high-calorie foods and beverages that result in energy imbalance are the most important contributors to the development of overweight and obesity in adolescents. In addition to their effect on immediate health problems, poor diet and physical activity patterns developed during adolescence increase the risk for several chronic diseases later in life including heart disease, type 2 diabetes, and osteoporosis. Anticipatory guidance to prepare adolescents for the physical changes of puberty and to promote adequate nutritional intake and participation in physical activities according to current recommendations is therefore essential.[1,3] This chapter reviews nutrition and physical activity issues for adolescents, current dietary and physical activity recommendations, and tools for supervising these aspects of adolescent health.

## COMMON NUTRITION AND PHYSICAL ACTIVITY CONCERNS OF ADOLESCENTS

There are considerable gaps between current dietary and physical activity practices of adolescents and recommendations for optimal health. National nutrition data indicate that many adolescents have marginal or insufficient intakes for several nutrients, including calcium, magnesium, zinc, iron, phosphorus, potassium, vitamins A, C, and E, and dietary fiber, and are consuming inadequate amounts of whole grains, fruits, vegetables, and fat-free or low-fat dairy foods.[4,5] Other dietary behaviors of concern among adolescents include skipping meals (especially breakfast), frequent intake of fast-food meals, and high intakes of energy-dense, nutrient-poor foods and sugar-sweetened beverages. Engaging in unhealthy weight-control behaviors also is a common problem, particularly among adolescent females. Adolescent females have the poorest dietary intakes of any group within the pediatric population.

Physical activity levels (PALs) of both males and females decline during adolescence, but the decline is particularly great among females.[3] Low PALs and highly sedentary leisure activities are common among adolescents, contributing to the growing prevalence of overweight. The prevalence of overweight among US adolescents has more than tripled over the past 30 years, and current estimates indicate that approximately 34% of adolescents are overweight or obese.[6] In contrast, fewer than 1% of adolescents develop anorexia nervosa, and bulimia nervosa affects fewer than 3% of the adolescent population.[7] However, these eating disorders also represent a significant cause of morbidity and mortality.[7] Other nutrition-related concerns among adolescents include the use of anabolic steroids and nonnutritional dietary supplements.

## CURRENT DIETARY RECOMMENDATIONS FOR HEALTHY ADOLESCENTS

Dietary recommendations for adolescents address what nutrients are required to maintain health, the amounts of various nutrients needed on a daily basis, the influence of growth and development on energy and nutrient needs, and how foods and beverages should be chosen to meet these recommendations. The following section considers each of these issues.

### MAJOR NUTRIENTS REQUIRED BY ADOLESCENTS FOR HEALTH

Nutrients required by the body to support normal adolescent growth, tissue maintenance, and ongoing health can be organized in to 6 categories (carbohydrates, proteins, fats, vitamins, minerals, and water). The first 3 categories, carbohydrates (chains of sugar molecules), proteins (chains of amino acids), and fats (glycerol and fatty acids), are energy-yielding nutrients. These nutrients provide the energy (kcal) to carry out basic functions of the body and to fuel activity. Vitamins and minerals are micronutrient chemical substances that do not provide energy but have specific roles in normal body functioning, such as enzyme and hormone activity.

Carbohydrates, certain amino acids, essential fatty acids (linoleic and alpha-linolenic), vitamins, minerals, and water are considered essential nutrients because they cannot be manufactured by the body or produced in sufficient amounts to meet demands. All adolescents need the same set of nutrients for growth and normal body functioning, but several factors, such as gender, body size, life stage, lifestyle habits, illness, pregnancy, lactation, and genetic characteristics influence the amount of each nutrient an individual needs to consume. Table 16-1 summarizes the major nutrients required for health, their functions in the body, dietary sources, and consequences of inadequate and excessive intakes.

**Table 16-1**

## Summary of Major Nutrients

| *Food Component* | *Function in Body* | *Dietary Sources* | *Consequences of Inadequate Intake* | *Consequences of Excessive Intake* |
|---|---|---|---|---|
| **Macronutrients** | | | | |
| Food energy | Metabolic functions: maintenance of body temperature, growth and repair of bones and tissue, and movement of muscles; body fat storage | Carbohydrate—4 kcal/g<br>Protein—4 kcal/g<br>Fat—9 kcal/g | Underweight, semistarvation, growth retardation | Contributes to the development of overweight |
| Water | Medium for most chemical reactions in the body; role in energy transformation, excretion of wastes, and regulation of temperature | Tap and bottled water, other nonalcoholic beverages | Dehydration | Rare |
| Carbohydrate | Energy source; stored as glycogen or converted to body fat | Simple carbohydrates: fruit, vegetables, milk<br>Complex carbohydrates: grain products and starchy vegetables | Ketosis | Contributes to excess energy intake and the development of overweight |
| Protein | Involved in most metabolic processes; essential for growth, development, and maintenance of body tissues; amino acids are structural elements of muscle, connective tissue, bone, enzymes, hormones, and antibodies | Lean meat, poultry, fish, eggs, fat-free or low-fat milk, cheese | Rare in the United States; protein-energy malnutrition or kwashiorkor | Excess protein intake is converted to body fat and may contribute to the development of overweight |

*(Continued)*

## Table 16-1 (Continued)

| *Food Component* | *Function in Body* | *Dietary Sources* | *Consequences of Inadequate Intake* | *Consequences of Excessive Intake* |
|---|---|---|---|---|
| Fat, fatty acids, cholesterol | Concentrated source of energy; carrier for the fat-soluble vitamins; structural and functional components of cell membranes | Linoleic acid: sunflower, soy, cottonseed, and safflower oils α-linolenic acid: canola, soybean, and flaxseed oils, walnuts | Clinical deficiencies of essential fatty acids and fat-soluble nutrients occur and are associated with poor growth, scaly skin, and a diminished immune response | Contributes to the development of overweight; may increase risk for cardiovascular disease later in life |
| Fiber | Bulk in diet; promotes health of digestive tract and normal elimination | Bran cereals, whole grains, many fruits and vegetables, legumes, nuts | Constipation | Potential to limit mineral absorption; may interfere with intake of adequate energy |
| **Micronutrients** | | | | |
| ***Minerals*** | | | | |
| Calcium | Important role in the development and maintenance of bones and teeth; needed for nerve activity, muscle contraction, and regulation of heart muscle function; aids in blood clotting | Dairy products, canned salmon and other fish with bones, calcium-set tofu, kale, broccoli, almonds | Decreased peak bone mass (may increase risk for osteoporosis later in life) | Interference with absorption of other minerals (eg, iron); kidney stones (rare); possible soft tissue calcification; constipation |
| Fluoride | Component of bones and tooth enamel | Fluoridated water, tea, shrimp, crab (also in fluoridated toothpastes and rinses) | Impaired dental health (eg, dental caries) | Mottled teeth; skeletal deformities |
| Iron | Carrier of oxygen in body; role in red blood cell formation; component of the muscle protein myoglobin; required for some energy-forming reactions | Liver, beef, poultry, fish/seafood, legumes, nuts and seeds, green leafy vegetables, whole and enriched grains | Microcytic anemia, pale appearance, reduced resistance to infection, atrophy of tongue epithelium, angular stomatitis, pica, impaired cognitive performance | Iron overload and tissue damage (in persons with genetic predisposition); impaired zinc absorption |
| Magnesium | Plays a role in the development and maintenance of bones; activates enzymes involved in most aspects of metabolism | Nuts, legumes, tofu, dark green vegetables, bran cereal, milk | Rare—muscle weakness and spasms, tremor, nausea, personality changes, anemia | Rare—paralysis of skeletal muscles |
| Phosphorus | Structural element of bones and teeth; component of cell membranes; participates in reactions of intermediary metabolism; acid-base regulation | Dairy products, meat, poultry, fish, eggs, other protein sources | Rare if protein and calcium nutrition are adequate; anorexia, lethargy, damage to the nervous system, osteomalacia, muscle weakness | Nutritional secondary hyperparathyroidism; reduced bone mass |

*(Continued)*

**Table 16-1 (Continued)**

| *Food Component* | *Function in Body* | *Dietary Sources* | *Consequences of Inadequate Intake* | *Consequences of Excessive Intake* |
|---|---|---|---|---|
| Potassium | Assists in muscle contraction; regulation of body fluid volume and acid-base balance; principal intracellular cation; required for protein and carbohydrate metabolism; potassium-rich diets lower blood pressure | Many fruits and vegetables, milk, yogurt, fish, pork | Weakness, irritability, mental confusion, cardiac arrhythmia | Cardiac arrhythmia |
| Sodium | Regulation with potassium of body fluid volume and acid-base balance; needed for muscle and nerve activity; principal extracellular cation | Table salt (sodium chloride), canned foods | Rare due to wide availability in foods | Hypertension in susceptible individuals |
| Zinc | Involved in the formation of proteins; component of insulin and many enzymes; role in wound healing, blood formation, general growth, and maintenance of all tissues | Meats, dairy products, nuts, whole grains | Growth failure and delayed sexual maturation, loss of taste and appetite, mental lethargy, slow wound healing, severe diarrhea, dermatitis | Relatively nontoxic; acute toxicities lead to tachycardia, hyperglycemia, and copper-deficiency anemia |
| ***Vitamins*** | | | | |
| Folate | Promotes the normal formation of red blood cells; required for reactions that synthesize proteins and nucleotides | Liver, dark green leafy vegetables, legumes, whole-grain cereals | Megaloblastic anemia, red and sore tongue, pallor, diarrhea, neural tube defects in offspring | May mask signs of a vitamin $B_{12}$ deficiency |
| Niacin | Central to energy metabolism of protein, carbohydrate, and fat; role in DNA repair | Liver and other meats, grains, legumes, peanuts (also dairy products and eggs as sources of tryptophan) | Dermatitis, fatigue, diarrhea/indigestion, nervous disorders, dementia (pellagra) | Low toxicity—side effects of clinical uses include flushing, headaches, tachycardia, nausea, diarrhea, impaired liver function |
| Riboflavin | Components of enzymes involved in metabolism of carbohydrates, protein, and fat; important role in biosynthesis of niacin from tryptophan; essential for activation of vitamins $B^6$ and folate | Dairy products, liver, and other meats, enriched and fortified cereals, grains | Cheilosis; angular stomatitis; fatigue; soreness and inflammation of mouth, lips, and tongue; peripheral neuropathy | No known toxicity |

*(Continued)*

**Table 16-1 (Continued)**

| *Food Component* | *Function in Body* | *Dietary Sources* | *Consequences of Inadequate Intake* | *Consequences of Excessive Intake* |
|---|---|---|---|---|
| Thiamin | Component of enzymes involved in release of energy from carbohydrates; supports growth and maintenance of nerve and muscle tissues | Pork and other meats, whole-grain and enriched grain products, legumes, milk | Anorexia, decreased muscle tone and motor weakness, cardiovascular and respiratory symptoms, neurological changes (beriberi) | Relatively nontoxic but massive doses may cause headaches, weakness, cardiac arrhythmia, and convulsions |
| Vitamin A (retinol) | Maintenance of healthy bones, teeth, hair, and mucous membranes; maintains vision; functions in reproduction and immune health | Preformed retinol: liver, fortified foods, eggs, milk, cheese<br>Carotene (provitamin): dark green leafy vegetables, yellow and orange vegetables, fruits | Increased susceptibility to infection, changes in eyes (keratomalacia) and skin, vision problems (night blindness, xeropthalmia), microcytic anemia, impaired growth | Teratogenic; chronic and acute overdoses produce toxicity symptoms such as nausea, headache, liver damage, dermatitis, and hair loss |
| Vitamin $B_6$ (pyridoxine) | Functions in metabolism of protein and glycogen; role in nervous system functioning; essential for conversion of tryptophan to niacin; supports normal growth | Meats, milk, eggs, legumes, fortified cereals, bananas, avocados, tomatoes, potatoes | Depression, confusion, convulsions | No effects associated with vitamin intake from food sources |
| Vitamin $B_{12}$ (cobalamin) | Required for formation of red blood cells, function of nervous system, and metabolism of protein and fat | Liver, red meat, fish and seafood, eggs, dairy foods, enriched cereals | Pernicious anemia; neurologic damage | None known—excess vitamin is rapidly excreted by the kidneys |
| Vitamin C (ascorbic acid) | Maintenance of healthy capillaries and gums; aids in iron absorption; functions in immune health; dietary antioxidant | Citrus fruits, other fruits, tomatoes, potatoes, dark green vegetables | Increased bruising and bleeding of skin and gums, weakness, slow recovery from infections (scurvy) | Gastrointestinal symptoms |
| Vitamin D | Needed for the absorption and use of calcium and phosphorus in bone formation, nerve function, and muscle activity | Fish, eggs, butter, some plant oils, vitamin D-fortified milk, margarines, cereals | Impaired mineralization of bones, bone pain, muscle weakness | Acute: weakness, nausea, anorexia, headache, cramps, vomiting<br>Chronic: calcification of soft tissue |
| Vitamin E ($\alpha$-tocopherol) | Antioxidant functions | Vegetable fats and oils, whole grains, wheat germ, nuts and seeds, eggs | Rare—neuropathological changes, enhanced fragility of red blood cells (hemolytic anemia) | Rare—at extremely high levels may antagonize actions of other fat-soluble vitamins |
| Vitamin K (phylloquinone, menaquinone) | Required for mechanisms that cause blood to clot when bleeding occurs; role in bone metabolism | Leafy green vegetables, liver, plant oils, margarine | Rare—increased bleeding, bruising; decreased calcium in bones | Rare—only with use of synthetic forms (ie, menadione) |

**AMOUNTS OF NUTRIENTS REQUIRED FOR HEALTH DURING ADOLESCENCE: DIETARY REFERENCE INTAKES**

Energy and nutrient needs are increased during adolescence to support rapid physiologic growth and development. Requirements parallel the rate of growth, with the greatest nutrient needs occurring during the period of peak height velocity. Nutrient requirements are also gender-specific after puberty due to differential changes in lean body mass and body fat mass composition in males and females, and the onset of menstruation in females. The Dietary Reference Intakes (DRIs)[8] are a set of 4 reference values useful for planning and evaluating the nutrient intakes of healthy people.

- Recommended Dietary Allowances (RDAs) represent goals for individual intake and are established at a level sufficient to meet the needs of nearly all persons (about 98%) in a particular life stage and gender group.
- Estimated Average Requirements (EARs) are reference values alternatively used to evaluate dietary intakes of populations and are established at a level sufficient to meet the needs of 50% of persons in a particular life stage and gender group.
- Adequate Intakes (AIs) are used in place of RDAs and EARs when there is not sufficient scientific evidence to support defining either of these.
- Tolerable Upper Intake Levels (ULs) represent the highest level of usual intake likely to pose no risk of adverse health effects for nearly all (about 98%) of individuals in a life stage and gender group. As intakes of a nutrient increase above the UL, the potential for adverse health effects increases.

Reference values for adolescents (Table 16-2 and Table 16-3) are categorized according to chronological age rather than developmental stage. Therefore, their use

**Table 16-2**

**Dietary Reference Intakes of Selected Nutrients for Adolescents[9-13]**

| *Life Stage Group* | *Males* | | *Females* | | *Pregnancy* | *Lactation* |
|---|---|---|---|---|---|---|
| | *9–13 y* | *14–18 y* | *9–13 y* | *14–18 y* | *≤18 y* | *≤18 y* |
| **Macronutrients** | | | | | | |
| Total water (L/d)* | 2.4 | 3.3 | 2.1 | 2.3 | 3.0 | 3.8 |
| Carbohydrate (g/d) | 130 | 130 | 130 | 130 | 175 | 210 |
| Protein (g/d) | 34 | 52 | 34 | 46 | 71 | 71 |
| Total fat (g/d) | ND | ND | ND | ND | ND | ND |
| Linoleic acid (g/d)* | 12 | 16 | 10 | 11 | 13 | 13 |
| α-Linolenic acid (g/d)* | 1.2 | 1.6 | 1.0 | 1.1 | 1.4 | 1.3 |
| Fiber (g/d)* | 31 | 38 | 26 | 26 | 28 | 29 |
| **Minerals** | | | | | | |
| Calcium (mg/d)* | 1,300 | 1,300 | 1,300 | 1,300 | 1,300 | 1,300 |
| Iron (mg/d) | 8 | 11 | 8 | 15 | 27 | 10 |
| Magnesium (mg/d) | 240 | 410 | 240 | 360 | 400 | 360 |
| Phosphorous (mg/d) | 1,250 | 1,250 | 1,250 | 1,250 | 1,250 | 1,250 |
| Zinc (mg/d) | 8 | 11 | 8 | 9 | 13 | 14 |
| **Vitamins** | | | | | | |
| Folate (μg/d)[a,b] | 300 | 400 | 300 | 400 | 600 | 500 |
| Niacin (mg/d)[c] | 12 | 16 | 12 | 14 | 18 | 17 |
| Riboflavin (mg/d) | 0.9 | 1.3 | 0.9 | 1.0 | 1.4 | 1.6 |

*(Continued)*

**Table 16-2 (Continued)**

| *Life Stage Group* | *Males* | | *Females* | | *Pregnancy* | *Lactation* |
|---|---|---|---|---|---|---|
| | *9–13 y* | *14–18 y* | *9–13 y* | *14–18 y* | *≤18 y* | *≤18 y* |
| Thiamin (mg/d) | 0.9 | 1.2 | 0.9 | 1.0 | 1.4 | 1.4 |
| Vitamin A (μg/d)[d] | 600 | 900 | 600 | 700 | 750 | 1,200 |
| Vitamin $B_6$ (mg/d) | 1.0 | 1.3 | 1.0 | 1.2 | 1.9 | 2.0 |
| Vitamin $B_{12}$ (μg/d) | 1.8 | 2.4 | 1.8 | 2.4 | 2.6 | 2.8 |
| Vitamin C (mg/d) | 45 | 75 | 45 | 65 | 80 | 115 |
| Vitamin D (μg/d)*[,e] | 5 | 5 | 5 | 5 | 5 | 5 |
| Vitamin E (mg/d) | 11 | 15 | 11 | 15 | 15 | 19 |
| Vitamin K* | 60 | 75 | 60 | 75 | 75 | 75 |

Source: Dietary Reference Intakes:The Essential Guide to Nutrient Requirements. Institute of Medicine, National Academies; 2006.

Note:This table presents Recommended Dietary Allowances (RDAs) and Adequate Intakes (AIs) where nutrients have an asterisk (*) after the name. RDAs and AIs may both be used as goals for individual intake. RDAs are set to meet the needs of almost all (97% to 98%) individuals in a group.

ND = Not determinable due to lack of data.

[a]As dietary folate equivalents (DFE). 1 DFE = 1 μg food folate = 0.6 μg of folic acid from fortified food or as a supplement consumed with food.

[b]In view of evidence linking folate intake with neural tube defects in the fetus, it is recommended that all women capable of becoming pregnant consume 400 μg from supplements or fortified food in addition to intake of food folate from a varied diet.

[c]As niacin equivalents (NE), 1 mg of niacin = 60 mg of tryptophan.

[d]As retinol activity equivalents (RAEs). 1 RAE = 1 μg retinol, 12 μg β-carotene, 24 μg α-carotene, or 24 μg β-cryptoxanthin. The RAE for dietary provitamin A carotenoids is twofold greater than retinol equivalents (RE), whereas the RAE for preformed vitamin A is the same as RE.

[e]As cholecalciferol, 1 μg cholecalciferol = 40 IU vitamin D. Requirement in the absence of adequate exposure to sunlight.

in practice should be informed by clinical judgment.[9-13] Nutritional requirements during the adolescent growth spurt compared to other stages of adolescence may be doubled. It is not necessary for individuals to achieve intakes of 100% of the RDA for every nutrient every day because the body stores some nutrients when they are consumed in excess for later use, such as energy-yielding nutrients and the fat-soluble vitamins A, D, E, and K.[8] In addition to intakes from food and beverages, nutrients coming from fortified foods and beverages and supplements need to be considered; the total intake from all of these sources should be determined and compared to reference values. Finally, assessments of individual intake need to take into account that nutrient intakes less than the RDA may be adequate for some individuals because these reference values are defined as adequate for nearly all individuals in a group.[8]

## THE INFLUENCE OF GROWTH AND DEVELOPMENT ON ENERGY AND NUTRIENT NEEDS

### Energy

In contrast to the established RDAs for nutrients, Estimated Energy Requirements (EERs) do not include a safety factor (Table 16-4). Energy intake must be balanced with energy expenditure to avoid excessive weight gain or weight loss. Established EER equations for adolescents represent the amount of energy required to maintain energy balance, plus a small allowance of energy to support growth and development. Energy requirements are greatest during periods of rapid growth. The energy needs of adolescent males are greater than those of adolescent females because during periods of growth they experience greater increases in height, weight, and lean body mass. Separate equations for adolescent males and females (ages 9–18 years) are therefore used to predict energy requirements based on age, weight, height, and usual physical activity with an allowance for growth of 25 kcal per day (see Box 16-1).[11]

**Table 16-3**

**Dietary Reference Intakes: Acceptable Macronutrient Distribution Ranges for Adolescents**

| *Macronutrient* | *Range (percentage of total energy)* |
|---|---|
| Carbohydrate | 45 to 65 |
| Added sugars | ≤25 |
| Protein | 10 to 30 |
| Fat | 25 to 35[a] |
| Saturated fatty acids | As low as possible[b] |
| Trans fatty acids | As low as possible[b] |
| Dietary cholesterol | As low as possible[b] |

[a]Approximately 10% of the total can come from longer-chain n-3 or n-6 fatty acids.

[b]While consuming a nutritionally adequate diet.

Dietary Reference Intakes: The Essential Guide to Nutrient Requirements. Institute of Medicine, National Academies; 2006.

**Box 16-1**

***Estimated Energy Requirement (EER) Equations for Adolescents (9–18 years)***

**EER for Males**

Male EER = 88.5 - (61.9 × age [years]) + PA × (26.7 × weight [kg] + 903 × height [m]) + 25 (kcal/day for energy deposition)

Sedentary PA = 1.00; Low active PA = 1.13

Active PA = 1.26

**EER for Females**

Female EER = 135.3 - (30.8 × age [years]) + PA × (10.0 × weight [kg] + 934 × height [m]) + 25 (kcal/day for energy deposition)

Sedentary PA = 1.00; Low active PA = 1.16

Active PA = 1.31

***Physical Activity Coefficients (PA)***

*Sedentary:* Less than 30 minutes a day of moderate physical activity in addition to daily activities

*Low active:* At least 30 minutes up to 60 minutes of daily moderate physical activity in addition to daily activities

*Active:* At least 60 minutes of daily moderate physical activity in addition to daily activities

Source: Dietary Reference Intakes: The Essential Guide to Nutrient Requirements. Institute of Medicine, National Academies; 2006.

**Table 16-4**

**Estimated Daily Energy (kcal) Needs for Adolescents, by Gender, Age, and Activity Levels[a]**

| | *Males* | | | *Females* | | |
|---|---|---|---|---|---|---|
| *Activity Level Age (years)* | *Sedentary* | *Low Active* | *Active* | *Sedentary* | *Low Active* | *Active* |
| **12** | 1,800 | 2,200 | 2,400 | 1,600 | 2,000 | 2,200 |
| **13** | 2,000 | 2,200 | 2,600 | 1,600 | 2,000 | 2,200 |
| **14** | 2,000 | 2,400 | 2,800 | 1,800 | 2,000 | 2,400 |
| **15** | 2,200 | 2,600 | 3,000 | 1,800 | 2,000 | 2,400 |
| **16** | 2,400 | 2,800 | 3,200 | 1,800 | 2,000 | 2,400 |
| **17** | 2,400 | 2,800 | 3,200 | 1,800 | 2,000 | 2,400 |
| **18** | 2,400 | 2,800 | 3,200 | 1,800 | 2,000 | 2,400 |
| **19–20** | 2,600 | 2,800 | 3,000 | 2,000 | 2,200 | 2,400 |

[a]Estimated for a person of average height who is at a healthy weight.

Source: MyPyramid: Steps to a Healthier You. US Department of Agriculture and the US Department of Health and Human Services. Available at: www.mypyramid.gov.

### Energy and Physical Activity Level

To accurately determine energy needs, it is necessary to determine an adolescent's level of physical activity. The formal definition of PAL is the ratio of total energy expenditure to basal energy expenditure.[11] Thus, the impact of any activity on PAL depends in part on determinants of basal energy expenditure including an individual's age and body size. Physical activity coefficients (PA) for computing EERs have been defined for 4 levels of physical activity, from lowest to highest energy expenditure: sedentary, low active, active, and very active.[11] Conducting a highly accurate assessment of PAL is complex; however, suggestions for approximating an adolescent's PAL are provided in Box 16-1.[14] To achieve the active PAL recommended for good health, at least 60 minutes of daily moderate-intensity activity is required. Physical activities are categorized by intensity in Table 16-5.[11,15]

### Acceptable Macronutrient Distribution Ranges

Acceptable Macronutrient Distribution Ranges (AMDRs)[11] provide guidance on the proportion of total energy that should be consumed as carbohydrate, protein, and fat to prevent chronic disease and ensure sufficient nutrient intake. The AMDRs for adolescents up to age 18 are 45% to 65% for carbohydrate, 10% to 30% for protein, and 25% to 35% for fat (see Table 16-3).[11] Although requirements for carbohydrate and fat are not influenced by growth beyond the increased requirement for energy intake during growth, protein requirements of adolescents are elevated during peak periods of growth. In preadolescence (9–13 years), the RDA for daily protein intake is 0.95 grams per kilogram, or about 34 grams per day.[11] The RDA in middle and late adolescence (14–18 years) is 0.85 grams per kilogram per day, about 52 and 46 grams per day for males and females, respectively.[11] National nutrition survey data indicate that most adolescents have more than adequate intakes of protein, but certain subgroups (eg, adolescents from food-insecure households, adolescents who severely restrict their energy intake, adolescents who follow a vegan diet) may still be at risk for low protein intake.[5] If protein intake is chronically poor during adolescence, linear growth may be reduced, sexual maturation delayed, and the accumulation of lean body mass compromised.

**Table 16-5**

**Selected Physical Activities of Moderate and Vigorous Intensity[11,15,19]**

| *Intensity* | *Activities* |
|---|---|
| **Moderate**<br>*Any activity that results in achieving 60% to 73% of peak heart rate[a]* | Active recreation, such as canoeing, hiking, skateboarding, rollerblading<br>Cycling (<10 mph)<br>Dancing<br>Golf (walking and carrying clubs)<br>Housework and yard work (eg, sweeping or pushing a lawn mower)<br>Swimming (slowly)<br>Tennis (doubles)<br>Walking briskly (3–4 mph, not race-walking)<br>Weightlifting (general, light) |
| **Vigorous**<br>*Any activity that results in achieving 74% to 88% of peak heart rate[a]* | Climbing hills<br>Cycling (>10 mph)<br>Dancing (high-impact, aerobic)<br>Jogging (<10-minute miles, race-walking, or running)<br>Jumping rope<br>Skating (ice or roller)<br>Skiing (water or downhill)<br>Sports such as soccer, ice or field hockey, or basketball<br>Swimming (continuous laps)<br>Tennis (singles)<br>Weightlifting (vigorous effort) |

[a]An estimate of a person's peak heart rate can be calculated by subtracting the person's age from 220 beats per minute.

**Micronutrients: Vitamins and Minerals**

Vitamin needs increase steadily from childhood into adolescence, but there is no evidence to indicate that the rapid growth that occurs during adolescence creates a high demand for fat- or water-soluble vitamins. Conversely, requirements for some minerals, such as iron, zinc, and calcium, are 2 to 3 times higher during the period of peak growth velocity than the average requirement in the second decade of life. The demand for iron is increased to support gains in lean muscle tissue requiring iron in the form of myoglobin and hemoglobin. In females, additional iron is also required after menarche to cover menstrual losses, which average 30 ml to 40 ml each menses. Zinc needs are similarly elevated due to gains in skeletal muscle and bone tissue where 90% of total body zinc is collectively stored. As a major component of bone mass, additional calcium is important to support skeletal growth; nearly half of peak bone mass is accumulated during adolescence.[2] Contrary to requirements for iron and zinc, which may be partially met by mobilizing body stores, increased calcium needs must be met entirely through increased dietary intake. Bone is the body's major nutrient reserve for calcium, and there is no other body store that may be used for bone mineralization. The most important dietary sources of calcium for US adolescents are milk and other dairy products, typically accounting for about 75% of calcium intake.[15] Additional key sources of calcium and sources of iron and zinc are noted in Table 16-1.

Although vitamin and mineral requirements are best met by a balanced, nutrient-dense diet, fortified foods or supplements are recommended for adolescents unable or unwilling to meet their nutritional needs through diet alone. For example, pregnant adolescents may need low-dose or prenatal vitamin-mineral supplements to achieve intake levels required for optimal fetal development, in addition to their own nutritional requirements for growth. In particular, vitamins and minerals needed by pregnant adolescents at higher levels than nonpregnant adolescents include folate, niacin, riboflavin, thiamin, vitamins A, $B_6$, and $B_{12}$, iron, magnesium, and zinc (see Table 16-2).[5,10-13] Other groups that may require supplements include adolescents who frequently skip meals, use substances such as tobacco and alcohol, or follow a strict vegan diet excluding all foods and beverages of animal origin. Nutrients of concern for adolescents following a vegan diet are protein, vitamins $B_6$, $B_{12}$, and D, iron, zinc, calcium, and the omega-3 fatty acids.[16]

## FOOD AND BEVERAGE SELECTION TO PROMOTE ADOLESCENT HEALTH

An underlying premise of the 2005 Dietary Guidelines for Americans (Dietary Guidelines), a set of science-based recommendations for promoting health and preventing chronic diseases, is that nutritional needs should be met primarily from foods and beverages. Most of the key recommendations in the Dietary Guidelines apply to adolescents, and some additional recommendations have been specifically developed for children and adolescents (Table 16-6). With the US Department of Agriculture (USDA) food guidance system, the recommendations

**Table 16-6**

**Selected Recommendations from the 2005 Dietary Guidelines for Americans[15]**

| *Target Behavior* | *Recommendations to Achieve* |
|---|---|
| **Adequate nutrients within energy needs** | • Consume a variety of nutrient-dense foods and beverages within and among the basic food groups while choosing foods that limit the intake of saturated and trans fats, cholesterol, added sugars, salt, and alcohol.<br>• Meet recommended intakes within energy needs by adopting a balanced eating pattern. |
| **Weight management** | • Maintain body weight in a healthy range by balancing energy from foods and beverages with energy expended.<br>• *Overweight children.* Reduce the rate of body weight gain while allowing growth and development. |
| **Physical activity** | • Engage in regular physical activity and reduce sedentary activities to promote health, psychological well-being, and a healthy body weight.<br>• Achieve physical fitness by including cardiovascular conditioning, stretching exercises for flexibility, and resistance exercises or calisthenics for muscle strength and endurance.<br>• *Children and adolescents.* Engage in at least 60 minutes of physical activity on most, preferably all, days of the week. |

*(Continued)*

**Table 16-6 (Continued)**

| *Target Behavior* | *Recommendations to Achieve* |
|---|---|
| **Food groups to encourage** | • Consume a sufficient amount of fruits and vegetables (2½–6½ cups or 5–13 servings daily) while staying within energy needs.<br>• Choose a variety of fruits and vegetables each day. In particular, select from all 5 vegetable subgroups (dark green, orange, legumes, starchy vegetables, and other vegetables) several times a week.<br>• Consume 3 cups per day of fat-free or low-fat milk or equivalent milk products.<br>• *Children and adolescents.* Consume whole-grain products often; at least half the grains should be whole grains with the rest of the recommended grains coming from enriched or whole-grain products. |
| **Fats** | • Consume <10% of energy from saturated fatty acids and <300 mg/day of cholesterol, and keep trans fatty acid consumption as low as possible.<br>• *Children and adolescents (4–18 years).* Keep total fat intake between 25% to 35% of energy, with most fats coming from sources of polyunsaturated and monounsaturated fatty acids, such as fish, nuts, and vegetable oils.<br>• When selecting and preparing meat, poultry, dry beans, and milk or milk products, make choices that are lean, low-fat, or fat-free.<br>• Limit intake of fats and oils high in saturated and/or trans fatty acids, and choose products low in such fats and oils. |
| **Carbohydrates** | • Choose fiber-rich foods, vegetables, and whole grains often.<br>• Choose and prepare foods and beverages with little added sugars or caloric sweeteners.<br>• Reduce the amount of dental caries by practicing good oral hygiene and consuming sugar- and starch-containing foods and beverages less frequently. |
| **Sodium and potassium** | • Consume <2,300 mg (approximately 1 tsp of salt) of sodium per day.<br>• Choose and prepare foods with little salt. At the same time, consume potassium-rich foods, such as fruits and vegetables. |

were designed to help Americans choose a diet that meets the RDAs, AIs, and AMDRs appropriate for their age, gender, and activity level. The Dietary Guidelines are also intended for use by policy makers, nutritionists, and other health care providers to assist in designing and implementing meal programs (eg, The National School Lunch Program), educational interventions, and health supervision activities.[15]

The USDA food guidance system, MyPyramid (Figure 16-1), provides food-based guidance that can be personalized to help individuals achieve the recommendations of the Dietary Guidelines and meet their total nutrient needs without consuming energy (kcal) or other dietary components (eg, trans fats) in excess. The 5 food groups of MyPyramid are (1) grains, (2) vegetables, (3) fruits, (4) milk, and (5) meats and beans. In addition, MyPyramid provides guidance on intake of

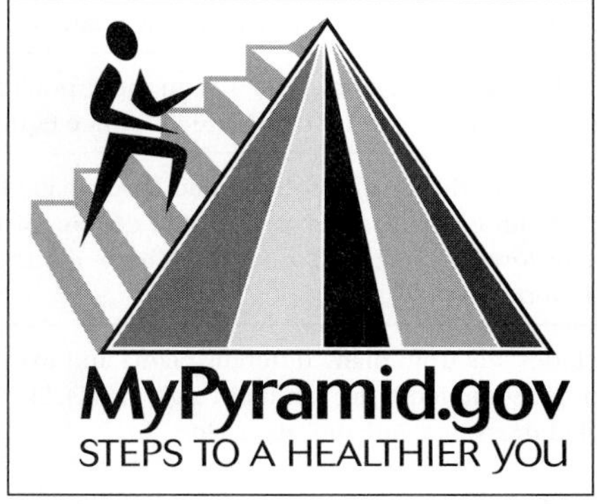


**FIGURE 16–1** MyPyramid, the USDA Food Guidance System. (MyPyramid: Steps to a Healthier You. US Department of Agriculture and the US Department of Health and Human Services. Available at: www.mypyramid.gov.)

oils, solid fats, and added sugars. Meal patterns developed to meet different levels of required energy intake are shown in Table 16-7. Meal patterns are based on the nutrients and energy that would be provided by consuming the most nutrient-dense forms of food and beverages (eg, lean meats, fat-free milk) within each food group. Individualized recommendations for adolescents needing more or less daily energy (kcal) and numerous tips and resources for nutrition education can be found on the USDA MyPyramid Web site.[17]

MyPyramid recommendations were designed to allow for the consumption of oils (eg, liquid plant oils and foods such as mayonnaise, certain salad dressings, and soft margarine that are "oil-like"), within the total energy budget. Dietary oils provide essential fatty acids and vitamin E but are also energy-dense and should be limited to avoid excess energy intake and weight gain. The recommended amount applies not only to oils added during home food preparation and at the table, but also to oils added to foods during processing.

**Table 16-7**

**Recommended Daily Food Intake Amounts for Selected Energy Levels[a]**

| | *Energy Level (kcal)* | | | | | | | | |
|---|---|---|---|---|---|---|---|---|---|
| ***Food group*** | ***1,600*** | ***1,800*** | ***2,000*** | ***2,200*** | ***2,400*** | ***2,600*** | ***2,800*** | ***3,000*** | ***3,200*** |
| Fruits in cups[b] | 1.5 | 1.5 | 2 | 2 | 2 | 2 | 2.5 | 2.5 | 2.5 |
| Vegetables in cups[c] | 2 | 2.5 | 2.5 | 3 | 3 | 3.5 | 3.5 | 4 | 4 |
| Grains in ounce equivalents[d] | 5 | 6 | 6 | 7 | 8 | 9 | 10 | 10 | 10 |
| Meats and beans in ounce equivalents[e] | 5 | 5 | 5.5 | 6 | 6.5 | 6.5 | 7 | 7 | 7 |
| Milk in cups[f] | 3 | 3 | 3 | 3 | 3 | 3 | 3 | 3 | 3 |
| Oils in teaspoons (5 ml)[g] | 5 | 5 | 6 | 6 | 7 | 8 | 8 | 10 | 11 |
| Discretionary energy allowance (kcal)[h] | 132 | 195 | 267 | 290 | 362 | 410 | 426 | 512 | 648 |

[a]Nutrient and energy contributions from each group are calculated according to the most nutrient-dense forms of foods in each group (ie, lean meats, fat-free milk).

[b]**Fruit group:** Includes all fresh, frozen, canned, and dried fruits and fruit juices. In general, a half-cup serving of fruit is equivalent to 1 medium piece of whole fruit, a half-cup of cut-up fruit, a quarter-cup of dried fruit, or 4 oz of 100% fruit juice.

[c]**Vegetable group:** Includes all fresh, frozen, and canned vegetables and vegetable juices. In general, a half-cup serving of vegetables is equivalent to a half-cup of raw or cooked vegetables, 1 cup of raw leafy greens, or 4 oz of 100% vegetable juice. Dark green and orange vegetables should be consumed often. See Table 16-8 for the recommended *weekly amounts* from each vegetable subgroup.

[d]**Grains:** Includes all foods made from wheat, rice, oats, cornmeal, and barley, such as bread, pasta, oatmeal, breakfast cereals, tortillas, and grits. In general, 1 slice of bread, 1 cup of ready-to-eat cereal, or a half-cup of cooked rice, pasta, or cooked cereal can be considered 1-oz equivalent (oz-eq) from the grains group. At least half of all grains consumed should be whole grains, consisting of the entire grain seed (eg, whole wheat, brown rice, oatmeal, whole-grain corn, whole rye).

[e]**Meats and beans:** In general, 1 oz of lean meat, poultry, or fish, 1 egg, 1 tablespoon of peanut butter, a half-cup of cooked beans, or a half-oz of nuts or seeds can be considered 1-ounce equivalent (oz-eq) from the meats and beans group.

[f]**Milk:** Includes all fluid milk products and foods made from milk that retain their calcium content, such as yogurt and cheese. This group does not contain foods made from milk that contain little or no calcium, such as cream cheese, cream, and butter. Most milk choices should be fat-free or low-fat. In general 1 cup of milk or yogurt, 1½ oz of natural cheese, or 2 oz of processed cheese can be considered 1 cup from the milk group.

[g]**Oils:** Includes fats from many different plants and from fish that are liquid at room temperature, such as canola, corn, olive, soybean, and sunflower oil. Some foods are naturally high in oils, like nuts, olives, some fish, and avocados. Foods that are mainly oil include mayonnaise, certain salad dressings, and soft margarine.

[h]**Discretionary energy allowance:** The remaining amount of energy in a food intake pattern after accounting for the energy needed for all food groups—using fat-free or low-fat forms of food with no added sugars.

Source: MyPyramid: Steps to a Healthier You. US Department of Agriculture and the US Department of Health and Human Services. Available at: www.mypyramid.gov.

**Table 16-8**

**Recommended Vegetable Subgroup Weekly Intake Amounts, in Cups[a] for Selected Energy Levels**

| *Energy (kcal) level* | *1,600* | *1,800* | *2,000* | *2,200* | *2,400* | *2,600* | *2,800* | *3,000* | *3,200* |
|---|---|---|---|---|---|---|---|---|---|
| Dark green vegetables (eg, broccoli, spinach, kale) | 2 | 3 | 3 | 3 | 3 | 3 | 3 | 3 | 3 |
| Orange vegetables (eg, carrots, acorn squash) | 1.5 | 2 | 2 | 2 | 2 | 2.5 | 2.5 | 2.5 | 2.5 |
| Legumes (eg, black beans, kidney beans, lentils) | 2.5 | 3 | 3 | 3 | 3 | 3.5 | 3.5 | 3.5 | 3.5 |
| Starchy vegetables (eg, corn, green peas, potatoes) | 2.5 | 3 | 3 | 6 | 6 | 7 | 7 | 9 | 9 |
| Other vegetables (eg, green beans, onions, celery) | 5.5 | 6.5 | 6.5 | 7 | 7 | 8.5 | 8.5 | 10 | 10 |

[a]All amounts are given as the recommended amount per week.

Source: MyPyramid: Steps to a Healthier You. US Department of Agriculture and the US Department of Health and Human Services. Available at: www.mypyramid.gov.

Discretionary energy is the energy remaining in an individual's EER after all foods and beverages (in their most nutrient-dense forms) needed to meet nutrient intakes have been consumed. Overweight adolescents desiring weight loss may choose not to consume all of their discretionary energy without compromising nutrient intake. Adolescents desiring weight maintenance can consume their discretionary energy allowance in different ways: (1) choosing more nutrient-dense foods from any food group that the food guide recommends; (2) choosing forms of some foods that contain fats or added sugars, such as whole milk or sweetened cereal; (3) adding fats, such as salad dressing or butter, or sweeteners such as syrup or table sugar, to foods or beverages; or (4) choosing foods or beverages that provide only fats or caloric sweeteners, such as candy or soft drinks. For most adolescents, the discretionary energy allowance is small, but allowances increase with increasing levels of physical activity.[14]

## PHYSICAL ACTIVITY RECOMMENDATIONS FOR HEALTHY ADOLESCENTS

In addition to enabling greater flexibility in food choices, regular physical activity promotes psychological well-being and reduces the risk of developing many chronic diseases in adulthood. Regular physical activity is associated with increased self-esteem and reduced levels of anxiety and depression.[18] Conversely, a sedentary lifestyle increases the risk for excess weight gain, heart disease, hypertension, type 2 diabetes, certain types of cancer, and osteoporosis.[15] The 2008 Physical Activity Guidelines for Americans and the Dietary Guidelines provide specific recommendations for physical activity during childhood and adolescence (see Table 16-6).[15,19] At least 60 minutes of moderate to vigorous physical activity is recommended on most, preferably all, days of the week above and beyond usual daily activities.

This amount of physical activity does not need to be completed at 1 time, but may be accumulated over the day in several short episodes (eg, 6 daily episodes of 10 minutes). Physical activities of moderate intensity involve exertion in which an adolescent can carry on a conversation comfortably while exercising. Vigorous physical activities represent a substantial challenge to an individual and result in significant increases in heart and breathing rate. Table 16-5 provides examples of both moderate and vigorous physical activities.[14,15] The Dietary Guidelines[15] also recommend reducing sedentary activities, such as watching television and playing video games. More specifically, the American Academy of Pediatrics (AAP)[20] encourages limiting time spent with television and other screen media to no more than 2 hours per day.

## DIETARY AND PHYSICAL ACTIVITY RECOMMENDATIONS FOR ADOLESCENTS WITH SPECIAL CONDITIONS OR DIETARY PRACTICES

Special conditions and dietary practices influence nutrition or activity recommendations for adolescents. Examples include overweight, eating disorders, pregnancy, hypertension, hyperlipidemia, iron deficiency anemia, type 2 diabetes, and vegetarianism. Table 16-9 provides a summary of criteria for evaluating these situations and key concerns and recommendations relevant to diet and physical activity.[7,17,21-31]

### RECOMMENDATIONS FOR NUTRITION AND PHYSICAL ACTIVITY SUPERVISION OF ADOLESCENTS

It is recommended that adolescents receive an annual preventive health assessment including nutrition and physical activity supervision.[24] An initial screening should include components addressing the adolescent's medical and psychosocial history, growth and development, nutritional status, dietary intake, and physical activity behaviors.[32] If nutritional risk factors are identified during the screening assessment, then a more comprehensive, in-depth evaluation is recommended, along with appropriate education to address identified risk factors. In addition to information obtained on history and physical examination noted previously, an in-depth nutrition evaluation should include a detailed assessment of diet and physical activity and a review of any available laboratory data.[32] All adolescents should also receive anticipatory guidance to promote positive attitudes and behaviors regarding healthy eating and physical activity. Tools for completing assessments of growth and development, nutritional status, dietary intake, and physical activity behaviors are discussed in the following sections.

**Table 16-9**

**Special Conditions and Dietary Practices**

| | *Criteria for Diagnosis or Evaluation* | *Key Nutrition Concerns and Recommendations* | *Key Physical Activity Concerns and Recommendations* |
|---|---|---|---|
| **Overweight and at risk for overweight**[24,30] (also see Chapter 79, Obesity) | • Overweight: BMI ≥85th but <95th percentile, based on age and gender<br>• Obese: BMI ≥95th percentile, based on age and gender | Using a staged approach, reduce or eliminate energy-dense foods to:<br>• Maintain weight if overweight, in the absence of weight-related complications<br>• Lose weight if obese at a rate no greater than 2 pounds per week | Using a staged approach, reduce time spent in sedentary activities and increase daily physical activity:<br>• Limit sedentary activities to ≤2 hours per day<br>• Gradually build up to ≥1 hour of daily physical activity |
| **Eating disorders** | | | |
| **Anorexia nervosa**[7,25] (also see Chapter 76, Anorexia Nervosa) | • Refusal to maintain body weight at or above a minimally normal weight for age and height<br>• Intense fear of gaining weight<br>• Disturbance in the way in which one's body weight or shape is experienced, undue influence of body weight or shape on self-evaluation, or denial of the seriousness of the current low body weight<br>• Amenorrhea in postmenarcheal females | Establish a set food plan to restore nutrition (starting with at least 1,200–1,500 kcal)<br>• Develop a contract for weight gain<br>• Add liquid supplements to diet if weight is not regained at an adequate rate | Restrict activity if weight is not regained at an adequate rate, vital signs are not stable, or heart rate is bradycardic |

*(Continued)*

**Table 16-9 (Continued)**

| | *Criteria for Diagnosis or Evaluation* | *Key Nutrition Concerns and Recommendations* | *Key Physical Activity Concerns and Recommendations* |
|---|---|---|---|
| **Bulimia nervosa**[7,28] (also see Chapter 77, Bulimia Nervosa) | • Recurrent episodes of binge eating<br>• Recurrent inappropriate, compensatory behavior to prevent weight gain, such as self-induced vomiting; misuse of laxatives, diuretics, enemas, or other medications; fasting; or excessive exercise<br>• Binge eating and inappropriate compensatory behavior both occur, on average, at least twice a week for 3 months<br>• Self-evaluation is unduly influenced by body shape and weight<br>• The disturbance does not occur exclusively during episodes of anorexia nervosa | • Establish a set food plan to provide adequate nutrition and energy for weight maintenance<br>• Ensure adequate fat and fiber intake to promote satiety<br>• Gradually reintroduce "forbidden foods" and social eating<br>• Monitor dietary intake along with relevant thoughts and feelings<br>• Increase knowledge of the futility of purging behaviors | Monitor physical activity and limit excessive exercise |
| **Eating disorder, not otherwise specified**[7,25] | Disorders of eating that do not meet the criteria for any specific eating disorder. Examples include:<br>• For females, all of the criteria for anorexia nervosa are met except that the individual has regular menses<br>• All of the criteria for bulimia nervosa are met except that the binge-eating and inappropriate compensatory mechanism occurs at a frequency of less than twice a week | See recommendations for the eating disorder most closely resembling presenting symptoms | See recommendations for the eating disorder most closely resembling presenting symptoms |
| **Binge eating disorder**[7,21] | Recurrent episodes of binge eating<br>The binge eating episodes are associated with 3 (or more) of the following:<br>• Eating much more rapidly than normal<br>• Eating until feeling uncomfortably full<br>• Eating large amounts of food when not feeling physically hungry<br>• Eating alone because of being embarrassed by how much one is eating<br>• Feeling disgusted with oneself, depressed, or guilty after overeating<br>• Marked distress regarding binge eating is present<br>• The binge eating occurs, on average, at least 2 days a week for 6 months<br>• The binge eating is not associated with the regular use of inappropriate compensatory behaviors | • Establish a set pattern of regular eating to displace binge eating<br>• Monitor dietary intake along with relevant thoughts and feelings | Establish a regular pattern of physical activity |

*(Continued)*

## Table 16-9 (Continued)

| | *Criteria for Diagnosis or Evaluation* | *Key Nutrition Concerns and Recommendations* | *Key Physical Activity Concerns and Recommendations* |
|---|---|---|---|
| **Hypertension**[22] (also see Chapter 118, Hypertension) | • Hypertension is defined as the average of 3 diastolic and/or systolic blood pressure readings ≤95th percentile, based on age, sex, and height<br>• Blood pressure readings between the 90th and 95th percentile represent a prehypertensive condition, which is an indication for lifestyle modification | • Prevent excess weight gain and if overweight, lose weight<br>• Increase intake of fresh vegetables, fresh fruits, fiber, and low-fat dairy<br>• Reduce sodium intake | • Participate in regular moderate physical activity (30–60 minutes per day)<br>• Restrict sedentary activity to <2 hours per day<br>• Limit participation in competitive sports if hypertension is uncontrolled and blood pressure is >99th percentile plus 5 mm Hg |
| **Pregnancy and lactation**[8,27] (also see Chapter 54, Pregnancy) | Warning signs of nutrition problems include age <16 years, a previous pregnancy, past or present eating disorder, underweight or overweight, inadequate or excessive weight gain during pregnancy, persistent nausea or vomiting, denial or refusal to accept the pregnancy, nutritional deficiencies, substance abuse, irregular meal patterns, poor appetite, and limited food resources | During pregnancy, increase energy intake to provide for increased needs and for energy deposition:<br>• Second trimester = adolescent EER + 160 kcal (8 kcal/week × 20 weeks) + 180 kcal<br>• Third trimester = adolescent EER + 272 kcal (8 kcal/week × 20 weeks) + 180 kcal<br>During lactation, adjust energy intake to provide for milk production and weight reduction:<br>• First 6 months = adolescent EER + 500 kcal – 170 kcal<br>• Second 6 months = adolescent EER + 400 kcal – 0 kcal<br>Consume an additional 25 grams per day of protein during pregnancy and lactation.<br>See Table 16-2 for recommendations regarding other nutrients. | • If physically active, continue to participate in moderate-intensity, rhythmical activities like walking, cycling, swimming, jogging, and dancing during pregnancy<br>• Avoid intense exercise and exercising for extended periods during pregnancy |
| **Hyperlipidemia**[31] (also see Chapter 81, Hyperlipidemia and Atherosclerosis) | • Borderline: Total blood cholesterol of 170–199 mg/dl; LDL cholesterol of 110–129 mg/dl<br>• Elevated: Total blood cholesterol of ≥200 mg/dl; LDL cholesterol of ≥130 mg/dl | • Consume a diet with <30% and ≥20% of total energy from fat<br>• Limit trans fatty acids to <1% of total energy<br>• Consume <7% of total energy from saturated fat<br>• Consume ≤200 mg per day of cholesterol<br>• Increase intake of soluble fiber | • Participate in at least 60 minutes of moderate to vigorous physical activity every day<br>• Limit sedentary activity to <2 hours per day |

*(Continued)*

**Table 16-9 (Continued)**

| | *Criteria for Diagnosis or Evaluation* | *Key Nutrition Concerns and Recommendations* | *Key Physical Activity Concerns and Recommendations* |
|---|---|---|---|
| **Iron deficiency anemia**[26] | **Males**<br>Hematocrit (%)<br>12–<15 years: ≤37.3<br>15–<18 years: ≤39.7<br>≥18 years: ≤39.9<br>Hemoglobin (g/dl)<br>12–<15 years: ≤12.5<br>15–18 years: ≤13.3<br>≥18 years: ≤13.5<br>**Females (nonpregnant and lactating)**<br>Hematocrit (%)<br>12–<15 years: ≤35.7<br>15–<18 years: ≤35.9<br>≥18 years: ≤35.7<br>Hemoglobin (g/dl)<br>12–<15 years: ≤11.8<br>15–<18 years: ≤12.0<br>≥18 years: ≤12.0 | • Increase intake of foods rich in iron and vitamin C (see Table 16-1)<br>• Add iron (ferrous sulfate) supplement to diet (60–120 mg per day)<br>• Avoid calcium supplements, dairy products, coffee, tea, and high-fiber foods within 1 hour of taking iron supplement | Anemia reduces physical endurance and performance |
| **Type 2 diabetes**[23,29] (also see Chapter 73, Diabetes Mellitus) | Classic symptoms of diabetes (eg, polyuria, polydipsia, unexplained weight loss) plus casual plasma glucose concentration ≥200 mg/dl, or fasting plasma glucose ≥126 mg/dl, or 2-hour plasma glucose ≥200 mg/dl during an oral glucose tolerance test | • Prevent excessive weight gain<br>• Decrease energy-dense, high-fat food and beverage choices | • Increase daily physical activity<br>• Decrease sedentary activity |
| **Vegetarianism**[16,27] | • Semi- or partial vegetarian: excludes red meat<br>• Lacto-ovo vegetarian: excludes meat, poultry, fish, seafood<br>• Lacto-vegetarian: excludes meat, poultry, fish, seafood, eggs<br>• Vegan: excludes all animal products including meat, poultry, fish, seafood, eggs, dairy products (and maybe honey)<br>• Macrobiotic: excludes meat, poultry, eggs, dairy, seafood (and maybe fish) | If all animal-derived food products are excluded from the diet, fortified foods or supplements should be included to provide for adequate intakes of protein, vitamins $B_6$, $B_{12}$, and D, iron, zinc, calcium, and omega-3 fatty acids | None applicable |

## MEASURES TO ASSESS GROWTH AND DEVELOPMENT

Assessment of growth and development should begin with accurate measurements of height and weight (see Chapter 9, Physical Examination and Laboratory Screening). Using these measurements, body mass index (BMI) should be calculated [(weight in kg) ÷ (height in $m^2$)] and plotted on age- and gender-appropriate Centers for Disease Control and Prevention 2000 growth charts.[33] A BMI <5th percentile indicates underweight, and the adolescent should receive full medical and nutritional evaluations. A BMI between the 85th and 94th percentile is labeled as overweight, and a BMI

≥95th percentile is labeled as obese for the purposes of documentation and risk assessment. A thorough physical examination and laboratory assessment for lipid abnormalities should be completed for all adolescents with a BMI ≥85th percentile. Additional laboratory testing to screen for nonalcoholic fatty liver disease and type 2 diabetes mellitus should be completed for adolescents with a BMI ≥95th percentile or other risk factors.[24] A staged approach to the treatment of overweight and obesity, including gradual changes in eating and activity behaviors, is recommended based on age, BMI, related comorbidities, parents' weight status, and progress in treatment (see Chapter 79, Obesity).[24]

### SCREENING MEASURES TO ASSESS NUTRITIONAL STATUS AND GENERAL HEALTH

Routine laboratory and screening tests such as hemoglobin, total cholesterol or blood lipids, and blood pressure should be reviewed during annual assessments. Abnormal findings indicating anemia, hyperlipidemia, or hypertension should be followed up appropriately (see Table 16-9). Additional laboratory tests such as a complete blood count with red blood cell indices, serum ferritin, or iron studies can help determine the cause of anemia. Adolescents with a nutritional anemia, hyperlipidemia, or hypertension should have an in-depth nutrition evaluation. Physical examination findings indicative of an eating disorder or malnutrition, such as calluses over the proximal interphalangeal joints (Russell sign), lanugo-type body hair, dry skin or lips, hypothermia, or bradycardia should also be followed up by an in-depth evaluation.[25]

## TOOLS AVAILABLE TO ASSESS DIETARY QUALITY AND MEAL PATTERNS

An initial dietary screening should evaluate usual eating patterns and assess for nutrition risk behaviors. Behaviors of concern include low dietary variety, inadequate fruit and vegetable intake, excessive intake of high-fat or high-sugar foods and beverages, a strict vegetarian or vegan meal pattern, frequent meal skipping, chronic dieting, binge eating and/or purging, other unhealthy weight-control behaviors, such as diet pill or laxative use, substance use, and the use of high-dose vitamin-mineral or nonnutritional supplements. A more detailed assessment of dietary intake should be completed if an adolescent reports 1 or more nutrition risk behaviors. Female adolescents who are pregnant, adolescents with inadequate food resources at home, and adolescents with a physical disability, chronic illness, or medical condition should also receive a more detailed assessment of dietary intake.

Food frequency questionnaires, 24-hour recalls, and food diaries or food records are all appropriate for use with adolescents to obtain a detailed assessment of dietary intake. Use of a 24-hour dietary recall is advantageous because information obtained can be directly entered into a dietary analysis program and reviewed with the adolescent as part of a counseling session. However, a recall record cannot be relied on to reflect usual intake, and its accuracy depends largely on the adolescent's memory. A registered dietitian or other skilled professional should complete the recall to enhance its accuracy as much as possible. Food records do not rely on memory and, if multiple days of intake are recorded, provide information more representative of usual intake. Unfortunately, recording food and beverage intake may influence the adolescent's selections and bias the information obtained. Skilled staff should also be employed to review food records for accuracy with the adolescent and evaluate the nutritional quality of reported intake. Although skilled staff are not required to administer food frequency questionnaires, questionnaires cannot be relied on to provide valid estimates of absolute intake for individuals and do not always provide information on meal patterning.[32] Sample nutrition screening questionnaires have been developed for practitioners by the Bright Futures health promotion initiative.[1] Examples of forms that might be used for more detailed nutrition assessments have also been published.[32]

## TOOLS AVAILABLE TO ASSESS PHYSICAL ACTIVITY AND INACTIVITY

Physical activity may be simply assessed in an initial screening by asking adolescents to report the number of days per week they participate in moderate and vigorous physical activities. Examples of moderate and vigorous physical activities might be provided to help prompt their memory (see Table 16-5). Adolescents should be similarly asked about their weekly participation in sedentary activities, such as watching television, using computers for purposes other than school work, and playing video games. After establishing the weekly frequency of these behaviors, additional questions may be used to assess their usual duration on weekdays and weekend days.

Adolescents not meeting the recommendations for physical activity or exceeding recommended limits for screen time should receive education and be offered strategies to improve their PAL. Excessive physical activity can also be unhealthy, and adolescents reporting intensive and unsupervised physical activity performed for extended periods of time should be further evaluated for an eating disorder. A number of questionnaires have been developed for the assessment of physical activity, including a brief questionnaire developed by the Bright Futures[3,34] health promotion initiative. In addition, strategies similar to those identified for conducting detailed dietary assessments may be used to comprehensively assess physical activity. For example, adolescents may be asked to recall their physical activity for the past few days or keep a log of their physical activity.

## SUMMARY

Nutrition and physical activity are major determinants of adolescent health. The development of healthful eating and activity behaviors plays a key role in supporting normal pubertal growth and development. Inadequacies and excesses in either of these domains can have a significant negative impact on adolescent growth, development, identity, and mental health. When inadequacies in 1 domain are combined with inadequacies in another domain, the results can be staggering, even life threatening. For example, inadequate physical activity combined with excessive energy consumption leads to obesity, with all of its associated morbidities. Likewise, anorexia nervosa is associated with excessive compulsive daily exercise and severe restriction of energy intake, with all of its associated morbidities and increased risk for mortality. On the positive side of this complex interplay, adolescents who maintain a regular pattern of physical activity, especially engaging in enjoyable exercise such as sports, and who establish a lifelong pattern of healthy eating, tend to enjoy better health both as adolescents and adults than adolescents who do not pay attention to nutrition and physical activity.

A strong understanding of nutritional needs and optimal physical activity during adolescence must be at the foundation of any recommendations a health care provider might make regarding these key determinants of health. Normal requirements for macro- and micronutrients described in this chapter may need to be modified depending on the intensity and demands of physical activity, as well as any health problems that an adolescent may have or want to avoid. Helpful resources for the reader interested in further information are offered in the following section.

## INTERNET RESOURCES

### AMERICAN ACADEMY OF PEDIATRICS POLICY STATEMENTS

- Policy Collections: aappolicy.aappublications.org/cgi/collection

### AMERICAN HEART ASSOCIATION

- Heart-healthy Recipes: www.deliciousdecisions.org/
- Heart-Smart Shopping Tools: www.heart.org/HEARTORG/GettingHealthy/NutritionCenter/HeartSmartShopping/Heart-Smart-Shopping_UCM_001179_SubHomePage.jsp

### BRIGHT FUTURES IN PRACTICE

- Nutrition: www.brightfutures.org/nutrition/pdf/index.html
- Physical Activity: www.brightfutures.org/physicalactivity/pdf/index.html

### CENTERS FOR DISEASE CONTROL AND PREVENTION

- Child and Teen Calculator: apps.nccd.cdc.gov/dnpabmi/Calculator.aspx
- 2000 CDC Growth Charts: www.cdc.gov/growthcharts/

### MATERNAL AND CHILD HEALTH LIBRARY

- Maternal and Child Health Library Knowledge Path: Physical Activity and Children and Adolescents: www.mchlibrary.info/KnowledgePaths/kp_phys_activity.html#overview
- Maternal and Child Health Library Knowledge Path: Child and Adolescent Nutrition: www.mchlibrary.info/KnowledgePaths/kp_childnutr.html

### NATIONAL HEART, LUNG, AND BLOOD INSTITUTE

- We Can! Ways to Enhance Children's Activity and Nutrition: www.nhlbi.nih.gov/health/public/heart/obesity/wecan/

### UNITED STATES DEPARTMENT OF AGRICULTURE

- MyPyramid Food Intake Patterns: www.mypyramid.gov/downloads/MyPyramid_Food_Intake_Patterns.pdf
- MyPyramid Food Intake Pattern Calorie Levels: www.mypyramid.gov/downloads/MyPyramid_Calorie_Levels.pdf
- MyPyramid Tracker: www.mypyramidtracker.gov/
- MyPyramid Plan for Moms: www.mypyramid.gov/mypyramidmoms/pyramidmoms_plan.aspx
- The Power of Choice: www.fns.usda.gov/TN/Resources/power_of_choice.html

### UNITED STATES DEPARTMENT OF HEALTH AND HUMAN SERVICES

- Dietary Guidelines Toolkit for Professionals: www.health.gov/dietaryguidelines/dga2005/toolkit/
- Food Sources of Shortfall Nutrients: www.health.gov/dietaryguidelines/dga2005/document/pdf/Appendix_B.pdf

- 2008 Physical Activity Guidelines for Americans Toolkit: www.health.gov/paguidelines/toolkit.aspx

## REFERENCES


1. Story M, Holt K, Sofka D, eds. *Bright Futures in Practice: Nutrition*. 2nd ed. Arlington, VA: National Center for Education in Maternal and Child Health; 2002

2. Spear B. Adolescent growth and development. *J Am Diet Assoc.* March 2002;102(3):S23–S29

3. Patrick K, Spear B, Holt K, Sofka D, eds. *Bright Futures in Practice: Physical Activity*. Arlington, VA: National Center for Maternal and Child Health; 2001

4. Cook A, Friday J. *Pyramid Servings Intakes in the United States 1999-2002, 1 Day*. Beltsville, MD: Agricultural Research Service, US Department of Agriculture; 2005

5. Moshfegh A, Goldman J, Cleveland L. *What We Eat in America, NHANES 2001-2002: Usual Nutrient Intakes from Food Compared to Dietary Reference Intakes.* Washington, DC: US Department of Agriculture, Agricultural Research Service; 2005

6. Ogden CL, Carroll MD, Flegal KM. High body mass index for age among US children and adolescents, 2003–2006. *JAMA.* 2008;299(20):2401–2405

7. American Psychiatric Association. *Diagnostic and Statistical Manual of Mental Disorders*. 4th ed. Text revision. Washington, DC: American Psychiatric Association; 2000

8. Institute of Medicine. *Dietary Reference Intakes: Applications in Dietary Planning*. Washington, DC: National Academy Press; 2003

9. Institute of Medicine. *Reference Intakes for Vitamin C, Vitamin E, Selenium, and Carotenoids*. Washington, DC: National Academy Press; 2000

10. Institute of Medicine. *Dietary Reference Intakes for Calcium, Phosphorus, Magnesium, Vitamin D, and Fluoride*. Washington, DC: National Academy Press; 1997

11. Institute of Medicine. *Dietary Reference Intakes for Energy, Carbohydrate, Fiber, Fat, Fatty Acids, Cholesterol, Protein, and Amino Acids*. Washington, DC: National Academy Press; 2002

12. Institute of Medicine. *Dietary Reference Intakes for Vitamin A, Vitamin K, Arsenic, Boron, Chromium, Copper, Iodine, Iron, Manganese, Molybdenum, Nickel, Silicon, Vanadium, and Zinc*. Washington, DC: National Academy Press; 2001

13. Institute of Medicine. *Dietary Reference Intakes for Thiamin, Riboflavin, Niacin, Vitamin $B_6$, Folate, Vitamin $B_{12}$, Pantothenic Acid, Biotin, and Choline*. Washington, DC: National Academy Press; 1998

14. US Department of Agriculture Center for Nutrition Policy and Promotion. MyPyramid food guidance system education framework. Available at: www.mypyramid.gov/professionals/pdf_framework.html. Accessed January 2010

15. US Department of Health and Human Services, US Department of Agriculture. Dietary guidelines for Americans 2005. Available at: healthierus.gov/dietaryguidelines. Accessed January 2010

16. Dunham L, Kollar L. Vegetarian eating for children and adolescents. *J Pediatr Health Care.* 2006;20:27–34

17. US Department of Agriculture. MyPyramid.gov. Steps to a healthier you. Available at: www.mypyramid.gov. Accessed January 2010

18. Calfas K, Taylor W. Effects of physical activity on psychological variables in adolescents. *Pediatr Exerc Sci.* 1994;6:406–423

19. US Department of Health and Human Services. 2008 physical activity guidelines for Americans. Available at: www.health.gov/paguidelines. Accessed January 2010

20. American Academy of Pediatrics Committee on Public Education. Children, adolescents, and television. *Pediatrics.* 2001;107(2):423–426

21. Fairburn C, Wilson G, eds. *Binge Eating: Nature, Assessment, and Treatment*. New York, NY: Guilford Publications; 1993

22. National High Blood Pressure Education Program Working Group on High Blood Pressure in Children and Adolescents. The fourth report on the diagnosis, evaluation, and treatment of high blood pressure in children and adolescents. *Pediatrics.* 2004;114(2):555–576

23. American Diabetes Association. Type 2 diabetes in children and adolescents. *Pediatrics.* 2000;105(3):671–680

24. Barlow SE and the Expert Committee. Expert Committee recommendations regarding the prevention, assessment, and treatment of child and adolescent overweight and obesity: summary report. *Pediatrics.* 2007;120(suppl 4):S164–S192

25. Rome ES, Ammerman S, Rosen DS, et al. Children and adolescents with eating disorders: the state of the art. *Pediatrics.* Jan 2003;111(1):e98–e108

26. Centers for Disease Control and Prevention. Recommendations to prevent and control iron deficiency in the United States. *MMWR.* 1998;47(No RR-3)

27. Story M, Stang J, eds. *Nutrition and the Pregnant Adolescent: A Practical Reference Guide*. Minneapolis, MN: Center for Leadership, Education, and Training in Maternal and Child Nutrition, University of Minnesota; 2000

28. Salvy SJ, McCargar L. Nutritional interventions for individuals with bulimia nervosa. *Eat Weight Disord.* December 2002;7(4):258–267

29. Gahagan S, Silverstein J, Committee on Native American Child Health and Section on Endocrinology. Prevention and treatment of type 2 diabetes mellitus in children, with special emphasis on American Indian and Alaska Native children. *Pediatrics.* 2003;112(4):e328–e347

30. Spear BA, Barlow SE, Ervin C, Ludwig DS, Saelens BE. Recommendations for treatment of child and adolescent overweight and obesity. *Pediatrics.* 2007;120(suppl 4):S254–S288

31. Daniels SR, Greer FR, Committee on Nutrition. Lipid screening and cardiovascular health in childhood. *Pediatrics.* 2008;122(1):198–208

32. Stang J. Assessment of nutritional status and motivation to make behavior changes among adolescents. *J Am Diet Assoc.* 2002;102(3):S13–S22

33. Centers for Disease Control and Prevention. 2000 CDC growth charts: United States. July 21, 2006; Available at: www.cdc.gov/growthcharts. Accessed February 2009

34. Krebs NF, Himes JH, Jacobson D, Nicklas TA, Guilday P, Styne D. Assessment of child and adolescent overweight and obesity. *Pediatrics.* 2007;120(suppl 4):S193–S228

SECTION 5

# Management Issues

# CHAPTER 17

## Complementary and Alternative Medicine

SUSAN M. YUSSMAN, MD, MPH • OLLE JANE Z. SAHLER, MD • MARILYN A. ROSEN, MLS

### DEFINITIONS

Complementary and alternative medicine (CAM) is a "group of diverse medical and health care systems, practices, and products that are not presently considered to be part of conventional medicine," according to the National Center for Complementary and Alternative Medicine (NCCAM), a division of the National Institutes of Health (NIH).[1] Conventional medicine may also be known as allopathy, Western, or mainstream medicine, and is practiced by an MD (medical doctor) or DO (doctor of osteopathy) and their allied health professionals, such as physical therapists, psychologists, and registered nurses.[1] Some health care providers practice CAM and conventional medicine.

*Complementary medicine* is the term referring to practices used with (complementing) conventional medicine, whereas *alternative medicine* is used instead of conventional medicine. An example of complementary medicine is using music therapy to lessen a patient's discomfort during a bone marrow biopsy, whereas an example of alternative medicine is using an herbal supplement to treat cancer instead of undergoing chemotherapy as prescribed by an oncologist. *Integrative medicine* combines treatments from conventional medicine and CAM for which there is evidence of safety and effectiveness. Integrative medicine emphasizes a collaborative approach to patient care that addresses the biological, psychological, social, and spiritual aspects of health and illness.[2]

The National Center for Complementary and Alternative Medicine (NCCAM) groups CAM practices into 5 domains. *Manipulative and body-based practices* are based on manipulation or movement of one or more body parts. Examples include chiropractic manipulation and massage therapy. *Mind-body medicine* uses a variety of techniques such as meditation, prayer, and creative arts therapy to enhance the mind's ability to affect bodily function and symptoms. Some techniques in this domain, such as patient support groups and cognitive–behavioral therapy, were once considered CAM but have now become a part of conventional medicine. Whole medical systems are built upon complete systems of theory and practice, often having evolved apart from and earlier than conventional medicine in Western Europe and the United States. Examples include naturopathy, homeopathy, traditional Chinese medicine, and Ayurveda. *Energy medicine* involves the use of energy fields and is divided into 2 areas. The first is bioelectromagnetic-based therapies that involve unconventional use of electromagnetic fields. The second is biofield therapies that affect energy fields that surround and penetrate the human body by applying pressure to or manipulating the body by placing the hands in or through these fields. Science has not yet established the existence of these fields. Examples of biofield therapies include *qi gong* and *reiki*. Finally, *biologically based practices* use substances found in nature, such as herbs, special diets, and vitamins in doses outside those used in conventional medicine.[1]

Dietary supplements fall within the domain of biologically based practices. Congress defined this term in the Dietary Supplement Health and Education Act of 1994 as a product (other than tobacco) taken by mouth that contains an ingredient intended to supplement the diet. Dietary ingredients may include vitamins, minerals, herbs, or other botanicals, amino acids, and substances such as enzymes, organ tissues, and metabolites. Dietary supplements come in many forms including extracts, concentrates, tablets, capsules, gel caps, liquids, and powders. A dietary supplement must be labeled as such on the front of the bottle; dietary supplements are considered foods, not drugs. Manufacturers do not have to provide the US Food and Drug Administration (FDA) with evidence that dietary supplements are safe or effective, and the FDA must prove that the product is not safe in order to restrict or remove it from the market.[3] Therefore, it is important to remember that "natural" may not necessarily mean "safe."

For example, dietary supplements containing ephedra alkaloids (also known as *ma huang*) had been known to cause adverse cardiovascular and central nervous system effects for more than 25 years.[4] However, it was not until 2004 that the FDA finally prohibited its sale.[5] Furthermore, because dietary supplements are biologically active, they may have interactions with other herbal products or prescription medications.

## CAM USE BY ADOLESCENTS

CAM is an increasingly popular therapeutic choice among American adults. In 1997, 42% of adults reported using CAM in 629 million office visits, exceeding the total visits to primary care physicians that year. Adults spent $21 billion on CAM professional services, with $12 billion paid out-of-pocket, exceeding the total out-of-pocket expenditures for US hospitalizations that year. Furthermore, they paid $27 billion on CAM therapies, exceeding the out-of-pocket expenditures for all US physician services that year.[6] In 2000, 62% of adults reported using CAM, with the most popular therapies being prayer and natural products.[7]

Most studies on CAM use have not included pediatric or adolescent populations. However, a national survey in 1996 demonstrated that 2% of parents reported that their children had visited a CAM provider and rarely disclosed this use to their conventional medical provider. The most common therapies used were spiritual healing, herbal remedies, and massage therapy. The most common providers visited were chiropractors and spiritualists.[8] Most other CAM use studies in children and adolescents have been limited to either subspecialty or convenience samples, demonstrating use ranging from 12% of private practice patients in Detroit,[9] to 70% of homeless teens in Seattle.[10]

Only a few studies have examined CAM use specifically by adolescents and young adults. A 2002 online survey demonstrated that 79% of teens 14 to 19 years of age had used CAM in their lifetime, with 49% having used CAM in the previous month. Forty-six percent had used dietary supplements in their lifetime, with 29% having used them in the past month. Factors associated with CAM use included being a female in the middle adolescent age group of 16 to 17 years old, and having a positive attitude toward CAM. Almost 10% of teens reported concurrent use of dietary supplements and prescription medications in the past month. The most common CAM therapies were home remedies (46%), expressive therapies (31%), faith healing (30%), and herbal remedies (23%). The most common herbal products were ginseng (17%), zinc (15%), Echinacea (14%), ginkgo (11%), weight loss supplements (11%), St John's wort (6%), creatine (5%), and ephedra (2%).[11]

It is unclear why adolescents use CAM, but they are more likely to do so if their parents or friends also use these therapies. Adults are more likely to try CAM because they feel that CAM combined with conventional medical treatments would help or that it would be interesting to try. Adults use CAM most often to treat back or neck problems, joint pain, colds, anxiety, and depression.[7]

Adolescents conceptualize using herbal products and nutritional supplements to *treat* illness, not to *prevent* illness. Adolescents tend to be most familiar with CAM therapies commonly used by people from their own cultural or ethnic background. Older suburban female teenagers and adolescents with chronic illness are more familiar with dietary supplements than other adolescents. Teens report rarely being asked about supplement use by their conventional medical provider and say they would be reluctant to disclose this use because their conventional health care providers are not educated about CAM or would not approve of them using it.[12]

## TREATMENTS

Healing systems outside of conventional medicine have relied heavily on empiricism rather than systematic investigation. Because the randomized controlled trial is a product of the second half of the 20th century, even most conventional medicine predates rigorous scientific validation. Much of conventional medicine is currently being scrutinized and reevaluated, similar to the evaluation studies that have just begun for CAM therapies. Most CAM therapies do not claim to treat emergency or major acute illness. Instead, in general, they are directed toward health promotion and illness prevention through stress reduction, exercise, and healthful eating.

Although there are many materials, including constantly updated Web sites that provide reliable information about CAM, there is no immediate solution to the problem that information, especially CAM information based on "scientific" study, is sparse. Table 17-1 outlines direct comparisons between pharmaceuticals and dietary supplements for some common adolescent complaints. However, it is rare to find these kind of data. Most researchers are currently studying the efficacy of a single CAM modality or supplement, not comparisons between modalities. Table 17-2 describes uses for some commonly used dietary supplements, acupuncture, and

## Table 17-1

### Common Adolescent Complaints: Comparison of Conventional and CAM Therapies

| *Condition* | *Rating* | *Most Effective Rx or OTC* | *Mechanism of Action* | *Rating* | *Most Effective Supplement* | *Mechanism of Action* | *Comparison* | *Supplement-Drug Interactions* |
|---|---|---|---|---|---|---|---|---|
| **Acne** | 1 | Benzoyl peroxide gel (effective) | Bacteriocidal, reduces oiliness of skin | 2 | Tea tree oil | May kill bacteria and fungi | As effective as 5% benzoyl peroxide; may be less irritating | • No known drug interactions<br>• Tea tree oil and lavender may be unsafe in prepubertal boys (hormone effects may cause gynecomastia) |
| **Attention deficit-hyperactivity disorder (ADHD)** | 2 | Atomoxetine | Increases norepinephrine (may increase suicidal ideation) | 3 | Lithium | Interacts with sodium ions to change neurotransmitter action; decreases impulsive–aggressive behavior; can be toxic | | • Can affect serotonin, do not take with dextromethorphan, ACE inhibitors, or NSAIDs.<br>• Can increase lithium levels.<br>• Calcium channel blockers and anticonvulsants can increase side effects. |
| | 2 | Dextroamphetamine | Stimulant | 3 | Zinc | Enzymatic activation; may modestly improve hyperactivity; does not improve attention deficit | May increase responsivity to stimulant therapy if zinc deficient | • May interfere with absorption of quinolones, tetracyclines, and penicillamine |
| | 2 | Methylphenidate | Stimulant | | | | | |

*(Continued)*

**Table 17-1 (Continued)**

| *Condition* | *Rating* | *Most Effective Rx or OTC* | *Mechanism of Action* | *Rating* | *Most Effective Supplement* | *Mechanism of Action* | *Comparison* | *Supplement-Drug Interactions* |
|---|---|---|---|---|---|---|---|---|
| **Anxiety** (Cognitive-behavioral therapy has been shown to be the BEST treatment for anxiety in most teenagers and adults.) | 2 | Paroxetine | Selective serotonin reuptake inhibitor | 3 | Kava (70% kavalactones) (nonaddictive) | Psychoactive anxiolytic | May be comparable to low-dose benzodiazepines | • Avoid using with any medication metabolized by cytochrome<br>• P450 in the liver<br>• Synergistic with alprazolam and central nervous system (CNS) depressants<br>• May decrease effectiveness of levodopa<br>• Do not use with any hepatotoxic agents |
| | 2 | Buspirone | Serotonin receptor agonist | | | | | |
| | 2 | Hydroxyzine | | | | | | |
| | 2 | Benzodiazepines (effective, but side effects may outweigh benefits, addictive) | GABAa modulator | | | | | |
| **Dysmenorrhea** | 1 | Ibuprofen (effective) | Reduces prostaglandin levels | 3 | Fish oil | Omega-3 fatty acids reduce inflammation and impair coagulation | | • Some contraceptives reduce triglycerides and decrease effectiveness<br>• May potentiate anticoagulants/antiplatelet drugs and antihypertensives<br>• Orlistat may decrease absorption of fish oil |

*(Continued)*

**Table 17-1 (Continued)**

| *Condition* | *Rating* | *Most Effective Rx or OTC* | *Mechanism of Action* | *Rating* | *Most Effective Supplement* | *Mechanism of Action* | *Comparison* | *Supplement-Drug Interactions* |
|---|---|---|---|---|---|---|---|---|
| **Dysmenorrhea** | | | | 3 | Vitamin E | | | • May potentiate anticoagulants/ antiplatelet drugs and increase absorption of cyclosporine<br>• Increases cytochrome P450 activity |
| **Chronic tension headache** | 1 | Amitriptyline | Inhibits serotonin and norepinephrine reuptake | 3 | Peppermint oil (possibly effective) | Muscle relaxant | | • Inhibits breakdown of cyclosporine<br>• Inhibits cytochrome P450 activity<br>• Enteric-coated peppermint preparations may cause heartburn when taken with $H_2$ blocker or proton pump inhibitor |
| | 1 | Mirtazapine (effective) | Noradrenergic and specific serotonin antidepressant (NaSSA) | | | | | |

**Key:**
1. Effective; 2. Likely Effective; 3. Possibly Effective

**Adapted from:** National Institutes of Health National Center for Complementary and Alternative Medicine. www.nccam.nih.gov

**Table 17-2**

## Common CAM Supplements and Therapies: Uses and Effectiveness

| *CAM Therapy* | *Rating* | *Effectiveness* | *Cautions*[a] |
|---|---|---|---|
| **Acidophilus (Lactobacillus)** | 2 | Childhood diarrhea caused by certain viruses | • Mild side effects include intestinal gas<br>• Avoid in people with impaired immunity (HIV/AIDS, s/p transplant)<br>• Effectiveness may be decreased by concurrent antibiotic therapy<br>• Oral use has been associated with hepatitis |
| | 3 | Diarrhea due to antibiotics | |
| | 3 | Diarrhea due to *C difficile* | |
| | 3 | Travelers' diarrhea | |
| | 3 | Ulcerative colitis when combined with bifido bacteria and streptococcus | |
| | 4 | Crohn disease | |
| | 4 | Lactose intolerance | |
| | 6 | Irritable Bowel Syndrome (IBS) | |
| | 6 | Urinary tract infection (UTI) | |
| | 6 | Canker sores | |
| | 6 | Acne | |
| | 6 | Improving immune system | |
| **Aloe vera** | 2 | Psoriasis when used topically | |
| | 6 | Wound healing | |
| | 6 | Healing skin sores | |
| | 6 | Burns | |
| **Aloe latex** | 2 | Constipation (stimulant laxative) | • Do not use with diabetes, inflammatory bowel disease, hemorrhoids, or renal problems<br>• Diarrhea may decrease absorption of medications |
| **Echinacea (coneflower)** | 3 | Treating common cold | • Can cause allergic reaction in people who are allergic to ragweed, mums, marigolds, or daisies<br>• Do not take if pregnant or breast-feeding, have pemphigus vulgaris, or autoimmune disease |
| | 3 | Preventing vaginal yeast infection | |
| | 4 | Preventing recurrent genital herpes | |
| | 6 | UTI | |
| | 6 | Migraine headaches | |
| | 6 | Chronic fatigue syndrome (CFS) | |
| | 6 | Eczema | |
| | 6 | ADHD | |
| **Creatine** | 3 | Improving athletic performance during brief, high-intensity exercise | • Water absorption into muscles may cause dehydration<br>• Do not use if breast-feeding, or with kidney disease or diabetes |
| **Evening primrose oil** | 3 | Breast pain | • Do not use if breast-feeding, with a bleeding disorder, seizure disorder, or schizophrenia |
| | 2 | Osteoporosis (when used with calcium and fish oils) | |
| | 4 | Premenstrual symptoms | |
| | 4 | ADHD | |
| | 4 | Eczema | |
| | 6 | Acne | |

*(Continued)*

**Table 17-2 (Continued)**

| CAM Therapy | Rating | Effectiveness | Cautions[a] |
|---|---|---|---|
| **Valerian** | 3 | Insomnia | • Long-term safety unknown<br>• Taper when discontinuing use after more than 4 weeks |
| | 6 | Depression | |
| | 6 | Anxiety | |
| | 6 | Headaches | |
| | 6 | Menstrual pain | |
| | 6 | CFS | |
| **St John's wort** | 2 | Mild to moderate depression | • Do not take for more than 2 months without medical supervision<br>• Do not take if breast-feeding, have bipolar disorder, schizophrenia, or major depression<br>• May decrease effectiveness of oral contraceptives; use second method of birth control<br>• Can potentiate effects of SSRIs if taken together |
| | 3 | Somatization disorder | |
| | 4 | Hepatitis C | |
| | 4 | HIV/AIDS | |
| | 6 | Migraine headaches | |
| | 6 | CFS | |
| | 6 | Obsessive–compulsive disorder | |
| | 6 | Seasonal affective disorder | |
| | 6 | ADHD | |
| **Acupuncture** | 1 | Nausea due to chemotherapy | • Should use only sterile needles and proper insertion techniques<br>• Acupuncturists are now licensed in most states<br>• Seek a practitioner certified by the National Certification Commission for Acupuncture and Oriental Medicine |
| | 1 | Postoperative nausea | |
| | 1 | Postoperative dental pain | |
| | 2 | Addiction | |
| | 2 | Fibromyalgia | |
| | 2 | Menstrual cramps | |
| **Chiropractic** | 2 | Low back pain | • Extremely low complication rate for manipulation (adjustment) of lower back<br>• Seek a practitioner with special training or experience in pediatric chiropractic techniques |
| | 3 | Neck pain | |
| | 3 | Headaches | |
| | 3 | Sports injuries | |

[a]In general no herb/supplement should be used during pregnancy or while breast-feeding without specific permission.

**Key:**

1. Effective; 2. Likely Effective; 3. Possibly Effective; 4. Possibly Ineffective; 5. Likely Ineffective; 6. Insufficient Evidence to Rate

**Adapted from**: National Institutes of Health National Center for Complementary and Alternative Medicine. www.nccam.nih.gov

chiropractic care. There are limited federal funds for CAM research. The 2009 proposed budget for the NCCAM is about $121 million, and has been flat for more than 5 years.[13]

## ROLE OF HEALTH CARE PROVIDERS

Most health care providers recognize the high level of patient interest in CAM. However, physicians report discomfort with CAM, not necessarily because they disapprove of its use, but because of their lack of knowledge and experience with it. They believe that they are not adequately educated to help patients and their families make decisions about referrals to CAM providers or for specific CAM therapies. A survey of members of the American Academy of Pediatrics (AAP) recently demonstrated that about one third of pediatricians had been asked about CAM by a patient or parent in the previous 3 months. Two thirds of pediatricians believed that CAM therapies could help patients, but three quarters were concerned about side effects or possible delay of conventional medical care. Only 20% routinely asked their patients about herb use, and fewer asked about other CAM practices. Fewer than 5% felt very knowledgeable about individual CAM therapies, and more than 80% requested more education about CAM.[14] The Institute of Medicine (IOM) has recognized the need for more CAM education and has recommended that health professional school curricula include information about safety, efficacy, and cost-effectiveness of CAM, with the goal of conventional health care providers being able to completely advise patients about CAM use.[15]

Although it is true that conventional medical practitioners are not fully informed about CAM modalities, this is also true of many areas of conventional medicine as well. However, providers perform risk–benefit analyses multiple times each day, weighing the severity of an illness, its curability using a particular therapy, degree of invasiveness and toxicity of a treatment, and the patient's ability to understand the risks and willingness to accept those risks. These principles underlie informed consent and are no different for a CAM modality than for a conventional treatment.

The argument can be made that there is less information about CAM modalities, which, in many instances, is true. However, it is important to remember that the term "evidence-based medicine," rooted in Archie Cochrane's book *Effectiveness and Efficiency* published in 1972, has been popularized not in response to the introduction of CAM but as a critique of Western medicine in general. A simple decision matrix about the use of any treatment, including CAM, shown in Table 17-3, weighs risks and benefits.

In general, clinicians don't ask and adolescents don't tell about their CAM use. This poor communication increases the potential risk for interactions with medications, undertreatment of conditions for which patients are self-medicating, or ingestion of potentially dangerous supplements. Openly asking patients and their families about CAM use may help open communication about much more sensitive adolescent topics. The overarching goal is integrated patient-centered care, where health professionals, conventional and nonconventional, work in an open and shared manner with patients taking into account patient individuality and psychosocial issues to enhance illness prevention and promote health.

**Table 17-3**

**Decision Matrix for Treatment**

| *BENEFIT* | *RISK* | |
|---|---|---|
| | *NO* | *YES* |
| YES | Recommend | Recommend if benefit outweighs risk |
| NO | Accept if social, emotional, cultural benefit outweighs cost | Discourage |

## INTERNET RESOURCES

The Internet is the most widely used source for gathering information today. Adolescents' first step in seeking health information on the Internet is to use a search engine. However, teens often feel the results are overwhelming in quantity and perplexing in quality.[16] Although there are many excellent health resources on the Internet, there are even more poor resources. So, what is a teen to do? We propose an acronym that may appeal to adolescents and, hopefully, clinicians alike: "You can trust a Web site if it's **COOL**!"

**C: Credentials**. Can you identify who wrote the information on the Web site, what their profession and education are? Are they physicians or other health professionals? Is there an identified Board of Directors or Review Board? Is there an "About Us" page with concrete details? Can you contact someone about the site? If not, the information on the Web site is suspect.

**O: Opinion**. Does the Web site give personal opinions or information based on credible evidence from medical research? Are the creators of the Web site trying to convince you of something, such as purchasing their product? Be skeptical of Web sites that promise "cures." Being aware of the Web address can help: *.edu* is an educational institution; *.org* is an organization; *.gov* is a government site; *.com* is commercial, meaning that they sell advertising space and want you to buy something from them or from their advertisers. Commerical sites are the least reliable for balanced and unbiased information.

**O: Out of date**. Are pages dated? Are the dates current? If there is a News section, does it include recent items? Information that guides you in making health decisions should be up to date.

**L: Links**. Links on a Web site should be active and accurate. Try several links. Broken links may indicate that the site is neglected. Sites will tout their credibility with awards they have won, which may also be links. The symbols to look for are the Health on the Net Foundation code (HONcode; www.hon.ch/HONcode/Conduct.html) and Utilization Review Accreditation Commission (URAC; www.urac.org) each of which denotes adherence with quality criteria.

The following are generally reliable and current Web sites. These sites, along with the quality evaluation criteria listed above, should help conventional medical providers and their patients navigate the plethora of CAM Web sites on the Internet. However, it is important to realize that findings summarized on many sites are not scientifically or rigorously vetted. As with all medications and therapies, use should be discussed with a medical practitioner who is knowledgeable about risks and benefits. Unfortunately, over the past several decades, health information from widely respected sources such as the FDA, peer-reviewed journals, and the pharmaceutical industry has proven to be less trustworthy and accurate than desirable. It is essential that consumers of all ages be reminded to approach all claims of efficacy with skeptical caution.

Scientific research in CAM is spearheaded by the federal government through NCCAM. Its Web site www.nccam.nih.gov lists not only current clinical trials and research but also explanations of various types of CAM therapies, statistics on CAM usage, tips on how to find a reliable CAM practitioner, information on herbs and dietary supplements (some items have links to MedlinePlus), and a live help line.

The National Library of Medicine, www.nlm.nih.gov, in 1998, believing that the Internet could be a credible source of health information, launched its consumer health information Web site, MedlinePlus medlineplus.gov/. Its current scope spans 700 to 800 conditions, more than 4,000 encyclopedia articles, more than 1,000 drugs, and there are 100 monographs on herbs and supplements. Health pages are comprised of links to reliable sources, such as government offices, professional associations, and charitable organizations. Topics include Alternative Medicine, Acupuncture, Chiropractic, and Herbal Medicine.

Bastyr University (Seattle, WA) offers graduate and undergraduate degrees in CAM science-based natural medicines. Its library Web site offers links to selected sites, ranging from the American Massage Therapy Association and the Harvard School of Public Health to Cochrane Library Reviews, the Drepung Loseling Monastery, World's Healthiest Foods, and the American Botanical Council, www.bastyr.edu/library/resources/online/bibliography.asp. The library is part of the National Network of Libraries of Medicine.

Other free Web sites specifically for herbal and dietary supplement information exist on the Internet. Memorial Sloan-Kettering Cancer Center, in the Integrative Medicine portion of its Web site, has created: About Herbs, Botanicals & Other Products, www.mskcc.org/mskcc/html/11570.cfm. Each monograph has 2 versions, one for health professionals and one for consumers, and is well referenced.

Fee-based CAM resources also provide detailed and pertinent information. The Natural Medicine Comprehensive Database, produced by the Therapeutic Research Center, which also creates "The Prescriber's Letter" and "The Pharmacist's Letter," contains more than 1,000 well-referenced monographs on herbs and dietary supplements that are updated daily at www.naturaldatabase.com. A patient information handout is a component of each entry. Commercial products are also listed by name with their full ingredients. Beginning in 2007, the database identified any product given the USP (United States Pharmacopeia) verified seal, which measures purity and overall quality.

AMED, Allied and Complementary Medicine Database, is produced by the Health Care Information Service of the British Library, www.bl.uk/reshelp/findhelpsubject/scitectenv/medicinehealth/amed/amed.html. It indexes articles from journals on such subjects as physiotherapy, palliative care, complementary medicine, and rehabilitation. Many of the journals are not indexed in other databases.

## REFERENCES

1. National Center for Complementary and Alternative Medicine. National Institutes of Health. What is CAM? Available at: nccam.nih.gov/health/whatiscam/. Accessed May 19, 2009

2. Osher Center for Integrative Medicine. University of California, San Francisco. Integrative medicine. Available at: www.osher.ucsf.edu/about/index.html Accessed May 19, 2009

3. Office of Dietary Supplements. National Institutes of Health. Dietary supplements: background information. Available at: ods.od.nih.gov/factsheets/Dietary Supplements.asp. Accessed May 19, 2009

4. Shekelle PG, Hardy ML, Morton SC, et al. Efficacy and safety of ephedra and ephedrine for weight loss and athletic performance: a meta-analysis. *JAMA*. 2003;289(12):1537–1545

5. US Food and Drug Administration. Final rule declaring dietary supplements containing ephedra alkaloids adulterated because they present an unreasonable risk. *Fed Reg* 21 CFR Part 119. 2/11/2004

6. Eisenberg D, Davis R, Ettner S, et al. Trends in alternative medicine use in the United States, 1990–1997: results of a follow-up national survey. *JAMA*. 1998;280(18):1569–1575

7. Barnes PM, Powell-Griner E, McFann K, Nahin RL. *Complementary and Alternative Medicine Use among Adults: United States, 2002. Advance Data from Vital and Health Statistics; no 343*. Hyattsville, MD: National Center for Health Statistics; 2004

8. Yussman SM, Auinger P, Weitzman M, Ryan SA. Visits to complementary and alternative medicine providers by children and adolescents in the United States. *Ambul Pediatr*. 2004;4(5):429–435

9. Sawni-Sikand A, Schubiner H, Thomas RL. Use of complementary/alternative therapies among children in primary care pediatrics. *Ambul Pediatr*. 2002;2(2):99–103

10. Breuner CC, Barry PJ, Kemper KJ. Alternative medicine use by homeless youth. *Arch Peds Adoles Med*. 1998;152(11):1071–1075

11. Wilson KM, Klein JD, Sesselberg TS, et al. Use of complementary medicine and dietary supplements by US adolescents. *J Adolesc Health*. 2006; 38(4):385–394

12. Klein JD, Wilson KM, Sesselberg TS, et al. Adolescents' knowledge of and beliefs about herbs and dietary supplements: a qualitative study. *J Adolesc Health*. 2005;37(5):409.e1

13. National Center for Complementary and Alternative Medicine. National Institutes of Health. Fiscal Year 2009 Budget Request. Available at: nccam.nih.gov/about/offices/od/directortestimony/0308.htm. Accessed May 19, 2009

14. Kemper KJ, O'Connor KG. Pediatricians' recommendations for complementary and alternative medical (CAM) therapies. *Ambul Pediatr*. 2004;4(6):482–487

15. Committee on the Use of Complementary and Alternative Medicine by the American Public, Board on Health Promotion and Disease Prevention, Institute of Medicine of the National Academies. *Complementary and Alternative Medicine in the United States*. Washington, DC: The National Academies Press; 2005

16. Gray NJ, Klein JD, Noyce PR, et al. The Internet: a window on adolescent health literacy. *J Adolesc Health*. 2005;37(3):243.e1

# CHAPTER 18

## Pain in Adolescents: Pathophysiology and Management

ÉLISE W. VAN DER JAGT, MD, MPH • OLLE JANE SAHLER, MD

### INTRODUCTION

Federal clinical practice guidelines have been published on the pain management of patients undergoing operative and medical procedures, those sustaining trauma, those with cancer,[1] and children and adolescents.[2] The American Academy of Pediatrics[3,4] also has issued guidelines related to the management of pain associated with procedures in patients with cancer or other diseases. In recognizing that the undertreatment of pain in children, adolescents,[5] and adults[6] is a serious public health issue, hospitals in the United States are required to have policies governing pain assessment and management as a condition for accreditation, and the 10-year period from 2001 to 2011 has been proclaimed the Decade of Pain Control and Research.[7]

Every adolescent health care practitioner should understand basic pain physiology, methods of pain assessment, and pain management options. Such basic knowledge, however, must be modulated by particular and distinctive developmental aspects of adolescents as they transition from childhood to adulthood. Just as there are unique aspects to neonatal and geriatric pain management, there are also aspects of adolescent pain peculiar to that age group that must be taken into consideration. This chapter includes current knowledge about the basic principles of pain assessment and pharmacologic management and addresses unique aspects of the adolescent with pain. More details about integrative medicine techniques to prevent or alleviate pain are described in the preceding chapter.

### DEFINITIONS

The International Association for the Study of Pain[8] defines pain as "an unpleasant sensory and emotional experience associated with actual or potential tissue damage or described in terms of such damage." More relevant in adolescent health care is McCaffery's[9] definition of pain as "whatever the experiencing person says it is, existing whenever and wherever the person says it does." These definitions emphasize that pain is a subjective experience mediated by physiologic and psychological factors. Underlying this concept is that only the adolescent with pain can know what his or her pain is like. The assessment and management of pain in adolescents is challenging, given the subjective nature of pain, the variable styles of communication, and the developmentally determined elements of the experience of pain. The report adolescents give about their pain, however, must be accepted by health professionals seeking to alleviate pain and its attendant suffering.

#### FEATURES OF PAIN

Pain may be described in terms of its duration, the source from which it emanates, and the pharmacologic response to treatment.

##### Duration of Pain

*Acute pain* is usually the result of an acute injury, disease process, procedure, or surgery and resolves once the underlying condition has been treated or improves, generally lasting less than 3 months. It is accompanied by physiologic findings such as tachycardia, increased blood pressure, mydriasis, pallor, and other physical findings related to sympathetic nervous system activity.

*Chronic pain* persists beyond the expected recovery time for acute pain (usually longer than 3 months), and instead of having associated signs of increased sympathetic symptoms is more commonly associated with sleep difficulties, loss of appetite, irritability, decreased motor and/or sexual function, and depression.

##### Origin of Pain

*Somatic pain* originates in bone, skin, ligament, and muscle and tends to be well localized; it is described as aching, throbbing, or gnawing.

*Visceral pain* originates in solid or hollow organs. It is caused by distension, traction, or ischemia and is poorly localized; it is described as cramping, colicky pressure, deep aching, or squeezing.

*Neuropathic pain* occurs secondary to dysfunction of the central or peripheral nervous systems and often is associated with neurologic deficit and/or abnormal sensation. It is often described as burning, electrical shock, hot, stabbing, shooting, itching, or tingling.

### Pharmacologic Management of Pain

*Tolerance* describes the need for escalating doses of medication to maintain an equal analgesic effect over time.

*Physical dependence* is the biologic response to chronic drug administration characterized by the onset of withdrawal symptoms when the drug is removed rapidly. For example, opioid withdrawal is characterized by tachycardia, hypertension, vomiting, diarrhea, diaphoresis, agitation, and even fever.

*Addiction* is a behavioral pattern of drug use characterized by a craving for and overwhelming involvement in obtaining and using a drug for pain control (see Chapter 179, Abuse of Prescription Drugs). Risk for addiction in medical use is low. This needs to be emphasized, particularly to parents of adolescents who have illnesses that cause pain. Nevertheless, because some adolescents may be at risk for abusing drugs, the potential for addictive behavior should be considered in this age group, particularly if there is a personal or family history of addictive behaviors or treated addictions.

*Pseudo-addiction* refers to chronic undermedication leading to behaviors that mimic addiction. Once the pain is adequately treated, the behaviors subside. This may be seen in chronic diseases, such as sickle cell disease, where the burden of pain is extremely high but there is a tendency for some clinicians to interpret pain relief-seeking behaviors as drug-seeking behaviors.

## ANATOMY AND PHYSIOLOGY OF PAIN

The peripheral and central nervous systems are involved in pain. The pain signal begins peripherally when nociceptors (primary neurons) are stimulated by mechanical, thermal, or chemical stimuli. This results in thinly myelinated, rapidly conducting "A-delta fibers" carrying impulses of well-localized, sharp ("first") pain, as well as slower-conducting unmyelinated "C fibers" carrying poorly localized, dull, aching, burning ("second") pain. These fibers synapse with secondary neurons in the dorsal horn of the spinal cord where they release glutamate, substance P, and other neurotransmitters. Central nervous system (CNS) descending fibers and dorsal horn interneurons usually inhibit the pain response by releasing norepinephrine, gamma-aminobutyric acid, serotonin, enkephalins, and other substances that interfere with the release of pain signal transmitters. The secondary neurons then cross to the opposite side of the spinal cord and ascend to the brainstem, midbrain, thalamus, and hypothalamus via the spinothalamic, spinomesencephalic, and spinoreticular tracts. From the thalamus there are projections to multiple subcortical and cortical areas, as well as the limbic system in the hippocampus and amygdala. Transmission of nociceptive signals into these areas results in the perception and interpretation of pain.

Central sensitization, a centrally mediated state of hyperexcitability, may significantly affect the status of pain perception as the brain receives and interprets nociceptive signals. Central sensitization occurs at the level of the dorsal horn where glutamate released from the primary afferent nociceptive neuron activates the alpha-amino-3-hydroxy-5-methyl-4-isoxazole propionic acid (AMPA) and N-methyl-D-aspartate (NMDA) receptors on secondary "wide-dynamic-range" neurons. Because this effect can be reduced by opioids, NMDA antagonists, and gabaminergic and alpha-2 antagonists, these modulators can be useful in pain management, especially before the nociceptive input reaches and sensitizes the upper-level brain structures. Local anesthetics, in particular, can help modulate control sensitization.

Because nociceptive signals ultimately reach the brainstem, the thalamic, hypothalamic, limbic systems, and subcortical, and cortical areas, a significant stress response results with measurable effects on respiratory, cardiovascular, metabolic, gastrointestinal, renal, and immune systems used in assessing the severity of pain. The stress response is mediated by the sympathetic nervous system and release of regulatory hormones that have an effect on the cardiovascular and other organ systems. Thus, pain can result in tachycardia, increased blood pressure, tachypnea, pallor, diaphoresis, hyperglycemia, increased antidiuretic hormone secretion, and other autonomic findings.

### MISCONCEPTIONS ABOUT PAIN

The assessment and treatment of pain can be hindered by numerous misconceptions. Patients particularly at risk of being misunderstood are adolescents who have a chronic illness, such as sickle cell disease; those with developmental delay who cannot communicate directly about their pain; and those with behavioral disorders where expressing the need for pain medication may be interpreted as manipulative and untruthful. Some of the most common misconceptions, along with the corresponding facts, are listed in Table 18-1.

## APPROACH TO PAIN ASSESSMENT IN THE ADOLESCENT

To treat an adolescent who has pain, the care provider must (1) understand and recognize the pathologic processes that might produce pain or discomfort, (2) be aware of the developmental differences at various stages of adolescence, because they may affect interpretation of pain and the way it is communicated, (3) know the

**Table 18-1**

**Common Misconceptions and Facts about Pain in Adolescents**

| *Misconception* | *Fact* |
|---|---|
| Children and adolescents will tell you when they are in pain. | Many children and adolescents will not admit that they are in pain for many reasons: fears or misperceptions about the cause of their pain, fear about side effects of medications, or feeling a need to be stoic about their pain. |
| The use of opioids for pain relief can lead to addiction and should be avoided. | It is extremely rare for addiction to occur as a result of using opioids for pain relief. Although physical dependence may occur after sustained use of opioids, this is not the same as addiction. |
| Objective/visible signs are necessary to verify existence and severity of pain. | A patient's self-report is the most reliable indicator of pain. Some patients with severe acute pain and many patients with chronic pain may not display any visible or overt signs. |
| Activity level is a good indicator for severity of pain. | Activity level may or may not be affected when someone is in pain. |
| Experience with pain leads to greater tolerance. | Assessing prior pain experiences is critical to understanding the patient's needs as this may affect coping with the current pain condition. |
| Mood has little effect on pain. | The meaning a person associates with pain can play a critical role in the pain experience. Anxiety, fear, and depression do not cause pain, but they can accentuate its perception and decrease coping ability. |
| Opioids should be limited in dying patients because they could hasten death. | The goal of pain management at the end of life is to achieve and maintain comfort. Good pain management is more likely to prolong life than to shorten it. Consultation with a palliative care specialist, anesthesia pain service, pastoral services, child life specialist, or bioethicist may be helpful. |
| Cultural practices and spiritual beliefs are not important in the management of pain. | Many cultural practices and spiritual beliefs can affect pain assessment and management. |

Adapted from Golisano Children's Hospital/Strong Memorial Hospital Pain and Sedation Resource Manual, 2001, with permission from the University of Rochester Medical Center.

psychosocial and historical background of the adolescent, (4) recognize the role of anxiety in causing and intensifying the pain experience, (5) know the adolescent's (and parents') goals for pain management, (6) understand the use of a variety of nonpharmacologic and pharmacologic treatment modalities, and (7) know when to obtain additional expertise. Pain assessment includes obtaining a detailed pain history, assessing the patient's physiologic variables affected by pain, and obtaining an objective measure of the adolescent's perception of pain.

## HISTORY

Although a complete pain history is frequently not possible in cases of acute pain, minimal data that should be obtained and recorded include the following: (1) time of onset and duration of pain, (2) events preceding, during, and immediately following pain onset, (3) location of pain, (4) radiation of pain to other areas of the body (with an emphasis on common sites of referred pain, such as to the top of the shoulder with diaphragmatic irritation or to the groin with kidney stones), (5) character of the pain (aching, sharp, burning, tingling, or pressure, using the adolescent's exact words when possible, "it feels like I'm being stabbed with a hot knife"), (6) intensity of pain on a numeric scale, including the peak and nadir, if not constant, (7) duration of pain and pain-free periods, if intermittent, (8) factors that relieve pain (eg, position, medications, or alternative therapies), and (9) any precipitants to pain (eg, movement, position, or eating).

The difference between an adolescent being awakened *because of pain* versus awakening for some other reason and *being aware of pain* is important, but often difficult practically. Adolescents experiencing pain often have a variety of reasons to sleep poorly. Although clinical dogma emphasizes that pain that awakens an adolescent from sleep is organic until proven otherwise, it is important to determine that the patient is awakened from a sound sleep *by the pain* itself.

In addition to the historical elements directly related to pain noted previously, the history should include a psychosocial assessment to identify vulnerabilities that might increase pain perception, such as anxiety or depression. Also, an understanding of the adolescent's psychosocial status provides clues to understanding and managing pain. For example, an adolescent who witnesses his or her grandfather having premortem chest pain may misinterpret his or her own chest pain. Assessing concerns and worries about pain informs management because anxiety tends to increase pain awareness, and pain often results in increased anxiety.

**PHYSIOLOGIC VARIABLES**

Especially with acute pain, there are physiologic effects: (1) increased resting heart rate, (2) increased blood pressure, (3) increased respiratory effort, including splinting, (4) pallor, (5) sweating, (6) hyperglycemia, (7) anorexia, and (8) mental status changes including irritability, agitation, crying, anxiety, or withdrawal. Variables often attributed to "emotional reactivity" have a physiologic basis.

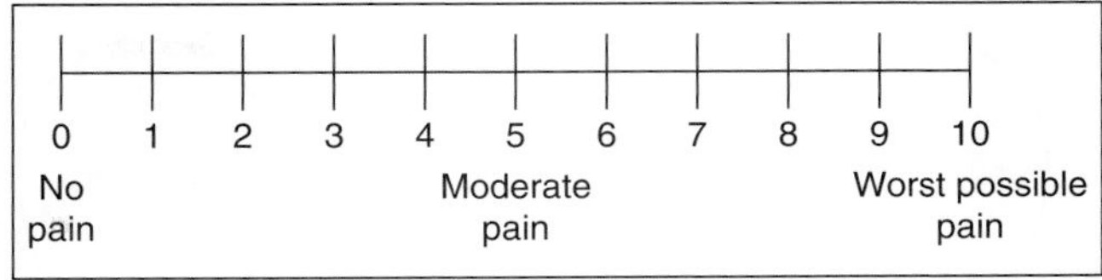


FIGURE 18-1 Numeric Scale for Pain Intensity (Teenagers and Young Adults).

**PATIENT PERCEPTION OF PAIN**

The most common objective measure of pain in adolescents is a validated numerical scale from 0 to 10 on which the adolescent identifies the number that best depicts the pain level (Figure 18-1). With developmental delays, the Revised Face, Legs, Activity, Cry, Consolability Scale (FLACC)[10] (Table 18-2) or the Faces Pain Scale-Revised[11] (Figure 18-2) can be used.

On the numeric pain scale, a score of < 3 is considered mild, 4 to 7 moderate, and 8 to 10 severe pain. Mild

**Table 18-2**

**Revised FLACC Scale (for Adolescents with Developmental Disabilities)**

| *Categories* | *0* | *1* | *2* |
|---|---|---|---|
| **Face** | No particular expression or smile | Occasional grimace or frown, withdrawn, disinterested, sad, appears worried | Frequent to constant quivering chin, clenched jaws, distressed-looking face, expression of fright/panic |
| **Legs** | Normal position or relaxed, usual tone and motion to limbs | Uneasy, restless, tense, occasional tremors | Kicking, or legs drawn up, marked increase in spasticity, constant tremors, jerking |
| **Activity** | Lying quietly; normal position; moves easily; regular, rhythmic respirations | Squirming, shifting back and forth, tense, tense/guarded movements, mildly agitated, shallow/splinting respirations, intermittent sighs | Arched, rigid or jerking, severe agitation, head banging, shivering, breath holding, gasping, severe splinting |
| **Cry** | No cry (awake or asleep) | Moans or whimpers; occasional complaint, occasional verbal outbursts, constant grunting | Crying steadily, screams or sobs, frequent complaints, repeated outbursts, constant grunting |
| **Consolability** | Content, relaxed | Reassured by occasional touching, hugging, or being talked to, distractible | Difficult to console or comfort, pushing caregiver away, resisting care or comfort measures |

Each of the 5 categories (F) Face (L) Legs (A) Activity (C) Cry (C) Consolability is scored from 0–2, which results in a total score between 0 (no pain) and 10 (maximum pain).

Document the total score by adding numbers from each of the 5 categories.

Modified with permission from Malviya S, Voepel-Lewis T, Burke C, Merkel S, Tait AR. The revised FLACC observational pain tool: improved reliability and validity for pain assessment in children with cognitive impairment. *Paediatr Anaesth*. 2006;16(3):258–265

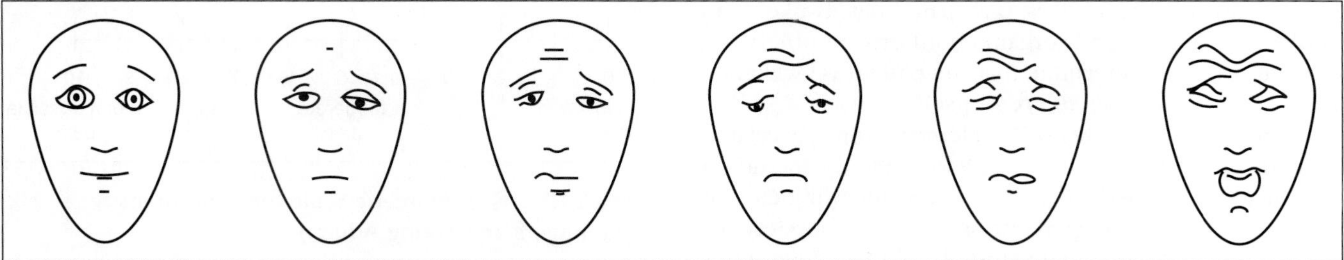

**FIGURE 18-2** Faces Pain Scale-Revised. (Reproduced from Hicks CL, von Baeyer CL, Spafford P, et al. Faces Pain Scale-Revised: Toward a common metric in pediatric pain measurement. *PAIN*. 2001;93:173–183, with permission from the International Association for the Study of Pain®. Further reproduction is prohibited.)

pain may be tolerated well. However, patients with a score of ≥4 should have a pain management plan developed and documented, even if the patient ultimately refuses pain treatment. One can ask the adolescent, "At what number would you like treatment." Few adolescents ask for specific pain treatment if their level of pain is 3 or less.

Documentation of an objective pain score provides a baseline and rationale for pain management and a means to determine how well pain is being relieved. Recorded numeric pain scores also enable different professionals providing health care to an adolescent to recognize changes over time, allowing them to adjust treatments in accordance with the patient's experience of pain. Despite such numeric measures, some health care providers make treatment decisions based on arbitrary rules ("He shouldn't still be having pain this long after surgery") or their own interpretation ("She doesn't act like her pain is an 8").

For inpatients, a record of a pain score with each set of vital signs emphasizes the importance of tracking pain control in the context of standard physiologic parameters. If blood pressure, heart rate, respiratory rate, and temperature are the first 4 vital signs, the pain score is sometimes called the "fifth vital sign."

## GENERAL PRINCIPLES OF PAIN MANAGEMENT

A number of general principles of pain management in adolescents are listed in Box 18-1. An important consideration in pain management is the differentiation between pain and suffering. Pain is a noxious feeling that occurs in the body, but suffering occurs at the level of the patient, or even the family, when pain is not relieved or its source is not known. Some pain conditions are associated with mental health diagnoses (see Chapter 183, Somatoform Disorders), but pain itself, especially if chronic or poorly understood, can also lead to depression and anxiety.

### Box 18-1

### *General Principles of Pain Management*

- Treat the adolescent who has pain rather than treating pain in the adolescent.
- Determine with the patient the goals of pain relief, which may not be the elimination of pain.
- Use a multimodal approach applied in a step-wise fashion as appropriate. Nonpharmacologic measures especially may be of profound benefit (see Chapter 17, Complementary and Alternative Medicine).
- Consider pain an emergency that needs to be assessed and managed quickly.
- Investigate the underlying cause of pain, but treat pain while the investigation is ongoing.
- Incorporate proactive treatment approaches because they are humane, improve pain physiology and pain relief, and avoid establishing negative conditioned responses to anticipated pain.
- Administer medications as early as possible rather than wait for pain to become established.
- Assess and reassess for response to planned management.
- Obtain additional expertise early in the course of continued or worsening pain.
- Provide continuous pain relief rather than alternating pain and pain relief cycles.

### NONOPIOID PHARMACOLOGIC OPTIONS

The World Health Organization (WHO) has developed a step-wise approach to pain management, illustrated in Figure 18-3. This approach begins with the least potent medications with the fewest side effects, then incrementally adds to the more potent lower-step drugs that have more side effects. Although there are some

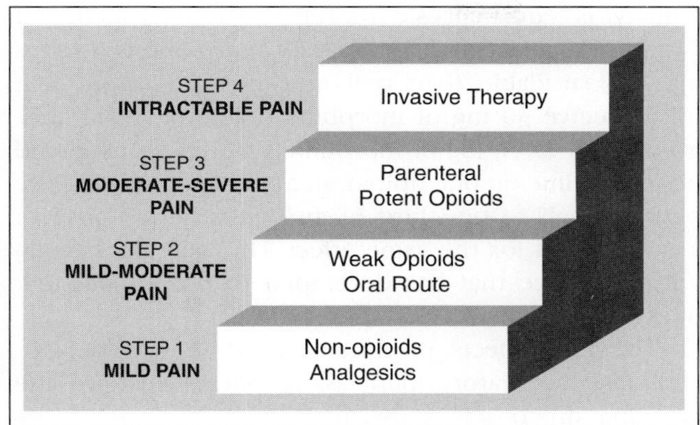


**FIGURE 18-3** World Health Organization (WHO) Steps of Analgesia. (Adapted with permission from World Health Organization. *Cancer Pain Relief and Palliative Care: Report of WHO Expert Committee.* 3rd ed. Geneva: WHO; 1996.)

limitations to this approach, especially for postsurgical pain where the oral route may not be possible or for cancer patients where rectal administration may be contraindicated, using an additive approach takes advantage of the synergistic effects of these medications and minimizes adverse effects. For example, use of a nonsteroidal medication with potent anti-inflammatory and analgesic properties enables the addition of an opioid at a low dose that further relieves pain but avoids adverse effects.

There are several classes of drugs that provide pain relief. They include prostaglandin synthesis inhibitors, weak and strong opioids, and adjunct medications (a mixture of medications including agents with a direct effect on the transmitters of the CNS).

### Prostaglandin Synthesis Inhibitors

These drugs interfere with nociception by inhibiting the synthesis of inflammatory prostaglandins centrally, and by spinal medication they may have an effect on NMDA receptors peripherally. They are weak analgesics compared to opiate agonists. Usually considered the first step of the analgesic stepped approach, proper administration, dose, and dosing regimen should be followed for optimal effect.

***Acetaminophen*** Acetaminophen is only available in oral and rectal form in the United States. After an initial oral loading dose of 20 mg/kg, standard dosing is 10 to 15 mg/kg every 4 to 6 hours up to 1,000 mg every 6 hours. No more than 90 mg/kg/day, or up to 4 gm/day in an adolescent or young adult, should be given because of effects on liver function. Higher doses do not result in more relief (ceiling effect). Rectal acetaminophen doses are usually higher, with a loading dose of 40 mg/kg and subsequent doses of 15 to 20 mg/kg. Unfortunately, the loading dose is frequently forgotten, resulting in a subtherapeutic level and a minimal or no effect. In addition, the use of rectal suppositories is often not acceptable and embarrassing for adolescents, but a patient should have the opportunity to decline the rectal route if the oral route is precluded.

***Nonsteroidal Anti-Inflammatory Drugs*** These drugs inhibit peripheral cyclo-oxygenase (COX), thereby decreasing prostaglandin synthesis and the production of inflammatory mediators, with reduction or elimination of nociceptive pain. Given their strong anti-inflammatory effects, these agents have a good analgesic effect when pain is mediated by inflammatory prostaglandins commonly present with musculoskeletal injury. The most commonly used agents in the United States are ibuprofen, ketorolac, naproxen, and tolmetin sodium. Diclofenac intramuscularly is used in other countries around the world, particularly for the management of fever.

These agents also have potential side effects, such as impaired mucin production (upper gastrointestinal bleeding), and clotting (platelet dysfunction), airway resistance (bronchospasm), and, in some studies, bone healing. In addition, nonsteroidal anti-inflammatory drugs (NSAIDs) may cause renal toxicity by inhibiting the release of intrarenal prostaglandins responsible for renal vasodilation and maintaining glomerular filtration during periods of decreased renal blood flow. This is more common with prolonged use of ketorolac, particularly with previous renal dysfunction. More selective cyclooxygenase inhibitors (COX-1 and COX-2) are less commonly used but are less likely to have NSAID side effects. Some contraindications to the use of nonsteroidal agents include peptic ulcer disease, renal failure, bleeding disorders, platelet dysfunction, and possibly asthma.

*Ibuprofen* is available as an oral preparation at a dose of 5 to 10 mg/kg every 6 to 8 hours up to 800 mg every 8 hours. It should be given with food to avoid gastritis. Peak analgesic effect is usually reached within 2 to 3 hours, although effects begin to occur in 20 minutes. Metabolism occurs in the liver via the cytochrome P450 system, with 5% to 10% excreted in the kidney.

*Ketorolac* may be given either orally or parenterally. It is particularly useful in patients who take nothing by mouth (NPO) after surgery and require adjunctive treatment for pain to reduce morphine requirements. It is effective for musculoskeletal, vaso-occlusive sickle cell crisis, and pleuritic pain. The intravenous (IV) or oral dose is 0.5 mg/kg up to 30 mg total, every 6 hours, for no more than 5 days; no additional analgesic effect is attained above a dose of 7.5 mg. Fixed dosing intervals for adolescents of parenteral ketorolac at 10 mg every 6 hours for up to 72 hours postoperatively can provide excellent pain control. Once oral medications can be given, ketorolac can be replaced with ibuprofen, an effective and less expensive alternative.

## OPIOIDS

Opioids are the mainstay of moderate to severe pain management. This class of drugs targets μ- and κ-receptors with effects that may be both therapeutic (blocking nociceptive input from μ-receptors) and adverse (κ-receptor). All opioids provide analgesia with varying degrees of sedation and similar side effects. Given an understanding of their pharmacology and kinetics, they can be easily interchanged; most may be given orally as well as parenterally, but with different times to peak effects and size of doses. Opiates vary considerably in terms of analgesic potency by weight and route of administration. Their interchangeability allows them to be given in varying amounts, but with equal analgesic effect (Table 18-3).

For example, because fentanyl is 100 to 150 times more potent than morphine, 1.0 microgram of IV fentanyl is "equianalgesic" to 100 to 150 micrograms of IV morphine. Likewise, because IV morphine is 3 times more bioavailable than oral morphine, an adolescent must receive 30 mg of morphine orally to obtain analgesia equal to 10 mg of morphine IV. After an extended period of time on one opioid, an adolescent may require only one-half to one-third of an equianalgesic dose of a new opioid for the same effect. This may have to do with tolerance that has developed to one opioid that does not carry over to the new opioid.

The side effects of opioids may be considerable, including respiratory depression/apnea, sedation and clouding of consciousness, hallucinations, nausea/vomiting, constipation (secondary to decreased peristalsis), generalized pruritus, hypotension (especially in intravascular, volume-depleted individuals), urinary retention, and miosis. One should treat opioid side effects as they arise rather than inadequately treat pain to avoid them. Often a change in the opioid will attenuate the adverse effects experienced. Otherwise, helpful ways to treat side effects include antiemetics for nausea (eg, ondansetron), antihistamines or low-dose naloxone for itching, and laxatives, colonic stimulants, or fiber for constipation.

**TABLE 18-3**

**Opioid Equianalgesic Doses for Adolescents**

| *Opioid* | *IV/IM* | *PO* | | |
|---|---|---|---|---|
| Morphine | 10 mg | 30 mg | | |
| Hydromorphone | 1.5 mg | 7.5 mg | | |
| Codeine | 120 mg (IM only) | 200 mg | | |
| Oxycodone | Not available | 20 mg | | |
| Hydrocodone | Not available | 30 mg | | |
| Fentanyl | 100 mcg (single dose) | 24-hour oral morphine | | Fentanyl patch |
| | 200 mcg (continuous IV infusion) | 45 mg | = | 12 mcg/hour |
| | | 90 mg | = | 25 mcg/hour |
| | | 180 mg | = | 50 mcg/hour |
| | | 360 mg | = | 100 mcg/hour |
| Methadone | 10 mg | To convert 24-hour oral morphine to 24-hour oral methadone, use the morphine:methadone ratio in the following chart, based on the daily dose of 24-hour oral morphine. | | |
| | | 24-hour oral morphine | | 24-hour oral morphine: methadone ratio |
| | | <30 mg | = | 2:1 |
| | | 31–99 mg | = | 4:1 |
| | | 100–299 mg | = | 8:1 |
| | | 300–499 mg | = | 12:1 |
| | | 500–999 mg | = | 15:1 |
| | | 1000–1299 mg | = | 20:1 |

### Weak Opioids

Codeine, oxycodone, and hydrocodone are weak opioids available in oral formulations. They are particularly useful to treat moderate pain. Because codeine's analgesic effect is due to the 10% of codeine metabolized to morphine, its potency is only one-tenth of morphine. Nausea and vomiting may occur with any weak opioid, but they are more common with codeine and less common with oxycodone or hydrocodone. Codeine, oxycodone, and hydrocodone are available in combination with acetaminophen (eg, Tylenol #2, 3, or 4, Percocet, and Vicodin, respectively) for synergistic analgesic effect (Table 18-4). Intramuscular codeine has been replaced by low-dose IV morphine. There are also slow-release oral preparations of oxycodone and hydrocodone useful for chronic pain. These synthetic codeine derivatives have high abuse potential and are used recreationally by some adolescents and young adults.

**Table 18-4**

**Opioid Drug Dosing for Adolescents**

| | *Parenteral* | | *Oral* | | |
|---|---|---|---|---|---|
| ***Drug*** | ***<50 kg*** | ***≥50 kg*** | ***<50 kg*** | ***≥50 kg*** | ***Preparations/Comments*** |
| Codeine | NR | NR | 0.5–1 mg/kg q 3–4 hours | 30–60 mg q 3–4 hours | Combination elixir:<br>• Codeine 12 mg/acetaminophen 120/5 ml<br>Combination tablets:<br>• Codeine 15 mg/acetaminophen 300 mg (Tylenol #2)<br>• Codeine 30 mg/acetaminophen 300 mg (Tylenol #3)<br>• Codeine 60 mg/acetaminophen 300 mg (Tylenol #4) |
| Oxycodone | Not available | Not available | 0.05–0.15 mg/kg q 4–6 hours | 10 mg q 4–6 hours | Immediate release tablets: 5 mg<br>Immediate release liquid: 20 mg/ml<br>Sustained release tablets: 10, 20, 40, 80 mg q 12 hour<br>Combination tablets: oxycodone/acetaminophen: 2.5/325; 5/325; 7.5/500; 10/650 mg (Percocet) |
| Hydrocodone | Not available | Not available | 0.2 mg/kg/dose q 4–6 hours | 5–10 mg q 4–6 hours | Combination tablets:<br>• Hydrocodone/acetaminophen 5/500 mg (Vicodin)<br>• Hydrocodone/ibuprofen 7.5/200 mg (Vicoprofen)<br>• Hydrocodone/acetaminophen 2.5/500; 5/500; 7.5/500 (Lortab) (use caution in renal disease) |
| Morphine | 0.05–0.1 mg/kg q 2–4 hours<br>Infusion: 0.02 mg/kg/hours | 5–10 mg q 2–4 hours<br>Infusion: 1–1.5 mg/hours | 0.3 mg/kg q 3–4 hours (IR or oral solution) | 15–30 mg q 3–4 hours (IR or oral solution) | Oral solution: 2 mg/ml; 4 mg/ml<br>Oral concentrate: 20 mg/ml<br>Immediate release tablets (IR): 10, 15, 30 mg<br>Sustained release tablets (SR): 15, 30, 60, 100, 200 mg q 12 hour |

*(continued)*

**Table 18-4 (continued)**

| | *Parenteral* | | *Oral* | | |
|---|---|---|---|---|---|
| ***Drug*** | ***<50 kg*** | ***≥50 kg*** | ***<50 kg*** | ***≥50 kg*** | ***Preparations/Comments*** |
| Hydromorphone | 0.015 mg/kg q 3-6 hours<br>Infusion: 0.004 | 1-2 mg IV/SC q 3-4 hours<br>Infusion: 0.2-0.4 | 0.03-0.08 mg/kg q 3-6 hours | 4-8 mg q 3-6 hours | Immediate release tablets: 2, 4, 8 mg<br>Immediate release liquid: 1mg/ml<br>May be used in renal disease |
| Fentanyl | 1-2 mcg/kg q 1-2 hours | 50-100 mcg q 1-2 hours | Available but absorption variable | Available but absorption variable | Transdermal patch: use only after total daily dose of parenteral fentanyl or morphine is determined |
| Methadone | Variable availability | Variable availability | 0.1-0.2 mg/kg q 6-8 hours | 2.5-10 mg q 8 hours | Use only in consultation with pain specialist due to very prolonged half-life (19 hours in children to 35 hours in adults) with repeated dosing. **Start with lower dose and adjust slowly if being used for chronic pain**. May accumulate easily, and dose adjustment is complex. |
| Tramadol | None | None | 50 mg (for pts >35 kg) q 3 hours | 50-100 mg q 3-6 hours | No studies in pediatric patients <35 kg 50 mg tablet only preparation available in United States. |

The dose of codeine is 0.5 to 1 mg/kg orally up to 30 to 60 mg per dose every 3 to 4 hours. Tablets containing a combination of codeine and acetaminophen have 300 mg of acetaminophen and codeine ranging from 7.5 to 60 mg per tablet. The elixir form contains 12 mg codeine and 120 mg acetaminophen in 5 ml. Oxycodone is prescribed at 0.05 to 0.1 mg/kg up to 5 to 10 mg per dose every 4 to 6 hours. Hydrocodone is prescribed at 0.05 to 0.15 mg/kg up to 5 to 10 mg per dose every 4 to 6 hours. Both come in combinations with fixed amounts of acetaminophen at 325 to 500 mg.

Tramadol is an opioid agonist that acts at the μ-receptor but also inhibits the reuptake of norepinephrine and serotonin in the CNS. A weak opioid with potency similar to codeine, tramadol is 75% bioavailable and is metabolized in the liver's P450 system. In the United States it is available only as a tablet, although it is manufactured in parenteral, liquid, and suppository formulations. There are few studies in pediatric patients, but in a study of adolescent patients recovering from orthopedic surgery, oral tramadol (1 tablet for patients 35 to 55 kg, 2 tablets for patients >55 kg) every 3 hours was effective.[12]

### Strong Opioids

***Morphine*** Morphine is the prototypic strong opioid. As a pure agonist stimulating the μ-receptor, its side effects are mediated by stimulation of κ-receptors as well as the release of histamine. Acute side effects include miosis, histamine release resulting in vasodilation and hypotension, urticaria and itching, nausea and vomiting, sedation, and suppression of ventilation. Hydration and antiemetics can minimize these side effects. Because hypoventilation may occur, respiratory status and underlying respiratory disorders should be recognized. Disturbing hallucinations may also occur with morphine.

Morphine can be infused *continuously*, at a starting dose of 0.02 mg/kg per hour. It can also be administered *intermittently* by IV at a starting dose of 0.1 mg/kg/dose every 2 to 4 hours, with peak effect in 20 to 30 minutes after administration. These doses are related to lean body mass, so obese adolescents should receive a lower dose than a lean individual of similar weight. If morphine is given too rapidly or at a high dose, apnea or respiratory depression may result. A safe and effective method to arrive at the 0.1 mg/kg initial dose, especially for morphine-naïve adolescents, is to deliver 5 divided doses of 0.02 to 0.03 mg/kg (up to 2 to 3 mg/dose) every 10 minutes and assess the effect of each dose. This decreases the risk of apnea while simultaneously treating the pain incrementally. The adolescent should be evaluated every 10 minutes with this protocol to ensure that the dosing schedule is not interrupted and the benefits of cumulative dosing are attained.

Oral dosing of morphine requires 3 times the amount used parenterally because it must first pass through the liver where it is metabolized into its active glucuronidated form. Thus, as illustrated in Table 18-3, an oral dose of 0.3 mg/kg of morphine is equianalgesic to 0.1 mg/kg IV morphine. Rapid-release oral form of morphine results in effect as early as 20 minutes after administration. Morphine may also be given intramuscularly, subcutaneously, and as slow-release oral formulations. To ensure the amount given will cover the duration of sustained release oral morphine, this slow-acting form should not be used until the total amount of short-acting morphine needed for pain relief has been determined.

***Hydromorphone*** Hydromorphone is a derivative of morphine that is 3 to 6 times more potent in providing excellent analgesia, but with fewer side effects, particularly nausea, pruritus, and sedation. For this reason, it is an excellent primary opioid, particularly in adolescents who already have significant nausea. Because there are no active metabolites it can also be used in the presence of renal failure. It may be given intravenously, intramuscularly, subcutaneously, orally, and as patient-controlled anaglesia (PCA). Peak effect is between 30 to 60 minutes after either an IV or oral dose.

A single IV dose of hydromorphone is 0.015 mg/kg (up to 2 mg maximum). Because the oral hydromorphone form has one-fourth the potency of the IV form, the oral dose is 0.03 to 0.08 mg/kg (up to 8 mg maximum every 6 hours, or 4 mg maximum every 3 hours).

***Fentanyl*** Much more potent (100- to 150-fold stronger) than morphine, fentanyl is a synthetic opiate agonist. Unlike morphine, fentanyl does not cause histamine release with secondary vasodilation and hypotension and is less likely to cause urticaria, pruritus, sedation, or nausea. Some adolescents experience nasal itching that disappears over time. Fentanyl has a rapid onset with an analgesic effect within 3 to 5 minutes, lasting less than one hour. Acute chest wall rigidity, rare in adolescents, is reversible with naloxone.

Fentanyl is administered in 1 to 2 mcg/kg doses IV every 1 to 2 hours. Although it can be given as a continuous IV or subcutaneous infusion at 2 to 10 mcg/kg per hour, associated hypoventilation requires this type of administration to be limited to intensive care-type settings.

For adolescents with chronic pain and difficult IV access, or for those who require slow weaning of narcotics, chronic fentanyl infusion subcutaneously can be as effective as intravenous use. Like morphine, fentanyl may be infused via a PCA pump. Fentanyl can also be delivered to adolescents with chronic pain by a transdermal patch, but this route takes 12 hours to reach a steady state, and fentanyl levels continue to be present 12 hours after patch removal. Patches come in different strengths; a 2 mcg/hour fentanyl patch will release the equivalent of 90 mg oral morphine per day. Fentanyl cannot be given orally, but transmucosal fentanyl (lollipops) has been used effectively, although up to one-third of patients experience nausea and vomiting with this form. Intranasal fentanyl, in combination with intranasal midazolam, has also been used with some success for procedural sedation. Intramuscular fentanyl is not recommended.

***Methadone*** Methadone is a long-acting opioid (half-life greater than 24 hours in adolescents) that can be given either parenterally or orally. Its main use is in long-term pain management (adolescents who are terminally ill, have cancer, or have significant chronic pain) or for slow withdrawal from opioids. Oral dosing 3 to 4 times a day precludes the need for an IV. In addition, it is useful for patients in renal failure because there is minimal renal excretion of methadone. Even with all these benefits, methadone dosing is complex. On a given dose, the full analgesic effect may not be reached for several days. In addition, the transition from shorter-acting opioids, such as morphine and fentanyl, can result in either under- or overdosing while attempting equianalgesic dosing.

Methadone is often used in adolescents to prevent opioid withdrawal symptoms after there has been a long course of shorter-acting narcotics. A loading dose is given over several days based on the total daily dosing of the shorter-acting narcotic. Then this is followed by a twice-daily dosing regimen with a decrease of 5% to 10% of the original dose every 3 to 5 days.

***Nalbuphine*** Nalbuphine is a mixed agonist–antagonist with antagonism toward the opioid μ-receptor and agonist activity at the κ-receptor. It competitively binds to the μ-receptor and displaces any bound opioids. Therefore, both the analgesic and side effects related to the μ-receptors are reversed: adolescents who have been taking opioids chronically may experience withdrawal symptoms, but the side effects of pruritus, nausea, vomiting, and intestinal motility impairment are reduced, although not consistently.[13,14] Stimulation of the κ-receptor results in significant analgesia independent of the μ-receptor effects. In addition, there appears to be a specific antianalgesic effect (in males) that can be reversed by low-dose morphine.[15,16]

## OPIOID REVERSAL AGENTS

Because opiates can cause respiratory depression and apnea, prescribing physicians need to be familiar with agents that can reverse these serious adverse effects. Opioid reversal agents should be targeted at life-threatening side effects while attempting to maintain analgesia. Analgesic effect reversal may result in severe pain, agitation, and acute signs of withdrawal, particularly with chronic opiate use.

Naloxone is the primary agent for reversing opioid-adverse effects. This drug is a pure μ-receptor nonselective antagonist and can reverse ventilatory and other adverse effects as well as analgesia. Its plasma elimination half-life is about 60 minutes so that frequent redosing may be necessary when opioids with longer half-lives have been used. Careful monitoring after naloxone is necessary to detect recurrence of a serious adverse effect. A starting dose of 2 to 5 mcg (0.002–0.005 mg)/kg IV push should be given with additional doses every 2 to 3 minutes until the adverse effect has been reversed. A reversal of adverse effects usually occurs within one minute of administration and may be abrupt. Repeat doses are often necessary over the following 30 to 60 minutes, depending on the opioid being reversed. If frequent repeat doses have to be given, a continuous naloxone infusion should be considered.

Naloxone has also been used effectively as a continuous infusion for the management of pruritus secondary to opioids, particularly morphine.[17,18] In low doses this is effective and does not appear to affect analgesia. An infusion should begin at 0.25 to 0.5 mcg/kg per hour (0.00025–0.0005 mg/kg per hour) and titrated to effect.

## PATIENT-CONTROLLED ANALGESIA

Patient-controlled analgesia is administered by a pump activated by the adolescent as needed to provide adequate pain control. For those with time-limited, severe, acute pain for known reasons, such as following surgery, PCA is an excellent option. Most adolescents desire to have control over their symptoms, and gaining a sense of mastery over the management (not necessarily elimination) of pain through PCA can significantly decrease anxiety. Patient-controlled analgesia also allows potent narcotic medications to be given safely and to control pain to the level the adolescent desires. Because respiratory depression is usually coupled with sedation with opioid use, adolescents generally do not administer additional medication once sedation is experienced, effectively precluding respiratory depression. There are studies demonstrating success with nurse- or parent-controlled analgesia using the same equipment for PCA, particularly in developmentally delayed and young patients,[19-21] but there is the possibility of either under- or overdosing with this mode of opioid delivery.

Although morphine is most commonly used in PCA and hydromorphone, fentanyl, and meperidine have all been used successfully, meperidine is not recommended because of the potential accumulation of normeperidine, a neurotoxic metabolite. Modern PCA pumps allow the clinician to program the pump to administer a constant, low-dose basal infusion rate (not controlled by the patient) in addition to small, preset boluses of an opioid administered with the push of a button, but no more frequently than a predetermined lockout period. During the lockout period, no additional opioid beyond the basal infusion rate is administered, regardless of how many times the button is pushed. The pump maintains a record of the number, frequency, and pattern of times of actual administration as well as "demands" when the patient pushes the button. These data inform dosing adjustments that may be needed.

Suggested dosing guidelines for morphine, hydromorphone, and fentanyl are shown in Table 18-5. Typically a loading dose is followed by maintenance dosing at 5- to 15-minute intervals. A background basal rate is optional and is used most frequently in situations where there is frequent breakthrough pain, where there might be concern about patient capacity, or during sleep so the patient does not need to wake up to give another minibolus of pain medication.

## ADJUVANT MEDICATIONS FOR PAIN CONTROL

Although opioids are excellent medications for treating nociceptive pain, neuropathic pain responds better to different types of drugs. Neuropathic is perceived as burning, shooting, or stabbing and is secondary to mechanical-, burn-, chemotherapy-, or radiation-induced trauma to nerves. Neuropathic pain is often present in terminally ill adolescent patients who have either undergone treatments that have had neurotoxic effects or have a disease process that directly affects the peripheral and/or CNS. Opioids are less effective in treating this type of pain and may result in the administration of very high doses of narcotic with serious adverse effects but little pain relief. More effective analgesics for neuropathic pain include tricyclic antidepressants such as amitriptyline, antiepileptics such as gabapentin or carbamazepine, antiarrhythmics such as mexiletine, alpha-2 antagonists such as clonidine, and topical anesthetics such as 4% lidocaine. Table 18-6 includes dosing and adverse side effects of adjuvant medications for neuropathic pain.

**Table 18-5**

**Patient-Controlled Analgesia Initial Dosing Guidelines in Adolescents[a]**

| | *Morphine PCA* | *Hydromorphone PCA* | *Fentanyl PCA* |
|---|---|---|---|
| **Adolescents ≥40 kg** | *Loading dose:* 0.1–0.2 mg/kg in 5 doses q5 minutes (0.02–0.04 mg/kg/dose) | *Loading dose:* 0.02–0.04 mg/kg in 5 doses q5 minutes (0.004–0.008 mg/kg/dose) | *Loading dose:* 1–2 mcg/kg in 5 doses q5 minutes (0.2–0.4 mcg/kg/dose) |
| | *Maintenance dosing:* 1 mg q5–15 minutes PCA, with or without basal infusion of 1–2 mg/hour so that total dose is ≤0.1 mg/kg/hour. Dose adjustments made in 0.5–1-mg increments | *Maintenance dosing:* 0.2 mg q5–15 minutes PCA, with or without basal infusion of 0.2–0.4 mg/hour. Dose adjustments usually made in 0.1–0.2-mg increments | *Maintenance dosing:* 10 mcg q5–15 minutes PCA, with or without basal infusion of 10–20 mcg/hour. Dose adjustments are usually made in 10–20-mcg increments |
| **Adolescents <40 kg** | *Loading dose:* 0.05–0.1 mg/kg in 5 doses q5 minutes (0.01–0.02 mg/kg/dose) | *Loading dose:* 0.01–0.02 mg/kg in 5 doses q5 minutes (0.002–0.004 mg/kg/dose) | *Loading dose:* 0.5–1 mcg/kg in 5 doses q5 minutes (0.1–0.2 mcg/kg/dose) |
| | *Maintenance dosing:* 0.02 mg/kg/hour basal infusion with 0.01–0.02 mg/kg intermittent dose at q10–15 minutes so that total hourly dose is ≤ 0.1 mg/kg/hour | *Maintenance dosing:* 0.004 mg/kg/hour basal infusion with 0.0015 mg/kg intermittent dose at q 5–15 minutes so that total hourly dose is ≤0.015 mg/kg/hour | *Maintenance dosing:* 0.2 mcg/kg/hour basal infusion, with 0.1 mcg/kg intermittent dose q5–15 minutes so that total hourly dose is ≤1 mcg/kg/hour |

[a]These are initial dosing guidelines. Dosing should be adjusted as necessary depending on pain scores. Except for respiratory depression, oversedation, and muscle rigidity, side effects should be treated rather than pain relief discontinued (eg, nausea or vomiting should be treated with ondansetron, droperidol, or promethazine; pruritus with diphenydramine or hydroxyzine; constipation with stimulant laxatives with/without stool softener).

### Regional and Spinal Anesthetics

To decrease the likelihood of unpleasant side effects and to provide more targeted pain relief, some adolescents with pain may be candidates for regional and/or spinal anesthetics, especially those who have had a surgical procedure with localized pain or those who have well-identified and severe regional pain. Epidural and intrathecal administration of medications to provide regional pain relief requires an experienced anesthesiologist or physician with similar skills. Common indications include pain following a thoracotomy, urologic, gynecologic, or peripheral vascular procedures, and orthopedic procedures involving the pelvis and lower extremities, as well as adolescents who have poorly controlled non-surgical regional pain. Contraindications for regional and spinal anesthesia include coagulopathy or infection in the skin area where the catheter is to be placed.

***Epidural catheters*** An epidural catheter is introduced percutaneously into the epidural space with the catheter tip resting adjacent to the location in the spinal cord from which nociceptive impulses from particular dermatomes enter the epidural space. Delivery of local anesthetic in a specific closed anatomic space provides significant pain relief in specific regions of the body. Thus, epidural catheters can be placed at the caudal, lumbar, and thoracic levels with continuous infusions to maintain a steady concentration of anesthetic/analgesic in the epidural space. A particularly useful additional option is patient-controlled epidural anesthesia (PCEA), in which miniboluses of anesthetic can be delivered by a pump.

The most commonly used agent for epidural blockade is bupivacaine (or more recently ropivacaine and lidocaine) in combination with either fentanyl, hydromorphone, or morphine, infused continuously on a pump with adjustments made while monitoring for side effects. Concentrations of drugs used are 10 times less than what would be used intravenously, and thus systemic side effects decrease significantly.

## Table 18-6

### Adjuvant Medications for Neuropathic Pain in Adolescents

| *Medication* | *Dosing* | *Comments* |
|---|---|---|
| **Tricyclic antidepressants** | | |
| Amitriptyline (po elixir, tablet) | Initial: 0.2–0.5 mg/kg (up to 10–25 mg) po qhs or divided into bid doses. Titrate increases by 0.25 mg/kg (up to 10–25 mg) every 5–7 days<br>Maintenance: 0.2–3.0 mg/kg (up to 10–150 mg) | Very sedating, anticholinergic side effects, drug levels available |
| Nortriptyline (po elixir, tablet) | See amitriptyline | Metabolite of amitriptyline with less anticholinergic and sedating effects, drug levels available |
| **Antiepileptics** | | |
| Carbamazepine (po suspension, tablets, chewables) | ≤12 yo: Initial, 10 mg/kg per day divided into bid doses (up to 100 mg/dose bid), increase 10 mg/kg per day, divided into bid doses each week<br>>12 yo: Initial, 200 mg po bid; increase 200 mg/day divided into bid doses each week (up to 2.4 g/day) | Many drug:drug interactions, blood dyscrasias, drug levels available |
| Gabapentin (po capsules only) | Initial: 5 mg/kg or 300 mg po qhs<br>Day 2: Increase to bid; Day 3: Increase to tid; titrate to effect or range of 8–35 mg/kg/day, up to 3600 mg/day | Sedating, no drug levels available |
| **Other medications** | | |
| Mexiletine (po tablets) | Initial: 2–3 mg/kg/day (up to 150–200 mg) po qd-tid; increase to 0.5 mg/kg (up to 25–50 mg) q 2–3 weeks<br>Maintenance: 2–8 mg/kg (150–400 mg) po qd-tid up to 1800 mg/day | Drug levels available, IV lidocaine trial may predict success<br>"Black Box warning" due to cardiac arrhythmias |
| Clonidine (po tablets; transdermal; IV form can be given epidurally or intrathecally) | Oral: 2–4 mcg/kg q 4–6 hours<br>Transdermal: delivers 0.1, 0.2, or 0.3 mg/day; calculate the total daily po dose to determine if the dose can be delivered by patch·<br>Epidural 0.5–2.0 mcg/kg/h | Change transdermal patch q 5–7 days; takes approximately 2 days to achieve therapeutic effect |

bid, twice a day; po, by mouth; qd, once a day; qhs, at bedtime; IV, intravenous; tid, 3 times a day

Modified from Galloway K, Yaster M. Pain and symptom control in terminally ill children. *Pediatr Clin North Am*. 2000;47:711–716, with permission from Elsevier.

Systemic side effects may still occur, however, depending on the amount of epidural medication infused. These effects are usually due to the opioid used and can be avoided by decreasing the opioid dose. Careful monitoring is required for hypotension, pruritus, nausea, and urinary retention (may require catheterization).

***Intrathecal medications*** Small amounts of opioids and/or local anesthetics can be injected directly into the intrathecal (subarachnoid) space through a percutaneous catheter. Opioids are effective for nonneuropathic nociceptive pain and are associated with far fewer side effects via this route. Local anesthetics are better than opioids for neuropathic pain and can be delivered intermittently or on a pump. Because the small unmyelinated pain fibers are more susceptible to block at lower doses of anesthetic than larger fibers that modulate touch and proprioception, and because they are much more susceptible than myelinated motor fibers, sensation and motor function are typically preserved with the intrathecal route of administration. Clonidine may also be given intrathecally and can be effective for neuropathic pain by blocking the release of norepinephrine from sympathetic fibers by stimulation of alpha-2 inhibitory presynaptic receptors.

***Regional Nerve Blocks*** If an adolescent experiences pain in a particular body region, peripheral nerves from these regions can be blocked with local anesthetics such as bupivacaine, lidocaine, ropivacaine, and mepivacaine. Examples of regional nerve blocks include femoral nerve block, brachial plexus block, digital blocks, and dorsal penile block.

## PROCEDURAL SEDATION AND ANALGESIA

### Types of Procedures Requiring Sedation/Analgesia

For some procedures, anxiolysis/sedation/analgesia is necessary based on the procedure itself, such as burn dressing changes. For example, adolescents with high levels of anxiety or with chronic diseases who have had multiple procedures in the past may benefit from sedation/analgesia, even for very brief or apparently "minor" procedures. For example, adolescents anxious prior to IV or urinary catheter placement may benefit from oral midazolam; those adolescents having a voiding cystourethrogram or nasogastric tube placement may benefit from IV propofol; patients who require insertion of a peripherally inserted central catheter may benefit from IV midazolam/fentanyl.

Typical procedures for which procedural sedation/analgesia is used include: lumbar puncture, bone marrow, upper and lower endoscopy, thoracentesis, bronchoscopy, chest tube insertion, central line placement, magnetic resonance imaging (MRI) and computed tomography (CT) scans, fracture reduction, burn dressing change, nerve conduction studies, and surgical wound dressing changes.

### Risk Assessment

The following increase the risk of a complication for procedural sedation:[22] (1) history of sleep apnea/snoring; (2) poor ability to open the mouth; (3) large tonsils/adenoids; (4) small/recessed mandible; (5) gastroesophageal reflux; (6) active pulmonary disease; (7) cardiac arrhythmias; (8) loose teeth; (9) recent intake of fluid/solids; and (10) distended abdomen. Of particular importance is that the adolescent has not eaten or had nonclear liquids (nothing by mouth; NPO) for at least 2 hours, with at least 6 hours NPO for solids and milk products, to minimize aspiration of stomach contents.

### Sedation Procedure Detail

It should be determined whether the patient requires minimal sedation (formerly called anxiolysis), moderate sedation, deep sedation, or anesthesia to accomplish the procedure. Standard definitions of these states are listed in Table 18-7.[23] Although listed as separate states, sedation is a continuum, and an adolescent can easily move from one state to another with a risk of adverse events occurring. If the patient is undersedated, the adverse event can include inability to accomplish the procedure and/or discomfort to the patient; if the patient is oversedated, the risk of respiratory or hemodynamic adverse events will be greater.

Topical anesthetics such as 4% lidocaine (L-MX), 2% lidocaine/2% prilocaine, and LET (lidocaine 4%, epinephrine 0.1%, tetracaine 0.5%) are useful in attenuating or even eliminating an initial needle puncture for giving intradermal/subcutaneous lidocaine before a procedure, such as a lumbar puncture or laceration repair.

Common medications used for procedural sedation either alone or in combination, are listed in Table 18-8. To allow for an objective assessment of the level of sedation, one should use a validated sedation scale such as the Ramsay Scale[24] or the University of Michigan Pediatric Sedation Scale.[25]

### Recovery from Procedural Sedation/Analgesia

Following the procedure, the adolescent should be allowed to return to the usual state of awareness spontaneously; no reversal agents should be given. In general, the aim should be arousability by 10 to 30 minutes after the procedure is over, and 99% to 100% full recovery within an hour. Careful monitoring during recovery is mandatory because adverse events can still occur during the recovery phase, particularly with some medications, such as ketamine or midazolam.

## INTEGRATIVE MEDICINE APPROACH TO PAIN MANAGEMENT IN THE ADOLESCENT

Our understanding that pain is a multidimensional, idiosyncratic, subjective experience mediated by both physiologic and psychologic factors leads naturally to the conclusion that a multimodal approach is critical for effective pain management. In an integrative medicine approach to pain management, the WHO Analgesic Ladder (see Figure 18-3) is expanded to explicitly include nonpharmacologic methodologies. These methodologies can substitute for, or enhance the effectiveness of, pharmacologic agents and can be used as adjunctive therapy on any step of the ladder.

**Table 18-7**

**Levels of Sedation**

| *Level* | *Description* |
|---|---|
| **Minimal sedation/(formerly anxiolysis)** | A drug-induced state during which patients respond normally to verbal commands. Although cognitive function and coordination may be impaired, ventilatory and cardiovascular functions are unaffected. |
| **Moderate sedation** | A drug-induced depression of consciousness during which patients respond purposefully to verbal commands, either alone or accompanied by minimal tactile stimulation. For older patients, this level of sedation implies an interactive state. |
| **Deep sedation/analgesia** | A drug-induced depression of consciousness during which patients cannot be easily aroused but respond purposefully after repeated or painful stimulation. The ability to independently maintain ventilatory function may be impaired. Patients may require assistance in maintaining a patent airway, and spontaneous ventilation may be inadequate. Cardiovascular function is usually maintained. A state of deep sedation may be accompanied by partial or complete loss of protective airway reflexes. |
| **General anesthesia** | A drug-induced loss of consciousness during which patients are not arousable, even by painful stimulation. Ability to independently maintain ventilatory function is often impaired. Patients often require assistance in maintaining a patent airway, and positive pressure ventilation may be required because of depressed spontaneous ventilation or drug-induced depression of neuromuscular function. Cardiovascular function may be impaired. |

From Coté CJ, Wilson S. Guidelines for monitoring and management of pediatric patients during and after sedation for diagnostic and therapeutic procedures: an update. *Pediatrics*. 2006;118:2587–2602.

**Table 18-8**

**Systemic Medications Commonly Used in Procedural Sedation/Analgesia**

| *Drug Class* | *Examples* |
|---|---|
| Benzodiazepines | Midazolam (oral, intranasal, intravenous, rectal) |
| Opioids | Morphine, fentanyl (intravenous) |
| Anesthetics | Ketamine (intramuscular, intravenous, oral, rectal) |
| Barbiturates | Pentobarbital (intravenous, oral, rectal), thiopental (rectal) |
| Hypnotics | Propofol (intravenous) – may result in general anesthesia at higher doses |
| Alpha-2 agonists | Dexmedetomidine (intravenous, buccal) |
| Other | Etomidate (intravenous) |

Purely alternative medicine (treatments used instead of conventional medicine) and purely conventional medicine (treatments used to the exclusion of any nonconventional therapies) can be viewed as polar ends of the spectrum of health care available to adolescents in the United States. Integrative medicine, in contrast, is defined as the proactive use of a mixture of appropriate conventional and nonconventional modalities that act synergistically to address the experience of pain from physical, sensory, emotional, cognitive, social, and spiritual perspectives. At its best, the development of a comprehensive integrative medicine pain management strategy will take into account the potential effects of prior pain experience, cognitive developmental level, cultural background, personal expectations and beliefs, and social context. The overarching principle is facilitation of the body's own innate ability to ameliorate the sensation of pain. To accomplish this, the patient must be an active participant in the pain management plan.

### Types of Complementary Therapies Used in Pain Management

Chapter 17 provides a detailed discussion of complementary and alternative therapies.

***Mind-Body Interventions*** Mind-body interventions such as meditation, hypnosis, prayer, biofeedback, and creative arts therapies, as well as some forms of cognitive behavioral therapy and social support, are used to modify the adolescent's understanding of how and why the pain is occurring. These modalities can also be used to help focus attention away from the pain to control how it is experienced in both intensity and duration.

A main premise of mind-body interventions is that mental activities such as perceptions, memories, expectations, and images can directly (via neurological processes) and indirectly (via behavior) transform pain processing.[26] Neuroimaging and electroencephalographic evidence is accumulating that demonstrates in real time how these mental activities have their effects on pain perception.[27,28]

Mind-body techniques can also address the emotional distress and functional disability associated with pain. In fact, lessening distress and disability is often the main target of such interventions. One way to accomplish this goal is to change the patient's expectation from experiencing "no pain" to reducing pain to the point of being functional despite lingering discomfort. This modified goal acknowledges that complete freedom from discomfort is often an unachievable goal, but managing the pain is a skill that can be learned successfully.

The most commonly used mind-body therapies for pain management are summarized in the following. The choice of modality in this category, as in any treatment design, is based on the adolescent's preference. This preference is typically formed by personal or family/friend experience, information from the media including the Internet, visceral reaction to a description of the therapy, and degree of personal willingness to invest time and energy to master the technique. That is, mind-body interventions require the active participation of the adolescent, and success will depend on his or her motivation to feel better versus the desire to maintain the symptom for secondary gain.

*Hypnosis* (all hypnosis is self-hypnosis) involves actively focusing attention in a way that transforms noxious sensations, apparently by reducing the sympathetic drive that can intensify the pain experience.[29] Although self-hypnosis has been used for some time in the treatment of acute pain, especially that associated with painful procedures, it has also been shown to be effective in chronic conditions such as headache.[30]

*Meditation*, like self-hypnosis and other mind-body techniques, is based on the notion that no individual can be in 2 incompatible states simultaneously (eg, both relaxed and anxious). Thus, mindfulness or transcendental meditation that promotes relaxation would be particularly useful in the management of pain that is exacerbated by stress or anxiety.

*Creative arts* include music, art, dance/movement, writing, and drama. Some of these therapies, such as music, can be used as distraction during an acute episode of pain, as during a painful procedure. They can also be used as a mechanism for self-expression to reduce the emotional elements (anxiety, tension, anger, guilt) of the pain experience that contribute to the development of chronic pain syndromes.

*Biofeedback-enhanced relaxation* training is the use of an external monitor that brings autonomic nervous system functioning (eg, heart rate, blood pressure, muscle tension) into conscious awareness. Deliberately gaining control over these "automatic" responses to stress through conscious awareness helps the adolescent attain a relaxed state. Like cognitive behavioral therapy (see Chapter 191), it is not a coping skill but an approach to learning a variety of behavioral and cognitive strategies to counteract the effects of stress and decrease the perception of pain. It should be noted that whether or not biofeedback, for example, truly enhances the effects of relaxation per se is being debated.[31] However, for today's adolescents who are enamored by electronic gadgets, computer-based biofeedback monitors, in particular, can provide the initial engagement essential to making a commitment to practicing relaxation techniques.

***Biologically Based Interventions*** Biologically based interventions are substances that occur in nature, such as herbs, and include botanicals, animal-derived extracts, vitamins, minerals, fatty acids, amino acids, proteins, enzymes, prebiotics and probiotics, and whole foods. Most biologically based therapies, or "natural remedies," have become part of the healing repertoire of the integrative clinician based on a long history of apparently beneficial effects on populations that have ingested or administered them topically over decades, if not centuries. A mechanism of action is known or has been postulated for many substances. A major concern about the use of biologicals is the variable potency of the preparations depending on the part of the plant used or part of the world from which the preparation was obtained. A second major concern is the potential interaction of a given substance with other biologicals or pharmaceuticals. Unlike pharmaceuticals, which are chemical preparations manufactured under strict conditions regulating purity and potency, most biologicals are considered "foods" and the regulations regarding manufacture/preparation are less regulated. Moreover, the addition of certain substances to the diet may inhibit or potentiate the action of other substances, increasing the possibility of severe harmful side effects. Teens should be counseled that natural does not necessarily mean safe.

The adolescent and the practitioner are advised to seek independent noncommercial information about the biological activity and potential interactions of any substance prior to its use. Resources for accessing this information are provided in Chapter 17.

A few of the more common and better studied biologically based nonpharmaceutical agents are:

*Magnesium*, a calcium channel-blocking agent, is a natural muscle relaxant and relieves pain by reducing nerve transmission and muscle contractibility. It is also an NMDA receptor antagonist and can reduce the neuropathic pain associated with, for example, headache and fibromyalgia.

*Conifer* is a COX and lipoxygenase inhibitor that can relieve inflammation and also reduce nausea and vomiting associated with chemotherapy or motion sickness.

*Omega-3 fatty acids* (DHA and EPA) are long-chained polyunsaturated fatty acids (PUFA) found in fish oil. Their anti-inflammatory effects are the result of competing with arachidonic acid for inclusion in the COX and lipoxygenase pathways. Analgesic effects have been demonstrated in such pain syndromes as dysmenorrhea, migraine, and sickle cell disease.

*Chamomile* has been found effective in the treatment of nausea, gastrointestinal spasms, and insomnia. The active component, apigenin, binds to GABA receptors in the CNS. The effect is much like administration of a benzodiazepine and can result in sedation. Like PUFA, chamomile inhibits the activities of COX and lipoxygenase, thus reducing production of the inflammatory prostaglandins and leukotrienes. Chamomile's antispasmodic effects on smooth muscle appear to be the result of blocking histamine release from mast cells.

***Manipulation Therapy*** Manipulation therapies include chiropractic, osteopathy, massage, exercise, and physical therapy. Exercise, physical therapy, and, increasingly, massage are now commonly used adjunctive therapies to relieve pain within the conventional medicine spectrum. They exert their effect primarily by altering the microenvironment of, for example, the spinal cord, muscles, deep tissues, and joints through increased circulation, direct muscle relaxation, and increased joint range of motion. In osteopathic and chiropractic manipulation, circulation of pain biomarkers (eg, beta endorphin, serotonin) is altered.[32] The stress-relieving effects of massage are believed to be due to activation of the parasympathetic nervous system.[33] Physical therapy and exercise restore function, improve endurance, and elevate mood.

***Alternative Medical Systems*** Alternative medical systems are complete medical systems in that they are self-contained and encompass all the healing elements thought necessary to provide treatment for all ailments. Two major examples are traditional Chinese medicine (TCM) and Ayurveda (Asian Indian medicine). In many instances, specific practices such as the use of particular herbs, certain massage techniques, acupuncture (TCM), or yoga (Ayurveda) have been adopted by people in other parts of the world as stand-alone treatments without necessarily adopting the foundational principles of the medical system as a whole. Both TCM and Ayurveda, like many medical systems, are based on balance. In TCM, it is the balance between yin (dark, slow, soft, cold, wet) and yang (light, fast, hard, warm, dry). In Ayurveda, the balance is among vata (wind/spirit/air), pitta (bile), and kappa (phlegm). In Greek, the sought-after balance is known as homeostasis.

*Homeopathy*, although included in the category of alternative medical systems, is limited to the use of diluted preparations of biologicals. A fundamental healing principle is the "Law of Similars," also known as "like cures like." That is, treatment consists of administering very highly diluted preparations of certain agents (eg, herbs) known to cause certain symptoms. The symptoms that develop (which are similar to those caused by the disease) are thought to neutralize and expel the original disease. The artificial disturbance or array of symptoms induced by administering the homeopathic preparations ends when dosing ends.

*Naturopathy* is also often listed under the heading of alternative medical systems. However, it is actually a philosophy of healing that emphasizes a natural approach and minimal use of surgery and drugs. Rather than being a system itself, naturopathy is an eclectic approach that uses self-healing therapies and modalities that stand alone or are part of another system. Thus, naturopaths, among other skills, can perform acupuncture, are trained herbalists, prescribe hydrotherapy, teach yoga or other movement therapies, and perform various types of massage. Such treatments as "synthetic" drugs, radiation, and major surgery are avoided. Prevention of disease or disability through stress reduction and a healthy diet and lifestyle are emphasized. The 6 ethical guidelines of naturopathy are (1) do no harm, (2) promote the self-healing power of nature, (3) remove the causes of illness rather than suppress symptoms, (4) encourage rational hope and self-responsibility for health, (5) treat each person as an individual, and (6) emphasize health as a means to promote well-being and prevent disease.

*Meditation-exercise* (yoga, QiGong) is used for relaxation and improved physical functioning. They are examples of specific therapeutic modalities that have been borrowed from whole medical systems as stand-alone treatments. Yoga is a traditional physical and mental discipline originating in India and is associated with meditative practices in Hinduism, Buddhism, and Taoism. Outside India, yoga is typically associated with "Hatha Yoga," which is characterized by postures and is used as a form of exercise. QiGong is a Chinese meditative practice that often uses slow graceful movements and controlled breathing to promote the circulation of Qi or "life force" within the body. QiGong, as a stand-alone treatment, is used to gain strength; improve health; balance the mind, body, and spirit; and reverse disease.

*Acupuncture*, or the insertion and manipulation of fine filiform needles at specific body points, can be used to relieve pain. Both the 1997[34] and 2006[35] reports from the National Institutes of Health (NIH) and a 2003 report from the WHO[36] have affirmed the safety and effectiveness of acupuncture in treating a variety of conditions including epigastric pain, lower back pain, and rheumatoid arthritis.

***Energy Therapies*** Energy therapies fall into 2 categories: the bioelectromagnetic-band therapies that involve the unconventional use of electromagnetic fields, and the biofield therapies that involve the energy fields that surround and penetrate the human body.[37]

Among these therapies, the biofield approaches such as *Reiki*, *Therapeutic Touch,* and *Healing Touch* are based on the goal of balancing the vital energy fields in the body, either by the laying on of hands or with non-touch interventions. Balancing these energetic forces is believed to restore health and to heal. The postulated mechanism of action for these modalities is the gate theory or the activation of life energy (Qi) that increases endogenous opioid production. Reiki treatment has been shown to decrease state anxiety and systolic blood pressure in association with an increase in salivary IgA levels.[38]

Table 18-9 lists suggestions for conventional and mind-body therapies that might be useful in managing the acute pain associated with procedures. An important tenant of treatment is that modalities can and should be combined to reach maximal effectiveness with minimal undesirable side effects.

**Table 18-9**

**Integrative Treatments to Manage Procedural Pain**

| *Type of Therapy* | *Example* |
|---|---|
| Mind-body | Hypnosis |
| | Music |
| | Distraction |
| | Guided imagery |
| | Relaxation |
| Biologically based | Aroma therapy (lavender, lemon balm) |
| Manipulation | Massage |
| Alternative medicine | Acupuncture |
| Energy | Reiki |
| | Therapeutic touch |

## SUMMARY

Although pain is a complex entity that even now is only incompletely understood, over the past 20 years pain has been recognized as a symptom that itself has physiologic consequences, and if not treated may cause significant morbidity and likely contributes to mortality. The convergence of new knowledge about pain in conjunction with the rise of health care quality improvement, patient/consumer rights, and the emphasis on quality of life has driven better assessment and management of pain. This chapter informs the reader about the general principles of pain assessment and management so that initial treatment for the adolescent in pain can be provided regardless of the underlying disease process. If there is a suboptimal response to initial treatment, it is essential that further pain management expertise be sought as soon as possible. Given the large arsenal of pain-relieving modalities currently in existence, adolescents and other patients should be provided these options, and adolescent health care providers should be strong advocates to ensure that this happens. An important complementary group of nonpharmacologic treatments from integrative medicine can enhance the effects of analgesic medications and can become the only method needed to manage milder chronic pain.

## REFERENCES

1. Acute Pain Management Guideline Panel. *Acute Pain Management: Operative or Medical Procedures and Trauma. Clinical Practice Guideline.* AHCPR Pub No 92-0032. Rockville, MD: Agency for Health Care Policy and Research, Public Health Service, US Department of Health and Human Services; February 1992

2. Acute Pain Management Guideline Panel. *Acute Pain Management in Infants, Children, and Adolescents: Operative Procedures*. Quick Reference Guide for Clinicians No 1b. AHCPR Pub No 92-0020. Rockville, MD:Agency for Health Care Policy and Research, Public Health Service, US Department of Health and Human Services; February 1993

3. Zeltzer LK, Altman A, Cohen D, LeBaron S, Munuksela EL, Schechter NL. American Academy of Pediatrics Report of the Subcommittee on the Management of Pain Associated with Procedures in Children with Cancer. *Pediatrics.* 1990;86 (5 Pt 2):826–831

4. Berde C, Ablin A, Glazer J, et al. American Academy of Pediatrics Report of the Subcommittee on Disease-Related Pain in Childhood Cancer. *Pediatrics.* 1990;86(5 Pt 2):818–825

5. Wolfe J, Grier HE, Klar N, et al. Symptoms and suffering at the end of life in children with cancer. *N Engl J Med.* 2000;342(5):326–333

6. Desbiens NA, Mueller-Rizner N, Connors AF Jr, Wenger NS, Lynn J. The symptom burden of seriously ill hospitalized patients. SUPPORT Investigators. Study to Understand Prognoses and Preferences for Outcome and Risks of Treatment. *J Pain Symptom Manage.* 1999;17(4):248-255

7. Loeser JD. The decade of pain control and research. *American Pain Society Bulletin.* 2003;13(3). Available at: www.ampainsoc.org/pub/bulletin/may03/article1.htm. Accessed April 13, 2010

8. Merskey H, Bogduk N. Part III: pain terms, a current list with definitions and notes on usage. *Classification of Chronic Pain.* 2nd ed. IASP Task Force on Taxonomy. Seattle, WA: IASP Press; 1994: 209-214. Available at: www.iasp-pain.org/AM/Template.cfm?Section=Pain_Definitions&Template=/CM/HTMLDisplay.cfm&ContentID=1728. Accessed April 13, 2010

9. McCaffery M, Beebe A. *Pain: Clinical Manual for Nursing Practice.* St Louis, MO: CV Mosby;1989

10. Malviya S, Voepel-Lewis T, Burke C, Merkel S, Tait AR. The revised FLACC observational pain tool: improved reliability and validity for pain assessment in children with cognitive impairment. *Paediatr Anaesth.* 2006;16(3):258-265

11. Hicks CL, von Baeyer CL, Spafford PA, et al. The Faces Pain Scale-Revised: toward a common metric in pediatric pain measurement. *Pain.* 2001;93:173-183

12. Tobias JD. Tramadol for postoperative analgesia in adolescents following orthopedic surgery in a third-world country. *Amer J Pain Management.* 1996;6:51-53

13. Nakatsuka N, Minogue SC, Lim J, et al. Intravenous nalbuphine 50 microg x kg(-1) is ineffective for opioid-induced pruritus in pediatrics. *Can Anaesth.* 2006;53(11):1103-1110

14. Yeh Y-C, Lin T-F, Lin F-S, et al. Combination of opioid agonist and agonist-antagonist: patient-controlled analgesia requirement and adverse events among different-ratio morphine and nalbuphine admixtures for postoperative pain. *Br J Anaesth.* 2008;101(4):542-548

15. Gear RW, Gordon NC, Hossaini-Zadeh M, et al. A subanalgesic dose of morphine eliminates nalbuphine anti-analgesia in postoperative pain. *J Pain.* 2008;9(4):337-341

16. Gear RW, Gordon NC, Miaskowski C, Paul SM, Heller PH, Levine JD. Dose ratio is important in maximizing naloxone enhancement of nalbuphine analgesia in humans. *Neurosci Lett.* 2003;351(1):5-8

17. Maxwell LG, Kaufmann SC, Bitzer S, et al. The effects of a small-dose naloxone infusion on opioid-induced side effects and analgesia in children and adolescents treated with intravenous patient-controlled analgesia: a double-blind, prospective, randomized, controlled study. *Anesth Analg.* 2005;100(4):953-958

18. Koch J, Manworren R, Clark L, Quinn CT, Buchanan GR, Rogers ZR. Pilot study of continuous co-infusion of morphine and naloxone in children with sickle cell pain crisis. *Am J Hematol.* 2008;83(9):728-731

19. Czarnecki ML, Ferrise AS, Jastrowski Mano KE, et al. Parent/nurse-controlled analgesia for children with developmental delay. *Clin J Pain.* 2008;24(9):817-824

20. Bainbridge D, Martin JE, Cheng DC, et al. Patient-controlled versus nurse-controlled analgesia after cardiac surgery—a meta-analysis. *Can J Anaesth.* 2006;53(5):492-499

21. Monitto CL, Greenberg RS, Kost-Byerly S, et al. The safety and efficacy of parent-/nurse-controlled analgesia in patients less than six years of age. *Anesth Analg.* 2000;91(3):573-579

22. Hoffman GM, Nowakowski R, Troshynski TJ, Berens RJ, Weisman SJ. Risk reduction in pediatric procedural sedation by application of an American Academy of Pediatrics/American Society of Anesthesiologists process model. *Pediatrics.* 2002;109(2):236-243

23. Coté CJ, Wilson S. Guidelines for monitoring and management of pediatric patients during and after sedation for diagnostic and therapeutic procedures: an update. *Pediatrics.* 2006;118(6):2587-2602

24. Malviya S, Voepel-Lewis T, Tait AR, Merkel S, Tremper K, Naughton N. Depth of sedation in children undergoing computed tomography: validity and reliability of the University of Michigan Sedation Scale (UMSS). *Br J Anaesth.* 2002;88(2):241-245

25. Ramsay MAE, Savege TM, Simpson BRJ, Goodwin R. Controlled sedation with alphaxalone-alphadolone. *Br Med J.* 2002;2:656-659

26. McGrath PJ, McAlpine L. Psychologic perspectives on pediatric pain. *J Pediatr.* 1993;122(5 Pt 2):S2-8

27. Goffaux P, Redmond W, Rainville P, Marchand S. Descending analgesia—when the spine echoes what the brain expects. *Pain.* 2007;130(1):137-143

28. Borsook D, Becerra LR. Breaking down the barriers: fMRI applications in pain, analgesia, and analgesics. *Mol Pain.* 2006;2:30

29. Lee LH, Olness KN. Effects of self-induced mental imagery on autonomic reactivity in children. *J Dev Behav Pediatr.* 1996;17(5):323-327

30. Hammond DC. Review of the efficacy of clinical hypnosis with headaches and migraines. *International J Clin Experimental Hypnosis.* 2007;55(2):207-219

31. NIH Technology Assessment Panel on Integration of Behavioral and Relaxation Approaches into the Treatment of Chronic Pain and Insomnia. *JAMA.* 1996;274(4):313-318

32. Degenhardt BF, Darmani NA, Johnson JC. Role of osteopathic manipulative treatment in altering pain biomarkers: a pilot study. *J Amer Osteopath Assoc.* 2007;107(9):387-400

33. Field T, Hernandez-Reif M, Diego M, Schanberg S, Kuhn C. Cortisol decreases and serotonin and dopamine increase following massage therapy. *Int J Neurosci.* 2005;115(10):1397-1413

34. National Institutes of Health. Acupuncture. *NIH Consensus Statement Online.* 1997;15(5):1-34. Available at: consensus.nih.gov/1997/1997Acupuncture107html.htm. Accessed March 14, 2010

35. National Institutes of Health, National Center for Complementary and Alternative Medicine. Acupuncture for pain. *NCCAM Newsletter.* 2009;May: 1-12.

36. World Health Organization. *Cancer Pain Relief in Palliative Care in Children*. Geneva, Switzerland: WHO Press; 1998. Available at: apps.who.int/bookorders/anglais/detart1.jsp?sesslan=1&codlan=1&codcol=15&codcch=459. Accessed March 14, 2010

37. Tan G, Craine MH, Bair MJ. Efficacy of selected complementary and alternative medicine interventions for chronic pain. *J Rehab Research & Development.* 2007;44(2):195–222

38. Wardell DW, Engebretson J. Biological correlates of Reiki touch(sm) healing. *J Adv Nurs.* 2001;33(4):439–445

# CHAPTER 19

## Palliative Care and Psychological Aspects of Death and Dying in Adolescence

OLLE JANE Z. SAHLER, MD • DAVID N. KORONES, MD • MARCIA LEVETOWN, MD • SARAH FRIEBERT, MD

## INTRODUCTION

This chapter focuses on the principles of pediatric palliative care (PPC) as a philosophy and system of care that extends throughout the course of an adolescent's life-limiting/life-threatening condition. This serves as a backdrop to how adolescents understand illness in general and their own terminal illness and death in particular. Especially important in this context is the role of the health care provider as the facilitator of a "good" death.

## ADOLESCENT PALLIATIVE CARE

Approximately 50,000 children and adolescents die in the United States each year. Of these, about 10,000 die after 1 year of age.

### EPIDEMIOLOGY OF DEATH IN ADOLESCENCE

Adolescents account for 25% of the annual deaths during childhood.[1] Most of these deaths are related to trauma, including motor vehicle crashes, drowning, suicide, and murder. Adolescent palliative care (APC) for these patients consists of addressing the often-overlooked bereavement needs of the surviving family and community. Unaddressed, the bereavement outcomes for families include high proportions of disability due to depression and anxiety and a poor rate of return to work.[2] Simple, time-limited interventions can be effective in preventing this outcome.[3]

### LIVING WITH A LIFE-THREATENING CONDITION

Adolescents living with chronic, life-threatening conditions frequently suffer for many years before their death related to cancer, congenital heart disease, cystic fibrosis, muscular dystrophy, AIDS, and an array of rare disorders. Most conditions are associated with social isolation, existential doubt, and family distress as well as significant pain, dyspnea, and asthenia, particularly in the later stages of illness. Patients and their families suffer when these issues are not addressed until the end of the child's life.[4–6]

### DEFINITION AND SCOPE OF PALLIATIVE CARE

Most adolescents with chronic conditions are cared for by hospital-based pediatric subspecialty groups as well as their primary care physician. Many require the involvement of multiple disciplines and agencies, many times resulting in fragmented and inconsistent care.

Palliative care (from the Latin, to *reduce or moderate*—in this case, the intensity with which a disease is experienced) is a philosophy and a system of care. It is designed to prevent and relieve suffering. Palliative care is often confused with "end-of-life" care. In keeping with the World Health Organization's construct of PPC, the American Academy of Pediatrics (AAP) recognizes that palliative care is care focusing on maintaining the best quality of life (QOL) possible for a child living with a chronic, complex, and/or life-threatening condition and his or her family. Palliative care, using this definition, seeks to minimize the physical, psychosocial, emotional, and spiritual suffering of those affected by life-threatening conditions and bereavement. Because no single health discipline is effective in addressing the spectrum of needs in its entirety, palliative care is best delivered by an interdisciplinary team including a trained physician, nurse, and chaplain and an expert in pediatric grief and communication such as a social worker, psychologist, or child life specialist. Together with involved primary care and subspecialty providers, team members collaborate in care, communicating their observations and therapeutic strategies as a cohesive whole.

Currently, palliative care is most often delivered at the end of life, in the pediatric specialty hospital. However, because QOL is the objective, palliative care should begin at the time of diagnosis, concurrently with disease-directed interventions. Regardless of prognosis or outcome, palliative care is most effective when introduced early to help the child and family cope with the loss of good health; fear of the future; questions of meaning; social isolation; and pain and other symptoms associated with the illness, treatments, and procedures. Palliative care is best delivered where the patient is most comfortable and should be available in the community as well as in institutions. In Figure 19-1, Feudtner and colleagues[7] illustrate how, when palliative care is seen as a complementary, concurrent component of care throughout the course of the illness, supportive care begins at presentation and evolves to bereavement care as the anticipated loss becomes a reality. Bereavement care continues until the loss is resolved, which may take months or years.

Efforts to bring APC into the mainstream of health care lag behind similar efforts for adults, even though the concept is hardly new. For example, the first pediatric hospice was created in England more than 100 years ago.[8] But it was not until the 1970s and 1980s that the effect of terminal illness on children and adolescents began to be explored.[9,10] A number of papers appeared in the 1980s about home care for children and adolescents with terminal illnesses, and the effect of a child's or adolescent's death on siblings and parents.[11,12]

Despite the fact that APC has been successfully developed in other countries[13] and that there is growing recognition of its importance in the United States, significant obstacles to widespread availability of APC remain. Many physicians and other health care providers are not taught the precepts of palliative care,[14] do not understand its appropriate role, and introduce it, if at all, late in the course of an adolescent's illness.[4,15,16]

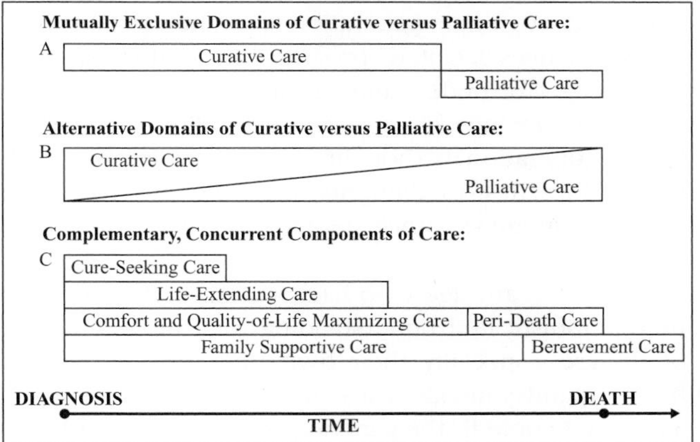


**FIGURE 19-1** Models of palliative care. (A) Abrupt transition to palliative care (all-or-nothing model). (B) Progressive transition to palliative care. (C) Enhanced model of family-focused palliative care extending into bereavement. (From Feudtner C, DiGiuseppe DL, Neff JM. Hospital care for children and young adults in the last year of life: a population-based study. *BMC Med.* 2003;1:3. ©2003 Feudtner et al; licensee BioMed Central Ltd. Available at: www.biomedcentral.com/1741-7015/1/3/abstract)

Even families present obstacles, as they, too, understand "palliative care" to be "care of last resort"[8] rather than care directed toward QOL.

Wolfe and colleagues[4] first demonstrated how poorly pain is managed in a study of symptoms of 103 children and adolescents who had died of cancer. Sixty percent of parents who were interviewed reported that their child/adolescent suffered from pain, and in only 20% of the cases did the parents feel that the pain was adequately treated. Parents reported similarly low success rates in treating nausea, vomiting, diarrhea, and fatigue. In another study, Contro and colleagues[5] surveyed attending physicians, residents, and nurses about their experience treating pain and other symptoms in dying children and adolescents. Approximately half of the physicians and a third of the nurses felt inexperienced treating symptoms in terminal conditions.

Although symptom treatment is only part of the palliative care mission, it is frequently the entry point for the team's involvement with the patient and family. The 2 overarching principles for physical symptom treatment should be discussed early in patient management because they provide reassurance that a primary goal of care will be patient comfort. The principles are: (1) symptoms will be addressed when they appear, not only when the final etiology of the symptom is known; and (2) symptom distress will be treated until it is resolved or is tolerable, according to the patient. It is important for families to know that nonpharmacologic mechanisms can be used with good effect for mild to moderate symptoms or as adjunctive therapy when symptoms are severe. It is also important for families to know that effective control of severe symptoms should be achieved using pharmacologic agents, beginning with low doses of medication, then titrating to comfort based on the medication chosen, the route of administration, and the speed with which its maximum effect is expected. Patients and families should be reassured that the dose can be escalated until the maximum dose is achieved or comfort occurs. If the maximum dose of a given medication is not beneficial at all, or if side effects are intolerable, then that medication will be discontinued and a new drug with a different mechanism of action will be substituted. However, if some, but not complete, symptom control is achieved at maximum doses without undue side effects, a compatible drug will be added to the regimen. Side effects will be anticipated and addressed, and medication regimens revisited regularly—especially as conditions and symptoms change—to avoid unnecessary or harmful polypharmacy. Patients and families often fear "addiction" so it is essential that they understand that physiologic tolerance or habituation is not addiction and that every step will be taken to avoid dependence. However, patient comfort is the foremost goal, and reliable reporting of symptom severity is critical to developing an effective management plan.

Discussion of end-of-life (EOL) issues is also a critical part of palliative care. In the study by Contro and colleagues,[17] 40% to 70% of hospital staff felt inexperienced talking to dying pediatric and adolescent patients and their families about forgoing disease-directed treatment or other limitations of medical intervention. Many families reported being given information by providers that seemed contradictory, and two-thirds recalled a provider making a careless or insensitive remark. In another study by Contro's group, 68 family members of 44 deceased children were interviewed and asked what were the most important aspects of their children's treatment and EOL care.[5] Recurrent themes included: (1) the importance of clinicians who were experienced, honest, and compassionate; (2) the importance of involving families in decision making; (3) the pain of insensitive remarks from health care providers; (4) the importance of how bad news is delivered; (5) the importance of including/involving siblings; (6) the importance of cultural sensitivity; (7) good pain control; and (8) the importance of bereavement follow-up.

Universal principles for APC have been established to emphasize that continuity of coordinated care is an essential component. These principles include: (1) palliative care programs should be available to all adolescents with life-threatening conditions, not just those for whom death is imminent; (2) care should be available to adolescents whether they are at home, in the hospital, or admitted to hospice; (3) disease-directed treatment and palliative care are not mutually exclusive and should be offered concomitantly; (4) the unit of care is the adolescent and his or her family; and (5) bereavement care should be offered.[18] Various organizations in the United States have helped translate these principles into functioning efforts, including the Children's International Project on Palliative/Hospice Services,[19] an initiative devoted to enhancing "the science and practice of pediatric hospice and palliative care, and to increase the availability of state of the art services to families" (www.nhpco.org/i4a/pages/index.cfm?pageid=3409&openpage=3409), and the Initiative for Pediatric Palliative Care,[20] a consortium that educates pediatric care providers about how to bring child and APC to their institutions (www.ippcweb.org/). In addition, the AAP[21] has called for the creation of child and APC services, education of trainees in palliative care, and research to improve understanding of the role of palliative care in the management of life-threatening diseases in children and adolescents. Many resources are becoming available to help practitioners address these issues (see Internet and Print Resources).

## ADOLESCENTS AND TERMINAL ILLNESS

Palliative care of adolescents requires an understanding of how adolescents typically develop their concepts of and communicate about health and illness, such as what it means to "be sick," the cause(s) of illness, and what to tell their friends. Health education can play a role in addressing each of these issues, especially for adolescents with terminal illness as it influences their understanding of death generally and with respect to their own death. Each of these issues will be addressed in the following sections.

### HOW ADOLESCENTS DEVELOP AN UNDERSTANDING OF HEALTH AND ILLNESS

In 1986, the First International Conference on Health Promotion defined child health as "the extent to which individual children or groups of children are able or enabled to (a) develop and realize their potential, (b) satisfy their needs, and (c) develop the capacities that allow them to interact successfully with their biological, physical, and social environments."[22]

What is the adolescent's conceptualization of health and illness? Studies of children and adolescents with a variety of illnesses and in a variety of cultures[23,24] have consistently found that the individual's understanding of illness develops in a step-wise process that evolves systematically and predictably. A useful framework for understanding this evolution is Piaget's theory of cognitive development.[25,26] Under this paradigm, both biologic and cognitive maturation and the accumulation of experiences facilitate progression to more sophisticated stages of understanding. Salient characteristics of each stage include the progressive ability to engage in logical (operational) thought, to separate internal realities (wishes, desires, thoughts) from the external world, and to distinguish other people's point of view from one's own.

People of any age who have a chronic illness have a more sophisticated understanding than healthy people of disease, especially their own, and their knowledge base expands quickly with increasing experience.[27,28] Similarly, people in the general population have a better understanding of "everyday" type illnesses—which they or a family member or friend have experienced—than they do of less common or esoteric illnesses.[29] However, even younger elementary school-aged children can benefit from appropriate, developmentally based instruction about relatively complicated conditions (eg, AIDS) without fearing that they will acquire or be harmed by the illness.[30-32] Thus, knowledge acquired from education plays a role in adolescents' understanding of illness. This augments knowledge gains that arise simply as a result of growing up or experience.

Adolescence is marked by the transition to formal operational thinking, which is the ability to clearly differentiate self from other, to have logical thought, and to be free of the need to respond to or be limited by immediate stimuli or real (concrete) objects (ie, to be able to hypothesize). Adolescents are also able to fill gaps in knowledge by reasoning from generalizations gleaned from their understanding of the concrete world. The most important feature of adolescence is the ability to understand that the source of an illness may be located within the body (host response), even though an external agent interacting with the body may be the ultimate cause of the illness. Thus, adolescents can understand the general principles of infection, health maintenance, and treatment. Adolescents also can define illness as an internal feeling of not being well even in the absence of external signs or symptoms.

## A SICK ADOLESCENT'S UNDERSTANDING OF ILLNESS

Adolescents process information about their own illnesses according to a predictable sequence of cognitive maturation[27] that is similar to their understanding of illness in general. Human causation (especially doing something "wrong") is followed by the germ theory, the differentiation of causes depending on the type of condition, and finally an interactional model in which physical or psychological susceptibility and external factors act together to cause illness. Although this sequence is no different from that of healthy individuals, having an illness can influence the rapidity with which adolescents pass through the various stages of understanding.

Crisp and colleagues[28] found that experience with a chronic illness (present for 3 or more months, involving repeated hospitalizations, or interfering with normal activity) increases understanding at a rapid rate. Interestingly, however, this greater sophistication does not necessarily generalize beyond the adolescent's specific condition. For example, patients with cancer do not necessarily know more than their healthy peers about the common cold.[28] A study by Krishnan and colleagues[33] raised the question of whether children with a chronic disease are resistant to learning about new medical information that has no bearing on their own illness.

## WHAT IS BEING "SICK"?

Typically a patient who has a congenital condition or one that arose early in life incorporates that illness into his/her identity. For example, a patient who had an amputation before the age of 18 months will likely draw a picture of him/herself as someone with 2 legs, 1 of which is the prosthesis. A patient who has the same amputation at a later age will draw a picture of him/herself with one whole leg and one leg that ends at the amputation site. The prosthesis may or may not appear in the picture; if it does, it is separate.

Also for example, the patient's perception of being "not sick" while having a chronic disorder like cystic fibrosis protects the patient from feeling different or having to continuously play the sick role. In fact, "forgetting" that he or she has a chronic disease and incorporating the condition into his/her self-perception serves as a useful adaptive mechanism rather than "denial" as a psychological defense mechanism. Being sick then becomes a state of having another, different condition (a "cold") that acutely changes activity for a defined period of time. Maladaptation arises when the patient denies an underlying condition that requires special treatments (eg, enzyme therapy, prophylactic antibiotic therapy), even when he or she is feeling "well." This is especially true when a teen must alter typical, everyday behaviors (eg, being with friends) to receive treatment (chest physiotherapy) in order to avoid some potential negative outcome (inspissated mucus plugging) in the (seemingly distant) future.

## DID I CAUSE MY ILLNESS?

Despite an advanced understanding of their own disease, adolescents may nevertheless continue to experience egocentric or magical thinking, especially about causation. In fact, even adults may experience such egocentrism ("I know that my child's cancer is caused by abnormal white blood cells, but I wonder if I did something to cause it"). Brewster[27] found that such magical thinking was especially likely to occur at times of great stress, when temporary regression to earlier developmental stages is common. This regression results in a state of "cognitive dissonance." For example, teens (and adults) may feel guilty for causing the malady despite "knowing better" and understanding logical explanations for illness causation.

In the mid-20th century, Gardner[34] hypothesized that guilt (feelings of having done something "bad") served to protect parents of children with severe physical illnesses against the feelings of overwhelming helplessness that would potentially result were they to believe that their child's condition was the result of mere chance. In this context, Gardner urged health providers to be wary of assuaging patient or parent guilt feelings too quickly, if such feelings serve a useful purpose in the search for meaning. Eliminating a defense is hazardous without a reasonable expectation that a more constructive concept will take its place. In the final analysis, the clinician hearing and understanding what the patient/parent is saying and why is more important than the patient/parent hearing and understanding what the clinician is saying.

## DISCLOSURE TO FRIENDS

The desire to not tell friends about a health condition is common, especially among preteens and early adolescents who worry about social acceptance. Teens who experience the acute onset of disease, such as the diagnosis of cancer, typically have little choice about disclosure because disfigurement (eg, alopecia, loss of a limb) is obvious and can lead to merciless taunting if no explanation is offered. In addition, news of a diagnosis of cancer spreads quickly. Although the community often reacts with compassion, its concern is tempered by misperceptions of what causes cancer and irrational fears about transmissibility. Positive social reintegration after hospitalization can be promoted through meetings with school personnel and classmates to explain the disease, the side effects of medication, the potential need for frequent hospitalizations, and the fact that cancer is not contagious. Under the best of circumstances, an entire homeroom will decide to have a head shaving party as a show of solidarity. Unfortunately, sometimes wigs or caps get pulled off and tossed around while other students cheer and jeer.

For the teenager with a chronic condition such as sickle cell anemia, social reintegration after hospitalization for a pain crisis is typically less formal. Frequently, because the teen insists on keeping the condition secret, there is no school management plan at all. Interestingly, the rise of HIV/AIDS has had a beneficial effect on disclosure of sickle cell disease. Because both are blood diseases, children with sickle cell disease, once reluctant, now prefer to disclose so that classmates will not assume that they have HIV/AIDS. In effect, they make their decision based on what they perceive as the "lesser of 2 evils."

For some teens, disclosure of their illness can become inescapable when they participate in sleepovers and class trips. Appliances such as colostomy bags become impossible to hide. Most teens are surprised when friends are curious, but also supportive.

## THE ROLE OF HEALTH EDUCATION

Health care personnel often assume that providing information will lead to greater understanding that then results in better adherence. This outcome is unusual, however, for several reasons: (1) adolescents have their own conceptualization of what is happening to them; (2) their ability to assimilate information may be limited by their general level of cognitive functioning; and (3) other factors, particularly emotional factors, may impede understanding.[27]

Although many different educational interventions have been tried to increase adherence, only modest improvements have been found and only in certain clinical outcomes. A recent meta-analysis of educational programs for children and adolescents with asthma found small to moderate gains in lung function, activity level, school attendance, and self-efficacy, and decreases in emergency department visits.[35] Such modest findings are fairly typical for educational interventions, especially among patients with chronic but nondisabling conditions. Clearly, new approaches are needed.

In contrast, children and adolescents diagnosed with potentially life-threatening illnesses such as cancer are interested in knowing about their disease and treatment.[22] Knowledge seems to reduce anxiety and depression and to increase self-esteem. For teenagers, increased knowledge leads to more trusting relationships with staff and enhanced coping with painful procedures. The process of information-sharing is not a one-time event; it extends over a series of sessions that address health status and any anticipated changes in treatment.

Differences between patients' views of cancer and asthma likely reflect the acuity, novelty, and perceived seriousness of the cancer diagnosis, as compared to the low-level chronicity and the perception that asthma is not a life-threatening condition. Motivation is a key element in learning. Helping patients understand the long-term seriousness of a particular condition is hampered by their limited ability to understand consequences that are not immediately observable. Concrete information (eg, viewing x-rays) and repeated experience may be helpful in hastening the process of understanding regardless of patient age.

## TEENS' UNDERSTANDING OF DEATH

Until the mid-1970s, it was unusual for pediatric patients to be given information about their illness. In particular, little was said about potentially fatal illnesses. Pioneering work by Spinetta and Bluebond-Langner,[9,36] among others, led to the discovery that pediatric patients who were uninformed about their illness, its treatment, and the prognosis felt lonely and isolated and had frightening fantasies about their condition. These findings have led to greater openness and more developmentally appropriate explanations about illness and about potential death to adolescents.

## DEVELOPMENT OF THE CONCEPT OF DEATH FROM CHILDHOOD THROUGH ADOLESCENCE

The acquisition of 4 basic cognitive concepts frames the stages of understanding death: irreversibility (death is permanent), inevitability or universality (all living things eventually must die), finality or nonfunctionality (dead people no longer have experiences or feelings), and causality (why a death occurs).[37]

Understanding the framework on which the adolescent's understanding of death is based helps explain why certain responses and ideations emerge under certain circumstances. For example, the child of age 4 watching other people cry at funerals begins to understand that death is a sad thing, but he/she is not sad in the absence of an understanding that death is irreversible. The child of age 5 or 6 will imagine death to be a ghost or scary creature that comes in the night to take you away when you die, making "going to sleep" or "on a trip" euphemisms something to be avoided at all costs. The child of age 7 or 8 may dig up the dead bird buried with great ceremony in the back yard in search of what "decomposition" means.

Preschool children are magical thinkers and may believe that their wishes make things happen, that they are the center of the universe, and that things that happen at the same time are connected as cause and effect. Children who are in elementary school have to see to believe, and it is not until early to mid-adolescence that youth begin to understand "what if."

Thus, adolescents entering the stage of formal operations can conceptualize the finality and inevitability of death. However, they also have a sense of personal invulnerability that makes it difficult for them to conceive of their own personal death (the "personal fable"). Their view of themselves as an integral part of a world adds further to their sense of invincibility: "If I'm this important, certainly I can't die." This type of thinking may account for risk-taking behaviors such as drinking and driving, 1 of the most common causes of death among 15- to 24-year-olds.

## PERSONAL DEATH

Like adults, adolescents with a chronic life-threatening illness vary in their readiness to talk about the end of their lives. Regardless of age, patients are likely to ask questions using language and imagery that reflects their understanding of death and any potential afterlife. Some wonder about impending death ("How will I feel when I die?"). Many wish to stop searching for a cure ("I'm so tired of being sick, but my mom doesn't want me to stop treatment"). Virtually all adolescents desire an open, honest discussion ("I'm not getting better, am I?"). Answering such questions is emotionally challenging for parents and health care providers. The involved adults may also incorrectly believe that discussion will provoke, rather than allay, fear and anxiety. Yet, speaking directly is the most effective way to explore the range of issues that preoccupy these needy children. Clarity about what question is being asked leads to the kind of reassurance we erroneously think we cannot give.

Question: "Doc, am I going to die?"

Answer: "You've been thinking about that. Tell me what you've been thinking."

Some patients fear pain ("Am I going to hurt?"). To which the provider can respond with: "We're here to give you whatever you need to be comfortable. You tell us if you want more medicine, a hug, or a visit from that puppy of yours. We don't want you to hurt at all."

Some patients are concerned with ritual. Questions like, "Will Dr. X and my nurses come to the funeral?" or "What will Heaven be like?" are seeking reassurance about the continuation of what is familiar and comforting. Comments like, "Promise me you won't cry a lot, Mom," reflect concern for others. Questions like, "Will you keep my pictures in the album?" are efforts to gain assurance that their life has been meaningful and that they will be remembered. Once you understand the question, it becomes easy to give true and heartfelt reassurance.

## END-OF-LIFE CARE

Many patients have difficulty expressing their preference for forgoing further disease-directed interventions. They are particularly concerned about disappointing their parents by not continuing to "fight." Interestingly, parents will often admit their own and their child's exhaustion. Helping parents express to the adolescent that he or she has endured a long and hard battle and is understandably physically and emotionally exhausted can be a turning point in setting appropriate goals for EOL care. Without permission to achieve personal goals rather than cure, patients will put themselves and their interests second, continuing to accept disease-directed interventions if they perceive that this is their parents' wish. The acceptance that accompanies mutual agreement about the next steps to be taken makes the dying process more peaceful and less terrifying for the entire family. Bereavement is enhanced in these cases.

Some adolescents are most concerned about the effect of their death on others. In particular, they worry about their parents and how they will deal with the loss. When asked, most patients, will state a preference to die at home, surrounded by friends and family, rather than in the hospital.[38] Most families try to accommodate their child's wish. However, clinicians should maintain the option of hospitalization if dying at home will be too physically and emotionally burdensome. A few teens will state a preference to die in the hospital. Typically, they worry that going home will be too difficult for their parents, especially their mother, and want to ensure that their family will get the support they need from hospital personnel.

Although there has been a major thrust over the past decade to proactively transition young adults with chronic illness to adult providers, young adults with chronic illness nearing the EOL represent a special population likely to benefit from continued pediatric care. Many may desire to be hospitalized on the pediatric service. If feasible, such accommodation is usually desirable and should be supported, rather than follow rigid age restrictions. The pediatric providers, who know the patient and family well, may be able to provide a higher degree of supportive care than is possible in a new environment.

## THE COMPETENCY OF MINORS TO MAKE MEDICAL DECISIONS

Most pediatric providers would agree that a 4-year-old with acute leukemia can decide which arm to use for intravenous (IV) insertion, but not whether an IV is needed. Most providers would also allow a 10-year-old the same option. What about the 14-year-old? Or the 17-year-old? Does it make any difference if this is a new diagnosis of cancer or the second relapse? Or the second relapse after stem cell transplantation? Does it make any difference if the patient and family agree or disagree? Or the physician agrees or disagrees?

Being considered to have the capacity to make a decision about treatment implies being able to understand the risks, benefits, and alternatives when choices are available and to express a choice between the alternatives; to demonstrate logical and rational reasoning; to make a "reasonable" choice; and to make a choice without coercion. Children in Piaget's preoperational stage are unable to reason beyond their own personal experience and are limited in their understanding of cause-and-effect relationships. During the concrete operational stage, children begin to think logically, but only about things that are physically present or that they have experienced. However, in the formal operational stage, adolescents show an intellectual capacity to reason, generalize beyond personal experience, deal with abstract ideas, and hypothesize or predict potential consequences of actions. Apart from inexperience, most individuals 14 years of age and older have the same capacities to process information as adults.[39] Bibace and Walsh[26] found that more than 40% of 11-year-old children understood that disease has a physiological basis. Thus, children begin to understand disease processes around the age of 11 and demonstrate the competence to make treatment decisions by the age of 14.

Virtually all states recognize the concept of the "emancipated minor" (eg, married, having served in the military, or living independently without parental financial support) as a person who is able to make his or her own health care decisions. The concept of the "mature minor" (an individual who is capable of fully appreciating the nature and consequences of a particular treatment) is, however, not recognized in all states, although it is part of Canadian law.[40] The concept of the mature minor is a higher standard than that of the emancipated minor because it demands specific knowledge and understanding, rather than mere circumstances, to grant decision-making rights. But what level of decision making is right for the teen who is not fully capable of complete understanding?

In adolescent decision making, with respect to EOL issues, the "proportionality" of a decision, for example, the withdrawing of medical interventions that are unduly burdensome, may be considered.[41] Proportionality refers to a "sliding scale" of competency: that is, the more important or serious the outcome, the higher the level of competency that should be required to make that decision. According to the AAP, "physicians and parents should give great weight to clearly expressed views of child patients regarding life-sustaining medical treatment, regardless of the legal particulars."[42] Similarly, the Society for Adolescent Health Medicine (SAHM)[43] has stated the general principle that an adolescent should have a major decision-making role in agreeing to participate in the research process. Although neither the AAP nor SAHM endorses sole decision making by the pediatric patient, the shift from "great weight" given to children's opinions to "major" decision making by adolescents reflects the growing influence of the child's wishes as he/she matures. Although most formal discussion of the capacity of pediatric patients to make informed decisions has centered on life-sustaining treatments and research participation, proponents of greater patient participation in decision making by younger patients have suggested that all clinical situations be opened for discussion at the policy-making level.[39]

Optimally, the adolescent participates with family and providers in all health care decisions, particularly those concerning life-sustaining medical treatment. Occasionally, the adolescent will disagree with his or her parents, physicians, or both. Under this circumstance, all parties should receive accurate information on prognosis, treatment options, and the clinical course with and without treatment. This is a situation in which a consultation by a hospital-based clinical ethics team can be invaluable. The physician should assess the adolescent's ability to comprehend and reflect on the choices available, to balance risks and benefits, and to understand the implications of his/her decisions. When an adolescent has the capacity to make competent health care decisions, the ethical physician should allow the adolescent the right to exercise autonomy.[39]

## SUMMARY

Although death and dying has always been a reality for some adolescents, palliative care for adolescents is a relatively new concept in US health care. Rather than referring to hospice-level services for which it is often mistaken, palliative care is about reducing symptoms and enhancing the QOL throughout the course of the illness, however long that might be. Palliative care programs consist of an interdisciplinary team of individuals focused on addressing specific issues as they arise, but also preventing symptoms through anticipatory work. For example, pain control is 1 of the most important aspects of palliative care, early in the course of the illness and at the EOL. However, patients, their parents, and loved ones often suffer because of pain that is not adequately treated. Learning nonpharmacologic skills and techniques to avert pain from intensifying, combined with the optimal use of analgesics administered early and in adequate doses, can improve the QOL not only for the adolescent, but also for those who are close to him or her. Knowing how teenagers understand illness and death, not only in the abstract but also as they apply to themselves as individuals, as well as their level of competence to make health care and EOL decisions, facilitates excellent palliative care to adolescents in a variety of health care settings.

Adolescents who are chronically or terminally ill often have important existential concerns and may delve deeply into religious or philosophical discussions. They may engage in harmful behaviors to express anger or retaliate at the unfairness of their fate, and often fear being forgotten. Skilled palliative care professionals can assist adolescents and families with the wide range of psychosocial, emotional, and existential suffering inherent in coping with a life-threatening illness. Teens who are devastatingly ill but who will recover need skills to integrate the experience into their self-concept. For chronically ill teens, support must adjust to their fluctuating understanding and processing of their situation with the goal of improving their self-efficacy and mastery. For teens who are dying, reassurances of how they will be remembered and celebrated and how they have left their mark on friends, family, and community may bring the ease and comfort that has been denied them during life.

## INTERNET AND PRINT RESOURCES

- ACT for Children: www.act.org.uk/; Symptom Control Manual available at: www.act.org.uk/page.asp?section=167&search=symptom+control+manual
- American Academy of Hospice and Palliative Medicine: www.aahpm.org
- Carter BS, Levetown M. *Palliative Care for Infants, Children, and Adolescents: A Practical Handbook.* Baltimore, MD: Johns Hopkins University Press; 2004
- Center to Advance Palliative Care: www.capc.org
- Children's Hospice and Palliative Care Coalition: www.childrenshospice.org/
- Glazer JP, Hilden JM, Yaldoo DT, eds. *Pediatric Palliative Care, an Issue of Child and Adolescent Psychiatry Clinics (The Clinics: Internal Medicine).* St. Louis, MO: Elsevier; 2006
- Goldman A, Hain R, Liben S, eds. *Oxford Textbook of Palliative Care for Children.* Oxford, England: Oxford University Press; 2006
- Initiative for Pediatric Palliative Care: www.ippcweb.org
- Kang T, Klick JC, Munson D, eds. *Pediatric Palliative Care, an Issue of Pediatric Clinics (The Clinics: Internal Medicine).* St. Louis, MO: Elsevier; 2007
- National Hospice and Palliative Care Organization (pediatric section of the Web site): www.nhpco.org/i4a/pages/index.cfm?pageid=3409

## REFERENCES

1. Martin JA, Kung HC, Mathews TJ, et al. Annual summary of vital statistics: 2006. *Pediatrics.* 2008;121(4):788–801

2. Oliver RC, Fallat ME. Traumatic childhood death: how well do parents cope? *J Trauma-Inj Infect Crit Care.* 1995;39(2):303–307

3. Oliver RC, Sturtevant JP, Scheetz JP, Fallat ME. Beneficial effects of a hospital bereavement intervention program after traumatic childhood death. *J Trauma-Inj Infect Crit Care.* 2001;50(3):447–448

4. Wolfe J, Grier HE, Klar N, et al. Symptoms and suffering at the end of life in children with cancer. *N Engl J Med.* 2000;342(5):326–333

5. Contro N, Larson J, Scofield S, Sourkes B, Cohen H. Family perspectives on the quality of pediatric palliative care. *Arch Pediatr Adolesc Med.* 2002;156(1):14–19

6. Hinds PS, Schum L, Baker JN, Wolfe J. Key factors affecting dying children and their families. *J Palliat Med.* 2005;8(suppl 1):S70–S78

7. Feudtner C, DiGiuseppe DL, Neff JM. Hospital care for children and young adults in the last year of life: a population-based study. *BMC Med.* 2003;1:3

8. Frader J, Morgan E, Levinson T, Morrow JSJM, Gilmer MJ, Carter BS. Barriers, education, and advocacy in palliative care.

In: Carter BS, Levetown M, eds. *Palliative Care for Infants, Children, and Adolescents*. Baltimore and London: The Johns Hopkins University Press; 2004:44–66

9. Bluebond-Langner M. *The Private Worlds of Dying Children*. Princeton, NJ: Princeton University Press; 1978

10. Nitschke R, Humphrey GB, Sexauer CL, Catron B, Wunder S, Jay S. Therapeutic choices made by patients with end-stage cancer. *J Pediatr.* 1982;101(3):471–476

11. Lauer ME, Camitta BM. Home care for dying children. A nursing model. *J Pediatr.* 1980;97(6):1032–1035

12. Lauer ME, Mulhern RK, Bohne JB, Camitta BM. Children's perceptions of their sibling's death at home or hospital: the precursors of differential adjustment. *Cancer Nurs.* 1985;21–27

13. Goldman A, Heller KS. Integrating palliative and curative approaches in the care of children with life-threatening illnesses. *J Palliat Care.* 2000;3(3):353–359

14. Hilden JM, Emanuel EJ, Fairclough DL, et al. Attitudes and practices among pediatric oncologists regarding end-of-life care: results of the 1998 American Society of Clinical Oncology Survey. *J Clin Oncol.* 2001;19(1):205–212

15. Sahler OJ, Frager G, Levetown M, Cohn FG, Lipson MA. Medical education: about end-of-life care in the pediatric setting: principles, challenges, and opportunities. *Pediatrics.* 2000;105(3):575–584

16. MacDonald N. Palliative care education: a global imperative. *Cancer Treat Res.* 1999;100:185–201

17. Contro NA, Larson J, Scofield S, Sourkes B, Cohen HJ. Hospital staff and family perspectives regarding quality of pediatric palliative care. *Pediatrics.* 2004;114(5):1248–1252

18. National Hospice and Palliative Care Organization. International project on palliative/hospice services (ChIPPS). Compendium of pediatric palliative care. 2000. Alexandria, VA: National Hospice and Palliative Care Organization. Ref Type: Pamphlet

19. Davies B, Lewandowski J, Levetown M, et al. ChIPPS Strategic Planning Summary; 2002

20. Center for Applied Ethics. The Initiative for Pediatric Palliative Care. 2003. Available at: www.ippcweb.org/ Accessed June 30, 2010

21. American Academy of Pediatrics Committee on Bioethics and Committee on Hospital Care. Palliative care for children. *Pediatrics.* 2000;106(2):351–357

22. Ottawa Charter for Health Promotion. Ottawa Charter for Health Promotion—First International Conference on Health Promotion; Nov 21, 1986

23. Perrin EC, Gerrity PS. There's a demon in your belly: children's understanding of illness. *Pediatrics.* 1981;67(6):841–849

24. Peltzer K, Promtussananon S. Black South African children's causal theories of their seizure disorders. *Child Care Health Dev.* 2003;29:385–393

25. Burbach DJ, Peterson L. Children's concepts of physical illness: a review and critique of the cognitive-developmental literature. *Health Psychol.* 1986;5:307–325

26. Bibace R, Walsh ME. Development of children's concepts of illness. *Pediatrics.* 1980;66:912–917

27. Brewster AB. Chronically ill hospitalized children's concepts of their illness. *Pediatrics.* 1982;69:355–362

28. Crisp J, Ungerer JA, Goodnow JJ. The impact of experience on children's understanding of illness. *J Pediatr Psychol.* 1996;21(1):57–72

29. Goldman SL, Whitney-Saltiel D, Granger J, Rodin J. Children's representations of "everyday" aspects of health and illness. *J Pediatr Psychol.* 1991;16(6):747–766

30. Shoemaker MR, Schonfeld DJ, O'Hare LL, Showalter DR, Cicchetti DV. Children's understanding of the symptoms of AIDS. *AIDS Educ Prev.* 1996;8(403):414

31. Schonfeld DJ. Teaching young children about HIV and AIDS. *Child and Adolescent Clinics of North America.* 2000;9: 375–387

32. Schonfeld DJ, O'Hare LL, Perrin EC, Quackenbush M, Showalter DR, Cicchetti DV. A randomized controlled trial of a school-based, multi-faceted AIDS education program in the elementary grades: the impact on comprehension, knowledge, and fears. *Pediatrics.* 1995;95:480–486

33. Krishnan B, Glazebrook C, Smyth A. Does illness experience influence the recall of medical information? *Arch Dis Child.* 1998;79(6):514–515

34. Gardner R. The guilt reaction of parents of children with severe physical disease. *Am J Psychiatry.* 1969;126:636–644

35. Richardson CR. Educational interventions improve outcomes for children with asthma. *J Fam Pract.* 2003;52(10): 764–766

36. Spinetta JJ. The dying child's awareness of death: a review. *Psychol Bull.* 1974;81(4):256–260

37. Schonfeld DJ. Talking with children about death. *J Pediatr Health Care.* 1993;7:269–274

38. Surkan PJ, Dickman PW, Steineck G, Onelov E, Kreicbergs U. Home care of a child dying of a malignancy and parental awareness of a child's impending death. *Palliat Med.* 2006;20(3):161–169

39. Doig C, Burgess E. Withholding life-sustaining treatment: are adolescents competent to make these decisions? *Can Med Assoc J.* 2000;162(11):1585–1588

40. Rozovsky LE. Children, adolescents, and consent. *The Canadian Law of Consent to Treatment*. 2nd ed. Toronto and Vancouver: Butterworths; 1997:61–75

41. Gaylin W. The competence of children: no longer all or none. *Hastings Cent Rep.* 1982;12:33–38

42. American Academy of Pediatrics, Committee on Bioethics. Guidelines on foregoing life-sustaining medical treatment. *Pediatrics.* 1994;93:532–536

43. Sigman G, Silber TJ, English A, Gans Epner JE. Confidential health care for adolescents: position paper of the Society for Adolescent Medicine. *J Adolesc Health.* 1997;21(6): 408–415

# CHAPTER 20

# Pharmacologic Considerations

BILL G. KAPOGIANNIS, MD

## OVERVIEW

The medical provider considering pharmacotherapy in caring for adolescents and young adults must begin with an understanding of the challenges inherent in working with this population and must become familiar with the fundamental objectives of pharmacologic therapy as well as the observed variations in pharmacologic parameters among youth. A brief overview of these elements follows.

### FACING THE CHALLENGES

Adolescence is a period that traverses numerous biobehavioral and cognitive, as well as physical developmental milestones in a person's life (Figure 20-1). The practicing clinician frequently confronts multiple challenges when approaching the pharmacologic management of an adolescent. Desires to achieve autonomy and independence and to fit in with one's peers often compete with basic principles of adherence to general clinical as well as pharmacologic management. Concomitant substance abuse and mood disorders may compound the difficulty. Administration of multiple medications must also be considered.

This chapter describes the fundamental principles a clinician should consider in the pharmacologic management of adolescents and highlights some of the anticipated challenges in this process that can ultimately improve patient outcomes.

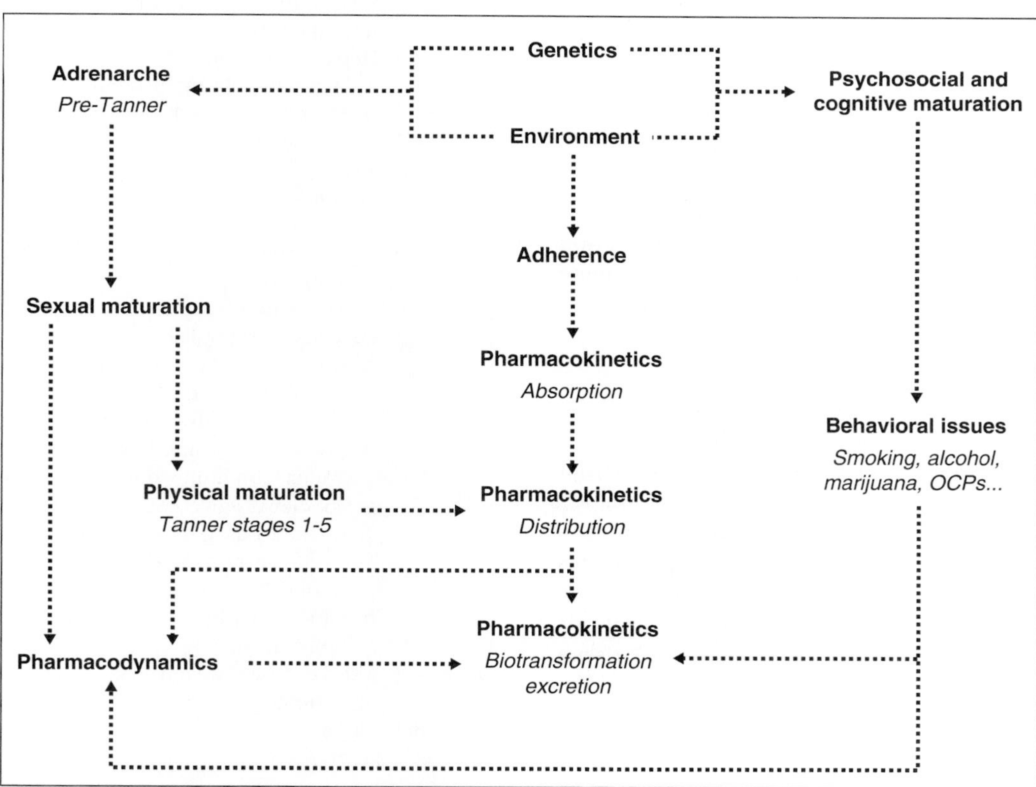


**FIGURE 20-1** Relationship of contributing factors in an adolescent's life to and their influence on various domains of clinical pharmacologic management. (Reprinted from Rogers AS. A research agenda for the study of therapeutic agents in adolescents. *J Adolesc Health.* 1994;15:672–674, with permission from Elsevier.)

### OBJECTIVES OF PHARMACOLOGIC THERAPY

It is important that the objectives of pharmacologic therapy in adolescents reconcile 5 major areas of consideration: (1) assessment of the need for therapy, (2) maximizing drug efficacy, (3) minimizing toxicity, (4) optimizing access and adherence to therapy, and (5) ensuring regimen acceptability to the patient. These will be discussed in more depth throughout the chapter.

### OBSERVED VARIATIONS IN PHARMACOLOGIC PARAMETERS IN ADOLESCENTS

In addition to the observed drug response variability intrinsic to medications and to human heterogeneity discussed below, adolescents introduce further convolution into this already complex equation. Various pubertal hormonal and physiologic changes during adolescence can manifest unpredictable pharmacologic parameters for some medications. These parameters do not possess any consistent direct relationship with an individual's age or metabolic function, making it difficult to scale up or down drug dosage based on data from pharmacokinetic (PK) studies of prepubescent children or adults. As a result, many medications will not require specific adjustment for this age group[1-4] whereas others would be frankly subtherapeutic or perhaps toxic if not carefully dosed.[5-7]

## CHOOSING A REGIMEN

The choice of a pharmacologic regimen should take into consideration drug variability as well as human heterogeneity as these elements can affect drug concentration in different tissue compartments and also the ultimate efficacy and toxicity of a drug in a given individual.

### DRUG VARIABILITY

Drug variability may be one of the considerations that determine the ultimate response an individual has to a given drug and encompasses numerous factors that include molecular steric interactions (size and shape), solubility at the site of absorption, degree of ionization, and relative lipid solubility.[8,9] These properties can affect trafficking of the medication between cellular compartments and thus affect drug concentrations as well as the ultimate efficacy at the targeted tissue compartments.

### HUMAN HETEROGENEITY

Human heterogeneity has recently become more recognized as a key determinant of the observed variability in treatment response to certain drugs between individuals and populations. Implicit within this concept of genetically mediated variation in drug response underlies a broad spectrum of possible mechanisms from accelerated or inhibited drug biotransformation to altered drug sensitivity at the tissue level. In addition, idiosyncratic reactions and certain disease states can contribute to this complex variation in treatment response. A more comprehensive list of sources contributing to this variation is presented in Box 20-1. Consequently, both medication efficacy and toxicity can be significantly affected by any combination of these variations.[10,11]

**Box 20-1**

***Sources of Variability in Drug Response and Toxicity Profile Attributable to Individual Characteristics***

I. Biological
   A. Physical
      1. Age
      2. Gender
      3. Tanner stage
      4. Gastrointestinal function
      5. Immune function
      6. Hepatic function
         a. Synthetic-plasma proteins
         b. Metabolic-cytochrome P450
      7. Renal function
   B. Acquired
      1. Pregnancy
      2. Lactation
      3. Disease states
      4. Immunization
   C. Pharmacogenetic
      1. Defective metabolism
         a. Slow inactivation of isoniazid
         b. Succinylcholine sensitivity
         c. Deficient parahydroxylation of phenytoin
         d. Bishydroxycoumarin sensitivity
         e. Phenacetin-induced methemoglobinemia
         f. Deficient N-glycosylation of amobarbital
         g. Impaired drug oxidation
      2. Altered receptor sites
         a. Coumadin resistance
         b. Glucose 6-phosphate dehydrogenase deficiency
      3. Altered drug transporters
         a. Antiepileptic resistance (MDR1 transporter)
II. Behavioral
   A. Exercise
   B. Diet
   C. Stress
   D. Substance abuse

**Box 20-1 (*continued*)**

1. Alcohol
2. Illicit drugs

E. Smoking

III. Environmental

A. Occupational exposures
B. Sunlight
C. Other medications
D. Barometric pressure
E. Circadian variation
F. Seasonal variation

Modified from Vesel E. Pharmacogenetics. In: Yaffe S, Aranda J, eds. *Pediatric Pharmacology: Therapeutic Principles in Practice.* 2nd ed. Philadelphia, PA: WB Saunders; 1992:29–44, with permission from Elsevier.

## CLINICAL PHARMACOLOGY

The word *pharmacology* is derived from the Greek word *pharmakologia*.[12] In the Greek language, *pharmakon* is defined as "poison" or "medicine" and *logia* is defined as "study." Hence, *pharmakologia* is the "study" of "poisons" or "medicines." Pharmacology is further subdivided into 2 major areas that are interrelated; PK and pharmacodynamics (Figure 20-2).[13] A thorough understanding of PK, pharmacodynamics, drug interactions, and their relevant applications to the care of the adolescent patient will ensure that all 5 previously discussed objectives of pharmacologic therapy can be met. Only key concepts are presented below as a comprehensive discussion of each of these areas is beyond the scope of this chapter. Key clinical pearls that will be helpful in the approach to pharmacologic management of adolescents are presented in Box 20-2.

### PHARMACOKINETICS AND DRUG DISPOSITION

Pharmacokinetics is defined as the science and study of the factors that determine the amount of drug at sites of biologic effect at various times after application of an agent to a biologic system.[14] Pharmacokinetics studies enable a clinician to best determine how, and to what extent a drug accumulates and is eliminated from the various tissue compartments of the body. The extent to which a drug concentrates in specific tissue compartments of the body is a function of (1) absorption, (2) distribution, (3) biotransformation, and (4) elimination of that agent (Figure 20-3).

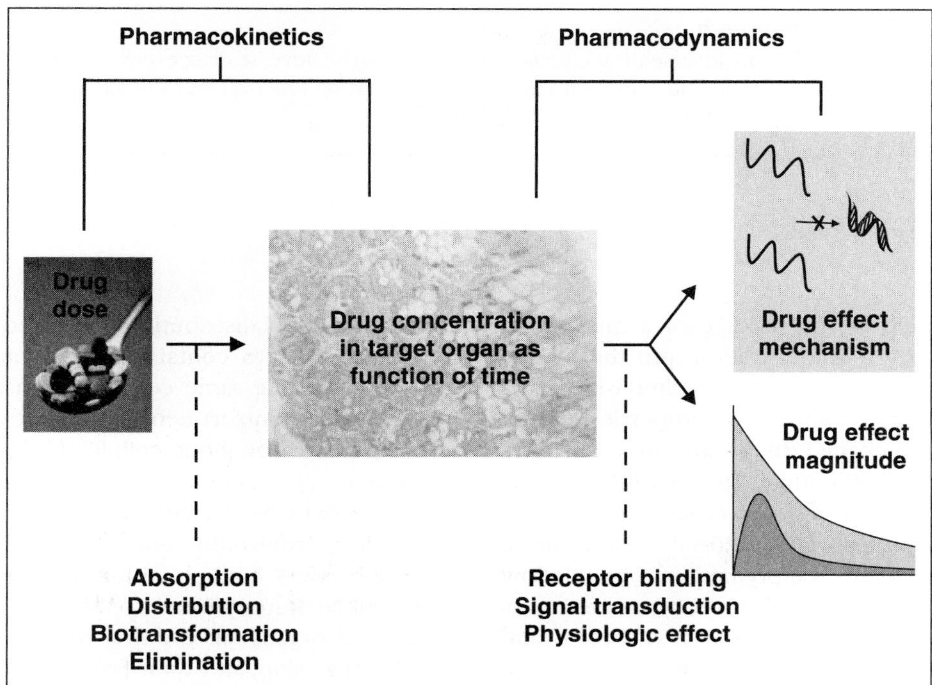


**FIGURE 20-2** The interactions of various aspects of pharmacokinetics and pharmacodynamics and their relationship to each other. (Modified from Brenner G. *Pharmacology Review*. Philadelphia, PA: WB Saunders; 2000:2, with permission from Elsevier.)

**Box 20-2**

***Clinical Pearls***

**Judicious Inaction**

Understand that the risk of beginning empiric therapy may outweigh the benefit of treatment in cases when there is significant diagnostic uncertainty.

**Thorough Drug History**

Ensure the absence of any gaps in histories obtained for the use of prescription, nonprescription, and illicit drugs so that therapeutic efficacy and toxicity monitoring are optimized and surprises are minimized.

**Pharmacologic Familiarity**

Agents whose pharmacokinetics, pharmacodynamics, and mechanisms of important drug interactions are well established are preferable to those newer, "in vogue" medications.

**Beware of Undiagnosed Pregnancy**

Adolescent pregnancy is commonly unplanned and unexpected. Agents with teratogenic potential should be used with extreme caution in this population.

**Treatment Goals and Endpoints**

Clearly define therapeutic endpoints and articulate them in the chart to encourage an almost reflexive and ongoing assessment of the success of an intervention.

**Beware of Pitfalls**

Exercise extreme caution when using drugs with narrow therapeutic indices and when in high-risk clinical scenarios where there are complex medical problems in which clinical parameters can change rapidly.

**Patient as Collaborator**

Engage and encourage the adolescent to consider the prescription as a contract between yourselves where both agree upon a schedule, endpoints, and toxicities, thus enhancing adherence and success of a safe intervention.

**Familiarize Yourself with Medwatch**

There is a paucity of information on adverse drug effects in adolescents. The adverse drug event reporting system is the fuel that drives postmarketing safety evaluation. Careful monitoring and reporting of such events in adolescents will ensure that adolescent-specific evaluation occurs if indicated.

### Absorption

*Absorption* is defined as the passage of a medication or drug from its site of administration into the plasma compartment.[15] The optimal route of administration is determined by the physiochemical properties of the drug and the natural characteristics and functionalities of the barriers it will encounter. *Bioavailability* designates the fraction of an ingested dose of a drug that gains access to the plasma (Figure 20-4)[15,16] and can be affected by gastric acidity, emptying time, blood flow and surface area, intestinal transit time, hepatic metabolism (first pass effect), diet, concurrent drug therapy, and certain disease states.[8] A treatment that requires rapid onset of action of a precise amount of drug would best be administered intravenously, avoiding physical barriers as well as the first pass effect that may lead to variable bioavailability.

### Distribution

The volume of distribution is defined as the volume of fluid required to contain the total amount of drug in the body at the same concentration as that present in the plasma compartment.[15] After absorption, the drug distributes throughout cellular body compartments at different rates and to variable extents depending on its physiochemical characteristics. These characteristics include permeability, and therefore solubility across tissue barriers, binding within tissue compartments and, pH and fat water partition.[17] The vasculature and highly perfused organs are the first to see the drug, followed by muscle, skin, and then fat, which may act as a long-term reservoir given its limited perfusion. Some tissue compartments may accumulate higher than expected concentrations of drug, given other driving factors such as pH gradients or binding to intracellular constituents

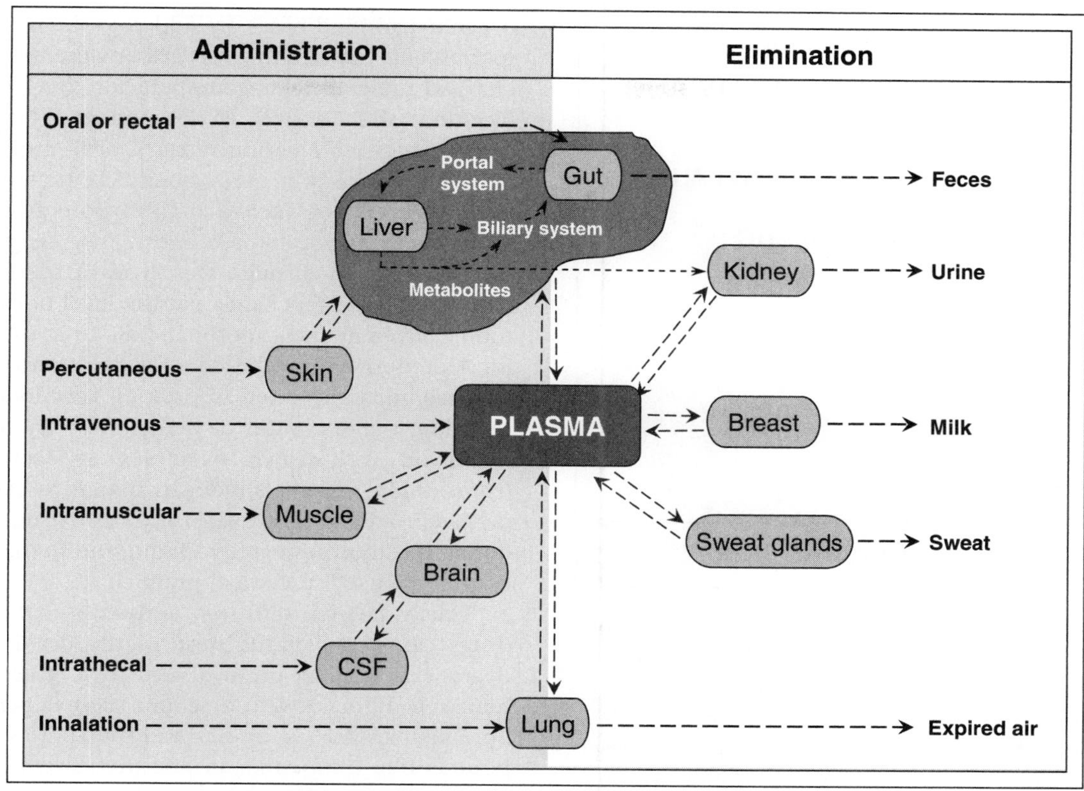


**FIGURE 20-3** Schematic representation of the pharmacokinetic processes of drug *absorption*, *distribution* to different tissue compartments, *biotransformation* in the liver and gut, and *elimination* via the kidneys and, less frequently, other organs. (Modified from Rang H. *Pharamacology.* 4th ed. New York, NY: Livingstone; 2001:68, with permission from Elsevier.)

(eg, digoxin, which binds to Na+, K+-ATPase in muscle), whereas others may have limited distribution owing to plasma binding. This latter phenomenon may lead to decreased drug clearance.[8]

### Biotransformation

*Biotransformation* or metabolism is 1 of the 2 principal mechanisms by which the body facilitates the elimination of most drugs, though this process per se does not eliminate drugs and may also affect the conversion of some prodrugs into their biologically active forms, releasing them into the bile to be reabsorbed from the intestine. It is important to recognize that although many enzyme systems that metabolize drugs are found in the liver, there are also those that can be found in other organs such as the kidney, lung, and gastrointestinal epithelium, and that these can exert clinically significant actions. These can be as profound as the well-known first pass effect (*presystemic metabolism*) that in some cases occurs at the level of the gut wall.[8,17] Metabolism allows many fat-soluble (lipophilic or nonpolar) drugs to be chemically altered into more water-soluble (hydrophilic or polar) molecules that are more readily excreted by the kidney. This process involves 2 kinds of biochemical reactions known as *phase I* and *phase II* reactions. *Phase I* reactions involve oxidation, reduction, and hydrolytic reactions that typically convert drug compounds into polar metabolites that can vary in activity from none to more than that of the parent compound. The well-known and dominant phase I oxidative system known as the cytochrome P-450 family metabolizes, to some degree, most drugs clinically used in humans. *Phase II* reactions result in the conjugation of a compound or its polar metabolite with an endogenous substrate such as glucuronate, glutathione, glucose, sulfate, or acetate. This process almost always results in the generation of a moiety that is pharmacologically inactive and less lipid-soluble than its precursor, enhancing its excretion in the urine or bile.

### Elimination

In addition to biotransformation-facilitated drug elimination, excretion of chemically unchanged drug into the urine or, less commonly, other body fluids, is the

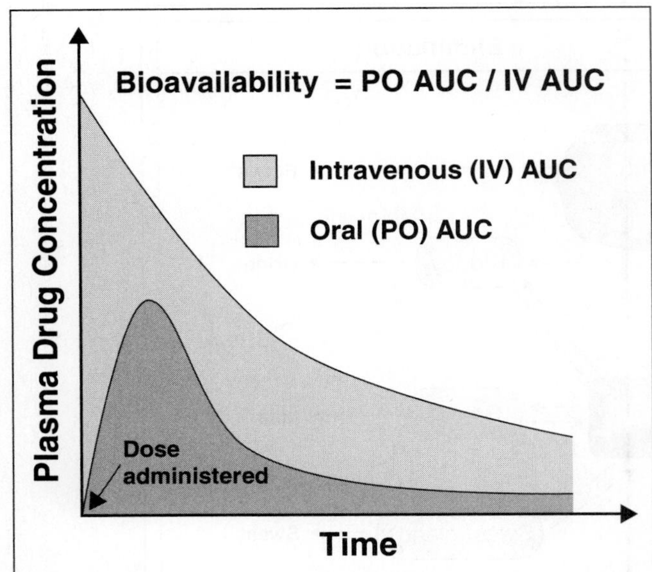


FIGURE 20-4 Graphic representation of the definition of bioavailability, which is defined as the fraction of the area under the curve (AUC) achieved from oral administration of the drug to that of intravenous administration. (Modified from Brenner G. *Pharmacology Review*. Philadelphia, PA: WB Saunders; 2000:8, with permission from Elsevier.)

other major mechanism of drug elimination. In urinary elimination, whether of unchanged or chemically modified compounds, there are 3 basic processes at play and involve (1) glomerular filtration, (2) *active* tubular secretion and reabsorption, and (3) *passive* diffusion across tubular epithelium. The efficiency of filtration is a function of the integrity of the glomerular unit, the glomerular filtration rate, which is dependent on renal blood flow, the size and charge of the molecule being filtered, and the extent to which it is bound to plasma proteins.[8] Drug therapy in the setting of decreased renal function can result in serious drug toxicity and may lead to many profound clinical consequences if not monitored carefully. This is particularly true for those drugs with narrow therapeutic indices, those that are highly protein bound, and in circumstances where a large percentage of the administered drug is excreted unchanged in the urine.[18] The peritubular capillaries of the proximal tubule receive up to 80% of the administered drug and actively secrete the drug molecules against an electrochemical gradient to the tubular lumen by 2 independent (one for acidic drugs and the other for organic bases, named organic cation [OCT] and anion transporter [OAT], respectively) and relatively nonselective carrier-mediated systems.[17,19] In these systems, various organic acids and bases are added to the drug molecule to facilitate transfer in a process where other similarly charged molecules can compete for transport.[8] Unlike filtration, such active carrier-mediated transport can achieve high elimination rates of drug molecules even if they are highly protein bound. Penicillin is a notorious example of such a highly protein-bound acidic drug that is slowly filtered and whose clearance is primarily achieved through this type of carrier-mediated active transport mechanism at the level of the proximal tubule. Probenecid is another acidic drug that competes for secretion within this same active transport process and has been exploited to prolong antibiotic action by retarding the secretion of penicillin.[19] There are many additional well-known examples of secreted acidic (furosemide, acetazolamide, hydrochlorothiazide, indomethacin, and methotrexate) and basic drugs (amiloride, dopamine, morphine, meperidine, and quinine) that are commonly used in clinical practice.

Finally, passive diffusion and reabsorption of some drugs can occur at the level of the distal tubule. The degree of tubular permeability to a given drug and hence its ultimate rate of elimination depend on how lipid soluble it is. Nonpolar and thus lipid-soluble compounds like thiopental, an anesthetic agent, have high tubular permeability and consequently are slowly eliminated because of the high degree of passive reabsorption that occurs. Elimination is further retarded by sequestration occurring in fat-rich tissue compartments that reflect the high volume of distribution for this drug, decreasing its availability to circulation and renal excretion. Conversely, more polar drugs like aminoglycosides and digoxin experience markedly decreased reabsorption by a phenomenon known as ion trapping in the renal tubule, which results in more rapid elimination compared to more lipid-soluble counterparts.[17] Tubular permeability to weak acids and bases is particularly vulnerable to extremes of urine pH and can be significantly decreased by alkalinizing and acidifying the urine, respectively.[8] This phenomenon has been exploited clinically for therapeutic advantages to hasten elimination of toxic drug levels such as in the treatment of aspirin overdose by the administration of intravenous bicarbonate.

In pharmacology, elimination is expressed as *clearance* and is defined as the volume of plasma containing the amount of a substance removed by all routes in unit time. Though multiple organs (see Figure 20-3) can contribute, the kidneys and liver are chiefly responsible for elimination of most drugs, and thus maintenance of perfusion to these organs is a vital determinant of drug clearance from the body. Elimination kinetics generally follow either a *dose-dependent* or *dose-independent* pathway. Dose-dependent kinetics

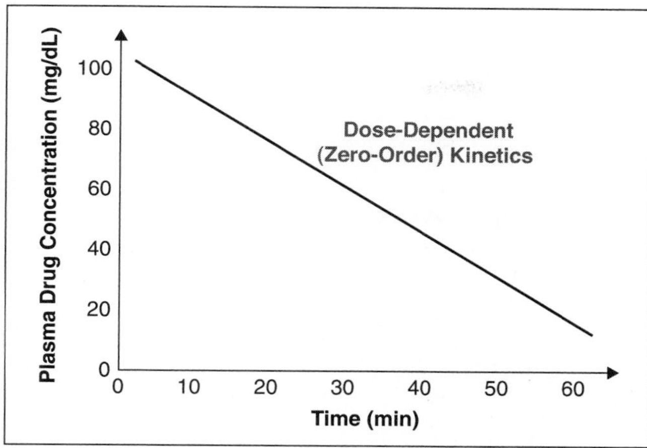


FIGURE 20-5 Graphic representation of Michaelis-Menten (zero-order) kinetics, which are dose-dependent and involve a saturable process where the amount of drug administered directly dictates the concentration of drug that is eliminated. (Modified from Brenner G. *Pharmacology Review*. Philadelphia, PA: WB Saunders; 2000:7, with permission from Elsevier.)

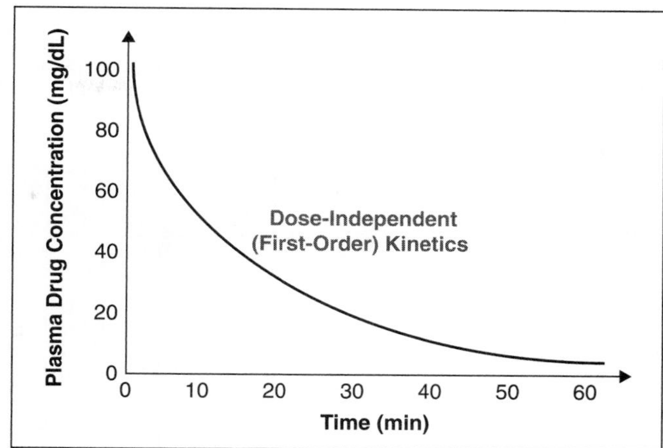


FIGURE 20-6 Graphic representation of dose-independent (first-order) kinetics where a constant percentage of drug is removed per unit time. (Modified from Brenner G. *Pharmacology Review*. Philadelphia, PA: WB Saunders; 2000:7, with permission from Elsevier.)

are also termed zero-order or Michaelis-Menten kinetics (Figure 20-5) and involve a saturable process whereby the amount of drug administered directly dictates the concentration of drug that is eliminated, making dosing of drugs that follow this kinetic pathway challenging. In this scenario, a given dose does not always result in a predictable plasma drug concentration, sometimes necessitating plasma drug-level sampling. As this metabolic pathway approaches saturation, even a small increment in dose administered can result in a large increase in plasma drug concentration. Simply put, all drugs can exhibit such zero-order kinetics in an overdose state; however, those that typically follow this kinetic pathway at therapeutic plasma concentrations include phenytoin, ethanol, propranolol, and aspirin. Most drugs are eliminated from the body following a dose-independent pathway, also called first-order kinetics and are cleared in a predictable manner by which a constant percentage of the drug is removed per unit time (Figure 20-6). Hence, this pathway allows for a more predictable determination of plasma drug concentration based on dosage. For drugs exhibiting such dose-independent kinetics, the *elimination half-life* ($t$) can be determined by plotting the exponential decay of drug in the plasma as a function of time and measuring the amount of time it takes for the plasma concentration of drug to decrease to half of the original amount (Figure 20-7). The $t$ is germane to the determination of time required to achieve plasma steady-state concentration (drug amount entering the system per unit time equals the amount leaving), the determination of time needed for plasma drug levels to decrease once administration is discontinued, and then ultimately for the calculation of the proper dosing interval to achieve the desired therapeutic plasma levels. It generally takes about 5 elimination half-lives to achieve steady-state plasma concentrations when dosing is based on an interval equivalent to the $t$ for that drug. Importantly, in an emergency, a loading dose is given to achieve therapeutic plasma levels more expediently because waiting to achieve steady-state concentrations is unacceptable in this scenario.

PK studies thus encompass all 4 processes of *absorption, distribution, biotransformation,* and *elimination*, and facilitate a practical understanding of how to best dose an agent, both in quantity and in frequency, for a given individual and for a specific disease process. To illustrate this, a urinary tract infection can easily be treated with relatively small doses of a fluoroquinolone antibiotic, whereas the same dose given for the treatment of meningitis may likely be ineffective or suboptimal at eradicating an infection by the same organism. This is because the antibiotic is well absorbed with high oral bioavailability and is distributed in high concentrations to the genitourinary tract for purposes of excretion[20] often exceeding the dose needed to inhibit growth of an organism, whereas the same is not true for the central nervous system, where a much higher dose would be required to achieve the same level of antibacterial activity.

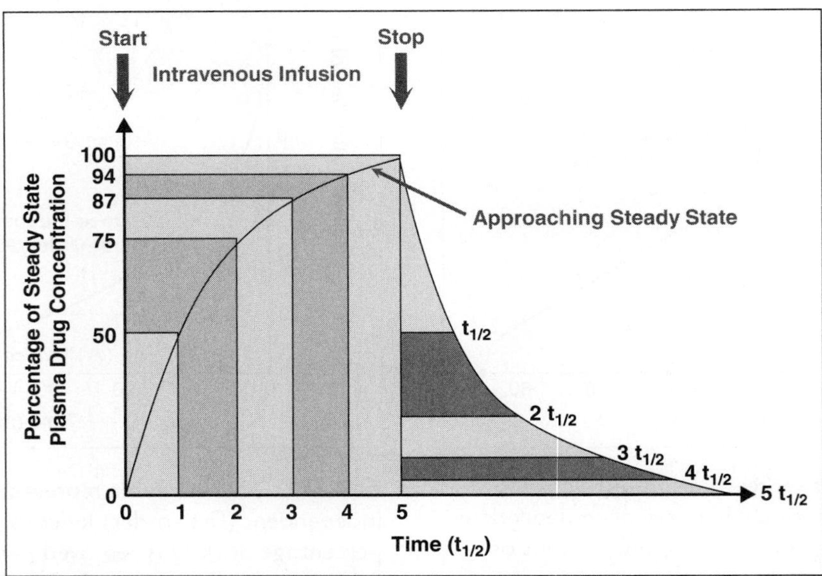


**FIGURE 20-7** Change in the percentage of steady-state plasma drug concentration after intravenous infusion is initiated and stopped over the course of time as represented by the drug elimination half-life (t). (Modified from Brenner G. *Pharmacology Review*. Philadelphia, PA: WB Saunders; 2000:9, with permission from Elsevier.)

## DRUG INTERACTIONS

Use of other medications concomitantly may affect any or all of the above functional pathways by varying mechanisms. *Absorption* of certain drugs may be impeded or enhanced by various agents such as chelating molecules (antacids → ↓ fluoroquinolone antibiotics), pH-altering agents (antacids, famotidine, or omeprazole → ↓ atazanavir), and emulsifiers (fatty foods → ↑ lopinavir/ritonavir). *Distribution* of a drug to a given tissue compartment may be increased or decreased depending on how much of it is nonselectively bound to plasma proteins (antiepileptic meds) and if there may be concomitant competition for binding by other drugs (bactrim → ↑ warfarin). *Biotransformation* can be upregulated by some agents (ethanol, rifampin, dexamethasone, clofibrate) while being downregulated by others (erythromycin, cimetidine, ketoconazole, grapefruit juice) via inductive or inhibitory effects they exert on hepatic cytochrome P450 enzymes, respectively.[21] Finally, *elimination*, and excretion in particular, may be affected by the above-discussed local acid-base alterations at the level of the renal tubule. Examples of exploiting this phenomenon for therapeutic benefit have been given above for purposes of prolongation of antibiotic action and treatment of drug overdoses. Examples of toxicity would include coadministration of methotrexate with aspirin, other salicylates or nonsteroidal anti-inflammatory agents (NSAIDs), all of which are commonly used in the treatment of rheumatologic diseases.

## PHARMACODYNAMICS

Pharmacodynamics is defined as the study of the actions and chemicals at all levels of organization of living material and of the handling of chemicals by the organism.[14] This encompasses 4 basic elements: (1) the biologic effects that chemicals manifest; (2) the sites at which and the mechanisms by which these effects are produced; (3) the magnitude of these effects; and (4) the factors that impact the safety and effectiveness of a pharmacologic agent. Put a different way, a drug engages its receptor, thereby initiating signal transduction, which triggers a cascade of events or chemical reactions that lead to a physiologic effect.[22] Furthermore, the ultimate physiologic response to the drug depends on the type of activity it exerts on its receptor (agonist, antagonist, combined or partial agonist) and whether the system it engages can undergo alterations in receptor density up- or down-regulating the numbers of drug receptors per cell and consequently exhibit either increased drug sensitivity or drug tolerance, respectively.[22] The latter phenomenon is termed tachyphylaxis and is essentially what is defined as pharmacodynamic tolerance. Finally, the magnitude of the physiologic effect is usually described by a dose–response relationship that is either graded (response per dose described by percentage of maximal response) (Figure 20-8a) or quantal (cumulative percentage of subjects exhibiting a defined all-or-none effect) (Figure 20-8b).[22] A thorough understanding of each of the previous 4 elements is integral to optimizing the pharmacologic management of every disease process.

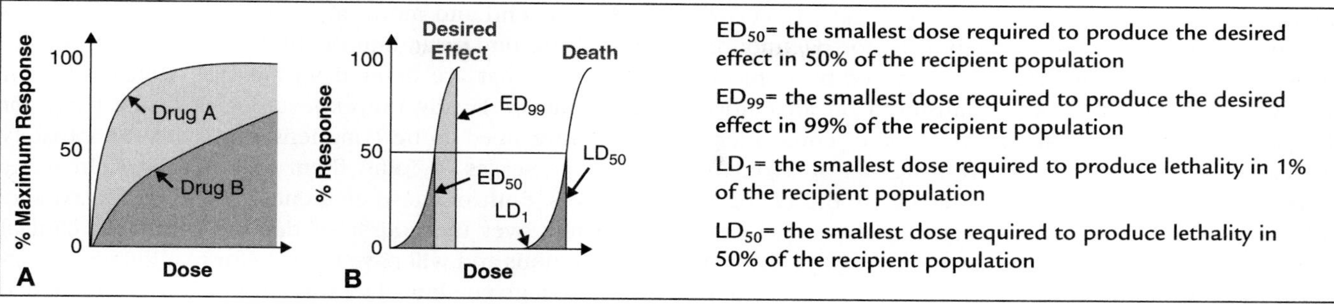


FIGURE 20-8 The magnitude of a drug's physiologic effect as described by either the (A) *graded* (response per dose is described by the percentage of maximal response) or (B) *quantal* (cumulative percentage of subjects exhibiting a defined all-or-none effect) dose–response relationship. (Modified with permission from Walsh C. *Levine's Pharmacology: Drug Actions and Reactions.* 7th ed. London: Informa Healthcare; 2005:189 and 207.)

## RELEVANCE TO ADOLESCENTS

There are numerous considerations that impact the discussed pharmacologic parameters when administering medications to an adolescent (Table 20-1). The rate of *absorption* but not the extent is usually affected by gastric emptying and, consequently, an adolescent's

**Table 20-1**

**Adolescent Conditions and Diseases Affecting Pharmacokinetics (PK)**

| *PK Parameter* | *Condition* | *Mechanism* | *Clinical Outcome* |
|---|---|---|---|
| **Absorption** | Eating disorders<br>*Bulimia*<br>*Anorexia nervosa* | Erratic intake, organ dysfunction, and electrolyte imbalance | Therapeutic failure, possible toxicity |
| **Distribution** | Obesity | Adipose serves as a reservoir for lipophilic agents | Prolonged clearance |
| | Malnutrition | Decreased fat, muscle mass, and plasma protein | Increased clearance with/without enhanced drug effect or toxicity |
| | Renal dysfunction | Decreased protein binding | Increased unbound drug in face of low serum levels |
| | Burns | Massive fluid shifts; cell membrane disruption; decreased serum albumin | Multifactorial |
| **Biotransformation** | Hepatic dysfunction<br>*Alcohol*<br>*Drug induced*<br>*Infectious*<br>*Steatosis* | Impaired metabolism | Possible toxicity |
| **Elimination** | Renal dysfunction | Accumulation of endogenous acids that compete/displace plasma protein-bound drug; accumulation of drugs >40% renally excreted | Enhanced drug effect/toxicity for drug >90% bound; toxicity profile depends on drug |
| | Burns | Renal blood flow and GFR decreased acutely | Possible toxicity |

*GFR*, glomerular filtration rate.

Data from Brater DC. Treatment of renal disorders and the influence of renal function on drug disposition. In: Melmon F, Morrelli H, Hoffman B, Nierenberg D, eds. *Melmon and Morrelli's Clinical Pharmacology: Basic Principles in Therapeutics.* 3rd ed. New York, NY: McGraw-Hill; 1992:270–308; and Bonate PL. Pathophysiology and pharmacokinetics following burn injury. *Clin Pharmacokinet.* 1990;18:118–130.

erratic eating behavior should have little effect on therapy where rapid onset of action is not paramount. Conversely, medications that are inactivated by stomach acidity should probably be administered on an empty stomach so that delayed emptying and consequent decreased bioavailability of active drug can be avoided. *Distribution* can be a variable affected by the changes in body size and composition characteristic of puberty. Lean body mass usually increases more in boys than in girls resulting in more relative body fat in girls compared to boys by late puberty and incumbent alterations in the volume of distribution of some drugs. The extent of *biotransformation* is dependent on multiple factors within a given individual (drug/toxin exposure, hepatic dysfunction, and pharmacogenetic capacity differences) and is only further complicated by pubertal hormonal and physiologic changes. Differences in drug metabolism and elimination are well documented between young children (toddlers and preteens) and adults;[23-28] however, there are limited data on the functional transition of a prepubertal child's drug metabolism to that of an adolescent, and consequently there are few mechanistic explanations of the phenotypic differences observed in some pharmacokinetic studies.[24,25,27,28] Only scant evidence to suggest potential Tanner stage-dependant, maturational biotransformation of some compounds such as caffeine, imipramine, and phenacetin has been uncovered.[29] *Elimination* and renal excretion have been suggested to have maturational variability also, as evidenced by data on decreased digoxin clearance when a child achieves Tanner stage 4 and 5 maturity.[30,31]

Finally, behaviors that result in substance use or other life circumstances specific to adolescents can complicate the management of many diseases common in this population. For example, a depressed teenager who is abusing alcohol may not necessarily be a good candidate for pharmacologic therapy with some medications given the potential for increased toxicity or further abuse. A seizure disorder in a sexually active teen who is taking oral contraceptives is a challenge to control with antiepileptic agents given the difficulty in establishing therapeutic levels.

## PHYSICIAN–PATIENT INTERACTIONS AND EXPECTATIONS

The relationship between a health care provider and an adolescent patient is one that can meet challenges. The astute clinician learns to navigate the relationship through these challenges by establishing some fundamental goals for both parties; first, both must realize the importance of building trust and confidence in each other. Second and more importantly, both must possess a realistic understanding of the boundaries inherent to this trust that are defined within the context of their relationship. Finally, the expectations of each party for the other need to be commensurate with the capacity each possesses to fulfill them to be realistic. In many patients, both of these elements can be cultivated successfully over the course of time and multiple clinical interactions and will pave the way for maximizing adherence to a given clinical treatment regimen. If confidence is not developed and expectations are unrealistic, simply providing a prescription to a youth will treat no one but the clinician.

Prescribing practices vary among clinicians depending on individual style; however, there are several key questions of paramount relevance that must be asked by every clinician, particularly in adolescent medicine, prior to prescribing a medication. Is the disease process you are managing acute or is it a chronic or pre-existing condition? Does it require pharmacologic therapy? Are there alternatives such as psychotherapy or lifestyle modifications that may be equally efficacious but are avoided because they are more labor intensive? If medications are required, is therapy a temporary intervention or will this require skill building for the adolescent to maximize his or her adherence to a more permanent lifestyle adaptation? If the youth has just been given a new diagnosis, can pharmacologic therapy be deferred without compromising the health of the youth while he or she adjusts to this news? Some chronic illnesses such as HIV infection have arbitrary criteria for treatment and can afford the adolescent and his or her doctor time to prepare for the long journey they embark on, whereas others such as type I diabetes do not allow for such luxuries without rapidly achieving the risk of potentially serious consequences. Furthermore, a prescription can be viewed as a commodity that is a necessary hallmark of a successful clinical encounter, often by both the prescriber as well as the recipient.[32] Hence, insight into this phenomenon is an additional consideration to weigh in the decision of whether a medication is clinically indicated.

Adherence is an absolutely essential component of any successful pharmacologic intervention. Challenges encountered in this area are one of the most frequent problems that frustrate many adolescent medicine specialists and are covered in more depth in Chapter 12, Adherence Issues. Developmental milestones normally experienced during adolescence[33] such as the desire to fit in with one's peers and the need to exercise autonomy and independence provide a difficult terrain for the clinician to navigate when pharmacologic treatment is considered. In this context, the chosen regimen

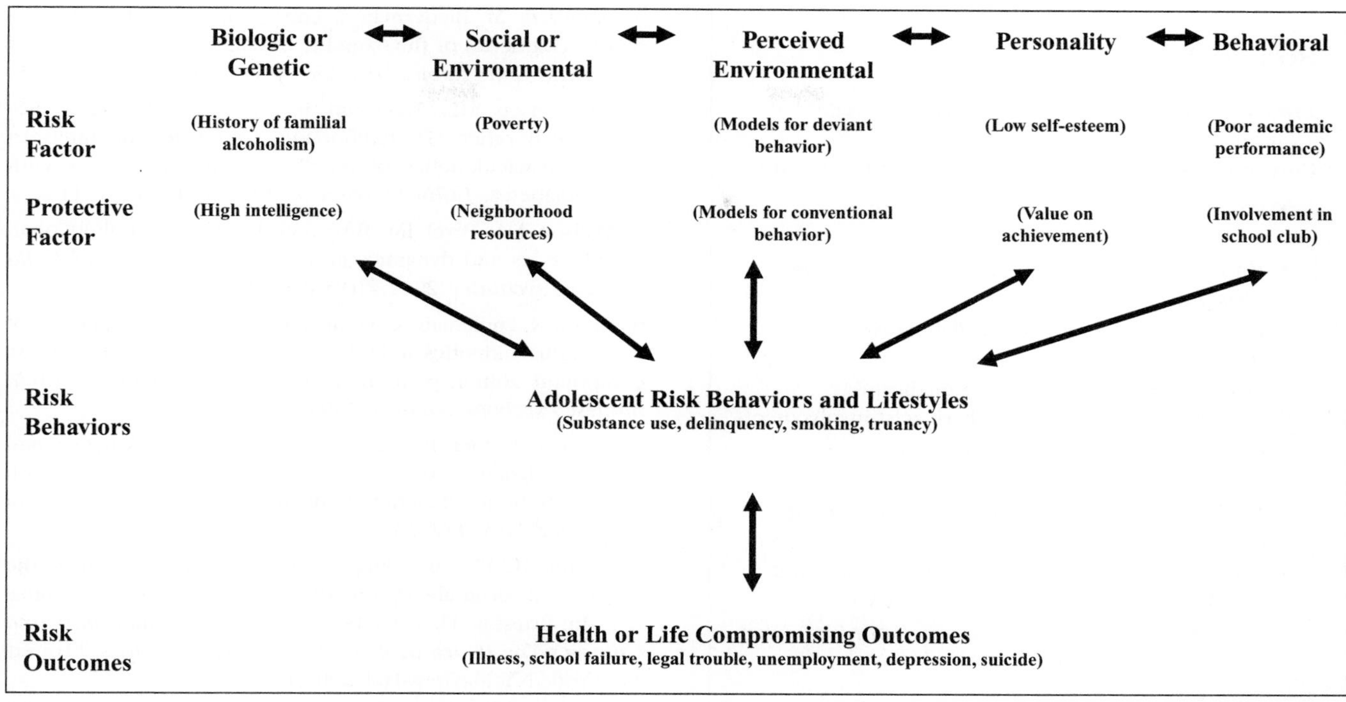


FIGURE 20-9 Interrelationships of various physical, social, behavioral and environmental factors and the resulting risk behaviors with their incumbent consequences. (Reprinted with permission from Jessor R. *New Perspectives on Adolescent Risk Behavior*. New York, NY: Cambridge University Press; 1998:4.)

may be onerous, embarrassing, or restricting in other ways that are perceived as limiting abilities to participate in usual "normal" activities.[34] Risk behavior is an additional milestone that entails a complex process of interrelated conceptual domains and also frequently complicates this goal (Figure 20-9).[35] Furthermore, it is common for youth to deny risk-taking behavior and the inherent consequences of "fitting in with the crowd." Compounding these issues can be comorbidities such as the use of illicit drugs and alcohol[36-39] and mood disorders[36,40] like depression and anxiety that can undeniably impair judgment, negatively affecting adherence to medications. Further complicating the adherence equation in many circumstances are issues of access to medications. Some conditions require medication treatments that are prohibitively expensive[32] and would result in the inadvertent disclosure of a diagnosis to the adolescent's caregiver, breeching delicately constructed bonds of trust and confidentiality between the clinician and the youth.[41] One such example is access to emergency contraception, whose broad availability in some foreign countries has had a profound effect in improving uptake[42,43] and reducing unplanned teen pregnancy,[44] though it remains a controversial topic in the United States.[45,46] These circumstances often require a multidisciplinary approach to identify alternative resources to subsidize the costs of these medications and to avoid breeching patient confidentiality by involving the caregiver either directly or indirectly via an insurance company. A recent international study has shown that the provision of vouchers for access to sexual and reproductive health services improved uptake of these services by adolescents in need.[47]

The final common pathway to a successful pharmacologic intervention in a teenager is based on identifying a regimen that will achieve the desired clinical therapeutic outcome and is acceptable to the youth. Issues to be considered in improving adherence (Box 20-3) are a medication's side effect profile, frequency and simplicity of dosing, and simplicity of integration into the adolescent's lifestyle.[32] Optimizing these key factors entails engaging the adolescent to participate actively in his or her care and requires fostering a collaborative relationship with the adolescent that will ultimately enhance adherence to a treatment regimen.

## Box 20-3

### *Improving Adolescent Adherence*

**Communication, Education, and Comprehension**

- Provide respectful and age-appropriate communication.
- *If youth is on medication, ask how he or she takes it.*
- Develop a satisfactory and collaborative relationship.
- Provide and encourage use of medication counseling and encourage pharmacist involvement.
- Give clear instructions, with most important information given first.
- *Support verbal instructions with easy-to-read information.*
- Assess patient's literacy and comprehension and modify educational counseling as needed.
- *Don't rely on patient knowledge about his or her disease, alone, to improve adherence.*

**Regimen Selection**

- Simplify regimen as often and whenever possible.
- Use optimal dosage form and schedule for each youth.

**Compliance Aids**

- Use behavioral techniques.
- *Goal setting, self-monitoring, cognitive restructuring, skills training, contracts, and positive reinforcement.*
- Use mechanical adherence aids as possible.
- *Sectioned pill boxes or trays, adherence packaging, color-coding.*
- Find solution for youth with physical or sensory disabilities.
- *No safety caps on bottles, use large type on labels and written material, place tape marks on syringes.*
- Judiciously enlist support and assistance from family or caregivers as appropriate.

Modified with permission from Buxton IL. Principles of prescription order writing and patient compliance. In: Brunton LL, Lazo JS, Parker KL, eds. *Goodman and Gilman's The Pharmacologic Basis of Therapeutics.* 11th ed. New York, NY: McGraw-Hill; 2006:1784.

## REFERENCES


1. Dutta S, Zhang Y, Conway JM, et al. Divalproex-ER pharmacokinetics in older children and adolescents. *Pediatr Neurol.* 2004;30(5):330–337

2. Marshall JD, Abdel-Rahman S, Johnson K, Kauffman RE, Kearns GL. Rifapentine pharmacokinetics in adolescents. *Pediatr Infect Dis J.* 1999;18(10):882–888

3. Labellarte M, Biederman J, Emslie G, et al. Multiple-dose pharmacokinetics of fluvoxamine in children and adolescents. *J Am Acad Child Adolesc Psychiatry.* 2004;43(12):1497–1505

4. Christensen ML, Meibohm B, Capparelli EV, Velasquez-Mieyer P, Burghen GA, Tamborlane WV. Single- and multiple-dose pharmacokinetics of pioglitazone in adolescents with type 2 diabetes. *J Clin Pharmacol.* 2005;45(10):1137–1144

5. Axelson DA, Perel JM, Birmaher B, et al. Sertraline pharmacokinetics and dynamics in adolescents. *J Am Acad Child Adolesc Psychiatry.* 2002;41(9):1037–1044

6. Dixon R, Engleman K, Kemp J, Ruckle JL. A comparison of the pharmacokinetics and tolerability of the novel antimigraine compound zolmitriptan in adolescents and adults. *J Child Adolesc Psychopharmacol.* 1999;9(1):35–42

7. Grub S, Delora P, Ludin E, et al. Pharmacokinetics and pharmacodynamics of saquixnavir in pediatric patients with human immunodeficiency virus infection. *Clin Pharmacol Ther.* 2002;71(3):122–130

8. Buxton IL. Pharmacokinetics and pharmacodynamics: the dynamics of drug absorption, distribution, action and elimination. In: Brunton LL, Lazo JS, Parker KL, eds. *Goodman and Gilman's The Pharmacologic Basis of Therapeutics.* 11th ed. New York, NY: McGraw-Hill; 2006:1–39

9. Walsh CT, Schwartz-Bloom RD. Factors modifying the effect of drugs in individuals: variability in response attributable to the conditions of administration. *Levine's Pharmacology: Drug Actions and Reactions.* 7th ed. London: Informa Healthcare; 2005:287–323

10. Rang HP, Dale MM, Ritter JM, Gardner P. Individual variation and drug interaction. In: Hunter L, Simmons B, eds. *Pharmacology.* 4th ed. New York, NY: Churchill Livingstone; 2001:750–760

11. Walsh CT, Schwartz-Bloom RD. Factors modifying the effect of drugs in individuals: variability in response attributable to the biologic system. *Levine's Pharmacology: Drug Actions and Reactions.* 7th ed. London: Informa Healthcare; 2005:259–286

12. Walsh CT, Schwartz-Bloom RD. The heritage of pharmacology. *Levine's Pharmacology: Drug Actions and Reactions.* 7th ed. London: Informa Healthcare; 2005:1–16

13. Brenner GM. Introduction to pharmacology. *Pharmacology Review.* Philadelphia, PA: WB Saunders; 2000:1–3

14. Walsh CT, Schwartz-Bloom RD. The scope of pharmacology. *Levine's Pharmacology: Drug Actions and Reactions.* 7th ed. London: Informa Healthcare; 2005:19–28

15. Rang HP, Dale MM, Ritter JM, Gardner P. Absorption and distribution of drugs. In: Hunter L, Simmons B, eds. *Pharmacology.* 4th ed. New York, NY: Churchill Livingstone; 2001:61–77

16. Brenner GM. Pharmacokinetics. *Pharmacology Review.* Philadelphia, PA: WB Saunders; 2000:3–11

17. Rang HP, Dale MM, Ritter JM, Gardner P. Drug elimination and pharmacokinetics. In: Hunter L, Simmons B, eds. *Pharmacology.* 4th ed. New York, NY: Churchill Livingstone; 2001:78–92

18. Brater DC. Treatment of renal disorders and the influence of renal function on drug disposition. In: Melmon F, Morrelli

H, Hoffman B, Nierenberg D, eds. *Melmon and Morrelli's Clinical Pharmacology: Basic Principles in Therapeutics*. 3rd ed. New York, NY: McGraw-Hill; 1992:270–308

19. Walsh CT, Schwartz-Bloom RD. How the actions of drugs are terminated. *Levine's Pharmacology: Drug Actions and Reactions*. 7th ed. London: Informa Healthcare; 2005:129–183

20. Petri WA. Sulfonamides, trimethoprim-sulfamethoxazole, quinolones, and agents for urinary tract infections. In: Brunton LL, Lazo JS, Parker KL, eds. *Goodman and Gilman's The Pharmacologic Basis of Therapeutics*. 11th ed. New York, NY: McGraw-Hill; 2006:1111–1126

21. Gonzalez FJ, Tukey RH. Drug metabolism. In: Brunton LL, Lazo JS, Parker KL, eds. *Goodman and Gilman's The Pharmacologic Basis of Therapeutics*. 11th ed. New York, NY: McGraw-Hill; 2006:71–91

22. Brenner GM. Pharmacodynamics. *Pharmacology Review*. Philadelphia, PA: WB Saunders; 2000:11–13

23. Evans WE, Relling MV, de Graaf S, et al. Hepatic drug clearance in children: studies with indocyanine green as a model substrate. *J Pharm Sci*. 1989;78(6):452–456

24. Evans WE, Crom WR, Stewart CF, et al. Methotrexate systemic clearance influences probability of relapse in children with standard-risk acute lymphocytic leukaemia. *Lancet*. 1984;1(8373):359–362

25. Crom WR, Relling MV, Christensen ML, Rivera GK, Evans WE. Age-related differences in hepatic drug clearance in children: studies with lorazepam and antipyrine. *Clin Pharmacol Ther*. 1991;50(2):132–140

26. Murry DJ, Crom WR, Reddick WE, Bhargava R, Evans WE. Liver volume as a determinant of drug clearance in children and adolescents. *Drug Metab Dispos*. 1995;23(10):1110–1116

27. Hughes W, McDowell JA, Shenep J, et al. Safety and single-dose pharmacokinetics of abacavir (1592U89) in human immunodeficiency virus type 1-infected children. *Antimicrob Agents Chemother*. 1999;43(3):609–615

28. Walsh TJ, Adamson PC, Seibel NL, et al. Pharmacokinetics, safety, and tolerability of caspofungin in children and adolescents. *Antimicrob Agents Chemother*. 2005;49(11):4536–4545

29. Lambert G, Kotake A, Schoeller D. The $CO_2$ breath tests as monitors of the cytochrome P450 dependent mixed function monooxidase system. In: MacLeod S, Okey A, Spielberg S, eds. *Developmental Pharmacology*. New York, NY: Alan R. Liss; 1983:119–145

30. Linday LA. Developmental changes in renal tubular function. *J Adolesc Health*. 1994;15(8):648–653

31. Linday LA, Drayer DE, Khan MA, Cicalese C, Reidenberg MM. Pubertal changes in net renal tubular secretion of digoxin. *Clin Pharmacol Ther*. 1984;35(4):438–446

32. Buxton IL. Principles of prescription order writing and patient compliance. In: Brunton LL, Lazo JS, Parker KL, eds. *Goodman and Gilman's The Pharmacologic Basis of Therapeutics*. 11th ed. New York, NY: McGraw-Hill; 2006: 1777–1786

33. Petersen A. Developmental issues in adolescent health. In: Coates T, Petersen A, Perry C, eds. *Promoting Adolescent Health: A Dialog on Research and Practice*. New York, NY: Academic Press; 1982:61–71

34. Hamburg B. Living with chronic illness. In: Coates T, Petersen A, Perry C, eds. *Promoting Adolescent Health: A Dialog on Research and Practice*. New York, NY: Academic Press; 1982:431–443

35. Jessor R. *New Perspectives on Adolescent Risk Behavior*. New York, NY: Cambridge University Press; 1998:1–10

36. Murphy DA, Marelich WD, Hoffman D, Steers WN. Predictors of antiretroviral adherence. *AIDS Care*. 2004;16(4): 471–484

37. Lucas GM, Gebo KA, Chaisson RE, Moore RD. Longitudinal assessment of the effects of drug and alcohol abuse on HIV-1 treatment outcomes in an urban clinic. *AIDS*. 2002;16(5): 767–774

38. Chesney MA, Ickovics JR, Chambers DB, et al. Self-reported adherence to antiretroviral medications among participants in HIV clinical trials: the AACTG adherence instruments. Patient Care Committee and Adherence Working Group of the Outcomes Committee of the Adult AIDS Clinical Trials Group (AACTG). *AIDS Care*. 2000;12(3):255–266

39. Cook RL, Sereika SM, Hunt SC, Woodward WC, Erlen JA, Conigliaro J. Problem drinking and medication adherence among persons with HIV infection. *J Gen Intern Med*. 2001;16(2):83–88

40. Williams PL, Storm D, Montepiedra G, et al. Predictors of adherence to antiretroviral medications in children and adolescents with HIV infection. *Pediatrics*. 2006;118(6):e1745–1757

41. Litt I. Adolescent health in the United States as we enter the 1980s. In: Coates T, Petersen A, Perry C, eds. *Promoting Adolescent Health: A Dialog on Research and Practice*. New York, NY: Academic Press; 1982:45–60

42. Moreau C, Bajos N, Trussell J. The impact of pharmacy access to emergency contraceptive pills in France. *Contraception*. 2006;73(6):602–608

43. American Academy of Pediatrics Committee on Adolescence. Emergency contraception. *Pediatrics*. 2005;116 (4):1026–1035

44. Persson E, Gustafsson B, Van Rooijen M. Subsidising contraception for young people in Sweden. *Plan Parent Eur*. 1994;23(1):2–4

45. Food and Drug Administration. Nonprescription Drugs Advisory Committee and the Advisory Committee for Reproductive Health Drugs. December 16, 2003. Available at: www.fda.gov/ohrms/dockets/ac/03/briefing/4015b1.htm. Accessed January 14, 2007

46. Food and Drug Administration. FDA issues not approvable letter to Barr Labs: outlines pathway for future approval. May 07, 2004. Available at: www.fda.gov/NewsEvents/Newsroom/PressAnnouncements/2004/ucm108296.htm. Accessed August 6, 2010

47. Meuwissen LE, Gorter AC, Knottnerus AJ. Impact of accessible sexual and reproductive health care on poor and underserved adolescents in Managua, Nicaragua: a quasi-experimental intervention study. *J Adolesc Health*. 2006;38(1):56

# CHAPTER 21

# Health Policy and Financing for Adolescent and Young Adult Health Services*

M. JANE PARK, MPH • CLAIRE BRINDIS, DrPH, MPH • TINA PAUL MULYE, MPH

## OVERVIEW

Adolescent health policies in the United States encompass a wide range of laws, regulations, and practices that influence health and well-being. These policies are shaped by myriad factors that underlie the US political process, including federalism, incrementalism, and civil rights and liberties.[1] This chapter provides an overview of adolescent health policy, with emphasis on the financing of health care services. Policies should be viewed in context of the unique health and developmental issues of adolescence.

By traditional markers, most adolescents are healthy: rates of hospitalization, chronic disease, and mortality are relatively low. Adolescents' health care needs stem largely from issues unique to this period of the life span. For example, as they grow increasingly independent, adolescents face choices in areas such as eating habits, exercise, driving, substance use, and sexuality. Adolescence presents an opportunity to foster healthy growth and development and to help young people make healthy choices. Unhealthy choices can have serious consequences for health, both in the short and long term. Policies to promote healthy choices must address not only individual adolescents, but also the family, school, and community contexts that shape adolescents' lives.

Data on adolescent health status show promising and discouraging news. Although trends have improved in many areas, concerns remain. Some encouraging trends appear to be leveling off—for example, homicide and suicide rates have changed little since the late 1990s and may be increasing.[2] As with the general population, rates of overweight and obesity are rapidly increasing. One in 5 adolescents experiences at least minor impairment due to mental or addictive disorders.[3] Large disparities persist in many areas, including disparities by race/ethnicity, gender, and income. Despite a 45% decrease in the homicide rate for black adolescent males between 1995 and 2005, they still have a rate 4 times that of all 15- to 19-year-old males.[2] American Indians/Alaskan Natives and whites continue to smoke at higher rates: 17% and 16% of 12- to 17-year-olds, respectively, reported past-month smoking, compared to 12% overall, in 2007.[4] These disparities point to the importance of recognizing and responding to the increasing diversity of America's youth. In young adulthood, these disparities persist and indicators for most areas of adolescent health worsen.[5] For example, 23% of 18- to 25-year-olds report drinking and driving, more than 7 times the rate for 12- to 17-year-olds (3%).[4]

Health policies can play a critical role in improving adolescent health, including policies that increase access to health care services. Ideally, services can help adolescents enter adulthood with the capacity to engage in healthy behaviors, avoid health-damaging behaviors, and negotiate the health care system as needed to manage their health. To be effective, the health care system must also deliver culturally competent care to meet the needs of an increasingly diverse adolescent population.

Health care services are particularly important for those with chronic conditions. Adolescents experience many conditions, ranging from mobility impairment to mental health and learning disorders, and, increasingly, obesity. Estimates of the size of the population for all children with special health care needs have ranged from 31%, where broad criteria are used, to 6%, where more restrictive definitions are used;[6] within the narrow range of 12- to 17-year-olds, 19% of youth have special health care needs.[7] Some conditions require complex, coordinated care. To ensure optimal functioning and well-being in adulthood, it is critical that these adolescents learn to manage their own health and health care as they transition to adulthood.

Several national organizations and agencies have created frameworks and recommendations to guide policy makers. One example is the 21 Critical Health Objectives for adolescents and young adults, identified by a national panel as part of *Healthy People 2010*, the nation's public health agenda (Box 21-1). In follow-up, 2 federal agencies—the Health Resources and Services Administration's Maternal and Child Health Bureau's Office of Adolescent Health, and the Centers for Disease Control and Prevention Division of Adolescent and School Health, have joined forces to create the National Initiative to Improve Adolescent and Young Adult Health. The initiative's goals include reducing health

**Box 21-1**

**Healthy People 2010 *21 Critical Health Objectives for Adolescents and Young Adults***

**Mortality**

- Overall death

**Unintentional Injury**

- Motor vehicle deaths
- Alcohol- and drug-related motor vehicle deaths and injuries
- Safety belt use
- Riding with a driver who has been drinking alcohol

**Violence**

- Homicide
- Physical fighting
- Weapon carrying

**Substance Abuse and Mental Health**

- Binge drinking
- Use of illicit substances (marijuana)
- Suicide deaths
- Suicide attempts that required medical attention
- Children and adolescents with disabilities who are sad, unhappy, or depressed
- Treatment among children with mental health problems

**Reproductive Health**

- Pregnancy
- HIV/AIDS diagnoses
- Chlamydia trachomatis infections
- Not sexually experienced/active or used condom

**Chronic Diseases**

- Tobacco
- Overweight or obese
- Vigorous physical activity

Source: Centers for Disease Control and Prevention, National Center for Chronic Disease Prevention and Health Promotion, Division of Adolescent and School Health. 21 Critical Objectives for Adolescent and Young Adult Health. Available at: cdc.gov/HealthyYouth/AdolescentHealth/NationalInitiative/pdf/21objectives.pdf. Accessed March 2006.

disparities and improving access to health care services, as well as achieving the 21 Critical Health Objectives.[8] Another example includes the many recommendations by professional medical associations. In 2004, the Society for Adolescent Medicine (SAM) issued an updated position paper on "Access to Health Care for Adolescents and Young Adults." That paper outlines 10 elements of high-quality, comprehensive health care for this age group: (1) health insurance coverage, (2) comprehensive coordinated benefits, (3) safety net providers and programs, (4) quality of care, (5) affordability, (6) consent and confidentiality, (7) compensation, (8) availability of trained and experienced health care providers, (9) visibility and flexibility of adolescent-oriented sites and services, and (10) coordination.[9] Despite the need for comprehensive and coordinated services, the health care system that finances and delivers these services is complex and fragmented, especially for those who are lower income or have special health care needs. A 2007 Institute of Medicine report, *Challenges in Adolescent Health Care,* identified 4 elements of a health care system that would serve adolescents well:

1. The system is adequately financed.
2. Adolescents have the skills to negotiate the system.
3. Preventable problems are prevented.
4. Chronic conditions are effectively managed and the transition to adult care is ensured.[10]

## HEALTH CARE EXPENDITURES AND UTILIZATION

Adolescents use health care services less frequently than adults, resulting in *per capita* expenditures about a third that of adults (about $799 vs $2,343 in 1997 dollars).[11] Dental services, physician ambulatory services, and inpatient hospital stays accounted for more than three-quarters of expenditures, whereas prescription medicine, ambulatory nonphysician services, and other services accounted for about a quarter of expenses in 1997 (Figure 21-1).[11] Expenditures vary among subpopulations. Adolescents from higher-income families have higher expenditures.[11,12] Not surprisingly, adolescents with disabilities also have higher expenditures accounting for only 4% of all adolescents, but 14% of all expenditures on adolescents.[11]

### TYPES OF HEALTH CARE VISITS

Reflecting their relatively low rates of disease and chronic conditions, primary care services dominate adolescents' health care utilization. Most adolescents depend on outpatient care. In 2005, most (87%) adolescents ages 12 to 17 in the United States had contact with a health care professional in the preceding year, and more than two-thirds (69%) had seen a provider within the previous 6 months.[13] Doctor's offices and health maintenance

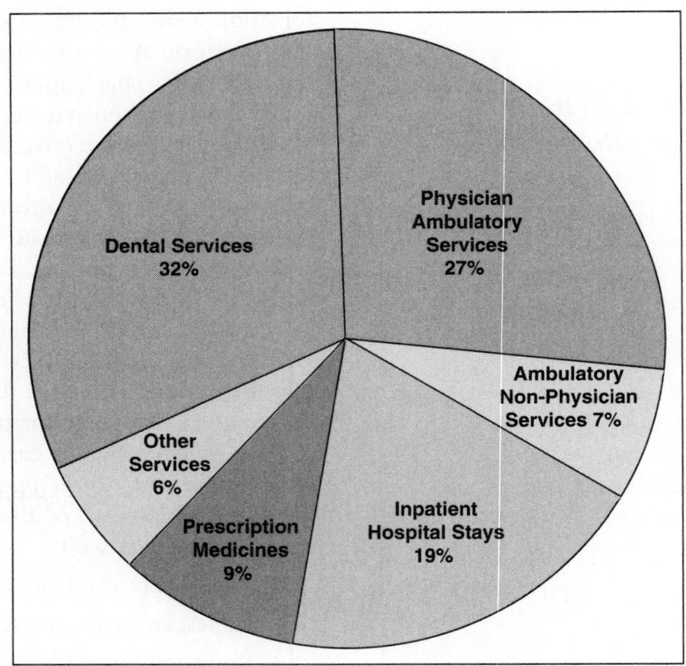


**FIGURE 21-1** Health care expenditures by type of services, ages 10–18, 1997. (Reprinted from Newacheck PW, Wong ST, Galbraith AA, Hung YY. Adolescent health care expenditures: a descriptive profile. *J Adolesc Health.* 2003;32:3–11, with permission from Elsevier.)

organizations (HMOs) serve as the most common source of usual care for adolescents, although nonpoor adolescents 13 to 17 years old are more likely to report this than poor adolescents (82% vs 68%). More than a quarter of poor adolescents ages 13 to 17 (28%) used a clinic or health center.[14] Relatively few adolescents are hospitalized, and adolescents account for a relatively small percentage of all hospital stays (<4%).[15] Pregnancy-related diagnoses are the leading cause of hospitalization, followed by injury and mental health diagnoses.[16] About 1 in 14 adolescents (5%) 12 to 17 years old had 2 or more visits to an emergency department (ED) in the past year.[13] Injury-related trauma is the most common ED diagnosis.[17]

## ADOLESCENTS WITH SPECIAL HEALTH CARE NEEDS

Children and adolescents with special health care needs use health care services, including inpatient and outpatient services, at higher rates than their peers without such needs. This population reports an average of 4.4 physician visits annually and 6.9 prescribed medications, compared with 1.8 and 1.2, respectively, for those without special needs. Hospitalization rates are also much higher among this population (89 vs 22 per 1,000).[7]

## DENTAL VISITS

Although most adolescents receive recommended visits, such as annual well visits and routine/preventive dental visits, many adolescents have unmet health needs; the poor and those with special health care needs are more likely to go without needed care. Professional organizations recommend an annual well visit and regular preventive dental visits.[18,19] A large percentage of adolescents have had a well visit in the prior year (66%).[20] National estimates of past-year routine/preventive dental visits vary widely, from 54% (for ages 13 to 17)[21] to 81% (for ages 12 to 17).[22] National data show great disparity by income. According to 2002 data, only 31% of adolescents in "poor" (income <100% of the federal poverty level: <$20,444 for a family of 4 in 2006) and "near-poor" (income 100%–200% of the federal poverty level: <$40,888) families received any dental service in the past year, compared to 52% of adolescents in families with higher incomes.[12] Unmet dental needs are common in adolescence. Untreated tooth decay is reported for 16% of 12- to 15-year-olds and 22% of 16- to 19-year-olds. Among 6- to 19-year-olds, those in poor families have more than twice the rate of untreated tooth decay as those from higher-income families (20% vs 8%).[23]

### MENTAL HEALTH VISITS

Data on treatment for mental health and substance abuse problems are more limited. Using a broad definition of mental health treatment, the 2004 National Survey on Drug Use and Health (NSDUH) estimates that 23% of 12- to 17-year-olds received treatment or counseling for emotional or behavioral problems in the preceding year. Asian youths were the least likely to report treatment (10%), whereas the rate for all other racial/ethnic groups ranged from 22% to 25%. More girls than boys 16 or 17 years old reported receiving treatment (27% vs 17%). The survey showed only slight differences by age group, income, and region of the United States.[24] The NSDUH estimates that 185,000 youths 12 to 17 years old received treatment at a specialty facility for illicit drug or alcohol abuse or dependence, a figure representing 8% of those needing treatment.[25]

### FOREGONE HEALTH CARE

Data on self-reported foregone care also suggest significant unmet need. Nearly 1 in 5 (19%) adolescents report foregone care, defined as not receiving care that adolescents thought "they should get." This figure is higher among certain adolescent populations. More than a third (35%) of adolescents with disabilities reported foregone care. Corresponding figures of foregone care for other conditions and risk factors include: frequent alcohol users, 30%; frequent smokers, 26%; sexually active adolescents, 25%; and overweight adolescents, 22%.[26]

## POLICIES SHAPING ACCESS TO CARE

Several factors influence an adolescent's ability to access health care. Among the most significant are policies related to insurance coverage of services and the ability of adolescents to seek health care on their own. In addition, policies related to quality of care can help to improve services that are provided by ensuring that certain standards are followed.

### INSURANCE OVERVIEW AND TRENDS

As with people of any age, ability to pay for services is a major factor influencing access to health care services for adolescents. Health insurance is strongly correlated with many indicators of access, with insured adolescents more likely to have a past-year visit, a usual source of care, and fewer unmet needs (Figure 21-2).[27-31] For example, in 2005 70% of adolescents 12 to 17 years old with full-year insurance coverage had a well visit in the previous year, compared to only 45% of adolescents with no or part-year coverage. Most adolescents (87%) had full-year insurance, according to these data: 66% had

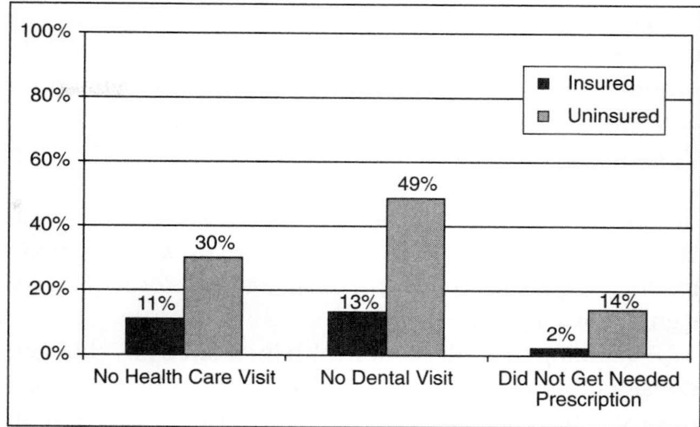


FIGURE 21-2 Access to care by insurance status (selected indicators), ages 12–17, 2005. (Data from Public Policy Analysis and Education Center for Middle Childhood, Adolescent, and Young Adult Health. National Health Interview Survey, 2005 [private data run].)

private insurance, primarily employer-sponsored; 20% had public insurance; and a small 1% had both public and private coverage.[20] By contrast, in 2003 only 77% of adolescents 12 to 17 years old had dental coverage.[22]

### MEDICAID AND STATE CHILDREN'S HEALTH INSURANCE PROGRAM (SCHIP)

Health care policies reflect the federal and incremental approaches that shape many US policies.[1] Medicaid and the State Children's Health Insurance Program (SCHIP), the primary sources of public coverage, are both federal–state programs that incrementally increase access to care for children and adolescents. Under the Medicaid program, established in 1965, the federal government matches state health care expenditures using a formula that varies by state. The program sets minimum benefits package and eligibility criteria and other regulations (eg, copayment restrictions). States have fairly wide latitude in expanding both benefits and eligibility criteria. Pathways to Medicaid eligibility are complex, involving a combination of income, condition, and participation in other social programs. For example, children and adolescents are generally automatically eligible for Medicaid if they qualify for the Supplemental Security Income (SSI) program, which supports low-income children and adolescents with disabilities. Over the past decade, to give states greater flexibility in administering their Medicaid programs, the federal government has allowed states to waive certain federal requirements. The Deficit Reduction Act, passed by Congress in 2006, allows states even more options with respect to federal requirements.[32]

The State Children's Health Insurance Program was established in the United States in 1997 to provide funding for states to extend insurance to poor children and adolescents. The State Children's Health Insurance Program is even more flexible than Medicaid, allowing states to use funds to expand their Medicaid program or create a separate program.[33] Because of the wide latitude that Medicaid and SCHIP gives states, public insurance programs for children and adolescents vary significantly by state.

Financing of adolescent health insurance has changed considerably over the past 15 years, reflecting 2 broad trends: a decrease in private coverage and an increase in public coverage. From 1989 to 2002 the percentage of adolescents with private coverage decreased from 73% to 65%. Over the same period, the percentage of adolescents with public coverage increased from 10% to 22%. Overall, the increase in public coverage has slightly offset the decrease in private coverage during this period, resulting in a small increase in coverage: from 86% to 88%.[34] The decline in private insurance is largely due to growth in the price of premium costs, as well as the increase in small and self-employed firms, which are less likely to provide insurance, and the decrease in larger firms more likely to provide insurance.[35] The increase in public insurance can be traced to 2 major federal initiatives. First, Congress enacted a series of Medicaid mandates from the mid-1980s to early 1990s, eventually requiring states to raise the income eligibility to cover all poor adolescents in 2001. Second, SCHIP's establishment in 1997 allowed many states to cover more poor and near-poor children and adolescents.[33]

## DISPARITIES IN HEALTH INSURANCE

### Hispanics

Although the insurance trend is encouraging, significant disparities in insurance remain. Hispanic adolescents are less likely to be insured compared to their white, non-Hispanic and black, non-Hispanic peers (75% vs 91% and 87%, respectively). Although Medicaid expansions and SCHIP have helped, only 77% of poor and near-poor adolescents are insured, compared to nearly 93% of adolescents from higher-income families.[20]

### Young Adults

Recent literature has highlighted the difficulties that adolescents face in securing insurance as they transition to young adulthood. In the late teen years, many adolescents lose eligibility for their family's employer-based insurance and/or Medicaid and SCHIP. According to 2002–2003 data, the percentage of young people without insurance more than doubled across increasing age from 9% for 17- or 18-year-olds, to 17% for 19- or 20-year-olds, to 23% for 21- to 22-year-olds.[36] Those adolescents and young adults who are not full-time students are particularly affected during this transition. Among those 19 to 23 years old in 2008, 39% of "non full-time students" lacked insurance compared to 17% of full-time students.[37]

### Adolescents with Special Health Care Needs

Securing insurance poses greater challenges for certain groups of adolescents, such as adolescents with special health care needs (ASHCN) and those in foster care. Although some mechanisms allow continuous coverage for these vulnerable groups in the late teen years, pathways to eligibility are complex and vary by state. Youth in the foster care system have a higher prevalence of physical and mental health problems. Most of these youth qualify for Medicaid by virtue of their foster care status but often lose eligibility at age 18, just as they lose support from the foster care system. Whereas some states take advantage of Medicaid options to extend coverage to age 21, most foster care youth in their late teens are left to negotiate the transition to adulthood without insurance coverage.[38] Similarly, ASHCN must contend with an array of state and federal laws that vary by condition and income. Many qualify for Medicaid through their participation in the children's SSI program. At age 18, adolescents must meet criteria for adult SSI to stay in the program. An estimated one-third of these adolescents fail to meet adult SSI criteria, which in turn jeopardizes their Medicaid eligibility.[39,40]

## UNDERINSURANCE: COST-SHARING AND BENEFITS

Although insurance coverage increases access, it does not ensure that adolescents actually obtain needed services. Copayments, for example, can pose barriers to care. Research on the general Medicaid population suggests that copayments deter the poor from securing basic services, which can lead to more expensive care, such as ED use and hospitalization.[41] Medicaid traditionally has not allowed copayments for recipients under age 18. However, the 2006 Deficit Reduction Act (DRA) law allows cost-sharing for some groups of children. Cost-sharing in the SCHIP program is capped at 5% of family income.[42]

Limited benefit packages also impede access to needed services, particularly services related to mental health and substance abuse disorders. In March 2006, the AAP proposed a comprehensive benefits package for the pediatric population.[43] The recommended benefits include many services relevant for adolescents, such as health supervision, reproductive health services, services for mental health problems and substance use disorders, and services for children and adolescents with special health care needs. A 2003 analysis of major private insurance plans in 48 states found inadequate coverage of many of these recommended services, including mental/behavioral health services such as treatment for anorexia nervosa and substance abuse.[44]

The 2 major public programs, Medicaid and SCHIP, differ tremendously in their respective benefits packages. In 1967, the federal government added a broad benefit to the Medicaid program, designed to promote healthy development. Titled Early and Periodic Screening, Diagnosis, and Treatment (EPSDT), this benefit offers children covered by Medicaid periodic screening to identify problems. State Medicaid programs are mandated to cover any services needed to rectify problems uncovered in the screen, whether or not the service is covered by a state's Medicaid program. Entitled Early and Periodic Screening, Diagnosis, and Treatment covers a range of services such as physical, occupational, and speech therapy, respiratory care, and mental health services, making the benefit particularly important for youth with disabilities. Adolescents who retain Medicaid eligibility at age 18 lose this benefit—a change that poses challenges to adolescents managing chronic conditions in the transition to young adulthood. The State Children's Health Insurance Program allows states considerable flexibility in defining the benefits package. By contrast, states have not been allowed to waive Medicaid's EPSDT benefit. In a major policy change, the DRA allows states to offer its Medicaid beneficiaries a "benchmark plan" (eg, a standard benefits package of a state's major insurer). If that plan's benefit does not include services that would have been covered by EPSDT, the law requires states to provide for "wrap-around coverage" to make coverage the equivalent of EPSDT. It is unclear how access to EPSDT services will be affected by this policy change.[32,45,46]

Underinsurance can pose special hardships for the ASHCN population. Among ASHCN with continuous past-year coverage, in 2001, 29% were classified as underinsured, by virtue of parent-reported inadequate coverage of benefits, costs, and/or providers. Those with inadequate insurance are more likely to report consequences affecting family finances and ability to access care.[47,48] About 1 in 5 youth with special health care needs are reported to have at least 1 unmet need (19%), difficulty receiving referrals for specialty care (23%), and family financial problems caused by the youth's health care needs (22%).[49]

## CONSENT AND CONFIDENTIALITY

In addition to the financing issues that affect access to care for people of all ages, the ability to consent to confidential services plays a special role for adolescents. Unlike younger children, adolescents are much more likely to need services for sensitive issues such as sexuality, sexually transmitted infections (STIs), substance use, and mental health. Research indicates that adolescents will forego needed care if confidentiality is not ensured.[50] Numerous medical and other professional associations, including the AMA, the American Academy of Family Practitioners (AAFP), the AAP, and SAM, support access to confidential care.[51] (See Chapter 11, Legal and Ethical Issues in Adolescent Health Care, for more information about consent and confidentiality.) The ability to secure confidential services encompasses 2 legal concepts: consent, the authority to seek services; and confidentiality, the guarantee that they will remain confidential. Reflecting the federal–state nature of US policies, consent and confidentiality laws vary tremendously by state. All states have some laws that allow adolescents to consent to care. These laws vary by type of service (eg, contraceptive care, substance abuse treatment) and status of the minor (eg, married, not residing with parents). At the federal level, regulations issued in 2002 about access to health care records (resulting from the 1996 Health Insurance Portability and Accountability Act) essentially reaffirm state confidentiality protections.[52]

In recent years, there have been legislative and regulatory attempts to repeal confidentiality laws, particularly laws relating to reproductive health services. This includes efforts to interpret mandatory reporting of abuse as requiring clinicians to report consensual sexual activity among adolescents.[53] A position paper issued jointly by SAM, AAP, AAFP, and the American College of Obstetricians–Gynecologists (ACOG) argued against these efforts, stating that existing abuse reporting laws are sufficient and increased reporting requirements may impede the delivery of needed confidential health care to adolescents involved in consensual sexual relationships. Outside the legal and regulatory realm, confidentiality can also be hampered by clinical practices, inability or unwillingness to offer confidential care, and billing procedures that inform parents of services received.[52]

## OPPORTUNITIES: QUALITY OF CARE INITIATIVES

Quality of care has received increasing national attention since the early 1990s, with several private organizations and public agencies creating measures to assess the performance of clinicians, health plans, and managed care organizations.[54] Initiatives addressing adolescents focus largely on preventive care.[55] The Health Plan Employer Data and Information Set (HEDIS), a widely used performance measurement tool, includes measures for adolescents that emphasize clinical preventive services. Measures include annual well visits that include anticipatory guidance, adolescent immunization, and chlamydia screening in sexually active females.[54,55] (Chapter 9, Physical Examination and Laboratory Testing, provides more information about preventive services). The Child and Adolescent Health Measurement Initiative has examined broader measures; researchers developed and tested an instrument measuring the provision of clinical preventive services, such as screening and counseling related to smoking, diet, weight, exercise, and emotional health.[56] Because quality of care provided to adolescents is also related to the training of professionals who render such care, the Institute of Medicine's Board on Children, Youth, and Families has recently emphasized that young people are best served by providers who understand the key developmental features, health issues, and overall social environment of adolescents (www.bocyf.org/ahc_brief.pdf; accessed September 12, 2009).

## OTHER HEALTH POLICIES

Policies outside the health care system, such as policies to reduce risky behaviors, can have a direct affect on adolescent health. These policies involve far fewer expenses than health care policies, yet still improve adolescent health outcomes. As with health care financing, these policies include state and federal roles in policymaking. In addition, public debates often involve issues of civil rights and liberties pertaining to minors. A key challenge is to create laws and regulations that reflect adolescents' developmental needs while recognizing the appropriate role of families, schools, and other institutions. Two areas of adolescent health related to such policies are: motor vehicle injury and sexuality. Other policies addressing areas such as violence, diet, exercise, substance use, and mental health have been less clearly defined.[57]

### Motor Vehicle Crashes and Graduated Driver's Licensing

Motor vehicle crashes are the leading cause of death in adolescence and young adulthood, accounting for 32% of mortality for 10- to 19-year-olds in 2005.[2] Fatal crashes among teens are more likely to occur at night and with multiple teen passengers. To address these risks, almost all states have adopted graduated driver's licensing (GDL), which phases in driving privileges, usually using a 3-stage process: (1) a learner's stage, where teens are supervised by adult licensed drivers; (2) an intermediate stage, often involving passenger and nighttime restrictions on unsupervised driving; and (3) full licensure. State GDL laws vary considerably from state to state in the length of each phase, the night hour restrictions, and the number of teenage passengers permitted. In some states, police are prohibited from stopping teens solely for violation of restrictions (secondary enforcement).[58] Evaluation of GDL programs demonstrates significant reduction in adolescent crash fatalities.[59] In addition, all 50 states have "zero alcohol tolerance" laws, making it illegal for those under age 21 to drive with any measurable amount of alcohol in their blood.[60]

### Adolescent Sexual Behavior

Adolescent sexual behavior has important implications for health and health care services. Rates of STIs peak in the late teen and young adult years and childbirth is by far the leading cause of adolescent hospitalization. Policies to address adolescent reproductive health frequently stir controversy. In addition to issues of confidential care raised earlier, policy makers have debated the role of abstinence and safer sex in sexuality education. Professional medical associations, including SAM, the AAP, and the AMA, recommend a "comprehensive" approach that includes abstinence as well as information about contraception and STI and HIV/AIDS prevention.[61-63] Evaluation research has identified comprehensive programs that delay adolescents' initiation of sexual relations and increase the use of protection. Moreover, research has consistently shown that information about safer sex does not increase adolescent sexual activity.[64]

## SUMMARY

Although adolescents tend to be relatively healthy on traditional measures of population health, neither health policy nor health financing is necessarily in alignment with prevention efforts related to the health risk behaviors in which some adolescents engage. Health policies can play a critical role in improving adolescent health, including those that increase access to, and reimbursement for, health care services, including those for immunizations and for chronic conditions. Such policies need to address not only individual adolescents but also the family, school, and community contexts that shape the lives of adolescents.

## REFERENCES

1. Brindis C, Ott M. Adolescents, health policy, and the American political process. *J Adolesc Health.* 2002;30:9–16

2. National Center for Injury Prevention and Control. Fatal injuries mortality reports [online database]. Available at: www.cdc.gov/ncipc/wisqars/default.htm. Accessed January 15, 2009

3. United States Public Health Service, Office of the Surgeon General. *Mental Health: A Report of the Surgeon General.* Rockville, MD: DHHS, US Public Health Service; 1999

4. Substance Abuse and Mental Health Services Administration. Results from the 2007 National Survey on Drug Use and Health: national findings. Available at: www.drugabusestatistics.samhsa.gov/nsduh.htm. Accessed January 15, 2009

5. Park MJ, Paul Mulye T, Adams S, Brindis CD, Irwin CE Jr. The health status of young adults in the US. *J Adolesc Health.* 2006;39:305–317

6. Newacheck P, Halfon N. Prevalence and impact of disabling chronic conditions in childhood. *Am J Public Health.* 1998;88:610–617. Taken from: *Pediatrics.* 2002;110(6):1315–1321

7. Newacheck P, Kim S. A national profile of health care utilization and expenditures for children with special health care needs. *Arch Pediatr Adolesc Med.* 2005;159:10–17

8. Centers for Disease Control and Prevention, National Center for Chronic Disease Prevention and Health Promotion, Division of Adolescent and School Health; Health Resources and Services Administration, Maternal and Child Health Bureau, Office of Adolescent Health; National Adolescent Health Information Center, University of California, San Francisco. *Improving the Health of Adolescents and Young Adults: A Guide for States and Communities*. Atlanta, GA: Centers for Disease Control and Prevention; 2004

9. Morreale MC, Kapphahn CJ, Elster AB, Juszczak L, Klein JD. Access to health care for adolescents and young adults: position paper of the Society for Adolescent Medicine. *J Adolesc Health.* 2004;35(4):342–344

10. Institute of Medicine. *Challenges in adolescent health care*. Workshop report. Washington, DC: The National Academies Press; 2007

11. Newacheck PW, Wong ST, Galbraith AA, Hung YY. Adolescent health care expenditures: a descriptive profile. *J Adolesc Health.* 2003;32(suppl 6):3–11

12. Simpson L, Owens PL, Zodet MW, et al. Health care for children and youth in the United States: annual report on patterns of coverage, utilization, quality, and expenditures by income. *Ambul Pediatr.* 2005;5:6–44

13. Bloom B, Dey AN, Freeman G. Summary health statistics for US children: National Health Interview Survey, 2005. *Vital Health Stat.* 2006;10(231):1–90. Available at: www.cdc.gov/nchs/data/series/sr_10/sr10_231.pdf. Accessed February 27, 2007

14. Maternal and Child Health Bureau. Child Health USA 2002. Rockville, MD: US Department of Health and Human Services, 2002. Available at: www.mchb.hrsa.gov/chusa02/main_pages/page_03.htm. Accessed August 7, 2006

15. Kozak LJ, Hall MJ, Owings MF. National Hospital Discharge Survey: 2000 annual summary with detailed diagnosis and procedure data. *Vital Health Stat.* 2002;13(153):1–194. Available at: www.cdc.gov/nchs/data/series/sr_13/sr13_153.pdf. Accessed December 6, 2006

16. MacKay AP, Fingerhut LA, Duran CR. *Adolescent Health Chartbook. Health, United States, 2000.* Hyattsville, MD: National Center for Health Statistics; 2000. Available at: www.cdc.gov/nchs/data/hus/hus00.pdf. Accessed April 27, 2010

17. Medical Expenditure Panel Survey. Summary data tables, household component summary tables [online tables]. Available at: www.meps.ahrq.gov/mepsweb/data_stats/quick_tables.jsp. Accessed April 27, 2010

18. Elster AB. Comparison of recommendations for adolescent clinical preventive services developed by national organizations. *Arch Pediatr Adolesc Med.* 1998;152:193–198

19. American Academy of Pediatric Dentistry. Reference manual 2005–2006, clinical guidelines: guideline on periodicity of examination, preventive dental services, anticipatory guidance, and oral treatment for children. Available at: www.aapd.org/media/Policies_Guidelines/G_Periodicity.pdf. Accessed February 28, 2007

20. Public Policy Analysis and Education Center for Middle Childhood, Adolescent, and Young Adult Health. National Health Interview Survey, 2005 [private data run]. Available at: www.cdc.gov/nchs/nhis.htm. Accessed March 2, 2006

21. Chu M. *Children's Dental Care: Periodicity of Checkups and Access to Care, 2003* [statistical brief 113]. Rockville, MD: Medical Expenditure Panel Survey, Agency for Healthcare Research and Quality; 2006. Available at: www.meps.ahrq.gov/mepsweb/data_files/publications/st113/stat113.pdf. Accessed December 6, 2006

22. Liu J, Probst JC, Martin AB, Wang J, Salinas CF. Disparities in dental insurance coverage and dental care among US children: The National Survey of Children's Health. *Pediatrics.* 2007;119:S12–S21

23. National Center for Chronic Disease Prevention and Health Promotion, Centers for Disease Control and Prevention. Fact Sheet: Key Findings from NHANES 1999–2002. Surveillance for Dental Caries, Dental Sealants, Tooth Retention, Edentulism, and Enamel Fluorosis, United States, 1988–1994 and 1999–2002. Available at: www.cdc.gov/mmwr/preview/mmwrhtml/ss5403a1.htm. Accessed August 9, 2010

24. Substance Abuse and Mental Health Services Administration. Results from the 2004 National Survey on Drug Use and Health: national findings. Available at: www.drugabusestatistics.samhsa.gov/nsduh.htm. Accessed December 7, 2006

25. Substance Abuse and Mental Health Services Administration. Substance use treatment need among adolescents: 2003–2004. *The NSDUH Report.* 2006;24:1–3

26. Ford CA, Bearman PS, Moody J. Foregone health care among adolescents. *JAMA.* 1999;282(233):2227–2234

27. Newacheck PW, Brindis CD, Cart CU, Marchi K, Irwin CE Jr. Adolescent health insurance coverage: recent changes and access to care. *Pediatrics.* 1999;104(2):195–202

28. Blackwell DL, Tonthat L. Summary health statistics for US children: National Health Interview Survey, 1998. *Vital and Health Stat.* 2002;10(208):1–45

29. Newacheck PW, McManus MA. Health insurance status of adolescents in the United States. *Pediatrics.* 1989;84(4):699–708

30. Newacheck PW, McManus MA, Brindis CD. Financing health care for adolescents: problems, prospects, and proposals. *J Adolesc Health Care.* 1990;11:398–403

31. Bartman BA, Moy E, D'Angelo LJ. Access to ambulatory care for adolescents: the role of a usual source of care. *J Health Care Poor Underserved.* 1997;8(2):214–226

32. Rosenbaum S, Markus A. *The Deficit Reduction Act of 2005: An Overview of Key Medicaid Provisions and Their Implications for Early Childhood Development Services.* New York, NY: The Commonwealth Fund; 2006. Available at: www.commonwealthfund.org/Content/Publications/Fund-Reports/2006/Oct/The-Deficit-Reduction-Act-of-2005-An-Overview-of-Key-Medicaid-Provisions-and-Their-Implications-for.aspx. Accessed August 9, 2010

33. Mann C, Rowland D, Garfield R. Historical overview of children's health care coverage. *Future Child.* 2003;13:31-53

34. Newacheck PW, Park MJ, Brindis CD, Biehl M, Irwin CE Jr. Trends in private and public health insurance for adolescents. *JAMA.* 2004;291(10):1231-1237

35. Holahan J, Cook A. Why did the number of uninsured continue to increase in 2005? Available at: www.kff.org/uninsured/upload/7571.pdf. Accessed December 3, 2006

36. Adams S, Newacheck P, Park MJ, Brindis CD, Irwin CE Jr. Health insurance across vulnerable ages: patterns and disparities from adolescence to the early 30's. *Pediatrics.* 2007;119(5);e1033-1039

37. Kriss JL, Collins SR, Mahato B, Gould E, Schoen C. Rite of passage? Why young adults become uninsured and how new policies can help, 2008 update. Available at: www.commonwealthfund.org/publications/publications_show.htm?doc_id=687669. Accessed January 15, 2009

38. English E, Stinnett AJ, Dunn-Georgiou E. *Health Care for Adolescents and Young Adults Leaving Foster Care: Policy Options for Improving Access.* Chapel Hill, NC: Center for Adolescent Health and the Law; San Francisco, CA: Public Policy Analysis and Education Center for Middle Childhood, Adolescent and Young Adult Health; 2006. Available at: www.cahl.org/PDFs/FCIssueBrief.pdf. Accessed December 7, 2006

39. Schulzinger R. *Youth with Disabilities in Transition: Health Insurance Options and Obstacles.* Gainesville, FL: Center for Policy and Partnerships, Institute for Child Health Policy; 2000. Available at: hctransitions.ichp.ufl.edu/policypapers/HealthInsuranceOptions.pdf. Accessed December 7, 2006

40. Bazelon Center for Mental Health Law. Moving on: An analysis of federal programs funding services for transition-age youth with serious mental health conditions. Available at: bazelon.org.gravitatehosting.com/LinkClick.aspx?fileticket=8Vesx_bWHBA%3d&tabid=104. Accessed August 9, 2010

41. Ku L, Wachino V. The effect of increased cost-sharing in Medicaid: a summary of research findings. Available at: www.cbpp.org/cms/?fa=view&id=321. Accessed April 27, 2010

42. Herz EJ. Medicaid cost-sharing under the Deficit Reduction Act of 2005 (DRA). Available at: file.wikileaks.org/file/crs/RS22578.pdf. Accessed August 9, 2010

43. American Academy of Pediatrics, Committee on Child Health Financing. Scope of health care benefits for children from birth through age 21. *Pediatrics.* 2006;117(3):979-982

44. Fox HB, McManus MA, Reichman MB. Private health insurance for adolescents: is it adequate? *J Adolesc Health.* 2003;32S:12-24

45. Rosenbaum S. Defined-contribution plans and limited-benefit arrangements: implications for Medicaid beneficiaries. Available at: www.gwumc.edu/sphhs/departments/healthpolicy/dhp_publications/pub_uploads/dhpPublication_5FCF8F52-5056-9D20-3D3E46549325343E.pdf. Accessed August 9, 2010

46. Williams B, Tolbert J. Aging out of EPSDT: issues for young adults with disabilities. Available at: www.kff.org/medicaid/upload/7491.pdf. Accessed December 7, 2006

47. Kogan MD, Newacheck PW, Honberg L, Strickland B. Association between underinsurance and access to care among children with special health care needs in the United States. *Pediatrics.* 2005;116(5):1162-1169

48. Honberg L, McPherson M, Strickland B, Gage JC, Newacheck PW. Assuring adequate health insurance: results of the National Survey of Children with Special Health Care Needs. *Pediatrics.* 2005;115(5):1233-1239

49. van Dyck PC, Kogan MD, McPherson MG, Weissman GR, Newacheck PW. Prevalence and characteristics of children with special health care needs. *Arch Pediatr Adolesc Med.* 2004;158:884-890

50. English A, Ford CA. More evidence supports the need to protect confidentiality in adolescent health care. *J Adolesc Health.* 2007;40:199-200

51. Morreale MC, Stinnett AJ, Downling EC, eds. *Policy Compendium on Confidential Health Services for Adolescents.* 2nd ed. Chapel Hill, NC: Center for Adolescent Health and the Law; 2005. Available at: www.cahl.org/web/index.php/policy-compendium-2005. Accessed April 27, 2010

52. Ford C, English A, Sigman G. Confidential health care for adolescents: position paper of the Society for Adolescent Medicine. *J Adolesc Health.* 2004;35:160-167

53. American Academy of Family Physicians, American Academy of Pediatrics, American College of Obstetricians and Gynecologists, and Society for Adolescent Medicine. Protecting adolescents: ensuring access to care and reporting sexual activity and abuse. *J Adolesc Health.* 2004;35:420-423

54. Brindis C, VanLandeghem K, Kirkpatrick R, Macdonald T, Lee S. *Adolescents and the State Children's Health Insurance Program (CHIP): Healthy Options for Meeting the Needs of Adolescents.* Washington, DC: Association of Maternal and Child Health Programs; San Francisco, CA: University of California, Policy Information and Analysis Center for Middle Childhood and Adolescence; and National Adolescent Health Information Center; 1999. Available at: policy.ucsf.edu/pubpdfs/SCHIP.pdf. Accessed February 27, 2007

55. Chung PJ, Lee TC, Morrison JL, Schuster MA. Preventive care for children in the United States: quality and barriers. *Ann Rev Public Health.* 2006;27:491-515

56. Bethell C, Klein J, Peck C. Assessing health system provision of adolescent preventive services: the Young Adult Health Care Survey. *Medical Care.* 2001;39(5):478-490

57. Public Policy Analysis and Education Center for Middle Childhood, Adolescent, and Young Adult Health. Tracking adolescent, health policy: an annotated list, 2008 update. Available

at: policy.ucsf.edu/pubpdfs/TrackingPolicy2008.pdf. Accessed January 15, 2009

58. Insurance Institute for Highway Safety. US licensing systems for young drivers. Available at: www.iihs.org/laws/state_laws/grad_license.html. Accessed February 27, 2007

59. Williams AF. Next steps for graduated licensing. *Traffic Injury Prevention.* 2005;6:199–201

60. National Highway Traffic Safety Administration. Alcohol and highway safety, 2001: a review of the state of knowledge. Available at: www.nhtsa.dot.gov/people/injury/research/AlcoholHighway/. Accessed March 2, 2007

61. American Academy of Pediatrics, Committee on Psychosocial Aspects of Child and Family Health, and Committee on Adolescence. Sexuality education for children and adolescents. *Pediatrics.* 2001;108(2):498–502

62. Santelli J, Ott MA, Lyon M, Rogers J, Summers D. Abstinence-only education policies and programs: position paper of the Society for Adolescent Medicine. *J Adolesc Health.* 2006;38(1):83–88

63. American Medical Association Council on Scientific Affairs. *Sexuality Education, Abstinence, and Distribution of Condoms in Schools* [Report 7, I-99]. Chicago, IL: American Medical Association; 1999

64. Kirby D. Comprehensive sex education: strong public support and persuasive evidence of impact, but little funding. *Arch Pediatr Adolesc Med.* 2006;160(11):1182–1184

---

*Since this chapter was completed in 2007, the health policy and financing landscape has changed significantly. Major health care reform legislation was enacted in March 2010. The federal Patient Protection and Affordable Care Act includes many provisions that will affect access to health care for adolescents. An analysis issued in August 2010, examines the legislation's provisions in several areas, including financial access, benefit package, adolescent health workforce, and special populations of adolescents and young adults.

The analysis, authored by Abigail English, JD of the Center for Adolescent Health and the Law, in partnership with the National Adolescent Health Information and Innovation Center at the University of California, San Francisco, is available at: nahic.ucsf.edu/downloads/HCR_Issue_Brief_Aug2010_Final_Aug31.pdf.

SECTION 6

# Office-Based Practice

# CHAPTER 22

## The Adolescent-Friendly Practice

ANDREA MARKS, MD

### WHAT IS AN ADOLESCENT-FRIENDLY PRACTICE?

An adolescent-friendly practice setting is a health care office in which adolescents feel at ease and secure to express feelings and beliefs, confident that their needs will be met, and where parents trust the judgment and intentions of the health care provider. Helping an adolescent feel comfortable and safe, and helping parents feel that their child is in good hands requires a complex set of interactions to "click" over time. The appearance of the practice setting, office policies and procedures, and the office personnel contribute to creating a place that is truly adolescent-friendly. Ultimately, the tone and quality of the one-to-one interaction between the teen and the primary health care provider will determine the success of these efforts.

### TRANSITIONING INTO ADOLESCENT/YOUNG ADULT CARE

Most adolescents in the United States receive their health care in the offices of pediatricians or family medicine practitioners. In many cases the health care providers and office staff have known the adolescent since birth. During the early childhood years, the primary relationship and most communication is with the child's parents. In an adolescent-friendly practice, the primary relationship needs to gradually shift toward being with the patient, generally some time during the preteen years, around age 10 to 12.

To emphasize the importance of this transition and to address any questions or concerns it entails, setting aside time for a family meeting with the preteen and parents to go over new "ground rules" is helpful. Probably the most important change that should occur is for the preteen to spend some *time alone with the health care provider* during office visits. This does not mean parents are suddenly totally excluded; the preteen is usually not quite ready for that, and surely the parents are not either. However, time alone between the preteen and health care provider helps the preteen learn to express his or her needs, explain his or her symptoms, and experience an independent relationship with the health care provider.[1,2]

Time alone with the preteen or adolescent requires a *change in the format of office visits*. For example, at a visit for an acute illness such as a sore throat and cough, it is helpful to first meet alone with the patient to take a history and perform an exam, and then invite parents in to review all findings and treatment recommendations. Parents are usually pleasantly surprised to hear how thoroughly their child handled the early part of the visit. If the visit is for an annual checkup, most of the visit should be alone with the patient, again to provide good practice in expressing his or her needs and also because some important issues require privacy to be discussed in a productive way. Generally it works well to meet with parents only at the end of the checkup, but sometimes parents prefer or request time at the beginning of the visit. Giving parents an opportunity to raise concerns early in the visit will avoid a list of problems at the end, when time has run out.

*Flexibility is key.* Many preteens are ready for this level of independence, but some are not. Some parents are proud and pleased to give their child time alone with the provider, but some feel uncomfortable not being present during the history-taking or physical examination. Transitioning into adolescent–young adult care may take several years, but the goal is to help the patient and family feel at ease with and trust the new way of doing things. Working parents may especially welcome the chance for their child to go for health care without them, yet they may appreciate a follow-up phone call later in the day or evening, if warranted.[3]

The most challenging and critical part of transitioning to adolescent care is a discussion with the patient and parents about *privacy and confidentiality*.[4] Private time and space for the patient and health care provider to talk and for the physical examination is not only respectful of the adolescent's autonomy but also fosters openness and connectedness with the provider, which in turn results in far better health care. Parents, however, may be wary of patient confidentiality, the assurance provided to the patient to "not tell" parents what is shared with the provider. And yet, there are many personal matters a teen would not discuss with his or her provider unless confidentiality, as well as privacy, were guaranteed.[5,6] Most parents and teens are comfortable with the concept that private matters may remain confidential unless such a serious situation arises that the teen absolutely needs the help and support of parents. Teens need to feel secure that the health care provider and their parents will not be speaking about them behind their back. This means that communication between the health care provider and parents may remain open, but the teen is consulted ahead of time if such communication must take place because a serious problem has surfaced. Likewise parents should feel free to call the health care provider about a concern they have and the adolescent should be told in advance that such an inquiry will be made. Ultimately, the provider's judgment of the limits to confidentiality considers what is in the best interest of the patient and family. The patient's age and maturity, ability to manage a problem independently, likelihood to follow up with the provider and, most importantly, the degree of seriousness of the matter at hand, factor into the provider's judgment whether to limit confidentiality in a particular clinical situation. Decision-making regarding patient confidentiality is often the most difficult and challenging part of adolescent health care, but because it is so key to a successful patient-provider relationship it is also the most gratifying to work through. Box 22-1 lists important changes involved in the transition into adolescent–young adult health care.

**Box 22-1**

***Key Elements of Transitioning into Adolescent–Young Adult Health Care***

- Time alone with the health care provider
- Change in format of office visits
- Flexibility involving parents
- Privacy and confidentiality

## DESIGNING AN ADOLESCENT-FRIENDLY OFFICE PRACTICE

The decision to create an adolescent-friendly environment within a setting that cares mainly for younger children or a multiage population requires a proactive approach to succeed. Of paramount importance is the realization by the health care provider that he or she *truly likes teens and young adults,* welcomes dealing with their unique set of health needs, and is willing to develop a setting, procedures, and policies that support the concept of providing comprehensive adolescent–young adult health care.[7] Despite the challenges involved, the decision to include a special focus on adolescent health care within a more general practice reaps potentially huge rewards and benefits. Once a teen recognizes the special care and attention he or she is receiving, you will have a friend for life; or at the very least, a devoted patient. Once comfortable within a practice setting, teens are by far the most interesting, engaging, and delightful people to know because they are more insightful and articulate than children and less formal and defensive than most adults.

In addition to recognizing positive feelings toward teens, which certainly helps, it also is *important to be practical*. The health care provider may have limited space, time, and even expertise to deal with adolescents' needs. However, a sincere affinity for this age group and a desire to become involved with their health care needs will provide an important initial impetus to establishing an adolescent-friendly setting, and over time a greater comfort and expertise will inevitably develop.[8–10]

The care of adolescents includes *primary care, specialized care,* and *collaborative care*. Primary care includes attention to acute illnesses, annual checkups, immunizations, counseling, and anticipatory guidance; specialized care addresses problems unique to adolescents including eating disorders, substance use, emotional disorders, school/peer/family-related problems, disorders of puberty, gynecologic concerns and sexuality-related care; collaborative care means working as part of a health care team with mental health, nutrition, medical subspecialty, and/or school-based professionals on behalf of a patient. Because most communities do not have specialists in adolescent medicine, other health care professionals must step into that role. Doing so in an adolescent-friendly practice setting will result in a far better outcome and greater professional satisfaction.

## THE TANGIBLES IN CREATING AN ADOLESCENT-FRIENDLY PRACTICE

The *office décor and milieu* first strike a young person who walks through the door. Are the colors, furnishings, wall hangings, magazines, brochures, and sounds conducive to adolescent comfort or are they more appropriate for babies and toddlers? Even if most of the office is typically "baby-friendly" it certainly is welcoming for adolescents to wait in a small room or area set up just for them. This does not require posters of rock or sports stars or loud popular music, but rather just some comfortable seats or couches, soft throw pillows, fun magazines, and good age-appropriate educational materials. An adolescent bulletin board is always handy and can even be used for teens to advertise their babysitting services to families with younger children.

The *front desk personnel* immediately set the tone, and a friendly greeting goes a long way to put the adolescent at ease. Again, it is not necessary for office staff to be a particular age or dress in a trendy style, but rather to speak to the adolescent with respect and with a smile. Although a glass-enclosed reception area provides greater privacy, it also creates a barrier to establishing a warm welcome.

*Waiting times* should be kept to a minimum, because the adolescent may feel awkward sitting among disparate-aged patients in a pediatric or medical office (hopefully not), but more importantly because teens these days are busy with homework, part-time jobs, after-school activities, or additional appointments.

A *consultation room*, even if small, is a must. Chatting in an examination room with an adolescent who feels awkward or embarrassed in a gown or half undressed is a great way to turn off any chance of having a meaningful conversation, especially about sensitive matters. All office visits, if possible, should begin with a conversation in a consultation room (with the adolescent in street clothes) before moving to the examination room. The *examination room* should not have wallpaper with monkeys or clowns, and should include an examination table long enough for the full length of a fully grown adolescent; if gynecologic examinations are performed, the exam table may be fitted with appropriate hide-away heel rests.

The *length of a visit* must be sufficient. It is extraordinarily difficult to address most adolescent issues in a very short visit; even if the doctor feels able to quickly determine the diagnosis and treatment, for example, of a sore throat, the teen generally needs, appreciates, and benefits from sufficient time to explain concerns and to absorb information. If the problem is more vague or complex, such as fatigue, headaches, nausea, abdominal pain, dizziness, or insomnia, then a half-hour visit is often needed to get a good feel for the problem, including possible psychosocial factors, to do an examination, and to explain findings and recommendations. *Annual checkups* may be completed in a half-hour, but new issues that come up will nearly always require a follow-up visit to explore further. *New patient visits*, which include a detailed history from parents and patients, as well as a complete physical examination, could easily take an hour. It works well to interview the parent(s) alone first (their chief complaint, any concerns about their child; patient's past medical history; family history; and a brief discussion about the adolescent in the family, with friends, and at school); then interview the adolescent alone about current-day health issues (chief complaint, concerns or worries; discussion of physical activity, nutrition, sleep, menstruation, general systems review; family, friends, school; and mood and health-risk behaviors including sexuality, smoking, substance use, and any abusive experiences) and do a complete physical examination; and finally provide feedback and discussion with the adolescent alone before inviting the parent(s) back into the consultation room for a review. Needless to say, at a visit this comprehensive, an hour goes by quickly.[11]

*Communicating with patients (and parents)* by phone, cell phone, text message, e-mail, fax, or snail mail are all options available to us these days. These methods greatly enhance opportunities for easy and confidential communication, but they can also inundate a busy provider with endless messages requesting a response. Gathering the appropriate data (numerous phone numbers and e-mail addresses) and deciding on ground rules for use of phones and cyberspace are important considerations to think through in advance. An office Web site can help transmit useful clinical and procedural information to patients and families and can be a time-saver for office staff as well as the health care provider.

Establishing a reasonable *fee system and coding* visits and procedures appropriately are necessary components of providing the best care for teens. Doctors cannot spend the time needed to provide comprehensive care to teens unless it is economically feasible. Health care providers need to become familiar with a variety of billing codes pertinent to adolescent health care, as discussed in the next chapter.[12] Box 22-2 lists the tangibles involved in designing an adolescent-friendly practice.

## THE INTANGIBLES IN CREATING AN ADOLESCENT-FRIENDLY PRACTICE

Ultimately it is the quality of the rapport between the adolescent and the health care provider that determines the success of their relationship. The adolescent

**Box 22-2**

***Tangibles of Designing an Adolescent-Friendly Office Practice***

- Office décor and milieu
- Front desk personnel
- Waiting times
- Consultation room
- Length of visit
- Communication by phone and e-mail
- Fee system and coding

**Box 22-3**

***Intangibles of Designing an Adolescent-Friendly Office Practice***

- Asking the right questions
- Respecting the adolescent's agenda
- Educating without judging
- Advising without criticizing
- Warmth and humor

must feel that the provider is interested, knowledgeable, and respectful. But how does one convey to patients, and adolescents in particular, that you understand, care about, and trust them? There is no simple answer to this question but rather many component parts.

*Asking the right questions* in an affable tone demonstrates interest, knowledge, and respect. A pleasant greeting ("How are you doing today?") and a little small talk help create a connection and relaxed mood. Discussing matters pertinent to the adolescent's life and lifestyle, ranging from how much sleep he or she gets to whether he or she feels satisfied with friendships, conveys the clinician's knowledge, understanding, and concern. Asking pertinent questions also conveys respect for the adolescent's capacity to tell his or her own story. It is critically important to not simply fire a list of questions, but rather to take the time to listen intently to answers, ask appropriate follow-up questions, and comment on or interpret what the adolescent has said.

*Respecting the adolescent's agenda and limits* engages the patient but doesn't overwhelm. After all, it is the patient's visit, not the health provider's. Allowing the adolescent to somewhat control the content and flow of the visit results in a comfortable patient who feels the visit was worthwhile and satisfying. By the same token, the clinician must be sure the time is used productively and that the adolescent doesn't totally avoid dealing with important issues at hand.

*Educating without judging* and *advising without criticizing* enhance the degree of acceptance the clinician's wisdom will receive and the likelihood that the adolescent will return for more. Teens are hungry for knowledge and guidance but distinctly sensitive to preaching that is overbearing or harsh.

*Warmth and a sense of humor* go far in enhancing a relationship that is inherently unequal in so many ways. These qualities are especially important if we are trying to help a teen, as we often are, with a matter that is potentially embarrassing or shameful, sad, extremely confusing, potentially serious, possibly illegal, or any combination of the above. Box 22-3 lists the intangibles involved in designing an adolescent-friendly office practice.

## GETTING TO KNOW THE PATIENT

It is much easier and more productive to care for a patient we know, and hopefully know well, than someone we have just met or with whom we have maintained a superficial relationship. Yet health care providers often do not have the time to get to know a patient, and teens generally do not respond well to rushed conversations in a noisy or chaotic environment. However, it is possible to get to know an adolescent if we take some time in a peaceful place, with the adolescent comfortable in street clothes, and ask a few key questions whether as part of a new patient visit, an annual checkup, or a visit initiated because of a specific complaint, such as headaches or fatigue.

*The 3 health basics are nutrition, sleep, and exercise*, and it is useful and enlightening to learn how the teen is doing in each of these realms. Useful questions can be: "Do you usually eat 3 meals a day and do you have any snacks? Have you ever been on a diet? Are you happy with your body the way it is now? How would you describe your appetite? What time do you generally go to bed on a school night? What time do you wake up on a school day? On weekends? Do you have any trouble falling asleep or staying asleep? Do you do any sports, physical activity, or exercise on a regular basis? Compared to other people your age do you think you have high, medium, or low amounts of energy?" An adolescent suffering from fatigue, headaches, abdominal discomfort, or excessive sadness or stress will almost always have difficulties in 1 or several of these areas.

We want to know how teens feel about their *relationships with family members and peers and their experiences at school*. Key questions can be: Do you have as many friends as you want or need? Do you like your friends? How would you describe your relationship with your mother (father)? Because no parent is perfect, if you could change 1 thing about your mother (father) or your relationship with your mother (father), what would that be? How do you like school? What do you like most about school? What do you like least? Do you have any idea what you would like to be when you grow up?

A review of *health risk behaviors* is always relevant, but questions should be carefully worded to be appropriate to the age and likely involvement of a particular teen. For the youngest or seemingly not experienced teen, questions can be more general about the kids at school or directed toward the teen's interests and beliefs rather than established behavior, such as: "Have you noticed that kids at school (or friends of yours) are starting to smoke cigarettes (or drink alcohol or use pot or hook up or have intercourse)? Are you curious about or interested in trying cigarettes (or alcohol or pot, etc)? If not now, do you think you will be interested sometime later in high school?" For the older or involved teen, more direct and specific questioning is appropriate. It is helpful to reassure the teen that the questions you are about to ask are asked of all your patients and are intended to help you get to know the teen and provide related counseling or health care, and that you hope they will be honest with you, but you understand that answering some of these questions may be difficult at first. It is also important to mention confidentiality and its limits; of course, you are in the best position to help a patient who trusts that you won't immediately pick up the phone and tell a parent what the teen just told you.

We want to know about a patient's *mood and general sense of well-being*. Helpful questions can be: "How would you describe your mood most of the time? Everyone gets into a bad mood or a funk sometimes; what are the kinds of things or situations that tend to put you in a bad mood? How would you describe yourself, not as your parents or teachers would describe you, but what is most important to you about yourself...your interests, your values, your personality traits?" Some adolescents will love this question and in a thoughtful, insightful, and honest way enjoy thinking about and expressing their answer; others, interestingly and importantly, seem to draw a blank. Some present a positive, negative, or mixed (often balanced) perspective of themselves. Box 22-4 summarizes the discussion topics effective in getting to know an adolescent patient.

**Box 22-4**

***Useful Discussion Topics for Getting to Know an Adolescent Patient***

- The 3 health basics: nutrition, exercise, sleep
- Relationships with family and peers; life at school
- Health risk behaviors
- Mood and general sense of well-being

## INVOLVING PARENTS IN THEIR ADOLESCENT'S CARE

When adolescent medicine first started as a field of practice in the 1950s, and as it became established during ensuing decades, the focus was so heavily on meeting the needs of the adolescent that parents often seemed to be forgotten in our teaching. In an effort to be loyal to and protective of adolescents and their needs and to respect the patient's confidentiality, the role and central importance of parents in their teens' lives, caring parents as well as those less involved, may have been inappropriately de-emphasized. That is no longer the case. Research has shown that adolescents who feel connected to their families and who involve parents in their health and health care decisions do better; they are happier, more secure, and partake in fewer health risk behaviors.[13] We no longer view adolescents and their parents as opposing forces to be reckoned with as adversaries. On the contrary, the health care provider can often help teens and parents work together toward a common goal, whether that is improving nutrition, dealing with problems at school, finding additional medical or mental health services, or negotiating privileges and responsibilities for the teen.

*What parents want* is for their teen to be healthy, content, and productive. They want to partner with their teen to maintain good health. Parents want their teen to feel better if he or she is ill or discontented. Most parents understand that teens need to become gradually more independent in all aspects of their lives, including decisions that affect their health and well-being.

*Adolescents want the same thing*. Most adolescents welcome parental involvement in optimizing their health and well-being. Most adolescents realize that they NEED their parents; not just financially, but in terms of support, advice, and love.

That doesn't mean the ideal is always achievable. As part of the struggle to become separate, to establish a unique and discrete identity, to deal with numerous and profound stresses (at home, with friends, and at school) teens may push parents away and not easily let them back in. Parents, in turn, may become overly critical, intrusive, controlling, even punitive. This pattern can cycle out of control until, in fact, teens and their parents truly are adversaries, whether the issue is the teen's weight, grades in school, use of cigarettes and alcohol, or choice of friends. The image of the sullen and angry teen and the intimidated and puzzled parent need not be the norm.

*In an adolescent-friendly medical practice*, it is critical that the teen and the parents feel at home. This is easily achieved by keeping in mind the ultimate goal of providing the teen the best health care possible while maintaining the trust of the parents. This may involve keeping parents informed, sometimes it will require their active participation, and sometimes family meetings will be needed to resolve conflicts. It is extraordinarily helpful if parents "buy in" to gradually giving their ever-maturing teen more independence, privacy, and confidentiality. The teenage years are a training ground for the future. Adolescents will benefit from and need the experiences of relating independently with health providers and making their own health decisions (hopefully wise ones) so that they will emerge from adolescence well prepared to care for themselves in the years beyond.

## REFERENCES


1. Marks A, Rothbart B. *Healthy Teens, Body and Soul: A Parent's Complete Guide to Adolescent Health*. New York, NY: Simon & Schuster; 2003

2. Prescott HM. *A Doctor of Their Own; A History of Adolescent Medicine*. Cambridge, MA: Harvard University Press; 1998

3. Hulbert A. *Raising America: Experts, Parents, and a Century of Advice About Children*. New York, NY: Alfred A. Knopf; 2003

4. Ford C, English A, Sigman G. Confidential health care for adolescents: position paper of the Society for Adolescent Medicine. *J Adolesc Health Care.* 2004;35(2):160–167

5. Marks A, Malizio J, Hoch J, Brody R, Fisher M. Assessment of health needs and willingness to utilize health care resources of adolescents in a suburban population. *J Pediatr.* 1983;102(3):456–460

6. Akinbami LJ, Gandhi H, Cheng TL. Availability of adolescent health services and confidentiality in primary care practices. *Pediatrics.* 2003;111:394–401

7. Marks A, Fisher M, Lasker S. Adolescent medicine in pediatric practice. *J Adolesc Health Care.* 1990;11(2):149–153

8. Gadomski A, Bennett S, Young M, Wissow LS. Guidelines for adolescent preventive services: the GAPS in practice. *Arch Pediatr Adolesc Med.* 2003;157:426–432

9. Ozer EM, Adams SH, Lustig JL, et al. Increasing the screening and counseling of adolescents for risky health behaviors: a primary care intervention. *Pediatrics.* 2005;115(4):960–968

10. Halpern-Felsher BL, Ozer EM, Millstein SG, et al. Preventive services in a health maintenance organization. *Arch Pediatr Adolesc Med.* 2000;154:173–179

11. Kaplan CP, Perez-Stable EJ, Fuentes-Afflick E, et al. Smoking cessation counseling with young patients: the practices of family physicians and pediatricians. *Arch Pediatr Adol Med.* 2004;158(1):83–90

12. Bradley J, Blythe MJ, eds. *Quick Reference Guide to Pediatric Coding and Documentation for Adolescent Medicine.* 2nd ed. Elk Grove Village, IL: American Academy of Pediatrics; 2005

13. Litt IF, ed. Parents and teens. *J Adolesc Health Care.* 2003;33(2, theme issue):59–132

# CHAPTER 23

# Documentation, Coding, and Billing

MICHAEL A. SPAULDING-BARCLAY, MD, MS • MARGARET J. BLYTHE, MD

Appropriate coding and reimbursement for services provided to adolescents and their families is dependent on accurate documentation of the encounter. Accuracy helps to justify provider charges and more importantly indicates the essential details of the medical care provided. This chapter reviews Procedural coding and Diagnosis coding, the documentation required to support code selection in outpatient and inpatient settings, common modifiers used, as well as the Medicare Resource-Based Relative Value Scale (RBRVS). After completing the chapter, those unfamiliar with issues of documentation and coding will have a foundation upon which to build their understanding; for those more knowledgeable, the discussion will provide a review and hopefully yield some coding "pearls."

## CODE SETS

There are 2 common types of code sets. *Current Procedural Terminology* (CPT) published by the American Medical Association (AMA) describes procedures and services performed by health care providers. Updated and released annually in October, the codes take effect January 1 of the following year. Codes in the *International Classification of Diseases*, currently the *Ninth Revision, Clinical Modification* (ICD-9-CM), published by the Department of Health and Human Services explain the disease or problem evaluated or treated (eg, abdominal pain) and/or define the medical necessity for a CPT procedure performed (eg, appendicitis, unqualified; appendectomy, uncomplicated). The ICD-9-CM codes are released in June, and become effective October 1 of that year.

### CPT CODES

In order to select the correct CPT code, providers must accurately define the encounter, as explained in the following sections.

#### Consult vs Office or Other Outpatient Visit

Consultations are frequently provided by specialists, but also may be provided by primary care physicians, when rendering an opinion (including initiating tests or treatments) but when not assuming total care for a patient. If care is transferred to the consulting physician, the office or other outpatient, or hospital care visit, codes should be used depending on the site of service. The rules for using consultation codes are strict but should be applied appropriately as the reimbursement rates are higher than the corresponding levels of outpatient or inpatient visit codes (Table 23-1). Consultation codes exist for both outpatient and inpatient services. Follow-up visits should use the established office or other outpatient (99211–99215) codes for the outpatient setting, or subsequent hospital care (99231–99233) codes for the inpatient setting. Be aware that CMS has stopped reimbursing for consultation codes, and many other insurers have begun also to not reimburse for them; alternatively, standard office or hospital (E/M) codes would be used.

**Table 23-1**

**The 3 Rs of Consultations**

| | |
|---|---|
| Request | From whom, documented by including request letter, or by note in the record. |
| Reason | Documented by including request letter, or by note in the record. |
| Report | Must send findings in writing back to the requesting source. This may be in the form of a letter or just a copy of office note. |

The request for the consultation usually comes from another physician but also may come from other "appropriate sources" such as a psychologist or therapist, school nurse, coach, the juvenile court system, or even a third-party payer seeking an opinion (if an insurance carrier is mandating the visit, the modifier 32 should be used). An example might be a high school coach who has noticed an athlete's decrease in performance associated with shortness of breath or chest pain.

Application of these codes cannot occur in situations where the patient or family is the requesting source. Office or other outpatient service visit codes should be used for those visits (CPT: 99201–99205 or 99212–99215).

Modified with permission from, Bradley J, Blythe MJ (eds). *Quick Reference Guide to Pediatric Coding and Documentation for Adolescent Medicine. A Companion to Coding for Pediatrics*. 2nd ed. Elk Grove Village, IL: American Academy of Pediatrics; 2005: 27.

### Outpatient vs Inpatient

Outpatient Services typically make up the majority of adolescent visits, and include observation codes for use in hospital "obs-hold" areas (Table 23-2). Additional critical care codes (CPT 99291-99292) may be utilized when life-preserving care is provided in the outpatient setting or office. Other codes (CPT: 99050-99060) are available to indicate services provided after posted hours or on an emergency basis. These codes are added to the regular Evaluation/Management (E/M) service codes or appropriate procedure codes. If a patient is seen in the emergency department (ED), the physician who bills ED codes is the treating physician (CPT: 99281-99285), while the primary care physician may report consultation codes or Outpatient Care Codes with ED as site of service. Other special codes are available for outpatient care that is provided in a home (CPT: new 99341-99345; established 99347-99350), nursing facility (CPT: initial 99304-99306; subsequent 99307-99310), and rest or custodial care facility (CPT: new 99324-99328; established 99334-99337).

Inpatient services include those provided for patients admitted to the hospital, with follow-up daily visits, and then discharged (Table 23-3). Other inpatient code possibilities include patients admitted and discharged on the same day. If a patient is admitted for observation but then gets admitted as an inpatient to the hospital later that same calendar day, the inpatient code for admission should include work done in observation. Two codes for the same day should not be submitted, unless the services were provided by different providers.

### New vs Established

A new patient is defined by CPT as one who "has not received any face-to-face professional services (professional services are "those face-to-face services rendered by a physician and reported by a specific CPT code[s]") from the physician or another physician of the same specialty who belongs to the same group practice" (or covering or on call physician) within the past 3 years. An established patient is one who has received any of these services. If a physician joins your group and "brings" some patients with him or her from the previous practice, those patients are considered "established" patients by CPT code. A patient who comes to see you for the first time as a referral from a physician of a different specialty (eg, surgeon for a pre-operative physical) may be treated as a consultation, a new patient, or even an established patient depending on the relationship you have with the surgeon (part of your large multi-specialty group or not), and how the contract with the multi-specialty group and payer source is structured. If unsure, consult your contract.

### Problem Based vs Preventive Care

The majority of visits to adolescent care providers are for problems or illnesses. Preventive care codes for "well" visits are assigned based on age and whether a patient is new or established (see Table 23-2).

### Cognitive vs Procedural

Cognitive codes are the most commonly billed codes by primary care physicians and sub-specialists alike. These are the standard CPT E/M codes 99201-99499 and reflect nonsurgical services for symptoms, problems, or disease diagnoses, and management. For primary care providers these codes also contain the preventive care codes.

Other codes utilized in an outpatient setting are procedural codes (CPT: 10021-69990) and typically describe minor surgical services and care. Medications are coded utilizing Healthcare Common Procedural Coding System (HCPCS) codes. Some common examples used in caring for adolescent patients are included in the following with a more complete list of procedures and medications presented in Table 23-4:

- Applying trichloroacetic acid (TCA) in the office to vulvar genital wart(s) is found in the surgery section (CPT 56501, Destruction of lesion(s), vulva; simple; 56515, extensive [eg, laser surgery, electrosurgery, cryosurgery, chemosurgery]).
- Albuterol aerosol treatment administration (CPT 94640 initial; use modifier 76 for successive treatments on the same day), with HCPCS code J7613 for the unit dose albuterol.
- Intramuscular ceftriaxone for pelvic inflammatory disease (CPT 96372 therapeutic injection) for the administration with HCPCS code J0696 for the ceftriaxone.

## ICD-9-CM CODES

The ICD-9-CM codes are used to identify the diagnosis, symptoms, conditions, problems, complaints, or other reason such as visits to screen for a condition (eg, sports physical, ICD-9-CM V70.3) for the patient encounter. Often attempts to save time in the name of office efficiency actually may be counterproductive in terms of identifying the most specific ICD-9-CM code for the condition being treated. For example, use of ICD-9-CM code Headache (784.0) for all headaches may be faster, but Headache, Migraine (346.9) suggests a more specific diagnosis and provides a more accurate medical record for the current provider as well as for a future provider who assumes that patient's care. In addition, payers may reject certain management and therapy options based on a lack of specificity of coding. For

## Table 23-2

### Common Outpatient Services

| Service | CPT Code | History | Physical Exam | Medical Decision Making | Time (mins) | 2010 NF Total RVUs | 2010 Facility Total RVUs |
|---|---|---|---|---|---|---|---|
| **Office Visit** | | | | | | | |
| New[a] | 99201 | PF | PF | SF | 10 | 1.08 | 0.69 |
| | 99202 | EPF | EPF | SF | 20 | 1.86 | 1.33 |
| | 99203 | D | D | LC | 30 | 2.71 | 2.02 |
| | 99204 | C | C | MC | 45 | 4.21 | 3.41 |
| | 99205 | C | C | HC | 60 | 5.28 | 4.41 |
| Established[b] | 99211 | — | — | — | 5 | 0.53 | 0.25 |
| | 99212 | PF | PF | SF | 10 | 1.08 | 0.68 |
| | 99213 | EPF | EPF | LC | 15 | 1.81 | 1.34 |
| | 99214 | D | D | MC | 25 | 2.71 | 2.06 |
| | 99215 | C | C | HC | 40 | 3.66 | 2.91 |
| **Preventive Care** | | | | | | | |
| 12–17 yr, new | 99384 | C | C | — | — | 2.97 | 2.15 |
| 12–17 yr, est | 99394 | C | C | — | — | 2.58 | 1.90 |
| 18–39 yr, new | 99385 | C | C | — | — | 2.97 | 2.15 |
| 18–39 yr, est | 99395 | C | C | — | — | 2.59 | 1.90 |
| **Consultation** | | | | | | | |
| | 99241 | PF | PF | SF | 15 | 1.35 | 0.93 |
| | 99242 | EPF | EPF | SF | 30 | 2.54 | 1.95 |
| | 99243 | D | D | LC | 40 | 3.47 | 2.72 |
| | 99244 | C | C | MC | 60 | 5.14 | 4.32 |
| | 99245 | C | C | HC | 80 | 6.28 | 5.36 |
| **Observation** | | | | | | | |
| Initial observation care | 99218 | D | D | SF | — | — | 1.76 |
| | 99219 | C | C | MC | — | | 2.93 |
| | 99220 | C | C | HC | — | | 4.11 |
| Subsequent observation care | 99224 | Interval | PF | Low/SF | 15 | | |
| | 99225 | Interval | EPF | MC | 25 | | c |
| | 99226 | Interval | D | HC | 35 | | |
| Discharge separate day | 99217 | — | — | — | — | — | 1.88 |

[a]Requires 3 of 3: History, Physical Exam, and Medical Decision Making

[b]Requires only 2 of 3: History, Physical Exam, and Medical Decision Making

[c]Code new for 2011, RVUs not available at time of print

C, comprehensive; D, detailed; EPF, expanded problem-focused; HC, high complexity; LC, low complexity; MC, medium complexity; NF, non-facility; PF, problem focused; RVU, relative value unit

**Table 23-3**

## Common Inpatient Services

| *Service* | *CPT Code* | *History* | *Physical Exam* | *Medical Decision Making* | *Time (mins)* | *2010 Facility RVUs* |
|---|---|---|---|---|---|---|
| **Hospital Visit** | | | | | | |
| Initial hospital care[a] | 99221 | D | D | SF | 30 | 2.64 |
| | 99222 | C | C | MC | 50 | 3.58 |
| | 99223 | C | C | HC | 70 | 5.27 |
| Subsequent hospital care[b] | 99231 | PF | PF | SF | 15 | 1.05 |
| | 99232 | EPF | EPF | MC | 25 | 1.90 |
| | 99233 | D | D | HC | 35 | 2.73 |
| Discharge | 99238 | — | — | — | < 30 | 1.87 |
| | 99239 | — | — | — | ≥ 30 | 2.74 |
| **Observation** | | | | | | |
| Observation or same day admit/ discharge hospital[c] | 99234 | D | D | SF | — | 3.59 |
| | 99235 | C | C | MC | — | 4.71 |
| | 99236 | C | C | HC | — | 5.84 |
| **Consultation** | | | | | | |
| | 99251 | PF | PF | SF | 20 | 1.37 |
| | 99252 | EPF | EPF | SF | 40 | 2.11 |
| | 99253 | D | D | LC | 55 | 3.22 |
| | 99254 | C | C | MC | 80 | 4.65 |
| | 99255 | C | C | HC | 110 | 5.62 |

[a]Requires 3 of 3: History, Physical Exam, and Medical Decision Making

[b]Requires only 2 of 3: History, Physical Exam, and Medical Decision Making

[c]Medicare payment policy requires that the same day admit/discharge codes (99234-99236) be used for patients who stay ≥ 8 hours in observation, otherwise use the initial observation codes only. Other payers are not required to adhere to this payment policy. Consult your local contract.

**Table 23-4**

## Common Procedures

| *Procedure* | *CPT Code* | *2010 NF RVUs* | *2010 Facility RVUs* |
|---|---|---|---|
| Aerosol treatment | 94640 | 0.38 | — |
| Aerosol/inhaler instruction | 94664 | 0.39 | — |
| Audiometry, screen | 92551 | 0.29 | — |
| Burn treatment, 1st degree | 16000 | 1.78 | 1.25 |

*(Continued)*

## Table 23-4 (Continued)

| *Procedure* | *CPT Code* | *2010 NF RVUs* | *2010 Facility RVUs* |
|---|---|---|---|
| Burn treatment, 2nd degree | 16020 | 2.10 | 1.49 |
| Chemocautery/granuloma | 17250 | 1.89 | 0.94 |
| Chemocautery/epistaxis | 30901 | 2.70 | 1.69 |
| Cerumen removal | 69210 | 1.30 | 0.88 |
| Digital block | 64450 | 2.67 | 1.86 |
| EKG, with interpretation | 93000 | 0.55 | — |
| EKG/interpretation only | 93010 | 0.25 | 0.25 |
| EKG tracing only | 93005 | 0.30 | — |
| Foreign body/subcutaneous | 10120 | 3.45 | 2.38 |
| Foreign body/removal/ear | 69200 | 3.11 | 1.48 |
| Foreign body/removal/nose | 30300 | 5.68 | 3.16 |
| Foreign body/removal/vagina | 57415 | 4.30 | 4.30 |
| Foreign body/corneal/conjunctival superficial | 65205 | 1.42 | 1.15 |
| Fracture/dislocation care—closed treatment only | | | |
| Metacarpalphalangeal dislocation | 26700 | 7.89 | 7.40 |
| Interphalangeal joint dislocation | 26770 | 6.72 | 6.20 |
| Radial shaft fracture | 25520 | 13.93 | 13.29 |
| Ulnar shaft fracture | 25530 | 6.28 | 5.68 |
| Phalangeal shaft fracture, proximal or middle | 26720 | 4.75 | 4.38 |
| Phalangeal fracture, distal | 26750 | 4.45 | 4.37 |
| Heme stool test | 82270 | — | — |
| Incision and drainage/simple | 10060 | 2.81 | 2.41 |
| Inject/asp joint/bursa small | 20600 | 1.40 | 1.04 |
| Inject/asp joint/bursa intermed | 20605 | 1.51 | 1.09 |
| Inject/asp joint/bursa large | 20610 | 1.98 | 1.32 |
| Injection tendon/ligament | 20550 | 1.49 | 1.10 |
| Lumbar puncture | 62270 | 4.07 | 2.13 |
| Lysis of labial adhesions | 56441 | 3.96 | 3.77 |
| Nail avulsion; single | 11730 | 2.45 | 1.47 |
| Pelvic exam under anesthesia | 57410 | — | 2.88 |
| Pulse oximetry | 94760 | 0.07 | — |
| Removal of skin tags | 11200 | 2.14 | 1.82 |
| Repair scalp/neck/axillae/genitalia/trunk/ext | 12001 | 3.85 | 2.76 |
| Suture/dermabond, simple ≤ 2.5 cm | 12002 | 4.10 | 3.06 |
| Suture/dermabond, simple 2.6–7.5 cm | | | |

*(Continued)*

**Table 23-4 (Continued)**

| *Procedure* | *CPT Code* | *2010 NF RVUs* | *2010 Facility RVUs* |
|---|---|---|---|
| Repair face/ears/eyelids/nose/lips | | | |
| Suture, simple ≤ 2.5cm | 12011 | 4.09 | 2.85 |
| Suture, simple 2.6–5.0 cm | 12013 | 4.51 | 3.25 |
| Skin biopsy, single | 11100 | 2.64 | 1.32 |
| Skin biopsy, each additional | 11101 | 0.86 | 0.67 |
| Spirometry, technical component | 94010-TC | 0.68 | — |
| Spirometry, professional component | 94010-26 | 0.23 | 0.23 |
| Splinting/strapping | | | |
| Finger splint | 29130 | 1.03 | 0.77 |
| Short arm splint | 29125 | 1.69 | 1.11 |
| Short leg splint | 29515 | 1.79 | 1.29 |
| Strapping ankle/foot | 29540 | 1.07 | 0.85 |
| Strapping elbow/wrist | 29260 | 1.30 | 0.98 |
| Strapping hand/finger | 29280 | 1.26 | 0.93 |
| Strapping shoulder | 29240 | 1.47 | 1.15 |
| Tympanometry | 92567 | 0.43 | 0.37 |
| Urine catheterization | 51701 | 1.65 | 0.78 |
| Vision screening | 99173 | 0.07 | — |
| Wart removal (1–14 warts) | 17110 | 2.78 | 1.77 |
| Wart removal (≥ 15 warts) | 17111 | 3.32 | 2.21 |
| **LABS** | | | |
| Arterial puncture | 36600 | 0.82 | 0.42 |
| Glucose/accuchek | 82962 | | |
| Hematocrit spun | 85013 | | |
| Hemoccult cards, 1–3 | 82270 | | |
| KOH smear (tissue) | 87220 | | |
| PPD | 86580 | 0.19 | — |
| Pregnancy test, urine | 81025 | | |
| Strep rapid screen | 87880 | | |
| UA automated w/microscopy | 81001 | | |
| UA dipstick automated w/o microscopy | 81003 | | |
| UA dipstick non-automated | 81002 | | |
| UA dipstick w/microscopy/non-auto | 81000 | | |
| Urine microalbumin | 82044 | | |
| Venipuncture > 3 years by physician | 36410 | 0.52 | 0.25 |
| Venipuncture by nurse | 36415 | — | — |
| Vital capacity, technical component | 94150 TC | 0.46 | |

**Table 23-4 (Continued)**

| *Procedure* | *CPT Code* | *2010 NF RVUs* | *2010 Facility RVUs* |
|---|---|---|---|
| Vital capacity, professional component | 94150 26 | 0.11 | |
| Wet mount | 87210 | | |
| **INJECTIONS** | | | |
| Admin of injectable, SQ/IM | 96372 | 0.59 | — |
| IV Infusion 1st hour | 96360 | 1.49 | — |
| IV Infusion each additional hour | 96361 | 0.42 | — |
| IV start | 36000 | 0.67 | 0.27 |
| Ceftriaxone, per 250 mg | J0696 | | |
| Depo provera 150 mg | J1055 | | |
| Imitrex, 6 mg | J3030 | | |
| Insulin, per 5 units | J1815 | | |
| Lidocaine HCI, per 10 mg for IV use | J2001 | | |
| Normal saline 1000 cc | J7030 | | |
| Phenergan up to 50 mg SQ/IM | J2550 | | |
| Toradol, per 15 mg | J1885 | | |
| **VACCINATIONS** | | | |
| Immunization administration | | | |
| First component, Pt ≤ 17 years w/counseling | 9046×1 | | |
| Each additional component, Pt ≤ 17 years w/ counseling | 9046×2 | | |
| Initial injection, Pt ≥ 18 years or no counseling | 90471 | 0.59 | — |
| Each additional injection, Pt ≥ 18 years or no counseling | 90472 | 0.30 | — |
| Initial oral/intranasal, Pt ≥ 18 years or no counseling | 90473 | 0.40 | — |
| Each additional oral/intranasal, Pt ≥ 18 years or no counseling. | 90474 | 0.26 | — |
| Hepatitis A vaccine, pediatric/adolescent dosage, 2 dose | 90633 | | V05.3 |
| Hepatitis B, pediatric/adolescent dosage, 3 dose | 90744 | | V05.3 |
| Human papillomavirus (HPV) vaccine, types 6, 11, 16, 18 (quadrivalent), 3 dose schedule, for intramuscular use | 90649 | | V04.89 |
| HPV vaccine, types 16 and 18, bivalent, 3-dose schedule for IM use | 90650 | | V04.89 |
| Influenza virus vaccine, split virus, preservative free, 3 years and older dosage | 90656 | | V04.81 |
| Influenza virus vaccine, split virus, 3 years and older dosage | 90658 | | V04.81 |
| Influenza virus vaccine, live, intranasal use | 90660 | | V04.81 |

(*Continued*)

## Table 23-4 (Continued)

| *Procedure* | *CPT Code* | *2010 NF RVUs* | *2010 Facility RVUs* |
|---|---|---|---|
| Measles, mumps, and rubella virus vaccine (MMR) | 90707 | | V06.4 |
| Meningococcal polysaccharide vaccine | 90733 | | V03.89 |
| Meningococcal conjugate vaccine, for IM use | 90734 | | V03.89 |
| Pneumococcal polysaccharide vaccine, 23-valent, adult or immunosuppressed patient dosage for use in individuals 2 years or older | 90732 | | V03.82 |
| Poliovirus vaccine (IPV), inactivated | 90713 | | V04.0 |
| Rabies vaccine, intramuscular | 90675 | | V04.5 |
| Tetanus Toxoid absorbed | 90703 | | V03.7 |
| Tetanus and diphtheria toxoids (Td) absorbed for use in individuals 7 years or older | 90718 | | V06.5 |
| Tetanus, diphtheria toxoids and acellular pertussis vaccine (Tdap) for use in individuals 7 years and older | 90715 | | V06.1 |
| Varicella virus vaccine | 90716 | | V05.4 |

Table includes information and codes adapted from *Current Procedural Terminology, Standard Edition*. American Medical Association, Chicago, IL, 2007 and *International Classification of Diseases, 9th Revision, Clinical Modification (ICD-9-CM)*. Department of Health and Human Services, 2007.

example, using ICD-9-CM code for Upper Respiratory Infection (URI), Acute (465.9) alone instead of URI, Acute (465.9) and Tachypnea (786.06) may result in payers refusing reimbursement for the pulse-oximetry (CPT 94760) obtained. Other reasons that providers should utilize codes with the highest level of specificity include improving accuracy for evaluating trends in health care diagnoses and services, and helping in future contract negotiations by documenting the complexity and number of diagnoses and services offered.

E codes are provided next as a way to categorize how an injury or poisoning occurred. E codes are never to be used as primary diagnoses, nor are they to be reported alone on a claim form. The primary ICD-9-CM code should be the actual injury or adverse effect that the patient presented with, followed by the E code to explain how this happened. For example, a 13-year-old presents with a dog bite to the left hand. The wound is open, but not considered complicated. Code 882.0 (open wound, hand w/o mention of complication) would be reported as primary along with E906.0 (dog bite) as secondary.

In order to aid providers in managing this balance of providing both accuracy and efficiency in selecting codes, superbills or routing slips pre-printed with the most commonly used ICD-9-CM codes may be used. In addition, providers may choose to use the annually updated American Academy of Pediatrics (AAP) *Pediatric ICD-9-CM Coding Pocket Guide* (an alphabetic listing of commonly used pediatric specific diagnosis codes, available in both a laminated version and a PDA version) to help. Some commonly used ICD-9-CM codes in adolescents are presented in Table 23-5.

## Table 23-5

### Common ICD-9-CM Codes for Adolescent Medicine

| *Diagnosis* | *ICD-9-CM Code* |
|---|---|
| **A** | |
| Abdominal pain, site unsp | 789.00 |
| Abdominal tenderness, site unsp | 789.60 |
| Abnormal findings, w/o diagnosis (examination, laboratory test) | 796.4 |
| Abnormal glucose | 790.29 |
| Abnormal periods (grossly) | 626.9 |

## Table 23-5 (Continued)

| *Diagnosis* | *ICD-9-CM Code* |
|---|---|
| Abnormal urination NEC | 788.69 |
| Abnormal weight gain | 783.1 |
| Abnormal weight loss | 783.21 |
| Abrasion, skin, multiple or unsp sites | 919.0 |
| Abscess, unsp site | 682.9 |
| Abuse child/adolescents | 995.50 |
| Abuse physical | 995.54 |
| Abuse sexual/rape | 995.53 |
| Acanthosis nigricans | 701.2 |
| Acne | 706.1 |
| Acute nasopharyngitis, common cold | 460 |
| ADD | 314.00 |
| ADHD | 314.01 |
| Adjustment reaction, adolescent | 309.22 |
| Alleged rape | V71.5 |
| Allergic reaction, NOS | 995.3 |
| Allergic rhinitis, cause unsp | 477.9 |
| Alopecia/hair loss, unsp | 704.00 |
| Amenorrhea/ovarian | 256.8 |
| Amenorrhea/primary, secondary | 626.0 |
| Anal fissure, tear | 565.0 |
| Anemia, iron deficiency | 280.1 |
| Anemia, unsp | 285.9 |
| Animal bite, unsp (report injury code as primary) | E906.5 |
| Annual pelvic/PAP | V72.31 |
| Anorexia nervosa | 307.1 |
| Anorexia | 783.0 |
| Anti-inflammatories, nonsteroidal long-term, current use | V58.64 |
| Anxiety (acute, stress) | 308.0 |
| Anxiety, unsp | 300.00 |
| Aphthous ulcer/stomatitis | 528.2 |
| Appendicitis | 540.1 |
| Assault sexual, rape, alleged | V71.5 |
| Asthma, acute exacerbation | 493.02 |
| Asthma, stable | 493.00 |
| Asthma, unspec. | 493.90 |
| Asthma, w/status | 493.01 |
| Ataxia | 781.3 |
| Athlete's foot | 110.4 |
| Athletic team examination | V70.3 |
| Autism | 299.00 |
| **B** | |
| Bacterial vaginosis | 616.10 |
| Balanitis | 607.1 |
| Bartholin gland, cyst | 616.2 |
| Bartholin gland, abscess | 616.3 |
| Beating/fight | E960.0 |
| Bee sting | 989.5 |
| Behavioral problems | V40.3 |
| Behavioral problems, unspec | V40.9 |
| Bell palsy | 351.0 |
| Bereavement | V62.82 |
| Bicycle accident | E826.9 |
| Bite, animal unsp | E906.5 |
| Bite, dog | E906.0 |
| Bite, human accidental | E928.3 |
| Bite, human intentional | E968.7 |
| Bite, refer to open wound by site or superficial injury by site | VARIES |
| Bite, rat | E906.1 |
| Bleeding, nose | 784.7 |
| Bloating, abdominal pain | 787.3 |
| Blurred vision | 368.8 |
| Body mass index, < 5th%ile | V85.51 |
| Body mass index, 5th < 85th%ile | V85.52 |
| Body mass index, 85th < 95%ile | V85.53 |
| Body mass index, ≥ 95th%ile | V85.54 |
| Boil, carbuncle, unsp | 680.9 |
| Bradycardia, sinus | 427.81 |
| Breast asymmetry | 611.9 |
| Breast lump/mass | 611.72 |
| Breast pain | 611.71 |
| Breast, problem, other | 611.79 |
| Bronchospasm, exercise-induced | 493.81 |
| Bulimia nervosa | 307.51 |
| Bulimia | 783.6 |
| Bunion | 727.1 |
| Burn, unspec site (multiple) first degree | 949.1 |
| Bursitis, other | 727.3 |

(*Continued*)

**Table 23-5 (Continued)**

| *Diagnosis* | *ICD-9-CM Code* |
|---|---|
| C | |
| Calcium dietary deficiency | 269.3 |
| Candidal vulvovaginitis | 112.1 |
| Carious teeth, unsp | 521.00 |
| Cellulitis/abscess, unsp site | 682.9 |
| Cerebral palsy, unsp | 343.9 |
| Cerumen, impacted (ear wax) | 380.4 |
| Cervicitis, chlamydial | 099.53 |
| Cervicitis, gonococcal | 098.15 |
| Cervicitis and endocervicitis | 616.0 |
| Chest pain, unsp | 786.50 |
| Chlamydia urethritis (STD) | 099.41 |
| Cholecystitis, acute | 575.0 |
| Chronic fatigue syndrome | 780.71 |
| Concussion w/LOC 30 min or less | 850.11 |
| Concussion w/LOC 31–59 min | 850.12 |
| Concussion w/LOC unspecified duration | 850.5 |
| Concussion w/o LOC | 850.0 |
| Conduct problems, adolescent onset | 312.82 |
| Condyloma acuminata | 078.11 |
| Congestion, nasal | 478.19 |
| Conjunctivitis, acute | 372.00 |
| Conjunctivitis, allergic | 372.05 |
| Constipation, unspec | 564.00 |
| Contact/exposure to STD | V01.6 |
| Contraceptive management, initiation, oral | V25.01 |
| Contraception, initiation, non-oral injection, device | V25.02 |
| Contraception management, emergency counseling & prescription | V25.03 |
| Contraceptive counseling/family planning | V25.09 |
| Contraception surveillance, unsp | V25.40 |
| Contraception surveillance, contraceptive pill | V25.41 |
| Contraception surveillance, intrauterine contraceptive device | V25.42 |
| Contraception surveillance, implantable subdermal contraceptive | V25.43 |
| Contraceptive surveillance, other specified (Injection) | V25.49 |
| Contusion (skin surface intact) | See Site |
| Convulsions, epilepsy unsp w/o mention of intractable epilepsy | 345.90 |
| w/intractable epilepsy | 345.91 |
| Corneal abrasion | 918.1 |
| Costochondritis | 733.6 |
| Cough variant asthma | 493.82 |
| Cough | 786.2 |
| Counseling, NOS | V65.40 |
| Counseling, dietary/nutrition | V65.3 |
| Counseling, exercise | V65.41 |
| Counseling, explanation/medication | V65.49 |
| Counseling, HIV | V65.44 |
| Counseling, injury prevention | V65.43 |
| Counseling, family disruption, military deployment | V61.01 |
| Counseling, family disruption, return from military deployment | V61.02 |
| Counseling, family disruption, divorce or legal separation | V61.03 |
| Counseling, family disruption, parent-child estrangement | V61.04 |
| Counseling, family disruption, child in welfare custody | V61.05 |
| Counseling, family disruption, child in foster or other care | V61.06 |
| Counseling, family disruption, death in the family | V61.07 |
| Counseling, family disruption, extended absence of family member | V61.08 |
| Counseling, family disruption, other | V61.09 |
| Counseling, medical for feared complaint/no disease found | V65.9 |
| Counseling, parent-child conflict, unsp | V61.20 |
| Counseling, parent-biological child problem | V61.23 |
| Counseling, parent-adopted child problem | V61.24 |
| Counseling, parent (guardian)-foster child problem | V61.25 |
| Counseling, phase of life problem | V62.89 |
| Counseling, school | V62.3 |

*(Continued)*

**Table 23-5 (Continued)**

| *Diagnosis* | *ICD-9-CM Code* |
|---|---|
| Counseling, specified reason tobacco | V65.49 |
| Counseling, STD prevention | V65.45 |
| Counseling, substance use/abuse | V65.42 |
| Counseling, victim of abuse NEC | V61.21 |
| Crabs, genital | 132.2 |
| Cramps, extremity, NEC | 729.82 |
| Cyst, ovary | 620.2 |
| Cystitis | 595.9 |
| **D** | |
| Dandruff | 690.18 |
| Dehydration | 276.51 |
| Delayed puberty, NEC | 259.0 |
| Dental abscess | 522.5 |
| Dental caries, unsp | 521.00 |
| Depression, NEC | 311 |
| Depression, anxiety | 300.4 |
| Depression, brief reactive/mood brief reaction | 309.0 |
| Dermatitis, atopic | 691.8 |
| Dermatitis, contact, NOS | 692.9 |
| Dermatitis, seborrheic | 690.10 |
| Dermatitis, sunburn | 692.71 |
| Diabetes mellitus type I, controlled | 250.01 |
| Diabetes mellitus type I, uncontrolled | 250.03 |
| Diabetes mellitus type II, controlled | 250.00 |
| Diabetes mellitus type II, uncontrolled | 250.02 |
| Diabetic ketoacidosis, uncontrolled | 250.13 |
| Diarrhea, NOS | 787.91 |
| Diarrhea/dysentery/infections | 009.2 |
| Dietary surveillance/counseling | V65.3 |
| Difficulty in walking | 719.7 |
| Dislocation, finger, closed | 834.00 |
| Disorder, eating unspec | 307.50 |
| Disorder, posttraumatic stress | 309.81 |
| Disturbance, sleep | 780.50 |
| Dizziness | 780.4 |
| Dog bite | E906.0 |
| Drowning/submersion | E910.9 |
| Drug overdose | 977.9 |
| Drug overdose, accidental | E858.9 |
| Drug overdose, intentional | E950.4 |
| DUB | 626.8 |
| Dysmenorrhea | 625.3 |
| Dyspnea | 786.09 |
| Dysuria | 788.1 |
| **E** | |
| Ear pierce, infection | 872.11 |
| Earache (otalgia), unsp | 388.70 |
| Earache, swimmers acute | 380.12 |
| Eating disorder, unspec | 307.50 |
| Eczema, NOS | 692.9 |
| Effusion/swelling, ankle | 719.07 |
| Effusion/swelling, elbow | 719.02 |
| Effusion/swelling, knee | 719.06 |
| Effusion/swelling, wrist | 719.03 |
| Electrolyte imbalance, NEC | 276.9 |
| Elevated blood pressure w/o hypertension | 796.2 |
| Emotional disturbance of childhood or adolescent, unspec | 313.9 |
| Enuresis, nocturnal | 788.36 |
| Epididymitis | 604.90 |
| Epilepsy, unsp | 345.90 |
| Epistaxis/nose bleed | 784.7 |
| Erythema multiforme, unsp | 695.10 |
| minor | 695.11 |
| major | 695.12 |
| Eustachian tube dysfunction | 381.81 |
| Exam for alleged rape | V71.5 |
| Exanthem (rash) | 782.1 |
| Excessive beginning periods | 626.3 |
| Excessive bleeding, menses | 626.2 |
| Exercise-induced broncho spasm | 493.81 |
| **F** | |
| Fatigue, other | 780.79 |
| Fatigue, chronic fatigue syndrome | 780.71 |
| Flat feet | 734 |
| Folliculitis | 704.8 |
| Follow-up exam | V67.x |
| Follow-up exam after STD treatment | V67.59 |
| Follow-up exam, pap smear | V67.01 |

(*Continued*)

**Table 23-5 (Continued)**

| *Diagnosis* | *ICD-9-CM Code* |
|---|---|
| Follow-up exam/recheck | V58.89 |
| Follow-up/unspecified | V67.9 |
| Foreign body, ear | 931 |
| Foreign body, nose | 932 |
| Foreign body, vagina | 939.2 |
| Fracture, ankle, closed, NOS | 824.8 |
| Fracture, clavicle, closed, unspecified | 810.00 |
| sternal end | 810.01 |
| shaft | 810.02 |
| acromial end | 810.03 |
| Fracture, coccyx, closed | 805.6 |
| Fracture, face bone NEC | 802.8 |
| Fracture, femoral neck | 820.8 |
| Fracture, femur, closed, unspecified | 821.00 |
| shaft | 821.01 |
| Fracture, fibula, unsp part, closed | 823.81 |
| Fracture, fibula, tibia, closed | 823.82 |
| Fracture, fibula, torus/buckle | 823.41 |
| Fracture, finger(s), (including thumb) closed, unsp | 816.00 |
| Fracture, foot, unsp, metatarsal bone(s), closed | 825.20 |
| Fracture, hand metacarpal bone(s), closed, site unsp | 815.00 |
| Fracture, humerus, closed, unsp | 812.20 |
| Fracture, lower end of forearm, unsp | 813.40 |
| Fracture, nasal bone, closed non-displaced | 802.0 |
| Fracture, phalanx (gnes) foot closed | 826.0 |
| Fracture, phalanx (gnes) of hand closed | 816.0 |
| Fracture, radius (alone), closed, unsp part | 813.81 |
| Fracture, radius, torus/buckle | 813.45 |
| Fracture, rib(s), closed, unspec | 807.00 |
| Fracture, skull | 803.00–803.99 |
| Fracture, tibia, unsp part, closed | 823.80 |
| Fracture, tibia, torus/buckle | 823.40 |
| Fracture, ulna (alone), unsp part, closed | 813.82 |
| Fracture, wrist, carpal bone, unsp, closed | 814.00 |
| **G** | |
| Gait abnormal/limp | 781.2 |
| Galactorrhea | 611.6 |
| Gambling problem | V69.3 |
| Ganglion of joint | 727.41 |
| Ganglion of tendon sheath | 727.42 |
| Ganglion, unsp | 727.43 |
| Gastritis, acute w/o mention of hemorrhage | 535.00 |
| Gastroenteritis and colitis, noninfectious, unsp | 558.9 |
| Gastroenteritis, colitis, enteritis, infectious | 009.0 |
| Gastroesophageal reflux (GERD) | 530.81 |
| Genital herpes, unsp | 054.10 |
| herpetic vulvovaginitis | 054.11 |
| herpetic ulceration of vulva | 054.12 |
| herpetic infection of penis | 054.13 |
| other | 054.19 |
| Genital pain, female | 625.9 |
| Genital pain, male, testicle, penis | 608.9<br>607.9 |
| Geographic tongue | 529.1 |
| Glucose tolerance test, impaired, fasting | 790.21 |
| Glucose tolerance test, impaired (oral) | 790.22 |
| Glycosuria | 791.5 |
| Gonococcal cervicitis, acute | 098.15 |
| Gonorrhea, acute urethritis, vulvovaginitis, acute, NOS | 098.0 |
| Grand mal epilepsy, w/o mention of intractable epilepsy | 345.10 |
| Gynecological exam, routine (PAP) | V72.31 |
| Gynecomastia | 611.1 |
| **H** | |
| Hallucinations | 780.1 |
| Hb-SS disease w/crisis | 282.62 |
| Hb-SS disease w/o crisis | 282.61 |
| Headache | 784.0 |
| Headache, migraine | See Migraine |
| Headache, tension | 307.81 |
| Hearing problem | V41.2 |

*(Continued)*

**Table 23-5 (Continued)**

| *Diagnosis* | *ICD-9-CM Code* |
|---|---|
| Hearing test, failed | 388.40 |
| Hearing test, following failed hearing screen | V72.11 |
| Heartburn | 787.1 |
| Heart murmur, NOS (not to be used for functional, benign) | 785.2 |
| Heat exhaustion, unsp | 992.5 |
| Helicobacter pylori | 041.86 |
| Hematuria (gross) | 599.71 |
| Hemorrhoids, uncomplicated, unsp | 455.6 |
| Hepatitis w/Infectious mononucleosis [Code Mono (075) first] | 573.1 |
| Hepatitis, unspec viral, w/o coma | 070.9 |
| Hepatitis, unspec | 573.3 |
| Hernia, inguinal, w/o mention of obstruction or gangrene, unsp | 550.90 |
| Herpes aoster/shingles w/o mention of complication | 053.9 |
| Herpes, senital | 054.10 |
| Herpes, labialis (simplex) | 054.9 |
| Herpetic gingivostomatitis | 054.2 |
| Hidradenitis (suppurative) | 705.83 |
| Hirsutism | 704.1 |
| HIV counseling | V65.44 |
| HIV infection w/o Sx | V08 |
| Hives/urticaria, unsp | 708.9 |
| Hoarseness | 784.42 |
| Homeless | V60.0 |
| Human papilloma virus (HPV) | 079.4 |
| Hydrocele, unsp | 603.9 |
| Hyperhidrosis/excessive sweating | 780.8 |
| Hyperinsulinemia | 251.1 |
| Hyperlipidemia, other and unsp | 272.4 |
| Hypertension, essential | 401.9 |
| Hypertrophy tonsils and adenoids | 474.10 |
| Hyperventilation syndrome | 306.1 |
| Hypochondriasis | 300.7 |
| Hypotension, unsp | 458.9 |
| Hypotension, orthostatic | 458.0 |
| Hypothyroidism, unsp | 244.9 |
| **I** | |
| Imperforate hymen | 752.42 |
| Impetigo | 684 |
| Indigestion | 536.8 |
| Infectious mono | 075 |
| Influenza w/other respiratory manifestations | 487.1 |
| Infrequent, menses | 626.1 |
| Ingestion/poisoning, unsp drug or medicinal substance | 977.9 |
| Ingrown nail/toenail | 703.0 |
| Inhalation, carbon monoxide, toxic effects | 986 |
| Injury, ankle, foot, NOS | 959.7 |
| Injury, arm (upper)/shoulder | 959.2 |
| Injury, eye | 921.9 |
| Injury, knee/leg | 959.7 |
| Injury, vaginal | 959.1 |
| Insect bite non-venomous | E906.4 |
| Insect bite w/infection | 919.5 |
| Insomnia | 780.52 |
| Irregular, menses, periods | 626.4 |
| Irritable bowel syndrome | 564.1 |
| **J** | |
| Joint pain (use 5th digit for site) | 719.4x |
| Joint swelling (use 5th digit for site) | 719.0x |
| JRA, chronic or unsp | 714.30 |
| JRA, acute | 714.31 |
| **K** | |
| Knife wound, intentional | E966 |
| Knife wound/accidental | E920.3 |
| Knock knee/genu valgum | 736.41 |
| **L** | |
| Labial adhesion | 623.2 |
| Laceration/bite/puncture face | 873.40 |
| Laceration/unspec | 879.8 |
| Laceration/vaginal | 878.6 |
| Lactase deficiency | 271.3 |
| Laryngitis | 464.0 |
| Learning problems | V40.0 |
| Lethargy | 780.79 |
| Leukocytopenia/leukopenia, unsp | 288.50 |

(*Continued*)

**Table 23-5 (Continued)**

| *Diagnosis* | *ICD-9-CM Code* |
|---|---|
| Lice, head | 132.0 |
| Lice, pubic | 132.2 |
| Light-headedness | 780.4 |
| Limp | 719.7 |
| Long-term use of medication as anticonvulsant, antireflux meds | V58.69 |
| Lordosis | 737.20 |
| Lymphadenitis, acute | 683 |
| Lymphadenitis, unspec | 289.3 |
| Lymphadenopathy | 785.6 |
| **M** | |
| Malingering | V65.2 |
| Malnutrition (calories) unspec | 263.9 |
| Marijuana, abuse, unsp | 305.20 |
| Mass, breast | 611.72 |
| Mass, scrotum | 608.89 |
| Mastalgia | 611.71 |
| Medical examination for camp/school | V70.3 |
| Menometrorrhagia | 626.2 |
| Menorrhagia (primary) | 626.2 |
| Menstruation, normal cycle | 626.5 |
| Menstruation, pubertal | 626.3 |
| Mental retardation, moderate | 318.0 |
| Mental retardation, severe | 318.1 |
| Mental retardation, profound | 318.2 |
| Mental retardation, unsp | 319 |
| Metrorrhagia | 626.6 |
| Migraine w/aura, w/o intractable migraine, w/o status migrainosus | 346.00 |
| Migraine, menstrual (use 5th digit to identify specific migraine) | 346.4x |
| Mittelschmerz | 625.2 |
| Molluscum contagiosum | 078.0 |
| Moniliasis, vulvovaginitis | 112.1 |
| Mononucleosis | 075 |
| Motor vehicle accident, unsp | E819.9 |
| Murmur, undiagnosed | 785.2 |
| Muscle cramps | 729.82 |
| Muscle spasm | 728.85 |
| Muscle weakness (generalized) | 728.87 |
| Mutilation, self-damaging behaviors | V69.8 |
| **N** | |
| Nail abnormality | 703.8 |
| Nail-stepped on | E920.8 |
| Nasopharyngitis, acute, common cold | 460 |
| Nausea (alone) | 787.02 |
| Nausea and vomiting | 787.01 |
| Near-syncope | 780.2 |
| Neutropenia, unsp | 288.00 |
| Night sweats | 780.8 |
| **O** | |
| Obesity, unsp | 278.00 |
| Obesity, morbid | 278.01 |
| Obsessive compulsive disorder | 300.3 |
| Oligomenorrhea | 626.1 |
| Onychomycosis | 110.1 |
| Oppositional defiant disorder | 313.81 |
| Osgood schlatter | 732.4 |
| Otalgia (ear pain) | 388.70 |
| Otitis media, unsp | 382.9 |
| Otitis media, chronic, serous | 381.10 |
| Otitis media, purulent, w/o rupture of ear drum | 382.00 |
| Ovarian cyst, unsp | 620.2 |
| Overweight | 278.02 |
| **P** | |
| Pain, abdominal (use 5th digit to specify locale) | 789.0x |
| Pain, ankle | 719.47 |
| Pain, back, unsp | 724.5 |
| Pain, breast | 611.71 |
| Pain, eye | 379.91 |
| Pain, hip | 719.45 |
| Pain, joint, site unsp | 719.40 |
| Pain, knee | 719.46 |
| Pain, limb/hand, foot | 729.5 |
| Pain, neck | 723.1 |
| Pain, pelvic (female) | 625.9 |
| Pain, rib | 786.50 |
| Pain, shoulder region | 719.41 |
| Pain, tooth | 525.9 |
| Pain, wrist | 719.43 |
| Palpitations | 785.1 |

*(Continued)*

**Table 23-5 (Continued)**

| *Diagnosis* | *ICD-9-CM Code* |
|---|---|
| Panic attack | 300.01 |
| PAP smear, abnormal, unsp | 795.09 |
| PAP smear, follow-up abnormal | V72.32 |
| PAP smear, follow-up | V67.01 |
| Parent brings in but could not find the problem | V71.89 |
| Paronychia, finger | 681.02 |
| Paronychia, toe | 681.11 |
| PCO (polycystic ovary) | 256.4 |
| Pectus excavatum | 754.81 |
| Pediculosis, body | 132.1 |
| Pediculosis, genital | 132.2 |
| Pediculosis, head | 132.0 |
| Pelvic inflammatory disease | 614.9 |
| Personal history of tobacco use | V15.82 |
| Petechiae | 782.7 |
| Petit mal epilepsy | 345.00 |
| Pharyngitis, acute | 462 |
| Phobic disorder | 300.20 |
| Physical abuse, hx of child physical/sexual abuse/rape | V15.41 |
| Pityriasis, alba | 696.5 |
| Pityriasis, rosea | 696.3 |
| Pityriasis, versicolor | 111.0 |
| PMS | 625.4 |
| Pneumonia | 486 |
| Polycystic ovaries | 256.4 |
| Polydipsia/excess thirst | 783.5 |
| Post traumatic stress disorder (PTSD) | 309.81 |
| Pregnancy/pregnant, incidental | V22.2 |
| Pregnancy exam or test, negative result | V72.41 |
| Pregnancy, counseling, other | V26.49 |
| Pregnancy, exam (test results pending) | V72.40 |
| Pregnancy exam or test, positive results | V72.42 |
| Premenstrual tension syndrome | 625.4 |
| Prescription refill noncontraceptive | V68.1 |
| Primary hypercoagulable state | 289.81 |
| Proteinuria | 791.0 |
| Proteinuria, postural | 593.6 |
| Pruritus, genital organs | 698.1 |
| Pseudotumor cerebri | 348.2 |
| Puberty status | V21.1 |
| Puberty, delayed | 259.0 |
| Puberty, precocious | 259.1 |
| Pyelonephritis, acute | 590.10 |
| **R** | |
| Rape | E960.1 |
| Rape, alleged | V71.5 |
| Rash, nonspecific | 782.1 |
| Reactive airway disease (asthma) | 493.90 |
| Reflex sympathetic dystrophy | 337. 20 |
| **S** | |
| Scabies | 133.0 |
| School avoidance (phobia) | 300.29 |
| Scoliosis | 737.30 |
| Screen for cholesterol | V77.91 |
| Screen for sickle cell | V78.2 |
| Screen for TB | V74.1 |
| Screen for thyroid | V77.0 |
| Scrotal/testicular mass | 608.89 |
| Sebaceous skin cyst | 706.2 |
| Seborrhea | 706.3 |
| Seizure, convulsions, NOS | 780.39 |
| Self-mutilation | 300.9 |
| Short stature | 783.43 |
| Shortness of breath | 786.05 |
| Sickle cell disease, unsp | 282.60 |
| Sickle cell disease, other, w/crisis | 282.69 |
| Sickle cell disease, other w/o crisis | 282.68 |
| Sickle cell thalassemia w/crisis | 282.42 |
| Sickle cell thalassemia w/o crisis | 282.41 |
| Sickle cell trait | 282.5 |
| Sickle cell/Hb-C disease w/crisis | 282.64 |
| Sickle cell/Hb-C disease w/o crisis | 282.63 |
| Sinusitis, acute | 461.9 |
| Skin infection, unspec | 686.9 |
| Skin mass/lump/nodule | 782.2 |
| Sleep disturbance | 780.50 |
| Somatization disorder | 300.81 |
| Sore throat, chronic | 472.1 |

(*Continued*)

**Table 23-5 (Continued)**

| *Diagnosis* | *ICD-9-CM Code* |
|---|---|
| Spasm, muscle | 728.85 |
| Spondylolisthesis | 756.12 |
| Sport/job/camp physical | V70.3 |
| Sprain/strain, ankle, unsp site | 845.00 |
| Sprain/strain, elbow, unsp site | 841.9 |
| Sprain/strain, foot/toe, unsp site | 845.10 |
| Sprain/strain, hand/finger, unsp site | 842.10 |
| Sprain/strain, knee, unsp site | 844.9 |
| Sprain/strain, lumbosacral | 846.0 |
| Sprain/strain, neck | 847.0 |
| Sprain/strain, wrist, unsp site | 842.00 |
| Sprain/strain/dislocation unspec | 848.9 |
| Status epilepticus | 345.3 |
| STD, contact | V01.6 |
| STD, counseling | V65.45 |
| STD, follow-up exam | V67.59 |
| STD screening, bacterial venereal diseases | V74.5 |
| STD, screening, HPV | V73.81 |
| STD, screening, other specified chlamydial | V73.88 |
| STD, screening, unsp chlamydial disease | V73.98 |
| STD, unspec | 099.9 |
| Stepped on nail | E920.8 |
| Steroids, long-term, current | V58.65 |
| Stress fracture, metatarsal | 733.94 |
| Stress fracture, other bone | 733.95 |
| Stress fracture, tibia or fibula | 733.93 |
| Stress, acute reaction to, other | 308.3 |
| Substance abuse counseling | V65.42 |
| Suicide attempt/risk/tendency | 300.9 |
| Suicide ideation | V62.84 |
| Sunburn | 692.71 |
| Suture removal | V58.32 |
| Syncope/fainting | 780.2 |
| Synovial cyst, unsp | 727.40 |
| Syphilis, genital, primary | 091.0 |
| **T** | |
| Tachycardia, unsp | 785.0 |
| TB screen (PPD) | V74.1 |
| TB test positive | 795.5 |
| Testicle torsion, unsp | 608.20 |
| Thalassemia, other | 282.49 |
| Throat pain | 784.1 |
| Thyroid enlargement/goiter | 240.9 |
| Tinea, capitis | 110.0 |
| Tinea, corporis | 110.5 |
| Tinea, cruris | 110.3 |
| Tinea, pedis | 110.4 |
| Tinea, versicolor | 111.0 |
| TMJ disorder, unsp | 524.60 |
| Tobacco use, hx of | V15.82 |
| Tonsillitis, acute | 463 |
| Tooth loss, trauma | 525.11 |
| Torticollis/wry neck, unsp | 723.5 |
| Tourette syndrome | 307.23 |
| Tremor | 781.0 |
| Trichomonal, vulvovaginitis | 131.01 |
| Trisomy 21/Down syndrome | 758.0 |
| Turner syndrome (XO) | 758.6 |
| **U** | |
| Underweight | 783.22 |
| Urethral discharge | 788.7 |
| Urethritis, gonococcal | 098.0 |
| Urethritis, non-STD | 598.8 |
| Urethritis, STD | 099.40 |
| URI, acute | 465.9 |
| Urinary complaints, SX | 788.9 |
| Urinary frequency | 788.41 |
| Urinary urgency | 788.63 |
| Urticaria/hives/unspec | 708.9 |
| UTI, site not specified | 599.0 |
| **V** | |
| Vaginal bleeding | 623.8 |
| Vaginal discharge, NOS | 623.5 |
| Varicocele | 456.4 |
| Vertigo/dizziness | 780.4 |
| Viral exanthem, unsp | 057.9 |
| Viral infection, unspec | 079.99 |
| Vision screen, failed | 368.9 |
| Vomiting (alone) | 787.03 |
| Vomiting, persistent | 536.2 |

*(Continued)*

**Table 23-5 (Continued)**

| *Diagnosis* | *ICD-9-CM Code* |
|---|---|
| Vulvovaginitis | 616.10 |
| Vulvovaginitis, candidal | 112.1 |
| Vulvovaginitis, trichomoniasis | 131.01 |
| **W** | |
| Warts, genital | 078.11 |
| Warts, other (common, flat) | 078.19 |
| Warts, plantar | 078.12 |
| Warts, unspec | 078.10 |
| Weight gain, abnormal | 783.1 |
| Weight loss | 783.21 |
| Well child | V20.2 |
| Wheezing | 786.07 |

Table includes information and codes adapted from *International Classification of Diseases, 9th Revision, Clinical Modification (ICD-9-CM)*. Department of Health and Human Services, 2007.

NEC, not elsewhere classified; ADD, attention-deficit disorder; ADHD, attention-deficit/hyperactivity disorder; NOS, not otherwise specified; DUB, dysfunctional uterine bleeding; STD, sexually transmitted disease; LOC, loss of consciousness; HIV, human immunodeficiency virus; TB, tuberculosis; PPD, purified protein derivative; TMJ, temporomandibular joint; URI, upper respiratory infection.

## CODING BASICS

This section provides a summary of the 1995 and 1997 Centers for Medicare and Medicaid Services (CMS) Documentation Guidelines for E/M Services. Documentation guidelines should not result in alteration of the type of care provided patients, but rather help ensure the recording of the details of care necessary to justify the CPT code selected: "If it is not documented, it did not happen." Resources that help with compliance in documenting may include the use of checklists, templates, and electronic medical records software.

Most visits in adolescent medicine come from the E/MCPT codes and are determined by the amount of work reflected in the documented history (H) and physical examination (PE), which then drives the medical decision making (MDM). These 3 components combine to determine the final level of the visit: problem focused, expanded problem focused (EPF), detailed (D), or comprehensive (C). Documenting non-applicable information in an effort to up-code is not appropriate (eg, pharyngitis in 13-year-old girl would likely not routinely require an extensive review of systems [ROS] or PE).

Using *time* to assign a code level is appropriate in some circumstances; specifically, if a visit is provided where counseling and/or coordination of care account for more than 50% of the provider face-to-face time with the patient. An example of use of time might be when a parent comes in alone to discuss the teen's condition or problem, using the teen's diagnosis or problem as the ICD-9-CM code. When using time, it is necessary to document the total time spent and the time spent providing the counseling and/or coordination of care. Nurse time in activities (eg, giving injections) is not included. However, for hospital encounters, "time" includes the total time spent at the patient's bedside, on the unit writing notes and communicating with staff (eg, nurses, residents) about the patient, and in other activities such as reading x-rays and electrocardiograms (EKGs). There are specific time requirements associated with each code (see Table 23-2 and Table 23-3). Not every type of E/M visit (eg, preventive care or emergency department visit codes) may use time to justify the code—only those where "typical times" are listed as part of the descriptor (ie, 99201-5, 99211-3, 99231-3, 99241-5, 99251-5, 99324-8, 99334-7, 99341-5, and 99347-50).

### HISTORY

Components of history include present illness (HPI), ROS, and past/family/social history (PFSH) (see Table 23-6). The following case serves as an example: A 14-year-old female adolescent established patient presents to your office with fever and abdominal pain. History includes an HPI with 2 problems. Four or more elements of each problem are documented (eg, fever pattern, severity, duration, use and response to anti-pyretics; location of abdominal pain, duration, limitation of activity; response to any treatment or medication); a ROS asking about symptoms from 2 or more but less than 10 systems (eg, urinary symptoms, vaginal discharge, last menstrual period (LMP) [genitourinary/gynecological], vomiting, diarrhea [gastrointestinal]); and a PFSH including elements from both the past history (current medications, previous history of urinary problems) and the social history (sexual activity status, possible ingestion of drugs or substances). This encounter would qualify as a detailed history.

### PHYSICAL EXAM

Physical exam may be documented by organ systems (1995 Medicare Documentation Guidelines) or by elements (1997 guidelines) (Table 23-7 and Table 23-8). The 1995 guidelines are generally more "primary care

**Table 23-6**

## Components of the History[a]

| *History* | *PF* | *EPF* | *D* | *C* |
|---|---|---|---|---|
| **History of Present Illness** | | | | |
| ___Location ___Quality ___Severity ___Duration ___Timing ___Context ___Modifying factors ___Associated signs/symptoms | 1 element | 1-3 elements | ≥ 4 elements | ≥ 4 elements |
| **Review of Systems (14 systems)** | | | | |
| ___Constitutional ___Eyes ___HENT ___Cardio ___Resp ___GI ___GU/GYN ___Musc ___Skin/breast ___Neuro ___Psych ___Endo ___Heme/Lymph ___All/Imm ___"all others neg" | None | 1 system | 2-9 systems | ≥ 10 systems |
| **Past/Family/Social History (PFSH)** | | | | |
| ___Past history (illness, injuries, operations, hospitalizations, medications, allergies, immunizations, nutrition, & treatments)<br>___Family history (current illnesses, health status/death of family members, specific diseases related to chief complaint, hereditary diseases)<br>___Social history (age-appropriate review patient's past and current activities: education, school; extracurricular activities; work; sexual history; use of: alcohol, tobacco, other) | None | None | 1 | 2 if established<br>3 if new<br>0 if patient hospitalized |

PF, problem focused; EPF, expanded problem focused; D, detailed; C, comprehensive

[a]OR ≥ 3 chronic or inactive conditions

**Table 23-7**

## Components of the Physical Exam

| *Year* | *Systems* | *PF* | *EPF* | *D* | *C* |
|---|---|---|---|---|---|
| 1995 Organ Systems | ___Constitutional ___Eyes ___ENT ___Neck ___Resp ___Cardio ___ Chest (breasts) ___GI ___GU ___ Skin ___Musculoskeletal ___Neuro ___Heme/lymph/imm ___Psych | 1 system | 2-4 systems | 5-7 systems | ≥ 8 systems |
| 1997 Elements | Allows the use of the general multisystem exam (Table 23-8) or single organ systems (not presented here) | 1-5 elements | 6-11 elements | 12-17 elements[a] | ≥ 18 elements[b] |

Modified and used with permission from Bradley, JF, *Coding for Pediatrics*. Elk Grove Village, IL: American Academy of Pediatrics; 2006: 78-80.

C, comprehensive, D, detailed; EPF, expanded problem focused; PF, problem focused

[a]Detailed exam includes ≥ 2 elements in each of 6 systems, or ≥ 12 elements from 2 systems

[b]Comprehensive exam includes ≥ 2 elements from 9 systems

**Table 23-8**

**1997 General Multisystem Examination Bulleted Elements**

| *Body Area* | *Bulleted Elements* |
|---|---|
| Constitutional | 1) Appearance; 2) Any 3 vital signs (BP, HR, RR, temp, wt, ht) |
| Eyes | 1) Lids & conj.; 2) Iris & pupil; 3) Ophthalmoscopy |
| ENT | 1) Ext ear & nose; 2) Ext. aud. canal & TMs; 3) Hearing; 4) Inner nose; 5) Lips, gums, teeth; 6) Oropharynx/mucosa/salivary/tongue/tonsils/hard & soft palate |
| Neck | 1) Appearance/symmetry/mass; 2) Thyroid |
| Cardiovascular | 1) Palpation; 2) Auscultation; 3) Carotid arteries; 4) Abdominal aorta; 5) Femoral arteries; 6) Pedal pulses; 7) Extremities for edema/varicosities |
| Respiratory | 1) Effort; 2) Palpation; 3) Percussion; 4) Auscultation |
| Breast | 1) Inspection; 2) Palpation breasts/axilla |
| GI | 1) Mass/tenderness; 2) Liver/spleen; 3) Hernia; 4) Anus/perineum/rectum; 5) Occult blood |
| GU | Male: 1) Penis; 2) Scrotal contents; 3) Prostate<br>Female: 1) External genitalia; 2) Urethra; 3) Cervix; 4) Adnexae; 5) Uterus; 6) Bladder |
| Musculoskeletal | 1) Gait and station; 2) Inspection/palpation of digits and nails; 3) Inspection/palpation, ROM, stability, strength/tone of 1 or more of the following areas: 1) Head and neck; 2) RUE; 3) LUE; 4) Spine/ribs/pelvis; 5) RLE; 6) LLE |
| Skin | 1) Inspection; 2) Palpation |
| Neuro | 1) Cranial nerves; 2) Reflexes; 3) Sensation |
| Heme/Lymph | Palpation of ≥ 2 areas: 1) Neck 2) Axilla 3) Groin 4) Other |
| Psychiatric | 1) Judgment/insight; 2) Orientation; 3) Mood/affect; 4) Recent/remote memory |

Table modified and used with permission from Bradley, *Coding for Pediatrics*. Elk Grove Village, IL: American Academy of Pediatrics; 2006: 78–80.

friendly;" however the 1997 guidelines may better address the needs of sub-specialists (cardiologists, dermatologists, etc) who may perform in-depth examinations on 1 or 2 organ systems, but not comprehensive general examinations. For the 14-year-old female with fever and abdominal pain, the provider would typically perform an examination covering several organ systems including documentation of vital signs, ears/nose/throat (ENT), neck, respiratory, cardiac, gastrointestinal, and genitourinary. By the 1995 guidelines, this examination is detailed.

## MEDICAL DECISION MAKING

The final criteria used in assigning the code to a service is MDM. Providers will recognize the MDM as the assessment and plan section of standard records—the differential diagnosis and the evaluation and treatment. There are 3 elements included in assigning the level of MDM for a visit: the number of diagnostic or management options, the amount or complexity of data to be reviewed, and the risk of the condition or its treatment to the patient (risk of morbidity and mortality) (Table 23-9 and Table 23-10). Two of these 3 elements must meet or exceed a level for it to be assigned for the MDM.

The level of risk of a condition or its treatment is determined by 3 sub elements: the risk of the problem or illness continuing undiagnosed or untreated until the next visit, the risk associated with the diagnostic procedures, and the risk of the management options (Table 23-11). The highest level of risk in any of these 3 sub-elements drives the assignment of the level of risk.

Again using the example of the febrile 14-year-old female presenting to the office, the patient presents with a new problem which required work-up (4 points, Table 23-10) and is "extensive." The work-up would include a complete blood count (CBC), urine pregnancy test, urinalysis and culture, and prescription for treatment (2 points, Table 23-10) and is "limited." Assessment of risk includes an acute new illness with systemic symptoms requiring labs and prescribed

**Table 23-9**

**Level of Medical Decision Making[a]**

| *Elements of MDM* | *Straightforward* | *Low* | *Moderate* | *High* |
|---|---|---|---|---|
| Diagnostic and management options | Minimal | Limited | Multiple | Extensive |
| Amount or complexity of data | None/minimal | Limited | Multiple | Extensive |
| Risk | Minimal | Low | Moderate | High |

[a]Two of 3 elements must meet the threshold to code the complexity of MDM.

**Table 23-10**

**Medical Decision Making**

| **Diagnostic and Management Options** | **Number × Points = Score** | |
|---|---|---|
| New problem with work-up | 4 | |
| New problem without work-up (max = 2) | 3 | |
| Established problem, not stable | 2 | |
| Established problem, improving | 2 | |
| Minor problem, self-limited (max = 3) | 1 | |
| **Total score for Diagnostic and Management Options[a]** | | |
| ***Amount or Complexity of Data*** | ***Points*** | ***Score*** |
| Labs: ordered or reviewed | 1 | |
| Radiology: ordered or reviewed | 1 | |
| Medicine: ordered or reviewed | 1 | |
| Independent visualization of tests (eg, x-ray, ECG) | 2 | |
| Review/discuss/summarize lab tests: | | |
| with performing MD | 1 | |
| with others, such as patient or parent(s) | 1 | |
| old records | 2 | |
| **Total score for Amount or Complexity of Data[b]** | | |
| ***Risk[c]*** | ***Level*** | |
| No medications; low-risk tests | Minimal | |
| Over-the-counter medications; more complex tests; risk of complications/morbidity is low | Low | |
| Prescription medications; moderate or high-risk tests or treatments | Moderate | |
| Administer or monitor potentially toxic medications; high-risk treatments or surgery | High | |

[a]Multiply the number of problems described by the points assigned. Sum into a total score to assign the level of MDM: 1 = minimal; 2 = limited; 3 = multiple; ≥ 4 = extensive.

[b]Sum the points assigned for the work-up into a total score to assign the level of MDM: ≤ 1 = minimal; 2 = limited; 3 = multiple; ≥ 4 = extensive

[c]See Table 23-11, "Elements of Risk," for further details.

**Table 23-11**

**Elements of Risk**

| *Risk*[a] | *Description* | *Presenting Problems* | *Diagnostic Procedures/Tests* | *Management Options* |
|---|---|---|---|---|
| Minimal | No meds; low-risk tests | • 1 self-limited, minor | • Lab tests requiring venipuncture<br>• CXR<br>• EKG or EEG<br>• U/A<br>• US | • Rest<br>• Gargles<br>• Elastic bandages<br>• Superficial dressing |
| Low | OTC meds; more complex tests; risk of complications, morbidity, or mortality is low | • 2 or more self-limited, minor<br>• 1 stable chronic<br>• Acute uncomplicated illness or injury (eg, acute gastroenteritis, cystitis, epistaxis, upper respiratory infection) | • Radiologic procedures (eg, barium study)<br>• Superficial needle bx<br>• Lab tests/arterial stick<br>• Skin bx | • Over-the-counter meds<br>• PT/OT referral<br>• IV fluids without additives<br>• Minor surgery without risk factors |
| Moderate | Rx meds; moderate or high-risk tests or treatments | • 2 or more stable, chronic (asthma, persistent or moderate)<br>• Undiagnosed new illness or injury with uncertain prognosis (eg, chronic abdominal pain)<br>• 1 or more chronic diagnosis with mild exacerbation/side effects (eg, mild persistent asthma)<br>• Acute illness with systemic symptoms (eg, pharyngitis with fever, vomiting; pneumonia; pyelonephritis)<br>• Acute complicated injury (eg, brief loss of consciousness) | • Lumbar puncture<br>• MRI<br>• Diagnostic endoscopy/no risk factors<br>• Deep needles or incisional bx<br>• CV imagining/contrast<br>• Obtain fluid from body cavity<br>• Imaging studies with contrast<br>• Foreign body removal<br>• Allergy testing<br>• Pelvic exam<br>• Mono test<br>• CBC<br>• Blood chemistries | • Prescription medications<br>• Referral to specialist<br>• IV fluids with additives<br>• Minor surgery with risk factors<br>• Closed treatment of fracture |
| High | Administer or monitor potentially toxic meds; high-risk treatments or surgery | • 1 or more chronic illnesses with severe exacerbation/side effects (eg, DKA)<br>• Acute or chronic illness/injury that pose a threat to life or bodily function (eg, meningitis, rape, or attempted suicide)<br>• Abrupt change in neurologic status (eg, status epilepticus) | • Diagnostic endoscopy/with risk factors<br>• Thoracentesis<br>• Paracentesis<br>• Bone marrow aspiration<br>• CT/MRI<br>• Imaging studies w/contrast | • Intravenous drug therapy requiring intensive monitoring<br>• Refer for elective surgery with risk factors<br>• Refer for emergency major surgery<br>• Parenteral controlled drugs<br>• Transfer to ICU<br>• Ventilator support |

[a]The highest level in any of the 3 components determines the level of risk.

Table modified and used with permission from Bradley JF, *Coding for Pediatrics*. Elk Grove Village, IL: American Academy of Pediatrics; 2006: 69–70.

medications; this is "moderate" risk. Thus the MDM of this encounter would be a summation of the presenting problem [extensive], work-up/treatment [limited], and risk [moderate] (Table 23-11). As 2 of the 3 elements of MDM must meet the threshold for assigning the level, this encounter would be considered "moderate." If the evaluation and treatment of this patient resulted in the need for IV medications, radiological evaluation, and referral for surgery, then the presenting problem [extensive], work-up/treatment [moderate], and risk [high] would result in "high" MDM.

## MODIFIERS

Modifiers are used to let payers know when special circumstances exist surrounding the provision of a service. The CPT modifiers are 2-digit numbers attached to the 5-digit CPT code being modified (eg, 99213-25). As the correct use of modifiers should increase reimbursements, providers should become acquainted with their use. Table 23-12 lists some of the common modifiers and provides brief examples of their use. A full list of modifiers is available in the CPT publication.

**Table 23-12**

**Common Modifiers**

| *Modifier* | *Description* | *Explanation* |
|---|---|---|
| 24 | Unrelated E/M service by the same physician during a postoperative period | When an E/M service was performed during a postoperative period for a reason(s) unrelated to the original procedure.<br>Ex: You treat a 14-year-old for a fractured clavicle. One week later, you see the patient again for shoulder pain from a new injury (a contusion). Because the second visit falls within the 90-day global payment period, attach this modifier to the E/M code for this visit. |
| 25 | Significant, separately identifiable E/M service by the same physician on the same day of the procedure or other service | When the patient's condition required a separate E/M service above and beyond the initial service provided (or the usual pre- and postoperative care associated with the procedure that was performed). The E/M service may be prompted by the symptom or condition for which the initial procedure of service was provided. As such, different diagnoses are not required for reporting of the E/M services on the same date. This modifier is NOT used to report an E/M service that resulted in a decision to perform surgery. |
| 26 | Professional component | When a procedure includes a technical component and a professional (physician) component, this modifier is used to indicate the physician component.<br>Ex: You read the results of an electrocardiogram (ECG) that was done at the hospital on your patient with tachycardia. Attach 26 to the CPT code for the ECG (CPT 93000), indicating that you only provided the reading (professional service) and did not provide the technical service of the ECG. |
| 51 | Multiple procedures | When multiple procedures (not E/M services) are performed at the same visit by the same provider. Note that this modifier is not to be used with "add-on" codes.<br>Ex: You drain a subungual hematoma from the thumb of a patient, and also remove a wart noted on his finger at the same visit. Code CPT 11740 (Evacuation of subungual hematoma) with ICD-9 927.3 (Crush injury finger), and then CPT 17000 51 (Destruction, benign lesion) with ICD-9 078.10 (wart, common). The modifier allows reimbursement for both procedures, although some payers will reimburse at a lower rate for the second procedure. |

(*Continued*)

**Table 23-12 (Continued)**

| *Modifier* | *Description* | *Explanation* |
|---|---|---|
| 52 | Reduced services | When a service or procedure is partially reduced or eliminated at the physician's discretion.<br>Ex.: A patient presents with a follow-up from an ear infection. During the previous encounter, the patient failed a tympanometry so the physician decides to repeat it on the affected (right) ear only. Report code 92567 with modifier 52 because the code refers to testing of both ears. |
| 57 | Decision for surgery | When identifying an E/M service that resulted in the initial decision to perform surgery. Most payers limit this to major procedures that have a 90-day global period.<br>Ex:You see a 15-year-old in consultation for leg pain after a month of cross-country running.An x-ray film reveals a fracture of the distal tibia, which you cast.You would report the E/M service for the evaluation portion (99241–99245) with modifier 57 attached to indicate the decision to perform the procedure (CPT 27824 Closed treatment of fracture, distal tibia). Both of these CPT codes would be linked to the same ICD-9 code (824.8 Fracture, tibia, closed, distal end). |
| 59 | Distinct Procedural Service | When a procedure is performed in addition to another significant and separately identifiable non-E/M service.<br>Ex: You see a patient who uses an inhaler for her asthma.The patient is found to be wheezing and you order a nebulizer (94640).You then ask your nurse to spend some time with the patient going over how she uses the inhaler and demonstrating the proposer technique (94664).You have to report the 94664 with modifier 59 to indicate it was a separate service from the nebulizer (94640). |
| 76 | Repeat procedure by same physician | When a procedure or service is repeated subsequent to the original procedure or service.<br>Ex: A patient presents with wheezing and shortness of breath. A nebulizer (94640) is administered. After the physician examines the patient, another nebulizer is ordered. Report the subsequent (repeat) nebulizer code 94640 with modifier 76. |

Table includes information modified and used with permission from Bradley J, Blythe MJ (eds). *Quick Reference Guide to Pediatric Coding and Documentation for Adolescent Medicine.A Companion to Coding for Pediatrics*. 2nd ed. Elk Grove Village, IL:American Academy of Pediatrics; 2005: 161–164.

## RESOURCE-BASED RELATIVE VALUE SCALE

The RBRVS has been used by CMS since 1992, when it was implemented to replace a system based on "usual and customary charges" for Medicare reimbursement for physician services. Under the RBRVS system, each provider service is assigned a number value defined as a relative value unit (RVU). The RVUs are determined by the CMS with input from the AMA/Specialty Society Relative Value Scale Update Committee (RUC). The physician fee schedule is published in the Federal Register each November (available at www.gpoaccess.gov/fr/index.html). The AAP also provides a summary of RBRVS at its web site (www.aap.org/visit/rbrvsbrochure.pdf).

The RBRVS is useful for physicians in several ways. For each service there is an associated pre-set value of "physician work" assigned, thus allowing negotiations with private payers for physician reimbursement to begin at the same number. In managed care or capitation environments, the RBRVS can assist in the calculation of per member per month cost estimates. The RBRVS can also be helpful for guiding individual physician reimbursements in profit-sharing environments where productivity is evaluated, as the RVU provides a measure of relative work completed regardless of specialty.

The RVU is calculated from 3 components associated with providing the service: the amount of physician work (~52%), the practice expense (~44%), and

**Box 23-1**

***Calculation of RVU***

Total RVU for 99213 =
(Work RVU × Work GPCI) + (Practice Expense RVU[a] × Practice Expense GPCI[a]) + (Malpractice Expense RVU × Malpractice Expense GPCI)
(0.97 × 0.986) + (0.80 × 0.918) + (0.05 × 0.599) = 1.72077 RVU
Total payment for 99213 = RVU × Medicare Conversion Factor
1.72077 × $36.0666 = $62.06

[a]Nonfacility expense based on the 2010 RVUs

2010 Medicare Conversion Factor in US Dollars: 1 RVU = $36.0666

GPCI, geographic practice cost index; RVU, relative value unit

GPCI for Indianapolis, IN

the professional liability/malpractice expense (~4%). As expenses vary according to location each component is multiplied by a geographic price cost index (GPCI). The total RVU is then multiplied by a conversion factor (CF) in dollars to determine the actual payment. Most payers (both public and private) have adapted at least some component of the CMS RBRVS system for calculation of physician reimbursements; however, this varies by payer and by service.

The practice expense component of the RVU will reflect either a nonfacility (eg, private doctor's office) or facility (eg, hospital or hospital outpatient clinic, skilled nursing facility, or outpatient surgery center) fee. A physician in private practice would collect the physician work, practice expense, and malpractice/liability components. In the hospital setting, the physician work and malpractice components of the service would usually be collected by the physician while the hospital where the care was provided would collect the practice expense component.

As an example, to calculate the reimbursement for the CPT E/M code 99213 (established outpatient visit) in Indianapolis, Indiana, use the formula in Box 23-1.

## CASE EXAMPLES IN CODING AND DOCUMENTATION

### CASE 1

A 17-year-old established patient presents to your office for her physical examination. You provide vision (using the Snellen chart) and urine dipstick screening, and perform a comprehensive history and PE. She has been sexually active since age 14 and is asymptomatic. A pelvic is included as a routine part of her examination. A Pap smear was obtained and sent to the appropriate laboratory, and a urine sample is sent for nucleic acid amplification tests for sexually acquired infection. Appropriate anticipatory guidance is given to the patient and her mother. Both the mother and teen want her to continue oral contraception. The physician counsels on and orders the third Hepatitis B vaccine. The nurse draws a CBC and gives the third Hepatitis B vaccination shot. A prescription is written for birth control pills. The CPT codes associated with this well visit (ICD-9-CM V20.2, well child check) include:

- 99394: Established patient 17-year-old preventive care visit; (note: includes pelvic exam)
- 99173: Screening test of visual acuity, quantitative, bilateral;
- 81002: Urinalysis, by dipstick or tablet reagent; nonautomated, without microscopy;
- 36415: Collection of venous blood by venipuncture per nurse;
- 9046x1: Immunization administration single component
- 90744: Hepatitis B vaccine, 3 dose schedule, intramuscular.

ICD-9-CM codes include:

- V20.2: Well child visit
- V25.41: Surveillance of previously prescribed contraceptive method; pills

If this patient had an additional problem identified and documented with treatment initiated (eg, dysmenorrhea, ICD-9-CM code 625.3), which would have required "a separate, identifiable visit" to assess and manage, then modifier 25 may be attached to the appropriate level of E/M visit (CPT 99212–99215).

### CASE 2

The 17-year-old female from Case 1 returns 3 months later for a sport physical and follow-up for her previously diagnosed dysmenorrhea. Choices for coding include:

- CPT 99394 (Established patient 17-year-old well adolescent visit) with ICD-9-CM V70.3 (Other medical examination for administrative purposes —sports competition);
- Appropriate CPT 99212–99215 with modifier 25 added for ICD-9-CM diagnosis code 625.3 (dysmenorrhea).

- Although this coding strategy accurately describes the service provided, most insurers only allow 1 "well" visit per year.

Or

- Appropriate CPT 99212–99215 with first ICD-9-CM diagnosis code 625.3 (dysmenorrhea) and second, V70.3 (sports physical). If her dysmenorrhea had completely resolved on medications, use ICD V67.59 (Unspecified follow-up examination) as the first diagnosis, with V70.3 as the second.

Or

- CPT 99080 (Special reports, more that the information conveyed in the usual medical communications or standard reporting form) alone without patient present. Most providers fill out the forms when requested if the patient has had a physical within the past school year. Reimbursement by insurers does not occur as most health plans consider sport physicals forms as "standard reporting forms."

**CASE 3**

The following case includes nongeographically adjusted RVUs to highlight the advantages to using specific CPT codes for procedures instead of just submitting CPT E/M codes (99212–99215) for procedures provided in the office (non facility). A 15-year-old male established patient is brought to the office unannounced and accompanied by his mother after suffering a hand and head injury at football practice the night before. He reports being dazed briefly but not losing consciousness. He reports a consistent headache since the injury. You see him immediately, in front of already scheduled patients. Your detailed history and PE revealed a large contusion on his lower cheek, but no evidence of obvious neurological sequelae. His 3rd finger is swollen and tender distally. Radiographs by the next door radiology service reveal a nondisplaced fracture of the distal phalanx that you treat with an aluminum finger splint. You spend a total of 55 minutes face-to-face with the patient and his mother, of which greater than 50% is spent in counseling (giving "concussion" instructions, ordering CT scan of brain, providing significant parental reassurance, and planning follow-up and return to activities). However, you must subtract the time spent performing the procedure, therefore the E/M service time is reduced and prolonged services are not appropriate. Suggestions for coding include:

- CPT 26750 (Closed treatment of distal phalangeal fracture, finger or thumb; without manipulation; 4.45 RVUs), with ICD-9-CM 816.02 (distal phalanx fracture);
- CPT 99214–25 (Established outpatient visit – based on your detailed history, PE, and moderate MDM for his head injury; 2.73 RVUs) with ICD-9-CM 850.0 (concussion w/o loss of consciousness); this service usually takes 25 minutes.
- CPT 99058 (Service(s) provided on an emergency basis in office, which disrupts other scheduled office services, in addition to basic service). No standard recognized RVUs have been assigned and reimbursement policies for CPT codes 99050–99060 vary among insurers.

Coding the fracture care as a procedure using the Medicare "global care package" and coding for the evaluation of the head injury utilizing modifier 25 results in higher RVUs for the provider (7.18) compared to coding only the E/M visit using time – even if one coded 99215 (the highest level available based on the 55 minutes spent with the patient), the total RVU is 3.68. When coding for procedures, providers need to be aware of the global period associated with the procedure. For this finger fracture, initial casting/splinting supplies, the application of the cast/splint, and follow-up visits for the next 90 days are all included in this global package (thus the higher RVUs). If you see the patient within this 90-day global period for a reason other than the fracture care (for example follow-up for the concussion), you will need to add modifier 24 (to report an E/M service provided for an unrelated condition during a global period) to the established other or outpatient visit code (CPT 99211–99215) as appropriate.

## SPECIAL SITUATIONS

In order to maintain consistency with CPT coding books and references, the word "physician" was used throughout the text; services are provided to adolescents by other skilled health care practitioners, including resident physicians, nurse practitioners, physician assistants, etc. Specific state scope of practice rules apply to billing when services are provided by resident physicians and non-physician providers, and readers are encouraged to seek out further education regarding these issues.

## REFERENCES

1. *Physicians' Current Procedural Terminology, Standard Edition*. Chicago, IL: American Medical Association; 2007

2. *ICD-9 CM Expert for Physicians Volumes 1&2*, 7th ed. Ingenix. St Anthony Publishing/Medicode; 2007

3. *International Classification of Diseases*, 9th Revision, Clinical Modification (ICD-9-CM). Department of Health and Human Services, 2007

4. Bradley J, Blythe MJ (eds). *Quick Reference Guide to Pediatric Coding and Documentation for Adolescent Medicine. A Companion to Coding for Pediatrics*, 2nd ed. Elk Grove Village, IL: American Academy of Pediatrics; 2005

5. Bradley JF, Salus T (eds). *Coding for Pediatrics 2006. A Manual for Pediatric Documentation and Reimbursement*, 11th ed. Elk Grove Village, IL: American Academy of Pediatrics; 2006

6. 1995 Documentation Guidelines for Evaluation & Management Services. Available at: www.cms.hhs.gov/MLNProducts/downloads/referenceI.pdf. Accessed November 2006

7. 1997 Documentation Guidelines for Evaluation & Management Services. Available at: www.cms.hhs.gov/MLNProducts/downloads/referenceII.pdf. Accessed November 2006

8. Federal Register. Centers for Medicare and Medicaid Services. Medicare program, physician fee schedule overview. Available at: www.cms.hhs.gov/PhysicianFeeSched/. Accessed August 17, 2010

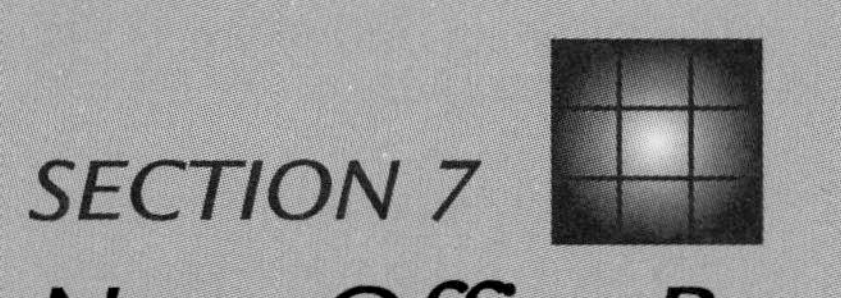

SECTION 7

# Non–Office-Based Practice Settings and Issues

## CHAPTER 24

## The Adolescent In-Patient Unit

KATHY SILVERMAN, DO • S. KENNETH SCHONBERG, MD

In a position statement published in 1996, the Society for Adolescent Medicine (SAM) advocated for the "establishment of adolescent inpatient units in both pediatric and general hospitals as an optimal approach to the delivery of developmentally appropriate health care to hospitalized adolescents."[1] Over a half-century has elapsed since the emergence of the first adolescent inpatient unit at the Boston Children's Hospital under the direction of J. Roswell Gallagher, yet the practice of dedicating a distinct area for the care of the hospitalized adolescent remains far from widespread. Although the exact number of adolescent units cannot be stated with certainty, surveys conducted in both 1968[2] and 1993[3] documented approximately 25 nonpsychiatric adolescent inpatient facilities, with other estimates being 40 to 60 such units in the United States.[3] In sharp contrast, the separation of hospitalized children from hospitalized adults, which dates back to the early 1900s, is now accepted without question as a minimal standard of care and is mandated by health code statutes that prohibit housing ill children with ill adults. Similarly, the need to further subdivide the pediatric population and create a distinct environment for newborns is in evidence throughout the nation in all hospitals that perform deliveries. At the other extreme of the life cycle, geriatric units have achieved wide prevalence and are designed to meet the physical and cognitive impairments of advancing age.

Those adolescent units that do exist range in capacity between 4 and 36 beds with a mean of approximately 20 beds and are most commonly associated with academic departments of pediatrics. Age limits vary, with most having lower limits of 10 to 13 years and upper limits of between 17 and 24 years of age.[3] Historically, brief-stay elective surgery, including plastic, ophthalmologic, and orthopedic procedures, accounted for a large number of adolescent admissions but that is no longer the case. In most centers, medical diagnoses now account for more than half of admissions,[4] particularly with the current and continuing emphasis on performing most elective surgery on an ambulatory basis. In addition, the diagnoses encountered on an adolescent unit vary both in relation to the community being served and the particular interests of the physicians admitting to the facility. Those units associated with urban medical centers with active emergency departments are prone to more acute conditions, including infectious illnesses and trauma. In those instances where the faculty has a particular interest or expertise in specific conditions, such as cystic fibrosis, eating disorders, or substance abuse, those conditions are likely to be disproportionately represented.

### DESIGN CONSIDERATIONS

Extant adolescent units vary greatly in size between 4 and 36 beds.[3] Ideally, the number of beds allocated should be based upon a historical assessment of the usual number of young people hospitalized on all floors within the medical center. However, such an ideal is rarely found as the number of adolescents hospitalized at any given time may vary greatly during the course of a year, with increased numbers often encountered during the winter months when infectious illnesses are more common. In addition, admissions for elective surgery, which could be scheduled to maintain a more constant census, are now less commonly performed on an inpatient basis, exposing the daily census to the mercy of less predictable and unscheduled acute conditions.

At times, adolescent units are established through the reallocation of pre existent space toward the exclusive use of admitted teenagers. At the other extreme, there is great flexibility in the design of an adolescent unit as the concept is incorporated into the architectural plans for a newly constructed children's hospital or other inpatient facility. As noted previously, there is great variability as to the number of beds within units. Ideally, the unit should be large enough both to accommodate all or most adolescents requiring admission to the medical center and to justify the expense of specialized personnel required to address the needs of hospitalized young people. Conversely, the unit should not be so large as to concentrate an unmanageable hoard of teenagers in a single location. Units of approximately 10 beds fit nicely within the design of most hospital floors and meet the criteria of not too big or too small.

The allocation of beds between single rooms and double rooms (housing more than 2 adolescents in one room is not a rational consideration) is at times dictated by architectural necessity rather than medical need or teenage preferences. Not dissimilar to preferences expressed when young people go off to college, when queried some teenagers prefer the privacy of a single room whereas others would opt for the companionship of a roommate.[5] In general, an equal division of total beds between double and single rooms best meets the desire to accommodate adolescent wishes and the occasional need to provide either medically based or behaviorally based isolation.

Room design must assure privacy. The pediatric practice of rooms windowed to the hall to allow for easier patient observation is unacceptable for adolescents, who should not be expected to dress, undress, and sleep in a "fish bowl." Rooms must allow for sufficient personal wardrobe space, particularly if dressing in "street clothes" is allowed or encouraged. Adolescent necessities, a telephone, and a television must be provided. When possible there should be computer and internet access to allow for diversion and to facilitate academic work for those who are hospitalized for more than a brief stay.

A "common room" or recreation area is a necessity to allow for socialization and escape from the incarceration of the hospital room. Recreational areas should be designed with the adolescent in mind. Optimally, such rooms should have computer, CD, and DVD capabilities. A microwave, to prepare snacks and popcorn, is a nice touch. A separate classroom to provide for the continuing education of teens who are hospitalized for extended periods of time is a worthwhile adjunct to bedside teaching. At times, the recreational area and the classroom can be one in the same and used for different purposes at different times of the day.

A further "adolescent unit" consideration is the location of elevators and stairways in relationship to the nursing station. Adolescents in particular may feel the need to explore their environment or escape the confines of the ward, and their ability to "elope" should be minimized. Similarly, the geography of the unit should minimize the potential that visitors—boyfriends and girlfriends—could come and go without being noticed. These considerations, although not motivated by child protection, are not dissimilar to those for a pediatric unit where access and egress from the floor must be controlled.

## PERSONNEL ISSUES

Having established an inpatient environment where a cohort of ill adolescents will receive care, it is necessary to surround them with a group of health professionals dedicated to meeting their needs. Although not mandatory, it is often best if the overall responsibility for the efficient functioning of the unit is vested in a medical director. Most designated units within a medical center, for example, intensive care units, dialysis units, and neonatal units, have a medical director responsible for overseeing the orderly function of the unit, arbitrating any disputes that may arise and achieving consensus among the various health professionals involved in care. Optimally, the medical director of an adolescent inpatient unit should be certified in the subspecialty or, at a minimum, have subspecialty training. As the care of hospitalized adolescents involves not only pediatricians but also internists, surgeons, and multiple adult and pediatric subspecialists, it is most often preferable that a physician director rather than a nurse represent the best interests of the unit and its patients.

Other professionals who should be a part of the core staff include a recreationist, a social worker and, if feasible, a psychiatrist or psychologist. A teacher, often available through the local school district, is a welcome addition and is at times mandated for facilities caring for children and adolescents. For each of these disciplines, the problems and needs of the hospitalized adolescent differ markedly from those encountered in children and adults. Hence, these professionals should be allowed to self-select on the basis of a willingness, even a passion, to work with teenagers and should, preferably, have prior training or work experience with adolescent populations.

In addition, the routine of the work week should allow for the conferencing and consultation necessary to transform a multidisciplinary group into an interdisciplinary team. Providing an office suite, which allows these individuals to work in close proximity to one another, their patients, and the physician staff, facilitates the informal communication and evolution of mutual respect, which maximizes the ability to address the complex psychosocial problems of the ill adolescent.

## GROUND RULES—ADMISSION POLICY

All hospital units have rules regarding admission criteria, patient behavior, and visiting hours; however, there is no circumstance where the clarity and enforceability of those rules is of greater importance than on an inpatient adolescent unit. Foremost is the hospital policy establishing the age limits of the unit. As noted previously, age limits on extant units vary, with most having lower limits of 10 to 13 years and upper limits ranging between 17 and 24 years of life.

Having set upper and lower limits, under which circumstances might they be ignored? Will younger but physically mature or precocious children be admitted to the adolescent unit? Will younger patients be accepted to the unit when "children's beds" are unavailable? Will older adolescents and young adults be allowed admission if they evidence either physical or cognitive delay? Will young people with chronic conditions who have been under pediatric care for years be allowed readmission to the adolescent unit even though they have aged beyond the upper limit? Will young adults who are terminally ill be allowed to spend their final days in a familiar environment even though they have "aged out"? None of these questions has a right or wrong answer, nor are they answered in the same way at all medical centers. The tendency to retain patients in a familiar environment under the continuing care of physicians that they may have known for years must be balanced against the risk of overprotecting and infantilizing chronically ill adolescents as they enter young adult life. The best interest of the patient should always be the final determinant, rather than physician convenience or parental preferences, but that best interest is not always clear.

Of particular importance are institutional rules of whether all patients who meet the age criteria must be admitted to the unit or if the decision as to where to house the patient will be left to the personal physician. If the medical center opts to allow for physician choice, the decision on where to admit is often based upon the convenience of the doctor, and there will be an impact upon not only daily census but also a concern that only or mostly behaviorally troublesome teens will be deemed best for the adolescent unit, changing the character and tone of the unit.

An additional concern relates to the range of diagnoses that will be allowed access to the unit or preferentially admitted to other areas of the hospital. Will adolescents be accepted for admission with primary psychiatric diagnoses and, if not, will exceptions be made if the possibility of an organic etiology for their psychosis cannot be excluded? Is the unit prepared to deal with the demands of treating teenagers with eating disorders or drug withdrawal syndromes? Where would it be best to hospitalize the pregnant adolescent who requires admission for a nonobstetrical condition such as asthma? How close to term might the pregnant teen be safely housed on a nonobstetric floor? Is the design of the unit suitable to the care of teenagers receiving chemotherapy or young people with cardiac conditions requiring telemetry? As always, the best interests of the patient are primary, and the necessity for advanced technology or specialized nursing care may suggest hospitalization on a unit better able to provide the needed care.

## GROUND RULES—WARD MANAGEMENT AND PATIENT BEHAVIOR

Adolescent environments function best with clear, enforceable rules, and this is particularly applicable to maintaining a milieu conducive to caring for young people who are ill. As the primary roles of the professionals working on an adolescent unit are to provide care and advocate for their young patients, the policing of the unit and the enforcement of rules may create an adversarial relationship, which is distasteful to many providers. As such, behavioral rules for the unit should evolve through achieving consensus among the disciplines staffing the unit with an understanding that, once agreed upon, enforcement of the rules is a shared responsibility.

Certain rules are obvious and require no discussion or debate. At one time smoking areas were common in hospitals, but current public health statutes prohibit smoking in virtually all health care facilities. Similarly, the use of illegal drugs, in particular marijuana and alcohol, which are common among adolescents, is not acceptable within a hospital setting. Prohibiting these behaviors is easy. Enforcing that prohibition is most difficult. Sniffing around for the telltale smell of tobacco or marijuana is understandingly abhorrent to most health professionals and often yields suspicion, which is short of absolute proof. Even when suspicion approaches or achieves certainty, other than saying stop, what are the enforcement alternatives? Eviction from the hospital is rarely an alternative. If the young person is so ill as to require hospitalization, it is neither easy nor safe to force discharge.

Other areas of concern are less straightforward. A cohort of teenagers walking around in their robes, nightgowns, and pajamas can be provocative. What is acceptable dress? Showing affection is a nice thing, but when is a little affection a little too much? What are the rules about visitors sitting on the patient's bed? Lying in the patient's bed? May the curtains be drawn when you have a visitor? What are the rules regarding patients visiting other patients and during what hours of the day or night? Emerging sexuality is a normal part of the journey from childhood to adulthood, but an interruption in that journey should take place during hospitalization.

Increasingly, both the design and rules of pediatric facilities have encouraged family-centered care. Certainly, allowing for the increased involvement of parents in the care of ill children and the facilitation of the opportunity to spend the night with a hospitalized child are worthwhile initiatives. The validity of extrapolating these practices to adolescents is uncertain. At the lower limits of the age group, the needs of a 10-year-old or a 13-year-old, particularly one who is ill, are little different than those of the younger child. At the other extreme of the age group, where achieving independence from parental control may be a difficulty for the chronically ill young adult, it may not be best to have your mother sleep in your room. Hence, no hard and fast rule regarding parents spending the night would appear as best for all adolescents of all ages with all conditions. The reality of these differing circumstances suggests a policy of flexibility, with the caution that flexibility easily deteriorates into inconsistency and chaos. Other cautions would include that consistency must be maintained when the supportive adult who wishes to spend the night in the room is the wife (or husband) of the older adolescent, and that if the supportive adult is of the opposite sex to the patient that they be housed in a single room (e.g., a teenage girl should not be asked to spend the night with someone else's father sleeping in the room).

Other rules that will require consideration include visiting hours and the number of visitors. If there are 20 adolescent patients and each has 2 adolescent visitors, that makes 60 adolescents in the unit. Should there be a "lights out" time, or should the adolescent be allowed to stay up all night (and sleep all day)? How loud is too loud for a "boom box"? This last question is a good example of how an ounce of common sense mixed with a tablespoon of humor is a good substitute for a pound of rules.

## DISADVANTAGES

Among the disadvantages of an adolescent inpatient unit are all those problems inherent in marshaling together a teenage assemblage that would otherwise be diffused throughout the hospital. The cost to the medical center of caring for these patients will increase. There is no economy in grouping teenagers together within the hospital. When teenagers are spread thinly throughout the hospital, their needs for special facilities, programs, and personnel are neither apparent nor obtainable and, therefore, are not addressed. Having gathered adolescent patients together, their needs become apparent and unavoidable.

As noted previously, a child life specialist with experience working with adolescents and a teacher need to be provided to minimize the tedium and educational disruption attendant upon a prolonged hospitalization. Social services and psychiatric support must be available. Each of these professionals will require office space and secretarial support, and a classroom and suitably equipped day room will be needed.

Crowd control and noise abatement become issues of concern. Although socialization, loud music, and uproar are normal adolescent behaviors, they can be unnerving to both the hospital staff and critically ill patients. Endeavoring to achieve adherence to guidelines on the number of visitors, noise control, permissible dress, and the limits of tolerable behavior is taxing to physicians and nursing personnel.

With teenagers parading about in nightgowns and robes, some sexual acting-out may occur. No one is surprised or alarmed when teenage counselors at a summer camp find a time and a place to rendezvous. However, there is some expectation that such behavior will not be attempted in a medical unit. Even if unit personnel are not dismayed by this sexual behavior, these acts are disquieting to parents, administrators, and visitors to the floor.

Having grouped adolescents together, one is still faced with heterogeneous and, at times, conflicting factions. Ten- and 12-year-olds are quite different from 18- and 21-year-olds, and an association between the youngest and oldest patients is not always a healthy happenstance.

Nurses skilled in the behavioral management of ill teenagers may be less prepared to render specialized postoperative care than their counterparts on an exclusively surgical or plastic surgery service. In addition, the sophisticated and expensive technology, such as cardiac telemetry, which can be incorporated into a unit that provides organ or disease-specific care, is economically impractical for an adolescent unit addressing the full spectrum of teenage conditions.

Finally, the concentration in a single hospital area of those behavioral problems of adolescents such as substance abuse, the consequences of promiscuous sexuality, and depression and suicidality may produce a volatile situation that would not have occurred if the same patients were diffused throughout the hospital.

## ADVANTAGES

Despite these disadvantages, an appropriately designed and staffed adolescent inpatient environment presents a multitude of opportunities not possible in a traditional hospital setting. The combination of an interdisciplinary staff attuned to the needs of the ill adolescent and an inpatient area designed specifically for the teenage patient can provide better support for the critically ill young person and expand the number of conditions that best lend themselves to inpatient treatment. Treatment can be undertaken in an atmosphere where the comfort of peers and the socialization of the group mitigate against the depression and regression that often accompany hospitalization.

Educational and recreational services can be provided that both ameliorate the boredom of the hospital day and aid in the overall evaluation of the adolescent. The assessment of behavioral problems can now be accomplished in a setting that allows observation of peer relationships within the confines of the hospital. The development of a team of health professionals that includes physicians, nurses, educators, and behavioralists allows for the efficient evaluation of the complex relationship between somatic and psychological illnesses. The provision of educational services permits evaluation and care to proceed without major disruption of schooling. Patients who require care over a period of weeks or months, as might be the case in conditions such as anorexia nervosa, can receive such care while participating in a full academic program.

Adolescents with problems for which admission to a traditional medical setting would be inappropriate or unacceptable can be made welcome in an adolescent unit. An example would be a young person who had attempted suicide but was at neither acute physiologic or behavioral risk. These patients have difficulty gaining admittance to inpatient psychiatric facilities or traditional medical settings and, in fact, the services to be offered such patients on those units are often inappropriate to their needs. Admission to an adolescent unit enables the teenager to receive medical care, social and psychiatric evaluation, and a cooling-off period prior to discharge back to an environment that precipitated the self-destructive behavior.[6]

The teenage victim of a sexual assault who requires medical attention is most often more comfortable and best cared for in an adolescent unit. The dying adolescent and his or her family can be better supported by a staff that has had the training and experience necessary to relate to this difficult situation. Teenagers with chronic illnesses, physical handicaps, and diseases secondary to substance abuse or sexuality most frequently require a multidisciplinary health team for their evaluation and management and are, at times, unwelcome on more traditional units.

In addition to offering improvements in patient care and comfort, clustering teenagers in a separate area facilitates educational and investigational opportunities. The training of house officers, nursing students, social workers, and other health care professionals in the care of ill teenagers is made feasible with the creation of an adolescent inpatient unit. The housing of all ill teenagers together facilitates the clinical investigation into both the types of problems that impact adolescents and the differing consequences of specific diseases upon this patient population.

## CONCLUSION

Despite the advocacy of the SAM for the "establishment of adolescent inpatient units in both pediatric and general hospitals as an optimal approach to the delivery of developmentally appropriate health care to hospitalized adolescents," and an initial flurry in the creation of such units some 50 years ago, most medical centers continue to admit teenagers to either pediatric or adult services. Although there are disadvantages associated with grouping adolescents together within the hospital, we believe that the advantages to be gained in not only patient care and comfort but also in the education of health professionals and the investigation of the nature and consequences of illness during the teenage years far outweigh the drawbacks. Even in the face of advancing technology that allows for and, at times, mandates hospitalization on very specialized disease- or organ-specific units, the concept of an age-specific unit for adolescents is worthy of continuing support. Certainly, for those medical centers hospitalizing large numbers of teenagers or with a responsibility for training health professionals in the care of adolescents, the establishment and maintenance of an inpatient unit specifically designed and staffed to deliver developmentally appropriate care to young people deserves strong consideration.

## REFERENCES


1. Society for Adolescent Medicine. Adolescent inpatient units: a position paper of the Society for Adolescent Medicine. *J Adolesc Health Care.* 1996;18:307–308

2. Rigg CA, Fisher RC. Some comments on current hospital medical services for adolescents. *Am J Dis Child.* 1970;120:193–196

3. Fisher M. Adolescent inpatient units. *Arch Dis Child.* 1994;70:461–463

4. Schonberg SK, Cohen MI. Emergence of an adolescent in-patient unit following the yellow brick road. *Montefiore Medicine.* 1978;3:4–8

5. Miller NO, Friedman SB, Coupey SM. Adolescent preferences for rooming during hospitalization. *J Adolesc Health.* 1998;23:89–93

6. Marks A. Management of the suicidal adolescent on a nonpsychiatric adolescent unit. *J Pediatr.* 1979;95(2): 305–308

# CHAPTER 25

# School-based Health Care

DORIS R. PASTORE, MD • MARTHA ARDEN, MD

Competing demands on the time of teens and their parents, lack of transportation or insurance, difficult-to-navigate appointment systems, concerns about confidentiality, and a lack of adolescent-friendly services keep many teens away from traditional health care practice settings. Nearly 18% of teens are uninsured, up to 25% have not had a visit to a health professional in the last year,[1] and many have difficulty accessing confidential services related to substance abuse, sexuality, or mental health care.[2] For this underserved population, the provision of health services in schools represents the perfect intersection of adolescent medicine and public health. Several models exist, with the school-based health center (SBHC) model being the most comprehensive. This chapter will address the unique strengths of the SBHC approach, update the latest information and concepts in the SBHC field, and review other approaches available in the school setting.

## DELIVERING NEEDS-FOCUSED CARE TO TEENS

Since the 1970s, more than 1,900 SBHCs have been developed. They currently serve approximately 1.2 million students, about 2% of students nationwide. Approximately half of all SBHCs serve those age 10 years or older, thus being able to reduce barriers to care for adolescents. School-based health centers are located in 43 states, as well as the District of Columbia. They are distributed among elementary schools (10%), high schools (33%), middle or middle/high schools (12%), and K–12 schools (17%). Most SBHCs are located in urban centers (57%), some are in rural settings (27%), and fewer are in suburban communities (16%).[3] School-based health center sites nationally are in schools where the race/ethnicity of the students are 37% Hispanic, 26% black, and 30% white. Full-time staffing by primary care nurse practitioners (NPs), physician assistants (PAs), or physicians is present in 60% of SBHCs, whereas part-time staffing (30 hours/week or less) occurs in the remainder. Mental health staff working full-time are found in 46% of programs, which is reduced from nearly 70% a few years ago.

The SBHC movement experienced its greatest expansion in the 1990s; high school sites are the most prominent among those SBHCs open 10 years or more. In 2002, a national definition of what constitutes a SBHC was adopted by the National Assembly on School-based Health Care (NASBHC). Key components of this definition include: (1) the presence of an interdisciplinary team of medical and mental health professionals that provide on-site and comprehensive medical, mental health, and age-appropriate health education services that address the most important health needs of students, and (2) a facility that is open every school day with staff working in collaboration with the school nurse and other service providers in the school and community.[4] According to this definition, the services may include but are not limited to, primary care for acute and chronic health conditions, mental health services, substance abuse services, case management, dental health services, reproductive health care, nutrition counseling, health education, and health promotion. All SBHCs must have a policy on parental consent, which is usually developed in conjunction with the local board of education. Although the model includes comprehensive care in its definition, a countrywide survey[3] conducted by the NASBHC in 2007–2008 found that there are currently 3 types of SBHCs: primary care (25%); primary care–mental health (40%); and primary care–mental health care plus (35%), in which a health educator, social services case manager, nutritionist, or dental health professional is also present. In 2001, the Society for Adolescent Medicine (SAM) published a position statement voicing support for the comprehensive SBHC model.[5]

The exact type of SBHC services provided on-site is developed in response to analyses of student need assessments as well as community resources. School-based health centers that treat adolescents use a variety of assessment tools, both for the individual student and school wide. These include instruments from the American Medical Association (AMA Guidelines for Adolescent Preventive Services [GAPS]), the American Academy of Pediatrics (*Bright Futures Guidelines*), and the United States Preventive Health Services Task Force (USPHSTF Guide to Clinical Preventive Services), and include a psychosocial and medical assessment. Common components across all SBHC sites include treatment for acute illness (96%), on-site asthma treatment (95%), prescriptions for medications (96%), physical examinations for sports (92%), and treatment of chronic illness (87%). School-based health centers aid in the treatment of chronic illnesses not only by providing direct medical care but also by being able to closely track follow-up and referral services.[6] Dental screenings take place in over half the SBHC programs (57%), whereas some provide on-site sealants (25%) and general dental care (25%). Kaplan et al[7] reported that elementary school students with access to an SBHC had a greater likelihood of having had a dental examination than those without such access.

School-based health centers may be more likely to provide adolescent preventive services, including services to promote reproductive health, compared to other types of medical services.[8] In one study, 80% of teens with access to SBHCs had at least one comprehensive health supervision visit compared to 69% for those without such access.[9] Review of the 1,051 sites completing the 2004–2005 census survey conducted by the NASBHC indicated that middle and high school students in schools with SBHCs were able to receive on-site pregnancy testing (80%), treatment for sexually transmitted infections (STIs) (68%), and HIV/AIDS counseling (64%). Most SBHCs do not dispense contraception (61%) but are able to provide family planning services such as birth control counseling (64%). Kiskar et al[10] found that SBHC sites that focused specifically on family planning demonstrated a delay in students' initiation of sexual activity compared with the trends of urban youths nationally. Kiskar et al[11] also found that a smaller percentage of students in schools with SBHCs had ever had sex but that seniors in these schools were no less likely to have had recent sexual intercourse compared with urban trends nationally. Furthermore, screening and treatment for chlamydia and gonorrhea in schools with SBHCs were associated with a decrease in prevalence (3.2% vs 6.4%) among males and a slight decrease among females.

When specific funding is available, school wide intervention programs can be implemented by SBHCs. Most commonly these have been related to asthma, with many sites utilizing the American Lung Association's "Open Airways for Schools" program, or a modification thereof. A more recent emphasis has been on prevention of diabetes mellitus type II and treatment of obesity. A recent survey demonstrated that 69% of 706 respondents were involved in classroom education on healthy eating and physical activity but that only 50% included measurement of body mass index (BMI) and provision of individual treatment.[12] Some sites are developing school health report cards to inform parents about their teen's medical status, including information on asthma treatment, blood pressure, vision, risk for obesity, and need for mental health follow-up.[13]

School-based health centers address mental health needs through several modalities, including individual and group counseling, crisis intervention, family therapy, and case management. In addition to mental health assessments (available in 96% of SBHCs) and crisis intervention (96%), the on-site mental health care professionals often are involved in grief and loss therapy (95%), conflict resolution/mediation (91%), tobacco use counseling (89%), substance abuse counseling (84%), and psychiatric consultation (58%). About 8% of programs report on-site, specialized drug and alcohol counselors. Weist et al[14] studied schools that contained school-based mental health clinics and reported that although students who received no mental health services during the academic year showed no change in mental health status, students treated at the clinics showed significant decreases in depression and improvements in self-concept from pre- and post self-report inventories. Another study has demonstrated that fewer students attending schools with SBHCs reported considering suicide compared to expected trends.

## COLLABORATION BETWEEN PUBLIC HEALTH AND EDUCATION

City school health programs in the United States have a long and illustrious history, beginning with the influx of large numbers of immigrants in the late 19th century, when New York City instituted vaccinations and Boston employed physicians to screen for infectious diseases in schools. By 1910, 337 city school systems had instituted some form of screening, many had physicians on staff, and school nursing programs peaked in the 1920s.

Over the last century, school health evolved from a focus on prevention of contagion to immunization documentation, screenings, and health education (1920s to 1950s), to provision of mandated services for students with disabilities (1960s and 1970s), to HIV/AIDS education (1980s), to the current emphasis on multifaceted health programs. Throughout the United States, school health services outside the comprehensive SBHC model remain uneven and underfunded.[15] Although 81% of school buildings have nurse's offices, the range of staffing may be from once weekly to a full-time health aide, licensed practical nurse, registered nurse, NP, or medical doctor. Fewer than 20% of schools are equipped with a glucometer or a nebulizer available for use by the general school population.

School-based health centers play several roles in supporting educational goals, although studying its effects is difficult due to great variation in defining and selecting outcome variables. Receiving direct, on-site medical services allows students to return to classes upon completion of treatment, such as after treatment of acute asthma.[16] One study demonstrated that elementary school students with asthma who had access to an SBHC missed 3 fewer days on average than those in a school without an SBHC and were 50% less likely to be hospitalized.[17] This study found no association by race/ethnicity or health insurance coverage. A 6-year study found that the risk of hospitalization for asthma dropped to less than half after the opening of an SBHC.[18] Furthermore, the risk of hospitalization decreased over time so that the potential cost savings was estimated as $970 per child. This represented a decrease in cost of hospitalization by more than 20%. Adams and Johnson[19] found that students in Atlanta in schools with SBHCs had lower total annual Medicaid expenditures for emergency department visits, inpatient hospital stays, and prescription drugs. They also found that 2 years after implementation of an SBHC, students had less than one half ($899) of total Medicaid expenditures than that of their counterparts in schools without centers ($2,360). Santelli et al[20] found a protective effect in terms of hospitalization among students with the longest tenure in the SBHC. Young et al[21] found that implementation of an elementary school SBHC resulted in a significant decrease in nonurgent emergency department visits. Key et al[22] found a similar decrease among 10- to 15-year-olds. Adams and Johnson[19] as well as Kaplan et al[23] have substantiated that SBHCs provide improved preventive care services to students and families who otherwise underutilize health promotion services.

McCord et al[24] found in an alternative high school that SBHC users had fewer absences than those who were not registered for the SBHC, and that students who used the SBHC were more likely to graduate or be promoted than students who did not use the service. In this same study, black males were more than 3 times as likely to stay in school if they had registered for the SBHC. Alternatively, Kisker[25] found no effect of SBHC participation on absences when compared to urban youths nationally. For students not doing well academically, SBHCs are able to assess for chronic illnesses, depression, and vision or hearing problems, as well as refer to the school support team for educational evaluations.

Nurses, health educators, nutritionists, and social workers provide critical education and skills-building training in the comprehensive SBHC setting. Health topics are addressed in individual counseling, small groups, classrooms, and school-wide settings. Health topics most frequently addressed by SBHCs include tobacco prevention and cessation (91%), violence prevention and conflict resolution (88%), and HIV/STI prevention (62%). Sites report that these figures represent a significant increase from 3 years ago when there was less funding for mental health staff. More recently, the use of sports physicals have offered a unique opportunity to screen and treat asymptomatic teens for STIs with the use of urine lipase chain reaction assays.

## PROVIDING INTERDISCIPLINARY AND SYSTEMS-BASED TRAINING

Since their inception, SBHC programs have traditionally served as sites for health care profession training activities, and in recent years the number of training experiences has increased due to a re-emphasis on involvement of pediatric training in community sites. Generally, the largest number of trainees has been in nursing. A report by Juszczak et al[26] found that in addition to medicine and nursing, the disciplines of social work, psychology, psychiatry, health education, and nutrition also utilized SBHCs for training. This report also noted that the range of time in training varied from a half-day introductory experience to an 80-day placement over several months. Fellows in adolescent medicine, psychology graduate students, and medical assistant students had the longest exposures, whereas medical students and residents had the shortest stays. Among the strengths that SBHCs presented in training were the ability to provide experiences without the usual ancillary support, as an example of health care on "the front lines." Trainees experience the intersection of public health mandates, health education concepts, collaboration with teachers, and programs for students with special needs.

Despite their unique advantages, SBHCs have generally not been introduced beyond the core biomedical content of ambulatory pediatric and family practice.[27] In response, a recent collaboration of several programs in the New York City area identified core competencies that can be taught in the SBHC setting and developed a comprehensive training model to assist in implementing a wide range of learning activities based on those competencies. The 8 core competencies identified by the 5 collaborative programs included (1) health assessment, risk reduction, and health promotion; (2) health care delivery systems; (3) advocacy; (4) legal and ethical issues; (5) cross-cultural competence; (6) interdisciplinary collaboration; (7) school health practice and education; and (8) oral health.[27]

Rotations in SBHCs expose trainees to different disciplines and a range of clinical experiences that contribute to fulfillment of Accreditation Council on Graduate Medical Education (ACGME) requirements along the 6 required educational domains of medical knowledge, patient care, practice-based learning and improvement, interpersonal and communication skills, professionalism, and systems-based practice. Trainees in SBHCs experience the practice of communication skills and interview techniques; the study of adolescent care and community pediatrics; exposure to schoolwide screenings; and interdisciplinary debriefings involving medical, mental health, and school staff. These experiences allow trainees to develop an understanding of the breadth and capabilities of all involved professions. Common didactic sessions offered in SBHC settings address topics such as screening in schools, consultation, health practices, sexuality education, and crisis management.

Systems-based care can be taught in the SBHC setting based on the level of interest and expertise of each student. A beginner-level trainee would learn how systems directly affect the SBHC patient, that is, how medical, reproductive, and mental health clinical care intersect with public health and education; a more intermediate-level trainee would be involved in SBHC clinical operations such as continuous quality improvement (CQI), case consultation, and implementation of specific subprograms; a more advanced trainee could be involved in system linkages with the back-up facility and community agencies and with larger programmatic issues such as billing, fund accounting, administration, and grant writing.

## ENSURING HIGH-QUALITY CARE

The 1998–1999 NASBHC Census survey of 806 SBHCs revealed information about professional standards of care, quality assurance measures, and components of quality assurance (QA) systems. Sites indicated that they most commonly (73%) used Medicaid Early Periodic Screening Diagnosis and Treatment (EPSDT) standards of care. The AMA GAPS was used for teens (41%), whereas the AAP Guidelines (60%) and the MCHB Bright Futures Guidelines (21%) were used more frequently in elementary grades.[30]

School-based health centers use a variety of evaluation tools to measure their quality of care and outcomes, including staff credentialing (85%), chart audits (84%), patient surveys (70%), parent surveys (44%), teacher surveys (40%), and computer surveys of student health (19%). A majority of health centers (65%) report using their own or their sponsoring agency's QA benchmarks, whereas others identify using Joint Commission on Accreditation of Healthcare Organizations (JCAHO), Healthcare Effectiveness Data and Information Set (HEDIS), or state-specific SBHC tools.

A notable CQI tool specific for comprehensive SBHCs has been designed by Juszczak, Pastore, and Reif with support from The Robert Wood Johnson Foundation's Making the Grade Initiative (now the Center for Health and Health Care in Schools). The development of this age-adjusted tool allows sponsors, funders, and providers to underscore the unique features of care that SBHCs provide. The sentinel conditions assessed at sites serving adolescents include the documentation of assessment, intervention plans, and level of follow-up among those at risk for alcohol use, personal violence, STIs, poor school performance, attention-deficient disorder, and depression, along with documentation of an annual comprehensive examination. In 2003, this tool was transferred to the NASBHC and has made available such resources as sampling plans, audit forms, and data management applications.[29] A similar tool is in development, that focuses on school sites that offer mental health services only.

## SCHOOL HEALTH CARE IN TRADITIONAL SETTINGS

Although SBHCs provide an excellent opportunity to provide easily accessible, high-quality, comprehensive, interdisciplinary care, they are not available to most adolescents. Nonetheless, the provision of more limited health care services in schools is an important adjunct to traditional medical care settings, especially when adolescents do not use available services. The focus of traditional school health care became mostly limited to screening and health education in the mid-20th century in response to concerns about parental autonomy, the focus of schools on basic education, and objections of some private physicians. Approximately 70% of pediatric residency programs use SBHCs for trainee education in school health, with other experiences also including court hearings, meetings with superintendents, and school health policy development. Of note, the 1990s were marked by an increase in resident discussions of topics such as "Primary Care in the School," "Health Problems of Athletes," and "School Athletics."[30]

Trainees in all disciplines need to be aware of local, state, and federal regulations governing educational and medical record information, particularly because it is estimated that 2.8 million students have learning disabilities and between 5% and 10% of all students receive special education services. Three federal laws, the Americans with Disabilities Act, the Individuals with Disabilities Education Act (IDEA), and Section 504 of the Rehabilitation Act of 1973 mandate that schools provide all students with the physical access and services they need to get an education. Last reauthorized by Congress in 2004, the IDEA secures an appropriate public education and related services to prepare students with disabilities for further education, employment, and independent living. The latest revision emphasizes "further education" and effective transition services for the older adolescent to promote eventually successful employment. The Family Educational Rights and Privacy Act (FERPA) protects the privacy of students' educational records, requiring written release except under certain specific conditions. As a medical facility, the SBHC also abides by Health Insurance Portability and Accountability Act (HIPPA) guidelines.

State and local health regulations have transformed schools into the site of public health services for children and adolescents. Even when services are not provided in the schools, immunization and entry requirements greatly increase use of other health care services. Similarly, school-based screening programs steer students to medical evaluations for suspected problems, and requirements for interscholastic sports send thousands of teens to their primary care providers annually.

Medical providers can become involved in school health care in a number of ways, providing health education, becoming involved in screening and planning, and helping to develop and institute health-related policies. Most school districts in the United States contract with a school physician, most often a local pediatrician or family practitioner, to serve these roles.

In the absence of SBHCs, school health services may include the following:

- Tracking of Immunizations: Schools play a major role in ensuring that school-age children are up to date with immunizations. In general, states establish immunization requirements in accordance with Centers for Disease Control and Prevention (CDC) recommendations, but there is variability in the requirements for, and enforcement of, newer and booster immunizations. The recent controversy regarding the mandating of human papillomavirus immunization for school attendance highlights the degree to which schools have become de facto centers of pediatric public health initiatives.

- Tracking of Physical Examinations: Many states require documentation of a recent physical examination upon entry to the school system and periodically throughout the school years. Required examinations for sports participation and work permits may be provided by physicians or mid-level providers contracting with the school system.

- First Aid: First aid services are universally provided by schools, but state requirements for staff training vary. Depending on the school district, first aid may be provided by nurses, health aides, coaches, physical education teachers, and even administrative staff members. Some states require defibrillators on-site and at athletic events.

- Screening: Screening requirements vary by state education regulations. In general, simple screening tests, with few false positives, for common, treatable conditions are suitable for in-school screening. Common examples include vision, hearing, height, weight, and scoliosis screening. In some states, data are compiled by schools and monitored by state education departments to ensure compliance.

- Administration of Medications: The 1991 IDEA requires the "least restrictive environment" for students who have disabilities. As a result, many students who in previous years would have been prevented from attending regular schools are now attending general education schools, which must provide appropriate accommodation. School nurses administer medications for chronic and acute conditions, check blood sugar levels for students with diabetes, and administer asthma nebulizers, while paraprofessionals and/or nurses are available throughout the school day for students who require more close monitoring.

- Emergency Care: School physicians often review and provide in-service training for schools regarding their emergency care policies as they relate to students with nut allergies, diabetes, and asthma.

- School Crisis Situations: School physicians are often members of the crisis intervention team, helping to organize or review intervention plans as they relate to threats to the physical safety of students, environmental crises, and bereavement. Emergency preparedness includes items such as plans for communication with parents; first aid supplies; medications; and adequate water and food for shelter-in-place.

School health policies have a major impact on adolescents, and community-based physicians may become involved in establishing and/or revising these policies. Most local school districts have policies regarding safety, accommodations for students with disabilities, physical and health education, athletic participation, and control and prevention of infection. In addition, the US Child Nutrition and WIC Reauthorization Act of 2004 established a requirement for all school districts to have a wellness policy addressing nutrition and the need to help prevent obesity to participate in the federal school lunch program. Other policies such as immunizations, screening, physical education, reproductive health, and HIV education are established at the state level.

At the local level, pediatricians often serve as consultants to schools and school districts to ensure that policies are consistent with AAP and other professional organization guidelines. The AAP *Red Book (Report of the Committee on Infectious Diseases)* is an excellent resource for immunization and infection control/prevention guidelines.

## FUTURE OF SCHOOL-BASED HEALTH CENTERS

The SBHC movement has evolved to play a vital role in providing specialized adolescent health services in the school setting. At the intersection of public health and education, SBHCs have an opportunity to assess, manage, and prevent the major medical, mental health, and reproductive issues facing adolescents. School-based health centers that provide comprehensive, continuous, age-appropriate care are an essential asset for health promotion, especially for otherwise underserved populations. School-based health centers also provide valuable training sites for health professionals in multiple disciplines. For most students in schools without SBHCs, local medical providers work with school nurses and other staff to provide for basic medical needs. The SBHC movement has been working to develop policies that can upgrade services in all schools based on the SBHC model.

## INTERNET RESOURCES

- GAPS: www.ama-assn.org/ama/pub/physician-resources/public-health/promoting-healthy-lifestyles/adolescent-health/guidelines-adolescent-preventive-services.shtml
- MCHB Bright Futures Guidelines: brightfutures.aap.org/
- USPSTF Guidelines to Clinical Preventive Services: www.ahrq.gov/clinic/uspstfix.htm#Recommendations
- American Lung Association Open Airways for Schools: www.lungusa.org/site/pp.asp?c=dvLUK9O0E~b=44142
- Americans with Disabilities Act (1990): www.ada.gov/pubs/ada.htm
- IDEA: idea.ed.gov/
- Section 504 of the Rehabilitation Act of 1973: www.section508.gov/index.cfm?FuseAction=Content~ID=15
- FERPA: www.ed.gov/policy/gen/reg/ferpa/index.html
- US Child Nutrition and WIC Reauthorization Act of 2004: www.fns.usda.gov/wic/
- Wellness Policy: www.fns.usda.gov/tn/healthy/wellness_policyrequirements.html

## REFERENCES


1. Newacheck PW, Hung YY, Park MJ, Brindis CD, Irwin CE Jr. Disparities in adolescent health and health care: does socioeconomic status matter? *Health Serv Res.* 2003;38:1235–1252

2. The Center for Health and Health Care in Schools. Available at: www.healthinschools.org. Accessed August 21, 2006

3. National Assembly on School-based Health Care. SBHCs: National Census School Year 2007-2008. Available at: www.nasbhc.org/atf/cf/%7Bcd9949f2-2761-42fb-bc7a-cee165c701d9%7D/NASBHC%202007-08%20CENSUS%20REPORT%20FINAL.PDF. Accessed November 8, 2010.

4. National Assembly on School-based Health Care. 2002. Available at: www.nasbhc.org. Accessed September 4, 2007

5. Pastore DR, Murray PJ, Juszczak L. SBHCs: a position paper for the Society of Adolescent Medicine. *J Adolesc Health.* 2001;(29):448–450

6. Hacker KA,Weintraub TA, Fried LE, Ashba J. Role of SBHCs in referral completion. *J Adolesc Health.* 1997;21(5):328–334

7. Kaplan DW, Brindis CD, Phibbs SL, Melinkovich P, Naylor K, Ahlstrand K. A comparison study of an elementary school-based health center: effects on health care access and use. *Arch Pediatr Adolesc Med.* 1999;153: 235–243

8. Blum RW, Beuhring T, Wunderlich M, Resnick MD. Don't ask, they won't tell: the quality of adolescent health screening in five practice settings. *Am J Public Health.* 1996;86:1767–1772

9. Kaplan DW, Calonge BN, Guernsey BP, Hanraham MB. Managed care and school-based health centers: use of health services. *Arch Pediatr Adolesc Med.* 1998;152: 25–33

10. Kisker EE, Brown RS. Do SBHCs improve adolescents' access to health care, health status, and risk-taking behavior? *J Adolesc Health.* 1996;18:335–343

11. Cohen DA, Nauami M, Martin DH, Farley TA. Repeated school-based screening for sexually transmitted diseases: a feasible strategy for reaching adolescents. *Pediatrics.* 1999;104(6):1281–1285

12. The Center for Health and Health in Schools. Childhood overweight and school health services survey results. Available at: http://www.healthinschools.org/Publications-and-Resources/Originial-Polls-and-Surveys/Web-Based-Surveys/Childhood-Overweight-and-School-Health-Services-Survey-Results.aspx. Accessed July 30, 2010

13. Pastore D. Report card on health, personal communication

14. Weist MD, Paskewita DA, Warner BS. Treatment outcomes of school-based mental health services for urban teenagers. *Community Ment Health J.* 1996;32:149–157

15. The Center for Health and Health Care in Schools. School health: where we've come from. Available at: http://www.healthinschools.org/~/media/Files/Presentations%20PPTs/washington.ashx. Accessed July 30, 2010

16. Pastore DR, Steed N, Maresca A. A two-year evaluation of walk-in visits to SBHCs for asthma-related complaints (poster presentation). Society for Adolescent Medicine meeting, Atlanta, GA; March 1998. See *J Adolesc Health.* 1998 meeting issue

17. Webber MP, Carpinello KE, Oruwariye T, Lo Y, Burton WE, Appel DK. Burden of asthma in inner-city elementary school children: do school-based health centers make a difference? *Arch Pediatr Adolesc Med.* 2003;157: 125–129

18. Guo JJ, Jang R, Keller KN, McCracken AL, Pan W, Cluxton RJ. Impact of school-based health centers on children with asthma. *J Adolesc Health.* 2005;37(4): 266–274

19. Adams EK, Johnson V. An elementary school-based health clinic: can it reduce Medicaid costs? *Pediatrics.* 2000;105:780–788

20. Santelli J, Kouzis A, Newcomer S. School-based health centers and adolescent use of primary care and hospital care. *J Adolesc Health.* 1996;19(4):267–275

21. Young T, D'angelo S, Davis J. Impact of a school-based health center on emergency department use by elementary school students. *J Sch Health.* 2001;71(5):196–198

22. Key JD, Washington EC, Hulsey TC. Reduced emergency department utilization associated with school-based clinic enrollment. *J Adolesc Health.* 2002;30(4): 273–278

23. Kaplan DW, Calonge BN, Guernsey BP. Managed care and school-based health centers: use of services. *Arch Pediatr Adolesc Med.* 1998;152(1):25–33

24. McCord MT, Klein JD, Joy JM, Fothergill K. School-based clinic use and school performance. *J Adolesc Health.* 1993;14:91–98

25. Kisker EE, Brown RS. Do SBHCs improve adolescents' access to health care, health status, and risk-taking behavior? *J Adolesc Health.* 1996;18:335–343

26. Juszczak L, Lear JG, Friedman SB. Back to school: training opportunities in school-based health centers. *J Adolesc Health.* 1995; 16(2): 101–104

27. Kalet A, Juszczak L, Pastore D, et al. Medical training in school-based health centers: a five school collaboration. *Acad Med.* 2007;82(5):458–464

28. Brindis CD, Klein J, Schlitt J, Santelli J, Juszczak L, Nystrom RJ. School-based health centers: accessibility and accountability. *JAH.* 2003;32(6)S1:96–107

29. Juszczak L, Pastore D, Reif C. Center for evaluation and quality. Continuous Quality Improvement (CQI) tool for SBHCs. National Assembly of School-based Health Care. Available at: http://www.nasbhc.org/site/c.jsJPKWPFJrH/b.2564543/apps/s/content.asp?ct=3875953. Accessed July 30, 2010

30. Bradford B. Resident education in school health. Available at: www.schoolhealth.org/article.cfm?contentID=34. Accessed September 4, 2007

# CHAPTER 26

# College Health

MARJORIE SEIDENFELD, MD

Going to college is a major milestone in an adolescent's advancement toward independence. It is often the first time the young person has lived away from home, and there are many decisions he or she will have to make that affect physical and mental health. Some adolescents enter college with chronic illnesses such as diabetes, which they will need to manage on their own. Others may develop an illness for which they must obtain care. Of course, many students also decide to engage in new behaviors that put their health at risk and may require help in dealing with the consequences of these behaviors. Other complicating factors include the common scenario where the student's primary care physician is hundreds or thousands of miles away, or where the student does not have the necessary health insurance to cover treatment.

For these reasons, it was long ago recognized that college students need specialized health care. In 1860, Edward Hitchcock, MD, became the medical director of the Department of Physical Education and Hygiene at Amherst College, making him the first official college health practitioner.[1] Four years later at both Mount Holyoke and Vassar, college health services were established,[1] and over time, many more colleges and universities opened health centers for their students. The providers at these colleges eventually recognized that they needed an association of their own in order to provide opportunities for collaboration on policies and standards of care. Thus, the American Student Health Association was created. The organization, which had its first annual meeting in 1920, eventually changed its name to the American College Health Association (ACHA). The organization has since grown, providing services and coordination of efforts for institutional and individual members, including medical providers, health educators, pharmacists, medical administrators, and mental health professionals.

## STRUCTURE OF COLLEGE HEALTH SERVICES

It is helpful to understand the administrative and financial frameworks of each college health service. There is a great deal of variability among health services, and a number of factors have a substantial affect on access and the availability of frequently sought services. Most college health services provide medical and mental health care and health education for students, but the scope and structure of college health services vary as much as the colleges themselves. Health services range from small, nurse-directed health centers to large, multidisciplinary medical and mental health practices. Many of the larger universities have dental, radiologic, pharmaceutical, and medical subspecialty services on site. Some have infirmaries that are open to students 24 hours. In addition, many have specialized health educators, as well as students who are trained as peer health educators, to provide individual sessions and health promotion initiatives on the general campus. Mental health services may be combined administratively and located with the medical center, or they may be independent.

From an administrative perspective, the college health service is complex. The budget is usually provided through the university, and expenses need to be justified to the college administration. This may result in the college dictating some policies for the medical practice. For example, health services in universities that are supported by certain religious groups may not permit contraceptive and abortion counseling and services.

Payment for services may be included in a "health service fee" charged to all students, may be paid per service rendered, may be a student health insurance plan, or may be covered by the parent's insurance plan. When parents are involved in the payment for services, issues of confidentiality may make it necessary for schools to have established procedures and policies within the health service to maintain patient confidentiality while still being able to obtain reimbursement for services.

## CONFIDENTIALITY

The issue of confidentiality is particularly delicate in college health. Providers have a legal obligation to protect the privacy of their patients not only from parents, but also from college administrators. This is often difficult because college administrators take their role of being *in loco parentis* quite seriously. Beyond the ethical and legal requirements to provide private and confidential care, students would likely be less inclined to use the health service if they perceived that their personal health information was readily available to faculty or administrators. Thus, when a health issue is affecting the student's academic performance or when a student needs to take a medical leave of absence from the college, it must be handled in a sensitive manner. Professors or a dean typically need to become informed of and involved in the health situation, but this should be done only after obtaining the expressed consent of the student. Of course, during a medical emergency when a student's life is in danger, the bond of confidentiality can be broken in order to assure safety. Most colleges have a written policy related to health and confidentiality that is given to students as they enter school. As much as possible, the boundaries of confidentiality are discussed in such a document.

## HEALTH PROBLEMS ON THE COLLEGE CAMPUS

The most prevalent medical conditions that students who visit a health service are diagnosed with are often parallel to those of older adolescents. Infectious illnesses, such as upper respiratory infections, gastroenteritis, pharyngitis, and conjunctivitis, occur with somewhat increased frequency because students often live in close, shared quarters. Infectious mononucleosis occurs in as many as 12 per 1,000 college students. Moreover, up to one-third become seropositive for Epstein-Barr virus during their college years because many students have not been previously exposed.[2] The health service provider is viewed as a sort of public health administrator on the college campus, keeping his or her eye on the trends of illness and doing his or her best to control contagious diseases.

At least 80% of college students are sexually active;[3] therefore, not unexpectedly, sexual health issues are another common reason for visiting the health service. Many of these visits are responsible, mature efforts to obtain contraception and seek appropriate information regarding disease prevention. However, because college students are testing their own limits and experimenting with their newfound freedom, they sometimes take risks involving sexual health. For example, about one-third of college students have had more than 6 sexual partners.[4] Moreover, when students also are experimenting with different licit and illicit substances and combined with sexual activity, there is an associated decreased use of condoms, resulting in unplanned pregnancies and sexually transmitted infections (STIs). Routine gynecologic examinations, contraceptive counseling, managing abnormal Papanicolaou smears, and providing emergency contraception are a large part of the college health practice.

Students who want to be tested for or who have symptoms of STIs comprise another common group of those who visit the health service. Among adolescents between the ages of 15 and 24 years, 4 million cases of STIs are diagnosed in the United States every year,[5] and many of these individuals are of college age. Although human papillomavirus (HPV) is the most common STI overall, chlamydia is the most common bacterial infection. Both infections may be insidious and may only be diagnosed on screening. According to a survey of college health services, 67% provide screening for students for chlamydia and gonorrhea on a routine basis.[6] Even though HIV infection is less common, screening for HIV is also performed frequently among college students. In addition to medical services for STI testing and treatment, a large proportion of health education efforts are directed toward increased awareness and prevention of STIs as well.

## IMMUNIZATIONS

Because so many students, particularly freshmen, are living in dormitories, it is crucial for them to have as much protection from infectious diseases as possible. For this reason, most college health services are diligent about requiring the submission of students' immunization records. Many schools have a policy of blocking the student's registration for classes unless documentation of all appropriate immunizations has been provided to the health service. The rules for which vaccines are required or recommended vary from state to state and college to college. Generally, the immunizations that are required (or, in some states, strongly recommended) are those recommended by the Centers for Disease Control and Prevention (CDC) childhood schedule.[7] A few are of particular note:

- Tdap (tetanus, diphtheria, and acellular pertussis—adolescent preparation): Due to the serious consequences of tetanus and diphtheria infections, the high rate of pertussis outbreaks reported among adolescents, and the development of an acellular pertussis vaccine with fewer side effects compared with the older preparation, it is recommended that Tdap be substituted for the tetanus-diphtheria (Td) booster used previously. If not given at the recommended age of 11 to 12 years, Tdap should be given prior to entry in college.
- MMR (measles, mumps, and rubella): In some states, 2 doses are required rather than merely recommended in order to register for college.

- Hepatitis A and B: Although the hepatitis B vaccine has been required for elementary and high schools, hepatitis A has only recently been recommended as a routine immunization in the United States.
- Varicella: This vaccine has been recommended for elementary and high school students who have not had the disease. It is important for college health practitioners to recognize, however, that even if a student has had the vaccine, it is still possible for him or her to acquire the disease, albeit in a milder form.
- Meningococcal: Strongly recommended by the Advisory Committee on Immunizations Practices of the CDC for incoming freshmen who will be living in dormitories. Some states require this vaccine for college admission. Other states mandate that students and their parents read information about meningitis and the vaccine and that they sign a waiver if they choose not to obtain this immunization.
- Influenza: This is recommended as an annual vaccine, particularly for those with chronic conditions. However, because students are living so closely together, it is ideal to immunize as many as possible each year to prevent a campuswide epidemic.
- HPV: A quadravalent vaccine (HPV types 6, 11, 16, and 18) and, more recently, a bivalent vaccine (HPV types 16 and 18) have been approved and recommended. Although directed at younger adolescents and preadolescents, it is being recommended for women up to age 26 years and, therefore, is still recommended for college-age women and, perhaps at some point, will be recommended for men as well (see Chapter 53, Sexually Transmitted Infections).

Most US students will have obtained most of their immunizations before attending college. However, it is more complicated with international students because their immunization histories will depend on the practices of their countries of origin. It may also be difficult to accurately assess immunization records written in different languages.

## TRAVEL MEDICINE

The number of students choosing to spend time in another country has risen dramatically over the years. Whether the student is spending a year abroad or participating in a remote work experience for only a few weeks, he or she may come into contact with dangerous infections that are preventable with the use of vaccines and other medications. Some college health services provide a travel clinic internally, whereas others refer to outside resources in their communities. One potential obstacle to this category of preventive care is the cost, which may be formidable for some vaccines and is not always covered by health insurance. Another challenge is the problem of needing to safely store vaccines that are not given frequently.

It is important to educate students about the urgency of preparing for travel, especially to less well-developed areas of the world. For guidance, practitioners and students can use the CDC's Web site (www. cdc.gov/travel/default.aspx), with its vast and timely travel information. Students may not think about the health aspects of their travel plans, so it is important for colleges that have travel-abroad programs to work closely with the school's health service to ensure that students begin the process early enough for all necessary immunization regimens to be completed on time. In addition to immunizations, other preventive approaches are commonly required, such as oral medication for malaria prophylaxis and education regarding prevention of traveler's diarrhea and dehydration. Knowledge about the local water supply and food-handling practices is crucial, and there are general principles that can be recommended in terms of hygiene. Issues such as sun exposure should also be discussed because students may not be aware of the high risk of getting sun poison in some areas of the world. Furthermore, some medications used for malaria prophylaxis, such as doxycycline, may result in photosensitivity, which can result in severe burns.

## CHRONIC ILLNESS AND DISABILITY

Many students who enter college bring with them a history of chronic illness. Depending on how it is defined, a chronic illness occurs in up to one-third of children, and more than 80% will carry their diagnosis to at least age 20.[8] The conditions most frequently seen include asthma, migraines, musculoskeletal disorders, seizure disorders, mental disorders, hearing impairments, and visual abnormalities. Although these are the most common conditions, the range of illness is wide, and the college health practitioner should be prepared for anything. It is helpful, if not essential, for the health service to maintain a referral base of subspecialists.

In some ways, the college health service functions as a transitional clinic for students with chronic illness. Typically, most adolescents in this category have been followed by a pediatrician or subspecialist in their hometowns. Although some students and their parents prefer to have these same physicians remain directly involved while they are at college, this is often not possible. Even if they are medically stable at the time of entry into college, the stress of a new environment, altered sleep and eating habits, and academic and social pressures may result in exacerbation of a chronic illness. It may be helpful for a student with a chronic illness to prospectively develop a relationship with either the college health provider or a local subspecialist with whom he or she can consult if experiencing new or recurrent symptoms related to his or her illness.

Based on the Americans with Disabilities Act of 1990, any college that receives federal funding must accommodate persons with disabilities. Most schools fall into this category and thus have resources for students with disabilities. Whether a student has a learning disability that necessitates an academic accommodation, or a physical disability for which he or she requires an exception to the standard living situation, colleges must provide provisions for these individuals to the extent that they are able. Generally, this requires close communication between the medical and mental health providers and the administrators responsible for providing these services. Occasionally, provisions are discussed and determined even before a student accepts admission to an institution.

## EATING DISORDERS

Eating disorders and disordered eating are common on university campuses. Anorexia nervosa occurs in about 1% of the adolescent population. Bulimia nervosa, while occurring in about 1% to 5% of the general adolescent population, can occur in up to 20% of college females. The incidence of these eating disorders has 2 peaks—1 during puberty and the other during the college years. The cause of this second peak is likely related to multiple factors. For some adolescents, being away from home may be stressful and may liberate them to try this new behavior. Other stressors include the social and academic pressures of college life. It is truly a serious problem for college health providers because it has a definite effect on the student, as well as on his or her immediate social circle, his or her professors, and the administrators of the college. The complexity of eating disorders and disordered eating requires a disproportionate amount of time on the part of providers and administrators alike.

Many college health services have established programs to identify and provide ongoing outpatient treatment for students with eating disorders. Because the multidisciplinary approach to treatment is most effective, many programs will involve a medical provider, psychotherapist, nutritionist, and a psychiatrist for medication management (if needed). Ideally, these providers should have an opportunity to meet regularly to discuss the student, or be in contact with each other to coordinate care. There should also be a member of the team who is responsible for communicating with the administration when, for example, there is a student whose status is so precarious as to necessitate a leave of absence. This situation may arise from either a medical abnormality, such as severe bradycardia, or a psychological disturbance that is interfering with the student's academic functioning. It is helpful for the program to have predetermined guidelines that require students to take medical leave for anorexia nervosa and bulimia nervosa. There should also be a system in place that mandates medical and psychological evaluations for students applying for readmittance after such a leave to determine their fitness to return. In addition, every college health service should have referral resources for possible day treatment (if available in the community) and inpatient treatment, if deemed necessary.

Another related disorder that occurs with significant frequency in college athletes is the female athlete triad, which includes disordered eating, amenorrhea, and osteoporosis. Because most colleges receive federal funding, they are subject to regulations passed in 1972, which require equal opportunities for men and women to participate in sports. This has facilitated a great increase in the number of women participating in varsity and intramural sports. In addition, many college women are involved in activities such as dance and running, which may be for their own fitness rather than for a collegiate sport. These female athletes are at higher risk than the general population for disordered eating,[9] which can lead to the other complications of the triad. Even though not all students will meet the criteria for anorexia nervosa or bulimia nervosa, they should still be considered at risk. A student diagnosed with the female athlete triad requires close coordination of care not only with the eating disorder team, but also with the coach/physical education person or, for example, the dance faculty member who supervises her activity.

## MENTAL HEALTH ISSUES

Among the many psychiatric diagnoses of students on college campuses, depression and anxiety disorders are the most common. Major depression occurs in approximately 4% to 8% of adolescents;[10] however, symptoms of depression occur with much greater frequency. One survey of 16,000 college students in the year 2000 showed that 44% were so depressed that it was difficult to function.[11] Another survey, the National College Youth Risk Behavior Survey, revealed that as many as 10% of college students had seriously considered suicide, and 1.5% had attempted suicide.[10]

One well-publicized case of a possible suicide was that of Elizabeth Shin, a student at the Massachusetts Institute of Technology (MIT).[12] The circumstances of her death were that she had had a history of depression and previous suicide attempts, which involved ingestions. Elizabeth's actual death was caused by a toxic ingestion, followed by her dorm room being lit into flames by an unattended candle. Her case gained notoriety because the court suggested that MIT administrators could be held liable for not preventing her death. This was a responsibility previously held only by individual mental health professionals. Because Elizabeth's case was settled out of court, there was no precedent established, but the case did generate much concern among college administrators that future decisions might hold them liable for completed suicides.

Another common mental health issue among students is anxiety disorder, which occurs in 8% to 9% of adolescents.[10] As previously stated, attending college can create an enormous amount of anxiety, even in well-adjusted adolescents. For those students with a predisposition to anxiety, the college experience can exacerbate this condition to a pathological degree, resulting in the manifestation of panic attacks, generalized anxiety disorder, social phobias, and obsessive-compulsive disorder.

Attention-deficit/hyperactivity disorder (ADHD), another condition with an effect on health and education, is being encountered more frequently than ever before by college health practitioners. Increasing numbers of students are entering college already having been started on medication for this disorder, and college health practitioners are finding it necessary to create policies on how to manage these students. Because most prescriptions for ADHD are controlled substances, students require renewal of their prescriptions every month, which creates a huge service need for mental health and general medical practitioners.

Because mental health services are needed by so many students, many colleges have counseling resources available on campus. At a minimum, most schools have local mental health practitioners that they use as referrals for students when they are struggling with psychological conditions.

## ALCOHOL AND SUBSTANCE ABUSE

Abuse of a substance, whether tobacco, alcohol, or illicit or prescription drugs, clearly involves both psychological and physiological consequences. For this reason, medical and mental health practitioners are often needed in the care of students with these problems.

Adolescents with the newfound freedom associated with college entry may believe that it is their first opportunity to test the limits of what they can do. They may also consider that they are impervious to the addictive properties or negative consequences of the various substances with which they are experimenting. Of course, this thinking only raises the likelihood of the risk. The ACHA, which conducts intermittent surveillance studies of student behavior, conducted a survey in the fall of 2008 that examined the most common substances of abuse—alcohol, tobacco, and marijuana. This survey revealed that 63% of students had used alcohol within the 30 days prior to the survey. Almost 4% admitted to driving after having had at least 5 drinks at a sitting, and 15% reported having had unprotected sex after drinking alcohol. The survey also revealed that 34% of college students had smoked cigarettes, with 17% having smoked cigarettes at least 1 day in the 30 days prior to the survey. Thirty-four percent had used marijuana, with almost 15% having used it in the 30 days prior to the survey. Perhaps most poignant was that when asked about factors that had an impact on their academic function, 4% of students answered alcohol use and 2% answered drug use.[13]

Although substance use has a significant effect on the individual, it also affects those surrounding him or her. Because many college students live in such close proximity, their behaviors take a toll on others. The intoxicated student might rely on his or her friends for help when he or she has vomited or passed out, or worse, when he or she needs to go to an emergency department. Friends may also be concerned about specific addictions in their peers, and may or may not be comfortable involving professional staff at the college. Likewise, college administrators, in conjunction with health services, usually struggle over policies concerning substance use in the dorms and the punishments that result. The concern is that if students are penalized for seeking self-help or help for a peer who is in need of emergency treatment, then they will be reluctant to do so and, as a result, someone may have a serious health consequence, or die. "Dry campuses" and "smokefree campuses" now exist throughout the United States in an attempt to minimize availability, and perhaps even the acceptability, of alcohol or cigarettes on campus.

## CONCLUSION

Although adolescents who are in college have many of the same health issues as other adolescents, caring for them is made somewhat more complicated because of the unique setting and the additional people who are responsible for them in the college environment. The college health provider must tread carefully between respecting the privacy of patients and being responsive to the responsibilities of faculty and administrators, as well as of parents on whom students are often still dependent financially and emotionally. In addition, the health provider is looked to as a public health administrator for the college, watching for trends in illness and working toward prevention of disease. Finally, the health needs of the college student include medical, psychological, and substance abuse factors as he or she is supported through the often exciting but stressful experience of college.

## REFERENCES

1. Patrick K. The history and current status of college health. In: Patrick K, ed. *Principles and Practices in Student Health*. Vol 3. CA: Third Party; 1992:504

2. Rimsza ME, Kirk GM. Common medical problems of the college student. *Pediatr Clin North Am.* 2005;52(1):9–24, vii

3. Greydanus DE, Rimsza ME, Matytsina L. Contraception for college students. *Pediatr Clin North Am.* 2005;52(1):135–161

4. Douglas K, Collins J, Warren C. Results from the 1995 National College Health Risk Survey (abstract). *J Am Coll Health.* 1997;46:55–67

5. Shafiti T, Burstein GR. An overview of sexually transmitted infections among adolescents. *Adolesc Med Clin.* 2004;15(2):201–214

6. Koumans EH. Sexually transmitted diseases services at US colleges and universities. *J Am Coll Health.* 2005;53(5): 211–217

7. Centers for Disease Control and Prevention. Recommended schedules for persons aged 0 through 18 years—United States, 2009. *MMWR. Morb Mortal Wkly Rep.* 57(51/52)

8. Greydanus DE, Rimsza ME, Newhouse PA. Adolescent sexuality and disability. *Adolesc Med.* 2002;13(2):223–247

9. Sundgot-Borgen J, Torstyeit MK. Prevalence of eating disorders in elite athletes is higher than in the general population. *Clin J Sport Med.* 2004;14:25–32

10. Brookman RR, Sood AA. Disorders of mood and anxiety in adolescents. *Adolesc Med Clin.* 2006;17(1):79–95

11. Kisch J, Leino V, Silverman MM. Aspects of suicidal behavior, depression, and treatment in college students: results from the Spring 2000 National College Health Assessment Survey. *Suicide Life Threat Behav.* 2005;35:3–13

12. Sontag D. Who was responsible for Elizabeth Shin? *New York Times Magazine.* NY ed. April 28, 2002;Section 6:57

13. American College Health Association. *American College Health Association—National College Health Assessment: Reference Group Executive Summary Fall, 2008.* Baltimore: American College Health Association; 2008

# CHAPTER 27

# Health Care of Incarcerated Adolescents

RONALD A. FEINSTEIN, MD • KEITH R. CRUISE, PHD, MLS

In 2003, law enforcement agencies in the United States reported 2.2 million arrests of youth younger than 18 years of age.[1] Of these, approximately 600,000 were processed through juvenile detention centers and almost 100,000 were placed in secure correctional facilities. In addition, many youth who commit crimes (even serious crimes) never enter the juvenile justice system but remain in the community under either formal or informal community supervision.[1,2] Consequently, developing a portrait of juvenile law-violating behavior from official records of youth in secure settings gives only a partial picture of the proportion of youth involved in illegal behaviors.

Delinquent youth represent a particularly high-risk and vulnerable population. Specifically in reference to medical needs, they tend to be disenfranchised from traditional health care services. There is a broad consensus across the professional literature that justice-involved youth are a multi-need population.[3,4] These young people are more likely to be victims of abuse and neglect, and to have medical, mental health, substance abuse, and educational problems compared with their nondelinquent peers. Major risk factors for behavior that may lead to involvement in the juvenile justice system have been identified and include cognitive delay or learning disabilities; substance use and abuse; mental health disorders; physical, sexual, or emotional abuse and trauma; and a host of family risk factors including parental substance use and abuse, parental history of incarceration, low levels of supervision and monitoring, and inconsistent parenting.[5]

Primary care providers and juvenile justice systems have an opportunity and responsibility to help improve the health of this underserved and vulnerable group of adolescents. This can be accomplished through: (1) a better understanding of the juvenile justice system, (2) early recognition of risk factors and referral of youth before contact with the juvenile justice system, (3) development and implementation of a cohesive network of services for youth during their involvement with the juvenile justice system, and (4) creation of a system that provides a continuation of services to youth following release from the juvenile justice system. Box 27-1 defines selected juvenile justice terms.

## HISTORY OF JUVENILE JUSTICE REFORM IN THE UNITED STATES

The 19th century was highlighted by a movement that changed the perception of children from one of being small adults to one of individuals with less than fully developed moral and cognitive capacities. The first juvenile court in this country was established in Cook County, IL, in 1899 and reflected the concerns of social reformers during the Industrial Revolution that adolescents warranted special protections from unsafe conditions and abuse in the workplace. Therefore under the doctrine of *parens patriae*, the first juvenile courts embodied an overarching philosophy of improving the welfare of youth through rehabilitation, and the court as a source of benevolent intervention.[1]

Juvenile courts developed throughout the United States during the 20th century. The rehabilitative mission was stated clearly in the laws that established these courts. Transfer decisions from the juvenile court evolved so that only if a juvenile court waived its jurisdiction in a case could a child/youth be tried as an adult within a criminal court. Transfer decisions were made on a case-by-case basis, and were thus within the realm of individualized justice.[1]

The focus on offenders and not offenses, on rehabilitation and not punishment, had substantial procedural effect on the court systems. The juvenile court system introduced a tremendous amount of flexibility in the justice system. Juvenile court judges had wide discretion to consider extralegal as well as legal factors in deciding how to dispose of a case, and provided for a less formal manner in which to handle cases. A range of dispositional options was available to judges in support of the rehabilitative ideal. Dispositions were tailored to "the best interests" of the youth. Treatment lasted until the youth was "rehabilitated" or became a legal adult.

During the second half of the 20th century, many individuals began to question the rehabilitative ideal and the overall effectiveness of the nation's juvenile court system. Beginning in the 1960s, the US Supreme Court issued a number of landmark decisions that

### Box 27-1

#### *Glossary of Selected Juvenile Justice Terms*

**Adjudication.** Legal hearing, similar to an adult trial, where allegations of delinquent conduct are presented. The end result is not a finding of guilt or innocence but a determination that the youth is delinquent or not delinquent.

**Child or Family in Need of Supervision (CHINS or FINS).** Legal designation that places a child, and/or the child's family, under the authority of the court with the purpose of providing interventions and services to reduce behaviors that place the youth at risk for future delinquent conduct.

**Delinquent.** Generally refers to an act committed by a youth, which if committed by an adult constitutes an offense under the statutes or ordinances of the state.

**Detention.** Placement of a youth, after arrest, into a secure facility awaiting a juvenile court hearing primarily based on a determination that placement of the youth in the secure facility is required to (a) protect others, property, or the child; (b) prevent the youth from absconding or not appearing for the juvenile court proceeding; (c) ensure that the youth who may lack adequate adult supervision will appear in court; or (d) because the youth is court-ordered to remain in detention as a result of a judicial court order.

**Disposition.** Legal hearing, similar to a sentencing hearing, after an adjudication hearing where the juvenile court judge determines the rehabilitation/service needs of the youth and custody status (ie, continued placement in the community under probation supervision, out-of-home placement in a residential treatment center or group home, out-of-home placement in a secure custody/juvenile center) of the youth.

**Forensic.** Relating to or dealing with the application of expert or scientific knowledge to the law. In the context of juvenile court proceedings, this includes court-ordered medical and mental health evaluations conducted by licensed professionals with the purpose of assisting the court.

**Informal Adjustment Agreement.** The process by which a youth is diverted from further juvenile court proceedings and agrees to a limited time period of supervision following the filing of a delinquency petition. If the youth satisfies the terms of the agreement, no further action on the delinquency petition is taken.

**Parole.** A period of time designated by the juvenile court during which the youth remains under the supervision of the court following a period of confinement, or placement, in a secure custody facility. During this period, the youth agrees to comply with a set of terms and conditions established by the court including regular meetings with juvenile court supervision personnel (ie, probation or parole officers).

**Probation.** A period of time designated by the juvenile court where the youth agrees to comply with a set of terms and conditions established by the juvenile court. These terms and conditions generally relate to participation in rehabilitation services with the goal of reducing further delinquent acts by the youth. Adherence generally is monitored by a juvenile court supervision officer (ie, juvenile probation officer).

**Status Offense.** An act committed by a juvenile that would bring him/her to court but is not a criminal act (ie, truancy, runaway).

**Transfer, or Waiver.** Refers to the legal process by which a youth is moved from juvenile court jurisdiction to the jurisdiction of the adult criminal court, often for serious felony charges.

resulted in a doctrinal shift by identifying juveniles as "persons" under the Constitution and granting juveniles greater due process protections.[1,6] Landmark decisions that reshaped the nation's juvenile courts are noted in the following:[1]

- 1966 (Kent vs US): courts must provide the "essentials of due process" in transferring juveniles to the adult system.
- 1967 (In re: Gault): in hearings that could result in commitment to an institution, juveniles have the right to (1) notice and counsel, (2) question witnesses, and (3) protection against self-incrimination.
- 1970 (In re: Winship): in delinquency matters, the state must prove its case beyond a reasonable doubt.
- 1971 (McKeiver vs Pennsylvania): jury trials are not constitutionally required in juvenile court hearings.
- 1975 (Breed vs Jones): waiver of a juvenile to criminal court following adjudication in juvenile court constitutes double jeopardy.
- 1977/79 (Oklahoma Publishing Co vs District Court/Smith vs Daily Mail Publishing Co): "press" may report juvenile court proceedings under certain circumstances.

- 1979 (Fare vs Michael C): juveniles have sufficient capacity to make decisions regarding 5th Amendment protections against self-incrimination.
- 1984 (Schall vs Martin): preventive "pretrial" detention of juveniles is allowable under certain circumstances.
- 2005 (Roper vs Simmons): 8th Amendment proscription against cruel and unusual punishments bars imposition of the death penalty for crimes committed by an offender under 18 years of age.

In addition to Supreme Court cases, the juvenile courts have been shaped by legislative acts of the US Congress. In 1968 legislation (Juvenile Delinquency Prevention and Control Act), Congress recommended that youth charged with a status offense be handled outside the court system. In 1974, the Juvenile Justice and Prevention Act required deinstitutionalization of status offenders and nonoffenders as well as the separation of juvenile delinquents from adult offenders. A 1980 amendment to this act required that juveniles be removed from adult jails and lock-up facilities.

In the 1980s, the pendulum began to swing toward law and order, and away from rehabilitation as the nation became increasingly concerned with the rise in juvenile crime. National arrest data indicate that juvenile crime steadily increased through the 1980s, and peaked in 1994.[1] During the 1990s, state legislatures shifted away from the doctrine of *parens patriae* toward a more punitive, crime-control model of juvenile justice. These legislative changes included:

- expanding standards for transfer/waiver of juveniles into the adult criminal justice system,
- lowering the maximum age of juvenile court jurisdiction,
- expanding sentencing options with a greater emphasis on determinant sentences for specific crimes, and
- allowing greater access to juvenile court records and limited opening of juvenile court proceedings balancing rehabilitation against public safety and protection of victims.

Currently, national juvenile crime rates are similar to or below those documented in the 1980s. Most state juvenile court systems seek a balanced approach between punishment and rehabilitation for juvenile offenders. Although juvenile crime seems to continue to trend downward, commentators have noted that roughly 10% to 15% of serious juvenile offenders account for most juvenile crime.[7] Juveniles continue to be processed through formal juvenile court proceedings at high rates, with a large percentage of these juveniles held in some form of out-of-home placement or secure confinement.[1] When youth are placed in the custody of the state, the state is obligated to provide appropriate care that broadly includes providing a safe environment, access to education, and a combination of medical and mental health care. Recent investigations by the US Department of Justice under the authority granted by the Civil Rights of Institutionalized Persons Act (CRIPA) suggest that many states experience difficulties in providing constitutionally protected levels of care.

## EPIDEMIOLOGY

In the United States in 2003, the population of youth ages 10 to 17 years was approximately 33 million.[1] Over the past 50 years, there have been dramatic changes in the rates of arrests, court appearances, and incarceration of juveniles. These changes probably reflect the changing attitudes toward juvenile justice in the United States and the effects of the evolution of the adolescent in our society.

Between 1994 and 2003, there was a significant drop in the arrest rate for most juvenile offenses. The most serious charges in almost half of all juvenile arrests were larceny-theft, simple assault, a drug abuse violation, disorderly conduct, or a liquor law violation. The female proportion of youth entering the juvenile justice system for law violations has continued to increase. Females accounted for 638,000 or 29% of total juvenile arrests. Black youth, who comprise 16% of the juvenile population, accounted for 27% of the total number of juvenile arrests.[1]

Law enforcement agencies refer approximately two-thirds of all arrested youth to a court with juvenile jurisdiction for further processing. Some cases are diverted from the juvenile justice system and others may be transferred to the adult court system. The net result was that in 2002 juvenile courts handled 1.6 million cases, which was an approximately 40% increase from the number of cases handled in 1985. Although older youth dominate delinquency caseloads, trends are similar for all age groups. Between 1985 and 2002, the overall delinquency caseload for females increased 92%, compared with a 29% increase for males. A disproportionate number of delinquency cases involved black juveniles. During 2002, blacks constituted 16% of the juvenile population but 29% of the delinquency caseload.

Long-term juvenile correctional facilities can vary from public to private, and from adult-like prisons to home-like environments. Nationally, nearly 92,000 youth are held in residential placement on any single day (October 2003).[1] Overall custody rates are higher for black youth (754/100,000) than for white youth (190/100,000).[1] Research shows that a significant amount of racial disparity exists throughout the juvenile justice system. The arrest rates for black youth are almost double that of white youth for every 100 individuals.[1] This disparity continues throughout the juvenile justice process so that in the end, whereas black youth comprise 16% of the youth population and are involved with 28% of the arrests, they account for 33% of cases that result in out-of-home placement.[1]

The rate of recidivism is high in juvenile correctional care facilities. Approximately 40% of youth appearing in juvenile court are repeat offenders. Repeat offenders tend to have committed more serious crimes and are younger at the time of their first offense than first offenders.

## MEDICAL ISSUES

Delinquent youth are frequently disenfranchised from traditional health care services. Involvement with the juvenile justice system offers an opportunity to deliver and coordinate medical care to a high-risk population of youth. Programs linking public and private health care providers with the correctional care system can provide juveniles with an opportunity to improve their overall well-being.[8]

Youth detained or confined in correctional care facilities have been shown to have numerous medical problems.[9,10] These conditions may have existed before incarceration; may be closely associated with legal problems; may have resulted from parental neglect, mental health problems, or physical, sexual, or drug abuse; or may develop within the institutional environment. Multiple studies over the past 3 decades have shown that incarcerated youth report a high rate of unmet health needs at the time of admission to a correctional facility. Only one-third of juveniles report having a regular source of medical care, only one-fifth report having a private physician, and half of juveniles report that their families would not be able to ensure follow-up of needed medical care upon release from a facility.

Delinquent youth are noted to have common conditions seen in a general adolescent population (ie, acne, asthma, sports injuries) but also a higher rate than the unincarcerated population of dental problems, sexually transmitted infections (STIs), and tuberculosis. In addition, many of the youth who are admitted to correctional facilities have medical problems that have not been properly tended to in the community because the youth has not sought medical treatment or follow-up. Such unmet needs involve old musculoskeletal problems and poor control of chronic illnesses such as asthma, hypertension, seizures, and diabetes. Additionally, juveniles often are not current on their immunizations.

Youth in correctional care facilities report having become involved in sexual activity at earlier ages and having a greater rate of STIs than other youth. As the number of females entering the juvenile justice system increases, the number who may be pregnant increases. At the present time, few cases of HIV infection or AIDS are being identified in juvenile correctional facilities. However, the population of juveniles is at high risk for developing HIV infection or AIDS in the future because of high rates of drug use, initiation of sexual activity at a young age, having multiple sexual partners, and inconsistent use of condoms.

Juveniles require significant amounts of medical care during their period of confinement. More than half sustain an injury. Half of those injuries are acquired through participation in sports or other recreational activities, but about 20% are associated with fighting, while an additional 20% are self-inflicted. Other common medical problems identified within the confined juvenile population include contagious diseases (ie, methicillin resistant staphylococcus aureus [MRSA]), frequent somatic complaints (ie, headaches, abdominal pain, and chest pain), menstrual problems, and skin conditions. Youth may be victims of sexual or physical abuse perpetrated by other inmates or staff. Such incidents may result from overcrowding, poor supervision or behavioral management, excessive use of restraints or isolation, or stress of confinement.

## MENTAL HEALTH ISSUES

Mental health professionals and juvenile justice personnel have recognized that justice-involved youth exhibit considerably high rates of mental health problems that warrant appropriate identification and intervention.[11] Historically, the prevalence of specific mental health problems was difficult to establish because studies used small samples and relied on varying definitions of mental illness, which limited the ability to generalize findings across studies.[12] More recently, a series of prevalence studies have been conducted with increased methodological rigor using structured diagnostic interviews based on *Diagnostic and Statistical Manual of Mental Disorder* (*DSM*)[13,15] criteria to obtain mental illness prevalence among juvenile offenders. These studies recruited male and female youth across race groups and examined disorder prevalence at multiple points in the juvenile justice system (eg, nonsecure group home or community residential placements, short-term detention centers, and long-term secure custody facilities).

Collectively, these studies indicate that approximately 70% of justice-involved youth meet diagnostic criteria for a mental health disorder. In general, extremely high rates of disruptive behavior disorders (eg, conduct disorder, oppositional defiant disorder) and substance use disorders (between 40% and 50%) have been found. In addition to externalizing problems, more than 20% of male and female youth are noted to suffer from mood and anxiety disorders. A significant finding from these studies is that high rates of mental health problems are not solely related to the presence of disruptive behavior disorders. For example, when conduct disorder was excluded, 60.9% of males and 70.0% of females in a large juvenile detention center still met diagnostic criteria for a mental disorder.[13] Similarly in a multistate, multisite prevalence study conducted by the National Center for Mental Health and Juvenile Justice (NCMHJJ),[14] 66.3% of youth met criteria for a mental health disorder after controlling for conduct disorder, and 61.8% continued to meet criteria after controlling for substance use disorders.

Averaged prevalence rates mask important findings regarding race and gender differences. In the NCMHJJ study, comparable rates of disruptive behavior and substance use disorders were found among male and female youth. However, rates of anxiety and mood disorders were much higher for female youth (29.2% and 56.0%, respectively) compared to male youth (14.3% and 26.4%, respectively). A gender comparison of youth at juvenile probation intake found similar results,[15] suggesting that such gender differences likely are found across all points of the juvenile justice system. Whereas females represent a much smaller percentage of justice-involved youth, these results suggest they warrant careful assessment given the high rates of mental health problems. Another key finding was that non-Hispanic white male and female youth had significantly higher rates of many disorders compared to black and Hispanic male and female youth. Researchers referred to higher prevalence rates for non-Hispanic white youth as "an important paradox" given the over-representation of male youth and youth of color in the juvenile justice system.[13] Finally, results from the NCMHJJ study confirmed that comorbidity (ie, combinations of mental health disorder—particularly mental health and substance use disorders) is the norm and not the exception. In this study more than 60% of the assessed youth met criteria for 3 or more mental health diagnoses, with the most common co-occurring diagnosis being a substance use disorder.

In summary, recent studies have confirmed that justice-involved youth across all levels of the juvenile justice system have much higher rates of mental health disorders compared to community youth and that high disorder rates are not simply due to the presence of behavioral and substance use problems. High rates of mood and anxiety disorders are present[6] with female youth being most likely to exhibit such internalizing problems. Paradoxically, non-Hispanic white youth appear more disordered than youth of color. This finding warrants further investigation to ascertain whether such results are due to measurement bias, true race differences, or a combination of both. Finally, assessment, intervention, and management of mental health disorders among justice-involved youth are often complicated by the presence of co-occurring disorders that necessitate multiple strategic mental health and psychiatric interventions.

## DEATH

Deaths of juveniles in custody are relatively rare. In 2002, 26 youth were reported to have died while in the legal custody of a juvenile facility.[1,16] There is concern that the risk of death to youth in a correctional facility is greater than for youth in the general population. However, data show that the death rate for youth in corrections is significantly lower than for youth in the population. Recent research has shown that suicide is an important cause of death in juvenile facilities, that deaths are more likely in facilities with larger minority populations, and that they are more likely to occur in locked sleeping rooms.[1,16]

## FINANCING ISSUES

Most funds used to pay for providing health care services to juveniles come from the same budget as those for operating the correctional facilities. Federal guidelines prohibit the portion of Medicaid dollars that comes from the federal government to be used for health services (medical or mental) within a correctional facility. A few states have used state Medicaid dollars to provide services for youth awaiting adjudication or for inpatient services. Some funding comes from county or state health departments, grants for pilot projects, or from services eligible for reimbursement from insurance companies.[17,18]

To control costs many facilities contract with local health care providers for services, purchase items, including medications, through state contracts, coordinate services with local health departments (eg, immunizations, STI screening, prenatal care), or work with the judicial system for the early release of youth with life-threatening or acute conditions (eg, newly diagnosed cancer). Unfortunately, financial constraints often limit the provision of comprehensive health care services to juveniles.[19]

## HEALTH CARE STANDARDS

The National Commission on Correctional Health Care (NCCHC),[20,21] a not-for-profit organization that comprises representatives from the fields of corrections, law, law enforcement, and medical, dental, and mental health care, has published standards for health services in juvenile detention and confinement facilities. The organization's primary purpose is to work with correctional facilities to assist in improving their systems for providing health care. Their standards are categorized into 6 sections: (1) administration, (2) managing a safe and healthy environment, (3) personnel, (4) care and treatment, (5) health records, and (6) medical-legal issues. Other organizations including the American Academy of Pediatrics, the American Medical Association, and the Society for Adolescent Medicine have published guidelines and policy statements regarding this population.[22,23]

In addition to promulgation of health care standards, best practice recommendations have been made concerning mental health screening, and assessment practices and blueprints have been made available that outline how state systems can design and implement model programs to meet the mental health needs of justice-involved youth.[24,25] Across these various guidelines a clear message emerges—all professionals working within the juvenile justice system (medical, dental, and mental health) must work in a collaborative manner with juvenile justice personnel, families, and the youth to address the multiple needs experienced by this population.

## SUMMARY

While this review highlights that many justice-involved youth are "healthy" and do not experience significant medical problems, medical professionals must be cognizant of the medical issues that arise from risky behaviors (sexual behavior and substance use) and the psychosocial stressors and economic factors that likely promote this group as disenfranchised from regular and consistent medical care. Finally, it is critical that all health care professionals working with justice-involved youth stay informed and sensitive to the myriad mental health needs of this population to refer youth appropriately and work collaboratively with psychiatric and psychological service providers.[26]

## INTERNET RESOURCES

- National Commission on Correctional Health Care: www.ncchc.org
- Office of Juvenile Justice and Delinquency Prevention: www.ojjdp.ncjrs.gov

## REFERENCES


1. Snyder HN, Sickmund M. *Juvenile Offenders and Victims: 2006 National Report*. Washington, DC: US Department of Justice, Office of Justice Programs, Office of Juvenile Justice and Delinquency Prevention

2. Parent DG. *Conditions of Confinement: Juvenile Detention and Corrections Facilities. Research Summary*. Washington, DC: Office of Juvenile Justice and Delinquency Prevention, US Department of Justice;1994

3. Corrado RR, Roesch R, Hart SD, Gierowski JK. *Multi-Problem Violent Youth: A Foundation for Comparative Research on Needs, Interventions, and Outcomes*. Washington, DC: IOS Press; 2002

4. Heilbrun K, Goldstein NES, Redding RE. *Juvenile Delinquency: Prevention, Assessment, and Intervention*. New York, NY: Oxford University Press; 2005

5. DeMatteo D, Marczyk G. Risk factors, protective factors, and the prevention of antisocial behavior among juveniles. In: Heilbrun K, et al, eds. *Juvenile Delinquency: Prevention, Assessment, and Intervention.* New York, NY: Oxford; 2005:19–44

6. Feld BC. Juveniles' waiver of legal rights: confessions, *Miranda*, and the right to counsel. In: Grisso T, Schwartz R, eds. *Youth on Trial: A Developmental Perspective on Juvenile Justice.* Chicago, IL: University of Chicago Press;2000:105–138

7. Krisberg B, Wolf AM. Juvenile offending. In: Heilbrun K, et al, eds. *Juvenile Delinquency: Prevention, Assessment, and Intervention*. New York, NY: Oxford; 2005:67–84

8. Anno BJ. Availability of health services for juvenile offenders: results on a national survey. *J Prison Jail Health.* 1984;4:77–90

9. Hein K, Cohen MI, Litt IF, et al. Juvenile detention: another boundary issue for physicians. *Pediatrics.* 1980;66:239–245

10. Bolin K, Jones D. Oral health needs of adolescents in a juvenile detention facility. *J Adolesc Health.* 2006;38:755–757

11. Cocozza JJ, Skowyra K. Youth with mental health disorders: issues and emerging responses. *Juvenile Justice.* 2000;3:3–13

12. Otto RK, Greenstein JJ, Johnson MK, et al. Prevalence of mental disorders among youth in the juvenile justice system. In: Cocozza JJ, ed. *Responding to the Mental Health Needs among Youth in the Juvenile Justice System*. Seattle, WA: National Coalition for the Mentally Ill in the Criminal Justice System; 1992:7–48

13. Teplin LA, Abram KM, McClelland GM, et al. Psychiatric disorders in youth in juvenile detention. *Archives of General Psychiatry.* 2002;59:1133–1143

14. Shufelt JL, Cocozza JJ. Youth with mental health disorders in the juvenile justice system: results from a multi-state prevalence study. 2006. Available at: www.ncmhjj.com/pdfs/publications/PrevalenceRPB.pdf. Accessed September 18, 2006

15. Wasserman G, McReynolds LS, Ko S, et al. Gender differences in psychiatric disorders at juvenile probation intake. *Am J Public Health.* 2005;95:131-137

16. Gallagher CA, Dorbin A. Deaths in juvenile justice residential facilities. *J Adolesc Health.* 2006;38:662-668

17. Cuellar AE, Kelleher KJ, Rolls JA, et al. Medicaid insurance policy for youths involved in the criminal justice system. *Am J Public Health.* 2005;95:1707-1711

18. Gupta RA, Kelleher KJ, Pajer K, et al. Delinquent youth in corrections: Medicaid and re-entry into the community. *Pediatrics.* 2005:1077-1083

19. Tennyson DH. Juvenile correctional system health care costs: a five-year comparison. *J Correct Health Care.* 2004;10:257-271

20. National Commission on Correctional Health Care. *Position Statement: Health Services to Adolescents in Adult Correctional Facilities: 1998.* Chicago, IL: National Commission on Correctional Health Care

21. National Commission on Correctional Health Care. *Standards for Health Services in Juvenile Detention and Confinement Facilities: 2004.* Chicago, IL: National Commission on Correctional Health Care

22. American Academy of Pediatrics, Committee on Adolescence. Health care for children and adolescents in the juvenile correctional care system. *Pediatrics.* 2001;107:799-803

23. Feinstein RA, Lampkin A, Lorish CD, et al. Medical status of adolescents at time of admission to a juvenile detention center. *J Adolesc Health.* 1998;22:190-196

24. Grisso T, Vincent G, Seagrave D. *Mental Health Screening and Assessment in Juvenile Justice.* New York, NY: Guilford;2005

25. Skowyra K, Cocozza J. A blueprint for change: improving the system response to youth with mental health needs involved in the juvenile justice system. 2006. Available at: www.ncmhjj.com/Blueprint/pdfs/ProgramBrief_06_06.pdf Accessed October 2, 2006

26. Lieberman A, Simkins S. Your patients in the juvenile justice system, and your role in their care and well-being. *Contemporary Pediatrics.* 2006;23:57-65

# CHAPTER 28

# Health Care of Adolescents in Military Settings

LT COL DALE M. AHRENDT, MD • COL ELISABETH M. STAFFORD, MD

*The views and opinions expressed are those of the authors and do not reflect the official policy or position of the Department of the Army, the Department of Defense, or the United States government.*

Adolescents and young adults in the military truly reflect the larger youth culture in which they live. Entering military service from around the nation and beyond, this population also presents a richness of diversity in geographic, racial, socioeconomic, and ethnic roots. The military culture in which they live also presents an environment with a unique set of challenges and influences. This is true for the young uniformed service members as well as for military family members who are adolescents or young adults.

The world has changed since the terrorist events of September 11, 2001, with the current engagement of tens of thousands of young service members in combat and other activities around the world. Additionally, as large-scale disasters occur, whether manmade or natural, service members stand at the ready to respond for rescue, stabilization, and recovery efforts whether at home or abroad. Given the nature of the occupation, risks to physical and mental health of the service member are inherent to military service. Parental service in the military affects the lives of adolescents within the military family at a time of critical psychosocial development as well.

A description of military cultural influences as it affects the lives of these young people is provided within this chapter, as well as a focus on health issues, the health care delivery system, history of adolescent medicine within the military, and consideration of future directions to better understand and optimize health care of adolescents and young adults in military settings.

## ADOLESCENTS AND YOUNG ADULTS IN UNIFORM

The defense of our nation falls largely on the shoulders of adolescents and young adults. Almost 50% of our active duty military service members are between the ages of 17 and 25 years old. This proportion has remained relatively stable over the last decade. The distribution varies from 67% of the Marines to 39% of the Air Force, with the Army and Navy falling in between at 44% of the total force. As of 2007, there were almost 632,000 troops age 25 or younger. The National Guard and Reserves include an additional 279,000 members of this age group, making up 30.6% of the total force (see Table 28-1).[1] Most of the enlisted members are recent high school graduates. Some completed a portion of their undergraduate education prior to leaving for military service. Motivation for joining military service is varied, including one or more of the following: desire to seek training opportunities; earn money to complete their education; gain more life experience before settling into a career path; patriotism; following in the footsteps of parents or other respected family or community members; and gain a sense of belonging to an organization with tradition and purpose. Whatever their reasons may be, the military is home to almost a million of our adolescents and young adults.

As these young people join the military, most of them have acquired the capacity for abstract thinking and future planning, with personal aspirations as previously described being expressed within the structure of a military setting. Of course, there are numerous

**Table 28-1**

**Active Duty and Reserve Troops in the US Military, Ages 17–25**

| *Branch* | *Enlisted* | *Officers* |
|---|---|---|
| Army | 221,802 | 12,263 |
| Navy | 138,556 | 6,511 |
| Marines | 121,207 | 3,276 |
| Air Force | 118,728 | 9,482 |
| Active Duty Total | 600,293 | 31,532 |
| Guard and Reserves | 274,713 | 4,377 |

Source: Department of Defense. *2007 Demographics: Profile of the Military Community*. Report Published by the Office of the Deputy Under Secretary of Defense (Military Community and Family Policy), under contract with ICF International.

adjustments that must be made that can be framed as early developmental milestones to be met by the new military recruit.[2] These include (1) disengagement from the family, (2) reflex, absolute obedience within a framework of lawful orders, (3) uniformity in appearance, and (4) subsuming personal identity within a group identity to build cohesion and efficacy, an accommodation that is critical to military mission accomplishment.

Although much attention has been given to the risk-taking behavior of high school-aged adolescents, research has shown that many of those behaviors become even more problematic after the age of 18. The 18- to 24-year-old age group has a mortality rate double that of the younger adolescent population, with unintentional injury being the leading cause of death. Seventy percent of injuries are due to motor vehicle crashes (MVCs), and almost a third of the fatal MVCs were caused by a driver who had been drinking alcohol. Substance abuse, cigarette smoking, heavy drinking and binge drinking, and unprotected sexual intercourse with subsequent sexually transmitted infections (STIs) are all behaviors seen with greater frequency in the young adult population as compared with younger adolescents. Mental health problems include suicide, with rates triple that of younger adolescents. This is the population entering the military, bringing many of these problems and risk behaviors with them.

As a tracking methodology, every 2 to 3 years over the past 20 plus years the military has been conducting a survey, the *Department of Defense Survey of Health Related Behaviors*. For many of these behaviors, the US military's higher accession standards mean a lower incidence. Some adolescents never make it through the enlistment and basic training process because of their underlying problems. Still, there remain critical issues for young people in the military. Of note, there are significant differences between the military cohort and civilian counterparts for some behaviors (Table 28-2).[3,4] By definition, all adolescents and young adults in the military are employed. As an organization, the military enforces higher standards of behavior for its members than most civilian employers or educational institutions. In addition, it maintains fitness standards that require a dedication to maintaining a healthier lifestyle. On the other hand, life in the military can also be more stressful than civilian life, with longer work hours, frequent moves, and sometimes dangerous assignments, often associated with separations from family members and social support networks. Being away from family and being on their own for the first time, which is true for many, means freedom to explore some behaviors they may not have been involved with in their younger years.

Significant health threats for young service members can be identified from review of the survey.[3] For young people in the military, binge drinking rates for the last 30 days, defined as 5 or more drinks on 1 occasion, are 53.8% for the 18- to 25-year-old age group. Heavy drinking, which is defined as 5 or more drinks on 1 occasion at least once a week for the last 30 days, is 26.1% in those age 20 or younger, and 28.4% in the 21- to 25-year-old group. As noted in Table 28-2, the rates are higher among males than females. Conversely, rates of illicit drug use are significantly lower in the military than in a comparable group of civilian adolescents and young adults. This can probably be attributed to multiple factors, including a zero tolerance policy for use, mandated random drug screening programs, and the personal motivations of the people who would choose a military career. Despite the low rates, drug use still exists, according to the surveys. It is important that health care providers screen for this and know how to address the issue when it arises. Cigarette use is similar to that seen in civilians in this age group. This is despite a health-promoting work environment that offers free smoking-cessation programs and encourages its members not to smoke. Even more concerning is the finding that of those military members who do smoke, about 31% started smoking *after* joining the military.

**Table 28-2**

**Risk Factor Comparisons between Military and Civilian Adolescents and Young Adults**

| *Risk Factor* | *Age 18–25* | *Military* | *Civilian* |
|---|---|---|---|
| Heavy alcohol use, last 30 days | Male | 32.2% | 17.8%[a] |
| | Female | 8.1% | 5.5%[a] |
| Any illicit drug use, last 30 days | Male | 5.8% | 20.8%[a] |
| | Female | 3.3% | 11.7%[a] |
| Cigarette smoking, last 30 days | Male | 45.4% | 42.2% |
| | Female | 26.5% | 30.3%[a] |

[a]Statistically significant difference between comparison groups at 95% confidence

Sources: Bray RM, Hourani LL, Rae KL, et al. *2002 Department of Defense Survey of Health Related Behaviors among Military Personnel.* Research Triangle Park, NC: RTI International; October 2003; and Park JM, Mulye TP, Adams SH, Brindis CD, Irwin CE. The health status of young adults in the United States. *J Adolesc Health.* 2006;39:305–317.

Not surprisingly, rates of sexual activity are higher among those in the 18- to 25-year-old age group than in those younger. It is important that as they become mature adults, responsible sexual habits are adopted. The survey of military personnel showed that 47.9% of those age 20 or younger who are unmarried used a condom at their last encounter, indicating that substantial numbers are at risk for STIs and unplanned pregnancy.

Significant mental health problems occur with some frequency in military personnel. The stressors associated with being in the military may exacerbate and bring these problems to light. Yet, identification of the mental health problems could result in disqualification from continued work in the military, so as a result, do not seek services. In the military survey, screening questionnaires have revealed the need for further evaluation in a significant number of adolescent and young adult members (Table 28-3). Screening for these issues during regular clinic visits is indicated.

Exercise rates are high in the military population, with 70.2% of all members reporting 20 minutes or more of strenuous exercise 3 or more times a week. Although the rates for the under-25 group alone are not available, it is reasonable to assume they are at least as good as the average for all age groups, if not better. In many ways the health care needs of the military population may be similar to that of athletes, with increased risk for musculoskeletal injuries. Weight is still an issue, with 23.8% of the 20 and younger group and 17.2% of the 21- to 25-year-old group being overweight; 10.5% and 6.5%, respectively, are underweight. Strictly regulated weight standards are a stressor for some service members and are a factor in unhealthy weight loss behaviors that must be proactively addressed. Seat belt use rates (92.1%) are higher than for their civilian counterparts (75%), and the number that wear helmets when riding a motorcycle are 82.1%, compared with an average of 58% nationally.

**Table 28-3**

**Identified Mental Health Needs in Military Adolescents and Young Adults**

| *Mental health need* | *Age group* | *Percentile* |
|---|---|---|
| Need evaluation for anxiety | 20 or younger<br>21–25 | 21.7%<br>20.7% |
| Need evaluation for depression | 20 or younger<br>21–25 | 27.1%<br>24.0% |
| Suicidal ideation in the past year | 20 or younger<br>21–25 | 9.1%<br>7.1% |

Sources: Bray RM, Hourani LL, Rae KL, et al. *2002 Department of Defense Survey of Health Related Behaviors among Military Personnel*. Research Triangle Park, NC: RTI International; October 2003

The physical requirements of a military job are more rigorous than for many civilian occupations. Active duty service members need to be capable of deploying to austere conditions and performing strenuous physical activities. The need to maintain this "military readiness" puts a focus on decreasing injuries and returning to functional status as soon after injury as possible. Again, this is similar to the health and fitness needs of an athlete. Members on flight status have additional requirements, as do those who work in sensitive areas. Impairment of any kind, whether from injury, mental health issues, or risk-taking behaviors including alcohol or substance use, can affect their ability to perform their mission. Physicians caring for this population need training to appropriately screen for adolescent risk-taking behaviors and address the problems before they have a detrimental effect on the service member's performance.

Although the military has a robust health system, there are some special problems that active duty members may face in accessing those services. The biggest issue is lack of privacy. As previously mentioned, random drug screening is done on all members, with the results reported to officials who administer the program. HIV screening tests are also done, with results, in the past, often leading to separation from the military or reassignment to different duties. The medical record itself is considered the property of the government. Many medical and mental health problems could result in a member's fitness for duty or ability to remain in the military challenged. Thus, it is not uncommon for military members to seek care outside of the system for issues they don't want documented in their medical record, such as evaluations for STIs. Although some privacy restrictions do apply to mental health records, not all members believe that such rules are enforced, and many are resistant to talk to a mental health professional for fear it could affect their military career. The resulting distrust that some military members may at times feel has the potential to affect the quality of care they receive.

A unique population of adolescents in the military is those at the military service academies, which are essentially unique university settings, including the US Military Academy, the US Naval Academy, and the US Air Force Academy. These are much more than colleges where students wear a uniform. The experience of young people at the academies is significantly different than that of their civilian counterparts. The entrance standard is high for all students, with each one expected to achieve academic excellence. In addition to their academic pursuits, they must also deal with the rigors of military training. The approximately 12,000 cadets of the military service academies are being molded into military leaders of tomorrow. Standards of conduct and professionalism are strictly enforced, adding to the challenges of undergraduate training. All of the stressors that affect other college students as many of them leave home for the first time also affect this group of students. However, here it is even more important than in the nonmilitary universities that risk-taking behaviors are not adopted. Sports also play an important role in the lives of many of these students. Physical fitness is even more heavily emphasized than it is in the regular military, and the health care needs of this population truly are that of an athlete. The physicians caring for these cadets must be able to meet all of these needs and ensure that the needs of the cadet, as well as those of the military, can be met.

Including almost 50% of the military population, from the basic trainees fresh from high school to young officers in the early stages of becoming our nation's military leaders, the roughly one million adolescents and young adults in the active duty military, guard, and reserve forces make up one of the largest single collections of post-high school populations in the United States. Recognizing the unique aspects of caring for an adolescent or young adult in the military setting and providing for those needs is an important task for the military leadership and the military medical system.

## COMBAT EXPOSURE AND MENTAL HEALTH

In the face of ongoing current conflicts in Iraq and Afghanistan, an extensive infrastructure of mental health monitoring and support has been integrated within the battle environment and on return home from combat service. Department of Defense policy mandates post-deployment health assessment within 30 days of return, and for those service members returning from a combat environment, subsequent reassessment within 4 to 6 months postreturn to further optimize mental health screening. A recent study by Hoge et al[5] demonstrated approximately 1 in 5 combat veterans returning from Iraq endorsing some mental health concern. Reports also indicate that symptoms often increase between initial homecoming and 3 to 4 months later.[6] Stigma associated with mental illness persists in the military community as it does within the larger society, and fewer than half of service members in these studies endorse seeking care. Young service members returning with a variety of injuries including burns, amputations, and traumatic brain injury also have attendant comorbid mental health conditions requiring optimized support for full rehabilitation.

## ADOLESCENTS AND YOUNG ADULTS IN MILITARY FAMILIES

Approximately 25% of children within military families of the active, reserve, and National Guard components currently serving are adolescents and young adults. The spectrum of challenges they face as they "serve" within military families make them a unique subpopulation to consider. The nature and severity of potential stressors for adolescents in military families can be contextualized within a framework of the following categories:

- Routine stressors: frequent moves; changes in school and social milieus, and routine separations from military parents, who often must go into the field or to sea to train for months at a time.
- Acute, severe stressors: wartime deployment of military parents; negative reactions from the surrounding civilian social structure regarding work the military child's parent is doing; and possible or actual injury or death of the military parent.
- Chronic, recurring, and severe stressors: living in remote, sometimes hostile foreign areas; accompanying threats or occurrences of terrorism.
- Complicating factors: effects of mental health problems such as attention-deficit/hyperactivity disorder (ADHD), oppositional defiant disorder, and depression, as well as developmental delays and physical abnormalities, upon already stressed families.[7]

In the 1970s, the term "military family syndrome" was coined to describe observations of the presumably deleterious effects of growing up within autocratic military families and communities.[8] This concept has not been borne out, however, by subsequent, more rigorous studies[9-11] comparing military-connected and civilian children for anxiety and other psychopathology. In contrast, the phrase "military brat" is a term often self-applied by adults as well as adolescents in military families reflecting "affectionate humor as well as identification" with growing up in a military family.[12]

A major challenge for many military families is the increased mobility, with relocations to new duty assignments that occur on average every 2 to 3 years. These new military assignments occur around the country and around the world, presenting the inevitable stressors of moving, leaving friends, schools, and pets behind, and adjusting to a new community. Typically this involves exposure to new cultures, languages, school systems, peer groups, and physical environments. As a result of this mobility, disruptions in education can occur: varied academic requirements in different states, different school-year calendars, different academic ranking schemes, and occasional requirements to move within the school year. In recent years, increasing attention has been given to providing greater support and stability to military-connected high school students, in particular, to address these challenges. Military family-oriented policies and programs have been developed to facilitate a more optimized education experience.[13–15]

Intermittent short and long separations from the military parent as a result of military training, deployments, and war present additional challenges. Obviously there are inherent dangers within the military service, with attendant concerns and anxiety regarding the physical safety of the military parent. Deployment can be defined as the assignment of military personnel to temporary, unaccompanied (by family members) duty away from the permanent duty station. There is a predictable pattern of emotional responses that family members, including adolescents, may experience with the deployment of the military parent, which may be expected and scheduled or may occur with short notice and without advance preparation of the family. Adolescents exhibit a range of reactions to the stresses of prolonged parental separation due to deployment. These may include irritability, anxiety, depression, attention-seeking, acting-out behaviors, or accelerated personal growth and maturation.[16,17] These reactions are dynamic and may wax and wane as the continued prolonged deployment presents new stressors within a personal, family, and community context. Deployment in the face of war brings clear concerns for the possible injury and death of a parent with which the adolescent must cope. Death and severe injury, whether physical or mental, can present catastrophic stressors for the adolescent and family. Military parents may also return from combat with unrecognized psychiatric illness including post-traumatic stress disorder, depression, substance abuse, and other disorders, all with potential for secondary traumatization of family members.[18]

These unique challenges for military-connected adolescents occur against the backdrop of meeting the universal developmental tasks of individuation from the family, body image consolidation, attainment of independence and autonomy, and psychosexual identity formation. Health care providers must be familiar with the unique challenges these adolescents and their families face and be prepared to provide anticipatory guidance to promote resiliency and optimized continued growth and development. Proactive screening and assessment of emotional distress is critical to early identification. This will allow early support interventions in times of anticipated stress due to relocations, deployment, parental injury, and death. Adolescents and their families can be directed to many military family support programs to facilitate resiliency building and adaptive coping.[19,20]

The health care issues of military-connected adolescents reflect the major health threats for adolescents in the US population at large. Obesity, as with their civilian counterparts, is a growing health issue for adolescents within military families. There are limited studies that make direct comparisons for risk behavior profiles between military connected adolescents versus the adolescent population at large. However, in a study of privacy issues for military adolescents, fewer risk-taking behaviors were identified for adolescents in a military family presenting for care in a clinic setting as compared with comparable Youth Risk Behavior Survey[21] state and national data. Medical records of adolescents in military families should be kept confidential by regulation for sensitive issues such as reproductive care, STI care, mental health issues and substance abuse, as guided by civil law and legal precedents. Where adolescent clinics exist, patients can make their own appointments, keep their records confidential, and see providers separately. Lesser degrees of privacy are afforded in general medicine clinics. Medical facilities have policies in place for the treatment of minors guided by standards of legal and medical practice within the state.

## ADOLESCENT MEDICINE IN THE MILITARY

Soon after Dr J. Roswell Gallagher established the first adolescent inpatient unit and clinic in Boston, the military followed suit in 1958 with the first adolescent clinic at Letterman Army Medical Center in San Francisco.[22] Under the leadership of then Major Frederick Biehusen, the first "adolescent medicine rotation" within a military pediatric residency training program was established.[23] Subsequently, one of the military pediatric residents, Captain Peter Patterson, requested and obtained the first Army-sponsored civilian fellowship and became one of Dr Gallagher's first adolescent medicine fellows at Children's Hospital Boston. This young visionary military physician went on to become the first consultant in adolescent medicine to the Army Surgeon General in 1973.[24] The military recognized the benefits of having physicians trained to meet the needs of adolescents and young adults under their care, and adolescent clinics were established in all major medical centers and many smaller community hospitals in the United States and overseas. In the early 1970s, school-based clinics were established in Europe. Both the Army and Navy have engaged in adolescent medicine fellowship training over the past 30 years. Since 2001, all military adolescent medicine training has been consolidated into a Triservice Adolescent Medicine Fellowship. This was established as a combined program at the Air Force and Army medical centers in San Antonio, Texas, and referred to as the San Antonio Uniformed Services Health Education Consortium (SAUSHEC) Adolescent Medicine Fellowship. This is the first new military adolescent medicine fellowship in the era of adolescent medicine subspecialty board certification and ACGME accreditation of fellowship programs. It includes a robust teaching program with 2 fellows per year and 5 core faculty adolescent medicine specialists. The military adolescent medicine fellowship currently represents 10% of the nation's adolescent medicine specialists in training.[25] It serves as a platform to:

1. Provide educational, training, and consultative support for adolescent medicine within the Department of Defense;
2. Conduct high-quality research addressing the unique health care needs of adolescents and young adults in the military, as well as family members who are adolescents;
3. Continue the tradition of developing future military medical leaders.

## MILITARY HEALTH CARE SYSTEM

Currently, adolescents being cared for in the military system are seen by many different types of health care providers in many possible settings. Lack of insurance coverage is not an obstacle, because all active duty members and their dependents have free access to care in military medical settings. Dependents of retired military members do have to pay an annual fee for full access to care, but the amount is minimal compared with civilian insurance rates. Most of the major medical centers have adolescent medicine clinics providing direct and consultative care for adolescents and young adults. All military pediatric trained providers have had formal training in the field of adolescent medicine, and many internal medicine and family medicine programs also include adolescent medicine experiences. The result is that most primary care providers have at least some training in dealing with this population. On review of scope of care provided to adolescents within the military health system, the most comprehensive care has been provided under adolescent medicine specialist and family practitioner supervision.[26] As a global military health care system, particular emphasis is given to preventive services and ongoing health promotion, which is generally well integrated into the health care of military-connected adolescents. Military policies have also been put in place, such as the Exceptional Family Member Program, to ensure that the special health and educational needs of adolescents are considered when a military service member comes up for new assignments. Considerations must be given to availability of scope of services that may be required for an adolescent with special needs at the new military assignment location.

The major disadvantages in the system are inconsistent protection of confidentiality and lack of uniform access to age-appropriate services. The medical record can at times come into the possession of the parent or guardian, such as when moving to a new assignment or medical visits outside of the military system. It is important that the provider makes the adolescent patient aware that absolute confidentiality of the medical record cannot be guaranteed. The other issue is access to appropriate care. Staff turnover can be frequent in a military setting, and new staff may not be aware of the regulations that give teenagers rights for accessing age-appropriate care, depending on policies and practices at previous duty locations. Adolescents may find themselves unable to book appointments or receive the confidential services they had received from previous providers or clinics.[26] Advocating for improvements in health care delivery systems with policies to break down barriers to appropriate care remains an important role of the military adolescent medicine specialist.

## FUTURE DIRECTIONS

What direction will military adolescent medicine take in the future? As the downsizing in total military personnel continues, the military health system must be more focused and efficient with finite resources, just as the larger military in general. Continued support for fellowship training is critical to ensure that adolescent medicine specialists have a place at the table for shaping ongoing optimization of the health and well-being of adolescents and young adults in military families and within the uniformed services. Expanding further into the care of our adolescents and young adults that are on active duty will benefit all. As the numbers of adolescent medicine board-certified physicians will not likely become a significant proportion of the military medical corps, it is important that these specialists are assigned to positions to teach the precepts of comprehensive care grounded in prevention and health promotion, to advocate for policies leading to population health improvement, and to guide health research priorities for this population. Training the providers who will provide care for these soldiers, sailors, airmen, and marines, and ensuring that policies and regulations are in place to enforce appropriate screening and that preventive services are accessible, are the challenges for the current group of military adolescent medicine physicians. Strategic assignment of military adolescent medicine specialists to military tertiary care centers with robust graduate medical education training programs for pediatrics, internal medicine, family practice, and other programs is key. Placing them in positions where they can provide oversight of the care of young service members at all military basic training sites and military service academies would also facilitate increased health care optimization for this group. Vigorous advocacy for this vision to expand comprehensive care for young uniformed service member and military family members continues with an ongoing focus on the preservation and extension of the rich history that is military adolescent medicine. This will remain the challenge of the next generation of military adolescent medicine physicians in the years to come.

## REFERENCES


1. Department of Defense. *2004 Demographics: Profile of the Military Community*. Washington, DC: The Office of the Deputy Under Secretary of Defense (Military Community and Family Policy), under contract with Caliber, an ICF consulting company. Available at www.armywifenetwork.com/wp-content/uploads/2009/03/military-community-profile.pdf. Accessed July 22, 2010

2. Hardoff D, Halevy A. Health perspectives regarding adolescents in military service. *Curr Opin Pediatr.* 2006;18:371-385

3. Bray RM, Hourani LL, Rae KL, et al. *2002 Department of Defense Survey of Health Related Behaviors among Military Personne*l. Research Triangle Park, NC: RTI International; October 2003. Available at www.tricare.mil/main/news/2002WWFinalReport.pdf. Accessed July 22, 2010

4. Park JM, Mulye TP, Adams SH, Brindis CD, Irwin CE. The health status of young adults in the United States. *J Adolesc Health.* 2006;39:305-317

5. Hoge CW, Castro CA, Messer SC, et al. Combat duty in Iraq and Afghanistan, mental health problems, and barriers to care. *N Eng J Med.* 2004;351:13-22

6. Hoge C, Auchterlonie J, Milliken C. Military mental health problems: use of the mental health services, and attrition from military services after returning home from deployment to Iraq or Afghanistan. *JAMA.* 2006;295:1023-1032

7. Hardaway T. Treatment of psychological trauma in children of military families. In: Webb NB, ed. *Mass Trauma and Violence Helping Families and Children Cope*. New York, NY: Guilford Press; 2004:259-282

8. Lagrone DA. The military family syndrome. *Am J Psych.* 1978;135:1040-1043

9. Jensen PS, Xenakis SN, Wolf P, et al. The "military family syndrome" revisited: by the numbers. *J Nerv Ment Dis.* 1991;179:102-107

10. Ryan-Wenger NA. Impact of the threat of war on children in military families. *Am J Orthopsych.* 2001;71:236-244

11. Watanabe HK, Jensen PS. Young children's adaptation to a military lifestyle. In: Martin JA, Rosen LN, Sparacino LR, eds. *The Military Family: A Practice Guide for Human Service Providers*. Santa Barbara, CA:Praeger; 2000:209-223

12. Wertsch ME. *Military Brats: Legacies of Childhood inside the Fortress.* New York, NY: Aletheia Publications; 1991

13. Keller MM. *US Army Secondary Education Transition Study.* Harker Heights, TX: Military Child Education Coalition; 2001

14. Department of Defense. In-state tuition. Available at: www.hrc.army.mil/site/education/InState/index.htm. Accessed September 18, 2009

15. Military Impacted Schools Association. Interstate compact on educational opportunities for military children. Available at: www.militaryimpactedschoolsassociation.org. Accessed September 18, 2009

16. Stafford EM, Grady BA. Military family support. *Pediatr Ann.* 2003;32:110-115

17. American Academy of Pediatrics. Support for military children and adolescents. Available at: www.aap.org/sections/unifserv/deployment/index.htm. Accessed May 18, 2010

18. Cozza SJ, Chun RS, Polo JA. Military children and families during Operation Iraqi Freedom. *Psych Quarterly.* 2005;76:371-378

19. Lemmon KM, Stafford EM. Recognizing and responding to child and adolescent stress: the critical role of the pediatrician. *Pediatr Ann.* 2007;36(4):225-231

20. Huebner AJ, Mancini JA. *Adjustments among Adolescents in Military Families When a Parent is Deployed.* West Lafayette, IN: Military Family Research Institute, Purdue University; 2005:1-50

21. Hutchinson JW, Stafford EM. Changing parental opinions about teen privacy through education. *Pediatrics.* 2005;116:966-970

22. Alderman EM, Rieder J, Cohen MI. The history of adolescent medicine. *Pediatr Res.* 2003;54:137-147

23. Biehusen F. The adolescent—a medical misfit. *US Armed Forces Medical Journal.* 1958;9:811-816

24. Schydlower M, Imai W. Adolescent medicine: practice and specialty training in the Army Medical Department. *J US Army Medical Department.* 1992;PB 8-92-7/8:14-15

25. Althouse LA, Stockman JA. Pediatric workforce: a look at adolescent medicine data from the American Board of Pediatrics. *J Pediatr.* 2007;150:100-102

26. Griffith JR, Schwab KA, Robinson A, et al. Physicians' perceptions of the status of adolescent health care within the military health system. *Military Medicine.* 1999;164:683-687

SECTION 8

# Special Populations of Adolescents

# CHAPTER 29

## Adolescents in Foster Care

MOIRA SZILAGYI, MD, PHD • SANDRA JEE, MD, MPH

### INTRODUCTION

Adolescents are a uniquely vulnerable subset of the population of young people in foster care, which is intended to be a temporary respite in which adolescents and their families receive appropriate services to allow for reunification. The passage of the Adoption and Safe Families Act in 1997 in the United States refocused the goals of foster care on the health, safety, and well-being of its charges. Because all children and teens need a sense of belonging in a family, permanency in a timely manner is a major goal of foster care, whether achieved through reunification with parents or relatives, adoption, or guardianship. When none of these are viable options for an adolescent in foster care, the system has to prepare the young person for independent living. In most states, emancipation from foster care occurs at 18 years of age; only a handful of states allow youth to remain in care until their 21st birthday.

**Table 29-1**

**Preteens and Youth in Foster Care in 2008, as Percentage of Foster Care Population**

| *Age (y)* | *Number (% of Foster Care Population)* |
|---|---|
| 11–12 | 34,743 (16.4%) |
| 13–15 | 78,767 (37.2%) |
| 16–18 | 91,376 (43.2%) |
| 19–20 | 6,837 (3.2%) |

Data from The AFCARS Report: Preliminary FY 2008 Estimates as of October 2009 (16). US Department of Health and Human Services, Administration for Children and Families, Administration on Children, Youth and Families, Children's Bureau. Available at: www.acf.hhs.gov/programs/cb/stats_research/afcars/tar/report16.htm. Accessed March 9, 2010.

### EPIDEMIOLOGY

Of the more than 700,000 young people in the United States who spend at least some time in foster care each year, almost half (46%) are preteens or adolescents. The most recent data from the Department of Health and Human Services Administration for Children and Families reveal that 463,000 children and adolescents were in foster care placement. Some teens entered foster care in infancy or childhood, whereas others entered foster care as adolescents. The age distribution of preteens and teens in care in the United States in 2008 is presented in Table 29-1.

Though 70% of the overall foster care population is removed from their family of origin because of abuse or neglect, a study in New York City indicated that only 29% of 11- to 15-year-olds were admitted for these reasons. The prevalence of child abuse and neglect among adolescents in foster care is most likely grossly underestimated. Many teens in foster care have experienced physical abuse, sexual abuse, and chronic neglect as younger children, although that history may not be well-documented.

Most teens enter foster care as "status offenders" because of acting-out behaviors. In many states, under family court authority a "person in need of supervision" (PINS) placement occurs when a person under 16 years of age is truant, incorrigible, ungovernable, or habitually disobedient and beyond the lawful control of a parent. Juvenile delinquent (JD) placement occurs when a 7- to

15-year-old is charged with engaging in an act that would be "criminal" if perpetrated by an adult; under this jurisdiction, a judge can order probation, confinement to juvenile detention facility, or placement in foster care. A juvenile offender (JO)—a 13- to 15-year-old youth charged with a felony—is not eligible for foster care placement due to the serious nature of the charge. Another major reason for foster care placement in adolescence is "voluntary placement." Less than 1% of foster care placements across all age groups fall into this category, but 43% of voluntary placements are for adolescents with major mental health problems who are in need of residential treatment. Families unable to afford this form of treatment may choose voluntary foster care placement as a means to access Medicaid funding for their teen's care.

In general, about half of children and teens in foster care are males, and minorities are overrepresented. The specific ethnic breakdown of adolescents in foster care is not known. Overall, minorities are overrepresented in foster care, with 58% being children of color, 30% white, and 15% Hispanic.

There are unique subpopulations of adolescents in foster care. Those with mental health diagnoses and substance-abusing teens, who are often in placement under PINS petitions, comprise perhaps the largest subsets. Other subpopulations with unique needs are pregnant or parenting teens, those with mental retardation and developmental delay, and lesbian/gay/bisexual/transsexual (LGBT) youth, some of whom have been evicted from their homes by their parents and have spent time homeless or living in shelters.

## RISK FACTORS FOR POOR LONG-TERM OUTCOMES

Adolescents in foster care often have experienced a multiplicity of adverse risk factors prior to foster care placement that predict and result in poor outcomes. Most of these adolescents come from families in which chaotic, impaired parenting in a disrupted family setting has been the norm. Impaired parenting is most commonly secondary to substance abuse, mental illness, cognitive impairment, and poor parenting skills. In addition, these families frequently experience domestic violence, homelessness, or transient housing. Teens in foster care are often from poor and disenfranchised households and have lived in neighborhoods rife with violence and criminal activity. School attendance tends to be meager, the quality of the education when they do attend school is regularly substandard, and the schools in which they are enrolled have high rates of failure and suspension. Further, limited access to normalizing activities and healthy adult role models reinforces a perception of a hopeless future. In addition, many have exhibited behavioral and mental health problems that result in criminal justice involvement and residential or group home placement.

Foster care, intended to be a window of opportunity for healing, may in fact have a negative effect on teens. Removal from the family of origin may be emotionally traumatic. This is especially true if the family has filed a PINS petition or voluntarily placed the teen in foster care, which the teen often interprets as rejection. Teens who have disclosed abuse or neglect may feel guilty for the ensuing family disruption. Ongoing separation and the uncertainty of when or if they will return to their family of origin can lead to depression and anxiety. Some teens have been the parental figure in their family of origin and may experience extreme anxiety about the welfare of their parents and siblings who remain together. Placement in residential or group home care often exposes the teen to peers whose lifestyles and choices are or have been unhealthy. In general, teens in foster care feel alienated from normal life and view themselves as less worthy than their peers.

## TYPES OF FOSTER CARE PLACEMENT

Preteens and young teens are more likely to live in foster family care or live with a relative who is a certified foster parent. Older teens, especially those with significant mental health or behavioral problems, are more likely to live in group homes or residential care, and are also likely to experience multiple transitions, moving among foster families, residential, group home, and inpatient psychiatric care settings. Treatment foster care, an evidence-based approach in which specially trained foster families provide mental health intervention in their homes with consultation and clinical support, is an alternative to residential placement. Improved foster care treatment outcomes include improvement in permanency, social skills, and behavior.

## HEALTH NEEDS

Many studies consistently demonstrate the significant physical and mental health problems of teens in foster care. These problems are noted upon entrance to foster care and have been documented years after a youth leaves foster care. Nearly half of youths formerly in foster care continue to have serious health problems and difficulty obtaining health coverage. Primary care for an adolescent in foster care should include not only assessments for physical and mental health status, but also ongoing screening for substance abuse and reproductive health concerns. The primary care physician needs to be aware of the increased educational needs of this population.

Adolescents in foster care are at a heightened risk for ongoing and emerging mental health problems. Prevalence studies find that 62% of youths in foster care have had the onset of a psychiatric disorder before entering the foster care system.[1] Another study showed that 94% of youths in foster care had used a mental health service in their lifetime, and 83% had used a mental health service in the past year; lifetime rates for inpatient psychiatric care (42%) and residential programs (77%) were also elevated. Youths in foster care use mental health services at exceedingly high rates, especially in comparison to Medicaid or Supplemental Security Income (SSI)-matched peers.[2,3] They are most commonly diagnosed with attention-deficit/hyperactivity disorder (ADHD)[4] and conduct disorder,[5] but also have been noted to have high levels of internalizing disorders. One study found that youths in foster care were 16 times more likely to have mental disorders and 8 times more likely to receive psychotherapeutic medications than SSI-matched peers not in foster care.[3] There is controversy over whether this represents an indication for medication or "chemical restraint" of behaviorally disruptive teens. It is unclear whether this high rate of service use is even sufficient to meet the manifold mental health needs of this population.

Primary care providers should be aware of important disparities in mental health care for this population. Of note, there are significant racial disparities in receipt of mental health care among adolescents in foster care. Although minorities are disproportionately overrepresented among those in foster care, black and Hispanic persons consistently receive fewer inpatient and outpatient mental health services.[6] Youths in foster care may be at increased risk for developing a psychiatric disorder because of: (1) a family history of psychiatric disorder, (2) a history of child abuse and neglect, (3) exposure to significant levels of violence within and outside the home, (4) the experience of disruptions in living situations, and (5) relationship losses.[1] As might be expected, older youths in foster care have disproportionately high rates of lifetime and past year psychiatric disorders. For this reason, young adults transitioning out of the foster care system have a particular need for initial and periodic mental health assessments, as recommended by joint policy statements from the American Academy of Pediatrics (AAP), the American Academy of Child and Adolescent Psychiatry, and the Child Welfare League of America.[7]

During adolescence, the possibility for high-risk behaviors to emerge, including abuse of illicit substances, should be anticipated. Adolescents who have struggled with unsuccessful placement settings may be particularly vulnerable to high-risk behaviors. Nearly one-third of respondents in a study of adolescents who had been in foster care for at least 1 year reported that they suffer from at least 1 substance use or affective disorder.[8] Lack of consistency in the home setting may predispose teens to experimental behaviors, particularly those who do not have the benefit of a positive peer social group or pro-social values.

Adolescent females in foster care are twice as likely as those not in foster care to become pregnant.[11] Because this has been reported more among youths in foster care who live in emergency shelters or group homes, it is unclear whether this rate might be affected by fragmentation of health care and social services.[9] Qualitative reports have also revealed that some adolescent females express an intention to become pregnant to fulfill a desire to love or to be loved. Lack of medical care continuity, coupled with lack of social supports, no sense of belonging in a family, and little hope for the future may create a synergistic effect contributing to elevated rates of pregnancy among teens in foster care. High-risk sexual behaviors and high rates of sexually transmitted infections (STIs) are common in adolescents in foster care. One study found that almost one-quarter of teens in foster care had been tested or treated for STIs, which is more than four times the national average in a comparative sample. The primary care provider will need to provide ongoing anticipatory guidance and surveillance for STIs and pregnancy.

## EDUCATION ISSUES

Youths placed in out-of-home settings are likely to come from disadvantaged families and neighborhoods. They have low educational status, limited employment experience, and struggle to build adult lives once they leave the foster care system. Societal expectations for an adult to lead a productive life often hinge on educational attainment. Unfortunately, for many youths in foster care, educational success is suboptimal. Studies have found that only 30% to 40% of older teens in foster care graduate from high school or obtain a general equivalency diploma (GED), although some samples of adolescents in family foster care have reported rates of 50% to 70%. College entrance rates are variable among youth formerly in foster care, but range from 2% to 11%. Older adolescents with the lowest rates of postsecondary education attendance have lived in restrictive placement settings, a marker for other concomitant mental health and delinquency problems. Some of this underachievement may be attributable to the impact of multiple placement changes on educational achievement. In 1 study, more than one-third reported having 5 or more school changes. High rates of school suspension and delayed school entry after placement in a new setting exacerbate the underachievement. However, there are also compelling data that school attendance and performance improve in foster care, particularly for younger adolescents and preteens.

Limited data exist on the educational experiences of adolescents in foster care. One qualitative study of 262 youths preparing for independent living found that fewer than half of teens reported involvement in extracurricular activities at school, and more than one-quarter reported dissatisfaction with the quality of their educational experience while in foster care.[10] The data are not encouraging: 73% of youths had been suspended at least once since the seventh grade, 58% had failed a class, and 29% had physical fights with students. Nearly half of respondents in 1 study reported having required special education services at some point during their educational career. In spite of these discouraging data, 70% of subjects expressed a desire to attend college. The desire for educational achievement was high even among those individuals who exhibited significant school behavior problems. Advocates for the adolescent in foster care should cultivate this desire for future success and facilitate the receipt of academic resources necessary for high school graduation and possibly continuation with postsecondary education or other vocational training.

## NORMALIZING ACTIVITIES

Adolescents in foster care lack exposure to normalizing activities, including extracurricular school activities and recreational opportunities such as sports, clubs, and music. Such activities can build self-efficacy and self-esteem, introduce the teen to appropriate adult role models and mentors, and teach relationship skills, teamwork, and cooperation. Work opportunities, which are often not readily available because of transportation barriers or frequent placement changes, can give the teen the ability to earn money while developing healthy work habits. Interviews with older adolescents in foster care suggest that more than one-third were employed and almost one-half had ever worked for pay. Most adolescents were employed at least half-time, and job training programs were integral to their employment.

## VISITATION WITH FAMILY

The goals of foster care are the achievement of health, safety, and permanency for children and teens. Reunification with family of origin remains the major means of achieving permanency, and visitation is the best predictor of reunification. In families where sexual abuse or severe physical abuse have been problems, reunification is unlikely unless the offender is removed from the home. Some families may reject the teen, especially if the teen's behaviors are seen as disruptive in the family. Similarly, rejection of a teen may occur if she or he discloses abuse or neglect that leads to removal of the children from the family, or an adult who provides financial support to the family. In such situations, the perpetrating adult is responible for those consequences, but the adolescent may be blamed for the breaking up of the family or the loss of household income. Teens may long for reunification, even when it is not possible. Other teens may choose to remain in foster care, particularly if they have a sense of belonging in their foster home. For a variety of reasons, some adolescents choose to remain connected to their parents and/or their siblings whereas others do not.

## OUTCOMES

Outcomes for youths who have spent time in foster care are variable. They include (1) return to biological parent(s), (2) reconnection with extended kin or birth family and siblings, (3) adoption by kin or foster parent caregiver, (4) elopement (the legal term for "running away"), (5) "aging out" of the system, and (6) transfer to a different foster care agency. It is likely that youths will experience more than 1 of these outcomes, which contribute to the instability of living in out-of-home care. Many youths will experience multiple foster home placements. In 1 study of 732 youths in foster care, one-quarter reported 5 or more foster home placements. Nearly half reported running away from out-of-home care (elopement), and nearly two-thirds of those who had run away had done so multiple times. In spite of high rates of attempted elopement, most youth report positive experiences with their out-of-home care and are generally satisfied with their experiences in foster care.

Approximately 20,000 adolescents in the United States leave the foster care system annually and attempt to live independently. As adolescents age out of foster care and transition to adulthood, they often lack the knowledge, resources, and skills for independence. Many find their way back to their family of origin despite years of separation because they have no sense of belonging in another family. The Chafee Foster Care Independence Act of 1997 provides states the opportunity to develop more extensive independent living programs to aid youth nearing emancipation, and many foster care agencies use this funding to continue programs for youth until they are 21 years old.

Youth and young adults who have spent time in foster care report many difficulties. The experience of complex, often multiple traumas prior to foster care result in poor, predictable long-term outcomes if such trauma is not adequately treated by appropriate mental health services and stable placement in a nurturing foster home. On the other hand, appropriate foster care placement and ancillary services may help resilient youth cope with their adverse life experiences despite early complex trauma. Because there are no longitudinal studies relating early life traumas, foster care experience, and long-term outcomes, information related to these areas usually is obtained from interviews with convenience samples of young adults who have a history of foster care placement.

Adolescents who age out of foster care often have continued difficulty finding or maintaining employment; 42% report 1 or more nights homeless within a year of leaving foster care at an average age of 18, and almost 20% report being homeless for a week or more.[12] Several investigative reports indicate high rates of homelessness and incarceration among adults with a history of foster care placement. Adults previously in foster care are less likely to be in intimate long-term relationships than their peers and have fewer friends. They also often idealize their birth parent and blame the child welfare system for the disintegration of their families. There is concern among professionals in the field that many of these individuals have not dealt with their grief and loss issues, and that many adults who experienced foster care when they were younger report lower expectations of self, poor self-concept, difficulty with regulating emotions, and difficulty with focusing attention or handling stress.

## IMPROVING OUTCOMES

Optimal outcomes for youths in foster care involve capitalizing on the youth's optimism to succeed in the future. An evidence-based approach to foster parent training and mentoring can have a positive impact on adolescent outcomes. Ultimately, laying the foundation for self-efficacy for adolescents in foster care involves attention to multiple domains: maximizing educational potential, offering job skills training, providing continuing mental health services, fostering independence through driving lessons and involvement in normalizing activities, and finding mentors and role models for teens and families. Though foster care seldom replicates the sense of belonging in a family that most adolescents grow up with, good caseworkers can foster the development of resilience by providing appropriate opportunities and services, supporting foster families with evidence-based interventions, and promoting a future orientation. The primary care provider may not be able to address all of these issues, but awareness of the complexity of challenges will help ensure the smoothest transition to late adolescence and early adulthood.

## REFERENCES

1. McMillen JC, Zima BT, Scott LD, Jr, Auslander WF, Munson MR, Ollie MT, et al. Prevalence of psychiatric disorders among older youths in the foster care system. *J Am Acad Child Adolesc Psychiatry.* 2005;44(1):88–95

2. Halfon N, Berkowitz G, Klee L. Mental health service utilization by children in foster care in California. *Pediatrics.* 1992;89(6 Pt 2):1238–1244

3. dosReis S, Zito JM, Safer DJ, Soeken KL. Mental health services for youths in foster care and disabled youths. *Am J Public Health.* 2001;91(7):1094–1099

4. Garland AF, Hough RL, McCabe KM, Yeh M, Wood PA, Aarons GA. Prevalence of psychiatric disorders in youths across five sectors of care. *J Am Acad Child Adolesc Psychiatry.* 2001;40(4):409–418

5. McCann JB, James A, Wilson S, Dunn G. Prevalence of psychiatric disorders in young people in the care system. *BMJ.* 1996;313:1529–1530

6. Snowden LR, Cuellar AE, Libby AM. Minority youth in foster care: managed care and access to mental health treatment. *Med Care.* 2003;41(2):264–274

7. American Academy of Pediatrics District II Task Force on Health Care for Children in Foster Care. *DICoEC, Adoption, and Dependent Care. Fostering Health.* Lake Success, NY: American Academy of Pediatrics District II; 2001

8. Courtney M, Terao S, Bost N. *Midwest evaluation of the adult functioning of former foster youth: conditions of youth preparing to leave state care.* Chicago, IL: Chapin Hall Center for Children, 2004:2–12

9. Ensign J. The health of shelter-based foster youth. *Public Health Nurs.* 2001;18(1):19–23

10. McMillen C, Auslander W, Elze D, White T, Thompson R. Educational experiences and aspirations of older youth in foster care. *Child Welfare League of America.* 2003; LXXXII(4):475–495

11. Bilaver LA, Courtney MA. Foster care youth. National campaign to prevent teen pregnancy. *Science Says.* 2006; 27:1–4

12. Pecora PJ, Williams J, Kessler RC, et al. *Assessing the Effects of Foster Care: Early Results of the Casey National Alumni Study.* Baltimore, MD: Annie Casey Foundation; 2003:25

# CHAPTER 30

# Immigrant Adolescents

JENNIFER JOHNSON, MD

Although the United States has always been a "nation of immigrants,"[1] today's immigrant adolescents are demographically very different from those of a generation ago. Immigrant youth born in foreign countries who come to the United States now come primarily from Latin America and Asia, not Europe as in the past. Most immigrant adolescents born in the United States have parents who came from Latin America. (The terminology used to describe immigrants is presented in Box 30-1.) Although most immigrants still settle in traditional immigrant-receiving states and communities, changes in geographic immigration patterns over the past 20 years have transformed American society and reshaped communities throughout the country.

This chapter presents demographic information, provides a framework for considering the effects of immigration on health and well-being, identifies challenges to health care access, reviews specific health issues in immigrant adolescents, and addresses the importance of culturally appropriate care. The relationship of race and ethnicity to adolescent health is discussed in a separate chapter.

Addressing immigrant adolescents as a distinct group poses challenges. Data and literature are sparse compared with other age groups. Demographic reporting most commonly encompasses children and adolescents in a single age group from 0 to 17 years. The diversity of immigrants' countries and cultures of origin is often not factored into studies; even nationally representative samples may not be of adequate size to do so. Studies are subject to confounding by the interrelationships of culture, race, ethnicity, economic status, and educational achievement. Acculturation, a key variable measured in a variety of ways, can be closely related to socioeconomic status. Differentiating acculturation effects from those linked to income and education remains a problem.

### Box 30-1

#### *Glossary*

**Documented immigrant.** Has legal documentation allowing him or her to live in and remain as a resident in host country.

**Undocumented immigrant.** Foreign-born noncitizen who comes to live in host country without legal documentation.

**Mixed-status family.** Family in which ≥1 parent does not have legal documentation but children are born in the United States and have citizenship.

**First-generation immigrant.** Foreign-born person with foreign-born parents.

**Second-generation immigrant.** Person born in the United States with at least 1 foreign-born parent.

**Asylee, refugee.** Person who seeks refuge due to fear of political, religious, or physical persecution in homeland. A *refugee* is an individual who applies for admission to the United States at an overseas facility; an *asylee* is one who applies for admission once within the United States or at a point of entry. Neither has the option to return to their country of origin.

## IMMIGRANTS IN THE UNITED STATES

Immigrants constitute the fastest-growing segment of the US population; more than 11 million immigrants entered the country in the 1990s. In 2007, 38 million foreign-born residents comprised 12.6% of the US population, the highest proportion since the 150-year low of 4.7% in 1970.[2] In 1960, 75% of the foreign-born population came from Europe, 9% from Asia, and 10% from North America.[3] At that time, no single country accounted for more than 15% of the total immigrant population.[2] In contrast, by the year 2000 more than 50% of the foreign-born population had been born in Latin America (30% in Mexico), with about 25% coming from Asia and 15% from Europe.[3]

About 11.8 million (31% of the total foreign-born population) were undocumented immigrants in 2007. This included 1.7 million children and adolescents <18 years of age and 1.9 million young adults 18 to 24 years of age.[4] A large group of undocumented immigrant children belong to families of migrant or seasonal workers. In the 2001–2002 school year, more than 190,000 students in grades 7 to 12 qualified for services in the US Department of Education Migrant Education Program.[5] At present, slightly fewer than 1 million legal immigrants and about half as many undocumented immigrants arrive in the United States each year. They come primarily from Mexico (57%) and other Latin American countries (23%).[6] In 2007, about 50,000 refugees were admitted to the United States, and 25,000 persons were granted asylum. In recent years, about 40% of refugees arriving in the United States were younger than 18 years of age, and just under 20% were 18 to 24 years of age. Thirty percent of asylees are younger than 25 years old.[7] Virtually all internationally adopted children, of whom there were 20,000 in 2007, are younger than 9 years of age.[8]

More than 20% of children ages 17 and younger in the United States today are children of immigrants. Of these, 85% are second-generation immigrants (born in the United States with at least 1 foreign-born parent), most of whom are Hispanic. These youth represent the first wave of a demographic shift that will lead, by the year 2030, to fewer than half of children in the United States being non-Hispanic white. About 60% of children of immigrants have a parent who is not a citizen.[9] Immigrant children not born in the United States represented 5.6% of 10- to 14-year-olds, 8.4% of 15- to 19-year-olds, and 15.3% of 20- to 24-year-olds in 2006.[10]

Since 1990, the same 6 states have had the highest numbers of foreign-born residents: California, New York, Texas, Florida, Illinois, and New Jersey. Together they account for two-thirds of all immigrants. These states also have the most children of immigrants. In California, children of immigrants make up nearly half of school children in both elementary and upper-level age groups.[11] In recent years, there have been large increases in immigrant populations in nontraditional receiving states. For example, the share of the foreign-born population increased by at least 50% from 2000 to 2007 in South Carolina, Nevada, Tennessee, Alabama, and Arkansas.[2] There have been significant increases in the percentage of school-aged youth who are second-generation immigrants in nontraditional states as well, creating new challenges for educational systems. Between 1990 and 2000, the proportion of children of immigrants in prekindergarten to fifth grade increased by 100% or more in 7 states, none of them in the "big 6" immigration states. This also applies to the 14 states that experienced the same proportional increase in 6th- to 12th-grade students.[11]

## ASSIMILATION AND ACCULTURATION

The terms *assimilation* and *acculturation* are used to describe immigrants' adaptation to life in a new country. These concepts are sometimes used interchangeably but are not identical. Acculturation can be described as an integrative process in which the attitudes, customs, behaviors, values, or beliefs of people from a culture are modified as a result of contact with a different culture. Each culture influences the other, hence references to the American "melting pot." Assimilation refers to a contrasting process in which a minority group is absorbed into the dominant culture. Traditionally, assimilation, as with European immigrants in the first half of the 1900s, results in increasing socioeconomic status and intermarriage in subsequent generations. With greater numbers of immigrants from Asia and Latin America in recent years, however, a different outcome is often being observed. This difference may be due to "segmented assimilation," in which the outcomes of the adaptation process depend upon the segment of the population to which assimilation occurs. Thus, children of immigrants who relocate into disadvantaged urban settings are placed at higher risk for "downward assimilation," whereas those placed in other settings may experience the opposite effect. The decreased social and economic advancement observed in many immigrant families recently may also be attributed to work force changes limiting the availability of blue-collar and union-supported jobs that helped previous generations of immigrants. Immigrants with few skills find work primarily in lower-paying, less secure jobs in the service industry, where there are few opportunities for advancement.

The challenges of adapting to a new culture are referred to as *acculturative stress*. These include language difficulties; adapting to new social structures; perceived or real discrimination based on skin color, language, clothing, or other characteristics; and cultural differences in family values and social roles. Acculturation is often more rapid in youth than in adults, creating an "acculturation gap" that can cause dissension and misunderstandings. Youth may be asked to translate or "culture broker" for their parents, thereby assuming a level of responsibility that may create additional stress. Parents may be less able to provide guidance and supervision as they themselves are adapting to a new culture and are not familiar with the risks encountered by their children.

Adolescent immigrants must integrate 2 cultures to develop their own cultural identity at the same time they are completing other developmental tasks of adolescence, including establishing a personal identity. Becoming competent in the new culture promotes academic success, whereas establishing a positive ethnic identity facilitates psychological well-being.[12] Maintaining connections to the native culture—dual cultural membership—helps bridge the acculturation gap. Despite advantages of a dual frame of reference, however, some youth may perceive themselves to be at the periphery of both cultures, not fully belonging to either.[13]

## IMMIGRANT YOUTH IN SCHOOLS

Nearly 1 in 5 middle and high school students is an immigrant. In 2000, 7% of those in 6th through 12th grades were first-generation immigrants, and 12% were second-generation immigrants.[11] Immigrants are less likely than native-born youth in native families to have graduated high school by age 19, as shown in Table 30-1. Those from Mexico, Central America, the Dominican Republic, Indochina, and Haiti are least likely to be graduates.[14]

The need for good English language skills presents the most obvious challenge to academic success. In 2000, 6% of 6th- to 12th-grade students were classified as "limited English proficient" (LEP). The US Census designates individuals as LEP if they speak a language other than English at home and speak English less than "very well." Two-thirds of LEP students lived in "linguistically isolated households," in which all household members older than 14 years of age are LEP. Contrary to expectations, more than half of these LEP students are second- or third-generation immigrants.[11]

Living in a linguistically isolated household is a factor associated with poor educational outcomes. Immigrant youth are disproportionately likely to experience other life circumstances that jeopardize educational outcomes, as illustrated in Table 30-1. Three additional variables are relevant: (1) having a mother who has not graduated from high school; (2) severe economic hardship (household income less than twice the poverty level); and (3) living in a single-parent family. Of non-Hispanic white children in native-born families, 35% experience 1 of these risk factors. Of all children in native-born families, the proportion is 44%, compared with 67% of children in immigrant families. When 2 risk factors are considered, the proportion of children in immigrant families (42%) is almost twice that of native-born families (24%). Lower parental education is associated with higher numbers of risk factors for both immigrants and nonimmigrants.[14]

First-generation immigrant youth in particular tend to grow up in environments less conducive to their development. They are more likely than second-generation immigrant children to belong to families of lower income and lower maternal educational achievement. Immigrants ≥2 years behind in school are most likely to be first-generation immigrants who come from families with low parental education.[14]

**Table 30-1**

**Demographic Characteristics of Youth in Immigrant versus Native-Born Families[14]**

| | *Native-Born (%)* | *Immigrant (%)* |
|---|---|---|
| 1 parent in home | 15.5 | 23.8 |
| ≥4 siblings <18 years of age | 13.6 | 18.1 |
| Someone other than a parent or dependent sibling living in home | 22.1 | 39.0 |
| Living in poverty | 14 | 21 |
| Behind in school at age 16 | 8 | 10 |
| High school graduate at age 19 | 79 | 72 |

## HEALTH STATUS, RISK, AND PROTECTIVE BEHAVIORS

Given the challenges encountered by immigrants and that immigration is commonly driven by the goal of enhancing social and economic well-being, it would be expected that health status is lower in immigrant than in native-born youth. In fact, based on a large number of indicators, the health of children in immigrant families appears to be better than those of native-born children in native families. In the 1994 National Health Interview Survey (NHIS),[15] immigrant youth had fewer acute and chronic health conditions and fewer school days missed from illness. Although the proportional differences were small, analysis of data from the 1995 National Longitudinal Study of Adolescent Health (Add Health)[16] indicated that first-generation immigrants in grades 7 through 12 reported better physical health than second-generation immigrants. Variables included general health, having missed school due to a physical or emotional problem in the past month, learning difficulties, obesity, and asthma. For youth from many, but not all, countries, this effect became more noticeable when analysis controlled for family and neighborhood context.

First-generation immigrant adolescents also appear to be less likely to engage in health risk behaviors.[15] In the aforementioned Add Health study,[16] foreign-born youth were less likely to have had sexual intercourse, engaged in delinquent or violent acts, and to have used controlled substances. Data analysis from the 1997 National Longitudinal Study of Youth[17] found that first-generation adolescents were less likely to participate in substance abuse and juvenile delinquency than third-generation youth. Of Hispanic youth in the same dataset, those who were foreign-born were less likely to have intercourse before age 18 but also less likely to use contraceptives consistently at age 17 if they were having intercourse. Effects for language, gender, and country of origin were observed; teens of Mexican origin were less likely to become sexually active.[18]

As with physical health, limited extant data suggest that the mental health and psychological adjustment of immigrant youth in general is at least as good as that of native-born children in native families.[14] In the 1994 Add Health[16] analysis cited previously, there was no difference between immigrants and nonimmigrants on measures of psychological distress or positive well-being. Youth with LEP or who were not fully acculturated to 2 cultures were most likely to have psychological adjustment problems.[15] Immigrant and especially refugee youth may have witnessed or experienced extreme harassment, violence (including rape), physical and mental torture, or other atrocities prior to arriving in the United States. Not surprisingly, rates of depression and posttraumatic stress disorder (PTSD) in such groups are high. Half of Khmer youth who experienced massive war trauma as children met criteria for PTSD; at 12-year follow-up, the prevalence was still 35%.[19]

## IMMIGRATION, ACCULTURATION, AND HEALTH

The *healthy immigrant effect* is a compelling explanation for findings of better-than-expected health status in immigrant populations. This phenomenon was first articulated in the mid-1980s as the "epidemiologic paradox" (also "Hispanic paradox"). The health status of the Hispanic population in the Southwest was noted to be similar to that of the non-Hispanic white population, even though their socioeconomic status—generally the best predictor of health status—was closer to that of the black population. Since then, this largely unexplained phenomenon has been particularly well documented in the Latino population, but the healthy immigrant effect has also been identified in children and adults in the United States as well as in immigrants in other countries.

Is the healthy immigrant effect attributable to preferential immigration of healthier populations? This does not appear to be the case, because acculturation ("Americanization") is generally associated with poorer health and health outcomes, higher rates of health risk behaviors, and lower levels of preventive behaviors. Well-being is generally found to be greater in foreign-born youth, declining across generations of immigrant families. The difference is greatest between the first and second generations (the "second-generation decline"). Factors that appear to be related to the decline in health status include changes in diet and lifestyle and limited access to health care.[16]

Findings regarding health-related behaviors and changes across generations in various populations of immigrants suggest that the healthy immigrant phenomenon varies by population and subpopulation. For example, analysis of 2001 data from a cross-sectional survey of adolescents in California found that, in the case of Asians, preventive health behaviors in successive generations either improved or remained better than those of non-Hispanic whites.[20]

## ACCESS TO CARE AND HEALTH SERVICES UTILIZATION

Access to health services is limited by lower rates of health insurance in immigrant families, fears that immigration status will have negative consequences when seeking medical care, and language and cultural barriers. Beliefs about causes, treatment, and prevention of illnesses may affect utilization of health services.

Lack of health insurance is a key factor in preventing immigrant children and youth from obtaining preventive as well as episodic health care services. In families below 200% of the federal poverty level, 48% of foreign-born immigrant children who are not citizens were uninsured in 2005, compared with 15% of US citizen children in native-born families.[21] In general, immigrant children do not lack health insurance because their parents are unemployed. Rather, disproportionate numbers of full-time wage earners in immigrant families do not have health benefits. A large share of immigrants is employed in low-income jobs and by businesses that do not provide health benefits. In addition, federal law denies virtually all legal immigrants eligibility for Medicaid and the State Children's Health Insurance Program (SCHIP) during their first 5 years in the United States. Thereafter, eligibility is limited by the factors used in its determination. Fewer than half of states currently provide health insurance coverage to legal immigrant children using state-only funds.[22]

Access to public insurance is even more difficult for undocumented immigrants. Federal law mandates that emergency treatment be available to all immigrants regardless of their status. In a few states, prenatal care is available to immigrants through the SCHIP. US-born children of all immigrants are, however, generally eligible for federal health insurance. Consequently, some members of a household may have health insurance, whereas others do not.[23] Even among those eligible, participation is greatly limited by lack of familiarity with public health programs and how to access services. Fear that information divulged about other family members could have negative consequences for their immigration status may prevent parents from applying for coverage for their eligible children. Immigrants have been found to be much less likely than citizens to use primary and preventive services as well as hospital, emergency, and dental services, even after controlling for the effects of race and ethnicity, income, insurance status, and health status.[24]

## HEALTH EVALUATION

### CONTEXT OF CARE

Virtually all who provide health care to adolescents have contact with immigrants, be they documented or undocumented, first or second generation. Cultural sensitivity, also known as cultural competency, is essential for all aspects of care, from establishing rapport to promoting adherence. More than a specific knowledge base, cultural competency can be considered an ongoing process that embodies respect for cultural differences, interest in learning about other perspectives, and acceptance of other world views. These concepts are discussed in detail elsewhere (Chapter 43, Cultural Considerations). The clinician elicits information about the patient's native culture, perceptions of health and illness, and use of religious and cultural traditions (including complementary and alternative medicine) in healing. Traditional cultural values should be considered strengths and reinforced as protective factors.

It is particularly important for the provider to understand the context of the patient's immigration. From what country, culture, and life circumstances did emigration occur? What are the details of the migration journey and resettlement process? Did the youth experience trauma, witness violence, live in a refugee camp? What is the youth's legal status? What support systems are available? Is the family intact or fragmented; what is the role of the family system in the patient's life? Have there been changes in social or economic status? What are the characteristics of the new school and community?[13]

### SCREENING PRIOR TO ARRIVAL IN THE UNITED STATES

All immigrant and refugee applicants must have a physical examination and mental status assessment as part of their application process. The medical examination focuses primarily on detecting certain serious contagious diseases that may be the basis for visa ineligibility. This "migration health assessment" is conducted overseas by a physician designated by the US Department of State to determine if medical conditions or mental disorders exist that would make the applicant inadmissible, need to be followed up after resettlement, or require the applicant to receive long-term institutionalization or maintenance income provided by the US government after resettlement. All immigrants and refugees 2 years of age and older applying for permanent visas in the United States must be screened for tuberculosis with a tuberculin skin test (and chest x-ray, when indicated). Serologic tests for syphilis and human immunodeficiency virus (HIV) infection with confirmatory tests for positives are also required of applicants 15 years of age and older. Applicants younger than 15 years of age are tested only if there is reason to suspect either of these diseases. Human immunodeficiency virus infection is no longer a cause for exclusion from the United States. Immigrants must show proof of having received recommended vaccines unless they are internationally adopted children younger than 11 years of age.

### HEALTH SCREENING AFTER ARRIVAL IN THE UNITED STATES

Initial assessment of health status for newly arrived documented and undocumented immigrants includes topics described in the previous section, "Context of Care." It is preferable that family or community members not be used as interpreters. As always when exploring sensitive topics, the clinician must be prepared to offer resources and support if the interview triggers strong emotional reactions. When conducting a physical examination, expectations regarding the sex of the provider, body areas to be examined, and the presence of a parent or third party during the examination may differ. Vision and hearing screening and a dental evaluation should be performed.

Screening for certain infectious diseases should be performed in individuals from countries with high prevalence. Common infectious diseases by geographic region are summarized in Table 30-2. Additional information is available from the Centers for Disease Control and Prevention (CDC) "Yellow Book,"[25] available online at wwwnc.cdc.gov/travel/content/yellow-book/home-2010.aspx. In general, laboratory testing should be performed as follows:

- Complete blood count (CBC) with differential
- Serum chemistries
- Serum lead level if ≤17 years of age and born or recently resided in a foreign country
- Hepatitis B serology (HbSAg, anti-HBs, anti-HBc) if from area with endemic hepatitis B infection (eg, Asia, Africa) (see Table 30-2).
- Hepatitis C serology if from area with endemic hepatitis C infection
- If sexually active or history of rape/sexual abuse, if indicated for clinical reasons, or if patient comes from a high-prevalence area (see Table 30-2), HIV antibody with confirmatory testing. This should be performed before any live vaccines are administered.

**Table 30-2**

**Infectious Disease Risk by Region of Origin**

| | *Tuberculosis* | *Hepatitis B* | *Intestinal Parasites*[a] | *Subacute, chronic, or latent infection* |
|---|---|---|---|---|
| Mexico and Central America | X | | X | Cysticercosis, Chagas disease, leishmaniasis |
| East Asia | X | X | X | Hepatitis C, schistosomiasis, liver flukes, paragonimiasis (lung flukes) |
| Southeast Asia | X | X | X | Other helminth infections (eg, paragonimiasis, opisthorchiasis, clonorchiasis) |
| South Asia | X | | X | Cysticercosis, visceral leishmaniasis, lymphatic filariasis, echinococcosis |
| Eastern Europe and Northern Asia | X[b] | X | | |
| Temperate South America | | | X | Cysticercosis, Chagas disease (from remote acquisition), echinococcosis, soil-associated fungal infections (eg, histoplasmosis, coccidiomycosis) in some countries |
| Tropical South America | X | | X | Schistosomiasis, leishmaniasis, Chagas disease, cysticercosis |
| Central, East, and West Africa | X | X | X | HIV, lymphatic filariasis, onchocerciasis, loiasis, schistosomiasis, echinococcosis, Hansen disease |
| North Africa | X | X | X | Hepatitis C, schistosomiasis, fascioliasis, echinococcosis |
| Southern Africa | X | | X | HIV, schistosomiasis |
| Middle East | X | | | Echinococcosis, cutaneous leishmaniasis, brucellosis |

Source: Centers for Disease Control and Health Promotion. Geographic distribution of potential health hazards to traveler. In: Arguin PM, Kozarsky PE, Reed C, eds. *CDC Health Information for International Travel 2008*. Philadelphia, PA: Elsevier Mosby; 2007.

[a]Most commonly strongyloidiasis

[b]Including multidrug-resistant tuberculosis

- Rapid Plasma Reagin (RPR) or Venereal Disease Research Laboratory (VDRL) for syphilis if sexually active or history of rape/sexual abuse; consider if treponemes prevalent in source country (eg, Liberia, Somalia)
- Examination of 3 stool specimens for the presence of ova and parasites.
- Targeted tuberculin testing in accordance with national guidelines. This includes those arriving ≤5 years previous from countries with a high incidence of tuberculosis.[26]
- Immunizations in accordance with national guidelines, the most recent of which are available at www.cdc.gov/vaccines. Mumps, rubella, varicella, hepatitis A, and human papillomavirus (HPV) are most likely to be inadequate.

## CONCLUSION

Immigrant adolescents will play a vital role in the future of the United States. Health care providers can play a role in facilitating social adaptation while also encouraging retention of bonds to their culture of origin to promote their health and well-being.

## REFERENCES


1. Kennedy JF. *A Nation of Immigrants*. Rev ed. New York, NY: Harper & Row; 1986

2. Terrazas A, Batalova J. Frequently requested statistics on immigrants in the United States. Washington, DC: Migration Policy Institute; 2009. Available at: www.migrationinformation.org/USfocus/print.cfm?ID=747. Accessed August 18, 2010

3. Migration Policy Institute. Foreign-born population by region of birth as a percentage of the total foreign-born population, for the United States: 1960 to 2008. Available at: www.migrationinformation.org/datahub/charts/fb.2.shtml. Accessed October 11, 2010

4. Hoefer M, Rytina N, Baker BC. Estimates of the unauthorized immigrant population residing in the United States: January 2007. Washington, DC: Office of Immigration Statistics, Policy Directorate, US Department of Homeland Security; 2008. Available at: www.dhs.gov/xlibrary/assets/statistics/publications/ois_ill_pe_2007.pdf. Accessed February 19, 2009

5. US Department of Education. Migrant education program annual report eligibility, participation, services (2001-02), and achievement (2002-03). Washington, DC: Office of the Planning, Evaluation, and Policy Development, Policy and Program Studies Service; 2006. Available at: www.ed.gov/rschstat/eval/disadv/migrant/annualreport/report.pdf. Accessed February 22, 2009

6. Passel GS, Capps R, Fix M. Undocumented immigrants: facts and figures. Fact sheet. Washington, DC: The Urban Institute; 2004. Available at: www.urban.org/UploadedPDF/1000587_undoc_immigrants_facts.pdf. Accessed February 4, 2009

7. Jefferys KJ, Martin DC. Refugees and asylees: 2007. Washington, DC: Department of Homeland Security, Office of Immigration Statistics; 2008. Available at: www.dhs.gov/xlibrary/assets/statistics/publications/ois_rfa_fr_2007.pdf. Accessed January 16, 2009

8. US Department of Homeland Security. Yearbook of immigration statistics: 2007. Washington, DC: US Department of Homeland Security, Office of Immigration Statistics; 2008. Available at: www.dhs.gov/xlibrary/assets/statistics/yearbook/2007/ois_2007_yearbook.pdf. Accessed February 7, 2009

9. Urban Institute. Children of immigrants: facts and figures. Washington, DC: Urban Institute; 2006. Available at: www.urban.org/Uploaded pDF/900955_children_of_immigrants.pdf. Accessed February 3, 2009

10. Pew Hispanic Center. Table 8. Nativity by sex and age: 2006. In: Statistical portrait of the foreign-born population in the United States, 2006. Washington, DC: Pew Hispanic Center; 2008. Available at: pewhispanic.org/files/factsheets/foreignborn2006/Table-8.pdf. Accessed January 5, 2009

11. Capps R, Fix M, Murray J, Ost J, Passel JS, Hernandez S. The new demography of America's schools: immigration and the No Child Left Behind Act. Washington, DC: Urban Institute; 2005. Available at: www.urban.org/url.cfm?ID=311230. Accessed February 10, 2009

12. Birman D, Weinstein T, Wing YC, Beehler S. Immigrant youth in US schools: opportunities for prevention. *Prevention Researcher.* 2007;14(4):14-17

13. Fong R. Immigrant and refugee youth: migration journeys and cultural values. *Prevention Researcher.* 2007;14(4):3-5

14. Hernandez DJ. Demographic change and the life circumstances of immigrant families. In: Behrman RE, Shields MK, eds. *Children of Immigrant Families: The Future of Children.* Princeton University and The Brookings Institution; 2004: 17-47

15. Committee on the Health and Adjustment of Immigrant Children and Families, National Research Council and Institute of Medicine. Health status and adjustment. In: Hernandez DJ, Charney E, eds. *From Generation to Generation: The Health and Well-Being of Children in Immigrant Families.* Washington, DC: National Academies Press; 1988: 59-110

16. Harris K. The health status and risk behaviors of adolescents in immigrant families. In: Hernandez D, ed. *Children of Immigrants: Health, Adjustment, and Public Assistance.* Washington, DC: National Academies Press; 1999:59-110

17. Bronte-Tinkew J, Moore KA, Capps RC, Zaff J. The influence of father involvement on youth risk behaviors among adolescents: a comparison of native-born and immigrant families. *Social Science Research.* 2006;35:181-209

18. McDonald JA, Manlove J, Ikramullah EN. Immigration measures and reproductive health among Hispanic youth: findings from the National Longitudinal Survey of Youth, 1997-2003. *J Adolesc Health.* 2009;44:14-24

19. Ellis BH, Betancourt TS. Children and adolescents. In: Walker PF, Barnett ED, eds. *Immigrant Medicine*. St Louis, MO: Saunders Elsevier; 2007:673-692

20. Allen ML, Elliott MN, Morales LS, Dimant AL, Hambarsoomian K, Schuster MA. Adolescent participation in preventive health behaviors, physical activity, and nutrition: differences across immigrant generations for Asians and Latinos compared with whites. *Am J Public Health.* 2007;97:337-343

21. Ku L, Lin M, Broaddus M. Improving children's health: a chartbook about the roles of Medicaid and SCHIP. 2007 ed. Washington, DC: Center on Budget and Policy Priorities; 2007. Available at: www.cbpp.org/schip-chartbook.htm. Accessed February 19, 2009

22. American Academy of Pediatrics. Committee on Community Health Services. Providing care for immigrant, homeless, and migrant children. *Pediatrics.* 2005;115:1095-1100

23. Kaiser Commission on Medicaid and the Uninsured. *Medicaid and SCHIP Eligibility for Immigrants.* Washington, DC: Henry J Kaiser Family Foundation; 2006

24. Ku L. *Why immigrants lack adequate access to health care and health insurance.* Washington, DC: Migration Policy Institute, Migration Information Source; 2006. Available at: www.migrationinformation.org/Feature/display.cfm?id =417. Accessed February 20, 2009

25. Centers for Disease Control and Health Promotion. Geographic distribution of potential health hazards to traveler. In: Kozarsky PE, Magill AJ, Shlim DR, eds. *CDC Health Information for International Travel 2010*. Philadelphia, PA: Elsevier Mosby; 2009. Available at: wwwnc.cdc.gov/travel/content/yellowbook/home-2010.aspx. Accessed October 11, 2010

26. Centers for Disease Control and Health Promotion. Controlling tuberculosis in the United States. *MMWR*. 2005:54(RR12):1–81

# CHAPTER 31

# Transition of Adolescents with Special Health Care Needs to Adulthood

PATIENCE H. WHITE, MD, MA

## INTRODUCTION

Transitions are part of normal, healthy development, and they occur throughout life. Currently, the transition from adolescence to adult independence is becoming longer and more challenging for all youth with and without special health care needs (SHCN). The increased need for postsecondary education to earn an adequate income has lengthened the time spent dependent on families. Those who do not go to college are subject to unstable job market participation and lower wages throughout life. Most young adults experience setbacks on the road to economic independence including unemployment and interruptions to their education and health insurance. Thus, all youth need networks of support in US society until they connect successfully with the labor force, which most commonly occurs in their mid-20s.

This chapter focuses on the key issues of health care transition that adolescent health care providers should know to plan, provide services, and create support systems for adolescents with SHCN. This chapter describes essential components of the transition in health care, the wishes of youth with disabilities and their families for their transition, and actions needed to meet requirements outlined in a consensus statement created by health care providers, families, and youth with SHCN to maximize a young person's lifelong functioning. With each of the 6 consensus statement requirements discussed in this chapter, tools are outlined to help the health care provider create a successful transition process for youth with SHCN in their practice.

## BACKGROUND

Children and adolescents with SHCN comprise 14% to 22% of the pediatric population and account for more than two-thirds of all health care expenditures for children. Like all adolescents, they deserve to be cared for in a developmentally appropriate environment. Having an SHCN can adversely affect the physical, mental, financial, and social well-being of adolescents and their families. Functional limitations are especially associated with increased health care needs, and the demands on the health care system grow as a youth becomes more physically and/or, in some instances, cognitively limited.[1] Healthy People 2010 goals include transition and aim to increase the number of states with systems of care for children and youth with SHCN.

Today most adolescents with SHCN live to age 21 years and older. Socioeconomic factors are being recognized as important determinants of health, whereas social inclusion and quality of life are the focus of outcome, not just survival.[2] Youth with SHCN experience the same transitions in life as those without disabilities, but they often need more extensive networks of support for their transition. Youth with SHCN often do not have these support networks because they are more likely to live in poverty and be in stressful family situations. In addition, many have benefited from government policies and programs, and transition can mean leaving the very programs on which they depend for health care.

The years from high school through the 20s can be the most challenging and consequential because they are a time of biological, emotional, and social change for the young person. Health and wellness are usually not the central focus of youth in their transition years, but good health is key to being successful in all other areas of transition: school to work, home to community, dependence through independence to interdependence, and pediatric to adult health care. Health care providers have a unique place in the transition process for youth with SHCN because of the regular contact they have with many of these young people and the close relationships that often occur with them and their families.

It is important to acknowledge that youth with SHCN will have varying capabilities and transition support needs. Some will be interdependent and manage their own health and health care like most adults without disabilities; others will need full-time support through legal avenues, and many will have arrangements between these 2 extremes. Timing and tempo of the transition process are essential to a successful transition that allows youth to assume adult roles. For some it will mean transferring their care from a pediatric health care professional to an adult-trained health care professional; for others it will mean a reorientation of clinical care relationships and roles within the same practice, such as in a family medicine practice.

The transition process gives youth with SHCN the time to learn and practice skills to:

- Optimize their outcomes
- Become more knowledgeable in staying well and about their SHCN
- Access systems of care
- Advocate for themselves and be informed decision makers—which will prepare them for the transition to adulthood systems and services

Transition is defined as "the purposeful, planned movement of youth from child-centered to adult-oriented systems."[3] Successful transition planning is the result of partnerships among the individual with SHCN, his or her family, school personnel, the health care system, local community and adult service organization representatives, and interested others. The ultimate outcome is maximizing lifelong functioning, participation in society, and human potential. Transition is the deliberate, coordinated provision of developmentally appropriate and culturally competent health care, including assessments, counseling, and referrals.

Successful transition include the following components:

- Self-determination
- Person-centered planning
- Preparation for adult health care
- Work/independence
- Inclusion in community life

## HEALTH CARE TRANSITION GOALS

The optimal goal of health care transition is to provide health care that is family-centered, continuous, comprehensive, coordinated, compassionate, and culturally competent in a health care system that is as developmentally appropriate as it is technically sophisticated.[4]

General principles of successful transitions are summarized in Box 31-1.

## OPTIMAL TIME FOR THE TRANSITION PROCESS TO BEGIN

There is often a debate as to when preparation for health care transition should begin and when transfer should occur. Age has been used as an anchor to discuss the transition process. Geeneen[5] surveyed parents and providers and found that they agreed that the average age youth with SHCN should be transitioned to an adult provider was 17. In contrast, providers thought they should engage adolescents in managing their own health at approximately 9.5 years, whereas the parents would wait until the age of 12 years. Providers felt they should see the youth independently for part of the visit at approximately age 12, and parents reported around age 14. Literature today suggests that the optimum time to begin the transition process is between ages 11 to 13 because youth are most engaged in the process before other issues of adolescence dominate their attention, such as peer group and social activities.[6]

### Box 31-1

### *General Principles of Successful Transitions of Youth with Special Health Care Needs (SHCN)*

1. Transition is a process, not an event. Planning should begin as early as possible on a flexible schedule that recognizes the young person's increasing autonomy and capacity for making choices. Transition to adult services should occur prospectively rather than during a crisis and when the young person's disease is stable and under control.
2. The transition process should begin at diagnosis and include long-term sequential planning toward goals of interdependence and self-management.
3. Coordination is essential among the many networks needed for integrated care such as health care, educational, vocational, and social service systems. It is particularly important to recognize the relationship between health and social outcomes as young people move into the employment system and, in the United States, into an employment-based health insurance system.
4. The roles of all involved will change. Preparing for and understanding these role changes are essential to the transition success of youth with SHCN. Pediatric and other health care professionals and the family should appreciate and acknowledge the young person's change in status as he or she moves from adolescence to adulthood.
5. Self-determination skills should be encouraged and taught throughout the transition process. Best practices for health care, as pointed out by the Institute of Medicine, call for a person-centered and asset-oriented approach that involves young people as decision makers during the entire transition process.

## TRANSITION PROCESS REQUESTS FROM YOUTH AND FAMILIES

To appropriately plan for the transition process, many researchers have asked teens with SHCN, their families, and health care professionals about their needs to be successful in this transition process.

**Box 31-2**

***Health Transition Issues***

- Learning to stay healthy
- Getting a good doctor who treats adults
- Having family members who expect me to be a successful adult
- Figuring out what accommodations I need and how to ask for them
- Finding out what could happen if my condition gets worse
- Finding out what to do in an emergency
- Figuring out how to get health insurance

Box 31-2 contains a representative list[7] of health transition issues reported by youth with SHCN.

In 2003, Geenen[5] surveyed parents of youth with SHCN. The top 10 transition activities parents requested included:

- Taking care of my child's health
- Taking care of my child's SHCN
- Coordinating my child's care with other health care professionals
- Helping my child get health insurance
- Helping to find an adult health care provider for my child
- Teaching my child to manage his or her own health
- Working with the school to coordinate care
- Discussing with my child how to take care of his or her health to be successful at work
- Connecting my child with other services in the community
- Screening my child for other mental health problems

In 2005–2006, a national telephone survey[8] of 40,804 families with youth with SHCN under the age of 18 found that only 48.8% of families with youth with SHCN ages 12 to 17 years stated their youth received the services necessary to make appropriate transitions to adult health care, work, and independence. Other results from this study included:

- 50.7% said their health care provider talked with them about having their child eventually see adult health care providers
- 46.2% said their health care provider talked with them about health care needs as their child becomes an adult
- 21.3% said their health care provider talked with them about how to obtain or keep health insurance coverage as their child becomes an adult
- 48.7% said their health care provider always encouraged their youth to learn about their health and medications

In addition, Lotstein[9] reported that, for youth with disabilities who aged out of Title V programs, 24% had no usual source of care, 27% had forgone medical needs, 39% had delayed care, and 40% had insurance gaps since turning 21 years of age. Of note, those who were in special education or who were currently on Supplemental Security Income (SSI) had fewer reported transition events (42% vs 78%).

## HEALTH CARE PROFESSIONALS' CURRENT EFFORTS IN TRANSITION

In 2002, a transition consensus statement was created by health care professionals and endorsed by their professional associations.[3] In 2005, a questionnaire reflecting components of the consensus statement was developed by the Healthy and Ready to Work National Center (HRTW) and completed by Educating Practices in Community Integrated Care (EPIC IC) Pennsylvania Medical Home Program, a statewide provider of medical home quality improvement programs for pediatric practices funded by the Maternal and Child Health Bureau (MCHB). One hundred percent of the 21 practices completed the questionnaire (146 pediatricians and 36 nurse practitioners) in 18 counties of the Commonwealth of Pennsylvania that are voluntarily participating in this project.[10]

The results listed in Box 31-3 show that practices are implementing only some of the consensus statement.

**Box 31-3**

***Results of HRTW[a] Questionnaire***

- 33% have a policy to transition youth, with the age of transfer being between 18–24 years
- 29% had an identified person with knowledge and skills to focus on transition issues for youth in the practice
- 19% discussed before age 18 the legal issues for adulthood surrounding medical decision making
- 31% had created transportable medical records for youth with SHCN
- 5% had developed individual transition plans
- 43% utilized preventive guidelines for adolescent care
- 24% assessed the youth and families' readiness for care
- 29% assisted in the plan for health insurance after age 18–21

[a]Healthy and Ready to Work

## AAP TRANSITION CONSENSUS STATEMENT: WHAT A HEALTH CARE PROVIDER CAN DO

In 2001, an MCHB-invited group of experts drafted a Consensus Statement on Health Care Transition for Young Adults with Special Health Care Needs[11] that outlined 6 critical requirements "that the medical profession needs to take to realize the vision of a family-centered, continuous, comprehensive, coordinated, compassionate, and culturally competent health care system that is as developmentally appropriate as it is technically sophisticated." This was endorsed in 2002 by the American Academy of Pediatrics (AAP), American Academy of Family Physicians (AAFP), and American College of Physicians-American Society of Internal Medicine (ACP-ASIM).

The 6 key requirements of the consensus statement are outlined in the following with suggested processes that the pediatric health care provider might adopt to improve quality of services around transition for the youth with SHCN in their practice.

### REQUIREMENT 1

Ensure that all young people with SHCN have an **identified health care professional** who attends to the unique challenges of transition and assumes responsibility for current health care, care coordination, and future health care planning. This responsibility is executed in partnership with other child and adult health care professionals, the young person, and his or her family.

### REQUIREMENT 2

**Identify the core knowledge and skills** required to provide developmentally appropriate health care transition services to youth with SHCN and make them part of training and certification requirements for primary care residents and physicians in practice. See Figure 31-1 for the HRTW Tool for core knowledge and skills for health care professionals.

### REQUIREMENT 3

**Prepare and maintain an up-to-date, portable, and accessible medical summary.** This information is critical for successful health care transition and provides the common knowledge base for coordination among health care professionals, yet it is often not available when the youth transfers to the adult provider and the youth is unable to discuss the basics of his or her condition at that first visit. This summary should include such information as patient's medical history and physical findings, hospitalizations, medical reports, medications, emergency numbers as well as power of attorney, levels of supports and communication supports if needed, along with cultural practices that might influence treatment plans. There is often a large medical record, so creating a concise 1-page medical summary will enable the youth once he or she is 18 years old (or family who before age 18 are acting as an agent of the minor child with SHCN) to quickly communicate with providers, home health services, and others the medical issues, provider contact information, medications, and diagnoses (includes ICD-9-CM codes). The 1-page summary should be available to youths, their circle of support, and their family, before age 18 or with their consent after age 18, by providing the record on a disc or flash drive. In preparing the 1-page summary, suggest that the youth, if capable, write a half-page summary of his or her history, as this prepares the youth to be able to succinctly tell others about his or her condition. An example of a 1-page summary template can be found on the www.hrtw.org Web site.

### REQUIREMENT 4

Create a **written health care transition plan by age 14** together with the young person and family. At a minimum, this plan should include what services need to be provided, who will provide them, and how they will be financed. This plan should be reviewed and updated annually and whenever there is transfer of care. Following are some initial components to consider:

**Develop a practice transition policy; put it in writing and make it visible.** An important first step to start the transition process is for a practice to develop a transition policy agreed upon by all key players to ensure consensus and mutual understanding of the processes involved and to provide a structure for evaluation. The policy should be posted for the youth and families to see.[12] A key component of such a policy is the preparation for transition of a health care timeline. As discussed previously, the process should start at the latest around the ages of 11 to 13 years so the youth has time to practice taking on responsibility for health and health care within his or her capabilities.

**Discuss differences in the cultures of pediatric and adult health care systems.** Preparation for transition before the transfer of care is central to success. Youth with SHCN and their families need support, encouragement, education, and time to practice essential skills to access the adult health care system. They find they have to negotiate 2 contrasting cultures and systems of health care: the pediatric and adult health care systems.[4] Table 31-1 outlines major differences in the 2 systems. The different approaches in the adult health care system and the timing for moving to the adult-oriented systems must be discussed with the young person and family so the young person can be knowledgeable about what to expect and be an integral part to the process.

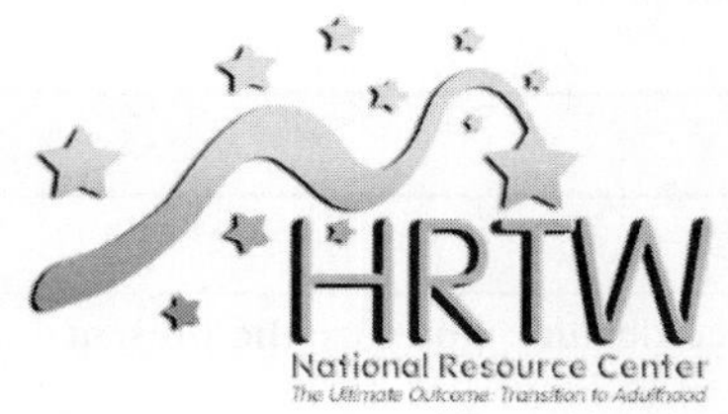


www.hrtw.org

## Checklist for Transition: Core Knowledge & Skills for Health Care Practices

### Core Knowledge & Skills Checklist for Practices

| | YES | NO |
|---|---|---|
| **POLICY** | | |
| 1. Dedicated staff position coordinates transition activities | | |
| 2. Office forms are developed to support transition processes | | |
| 3. CPT coding is used to maximize reimbursement for transition services | | |
| 4. Legal health care decision making is discussed prior to youth turning 18 | | |
| 5. Prior to age 18, youth sign assent forms for treatments, whenever possible | | |
| 6. Transition policy states age youth should no longer see a pediatrician is posted | | |
| **MEDICAL HOME** | | |
| 1. Practice provides care coordination for youth with complex conditions | | |
| 2. Practice creates an individualized health transition plan before age 14 | | |
| 3. Practice refers youth to specific family or internal medicine physicians | | |
| 4. Practice provides support and confers with adult providers posttransfer | | |
| 5. Practice actively recruits adult primary care/specialty providers for referral | | |
| **FAMILY/YOUTH INVOLVEMENT** | | |
| 1. Practice discusses transition after diagnosis, and planning with families/youth begins before age 10 | | |
| 2. Practice provides educational packet or handouts on transition | | |
| 3. Youth participates in shared care management and self-care (call for appt/Rx refills) | | |
| 4. Practice assists families/youth to develop an emergency plan (health crisis and weather or other environmental disasters) | | |
| 5. Practice assists youth/family in creating a portable medical summary | | |
| 6. Practice assists with planning for school and/or work accommodations | | |
| 7. Practice assists with medical documentation for program eligibility (SSI, VR, College) | | |
| 8. Practice refers family/youth to resources that support skill-building: mentoring, camps, recreation, activities of daily living, volunteer/paid work experiences | | |
| **HEALTH CARE INSURANCE** | | |
| 1. Practice is knowledgeable about state-mandated and other insurance benefits for youth after age 18 | | |
| 2. Practice provides medical documentation when needed to maintain benefits | | |
| **SCREENING** | | |
| 1. Exams include routine screening for risk-taking and prevention of secondary disabilities | | |
| 2. Practice teaches youth lifelong preventive care, how to identify health baseline and report problems early; youth know wellness routines, diet/exercise, etc. | | |

The HRTW National Resource Center believes these skills apply to all youth with and without a diagnosis.

The HRTW National Resource Center is headquartered at the Maine State Title V CSHN Program and is funded through a cooperative agreement (U39MC06899-01-00) from the Integrated Services Branch, Division of Services for Children with Special Health Needs (DSCSHN) in the Federal Maternal and Child Health Bureau (MCHB), Health Resources and Services Administration (HRSA), Department of Health and Human Services (DHHS). Activities are coordinated through the Center for Self-Determination, Health, and Policy at the Maine Support Network. The Center enjoys working partnerships with the Shriners Hospitals for Children and the KY Commission for CSHCN.



**FIGURE 31-1** Checklist for Transition: Core Knowledge and Skills for Health Care Practices. (Courtesy of the HRTW National Resource Center)

**Table 31-1**

**Cultural Differences between Pediatric and Adult Health Care**

| | *Pediatric* | *Adult* |
|---|---|---|
| Age-related | Growth and development, future focused | Maintenance/decline: Optimize the present |
| Focus | Family | Individual |
| Approach | Paternalistic, proactive | Collaborative, reactive |
| Shared decision making | With parent | With patient |
| Services | Entitlement | Qualify/eligibility |
| Nonadherence | Greater assistance | Less tolerance |
| Procedural pain | Lower threshold of active input | Higher threshold for active input |
| Tolerance of immaturity | Higher | Lower |
| Coordination with federal systems | Greater interface with education | Greater interface with employment |
| Care provision | Interdisciplinary | Multidisciplinary |
| Number of patients with special needs in practice | Fewer | Greater |

Adult-oriented systems focus on the individual, not the family unit, and are rarely structured to provide multidisciplinary care. A surprise to youth with SHCN and their families is that in the pediatric practice they make up a small percentage of a pediatrician's practice, whereas in the adult system they are more like most people in an adult practice, as the majority have chronic illnesses. Thus youth with SHCN must become excellent advocates to have their needs addressed in the new adult setting and be ready to discuss their health issues without the parent unless they have a legally appointed health guardian or health surrogate. The pediatric health care professional should discuss these differences and strategize how the youth and family will negotiate these differences and add the skills required to the youth's transition plan.

The transition plan should include changing roles and skills to be acquired by the youth and family and coordinate the skill development with activities in the youth's individual education plan at school if available.

Care coordination is essential to the medical home and a successful transition process. Developing a common medical transition plan among all providers can help in this process. See the AAP policy statement and other resources on care coordination for a more detailed discussion of the pediatrician's role.[13-15] In light of the differences in the 2 approaches of pediatrics and adult health care outlined previously and the youth's self-management capability, develop a transition plan that matches the demands of the new system to the skills needed. If the demands match the youth's skills, there will be far less anxiety on behalf of the youth and family as they move through the transition process. See Figure 31-2 and Figure 31-3 for youth and parent skills questionnaires to include in a transition plan. Also consider offering the AAP pamphlet "Tips for Parents of Adolescents" to parents to reinforce with them that their adolescent with SHCN is a teenager first and a teenager with SHCN second.

Other areas to include in a transition plan are listed in Box 31-4.

**REQUIREMENT 5**

Apply the same **guidelines for primary and preventive care** including mental health for all adolescents and young adults, including those with SHCN, recognizing that young people with SHCN may require more resources and services than other young people to optimize their health. Examples of such guidelines include the American Medical Association's Guidelines for Adolescent Preventive Service, the AAP's *Bright Futures: Guidelines for Health Supervision of Infants, Children, and Adolescents*, and the US Public Health Service's Guide to Clinical Preventive Services.

**REQUIREMENT 6**

Ensure affordable, **continuous health insurance coverage** for all young people with SHCN throughout adolescence and adulthood. This insurance should cover appropriate compensation for (1) health care transition

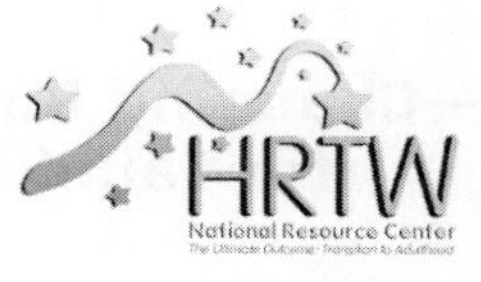


www.hrtw.org

**Transitions—Changing Role for Youth**

| **Health & Wellness 101 The Basics** | **Yes** I do this | I want to do this | I need to learn how | Someone else will have to do this - Who? |
|---|---|---|---|---|
| 1. I understand my health care needs, and disability and can explain my needs to others. | | | | |
| 2. I can explain to others how our family's customs and beliefs might affect health care decisions and medical treatments. | | | | |
| 3. I carry my health insurance card everyday. | | | | |
| 4. I know my health and wellness baseline (pulse, respiration rate, elimination habits). | | | | |
| 5. I track my own appointments, prescription refills, and expiration dates. | | | | |
| 6. I call for my own doctor appointments. | | | | |
| 7. I call in my own prescription refills. | | | | |
| 8. Before a doctor's appointment I prepare written questions to ask. | | | | |
| 9. I know I have an option to see my doctor by myself. | | | | |
| 10. I carry my important health information with me everyday (ie, medical summary, including medical diagnosis, list of medications, allergy info, doctor's numbers, drug store number, etc). | | | | |
| 11. I have a part in filing my medical records and receipts at home. | | | | |
| 12. I pay my co-pays for medical visits. | | | | |
| 13. I co-sign the "permission for medical treatment" form (with or without signature stamp, or can direct others to do so). | | | | |
| 14. I know my symptoms that need quick medical attention. | | | | |
| 15. I know what to do in case I have a medical emergency. | | | | |
| 16. I help monitor my medical equipment so it's in good working condition (daily and routine maintenance). | | | | |
| 17. My family and I have a plan so I can keep my health care insurance after I turn 18. | | | | |

**FIGURE 31-2** Youth Skill Questionnaire. (Courtesy of the HRTW National Resource Center)

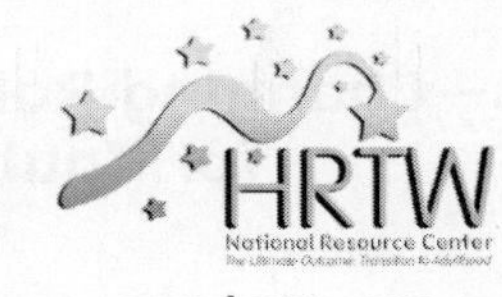


www.hrtw.org

## Transitions—Changing Role for Families

| **Health & Wellness 101 The Basics** | **Yes** my child/ youth can do this | I want my child/ youth to do this | I need to learn how to teach my child/ youth | Someone else will have to do this for my child/youth- Who? |
|---|---|---|---|---|
| 1. My child/youth understands his/her health care needs and disability and can explain needs to others. | | | | |
| 2. My child/youth can explain to others how our family's customs and beliefs might affect health care decisions and medical treatments. | | | | |
| 3. My child/youth carries his/her health insurance card with him/her. | | | | |
| 4. My child/youth knows his/her health and wellness baseline (pulse, respiration rate, elimination habits). | | | | |
| 5. My child/youth tracks appointments, prescription refills, and expiration dates. | | | | |
| 6. My child/youth call to make his/her own doctor appointments. | | | | |
| 7. My child/youth calls in his/her prescription refills. | | | | |
| 8. Before a doctor's appointment my child/youth prepares written questions to ask. | | | | |
| 9. My child/youth is prepared to see the doctor by him/herself. | | | | |
| 10. My child/youth carries his/her important health information everyday (ie, medical summary, including medical diagnosis, list of medications, allergy info, doctor's/drug store numbers, etc). | | | | |
| 11. My child/youth helps file medical records and receipts at home. | | | | |
| 12. My child/youth pays co-pays for his/her medical visits. | | | | |
| 13. My child/youth co-signs the "permission for medical treatment form" (with or without signature stamp, or can direct others to do so). | | | | |
| 14. My child/youth knows his/her symptoms that need quick medical attention. | | | | |
| 15. My child/youth knows what to do if they have a medical emergency. | | | | |
| 16. My child/youth knows how to monitor medical equipment so it's in good working condition (daily and routine maintenance). | | | | |
| 17. My child/youth and I have discussed a plan to be able to continue health care insurance after they turn 18. | | | | |

**FIGURE 31-3** Parent Skill Questionnaire. (Courtesy of the HRTW National Resource Center)

**Box 31-4**

***Key Areas to Include in a Transition Plan***

- Plan when to discuss legal health care decision making before age 18, including the issue of guardianship. Ask the youth to give assent before he or she is required to give consent. Be mindful of the adolescent's desire for confidentiality.
- Help youth provide a concise medical report including knowledge about his or her condition and what happened since the last visit. Ask the youth to prepare 5 questions for the next doctor's visit. The www.hrtw.org Web site has examples of a reporting sheet by systems, and how to prepare 5 questions for the doctor's visit.
- Plan when the youth will start seeing his or her health care provider alone. An important correlation in transition studies is that youth seen alone during health care visits are more likely to take charge of taking medications, a key to self-management.
- Create an emergency plan so youth and their families are prepared for a medical emergency. Youths should use ICE (in case of emergency) designation in their cell phone with the appropriate numbers and medications/allergies listed after the ICE designation. As most youths carry a cell phone, this is the first place the emergency personnel will look for important numbers and information. Check that the person whose number is listed is up to date with the youth's medical condition.
- Outline steps for health promotion. Regular exercise and good nutrition are essentials to good health. Youth with SHCN have similar rates of obesity and risky behaviors (tobacco and alcohol use) as people without disabilities.
- Outline educational goals. Pediatricians should help youth with SHCN attain the highest level of education as possible, because educational success is related to health outcome, and attending postsecondary education increases the likelihood of attaining adult social roles among young adults with childhood disabilities.
- Outline career/work goals. Attendance, as well as volunteer and paid jobs during high school, improve success in the workplace. Emphasize the importance of being on time for school, volunteer activities, and appointments as this translates to employment skills needed to maintain a job. Be sure to encourage, if culturally appropriate, the youth with SHCN to participate in chores at home like others in the household. Allowing the youth not to have expectations/obligations for participation as other children in the family can send the wrong message that "I do not have to do what others do."
- Discuss transportation issues and plan when the youth will come to the appointment alone, if appropriate.
- Help the adolescent and family find an adult primary care practice and plan a visit to that practice or plan a joint visit with the adult provider. To help the youth see what the adult health care system is like, plan an observational visit a year or more before the actual date of transfer so the youth and family can see what the adult system will require and then return to the pediatric provider to assess the level of skills still needed to be successful. This also gives the youth and family the opportunity to choose the adult provider when the youth is medically stable. Alternatively, plan a joint visit with an adult provider so that there can be verbal transfer of medical information as well as the medical record and discussion of remaining skills needed to be accomplished from the original transition plan.[16] In addition, if needed, discuss with the youth and the adolescent's subspecialty care providers a plan for transition to an adult specialty care provider at a different time than the transfer to the primary care provider. If the health care provider keeps the youth's list of transition skills attained, the portable medical summary, and the transition plan up to date, these documents can become the health passport that the adolescent can present to the adult provider at his or her introductory visit.

planning for all young people with SHCN, and (2) care coordination for those who have complex medical conditions. Be sure to have the family become familiar with the options and their requirements, such as being a student or remaining an adult disabled child.

## CONCLUSION

Adolescents with SHCN want a full range of possibilities to participate in adult society and will require a coordinated system of care to support them in this goal. Although federal and state mandates exist through some programs, these can change when the adolescent ages out of the program and overall outcomes for youth with SHCN continue to be less than optimal. The challenge for all health care providers is to take steps to prepare youth and their families with the knowledge and skills necessary to promote self-determination and successful navigation of adult systems of care. With or without all of us, teens with SHCN will grow up and move on. An important part of the practitioner's job is to prepare adolescents for the next step toward a healthy and successful adulthood.

## REFERENCES

1. Nageswaran S, Silver E, Stein R. Association of functional limitation with health care needs and experiences of

children with special health care needs. *Pediatrics.* 2008;121: 994-1001

2. Schidlow DV, Fiel SB. Life beyond pediatrics: transition of chronically ill adolescents from pediatric to adult health care systems. *Med Clin North Am.* 1990;74:1113-1120

3. American Academy of Pediatrics, American Academy of Family Physicians, American College of Physicians—American Society of Internal Medicine. A consensus statement on health care transitions for young adults with special health care needs. *Pediatrics.* 2002;110(6 Pt 2):1304-1306

4. Rosen DS, Blum RW, Britto M, Sawyer SM, Siegel DM, and Society for Adolescent Medicine. Transition to adult health care for adolescents and young adults with chronic conditions: position paper of the Society for Adolescent Medicine. *J Adolesc Health.* 2003;33(4):309-311

5. Geenen SJ, Powers LR, Sells W. Understanding the role of health care providers during the transition of adolescents with disabilities and special health care needs. *J Adolesc Health.* 2003;32:225-233

6. Wolf-Branigin M, Schuyler V, White P. Improving quality of life and career attitudes of youth with disabilities: experiences from the Adolescent Employment Readiness Center. *Res Soc Work Pract.* 2007;17:324-333

7. National Youth Leadership Network. 2002 Research Brief: what youth with disabilities say is important for building a successful life. Available at: www.nyln.org/experts/htmls/2002researchbrief.htm. Accessed October 1, 2009

8. National Survey of Children with Special Health Care Needs Data Resource Center. 2005/06 CSHCN Survey. Available at: www.cshcndata.com. Accessed July 28, 2009

9. Lotstein DS, Inkelas M, Hayes RD, Halfon N, Brook R. Access to care for youth with special health care needs in transition to adulthood. *J Adolesc Health.* 2008;43:23-29

10. White PH, Turchi RM, Hackett P, Gatto M. Preparing children and youth with special health care needs for adult health care: progress of general pediatricians translating national transition policy into practice. *Presented at: the Pediatric Academic Society meeting*, May 2006

11. American Academy of Pediatrics, American Academy of Family Physicians, American College of Physicians-American Society of Internal Medicine. A consensus statement on health care transitions for young adults with special health care needs. *Pediatrics.* 2002;110:1304-1306

12. McDonogh JE, Shaw KL, Southwood TR. Translating policy into practice. Development of a transitional care policy for youth with chronic illness. *J Exp Rheumatol.* 2005;23:S88

13. Council on Children with Disabilities. Care coordination in the medical home: integrating health related systems of care for children for children with special health care needs. *Pediatrics.* 2005;116:1238-1244

14. Johnson CP, Kastner TA, and the Committee/Section on Children with Disabilities. Helping families raise children with special health care needs at home. *Pediatrics.* 2005;115:507-511

15. Bodenheimer T. Coordinating care—a perilous journey through the health care system. *NEJM.* 2008;258:1064-1071

16. Kipps S, Bahu T, Ong K, et al. Current methods of transfer of young people with Type I diabetes to adult services. *Diabetic Medicine.* 2002;19:649-654

# CHAPTER 32

# Solid Organ Transplantation

GINA S. SUCATO, MD, MPH • PAMELA J. MURRAY, MD, MHP • BEVERLY KOSMACH-PARK, DNP

## INTRODUCTION

The number of successful pediatric organ transplants has increased steadily since they were first performed in the 1960s. In 2008, nearly 2,000 pediatric solid-organ transplants (SOTs) were performed in the United States, including kidney (39%), liver (31%), heart (19%), intestine, pancreas, pancreas/kidney, lung, and heart/lung.[1] As survival has increased, a growing number of pediatric transplant recipients have achieved stable graft function and have returned to their communities, schools, and extracurricular activities. Following the early postoperative period that requires close follow-up with the transplant center, patients have returned to the care of their primary care providers (PCPs) for routine medical needs. The aim of this chapter is to review the issues involved in providing routine medical care to the adolescent SOT recipient. Supplemental information can be found in the Internet resources listed in Box 32-1. The importance of collaboration and routine communication with the transplant center is emphasized.

### Box 32-1

### *Internet Resources*

- Children's Organ Transplant Association: www.cota.org
- American Liver Foundation: www.liverfoundation.org
- National Kidney Foundation: www.kidney.org
- International Society for Heart and Lung Transplantation: www.ishlt.org
- International Transplant Nurses Society: itns.org/education (Excellent resource for patient education materials)
- American Society of Transplantation: www.a-s-t.org
- MyHealth Passport: www.sickkids.on.ca/myhealthpassport (Web-based program that produces an individualized wallet-sized card for transplant patients that contains important medical information)

## PRIMARY CARE OF THE TRANSPLANT RECIPIENT

In the immediate post-transplantation period, pediatric SOT recipients are closely monitored by the transplant team. Consequently, the first post-transplantation primary care visit may not occur for at least 3 to 6 months after transplantation. At this visit, the patient's and family's understanding of life post-transplantation should be assessed, and the balance of responsibility for care between the adolescent and parent(s) should be determined. Discussion topics for this visit are listed in Box 32-2, and key issues for ongoing primary care of SOT recipients are listed in Box 32-3.

### Box 32-2

### *Agenda for First Primary Care Visit after Transplantation*

- Post-transplant course: Ask the patient/family about the transplant procedure and early postoperative period to assess what they know about the transplant process, signs and symptoms of complications, and their understanding of existing complications and treatment.
- Medications: Review all medications with the adolescent, asking about dosage, administration method, rationale for use, and adherence. Ask the patient to describe the most common side effects of each medication. Confirm that the patient is enrolled with a local or mail-order pharmacy that can continue to fill prescriptions. Discuss how new medications or additional refills will be ordered through either the transplant center or primary care provider (PCP).
- Rejection: Ask the adolescent/parent about the recipient's history of rejection, symptoms of rejection, treatment required, and response.
- Laboratory tests: Discuss the method for obtaining laboratory work in the community and sending results to the transplant center. Discuss how lab results will be communicated to the

*(Continued)*

## Box 32-2 (Continued)

transplant center, the PCP, and the patient/family. Discuss how any subsequent treatments will be decided between the PCP and transplant center and how treatment plans will be communicated.

- Routine calls: Discuss the most common symptoms/illnesses that may occur, when the patient/family should call, and whom to call. Provide contact numbers.
- Emergency situations: Discuss the most common emergencies, when to call the PCP office, and when to call 911.
- Reintegration plans: Discuss the adolescent's plans for returning to school, work, and community activities.
- Risk-taking behaviors: Discuss the risks of smoking, alcohol use, and drug use.
- Sexuality: Issues related to sexuality should be discussed confidentially with the adolescent. Education regarding puberty, sexually transmitted infections, and birth control methods should be provided. The adolescent must also understand that although pregnancy is generally successful after transplantation with appropriate planning and follow-up, some medications may be harmful to the developing fetus. Unplanned pregnancies may carry a higher risk for problems. In cases of genetic disorders, the adolescent should be aware of the risks of inheritance.

## Box 32-3

### *Key Issues for Primary Care of SOT Recipients*

- A complete yearly physical examination is indicated and should include careful examination of the skin, oropharyngeal mucosa, anogenital area, and a pelvic examination with a Pap smear in sexually active female patients.
- All suspicious skin and mucosal lesions should be promptly referred for further evaluation.
- Patients and household contacts should be vaccinated to the fullest extent possible.
- Medication adherence is challenging for all patients. Nonadherence, sometimes accompanied by taking excess doses prior to appointments and/or laboratory testing, should always be considered for unexplained symptoms.
- Graft rejection is often asymptomatic, so patient adherence with routine surveillance for rejection is vitally important.

## Box 32-3 (Continued)

- Time alone with the patient at each visit will encourage disclosure of confidential concerns.
- Sexual activity and fertility are likely, and hormonal methods provide the most effective contraception.
- Transition to the adult health care system requires adequate time and preparation. Adolescents should be encouraged to take increasing responsibility for their care, and discussion about transition to adult services should begin early.
- Good communication with the transplant center is of paramount importance.

Additionally, a timeline should be developed for the patient to gradually assume personal responsibility for medical care, including making appointments, obtaining and taking prescription medicines, and communicating with the transplant center. The ultimate goal of this timeline should be the transition to adult medical care. Discussing this goal early imparts a strong message to the adolescent that long-term survival and development into a self-sufficient adult are anticipated. For further discussion of transition of transplant recipients to adult care, see the excellent review of this topic by Bell and colleagues.[2]

## ROUTINE HEALTH MAINTENANCE IN ADOLESCENCE

### PUBERTAL GROWTH

The chronic organ failure that typically precedes transplantation can lead to growth retardation and pubertal delay. After transplantation, catch-up growth may occur, but it is not universal and is often incomplete;[3] transplant recipients frequently experience a delay in pubertal onset of 1 to 2 years.[4] The tempo of pubertal development and final adult height vary according to age at transplantation, type of organ transplanted, long-term organ function, steroid exposure, and treatment with growth hormone. However, final adult height is below target in a large proportion of SOT recipients, most notably those with renal transplants.[5]

### NUTRITION

Within several days after transplantation, most patients are able to tolerate a regular diet. Dietary restrictions are rare but occasionally are required to manage medication-induced hyperglycemia, hypertension, or weight reduction. In cases of hyperkalemia, a common side effect of tacrolimus (discussed below), treatment includes fludrocortisone and a limit on potassium-rich foods.

Immunosuppressed patients have a greater risk of contracting food-borne illnesses. Transplant recipients are advised to avoid foods at high risk for contamination such as raw fish and unpasteurized dairy and juice products. Transplant recipients should also avoid eating from salad bars and buffets because of possible contamination or poor temperature control. In addition, grapefruit must be eliminated from the diet because it inhibits the cytochrome P450 system, interfering with the metabolism of tacrolimus and cyclosporine section. Ingestion of grapefruit or grapefruit juice increases levels of these medications and thus increases risk of immunosuppressive toxicity.[6]

### IMMUNIZATIONS

Prior to transplantation, every effort should be made to fully immunize potential transplant recipients according to current pediatric recommendations, both to prevent subsequent severe infections and because vaccine-induced immunity may be suboptimal after transplantation. Live vaccines should be given at least 4 weeks prior to transplantation.[7] Because timing of cadaver organ donation is often unpredictable, vaccinations should be given as soon as a patient is considered a transplant candidate. If transplantation occurs shortly after administration of varicella vaccine, antiviral treatment can be used to prevent vaccine-related disease. With regard to the new herpes zoster (shingles) vaccine, further data are needed to determine its efficacy in pretransplant patients.[8]

Following transplantation, live vaccines are generally contraindicated. Recent data suggest that varicella vaccine may be safe in carefully selected posttransplant patients;[8] however, this should not be undertaken without expert consultation. Household members should receive standard live vaccines against measles, mumps, and rubella (MMR), varicella, and rotavirus, but they should receive only inactivated polio and influenza vaccines.

Although vaccination efficacy is lower in transplant recipients than in nonimmunosuppressed patients, vaccines still offer these patients protection, and all routine inactivated vaccines (human papillomavirus [HPV], meningococcus, hepatitis A and B, and tetanus, diphtheria, and acellular pertussis [Tdap]) should be administered once the patient's immunosuppression has been decreased, usually by 6 months post-transplantation.[7] Although data are not available on the immunogenicity of HPV vaccines in transplant recipients, it may be particularly beneficial to this group of patients as they are more likely than immunocompetent patients to have high-risk oncogenic HPV subtypes 16 and 18.[9] Current recommendations are to immunize females; however, the vaccine is now also approved for use in males, so future recommendations are likely to include immunizing males as well. Transplant recipients should also receive the pneumococcal vaccine and the annual inactivated influenza vaccine.[10]

### EYE AND DENTAL CARE

Transplant recipients should have routine ophthalmologic examinations with attention to the increased risk for glaucoma and cataract formation associated with a history of steroid use. Routine dental care is also critical because optimal oral hygiene is more important than prophylactic antibiotics to reduce the risk of infective endocarditis (IE). Most transplant centers responding to a 2002 survey on dental care advised prophylactic antibiotics prior to all dental procedures, not just invasive procedures, for all organ transplant recipients.[11] However, this survey has not been updated since the publication of the new 2007 American Heart Association Guidelines[12] on the prevention of IE, which specify antibiotic prophylaxis only for cardiac transplantation recipients who develop cardiac valvulopathy. Specific recommendations for prophylactic antibiotics prior to procedures should be made in collaboration with the patient's transplant team.

## ROUTINE HEALTH MAINTENANCE OF TRANSPLANT-RELATED ISSUES

### MANAGING IMMUNOSUPPRESSION

Immunosuppression for the patient who has received an SOT is lifelong. Immunosuppressive protocols vary by center and by type of organ transplanted. In most cases, the primary management of immunosuppressive regimens remains the responsibility of the transplant center. However, the PCP has an essential role in assessing for stable immunosuppressive drug levels, adverse drug reactions, complications related to immunosuppression, and adherence.

The goal of immunosuppressive therapy is to maintain the lowest acceptable level of immunosuppression that results in stable function of the transplanted organ with minimal side effects. The most common maintenance immunosuppressive agents are cyclosporine and tacrolimus (formerly known as FK-506). These medications, classified as calcineurin inhibitors, have similar mechanisms of action that inhibit T-cell-mediated rejection.[13] Although both of these medications carry significant side effects, tacrolimus is associated with a more favorable cardiovascular disease risk profile and improved cosmetic appearance.[14] In patients with stable organ function, decreasing the dosage of immunosuppression can lessen side effects. Corticosteroids continue to be included in immunosuppressive regimens, but there is growing evidence of the effectiveness of steroid-sparing regimens to avoid the long-term side effects of steroids.[13] See Table 32-1 for a list of common side effects of immunosuppressive medications.

In prescribing medications for routine illnesses, PCPs should be aware that some medications commonly prescribed in pediatric practice may interfere with therapeutic levels of tacrolimus and cyclosporine. Levels not within the acceptable range for an organ or a specific time posttransplantation may result in an increased risk for rejection, infection, and/or drug-related toxicities.

**Table 32-1**

**Common Immunosuppressive Agents: Adverse Effects[13,15,16]**

| *Agent* | *Side effects* |
|---|---|
| Cyclosporine | • Hypertension |
| | • Neurotoxicity (headache, seizure, tremor, paresthesia) |
| | • Gastrointestinal disturbance (nausea, diarrhea, abdominal discomfort) |
| | • Nephrotoxicity |
| | • Hirsutism |
| | • Gingival hyperplasia |
| | • Hepatotoxicity |
| | • Hyperkalemia, hypomagnesemia, hyperuricemia |
| | • Myositis |
| | • Lymphoproliferative disorder |
| Tacrolimus | • Hypertension |
| | • Neurotoxicity (headache, seizure, tremor, hyperesthesia, photophobia, confusion, persistent coma, insomnia, dysarthria) |
| | • Gastrointestinal disturbance (nausea, diarrhea, abdominal discomfort) |
| | • Nephrotoxicity |
| | • Glucose intolerance/diabetes |
| | • Hyperkalemia |
| | • Lymphoproliferative disorder/lymphoma |
| | • Alopecia |
| Corticosteroids | • Hypertension |
| | • Neurotoxicity (headache, seizure, vertigo, insomnia, pseudotumor cerebri) |
| | • Gastrointestinal disturbance (nausea, vomiting, peptic ulcer) |
| | • Glucose intolerance/diabetes |
| | • Muscle weakness |
| | • Pituitary–adrenal axis suppression |
| | • Cushing syndrome |
| | • Growth suppression |
| | • Osteopenia/osteoporosis/fractures/aseptic necrosis of bone |
| | • Dermatological complications (acne, skin atrophy) |
| | • Cataracts, glaucoma |
| | • Hyperlipidemia |
| | • Hypokalemia |
| | • Edema |
| | • Impaired wound healing |
| | • Polyphagia, obesity |
| | • Emotional lability, psychosis |

Also, use of calcineurin inhibitors can result in impaired renal function, so it is important to be aware of the additive nephrotoxicity that may occur with simultaneous administration of other potentially nephrotoxic medications such as acyclovir, aminoglycosides, nonsteroidal anti-inflammatory drugs, or intravenous radiocontrast.[14] Cyclosporine and tacrolimus are metabolized in the liver by the cytochrome P450 system; thus, serum levels are decreased when cytochrome P450 is induced and are increased when cytochrome P450 is inhibited. See Table 32-2 for the most common drug interactions with cyclosporine and tacrolimus. Table 32-2 is not

**Table 32-2**

**Medication Interactions[a] with Cyclosporine and Tacrolimus[13,14,15,17]**

| | ***Medications That Decrease Immunosuppressant Levels*** | ***Medications That Increase Immunosuppressant Levels*** |
|---|---|---|
| Antimicrobials | • Clindamycin<br>• Antituberculosis agents (rifampin, isoniazid)<br>• Nafcillin<br>• Trimethoprim<br>• Sulfadiazine | • Ciprofloxacin and ofloxacin (but not levofloxacin or moxifloxacin)<br>• Metronidazole<br>• Antifungal agents[b] (ketoconazole, fluconazole, clotrimazole, and itraconazole)<br>• Macrolide antibiotics (erythromycin,[c] clarithromycin, azithromycin)<br>• Dapsone<br>• Chloramphenicol |
| Antiepileptics | • Phenytoin<br>• Carbamazepine<br>• Primidone<br>• Barbiturates (Phenobarbital)<br>• **No change with benzodiazepines, valproic acid, or topiramate** | |
| Calcium channel blockers | | • Verapamil<br>• Diltiazem<br>• Nicardipine<br>• Nifedipine |
| Herbal supplements | • St John's wort (*Hypericum perforatum*) | |
| Food | — — | • Grapefruit |
| Other medications | • Orlistat<br>• Octreotide<br>• Cholestyramine<br>• Aluminum/magnesium hydroxide antacid preparations[d]<br>• Magnesium oxide, magnesium gluconate<br>• Sodium bicarbonate | • Protease inhibitors<br>• Danazol<br>• Corticosteroids<br>• Cimetidine<br>• Metoclopramide, cisapride<br>• Omeprazole<br>• Lovastatin, simvastatin<br>• Ethinyl estradiol (found in combined hormonal contraception) |

[a]Both cyclosporine and tacrolimus are metabolized by the cytochrome P-4503A pathway.[14] Therefore, data for an interaction with either of these medications have been interpreted to indicate an interaction with both.

[b]Antifungal agents increase cyclosporine to the extent that a cyclosporine dose reduction of 80% (with close monitoring of levels) has been recommended during antifungal therapy.[18]

[c]Interaction most pronounced with erythromycin.

[d]Tacrolimus levels are reduced by the magnesium component in many common antacid products such as Mylanta, Gaviscon, and Milk of Magnesia.

exhaustive; individual therapeutic drug management decisions should be made in consultation with the patient's transplant team and a clinical pharmacologist when necessary.

**MONITORING FOR REJECTION**

Rejection is an inflammatory immune response in which the immune system of the host recognizes the allograft as foreign. Acute cellular rejection is primarily a T-cell-mediated event, which occurs most commonly during the first 6 months after transplantation. Acute rejection is usually reversible. Chronic rejection occurs over an extended period of time and involves a combination of cellular and humoral immune responses. Chronic rejection is generally unresponsive to increased immunosuppressive therapy and the graft may subsequently be lost.[19] The PCP can assist the transplant center staff in evaluating the patient for signs and symptoms of rejection through physical examination and/or assessment of laboratory values. Signs and symptoms of rejection are listed in Table 32-3. Although there are specific symptoms associated with rejection of the kidney, liver, and heart, rejection can be asymptomatic, particularly in the early stages, underscoring the need for routine surveillance. Surveillance for rejection is organ specific and varies by center.

Biopsy of the graft is the diagnostic gold standard used to establish a definitive diagnosis of rejection prior to treatment. Patients suspected of having rejection are usually asked to return to the transplant center for evaluation and management. In some cases, biopsies may be performed at the patient's local hospital and the tissue sent to the transplant center for review by a pathologist who specializes in transplantation. Following diagnosis by biopsy, a treatment plan will be initiated by the transplant center with follow-up by the PCP.

Rejection in cardiac recipients is usually asymptomatic until severe enough to cause symptoms of heart failure. Therefore special attention must be paid to nonspecific symptoms, such as fever, which could be an early symptom of rejection. Acute onset heart failure may cause painful liver distension leading to abdominal pain, nausea, and anorexia. This should not be confused with gastroenteritis. When graft dysfunction has ensued,

**Table 32-3**

**Signs and Symptoms of Organ Rejection**

| | *Liver* | *Kidney* | *Heart* |
|---|---|---|---|
| Constitutional | • Fever<br>• Lethargy, fatigue, malaise<br>• Anorexia<br>• Jaundice, itching | • Fever<br>• Lethargy, fatigue, malaise<br>• Anorexia<br>• Weight gain | • Fever<br>• Lethargy, fatigue, malaise<br>• Anorexia<br>• Weight gain |
| Gastrointestinal | • Abdominal tenderness<br>• Acholic stools<br>• Elevated ALT, AST, GGTP, bilirubin, alkaline phosphatase<br>• Ascites | | • Abdominal tenderness<br>• Hepatomegaly<br>• Vomiting |
| Renal | • Bile-stained urine | • Oliguria<br>• Elevated BUN and creatinine, proteinuria<br>• Tenderness at graft site | |
| Cardiac | | • Hypertension<br>• Edema, particularly of lower extremities | • Shortness of breath<br>• Edema<br>• Tachycardia, gallop rhythm, raised JVP<br>• Cardiomegaly<br>• New onset arrhythmia |

ALT, alanine aminotransferase; AST, aspartate aminotransferase; GGTP, gamma-glutamyl transpeptidase phosphate; BUN, blood urea nitrogen; JVP, jugular venous pressure

there will often be a gallop rhythm as well. However, advanced rejection may also occur without symptoms or abnormalities on the physical examination, blood testing, or echocardiography.[20] Therefore, cardiac biopsies form the basis for routine screening for rejection following cardiac transplantation in most centers. Cardiac biopsies are typically performed as outpatient procedures every few weeks in the early posttransplant period and with decreasing frequency as the risk of rejection diminishes.

Chronic rejection in the heart transplant recipient usually takes the form of a diffuse coronary artery vasculopathy that develops many years after transplantation. It is a progressive condition that results in graft loss with no treatment other than retransplantation. Chronic rejection may be detected by routine coronary arteriography, which is performed every 1 to 2 years after transplantation. Syncope may be the first manifestation of chronic rejection, but sudden death can also occur. Both are probably caused by cardiac arrhythmia secondary to cardiac ischemia. Thus, syncope or presyncope in pediatric heart transplant recipients requires immediate evaluation at the transplant center.

### ASSESSING FOR INFECTION

Maintenance of the transplanted organ requires that the immune system be adequately suppressed to prevent rejection and yet sufficiently competent to resist infection. As a result, infectious complications remain a major source of morbidity and mortality. Key principles in the assessment of infection are listed in Box 32-4. The risk of infection after transplantation depends on several factors, including the type of organ transplanted, the degree of immunosuppression, environmental exposures, and the sequelae of invasive procedures.[21] As summarized by Fonseca-Aten and Michaels,[21] infections in transplant recipients can be categorized by time periods post-transplant. Early infections most commonly occur at 0 to 30 days post-transplantation, intermediate infections occur between 1 and 6 months post-transplantation, and late infections present most commonly beyond 6 months post-transplantation.

**Box 32-4**

***Key Principles in the Assessment of Infection***

- Transplant patients have a lifelong risk of unusual or covert infection.
- All fevers require prompt and thorough evaluation.
- Vague constitutional symptoms may signify common community-acquired infection. However, the possibility of rejection, infection with cytomegalovirus (CMV) or Epstein-Barr virus (EBV), or side effects of immunosuppressive medications must always be considered.
- Vomiting and diarrhea may decrease medication absorption and result in subtherapeutic levels of immunosuppression.
- Any increase in immunosuppression warrants increased surveillance for immunosuppressive drug toxicity and infection.

Early infections are often the result of a pre-existing chronic illness or infection, a typical postoperative infection, or a nosocomial infection.[21] Early infections are less commonly encountered by the PCP because the transplant recipient may be hospitalized, or still residing near the transplant center during this time period. However, the PCP may be the first clinician to detect intermediate and late viral pathogens and opportunistic infections. Common intermediate infections are discussed in further detail in the following sections. Late infections, which are usually community-acquired viruses, vary based on allograft function and degree of immunosuppression. Patients with good allograft function and low-dose maintenance immunosuppression tend to acquire infections similar to those seen in otherwise healthy children.[22]

Transplant recipients are susceptible to a number of infections, including bacterial infections with multidrug-resistant bacteria, opportunistic fungal infections with organisms such as candida and aspergillus, and viral infections including herpes viruses and community-acquired respiratory viruses. All of these can lead to more severe disease in transplant recipients. Diagnosing infection in the transplant recipient can be challenging, and knowledge of the patient's baseline temperature and leukocyte count can be helpful.[17] Recommendations for evaluation of the pediatric transplant recipient with suspected infection are provided in the excellent review by Keough and Michaels,[23] which offers detailed guidance for evaluation, categorized by presenting symptoms. Recent exposure to high-dose immunosuppression, such as that used for the treatment of rejection, can increase the risk of infection compared to the use of maintenance immunosuppression.[17] Collaboration with the transplant center is always advised. Although some of the initial evaluation, and occasionally the treatment, for infection may be conducted locally, serious infections usually necessitate a patient's return to the transplant center for further evaluation and management.

#### Cytomegalovirus

Although its incidence and mortality have been reduced by the use of ganciclovir and valganciclovir prophylaxis, cytomegalovirus (CMV) remains an important source of morbidity for transplant recipients. This disease presents with a wide range of clinical manifestations, including fever, malaise, leukopenia, thrombocytopenia, and mild atypical lymphocytosis. Invasive disease may result in injury of the transplanted organ.[21] For diagnosis and therapeutic monitoring, assays that quantify CMV-DNA by polymerase chain reaction are becoming the test of choice. Treatment for CMV disease includes intravenous ganciclovir and the judicious reduction of immunosuppression.[21]

#### Epstein-Barr Virus-Associated Lymphoproliferative Disorders

Epstein-Barr virus (EBV) and associated post-transplant lymphoproliferative disorders comprise a range of conditions from a nonspecific viral illness to post-transplantation lymphoproliferative disorder (PTLD), which may ultimately progress to lymphoma. Primary EBV infection (after transplantation of an organ from an EBV-positive donor to an EBV-negative recipient) increases the risk of PTLD.[21] Symptoms and findings suggestive of EBV disease/PTLD include fever, lethargy, gastrointestinal disturbances, lymphadenopathy, pharyngitis, and organomegaly. Diagnostic evaluation includes a thorough history and physical examination, quantitative EBV assays, and imaging of the chest, abdomen, and pelvis. Treatment typically involves reduction or temporary cessation of immunosuppression. Because early treatment of EBV is vital to a successful recovery, evaluation should always be conducted in collaboration with the transplant center.

#### Opportunistic Infections

*Pneumocystis jiroveci* (formerly *Pneumocystis carinii)* pneumonia should always be considered in transplant recipients with fever and lower respiratory tract symptoms. Fortunately, it is rarely seen because of the widespread use of prophylactic trimethoprim-sulfamethoxazole. Further discussion of opportunistic pathogens in SOT recipients can be found in a recent review.[17]

## ADOLESCENT LIFESTYLE AFTER TRANSPLANTATION

### RESUMPTION OF USUAL ACTIVITIES

Within 2 or 3 months post-transplant, most patients are ready to attend school for a few hours each day, gradually returning to full school participation. To date, studies of intellectual functioning in adolescent SOT recipients are limited and results are variable. However, given the possibility for developmental delay and learning disabilities,[24] families should maintain a low threshold in requesting additional academic testing in these patients.

Physical activity is encouraged as soon as tolerated. Heart transplant recipients may resume all activities after 2 months post-transplantation. Kidney and liver transplant recipients may also resume normal activities but should avoid heavy lifting and activities that stretch or put pressure on the abdomen for 3 to 6 months.[25] Many transplant centers advise that vigorous contact sports such as football, hockey, and wrestling be avoided. With these exceptions, as soon as patients feel able to do so, they should be permitted to participate in camps and noncontact sports. Adolescents who meet their state's requirements for driving can apply for a driver's permit and learn to drive. Licensed drivers may resume driving 2 months after transplantation.[26]

Pet ownership is permitted by most transplant centers provided the pets have routine veterinary checkups, all required vaccinations, and are treated promptly for any illnesses. Transplant recipients should avoid contact with the pet's bodily fluids and feces and should not change cat litter. Good hand washing should be emphasized when interacting with pets. The following pets should be avoided and are considered high-risk animals by the Centers for Disease Control and Prevention[27] for people who are immunosuppressed: reptiles, including lizards, snakes, and turtles; baby chicks and ducklings; and exotic pets, including monkeys. Some transplant centers also restrict amphibians (frogs), hamsters, guinea pigs, and caged birds as pets in the home.

### NONADHERENCE

Although patients receiving transplants as adolescents have excellent 1-year graft and patient survival, long-term outcomes (>5 years post-transplant) for this group are significantly worse than those receiving their transplant at a younger age.[28] Nonadherence plays a significant role in the poor outcomes of some adolescents following SOT. It is estimated to be a factor in 14% to 35% of graft losses and 33% to 73% of late acute rejection episodes in pediatric renal, liver, and heart transplant recipients.[28] The PCP has an important role in encouraging and monitoring adherence and in suggesting interventions to meet psychosocial needs of the adolescent. In the setting of stable graft function, every effort should be made to reduce the burden and stigma of medications. In many transplant recipients, this can be accomplished by decreasing the number of medication dosing times, using daily or twice daily dosing whenever possible; prescribing medications with longer half-lives to require less rigid adherence to timing; discontinuing minimally effective medications; and/or decreasing dosages of medications that may affect physical appearance. Treatments for side effects, such as steroid-induced acne, should be pursued. Counseling, peer support, and psychosocial support are interventions that can help adolescents adapt and cope with the chronicity of transplantation.

### DEVELOPMENTAL ISSUES

Transplantation offers many adolescents the opportunity for improved health and well-being—in some cases for the first time. However, patients must adhere to a strict regimen of medication and monitoring and must live with the long-term threat of rejection. These challenges are superimposed on the ongoing developmental tasks of adolescence. For example, the task of establishing independence from parents must be balanced with the need for parental assistance with medical care. For some patients, body image may be adversely affected by poor growth, surgical scars, or changes in appearance caused by medications. It is also common for adolescents to go through periods of experimentation and risk-taking. However, the consequences of risk-taking behaviors can be more dire for transplant recipients, particularly if they involve poor adherence with medications and medical follow-up. Identifying the need for ongoing psychosocial support services for both the patient and the family is an important role of the PCP.

Another important developmental task of adolescence is establishing a psychosexual identity. Although adolescents with chronic disease may be perceived as having fewer romantic and sexual desires than healthy adolescents,[29] it should nonetheless be remembered that young transplant recipients are often sexually active and that neither transplantation nor immunosuppressive medications preclude fertility in males or females.[30] It is critical that PCPs speak confidentially with their adolescent patients to identify those who are, or may soon become, sexually active and to help them prevent an unplanned and potentially high-risk pregnancy. When pregnancy is desired, conception should be deferred for at least the first 12 months after transplantation[31] and should include preconceptual care from an obstetrician with expertise in this area.

### CONTRACEPTIVE METHOD CHOICE

For those adolescents who are not abstinent, hormonal contraception is more effective than condoms alone and can be recommended for appropriately selected transplant recipients.[32] For patients reporting unprotected sexual intercourse within the previous 5 days, emergency contraception can prevent up to 85% of pregnancies. The preferred regimen for adolescents is a single dose of levonorgestrel 1.5 mg,[33] which has no medical or pharmacological contraindications. Emergency contraception is sold as Plan B in pharmacies and is now available to patients 17 years and older without a prescription. Patients younger than 17 years can be provided with an advance prescription to have immediately available should the need arise.[33] For guidance prescribing an ongoing method of contraception, see the recent detailed discussion of contraceptive use in adolescent transplant recipients.[34]

### SEXUALLY TRANSMITTED INFECTIONS

Similar to all sexually active adolescents, transplant recipients are at high risk for sexually transmitted infections (STIs) and should undergo routine screening every 6 months or whenever there are complaints of vaginal or penile discharge, dysuria, or other genitourinary symptoms. Screening for STIs should include specific laboratory testing for gonorrhea and chlamydia; visual inspection for signs of herpes simplex virus, genital warts, and molluscum contagiosum; serologic testing for HIV, syphilis, and hepatitis C; and in females, microscopic evaluation of vaginal discharge for trichomonas, bacterial vaginosis, and yeast. The PCP should have a low threshold for empiric treatment of STIs in immunosuppressed adolescents with genitourinary symptoms.

Among transplant recipients, the risk of HPV-related anogenital cancer is 10 to 20 times higher than in the general population.[35] Early identification of HPV-related precancerous lesions can be accomplished by visual inspection of the vulva and penis and Pap smear screening performed according to American Cancer Society[36] guidelines for immunocompromised patients. Among adolescent transplant recipients, Pap smear screening should be considered at least annually beginning with the onset of sexual activity.

## CONCLUSION

The PCP plays a vital role in monitoring the adolescent transplant recipient's outpatient health status. Therefore it is imperative that the PCP have an efficient method of routinely communicating with the transplant center. The primary contact for the PCP is typically the transplant coordinator, who is usually a registered nurse. Although the early postoperative period requires close scrutiny and attentive medical management and may seem to be the period most crucial to survival, long-term follow-up through the teamwork of transplant physicians, transplant coordinators, PCPs, patients, and their families is imperative for a successful outcome.

## REFERENCES

1. Organ Procurement and Transplantation Network. Available at: optn.transplant.hrsa.gov/Data/. Accessed May 17, 2010

2. Bell LE, Bartosh SM, Davis CL, et al. Adolescent transition to adult care in solid organ transplantation: a consensus conference report. *Am J Transplant.* 2008;8(11):2230–2242

3. Schaefer F. Growth and puberty. In: Fine RN, Webber SA, Olthoff KM, Kelly DA, Harmon WE, eds. *Pediatric Solid Organ Transplantation*. 2nd ed. Malden, MA: Blackwell Publishing; 2007:403–411

4. Sucato GS, Murray PJ. Gynecologic issues of the adolescent female solid organ transplant recipient. *Pediatr Clin North Am.* 2003;50(6):1421–1542

5. Fuqua JS. Growth after organ transplantation. *Semin Pediatr Surg.* 2006;15(3):162–169

6. Mertens-Talcott SU, Zadezensky I, De Castro WV, Derendorf H, Butterweck V. Grapefruit-drug interactions: can interactions with drugs be avoided? *J Clin Pharmacol.* 2006;46(12):1390–1416

7. Lopez MJ, Thomas S. Immunization of children after solid organ transplantation. *Pediatr Clin North Am.* 2003;50(6): 1435–1449, ix–x

8. Avery RK, Michaels M. Update on immunizations in solid organ transplant recipients: what clinicians need to know. *Am J Transplant.* 2008;8(1):9–14

9. Brown MR, Noffsinger A, First MR, Penn I, Husseinzadeh N. HPV subtype analysis in lower genital tract neoplasms of female renal transplant recipients. *Gynecol Oncol.* 2000;79(2):220–224

10. Verma A, Wade JJ. Immunization issues before and after solid organ transplantation in children. *Pediatr Transplant.* 2006;10(5):536–548

11. Guggenheimer J, Mayher D, Eghtesad B. A survey of dental care protocols among US organ transplant centers. *Clin Transplant.* 2005;19(1):15–18

12. Wilson W, Taubert KA, Gewitz M, et al. Prevention of infective endocarditis. Guidelines from the American Heart Association: A guideline from the American Heart Association Rheumatic Fever, Endocarditis, and Kawasaki Disease Committee, Council on Cardiovascular Disease in the Young, and the Council on Clinical Cardiology, Council on Cardiovascular Surgery and Anesthesia, and the Quality of Care and Outcomes Research Interdisciplinary Working Group. *Circulation.* 2007;116:1736–1754

13. Agarwal A, Pescovitz MD. Immunosuppression in pediatric solid organ transplantation. *Semin Pediatr Surg.* 2006;15(3):142–152

14. Gaston RS. Current and evolving immunosuppressive regimens in kidney transplantation. *Am J Kidney Dis.* 2006;47(4, suppl 2):S3–S21

15. McGhee BH, Schmitt C, Phuong-Tan N, et al., eds. *Pediatric Drug Therapy Handbook and Formulary 5th ed.* Hudson, OH: Lexi-Comp Inc; 2007

16. Smith JM, Nemeth TL, McDonald RA. Current immunosuppressive agents: efficacy, side effects, and utilization. *Pediatr Clin North Am.* 2003;50(6):1283–1300

17. Fischer SA. Infections complicating solid organ transplantation. *Surg Clin North Am.* 2006;86(5):1127–1145, v–vi

18. Danovitch G. Immunosuppressive medications and protocols for kidney transplantation. In: Danovitch G, ed. *Handbook of Kidney Transplantation*. Boston, MA: Little Brown; 1992

19. Bartucci MR, Seller MC. The immunology of transplant rejection. In: Sigardson-Poor KM, Haggerty LM, eds. *Nursing Care of the Transplant Recipient*. Philadelphia, PA: WB Saunders; 1990

20. Mena C, Wencker D, Krumholz HM, McNamara RL. Detection of heart transplant rejection in adults by echocardiographic diastolic indices: a systematic review of the literature. *J Am Soc Echocardiogr.* 2006;19(10):1295–1300

21. Fonseca-Aten M, Michaels MG. Infections in pediatric solid organ transplant recipients. *Semin Pediatr Surg.* 2006;15(3):153–161

22. Their M, Holmberg C, Lautenschlager I, Hockerstedt K, Jalanko H. Infections in pediatric kidney and liver transplant patients after perioperative hospitalization. *Transplantation.* 2000;69(8):1617–1623

23. Keough WL, Michaels MG. Infectious complications in pediatric solid organ transplantation. *Pediatr Clin North Am.* 2003;50(6):1451–1469, x

24. Baum M, Freier MC, Chinnock RE. Neurodevelopmental outcome of solid organ transplantation in children. *Pediatr Clin North Am.* 2003;50(6):1493–1503, x

25. McNamara D, Pike N, Gettys C, et al. Organ transplants. In: Jackson PL, Vessey JA, eds. *Primary Care of the Child with a Chronic Condition*. 2nd ed. St Louis: Mosby; 1996

26. Kosmach B, Lawrence K, Klein M. Solid organ transplantation. In: Jackson PL, Vessey JA, eds. *Primary Care of the Child with a Chronic Condition*. 4th ed. St Louis: Mosby; 2003

27. Centers for Disease Control and Prevention. Organ transplant patients: pet safety tips. Healthy pets healthy people. Available at: www.cdc.gov/healthypets/bonemarrow_transplant.htm. Accessed June 20, 2007

28. Dobbels F, van Damme-Lombaert R, Vanhaecke J, De Geest S. Growing pains: non-adherence with the immunosuppressive regimen in adolescent transplant recipients. *Pediatr Transplant.* 2005;9(3):381–390

29. Valencia LS, Cromer BA. Sexual activity and other high-risk behaviors in adolescents with chronic illness: a review. *J Pediatr Adolesc Gynecol.* 2000;13(2):53–64

30. Armenti VT, Radomski JS, Moritz MJ, Philips LZ, McGrory CH, Coscia LA. Report from the National Transplantation Pregnancy Registry (NTPR): outcomes of pregnancy after transplantation. *Clin Transpl.* 2000:123–134

31. McKay DB, Josephson MA, Armenti VT, et al. Reproduction and transplantation: report on the AST Consensus Conference on Reproductive Issues and Transplantation. *Am J Transplant.* 2005;5(7):1592–1599

32. Lessan-Pezeshki M, Ghazizadeh S, Khatami MR, et al. Fertility and contraceptive issues after kidney transplantation in women. *Transplant Proc.* 2004;36(5):1405–1406

33. Gold MA, Sucato GS, Conard LA, Hillard PJ. Provision of emergency contraception to adolescents. *J Adolesc Health.* 2004;35(1):67–70

34. Sucato GS, Murray PJ. Developmental and reproductive health issues in adolescent solid organ transplant recipients. *Semin Pediatr Surg.* 2006;15(3):170–178

35. Adami J, Gabel H, Lindelof B, et al. Cancer risk following organ transplantation: a nationwide cohort study in Sweden. *Br J Cancer.* 2003;89(7):1221–1227

36. Saslow D, Runowicz CD, Solomon D, et al. American Cancer Society guideline for the early detection of cervical neoplasia and cancer. *CA Cancer J Clin.* 2002;52(6):342–362

SECTION 9

# Family Relationships

## CHAPTER 33

# Communication Between Parents and Adolescents

ARTHUR L. ROBIN, PhD

"My parents don't understand me." "Their rules are unfair—why should I have an earlier curfew than my friends?" "They lecture about responsibility and make me do these ridiculous chores." How often has a pediatrician heard such complaints from adolescents?

"My teen talks disrespectfully." "Every time we talk, we argue." "He should do what I say without asking any questions." "If you give her an inch, she will take a yard and really end up in trouble." "I try to discipline her, but my wife lets her off easy." How often has a pediatrician heard such complaints from parents?

Practitioners caring for adolescents need a developmentally based framework within which to conceptualize and intervene to change the parent–teen relationship problems inherent in these laments. A behavioral family systems model provides such a framework and intervention.[1-3] Early to middle adolescence is a time when individuals separate from parents and assume personal responsibility for their own behavior. As a normal part of the individuation process, the young adolescent will argue and disobey parental rules. Three factors in the family's reaction to these individuation-related conflicts affect whether clinically significant conflict will occur: (1) skill, (2) beliefs, and (3) family structure.

Skill encompasses communication, problem solving, and behavior management. When faced with "You don't understand me," the effectively communicating parent employs active listening to draw out the teen: "So you feel misunderstood. Tell me how." As the teen recites a litany of complaints, the parent continues to employ active listening along with "I" statements to respond in a nonaccusatory fashion. Then, the parent coaches the teen to use active listening to understand the parental viewpoint. The ineffectively communicating parent gets defensive and responds with accusations and criticisms, heating the discussion up, which usually culminates in an unproductive argument. When faced with, "Why do I have to have an earlier curfew than all of my friends," the highly skilled parent engages the adolescent in a mutual problem-solving discussion including clear definitions of the problem, creative brainstorming of a variety of solutions, and negotiating a compromise solution that meets everyone's needs. Then, the parent and teen together establish positive incentives for complying with the agreement and punishments for failure to comply. The parent who is not able to apply effective problem-solving skills unilaterally decrees an early curfew and lectures to the teen in an autocratic way about the virtues of an early curfew. The teen tunes out the parent and disobeys the curfew, resulting in unrealistic punishments such as "you're grounded for life."

Rigid beliefs, unreasonable expectations for obedience, and doom and gloom projections of the ruinous consequences of granting teens more freedom elicit angry affect and impede rational resolution of parent–teen conflicts. For example, consider the belief, "If you give her an inch, she will take a yard and really end up in trouble." Applied to curfew, this might be: "If I let her stay out late, she will become pregnant, an alcoholic, or a drug addict." For a small number of adolescents, this is a true statement, not an extreme belief, but for most it is unrealistic. A parent who adheres to this belief will become upset if his or her daughter asks for a curfew extension and will be unlikely to engage in a meaningful discussion of the issue. A great deal of conflict will occur, quite possibly resulting in the teen disobeying the current curfew. Adolescents may also adhere to extreme beliefs. "My parents' rules are unfair; they are going to ruin my life. I deserve complete freedom." This is the most common extreme belief for teens. Who said freedom is a birthright rather than a privilege earned by demonstrations of responsibility? Teens who adhere to such beliefs get into more conflict with their parents than teens who are more reasonable in their beliefs.

Family structure refers to the clarity of the power hierarchy in the family. Parents are supposed to be in charge of children, even teenagers, although they should be gradually letting go of their control over the course of adolescence. The adults in the family (parents, caretakers, etc) are supposed to work as a team in parenting, not be divided or manipulated by the teenager. When the practitioner hears a parent say, "I try to discipline her, but my wife lets her off easy," the family has structural problems. If this is an accurate description, then the mother is siding with her daughter against the father; parental authority is diluted and the teen can get away with misbehavior. If a teenager says about her divorced parents, "They put me in the middle and force me to take sides," the family has structural problems—this all too commonly occurs during and after a divorce.

## ANTICIPATORY GUIDANCE

What can the practitioner do to help parents and adolescents acquire positive skills, reasonable beliefs, and appropriate hierarchies in the family structure before problems arise? Box 33-1 puts these dimensions into a series of principles for parenting the adolescent. During an annual physical examination in early adolescence, the practitioner can distribute and review Box 33-1 with the family. The family should be invited to use these principles as the basis for dealing with conflicts that arise.

### Box 33-1

### *Principles for Parenting the Adolescent*

1. Facilitate appropriate independence seeking.
2. Divide the world of issues into negotiable and non-negotiable issues. Consistently enforce the rules regarding non-negotiable issues, which are bottom line rules for living in a civilized society.
3. Involve the adolescent in negotiating mutually satisfactory solutions to all other issues.
4. Actively monitor the adolescent's behavior outside the home.
5. Use consequences wisely.
6. Maintain good communication.
7. Focus on the positive.

- **Facilitate appropriate independence seeking**. Because becoming independent from the family is the primary developmental task of adolescence, parents need to look for opportunities to gradually give their adolescents more freedom in return for demonstrating responsibility. A parent might divide freedom to do a certain activity into small units and move onto the next step after the teenager has demonstrated responsibility on the last step. Consider the freedom to stay at home overnight for a weekend while parents go out of town. The responsibilities would be taking proper care of the house, for example, nothing left unlocked, nothing missing, lawn watered and pets fed, no wild parties. The parent might break this freedom into smaller units, for example, staying in the house for a few hours, an evening, a night, 2 nights. As the adolescent successfully accomplishes each step, the parent moves on to the next step. If the adolescent makes a mistake, parents need to pull back part way, not all the way; after a reasonable period of time has transpired, they again need to give a little more freedom in exchange for responsibility.
- **Divide the world of issues into 2 categories: non-negotiable and negotiable. For the non-negotiable issues, establish "the bottom line" rules for living in the family and enforce them consistently.** There is an important distinction between issues that can be handled democratically and those that cannot. Each parent has a small set of bottom line issues that relate to basic rules for living in civilized society, values, morality, and legality, which are not subject to negotiation. Such issues usually include drugs, alcohol, aspects of sexuality, religion, and perhaps several others. Parents need to clearly list and present to the teenager those issues that are non-negotiable. Then they need to enforce the rules around these issues consistently and fairly through the wise use of consequences.
- **Negotiate all other issues that are not bottom lines with the adolescent.** Parents need to involve their teenagers in decision making regarding the issues that can be negotiated. This is the single most important principle of parenting an adolescent and is 1 of the primary methods of shaping responsible independence behaviors. Teenagers are more likely to adhere

to rules and regulations that they helped to create. Furthermore, they may have novel and creative perspectives on issues because of their youth and unique position in the family. Often, their perspectives lead them to suggest novel solutions. Parents need to remember, however, that involvement in decision making doesn't necessarily mean being an equal partner with parents and certainly does not mean dictating to parents. Parents may retain the ultimate veto. Problem-solving training, discussed later in this chapter, is the technique used to accomplish this goal.

- **Actively monitor the adolescent's behavior outside the home.** Parents should always know the answer to 4 basic questions: (1) Whom are your adolescents with? (2) Where are they? (3) What are they doing? (4) When will they be home? Research has shown that parents who cannot consistently answer these 4 questions have adolescents who are at risk for drifting into deviant peer groups, substance abuse, and delinquency.[4] Parents should also develop clear "street rules" for how they expect their adolescents to conduct themselves in the community outside of the home. In this day of cell phones and instant communication, teenagers should be expected to call their parents periodically.
- **Use consequences wisely.** Parents need to become experts at behavior management to enforce their bottom line rules, monitor and structure effectively, and discipline consistently.[1] First, they should *use incentives before punishments*. It is a knee-jerk reaction for parents to ground an adolescent until the end of the next marking period upon receiving a bad report card. Parents commonly load on immense punishments until they have used up all of their ammunition and the adolescent has little else to lose by misbehaving. Furthermore, many punishments that initially seem fitting turn out to be impractical to enforce. When parents wish to modify a behavior such as poor study habits, first they need to ask what positive habits they wish to see the adolescent perform, and then ask next how can they reinforce that positive behavior. Only after using positive incentives for several weeks should they select a punishment for the negative behavior. Second, they should *strive for consistency*. Parents often give up easily on behavior change interventions at the first sign of failure. Smart adolescents incessantly bicker with their parents, sometimes wearing them down to the point where the parents back off. Parents must stick with their interventions and demands. "Divide and conquer" is also a motto of many adolescents, who have learned that if they can get Mom and Dad to disagree, then they can avoid unpleasant effort and/or discipline. The practitioner should encourage mothers and fathers to work as a team. Third, they should *act, don't yak*. Many parents repeat themselves incessantly when their adolescents fail to comply with their requests. Adolescents quickly learn that Mom or Dad are "all talk, no action." The practitioner should encourage parents to talk during family meetings, but after the rules and consequences have been clearly stated, administer the consequences, don't repeatedly remind the teen to adhere to the rule.
- **Maintain good communication.** Parents need to make themselves available to listen when their adolescents wish to talk, but don't expect the adolescent to confide regularly in them. Parents and adolescents need to learn effective skills for listening to each other and expressing their ideas and feelings assertively but without putting down or hurting each other.
- **Focus on the positive.** When in the throes of conflict dealing with a defiant adolescent, it is difficult for parents to seriously think about being positive. However, it is important to remind parents to *be their adolescent's cheerleading squad*. Adolescents need unconditional positive regard and focused positive time with their parents. They also need their parents to spend focused time with them; busy parents may not have a great deal of focused time to give, but it is the quality rather than the quantity of focused time that really matters. The author often prescribes "1 on 1 time" as an exercise to increase focused positive parent–teen interaction.[1] The parent invites the adolescent to pick an activity and engage in the activity with the parent for 20 minutes, during which the parent refrains from ordering, directing, criticizing, commanding. The parent is simply there to engage in the activity as the adolescent wishes. Parents are encouraged to do "1 on 1 time" 5 to 6 times per week.

A second important aspect of focusing on the positive is for parents to *encourage their adolescent to build on his/her strengths*. Parents should help the teenager identify those, hobbies, artistic pursuits, sports, and activities that are pockets of strength, and help them pursue and succeed at those interests, even if it creates some inconvenience for the parents.

The adolescent medicine practitioner should advise the parents to keep copies of this list where they can often view it, for example, posted on the refrigerator, programmed into personal digital assistants (PDAs), cell phones, or computers. When they are faced with a problem situation with their adolescent and don't know how to respond, they should review this list of principles and derive a response from the list.

## ASSESSMENT

At regular intervals when adolescents come to the office for routine medical care, the practitioner should conduct a brief interview with the adolescent and parents together to assess their communication skills, problem solving, beliefs, and family structure. This interview should be used to provide brief counseling during the office visit or referral for mental health services. The practitioner might ask the following questions:[1]

- In general, how well do you get along?
- In the past 2 weeks, how many arguments have you had? Pick a recent argument. Give me a "blow-by-blow" description of what happened.
- What topics do you disagree about? How much anger is involved in these disagreements?
- What do you like and what do you dislike about the way your parent/teen communicates with you?
- When you have a disagreement about something such as chores, homework, or video games, how do you work it out?
- (To parents) If you give your teenager more freedom, what do you think will happen? How much obedience do you expect from your teenager?
- (To teenager) How unfair are your parents' rules compared with the rules at your friends' houses? How much freedom should someone your age be given?
- Do family members take sides against each other? Who takes sides against whom? What problems does this create?

Substantial problems in any of these areas would be an indication for family therapy. Specifically, questions 1 through 4 address general relationship problems and communication. Problems in these areas would be an indication for communication training. Question 5 addresses conflict resolution. Problems in this area would be an indication for problem-solving training. Questions 6 and 7 address extreme beliefs. Problems in these areas would be an indication for cognitive restructuring. Question 8 addresses family structure. Substantial problems in this area would be an indication for structural family therapy approaches.

## INTERVENTION

A behavioral family systems intervention enhances positive communication, teaches problem-solving skills, corrects distorted belief systems, and corrects problems in family structure. Each component of this intervention will be described. Some of these techniques could be implemented in an adolescent medicine office setting; others will require referral to a mental health professional.

### TEACHING COMMUNICATION SKILLS

In a meeting with the parent and adolescent together, the practitioner distributes copies of Table 33-1 and conducts a didactic review of these negative communication habits to increase the family's awareness of them. Family members are asked to indicate how often each negative response occurred within the past few days. Second, the practitioner teaches the family to "dialogue" with each other. The parent and teen take turns being the speaker and the listener. The speaker's job is to pick a topic and make clear, concise, nonaccusatory statements of his/her opinions and feelings about this topic to the listener; after each statement, the speaker pauses for a reaction from the listener. The listener's job is to look at, and attentively listen to, the speaker. When the speaker pauses, the listener paraphrases the speaker's statement without adding any of his/her own opinions or ideas. Then, the speaker verifies whether the paraphrase was correct. After 4 or 5 statements, the dyad reverse roles and again practice the dialogue.

Third, the practitioner instructs the family in ways to correct the specific negative communication habits identified during the didactic review. For example, consider a father who lectures his daughter in an accusatory, critical manner: "You are so irresponsible about your homework. You are old enough to do it without nagging. How will you ever get through college? How will you ever hold down a job? This is a basic issue for your future." The practitioner might discuss with the father the negative effect of his communication, suggesting a more positive alternative: "I am very upset about your incomplete and missing homework. I want to help you solve this problem. I'm worried about your future."

Family members then rehearse the positive communication skills in the office during a problem-solving

**Table 33-1**

**Negative and Positive Communication Skills**

| *Check if Your Family Does This:* | *More Positive Way to Do It:* |
|---|---|
| ___ Call each other names | Express anger without hurt |
| ___ Put each other down | "I" statements: "I'm upset that…" |
| ___ Interrupt each other | Take turns and keep it short |
| ___ Criticize all the time | Point out the good and the bad |
| ___ Get defensive when attacked | Listen, then calmly disagree |
| ___ Give a lecture | Tell it straight and short |
| ___ Use big words | Stick to simple words |
| ___ Dredge up the past | Stick to the present |
| ___ Talk in a sarcastic tone | Talk in a normal tone |
| ___ Get off the topic | Stick to the topic |
| ___ Think the worst | Keep an open mind |
| ___ Command, order | Ask nicely |
| ___ Look away from the speaker | Look at the speaker |
| ___ Slouch | Sit up attentively |
| ___ Give the silent treatment | Say it if you feel it |
| ___ Deny you did it | Take responsibility for your actions |
| ___ Nag about small mistakes | Overlook small things |

discussion. Specific negative responses would be corrected through feedback, instructions, demonstrations of positive responses, and requests to rehearse the positive responses. Family members also should practice the communication skills at home.

## TEACHING PROBLEM-SOLVING SKILLS

Problem solving is an approach to resolving negotiable issues through mutual discussion and compromise. The practitioner should distribute the problem-solving outline in Box 33-2 to the family and explain that s/he will serve as a mediator, guiding the family to discuss a problem using the problem-solving steps. Each step is explained to the family; each family member is given a chance to perform the step, with coaching and feedback from the practitioner.

**Box 33-2**

***Problem-Solving Outline for Families***

I. Define the problem
   A. Tell the others what they do that bothers you and why
   B. Start your definitions with an "I"; be short, clear, and don't accuse
   C. Ask the other to paraphrase your definition to see whether you got your point across
   D. If they understood you, go on; if not, repeat your definition

II. Generate a variety of alternative solutions
   A. Take turns listing solutions
   B. Follow 3 rules:
      1. List as many ideas as you can
      2. Don't evaluate ideas
      3. Be creative; anything goes
   C. One person writes down ideas to keep track of them

III. Evaluate the ideas and decide upon the best one
   A. Take turns saying whether you like each idea and what would happen if you followed it
   B. Vote "Yes" or "No" for each idea and record your vote in writing next to the idea
   C. Look for ideas voted "Yes" by everyone
   D. Select 1 of these ideas or combine several
   E. If none were voted "Yes" by everyone, negotiate a compromise
      1. Select an idea voted "Yes" by 1 parent and the adolescent
      2. List as many possible compromises as you can
      3. Evaluate the compromises as you did the original ideas
      4. Try to reach an agreement

IV. Plan to implement the selected solution
   A. Decide who will do what, where, how, and when
   B. Decide who will monitor adherence with the solution
   C. Decide upon the consequences for adherence or nonadherence
      1. Rewards for adherence
      2. Penalties for nonadherence

A topic of mild to moderate intensity is appropriate for this first problem-solving discussion. It is important for the practitioner to maintain neutrality, not siding with any 1 family member, and to keep the family on task, interrupting when irrelevant comments are made and redirecting the family members to the steps of problem solving. By the end of 30 to 40 minutes, the family can usually reach an agreement to implement a particular solution. The practitioner sends them home to do so and has them report back at the next session. If the family members verify that the solution worked, a new problem is discussed. If not, the original problem is renegotiated. Family members also are encouraged to practice problem-solving and communication skills at home. The practitioner can ask the family to schedule a regular meeting to practice the steps of problem solving.

### CORRECTING DISTORTED BELIEF SYSTEMS

Cognitive restructuring with parents and adolescents consists of 4 steps: (1) identify the extreme thought; (2) provide a logical challenge to it; (3) identify alternative, more realistic thoughts; and (4) collect evidence to disconfirm the extreme thought and confirm the reasonable thought. Unlike problem solving, which follows an outline in a psycho-educational manner, implementing the steps of cognitive restructuring requires clinical training and supervised experience.

The steps of cognitive restructuring will be illustrated through the case of 14-year-old Andrew Jones and his mother, who sought family therapy for parent–adolescent conflict. Andrew complained that his mother incessantly nagged him about completing homework and chores; Mrs Jones responded that she was teaching him to be responsible, as any parent should. Arguments frequently occurred. The therapist suspected that extreme thinking was contributing to this conflict.

Extreme beliefs come to light in several ways: (1) a family member openly states an extreme belief; (2) a family member resists compromise during a problem-solving discussion; or (3) a therapist asks the family to imagine a typical parent–teen interaction and report on their cognitions. The therapist asked Mrs Jones what was the worst thing that might happen if she stopped nagging Andrew about his homework, and when she replied, continued to ask, "What would happen next?" She indicated that Andrew would fail his classes, fail to graduate from high school, fail to get a good job, fail to live independently, and end up an unemployed burden on her and her husband. Thus, her extremely ruinous thinking was clearly identified.

Second, the therapist tactfully provided a logical challenge to the extreme thought. The therapist asked Mrs Jones, "Is it remotely possible that Andrew is now mature enough to get at least some of his homework done without your frequent reminders?" She was skeptical, but conceded that it was a remote possibility. Third, the practitioner suggested a more reasonable belief: "So what we are saying is that Andrew may complete homework successfully without nagging."

Fourth, the therapist proposed an experiment to test the reasonable versus unreasonable belief. Such experiments often include collecting data from other parents about normative behavior for teens in the community or implementing a solution to the problem on a trial basis. In this case, the therapist proposed to Mrs Jones that she stop nagging Andrew about homework for one month and check with his teachers weekly to see how much of his homework was turned in. The therapist also talked to Andrew privately and told him that this was his 1 chance to get his mother off his back; he must turn in all of his homework if he expected her to stop nagging him. Mother and son agreed to the experiment. Andrew turned in 90% of his homework and nagging decreased. Mrs Jones' unreasonable belief about Andrew's getting failing grades if she stopped nagging was disconfirmed; the therapist would have to deal with her other unreasonable beliefs later.

### ADDRESSING FAMILY STRUCTURE

Common family structure problems include parents not working well as a team in disciplining an adolescent, 1 parent taking sides with the adolescent against the other parent, or 2 parents putting the adolescent in the middle. Structural interventions often require specialized family therapy training and are best conducted by referral to a mental health professional. An illustration will be given for the case of 2 parents not working consistently as a team. The therapist might ask the family to discuss an issue such as curfew and tell the parents that teamwork will be reinforced. The therapist then praises the parents for each statement they make backing each other up; any time 1 parent disagrees with the other in front of the teen, the therapist stops the discussion, points out the problem, and asks the offending parent to back up the other parent's position. The therapist continues to provide such feedback and correction over the course of many therapy sessions, gradually helping the parents discipline consistently. Other problems in family structure are similarly targeted for change through feedback, behavior rehearsal, and correction during future therapy sessions.

## CONCLUSION

Using a behavioral family systems model, the practitioner who understands that parents and teenagers need knowledge and skills to negotiate the process of adolescent individuation can be extremely helpful to families through anticipatory guidance and intervention. Skill training in family communication and problem solving can be done within a primary care adolescent medicine setting. Cognitive restructuring of unreasonable beliefs and interventions to change family structure are more difficult to achieve without special training in psychology and often require referral to a specialist. The anticipatory guidance suggestions and interventions discussed in this chapter have been subjected to empirical scrutiny over the past 30 years and been have found to be effective.[1-3,5]

## REFERENCES

1. Robin AL, Foster SL. *Negotiating Parent-Adolescent Conflict: A Behavioral Family Systems Approach.* New York, NY: Guilford Press; 1989

2. Barkley RA, Edwards G, Robin AL. *Defiant Teens: A Clinician's Manual for Assessment and Family Intervention.* New York, NY: Guilford Press; 1999

3. Robin AL. *ADHD in Adolescents: Diagnosis and Treatment.* New York, NY: Guilford Press; 1998

4. Patterson GR, Forgatch M. *Parents and Adolescents Living Together: Part I. The Basics.* Eugene, OR: Castalia Press; 1987

5. Barkley RA, Edwards R, Laneri M, Fletcher K, Metevia L. The efficacy of problem-solving communication training alone, behavior management training alone, and their combination for parent-adolescent conflict in teenagers with ADHD and ODD. *J Consult Clin Psychol.* 2001;69:926–941

# CHAPTER 34

# Parenting the Adolescent

LAURENCE STEINBERG, PHD

## INTRODUCTION

Family relationships are most likely to change during transitional periods in the child's development, and adolescence is certainly a time of dramatic and often challenging transformations in relations among family members. The biological, intellectual, and psychosocial changes of adolescence reverberate throughout the family, often upsetting a peaceful equilibrium that characterized the middle childhood years. When surveyed, parents typically list adolescence as the most challenging period in the child's development, and this is reported by parents whose children are not yet teenagers, by those whose children are in the midst of adolescence, and by those whose children are young adults.[1]

A quick glance at the titles of books aimed at parents of teenagers reveals that most writers portray adolescence as an unhappy and tumultuous time for the family, a picture that is not borne out by research on parents and teenagers, however. Although many families do find the period to be one of marked transformation in parent–child relations, most teenagers and parents report that they get along well, feel close, and respect each other.[2]

In other words, adolescence is a time during which family relationships are altered rather than jeopardized. Research shows quite clearly that most families who experience serious problems during adolescence had problems during earlier periods of the child's development. In the minority of families in which serious difficulties do arise for the first time in adolescence, the problems usually have less to do with adolescence per se than with other factors that may be impinging on the family at that time, such as marital difficulties, financial strain, relocation, or physical illness.[2]

Parents who have enjoyed close and satisfying relationships with their children during the elementary school years should not go into adolescence expecting things will fall apart as soon as their children become teenagers, despite what many popular parenting books imply. In fact, there is some evidence that this expectation can easily become a self-fulfilling prophecy, whereby parents who expect the worst change their behavior in ways that actually bring out the worst in their adolescents.[3] The parent who treats a teenager with unwarranted suspicion may alienate the adolescent to the point where he or she pulls away and disengages from the family, confirming parents' worst fears.

One reason that parents describe adolescence as a challenging time is that they are often unprepared for the normative changes in their child's behavior and in family relationships that occur during this transitional period. Most parents do not realize, for example, that the most dramatic changes in family relationships occur relatively early in the period—sometimes before the child technically has become a teenager. This is particularly the case for parents of girls. Studies indicate that the peak period of change in the parent–child relationship is around age 13 or 14 years in the case of sons, but between 11 and 12 years in the case of daughters.[4] The most challenging time for parents, therefore, is likely to be when their child is in middle or junior high school, not high school, as many parents expect.

In addition, although most parents refer to books on infancy during their child's early years, few refer to guides about adolescent development. As a result, the major developments of the period are often misunderstood. This is unfortunate because good sources of information do exist, and parents who understand adolescence is a developmental period are more likely to have a satisfying relationship with their child. A well-developed body of scientific literature on parenting during adolescence does exist that provides clear guidelines about what parents should expect and what they should do.[5-7]

## CHANGES IN PARENT–CHILD RELATIONSHIPS IN ADOLESCENCE

Psychologists who study parent–child relationships point to 3 main changes that occur during the transition into adolescence.[8,9] First, there is a temporary increase in the frequency of bickering over mundane matters—the tidiness of the adolescent's bedroom, the adolescent's appearance, or how the adolescent spends free time. (One remarkable finding from studies of families with teenagers is that the points of conflict between parents and teenagers have not changed in at least a half-century; fashions may come and go, but quarreling over the adolescent's choice of clothing, cosmetics, or hairstyle is virtually inevitable.[2]) The main reason for this increase is that the adolescent's ideas about parental authority are changing, largely because he or she is becoming more cognitively sophisticated and able to tell the difference between a rule that has some logic behind it and one that seems arbitrary. As a consequence, what had previously been seen as legitimate assertions of parental control are now experienced by the teenager as unfair or intrusive. Adolescents do not reject all parental authority as illegitimate, but they will challenge their parents to explain their decisions and distinguish between matters of genuine importance (on which they will generally defer to parents' authority) and those that most likely reflect personal taste (on which they generally will assert their rights to control this aspect of their lives).[10] As parents and teenagers renegotiate what the adolescent is and is not allowed to decide on his or her own, the squabbling generally stops.

Second, there is usually a slight decline in intimacy between parents and children as they mature into adolescence. Young adolescents often are reluctant to be physically affectionate toward their parents in public or, for that matter, to even be seen with them in public. Teenagers become increasingly likely to turn to peers as confidantes and less likely to confide in parents, even in families in which close relationships had been the norm during childhood. They are more likely to choose to spend time with friends than family members and may complain about having to participate in family activities. Many adolescents go through a period during which they "de-idealize" their parents, criticizing them whenever possible, dismissing their opinions as dated, and questioning their values and beliefs. It is important that parents understand that this is both normal and reflective of the adolescent's need to establish emotional autonomy from his or her parents. Although many parents are distressed by this distancing, they need to keep in mind that it has nothing to do with them personally; it is more about what they symbolize (the teenager being someone's child) than who they are. Trying to act like a child's friend, rather than a parent, in an effort to deflect this criticism is unlikely to work and will only serve to undermine the parent's authority.[7]

Finally, there is usually a renegotiation of the balance of power in the family, with the adolescent striving for more independence from parental control. This has many manifestations, including an increase in the adolescent's desire for privacy; more frequent requests for greater decision-making autonomy over things such as curfew, schoolwork, free time, and expenditures; and a sharp increase in the sheer amount of time adolescents spend away from parental supervision. In healthy families, these matters are negotiated gradually over time, with an open and respectful exchange of ideas and opinions. Adolescents, like adults, appreciate being given their "day in court," even if they ultimately do not get their way. Most teenagers are far more reasonable than their parents believe or expect them to be, as long as they are treated with respect. Many disagreements can be handled effectively through collaborative problem solving, where both the parent and the teenager are involved in coming up with a suitable solution with which both can live.[11]

## STYLES OF PARENTING

Despite these broad generalizations about the ways in which family relationships change during adolescence, there are wide variations among families in how they approach child rearing and discipline. Psychologists refer to this as "parenting style"—the general way in which parents interact with their adolescent. Parenting style is important because research has shown that the same parental behavior may have different effects on the adolescent depending on the parents' style. Two parents, for example, may monitor their child's schoolwork, but an adolescent whose parents do this in a way that is rigid and autocratic will react much differently than one whose parents approach the same task in a warm and supportive fashion.[2]

In characterizing parents' style, psychologists generally focus on 2 aspects of the parent's behavior toward the adolescent: responsiveness and "demandingness." Responsiveness refers to the degree to which the parent responds to the child's needs in an accepting, supportive manner. Demandingness refers to the extent to which the parent expects and demands mature, responsible behavior. Because responsiveness and demandingness are more or less independent of each other—that is, it is possible for a parent to be demanding without being responsive and vice versa—psychologists who study parenting look at various combinations of these dimensions. This has yielded a system for classifying parents that is helpful in understanding the ways in which adolescents are affected by different family environments.[5]

Parents who are both responsive and demanding are labeled *authoritative*. *Authoritative parents* are warm but firm. They set standards for the child's conduct but form expectations that are consistent with the child's developing needs and capabilities. Although they place a high value on the development of autonomy and self-direction, they assume ultimate responsibility for their child's behavior. Authoritative parents deal with their child in a rational, issue-oriented manner, frequently engaging in discussion and explanation with their children over matters of discipline. Authoritative parents strive to raise children who are self-reliant and who have a strong sense of initiative.

Parents who are very demanding but not responsive are called *authoritarian*. *Authoritarian parents* place a high value on obedience and conformity. They tend to favor more punitive, absolute, and forceful disciplinary measures. Verbal give-and-take is not common in authoritarian households because the underlying belief of authoritarian parents is that the child should accept without question the rules and standards established by the parents. They tend not to encourage independent behavior and, instead, place a good deal of importance on restricting the child's autonomy. Authoritarian parents place a premium on obedience.

A parent who is very responsive but not at all demanding is referred to as *indulgent*. *Indulgent parents* behave in an accepting, benign, and somewhat more passive way in matters of discipline. They place relatively few demands on the child's behavior, giving the child a high degree of freedom to act as he or she wants. Indulgent parents are more likely to believe that control is an infringement on the child's freedom that may interfere with the child's healthy development. Instead of actively shaping their child's behavior, indulgent parents are more likely to view themselves as resources that the child may or may not use. Indulgent parents tend to be especially concerned with raising children who are happy.

Parents who are neither demanding nor responsive are labeled *indifferent*. *Indifferent parents* try to do whatever is necessary to minimize the time and energy they must devote to interacting with their child. In extreme cases, indifferent parents may be neglectful. They know little about their child's activities and whereabouts, show little interest in their child's experiences at school or with friends, rarely converse with their child, and seldom consider their child's opinion when making decisions. Rather than raising their child according to a set of beliefs about what is good for the child's development (as do the other parent types), indifferent parents are "parent centered"—that is, they structure their home life primarily around their own needs and interests.

## BASIC PRINCIPLES OF GOOD PARENTING

Although we do not ordinarily think of parenting as a scientific enterprise, there is a great deal of systematic research on the links between different types of parenting and children's and adolescent's development, adjustment, and behavior.[7] Basically, good parenting boils down to several fundamental principles, and parents who follow these principles will facilitate their adolescent's healthy development and promote more positive family relationships. First, treat your teenager warmly and affectionately, even during periods when he or she seems to be pulling back. Do not make the mistake of pulling back in return. Second, have clearly articulated expectations for mature and responsible behavior, and enforce them consistently. If you and your spouse disagree, try to find common ground and be consistent with each other. This is just as important—perhaps even more so—for divorced parents as it is for married ones. Third, strive to balance your desire to be in control with your teenager's natural need for independence. Do not make an issue out of every little thing, and do not make or enforce rules just for the sake of showing your child who is in charge; if parents save unilateral assertions of their authority for things that really matter, adolescents are more likely to pay attention and comply. Discipline rationally, and explain your decisions to your child. Finally, treat your child with respect. Ask his or her opinions, engage in real conversations rather than perfunctory ones, and give your child the benefit of the doubt. Do not spy on your child; instead, ask questions on issues about which you are concerned. Parents often complain that their teenager does not open up to them, but it is hard to open up with someone whose main way of conversing is via an interrogation or a lecture.[11]

## IMPACT OF PARENTING ON ADOLESCENT DEVELOPMENT

Few areas of research in the field of adolescent development have received as much attention as the link between what parents do and how adolescents turn out, and the findings of this work are amazingly consistent.[2,8,9] Generally, young people who have been raised in authoritative households are more emotionally mature than peers who have been raised in authoritarian, indulgent, or indifferent homes. Adolescents raised in authoritative homes are more responsible, more self-assured, more adaptive, more creative, more curious, more socially skilled, and more successful in school. Adolescents raised in authoritarian homes, in contrast, are more dependent, more passive, less socially adept, less self-assured, and less intellectually curious. Adolescents raised in indulgent households are often less mature, more irresponsible, more conforming to their peers, and less able to assume positions of leadership. Adolescents raised in indifferent homes are often impulsive and more likely to be involved in delinquent behavior and in precocious experiments with sex, drugs, and alcohol. Parenting that is indifferent, neglectful, or abusive has been consistently shown to have harmful effects on the adolescent's mental health and development, leading to depression and a variety of behavior problems including, in cases of physical abuse, aggression toward others. Severe psychological abuse (excessive criticism, rejection, or emotional harshness) appears to have the most deleterious effects. The evidence linking authoritative parenting and healthy adolescent development is remarkably strong, and it has been found in studies of a wide range of ethnicities, social classes, and family structures, not only within the United States but also around the world. In addition, educational programs designed to teach parents how to be more responsive and more demanding have been effective in fostering healthy adolescent development and behavior.[2]

Why is authoritative parenting associated with healthy adolescent development? First, authoritative parents provide an appropriate balance between restrictiveness and autonomy, giving the adolescent opportunities to develop self-reliance while providing the sorts of standards, limits, and guidelines that developing individuals need. Second, because authoritative parents are more likely to engage their children in verbal give-and-take, they are likely to promote the sort of intellectual development that provides an important foundation for the development of psychosocial maturity. Third, because authoritative parenting is based on a warm parent–child relationship, adolescents are more likely to identify with, admire, and form strong attachments to their parents, which leaves them more open to their parents' influence. In contrast, adolescents who are raised by nonauthoritative parents often end up having friends their parents disapprove of, including those involved in problem behaviors.[5]

## IMPACT OF ADOLESCENCE ON PARENTS' MENTAL HEALTH

The challenging nature of the adolescent transition sometimes takes its toll on parents' mental health. In fact, many studies indicate that as a developmental period, adolescence may actually be more stressful for parents than teenagers. It is not hard to see why: the frequent bickering and squabbling is unpleasant, the adolescent's distancing and de-idealization hurts parents' feelings, and the renegotiation of rules about independence can be upsetting because parents must relinquish some of their power over things they previously controlled. Perhaps not surprisingly, research shows that a substantial proportion of parents (more often mothers than fathers) report an increase in feelings of depression, anxiety, dissatisfaction, and self-doubt as their children mature into and through early adolescence. Studies have also shown that the period of time surrounding a child's transition into adolescence is usually the lowest point in marital satisfaction for both husbands and wives.[12]

Research also suggests a number of things that parents can do to protect their mental health during this time.[12] It is especially important that parents have other interests and sources of fulfillment, such as a satisfying job, an intimate marriage, or a rewarding hobby or community activity; parents who report sources of life satisfaction in addition to being a parent fare better during adolescence than those who do not. Second, it is helpful for parents to understand the basics of adolescent development, which will enable them to put some of their child's behavior into perspective and interpret it correctly. Third, it helps to go into adolescence with positive expectations. Finally, practicing the principles of authoritative parenting will lead to a teenager's healthier psychological development, which will make parenting that much easier.

## WHEN TO SEEK HELP

Because adolescence has been stereotyped as a time of inherent difficulty, many parents are unsure about when an apparent problem is really a problem and when it is part of normal adolescent development. If signs of a problem are obvious (eg, a teenager talks about suicide, shows signs of being physically or sexually abused by someone, has committed an act of violence, is abusing alcohol or drugs), the parent should seek help immediately for their adolescent. For less clear-cut situations, a good rule of thumb is that the adolescent and family should probably seek help if there is a noticeable and worrisome change in the teen's behavior (eg, a sharp decline in school performance, a marked decrease in socializing with friends, a significant increase in irritability or sadness, signs of recklessness) or in the parent's relationship with the teen (eg, frequent arguments that escalate beyond bickering) that persists for more than 2 weeks. The parent can be advised to start by simply asking their child whether something is troubling him or her and if it would be helpful to talk to you or someone else about it. If the parent or teen ask for help, it is best to start with their teen's primary care practitioner. If the primary care provider feels the problem is beyond their scope, the teen and family may need to seek the help of an expert who has specific experience with adolescents.[11]

## REFERENCES

1. Steinberg L, Silk J. Parenting adolescents. In: M. Bornstein, ed. *Handbook of Parenting: Volume 1. Children and Parenting*. 2nd ed. Mahwah, NJ: Erlbaum; 2002:103–133

2. Steinberg L. We know some things: adolescent-parent relationships in retrospect and prospect. *J Res Adolesc.* 2001;11: 1-20

3. Jacobs J, Chin C, Shaver K. Longitudinal links between perceptions of adolescence and the social beliefs of adolescents: are parents' stereotypes related to beliefs held about and by their children? *J Youth Adolesc.* 2005;34:61-72

4. Granic I, Hollenstein T, Dishion TJ, Patterson GR. Longitudinal analysis of flexibility and reorganization in early adolescence: a dynamic systems study of family interactions. *Dev Psychol.* 2003;39:606-617

5. Steinberg L. *Adolescence*. 8th ed. New York: McGraw-Hill; 2008

6. Lerner R, Steinberg L, eds. *Handbook of Adolescent Psychology.* 3rd ed. New York: Wiley; 2009

7. Steinberg L. *The Ten Basic Principles of Good Parenting*. New York: Simon & Schuster; 2005

8. Laursen B, Collins WA. Parent-child relationships during adolescence. In: Lerner R, Steinberg L, eds. *Handbook of Adolescent Psychology*. New York: Wiley; 2009

9. Collins WA, Steinberg L. Adolescent development in interpersonal context. In: Damon W, Lerner R, eds. Eisenberg N, vol ed. *Social, Emotional, and Personality Development: Handbook of Child Psychology*. New York: Wiley; 2006: 1003-1067

10. Smetana J. Adolescent-parent conflict: resistance and subversion as developmental process. In: Nucci L, ed. *Conflict, Contradiction, and Contrarian Elements in Moral Development and Education*. Mahwah, NJ: Erlbaum; 2005:69-91

11. Steinberg L, Levine A. *You and Your Adolescent: A Guide for Ages 10 to 20*. Rev ed. New York: HarperCollins; 1997

12. Steinberg L, Steinberg W. *Crossing Paths: How Your Child's Adolescence Triggers Your Own Crisis*. New York: Simon & Schuster; 1994

# CHAPTER 35

# Divorce, Separation, and Blended Families

SANDRA J. KAPLAN, MD

*Dr. Sandra Kaplan passed away on July 23, 2010. For nearly 30 years, she oversaw the clinical, teaching, and research efforts of the Division of Child and Adolescent Psychiatry at North Shore University Hospital in New York. She was a superb and dedicated clinician, an inspiring teacher, and a beloved colleague. She will be sorely missed.*

## INTRODUCTION

This chapter presents an overview of the divorce/family dissolution process and its effect on adolescents. Divorce is defined as a dissolution of marriage decreed by a court. It indicates that a valid marriage no longer exists and that both parties are free to remarry. It provides for the division of property between parents and for their postdivorce financial responsibilities. When married parents divorce or when unmarried parents dissolve their relationships, state courts render legal documents that authorize custody of children under 18 years of age and the support of the children.[1] The term "family dissolution" is used in this chapter to refer to the separation of parents who did not marry.

There are different types of child custody. Legal custody refers to the right and responsibility to make decisions for a child. Physical or residential custody indicates with whom a child will reside. Joint custody refers to parents making major decisions (ie, pertaining to education, health care, and religion) about their children together. Sole custody refers to one parent having the right to make major decisions about a child. Courts authorize plans for parenting (child access/visitation) times for the noncustodial parent unless it has been determined that the safety of a child would be compromised by access to a parent.[1]

Child support, including each parent's financial responsibilities following divorce or family dissolution, is authorized either by agreement between the parents or by a court order. Although federal and state laws authorize collection of child support from parents who do not voluntarily pay, the Census Bureau,[1] has reported that only about half of the parents entitled to do so received the full amounts that were due.

Divorce litigation occurs if adults dissolving their marriages do not agree on child custodial issues or financial matters. The American Bar Association estimates that 5% or fewer divorces involve litigation over child custody. Divorces that involve custody or legal disputes often involve recurrent litigation as children grow. When child custody decisions are made by judges and have not been made by agreements between parents, judges utilize a concept to make determinations based on "the Best Interests of the Child." The "Best Interests Standard" refers to the responsibilities of courts to decide cases involving child custody in ways that ensure the well-being of children. During child custody cases, children and adolescents may be interviewed in chambers by judges who also hear evidence in court hearings and then determine custody based on multiple factors.[2]

Factors considered by judges when determining custody include the child's age and gender, and relationships with each of the parents, the siblings, and others who will affect his or her well-being. Also considered are each parent's wishes, the child's wishes (particularly for teenagers); each parent's willingness and ability to care for a child and cooperate with the other parent; the child's adjustment to home, school, and community; the parents' adjustment; and evidence of interpartner domestic violence (between parents) or of child abuse or neglect.[1]

Attorneys are usually involved during divorce/family dissolution child custody and financial legal proceedings. They usually represent the parents but may also represent adolescents or younger children. If a parent is unable to afford an attorney, some states have resources to appoint and pay an attorney. Parents may also represent themselves, in which case they are referred to as "pro se litigants" (meaning "for oneself"). Attorneys for children and adolescents are called law guardians. Law guardians may be appointed by judges and paid for by parents or by states, depending on family income, and are charged with looking out for the best interests of the child or adolescent during the course of the proceedings.[2] A forensic mental health consultant may also be appointed by a judge to provide information about an adolescent and his or her family to assist in the determination of the "best interests of the child" during custody trials.

## PREVALENCE OF DIVORCE/FAMILY DISSOLUTION

Results of the 2001 United States Census indicate that 41% of men and 39% of women ages 50 to 59 have been divorced. Fifty-five percent of American children younger than age 18 were found to have spent time living in a single-parent family, usually led by a mother. Half of their mothers were single because of divorce. Approximately 50% of divorced women remarry within 4 years. Divorce rates of remarried families are greater than for first marriages. Nearly 10% (3.6 million) of all households with children younger than age 18 in the United States include stepparents, stepsiblings, or half siblings, and 15% (10.6 million) of children in the United States live in these households.[3]

## DIVORCE-ASSOCIATED FAMILY STRESSFUL EVENTS AND CIRCUMSTANCES

The dissolution of families by parental divorce, or by parents who have never been married living separately, increases the risk of adolescents having developmental and mental health problems due to various factors. Economic, community, and residential stressors for adolescents and children often are associated with divorce/family dissolution. Mothers often have resultant decreased incomes, which necessitates moves of residences and changes in schools for adolescents. The adolescent's new and less expensive home is often in a community with increased crime to which the adolescent is then exposed.[4]

In addition to the previously mentioned stressors related to economic factors, adolescents are often exposed to parents who have individual mental health problems, before and after the divorce/family dissolution,[5] and distress and conflict pertaining to their relationships with each other. Parental mental health problems, as well as distress about and conflict during their relationships with each other, have been found to be associated with diminished parenting.[6] Divorce and family dissolution have been associated with increased rates of maternal depression, particularly in those who have economic hardship.[3] Maternal depression has been found to increase the risk of adolescents having anxiety disorders, and maternal and paternal parental depression have been found to predict adolescent conduct disorders and depression.[7] Parental depression has been found to be associated with coercive and impulsive parenting behaviors, reduced use of negotiations and warmth with children and adolescents, and false beliefs and miscommunication in the family.[8] Alcohol abuse by parents has been associated with marital conflict and particularly with domestic violence between parents. Parental alcohol abuse has been found to increase the risk of adolescent alcohol dependence.[9]

Divorce is also associated with the loss of fathers, because of lack of contact, for up to 25% of children and adolescents 2 to 3 years after their parents' marriage is dissolved.[10] The loss of a parent before adulthood is also a well-known risk factor for mental health problems.[11]

## DEVELOPMENTAL ISSUES FOR THE ADOLESCENT

The effect of divorce/family dissolution on adolescents varies with the age of the teen. Young adolescents (ages 12–15 years) are often concerned about peer relationships and status within their peer group and may respond to the breakup of their families with feelings of shame and isolation. Also, young adolescents are at a stage in development in which they are being left alone by their parents more often, and for longer periods. If not adequately supervised, they, as well as older adolescents, may have increased vulnerability to drug and alcohol use, early sexual relationships, teen pregnancy, and truancy. Divorce, which is often associated with decreased parental availability to supervise adolescents, puts adolescents in this age group at increased risk.[2]

Older adolescents (ages 15–19 years) tend to socialize with a few close friends and have romantic relationships. They also explore interests and make future educational and career plans. Supervision by parents ensures their safety and security as they consolidate their identities and become increasingly independent of their families.[2] Divorce may affect adolescents in this age group by making them feel rejected by their parents, particularly the parent who initiated the divorce/family dissolution. The confidence of these teenagers may become impaired and they may fail to achieve their potential, making impulsive decisions about their futures without parental guidance and support. Older adolescents may also be fearful about their abilities to achieve educational and career goals because of the lack of financial support that often follows divorce/family dissolution.[12]

Adolescents often become judgmental of their parents as they strive for independence and achieve increased ability to think critically. Some adolescents may hold one parent more responsible for the failure of the marriage or relationship than the other, and then form an alliance with the rejected parent. The extreme version of this alliance with one parent and rejection of the other is termed "the alienated child," which can also involve teens and preteens.[13] Adolescents may experience intense grief about their parents' divorce/separation. This may result in a decreased ability to concentrate and to an increase in risk-taking behaviors.[12]

## PHYSICAL HEALTH ISSUES FOR THE ADOLESCENT

Studies have shown that adolescents from divorced families do not have more health care visits than adolescents from intact families. However, adolescents who perceive the divorce experience negatively are found to have more health care visits and somatic complaints than adolescents who do not find the divorce experience to be as negative.[14]

## MENTAL HEALTH EFFECTS ON THE ADOLESCENT

Male and female adolescents of divorced families have been found to have more internalizing (emotional) and externalizing (behavioral) problems than do adolescents from intact families.[15] Adolescents and children who had problems prior to the divorce/dissolution of their families have been found to have an increase in these problems following the divorce.[16]

Exposure to a parental divorce during adolescence has been found to predict the presence of emotional disorders when these adolescents become adults.[17] Teenagers who experienced divorce of their parents before age 15 were found to be particularly vulnerable to having depressive symptoms compared with teenagers of the same ages whose parents did not divorce.[18] Females whose parents divorced when they were children had increased symptoms of anxiety and depression as adolescents. Decreased contact with fathers following divorce was found to be associated with increased symptoms of anxiety and depression in male adolescents.[19]

## ACADEMIC ISSUES FOR THE ADOLESCENT

In a meta-analysis of 67 studies of divorce, Amato[20] found that children of divorce had lower average levels of cognitive achievement even a decade after the divorce. Male and female adolescents who experienced divorce had poorer grades compared with adolescents from intact families.[15] Among adolescents who experienced a divorce, females had a greater risk of dropping out of high school than did males.

In an analysis of responses of more than 17,000 students in junior and senior high school to an adolescent health study, 30% of adolescents living with a single parent reported that they had repeated a grade, and 40% reported that they had been suspended. Both of these figures were greater than those found for adolescents who had lived continuously with both parents. This survey also found that 45% of teenagers between 12 and 18 years of age did not live with both biological parents.[4]

Following divorce/family dissolution, greater paternal involvement in an adolescent's schoolwork was found to be associated with increased school performance.[21] Paternal contact, coupled with the father paying child support, was found to predict successful high school completion and college attendance by adolescents of divorce.[22]

## PARENTAL REMARRIAGE AND THE IMPACT ON ADOLESCENTS

Adolescents are affected by their parents' remarriages. Early adolescents and those adolescents who have lived with single parents longest were found to have increased behavioral and emotional problems following parental remarriage. Female adolescents were found to benefit less from exposure to stepfathers than did male adolescents.[22]

Adding a stepfather to a household usually improves adolescents' standards of living. However, adolescents who have had much autonomy in a single-parent household may resent supervision by a step-parent and may react with hostility to their step-parents' authority. Adolescents may also experience loyalty conflicts, and may fear that becoming emotionally close to a step-parent may imply that they are betraying their nonresident parent. Some teenagers may become jealous after a parent remarries because they then need to share parental time with the step-parent and any children from a previous relationship. The remarriage of a parent may also end the adolescent's hopes for a reunion of his or her parents.[23] The safety of adolescents within families has also been found to be affected by parental remarriage, as stepfathers have been found to be overrepresented in documented cases of child abuse.[24]

## ADOLESCENTS' PERCEPTIONS OF DIVORCE/FAMILY DISSOLUTION AND CUSTODY

Adolescents' views of custody arrangements merit important consideration by parents who agree on plans for parenting teens and by judges who order parenting plans when parents do not agree. Kelly and Emery[10] reported that adolescents and younger children have greater satisfaction and closeness in shared/joint custody arrangements than they do if sole physical custody is given to a single parent. They also found that children want fathers to be emotionally supportive, affectionate, and actively engaged in their lives. This same study reported that children often want to distance themselves from fathers or mothers who are rigid and inflexible, angry and demeaning, self-centered and demanding. In contrast, when the child's input is taken into account, arrangements are more often viewed as fair, and this results in increased child and adolescent satisfaction.[10]

## ADOLESCENT RESILIENCE AND DIVORCE

Most adolescents and children whose parents divorce do not have long-lasting problems. Those who seem to be most resilient are those who did not have problems before the divorce of their parents, and who were exposed to diminished conflict and violence between their parents following the divorce. In addition, adolescent resilience is associated with exposure to high-quality parenting, as well as access to both parents following the divorce, and without conflict between the parents regarding parental access. Positive psychological adjustment of the custodial parent, combined with high-quality parenting, has been found to be particularly protective. Protective parenting qualities have been reported to include warmth, emotional support, adequate monitoring, provision of authoritative discipline, and age-appropriate expectations of adolescents.[23]

## FUTURE ADJUSTMENT OF ADOLESCENTS FOLLOWING DIVORCE/FAMILY DISSOLUTION

Adolescents of divorced families are more likely than adolescents from intact families to drop out of school and become pregnant.[25] As young adults, adolescents of divorce are also less likely than teens from intact families to attend or complete college and to be employed. They are more likely to be on welfare, to have problems with parents, siblings, and significant others, and to become divorced as adults than are adolescents from intact families.[25]

## INTERVENTIONS TO MINIMIZE STRESS AND ENHANCE FUNCTIONING DURING DIVORCE/ FAMILY DISSOLUTION

Kelly and Emery[10] reported that the primary goal of interventions for dissolving families is the prevention of conflict between parents, and diverting the parents from engaging in custody litigation. They recommend early interventions, including parent custody education and mediation, which focus on containing conflicts between the parents and on the formulation of parenting plans that will benefit the children and adolescents in the family. They also recommend collaborative lawyering (ie, attorneys, accountants, and mental health professionals collaborating to help the family), judicial settlement conferences, the use of parenting coordinators or arbitration programs for chronically litigating parents, and family and group therapy for children and parents.[10]

Kelly and Emery[10] recommend that custody mediation emphasize conflict reduction, meeting adolescent and parental needs, and settlement. They reported that use of mediation is associated with more positive effects, such as enhanced parent-child and parent-parent relationships and more sustained contact between the children/adolescent and his or her parents, than when mediation is not utilized.

Divorce education programs for parents may be provided or accredited by courts. State offices of court administration are resources for locating such programs. Parent education programs discuss such issues as the legal process surrounding divorce, child and adolescent development, communication between the divorcing parents, and between parents and adolescents. A treatment program for mothers focusing on enhanced communication with their children has been found to improve the functioning of adolescents after divorce.[26]

The American Academy of Pediatrics[27] has a number of resources for the practitioner as well as for teens and parents of divorcing/separating families. This guidance includes discussions on adolescent development, divorce stressors and effects, and communication between parents and between parents and children about information pertaining to divorce. Adolescent medicine practitioners are uniquely positioned to advocate for optimum adolescent development and future functioning in teens whose parents are divorced or separated. Anticipatory guidance urging both parents to support their teen's relationship with and access to the other parent, and encouraging parents to prevent their adolescent's exposure to parental conflict provides much protection during the teenage years and ensures a more positive adulthood.

## REFERENCES

1. American Bar Association. Division for Public Education. Available at: www.abanet.org/publiced/resources/home.html. Accessed March 1, 2007

2. Center on Children and the Law, State Justice Institute. *A Judge's Guide: Making Child-Centered Decisions on Custody Cases*. American Bar Association; 2001

3. Kreider RM. *Number, Timing, and Duration of Marriages and Divorces, 2001.* US Census Bureau. US Department of Commerce—Economics and Statistics Administration; 2005

4. Amato PR. The impact of family formation change on the cognitive, social, and emotional well-being of the next generation. *The Future of Children.* 2005;15:75-96

5. Whisman MA, Uebelacker LA, Weinstock LM. Psychopathology and marital satisfaction: the importance of evaluating both partners. *J Consulting and Clinical Psych.* 2004;72: 830-838

6. Peris TS, Emery RE. A prospective study of the consequences of marital disruption for adolescents: predisruption family dynamics and postdisruption adolescent adjustment. *J Clin Child Adolesc Psychol.* 2004;33:694-704

7. Ohannessian CM, Hesselbrock VM, Kramer J. The relationship between parental psychopathology and adolescent psychopathology: an examination of gender patterns. *J Emotion Behav Dis.* 2005;13:67-76

8. Solantaus-Simula T, Punamaki RL, Beardslee WR. Children's responses to low parental mood II: associations with family perceptions of parenting styles and child distress. *J Am Acad Child Adolesc Psych.* 2002;41:287-295

9. Chassin L, Pitts S, DeLucia C, Todd M. A longitudinal study of children of alcoholics: predicting young adult substance abuse disorders, anxiety, and depression. *J Abnorm Psych.* 1999;108:106-119

10. Kelly J, Emery R. Children's adjustment following divorce: risk and resilience perspectives. *Family Relations.* 2003;52:352-362

11. Worden WJ, Davies B, McCown D. Comparing parent loss with sibling loss. *Death Studies.* 1999;21:1-15

12. Wallerstein JS, Lewis JM, Blakeslee S. *The Unexpected Legacy of Divorce: A 25-Year Landmark Study*. New York, NY: Hyperion; 2000

13. Johnston JR. Parental alignments and rejection: an empirical study of alienation in children of divorce. *J Amer Acad Psych Law.* 2003;31:158-170

14. Luecken LJ, Fabricius WV. Physical health vulnerability in adult children from divorced and intact families. *J Psychos Res.* 2003;55:221-228

15. Lansford JE, Malone PS, Castellino DR, et al. Trajectories of internalizing, externalizing, and grades for children who have and have not experienced their parents' divorce or separation. *J Family Psych.* 2006;20:292-301

16. Cherlin A, Furstenberg Jr F, Lindsay P, et al. Longitudinal studies of the effects of divorce on children in Great Britain and the United States. *Science.* 1991;252:1386-1389

17. Chase-Lansdale PL, Cherlin AJ, Kiernan KE. The long-term effects of parental divorce on the mental health of young adults: a developmental perspective. *Child Devel.* 1995;66: 1614-1634

18. Ge X, Natsuaki MN, Conger RD. Trajectories of depressive symptoms and stressful events among male and female adolescents in divorced and non divorced families. *Devel Psychopath.* 2006;18:253-273

19. Storksen I, Roysamb E, Mourn T, Tambs K. Adolescents with a childhood experience of parental divorce: a longitudinal study of mental health and adjustment. *J Adolesc.* 2005;28:725-739

20. Amato PR. Children of divorce in the 1990s: an update of the Amato and Keith (1991) meta-analysis. *J Family Psych.* 2001;15:355-370

21. Nord CW, Brimhall D, West J. *Fathers' Involvement in Their Children's Schools*. Washington, DC: National Center for Education Statistics; 1997

22. Menning CL. The absent parents are more than money: the joint effects of activities and financial support on youths' educational attainment. *J Family Iss.* 2002;23:648-671

23. Hetherington EM, Kelly J. *For Better or for Worse: Divorce Reconsidered*. New York, NY: Norton; 2002

24. Margolin L, Craft JL. Child abuse by caretakers. *Ethol Sociobio.* 1989;38:450-455

25. Hetherington EM, Stanley-Hagan M. The adjustment of children with divorced parents: a risk and resiliency perspective. *J Child Psychol.* 1999;40:129-140

26. Wolchik SA, Sandler IN, Millsap RE, et al. Six-year follow-up of preventive interventions for children of divorce: a randomized controlled trial. *JAMA.* 2002;288:1874-1881

27. Cohen GJ. American Academy of Pediatrics. Helping children and families deal with divorce and separation. *Pediatrics.* 2002;110:1019-1023

# CHAPTER 36

# Adoption and Adolescence

LISA ALBERS PROCK, MD, MPH

Adolescents with a history of adoption are a heterogeneous group; the reasons they join their adoptive families and the characteristics of those adoptive families are variable. Secular trends also affect the practice of adoption and are continuously changing. Specifically, children with a history of adoption in the 21st century will be growing up in a society with quite different expectations of open communication throughout the adoption process and different approaches to supporting the emotional health of adoptees (including a possible search for the birth family) than individuals with a history of adoption in previous generations. When working with adolescents and their families, providers should understand the effects of adoption history on the child's current health and presentation. Clearly, each child, family, and adoption experience is unique.

> **Box 36-1**
>
> ***Age of Child at Adoption Varies with Type***
>
> **Domestic private adoption** typically leads children to join their families during the newborn period. **Intercountry adoptees** most commonly join their families between 9 and 24 months of age (with a substantial minority being preschoolers, school-aged children, and even adolescents). Children adopted from the **US foster care system** have a mean age of 6.6 years at the time of joining their adoptive families.

## EPIDEMIOLOGY OF ADOPTION IN THE UNITED STATES

Approximately 120,000 nonrelated children have been adopted by families in the United States annually for at least the past 2 decades. More than 1.5 million children under 18 years of age (~2% of US children) have a history of adoption. Although the number of children affected by adoption over the past several decades has remained relatively stable, the preadoptive conditions for children entering the adoption process are continually changing.

Current estimates suggest that of the more than 100,000 children adopted in the United States by nonrelatives in 2007 and 2008 (excluding children adopted by extended family members in kinship adoptions or by stepparents), 25,000 to 30,000 were adopted via domestic private adoptions; 18,000 to 20,000 were adopted via intercountry adoption; and more than 50,000 were adopted via the domestic public system.[1] The age of a child at adoption is correlated with the type of adoption process involved (Box 36-1).

Over the past 4 decades, the relative number of infants available for domestic infant adoption in the United States has declined dramatically due to greater acceptance of single parenting along with increased access to family planning and abortion services. The past 2 decades were marked by a dramatic increase in adoption of children from other countries by families in the United States. More recently, however, there has been a decline in intercountry adoptions due to the implementation of intercountry adoption standards established by the Hague Convention in 1993. This convention has been accepted by the United States and more than 100 other countries. The convention defines minimum rights and procedures for intercountry adoptions and has led to closer regulation and integration of agencies and governments involved in the process.

## TERMINOLOGY

Although adoption of children into families has occurred for thousands of years, sensitivity to all individuals involved in the adoption process and related care in the use of terminology is a far more modern event. For example, discussing children who are **placed for adoption** rather than "given up for adoption" honors the planning process leading to the legal event of a child permanently joining a family. The term **adoption triad** is commonly used to describe those affected by adoption including **birth parents, adoptive parents,** and the **adoptee** or **adopted person**. Terms such as "real" or "natural" parent are best avoided as they may be considered pejorative to the adoptive parents. Although most adoptions from previous generations are best described as **closed** with respect to communication between adoptive and birth families, the current trend with domestic infant adoption, public adoptions, and even international adoption has increasingly been toward **openness with respect to communication in adoption**.

## OPENNESS IN ADOPTION: FACTORS PREDICTING SUCCESS

Communication between birth and adoptive families participating in "open adoptions" ranges along a spectrum from sharing letters and photographs between adoptive and birth families several times per year to telephone or in-person contact between triad members. In addition, some adoption arrangements that begin as closed arrangements may change with respect to degree of contact between triad members over time (eg, intercountry adoptions). Although all adoption triads are unique, research suggests that desired openness within the context of an adoption arrangement is greatly facilitated by adoptive and birth parents who demonstrate commitment, communication, flexibility, and mutual respect.[2] In 1 follow-up study of adolescents with a history of adoption, a higher degree of contact with birth parents resulted in higher satisfaction with contact status than in those with lesser or no contact.[3] In addition, although many children did not have interactions with their birth father, contact with a birth father was correlated with increased satisfaction with the adoption. However, most research looking at "openness" in adoption was conducted with healthy infants and their voluntarily relinquishing parents; it is unclear how the dynamics of an open adoption would work for any given child at various stages. Evidence suggests that open adoption is definitely not helpful if a parent is actively using substances, is violent, or is abusive toward a child or adolescent.

## IDENTITY DEVELOPMENT AND ADOPTION

A crucial and healthy task for all adolescents is working to develop a "sense of self." For adopted adolescents, an interest in and attempts to integrate the adoption history into their life story is quite normal. Adolescents may exhibit a range of responses to their adoptive history; some children/adolescents/young adults with a history of adoption are intensely interested in contact with their birth family whereas others show little interest in this topic. Adoption across racial lines, by single parents, or by same sex couples may add another layer of consideration with respect to identity development (Box 36-2).

### Box 36-2

### *Identity Development—Pointers for Providers and Adoptive Parents*

- Identity development is complex and is affected by factors that may be unique to the individual (eg, temperament, self-esteem), the family (eg, child/parent relationships, parental attitudes about adoption), and the community (eg, school, peers, birth family).
- Parents can assist their child's healthy and positive integration of the adoption history with a communication style that is open, supportive, and empathic.
- Access to information about one's birth family and adoptive circumstances generally facilitates positive adoptive identity development.
- For transracially adopted children, exposure to positive role models of the same race as the adoptee and the same socioeconomic status as the adoptive family is protective with respect to identity development.

Regardless of the age at the time of joining their family via adoption and the quality and length of any positive or negative preadoptive experiences, adolescents may be interested in many aspects of their history, including understanding the specific circumstances leading to their adoption for both their adoptive and birth parents; who they most resemble physically from their birth family; what, if any, medical and/or mental health concerns their birth family members may have and what the implications are for them in the future; and what members of their birth family have done and are currently doing with respect to education, careers, and family relationships.

Parents who adopt a child of a different race than themselves especially may benefit from explicit education about the prevalence of racism in society and the typical trajectory of racial identity development in all individuals. Especially for successful adults who have not experienced the effects of racism themselves, understanding the role race plays in the perceptions of others about a specific child, adolescent, or young adult is critical to optimally parenting a transracially adopted child.[4]

Transracial adoption can add an additional facet to identity development and can have relevance for all members of the adoption triad. Transracial adoption has a long history of controversy, with research prior to the past decade most often focused on black children adopted into white families. However, the racial mix of many families has become far more complex over the past several decades, in large part due to international adoption. Research often focuses on the effect of racial and ethnic experiences, rather than on how adolescent and young adult adoptees act on their environment to negotiate identities and their place in society.

Based on a review of the literature, Lee[5] has described 4 patterns or strategies that adopted children and their families may pursue with respect to racial/cultural identity development:

1. **Cultural assimilation:** adoptive parents reject or downplay differences
2. **Enculturation:** adoptive parents acknowledge differences within the family while promoting the child's learning about his/her birth culture and heritage
3. **Racial inculcation:** adoptive parents teach coping skills to facilitate their child's capacity to deal effectively with racism and discrimination
4. **Child choice:** adoptive parents provide children with cultural opportunities but ultimately abide by their children's interests

Longitudinal studies based on parent report suggest that adjustment problems are no more common in adulthood for children with a history of transracial adoption than for those with inracial adoptions. One 19-year follow-up study of transracial adoptees suggested that females were typically better adjusted than males and that Asian adoptees fared better than white or black adoptees.[6]

## DEVELOPMENTAL, BEHAVIORAL, AND MENTAL HEALTH CONCERNS

Research and clinical experience demonstrate that adoption of a child leads to many rewards and challenges for children and their parents. Research is unequivocal in supporting the benefits of adoption into a permanent family for children whose birth parents are unwilling or unable to care for them.[7,8] It is clear that most adopted individuals are well adjusted; however, it is also known that children and adolescents with a history of adoption (especially children adopted later in life) are overrepresented in inpatient and outpatient mental health settings.[9] Adopted children are reported to have an increased risk of learning, developmental, and emotional difficulties.[10,11] Population-based studies report an elevated risk for psychological maladjustment in adopted children compared with representative samples of nonadopted children.[12] A recent meta-analysis reported significantly more behavioral problems (based on questionnaire assessments—not clinical evaluations) among adoptees compared with nonadoptees, although the effect sizes were small.[13] In-depth clinical interviews of adolescent adoptees living in Minnesota and their parents also found that although most individuals adopted as infants are well adjusted and psychologically healthy, a subset of adoptees did present with an increased risk of externalizing behaviors.[10]

Many cognitive, behavioral, and mental health difficulties affecting children and adolescents with a history of adoption and their families may result from difficulties directly related to preadoptive factors. In fact, most serious developmental, learning, or emotional concerns for individuals with a history of adoption may have little to do with the adoptive family situation or dynamics and primarily can be linked to genetic, prenatal, perinatal, or other preadoptive experiences for a child, which are often not known at the time of adoption (Table 36-1).

**Table 36-1**

**Potential Preadoptive Factors that May Affect a Child's Developmental, Behavioral, and Emotional Status Postadoption**

| *Risk Category* | *Example of Known Risk Factor* |
|---|---|
| Birth family genetics | Schizophrenia |
| | Bipolar disorder |
| | Attention-deficit/hyperactivity disorders |
| | Alcohol |
| Prenatal exposures | Cocaine |
| | Prescription medications |
| | Prematurity |
| Perinatal experiences | Birth trauma |
| | Congenital infections |
| | Orphanage |
| Early childhood | Foster care |
| Environment | Lack of caring caregiver |
| | Lack of consistent environment |
| | Malnutrition |
| Poor health | Inadequate medical care |
| | Isolated neglect |
| | Physical abuse |
| Critical events | Sexual abuse |
| | Chronic neglect/chaos |
| | Multiple placements |

As would be expected regardless of an adoptive history, children with a history of prenatal substance exposure or preplacement deprivation are known to be at increased risk of having later social, cognitive, and emotional difficulties.[14,15] Older age at adoption has been correlated with greater developmental and behavioral challenges as well—likely related to the increased time of exposure to negative preadoptive factors.[16]

## ADOPTION MYTHS AND REALITIES

Adolescents or their parents may have questions about the affect of adoption on many aspects of an individual's long-term health and development, which may or may not come up during routine adolescent visits. At some point prior to or during adolescence, most adoptees or their adoptive parents will likely address the following questions:

### 1. WHEN IS THE "RIGHT" TIME TO DISCUSS MY CHILD'S HISTORY OF ADOPTION? IS THERE INFORMATION I SHOULD NOT SHARE?

Parents often begin discussing the history of adoption with the child shortly after the adoption process—even if this was an infant adoption. This approach allows parents to decrease their own anxiety about discussing the topic—as often a child's history of adoption into the family is linked with the parents' history of infertility and the acknowledgment that they will not have a biological connection with their child. Rather than having a solitary and isolated discussion of the history of adoption when the child can understand all of the details, most experts recommend presenting information about the history as the child asks and is able to understand it.[17,18] Families may find the use of a "life book" helpful in documenting the facts about their child's history as they learn them, and for having an ongoing discussion about that history. Sensitive information, such as birth parent substance abuse, incarceration, or mental health concerns, is best shared when children are old enough to understand the implications.

As a result of this approach, most children enter adolescence knowing most of the facts of their adoptive history and can begin to integrate what they know into their sense of self. For those children who have not been told of their adoption history before their teenage years, it is best that this key information be shared within the context of a professional therapeutic relationship, given the potential that emotionally charged material will be revealed in this life-changing discussion.

In addition to conversations between parents and their child about the history of adoption, families often struggle with "how much of their child's history to share" with extended family members, friends, schools, providers, and others who know their child. Ultimately there is no correct decision whether to "share or not share" information about a child's history beyond immediate family members. Key information about a child's history can be shared as needed to assist providers in understanding a child's struggles without providing sensitive details about the birth family history. Adoption professionals emphasize the importance of differentiating privacy (not sharing all information regarding a child's history with everyone) from secrecy (not sharing key information about one's own history with an adopted individual) when considering with whom to share adoptive information.[17,19]

### 2. WHAT SHOULD WE KNOW ABOUT "SEARCH AND REUNION" BETWEEN ADOPTEES AND BIRTH FAMILIES?

Generally the process of "searching" for one's birth family cognitively begins prior to adolescence with a natural curiosity about birth family members, but it may take on increased importance during adolescence in concert with other identity considerations. Although searching for birth parents is by no means universal, trends suggest an increase in the prevalence of adopted individuals searching for more information about their birth family and circumstances. Although some birth parents do search for their birth children, more typically it is the adopted person who initiates contact with birth parents. Adoptive parents are encouraged to allow their children to take the lead in the process but may be asked for assistance. Once a birth parent or birth sibling has been "found," individuals may continue the process and meet in person, known as a "reunion." A variety of factors may influence the outcome of a reunion, including the emotional stability and security of both the adopted and the birth relatives. In 1 follow-up study of adult adoptees up to 8 years postreunion, most adoptees reported that the search and contact experience was satisfying and worthwhile and helped to answer questions about their origins, background, and reasons for being placed; adoptive parents typically reported a fear of potential loss associated with "sharing their child," whereas 94% of birth mothers reported that they were pleased that the adopted adult had contacted them.[20,21]

Many individuals who search for information about, or a reunion with, their birth parents do not seek or want interference from professionals. However, clinicians should be knowledgeable about the process to help serve as a resource if needed. It is important to realize that many adoptees may be interested in searching but may feel guilty or disloyal to their adoptive family because of this desire. There are also very few social guidelines for negotiating a search and reunification process and all members of the triad may benefit from professional support.

### 3. DOES MY CHILD'S INTEREST IN SEARCHING FOR HIS OR HER BIRTH PARENTS/FAMILY SUGGEST DISCONTENT WITH OUR FAMILY?

Adopted parents frequently wonder if their child's interest in searching for the birth family suggests dissatisfaction with the adoptive family.[22] Although adopted persons who have had a negative adoptive experience are more likely to remain in contact with their birth mother after a reunion, those who described positive adoption experiences are just as likely to search for their birth family. In other words, although many people with a history of adoption do feel a need to know about their genetic and genealogical background, this desire does not supersede or supplant important relationships formed with their adoptive families.

### 4. IS THIS "NORMAL"—OR DOES MY CHILD/ FAMILY NEED HELP?

An interest in searching for adoptive family and developing one's own style and persona is typical for anyone with a history of adoption; but certainly this process may lead to emotional distress for children and their parents. Although individual counseling is sometimes indicated, family therapy may more often be a helpful approach to addressing the challenges being faced by all of the family members. In general, adoptive families may benefit from professional assistance if their children are presenting with emotional distress or functional impairment in the home and school settings or if they present with "acting out" behaviors that put themselves or others at risk.

## INTERNET AND PRINT RESOURCES

- Domestic Adoption—Adoptive Families. www.adoptivefamilies.com/domestic_adoption.php. Accessed November 12, 2009.
- Safeguarding the Rights and Well-Being of Birth Parents in the Adoption Process. Smith, S. Revised January, 2007. Evan B. Donaldson Adoption Institute. www.adoptioninstitute.org/research/2006_11_birthparent_wellbeing.php. Accessed November 12, 2009.
- US Department of Health and Human Services Administration for Children and Families. www.acf.hhs.gov/index.html. Accessed November 12, 2009.
- Tatum B. *Why Are All the Black Kids Sitting Together in the Cafeteria?* New York, NY: Basic Books; 1997.
- Pavao J. *The Family of Adoption*. Boston, MA: Beacon Press; 2005.

## REFERENCES

1. Adoptive Families. Domestic adoption. Available at: www.adoptivefamilies.com/domestic_adoption.php. Accessed November 12, 2009

2. Neil E, Beek M, Schofield G. Thinking about and managing contacts in permanent placements: the differences and similarities between adoptive parents and foster care. *Clin Child Psychol Psychiatry.* 2003;8:401-418

3. Grotevant H, McCroy R. The Minnesota/Texas adoption research project: implications of openness in adoption for development and relationship. *Appl Devel Sci.* 1997;1:168-186

4. Tatum B. *Why Are All the Black Kids Sitting Together in the Cafeteria?* New York, NY: Basic Books; 1997

5. Lee R. The transracial adoption paradox: history, research, and counseling implications of cultural socialization. *Counseling Psychologist.* 2003;31:711-744

6. Brooks D, Barth R. Adjustment outcomes of adult transracial and inracial adoptees: effects of race, gender, adoptive family structure, and placement history. *Am J Orthopsychiatry.* 1999;69:87-102

7. Brodzinsky DM, Pinderhughes EE. Parenting and child development in adoptive families. In: Bornstein M, ed. *Handbook of Parenting: Vol 1. Children and Parenting*. Mahwah, NJ: Lawrence Erlbaum Associates; 2002:279-311

8. Van IJzendoorn MH, Juffer F. The Emanuel Miller Memorial Lecture 2006: adoption as intervention. Meta-analytic evidence for massive catch-up and plasticity in physical, socio emotional, and cognitive development. *J Child Psychol Psychiatry.* 2006;47:1228-1245

9. Haugaard J. Is adoption a risk factor for the development of adjustment problems? *Clin Psychol Rev.* 1998;18(1):47-69

10. Keyes M, Sharma A, Elkins IJ, et al. The mental health of US adolescents adopted in infancy. *Arch Pediatr Adolesc Med.* 2008;162:419-425

11. Nickman SL, Rosenfeld AA, Fine P, et al. Children in adoptive families: overview and update. *J Am Acad Child Adolesc Psychiatry.* 2005;44(10):987-995

12. Verhulst FC, Althaus MS, Bieman HJ. Problem behavior in international adoptees, I: an epidemiological study. *J Am Acad Child Adolesc Psychiatry.* 1990;29(1):94-113

13. Juffer F, van IJzendoorn MH. Behavior problems and mental health referrals of international adoptees: a meta-analysis. *JAMA.* 2005;293(20):2501–2515

14. Beckett C, Maughan B, Rutter M, et al. Do the effects of early severe deprivation on cognition persist into early adolescence? Findings from the English and Romanian adoptees study. *Child Dev.* 2006;77(3):696–711

15. Nulman I, Rovet J, Greenbaum R, et al. Neurodevelopment of adopted children exposed in utero to cocaine: the Toronto Adoption Study. *Clin Invest Med.* 2001;24(3):129–137

16. Sharma AR, McGue M, Benson P. The emotional and behavioral adjustment of United States adopted adolescents, part II: age at placement. *Child Youth Serv Rev.* 1996;18(1-2): 101–114

17. Pavao J. *The Family of Adoption*. Boston, MA: Beacon Press; 2005

18. Brodzinsky DM, Schecter MD, Henig RM. *Being Adopted: The Lifelong Search for Self.* New York, NY: Doubleday; 1992

19. Brodzinsky DM, Smith DW, Brodzinsky AB. *Children's Adjustment to Adoption: Developmental and Clinical Issues.* Thousand Oaks, CA: Sage Publications; 1998

20. Howe D, Feast J. The long-term outcome of reunions between adult adopted people and their birth mother. *Br J Soc Work.* 2001;31:351–368

21. Wrobel G, Grotevant H, McRoy R. Adolescent search for birthparents: who moves forward? *J Adolesc Res.* 2004;19:132–151

22. Muller U, Perry B. Adopted persons' search for and contact with their birth parents I: who searches and why? *Adoption Q.* 2001;4:5–37

# CHAPTER 37

# Adolescents with Lesbian or Gay Parents

CHARLOTTE J. PATTERSON, PhD • RACHEL G. RISKIND, MA

How does parental sexual orientation affect adolescent development, if at all? This question has been posed in the context of legal and policy matters such as foster care, adoption, and custody proceedings and also from a conceptual standpoint. Some scholars argue that parental sexual orientation may affect adolescent issues such as exploration of sexuality and entrance into a larger peer group. Awareness of these discussions and of relevant empirical findings may help pediatricians who work with adolescents.

Families of adolescents with lesbian or gay parents may have been formed in a number of ways. Some adolescents began life in the context of a heterosexual marriage that later dissolved when 1 or both partners identified themselves as lesbian and/or gay. Other adolescents may have been conceived and born to parents already identified as lesbian or gay. Still others may have been adopted by lesbian or gay parents or they may be living with lesbian or gay foster parents. Thus, the families of adolescents with lesbian or gay parents are themselves a diverse group.

In the United States today, the legal environments of families with lesbian and gay parents are also varied, and these variations may have an effect on adolescents' social experiences.[1] In some parts of the country, an adolescent's same-sex parents may be legally married or may have completed adoptions that provide legal recognition of both parents. In other parts of the country, these options may not be available. To some degree, the social experiences of youth may reflect their legal and policy climates. For example, it is possible that children of married same-sex parents might experience less stigma than children of unmarried same-sex parents, or that children with legal connections to both parents might cope better with dissolution of their parents' relationship.

## HISTORY OF RESEARCH

Substantial literature on the development and adjustment of children with lesbian and gay parents has emerged over the past 25 years. Both longitudinal and cross-sectional studies, in the United States and abroad, have found that children of lesbian and gay parents are well adjusted and develop in ways similar to other children.[2-4] Many areas have been studied, including adjustment at home, at school, with peers, and in other domains. In all of these areas, the strength of parent–child relationships has been a more important predictor of adjustment than parental sexual orientation.[3]

Many mainstream professional organizations recognize the strength of these findings in official statements. For instance, after a careful review of the research findings, the American Psychological Association[5] has gone on record opposing "any discrimination based on sexual orientation in matters of adoption, child custody and visitation, foster care, and reproductive health services." After its review of research in this area, the American Academy of Pediatrics (AAP)[4] similarly recognized "that a considerable body of professional literature provides evidence that children with parents who are homosexual can have the same advantages and the same expectations for health, adjustment, and development as can children whose parents are heterosexual." These and other mainstream professional groups, including the American Bar Association, the Child Welfare League of America, and the National Association of Social Workers, have based their policies on findings from social science research suggesting that parental sexual orientation is not a good predictor of parenting ability or child adjustment.

The fact that youngsters with lesbian or gay parents appear to be developing in positive ways should not suggest that they never experience difficulties. Like other members of stigmatized minority groups, the offspring of lesbian and gay parents sometimes encounter antigay bigotry and discrimination.[6,7] This experience is likely to be more common in some environments than in others, but evidence for the impact of such experiences on overall adjustment is lacking.

Most studies to date have focused on young children, with less research conducted on *adolescent* offspring of lesbian or gay parents. Some writers argue for caution when generalizing the results of research conducted with young children to adolescents.[4] Because adolescence is a time when personal identity, peers, and dating are likely to be salient, this is a key period to examine development of youth with nonheterosexual parents.

A small body of research focuses on the development of adolescent offspring in families headed by lesbian couples. Some studies compare adolescents with lesbian mothers to those with heterosexual mothers. For example, Huggins[8] reported a study of 18 adolescents with divorced heterosexual and 18 with divorced lesbian mothers in which she found no differences in adolescent self-esteem as a function of mothers' sexual orientation. No reliable differences have been reported between adolescents reared by lesbian parents and those reared by heterosexual parents. It should be noted that there is research on children of gay fathers, which are generally consistent with the findings for children of lesbian parents, but to date there has been no published research on adolescents raised by gay fathers.

Some studies have focused on individual differences among those with lesbian or gay parents. For instance, O'Connor[9] studied 11 young men and women who were the offspring of divorced or separated lesbian mothers. Her participants expressed strong loyalty and protectiveness toward their mothers, but some also described worries about losing friends or being judged by others because of their mothers' sexual orientation. Gershon, Tschann, and Jemerin[10] studied self-esteem, perception of stigma, and coping skills among 76 adolescent offspring of lesbian mothers. They reported that among adolescents with lesbian mothers, those who perceived more stigma related to having a lesbian mother had lower self-esteem in a number of areas, such as social acceptance and self-worth.

Tasker and Golombok's[11] longitudinal study included a slightly older population, consisting of 23 young adult offspring of lesbian mothers and a matched group of 23 young adult offspring of heterosexual mothers. In this generally well-adjusted sample, young men and women reared by lesbian mothers were no more likely than those reared by heterosexual mothers to experience depression or anxiety or to have sought professional help for psychiatric problems. They reported having close friendships during adolescence and were no more likely to remember peer group hostility than those from other families.

The Tasker and Golombok study also focused on the development of sexual identity. These authors distinguished among sexual attractions (ie, to whom is a person sexually attracted), sexual behaviors (ie, with whom a person participates in sexual activities), and sexual identity (ie, identification as lesbian, gay, or heterosexual). Tasker and Golombok's results showed that although offspring of lesbian mothers were no more likely to report same-sex sexual attractions than those from heterosexual families, they were more likely to have been involved in a same-sex sexual relationship. The offspring of lesbian mothers were, however, no more likely than those with heterosexual mothers to identify themselves as lesbian or gay. As intriguing as they are, these results were derived from a small, nonrepresentative sample, so they should be considered preliminary in nature.

## RESEARCH BASED ON REPRESENTATIVE SAMPLES

Review of earlier research indicated a need to study a more comprehensive set of outcomes for adolescents who live with same-sex parents. The National Longitudinal Study of Adolescent Health (known as Add Health) provided an opportunity for such research. The Add Health study assessed adolescent adjustment in a near-representative sample of American adolescents. Assessments focused on many topics, including aspects of adolescents' psychosocial well-being, school functioning, romantic relationships and behaviors, risky behaviors such as substance use, and peer relations. This study also examined family and relationship variables, including parents' assessment of the quality of the parent–teen relationship as well as adolescents' perceptions of parental warmth, care from adults and peers, integration into the neighborhood, and autonomy. The Add Health database thus afforded a broad overview of adolescent adjustment.

A series of studies by Patterson and her colleagues[12-14] drew upon data from Add Health to assess adjustment among adolescent offspring of same-sex parents and to explore individual differences in adjustment and behavior within this group. The sample included 88 families, half of whom were headed by mothers with female partners and half of whom were headed by other-sex couples. This group of families was demographically similar to the population from which it was drawn. Thus, research compared adolescents living with same-sex couples to a matched group of those living with other-sex couples on a broad range of outcomes.

Findings revealed that adolescents living with same-sex couples were no different in their overall adjustment than those living with other-sex couples. For instance, on self-report measures of well-being, such as measures of self-esteem, there were no reliable differences between those living with same-sex couples and those living with other-sex couples. On measures of depression and anxiety, there were likewise no differences. Adolescents' self-reported adjustment did not vary as a function of family type.[12]

Relationships within the family were also unrelated to family type.[12] For instance, adolescents were asked to report on the warmth and closeness of their relationships with parents, and no differences in this regard emerged between those living with same-sex couples and those living with other-sex couples. The same kinds of results were obtained from parental reports on the closeness of their relationships with adolescents. In short, no differences in the qualities of family relationships were attributable to family type.[12]

Peer relations—especially romantic relationships—are particularly important in adolescence, and data revealed no differences in this regard between those living with same-sex and other-sex couples.[14] For instance, adolescent reports about closeness and other qualities of peer relationships were unrelated to family type. Similarly, peer reports on the popularity of adolescents in the study were unrelated to family type. An adolescent's likelihood of participating in a romantic relationship in recent months or of becoming sexually active were likewise unrelated to family type. The likelihood of peer victimization was also unrelated to family type.[13] In summary, peer relations were not significantly associated with family type in this sample.[14]

The Add Health data also explored questions about substance use and delinquent behavior. Results showed that adolescents living with same-sex couples were no more and no less likely than those living with other-sex couples to report using alcohol, tobacco, or other drugs. Self-reported delinquent behavior such as vandalism and shoplifting was also unrelated to family type in this sample. Overall, the similarities in adjustment among adolescents living with same-sex and other-sex couples were remarkable.

If parental sexual orientation is not a good predictor of adolescent outcomes, what is a strong predictor? A substantial body of research indicates that parenting style influences effectiveness of parents' efforts to socialize both children and adolescents.[15] In particular, a warm, accepting style of parenting is related to optimal outcomes for adolescents, especially if it is combined with appropriate limit-setting and monitoring of adolescent behavior. An association between parental warmth and positive outcomes has been found for adolescents from a wide variety of ethnic, socioeconomic, and family structure backgrounds,[15] and by researchers working with a variety of methodological approaches.

As expected on the basis of earlier research with children, adolescent adjustment was strongly related to qualities of parent–adolescent relationships in the Add Health sample.[12-14] For example, adolescents who described closer relationships with their parents were less likely to be depressed, and they did better in school.[12] Those describing closer relationships with their parents were also more likely to report having strong friendships with peers and were described by others as being more central to peer networks.[14] They were less likely to report using tobacco, alcohol, and marijuana or engaging in delinquent behavior.[13] Overall, the qualities of adolescent relationships with their parents were strongly associated with many important outcomes, and adolescent behavior and adjustment were much more closely associated with the qualities of family relationships than with family type.

## CONCLUSION

Research results to date provide no evidence that parental sexual orientation has a measurable impact on child or adolescent development. In fact, when considering youth development, research findings suggest that the qualities of the relationships adolescents enjoy with their parents are more important than parental sexual orientation.

Some might be tempted to dismiss the results reported in this research with the saying that "one cannot prove the null hypothesis." In other words, one cannot prove that adolescents with lesbian or gay parents are identical to those with heterosexual parents. To react in this way, however, would be to miss the central message of the research findings. Whether or not a measurable impact of parental sexual orientation on adolescent development is ultimately identified, the main conclusions from research to date will remain. Whatever associations between adolescent outcomes and parental sexual orientation exist, they seem less important than those between adolescent outcomes and qualities of family relationships.

These conclusions have important ramifications for policy and legal issues currently the subject of vigorous public debate.[1] For instance, as the AAP[4] has recognized, findings provide no support for those who would make lesbian or gay adults ineligible to become adoptive or foster parents. Similarly, results of research provide no empirical rationale for depriving lesbian mothers or gay fathers of custody or visitation when these are contested on grounds of parental sexual orientation.[1] As the research findings are increasingly made available to legislators and judges by way of policy statements, amicus briefs, and related strategies, they are also becoming part of the public discourse on these issues.

Findings of this research are also of great interest from a theoretical standpoint. If adolescents with same-sex parents fare as well as those with other-sex parents, as appears to be the case, then traditional ideas about gender development may need to be reconsidered. Data on adolescents with lesbian and gay parents suggest that it is the quality of parenting rather than the gender or sexual orientation of parents that is significant for youngsters' development.[3]

In summary, it does not appear that the development of adolescents with lesbian or gay parents is disadvantaged in significant ways. Pediatricians should be sensitive to discrimination and other issues that can accompany minority status, but they should not assume that any problems experienced by an adolescent stem from parental sexual orientation.

## REFERENCES

1. Patterson CJ. Lesbian and gay family issues in the context of changing legal and social policy environments. In: Bieschke KJ, Perez RM, DeBord KA, eds. *Handbook of Counseling and Psychotherapy with Lesbian, Gay, Bisexual and Transgender Clients.* 2nd ed. Washington, DC: American Psychological Association; 2007

2. Patterson CJ. Sexual orientation and family life: a decade review. *J Marriage Fam.* 2000;62:1052–1069

3. Patterson CJ. Children of lesbian and gay parents. *Curr Dir Psychol Sci.* 2006;15:241–244

4. Perrin EC, Committee on Psychosocial Aspects of Child and Family Health. Technical report: co-parent or second-parent adoption by same-sex partners. *Pediatrics.* 2002;109:341–344

5. American Psychological Association. *Resolution on Sexual Orientation, Parents, and Children.* Washington, DC: American Psychological Association; 2004

6. Gartrell N, Deck A, Rodas C, Peyser H, Banks A. The National Lesbian Family Study: 4. Interviews with the 10-year-old children. *Am J Orthopsychiatry.* 2005;75:518–524

7. Goldberg AE. (How) does it make a difference? Perspectives of adults with lesbian, gay, and bisexual parents. *Am J Orthopsychiatry.* 2007;7:550–562

8. Huggins SL. A comparative study of self-esteem of adolescent children of divorced lesbian mothers and divorced heterosexual mothers. In: Bozett FW, ed. *Homosexuality and the Family.* New York, NY: Harrington Park Press; 1989:123–135

9. O'Connor A. Voices from the heart: the developmental impact of a mother's lesbianism on her adolescent children. *Smith Coll Stud Soc Work.* 1993;63:281–299

10. Gershon TD, Tschann JM, Jemerin JM. Stigmatization, self-esteem, and coping among the adolescent children of lesbian mothers. *J Adolesc Health.* 1999;24:437–445

11. Tasker FL, Golombok S. *Growing Up in a Lesbian Family: Effects on Child Development.* New York, NY: Guilford Press; 1997

12. Wainright JL, Russell ST, Patterson CJ. Psychosocial adjustment, school outcomes, and romantic relationships of adolescents with same-sex parents. *Child Development.* 2004;75:1886–1898

13. Wainright JL, Patterson CJ. Delinquency, victimization, and substance use among adolescents with female same-sex parents. *J Fam Psychol.* 2006;20:526–530

14. Wainright JL, Patterson CJ. Peer relations among adolescents with female same-sex parents. *Dev Psychol.* 2008;44:117–126

15. Collins WA, Steinberg L. Adolescent development in interpersonal context. In: Damon W, Lerner RM, Eisenberg N, eds. *Handbook of Child Psychology, Volume 3: Social, Emotional, and Personality Development.* 6th ed. New York, NY: Wiley; 2006

# CHAPTER 38

## Family Systems Approaches to Adolescent Health and Illness

MARY SPAGNOLA-MARSH, PhD • ANTHONY R. PISANI, PhD • SUSAN H. McDANIEL, PhD

### INTRODUCTION

Medical family therapy (MedFT) is an approach to psychotherapy that includes attention to health and illness and emphasizes collaboration between behavioral and biomedical health professionals in the care of patients and their families.[1,2] MedFT is a practical application of the biopsychosocial model[3–5] and family systems theory[3,6] in psychotherapy. Family systems medicine (FSM) applies these same principles outside of formal psychotherapy in routine health care. Adolescent health professionals across a spectrum of settings can draw upon the principles of FSM and MedFT to achieve patient health care goals.

Practitioner roles and patient and family needs determine how these principles are applied. Physicians and nurses generally apply FSM in the direct medical care of an adolescent in consultation with family members and in collaborative referral. Mental health professionals use MedFT in direct psychotherapy intervention and collaboration with the health care team. Doherty and Baird's[7] 5 levels of physician involvement with families provide a helpful guide for thinking about how an adolescent health professional might incorporate techniques and principles of FSM and MedFT (Table 38-1). Almost all adolescent health professionals are proficient in FSM, which includes level 2 (information and collaboration with families) and level 3 (dealing with feelings and support of the patient and family members). Some medical providers have had family systems training during their professional education and are proficient in level 4 (family assessment/counseling).[2] At level 4, the practitioner takes an active role in helping families identify and address dynamics that adversely affect their patients. Level 5 is MedFT and requires specialty family therapy training—several years of didactic and supervised psychotherapy experience. (Information about an annual 5-day training experience in MedFT for health and mental health professionals is available at: www.urmc.rochester.edu/smd/psych/educ_train/family/MFTI.cfm.)

With this understanding in mind, the goal of this chapter is to familiarize adolescent health professionals with the conceptual and practical aspects of MedFT. This chapter includes an overview of MedFT, its origins, and supporting evidence; a discussion of medical illness and normal adolescent development and how FSM and MedFT might help families and practitioners navigate this challenging intersection; case

**Table 38-1**

**Levels of Family Involvement**

| *Level* | *Description* |
|---|---|
| 1 | Minimal contact<br>Families are dealt with for practical or legal reasons. One-way communication prevails. |
| 2 | Information and collaboration<br>Communicate information clearly to patients and families. Elicit questions and areas of concern, and generate mutually agreed-upon action plans. |
| 3 | Feelings and support<br>Demonstrate empathic listening and elicit expressions of feelings and concerns from patients and families. Normalize feelings and emotional reactions to illness. |
| 4 | Family assessment/counseling<br>Assess the relationship between the illness problem and family dynamics. If the problem is not complex or longstanding, work with the family to achieve change. If the problem is entrenched or family counseling is not effective, make a referral and educate the family and therapist about what to expect. Continue to collaborate. |
| 5 | Medical family therapy<br>Medical family therapy is intensive specialty care delivered by professionals with advanced psychotherapy training. Physicians or other medical providers should collaborate closely on those patients with whom they have active involvement. |

Adapted with permission from Doherty WJ, Baird MA. Developmental levels in family-centered medical care. *Family Medicine*. 1986;18(3):153.

example that illustrate the application of MedFT to practice, including diabetes, eating disorders, and somatic depression; and a brief guide to referral and collaboration.

## MEDICAL FAMILY THERAPY: SCIENTIFIC, CONCEPTUAL, AND HISTORICAL ROOTS

### SCIENTIFIC ROOTS: FAMILIES, SYSTEMS, AND HEALTH

There is substantial evidence that family relationships, physical illness, and other health outcomes are interconnected.[2,8-12] Family variables have as strong a relationship with physical health as other, traditional medical risk factors, such as cigarette smoking.[13] Adolescent health researchers have also found a relationship between family functioning and adolescent health.

The affective environment in the home predicts health outcomes across a range of illnesses and health risks.[14-18] Among adolescents with diabetes, parental attitudes of acceptance predict greater health care-related self-efficacy and fewer depressive symptoms,[19] and critical parenting, along with externalizing behavior problems, are associated with higher levels of hemoglobin A1c (HbA1c).[20] Parent and family connectedness protects against suicide attempts in adolescence, regardless of ethnicity or gender.[21] Conversely, problematic family relations adversely affect treatment of anorexia nervosa, leading to lower rates of remission of adolescents following family therapy for the condition.[22] Emotionally meaningful family rituals (such as regular mealtimes) are predictors of health and adjustment in adolescents across various health conditions; asthma,[23] neurofibratosis 1,[24] as well as substance use and sexual activity,[14] all are affected by these family dynamics. Mechanisms for the connection between family functioning and health are complex and often indirect, but the relationships are consistent and generally moderate to strong, especially for health conditions for which treatment requires significant alterations in lifestyle.

### Conceptual and Historical Roots

Engel[4,25] foreshadowed scientific discoveries regarding the interdependence of biological, psychological, individual, family, and community systems. Drawing on general systems theory,[26] he described the biopsychosocial model. The biopsychosocial approach promotes a holistic view of illness as residing simultaneously at multiple levels of life—from action at the molecular level up to interaction with the surrounding culture and society. Engel developed the biopsychosocial model partly in response to reductionist versions of the biomedical model, which neglected the person and context of disease and illness in favor of a biological viewpoint.

Around the time that Engel was developing his systems approach to illness and health, family theorists and therapists were drawing on general systems theory to understand change, health, and dysfunction in human behavior and relationships. Family systems theory posits that the whole (the family) is more than a simple sum of its parts (the family members) and that assessment and intervention in family processes and structures can produce a lasting change in the symptoms and behaviors observed in individual family members.

Family systems medicine[2] and MedFT[1] joined the biopsychosocial model with family systems theory. These interdisciplinary approaches came from efforts among family therapists and family physicians working in tandem to care for individuals with complex medical and behavioral health problems. These family systems-based health and mental health approaches focus health care providers and families on the interplay between health and relationships and propose techniques to address the interaction.

An underlying premise of family-oriented care, supported by the research cited previously, is an ecological approach to illness in which it is assumed that illness in one family member affects the entire family and family dynamics also influence the course of disease for the patient. For example, Patterson[27] cautioned that chronic illness draws a disproportionate amount of family energy and resources to the individual with the illness, sometimes at the expense of other family members. One person experiences the physical aspect of an illness, but no one in the family is untouched.

### Goals: Agency and Communion

The overarching goal of family systems approaches to health care is to increase *agency* and *communion*.[1] **Agency** refers to the sense that individuals can and should make personal choices when dealing with their own illness, treatment, and the health care system delivering that treatment. For example, an adolescent health care professional asks a 15-year-old female with asthma which type of delivery system for her daily, inhaled corticosteroid she thinks would best suit her lifestyle. Or, an adolescent with diabetes conducts an Internet search about new insulin pump technology. Because adolescents are often preoccupied with their own independence, agency is relevant to the developmental needs of adolescent patients. Supporting agency is central to success with this patient category.

**Communion** refers to the goal of being cared for, connecting with others, and feeling supported by family and community members when experiencing illness or navigating the health care system. Because the development of autonomy is salient in adolescence, most health care professionals are highly attuned to the need for agency. Support for communion, on the other hand, can get lost. In pediatrics, for example, parents are sometimes excluded from key aspects of the care process once their child has made the transition to having privacy for his or her physical examination or has reached the age of majority. Family systems medicine and MedFT advocate for ongoing assessment of the balance between agency and communion. This balance is important in the care of adolescents because the role parents and family members play may be harder to detect than with a younger child.

For example, the parents of Jo, a teenage athlete with asthma, cheer her from the bleachers while she plays soccer. They watch the game, but also her breathing, prepared to run to the sidelines with a rescue inhaler if needed. The girl does not perceive this as parental support of her illness. If asked, she would deny knowing that her parents bring an inhaler with them. She thinks she doesn't need that kind of support, but her parents are not yet convinced. Like many adolescents, Jo overestimates the degree of her separation from family support. As health care providers, we run the risk of doing the same. Careful attention to the balance between agency and communion can be a good antidote, helping remind the family and health care team that physical and psychological health do not rest with either complete independence or complete reliance on family members, rather with a balance of each.[28]

## ADOLESCENCE: A TIME OF INDIVIDUATION AND CONNECTEDNESS

As noted throughout this textbook, adolescence is a time of physical, emotional, cognitive, and social changes. Development in these domains may be asynchronous and unpredictable. Yet there are basic commonalities of the adolescent experience. Common developmental tasks of adolescence include increased intimacy of peer and romantic relationships, a maturing sexual identity, and increasingly focused educational/vocational goals. Developing independence from the family while maintaining emotional closeness (individuation) is also a goal. The complication of illness makes individuation a challenging developmental task for adolescents and their families. In this chapter, we focus on individuation as a developmental process relevant to family functioning, adolescent health, FSM, and MedFT.

## INDIVIDUATION

Although the term individuation may indicate a process by which adolescents pull away from family, move toward friends, and autonomously forge their own identity, nothing could be further from the truth. Individuation is relational and systemic; it takes place within the context of the family and requires negotiation, adaptation, and flexibility from all family members to be successful. Because the family is a system, this process stimulates changes beyond the adolescent—in the nature of family relationships.[2]

### Conflict and Closeness

Blos[29] argued that parent–child conflict spurs the progression toward individuation. Popular cultural myths portray adolescence as a time fraught with turmoil and rejection of parental beliefs and values, a time of "storm and stress." The truth is less dramatic—most adolescents report that they feel close to their parents, value their beliefs, and respect their opinions.[30]

This does not mean there is no conflict. In fact, moderate conflict with warmth and support for increased autonomy are important for healthy individuation. Moderate conflict paired with support indicates better adjustment in adolescents than either no conflict at all or high conflict.[31] Observational studies have found that families can encourage higher self-esteem, psychosocial competence, and reduced depression by allowing adolescents to express independent thoughts while simultaneously maintaining connection and warmth.[32–35]

### Family Roles, Individuation, and Illness

Family relationships are altered as individuation is negotiated. Progressing from childhood to adulthood, the adolescent takes on increasing responsibility in her or his own health care decisions and behaviors. Along with this responsibility comes the necessity to develop the skills needed to manage illness and treatment. Viner[36] described this as part of the wider developmental transition toward autonomy. The movement toward increasing autonomy of health behavior exists alongside a continued connectedness with parents, as there is still a need for their support during the transition.[34,37] It is no longer appropriate for parents to take *full* responsibility for all health care decisions, yet adolescents are rarely ready to assume full responsibility themselves. In addition, the nature of the support might differ, with instrumental support (administering medications) being gradually replaced by emotional support (discussing the pros and cons of a new treatment). It can be difficult for parents to recognize when to provide more support and when to provide less.

By the time a child reaches adolescence, his or her family may already have practice negotiating the balance between support and independence. For example, children with asthma may be taught to recognize when they are having trouble breathing during the preschool years, to learn how to use the inhaled medication with assistance during the early school years, and to take their rescue medication independently during gym class in the later school years. Ideally, parents will have gradually assisted their child throughout their development to engage in aspects of their own health care.

## THE FAMILY, MEDICAL ADHERENCE, AND THE TRANSFER OF RESPONSIBILITY

Unfortunately, the shift in balance of responsibility from parents to adolescents does not necessarily predict adherence with recommended medical treatment. McQuaid and colleagues[38] found that adherence to asthma medication was inversely related to age, despite its positive association with illness knowledge and reasoning. Increased agency by itself does not mean increased adherence.

Reasons for decreased adherence vary. The adolescent may have made a conscious decision not to adhere, or may decide to test the limits of the prescribed treatment regimen. Poor adherence may result from a desire to participate more fully in peer activities limited by medications and prevention measures. Limited insight related to cognitive development may have an impact.[39] These explanations cast poor adherence as common and normal in the process of individuation. Optimally, an increase in adherence follows this stage.

As an alternate explanation, medical illness in the adolescent may compromise, and may be compromised by, individuation. This is a greater cause for concern. For adolescents preoccupied with asserting independence from their family at the cost of connectedness, reduced adherence may be used as a tool to express anger or resentment.[40] By asserting independence in their health care decisions, adolescents may react against parents who grant less autonomy in general. It may also be a reaction related to resentment for having the illness. Although such behavior is often interpreted as "independence," it is actually a manifestation of "counterdependence," doing the opposite of what is prescribed.

Shaw[40] describes a pattern in which the adolescent adheres poorly and denies doing so. The goal of this behavior is to pull parents into the role of primary responsibility for their health care. In this respect, poor adherence may be a way to signal the need for more connectedness. Another (and more optimistic) explanation is that this difficult role transition requires a period of experimentation. The adolescent may eventually get back on track; skipping doses, making poor dietary choices, and ignoring symptom triggers can be part of a learning process.

## FAMILY-ORIENTED HEALTH CARE FOR ADOLESCENTS

Coordinated, shared responsibility for health care (including a health care professional, family members, and the adolescent) with periodic renegotiation of responsibility is ideal.[41] There is no particular age that should mark the shift to more autonomous care. It depends on an adolescent's individual level of readiness as well as the complexity of disease management. Poor adherence in the context of adolescent individuation often has many underlying factors. The process of individuation and subsequent illness-related outcomes is likely to be bidirectional or transactional, with each having an influence on the other.

Despite increasing autonomy in the teen years (more time spent with peers and greater involvement in school activities), the family continues to play a major role in the daily lives of adolescents. Most adolescents remain under parental guardianship and control, and most value their parents' opinions on important matters.[30,32] Yet health care providers often see adolescent patients alone. In many cases, adolescents may prefer to discuss private health matters (such as sexual behavior, substance use, or mental health concerns) with their physician and not their parents. This is developmentally appropriate. Private, individual meetings with adolescents may also be a well-intentioned attempt to involve adolescents in responsible self-care, communicating they should be ready to take charge of their own disease management. It may be that family will not be brought in until there is a health problem resulting from the illness or its treatment. But involving the larger family unit early may prevent and address illness-related problems.

Although the focus has been on medical adherence and individuation, including the family of an adolescent is helpful during initial diagnosis to address illness-related sibling difficulties and school or peer problems, among others. A family systems approach is not "1 more thing to add on" and does not generally pose threats to the already brief time physicians have with patients, as it can be integrated into a routine office visit. If the physician identifies an area of concern that would benefit from MedFT, a referral or consultation request may be made.

# MEDICAL FAMILY THERAPY CASE ILLUSTRATIONS

Core concepts and strategies for family systems interventions are (1) support for agency and communion, (2) collaboration with family members and treatment teams, and (3) attention to individual and family developmental issues. In the next section, 3 case-based interventions—for type I diabetes mellitus, anorexia nervosa, and somatic depression—highlight these concepts and strategies.

## CASE #1: RESTORING THE BALANCE BETWEEN COMMUNION AND ADOLESCENT AGENCY: TYPE I DIABETES MELLITUS

### Referral

A 15-year-old Mexican-American boy, Manuel, was referred by his physician, Dr Boyer, for difficulty following his diabetes management plan. Manuel was nonadherent with tracking blood glucose and carbohydrate intake, and with self-administering insulin. His physician reported that Manuel's HbA1c had been consistently high, putting the boy at risk for premature diabetes-related health problems.

### Background

Manuel and his mother agreed to consult with a medical family therapist. At first, Manuel spoke reluctantly about his illness. He reported feeling "just fine," stated that he took his medicine correctly, tracked his glucose "sort of" and "most of the time." Manuel's mother disagreed and added that Manuel "never" does what she asks him to.

In gathering family history, the therapist learned that Manuel's father died from diabetes-related complications the previous year. Prior to that, his father and his brother Gus had taken primary responsibility for Manuel's disease management. After his father's death, Manuel was given responsibility for his care. This coincided with starting high school. According to his mother, "We felt at that time that since Manuel was in high school, he was old enough to do this on his own." Unfortunately, this was the same year Gus moved from the family home to his own apartment.

### Treatment Approach

Medical family therapy seeks to find solutions within the family and to restore proper balance between agency and communion. In this case, Manuel's sense of agency was unsupported by communion and therefore failed to bring about desired health outcomes. Because Gus had once supported Manuel's diabetes management, the medical family therapist asked the family to invite him to the next session. Gus revealed that he motivated his brother to manage his diabetes by spending time with him. He would play football with him only on the condition that his glucose reading was stable and low. Manuel denied that he was motivated by that strategy but acknowledged that it was easier and more fun in the house when Gus was there. It was easier to manage his diabetes when his brother "bugged him" at the end of the day. After brainstorming, Gus said he would call Manuel after school to go through his "checklist" and that they would do something together on the weekend.

This case provides an example of improving Manuel's adherence by increasing his sense of *communion.* Manuel needed to feel closer to his family and to involve his brother in his care once again. The family responded by accommodating his need for care. However, the circle of support would be incomplete if it did not loop back to the referring physician. The therapist and physician spoke the day after Manuel's next medical appointment. Dr Boyer reported that Manuel's glucometer data indicated lower blood glucose levels over the past several days. Together they 2 decided to support Gus' continued involvement by calling him from Manuel's exam room at every visit.

## CASE #2: ATTENTION TO INDIVIDUAL AND FAMILY DEVELOPMENTAL PROCESSES: ANOREXIA NERVOSA

### Referral

Nearing the end of her inpatient treatment for anorexia nervosa, 14-year-old Alicia, and her parents, Ellen and David, were referred by her physician for MedFT. During her inpatient stay, Alicia gained 10 lbs. She protested and said she would restrict her eating and lose the weight as soon as she was discharged. Her parents were unsure that they would be able to maintain the structure and support of the hospital environment and were afraid that her progress would be reversed at home, as she had threatened would happen.

### Background

Alicia's parents first noticed symptoms the summer before her freshman year in high school, when Alicia was anxious about making new friends and leaving her small, private school for a large, public school. That same summer, Alicia's parents argued often about David's increase in hours at work that made him unavailable for family activities. Her sister had also moved out of the house to begin college. Shared family dinners and activities together on weekends had ceased. Alicia increased her ballet practices to 5 times a week, and began running to "get in shape." She began a "healthy, vegetarian diet." Prior to her illness, Alicia had always been concerned with doing what was right. Her parents had never found it necessary to enforce rules because Alicia never broke them, being described as "self-disciplining" by her parents. When she became symptomatic, Alicia "was a different person"—defiant and demanding of her parents' attention and neglectful of friends. As school began, Alicia dropped from 115 to 90 lbs and was hospitalized.

### Treatment Approach

In part, Alicia's illness was a response to a perceived "push" toward independence. Recent life events separated her, emotionally and physically, from family members. This coincided with a desire to stay connected with her family because she was apprehensive about establishing new peer relationships. Although it may not have been apparent to Alicia, increased time spent at home and restrictive eating acted as a signal to her family members, eliciting concern and caregiving. While approaching increased autonomy, Alicia still desired continued closeness with her family. By refusing to eat, Alicia's behavior prompted her parents to re-establish a caregiving role by focusing on her needs and becoming responsible for her physical wellness.

As Alicia prepared for discharge, the medical family therapist addressed Ellen and David's concerns. He learned about the family's schedule, routines, and mealtime habits. An important component of home-based follow-up care was to prescribe a consistent family meal each day. During the meal, Ellen and David were to replicate the structure and expectations of her therapeutic meals in the hospital. While Alicia was still an inpatient, the medical family therapist met with the family and medical staff during a therapeutic meal. She coached family members on handling Alicia's attempts to restrict her eating and to create conflict at the table. She emphasized a warm, supportive atmosphere with structure, clear expectations for behavior, and calm consistency in response to expected resistance by Alicia regarding normal eating.

During the next meeting, the family shared a meal in the hospital. Ellen and David practiced their roles as monitors of their daughter's food choices and intake. They were supported by the medical family therapist and hospital staff, learning to normalize family mealtime while adhering to treatment goals. Following discharge, the family continued weekly outpatient appointments. They encouraged Alicia to be more independent during meals by reducing their roles as meal monitors as she gained weight. They also allowed her to gradually resume activities as she continued to demonstrate increasing competence in self-care.

Mealtimes presented a point of entry to address developmentally based issues related to Alicia's eating disorder and overall family functioning. The mealtime intervention was effective in 3 ways: (1) it promoted healthy eating and behavioral goals of recovery related to Alicia's physical condition; (2) it supported individuation and reintroduced Ellen and David's parenting roles; and (3) it brought the family back together, both physically and emotionally, as dinnertime became a meaningful, shared routine. Alicia also made progress in her peer relationships. She made new friends at school and enjoyed activities with peers away from home without losing her sense of connection with her parents. The family continued to make dinnertime a priority, even after recovery was well underway.

## CASE #3: INTRODUCING A MEDICAL FAMILY THERAPIST IN CASES OF DEPRESSION WITH SOMATIZATION

### Referral

Sixteen-year-old Samuel presented with both of his parents for an infectious diseases consultation at the request of his primary care pediatrician when the boy failed to recover as expected from what seemed to be a flu-like illness. He had not returned to school after being sick because "I never got my energy back." Sam complained of dizziness and diffuse stomach and head pain, which overtook him at unpredictable moments each day. The pediatrician found no organic explanation for the persistent symptoms and referred the boy to an infectious disease specialist in response to parental pressure for a second opinion.

### Infectious Diseases Consultation

The parents vocalized surprise, worry, and frustration to the specialist. Sam had never had any medical or school-related problems. Samuel's grandfather died of "belly cancer" when Sam's father was a teenager; Sam's father asked if Sam could be tested to make sure he didn't have the same thing. On interview, Sam was cooperative but distant and lethargic. He stated that he wanted to go back to school but couldn't because of pain, fatigue, and dizziness. His parents reported that Sam would sleep in his room all day and stay up at night listening to music. They could see him feeling more and more down as the illness dragged on with no medical explanation or useful treatment.

The infectious diseases specialist suggested a medical family therapist. "The good news is that I'm fairly certain this sickness will not progress into anything worse. All of the tests have normalized, which means that it's not life threatening. Based on my physical examination and the complete picture of his illness, I expect Sam to fully recover. However, we're at the edge of what we understand medically. Although we continue to explore what's causing this and how to treat it, I'd like to invite Dr Ganson to our next visit. He is a medical family therapist who specializes in the type of stress that accompanies a prolonged, unexplained illness."

The family was amenable and returned for 2 joint visits with the infectious diseases specialist and the medical family therapist. At the first visit, the medical family therapist helped the family generate a family tree focused on medical illness and coping. A key theme was "how do people in your family handle adversity." The boy was given the task of tracking his symptoms and how he coped with them. At the second visit, the boy reported some symptom relief and the experience of "learning to live with adversity." His parents supported his courage and together began to make plans for return to school the next week. Shortly thereafter, the symptoms remitted and Sam returned to his previous level of functioning and achievement.

### Reflection

Two core tenets of MedFT are to respect the patient's defenses and to consider the biopsychosocial

**Table 38-2**

**Steps in Making a Successful Referral: Collaboration with the Medical Family Therapist**

| *Step* | *Action* | *Example* |
|---|---|---|
| 1 | Clarify the consultation or referral question in your mind | "I need to bring someone into this case to help family members accept and adjust to Leila's diagnosis of sickle-cell anemia." |
| 2 | Refer to a therapist you know and trust | "I have been familiar with Dr Pavone's work with obese adolescents for a long time. She should be able to help Greg's family to promote healthy eating patterns." |
| 3 | Consult with the intended therapist as early as possible prior to presenting to the family | "Dr Thompson, I have a family I am seeing that I think would benefit from seeing you. Can we discuss?" |
| 4 | Make explicit the medium, frequency, and depth of information you desire after the therapist begins work with the family | "I prefer that we communicate briefly by e-mail biweekly just to update each other. But let's agree to talk over the phone if something more pressing emerges." |
| 5 | Identify your preferences for collaborative style (eg, timeliness of feedback, provision of the treatment plan) | "I prefer that we provide each other with notes and treatment reports through the hospital's electronic system. We should also work together on developing the treatment plan so that we can support each other's goals for this family." |
| 6 | Clarify your level of availability with the case | "I have a very full caseload right now, and this patient has continued with problem behavior, despite the progress she's made with her illness. I'd like you to take the lead on helping this family deal with this behavior." |
| 7 | Negotiate and clarify roles in the collaborative process | "I'd prefer that I meet with the Harris family twice a month for medical monitoring of her symptoms, and that you help them incorporate her treatment into everyday life by meeting with them weekly." |

Adapted from McDaniel SH, Campbell TL, Hepworth JE, Lorenz A. *Family-Oriented Primary Care*. 2nd ed. New York, NY: Springer; 2005, with kind permission of Springer Science+Business Media.

complexity of illness. These collaborating professionals viewed the symptoms from the patient's perspective, took ownership of the failure to explain the symptoms, and invited a discussion of stress without implying it was causative. Note that this approach will generally fall flat if employed as a mere "strategy" to get the family to agree to see a mental health professional. In our experience, patients and family will immediately recognize artifice and react negatively. In contrast, adolescents respond to genuine humility and a view of the illness that respects their experience and expertise.

## REFERRAL AND COLLABORATION

The previous case offered an example of artful referral for behavioral health care. In this case, a medical family therapist was available on the same health care team. The same principles apply in settings where this preferred arrangement has not yet been established. Tables 38-2 and 38-3 provide additional guidance for successful referral and collaboration. Table 38-2 provides recommendations and examples for professional communication; Table 38-3 does the same for communication with families.

## CONCLUSION

Family systems approaches are well suited for adolescent health care because relationship renegotiation is central to this developmental period. Adolescent health care professionals can apply family systems principles across a spectrum of care—from FSM in routine visits that include and involve key family members to referral and collaboration with medical family therapists on cases requiring intensive family intervention.

**Table 38-3**

**Presenting Consultation with a MedFT to Family Members**

| Step | Action | Example |
|---|---|---|
| 1 | Use the language and beliefs about the illness of the patient and family | "You're worried about my prescribing birth control pills for your daughter's severe menstrual pain, and that this may give her permission to have sex. This is an important issue. I work with someone who may be helpful in sorting out these concerns. She has worked with many parents of teens who grapple with tough decisions like these." |
| 2 | Refer to "evaluation," "consultation," or "counseling" | "Many families have trouble with learning how to help their teen manage their asthma. I'd like to ask Dr. Weaver to consult with us on this. She specializes in helping families facing an illness like asthma." |
| 3 | Refer to the specialist as a "counselor" or an "expert" who "helps families with difficulties like the one yours is facing" | "Dr Su is trained in a special form of relaxation exercises that have worked with many families of adolescents who have colitis." |
| 4 | Elicit family support for the referral | "You told me that it's important to your family that Eric can join the family in their weekly hikes and physical activities. There is someone here who specializes in helping families get back to normal life after the type of surgery your son has had." |
| 5 | Have the patient or family call the therapist before they leave your office | "I think it would be a good idea to contact Dr Vishal right now—then you won't have to try to fit it in this week." |
| 6 | Avoid a battle if the family resists the referral | "I can see you would rather pursue another option right now. Let's discuss some other possibilities." |
| 7 | Support treatment with the behavioral health specialist | "You didn't understand why Dr Munoz would have the whole family come to a visit to discuss Ellie's refusal of treatment. Maybe it would help to ask her why she thinks it will help. Another idea may be to all meet together for a few minutes to discuss this when you come to your next appointment with her." |

Adapted from McDaniel SH, Campbell TL, Hepworth JE, Lorenz A. *Family-Oriented Primary Care*. 2nd ed. New York, NY: Springer; 2005, with kind permission of Springer Science+Business Media.

## REFERENCES

1. McDaniel SH, Hepworth J, Doherty WJ. *Medical Family Therapy: A Biopsychosocial Approach to Families with Health Problems*. New York, NY: BasicBooks; 1992

2. McDaniel SH, Campbell TL, Hepworth JE, Lorenz A. *Family-Oriented Primary Care.* 2nd ed. New York, NY: Springer; 2005

3. Bowen M. *Family Therapy in Clinical Practice*. New York, NY: Aronson; 1978

4. Engel GL. The need for a new medical model: a challenge for biomedicine. *Science.* 1977;196(4286):129

5. Frankel RM, Quill TE, McDaniel SH. *The Biopsychosocial Approach: Past, Present, and Future*. Rochester, NY: University of Rochester Press; 2003

6. Mikesell RH, Lusterman DD, McDaniel SH. *Integrating Family Therapy: Handbook of Family Psychology and Systems Theory*. Washington, DC: American Psychological Association; 1995

7. Doherty WJ, Baird MA. Developmental levels in family-centered medical care. *Family Medicine.* 1986;18(3):153

8. Campbell TL. The effectiveness of family interventions for physical disorders. *J Marital Fam Ther.* 2003;29(2):263-281

9. Gallo LC, Troxel WM, Kuller LH, Sutton-Tyrrell K, Edmundowicz D, Matthews KA. Marital status, marital quality, and atherosclerotic burden in postmenopausal women. *Psychosom Med.* 2003;65(6):952-962

10. Kiecolt-Glaser JK, Loving TJ, Stowell JR, et al. Hostile marital interactions, proinflammatory cytokine production, and wound healing. *Arch Gen Psychiatry.* 2005;62(12):1377-1384

11. Repetti RL, Taylor SE, Seeman TE. Risky families: family social environments and the mental and physical health of offspring. *Psychol Bull.* 2002;128(2):330-366

12. Weihs K, Fisher L, Baird M. Families, health, and behavior: a section of the commissioned report by the Committee on Health and Behavior: research, practice, and policy, Division of Neuroscience and Behavioral Health and Division

of Health Promotion and Disease Prevention, Institute of Medicine, National Academy of Sciences. *Fam, Syst, & Health.* 2002;20(1):7–46

13. House J, Landis K, Umberson D. Social relationships and health. *Science.* 1988;241(4865):540–545

14. East PL, Khoo ST. Longitudinal pathways linking family factors and sibling relationship qualities to adolescent substance use and sexual risk behaviors. *J Fam Psychol.* 2005;19(4):571

15. Franko DL, Thompson D, Affenita SH, Barton BA, Striegel-Moore RH. What mediates the relationship between family meals and adolescent health issues? *Health Psychol.* 2008;27(2 suppl):S109–S117

16. Kaugars AS, Klinnert MD, Bender BG. Family influences on pediatric asthma. *J Pediatr Psychol.* 2004;29(7):475–491

17. Landolt MA, Grubenmann S, Mueli M. Family impact greatest: predictors of quality of life and psychological adjustment in pediatric burn survivors. *J Trauma.* 2002;53:1146–1154

18. Palermo TM, Putnam J, Daily S. Adolescent autonomy and family functioning are associated with headache-related disability. *Clin J Pain.* 2007;23(5):458–465

19. Butler JM, Skinner M, Gelfand D, Berg CA, Wiebe DJ. Maternal parenting style and adjustment in adolescents with type I diabetes. *J Pediatr Psychol.* 2007;32(10):1227–1237

20. Duke DC, Geffken GR, Lewin AB, Williams LB, Storch EA, Silverstein JH. Glycemic control in youth with type 1 diabetes: family predictors and mediators. *J Pediatr Psychol.* 2008;33(7):719–727

21. Wagman-Borowsky I, Ireland M, Resnick MD. Adolescent suicide attempts: risks and protectors. *Pediatrics.* 2001;107: 485–493

22. Lock J, Couturier J, Bryson S, Agras S. Predictors of dropout and remission in family therapy for adolescent anorexia nervosa in a random clinical trial. *Int J Eat Disord.* 2006;39(8):639–647

23. Markson S, Fiese BH. Family rituals as a protective factor for children with asthma. *J Pediatr Psychol.* 2000;25(7): 471–480

24. Reiter-Purtill J, Schorry EK, Lovell AM, Vannatta K, Gerhardt CA, Noll RB. Parental distress, family functioning, and social support in families with and without a child with neurofibromatosis 1. *J Pediatr Psychol.* 2008;33(4):422–434

25. Engel GL. The clinical application of the biopsychosocial model. *Am J Psychiatry.* 1980;137:535–544

26. Von Bertalanffy L. *General Systems Theory: Foundations, Development, Applications*. New York, NY: WW Norton; 1968

27. Patterson JM. Integrating family resilience and family stress theory. *J Marriage Fam.* 2002;64(2):349–360

28. Helgeson VS. Relations of agency and communion to well-being: evidence and potential explanations. *Psychological Review.* 1994;116:412–428

29. Blos P. When and how does adolescence end? Structural criteria for adolescent closure. *Adolescent Psychiatry.* 1997;5:5–17

30. Allen JP, Land D. Attachment in adolescence. In: Cassidy J, Shaver RP, eds. *Handbook of Attachment: Theory, Research, and Clinical Applications*. New York, NY: Guilford; 1999:319–335

31. Adams R, Laursen B. The organization and dynamics of adolescent conflict with parents and friends. *J Marriage Fam.* 2001;63(1):97–110

32. Allen JP, Land D. Autonomy and relatedness in family interactions as predictors of expressions of negative adolescent affect. *J Res Adolesc.* 1994;4(4):535

33. Allen JP, Leadbeater BJ, Aber JL. The development of problem behavior syndromes in at-risk adolescents. *Dev Psychopathol.* 1994;6:323–342

34. Grotevant HD, Cooper CR. Patterns of interaction in family relationships and the development of identity exploration in adolescence. *Child Dev.* 1985;56(2):415–428

35. Walker LJ, Taylor JH. Family interactions and the development of moral reasoning. *Child Dev.* 1991;62(2):264–283

36. Viner R. Transition from paediatric to adult care. Bridging the gaps or passing the buck? *Arch Dis Child.* 1999;81(3):271–275

37. Grotevant HD, Cooper CR. Individuation in family relationships: a perspective on individual differences in the identity of role-taking in adolescence. *Hum Devel.* 1986;29:82–100

38. McQuaid EL, Kopel SJ, Klein RB, Fritz GK. Medication adherence in pediatric asthma: reasoning, responsibility, and behavior. *J Pediatr Psychol.* 2003;28(5):323–333

39. Tucker LB, Cabral DA. Transition of the adolescent patient with rheumatic disease: issues to consider. *Pediatr Clin North Am.* 2005;52(2):641–652

40. Shaw RJ. Treatment adherence in adolescents: development and psychopathology. *Clin Child Psychol Psychiatry.* 2001;6(1):137–150

41. Rosen DS, Blum RW, Britto M, Sawyer SM, Siegel DM. Transition to adult health care for adolescents and young adults with chronic conditions: position paper of the Society for Adolescent Medicine. *J Adolesc Health.* 2003;33(4):309–311

# CHAPTER 39

## Peers

DENYELLE B. KENYON, PhD • MARTHA Y. KUBIK, PhD, RN • RENEE SIEVING, PhD, RN

### CONCEPTUAL FRAMEWORK FOR UNDERSTANDING PEER INFLUENCE

Health behavior theories, such as Bandura's social cognitive theory (SCT) and Bronfenbrenner's ecological model provide a conceptual framework for understanding the influence of peers on adolescent health behavior. According to SCT, behavior is a result of a dynamic, interactive process known as "reciprocal determinism," whereby personal, behavioral, and environmental factors interact simultaneously to determine individuals' behavior.[1] An important SCT concept, observational learning, represents the ability to learn from the actions and reinforcement given by others, and recognizes the environment as an important source of role models. Also referred to as vicarious experience, observational learning is a component of several other SCT concepts, including individuals' expectations for behavior and self-efficacy, and is important to understanding the powerful influence of peers on adolescent behavior.

Similar to SCT, ecological models specify that behavior is influenced by intrapersonal, social, and cultural factors, as well as physical environments.[2,3] Ecological theory explicitly recognizes that social and cultural factors and physical environments can directly influence health behavior without mediating changes in individual beliefs, skills, attitudes, or knowledge. For example, providing supervised pro-social activities for youth can reduce opportunities for engaging in risky health behaviors that are not dependent on altering individuals' attitudes and beliefs about risky behavior.[4]

Bronfenbrenner[2,3] conceptualized the environment as consisting of four systems where individuals interact with the environment in a reciprocal fashion; interactions occur both within and between systems. As described by Bronfenbrenner, the *microsystem* consists of interpersonal interactions in specific settings, such as family and peer gatherings, such that the effects of role modeling and peer influence are evident at this level. At the level of the *mesosystem*, interactions occur between settings, such as family and peer group, and the quality and strength of the relationships within each setting influence the sustainability of a behavior. The *exosystem* encompasses the influence of media, laws, and policies, whereas the *macrosystem* represents the overarching social system within which the other systems exist, exerting influence over individuals and settings via economic factors, cultural beliefs, and values.

Perry[5] offers a framework for understanding the social environment of adolescents and adolescent health behavior that incorporates aspects of both social cognitive and ecological theory. Perry[5] conceptualizes the adolescent's social environment as consisting of three levels of influence. Parents, siblings, and best friends represent the most proximal level of influence, followed by a second level that consists of peers and other significant adults and, finally, the most distal level, which includes the powerful influence of cultural and media messages, along with policies and practices. Each level influences adolescent behavior via key social-environmental factors including normative expectations, role models, social support, and opportunities to practice or engage in a behavior. Social-environmental factors, recognized as powerful predictors of adolescent behavior, are the mechanisms by which peers influence adolescent health behaviors. Thus, these social-environmental factors require careful consideration when planning interventions to positively influence adolescents.[5]

## TYPES OF PEER INFLUENCE

With the development of autonomy from parents, adolescents spend increasingly more time with their peers. Although this shift represents a natural and expected progression, it occurs at a time when adolescents are faced with difficult choices regarding behaviors that may or may not be health-enhancing. Thus, it is important to consider the types of influence peers may exert on young people's health behaviors.

### MODELING

A fundamental component of SCT,[1] role modeling, is recognized by Perry[5] as a key social-environmental factor that influences adolescent behavior. Role models can include adults and peers and may be persons known to the adolescent, such as teachers, relatives, friends, and classmates, or not known, such as athletes and media stars. Peers in particular are influential role models during adolescence, modeling many behaviors that may or may not be health-enhancing. Along with modeling a behavior, peers also model consequences of a behavior that may include reward or punishment, with consequences serving to positively or negatively reinforce adoption of the behavior by others. For example, a group of adolescents smoking and laughing together may be perceived by other teens as "cool" and "fitting in" and increase the likelihood that the younger teens may smoke (negative modeling and reinforcement). Conversely, girls observing other girls with a range of athletic abilities playing a sport and receiving encouragement from parents and teachers may be prompted to try the sport (positive modeling and reinforcement).

### SETTING GROUP NORMS

As described by Perry,[5] normative expectations include an adolescent's perception of what they ought to do, what is acceptable to do, and what others are doing. Importantly, perception of the prevalence of a behavior may or may not be accurate; overestimation of a behavior increases the likelihood that a risky behavior, such as smoking, alcohol use, or unprotected sexual activity, will be adopted.[5] Peer influence often plays out in the setting of peer group norms, with the establishment of a standard of behavior for group members and for teens aspiring to be group members. Group norms may be dictated by distal influences, such as culture and media, or be the result of more proximal influences, such as the behavior of a group of close friends. Indeed, research suggests that females react more to the norms of close friends (proximal influence), whereas males respond more to the norms exhibited by the larger peer group (distal influence).[6]

### STRUCTURING OPPORTUNITIES

Another key social-environmental factor is opportunities, defined as whether a behavior is possible, or conversely, what barriers exist to engaging in a behavior.[5] Opportunities and barriers are often found in adolescents' physical environment, such as availability of sports teams or neighborhood parks. Peer influence is evident in the opportunities offered young people and whether they are sustainable.[6] For example, availability of fresh fruits and vegetables at school, home, and friends' homes provides adolescents opportunities to consume healthy foods in supportive environments among friends and peers who are choosing the same foods. In other words, through these opportunities, healthy dietary practices become acceptable and a peer group norm.

### PEER PRESSURE

Peer pressure is defined as a direct effort to shape the attitudes or behavior of an adolescent.[6] Peer pressure can either be a negative or positive influence. Susceptibility to peer pressure peaks around age 14.[7] In fact, many adolescents report that their friends influence them *not* to engage in sexual activity or drug use,[6] and drinking behavior has been found to be more strongly influenced by peers than parents.[6] The ecological model suggests that the reason peers have a greater influence than parents is because peers have a more proximal influence on drinking during adolescence.[2,3]

Oftentimes, peer pressure is blamed for the negative behaviors of adolescents, such as risky sexual activity or drug use, and is the focus of many intervention strategies. Because peer pressure has a known negative connotation, adolescents often deny that their friends exert pressure on them to become involved in deviant behavior or have sex. In reality, Brown and colleagues[6] found that adolescents adamantly denied feeling any peer pressure, but then went on to describe situations of obvious peer influence. Therefore, interventions that solely focus on negative peer pressure and teach adolescents to "just say no" may be wholly ineffective.

Moreover, the influence of peers is not simplistic—because peer relations by nature are reciprocal, influence is bidirectional. Peer relations are inherently equal and are unlikely to have a power differential like the parent–adolescent relationship.[6] Therefore, the influence of peers is not as simple as a "bad" teen pressuring a "good" teen to engage in a negative behavior. Researchers have examined differences in susceptibility and found that adolescents are more susceptible to peer influence when they are in the company of acquaintances rather than with closer friends.[6] In other words, adolescents may be more susceptible to peer pressure when trying to gain new friendships or belonging to a crowd.

### PEER INFLUENCE VS PEER SELECTION

Peer influence has been linked to adolescent health behaviors such as delinquent behavior, substance use, violence, and sexual activity.[6–8] One reason it is difficult to discern how peers influence adolescent health is that young people select like-minded peers to be friends with, as in the saying "birds of a feather flock together." In the peer literature, this idea is termed "selection effects," the tendency of adolescents to choose friends who already share their interests, values, and personality dynamics.[9,10] Indeed, selection effects interact with the influence of peer pressure because some research suggests that adolescents who are most susceptible to peer pressure are those who are most likely to select peers already engaged in antisocial behavior.[7]

Research on delinquency has suggested that girls are more susceptible to negative peer influence than boys, whereas other research has found that boys are more influenced by same-sex peers, and girls are more influenced by their male peers.[8] Furthermore, recent analyses suggest that peer influence is weaker among adolescents who are satisfied with their relationships with parents.[10] In other words, poor relationships with parents may exacerbate peers' negative influence on problem behavior.[6]

A body of research by Dishion and colleagues[8,11] on delinquency training has implicated a causal role of peers in increasing antisocial behavior. This research found that interventions that placed boys with conduct disorder together into interventions led the youth to engage in more delinquency and drug use.[8,11] In sum, although we cannot ignore the powerful impact of peers, we must remember the complicated nature of peer relations and how other interactive contextual factors can influence adolescent behavior.[2,3]

### CONNECTIONS BETWEEN PEER AND PARENT INFLUENCES

Although adolescents spend increasing amounts of time with their peers during adolescence, parents still remain a strong influence in adolescents' lives. For example, parents generally influence long-term issues (like career choices and moral issues), whereas peers influence adolescents in terms of appearances and style.[12] A part of parents' influence on adolescent behavior may be indirect, through influencing adolescents' choices of friends.[2,3] Research has shown that when parents facilitate their early adolescents' friendships, they had greater intimacy and companionship in those new friendships.[7] Other research has shown that when parents used high levels of guiding peer relationships (communicating values, expectations for, and possible consequences of friendships), adolescents were more likely to select friends with higher grades.[7] On the other hand, Mounts[7] found that parental monitoring or prohibiting had little influence on adolescents' selection of friends. In sum, a growing research body has demonstrated that parents can influence their children's peer relationships, but that parental influence has its limits.

## LEVELS OF PEER INFLUENCE

### BEST FRIENDSHIPS

The positive qualities of friendships, such as closeness, supportiveness, intimacy, and disclosure, increase across adolescence.[12] Indeed, having a mutual best friendship has been found to be an extremely protective factor. Holding positive friendships has been found to decrease the effects of negative family and peer experiences.[9] For example, having a best friend protects against peer victimization,[11] as well as the negative outcomes associated with being victimized.[13] Friendships that have high levels of support, security, stability, intimacy, and lack of conflict have been associated with higher rates of self-esteem, and lower delinquent behavior, hostility, school problems, anxiety, and depression.[9,13]

However, not all influence from best friends is positive. Some research suggests that adolescents' close friends may promote unhealthy coping behaviors (such as partying and reckless driving) and other risky health behaviors such as tobacco use.[9] Similarly, recent analyses with a nationally representative sample demonstrated a significant (but small) effect of close friends on adolescents' binge drinking and sexual behavior.[10] In other words, when adolescents' close friends engaged in binge drinking or sexual activity, their likelihood of binge drinking or having sex increased. Therefore, the influence of close friends may enhance health for some adolescents and worsen it for others.

### ROMANTIC RELATIONSHIPS

Dating and romantic relationships are a significant aspect of adolescents' social world.[12] Initial interactions with opposite-sex peers often first occur in mixed-sex contexts during early adolescence, and romantic relationships become relatively stable during middle adolescence.[12] Romantic relationships during adolescence can have both negative and positive effects on adolescents' health. For example, key features of attractiveness in the United States are physical appearance (especially for girls) and athletic prowess (especially for boys), which may promote healthy behaviors such as good nutrition and exercise.[9] On the other hand, attainment of physical beauty may prompt some adolescent girls to diet, making them susceptible to eating disorders; other adolescents, particularly boys, may take steroids to build their athletic performance.[9] Other negative outcomes of relationships may occur when the relationship dissolves, such as heavy drinking and depression.[9] Furthermore, romantic relationships and sexual activity may be especially stressful for bisexual, homosexual, or questioning adolescents. Research has found that these youth are particularly vulnerable for ridicule and ostracism by peers, and have comparatively higher rates of drug and alcohol use, depression, suicide attempts, and running away than their heterosexual peers.[9]

### PEER GROUPS

Peer groups, also known as cliques, are small groups of friends (usually 6 to 12) who share activities.[12,13] Cliques are fairly homogenous, and members are likely to be of the same age, ethnicity, socioeconomic status, and gender (during early adolescence).[12] Research has found that less than half of adolescents belong to a clique; girls are more likely to be members than boys.[12] These peer groups are usually stable in membership, and increase in stability across adolescence.[13]

### SOCIAL CROWDS

Crowds are defined as labels that describe stereotypical reputations, behaviors, and personality traits.[12,13] Crowd membership is based on reputation rather than an adolescent's active participation.[13] Crowds provide a context to develop identity, and help channel adolescents into friendships with similar peers.[12,13] Examples of crowds are jocks, preppies, brains, normals, emos, druggies, and nerds.[13] Adolescents' views about other crowds depends on what crowd they themselves are in. For example, a jock may believe that preppies are friendly, whereas a druggie may think that preppies are stuck up.[13]

Various health behaviors, such as alcohol, tobacco, and other drug use, delinquent behavior, sexual activity, academic achievement, and emotional health are associated with different crowds.[9] Research has found that some risky health behaviors (eg, alcohol use) are more common in high status groups (eg, elites, popular blacks).[9] Up to half of young people are outside the crowd system or float among several groups, and outsiders who wish to be part of a group are more likely to be smokers and have poor self-esteem and higher anxiety.[9] In sum, crowds are a salient facet of peer relationships that have important implications for adolescent health.

## TAPPING THE POWER OF PEERS: INVOLVING PEERS IN HEALTH PROMOTION

Because peer influence is a central theme of adolescence, structuring positive peer influence may be critical to the success of health promotion efforts.[14] Effective peer involvement programs empower young people to take charge of their social environments and to create healthier norms and values for their generation.[5] A rationale for peer involvement in health promotion programs emerges from themes highlighted previously in this chapter. At the *social environment* level, peer involvement can leverage the power of peer role modeling, peer social support, and peer norms in supporting healthy behaviors. At the *individual level*, messengers who use the same language and who face similar concerns and pressures as the targeted youth increase credibility of health-related messages.[15,16] At the level of *behavior*, peer involvement can be utilized to model new skills, intentions, and healthy behaviors.

How can adolescent health professionals enlist the positive qualities of youth's peer interactions to create effective peer involvement programs? To address this question, we provide an overview of types of effective peer involvement programs. We articulate principles for designing effective peer involvement programs. Finally, we highlight challenges to consider in implementing peer involvement programs.

### TYPES OF PEER INTERVENTION PROGRAMS

As noted in Table 39-1, several types of peer involvement programs have been evaluated in the context of adolescent health programs focused on sexuality education, substance use, and violence prevention.[5] Research suggests that peer involvement programs can be effective in bringing about positive health behavior change in adolescents.[17] Effective peer involvement programs tend to be theory-based, highly structured, and led by well-trained peers.[15]

Students Together Against Negative Decisions (STAND) is a peer leader program promoting both abstinence and sexual risk reduction among adolescents in the rural South. Through 28-session training, STAND prepares teens to initiate one-on-one conversations with their peers about sexual risk reduction. STAND peer leaders contract with the program to engage in a minimum number of conversations each week. Throughout high school, peer leaders also participate in the STAND Club (monthly reflection and planning gatherings) and facilitate a range of formal group activities. Teens are selected for STAND based on peer- or self-nominations. STAND has been linked to improvements in condom

**Table 39-1**

**Types of Peer Involvement Programs**

| | |
|---|---|
| Peer leadership programs | Peers are elected by classmates to lead prevention programs. Successful programs include extensive training of peer leaders, concrete activities, rehearsal, an adult coordinator, and reinforcements. |
| Peer counseling, peer mediation programs | Peers help others who have social and behavioral problems. Successful programs include extensive training (eg, a separate school course) and ongoing supervision from an adult counselor. |
| Peer participation, peer action programs | Peers volunteer to create, plan, and implement programs in their schools or communities concerning a particular goal. Successful programs include skill training, advocacy training, funding, and adult involvement. |

use consistency, both among STAND peer leaders and among sexually active students in the STAND intervention county.[18]

Project Northland, a community-wide intervention study to reduce youth alcohol use during middle school and high school, has implemented and evaluated multiple types of peer involvement programs.[14] During seventh and eighth grades, *peer leaders* are elected by classmates, trained by field staff, and co-facilitate classroom curricula with teachers. In addition, students volunteer in seventh and eighth grades to form groups to plan alcohol-free social activities facilitated by adult volunteers. These *peer participation groups* resulted in lower alcohol use among teens that were active in planning. During 11th and 12th grades, youth volunteer to be members of *peer action teams*. These teams work outside of school with adult coordinators on projects that affect alcohol availability and use by high school students, such as local alcohol access ordinances.

## PRINCIPLES FOR DESIGNING EFFECTIVE PEER INVOLVEMENT PROGRAMS

Several principles can be used to guide the design of effective peer involvement programs. *First, peer involvement programs should reflect adolescent participants' developmental level.* Cognitive, social, and psychological capacities of the young people involved should guide the development of peer leadership activities. For example, while young adolescent peer action teams may take on concrete projects with intensive adult support, older adolescent peer action teams can take on more complex projects with less logistical coaching from adults. *Second, peer involvement programs should be voluntary and structured (with rules, expectations, and goals) in ways that promote pro-social engagement with peers.* For young people, motivation to become involved in voluntary programs may come through small incentives, opportunities to choose among activities, or formal course credit. STAND illustrates the success of structured and voluntary programs. Although recruited by adults, STAND peer leaders volunteer their time. Youth who volunteer are given a clear and concise program goal: promote abstinence for all teens and safer sex for those who choose to be sexually active. In training, STAND peer leaders are taught to assess a person's stage of change and to deliver health messages tailored to that stage. Throughout their training, STAND peer leaders are reminded that they should refer peers with substantial problems to proper counselors. *Third, peer involvement programs must be carefully structured to promote pro-social skills and behaviors.* In Project Northland, peer leaders are provided opportunities and support they need to have a positive effect on their peers. Youth in leadership roles participate in formal trainings, that provide ample time to learn about the rationale for the program, recognize the importance of their roles, become skilled in implementing particular program elements, consider potential implementation problems and ways to deal with those problems, and become committed to their roles and goal of the program. In addition to learning about the dangers of adolescent alcohol use, peer leaders gain skills that enable them to address alcohol use problems in positive ways, such as by planning and promoting alcohol-free social activities for their peers. Youth action team members are equipped with specific skills and support needed to have an effect on the broader community, such as knowledge and skills needed to address policies concerning access to alcohol within the community. The pro-social skills that peer leaders learn by participating in Project Northland can have positive effects on their peers, their community, and their own developing identities.[19]

## CHALLENGES IN IMPLEMENTING PEER INVOLVEMENT PROGRAMS

While programs for youth that are developed and implemented through youth-adult partnerships may be highly effective in building adolescents' skills and preventing health risk behaviors, several real challenges exist in implementing peer involvement programs. First, logistics are often problematic. Transportation, scheduling, and arranging releases from regular classes for peer leaders create challenges for many peer involvement programs.[16] Second, if peers themselves are high-risk, they may convey undesirable messages. There is growing consensus that peer involvement programs, in which high-risk or marginalized youth are leaders, can actually facilitate development of problem behaviors when interactions among youth reinforce antisocial behaviors and subvert pro-social norms. Even well-designed programs must be carefully implemented and actively structured by adults to support conventional norms and reinforce pro-social behaviors.[19] In light of the understanding that it is often peer leaders who benefit most from peer involvement programs, working with high-risk or marginalized youth as peer leaders requires a particular programmatic emphasis on the development of youth leadership skills.[20] Third, the sustainability of peer involvement programs is particularly challenging. While adults can offer programs for long periods of time, peers do not remain peers of a targeted age group for long. This means that programs must continually recruit and train new cohorts of peer leaders.[16] Another sustainability issue involves the reality that peer involvement programs are not the norm in most organizations. Therefore, if a peer involvement program has been initiated outside of an organization, a representative from the organization should be sought out to act as a liaison between program coordinators and peer leaders. This person should be committed to the peer program and involved in training and ongoing support of peer leaders. A formal commitment from the organization should be sought, should the program prove successful. Finally, peer involvement programs generally require additional adult staff and specific curricula, and thus may be more costly to implement than adult-led programs. However, the costs have been far outweighed by what the teens learned from being peer leaders and from the positive impact they have on their peers.[21]

## CONCLUSION

Both research and theory demonstrate that peers are an important influence in adolescents' social world. Peer influence has an undeniable effect on adolescent health. Diverse aspects of adolescents themselves, as well as the crowds, cliques, friendships, and romantic relationships they hold, have implications for their behaviors. In this chapter, we detailed these peer influences and the benefits of utilizing peers in programmatic efforts to promote healthy behaviors during adolescence.

## INTERNET RESOURCES

- A Clearinghouse of information and resources on adolescent issues: www.focusas.com/PeerInfluence.html
- Teen Link resource guide links to books and journal articles on peers: teenlink.education.umn.edu
- Princeton Center for Leadership Training offers peer leadership training programs: www.princetonleadership.org

## REFERENCES

1. Bandura A. *Social Foundations of Thought and Action: A Social Cognitive Theory*. Upper Saddle River, NJ: Prentice-Hall, Inc.; 1986

2. Bronfenbrenner U. *The ecology of human development experiments by nature and design*. Cambridge, MA: Harvard University Press; 1979

3. Bronfenbrenner U. Ecology of the family as a context for human development: Research perspectives. *Dev Psychol.* 1986;22:723–742

4. Cohen DA, Scribner RA, Farley TA. A structural model of health behavior: A pragmatic approach to explain and influence health behaviors at the population level. *Preventive Medicine: An International Journal Devoted to Practice and Theory.* 2000;30:146–154

5. Perry CL. *Creating health behavior change: How to develop community-wide programs for youth*. Thousand Oaks: Sage Publications, Inc.; 1999

6. Brown B, Theobald W. How peers matter: A research synthesis of peer influences on adolescent pregnancy prevention. In: *Peer Potential: Making the Most of How Teens Influence Each Other*. Washington, DC: National Campaign to Prevent Teen Pregnancy; 1999:27–80

7. Mounts NS. Parental management of adolescent peer relationship: What are its effects on friend selection? In: Kerns K, Contreras J, Neal-Barnett A, eds. *Family and peers: Linking two social worlds*. Westport, CT: Praeger Publishers; 2000:169–193

8. Gifford-Smith M, Dodge KA, Dishion TJ, McCord J. Peer influence in children and adolescents: Crossing the bridge from developmental to intervention science. *J Abnorm Child Psychol.* 2005;33:255–265

9. Brown BB, Dolcini MM, Leventhal A. Transformations in peer relationships at adolescence: Implications for health-related behavior. In: Schulenberg J, Maggs JL, Hurrelmann K, eds. *Health Risks and Developmental Transitions during Adolescence*. New York, NY: Cambridge University Press; 1997: 161–189

10. Jaccard J, Blanton H, Dodge T. Peer influences on risk behavior: An analysis of the effects of a close friend. *Dev Psychol.* 2005;41:135–147

11. Deater-Deckard K. Annotation: Recent research examining the role of peer relationships in the development of psychopathology. *J Child Psychol Psychiatry.* 2001;42:565–579

12. Smetana JG, Campione-Barr N, Metzger A. Adolescent development in interpersonal and societal contexts. *Annu Rev Psychol.* 2006;57:255–284

13. Meece D, Laird RD. The importance of peers. In: Villarruel FA, Luster T, eds. *The Crisis in Youth Mental Health: Critical Issues and Effective Programs*. Vol 2. Westport, CT: Praeger Publishers/Greenwood Publishing Group; 2006:283–311

14. Perry C, Williams CL, Komro KA, et al. Project Northland: Long-term outcomes of community action to reduce adolescent alcohol use. *Health Educ Res.* 2002;17:117–132

15. Caron F, Godin G, Otis J, Lambert LD. Evaluation of a theoretically based AIDS/STD peer education program on postponing sexual intercourse and on condom use among adolescents attending high school. *Health Educ Res.* 2004;19:185–197

16. Philliber S. In search of peer power: A review of research on peer-based interventions for teens. In: *Peer Potential: Making the Most of How Teens Influence Each Other*. Washington, DC: National Campaign to Prevent Teen Pregnancy; 1999:81–111

17. Harden A, Oakley A, Oliver S. Peer-delivered health promotion for young people: a systematic review of difference study designs. *Health Educ J.* 2001;60:339–353

18. Smith M, Dane F, Archer M, Devereaux R, Katner H. Students Together Against Negative Decisions (STAND): Evaluation of a school-based sexual risk reduction intervention in the rural South. *AIDS Education and Prevention*. 2000;12:49–70

19. Karcher MJ, Brown BB, Elliott DW. Enlisting peers in developmental interventions: Principles and practices. In: Hamilton SF, Hamilton MA, eds. *The Youth Development Handbook: Coming of Age in American Communities*. Thousand Oaks, CA: Sage Publications, Inc; 2004:193–215

20. Shiner M. Defining peer education. *J Adolesc.* 1999;22:555–566

21. Black DR, Tobler NS, Sciacca JP. Peer helping/involvement: An efficacious way to meet the challenge of reducing alcohol, tobacco, and other drug use among youth? *J Sch Health.* 1998;68:87–93

# CHAPTER 40

# Socioeconomic Status

ELIZABETH ALDERMAN, MD • ALWYN COHALL, MD

*The authors would like to thank Sheila Dini, MPH (Research Assistant, Harlem Health Promotion Center) and Janice Cooper, MD (Director, National Center for Children in Poverty) for all their help in preparing this manuscript for publication.*

## INTRODUCTION

On a typical afternoon in a major metropolitan region, 2 health providers prepare to start their clinical sessions. One sees youth from a primarily lower socioeconomic status (SES) community in an urban hospital clinic. The other provides care for more affluent youth in a suburban, private practice setting. The casual observer might expect that the former may encounter youth with more health problems and who are engaged in significantly more risk-taking behaviors than the latter. In reality, however, the distribution of health concerns and risks may be more varied than conventional wisdom might hold.

The adult literature suggests that a graded relationship exists between socioeconomic status and health, that is, better educated and more financially secure individuals usually enjoy a better standard of health.[1] Disparities in health status are most profoundly noted between individuals in the lowest and highest SES, as measured by mortality rates, various chronic and acute health concerns, and individual perceptions of health.[2-4] In large part, mortality among adults can be attributed to cancer and cardiovascular diseases. Factors related to development of these chronic diseases may include smoking, sedentary lifestyles, and improper nutrition. Initiation of behaviors that lead to these behaviorally related health problems may start during adolescence.[5]

Adolescents from lower SES backgrounds are disproportionately affected by a variety of economic and social contextual factors that may confer upon them a degree of "vulnerability" that may contribute to the initiation and maintenance of improper health habits and risk-taking behaviors. However, despite being dealt a "stacked hand," many youth from impoverished circumstances manage to break free of the intense, gravitational pull of poverty to become productive members of society. Conversely, although wealth and social standing provide some degree of insulation from harm, affluent adolescents can be involved in health-compromising and risk-taking behaviors that may also affect their health and longevity.

This chapter provides a descriptive profile of the distribution of SES among adolescents, discuss issues related to measurement of SES, and discuss the various ways in which SES may affect health status. Subsequently, we offer suggestions that may help support healthy transitions into adulthood for all adolescents and their families.

## DISTRIBUTION OF SOCIOECONOMIC STATUS

According to 2005 Census figures, real median income in the United States did not change appreciably from previous years.[6] Real median income in 2005 was $46,326. Although there were no statistically significant differences between racial groups, Asian Americans families had the highest median income and black families the lowest. Families with 2 married persons had higher median incomes than single male head of family and single woman head of family. The poverty rate has remained essentially the same at 12.6% and the federal poverty level for a family of 4 was $19,350. The National Center for Children in Poverty Web site states that for children 12 to 18 years of age, 58% Latino, 57% black, 24% Asian American, and 24% white are living in low-income families. Whereas black and Latino adolescents are disproportionately low income, whites comprise the largest group of low-income children ages 12 to 18 years. Adolescents of immigrant parents and adolescents living in the south and west are more likely to be living in low-income families.[7]

Income in the 90th percentile has increased by 13% and income at the lowest 10th percentile has increased by 23%. The highest quintile of income was $91,705 with most of those families living in the suburbs. There are no statistics that specifically relate to numbers of adolescents living in poverty, affluence, middle, or working class. However, these Census figures give a broad view of SES of families living in the United States during the first decade of the third millennium.[6]

## MEASUREMENT OF SOCIOECONOMIC STATUS

Because most adolescents are not financially independent and are usually members of a family, it is more useful to assess the SES of the family unit rather than the individual adolescent.[8] This presents a challenge because it is the exceptional adolescent who knows true family income, particularly in households without fathers. A study by Currie, Elton et al[9], surveying Scottish school children ages 11 to 15 years, found that 20% were unable to provide an adequate response when asked their father's occupation. Thus, obtaining information about SES often involves sources other than the adolescent.

Further, SES is a complex variable with multiple contributing factors and encompasses much more than simply measuring income.[10] It has been suggested that using wealth (accumulation of assets, real estate, stocks, bonds, business holdings, inheritance, etc.) as well as dividing income by family size might give a clearer picture of a family's financial standing. A family of 4 with an income of $50,000 may have relatively more resources at its disposal (income-to-needs ratio) than a family of 6.[11] Family composition is also important, in addition to size. Families with two parents usually enjoy a higher standard of living than those headed by a single parent. Additionally, parental educational attainment and occupational status are important to assess. In general, parents holding a college or graduate degree make more money and have more assets than parents with a high school degree or less. Finally, others argue that the SES of the family's neighborhood is relevant. A low SES family living in an area of concentrated and circumscribed poverty may be exposed to harsher environmental influences and have less access to resources than one of similar means but living in or near a more moderate SES community.[12]

## IMPACT OF SOCIOECONOMIC STATUS ON ACCESS TO CARE

Access to quality health care is a key factor in identifying, addressing, and possibly preventing risk-taking behaviors among adolescents. Health insurance coverage and SES are tied closely to access to care. Approximately 12% of adolescents were uninsured in 2002 (a decrease from 14% in 1995).[13] Although improvements were noted in insurance coverage of youth in lower socioeconomic families as a result of expansion of Medicaid and SCHIP programs, still close to 20% of poor adolescents and 19% of near-poor adolescents were without insurance coverage in 2002. By contrast, only 6.3% of youth in middle- and higher-income families lacked insurance coverage in 2002.[13]

In a study comparing poor adolescents to their peers in middle and higher SES income levels, disparities are noted with respect to health status, usual source of care, and access to and utilization of services. Despite being eligible for either Medicaid or SCHIP, poor adolescents were 5 to 6 times more likely to be uninsured. Additionally, disparities were similarly noted with respect to health status, access to, use of, and satisfaction with care.[14] However, although ensuring a level playing field is important, further analysis indicated that disparities in access and utilization continued to exist, even after controlling for insurance coverage, suggesting the need to examine and address other contextual factors such as transportation, child care, provider availability, and cultural competence.

Although poor youth are at greatest risk for being uninsured, changes in the economy have affected middle-income families as well. For example, as technology and manufacturing firms downsize, jobs—with insurance as a fringe benefit—are lost. Parents going from these types of jobs to temporary positions or those in the service sector may find themselves without insurance benefits or with benefits that do not extend to their dependent children.[13]

## SOCIOECONOMIC STATUS AND DIFFERENTIAL HEALTH OUTCOMES

Although SES remains an elusive and imprecise construct to pin down accurately, it has been used extensively in the literature, particularly as it relates to addressing health disparities. As noted previously, due to the disproportionate representation of minorities in the lower SES strata, there has been a tendency to equate race/ethnicity with SES and in some cases to use race/ethnicity as a proxy for SES. However, there now is a growing body of evidence encouraging researchers to go beyond this association and to take another look at other factors that may contribute to disparities in health outcomes. For example, among adults, lower SES individuals experience poor health outcomes and report perceptions of poorer health. One would expect that as SES (as measured by income and education) improved, differences in health outcomes between blacks and whites would be attenuated. However, college-educated, higher SES blacks still experience poorer health status and perceive themselves to be less healthy than their white counterparts. The "diminishing returns" hypothesis suggests that factors related to persistent and pervasive racial discrimination preclude blacks from enjoying the same social status benefits as whites of similar educational levels. Reduced income, restricted housing (and neighborhood) choices, etc. may cause psychological distress and chronic stress that, through primary (excess release of cortisol and catecholamines) or secondary (inadequate or overwhelmed coping mechanisms) pathways, may affect health outcomes.[15]

Similar findings have been noted among populations of adolescents.[16] In a high school-based study of 1,200 adolescents, social disadvantage was found to be associated with increased stress. A social hierarchy was noted, as youth from moderate and higher SES families reported less stress than their lower SES peers. However, similar advantages were not noted for blacks youth, underscoring the importance of race.[16] McGrath and colleagues[17] found that youth living in lower SES communities in general and black youth in particular had increased heart rate and blood pressure measurements. These findings correlated more closely with race and neighborhood measures of SES rather than individual measures of SES. Explanations offered include that youth from lower SES neighborhoods and black adolescents experienced chronic stressors in their neighborhoods that led to a heightened sense of arousal, which consequently lead to increases in heart rate and blood pressure.

This underscores the importance of considering race/ethnicity in addition to SES. As noted by Navarro,[18] "...the issue is not race or class, the issue is race and class." Goodman and colleagues[16] suggest that race/ethnicity and SES should not be considered as "risk factors" (implying causation) but "risk markers" (suggesting that a range of social contextual issues be explored).

## SOCIOECONOMIC STATUS AND ADOLESCENT HEALTH STATUS

"When the world is harsh and challenging, health consequences accrue."[16] Clearly, an adolescent living in a neighborhood of crumbling tenements, where diesel buses belch out noxious fumes, where drug dealers flash pills, pots, and pistols, and where basketball hoops are made out of square milk crates, is exposed more consistently and to a deeper degree of health threats than youth living in more comfortable settings with better resources. Socioeconomic factors clearly play a role in outlining the framework of an adolescent's world. However, filling out the details of that framework is much more complex. Other important factors besides SES and race/ethnicity may play roles in mediating behavior.

For example, the ADDHealth survey, a large national study of several thousand adolescents, examined multiple health-related behaviors such as cigarette use, alcohol use, suicidal thoughts and attempts, weapon-related violence, and sexual intercourse. Although youth in lower SES groups reported higher involvement in cigarette use, suicidal thoughts and attempts, weapon-related violence, and sexual intercourse, youth in higher SES groups reported greater involvement in alcohol abuse. Further, whereas SES appears to contribute to risk-taking behavior, its effect may be mediated by other contextual factors such as race, gender, and family structure. For example, white youth smoke more cigarettes than blacks or Hispanic youth, females were more likely to report suicidal thoughts and attempts, and youth in single-parent families were more likely to drink than those in 2-parent families. However, when taken together, race/ethnicity, family structure, and income appear to be only weak predictors in explaining youth risk behaviors.[19]

If these factors seem to only be partially explanatory for adolescent involvement in risk-taking behaviors, can we delve deeper below the surface and come up with better explanations that also may set the stage for planned interventions?

"Social scientists have come to regard problem behaviors largely as emerging from an interaction or fit between adolescents and their environments rather than an intrinsic or fixed set of attributes of the adolescents themselves. From this vantage point, adolescent problem behavior appears to result from a mismatch between the needs of the child and the opportunities provided by the social context."[12]

Let us assume for the moment that all children (and adolescents) start off with similarities in terms of basic needs and expectations for future success. The interaction between children, their social networks (families, peers, etc.), and the communities in which they live may play significant roles in whether these needs and expectations are successfully met. In general terms, the availability of sufficient community resources (social capital) and the presence of strong connections between youth and these resources seem to be protective against problem behaviors; attenuated social connections and inadequate community resources seem to be contributory.[20] Socioeconomic status may affect both the availability of community resources and the ability of youth to connect with them in a meaningful and sustained fashion.

Social capital builds on the concept that both the quantity (number of community resources such as educational, social, and recreational organizations) and the quality (types of interactions—trust, reciprocity cooperation—among organizations and their constituents) of community resources affect behavior and ultimately health status. In general, more is better. A significant amount of adolescent risk-taking behavior occurs between 3 pm to 9 pm when youth tend to be unsupervised and unchaperoned.[21] Conversely, adolescents actively involved in recreational or cultural activities, supported and monitored by adult mentors, and involved with positive peers have increased opportunities for selection of prosocial choices.[22]

Youth in more affluent communities may have access to more resources and may experience fewer and less prolonged exposure to certain stressors but nonetheless experience contextual issues that affect their involvement in risk-taking behaviors.

Robert Coles[23] was one of the first behaviorists to describe the developmental and emotional problems of affluent youth. He coined the term "entitlement" and defined it as the class-bound prerogative of money and power. On interviewing adolescents from affluent families across the United States, Coles found many to have an exaggerated sense of social class and power that they felt exempted them from following rules and laws. In her book *The Price of Privilege*, psychologist Madeline Levine discusses "the culture of affluence" that stresses materialism rather than having fulfilling relationships with people. This creates a culture of competition rather than cooperation. Sometimes, parents in affluent and middle-class families make childhood and adolescence a "hard act to follow."[24] This may create an expectation of a perfect life without developing the ambition and self-confidence that would allow attainment of success in his or her own right.

The "silver spoon syndrome" has been attributed to the emotional deprivation wealthy adolescents may experience when their parents are not at home parenting but are excessively committed to professional or social endeavors. In some of these families, there are few family-centered interactions and activities as the parents' social demands interfere with the family's daily routines.[25] Parents try to compensate by deluging their children with gifts and unlimited funds.[26] Adolescents who have everything monetarily may become jaded; nothing is new to them, and there is nothing to strive for or to be surprised with. Others may become overwhelmed with all they have and may become incapable of making choices.[23]

Thus, it may be more useful to conceptualize contemporary threats to adolescent well-being as existing along a continuum as compared to being clustered in one stratum. A multitude of factors (individual, familial, and neighborhood) may contribute or mitigate responses to these threats. For example, strong connections between parents and adolescents have been associated with fewer adolescent risk-taking behaviors. Parental monitoring may be a concrete example of how this connection between parent and teen can be advantageous, regardless of SES status of the family. Lower SES parents, particularly those who are single head-of-households, may be overwhelmed by the pressures of trying to make ends meet and consequently less available to consistently plan and monitor the activities of their adolescents. Furstenburg has demonstrated that on the other hand, knowing the risks inherent in living in lower SES communities, these parents may be hypervigilant and tightly structure their teens' lives, even arranging for involvement in pro-social activities within their own communities or in more affluent communities with fewer dangers and more bountiful resources.[12]

Similarly, more affluent parents may spend extensive periods of time working outside of the home to maintain the family's lifestyle, which may make monitoring difficult. Additionally, they may be lulled into a false sense of security by virtue of their distance (geographic, as well as social) from "high-risk" communities, and may consequently be less vigilant. On the other hand, they may be realistic about the issues confronting all youth, regardless of SES status, and have the financial capabilities and community resources available to provide a range of supportive and creative services for their children.

## PROMOTING ADOLESCENT HEALTH

In light of the previous section, Blum and others[19] have called for a careful approach to developing interventions and services that have the best chances of assisting a broad array of adolescents. Although certainly leveling the playing field in terms of family income and educational attainment are important societal goals in and of themselves, they may still not result in optimal health status improvement for youth, as witnessed by the health-compromising behaviors of affluent youth. Rather, a more manageable, concrete approach to improving adolescent health status and reducing risk-taking behaviors may include: (a) improving access to comprehensive, confidential health services for all youth; (b) identifying and supporting youth assets through coordination with social institutions; and (c) improving communication and strengthening connections between youth and their families. For example, Youngblade[27] found that adolescents in communities with greater social capital (schools, houses of worship, access to health providers, family planning clinics, etc.) had lower odds of risky behavior, greater odds of health care utilization, and lower expenditures for health care. Thus, social capital may improve health outcomes by (a) establishing cohesive social conditions that promote health directly, (b) fostering protective behaviors and reducing risky behaviors, and (c) promoting access to public health services.[28] The next section outlines recommendations for improving resources for youth in more detail.

## RECOMMENDATIONS

Improving access to care, identifying and supporting youth assets, and strengthening connections between youth and families are 3 broad strategies for promoting adolescent health. Activities for achieving these broad objectives are described next.

### INCREASE SCHIP AND MEDICAID ENROLLMENT

As noted previously, a differential in health care utilizations exists between lower and higher socioeconomic families with respect to access to care. Health insurance coverage is an important mediating factor. A recent study in New York state comparing access to care of uninsured youth prior to and 1 year following enrollment in SCHIP found the program to significantly increase the percentage of youth who have a usual and customary service provider (81.9% to 94.9%). Additionally, the program demonstrated effectiveness in increasing the percentage of youth (ages 12 to 18) reporting both preventive care (68.9% to 72.6%) and continuity of care visits (47.4% to 90.2%) while reducing the percentage of youth reporting unmet health needs (37.4% to 18.1%).[29]

However, although improvements have been made creative strategies are needed to enhance enrollment of those youth who are eligible for services but remain marginalized. With current health care reform, this issue may be moot but providers still need to make sure that youth have the information for enrollment into health insurance plans.

In addition to increasing enrollment for eligible teens, consideration needs to be given toward expanding eligibility, particularly for (a) middle-income youth whose parents have lost their commercial insurance, and (b) the young adult population. The former category has been briefly discussed previously; in the terms of the latter, the situation is also problematic. Once an adolescent reaches age 19, SCHIP benefits are terminated. Adolescents in higher SES families who are covered by their parents' commercial insurance plans face a similar fate if they are not enrolled in college full-time. Often, if they enter the workforce at this juncture, their first jobs may pay low salaries and have minimal, if any, benefits. Consequently, adolescents and young adults (ages 19 to 29) are more than twice as likely as children and youth ages 18 and younger to be uninsured (30% vs 12%).[30] Thus, consideration should be given to increasing Medicaid/SCHIP coverage to at least age 23 for those with incomes below 100% of poverty, the largest group (2.7 million) of uninsured young adults in this age group. Additionally, for those young adults whose parents have commercial insurance products, private insurers should consider extending their coverage limits to at least the age of 23 as well. Current health care reform provides for the ability of young adults up until age 26 to enroll in their parents' insurance plans, which will ameliorate this problem for many youth. Such an expansion would assist an additional 500,000 to 800,000 young adults.[31]

New York is an example of one state that has attempted to address these concerns by developing 2 insurance plans-Family Health Plus and Healthy NY, that provide coverage for working families with dependent children (up to age 23), as well as young adults (> over age 19) living independently. Family Health Plus is solely government-funded and requires no monthly premium from subscribers.[32] Healthy NY offers reduced cost coverage through government subsidy, designed to supplement services not provided through subscribers' existing health maintenance organizations (HMOs). Healthy NY benefits must be purchased through HMOs, with premiums costing more than $200 per month for an individual.[33]

### INCREASE SUPPORT FOR AND NUMBER OF SCHOOL-BASED AND SCHOOL-LINKED HEALTH CLINICS

Since their inception in the early 1970s, the number of school health clinics has increased substantially to about 1,500 sites nationwide[34] (Chapter 25). These clinics frequently act as "safety nets" to provide quality, comprehensive services for youth in communities lacking an adolescent-friendly primary care infrastructure. Although the number of clinics have increased, there are still many more schools and students that could benefit from having additional resources in their settings. In fact, school-based clinics in suburban schools and private schools would achieve the same purpose as having such in public, urban schools. Additionally, funding support for the clinics should be expanded to allow for an increase in services.

### IMPROVE COMPETENCIES OF PRIMARY CARE PROVIDERS

Adolescents are generally regarded as the "least favorite" age group that primary care providers like to see. In large part this is because of a lack of familiarity with teens and minimal training during medical school and residency.[35] Although adolescent medicine specialists exist, their numbers are relatively small. Thus, to improve service delivery to this age cohort, it is imperative that improvements in training be made at all levels (students, residents, and physicians currently in practice) and in various settings, not only urban medical school clinics. In addition to improving their skills in providing basic medical care to this age group, providers should receive training on how to counsel parents and link families to appropriate community resources.

### IMPROVE SCREENING AND DELIVERY OF PREVENTIVE HEALTH SERVICES

Closely related to increasing insurance coverage for youth and improving provider competencies is the need to improve screening and delivery of preventive health services. All adolescents need to be screened for health risk behaviors regardless of their SES. Whereas lower SES youth may lack access to care or receive fragmented services in emergency departments, youth in affluent communities may also receive suboptimal care. Confidentiality is the cornerstone of effective adolescent service delivery, no matter what the setting. The problem is that in affluent communities, some providers may underestimate the degree of risk-taking generated among their clientele. Additionally, when the health care provider plays golf with the parents of the adolescent, it is hard to convince the teen that answers to questions related to substance use or sexual activity may be held in confidence. Due to parental closeness to the practitioner, questions related to such "uncomfortable issues" may not be raised by either the youth or the provider, and thus the adolescent does not receive needed guidance or help. However, as described previously, adolescents from affluent families participate in substance use, sexual activity, and delinquent behaviors.

### IMPROVE MENTAL HEALTH BENEFITS

Regardless of SES, no family and no adolescent is exempt from learning disabilities attention-deficit/hyperactivity disorder (ADHD) or stress. Although most commercial and governmental insurance plans adequately cover medical services, significant gaps exist with respect to mental health coverage.[36] Outpatient and inpatient benefits may be limited or restricted. Whereas more affluent families may be better positioned in the short run to use family resources to support mental health services, few families are prepared to handle long-term chronic care costs. Thus, a need exists to establish equity between coverage for medical services and mental health/substance abuse care, and strategies should be developed to encourage both SCHIP and managed care plans to expand coverage accordingly.[37]

### IDENTIFY AND SUPPORT YOUTH ASSETS

Although it is critically important that we identify youth involved in risk-taking behaviors so that appropriate services can be provided, it is also important to balance this discovery with a comparable search for youth assets. The Urban Institute reports that even among high risk-takers (youth engaged in 5 or more risky behaviors), 81% also engage in at least one positive behavior, and 49% in at least 2 positive behaviors.[38] Identifying and supporting these positive behaviors may help reduce those behaviors that may lead to health consequences.

### IMPROVE CONNECTIONS WITHIN SCHOOLS

Another area in need of focused consideration centers on the relationship between adolescents and their schools. There is an almost linear relationship between academic achievement, employment, income, and social standing. Whereas race and gender may mediate, to some degree, the impact of social class on health status, nonetheless education remains important to one's eventual life trajectory. Beyond academic performance, however, are the important health educational, social, and cultural functions embodied within schools. Schools can be an important mechanism for educating youth about healthier behaviors. Unfortunately, most schools do not have certified health education instructors and give scant space in the curriculum for cohesive and comprehensive health education. Thus, important opportunities for health promotion are being lost.

With respect to building connections, the ADD-Health surveys suggest that youth with strong connections to school, regardless of other factors (race, SES, etc.), have better health outcomes than those with weaker connections.[19] Although building and maintaining those connections is easier in communities where class size is small, teachers are well-paid, and both in-school and after-school cultural and recreational programs abound, low-income communities are creatively strengthening connections between youth and schools. Strategies include breaking up large, impersonal schools into smaller "houses," often organized around a particular theme or interest, or establishing new charter schools. In both instances, connections are improved due to reduction in class size and recruitment of highly motivated instructors.

### IMPROVE CONNECTIONS BETWEEN YOUTH AND COMMUNITY PROGRAMS

In addition to strengthening the connections between youth and schools, examining ways to keep youth occupied once the school day ends is important. Going home to an empty house with nothing to do but play video games or surf the Web is often an open invitation for engaging in health-compromising behaviors. Institutions such as the YMCA, the Boys and Girls Clubs, as well as faith-based institutions, have historically provided safe havens and opportunities for adolescents to engage in prosocial activities with their peers and adult mentors. Just as providers have listings of referral sources for orthopedists or endocrinologists, they should similarly know what resources exist for parents of adolescents in the communities they serve and be prepared to facilitate referrals and linkages.

### STRENGTHEN CONNECTIONS BETWEEN YOUTH AND FAMILY

Perhaps the most important variable shown to consistently make a difference in the lives of youth is the connection between them and their parents or guardians. However, in contrast to the amount of support services available to new parents and parents of toddlers, relatively little information and advice is disseminated to parents of adolescents through school, community, or health settings. Therefore, we suggest that as part of the enhancement of competencies described here, practitioners learn how to provide support and counseling to parents as well as adolescents. In some cases, that may consist of simple encouragement and reinforcement for doing a good job in communicating with their teens. In other cases, more extensive work may need to be done to help parents identify adequate schools and community resources for their teens.

Additionally, providers, no matter what types of families they see in their practice, need to teach parents to monitor the social and educational activities of their adolescent children. By paying attention to the everyday activities of adolescents, parents will be aware of a problem before it escalates. Practitioners should empower parents to be diligent while not compromising the gradual "letting go" as adolescents strive for independence. Parents should be advised that they cannot be "too busy" and that parental involvement in keeping their adolescent child safe is just as important as such parental involvement for a toddler or school-age child.

Practitioners should be prosocial in the communities where they practice and serve as a resource for schools, community organizations, and religious houses. In an affluent community, that may entail giving talks to groups about the fact that affluent youth may be participating in high-risk behaviors and how parents and teachers can be attuned to the warning signs of such behaviors. In a community where most families are impoverished, the practitioner might wish to give talks about what resources exist for adolescents and their families in terms of preventing high-risk behaviors or addressing such behaviors. In both cases, the practitioner can help build social capital for youth and their families no matter what socioeconomic group they fall into.

## CONCLUSION

Socioeconomic status is an important construct for providers working with adolescents and their families to understand and use appropriately. In and of itself, it does not predict or preclude behaviors. However, it may affect the degree to which adolescents and their families are exposed to and develop responses to important social influences. As such, it is one of many factors that providers should keep in mind when assessing youth and providing them with guidance and support. Additionally, helping communities create and coordinate a network of resources and assisting youth and their parents to identify and utilize these resources consistently may play a role in improving adolescent health-promoting behaviors.

## REFERENCES

1. Adler NE, Ostrove JM. Socioeconomic status and health: what we know and what we don't. *Ann N Y Acad Sci*. 1999;896: 3-15

2. Krieger N, Chen JT, Waterman PD, Rehkopf DH, Subramanian SV. Painting a truer picture of US socioeconomic and racial/ethnic health inequalities: the Public Health Disparities Geocoding Project. *Am J Public Health*. 2005;95(2):312-323

3. Benson V, Marano MA. Current estimates from the National Health Interview Survey, 1992. *Vital Health Stat*. 1994;10(189):1-269

4. Kennedy BP, Kawachi I, Glass R, Prothrow-Stith D. Income distribution, socioeconomic status, and self-rated health in the United States: multilevel analysis. *BMJ*. 1998; 317(7163): 917-921

5. Eaton DK, Kann L, Kinchen S, Ross J, Hawkins J,Harris WA, et al. Youth risk behavior surveillance-United States, 2005. *MMWR Surveill Summ*. 2006;55(5):1-108

6. US Census Bureau. Income, poverty, and health insurance coverage in the United States, 2005. Available at: www.census.gov/prod/2006pubs/p60-231.pdf. Accessed September 6, 2007

7. National Center for Children in Poverty (NCCP) Analysis of the US Current Population Survey. Annual social and economic supplement, March 2008. Available at: www.nccp.org. Accessed September 6, 2007

8. Santelli JS, Lowry R, Brener ND, Robin L. The association of sexual behaviors with socioeconomic status, family structure, and race/ethnicity among US adolescents. *Am J Public Health*. 2000;90(10): 1582-1588

9. Currie CE, Elton RA, Todd J, Platt S. Indicators of socioeconomic status for adolescents: the WHO Health Behaviour in School-aged Children Survey. *Health Educ Res*. 1997;12(3):385-397

10. Krieger N, Williams DR, Moss NE. Measuring social class in US public health research: concepts, methodologies, and guidelines. *Annu Rev Public Health*. 1997;18: 341-378

11. Cubbin C, Smith GS. Socioeconomic inequalities in injury: critical issues in design and analysis. *Annu Rev Public Health*. 2002;23:349-375

12. Furstenberg F, Cook T, Eccles J, Elder G, Sameroff A. *Managing to Make It: Urban Families and Adolescent Success*. University of Chicago Press; 1999

13. Newacheck PW, Park MJ, Brindis CD, Biehl M, Irwin CE, Jr. Trends in private and public health insurance for adolescents. *JAMA*. 2004;291(10):1231-1237

14. Newacheck PW, Hung YY, Park MJ, Brindis CD, Irwin CE, Jr. Disparities in adolescent health and health care: does socioeconomic status matter? *Health Serv Res*. 2003;38(5):1235-1252

15. Farmer MM, Ferraro KF. Are racial disparities in health conditional on socioeconomic status? *Soc Sci Med*. 2005;60(1): 191-204

16. Goodman E, McEwen BS, Dolan LM, Schafer-Kalkhoff T, Adler NE. Social disadvantage and adolescent stress. *J Adolesc Health*. 2005;37(6):484-492

17. McGrath J, Matthews K, Brady S. Individual versus neighborhood socioeconomic status and race as predictors of adolescent ambulatory blood pressure and heart rate. *Soc Sci Med*. 2006.

18. Navarro V. Class and race: life and death situations. *Monthly Review*. 1991;43:1-13

19. Blum RW, Beuhring T, Shew ML, Bearinger LH,Sieving RE, Resnick MD. The effects of race/ethnicity, income, and family structure on adolescent risk behaviors. *Am J Public Health*. 2000;90(12):1879-1884

20. Benson PL, Leffert N, Scales PC, Blyth DA. Beyond the "village" rhetoric: creating healthy communities for children and adolescents. *Appl Dev Sci*. 1998;2:138-169

21. Carnegie Council on Adolescent Development. *Task Force on Youth Development and Community Programs. A Matter of Time: Risk and Opportunity in the Nonschool Hours*. New York: Carnegie Corporation; 1996

22. Vesely SK, Wyatt VH, Oman RF, Aspy CB, Kegler MC, Rodine S, et al. The potential protective effects of youth assets from adolescent sexual risk behaviors. *J Adolesc Health*. 2004;34(5):356-365

23. Coles R. *Privileged Ones: The Well-Off and Rich in America* (Children of Crisis, Vol 5). Boston, MA: Little Brown & Co; 1977

24. Levine M. *The Price of Privilege: How Parental Pressure and Material Advantage Are Creating a Generation of Disconnected and Unhappy Kids.* New York: Harper Collins; 2006

25. Wise PH, Schor L. The neighborhood-poverty, affluence and violence. In: Levine MD, Carey WB, Crocker AC, eds. *Developmental-Behavioral Pediatrics*. 22nd ed. Philadelphia, PA: B Saunders, Co;1992:160-170

26. Shine WA. Affluent adolescents. *J Dev Behav Pediatr*. 1992;13(1):50-52

27. Youngblade LM, Curry LA, Novak M, Vogel B, Shenkman EA. The impact of community risks and resources on adolescent risky behavior and health care expenditures. *J Adolesc Health*. 2006;38(5):486-494

28. Crosby RA, Holtgrave DR. The protective value of social capital against teen pregnancy: a state-level analysis. *J Adolesc Health*. 2006;38(5):556-559

29. Szilagyi PG, Dick AW, Klein JD, Shone LP, Zwanziger J, McInerny T. Improved access and quality of care after enrollment in the New York State Children's Health Insurance Program (SCHIP). *Pediatrics*. 2004;113(5): e395-404

30. Collins S, Schoen C, Tenney K, Doty M, Ho A. Rite of passage? Why young adults become uninsured and how new policies can help. *Issue Brief (Commonw Fund)*. 2005;649:1-12

31. Glied S, Gould D. Analysis of the March 2003 Annual Social and Economic Supplement to the Current Population Survey.

32. New York State Department of Health, Family Health Plus. What is Family Health Plus? Available at: www.health.state.ny.us/nysdoh/fhplus/. Accessed March 7, 2007

33. New York State Insurance Department. HMOs and rates by county. Available at: www.HealthyNY.com. Accessed March 3, 2007

34. Lear JG. School-based health centers: a long road to travel. *Arch Pediatr Adolesc Med*. 2003;157(2):118-119

35. Verhoeven V, Bovijn K, Helder A, Peremans L, Hermann I, Van Royen P, et al. Discussing STIs: doctors are from Mars, patients from Venus. *Fam Pract*. 2003;20(1):11-15

36. Fox HB, McManus MA, Reichman MB. Private health insurance for adolescents: is it adequate? *J Adolesc Health*. 2003;32(6 Suppl):12-24

37. American Academy of Pediatrics. Insurance coverage of mental health and substance abuse services for children and adolescents: a consensus statement. *Pediatrics*. 2000;106 (4):860-862

38. Lindberg L, Boggess S, Porter L, Williams S. *Teen Risk-Taking: A Statistical Portrait*. Washington, DC: US Department of Health and Human Services; June 2000

# CHAPTER 41

# The Media

VICTOR C. STRASBURGER, MD

*True, media violence is not likely to turn an otherwise fine child into a violent criminal. But, just as every cigarette one smokes increases a little bit the likelihood of a lung tumor someday, every violent show one watches increases just a little bit the likelihood of behaving more aggressively in some situation.*

—Psychologists Brad Bushman and L. Rowell Huesmann[1]

*One erect penis on a US screen is more incendiary than a thousand guns.*

—Newsweek critic David Ansen[2]

*Whether we like it or not, alcohol advertising is the single greatest source of alcohol education for Americans.*

—Representative Joe Kennedy (D-MA)[3]

*Research shows that virtually all women are ashamed of their bodies. It used to be adult women, teenage girls, who were ashamed, but now you see the shame down to very young girls—10, 11 years old. Society's standard of beauty is an image that is literally just short of starvation for most women.*

—Best-selling author Mary Pipher[4]

Physicians who treat adolescent patients need to realize that the media influence virtually every concern that they or the teens' parents might have about adolescence—sex, drugs, violence, suicide, school problems, obesity, eating disorders, even sleep. Failure to appreciate a teenager's cultural milieu may result in a physician's inability to treat a basic problem like obesity or a failure to understand a teenager's problems at home or in school. Two simple questions are all that are needed during a routine history and physical examination: (1) How much time do you spend daily with all electronic media? (2) Is there a TV set or an Internet connection in your bedroom?[5] Granted, physicians who see adolescents are under increasing pressure to do more counseling in less time, for less reimbursement. But asking 2 questions about media use will consume only about 15 seconds worth of time in the office and may be a clue to many significant problems and their potential solutions.

Practitioners also need to be aware that young children are uniquely susceptible to media influence but that their behavior may not show that influence until they are adolescents or young adults.[6] Therefore, when thinking about media effects, the entire range of childhood through adolescence must be considered.

## SCOPE OF MEDIA USE AMONG TEENS

Media represent the most significant cultural influence on teenagers in their lives. Teens are surrounded by media daily and spend more time with a variety of different media than they do in any other activity except for sleeping. By the time today's teenagers reach age 70, they will have spent 7 to 10 years of their lives watching television alone.[6] Multitasking only adds to the potential effect. A 2009 survey of more than 2,000 3rd through 12th graders found that young people spend an average of more than 7 hours per day with a variety of different media (see Figure 41-1).[7] Television remains the predominant medium, even for teenagers, but they tend to branch out into computer games, music, music videos, and movies as well (see Figure 41-1).[7] One of the biggest problems is that two-thirds of American children and teens have a television set in their own bedroom, one-half have a VCR or DVD player, one-half have a video game console, and nearly one-third have a computer. Bedroom media increases screen time (see Figure 41-1).[7] Despite general concerns about "new media," there are currently no behavioral studies available on teens' use of iPods or cell phones. In addition, "old media" are now playing on cell phones, and in the near future, TV shows and movies will be playing on personal Internet devices as well.

## HOW ARE ADOLESCENTS INFLUENCED BY THE MEDIA?

For teenagers seeking the answers to such crucial questions as, "Who am I?" "What am I going to do when I grow up?" "When should I start having sex?" "Should

I use drugs?" the media provide all the answers that parents, sex education, and drug prevention education often do not. Because of the prevalence of casual sex and drug use in the media, teenagers get the impression that such behaviors are "normative"—ie, "everyone's doing it." In fact, studies show that teenagers routinely overestimate the number of their peers who are having sex, for example.[8] In this way, the media function as a kind of "super-peer," exerting an extraordinary amount of pressure on teenagers to have sex, use drugs, or use violence as an acceptable solution to problems.[8,9] The media offer teenagers a variety of "scripts" for dealing with important issues—gender identity, conflict resolution, sexual gratification, stress, parents, school, etc. Although teenagers acknowledge the potential power of the media to influence behavior, they believe that the media influence everyone else but themselves—the so-called third-person effect that is well documented in literature (and applies to adults as well) (see Figure 41-2).[10]

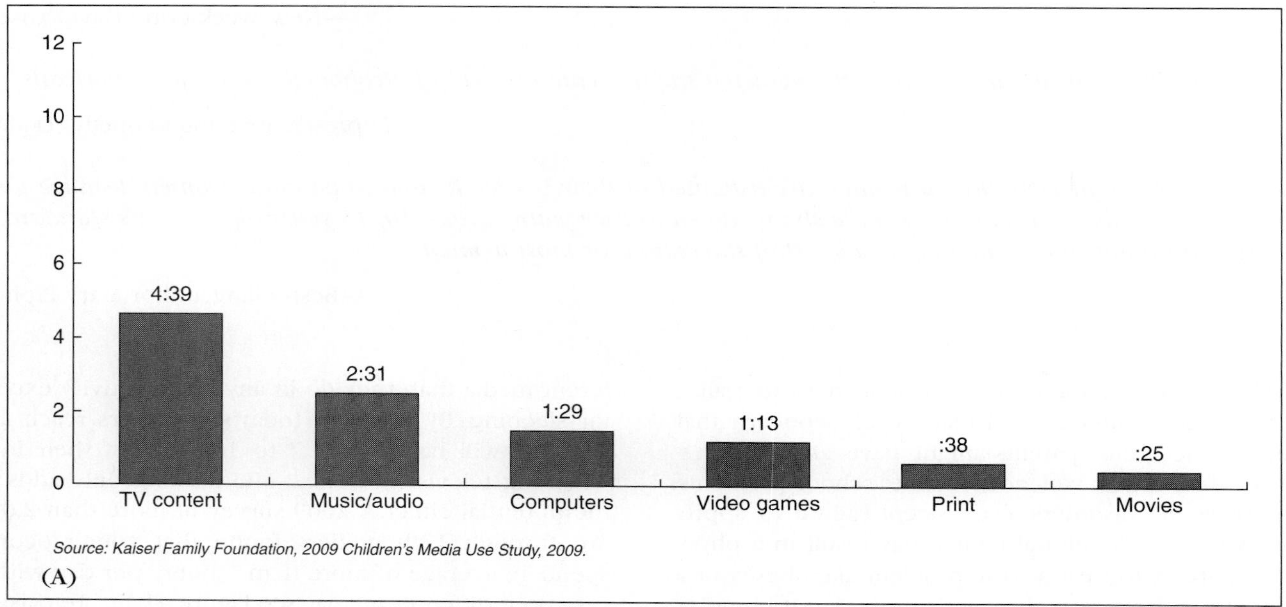


Source: Kaiser Family Foundation, 2009 Children's Media Use Study, 2009.

(A)

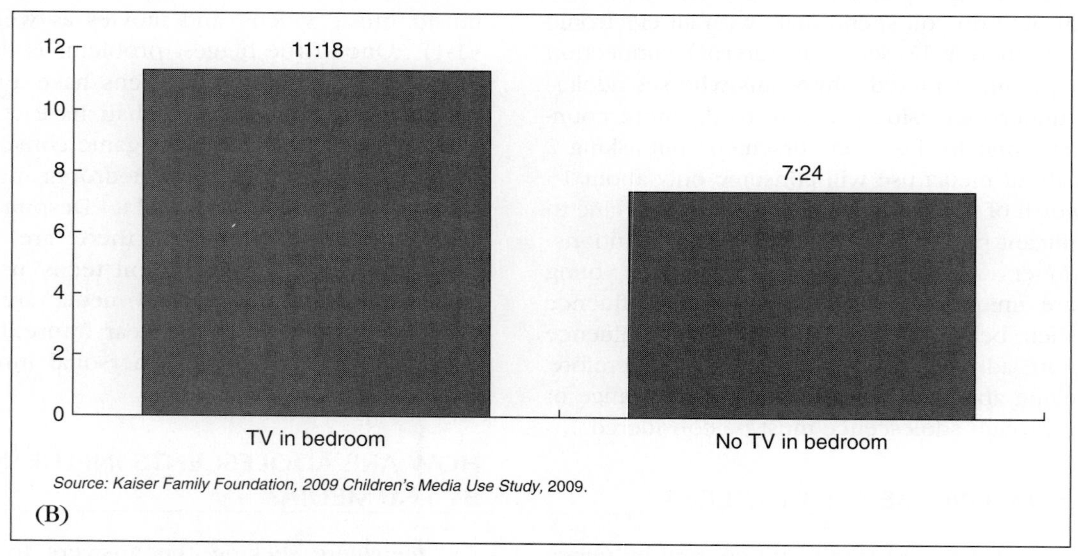


Source: Kaiser Family Foundation, 2009 Children's Media Use Study, 2009.

(B)

**FIGURE 41-1** *(Continued)*

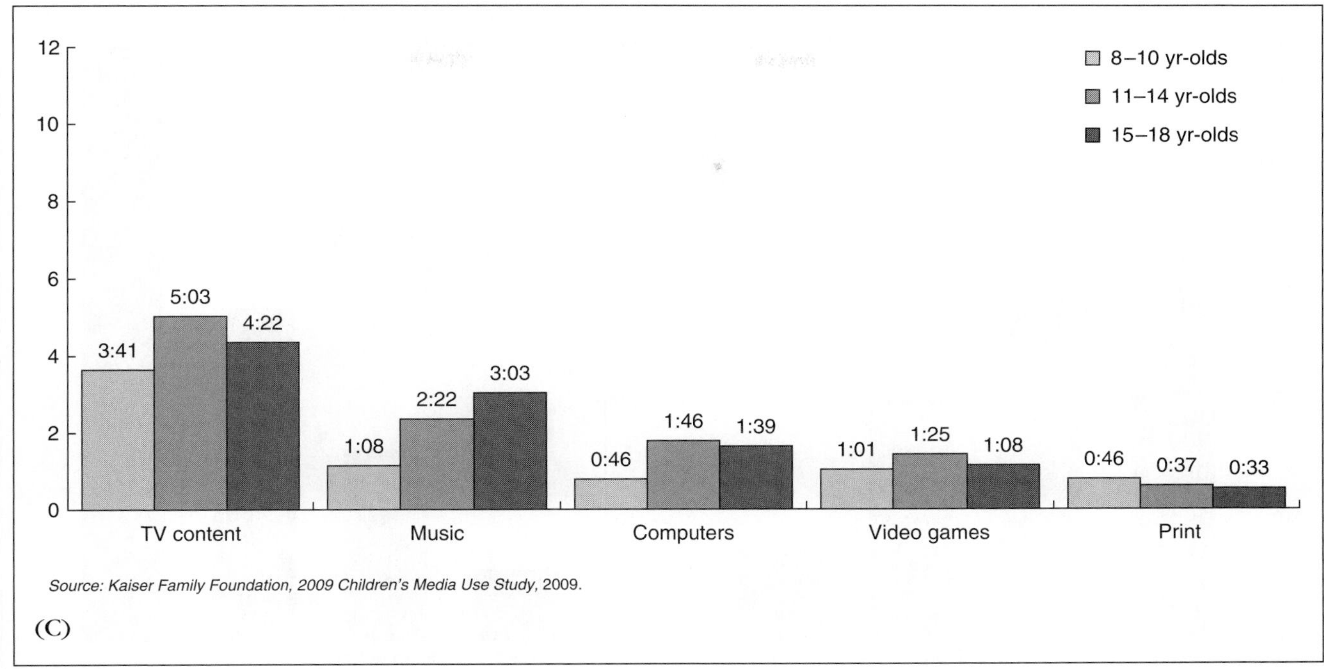


**FIGURE 41-1** Media Use among 8-18 year-olds. (A) Total time spent with media is > 7 hours per day. (B) Presence of a TV set in the bedroom increases total daily media time to >11 hours per day. (C) Even among older adolescents, television remains the predominant medium. (From Rideout V. *Generation M²: Media in the lives of 8- to 18-Year-olds*. Menlo Park, CA: Kaiser Family Foundation, 2010. Reprinted with permission from the Henry J. Kaiser Family Foundation.)

## MEDIA VIOLENCE

Of all the research in the past 60 years on media, studies on media violence and its connection to real-life aggressive behavior are, by far, the most numerous and most compelling. As 1 leading researcher suggests, there should no longer be any controversy that a cause-and-effect connection exists.[11] More than 3,500 reports, including 1,000 research studies, have been done; fewer than 30 studies have found no relation.[12] But social science research is not like medical research: teasing out behavioral effect from ubiquitous influences like media is extraordinarily difficult. Like smoking, media violence is a negative environmental influence. As with smoking, not all who partake are affected. But the connection between media violence and real-life aggression is nearly as strong as the connection between smoking and lung cancer, and given the difficulties of doing social science research, this finding is quite striking (Figure 41-3).[1,6] The effect size is significant: approximately 10% to 30% of violence in society can be attributed to the impact of media violence.[1,6] The research shows that children and teenagers are most likely to be affected because they learn at an early age from the media that violence is an acceptable solution to everyday problems.[6,13,14] Several longitudinal studies have shown that young children exposed to a lot of media violence are much more likely to exhibit aggressive behavior as teenagers.[14-17] A study in the 1960s of 875 third graders found that exposure to TV violence was highly predictive of aggressive behavior 11 and 22 years later.[15] The researchers concluded that young people learn their attitudes about violence at a very young age (age 8 or younger) and, once learned, their attitudes are difficult to modify.[15] A similar study of 707 children aged 1 to 10 years found that time spent watching television was a significant risk factor for adolescent boys.[16] And a 15-year study in 1977 found that viewing violent media at the ages of 6 to 9 was predictive of adolescent aggression and even criminal behavior and spousal abuse in adulthood.[17]

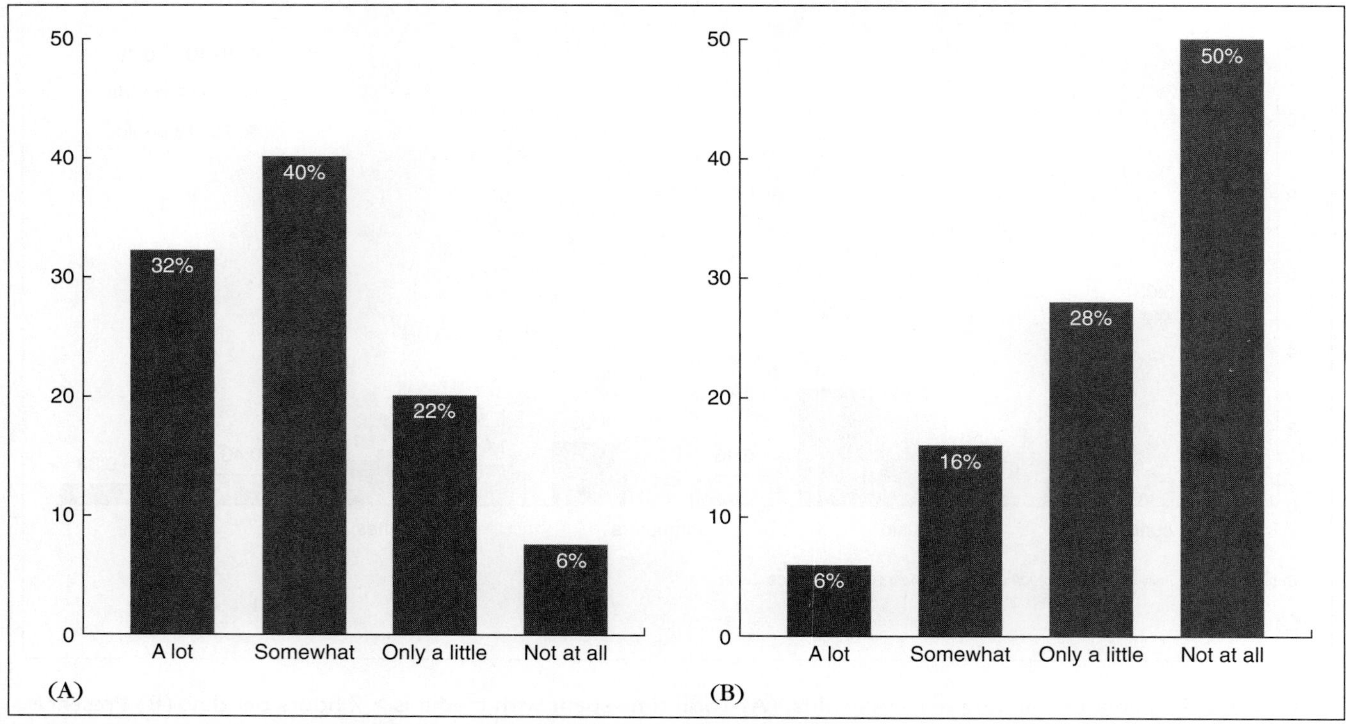


**FIGURE 41-2** The third-person effect. (A) Respondents were asked how much, if at all, they think sexual behaviors on television influence sexual behaviors of teens their age; (B) Respondents were asked how much, if at all, they think sexual behaviors on television influence their own sexual behavior. (From *Teens say sex on television influences behavior of peers—news release,* The Henry J. Kaiser Family Foundation, May 2002. This information was reprinted with permission from the Henry J. Kaiser Family Foundation.)

Violent video games are another concern.[18,19] Interactive media may have even more profound effects on aggressive attitudes and behavior than passive media like television. In 3 recent studies comparing the effects of video games with television and movies, the effect of interactive media was stronger.[19] Many studies have found that violent video games can lead to increases in aggressive thoughts and behavior and decreases in prosocial behavior.[18,20,21] In addition, new media give youth the opportunity to behave aggressively through Internet bullying and harassment.[22]

Research on media violence has been conducted since the 1950s, yet the American government, Hollywood, and the American public seem unconvinced. Why? Part of the reason may be found in the fact that exposure to media violence results in the desensitization of virtually everyone who views it.[6,13] The other dangerous aspect of American media violence is its glorification of guns[6,23] and its obsession with "good guys versus bad guys." The notion of "justifiable violence" is the most prevalent aspect of American media violence and the most powerfully reinforcing.[23] It may help explain the motives behind many of the schoolyard shooters in the 1990s.[23]

## SEX AND THE MEDIA

In the absence of effective sex education at home or in school, the media have become the leading sex educator in America today.[8,24] This is not a healthy situation, given that more than 75% of all prime-time shows contain sexual content, teen shows having even more sexual content than adult shows (see Figure 41-4). Furthermore, 10% of shows portray or imply sexual intercourse, but only 14% of shows with sexual content mention any risks or responsibilities of having sex (see Figure 41-4).[25] American television is not the most sexually graphic medium in the world. Other countries display far more nudity, for example. But American television is the most sexually suggestive medium in the world.[8,24] Sex is used to sell everything from shampoo to cars, from vacations to hamburgers. Sex is most often portrayed as a sport, with no risks of sexually transmitted

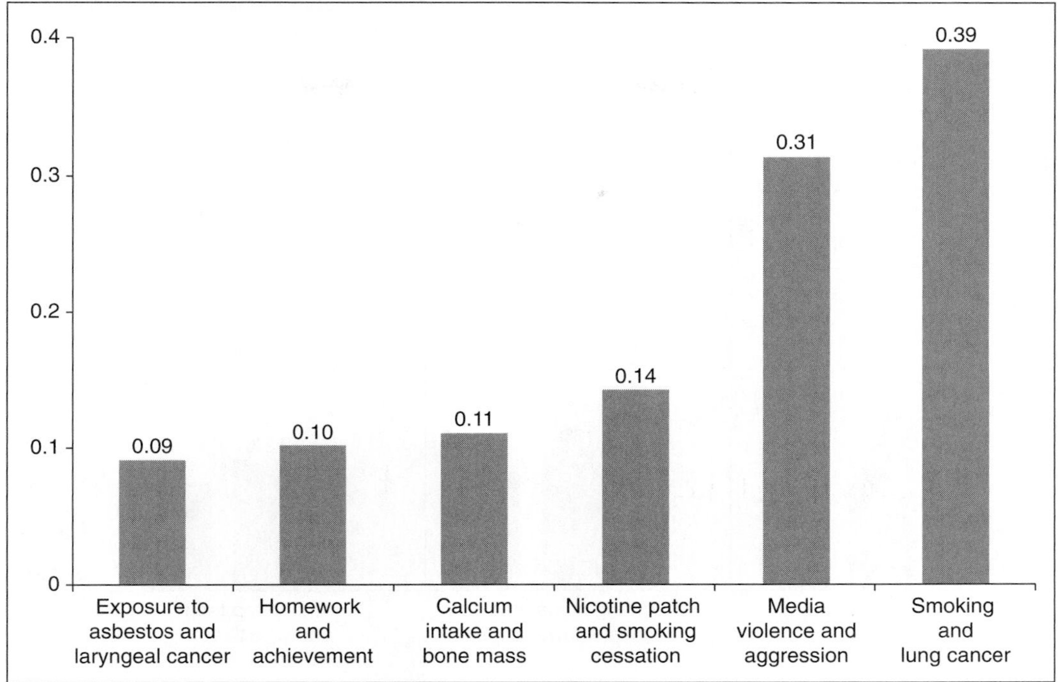


**FIGURE 41-3** The violence effect. How does media violence compare with other widely accepted public health risks? (Adapted from Bushman BJ, Huesmann LR. Effects of televised violence on aggression. In: DG Singer, JL Singer, eds. *Handbook of Children and the Media.* Thousand Oaks, CA: SAGE Publications; 2001. Used with permission.)

infections or pregnancy. Again, the most powerful and worrisome aspect is the "normative behavior" conveyed, and prime-time television makes it seem like everyone is having sex.

What affect does all of this sexual content have on teenagers? As abstinence-only sex education expands—despite its lack of documented effectiveness[26,27]—the media have become the primary source of information about sex for teenagers by default.[28,29] A 2004 national survey of 15- to 17-year-olds found that the media far outranked parents or schools as a source of information about birth control, for example.[30] Teenagers' beliefs about how males and females behave in romantic relationships can be shaped by the media they view.[31,32] The Internet is also becoming an important source of sexual information and pornography.[29,33-35] In a national sample of 1,500 10- to 17-year-olds, nearly half of the Internet users had been exposed to online pornography in the previous year.[34] Unwanted sexual solicitations and online harassment are not uncommon,[34] although they may not be as frequent as parents fear.[36] Social networking sites and home pages enable teenagers to present themselves publicly, sometimes in very sexually suggestive ways.[29] One national survey found that up to 20% of teens are involved in sexting.[37]

What about the effect of sexual content on teenagers' sexual behavior?

- Researchers have found modest but significant associations between sexual content and

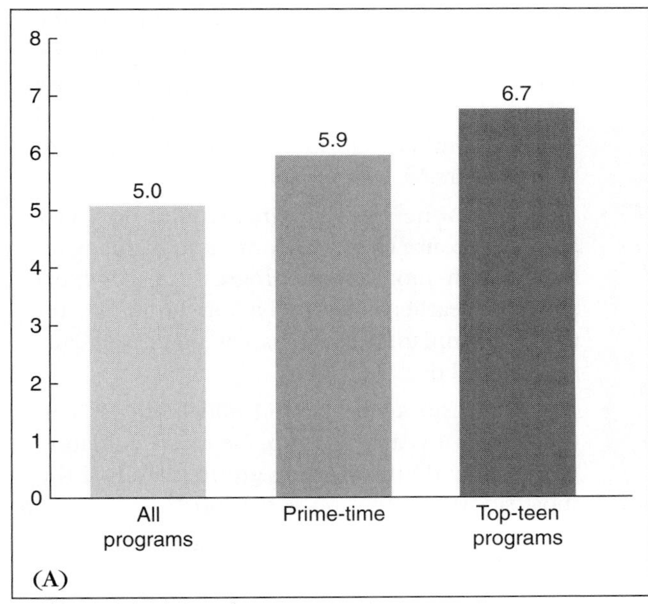


**FIGURE 41-4** *(Continued)*

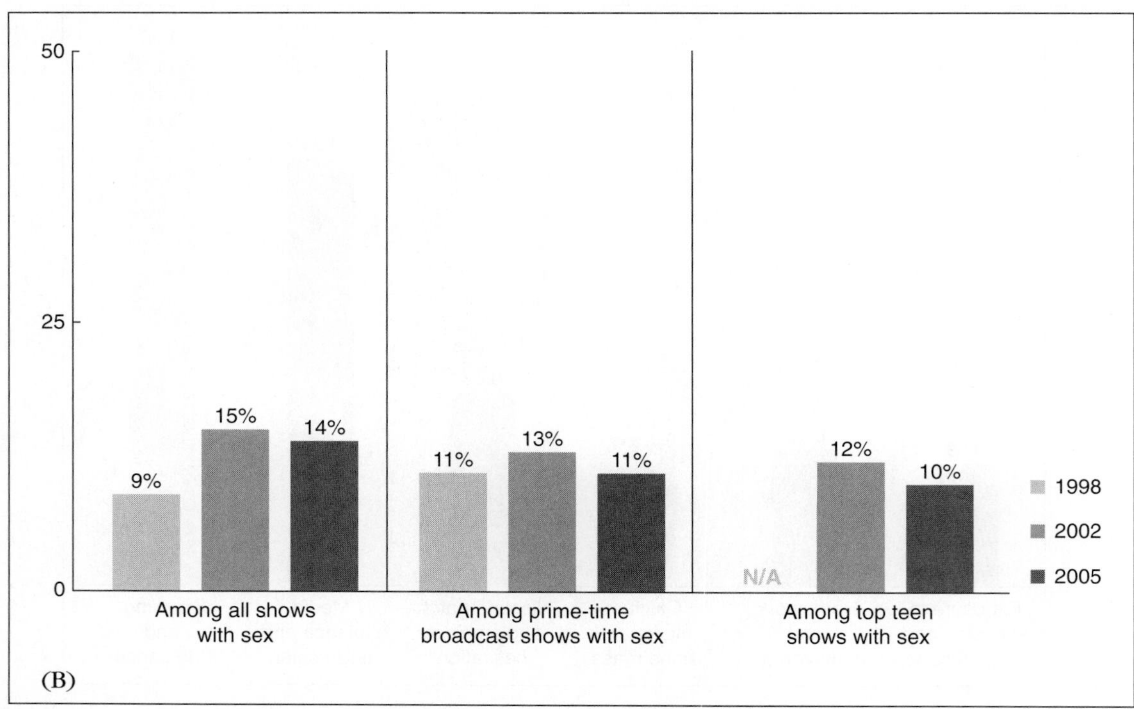


**FIGURE 41-4** Sexual content in television programs. (A) Among shows in 2005 with sexual content, the number of sex-related scenes per hour; (B) Among all shows with sexual content, the percentage that also include references to risks or responsibilities, over time. (From *Sex on TV 4* (#7398), The Henry J. Kaiser Family Foundation, November 2005. This information was reprinted with permission from the Henry J. Kaiser Family Foundation.)

earlier onset of sexual behavior, particularly with exposure to pornography.[29] In a sample of middle school youth, exposure to sexually explicit (X-rated) content predicted perpetration of sexual harassment (for males), more permissive sexual norms, having oral sex, and engaging in sexual intercourse during high school years.[32]

- Also, several new longitudinal studies now link heavy exposure to sexual content in mainstream media with more rapid progression of sexual activity,[28] earlier coital behavior,[38] and greater risk for unplanned pregnancy[39] and sexually transmitted disease.[40]
- In a RAND survey of nearly 1,800 12- to 18-year-olds with a 1-year follow-up, the risk of initiating intercourse doubled in the group watching the most sexual content on television.[38]
- In the most comprehensive study to date, researchers in North Carolina conducted a 2-year longitudinal study of more than 1,000 12- to 14-year-olds and compiled a "media diet" for each, comprising their use of television, movies, music, and magazines. Again, a twofold risk of sexual intercourse for white teens exposed to a heavy diet of sexy media was found.[41]

One explanation for this relationship may lie in the role of media as a "super peer" that provides adolescent audiences with a consistent message that sex is normative and risk-free.[8] By contrast, parents' influence may be protective.[42,43] A longitudinal study of nearly 1,000 adolescents and their parents found that teens whose parents limit their TV viewing are less likely to engage in early sex.[42]

This is not easy research to do. The fact that there are 1,000 studies on media violence but only a half dozen on sexual activity and the media is striking. However, there are dozens of other correlational studies on sexual attitudes and behaviors that contribute as well:

- Teens who watch a lot of soap operas are less likely to believe that they should use birth control if their favorite characters do not use it.[44]

- Earlier sexual intercourse is correlated with a preference for Music Television (MTV),[45] music videos,[46] rap or hip-hop music,[47,48] reading women's magazines,[49] and X-rated movies.[40]

What *is* clear is that the media *could* serve as an important access point for teenagers about birth control, but they fail, almost entirely, to do so. The United States remains the only Western nation that still subscribes to the myth that making birth control available to teenagers will make them sexually active at a younger age.[8] In fact, there are now 8 peer-reviewed studies that document that making condoms available in school-based health clinics, for example, does nothing more than increase the use of condoms for those teens who begin having sex.[8] Currently, 3 of the 6 major networks refuse to air advertisements for condoms, and 3 other networks reject ads for birth control pills. In 2007, CBS and FOX refused to air a commercial for Trojan condoms because it mentioned pregnancy prevention.[50] Meanwhile, ads for Viagra, Cialis, and Levitra—with their prominent mention of "4-hour erections"—are nearly ubiquitous. Between January and October of 2004 alone, drug companies spent nearly $350 million advertising drugs for erectile dysfunction.[51] Although one might argue that these ads are targeted to an older population, adolescents are flooded with these messages as well, so American media can hardly be considered "abstinence-only."

## DRUGS AND THE MEDIA

American advertisers spend virtually nothing to advertise contraceptives, but they do spend more than $20 billion a year advertising tobacco, alcohol, and prescription drugs.[52] "Just say no" has become "Just say yes."

Of that $20 billion, more than half is spent on tobacco advertising—$11.2 billion a year—which may have more effect than peers or family.[53] Because half of smokers begin by age 13 and 90% by age 19, targeting teenagers is inevitable. Two large studies have found that one-third of all adolescent smoking can be attributed to the influence of tobacco advertising and promotions.[54,55] Alcohol advertising accounts for nearly $6 billion a year,[56] and the average American teenager sees 2,000 alcohol ads per year on television alone.[52] Again, several studies have shown an effect of such ads on children's and adolescents' intentions to drink.[6,57-59] As with other advertising, alcohol advertising frequently uses sex to sell, or depicts alcohol use as "normative" behavior (see Figure 41-5).

Finally, another $4 billion is spent on prescription drug advertising.[60] Drug companies now spend more

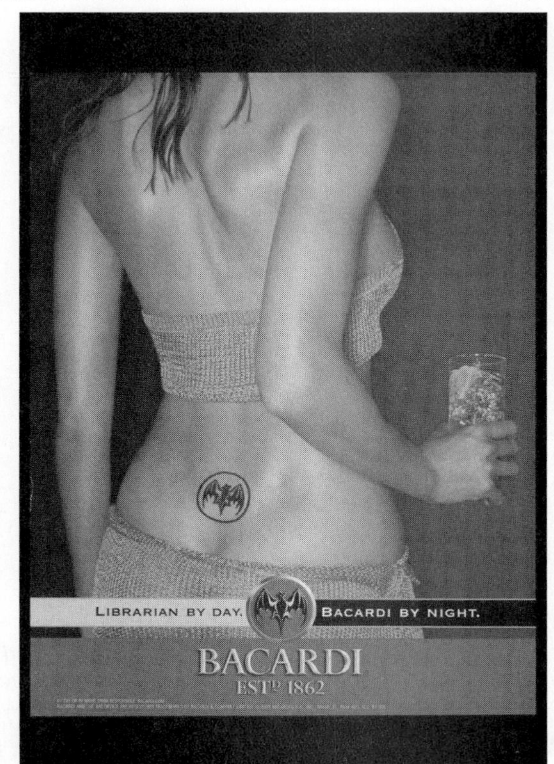


(A)

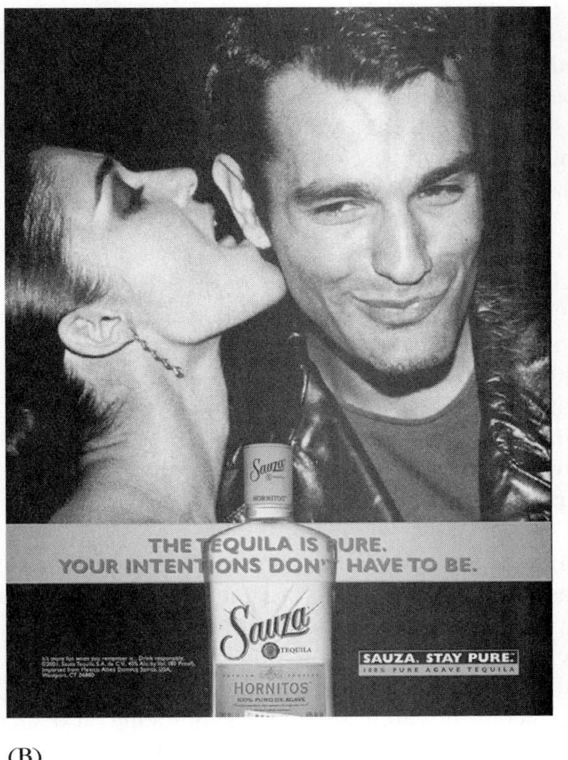


(B)

**FIGURE 41-5** Alcohol ads. (A) Sexy; (B) Normative.

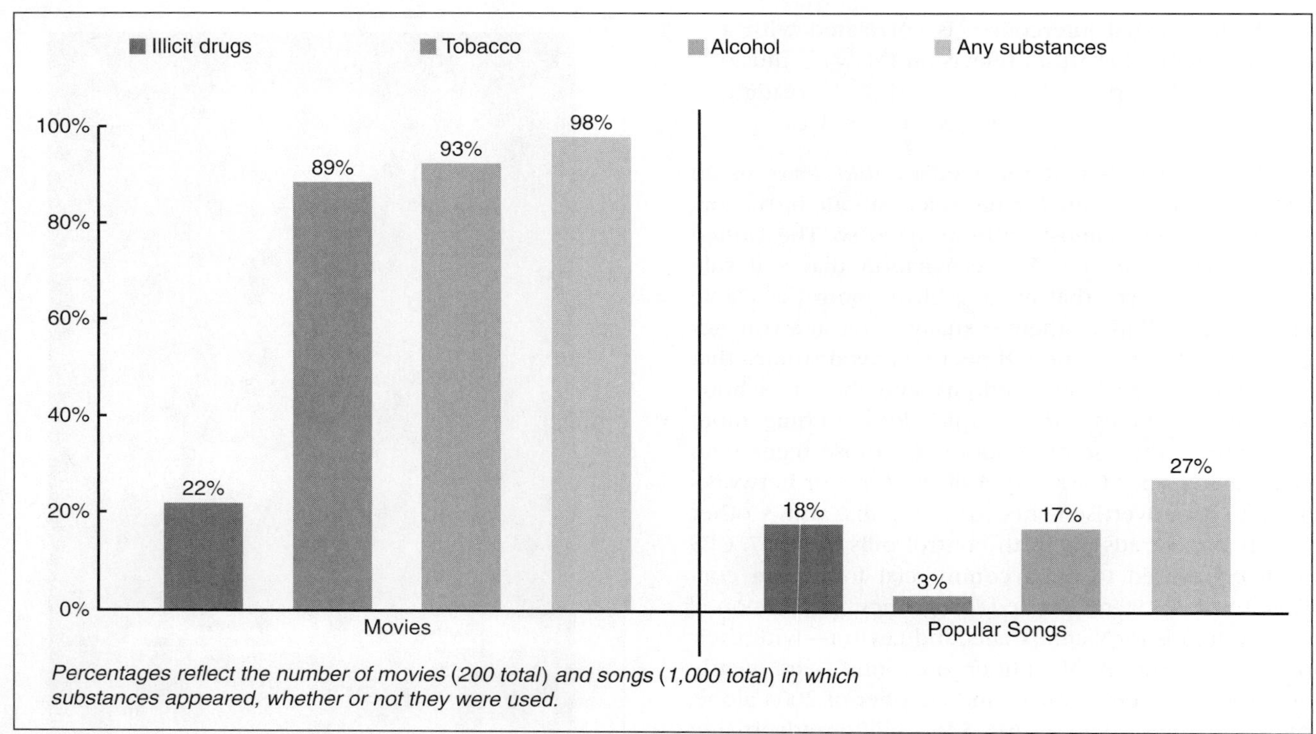


**FIGURE 41-6** Drugs in Popular Movies and Songs. (From Roberts DF, Henriksen L, Christenson PG. *Substance use in popular movies and music*. Washington, DC: Office of National Drug Policy Control, 2000.)

than twice as much on marketing as they do on research and development. Young people clearly get the message that there is a drug to cure every ailment.

Drug advertising is only part of the picture, however. Children and adolescents are also inundated with drug-related content on television, in popular movies, and in popular music (Figure 41-6).[61-63] After a number of years where awareness and social pressures resulted in a clear decrease, smoking cigarettes seems to be making a comeback in the media, with nearly one-quarter of shows on television featuring smoking and 85% of the 250 top-grossing movies from 1988 to 1997.[64] In particular, the rate of smoking on the big screen far outstrips the rate in real life (which answers Hollywood's frequent argument that movies simply "mirror" what is happening in society).[64] On prime-time television, 71% of shows depict alcohol use, whereas 93% of movies contain scenes with alcohol.[61,62] By comparison, drugs like marijuana, inhalants, cocaine, and ecstasy are rarely depicted on television or in the movies. Yet, nearly all of the federal government's antidrug efforts have focused on illegal drugs, not legal ones.

Recent research shows that smoking and alcohol scenes on television and in movies may be particularly powerful in interesting young people to begin experimenting with cigarettes and alcohol.[65-70] Children and teens who watch more than 4 hours of television per day are 5 times more likely to start smoking than those who watch less than 2 hours per day,[66] and exposure to R-rated movies doubles the risk of new smoking among teens, independent of whether their parents smoke.[67-69]

Again, new technologies—the Internet, social networking sites, even cell phones—offer problematic opportunities for teen drug exposure.[59,71] A variety of Internet Web sites sell tobacco products.[3,72] One national survey of more than 1,000 youths ages 14 to 20 found that 2% reported having purchased alcohol online and 12% reported having a friend who did so.[73] Popular beer brands use "advergames" to entice a younger audience.[74] Prescription drugs can also be purchased online with minimal difficulty. Teens also see considerable alcohol and drug content in online videos[75] and in social networking sites,[76] where 1 study found that 40% of profiles referenced substance abuse.[77]

## OBESITY, EATING DISORDERS, AND THE MEDIA

In the past decade, an increased appreciation has emerged of the media's effect on obesity and eating disorders among children and adolescents. How much do the media contribute to obesity? The answer is: significantly, but the research is sometimes complicated. Certainly, the advertising part of the equation is easy: Americans spend more on fast food ($110 billion) than they do on higher education, computers, or cars.[78] Every day, throughout the world 45 million people eat at McDonald's.[78] Half of the nearly 40,000 ads that children and teens see on television every year are for fast food or high-calorie snacks or sugared cereals.[79] Advertising for food does not stop at school doors anymore either. There are more than 4,500 Pizza Huts and 3,000 Taco Bells in school cafeterias around the country.[52] New research shows that soft drink consumption may contribute substantially to obesity,[80] yet many school districts still have lucrative contracts to include sodas and juices in vending machines.[81]

The relationship between TV viewing and obesity is, unfortunately, not quite as clear. A number of good studies have found a significant association between TV viewing and obesity.[6,82,83] However, nearly all have been correlational studies, not longitudinal ones, meaning that the results could simply be reflecting greater sedentary habits of obese children or teens. One study found that children with a TV set in their bedroom have a 30% increased risk of being overweight (body mass index >85th percentile).[84] The most intriguing study was an intervention to reduce media time over a 6-month period, which resulted in significant decreases in all measures of adiposity.[85] Part of the problem is that researchers still do not know exactly how the media affect obesity.[86-88] Is it because media use displaces other, more active pursuits? Is it because TV viewing exposes young people to advertising for fast food and unhealthy food? Is it because screen time increases snacking and unhealthy food choices? Or is it the affect on sleep? The answer is probably "all of the above," but at the moment, the research is unclear.

At the opposite end of the spectrum, the media's contribution to abnormal body self-image among young girls and to eating disorders is being increasingly well defined.[89] To a great extent, the media define "what is thin," "what is cool," "what is hot" in teenage society. In the 1950s, Marilyn Monroe wore a size 14 dress. Now, the average media model weighs 23% less than the average American woman.[6] Preteen and teen girls are bombarded with images of anorectic models and movie stars (Figure 41-7) and discussions in teen magazines about dieting and fat. The effect is enormous. Nearly one-third of third-grade girls have dieted; 60% of sixth-grade girls have dieted.[90] As many as half of normal-weight teenage girls consider themselves overweight or fat.[90] Many studies have found that the media contribute to the development of abnormal body self-image among young girls. For example:

- Two studies, each with nearly 7,000 9- to 15-year-olds, found that girls who wanted to look like television or movie stars were twice as likely to have weight concerns, be dieters, or be engaged in purging behavior.[91,92]
- A study of 600 girls in 5th to 12th grades found that more than two-thirds said their ideal body shape was influenced by the fashion magazines they read.[93]
- A study of nearly 1,000 ninth-grade girls found a correlation between watching a lot of music videos and concerns about appearance and weight.[94]

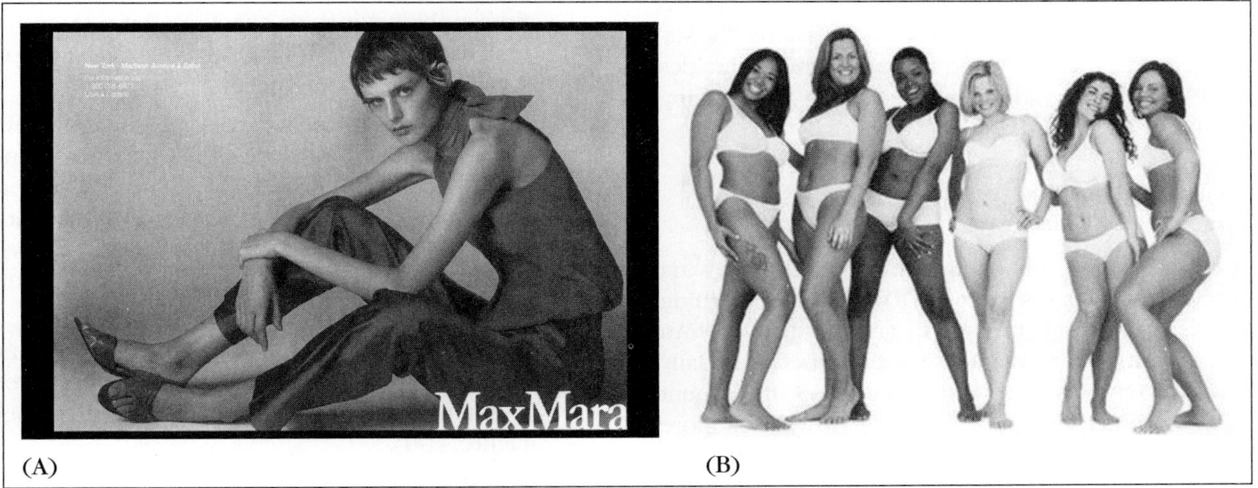


FIGURE 41-7 Compare the anorectic-looking model in (A) with the healthier body types portrayed in Dove's "Campaign for Real Beauty" ad in (B).

Given these studies, and the fact that an abnormal body self-image is a key ingredient in the development of an eating disorder, is it possible that the media cause eating disorders in teenagers? There are several intriguing studies, but they do not yet rise to the level of cause-and-effect:

- A recent study of more than 10,500 athletes and nonathletes found that approximately 30% of adolescent females and males are concerned about their muscle definition, and that 2% to 5%, respectively, have tried products to change their muscle mass.[95]
- A study of nearly 3,000 Spanish 12- to 21-year-olds found that those who read girls' magazines over a 19-month period had twice the risk of developing an eating disorder.[96]
- A naturalistic study of the effect of introducing American TV shows like "Beverly Hills 90210" into the Pacific isle of Fiji found that 15% of teen girls reported vomiting to control their weight after American shows were introduced, compared with only 3% beforehand.[97] In addition, nearly 75% reported feeling "too big or fat" after American television arrived.

## OTHER MEDIA EFFECTS

### SUICIDE

Several studies have found that media coverage of suicide and made-for-TV movies about suicide can result in an increase in teen suicides.[98] Even sensitively made films result in an increase.[98] This "suicide contagion" is far stronger in adolescents than in adults. The Centers for Disease Control and Prevention have issued guidelines for reporting suicide in the media, asking TV stations and newspapers to avoid sensationalizing suicides (eg, Kurt Cobain, the well-known rock star) or glorifying the person involved.[99]

### SCHOOL PERFORMANCE AND LEARNING PROBLEMS

The possibility of a connection between TV viewing and attention-deficit disorder (ADD) or other learning disabilities is currently an issue of great controversy. An initial report in 2004 found an association between daily hours of TV viewing at ages 1 to 2 years and subsequent attentional problems at the age of 7.[100] However, a more recent report examining 59 children with ADD and 106 comparison children actually found that the latter had more impairment in their cognitive processes after viewing television than the former.[101] At least 4 studies have found an effect on academic performance,[102-105] especially if there is a TV set in the child's or teen's bedroom.[104]

Many teenagers get far fewer than the 8 to 9 hours of sleep per night that they need, and media use has been associated with a variety of sleep disturbances, including sleep deprivation, fatigue, and neurocognitive impairment.[106] In turn, inadequate sleep has been associated with poor school performance, obesity, accidents and injuries, and aggressive behavior.[106]

## IMPROVING MEDIA FOR ADOLESCENTS

### HOLLYWOOD'S ROLE

An editorial cartoon shows the famous "Hollywood" sign being transformed into "Notmyfaultywood." Traditionally, Hollywood has resisted and resented any pressure from public health groups to make movies or television less violent, less sexually suggestive, or less drug-oriented.[6] Frequently, writers, directors, and producers cite First Amendment concerns, although the American Academy of Pediatrics[107] and many other organizations have specifically ruled out censorship as a solution. Hollywood and TV network moguls need to accept the fact that the media are a powerful teacher of children and adolescents and that research is quite convincing on this point. In return for the free use of the airwaves (TV) or the millions of dollars in profit made (movies), the entertainment industry needs to accept the fact that it has a public health responsibility.

### WHAT, SPECIFICALLY, COULD BE DONE?

- Decreases in cigarette smoking in movies. This could entail having movie sets designated as nonsmoking zones or changing the ratings system used by the Motion Picture Association of America (MPAA) (Figure 41-8).
- Less gratuitous violence in movies and on television. One study of popular PG-13 movies found that nearly 90% contained violence.[108] The consequences of violence and the effect of violence on families and society need to be shown. Gunplay needs to be severely curtailed in media that are popular with young people.
- More discussion of responsible sexuality and birth control on television, including advertisements for birth control products (see Figure 41-9).
- Creation of a universal ratings system that would apply to television, movies, video games, and music.[109] Currently, each medium has its

R

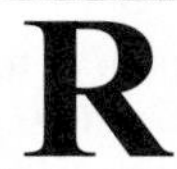

**RESTRICTED**

UNDER 17 REQUIRES ACCOMPANYING PARENT OR ADULT GUARDIAN

**STRONG LANGUAGE AND TOBACCO USE**

***"R" FOR RESPONSIBLE. The MPAA claims the First Amendment is the reason it won't rate smoking "R." But it R-rates offensive but perfectly legal language now. Surely it doesn't consider its own age-classification system censorship? After all, the First Amendment prohibits the government from banning movies, not voluntary, responsible rating choices by the studio-controlled MPAA.***

FIGURE 41-8 Many public health organizations have called for an automatic R rating to be given for movies in which any amount of significant smoking is depicted. The MPAA responded that it would "consider" smoking in its ratings assignments but that no rating would be automatic. (Copyright © SmokeFreeMovies.org. Reprinted with permission.)

"I didn't use one because I didn't have one with me."

GET REAL
If you don't have a parachute, don't jump, genius.

TROJAN
Helps reduce the risk

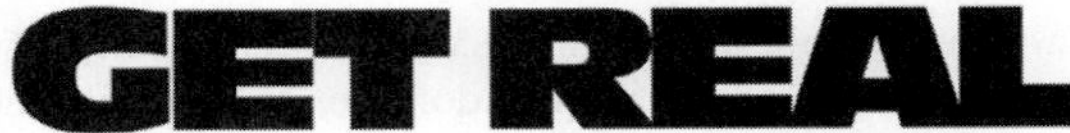

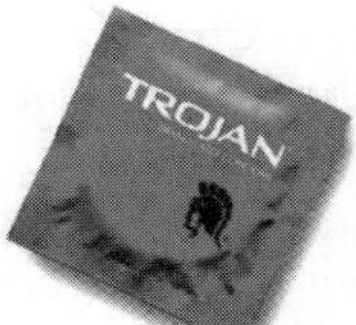

FIGURE 41-9 Condom ad depicting responsible sexuality and birth control.

own ratings system, often done in secret or by the producers themselves. The current system is unworkable, inaccurate, and not useful to parents.[109]

- More dialogue between public health activists and the creative community in Hollywood.

**MADISON AVENUE'S ROLE**

The United States is unique in spending $250 billion a year on advertising—more than twice the second-place nation (Japan). Clearly advertising works or advertisers wouldn't spend so much money on it! But it needs to be made healthier from a public health perspective. This means elimination of or severe restrictions on ads for unhealthy snack foods and fast food on shows that target children and adolescents. It also means that there should be a closer look at the types of models used in print and TV ads. In the United Kingdom, the British Medical Association[110] sponsored a meeting of advertisers, representatives from the entertainment industry, and public health activists. They all agreed to voluntary restrictions on the use of anorectic models and actresses in mainstream media.

**THE FEDERAL GOVERNMENT'S ROLE**

Traditionally, the government has been reluctant to intervene in the "free marketplace," even when there is ample evidence that intervention is necessary (eg, cigarette advertising). Scores of laws have been introduced in Congress, but they are usually followed by a flood of political donations from industries that would be affected. Legislation that would directly improve adolescents' health includes the following:

- A ban in all media on tobacco advertising. Several European countries already do this.
- Restrictions on alcohol advertising to "tombstone" advertisements (ie, only the product is shown, not the sexy beach babes or funny lizards).
- A law that would mandate media education for all K–12th-grade students.
- A law that would mandate a media component for all sex education and drug prevention programs in schools.
- Increased funding for basic media research.

**THE ROLE OF SCHOOLS**

Schools need to recognize the importance of media in students' lives. They could do so by teaching media literacy,[111] incorporating media education principles into existing sex and drug education programs, and using media more creatively. For example, for the past 50 years or so, middle school preteens and teens have had to read "Romeo and Juliet" as their first exposure to Shakespeare. The problem with that is (1) it is a play about 2 teens who have sex and then commit suicide, and (2) Shakespeare never wrote his plays to be read—he wrote them to be performed and seen. There are now a half-dozen good versions of "Romeo and Juliet" on DVD and videotape. If the play must be taught, it can be viewed, not read. Similarly, anyone trying to teach about the American Civil War would be foolish not to assign Ken Burns' extraordinary "Civil War" series as homework. Finally, with the nearly universal availability of the Internet, the need to memorize arcane historical facts should become a thing of the past.

## THE ROLE OF PARENTS

As with schools, parents need to recognize the incredible power of the media to teach and shape attitudes and behaviors. Closely controlling media at a young age may pay rich dividends when children become adolescents. This is especially true of exposure to media violence at a young age. But, by far, the most effective means of controlling media is to avoid placing a TV set in a child's bedroom. Parents also need to recognize the increasing evidence that exposing children and teens to R-rated movies may increase their risk of smoking and drinking[112] and of early sexual intercourse.[41]

## THE ROLE OF PRACTITIONERS

Besides the 2 key questions discussed at the beginning of this chapter, practitioners need to advise parents about how to control adolescents' media use (eg, avoiding TV sets and Internet connections in bedrooms), how to use media wisely (eg, co-view, and use a sexy scene to open a discussion about teen sex), and how to encourage schools to implement media education programs. Adolescents who have conduct disorders, learning problems, or are obese may merit a more detailed media history and counseling. To date, practitioners have been woefully reluctant to do any of these things.[24] Is it because they, themselves, do not watch much television? Is it because they remember a "gentler, kinder" media? Or is it because they already have a list of 20 topics to counsel parents and teens about, and the media are #21 on the list? New research shows that even brief counseling about media can be extremely effective.[113] More research will be needed to understand practitioners' reluctance to deal with the issue of the media, despite the fact that the media have a considerable impact on adolescents' lives and health.[114]

## REFERENCES


1. Bushman BJ, Huesmann LR. Effects of televised violence on aggression. In: Singer DG, Singer JL, eds. *Handbook of Children and the Media.* Thousand Oaks, CA: Sage; 2002:223-254

2. Ansen D. A handful of tangos in Paris. *Newsweek.* September 13, 1999:66

3. *American Medical News.* April 20, 1992

4. Schneider KS. Mission impossible. *Parade magazine.* June 3, 1996

5. Strasburger VC. The importance of media in child health. *Arch Dis Child.* 2009;94:655-657

6. Strasburger VC, Wilson BJ, Jordan A. *Children, Adolescents, and the Media.* 2nd ed. Thousand Oaks, CA: Sage; 2009

7. Rideout V. Generation M$^2$: Media in the lives of 8- to 18-Year-olds. Menlo Park, CA: Kaiser Family Foundation, 2010.

8. Strasburger VC. Adolescents, sex, and the media: oooo, baby, baby—a Q&A. *Adolesc Med.* 2005;16:269-288

9. Brown JD, Halpern CT, L'Engle KL. Mass media as a sexual super peer for early maturing girls. *J Adolesc Health.* 2005;36:420-427

10. Kaiser Family Foundation. *Teens, Sex, and TV.* Menlo Park, CA: Kaiser Family Foundation; 2002

11. Anderson C, Berkowitz L, Donnerstein E, et al. The influence of media violence on youth. *Psychol Sci Public Interest.* 2003;4:81-110

12. Wartella E, Olivarez A, Jennings N. Children and television violence in the United States. In: Carlsson U, von Feilitzen C, eds. *UNESCO International Clearinghouse on Children and Violence on the Screen.* Goteborg, Sweden: UNESCO; 1998:55-62

13. Hogan MJ. Adolescents and media violence: six crucial issues for practitioners. *Adolesc Med Clin.* 2005;16:249-268

14. Bushman BJ, Huesmann LR. Short-term and long-term effects of violent media on aggression in children and adults. *Arch Pediatr Adolesc Med.* 2006;160:348-352

15. Huesmann LR, Eron LD, Lefkowitz MM, et al. Stability of aggression over time and generations. *Dev Psychol.* 1984;20:1120-1134

16. Johnson JG, Cohen P, Smailes EM, et al. Television viewing and aggressive behavior during adolescence and adulthood. *Science.* 2002;295:2468-2472

17. Huesmann LR, Moise-Titus J, Podolski C, et al. Longitudinal relations between children's exposure to TV violence and their aggressive and violent behavior in young adulthood: 1977-1992. *Dev Psychol.* 2003;39:201-221

18. Anderson CA, Gentile DA, Buckley KE. *Violent Video Game Effects on Children and Adolescents: Theory, Research, and Public Policy.* New York, NY: Oxford University Press; 2007

19. Funk J. Video games. In: Strasburger VC, Wilson BJ, Jordan AB. *Children, Adolescents, and the Media*, 2nd ed. Thousand Oaks, CA: Sage; 2009:435-470

20. Anderson CA, Carnagey NL, Flanagan M, Benjamin AJ, Eubanks J, Valentine JC. Violent video games: specific effects of violent content on aggressive thoughts and behavior. *Advances in Experimental Social Psychology.* 2004;36:199-249

21. Anderson CA, Sakamoto A, Gentile DA, et al. Longitudinal effects of violent video games aggression in Japan and the United States. *Pediatrics.* 2008;122: e1067-e1072

22. Ybarra M, Mitchell K. Prevalence and frequency of Internet harassment instigation implications for adolescent health. *J Adol Health.* 2007;41:189-195

23. Strasburger VC, Grossman D. How many more Columbines? What can pediatricians do about school and media violence? *Pediatr Ann.* 2001;30:87-94

24. Strasburger VC. "Clueless": why do pediatricians underestimate the media's influence on children and adolescents? *Pediatr.* 2006;117:1427-1431

25. Kunkel D, Eyal K, Finnerty K, et al. *Sex on TV 3*. Menlo Park, CA: Kaiser Family Foundation; 2005

26. Santelli J, Ott MA, Lyon M, et al. Abstinence and abstinence-only education: a review of US policies and programs. *J Adolesc Health.* 2006;38:72-81

27. Kohler PK, Manhart LE, Lafferty WE. Abstinence-only and comprehensive sex education and the initiation of sexual activity and teen pregnancy. *J Adolesc Health.* 2008;42:344-351

28. Hennessy M, Bleakley A, Fishbein M, Jordan A. Estimating the longitudinal association between adolescent sexual behavior and exposure to sexual media content. *J Sex Res.* 2009;46:1-11

29. Brown JD, Strasburger VC. From Calvin Klein, to Paris Hilton and MySpace: adolescents, sex, and the media. *Adolesc Med: State Art Rev.* 2007;18:484-507

30. Kaiser Family Foundation/*Seventeen* Magazine. *Sex Smarts: Birth Control and Protection.* Menlo Park, CA: Kaiser Family Foundation; 2004

31. Tolman DL, Kim JL, Schooler D, Sorsoli CL. Rethinking the associations between television viewing and adolescent sexuality development: bringing gender into focus. *J Adol Health.* 2007;40:e9-e16

32. Brown JD, L'Engle KL. X-rated: sexual attitudes and behaviors associated with US early adolescents' exposure to sexually explicit media. *Communication Research.* 2009;36:129-151

33. Donnerstein E. The Internet. In: Strasburger VC, Wilson BJ, Jordan AB, eds. *Children, Adolescents, and the Media.* 2nd ed. Thousand Oaks, CA: Sage; 2009

34. Wolak J, Mitchell K, Finkelhor D. Unwanted and wanted exposure to online pornography in a national sample of youth Internet users. *Pediatrics.* 2007;119:247-257

35. Mitchell KJ, Wolak J, Finkelhor D. Trends in youth reports of sexual solicitations, harassment, and unwanted exposure to pornography on the Internet. *J Adolesc Health.* 2007;40:116-126

36. Ybarra ML, Mitchell KJ. How risky are social networking sites? A comparison of places online where youth sexual solicitation and harassment occurs. *Pediatrics.* 2008;121:e350-e357

37. National Campaign to Prevent Teen and Unplanned Pregnancy. *Sex and Tech.* Washington, DC: National Campaign to Prevent Teen and Unplanned Pregnancy; 2008

38. Collins RL, Elliott MN, Berry SH, et al. Watching sex on television predicts adolescent initiation of sexual behavior. *Pediatrics.* 2004;114:e280

39. Chandra A, Martino SC, Collins RL, et al. Does watching sex on television predict teen pregnancy? Findings from a National Longitudinal Survey of Youth. *Pediatrics.* 2008;122:1047-1054

40. Wingood GM, DiClemente RJ, Harrington K, et al. Exposure to X-rated movies and adolescents' sexual and contraceptive-related attitudes and behavior. *Pediatrics.* 2001;107:1116-1119

41. Brown JD, L'Engle KL, Pardun CH, et al. Sexy media matter: exposure to sexual content in music, movies, television, and magazines predicts black and white adolescents' sexual behavior. *Pediatrics.* 2006;117:1018-1027

42. Bersamin M, Todd M, Fisher DA, Hill DL, Grube JW, Walker S. Parenting practices and adolescent sexual behavior: a longitudinal study. *J Marriage Fam.* 2008;70:97-112

43. Fisher DA, Hill DL, Grube JW, Bersamin MM, Walker S, Gruber EL. Televised sexual content and parental mediation: influences on adolescent sexuality. *Media Psychology.* 2009;12:121-147

44. Corder-Bolz C. Television and adolescents' sexual behavior. *Sex Education Coalition News.* 1983;3:40

45. Peterson RA, Kahn JR. Media preferences of sexually active teens. Presented at: the Annual Meeting of the American Psychological Association; August 1984; Toronto, Canada

46. Strouse JS, Buerkel-Rothfuss N, Long EC. Gender and family as moderators of the relationship between music video exposure and adolescent sexual permissiveness. *Adolescence.* 1995;30:505-521

47. Primack BA, Douglas EL, Fine MJ, Dalton MA. Exposure to sexual lyrics and sexual experience among urban adolescents. *Am J Prev Med.* 2009;36:317-323

48. Martino SC, Collins RL, Elliott MN, Strachman A, Kanouse DE, Berry SH. Exposure to degrading versus nondegrading music lyrics and sexual behavior among youth. *Pediatrics.* 2006;118:e430-e431

49. Pazos B, Fullwood EU, Allan MJ, et al. Media use and sexual behaviors among Monroe County adolescents. Presented at: the Annual Meeting of the Society for Adolescent Medicine; March 2001; San Diego, CA

50. Newman AA. Pigs with cell phones but no condoms. *New York Times*. June 19, 2007

51. Snowbeck C. FDA tells Levitra to cool it with ad. Business News, Post-Gazette.com. Available at: www.post-gazette.com/pg/05109/490334.stm. Accessed April 19, 2006

52. Strasburger VC, Jordan AB, Donnerstein E: Child and adolescent health and the media. Pediatrics. 2010;125:756-767.

53. Federal Trade Commission. *Cigarette Report for 2001.* Washington, DC: FTC;2003

54. Pierce JP, Choi WS, Gilpin EA, et al. Industry promotion of cigarettes and adolescent smoking. *JAMA.* 1998;279:511-515

55. Biener L, Siegel M. Tobacco marketing and adolescent smoking: more support for a causal inference. *Am J Public Health.* 2000;90:407-411

56. Center on Alcohol Marketing and Youth. Alcohol advertising and youth. Washington, DC: CAMY; 2003. Available at: www.camy.org. Accessed April 19, 2006

57. Grube JW, Waiters E. Alcohol in the media: content and effects on drinking beliefs and behaviors among youth. *Adolesc Med Clin.* 2005;16:327-343

58. Henrickson L, Feighery EC, Schleicher NC, Fortmann SP. Receptivity to alcohol marketing predicts initiation of alcohol use. *J Adolesc Health.* 2008;42:28-35

59. Borzekowski DLG, Strasburger VC. Tobacco, alcohol, and drug exposure. In: Calvert S, Wilson BJ, eds. *Handbook of Children and the Media.* Boston, MA: Blackwell; 2008:432–452

60. Rubin A. Prescription drugs and the cost of advertising them, November 6, 2004. Available at: www.therubins.com. Accessed April 19, 2006

61. Christenson PG, Henriksen L, Roberts DF. Substance use in popular prime-time television. Washington, DC: Office of National Drug Control Policy; 2000. Available at: www.whitehousedrugpolicy.gov. Accessed April 19, 2006

62. Roberts DF, Henriksen L, Christenson PG. Substance use in popular movies and music. Washington, DC: Office of National Drug Policy Control; 2000. Available at: www.whitehousedrugpolicy.gov. Accessed April 19, 2006

63. Primack BA, Dalton MA, Carrol MV, Agarwal AA, Fine MJ. Content analysis of tobacco, alcohol, and other drugs in popular music. *Arch Pediatr Adolesc Med.* 2008;162:169–175

64. Sargent JD, Beach ML, Dalton MA, et al. Effect of seeing tobacco use in films on trying smoking among adolescents. *BMJ.* 2001;232:1394–1397

65. Charlesworth A, Glantz SA. Smoking in the movies increases adolescent smoking: a review. *Pediatrics.* 2005;116:1516–1528

66. Gidwani PP, Sobol A, DeJong W, et al. Television viewing and initiation of smoking among youth. *Pediatrics.* 2002;110: 505–508

67. Sargent JD, Beach ML, Adachi-Mejia AM, et al. Exposure to movie smoking: its relation to smoking initiation among US adolescents. *Pediatrics.* 2005;116:1183–1191

68. Jackson C, Brown JD, L'Engle KL. R-rated movies, bedroom televisions, and initiation of smoking by white and black adolescents. *Arch Pediatr and Adolesc Med.* 2007;161:260–268

69. Titus-Ernstoff L, Dalton MA, Adachi-Mejia AM, Longacre MR, Beach ML. Longitudinal study of viewing smoking in movies and initiation of smoking by children. *Pediatrics.* 2008;121: 15–21

70. Hanewinkel R, Sargent JD. Longitudinal study of exposure to entertainment media and alcohol use among German adolescents. *Pediatrics.* 2009;123:989–995

71. Office of National Drug Control Policy. Teen online exposure: a snapshot of data. Washington, DC: ONCDP; 2008. Available at: www.TheAntiDrug.com. Accessed August 6, 2009

72. Jenssen BP, Klein JD, Salazar LF, Daluga NA, DiClemente RJ. Exposure to tobacco on the Internet: content analysis of adolescents' Internet use. *Pediatrics.* 2009;124:e180–e186

73. Leinwand D. Teens not rushing online to buy wine, survey shows. *USA Today.* August 9, 2006. Available at: www.usatoday.com/tech/news/2006-08-09-survey-online-alcohol_x.htm. Accessed July 5, 2009

74. Montgomery KC, Chester J. Interactive food and beverage marketing: targeting adolescents in the digital age. *J Adolesc Health.* 2009;45(3S):S18–S29

75. Center on Alcohol Marketing and Youth. *Clicking with Kids: Alcohol Marketing and Youth on the Internet.* Washington, DC: CAMY; 2004

76. Moreno MA, Briner LR, Williams A, Walker L, Christakis DA. Real use or "real cool": adolescents speak out about displayed alcohol references on social networking websites. *J Adolesc Health.* 2009;44:S22

77. Moreno MA, Parks MR, Zimmerman FJ, Brito TE, Christakis DA. Display of health risk behaviors on MySpace by adolescents. *Arch Pediatr Adolesc Med.* 2009;163:27–34

78. Schlosser E. *Fast Food Nation.* Boston, MA: Houghton Mifflin;2001

79. McGinnis JM, Gootman J, Kraak VI, eds. *Food Marketing to Children and Youth: Threat or Opportunity?* Washington, DC: The National Academies Press; 2006

80. Giammattei J, Glix G, Marshak HH, et al. Television watching and soft drink consumption: associations with obesity in 11- to 13-year-old school children. *Arch Pediatr Adolesc Med.* 2003;157:882–886

81. Molnar A. School commercialism and adolescent health. *Adolesc Med Clin.* 2005;16:447–461

82. Dietz WH, Robinson TN. Overweight children and adolescents. *New Engl J Med.* 2005;20:2100–2109

83. Jordan AB, Strasburger VC, Kramer-Golinkoff EK. Does adolescent medial cause obesity and eating disorders? *Adolesc Med State Art Rev.* 2008;19:431–449

84. Dennison BA, Erb TA, Jenkins PL. Television viewing and television in bedroom associated with overweight risk among low-income preschool children. *Pediatrics.* 2002;109:1028–1035

85. Robinson TN. Reducing children's television viewing to prevent obesity: a randomized controlled trial. *JAMA.* 1999;282:1561–1567

86. Dixon HG, Scully ML, Wakefield MA, White VM, Crawford DA. The effects of television advertisements for junk food versus nutritious food on children's food attitudes and preferences. *Social Science & Medicine.* 2007;65:1311–1323

87. Jordan AB, Robinson TN. Children, television viewing, and weight status: summary and recommendations from an expert panel meeting. *Ann Am Acad Pol Soc Sci.* 2008;615:119–132

88. Brownell KD, Schwartz MB, Puhl RM, Henderson KE, Harris JL. The need for bold action to prevent adolescent obesity. *J Adolesc Health.* 2009;45:S8–S17

89. Hogan MJ, Strasburger VC. Body image, eating disorders, and the media. *Adolesc Med State Art Rev.* 2008;19:521–546

90. Krowchuk DP, Dreiter SR, Woods CR, et al. Problem dieting behaviors among young adolescents. *Arch Pediatr Adolesc Med.* 1998;152:884–888

91. Field AE, Cheung L, Wolf AM, et al. Exposure to the mass media and weight concerns among girls. *Pediatrics.* 1999;103:e236

92. Field AE, Javaras KM, Aneja P, et al. Family, peer, and media predictors of becoming eating disordered. *Arch Pediatr Adolesc Med.* 2008;162:574–579

93. Field AE, Camargo CA Jr, Taylor CB, et al. Relation of peers and media influences to the development of purging behaviors among preadolescent and adolescent girls. *Arch Pediatr Adolesc Med.* 1999;153:1184–1189

94. Borzekowski DLG, Robinson T, Killen JD. Does the camera add 10 pounds? Media use, perceived importance of appearance, and weight concerns among teenage girls. *J Adolesc Health.* 2000;26:36–41

95. Field AE, Austin SB, Carmargo CA Jr. Exposure to the mass media, body shape concerns, and use of supplements to improve weight and shape among male and female adolescents. *Pediatrics.* 2005;116:e214–e220

96. Martinez-Gonzalez MA, Gual P, Lahortiga F, et al. Parental factors, mass media influences, and the onset of eating disorders in a prospective population-based cohort. *Pediatrics.* 2003;111:315–320

97. Becker AE. Eating behaviours and attitudes following prolonged exposure to television among ethnic Fijian adolescent girls. *Br J Psychiatry.* 2002;180:509–514

98. Gould M, Jamieson P, Romer D. Media contagion and suicide among the young. *Am Behav Sci.* 2003;46:1269–1284

99. Centers for Disease Control and Prevention. Guidelines for reporting suicide in the media. Available at: www.afsp.org. Accessed April 19, 2006

100. Christakis DA, Zimmerman FJ, DiGiuseppe DL, et al. Early television exposure and subsequent attentional problems in children. *Pediatrics.* 2004;113:708–713

101. Acevedo-Polakovich ID, Lorch EP, Milich R, et al. Disentangling the relation between television viewing and cognitive processes in children with attention-deficit/hyperactivity disorder and comparison children. *Arch Pediatr Adolesc Med.* 2006;160:354–360

102. Hancox RJ, Milne BJ, Poulton R. Association of television viewing during childhood with poor educational achievement. *Arch Pediatr Adolesc Med.* 2005;159: 614–618

103. Zimmerman FJ, Christakis DA. Children's television viewing and cognitive outcomes: a longitudinal analysis of national data. *Arch Pediatr Adolesc Med.* 2005;159:619–625

104. Borzekowski DLG, Robinson TN. The remote, the mouse, and the no. 2 pencil: the household media environment and academic achievement among third grade students. *Arch Pediatr Adolesc Med.* 2005;159:607–613

105. Sharif I, Wills TA, Sargeant JA. Effect of visual media use on school performance: a prospective study. *J Adolesc Health.* 2010;46(1):52–61

106. Zimmerman FJ. *Children's media use and sleep problems: issues and unanswered questions*. Menlo Park, CA: Kaiser Family Foundation; 2008

107. American Academy of Pediatrics. Media violence. *Pediatrics.* 2009;124:1495-1503

108. Webb T, Jenkins L, Browne N, Afifi AA, Kraus J. Violent entertainment pitched to adolescents: an analysis of PG-13 films. *Pediatrics.* 2007;119:e1219–e1229

109. Gentile DA, Humphrey J, Walsh DA. Media ratings for movies, music, video games, and television: a review of the research and recommendations for improvements. *Adolesc Med Clin.* 2005;16:427–446

110. British Medical Association. *Eating disorders, body image, and the media*. London: BMA; 2000

111. McCannon B. Media Literacy/Media Education: Solution to Big Media? In: Strasburger VC, Wilson BJ, Jordan A. *Children, Adolescents, and the Media*, 2nd ed. Thousand Oaks, CA: Sage; 2009:519–569

112. Longacre MR, Adachi-Mejia AM, Titus-Ernstoff L, Gibson JJ, Beach ML, Dalton MA. Parental attitudes about cigarette smoking and alcohol use in the Motion Picture Association of America rating system. *Arch Pediatr Pediatr Med.* 2009;163:218–224

113. Barkin SL, Finch SA, Ip EH, et al. Is office-based counseling about media use, timeouts, and firearm storage effective? Results from a cluster-randomized, controlled trial. *Pediatrics.* 2008;122:e15–e25

114. Strasburger VC. Why do adolescent health researchers ignore the influence of the media? *J Adolesc Health.* 2009;44:203–205

# CHAPTER 42

# Computers, Technology, and the Internet

DAVID PAPERNY, MD

Electronic technology, electronic medical records, the Internet, and communication media can have a dramatic impact on adolescent health and wellness.[1] There are now advances in adolescent health communications, screening and assessment, and applications of video and multimedia for health education and promotion. Media-capable adolescents can use technology to benefit their health, particularly if they have a physician who collaborates with them. Computers and the Internet can provide immediate up-to-date health information for both adolescents and adults.

In the current climate, there is a need to more effectively provide health education in less time, which can be facilitated by media-based approaches. Office-based communication technologies, both on the Internet and using multimedia, are becoming an expected practice standard. This is due to increased availability and lower cost, as well as to the usefulness of computer technology in marketing a practice and facilitating communications with adolescent patients. Computer use is an area of competence that affects the ability to care for adolescents effectively and to compete in the health care marketplace.

## CLINICAL COMMUNICATIONS WITH PATIENTS

Adolescents are well versed in high-tech communications, and this ability can facilitate their health care. Confidential medical questions and appointment reminders are common uses. Although e-mail or secure electronic messaging and text messaging to a cell phone are useful for adolescent communications, text messages to cell phones are not secured by password protection. Electronic messaging between clinicians and patients creates no office visit charge and no confidential billing concerns, eliminating some issues but creating others. Most adolescents carry cell phones capable of reminders, alarms, and text messaging; playing music and sound; sending and receiving photos, video, and still photography; and providing Internet access. Podcasts (media files) are a new form of sharing audio, video, and other health education information that adolescents are becoming familiar with.

### E-MAIL AND SECURE MESSAGING WITH ADOLESCENT PATIENTS

More than 75% of all patients say that e-mail messaging improves access to their clinician. For clinicians and adolescents, e-mail can be more efficient than office visits and phone calls.[2,3] Like telephone calls, e-mail is usually not encrypted or authenticated, but it is usually password protected, making it especially useful for confidential messaging. However, not all e-mail is handled in ways consistent with the HIPAA (Health Insurance Portability and Accountability Act) or e-Risk standards. Therefore safe, effective, and convenient use of personal e-mail with adolescent patients requires preplanning with appropriate policies and procedures in place. Secure medical messaging is available from several Internet services that collect a small fee. When using these services, one should always use an e-mail signature, which includes the clinician's name, address, phone and fax numbers, an e-mail address for patient use, and disclaimers such as: *"In case of emergency…."* Text messages to a patient's cell phone cannot be "safety-proofed" or authenticated for health care purposes. Boxes 42-1 and 42-2 describe acceptable uses for patient e-mail, as well as administrative and legal guidelines. Legal and financial issues must be considered by those clinicians who choose to provide e-mail access to their patients.

**Box 42-1**

***Acceptable Uses for Patient E-Mail***

- General, nonurgent questions
- Forms and documentation requests
- Prescription refills (particularly if confidential, such as contraceptives)
- Patient management (ie, blood sugar readings or peak flow meter readings)
- Appointment reminders, lab and test results (particularly if confidential)
- Confidential and sensitive issues such as contraception questions

**Box 42-2**

***Administrative and Legal Guidelines for Patient E-Mail***

- Put e-mail guidelines, policies, and rules in writing and have the patient sign them, including consent for electronic communications
- Specify terms for "escalation" to telephone and an agreement to only use the e-mail for medical communications and to not share the clinician's e-mail address
- Include disclaimer for equipment failures, data back-up loss, limited security protocols, and lack of encryption
- Require patient identification as a medical record number or birth date, as well as an acknowledgment, in every message

**Box 42-3**

***File Types That Can Be Given to Adolescents in the Office or Provided on the Physician's Web Site***

**.doc = document** (word processing) files for handouts and personal information

**.txt = document** (text) files for handouts and personal information (virus-free, easy to e-mail)

**.jpg = photo files** (health education, photos of findings sent to office by e-mail)

**.mp3 = audio files** (health education podcasts and downloads)

**.mpg = video** (MPEG-1) files (health education podcasts and downloads)

### INTERNET PATIENT COMMUNICATIONS AND THE PHYSICIAN'S WEB SITE

A clinician's professional Web site can offer information about the clinician's practice and include a variety of functions for patient use. There are many Web site providers, but health care providers can create their own at very low cost using templates. Adolescents regularly use the Internet to find health information, and a provider's site can link to credible Internet sites recommended for adolescents to obtain health education and information. The office/clinic Web site can also offer access to patients' personal health records (available information linked to their problem list, medications, allergies, and immunizations via an electronic medical record). Three quarters of Internet users have reported that they want this online information, as well as the ability to obtain test results and transfer medical histories to new health providers.

Digital health information files can be downloaded from the clinician's Web site, and this information can also be given to the patient in the office using various media. Adolescents can accept media files (see Box 42-3) onto an MP3 player, iPod, burned CD, or USB memory stick. Files can also be "beamed" to a patient's cell phone.

### TELEMEDICINE

As suggested in Box 42-3, patients can e-mail photos of signs and visual findings to clinicians and can also communicate with webcams (live video) via the Internet. For certain consultations and situations, where a physical examination can be deferred, remote video now enables providers to interview, assess, and counsel adolescents as if they were in their presence. According to the clinician's comfort level, it is feasible to communicate with adolescent patients via digital photos using e-mail or online real-time video. The clinician can "see" the patient, make recommendations, and give advice and health education. This can help with case management and compliance with follow-up visits and can save both the adolescent and the clinician time and expense.[4] Various records, forms, and health education media can be e-mailed to patients as attachments. Virtual reality technology and remote medical monitoring devices are now available to facilitate patient reporting and transfer of medical data.

## COMPUTERIZED HEALTH SCREENING AND ASSESSMENT

Early risk and problem detection, prompt assessment, and personalized intervention are the keys to optimal adolescent health promotion. Computers can help in the evaluation of health needs and concerns. They can also improve reliability and timeliness of health care, enhance case management, and help physicians make sounder medical decisions. Information technology can increase the capacity of the clinic or office to provide more cost-effective services to adolescents.[5] Educators and allied health professionals, using expert health assessment software and educational technology (Box 42-4) and working together with a physician, can expand the capacity to cost-effectively deliver more comprehensive services to at-risk adolescents.[6]

Written screening questionnaires and computerized health assessments improve services for adolescents.[7] Psychosocial,[8] behavioral, and medical[9] history-taking is easily automated. Adolescent patients often prefer

**Box 42-4**

***Capabilities of Expert Health Assessment Software***

- Obtain a complete health and behavioral risk history
- Identify and prioritize problem areas and health needs
- Provide specific health advice, local referrals, and need-specific anticipatory guidance
- Administer pertinent health education videos
- Print specific, customized educational materials
- Provide a prioritized problem list for the physician's use

interactive computer-assisted interviews and educational software programs rather than direct human interventions about sensitive topics. Adolescents readily reveal sensitive information to computers. In a 1983 study, more than 100 adolescent girls completed a computer-assisted self-interview (CASI) about sexual behavior, and when compared to a self-administered questionnaire and face-to-face interview, results showed they preferred and were more comfortable with the computerized interview.[10]

### COMPUTER-ASSISTED SELF-INTERVIEW

A comprehensive health interview and appropriate counseling can be done with an expert interactive software system using sophisticated rule-based algorithms for branching and decision making.[11] Interview logic proceeds in the format of a trained history-taking clinician. Algorithms, branching, and clinical logic programming ask questions based on the adolescent's responses, which also determine educational feedback that is provided. An automated interview minimizes discomfort, denial, worries about confidentiality, and other interpersonal barriers and concerns. Computer-assisted self interview with health assessment can be administered with a dedicated office computer or network terminal, a telephone response system from home, or over the Internet. Many Internet health services offer various adolescent health risk appraisals (HRAs), which vary in behavioral assessment sophistication and educational feedback capabilities.

A study of 800 adolescents compared CASIs with and without the expectation to share printed results of their responses to sensitive questions with their clinician.[7] The 2 computer groups (expected to be shared vs anonymous) were similar in sensitivity and were equally better in detecting sensitive issues than the matched written questionnaire (expected to be shared). This suggested superiority of CASI over written questionnaires in detecting sensitive issues. The computer was perceived as anonymous and nonjudgmental compared with the perception of verbal admission of risky behaviors with possible physician disapproval as a barrier.

Further research with more than 4,000 adolescents doing CASI assessments evaluated their opinions and self-reports on the computer interview process.[12] Results were that 85% of adolescents reported they were totally honest and accurate; 8% said they were not completely honest; 5% said they couldn't understand some of the questions; and 2% said they were pretty inaccurate. The computer was a preference for 89%, with only 5% preferring a personal interview and 6% a written questionnaire. The studies suggested that adolescents want to divulge sensitive information in the health setting and that the "impersonal" method of obtaining it by computer is easy, protects them from embarrassment and judgment, and saves interviewer time.

Computerized health history questions can generate educational feedback when associations between responses are provided by such expert systems. The resulting personalized feedback can facilitate higher-level interventions that would usually be too time-consuming and impractical to attain in a busy clinical setting.

## THE INTERNET

The predominant media of different eras have always affected the community life and social relationships of adolescents (Table 42-1). Today's digital media culture, dominated by the Internet, creates a social milieu in which many adolescents live worldwide. There are billions of sites with online content from around the world, including those from nonprofit organizations, museums, libraries, educational institutions, and government agencies.

**Table 42-1**

**Effects of Media on the Community Life and Social Activity**

| *Media* | *Era* | *Predominant Social Activity* |
|---|---|---|
| Telephone | Early 1900s | Farm, industry |
| Television | 1960s | Family, school |
| Videotape | 1970s | Rock concerts |
| Computer | 1980s | Parties |
| Cell phone | 1990s | Networking |
| Internet | 2000s | Digital media culture |

**Box 42-5**

***Close Online Friendships during the Past Year***[15]

70% were with same-age peers
71% crossed gender lines
74% were known to parents
32% were initiated by introductions from friends/family
70% had offline contact by mail/phone
41% had face-to-face meetings

For adolescents, however, communication is the most popular Internet use. This includes e-mail, interactive games, text messaging with friends, and real-time chatting. These activities provide both individual and group connectedness and social networking of an unprecedented nature.[13] Dedicated social networking Web sites include MySpace, Facebook, and blogs on YouTube. Adolescents frequently display risk behavior information on such public Web sites.[14] Online Internet relationships are the rule; in a study[15] of 1,500 American adolescents, 14% of all youths reported close online friendships during the past year (Box 42-5).

## INTERNET SITES FOR HEALTH INFORMATION

At least 3 of 4 adolescents report using the Internet to obtain personal health information, and 2 of 3 use it to obtain health information for school-related projects.[16] Adolescents access online health information more often than they check sports scores, purchase merchandise, download music, play games, or participate in chat rooms.[17] About 1 in 5 seeks help on the Internet for emotional problems.[18] Adolescents need to know that anybody's material and any opinion can be posted online and that the information may not be valid or correct. Table 42-2 provides a list of useful and reliable Internet sites containing health information for adolescents.

## PROTECTING ADOLESCENTS FROM INTERNET AND TECHNOLOGY RISK

Although much has been said in the media about exposure of adolescents to online sexual predators, not enough emphasis has been placed on the time spent in front of TV screens and computer monitors, displacing adolescents from other social and physical activities. Adolescent obesity is directly linked to such sedentary activity. Online gaming addiction is a serious behavioral problem, affecting adolescent males in particular. "Sex" is the most searched word on the Internet, and exposure to sexual, violent, and potentially harmful media content

**Table 42-2**

**Internet Sites with Health Information for Adolescents**

| *Web Site* | *Sponsor* | *Information* | *URL* |
|---|---|---|---|
| Teen Health | Nemours Foundation | Physical and mental health issues | www.TeensHealth.org |
| Go Ask Alice | Columbia University | Various health | www.goaskalice.columbia.edu |
| National Institute on Drug Abuse | National Institutes of Health | Information on drug abuse | www.nida.nih.gov |
| Teen Matters | So. Carolina Share | Mental health | www.Teen-Matters.com |
| Teen Growth | TeenGrowth.com, Florida | Health and safety | www.TeenGrowth.com |
| SAHM | Society for Adolescent Health and Medicine | Parents and adolescents | www.adolescenthealth.org |
| National Library of Medicine | National Institutes of Health | Medical information | www.ncbi.nlm.nih.gov/PubMed/ |
| AAP | American Academy of Pediatrics | Providers, parents, and adolescents | www.aap.org |
| Bright Futures Guidelines | Bright Futures/AAP | Providers, parents, and adolescents | www.brightfutures.org/index.html |
| TeenHealthFX | Atlantic Health/Goryeb Children's Hospital | Information on health, body, relationships/sexuality | www.TeenHealthFX.com |

is commonplace; yet pornography constitutes less than 2% of the Web. There is, however, some online exposure to predators and relatively limited amount of online access to alcohol, tobacco, and drugs.

Exposure to inappropriate or harmful online relationships can result in unwanted sexual solicitations (1 in 5 teens have experienced this)[17] as well as cyberbullying. Cyberbullies use online social cruelty to intimidate and exert control and power by spreading online rumors and threats, forwarding private e-mails, and posting sensitive photos or videos of others on a Web site or sending them via e-mail.[19] Referred to as electronic bullying, it also includes bullying through text messaging, in a chat room, or through digital messages or images sent to a cell phone. Almost half of electronic bully victims report not knowing the perpetrator's identity. Adolescents need to be aware that sending or downloading photographs of a sexual nature of themselves or friends under age 18 may be a violation of federal child pornography laws, which carries severe penalties.

Parents set rules for how their children should deal with strangers and which TV, movies, or videos they are allowed to watch. They should also have a set of rules for children of all ages regarding Internet use that does not allow surfing the Internet to take the place of homework, spending time with family and friends, and pursuing other interests. Parents should provide these guidelines and consider having an adolescent sign an *online use contract* (Boxes 42-6 and 42-7). Parents should control online access to obscene, pornographic, violent, racist, and other offensive material and discuss what is considered inappropriate. They can place the computer in a public area, such as the living room, and use filtering software to block specific, inappropriate Internet sites. It is also important to teach children to resist ads and solicitations, especially anything from outside their country.

**Box 42-6**

***Purposes of Online Use Contract***

Defines appropriate and inappropriate information exchange.

Specifies when to contact a parent about a problem.

Sets limits on the amount of time the adolescent can spend online each day or week (agree to use a timer).

Links online/computer time to physical activities and health monitoring.

Ensures the adolescent knows that people online are not always who they say they are and that online information is not private.

**Box 42-7**

***Prohibitions Specified on the Online Use Contract***

Revealing personal information—name, address, telephone number, location, birthday, other identifying information.

Using a credit card online—without parent permission.

Sharing passwords, even with friends.

Arranging or requesting a personal meeting with someone met online—without parent present.

Responding to uncomfortable or distasteful messages.

Sending obscene or threatening messages.

Health advice should include when not to use electronic and mobile devices (eg, cell phones in the car). Distraction from focused activities (such as driving) by the use of music players, cell phones, and text messaging poses significant health risks. Such technology-related risks are rarely addressed in medical screenings, yet identification and guidance in reducing these behaviors is appropriate.

## HEALTH PROMOTION AND HEALTH EDUCATION USING INTERACTIVE MULTIMEDIA

Recommendations for content and delivery of preventive services for adolescents, including *Guidelines for Adolescent Preventive Services (GAPS)*,[20] published in 1994, and *Bright Futures, Guidelines for Health Supervision of Infants, Children, and Adolescents,*[21] recently updated in 2008, emphasize behavioral and psychological components. They recommend annual health supervision visits during adolescence and stress screening and counseling for problem behaviors—a time-intensive endeavor. Research on the effectiveness of comprehensive adolescent preventive services to improve adolescent health[22] suggests that even limited behavioral change and risk reduction have profound effects on the lives of adolescents.[23,24]

Every opportunity should be used to identify high-risk adolescents and to administer and reinforce health promotion messages by offering adolescents health education using the most familiar media—*television, video, and computers*. We normally speak with adolescents to communicate medical advice, but understanding, acceptance, assimilation, and retention of verbal advice varies widely,[25] as does adherence with health recommendations. Because health advice and education are time intensive, providers should consider combinations of allied health personnel, such as health educators and peer counselors, and working with screening and educational information technology to offer interventions and health promotion.[6]

Interactive multimedia is the use of software to *control various media output and feedback* so that the *branching and decision making of the process continually depends on the learner's choices or responses.* Interactive video and multimedia for training and education produce strong reinforcement that helps trainees learn twice as fast as standard instruction. Information is quickly and easily understandable and keeps adolescent attention focused, and feedback provides ongoing, personalized reinforcement that is highly motivating. Interactive technology reduces learning time by 50% and improves retention of material by more than 25%.[26] It requires no clinician time and is delivered privately and consistently, any time in the office or clinic, and can then be reviewed at home.

## THE USE OF VIDEO MEDIA AND DVDS IN HEALTH EDUCATION

Clinicians provide guidance by repeatedly presenting standardized health information to adolescents, and there is a need to use video (the precursor to interactive multimedia) as an enhancement to the spoken and printed word. Video can enable clinicians to demonstrate home management techniques, can validate medical advice for skeptical adolescents, and can dramatize consequences that they should anticipate from high-risk health choices. Problem-based and anticipatory guidance may be provided by a variety of information technology and media within the clinic setting (audio, video, interactive multimedia). Current, easy-to-use storage media (CD-ROM and DVD) allow dissemination of huge amounts of information to educate patients both in the office or clinic and at home.

The requirements of useful health videos are (1) succinctness of presentations, (2) understandable scripts, (3) evaluation of outcomes and results, and (4) ease of administration. Video is ubiquitous for adolescents worldwide. In the medical setting, current digital compact videodisks and DVDs eliminate the problems of cumbersome videotapes. Digital video files (MPEG-1) and streaming video from the Internet can be shown on any office computer terminal.

Video-enhanced health education and video reinforcement of medical advice has proven effective with adolescents. A video efficacy study[27] of 600 adolescents compared video watchers to handout readers and evaluated knowledge items learned from the content; video watchers had 57% more knowledge improvements than handout readers. In a pediatric study, medical adherence improved by 50% when medical advice was followed by video viewing.[28] Adherence was 65% when the patient was counseled by the physician alone, 60% when counseled by the physician and given a handout, and 90% when counseling by the physician was followed by video viewing. Adolescents improved asthma self-management skills with training from an interactive video-DVD used in an emergency department.[29]

Health education videos can teach the basics, allowing more advanced use of professional or educator time to evaluate understanding and readiness for behavior change. With the need for more efficient use of physician time while also meeting more educational standards and requirements, video can be a useful tool. Video scripts placed into the medical record constitute superior documentation of information provided to patients.

## COMPUTER-ASSISTED INSTRUCTION HEALTH EDUCATION GAMES

Technology can also help adolescents evaluate the consequences of their health behavior choices. Computer-assisted instruction (CAI) health games teach informed decision making without embarrassment or real consequences of poor health choices. They influence patient attitudes, beliefs, feelings, and knowledge, even on sensitive health subjects.[30] Animated-action computer games and interactive training programs capture and hold attention by presenting situations and scenarios that simulate outcomes, creating the effect of reality. Adolescent risk-taking and reality testing is modified by exploring alternative choices and health outcomes and then experiencing consequences of the choices. Interactive CAI games allow adolescents to role-play desired behaviors and practice appropriate decision-making skills. They have been shown to reduce counseling time and facilitate acceptance and retention of critical health concepts.[30]

## REFERENCES

1. Paperny DM. Computers and information technology: implications for the 21st century. *Adolesc Med State Art Rev.* 2000;11(1):183–202

2. Liederman E, Morefield C. Web messaging: a new tool for patient–physician communication. *J Am Med Inform Assoc.* 2003;10:260–270

3. Gerstle R, AAP Task Force on Medical Informatics. E-mail communication between pediatricians and their patients. *Pediatrics.* 2004;114(1):317–321

4. Tidwell J. House calls of the future. *Modern Maturity.* 1998;41R(6):8

5. Elster AB. Confronting the crisis in adolescent health: visions for change. *J Adolesc Health.* 1993;14(7):505–508

6. Paperny DM, Hedberg V. Computer-assisted health counselor visits: a low-cost model for comprehensive adolescent

preventive services. *Arch Pediatr Adolesc Med.* 1999;153 (1):63-67

7. Paperny DM, Aono JY, Lehman RM, et al. Computer-assisted detection and intervention in adolescent high-risk health behaviors. *J Pediatr.* 1990;116(3):456-462

8. Greist J. A computer interview for suicide risk prediction. *Am J Psychiatr.* 1973;130:1327

9. Grossman S. Evaluation of computer-acquired patient histories. *JAMA.* 1971;215:1286

10. Millstein S, Irwin C. Acceptability of computer-acquired sexual histories in adolescent girls. *J Pediatr.* 1983;103(5):815-819

11. Rathbun J. Development of a computerized alcohol screening instrument for the university community. *J Am Coll Health.* 1993;42(1):33-36

12. Paperny DM. Computerized health assessment and education for adolescent HIV and STD prevention in health care settings and schools. *Health Educ Behav.* 1997;24(1):54-70

13. Klein JD, Graffle Havens C, Rhomas R, et al. *The Impact of Cyberspace on Teen and Young Adult Social Networks.* Toronto, Ontario, Canada: Pediatric Academic Societies; 2007

14. Moreno M, Parks M, Zimmerman F, et al. Display of health risk behaviors on MySpace by adolescents. *Arch Pediatr Adolesc Med.* 2009;163(1):27-34

15. Mitchell KJ, Finkelhor D, Wolak J. Risk factors for and impact of online sexual solicitation of youth. *JAMA.* 2001;285(23)1-4

16. Borzekowski DL, Rickert VI. Adolescent cybersurfing for health information: a new resource that crosses barriers. *Arch Pediatr Adolesc Med.* 2001;155(7):813-817

17. Borzekowski DL. Adolescents' use of the Internet: a controversial, coming-of-age resource. *Adolesc Med Clin.* 2006;17(1):205-216

18. Gould MS, Munfakh JL, Lubell K, et al. Seeking help from the Internet during adolescence. *J Am Acad Child Adolesc Psychiatry.* 2002;41(10):1182-1189

19. Kowalski RM, Limber SP. Electronic bullying among middle school students. *J Adolesc Health.* 2007;41(6 suppl 1):S22-S30

20. Elster AB, Kuznets NJ. *AMA Guidelines for Adolescent Preventive Services (GAPS): Recommendations and Rationale.* Baltimore, MD: Williams and Wilkins; 1994

21. Hagan JF, Shaw JS, Duncan PM, eds. *Bright Futures: Guidelines for Health Supervision of Infants, Children, and Adolescents.* 3rd ed. Elk Grove Village, IL: American Academy of Pediatrics; 2008

22. Halpern-Felsher BL, Ozer EM, Millstein SG, et al. Preventive services in a health maintenance organization: how well do pediatricians screen and educate patients? *Arch Pediatr Adolesc Med.* 2000;154(2):173-179

23. Gans JE, Alexander B, Chu RC, Elster AB. The cost of comprehensive preventive medical services for adolescents. *Arch Pediatr Adolesc Med.* 1995;149:1226-1234

24. Downs SM, Klein JD. Clinical preventive services efficacy and adolescents' risky behaviors. *Arch Pediatr Adolesc Med.* 1995;149:374-379

25. Bartlett EE. Effective approaches to patient education for the busy pediatrician. *Pediatrics.* 1984;74(suppl):920-923

26. Schwier R. *Interactive Video.* Englewood Cliffs, NJ: Educational Technology Publications; 1987

27. Paperny DM. Automated adolescent preventative services using computer-assisted video multimedia. *J Adol Health.* 1994;15(1):66

28. Paperny DM. Pediatric medical advice enhanced with use of video. *Am J Dis Child.* 1992;146(7):785-786

29. Boychuk R, DeMesa C, Kiyabu K, et al. Change in approach and delivery of medical care in children with asthma: results from a multicenter emergency department educational asthma management program. *Pediatrics.* 2006;117(4):S145-S151

30. Paperny DM, Starn JR. Adolescent pregnancy prevention by health education computer games: computer-assisted instruction of knowledge and attitudes. *Pediatrics.* 1989;83(5):742-752

31. Krishna S. Clinical trials of interactive computerized patient education: implications for family practice. *J Fam Pract.* 1997;45(1):25-33

# CHAPTER 43

# Cultural Considerations in Adolescent Health Care

CHERYL M. KODJO, MD, MPH • KATHRYN CASTLE, PhD

## INTRODUCTION

The United States will experience a considerable shift in the racial and ethnic composition of the adolescent population within the next 30 to 40 years.[1] Due to these demographic changes and the strong influence of racial and ethnic factors on health-damaging and health-promoting behaviors, as well as access to and utilization of health services, it is imperative that culturally competent care becomes the norm in providing clinical adolescent health services.

Becoming culturally competent in the context of health care requires the clinician to develop a level of self-knowledge and self-reflection often not included in the training of health care professionals who serve adolescents. Common perceptions include the beliefs that cultural competence cannot be taught or learned, or that content is only about subjective feelings that the clinician already has; or that the clinician already understands the population being served and does not require additional training. There is a growing number of clinicians who are open to the context of culture and fully incorporate it into the services they render.

Following a discussion of the development and importance of cultural competence within adolescent medicine practice, this chapter defines the term and its essential features. Practical issues in cultural competence are explored through case examples in which more comprehensive care to the patient and family can be provided. Information contained herein emphasizes that, regardless of attitudes, knowledge and skills can be acquired, practiced, and honed in the process of becoming a more culturally competent clinician.

## DEVELOPMENT OF CONCEPTS RELATED TO CULTURAL COMPETENCE

Betancourt[2] has pointed out that substandard competence in other areas of clinical medicine is not acceptable, and cultural competence should not be an exception. A clinician who ignores culture in the evaluation and treatment of an adolescent because it is not a biological variable does so at the risk of ignoring or, worse, suppressing important social data about patients.

### IMPORTANCE OF CULTURAL COMPETENCE IN ADOLESCENT HEALTH CARE

The child and adolescent population of the United States is in the midst of a rapid change in demographics. Figure 43-1 compares the demographics of adolescents with adults. The immigrant child population is the fastest-growing portion of the child population.[3] In contrast to the white European and English-speaking populations that migrated to the United States in the early 20th century, families from the Caribbean, Africa, and Asia now constitute significant immigrant groups. Noteworthy is the rapidly growing Latino population as immigrants from Mexico and Central America settle and raise their families in the United States, and similar to other immigrants, look for greater economic opportunities or seek safety from conflict in their homeland.

Given the change in the cultural makeup of the United States, health care clinicians are being challenged to provide cross-cultural care that is sensitive, effective, and meets the needs of the patient and family. Cross-cultural care requires clinicians to be open and to understand the diverse cultural dynamics that play into the patient–clinician encounter such as: (1) variation in the perception of illness; (2) diverse belief systems around health; (3) differences in help-seeking behaviors; and (4) preferences in approaches to health care. Therefore, cultural competence is not merely an issue of "doing the right thing," it is an important vehicle for patient satisfaction, safety, and improved health outcomes.

The Institute of Medicine[4] issued a monograph in 2002 that detailed disparities in health and health care among Americans related specifically to being a member of a racial or ethnic minority. This report, "Unequal Treatment," focused primarily on adult health conditions, but there are well-known examples in adolescent health as well (eg, immunization, asthma, and pregnancy) related to racial and ethnic minority status, largely mediated by poverty. The current population estimate is that there will be 64 million adolescents living in the United States by the year 2020; of these, 40% will belong to a minority group. If present trends continue, the adolescent population will become more diverse, with non-Hispanic whites, currently the majority group, comprising less than 50% of the projected population by 2040.[5]

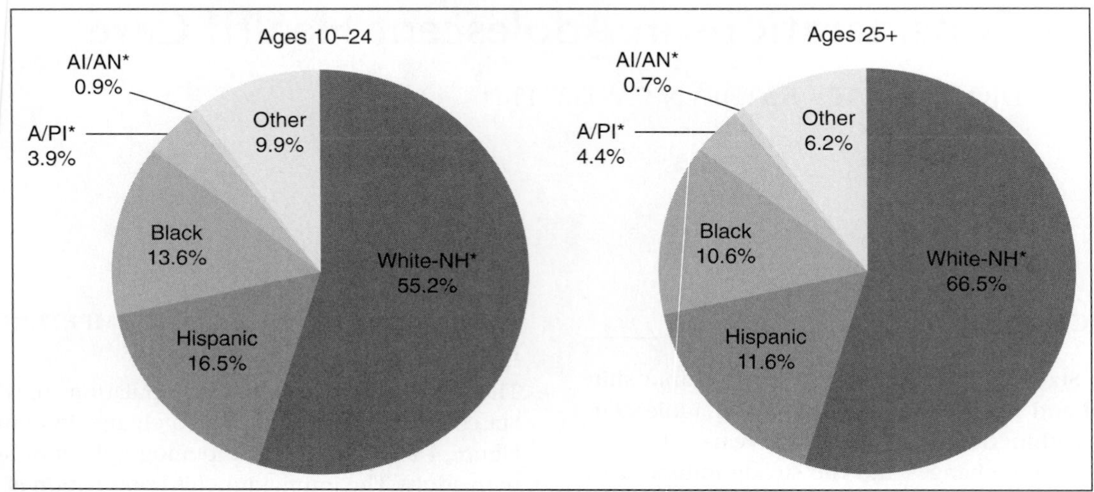


**FIGURE 43-1** US population by age group and race/ethnicity, 2006. NH, non-Hispanic; AI/AN, American Indian/Alaskan Native; A/PI, Asian/Pacific Islander. (From National Adolescent Health Information Center. *Fact Sheet on Demographics: Adolescents & Young Adults.* San Francisco, CA: NAHIC, University of California, San Francisco; 2008.)

One in 5 children and adolescents lives in poverty, black and Hispanic adolescents being most affected. Poor adolescents and those without insurance for other reasons are more likely to seek routine health care from a hospital emergency department, as well as perform poorly in school because they miss school due to illness. Poor adolescents also experience more health problems, perceive their health to be fair to poor, and have higher rates of pregnancy, cigarette use, delinquency, depression, and victimization.[6] Cultural competence is 1 vehicle, along with increased access and insurance coverage, that can improve health outcomes for poor adolescents through improved communication, and increased trust, and understanding, between the patient and clinician.[7]

## DEFINITION AND FEATURES OF CULTURAL COMPETENCE

Culture is defined as a pattern of behaviors, such as thought, speech, action, beliefs, customs, values, and morals shared by a group of people based on factors such as race, ethnicity, religion, social group, sexual orientation, or socioeconomic status.[8] Culture is continually influenced by social conflicts, social transformations, and differentials in power (perceived or actual). Some of the variance across cultural groups can be affected by immigration, family structure, educational attainment, and socioeconomic status. In addition, some adolescent social groups can be defined by age, generation, ableness, and literacy. Social groupings in school tend to have cultural features related to social identity development. For example, "jocks," "nerds," "preppies," "goths," "druggies," and "emos" are labels in the lexicon of many adolescents in school. They represent subcultures characterized by the way they communicate, the clothes they wear and how they wear them, the types of music they enjoy, and what they value.

Cultural competence acknowledges and incorporates culture as a defining feature of every adolescent patient. It includes (1) ongoing assessments of cross-cultural interactions, (2) vigilance regarding the dynamics that result from cultural similarities and differences, (3) the expansion of cultural knowledge, and (4) the adaptation of services to meet various cultural needs.[9] Being culturally competent implies that the clinician does not treat all patients the same, given the varied cultural dynamics each adolescent brings to the health care encounter.

The concept of cultural competence has come slower to medicine than to other professional disciplines who provide health care services to adolescents, such as nursing, psychology (both clinical and counseling), and social work, each of which includes it in their training and literature. The nomenclature for cultural competence has evolved over the last 2 decades from cultural awareness to cultural sensitivity to cultural competence. Other terms such as cultural "effectiveness" and cultural "humility"[10] are currently being used; the former term implies that including cultural considerations improves the outcome of clinical interactions, whereas the latter term emphasizes that culture is not hierarchical or rank-ordered. In this regard, the most skilled clinicians are continually engaged in *becoming* more culturally competent with no endpoint in the process sought or possible. As an ongoing process, it builds on dialogue with adolescents and their families grounded in clinician self-reflection.

Because of its familiarity to most clinicians, the term "cultural competence" is used in this chapter for the purposes of this discussion. Regardless of the term used, the key features of cultural competence include *empathy*, *curiosity*, and *respect*, with which comes a heightened understanding and appreciation of the social context of the adolescent.

## ATTITUDES, KNOWLEDGE, AND SKILLS ASSOCIATED WITH CULTURAL COMPETENCE

The elements of a clinician becoming more culturally competent include (1) increasing self-awareness and receptivity (**attitudes**) to diverse patient populations; (2) understanding the importance of cultural variation (**knowledge**) in the expression of and meaning of illness and treatment to patients of diverse backgrounds; (3) increasing clinical excellence in terms of the ability to deliver culturally competent care (**skills**) to a diverse group of patients, including the ability to establish strong collaborative alliances with patients.[11,12]

### ATTITUDES

All prominent cultural competence models and theories endorse the need for the clinician to first grasp a broad concept of "culture" and then apply this construct to examining (self-awareness, self-knowledge) their own assumptions, biases, stereotypes, and responses. It is vital to examine the concept of "culture," to illuminate the connections between worldview, beliefs, norms, and behaviors related to health, illness, and care-seeking in different populations. In this regard, clinicians should begin to explore how their own cultures, including the cultures of their discipline, inform their perceptions and behaviors. Probing self-directed questions that facilitate increasing awareness in this regard include the following:

- Are you aware and mindful of your own cultural beliefs, values, and behaviors?
- How do these affect your interactions with patients?
- If you cannot manage your biases for the sake of the patient, do you recognize that limitation and defer to a colleague?
- Do you understand the dynamics of difference? This is a particularly important point for physicians, given how much power is bestowed upon them by authority within the health care system. If you believe that a particular treatment is best for an adolescent, but the adolescent does not agree based on cultural differences, despite the power differential between you and the adolescent, do you respect and work within that context to arrive at a compromise that does not adversely affect the overall care of the patient?

### KNOWLEDGE

Information about local and national demographics need to be part of the general knowledge base of the practitioner. This includes attention to specific populations, immigration, changing demographics, and health disparities. Clinicians aware of the kinds and degrees of disparities in health status, health care access, and preventive strategies across racial, ethnic, and other factors related to culture are able to anticipate issues that might otherwise not be considered in providing health care to an adolescent. Cultural knowledge is shaped by integrating lessons learned from colleagues and patients with whom we providers interact. It is important, however, for providers to be aware of the limits of their knowledge regarding a particular culture and to seek assistance from those more knowledgeable. For small groups of immigrant populations sponsored by a social agency or faith community, the sponsoring entity generally can provide such information. If such a resource is not available locally, 1 potential resource in this regard is the adolescent himself or herself. Patients may be honored to have their physician ask them about elements of their culture that might enhance or impede health care for the adolescent. This also can enhance the therapeutic relationship.

### SKILLS

Skills (eg, communication), in combination with a strong knowledge base, enable the clinician to assess his or her own responses, biases, and cultural preconceptions on an ongoing basis. Clinicians should consistently utilize communication tools and strategies for eliciting patients' social, family, and medical histories, as well as patients' health beliefs, practices, and explanatory models. Communication skills for fostering positive therapeutic alliances with diverse patients are also important. These include ways to assess an adolescent's expectations around levels of interactive formality with clinicians, valuing and incorporating the adolescent's beliefs and understanding into diagnosis, treatment options, and negotiating conflicting patient/provider perspectives when necessary. To become a more culturally competent clinician, 1 needs to adapt to diversity, and the needs and preferences of patients, and remain open to different approaches to a given problem.

In addition, as previously noted cultural competence involves empathy, curiosity, and respect. Although being aware of the history and health beliefs and practices of a particular cultural group can provide a foundation for understanding, this knowledge needs to be carefully balanced when dealing with an individual adolescent. There is often as much diversity within a cultural or ethnic group as there is across such groups. Labeling an adolescent "Latino" provides little information regarding that particular adolescent. Assumptions emanating from stereotyping are best avoided to accommodate recognition of diversity within groups.

## PRACTICAL ISSUES IN BECOMING MORE CULTURALLY COMPETENT

The attitudes, knowledge, and skills discussed previously help frame cultural competence working with adolescents in a variety of clinical settings. Practical behaviors described in the following can move the health care provider toward becoming more culturally competent.

### KEY ELEMENTS AND QUESTIONS

With the previously noted qualities of empathy, curiosity, and respect grounding all clinical interactions, there are a number of specific behaviors that support clinical competence.

#### Exploring the Meaning of Illness

Patients who have difficulty expressing their beliefs and fears can be encouraged to communicate through respectful questioning (see Box 43-1). Clinicians can expedite an encounter by joining with the patient to set an agenda for the visit to meet his or her needs. Enquiring about the role of integrative medicine may shed light on an adolescent's guiding model for health or illness. This section will highlight how the clinician can go about asking such questions to facilitate the visit.

**Box 43-1**

***Exploring the Meaning of Illness***

**Explanatory model**[10]

- What do you think has caused your problem? What do you call it?
- Why do you think it started when it did?
- How does it affect your life?
- How severe is it? What worries you the most about it?
- What kind of treatment do you think would/would not work for you? Why?

**The patient's agenda**

- How can I be most helpful to you?
- What is most important for you?

**Illness behavior**

- Have you seen anyone else about this problem besides a "physician"?[a]
- What non-medical remedies or treatment have you tried for your problem?
- Who advises you about your health?

From material cited in Carrillo JE, et al. Cross-cultural primary care: a patient-based approach. *Ann Intern Med*. 1999; 130(10):829–834.

[a]Note: Any health care clinician can be referenced here (eg, nurse, psychologist, dietitian, or social worker).

***CASE SCENARIO #1*** *A 17-year-old black female with epilepsy presents for an initial primary care visit. With the goal of not having any more seizures at school in front of friends, she has increased her anticonvulsant dose without the knowledge or advice of any adult. Because of an active seizure disorder, she is unable to get her driver's permit and is transported by her family and friends. She also worries she will not be able to have children because she remembers the neurologist counseling her about the teratogenic effects of her medications.*

This reflects the culture of a chronic, episodically disabling illness. Questions such as, "How does this illness affect your life?" and "What worries you the most about it?" would demonstrate an interest in issues that she might not otherwise mention in a visit. For this patient, her seizure disorder—her disability—has given her unwanted visibility. Because of the unpredictability of having a seizure and because it makes her different from peers, she has gone to great (inadvisable) lengths to attempt to control it herself.

The clinician can help this patient achieve her goal of better seizure control by emphasizing adherence to the prescribed medication regimen as the best means to achieve normalcy. Counseling regarding reproductive potential with new medication options may be reassuring.

***CASE SCENARIO #2*** *A 16-year-old white male presents for a health supervision visit that was scheduled by his mother. He becomes more anxious during a psychosocial assessment. When the physician notes this, the adolescent asks about sexually transmitted infection (STI) testing. The physician then asks if the patient always wears a condom when he has sex with his girlfriend. The patient then says, "You're right, I've only had sex once, I wore a condom and I don't have any symptoms. I don't need testing, I just wanted to know if I could get it here if I needed it."*

This scenario presents 2 issues: conflicting agendas and false assumptions. The first problem was that the parent and physician were focused on conducting a health supervision visit, whereas the adolescent had another agenda. Starting with "How can I be most helpful to you today?" might have helped uncover the patient's "hidden" agenda. The disconnection between physician and adolescent was heightened by the physician assuming that the boy was heterosexual. In fact, the boy had engaged only in same-sex behavior and was worried that he might have acquired an infection. Openness by his physician to this concept might have enabled the question to be asked, "Have you had sex with males, females, or both females and males?" An honest answer to this question could have led to a more in-depth discussion about sexual orientation, coming out, safe relationships and safe sex.

***CASE SCENARIO #3*** *A 15-year-old girl and her mother seek help for chronic abdominal pain and malaise preventing her from attending school for 6 weeks. The patient has seen gastroenterology and gynecology specialists, and their evaluations have been "negative." The mother is relieved to know the pain is not caused by a serious medical problem, but she has questions about how to manage her daughter's pain. She has been prescribed narcotics that resulted in constipation and further exacerbation of abdominal pain.*

Rather than order more tests or explore other medical explanations for the pain, the culturally competent clinician respectfully asked the mother and daughter to share their ideas about possible pain management options. This not only reflected the openness of the clinician to a different approach, but also gave the clinician a sense of the family's openness. Questions such as, "What non medical remedies or treatments have you tried?" facilitate discussion about how patients can help themselves. Asking about and coordinating care with integrative clinicians or traditional healers can be validating to family and encourage complementary approaches to a health condition. The patient's brother suffered from migraine headaches and responded well to biofeedback. Some proposed therapies included biofeedback and acupuncture. The family also accepted a referral to a psychotherapist for continued care.

### Social Context "Review of Systems"

The adolescent's social context can affect his or her clinical presentation. For example, poverty is a significant barrier to accessing health care and is negatively correlated with self-perceived well-being. Box 43-2 lists questions regarding resources, change in environment, social supports, and literacy that can open communication. Understanding such social factors can increase the clinician's appreciation of the challenges encountered by patients. The following are case scenarios that highlight this element of culturally competent care.

## Box 43-2

### *Social Context "Review of Systems"*

**Control over environment**

- Is money a big problem in your life? Are you ever short of food or clothing?
- How do you keep track of appointments? Are you more concerned about how your health affects you right now or how it might affect you in the future?

**Change in environment**

- What is your country (city, town) of origin?
- What made you decide to come to this country (city, town)? When did you come?
- How have you found life here compared to life in your country (city, town)? What was medical care like there compared with here?

**Social stressors and support network**

- What causes the most difficulty or stress in your life? How do you deal with this?
- Do you have friends or relatives that you can call for help? Who are they? Do they live close to you?
- Are you involved in a religious or social group? Do you feel that God (or a higher power) provides a strong source of support in your life?

**Literacy and language**

- Do you have trouble reading your medication bottles or appointment slips?
- What language do you speak at home? Do you ever feel that you have difficulty communicating everything you want to say to the doctor or staff?

From material cited in Carrillo JE, et al. Cross-cultural primary care: a patient-based approach. *Ann Intern Med*. 1999;130(10)829–834.

***CASE SCENARIO #4*** *A 12-year-old biracial female presents for evaluation of obesity. Her mother has been unemployed for 6 months and has not had health insurance for herself for 4 years. The health care provider would like to refer the patient and mother to an effective weight management program that costs $800 and is not covered by insurance, but hesitates to do so because of the mother's financial situation.*

It is important to not make assumptions about what families can or cannot do in providing care for an adolescent; families may have resources not readily apparent to the clinician. Information about the weight management program was presented to this patient and her mother. However, the mother reported that she was barely getting by with the monthly income she receives for rent, utilities, and groceries. Fortunately, most of the cost was deferred through advocacy work with the insurance companies, social service agencies, and a grant program for patients.

***CASE SCENARIO #5*** *A 14-year-old male with sickle cell disease who emigrated from Jamaica 2 years ago presents with an adjustment reaction and conflict with his mother. As an undocumented resident she has had a dramatic change in earnings compared with her income in Jamaica. The family emigrated seeking better health care for the boy.*

As a recent immigrant, this adolescent found himself in a "cultural warp" between 2 worlds. He mourned the loss of his life in Jamaica, while also being confronted daily with the unpredictability of his family life in a new country. His mother had to work jobs that paid "under the table," which sometimes meant that his mother needed to move away for months at a time, leaving the patient with other family members.

Questions such as, "Tell me what brought you to this country" and "What was life like for you in your country?" can elicit information about place and family of origin, changes in socioeconomic status, and acculturation. Let the patient tell his or her story to answer these questions.

Regarding psychological intervention in this case, community resources such as a charity, church, or civic organization might provide counseling for immigrants regardless of status. Building trust with an immigrant family, particularly of illegal status, is key for services to be utilized without fear of consequences.

***CASE SCENARIO #6*** *A 19-year-old black young adult is dealing with the second recurrence of his cancer. He is admitted to the hospital. Both parents are vigilant and at the bedside. Various family and church members come pray for him. The number of visitors becomes more of an issue as the patient develops neutropenia and requires isolation.*

This family was connected to its church and spirituality was also important to this young man. He had taken on many active roles in the church, including maintaining the property and helping some elderly parishioners. These parishioners, in turn, visited him to lay on hands to facilitate prayer and healing.

Questions such as, "Where do you get support in times like this?" would uncover this family's religious beliefs and connectedness to its church community. This understanding also would help the clinician anticipate expectations and challenges around visitation.

The family, pastor, and hospital staff collaborated to maintain universal infectious precautions. In this case, the pastor was key because he had the respect and power to communicate with the parishioners the importance of adhering to the protocol that had been advised by the treatment team.

***CASE SCENARIO #7*** *A 17-year-old girl presents for her third human papillomavirus (HPV) vaccine dose, having received the first 2 doses in the Dominican Republic, from which she immigrated with her grandmother 9 months ago. She speaks some English and is in bilingual classes in high school. The clinician speaks some functional Spanish, but communicated through an interpreter. When asked about her goals, she says she wants to get a job after high school.*

If an interpreter had not been used, the clinician's communication might have been limited and a discussion about the patient's decision to get a job following graduation and provide counseling would not have been possible. Through the interpreter, the clinician was able to counsel the patient about opportunities and career possibilities.

Knowing the preferred language of the patient allows a professional interpreter to be scheduled. Using family members as interpreters, despite convenience and availability, should be avoided. Family members may not be fluent in the language of the provider, may not be familiar with medical terminology, may be selective in the information they share between provider and patient, and may alter the dynamics between provider and patient. Even in the absence of these impediments, adolescent patients may not fully disclose symptoms or behaviors to aid in diagnosis and treatment. Therefore, the standard of care is to use a professional interpreter if available in person. Telephone and Web-based services are also available. Resources such as "Working with an Interpreter: Stronger Outcomes Tips" address communicating with a patient through an interpreter (www2.massgeneral.org/interpreters/working.asp).

### Cross-Cultural Negotiation

The final phase to the patient encounter is negotiating a treatment plan. This final case exemplifies differences in explanatory models for illness, the influence of family members, and the need to bridge gaps. Box 43-3 includes action steps to create a shared understanding and agreement or, at the very least, an acknowledgment of clinician's and families' boundaries.

***CASE SCENARIO #8*** *A 16-year-old boy with an eating disorder is in relapse. He has required an inpatient level of care in the past and may require it again. His family is ambivalent about next steps in his care, and several consultants have added their perspective to the treatment recommendations. A family meeting is arranged.*

The family's explanatory model was that the patient was being willful in his relapse. Family members generally felt disempowered and at the whim of their son's eating disorder. The patient, on the other hand, believed that engaging in restrictive eating was the only way to control his anger toward his parents.

## Box 43-3

### *Negotiation*

**Negotiating explanatory models**[14,15]

- Explore patient's explanatory model.
- Determine how the explanatory model differs from the biomedical model and how strongly the patient adheres to it.
- Describe the biomedical explanatory model in understandable terms, using as much of the patient terminology and conceptualization as necessary.
- Determine the patient's degree of understanding and acceptance of the biomedical model as it is described.
- If conflict remains, re-evaluate core cultural issues and social context (eg, bring in family members or maximize interpretations).

**Negotiating for management options**

- Describe specific management options (tests, treatments, or procedures) in understandable terms.
- Prioritize management options.
- Determine patient priorities.
- Present a reasonable management plan.
- Determine the patient's level of acceptance of this plan (do not assume acceptance—inquire directly).
- If conflict remains, focus negotiation on higher priorities.

From material cited in Carrillo JE, et al. Cross-cultural primary care: a patient-based approach. *Ann Intern Med*. 1999;130(10):829:834.

The family meeting gave the treatment team a chance to re-explore with the family its conceptualization of the eating disorder and to provide an alternative framework for his behaviors. It also provided an opportunity to review ethical standards with the patient regarding how long the clinicians could support his engagement in a support group without improvement in his physical health. The patient and family agreed to start a new medication as well as an additional psychotherapeutic modality.

This case was unhindered by real conflict, time pressure, or imminent health risk. Difficult negotiations often are characterized by adherence to absolutes on the part of the clinician, patient, family, or all parties. Even what appears to be absolute can be relative and leave room for negotiation and compromise. Involving a family, religious, or community leader can also help broker a difficult negotiation. And sometimes, despite brokers, there is an impasse requiring legal intervention if it is a matter of imminent harm to a minor.

## AT THE SYSTEMS LEVEL

There are potential cultural competence interventions at the systems level as well. The cornerstone for any system (whether a private office, group practice, school-based clinic, or hospital) is the acknowledgment, by the system, that culture is a dominant force in shaping behaviors, values, and institutions. There needs to be acceptance that cultural differences exist and can affect service delivery. It also must be understood that diversity within cultures is as important as diversity between cultures.

A system can demonstrate its value for diversity in hiring practices of clinicians and office staff. It can support cultural competence training of office staff to enhance quality of care provided at every point of the patient encounter. The institution can provide educational materials and display posters in different languages. Techniques like culturally competent health promotion, interpreter services, training and accommodations and time and space for self-reflection, can communicate value for diversity within the practice or system.[7]

Cultural competence can be evaluated in several ways. For example, evaluations and/or satisfaction surveys from patients, families, and staff, otherwise known as 360° evaluations, in a busy pediatric practice can provide useful feedback that prompts change in behavior. Observation, 1 of the best tools for evaluating clinician behavior, can be performed using either standardized patients or actual patients. Observed role-plays with standardized patients are used in medical school settings to provide students with formative feedback to improve interviewing skills. Observation of actual patients or unidentified standardized patients, similar to the observation model used in education, captures clinician behavior in real time under usual clinical conditions.

## SUMMARY

Cultural competence in adolescent health care is critical in view of the ever-changing demographics of the United States. Becoming a culturally competent clinician requires the fundamental attitudes of empathy, curiosity, and respect constantly being reshaped by self-reflection. Clinicians can develop their skills by incorporating key questions into their interviews with patients. Practitioners can take cultural competence to the next level by reviewing and modifying office and systems practices to reflect a value for diversity within our staff, educational materials, and health promotion. Ongoing evaluation of the individual clinician and the health care system can identify areas or dimensions for further development.

## INTERNET RESOURCES

These resources provide guidance on how to facilitate cross-cultural and cross-lingual patient interactions:

- Culture Clues at: depts.washington.edu/pfes/cultureclues.htm.
- CulturedMed at: culturedmed.sunyit.edu/.
- DiversityRx at: www.diversityrx.org/.
- The Manager's Electronic Resource Center at: ethnomed.org.
- National Center for Cultural Competence at: nccc.georgetown.edu.
- US Department of Health and Human Services. National Standards for Culturally and Linguistically Appropriate Services in Health Care. Final Report, March 2001 at: minorityhealth.hhs.gov/assets/pdf/checked/finalreport.pdf.
- Working with an Interpreter: Stronger Outcomes Tips at: www2.massgeneral.org/interpreters/working.asp.

These resources provide tools to evaluate clinicians, offices, and larger health systems on cultural competence practices:

- Cultural Competence Health Practitioner Assessment at: www11.georgetown.edu/research/ gucchd/nccc/features/CCHPA.html.
- Cultural Competency Organizational Assessment—360 (COA 360) at: apps2.jhsph.edu/coa360.

## REFERENCES

1. Frable D. Gender, racial, ethnic, sexual, and class identities. *Annu Rev Psychol.* 1997;48:139–162

2. Betancourt JR. Cultural competence and medical education: many names, many perspectives, one goal. *Academic Medicine.* 2006;81:499–501

3. Suarez-Orozco MM. Everything you ever wanted to know about assimilation but were afraid to ask. *DAEDALUS.* 2000;129:1–30

4. Smedley B, Stith AY, Nelson AR. *Unequal Treatment: Confronting Racial and Ethnic Disparities in Health Care.* Washington, DC: National Academic Press; 2002

5. Ozer EM, Park J, Paul T, Brindis CD, Irwin CE. *America's Adolescents: Are They Healthy?* San Francisco, CA: National Adolescent Health Information Center; 2003

6. Elster A, Jarosik J, Van Geest J, Fleming M. Racial and ethnic disparities in health care for adolescents: a systematic review of the literature. *Arch Pediatr Adolesc Med.* 2003;157:867–874

7. Brach C, Fraser I. Can cultural competency reduce racial and ethnic health disparities? A review and conceptual model. *Med Care Res Rev.* 2000;57:181–217

8. Cross T, Bazron B, Dennis K, Isaacs M. *Towards a Culturally Competent System of Care, Volume 1.* Washington, DC: Georgetown University Children Development Center, CASSP Technical Assistance Center; 1989

9. Lavizzo-Mourey R, Mackenzie E. Cultural competence: essential measurement of quality for managed care organizations. *Ann Intern Med.* 1996;124:919–926

10. Tervalon M, Murray-Garcia J. Cultural humility versus cultural competence: a critical discussion in defining physician training outcomes in multicultural education. *J Health Care Poor Underserved.* 1998;9:117–125

11. Pedersen P. *A Handbook for Developing Multicultural Awareness.* Alexandria, VA: American Association for Counseling and Development; 1988

12. Hansen ND, Pepitone-Arreola-Rockwell F, Greene AF. Multicultural competence: criteria and case examples. *Professional Psychology: Research & Practice.* 2000;31:625–660

13. Kleinman A, Eisenberg L, Good B. Cultural, illness, and care: clinical lessons from anthropologic and cross-cultural research. *Ann Intern Med.* 1978;88:251–258

14. Botelho RF. A negotiation model for the doctor–patient relationship. *Family Practice.* 1992;9:210–218

15. Katon W, Kleinman A. Doctor–patient negotiation and other social science strategies in patient care. In: Eisenberg L, Kleinman A, eds. *The Relevance of Social Science for Medicine.* Boston: Reidel; 1980:253–279

# CHAPTER 44

# Religion and Spirituality

KENNETH J. STEINMAN, PhD, MPH

Twenty years ago, few people interested in adolescent health were writing or reading about religion. Three quarters of college textbooks on adolescent development did not mention the subject[1] and only 12% of empirical studies in adolescent health journals considered religion's influence.[2] Recent years, however, have seen first editions of prominent texts with titles such as *Handbook of Religion and Health,*[3] as well as National Institutes of Health[4] program announcements supporting research on youth and religion. Meetings of the Society for Adolescent Health and Medicine, the Society for Research in Child Development, and the Society for the Scientific Study of Religion now sponsor sessions, and even entire preconferences devoted to adolescents and religion.

This flurry of activity is exciting yet bewildering. Despite growing interest in the topic, many people who research or provide health care for adolescents lack a framework for understanding what religion is and how it might influence young people. The aim of this chapter is to provide such a framework. Because more comprehensive reviews of the literature already exist,[3,5] this chapter references only a few studies to provide the reader with an introduction to the topic and a means of contextualizing results from future research in the area. Also, this volume's devotion to adolescents requires that this chapter focus largely on religion's influence on *behavior*. Some of the most compelling illustrations of the religion–health connection involve studies of adult chronic disease and all-cause mortality. Yet because mortality and chronic disease are less appropriate indicators of adolescent health, this chapter aims to examine how different aspects of religion influence young people's risk behaviors.

The chapter is organized into 3 sections. The first section presents a framework for defining religiosity and integrating its different dimensions. The second section reviews how adolescents' religiosity influences their risk behaviors. The third section discusses implications for adolescent health researchers and health care providers applying this knowledge in practice.

## WHAT IS RELIGIOSITY?

In the tradition of psychology and theologian Paul Tillich, Pargament,[6] defines religion as "a search for significance in ways related to the sacred" (p 204). This definition implies dimensions of both belief (ie, "significance") and practice (ie, "a search"). Writing from a different perspective, sociologists highlight religion's communal nature—that practices and beliefs only constitute a religion when they are shared within a community of affiliated members. Thus, religion may be organized around 3 broad dimensions: beliefs, practices, and affiliation. Within this classification, researchers with a clinical focus often employ the term "religiosity" rather than "religion" as an individual-level variable that exists and changes within each person. In contrast, "religion" may also refer to patterns of belief and behavior that occur across communities, societies, and higher levels of social organization.

### BELIEFS

Beliefs refer to one's cognitive and affective understanding of the world. In a religious context, theologians describe this distinction as "believing that" versus "believing in." In the cognitive realm, individuals develop specific conceptions of oneself (eg, "... *that* I can choose between right and wrong"), the world (eg, "... *that* alcohol use is immoral"), and God (eg, "... *that* God punishes those who sin"). Yet it is often difficult to distinguish certain beliefs as "religious." Whereas the content of certain topics (eg, God, the afterlife) might be considered religious, most beliefs about oneself and the world are less easily classified. For example, a teen who believes that premarital sex is wrong may be more likely to explain his or her belief based on a friend's unintended pregnancy or his or her own regretted experience than to cite a passage from Leviticus. Rather than classify some beliefs as religious and others as not, a person's "religious" beliefs may be best understood as an "everyday theology" that influences and is influenced by a larger belief structure.

Beyond the content of specific beliefs, believing *in* something represents an individual's affective connection. Some youth, for example, report feeling close to God, their coreligionists, or even all of humanity. With its emphasis on feeling a connection beyond oneself, the affective dimension of religious beliefs parallels some definitions of spirituality. Despite popular belief that many teenagers consider themselves "spiritual" but

**Table 44-1**

**Prevalence of Religious Beliefs, Practices, and Affiliation among US Youths, 13–17 Years Old**

| | *Prevalence* |
|---|---|
| ***Beliefs*** | |
| Believe in God | 84% |
| Believe in a judgment day, where God will reward some and punish others | 71% |
| Definitely believe in existence of angels | 63% |
| Definitely believe in existence of demons or evil spirits | 41% |
| ***Spirituality*** | |
| Feel very/extremely close to God | 36% |
| ***Practices*** | |
| Attend worship services at least weekly | 40% |
| Currently involved in a religious youth group | 38% |
| Pray alone at least weekly | 65% |
| Listen to religious radio programs, CDs, or tapes (past year) | 51% |
| ***Affiliation*** | |
| Belong to a religious denomination | 82% |
| Family talks about God, scripture, prayer, or other religious or spiritual things together at least weekly | 45% |
| Have very similar religious beliefs to mother | 41% |
| Mean number of 5 closest friends who hold same religious beliefs as teen | 2.6 |

Data from National Study of Youth and Religion[7]

not "religious," youths who feel close to God (or, alternatively, a transcendent being) also tend to endorse traditional religious beliefs and conventional practices. Results from the *National Study of Youth and Religion* (NSYR),[7] a recent study of 13- to 17-year-olds, found that an overwhelming majority (84%) believe in God and 48% have had no doubts in the past year (see Table 44-1). Yet only one-third of youth (36%) report feeling very close to God. In summary, many American youths agree with conventional religious beliefs, yet only some also report a depth of religious feeling.

## PRACTICES

Scholars typically identify 2 types of religious practices: private and public. Private religious practices include activities individuals engage in outside of organizational contexts, such as personal prayer, reading religious texts, consuming religious media, and reciting grace before or after meals. To some extent, such activities typify more devout individuals whose religious involvement is motivated by personal (or to use another term, "intrinsic") factors. Yet private religious practices are often undemanding to perform: It is relatively easy, for instance, to listen to gospel music on the way to school or utter a brief prayer before taking an exam.

Public religious practices are activities that occur in an organizational context. Perhaps the most common measure of religiosity is "How often do you attend religious services?" Despite the limited scope and documented overreporting of this single item on surveys, it is associated with a surprisingly wide range of outcomes. Other examples of public religious activity include religious summer camp, youth group activities, Bible study classes, and Sunday school.

Given the wide range of activities sponsored or based in congregations, it can be difficult to classify "public" activities as either religious or nonreligious. Two youths working in a church's food pantry, for instance, may do so for different reasons and may attribute different meanings to the experience. Even attending worship services is, for many people, more of a social than religious activity. Thus, some researchers frame public religious practices, along with academic and other extracurricular activities, as part of a larger dimension of adolescents' "prosocial" behavior.[1,8] In this sense, going to church resembles writing for the student newspaper, joining the 4-H club or participating in the school band. Although there is much to recommend this view, some scholars argue that public religious activity represents a qualitatively different type of experience for youth. Religious activities, for instance, can provide youth with a coherent belief structure in which to understand the meaning of their work.[9] In addition, prosocial behavior performed in a religious context may be more likely to afford access to a social network of religiously oriented peers.

Public and private religious practices are remarkably common among adolescents in the United States. More than 40% of youths report attending religious services at least weekly, and 45% say they would attend weekly even if it were totally up to them.[7] At the other end of the spectrum, 18% report that they never attend services. Participation in other religious activities is also common, with 38% of young people reporting current involvement in a youth group. Many youth also regularly pray on their own (65%) and listen to religious music (51%).

## AFFILIATION

If asked,"Why are you (Jewish/Lutheran/Greek Orthodox, etc)?" many teens simply respond, "Because my parents are." This underscores the importance of affiliation for understanding religion. Religion is not only what one thinks, feels, and does, it also reflects a network of family and community relationships. Prior to adapting any religious beliefs or practices, individuals are born into a social world of family, neighbors, and community. The structure and content of these relationships form an essential component of what it means to be religious.

Religious denomination is a common, if imprecise, means of distinguishing different types of affiliation. In the United States, 82% of adolescents (and a similar proportion of adults) report belonging to some religious denomination—a figure much higher than in Canada or other Western industrialized countries. Nonetheless, many youths' identification with a particular denominational label is weak and transient. The frequency of intermarriage across denominations and changes in individuals' religious affiliation over the life span suggest that many adolescents grow up in homes with multiple and changing religious affiliations. A youth, for example, might be active in a local Methodist youth group but report his religion as "Church of God" because of the congregation where he usually attends services with his mother (raised Baptist) and father (raised unaffiliated).

In research on adolescent risk behaviors, denominational differences often reflect the confounding effects of other demographic variables such as income, ethnicity, and region. Catholic youth, for example, are disproportionately Latino; Jewish youth are more likely to live in or near urban areas and come from families with higher household incomes. Yet even after accounting for such confounders, researchers often detect certain denominational differences: Teenagers from conservative Protestant denominations (eg, Pentecostal, Baptist)

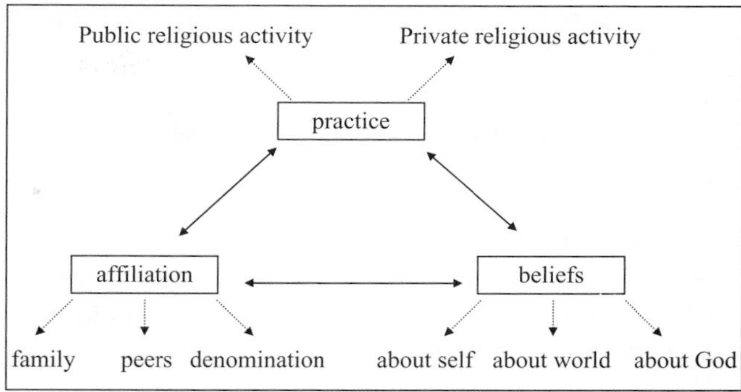


**FIGURE 44-1** Model of adolescent religiosity.

and Latter Day Saints (ie, Mormons), for example, tend to report lower rates of alcohol and other drug use. They also report later debut of sexual intercourse, but they are also be less likely to use consistent, effective contraception. Another consistent finding involves unaffiliated youth, who are more likely to engage in risky behaviors compared to other youth.

## AN INTEGRATED FRAMEWORK

Whereas beliefs, practices, and affiliation represent different dimensions of religiosity, they nonetheless remain highly interrelated (see Figure 44-1). Just as an individual's family, friends, and denomination may initially influence his or her religious beliefs, beliefs may also influence his or her relationship with family and the friends and denomination with which he or she chooses to affiliate. Other reciprocal (ie, transactional) relationships exist among all 3 dimensions of beliefs, practices, and affiliation. Such interrelatedness complicates statistical analyses of religious variables. Multivariate analyses, for example, aim to estimate the unique effects of specific variables on an outcome while controlling for the effects of other variables. The greater the association among the predictor variables, however, the more difficult it is to isolate the unique effects of each.

One approach to summarizing how these different dimensions relate to one another is to examine how different patterns cluster within individuals. Teenagers who attend worship services each week, for example, also tend to participate in youth group activities, believe in God, and report denominational affiliation. Rather than trying to isolate the unique contribution of each dimension of religion, some scholars classify individuals into different groups based on their responses to a variety of questions. Using NSYR data, Smith[7] identified 4 different "religious types" of adolescents:

1. **Devoted adolescents** (8%) report frequent attendance at services and involvement in other religious activities. They also tend to endorse

traditional religious beliefs, pray frequently on their own, and report that religion is an important part of their lives.

2. **Regular attenders** (27%) are the most common type. They regularly attend services but are only moderately devout in their beliefs and private behavior.
3. **Sporadic attenders** (17%) resemble regular attenders, except that they attend religious services only occasionally.
4. **Disengaged** (12%) youth rarely if ever attend religious services and report low levels of commitment to religious beliefs and affiliation.

Using such a classification scheme may represent a more promising approach to assessing the broad nature of how religion influences adolescents' lives. Yet it too is not without limitations. First, many youth (36% in the NSYR data) do not fit into 1 of the 4 types (eg, youths who attend services regularly yet do not believe in God). Moreover, young people often switch types from year to year. In particular, devoted and disengaged youth may be more likely to remain stable over time compared to regular and sporadic attenders. One longitudinal study of black high school students found that 59% of disengaged youth and 45% of devoted youth remained in the same pattern over 3 years, compared to only 27% of sporadic attenders and 15% of regular attenders.[11] Such person-centered analyses remain uncommon, however, and research is needed to understand how patterns of religiosity change during adolescence.

## HOW DOES RELIGIOSITY INFLUENCE RISK BEHAVIOR?

Considerable evidence suggests that religion is negatively associated with a variety of adolescent health behaviors, such as early coital debut, substance use, violent behavior, and seat belt use.[3,5,12] Despite the strength of the bivariate association of religiosity with different risk behaviors, such effects often disappear in multivariate models that account for other influences such as parents, peers, and personality. Such a finding requires describing how the effects of religiosity on risk behaviors can be integrated into a more general model of adolescent risk behaviors.

Adolescent risk behaviors are shaped by 2 forces: a youth's propensity to engage in specific behavior (see Figure 44-2, vector *a*) and his or her opportunity to do so (vector *b*).[10] The concept of "propensity" comprises a range of intrapersonal characteristics youths carry with them across different environments (eg, home, school, work). Factors like personality traits (eg, sensation-seeking), beliefs about behavior (eg, "what will happen if I do [not] act?"), and values they place on those outcomes (eg, "how much do I care about being popular?") all influence an individual's propensity to engage in a specific behavior (vector *c*).

Of course not all youths with a propensity to engage in risky behavior actually do—for instance, the number of 14-year-old boys willing to have unprotected sexual intercourse is much greater than the number who actually do. Risk behavior requires opportunity (vector *b*).

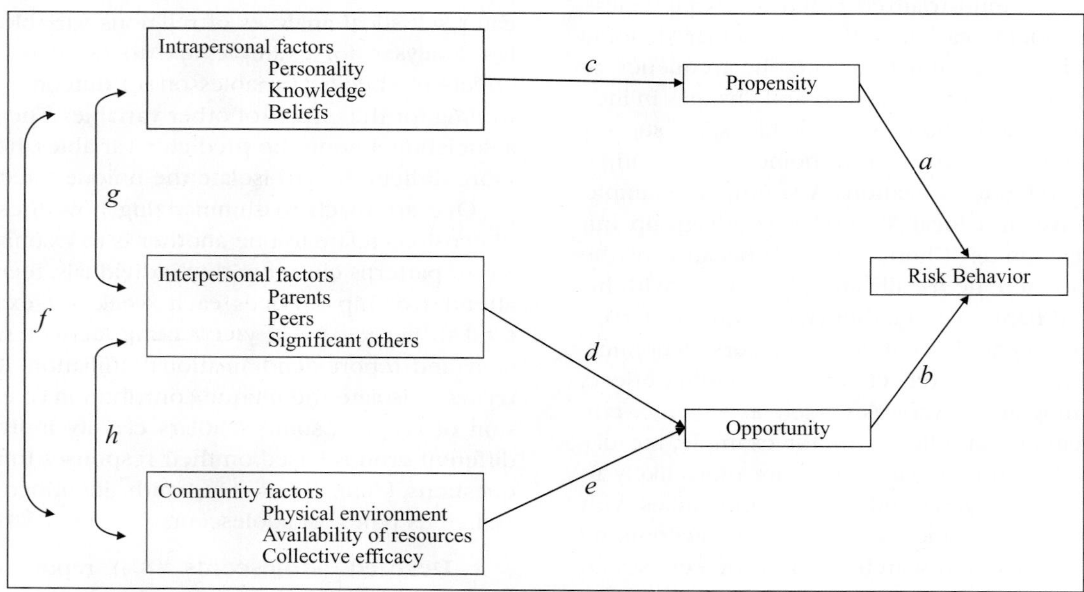


**FIGURE 44-2** Model of adolescent risk behavior.

Because most adolescent risk behaviors are inherently or typically interpersonal, peers have a tremendous influence on opportunities for risk behavior. Risky sex and interpersonal violence, for instance, require at least 2 people, whereas most teenage drug and alcohol use occurs in groups. Thus, youths' opportunity to engage in risk behavior depends on the peers with whom they socialize (vector *d*). Similarly, parents influence youths' opportunity to engage in risk behavior by choosing which schools they attend, monitoring friends, setting curfews, and so on. At another level, community-level factors shape opportunity (vector *e*). Access to contraception, availability of extracurricular activities, and community norms about teenagers' unsupervised free time can all influence youths' risk behavior opportunities.

Beyond their direct effects on risk behavior, intrapersonal, interpersonal, and community-level risk factors in the Figure 44-2 model also operate indirectly (vectors *f, g, h*). An adolescent's personality, for instance, may influence who his or her peers are, which in turn, may affect his or her opportunities for risk behavior. Similarly, peers may influence beliefs, and consequently, propensity for risk behavior. This model is broad and flexible enough to account for a number of direct and indirect effects on risk behavior across multiple levels of organization.

The 3 dimensions of religiosity—belief, practice, and affiliation—could fit into this model in many ways. Rather than describe all possible pathways, this chapter highlights a few to illustrate the complexity of religiosity.

## BELIEFS

Beliefs about the consequences of one's behavior are central constructs in most theories of health behavior, and numerous studies suggest religiosity can shape such beliefs. Most traditions, for instance, explicitly discourage certain risk behaviors (eg, extramarital sex) and describe the consequences of disobedience. Thus, the more teens believe that God (1) disapproves of extramarital sexual activity; (2) is aware of and cares about their individual behavior; and (3) punishes transgressions, the less likely they are to engage in it. As noted in Figure 44-2, beliefs (including those influenced by religion) may also operate indirectly. Young people seek out and maintain friendships with peers who share similar characteristics. Thus, a young woman who endorses the beliefs listed previously is more likely to spend time with peers who think similarly. In so doing, she reduces opportunities to engage in the behavior.

## PRACTICES

In adolescent risk behavior studies, public religious activity (eg, attending religious services) is the most frequently employed measure of adolescent religiosity, with published studies overwhelmingly showing a salutary effect.[12] In practice, however, it is unclear why, for instance, sitting through 2 to 3 hours of religious services each week is beneficial. It is more useful to view survey measures of public religious activity as a proxy for a range of other phenomena that are more difficult to measure. Teens' public religious activity may indicate exposure to messages discouraging risky behavior; access to youths and adults who endorse these messages; or affective or spiritual experiences that clarify and reinforce beliefs. Because most youth attend services with family members, public religious activity may also reflect the state of parent–child relations within the family.

This view of public religious activity differs from that of congregations and parents who encourage teens' participation as a means to address risky behavior—simply sitting in a sanctuary is unlikely to have much of an effect. Rather, content and context of such experiences may be most influential.

## AFFILIATION

Each adolescent's family represents an important dimension of religiosity and its influence on risk behavior. Family members can indirectly influence a youth's propensity by shaping, for instance, beliefs. Despite popular images of the rebellious teen, most young people resemble their parents' religious beliefs and practices.[7] Whereas religious similarity may strengthen the quality of parent–child relationships,[13] these effects can be understood as the relative absence of discord. In other words, parents and children whose religiosity is more similar than average are not necessarily better off than families that experience an average degree of similarity. It may be that only large differences in religiosity between parents and children exacerbate strained relations and increase youths' likelihood of risk behavior.

Spending time with peers in a religious context may limit a teen's opportunities for risk behavior. Such networks may involve greater adult supervision, as well as a greater proportion of youth who discourage alcohol, drugs, sex, and so on. Empirical evidence supporting or refuting this hypothesis remains sparse, as few studies directly examine the effects of religious peer networks. Part of the challenge is accounting for youths' affiliation with different peer networks in different contexts. A teenager may have 1 group of friends at school and a very different group at church. To the extent that these networks differ, youth are apt to behave differently among different groups of friends.

## PERSONALITY

Religiosity is, of course, not the only important influence on adolescents' risk behavior. Personality traits, for instance, are noteworthy for their association with both religiosity and risk behavior. Unlike other pathways described previously, it is difficult to argue that religiosity *affects* personality, which in turn alters the propensity for risk behavior. A more compelling model may be that an observed association between religiosity and risk behavior is spurious; that is, it is due to their both being influenced by certain personality traits. Traits like impulsivity or sensation-seeking may independently undermine religious involvement and contribute to risky behavior. Because personality traits are often heritable, these effects are compounded within families where, for instance, an introverted teen lives with introverted parents, all of whom are particularly receptive toward religiosity and uninterested in risky behavior. Studying and disentangling effects of personality from parenting and religiosity is challenging because it is impractical and unethical to randomly assign (from birth!) youth to families of different levels of religiosity.

## IMPLICATIONS FOR ADOLESCENT HEALTH RESEARCHERS AND HEALTH CARE PROVIDERS

Many researchers and practitioners express interest in adolescent religiosity as a potential protective factor against a range of risk behaviors and adverse health consequences. Their (often unstated) assumption is that changing a youth's religiosity in certain ways should lead to better health outcomes. Yet applying this knowledge in practice raises serious challenges. One concern is that we simply do not yet know enough about adolescent religiosity and health. Even the most rigorous, longitudinal studies on the subject of health are observational. To date, few if any intervention studies suggest that changing youths' religiosity will yield desirable outcomes. Without such findings it would be irresponsible to issue recommendations on changing religiosity without understanding the range of likely effects.

Another concern relates to the legal and ethical issues associated with prescribing religion.[14] Most health care providers can articulate why they have the right to encourage kids to exercise and avoid smoking. Yet most would justifiably balk if asked to promote religious services or encourage families to join a Mormon or Seventh Day Adventist congregation. Promoting religion in this way would undermine individual and community autonomy, fundamental values of Western medicine, and secular democracy.

So what should we do? Clinicians should recognize the potentially powerful influence religiosity can have in some young people's lives. In some cases, understanding a young person's religious beliefs, practices, and affiliation may yield valuable insight into health and well-being. Currently, a growing number of guides suggest when and how to incorporate such discussions into the patient–provider encounter, although most are geared toward adults.[15]

A longer-term suggestion is the need to develop partnerships among congregations, educational institutions, and health care providers. Whereas providers and schools are not in the business of changing individuals' religiosity, congregations are. By forming partnerships, we can study and develop evidence-based recommendations for how congregations can improve their ability to contribute to healthy development. By building such trusting relationships, we can also enable congregations to examine and consider how their activities may be harmful to some teens (eg, lesbian, gay, bisexual youth).

Religion is important to many young people and it elicits strong feelings among researchers and providers. Creating and applying knowledge in this area requires a respect for religion as well as a commitment to critical scholarship and improving health.

## REFERENCES

1. Thomas DL, Carver C. Religion and adolescent social competence. In Gullota TP, Adams GR, Montemayer R, eds. *Developing Social Competency in Adolescence: Advances in Adolescent Development*. Newbury Park, CA: Sage; 1990:195–219

2. Weaver AJ, Samford JA, Morgan VJ, Lichton AI, Larson DB, Garbarino J. Research on religious variables in five major adolescent research journals: 1992 to 1996. *J Nerv Ment Dis.* 2000;188:36–44

3. Koenig HG, McCullough ME, Larson DB. *Handbook of Religion and Health.* New York, NY: Oxford University Press; 2001

4. National Institutes of Health. The influence of religiosity and spirituality on health risk behaviors in children and adolescents (R01). 2007. Available at: grants.nih.gov/grants/guide/pa-files/pa-07-181.html. Accessed July 1, 2007

5. Regnerus MD. Religion and positive adolescent outcomes: a review of research and theory. *Rev Relig Res.* 2003;44:394–413

6. Pargament KI. Of means and ends: religion and the search for significance. *Int J Psychol Relig.* 1992;2:201–229

7. Smith C, Denton M. *Soul Searching: The Religious and Spiritual Lives of American Teenagers.* New York, NY: Oxford University Press; 2005

8. King PE, Furrow JL. Religion as a resource for positive youth development: religion, social capital, and moral outcomes. *Dev Psychol.* 2004;40:703–713

9. Youniss J, McLellan JA, Yates M. Religion, community service, and identity in American youth. *J Adolesc.* 1999;22:243–253

10. Brynes JP. Changing views on the nature and prevention of adolescent risk-taking. In Romer D, ed. *Reducing Adolescent Risk: Toward an Integrated Approach*. Thousand Oaks, CA: Sage; 2003:11–17

11. Steinman KJ, Zimmerman MA. The social context of religious activity among African-American adolescents: influences on sexual behavior and substance use. Conference of the International Center for the Integration of Health and Spirituality, National Institutes of Health, Bethesda, MD, April 2003

12. Rew L, Wong YJ. A systematic review of associations among religiosity/spirituality and adolescent health attitudes and behaviors. *J Adolesc Health.* 2006;433-442

13. Mahoney A, Pargament KI, Tarakeshwar N, Swank AB. Religion in the home in the 1980s and 1990s: a meta-analytic review and conceptual analysis of links between religion, marriage, and parenting. *J Fam Psychol.* 2001;15:559-596

14. Sloan RP, Bagiella E, VandeCreek L, et al. Should physicians prescribe religious activities? *N Engl J Med.* 2000;342:1913-1916

15. Koenig HG. *Spirituality in Patient Care: Why, How, When, and What.* Radnor, PA: Templeton Foundation Press; 2002

# CHAPTER 45

# Cults and Adolescents

CURREN WARE, MD, MSED

## INTRODUCTION

Although adolescent involvement in cult-like groups has been in decline, it remains a concern for parents of involved youth, and to physicians, psychologists, and others because of perceived risks to physical and mental health. Though there remains a lack of consensus over what constitutes a "cult," the most disturbing potential effects on young people, including isolation from family and friends and interruption of traditional pursuits of education and employment, can have a significantly negative effect on healthy adolescent development. Despite the commonly pejorative treatment of cult-like groups, they are appealing to some adolescents because at a time of life when the adolescent may be floating and without clear direction, joining a cult may meet the developmental needs of belonging and fulfilling a sense of purpose in life. In some groups, there is a risk of exploitation, financial and sexual (although some have questioned whether these risks are greater for the youth in most of these groups than for youth who do not belong to these groups). Notwithstanding the isolation from family that frequently follows involvement in a cult, research indicates that parents retain significant influence when they can maintain a positive relationship with their child.

## DEFINITION OF TERMS

There is no consensus on what constitutes a "cult."

Webster's defines a cult as (1) adherents of an exclusive system of religious beliefs and practices, (2) an interest followed with exaggerated zeal: "He always follows the latest fads"; "it was all the rage that season," and (3) a system of religious beliefs and rituals.

This is a relatively nonjudgmental definition; however, in the United States the term "cult" has taken on a pejorative meaning with implications that such groups hold beliefs that are unacceptably outside the mainstream and may exploit members emotionally, financially, and sometimes sexually. In an attempt to ameliorate the bias implicit in the term "cult," these groups are sometimes referred to as "new religious movements."

Adding to the confusion and imprecision of the terminology, not all groups referred to as cults are religious or spiritual in character; there are groups in which participants are perceived to have an inordinate devotion to a charismatic leader or to a specific philosophy or worldview, usually isolating members from the broader society, particularly their families. Several of these nonreligious groups developed around psychotherapeutic schools or intensive residential substance abuse programs such as *est* and Synanon and have exerted a compelling appeal by promising adherents more control over their lives, greater productivity, and happiness—the same promise as mainstream psychotherapy.

Members of cults commonly view their particular group as the apex of history, frequently with devotion to a specific charismatic person. Some cults take on an evangelical character, with members feeling that they have the "one true way" and developing a commitment to convert and save others.

Given the lack of consensus over what constitutes a cult, it is more useful to conceptualize cults on a continuum from those that are most controlling and psychologically abusive at one extreme to those that are relatively benign at the other end. It may be helpful to abandon the terminology of "cult" and instead describe the specific concerns of young people's loss of contact with family, withdrawal from pursuit of education and employment, the undue influence of leaders on the group, and the risk of exploitation or abuse.[1]

## SOME HISTORICAL FEATURES

Religious and spiritual cults have existed throughout history. In fact, the starting point for essentially all religions is a charismatic leader and a band of devoted followers with a simple organizational structure and unifying belief system—essentially, a cult. Historically, many contemporary religious groups such as Mennonites, Mormons, Shakers, Jehovah's Witnesses, Quakers, and Jews have been labeled by their detractors as "cults." Non-Western religions, such as Hinduism and Buddhism, though they have hundreds of millions of adherents, are sometimes referred to as "cults" by members of dominant American mainstream religions. Some groups referred to as "cults" derive from established churches or religions, or sects of churches or religions, frequently with a fundamentalist character.

Contemporary groups sometimes referred to pejoratively as cults, such as the Church of Scientology, the Unification Church, and others, come into conflict with established religious groups by competing for members and challenging established beliefs, and with parents by providing an alternative structure for spiritual expression from that of the family. Given the diversity of religious and spiritual expression in the United States, it is impossible to distinguish between the practices and beliefs of "accepted" religious groups and of "cults," and the distinction can be arbitrary and more a reflection of personal bias or social prejudice than science.

In the United States during the 1960s, many cults, embedded in a flourishing youth culture, attracted adherents, predominately adolescents and young adults. There has been a waning of popularity of cults since the 1960s due to several factors including greater caution on the part of groups to recruiting minors without parental consent, well-publicized tragedies of multiple deaths associated with some groups, and the deaths of many of the original charismatic leaders.[2]

Over the last several decades, there have been a number of famous tragedies involving cult groups. These include followers of charismatic leader Jim Jones from San Francisco's Peoples Temple, who committed mass suicide in Jonestown, Guyana, resulting in 914 deaths (including 274 children) in 1978; the Branch Davidians, an apocalyptic split-off from the Seventh Day Adventists in Waco, Texas, who underwent a siege by the federal government in 1993, driven in large part by allegations of sexual abuse of children, resulting in about 80 deaths by inflicted injury and suicide; and the Heaven's Gate mass suicide in 1997, resulting in 39 deaths. The Heaven's Gate suicides were driven by a belief that their souls would be transported to a spaceship behind the Hale-Bopp comet. Unlike most cult-like groups constituted for the most part of single young adults, many of the members of the mentioned groups were adults who left spouses and children behind; the Heaven's Gate group included a 72-year-old member and a member who had belonged for almost 20 years. Although adolescents without parental accompaniment were generally not involved in these groups, there were a number of children and adolescents who accompanied their parents and died; adolescents were not organizers of any of these events. It should be emphasized that these incidents are notable more for their exceptional tragic consequences than as representative examples of cults.

More recently, in 2006, 2007, and 2008 members of several fundamentalist offshoots of the Mormon Church, in particular the Fundamentalist Church of Jesus Christ of Latter Day Saints in Texas, have made allegations of child sexual molestation through arranged polygamous marriages of young teen girls to middle-aged and elderly adult leaders resulting in coercive sexual relationships, some resulting in pregnancy. A 2008 case resulted in the removal of 416 children to Child Protective Services (CPS), although many of the allegations were ultimately unsubstantiated. One should not forget, however, that the sexual exploitation of children has not been limited to marginalized religious sects, but has occurred as well in mainstream religions, including the Catholic Church.

## PREVALENCE

The prevalence of participation in cults is unknown but estimates have run from 2 million to 5 million Americans involved in 2,000 to 5,000 cultic groups.[1] Numbers of adolescents are not known. An interesting study from 1993 noted that 2.2% of surveyed primary care physicians reported that either they or an immediate family member had been involved in a cult.[3]

## ADOLESCENT DEVELOPMENT AND ATTRACTION TO CULTS

During adolescence, young people become capable of an increasing engagement in abstract thought and conceptualization, and many develop a great intellectual curiosity, an interest in spiritual issues or in politics, and become open to new ideas.

Young people are commonly impatient with and critical of established values and behaviors of the broader society. They may feel that they have a unique sense of clarity about social problems, and solutions may also seem clear and simple. They challenge established ideas, assumptions, and customs. Young people lack the experience of adults, but they also may appear to lack many of the biases and the resignation to the status quo. It is difficult for many young people, despite a passionate pursuit of truth, to distinguish between fantasy and reality, and they may become susceptible to ideas that offer a new and unique explanation for complex problems.[4]

This fresh ability to think abstractly, the desire to confront social injustices, and impatience with the established order has fueled young people's involvement in the important social movements that have shaped our history, such as the political and social movements for women's suffrage and equality, for civil rights, and for peace. Idealism and striving for a better world leads some young people to join the Peace Corps, Americorps, political groups, or service organizations. Young people usually have fewer responsibilities than adults and more expendable time to direct toward social causes perceived as intrinsically meaningful.[5]

Adolescents and young adults commonly experience a period of aimlessness and lack of clear goals. At the same time, they may experience pressure from parents and others to define themselves and are told to "do something with your life." These pressures and demands can have unintended consequences, including developing a drive to escape to what may appear to be the safety of a cult-like group. Involvement in a cult offers a confused or isolated adolescent or young adult a respite from conventional pressures of education or working, as well as an opportunity to simultaneously drop out and belong. Few young people who join cults take into account future conventional responsibilities such as rearing children, maintaining ties with family, or pursuing an education or career path.[5] It should be noted that this is true as well for many young people who do not join cults.

An openness to fresh ideas and a desire to change the world make many young people vulnerable to organizations, ideologies, or charismatic leaders who promise a vision of a better world and meet emotional needs for a sense of purpose and meaning in life, fulfillment of spiritual needs, a sense of deep personal connection with peers, and frequently a charismatic adult—resembling in many ways a surrogate family. Joining may seem irresistible.[4]

Not all adolescents are equally susceptible to involvement in cults. Studies[6] have indicated that many young people involved in cults come from relatively high socioeconomic strata families that seem to have been democratic and egalitarian, without clearly identified dysfunction or problems. A 1986 literature review of cults[3] found that young people's attraction to cults had been strengthened by the group's clearer definition of rules than what existed in the family. Vulnerability to joining a cult because of a young person's developing independence, need for a sense of meaning, desire for community and intense peer attachment, and desire for spiritual fulfillment can be interpreted not so much as a reflection of family dysfunction or difficulty but rather as a way for the young person to meet unmet needs.[3] The majority of recruits are idealists seeking someone or something in which to believe. They tend to be smart and lonely young people but naïve and without "street smarts."[2]

Some studies identify beneficial experiences that may result from joining a cult-like group (Box 45-1). For example, some report that joining a particular cult helped youth cope with separating from their parents.[7] In a study of the Meher Baba cult, participants and observers reported that members decreased their use of illicit drugs.[8] In fact, in many cults the expectations for behavior, the communal nature of living arrangements, and the emphasis on a higher purpose resemble models of substance abuse treatment programs. Other studies indicate that members may experience enhanced self-esteem[9] and greater social poise.[10]

Joining a cult-like group may meet a young person's emotional and developmental needs and may be associated with a perception of a deep spiritual, or conversion, experience. Given the diversity of religious beliefs in the United States, and indeed in the world, belief systems are endlessly debatable, and it is generally not the content of the belief system that is specifically damaging (Box 45-2). What is damaging, whether from a small cult-like group or any other religious or spiritual group, is the use of deception and manipulation, the suspension of contact from one's family and friends, and the displacing of loyalties from the family of origin.[5]

**Box 45-1**

***Developmental Needs Met by Cult-Like Groups***

- Supporting separation from family of origin
- Respite from family pressures
- Development of sense of purpose and meaning in life
- Peer relationships and peer acceptance
- Expression of spiritual beliefs
- Increased structure and rules for life
- Reconstruction of surrogate family

**Box 45-2**

***Potential Negative Effects of Youth Involvement in Cult-Like Groups***

- Loss of contact with and isolation from family of origin and mainstream society
- Removal from traditional pathways of education, employment, and career development
- Risk of financial exploitation
- Risk of sexual exploitation

## PARENTAL RESPONSES TO YOUTH INVOLVEMENT

Parents frequently express an understandable and intense concern that their child has been taken out of conventional social networks and productive career paths. Parents may become very angry, feeling that their child has become "brainwashed." The intensity of parental reactions may in some cases be representative of preexisting conflict and estrangement. Angry responses of parents and the alienation of children can lead to a vicious spiral in which family relationships further deteriorate.[5,11] Parents may inadvertently inhibit the willingness of a young person to leave their new peer group through their lack of appreciation of growing adolescent autonomy, the intensity of their reactions, and highly critical remarks. Although outside observers, including family members of group participants, may feel that a particular group meets their criteria for a "cult," if they have an interest in maintaining communication with the participant it is more helpful, in their communication, to consider the specific and harmful practices of a particular group rather than utilize labels.[1]

Minor children require parental or guardian consent to live with other adults. If the parent does not give consent for a minor to live with a particular group, the parents have recourse to intervention through the police or through CPS.

## GROWING UP IN A CULT

As groups have aged, children have grown up in cults and have had widely varied experiences. Many live in a communal, protective, and caring environment and have a remarkably low behavioral risk profile. Many, on the other hand, grow up socially removed from other children and youth and have not attended public schools; some lack any formal schooling at all. In some cases, children have been subjected to harsh physical punishment and maltreatment or sexually abused, leading to reports to CPS when it is detected in a medical or mental health setting. Child abuse investigations can be exceedingly difficult because the group participants may view themselves as objects of religious persecution, and the vigilance and suspicion that many people harbor toward these groups can lead to speculative and inaccurate allegations. Although the First Amendment to the US Constitution protects the right to freedom of religious belief, freedom of religion is not a defense against an accusation of child abuse.[2]

Some sects of religious groups, frequently with a fundamentalist orientation, allow or encourage the "marriage" of minor females to adult men, sometimes in polygamous relationships. As with other types of child sexual abuse, physicians and other mandated reporters of child abuse are obligated to contact CPS or the police, consistent with state and federal legislation, when these situations come to their attention.

## PSYCHOLOGICAL CORRELATES

There are several studies reviewing personality and psychopathology of members of specific cults. In a 1987 study of Hare Krishna members and nonmembers,[1,12] Hare Krishna members were found to be somewhat more compulsive and less trusting than nonmembers; however, scores were within the normal range on a standardized test, and these characteristics may have reflected the compulsivity required for rituals in the group and an understandable perception that their group was viewed critically by society. A 1990 study[9] using a standardized scale found that members of the Rajneeshpuram commune participated in more self-exploration and had lower social anxiety and higher self-esteem than a control group. This may not be surprising given that the tenets of the group include striving for self-exploration, self-acceptance, personal growth, and the taking of personal responsibility. Although most studies seem to indicate that adolescent cult members are reasonably well-adjusted psychologically relative to other youth, and that they do not have conspicuous psychopathology, most studies are small and do not use standardized scales so that findings cannot be generalized.[1]

Interestingly, psychological problems of young people involved in cults seem more likely to emerge after they leave: participants may need to cope with loss and readjustment after leaving a group to which they had been deeply committed; they may only realize the stress they had been under after they leave; their family of origin may not offer the closeness and support of the surrogate family they left; and they may have been shielded from the negative perception of their group while involved but experience it intensely once they leave.[1]

## LEAVING CULTS

There are 3 basic processes through which individuals leave cults. Most commonly, they just walk away from the group; secondly, they may receive intensive exit counseling; or finally, they may be subjected to "deprogramming." The latter essentially involves an involuntary kidnapping (sometimes of young adults) with subjects receiving hours of lectures about their group in an attempt to change their

**Table 45-1**

**Approaches to Leaving Cults**

| *Type* | *Prevalence* | *Comments* |
|---|---|---|
| Voluntary attrition | Most common | Most common if member maintains close relationship with family |
| Intensive exit counseling | Infrequent | May be helpful in adjusting to loss of benefits of group (sense of purpose, close friendships) |
| Deprogramming | Very uncommon | Potential for deep estrangement from family<br>Raises issues of religious freedom and civil liberties |

thoughts and beliefs (Table 45-1). The parents of adult children may attempt to be appointed conservators and seek support from the mental health professions. When deprogramming fails, the young person in most cases is predictably far more estranged from the family. Although "deprogramming" has received a great deal of publicity, it is used far less frequently than in the past, and the vast majority of people who leave cults do not go through a deprogramming process.

Deprogramming raises important civil liberties issues. The First Amendment of the US Constitution guarantees freedom of religion, and historically it is interpreted to include the protection of the rights of unpopular faiths. It is often difficult to distinguish religions from cults: One person's cult may be another person's valid religion. There have been attempts to involve the medical and mental health professions in coercive deprogramming by defining involvement in a cult as a manifestation of "mental illness" and a justification for establishment of adult conservatorship and removal of individual liberties.[13]

An interesting study looking at cult attrition and family relations found that if the family had a negative attitude about joining a cult, family closeness was highly influential in a young person leaving the cult. However, if relations with the family were not close, parental attitudes toward the young person joining the cult were unrelated to voluntarily leaving. Children of parents who held a positive attitude toward the cult were more likely to remain with the cult. In this study, parental disapproval of a son or daughter's involvement was found to be the most important variable in explaining disaffiliation, particularly among those youth who expressed a smooth adolescent experience and close relationships with parents before joining. The family can retain an influence over the decision of young people to leave a cult through maintaining viable relationships during the period of involvement.[5]

## SOME PRACTICAL GUIDELINES FOR WORKING WITH YOUTH INVOLVED IN CULTS

Clinicians who interact with children growing up in cult-like groups are advised to assess their own biases, to treat the young person, his or her parents, and the affiliated group nonjudgmentally, and to address the health and behavioral concerns matter-of-factly.

Regardless of personal biases and beliefs, clinicians need to maintain a respectful and nonjudgmental approach toward the group. If the youth is interested in sharing information, a calm curiosity may encourage disclosure of information. As with other young people, inquire about interests and activities and about contact and relationships with family. Many ostensibly cult-like groups provide clear guidelines for behavior of involved young people, including proscriptions against alcohol and drug use. As with other young people, do not make assumptions about sexual orientation or behaviors; young people involved in cults require the same spectrum of reproductive health choices as other youth. As with other young people, if there is a disclosure or reasonable suspicion of child maltreatment, sexual abuse, or endangerment, CPS must be notified; if a minor cannot be returned because of imminent danger, the police need to be notified. There is no evidence that child maltreatment is either intrinsic to cult-like groups or more prevalent than in general society.

Parents should be advised to maintain frequent contact with their children, demonstrate an interest in their activities, and honestly express their concerns about their future. Parents who appreciate their young adult child's need for an independent identity, realize the needs that the group may be meeting in his or her development, and continue to welcome their child home have the best chance of preserving a relationship and maintaining influence on their child's future decisions. Overreacting, being overly confrontational, and attempting or threatening to attempt coercive measures each run a risk of creating great damage to the relationship that may last for years and reduce parental ability to influence future decisions.

## REFERENCES


1. Aronoff J, Lynn JL, Malinoski P. Are cultic environments psychologically harmful? *Clin Psychol Rev.* 2000;20(1):91–111

2. Schwartz LL, Kaslow FW. The cult phenomenon: a turn of the century update. *Am J Fam Ther.* 2001;29:13–22

3. Lottick EA. Survey reveals physicians' experiences with cults. *Pennsylvania Medicine.* 1993;96:26–28

4. Hunter E. Adolescent attraction to cults. *Adolescence.* 1998;131:7014

5. Wright WA, Piper ES. Families and cults: familial factors related to youth leaving or remaining in deviant religious groups. *J Marriage Fam.* 1986;48(1):15–25

6. Andron S. Our gifted teens and the cults. *Gifted, Creative, Talented Children.* 1983;26:32–33

7. Levine SV. Radical departures. *Psychology Today.* 1984;8: 21–27

8. Robbins T, Anthony D. Getting straight with Meher Baba: a study of drug rehabilitation, mysticism, and post-adolescent role conflict. *J Sci Study Relig.* 1972;11:122–140

9. Latkin CA. Self-consciousness in members of a new religious movement: the Rajneeshees. *J Soc Psychol.* 1990;130:557–558

10. Sunberg ND, Latkin CA, Littman RA, Hagan RA. Personality in a religious commune: CPIs in Rajneeshpuram. *J Pers Assess.* 1990;55:7–17

11. Beckford JA. A typology of family responses to a new religious movement. *Cults and the Family.* Boston, MA: Haworth. 1982:41–56

12. Weiss AS, Comrey AL. Personality characteristics of Hare Krishnas. *J Pers Assess.* 1987;51:399–413

13. Davis DS. Joining a "cult": religious choice or psychological aberration? *J Law Health.* 1996–1997;11:145

# CHAPTER 46

## Environmental Health

SOPHIE J. BALK, MD

Environmental health is the field of science that concerns how the environment influences human health and disease. Pediatric environmental health (PEH) focuses on the fetus, infant, child, and adolescent. Environmental health hazards include naturally occurring and man-made physical, chemical, and biological contaminants in air, water, food, and soil. Secondhand smoke (SHS), lead, mercury, pesticides, and ionizing radiation are examples of environmental hazards with well-known adverse health effects. The environment also includes the physical structures where people live, work, and play. More broadly still, the social environment encompasses factors such as diet and exercise, socioeconomic status, and other societal influences that may affect health. There is also increasing recognition that gene–environment interactions can shift the balance between health and disease. As is often quoted, "Genetics loads the gun ... but environment pulls the trigger."[1] Our knowledge about PEH has expanded greatly in the past 2 decades. Research has shed light on the relationship of health and developmental conditions to toxicants (toxicant refers to a chemical agent; toxin is used for a biological agent such as botulinum toxin), but many questions remain unanswered.

This chapter reviews why adolescents may be more susceptible to environmental hazards when compared to adults. Taking an environmental history during well adolescent exams follows in this chapter, highlighting key issues. The chapter then discusses the history needed if there are symptoms possibly relating to an environmental exposure.

Although the environment may be broadly defined, the chapter focuses on chemical and physical hazards.

## DEVELOPMENTAL CONCERNS—THE INCREASED SUSCEPTIBILITY OF ADOLESCENTS TO ENVIRONMENTAL TOXICANTS

Most PEH literature highlights the increased susceptibility of fetuses, infants, and young children to the effects of environmental toxicants. Compared to adults, children at these early life stages are at risk because of increased exposures (including behavioral factors such as the toddler's normal hand–mouth and hand–object behaviors) and increased vulnerabilities (including rapid development of sensitive organ systems). Compared to adults, people exposed early usually have a long life ahead of them ("greater shelf life"), during which time the adverse effects of exposures may be expressed. The concept of special susceptibility has been extended to adolescents relatively recently; there are few data, however, on adolescent exposures and resulting consequences on organ systems.[2]

### ADOLESCENT EXPOSURES

Adolescents have greater physiologic need for fluids and calories because of rapid growth. They may be exposed to more toxicants per pound of body weight compared to adults (although less so than are infants and toddlers).[3] With increased energy needs, there is more need for oxygen,[4] possibly resulting in increased exposure to contaminants in the air.

Adolescents live, work, and play in a variety of settings. Most environmental exposure issues focus on occupational settings (Chapter 47, Adolescents at Work), where adolescents may encounter chemicals. For example, adolescents working in agriculture often are exposed to pesticides; although children under 16 are legally restricted from handling or applying pesticides with certain warning labels (ie, danger, poison, warning), they can be employed in harvesting after pesticides are applied. Rules are less stringent for teens working on family farms and businesses.[2] Teens can be exposed through their hobbies, model building, woodworking, ceramics, arts and crafts, and shop activities in school and at home. Chapter 178 on Hallucinogens, Club Drugs, and Inhalants discusses the dangers of inhalants in more detail. Exposures may occur in dormitories in boarding schools or colleges. Behavioral factors are relevant as teens become independent, work, and gain freedom from parental authority. Because they may not consider cause and effect in the same way adults do, they may engage in risky behaviors including becoming exposed to environmental hazards at work and elsewhere.[4]

**ADOLESCENT VULNERABILITIES**

The concept of critical periods of vulnerability or critical windows of exposure, derived from the field of teratology, was originally defined as a "highly susceptible period of organogenesis." This idea was at first applied to the fetus, but more recently the importance of exposure timing has extended to the postnatal period, including the teenage years.[5] There is concern that the delicate processes governing rapidly growing and developing organ systems are subject to derangement—including an increased risk of cancer—when a person is exposed to toxic substances. Each organ system may have periods in development of heightened susceptibility to the effects of chemicals and drugs, and these periods may vary depending on the system. Adolescence is characterized by many changes including rapid skeletal growth and bone mineralization; changes in the immune system including thymic involution; and a growth spurt in lung function.[2] Sexual maturation occurs during adolescence, with complex changes in endocrine function. Developmental exposure to environmental compounds with estrogenic properties (such as pesticides) or other hormonal properties may result in endocrine disruption. An endocrine disruptor is an exogenous agent that interferes with the synthesis, storage/release, transport, metabolism, binding, action, or elimination of natural blood-borne hormones responsible for the regulation of homeostasis and the regulation of developmental processes.[6]

The central nervous system (CNS) continues to grow and develop. This is characterized by differentiation of many cell types, migration of cells, formation of connections, periods of cell death, trimming ("pruning") of connections, and other factors. Studies of the maturation of gray matter density show a prepubertal increase followed by postpubertal loss during adolescence and early adulthood. Magnetic resonance imaging data confirm that the brain changes until the late teens and early 20s, with higher-order association cortices maturing after lower-order somatosensory and visual cortices.[7] There are increases in dopamine content in the prefrontal cortex to peak levels well above those seen earlier or later in life; changes in serotonin levels and other neurotransmitters also occur.[8]

Adolescents' increased susceptibility to tobacco dependence (Chapter 173, Tobacco) is an example of the critical windows concept. Animal and human studies suggest that the adolescent CNS is more vulnerable to nicotine dependence compared to adults. Adolescents may become dependent easily, often before the onset of daily smoking.[9,10] Individuals who begin smoking during adolescence are more likely to become dependent, progress to daily smoking, continue to smoke for a greater number of years, and smoke more heavily as adults. These observations suggest that juvenile-onset nicotine dependence represents a more serious disruption of neurological functioning compared to adult-onset dependence.[10] There is mounting evidence that adolescents are differentially sensitive to the acute and chronic effects of ethanol (Chapter 174, Alcohol). Ethanol exposure during adolescence may alter the normal trajectory of human brain development in long-lasting and perhaps permanent ways[11] not seen in adults. On the other hand, the developmental changes occurring in the adolescent brain may represent a window for "unusual plasticity and recovery."[12,13]

A few examples illustrate adolescents' greater susceptibility to environmental toxicants compared to adults, resulting in increased cancer risk. Adult lung-cancer risk may be increased as a result of secondhand smoke exposure in childhood and adolescence.[14,15] Adolescents are at higher risk of skin cancer after exposure to ultraviolet (UV) radiation,[16] illustrating the sensitivity of their skin and immune system. Adolescents are more susceptible to the effects of ionizing radiation, as demonstrated by the effects of the 1986 meltdown of the nuclear reactor in Chernobyl, Ukraine, which resulted in heavy contamination with plutonium, cesium, and radioactive iodine. Almost 17 million people were exposed to excess radiation. Four years after exposure, a large number of cases of thyroid cancers in adolescents and in children began to emerge, underscoring the special vulnerability at young ages to the effects of radioiodine.[17]

Although information about exact timing and periods of sensitivity is limited,[5] it is likely that many other effects will be discovered as researchers investigate adolescent exposures. In the meantime, clinicians can use available information to ensure the healthiest environment possible for their adolescent patients.

## ENVIRONMENTAL HISTORY

Physicians can ask about home, school, and work situations to identify, reduce, and prevent exposures. An environmental history is a basic part of the medical history; no matter what the patient's age, it is important for physicians to find out about the patient's physical surroundings and exposures. The American Academy of Pediatrics (AAP) Committee on Environmental Health (COEH) recommends that pediatricians review 6 basic areas on health supervision visits: (1) where the child lives or spends time; (2) exposure to SHS; (3) water sources; (4) exposures from food; (5) exposure to UV radiation; and (6) exposures related to parents' and teens' occupations.[18] Additionally, environmental hazards in the community—such as the presence in the community of a nuclear power facility—deserve special attention. Table 46-1 summarizes elements of this history adapted for adolescents. A few issues, discussed here with suggestions for anticipatory guidance, have special relevance to adolescents and their parents.

**Table 46-1**

## Elements of an Environmental History Adapted for Well Adolescent Care

| *Area* | *Key Points* | *Advice/Abatement* | *Comment* |
|---|---|---|---|
| 1-Where the Teen Lives or Spends Time | Dwelling type: Apartments, private homes may have high radon levels on lower floors, or friable asbestos. | Test for radon as recommended by US EPA. Test for asbestos by inspection and/or lab testing; have certified contractors do removal if needed. | Consider home, school dormitories, other living settings. |
| | Age/condition: Pre-1970s buildings may have lead paint; water damage may promote mold growth. | Test blood of young children, or other people at risk, for lead Promptly repair water leaks and remove mold. | Lead poisoning results in neurodevelopmental damage Mold exposure may worsen asthma, allergies. |
| | Heating sources: malfunctioning heaters may emit CO; wood stoves may emit irritants. | Test heating equipment as per manufacturer's instructions Install CO detectors in each sleep area. | Include CO questions when evaluating headaches, nausea, fatigue; inquire about heating sources when evaluating asthma. |
| | School exposures. | Many hazards may be found in school buildings; many built on less desirable land; many unhealthy with poor air quality. | Ask about exposures at school when investigating symptoms. |
| 2-Secondhand Smoke (SHS) Exposure | SHS exacerbates asthma; long-term health effects include increased risk of lung cancer. | Ask about SHS exposure when asking about active smoking; include in preconception counseling. | Urge teens to advocate for their own clean air at home, work, elsewhere. |
| 3-Water Source | Teen mothers should be informed that contaminated water may affect infants. They should not overboil water (>1 minute) as this may concentrate contaminants. | Municipal tap water can be tested for lead; well water should be tested for nitrates. | |
| 4 - Dietary Exposures | Organic mercury contamination of fish is a preconception and prenatal concern. | Educate teens about fish high in mercury, PCBs, and safe alternatives. | Weigh risks and benefits; fish may be major protein source. |
| 5-Ultraviolet (UV) Radiation | Sunburns increase skin cancer risk, including melanoma; artificial tanning (eg, tanning salons) also increases risk. | Outdoor activities encouraged but no sunburning; avoid peak sun exposure times (10 am–4 pm); use sunscreen with SPF of at least 15, wear clothes, hats, sunglasses. Avoid tanning salons. | Specifically target high-risk teens: those with a family history of melanoma; light skin and eyes, nevi, freckling. |

*(Continued)*

**Table 46-1 (Continued)**

**Elements of an Environmental History Adapted for Well Adolescent Care***

| *Area* | *Key Points* | *Advice/Abatement* | *Comment* |
|---|---|---|---|
| 6-Occupational and Paraoccupational Exposures | Ask about teen occupation when authorizing work permits (working papers); ask about parents' occupations (brought-home, paraoccupational exposures). | Use visits for work permits to counsel about possible job hazards (potential for unintentional injury and/or environmental exposure). | High-risk teens include those exposed to pesticides because of work in farms and agriculture. |
| 7-Community Issues | Teens may live, work, or play near hazards in their community. | Ask about proximity to industrial plants, dump sites, agricultural exposures, nuclear power plants. | People living in homes and schools near nuclear plants should have potassium iodide (KI) available. |

*Adapted from American Academy of Pediatrics. *Pediatric Environmental Health*. Etzel RA and Balk SJ, eds. 2nd ed. Elk Grove Village, IL: American Academy of Pediatrics; 2003. Consult the text of this chapter and *Pediatric Environmental Health* for additional information.

## 1. WHERE THE TEEN LIVES OR SPENDS TIME—INDOORS

Exposure to carbon monoxide and radon are of particular concern.

### Carbon Monoxide

Unintentional carbon monoxide (CO) poisoning causes hundreds of deaths in the United States each year. Sources of CO include unvented kerosene and propane gas space heaters, leaking chimneys and furnaces, wood stoves, fireplaces, and gas appliances.

***Anticipatory Guidance*** Chimneys should be inspected and cleaned annually. Combustion appliances must be properly installed, maintained, and vented according to the manufacturers' instructions. Parents should install CO detectors that meet Underwriters Laboratories most recent standards in every sleeping area and should never ignore an alarming CO detector.[18]

### Radon

Radon is a leading—and preventable—cause of lung cancer in the United States, with 10% of lung cancers attributable to radon. The risk of developing lung cancer as a result of radon exposure increases with radon concentration and years of exposure.[19]

***Anticipatory Guidance*** Parents can be informed that the US Environmental Protection Agency (EPA) recommends testing homes below the third floor for radon and that radon testing be done before buying or selling a home.[20] Radon testing and remediation are generally affordable.

## 2. EXPOSURE TO SECONDHAND SMOKE

Secondhand smoke exposure has serious acute and chronic adverse health effects—including coughing, phlegm production, and reduced lung function—on nonsmokers. In 2005, estimates were that SHS exposure kills more than 3,000 adult nonsmokers annually from lung cancer and approximately 46,000 from coronary heart disease.[21] Although these deaths occur in adults, the effects of are cumulative and no one, including teens, should be exposed. Pregnant women (including pregnant teens) who are nonsmokers and exposed to SHS increase their risk of having a child of lower birth weight. Secondhand smoke exposure is linked to premature delivery.[21]

Chemicals found in SHS such as nicotine, CO, and tobacco-specific carcinogens can be detected in body fluids of exposed nonsmokers. In 2005, the Centers for Disease Control and Prevention (CDC) released the Third National Report on Human Exposure to Environmental Chemicals that found that the median level of cotinine (a metabolite of nicotine) in nonsmokers had decreased across the life stages. In children, cotinine levels decreased by 68%; in adolescents by 69%; and in adults by 75% when samples collected between 1999 and 2002 were compared with samples collected a decade earlier. These dramatic declines added further evidence that smoking restrictions in public places and workplaces are effective.[21] Unfortunately, many people continue to be exposed at work and in the home, a setting not regulated by public health authorities.

***Anticipatory Guidance*** It is the standard of care to ask teens about their personal smoking behavior and to counsel them to quit smoking. Clinicians should add questions about teens' exposure to SHS and advise them to advocate for their own clean air at home, work, and elsewhere because "there is no risk-free level of exposure to secondhand smoke."[21] Pediatricians involved in preconception care should counsel teens who are contemplating pregnancy to avoid SHS.

## 3. WATER SOURCES

Adolescent mothers should be informed that contaminated water may affect infants. Tap water may contain lead; well water may contain nitrates.

***Anticipatory Guidance*** Municipal tap water can be tested for lead; well water should be tested for nitrates. Water should not be boiled for more than one minute because this practice may concentrate contaminants.

## 4. DIETARY EXPOSURES: MERCURY AND OTHER FISH CONTAMINANTS

Mercury, a toxicant with neurologic and other effects, occurs in elemental, inorganic, and organic forms. Organic mercury contamination of fish is relevant to adolescents mainly because of preconception and prenatal concerns. Fish is an excellent source of protein and can be high in omega-3 fatty acids. However, mercury in water can contaminate fish and subsequently people who ingest the fish. Mercury from natural and combustion sources enters the air, falls into bodies of water, and is methylated by aquatic organisms into organic methylmercury. It is taken up by fish where it accumulates in fish muscle. Large predator fish, including swordfish and tuna, feed on smaller fish and accumulate the most mercury. People eating mercury-containing fish accumulate the mercury over time. Fetuses and young children are most susceptible to mercury's neurotoxic effects. In 2000, it was estimated that 60,000 American children born each year may suffer from learning disabilities due to prenatal mercury exposure.[22]

Polychlorinated biphenyls (PCBs) have neurotoxic and other adverse health effects. They accumulate in the fat of fatty fish such as salmon.

***Anticipatory Guidance*** Adolescents who may become pregnant should know about the effects of consuming mercury-containing fish. Pregnant teens, nursing mothers, and young children should completely avoid shark, tilefish, swordfish, and king mackerel because of high levels of methylmercury; they should limit consumption of other mercury-containing fish.[22,23] Healthier fish choices can be made. Several Web sites, including the Oceans Alive campaign of Environmental Defense Fund, list best and worst alternatives with regard to mercury and PCBs.[24] Mercury levels can decrease over time, although it may take more than a year for mercury levels to drop significantly. In addition to recommending a folic acid-containing vitamin to pregnant teens to prevent neural tube defects in their offspring, pediatricians should counsel teens who may become pregnant to avoid fish with high levels of mercury and PCBs.

## 5. SUNLIGHT AND ARTIFICIAL UV RADIATION EXPOSURE

Exposure to the UV portion of the sunlight spectrum can harm the skin, immune system, and eyes (including cataract formation and ocular melanoma). Skin effects include sunburn, tanning (a protective response to UV radiation), skin aging, photosensitivity, and skin cancer. Skin cancer is the most common cancer in the United States. More than 1 million new cases occur each year and the incidence is rising. Most skin cancers are basal cell carcinomas (BCC)—800,000 to 900,000 occur in the United States annually. Approximately 200,000 to 300,000 of squamous cell carcinoma (SCC) occur annually. UV radiation exposure, the main environmental cause of skin cancer, is linked to the development of BCC, SCC, and melanoma. Generally, BCC and SCC are found on maximally exposed areas such as the face and arms. Basal cell carcinoma and SCC do not usually result in fatalities unless they are left untreated.

Melanoma comprises just 3% of all skin cancers, but causes most of skin cancer fatalities. The American Cancer Society predicted that in 2010 there would be 68,130 new melanoma cases with 8,700 deaths.[25] The incidence of melanoma increased dramatically during the last century, possibly due to the decrease in the earth's protective ozone layer, changing patterns of dress favoring more skin exposure, more opportunities for leisure activities in sunny areas, and other factors. People at highest risk have light skin and light eyes and sunburn easily. Melanoma affects primarily older white men but also occurs in teenagers and young adults; it is the second most common cancer of women in their 20s and the third most common cancer of men in their 20s.[26] When detected early, melanoma has an excellent prognosis. Metastatic melanoma has a grave prognosis, however, with few if any successful treatment options. Clinicians' efforts must therefore focus on prevention and early detection. Chapter 147, Adolescent Dermatology, discusses melanoma in detail.

Whereas SCC is linked to cumulative sun exposure, melanoma is linked to intense or brutal sun exposure. Intense sun exposure during childhood and adolescence, enough to cause a blistering sunburn, is linked with an increased risk of melanoma later in life, illustrating heightened susceptibility at young ages. People with large numbers of nevi (moles) and those with dysplastic nevi also are at higher risk.

### Artificial Sources of UV Radiation—Tanning Salons

More and more young people use tanning salons. In the United States in 2003, 26% of people under 25 visited a tanning salon compared to 8% in 1996. Between 32% and 55% of college students used tanning salons; 6% to 44% of high school boys and 30% to 70% of high school girls used tanning salons. The indoor tanning industry generated $5 billion in annual revenues, up from $1 billion in 1992.[27]

A recent review by the International Agency for Research on Cancer (IARC) revealed that there is a 75% increase in risk of melanoma and SCC for people who use sunbeds in their teens. Data suggested detrimental effects on the skin's immune response and possibly on the eyes (ocular melanoma). No positive effects were found. Artificial tanning conferred little if any protection against solar damage to the skin, nor did using indoor tanning facilities provide protection against vitamin D deficiency. The IARC concluded that "effective action to restrict access to artificial tanning facilities (solariums, tanning salons, tanning parlors) to minors and young adults should be strongly considered."[28]

Federal regulations govern the manufacture of tanning equipment; once manufacturers sell the equipment, states regulate their use. Legislation for salon operators varies by state; as of November 2010, more than 60% of states had regulated the use of tanning facilities by minors.[29] Some states prohibit minors' access to tanning booths without parental consent; others require warning signs in visible locations. Enforcement of regulations varies. Advocates of restricting minors' access to tanning salons argue that our society protects teens from using alcohol and smoking until a certain age but we do not generally protect them from using tanning parlors. The American Academy of Dermatology recently issued a recommendation that no person under 18 use a tanning facility. Indoor tanning is so troubling because it is so unnecessary—it is not associated with sports activities but instead is purely cosmetic, resulting in teenagers putting their health at risk.[30]

***Anticipatory Guidance*** Sun protection messages are best delivered in the context of promoting outdoor physical activity in a sun-safe manner. Teens should be strongly discouraged from sunburning, particularly if they have light skin and light eye color. If possible, activities should be timed to limit or avoid sun exposure during peak sun hours (10 am–4 pm). Teens should generously apply a broad-spectrum (UVA and UVB protection) sunscreen with a sun protection factor (SPF) equal to or more than 15 before going outside, and reapply often especially after swimming or sweating. They should wear protective clothing, brimmed hats, and sunglasses whenever feasible, seek shade whenever possible, and use caution near water, snow, and sand because they reflect sunlight.[31] Teens should be strongly discouraged from using tanning salons. If they feel that a tanned skin looks healthier or more attractive, they may use a sunless self-tanning product—but they must continue to use sunscreen with it.

## 6. OCCUPATIONAL AND PARAOCCUPATIONAL EXPOSURES

Adolescents may be directly exposed to environmental hazards at work. Exposures include UV radiation with outdoor work, SHS encountered in restaurants and bars, pesticides from lawn-care and farm work, and noise from operating equipment. Teens may be also exposed when parents bring home toxicants on work clothes and shoes, Paraoccupational exposures, also referred to as brought-home exposures, resulting in "fouling one's own nest".

***Anticipatory Guidance*** Pediatricians may ask about an adolescent's occupation when authorizing work permits (working papers); this provides the opportunity to give advice about avoiding or minimizing exposure.

## 7. COMMUNITY ISSUES—PLANNING FOR A RADIATION DISASTER

The events of September 11, 2001, resulted in greater awareness that a radiation disaster is possible as an intentional terrorist act or unintentional occurrence such as a nuclear power plant malfunction. Radioiodines are common by-products of nuclear power plant activities, and are likely to be emitted after a power plant incident. Infants, children, and adolescents will be especially vulnerable to the carcinogenic effects of radioiodine after such a disaster. Treatment with potassium iodide (KI)[32] immediately before, during, or shortly after exposure to radioiodine is the cornerstone of treatment to prevent thyroid cancer. Potassium iodide floods the thyroid, blocking uptake of inhaled or ingested radioiodines. When taken promptly after a radioiodine release and at proper dose, KI is effective in preventing radiation-induced thyroid effects. Potassium iodide the same compound used in smaller quantities to iodize table salt, is available without a prescription.[17]

***Anticipatory Guidance*** The US Food and Drug Administration recommends that KI be administered only after certain levels of radioiodine exposure. Compared to adults, the radiation threshold for administering KI

**Table 46-2**

**Guidelines for Potassium Iodide (KI) Administration[a]**

| *Age* | *Exposure Gy (rad)* | *KI Dose (mg)* |
|---|---|---|
| >40 years of age | >5 (500) | 130 |
| 18–40 years of age | ≥0.1 (10) | 130 |
| Adolescents 12 through 17 years of age[b] | ≥0.05 (5) | 65 |
| Children 4 through 11 years of age | ≥0.05 (5) | 65 |
| Children 1 month through 3 years of age[c] | ≥0.05 (5) | 32 |
| Birth through 1 month of age | ≥0.05 (5) | 16 |
| Pregnant or lactating women | ≥0.05 (5) | 130 |

[a]KI is useful only after exposure to a radioiodine. KI is given once only to pregnant women and neonates unless other protective measures (evacuation, sheltering, and control of the food supply) are unavailable. Repeat dosing should be on the advice of public health authorities.

[b]Adolescents weighing more than 70 kg should receive the adult dose (130 mg).

[c]KI from tablets or as a freshly saturated solution may be diluted in water and mixed with milk, formula, juice, soda, or syrup. Raspberry syrup disguises the taste of KI the best. KI mixed with low-fat chocolate milk, orange juice, or flat soda (eg, cola) has an acceptable taste. Low-fat white milk and water did not hide the salty taste of KI.

Adapted from US Food and Drug Administration, Center for Drug Evaluation and Research. *Guidance Document: Potassium Iodide* as a *Thyroid Blocking Agent in Radiation Emergencies.* Available at: www.fda.gov/downloads/Drugs/GuidanceComplianceRegulatoryInformation/Guidances/ucm080542.pdf. Accessed February 24, 2010.

is lower for infants, children, and teens (Table 46-2). It should be immediately available in homes, child care settings, and schools located within 10 miles of a nuclear power plant; many authorities recommend a wider radius. Potassium iodide is available over the counter; information about obtaining KI is available.[32]

## TAKING AN EXPOSURE HISTORY WHEN A SYMPTOM MAY BE RELATED TO AN ENVIRONMENTAL EXPOSURE

Making the connection between a disease and an environmental exposure requires a high index of suspicion. Illnesses caused by environmental agents often present as common medical problems. Most clinicians will think about SHS exposure when a patient has respiratory problems such as asthma. Lead poisoning is in the differential diagnosis of coma, seizures, developmental delay, irritability, and constipation. Poisoning from certain types of pesticides may present with headache, dizziness, and diarrhea. It is critical (and may be life-saving) to consider CO poisoning when there is fatigue, headache, dizziness, weakness, nausea, or vomiting, especially when more than one family member has symptoms. Clinicians must keep in mind the particular environmental hazards that exist in their community. For example, pesticide exposure is common in agricultural areas. The patient's country of origin or travel to foreign countries may be relevant. For example, children (including adolescents) in one family were poisoned by lead as a result of ingesting spices purchased from a street vendor during a trip to the Republic of Georgia.[33] Box 46-1 lists basic questions for an exposure history.

## CONCLUSION

Adolescents, because of their rapid growth and development and increased exposures, may be more susceptible to environmental hazards compared to adults. An environmental history is an important part of a complete well adolescent visit. Because pediatricians are urged to provide advice on hundreds of topics.[35] it may seem daunting to add an environmental history to an already long list of topics to be discussed with teenagers. This is, however, a worthwhile endeavor. Pediatricians may play an important role in identifying teen exposures and providing anticipatory guidance to prevent or minimize those exposures.

## INTERNET RESOURCES

### RESOURCES/SEARCH ENGINES

- Google US Government Search (www.google.com/ig/usgov). Specialized search within Google with results limited to US federal, state, and local government Web sites.

## Box 46-1

### *Questions for Exposure History*

The etiology of symptoms and signs may not be obvious; a systematic approach includes questions such as:

- EXPOSURES AT HOME, SCHOOL, OR WORK: Has there been any exposure to metals, dusts, fibers, fumes, chemicals (including pesticides, cleaning agents), biologic hazards, radiation, noise, or vibration? Have there been any changes at home, school, or work such as renovation or remodeling? Have there been any spills or hazardous waste incidents?
- HOBBIES: Is the adolescent involved with activities such as painting, sculpting, welding, woodworking, piloting, auto repair, shooting, stained glass making, ceramics, or gardening?
- WHO: Are others similarly affected?
- WHAT: What are the symptoms?
- WHEN: Are symptoms better/worse on weekdays or weekends? What time of day? During a particular week or season?
- WHERE: Do symptoms subside or worsen in a particular location such as home, a particular room, at school or work? During specific activities such as hobby activities or arts and crafts?
- WHY: Teens and/or parents' theories of what is happening

Adapted from Frank A, Balk SJ. Taking an exposure history. In: *Case Studies in Environmental Medicine*. Agency for Toxic Substances and Disease Registry, DHHS, October 1992 and American Academy of Pediatrics. *Pediatric Environmental Health*. Etzel RA and Balk SJ, eds. 2nd ed. Elk Grove Village, IL: American Academy of Pediatrics; 2003.

- EPA Children's Health Protection Environmental Hazard Search (yosemite.epa.gov/ochp/ochpweb.nsf/frmChemicals). Focused search that yields results from government and nongovernment sites for common environmental hazards. Also contains links to related sites.

## SPECIALIZED DIRECTORIES

- MedlinePlus Health Topic: Environmental Health (www.nlm.nih.gov/medlineplus/environmentalhealth.html). Authoritative information covering environmental health from the National Library of Medicine (NLM), the National Institutes of Health (NIH), and other government agencies and health-related organizations. There is a special children's section and a link to a preset MEDLINE/PubMed search for recent research articles on environmental health.
- Public Health Partners Children's Environmental Health World Wide Web Sampler (www.phpartners.org/cehir/sampler.html). A collaboration of US government agencies, public health organizations, and health sciences libraries with an extensive directory of pediatric environmental health Web sites that goes beyond government sites and includes academic and nongovernmental sites.

## CLINICAL AND EDUCATIONAL RESOURCES

- Pediatric Environmental Health Specialty Unit (PEHSU) (www.aoec.org/PEHSU.htm). National network of CDC-supported specialty units that provide PEH education and consultation for health professionals, parents, government agencies, and others.
- AAP Council on Environmental Health (COEH) (www.aap.org/visit/cmte16.htm). The committee responsible for developing national AAP policy and furthering PEH education.
- *Pediatric Environmental Health* 2nd ed. (www.nfaap.org/netforum/eweb/dynamicpage.aspx?site=nf.aap.org&webcode=aapbks_productdetail&key=17837ee5-f0fd-4486-9bcc-64f986b0f703). AAP comprehensive handbook, written for clinicians, on PEH.
- ATSDR Case Studies in Environmental Medicine. Self-guided educational modules covering a number of common issues including three related to PEH:
    - Pediatric Environmental Health Overview (www.atsdr.cdc.gov/HEC/CSEM/pediatric/index.html)
    - Taking an Environmental History (www.atsdr.cdc.gov/HEC/CSEM/exphistory/index.html)
    - Environmental Triggers of Asthma (www.atsdr.cdc.gov/HEC/CSEM/asthma/index.html)
- National Environmental Education and Training Foundation (NEETF) (www.neetf.org). National nonprofit organization with many PEH educational initiatives, including Powerpoint presentations.

## OTHER RESOURCES

- Healthy Schools Network (www.healthyschools.org). National organization dedicated to assuring that children and school employees have environmentally safe and healthy schools.

- Medical–Legal Partnership for Children (www.mlpforchildren.org). National program that partners pediatric clinicians with lawyers was founded at Boston Medical Center and Boston University School of Medicine and has been replicated across the country.

- Balk SJ, Forman JA, Johnson CL, Roberts JR. Safeguarding Kids from Environmental Hazards. *Contemporary Pediatrics* March 2007.

## REFERENCES

1. Olden K. Fiscal Year 2006 budget request. Available at: www.nih.gov/about/director/budgetrequest/fy2006directorsbudgetrequest.htm

2. Golub MS. Adolescent health and the environment. *Environ Health Perspect.* 2000;108:355–362

3. Moya J, Bearer CF, Etzel RA. Children's behavior and physiology and how it affects exposure to environmental contaminants. *Pediatrics*. 2004;113:996–1006

4. Bearer CF. How are children different from adults? *Environ Health Perspect*. 1995;103(S):7–12

5. Selevan SG, Kimmel CA, Mendola P. Identifying critical windows of exposure for children's health. *Environ Health Perspect*. 2000;108(S):451–455

6. Cooper RL, Kavlock RJ. Endocrine disruptors and reproductive development: a weight-of-evidence review. *J Endocrinol*. 1997;152:159–166

7. Gogtay N, Giedd JN, Lusk L, et al. Dynamic mapping of human cortical development during childhood through early adulthood. *PNAS*. 2004;101:8175–8179

8. Crews FT, Braun CJ, Hoplight B, Switzer III RC, Knapp DJ. Binge ethanol consumption causes differential brain damage in young adolescent rats compared with adult rats. *Alcoholism: Clin Exp Res*. 2000;24:1712–1723

9. DiFranza JR, Rigotti NA, McNeill AD, et al. Initial symptoms of nicotine dependence in adolescents. *Tobacco Control*. 2000;9:313–319

10. DiFranza JR, Savageau JA, Rigotti NA, et al. Development of symptoms of tobacco dependence in youths: 30-month follow-up data from the DANDY study. *Tobacco Control*. 2002;11:228–235

11. Barron S, White A, Swartzwelder HS, et al. Adolescent vulnerabilities to chronic alcohol or nicotine exposure: findings from rodent models. *Alcoholism: Clin Exp Res*. 2005;29:1720–1725

12. Spear LP. Assessment of adolescent neurotoxicity: rationale and methodological considerations. *Neurotoxicol and Teratol*. 2007;29:1–9

13. Adams J, Barone Jr S, LaMantia A, et al. Workshop to identify critical windows of exposure for children's health: neurobehavioral work group summary. *Environ Health Perspect*. 2000;108(S3):535–544

14. Janerich DT, Thompson WD, Varela LR, et al. Lung cancer and exposure to tobacco smoke in the household. *New Eng J Med*. 1990;323:632–636

15. Centers for Disease Control and Prevention. Secondhand smoke exposure among middle and high school students, Texas, 2001. *MMWR*. 2003;52(8):152–154

16. Whiteman DC, Whiteman CA, Green AC. Childhood sun exposure as a risk factor for melanoma: a systematic review of epidemiologic studies. *Cancer Causes Control*. 2001;12: 69–82

17. Balk SJ, Miller RW, Shannon MW, AAP Committee on Environmental Health. Radiation disasters and children. *Pediatrics*. 2003;111:1455–1466

18. American Academy of Pediatrics. *Pediatric Environmental Health*. Etzel RA, Balk SJ, eds. 2nd ed. Elk Grove Village, IL: American Academy of Pediatrics; 2003

19. Chen J. Estimated risks of radon-induced lung cancer for different exposure profiles based on the new EPA model. *Health Physics*. 2005;323–333

20. US Environmental Protection Agency. A citizen's guide to radon: the guide to protecting yourself and your family from radon. Available at: www.epa.gov/radon/pdfs/citizensguide.pdf. Accessed October 5, 2010

21. US Department of Health and Human Services. The health consequences of involuntary exposure to tobacco smoke: a report of the Surgeon General — executive summary. US Department of Health and Human Services, Centers for Disease Control and Prevention, Coordinating Center for Health Promotion, National Center for Chronic Disease Prevention and Health Promotion, Office on Smoking and Health; 2006

22. National Research Council. Toxicological effects of methylmercury. Available at: www.nap.edu/books/0309071402/html. Accessed September 7, 2007

23. US Environmental Protection Agency. What you need to know about mercury in fish and shellfish. Available at: www.epa.gov/waterscience/fish/Methylmercury Brochure.pdf. Accessed September 7, 2007

24. Environmental Defense. Buying guide: becoming a smart seafood shopper. Available at: www.edf.org/article.cfm?contentID=4021. Accessed October 5, 2010

25. American Cancer Society. How many people get melanoma skin cancer? Available at: www.cancer.org/Cancer/SkinCancer-Melanoma/OverviewGuide/melanoma-skin-cancer-overview-key-statistics. Accessed October 5, 2010

26. Wu X, Groves FD, McLaughlin CC, Jemal A, Martin J, Chen VS. Cancer incidence patterns among adolescents and young adults in the United States. *Cancer Causes Control*. 2005;16:309–320

27. Levine JA, Sorace M, Spencer J, Siegel D. The indoor UV tanning industry: a review of skin cancer risk, health benefit claims. *J Am Acad Dermatol.* 2005;53:1038–1044

28. International Agency for Research on Cancer. Sunbed use in youth unequivocally associated with skin cancer. Press Release No. 171, November 29, 2006. Available at: www.iarc.

fr/ENG/Press_Releases/pr171a.html. Accessed September 7, 2007

29. National Conference of State Legislatures. Tanning restrictions for minors. A state-by-state comparison. Available at: www.ncsl.org/default.aspx?tabid=14394. Accessed November 23, 2010.

30. Lim HW, Cyr WH, DeFabo E, et al. American Academy of Dermatology. Scientific and regulatory issues related to indoor tanning. *J Am Acad Dermatol*. 2004;51:781-784

31. National Council on Skin Cancer Prevention. Skin cancer prevention tips. Available at: www.skincancerprevention.org/Tips/tabid/54/Default.aspx. Accessed September 7, 2007

32. US Food and Drug Administration, Center for Drug Evaluation and Research. *Frequently Asked Questions on Potassium Iodide (KI)*. Rockville, MD: Center for Drug Evaluation and Research; Updated March 6, 2006. Available at: www.fda.gov/Drugs/EmergencyPreparedness/BioterrorismandDrugPreparedness/UCM072265. Accessed October 5, 2010

33. Woolf AD, Woolf NT. Childhood lead poisoning in two families associated with spices used in food preparation. *Pediatrics*. 2005;116:314-318

34. Frank A, Balk SJ. Taking an exposure history. In: *Case Studies in Environmental Medicine*. Agency for Toxic Substances and Disease Registry, DHHS, October 1992

35. Belamarich PF, Gandica R, Stein REK, Racine AD. Drowning in a sea of advice: pediatricians and American Academy of Pediatrics policy statements. *Pediatrics* 2006;118:e964-e978

# CHAPTER 47

# Adolescents at Work

JOHN ROWLETT, MD

*Employment is nature's physician, and is essential to human happiness.*
—Galen, Greek Physician (130–c. 201)

## HISTORY

It has long been agreed that it is beneficial for adolescents to enter the work force. The nature and extent of this entry is variable, and recent decades have seen tremendous changes in both the types of employment youth seek and the reasons they choose to work. Whereas some youth work to assist the family business, many work simply to provide money for discretionary spending. Child labor has been part of the world's culture for the entirety of recorded history. Similarly, children and especially adolescents have been an integral part of the US labor force for centuries.

## DEMOGRAPHICS

According to US Department of Labor[1] estimates, about 45% of 16- to 17-year-olds worked at some time during the year (school year, summer, or both); self-reported surveys of high school students report employment rates as high as 80%. Estimates are that 70% to 80% of youth have worked for pay at some time during their high school years. More than half of working teens are employed in the retail industry (25% by restaurants); other popular jobs include service industries, stock handlers, laborers, administrative support, farming forestry, and fishing. Self-employment is common among youth (eg, babysitting, small jobs in neighborhoods, lawn services). Popular fast-food chain restaurants offer youth a wide range of employment opportunities ranging from full-time jobs to part-time weekend hours. These firms usually require minimal skill sets for initial employment, and motivated workers can obtain management experience more rapidly than with traditional industries. Teens are frequently able to keep these initial jobs for several years as they continue their education.

Employment of teens is cyclical and sensitive to changes in the overall work force. Teen employment expands most rapidly during strong, steady employment growth. Separate from this, recent trends have demonstrated that despite available jobs, fewer teens are choosing to work. The 2004 summer male teen employment rate was the lowest ever recorded, falling more than 20 percentage points from the value in the late 1970s, when 60% of teens had jobs. Working youth change jobs frequently in response to their personal needs and those of employers and the job market. Unlike in the past, most US teens work for personal rather than family money. Teens whose parents work are more likely to work than those whose parents are unemployed. For adolescent males, parental unemployment is the strongest predictor of youth unemployment. White teens are twice as likely (40%) to work as black teens. Teen employment rates increase (in the United States) with increasing household income. One in 3 youth with annual household incomes less than $20,000 work, whereas more than half of those from households with annual incomes less than $100,000 are employed (exception is high-income Asian families, whose children are less likely to work). When youth from low-income families work, they are more likely to be employed in more dangerous jobs (agriculture, construction) and their wages are more likely to contribute to household income (accounting for up to 10% of the household income) than personal expenses.[2]

Work begets work—80% of teens with more than 6 months work in the previous year are likely to be employed. Youth employment lays the foundation for adult work and has substantial effects on the wages and annual earnings of young men and women; those who acquire limited work experience in their late teens and early 20s cannot command high wages in the labor market, and their limited wage prospects reduce the economic incentive for them to seek employment. Teen dropouts from low-income families are at greatest risk of year-round joblessness. Lower-income youth may not have access to transportation, may not live near jobs, may need to provide unpaid market work (child care, housekeeping), and may be less successful in finding work when they seek it. Youth in impoverished neighborhoods often experience difficulty finding jobs with local businesses because of the usually unfounded fear that they may be involved in illegal activities. Additional barriers to employment include availability of jobs, language difficulties, lack of parental support, difficulty with peer relationships, behavioral problems, and parental divorce.

## BENEFITS OF WORKING

Employed youth report many positive benefits from working (Box 47-1). In addition to reporting increased disposable income, youth who work report increased self-esteem, independence, and responsibility. Adolescent employment provides opportunities to acquire valuable skills such as attendance, punctuality, and customer service. Youth who work fewer than 20 hours per week report higher levels of postsecondary education. Further, as adults, workers who were employed as teens report lower unemployment rates and earn higher wages.

> **Box 47-1**
>
> ***Potential Benefits of Youth Employment***
>
> 1. Increased monetary resources
> 2. Introduction or exposure to potential careers
> 3. Improved socialization and networking
> 4. Enhanced self-esteem and self-confidence
> 5. Increased independence and autonomy
> 6. Improved time management

## RISKS OF WORKING

Adolescent employment is not without measurable risks. There seems to be a threshold, roughly 20 hours per week, for youth to work without untoward consequences. Increased work is associated with more time in unstructured social activities and less time in sports and school activities. With less time available for studying, grades tend to decline with increasing hours worked; this decline is similar in both sexes but more pronounced among black youth. Youth who work more than 20 hours per week frequently report negative consequences including increased substance use and abuse, inadequate time with friends, family, and deficiencies of sleep and exercise. Further, youth who report working more than 20 hours per week are less likely to attain postsecondary education.

There is growing agreement that work intensity (ie, longer hours) fosters underage drinking and other substance use. Based on data from the National Longitudinal Study of Adolescent Health,[3] the effect of work intensity on substance use seems to be mostly limited to white males who work more than 15 hours per week; work intensity is not consistently related to alcohol, cigarette, and marijuana use among minority adolescents. Adolescents who work more than 20 hours per week are more likely to have an earlier sexual debut; working more than 31 hours per week is associated with an increased rate of binge drinking in both sexes, though the association is somewhat weaker in youth from lower-income families.[3]

## APPLICABLE LAWS AND REGULATIONS

The first effective child labor law in the United States was passed in Massachusetts in 1836; it required that children younger than age 15 years employed in manufacturing spend at least 3 months each year in school. In 1908, President Taft signed legislation that created the Children's Bureau within the Department of Labor whose stated purpose was to investigate and report "upon all matters pertaining to the welfare of children and child life among all classes of our people." Included in this charge was oversight of child employment. The Fair Labor Standards Act (FLSA) was enacted in 1938 and applied to all industries engaged in interstate commerce. The FLSA established minimum ages for work and delineated jobs that children could not perform (Box 47-2 and Box 47-3). The FLSA established guidelines for the hours that youth could work during the school year and summer; it has remained the foundation for current child labor laws (Box 47-4). Additional

> **Box 47-2**
>
> ***Jobs Banned for Youth Younger than 18 Years of Age (Nonagricultural)***[6]
>
> 1. Working with explosive and radioactive materials
> 2. Operating motor vehicles or working as outside helpers on motor vehicles
> 3. Mining activities
> 4. Operating most power-driven woodworking and certain metalworking machines
> 5. Operating power-driven bakery, meat processing, and paper products machinery including meat slicers and most paper balers and compactors
> 6. Operating various types of power-driven saws and guillotine shears
> 7. Operating most power-driven hoisting apparatuses, such as manual elevators, forklifts, and cranes
> 8. Most jobs in slaughtering and meatpacking establishments
> 9. Most jobs in excavation, logging, sawmilling, roofing, wrecking, demolition, and ship-breaking
> 10. Most jobs in the manufacturing of bricks, tiles, and similar products

## Box 47-3

### *Jobs Banned for Youth Younger than Age 16 in Agricultural Work*

1. Operating a tractor of 20 horsepower or connecting or disconnecting an implement or any of its parts to or from such a tractor
2. Operating or assisting to operate any of the following machines: corn picker, cotton picker, grain combine, hay mower, forage harvester, hay baler, potato digger, mobile pea viner, feed grinder, crop dryer, forage blower, auger conveyor, the unloading mechanism of a gravity-type self-unloading wagon or trailer, trencher, forklift, potato combine, power post hole digger, power post driver, nonwalking-type rotary tiller, and power-driven circular, band, or chainsaws
3. Working on a farm in a yard, pen, or stall occupied by a bull, boar, or stud horse maintained for breeding purposes; or a sow with suckling pigs; or a cow with a newborn calf
4. Felling, buckling, skidding, loading, or unloading timber with a butt diameter of more than 6 inches
5. Working from a ladder or scaffold at a height of more than 20 feet
6. Driving a bus, truck, or automobile when transporting passengers, or riding on a tractor as a passenger or a helper
7. Working inside fruit, forage, or grain storage designed to retain an oxygen-deficient or toxic atmosphere; in an upright silo within 2 weeks after silage has been added

US Department of Labor. Jobs restrictions. Available at: www.dol.gov/elaws/esa/flsa/docs/hazardous.asp. Accessed April 20, 2010

## Box 47-4

### *Hours Restrictions (Agricultural and Nonagricultural) (Additional Local and State Laws May Apply)*[6]

**Agricultural:**

- 16 years and older:
  - May work on any day, for any number of hours, and in any job in agriculture
- 14–15 years:
  - Can work in agriculture on any farm but only during hours when school is not in session and in nonhazardous jobs
- 12–13 years:
  - Can work only with written permission from parents
- Under 12 years
  - Only can work if small farm with fewer than 500 "man days" in the previous quarter, with same restrictions as 12–13 y/o

**Nonagricultural:**

- 18 years and older:
  - May perform any job, hazardous or not, for unlimited hours
- 16–17 years:
  - Nonhazardous jobs for unlimited hours
- 14–15 years:
  - May work outside school hours in various nonhazardous jobs
  - May work after 7 am until 7 pm (9 pm from June 1–Labor Day)
  - Cannot work more than 3 hours a day on school days, including Friday
  - Cannot work more than 18 hours a week during school weeks*
  - Cannot work more than 8 hours a day on nonschool days
  - Cannot work more than 40 hours a week when school is not in session

*Youth enrolled in an approved work experience and career exploration program may be employed for up to 23 hours during school weeks and 3 hours on school days (including school hours).

local, state, and federal laws aimed at protecting youth at work have been enacted; most problems associated with youth employment are from lack of adherence to existing legislation rather than legislative deficiencies. Nearly 40% of teens under age 16 report having worked after 7 pm on a school night—a clear violation of applicable federal law. Even though prohibited by law, 52% of males and 43% of females under 18 years report having performed greater than or equal to 1 dangerous task (eg, using a box crusher, slicer, paper baler).[4] Youth workers without work permits are more likely to perform hazardous tasks, use dangerous equipment, and receive less health and safety training than those with permits.[5] There are limited exemptions for time of day and hours that a child can work in a family-owned business; there are no exemptions from safety standards. There are limited exemptions from some hazardous jobs for youth older than age 16 enrolled in specific approved apprentice programs. The Child Work Experience and Career Exploration Program (WECEP) is an exempt program that permits 14- and 15-year-olds to work in otherwise prohibited jobs. It is designed to provide a work experience and career exploration program, especially for youth at risk for leaving school, and permits the employment of 14- to 15-year-olds during school hours and for up to 23 hours/week during the school year. Child labor rules do not apply to youth actors, newspaper delivery (though door-to-door sales by teens are prohibited in an increasing number of states and restricted in many others), and limited other occupations. Specific exemptions are found at the referenced resources (www.dol.gov/elaws).

## OCCUPATIONAL INJURIES AND DEATHS

For the year 2005, the Bureau of Labor Statistics (BLS) recorded 5,702 fatal occupational injuries in the United States. Men, though comprising only 54% of the work force, were 93% of the victims. A total of 166 US youth younger than age 20 died of occupational injuries in 2005. For each fatality, it is estimated there are 1,000 injuries that require medical attention; unreported injuries may be threefold higher. The injury rate for youth workers is more than twice that of comparable adult workers. Motor vehicle accidents account for nearly 50% of all adolescent occupational fatalities. These deaths include workers who were drivers or passengers in vehicles or bicyclists/pedestrians involved in motor vehicle crashes; it does not include youth who died while traveling to or from work. About one-sixth of adolescent occupational deaths are from homicide. Increased risk for death includes working alone or in small numbers, handling cash, deliveries, and working late evening or early morning hours.

More than 1 million children and adolescents live and work on family farms. About 40% of adolescent occupational fatalities occur in agricultural employment (vehicular and heavy machinery accidents, drowning, and electrocutions). Young agricultural workers are 4 times more likely to be fatally injured. The most common injuries on farms include fractures, cuts, and lacerations of the head and extremities. In addition to machinery, many injuries are due to animals (horses for girls, cattle for boys). Strategies for preventing agricultural injuries in adolescent workers are detailed in Box 47-5.

Adolescents working in construction are at greater risk than their adult counterparts; construction injuries are second only to those in agriculture in number of fatal injuries. One study[7] found that among youth construction workers with work permits (implying parental and employment involvement and required in 40 states for youth younger than 18 years), safety violations are common (15% were younger than 16 years, 84% reported performing at least 1 clearly prohibited task, and almost 50% reported performing 3 or more prohibited tasks); it is likely that the rate of violations by youth without work permits is even higher.

### Box 47-5

### *Prevention of Agricultural Injuries in Adolescent Workers*

1. Parents, teens, and employers should be informed of the risk of agricultural injuries and effective prevention measures, including the following:
   a. Ensuring that rollover protective structures and seat belts on tractors and all farm equipment are used at all times by all riders.
   b. Proper storage of farm chemicals.
   c. Provision of hearing protection equipment.
2. Appropriate training and supervision.
3. Appropriate safety and first-aid equipment and training, including EMS access.
4. Children younger than 16 should not operate any farm vehicles, including all-terrain vehicles. Individuals between 16 and 18 should have a driver's license and should have received formal farm vehicle safety training.
5. Riders should not be permitted in any area of a vehicle not approved for passengers, including the racks of ATVs, fenders of tractors, and cargo areas of trucks.
6. Existing laws regarding youth agricultural workers should be followed and enforced when necessary.

Source: Committee on Injury and Poison Prevention and Committee on Community Health Service. Prevention of agricultural injuries among children and adolescents. *Pediatrics*. 2001;108:1016–1019

Major injuries and deaths are more likely to occur at small firms exempt from federal enforcement of child labor laws; half of these fatalities were in apparent violation of existing child labor laws.[8] Historically, more than three-fourths of all fatal occupational injuries of youth involved activities in violation of the FLSA.[9] Factors contributing to young worker deaths are listed in Box 47-6.

Nonfatal occupational injuries among adolescents are tracked by the Department of Labor and have been trending downward for the past decade. As most youth are employed in the retail industry, it is not surprising that it is within this sector that most injuries occur. More than 25,000 teenagers are injured annually while working in the fast-food industry. The majority of these injuries are from minor falls, cuts, and burns to the hands and extremities. Factors that place adolescents at increased risk for injury include working outside of the usual assignment in areas in which they are unfamiliar, untrained, and/or unsupervised; lack of physical and/or emotional maturity; lack of (or failure to use) appropriate

**Box 47-6**

***Factors Contributing to the Deaths of Young Workers***

1. Inadequate supervision
2. Inadequate training and preparation for selected task(s)
3. Failure to recognize hazardous or potentially hazardous work situations
4. Absent or ineffective workplace safety programs, particularly those appropriate for young workers
5. Inadequate training and experience to handle emergencies
6. Lack or failure to use personal protective equipment
7. Failure of employers to provide equipment with safety features
8. Assignment of incidental tasks for which the youth worker is inadequately trained (or they may have taken upon themselves to perform the task)
9. Inadequate knowledge and/or adherence to applicable child labor laws (by child, employer, and/or parents)

Source: NIOSH Alert. *Preventing Deaths, Injuries, and Illnesses of Young Workers*. NIOSH Publication 2003-128, July 2003. Available at: www.cdc.gov/niosh/docs/2003-128/2003128.htm. Accessed May 18, 2008

personal protective gear; and lack of understanding of their legal rights (and those of their employer). Additional factors that may contribute to injuries include unsafe equipment, trying to "speed up," and fear or retribution if they report violations and unsafe practices. Teenagers in the retail industry experience greater workplace violence (mostly robberies) than other workers; risk factors include working alone and at night.[10]

Safety programs such as "Youth@work" require adequate time and funding in schools and need to alert teachers and other effective partners to their importance. Programs aimed at promoting youth worker safety should be targeted at not only large firms but also small "Mom and Pop" operations.

## THE CHANGING WORKPLACE

Today's youth face an ever-changing job market. Although some factors, such as the impending retirement of more than 75 million baby boomers, will create a huge void in the work force, other changes such as the marked increase in immigration work against teen employment opportunities. Teens face increased competition from older workers who often lack the educational and/or market skills to progress in traditional and emerging markets; youth not in school do not fare nearly as well in the job market.

After initial employments in long-established teenage jobs, tomorrow's workers will face increased competition from emerging markets. Just as it would have been difficult in 1975 to predict jobs that are emerging in the Internet and information industries, it has been postulated that the top 5 jobs for the 2030s have not even been created. It is crucial that youth develop the necessary skills to compete in both the national and international job markets. Increased college attendance will be critical; among 2004 US high school graduates, young women (72%) were more likely than young men (51%) to enroll in college. The US education ranking among the world's most developed nations is dichotomous. Although ranking first in education of adults aged 45 to 64 years, the United States falls to sixth for the 35- to 44-year-old age group, ninth for 25 to 34, and is at least 15th in the education of those aged 18 to 24. About 80% of US youth graduate from high school with a traditional diploma; an additional 7% achieve a GED by age 24. By comparison, 97% of Hungarian youth and 94% of Japanese youth graduate high school. There is disparity by race, with 92% of Asian, 91% of non-Hispanic white, 82% of black, and 66% of Hispanic youth earning a high school diploma. Among 29 developed industrialized nations, US high school students ranked 15th in reading, 20th in science, and 24th in mathematics. Job opportunities for dropouts are becoming increasingly scarce and competition from displaced adult workers and immigrants is intense. During the 1990s, 13.65 million new immigrants accounted for 40% of the increase in population. Up to half of the immigrant population is undocumented, therefore results/data are incomplete. This population shift is significant for US adolescents as 50% of the working-age immigrants are under age 30; 70% of the immigrants between ages 25 and 34 are participating in the work force. Immigrants now comprise 15% of the US work force (increased from 8% in 1980) and account for 65% of the increase in the nation's civilian work force between 2000 and 2005. Thirteen US states report that 100% of the growth in employment between 2000 and 2005 was attributable to immigrant workers; an additional 14 states report more than 64% of the work force increase was from immigrant workers. Of these, 65% are high school graduates and 40% have further training, 27% with a bachelor's degree or higher. Of immigrants without high school diplomas, 87% are employed. By comparison, for native-born US citizens, only 57% of high school dropouts were employed. There is a wide variation of the educational status of immigrants. Fifty percent of Latin American immigrants have failed to graduate from high school and only 10% have graduated from college. This contrasts with Asian immigrants, 92% of whom have graduated from high school and 65% of whom have college degrees.[11] The end result of these changes has a major effect on employment opportunities for US youth. Limited research suggests that young immigrant workers are often preferred by employers to poorly educated native-born workers, especially from inner-city neighborhoods with high poverty rates. Those with less education, teenagers, and black males suffer employment declines as a result of the recent tide of immigration. Each 1% increase in the immigrant labor force results in a 1.2% decrease in the youth labor market with a far greater effect for less educated youth.[11]

## EMPLOYMENT AND SPECIAL NEEDS YOUTH

Continued advances in treatments for medical disorders including cancer, congenital heart disease, trauma, extreme prematurity, and other diseases have increased the number of adolescents who desire to enter the work force. Previously thought to be unemployable, with appropriate educational and social support many of these youth are able to find meaningful work. A 2000 (and reaffirmed in 2005) policy statement from the American Academy of Pediatrics[12] states that pediatricians are key to the successful vocational integration of children with disabilities; major strategies are summarized in Box 47-7.

All youth, including those with disabilities, are exposed to workplace issues beginning at young ages.

> **Box 47-7**
>
> ***Selected Roles of the Pediatrician in Transition from School to Work in Adolescents with Disabilities and Chronic Illness***[a]
>
> 1. Establishing a medical home
> 2. Helping the parents (and child) focus on realistic but progressive goals
> 3. Assessing a child's strengths and abilities (not just disabilities)
> 4. Begin planning transition early (by age 14)
> 5. Discussing (with youth and parents) pertinent medical information with the IEP team
>
> [a]Link to complete list in references.

Special needs youth should be realistically counseled about their potentials and limits, as well as those of particular vocations. Vocational education can be promoted through the identification of successful role models, volunteer activities, internship and shadowing experiences, summer jobs, and industry tours.

Multiple federal laws have sought to improve employment opportunities for special needs youth. The Individuals with Disabilities Education Act (IDEA) of 1990 and 1997 mandates that transition planning be a part of each student's individual education plan (IEP) and that it must begin no later than 14 years of age. The Americans with Disabilities Act (ADA) of 1990 requires employers (with more than 15 employees) to make "reasonable" accommodations for special-needs employees. Further information is available at www.eeoc.gov.

The combination of multiple programs (occupational therapy, physical therapy, medical services, schools, communities) effectively increases the employability of adolescents with chronic disease and disability. Accurate assessment of an adolescent's function and social readiness is essential to proper vocational placement; tools that assist in this have been developed.[13] Early inclusion into transition programs and vocational education classes is effective in increasing long-term employability. Most universities and technical/vocational schools, as well as local, state, and federal vocational offices, are available to assist those with disabilities and special needs in developing and implementing effective educational and employment goals.

## WORKSITE HEALTH PROMOTION

Many employers have effective worksite health promotions that, in addition to decreasing on-the-job injuries and meeting mandatory monitoring (eg, OSHA), aim to improve the overall health of employees. Adolescents may benefit from popular programs aimed at increasing physical activity, controlling diet, quitting smoking, screening for cancer, and others. Adolescents in workplaces where smoking is prohibited have been shown to be one-third less likely to smoke than employed peers who work in smoking-tolerant environments.[14] This must be balanced against other data suggesting that working actually increases the rate of smoking among adolescents.

## ROLE OF THE HEALTH CARE PROVIDER

Work is a crucial component of the lives of many adolescents. Health care providers should be knowledgeable about the specific types of employment common

**Box 47-8**

***The Adolescent Occupational History***

1. What sort of employment?
2. How many hours per week? When do you work?
3. Reasons and motivations for work?
4. What sort of supervision is provided?
5. Safety issues
   a. Exposure to chemicals, machines, toxins
   b. Need for specialized safety training
   c. Need for safety equipment (eye/ear/sun protection)
   d. Any work-related injuries?
   e. Basic first-aid knowledge and availability of kit
6. Effect of work on:
   a. Academic performance
   b. Sleep
   c. Family and friends

in their community. Familiarity with common types of employment and associated risks/benefits is essential in providing appropriate guidance and supervision. Youth who live and work in rural areas may have different risks and needs than urban and suburban youth. Occupational history is valuable in identifying potential risks to the working adolescent and should be included as part of the routine health maintenance visit. Key elements of the occupational history are reviewed in Box 47-8.[15] Teens who seek pre-employment physicals should be informed about risks and benefits of employment. Physicians should advise youth and parents of appropriate labor laws and should encourage and approve only legal employment. Emergency department personnel should be suspicious of unexplained work-related injuries, especially those involving cuts to the hand; authorities should be notified if violations are suspected.

## INTERNATIONAL YOUTH EMPLOYMENT ISSUES

Unsafe and unsanitary working conditions in developing countries pose a myriad of short- and long-term risks to youth workers. Unlike most adolescents in the United States, youth workers in developing countries work to earn money for basic necessities. These youth face hazards mirroring historic problems once faced in more developed countries. Long hours for minimal pay in unsafe and unsanitary working conditions are common. Major risks include issues of personal safety, occupational safety, personal hygiene, and exposure to toxins with immediate and distant (carcinogens) effects. Indian children and adolescents who weave carpets spend up to 14 hours a day squatting with only 1 break; higher rates (than nonworking peers) of malnutrition, respiratory disease, inadequate immunization, and other morbidities have been demonstrated among these youth.[16] Less than 20% of working children and adolescents in India continue their education. Exposures to toxic chemicals and fumes contribute to premature disability and death. Physical cruelty and compromised personal safety are brutal realities for many international youth workers. Many of these youth labor in unsafe conditions for miniscule pay to manufacture goods destined for developed nations. Child laborers in Calcutta work in abject poverty and like other child and adolescent laborers are deprived of educational and recreational opportunities. This may lower aspirations and blunt mental faculties. Higher rates of smoking, malnutrition, injuries, and physical abuse are reported in children and adolescents working in some developing nations. In developing nations the short-term risks are related to personal safety and exposures. Children and adolescents orphaned by the HIV/AIDS epidemic in Africa have been prematurely pushed into employment. Reform in these areas arises from social, political, and economic pressures, but it is slow in coming.

## INTERNET RESOURCES

### COMPREHENSIVE REVIEWS

- Sum A, Barnicle T, Khatiwada I, et al. Educational and Labor Market Outcomes for the Nation's Teens and Young Adults Since the Publication of America's Choice: A Critical Assessment. National Center on Education and the Economy, 2006. Available at: www.skillscommission.org Accessed May 18, 2008.
- Protecting Youth at Work: Health, Safety, and Development of Working Children and Adolescents in the United States (1998) Commission on Behavioral and Social Sciences and Education. Available at: books.nap.edu/openbook.php?record_id=6019&page=R1. Accessed May 18, 2008.
- Report on the Youth Labor Force: Alexis Herman (DOL) June 2000. Available at: www.bls.gov/opub/rylf/rylfhome.htm. Accessed August 26, 2010.

**DISABLED YOUTH**

- American Academy of Pediatrics Policy Statement on the Role of the Pediatrician (physician) in Transitioning Children and Adolescents with Disabilities and Chronic Illness from School to Work or College. Available at: aappolicy.aappublications.org/cgi/reprint/pediatrics;106/4/854. Accessed May 18, 2008.
- US Equal Employment Opportunity Commission. Information Regarding Employment of Disabled Youth (and Other). Available at: eeoc.gov/. Accessed May 18, 2008.

**EMPLOYER RESOURCES**

- US Department of Labor. Information for Employers of Youth Workers. Available at: www.youthrules.dol.gov/employers/default.htm. Accessed May 18, 2008.
- US Department of Labor, Occupational Safety and Health Administration (OSHA). Information for Employers of Teen Workers. Available at: www.osha.gov/SLTC/teenworkers/employers.html. Accessed May 18, 2008.
- US Department of Labor, Job Corps. Available at: jobcorps.dol.gov/hire.htm. Accessed May 18, 2008.
- US Department of Labor, Fair Labor Standards Act. Applicable laws and references, available at: www.dol.gov/elaws. Accessed May 18, 2008.

**FARM SAFETY/AGRICULTURAL ISSUES**

- National Children's Center for Rural and Agricultural Health and Safety Resources. Available at: www.marshfieldclinic.org/nccrahs/default.aspx?page=nccrahs_resources. Accessed June 17, 2010.
- AAP Policy Statement. Prevention of Agricultural Injuries among Children and Adolescents. Available at: aappolicy.aappublications.org/cgi/reprint/pediatrics;108/4/1016.pdf. Accessed May 18, 2008.
- Farm Safety for Just Kids. Available at: www.fs4jk.org/. Accessed May 18, 2008.

**FEDERAL WORK LAWS/REQUIREMENTS**

- US Department of Labor. Child Labor Laws Advisor for Compliance with the Fair Labors Standards Act (FLSA). Available at: www.dol.gov/elaws/esa/flsa/cl/default.htm. Accessed May 18, 2008.

**IMMIGRANTS**

- National Center on Education and the Economy. Paper on Educational and Labor Market Outcomes for Teens and Young Adults, includes immigrant data. Available at: www.skillscommission.org/pdf/commissioned_papers/Education%20and%20Labor%20Market%20Outcomes.pdf. Accessed May 18, 2008.
- US Department of Labor, Bureau of Labor Statistics. Injuries, Illnesses, and Fatalities. Available at: www.bls.gov/iif. Accessed May 18, 2008.
- Federal Network for Young Worker Safety and Health. Available at: www.cdc.gov/niosh/fedNet/. Accessed May 18, 2008.
- National Institute for Occupational Safety and Health. Worker Health Chartbook 2004. Available at: www.cdc.gov/niosh/docs/2004-146/. Accessed June 17, 2010.

**PARENT RESOURCES**

- Occupational Safety and Health Administration. Information for Parents of Teen Workers. Available at: www.osha.gov/SLTC/teenworkers/parents.html. Accessed May 18, 2008.
- US Department of Labor. Information for Parents Regarding Youth Employment Regulations. Available at: www.youthrules.dol.gov/parents/default.htm. Accessed May 18, 2008.
- US Department of Labor. Information for Parents on Job Corps Opportunities (for Students). Available at: www.jobcorps.gov/parents.aspx. Accessed August 26, 2010.

**STATE WORK LAWS/REQUIREMENTS**

- US Department of Labor. Information for Specific State Laws Governing Youth Employment. Available at: www.dol.gov/whd/state/state.htm. Accessed June 17, 2010.

**TEEN RESOURCES**

- NIOSH Information on Job Safety for the Youth Worker. Available at: www.cdc.gov/niosh/adoldoc.html. Accessed May 18, 2008.
- Occupational Safety and Health Administration. Information for Teen Workers. Available at: www.osha.gov/SLTC/teenworkers/teenworkers.html. Accessed May 18, 2008.

- US Department of Labor. Information for Youth on Employment Regulations. Available at: www.youthrules.dol.gov/teens/default.htm. Accessed May 18, 2008.
- Youth at Work, Web site of the US Equal Employment Opportunity Commission, contains information regarding the rights and responsibilities of youth workers. Available at: youth.eeoc.gov/. Accessed May 18, 2008.
- US Department of Labor. Information on Job Corps Opportunities for Students Both Before and After Graduation. Available at: www.jobcorps.gov/youth.aspx. Accessed August 26, 2010.

## REFERENCES

1. Committee on the Health and Safety Implications of Child Labor, National Research Council, and Institute of Medicine. *Protecting Youth at Work: Health, Safety, and Development of Working Children and Adolescents in the United States*. Washington, DC: National Academy Press;1998

2. Johnson DS, Lino M. Teenagers: employment and contributions to family spending. *Mon Labor Rev.* 2000;9:15-25

3. Johnson MK. Further evidence on adolescent employment and substance use: differences by race and ethnicity. *J Health Soc Behav.* 2004;45:187-197

4. Runyan CW, Schulman M, Dal Santo J, et al. Work-related hazards and workplace safety of US adolescents employed in the retail and service sectors. *Pediatrics.* 2007;119:526-534

5. Delp D, Runyan CW, Brown M, et al. Role of work permits in teen workers' experiences. *Am J Ind Med.* 2002;41:477-482

6. US Department of Labor. Jobs restrictions. Available at: www.dol.gov/elaws/esa/flsa/docs/hazardous.asp. Accessed April 20, 2010

7. Runyan CW, Dal Santo J, Schulman M, et al. Work hazards and workplace safety violations experienced by adolescent construction workers. *Arch Pediatr Adolesc Med.* 2006;160:721-727

8. Suruda A, Philips P, Lillquist D, Sesek R. Fatal injuries to teenage construction workers in the US. *Am J Ind Med.* 2003;44:510-514

9. Dunn KA, Runyan CW. Death at work among children and adolescents. *AJDC.* 1993;146:1044-1047

10. Runyan CW, Bowling JM, Schulman M, Gallagher SS. Potential for violence against teenage workers in the United States. *J Adolesc Health.* 2005;36:267.e1-5

11. Khatiwada I, Sum A, Barnicle T. New foreign immigrant workers and the labor market in the US: The contributions of new immigrant workers to labor force and employment growth and their impact on native born workers, 2000 to 2005. National Center on Education and the Economy, 2006. Available at: www.skillscommission.org. Accessed August 26, 2010

12. American Academy of Pediatrics, Committee on Children with Disabilities. The role of the pediatrician in transitioning children and adolescents with developmental disabilities and chronic illnesses from school to work or college. *Pediatrics.* 2000;106:854-856

13. Avjian SK, Wills JB, Hixson D, White P. Assessing adolescent function. *Clin Man.* 1991;11:60-65

14. Farkas AJ, Gilpin EA, White MM, Pierce JP. Association between household and workplace smoking restrictions and adolescent smoking. *JAMA.* 2000;284:717-722

15. Rubenstein H, Sternbach MR. Protecting the health and safety of working teenagers. *Am Fam Physician.* 1999;60:575-587

16. Joshi SK, Sharma U, Sharma P, et al. Health status of carpet-weaving children. *Indian Pediatr.* 1994;31:571

# CHAPTER 48

# Disasters

ROBIN H. GURWITCH, PhD • DAVID J. SCHONFELD, MD

Disasters challenge our world views and undermine our sense of safety, security, and stability. These events include natural disasters (eg, weather-related) and man-made disasters (eg, acts of terrorism, industrial, or transportation accidents), which frequently touch the lives of adolescents. Disasters are widely covered by all types of media including television and the Internet, and are topics of discussion in families as well as at school and among friends. Increasing world concern about terrorist attacks with weapons of mass destruction add to the focus on disasters and their effect. Communities, hospitals, and schools participate in drills to prepare for and respond to disasters. Adolescents and adults may find implications of these drills and exercises troubling; false alarms that result from a heightened state of alert may result in significant reactions, some of which may persist long after risks have been found to be unsubstantiated.

Acts of terrorism, the goals of which are to terrorize and undermine the sense of safety and security of a population much larger than the direct victims, result in psychological consequences more prevalent and long-lasting than those seen after other disasters.[1,2] However, no matter the type of disaster, children are recognized as a vulnerable population at high risk for psychological consequences and behavioral difficulties in the aftermath of the event.[3] Within this population, adolescents may be at particularly high risk as the normal developmental challenges that they face may interact with how they respond to the disaster. Adolescents are developing their sense of personal identity. They are no longer an extension of their parents or caregivers, and they strive for independence. They are beginning to consider their place in the world around them as well as their place in the future. Perceptions of the world as unsafe or hostile are particularly challenging to adolescents contemplating venturing out on their own. For this reason, particular attention should be paid in the aftermath of a major crisis to high school juniors and seniors to minimize the negative effect of the event on their career choices, which may have lifelong ramifications. Because of their developmental stage, adolescents may be less likely than younger children to share concerns or seek help from adults.[4,5] Therefore, understanding how disasters affect adolescents is essential to the health care professional's ability to help them cope and to increase their resilience in the face of such events.

## REACTIONS TO DISASTERS

Reactions to disasters can be conceptualized in 4 domains: emotional, cognitive, behavioral, and physiological.[6,7]

### EMOTIONAL CONCERNS

Emotional concerns center on worries and fears. In a study of middle and high school students 7 weeks after the terrorist bombing in Oklahoma City, 60% of respondents expressed continued worry about their personal safety and the safety of their families.[8] Adolescents have a well-developed sense of empathy. Their worry extends beyond personal safety and security to the safety and security of others, even those they do not know, encompassing their community and beyond. The threat of war and ongoing conflicts adds new worries and fears for many adolescents. They may worry about the consequences of war on soldiers and on innocent civilians. In the United States, because the average age of many in the military is approximately 20 years of age, adolescents may identify with the soldiers and see their future as closely aligned with military service. Adolescents also may have siblings, relatives, or acquaintances deployed to respond to conflicts. Worry about reoccurrence exists no matter what type of disaster is experienced. For example, with each rainstorm, adolescents who have been affected by hurricanes, tornadoes, or floods may worry that another catastrophic event will occur. Or, they may fear going into a tall building if a similar building was destroyed in a terrorist attack.

Adolescents who have experienced the death of a family member or friend also have needs related to bereavement support; bereavement, rather than trauma, may be the predominant issue for a particular individual.[5,9] Adolescence is an especially difficult time for adjustment to the loss of a parent, even outside of the context of a disaster. Parental death generally results in a range of other stressors, including financial and practical challenges, which further complicate adjustment for surviving family members.[10]

If a disaster results in relocation of adolescents and their families, additional concerns may be present.[7] Peers are extremely important to this age group.[2] With displacement comes worry about friends left behind. As adolescents are more concerned than other age groups about "fitting in" with peers, they may be particularly anxious about their reception in a new school environment. If they were previously involved in school or extracurricular activities, relocation could result in worry about continued involvement in these activities in a new school and community.

Adolescents may experience guilt or shame in the face of disaster.[6] They may believe actions they took or did not take could have changed the outcome. Could she have reduced family stress if only she had taken important papers from the home as the family evacuated in the wake of a hurricane? If he had not argued with his father, would he not have been at work early when the terrorist attacks occurred? They may also feel guilt if the family is stressed after the event, believing they are wholly or partially responsible for how the family is faring. Or they may experience survivor guilt if they were less directly affected than their peers. Shame may lead survivors to be reluctant to identify themselves as part of the affected group, to the point that they fail to avail themselves of physical resources and emotional supports so that they are not perceived as a "victim." When a disaster is man-made, adolescents may seek someone to blame for its aftermath. This blame may be directed to groups, including governments, organizations, and faith- or culture-based groups. Adolescents may express these feelings through hate talk or action. If the adolescent (or a family member) is a member of the group receiving negative attention or blame after a disaster, feelings of guilt and shame may be magnified.[2]

**Table 48-1**

**Potential Academic Consequences of Disasters on Adolescents**

| *Academic Consequences* | *Contributing Factors* |
|---|---|
| Decreased cognitive function and academic achievement | • Decreased concentration<br>• Sleep problems<br>• Depression<br>• Anxiety |
| Increased absenteeism | • School avoidance<br>• Family stressors |
| Increased suspensions and expulsions | • Social regression<br>• Irritability<br>• Substance abuse |
| Decreased rates of graduation | • Decreased academic achievement<br>• Increased absenteeism<br>• Increased suspensions and expulsions |

## COGNITIVE REACTIONS

Cognitive reactions after a disaster are often expressed as a focus on the event.[7] Adolescents may repeatedly talk about the disaster, their roles, and the roles and actions of others. Thoughts about the disaster may intrude on other thoughts, or adolescents may experience memories or flashbacks of the disaster, both of which increase feelings of vulnerability and distress. The cognitive effects of disasters may cause difficulty with concentration, attention, learning new material, and remembering past information. Consequences of these reactions may be seen in school performance, with adolescents showing a brief decline in grades after a disaster. As noted in Table 48-1, there are a range of academic consequences of disaster on adolescents, especially in the absence of interventions. Taking time in schools to help children adjust to a disaster and its aftermath is essential to promote academic achievement and decrease the likelihood of academic failure and dropout. Adolescents may also forget chores or not complete them as well as before the disaster. They may have trouble making decisions, especially good ones. Younger children may turn to parents for help, but as teens work toward independence, they may be hesitant to ask for assistance or opinions from adults.

## BEHAVIORAL REACTIONS

Behavioral reactions after disaster are, perhaps, the responses most readily noted by adults. Increased irritability, excitement about the event, and decreased cooperation with family, teachers, and friends are common. Adolescents may have changes in health behaviors, such as sleeping, eating, and performance of daily activities. They may have trouble falling or staying asleep or have sleep punctuated by nightmares. Appetite may change in either direction, resulting in weight gain or weight loss.[7] Adolescents may withdraw from activities they enjoyed before the disaster. These include time spent with friends and family as well as extracurricular activities such as sports, dance, youth groups, or other structured programs. They may appear indifferent to activities around them. Adolescents may also appear uninterested in the disaster and its aftermath. This reaction may be seen when they are unsure how to discuss the event with adults.[5] Adolescents may react to a disaster by taking a "live for today" approach;[9] some will begin to engage or increase participation in high-risk behaviors such as substance use, drinking, promiscuity, and/or reckless driving. Depression and fascination with death may also be seen. Given the difficulty in making sound decisions in the aftermath of a disaster and concern about the future following a disaster, adolescents are at increased risk for suicidal ideation and intent.[7]

#### PHYSIOLOGIC RESPONSES

Physiological responses to disaster experienced by adolescents can present as hypervigilance to the world around them. The startle response may be heightened, adding to a feeling of being "on edge." Adolescents may react to disasters with increased somatic concerns, complaining of headaches, stomachaches, and vague aches and pains, as well as increased fatigue.[7,9] In the setting of potential exposure to biological, chemical, or radioactive agents, where physical consequences may be delayed or not readily apparent, extent and duration of worry and concern about physical health can increase.[11] It may be physiological reactions to disaster that prompt parents and caregivers to seek a health care consultation (Box 48-1).

### MEDIATING FACTORS

Adolescents' responses to disaster may be mediated by several factors. Dose exposure to the disaster is one of the best predictors of outcome, with adolescents experiencing direct exposure, threat to life, and injury or death of family members generally having the greatest number of reactions.[7] However, indirect exposure through concentrated exposure to media coverage is also correlated with increased reports of symptoms in children of all age groups. This correlation was found following the terrorist attack in Oklahoma City[13] and the attacks in New York City on September 11, 2001.[1,14] Loss, including pets, belongings, and home, is associated with increased symptoms. The time adolescents are separated from family after the disaster, as well as the time it takes to re-establish routines and activities, may also mediate reactions. It is important for health care professionals to evaluate for pre-existing problems in emotional functioning and prior exposure to trauma; both place adolescents at greater risk for difficulties after a disaster. In a survey of New York City children after the September 11 attacks, 64% reported a *prior* traumatic event, with 27% having experienced the death of a family member through violence or an accident prior to September 11, 2001.[15] Although adolescence is when children become increasingly independent of adult influences, parents still remain a major influence in their lives. As parental distress and coping after disaster is one of the best predictors of how children will respond,[1,9] addressing the effect of the disaster on *all* family members is important to minimize the toll of the disaster on adolescents.

**Box 48-1**

***Adolescent Reactions after a Disaster***

**Emotional**

- Worries and fears
- Anxiety
- Guilt, shame
- Blame
- Concern about the future

**Behavioral**

- Changes in sleep, appetite, and exercise
- Withdrawal from family, friends, and activities
- Irritability
- Decreased school performance
- School avoidance
- Engagement in high-risk behaviors
- Depression with possible suicidal ideation or intent

**Mediating factors after disaster[1,9,12]**

- Degree of exposure
- Loss
- Evacuation/relocation
- Prior trauma
- Prior functioning
- Disruption of routine
- Separation from family
- Parental adjustment
- Support systems

**Cognitive**

- Focus on the event
- Intrusive thoughts and flashbacks
- Problems with attention and concentration
- Problems with memory
- Difficulty making decisions

**Physiological**

- Hypervigilance
- Increased startle response
- Increased arousal
- Numbness of emotions
- Increased somatic complaints

## ROLES OF THE HEALTH CARE PROVIDER

Health care providers can play a key role in reducing the negative psychological effect of a disaster on adolescents and their families.[5,6,16] One goal is to help adolescents understand the event. To do so, it is important to provide basic information about the event but without unnecessary graphic details. Although it is generally not appropriate to force conversations with adolescents who are reluctant to talk, waiting for adolescents to discuss the disaster and any related difficulties they may be experiencing may result in *no* discussion at all. Talk about the disaster and ask adolescents what they know or have heard and what they think about the information. Follow this discussion by asking if there is anything they would like to know; answer with honesty in an age-appropriate manner. Use this discussion to reinforce a sense of safety and security. Share what is being done by various systems (eg, government, community, and schools) to prevent recurrence of the event and to help recovery efforts. Help adolescents identify at least one action they can take to help others. Resilience is enhanced when children and adolescents, even those directly affected, help others.[17]

Adolescents may be concerned about reactions to a disaster, believing they are "going crazy" or something is terribly wrong with them. As such, psychoeducation about common reactions after disaster is essential to aiding in recovery.[6] Because concentration and attention may be compromised, a handout about reactions they can review at a later time may increase the likelihood they will benefit from psychoeducational efforts. Parents also may benefit from a discussion of reactions and receiving printed materials. This will help them better understand adolescents' behaviors and may help parents with their own recovery. Parents generally underestimate children's reactions to disaster.[18] One reason for this may be lack of knowledge about what reactions to look for after the event; discussion can promote accurate identification. As some reactions cannot be seen (eg, numbness, hyperarousal), establishing open communication and creating an environment that encourages disclosure is particularly important. If parents are distressed by their own reactions, they may have more difficulty seeing distress in their children; if parents are overly distressed, children, particularly adolescents, may also try to hide their reactions to decrease parental worries. Talking with adolescents and parents about common reactions and the importance of discussing feelings can facilitate communication and early identification of problems and convey to families concern and a willingness to help.

Even in the best of times, adolescence can be trying for many parents and adolescents; it may be doubly so after a disaster. Encourage parents to be more patient and attentive to their adolescents after a disaster. Connecting adolescents with support systems they have used in the past can be another important intervention. Help adolescents identify individuals and activities that have been important to them in the past. These may include friends, relatives, teachers, their pediatrician, faith-based leaders, and coaches. Encourage involvement in extracurricular activities they enjoyed before the disaster. Recognize that although adolescents may not want to participate in these activities after a disaster, participation (behavior) is often the catalyst to changes in their emotional state (feelings). Assess prior coping strategies and encourage positive coping skills that were effective after other difficult life events. These may include spending time with friends, talking to parents or other trusted adults, journaling or drawing, exercise, setting small goals for each day, and relaxation techniques (eg, deep muscle relaxation, breathing exercises, yoga, and meditation). Relaxation skills are beneficial in reducing the anxiety and physiological arousal common after disasters. Children with positive coping strategies and self-efficacy can experience psychological growth after traumatic experiences. Such posttraumatic growth is likely to occur only when children have sufficient internal and external resources and adequate supports.

Listen to what adolescents want to say, without judgment. Validate their emotions, unless they are destructive, such as hate toward people/faith/ethnicity. Understand that hate may be expressed following a terrorist event or man-made disaster and may mask extreme fear or sadness. Help adolescents understand that perpetrators of a terrorist attack are generally a small group and not indicative of an entire people. Tolerate the retelling of their experiences. They may voice feelings of guilt, shame, or blame that need to be considered and addressed. Listen for inaccurate understanding of events or misperceptions. Health care professionals must correct these misunderstandings in a truthful and age-appropriate manner. Although most adolescents can be supported after disaster and will be resilient with this support, some adolescents may benefit from health care professionals with expertise in disaster and trauma-related services. There continues to be a stigma associated with receiving care for mental health concerns, even in the aftermath of a crisis event. Talk to the adolescent and family about their thoughts and help them understand the reasons for your recommendation. Adolescents with more marked adjustment difficulties may benefit from a specialized, evidence-based intervention, such as Trauma-Focused Cognitive Behavioral Therapy.[1] Other warning signs suggesting a referral include the symptoms of post-traumatic stress disorder (PTSD),[20] direct exposure to the disaster, re-experiencing the disaster, feelings of numbness, avoidance of disaster reminders, hypervigilance, and a decrease in social and school functioning. Although most adolescents may experience reactions to disaster similar to individual symptoms of PTSD (eg, sleep problems or active avoidance of talking or thinking about the event) most do not meet the full criteria for the diagnosis, which includes the specification that symptoms last more than one month.[20] Clearly, immediate intervention is warranted if the adolescent has significant depression with suicidal ideation or intent.

Helping adolescents after a disaster includes providing their families with information about resources and services. These are generally available through community agencies and school systems. It is important for health care professionals to know about these resources, including having materials available for distribution. Talk to parents about minimizing re-exposure to the disaster, such as with excessive visits to disaster sites or extensive attention to disaster-related media coverage. Consider asking adolescents how their peers are reacting to and coping with the events; this may be less threatening than direct inquiry about their own feelings and behaviors. These actions will improve communication, which is important at all times but especially after a disaster. Explain to parents that reactions may wax and wane over time, with a likely increase at times such as anniversaries and holidays. Preparing for these events in advance may help attenuate distress and reinforce recovery efforts.

Health care providers can play an important role by helping individual adolescents and families under their care in the aftermath of a disaster; they can also play a critical role in fostering supports outside of the office or clinic setting. Health care professionals are encouraged to take an active role in school and community preparedness, response, and recovery efforts, lending n about the overall needs of children and adolescents in the face of disaster.[21] Disasters have become part of our changing world; taking an active role in decreasing the adverse effect on adolescents can help increase their adjustment today and their resilience in the future.

## INTERNET RESOURCES

1. American Academy of Pediatrics. Children and Disasters: www.aap.org/terrorism
2. National Center for School Crisis and Bereavement: www.cincinnatichildrens.org/school-crisis
3. Listen, Protect, and Connect: Psychological First Aid for Children and Parents: www.ready.gov/kids/_downloads/PFA_Parents.pdf

## REFERENCES


1. Gurwitch RH, Sitterle KS, Young BH, et al. Helping Children Cope with Disasters and Terrorism. In: LaGreca A, Silverman W, Vernberg E, Roberts M (eds). The Aftermath of Terrorism. Washington DC: American Psychological Association Press; 2002:327–357

2. Schonfeld D. Helping children deal with terrorism. In: Osborn L, DeWitt T, First L, Zenel J, eds. *Pediatrics.* Philadelphia, PA: Elsevier Mosby; 2005:1600–1602

3. IOM (Institute of Medicine. Preparing for the Psychological Consequences of Terrorism: A Public Health Strategy. The National Academics Press 2003.

4. American Academy of Pediatrics. Pediatric Terrorism and Disaster Preparedness: A Resource for Pediatricians. Foltin GL, Schonfeld DJ, Shannon MW, editors. AHRQ Publication No. 06(07)-0056. Rockville, MD: Agency for Healthcare Research and Quality. October 2006. Available at: www.ahrq.gov/research/pedprep/pedresource.pdf. Accessed September 14, 2007.

5. Schonfeld D. Supporting adolescents in times of national crisis—potential roles for adolescent healthcare providers. *J Adolesc Health.* 2002;30:302–307

6. Schonfeld D, Gurwitch R. Addressing disaster mental health needs of children: Practical guidance for pediatric emergency healthcare providers. *Clin Pediatr Emerg Med.* 2009;10:208–215

7. LaGreca A, Silverman W, Vernberg E, Roberts M, eds. *Helping Children Cope with Disasters and Terrorism.* Washington, DC: American Psychological Association Press; 2002

8. Pfefferbaum B, Nixon S, Krug R, et al. Clinical Needs Assessment of Middle and High School Students Following the 1995 Oklahoma City Bombing. *Am J of Psychiatry* 1999; 156:1069–1074

9. Schonfeld D. Supporting children after terrorist events: potential roles for pediatricians. *Pediatr Ann.* 2003;32:3:182–187

10. Schonfeld D, Quackenbush M. *The grieving student: a teacher's guide.* Baltimore, MD: Brookes Publishing; 2010

11. Hu Y, Adams RE, Boscarino JA, et al. Training Needs of Pediatricians Facing the Environmental Health and Bioterrorism Consequences of September 11$^{th}$. The Mount Sinai Journal of Medicine 2006;73(8):1156–1164

12. Thienkrua W, Cardozo BL, Chakkraband MLS, et al. Symptoms of Posttraumatic Stress Disorder and Depression Among Children in Tsunami-Affected Areas in Southern Thailand. *JAMA.* 2006:296(5):549–559

13. Pfefferbaum B, Nixon SJ, Tivis RD, et.al. Television Exposure in Children After a Terrorist Incident. *Psychiatry.* 2001;64:202–11

14. Madrid PA, Grant R, Reilly MJ, et al. Challenges in Meeting Immediate Emotional Needs: Short-term Impact of a Major Disaster on Children's Mental Health: Building Resiliency in the Aftermath of Hurricane Katrina. *Pediatrics.* 2006;117: S448–S453

15. Hoven C, Duarte C, Lucas C, et al. Psychopathology among New York City Public School children 6 months after September 11. *Arch Gen Psychiatry* 2005;62:545-552

16. Hagan J and the Committee on Psychosocial Aspects of Child and Family Health and the Task Force on Terrorism. Psychosocial implications of disaster or terrorism on children: a guide for the pediatrician. *Pediatrics*. 2005;116(3):787-795

17. American Psychological Association. *Resilience for Teens: Got Bounce?* (2003) available at www.apa.org/helpcenter/bounce.aspx. Accessed from APA Psychology Help Center, July 14, 2010

18. Vogel JM, Vernberg EM. Part 1: Children's Psychological Responses to Disasters. *J Clin Child Psychol*. 1993;22:464-84

19. Cohen JA, Mannarino AP, Deblinger E. *Treating Trauma and Traumatic Grief in Children and Adolescents*. New York: The Guilford Press; 2006

20. American Psychiatric Association. *Diagnostic and Statistical Manual of Mental Disorders*. Fourth Edition, Text Revision. Washington, DC: American Psychiatric Association; 2000

21. Schonfeld D, Lichtenstein R, Pruett MK, Speese-Linehan D. *How to Prepare for and Respond to a Crisis*. 2nd ed. Alexandria, VA: ASCD; 2002

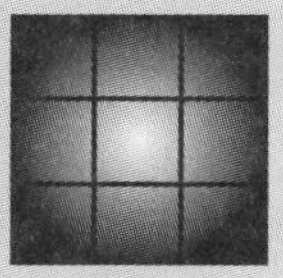

# Part 2

# Adolescent Sexuality and Reproductive Health

# SECTION 1
# Sexuality

## CHAPTER 49

## Adolescent Sexual Behaviors

MICHELLE FORCIER, MD, MPH • ROBERT GAROFALO, MD

### INTRODUCTION

Sexuality is a part of normal human development as teens grow into healthy whole adults. For some parents and pediatricians, acknowledging that adolescents are sexual, and often engaged in sexual activity, can be difficult and uncomfortable. However, it is important that health care professionals provide accurate and comprehensive information, as well as nonjudgmental support and care, so that teens undergoing this maturational process can make healthy and safe decisions. Nationwide, sexual activity is a prevalent and important part of teens' lives, with more than 46.8% of teens in grades 9 to 12 reporting having had sex and 33.9% reporting current sexual activity (ie, having sexual intercourse in the last 3 months).[1]

To understand adolescent sexual development, it is important to recognize that an individual's sexuality encompasses his or her unique emotional and cognitive understanding of many factors including hormonal and intellectual development; interpersonal and social environments of peers, family, school, and neighborhood; and broader sociocultural values that affect decision making and the expression of sexual behaviors.[2] During the teen years, youth priorities shift to increased sexual feelings and behaviors, increased importance of peer relationships, and decreased reliance on the parent and family unit. Although risk-taking and risky behaviors, including an exploration of sexuality or sexual activity, may be part of normal adolescent development, there exist multiple opportunities to educate and inform teens in their healthy decision making along the way. Understanding the natural range of sexual expression, from preadolescent childhood sexual curiosity to physical and hormonal maturation to increased curiosity, experimentation, and exploitation to responsible and expressive sexual demonstrations of intimacy of the young adult can help a provider provide developmentally appropriate advice and guide teens to develop strategies toward healthy sexuality.

### ADOLESCENT SEXUAL DEVELOPMENT

General adolescent development is frequently divided into 3 stages based loosely on chronologic age and level of functioning: early, middle, and late adolescence. One of the tasks for healthy adolescent development is the acquisition of a mature and responsible sexual identity including both an expression of sexual behaviors and the capacity for meaningful intimate relationships. Early adolescence (ages 10–14) coincides with the onset of puberty and typically involves preoccupations and insecurities surrounding the physical changes occurring with their own body and an egocentric approach to sexuality. Sexual curiosity and exploration may lead to sexual experimentation with masturbation or early sexual activity with same- or opposite-gender sexual partners.

Middle adolescents (ages 14–17) complete the physical changes of puberty and begin to have more romantic relationships characterized by serial monogamy or having several partners at once and over brief periods of time. Middle teens can begin to imagine the consequences of their actions but still may not fully understand them. Because of this, teens in middle adolescence often engage in experimental and risk-taking behaviors such as substance use and sexual activity.

Late adolescents (ages 17 and up) begin to have a more mature social and emotional view of their sexuality as well as more clearly defined gender roles. Late adolescents prioritize romantic relationships, where communication, intimacy, and support have a greater role than just sexual behaviors.

## CONFIDENTIALITY, RIGHTS, AND COUNSELING MINORS ON SEXUAL HEALTH ISSUES

Teens place significant and appropriate importance on the ability to seek and receive confidential health care. Public health policy routinely recognizes the importance of teen priorities as well as the reality that many teens will not seek necessary services if they are required to inform and involve a parent. At present, all 50 states allow youth to consent to confidential services for sexually transmitted infections (STIs). Almost 50% of states explicitly safeguard teens' rights to contraception, whereas other states affirm rights for certain categories of care and for certain subgroups of youth. In states with limited or no policies, decisions regarding parental involvement are typically left to the provider's discretion, based on promoting best interests and safety for the minor.[3] For a more in-depth discussion of confidential care of adolescents, refer to Chapter 11, Legal and Ethical Framework.

The pediatrician can play an important role in the safe and healthy development of an adolescent's sexual identity, including educating and empowering teens regarding sexual decision making and helping them navigate the challenges involved with becoming sexually active. Ensuring a safe and confidential place for care, honest and open communication, and accurate and developmentally appropriate education are essential in helping teens transition from childhood to young adulthood. Teens expect health care providers to not only be knowledgeable counselors regarding sexual health, but they also expect providers to initiate and direct these conversations even if unprompted.

## RANGE OF ADOLESCENT SEXUAL BEHAVIORS

Sexual behaviors in teens include a range of activities from kissing, petting, and fondling to oral, anal, and vaginal sex. Table 49-1 describes sources of information and data on sexual behavior of adolescents in the

**Table 49-1**

**Sources of Information and Data on Sexual Behaviors of Youth in the United States**

| *Source/Web Site* | *Survey Years* | *Survey Type*[a] | *Age (yrs)/Grade Gender, Location* |
|---|---|---|---|
| National Survey of Young Women (NSYW) www.socio.com/srch/summary/daappp/dap01.htm | 1971,1976, 1979 | Cross-sectional (IA,SA,PP) | 15-19 Females, Urban households |
| National Survey of Young Men (NSYM) www.socio.com/srch/summary/daappp/dap45.htm | 1979 | Cross-sectional (IA,SA,PP) | 17-21 Males, Urban households |
| National Survey of Family Growth (NSFG) www.cdc.gov/nchs/nsfg.htm | 1982,1988,1995 | Cross-sectional (IA, SA, PP- 82-88) CAPI, ACASI (95,02-03) | 15-44 Females, Males (02-03) Households |
| National Survey of Adolescent Males (NSAM) www.urban.org/publications/403709.html | 1988,1990-1, 1995 | Panel (IA,SA,PP-88, 90-1); (IA, SA, PP, ACASI- 95) | 15-19 Males Households |
| Youth Risk Behavior Survey (YRBS) www.cdc.gov/nccdphp/dash/yrbs/index.htm | 1991-present (biennial) | Cross-sectional (SA,PP) | Grades 9-12 Females/ Males, Schools |
| National Longitudinal Study of Adolescent Health www.cpc.unc.edu/projects/addhealth/ | 1994-5, 1996, 2001-2 | Panel (IA, SA, PP, CAPI, ACASI) | Grades 7-12 Females/ Males, Schools |

[a]Survey types include: IA, interviewer administered; SA, self-administered; PP, paper-and-pencil questionnaire; CAPI, computer-assisted personal interview (administered by an interviewer); ACASI, audio computer-assisted self-interview (self-administered).

Adapted by permission from BMJ Publishing Group Limited. (*Sexually Transmitted Infections*, Biddlecom AE, 80, ii75, 2004)

United States. Although vaginal–penile intercourse, with its inherent risks for pregnancy and STIs, has been the most well-researched, many of these other sexual behaviors may serve as a prelude to intercourse or as a substitute for intercourse for teens wishing to preserve their virginity. Studies evaluating teen sexual behaviors are fraught with problems regarding reliability and consistency of reported behaviors, definitions and understanding of specific behaviors, difficulties in measuring activities and the effect of these activities on their current and future lives. Many studies indicate high levels of inconsistent reporting for sensitive, sexually related behaviors including dating, first sexual intercourse, virginity, risk for STIs, and experiences with abortion.[4–7] Although trends in sexual activity can be demonstrated by statistics, it is a clinician's understanding of the multifaceted nature and complexity of sexual behaviors that helps teens explore their sexual identity in ways that are respectful, healthy, and safe.

## MASTURBATION

Masturbation, or the touching of one's genitals for sexual pleasure and arousal, is a normal part of sexual development in children of all ages, starting as early as in utero.[8] As long as youth do not masturbate inappropriately, in public, or so that it otherwise interferes with other tasks of adolescence, it is considered a normal healthy sexual behavior.[9] Males masturbate more frequently than females at rates ranging from 58% to 90%, versus about 40%, respectively.[10-12] However, there seems to be either no gender difference in age of initiation of masturbating behaviors or even perhaps some evidence that females may begin masturbating at an earlier age than boys.[10] Masturbation has been positively correlated to sexual self-esteem[10] but has not been found to be either beneficial or harmful to overall sexual adjustment in young adulthood.[12] Mutual masturbation, or masturbating a partner, as a trend seems to have increased in the 1990s.[13] Fifty-three percent of US adolescent males ages 15 to 19 report having been masturbated by a female, which represents a 40% rise since 1988. The degree of increase is most pronounced in 15- to 16-year-olds and among older males who have not yet engaged in vaginal intercourse. In 1995, more than half of males ages 15 to 19 reported being masturbated by a female partner.[13] It is interesting to note that despite the fact that masturbation is a normal behavior that is part of the healthy developmental process for many teens, much of the current literature on this behavior focuses on pathology, such as masturbation associated with neurologic or psychiatric disorders.[14-16]

## PETTING

The only available data regarding adolescents and petting behavior dates to a 1979 survey of sexual behaviors. Ninety-one percent of girls said they had their breasts touched by a boy. The percentage of boys who had touched a girl's breast increased throughout adolescence from 48% at age 13 to 73% by age 15, and 90% by age 18.[17] Again, despite this being relatively common in adolescence and a normal part of adolescent sexual exploration, there is little in the literature documenting the role that this behavior might have on adolescent sexual development. Both petting and masturbation are also remarkable for sexual behaviors that generally do not increase the risk for STIs.

## ORAL SEX

Oral sexual activity (including kissing, licking, or sucking on the penis, scrotum, vagina, or anus) is one of the most common forms of sexual expression among teens, often precedes vaginal intercourse, and may not be viewed by teens as sex but more simply as a way to gain sexual pleasure and intimacy without losing one's virginity.[18–21] More adolescents have had oral sex than vaginal sex, and few use barrier protection despite some risk for the acquisition of a number of STIs (eg, herpes, gonorrhea, etc). Overall, most studies suggest that there are few gender differences in either giving or receiving oral sex. The prevalence of receiving oral sex approaches one-half of male teens 15 to 19 years old, while the prevalence of giving oral sex is approximately 40%.[13] In a recent study with ninth graders, 19.6% reported having oral sex whereas only 13.5% had vaginal sex, and more early teens intended to have oral sex in the next 6 months (31.5% vs 26.3%).[18] The teens in this study believed that oral sex was more acceptable for their age group, for dating, and for more casual partnering than vaginal sex. Rates of self-reported oral sex in 12- to 25-year-olds doubled among males (16%–32%) and more than doubled among females (14%–38%) in the last 5 to 10 years.[22] Shifts in oral sex trends from 1988 to 1995 have not been striking except for trends in the black community, where black males almost doubled in reporting receiving oral sex (increasing from 25%–57%). Similar values are seen in other races.[13]

Although teens have realistic perceptions of negative health outcomes involved in vaginal–penile sex, such as pregnancy, chlamydia, and HIV, they are likely to underestimate the risk of disease associated with oral sex. In fact some teens incorrectly assume that there are no risks for STI transmission from oral sex.[18] Although teens' assessment of lower STI risk from oral sex is to some extent accurate, particularly for HIV, oral sex is an efficient mode of transmission for most other STIs including gonorrhea, herpes, syphilis, and chlamydia. With regard to HIV risk, cases of transmission from oral sex have been reported, but the risk for transmission from oral sex is dramatically lower than for vaginal or anal sex.[23,24] When counseling teens about health risks associated with oral sex it is important for clinicians to remember that teens almost never use condoms for oral sex, with only 4% of teens reporting condom use with first oral sex experience.[25] Incorporating other risk-reduction strategies, such as not brushing one's teeth after oral sex and not ejaculating in someone's mouth (or having someone ejaculate in yours), can be important in reducing incidence of disease.

## ANAL SEX

Anal sex is a relatively common form of sexual activity for both male and female teens, and one that has a significantly increased risk for STIs, including HIV. In a 1995 survey, 11% of US teens ages 15 to 19 engaged in rectal sexual intercourse.[13] From 1995 to 2002, anal sex practices among young women increased from 3% to 5.5%, but less so than oral sex.[22] Like oral sex, females who practice anal sex seems less likely to use condoms than those involved in vaginal-penile intercourse, perhaps related to the elimination of concerns about unwanted pregnancy. A 2005 study[25] reports as few as 1 in 3 female teens used condoms when engaging in their first episode of anal sex. In 1988, up to 6% of young males reported oral or anal sexual activity with another male.[6,26] Among all teen males, particularly young men who have sex with other men (MSM), inconsistent condom use for anal sex continues to be observed with some frequency, and this risky sexual behavior is believed in part to have fueled the rising HIV epidemic in this particular subpopulation of youth.[27-29]

## VAGINAL INTERCOURSE

More than half of adolescent females and nearly two-thirds of adolescent males have had vaginal intercourse by their 18th birthday[30] (Table 49-2). Among high school students, reported prevalence of current sexual activity (defined as sex in the last 3 months preceding the survey) did not change significantly between 1991 and 2001, fluctuating between 33% to 40% for females

**Table 49-2**

**Summary of Percentage of High School Students Who Engaged in Sexual Behaviors, by Sex, Race/Ethnicity, and Grade from the Youth Risk Behavior Survey, United States, 2009**

| *Category* | *Ever Had Sexual Intercourse* | | *Had First Sexual Intercourse before Age 13 Yrs* | | *Had Sexual Intercourse with >4 Persons during Their Life* | |
|---|---|---|---|---|---|---|
| | *Female (%)* | *Male (%)* | *Female (%)* | *Male (%)* | *Female (%)* | *Male (%)* |
| Race | | | | | | |
| White[a] | 44.7 | 39.6 | 2.2 | 5.0 | 10.0 | 11.0 |
| Black[a] | 58.3 | 72.1 | 5.6 | 26.8 | 18.0 | 39.4 |
| Hispanic | 45.4 | 52.8 | 3.7 | 11.1 | 10.4 | 18.0 |
| Grade | | | | | | |
| 9 | 29.3 | 33.6 | 3.6 | 12.0 | 6.3 | 11.1 |
| 10 | 39.6 | 41.9 | 3.6 | 7.7 | 7.6 | 15.3 |
| 11 | 52.5 | 53.4 | 2.7 | 8.0 | 12.9 | 17.5 |
| 12 | 65.0 | 59.6 | 2.2 | 6.2 | 19.1 | 22.7 |

[a]Non-Hispanic

Adapted from Centers for Disease Control and Prevention. Youth Risk Behavior Surveillance–United States,2009. Surveillance Summaries, June 4, 2010. *MMWR*. 2010;59(SS-5).

and 33% to 38% for males.[4] Trends since 1979 have found no significant increase in the average number (6) of sex partners among US adolescents, but this is higher than found in European teens.[31,32] The 2006 Youth Risk Behavior Survey indicates that the average number of students having 4 or more partners in their lifetime approximated 14%.[1] Certain personal characteristics, such as early childhood sociability, higher-quality here friendships, earlier initiation of romantic relationships, more frequent use of alcohol in middle adolescence, more mature appearance, and physical attractiveness is associated with number of lifetime sexual partners.[33]

## COMMON ISSUES RELATED TO SEXUAL RISK-TAKING IN ADOLESCENTS

Although it is normal and healthy for adolescents to begin exploring their sexuality as teens, there are issues common to this age group that put them at higher risk for adverse outcomes related to their sexual activities. These issues include early sexual debut, inconsistent contraception, and inconsistent condom use.

### EARLY SEXUAL DEBUT AND ABSTINENCE

Our youngest teens are those most at risk for adverse consequences of early sexual activity. Data from the 2009 Youth Risk Behavior Survey indicates that 5.9% of teens have sex before the age of 13.[1] Five percent of girls and 17% of boys in the fifth grade (age 11) have reported being sexually active. Sixty-six percent of fifth-grade girls and 87% of boys intended to have sex if they were "going with" someone they "liked a lot."[34] Among 14- to 15-year-olds, 12% to 13% of all adolescents have reported ever having intercourse. Adolescent females, especially younger teens, who are romantically involved with older partners are more likely to have intercourse and at younger ages than females partnering with same-age teen males.[35]

Overall, earlier sexual debut has been linked to multiple factors including male gender; black race; early puberty and high levels of testosterone; early use of alcohol, tobacco, and other substances; school problems and poor academic performance; delinquency, physical aggression and fighting; having sexually active friends and siblings; identifying as gay or bisexual; involvement in alcohol and drug use; not overweight; weak self-concept and low self-esteem; parent's marital discord and divorce or being in a single-parent family; lower socioeconomic status and family income; disadvantaged neighborhoods; lesser parental supervision and parents modeling high-risk and permissive attitudes about sex.[30,36-38] Early debut also has been linked to coercive or forced sexual activity and has been shown to have an association with increased risk of pregnancy and STI.[30] Protective factors for delaying sexual activity include better-educated parents; supportive family relationships; greater but not excessively controlling parental supervision; having sexually abstinent friends; getting good grades at school; and attending church or expressing religiosity.[30] Having a more sophisticated and realistic understanding of sexual responsibilities and outcomes, having lower expectations of positive outcomes, not involving peers in sexual relationships, and having better refusal skills have also been associated with delaying sexual debut.[39]

Virginity pledges and other public or private affirmations of religiosity and morals are a relatively new cultural phenomena in adolescent sexual behavior. Approximately 1 in 10 adolescents are classified as "reconstructed virgins," that is, teens who reported ever being sexually active in an initial interview and then deny this in subsequent interviews. This percentage is in line with other US studies[25,40] that have estimated between 5% and 12% of teens are "virgins again." Virginity pledges seem to have some effect on adolescent sexual behaviors, as adolescents who pledge their virginity tend to delay sexual debut and marry earlier than those who do not take a pledge. The research demonstrates that not all virginity pledgers wait until marriage to have their first sexual experience. According to one source, 88% of pledgers versus 99% of nonpledgers report vaginal intercourse before marriage.[25,41] Although public virginity pledges may not have a significant or consistent long-term affect on abstinence, private pledges or promises to delay sexual activity until an older age do seem to reduce rates of vaginal and oral sex before marriage.[42]

It is interesting to note that many teens who make virginity pledges do not consider oral or anal sexual activities as breaking virginity vows and so are consistently overrepresented among teens having oral or anal sex. Thirteen percent of consistent virginity pledgers reported having oral sex with one or more partners as compared to 2% of nonpledgers in a 2005 study. In this same study, 0.7% of nonpledgers report anal and no vaginal intercourse, compared with 1.2% for pledgers who had anal intercourse. These findings were particularly significant for males, with 4% of male pledgers engaging in anal intercourse as compared to 1% of male nonpledgers.[25] Despite data demonstrating that most virginity pledgers transition to first sex later, have sex less frequently, have fewer partners, and have fewer nonmonogamous partners, there seem to be no significant differences in rates of STIs between pledgers and nonpledgers. This phenomena may be explained by pledgers being less prepared and knowledgeable about sexuality, and therefore less likely to use condoms at first intercourse. As condom use at first intercourse can be a significant predictor for later consistent use, this risk for STIs may persist into subsequent sexual activity. Other data suggest that pledgers may be less aware of their STI risk and status, and report being less likely to see a physician regarding STI no matter what level of sexual activity they are involved in.[25] These findings underscore the importance of careful history-taking and highlight the need for education, specifically safer sex and STI prevention education for all teens regardless of their current virginity status.

### CONTRACEPTION FAILURES AND PREGNANCY

Sexually active teens who do not use contraception have a 90% chance of becoming pregnant in a year.[43] A more in-depth discussion of adolescent pregnancy may be found in Chapter 54. Although 9 out of 10 young women and their partners say they do use methods of contraception, many or most of them do not always use them consistently or correctly.[44] As many as 7 of 10 teen pregnancies occur while teens are not using any contraception. The remainder occur when teens incorrectly or intermittently use contraception. Teens' sexual encounters are often unplanned and sporadic, such that risk assessment and planning for protection is not typically well thought through in advance. Not only do teens neglect to use contraception at first sex, they delay starting regular contraceptive practices for on average up to a year. Reported reasons for the delay include procrastination, not thinking they could get pregnant, ambivalence about being sexually active, ambivalence about using contraception or wanting a pregnancy, and concerns about confidentiality when obtaining medical services. One of 3 teens makes a first family planning appointment in response to being concerned about a pregnancy, highlighting the importance of early education and counseling regarding family planning options.[30]

In the United States, there are approximately 800,000 teen pregnancies annually. In fact, 10% of all women ages 15 to 19 have an unintended pregnancy annually. Teen pregnancy occurs in up to 19% of teens who are sexually active.[45] By age 18, 25% of all US females will have been pregnant at least once.[46] Seventy-eight percent of all teen pregnancies are unplanned, accounting for one-quarter of all accidental pregnancies annually.[47] Of those young women experiencing an early pregnancy, national statistics demonstrate that approximately half opt to continue the pregnancy, with most (98% or more) of these teens planning to parent themselves. Approximately one-third of teens choose to terminate their pregnancies and another 15% of teen pregnancies end in miscarriage.[48]

Rates of teen childbearing have fallen steeply from the 1950s, from an all-time high of 96 births per 1,000 women aged 15 to 19, to 49 births per 1,000 in 2000. This trend is observed among teens of all ages and races. Nonmarital births among all ages, however, increased significantly from the 1950s from 13% to 79% in 2000. Declines in adolescent birth rates are most likely due to decreased pregnancy rates, with some evidence suggesting that three-quarters of the drop can be attributed to improved contraception methods and one-quarter of the drop due to increased rates of sexual abstinence.[49,50] In a study of sexual trends from 1991 to 2001, declines in the withdrawal method of contraception (20% to 13%), and in using no method of contraception (17%–13%), as well as increased condom use for contraception (40%–51%) may also have contributed to improved teen family planning.[51]

### INCONSISTENT CONDOM USE: HIGHEST RATES OF SEXUALLY TRANSMITTED INFECTIONS

As many as 1 in 4 sexually experienced teens in the United States acquire an STI, such that there are approximately 3 million STIs diagnosed in teens each year.[52] Chapter 53 contains a full discussion of STIs. As of the mid-1990s, the United States ranked in the top 3 for highest reported rates of syphilis, gonorrhea, and chlamydia among 15- to 19-year-olds in the developed world.[53] Younger age at first intercourse predicts higher risk of acquiring an STI during adolescence but is not necessarily linked with risk in the young adult years.[54] Chlamydia rates are highest and rising in women 15 to 19 years old, increasing 9.8% from 2,982.5 per 100,000 to 3,275.8 per 100,000 population in 2008. Gonorrhea rates decreased in 2008 for the first time in 4 years, dropping by 1.3% in 15- to 19-year-olds and 2.5% in 20- to 24-year-olds. Young women 15 to 19 years had the highest rates of gonorrhea (636.8/100,000).[55] HIV rates for persons ages 15 to 19 and 20 to 24 increased between 2005 and 2008.[4,56] All sexually active adolescents are at risk of contracting STIs; however, risk is not distributed equally across demographic groups. Young women bear a disproportionate amount of the burden of these infections diagnosed during the teen years. Adolescent and young adult MSM are at increased risk for a number of STIs, including HIV, in comparison to heterosexual male youth. Teens from racial/ethnic minority groups, particularly black youth, are also at increased risk for the acquisition of STIs.

Adolescents are one of the age groups most at risk for contracting HIV, with sexual transmission accounting for the overwhelming majority of new cases. HIV transmission is especially common among MSM and heterosexual females, many of whom have sexual relations with older men.[57] Worldwide, 5 adolescents and young adults, ages 10 to 24 years become HIV infected every minute.[58] In the last 10 years, the proportion of female adolescent AIDS cases has tripled, rising from 14% to 46% from 1987 to 1996.[59] Unlike adults, where almost 70% of new HIV infections occur in males, adolescents are the only age demographic where new HIV infections in young women roughly approximates new infections among men. Despite these statistics, the 2009 Youth Risk Behavior Survey indicates that only 12.7% of high school students have been tested for HIV, with testing rates higher in female and older students.[1]

Regarding trends in STI prevention and safer sexual behaviors, condom use at first intercourse and current condom use has increased from the 1980s to 2000, regardless of gender.[4] Condom use at sexual debut increased between 1988 and 1995, from 50% to 70% of females and 55% to 69% of males. Condom use at last sex increased from 31% to 38% in females and 53% to 64% in males. The ability to obtain free condoms from service providers predicted greater condom self-efficacy and personal responsibility but was only linked to greater consistency of use if the teen had visited the clinic for the purposes of obtaining condoms.[60] Nationally, most data suggest that of the one-third of currently sexually active high school students, 63% report that either they or their partner used a condom during their last sexual intercourse, and condom use was more common in the younger grades than in older grades (9th grade 74.5%; 10th grade 65.3%; 11th grade 61.7%; and 12th grade 55.4%).[1]

## THE HEALTH CARE PROVIDER'S ROLE IN PREVENTION

Teens generally describe getting their sexual health information from both parents and professionals. Anywhere from one-third to one-half of teens get sexual health information from their parents.[56,61] Teens say that parental sexual education is generally focused on menstruation, whereas sources in educational settings tend to focus on STI prevention. Of note, 26% of girls received their first formal reproductive education during or after sexual debut.[62] Screening for associated risk behaviors such as substance use and violence, the sequelae of risk-taking, and appropriate anticipatory guidance may reduce risks and provide accurate information and tools for teens to make healthier sexual decisions (Table 49-3).

**Table 49-3**

**Summary of Percentage of High School Students Who Drank Alcohol or Used Drugs before Last Sexual Intercourse, Were Ever Taught in School about HIV Infection or AIDS, and Who Were Tested for HIV by Sex, Race/Ethnicity, and Grade—from the Youth Risk Behavior Survey, United States, 2009**

| *Category* | *Alcohol or Drug Use before Last Sexual Intercourse* | | *Taught in School about HIV or AIDS* | | *Tested for HIV* | |
|---|---|---|---|---|---|---|
| | *Female (%)* | *Male (%)* | *Female (%)* | *Male (%)* | *Female (%)* | *Male (%)* |
| Race | | | | | | |
| White[a] | 18.2 | 28.0 | 89.6 | 87.8 | 13.2 | 9.1 |
| Black[a] | 15.2 | 20.8 | 86.9 | 85.2 | 25.1 | 17.6 |
| Hispanic | 15.0 | 22.6 | 83.2 | 83.2 | 12.4 | 12.4 |
| Grade | | | | | | |
| 9 | 23.5 | 25.9 | 84.6 | 81.8 | 8.2 | 8.9 |
| 10 | 18.1 | 26.5 | 87.7 | 86.9 | 12.0 | 9.2 |
| 11 | 14.7 | 25.9 | 89.9 | 88.9 | 16.4 | 12.5 |
| 12 | 15.2 | 25.8 | 89.4 | 89.1 | 23.5 | 13.7 |

[a] Non-Hispanic

Adapted from Centers for Disease Control and Prevention. Youth Risk Behavior Surveillance–United States, 2009. Surveillance Summaries, June 4, 2010. *MMWR*. 2010;59(SS-5).

The Society for Adolescent Health and Medicine (SAHM) recognizes that since the 1996 Section 510 of the Social Security Act, when the federal government expanded its funding and support for abstinence-only programs, many school- and public health-based programs promote only abstinence outside of marriage at any age and have a restrictive and often inaccurate focus on contraception, sexual orientation, and gender identity among other aspects of human sexuality. Abstinence-based curricula often indicate that contraceptives may not be discussed except to emphasize failure rates and that homosexuality is portrayed as unnatural and deviant behavior.[63] Two reviews evaluating the evidence and outcomes of abstinence-only programming indicate that they have had no efficacy in delaying sexual debut.[64–66] Abstinence-only education is of great national importance because more than one-third of all local US school districts that have policies on sexuality education require that an abstinence-only education option for unmarried people be presented, and that contraception not be presented or must be presented only as an ineffective option in preventing pregnancy. Fifty-five percent of southern school districts have abstinence-only curricula compared to lower numbers in other parts of the country and demonstrate higher birthrates than the national average.[49]

It is important that providers ensure access to sexual health information to their adolescent patients as they might be the only source of accurate and comprehensive education, in addition to offering preventive services. The SAHM 2006 position paper on abstinence-only education policies and programs suggests that not only do health providers have an ethical obligation to provide accurate health information but that "current abstinence only legislation is ethically problematic as it excludes accurate information about contraception, misinforms by overemphasizing or misstating risks of contraception, fails to require the use of scientifically accurate information while promoting approaches of questionable value" and discriminates against youth who identify as sexual minorities (ie, lesbian, gay, bisexual, transgender, queer, etc).[67]

## SUMMARY

As sexuality is a predictable stage in the normal development of teens and young adults, health care providers for adolescents have a professional obligation to be knowledgeable and proactive in initial screening and management of common sexual health issues. Providers should fully understand federal and local laws regarding minors' access to and ability to consent to reproductive health services in their community. They should strive to be comfortable in initiating sexual health discussions, preserve some measure of privacy for these youth, and conduct regular risk assessment and screening in sexual health matters for their adolescent patients. The health care provider's ability to listen to and hear teens, to accurately provide helpful information and to help teens access necessary community resources will help them effectively serve their teen patients' need for confidential and comprehensive sexual health care.

## REFERENCES


1. Centers for Disease Control and Prevention. *Youth risk behavior surveillance—United States, 2005. CDC Division of Adult and Community Health.* June 4, 2010;59(SS-5):1–148

2. Nelson EE, Leibenluft E, McClure EB, Pine DS. The social re-orientation of adolescence: a neuroscience perspective on the process and its relation to psychopathology. *Psychol Med.* 2005;35(2):163–174

3. Dailard C, Turner RC. Teenagers' access to confidential reproductive health services. *The Guttmacher Report on Public Policy,* November 2005

4. Biddlecom AE. Trends in sexual behaviors and infections among young people in the United States. *Sexually Transm Infect.* 2004;80(S2):ii74–79

5. Fu H, Darroch JE, Henshaw SK, et al. Measuring the extent of abortion underreporting in the 1995 National Survey of Family Growth. *Fam Plan Perspect.* 1998;30:128–133, 138

6. Turner CF, Ku L, Rogers SM, et al. Adolescent sexual behavior, drug use, and violence: increased reporting with computer survey technology. *Science.* 1998;280:867–873

7. Sexual behavior by personal interview and audio computer-assisted self-interviewing: analyses of the 1995 National Survey of Family Growth. *Sociology Methods Res.* 2002;31:3–26

8. Meizner I. Sonographic observation of in utero fetal "masturbation." [Case Reports. Letter] *J Ultrasound Med.* 1987;6:111

9. Leung AK, Robson WL. Childhood masturbation. *Clin Pediatr.* 1993;32:232–241

10. Smith AM, Rosenthal DA, Reichler H. High schoolers masturbatory practices: their relationship to sexual intercourse and personal characteristics. *Psychol Rep.* 1996;79:499–509

11. Sorenson RC. *Adolescent Sexuality in Contemporary America.* New York, NY: World Publishing; 1973

12. Leitenberg H, Detzer MJ, Srebnik D. Gender differences in masturbation and the relation of masturbation experience in preadolescent and/or early adolescence to sexual behavior and sexual adjustment in young adulthood. *Arch Sex Behav.* 1993;22:87–98

13. Gates GJ, Sonenstein FL. Heterosexual genital sexual activity among adolescent males: 1988–1995. *Fam Plan Perspect.* 2000;32:295–297, 304

14. Albertini G, Polito E, Sara M, Di Gennaro G, Onorati P. Compulsive masturbation in infantile autism treated by mirtazapine. [Case Reports. Journal Article] *Pediatr Neuro.* 2006;34:417–418

15. Lopez-Meza E, Corona-Vazquez T, Ruano-Calderon LA, Ramirez-Bermudez J. Severe impulsiveness as the primary manifestation of multiple sclerosis in a young female. [Case Reports. Journal Article] *Psychiatry Clin Neurosci.* 2005;59:739–742

16. Bodensteiner JB, Sheth RD. Masturbation in infancy and early childhood presenting as a movement disorder. [comment]. *Pediatrics.* 2006;117:1861; author reply 1861–1862

17. Hass A. *Teenage Sexuality: A Survey of Teenage Sexual Behavior*. Los Angeles, CA: Pinnacle Books; 1979

18. Halpern-Felsher BL, Cornell JL, Kropp RY, Tschann JM. Oral versus vaginal sex among adolescent: perceptions, attitudes, and behavior. *Pediatrics.* 2005;115:845–851

19. Gerbert B, Herzig K, Volberding P, Stansell J. Perceptions of health care professionals and patients about the risk of HIV transmission through oral sex: a qualitative study. *Pediatric Education and Counseling.* 1999;38:49–60

20. Remez L. Oral sex among adolescents: is it sex or is it abstinence? *Fam Plan Perspect.* 2000;32:298–304

21. Sanders SA, Reinisch JM. Would you say you "had sex" if...? *JAMA.* 1999;281:275–277

22. Mosher WD, Chandra A, Jones J. Sexual behavior and selected health measures: men and women 15–44 years of age, United States, 2002. *Advance Data from Vital and Health Statistics,* No. 362, September 15, 2005

23. Vittinghoff E, Douglas J, Judson F, McKirnan D, MacQueen K, Buchbinder SP. Per-contact risk of human immunodeficiency virus transmission between male sexual partners. *Am J Epidem.* 1999;150:306–311

24. Rothenberg RB, Scarlett M, del Rio C, Reznik D, O'Daniels C. Oral transmission of HIV. *AIDS.* 1998;12:2095–2105

25. Brückner H, Bearman P. After the promise: the STD consequences of adolescent virginity pledges. *J Adolesc Health.* 2005;36:271–278

26. Ku L, Sonenstein FL, Pleck J. Young men's risk behaviors for HIV infection and sexually transmitted diseases, 1988 through 1991. *Am J Public Health.* 1993;83:1609–1615

27. Celentano DD, Valleroy LA, Sifakis F, et al for the Young Men's Survey Study Group. Associations between substance use and sexual risk among very young men who have sex with men. *Sex Transm Dis.* 2006;33:265–271

28. Killebrew M, Garofalo R. Talking to teens about sex, sexuality, and sexually transmitted infections. *Pediatric Annals.* 2002;31:566–572

29. Clatts MC, Goldsamt LA, Yi H. Drug and sexual risk in four men who have sex with men populations: evidence for a sustained HIV epidemic in New York City. *J Urban Health.* 2005;82(Suppl 1):i9–17

30. Moore KA, Miller BC, Sugland BW, Morrison DR, Glei DA, Blumenthal C. From beginning too soon: Adolescent sexual behavior, pregnancy, and parenthood: a review of research and interventions. *Report prepared by Child Trends Inc. for Office of Assistant Secretary for Planning and Evaluation, US DHHS.* Washington, DC. June 1995

31. Santelli JS, Lindberg LD, Abma J, et al. Adolescent sexual behavior: estimates and trends from four nationally representative surveys. *Fam Plan Perspect.* 2000;32:156–165, 194

32. Brener N, Lowry R, Kann L, et al. Trends in sexual risk behaviors among high school students—United States, 1991–2001. *MMWR.* 2002;51:856–859

33. Zimmer-Gembeck MJ, Siebenbruner J, Collins WA. A prospective study of intra-individual and peer influences on adolescent's heterosexual romantic and sexual behavior. *Arch Sexual Behav.* 2004;33:381–394

34. Rose A, Koo HP, Bhaskar B, Anderson K, White G, Jenkins RR. The influence of primary care providers on the sexual behavior of early adolescents. *J Adolesc Health.* 2004;37:135–144

35. Kaestle CE, Morisky DE, Wiley DJ. Sexual intercourse and the age difference between adolescent females and their romantic partners. *Perspect Sex Reprod Health.* 2002;34:304–309

36. Santelli JS, Kaiser J, Hirsch L, Radosh A, Simkin L, Middlestadt S. Initiation of sexual intercourse among middle school adolescents: the influence of psychosocial factors. *J Adolesc Health.* 2004;34:200–208

37. Garofalo R, Wolf RC, Kessel S, Palfrey SJ, DuRant RH. The association between health risk behaviors and sexual orientation among a school-based sample of adolescents. *Pediatrics.* 1998;101:895–902

38. Garriguet D. Early sexual intercourse. *Health Reports.* 2005;16:9–18

39. O'Donnell L, Myint UA, O'Donnell CR, Stueve A. Long-term influence of sexual norms and attitudes on time of sexual initiation among urban minority youth. *J Sch Health.* 2003;73:68–75

40. Upchurch DM, Lillard LA, Aneshensel CS, et al. Inconsistencies in reporting the occurrence and timing of first intercourse among adolescents. *J Sexual Res.* 2002;39:197–206

41. Rostosky SS, Regnerus MD, Wright ML. Coital debut: the role of religiosity and sex attitudes in the Add Health Survey. *J Sex Res.* 2003;40:358–367

42. Bersamin MM, Walker S, Waiters ED, Fisher DA, Grube JW. Promising to wait: virginity pledges and adolescent sexual behavior. *J Adolesc Health.* 2005;36:428–436

43. Harlap S, Kost K, Forrest JD. *Preventing Pregnancy, Protecting Health:A New Look at Birth Control Choices in the United States.* New York, NY: AGI; 1991

44. The Alan Guttmacher Institute. *Sex and America's Teenagers*. New York; AGI: 1994;19–20

45. The Alan Guttmacher Institute. Teenage pregnancy: overall trends and state by state information. New York; AGI; 1999:5

46. Lerner RM. *Youth in Crisis: Challenges and Options for Programs and Policies.* Thousand Oaks, CA: Sage Publications; 1995

47. Henshaw SK. Unintended pregnancy in the United States. *Fam Plan Perspect.* 1998;30(1):24–29, Table 49-1

48. The Alan Guttmacher Institute. US teenage pregnancy statistics with comparative statistics for women aged 20-24. Available at: www.guttmacher.org/pubs/teen_stats.pdf. Accessed February 19, 2004

49. Boonstra H. *Teen Pregnancy: Trends and Lessons Learned. The Guttmacher Report on Public Policy.* New York, NY: Alan Guttmacher Institute; 2002

50. Darroch J, Singh S. Why is teenage pregnancy declining? The roles of abstinence, sexual activity, and contraceptive use. Occasional Report, New York, NY: Alan Guttmacher Institute; 1999, No. 1

51. Santelli JS, Abma J, Ventura S, et al. Can changes in sexual behaviors among high school students explain the decline in teen pregnancy rates in the 1990? *J Adolesc Health.* 2004;35:80-90

52. The Alan Guttmacher Institute. *Sex and America's Teenagers*. New York, NY: AGI; 1994:38

53. Panchaud C, Singh S, Feivelson D, Darroch JE. Sexually transmitted diseases among adolescents in developed countries. *Fam Plan Perspect.* 2000;32:24-32, 45

54. Kaestle CE, Halpern CT, Miller WC, Ford CA. Young age at first sexual intercourse and sexually transmitted infections in adolescents and young adults. *Am J Epidemiology.* 2005;161:774-780

55. Centers for Disease Control and Prevention. 2008 Sexually Transmitted Disease Surveillance. STDs in Adolescents and Young Adults. Available at: www.cdc.gov/std/stats08/adol.htm. Accessed November 23, 2010.

56. Centers for Disease Control and Prevention. Diagnoses of HIV infection and AIDS in the United States and Dependent Areas, 2008. HIV Surveillance Report, Volume 20. Available at: http://www.cdc.gov/hiv/surveillance/resources/reports/2008report/. Accessed November 23, 2010.

57. Centers for Disease Control and Prevention. *Adolescents and HIV/AIDS: facts*. Atlanta, GA: Centers for Disease Control and Prevention, March 1998

58. US Department of Health and Human Services. *Healthy People 2000, progress review (HIV infection)*. Washington, DC: US Department of Health and Human Services, Public Health Service, July 8, 1997

59. Joint United Nations Programme on HIV/AIDS. UNAIDS press release: new report finds five young people infected with HIV every minute, April 22, 1998.

60. Parkes A, Henderson M, Wight D. Do sexual health services encourage teenagers to use condoms? A longitudinal study. *J Fam Plan Repro Health Care.* 2005;31:271-280

61. Hutchinson MK, Cooney TM. Patterns of parent-teen sexual risk communication: implications for intervention. *Family Relations.* 1998;47:185-194

62. Ancheta R, Hynes C, Shrier LA. Reproductive health education and sexual risk among high-risk female adolescents and young adults. *J Pediatr Adolesc Gyn.* 2005;18:105-111

63. Committee on Government Reform-Minority Staff. *The Content of Federal Funded Abstinence-only Education Programs*. Washington, DC: US House of Representatives; 2004

64. Kirby D. *Emerging Answers: Research Findings on Programs Designed to Reduce Teen Pregnancy*. Washington, DC: National Campaign to Prevent Teen Pregnancy; 2001

65. Devaney B, Johnson A, Maynard R, Trenholm C. *The Evaluation of Abstinence Education Programs Funded under Title V Section 510: Interim Report to Congress on a Multisite Evaluation*. Princeton, NJ: Mathematica Policy Research, Inc; 2002

66. Manlove J, Romano-Papillo A, Ikramullah E. *Not Yet: Programs to Delay First Sex among Teens*. Washington, DC: National Campaign to Prevent Teen Pregnancy; 2004

67. Santelli J, Ott MA, Lyon M, Rogers J, Summers D. Abstinence-only education policies and programs: a position paper of the Society for Adolescent Medicine. *J Adolesc Health.* 2006;38:83-87

# CHAPTER 50

# Issues Affecting Gay, Lesbian, and Bisexual Youth

WAYNE SELLS, MD, MPH • GARY REMAFEDI, MD, MPH

## GENERAL DESCRIPTION

The issues of adolescent gender identity and sexual orientation are relatively new to medical providers. In 1973, the American Psychiatric Association (APA) removed homosexuality from the *Diagnostic and Statistical Manual of Mental Disorders*.[1] In 1983, the American Academy of Pediatrics (AAP) formally recognized the importance of the topic and the responsibility of health care providers to meet the needs of homosexual youth.[2] Gay, lesbian, and bisexual (GLB) youth are affected by many of the same issues encountered by their heterosexual counterparts. However, there are many experiences that are unique to GLB adolescents and young adults. Health care providers play an important role facilitating a healthy transition from adolescence to adulthood. This chapter reviews some of the important issues affecting GLB youth.

## DEFINITIONS

The acronyms GLBTQ (gay, lesbian, bisexual, transgender, and questioning or queer) and GLBT (gay, lesbian, bisexual, transgender) are frequently used to reference GLB youth. Though at times it is convenient to combine these populations, each has unique issues. Some GLBT youth enter adulthood without any significant consequences, and others have a much more eventful transition.

Sexual orientation includes attractions, fantasies, self-identification, and sexual behavior; and it should be viewed on a continuum between absolute homosexuality and heterosexuality. Homosexuality has been defined as a "persistent pattern of homosexual arousal accompanied by a persistent pattern of absent or weak heterosexual arousal."[3] The term "gay" usually refers to homosexual males, but it may include homosexual females and bisexual individuals. "Lesbian" refers to homosexual females. Bisexual individuals are attracted to both males and females. Transient ambiguity about sexual orientation or "questioning" is relatively common among younger adolescents. With appropriate support and information, most youth resolve any uncertainty concerning their sexual orientation by late adolescence.

Gender identity is a person's innate sense of being female or male. A transgender individual is a person whose birth gender does not match their psychological gender identity. A more in-depth discussion of transgender youth may be found in Chapter 51, Transgendered Youth. A transsexual is a person who is in the process of transitioning physical appearance to be more consistent with gender identity. The transitioning process can involve medications such as hormones, surgical intervention (ie, sexual reassignment surgery), cosmetic interventions, or any combination of these interventions. Intersex (also referred to as a disorder of sexual development) specifically refers to individuals whose genitalia or secondary sexual characteristics are neither exclusively male nor female. Some intersex individuals experience gender identity dysphoria. A transvestite is a person who derives sexual pleasure from cross-dressing or wearing the clothing of the opposite gender. Transvestites may be heterosexual, homosexual, or bisexual in their orientation.

## EPIDEMIOLOGY

Although homosexuality has been documented in most societies throughout history, the visibility of homosexual people is related to societal attitudes. The exact prevalence of homosexuality among adolescents is unknown, as is the prevalence of same-sex experiences. One of the earliest studies of homosexual behaviors reported that 37% of males and 13% of females have had at least one same-sex experience resulting in orgasm.[4,5] A more recent study of persons 16 to 19 years old found that 17% of males and 6% of females reported at least one sexual experience with someone of the same gender.[6]

A large population-based study of almost 35,000 junior and senior high school students in Minnesota evaluated sexual fantasies, behaviors, attractions, and identity. The survey found that 25% of the 12-year-old students were unsure of their sexual orientation, with the proportion decreasing to 5% by age 18. The overall proportion of youth who reported predominantly homosexual attractions was 5%. The proportion reporting predominantly homosexual attractions increased with age, peaking at 6% among 18-year-old males. The prevalence of reported same-gender sexual experiences was constant at 1% for females and increased from 0.4% to 3% from males between the ages of 12 and 18 years. Only 1% of youth described themselves as homosexual or bisexual.[7]

A later study using Massachusetts Youth Risk Behavior Survey (YRBS) data of 9th- to 12th-grade students found that 3% self-identified as GLB, and 1% reported being unsure of their sexual orientation. Overall, 2% reported same-gender sexual experiences.[8] These studies demonstrate the discrepancy between sexual attractions, behavior, and self-identification. Thus, it is important for health care providers to recognize that a relatively large proportion of youth may have questions about their sexual feelings, and fewer report same-gender sexual attractions or identify as GLB.

## ETIOLOGY

Although no one theory completely explains human sexual orientation, those that have been proposed include environmental, hormonal, and genetic influences.[9]

### ENVIRONMENTAL THEORY

There is no scientific evidence that environmental stressors, sexual abuse, abnormal parenting, or other adverse experiences determine sexual orientation.[10,11] However, environment may affect the expression of genetic predisposition by influencing social behavior. Societal attitudes toward homosexuality, as well as access to healthy role models, are important to GLBT youth.

### HORMONAL THEORY

A biological model involving the influences of hormones on homosexuality has been proposed. Studies have failed to find consistent differences in sex hormone levels between heterosexual and homosexual adults. However, an increased incidence of homosexuality in women with congenital adrenal hyperplasia has been observed despite early diagnosis and treatment.[12] Such evidence suggests that prenatal androgen exposure influences sexual orientation, even in the absence of differences in postnatal sex steroid levels. Neuroanatomical, -physiological, and -behavioral differences between heterosexual and homosexual individuals have been reported.[11] Thus, it has been hypothesized that factors that affect early development affect the structure and function of the brain and, in turn, influence sexual orientation.

### GENETIC THEORY

More recent evidence suggests that homosexuality is influenced by genetics. The clustering of homosexuality within families frequently exceeds that of the general population. A higher concordance of homosexuality among monozygotic twins compared to dizygotic twins has been reported, but varies widely.[13] One study that has not been duplicated reported an association with male homosexuality and loci on the X chromosome.[14]

## STAGES IN THE ACQUISITION OF GAY/LESBIAN IDENTITY

Troiden[15] summarized the 4 stages of development in the acquisition of the gay/lesbian identity as sensitization, identity confusion, identity assumption, and commitment.

### STAGE I: SENSITIZATION

Sensitization usually occurs prior to puberty. During this stage, the child senses being different from same-sex peers but does not understand the reason for these feelings.

### STAGE II: IDENTITY CONFUSION

Homosexual feelings and behaviors may create uncertainty and confusion with regard to sexual orientation. Some adolescents try to ignore these behaviors or feelings, whereas others view them as temporary. Some seek counseling to help them cope with their feelings, and others remain socially isolated.

### STAGE III: IDENTITY ASSUMPTION

During this stage, the adolescent is able to resolve confusion about sexual orientation and discuss sexual identity with others. Youth frequently discuss sexual identity with close friends before talking openly with parents or professionals. This process is known as "coming out." Identity assumption may happen during adolescence, young adulthood, or much later.

### STAGE IV: COMMITMENT

This stage involves the individual experiencing self-acceptance, emotional intimacy, and unwillingness to alter one's sexual identity. At the point of acceptance, homosexual identity is no longer a description of a behavior but an integrated component of self-concept.

## PSYCHOLOGICAL STRESSORS

Coming out, or disclosing one's sexual orientation, may cause significant distress for the youth and their families. Family rejection or disapproval is commonly experienced. The stigma and isolation associated with homosexuality can adversely affect the normal developmental process.

Real or perceived lack of social support from families, friends, and communities can result in poor self-esteem and difficulty developing appropriate relationships.

Some youth experience physical or emotional abuse from their family, and some are forced to leave their homes. Although the proportion of GLB youth who become homeless is unknown, GLBT teens appear to be overrepresented among homeless and runaway youths in the United States.[16] With limited educational or vocational skills, it is not surprising that some youth resort to illegal activities including engaging in sex for survival.

### INTERNALIZED AND EXTERNALIZED HOMOPHOBIA

Homophobia is an irrational hatred or distorted fear of homosexuality or homosexual individuals that may present as general discomfort or prejudice. Externalized homophobia is the expression of these attitudes that might be manifested by psychological or physical abuse. During adolescence, peers are important in a youth's personal and social development. Isolation, stigma, or disapproval from friends or family may be internalized, contributing to poor self-image, self-destructive behaviors, and the abandonment of educational or vocational goals.

### VIOLENCE AND SCHOOL SAFETY

A healthy adolescent transition from childhood to adulthood depends on the support from families, peers, school, and communities. Unfortunately violence, victimization, discrimination, and harassment are commonly experienced by GLBT individuals. In a study of 194 GLB youths between the ages of 15 and 21, more than 80% reported some form of victimization due to sexual orientation. Victimization was pervasive and frequently occurred in multiple settings including school, work, community, and home environments.[17] A national study found that youth who reported same- or both-sex attractions were more likely to have been subjected to extreme forms of violence and to have witnessed violence than youth who reported heterosexual attractions.[18]

School is an important place where youth can develop safe and supportive relationships with teachers and peers. However, for many GLBT youth school-related violence and victimization are unfortunately common. As a result, GLBT youth are at risk for academic underachievement and school avoidance. Thus, it is not surprising that school dropout rates have been reported to be higher for GLBT youth than for the general population.

Violence also may be associated with other health risk behaviors. A school-based study of 9th to 12th graders in Massachusetts and Vermont examined the association between at-school victimization and substance use, suicidality, and sexual behaviors. Gay, Lesbian, and Bisexual youth who reported victimization at school also reported significantly higher levels of substance use, suicidality, and sexual risk behaviors than their heterosexual peers.[19] Protecting vulnerable youth in all social and community environments should be a high priority to reduce other health risk behaviors.

## HEALTH CARE ISSUES AND DISPARITIES

Significant health disparities exist for GLBT youth, but they have been largely ignored by public health systems. Many of these disparities stem from the stigma associated with sexual identity, and they are compounded by the youths' inability to effectively advocate for themselves. Although the condition of homosexual youth in contemporary society has not been systematically evaluated, they are disproportionately affected by problems of suicide, eating disorders, tobacco and substance abuse, HIV/AIDS, and STIs.

### DEPRESSION AND SUICIDE

The stigma of homosexuality, in conjunction with a sense of isolation in an openly hostile environment, may result in depression and/or suicide attempts—particularly during the periods of identity confusion or early identity assumption. Multiple studies using a variety of methods and sampling strategies have tried to determine the degree to which same-gender sexual orientation is a risk factor for suicide.

In a large, population-based study of Minnesota junior and senior public high school students, 28% of bisexual and homosexual males—compared to 4% of heterosexual males—reported suicide attempts.[20] The Massachusetts YRBS found that bisexual and homosexual males were 3 times more likely than their heterosexual peers to have attempted suicide. Data from the National Longitudinal Study of Adolescent Health revealed that youth with same-gender sexual attractions and relationships were more than twice as likely as their same-sex peers to attempt suicide. The study also found that youth with homosexual attractions and relationships reported higher levels of depression, victimization, and alcohol abuse than their heterosexual peers. Although most gay (85%) and lesbian (72%) youth reported no suicidal behaviors, the study concluded that a significant proportion remained at high risk.[21] Thus, it is important for providers to inquire about suicidal behaviors, especially among those with known risk factors, including depression, alcohol or substance abuse, victimization, lack of social support, school failure, family problems, homelessness, and prior suicidal behavior.

## EATING DISORDERS

It also is important for providers to screen GLBT youth for eating disorders. In a large population-based study of 7th to 12th grade students, homosexual and bisexual males were more likely than heterosexual males to report poor body image (28% vs 12%), frequent dieting (9% vs 6%), binge eating (26% vs 11%), and vomiting (12% vs 4%). Homosexual and bisexual females were more likely than their heterosexual peers to report a positive body image, with no significant differences in frequent dieting, binge eating, or purging behavior.[22]

Likewise, the statewide Massachusetts YRBS found gay and bisexual adolescent males and those with same-gender sexual experiences were significantly more likely than heterosexual adolescent males to have fasted (21% vs 6%), vomited, or used laxatives (22% vs 4%) and diet pills (19% vs 4%) to lose weight.[23] A large national cohort study found that gay and bisexual male adolescents were more likely than their heterosexual peers to report binge eating and to emulate media images.[24]

## TOBACCO AND SUBSTANCE ABUSE

Rates of tobacco and other substance use among gay, lesbian, and bisexual youths generally exceed that of their heterosexual peers. Studies of teens and young adults consistently have found higher smoking rates among GLB youth than in the general population.[16,25,26] In the Massachusetts and Vermont YRBS, GLB youth were more likely to report tobacco use than their heterosexual peers. Gay, lesbian, and bisexual youth were more likely to initiate smoking prior to their 13th birthday (48% vs 23%) and to smoke at school (37% vs 18%), and nearly twice as likely to have smoked in the past 30 days (59% vs 35%).[27] Although the research concerning the use of tobacco among GLBT youth is expanding, currently little is known about successful smoking prevention and cessation programs for these populations.

Some GLBT youth use substances to numb the pain of rejection, condemnation, or isolation. A large convenience sample of young gay and bisexual males reported considerably higher rates of problematic substance use, compared to a normative sample of high school students (19% vs 9%).[28] In the Massachusetts and Vermont YRBS, GLB youth were more likely to report alcohol and substance use than their heterosexual peers. They were significantly more likely to initiate marijuana use prior to age 13 (34% vs 9%), and more likely to report use in the past 30 days (54% vs 31%) than their heterosexual peers. They also were significantly more likely to initiate cocaine use prior to age 13 (17% vs 1%), and more likely than their heterosexual peers to use in the past 30 days (25% vs 3%). Gay, lesbian, and bisexual youth were significantly more likely to report injection drug use (22% vs 2%) and more likely to report sharing needles (16% vs 1%) than their heterosexual peers.[27] For many GLBT youth, increased substance use may be associated with increased risk of STIs/HIV, truancy, and homelessness.

## HIV/SEXUALLY TRANSMITTED INFECTIONS

As previously discussed in this chapter, sexual behaviors may be inconsistent with a youth's sexual identity. Youth who identify as heterosexual also may have same-gender sexual activity. It is sexual behavior, not orientation, that places youth at risk for HIV and STIs. Although STIs are less prevalent among women who exclusively have sex with women, lesbians are not immune. In fact, one study involving lesbian and bisexual adolescents found higher pregnancy rates and—among sexually experienced adolescents—higher rates of prostitution than among heterosexual or unsure adolescents.[29] The perception of providers and youth that lesbians are universally low risk can create barriers to appropriate STD screening and routine Pap smears.

Regardless of perceived sexual orientation, young men who have unprotected sexual intercourse with men continue to face significant risk of acquiring STIs. Although fewer than 3% of male US high school students report same-gender sexual experiences, men having sex with men (MSM) accounted for 48% of all new cases of HIV/AIDS diagnosed in 2004.[30]

Men who have unprotected receptive genital-anal intercourse with men are at risk for hepatitis B, HIV, and proctocolitis caused by chlamydia, gonorrhea, syphilis, human papillomavirus (HPV), and cytomegalovirus (CMV). Men who have receptive oral-anal intercourse with men are at increased risk for colitis and enteritis caused by *Salmonella, Shigella, Campylobacter, Entamoeba*, CMV, and other enteric pathogens. Those who have insertive genital-anal sex are at risk for gonococcal and nongonococcal urethritis. Unprotected genital-oral sex is common among MSM and may be associated with the transmission of hepatitis A and B, gonorrhea, herpes simplex virus (HSV) 1 and 2, and HPV.[31] They also are at risk of genital ulcers, both painless (eg, syphilis, granuloma inguinale) and painful (eg, HSV, chancroid, and lymphogranuloma venereum).

STIs, especially ulcerative diseases such as syphilis and HSV, facilitate the transmission of HIV.[32] Men who have sex with men who are infected with HPV are at significant risk for anal cancer, especially if they are immunocompromised. Comprehensive prevention plans must offer primary, secondary, and tertiary interventions to reduce STIs. Although extensive discussion about STIs is beyond the scope of this chapter, the "2006 Sexually Transmitted Diseases Treatment Guidelines" provide comprehensive information on the diagnosis and treatment of STIs, including issues unique to GLBT youth.[33] A full discussion of sexually transmitted infections in adolescents may be found in Chapter 53, Sexually Transmitted Infections.

## HELPFUL INTERVENTIONS AND RESOURCES

Organizational policies and position statements regarding GLBT youth are important for providers, adolescents, and young adult clients alike. These policies provide clinical guidelines, facilitate the training of providers, and help prevent harmful practices. The following organizations have issued policies or guidelines regarding the care of homosexual youth.

- **American Academy of Pediatrics (AAP)** issued its first policy statement on adolescent homosexuality in 1983. The policy was last updated in 2004. The AAP reaffirmed the responsibility of physicians to provide comprehensive health care and anticipatory guidance in a supportive and safe environment to all adolescents, including GLBT youth.
- **American Psychological Association (APA)** first adopted a resolution that opposed the portrayal of homosexuality as a mental illness in 1975. Since that time, the APA has strived to provide health professionals with the information needed to evaluate and treat GLB adolescents and adults. In 2000, the APA published its "Guideline for Psychotherapy with Lesbian, Gay, and Bisexual Clients"[34] that addresses attitudes toward homosexuality and bisexuality, relationships with families, issues of diversity, and the importance of education.
- **Society for Adolescent Health and Medicine (SAHM)** published a position paper on abstinence-only sexual education policies and programs, describing them as flawed from the viewpoints of science and medical ethics. The paper states that abstinence-until-marriage programs exclude and discriminate against GLBT youth because federal law limits marriage to opposite-sex partners.[35] Abstinence-only educational programs often ignore issues that are important to GLBT youth and stigmatize homosexuality as unnatural and deviant behavior.[36]

### ACCESS TO APPROPRIATE HEALTH CARE

All adolescents and young adults need access to comprehensive health care. Primary care providers can help discuss questions about sexual orientation and activity in a safe, confidential setting. Although it is not the provider's responsibility to identify or label youth as GLBT, providers play an important role in creating an environment where personal issues can be addressed in a sensitive and confidential manner. Successful interventions must focus on prevention and early intervention to promote health and well-being.

### HIV/STI PREVENTION

Diffusion of Effective Behavioral Interventions (DEBI) is a national program sponsored by the Centers for Disease Control and Prevention (CDC) that provides training and technical assistance on evidence-based HIV/STI interventions. The DEBI program works in collaboration with community-based partners to coordinate the dissemination of programs with demonstrated effectiveness. The DEBI project has recognized 2 interventions that have been effective in preventing HIV infections among young MSM.[37]

One such successful program for young gay and bisexual men is **Mpowerment.** The key elements include (1) development and leadership by a core group of young gay men, (2) outreach activities in venues where young gay men are frequently encountered, (3) social events to promote community-building among young gay men, and (4) peer-based distribution of information to spread safer sex norms.[38] Mpowerment has been successful in decreasing rates of unprotected anal intercourse.[39]

**Street Smart** is an intensive program developed for runaway and homeless youth. The program's focus is to increase safer sex behaviors and to reduce substance use. The shelter-based program involves eight sessions with 4 major components: improved access to health resources, improved access to condoms, training staff, and training for youth. The program helps youth improve social skills, solve problems, identify triggers for risky behavior, and reduce harmful behaviors. Street Smart has been successful in increasing condom use among homeless and runaway youth.[40]

### TOBACCO CESSATION

Programs for the prevention and cessation of tobacco use among GLBT youth are in development. A recent qualitative study evaluating prevention and cessation efforts from young people's perspective recommended that programs should involve GLBT adolescents in the planning and implementation process, support healthy psychosocial development, engage adolescents in enjoyable activities, address psychosocial and cultural issues associated with tobacco use, and offer pharmacological smoking cessation aids.[41]

## SOCIAL SUPPORT

Gay and lesbian youth need the opportunity to mature in a supportive environment. Health care providers may serve as an important resource for both youth and their families as they develop safe and supportive social networks.

### YOUTH

Social support is a critical component of any prevention effort that focuses on GLBT youth, creating opportunities to develop friendships and social networks in safe environments. Gay–straight alliances (GSAs) have become increasingly popular. It is estimated that more than 3,000 schools have student-organized and student-run clubs that focus on GLBT issues.[42] Advocates for GLBT youth have successfully argued that the Federal Equal Access Act (20 U.S.C. §§ 4071–74) requires public secondary schools that offer noncurriculum clubs also to allow GSAs or risk losing federal funding.[43]

### INFORMATION FOR THE FAMILY

Parents and family members of GLBT teens may experience a full range of emotions—including fear, guilt, anger, and grief—when youth disclose their sexual orientation. It is important for primary care providers to explore these feelings. The provider may be able to help the family accept homosexuality as a normal variation of sexual orientation. Most states have local chapters of Parents, Families, and Friends of Lesbians and Gays (PFLAG) that are important resources for families.

### SAFETY

All children have the right to grow up in a safe environment. Schools must provide a setting free of bullying, verbal abuse, and physical violence. Ensuring safety would likely improve educational outcomes and reduce health risk behaviors. In addition to schools, there is a need to reform other institutions that exclude GLBT youth from activities, occupations, and social institutions. Assuring safety in communities is of the highest priority.

### COMMUNITY AWARENESS AND CAPACITY BUILDING

The general public can become more aware of issues affecting GLBT youth through the publication of well-designed research. Programs that address health problems that adversely affect GLBT youth (eg, STIs/HIV, substance abuse, suicide) will need to be designed, proven successful, and replicated to improve the health and well-being of this vulnerable population.

Well-informed professionals play an important role in working with schools and community leaders to advocate for GLBT youth, providing factual information about sexual orientation and raising community awareness about important issues. Health professionals also can help establish school and community-based support groups, as well as HIV/AIDS prevention efforts. With appropriate support from communities, school, family, and friends, GLBT youth have the same opportunity as others to lead healthy, happy, and productive lives.

## INTERNET RESOURCES

### TEENS AND YOUNG ADULTS

- Advocates for Youth: www.advocatesforyouth.com
- Bisexual Resource Center: www.biresource.org
- Gay, Lesbian, and Straight Educational Network: www.glsen.org/templates/index.html
- National Gay and Lesbian Task Force: www.thetaskforce.org/index.cfm
- National Youth Advocacy Coalition: nyacyouth.org

### PARENTS

- Parents, Families, and Friends of Lesbians: www.pflag.org

### PROFESSIONAL

- Sexually Transmitted Diseases Treatment Guidelines, 2006: www.cdc.gov/std/treatment/default.htm

## REFERENCES

1. American Psychiatric Association. *Diagnostic and Statistical Manual of Mental Disorders.* 4th ed. Washington, DC: American Psychiatric Association; 1994

2. American Academy of Pediatrics, Committee on Adolescence. Homosexuality and adolescence. *Pediatrics.* 2004;113(6):1827–1832

3. Spitzer RL. The diagnostic status of homosexuality in DSM-III: a reformulation of the issues. *Am J Psychiatry.* 1981;138:210

4. Kinsey AC, Pomeroy WB, Martin CE. *Sexual Behavior in the Human Male.* Philadelphia, PA: WB Saunders; 1948

5. Kinsey AC, Pomeroy WB, Martin CE. *Sexual Behavior in the Human Female.* Philadelphia, PA: WB Saunders; 1953

6. Sorenson RC. *Adolescent Sexuality in Contemporary America.* New York, NY: World Publishing; 1973

7. Remafedi G, Resnick M, Blum R, et al. Demography of sexual orientation in adolescents. *Pediatrics.* 1992;89:714–721

8. Garofalo R, Wolf RC, Wisslow LS, Woods ER, Goodman E. Sexual orientation and risk of suicide attempts among a

representative sample of youth. *Arch Pediatr Adolesc Med.* 1999;153:487-493

9. Perrin EC. *Sexual Orientation in Child and Adolescent Health Care*. New York, NY: Kluwer Academic/Plenum Publishers; 2002

10. Friedman RC, Downy JL. Homosexuality. *N Engl J Med.* 1994;331:923-930

11. Stronski Huwiler SM, Remafedi G. Adolescent homosexuality. *Adv Pediatr.* 1998;45:107-144

12. Dittmann RW, Kappes ME, Kappes MH. Sexual behavior in adolescent and adult females with congenital adrenal hyperplasia. *Psychoneuroendocrinology.* 1992;17 (2/3): 153-170

13. Hershberger SL. Biological factors in the development of sexual orientation. In: D'Angelli A, Patterson C, eds. *Lesbian, Gay, and Bisexual Identities and Youth: Psychological Perspectives*. New York, NY: Oxford University Press; 2001: 27-51

14. Hamer DH, Hu S, Magnuson VL, et al. A linkage between DNA markers on the X chromosome and male sexual orientation. *Science.* 1993;261:321

15. Troiden RR. Homosexual identity development. *J Adolesc Health Care.* 1988;9:105-113

16. Remafedi G. Adolescent homosexuality: psychosocial and medical implications. *Pediatrics.* 1987;79 (3):331-337

17. Pilkington NW, D'Augelli AR. Victimization of lesbian, gay, and bisexual youth in community settings. *J Community Psychology.* 1995;23:34-56

18. Russell ST, Franz BR, Driscoll AK. Same-sex romantic attraction and experiences of violence in adolescence. *Am J Public Health.* 2001;91 (6):903-906

19. Bontempo DE, D'Augelli AR. Effects of at-school victimization and sexual orientation on lesbian, gay, or bisexual youths' health risk behavior. *J Adolesc Health Care*. 2002;30:364-374

20. Remafedi G, French S, Story M, Resnick MD, Blum R. The relationship between suicide risk and sexual orientation; results of a population-based study. *Am J Public Health.* 1988;88(1):57-60

21. Russell ST, Joyner K. Adolescent sexual orientation and suicide risk: evidence from a national study. *Am J Public Health.* 2001;91(8):1276-1281

22. French SA, Story M, Remafedi G, Resnick MD, Blum RW. Sexual orientation and prevalence of body dissatisfaction and eating disordered behaviors: a population-based study of adolescents. *Int J Eat Disord.* 1996;19(2):119-126

23. Massachusetts Department of Education. *1999 Youth Risk Behavior Survey*. Massachusetts Department of Education; 2000

24. Austin SB, Zihadeh N, Kahn JA, Camargo CA, Colditz GA, Field AE. Sexual orientation, weight concerns, and eating-disorder behaviors in adolescent girls and boys. *J Am Acad Child Adolesc Psychiatry*. 2004;43(9):1115-1123

25. Ryan H, Wortly PM, Easton A, Pederson L, Greenwood G. Smoking among lesbians, gays, and bisexuals: a review of the literature. *Am J Prev Med.* 2001;21(2):142-149

26. Rosario M, Hunter J, Gwadz M. Exploration of substance use among lesbian, gay, and bisexual youth: prevalence and correlates. *J Adolesc Research.* 1997;12 (4):454-476

27. Garofalo R, Wolf RC, Kessel S, Palfrey SJ, DuRant RH. The association between health risk behaviors and sexual orientation among a school-based sample of adolescents. *Pediatrics.* 1988;101(5):895-902

28. Winters KC, Remafedi G, Chan BY. Assessing drug abuse among gay-bisexual young men. *Psychology of Addictive Behaviors.* 1996;10(4):228-236

29. Saewyc E, Bearinger L, Blum R, Resnick M. Sexual intercourse, abuse, and pregnancy among adolescent women: does sexual orientation make a difference? *Fam Plann Perspect.* 1999;31(3):127-131

30. Centers for Disease Control and Prevention. *HIV/AIDS Surveillance Report, 2004*. Volume 16. Atlanta, GA: US Department of Health and Human Services, Centers for Disease Control and Prevention; 2005:1-45

31. Edwards S, Carne C. Oral sex and the transmission of viral STIs. *Sex Transm Inf.* 1998;74:6

32. Stamm WE, Handsfield HH, Rompalo AM, Ashley RL, Roberts PL, Corey L. The association between genital ulcer disease and acquisition of HIV infection in homosexual men. *JAMA.* 1988;260(10):1429-1433

33. Centers for Disease Control and Prevention. Sexually transmitted diseases treatment guidelines, 2006. *MMWR.* 2006;55: 1-93

34. American Psychological Association. Guidelines for psychotherapy with lesbian, gay, and bisexual clients. *APA Online.* 2006;1-27

35. Abstinence-only education policies and programs: A position paper of the Society for Adolescent Medicine. *J Adolesc Health*. 2006;38:83-87

36. Kempner ME. *Toward Sexually Healthy America: Abstinence-Only-Until-Marriage Programs That Try to Keep Our Youth "Scared Chaste."* New York, NY: Sexuality Information and Education Council of the United States; 2001

37. Centers for Disease Control and Prevention. Diffusion of effective behavioral interventions. Available at: www.cdc.gov/hiv/topics/research/prs/prs_rep_debi.htm. Accessed August 8, 2006

38. Centers for Disease Control and Prevention. The Mpowerment Project: A community-level HIV prevention intervention for young gay men. Available at: www.cdc.gov/hiv/topics/prev_prog/rep/packages/mpower.htm. Accessed May 29, 2008

39. Kegeles SM, Hays RB, Pollack LM, Coates TJ. Mobilizing young gay and bisexual men for HIV prevention: a two-community study. *AIDS*. 1999;13:1753-1762

40. Rotheram-Borus MJ, Song J, Gwadz M, Lee M, Rossem RV, Koopman C. Reductions in HIV risk among runaway youth. *Prevention Science.* 2003;4(3):173–187

41. Remafedi G, Carol H. Preventing tobacco use among lesbian, gay, bisexual, and transgender youths. *Nicotine and Tobacco Research.* 2005;7(2):249–256

42. Jennings K. Gay, Lesbian and Straight Education Network. Available at: www.glsen.org/cgi-bin/iowa/all/about/history/index.html. Accessed August 16, 2006

43. Wall L. ACLU sues Klein school on behalf of lesbian student. *Houston Chronicle;* 2003

# CHAPTER 51

# Medical Treatment of the Transgender Adolescent

NORMAN P. SPACK, MD • LAURA EDWARDS-LEEPER, PHD

## TERMINOLOGY

*Transgender* is not a formal diagnosis but a term that describes individuals whose gender identity is different from their biological sex. Gender identity disorder (GID) is the formal diagnostic label used in the *Diagnostic and Statistical Manual of Mental Disorders*, 4th Edition, Text Revision (*DSM-IV-TR*) to describe these individuals.[1] *Transsexual* is often used interchangeably with *transgender*, especially when referring to adults, but the term also identifies individuals who desire to make their anatomy congruent with their gender identity. Because each term may be offensive to some, it is often best to ask patients how they wish their condition to be called.

In general, *gender* refers to the psychological and societal aspects of being male or female and *sex* refers to the physical aspects. *Gender identity* refers to one's inherent sense of being male or female, regardless of anatomic makeup, and it should not be confused with sexual orientation, which refers to the individuals to whom one is sexually or romantically attracted (ie, to one's heterosexuality, homosexuality, or bisexuality). *Gender dysphoria* refers to the discomfort individuals experience with their biological sex and/or with the gender role assigned to it. *Male-to-female (MTF)* and *female-to-male (FTM)*, terms that capture the social and physical transitions, have been supplanted in the transgender community with *affirmed female* or *trans-woman* and *affirmed male* or *trans-man*, terms that reflect the belief that the brain (or soul) has always known the transgender individual's gender identity.

### ETIOLOGY

Gender identity disorder does not result from a dysfunctional family system, childhood abuse or trauma, or an emotional disorder. However, the debate continues about whether GID should continue to be considered a psychiatric disorder and included in the next edition of the *DSM*. Although no known anatomical or biochemical disorders exist in transgender individuals, some evidence suggests a biological explanation for transgenderism. For a review of the potential impact of hormones on gender identity, see Gooren.[2] A recent study conducted by Hare et al[3] found a possible genetic link for affirmed females.

## PSYCHOLOGICAL CONSIDERATIONS

Prior to receiving a medical intervention, many transgender adolescents are considerably depressed, anxious, or both. Many engage in self-harming behavior and report suicidal ideation and attempts.[4] They often exhibit low self-esteem and a lack of self-worth and report being socially isolated or bullied by peers and adults. Psychological problems typically intensify when transgender children reach puberty, at which point they cannot escape the reality of their biological sex, which is at odds with their gender identity. Although there are cases of comorbid psychiatric disorders (eg, depression, anxiety), these psychological symptoms are often a result of the discomfort transgender individuals feel in their own bodies and the social rejection they experience. It is common for these symptoms to decrease and even disappear after the adolescent begins a social or physical transition. Diagnoses of major disorders, especially mood disorders (eg, major depressive disorder, bipolar disorder) should therefore be re-evaluated.

Most adolescents seeking treatment have experienced gender dysphoria from an early age. Some report not having the courage to express this discomfort openly until later because of shame, embarrassment, or fear of others' reactions. A subset of transgender adolescents does not report gender dysphoria in early childhood. This atypical gender development should be evaluated carefully, but it does not preclude consideration of medical treatment. Bradley and Zucker[5] noted that preadolescent children with GID are likely to "desist" from a transgender identity as they enter adolescence; most go on to identify as gay or lesbian. Adolescents who present with persistent GID from childhood are more likely to be transgender in adolescence and adulthood.[6]

### PRESENTATION OF TRANSGENDER YOUTH

Transgender adolescents often appear androgynous, but those who have already socially transitioned may present convincingly as the other gender, wearing clothes more appropriate for the other sex, including underwear. Biological females may present with tightly bound breasts, and/or multiple layers to hide breasts, and a short haircut. Biological males may present with long hair and may have folded their genitalia to hide or avoid contact with their phallus or testicles. The further into puberty, the more difficult it is for an individual to "pass" as the desired gender without the help of a medical intervention.

**RECOMMENDED ASSESSMENT**

The Amsterdam Gender Clinic for Adolescents and Children, Free University Medical Center, has developed a protocol for evaluating and treating adolescents with gender dysphoria now being followed or adapted in several countries, including the United States, Belgium, Norway, and several provinces in Canada.[7] The protocol follows the recommended procedure outlined in the *Standards of Care* of the World Professional Association of Transgender Health (WPATH),[8] formerly known as the "Harry Benjamin Society Standards."

Initial assessment requires the involvement of a child/adolescent mental health professional. Child/adolescent psychiatrists, psychologists, and social workers have not necessarily had training or experience with issues related to transgenderism, nor are many mental health professionals who specialize in transgender issues for adults appropriate for adolescents. Thus, the mental health provider should be trained in child/adolescent development, gender identity development, and the recommended best practices for treating transgender youth. This relationship will help patients and their families clarify whether the patient is transgender, a process that may require many sessions over the course of multiple months or even years. Throughout the process, the mental health professional can encourage patients and families to understand and accept behaviors that fall outside cultural norms for biologic sex, emphasizing that gender nonconformance is possible without necessarily having to alter one's gender identity or body. The therapist can also help families advocate for their children in school and in the community, writing letters of support and advising school counselors.

If it is determined that the preadolescent or adolescent fulfills the *DSM-IV-TR* criteria for GID, the mental health provider's role shifts to supporting the patient and family in deciding whether a formal social and/or physical transition is in the patient's best interest. Ideally, the mental health professional connects the family with a comprehensive, interdisciplinary clinic to provide further evaluation. The importance of a long-term relationship with a qualified and supportive mental health professional cannot be overstated.

The initial evaluation in an interdisciplinary medical clinic is usually completed by a psychologist and includes the following:

- A comprehensive clinical interview with the adolescent and parent(s) together and individually to obtain extensive information about the following: (a) adolescent's gender identity development, (b) psychosexual functioning, (c) current wishes regarding medical interventions, (d) body image concerns, (e) mental health history and current status, (f) information about the family system, psychiatric history, and support, (g) school/educational information, and (h) social history/peer relationships.
- A battery of measures to formally assess the adolescent's gender identity.
- A battery of measures to formally assess the adolescent's psychological functioning.

This evaluation aims to determine whether the following 4 key criteria are met:

- Fulfillment of the *DSM-IV-TR* criteria for a GID diagnosis.
- The absence of any underlying, untreated psychiatric disorders.
- Agreement to continue participating in ongoing, supportive psychotherapy.
- The presence of a supportive family system.

If the criteria are met, the patient should be referred to a pediatric endocrinologist or adolescent medicine specialist for the next part of the evaluation to determine if the patient is a candidate for medical intervention.

## MEDICAL INTERVENTION

In the United States, parental approval for medical intervention is necessary for patients under 18 years of age unless the patient meets the legal standards of an emancipated minor. The age of informed consent may differ in other countries. The percentage of gender dysphoric children who ultimately pursue a medical intervention is unknown. There is variability among gender dysphoric adolescents regarding the medical intervention they wish to pursue.[9] Patients may be ambivalent about receiving medical intervention at the outset but may later change their mind, or they may question their gender identity but not request medical intervention. Some may experience gender concerns in conjunction with a coexisting condition, such as a pervasive developmental disorder, which requires more extensive evaluation. The transgender adolescent experiences a state of undesired and seemingly precocious puberty. The reaction to the onset of puberty is an important diagnostic tool. Transgender youth are often so distressed by physical changes that they are at risk for self-harm, including suicide. If breast budding or increased spontaneous erections are not perceived by the patient as noxious, the diagnosis of transgenderism should be questioned.

Given that specialists in adolescent medicine incorporate all aspects of patient care into a physical, social, educational, psychological, and sexual developmental model, they are uniquely positioned to guide and treat the gender dysphoric patient who expresses cross-gender feelings and the transgender patient who qualifies for medical intervention. Although the transgender population may be new to physicians who care for adolescents, the treatment itself involves familiar hormonal therapy. Gonadotropin-releasing hormone analogues are now the intervention of choice in selected Tanner stage 2 transgender youth, according to the Endocrine Society guidelines.[10] They are used routinely to treat central precocious puberty (CPP) and endometriosis; sex hormones are used routinely to offset medical deficiencies caused by cancer and other conditions. If a physician does not feel comfortable treating, rather than put the patient off indefinitely, the patient should be referred to another physician or center. A growing number of young pediatric endocrinologists are becoming familiar with treatment protocols for transgender youth, and the number of specialized centers is increasing.

Genetic females at Tanner stage 2 breast development (usually age 10–12 years) and Tanner stage 2 males with testicular volumes 4 to 6 cc (usually age 12–14 years) are potential candidates for fully reversible intervention using GnRH analogues to suppress further puberty.[11,12] By Tanner 2 the patient has experienced transient rises in sex steroids. Gonadotropin-releasing hormone analogue treatment prolongs the diagnostic phase similar to the real-life experience of living in the affirmed gender.[12,13] Pubertal suppression provides time for the patient to continue meeting with his or her psychotherapist without the intense distress caused by the physical effects of puberty to determine whether cross-gender identity is persistent and whether a full physical transition is ultimately in his or her best interest. This intervention also allows the clinician to assess how the adolescent functions when unwanted secondary sex characteristics are suppressed. If prior psychological distress decreases significantly, the source of distress likely can be attributed to gender dysphoria. Finally, delaying puberty allows for a more natural physical transition to the other gender at a later time, as the individual's body remains in a neutral, early pubertal state. If the patient decides *not* to transition to the opposite sex, pubertal suppression can be discontinued, genetic puberty will resume,[14] and the patient will inevitably attain full maturation.

Patients taking puberty-blocking drugs who choose to continue with medical intervention, as well as patients who have completed or nearly completed puberty, may be candidates for cross-sex hormone therapy if there are no contraindications. Parents and the patient should be aware of the effects and side effects of cross-sex hormones.[15,16] Cross-sex hormone therapy (estrogen or testosterone) has irreversible effects: estrogen diminishes sperm production in males, and testosterone causes females to stop ovulating and menstruating. As with all sex hormone addition or substitution therapy, patients should be closely monitored for side effects. Regrettably, many transgender adolescents, marginalized by their families and victimized in schools, seek relief by running away from home and dropping out of school. Separated from their families, they no longer have access to health care and on the streets, sex steroids are easily available. Needle-sharing when using these steroids poses life-threatening risks and medical intervention is rarely sought. Street life may result in involvement in criminal activity, including the sex industry, for survival.

## FULLY REVERSIBLE PUBERTAL SUPPRESSION WITH GnRH ANALOGUES

Gonadotropin-releasing hormone analogues suppress gonadotropin release and, thereby, gonadal testosterone or estrogen. They arrest puberty and cause breast and testicular regression while allowing linear growth and bone mineral density accretion at a prepubertal rate.[7] Virtually all external physical differences between the sexes, with the exception of genitalia, can be eliminated. Genotypic females who are treated in earliest puberty with the GnRH analogue will not need mammoplasties and will not menstruate, and they will gain a more normative masculine height and bone structure. Genotypic males treated with the GnRH analogue will not need electrolysis, will not develop a deepened voice or Adam's apple, and will not experience virilization of the facial bones; and they will develop a more typically feminine bone structure, including smaller hands and feet, and a more normative female height. A long duration of GnRH analogue use beginning at Tanner stage 2 does not render patients osteopenic or dwarfed, as once feared. Patients in the Amsterdam study grew at a pubertal rate while retaining potential for epiphyseal growth. Bone mineral density also progressed at a prepubertal rate but normalized 2 years after initiation of cross-sex steroids.[7] In the United States, CPP is the only US Food and Drug Administration (FDA) indication for GnRH analogue use in children; any other use is considered "off-label" (Table 51-1 and Box 51-1). The coauthor (NPS) has used these medicines for off-label diagnoses and has used off-label medications for transgender youth for more than a decade.

## PARTIALLY REVERSIBLE THERAPY WITH CROSS-SEX HORMONES

Clinical judgment is necessary to determine the age at which to administer cross-sex hormone therapy. The

**Table 51-1**

**Hormonal Treatment for Pubertal Suppression**

| *Drug* | *Dose* | *Pros* | *Cons* |
|---|---|---|---|
| **FDA-approved GnRH analogues for pediatric use** | | | |
| Leuprolide | 11.25–15 mg IM q28 days<br>q3–4 month preparations may be effective but require closer monitoring of LH, FSH, and sex steroids. | 30-yr successful history of use in central precocious puberty including successful bone density[17] and fertility after years of use[18] | May take 3–4 months to suppress LH and FSH following initial agonist action, which transiently increases sex steroids and may initiate/perpetuate menses;[19,20] painful injection, occasionally causing sterile abscesses<br>Must check efficacy q3–4 months: draw LH/FSH with estradiol or testosterone level 45 minutes postinjection<br>15 mg q28 days may not suppress; may need to increase frequency to q21days |
| Nafarelin | 2 sprays (200 μg/spray) each nostril bid. | Ease of use, painless; a 50% dose may work | Absorption variability, especially with nasal congestion |
| Histrelin implant[21] | Placed via tiny subcutaneous incision in medial surface of upper arm, secretes drug for a year | Ease of care after insertion<br>Powerful: an agonist for <14 days then profoundly suppressive<br>Drug is not new—just a new delivery system | Implant must be replaced annually<br>No long-term data on product |
| **Non-FDA approved GnRH analogues (no option for insurance coverage in the US)** | | | |
| Triptorelin (commonly used in Europe) | 3.75 mg IM repeated 14 days later, then q28 days | Most-studied analogue in transgender adolescents (used in Netherlands)[7] | Not available in US; may be ordered from Canada |
| **Other options to suppress puberty, if GnRH analogue not obtainable** | | | |
| Medroxyprogesterone | High daily dose (40–80 mg po qd) or via depot injection (Depo Provera IM q3 months) to suppress gonadotropins | Inexpensive, long history of use (the only available treatment for CPP before replaced by GnRH analogues in the 1970s)<br>Often suppresses menarche | Growth suppression, lower bone mineral density (BMD)[22,23]<br>Potential adrenal suppression, hypertension, Cushing appearance, fluid retention, weight gain, alopecia, acne |
| Combination | Tamoxifen[24]<br>20 mg qd to block estrogen at receptor + norethindrone<br>0.35 mg qd, a daily progestin, to suppress gonadotropins | Suppresses breast development and delays menarche<br>Inexpensive | Useful for only 12–18 months |

Note: All GnRH analogues are extremely expensive (at least $350 per month, rarely covered by insurance).
CPP, central precocious puberty; FDA, Food and Drug Administration; FSH, follicular stimulating hormone; LH, luteinizing hormone.

WPATH Standards of Care, currently under revision, now recommend consideration of hormones at age 16. However, if a genotypic male is destined to be extremely tall for a woman, the clinician may want to individualize the timing of estrogen via earlier use to close epiphyses (see Eugster et al[24] for similar treatment of precocious puberty).[7] If a genotypic female is destined to be extremely short, the clinician may want to promote virilization via 5 mg of

**Box 51-1**

***Tests to be Done in Conjunction with Pubertal Suppression***

Pre-suppression

- Bone age
- Accurate height/weight/body proportions (span, upper:lower segment)
- BMD of hip and spine
- Hgb
- Fasting lipids
- AM: LH, FSH, estradiol/testosterone, AST, ALT, prolactin (genetic females)

Mid/Postsuppression

- Annual bone age and BMD
- LH
- FSH
- Estradiol or testosterone levels every 3-4 mos

ALT, alanine aminotransferase; AST, aspartate aminotransferase; BMD, bone mineral density; FSH, follicular stimulating hormone; LH, luteinizing hormone

daily oral oxandrolone, a nonaromatizable androgen that keeps growth plates open (see Nilsson et al[25] for similar treatment of Turner syndrome).

In the Dutch protocol, GnRH analogues are used continuously to suppress endogenous sex hormones whereas cross-sex hormones are slowly increased in a manner comparable to normal puberty. Analogues are thus maintained until gonadectomy.[7] Although this may be an optimal form of therapy, the cost may be prohibitive in countries where insurance does not cover the drugs.

For physical virilization, testosterone enanthate or cypionate can be initiated at 25 to 50 mg every 2 weeks for a month and then increased to 50 mg weekly, which is a final dose for most affirmed males. Weekly dosing is the key to maintaining stable testosterone levels in the 300 to 500 ng/dl range, which suppresses menses, increases libido, and gradually increases clitoral length. Testosterone patches and gels, although popular with hypogonadal genotypic males, are associated with breakthrough vaginal bleeding in affirmed males with retained ovaries because absorption of these preparations is variable. Few patients will self-administer deep intramuscular dosing weekly, but subcutaneous injections are equally effective and virtually painless. The bottle should be hand-warmed for several minutes and the dose delivered via a 3-cc syringe and 25-gauge 5/8-inch needle, preferably into the lateral buttock (personal written communication from the late John Crawford, MD, January 2004). The site should be rubbed to disperse the injected dose. On weekly therapy, testosterone levels can be drawn at any time. Hemoglobin levels should be checked for polycythemia[26] (>16.5 gm/dl). Blood pressure and acne may increase. Lipids assume a riskier male profile, with lowering of high-density lipoprotein (HDL) cholesterol, and body fat redistributes to the abdominal/visceral male pattern associated with cardiovascular risk.[27]

Virilizing the face and hair of the genotypic female is relatively simple through the use of testosterone, but time is not on the side of the genotypic male who affirms a female identity and has gone to Tanner stage 4 or beyond. The rate of growth and thickness of facial hair can be attenuated with the potassium-sparing diuretic spironolactone due to its mild blockade of the androgen receptor.[28] A dose of 50 to 100 twice a day is adequate, although the effects on nascent facial hairs may not be noted for 3 to 6 months. Patients must be cautioned not to take spironolactone if they have insufficient fluid intake or excess output, lest they become dehydrated and/or hyperkalemic. Treated patients should have AST, ALT, and electrolytes drawn every 3 to 4 months.

Feminization in a mature genotypic male through estrogen poses unique challenges. If the patient is less than Tanner stage 4, estrogen will rapidly close the epiphyses and growth will cease. If GnRH analogue use is ongoing, spironolactone is unnecessary and usual replacement estrogen doses will suffice. However, in the absence of GnRH analogue, estrogen doses 4 to 6 times greater than those required to feminize an agonadal but otherwise normal female are needed to reduce the genotypic male's serum testosterone level to the desired low-adult female range. Although there are many options, including injections and patches, oral 17-beta estradiol has the advantage of low thrombogenic risk and is measurable via most estrogen assays. Daily doses of 4 to 6 mg per day are often required and repeat testosterone levels need to be checked. If the testosterone levels are not suppressed, bothersome erections will persist and breast development will be retarded. There is debate as to whether breast development is enhanced by the addition of progesterone in daily doses of 100 mg of "micronized" progesterone or 5 mg of medroxyprogesterone for 1-2 years.[29,30]

Estrogen-treated affirmed females will have hemoglobins 4 to 5 gm/dl lower than males due to the reduction in secreted testosterone, which stimulates bone marrow red blood cell (RBC) production. They will also develop higher HDLs and a redistribution of body fat from the abdomen to hips and thighs. Testes will shrink and soften. Because thromboembolism is the most serious risk associated with estrogen, patients should be cautioned not to smoke. If more than several days of immobilization are anticipated, estrogen should be stopped 3 weeks previously.

### IRREVERSIBLE THERAPY

The affirmed male presenting with full B-cup breasts with an inframammary fold who requests mammoplasty may require bilateral subcostal incisions with relocation of the nipples. Only a few surgeons perform this procedure. A plastic surgeon skilled in gynecomastia surgery can perform a more aesthetic procedure on a patient with smaller breasts using a single subareolar incision on each side. Breast surgery has been performed in the United States on patients under age 16, but gonadectomy or genital surgery is not offered until the age of legal informed consent, usually 18.[11] All surgeons require letters of approval from the treating physician and all mental health professionals involved with the patient.

### ADDITIONAL CONSIDERATIONS

In order to reach the point of providing medical care for a transgender adolescent, the adolescent must trust and respect the physician and feel comfortable in the health care setting. To that end, the physician should consider the following suggestions:

1. Create safe, private, confidential, respectful environments and relationships.
2. Know what to call the individual, ie, what pronouns to use and whether to use a given name or a name assumed by the adolescent that better reflects his or her true identity.
3. Establish policies and procedures and education programs in the clinic/office setting that all staff should follow with regard to transgender adolescents (eg, avoid the situation in which the physician calls the adolescent Joe, but the nurse calls him Joanne because that is the name in the medical record).
4. Permit the transgender patient to be dressed for the physical examination according to his or her affirmed gender (ie, MTF permitted to wear gowns and underpants; FTM permitted to wear t-shirts (no bra) and underpants).

Helping transgender adolescents express who they are by environment and medical modification is one of the most satisfying interventions that an adolescent's physician can perform; it can be a challenge and the opportunity of a lifetime.

## INTERNET AND PRINT RESOURCES

- Brill S, Pepper R. *The Transgender Child: A Handbook for Families and Professionals*. San Francisco, CA: Cleis Press, Inc; 2008
- Brown ML, Rounsley CA. *True Selves: Understanding Transsexualism*. San Francisco, CA: Jossey-Bass Publishers; 1996
- Ettner R, Monstrey S, Eyler AE (eds.). *Principles of Transgender Medicine and Surgery*. New York, NY: The Haworth Press; 2007
- Gender Identity Resource and Education Society of UK (GIRES): www.gires.org.uk
- Gender Spectrum Education and Training: www.genderspectrum.org
- International Foundation for Gender Education: www.ifge.org
- Parents, Families, and Friends of Lesbians and Gays (PFLAG): community.pflag.org
- Trans Youth Family Allies (TYFA): imatyfa.org
- World Professional Association for Transgender Health (WPATH): www.wpath.org

## REFERENCES

1. American Psychiatric Association. *Diagnostic and Statistical Manual of Mental Disorders,* Fourth Edition, Text Revision (DSM-IV-TR). Washington, DC: APA; 2001

2. Gooren L. The biology of human psychosexual differentiation. *Hormones and Behav.* 2006;50:589–601

3. Hare L, Bernard P, Sanchez FJ, et al. Androgen receptor repeat length polymorphism associated with male-to-female transsexualism. *Biol Psychiatry.* 2009;65(1):93–96

4. Grossman AH, D'Augelli AR. Transgender youth and life-threatening behaviors. *Suicide Life Threat Behav.* 2007;37(5):527–537

5. Bradley SJ, Zucker KJ. Gender identity disorder: a review of the past 10 years. *J Am Acad Child and Adolescent Psych.* 1997;35:872–880

6. Zucker KJ, Bradley SJ. *Gender Identity Disorder and Psychosexual Problems in Children and Adolescents*. New York, NY: Guilford Press; 1995

7. Delemarre-van de Waal HA, Cohen-Kettenis PT. Clinical management of gender identity disorder in adolescents: a protocol on psychological and paediatric endocrinology aspects. *Eur J Endocrinol.* 2006;155(suppl 1):S131–S137

8. Harry Benjamin International Gender Dysphoria Association (HBIGDA). Standards of care for gender identity disorders, sixth version. *J Psych Hum Sexuality.* 2001;13:1

9. De Vries ALC, Cohen-Kettenis PT, Delemarre-van de Wall H, Holman CW, Goldberg J. *Caring for transgender adolescents in BC: suggested guidelines.* 2006. Available at: transhealth.vch.ca/resources/library/tcpdocs/guidelines-adolescent.pdf Accessed January 7, 2009

10. Hembree WC, Cohen-Kettenis P, Delemarre-van de Waal HA, et al. Endocrine treatment of transsexual persons: an Endocrine Society clinical practice guideline. *J Clin Endocrinol Metab*. 2009;94:3132–3154

11. Meyer W, Bockting WO, Cohen-Kettenis P, et al. *The Harry Benjamin International Gender Dysphoria Association's Standards of Care for Gender Identity Disorders*, 6th ed. Available at: wpath.org/Documents2/socv6.pdf. Accessed December 10, 2008

12. Houk CP, Lee PA. The diagnosis and care of transsexual children and adolescents: a pediatric endocrinologist's perspective. *J Pediatr Endocrinol Metab.* 2006;19:103–109

13. Cohen-Kettenis PT, Delemarre-van de Waal HA, Gooren LJG. The treatment of adolescent transsexuals: changing insights. *J Sex Med.* 2008;5:1892–1897

14. Manasco PK, Pescovitz OH, Feuillan PP, et al. Resumption of puberty after long-term luteinizing hormone-releasing hormone agonist treatment of central precocious puberty. *J Clin Endocrinol Metab.* 1988;67:368–372

15. De Sutter P. Reproduction and fertility issues for transpeople. In: Ettner R, Monstrey S, Eyler AE, eds. *Principles of Transgender Medicine and Surgery*. New York, NY: Haworth Press; 2007:209–221

16. De Sutter P. Gender reassignment and assisted reproduction: present and future reproductive options for transsexual people. *Hum Reprod.* 2001;16:612–614

17. Van Der Sluis IM, Boot AM, Krenning EP, Drop SLS, de Muinck Keizer-Schrama SMPF. Longitudinal follow-up of bone density and body composition in children with precocious or early puberty before, during, and after cessation of GnRH agonist therapy. *J Clin Endocrinol Metab.* 2002;87(2):506–512

18. Tanaka T, Niimi H, Matsuo N, et al. Results of long-term follow-up after treatment of central precocious puberty with leuprorelin acetate: evaluation of effectiveness of treatment and recovery of gonadal function. The TAP-144-SR Japanese study group on central precocious puberty. *J Clin Endocrinol Metab.* 2005;90(3):1371–1376

19. Tuvemo T. Treatment of central precocious puberty. *Expert Opin Investig Drugs.* 2006;15:495–505

20. Roth C. Therapeutic potential of GnRH antagonists in the treatment of precocious puberty. *Expert Opin Investig Drugs.* 2002;11:1253–1259

21. Eugster EA, Clarke W, Kletter GB, et al. Efficacy and safety of histrelin subdermal implant in children with central precocious puberty: a multicenter trial. *J Clin Endocrinol Metab.* 2007;92:1697–1704.

22. US Food and Drug Administration. New warning on Depo-Provera contraceptive injection. Available at: www.accessdata.fda.gov/scripts/cdrh/cfdocs/psn/printer.cfm?id=291. Accessed July 22, 2010

23. Scholes D, LaCroix AZ, Ichikawa LE, Barlow WE, Ott SM. Change in bone mineral density among adolescent women using and discontinuing depot medroxyprogesterone acetate contraception. *Arch Pediatr Adolesc Med.* 2005;159(2): 139–144

24. Eugster EA, Rubin SD, Reiter EO, et al. Tamoxifen treatment for precocious puberty in Mccune Albright syndrome: a multicenter trial. *J Pediatr.* 2003;143:60–66

25. Nilsson KO, Albertsson-Wikland K, Alm J, et al. Improved final height in girls with Turner's syndrome treated with growth hormone and oxandrolone. *J Clin Endocrinol Metab.* 1996;81:635–640

26. Alexanian R, Vaughn WK, Ruchelman MW. Erythropoietin excretion in man following androgens. *J Lab Clin Med.* 1967;70(5):777–785

27. Bhasin S, Cunningham GR, Hayes F, et al. Testosterone therapy in adult men with androgen deficiency syndromes. *J Clin Endocrinol Metab.* 2006;91:1995–2010

28. Rose LI, Underwood RH, Newmark SR, Kisch ES, Williams GH. Pathophysiology of spironolactone-induced gynecomastia. *Ann Intern Med.* 1977;87(4):398–403

29. Tangpricha V, Ducharme SH, Barber TW, Chipkin SR. Endocrinological treatment of gender identity disorders. *Endocrine Practice.* 2003;9(1):12–21

30. Gooren LJ, Giltay EJ, Bunck MC. Long-term treatment of transsexuals with cross-sex hormones: extensive personal experience. *J Clin Endocrinol Metab.* 2008;93(1):19–25

# CHAPTER 52

# Contraception

MARGARET MARY POLANECZKY, MD

Despite declines in the rates of teenage sexual activity since the 1980s, most adolescents will have had sexual intercourse by the time they graduate from high school, and each year approximately 75,000 pregnancies occur among teens in the United States. Thus, the provision of contraceptives remains an important component of medical care for the sexually active adolescent.

## ADOLESCENT CONTRACEPTIVE USE

Most sexually active adolescents use birth control. About three fourths of adolescents will use some form of birth control (usually a condom) at first intercourse, and at most recent intercourse, 83% of teen girls and 91% of boys report using some form of contraception.

The most popular form of contraception in teens is the condom, which is used by 66% of sexually active girls and 71% of sexually active boys ages 15 to 19 years at last intercourse. Despite its popularity, condom use can be inconsistent, with only 50% of girls and 71% of boys reporting use every time they had sex. Highly effective hormonal contraception is used at last reported intercourse by 40% of teen girls ages 15 to 19 years, and about 20% will combine a hormonal method with condoms.[1]

Why do some teens use contraception and others do not? The factors are complex, including the context of the relationship and personal attitudes toward contraception and pregnancy. Young women tend to use effective contraception more often the longer they are in a relationship, but less often if that relationship is perceived as romantic rather than just with someone whom they like. Contraceptive use is lower among girls in sexual relationships with males whom they meet outside school, family, or friends, and in relationships with violent partners. Girls who discuss birth control with their partners before having sex and who use hormonal contraception are more likely to continue to use contraception. Interestingly, contraceptive use is lowest among young women who hold ambivalent attitudes about pregnancy (as opposed to being for or against this idea), and, not surprisingly, highest among those who hold favorable attitudes about contraception. Also not surprising is that adolescents who do well academically and anticipate future successes are more likely to use effective contraception.

Programs that provide clear messages about abstinence, sex, and contraceptive use are associated with more consistent condom and contraceptive use among teen participants, as are those programs that actually provide contraception. Abstinence-only education has little to no impact on delaying sexual activity or number of sexual partners.[2-3] A good parent–child relationship that includes discussion about sex and contraception may delay the onset of sexual activity and increase the use of effective contraception when sexual activity does occur. Supporting this is the fact that most adolescents attending family planning clinics overwhelmingly report good relationships with their parents and parental knowledge about their use of contraception.

There are no data to support the notion that providing contraception to adolescents encourages sexual activity, or conversely, that denying contraception prevents or delays sexual activity. Teens living in countries with easy access to contraception have sexual activity rates no higher than those in the United States, but they are more likely to use contraception and less likely to become pregnant. Data from school-based clinics show that the provision of referral for contraceptive services does not increase rates of sexual activity among students in those schools.

The most important protective factor against teen pregnancy is a high-quality parent–child relationship, not access to contraception. Teens who report good relationships with their parents are far more likely to delay sexual activity and are more likely to use contraception when they do become sexually active.[4]

## LEGAL CONSIDERATIONS

There is considerable variability in state laws regarding provision of contraceptive services to minors. As of 2011, 21 states and the District of Columbia allow all minors to access these services, 25 states permit minors who meet certain circumstances (eg, being married or a parent, with a physician referral or with health hazards related to pregnancy), and 4 states have no policy on contraceptive services for minors.

## CONTRACEPTIVE EFFICACY

Contraceptive method efficacy is defined as the percentage of users experiencing a pregnancy within the first year of use. Failure rates are defined as occurring either with perfect use (method failures) or typical use (user failures *plus* method failures) (Table 52-1).

For most contraceptive methods, typical use efficacy rates are lower than perfect use rates, due to nonadherence and misuse. Factors associated with contraceptive nonadherence among adolescents include lack of parental involvement in contraception, low self-esteem and self-efficacy, perceived and real side effects, low educational goals, and inner-city versus suburban residency. Teenage girls whose dysmenorrhea decreases as a result of using hormonal contraception are more likely to continue their method and be adherent with its use.[5] Longer-acting methods may have better efficacy among adolescents because they are less dependent on user behavior. However, the need for repeat visits or refills may still pose a problem for teens who use these methods.

### BALANCING CONTRACEPTIVE EFFICACY AND SEXUALLY TRANSMITTED INFECTION PROTECTION

The ideal contraceptive would be 100% effective at preventing pregnancy and also provide protection against sexually transmitted infections (STIs). Unfortunately, that perfect method does not exist. Condoms, although highly effective against STIs, have typical failure rates of 15%, indicating that typical use is not perfect. In addition, among teens who report themselves as condom users, only about half use condoms consistently, indicating that they remain at significant risk for both pregnancy and STIs.

Although the combined use of condoms and spermicide can be close to 100% effective at preventing pregnancy, spermicide use is associated with higher rates of genital ulcers and HIV acquisition in exposed users. Hormonal methods, which can come close to 100% efficacy with perfect use, provide no protection against the acquisition of STIs, and may actually increase the risk of acquiring certain infections such as chlamydia and HIV when exposed.[6] There has been renewed interest in the diaphragm and cervical cap as methods that may provide dual protection against STIs and HIV.

The current recommendation is to combine barrier and hormonal methods, the so-called "belt plus suspenders" or dual-method approach. Dual use is becoming increasingly popular. In fact, it is used more often by teens than adults, even though, unfortunately, it is still quite uncommon. Twenty percent of teenage girls overall who used birth control the last time they had

**Table 52-1**

**Contraceptive Efficacy**

| | ***% of Women Experiencing an Unintended Pregnancy within the First Year of Use*** | |
|---|---|---|
| ***Method*** | ***Typical Use*** | ***Perfect Use*** |
| No method | 85 | 85 |
| Spermicides | 28 | 18 |
| Fertility awareness-based methods | 24 | |
| Standard Days method | | 5 |
| TwoDay method | | 4 |
| Ovulation method | | 3 |
| Symptothermal method | | 0.4 |
| Withdrawal | 22 | 4 |
| Sponge | | |
| Parous women | 24 | 20 |
| Nulliparous women | 12 | 9 |
| Condom | | |
| Female | 21 | 5 |
| Male | 18 | 2 |
| Diaphragm | 12 | 6 |
| Combined pill and progestin-only pill | 9 | 0.3 |
| Evra patch | 9 | 0.3 |
| NuvaRing | 9 | 0.3 |
| Depo-Provera | 6 | 0.2 |
| Intrauterine contraceptives | | |
| ParaGard (copper T) | 0.8 | 0.6 |
| Mirena (LNG) | 0.2 | 0.2 |
| Implanon | 0.05 | 0.05 |
| Female sterilization | 0.5 | 0.5 |
| Male sterilization | 0.15 | 0.10 |

Source: Trussell J. Contraceptive efficacy. In: Hatcher RA, Trussell J, Nelson AL, Cates W, Kowal D (eds). *Contraceptive Technology: Twentieth Revised Edition*. New York, NY: Ardent Media; 2011.

sex report using this strategy for protection against both pregnancy and STIs. Dual-method use is much lower among sexually active high school students, with rates of about 8%.[1,7]

Although the concern remains that hormonal contraceptive use leads to decreased condom use, relationship factors appear to play a more important role than the method itself in the decision to use or not use a condom.[8]

## HORMONAL CONTRACEPTION—GENERAL PRINCIPLES

Hormonal contraceptives remain the most effective methods for adolescents. All methods contain a progestin with or without estrogen, and are available as pills, patches, vaginal rings, subdermal implants, and injections. Each method has its risks and benefits, although long-acting methods in general will be more effective than pills due to guaranteed compliance. Continuation rates, however, for all but implants are about the same.

### CHOICE OF HORMONAL CONTRACEPTIVE METHOD

Any healthy, sexually active adolescent female is a candidate for hormonal contraception. Younger postmenarchal adolescents can safely use estrogen-containing and low-dose progestin-only methods without adverse effects on growth or maturation of the hypothalamic-pituitary-ovarian axis (Table 52-2). When considering the use of Depo-Provera in the younger adolescent, its effects on bone mass need to be considered and weighed against the risks of pregnancy and other potential benefits. Many adolescents with chronic medical conditions can safely use hormonal contraception (Box 52-1).

Counseling is important to determine which method is best. Issues to be considered include prior contraceptive experience, previous side effects, fears and concerns, the need for privacy, cost, availability, potential partner issues, other medical issues, maturity, presence of menstrual abnormalities, and the potential need for other nongynecologic benefits of hormonal contraception.

When considering pill use, try to have the adolescent realistically assess her own ability to remember to take a pill every day, a task that is not easy, even for adults. Explore the use of cell phone, e-mail, or instant message reminders, or enlist the partner or parent to assist with daily adherence. Review strategies for dealing with missed pills and refills. Good candidates for oral contraceptives are those adolescents who believe that they can reliably take a pill every day, particularly those who have taken other daily medications successfully in the past. Those who have trouble swallowing pills may want to try a chewable contraceptive (Ovcon), or consider the patch, ring, implant, or injectable.

**Table 52-2**

**Choosing a Hormonal Method**

| *Issue* | *Options* |
|---|---|
| Contraindication to estrogen | Progesterone-only pill, Depo-Provera, implant |
| Poor compliance with pills | Ring, patch, implant, Depo-Provera |
| Estrogen-related side effects (nausea, breast tenderness) | 10 μg/20 μg pill, contraceptive vaginal ring, progestin-only pill, Depo-Provera, implant |
| Migraine headaches | 10 μg/20 μg monophasic pill, contraceptive vaginal ring |
| Menstrual migraines (worsening of migraine headaches at the time of menses) | 10 μg/20 μg pill with shortened placebo interval, any other 10 μg/20 μg monophasic pill or NuvaRing, either continuously (so no days off) or with the estrogen patch on pill-free days |
| Minimization of androgenic side effects and lipid effects | Any pill containing a third-generation progestin, drospirenone, low-dose norethindrone, or ethynodiol diacetate NuvaRing, patch |
| Premenstrual syndrome | Ethinyl estradiol/drospirenone |
| Breakthrough bleeding | Monophasic or triphasic 30- to 35-μg pill<br>Levonorgestrel, pill, NuvaRing, or patch |

**Box 52-1**

***Use of Hormonal Contraceptives in Adolescents with Special Medical Conditions***

Use of hormonal contraceptives is generally safe, even in adolescents with chronic medical conditions.

- Diabetes: Hormonal contraception is safe for adolescent patients with well-controlled diabetes who have no end-organ or vascular involvement.
- Postpartum: Estrogen-containing methods should be avoided during the first 2–3 weeks postpartum because this period is associated with increased risk of thrombosis.
- Breast-feeding: Consider progestin-only methods, which are lactogenic. After breast-feeding is well established, estrogen-containing combination methods can be used.
- Hypertension: If blood pressure is well controlled, estrogen-containing contraceptives are appropriate with careful monitoring. If hypertension occurs, consider progestin-only pills (POPs) or other progestin-only methods.
- Migraine headache: Avoid estrogen use in migraineurs with focal neurologic symptoms. For adolescents who have migraines without neurologic symptoms, monitor for increasing frequency of headaches and discontinue if headaches increase in frequency or intensity. Consider a monophasic pill or shortened placebo interval pill. Stress adherence with daily pill-taking to avoid estrogen withdrawal headaches, and consider the longer-acting combination methods if this is problematic. POPs and progestin-only hormonal methods may also exacerbate migraines.
- Hyperlipidemia: Consider a third-generation combined oral contraceptive (potentially less effect on lipids). Monitor closely.
- Biliary tract disease: Active disease contraindicates the use of estrogen-containing contraceptives. History of prior cholecystectomy does not.
- Hepatitis: Estrogen-containing contraceptives are contraindicated in active liver disease, but are safe in chronic hepatitis B or C carriers if liver enzymes are normal.
- Sickle cell anemia: Both estrogen-containing and progestin-only methods are safe, and any formulation can be used. The mechanism for ischemia in sickle cell anemia is not related to abnormalities in the thrombotic cascade. Consider Depo-Provera for these patients because it has been shown to stabilize the red cell membrane and lead to decreased frequency of sickle crises. This effect has not been shown with other progestins.
- Seizure disorders: Adolescents with seizure disorders can safely use hormonal contraceptives. However, interactions with antiseizure medication must be considered, and higher doses of oral contraceptives may be needed to ensure adequate contraceptive effect.

Sources: Gittes EB, Strickland JL. Contraceptive choices for medically ill adolescents. *Adolesc Med Clin*. 2005;16(3):635–644; Curtis KM, Chrisman CE, Peterson HB. The WHO Programme for Mapping Best Practices in Reproductive Health. Contraception for Women in Selected Circumstances 2002. *Obstet Gynecol.* 2002;99:1100–1112.

In considering progestin-only methods, the patient's tolerance for unpredictable or irregular bleeding needs to be frankly discussed, as well as weighed against the potential benefits of these methods and her previous experiences with oral contraceptives.

For patch users, review what to do if the patch comes off, if the weekly day for patch change is forgotten or missed, or the day for starting a new month is missed. Again, having a system for reminders is worth considering.

Ring users need to be informed as to what to do when they have their menses, what they will do with their ring when having intercourse, and what to do if the ring falls out.

## BODY WEIGHT AND HORMONAL CONTRACEPTION

Several studies in the past decade have suggested that hormonal contraceptive efficacy may be lower in overweight women; however, the data are insufficient to make any broad conclusions. In a retrospective study of pill users, failure rates ranged from 5.2 per 100 person-years of use for 30-μg pills to 6.8 per 100 person-years for 20-μg pills.[9] The data are insufficient to recommend any changes in prescribing patterns at this point in time. However, until better data are available, there is no harm in instructing heavier teens to use a back up method if they miss a pill.

For the contraceptive patch, it has been shown that for women weighing more than 90 kg, the failure rate is significantly higher, about 6 per 100.[10] No data regarding weight and efficacy have been reported for the ring. Implanon is effective in women weighing as much as 100 kg, but has not been studied in women over this weight, and levels of etonogestrel (ENG) are known to be inversely related to body weight. Depo-Provera efficacy is not affected by body weight, but this method is associated with weight gain.

It is important to remember that hormonal methods remain superior to barrier methods in preventing pregnancy in teens of all weights, and that ultimately, it is adherence that has the biggest impact on pregnancy rates.

## INITIATING HORMONAL CONTRACEPTION

Before initiating hormonal contraception, a detailed medical and family history should be taken. Breast and pelvic examinations can be performed at that time as well, or deferred to a later time if the patient requests it and the clinician believes that it is appropriate. It is not mandatory to perform a pelvic examination on a girl prior to beginning hormonal contraception. If STI screening is necessary, urine-based testing can be performed if the pelvic exam is deferred. Urine pregnancy testing, if available, can be useful in teens already having unprotected sex.[11]

Typically, hormonal contraceptive methods are started on or close to the first day of the menses. Pill, patch, and ring users can be given a prescription or their medication, and instructed to start their method on the first day of the subsequent menses. Injection and implant users are instructed to return as close to the onset of their next menses as possible to begin their method. By starting at the onset of the menses, efficacy begins almost immediately, and a nonpregnant state is generally assured if the menses is normal and on time. If for any reason, the menses is not normal, advise the teen to undergo pregnancy testing before starting her method.

The Sunday start method allows for menses-free weekends during pill, patch, or ring use. Users start their method on the first Sunday after the onset of the menses, even if still bleeding. If the menses begins on Sunday, she starts that same day. Condoms or spermicide should be used as a back up method if intercourse occurs anytime within the first week of use. Sunday start may be confusing for some teens, and could risk pregnancy if a back up method is not used as instructed. The Quick Start method of contraceptive initiation allows teens with a normal menstrual history and a negative pregnancy test to begin the pill, patch, or ring on the same day as their office visit, regardless of where they are in their menstrual cycles (Figure 52-1). If unprotected intercourse has recently occurred, emergency contraception can be given first.

Quick Start may hold distinct advantages over other methods of initiation, given that up to one fourth of adolescents may fail to start hormonal contraception on their own after leaving the office with a prescription. It has been shown that adolescents who use the Quick Start method have higher rates of method continuation at 3 months compared with those using traditional start methods. The side effect profile, efficacy, and safety are similar to the Sunday start method, and bleeding patterns are comparable.[12–13] Adolescents using the Quick Start method should be advised to return for pregnancy testing if their first menses is late, and pregnancy may be diagnosed at that point without concerns about teratogenicity. Reliable use of back up contraception during the first week of hormone use practically eliminates even this risk.

Teens initiating long-acting contraceptives such as Depo-Provera (DPMA) or implants may also be considered candidates for immediate initiation of their method. In these teens, however, a follow-up pregnancy test is used to confirm absence of pregnancy at 3 weeks after method initiation. Alternatively, a Quick Start bridge method such as oral contraceptives or the vaginal ring can be given until either the menses occurs or a nonpregnant state is assured and the long-acting method started. Users of bridge methods, however, will have higher rates of pregnancy than those who immediately initiate Depo-Provera.

Adolescents who are switching between highly effective hormonal methods, and who are adherent to these methods may start their new method any day in the cycle. However, they should be advised that this may alter the date their menses occurs according to the new method cycle they are starting.

Postpartum adolescents who are breastfeeding can start progestin-only methods immediately after giving birth because these methods do not impart an increased risk of clotting and are lactogenic. Use of estrogen-containing methods should be avoided until at least 6 to 8 weeks postpartum because there is an elevated risk for clotting during this time. Adolescents who are not breastfeeding and who have not begun effective contraception by 6 weeks postpartum may have ovulated, and should adhere to the Quick Start or same-day start methods. Post-abortion adolescents may start their hormonal method immediately after their abortion. Diaphragms or cervical caps may be fitted at any time in the cycle or after a first-trimester abortion, but should be delayed for 6 weeks postpartum or after second-trimester abortion.[14]

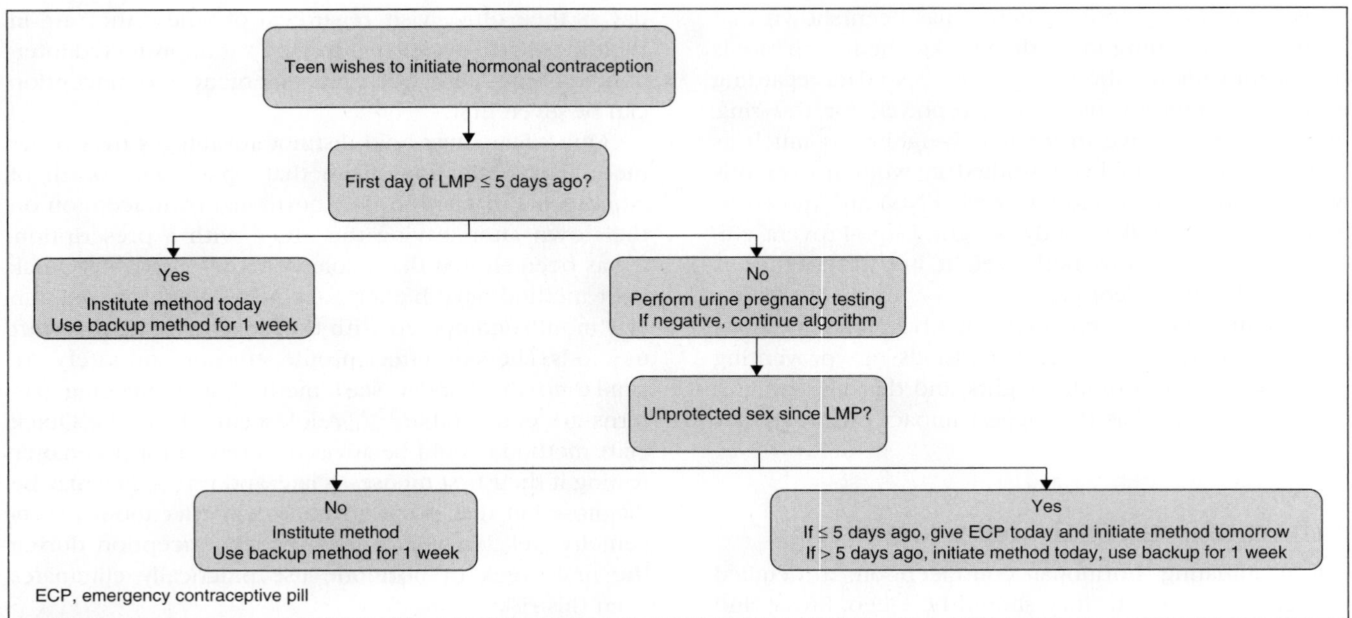


**FIGURE 52-1** Quick Start algorithm for initiating hormonal contraception. This algorithm is best used for teens initiating the pill, patch, or ring. For teens who want to start implants and injectables, and who have had unprotected sex since their last menstrual period (LMP), consider giving the pill, patch, or ring according to the Quick Start algorithm as a bridge method. Have patient return with first menses to initiate longer-acting method. Teens who have had unprotected sex since their LMP and have a negative urine pregnancy test may still be pregnant, and should be advised to return for pregnancy testing if their menses does not occur when expected. (Adapted from Hatcher RA, Zieman M, Cwiak C, Darney PD, Crenin MD, Stosur HR. *A Pocket Guide to Managing Contraception.* Tiger, GA: Bridging the Gap Foundation; 2005:135; and from Lesnewski R, Prine L. Initiating hormonal contraception. *Am Family Physician.* 2006;74:105–112.)

## ORAL CONTRACEPTIVES

Of the 3.1 million teenage women who use contraceptives, 53% rely on the pill.[15] Newer, longer-acting methods such as injectables, patches, and vaginal rings are becoming increasingly popular choices, but for the moment, appear to be supplanting pill use rather than increasing hormonal contraceptive use overall.

Oral contraceptives are safe and highly effective at preventing pregnancy.[16] Oral contraceptives are either combination pills (combined oral contraceptives [COCs]), containing both estrogen and progestin, or progestin-only pills (POPs). Most adolescents use combination pills. Oral contraceptives prevent pregnancy primarily by inhibition of ovulation (an effect of the progestin and estrogen components of the pill) and thickening of the cervical mucus (a progestin effect). The progestin component of the pill is responsible for most of the pill's contraceptive effect. The addition of estrogen adds efficacy by increasing the inhibition of ovulation and has an important role in providing regular bleeding pattern throughout the cycle. Secondary effects of the pill, such as thinning and deciduation of the endometrium and impairment of tubal motility, are likely to be less important, given the profound effects on ovulation and cervical mucus.[17]

### ORAL CONTRACEPTIVE FORMULATIONS

All currently marketed COCs contain either ethinyl estradiol (EE) or mestranol as the estrogen component, in doses typically ranging from 20 to 40 µg. One higher-dose pill containing 50 µg of mestranol is available, but it is used only for treatment of dysfunctional bleeding and when higher estrogen doses are needed due to interaction with other medications. All currently marketed COCs have similar efficacy.[18]

Progestins may be classified by generations (the order in which they were introduced into the marketplace), by steroid backbone (gonane or estrane), or by binding affinity to androgen receptors (androgenicity). In a recent Cochrane Review, second- and third-generation progestins were shown to be more acceptable than first-generation progestins (Table 52-3).

**Table 52-3**

**Progestins in Oral Contraceptives**

| *Progestin Grouping* | *Progestin* | *Relative Androgenicity*[a] |
|---|---|---|
| First generation (estrane) | Norethindrone (acetate) | ++ |
| | Ethynodiol diacetate | ++ |
| Second generation (gonane) | Levonorgestrel | +++ |
| | Norgestrel | +++ |
| Third generation (gonane) | Desogestrel | + |
| | Norgestimate | + |
| Other | Drospirenone | – |

[a]Refers to the relative androgenicity of the progestin component alone and in vitro. Androgenicity is defined as the relative binding affinity of a given progestin for testosterone receptors in an in vitro binding assay. It does *not* relate to overall androgenicity of the pill containing that progestin, and does not take into account changes in androgenicity with increasing or decreasing doses of progestin.

Combined oral contraceptives are available in multiple formulations (Table 52-4) and may be classified as monophasic (fixed dose throughout the cycle), biphasic, or triphasic (variable dose throughout the cycle). Pills were initially phased in order to decrease the overall monthly hormonal dose and the incidence of side effects without impacting efficacy. A recent Cochrane Review indicated no important differences among monophasic, biphasic, or triphasic preparations, although levonorgestrel preparations were associated with superior cycle control compared to norethindrone-containing preparations.[19–21]

Shortened placebo intervals have been recently formulated to reduce the incidence of estrogen withdrawal symptoms such as headache, and to minimize ovarian follicular recruitment during the placebo interval, theoretically improving efficacy in typical users and lessening the incidence of ovarian cysts. Pills are also available with every-3-month cycling (Seasonale, Seasonique), as well as a pill designed to completely eliminate withdrawal menstrual flow (Lybrel). These pills may be helpful in adolescents with severe menstrual symptoms that do not respond to standard dosing regimens. Any pill, however, can be taken in this manner.

Generic substitutions are available for most older pills, and although theoretical concerns exist that lower-dose generics may have less EE than studied, no data exist that

**Table 52-4**

**Oral Contraceptive Formulations**

| *Brand Name* | *Estrogen* | *Progestin* | *Cycle* | *Other* |
|---|---|---|---|---|
| Lo-Loestrin FE | 10 μg EE × 24<br>10 μg EE × 2 | 1 mg NA × 24 | Monophasic<br>Shortened Placebo | |
| Loestrin 1/20<br>Junel 1/20 | 20 μg EE | 1 mg NA | Monophasic | |
| Alesse<br>Levlite | 20 μg EE | 0.1 mg LNG | Monophasic | |
| Loestrin 24Fe | 20 μg EE | 1 mg NA | Monophasic<br>Shortened placebo | |
| Yaz | 20 μg EE | 3.0 mg DRSP × 24 | Monophasic<br>Shortened placebo | PMDD indication |
| Mircette, Apri | 20 μg EE × 21<br>10 μg EE × 5 | 0.15 mg DSG × 21 | Monophasic<br>Shortened placebo | |
| Estrostep | 20 μg EE × 7<br>30 μg EE × 7<br>35 μg EE × 7 | 1 mg NA | Triphasic | Acne indication |
| Ortho Tri-Cyclen Lo | 25 μg EE | 0.18 mg NGM × 6<br>0.215 mg NGM × 5<br>0.25 mg NGM × 10 | Triphasic | |

*(Continued)*

## Table 52-4 (Continued)

| *Brand Name* | *Estrogen* | *Progestin* | *Cycle* | *Other* |
|---|---|---|---|---|
| Levlen | 30 µg EE | 0.15 LNG | | |
| Lo Ovral | 30 µg EE | 0.3 mg NG | Monophasic | |
| Loestrin 1.5/30<br>Junel 1.5/30 | 30 µg EE | 1 mg NA | Monophasic | |
| Yasmin | 30 µg EE | 3.0 mg DRSP | Monophasic | |
| Seasonale | 30 µg EE | 0.15 mg LNG | Monophasic<br>Extended cycle | |
| Tri-Levlen<br>Triphasil | 30 µg EE<br>40 µg EE<br>30 µg EE | 0.05 LNG × 6<br>0.075 × 5<br>0.125 mg LNG × 10 | Triphasic | |
| Ortho-Novum 1/35<br>Genora 1/35<br>Nelova 1/35<br>Necon 1/35 | 35 µg EE | 1 mg N | Monophasic | |
| Ortho-Novum 7/7/7 | 35 µg EE | 0.5 mg N × 7<br>0.75 mg N × 7<br>1 mg N × 7 | Triphasic | |
| Ortho-Novum 10/11 | 35 µg EE | 0.5 mg N × 10<br>1 mg N × 11 | Biphasic | |
| Ortho-Cyclen | 35 µg EE | 0.25 mg NGM | Monophasic | |
| Ortho Tri-Cyclen<br>TriNessa<br>Tri-Sprintec | 35 µg EE | 0.18 mg NGM × 6<br>0.215 mg NGM × 5<br>0.25 mg NGM × 10 | Triphasic | Acne indication |
| Ovcon 35 | 35 µg EE | 0.4 N | Monophasic | Chewable |
| Modicon | 35 µg EE | 0.5 mg N | Monophasic | |
| Demulen 1/35<br>Zovia 1/35 | 35 µg EE | 1 mg EDA | Monophasic | |
| Ovcon 50 | 50 µg EE | 1 mg N | Monophasic | |
| Ovral | 50 µg EE | 0.5 mg NG | Monophasic | |
| Demulen 1/50<br>Zovia 1/50 | 50 µg EE | 1 mg EDA | Monophasic | |
| Ortho-Novum 1/50<br>Necon 1/50<br>Norinyl 1/50 | 50 µg M<br>(equivalent<br>EE 1/35) | 1 mg N | Monophasic | |
| Micronor[a] | — | 0.35 mg N | Continuous | POP |
| Ovrette[a] | — | .075 mg NG | Continuous | POP |

[a]Progesterone-only preparations

DRSP, drospirenone; DSG, desogestrel; EDA, ethynodiol diacetate; EE, ethinyl estradiol; LNG, levonorgestrel; M, mestranol; N, norethindrone; NA, norethindrone acetate; NG, norgestrel; NGM, norgestimate; PMDD, premenstrual dysphoric disorder; POP, progestin-only pill.

For a more complete listing of available oral contraceptives, see Hatcher RA, Trussell J, Cates W, et al. *Contraceptive Technology: Twentieth Revised Edition.* New York, NY: Ardent Media; 2011.

## Box 52-2

### *Patient Instructions for Birth Control Pills*

Take your pill every day, preferably at the same time.

- *If you miss 1 active pill,* take it as soon as you remember. Take the next pill at your regular time. This means you may take 2 pills in 1 day. You do not need to use a back up birth control method if you have sex.
- *If you miss 2 active pills in a row,* take 2 pills on the day you remember and 2 pills the next day. Then take 1 pill a day until you finish the pack. *Use a condom if you have sex within the next 7 days.*
- *If you miss more than 2 pills,* throw out the pack of pills and start a new pack that day. *Use a condom if you have sex within the next 7 days.*

*If you miss 1 or more pills, you may have bleeding. This is expected, and you should not stop your pills.*

Call your doctor immediately if you have

- Severe stomach or chest pain
- Trouble breathing
- Unusual, severe, or worsening headaches
- Difficulty seeing
- Leg pain or swelling

*The birth control pill does not protect against HIV (AIDS) or STIs. Regardless of contraceptive method, use a condom.*

indicate they are less effective than branded pills. Few head-to-head comparisons between formulations exist, and for the typical pill user, any modern low-dose pill will be safe and effective. Trial and error will determine individual tolerability, and clinicians should not hesitate to change brands or formulation to increase patient satisfaction or increase availability and affordability.

Instructions for pill users are shown in Box 52-2.

### PROGESTIN-ONLY PILLS

Progestin-only pills differ somewhat from estrogen-containing oral contraceptives. Although their mechanism of contraceptive action is similar, the absence of the estrogen component means that there is less suppression of follicular development than with combination pills. The failure rate of POPs is about 5% (compared with 0.1% for combination COCs). Progestin-only pills do not "cycle" per se; they are taken continuously, with no placebos or pill-free days. Irregular bleeding is fairly typical during POP use, although light regular bleeding is the most common pattern seen. The half-life of POPs is short, making it extremely important to take the pill at the same time every day. Because the overall hormonal dose is lower, backup contraception is recommended if only 1 pill is missed. Although ectopic pregnancy rates among users of POPs are extremely low compared to nonusers of contraception, when pregnancy does occur in users of progestin-only methods, the risk of ectopic pregnancy is increased. Despite these seeming disadvantages, POPs provide a major advantage over estrogen-containing methods in that there are almost no contraindications to their use. They provide an important alternative for pill users who cannot take or tolerate the estrogen component of COCs.[22]

### BENEFITS OF ORAL CONTRACEPTIVES

For the healthy adolescent, the benefits of hormonal contraceptives far outweigh the associated risks[23] (Box 52-3). Younger postmenarchal adolescents can safely use hormonal contraceptives without adverse effects on the developing hypothalamic-pituitary axis.

Oral contraceptives are first-line therapy for primary dysmenorrhea.[24] They are also effective treatment for the pain associated with ovulation (mittelschmerz) and endometriosis and prevent the formation of functional ovarian cysts. Extended cycle or shortened placebo interval pills may provide additional advantages for these conditions, although there are no data comparing these pills to standard cycling for such indications.

All COCs have the potential to improve acne and hirsutism by decreasing free testosterone levels. This occurs through suppression of ovarian testosterone production and increase in hepatic production of sex hormone-binding globulin. Although only two pill manufacturers have obtained a prescribing indication

## Box 52-3

### *Benefits of Oral Contraceptives*

- Treatment of dysmenorrhea
- Treatment of endometriosis
- Shorter, lighter menses
- Improvement in acne
- Improvement in hirsutism
- Treatment of PMDD
- Prevent mittelschmerz
- Prevent functional ovarian cysts
- Prevention of ovarian cancer
- Prevention of endometrial cancer
- Prevention of osteoporosis
- Treatment of fibrocystic breast disease
- Treatment of perimenstrual mastalgia

for acne, any combination pill might be expected to have this benefit. In theory, a less androgenic progestin may be preferable, but there are no data to support this. Drospirenone has a theoretical advantage due to its potential inhibition of 5-alpha reductase in the skin, but no comparative data between drospirenone-containing pills and other COCs are available.[25,26]

Use of COCs reduces the risks of ovarian and endometrial cancer. The risk reduction in ovarian cancer is 30% for 4 years of use, 60% for 5 to 11 years, and 80% after 12 or more years. For endometrial cancer, the risk reduction is 40% at 2 years and 60% with 4 years or more of use.[27]

Although multiple retrospective and cross-sectional studies in adult women have demonstrated a positive association between prior oral contraceptive pill (OCP) use and bone mass at menopause, more recent studies of bone mass in adolescents suggest that users of 20-μg pills may have lower rates of bone gain compared to nonusers. Thus, the benefits of "ultra low-dose" pills in terms of reduced nausea and breast tenderness need to be balanced against the potential for lower bone gains in growing adolescent users. COC use has not been shown to increase bone mass in anorectic adolescents. Use of COCs in young women with hypothalamic amenorrhea and normal weight has not been as well studied, but it seems reasonable to use COCs in this group.[28]

One COC containing drospirenone (Yaz) has been shown to be effective in the treatment of PMDD, perhaps as a result of its antiandrogenic and diuretic effects.[29] Other COCs are in clinical trials for this indication. Combined oral contraceptives have also been shown to decrease the symptoms of fibrocystic breast disease.[30]

## RISKS OF ESTROGEN-CONTAINING ORAL CONTRACEPTIVES

The only significant risk of oral contraceptive use in the otherwise healthy, low-risk adolescent is thromboembolic disease such as primary deep vein thrombosis (DVT). The risk in COC users younger than 35 years is about 15 per 100,000. These risks are higher among smokers and carriers of inherited thrombophilic disorders, the most common of which is the factor V Leyden mutation.[31]

Estrogen-containing contraceptive users should be advised to notify their physician immediately if they have chest pain, shortness of breath, new-onset headache, or leg pain associated with swelling, redness, or heat, which may indicate presence of a clot. It may be worthwhile to warn all pill users against prolonged immobilization on long plane flights, a factor additive to pill use in thrombotic risk. Common sense strategies worth discussing for long flights include drinking adequate water, avoiding caffeine and alcohol, moving about the plane, and deplaning during layovers.

Oral contraceptive pills containing the third-generation progestins desogestrel and gestodene (not available in the United States) may be associated with DVT risk twice as high as that associated with pills containing norethindrone and levonorgestrel.[32] No increased risk for thrombosis has been reported in users of progestin-only contraceptive pills or other progestin-only methods.

Although multiple epidemiologic studies report an association between long-term oral contraceptive use and cervical cancer, most of these did not control for human papilloma virus (HPV) infections, now known to be causative in these cancers. It is unlikely that oral contraceptives are an independent cause of cervical cancer, although estrogens may act as cofactors for dysplasia among chronic carriers of HPV infection.[33] An effective vaccine against HPV is now available and recommended for adolescents.

The risk of cervical infection with chlamydia and gonorrhea may be increased in pill users who fail to use condoms due to an increase in cervical ectopy. A recent study has shown that oral contraceptives do not protect against pelvic inflammatory disease (PID) with typical use.[34]

Other risks associated with COC use are confined to certain population subgroups. For example, the risk of myocardial infarction is increased in users with hypertriglyceridemia. Estrogen-induced cholestatis may exacerbate underlying gallbladder disease. Although earlier pills containing high doses of estrogen were reported to affect carbohydrate metabolism and insulin sensitivity in women with diabetes or glucose intolerance, currently used low-dose pills do not do so. Benign liver tumors have been associated with older high-dose OCPs, but none have been reported to date with currently used low-dose (35 μg or lower) pills. Pseudotumor cerebri, a common disorder in women of reproductive age, has been reported in users of most hormonal methods and is relatively common in pregnancy. Although oral contraceptives do not appear to cause this condition, they can exacerbate it and should be discontinued if this condition is diagnosed. See Box 52-4 for contraindications to COC use.

## DRUG INTERACTIONS WITH ORAL CONTRACEPTIVES

Drug interactions with oral contraceptives fall into 2 categories: drugs that affect oral contraceptive efficacy, and drugs whose metabolism is affected by oral contraceptives. The major class of drugs that interact with oral contraceptive use are those that induce hepatic cytochrome P450 enzymes, which cause increased metabolism of the estrogen and/or progestin component

## Box 52-4

### *Contraindications to Oral Contraceptives*

- History of active thromboembolic disease or hypercoagulable state[a]
- Cerebrovascular or coronary artery disease[a]
- Known or suspected carcinoma of the breast
- Carcinoma of the endometrium or other known or suspected estrogen-dependent neoplasia
- Undiagnosed abnormal genital bleeding
- Cholestatic jaundice of pregnancy or jaundice with prior pill use
- Hepatic adenomas or carcinomas; active liver disease
- Known or suspected pregnancy

[a]May consider progestin-only pills.

of the pill, and lead to lower blood levels and decreased efficacy. Other possible mechanisms of interference include drugs that affect serum protein binding and thus free hormone levels, and those that affect absorption of the drug in the gastrointestinal (GI) tract.

#### Anticonvulsants

Phenobarbital and phenytoin are the most commonly discussed, although primidone, carbamazepine, topiramate, and ethosuximide have been reported as well. These drugs induce liver enzymes and lower hormone levels. The effect is so pronounced in implant users that these methods should not be used. Consider prescribing high-dose (50 µg ethinyl estradiol) oral contraceptives or the patch in adolescents taking these medications, reducing the pill-free interval, or eliminating it altogether. If breakthrough bleeding occurs despite these regimens, then contraceptive efficacy is likely to be compromised, and an alternative method should be used. The metabolism of Depo-Provera is not affected by anticonvulsants, and Depo-Provera can lower seizure frequency in some cases. (Note: Valproic acid does *not* affect oral contraceptive metabolism or efficacy.)[35]

#### Antibiotics

Numerous case reports and uncontrolled retrospective studies have implicated antibiotic use, most often ampicillin and tetracyclines, in reducing oral contraceptive efficacy, presumably through effects on enterohepatic recirculation. It is theorized that certain individuals may be predisposed to this interaction due to a combination of low bioavailability of ethinyl estradiol, a large enterohepatic recirculation, and susceptible intestinal flora. However, no pharmacokinetic data exist to support these claims for any antibiotic other than rifampin (a known cytochrome P450 inducer) and griseofulvin (mechanism unknown, but probably hepatic enzyme induction).[36] Current expert opinion is that short-term antibiotic use does not reduce oral contraceptive efficacy. However, if breakthrough bleeding or diarrhea occur, a backup barrier method of contraception can be used short term. Adolescents using antibiotics long term can preferentially use 30- to 35-µg pills; if breakthrough bleeding occurs, a higher dose (50-µg) pill may be prescribed.

#### St John's Wort

St John's wort has been shown to induce hepatic cytochrome P450, and hormonal contraceptive users should be advised against using St John's wort.[37]

#### Vitamin C

Several studies have shown that high-dose vitamin C (1 g or more daily) may increase hormonal levels in oral contraceptive users, although other studies refute this finding.[38] Ascorbic acid remains listed in the package insert as an interacting medication.

#### Antacids

Antacids may interfere with the absorption of oral contraceptives if taken within 3 hours of pill ingestion.

#### Theophylline

Numerous well-done pharmacokinetic studies have documented that oral contraceptives reduce clearance of theophylline by as much as 50%. Theophylline doses should be lowered accordingly. The same effect is noted with caffeine.

#### Analgesics and Corticosteroids

Oral contraceptive use appears to lower aspirin levels. Chronic acetaminophen use can lead to increased ethinyl estradiol levels in OCP users. Oral contraceptives may lead to decreased clearance and prolonged elimination of certain anti-inflammatory corticosteroids, notably hydrocortisone, prednisone, and prednisolone.

#### Benzodiazepines

Oral contraceptives can decrease clearance of benzodiazepines such as diazepam, alprazolam, nitrazepam, and chlordiazepoxide.[39]

#### Antiretrovirals

Most antiretrovirals used to treat HIV infection have interactions with medications using the cytochrome P450 system. Ritonavir decreases EE levels by as much as 40%, and alternative contraception is recommended. Nevirapine and nelfinavir are presumed to act similarly. Indinavir can raise EE levels, which could increase side effects.[40]

## EFFECTS OF ORAL CONTRACEPTIVES ON LABORATORY TESTS

Combined oral contraceptives affect certain hematologic parameters. These include an increase in prothrombin factors VII, VII, IX, and X, and norepinephrine-induced platelet aggregation and a decrease in anti-thrombin 3 levels. Thyroid-binding globulin (TBG) levels are increased, so that total thyroid hormone levels are increased. However, T3-resin uptake is decreased, reflecting the elevated TBG, and the free T4 concentration remains unchanged. Glucose levels are not affected. Serum folate levels may be lowered in users of COCs.[41]

## SIDE EFFECTS OF ORAL CONTRACEPTIVES

The experience of side effects, and the fear that accompanies them, is a major reason for contraceptive noncompliance and method discontinuation among adolescent pill users.[42] It is worthwhile to spend the time at the pill start visit to review these possible side effects and to encourage adolescents not to discontinue their pills when side effects occur until they speak to their provider.

### Breakthrough Bleeding

Irregular bleeding or spotting is common in the first few cycles of pill use, ranging from 10% to 30% of cycles, depending on the pill. Bleeding rates are higher in pills with 20 µg EE than in those with 30 to 35 µg. Common causes of breakthrough bleeding include missed pills, drug interactions, and infection with chlamydia. Most breakthrough bleeding will resolve over time, especially if nonadherence is the cause. Changing to a monophasic pill, a higher-dose pill if the patient is on a 20-µg pill, a different progestin, or a shorter placebo interval pill are acceptable strategies for dealing with persistent breakthrough bleeding. Levonorgestrel- and norgestimate-containing pills have been associated with low rates of breakthrough bleeding. If breakthrough bleeding continues to be a concern, a pelvic ultrasound can be performed to rule out underlying pathology such as endometrial polyps or fibroids (rare in adolescents). If adherence continues to be a problem, consider a longer-acting hormonal method such as the NuvaRing or the patch.

### Amenorrhea

Amenorrhea occurs in about 6% of COC users, more often after prolonged use. Once pregnancy is ruled out, reassurance is all that is necessary. If a 20-µg pill is being used, changing to a higher dose or giving a 6-week course of supplemental estrogen may resolve the problem. For teens who are not sexually active, a month or 2 off the pill should resolve the problem.

### Weight Gain

Studies of modern low-dose pills have failed to show significant weight changes in pill users when compared with those on placebo or using other nonhormonal methods. Changing to a different progestin or lower-dose pill may help the adolescent who gains weight because of fluid retention or experiences an undesired increase in breast size or appetite.

### Headache

Worsening or new-onset migraine with neurologic or visual symptoms is an indication for discontinuing the pill. Typical migraine or more frequent migraines in the pill-free interval may be due to estrogen withdrawal, and can be managed by lowering the dose or switching to a monophasic preparation or one with a shortened placebo interval. Other causes of headache such as tension headache, sinusitis, or allergies, or migraines that do not start or worsen on the pill should be managed individually, and do not mandate a change in contraceptive.

### Nausea

Although this side effect tends to occur more often in the beginning of a pill pack and resolve with time, many adolescents will discontinue their pills in the first cycle if this side effect occurs. It is important that they be advised to take the pill with food and not in the morning on an empty stomach. Changing to a lower-dose pill, a pill with a shorter placebo interval, or the vaginal ring may resolve the problem. For refractory cases, consider a POP. Nausea that is severe, persistent, or does not resolve in the pill-free interval should be evaluated because it is most likely due to other causes.

### Breast Tenderness

Breast tenderness is usually confined to the first few cycles of pill use. Assuming it is bilateral and not associated with breast pathology, changing to a 20-µg pill can help. Use of a supportive bra and elimination or decrease in caffeine may help. Evening primrose oil, 1,000 mg daily, has been shown in placebo-controlled trials to be effective for cyclic mastalgia, although it has not specifically been studied in oral contraceptive users.

### Chloasma

Both estrogens and progestins may cause irregular pigmentation of sun-exposed skin in susceptible individuals. Although skin-lightening agents can be used to fade the pigmented areas, it is probably best to change to a nonhormonal method.

### Contact Lens Problems

Wearers of older hard contacts may notice problems due to increased fluid retention in the eye. This problem is less frequent with soft lenses.

### Depression or Mood Changes

Mood may improve or worsen while taking oral contraceptives, and the cause is more often unrelated to pill use. Changing or lowering the estrogen or progestin dose may be helpful if the pill is the only cause. If premenstrual syndrome (PMS) is the issue, changing to Yaz may be therapeutic. For severe cases, a cycle off may be necessary to determine whether the pill is causative. Abstinence or the use of a barrier method of contraception should be strongly encouraged during that cycle.

## EMERGENCY CONTRACEPTIVE PILLS

Emergency contraceptive pills (ECPs) are high doses of progestin with or without estrogen given within a short period of time after unprotected intercourse in an attempt to prevent pregnancy. Emergency contraceptive pills act by preventing or delaying ovulation and impairing corpus luteum function. Other proposed mechanisms of action are theoretical. Emergency contraceptive pills will not interrupt an implanted pregnancy and are not teratogenic if pregnancy has already occurred.

The efficacy of ECPs ranges from 80% to 85%, and if used after all contraception failures, could prevent up to 50% of unplanned pregnancies and reduce abortion rates by as much as 70%.

The only contraindications to ECP use are known or suspected pregnancy, hypersensitivity to the product's components, or undiagnosed genital bleeding. Pregnancies conceived despite ECP use have no increase in anomalies or adverse outcomes. Side effects are transient and minor, and include nausea and vomiting, breast tenderness, headache, dizziness, and fatigue.

Progestin-only ECPs are preferred because they are more efficacious and have fewer side effects than combination (or Yuzpe) regimens (Table 52-5). The incidence of nausea and vomiting are 23% and 6%, respectively.

If the progestin-only ECPs (Plan B) are unavailable, the Yuzpe regimen can be used. This method uses 1 of 10 different combination oral contraceptives or a prepackaged product called Preven. Nausea occurs in up to 50% of users, with vomiting in 12% to 22%. Consider prescribing an antiemetic along with the Yuzpe regimen.

Plan B has been approved for over-the-counter sale in women older than 17 years, but younger adolescents require a prescription. In nine states (Alaska, California, Hawaii, Maine, Massachusetts, New Hampshire, New Mexico, Washington, and Vermont), adolescents of any age can obtain ECP directly from a participating pharmacy without a doctor's prescription.

Adolescents presenting for ECPs do not need a special examination—a health history will suffice, along with pregnancy testing if preexisting pregnancy is suspected. It is also appropriate (and encouraged) to give prescriptions over the phone for patients who call. Adolescents using barrier methods can be given an anticipatory prescription or packet of ECPs, along with instructions for their use. They should be counseled to call the office after ECP use to arrange appropriate follow-up care. Two large European studies have shown that patients who receive a prescription or package of ECPs to have on hand at home are significantly more likely to use emergency contraception than those given education alone, and do not abuse the method or use it repeatedly. It is important to note, however, that young women who request or use emergency contraception are at high risk for pregnancy in the year following ECP use and, therefore, require contraceptive counseling.[43]

In about half of ECP users, the subsequent menses is either early (if ECP is taken in the follicular phase) or

**Table 52-5**

**Emergency Contraceptive Pill Dosing**

| *Type of ECP* | *Dosing* |
|---|---|
| **Progestin-only method** | |
| Levonorgestrel 0.75 mg (Plan B, Next Choice) | 1 pill q 12 hours × 2 doses |
| Levonorgestrel 1.5 mg (Plan B One Step) | 1 pill × 1 dose |
| **Yuzpe regimen** | |
| Preven | 2 pills q 12 hours × 2 doses |
| Ovral, Ogestrel | 2 white pills q 12 hours × 2 doses |
| Alesse, Levlite | 5 pink pills q 12 hours × 2 doses |
| Aviane | 5 orange pills q 12 hours × 2 doses |
| Nordette, Levlen | 4 light-orange pills q 12 hours × 2 doses |
| Levora, Lo/Ovral, Low-Ogestrel | 4 white pills q 12 hours × 2 doses |
| Triphasil, Tri-Levlen | 4 yellow pills q 12 hours × 2 doses |
| Trivora | 4 pink pills q 12 hours × 2 doses |

delayed (if taken in the luteal phase). Most will bleed normally, and 98% will menstruate within 21 days; if not, pregnancy is a concern.

An excellent ECP resource for patients and providers is the Emergency Contraception Hotline (1-800-not-2-late) and Web site (ec.princeton.edu).

## LONG-ACTING HORMONAL CONTRACEPTIVES

The OCP has some drawbacks for women of all ages, the major one being that users must take it every day to optimize its contraceptive benefits. Newer hormonal methods, which include the contraceptive injectable, implant, patch, and vaginal ring are formulations designed to circumvent the need for daily adherence. All have modes of action similar to the oral contraceptive and ideal efficacy rates very close to 100%, and, like the oral contraceptive pill, they are extremely safe. For adolescents who have problems remembering to take a pill every day, or who desire the convenience of a long-acting method, these new methods provide a welcome alternative to the pill.

### DEPOT MEDROXYPROGESTERONE ACETATE (DEPO-PROVERA)

Depo-Provera is 150 mg of the progestin medroxyprogesterone acetate, given as an intramuscular injection once every 3 months in either the deltoid or gluteal muscle. The injection site should not be massaged because duration and efficacy could be reduced. The protocol to follow if more than 13 weeks has elapsed since the last injection includes: (1) an initial negative urine pregnancy test prior to repeat injection; (2) administration of a repeat injection; and (3) if the teen has not been sexually active in the past 3 weeks, a prescription for a bridge method until a second negative pregnancy test is obtained in 3 weeks, and then a repeat injection. If the decision is made to offer the late injection immediately in a teen who is sexually active, she should be advised of the risk of pregnancy and have another pregnancy test in 21 days to confirm absence of pregnancy. As would be expected for a progestin, DMPA prevents pregnancy by inhibiting ovulation and thickening cervical mucus. However, its effect on the hypothalamic-pituitary axis is more profound than other progestin-only methods, resulting in increased suppression of ovulation and follicular development, and in some cases, lowering of estrogen production by the ovary.

Depo-Provera is an extremely effective, safe, and well-tolerated contraceptive.[44] Side effects are typical for a progestin-only method, with menstrual alterations predominating. Amenorrhea is the predominant bleeding pattern, with 80% of users being amenorrheic by 2 years of use. Prior to this time, irregular bleeding and spotting can be problematic, particularly in the first few months to year of use.[45] Bleeding can occasionally be heavy, but it is unlikely to cause anemia. Intolerance of menstrual changes is a major reason for discontinuation within the first year of DMPA use, but structured, anticipatory counseling has been shown to increase continuation rates among women experiencing this side effect. 46 Treatment options for irregular bleeding include giving COCs for 7 to 21 days, Ibuprofen (600–800 mg/day) for 10 to 14 days or adding cyclical estrogen (2 mg ethinyl estradiol, 0.65–1.25 mg conjugated estrogen or 0.1 mg 17 B estradiol patch) for 25 days per month. Although giving the next DMPA injection earlier is often suggested, in a study of adolescent DMPA users, this did not impact bleeding patterns and resulted in more weight gain. Persistent or severe bleeding should prompt investigation for other underlying causes. Weight gain was reported in the clinical trials of DMPA, on average 5 lbs in the first year and 8 lbs in the second, although not all women gain weight during DMPA use. Weight gain has also been reported among adolescent DMPA users; however, in small controlled trials, it was not statistically different from users of other hormonal methods. Although mood changes were reported in initial experiences, subsequent studies refute that this effect is not seen in DMPA users any more than in other hormonal methods.

Depo-Provera suppresses ovarian follicular development, and estradiol levels are suppressed to early follicular phase levels. Significant declines in bone mass can occur during DMPA use by adolescents, with declines at the hip averaging 3% at 1 year and 7% at 3 years, as compared with an increase of 1% to 2% among control teens. The bone loss appears, however, to be reversible, with full recovery of lumbar spine bone density at about one year and return to baseline at the femoral neck in about 4 years post DMPA discontinuation.[46] As a result, some experts advise against DMPA use until after age 15 years, when most bone has been laid down. Others recommend that the potential risk of bone loss in younger sexually active teens needs to be balanced against the patient's risk of pregnancy if she fails to use an effective contraceptive method. All DMPA users should be advised to get the recommended daily requirements of calcium and vitamin D, to exercise regularly, and to avoid cigarette smoking, which is another risk factor for bone loss.[47]

Overall, DMPA use does not affect fertility, but the return to fertility is delayed among users of DMPA as compared with those discontinuing pills or barrier methods, a fact that can be seen as an advantage among adolescent users. The mean interval from injection to the return to ovulation is 4.5 months, but ovulation may occur as little as 14 weeks after the last injection.

The only reported medication interaction with DMPA is with aminoglutethimide, making it an excellent choice for teens on medication that may interfere with other hormonal methods. It is safe to use DMPA in adolescents at risk for clotting or with liver disease because it may lessen the frequency of sickle cell crises and seizures. Depo-Provera is safe to use in lactating women and can be initiated immediately following delivery or abortion.

## TRANSDERMAL CONTRACEPTIVE PATCH (ORTHO EVRA)

Ortho Evra is a 4.5-cm patch containing 0.75 mg EE and 6 mg norelgestromin. Norelgestromin is the active metabolite of norgestimate, a progestin used in oral contraceptives. The patch is applied to the lower abdomen, buttocks, upper outer arm, or upper torso (not the breast), and is changed once a week for 3 weeks, followed by a patch-free week to allow for menses.

In a large multicenter adult clinical trial, pregnancy rates with the patch are 1.2 per 100 women-years of use (Pearl index), compared with 2.2 pregnancies in oral contraceptive users. Importantly, although women weighing more than 196 lbs constituted less than 3% of the study population, they had one third of the pregnancies, suggesting that the patch may be less effective in women weighing more than 196 lbs.[48]

The mechanism of action of the patch is similar to COCs. Due to its transdermal delivery mechanism, direct comparison of dose levels with oral contraceptives is not meaningful. However, comparison of pharmacokinetics reveals that although peak concentrations of EE are 35% higher in pill users, overall EE exposure (area under the curve) is 60% higher for patch users.[49] Given that the risk of thromboembolism in estrogen users is dose dependent, there are concerns as to whether the higher EE levels in the patch translate into higher risks for venous thromboembolism in patch versus pill users. Three case-control studies to date have conflicting results. One study (abstract only) found a twofold increase risk for thromboembolism among users of the patch compared with users of a 35-µg pill containing norgestimate.[50] The other two studies found no increased risk of either thromboembolism or central venous sinus thrombosis in patch users.[51,52] The potential risk for thrombotic side effects should be balanced against the need for effective contraception in any teen prescribed the patch.

About 20% of patch users experience breakthrough bleeding in the first cycle, although this decreases over time to less than 10%. In a trial of adult women, adherence with the patch was significantly better than with pills; overall, 89% of cycles in patch users had perfect adherence, compared with 70% of pill cycles. The patch was well tolerated, with a safety and side effect profile similar to oral contraceptives, with the exception of breast tenderness, which was higher in the patch group, and patch site reactions.

Smaller studies in adolescents suggest that the patch is well accepted in this age group, with good short-term adherence.[53-55] Two studies published to date report higher patch detachment rates among teen users than in the adult clinical trials. It is important to counsel teens on what to do if a patch detaches and to give them a prescription for an extra patch if this occurs (Box 52-5).

The patch is an appropriate contraceptive method for adolescents who have problems remembering to take a pill every day or who need higher estrogen doses because of interaction with other medications. Heavier adolescents may experience lower efficacy rates. Visibility of the patch could be problematic for adolescents who need confidentiality. The potential for increased thromboembolism should be weighed against the risks of pregnancy and the need for effective contraception in any adolescent using the patch. Contraindications are the same as for the COCs.

## CONTRACEPTIVE VAGINAL RING (NUVARING)

The contraceptive vaginal ring is a soft, flexible, nonbiodegradable transparent ring approximately 2 inches in diameter. The ring is worn for 3 weeks (21 days), during which time it releases on average 0.120 mg of ENG and 0.015 mg of EE per day. The ring is then removed for 7 days to allow for menses. A new ring is then inserted for the next cycle.

The vaginal ring is initiated by the user within 5 days of the menses. It can be worn while menstrual bleeding is still occurring and during intercourse. User satisfaction is high. The ring does not have to be fitted, and its exact positioning within the vagina is not critical for efficacy, so it cannot be incorrectly inserted. There is no increase in vaginal infections during ring use, and concurrent tampon use does not affect efficacy.

The ring inhibits ovulation in a manner similar to oral contraceptives, with failure rates of 6.5 pregnancies per 100 women-years (Pearl index).[56] Comparison of pharmacokinetics shows that EE exposure in users of the ring (as measured by area under the curve) is 3.4 times lower than in patch users and 2.1 times lower than in users of a 30-µg pill, with less variation in levels than with the patch or the pill.[49] Despite this, ovulation inhibition in ring users is similar to that in 30-µg pill users. Breakthrough bleeding rates are very low—less than 10%—and close to 100 versus users have regular withdrawal bleeding, a profile better than

**Box 52-5**

***Instructions for Contraceptive Patch Users***

If a patch is partially or completely detached:

- If detached for less than 24 hours, try to reapply the patch to the same place or replace it with a new patch immediately. No backup contraception is needed. Your "patch change day" will remain the same.
- If detached for more than 24 hours, or if you are not sure how long the patch has been detached, stop the current contraceptive cycle, and start a new cycle immediately by applying a new patch. backup contraception must be used for the first week of the new cycle. You now have a new patch change day.
- A patch should not be reapplied if it is no longer sticky, has become stuck to itself or another surface, has other material stuck to it, or has previously become loose or fallen off. If a patch cannot be reapplied, a new patch should be applied immediately. Supplemental adhesives or wraps should not be used to hold the Ortho Evra patch in place.

If you forget to start your patch at the beginning of a new cycle, you may not be protected against pregnancy.

You should never be off the patch for more than 7 days.

Apply the patch as soon as you remember. Use backup contraception for the first week of the new cycle.

If you forget to change your patch:

- If it is less than 48 hours late, you can apply a new patch immediately and still be protected against pregnancy. You now have a new patch change day.
- If your patch change is more than 48 hours past due, apply a new patch immediately, but use Backup contraception for the next week. You now have a new patch change day.

Call you doctor immediately if you have:

- Severe stomach or chest pain
- Trouble breathing
- Unusual, severe, or worsening headaches
- Difficulty seeing
- Leg pain or swelling

The patch does not protect against AIDS or STI.

Always use a condom.

that seen with oral contraceptive users in comparison studies.[57,58] More than 90% of cycles were completely adherent.

Interactions with medications are similar as for oral contraceptives. In addition, the use of vaginal antifungal preparations raises EE and ENG levels by about 17%, but efficacy is not affected. Water-based lubricants and non-oxyl-9 also do not affect efficacy.[59]

The safety profile and contraindications for the ring are similar to that of COCs. For teens who are comfortable with inserting and removing a vaginal device, the vaginal ring is a safe, effective, and private option for contraception.

### CONTRACEPTIVE IMPLANT (IMPLANON)

Although there are several contraceptive implants available worldwide, only Implanon is currently marketed in the United States. Norplant, a 6-rod levonorgestrel implant with five years of efficacy, was US Food and Drug Administration (FDA) approved in the United States in 1991. The method was initially well accepted by adolescents, with significantly higher continuation rates than oral contraceptives. However, widespread adverse publicity related to the known side effects of the progestin-only formulation, as well as to removal problems, led to a decline in popularity of the method. The manufacturer discontinued marketing of the method in the United States in 2002.

Implanon is a single-rod, progestin-only implant providing 3 years of highly safe and effective contraception. Each Implanon rod consists of an ethylene vinylacetate (EVA) copolymer core, containing 68 mg of the synthetic progestin ENG, surrounded by an EVA copolymer skin. The release rate gradually declines from a high of 60 to 70 μg/day in weeks 5 to 6, to 25 to 30 μg/day at the end of year 3 of use.[60]

Implanon is highly effective, with pregnancy rates less than 1%. Method failures have been reported because of improper placement of the rod. Implanon acts to prevent pregnancy through inhibition of ovulation (in one study, 100% inhibition in the first 2.5 years), thickening of cervical mucus, and effects on the endometrium. Because ENG levels are inversely related to body weight, the method may be less effective in heavier women and has not been studied as of yet in women weighing more than 130% of ideal body weight.

Side effects with Implanon are those expected with a progestin-only contraceptive, the most common of which is unpredictable bleeding. Most users will have either amenorrhea (about 20%) or infrequent bleeding (34%), but prolonged bleeding occurs in 18% of users and frequent bleeding in 8%. For a given user, any pattern is possible, and previous patterns do not necessarily predict future bleeding frequency in any given individual. Overall, 11% of users in the US clinical trials discontinued Implanon due to bleeding. Other reasons for discontinuation include weight gain, acne, mood changes, and headache, none accounting for more than a 3% discontinuation rate. Insertion site complications, although possible, are rare, although 5% of subjects report pain at the site afterward.[60]

Drug interactions with Implanon are similar to those for oral contraceptives. There are few contraindications to Implanon use, although use of medications that affect the cytochrome P450 system, particularly anticonvulsants, protease inhibitors, and St John's wort, can impair efficacy. Use of ketoconazole or itraconazole may increase hormone levels.

The FDA has mandated that prescribers of Implanon receive training in insertion and removal, and that, where appropriate, their first insertion be supervised. Because the method is not radiopaque, suitable methods to locate a nonpalpable rod include ultrasound with a high-frequency linear array transducer (≥10 mHts) or magnetic resonance imaging. If these fail, serum levels can be sent to the manufacturer.

Implanon is a suitable contraceptive for any adolescent requiring safe, long-term, and effective contraception who has no contraindications and who is prepared for, and can tolerate, unpredictable bleeding. The method does not protect against AIDS or STIs, so users should be advised to use a condom. Return to fertility is immediate on removal of Implanon. Implanon is latex free.

## BARRIER CONTRACEPTION

Barrier contraception has advantages and disadvantages when used by adolescents. It is an extremely safe method with relatively few contraindications or side effects and no interaction with medications. With the exception of the contraceptive diaphragm or cervical cap, they are readily and widely available over the counter or via the Internet, and do not require either a prescription or a visit to a heath care provider to obtain them. Barrier methods are effective when used consistently and properly, and they can provide protection against STIs (the condom more so than the diaphragm or cap).

The primary disadvantage of barrier methods is that their efficacy relies on use with each and every act of intercourse, and on some degree of partner cooperation. Their efficacy will be highest in mature adolescent couples who are highly motivated to avoid pregnancy. For others, hormonal methods have lower failure rates. Condom use, however, should always be encouraged to prevent STIs, even in users of hormonal contraception.

### MALE CONDOMS

Despite the widespread availability of more effective hormonal contraceptives, condoms are the most popular contraceptives used by adolescents. This is most likely due to their over-the-counter availability, relatively low cost per use, ease of use and travel, and lack of side effects.

Frequency of condom use with intercourse among adolescents appears to be related to the quality of the relationship. Overall, condom use declines as frequency of sexual activity increases, and among girls, condoms are used less as they become more attached to a main partner. However, this may reflect perceived risks of STIs rather than pregnancy because hormonal contraceptive use increases with duration of relationship and female age. Although educational efforts increase intent to use condoms, intent does not always translate to consistent use or lowered rates of pregnancy or STIs. Effective parent–child communication increases condom use; adolescents whose mothers discussed condoms with them before their first sexual encounter were three times more likely to use condoms at first intercourse, and teens who used condoms the first time they had sex were 20 times more likely to use them subsequently.[61,62]

Condoms act as mechanical barriers to sperm, bacteria, and viruses. They are available in both latex and polyurethane, in a variety of sizes, and with amenities such as flavoring and ribbing. Latex condoms are preferred; however, due to allergies, users may prefer polyurethane varieties. Polyurethane condoms may require more lubricant and have slightly higher breakage rates than latex condoms, but contraceptive efficacy is similar. Latex condom users should not use oil-based lubricants or vaginal products because they may degrade the latex. This includes most vaginal antifungal and antibacterial medications used to treat vaginitis. Metronidazole gel, but not tablets or cream, is safe to use with condoms. (See Table 52-6.)

Condom manufacturers are regulated by the FDA, which mandates quality testing via water leak test, in which the condom is filled with 300 mL of water and examined for leaks. Breakage rates must be less than 4 per 1,000 and average 2.3 per 1,000 among batches that pass inspection. Foreign-made condoms must maintain the same standards to pass through US customs and have significantly higher chance of failing inspection than those made in the United States.

If used perfectly, the failure rate of condoms in preventing pregnancy is 3%; typical failure rates are closer to 15%, but this latter number may be inflated due to overreporting of condom use in surveys by those who become pregnant using no contraception.[18] Condom technique and breakage rates among males improves with experience. Still, up to 40% of college-age males

## Table 52-6

### Lubricant Use and Latex Male Condoms

| *Safe with All Condoms* | *Unsafe with Latex Condoms* |
|---|---|
| • Aloe-9 | • Aldara cream |
| • Aqualube | • Baby oils |
| • Astroglide | • Bag balm |
| • Corn Huskers lotion | • Clindamycin 2% vaginal cream and suppositories |
| • deLUBE | • Cold cream |
| • Durex lubricant | • Edible oils |
| • ForPlay | • Head and body lotions |
| • Glycerin | • ID brand cream lubricant |
| • Gynol II | • Massage oils |
| • H-R lubricating jelly | • Mineral oil |
| • K-Y lubricating jelly | • Petroleum jelly |
| • I-D brand Glide, Juicy Lube, Millennium, Pleasure, and Sensation | • Rubbing alcohol |
| | • Shortening |
| | • Suntan oil and lotions |
| • Pjur lubricants | • Vegetable or cooking oils |
| • PrePair | • Whipped cream |
| • Probe | • Metronidazole tablets and cream |
| • Silicone lubricant | |
| • Water and saliva | • Gynazole, Monistat, Terazol, and other vaginal antifungals |
| • Wet | |
| • Metronidazole gel | |

Data adapted from Planned Parenthood and from Hatcher RA, Zieman M, Cwiak C, Darney PD, Crenin MD, Stosur HR. *A Pocket Guide to Managing Contraception*. Tiger, GA: Bridging the Gap Foundation; 2005.

## Box 52-6

### *Instructions for Condom Use*

- Store condoms at room temperature. Condoms kept in glove compartments or wallets deteriorate quickly.
- Check the expiration date, and do not use if it has passed because older condoms may be brittle and break.
- Do not use fingernails, teeth, or sharp objects to open the condom wrapper.
- Do not unroll the condom before putting it on.
- Unroll the condoms right-side up on an erect penis before any vaginal, rectal, or oral penetration. If the condom is accidentally put on upside down, discard it and use a new condom because preejaculate may have already contaminated the condom.
- Roll the condom down completely to the base of the penis.
- If a vaginal lubricant is required, a commercially available water or silicone-based product should be used (eg, K-Y jelly, Pjur, Astroglide). Read the label to be sure that it is compatible with condoms.
- Do not use oil-based products (eg, mineral oil, food oils, cold cream, petroleum jelly) with condoms. They may degrade the latex and increase breakage.
- Squeeze the air out of the tip of the condom and leave room at the tip. This allows room for the semen ("cum").
- Following ejaculation, the male should immediately withdraw his penis while it is still erect. Hold the condom in place at the base of the penis before withdrawing (pulling out) after sex.
- Do not reuse the condom.

reporting incorrect technique within the previous 3 months of condom use, reinforcing the need for continued review and reinforcement of technique.[66] See Box 52-6 for instructions on correct condom use. Spermicidal lubrication does not increase the contraceptive efficacy of condoms and may increase the risk of HIV transmission if exposure occurs; thus, it is not recommended.

Teens using condoms for birth control should be advised of the availability of emergency contraception, and considerations should be given to advance prescription of ECPs.

#### FEMALE CONDOM

The female condom is a soft but strong polyurethane pouch 15 cm long and 7 cm wide, containing two flexible rings—one ring is used to insert the condom and rests behind the female pubic bone, similar to a diaphragm placement, to hold the condom in place. The outer ring remains outside the vagina, partially covering the vulva and facilitating removal of the condom. The female condom is prelubricated with a silicone lubricant, and additional lubricant is supplied with the condom. It does not contain spermicide. Vaginal penetration occurs inside the condom.

A new female condom (FC2) composed of a nitrite material has been recently released for mass distribution at low cost, and has similar efficacy and characteristics otherwise to the polyurethane condom. Female condoms are widely used in countries that promote its use, but are much less popular in the United States, where acceptance has been limited.

The female condom is an effective barrier against sperm, as well as bacterial and viral STIs. Pregnancy rates reported with female condom use range from 3% to 15% and seem to be related to both user- and relationship-specific factors.[64] In studies measuring vaginal levels of prostate-specific antigen, semen exposure occurs on 7% to 21% of uses, and is correlated to both intensity of intercourse and reported problems with using the condom.[65] Semen exposure is higher in women of lower income levels, if there is a large disparity between vaginal and penile size, and in relationships of less than 2 years' duration.[66]

One major advantage over the male condom is that it is a female-controlled method, although males resistant to condom use are generally also resistant to female condom use. Other advantages over male condoms are that the female condom is stronger, does not deteriorate with time and temperature, can be used with either water- or oil-based lubricants, does not require an erect penis, can be inserted up to 8 hours prior to intercourse, and does not need to be removed immediately after ejaculation. Compared to the male condom, the female condom also covers the base of the male penis, as well as the vulvar vestibule and a variable portion of the labia. It should not be used concurrently with a male condom.

Disadvantages of the female condom include its higher cost compared to male condoms, and the need to use it with every act of intercourse. New users may need practice to become comfortable with the method. The method can make noise during use, but this is diminished with additional lubricant. Although most young women have heard about the female condom, most prefer male condoms, and concerns about inserting it properly appears to be a barrier to its use among inner-city teens in the United States.

## CONTRACEPTIVE DIAPHRAGM, CERVICAL CAP, AND SPONGE

The combination of an intravaginal barrier with a spermicide has been recognized for centuries by women as a means of preventing pregnancy. One need only compare the modern sponge or diaphragm to the centuries-old practice of inserting a lemon or pomegranate half into the vagina to realize that our modern methods are no more than a perfection of these tried and true homemade remedies.

### Diaphragm

The diaphragm is a dome-shaped cup made of either rubber or latex that serves essentially as a holder for spermicide in the vagina. Spermicidal creams and jellies manufactured especially for the diaphragm or cap should be used. After applying spermicide to the inside of the diaphragm, the diaphragm is inserted into the vagina, where it sits snugly behind the pubic symphysis, covering the cervix and providing effective contraception for up to 6 hours. The diaphragm may be inserted up to 6 hours prior to intercourse and must remain in the vagina for at least 6 hours after intercourse has occurred. It should not remain in place for longer than 24 hours due to the risk of infection or toxic shock. After removal, the diaphragm is washed with mild soap and water, rinsed, dried, and stored in its protective container. Perfect use failure rates for the diaphragm are 6%, with more typical rates of 16%.[18]

The diaphragm should be refitted if a woman gains or loses 10 lbs, and current size confirmed at every annual visit. It should be replaced every 2 years.

The diaphragm comes in sizes from 50 to 95 mm, requires a prescription, and must be fitted by a trained health professional. Various styles are available. The thin, flat spring diaphragm is best suited for a nulliparous individual with firm vaginal tone. Arcing spring (All-flex) diaphragms are suitable for almost any woman and accommodate to the angle of the vagina under the pubic arch during insertion. Coil spring diaphragms have a single point of flexure, making them easy to insert, and may be an option for women with more lax vaginal tone. Wide seal diaphragms may be appropriate for women unable to hold a seal with the other varieties. Some women, due to vaginal anatomy or previous childbearing, should not use the diaphragm because it does not sit snugly enough in the vagina to stay in place during intercourse. For these women, the cap may be an option. A diaphragm introducer is available and may be used by women who prefer it.

Diaphragm use may increase the incidence of bacterial vaginosis and urinary tract infections (UTIs). Contraindications include spermicidal or latex allergy (except for the silicone diaphragm) or history of toxic shock. The same precautions as with latex condoms exist for use of vaginal creams and lubricants, namely, to avoid oil- and cream-based products that may deteriorate latex.

### Cervical Cap

The cervical cap differs from the diaphragm in that it fits directly over the cervix, where it is held in place by mild vacuum forces, and does not depend on vaginal tone to hold it in place. Additional spermicide is not required if repeated intercourse occurs within 6 hours.

The Prentif cap is currently unavailable in the United States. The FemCap is a nonlatex sailor hat–shaped cap that has a handle that facilitates removal. It comes in three sizes: small for nulliparous women, medium for parous women who have not had a vaginal delivery, and large for women who have had a vaginal delivery in the past. Pregnancy rates at 12 months were 23%, and ranged from 14% among users of the two smaller sizes to 29% in parous users of the largest size.[67-68]

Lea's Shield is a one-size silicone cervical cap containing both a strap for removal and a one-way valve that acts to vent the air between the device and the shield, allowing for a tight fit. The shield differs from the cap in that it relies on the upper vagina rather than the cervix to hold it in place. Spermicide is used similarly to the diaphragm. The shield must be kept in place for 8 hours after intercourse, for up to 48 hours. Unlike the diaphragm, it does not need to be fitted, and it is not affected by vaginal length or lower vaginal dimensions. First-year failure rates are 15%.[69] The incidence of may be increased among users of the shield. The only contraindications are spermicidal allergies or history of toxic shock.

A Cochrane Review of the diaphragm versus cervical cap found that although the Prentif cap was as effective as the diaphragm in preventing pregnancy, the FemCap is not, with 6-month pregnancy rates almost twice that of the diaphragm. Nulliparous women have lower failure rates than multiparous women using the cervical cap.[70] Lea's Shield was not considered in this review.

### Contraceptive Sponge

The sponge, off the US market for more than a decade due to lack of a manufacturer, was reapproved for use in the United States in 2005, and is currently available over the counter. The sponge is a small soft sponge impregnated with 1 g nonoxyl-9 spermicide; it acts as a reservoir for spermicide, a trap for sperm and semen, and a barrier between the sperm and the cervix. Moistening the sponge with water just prior to insertion into the vagina activates the spermicide, which remains effective in the vagina for up to 24 hours. The sponge must remain in place for at least 6 hours after the last intercourse that occurs during that time, after which it is removed and discarded.[71] According to a recent Cochrane Review, the sponge is less effective than the diaphragm, with failure rates of 17.4% to 24.5% at 1 year, compared with rates of 10.9% to 12.8% for diaphragm users. There are no direct comparison data comparing sponge and condom failure rates. Continuation rates at 1 year are lower with the sponge than the diaphragm.[72]

Contraindications to the sponge include sensitivity to sulfa, nonoxyl-9, or polyurethane, or a history of toxic shock. The sponge does not protect against HIV transmission, and, like other spermicides, may increase the risk of vulvitis and genital ulcers in frequent users.

One major advantage to the sponge in teenagers is that it is a female-controlled method that is available over the counter. Disadvantages are its relatively lower efficacy compared to hormonal methods, the need for use with every act of intercourse, lack of HIV protection, and issues related to messiness or removal difficulties. Combining the sponge with a condom may circumvent many of these negatives.

## SPERMICIDES

Spermicides consist of a base (foam, gel, cream, suppository, film, or tablet) and a spermicidal chemical, which in the United States is currently nonoxyl-9. Nonoxyl-9 acts as a surfactant to break down the sperm membrane. To be effective, spermicides must be inserted into the vagina prior to penile penetration. Films and suppositories require 10 to 15 minutes to dissolve and disperse in the vagina before intercourse can be initiated, whereas foams, gels, and creams are effective immediately. Efficacy in the vagina lasts up to 1 hour, after which reapplication is necessary if ejaculation has not occurred or intercourse recurs. Efficacy studies of spermicides suffer from poor design and high rates of loss to follow-up, so that reliable data are not available for most products. In a recent Cochrane Review, efficacy was related more to user characteristics and nonoxyl-9 dose (doses of 100–150 mg being 85% effective compared with 78% efficacy for 52.5-mg doses) than to choice of vehicle.[73]

Possible side effects from spermicides include vaginal odor, local irritation, allergic reactions, and possible increase in UTIs. Nonoxyl-9 spermicides do not prevent HIV transmission; in fact, they increase transmission by causing genital sores in women who use them very frequently due to irritation of the vaginal mucosa.[74] If spermicide is used, use of a condom with it is the safest choice.

## INTRAUTERINE DEVICES

The intrauterine device (IUD) is a device that is placed into the uterus to prevent pregnancy. Two IUDs are currently available in the United States: the copper T (Cu-T or ParaGard) and the levonorgestrel (Lng-IUD or Mirena). The Cu-T prevents fertilization by inhibiting sperm mobility and stimulating a cytotoxic inflammatory reaction that is spermicidal, and by changing the intrauterine environment to make it more hostile for implantation. The Lng-IUD acts by thickening the cervical mucus, thinning the endometrium, and, less frequently, inhibiting ovulation. Intrauterine devices are generally inserted during the menses, but act as highly effective emergency contraception if inserted any other time in the cycle. The Cu-T is approved for 12 years of use and the Lng-IUD for 5 years.[75,76]

The IUD is a highly effective, long-acting contraceptive. Advantages are that it is long term, easy to use, and safe for breast-feeding mothers. Users of both IUDs may experience cramping and menstrual disturbances. The Lng-IUD reduces menstrual flow, leading to amenorrhea over the long term, although bleeding may be more frequent and irregular at first. The Cu-T may cause increased menstrual flow. Users of IUDs have higher rates of bacterial vaginosis.

Although older IUDs were associated with pelvic infections, the currently marketed IUDs do not impart an infection risk beyond that associated with the procedure itself, which is limited to the first 4 to 6 weeks after insertion. These infection rates are exceedingly low, so low that prophylactic antibiotics for insertion are not routinely necessary. Modern IUDs do not impair future fertility.[77,78]

The levonorgestrel IUD is well-tolerated in adolescents using it for treatment of menorrhagia and dysmenorrhea.[79] Although there is limited data on use and acceptability of the IUD for contraception in adolescents, the method has obvious benefits in this population and can be considered a first line method for most adolescents.[80, 81, 82]

The levonorgestrel IUD may have advantages over the copper IUD in teens who have menorrhagia or dysmenorrhea. Screening for and treatment of gonorrhea and chlamydia should be done prior to IUD insertion; alternatively, prophylaxis with 1 gram of azithromycin can be given for the insertion procedure. Pre-medication with NSAIDs may help with insertion discomfort. Expulsion rates are about 3-4% for the levonorgestrel IUD in both nulliparous and parous users, while the copper IUD appears to have higher expulsions rates among nulliparas.

Intrauterine devices do not protects against HIV or STIs.

## CONCLUSION

There are many safe and effective options for contraception for the sexually active adolescent. Although use of contraception has increased, unplanned pregnancy remains a problem. Myths and concerns about safety remain an obstacle to increased uptake of effective methods. Patient counseling is a critical component of the provision of contraception to adolescents.

## INTERNET RESOURCES

- Alan Guttmacher Institute (www.guttmacher.org/): A nonprofit organization focused on sexual and reproductive health research, policy analysis, and public education.
- American College of Obstetrics and Gynecology (www.acog.org): Contraceptive and adolescent reproductive health information for clinicians.
- ARHP Adolescent Health Clinical Publications and Resources (www.arhp.org/topics/adolescent-health/clinical-publications-and-resources): Resources for reproductive health professionals who work with adolescents.
- ARHP Contraception Clinical Resources and Publications (www.arhp.org/topics/contraception/clinical-publications-and-resources)
- Emergency Contraception Web site (ec.princeton.edu/for-providers.html): Operated by Princeton University's Office of Population Research and the Association of Reproductive Health Professionals.
- Kaiser Family Foundation Daily Reproductive Health Report (www.kaisernetwork.org/daily_reports/rep_repro.cfm): An e-mail daily report on issues related to reproductive health.
- Managing Contraception (www.managing contraception.com).
- The National Campaign to Prevent Teen Pregnancy www.thenationalcampaign.org.
- Planned Parenthood Federation of America (www.ppfa.org).
- ReproLine (www.reproline.jhu.edu/).
- World Health Organization (www.who.int/reproductive-health/publications/spr/index.htm): Free full-text (pdf and html) access to *Medical Eligibility Criteria for Contraceptive Use*, 3rd ed (2004) and *Selected Practice Recommendations for Contraceptive Use*, 2nd ed (2004).

## REFERENCES


1. Abma JC, Martinez GM, Copen CE. Teenagers in the United States: sexual activity, contraceptive use, and childbearing, National Survey of Family Growth 2006–2008. National Center for Health Statistics. *Vita Health Stat*. 2010;23(30)

2. Kirby D. *No Easy Answers: Research Findings on Programs to Reduce Teen Pregnancy*. Washington, DC: The National Campaign to Prevent Teen Pregnancy; 1997

3. Trenholm C, Devaney B, Fortson K, Quay L, Wheeler J, Clark M. *Impacts of Four Title V, Section 510 Abstinence Education Programs: Final Report*. Princeton, NJ: Mathematica Policy Research, Inc.; April 2007

4. Klein JD,. The Committee on Adolescence. Adolescent pregnancy: current trends and issues. *Pediatrics*. 2005;116: 281–286

5. Dardano KL, Burkman RT. Contraceptive compliance. *Obstet Gynecol Clin North Am*. 2000;27:933–941

6. Morrison CS, Bright P, Wong EL, et al. Hormonal contraceptive use, cervical ectopy, and the acquisition of cervical infections. *Sex Transm Dis*. 2004;31(9):561–567

7. Santeli JS, Lindberg LD, Finer LB, Singh S. Adolescent pregnancy in the United States: the contribution of abstinence and improved contraceptive use. *Am J Public Health*. 2007;(1):1–7

8. Woods JL, Shew ML, Tu W, Ofner S, Ott MA, Fortenberry JD. Patterns of oral contraceptive pill-taking and condom use among adolescent contraceptive pill users. *J Adolesc Health*. 2006;39:381–387

9. Holt VL, Scholes D, Wicklund KG, Cushing-Hagan KL, Daling JR. Body mass index, weight, and oral contraceptive failure risk. *Obstet Gynecol*. 2005;105:46–52

10. Forinash AB, Evans SL. New hormonal contraceptives: a comprehensive review of the literature. *Pharmacotherapy*. 2003;23:1573–1591

11. Stewart FH, Harper CC, Ellertson CE, Grimes DA, Sawaya GF, Trussell J. Clinical breast and pelvic examination requirements for hormonal contraception: current practice vs evidence. *JAMA*. 2001;285:2232–2239

12. Westhoff C, Kerns J, Morroni C, Cushman LF, Tiezzi L, Murphy PA. Quick Start: novel oral contraceptive initiation method. *Contraception*. 2002;66:141–145

13. Westhoff C, Morroni C, Kerns J, Murphy PA. Bleeding patterns after immediate vs conventional oral contraceptive initiation: a randomized, controlled trial. *Fertil Steril*. 2003;79:322–329

14. Lesnewski R, Prine L. Initiating hormonal contraception. *Am Family Physician*. 2006;74:105–112

15. Mosher WD, Martinez GM, Chandra A, Abma JC, Willson SJ. Use of contraception and use of family planning services in the United States: 1982–2002. *Adv Data*. 2004;10:1–36

16. World Health Organization (WHO). *Medical Eligibility for Contraceptive Use*. 3rd ed. Geneva: WHO; 2004

17. Rivera R, Yacobson I, Grimes D. The mechanism of action of hormonal contraceptives and intrauterine contraceptive devices. *Am J Obstet Gynecol*. 1999;181(5 pt 1):1263–1269

18. Hatcher RA, Trussell J, Stewart F, et al. *Contraceptive Technology*. 18th rev ed. New York: Ardent Media; 2005

19. Van Vliet HA, Grimes DA, Helmerhorst FM, Schulz KF. Biphasic versus monophasic oral contraceptives for contraception: a Cochrane Review. *Hum Reprod*. 2002;870–873.

20. Van Vliet HA, Grimes DA, Helmerhorst FM, Schulz KF. Triphasic versus monophasic oral contraceptives for contraception. *Cochrane Database Syst Rev*. 2001; (2). Art. No.: CD003553. DOI: 10.1002/14651858.CD003553

21. Van Vliet HA, Grimes DA, Helmerhorst FM, Schulz KF. Biphasic versus triphasic oral contraceptives for contraception. *Cochrane Database Syst Rev*. 2006;19;3:CD003283

22. Burkett AM, Hewitt GD. Progestin-only contraceptives and their use in adolescents: clinical options and medical indications. *Adolesc Med Clin*. 2005;1:553–567

23. Ornstein RM, Fisher MM. Hormonal contraception in adolescents: special considerations. *Paediatr Drugs*. 2006;8:25–45

24. Harel Z. Dysmenorrhea in adolescents and young adults: etiology and management. *J Pediatr Adolesc Gynecol*. 2006;19:363–371

25. Arowojolu AO, Gallo MF, Grimes DA, Garner SE. Combined oral contraceptive pills for treatment of acne. *Cochrane Database Syst Rev*. 2004;(3):CD004425

26. Rosenfield RL. Clinical practice: hirsutism. *N Engl J Med*. 2005;353(24):2578–2588

27. Blackburn RD, Cunkelman JA, Zlidar VM. Oral contraceptives—an update. *Population Reports*. Series A, No. 9. Baltimore: The Johns Hopkins University School of Public Health, Population Information Program; Spring 2000. Available at: www.infoforhealth.org/pr/a9/a9.pdf. Accessed September 1, 2009

28. DiVasta AD, Gordon CM. Bone health in adolescents. *Adolesc Med Clin*. 2006;17(3):639–652

29. Pearlstein TB, Bachmann GA, Zacur HA, Yonkers KA. Treatment of premenstrual dysphoric disorder with a new drospirenone-containing oral contraceptive formulation. *Contraception*. 2005;72(6):414–421. Epub November 2, 2005

30. Kaunitz AM. Oral contraceptive health benefits: perception versus reality. *Contraception*. 1999;59(1 suppl):29S-33S

31. Creinin MD, Lisman R, Strickler RC. Screening for factor V Leiden mutation before prescribing combination oral contraceptives. *Fertil Steril*. 1999;72(4):646–651

32. Gomes MP, Deitcher SR. Risk of venous thromboembolic disease associated with hormonal contraceptives and hormone replacement therapy: a clinical review. *Arch Intern Med*. 2004;164(18):1965–1976

33. Smith JS, Green J, Berrington de Gonzalez A. Cervical cancer and use of hormonal contraceptives: a systematic review. *Lancet*. 2003;361(9364):1159–1167

34. Ness RB, Soper DE, Holley RL, et al. PID Evaluation and Clinical Health (PEACH) Study Investigators. Hormonal and barrier contraception and risk of upper genital tract disease in the PID Evaluation and Clinical Health (PEACH) study. *Am J Obstet Gynecol*. 2001;185(1):121–127

35. Zupanc ML. Antiepileptic dregs and hormonal contraceptives in adolescent women with epilepsy. *Neurology*. 2006;66:S37–S45

36. Dickinson BD, Altman RD, Nielsen NH, Sterling ML, for the Council on Scientific Affairs, American Medical Association. Drug interactions between oral contraceptives and antibiotics. *Obstet Gynecol*. 2001;98:853–860

37. Pfrunder A, Schiesser M, Gerber S, Haschke M, Bitzer J, Drewe J. Interaction of St John's wort with low-dose oral contraceptive therapy: a randomized controlled trial. *Br J Clin Pharmacol*. 2003;56(6):683–690

38. Zamah NM, Humpe lM, Kuhnz W, Louton T, Rafferty J, Back DJ. Absence of an effect of high vitamin C dosage on

the systemic availability of ethinyl estradiol in women using a combination oral contraceptive. *Contraception*. 1993;48(4): 377–391

39. Office of AIDS Research Advisory Council. Guidelines for the use of antiretroviral agents in HIV-1-infected adults and adolescents. January 29, 2008. Available at: www.aidsinfo.nih.gov/ContentFiles/AdultandAdolescentGL.pdf. Accessed June 11, 2008

40. Cerel-Suhl SL, Yeager BF. Update on oral contraceptive pills. *Am Family Physician*. 1999;60:2073

41. Hatcher RA, et al. *Contraceptive Technology*. 18th revised ed. New York: Ardent Media; 2005

42. Sher PP. Drug interference with laboratory tests—oral contraceptives. *Drug Ther (NY)*. 1977;2:61–63

43. Gold MA, Sucato GS, Conard LA, Adams Hillard P. Provision of emergency contraception to adolescents: position paper of the Society for Adolescent Medicine. *J Adolesc Health*. 2004;25 (1):66–70

44. Westoff C. Depot-medroxyprogesterone acetate injection (Depo-Provera): a highly effective contraceptive option with proven long-term safety. *Contraception*. 2003;68(2): 75–87

45. Belsey EM. The association between vaginal bleeding patterns and reasons for discontinuation of contraceptive use. *Contraception*. 1988;38(2):207–225

46. Harel Z, Johnson CC, Gold MA, et al. Recovery of bone mineral density in adolescents following the use of depot medroxyprogesterone acetate contraceptive injections. *Contraception*. 2010 Apr;81(4):281–29

47. Curtis KM, Martins SL. Progestogen-only contraception and bone mineral density: a systematic review. *Contraception*. 2006;73(5):470–487

48. Forinash AB, Evans SL. New hormonal contraceptives: a comprehensive review of the literature. *Pharmacotherapy*. 2003;23(12):1573–1591

49. van den Heuvel MW, van Bragt AJ, Alnabawy AK, Kaptein MC. Comparison of ethinylestradiol pharmacokinetics in three hormonal contraceptive formulations: the vaginal ring, the transdermal patch, and an oral contraceptive. *Contraception*. 2005;72(3):168–174

50. Cole JA, Norman H, Doherty M, Walker AM. Venous thromboembolism, myocardial infarction, and stroke among transdermal contraceptive system users. *Obstet Gynecol*. 2007;109(2 pt 1):339–346

51. Jick SS, Jick H. Cerebral venous sinus thrombosis in users of four hormonal contraceptives: levonorgestrel-containing oral contraceptives, norgestimate-containing oral contraceptives, desogestrel-containing oral contraceptives and the contraceptive patch. *Contraception*. 2006;74(4):290–292. Epub July 7, 2006

52. Jick SS, Kaye JA, Russmann S, Jick H. Risk of nonfatal venous thromboembolism in women using a contraceptive transdermal patch and oral contraceptives containing norgestimate and 35 microg of ethinyl estradiol. *Contraception*. 2006;73(3):223–228. Epub January 26, 2006

53. Rubinstein ML, Halpern-Felsher BL, Irwin CE Jr. An evaluation of the use of the transdermal contraceptive patch in adolescents. *J Adolesc Health*. 2004;34 (5):395–401

54. Logsdon S, Richards J, Omar HA. Long-term evaluation of the use of the transdermal contraceptive patch in adolescents. *Sci World J*. 2004;4:512–516

55. Harel Z, Riggs S, Vaz R, Flanagan P, Dunn K, Hare lD. Adolescents' experience with the combined estrogen and progestin transdermal contraceptive method Ortho Evra. *J Pediatr Adolesc Gynecol*. 2005;18(2):85–90

56. Dieben TO, Roumen FJ, Apter D. Efficacy, cycle control, and user acceptability of a novel combined contraceptive vaginal ring. *Obstet Gynecol*. 2002;100 (3):585–593

57. Vree M. Lower hormone dosage with improved cycle control. *Eur J Contracept Reprod Health Care*. 2002;7 (suppl 2):25–30; discussion 37–39

58. Bjarnadottir RI, Tuppurainen M, Killick SR. Comparison of cycle control with a combined contraceptive vaginal ring and oral levonorgestrel/ethinyl estradiol. *Am J Obstet Gynecol*. 2002;186(3):389–395

59. Haring T, Mulders TM. The combined contraceptive ring NuvaRing and spermicide co-medication. *Contraception*. 2003;67:271–272

60. Funk S, Miller MM, Mishell DR, Archer DF, Poindexter A, Schmidt D, et al, for The Implanon US Study Group. Safety and efficacy of Implanon, a single-rod implantable contraceptive containing etonogestrel. *Contraception*. 2005;71(5): 319–326

61. Sayegh MA, Fortenberry JD, Shew M, Orr DP. The developmental association of relationship quality, hormonal contraceptive choice, and condom non-use among adolescent women. *J Adolesc Health*. 2006; 39(3):388–395

62. Miller KS, Levin ML, Whitaker DJ, Xu X. Patterns of condom use among adolescents: the impact of mother–adolescent communication. *Am J Public Health*. 1998;88 (10):1542–1544

63. Crosby RA, Sanders SA, Yarber WL, Graham CA, Dodge B. Condom use errors and problems among college men. *Sex Transm Dis*. 2002;29(9):552–557

64. Trussel J. Contraceptive efficacy of the Reality female condom—a critical review of the literature. *Contraception*. 1998;58(3):147–148

65. Macaluso M, Lawson ML, Hortin G, Duerr A, Hammond KR, Blackwell R, et al. Efficacy of the female condom as a barrier to semen during intercourse. *Am J Epidemiol*. 2003;157(4):289–297

66. Lawson ML, Macaluso M, Duerr A, et al. Partner characteristics, intensity of the intercourse, and semen exposure during use of the female condom. *Am J Epidemiol*. 2003;157(4): 282–288

67. FDA Femcap Approval. Information. FemCap - P020041. March 28, 2003. Available at:www.accessdata. fda.gov/scripts/

cdrh/cfdocs/cftopic/pma/pma.cfm?num=p020041. Accessed October 13, 2009

68. Mauck C, Callahan M, Weiner DH, Dominik R. A comparative study of the safety and efficacy of FemCap, a new vaginal barrier contraceptive, and the Ortho All-Flex diaphragm. The FemCap Investigators' Group. *Contraception*. 1999;60(2):71–80

69. Mauck C, Glover LH, Miller E, et al. Lea's Shield: a study of the safety and efficacy of a new vaginal barrier contraceptive used with and without spermicide. *Contraception*. 1996;53(6):329–335

70. Gallo MF, Grimes DA, Schulz KF. Cervical cap versus diaphragm for contraception. *Cochrane Database Syst Rev*. 2002;(4):CD003551

71. Yranski PA, Gamache ME. New options for barrier contraception. *J Obstet Gynecol Neonatal Nurs*. 2008;37(3): 384–389

72. Kuyoh MA, Toroitich-Ruto C, Grimes DA, Schulz KF, Gallo MF. Sponge versus diaphragm for contraception: a Cochrane Review. *Contraception*. 2003;67(1):15–18

73. Grimes DA, Lopez L, Raymond EG, Halpern V, Nanda K, Schulz KF. Spermicide used alone for contraception. *Cochrane Database Syst Rev*. 2005;(4). Art. No.: CD005218. DOI: 10.1002/14651858.CD005218.pub2

74. *WHO/CONRAD Technical Consultation on Nonoxynol-9: Summary Report*. Geneva: World Health Organization (WHO); October 9–10, 2001. Available at: www.aegis.com/files/who/N9_meeting_report.pdf. Accessed September 1, 2009

75. Rivera R, Yacobson I, Grimes D. The mechanism of action of hormonal contraceptives and intrauterine contraceptive devices. *Am J Obstet Gynecol*. 1999;181(5, pt 1):1263–1269

76. Johnson BA. Insertion and removal of intrauterine devices. *Am Fam Physician*. 2005;71(1):95–102

77. Hov GG, Skjeldestad FE, Hilstad T. Use of IUD and subsequent fertility—-follow-up after participation in a randomized clinical trial. *Contraception*. 2007;75(2):88–92. Epub November 14, 2006

78. Doll H, Vessey M, Painter R. Return of fertility in nulliparous women after discontinuation of the intrauterine device: comparison with women discontinuing other methods of contraception. *BJOG* 2001;108:304–314

79. Aslam N, Blunt, S, Latthe, P. Effectiveness and tolerability of levonorgestrel intrauterine system in adolescents. *J Obstet Gynecol*. 2010;30(5):489

80. ACOG.ACOG Committee Opinion No. 392, December 2007. Intrauterine device and adolescents. *Obstet Gynecol*. 2007 Dec;10(6):1493

81. Yen S, Saah T, Hillard PJ. IUDs and adolescents–An under-utilized opportunity for pregnancy prevention. *J Pediatr Adolesc Gynecol*. 2010;23(3):123-128.

82. Lara-Torre E, Spotswood L, Correia N, Weiss PM. Intrauterine contraception in adolescents and young women: a descriptive study of use, side effects, and compliance. *J Pediatr Adolesc Gynecol*. 2011;24(1):39-41.

# CHAPTER 53

## Sexually Transmitted Infections

TANYA KOWALCZYK MULLINS, MD, MS • PAULA K. BRAVERMAN, MD

### OVERVIEW OF SEXUALLY TRANSMITTED INFECTIONS (STIs) IN ADOLESCENTS

Adolescents have the highest risk of sexually transmitted infections (STIs) of any sexually active age group.[1] Biological, behavioral, and developmental factors, as well as issues related to access to health care, contribute to this increased risk.

#### BIOLOGICAL FACTORS

Adolescent women have an increased biological susceptibility to STIs due to the presence of the cervical ectropion. The ectropion is an area of columnar epithelium that is generally present within the endocervix in adult women but can be located on the exocervix of healthy adolescent women. The area between the normal squamous epithelium of the exocervix and the columnar epithelium is the transition zone, which is an area of active squamous metaplasia. Many STI pathogens have an increased tropism for the transition zone and columnar epithelium. Lack of cervical immunity may also contribute to the increased risk of STIs as most adolescents are newly exposed to STIs and thus do not have protective immunity.[2]

#### BEHAVIORAL FACTORS

Younger age at first intercourse is associated with an increased number of STIs, although this effect diminishes with time after sexual initiation.[3] Adolescents are also more likely to engage in risky sexual behaviors. These include poor use of condoms[4] and substance use during sexual encounters, which increase the likelihood of poor decision making. In addition, although teens are generally monogamous[3] adolescent sexual relationships are usually shorter in duration than those of adults, leading to more sequential sexual partners and increased chances for exposure to STIs. Some subpopulations of adolescents have higher rates of STIs, including those in juvenile justice centers, injection drug users, and patients attending STI clinics.

#### DEVELOPMENTAL FACTORS

Adolescence is characterized by a sense of invulnerability to negative outcomes, including STIs. Many adolescents are woefully unaware of the risks associated with sexual activity, and many have never had frank discussions with a trusted adult about self-protection, including condom use. In one study, even when confronted with the reality of an STI diagnosis, 81.3% of a group of teen women studied characterized themselves as being at "little or no risk" of acquiring STIs.[5]

#### HEALTH CARE ACCESS

Factors related to accessing the health care system also play a role in the increased risk of STIs in adolescents. Fear of disclosure of sexual activity to parents may prevent teens from seeking medical care. Inability to pay for medical services and lack of access to teen-friendly clinics are also contributing factors.[4] Further, many teens are not aware that they are legally entitled to confidential STI-related health care.

#### PROTECTIVE FACTORS

In general, parental monitoring, open communication between teens and parents, and a high degree of parental supervision are protective against risk-taking behaviors in teens, including substance use, sexual activity, and delinquency.[6] In one study, teens who reported higher levels of perceived parental supervision were less likely to have gonorrhea or chlamydia.[7] In another study, adolescents with higher grades in high school and greater perceived parental disapproval of sex were less likely to be diagnosed with STIs in early adulthood.[8]

### TAKING A SEXUAL HISTORY

When assessing an adolescent presenting with complaints suggestive of genital infection, a nonjudgmental, open manner and absence of medical jargon goes a long way in establishing rapport. It is often helpful to discuss confidentiality issues proactively with the adolescent to build trust. Adolescents in general are honest even when asked personal questions. Assessment should include age at first intercourse, number of partners, age of partners, types of sexual activity (oral, vaginal, digital, anal), condom use with specific types of intercourse, and previous personal or partner history of STIs. In addition to genital and systemic symptoms, pharyngeal and anorectal symptoms should be discussed because many STIs can infect these areas, and adolescents may be less likely to use condoms during oral or anal intercourse. Sexually active adolescent women who complain about urinary symptoms (eg, dysuria) should be evaluated for urinary tract infection (UTI) and STIs. Sexually transmitted infections may cause dysuria, mimicking symptoms of UTI, and UTI and STI may coexist.[9]

## NEW DEVELOPMENTS IN STI TESTING

Recent developments in laboratory tests available for STIs have dramatically changed the ability of clinicians to detect these infections. The bacterial STIs that are most commonly included in screening are *Neisseria gonorrhoeae* (GC) and *Chlamydia trachomatis* (CT). Cultures for GC and CT had been the gold standard in the past. Chlamydia culture results are dependent on the skill and performance characteristics of the laboratory performing the test.[10] The sensitivity of chlamydia culture is 50% to 85%,[11] although the specificity is somewhat greater. Gonorrhea culture reaches a 69.8% to 92.6% sensitivity and 100% specificity.[11] Because of the high specificity of culture and lack of false-positive results, culture has historically been the only acceptable method of identification in legal cases. Other available testing methods have included nucleic acid hybridization tests, direct fluorescent antibody tests (CT only), and enzyme immunoassays. In general, these tests are not as sensitive as culture tests and can produce false-positive results. Non-culture tests are most accurate in high-prevalence populations because as the prevalence of a disease increases, the number of false-positive results decreases.

The latest developments in testing methodology include nucleic acid amplification tests (NAATs), which do not require viable organisms and have improved sensitivity and specificity when compared to culture, especially in the case of CT infection. These methods include polymerase chain reaction (PCR), strand displacement amplification, and transcription-mediated amplification. Many of the NAAT methods may be used not only on endocervical or urethral samples but also on first voided urine samples, providing a less invasive and more acceptable means for routine asymptomatic STI screening. The Aptima 2 assay (Gen Probe, San Diego, CA) and the BD ProbeTec *Chlamydia trachomatis/Neisseria gonorrhoeae* (CT/GC) $Q^x$ Amplified DNA Assays (BD, Franklin Lakes, NJ) have also been approved for use with clinician or patient-obtained vaginal swabs, alleviating the need for a speculum examination.[12,13]

Spigarelli and Biro[11] reviewed the literature on NAATs and found that NAATs have better sensitivity than culture for detection of CT. In the same review, cervical specimens are more sensitive than urine specimens for women, whereas urine specimens for men are comparable or more sensitive than urethral specimens (Table 53-1). Specific testing strategies for GC, CT, and other pathogens of interest are discussed in the subsequent sections.

**Table 53-1**

**Test Characteristics of Nucleic Acid Amplification Tests (NAATs)[11]**

| | *Sensitivity (%)* | *Specificity (%)* |
|---|---|---|
| **Chlamydia** | | |
| Cervix | 92.8–98.4 | 97.9–99.7 |
| Urine (female) | 83.9–96.8 | 98.3–99.5 |
| Urethra (male) | 85.7–94.6 | 97.6–99.3 |
| Urine (male) | 93.5–96.3 | 98.8–99.2 |
| **Gonorrhea** | | |
| Cervix | 96.1–99.2 | 98.7–99.6 |
| Urine (female) | 83.3–91.3 | 98.5–99.4 |
| Urethra (male) | 98.4–99.0 | 96.5–99.2 |
| Urine (male) | 95.8–98.2 | 99.2–99.4 |

## ULCERATIVE GENITAL LESIONS

Several STIs are characterized by genital ulcers, including herpes simplex virus (HSV), syphilis, chancroid (*Haemophilus ducreyi*), and lymphogranuloma venereum (LGV). In the United States, the assessment of a genital ulcer usually includes evaluation for syphilis, HSV and *H ducreyi*, as these are the most common genital ulcer diseases in this country. The prompt evaluation and treatment of genital ulcers is imperative as human immunodeficiency virus (HIV) transmission is enhanced via disruptions in the skin and mucosal surfaces.

### HERPES SIMPLEX VIRUS

#### Epidemiology

Two types of HSV infect humans: HSV-1 and HSV-2. Seroprevalence studies indicate that HSV infection varies by type and age. In the National Health and Nutrition Examination Survey (NHANES) 1999–2004, seroprevalence of HSV-1 in 14- to 19-year-olds was 39%, increasing to 54.4% in 20- to 29-year-olds. HSV-2 seroprevalence was 1.6% in 14- to 19-year-olds and 10.6% in 20- to 29-year-olds.[14]

Herpes episodes may be categorized as primary (true first episode of infection with no evidence of prior HSV exposure on serologic testing); nonprimary (first clinical episode of HSV in a patient with serologic evidence of past HSV infection, indicating past subclinical episodes); and recurrent (episode of HSV in a patient with a past history of symptomatic HSV infection). HSV-1 infection has classically been associated with herpetic gingivostomatitis, contracted via kissing or contact with oral secretions, and HSV-2 with genital HSV infection, contracted via genital-genital sexual contact. However, an increasing proportion of genital herpes infections are associated with HSV-1, which has been linked to receptive oral sex. The increasing proportion of genital HSV-1 infection compared with HSV-2 may be due to changing trends in sexual behavior.[15] Overall, HSV-1 genital infection is associated with a decreased number of recurrences and decreased viral shedding compared to HSV-2.[4]

### Biology/Pathophysiology

HSV-1 and HSV-2 are members of the herpes virus family. Acquisition of infection occurs following close contact of mucosal areas or abraded or injured skin with an individual who is shedding the virus. Once infection is established, the virus travels along sensory nerves to the nerve root ganglia and enters a latent phase. Subsequently, the virus may become reactivated and cause recurrent disease.[16]

### Clinical Presentation

Symptomatic genital HSV infection classically presents with clusters of multiple small painful vesicles or ulcers (Figure 53-1).[4,16] Lesions also may be atypical, appearing as linear ulcerations or fissures[16] and may last 4 to 15 days.[4,16] Other presenting symptoms include dysuria, discharge, pain, pruritis, or inguinal lymphadenopathy. HSV cervicitis is common in women with the first genital HSV outbreak. Primary HSV outbreaks are often associated with systemic symptoms including fever, malaise, and myalgias.[16] The natural history of genital herpes includes a pattern of outbreaks that generally become less frequent over time. Recurrent HSV is often associated with prodromal symptoms, most often tingling or pain in the affected area. Both HSV strains may lead to recurrences and viral shedding, which can be symptomatic or asymptomatic.[4]

(A)

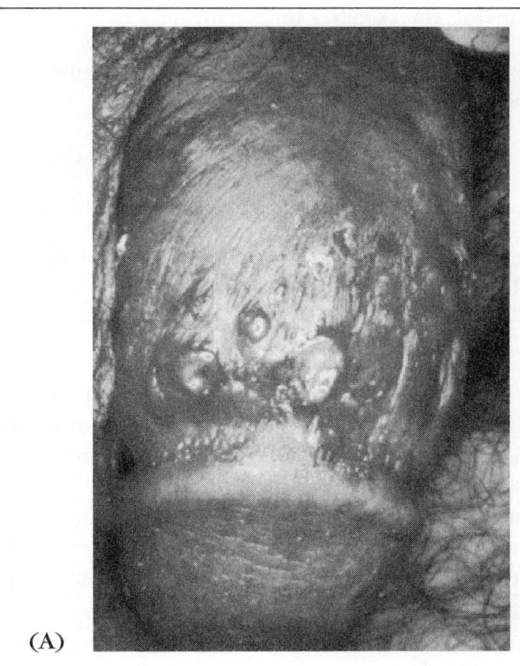

(B)

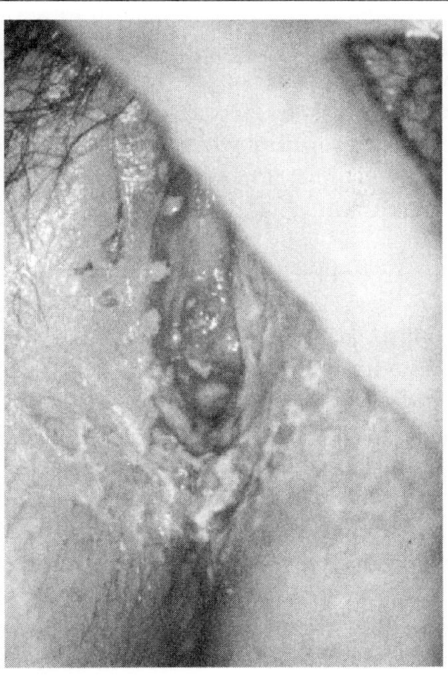

**FIGURE 53-1** Herpes Simplex Virus (HSV). (A) Primary HSV in a male patient. (B) Primary HSV in a female patient. (From Centers for Disease Control and Prevention (CDC), Training and Health Communication Branch of the Division of STD Prevention, National Center for HIV/AIDS, Viral Hepatitis, STD, and TB Prevention. Available at: www.cdc.gov/std/training/clinicalslides/slides-dl.htm.) (See color insert)

### Complications

Complications of genital HSV infection include aseptic meningitis, transverse myelitis, autonomic nervous dysfunction, pharyngeal HSV, disseminated HSV, and bacterial superinfection of HSV lesions. Aseptic meningitis is generally caused by HSV-2, whereas oral HSV-1 is associated with encephalitis.[16] In addition, prenatal and neonatal infection may occur, particularly if primary infection occurs during late pregnancy. The risk of transmission to a fetus is decreased during recurrent HSV infection as compared to primary episodes due to the protective effect of maternal antibodies.[4]

### Diagnosis

Because genital HSV infection can be caused by either HSV-1 or HSV-2, the Centers for Disease Control and Prevention (CDC) recommends laboratory testing of herpetic lesions to identify the infecting strain. Although HSV culture of suspicious lesions is preferred, this methodology is less reliable once lesions have begun to heal or for recurrent episodes. In these cases, although not currently FDA-approved for use in the diagnosis of genital HSV, PCR is more sensitive. HSV PCR may only be available from reference laboratories, which may have different validation procedures and levels of testing for sensitivity and specificity. Use of Tzanck preparation or other methods to detect cellular changes are not recommended. Type-specific HSV serology is available and may be useful in patients with HSV recurrences or in those with a clinical diagnosis of HSV who are culture negative. Serology is not recommended for screening of asymptomatic individuals. One potential exception would be in HSV-discordant couples to determine if one of the partners is at risk for primary infection.[4]

### Treatment/Management

Medical management of genital HSV infection decreases clinical symptoms during an outbreak as well as viral shedding and transmission to sexual partners. For the initial episode, therapy generally begins with acyclovir, famciclovir, or valacyclovir for 7 to 10 days. For recurrent episodes, these medications may be used intermittently during outbreaks or as daily suppressive therapy. The CDC recommends that patients be counseled about the availability of both therapies. Intermittent therapy is generally started when the patient first notes prodromal symptoms or lesions, preferably within 24 hours, and is given for a shorter course than for initial episodes. Valacyclovir, which is given as a single daily dose, may be preferred by some patients. Daily suppressive therapy decreases the frequency of HSV outbreaks and decreases asymptomatic viral shedding.[4] Use of daily valacyclovir by HSV-2 infected individuals is associated with decreased transmission to partners, decreased number of recurrences, and decreased number of days of detectable viral shedding. (See Box 53-1 for recommended treatment of HSV.)

Because ulcerative genital diseases are associated with an increased risk of HIV acquisition, patients who are diagnosed with HSV should also receive HIV testing. The CDC strongly encourages thorough counseling of patients with newly diagnosed HSV, as this diagnosis can be emotionally difficult. Counseling should include discussion of the natural history of the infection, therapy options, asymptomatic viral shedding, partner notification, risks of HSV during pregnancy, and avoidance of intercourse when lesions or prodromal symptoms are

## Box 53-1

### *Herpes Simplex Virus Treatment*

**First Episode:**

Acyclovir 400 mg orally 3 times daily for 7–10 days
OR
Acyclovir 200 mg orally 5 times daily for 7–10 days
OR
Famciclovir 250 mg orally 3 times daily for 7–10 days
OR
Valacyclovir 1 gram orally 2 times daily for 7–10 days

**Daily Suppressive Therapy:**

Acyclovir 400 mg orally 2 times daily
OR
Famciclovir 250 mg orally 2 times daily
OR
Valacyclovir 500 mg orally 1 time daily
OR
Valacyclovir 1 gram orally 1 time daily

**Episodic Therapy for Recurrences:**

Acyclovir 400 mg orally 3 times daily for 5 days
OR
Acyclovir 800 mg orally 2 times daily for 5 days
OR
Acyclovir 800 mg orally 3 times daily for 2 days
OR
Famciclovir 125 mg orally 2 times daily for 5 days
OR
Famciclovir 1 gram orally 2 times daily for 1 day
OR
Famciclovir 500 mg once, then 250 mg 2 times daily for 2 days
OR
Valacyclovir 500 mg orally 2 times daily for 3 days
OR
Valacyclovir 1 gram orally 1 time daily for 5 days

Source: CDC. Sexually transmitted diseases treatment guidelines, 2010. *MMWR*. 2010;59:21–22

present. HSV-discordant couples should be counseled to avoid intercourse when active lesions are present, and to consistently use condoms. HSV vaccines are under development, although none are currently available commercially.

## SYPHILIS (*TREPONEMA PALLIDUM*)

### Epidemiology

In 2008, the rate of primary and secondary syphilis in 15- to 19-year-olds was 4.6 per 100,000 and 11.4 per 100,000 in 20- to 24-year-olds. The highest rate of primary and secondary syphilis are in women aged 20 to 24 and men aged 20 to 24. Syphilis is more common in black men, and those residing in the Southern region of the United States.[17] Overall, the rates of primary and secondary syphilis declined through the 1990s; however, between 2001 and 2008, there was an increase in the rate of primary and secondary syphilis. Between 2007 and 2008, the rate of primary and secondary syphilis increased by 18.4%, with a 15.2% increase in men and a 36.4% increase in women.[17] Recent epidemiologic studies demonstrate that much of this increase can be attributed to the rise in syphilis cases in men who have sex with men, possibly due to poor adherence with safer sex recommendations.[18,19]

### Biology/Pathophysiology

Syphilis is caused by the spirochete *Treponema pallidum* (Figure 53-2), and humans are the only host for this pathogen.[20] In adolescents, syphilis infection is generally acquired via sexual contact with the highly infectious cutaneous lesions.[21]

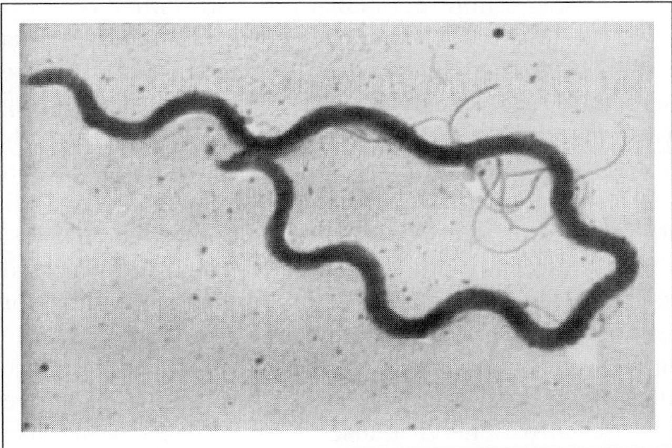

FIGURE 53-2 Syphilis: *Treponema pallidum* organism. (From Centers for Disease Control and Prevention (CDC), Training and Health Communication Branch of the Division of STD Prevention, National Center for HIV/AIDS, Viral Hepatitis, STD, and TB Prevention. Available at: www.cdc.gov/std/training/clinicalslides/slides-dl.htm.)

### Clinical Presentation

The average incubation period for syphilis is 3 weeks with a range of 10 to 90 days.[21] Syphilis occurs in several stages: primary, secondary, latency, and tertiary.

Primary syphilis is characterized by one or more painless indurated genital ulcerations (chancres) (Figure 53-3) that are filled with infectious spirochetes. Associated regional adenopathy is common.[20] The chancre is generally 1 to 2 cm in diameter and resolves in 3 to 6 weeks, even without antibiotic therapy.[22] Two to 10 weeks after appearance of the chancre and following systemic dissemination of treponemes, signs of secondary syphilis develop. Dermatologic manifestations include a maculopapular, reddish, slightly scaly skin rash that involves the palms and soles (Figure 53-4) and characteristic mucous membrane lesions that appear as raised gray papules in the moist regions of the body such as the groin or axilla. These lesions are called condyloma lata and are the result of hyperplasia of the epidermis in response to the infection.[20,22] Other accompanying systemic symptoms may include malaise, fever, weight loss, and lymphadenopathy. Secondary syphilis also spontaneously resolves after 3 to 12 weeks, and the patient enters the asymptomatic latency phase. During this stage, infection can only be diagnosed with serologic testing.[22] Early latent syphilis lasts for 1 to 2 years, during which time patients may relapse into active secondary syphilis. Patients in the late latent phase do not relapse.[23]

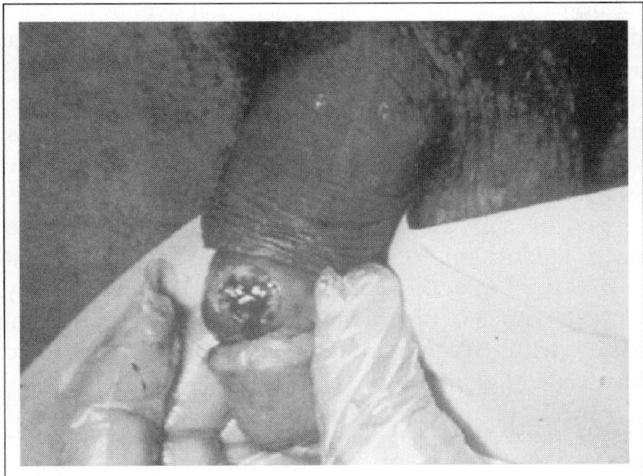

FIGURE 53-3 Primary syphilis: Chancre on penis. (From Centers for Disease Control and Prevention (CDC), Training and Health Communication Branch of the Division of STD Prevention, National Center for HIV/AIDS, Viral Hepatitis, STD, and TB Prevention. Available at: www.cdc.gov/std/training/clinicalslides/slides-dl.htm.) (See color insert)

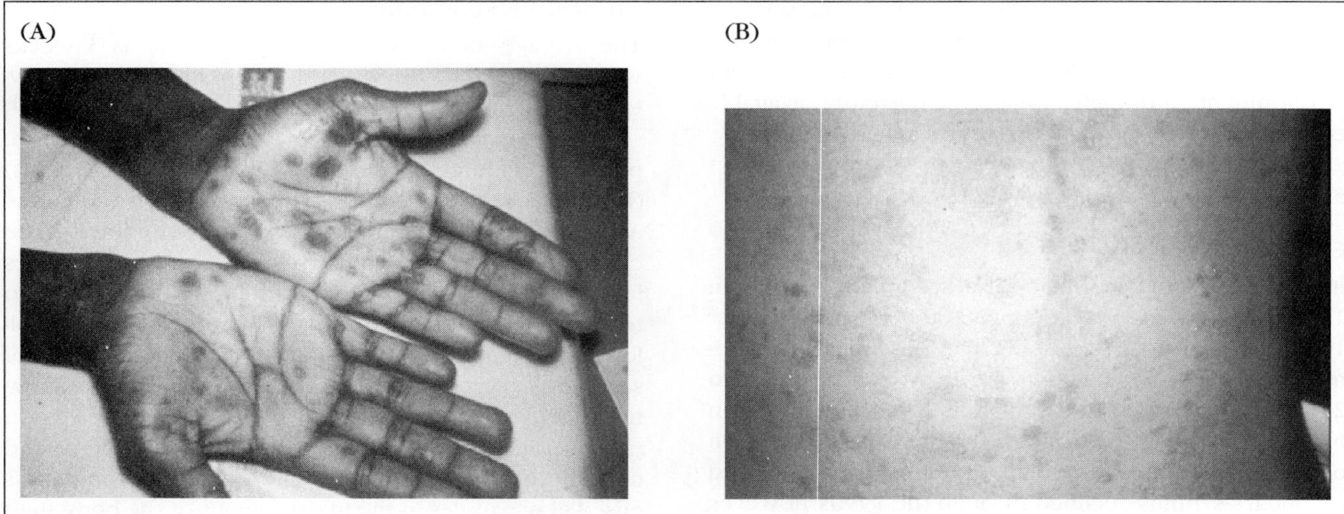


**FIGURE 53-4** Secondary syphilis. (A) Characteristic rash on palms of hands; (B) Characteristic maculopapular slightly scaly rash on the trunk. (From Centers for Disease Control and Prevention (CDC), Training and Health Communication Branch of the Division of STD Prevention, National Center for HIV/AIDS, Viral Hepatitis, STD, and TB Prevention. Available at: www.cdc.gov/std/training/clinicalslides/slides-dl.htm.) (See color insert.)

Tertiary syphilis occurs after a variable length of time and affects multiple systems, including the central nervous system, eyes, cardiovascular system, skin/connective tissue, and bone. Focal areas of necrosis, known as gummas, may occur anywhere in the body, particularly in the skin, soft tissues, and bones.[23] Cardiovascular syphilis may involve the myocardium, aorta, aortic valve, or coronary arteries.[23] Progressive visual loss due to optic atrophy can occur. Neurologic involvement may include meningitis, meningoencephalitis, cerebrovascular syphilis, meningovascular syphilis of the spinal cord, and tabes dorsalis. Tabes dorsalis is characterized by shooting pains, paresthesias, and decreased deep tendon reflexes.[23] Neurosyphilis may occur at any stage of infection and should be considered in any patient who has neurologic complaints. Patients coinfected with HIV are more likely to have neurologic involvement earlier in the course of the disease.[4]

### Complications

In addition to complications of tertiary syphilis noted previously pregnant women may transmit syphilis to the unborn fetus, leading to congenital infection in the newborn. Fetal transmission may occur at any stage but is most likely during the primary and secondary stages (60% to 100% transmission). Syphilis during pregnancy may also result in stillbirth, spontaneous abortion, or perinatal death.[21]

### Diagnosis

Definitive diagnosis of syphilis is made by direct visualization of treponemes with darkfield microscopy or direct fluorescent antibody testing for treponemes in body fluid or tissue samples. As these techniques are generally unavailable, most diagnoses are presumptive and made by serological testing. Blood samples are first tested using a nontreponemal test with either Venereal Disease Research Laboratory [VDRL] or rapid plasma reagin [RPR]. Patients who are positive on one of these screening tests must then have confirmatory testing with a treponemal test: fluorescent treponemal antibody absorbed [FTA-ABS] or *T pallidum* particle agglutination [TP-PA]. Treponemal tests generally remain positive for life even after treatment. However, nontreponemal test results correlate with disease activity and are reported as an antibody titer that is followed to monitor for response to treatment. HIV-infected individuals may have inconsistent titers that can be more difficult to interpret. Because of the association of HIV with genital ulcerative disease, all patients diagnosed with syphilis should also be tested for HIV.[4]

Evaluation for neurosyphilis should be done in patients with 1) neurologic or ophthalmologic complaints or related physical findings, 2) active tertiary syphilis, or 3) failure to respond to appropriate antibiotic therapy. No single laboratory study provides the diagnosis of neurosyphilis. Therefore, a combination of tests are used, including serologic testing, cerebrospinal fluid (CSF) studies (white blood cell count and protein), and reactive VDRL on CSF. Because the VDRL on CSF alone is not sensitive for neurosyphilis, testing with FTA-ABS on CSF may be necessary in conjunction with the VDRL.[4]

#### Treatment/Management

Intramuscular benzathine penicillin G is the treatment of choice for primary, secondary, and latent syphilis. (See Box 53-2 for treatment.) The specific treatment regimen is determined by the stage of infection. Oral penicillin is not considered an appropriate treatment regimen. Because penicillin is the only treatment available for pregnant women, those with penicillin allergy should be referred for skin testing and desensitization. Follow-up serologic titers should be performed at a minimum of 6 and 12 months after treatment with the same non-treponemal serologic test initially performed at diagnosis. Titers should fall by fourfold or by two dilutions (eg, 1:16 to 1:4) to indicate appropriate response to therapy.

> **Box 53-2**
>
> ***Syphilis Treatment***
>
> **Primary and Secondary and Early Latent:**
>
> Benzathine penicillin G 2.4 million units IM once
> In penicillin allergy:
> Doxycycline 100 mg orally 2 times daily for 14 days
>
> OR
>
> Tetracycline 500 mg orally 4 times daily for 14 days
>
> **Late Latent or Latent Unknown Duration or Tertiary:**
>
> Benzathine penicillin G 2.4 million units IM weekly for 3 weeks
> In penicillin allergy:
> Doxycycline 100 mg orally 2 times daily for 28 days
>
> OR
>
> Tetracycline 500 mg orally 4 times daily for 28 days
>
> **Neurosyphilis:**
>
> Aqueous crystalline penicillin G 3–4 million units IV every 4 hours (or as a continuous infusion) for 10–14 days
>
> OR
>
> Procaine penicillin 2.4 million units IM daily for 10–14 days WITH probenecid 500 mg orally 4 times daily for 10–14 days
>
> Source: CDC. Sexually transmitted diseases treatment guidelines, 2010. *MMWR*. 2010;59:29–32

Symptoms that fail to resolve or titers that fail to fall fourfold by 6 months after treatment indicate treatment failure or reinfection. One-third to two-thirds of patients treated for primary or secondary syphilis experience the Jarisch-Herxheimer reaction characterized by fever, joint complaints, headache, and chills. This reaction, which is secondary to lysing of the treponemes, generally begins 4 to 6 hours after administration of antibiotics and lasts less than 24 hours. Treatment consists of appropriate symptomatic care.[4,22]

Neurosyphilis is treated with intravenous aqueous crystalline penicillin G or intramuscular procaine penicillin. CSF should be evaluated for improvement in pleocytosis at 6 months after treatment, with repeated CSF examination for white blood cell count every 6 months until the pleocytosis completely resolves. Retreatment should be considered if the CSF white blood cell count does not start to fall by 6 months or does not return to normal by 2 years post-treatment.[4]

In non-pregnant patients who are allergic to penicillin, alternative treatment regimens for primary and secondary syphilis or early latent syphilis include doxycycline twice daily for 14 days or tetracycline 4 times daily for 14 days. Doxycycline twice daily for 28 days or tetracycline 4 times daily for 28 days are alternatives for use in penicillin-allergic patients with late latent syphilis, tertiary syphilis without neurologic involvement, or syphilis of unknown duration.[23] Single-dose azithromycin (2 grams orally) has been used in developing countries and has equivalent cure rates at 9 months in patients with primary or presumed early latent syphilis.[24] However, strains of *T pallidum* resistant to macrolides have been documented across the globe.[4,24,25] Alternative regimens have not been extensively studied and any patient treated with a second-tier regimen should be closely followed.[4]

### CHANCROID (*HAEMOPHILUS DUCREYI*)

#### Epidemiology

Chancroid is an uncommon disease in industrialized countries but is endemic in other parts of the globe. It is strictly sexually transmitted, and men are more often affected than women. Localized outbreaks of chancroid do occur in areas of the United States.[26] In 2008, 25 cases of chancroid, from 9 states, were reported to the CDC.[17] Chancroid can occur as a co-infection in patients with syphilis or HSV.[4]

#### Biology/Pathophysiology

*H ducreyi* is a gram-negative facultative anaerobe. Infection occurs following exposure of damaged skin or mucous membranes to an infected partner.[26]

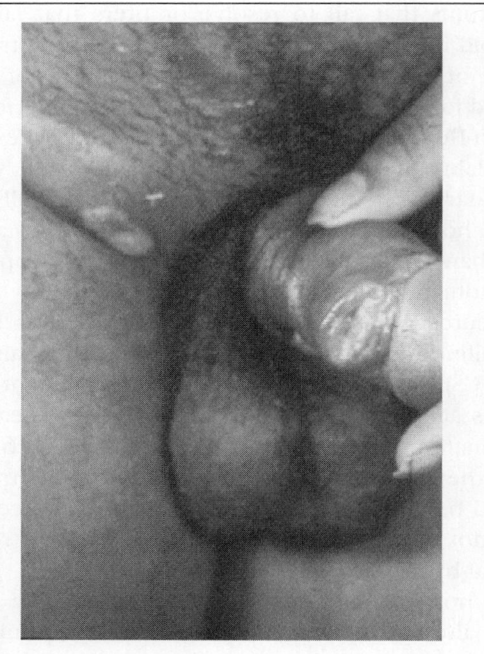

FIGURE 53-5 Chancroid: Male with penile lesion and regional adenopathy. (From Centers for Disease Control and Prevention (CDC), Training and Health Communication Branch of the Division of STD Prevention, National Center for HIV/AIDS, Viral Hepatitis, STD, and TB Prevention. Available at: www.cdc.gov/std/training/clinicalslides/slides-dl.htm.) (See color insert.)

### Clinical Presentation

After a 4- to 7-day incubation period, a tender papule arises that develops into the painful, sharply demarcated genital ulcer of chancroid. Patients may present with complaints related to the ulcer or with painful unilateral inguinal adenopathy (Figure 53-5). Female patients may complain of dysuria, vaginal discharge, or painful intercourse. The adenopathy may progress to spontaneous drainage and lead to significant soft tissue destruction.[26]

### Complications

Without appropriate antibiotic therapy, chronic drainage of enlarged lymph nodes may occur associated with destruction of the overlying skin and soft tissues.[26]

### Diagnosis

The definitive diagnosis of chancroid is made by culture, although this diagnostic technique is less than 80% sensitive. No FDA-cleared PCR test is available. More commonly, "probable" diagnosis is made by: 1) clinical findings consistent with chancroid, including presence of one or more painful genital ulcers; 2) negative studies for syphilis; and 3) negative HSV testing of the ulcer.[4]

**Box 53-3**

***Chancroid* (Haemophilus ducreyi)**

***Treatment***

Azithromycin 1 gram orally once

OR

Ceftriaxone 250 mg IM once

OR

Ciprofloxacin 500 mg orally 2 times daily for 3 days

OR

Erythromycin base 500 mg orally 3 times daily for 7 days

Source: CDC. Sexually transmitted diseases treatment guidelines, 2010. *MMWR*. 2010;59:19

### Treatment/Management

Chancroid may be treated with one dose of oral azithromycin, a 3-day course of oral ciprofloxacin, a 7-day course of oral erythromycin, or one dose of intramuscular ceftriaxone. (See Box 53-3 for medical treatment of chancroid.) Patients should return for evaluation within 1 week of treatment. Symptomatic improvement generally occurs by 3 days after initiation of appropriate antibiotics. However, large areas of infection may take several weeks to heal completely, and fluctuant adenopathy may require surgical drainage.[4]

## LYMPHOGRANULOMA VENEREUM

### Epidemiology

Lymphogranuloma venereum (LGV) is uncommon in the United States and other industrialized nations, occurring most frequently during episodic outbreaks. No national data on LGV are available for the United States. However, in 2003 to 2004 the Netherlands identified more than 90 cases of LGV in men who have sex with men (MSM).[27] Cases of LGV were also reported in MSM in 2003 to 2004 in Canada. Several of these patients were co-infected with HIV and were initially misdiagnosed as having inflammatory bowel disease.[28]

### Biology/Pathophysiology

LGV is caused by *Chlamydia trachomatis* serovars L1, L2, and L3. Infection generally begins via abrasions or breaks in the skin or mucous membranes. The primary pathology of LGV is lymphangitis with surrounding inflammation of lymphatic vessels and lymph nodes.[29]

### Clinical Presentation

Most commonly, LGV presents as a self-limited genital ulcer with unilateral and less commonly bilateral painful inguinal or femoral adenopathy.[4] Adenopathy develops up to 6 months following initial infection and affected lymph nodes continue to enlarge and may rupture through the skin, causing drainage of the infected area. Patients with LGV may also have symptoms of urethritis or cervicitis, and there may be infection of the rectum leading to rectal discharge, ulceration, and abscesses.[29]

### Complications

Healing of genital infections can be associated with fibrosis leading to lymphatic obstruction and enlargement of the genitals. Pelvic adhesions may occur in women, and rectal infection may lead to stricture or fistula formation.[29]

### Diagnosis

Identification of the organism by culture, direct immunofluorescence, or nucleic acid detection is not readily available in most laboratories, and results may not be specific for the *Chlamydia* serovars that cause LGV. However, when clinical findings consistent with LGV are present, *Chlamydia* serology, with a complement fixation titer greater than 1:64, can support the diagnosis of LGV.[4]

### Treatment/Management

Lymphogranuloma venereum is treated with doxycycline for 21 days. Alternatively, erythromycin for 21 days may be used. (See Box 53-4 for treatment of LGV.) Aspiration or incision and drainage of affected lymph nodes may be necessary.[4]

**Box 53-4**

***Lymphogranuloma venereum Treatment***

**Recommended:**

Doxycycline 100 mg orally 2 times daily for 21 days

**Alternative:**

Erythromycin base 500 mg orally 4 times daily for 21 days

Source: CDC. Sexually transmitted diseases treatment guidelines, 2010. *MMWR*. 2010;59:26

## URETHRITIS/CERVICITIS/PROCTITIS

Urethritis and cervicitis may be caused by a number of pathogens, including GC, CT, *Mycoplasma genitalium*, and *Trichomonas vaginalis*. Proctitis may be caused by gonorrhea, chlamydia, HSV, LGV, and syphilis.

Urethritis is associated with complaints of dysuria and penile discharge in men, and dysuria in women. In men, diagnostic criteria for urethritis include purulent urethral discharge or an increased number of white blood cells on Gram stain of a urethral swab or in a first void urine sediment. Presence of leukocyte esterase in first void urine of men is also considered evidence of urethritis.[4] Laboratory testing for GC and CT should be part of the initial evaluation. For empiric treatment of nongonococcal urethritis, the CDC recommends use of azithromycin or doxycycline (see Box 53-5). Based on potential etiologic agents, patients with persistent nongonococcal urethritis following appropriate first-line treatment should be treated with azithromycin 1 gram orally once (if not used in the initial treatment) in combination with either metronidazole 2 grams orally once or tinidazole 2 grams orally once.[4]

Cervicitis may present with dyspareunia, vaginal discharge, abnormal vaginal bleeding, or postcoital bleeding. Women with cervicitis may also have

**Box 53-5**

***Empiric Treatment of Nongonococcal Urethritis***

**Recommended:**

Azithromycin 1 g orally once

OR

Doxycycline 100 mg orally 2 times daily for 7 days

**Alternatives:**

Erythromycin base 500 mg orally 4 times daily for 7 days

OR

Erythromycin ethylsuccinate 800 mg orally 4 times daily for 7 days

OR

Ofloxacin 300 mg orally 2 times daily for 7 days

OR

Levofloxacin 500 mg orally 1 time daily for 7 days

**Recurrent or Persistent Urethritis:**

Metronidazole 2 g orally once

OR

Tinidazole 2 g orally once

WITH:

Azithromycin 1 g orally once (if not used in initial treatment)

Source: CDC. Sexually transmitted diseases treatment guidelines, 2010. *MMWR*. 2010;59:42

**Box 53-6**

***Empiric Treatment of Cervicitis***

Azithromycin 1 g orally once

OR

Doxycycline 100 mg orally 2 times daily for 7 days
Consider concurrent treatment for gonorrhea in areas of high gonorrhea prevalence.

Source: CDC. Sexually transmitted diseases treatment guidelines, 2010. *MMWR*. 2010;59:44

symptoms of urethritis. The CDC diagnostic criteria for cervicitis include purulent or mucopurulent discharge or cervical friability. Women with cervicitis should also be examined for signs of pelvic inflammatory disease (discussed later). Following appropriate testing for gonorrhea or chlamydia, empiric antibiotic therapy should be provided for high-risk individuals. The CDC recommendations for empiric treatment of cervicitis include azithromycin or doxycycline (see Box 53-6). Concurrent therapy for gonorrhea is suggested in areas with greater than 5% gonorrhea prevalence.[4]

Proctitis is inflammation of the distal 10 to 12 cm of the rectum, and both men and women can be affected with complaints of rectal pain, pain with defecation, or rectal discharge. Generally, patients with proctitis have a history of receptive anal sex. Evaluation includes anoscopy and appropriate laboratory studies for potential pathogens. The empiric treatment of proctitis includes intramuscular ceftriaxone and oral doxycycline (see Box 53-7).[4]

### *NEISSERIA GONORRHOEAE*

#### Epidemiology

In 2008, the rate of GC was highest in women aged 15 to 19 years (636.8 cases per 100,000) and in men aged 20 to 24 years (433.6 cases per 100,000). In 20- to 24-year-old women, the rate of GC was 608.6 cases per 100,000 and in 15- to 19-year-old men, the GC rate was 278.3 cases per 100,000. *Neisseria gonorrhoeae* is more common in blacks.[17] In incarcerated adolescents, the prevalence of GC was 2.9% overall, with higher rates in women than men.[30] Co-infection with CT is common. In one study of urban high school students, of those infected with GC, 42.7% were co-infected with CT.[31]

**Box 53-7**

***Acute Proctitis Treatment***

Ceftriaxone 250 mg IM once
AND
Doxycycline 100 mg orally 2 times daily for 7 days

Source: CDC. Sexually transmitted diseases treatment guidelines, 2010. *MMWR*. 2010;59:88

#### Biology/Pathophysiology

*Neisseria gonorrhoeae* is a gram-negative intracellular diplococcus (Figure 53-6) that infects the noncornified epithelium of the genitourinary tract, rectum, oropharynx, and conjunctiva. The pathogen attaches to epithelial cells by pili. Genital GC generally causes local infection of the urethra, vagina, and cervix, but may ascend into the upper genital tract in women, infect the testicles and prostate in men, or disseminate.[32] Recently, an increasing number of GC strains have become resistant to fluoroquinolones. These strains are more common in MSM or in individuals who acquired GC infections in Europe, the Middle East, Asia, or the Pacific.[4] Antibiotic resistance may be either chromosomally mediated or plasmid mediated.[4,33]

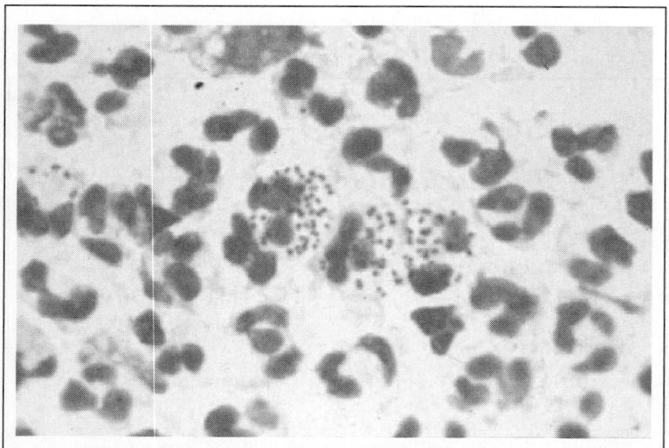

**FIGURE 53-6** Gonorrhea (GC): Gram stain of urethral discharge demonstrating gram-negative intracellular diplococci. (From Centers for Disease Control and Prevention (CDC), Training and Health Communication Branch of the Division of STD Prevention, National Center for HIV/AIDS, Viral Hepatitis, STD, and TB Prevention. Available at: www.cdc.gov/std/training/clinicalslides/slides-dl.htm.)

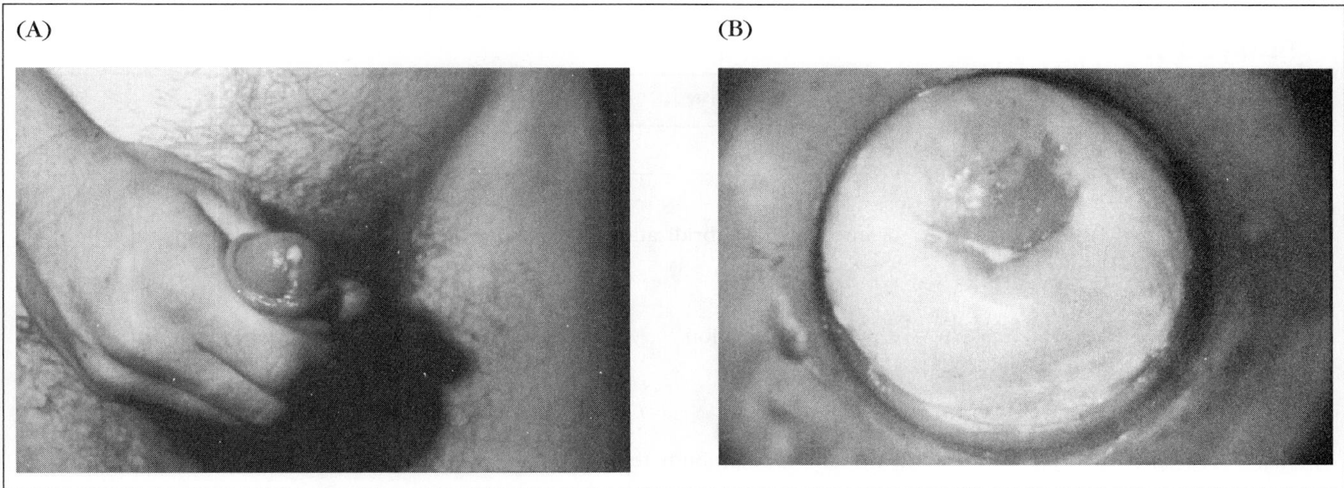


**FIGURE 53-7** Gonorrhea (GC). (A) Male with gonococcal urethritis; (B) Gonococcal cervicitis. (From Centers for Disease Control and Prevention (CDC), Training and Health Communication Branch of the Division of STD Prevention, National Center for HIV/AIDS, Viral Hepatitis, STD, and TB Prevention. Available at: www.cdc.gov/std/training/clinicalslides/slides-dl.htm.) (See color insert.)

### Clinical Presentation

*Neisseria gonorrhoeae* infection may be symptomatic or asymptomatic. Following an incubation period of 1 to 14 days, men develop symptoms of penile discharge and dysuria, with possible erythema and edema of the meatus. Women generally complain of vaginal discharge, dysuria, or abnormal vaginal bleeding (Figure 53-7). Rectal infection may occur in individuals who practice receptive anal sex. Pharyngeal infection, which is often asymptomatic and self-resolving, has been reported in men and women who participate in oral sex, and GC conjunctivitis has been found in adolescents and young adults.[32]

### Complications

In men, complications of GC include epididymitis, prostatitis, inflammation of the seminal vesicles, or infection of Cowper or Tyson glands. In women, GC infection may result in pelvic inflammatory disease or abscess of the Bartholin glands, as well as pregnancy complications including spontaneous abortion, premature rupture of membranes, or premature delivery. Transmission of infection to a neonate can cause gonococcal ophthalmic disease or pharyngeal infection.[32] Both men and women may develop disseminated gonorrhea infection (DGI), characterized by tender pustular skin lesions that can become necrotic ulcers (Figure 53-8) and asymmetric arthralgias, tenosynovitis, and arthritis. Dissemination of GC occurs via the bloodstream, and may be associated with cardiac involvement or meningitis.[4,32] Disseminated gonorrhea infection is more likely in patients with certain complement deficiencies.[32]

### Diagnosis

Although it has a low sensitivity, visualization of gram-negative intracellular diplococci on a urethral smear is diagnostic of GC infection in males. Gram stain of cervicovaginal secretions in women is not diagnostic of GC infection. In 2002, the CDC published recommendations

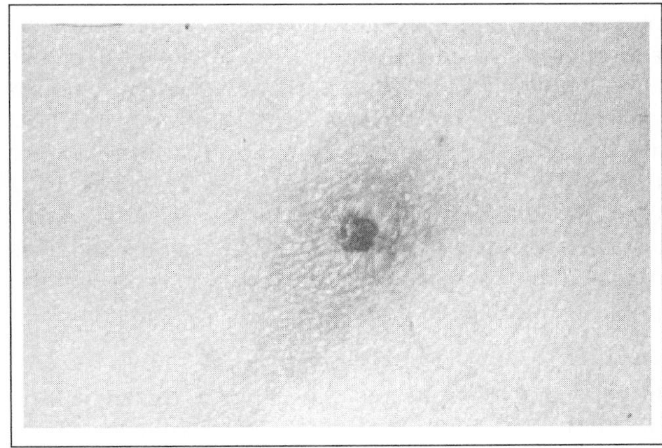

**FIGURE 53-8** Gonorrhea (GC). Disseminated gonorrhea skin lesion. (From Centers for Disease Control and Prevention (CDC), Training and Health Communication Branch of the Division of STD Prevention, National Center for HIV/AIDS, Viral Hepatitis, STD, and TB Prevention. Available at: www.cdc.gov/std/training/clinicalslides/slides-dl.htm.) (See color insert.)

**Table 53-2**

**Screening Tests for Gonorrhea and Chlamydia**

| *Disease* | *Women* | *Men* |
|---|---|---|
| Gonorrhea | • Endocervical culture<br>• Endocervical NAAT or nucleic acid hybridization<br>• Urine NAAT | • Intraurethral culture if acceptable<br>• Intraurethral NAAT or nucleic acid hybridization if acceptable<br>• Urine NAAT |
| Chlamydia | • Endocervical NAAT if pelvic examination acceptable<br>• Urine NAAT<br>• Endocervical unamplified nucleic acid hybridization or direct fluorescent antibody test<br>• Endocervical culture | • Intraurethral NAAT if acceptable<br>• Urine NAAT<br>• Intraurethral non-NAAT test or culture |

NAAT, nucleic acid amplification testing

Source: CDC. Screening Tests to Detect *Chlamydia trachomatis* and *Neisseria gonorrhoeae* Infections, 2002 *MMWR*.2002;51.

regarding testing for GC.[10] These recommendations are aimed at maximizing sensitivity while minimizing false-positive results. In order of preference, the recommendations for testing in men is an intraurethral swab specimen for culture or a NAAT, followed by nucleic acid hybridization test on an intraurethral swab or NAAT on a urine sample. For women, the recommended tests are endocervical swab specimens for culture or NAAT followed by a nucleic acid hybridization test on an endocervical specimen. NAAT of urine specimens is also acceptable, although it is less sensitive than NAAT on an endocervical sample[10] (Table 53-2). The Gen-Probe Aptima 2 assay (Gen-Probe, San Diego, CA) and the BD ProbeTec *Chlamydia trachomatis/Neisseria gonorrhoeae* (CT/GC) $Q^x$ Amplified DNA Assays (BD, Franklin Lakes, NJ) are FDA-approved for detection of GC using specimens obtained by vaginal swab.[12,13] However, only culture provides information about antibiotic susceptibilities.[4]

### Treatment/Management

In general, uncomplicated gonorrhea is treated with a one-time intramuscular dose of ceftriaxone or, if not an option, single-dose oral cefixime. (See Box 53-8 for guidelines on treatment of GC.) Because of rising rates of antibiotic resistance, as of April 2007 the CDC no longer recommends the use of quinolone antibiotics for treatment of gonorrhea infections in the United States.[33,34] Further information on antimicrobial resistance can be found at the Web site for the CDC Gonococcal Isolate Surveillance Project (GISP)

**Box 53-8**

***Gonorrhea* (Neisseria gonorrhoeae) *Treatment***

**Cervix, Urethra, Rectum:**

Ceftriaxone 250 mg IM once

OR, IF NOT AN OPTION,

Cefixime 400 mg orally once

PLUS

treatment for chlamydia with azithromycin 1 g orally once

OR

doxycycline 100 mg orally 2 times daily for 7 days

**Alternative:**

Single-dose cephalosporin (such as ceftizoxime 500 mg IM once, or cefoxitin 2 grams IM once with probenecid 1 gram orally once, or cefotaxime 500 mg IM once)

**Pharyngeal Infection:**

Ceftriaxone 250 mg IM once

PLUS

treatment for chlamydia with azithromycin 1 g orally once

OR

doxycycline 100 mg orally 2 times daily for 7 days

Source: CDC. Sexually transmitted diseases treatment guidelines, 2010. *MMWR*. 2010;59:50–51

**Box 53-9**

***Disseminated Gonococcal Treatment***

**Recommended:**

Ceftriaxone 1 g IM or IV daily

**Alternatives:**

Cefotaxime 1 g IV every 8 hours

OR

Ceftizoxime 1 g IV every 8 hours
Parenteral therapy for 24–48 hours after clinical improvement begins, then change to one of the following regimens to provide at least 7 days of antibiotic therapy:
Cefixime 400 mg orally 2 times daily

**Gonococcal Meningitis or Endocarditis:**

Ceftriaxone 1–2 g IV every 12 hours
Consultation with a specialist

Source: CDC. Sexually transmitted diseases treatment guidelines, 2010. *MMWR*. 2010;59:53

(www.cdc.gov/std/gisp). In all patients diagnosed with GC, concurrent treatment for CT should be provided because this co-treatment may slow the development of further antibiotic resistance in GC. Test of cure is not needed following a recommended regimen.[4] Testing for GC with NAAT less than 3 weeks following treatment may lead to false-positive results.

Intramuscular or intravenous ceftriaxone is the recommended treatment for disseminated GC without endocarditis or meningitis (see Box 53-9). Parenteral therapy for DGI is generally continued for 24 to 48 hours after clinical improvement begins, at which time patients may be transitioned to an oral regimen. Treatment of complicated disseminated GC should be managed in conjunction with a specialist.[4]

### *CHLAMYDIA TRACHOMATIS*

#### Epidemiology

*Chlamydia trachomatis* is the most commonly reported infectious disease in the United States.[4] Overall, the rate of CT infection has been increasing since 1987, and it is more prevalent in areas of the southern United States and among African-Americans. In 2008, the rate of CT in the United States was 3275.8 cases per 100,000 in adolescent women aged 15-19 years and 3179.9 per 100,000 in women aged 20 to 24 years. In men aged 15 to 19 years, the CT rate was 701.6 per 100,000, whereas men aged 20-24 years were in the highest-risk age group with a rate of 1056.1 per 100,000.[17] Among individuals aged 16 to 24 years entering the National Job Training Program, 13.1% of women and 7.9% of men were infected with CT whereas 14.2% of adolescent women in juvenile detention centers had chlamydia in 2006.[18] Co-infection with GC is common. In a study of high school students, 11.1% of those with CT were co-infected with GC.[31]

#### Biology/Pathophysiology

*Chlamydia trachomatis* is a gram-negative, obligate intracellular bacterium that infects the epithelium of the urogenital tract or rectum. It exists in 2 phases during its lifecycle. The elementary bodies invade the host cells, and then become intracellular active reticulate bodies. Adolescent women are at particular risk for CT infection due to the presence of the cervical ectropion. *Chlamydia trachomatis* infects the exposed columnar epithelial cells that comprise the ectropion.[35]

#### Clinical Presentation

*Chlamydia trachomatis* is commonly asymptomatic in both sexes and may persist for months to years.[35] Following a 1- to 3-week incubation period, men may complain of dysuria or penile discharge, which is often less copious than that seen with GC.[35] Women with CT may complain of symptoms suggestive of UTI, such as dysuria,[9] as well as abnormal vaginal discharge or bleeding due to cervical friability.[35]

#### Complications

Reactive arthritis, formerly known as Reiter syndrome, (comprising conjunctivitis, arthritis, and urethritis) occurs as a complication of CT infection, especially in HLA-B27-positive individuals.[36] Men are more often affected than women.[35] Other complications in men include epididymitis, prostatitis, and proctitis, and additional complications in women include abscess of the Bartholin gland, pelvic inflammatory disease, and perihepatitis.[35] Pregnant women may also transmit CT to newborns during vaginal birth, leading to CT conjunctivitis and pneumonia in the perinatal period.[4,37]

#### Diagnosis

The CDC recommends routine yearly CT screening of all sexually active women aged 25 years or younger.[4] In 2002, the CDC published recommendations regarding testing for CT.[10] In women, the preferred diagnostic test is NAAT of an endocervical swab sample. NAAT of a first voided urine sample can be performed if a pelvic examination is not done. Unamplified nucleic acid hybridization testing, enzyme immunoassay, or direct fluorescent antibody testing of an endocervical sample is also satisfactory but not as sensitive as NAAT. Culture of an endocervical sample is the least preferred method of diagnosis in women. The recommended testing modality in men is

NAAT of an intraurethral swab or urine sample. Intraurethral swabs may also be tested by non-NAAT or culture if other methods are unavailable[10] (see Table 53-2). The Aptima 2 Assay is FDA-approved for detection of CT using specimens obtained by vaginal swab.[12]

### Treatment/Management

*Chlamydia trachomatis* is generally treated with a single dose of oral azithromycin or one week of twice daily doxycycline. Recommended treatment for CT is given in Box 53-10. The CDC supports presumptive treatment of CT in patients diagnosed with GC infection. Single-dose observed azithromycin therapy may be most cost-effective when compliance with an outpatient regimen is in question. Test of cure following recommended therapies is not necessary unless noncompliance or reinfection is suspected. Furthermore, testing for CT with NAAT less than 3 weeks following treatment may lead to false-positive results. Women with a history of CT infection should be rescreened 3 to 12 months after treatment due to the high rates of reinfection.[4] In a recent study, only 75% of adolescent women treated for CT reported notifying their partners of their need for evaluation and treatment.[38]

## *MYCOPLASMA GENITALIUM*

Growing evidence in the literature supports a role for *Mycoplasma genitalium* as a cause of nongonococcal urethritis (NGU) and cervicitis.

> **Box 53-10**
>
> ***Chlamydia* (Chlamydia trachomatis) *Treatment***
>
> **Recommended:**
>
> Azithromycin 1 g orally once
>
> OR
>
> Doxycycline 100 mg orally 2 times daily for 7 days
>
> **Alternatives:**
>
> Erythromycin base 500 mg orally 4 times daily for 7 days
>
> OR
>
> Erythromycin ethylsuccinate 800 mg orally 4 times daily for 7 days
>
> OR
>
> Ofloxacin 300 mg orally 2 times daily for 7 days
>
> OR
>
> Levofloxacin 500 mg orally 1 time daily for 7 days
>
> Source: CDC. Sexually transmitted diseases treatment guidelines, 2010. *MMWR*. 2010;59:45

### Epidemiology

*M genitalium* has been associated with NGU in men.[39-42] In one study, 14% of men presenting for evaluation of urethritis were found to have *M genitalium* alone, with similar prevalence in heterosexual men and MSM.[43] In a review of the literature, Deguchi and Maeda[44] found that *M genitalium* was associated with 18.4% to 45.5% of nonchlamydial NGU. Taylor-Robinson found *M genitalium* significantly associated with NGU in a review of 17 studies. Further review of 10 of these studies demonstrated that *M genitalium* was associated with nonchlamydial NGU as well.[45]

*M genitalium* has been associated with microscopic cervicitis and urethritis in women[39] as well as with endometritis, independent of co-infection with GC or CT.[46] In one study in women, *M genitalium* was associated with a 3.3-fold increased risk of mucopurulent cervicitis. That study demonstrated an association between *M genitalium* and a younger age at sexual debut as well as multiple new partners in the preceding month.[47] In another study, male partners of women with *M genitalium* were found to be infected with this pathogen at a rate similar to the rate of CT infection in male partners of women with diagnosed CT.[48]

### Biology/Pathophysiology

*M genitalium* is a flask-shaped bacterium. It was first isolated in the early 1980s from urethral swabs of men and subsequently has been isolated from the urinary, genital, rectal, and respiratory tracts.[45] Newborns are frequently colonized by this organism at birth, but after puberty, colonization is primarily through sexual contact. Rates of colonization increase with a greater number of sexual partners.[49]

### Clinical Presentation

Clinical symptoms and signs of *M genitalium* infection in women are similar to those found in patients infected with CT,[48] although men with *M genitalium* may exhibit more symptoms of urethritis than those with CT infection.[50]

### Complications

Although *M genitalium* has been associated with endometritis,[46] most other common STI complications (eg, prostatitis, epididymitis, reactive arthritis) have not been conclusively linked to *M genitalium* infection.[49]

### Diagnosis

Diagnosis of *M genitalium* is difficult, and standardized tests are not available. *M genitalium* is not generally amenable to culture, and most research studies have utilized PCR testing of urethral, cervical, or urine samples.[51] In a study comparing optimal methods of specimen collection, PCR of first voided urine was superior to urethral swab sampling in men and cervical sampling in women.[51]

### Treatment/Management

A single oral dose of 1 gram of azithromycin has been recommended by the CDC for treatment of *M genitalium*.[4] Doxycycline 100 mg orally twice daily for 1 week has also been efficacious.[44]

## *UREAPLASMA UREALYTICUM*

Evidence supporting a role for *U urealyticum* in NGU is somewhat more contradictory. In men with NGU, *U urealyticum* was more common than in those without urethritis.[41] However, Totten and colleagues[40] found no association between *U urealyticum* and NGU. In a separate study, *U urealyticum* was associated with the development of chronic symptomatic NGU and with urethritis following appropriate treatment for other pathogens.[42] Newborn infants may be colonized with *U urealyticum*, and during puberty colonization has been linked with sexual activity.[49] Diagnosis of *U urealyticum* is hampered by a lack of standardized tests. Some *U urealyticum* strains are resistant to tetracyclines and thus may not be adequately treated with a course of doxycycline given for treatment of urethritis.[4]

## PELVIC INFLAMMATORY DISEASE

Pelvic inflammatory disease (PID) is classically described as an ascending polymicrobial infection of the upper genital tract in women.[4,52]

### Epidemiology

The CDC estimates that more than 1 million cases of PID occur in the United States per year, leading to infertility in approximately 100,000 women annually. In addition, PID is a causative factor in more than 150 deaths per year in the United States alone. Although these numbers are sobering, in two-thirds of cases PID is not recognized by the woman or her provider. All PID statistics are estimates, as PID, unlike gonorrhea or chlamydia, is not a reportable disease.[53] Pelvic inflammatory disease is most common in sexually active adolescent women, who have a 7- to 10-fold greater risk of PID than women in their 20s.[54] In a study of PID in an outpatient adolescent clinic, Kelly and colleagues[55] found an incidence of 9.7%. Of these cases, 47% of women had recurrent disease with at least one prior or one subsequent diagnosis of PID, and 27% had had three or more episodes of PID.

### Biology/Pathophysiology

Pelvic inflammatory disease most often occurs as a complication of GC or CT, although other pathogens have been implicated, including anaerobic bacteria, *Gardnerella* species, *Haemophilus influenza*, enteric gram-negative rods, *Mycoplasma* species, *U urealyticum*, and cytomegalovirus.[4] Pelvic inflammatory disease is a polymicrobial ascending infection resulting in endometritis, salpingitis, and oophoritis.[4,52]

Bacterial vaginosis (BV) is commonly found in patients with PID, but it remains unclear whether BV organisms lead to PID or merely ascend to the upper tracts in the wake of an initial GC or CT infection.[56]

### Clinical Presentation

The clinical presentation of PID ranges from very mild cases that are difficult to diagnose to florid acute cases requiring hospitalization and intravenous antibiotic therapy. Patients often present with complaints of lower abdominal pain and vaginal discharge and may also experience fever, nausea, vomiting, worsening pain with ambulation, abnormal vaginal bleeding, dyspareunia, or right upper quadrant abdominal pain.[53]

### Complications

Perihepatitis (Fitz-Hugh-Curtis syndrome) is a perihepatic inflammatory condition associated with PID. Patients present with right upper quadrant tenderness on examination, sometimes associated with right shoulder pain due to referred pain from irritation of the right diaphragm. In some cases, the initial presentation of PID may have been missed and the patient only presents with right upper quadrant pain. The exact mechanism of pathogen spread is unclear, although direct spread along the paracolic region has been proposed. Serum transaminases may be normal or mildly elevated. Characteristic "violin-string" adhesions may be seen on laparoscopy and may require surgical lysis if symptoms do not improve with appropriate antibiotic therapy.[57]

Tubo-ovarian abscess (TOA) is another acute complication of PID. On ultrasound, TOA appears as a large adnexal mass with poor differentiation between structures and an increased amount of free fluid in the pelvis.[58]

Infertility, chronic pelvic pain, and ectopic pregnancy are long-term complications of PID. The risk of these long-term sequelae increases with an increasing number of PID episodes.[52,53] The risk of tubal occlusion escalates with each episode of PID, with a rate of 8% to 12.8% after 1 episode of PID, 19.5% to 35.5% after 2 episodes, and 35.5% to 40% after 3 or more episodes.[54]

### Diagnosis

Diagnosis of PID primarily rests on clinical examination, with use of laboratory studies to support the diagnosis. The criteria for clinical diagnosis of PID were last revised in 2002 and are published by the CDC in the Sexually Transmitted Diseases Treatment Guidelines.[4,59] In the past, the diagnosis of PID required the presence of cervical motion tenderness and uterine or adnexal tenderness.[60] Concern for missing subtle cases of PID led to a broadening of the diagnostic criteria, which currently include cervical motion tenderness or uterine tenderness or adnexal tenderness.[4] The clinical diagnosis of PID reaches a positive predictive value of 65% to 90% for salpingitis when compared to laparoscopy (gold standard).[53] Laparoscopy is not indicated for the clinical diagnosis of PID and is more often reserved for diagnostic evaluation in complicated cases.[4]

Practitioners are cautioned to have a low threshold for treatment of PID, particularly in young sexually active women who have no other cause for the presenting complaints. Please refer to Box 53-11 for the diagnostic criteria for PID. Because PID is a polymicrobial disease, negative laboratory tests for cervical gonorrhea and chlamydia do not rule out PID. In a review of the literature, Westrom and Eschenbach[53] found that only 29% of PID cases had positive cervical cultures for CT and only 26% of cases had positive cervical GC cultures. In addition, although not diagnostic, ultrasound findings including endometrial thickening and distended, thick-walled fallopian tubes can support the other clinical criteria.[58]

### Box 53-11

#### *Diagnostic Criteria for Pelvic Inflammatory Disease*

**Minimum Criteria:**

Cervical motion tenderness

OR

Uterine tenderness

OR

Adnexal tenderness

**Supportive Findings (not required for diagnosis):**

Fever (oral temperature >101°F [38.3°C])
Abnormal cervical or vaginal discharge
Increased number of white blood cells on wet mount of vaginal fluid
Elevated erythrocyte sedimentation rate (ESR)
Elevated C-reactive protein (CRP)
Laboratory documented *N gonorrhoeae* or *C trachomatis* cervical infection

Source: CDC. Sexually transmitted diseases treatment guidelines, 2010. *MMWR*. 2010;59:64

### Treatment/Management

The goals of treatment for PID are twofold: to cure the immediate infectious process and to prevent short and long-term sequelae. No difference has been found in either short- or long-term outcomes when comparing inpatient and outpatient therapy for PID in any group, including adolescents.[61] The CDC criteria for hospitalization for PID treatment may be found in Box 53-12.

### Box 53-12

#### *Suggested Hospitalization Criteria for PID Treatment*

Inability to rule out surgical emergencies (eg, appendicitis)
Pregnancy
Failure to improve on appropriate outpatient antibiotic therapy
Patient unable to tolerate or follow outpatient regimen
Severe illness, including nausea, vomiting, significant fever
Tubo-ovarian abscess (TOA)

Source: CDC. Sexually transmitted diseases treatment guidelines, 2010. *MMWR*. 2010;59:65

Outpatient management of PID is found in Box 53-13. For patients treated with an outpatient regimen, follow-up pelvic examination in 48 to 72 hours should be performed to evaluate for clinical improvement. If clinical improvement has not occurred, hospitalization and intravenous (IV) antibiotics may be indicated.[4]

### Box 53-13

#### *Outpatient Treatment of Pelvic Inflammatory Disease*

Ceftriaxone 250 mg IM once
PLUS
Doxycycline 100 mg orally 2 times daily for 14 days

OR

Cefoxitin 2 g IM once with concurrent probenecid 1g orally once
PLUS
Doxycycline 100 mg orally 2 times daily for 14 days

OR

Other parenteral 3rd generation cephalosporin (such as ceftizoxime or cefotaxime)
PLUS
Doxycycline 100 mg orally 2 times daily for 14 days
For all of the above regimens, the addition of Metronidazole 500 mg orally 2 times daily for 14 days should be considered for additional anaerobic coverage.

Source: CDC. Sexually transmitted diseases treatment guidelines, 2010. *MMWR*. 2010;59:66

**Box 53-14**

***Inpatient Parenteral Treatment of Pelvic Inflammatory Disease***

**Regimen A:**

Cefotetan 2 g IV every 12 hours OR Cefoxitin 2 g IV every 6 hours
PLUS
Doxycycline 100 mg orally or IV every 12 hours
**Doxycycline should be administered orally whenever possible to avoid pain during IV infusion.**

**Regimen B:**

Clindamycin 900 mg IV every 8 hours
PLUS
Gentamicin 2 mg/kg body weight as a loading dose IV or IM, with maintenance dose of 1.5 mg/kg every 8 hours thereafter. Single daily dosing with 3 to 5 mg/kg also can be used.

**Alternative Regimens:**

Ampicillin/Sulbactam 3 g IV every 6 hours
PLUS
Doxycycline 100 mg orally or IV every 12 hours
**Following 24–48 hours of clinical improvement, patients may be switched to one of the following oral antibiotic regimens:
Doxycycline 100 mg orally 2 times daily to complete 14-day course

OR

Clindamycin 450 mg orally 4 times daily to complete 14-day course

Source: CDC. Sexually transmitted diseases treatment guidelines, 2010. *MMWR*. 2010;59:65

Inpatient treatment of PID is found in Box 53-14. For hospitalized patients, IV antibiotic therapy is administered for 24 to 48 hours or until clinical improvement occurs. Antibiotic therapy for TOA must include adequate coverage for anaerobic organisms, which predominate in the abscess (see Box 53-15).

## VAGINITIS

A comprehensive differential diagnosis of vaginal discharge is presented in Chapter 116, Urinary Tract Infections in Adolescents. Vaginitis is irritation or inflammation of the vagina. Infectious causes include *Trichomonas vaginalis*, BV, and vulvovaginal candidiasis (VVC), which are discussed next.

**Box 53-15**

***Antibiotic Management of Tubo-Ovarian Abscess***

Hospitalization
Administration of a recommended parenteral PID treatment regimen with anaerobic coverage
Following 24–48 hours of clinical improvement, change to oral antibiotics.

- For Parenteral PID treatment Regimen A:
  - Clindamycin or metronidazole with doxycycline (to improve anaerobic coverage) to complete 14-day course
- For Parenteral PID Treatment Regimen B:
  - Clindamycin to complete 14-day course

Source: CDC. Sexually transmitted diseases treatment guidelines, 2010. *MMWR*. 2010;59:65

### VULVOVAGINAL CANDIDIASIS

#### Epidemiology

Vulvovaginal candidiasis is a common diagnosis among adolescent women. Three out of 4 adult women report having had at least one episode of VVC, and 40–45% report 2 or more lifetime episodes.[4] Risk factors for VVC include pregnancy, poorly controlled diabetes mellitus, recent antibiotic use, receptive oral sex, and increased frequency of sexual activity.[62–64] HIV-infected women have higher rates of colonization with yeast species. Uncomplicated VVC occurs in immunocompetent patients, accounts for 80% to 90% of VVC, is sporadic, is mild to moderate in severity, and is generally caused by *Candida albicans*. Complicated VVC occurs in patients with underlying medical problems, such as immunocompromise, diabetes mellitus, and pregnancy. Recurrent VVC (defined as 4 or more episodes in 1 year) occurs in 10% to 20% of women with a history of VVC and can involve non-*C albicans* yeast species.[4]

#### Biology/Pathophysiology

Most uncomplicated VVC is caused by overgrowth of *C albicans*.[4,62,65] However, one fifth of women are colonized by *C albicans* without any signs or symptoms of infection.[62] The initial source of VVC is unclear; VVC may result from yeast translocation from the rectum or perineum during sexual intercourse.[62] Non-*C albicans* species are more common in patients with complicated VVC, and these strains may be more resistant to standard treatment regimens.[4,62,63]

### Clinical Presentation

Vulvovaginal candidiasis in women often presents with vaginal or vulvar irritation, redness, external dysuria, and a thick vaginal discharge. On examination, the vulva and labia are often edematous and erythematous, and fissures may be present in severe cases.[4,62,63] Symptoms may worsen immediately prior to the menstrual period.[62] Men may present with erythema and irritation of the penis.[4,62]

### Complications

HIV-infected women with VVC have higher HIV RNA levels in cervicovaginal secretions when compared with HIV-infected women without VVC.[66] In addition, one study found an association between VVC and acquisition of HIV infection.[67]

### Diagnosis

Direct microscopic examination of vaginal discharge is the most common method of diagnosis of VVC. Diagnosis can be aided by the addition of 10% potassium hydroxide (KOH) solution, which removes other cells and debris that may obscure the yeast. Visualization of pseudohyphae or blastospores confirms diagnosis of VVC; however, up to half of patients with VVC will have a negative wet mount. In general, white blood cells are not increased in the vaginal discharge. In patients with symptoms highly suggestive of VVC but with a negative microscopic examination of vaginal saline wet mount, fungal culture for *C albicans* can be performed to confirm the diagnosis. Culture should not be routinely performed on asymptomatic women as *C albicans* is part of the normal vaginal flora.[4,62,63,68] In addition, culture with speciation of yeast can be useful for patients with recurrent VVC.[4] Antimicrobial resistance testing is not widely available.

### Treatment/Management

Treatment regimens for uncomplicated VVC are listed in Box 53-16. Cure rates for oral fluconazole versus topical azole therapy are equivalent.[4,62,69] The most common reported side effect for topical azoles is superficial burning or irritation at the application site. Oral fluconazole treatment has been associated with gastrointestinal upset, headache, and medication interactions.[4,63] Patients should be advised that creams and suppositories may weaken latex condoms. There are currently no recommendations for the treatment of male partners of women with VVC. Males with balanitis should receive a course of topical antifungal therapy. Pregnant women may be treated with topical azoles for a total of 7 days.[4] Clotrimazole and miconazole are recommended as treatment of choice in pregnancy, with nystatin as the preferred alternative therapy. Oral therapy is contraindicated in pregnancy.[4]

**Box 53-16**

***Treatment of Vulvovaginal Candidiasis***

**Select one of the following regimens:**

- Butoconazole 2% cream 5 g intravaginally once daily for 3 days
- Butoconazole 2% cream 5 g (Butoconazole 1-sustained release) intravaginally once
- Clotrimazole 1% cream 5 g intravaginally once daily for 7-14 days
- Clotrimazole 2% cream 5 g intravaginally once daily for 3 days
- Miconazole 2% cream 5 g intravaginally once daily for 7 days
- Miconazole 4% cream 5 g intravaginally once daily for 3 days
- Miconazole 100 mg vaginal suppository intravaginally once daily for 7 days
- Miconazole 200 mg vaginal suppository intravaginally once daily for 3 days
- Miconazole 1200 mg vaginal suppository intravaginally once
- Nystatin 100,000-unit vaginal tablet intravaginally once daily for 14 days
- Tioconazole 6.5% ointment 5 g intravaginally once
- Terconazole 0.4% cream 5 g intravaginally once daily for 7 days
- Terconazole 0.8% cream 5 g intravaginally once daily for 3 days
- Terconazole 80 mg vaginal suppository intravaginally once daily for 3 days
- Fluconazole 150 mg orally once

Source: CDC. Sexually transmitted diseases treatment guidelines, 2010. *MMWR*. 2010;59:61

For patients with complicated VVC, the course of treatment with topical agents should be extended to 10 to 14 days.[68] Alternatively, oral fluconazole may be used every 3 days for 3 doses total. Maintenance therapy for VVC may then be initiated with oral fluconazole once weekly or topical clotrimazole 200 mg twice weekly (or 500 mg once weekly) for 6 months. One-third to one-half of women with recurrent VVC will experience a recurrence when maintenance therapy is stopped.[4,68]

## BACTERIAL VAGINOSIS

### Epidemiology

Because BV is not a reportable disease, there are limited data regarding prevalence. Data from NHANES 2001–2004 demonstrated BV prevalence of 23.3% in 14- to 19-year-old women and 31.1% in 20- to 29-year-old women. There was no significant difference in report of vaginal symptoms between those women with BV and those without BV.[72] BV has been associated with race/ethnicity (more common in black and Mexican-American women), increased number of lifetime partners, previous female partner, lower educational attainment, poverty, a history of pregnancy, stress, higher body mass index (BMI), douching, and smoking.[4,71] Because BV increases with the number of lifetime partners, other STIs may co-occur with BV. In addition, BV is associated with sexual assault and can be detected 1–2 weeks after the assault episode.[72,73]

### Biology/Pathophysiology

Bacterial vaginosis represents polymicrobial overgrowth and replacement of the peroxide-producing lactobacilli that are normally present in the vagina with *Gardnerella vaginalis*, *Mycoplasma hominis*, *Mobiluncus* species, and various anaerobic bacteria (including *Prevotella* spp, *Peptostreptococcus*, *Porphyromonas* spp, *Bacteroides* spp, and *Fusobacterium* spp).[4,71] The characteristic odor of BV is thought to be due to amine production by these bacteria. Newer molecular techniques have also identified several newly described species of BV-associated bacteria.[74]

### Clinical Presentation

Most symptomatic women complain of malodorous discharge; however, more than 50% of women who meet criteria for BV are asymptomatic.[71] The vaginal discharge is often described as thin, white, and adherent to the vaginal walls.[4,71]

### Complications

In pregnant women, BV has been associated with premature rupture of membranes, preterm birth, and amniotic infection.[4,71] As BV is not spontaneously cleared during pregnancy,[71] the CDC recommends treatment of BV in any pregnant patient who has a history of preterm birth.[4] BV has also been associated with abdominal wound infection after cesarean section, as well as post partum endometritis. In nonpregnant women, the relationship between BV and PID remains unclear (see PID section). However, BV has been associated with irregular vaginal bleeding.[71]

### Diagnosis

The diagnosis of BV can be made in several different ways. Using Amsel's criteria, BV is diagnosed if 3 of the following 4 factors are present: 1) thin white discharge adhering to the walls of the vagina; 2) vaginal pH of greater than 4.5; 3) characteristic "fishy" odor following addition of 10% KOH to a sample of vaginal fluid ("whiff test"); and 4) presence of clue cells on microscopic examination of vaginal fluid (must be 20% or more of the total epithelial cells). Clue cells are vaginal epithelial cells that have a stippled appearance due to adherent bacteria (such as *G vaginalis* or various anaerobes).[4] Neutrophils are generally absent on saline wet mount examination of vaginal fluid.

Gram stain examination of vaginal fluid is considered the gold standard for BV diagnosis and is performed by scoring for the presence or absence of various morphologic forms of bacteria.[4,75] More recently, DNA probe testing for *G vaginalis* and card tests for amines produced by the BV-related bacteria have become commercially available. Culture for *G vaginalis* is not useful because women without BV may be colonized by this bacterium. Cervical Papanicolaou (Pap) testing is also not useful in the diagnosis of BV.

### Treatment/Management

Recommended treatment regimens for BV are listed in Box 53-17. Of note, in the most recent guidelines single-dose treatment with oral metronidazole is no longer recommended. The CDC recommends that all symptomatic women be treated for BV. Women who

## Box 53-17

### *Treatment of Bacterial Vaginosis*

**Treatment of Non-pregnant Women**

Metronidazole 500 mg orally 2 times daily for 7 days

OR

Metronidazole 0.75% gel 1 applicator (5 grams) intravaginally nightly for 5 days

OR

Clindamycin 2% cream 1 applicator (5 grams) intravaginally nightly for 7 days

**Alternative Regimens for Non-pregnant Women**

Clindamycin 300 mg orally 2 times daily for 7 days

OR

Clindamycin 100 mg ovules intravaginally nightly for 3 days

OR

Tinidazole 2 g orally once daily for 2 days

OR

Tinidazole 1 g orally once daily for 5 days

**Treatment of Pregnant Women**

Metronidazole 500 mg orally 2 times daily for 7 days

OR

Metronidazole 250 mg orally 3 times daily for 7 days

OR

Clindamycin 300 mg orally 2 times daily for 7 days

Source: CDC, CDC. Sexually transmitted diseases treatment guidelines, 2010. *MMWR.* 2010;59:57-58

are undergoing cervical or uterine instrumentation (ie, abortion or placement of an intrauterine contraceptive device) should be treated for BV to prevent endometritis. In addition, any pregnant woman with a history of preterm delivery should be treated for BV regardless of the presence of symptoms. Pregnant women should not be treated with intravaginal clindamycin due to reports of possible adverse pregnancy outcomes when used during the second half of pregnancy.[76] Patients treated with oral metronidazole may experience nausea, gastrointestinal upset, or a metallic taste, and should be counseled to avoid alcohol during treatment and for 24 hours after completing the treatment course to prevent a disulfiram-like reaction. Patients receiving intravaginal clindamycin for BV treatment should be advised that the oil-based cream may weaken latex condoms.[4] Recurrence of BV is common, and currently no regimen is recommended by the CDC for suppressive therapy. One placebo-controlled trial of suppressive therapy using metronidazole intravaginal gel demonstrated decreased rates of recurrence.[77] Treatment of sexual partners and yogurt-based therapies have not been shown to cure BV or prevent recurrences.

## *TRICHOMONAS VAGINALIS*

### Epidemiology

*Trichomonas vaginalis* is not a reportable infection. According to the National Disease and Therapeutic Index (NDTI), an estimated 200,000 initial medical visits in 2006 in women were attributable to *T vaginalis* infection.[78] Up to 50% of women presenting with vaginal symptoms are infected with *T vaginalis*.[79] In one study of adolescents, 18% of participants were diagnosed with *T vaginalis*.[80] In an analysis of national US data in young adults, the overall prevalence of *T vaginalis* diagnosed by PCR was 2.3% (2.8% in women and 1.7% in men).[81] Among men, 4.5–17.3% of STI clinic patients had *T vaginalis* infection detected by molecular techniques (transcription mediated assay and PCR).[82,83] In women, African-American race, multiple sexual partners, and substance use are associated with trichomoniasis.[84]

### Biology/Pathophysiology

*T vaginalis* is a parasitic protozoan that is transmitted through sexual intercourse. *T vaginalis* attaches to vaginal epithelial cells, causing local inflammation and cellular damage. The characteristic discharge associated with *T vaginalis* likely results from both host defense mechanisms and the release of enzymes from the invading protozoa.[84] In women, *T vaginalis* may infect the vagina, urethra, endocervix, and Bartholin and Skene glands. In men, the urethra is the primary site of infection.[84]

### Clinical Presentation

*T vaginalis* vaginal discharge is classically described as copious, "frothy," and yellow-green in color.[4,84] Many women also have vulvar irritation and pruritis resulting from the profuse discharge.[4] Punctate hemorrhages may be seen on the ectocervix ("strawberry cervix" or colpitis macularis). However, this highly specific finding is only present in less than 5% of infected women.[84] Men may describe urethral discharge or dysuria. However, many women and most men are asymptomatic. [84]

### Complications

In women, *T vaginalis* infection is associated with preterm delivery, preterm rupture of membranes during pregnancy, low birth weight, and possibly upper reproductive tract infection.[4,84] Some studies in men have demonstrated a possible relationship between untreated *T vaginalis* infection and epididymitis, prostatitis, and abnormal sperm morphology.[84]

### Diagnosis

Microscopic examination of vaginal discharge demonstrating motile flagellated organisms is the most common method of diagnosing *T vaginalis* infection in women. Samples must be evaluated immediately after collection.[4,84] However, the sensitivity of saline wet mount for detection of *T vaginalis* is 68% (range 15–98%), with a specificity of 99.9% (range 98–100%).[85] Furthermore, although cervical Pap testing can also identify *T vaginalis*, the sensitivity and specificity are somewhat lower (sensitivity 58% with range 32–89%; specificity 97% with range 32–89%), and Pap smear is not recommended as a diagnostic modality.[85] Culture of *T vaginalis* is the gold standard but requires 3 to 5 days of incubation before results are available. Culture is recommended for women who are suspected of having *T vaginalis* infection but who have a negative microscopic examination of vaginal discharge.[4] Two commercially available point-of-care rapid tests are available for detection of *T vaginalis*, both with sensitivity greater than 83% and specificity more than 97%. One test uses immunochromatography whereas the other uses a nucleic acid probe.[4] Use of NAATs for *T vaginalis* detection requires individual labs to perform necessary CLIA verification testing.

Diagnosis of *T vaginalis* in males is somewhat more problematic. Saline microscopic examination of urinary sediment is of little utility in men, and neither rapid *T vaginalis* test is approved for use in men. The primary diagnostic method in men is culture of a urethral swab sample.[4,85] The InPouch TV test (*T vaginalis* culture) is approved for use with spun urine sediment in men.[86]

**Box 53-18**

***Treatment of Trichomoniasis***

Metronidazole 2 g orally once

OR

Tinidazole 2 g orally once

**Alternative Regimen**

Metronidazole 500 mg orally 2 times daily for 7 days

Source: CDC. Sexually transmitted diseases treatment guidelines, 2010. *MMWR*. 2010;59:59

### Treatment/Management

The treatment of *T vaginalis* is listed in Box 53-18. Ninety to 95% of patients successfully respond to metronidazole, whereas the cure rate for tinidazole is 86% to 100%. Metronidazole intravaginal gel is not recommended because it does not penetrate the periurethral glands and cures the infection less than 50% of the time. Although there are reports of metronidazole and tinidazole resistance, most patients with persistent or recurrent symptoms have experienced reinfection. Metronidazole resistance has been found in 2% to 9.6% of *T vaginalis* isolates.[4,87] Most resistant isolates can be effectively treated with single-dose tinidazole or a 7-day course of metronidazole. Patients should be counseled to avoid drinking alcohol for 1 day after completing metronidazole treatment and for 3 days after completing tinidazole treatment to avoid a disulfiram-like reaction.[4] Sexual partners should also be treated, and patients should be screened for other STIs. For pregnant women, single-dose metronidazole may be used. However, tinidazole should be avoided.

## HUMAN PAPILLOMAVIRUS

Human papillomavirus (HPV) infection causes asymptomatic genital infection, genital warts, and genital precancerous lesions and malignancies of the cervix, vulva, vagina, penis, and anus. This section focuses primarily on HPV infection and genital warts. For more detailed information regarding cervical cytology, please see Chapter 60, Management of Abnormal Pap Smears in Adolescent Women.

### EPIDEMIOLOGY

The CDC estimates that half of sexually active individuals will contract HPV in their lifetime.[88] Two nationally representative studies have demonstrated a high prevalence of HPV in adolescent and young adult women. Among women participating in NHANES 2003–2004, the HPV prevalence was 24.5% in 14- to 19-year-olds and increased to its peak at 44.8% in 20- to 24-year-olds.[89] In a separate study of women in the National Longitudinal Study of Adolescent Health (AddHealth), HPV prevalence in this group of 19- to 24-year-old women was 26.5%.[90] Among sexually active 18- to 59-year-old adults participating in NHANES 1999–2004, 5.6% reported ever having been diagnosed with genital warts.[91,92] Risk factors for HPV acquisition in women include increased number of sexual partners, frequency of intercourse, younger age at first intercourse, and presence of warts on the partner.[93-95] For males, number of sexual partners and poor condom use are associated with HPV infection.[93] Conflicting results have been found regarding a possible association between HPV infection and smoking or oral contraceptive use. Condoms appear to provide some protection in both men and women.

The high rate of HPV in young adult women has been demonstrated in studies of college students. In one study of college women, the average annual incidence of HPV infection was 14%, with a median duration of 8 months for newly acquired infections. Over the course of 3 years, 60% of the women had contracted HPV. Infections persisting longer than 6 months were associated with older age, high-risk HPV type, and infection with multiple HPV types.[94] In a separate study of college-age women with one lifetime male sexual partner, the 12-month cumulative incidence of HPV infection after coitarche was 28.5%. The cumulative incidence of HPV infection increased to 39.2% at 2 years after coitarche and 49.1% at 3 years. Greater number of partner's previous sexual partners was associated with an increased risk of incident HPV infection.[96]

### BIOLOGY/PATHOPHYSIOLOGY

More than 100 different strains of HPV have been identified, and approximately 30 of these infect the human genital tract. Different HPV types have been linked to different clinical presentations, with types 6 and 11 classically causing at least 90% of genital warts ("low-risk types") and types 16, 18, 31, 33, and 35 associated with genital tract dysplastic lesions, abnormal cervical cytology, and cancers ("high-risk types").[4,97] Human papillomavirus types 16 and 18 cause approximately 70% of cervical cancers.[97] HPV infects squamous epithelium, causing characteristic microscopic changes.[93] HPV also preferentially infects the cells of the transformation zone of the cervix, which is on the more exposed exocervix of adolescent women (compared to adult women) and is an area of active squamous metaplasia, during which HPV can be incorporated. Once an individual is exposed, viral shedding may be cleared by the host or may persist. Persistence of the infection is believed to be one of the key factors in progression to complications of HPV infection, including abnormal cytology and cancer.

**CLINICAL PRESENTATION**

Human papillomavirus infection is frequently subclinical but also may present as clinically apparent genital warts. Generally, warts are asymptomatic, although occasionally patients may note itching, pain, or friability. Visualized warts may be flat, papular, or pedunculated and can be located in the urethra or on the penis, scrotum, or perianal area of men, and on the vulva, perineum, vagina, cervix, periurethral, or perianal area in women (Figure 53-9). Genital warts may also be found perioraly.[4,93] The differential diagnosis of genital warts includes condyloma lata (secondary syphilis) and molluscum contagiosum.

**COMPLICATIONS**

Abnormal cervical cytology and progression to invasive cervical cancer are known complications of HPV infection. In addition, HPV infection has been linked to anal cancers (particularly in MSM and patients who are HIV-infected), as well as vulvar, vaginal, and penile cancers. The presence of a transformation zone in the anus, similar to that found in the cervix, is a factor in the development of anal cancer attributable to HPV.[98] Bacterial superinfection of lesions is possible in excoriated areas. In addition, there is a risk of HPV transmission from an infected pregnant woman to the neonate, resulting in recurrent respiratory papillomatosis.[4]

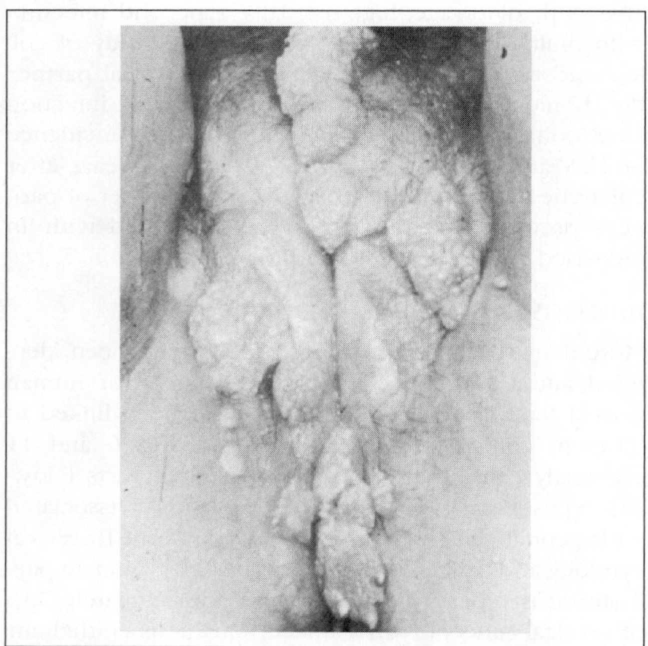

**FIGURE 53-9** Human papillomavirus (HPV). Condyloma acuminata of vulva. (From Centers for Disease Control and Prevention (CDC), Training and Health Communication Branch of the Division of STD Prevention, National Center for HIV/AIDS, Viral Hepatitis, STD, and TB Prevention. Available at: www.cdc.gov/std/training/clinicalslides/slides-dl.htm.) (See color insert.)

**DIAGNOSIS**

The diagnosis of genital warts is usually made strictly on visual inspection, and biopsy can be performed for diagnostic dilemmas. Human papillomavirus typing should not be performed for diagnostic purposes in patients with genital warts. Although application of a 3% to 5% acetic acid solution should not be used to screen for subclinical HPV infection,[4] it is commonly used to guide colposcopic examination.

**TREATMENT/MANAGEMENT**

The goal of therapy for genital warts is patient comfort. There is no evidence that wart treatment leads to eradication of the virus or decreased transmission of HPV to sexual partners. Genital warts may spontaneously resolve without treatment. In addition, warts may recur after initial successful treatment, particularly in the first 3 months following therapy. Thus, the decision to treat and the method of treatment should be made in consultation with the patient.[4] Treatment for external genital warts may be patient-applied, such as podofilox, imiquimod, or sinecatechins ointment, or clinician-applied, such as cryotherapy, podophyllin resin, trichloroacetic acid (TCA), bichloroacetic acid (BCA), surgical removal, intralesional interferon, or laser surgery. Treatment guidelines for HPV-related warts are summarized in Box 53-19.

As with HSV, the diagnosis of HPV can be emotionally difficult for some patients. Counseling regarding HPV should take place at the time of diagnosis and include the prevalence of the virus, the difficulty in determining the exact source partner, and the possibility of spontaneous regression as well as recurrences following treatment.[4]

Two vaccines for the prevention of HPV have recently been evaluated. A bivalent, preventive, HPV vaccine against HPV 16 and 18 has demonstrated a vaccine efficacy of 100% for cervical intraepithelial neoplasias caused by these 2 types of HPV at 4.5 years of follow-up.[99] The vaccine, which received FDA approval in 2009, is approved for use in females age 10 to 25 years and is administered as a 3-dose series at 0, 1, and 6 months. A quadrivalent preventive HPV vaccine, against HPV types 6, 11, 16, and 18, received FDA approval in 2006. The vaccine comprises non-infectious HPV virus-like

## Box 53-19

### *Genital Wart Therapy*

**External Genital Warts**

*Patient Applied:*

*Podofilox 0.5% solution or gel* to visible warts 2 times daily for 3 days, then rest for 4 days. Repeat up to 4 cycles. Total daily volume of podofilox used should be less than 0.5 mL and total wart area less than 10 $cm^2$

OR

*Imiquimod 5% cream* 1 time daily to visible warts at bedtime 3 times per week for up to 16 weeks. Wash off cream 6–10 hours after application.

OR

*Sinecatechins 15% ointment* 0.5 cm ribbon to each wart 3 times daily for up to 16 weeks

*Provider Applied:*

*Cryotherapy* with liquid nitrogen or cryoprobe every 1–2 weeks

OR

*Podophyllin resin 10–25%* in compound tincture with benzoin to visible warts weekly. Apply a small amount and allow to air-dry. Do not apply to open lesions. Do not use more than 0.5 mL or treat an area larger than 10 $cm^2$ per session. May be washed off 1–4 hours later.

OR

*Trichloroacetic acid (TCA) or bichloroacetic acid (BCA) 80–90%* applied to visible warts weekly as needed. Apply a small amount and allow to air-dry and develop a "white frosting."

OR

Surgical removal

Alternative treatment of external genital warts: intralesional interferon or laser surgery

**Cervical Warts**

Consult specialist

**Vaginal Warts**

Cryotherapy with liquid nitrogen

OR

TCA or BCA 80–90% as above for external genital warts

**Urethral Meatus Warts**

Cryotherapy with liquid nitrogen

OR

Podophyllin resin 10–25% as above for external genital warts

**Anal Warts**

Cryotherapy with liquid nitrogen

OR

TCA or BCA 80–90% as above for external genital warts

OR

Surgical removal

Source: CDC. Sexually transmitted diseases treatment guidelines, 2010. *MMWR*. 2010;59:71–72

particles and has shown 100% efficacy in prevention of high-grade cervical intraepithelial neoplasias and adenocarcinoma in situ caused by the HPV types in the vaccine. It was nearly 100% effective against the targeted HPV strains that cause genital warts.[97] Stable detectable levels of antibodies against HPV types 6, 11, 16, and 18 were present for at least 5 years.[100] This vaccine consists of 3 total doses given at 0, 2, and 6 months. The quadrivalent HPV vaccine is licensed for use in females and males aged 9-26 years for prevention of genital warts, cervical cancer, anal cancer, vulvar cancer, vaginal cancer, and anogenital precancerous lesions of the cervix, anus, vulva, and vagina. The Advisory Committee on Immunization Practices (ACIP), a branch of the CDC, has recommended routine immunization of all 11- and 12-year-old girls, and catch-up vaccination of 13- to 26-year-olds.[101] Girls can also be vaccinated as young as age 9 at the discretion of the provider. Although there are currently no recommendations for routine HPV vaccination in males, use of the vaccine is approved and permitted in males. The Society for Adolescent Health and Medicine,[102] the American Academy of Pediatrics,[103] the American College of Obstetricians and Gynecologists,[104] the American College of Physicians,[105] and the American Academy of Family Physicians[106] have issued position statements in support of this vaccine.

## *PHTHIRUS PUBIS* (PUBIC LICE)

### EPIDEMIOLOGY

There are no well-published incidence or prevalence rates for pubic lice. Although pubic lice are primarily transmitted through sexual contact, sharing of infected clothing or bedding is another modality. Populations at high risk for pubic lice are those at risk for other STIs, particularly adolescents and young adults. Pubic lice are rarely found in people older than age 35.[107]

### BIOLOGY/PATHOPHYSIOLOGY

The primary hosts for these ectoparasites are humans, although pubic lice have been found on dogs. Lice have a life span of approximately 24 hours, making fomite transmission unlikely. Localized pruritis occurs following allergic sensitization to the lice and is generally seen 5 days after initial infestation.[107]

### CLINICAL PRESENTATION

Patients most often present with itching, rash, or visible lice or nits, which are the eggs attached to hair shafts (Figure 53-10). In addition to the pubic region, infestations may affect facial hair, axillary areas, eyelashes, or eyebrows.[108,109]

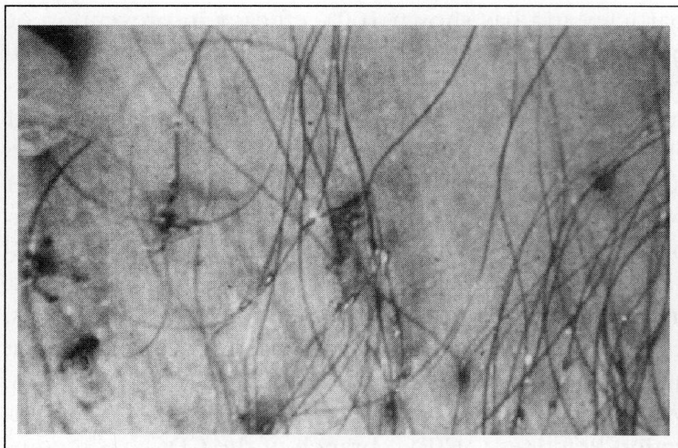

FIGURE 53-10 Pubic lice. (From Centers for Disease Control and Prevention (CDC), Training and Health Communication Branch of the Division of STD Prevention, National Center for HIV/AIDS, Viral Hepatitis, STD, and TB Prevention. Available at: www.cdc.gov/std/training/clinicalslides/slides-dl.htm.) (See color insert.)

**Box 53-20**

***Treatment of* Phthirus pubis *(Pubic lice)***

**Recommended:**

Permethrin 1% cream rinse applied to affected areas and washed off after 10 minutes

OR

Pyrethrins with biperonyl butoxide applied to affected areas and washed off after 10 minutes

**Alternative Regimens:**

Malathion 0.5% lotion applied for 8–12 hours and then washed off

OR

Ivermectin 250 mcg/kg orally repeated in 2 weeks

Source: CDC. Sexually transmitted diseases treatment guidelines, 2010. *MMWR*. 2010;59:88

### COMPLICATIONS

Local bacterial superinfection may occur in excoriated areas.

### DIAGNOSIS

Diagnosis is made through direct visualization of living lice or nits on the hair shaft.

### TREATMENT/MANAGEMENT

Treatment of pubic lice is accomplished with topical permethrin or pyrethrins with biperonyl butoxide (Box 53-20). In addition, all washable items that have been in contact with the patient should be washed in hot water or items removed from patient contact for at least 72 hours. Any sexual partners in the preceding 30 days should also be treated. Patients should also be evaluated for other concurrent STIs.[4]

## PREVENTION ISSUES

### PREVENTION FOLLOWING SEXUAL ASSAULT

Assessment of the post-assault patient should include consideration of potential STI exposure. During the initial examination of the post-assault patient, specimens for GC and CT should be taken from any sites of attempted or successful penetration (eg, pharynx, rectum, vagina) using culture or an FDA-approved NAAT. Regardless of the test used, providers should be aware of the possibility of false positive or false negative results and consider whether further confirmatory testing is warranted. Trichomonas culture or point-of-care-testing should also be obtained. Wet mount of vaginal secretions should be performed for diagnosis of vaginal candidiasis, bacterial vaginosis, and trichomoniasis. Baseline serum testing for HIV, hepatitis B, and syphilis should also be sent.

Because of difficulties ensuring follow-up for these individuals, prophylactic administration of antibiotics is generally recommended for victims of sexual assault. If the victim has not been vaccinated against hepatitis B, the hepatitis B vaccine series should be initiated. Hepatitis B immunoglobulin does not have a role in this setting. Empiric antibiotic treatment should include treatment for CT, GC, and trichomonas. The CDC-recommended empiric antibiotic regimen consists of intramuscular (or oral cefixime) oral metronidazole, and either one dose of oral azithromycin or 7 days of oral doxycycline (Box 53-21).[4]

Follow-up assessment should be done at 1 to 2 weeks post assault with repeat STI testing if antibiotic prophylaxis was not provided at the time of initial presentation. If prophylactic therapy was completed, STI testing is indicated only if the patient is symptomatic. Syphilis and HIV serologies should be repeated at 6 weeks, 3 months, and 6 months after assault if the assailant's serologic status is unknown.[4]

The provision of post exposure prophylactic medication for HIV is more complex. Consideration of the possible HIV status of the assailant is necessary. Victims are at increased risk of HIV transmission if vaginal or anal penetration occurred (particularly if grossly traumatic), several assailants were involved, ejaculation onto

**Box 53-21**

***Empiric Post sexual Assault Antibiotic Prophylaxis***

**Recommended:**

Ceftriaxone 250 mg IM once or Cefixime 400 mg orally once
PLUS
Metronidazole 2 g orally once
PLUS
Azithromycin 1 g orally once
OR
Doxycycline 100 mg 2 times daily for 7 days

Source: CDC. Sexually transmitted diseases treatment guidelines, 2010. *MMWR*. 2010;59:91

mucous membranes occurred, or genital or mucosal lesions were present on the assailant or the victim. The CDC recommends consultation with an HIV specialist if post exposure prophylaxis is being considered.[4]

### PARTNER NOTIFICATION AND TREATMENT

In the case of any STI, partner treatment is essential, to prevent infectious sequelae in the partner as well as to prevent reinfection of the treated patient. Evaluation and treatment is imperative for any sexual partner within 60 days of symptom onset (or the last sexual partner if most recent sexual activity was greater than 60 days prior to symptoms). Various methods of partner notification are used, including patient directed, clinician directed, anonymous notification, and expedited partner treatment (where legally permitted). Abstinence from sexual activity for 7 days is generally encouraged following treatment for most STIs. Partners should be screened for other common STIs in addition to those specifically diagnosed and HIV testing should be offered.[4]

### ROLE OF CONDOMS

Evaluation and treatment of STIs includes counseling about behavior changes to prevent future infections. Although condoms may not be as effective for some STIs (eg, HSV, HPV, pubic lice), latex condom use has been shown to prevent transmission of most bacterial STIs and HIV. Other types of condoms available include polyurethane condoms and "natural" condoms (eg, lamb cecum). Although polyurethane condoms are more costly and may slip or break more easily than latex condoms, the level of protection against STIs is similar. Natural condoms, however, provide no protection against viral STIs due to the presence of large pores.[110] Condoms should be used with all types of sexual activity, including oral, anal, and vaginal intercourse. Proper condom use should be discussed with any adolescent presenting for evaluation and treatment of a possible STI. Although in 1 study only 16% of adolescents used condoms correctly and consistently, when condoms were used properly adolescents were protected from both CT and GC.[111] In addition, condom use should be discussed and encouraged at every well visit with adolescents, regardless of current sexual activity. Demonstration of correct condom use and provision of written materials may also be helpful. Many centers treating adolescents offer free condoms to patients, recognizing that barriers to condom use may include lack of condoms or embarrassment when purchasing condoms.

### STI SCREENING IN ADOLESCENTS

The US Preventive Services Task Force has issued official recommendations for annual CT screening of all sexually active women age 24 years and younger and GC screening for women at high risk for GC infection. These recommendations would include all adolescents.[4] Annual GC and CT screening may be considered in sexually active men. No optimal screening interval has been established, although many providers screen for GC and CT in male and female teens every 6 to 12 months. In areas of high prevalence, routine screening for trichomonas may be considered. Given that many GC, CT, and trichomonas infections are clinically silent, routine screening is one way to decrease the number of asymptomatic transmissions and the frequency of negative sequelae, such as PID. See Table 53-2 for recommended screening tests for GC and CT.

## REFERENCES

1. Centers for Disease Control and Prevention. Sexually transmitted disease surveillance, 2003. Atlanta, GA: US Department of Health and Human Services, 2004 (vol 2004)

2. Shrier LA. Sexually transmitted diseases in adolescents: biologic, cognitive, psychologic, behavioral, and social issues. *Adolesc Med Clin*. 2004;15:215–234

3. Kaestle CE, Halpern CT, Miller WC, Ford CA. Young age at first sexual intercourse and sexually transmitted infections in adolescents and young adults. *Am J Epidemiol*. 2005;161:774–780

4. Centers for Disease Control and Prevention. Sexually transmitted diseases treatment guidelines, 2010. *MMWR*. 2010;59:1–110

5. Ethier KA, Kershaw T, Niccolai L, Lewis JB, Ickovics JR. Adolescent women underestimate their susceptibility to sexually transmitted infections. *Sex Transm Infect*. 2003;79:408–411

6. DeVore ER, Ginsburg KR. The protective effects of good parenting on adolescents. *Curr Opin Pediatr*. 2005;17:460–465

7. Bettinger JA, Celentano DD, Curriero FC, Adler NE, Millstein SG, Ellen JM. Does parental involvement predict new sexually transmitted diseases in female adolescents? *Arch Pediatr Adolesc Med*. 2004;158:666-670

8. Ford CA, Pence BW, Miller WC, et al. Predicting adolescents' longitudinal risk for sexually transmitted infection: results from the National Longitudinal Study of Adolescent Health. *Arch Pediatr Adolesc Med*. 2005;159:657-664

9. Huppert JS, Biro FM, Mehrabi J, Slap GB. Urinary tract infection and Chlamydia infection in adolescent females. *J Pediatr Adolesc Gynecol*. 2003;16:133-137

10. Centers for Disease Control and Prevention. Screening tests to detect Chlamydia trachomatis and Neisseria gonorrhoeae infections—2002. *MMWR*. 2002;51

11. Spigarelli MG, Biro FM. Sexually transmitted disease testing: evaluation of diagnostic tests and methods. *Adolesc Med Clin*. 2004;15:287-299

12. Gen-Probe.Aptima Combo 2 Assay Package Insert. Available at: www.gen-probe.com. Accessed June 3, 2008

13. BD. BD ProbeTec. *Chlamydia trachomatis/Neisseria gonorrhoeae* CT/GC) Q$^x$ Amplified DNA Assays Package Insert. Available at: www.bd.com. Accessed January 25, 2010

14. Xu F, Sternberg MR, Kottiri BJ, et al. Trends in herpes simplex virus type 1 and type 2 seroprevalence in the United States. *JAMA*. 2006;296:964-973

15. Cherpes TL, Meyn LA, Hillier SL. Cunnilingus and vaginal intercourse are risk factors for herpes simplex virus type 1 acquisition in women. *Sex Transm Dis*. 2005;32:84-89

16. Corey L, Wald A. Genital Herpes. In: Holmes KK, Sparling PF, Mardh P-A, et al, eds. *Sexually Transmitted Diseases*. New York: McGraw-Hill Health Professions Division; 1999

17. Centers for Disease Control and Prevention. *Sexually Transmitted Disease Surveillance, 2008*. Atlanta, GA: US Department of Health and Human Services. November 2009

18. Centers for Disease Control and Prevention. Trends in Reportable Sexually Transmitted Disease in the United States, 2006. Available at: www.cdc.gov/std/stats06/trends2006.htm. Accessed October 7, 2010.

19. Peterman TA, Heffelfinger JD, Swint EB, Groseclose SL. The changing epidemiology of syphilis. *Sex Transm Dis*. 2005;32:S4- S10

20. Woods CR. Syphilis in children: Congenital and acquired. *Semin Pediatr Infect Dis*. 2005;16:245-257

21. American Academy of Pediatrics. Syphilis. In: Pickering LK, Baker CJ, McMillan J, Long S, eds. *Red Book: 2006 Report of the Committee on Infectious Disease*. 27th edition. Elk Grove Village, IL: American Academy of Pediatrics: 2006: 631-644

22. Musher DM. Early syphilis. In: Holmes KK, Sparling PF, Mardh P-A, et al, eds. *Sexually Transmitted Diseases*. New York: McGraw-Hill Health Professions Division; 1999.

23. Swartz MN, Healy BP, Musher DM. Late syphilis. In: Holmes KK, Sparling PF, Mardh P-A, et al, eds. *Sexually Transmitted Diseases*. New York: McGraw-Hill Health Professions Division; 1999

24. Riedner G, Rusizoka M, Todd J, et al. Single-dose azithromycin versus penicillin G benzathine for the treatment of early syphilis. *N Engl J Med*. 2005;353:1236-1244

25. Holmes KK. Azithromycin versus penicillin G benzathine for early syphilis. *N Engl J Med*. 2005;353:1291-1293

26. Ronald AR, Albritton W. Chancroid and *Haemophilus ducreyi*. In: Holmes KK, Sparling PF, Mardh P-A, et al, eds. *Sexually Transmitted Diseases*. New York: McGraw-Hill Health Professions Division; 1999

27. van de Laar MGW, Gotz HM, de Zwart O, et al. Lymphogranuloma venereum among men who have sex with men Netherlands, 2003-2004. *MMWR*. 2004;53:985-988

28. Tinmouth J, Rachlis A, Wesson T, Hsieh E. Lymphogranuloma venereum in North America: case reports and an update for gastroenterologists. *Clin Gastroenterol Hepatol*. 2006;4: 469-473

29. Perine PL, Stamm WE. Lymphogranuloma venereum. In: Holmes KK, Sparling PF, Mardh P-A, et al, eds. *Sexually Transmitted Diseases*. New York: McGraw-Hill Health Professions Division; 1999

30. Kahn RH, Mosure DJ, Blank S, et al. Chlamydia trachomatis and Neisseria gonorrhoeae prevalence and coinfection in adolescents entering selected US juvenile detention centers, 1997-2002. *Sex Transm Dis*. 2005;32:255-259

31. Nsuami M, Cammarata CL, Brooks BN, Taylor SN, Martin DH. Chlamydia and gonorrhea co-occurrence in a high school population. *Sex Transm Dis*. 2004;31:424-427

32. Hook EW, Handsfield HH. Gonococcal infections in the adult. In: Holmes KK, Sparling PF, Mardh P-A, et al, eds. *Sexually Transmitted Diseases*. New York: McGraw-Hill Health Professions Division: 1999

33. Centers for Disease Control and Prevention. *Sexually Transmitted Diseases Treatment Guidelines, 2006*: Fluoroquinolones no longer recommended for treatment of gonoccocal infections. *MMWR*. 2007;56:332-336

34. Centers for Disease Control and Prevention. Updated recommended treatment regimens for gonococcal infections and associated conditions-United States, April 2007. Available at: www.cdc.gov/std/treatment/2006/GonUpdateApril2007.pdf. Accessed June 3, 2008

35. Stamm WE. Chlamydia trachomatis infections of the adult. In: Holmes KK, Sparling PF, Mardh P-A, Lemon SM, Stamm WE, Piot P, Wasserheit JN, eds. *Sexually Transmitted Diseases*. New York: McGraw-Hill Health Professions Division, 1999

36. McCormack WM, Rein MF. Urethritis. In: Mandell GL, Bennett JE, Dolin R, eds. *Principles and Practice of Infectious Diseases*. Philadelphia, PA: Churchill Livingstone; 2005

37. American Academy of Pediatrics. Chlamydia trachomatis. In: Pickering LK, Baker CJ, McMillan J, Long S, eds. *Red Book: 2006 Report of the Committee on Infectious Diseases*. 27th edition. Elk Grove Village, IL: American Academy of Pediatrics, 2006:252-257

38. Lim SW, Coupey SM. Are adolescent girls with Chlamydia infection notifying their partners? *J Pediatr Adolesc Gynecol*. 2005;18:33-38

39. Anagrius C, Lore B, Jensen JS. Mycoplasma genitalium: prevalence, clinical significance, and transmission. *Sex Transm Infect*. 2005;81:458-462

40. Totten PA, Schwartz MA, Sjostrom KE, et al. Association of Mycoplasma genitalium with nongonococcal urethritis in heterosexual men. *J Infect Dis*. 2001;183:269-276

41. Deguchi T, Yoshida T, Miyazawa T, et al. Association of Ureaplasma urealyticum (biovar 2) with nongonococcal urethritis. *Sex Transm Dis*. 2004;31:192-195

42. Horner P, Thomas B, Gilroy CB, Egge M, Taylor-Robinson D. Role of Mycoplasma genitalium and Ureaplasma urealyticum in acute and chronic nongonococcal urethritis. *Clin Infect Dis*. 2001;32:995-1003

43. Gambini D, Decleva I, Lupica L, Ghislanzoni M, Cusini M, Alessi E. Mycoplasma genitalium in males with nongonococcal urethritis: prevalence and clinical efficacy of eradication. *Sex Transm Dis*. 2000;27:226-229

44. Deguchi T, Maeda S. Mycoplasma genitalium: another important pathogen of nongonococcal urethritis. *J Urol*. 2002;167:1210-1217

45. Taylor-Robinson D. Mycoplasma genitalium—an update. *Int J STD AIDS*. 2002;13:145-151

46. Cohen CR, Manhart LE, Bukusi EA, et al. Association between Mycoplasma genitalium and acute endometritis. *Lancet*. 2002;359:765-766

47. Manhart LE, Critchlow CW, Holmes KK, et al. Mucopurulent cervicitis and Mycoplasma genitalium. *J Infect Dis*. 2003;187:650-657

48. Falk L, Fredlund H, Jensen JS. Signs and symptoms of urethritis and cervicitis among women with or without Mycoplasma genitalium or Chlamydia trachomatis infection. *Sex Transm Infect*. 2005;81:73-78.

49. Taylor-Robinson D, Ainsworth JG, McCormack WM. Genital mycoplasmas. In: Holmes KK, Sparling PF, Mardh P-A, et al, eds. *Sexually Transmitted Diseases*. New York: McGraw-Hill Health Professions Division; 1999

50. Falk L, Fredlund H, Jensen JS. Symptomatic urethritis is more prevalent in men infected with Mycoplasma genitalium than with Chlamydia trachomatis. *Sex Transm Infect*. 2004;80:289-293

51. Jensen JS, Bjornelius E, Dohn B, Lidbrink P. Comparison of first void urine and urogenital swab specimens for detection of Mycoplasma genitalium and Chlamydia trachomatis by polymerase chain reaction in patients attending a sexually transmitted disease clinic. *Sex Transm Dis*. 2004;31:499-507

52. Pletcher J, Slap GB. Pelvic inflammatory disease. In: Neinstein L, ed. *Adolescent Health Care: A Practical Guide*. Philadelphia: Lippincott, Williams, & Wilkins: 2002

53. Westrom L, Eschenbach D. Pelvic inflammatory disease. In: Holmes KK, Sparling PF, Mardh P-A, et al, eds. *Sexually Transmitted Diseases*. New York: McGraw-Hill Health Professions Division; 1999

54. Emans SJ. Sexually transmitted diseases: Gonorrhea, Chlamydia trachomatis, pelvic inflammatory disease, and syphilis. In: Emans SJ, Laufer MR, Goldstein DP, eds. *Pediatric and Adolescent Gynecology*. New York: Lippincott-Raven Publishers; 1998

55. Kelly AM, Ireland M, Aughey D. Pelvic inflammatory disease in adolescents: high incidence and recurrence rates in an urban teen clinic. *J Pediatr Adolesc Gynecol*. 2004;17:383-388

56. O'Brien RF. Bacterial vaginosis: many questions-any answers? *Curr Opin Pediatr*. 2005;17:473-479

57. Peter NG, Clark LR, Jaeger JR. Fitz-Hugh-Curtis syndrome: a diagnosis to consider in women with right upper quadrant pain. *Cleve Clin J Med*. 2004;71:233-239

58. Lambert MJ, Villa M. Gynecologic ultrasound in emergency medicine. *Emerg Med Clin North Am*. 2004;22:683-696

59. Centers for Disease Control and Prevention. Sexually transmitted diseases treatment guidelines 2002. *MMWR*. 2002;51

60. Centers for Disease Control and Prevention. Guidelines for the treatment of sexually transmitted diseases. *MMWR*. 1998;47:79-86

61. Ness RB, Soper DE, Holley RL, et al. Effectiveness of inpatient and outpatient treatment strategies for women with pelvic inflammatory disease: results from the Pelvic Inflammatory Disease Evaluation and Clinical Health (PEACH) Randomized Trial. *Am J Obstet Gynecol*. 2002;186:929-937

62. Sobel JD. Vulvovaginal candidiasis. In: Holmes KK, Sparling FP, Stamm WE, et al, eds. *Sexually Transmitted Diseases*. 4th ed. New York: McGraw-Hill Medical Professions Division; 2008:823-838

63. Nyirjesy P. Vaginitis in the adolescent patient. *Pediatr Clin North Am*. 1999;46(4):733-745, xi

64. Foxman B. The epidemiology of vulvovaginal candidiasis: risk factors. *Am J Public Health*. 1990;80 (3):329-331

65. Holland J, Young ML, Lee O, SCAC. Vulvovaginal carriage of yeasts other than *Candida albicans*.*Sex Transm Infect*. 2003;79 (3):249-250

66. Spinillo A, Zara F, Gardella B, Preti E, Mainini R, Maserati R. The effect of vaginal candidiasis on the shedding of human immunodeficiency virus in cervicovaginal secretions. *Am J Obstet Gynecol*. 2005;192 (3):774-779

67. Martin HL Jr, Nyange PM, Richardson BA, et al. Hormonal contraception, sexually transmitted disease, and risk of heterosexual transmission of human immunodeficiency virus type 1. *J Infect Dis*. 1998;178(4):1053-1059

68. Sobel JD, Faro S, Force RW, et al. Vulvovaginal candidiasis: epidemiologic, diagnostic, and therapeutic considerations. *Am J Obstet Gynecol*. 1998;178(2):203-211

69. Watson MC, Grimshaw JM, Bond CM, Mollison J, Ludbrook A. Oral versus intra vaginal imidazole and triazole antifungal agents for the treatment of uncomplicated vulvovaginal candidiasis (thrush): a systematic review. *BJOG*. 2002;109(1):85-95

70. Koumans EH, Sternberg M, Bruce C, et al. The prevalence of bacterial vaginosis in the United States, 2001-2004; associations with symptoms, sexual behaviors, and reproductive health. *Sex Transm Dis*. 2007;34 (11):864-869

71. Hillier SL, Marazzo J, Holmes KK. Bacterial vaginosis. In Holmes KK, Sparling PF, Stamm WE, et al, eds. *Sexually Transmitted Diseases*. 4th ed. New York: McGraw-Hill Medical; 2008:737–768

72. Glaser JB, Schachter J, Benes S, Cummings M, Frances CA, McCormack WM. Sexually transmitted diseases in postpubertal female rape victims. *J Infect Dis*. 1991;164(4):726–730

73. Jenny C, Hooten TM, Bowers A, et al. Sexually transmitted diseases in victims of rape. *N Engl J Med*. 1990;322(11): 713–716

74. Fredricks DN, Fiedler TL, Marazzo JM. Molecular identification of bacteria associated with bacterial vaginosis. *N Engl J Med*. 2005;353(18):1899–1911

75. Nugent RP, Krohn MA, Hillier SL. Reliability of diagnosing bacterial vaginosis is improved by a standardized method of Gram stain interpretation. *J Clin Microbiol*. 1991;29(2):297–301

76. Joesoef MR, Hillier SL, Wiknjosastro G, et al. Intravaginal clindamycin treatment for bacterial vaginosis: effects on preterm delivery and low birth weight. *Am J Obstet Gynecol*. 1995;173(5):1527–1531

77. Sobel JD, Ferris D, Schwebke J, et al. Suppressive antibacterial therapy with 0.75% metronidazole vaginal gel to prevent recurrent bacterial vaginosis. *Am J Obstet Gynecol*. 2006;194(5):1283–1289

78. Centers for Disease Control and Prevention. Sexually Transmitted Disease Surveillance 2006: Other STDs. Available online at www.cdc.gov/std/stats06/default.htm. Accessed October 7, 2010

79. Krieger JN, Alderete JF. *Trichomonas vaginalis* and Trichomoniasis. In: Holmes KK, Sparling PF, Mardh P-A, et al, eds., *Sexually Transmitted Diseases*, 3rd ed. New York: McGraw-Hill Health Professions Division; 1999:587–604

80. Huppert JS, Biro F, Lan D, Mortensen JE, Reed J, Slap GB. Urinary symptoms in adolescent females: STI or UTI? *J Adolesc Health*. 2007;40(5):418–424

81. Miller WC, Swygard H, Hobbs MM, et al. The prevalence of trichomoniasis in young adults in the United States. *Sex Transm Dis*. 2005;32(10):593–598

82. Hardick A, Hardick J, Wood BJ, Gaydos C. Comparison between the Gen-Probe transcription-mediated amplification *Trichomonas vaginalis* research assay and real-time PCR for *Trichomonas vaginalis* detection using a Roche LightCycler instrument with female self-obtained vaginal swab samples and male urine samples. *J Clin Microbiol*. Nov 2006;44(11): 4197–4199

83. Schwebke JR, Hook EW III. High rates of *Trichomonas vaginalis* among men attending a sexually transmitted diseases clinic: implications for screening and urethritis management. *J Infect Dis*. 2003;188(3):465–468

84. Hobbs MM, Sena AC, Swygard H, Schwebke J. *Trichomonas vaginalis* and Trichomoniasis. In: Holmes KK, Sparling PF, Stamm WE, et al, eds. *Sexually Transmitted Diseases*, 4th ed. New York: McGraw-Hill Medical Professions Division; 2008: 772–793

85. Wiese W, Patel SR, Patel SC, Ohl CA, Estrada CA. A meta-analysis of the Papanicoulaou smear and wet mount for the diagnosis of vaginal trichomoniasis. *Am J Med*. 2000;108(4): 301–308

86. Biomed Diagnostics. InPouch TV Package Insert (*Trichomonas vaginalis* Test). Available at: www.biomed-diagnostics.com/files/100-001%20TV%20Insert%20Rev%20J.pdf. Accessed October 7, 2010

87. Schwebke JR, Barrientes FJ. Prevalence of *Tribomonas vaginalis* isolates with resistance to metronidazole and tinidazole. *Antimicrob Agents Chemother*. 2006;50 (12):4209–4210

88. Centers for Disease Control and Prevention. Genital HPV Infection. Available at www.cdc.gov/std/HPV/STDFact-HPV.htm. Accessed October 7, 2010

89. Dunne EF, Unger ER, Sternberg M, et al. Prevalence of HPV infection among females in the United States. *JAMA*. 28, 2007;297(8):813–819

90. Dempsey AF, Gebremariam A, Koutsky LA, Manhart L. Using risk ractors to predict human papillomavirus infection: implications for targeted vaccination strategies in young adult women. *Vaccine.*, 2008;26 (8):1111–1117

91. Dinh TH, Sternberg M, Dunne MF, Markowitz LE. Genital warts among 18–59-year-olds in the United States, National Health and Nutrition Examination Survey, 1999–2004. *Sex Transm Dis*. 2008;35(4):357–360

92. Dinh TH, Sternberg M, Dunne EF, Markowitz LE. Erratum: Genital warts among 18–59-year-olds in the United States, National Health and Nutrition Examination Survey, 1999–2004. *Sex Transm Dis*. 2008;35(8):772–773

93. Koutsky LA, Kiviat NB. Genital Human Papillomavirus. In: Holmes KK, Sparling PF, Mardh P-A, et al, eds. *Sexually Transmitted Diseases*. New York: McGraw-Hill Health Professions Division; 1999

94. Ho GY, Bierman R, Beardsley L, Chang CJ, Burk RD. Natural history of cervicovaginal papillomavirus infection in young women. *N Engl J Med*. 1998;338:423–428

95. Moscicki AB, Hills N, Shiboski S, et al. Risks for incident human papillomavirus infection and low-grade squamous intraepithelial lesion development in young females. *JAMA*. 2001;285:2995–3002

96. Winer RL, Feng Q, Hughes JP, et al. Risk of female human papillomavirus acquisition associated with first male sex partner. *JID*. 2008;197:279–282

97. Centers for Disease Control and Prevention. HPV Vaccine Information for Clinicians. Available at: www.cdc.gov/std/HPV/STDFact-HPV-vaccine-hcp.htm. Accessed August 7, 2008

98. Partridge JM, Koutsky LA. Genital human papillomavirus infection in men. *Lancet Infect Dis*. 2006;6:21–31

99. Harper DM, Franco EL, Wheeler CM, et al. Sustained efficacy up to 4.5 years of a bivalent L1 virus-like particle vaccine against human papillomavirus types 16 and 18: follow-up from a randomized control trial. *Lancet*. 2006;367:1247–1255

100. Olsson SE, Villa LL, Costa RL, et al. Induction of immune memory following administration of a prophylactic quadrivalent human papillomavirus (HPV) types 6/11/16/18 L1 virus-like particle (VLP) vaccine. *Vaccine,* 2007;25(26):4931-4939

101. Markowitz LE, Dunne EF, Saraiya M, et al. Quadrivalent Human Papillomavirus Vaccine: Recommendations of the Advisory Committee on Immunization Practices (ACIP). *MMWR Recomm Rep*. 2007;56(RR-2):1-24

102. Friedman LS, Kahn J, Middleman AB, Rosenthal SL, Zimet GL. Human Papillomavirus (HPV) Vaccine: A Position Statement of the Society for Adolescent Medicine. *J Adolesc Health*. 2006;39(4):620

103. American Academy of Pediatrics. Prevention of human papillomavirus infection: provisional recommendations for immunizations of girls and women with quadrivalent human papillomavirus vaccine. *Pediatrics*. 2007;120(3):666-668

104. American College of Obstetrics and Gynecology (ACOG). Committee Opinion No. 344: Human papillomavirus vaccination. *Obstet Gynecol*. 2006;108(3Pt 1): 699-705

105. American College of Physicians. Recommended adult immunization schedule: United States, October 2007-September 2008. *Ann Intern Med*. 2007;147(10):725-729

106. American Academy of Family Physicians. Recommended Immunization Schedule for Persons Aged 7-18 Years-US, 2008. Available at: www.aafp.org/online/etc/medialib/aafp_org/documents/clinical/immunization/adolescenimmsched.Par.0001.File.dat/2010AdolescentImmunizationschedulefinal121709.pdf. Accessed October 7, 2010

107. Billstein SA. Pubic Lice. In: Holmes KK, Sparling PF, Mardh P-A, et al, eds. *Sexually Transmitted Diseases*. New York: McGraw-Hill Health Professions Division; 1999

108. Centers for Disease Control and Prevention. Pubic "Crab" Lice. Available at: www.cdc.gov/lice/pubic/factsheet.htm. Accessed on August 7, 2008

109. Orion E, Matz H, Wolf R. Ectoparasitic sexually transmitted diseases: scabies and pediculosis. *Clin Dermatol*. 2004;22:513-519

110. Kane ML, Rosen DS. Sexually transmitted infections in adolescents: practical issues in the office setting. *Adolesc Med Clin*. 2004;15:409-421

111. Paz-Bailey G, Koumans EH, Sternberg M, et al. The effect of correct and consistent condom use on chlamydial and gonococcal infection among urban adolescents. *Arch Pediatr Adolesc Med*. 2005;159:536-542

# CHAPTER 54

## Adolescent Pregnancy

CATHERINE STEVENS-SIMON, MD • JEANELLE SHEEDER, MSPH

*Dr. Catherine "Cassie" Stevens-Simon passed away in November 2007 after a long battle with cancer. We would like to acknowledge her life-long dedication to pregnant adolescents and their families and to the Colorado Adolescent Maternity Program, which she founded. She is greatly missed and we hope to continue her legacy of caring for adolescent mothers and their families.*

### HISTORICAL PERSPECTIVE

Adolescent pregnancy is a complex issue in the United States. Furstenberg[1] describes it as "conspicuously invisible" during the 1960s. With 1 in 10 American teenagers conceiving, it was extremely common. However, it was not considered a public health problem in need of governmental oversight.[1] Two factors led Americans to re-examine this view; social disapproval of the rapidly rising rate of nonmarital births to adolescents, and the development of a scientific evidence base that demonstrated the taxpayers' stake.[2] Concern has waned since the early 1990s due to the decline in teen births and the erosion of the evidence base.[3] The perception that fewer teenagers are conceiving and that doing so need not become a costly biopsychosocial problem has fostered a sense of complacency that is difficult to justify empirically.[3] Up until 2006, the teen pregnancy rate was the lowest in 20 years and the teen birth rate the lowest ever recorded in the United States.[4] However, in the last few years, the rate has risen again. American teenagers are still more likely to conceive than teenagers in other developed countries.[5] This would not be troubling if the effects of having a child during adolescence were positive or neutral. However, in the United States, annual expenditures for women who become pregnant during their teens and their children total $6 billion.[2] The view that early childbearing is responsible for this has encountered strong opposition from researchers who contend that given the problems of urban youth, deferring childbearing is unlikely to have a substantial impact on these expenditures.[1] However, with 1 in 20 American girls conceiving before 20 years of age, if the effect of early childbearing is even marginally negative, the public health repercussions would be enormous.

It is difficult to measure the socioeconomic consequences of adolescent childbearing. Controversy arises because unobserved differences in adolescents' preferences and opportunities affect their likelihood of bearing children and their health and socioeconomic success. Taking this self-selection process into account reduces the negative consequences of early childbearing.[1-3] However, with 50% of the psychosocially lowest risk teenage mothers having serious school and substance abuse problems and another 40% in trouble with the law,[6] it is far from evident that adolescent pregnancy is "neither a potent nor a permanent cause of long-term poverty and disadvantage among women who would have otherwise escaped this fate had they only waited to have their first child."[1] Rather, it seems that expectations for the performance of teenage mothers have eliminated their social obligation to be successful. To wit, "... for someone tottering on the brink of school dropout with no real likelihood of going to college, an untimely pregnancy if not a salvation as some have claimed, is certainly not a disaster either."[1] When school dropout and reliance on public assistance are expected, taking classes toward a graduate equivalency degree is heralded as a success. Elsewhere around the globe the increased importance placed on higher education motivates young women to obtain job skills before starting families.[5] Only in the United States, where teenage childbearing is portrayed as an appropriate, adaptive response to the debilitating circumstances of urban poverty do young women routinely fail to appreciate the importance of doing so.

Failure to distinguish between teenagers who are willing to become pregnant and those who are not has also contributed to this disconnect between the facts and perceptions about teenage childbearing in the United States.[7] Teenagers who seek therapeutic abortions consistently fare better than socioeconomically similar young women who miscarry or become mothers.[3] Thus analyses that do not take childbearing intentions into account seriously underestimate the negative impact of teenage pregnancy on young Americans.[7] Although it was overly pessimistic to conclude that "when a 16-year-old girl has a child, 90% of her life's script is written for her,"[3] there is still substantial evidence that teenage childbearing is a public health problem worthy of prevention.

### EPIDEMIOLOGY

#### PREVALENCE

For 50 years there has been a steady global decline in the pregnancy rate.[5] Except for a 6-year increase in the late 1980s and early 1990s, the US teen pregnancy, abortion, and birth rates have also been declining, in that order.[8] However, US teen pregnancy rates have increased in the last few years. During the height of the baby boom, 10% of American teenagers gave birth, compared with 5% today. Nonetheless, most teen pregnancies and half of teen births are still unplanned.[2] The rate of second and higher-order teen pregnancies has also declined, albeit less rapidly than the rate of first teen pregnancies.[9] Currently, approximately 1 in 5 teen births are to young women who already have children.[9] Because repeat teen pregnancy is associated with a host of adverse maternal and child outcomes, these young women contribute disproportionately to the magnitude and cost of adolescent childbearing in the United States.[9] Just more than half of teen pregnancies end as live births. Approximately a third end in therapeutic abortion, and the rest abort spontaneously or end as ectopic or molar pregnancies.

In 2004, the teen birth rate was less than half the rate in 1957 when teen births peaked, and 33% lower than the rate in 1991 when teen births reached a 20-year high.[4] Although global, societal-level factors have undoubtedly been contributory, in the United States the adolescent fertility decline has been more rapid than the general fertility decline.[4,5] The explanation for these trends is complex.[8] Over the last decade there has been a decrease in sexual activity and fecundity among American adolescents.[8] Teenagers are delaying the initiation of sexual activity, and those who are sexually active are using a more effective mix of contraceptives, particularly at coitarche. Although decreased sexual activity has undoubtedly contributed to the decline in the US teen pregnancy rate, nearly 60% of American high school seniors are still sexually active. With a 9 in 10 chance that those who do not use contraception will conceive within a year, the decline in the US teen pregnancy rate is likely to continue to lag behind other Western countries until their approach to teen sexuality is adopted.[5,10] Indeed, coincident with the shift from comprehensive sex education to abstinence-only programs, the rate of decline in sentinel teen sexual risk-taking behaviors leveled off to insignificant.[11]

## RISK FACTORS AND PRODROMAL SYMPTOMS

Pregnant and parenting teenagers are not a homogenous group. Nonetheless, it is useful to identify shared demographic, psychosocial, and behavioral characteristics as they can be used to guide the development of etiological theories and target prevention interventions. Variables from numerous domains are associated with a heightened probability of conception during adolescence (Box 54-1). They can be divided into "generic" and "pregnancy-specific" subgroups to differentiate between characteristics associated with an increase in the odds of engaging in socially deviant behavior and characteristics that increase vulnerability to pregnancy. Because these 2 types of risk factors probably involve different etiological mechanisms, they may inform prevention theories and interventions differently. Although detailed reviews have been published,[12] there is nothing intrinsic about any of these factors that necessarily leads teenagers to engage in unprotected rather than protected sexual intercourse, and only a few are modifiable. Thus, despite a wealth of correlational data, efforts to target prevention interventions continue to suffer from the poor predictive capacity the factors in Box 54-1 have for conception. Although this has also created the impression that rational decision-making frameworks are of limited value in predicting teenagers' reproductive health behavior, few teen pregnancies are random events that can be attributed to contraceptive method failures or brief hiatuses in contraceptive

### Box 54-1

### *Risk Factors for Teen Pregnancy*

| *Generic* | *Pregnancy-specific* |
|---|---|
| Poverty | Precocious physical development |
| Minority race/ethnicity | Precocious sexual development |
| Not living with either biologic parent | Teen pregnancy socially normative |
| Growing up in a single-parent home | Religious prohibition on teen sex |
| Dysfunctional family | Boyfriend wants a baby |
| Childhood victimization | Deep romantic relationship |
| Unconventional/socially deviant behavior | Older, adult male partner |
| Poor self-esteem/mastery | Coercive sexual relationship |
| Depression/stress | Recent sexual debut |
| School failure | Prolonged sexual activity |
| No future plans | No contraception at sexual debut |
| No affiliation with conventional institutions | Request for pregnancy test |

use that are beyond user control.[13] Rather, most occur within the context of ongoing intimate relationships when events conspire to make the perceived burdens of using contraception outweigh the perceived benefits.[13,14] Under these circumstances, teen couples are more likely to become pregnant because they do not have any reason to try to avoid conceiving than because they have reasons to try to do so.[13] Absence of negative expectations is an important prodromal symptom because it fosters compliancy. This leaves teenagers cognitively susceptible to problems like pregnancy that require action to avoid. Other prodromal symptoms include the belief that pregnancy will not occur even if contraception is not used, that contraceptives are unsafe and cumbersome, and that women should not plan ahead for sex. Appreciation that it is these common misperceptions that undermine the motivation to use contraception at this age has altered professional understanding of the developmental processes that operate against responsible sexual behavior and have facilitated efforts to target prevention interventions because these warning signs are modifiable and more potent predictors of conception than the risk factors listed in Box 54-1.

## WHAT MAKES TEEN PREGNANCY DIFFERENT?

### THE MOTHER

Young maternal age is a complex biopsychosocial obstetrical risk factor.[15] Pregnant teenagers are in better physical condition, suffer from fewer chronic diseases, and engage in fewer unhealthy behaviors than socioeconomically similar pregnant adults. However, despite decades of research, young American women who conceive before 18 years of age give birth to disproportionately large numbers of premature infants who are prone to costly neonatal complications and childhood disabilities. This paradox is not evident in traditional societies, where early childbearing is characteristic of the most rather than least financially advantaged members. However, in the United States age is usually confounded by characteristics that predispose women of all ages to adverse pregnancy outcomes. When these factors are taken into account, young maternal age is only an independent risk factor for 2 obstetrical complications: gastroschisis and preterm delivery. The minority of teenagers who conceive prior to 16 years of age and/or within 2 to 3 years of menarche are at highest risk. For this subgroup, the etiology of the risks associated with childbearing are also biologic. As previously reviewed, puberty interacts with and exacerbates many of the risk factors listed in Box 54-2.[15]

**Box 54-2**

***Risk Factors for Preterm Delivery***

| ***Sociodemographic*** | ***Behavioral*** |
|---|---|
| Age | Adequacy of prenatal care |
| Race | Concurrent sexual relationships/serial monogamy |
| Educational achievement | Tobacco and substance use |
| Health literacy | Socially deviant and problem behaviors |
| Socioeconomic status | Diet |
| Marital status | Activity |
| ***Physiologic*** | ***Psychological*** |
| Maternal size/body composition | History of abuse |
| Rate of maternal weight gain | Poor support |
| Subfecundity | Problem people |
| Vaginal bleeding | Desired pregnancy |
| Alkaline vaginal pH | Exposure to violence |
| Short cervix | Older, nonteen father of baby |
| Obstetric complications | Stress and depression |
| Lower genital tract infections | Poor psychological resources/mastery |
| Trauma | Developmental conflicts |

The onset of menarche does not mark the cessation of growth or the attainment of physical, reproductive, cognitive, or psychosocial maturity.[15] Because the maternal growth that takes place during adolescent pregnancies is measured in tenths of millimeters, it is unlikely that the additional caloric demands deprive the fetus of nutrients. Rather, studies of still-growing pregnant humans and animals suggest that the low level of luteal-phase progesterone and selective deficit of central body fat stores characteristic of the first 2 to 3 postmenarcheal years could compromise placentation by creating a metabolic environment that favors maternal fat deposition over placental growth. The fat component of the weight gained early in gestation corrects deficits in maternal stores and is a significant predictor of infant birth weight among young adolescents but not older American women. However, excessive weight gain early in gestation can adversely affect insulin metabolism, compromise placentation, and increase the risk of preterm delivery and maternal obesity.[15] In the United States, gestational weight gain recommendations are based on body mass index (BMI); women are classified as under, average, and overweight. Weight gain in excess of the recommended level increases the risk of maternal obesity without benefit to the fetus. Because the BMI cut-points for under, average, and overweight increase during adolescence, basing gestational weight gain recommendations for adolescents on the adult BMI scheme could overestimate their nutritional needs and put them at risk for postpartum obesity. The authors found that basing weight gain recommendations for pregnant adolescents on their age-specific BMI percentiles minimizes postpartum weight retention without compromising fetal growth.

In addition to the maturation of the hypothalamic-pituitary-gonadal axis and body fat stores, the reproductive organs grow and the vaginal fluids become more acidic for 2 to 3 years after women are able to conceive.[15] Teenagers who conceive prior to 16 years of age are significantly more likely to have the critically short cervixes associated with an increased risk of preterm labor. Vaginal alkalinity exacerbates this anatomical situation by increasing vulnerability to lower genital tract infections, and enhancing the virulence of the inflammatory response to them. Serially monogamous sexual relations further increase the risk of infection, which is an especially important cause of early preterm deliveries that adolescents are prone to. When present prior to conception it impedes placentation. Later in gestation it weakens the placental membranes. Screening for and treating genitourinary tract infection mitigates this risk. However, when used indiscriminately, prophylactic antibiotics increase colonization with resistant microorganisms and foster concerns about partner fidelity without reducing the risk of preterm delivery.[16]

Psychological stress is another arena in which the normal developmental changes associated with puberty and adolescence could exacerbate the risk of preterm delivery.[15] Chronic exposure to circumstances that the mother finds stressful is most detrimental. Superimposing pregnancy on adolescence creates unique stresses. In addition to the conflicts that inevitably arise between these competing developmental needs, the circumstances antedating teen pregnancies are often extremely stressful. The mechanisms underlying the association between maternal psychological stress and preterm delivery are speculative.[15,17] Stress may increase the risk of preterm delivery indirectly by decreasing appetite or fostering adverse habits. Alternatively, stress could suppress the hypothalamic-pituitary-gonadal axis and impede placentation, alter maternal carbohydrate metabolism and reduce insulin resistance, stimulate placental vasoconstriction and decrease blood flow to the fetus, weaken the maternal immune response to lower genital tract infections, and trigger the precocious release of neuropeptides that accelerates parturition. Helping women cope with stressful aspects of their lives improves psychological well-being, reduces adverse health habits, slows the process of preterm cervical maturation, and decreases the risk of lower genital tract infection and preterm delivery.[15,16] During adolescence, adequate support from the father, maternal grandmother, or a primary confidant is especially important. Teenagers who lack or reject the support of these key people often turn to mood-altering substances, peer-dominated support networks, or enter into liaisons with older males for solace.

## THE FATHER

Comparatively little is known about the men who father adolescent pregnancies.[12,18] Much of the information about them is suspect because it has been obtained from teenage mothers. Although we do not have a clear description of these young men, regardless of age, demographically and psychosocially they resemble their teenage partners. They have significantly more academic, financial, and behavioral problems and are also more likely to have experienced abuse and domestic violence as children, to abuse alcohol and illicit drugs, to have concurrent sexual relationships and sexually transmitted infections (STIs) and to mistreat their intimate partners. Thus, there are more similarities between groups of adult and adolescent men who father the babies of teen mothers than between groups of adult men who father the babies of teen and adult women.

Adolescent girls are often attracted to older males because they appear more successful economically and more supportive than their teenage counterparts. However, the perceived benefits of these partnerships are dubious at best. Teen mothers who partner with adult males are more likely to engage in risky social and sexual behavior for nonautonomous reasons, drop out of school, become socially isolated and estranged from their families, and plan repeat pregnancies during adolescence.[18] Pre-existing differences between teenagers who choose older and same-aged partners are as likely to be etiologic as the age difference between partners. Nonetheless, in the mid-1990s public concern galvanized efforts to use statutory rape laws as a deterrent to this "predatory behavior." Interest in this approach to the prevention of teen pregnancy waned with the realization that because most teen mothers are 18 to 19 years old, inappropriately older adult males are only responsible for 5% to 8% of teen pregnancies in the United States.[19] Concern that the threat of prosecution might discourage minor teenagers in supportive, culturally sanctioned relationships with adult males from seeking care further dampened enthusiasm for this strategy.[19]

## THE CHILD

The high incidence of medical and social problems among infants and children of adolescent mothers emphasizes the necessity of attending closely to both their physical and psychosocial development. Toddlers who are not responding verbally, and children who are failing in school must be identified before they become angry, frustrated adolescents who leave high school and become parents.

During the neonatal period these children are at increased risk for morbidity and mortality because they are often premature.[12,18,20] During infancy, childhood, and adolescence most grow normally but are at high risk for developmental delay, intellectual impairment, and behavioral problems (Table 54-1).[12,18,20] These deficits are most noticeable among normal birth weight, term infants. A similar pattern of disability has been reported when preterm infants and infants exposed to illicit drugs in utero are raised in socioeconomically disadvantaged environments.[21]

Children who are raised in extended families are less apt to exhibit the medical problems and intellectual deficits of children who are raised primarily by their teenage mothers. However, there is no evidence that the presence of an adult in the home has a direct, beneficial effect on child development.[20] Indeed, the children of older adolescent mothers fare worse when reared simultaneously by their mothers and grandmothers.[18,20] Thus, the same personal attributes that enable some adolescent mothers to elicit the daily support of adults in their environment may also make them more nurturing parents.

Teenage mothers tend to reinforce vocalizations less and take a more negative, punitive approach to childrearing than adults. However, no studies have shown that their atypical and unconventional mothering behaviors contribute to the problems their children encounter.[20] Rather, the available empiric data suggest that poverty and social deprivation are more important determinants of these children's performance than maternal age. Thus it is apt to be more expedient to encourage teen parents and their children to enroll in programs that remediate the shortcomings of their environment, rather than enforce policies that mandate adult supervision in the home.

**Table 54-1**

**Problems of Children of Adolescent Mothers**

| | *Medical* | *Psychosocial* |
|---|---|---|
| Infants | • Under- and over-nutrition<br>• Growth delay<br>• Prematurity and its sequelae<br>• Hospitalization and death from accidental trauma and acute infections<br>• Sudden infant death syndrome | • Developmental delay<br>• Neglect/abandonment<br>• Nonaccidental trauma |
| Children | • Accidental trauma and poisoning<br>• Minor acute infections<br>• Under- and over-nutrition<br>• Hospitalization and death from poorly controlled chronic disease such as asthma<br>• Hospitalization and disability from exposure to environmental toxins such as lead | • Intellectual deficits<br>• Attention-deficit disorder and other behavior problems<br>• Truancy, school failure, and grade retention<br>• Nonaccidental trauma<br>• Stress related to family and environmental violence<br>• Fighting |
| Adolescents | • Over-nutrition<br>• Accidental trauma<br>• Hospitalization and death from poorly controlled chronic disease such as asthma | • Intellectual deficits<br>• Mental health problems such as depression<br>• Socially deviant/violent behavior problems such as substance abuse and fighting<br>• Legal problems/jailing<br>• Truancy, school failure, and withdrawal<br>• Removal from parental custody<br>• Unplanned pregnancy |

## PREVENTION

### PRIMARY

Primary prevention interventions target the teenage population as a whole. The goal is to change cultural attitudes that favor early sexual activity as a means of achieving emotional closeness and early childbearing as a means of individuating and achieving adult status. These programs fall into 3 categories: abstinence-only, comprehensive sex education, and youth development. Abstinence-only programs are based on the premise that any sexual activity outside of marriage is morally reprehensible.[10] Discussions about contraceptives and prophylactics are forbidden on the grounds that they are unnecessary and apt to send a mixed message to teenagers about the acceptability of premarital sexual intercourse. Abstinence-only education delays the onset of sexual activity but does not prevent teenagers from becoming pregnant or acquiring STIs and may actually be counterproductive in this regard.[10] By contrast, addressing abstinence and contraceptives in the same curriculum increases the use of both without promoting nonmarital sexual activity.[10]

Comprehensive sex education is based on the premise that sexual activity is part of normal development. Accordingly students learn that abstinence, dual protection, contraceptives, and unprotected intercourse from a continuum of protection against pregnancy and STIs within all of their interpersonal relationships.

Youth development programs are based on the premise that the morbid consequence of risky adolescent sexual behavior can be prevented by addressing the shared, "nonsexual" antecedents of social deviance.[22] These programs can prepare young, socially disadvantaged children to assume productive adult roles, but there is no evidence that promoting attachment to conventional institutions such as family, school, and church, emulating successful role models, or engaging in voluntary community service prevents more early childbearing than simply discouraging unprotected sexual activity.[23]

Because most teenagers spend more time in school than medical offices and clinics, schools are the usual setting for primary prevention interventions. The use of school curricula to promote safe sexual behavior has met with variable success. However, even when knowledge-based sex education programs are grounded in theories of human behavior and linked to school or community-based clinics or youth development programs, they do not prevent teen pregnancy.[24] There is nothing intrinsic about goal setting, academic achievement, or family discourse that necessarily makes teenagers want to avoid pregnancy. Hence, in communities where early childbearing and single motherhood are normative, even family-oriented teenagers who go to school and church grow up believing that these are acceptable models compatible with the lifestyles they envision for themselves. In these settings it is less important to encourage teenagers to formulate conventional educational and career goals than to ensure that they understand that pregnancy prevention is not an end in itself, but a means of obtaining what they want most for themselves in life. Pediatric health care providers can assist by using the questions in Box 54-3 to identify the specific aspects of their teenage patients' lives that make pregnancy an acceptable life course event. In addition, when confronted with a sexually active, noncontraceptive-using teenage patient, providers should not assume that pregnancy prevention is desired. The numerous factors that undermine contraceptive vigilance (Table 54-2) should be reviewed systematically with patients and used to formulate a differential diagnosis for their risky sexual behavior.

**Box 54-3**

***Life Domain-Specific Expectations about the Effects of Teen Pregnancy***

**Future Plans**

Would having a (another) baby now get in the way of your future plans, make it hard for you to do what you want to do with your life, or be a burden on you?[a]

**Self-esteem**

Would you be disappointed in yourself, think less highly of yourself, or like yourself less if you had a (another) baby now?

**Boyfriend relations**

Would having a (another) baby now cause trouble between you and your boyfriend and drive you apart?

**Autonomy**

Would having a (another) baby now force you to move out of your home and get your own place before you are ready to do so or make it harder for you to move out when you are ready to live independently?

**Peer relations**

Would having a (another) baby now make it harder for you to fit in and do things with your friends?

**Family relations**

Would having a (another) baby now be a burden on your family and make them unhappy with you?

[a]Teenagers who do not give a "Yes" response are at an increased risk for pregnancy because they have no reason to avoid it.

**Table 54-2**

**Differential Diagnosis for Inconsistent Contraceptive Use**

| *Reason for Nonuse* | *Counseling Strategy* |
|---|---|
| **Not ready to try to prevent pregnancy** | |
| • Consciously seeking pregnancy<br>• Not consciously seeking pregnancy, but does not mind having a baby | Dispel misperceptions about the opportunity costs of early childbearing and burdens of prevention |
| **Does not believe that she will become pregnant if she does not use contraception** | |
| • Thinks she is sterile<br>• Thinks her partner is sterile<br>• Thinks natural family planning methods are adequate | Dispel the misperceptions that develop when a woman does not become pregnant after several episodes of unprotected sexual intercourse or when one or both partners have had experiences such as being sexually abused or treated for a sexually transmitted disease or abnormal Pap test |
| **Does not believe that contraceptives are safe or feels that the benefits of using them do not outweigh the medical risks** | |
| • Has experienced side effects or had negative experiences<br>• Has heard about side effects or negative experiences | Dispel the misperceptions that develop when information about contraceptives and contraceptive safety is obtained from friends, relatives, and the media |
| **Does not anticipate that she is going to have sexual intercourse and/or is unwilling or psychologically unable to prioritize pregnancy prevention** | |
| • Cultural taboos and moral prohibitions against premarital sex deter conscious decision making about reproductive behavior<br>• Early childbearing is the cultural norm, prevention is not a priority because teen pregnancy is not perceived to be an important obstacle to attaining economic self-sufficiency or a desirable lifestyle | Dispel passive, fatalistic attitudes about pregnancy planning and misperceptions about the relative importance of postponing childbearing beyond adolescence in the 21st century |
| **Unable to overcome logistical barriers** | |
| • Infrastructure problems: time, transportation, and finances<br>• Superstructure problems: embarrassment about obtaining and negotiating contraception use and being too intoxicated to do so | Barrier-specific |

## SECONDARY

Secondary prevention begins at conception. The goal is to prevent medical and psychosocial morbidity among adolescent parents and their children by providing early consistent, comprehensive prenatal and postpartum care.[15,25] Few pediatric health care professionals provide obstetrical care. However, they have an important role in diagnosis, options counseling, follow-up, and subsequent care of adolescent mothers and their children.

### Diagnosis

A high index of suspicion may be needed to avoid missing the diagnosis of pregnancy in the adolescent. First-trimester vaginal bleeding occurs in more than a third of cases,[15] and young women who wish to conceal their pregnancies may initially even deny sexual activity. Therefore, when pregnancy is suspected, it is important to interview the adolescent in private, reaffirm confidentiality, be direct, and perform a blood or urine pregnancy test (hCG). The trophoblast begins to produce hCG at implantation. Pregnancy can be reliably diagnosed at an hCG concentration of 10 mIU/mL in the blood and 30 to 50 mIU/ml in the urine. This usually occurs within 2 to 3 days of implantation or 5 or 6 days after ovulation. However, because the interval between ovulation and implantation ranges from 6 to 12 days, 10% of conceptions are undetectable on the first day of the missed period.[26] The serum pregnancy test is quantitative and more sensitive and reliable than the urine. Nonetheless, when performed in a medical

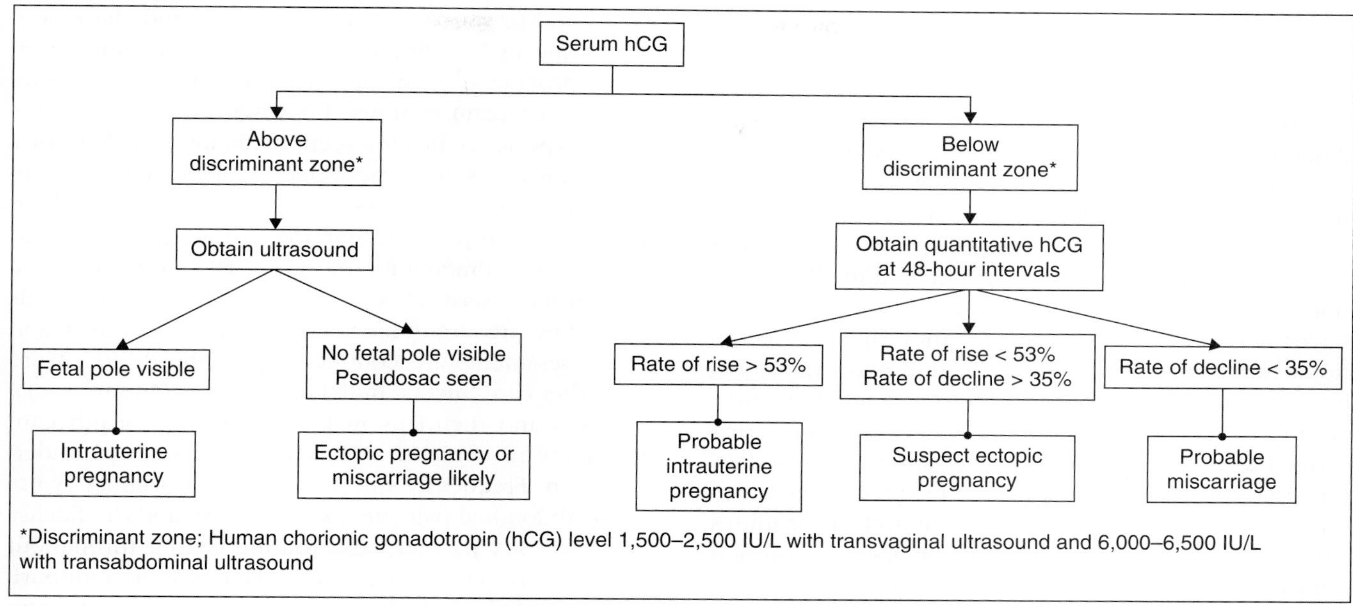


**FIGURE 54-1** Evaluation of suspected ectopic pregnancy

office or clinical laboratory, false-positive urine pregnancy test results are rare. This cannot be said of home pregnancy test kits.[27] They are unreliable, and because only a minority of teenagers seeks contraceptives after obtaining a negative result at home, home pregnancy test takers are at higher-than-average risk for conception.[27] Thus their use should not only be discouraged but regarded as a red flag.

A positive pregnancy test in the absence of uterine enlargement should raise suspicion of miscarriage or ectopic pregnancy, especially in patients who report irregular or abnormal menstrual bleeding, unilateral abdominal or pelvic pain, and in patients whose medical histories reveal conditions that impede the migration of the fertilized ovum to the uterus such as smoking, pelvic inflammatory disease, or the use of an intrauterine device or progesterone-only contraceptive. If the diagnosis of ectopic pregnancy is entertained, a serum hCG level and transvaginal ultrasound study should be obtained and an obstetrician consulted. Ectopic pregnancy remains the leading pregnancy-related cause of death in the first trimester and accounts for approximately 12% of all pregnancy-related deaths in the United States.[28] The concept of the "discriminatory cut-off," or the hCG level at which a normal intrauterine pregnancy can be visualized by ultrasound, is critical to the diagnosis and management of suspected ectopic pregnancies (Figure 54-1).[28] If diagnosed early, patients can be treated medically or with minimally invasive surgery, but hemodynamically unstable patients require laparotomy.[28] A positive pregnancy test in the presence of excessive uterine enlargement should raise suspicion of a multiple gestation or molar pregnancy, especially in patients who develop hyperemesis or preeclampsia during the first trimester. A serum hCG level and ultrasound should be obtained and an obstetrician consulted. Neoplastic transformation occurs in up to a third of cases. Although obstetric referral is a necessity, the pediatric health care provider should remain involved as teenagers who experience a pregnancy loss often become depressed and many become pregnant again during adolescence.

### Options Counseling

The adolescent should be informed of her pregnancy in private and management options presented nonjudgmentally in the context of her future career and family plans. Health care providers who strongly support or oppose a particular option should refer their pregnant patients to a neutral provider who can present the risks and benefits of obtaining a therapeutic abortion, relinquishing the baby following birth, or keeping and raising the infant. Although confidentiality must be maintained, it is prudent to encourage younger adolescents to share the decision-making process with a parent or trusted adult. However, this does not mean that adult involvement should be a prerequisite for care. The health care provider should know their state's laws regarding confidential care of the pregnant adolescent.

### Termination

Health care providers who work with sexually active adolescents must familiarize themselves with the laws governing the right to therapeutic abortion as they differ from state to state. Chapter 56 provides a more comprehensive discussion of abortion. Several abortion procedures are available.[29] First-trimester abortion is a low-risk, outpatient procedure. Most women undergo dilation and suction curettage or obtain a medical abortion. Teenagers do well with both, and generally suffer fewer complications than adults. After the 12th gestational week, abortion requires dilation and evacuation, intact dilation and extraction, or prostaglandin induction. Hospitalization is usually necessary for abortions performed after the 16th week of gestation. With modern techniques there is no overall risk of cervical incompetence or subsequent miscarriage. Multiple procedures may increase the risk. However, therapeutic abortion contributes less to cervical incompetence than precipitous delivery and the surgical treatment of abnormal Pap smears.

Although therapeutic abortion is far safer than pregnancy, the risk of death increases exponentially after the 8th week of gestation. Thus, delay in obtaining the procedure is the primary cause of abortion-related mortality in the United States.[29] Failure to recognize pregnancy, difficulty accessing services due to decreased physician training and social acceptability, and laws mandating fixed waiting periods and parental notification significantly increase the need for second-trimester procedures, especially in minors.[29,30]

There have been anecdotal reports of poor psychological outcomes and anniversary suicide reactions following therapeutic abortions, particularly among adolescents who are coerced or persuaded to abort against their will. However, adolescents who are provided with adequate pre- and postabortion counseling do as well or better than their parenting peers.[12] Most subsequently use contraceptives, avoid additional pregnancies, and complete their educations.[3]

### Continuation

Adolescents who decide to continue the pregnancy have the options of parenting the child after birth, having the child placed in foster care, or putting the child up for adoption. These should all be presented as options when counseling a pregnant adolescent.

Adolescents who choose to continue their pregnancies should be referred for prenatal care. Referral to a comprehensive adolescent-oriented maternity program designed to meet their unique nutritional, psychosocial, and educational needs is preferable.[12,15,16] Because adolescents who conceive when they are younger than 16 years of age are more apt to be under psychological stress and to start pregnancy with low body fat stores, they typically benefit more than older adolescents from these programs.[15] Care is usually provided by a multidisciplinary team composed of physicians with subspecialty experience in adolescent medicine and obstetrics, nurse midwives and practitioners, social workers, dietitians, and case managers who are capable of making home visits. To promote staff–patient interaction and to facilitate implementation of individual care plans, clinic appointments are scheduled at more frequent intervals than they are in adult-oriented obstetric settings, and risk assessments are conducted periodically to ensure that the care meets individual needs. On-site social workers and dietitians make it easier for health care providers to contend with maternal stress and undernutrition. Frequently questioning about vaginal symptoms, abdominal pain, new sex partners, and the fidelity of steady sex partners and routine testing throughout gestation facilitates the early diagnosis of genitourinary tract infections. Because teenagers cannot be randomly assigned to adolescent- and adult-oriented care, the best evidence that the improved pregnancy outcomes of adolescents enrolled in these programs does not simply reflect a bias toward healthier, more highly motivated young women using these services comes from randomized controlled trials that demonstrate that when the individual components are administered selectively to pregnant women with specific, modifiable risk characteristics, they experience fewer obstetrical complications.[16]

The first encounter with an adolescent who chooses to continue her pregnancy provides an opportunity to start prenatal vitamins including folic acid, discuss health behaviors, nutrition, and risks of STIs, and promote breastfeeding. Adolescent parenting decisions, such as choice of infant feeding, may be effectively addressed throughout the prenatal period. Multidisciplinary programs that utilize group sessions, peer role models, and teen-friendly education activities enhance compliance with prenatal care and adoption of healthy behaviors.[31] Such programs are effective in lowering rates of preterm delivery, low birth weight infants and cesarean sections, and in increasing rates of breastfeeding and identification of a pediatric health provider.

### Follow-up

Regardless of the management option selected, adolescents who have been pregnant are at a greater risk for conception and the acquisition of STIs than their nulliparous peers.[32] Hence a postpartum checkup 6 to 8 weeks after delivery and counseling about dual protection and safe partner selection are a necessity. However, ongoing primary health care should be provided by a health care professional who can address future gynecological concerns and common adolescent medical and mental health problems.

### Adoption

Fewer than 5% of teen mothers voluntarily place their children with adoptive families.[12] Hence it is difficult to determine the long-term ramification of this management option. However, for young people who are morally opposed to or who are unable to obtain a therapeutic abortion but have plans for the future that do not include adolescent parenthood, adoption may be the ideal solution to an otherwise devastating dilemma.

## CARING FOR THE ADOLESCENT MOTHER

The pediatric health care provider is often the only health care professional who sees new mothers at regular intervals following delivery. Some offer primary health care services to the adolescent mothers of infants in their practices. Studies indicate that young mothers who are cared for with their infants receive more regular care, are more adherent with contraceptive prescriptions, and postpone second pregnancies for longer periods of time than their peers who receive medical care in other settings.[25,33] Other pediatric health care providers refer the adolescent mothers in their practice to clinics that offer special adolescent-oriented health care services. Even if health care is not provided for the adolescent mother, pediatric caregivers should inquire at each well baby visit about the young mother's plans for breast-feeding, use of contraceptives, school and work attendance, future career and family plans, exposure to violence and STIs, self-esteem and mastery, level of stress and symptoms of depression, and support network structure and function. It is estimated that during the first 6 postpartum months as many as 50% of adolescent mothers experience depressive symptoms that are severe enough to interfere with their daily lives, and 20% are physically abused or assaulted. Yet most cases are never diagnosed or treated. Worries about maternal self-efficacy and stress related to the demands of homemaking and childrearing are the most common precipitants. Factors such as inadequate social support, the birth of an abnormal, preterm, or low birth weight baby, rapid repeat pregnancy, and educational deficits that preclude gainful employment and necessitate long-term welfare dependency tend to exacerbate the situation and contribute to the high rate of separation among adolescent couples.[12,20] Whereas mild cases may be responsive to social support, young families with multiple problems should be referred to comprehensive adolescent parenting programs. For a full discussion of the adolescent parent, refer to Chapter 55, Adolescent Parenthood.

## SUBSEQUENT CONCEPTIONS

Among the numerous factors that threaten the success of teenage mothers and their children, the birth of a second child during the first 2 postpartum years is pivotal.[9] Complications ranging from an increased likelihood of prematurity, accidental/nonaccidental trauma, and social deviance in the next generation, to a decreased likelihood of high school graduation and economic self-sufficiency among parents have been reported.[9] Most new teenage mothers want to avoid conception. They have aspirations for their futures that are as incompatible with closely spaced childbearing like their never-pregnant peers, and begin using contraception after delivery.[33,34] However, this heightened contraceptive vigilance tends to wane rapidly in daily living environments that are conducive to first teen pregnancies. As a result, the repeat conception rate averages 5% 6 months after delivery and rises exponentially to 20% to 25% at 12, and 30% to 35% at 24 months postpartum.[9] Even among teenage mothers who are enrolled in comprehensive, multidisciplinary programs that provide access to contraceptives and promote their use as a means of achieving personal goals, the risk of repeat conception is as high during the first 6 postpartum months as the risk of first pregnancy in the adolescent population as a whole.[34] Because the majority of repeat pregnancies occur during the 5 years following the first, long-acting contraceptives are an attractive short-term solution. These agents provide a unique window of opportunity during which teenagers can be helped to develop personal reasons for remaining nonpregnant.[33] Convincing teenage mothers that having numerous, closely spaced children will not solve the multitude of problems that discrimination and social deprivation create in their lives is a difficult task best accomplished within the context of the strong, long-term relationships home visitors form with them.[9,34] To be maximally effective, counseling should be initiated during the first pregnancy and be part of every pre- and postnatal visit. Teens should not leave the postpartum unit without contraceptive supplies, as most resume sexual activity soon after delivery. However, because they cannot be case managed into nonexistent family planning services, home visitors may be unable to help them overcome the system-related barriers that make it difficult to continue to use contraception consistently.[34] Programs that provide medical care for adolescent parents and their children were developed to meet this need and to provide teenagers with the encouragement they need to pursue goals that make them want to use the contraceptive supplies they are given to postpone childbearing beyond adolescence.[25,33]

## TERTIARY PREVENTION

Tertiary prevention interventions target the siblings and offspring of teenage mothers. The goal is to prevent the transmission of early childbearing and associated morbidities to the next generation by helping families who have experienced a teen pregnancy avoid others.[35] Because these families typically share numerous characteristics that foster negative attitudes about contraception and positive feelings about having babies, the younger, 12- to 14-year-old sisters and daughters of teen mothers are 2 to 3 times more likely than their peers to conceive during adolescence. They are a particularly attractive target population because pivotal events like an unplanned teen pregnancy tend to leave families open to change. Moreover, the middle school years are decisive in the formation of lifelong sexual and contraceptive behavior. Few younger sisters and daughters of teen mothers want or plan to become teen parents. However, most lack the role models and daily living experiences that foster an innate resolve to remain nonpregnant. Tertiary intervention programs provide the necessary additional prompting.[35] Family involvement is crucial so the teens receive the same messages from the program and home. Moreover, establishing channels of communication that make it easy for teens to share their daily experiences with their parents minimizes the need for the direct monitoring these parents find so difficult to implement.[36]

## FUTURE RESEARCH

This chapter highlights some of the most glaring gaps in our knowledge about adolescent pregnancy and parenthood, and points out the research dilemmas and controversies that remain. Observational studies have generated a wealth of correlation data. However, their design precludes inferences about causality. Effective intervention requires an understanding of causal mechanisms. Thus it is imperative that future investigators address testable hypotheses, perform sample-size calculations, and employ multivariate analytical techniques. It may be most expedient to focus on high-risk subgroups, such as the siblings and children of teen parents, teenagers with negative pregnancy tests, and teenagers who have been pregnant before. Because the rates of pregnancy are 2 to 3 times higher within these subgroups, the efficacy of interventions can be tested more rapidly. In addition, the central role that the adolescent male plays in the contraceptive decisions that antedate adolescent conceptions highlights the importance of studying their attitudes toward pregnancy and parenthood. Effective treatment of the immediate morbidity associated with adolescent childbearing requires that we learn more about the etiologic mechanisms underlying the effects that fetal programming and adolescent pubertal, cognitive, and psychosocial development have on female reproductive performance. Thus it is imperative that risk assessments based on maternal age be replaced by objective, quantifiable measures of modifiable characteristics of puberty and adolescence that have biologically plausible links to prematurity and that intervention be based upon testable hypotheses regarding the elimination of the most prevalent risk factors. Adolescent pregnancy is a complex problem; simple answers and solutions are unlikely. Unless these rigorous research tactics are adopted, there is little hope of decreasing the preterm delivery rate and interrupting the cycle of poverty associated with adolescent childbearing in the United States. Early childbearing adversely affects the health and socioeconomic well-being of mothers and children. However, without societal changes we should not expect that simply postponing would-be adolescent conceptions will eliminate the problems associated with childbearing at this age.

## REFERENCES

1. Furstenberg FF. Teenage childbearing as a public issue and private concern. *Ann Rev Sociol.* 2003;29:23–29

2. Maynard RA. Kids having kids. A Robin Hood Foundation Special Report on the Costs of Adolescent Childbearing. Washington, DC: Urban Institute; 1996

3. Hoffman SD. Teenage childbearing is not so bad after all… or is it? A review of the new literature. *Fam Plann Perspect.* 1998;30:236–239

4. Hoyert DL, Mathews TJ, Menacker F, Strobino DM, Guyer B. Annual summary of vital statistics: 2004. *Pediatrics.* 2006;117:168–183

5. Singh S, Darroch JE. Adolescent pregnancy and childbearing: levels and trends in developed countries. *Fam Plann Perspect.* 2000;32:14–23

6. Oxford ML, Gilchrist L, Lohr MJ, Gillmore MR, Morrison DM, Spieker SJ. Life course heterogeneity in the transition from adolescence to adulthood among adolescent mothers. *J Res Adolesc.* 2005;15:479–504

7. Stevens-Simon C, Lowy R. Is teenage childbearing an adaptive strategy for the socioeconomically disadvantaged or a strategy for adapting to socioeconomic disadvantage? *Arch Pediatr Adolesc Med.* 1995;149:912–915

8. Stevens-Simon C, Kaplan D. Teen childbearing trends: which tide turned when and why? *Pediatrics.* 1998;102:1205–1206

9. Klerman LV. *Another Chance: Preventing Additional Births to Teen Mothers*. The National Campaign to Prevent Teen Pregnancy; 2004

10. Santelli J, Ott MA, Lyon M, Rogers J, Summers D, Schleifer R. Abstinence and abstinence-only education: a review of US policies and programs. *J Adolesc Health.* 2006;38:72–81

11. Advocates for Youth. Trends in sexual risk behavior among high school students—United States 1991 to 1997 and 1999 to 2003. Available at: www.advocatesforyouth.org/index.php?option=com_content&task=view&id=459&Itemid=336. Accessed October 8, 2010

12. Stevens-Simon C, McAnarney ER. Pregnancy. In: Greydanus DE, Wolraich ML, eds. *Behavioral Pediatrics*. New York, NY: Springer-Verlag; 1992

13. Stevens-Simon C, Beach R, Klerman LV. To be rather than not to be, that is the problem with the question. *Arch Pediatr Adol Med.* 2001;155:1298–1300

14. Jones RK, Darroch JE, Henshaw SK. Contraceptive use among US women having abortions in 2000–2001. *Perspect Sex Reprod Health.* 2002;34:294–303

15. Stevens-Simon C, Beach R, McGregor JA. Do incomplete pubertal growth and development predispose teenagers to preterm delivery? A template for research. *Am J Perinatol.* 2002;22:315–323

16. Stevens-Simon C, Orleans M. Low-birth weight prevention programs: the enigma of failure. *Birth.* 1999;26:184–191

17. Wadhwa PD, Culhane JF, Rauh V, Barve SS. Stress and preterm birth: neuroendocrine, immune/inflammatory, and vascular mechanisms. *Matern Child Health J.* 2001;5:119–125

18. Elfenbein DS, Felice ME. Adolescent pregnancy. *Pediatr Clin North Am.* 2003;50:781–800

19. Donovan P. Can statutory rape laws be effective in preventing adolescent pregnancy? *Fam Plann Perspect.* 1997;29:30–34

20. Stevens-Simon C, McAnarney ER. The teenage parent. In: Hoekelman RA, Friedman SB, Nelson NM, Seidel HM, eds. *Primary Pediatric Care*. New York, NY: Mosby; 2000

21. Saigal S, Stoskopf B, Streiner D, et al. Transition of extremely low-birth-weight infants from adolescence to young adulthood: comparison with normal birth-weight controls. *JAMA.* 2006;295:667–675

22. Roth J, Brooks-Gunn J. Promoting healthy adolescents: synthesis of youth development program evaluations. *J Res Adol.* 1998;8:423–459

23. Guilamo-Ramos V, Litardo HA, Jaccard J. Prevention programs for reducing adolescent problem behaviors: implications of the co-occurrence of problem behaviors in adolescence. *J Adol Health.* 2005;36:82–86

24. Guyatt GH, DiCenso A, Farewell V, Willan A, Griffith L. Randomized trials versus observational studies in adolescent pregnancy prevention. *J Clin Epidemiol.* 2000;53:167–174

25. Stevens-Simon C, Fullar SA, McAnarney ER. Teenage pregnancy: caring for adolescent mothers with their infants in pediatric settings. *Clin Pediatr.* 1989;28:282–283

26. Wilcox AJ, Baird DD, Dunson D, McChesney R, Weinberg CR. Natural limits of pregnancy testing in relation to the expected menstrual period. *JAMA.* 2001;286:1759–1761

27. Kelly L, Sheeder J, Stevens-Simon C. Teen home pregnancy test takers: more worried or more wishful? *Pediatrics.* 2004;113:581–584

28. Seeber BE, Barnhart KT. Suspected ectopic pregnancy. *Obstet Gynecol.* 2006;107:399–413

29. Stubblefield PG, Carr-Ellis S, Borgatta L. Methods for induced abortion. *Obstet Gynecol.* 2004;104:174–185

30. Crosby MC, English A. Mandatory parental involvement/judicial bypass laws: do they promote adolescents' health? *J Adolesc Health.* 1991;12:143–147

31. Grady MA, Bloom KC. Pregnancy outcomes of adolescents enrolled in a Centering Pregnancy program. *Midwifery Womens Health J.* 2000;49(5):412–420

32. Meade CS, Ickovics JR. Systematic review of sexual risk among pregnant and mothering teens in the USA: pregnancy as an opportunity for integrated prevention of STD and repeat pregnancy. *Soc Sci Med.* 2005;60:661–678

33. Stevens-Simon C, Kelly L, Kulick R. A village would be nice but it takes a long-acting contraceptive to prevent repeat adolescent pregnancies. *Am J Prevent Med.* 2001;21:60–65

34. Gray S, Sheeder J, O'Brien R, Stevens-Simon C. Having the best intentions is necessary but not sufficient: why home visitation does not prevent more second teen pregnancies. *Prev Sci.* 2006;7:389–395

35. Stevens-Simon C. Participation in a program that helps families with one teen pregnancy prevent others. *J Pediatr Adolesc Gynecol.* 2000;13:167–169

36. Resnick MD, Bearman PS, Blum RW, et al. Protecting adolescents from harm. *JAMA.* 1997;278:823–832

# CHAPTER 55

# Adolescent Parenthood

KAROLYN KABIR-GREHER, MD • CATHERINE STEVENS-SIMON, MD

*Catherine "Cassie" Stevens-Simon, MD, passed away in November 2007 after a long battle with cancer. We would like to acknowledge her life long dedication to pregnant adolescents and their families and to the Colorado Adolescent Maternity Program, which she founded. She is greatly missed and we hope to continue her legacy of caring for adolescent mothers and their families.*

## OVERVIEW

Adolescent parenthood is commonly viewed as a risk factor for suboptimal childrearing practices and outcomes.[1,2] The supportive evidence is circumstantial and substantially weakened by statistical controls for appropriate confounders. For example, maternal stress and common life situations (ie, depression, inadequate support, and exposure to violence) are far more detrimental to good parenting than the risk factors that are usually considered (ie, poverty, undereducation, and health illiteracy). There is also considerable variability in the functioning in this population. Adolescents become pregnant for many reasons, some conscious, others subconscious. Like older women, those who conceive for reasons other than the desire to mother are less attentive to their children and take a more negative, physically punitive approach to childrearing. Furthermore, the teen's cognitive abilities are less likely to allow them wise choices of suitable intended mates.[1]

A generally negative impression of adolescent parents prevails because it is socially plausible in settings where drinking laws and other statutes restrict the level of social participation by age. This practice reflects the collective conviction that younger members of society are not sufficiently cognitively and psychosocially mature to assume the responsibilities associated with these activities.[3] The job of the 21st-century American parent is at least as complex as drinking alcohol responsibly.[1-3] Moreover, parenting style is as robust a predictor of cognitive, behavioral, and emotional problems in children as drinking style is of automobile accidents.[1-3] Historically, adolescents have not been sufficiently cognitively and psychosocially mature to assume the responsibilities of either activity, and traffic fatalities and dysfunctional development of offspring invariably result.[1-3] Many of the problems that arise when adolescents try to parent can be attributed to the circumstances that surround their conceptions, sociocultural influences, their psychological status, and comorbidities that have the potential to bolster or undermine the childrearing efforts of individuals of all ages.[1-3] Yet, it is only logical that unique conflicts should arise when two such life-altering events as adolescence and pregnancy are superimposed. It is also plausible that these conflicts, cognitive and psychosocial immaturity, and the lack of worldly experience associated with young maternal age should adversely affect the quality of parenting adolescents are able to provide and, in so doing, make a unique contribution to the behavioral problems, cognitive impairment, and school failure reported among their offspring.

Accordingly, the disproportionately high rate of the medical and social pathology among the children of adolescent mothers is typically attributed to parental immaturity and corresponding ineptitude.[1,2] The problem is proving that this is true. Studies of the consequences of adolescent parenthood have been hampered by the lack of convincing animal models and the unacceptability of randomized controlled trials. The alternative, reliance on statistical methods to control for potential confounders, also is problematic. On one hand, investigators run the risk of missing important age-related differences by overcontrolling their models. On the other hand, it is difficult to know if apparent age-related differences are real or a reflection of unrecognized observing biases.

These methodological problems are too fundamental to be resolved anytime soon. Thus, the safest assumption is that age-related differences in parenting abilities are as robust as age-related differences in drinking readiness. Although far from unanimous, the available empirical data support this inference.[1,2] However, it is not until the strong physiological risks associated with characteristics such as prematurity are removed and known confounders are controlled that the more subtle adverse effects of young maternal age on infant survival and child development become evident.[1,2,4]

Accordingly, researchers who study the causes of childhood cognitive delay and psychosocial dysfunction have increasingly accepted the idea that young maternal age is more of a social than a biological construct.[1,2] However, there are equally plausible organic explanations for the propensity the children of adolescent mothers exhibit for disruptive behavior and their vulnerability to school failure, infection, and premature death.[5-8] Due to the emphasis on modifiable psychosocially mediated mechanisms, the impact of innate physiology is rarely considered. For example, the disproportionate number of adolescent parents who are afflicted by inheritable psychological and behavioral disorders in the United States[9] suggests that some of the problems these children exhibit could be genetically mediated. Alternatively, the elevated risk of stress and exposure to environmental toxicants such as nicotine and lead among adolescent mothers could be contributory.[5-8] Such in utero exposures can permanently alter the structure and functioning of the developing brain and immune system.[5-8] Thus, it may be problematic to assume that increased support for adolescent parents will mitigate their children's medical and psychosocial problems.

## DEVELOPMENTAL CONTEXT

Adolescence is typically described as a three-stage process. Each stage has its own characteristics and developmental tasks that must be taken into account when formulating expectations for adolescent parents.[1] An exhaustive review of adolescent development is beyond the scope of this chapter, and the reader is referred to Chapter 4, "Physical Growth and Development," for that information. Rather, certain characteristics have been selected as examples of the ways in which adolescence might interact with and exacerbate widely accepted risk factors for dysfunctional parenting. As we shall discuss, well-designed, age-specific interventions based on an understanding of the mechanisms underlying the effects that adolescent cognitive and psychosocial development have on parenting performance can help families resolve conflicts and promote the healthy development of all members. Bad interventions are apt to only exacerbate the situation. To minimize the likelihood of such paradoxical outcomes, research and policy addressing this topic should reflect the dual needs of adolescent parents to gain knowledge and expertise to fulfill their role as parents and to move through their adolescence in concert with their peers.

During early adolescence, the major task for 12- to 14-year-olds is to come to terms with a new body shape. Young people at this stage of development are very self-conscious. Because most are still adjusting to their mature body image, the physical changes of pregnancy can provoke embarrassment, anger, and resentment. These feelings may be verbalized as "My baby is mean and hurts me when he kicks." Psychologically, young adolescents are concrete thinkers who adhere to a black and white code of ethics and have little understanding of moral concepts beyond right and wrong. This makes compromise difficult and authoritarian parenting and unrealistic expectations for infant behavior likely. The unanticipated claims a baby who does not eat, sleep, and play with its mother and the demand the baby makes can also provoke anger and resentment. These feelings may be verbalized as "My baby is bad; he wakes me up to eat and sleeps when I want to play." Socially, young adolescents are beginning to separate from their parents. However, when stressed, they typically still look first to their parents for support and advice. Thus, it is not uncommon for them to compete with their infants for attention. While it is appropriate for young people at this stage of development to share much of the responsibility for parenting with their parents or other adults, professionals need to be aware of the potential for regression and enmeshment. This often manifests as school avoidance and somatization disorders.

During middle adolescence, the major tasks for 15- to 17-year-olds are the formation of a personal identity and separation from family. Young people at this stage of development are concerned about their appearance, but are less self-conscious. Rather, middle adolescents tend to be egocentric, narcissistic risk-takers who thrive on experimentation and independence and exude invincibility as they strive to become self-sufficient members of society. This makes it difficult for them to separate their own needs and feelings from those of others. They are impulsive and prone to fantasy. Because activities such as talking to children and reinforcing their vocalizations tend to be regarded as childish at this age, middle adolescents provide lower quality, less consistent, and less stimulating homes and learning environments for their children than older parents, and often overuse physical punishment. Many middle adolescents also have idealized and unrealistically positive expectations about the changes motherhood will make in their lives; disappointment from overestimation of support and positive consequences compounds parenting stress.[10,11] Although cognitively middle adolescents are becoming less-concrete thinkers, they still have difficulty anticipating the negative consequences of their actions, envisioning alternative solutions, and reasoning about probabilities. As a result, they, too, tend to be rigid, authoritarian parents who favor negative physical over positive verbal modalities when interacting with their children and have trouble protecting their children from illness, accidents, and injury. Socially, the middle adolescent must become her own person. This requires experimentation with different roles and identities. Hence, girls at this stage of development tend to be especially reluctant to assume the identity of mother. The increased need for family support, restricted time with peers, and limitations on mobility and activities can make pregnancy and parenthood intolerable. Young people at this stage of development would still benefit from sharing much of the responsibility for parenting with their parents and other adults. However, accepting assistance from her mother returns the middle adolescent to a dependent role precisely when she is seeking independence. Offers of help may be misinterpreted as intrusions or efforts to limit freedom and autonomy. To avoid regressing, some middle adolescents detach themselves from their families and the adult world and refuse to ask for help or take advice. The social isolation that inevitably ensues often manifests as depression and conduct disorders. Alternatively, observing the competence of older mothers can undermine the middle adolescent's confidence in her own ability to mother. In this case, regression and disengaged parenting are likely outcomes.

During late adolescence, the major task for 18- to 21-year-olds is the formation of a life plan for the future. Young people at this stage of development tend to be less concerned about their bodies, identities, and peers' opinions. By engaging in experimental and risk-taking behaviors, they mature psychosocially and cognitively; most lose their narcissistic feelings of personal omnipotence. They also acquire the ability to consider needs other than their own, a developmental milestone that is a prerequisite for forming intimate, mutually respectful relationships with partners and children. As they begin to develop a sense of their future, they learn to reason abstractly and think causally. These new skills diminish the need for risky experimentation. Establishing a sense of personal identity frees late adolescents from concern about threats to their independence. This allows them to seek the advice of their parents and other adults. Envisioning alternatives makes it possible for late adolescents who are adequately supported to learn to become authoritative rather than authoritarian or rejecting parents. Late adolescence is such a relief after middle adolescence that it is easy to overlook limitations. Indeed, in traditional societies, where childrearing is a simpler task and young people perceive other adult roles as inaccessible or undesirable, becoming a parent during late adolescence is rarely problematic for mothers or their offspring.[12] Yet, the tendency late adolescents have of slipping into magical, concrete thinking, especially in emotionally charged situations or when surrounded by peers, emphasizes their ongoing need for guidance in the parenting arena.

## REPERCUSSIONS

Adolescent parenthood need not be a permanent cause of poverty and social disadvantage for the mother and her children.[13] However, as discussed in Chapter 54, "Adolescent Pregnancy," it often is. By having children, adolescents decrease their chances of graduating from high school, marrying, and becoming productive members of their communities.[2] There is also substantial evidence that the social isolation and stress associated with childbearing at this age decreases the quality of the parents' lives and undermines their emotional well-being by fostering poor self-esteem, stress, and depression.[1,2,10,11] The negative, intolerant attitudes about children and their behavior that ensue breed authoritarian, disengaged, and occasionally neglectful and abusive parenting.[1,2] As a group, adolescent parents fit the profile for dysfunctional parents (Box 55-1). Their preference for physical over verbal punishment and their propensity to use negative rather than positive epitaphs when describing their children and their behavior is also concerning. Accordingly, they typically score high on objective tests of child abuse potential. Although few adolescent parents are intentionally abusive or neglectful, their approach to parenting fosters aggression in children and increases their risk of experiencing medical, cognitive, psychiatric, and behavioral problems.[2] As we discuss in this section, these risks are inversely related to the quality of the relationship between adolescent parents, their intimate partners, and their own parents and directly related to the innate characteristics of their child.

### Box 55-1

### *Characteristics that Contribute to Dysfunctional Adolescent Parenting*

Young age
Rigidity
Impulsivity
Low cognitive capacity
Undereducation and poor health literacy
Unrealistic expectations
Poor self-esteem, stress, and depression
Poor support and social isolation
Unmarried status
Poor interpersonal relations
Childhood abuse and exposure to violence
Domestic and intimate partner violence
Substance abuse
Poverty and underemployment

During the neonatal period (the first 28 days of life), the children of adolescent mothers are at increased risk for morbidity and mortality because they are small and often preterm.[6] Young maternal age is an independent predictor of prematurity, but not of infant survival for gestational age; the excess morbidity and mortality reported among their newborns is entirely explained by the strong physiological risks associated with prematurity. By contrast, studies spanning three decades demonstrate an independent, essentially linear relationship between maternal age and the risk for postneonatal morbidity and mortality.[4] The disproportionately high incidence of preventable hospitalizations and deaths from accidents and infectious diseases and the increased risk of sudden infant death syndrome are most evident among the normal birth weight, term infants of adolescent mothers. Additionally, adolescents traditionally have had the lowest breastfeeding rates, even after controlling for income, education, and lack of prenatal care.[26] Lack of breastfeeding leads to additional health risks affecting the mother and her infant.[27] Collectively, these findings strongly suggest that lack of adequate knowledge of child development, inappropriate parenting practices, and failure to adhere to medical recommendations are responsible for the excess risk of death and disease.[1,2,4]

Findings regarding the prevalence of the medical and social problems listed in Box 55-2 vary in relation to the age of the child and the other variables included in the analysis. Studies of infants and younger children and studies that control for maternal stress and educational status generally demonstrate the fewest differences between the offspring of adolescent and adult mothers.[1,2] Like the effects of prematurity and in utero exposure to illicit substances,[14] the subtle effects of young maternal age are obscured by the more potent effects of environmental stress and privation. Negative findings are most likely early in life because performance demands are minimal and the achievement of developmental milestones is usually compromised by the innate characteristics of the child. Hence, the subtle differences between the offspring of adolescent and adult mothers are easy to overlook at this age. However, they become painfully evident as these children age and the complexity of the demands placed on them increases. This, too, is consistent with the results of studies of premature infants and infants who are exposed to illicit substances in utero.[14] Accordingly, the negative effect of small, age-related differences in parenting style may not be evident until the overwhelming effects of environmental deprivation are removed and the offspring are sufficiently cognitively and psychosocially mature to undergo sophisticated neuropsychological testing. Thus, the results of studies that end before children are old enough to be expected to meet the demands of 21st century American society must be interpreted cautiously.

**Box 55-2**

***Common Medical and Psychological Problems Among the Children of Adolescent Mothers***

| *Medical* | *Psychological* |
|---|---|
| Growth retardation/ low birth weight | Developmental delay |
| Prematurity | Neglect |
| Infant death | Behavior problems/ substance use |
| Sudden infant death syndrome | School failure and withdrawal |
| Minor acute infections | Underemployment/ poverty |
| Accidents/injury/ poisoning | Unplanned pregnancy |
| Undertreament of chronic diseases | Interpersonal violence |

Because of the emphasis on these psychosocially mediated mechanisms, there has been a tendency to overlook the evidence that in utero exposure to the hormonal changes associated with maternal anxiety and depression sensitizes the fetal hypothalamic-pituitary-adrenal axis and damages the developing hippocampus in ways that are associated with long-term behavioral, emotional, and cognitive problems.[5-7] Although the children of adolescent mothers have not been studied, neuro-imaging studies of stressed adults and children demonstrate decreased hippocampal volumes.[6] Despite the tremendous postnatal growth of the human brain, aberrant behavior that cannot be explained by other physiological and sociodemographic risk factors has been documented in newborns, infants, toddlers, and preschool and school-aged children who were exposed to maternal stress and depression in utero.[7] Thus, on balance the vulnerability of the fetal brain to insults seems to outweigh its plasticity. In utero exposures to stress might also compromise the development of the immune system and make these infants more susceptible to infections and related morbidities and mortality.[5]

## MANAGEMENT

The high incidence of medical and social problems noted in adolescent-headed families emphasizes the necessity of attending closely to the physical and psychosocial development of all members. In this section, we focus on the needs of adolescent mothers and their children. However, adolescent fathers who want to be actively involved with their children need the same support as mothers.[2] Few of these young men are prepared for fatherhood and as discussed in Chapter 54, Adolescent Pregnancy, as a group they exhibit more academic, substance abuse, and conduct problems than their nonparenting peers. Even if the adolescent father is not available personally, he may want members of his extended family to support the mother and his child.

Over the last five decades, most of the research and interventions aimed at improving the quality of interactions between adolescent parents and their children has been guided by a conceptual model that includes the influence of immutable age-related limitations on cognitive and psychosocial functioning and modifiable enhancers and buffers.[1,2,15-17] However, because intervention has been based on circumstantial evidence derived from observational studies, association is frequently equated with causation when therapeutic strategies are designed.

For example, controlling statistically for factors that adversely affect health-seeking behavior and adherence with medical recommendations (ie, undereducation and poor health literacy) reduces the negative impact of young maternal age on the health and well-being of children. Accordingly, the provision of remedial parenting education has been the thrust of many interventions. These programs increase adolescent knowledge about child development and appropriate disciplinary measures but do not consistently eliminate education-related disparities in parenting behavior and child outcomes. Indeed, the literature suggests that knowledge only partially explains the association between traditional educational milestones and health.[18] Achievements such as high school graduation are epidemiological markers for cognitive and psychosocial characteristics (ie, the ability to think causally or facility in acquiring self-management skills) that are the key determinants of health.[18] Thus, during adolescence undereducation may be a less remedial cause of dysfunctional parenting than is generally assumed; the only way to fill the void created by a 16-year-old mother's lack of a high school diploma is direct supervision by an individual who has had time to develop the cognitive skills associated with this educational milestone.

In contrast, effective programs using teen-friendly, positive role models have been effective in promoting healthy behaviors such as breastfeeding continuation.[28,29] Home visitation is another strategy to provide ongoing, family-centered, support resulting in increased parenting skills and optimal breastfeeding outcomes.[30] Competence in parenting enhances self-esteem and does not necessarily involve independent child rearing. Shared parenting among multiple generations in the home may be viewed as positive when grandparents and great-grandparents are supportive of the adolescent parenting style and empower the adolescent to make good decisions on behalf of their child.[31] Multidimensional programs offering home visitations with peer mentors and role-modeling using instructional video tapes or DVDs have also been effective in establishing optimal feeding practices by adolescent mothers.[32]

Similarly, the results of numerous studies demonstrate that social support helps women cope with stress and depression and improves their parenting behavior.[1,2,10,11,19] The individuals who most frequently provide support to adolescent mothers are their mothers and the men who father their babies.[1,2,19] Accordingly, when late adolescent parents choose to live together and early and middle adolescent parents choose to live with their own parents or other supportive family members, their children are more likely to survive infancy, less likely to be maltreated and hospitalized, and less apt to experience behavioral, academic, and health problems.[1,2] These findings have generally been interpreted as evidence that the presence of a parenting partner or mature adult in the home has a direct beneficial effect on the development of the children of adolescent mothers. Hence, program planners and policy makers have tried to replicate them by legislating that adolescent parents should adopt them and by offering or mandating supplemental in-home support.[15-17,20] However, social support is not a unitary construct that exerts a uniformly positive effect on outcomes. Correspondingly, these efforts have never had the same positive effects as the support provided by a voluntarily cohabitating partner or parent.[1,2,15-17,21-23] Involving other individuals can lessen the stress that precipitates authoritarian and disengaged parenting.[2,17] However, there is also evidence that the presence of a naturally supportive relationship with a partner or parent is a marker for personal characteristics that are the key determinants of the way adolescents interact with their children. These data suggest that it is not only the amount or content of the support the adolescent mother receives but also her own personality that determines whether support helps or hinders. Evidence that in multigenerational families the quality of mothering, grandmothering, and child behavior is inversely related to the age of the adolescent mother supports this inference.[2,22] The children of early and middle adolescent mothers fare better when they are reared simultaneously by their mothers and grandmothers, but the children of late adolescent and young adult mothers fare worse in this setting because it is not a developmentally appropriate arrangement. Thus, during adolescence, the absence of a supportive parenting partner may be a less remedial cause of dysfunctional childrearing behavior than is generally assumed. Encouraging adolescent mothers to identify an adult confidant might fill the void. At a minimum, when relations with their mothers and their babies' fathers are strained, there would be another supportive adult to turn to for solace. This is clearly preferable to mood-altering substances and peers and older males who often exacerbate their stress by mistreating them and luring them into risk-taking activities. In addition, by focusing on the skills required to transform daily interactions into supportive interpersonal relationships, adolescents may learn how to elicit the support they need from their environment. Finally, all efforts to augment the support adolescent parents receive are likely to be more effective if they are accompanied by interventions that minimize exposure to objectively stressful events such as the birth of a second child during the first two postpartum years. As discussed in Chapter 54, Adolescent Pregnancy, this is an important end-point for intervention as complications ranging from an increased likelihood of prematurity, accidental/nonaccidental trauma, and social deviance in children to a decreased likelihood of high school graduation and economic self-sufficiency among parents have been reported.[2,23]

In randomized controlled trials, home visiting by nurses and volunteers is the only strategy that has been found to help adolescent parents and their families effect an appropriate balance between parental duties and peer, school, and social responsibilities.[17] Including parents and partners improves compliance with home visits and may prevent the untoward outcomes that have occasionally been observed when intervention disrupts the naturally supportive relationships that guide the manner in which child care responsibilities are shared within families.[21] However, the efficacy of home visitation is proportional to its intensity. This raises concerns about generalizing from the apparent success of randomized trials to real world settings where the costs of providing the requisite number of visits by qualified individuals are often prohibitive. Yet, there is no good-quality empirical evidence from randomized controlled trials that intervention strategies such as community- and faith-based support groups for new parents, alternative schools with child care and flexible hours, and comprehensive, multidisciplinary programs that provide simultaneous medical care and social services to adolescent parents and their children are beneficial.[2,15-17] Our review of this vast literature suggests programs are more apt to be effective if they incorporate the characteristics listed in Box 55-3. Accordingly, adding home visitation to programs that provide medical care to adolescents and their children may be optimal for treating such intractable problems as repeat adolescent pregnancy, delinquent immunizations, and noncompliance with safety recommendations.[23] However, further study is needed to prove that this is true.

**Box 55-3**

***Common Elements of Successful Adolescent Parenting Interventions***

- Contact between parents and providers starts before the child is born; health centers in which pediatricians and obstetricians are housed in close quarters are ideal.
- Contact between parents and providers is frequent and intensive enough to foster a strong, long-term, mutually caring and respectful therapeutic relationship; home visits are ideal.
- The infrastructure reduces fragmentation of health and social service care; two-generation clinics where both adolescent parents and their children can receive care are ideal.
- The therapeutic agenda considers the numerous interacting causes of adverse adolescent parenting experiences and outcomes; a broad ecological approach is ideal.

## CONCLUSIONS

Adolescent parenthood remains a source of social, economic, and political concern in the United States because there is substantial evidence that by limiting the educational achievements and vocational opportunities of successive generations, it both contributes to the impoverishment of one of the most socioeconomically disadvantaged segments of American society and promotes intergenerational transmission of this socioeconomic disadvantage. Well-designed research is required to determine the nature and extent of health and mental health problems associated with childbearing at this age and their responsiveness to intervention. The experiences and misadventures of prior investigators demonstrate that when causal sequences are misinterpreted, interventions are inappropriate and unsuccessful, and well-intentioned policies do not lead to overall improvements in adolescent parenting behavior and offspring outcomes.

Although adolescence and early parenthood can be times of tremendous stress, not all adolescent parents and their children have problems negotiating this tumultuous period. Indeed, with time and patience, most young parents can be taught about their needs and their children's needs and the variety of appropriate responses to meet those needs. Accordingly, professionals who have worked with adolescent parents are often impressed by their strengths and their ability to learn how to be effective parents when they receive adequate instruction. Studies comparing the outcomes of the children of adolescent mothers to the children of older mothers reveal that in addition to the obvious maternal factors related to age and immaturity, significant predictors of adverse outcome can be broadly categorized as sociodemographic (ie, poverty, undereducation, and single parenthood), maternal mental health (ie, stress, depression, and poor self-esteem), and child (prematurity, intrauterine growth retardation, and intrauterine exposure to stress and environmental toxicants). Maternal responsivity as assessed by positive maternal-child interactions can modulate the adverse effects of sociodemographic and innate child risk factors on the performance of children.[2,17] However, even when the quality of the maternal-child interactions is taken into account, adverse outcomes as assessed by indicators such as grade retention and need for special education remain high in this population.[1,2] Thus, some effort must be made to change the environment the children are reared in. Identifying and treating toddlers who are not responding verbally and children who are failing in elementary school prevents them from becoming angry, frustrated adolescents who leave high school and become parents.[17,24] However, most children of adolescent mothers develop normally during infancy and the toddler period. Hence, few are identified as being in need of remedial services until they enter school and more complex learning, performance, and conduct demands are placed them. This "waiting to fail" model makes it difficult for the children to catch up and almost guarantees that they will develop the behavioral problems, poor self-esteem, anxiety, and depression that fosters school drop-out and early childbearing. Thus, it may be most expedient to encourage adolescent parents and their children to enroll in programs that remediate the shortcomings of their living environments. These programs offer adolescent parents choices about their behavior but alter the environment in which they make decisions by communicating a cost-benefit relationship that makes the recommended activities the most advantageous. Further study is needed, but theories of human behavior suggest that this strategy is apt to be more effective than the legal and educational approaches that have been tried.

## REFERENCES


1. Flanagan P. Teen mothers: countering the myths of dysfunction and developmental disruption In: Garcia Coll C, Surrey J (Eds). *Mothering Against the Odds: Diverse Voices of Contemporary Mothers*. New York: Guilford Press; 1998

2. Elfenbein DS, Felice ME. Adolescent pregnancy. *Pediatr Clin North Am*. 2003;50:781–800

3. Federal Uniform Drinking Age Act. Public Law 98-363; 1984

4. Markovitz BP, Cook R, Flick LH, Leet TL. Socioeconomic factors and adolescent pregnancy outcomes: distinctions between neonatal and post-neonatal deaths? *BMC Public Health*. 2005;255:79

5. Wadhwa PD, Culhane JF, Rauh V, Barve SS. Stress and preterm birth: neuroendocrine, immune/inflammatory, and vascular mechanisms. *Matern Child Health J*. 2001;5:119–125

6. Carrion VG, Weems CF, Reiss AL. Stress predicts brain changes in children: a pilot longitudinal study on youth stress, posttraumatic stress disorder, and the hippocampus. *Pediatrics*. 2007;119:509–516

7. Van den Bergh BR, Mulder EJ, Mennes M, Glover V. Antenatal maternal anxiety and stress and the neurobehavioural development of the fetus and child: links and possible mechanisms. A review. *Neurosci Biobehav Rev*. 2005;29:237–258

8. Ernst M, Moolchan ET, Robinson ML. Behavioral and neural consequences of prenatal exposure to nicotine. *J Am Acad Child Adolesc Psych*. 2001;40:630–641

9. Trad PV. Mental health of adolescent mothers. *J Am Acad Child Adolesc Psych*. 1995;34:130–142

10. Quinlivan JA, Luehr B, Evans SF. Teenage mother's predictions of their support levels before and actual support levels after having a child. *J Pediatr Adolesc Gynecol*. 2004;17:273–278

11. Frost JJ, Oslak S. Teenagers' pregnancy intentions and decisions: A study of young women in California choosing to give birth. New York: Alan Guttmacher Institute, 1999

12. Way S, Finch BK, Cohen D. Hispanic concentration and the conditional influence of collective efficacy on adolescent childbearing. *Arch Pediatr Adolesc Med*. 2006;160:925–930

13. Furstenberg FF. Teenage childbearing as a public issue and private concern. *Annu Rev Sociol*. 2003;29:23–29

14. Kilbride HW, Thorstad K, Daily DK. Preschool outcome of less than 801-gram preterm infants compared with full-term siblings. *Pediatrics*. 2004;113:742–747

15. Coren E, Barlow J, Stewart-Brown S. The effectiveness of individual and group-based parenting programs in improving outcomes for teenage mothers and their children: a systematic review. *J Adolesc*. 2003;26:79–103

16. Akinbami LJ, Cheng TL, Kornfeld D. A review of teen-tot programs: comprehensive clinical care for young parents and their children. *Adolescence*. 2001;36:381–393

17. Olds DL. Prenatal and infancy home visiting by nurses: from randomized trials to community replication. *Prev Sci*. 2002;3:153–172

18. DeWalt DA, Berkman ND, Sheridan S, Lohr KN, Pignone MP. Literacy and health outcomes: A systematic review of the literature. *J Gen Int Med*. 2004;19:1228-1239

19. Logsdon MC, Gagne P, Hughes T, Patterson J, Rakestraw V. Social support during adolescent pregnancy: piecing together a quilt. *J Obstet Gynecol Neonatal Nurs*. 2005;34:606-614

20. US House of Representatives. *Personal Responsibility and Work Opportunity Reconciliation Act of 1996. Conference Report HR 3734.* Washington, DC: US Government Printing Office; 1996. Report No. 104; 725

21. Duggan AK, Fuddy L, Burrell L, et al. Randomized trial of a state-wide home visiting program to prevent child abuse: impact in preventing child abuse and neglect. *Child Abuse Negl*. 2004;28:597-622

22. Black MM, Papas MA, Hussey JM, et al. Behavior and development of preschool children born to adolescent mothers: risk and 3-generation households. *Pediatrics*. 2002;109:573-580

23. Stevens-Simon C, Kelly L, Kulick R. A village would be nice but it takes a long acting contraceptive to prevent repeat adolescent pregnancies. *Am J Prevent Med*. 2001;21:60-65

24. Institute of Medicine. *From Neurons to Neighborhoods: The Science of Early Childhood Development*. Washington, DC: National Academies Press; 2000

25. Rothschild M. Carrots, sticks and promises: A conceptual framework for the management of public health and social issues behaviours. *J Market*. 1999;63:24-37

26. Feldman-Winter L, Shaikh U. Optimizing breastfeeding promotion and support in adolescent mothers. *J Hum Lact*. 2007;23(4):362-7

27. Ip S, Chung M, Raman G. *Breastfeeding and Maternal and Infant Health Outcomes in Developed Countries*. Rockville, MD: Agency for Healthcare Research and Quality; April 2007. AHRQ Publication No. 07-E007

28. Grady MA, Bloom KC. Pregnancy Outcomes of Adolescents Enrolled in a Centering Pregnancy Program. *Midwifery Womens Health J*. 2000;49(5):412-420

29. Pierre N, Emans SJ, Obeidallah DA. Choice of Feeding Method of Adolescent Mothers: Does Ego Development Play a Role? *J Pediatric Adolesc Gynecol*. 1999;12:83-89

30. Barlow A, Varipatis-Baker E, Speakman K. Home-visiting Intervention to Improve Child Care Among American Indian Mothers. *Arch Pediatric Adolesc Med*. 2006;160:1101-1107

31. Oberlander SE, Black MM, Starr RH. African American adolescent mothers and grandmothers: A multigenerational approach to parenting. *Am J Community Psychol*. 2007;39:37-46

32. Black MM, Siegel EH, Abel Y, Bentley ME. Home and Videotape Intervention Delays Early Complementary Feeding Among Adolescent Mothers. *Pediatrics*. 2001; 107(5):e67

# CHAPTER 56

# Abortion in Adolescents

ANNE DAVIS, MD, MPH

## EPIDEMIOLOGY OF ADOLESCENT PREGNANCY AND ABORTION

Each year in the United States, about 800,000 adolescents aged 19 years or younger become pregnant.[1] Adolescent pregnancy and childbearing are associated with adverse health and social consequences for young women and their children. Teenage parenthood is linked to educational underachievement, poverty, welfare dependence, domestic violence, and poor social relationships.[2] Higher rates of pregnancy occur in older (18–19 years) rather than younger (<18 years) adolescents and among black and Hispanic than white adolescents.[3] Adolescent pregnancy, birth, and abortion rates have been declining steadily since a peak in 1990 among adolescents of all ages and races[3] (Figure 56-1). Increased use of contraception and decreased rate of sexual activity among teens contributed to this decline.[4] An upturn was seen in 2006. However, the recent US adolescent pregnancy rate is still substantially higher than rates in other developed countries.[5]

In the United States, 4 out of 5 pregnancies in teenagers are unintended, and about one-third of all adolescent pregnancies end in induced abortion.[3] Most adolescents obtain abortions during the first trimester of pregnancy. However, on average adolescents obtain abortions later in pregnancy than adults; 1 survey study found that minors younger than 18 years old underwent abortion about a week later than older women.[6] Delays may be due to physiologic or social reasons. Adolescents may not recognize the signs and symptoms of pregnancy, and may not realize amenorrhea indicates pregnancy if they have irregular menstrual cycles. Additionally, adolescents may be unsure where to seek assistance or may deny pregnancy due to fear of repercussions from family or a partner.

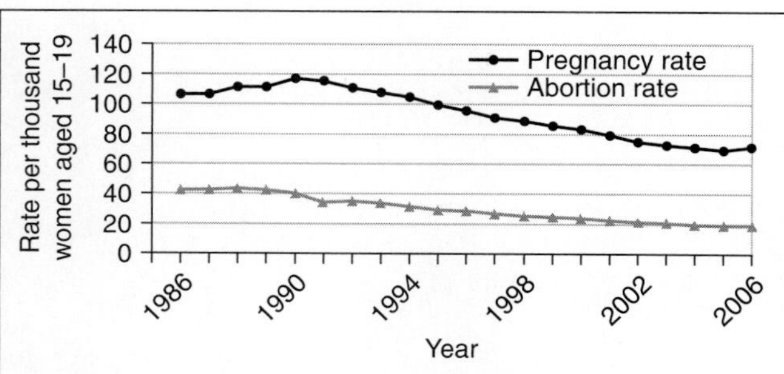


**FIGURE 56-1** Pregnancy and abortion rates over time among adolescents aged 15 to 19 years. The rate is per 1,000 adolescents aged 15 to 19 years old. The squares represent the pregnancy rate and the diamonds represent the abortion rate. (Data based on a report from the Guttmacher Institute. Available at: www.guttmacher.org/pubs/USTPtrends.pdf. Accessed April 13, 2010.)

## ABORTION AND DECISION MAKING

Adolescents faced with unintended pregnancy give several reasons in their decision to have an abortion. Reasons are similar across diverse groups of young women. Adolescents feel unprepared for motherhood psychologically and financially, and are concerned that childbearing will adversely affect educational attainment, career opportunities, and personal relationships with partners and family members.[2] Research supports these concerns by demonstrating better educational outcomes among adolescents choosing abortion compared with those continuing pregnancy. One study[7] found that those undergoing abortion were more likely to complete high school than those who carried their pregnancies to term. Another 25-year longitudinal study found that those adolescents undergoing abortion achieved higher levels of education than those carrying to term, even after adjustment for family, social, and educational differences.[6]

## ACCESS TO ABORTION AND PARENTAL INVOLVEMENT

The availability of affordable abortion services determines if a young woman may obtain an abortion and how quickly. Barriers to care may particularly affect those adolescents with limited resources compared with adults. Obtaining care may require significant travel because most counties in the United States (>80%) have no abortion provider. In most states, abortion is not covered by state Medicaid programs, so poor teens may have difficulty raising funds for the cost of care. Consequent delays experienced by adolescents lead to increased costs; later abortions are more complex and more expensive.

Most states require parental involvement in an adolescent's decision to have an abortion. In some states, one or both parents must be notified; in other states, one or both parents must provide consent. All of the states that require parental involvement also have alternative guidelines when minors believe involving their parents would not be in their best interest. Some allow a minor to obtain an abortion if another adult relative is involved in the decision. Others have a judicial bypass procedure whereby a minor may obtain an abortion after obtaining approval from a court. Local statutes change frequently in some states; providers should be aware of current relevant regulations.[8] Most pregnant adolescents consult a parent in their decision to have an abortion regardless of local laws.[9]

Parental involvement legislation assumes that pregnant minors are not competent to make informed decisions. However, most adolescents can understand the risks and benefits of medical procedures as well as adults and are able to make independent decisions about their medical care.[10] Mandating parental involvement in this decision-making process creates delays, leads to later abortion, and in some cases places teens at risk of physical violence or being forced to leave home.[9] National medical organizations including the American Medical Association, the American Academy of Pediatrics, and the American College of Obstetricians and Gynecologists reached a consensus that minors should be strongly encouraged to discuss their pregnancies with their parents but should not be required to involve their parents in the decision to have an abortion.[10]

## BEFORE THE ABORTION

As a first step, the diagnosis of pregnancy should be confirmed. Especially in adolescence, amenorrhea or menstrual delay is not necessarily indicative of pregnancy. Sensitive, accurate urine human chorionic gonadotropin (hCG) kits are widely available and obviate the need for a serum test. A physical examination or ultrasonography (vaginal or abdominal) should be performed to estimate gestational age. Examination of pregnant adolescents should include screening for sexually transmitted infections (STIs), especially *Chlamydia trachomatis*, because teens having unprotected intercourse are at risk of STIs. Rhesus status should be determined, and a complete blood count may be helpful for hemoglobin status. Counseling regarding choice of contraception can begin prior to the abortion procedure. A plan for contraception should be in place because teens may not return for follow-up care after their abortion is complete.

## EARLY ABORTION: CHOOSING THE RIGHT TREATMENT

Early in pregnancy, both surgical and nonsurgical (medication) approaches are available. Health care providers who counsel pregnant adolescents should be aware of the differences between surgical and medication abortion. Overall, adolescents and their parents or guardians can be reassured that both approaches generally are safe and effective.

### SURGICAL ABORTION

Surgical methods are well established and currently more widely available than medication abortion. The surgical method is commonly referred to as D and C, or dilatation and curettage. The cervix is dilated (opened) mechanically or using medication (prostaglandins), and then a sterile suction curette is placed in the uterine cavity and attached to a source of suction to remove the products of conception. Suction curettage has replaced sharp curettage as the preferred method of early abortion in the United States. Suction may be achieved manually using a handheld, nonelectric aspirator (manual vacuum aspiration or MVA) or with an electric source of suction (electric vacuum aspiration or EVA). Suction curettage can be performed effectively by an experienced clinician as early as 5 weeks from the last menstrual period.

A range of anesthesia options are available for early surgical abortion. Local anesthesia is often acceptable and usually includes an oral medication for uterine cramping, such as a non-steroidal anti-inflammatory drugs (NSAIDs), combined with a paracervical block using a local anesthetic such as lidocaine. Some providers supplement this regimen with oral anxiolytics or narcotics. Most experienced clinicians believe that reassurance and support during the procedure increase the acceptability of local anesthesia. Intravenous agents for moderate or deep sedation can also be provided by qualified personnel. Adequate respiratory support, especially in obese patients, prevents hypoventilation and hypoxia, which are rare but important causes of abortion-related mortality when deep sedation is used. Anesthesia choice for adolescents includes all the modalities mentioned here.

## MEDICATION ABORTION

Nonsurgical, or medication (medical) abortion refers to complete expulsion of the products of conception without surgical intervention. Medication abortion is becoming more widely available in the United States, and an increasing proportion of women are choosing this approach. The most commonly used regimen is mifepristone followed by misoprostol. This combination was approved by the US Food and Drug Administration (FDA) for abortion in 2001. Mifepristone is a potent progesterone antagonist that leads to decidual necrosis and detachment of the trophoblast. Misoprostol is a synthetic prostaglandin E1 analogue that causes uterine contractions, cervical softening, and expulsion of the products of conception. Neither mifepristone nor misoprostol alone provides satisfactory efficacy. Injectable methotrexate may also be used with misoprostol for medication abortion; this alternative regimen, however, has not received FDA approval. Methotrexate is an antimetabolite that interferes with cell division and is also effective in the treatment of ectopic pregnancy. Mifepristone and misoprostol are not recommended for the treatment of ectopic pregnancy.

There are numerous published protocols for use of mifepristone and misoprostol. All protocols share these similarities: (1) first, mifepristone is administered orally by the health care provider, (2) next, misoprostol is administered by the oral, vaginal, sublingual, or buccal route 6 to 72 hours later, (3) bleeding and contractions occur, and (4) patients return for follow-up to ensure complete abortion using repeat ultrasound or serial hCG testing. In most protocols, women self-administer misoprostol at home. Bleeding heavier than menses usually occurs for 1 or 2 days after misoprostol; lighter bleeding and spotting may persist until the next spontaneous menses.[11] Most providers encourage use of NSAIDS for pain control; some also prescribe narcotic analgesics. Several small studies have demonstrated that most adolescents choosing medical abortion found the process highly acceptable.[12,13]

Medication abortion is an option for nearly all healthy adolescents seeking abortion in early pregnancy. Absolute contraindications are few: suspicion of ectopic pregnancy, current anticoagulation or clotting disorder, and known allergy to mifepristone or misoprostol. In choosing an abortion technique for adolescents, other factors may be relevant. Medication abortion requires (1) some privacy because the process includes bleeding and passage of clots, (2) follow-up care to ensure the abortion is complete with a repeat ultrasound examination or beta hCG level, and (3) access to emergency care.

Medication abortion is highly effective. Published success rates indicate that complete expulsion rates of greater than 95% can be achieved with a variety of protocols. The highest success rates occur when medication abortion is administered at 7 weeks or less from the last menstrual period, with modest decreases in efficacy from 7 to 9 weeks from the last menstrual period. Most abortion providers in the United States who offer medication abortion limit its use to 9 weeks or less from the last menstrual period. Most published efficacy data do not report separate success rates for adolescents and adults. In small studies of adolescents receiving medical abortion, success rates are comparable to those observed in older women.[12]

## SECOND TRIMESTER ABORTION

Dilatation and suction curettage may be used until early in the second trimester. After about 14 weeks from the last menstrual period, dilatation and evacuation (D and E) is used for surgical abortion. Adequate dilatation for evacuation of fetal tissue requires opening the cervix gradually to a greater diameter than in the first trimester. This is usually accomplished using an osmotic cervical dilator such as laminaria over a period of 1 to 2 days. Laminaria are dried natural fibers that soften and open the cervix gradually as they expand. After dilatation, a narrow forceps and suction are used to remove the fetal parts and placental tissue. Prostaglandins may be used as an alternative to or adjunct to laminaria early in the second trimester. Adolescents and their parents are often concerned about the effect of abortion, particularly in the second trimester, on future pregnancy. Gradual cervical dilatation before D and E with laminaria over 1 or 2 days, even to several centimeters, does not increase the risk of premature labor or preterm delivery.[14]

In the second trimester, labor induction may also be used for abortion. Most abortions in the second trimester of pregnancy in the United States are done by D and E. For an induction abortion, medications such as prostaglandins are used to induce labor, and the fetus is expelled similar to birth. Whether surgical or medical abortion is chosen may depend on what is available. In some settings, adolescents may only have induction or D and E available to them.

## SAFETY OF ABORTION

In the United States, abortion is common and very safe. Nearly 45% of American women will have at least one abortion, and abortion is among the most common surgical procedures performed in the United States. The risk of serious morbidity and mortality related to abortion has declined dramatically since legalization. Women undergoing abortion face about one-tenth the risk of death as women having live birth.[15] There is a clear relationship between the safety of abortion and gestational age. With advancing pregnancy, the risk of morbidity and morality related to abortion also increase.[16] The overall safety of abortion is comparable for adolescents and older women.[16] Some adolescents will experience preventable, increased risk from abortion due to delays in obtaining care requiring procedures at more advanced gestational ages.

Morbidity related to surgical abortion includes infection, hemorrhage at the time of the procedure or later, failed abortion with an ongoing pregnancy, an incomplete procedure or hematometra requiring repeat aspiration, and uterine perforation. In most large series, rates of any of these complications are about 1% to 2% or less. Mortality from abortion-related causes include infection, hemorrhage, embolism, and complications of anesthesia.[16] Adolescents, as well as older women, vastly overestimate the risk associated with abortion.[17] Providers counseling adolescents should reassure teens choosing abortion that the procedure is safe.

The safety of medical abortion is also well established. Medical abortion has been used safely by millions of women in more than 50 countries since the 1980s. Early data indicated that risks included ongoing pregnancy (1%–5% depending on the regimen used and gestational age), incomplete expulsion of the products of conception (1%–3%), bothersome, persistent bleeding requiring D and C (1%), and very rarely, heavy bleeding leading to emergent D and C, transfusion, or both (1/1,000). Infection following medical abortion is very rare. Fatal cases of infection due to *Clostridium sordellii* following mifepristone and misoprostol for medical abortion have been reported. The risk factors for clostridial infection are unclear; it has also occurred after miscarriage, birth, and nonpregnancy-related events. Adolescents and providers should be vigilant for any signs of infection. The risk of clostridial infection is exceedingly small, less than 1 in 100,000 US women undergoing medical abortion.[18]

## LONG-TERM SAFETY OF ABORTION

Adolescents and those who care for them should be reassured that abortion does not lead to problems in future pregnancies. Uncomplicated vacuum aspiration abortion does not increase the risk of breast cancer, infertility, miscarriage, ectopic pregnancy, early pregnancy failure, or birth defects.[19] Reassurance during counseling is especially important; many women and adolescents overestimate the risks of abortion to their current and future health.[17]

The mental health of pregnant adolescents is an important concern for parents and health care providers. In an attempt to identify independent effect of abortion on mental health, some researchers have compared women undergoing abortion to those continuing pregnancies. Such comparisons can only isolate the effect of abortion if the pre-existing psychosocial situations of those choosing abortion and those continuing pregnancy are accounted for. Overall, existing research demonstrates no clear evidence that abortion itself increases the risk of poor psychological outcomes. On the contrary, studies of short-term outcomes show that most women and adolescents experience improvements in psychological health after abortion.[20] In one study with 2-year follow-up, adolescents showed no decline in psychological functioning after abortion compared to before abortion.[21]

## CONTRACEPTION AFTER ABORTION

Most adolescents who undergo abortion have minimal if any experience with contraception, and therefore will need careful counseling regarding selection of a method. One large study among adolescents obtaining abortions found that about half reported using no method of contraception when they became pregnant.[22] In some studies, teens shifted their choice of contraception away from barrier methods toward more effective hormonal methods after abortion.[23,24] Unfortunately, discontinuation rates for hormonal methods are high among teenagers even after abortion, and repeat pregnancy is not uncommon.[25]

Contraception after abortion should be initiated immediately. Ovulation and pregnancy are possible before the first normal menstrual period. Delaying initiation undoubtedly contributes to the substantial number of teens who will experience repeat unintended pregnancy after abortion. Medical decision making regarding contraception after abortion is the same as starting contraception at any other time. Unlike after term birth where thrombosis is a consideration, no delay is required for initiation of estrogen-containing methods after abortion in the first or second trimester.[26] All teens initiating contraception should be aware that irregular bleeding is expected after abortion regardless of contraceptive method. Heavy bleeding is not expected, however, and should prompt evaluation. Sexually active teenagers should be strongly encouraged to use condoms for STI prevention whatever their method of contraception.

## REFERENCES

1. Centers for Disease Control and Prevention. National and state specific pregnancy rates among adolescents. *MMWR.* 2000;49:605-611

2. Fergusson DM, Boden JM, Horwood LJ. Abortion among young women and subsequent life outcomes. *Perspect Reprod Sexual Health.* 2007;39:6-12

3. Guttmacher Institute. *US Teenage Pregnancy Statistics. National and state trends and trends by race and ethnicity.* New York, Guttmacher Institute; 2006.

4. Santelli JS, Lindberg LD, Finer LB, Singh S. Explaining recent declines in adolescent pregnancy in the United States: the contribution of abstinence and improved contraceptive use. *Amer J Public Health.* 2007;97:150-156

5. Singh S, Darroch JE. Adolescent pregnancy and childbearing: levels and trends in developed countries. *Fam Plan Perspect.* 2000;32:14-23

6. Finer LB, Frohwirth LF, Dauphinee LA, Singh S, Moore AM. Timing of steps and reasons for delays in obtaining abortions in the United States. *Contraception.* 2006;74:334-344

7. Zabin LS, Hirsch MB, Emerson MR. When urban adolescents choose abortion: effects on education, psychological status, and subsequent pregnancy. *Fam Plan Perspect.* 1989;21:248-255

8. Guttmacher Institute. Parental involvement in minors' abortions. Available at: www.guttmacher.org/statecenter/spibs/spib_PIMA.pdf. Accessed April 27, 2010

9. Henshaw SK, Kost K. Parental involvement in minors' abortion decisions. *Fam Plan Perspect.* 1992;24:196-207

10. American Academy of Pediatrics. The adolescent's right to confidential care when considering abortion. *Pediatrics.* 1996;7:746-751

11. Davis AR, Westhoff C, DeNonno L. Bleeding after early abortion with mifepristone or manual vacuum aspiration (MVA). *JAMWA.* 2000;55:141-144

12. Phelps RH, Schaff EA, Fielding SL. Mifepristone abortion in minors. *Contraception.* 2001;64(6):339-343

13. Creinin MD, Wiebe E, Gold M. Methotrexate and misoprostol for abortion in adolescent women. *J Ped Adolesc Gynecol.* 1999;12:71-77

14. Chasen ST, Kalish RB, Gupta M, Kaufman J, Chervenak FA. Obstetric outcomes after surgical abortion at ≥ 20 weeks' gestation. *AJOG.* 2005;193(3 Pt 2):1161-1164

15. Grimes DA. Estimation of pregnancy-related mortality risk by pregnancy outcome, United States, 1991 to 1999. *AJOG.* 2006;194(1):92-94

16. Bartlett LA, Berg CJ, Shulman HB, et al. Risk factors for legal induced abortion-related mortality in the United States. *Obstet Gynecol.* 2004;103(4):729-737

17. Gold MA, Coupey SM. Attitudes of inner-city adolescents toward medical and surgical abortion. *J Ped Adol Gyn.* 1998;11(3):127-131

18. Fischer M, Bhatnagar J, Guarner J, et al. Fatal toxic shock syndrome associated with Clostridium sordellii after medical abortion. *New Eng J Med.* 2005;353(22):2352-2360

19. Hogue CJ, Cates W Jr, Tietze C. The effects of induced abortion on subsequent reproduction. *Epidemiol Rev.* 1982;4:66-94

20. Pope LM, Adler NE, Tschann JM. Postabortion psychological adjustment: are minors at increased risk? *J Adol Health.* 2001;29(1):2-11

21. Zabin LS, Hirsch MB, Emerson MR. When urban adolescents choose abortion: effects on education, psychological status, and subsequent pregnancy. *Fam Plann Perspect.* 1989;21(6):248-255

22. Jones RK, Darroch JE, Henshaw SK. Contraceptive use among US women having abortions in 2000-2001. *Perspec Sex Reprod Health.* 2002;34(6):294-303

23. Truong HM, Kellogg T, McFarland W, Kang MS, Darney P, Drey EA. Contraceptive intentions among adolescents after abortion. *J Adol Health.* 2006;39(2):283-286

24. Paukku M, Quan J, Darney P, Raine T. Adolescents' contraceptive use and pregnancy history: is there a pattern? *Obstet Gynecol.* 2003;101(3):534-538

25. Blumenthal PD, Wilson LE, Remsburg RE, Cullins VE, Huggins GR. Contraceptive outcomes among post-partum and post-abortal adolescents. *Contraception.* 1994;50(5):451-460

26. Reproductive Health and Research. *Medical Eligibility Criteria for Contraceptive Use,* 3rd ed. Geneva, Switzerland: World Health Organization; 2004

# CHAPTER 57

# Sexual Dysfunction

ALWYN T. COHALL, MD • DIANE DI MAURO, PhD

## ADOLESCENT PSYCHOSEXUAL DEVELOPMENT

There are several developmental tasks that adolescents must complete on the pathway toward adulthood, such as emancipation from parents, development of abstract reasoning, achievement of moral identity, development of plans for the future, and acquisition of the means for making those plans come true. Just as important are the tasks of psychosexual development.

Sarrel and Sarrel[1] posit that to become a "sexually healthy" adult, several "mini-tasks" must be completed. These include (1) the development of a positive gender-specific body image that is relatively free from distortion, (2) acceptance of oneself as a sexual person, (3) resolution of gender identity conflicts and determination of sexual orientation, (4) the ability to make personally and socially responsible sexual decisions, and (5) a gradually increasing ability to experience eroticism as one aspect of intimacy.

Failure to completely master these tasks may impair sexual functioning. There are many obstacles to negotiate during psychosexual development; relatively few teens approach their first sexual experiences with a knowledge and acceptance of their capacity for sexual expression. Early sexual exploration is typically covert and rushed.

Mixed parental, peer, religious, and cultural messages can foster confusion and guilt. Combined with sexual ignorance, identity concerns, relationship issues, and performance demands, the situation is ripe for the development of sexual problems.

Scattered case reports and studies[2-6] provide insight into adolescent sexual complaints, but it is not possible to determine the true incidence or prevalence of sexual dysfunction among sexually active teens because there have been no population-based studies of this age group. In the absence of such data, we must guardedly use extant adolescent studies in conjunction with those studies involving adults to estimate the dimensions of the problems affecting teenagers. Before the psychosexual dysfunctions listed in the *Diagnostic and Statistical Manual of Mental Disorders, Fourth Edition* (*DSM-IV*)[7] can be described, it is important to frame the discussion within the context of the sexual response cycle.

## HUMAN SEXUAL RESPONSE

In their pioneer 1966 volume, Masters and Johnson[8] provided the first clear description of the physiology of the human sexual response. Their findings were based on observations of 694 men and women aged 18 to 89 years during more than 7,000 cycles of sexual response. Table 57-1 presents a summary of each phase of the cycle. During the sexual response cycle, complementary physiologic changes occur in both sexes. There is a noted increase in heart rate, blood pressure, genital vasocongestion, muscle tension, breathing rate, and skin flush. Orgasmic contractions occur at the same 0.8-second interval for both men and women. The only substantial sex differences identified by Masters and Johnson concern ejaculation (women do not experience ejaculation) and multiple orgasm (men do not experience multiple orgasm). A critical contribution has been Masters and Johnson's debunking of the vaginal orgasm myth: *all* female orgasms are the result—directly or indirectly—of clitoral stimulation.

Kaplan[9] conceptually simplified Masters and Johnson's model and speaks in terms of a biphasic model of sexual response. She states that the sexual response consists of 2 distinct and relatively independent components: (1) a general vasocongestive reaction (arousal), which is controlled by the parasympathetic system; and (2) reflexive clonic muscular contractions (orgasm), which are controlled by the sympathetic system. Because the 2 components are controlled by different parts of the central nervous system, 1 component can be inhibited or impaired while the other functions normally.

## CONCEPTUALIZING SEXUAL PROBLEMS

Before specific dysfunctions and possible etiologic factors can be discussed, establishing a general framework for evaluating sexual difficulties is in order. When problems of sexual functioning are conceptualized, it is useful to distinguish between ***primary*** and ***secondary*** dysfunctions. In the former case, the individual has never experienced a period of normal functioning; in the latter, a period of adequate functioning occurred prior to the

**Table 57-1**

**Sexual Response Cycle**

| | *Desire* | *Arousal* | *Orgasm* | *Resolution* |
|---|---|---|---|---|
| Subjective recognition | Cognitive perception | Female: vaginal lubrication | Female: genital throbbing | Relaxation |
| | | Male: erection | Male: emission, ejaculation | Detumescence in male |
| Primary physiologic process | Hormonal | Genital vasocongestion | Muscular contraction | |

development of the sexual dysfunction. Also, it is fairly common for multiple sexual problems to coexist—for instance, low desire may develop in association with erectile failure, or an individual with orgasm difficulty may also experience problems with arousal.

## PREVALENCE

The sexual dysfunctions "*are characterized by disturbance in sexual desire and in the psychophysiological changes that characterize the sexual response cycle and causes marked distress and interpersonal difficulty.*"[7] How common are sexual dysfunctions? The *DSM-IV* acknowledges that there are few systematic epidemiological data regarding the prevalence of various sexual dysfunctions, "and these studies show extremely wide variability, probably reflecting differences in assessment methods, definitions used, and characteristics of sampled populations."[7] However, as Heiman[10] reported in her recent overview on the topic, "it is likely that sexual problems are highly prevalent in both sexes." Community samples estimates range from 10% to 52% of [adult] men and 25% to 63% of [adult] women.[11-14] The National Health and Social Life Survey (NHSLS),[15] a 1992 national probability sample of 1,410 men and 1,749 women between the ages of 18 and 59 years living in US households, reported the prevalence of sexual dysfunction to be 43% for women and 31% for men. Specifically, among adolescents and young adults (ages 18–29), 14% of males and 32% of females expressed low sex desires; 7% of males and 26% of females reported difficulties achieving orgasm; 30% of males reported premature ejaculation, and 19% of females reported difficulty becoming lubricated.[15]

## ETIOLOGICAL CONTEXT OF SEXUAL DYSFUNCTIONS

Heiman emphasizes the importance of considering the significant mitigating factors involved in any clinical diagnosis of sexual dysfunction. Among adults, sexual dysfunctions are often correlated with other health conditions, particularly those dealing with the cardiovascular system, common diseases (diabetes, high blood pressure, heart disease), health habits (cigarette smoking and possibly high alcohol consumption), and mental health (anxiety, depression).[10]

To help the reader discern the multitude of factors contributing to sexual dysfunction among adolescents, we outline 3 major categories: **clinical** (conditions, diseases, medications, and substances that affect physical, mental, and sexual health); **psychosocial** (family and societal influences that shape sexual behavior); and **interpersonal** (effect of relationships on sexual expression).

### Clinical

The search for the cause of sexual dysfunction should always address possible organic factors. The likelihood of organic contributions tends to vary with the specific disorder. In males, physiologic factors are rarely implicated as a reason for premature ejaculation. Organic causes are more likely in erectile difficulties,[16] although psychic impotence is the usual reason for erectile dysfunction (ED) among adolescent males.[5] In general, conditions associated with low levels of circulating testosterone—or more precisely, its active metabolite, dihydrotestosterone—may cause problems with erection because testosterone is essential for the achievement of adequate erectile function (Table 57-2). Conditions associated with increased levels of prolactin may similarly

**Table 57-2**

**Definition of Selected Psychosexual Dysfunctions According to the *DSM-IV***

| *Dysfunction* | *Response Cycle Phase* | *Definition* |
|---|---|---|
| Hypoactive sexual desire disorder | Desire | A persistent and pervasive inhibition of sexual desire usually accompanied by an absence of sexual fantasies |
| Sexual arousal disorder | Arousal | A recurrent and persistent inability to attain or maintain an erection or lubrication-swelling response<br>(*Note:* "Sexual excitement" here has a physical, not merely psychic, meaning) |
| Male orgasmic disorder | Orgasm | A recurrent or persistent delay in or absence of orgasm following a normal sexual excitement phase; the clinician must take into account whether the stimulation is adequate in focus, intensity, and duration |
| Female orgasmic disorder | Orgasm | A recurrent or persistent delay in or absence of orgasm following a normal sexual excitement phase; the clinician must take into account the women's sexual experience, whether her orgasmic capacity is less than would be reasonable for her age, and the adequacy of sexual stimulation<br>(*Note:* Many women can experience orgasm during noncoital stimulation but not during vaginal intercourse in the absence of direct clitoral stimulation) |
| Premature ejaculation | Orgasm | The recurrent onset of orgasm and ejaculation with minimal sexual stimulation before, on, or shortly after penetration and before the person wishes it. The clinician must take into account factors that affect duration of the excitement phase, such as age, novelty of the sexual partner or situation, and recent frequency of sexual activity |
| Dyspareunia | Not part of cycle | Genital pain associated with sexual intercourse |
| Vaginismus | Not part of cycle | A condition that involves involuntary contraction of the perineal muscles surrounding the outer third of the vagina when vaginal penetration with penis, finger, tampon, or speculum is attempted |

be problematic because prolactin interferes with the bioactivity of testosterone.[17]

Vascular occlusion or diversion of blood supply to the pelvic organs can also result in erectile problems[18] and probably lubrication/swelling difficulties in females. Similarly, conditions resulting in sensory neuropathy may decrease genital sensation and sensory feedback. Autonomic neuropathy may prevent adequate maintenance of the venous constriction needed to keep the corpora cavernosa engorged to maintain an erection. It may also impair arousal in females. Infections of the prostate gland in males (usually secondary to gonorrhea or chlamydia) may also be implicated in ED and premature ejaculation.[3] In a study of 40 young men between the ages of 14 and 19 presenting with ED, 74% had a physical problem and 60% had an underlying vascular abnormality. Thirty-seven percent gave a history of perineal trauma and 15% reported penile trauma, 7% had a history of diabetes or hypercholesterolemia.[19]

In females, local irritation secondary to vaginal infections may contribute to the development of vaginismus. Internal genital tract abnormalities, endometriosis, or infections involving the cervix, uterus, or fallopian tubes may cause discomfort or pain during intercourse. Vaginismus may then develop as a protective measure in cases involving these internal genital tract abnormalities[9] (see Table 57-3).

**Table 57-3**

## Clinical Causes of Sexual Dysfunction

| *Classification* | *Disorder/Cause* | *Possible Effect on Functioning* |
|---|---|---|
| Cardiovascular | Aortic coarctation; internal iliac/pudendal artery stenosis; thrombosis of arteries or veins of penis | Impairment of erection in men |
| Metabolic | Sickle cell disease; chronic cardiac, pulmonary, renal, and hepatic disorders; autoimmune diseases; cancer; anemia | May decrease libido and impair arousal response in men and women |
| Endocrine | Addison disease; hypoprolactinemia; hypothyroidism; hypogonadism; Cushing syndrome; Klinefelter syndrome; acromegaly; diabetes mellitus | May decrease libido and impair arousal response in men and women |
| Systemic infections | Infectious mononucleosis; hepatitis; HIV | May decrease libido and impair arousal response in men and women; among HIV-infected males, low testosterone levels have been noted |
| Local genital disease | Penile trauma; priapism; chordee; phimosis; hypospadias; bilateral orchitis due to mumps; balanitis | May decrease libido and impair arousal in men |
| | Urethritis; prostatitis; urethral pathology | Impaired arousal, premature ejaculation |
| | Vulval and vaginal pathology; endometriosis; pelvic inflammatory disease; prolapse of the uterus; ovarian and uterine cysts and tumors | Dyspareunia and consequent decrease in libido; vaginismus; orgasm may be unaffected |
| | *Neisseria gonorrhoeae; Chlamydia trachomatis* | Decreased libido, impaired arousal in men and women |
| Neurologic | Spinal cord injury; peripheral neuropathy (metabolic drug-induced); epilepsy; cardiovascular accident; head injury; spinal bifida; cerebral palsy; muscular dystrophy; multiple sclerosis; syringomyelia | May affect arousal and/or orgasm response in men and women |
| | Surgery or trauma of sacral or lumbar cord; cauda equina; pelvic sympathetic nerves | May cause increase or decrease in libido and changes in sexual behavior in men and women |
| Medication/drugs | Sedatives (narcotics, tranquilizers, alcohol) | May impair arousal and orgasm; in acute doses, increased libido |
| | Stimulants (amphetamines, cocaine) | May increase libido, impair orgasm |
| | Antidepressants (ex: SSRI, fluoxetine, paroxetine, sertraline) | May decrease libido, impair arousal, impair orgasm |
| | Antipsychotics (ex: haloperidol, decanoate, riperidone, olanzapine) | May decrease libido, impair arousal, impair orgasm |
| | Antihypertensives (ex: propranolol, hydrochlorothiazide) | May impair arousal |
| | Chemotherapeutic agents (cisplatin) | May decrease libido |
| | Antiretroviral medications for HIV | May decrease libido |
| | Hormonal contraceptives | May decrease libido |
| Eating disorders | Anorexia nervosa, bulimia nervosa | |
| | Overweight, obesity | Decreased libido may be noted |

There are rarely organic causes for primary or secondary orgasmic phase disorder or for primary excitement phase dysfunctions, but secondary excitement phase dysfunctions may be caused by many factors. The recent development of a systemic medical illness may leave the patient temporarily denervated and unable to participate fully in sexual relations. Dyspareunia, occurring secondary to infections with sexually transmitted infections (STIs), may cause the patient to suppress the desire to have sex. Invasive surgical procedures and concomitant scarring can affect a teenager's sense of attractiveness and body integrity, which subsequently can have an effect on sexual feelings.[5]

Medication that affects parasympathetic or sympathetic systems may interfere with arousal or orgasm responses, presumably in both sexes; however, there has been little research on such effects in females.[9] Table 57-3 presents a more complete review of organic causes.

Of all the medications listed previously, the 2 categories with the greatest potential to affect adolescent functioning include hormonal contraceptive agents and antidepressants. This is secondary to the degree to which these medications are prescribed to reduce unintended pregnancies and address depression respectively.

***Hormonal Contraceptive Agents*** In addition to barrier methods, hormonal contraceptive methods are prescribed to young women to reduce the potential for unintended pregnancy. Although hormonal contraceptive methods have been described as contributing to reduced sexual desire, review of the literature reveals mixed results (ie, some studies suggest no change, others report an increase in libido).[20]

***Antidepressants*** Mental health conditions are common among adolescents. For example, it is estimated that 8.8% of youths aged 12 to 17 years (2.2 million persons) experienced at least one major depressive episode (MDE) in the past year.[21]

Depression has been linked to difficulties in sexual functioning.[9] At times, it may be difficult to assess whether depression or anxiety are primarily or secondarily implicated in the development of such sexual dysfunctions as loss of desire, arousal difficulties, or premature ejaculation. Additionally, medications used to treat depression may be implicated in lowering libido or delaying ejaculation among adults. For example, the incidence of selective serotonin reuptake inhibitor (SSRI)-induced sexual dysfunction may range from 30% to 58%[22,23] and may affect males more than females.[24] However, although the potential exists for similar findings to be noted among depressed adolescent patients, specific data are lacking. In 1 report of 5 male adolescents taking SSRIs, 2 patients reported "no change" in sexual functioning, 2 reported impaired sexual functioning, and 1 reported "improved" functioning (delayed ejaculation). Additionally, over an 11-year period, only 8 MedWatch reports have been filed regarding SSRI-induced sexual dysfunction among adolescents. It is not clear whether the lack of reporting is due to a difference in how these medications affect adolescents, or is a result of failure to query youth about sexual functioning, and thus represents underreporting.[25]

Similarly, patients treated for schizophrenia or schizoaffective disorder with antipsychotic medications (quetiapine, olanzapine, or risperidone) may experience sexual dysfunction as well.[26]

***Substance Use*** In addition to prescribed medications, there is evidence to suggest that youth with depressive symptoms may self-medicate with various substances.[27]

In 2007, according to the Monitoring the Future Study,[28] which tracks national prevalence of substance use among adolescents, the percentage of 10th graders who had at least 1 drink of alcohol on one or more occasions in the past 30 days was 29%; 12% smoked cigarettes; 22% used marijuana; 3% used cocaine; 6.4% used amphetamines; and 1.5% reported methamphetamine use.

In addition to their intended effects, these substances may also affect sexual functioning. Nicotine has been correlated with an increase in ED among males. A meta-analysis of several large studies revealed that 40% of impotent men are current smokers as compared to 28% of males in the general population.[29] Nicotine exerts an effect on the vascular system and may play a synergistic role in affecting men for whom hypertension and/or diabetes are primary risk factors. Again, although these figures represent a primarily older, adult population, 80% to 90% of smokers initiate this behavior during adolescence.[30]

Alcohol and drugs can temporarily distance the adolescent from environmental and intrapsychic problems. In addition, many adolescents believe that mood-altering substances may have aphrodisiac properties. However, the psychologically disinhibiting effects of small amounts of alcohol may also yield to an erectile or a lubrication deficit as the quantity of alcohol builds up in the body. Although many cocaine/crack users report an initially elevated sex drive and level of sexual stamina associated with drug use, these reported effects diminish over time as the quest for the drug overrides all other concerns. Male users of methamphetamine report heightened sexual arousal and desire but reduced capacity to perform due to ED. To counteract this, methamphetamine users may combine crystal meth with Viagra. The combination of a mood-altering substance that increases sexual desire with a medication that allows for unabated erections may set the stage for repeated and/or multiple sexual encounters, which are often risky, thereby predisposing youth to STIs and HIV.

***Eating Disorders*** It is estimated that 5% to 10% of adolescent and young adult females may have an eating disorder (anorexia nervosa, bulimia nervosa, or atypical eating disorder).[31] Studies also indicate that individuals with eating disorders may have less desire to have sex and may have a more negative affect during sex.[32]

***Obesity*** Among children aged 6 through 19 years in 1999 to 2002, 31.0% were at risk for overweight or obesity and 16.0% were overweight.[33] Although being overweight or obese is not a deterrent to a satisfactory sex life, excessive weight can be an obstacle for some. Concerns about body image, hygiene, and perceived size of genitalia may affect self-esteem and social relationships. Conversely, some overweight and obese teens may be hypersexual, in part due to a desire for acceptance and nurturance.

### Psychosocial

Prioritizing sexual health and conceptualizing positive adolescent sexual development is a relatively new approach within the public health fields.[34,35] In rejecting a more traditional, proscriptive view of adolescent sexuality—one that assumes its primary task as identifying risk statuses and emphasizing the negative consequences of sexual activity for adolescents—this perspective seeks to identify potential patterns of sexual health by focusing on the variability in *meanings* and *understandings* of sexual behavior among youth. It prioritizes the central role culture and sexuality play in shaping romantic relationships and the links between specific characteristics of adolescent romantic relationships and adolescent sexual health. Although research in public health has been conducted on the precursors and consequences of adolescent sexual behavior, less is known about what constitutes relational and sexual self-efficacy, or a mature adolescent competence related to intimacy and sexual relationships—a significant precursor to sexual health and functioning for this population. In general, such competence consists of the ability to appropriately identify and express sexual needs, engage in empathetic mutuality with one's sexual partner, and seek out and maintain romantic relationships that are emotionally and physically healthy and satisfying for both partners.

***Early Conditioning*** Children who grow up in a sex negative, morally repressive environment are likely to experience guilt and anxiety about their bodies, their sexual thoughts, their sexual feelings, and, ultimately, their sexual behavior. Those who learn that sex is sinful or "dirty" carry a burden that may impede the natural and mature expression of sexual feelings. Evidence indicates that individuals with high levels of "sex guilt" have less knowledge about sex, use condoms and other contraception less frequently, and find it more difficult to communicate about sex.[36] Sex guilt also has been specifically implicated in the development of sexual dysfunction.[37] The role of parents or primary caretakers is a significant factor here; in addition to the sexual information, support, and guidance they provide to their developing adolescent children, the approach with which they provide this support/information is crucial. According to cross-cultural research by Schalet,[38] American parents typically have a "dramatization" view of adolescent sexuality, one in which adolescent sexuality is seen as a psychological, medical, or familial "drama." This view categorizes teens' sexual urges as overpowering and difficult to control, and as a result typically circumscribes their access to information about sexuality and adopts a proscriptive view toward adolescent sexual behavior and relationships. A more "normalizing" view by comparison treats adolescents as the owners of their own bodies and the agents of their own sexual behaviors.[38] It is accompanied by a commitment to provide them with guidance and access to the information and resources they need to exercise this agency over their sexual behaviors. Providers can play significant roles in providing information to both parents and adolescents about healthy sexual development (see resource section at the end of this chapter) and can facilitate meaningful dialogue between parties about this important topic.

***Sexual Abuse and Coercion*** Unwanted sexual advances or peer pressure to initiate sexual intercourse can have a negative effect on the development of relational competence—experiences that have been increasing over the past decade, although the pressure is qualitatively different for males and females. Some sobering statistics in this regard are:

- 13% of young men ages 13 to 18 cited pressure from their friends, and 8% of women of the same ages cited pressure from a partner when asked why they had sexual intercourse for the first time.[39] Similarly, 47% of teens who had experienced sexual intimacy said they felt pressure to do something they weren't ready to do.[39]
- In 2001, the National Crime Victimization Survey[40,41] estimated that 248,000 people were raped or sexually assaulted. Approximately 44% of rape victims are under age 18. Additionally, girls ages 16 to 19 are 4 times more likely than the general population to be victims of rape, attempted rape, or sexual assault.

- It has been estimated that 33% of females and 5% to 10% of males under the age of 18 have been victimized by sexual abuse.[42,43]

Many survivors of sexual abuse experience long-term disturbances in sexual functioning. Among females, common disturbances include low sexual desire, difficulties with arousal, and achieving orgasm.[44] Additionally, in some cases there is an increased susceptibility toward "revictimization." Women with a history of childhood sexual abuse were 2.4 times more likely to experience rape and attempted rape as adults.[45] Additionally, 1 study reports female sexual abuse survivors as 7 times more likely to engage in high-risk behaviors for HIV such as intravenous drug use and unprotected anal sex.[46] The timing of the assault along the developmental trajectory appears to be important also. As compared to women who had experienced sexual assault as adults, female child sexual abuse survivors reported greater difficulties with low sexual desire, achieving orgasm, and feeling anxious or guilty about sex.[47]

With respect to male sexual abuse survivors, ED has been noted along with a range of behaviors that "...incorporate painful sexual experiences into their sexual repertoire (such as the pairing of sexual arousal with choking)."[48]

***Sexual Minority Youth*** Although the process of becoming comfortable with one's sexuality is often difficult for heterosexual youth, the prevailing social stigma against homosexuality sometimes makes the process even more difficult for gay youth.[49] Facing disapproval, discrimination, and even physical abuse, some youth may try to deny same sex attractions and may even aggressively pursue opposite sex relationships. In some cases, youth may even become involved in a pregnancy to show positive proof of "normalcy." Intrapsychic conflict, however, may contribute subsequently to performance difficulties and lack of sexual fulfillment. Additionally, even those youth who are comfortable with their sexual orientation may experience sexual difficulties; in some cases due to sex guilt, and in other cases due to comorbid depression that may be addressed through substance use.[50] Considerate clinicians can assist youth in identifying and addressing sources of conflict. However, although welcoming support from health providers, many lesbian, gay, bisexual, transgender, questioning youth report rarely being asked about their sexual orientation during clinical encounters.[51]

***Media*** Adolescents face conflicting and confusing sexual messages from society at large. They are guided by media portrayals of sexuality on film and television that are often stereotyped and idealized. Sex is not only normative but frequent and free of consequences (such as STIs, HIV, and pregnancy).[52] This "fantasy" is further accentuated when youth view soft-core pornography, available on many cable television channels. Unrealistic and misconceived expectations may be shaped by exposure that can contribute to anxiety about performance. In a survey of more than 500 adolescents, almost three-fourths believed that sexual content on television influenced teen behaviors.[53]

It is critically important that youth receive balanced information and are helped to form more realistic expectations for sexual behaviors. Schools could provide parents with assistance in this regard. However, sexuality education in the United States has historically been, and still remains, a form of social control of sexuality for adolescents[54]—one that currently has nationwide taken the form of abstinence-only education in which accurate information and resources regarding contraception and STIs are absent. In the absence of comprehensive sex education and given the prevalence of ignorance and misconceptions about sexuality among adolescents, the burden lies with the clinician to provide the young people with whom they work (via private sessions, young clinics, and discussion groups, etc) with age-appropriate information about taking care of their sexual health, including contraception, physical anatomy, and bodily functions, and to help them acquire skills to resist social and peer pressure, assess potentially dangerous situations, and make responsible decisions.

***Internet*** The Internet, as a relatively new source of sexual information and dating for young people, holds possibilities, promises, and problems. The Internet has become a primary communication venue for young people, who typically are early adopters of all new technology. Although it provides unfettered access to a wide range of information, accurate and inaccurate, the Internet has become a primary source for young people to meet potential partners, develop friendships and intimate relationships with others, and access explicit sexual imagery and text. Although its anonymous character allows adolescents to bypass traditional sources of information and easily and quickly gain answers to their sexual questions, it also places adolescents at risk for unsolicited, potentially dangerous exchanges (especially for young adolescents) and perpetuates, via its pornographic component, significant misinformation and myths regarding sexual functioning and anatomy. Seventy percent of all 15- to 17-year-old adolescents who have used the Internet report having viewed pornographic material.[55]

The interactive potential of the Internet also lends itself to developing effective online sexual health interventions for adolescents.[56] This potential is especially useful to health care practitioners and clinicians who can guide their adolescent patients toward accurate, responsible Web sites (see the Web site listed at the end of this chapter) geared toward young people and monitored by reputable experts and educators. These Web sites can provide effective sexual health education by providing adolescents with immediate, customized feedback, measuring risk assessment, facilitating decision making, and providing online peer support networks through peer advisers, chat rooms, and message boards.

### Interpersonal

Little is known of the ways adolescents experience the emergence of their sexual and romantic feelings, or of their ability to navigate sexuality and how these abilities affect their transition to adulthood and their capacity to form healthy and fulfilling relationships as adults.[34] Less is known about the connections between adolescent intimate relationships and sexual behavior, and we have little information on the factors, conditions, and situations that may be associated with relational and sexual empowerment. Sexual behavior/relationships between adolescents are typically characterized by poor or absent communication, and as a consequence the sexual exchange is often based on unverified assumptions of the other's sexual attitudes, preferences, and tastes. Traditional gender scripts are typically at play in which the male may assume the role of the sexual expert—(leading to male performance anxiety and erectile difficulties)—and the female the passive recipient, preventing her from taking responsibility for her own pleasure and desire. Lack of basic information about sexual functioning is also a significant obstacle—for instance, female and male teens are not familiar with the role of the clitoris in self-functioning, and many young men indoctrinated with "knowledge of the street" develop deep feelings of insecurity after hearing about the exploits of peers who can "stay hard for hours (naturally)" during love-making when, in actuality, the average male ejaculates within 2 to 3 minutes of intromission.[57]

Additionally, for many adolescent girls, expressing sexual desire is a more complicated issue. Tolman's[35] research on adolescent girls and their experiences with relationships and sexuality refers to the "missing discourse of desire" among girls; they do not speak of sexual pleasure or desire when discussing their sexual relationships. Being unable to verbalize desire may perhaps denote difficulty or inability to recognize themselves as equal, desiring partners in their relationships with others.

Helping teens articulate concerns and improve verbal and nonverbal sexual communication skills can go a long way toward improving their sexual functioning.

## ASSESSMENT ISSUES

Adolescents rarely present at a clinician's office with a chief complaint of sexual dysfunction. Many teens (and adults) feel uncomfortable talking about sexual issues and tend not to volunteer information not specifically elicited. The ease with which the clinician discusses sex will help set the pace for the adolescent. Assurances of confidentiality, acknowledgment of potential patient (and clinician) discomfort in discussing the subject, and validation of the importance of the discussion are important initial steps in the evaluation. As with many sensitive topics, once the subject of sexual difficulties is broached, the adolescent often feels a tremendous sense of relief that he or she has found someone to talk to about these concerns. Although it is useful for all youth to be queried about attitudes toward, and performance during sex, the busy provider is encouraged to pay particular attention to patients with histories of chronic illness, psychiatric disorders, and substance use. Additionally, any patient for whom particular concerns have been noted with respect to sex (ie, multiple STIs, pregnancies, difficulty in adherence to contraceptive methods) should be specifically evaluated.

A detailed sexual history should be obtained, which should address the adolescent attitude toward sex in general, that is, the meaning and importance of sex in the context of their life. A developmental framework is important to keep in mind, as sex may be less of a focus for early adolescents than for their middle and late adolescent peers. Related areas of exploration may include perceived parental and peer values toward sex and sources of information (and influences) about sex (media, Internet, peers, and family).

Additional areas to review include sexual initiation, profile of sexual partners, experiences with STIs/HIV and pregnancy, attitudes toward and use of condoms and contraceptive agents. Subsequently, the provider should steer the conversation toward a specific exploration of concerns about sex (desire, performance, etc). Table 57-4 provides suggested queries. When an assessment of sexual dysfunction is performed, it is useful to work from the general (eg, attitudes about sexuality toward the same and opposite sex, current activity, satisfaction with sex life, etc) toward more specific concerns (eg, sexual practices, arousal, orgasm). It is also important to explore the context surrounding the sexual experience (for example: does a problem occur with 1 specific partner or with all partners? Does a problem also occur during masturbation? Are substances used prior to a sexual act?) When talking to adolescents about sex, the clinician must make sure the terms that are used are clearly understood. The authors recommend using formal vocabulary and then inviting the

**Table 57-4**

## Approach to Eliciting Sexual Concerns

| *Content Area* | *Query* |
|---|---|
| Introduction to discussion about sex function | "Ok, ___, now that we've spent some time talking about sex, STIs/HIV, and ways to protect yourself and your partner/s, I wanted to shift the conversation a bit. Many of the young people who I work with say that sex is enjoyable and pleasurable, but sometimes they have questions or concerns about their feelings about sex, in general, or about their performance during sex. Do you have any questions or concerns that you'd like to share today?" |
| Specific probes for males to elicit concerns | "Some guys worry about not being 'in the mood,' getting/staying hard, or ejaculating ('cumming') too quickly, especially when they are trying to use a condom. Have you had any concerns about this, or anything else?" <br> *Probe for: onset, frequency, and situational context of concerns (ie, When did this start? How did this start? How often does this happen? Under what circumstances, and with whom (or what type of partners?)* |
| Specific probes for females to elicit concerns | "Some girls worry about not being 'in the mood' for sex, or feel very dry or uncomfortable during sex, or are not sure what an orgasm is. Have you had any concerns about this, or anything else?" <br> *Probe for: onset, frequency, and situational context of concerns* |
| Evaluation | If not already done, conduct assessment of medical and psychiatric history; review of systems; review of prescription and nonprescription medications (including substance use) |
| Specific probes for etiology | "Have you had any sexual experiences that were disturbing to you, or that you felt you had to keep secret?" <br> *Probe for: sexual abuse, sexual assault, dating violence, etc* |

adolescent to let the clinician know what terms are most comfortable for him or her.

During the discussion, if the existence of a problem is disclosed by the adolescent, information should be obtained on its parameters: onset, duration, and situational/global dimensions. In addition, it is important to attend to the adequacy of stimulation and other contextual factors. The clinician should be clear about determining whether the dysfunction is primary or secondary. Client characteristics such as general physical and mental health, cultural/religious background, and use of prescription and nonprescription drugs, need to be taken into account.

It should be noted that in many cases information about sexual dysfunction may be difficult to obtain. Many young people may be embarrassed, angry, or afraid to share intimate details of their life and history. However, providing a safe and open environment to discuss sensitive issues will allow the adolescent to eventually become forthcoming. Even if the initial probe seems negative, it sets the stage for future conversations and alerts the adolescent that it is "OK" to discuss these types of concerns in the office setting. For those youth who do reveal concerns, following the assessment outlined previously, the provider will have a basic sense for factors contributing to the initiation and maintenance of the dysfunction. This will shape the development of the treatment plan discussed in the following.

## TREATMENT ISSUES

It would be difficult for anyone to ignore the plethora of media advertisements for ED medications, let alone adolescents and young adults who spend on average 3 hours daily watching television.[58] It is conceivable that males with perceived (or actual) concerns about ED may be interested in using these products. One study of adolescent/young adult males reported that 13% experienced ED but rarely discussed this with medical providers, and 6% used ED medications, most often not under medical supervision (frequently obtained over the Internet) and often mixed with recreational drugs.[59] Again, this heightens the need for practitioners to conduct thorough and detailed histories with their patients and provide appropriate evaluation, education, counseling, and support.

In many cases, if an organic cause for the dysfunction is identified, it may be remediable through medical or surgical treatment. In the case of drug-induced problems, discontinuation or switching to an alternate medication may be indicated (eg, if appropriate, switching from fluoxetine or paroxetine to bupropin). If practical concerns (eg, lack of correct information about duration of sexual activity, or anxiety regarding condom use) are the issue, the clinician may discover that providing basic sexual information and helping adolescents view their sexual experiences as normal can substantially reduce concerns and enhance sexual functioning (see Web sites following for resources). In terms of the latter concern, educational practice sessions using a condom model may be beneficial to build competence.

If sexual difficulties (eg, lack of vaginal lubrication, failure to sustain an erection) are related to poor communication within a relationship, the provider may want to hold couples sessions to help teens improve verbal and nonverbal sexual communication skills that may assist in articulating needs and desires, particularly with respect to foreplay and clitoral stimulation. Additionally, work with couples may enhance the ability of males to not only identify the sensations that precipitate ejaculation but to facilitate communication with partners of the need to temporarily reduce or stop stimulation. Further, the provider may want to encourage the couple to use condoms. In addition to protecting against infection and pregnancy, they also reduce stimulation and premature ejaculation (provided issues noted previously related to putting on a condom are addressed). It should also be noted that "off-label" use of SSRIs to delay premature ejaculation has been used with adults, but in the absence of clinical symptoms of depression, some of the strategies discussed previously should be considered initially.

Addressing more detailed psychosocial issues (eg, depression, substance use, sexual victimization) may be far more complex, and in this regard the clinician may require consultation with a substance abuse counselor or mental health therapist.

## CONCLUSION

Adolescent medicine clinicians are the front-line forces in addressing the physical, psychological, and psychosexual problems of young adults. By incorporating an assessment of sexual functioning into the standard physical examination, the clinician can play a crucial role, not only in providing basic sexual information, but also in fostering the development of healthy, satisfying sexual expression. In addition, early identification and referral of those young people who need further counseling and treatment may prove beneficial in reducing future sexual morbidity.

## INTERNET RESOURCES

- **Advocates for Youth** (www.advocatesforyouth.org.) Established in 1980 as the Center for Population Options, Advocates for Youth champions efforts to help young people make informed and responsible decisions about their reproductive and sexual health. Advocates believes it can best serve the field by boldly advocating for a more positive and realistic approach to adolescent sexual health. See Advocates for Youth handouts: Adolescent Sexual Behavior I: Demographics; Adolescent Sexual Behavior II: Socio-Psychological Factors by Katie Dillard, 2002.
- **Go Ask Alice!** (www.goaskalice.columbia.edu.) Go Ask Alice! is a health Q&A Internet service, providing readers with reliable, accessible, culturally competent information and a range of thoughtful perspectives so that they can make responsible decisions concerning their health and well-being.
- ***Sex, Etc*** (www.sexetc.org) *Sex, Etc* is an award-winning national magazine and Web site on sexual health that is written by teens for teens. It is part of the Teen-to-Teen Sexuality Education Project developed by Answer (formerly the Network for Family Life Education), a leading national organization dedicated to providing and promoting comprehensive sexuality education.
- **SIECUS** (www.siecus.org) SIECUS provides information and training opportunities for young people, educators, health professionals, parents, and communities across the country to ensure that people of all ages, cultures, and backgrounds receive high-quality, comprehensive education about sexuality.

## REFERENCES

1. Sarrel LJ, Sarrel P. *Sexual Unfolding*. Boston: Little, Brown; 1979

2. Farrow JA. An approach to the management of sexual dysfunction in the adolescent male. *J Adolesc Health Care*. 1985;6:397–400

3. Johnson RL, Stanford P. Sexual dysfunctions in adolescent males with prostatic enlargement. *J Curr Adolesc Med.* 1980;2:31-35

4. Miller GD, Cirone J. Sexual dysfunction in college sexuality course attenders and course treatment benefits. *J Am Coll Health.* 1978;27:107-108

5. Greydanus DE, Demarest MS, Sears JM. Sexual dysfunctions in adolescents. *Semin Adolesc Med.* 1985;1:177-187

6. Haas A. *Teenage Sexuality: A Survey of Teenage Sexual Behavior*. New York, NY: Macmillan; 1979

7. American Psychiatric Association. *The Diagnostic and Statistical Manual of Mental Disorders*, 4th ed. Washington, DC: American Psychiatric Association; 1994

8. Masters WH, Johnson VS. *Human Sexual Response*. Boston: Little, Brown; 1966

9. Kaplan HS. *The New Sex Therapy*. New York, NY: Brunner-Mazel; 1974

10. Heiman JR. Sexual dysfunction: overview of prevalence, etiological factors, and treatments—statistical data included. *J Sex Res.* 2002;39(1):73-78

11. Feldman HA, Goldstein I, Hatzichristou DG, Krane RJ, McKinlay JB. Impotence and its medical and psychosocial correlates: results of the Massachusetts Male Aging Study. *J Urology.* 2004;151:54-61

12. Frank E, Anderson C, Rubenstein D. Frequency of sexual dysfunction in "normal" couples. *N Engl J Med.* 1978;229:111-115

13. Rosen RC, Taylor JF, Leiblum SR, Bachman GA. Prevalence of sexual dysfunction in women: results of a survey of 329 women in an outpatient gynecological clinic. *J Sex Marital Therapy.* 1993;19:171-188

14. Spector IP, Carey MP. Incidence and prevalence of the sexual dysfunctions: a critical review of the empirical literature. *Arch Sexual Beh.* 1990;19:389-408

15. Laumann EO, Paik A, Rosen RC. Sexual dysfunction in the United States: prevalence and predictors. *JAMA.* 1999;281:537-544

16. Krauss D. The physiologic basis of male sexual dysfunction. *Hosp Pract.* 1983;2:193-222

17. Frank S, Jacobs HS, Martin N, Narbarro JD. Hyperprolactinaemia and impotence. *Clin Endocrinol.* 1978;8:277-287

18. Jevitch MJ. Vascular noninvasive diagnostic techniques. In Krone RJ, Sirosky MB, Goldstein I, eds. *Male Sexual Dysfunction*. Boston, MA: Little, Brown; 1983

19. Edelson E. ED in teenagers: it's not necessarily psychological. RNWeb. Mar 1, 2006. Available at: www.modernmedicine.com/modernmedicine/article/articleDetail.jsp?id=310587. Accessed June 18, 2010

20. Davis AR, Castaño PM. Oral contraceptives and libido in women. *Annu Rev Sex Res.* 2004;15:297-320

21. National Survey on Drug Use and Health. The NSDUH Report. Depression and the initiation of alcohol and other drug use among youths aged 12 to 17. May 2007. Available at: www.oas.samhsa.gov/2k7/newUserDepression/newUserDepression.htm. Accessed September 20, 2007

22. Janicak PG, Davis JM, Preskorn SH, Ayd FJ. *Principles and Practice of Psychopharmacology.* 3rd ed. Philadelphia, PA: Lippincott Williams & Wilkins; 2001

23. Montejo-Gonzalez AL, Liorca G, Izquierdo JA, et al. SSRI-induced sexual dysfunction: fluoxetine, paroxetine, setraline, and fluvoxamine in a prospective, multicenter, and descriptive clinical study of 3,444 patients. *J Sex Marital Ther.* 1997;23:176-194

24. Kennedy SH, Fulton KA, Bagby RM, et al. Sexual function during bupriopion or paroxetine treatment of major depressive disorder. *Can J Psychiatry*. 2006;51:234-241

25. Scharko AM. Selective serotonin reuptake inhibitor-induced sexual dysfunction in adolescents: a review. *J Am Acad Child Adolesc Psychiatry.* 2004;43:1071-1079

26. Byerly MJ, Nakonezny PA, Bettcher BM, et al. Sexual dysfunction associated with second-generation antipsychotics in outpatients with schizophrenia or schizoaffective disorder: an empirical evaluation of olanzipine, risperidone, and quetiapine. *Schizophr Res.* 2006;86:244-250

27. Kelder SH, Murray NG, Orpinas P, et al. Depression and substance use in minority middle-school students. *Am J Public Health*. 2001;91:761-766

28. Johnston LD, O'Malley PM, Bachman JG, Schulenberg JE. *Various stimulant drugs show continuing gradual declines among teens in 2008, most illicit drugs hold steady*. University of Michigan News Service: Ann Arbor, MI; December 11, 2008 Available at: www.monitoringthefuture.org/pressreleases/08drugpr.pdf. Accessed April 20, 2009

29. Tengs TO, Osgood ND. The link between smoking and impotence: two decades of evidence. *Preventive Medicine.* 2001;32:447-452

30. Lynch BS, Bonnie RJ, eds. *Growing Up Tobacco Free: Preventing Nicotine Addiction in Children and Youth*. Washington, DC: National Academy Press; 1994

31. Neinstein LS, Mackenzie RG. Anorexia nervosa and bulimia nervosa. In Neinstein L, ed. *Adolescent Health Care: A Practical Guide*. 4th ed. Philadelphia, PA: Lippincott Williams & Wilkins; 2002

32. Morgan CD, Wiederman MW, Pryor TL. Sexual functioning and attitudes of eating-disordered women: a follow-up study. *J Sex Marital Ther.* 1995;21(2):67-77

33. Hedley AA, Ogden CL, Johnson CL, Carroll MD, Curtin LR, Flegal KM. Prevalence of overweight and obesity among US children, adolescents, and adults, 1999-2002. *JAMA.* 2004;16;291(23):2847-2850

34. Russell S. Conceptualizing positive adolescent sexuality development. *Sex Res Social Policy.* 2005;2:4-12

35. Tolman DL. *Dilemmas of Desire: Teenage Girls Talk About Sexuality*. Cambridge, MA: Harvard University Press; 2002

36. Mosher DL. The meaning and measurement of guilt. In Izard CE, ed. *Emotions in Personality and Psychopathology*. New York, NY: Plenum Press; 1979

37. Nowinski JK. Sex therapy: principles and practice. In: Olden CJ, Alcaparras SS, Strider FD, Graber IF, eds. *Applied Techniques in Behavioral Medicine*. New York, NY: Grune & Stratton; 1981

38. Schalet A. Must we fear adolescent sexuality? *Med Gen Med.* 2004;6(4):44

39. Kaiser Family Foundation. *The Kaiser Family Foundation/YM 1998 National Survey of Teens: Teens Talk about Dating, Intimacy, and Their Sexual Experiences*. Menlo Park, CA: Kaiser Family Foundation: 1998

40. Rennison C. *Criminal Victimization in the United States 2001: Changes 2000-2001 with Trends 1993-2001*. Washington, DC: Bureau of Justice Statistics, US Department of Justice; 2002

41. Greenfeld L. *Sex Offenses and Offenders: An Analysis of Data on Rape and Sexual Assault*. Washington, DC: Bureau of Justice Statistics, US Department of Justice; 1997

42. Wyatt GE, Loeb TB, Romero G, et al. The prevalence and circumstances of child sexual abuse: changes across a decade. *Child Abuse Negl.* 1999;23:45-60

43. Finkelhor D. Current information on the scope and nature of child sexual abuse. *Future Child.* 1994;4(2):31-53

44. Kinzl J, Mangweth B, Traweger C, Bibel W. Sexual dysfunction in males: significance of adverse childhood experiences. *Child Abuse Negl.* 1996;20:759-766

45. Wyatt GE. The sociocultural context of African-American and White American women's rape. *J Soc Issues.* 1992;48:77-91

46. Bensley LS, Van Eenwyk JV, Simmons KW. Self-reported childhood sexual and physical abuse and adult HIV-risk behaviors and heavy drinking. *Am J of Prev Med.* 2000;18:151-158

47. Mackey TF, Hackey SS, Weissfeld LA, Ambrose NC. Comparative effects of sexual assault on sexual functioning of child abuse survivors and others. *Issues Ment Health Nurs.* 1991;12:89-112

48. Loeb TB, Williams JK, Carmona JV, et al. Childhood sexual abuse: associations with the sexual functioning of adolescents and adults. *Ann Rev Sex Res.* 2002;13:307-345

49. Hunter J, Mallon G. Lesbian, gay, and bisexual adolescent development: dancing with your feet tied together. In: Green B, Croom GL, eds. *Education, Research, and Practice in Lesbian, Gay, Bisexual, Transgendered Psychology: A Resource Manual*. Thousand Oaks, CA: Sage Publications; 2002: 226-243

50. Garofalo R, Wolf RC, Kessel S, Falfrey J, DuRant RH. The association between health risk behaviors and sexual orientation among a school-based sample of adolescents. *Pediatrics* 1998; 101;895-902

51. Hunter J, Cohall R, Castrucci B, Ellis J. Lesbian, gay, bisexual and transgender adolescent perceptions of medical providers. Oral presentation:American Public Health Association Annual Meeting; October, 2001

52. Kunkel D, Eyal K, Finnerty K, Biely E, Donnerstein E. *Sex on TV*. Menlo Park, CA: Kaiser Family Foundation; 2005

53. Kaiser Family Foundation. *Teens, Sex and TV*. Menlo Park, CA: Kaiser Family Foundation; 2002

54. Moran J. *Teaching Sex: The Shaping of Adolescence in the 20th Century*. Boston, MA: Harvard University Press; 2000

55. Rideout V. *GenerationRx.com: How Young People Use the Internet for Health Information*. Menlo Park, CA: Kaiser Family Foundation; 2001

56. Isaacson N. An overview of the role of sexual health organizations, corporations, and government in determining content and access to online sexuality education for adolescents. *Sexuality Research and Social Policy* 2006;3:24-36

57. Kinsey AC, Pomeroy WE, Martin CE. *Sexual Behavior in the Human Male*. Philadelphia, PA: WB Saunders; 1948

58. Woodard EH, Gridina N. *Media in the Home 2000: The Fifth Annual Survey of Parents and Children*. The Annenberg Public Policy Center; 2000

59. Musacchio NS, Hartrich M, Garofalo R. Erectile dysfunction and Viagra use: what's up with college-age males? *J Adolesc Health.* 2006;39:452-454

SECTION 2

# Reproductive Health

## CHAPTER 58

# Physiology of Menstruation

JOSEPH S. SANFILIPPO, MD • JENNIFER DIETRICH, MD • S. PAIGE HERTWECK, MD

The earliest physiological beginnings of the menstrual cycle occur during fetal development, 10 to 12 weeks after conception. In humans, sexual dimorphism begins at this point, resulting in male and female sexual differentiation. As early as 10 weeks of gestational age, hypothalamic production of gonadotropin-releasing hormone (GnRH) has been noted in the fetal circulation.[1] Although GnRH is known to have a role in pubertal/menarchal development, the exact "trigger" for the onset of puberty remains a point of controversy. Whether puberty represents a change in the sensitivity to negative feedback at the hypothalamic level, the presence of critical lean body mass, or enhanced (ie, increased) pulsatile secretion of GnRH, with subsequent increases in both follicle-stimulating hormone (FSH) and luteinizing hormone (LH), remains to be determined.[2-4] The usual sequence of pubertal milestones includes thelarche, adrenarche, peak growth velocity, and, finally, menarche.

## HORMONAL PATTERNS OF THE FIRST MENSTRUAL CYCLES

Hypothalamic development, as it pertains to reproductive neuroendocrinology, primarily involves development of the median eminence and medial preoptic area. Neurons containing GnRH are present in both of these segments of the hypothalamus. The gonadostat, the physiological structure composed of the hypothalamic median eminence and medial preoptic area, serves as the primary site of GnRH release. This region of the brain is associated with the pulsatile efflux of GnRH that occurs every 60 to 90 minutes. Hypothalamic output is delicately balanced, in such a way that neural input into this region is received from serotonergic, noradrenergic, and dopaminergic pathways.

Gonadotropin-releasing hormone, a decapeptide, is released into the portal system; the releasing hormone is then delivered to the anterior pituitary gland, with a resultant release of the glycoprotein hormones FSH and LH. Both gonadotropins exit the pituitary and enter the bloodstream, through which they are ultimately delivered to the ovarian follicle apparatus, with resultant stimulation of preantral follicles. A composite view of the relationship among FSH, LH, and estradiol is presented in Figure 58-1. Oocytes are recruited, after which a dominant follicle is selected to provide primary governance during that particular menstrual cycle. Once ovulation occurs, a corpus luteum is formed on the ovary at the site where the ovum was extruded. Formation of the corpus luteum is characterized by production of progesterone.

The circulating gonadotropin levels throughout a woman's life from conception to adolescence are highlighted in Figure 58-2. A nadir of circulating gonadotropin (FSH and LH) levels occurs at 4 to 8 years of age, followed immediately by a prepubertal pattern of gonadotropin production. This prepubertal period is characterized by unique nocturnal LH surges,[5] in large part associated with rapid eye movement sleep.

Knowledge of this preliminary information enables the clinician to understand how persistent endocrine patterns observed in the course of early puberty (ie, anovulation) may explain pathological conditions during an adult's life, such as polycystic ovarian disease.[6,7]

Figure 58-3 and Figure 58-4 depict comparisons of the hypothalamic-pituitary-ovarian axis of the fetus with those of the prepubertal and late pubertal patient. Apter and Vihko[8] noted that, under normal circumstances, the first endocrinologic change recorded in the immediate premenarchal period at 7 years of age is an increase in serum dehydroepiandosterone

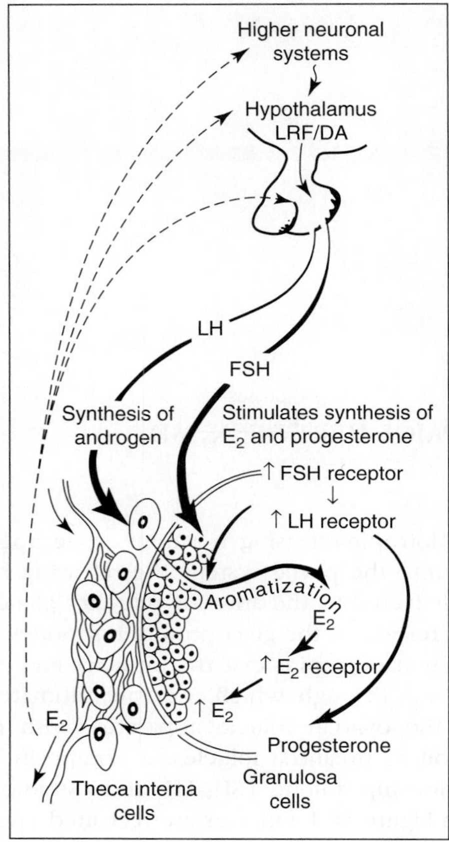


FIGURE 58-1 Composite view of the relationship between follicle-stimulating hormone (FSH), luteinizing hormone (LH), and estradiol ($E_2$) during the menstrual cycle. *LRF*, luteinizing hormone–releasing factor; *DA*, dopamine. (From Yen SSC, Jaffee RB, eds. *Reproductive Endocrinology: Physiology, Pathophysiology, and Clinical Management.* Philadelphia: WB Saunders; 1978, with permission from Elsevier.)

concentrations complemented by an elevation of testosterone levels (Figure 58-5). In the immediate postmenarcheal period, there is a predominance of FSH in the circulation.[9] Once regular ovulatory cycles are established, an adult FSH-to-LH ratio evolves. Follicle-stimulating hormone seems to be the primary hormone involved in ovum recruitment, with the selection of a dominant follicle usually around cycle day 6 or 7 and a subsequent rapid increase in the circulating concentration of estradiol. Serum testosterone and androstenedione levels closely parallel that of estradiol throughout the menstrual cycle.[10]

## REGULATION OF THE MENSTRUAL CYCLE

The menstrual cycle is the result of tightly coordinated cycles of stimulatory and inhibitory signals that ultimately result in the release of a single mature oocyte recruited from a pool of hundreds of thousands of primordial oocytes. Multiple factors contribute to the regulation of this process, including hormones and paracrine and autocrine factors that are still being identified. The cyclic changes in the primary pituitary and gonadal hormones are seen in Figure 58-6.[11]

### PHASES OF THE MENSTRUAL CYCLE

The menstrual cycle, in essence, is composed of 3 components: the follicular, ovulatory, and luteal phases. The first day of menses represents the first day of the cycle; then the cycle is divided into the follicular and luteal phase, with the time of ovulation being the defining moment separating the 2 phases (Figure 58-7). The follicular phase begins with the onset of menses and ends with the LH surge. The luteal phase begins with the LH surge and ends at the onset of the next menses.

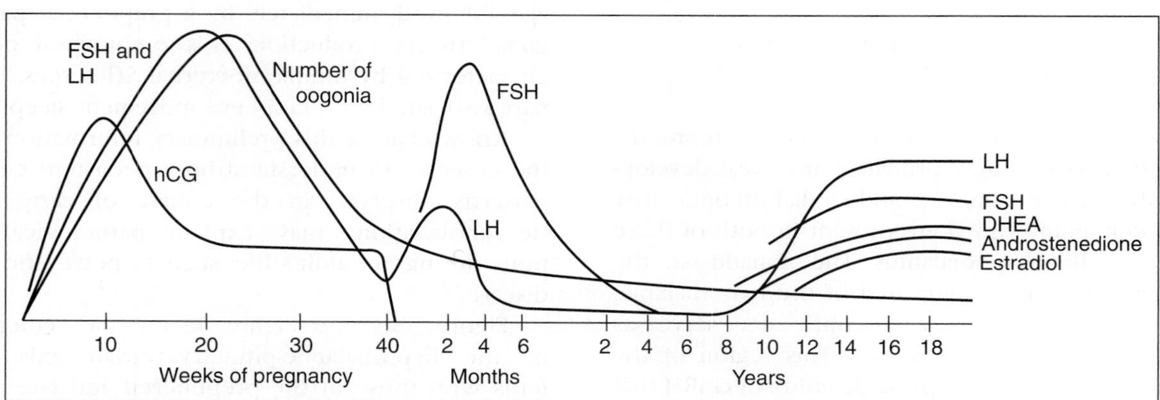


FIGURE 58-2 Serum levels of follicle-stimulating hormone (FSH), luteinizing hormone (LH), human chorionic gonadotropin (hCG), dehydroepiandrosterone (DHEA), androstenedione, and estradiol in females from prenatal state to 18 years of age. (From Speroff L, Fritz MA. *Clinical Gynecologic Endocrinology and Infertility.* 4th ed. Baltimore: Williams & Wilkins; 2005:179, with permission from Wolters Kluwer Health.)

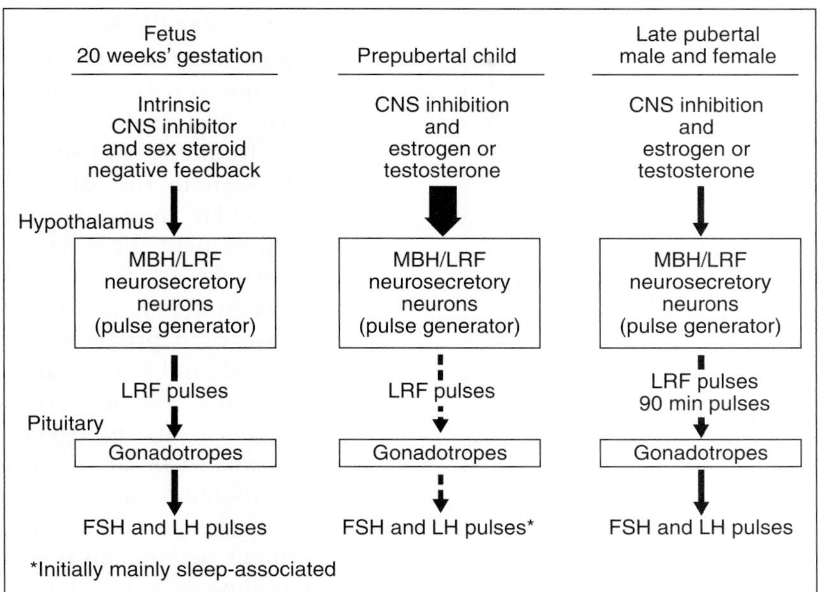


**FIGURE 58-3** Changes in activity of the medial basal hypothalamic pulse generator during development and the effect on pituitary gonadotropes. It is hypothesized that functional gonadotropin-releasing hormone (GnRH) insufficiency of a prepubertal child is a consequence of central nervous system (CNS) restraint by sex steroid–dependent and –independent mechanisms. *MBH*, medial basal hypothalamus; *LRF*, luteinizing hormone–releasing factor. (Modified from Reiter EO. Neuroendocrine control processes. *J Adolesc Health Care*. 1987;8:479–491, with permission from Elsevier.)

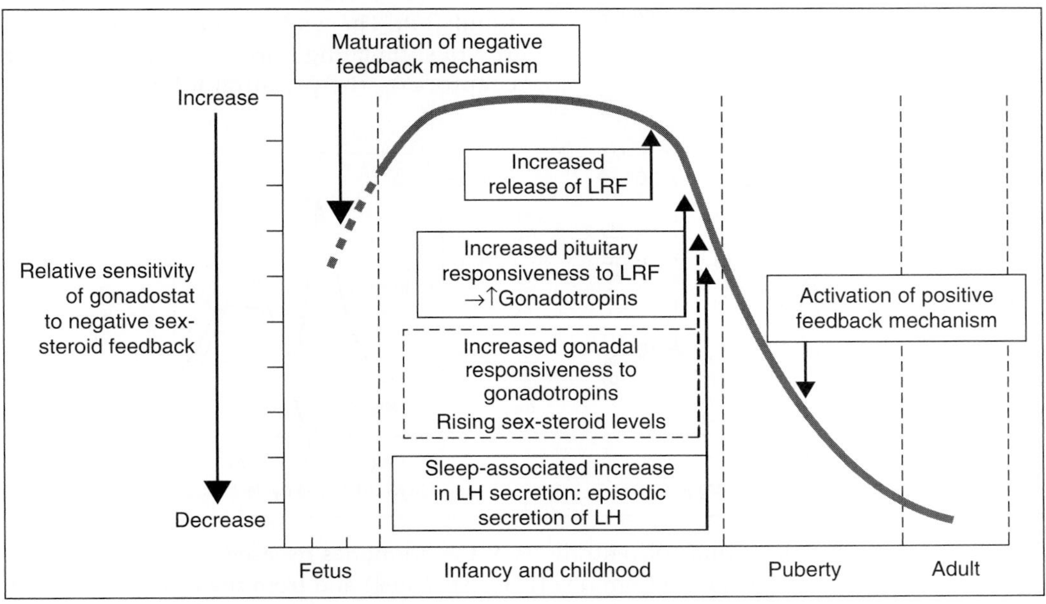


**FIGURE 58-4** Change in the set point of hypothalamic (gonadotropin-releasing hormone [GnRH]) luteinizing hormone–releasing factor (LRF) and in pulse-generator pituitary gonadotrope unit (gonadostat) (denoted by dashed and solid line) and maturation of negative and positive feedback mechanisms from fetal life to adulthood in relation to normal changes of puberty. (From Grumbach MM, et al. Hypothalamic-pituitary regulation of puberty in man: evidence and concepts derived from clinical research. In: Grumbach MM, Grave GD, Mayer FE, eds. *Control of the Onset of Puberty*. New York: John Wiley; 1974:115–166, with permission from Wolters Kluwer Health.)

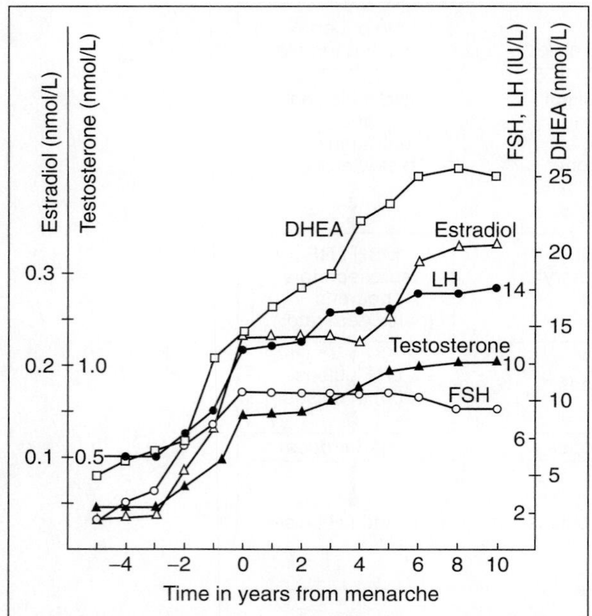


FIGURE 58-5 Serum concentrations of follicle-stimulating hormone (FSH), luteinizing hormone (LH), dehydroepiandrosterone (DHEA), estradiol, and testosterone in relation to time since menarche (no. of observations = 410). First points at −5 years include all subjects 7.3 to 5 years before menarche. Last points at 10 years include all subjects more than 8 to 12.7 years since menarche. Postmenarchal specimens were drawn on days 6 to 9 of the cycle. (From Flamigni C, Venturoli S, Givens JR, eds. *Adolescence in Females*. Chicago: Mosby-Year Book; 1985:218, with permission from Elsevier.)

**Early Follicular Phase**

The early follicular phase is the time of lowest ovarian hormonal output of estradiol and progesterone (Figure 58-7). The decrease in negative feedback from estradiol and progesterone and inhibin A levels seen in the late luteal phase result in an early follicular increase in GnRH pulse frequency and a subsequent increase in FSH concentrations of approximately 30%.[12] The increase in FSH is required for the recruitment of the primordial follicles, 1 of which will then progress though the stages of preantral, antral, and preovulatory follicle development. The primordial follicle, surrounded by a single layer of granulosa cells, is characterized by an oocyte, which seems to be arrested in the dictyotene phase of the diplotene stage of meiotic prophase. It progresses to the preantral state, during which oocyte enlargement occurs and the zona pellucida develops. The granulosa cells proliferate, complemented by the development of the theca layer during this developmental phase. Growth of the preantral follicle seems to directly depend on FSH and LH and correlates with increased production of estrogen. The key events in preantral follicle development are (1) initial recruitment and growth independent of gonadotropin influences, (2) response to FSH stimulation as the follicle begins to grow, and (3) FSH-induced aromatization of androgens in the granulosa cells, which appear to be transported from the thecal cells in response to FSH stimulation. The end product is estradiol production; growth-stimulating hormone and estradiol induce FSH receptors on the preantral follicle.

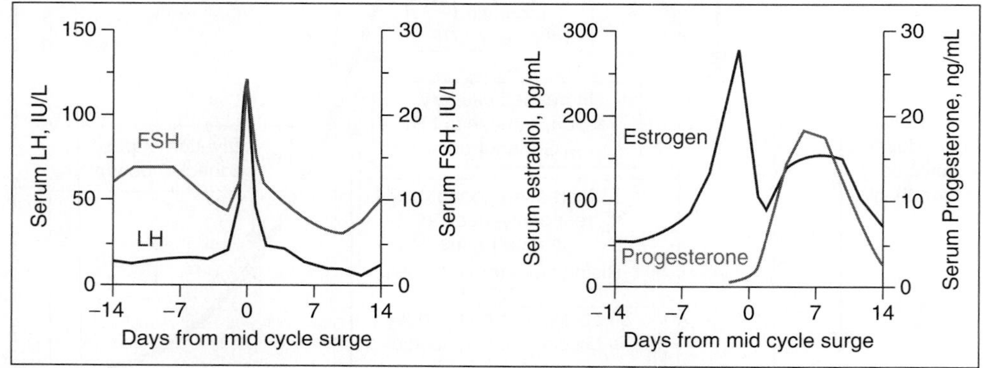


FIGURE 58-6 Sequential changes in the serum concentrations of the hormones released from the pituitary (follicle-stimulating hormone [FSH] and luteinizing hormone [LH]; left panel) and from the ovaries (estrogen and progesterone; right panel) during the normal menstrual cycle. By convention, the first day of menses is day 1 of the cycle (shown here as day −14). The cycle is then divided into 2 phases: the follicular phase is from the onset of menses until the LH surge (day 0); and the luteal phase is from the peak of the LH surge until the next menses. To convert serum estradiol values to pmol/L, multiply by 3.67, and to convert serum progesterone values to nmol/L, multiply by 3.18. (Reproduced with permission from: Dubin, AM. Supraventricular tachycardia in children: AV reentrant tachycardia (including WPW) and AV nodal reentrant tachycardia. In: UpToDate, Basow, DS (Ed), UpToDate, Waltham, MA 2010. Copyright © 2010 UpToDate, Inc. For more information visit www.uptodate.com.)

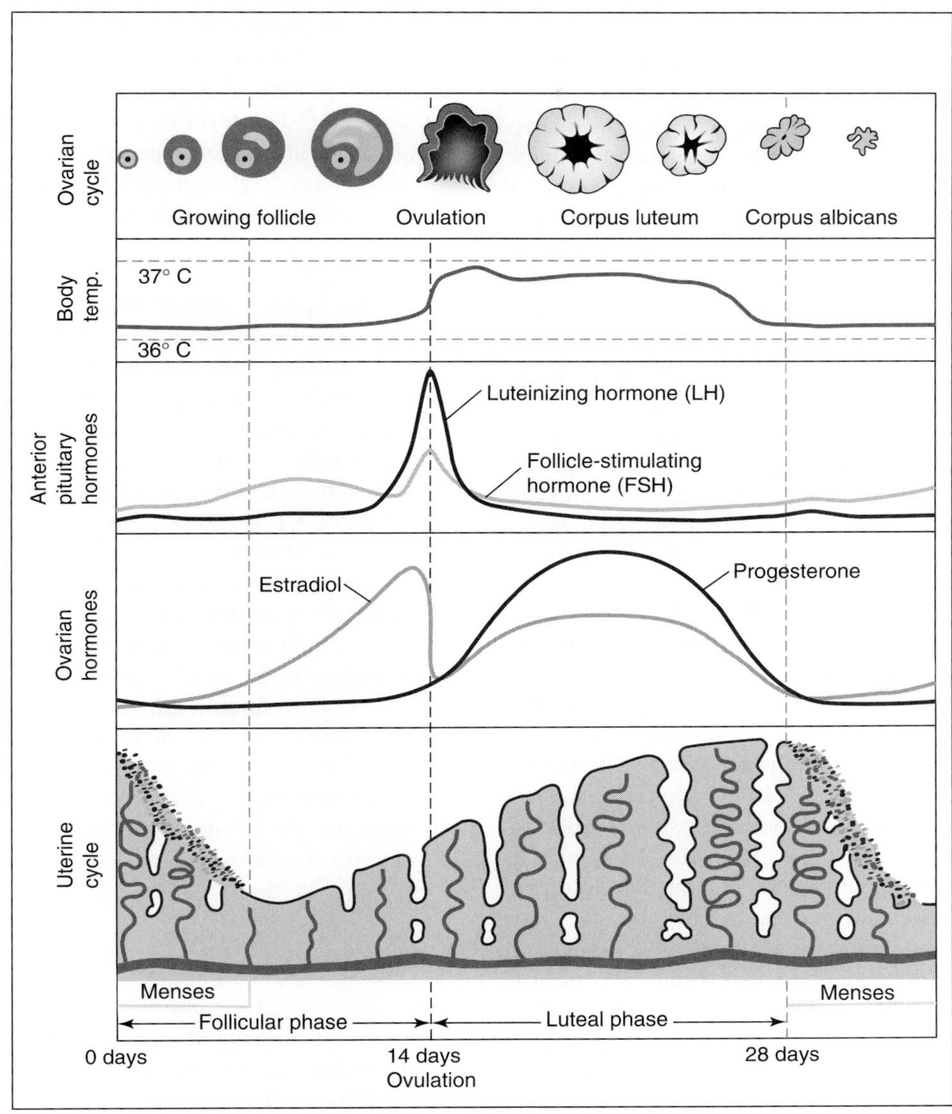


**FIGURE 58-7** Menstrual cycle. (Reproduced with permission from Welt, CK. Normal menstrual cycle. In: UpToDate, Basow, DS (Ed), UpToDate, Waltham, MA 2010. Copyright © 2010 UpToDate, Inc. For more information visit www.uptodate.com.)

Inhibin B is secreted by the recruitable pool of small follicles, and the level is maximal in this phase and may play a role in suppressing the FSH rise at this time in the cycle.[13] Luteinizing hormone pulse frequency increases during this time from 1 pulse every 4 hours in the late luteal phase to 1 pulse every 90 minutes in the early follicular phase.[14] Interestingly, LH pulses slow or cease during sleep in the early follicular phase.

### Midfollicular Phase

The next stage of development is the formation of the antral follicle. The increasing FSH levels gradually stimulate folliculogenesis and estradiol production, leading to growth of the follicular cohort selected that cycle. As several follicles grow to the antral stage, their granulosa cells hypertrophy, divide, and produce increasing estradiol initially via FSH stimulation of aromatase and then from inhibin A from the granulosa cells in the ovaries. This increase in estradiol production causes negative feedback on the hypothalamus and pituitary that results in suppression of serum FSH and LH concentrations and on LH pulse amplitude. In contrast, the GnRH pulse generator speeds up to a mean pulse frequency of 1 per hour compared to the 1 per 90 minutes seen in the early follicular phase. This GnRH stimulation is believed to be due to the release of negative feedback effects of progesterone from the previous luteal phase.

### Late Follicular Phase

By the late follicular phase, a dominant follicle is "selected" from the original primordial follicle cohort, which is near 1,000, and is initiated each cycle before antral follicle development. Exactly how the dominant follicle is selected remains a question of continued research and fascinating inquiry. Once the dominant follicle is selected, usually on cycle day 6 or 7 in the typical 28-day cycle, this follicle becomes responsible for the production of large quantities of estradiol and inhibin A that increases daily during the week before ovulation. As the dominant follicle is selected, FSH induces LH receptors in the ovary and increases ovarian secretion of intrauterine growth factors such as insulin-like growth factor-I (IGF-1). This activity enhances the dominant follicle's response to both FSH and LH. Serum FSH and LH levels fall at this time due to the negative feedback effect of estradiol released from the ovary (see Figure 58-7).

### Luteal Phase: Midcycle Surge and Ovulation

Serum estradiol levels rise until they reach a peak approximately 24 hours before ovulation. Exposure to this large quantity of estradiol (±200 pg/mL for at least 36 hours) creates a unique neuroendocrine phenomenon: the midcycle surge.[15] This surge represents a sudden switch from negative feedback control of LH secretion by ovarian estradiol and progesterone to a sudden positive feedback, resulting in a 10-fold increase in LH levels and a smaller rise in FSH levels (see Figure 58-7). Also at this time, the frequency of LH pulses continue at approximately 1 per hour, but the amplitude increases dramatically. This switch from negative to positive feedback of LH release is poorly understood. It would appear that there is an increase in GnRH receptors at the level of the pituitary or that they are modulated in some way to contribute to the pituitary response to GnRH, as there is probably no change in GnRH input on the pituitary.[16] Gonadotropin-releasing hormone release causes a large LH surge and a smaller FSH release, resulting in ovulation within approximately 36 hours of the GnRH surge. The remaining cohort of original follicles undergoes atresia, primarily as a result of the predominant androgenic steroidal milieu.

### Ovulation

Ovulation is a direct response to the LH surge. As LH levels in the circulation rise and the quantity of the lipoprotein hormone in the ovarian apparatus increases, LH overcomes the local inhibitory action of oocyte maturation inhibitor and utilization inhibitor, both of which facilitate extrusion of the ovum. Progesterone contributes to enhanced distensibility of the follicle wall. Follicular wall distensibility is complemented by smooth muscle contraction at the level of the ovary. Digestion of collagen takes place in the follicular wall in response to the proteolytic enzymes, collagenases, and plasmin. In addition, histamine has been associated with ovulation in animal models, although its role in humans remains to be defined.[17] The level of prostaglandin in the follicular fluid peaks just before the release of the ovum.[17] Furthermore, prostaglandin synthetase inhibitors have an adverse effect on ovum release.[18]

### Luteal Phase

The luteal phase is characterized by the release of progesterone from the corpus luteum in response to LH stimulation. Luteinizing hormone is released from the pituitary in a pulsatile manner progressively slowing LH pulses down to 1 pulse every 4 hours; progesterone levels seem to reflect this pattern of response.[19] Low-density lipoprotein (LDL)-cholesterol provides the precursor for progesterone production. The enzymatic machinery of the corpus luteum allows cholesterol to be converted to pregnenolone and, ultimately, to progesterone. Peak levels of progesterone occur on cycle days 20 to 22 of the 28-day cycle. In general, the luteal phase lasts 14 days; however, a range of 12 to 17 days is considered normal.[20]

The corpus luteum appears to decline approximately 10 days after ovulation. The exact mechanism that initiates this decline is not understood. If fertilization does occur, human chorionic gonadotropin (hCG) seems to continue to stimulate the LH receptors because there seems to be 1 receptor that responds to either LH or hCG.[21]

## MENARCHE

The median age for the first period or menarche is 12.43 years.[22] Ten percent of females are menstruating by age 11.11 years and 90% by age 13.75 years. Black and Hispanic females have a younger median age at menarche (12.06 and 12.25 years, respectively) than do non-Hispanic white females.[22]

Menarche typically occurs within 2 to 3 years of breast budding (thelarche) at Tanner stage IV breast development and is rare before Tanner stage III breast development.[23] The interval between thelarche and menarche is longer (closer to 3 years) in those girls with earlier thelarche than those in whom thelarche occurs later (closer to a 2-year interval). By 15 years of age, 98% of girls have experienced menarche.[22,24,25]

Although primary amenorrhea (absence of menarche) has been traditionally defined as no menses by age 16, if the more statistically proven age of 13 or 14 is used when determining when to clinically evaluate patients, many diagnosable and treatable disorders can and should be detected earlier. Clinically, any adolescent who has not reached menarche by age 15, or within 3 years of thelarche, should undergo evaluation. Accordingly, any adolescent without breast development by age 13 should also undergo evaluation.[26]

## CYCLE LENGTH

The first menstrual cycle typically lasts from 2 to 7 days. The interval between menstrual cycles can be somewhat irregular during adolescence, with the median length of first cycle after menarche being 34 days, and 39% of cycle lengths exceeding 40 days. There is considerable variability, with 10% of females having 60 days between their first and second menses and 7% having a first cycle interval of 20 days.[27] Despite this variability, even within the first gynecologic year, most cycles occur between 21 and 45 days apart with only 2% occurring more than 90 days apart.[28] Most prolonged intervals tend to occur within the first 3 years of menarche, with the trend toward shorter and more regular cycles with increasing age. By the third year after menarche, most menstrual cycles are 21 to 34 days long, as is typical in adults.[24,27] Table 58-1 summarizes the normal menstrual cycle.

## OVULATION

Early menstrual life is characterized by anovulatory cycles.[29] The frequency of ovulation is related both to age at menarche and the time since menarche,[29–31] with early menarche being more associated with early ovulation. When menarche occurs younger than age 12, 50% of cycles are ovulatory in the first gynecologic year (the first year after menarche). In contrast, it may take up to 8 to 12 years for girls with later menarcheal onset to develop ovulatory cycles. Regardless of ovulation, most cycle intervals range from 21 to 45 days, even in the first gynecologic year, with the 5th percentile for cycle length being 23 days and the 95th percentile being 90 days. Intervals longer than 90 days are statistically uncommon. Cycles on the longer range of normal are more commonly seen in the first gynecologic year, with the trend toward shorter and more regular cycles with increasing age. By the third year after menarche, 60% to 80% of cycles are 21 to 34 days apart, which is more typical of adult cycles. By the sixth gynecologic year, at or around the age of 19, a woman's cycle is typically established.[27,32,33]

**Table 58-1**

**Normal Menstrual Cycles in Young Females**

| | |
|---|---|
| Menarche (median age) | 12.43 years |
| Mean cycle interval | 32.2 days between cycles in the first gynecologic year |
| Menstrual cycle interval | Range 21–45 days |
| Menstrual flow in length | ≤7 days |
| Menstrual product use | 3–6 pads/tampons per day |

## REFERENCES


1. Kaplan S, Grumbaugh M. Physiology of puberty. In: Flamigni C, Givens J, eds. *The Gonadotropins: Basic Science and Clinical Aspects in Females.* New York: Academic Press; 1982:167

2. Grumbach MM, Roth JC, Kaplan SL, et al. Hypothalamic-pituitary regulation of puberty in man: evidence and concepts derived from clinical research. In: Grumbach MM, Grave GC, Mayer FE, eds. *Control of the Onset of Puberty*. New York: John Wiley; 1974:115

3. Freisch RE, McArthur J. Menstrual cycles: fatness as a determinant of minimum weight for height necessary for the mainenance or onset. *Science.* 1974;185:949–951

4. Neinstein LS. Menstrual problems in adolescence. *Med Clin North Am.* 1990;74:1181–1203

5. Roth J, Kelch R, Kaplan S, Grumbach M. FSH and LH response to luteinizing hormone-releasing factor in prepubertal and pubertal children, adult males, patients with hypogonadotropic and hypertropic hypogonadism. *J Clin Endocrinol Metab.* 1972;35(6):926–930

6. Yen SS. The polycystic ovary syndrome. *Clin Endocrinol.* 1980;12(2):177–207

7. Rosenfeld R. The ovary and female sexual maturation. In: Kaplan SA, ed. *Clinical Pediatric and Adolescent Gynecology*. Philadelphia: WB Saunders; 1982

8. Apter D, Vihko R. Hormonal patterns of the first menstrual cycles. In: Flamigni C, Venturoli S, Givens J, eds. *Adolescence in Females*. Chicago: Mosby–Year Book; 1985

9. Apter D, Pakarien A, Vihko R. Serum prolactin, follicle-stimulating hormone and luteinizing hormone during puberty in girls and boys. *Acta Paediatr Scand.* 1978;67:417–423

10. Apter D. Serum steroids and pituitary hormones in female puberty: a partly longitudinal study. *Clin Endocrinol (Oxf).* 1980;12:107–120

11. Welt CK. The normal menstrual cycle. Available at: www.uptodate.com. Accessed September 21, 2007

12. Hall JE, Schoenfeld DA, Martin KA, Crowley WF Jr. Hypothalamic gonadotropin-releasing hormone secretion and follicle-stimulating hormone dynamics during the luteal-follicular transition. *J Clin Endocrinol Metab.* 1992;74:600–607

13. Weit CK, McNicholl DJ, Taylor AE, Hall JE. Female reproductive aging is marked by decreased secretion of dimeric inhibin. *J Clin Endocrinol Metab.* 1999;84:105–111

14. Filicori M, Santoro N, Merriam GR, Crowley WF Jr. Characterization of the physiological pattern of episodic gonadatropin secretion throughout the human menstrual cycle. *J Clin Endocrinol Metab.* 1986;62:1136–1144

15. Adams JM, Taylor AE, Schoenfeld DA, et al. The midcycle gonadotropin surge in normal women occurs in the face of an unchanging gonadotropin-releasing hormone pulse frequency. *J Clin Endocrinol Metab.* 1994;79: 858–864

16. Martin KA, Welt CK, Taylor AE, et al. Is GnRH reduced at the midcycle surge in the human? Evidence from a GnRH-deficient model. *Neuroendocrinology.* 1998;67:363–369

17. Lumsden MA, Kelly RW, Templeton AA, van Look PF, Swanston IA, Baird DT. Changes in the concentrations of prostaglandins in preovulatory human follicles after administration of hCG. *J Reprod Fertil.* 1986;77(1):119–124

18. O'Grady J, Caldwell B, Auletta F, Speroff L. The effects of an inhibitor of prostaglandin synthesis (indomethacin) on ovulation, pregnancy, and pseudopregnancy. *Prostaglandins.* 1972;1:97–106

19. Saracoglu OF, Askel S, Yeoman RR, Wiebe RH. Endometrial estradiol and progesterone receptors in patients with luteal phase defects and endometriosis. *Fertil Steril.* 1985;43:851–855

20. Lenton E, Langren B, Sexton L. Normal variation in the length of the luteal phase of the menstrual cycle: identification of the short luteal phase. *Br J Obstet Gynecol.* 1984;91:685–689

21. Rao CV, Griffin LP, Carman FR Jr. Gonadotropin receptors in human corpora lutea of menstrual cycle and pregnancy. *Am J Obstet Gynecol.* 1977;128:146–153

22. Chumlea WC, Schubert CM, Roche AF, et al. Age at menarche and racial comparisons in US girls. *Pediatrics.* 2003;111:110–113

23. Marshall WA, Tanner JM. Variations in pattern of pubertal change in girls. *Arch Dis Child.* 1969;44:291–303

24. American Academy of Pediatrics Committee on Adolescence, American College of Obstetricians and Gynecologists, and AAP Committee on Adolescent Health Care. Menstruation in girls and adolescents: using the menstrual cycle as a vital sign. *Pediatrics.* 2006;118:2245–2250

25. Chandra A, Martinez GM, Mosher WD, Abma JC, Jones J. Fertility, family planning, and reproductive health of U.S. women: Data from the 2002 National Survey of Family Growth. National Center for Health Statistics. Vital Health Stat 23(25). 2005. Available at: www.cdc.gov/nchs/data/series/sr_23/sr23_025.pdf. Accessed March 29, 2010

26. Reindollar RH, Byrd JR, McDonough PG. Delayed sexual development: a study of 252 patients. *Am J Obstet Gynecol.* 1981;140:371–380

27. World Health Organization Task Force on Adolescent Reproductive Health. World Health Organization multicenter study on menstrual and ovulatory patterns in adolescent girls. II. Longitudinal study of menstrual and ovulatory patterns on early postmenarchal periods, duration of bleeding episodes and menstrual cycles. *J Adolesc Health Care.* 1986;7:246–244

28. Treloar AE, Boynton RE, Behn BG, Brown BW. Variation of the human menstrual cycle throughout reproductive life. *Int J Fertil.* 1967;12:77–126

29. Venturoli S, Porcu E, Fabbri R, et al. Longitudinal evaluation of the different gonadatropin pulsatile patterns in anovulatory cycles of young girls. *J Clin Endocrinol Metab.* 1992;74:836–841

30. Apter D, Vihko R. Early menarche, a risk factor for breast cancer indicates early onset ovulatory cycles. *J Clin Endocrinol.* 1983;57:82–86

31. Vihko R, Apter D. Endocrine characteristics of adolescent menstrual cycles: impact on early menarche. *J Steroid Biochem.* 1984;20:231–236

32. Widhom O, Kantero RL. A statistical analysis of the menstrual cycles of 8,000 Finnish girls and their mothers. *Acta Obstet Gynecol Scand Suppl.* 1971;14(14):1–36

33. Hickey M, Balen A. Menstrual disorders in adolescence: investigation and management. *Human Reprod Update.* 2003;9:493–504

# CHAPTER 59

# Perineal and Vaginal Abnormalities

DIANE F. MERRITT, MD

## INITIAL GYNECOLOGY VISIT AND PELVIC EXAM

Adolescent girls should receive an initial reproductive health visit with their primary provider, adolescent specialist, or gynecologist between the ages of 13 and 15, followed by annual visits. Care should be delivered according to the patient's stage of physical, sexual, psychological, and cognitive development. The initial visit generally does not include a pelvic examination, but is an opportunity to establish rapport, ensure confidentiality, review menstrual and developmental issues, and address behavioral issues such as eating disorders, tobacco use, alcohol and drug use, motor vehicle safety, physical fitness, early sexual activity and safe sex, prevention of sexually transmitted infections (STIs), violence/abuse, date rape, mood swings/depression, and school performance.[1–4]

Many women equate a visit to the gynecologist with a speculum examination and Pap smear. In the adolescent population, a speculum examination is rarely required. An external genital examination should be performed for the purpose of patient education or when indicated by the medical history, such as pubertal aberrancy, abnormal bleeding, vaginal discharge, or vulvar irritation. If the patient has had sexual intercourse, screening for STIs is appropriate and important, and may be accomplished by collecting urine or vaginal swabs for gonorrhea and chlamydia nucleic acid amplification testing (NAAT), as well as by endocervical specimen collection.[5] Young women should have their first Pap test at age 21, unless they are immunocompromised (ie, HIV-positive or an organ transplant recipient) and sexually active. In this circumstance, the initial Pap test is done following the onset of sexual activity, repeated at 6 months, and thereafter at 1-year intervals.[6]

The initial reproductive health examination presents an invaluable opportunity to educate an adolescent about her personal genital anatomy. If the teen is amenable, offer her a hand-held mirror to enable her to follow the examination, learn the correct medical terms, and empower her to ask questions about her anatomy. While positioned upright with her head elevated and her feet in stirrups, the patient is directed to inspect her perineum while the examiner reviews the names and locations of her mons, labia majora, labia minora, clitoris, urethral orifice, hymen, vagina, and rectum. Furthermore, this provides a valuable opportunity to discuss hygiene with the patient, specifically cleaning accumulated secretions and exfoliated skin between the folds of the labia majora and minora and wiping front to back after voiding to prevent contamination of the urethra or vagina with fecal pathogens and subsequent development of vulvovaginitis or urinary tract infections.

If a speculum examination is necessary, use an instrument appropriate in size for an adolescent. The standard Graves speculum is too wide for young teens and the shorter 3-inch speculum is rarely useful because of its inadequate length. A Huffman speculum (½ in × 4 ¼ in) or slightly larger Pederson speculum (⅞ in × 4 ½ in) can be used to visualize the vagina and cervix. Warming the speculum is usually appreciated by patients. The examiner should explain the steps of the examination prior to and during the bimanual or speculum exams. A bimanual examination to evaluate the uterus and ovaries is accomplished by placing one lubricated digit in the vagina and the other hand on the abdomen. If an adolescent declines a vaginal exam, a recto-abdominal exam may yield useful assessment of the uterus, adnexa, or pelvic masses. If a pelvic mass is detected, or if there is concern for pelvic pathology, young patients generally tolerate a non-invasive transabdominal pelvic ultrasound examination of the internal genital structures. Use of intravaginal probes for sonographic evaluation of the pelvis must be individualized.

## HYMEN

The hymen is derived from the junction of the sinovaginal bulbs with the urogenital sinus.[7] There are many variations of normal hymeneal anatomy. The orifice may be central or located just beneath the urethral meatus. Failure of apoptosis may result in multiple small openings, overlying bands or webs of tissue, or hymeneal septum. Anatomic variations of hymeneal anatomy are illustrated in Figure 59-1.

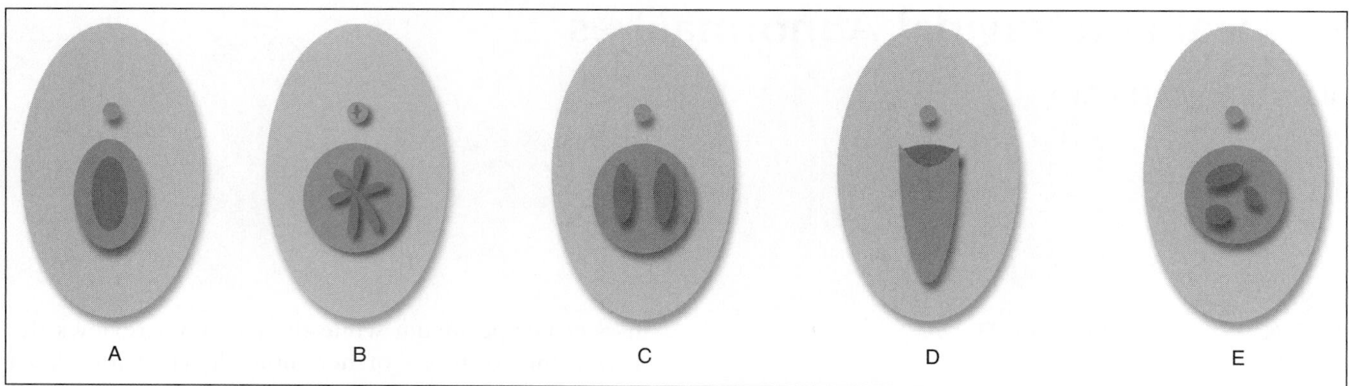


**FIGURE 59-1** Variations of hymenal anatomy. (A) Normal central hymenal orifice; (B) Normal fimbriated hymen; (C) Hymen with midline septum; (D) Thick posterior hymen; (E) Cribiform hymen.

The edges of the hymen in the prepubertal child may be smooth or ruffled (fimbriated), but in the nonestrogenized state the hymen is thin and easily torn if there is blunt forceful penetration that exceeds the ability of the hymen to stretch. The effect of estrogen at puberty is dramatic; the hymen changes to a pale pinker color and the tissue becomes thickened and moist as well as more elastic.

Some variations of hymeneal anatomy may make placement of a tampon or first coitus painful, difficult, or impossible. The patient with a cribriform hymen, thick posterior hymen, or hymeneal septum may require surgical revision to enable use of tampons or vaginal intercourse. The American College of Obstetricians and Gynecologists (ACOG) Committee on Adolescent Health recommends that the first gynecologic visit occur at age 13 to 15.[1,3] When an external genital examination is performed at this time, variations in hymeneal anatomy can be detected and discussed. Some adolescents who need instruction in the placement of a tampon can be given a demonstration during their own external genital examination while they are able to watch or using a pelvic model. Adolescents should be reminded that tampons should be changed every 4 to 6 hours to prevent toxic shock syndrome (TSS), a rare but dangerous condition that can develop when women use highly absorbent tampons inappropriate for their flow or do not change their tampon for extended periods of time.[8] Symptoms include fever, extensive rash resembling a sunburn, vomiting, diarrhea, myalgia, and hypotension. Toxic shock syndrome is treated with IV antibiotics and fluids with electrolytes and can be prevented by using tampons with the correct absorption for the patient's flow, changing tampons on a frequent basis, and using pads at night. Once a patient is treated for TSS due to superabsorbent or prolonged tampon use, there are no official guidelines or recommendations on future use of tampons by the Centers for Disease Control, according to the Chief of the Prevention and Response Branch Division of Health Quality Promotion (L. Clifford McDonald, MD, FACP, personal communication, July 2010).

The hymen may have variable configurations, including a septum that makes tampon placement and intercourse difficult. Sometimes it is difficult to determine if the patient has a hymeneal septum or longitudinal vaginal septum. If a moistened cotton swab is placed inside the vagina and it is easily visible through the other openings, the patient has a hymeneal septum. If the cotton swab seems to disappear into the vagina and cannot be seen from the other opening(s), a longitudinal vaginal septum should be considered (see Figure 59-2). A longitudinal vaginal septum is usually associated with uterine didelphis. A transverse vaginal septum may be complete or perforate.

Patients with an imperforate hymen who have begun to menstruate may present with normal secondary sexual development and amenorrhea due to the obstructed outflow. The menstrual fluid may collect, causing a hematometria (uterus), hematocolpos (vagina), and hematosalpinges (fallopian tubes). These teens may have cyclic lower abdominal pain, back pain, urinary retention, and constipation or tenesmus. Pelvic endometriosis is associated with obstruction of menstrual flow. The obstructed hymen appears as a bulging blue membrane in the "classic presentation" of imperforate hymen. This bulging membrane will distend further with Valsalva maneuvers (straining). If this bulging membrane is not seen, the clinician must consider other possible diagnoses such as a transverse vaginal septum or vaginal agenesis, or cervical agenesis (Figure 59-3). A rectal examination is helpful if a bulging mass can be appreciated. This enables the examiner to determine if a hematocolpos is present and distance to the perineum.

If an imperforate hymen is diagnosed, the patient will need surgical excision of the hymen to give the accumulated menstrual fluid a proper outlet. A central portion

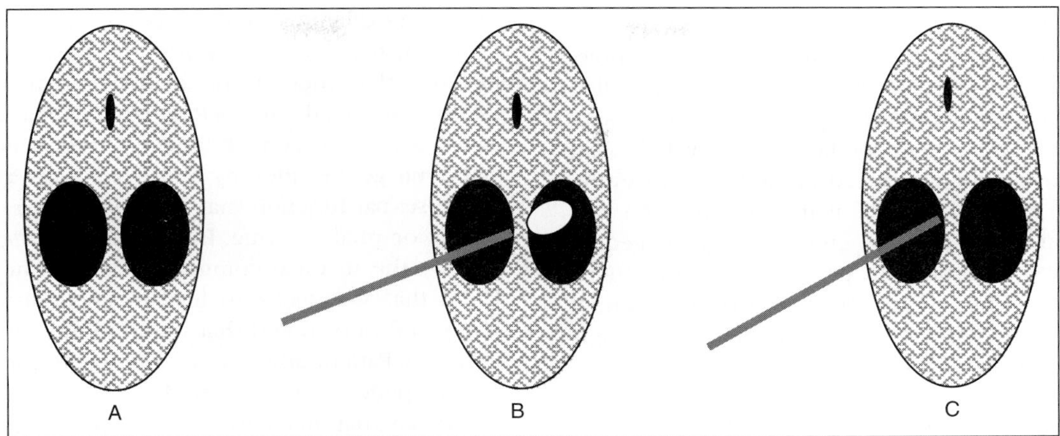


**FIGURE 59-2** How to determine if a septum is at the hymen or extends the length of the vagina (A). Place a moistened cotton swab through 1 of the hymeneal orifices. (B) If easily visible through the second opening, the septum is at the hymen. (C) If unable to see the cotton swab, a longitudinal vaginal septum is likely.

of the hymen is resected, taking care to avoid the urethra, and allowing menstrual fluid collection to drain. The surgical goal is to drain the menstrual fluid and create a permanent outflow tract that will not stenose.

## VULVA

In approaching the initial adolescent gynecologic examinaton it is important to begin with examining the external appearance of the genitalia. Appreciation of the many variations of normal labial anatomy and the changes the labia undergo with the onset of puberty is essential, and reassuring young women regarding their own anatomy is often necessary. Furthermore, it is also important to be conscious of the popular practice of body modification, specifically genital piercing, tattoos, and the increasing trend of pubic hair styling, particularly total pubic hair removal, and its implications for genital health in the adolescent population. Folliculitis, abscesses, and methicillin-resistant *Staphylococcus aureus* (MRSA) infections are seen as consequences of razor burn and ingrown hairs associated with pubic hair shaving.

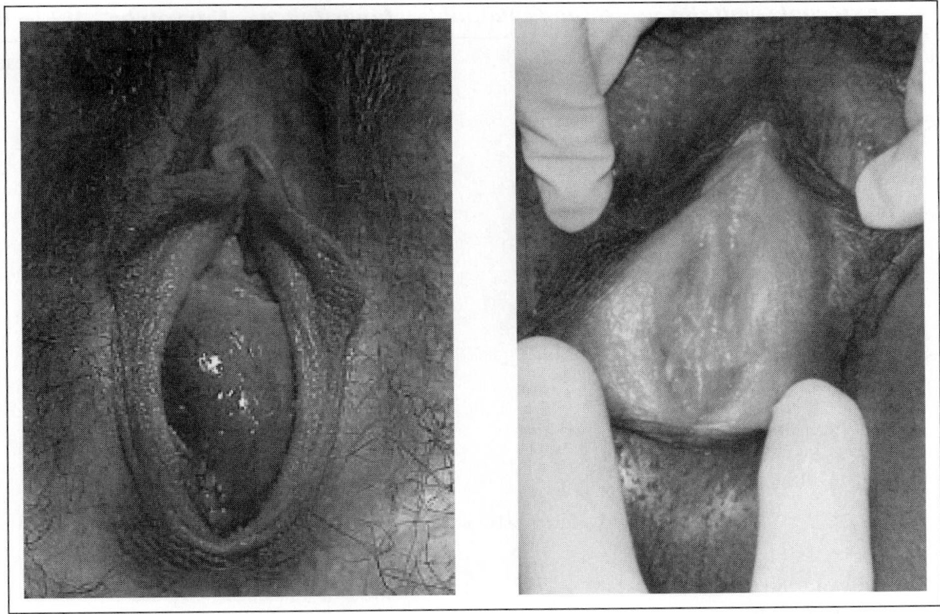

**FIGURE 59-3** Imperforate hymen vs vaginal agenesis. (Photographs courtesy of Diane F. Merritt, MD.) (See color insert.)

## ANOMALIES OF THE VULVA

Major vulvar anomalies that present in infancy as ambiguous genitalia may signal life-threatening disorders like salt-wasting congenital adrenal hyperplasia. In these special cases there are urgent medical and psychological issues that need to be addressed immediately. In evaluating children with ambiguous genitalia it is important to involve a medical team of endocrinologists, geneticists, urologists, gynecologists, psychologists, and social services. The parents should be told that the genital development is incomplete and that additional testing is necessary to determine the baby's sex.[9,10]

## AMBIGUOUS GENITALIA

Female fetuses exposed to androgens in utero will have ambiguous genitalia at birth (Table 59-1). The spectrum of appearance may range from complete fusion of the labioscrotal folds and a phallic urethra, to clitoromegaly and partial fusion of the labioscrotal folds, to normal genitalia at birth with early pubic hair or clitoromegaly in childhood.[9,11] Whenever there appears to be labioscrotal fusion or clitoral enlargement, a referral to an experienced pediatric specialist (endocrinologist and pediatric gynecologist or urologist) is appropriate. Children with intersex disorders (1 per 2,000 live births) present an interesting dilemma as there is controversy about genital reconstructive surgery. It is the position of intersex societies that there is no evidence that a feminizing genitoplasty leads to better psychological outcomes than leaving the genitals intact. There is no guarantee that adult gender identity will develop as assigned, and future sexual function may be altered by removing the clitoris or phallic tissue. In the past, intersex was handled by the medical community as a pathological condition that was likely to lead to great distress for the family and person and that required immediate medical attention. Patient advocate groups are hoping to shift to a more patient-centered model where intersex is considered an anatomical variation from the "standard" male and female types; just as skin and hair color vary along a wide spectrum. In this model, gender assignment is neither a medical emergency nor social pathology.[10]

## HYPERTROPHY OF THE LABIA MINORA

With the onset of puberty the labia minora begin to thicken and elongate under the influence of steroid hormones. Although most young women can be reassured that this is a normal pubertal change, for some girls this growth is unexpected and bothersome. At the time of the initial genital examination, it is useful to reassure

**Table 59-1**

**Differential Diagnosis of Ambiguous Genitalia**

| *Syndrome* | *External Genitalia* | *Gonads Palpable* | *Inheritance* | *Karyotype* | *Müllerian Structures* |
|---|---|---|---|---|---|
| Congenital adrenal hyperplasia | Labioscrotal fusion + clitoromegaly | – | Autosomal recessive | XX or XY | XX present; XY absent |
| Complete androgen insensitivity | Female | +/– | X-linked recessive | XY | Absent |
| Incomplete androgen insensitivity | Labioscrotal fusion + clitoromegaly | +/– | X-linked recessive | XY | Absent |
| 5-alpha reductase deficiency | Female, masculinized at puberty | + | | XY | Absent |
| Leydig cell agenesis or hCG/LH receptor defect | Labioscrotal fusion + clitoromegaly | +/– | | XY | Absent |
| Aromatase deficiency | Labioscrotal fusion + clitoromegaly | – | | XY | Absent |
| XY gonadal dysgenesis | | +/– streak | | XY | Present |
| Elevated maternal androgens | Labioscrotal fusion + clitoromegaly | – | Unrelated | XX | Present |

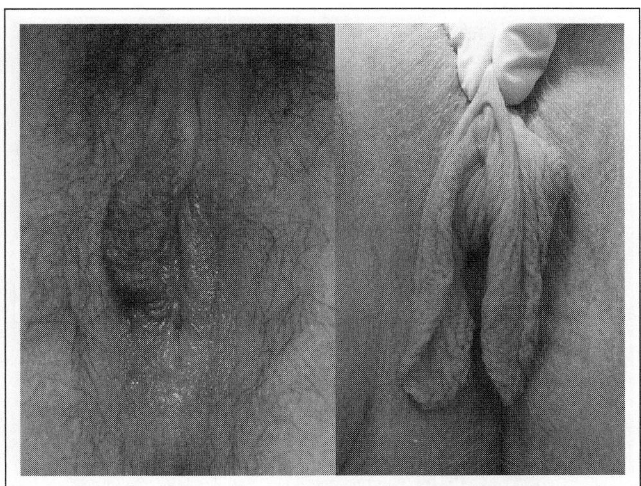

FIGURE 59-4 Normal labial variant (asymmetry) vs labia that required surgery. (Photos courtesy Diane F. Merritt, MD.) (See color insert.)

teens that the labia minora mature during puberty, and growth of these structures is normal. Although labial symmetry is usual, asymmetry is a common normal variant. It is appropriate to reassure the teen that asymmetric labia minora require no surgical intervention. Sometimes the disparity between the sizes of asymmetric labia distresses a teen, who may even request plastic surgical correction. Subjective complaints may include local irritation, discomfort while walking, running, or sitting, difficulties with personal genital hygiene, dyspareunia, and aesthetic concerns about the asymmetry or size of the labia. There are no established criteria for plastic surgery involving the labia. Teens may be more focused on this area because they are beginning to use tampons and sanitary supplies, and because of the current fashion of pubic hair removal. ACOG does not support aesthetic surgery of the genital area because of the risks of infection, loss of innervation, and lack of outcome data to support such surgery. Medically indicated surgical procedures may include reversal or repair of genital cutting or treatment of medically significant labial hypertrophy (Figure 59-4).[12]

### GENITAL PIERCING, TATTOOING, AND PUBIC HAIR STYLING

The practice of tattooing and genital piercing has dedicated Web sites that teens may access. If the clitoral hood and/or the labia minora are pierced, these sites may take as long as 6 to 8 weeks to heal. Women with genital piercing may develop bleeding, infection, allergic reactions, keloids, and scarring. Sexually active persons with genital piercings should be counseled that jewelry may compromise the use of barrier contraception, causing condoms or diaphragms to break or become dislodged during sex.[13] Tattooing can result in hypersensitivity reactions and local skin infections.[13,14] Pubic hair can be removed by shaving, depilation, and waxing or laser therapy. Young athletes, dancers, and swimmers often remove pubic hair that may show at the bikini line. Bikini waxing is often practiced by adolescents, and recently total pubic hair removal by shaving has gained in popularity. Skin infections from ingrown hairs and folliculitis are common complications of this practice, and may lead to abscesses and MRSA infections.

### NON SEXUAL GENITAL ULCERS

Acute non sexually-related genital ulcers are very painful, single or multiple lesions, and can be up to a centimeter in diameter or larger. They usually begin as painful red areas, develop into an ulcer with sharply demarcated edges and a purulent or necrotic base, and usually present associated with systemic viral symptoms and painful urination. A thorough sexual history should be taken to rule out any STI, but the lesions do not resemble herpetic infections, and if obtained, herpes simplex virus (HSV) cultures will be negative. If the patient cannot urinate due to pain or swelling, admission to the hospital and placement of a Foley catheter are necessary to avoid urinary retention.[15] Acute genital ulcers can be treated with topical anesthetics, pain management, and antibiotics if bacterial infection is present, and generally resolve in about 7 to 14 days. Patients with recurrent genital ulcers should undergo an autoimmune work-up to exclude Behçet disease or inflammatory bowel disorders.

### TUMORS OF THE VULVA

Most of the tumors of the vulva are related to the epidermis or other epidermal appendages as listed in Box 59-1. They are often slow-growing and asymptomatic. Excision of these lesions is based on symptoms. Painful enlargement of the Bartholin glands may require surgical drainage or marsupialization.

## VAGINA

### VAGINAL ANOMALIES

Vaginal anomalies include transverse and longitudinal septa, obstruction of a hemi-vagina, and partial or complete agenesis. Patients with vaginal anomalies often present in adolescence with a variety of complaints related to menstruation, commonly cyclical abdominal pain with or without vaginal bleeding, or primary amenorrhea.

**Box 59-1**

***Vulvar Tumors***

- Acrochordon (fibroepithelial polyp)
- Angiokeratoma
- Bartholin and Skene duct cysts
- Endometriosis
- Epidermal inclusion cysts
- Fibroma, fibromyoma, dermatofibroma
- Hidradenoma
- Hemangioma
- Lipoma
- Lymphangioma
- Mucous cysts
- Myxoma
- Neuroma
- Papillomatosis
- Pyogeneic granuloma
- Sebaceous glands
- Sebaceous gland hyperplasia
- Seborrheic keratosis

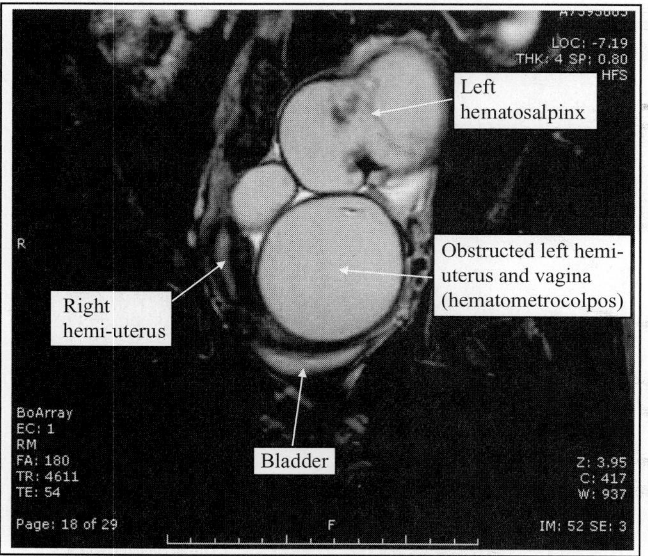


**FIGURE 59-5** Uterine duplication disorder with normal right uterus and vagina, and left hematometrocolpos, left hematosalpinx.

A transverse vaginal septum is 1 of the least common Müllerian duct anomalies, occurring with a frequency of 1 case in 70,000 females. The transverse vaginal septum results from failure of fusion or canalization of the urogenital sinus and Müllerian duct derivatives. A transverse vaginal septum can divide the vagina into 2 segments and result in a shortened functional vagina. Most are located in the upper vagina (46%), followed by the middle vagina (40%), and the inferior vagina (14%).[16] The septum can be perforate or imperforate. If the septum is perforate, the patient may menstruate normally or retain menstrual fluid with a resulting persistent brown drainage following menses. If imperforate, the patient may develop a hematocolpos and a symptomatic pelvic mass. If the septum is low, a tampon may not fit comfortably. Such patients are best diagnosed by ultrasound or magnetic resonance imaging (MRI). Surgical correction necessitates full resection of the transverse septum and may require preoperative dilation of the distal vagina to minimize the amount of tissue to be resected and decrease the need for a graft to bridge the distance from the upper to lower vagina. Such procedures should be carried out by a gynecologist surgeon with expertise in Müllerian anomalies to avoid complications. If there is a high obstruction, an inexperienced surgeon may not be able to locate the hematocolpos, or if incompletely drained, bacteria can multiply in a contaminated hematocolpos and result in sepsis. Morbidities, including sepsis and death, have been reported in failed attempts to properly maintain a surgically created patient outflow tract.[17,18]

A longitudinal vaginal septum is usually associated with a uterine duplication disorder (didelphic uterus) (Figure 59-5). Patients with this anomaly may present complaining that a single tampon does not provide adequate hygiene, or may have dyspareunia or sustain a traumatic laceration with coitus. Once the anomaly is diagnosed and explained, some patients with this condition will be able to place 2 tampons, 1 in each vagina, during their period. Removal of the longitudinal septum may be offered to women who have persistent dyspareunia or other difficulties.[10] Outlet obstruction of a hemivagina is frequently associated with renal agenesis on the ipsilateral side. Because the contralateral vagina is patent, the patient may present with normal menses, which become increasingly painful. The patient may present with presence of a mass bulging into the vagina, or urinary obstruction. Surgical correction is accomplished by resecting as much vaginal septum as possible to allow drainage of the obstructed uterus and vagina.[19] Figure 59-6 illustrates normal and abnormal uterine anatomy.

Vaginal and uterine agenesis (Mayer Rokitanasky Küser Hauser [MRKH] syndrome) occurs once in every 4,000 to 5,000 births.[16] Vaginal agenesis is second to gonadal dysgenesis as a case of primary amenorrhea. The patient usually presents with normal secondary

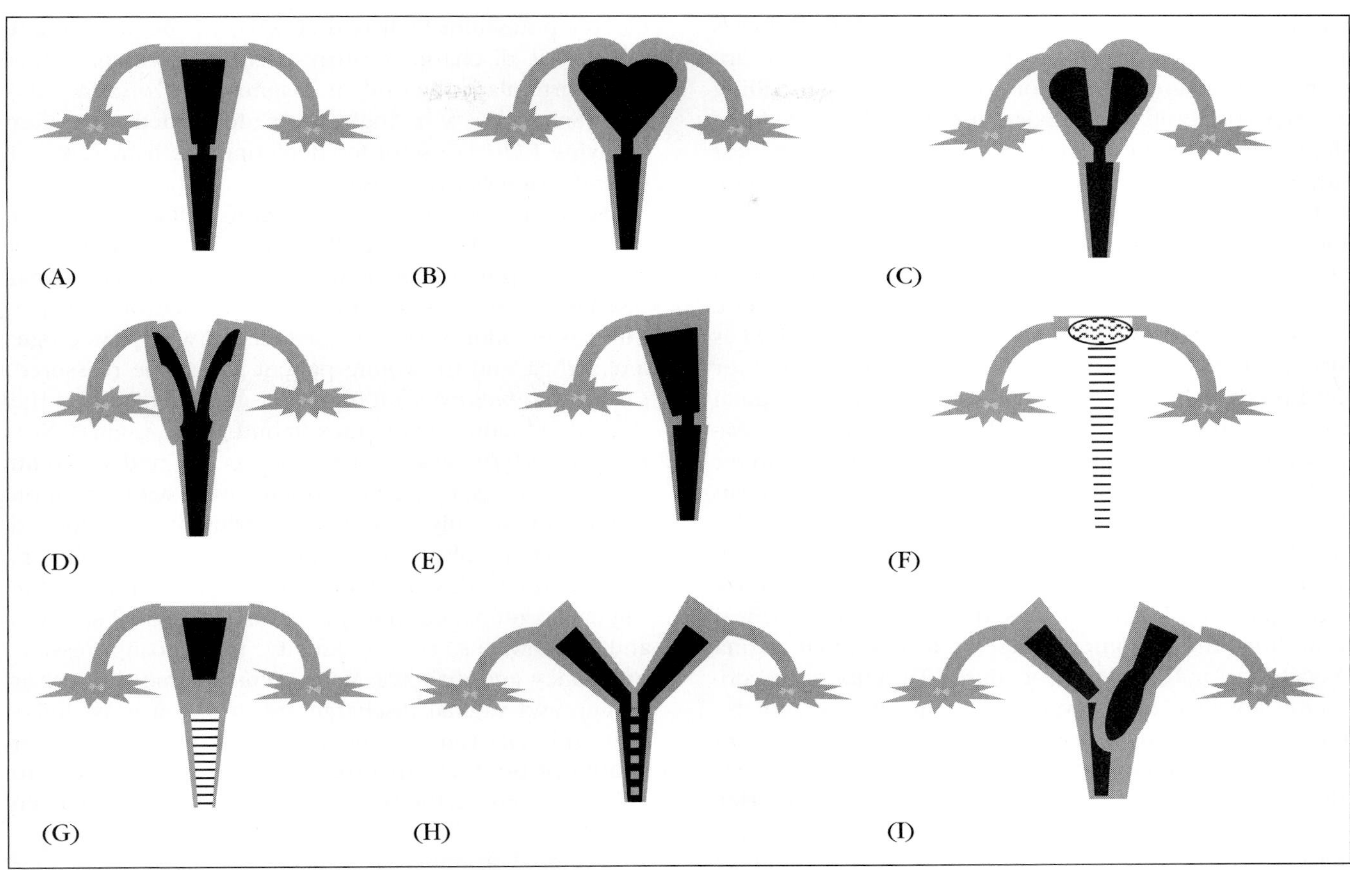


**FIGURE 59-6** Normal and abnormal uterine anatomy. (A) Normal uterus and vagina; (B) Arcuate uterus; (C) Septate uterus; (D) Bicornuate uterus; (E) Unicornuate uterus; (F) Agenesis of uterus and vagina; (G) Cervico-vaginal agenesis; (H) Didelphic uterus with or without longitudinal vaginal septum; (I) Didelphic uterus with obstructed hemivagina.

sexual development because the ovarian steroid production is normal. When there is rudimentary uterine development, the patient may present with cyclic pain if there is any endometrial proliferation. The MRKH syndrome is often associated with renal, skeletal, and otic anomalies. The precise genetic cause for this condition is yet to be determined, but several genetic mutations are being considered. Counseling patients with congenital anomalies of the reproductive tract requires that the clinician be sensitive, tactful, compassionate, knowledgeable, and professional. The patient and her family deserve a thorough and clear explanation. While patient autonomy is to be preserved, a sensitive and experienced clinician should deliver this diagnosis and implications for future fertility in digestible pieces, and in language that the patient and family can understand, with sufficient time available for questions. When this diagnosis is made in a young child or teen, the parents or guardians can be informed privately and prior to discussions with the patient. Once the parents have had the opportunity to be informed and understand the diagnosis and implications for future fertility, they may be in the best position to be supportive as their daughter is informed by her medical professional. Supportive family members should be included in this discussion with the patient's permission. Each patient should be reassured that she has normal ovaries, and normal female hormones. She will be able, if and when she chooses, to lead a sexually fulfilling life and parent children. When the patient is able to participate in the use of vaginal dilators to create a neovagina, this is a good nonsurgical option. It is important to note that the patient must be motivated to adhere to the daily regimen of dilation and familiar with her own anatomy before beginning. Patients should be seen regularly, and progress should be assessed with the gradual increase in size of the dilators until a neovagina adequate for most sexual practices is achieved, usually over the course of 2 to 4 weeks. Occasionally a patient requires a surgical procedure to create a neovagina. There are many options for the surgeon to implement depending on expertise, and there exists a debate if procedures should be done in infancy or after puberty. The best surgical results occur with the initial procedure, limiting subsequent surgeries and the chance for infection and scarring. A McIndoe vaginoplasty involves creation of a neovaginal space and the insertion of a custom vaginal mold covered with a split-thickness skin graft. The mold is removed after 1 week, and the patient is instructed to use a soft rubber mold for 6 weeks or until the incisions have healed successfully.[16,20] Vaginal dilators will need to be placed to maintain the neovagina until the graft has matured. Many clinicians prefer to defer creation of a neovagina until the young woman is ready to become sexually active, to decrease the likelihood of stenosis of the neovagina. Other surgical options include transposition of intestinal segments, and laparoscopic procedures that draw the perineal tissue into the abdomen to create a functional vagina (Vecchietti or Davydov procedure). Patients with congenital absence of the vagina and uterus will not be able to become pregnant, but they can, through assisted reproductive technology, have their eggs harvested, fertilized, and implanted into a willing gestational carrier. Research on the long-term outcomes of women with neovaginas is needed to determine if sexual function and satisfaction are best served by different options of surgical creation or dilator therapy. Assisted reproductive technologies offer an alternative to parent children. To date, the children of these women do not seem to have a greater risk than the general population for Müllerian anomalies.[21]

## VAGINAL INFECTIONS

Measurement of vaginal pH is the most important finding when diagnosing a vaginal infection. Under the influence of estrogen, the normal vaginal epithelium cornifies and produces glycogen, which acts as a substrate for lactobacilli. These bacteria produce hydrogen peroxide and lactic acid, maintaining the normally acidic vaginal pH. This acidic environment is protective against infection from a number of pathogens. Vaginal pH may be altered (usually to a higher pH) by contamination with lubricating gels, semen, douches, and intravaginal medications. Saline microscopy should be performed to look for candidal buds or hyphae, motile trichomonads, epithelial cells studded with adherent coccobacilli (clue cells), and polymorphonuclear cells (PMNs). The saline should be at room temperature and microscopy should be performed within 10 to 20 minutes of obtaining the sample to reduce the possibility of loss of motility of any trichomonads. The addition of 10% potassium hydroxide (KOH) to the wet mount of vaginal discharge destroys cellular elements, thus it is particularly helpful in diagnosing *Candida* vaginitis. Smelling ("whiffing") the slide immediately after applying KOH is useful for detecting the fishy (amine) odor of bacterial vaginosis.

Some prepubertal and pubertal adolescents may become concerned by a clear, mucous discharge. This is actually physiologic leukorrhea, the normal vaginal discharge that occurs under the influence of estrogen. There is no odor or irritation associated with physiologic leukorrhea, and the young patient should be reassured. *Candida albicans* is a fungus that normally lives on the skin and mucous membranes (mouth, nose, vagina). Normally, *Candida* causes no symptoms but under certain clinical settings, may cause itching, pain with urination or intercourse, vulvar soreness or irritation, or reddened and swollen vulvar and vaginal tissues. Risk factors include antibiotics that alter the bacterial flora of the vagina, hormonal contraceptives, use of vaginal sponges and diaphragms, sexual activity, immunosuppression, pregnancy, and diabetes. Many teens assume that vulvar itching and vaginal discharge are due to a yeast infection and self-diagnose and treat with over-the-counter antifungal products. Incorrect self-diagnosis can lead to delay in receiving the proper treatment and may worsen symptoms.

Bacterial vaginosis is usually associated with poor hygiene and the presence of fecal pathogens in the vagina. The vaginal pH will be elevated, and clue cells in the absence of lactobacilli can be seen on a vaginal wet mount. Sexually transmitted infections may present as vulvovaginal irritation. Trichomonads may be diagnosed by an elevated vaginal pH and seen on microscopic evaluation. Contact and allergic vaginitis can result from use of perfumed soaps, bubble baths, perfumed feminine hygiene products, and self-treatment with topical agents for itching. Screening questions should reference hygiene practices (type of soap used, direction of wiping motion employed). Patients should be encouraged to eliminate perfumed soaps and bubble baths. If the adolescent has poor hygiene, she should be reminded to cleanse between the folds of the labia when bathing, wipe only front to back after bowel movements and urination, and if problems persist, use wet wipes after bowel movements. The clinical examination should include an external inspection of the perineal area, including the vaginal introitus via lateral traction of the labia majora. Table 59-2 describes the clinical diagnosis of vaginal discharge.

## VAGINAL FOREIGN BODIES

The most common foreign body found in the adolescent's vagina is the forgotten tampon or portion of

**Table 59-2**

**Clinical Diagnosis of Vaginal Discharge**

| *Clinical Setting* | *pH* | *Findings* | *Saline Microscopy* |
|---|---|---|---|
| Normal prepubertal girl or postmenopausal woman | 4.7 or more | Scant vaginal discharge | Parabasal cells, scant WBC, and bacteria |
| Normal reproductive age adolescent and woman | 4.0–4.5 | Normal vaginal discharge consists of 1 to 3 mL fluid (per 24 hours), which is white or transparent, thick, and mostly odorless | Abundant lactobacilli (rods) and squamous cells |
| *Candida vaginitis* | 4.0–4.5 | Pruritis, soreness, change in discharge, dyspareunia, valvular erythema, edema, fissure | Pseudohyphae and budding yeast; addition of 10% KOH will allow the hyphae to be seen more easily |
| Trichomonas | 5.0–6.0 | Malodorous, purulent discharge, dyspareunia | Motile trichomonads; if microscopy negative, perform culture or rapid antigenucleic acid amplification tests |
| Bacterial vaginosis | Above 4.5 | Malodorous discharge, addition of 10% KOH = + whiff test | Loss of rods; increased coccobacilli; clue cells (<90%) |

a condom that broke or slipped off as the penis was removed. Patients with retained tampons will present with a foul-smelling discharge and are at risk for TSS. Prompt removal is necessary, and often requires placement of a speculum to visualize the object, which can be grasped with a uterine dressing forceps or sponge stick and drawn into an examination glove to minimize the odor associated with the bacterial overgrowth. Individuals who are mentally ill may place objects out of curiosity. "Body packing" of latex condoms or plastic bags of illicit drugs for trafficking may have devastating outcomes if the containers rupture, leading to vaginal absorption and a drug overdose. Foreign objects may be introduced for sexual stimulation, and become lodged and difficult to remove. The patient may be reluctant to disclose her true story and may have tried many times to personally remove the object without success. This leads to a delay in the diagnosis and the patient may present complaining of a vaginal discharge, bleeding, or pain. Blunt objects can be grasped and removed as the patient bears down. Intravenous sedation or general anesthesia may be need to enable the patient to relax and provide better exposure and visualization. Sharp objects should not be grasped blindly, but removed under direct visualization to limit injury to the vaginal walls and adjacent bladder and rectum.

## GENITAL TRAUMA

### STRADDLE INJURIES

Vulvar trauma usually occurs as the result of straddle injuries. A straddle injury can result from falling upon the frame of a bicycle, climbing a fence, playground equipment, or piece of furniture, entering or exiting a swimming pool (especially above-ground pools) or bathtub. The soft tissues of the vulva are compressed between the object and the pubic symphysis and pubic rami. Nonpenetrating injuries usually involve the mons, clitoris, and labia, and they often result in hematomas, linear lacerations, and abrasions. If the clinician is unable to fully assess or repair the injuries in a conscious patient, an examination under anesthesia is indicated.[22]

Vulvar hematomas can be very painful and may prevent an adolescent from urinating because of pain and swelling. If the hematoma is not large, and the perineal anatomy is not distorted, and the patient has no difficulty emptying her bladder, manage the patient with immediate application of ice packs and bed rest. If the adolescent has a large vulvar hematoma and is unable to void, place an indwelling urinary catheter, and continue bladder drainage until the swelling resolves.

Very large vulvar hematomas that distort the vulvar anatomy may dissect into the loose areolar tissue along the vaginal wall and along the fascial planes overlying the symphysis pubis and lower abdominal wall. Pressure from an expanding hematoma can cause necrosis of the skin overlying the hematoma. Evacuate the hematoma to reduce pain, hasten recovery, and prevent necrosis, tissue loss, and secondary infection. Incise large vulvar hematomas at the medial mucosal surface near the vaginal orifice. Debride the wound of all devitalized tissue. In an attempt to shorten the patient's convalescence, ligate bleeding vessels and place absorbable mattress sutures to control bleeding. Place a closed system drain, which prevents reaccumulation of blood to reduce pain and reduce the risk of bacterial growth.[22]

## VAGINAL INJURIES

### Coital-Related Vaginal Injuries

Although the vagina can be injured accidentally, clinicians should suspect consensual intercourse or sexual assault when an adolescent presents with vaginal trauma. Predisposing factors for coital injury include initial coitus, resumption of intercourse after a long abstinence, congenital anomalies of the vagina, unusual coital positions that permit deep penetration, concomitant inebriation or drug use by either partner, brutality, violence, and use of a foreign object. The patient may feel uncomfortable explaining her injuries, and initially she may offer a misleading clinical history. Failure to perform a proper pelvic examination to evaluate vaginal bleeding will compound the error and lead to a delay in diagnosis and treatment.

Adolescents who sustain vaginal lacerations from coitus may present with sharp vaginal pain, profuse or prolonged vaginal bleeding, and shock. Because digital vaginal examination is inadequate to assess injuries of this nature, the clinician must inspect the vagina with a speculum. The most frequent types and sites of injury in rape victims include tears and abrasions of the posterior fourchette, tears and abrasions of the labia minora, tears of the fossa navicularis, and lacerations and ecchymosis of the hymen. Minor lacerations of the introitus and lower vagina also can occur with initial coitus.

Minor lacerations can be repaired under local anesthesia. Vaginal wall injuries can be managed with vaginal packing until a more definitive repair can be done. Adolescents who are subjected to blunt, penetrating, forceful trauma usually sustain lacerations in the posterior aspect of the hymen. Deep lacerations must be evaluated and treated under general anesthesia. Lateral vaginal wall and posterior fornix lacerations can occur. In serious cases, the cervix may be avulsed from its attachment to the vagina, and the penis or other object being thrust into the vagina may enter the peritoneal cavity. The bowel, omentum, or fallopian tubes may eviscerate through the laceration. These patients present with vaginal bleeding and may be at risk of morbidity or death from exsanguination.

### Noncoital-Related Vaginal Injuries

Crush injuries resulting from motor vehicle crashes and falls can produce pelvic fractures. As a result, sharp spicules of bone may penetrate the vagina and lower urinary tract. Accidental penetrating injuries can affect the vagina if a patient falls on a pointed object. Resultant injuries include lacerations of the fourchette, hymen, and vagina or rectum.

There also are reports of high-pressure insufflation injuries that resulted when females fell off jet skis and water skis, slid down water slides, and came in direct contact with pool or spa jets.[23-25] As pressurized water enters the vagina, the walls may overdistend and tear. These patients will present with vaginal bleeding. Such injuries may produce no sign of external trauma, and only careful vaginal examination (often under anesthesia) will reveal the true extent of injury and cause of bleeding. Counsel patients who participate in water sports that they can prevent vaginal injuries by using protective clothing such as wet suits or cutoff jeans while water or jet skiing, and by keeping their feet together when entering the water on a slide.

### Assessing Vaginal Injuries

If you determine that an adolescent's injury extends above the hymen but you cannot assess the true extent of the injury or repair it, you must perform a complete examination under general anesthesia. Every hospital should have a defined protocol for collection of forensic evidence in cases of alleged sexual assault. It is important to provide a clear description of the injuries and maintain the chain of evidence until collected by legal authorities.

If a Huffman or Pederson vaginal speculum is too large for a young adolescent, use a cystoscope and saline irrigation to visualize the vagina and determine the extent of vaginal injuries. Gently hold the labia together to distend the vagina with saline and facilitate careful inspection.

### Repairing Vaginal Injuries

The importance of using a suitable light source and proper positioning, and obtaining her complete cooperation (which may require sedation or anesthesia) cannot be overemphasized. Perforations into the peritoneal cavity mandate an exploratory laparotomy or laparoscopy to determine if other structures, such as the bowel or blood vessels, have been injured. In the young adolescent who has a small-caliber vagina, begin repair of lacerations with the deepest (most distal from the introitus) vaginal injuries first, and end repair with introital lacerations to allow for maximum working space and visualization. Postoperative application of topical estrogen cream to injuries of the mucosal surfaces of the vagina and introitus may decrease formation of granulation tissue and promote healing without stricture.

### URETHRAL INJURIES

In contrast to the urethra in the male, the female urethra is short, not rigidly fixed on the pelvic floor, and usually protected from injury. High-speed motor vehicle crashes are the most common scenario in which pelvic fractures and deceleration injuries lead to bladder and urethral trauma in the adolescent. Indicators of urethral disruption are blood at the introitus or urethral meatus, inability to void in a conscious patient, and gross hematuria.

Primary repair of the urethral injury is preferable to delayed repair and should be performed by a clinician with urologist expertise. Failure to promptly diagnose and properly repair urethral injuries may result in urinary incontinence, urethral stricture, and vesicovaginal or urethrovaginal fistulas. A prompt cystoscopic evaluation for partial urethral injury is in order for a patient who experiences difficulty with voiding or develops vulvar edema (due to extravasation of urine) after removal of a urinary drainage catheter following pelvic fracture.[22]

### GENITAL BURNS

Because the perineum is hidden between the thighs, it is generally protected from burn injuries. When they occur, burns of the female genitalia and perineum are most likely to be associated with extensive burns involving one-third to one-half of the total body surface area, which carry a 30% to 70% mortality rate. The most common burn in adults is by flame, whereas children usually are scalded by liquids or immersion. The management of genital and perineal burns includes short-term urinary diversion for comfort and hygiene, topical application of antimicrobials (silver sulphadiazine), and skin grafting, which is used only for full-thickness loss. In cases of perineal burns, contractures can be prevented with use of thigh abduction, hip exercises, early ambulation, and pressure garments. Scarring as a result of perineal burns affects skin texture, pigmentation, and pliability. The ability of a patient who has sustained burns to maintain hygiene with micturition and defecation may be compromised and can have a devastating effect on sexuality and body image.

## PSYCHOLOGICAL FACTORS

The ability to bear children and have sexual relations in the future is a topic that should specifically be addressed with adolescents who have had genital injuries. When appropriate, offer reassurance of reproductive capacity, as these concerns will not always be verbalized by a patient or her family members. Adolescents who have sustained sexual assault may suffer from sleep disturbances, nightmares, flashbacks, anxiety, and anger. Depression is common, and often is compounded by feelings of guilt and shame. Offer specific referrals for professional counseling to those who have been sexually assaulted.

## CONCLUSIONS

As young girls progress through puberty, many physical changes occur in the perineum, vulva, and vagina. Reassurance about normal pubertal changes should be incorporated into all routine preventive care visits for adolescents. ACOG advocates performing the initial reproductive health visit at ages 13 to 15, and presents a golden opportunity for the provider to educate the patient and answer questions and concerns; and identify health risk behaviors. Adolescent gynecology is a unique specialty that fills an important need in reproductive health. The American Academy of Pediatrics (AAP) has an appointed Committee on Adolescence that addresses the special health care needs of adolescents and promotes the pediatrician as their optimal source of health care. This committee works closely with the Section on Adolescent Health. Subspecialty training in adolescent medicine is available. The ACOG Committee on Adolescent Health Care guides ACOG activities designed to improve adolescent physical, psychological, reproductive, and sexual health and development. This committee also aims to improve access to primary and preventive care, including comprehensive reproductive health care for adolescents of all socioeconomic backgrounds. Fellowships in pediatric and adolescent gynecology are available at several centers. Other professional organizations include the North American Society for Pediatric and Adolescent Gynecology and the Society of Adolescent Health and Medicine. Following the recommendations and clinical guidelines of these committees and professional organizations assures clinical practice standards are of the highest quality.

## INTERNET RESOURCES

- American Academy of Pediatrics: www. aap. org
- American College of Obstetricians and Gynecologists: www. acog. org

- North American Society for Pediatric and Adolescent Gynecology: www. naspag. org
- Society for Adolescent Health and Medicine: www. adolescenthealth. org

## REFERENCES


1. American College of Obstetricians and Gynecologists. Primary and preventive health care for female adolescents. *Tool Kit for Teen Care.* Washington, DC: ACOG; 2009

2. Hewitt GD.The young woman's initial gynecologic visit. *The Female Patient.* 2006;31(9):25–29

3. American College of Obstetricians and Gynecologists. Initial reproductive health visit. Committee Opinion No. 460. *Obstet Gynecol.* 2010;116:240–243

4. Emans SJ. Office evaluation of the child and adolescent. In: Emans SJ, Laufer MR, Goldstein DP, eds. *Pediatric and Adolescent Gynecology*. 5th ed. Philadelphia, PA: Lippincott Williams & Wilkins; 2005

5. The Association of Public Health Laboratories and the Centers for Disease Control and Prevention. Laboratory diagnostic testing for *Chlamydia trachomatis* and *Neisseria gonorrhoeae* expert consultation meeting summary report. January 13–15, 2009. Available at: aphl.org/aphlprograms/infectious/std/documents/ctgclabguideliesmeetingreport.pdf. Accessed June 28, 2010

6. American College of Obstetrics and Gynecology. ACOG Practice Bulletin No. 109: Cervical cytology screening. *Obstet Gynecol.* 2009;114(6):1409–1420

7. Sadler TW. *Langman's Medical Embryology.* 11th edition. Philadelphia, PA: Lippincott Williams & Wilkins; 2010

8. Schuchat A, Broome CV. Toxic shock syndrome and tampons. *Epidemiol Rev.* 1991;13:99–112

9. Holm I. Ambiguous genitalia in the newborn. In: Emans SJ, Laufer MR, Goldstein DP, eds. *Pediatric and Adolescent Gynecology*. 5th ed. Philadelphia, PA:Lippincott Williams & Wilkins; 2005

10. Consortium on the Management of Disorders of Sex Development. *Clinical Guidelines for the Management of Disorders of Sexual Development*. Rohnert Park, CA: Intersex Society of North America; 2006. Available at: www.dsdguidelines.org/files/clinical.pdf. Accessed June 28, 2010

11. Nimkam S, Lin-Su K, New MI. Steroid 21 hydroxylase deficiency congenital adrenal hyperplasia. *Endocrinol Metabol Clin North Am.* 2009;38(4):699–718

12. American College of Obstetricians and Gynecologists. Vaginal "rejuvenation" and cosmetic vaginal procedures. ACOG Committee Opinion No 378. *Obstet Gynecol.* 2007;110:737–738

13. Braverman PK. Body art: piercing, tattooing, and scarification. *Adolesc Med Clinic.* 2006;17:505–519

14. Meltzer DI. Complications of body piercing. *Am Fam Physician.* 2005;72:2029–2034

15. Farhi D, Wendling J, Molinari E. Non sexually related acute genital ulcers in 13 pubertal girls. *Arch Dermatol.* 2009;145(1):38–45

16. Edmonds DK. Congenital malformations of the genital tract and their management. *Best Pract Res Clin Obstet Gynaecol.* 2003 Feb;17(1):19–40

17. Casey AC, Laufer MR. Cervical agenesis: septic death after surgery. *Obstet Gynecol.* 1997;90:706

18. Cooper AR, Merritt DF. Novel use of tracheobronchial stent in a patient with uterine didelphys and obstructed hemivagina. *Fertil Steril.* 2010;93:900–903

19. Smith NA, Laufer MR. Obstructed hemivagina and ipsilateral renal anomaly (OHVIRA) syndrome: management and follow-up. *Fertil Steril.* 2007;87:918–922

20. Laufer MR, Goldstein DP, Hendren WH. Structural abnormalities of the female reproductive tract. In: Emans SJ, Laufer MR, Goldstein DP, eds. *Pediatric and Adolescent Gynecology*. 5th ed. Philadelphia, PA: Lippincott Williams & Wilkins; 2005:386

21. Rackow BW, Arici A. Reproductive performance of women with Müllerian anomalies. *Curr Opin Obstet Gynecol.* 2007;19:229– 237

22. Merritt DF, Rimsza ME, Muram D. Genital injuries in pediatric and adolescent girls. In: Sanfilippo JS, Muram D, Dewhurst J, Lee P, eds. *Pediatric and Adolescent Gynecology*. 2nd ed. Philadelphia, PA: WB Saunders; 2001

23. Niv J, Lessing JB, Hartuv J, et al. Vaginal injury resulting from sliding down a water chute. *Am J Obstet Gynecol.* 1992;166(3):930–931

24. Haefner HK, Anderson F, Johnson MP. Vaginal laceration following a jet-ski accident. *Obstet Gynecol.* 1991;78:986–988

25. Perlman SE, Hertweck SP, Wolfe WM. Water-ski douche injury in a premenarcheal female. *Pediatrics.* 1995;96:782–783

# CHAPTER 60

# Cervical Findings and the Papanicolaou Smear

JUDITH T. BURGIS, MD • JANICE L. BACON, MD

## INTRODUCTION

The uterine cervix sits in a unique position. It is accessible, to the physician for screening and evaluation and to infectious agents that may act locally or set up a well-described spectrum of disease, ranging from local infection to invasive cancer.

## EMBRYOLOGY

The cervix develops from 2 embryonic sites. Most come from the Müllerian ducts, which also serve as the beginning of the uterus and adnexa. The remainder comes from the urogenital sinus, which is also the origin of the lower two-thirds of the vagina. At 16 weeks' gestation, the urogenital plate expands to meet the Müllerian ducts. The cervix then undergoes cavitation. The centrally hollow cervix is lined with columnar epithelium. The urogenital plate is lined with stratified squamous epithelium. Where the 2 meet is an important cytologic landmark, the squamocolumnar junction. The position of the squamocolumnar junction varies in fetal and postnatal life. Its position is influenced by sex steroids. In fact, prenatal exposure to exceptionally high levels of estrogen is believed to be responsible for deformations of the cervix, including the hood and the collar, or the cockscomb abnormality.[1,2]

## ANATOMY AND HISTOLOGY

The cervix is the inferior extension of the uterus. Its name comes from the Latin word for "neck." The lower portion of the cervix extends into the vagina and thus is accessible for examination. The upper portion of the cervix extends from the vaginal fornix to the lower uterine segment. In the nulliparous patient, the cervix makes up 50% of the uterine volume. It is approximately 3 cm in length and 2.5 cm in diameter. The size and shape of the cervix varies with age, parity, and hormonal state. The opening in the cervix, visible in the vagina, is called the external os. The portion exterior to the external os is called the ectocervix. The cervix extends to the uterus via the endocervical canal, ending at the internal cervical os.[1,2]

Blood is supplied from the internal iliac arteries. Cervical and vaginal branches supply the cervix via the uterine artery. Venous drainage parallels the arterial supply. Lymphatic drainage is through the common internal and external iliac nodes, the obturator, and the parametrial nodes. The cervix is supported by parametrial soft tissue and the cardinal and uterosacral ligaments. These attach to the lateral and posterior cervix and extend to the bony pelvis.[2]

Most of the cervix is covered with stratified squamous epithelium, which is pale pink and opaque. As the squamous epithelium matures, the cells enlarge while the nuclei decrease in size. Squamous maturation is influenced by ovarian hormones. Estrogen promotes maturation, glycogenation, and desquamation. Progesterone inhibits superficial maturation. Understanding the influence of ovarian hormones explains the atrophic appearance of the cervix after menopause or after prolonged exposure to progestins, as with progesterone-only contraceptives used by many adolescents.[1-3]

After maturation, there are 4 distinct cell layers: the basal or germinal layer, the parabasal or prickle cell layer, the intermediate or navicular layer, and the superficial or stratum corneum layer. The basal and superficial cells are the easiest to identify.[1]

Columnar epithelium lines the portion of the cervix from the squamocolumnar junction to the lower uterine segment. This comprises the endocervix. This epithelium is also referred to as glandular, and it secretes mucin. The cells are single layer and invaginate, forming crypts and channels. Grossly, this epithelium looks grainy and red when compared with the squamous epithelium.[1]

The squamocolumnar junction is the area where the squamous and the columnar epithelium meet. It is generally located on the ectocervix, although the location varies with age and hormonal status. The cervical transformation zone is an area of squamous metaplasia. In this area, columnar epithelium is replaced with squamous epithelium. Estrogen and increasing acidity are believed to be "triggers" for metaplasia. The transformation zone is important because essentially all cervical neoplasia arises within this area.[2,4]

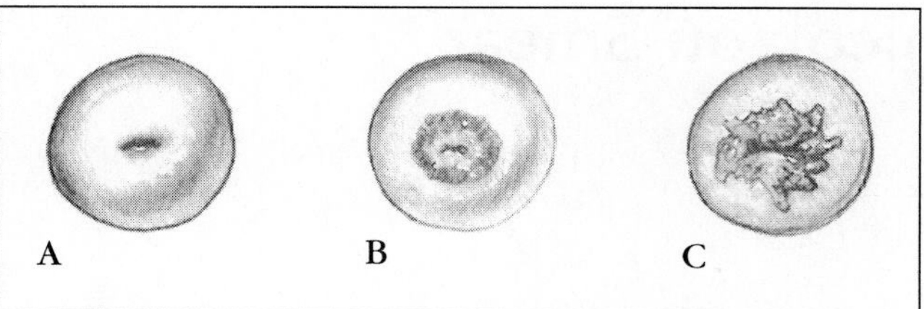


FIGURE 60-1 Appearance of cervix. (A) Normal, nulliparous cervix (B) Ectropion (C) Erosion

The healthy ectocervix is smooth and pink, whereas the columnar epithelium adjacent to the external os is grainy and red. The cervix may be reddened when infected. Infection also is associated with loss of epithelium or erosion. This is frequently seen as bleeding when the cervix is sampled. Cervicitis also is associated with a spotted or "strawberry" appearance of the ectocervix. Chapter 53, Sexually Transmitted Infections, discusses cervicitis. The cervix may have condyloma present. Condyloma appear as flat or bulky warts and represent human papillomavirus (HPV) infection. Cervical intraepithelial neoplasia (CIN) is not visible on routine examination. Endocervical polyps may appear through the external cervical os. Polyps are innocuous, inflammatory tumors comprising fibromuscular stroma, dilated mucous glands, inflammation, and squamous metaplasia. They are uncommon in adolescents and are treated by simple excision. Figure 60-1 illustrates cervical findings.[1,3]

## METHODS OF EXAMINATION

The vaginal portion of the cervix may be examined by inspection and palpation. The cervix is visualized by using a vaginal speculum and light. This approach facilitates specimen collection for cytology and culture. This approach also is used to evaluate abnormal cytology. Called colposcopy, this technique uses magnification and solutions (acetic acid and iodine) to locate abnormal areas and facilitate biopsy. Colposcopy is used in adolescents with persistently abnormal screening tests or screening tests that suggest high-grade abnormalities.

The cervix is palpated by the examiner's fingers. Palpation may help discover tenderness or texture of lesions discovered on inspection.

### THE PAPANICOLAOU TEST

The classic monograph demonstrating the value of cervical and vaginal cytology was published in 1943. The use of the Papanicolaou (Pap) test, credited to George Papanicolaou, MD, has been responsible for a 70% decline in invasive cervical cancer in developed countries. Cervical cytology or performance of the Pap test is the most effective screening tool in modern times.[2,4]

A Pap test is performed to sample the transformation zone and the endocervical canal. The sensitivity of the test is best using a liquid-based medium. Liquid-based, thin-layer technology was developed to address the limitations of conventional Pap smears.[4] By mixing cells in liquid media, an even distribution is created, enhancing the ability of a test to detect abnormalities.[4] After visualizing the cervix, a spatula is used to scrape the ectocervix. The spatula is placed into the liquid media. A cytobrush is placed in the endocervix, rotated 90 degrees, and removed. The cytobrush also is placed into the liquid media. The brush and spatula are rotated in the liquid media to facilitate cell transfer to the liquid media. The liquid vial is sent for cytologic examination. This media may be used for gonorrhea and chlamydia testing in some laboratories, making it ideal for use in adolescents.

Cervical cancer screening should begin at age 21 regardless of the age of sexual debut. Following screening recommendations helps avoid overtreatment of adolescents. Initiation of screening at age 21 does not seem to change the rate of cervical cancer within these young women. Screening should also be deferred to young women at age 21 if:

1. they have had past normal screening Pap tests, and
2. past Pap tests have been interpreted having atypical squamous cells of undetermined significance (ASC-US), low-grade squamous intraepithelial lesion (LSIL), or CIN 1 with subsequent to normal Pap tests after these findings.

Adolescent women younger than age 21 who have received past Pap screening results interpreted as high-grade squamous intraepithelial lesion (HSIL), atypical glandular cells (ASC-H), CIN 2 or 3 or greater, should receive further evaluation. However, once an ongoing process has resolved, Pap testing may again be deferred to age 21.[5,6]

The Bethesda System is used to classify cervical cytology (Box 60-1). In adolescent women, the reported rates of atypical squamous cells of undetermined significance (ASCUS) range from 7% to 16%, LSIL from 3% to 13%, and HSIL from 0.2% to 30%, thus making cervical dysplasia a relatively common disorder in young women. However, because cervical cancer is exceedingly rare, the emphasis is on conservative management for teens.

### Box 60-1

***The 2001 Bethesda System (Abridged)***

**SPECIMEN ADEQUACY**

- Satisfactory for evaluation (note presence/absence of endocervical/transformation zone component)
- Unsatisfactory for evaluation ... (specify reason)
  - Specimen rejected/not processed (specify reason)
  - Specimen processed and examined, but unsatisfactory for evaluation of epithelial abnormality because of (specify reason)

**GENERAL CATEGORIZATION (optional)**

- Negative for intraepithelial lesion or malignancy
- Epithelial cell abnormality
- Other

**INTERPRETATION/RESULT**

- **Negative for intraepithelial lesion or malignancy**
  - Organisms
    - *Trichomonas vaginalis*
    - Fungal organisms morphologically consistent with *Candida* species
    - Shift in flora suggestive of bacterial vaginosis
    - Bacteria morphologically consistent with *Actinomyces* species
    - Cellular changes consistent with herpes simplex virus
  - Other non-neoplastic findings (optional to report; list not comprehensive)
    - Reactive cellular changes associated with inflammation (includes typical repair)
    - Radiation
    - Intrauterine contraceptive device
  - Glandular cells status posthysterectomy
  - Atrophy
- **Epithelial cell abnormalities**
  - **Squamous cells**
    - Atypical squamous cells of undetermined significance
    - Cannot exclude high-grade squamous intraepithelial lesion (HSIL)
    - Low-grade squamous intraepithelial lesion encompassing human papillomavirus/mild dysplasia/cervical intraepithelial neoplasm (CIN) 1
    - HSIL encompassing moderate and severe dysplasia, carcinoma in situ; CIN2 and CIN3
    - Squamous cell carcinoma

### Box 60-1 (continued)

  - **Glandular cells**
    - Atypical glandular cells (AGCs) (specify endocervical, endometrial, or not otherwise specified)
    - AGCs, favor neoplasia (specify endocervical or not otherwise specified)
    - Endocervical adenocarcinoma in situ
    - Adenocarcinoma
- Other (list not comprehensive)
  - Endometrial cells in a woman ≥ 40 years

**AUTOMATED REVIEW AND ANCILLARY TESTING (include as appropriate)**

**EDUCATIONAL NOTES AND SUGGESTIONS (optional)**

---

Adapted with permission from Solomon D, Davey D, Kurman R, et al. The 2001 Bethesda System: terminology for reporting results of cervical cytology. *JAMA*. 2002;287(16):2114–2119. 

The etiology of cervical cancer and its precursor lesions is HPV, which is a DNA virus that infects epithelial cells. There are more than 100 types of HPV, with 40 of those types infecting the genital areas. Most HPV infections are transient, and viral DNA is absent 1 to 2 years after infection. Persistent HPV infection can occur, and it is this persistent infection with oncogenic HPV that dramatically increases risk for high-grade cervical lesions and cervical cancer.

The genital types of HPV are divided into low- and high-risk types, depending on their association with cancer. An HPV infection is acquired by most people in late adolescence, coinciding with the onset of sexual activity (Box 60-2). Approximately half the genital types are "high risk." These types include HPV 16, 18, 31, 33, 35, 39, 45, 51, 52, 56, 58, 59, 68, 73, and 82. The HPV 16 and 18 are the most common types found in HPV infection, and they are found in 70% of cervical cancer throughout the world. Low-risk types include HPV 6, 11, 40, 42, 43, 44, 54, 61, 70, 72, 81, and CP6108. These types are responsible for genital warts, atypical Pap tests, and low-grade abnormalities. They are not associated with high-grade abnormalities or cervical cancer.

The HPV is spread primarily through sexual contact. The virus infects basal cells in stratified squamous epithelium. Infection seldom disrupts cell function, but HPV also fails to invoke an aggressive host immune response. In most instances, HPV genomes reside as

**Box 60-2**

***Mechanisms of Human Papillomavirus (HPV) Transmission and Acquisition***

**Sexual contact**

- Sexual intercourse
- Genital-genital, manual-genital, oral-genital
- Genital HPV infection in virgins is rare, but may result from nonpenetrative sexual contact

**Nonsexual routes**

- Mother to newborn (vertical transmission; rare)
- Fomites (eg, undergarments, surgical gloves, biopsy forceps): hypothesized but not well documented

circular episomal DNA. This DNA may become integrated into human DNA in high-grade abnormalities and cervical cancers. Still, most HPV infections clear spontaneously, and invasive cervical cancer is rare in those younger than 21 years (Box 60-3).

**Box 60-3**

***Risk Factors for Human Papilloma Virus Infection***

| *Women* | *Men* |
|---|---|
| • Young age (peak age group 20–24 years)<br>• History of herpes simplex or chlamydia infections<br>• Lifetime number of sex partners<br>• Early age of first sexual intercourse<br>• Male partner sexual behavior<br>• Smoking<br>• Oral contraceptive use<br>• Uncircumcised male partners<br>• Diseases that compromise the immune system | • Young age (peak age group 25–29 years)<br>• Lifetime number of sex partners<br>• Being uncircumcised<br>• Failure to use condoms<br>• Diseases that compromise the immune system |

## NATURAL HISTORY OF HUMAN PAPILLOMAVIRUS IN ADOLESCENT GIRLS

The increased use of screening for cervical cancers by the Pap test has led to a decreased incidence of cervical cancer in areas where screening programs are in place. It has also led to an increase in detection of CIN. It is now well established that HPV is the cause of almost all cases of cancer of the cervix.

At any time, the prevalence of HPV in the general population is 14% to 35%,[7] and it is even more prevalent in adolescent women.[8,9] Of new HPV infections, 74% occur among sexually active women (in the United States, ages 15–24).[10] Sexual activity at a young age, multiple partners, and concurrent genital infections contribute to the rising detection of cervical cytologic abnormalities in adolescent women (Box 60-4). Woodman et al[8] noted that 28% of adolescents undergoing Pap testing showed cytologic abnormalities, and 33% who are HPV positive developed cervical dysplasia.

These findings make HPV the most commonly diagnosed sexually transmitted infection (STI) in young sexually active patients.

Despite the high frequency of infection, most HPV infections are transient, especially in younger women with intact immune systems. Ho et al[9] followed the natural history of cervical/vaginal HPV in young college females, showing a median duration of infection of 8 months for high-risk HPV types and shorter times for low-risk types. Up to 90% of HPV infections in adolescent patients with an intact immune system resolve within 24 months.[11]

Most adolescent women with HPV infections do not have abnormal cervical cytology. Tarkowski et al[12] studied 312 adolescents with HPV infections, and more than 50% showed normal cervical cytology. Persistent viral infections, however, are associated with the greatest risk for genital pathology.

Low- and high-risk HPV types are associated with CIN.[13] HPV infections, frequently high-risk types, are also associated with dysplasia of the vagina and vulva,

**Box 60-4**

***Risk Factors for Cervical Dysplasia in Adolescent Women***

- Early sexual activity
- Increased number of sexual partners
- No prior history of HPV exposure
- Vaginal/cervical inflammation or sexually transmitted infections
- Large cervical ectropion

**Box 60-5**

***Genital Pathologies Caused by Human Papillomavirus***

- Cervical dysplasia or cancer (squamous and adenocarcinoma), including endocervix
- Vaginal dysplasia and malignancy
- Vulvar dysplasia and malignancy
- Anorectal malignancy
- Penile cancer
- Laryngeal papillomatosis

as well as malignancies of the vagina, vulva, penis, anal areas, and oral-pharyngeal tissues (Box 60-5).

Recent attention has focused on the management of abnormal Pap test findings in adolescent women. The hallmark of care in adolescent women is conservative management to minimize the risk of long-term morbidity and maximize future child-bearing potential. Although HPV testing was previously recommended for some populations for screening or follow-up, HPV testing is not recommended at any time for adolescent women. HPV testing is not appropriate as any part of screening, triage, or subsequent Pap testing. There is also not a role for HPV testing before administering the HPV vaccine.[11]

## MANAGEMENT OF ABNORMAL TESTS

Initial management strategies for adolescent women with abnormal Pap tests may be addressed according to cytologic interpretations (Table 60-1). These are based on 2006 consensus guidelines by the American Society of Colposcopy and Cervical Pathology.[14–16]

After initial management of an abnormal Pap test, a return to negative results should prompt a return to screening again at age 21.

For persistent abnormal Pap testing, see Table 60-2 for recommendations.

## OTHER CERVICAL CYTOLOGY ABNORMALITIES

The Bethesda Pap classification offers information about cytologic abnormalities other than squamous cell disease. It also comments on the adequacy of sampling the transformation zone and the presence of endocervical cells. The glandular cell category of Pap smear interpretation encompasses endometrial cells or other cells of pelvic origin (fallopian tube or ovary), if present, as well as commenting on the endocervical cell findings. Endocervical cells are categorized as negative for malignancy or with atypical findings worrisome for neoplasm, endocervical adenocarcinoma in situ (AIS), or adenocarcinoma.

**Table 60-1**

**Initial Management of Abnormal Pap Tests in Adolescent Women**

| *Diagnosis* | *Recommendations for Adolescent Women* |
|---|---|
| ASCUS/LSIL | Repeat cytology at 12-month intervals for 2 years |
| CIN 1 | Colposcopy only for worsening Pap results within 2 years |
| ASC-H | Colposcopy |
| HSIL | Colposcopy with endocervical sampling |
| AGUS | Colposcopy with endocervical sampling |
| | Endometrial evaluation for adolescent women with dysmenorrhea, obesity, abnormal uterine bleeding, or other suspicion of uterine malignancy |

AGUS, atypical glandular cells of undetermined significance; ASC-H, atypical squamous cells cannot exclude high-grade lesion; ASCUS; atypical squamous cells of undetermined significance; CIN, cervical intraepithelial neoplasia; HSIL, high-grade squamous intraepithelial lesions; LSIL, low-grade squamous intraepithelial lesions

Women of all ages, including adolescents, should undergo colposcopy and endocervical sampling when atypical glandular cells are reported on the Pap smear. This should be part of the initial evaluation with colposcopy-directed biopsies of any abnormal areas noted. Most atypical glandular cell interpretations are associated with squamous cell abnormalities rather than glandular abnormalities in the endocervix. If colposcopy and endocervical sampling reveal negative histologic findings, selected patients may be referred for ultrasound of the pelvis and possible endometrial biopsy. This may also be an initial step if endometrial cell abnormalities are reported on the Pap smear. Adolescents with chronic anovulatory conditions may be at increased risk of endometrial pathology, including endometrial hyperplasia. However, malignancy of the cervix is extremely rare in women younger than 21 years.

Pap smears obtained in the immediate proximity of a menses or when any spotting or bleeding occurs may yield endometrial cells without atypical findings.

Carcinoma in situ/severe dysplasia has been reported only in a small number of adolescents. Therapy is oriented toward ablative (laser) or excisional therapies (electroexcision procedures and cold knife cone) according to the disease location, extent, and concurrent medical disease.

**Table 60-2**

**Management of Persistent Abnormal Pap Testing in Adolescent Women**

| *Diagnosis* | *Recommendations* |
|---|---|
| ASCUS/LSIL | Repeat cytology every 12 months for 2 years |
| CIN 1 | Colposcopy only for cytologic diagnosis of HSIL or persistent abnormal results after 2 years* |
| ASC-H | Colposcopic evaluation with biopsy of abnormalities. Repeat Pap testing every 6 months if ASCUS, LSIL, or CIN1. Repeat colposcopy for greater cytologic abnormalities. |
| HSIL | Colposcopy with endocervical sampling with biopsies as needed |
| | Biopsy diagnosis less than CIN2 or 3 may be followed by colposcopy and Pap testing at 6-month intervals |
| | Biopsy diagnosis of CIN 2 may be individualized to continued observation |
| | Persistent HSIL after 1 year warrants repeat colposcopy, endocervical sampling, and colposcopy of the vagina |
| | Diagnostic excisional procedure for HSIL persisting for more than 24 months |

* Persistent cytologic diagnosis of CIN 1 after 2 years should be individualized with emphasis on conservative care and annual cytologic tests.
Note: "See and treat" loop electroexcision procedures are never recommended in adolescent women.

## ADOLESCENTS WITH SPECIAL NEEDS: PAP TEST MANAGEMENT IN SPECIAL GROUPS

Sexually active adolescents with immunosuppression represent a special group of young women warranting close evaluation and monitoring of Pap smear abnormalities. Diseases originating from HPV may have altered rates of "progression" or a higher disease state at diagnosis, and a medical condition associated with immunosuppression may be permanent (solid organ transplant) or transient (HIV disease).

Initial cytologic assessment recommendations are cytology testing twice in the year of diagnosis and annually thereafter.[17] The current recommendations for management of abnormal cervical cytology in women with HIV can be reviewed at: www.cdc.gov/mmwr/preview/mmwrhtml/rr5804a1.htm.[6] Other conditions of immunocompromise are listed in Box 60-6.

Patients with any of the above conditions should have cytologic testing twice during the year of initiation of sexual activity, regardless of age. Annual evaluation after the first year may be performed if test results are negative. Pregnant adolescents do not warrant a change in screening practices.[17]

Teens with physical or cognitive disabilities may not often be questioned about sexual activity and the associated risk of abnormal cervical cytology. These teens, however, do participate in the same social maturation process and experience the same pressures for sexual experimentation. In addition, the medical needs of these teens may restrict their access to health care providers and contraception, or barrier protection against STIs. Cervical cytology screening should be obtained at age 21.

Cytological abnormalities in teens with disabilities should be managed by the same guidelines noted previously, with special consideration given to pain management, physical positioning, and awareness of other medical needs.

**Box 60-6**

***Conditions of Immunocompromise***

Solid organ transplant
Bone marrow transplant
Chemotherapy (malignancy, autoimmune disease)
Chronic steroid administration
Sickle cell disease
Renal failure
Advanced stage autoimmune disease

## PREVENTING CERVICAL DYSPLASIA

The essentials of decreasing the risk of CIN parallel the prevention of genital infections in general. Sexually transmitted infections may allow open access through the skin for the entrance of the HPV. Data are also accumulating regarding the entrance of the HPV into humans via the hair follicle.

In 2006, the first vaccine effective in preventing the most common types of HPV associated with genital warts and cervical/endocervical dysplasia was approved by the US Food and Drug Administration and released for administration. Knowledge of the etiology of HPV as the causative factor in cervical cancer is clearly accepted. No other cancer in humans has yet been shown to have such a specific etiology. HPV 16 and 18 are found in more than two-thirds of cervical carcinomas worldwide.

The current vaccines are a quadrivalent vaccine of viruslike particles from HPV types 6, 11, 16, and 18 produced in *Saccharomyces cerevisiae* (baker's yeast), with an amorphous aluminum adjuvant to enhance immune response or a bivalent vaccine with components of HPV 16 and 18. Each vaccine is available in 0.5-cc single-dose vials or injections and administered in 3 injections.

Phase II and III trials administered the vaccine to females ages 9 to 26 from the general population, and to an HPV-naïve population. The determination of the presence of HPV was made by serum assays and polymerase chain reaction studies. Sampling of the general population included women who may have had a history of prior HPV exposure. Study results revealed 100% efficacy of the vaccines against HPV 16 and 18 in patients with no prior exposure to these HPV types. In addition, the quadrivalent vaccine provides efficacy against HPV types 6 and 11, which are involved with 90% of genital warts. There was no protection from diseases caused by HPV types for which the patients were seropositive at baseline entrance into the study. Future studies are evaluating the possibility of protection against other HPV subtypes in the same epitope (those with very similar DNA compositions), and the studies will provide information about the need for vaccine boosters. Thus the vaccines may be able to provide more benefit than currently anticipated.[18,19]

Although uncommon in adolescents, the vaccine also is expected to reduce vulvar intraepithelial neoplasia (VIN) and vaginal intraepithelial neoplasia (VAIN). The degree of disease protection offered is less than that of CIN because not all VIN and VAIN is due to HPV infection. Most recently, the quadrivalent vaccine has been approved for males to assist with prevention of genital warts.

Future studies of vaccines and genital malignancy will focus on prophylactic and therapeutic formulations.

## REFERENCES


1. Wright TC, Ferenczy A. Anatomy and histology of the cervix. In: Kurman RJ, ed. *Blaustein's Pathology of the Female Genital Tract*. New York: Springer-Verlag; 2002:207–223

2. Droegemueller W. Reproductive anatomy: gross and microscopic, clinical correlations. In: Stenchever MA, Droegemueller W, Herbst AL, Mishell DR, eds. *Comprehensive Gynecology*. St. Louis, MO: Mosby; 2001:44–46

3. Crum CP. The female genital tract. In: Cotran RS, Kumar V, Collins T, eds. *Robbins Pathologic Basis of Disease*. Philadelphia: WB Saunders; 1999:1047–1048

4. Spitzer M, Johnson C. The Papanicolaou smear. In: Apgar BS, Brotzman GL, Spitzer M, eds. *Colposcopy: Principles and Practice*. Philadelphia: WB Saunders; 2002:41–59

5. Barnholtz-Sloan J, Patel N, Rollison D, Kortepeter K, MacKinnon J, Giuliano A. Incidence trends of invasive cervical cancer in the United States by combined race and ethnicity. *Cancer Causes Control*. 2009;20:1129–1138

6. American College of Obstetricians and Gynecologists (ACOG). ACOG Committee Opinion No 463: Cervical Cancer in Adolescents: Screening, Evaluation, and Management. *Obstet Gynecol* 2010;116:469–472

7. American College of Obstetrics and Gynecology. Human Papilloma Virus. Washington, DC: ACOG; April 2005. ACOG Practice Bulletin No 61

8. Woodman CB, Collins S, Winter H, et al. Natural history of cervical human papillomavirus infection in young women: a longitudinal cohort study. *Lancet*. 2001;357:1831–1836

9. Ho GY, Bierman R, Beardsley L, et al. Natural history of cervicovaginal papillomavirus infection in young women. *N Engl J Med*. 1998;338:423–428

10. Weinstock H, Berman S, Cates W Jr. Sexually transmitted diseases among American youth: incidence and prevalence estimates, 2000. *Perspect Sex Reprod Health*. 2004;36:6–10

11. Moscicki AB, Schiffman M, Kjaer S, Villa LL. Chapter 5: Updating the natural history of HPV and anogenital cancer. *Vaccine*. 2006;24 (Suppl 3):S3/42–51

12. Tarkowski TA, Koumans EH, Sawyer M, et al. Epidemiology of human papillomavirus infection and abnormal cytologic test results in an urban adolescent population. *J Infect Dis*. 2004;189:46–50

13. Burd EM. Human papillomavirus and cervical cancer. *Clin Microbiol Rev*. 2003;16:1–17

14. Wright TC Jr, Massad LS, Dunton CJ, Spitzer M, Wilkinson EJ, Solomon D. 2006 Consensus Guidelines for the Management of Women with Abnormal Cervical Screening Tests. 2006 ASCCP-Sponsored Consensus Conference [published erratum appears in *J Low Genit Tract Dis* 2008;12:255]. *J Low Genit Tract Dis* 2007; 11:201–222

15. American Society for Colposcopy and Cervical Pathology. Management of women with atypical squamous cells of undetermined significance (ASC-US). Hagerstown, MD: ASCCP; 2007. Available at: www.asccp.org/pdfs/consensus/algorithms_cyto_07.pdf. Accessed August 10, 2010

16. American Society for Colposcopy and Cervical Pathology. Management of women with a histological diagnosis of cervical intraepithelial neoplasia grade 1 (CIN1) preceded by ASC-US, ASC-H, or LSIL cytology. Hagerstown, MD: ASCCP; 2007. Available at: www.asccp.org/pdfs/consensus/algorithms_hist_07.pdf. Accessed August 10, 2010

17. Kaplan JE, Benson C, Holmes KH, Brooks JT, Pau A, Masur H. Guidelines for prevention and treatment of opportunistic infections in HIV-infected adults and adolescents: recommendations from CDC, the National Institutes of Health, and the HIV Medicine Association of the Infectious Diseases Society of America. Centers for Disease Control and Prevention; National Institutes of Health; HIV Medicine Association of the Infectious Diseases Society of America. *MMWR Recomm Rep* 2009;58:1207;quiz CE1-4

18. Centers for Disease Control and Prevention. HPV Vaccine. Atlanta: CDC; February 4, 2010. Available at: www. cdc.gov/vaccines/vpd-vac/hpv/default.htm. Accessed April 13, 2010

19. Merck & Co., Inc. Prescribing Information for GARDASIL. Whitehouse Station, NJ: Merck & Co., Inc.; 2009. Available at: www.merck.com/product/usa/pi_circulars/g/gardasil/gardasil_pi.pdf. Accessed April 13, 2010

# CHAPTER 61

# The Uterus and Adnexa

ERICA J. GIBSON, MD • ELIZABETH ALDERMAN, MD

## DEVELOPMENT AND ANATOMY

In the female fetus, the uterus, fallopian tubes, and ligaments are embryologically derived from the paramesonephric or Müllerian ducts whereas the ovaries develop from the undifferentiated gonads. In the postmenarchal nulliparous girl, the uterus is a pear-shaped, hollow, fibromuscular midline pelvic organ that normally measures 8 cm × 5 cm × 2.5 cm. It is divided anatomically into 2 parts, the fundus, which is the body of the uterus, and the cervix, which is approximately 3.5 cm in length and partially intravaginal.

The position of the uterus in the pelvis is usually anteverted and anteflexed, although an axial or retroflexed uterus are normal variants. The adnexa consist of the ovaries, fallopian tubes, round ligament, and ovarian ligament. Both the uterus and adnexa should be palpable on a bimanual examination in an adolescent, although assessment may be limited in an obese adolescent.

## THE UTERUS

### CONGENITAL ANOMALIES

Congenital anomalies of the uterus may be a result of abnormal fusion, canalization, or resorption of the paired Müllerian ducts during embryogenesis.[1] The exact prevalence of uterine anomalies is probably more common than suspected, as they are usually asymptomatic and most often discovered in women with infertility. A 1998 review of 22 studies involving universal screening for uterine malformations found that 1 in 29 infertile women had uterine anomalies whereas only 1 in 594 fertile women had them.[2]

The American Fertility Society Classification of Müllerian Anomalies is pictured in Figure 61-1.[3] The most common defects result in a bicornuate or septate uterus. Bicornuate uterus develops secondary to partial failure of fusion of the paired Müllerian ducts. Septate uterus results from failure of septal resorption after the ducts have

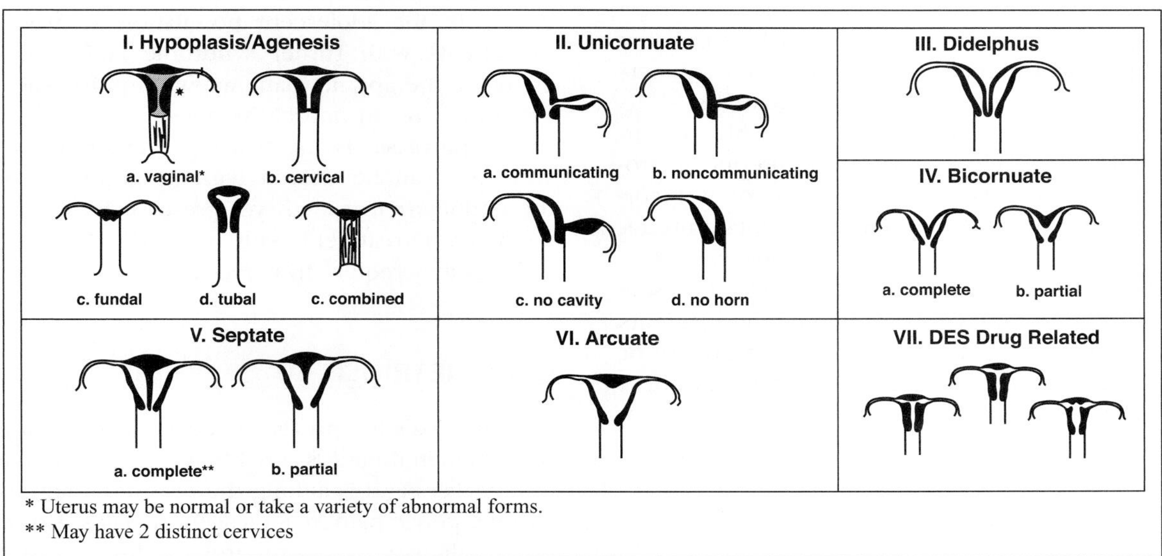


FIGURE 61-1 The American Fertility Society Classification of Müllerian Anomalies. (Copyright 2010 by the American Society for Reproductive Medicine. All rights reserved. No part of this presentation may be reproduced or transmitted in any form or by any means, electronic or mechanical, including photocopying, recording or by any information storage and retrieval system without permission in writing from the American Society for Reproductive Medicine, 1209 Montgomery Highway, Birmingham, AL 35216.)

already fused. Other less common types of uterine anomalies include didelphic, unicornuate, and arcuate uterus.[1] Less commonly seen now is a hypoplastic or T-shaped uterus first identified in women exposed to diethylstilbestrol in utero between 1945 and 1971. A didelphys uterus results from complete nonfusion of the Müllerian ducts, unicornuate uterus is due to arrest of one Müllerian duct, and arcuate uterus is a single uterus with a convex or flat uterine fundus (this is often considered a normal variant). If there are 2 uterine cavities, 1 of the 2 sides is usually more developed than the other, and a unicornuate uterus often has a rudimentary horn. Abnormal uteri may or may not be associated with single or double cervices. Müllerian anomalies may be associated with multiple other congenital abnormalities. Congenital urinary tract anomalies are the most common and most frequently include ipsilateral renal agenesis. Skeletal and cardiac anomalies and inguinal hernia of the adnexa have also been identified.[1] A thorough evaluation of other malformations must be conducted in all patients presenting with a Müllerian anomaly.[4]

Adolescents with uterine anomalies usually present with acute or chronic pelvic pain.[5] Other presentations include menstrual disorders, abnormal vaginal bleeding or discharge, endometriosis, and recurrent miscarriages or infertility.

Diagnosis of uterine anomalies may be made by transabdominal and transvaginal ultrasound with increased sensitivity and specificity if new 3-dimensional techniques are used. Magnetic resonance imaging (MRI) is considered the gold standard for diagnosis and has the added benefit of enabling visualization of the urinary tract for coexistent anomalies.[6] Hysterosalpingography, hysteroscopy, and laparoscopy may be useful adjuncts to delineate a more complicated uterine anatomy.

Numerous surgical techniques are available now to correct uterine anomalies; in particular, uterine metroplasty can unify the endometrial cavity of a bicornuate uterus or remove the septum in a septate uterus. Although conception is possible with uterine anomalies, patients may be at greater risk for abnormal fetal presentation, preterm labor, and cervical malfunction.[1] Patients may require hysteroscopic intervention, metroplasty, or other assisted reproductive technologies to ensure a healthy pregnancy and delivery.

## UTERINE MASSES

### BENIGN UTERINE MASSES: MYOMAS

The most common uterine mass other than pregnancy in an adolescent female is the benign myoma or fibroid. Malignant tumors are very rare. Although myomas are the most common solid pelvic tumor in women, they are uncommon in adolescence. A myoma is a discrete, firm growth of smooth muscle in the uterus that may be in the myometrium, within the endometrium, or on the surface of the uterus. They may be single or multiple and most often are asymptomatic. Excessive menstrual bleeding and secondary dysmenorrhea are often the only symptoms of a myoma in adolescent patients. Bleeding unassociated with menses is seldom seen. Occasionally, myomas may cause lower abdominal pain secondary to infarction, infection, or torsion. In general, adolescent patients do not require surgical intervention for dysfunctional uterine bleeding, pain, or mass effect secondary to myomas. As adults, myomectomy may be necessary for the previous issues or if myomas are interfering with fertility. Hysterectomy may be considered in women who are postchildbearing or postmenopausal depending on the severity of symptoms.

### MALIGNANT UTERINE MASSES

Malignant uterine masses are exceedingly rare in the pediatric and adolescent age group, although a study of nonovarian female genital tract tumors in children showed 21% were uterine cancers.[7] This same study noted that cancer of the uterus was more lethal than other nonovarian tumors. The most common uterine malignancies identified were rhabdomyosarcoma, botryoid, and mixed mesenchymal type.[7] Surgery, radiation, and chemotherapy with vincristine, actinomycin, and cyclophosphamide continue to be the most effective treatment for uterine malignancies.[8]

Endometrial carcinoma, although the most common malignancy of the female genital tract in mature women, is rare in the adolescent population. It may be seen in patients with Turner syndrome taking unopposed estrogen therapy, in patients with polycystic ovarian syndrome, or in morbidly obese patients.[9] Endometrial hyperplasia is the usual precursor to carcinoma, and both can be treated with progestins to suppress the endometrial growth yet preserve fertility in young women.[9] If treatment with progestins is unsuccessful, patients may require hysterectomy.

## ENDOMETRIOSIS

Endometriosis has previously been viewed as a problem of women in their 20s and 30s. It is now known to occur in teenagers and is among the most common causes of chronic pelvic pain in adolescent females. Although it is not a malignancy, it is a progressive disease that presents a variety of clinical challenges.

### ETIOLOGY

Endometriosis is the presence and growth of endometrial glands and stroma in an atypical location outside of the uterus. The pathophysiologic origin of endometriosis is probably multifactorial. Current theories of causation include retrograde menstruation, coelomic metaplasia, activation of "embryonic rests," lymphatic and vascular metastases, immunologic changes, genetic predisposition, and iatrogenic dissemination. Adolescents in particular need to be evaluated for obstructive anomalies of the reproductive tract, which have been found to greatly increase the incidence of endometriosis.[10]

The pain of endometriosis is caused by swelling and bleeding of the endometrial implants consequent to hormonal stimulation during the menstrual cycle. Most endometrial implants are in the dependent areas of the pelvis, and the ovaries are the most common sites of involvement. If ovarian endometriomas (hemorrhagic or chocolate cysts) develop on the ovaries they may burst, causing severe acute abdominal pain, but this is far less common in adolescent patients than in adults. The anterior and posterior cul-de-sacs, the uterosacral, round, and broad ligaments, and the pelvic peritoneum overlying the uterus are additional frequent sites of endometrium implantation. Endometriosis has been identified in any number of locations throughout the anterior peritoneum, including along the bladder and bowel; far-reaching sites in the remainder of the body have also been found.

Endometriosis has come to be recognized as a more common problem in adolescent women than previously realized. In a 2003 review by Attaran and Gidwani,[11] endometriosis was found at rates of 20% to 73% in multiple studies of chronic pelvic pain in adolescents. It is important to note that the presentation of endometriosis differs in adolescents from that in older women. Although adults present with cyclic pelvic pain and infertility, adolescents tend to present with cyclic and/or acyclic chronic pelvic pain. They are also more likely to have associated bowel and bladder symptoms.[12] Girls with a first-degree relative who has endometriosis seem to have a sevenfold increased risk for this disorder.[13]

## DIAGNOSIS

The chronic pelvic pain of endometriosis often coincides with the menstrual cycle. Most girls have cyclic pain just prior to or during menses that may cause severe dysmenorrhea. The pain is usually severe enough to prevent normal activities such as school attendance. Less commonly, the pain may occur midcycle or may have no relation to the menstrual cycle. Other gynecologic symptoms associated with endometriosis in adolescents include irregular menses, dyspareunia (usually with deep penetration), brownish vaginal discharge, and infertility. Gastrointestinal complaints such as constipation, nausea, vomiting, diarrhea, or pain on defecation prior to or during menstruation are also common. In addition, a girl may complain of urinary tract symptoms of frequency, dysuria, and hematuria.

On physical examination, most girls with endometriosis have generalized abdominal tenderness, but many also have evidence of localized pain.[11] Tenderness of the posterior cul-de-sac or rectovaginal pouch is common, but it is rare in adolescent patients to palpate the nodules or masses of endometriosis associated with adult patients.[14] Most adolescents will have a normal pelvic examination because their disease is usually minimal. One of the primary goals of a physical examination and bimanual or rectal-abdominal examination is to rule out any other abnormalities of the uterus or adnexa. Laboratory studies should be done to rule out pregnancy, infection, or chronic disease. Ultrasound is helpful to initially identify other possible causes of pelvic pain such as ovarian torsion, cysts, tumors, or anatomic anomalies.

## MANAGEMENT

Initial management of suspected endometriosis should include a trial of nonsteroidal anti-inflammatory drugs (NSAIDs) and low-dose oral contraceptives (OCPs). Any adolescent female with persistent pelvic symptoms who fails management with NSAIDs or OCPs for 3 to 6 months should be considered for laparoscopy.[15] The goal of laparoscopy is to diagnose, stage, and treat endometriosis. It is vital that surgical treatment of adolescent patients be done by a surgeon trained in identifying the endometrial lesions in adolescents, as they often look far different than lesions found in adults. Most surgeons recommend that if no obvious lesions are found, biopsies should be taken from the posterior cul-de-sac to rule out microscopic disease. Laufer et al[12] found that 69% of patients with chronic pelvic pain refractory to NSAIDS and OCPs had evidence of endometriosis on laparoscopy.

The most commonly used system for classifying endometriosis at the time of laparoscopy has been proposed by the American Fertility Society and is pictured in Figure 61-2.[16] This system defines 4 stages of disease: minimal, mild, moderate, and severe. Staging is based on a weighted point system that describes size and position of the endometrial implants in the peritoneum and ovaries. It also describes size and position of adhesions on the ovaries and fallopian tubes. Endometriosis of the bowel, urinary tract, vagina, cervix, skin, and other organs is designated as "additional endometriosis."

In a 1995 study by Laufer et al[12] of the 32 of 46 patients found to have endometriosis on laparoscopy, 77% of patients were found to have stage I disease, whereas 22% were found to have stage II disease, further supporting previous studies that adolescents usually have minimal disease responsible for their pelvic symptoms. Adults who may have had endometriosis from time of menarche typically present with infertility caused by long-term

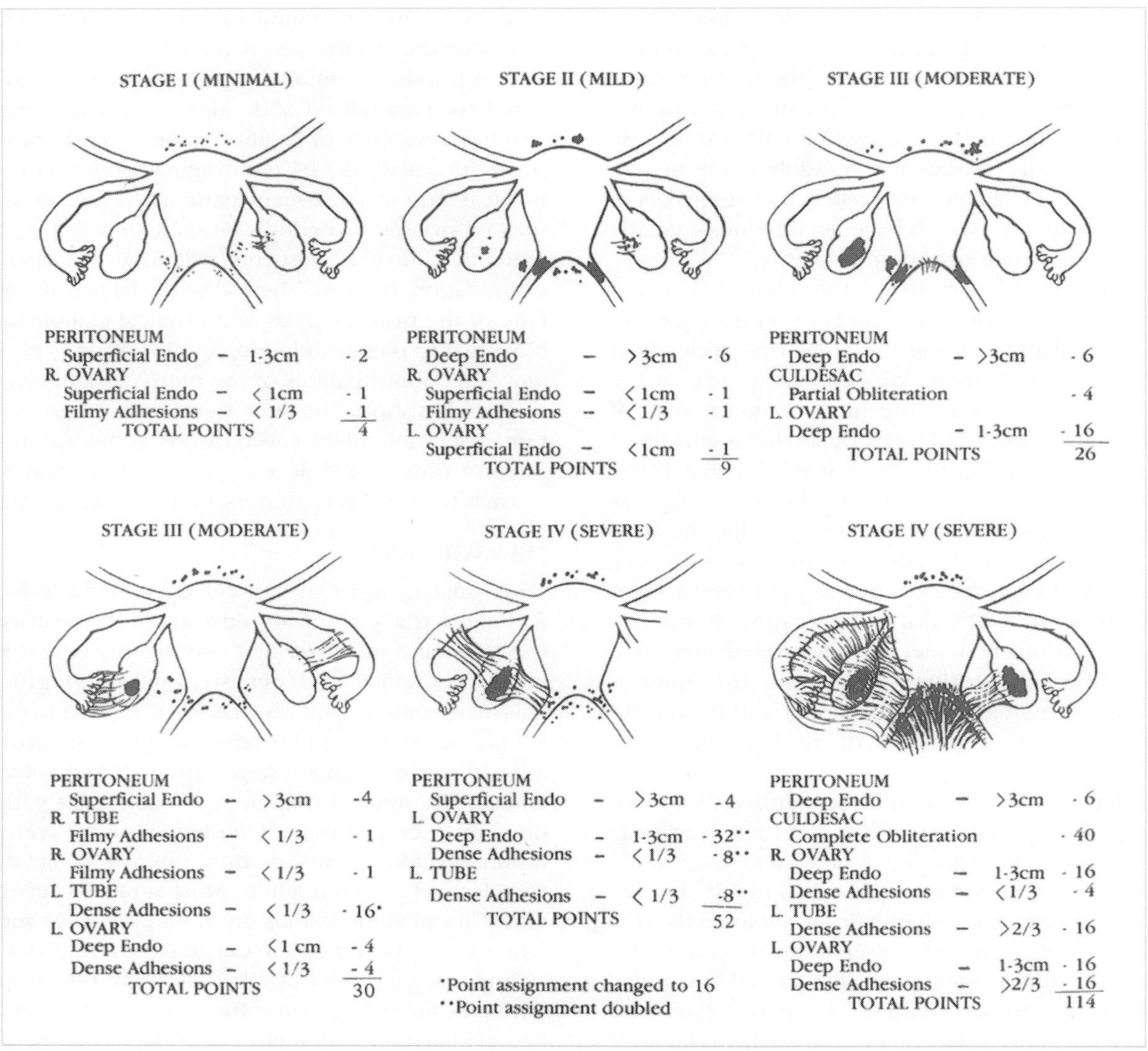


**FIGURE 61-2** American Society for Reproductive Medicine Revised Classification of Endometriosis. (Copyright 2010 by the American Society for Reproductive Medicine. All rights reserved. No part of this presentation may be reproduced or transmitted in any form or by any means, electronic or mechanical, including photocopying, recording or by any information storage and retrieval system without permission in writing from the American Society for Reproductive Medicine, 1209 Montgomery Highway, Birmingham, AL 35216.)

peritubal endometriosis and adhesions resulting in tubal obstruction or impaired tubal motility. It is important to note that mild or minimal disease has been associated with infertility in some instances.[10]

Surgical techniques for treatment of endometriosis include laser vaporization, coagulation, and resection. Subsequent to surgical treatments in adolescents, Laufer, Sanfillipo, et al[5] recommend adjuvant medical management to suppress further disease and to control pain. Initially, they recommend continuous hormonal contraceptives for women younger than 16 years with consideration of a gonadotropin-releasing hormone (GnRH) agonist for women older than 16 years. The goals of pharmacologic treatment are to shrink the endometrial lesions and activity. Continuous combined hormonal contraception creates a state of "pseudopregnancy" that suppresses implant activity and may be used in the form of monophasic oral contraceptives, the contraceptive patch, or the vaginal ring. Progestin-only oral contraceptives or intramuscular (IM) depot-medroxyprogesterone acetate may be used for patients who do not tolerate or have a contraindication to using combined hormonal contraception, but effectiveness has been found to be variable. The side effects of progestins include irregular menstrual bleeding and weight gain, which are often difficult for adolescents to tolerate. Gonadotropin-releasing hormone agonists, such as IM leuprolide (11.25 mg IM every 3 months) or intranasal nafarelin (1 puff twice daily), may be used to create a low estrogen state by decreasing follicular stimulating hormone and luteinizing hormone.[17] It is important for patients to know that GnRH-a treatment will result in an initial stimulatory phase prior to downregulation that will worsen symptoms with an initial withdrawal bleed 21 to 28 days after the initiation of therapy.[10] Side effects of nafarelin and leuprolide therapy are the same as symptoms of menopause (hot flashes, osteoporosis, decreased libido, vaginal dryness).[18] To counteract these side effects, additional estrogen may be necessary. Alternative treatment regimens, although unpopular with adolescents because of the side effects, are androgens, such as danazol, and synthetic progestins. These agents cause atrophy of endometrial implants and interrupt ovarian follicle development by creating an antiestrogen state. Side effects of androgens include irregular menses, virilization with hirsutism, acne, deep voice, and weight gain.

In severe or persistent disease, repeat laparoscopy may be required. Laparotomy is rarely required due to advances in laparascopic technique. Additional possible interventions include presacral neurectomy to relieve pain and uterine suspension to correct retroversion. Girls with endometriosis require periodic re-evaluation, at approximately 6-month intervals, to monitor progress and assess for side effects of medication. A serologic marker, CA-125, may correlate with disease activity in endometriosis and may be useful in monitoring response to treatment.[19]

### PROGNOSIS

The prognosis for control of disease and future fertility of adolescent girls with endometriosis is quite good. Most adolescents have minimal disease that is responsive to available therapies. The challenge for the clinician is to make the diagnosis early to prevent chronic pelvic pain and to preserve future fertility. In working with the adolescent, the clinician must be mindful of the side effects of the medications used to treat endometriosis because compliance may be the key to attaining a cure.

## THE ADNEXA

### OVARIAN CYSTS

#### Etiology

Girls in early or midpuberty may have enlarged ovaries with multiple small cysts that are considered a normal variant. The average physiologic ovarian follicle is usually less than 3 cm in diameter.[20] As fluid accumulates in preformed ovarian cavities functional ovarian cysts may form and are quite common in postmenarchal adolescents.[21] Most ovarian cysts are follicular cysts, which are a result of the failure of the maturing follicle to ovulate and involute.[22] Such cysts contain clear fluid and are often small, asymptomatic, and resolve spontaneously. On some occasions, however, they may enlarge to 6 to 8 cm then torse or rupture, causing acute abdominal pain.[10] Other types of functional ovarian cysts include postovulatory corpus luteum cysts that rarely exceed 5 cm in diameter but tend to be more symptomatic than follicular cysts and theca luteum cysts, which are usually multiple.[21] Hemorrhagic cysts, known also as endometriomas or chocolate cysts, may be associated with endometriosis. Symptoms of ovarian cysts include acute or chronic abdominal pain due to torsion, rupture or hemorrhage, menstrual abnormalities, constipation, or urinary symptoms.

#### Diagnosis

An adnexal mass may be palpated on the bimanual examination, but a pelvic ultrasound is important to determine size, appearance, and how to guide subsequent management. On ultrasound, nonhemorrhagic cysts appear to be smooth and unilocular.[20] Hemorrhagic cysts contain internal debris. Size and appearance of the cyst should be correlated to the menstrual cycle.

#### Management

Most follicular cysts resolve spontaneously in a few months.[10] Large cysts are defined as those greater than 5 cm in diameter. If a patient has a large or symptomatic cyst determined to be simple on ultrasound, a trial of OCPs may be considered to prevent further cyst formation. A low-dose estrogen/progestin formulation of OCPs is appropriate in these cases to suppress the hypothalamic–ovarian axis. A monophasic OCP with a 35 μg formulation of estrogen should be prescribed because extremely low-dose OCPs, and progestin-only OCPs are not likely to sufficiently suppress the pituitary axis.[21] The patient should be followed clinically and examined monthly. A repeat ultrasound is recommended 8 to 10 weeks into treatment to re-evaluate the appearance of the cyst. The ultrasound should be done at the beginning of the menstrual cycle before the possible formation of new follicular cysts.

Although surgical intervention for cysts is controversial, most specialists recommend laparoscopic drainage of the cyst or cystectomy if the cyst is greater than 8 cm. Intervention is also recommended if a cyst persists for more than 3 to 4 months, continues to grow, is solid on ultrasound, or is severely symptomatic.[21] Postsurgery, patients are usually placed on monophasic oral contraceptive pills to prevent future cyst development.

### ADNEXAL TUMORS

Ovarian and adnexal masses account for 1% of all pediatric neoplasms but comprise almost 70% of all pediatric gynecologic malignancies. Only 10% to 30% of ovarian masses are malignant.[9] Germ cell tumors (GCT) are the most common ovarian histologic type tumor diagnosed in adolescents age

15 to 19 years (54%).[9] These include benign mature cystic teratomas and the 2 most common malignant tumors, the endodermal sinus tumor and the dysgerminoma.

**Benign Mature Cystic Teratoma or Dermoid Cyst**

Benign mature cystic teratomas or dermoid cysts are the most common ovarian germ cell neoplasm in adolescent females.[23] These benign neoplasms may contain any descendent of endoderm, ectoderm, or mesoderm, enclosed in a thick capsule of squamous epithelium. Common components of teratomas include hair, thyroid tissue, teeth (which can be visualized on plane radiograph), sebaceous glands, sebum, and choroid plexus. Their average size is 10 cm in diameter, so they often present as an abdominal mass. Another common presentation is abdominal pain due to torsion of the ovarian pedicle, or rarely, rupture of the thick capsule. They may also be asymptomatic. Teratomas do not have a distinct appearance on ultrasound, but pelvic CT scan or MRI may further characterize the cyst.[24] Dermoid cysts have an increased risk of ovarian torsion and should be resected from the ovary, if possible, to preserve future reproductive function. Use of laparoscopy versus laparotomy to achieve this remains a controversial subject. Because 15% of all ovarian teratomas appear bilaterally, the opposite ovary should be visually inspected. Several large studies have shown that biopsy or removal of the nonaffected ovary is not efficacious.[25] It should be noted that the rare immature cystic teratoma or struma ovarii is malignant and requires resection and chemotherapy.

**Malignant Tumors**

Ovarian germ cell tumors (GCT) are the most common ovarian malignancies in the pediatric population. Endodermal sinus tumors are the most common GCT in pediatrics, closely followed by dysgerminomas. Endodermal sinus tumors originate from extra embryonic germ cells and produce alpha-fetoprotein (AFP), which can serve as a useful tumor marker in the course of therapy. They present at the median age of 18 years with one-third of patients presenting in the premenarchal period.[9] Dysgerminomas are usually unilateral, but 15% are bilateral.[25] They have no specific tumor markers, but patients may have an elevated human chorionic gonadotropin (HCG) and lactic dehydrogenase.

Ultrasound evaluation suggestive of a malignant adnexal mass includes large size, complex appearance, the presence of loculations, and fluid in the posterior cul-de-sac.[9] In general, treatment of pediatric ovarian malignancies includes resection and postoperative chemotherapy with bleomycin, etoposide, and cisplatin (BEP). Although radiation therapy was used in the past for some ovarian malignancies, it has been virtually abandoned secondary to subsequent infertility and tissue scarring. Radiation is now considered only in disease recurrence.

The first step in treating ovarian carcinoma is a staging laparotomy. If the tumor is localized to one ovary, then unilateral salpingo-oopherectomy is performed with removal of the para-aortic and ipsilateral lymph nodes, as there is a great risk of spread to the retroperitoneal lymph nodes. Sampling of the diaphragm, peritoneal washings, and omentectomy are also performed at that time. Box 61-1 describes the Federation of Gynecology and Obstetrics[26] staging system for ovarian cancer.

Other ovarian carcinomas that may be found in adolescent girls include the immature teratoma, embryonal carcinoma, mixed germ cell carcinoma, gonadoblastoma, sex cord-stroma tumors of the ovary, juvenile granulosa cell tumors, and epithelial ovarian tumors. Immature teratomas often have elevated AFP whereas embryonal carcinomas often have elevated AFP and beta human chorionic gonadotropin (BHCG). Again, after surgical resection, chemotherapy with BEP has been shown to produce the best outcome.

## Box 61-1

### *Staging of Ovarian Carcinoma*

Stage I. Growth limited to the ovaries

Stage II. Growth involving one or both ovaries with pelvic extension

Stage III. Tumor involving one or both ovaries with the peritoneal implants outside the pelvis and/or positive retroperitoneal or inguinal nodes. Superficial liver metastases equal Stage III. Tumor is limited to the true pelvis but with histologically verified malignant extension to small bowel or omentum

Stage IV. Growth involving one or both ovaries with distant metastasis. If pleural effusion is present, there must be positive cytologic test results to consider staging at Stage IV. Parenchymal liver metastases equals Stage IV

Adapted from International Federation of Gynecology and Obstetrics. Changes in definitions of clinical staging for carcinoma of the cervix and ovary. *Am J Obstet Gynecol*. 1987;156:236.

## PELVIC PAIN

Acute and chronic pelvic pain are common complaints in adolescent patients. A full evaluation of pelvic pain must rule out pathologic processes of the uterus or adnexal

**Box 61-2**

***Gynecologic Causes of Acute Abdominal Pain in Adolescent Females***

Rupture of ovarian cyst
Hemorrhagic ovarian cyst
Pelvic inflammatory disease
Dysmenorrhea
Hydrosalpinx
Torsion of ovary
Intrauterine pregnancy
Ectopic pregnancy
Threatened abortion
Pelvic thrombophlebitis
Ovarian tumor
Endometriosis

organs. The differential diagnosis of pelvic pain includes not only the gynecologic, but urologic, gastrointestinal, neurologic, and musculoskeletal systems. Psychiatric or psychosocial influences on pain must also be evaluated. If an evaluation for an organic etiology of pelvic pain is negative then functional causes of pain must be considered. Box 61-2 and Box 61-3 list the gynecologic causes of acute and chronic pelvic pain. Many of these entities have been discussed in detail throughout this chapter. Pelvic inflammatory disease is described in Chapter 53, STIs. Pregnancy and its complications are discussed in Chapter 54, Pregnancy.

**Box 61-3**

***Gynecologic Causes of Chronic Abdominal Pain in Adolescent Females***

Ovarian cyst
Mittelschmerz
Endometriosis
Fibroids
Genital tract malformation
Chronic pelvic inflammatory disease
Adhesions secondary to pelvic inflammatory disease
Postoperative adhesions
Pelvic serositis
Pelvic congestion

### HISTORY/PHYSICAL EXAMINATION

It is important, when eliciting a history of pelvic pain, to determine the quality and chronology of events. Chronic pelvic pain can be defined as continuous or intermittent pain for at least 3 months. Specific information must be clarified, including characteristics of the pain, intensity, timing, location, and radiation.[27] Basic information regarding bowel and bladder habits should be elicited. A menstrual history including menarche, cycle length, duration of bleeding, and relationship of the pain to the menstrual cycle is important. Is the pain related to menses at all and if so does it occur midcycle or with menses? If pain is related to menses has it responded to nonsteroidal anti-inflammatory (NSAID) medication or combined hormonal contraception? A sexual history including possible exposure to sexually transmitted infections or dyspareunia is also important. Family history should be reviewed for endometriosis, depression, connective tissue disorders, uterine or ovarian cancer because a patient may be at higher risk for these diagnoses with a positive family history. Any exposure to sexual/physical abuse or substance use should also be elicited as this can often lead to chronic pain syndromes. Exploring psychosocial factors should examine the impact of the discomfort on activities of daily living, in particular school attendance, sleep, exercise, and social participation.

Adolescent girls with pelvic pain require a physical examination with special attention to the abdomen, musculoskeletal system, pelvic organs, and rectum. Initially, a patient should be asked if she can localize her discomfort to one specific area, as this is more frequently associated with an organic pathology.

Abdominal examination should include evaluation for masses, scarring, and hernias. Musculoskeletal examination should rule out scoliosis, lordosis, kyphosis, and trigger points using a single finger.[28] All sexually active females should have a complete external and internal pelvic examination to evaluate for discharge, lesions, masses, abnormal anatomy, or trigger points. A single-digit bimanual examination may be done in a virginal female if tolerated. A rectoabdominal examination should be done in all patients to evaluate for pain or nodularity of the posterior cul-de-sac.

### DIAGNOSIS

The diagnostic work-up for pelvic pain usually includes a pregnancy test, complete blood count with differential, sedimentation rate, urinalysis, urine culture, gonorrhea, and chlamydia tests if the girl is sexually active. A pelvic ultrasound is helpful especially if the patient cannot tolerate a bimanual examination or if a mass or ovarian torsion is suspected. An MRI is the most appropriate test for suspected genital anomalies. Diagnostic laparascopy is often a last resort in cases of persistent chronic pelvic pain. Management of pelvic pain will depend on the specific cause revealed in the evaluation.

In a study at Children's Hospital Boston, 121 adolescent girls were evaluated via laparoscopy for acute abdominal pain.[29] The most common diagnoses were ovarian cyst, acute salpingitis, no pathology, appendicitis, and ovarian torsion. A similar study of adolescent females undergoing laparoscopy for chronic pelvic pain at Children's Hospital Boston revealed endometriosis, no organic disease, postoperative adhesions, serositis, and ovarian cysts to be the most prevalent causes of pain.[29]

Diagnosing chronic pelvic pain in adolescent females is often a source of frustration for both the adolescent and the physician. Frequently, families are distressed secondary to ongoing interruptions of daily life and school attendance. An integrated approach to both physiologic and psychosocial contributions is vital to the evaluation.[28] Establishing a sound and open rapport with families is the most important part of a successful evaluation and treatment plan.

## REFERENCES

1. Heller D. Diseases manifesting in the upper genital tract in children and adolescents: a review. *J Pediatr Adolesc Gyn.* 2006;19:3-9

2. Nahum GG. Uterine anomalies. How common are they, and what is their distribution among subtypes? Abstract. *J Repro Med.* 1998;43(10):877-887

3. The American Fertility Society. *The American Fertility Society Classification of Müllerian Anomalies*. Birmingham, AL: American Society for Reproductive Medicine; 2006

4. Edmonds DK. Sexual developmental anomalies and their reconstruction: upper and lower tracts. In: Sanfilippo JS, Muram D, Lee PA, Dewhurst J, eds. *Pediatric and Adolescent Gynecology*. Philadelphia, PA: WB Saunders; 1994: 535-566

5. Pinsonneault O, Goldstein DP. Obstructing malformations of the uterus and vagina. *Fertil Steril.* 1985;44:241-247

6. Syed I. Uterus, mullerian duct abnormalities. *Emedicine.* Available at: www.emedicine.com/radio/topic738.htm. Accessed November 22, 2010

7. La Vecchia C, Draper GJ. Childhood nonovarian female genital tract cancers in Britain, 1962-1978. Descriptive epidemiology and long-term survival. *Cancer.* 1984;54:188-192

8. Hicks ML, Piver MS. Oncologic problems. In: Sanfilippo JS, Muram D, Lee PA, Dewhurst J, eds. *Pediatr Adolesc Gyn*. Philadelphia, PA: WB Saunders; 1994:601-616

9. Stepanian M, Cohn DE. Gynecologic malignancies in adolescents. *Adolesc Med Clin.* 2004;15:549-568

10. Emans SJ, Laufer MR, Goldstein DP. *Pediatric and Adolescent Gynecology*. 5th ed. Philadelphia, PA: Lippincott Williams & Wilkins; 2005

11. Attaran M, Gidwani G. Adolescent endometriosis. *Ob Gyn Clin N Am.* 2003;30:379-390

12. Laufer MR, Goitein L, Bush M, Cramer DW, Emans SJ. Prevalence of endometriosis in adolescnt women with chronic pelvic pain not responding to conventional therapy. *J Pediatr Adolesc Gyn.* 1997;10:199-202

13. Simpson JL, Elias S, Malinak LR, et al. Heritable aspects of endometriosis: I. Genetic studies. *Am J Obstet Gynecol.* 1980;137:327-331

14. Batt RE, Mitwally MFM. Endometriosis from thelarche to midteens: pathogenesis and prognosis, prevention and pedagogy. *J Pediatr Adolesc Gyn.* 2003;16(6):337-347

15. Laufer MR, Sanfilippo J, Rose G. Adolescent endometriosis: diagnosis and treatment approaches. *J Pediatr Adolesc Gyn.* 2003;16:S3-S11

16. American Society for Reproductive Medicine. *American Society for Reproductive Medicine Revised Classification of Endometriosis*. Birmingham, AL: American Society for Reproductive Medicine; 2006

17. Henzl MR, Corson SC, Moghissi K, et al. Administration of nasal nafarelin as compared with oral danazol for endometriosis. *N Engl J Med.* 1988;318:485-489

18. Lu PT, Ory SJ. Endometriosis: current management. *Mayo Clin Pro.* 1995;70:453-463

19. Barbieri RL. CA-125 in patients with endometriosis. *Fertil Steril.* 1986;45:767-769

20. Surratt JT, Siegel MJ. Imaging of pediatric ovarian masses. *RadioGraphics.* 1991;11:533-548

21. Powell JK. Benign adnexal masses in the adolescent. *Adolesc Med Clin.* 2004;15:535-547

22. Murray S, London S. Management of ovarian cysts in neonates, children, and adolescents. *Adolesc Pediatr Gynecol.* 1995;8:64-70

23. Jones HW. Germ cell tumors of the ovary. In: Jones HW, Wentz AC, Burnett LS, eds. *Novak's Textbook of Gynecology*. 11th ed. Baltimore, MD: Williams & Wilkens; 1988

24. Laing FC, Van Dalsem VF, Marks WM, et al. Dermoid cysts of the ovary: their ultrasonographic appearances. *Ob Gyn.* 1981;57(1):99-104

25. Woodruff JD, Protos P, Peterson WF. Ovarian teratomas. *Am J Obstet Gynecol.* 1968;102:702-715

26. Tsai JY, Saigo PE, Brown C, La Quaglia MP. Diagnosis, pathology, staging, treatment, and outcome of epithelial ovarian neoplasia in patients age (21 years). *Cancer.* 2001;19(11):2065-2070

27. Song AH, Advincula AP. Adolescent chronic pelvic pain. *J Pediatr Adolesc Gyn.* 2005;18:371-377

28. Holland-Hall CM, Brown RT. Evaluation of the adolescent with chronic abdominal or pelvic pain. *J Pediatr Adolesc Gyn.* 2004;17:23-27

29. Goldstein DP. Acute and chronic pelvic pain. *Ped Clin North Am.* 1989;36(3):573-580

# CHAPTER 62

# Amenorrhea

GERI HEWITT, MD

## INTRODUCTION

Amenorrhea is the absence or abnormal cessation of menses for greater than 3 months.[1] Primary amenorrhea occurs in the absence of menarche; other secondary sexual characteristics including breast development and axillary/pubic hair may or may not be present depending on the underlying etiology. Secondary amenorrhea occurs after the completion of the pubertal process and menarche; all patients with secondary amenorrhea will have mature breast development as well as axillary/pubic hair. Secondary amenorrhea is much more common than primary amenorrhea.

The World Health Organization (WHO) has developed a framework describing and categorizing the causes of amenorrhea; these descriptive categories are helpful references when evaluating patients. World Health Organization group I includes patients with no evidence of endogenous estrogen production, normal or low follicle-stimulating hormone (FSH) levels, normal prolactin levels, and no evidence of a lesion in the hypothalamic–pituitary region. World Health Organization group II includes patients with evidence of estrogen production and normal levels of prolactin and FSH. Lastly, WHO group III includes patients with elevated serum FSH levels indicating gonadal failure.[2] Although primary and secondary amenorrhea share some clinical similarities and common etiologies, they will be discussed separately for educational purposes. Although less common than secondary amenorrhea, primary amenorrhea represents a more complex paradigm and will be reviewed first.

## PRIMARY AMENORRHEA

### EVALUATION

Historically, patients were diagnosed with primary amenorrhea and an evaluation was initiated if they were 16 years old with the absence of menarche. As more recent research has enhanced our understanding of normal timing of pubertal onset, newer recommendations suggest the evaluation should begin sooner. The current standard is to initiate an evaluation if a patient reaches 15 years of age (2 standard deviations above the mean age for menarche of 13 years) with normal secondary sexual characteristics and has not begun menstruating.[3] Other clinical scenarios that require evaluation include girls who begin breast development prior to 10 years of age and who have not begun menstruating within 5 years of thelarche (for example, breast bud development at age 9 with the absence of menses at age 14) and girls who have not yet begun breast development by age 13.[3]

Like all complicated medical evaluations, the evaluation of primary amenorrhea should begin with a history. Several key elements that need to be explored include the timing and age of linear growth, age of thelarche and pubarche, as well as the presence of lower abdominal pain, galactorrhea, or headache. Family history of any genetic abnormalities should also be ascertained.

The physical examination in patients presenting with primary amenorrhea is crucial and will often reveal the cause. Height and weight should be obtained and plotted on a growth curve. Short stature may suggest Turner syndrome 45, XO or a chromosomal mosaic variant (ie, 46,XX/45,XO). Although more commonly associated with secondary amenorrhea, extremes in weight can also delay or abolish menarche. Assessing breast development is important; thelarche ensures evidence of endogenous estrogen production. True breast development (palpable breast bud, areola papilla complex) should be differentiated from simply fatty tissue. Axillary and pubic hair should be assessed; scant or absent axillary or pubic hair may suggest either androgen insensitivity syndrome (AIS) or 46,XY gonadal dysgenesis (Swyer syndrome). Evaluation of the external genitalia should answer 2 important questions. First, is there evidence of a patent vagina, meaning an introital opening is present? An obstruction in the vaginal outflow tract, such as an imperforate hymen or transverse vaginal septum (Figure 62-1) will result in an absence of menstrual flow. Simply passing a swab through the vaginal opening and identifying a 3- to 4-cm vagina will rule out the possibility of these abnormalities. Secondly, has there been estrogenization of the vagina and labia from its prepubertal state? This represents additional evidence supporting endogenous estrogen production. When the prepubertal vagina becomes estrogenized,

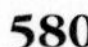

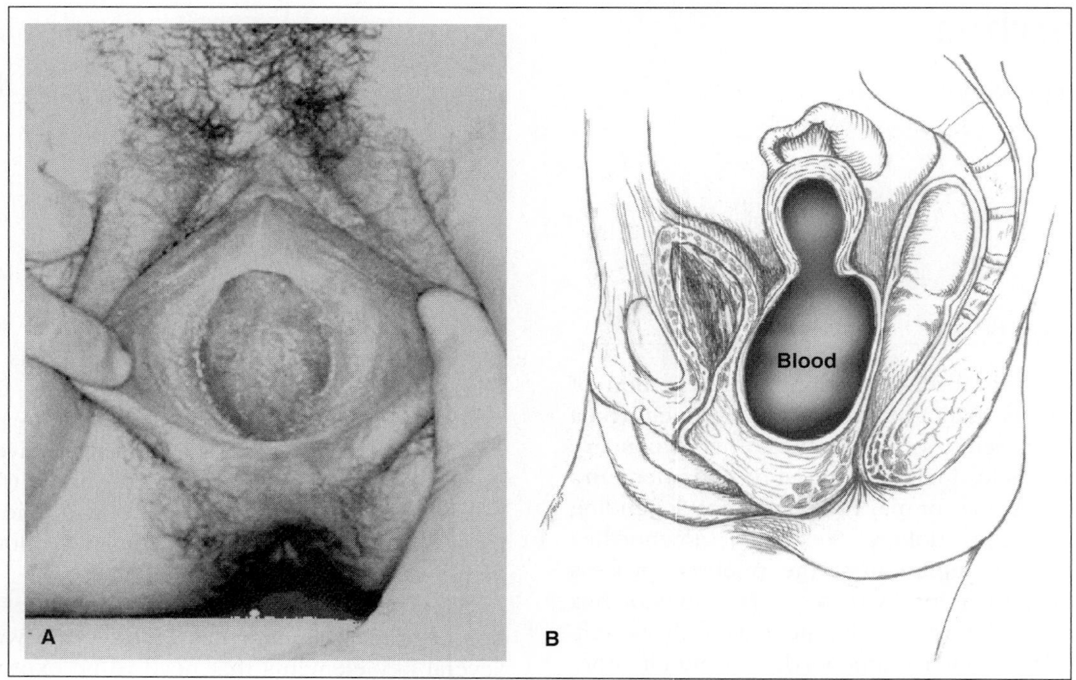


FIGURE 62-1 Imperforate hymen. (A) Classic appearance of the bulging, blue-domed, translucent membrane. (See color insert.) (B) Diagram of hematometra and hematocolopos with imperforate distal transverse vaginal septum. (Image reprinted with permission from eMedicine.com, 2010. Available at: emedicine.medscape.com/article/269050-media.)

the vaginal mucosa becomes moist, pink, and rugated; it loses its smooth, pale, prepubertal appearance. Another crucial element of the physical examination is to evaluate the length of the vagina and determine whether the uterus is present, eliminating the diagnosis of CAUV (congenital absence of the uterus and vagina) or AIS. This is typically accomplished with a gentle bimanual examination; a rectal examination can also be useful to verify the presence of the uterus. All elements of the physical examination should be complete and accurate before turning attention toward ordering or interpreting laboratory values or radiological imaging studies.

Initial laboratory work should include a serum beta human chorionic gonadotropin level (BHCG) if the patient is sexually active, FSH, TSH (thyroid-stimulating hormone), and prolactin (Box 62-1). A negative serum BHCG eliminates the possibility of pregnancy in the sexually active patient with amenorrhea. An elevated FSH level is indicative of ovarian failure (primary hypogonadism). The ovaries may fail prior to the onset of puberty or at any point during the pubertal process. Some patients with gonadal failure will achieve significant stature and breast development prior to ovarian failure; others will have short stature and absent breasts, depending on at what point estrogen production is diminished or halted. Patients diagnosed with elevated FSH require a karyotype to rule out Turner

**Box 62-1**

***Evaluation of Primary Amenorrhea***

History
Physical examination
BHCG
TSH
Prolactin
FSH
Pelvic ultrasound (if indicated to determine uterine structure)
Karyotype (if FSH elevated)
Brain MRI (if increase prolactin, delayed puberty, or low FSH)

Adapted with permission from The Practice Committee of the American Society for Reproductive Medicine. Current evaluation of amenorrhea. *Fertil Steril.* 2004;82(1):266-272.

syndrome (45,XO) or a mosaic variant of the same (45, XO/46,XX), as well as 46, XY gonadal dysgenesis. If any Y chromosomal material is identified in patients with primary hypogonadism, either in pure or mosaic form, the patient should be referred for immediate gonadectomy due to the malignant potential of the gonads. Normal FSH levels suggest that the hypothalamic-pituitary-gonadal axis is intact, and that anatomic variations such as outflow tract obstructions or congenitally absent organs are causing the lack of menstruation. Low FSH levels are indicative of hypothalamic or pituitary causes of amenorrhea. Examples of hypothalamic amenorrhea include eating disorders and craniopharyngiomas; the hypothalamus is not stimulating the pituitary to secrete FSH in normal levels. Pituitary causes resulting in decreased FSH production and amenorrhea include hormone-secreting pituitary tumors or, alternatively, mutations in the FSH receptor. The TSH is useful to rule out subclinical hypothyroidism, even in patients who are asymptomatic. If elevated, a work-up for hypothyroidism should be initiated. In the absence of hypothyroidism, an elevated serum prolactin prompts further evaluation to rule out a pituitary prolactinoma or medication use associated with elevated serum prolactin levels. In primary hypothyroidism, the elevated hypothalamic TSRH levels can stimulate increased secretion of prolactin from the pituitary, resulting in hyperprolactinemia.

Ultrasound and magnetic resonance imaging (MRI) imaging may be indicated in patients with primary amenorrhea. Pelvic ultrasound can be useful to identify the presence or absence of a uterus. Additionally, the ultrasound can reveal whether the ovaries have follicles and appear to be hormonally active, the size and shape of the uterine structure, and if the endometrial lining of the uterus appears to be stimulated by endogenous estrogen production. In cases of outflow tract obstruction, the level of obstruction (imperforate hymen, vaginal agenesis, cervical agenesis, and noncommunicating uterus) can often be identified. Renal ultrasound may be indicated for patients diagnosed with congenitally absent or abnormal uteri because those patients are at increased risk of renal abnormalities. A pelvic MRI may be useful to further delineate a Müllerian abnormality. Figure 62-2 demonstrates a pelvic MRI with hematocolpos. Brain MRI should be considered for patients with significantly elevated serum prolactin levels to investigate the possibility of a prolactinoma or other hypothalamic or pituitary tumors or abnormalities (such as empty sella syndrome). Some experts would recommend brain evaluation with MRI in all patients with hypogonadism and delayed puberty to rule out tumors.[4]

### Hypergonadotrophic Hypogonadism

The single most common cause of primary amenorrhea is ovarian failure caused by gonadal dysgenesis (Box 62-2).[5]

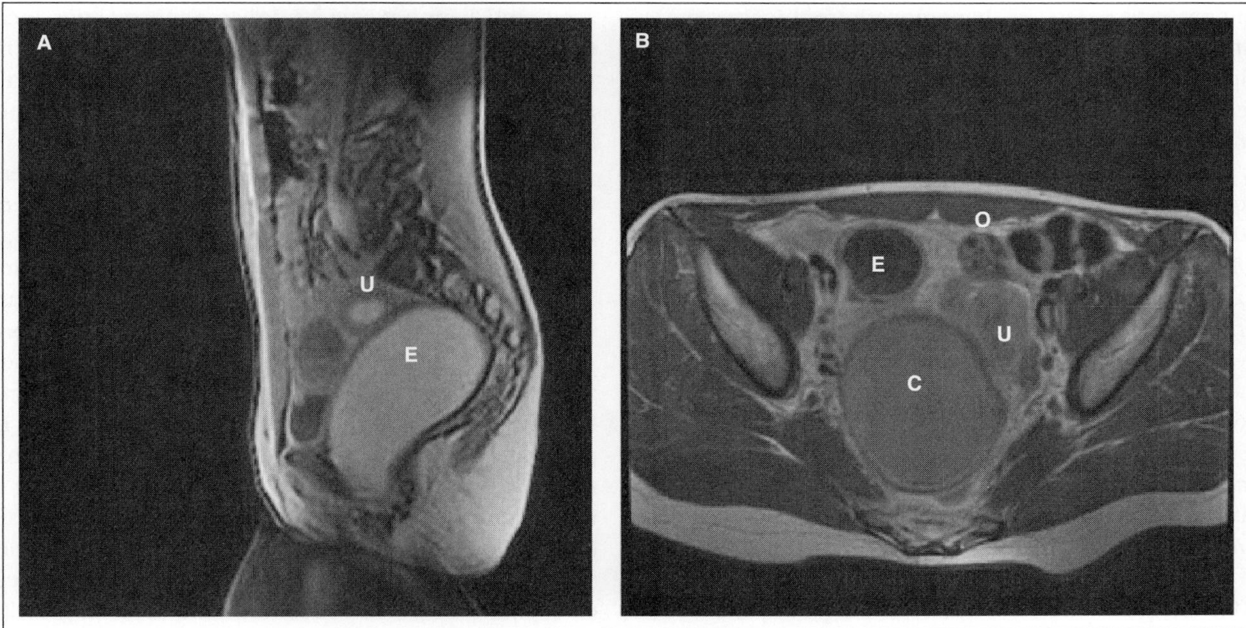


FIGURE 62-2 Pelvic MRI. U: right-sided uterus with hematometra, C: hematocolpos. (Reprinted from Hollander MH. Unilateral renal agenesis and association Müllerian anomalies: a case report and recommendations for pre-adolescent screening. *J Pediatr Adolesc Gynecol*. 2008;21:151–153, with permission from Elsevier.)

**Box 62-2**

***Common Causes of Primary Amenorrhea***

- Breast development present
  - CAUV (Congenital absence of uterus and vagina)
  - AIS (androgen insensitivity syndrome)
  - Vaginal septum
- Imperforate hymen
- Constitutional delay
- No breast development: high FSH
  - Gonadal dysgenesis
    - 46,XX
    - 46,XY
  - Abnormal or mosaic karyotype
- No breast development: low FSH
  - Constitutional delay
  - Prolactinomas
  - Kallmann syndrome
  - Other central nervous system lesions
  - Stress, weight loss, anorexia nervosa
  - Polycystic ovary syndrome
  - Congenital adrenal hyperplasia

Modified from The Practice Committee of the American Society for Reproductive Medicine. Current evaluation of amenorrhea. *Fertil Steril.* 2004;82:266-272, with permission from Elsevier.

Patients with gonadal failure will have elevated FSH levels, commonly referred to as hypergonadotrophic hypogonadism (WHO group III). The gonads can fail at any time during development, from failure in utero through failure at the end of the pubertal process just prior to menarche. Patients can express varying degrees of breast development depending on when in the pubertal process the gonads fail. Patients with an elevated FSH, indicating gonadal failure, all require determination of their karyotype. This is crucial to help differentiate the diagnosis, as well as to eliminate the presence of any Y chromosomal material, which increases risk of malignant transformation of the gonads. The largest number of patients with ovarian failure have Turner syndrome (45,XO), followed by 46,XX gonadal dysgensis, and rarely, 46,XY gonadal dysgenesis. Each of these clinical entities will be discussed separately.[5]

Turner syndrome represents the leading cause of patients undergoing primary ovarian failure. These patients can have the classic form of Turner syndrome (45,XO) or they can have a mosaic variant (45,XO/46,XX or 45,XO/46,XY); the mosaic variants account for the majority of cases of Turner syndrome.[5] The underlying defect in patients with Turner syndrome is the accelerated loss of ovarian germ cells. The ovarian determinant genes are found on the short arm of the X chromosome; patients with Turner syndrome do not have a full complement of both short arms of the X chromosome, resulting in accelerated loss of ovarian germ cells and eventually loss of ovarian function. This loss of ovarian function can occur anytime from in utero until after the onset of the first menses. Some patients will have enough ovarian function for a normal pubertal process culminating in regular, ovulatory menstrual cycles, for a significant portion of the adolescent and young adult life prior to the ovarian failure and subsequent amenorrhea. Fewer than 5% of patients with Turner syndrome will ever achieve a spontaneous pregnancy prior to ovarian failure.[6] Once the germ cells have been depleted, the ovary has only the remaining connective tissue stroma, which is hormonally inactive and does not contain follicles; these ovaries are now abnormal in appearance and are often referred to as "streak gonads." If the patient's karyotype reveals any Y chromosomal material, the gonad should be removed immediately to eliminate the possibility of malignant transformation, most commonly the development of gonadoblastomas and malignant germ cell tumors.[7] Unlike patients with AIS these gonads are not hormonally active; there is no clinical advantage to waiting for further pubertal development prior to removal.

Turner syndrome patients (Figure 62-3) have variable clinical stigmata including cardiovascular anomalies, renal abnormalities, high arched palate, low hair line, webbed neck, multiple pigmented nevi, short fourth metacarpals, shield chest, increased carrying angle of the arms, and lymphedema.[5] Cardiac abnormalities include the presence of coarctation of the aorta in up to 30% of patients.[6] Because of the risk of developing dilation and rupture of the ascending aorta, these patients should have a cardiac echocardiogram every 3 to 5 years.

Gonadal failure in the presence of a normal female karyotype (46,XX) can be either acquired or inherited. A relatively common acquired cause of primary ovarian failure in patients with a normal karyotype is autoimmune in nature. Along with the primary amenorrhea, they are at increased risk of developing other autoimmune abnormalities including Hashimoto thyroiditis, hypoparathyroidism, adrenal insufficiency, and pernicious anemia. Ovarian biopsy is not indicated for diagnostic purposes; there is no practical way to confirm the diagnosis. There is currently no validated serum antibody marker to confirm the clinical diagnosis of autoimmune premature ovarian failure (POF). However, when it is suspected, patients should be screened regularly for hypothyroidism and other endocrinopathies. Currently recommended screening includes TSH, thyroid autoantibodies, fasting glucose, and electrolytes.[1,2] Screening for adrenal insufficiency can be done with either an adrenocorticotropic hormone (ACTH) stimulation test or a random serum cortisol level.

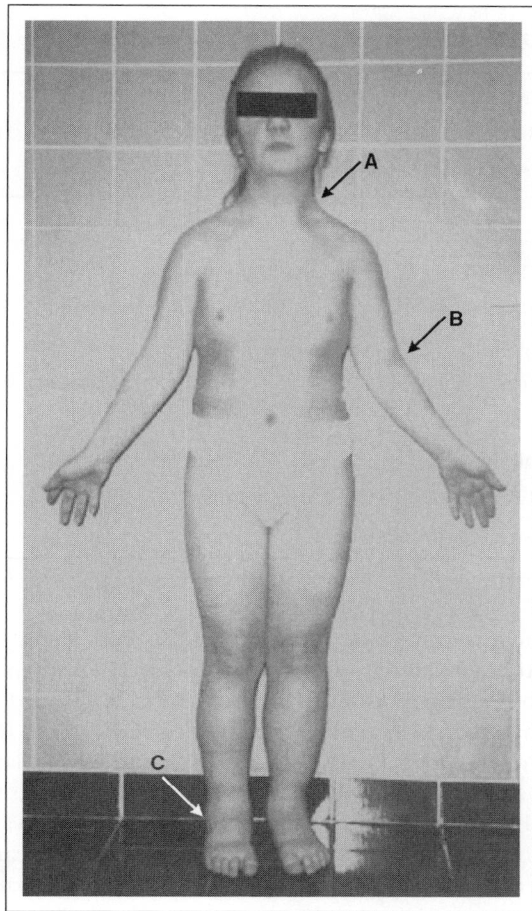


FIGURE 62-3 Photo of patient with Turner syndrome. The arrows point to some of the classical features of Turner syndrome: (A) short webbed neck; (B) cubitus valgus; (C) lymphedema. (Reprinted by permission from Macmillan Publishers Ltd: Gawlik A, Malecka-Tendera E. Hormonal therapy in a patient with a delayed diagnosis of Turner syndrome. *Nat Clinical Pract Endocrinol & Metab.* 2008;4:173–177, copyright 2008.)

Other acquired causes of POF include iatrogenic etiologies such as chemotherapy and radiation used for treatment of various malignancies. The impact of radiation on ovarian function depends on the age of the patient at the time of the exposure as well as the quantity and location of the exposure. Chemotherapeutic agents vary in terms of their potentially toxic effects on the ovary; alkylating agents are thought to be the most harmful. Ovarian failure due to iatrogenic exposure to chemotherapy and radiation can be transient, with some patients recovering ovarian function over time. Patients who present with abnormal vaginal bleeding should be evaluated for resumption of ovarian function by ordering a serum FSH; resumption of ovarian function is confirmed when the FSH is no longer elevated.

Patients with a normal karyotype may have a genetic as opposed to chromosomal etiology of their primary amenorrhea. Genetic disorders, such as myotonia dystrophica, ataxia telangiectasia, galactosemia, and mucopolysaccharidoses, have been associated with primary ovarian failure.[8]

Girls with POF regardless of the etiology should be placed on hormone replacement therapy to promote and maintain secondary sexual characteristics and reduce the risk of developing osteoporosis. Patients should continue with combination estrogen and progestin hormone replacement therapy until the natural age of menopause, which is around age 50. If ovarian failure occurs prior to acquisition of normal breast development, the therapy should begin with low doses of estrogen to promote breast development; progestins are then added only after the breast mound and areola are appropriately developed.[9]

After the acquisition of breast development, a patient may either take combination hormone replacement therapy or oral contraceptive pills. Patients and their families often have concerns about the use of hormones at a young age or for extended periods of time. The dose of hormones used in traditional hormone replacement therapy is much lower than the level of hormones they would be exposed to through endogenous production from normally functioning ovaries. Additionally, many of the risks associated with hormone replacement therapy are age dependent; younger patients face fewer risks. Lastly, avoiding hormone replacement therapy in patients with POF has a significant risk of bone loss and could have a negative impact on development and maintenance of normal secondary sexual characteritics and sexual functioning.

The most uncommon karyotype found in patients with primary amenorrhea and hypergonadotrophic hypogonadism is 46,XY (Swyer syndrome). These patients have testes that have failed (streak gonads) and therefore do not produce testosterone and Müllerian inhibiting factor (MIF). This germ cell depletion is complete before birth. The lack of testosterone results in female external genitalia and the lack of acquisition of normal secondary sexual characteristics; the lack of MIF results in the development of a normal uterus, fallopian tubes, and vagina. The absence of ovaries results in a lack of endogenous estrogen and, therefore, breast development. Because of the presence of the Y chromosome, these patients are often tall, and their gonads should be removed because of their malignant potential.

### Eugonadism

Patients with normal ovarian function (eugonadism, FSH normal) will often have an abnormality associated with the outflow tract (WHO group II). The hypothalamic-pituitary-ovarian axis is intact, resulting in normal secondary sexual characteristics and normal serum hormone levels. The absence of menarche is due to absence of endometrial lining to produce menses or an obstruction blocking the egress of the menstrual flow. Patients who do not have a uterus or endometrial lining will be relatively asymptomatic, except for the lack of menarche. Because an absent uterus can be associated with a shortened, blind vagina, these patients may complain of excessive pain when trying to initiate sexual intercourse. If a patient has endometrial tissue that is stimulated with estrogen, she will produce menstrual blood. Any abnormality that results in a blockage of menstrual egress can result in amenorrhea and cramping, cyclic, lower abdominal pain. The lower abdominal pain is due to the accumulation of blood in the vagina (hematocolpos) or uterine cavity (hematometra). Imperforate hymen represents the most common type of an outflow tract obstruction and can usually be identified on physical examination by visualizing the intact hymenal membrane between the labia. Having the patient cough or bear down (or even move down the examination table) will cause the hymenal membrane to bulge and help confirm the diagnosis. Patients should be referred for a relatively simple surgical correction (hymenectomy) after which they will experience immediate menstrual egress and relief of their symptoms. Imperforate hymen is an isolated lesion, not associated with other Müllerian abnormalities. Transverse vaginal septum and cervical stenosis/agenesis also block menstrual egress and require more complex surgical intervention. Congenitally abnormal uteri that have endometrial tissue but are not appropriately connected to an open vagina produce similar symptoms and also require surgical intervention. These abnormalities can usually be readily identified with radiological imaging procedures.

### Congenital Absence of the Uterus and Vagina (CAUV) and Androgen Insensitivity Syndrome (AIS)

The differential diagnosis in patients with primary amenorrhea who present with breast development and an absent uterus with a shortened, blind vagina consists of 2 possibilities; Müllerian agenesis leading to CAUV and androgen insensitivity (Table 62-1). CAUV is the second most common cause of primary amenorrhea.[5] It has been known by the name Mayer-Rokitansky-Kuster-Hauser syndrome in deference to those who first described aspects of the symptoms. Normally during intrauterine development, 2 Müllerian structures fuse in the midline; canalization then results in a normal midline single uterine cavity and a vagina of appropriate length. CAUV is considered a failed fusion defect and absence of vaginal canalization. These patients have no midline uterine structure but do have normal ovaries and fallopian tubes bilaterally. In addition to the aberrant pelvic structures, CAUV is associated with an increased risk of renal and skeletal abnormalities. Nearly 30% of these patients have renal anomalies, most commonly unilateral renal agenesis. From 12% to 50% of patients have skeletal abnormalities, most commonly scoliosis.[10] A vagina of normal length to accommodate sexual activity can be created by using vaginal dilators in a motivated patient at the appropriate developmental age. Rarely is surgical intervention in the form of vaginal neoplasty required. Because the ovaries are functioning normally, patients with CAUV can have their own biologic children through in vitro fertilization using a surrogate gestational carrier. These patients have the normal female karyotype, 46XX.

**Table 62-1**

**Congenital Absence of the Uterus and Vagina (CAUV) and Androgen Insensitivity Syndrome (AIS)**

| | *CAUV* | *AIS* |
|---|---|---|
| Karyotype | 46,XX | 46,XY |
| Gonads | ovaries | testes |
| Breasts | present | present |
| Uterus | absent | absent |
| Testosterone | female | male |
| Pubic hair | yes | no |
| Stature | normal | tall |
| Associated abnormalities | yes | no |

Like patients with CAUV, patients with AIS have normal breast development during puberty, but never menstruate; they also lack a uterus and have a shortened vagina. Unlike patients with CAUV, patients with AIS have a normal male karyotype, 46XY. Because of this, the gonads are testes that produce normal male quantities of both testosterone and MIF. The primary defect in AIS is an androgen receptor gene mutation that causes the receptor's inability to respond to the testosterone signal. This results in a lack of masculinization of the external genitalia in utero and a lack of male secondary sexual characteristics at the time of puberty. The MIF appropriately inhibits the development of the uterus and vagina. Increasing testosterone levels at puberty results in breast development as the testosterone is converted to estrogen. Because the testosterone receptor is defective, there is little if any pubic hair development. AIS patients are typically taller than their female peers because they have a male karyotype. The gonads require surgical removal once breast development is complete to avoid malignant transformation (seminoma). Like patients with CAUV, a vagina with appropriate length to accommodate sexual activity can be created either through vaginal dilators or surgical intervention if the dilators fail.

### Hypogonadotrophic Hypogonadism

Patients with primary amenorrhea and hypogonadotrophic hypogonadism will typically present with delayed puberty. These patients have low levels of FSH; the underlying etiology is either interruption in GnRH secretion from the hypothalamus or the FSH secretion from the pituitary. Congenitally acquired abnormalities include both the third most common cause of primary amenorrhea, idiopathic hypogonadotrophic hypogonadism (IHH),[5] and Kallmann syndrome. Patients with IHH have low levels of gonadotrophins (FSH and LH) but may respond to treatment with pulsatile GnRH, secreting normal levels of FSH and LH, subsequently stimulating steroidogenesis and follicular activity. Some patients who do not respond to GnRH stimulation will respond to exogenous FSH and LH culminating in folliculogenesis and ovulation. The latter patients are thought to have mutations in the GnRH receptor gene.[5] Some patients with isolated deficiency of GnRH production have Kallmann syndrome. These patients present with hypogonadotrophic hypogonadism, hyposmia or anosmia, midline facial defects, and occasionally, renal agenesis.[5] Some patients with Kallmann syndrome have mutations in an X-linked recessive gene (KAL gene), which encodes an adhesion molecule. Due to lack of the adhesion protein, GnRH-containing neurons do not migrate from the olfactory placode to the medial basal hypothalamus during fetal development.[11] The hypogonadotrophism is due to the anatomic variation.

Another cause of hypogonadotrophic hypogonadism and primary amenorrhea is constitutional delay of puberty. These patients will undergo puberty at a time greater than 2.5 standard deviations from the mean. They typically present at age 13 to 16 with little evidence of pubertal change (Tanner II breast development), shorter than their peers, with delayed bone ages and suppressed estradiol and gonadotrophin levels. Family history of late puberty may be elicited from either the mother or the father. Pelvic ultrasound will typically show multiple small ovarian follicles, consistent with early puberty, and if given a GnRH stimulation test, they will generate a pubertal response, with greater LH release than FSH. These patients do eventually enter puberty, typically when their bone age reaches age 9 to 11 years. The diagnosis is confirmed once the patient experiences menarche; exclusion of more worrisome diagnoses is important and justifies an appropriate evaluation.[5]

Several acquired abnormalities can result in hypogonadotrophic hypogonadism and primary amenorrhea by interfering with either GnRH production or gonadotrophin secretion. Several endocrine disorders, including Cushing syndrome, hypothyroidism, and congenital adrenal hyperplasia, can all interfere with gonadotrophin production. Diagnosis and treatment of the underlying disorder allows for return of normal gonadotrophin production, steroidogenesis, and pubertal development. Pituitary tumors can also cause hypogonadotrophic hypogonadism and pubertal delay. As mentioned earlier, some experts advocate brain imaging studies on all patients with pubertal delay and primary amenorrhea to increase identification of these tumors.[4] Prolactinomas are the most common pituitary tumor implicated and typically present once puberty has been initiated. Increased estrogen production in early puberty is thought to increase production of prolactin; the prolactinoma is thought not to delay the pubertal process, but rather to stop a normally timed puberty. Prolactinomas are typically slow-growing tumors identified by MRI in patients found to have elevated serum prolactin levels. Patients may present with oligomenorrhea (if menses have been established) or amenorrhea, as well as galactorrhea. Most prolactinomas are successfully treated medically with a dopamine agonist, and once normal serum prolactin levels are attained, the pubertal process and normal menarche/menses ensues. Craniopharygioma is another pituitary tumor that can cause destruction of the pituitary and suprasellar regions resulting in decreased gonadotrophin production. It typically presents before the onset of puberty and delays the pubertal process. These tumors can be aggressive in their growth or more indolent, in which case they may not present until later adolescence or early 20s. The tumor is highly calcified making it easily visible on radiological imaging studies. Other systemic diseases that can diminish gonadotrophin release include malabsorptive bowel disease, poorly controlled diabetes, poorly controlled rheumatoid arthritis, and eating disorders, particularly anorexia nervosa.[5] Part 3, Section 2, Eating Disorders, provides an in-depth discussion of menstrual disorders in such patients.

## SECONDARY AMENORRHEA

Secondary amenorrhea is much more common than primary amenorrhea. An evaluation for secondary amenorrhea should be initiated when a patient has not had spontaneous menses for more than 3 months or has had fewer than 9 menses over the previous year (Box 62-3).[5] The differential diagnosis and evaluation of a patient

**Box 62-3**

***Evaluation of Secondary Amenorrhea***

History
Physical examination
Pregnancy test
TSH, prolactin
Testosterone, DHEAS if clinical evidence of hyperandrogenism
Progestin challenge
FSH if negative progestin challenge

with secondary amenorrhea is much less complex than that of a patient with primary amenorrhea (Box 62-4). Already, the patient has successfully completed menarche, and therefore the clinician can feel confident that the patient has had a normal pubertal process.

The history and physical examination should be directed in an attempt to discover or rule out various etiologies of secondary amenorrhea. The history should elicit the highlights of the patient's pubertal process and when menarche occurred as well as the menstrual cycle pattern to date. Other important historical points to note include any significant change in weight, male patterned hair growth, worsening acne, breast discharge, changes in sleep patterns or mood and affect, and current medications including recent use of hormonal contraception. Lifestyle issues that are important to explore include dietary habits, exercise intensity, whether sexual activity has been initiated, and stressors at home, school, work, or with other relationships. Physical examination should begin with both weighing and measuring the patient to determine her percentage of ideal body weight, or alternatively, her body mass index (BMI). Other physical signs associated with eating disorders can include loss or thinning of hair, lanugo, and dental erosion. An evaluation of skin looking for striae, acne, hirsutism, or *Acanthosis nigricans* should be completed. The thyroid should be palpated to evaluate for enlargement or nodules; breast examination should be performed to evaluate for galactorrhea. If the patient is sexually active, a pelvic examination may be indicated to assess the possibility of pregnancy, screen for sexually transmitted infection, and obtain a Pap smear, if indicated.

If the patient reports a history of sexual activity or if sexual activity is suspected, a urine or serum pregnancy test should be performed to rule out pregnancy. Pregnancy is the most common cause of secondary amenorrhea in sexually active girls. If the pregnancy test is positive, appropriate referral should be made. A negative pregnancy test in a sexually active patient is an important opportunity to discuss and initiate contraception, if appropriate.

Once the possibility of pregnancy has been eliminated, initial laboratory evaluation should include a TSH and prolactin. If the patient has any clinical evidence of hyperandrogenism (hirsutism or acne), then testosterone and dehydroenpiandrosterone sulfate (DHEAS) should be ordered as well. Testosterone is produced by the ovary; DHEAS is produced by the adrenal gland. A progestin challenge should be initiated as well once pregnancy has been ruled out while waiting for the laboratory results. A progestin challenge is a diagnostic and potentially therapeutic step. There are many different ways to prescribe progestins for a progestin challenge; 1 commonly used regimen is medroxy-progestone acetate 10 mg by mouth each day for a total of 10 days. It is very important not to use oral contraceptive pills for a progestin challenge because they contain an estrogen, ethinyl estradiol. The patient is instructed to note any vaginal bleeding experienced either while taking the medication or during the week following completion of the 10-day course. Any visible bleeding constitutes a positive progestin challenge. A positive progestin challenge suggests 2 things: (1) ample production of endogenous estradiol to stimulate the endometrial lining, and (2) an endometrial lining that responds appropriately

**Box 62-4**

***Common Causes of Secondary Amenorrhea***

- Low or normal FSH
  - Weight loss, anorexia nervosa, excessive exercise
  - Hypothalamic amenorrhea/nonspecific
  - Polycystic ovary syndrome
  - Hypothyroidism
  - Cushing syndrome
  - Pituitary tumor
- High FSH
  - Gonadal failure
  - 46,XX
  - 46,XY
  - Abnormal karyotype
- Hyperprolactinemia
- Anatomic
  - Endometrial adhesions (Asherman syndrome)
- Hyperandrogenic state
  - Ovarian tumor/adnexal tumor
  - Late-onset congenital adrenal hyperplasia

Modified from The Practice Committee of the American Society for Reproductive Medicine. Current evaluation of amenorrhea. *Fertil Steril.* 2004;82:266–272, with permission from Elsevier..

to estrogen and progestin stimulation. A negative progestin challenge suggests either that there is inadequate endogenous estrogen production to stimulate the endometrium or that the endometrium has been damaged in some way (for example, scar tissue formation after a dilatation and curettage, also known as Asherman syndrome).

For many patients, results of the history, physical examination, labs, and progestin challenge will confirm the correct diagnosis. An abnormal TSH should prompt a complete evaluation for thyroid disease. Hypothyroidism, more commonly than hyperthyroidism, can lead to menstrual cycle changes including oligomenorrhea and amenorrhea. Once the underlying thyroid condition has been corrected and the patient is euthyroid, normal ovulatory menstrual cycles will resume.

Patients with hyperprolactinemia may present with galactorrhea in addition to menstrual cycle abnormalities. Hyperprolactinemia has a wide range of etiologies, some more serious than others. Both hyperprolactinemia and thyroid disease are seen more commonly in patients with chronic anovulation with hyperandrogenism, or polycystic ovarian syndrome (PCOS). Also, numerous medications, most commonly psychotropic medications, can cause hyperprolactinemia. A significantly elevated serum prolactin level warrants central nervous system (CNS) imaging with MRI to evaluate for lesions such as prolactinomas or craniopharyngiomas (both discussed with primary amenorrhea). A prolactinoma less than 10 mm in size is called a microadenoma and responds well to medical intervention with a dopamine agonist. Medical management is indicated for ovulation induction or for breast symptoms (pain, swelling, galactorrhea). Patients whose only symptoms are menstrual cycle abnormalities and are not trying to achieve pregnancy can be managed long term with oral contraceptive pills or cyclic progestins to regulate the menstrual cycles. They do not need to be maintained on a dopamine agonist long term.[4] The CNS imaging study is most important to identify macroadenomas (prolactinomas >10 mm) or other significant pituitary or hypothalamic lesions. Most macroadenomas are successfully managed medically and rarely require surgical intervention.

Elevated serum testosterone levels in addition to menstrual cycle irregularities suggest the diagnosis of chronic anovulation with hyperandrogenism, or PCOS. Women with PCOS have a positive progestin challenge due to stimulation of the endometrium by estrone, an estrogen produced peripherally by the aromatization or androstenedione. Patients with PCOS are more likely to experience central obesity, and an important element of management includes weight loss/control. In addition to obesity, patients with PCOS are more likely to experience hirsutism, acne, endometrial hyperplasia or cancer, infertility, diabetes, and hyperlipidemia. Immediate needs for women first diagnosed with PCOS typically include a medical regimen to initiate regular withdrawal bleeds, using either oral contraceptive pills or cyclic progestins, and medications to help with the androgenic side effects such as oral contraceptive pills, spironolactone, cosmesis for hirsutism, or topical acne medications. Polycystic ovarian syndrome is discussed more completely in Chapter 65. Although PCOS is the most common cause of hyperandrogenism and amenorrhea in girls, it is important to rule out other less likely causes such as late onset congenital adrenal hyperplasia or Cushing syndrome.

A negative progestin challenge in a girl with secondary amenorrhea suggests lack of endogenous estrogen production. Alternatively, a patient may have had damage to the uterine lining during a dilation and curettage, much less common in the age group compared to adult women. To determine whether the lack of endogenous estrogen production is due to either ovarian failure or a lack of appropriate signal from the pituitary or hypothalamus, a serum FSH should be ordered. An elevated serum FSH confirms POF, as discussed earlier in the chapter. All girls diagnosed with POF require a karyotype to identify any Y chromosomal material, which would require gonadectomy because of malignant potential. Women with POF should receive standard combination hormone replacement therapy (not oral contraceptive pills) until the age of a normal menopause (around 50 years) to minimize bone loss; they also require monitoring for other autoimmune-related endocrinopathies.

A negative progestin challenge with a normal or low FSH suggests a hypothalamic cause of the amenorrhea. Common hypothalamic causes of secondary amenorrhea in girls include stress, anorexia nervosa, and excessive exercise. For patients undergoing extreme stress that has resulted in a disruption of the menstrual cycle, removing them from the stressful environment will typically result in the resumption of menses. The female athlete triad is characterized by amenorrhea, decreased bone mineral density or osteopenia, and disordered eating (see Chapter 78, The Female Athlete Triad). These patients typically have low body weight/body fat and a history of excessive exercise leading to disruption of menstrual cycles. Girls with the female athlete triad have some form of disordered eating, but they do not necessarily exhibit the altered body image seen in anorexia nervosa. The female athlete triad represents a negative energy balance in which the patient is chronically expending more energy exercising than she is consuming with eating, resulting in low body weight and menstrual cycle disruption. If the amenorrhea persists for an extended period of time, these patients are at increased risk for bone loss and osteopenia. Their excessive weight-bearing exercise does not make up for the lower estrogen levels seen with amenorrhea, resulting in a risk of bone loss. Patients need to be counseled to correct the negative energy imbalance by either consuming more calories or exercising less vigorously, working toward resumption of menses. If the amenorrhea persists, hormone replacement therapy in addition to calcium supplementation may be considered to try to minimize bone loss; although currently there is no evidence to support that hormone replacement therapy will protect the bone.

Anorexia nervosa is a life-threatening medical condition that may present with amenorrhea. Patients with anorexia nervosa and amenorrhea are at increased risk of bone loss and osteopenia. Therapy should be directed at treating the eating disorder with weight restoration and mental health support. Most patients will resume menstruating when reaching a more normal weight, a sign of health. If patients experience amenorrhea for extended periods of time, again, hormone replacement therapy can be considered to help minimize bone loss with the understanding that there is no evidence that hormone replacement therapy will be protective.

## REFERENCES

1. *Stedman's Medical Dictionary.* 27th ed. Philadelphia, PA: Lippincott Williams & Wilkins; 2000

2. Insler V. Gonadotropin therapy: new trends and insights. *Int Fertil.* 1988;33:85–97

3. Herman-Giddens ME, Slora EJ, Wasserman RC, et al. Secondary sexual characteristics and menses in young girls seen in office practice; a study from the Pediatric Research in Office Settings network. *Pediatrics.* 1997;99:505–512

4. Speroff L, Fritz MA. *Clinical Gynecologic Endocrinology and Infertility.* 7th ed. Baltimore, MD: Williams & Wilkins; 2005

5. Timmreck LS, Reindollar RH. Contemporary issues in primary amenorrhea. *Obstet Gynecol Clin N Amer.* 2003;30:287–302

6. Reindollar RH, Byrd JR, McDonough PF. Delayed sexual development; a study of 252 patients. *Am J Obstet Gynecol.* 1981;140(4):372–380

7. Manuel M, Katayama PK, Jones HW Jr. The age of occurrence of gonadal tumors in intersex patients with a Y chromosome. *Am J Obstet Gynecol.* 1976;124:292–300

8. Simpson JL, Rajkovic A. Ovarian differentiation and gonadal failure. *Am J Genet.* 1999;89(4):186–200

9. Rebar RW, Connolly HV. Clinical features of young women with amenorrhea. *Fertil Steril.* 1990;53:804–810

10. Griffin JE, Creighton E, Madden JD, et al. Congenital absence of the vagina: the Mayer-Rokitansky-Kuster-Hauser syndrome. *Ann Int Med.* 1976;85:224

11. Layman L. Molecular basis of human hypogonadotropic hypogonadism. *Mol Genet Metab.* 1999;68:191–198

12. The Practice Committee of the American Society for Reproductive Medicine. Current evaluation of amenorrhea. *Fertil Steril.* 2004;82(1):266–272

# CHAPTER 63

# Menstrual Disorders: Dysmenorrhea and Premenstrual Syndrome

ALEXANDRA S. CAREY, MD • PAMELA J. MURRAY, MD, MHP

## INTRODUCTION

There is a wide array of menstrual disorders in adolescent females, most of which cause substantial morbidity and are often poorly understood by the patient. The specific disorders that are addressed in this chapter, Dysmenorrhea and Premenstrual Syndrome (PMS), have very different etiologies, yet both are associated with ovulatory cycles. This is in contrast to disorders such as dysfunctional uterine bleeding or oligomenorrhea, which are associated with anovulatory cycles. Refer to chapters 62, Amenorrhea, and Chapter 64, Abnormal Uterine Bleeding, for an in-depth discussion of these menstrual disorders.

Dysmenorrhea and PMS are linked to very specific times in the menstrual cycle. Dysmenorrhea occurs during the first days of the menstrual cycle, in the early follicular phase, while PMS occurs in the luteal phase. Both disorders are common complaints, and proper diagnosis, targeting specific symptoms, will optimize treatment and improve the quality of life for the adolescent.

## DEFINITION

Dysmenorrhea, defined as "difficult menstrual flow," is the most common gynecologic complaint in female adolescents. *Primary dysmenorrhea* is recurrent lower abdominal or pelvic pain that occurs just before and with menstruation without pelvic pathology. Typically, symptoms begin in the first 3 years after menarche and are associated with ovulatory menstrual cycles. Classic symptoms of dysmenorrhea include crampy lower abdominal pain, which may radiate to the lower back or thighs, and occur within several hours of menses and lasts several hours to days. However, symptoms may begin as early as 2 days before and continue throughout menstruation. Primary dysmenorrhea is also associated with nonpelvic symptoms, as listed in Box 63-1. *Secondary dysmenorrhea* is recurrent pelvic or abdominal pain that occurs secondary to pelvic pathology. Box 63-2 lists the differential diagnosis of secondary dysmenorrhea.

### Box 63-1

### *Nonpelvic Symptoms of Primary Dysmenorrhea*

Nausea
Vomiting
Diarrhea
Backache
Leg pains
Breast tenderness
Headache
Fatigue
Sleep disturbances
Increased or altered appetite
Dizziness
Nervousness
Syncope

## EPIDEMIOLOGY

Dysmenorrhea usually occurs after ovulatory cycles are established (see Box 63-3). However, symptoms of dysmenorrhea can accompany anovulatory cycles, particularly if heavy bleeding and clots are present. Studies of dysmenorrhea in adolescent females have shown its prevalance to be from 20% to 90%.[1] The wide variation is due, in part, to inconsistent definitions of dysmenorrhea. The prevalence of severe dysmenorrhea is lower but can range from 14% to 42%, with Hispanic females having the highest prevalence.[2,3] Dysmenorrhea is the leading cause of recurrent school or work absences; however, relatively few adolescents seek medical care for their discomfort.[3,4] Moreover, most are unaware that nonsteroidal anti-inflammatory drugs (NSAIDs) are an effective treatment option.[5] One study found that of adolescents who self-medicate with over-the-counter (OTC) preparations, 57% used subtherapeutic doses.[6] Another study found that 98% of adolescents used nonpharmacologic methods to treat their dysmenorrhea (heat, rest, distraction) with perceived efficacy of 40%

**Box 63-2**

***Differential Diagnosis of Secondary Dysmenorrhea***

**Gynecologic causes**

Endometriosis

Infection (STI or postinstrumentation)
- Pelvic inflammatory disease (PID)
- Endometritis
- Asherman syndrome

Pregnancy-related complications
- Incomplete or threatened abortion
- Ectopic pregnancy

Ovarian cyst or mass
- Ruptured, torsed, or hemorrhagic cyst

Congenital Müllerian malformations (partial or unilateral obstruction)

Distal outflow tract obstruction
- Imperforate hymen
- Complete transverse vaginal septum

Pelvic adhesions

**Nongynecologic causes**

Gastrointestinal disturbances (may be present with or be exacerbated by menses)
- Constipation
- Irritable bowel syndrome (IBS)
- Inflammatory bowel disease (IBD)
- Lactose intolerance
- Giardiasis or other parasitic infections
- Celiac disease

Musculoskeletal pain
- Inflammatory process of the lower back, pelvis, or hip
- Anatomic disorders of the lower back, pelvis, or hip
- Trauma
- Tumor
- Abdominal wall trigger points in fibromyalgia

Genitourinary abnormalities
- Cystitis or pyelonephritis
- Urethral obstruction
- Calculi
- Interstitial cystitis

Psychogenic
- History of sexual or physical abuse
- History of trauma

Rare causes of pelvic pain
- Meckel diverticulum
- Midgut malrotation
- Henoch-Schönlein purpura
- Acute intermittent porphyria
- Uteropelvic junction obstruction

**Box 63-3**

***The Relationship between the Age of Menarche and Ovulation***

The earlier the age of menarche, the shorter the interval to regular ovulation:
- Menarche <11: 50% cycles ovulatory in 6 months
- Menarche 11–14: 50% cycles ovulatory in 2 years
- Menarche >14: 50% cycles ovulatory in 4.5 years

Source: Apter D, Vihko R. Early menarche, a risk factor for breast cancer, indicates early onset of ovulatory cycles. *J Endocrinol Metab.* 1983;57:82–86.

**Box 63-4**

***Risk Factors Associated with Increased Severity of Dysmenorrhea***

Evidence-based support
- Earlier age at menarche
- Longer menstrual flow
- Heavier menstrual flow
- Nulliparity
- Younger age
- Diet low in consumption of omega-3 fatty acids
- Smoking[a]

Possible associations
- Obesity
- Alcohol consumption
- Mood disorders

[a]Associated with longer duration of symptoms more than increased severity.

or less.[7] Numerous studies have examined risk factors for dysmenorrhea, and those associated with increased severity are listed in Box 63-4. Notably, improvement of symptoms is more likely in women who bear children.[8]

## PATHOPHYSIOLOGY

The prostaglandin (PG) pathway has a central role in the pathophysiology of primary dysmenorrhea. Chan and Hill[9] found $PGF_2$ activity in menstrual fluid was twice as high in women with dysmenorrhea compared to those without symptoms. Prostaglandins are formed in the secretory endometrium during ovulatory cycles and there is a major increase in PG release within the first 2 days after menses onset. The specific prostaglandins

### Box 63-5

### *Questions to Be Included in History-Taking and Review of Symptoms*

- Menstrual history
  - Age at menarche
  - Menstrual timing, duration, and regularity
  - Bleeding quantity and pattern
  - Change in pattern over time
- Specific questions related to menstrual pain
  - Onset of pain in relation to menarche
  - Onset, duration, quality, and severity of cramps
  - Other menstrual or premenstrual symptoms
  - Degree to which pain/symptoms interfere with life
    - Days of school or work missed
    - Frequency and number of days missed
    - Missing or limited participation in activities or social events
  - Response to interventions/medicines used
  - Dose, frequency, and initiation of medications or other treatments used
- Sexual history/sexual activity
  - History of sexually transmitted infections including PID, gonorrhea, or chlamydia
  - History of pregnancy and outcomes
  - Recent unprotected sex (pregnancy and infection risk)
  - Contraceptive and/or condom use
  - Current symptoms of STIs
  - Pain with sexual behaviors or positions
- Past medical history/other symptoms
  - History of abdominal or pelvic surgery
  - History of gastrointestinal disease or symptoms
  - History of cystitis, known urinary tract anomalies, or genitourinary symptoms
  - History of musculoskeletal trauma or complaints
  - Diet and exercise patterns
  - Psychosocial profile (HEADSS history):
    - H: Home environment
    - E: Education - School performance and absenteeism
    - A: Activities - Involvement in extracurricular activities/employment
    - D: Drugs - Tobacco use or use/abuse of alcohol or illicit drugs
    - S: Sexual history, including history of abuse
    - S: Suicidality and mental health screen as well as family history of these
  - History of menstrual cramps in female relatives
  - History of endometriosis in first-degree female relatives

involved in dysmenorrhea are $PGE_2$ and $PGF_2$, which are cyclo-oxygenase metabolites of arachidonic acid, an omega-6 fatty acid. At the end of the luteal phase, omega-6 fatty acids are released from cell wall phospholipids. This leads to a cascade of PG and leukotriene release in the uterus, which causes an inflammatory response characterized by hypercontractility and uterine ischemia. Clinically, this manifests as crampy pain and other PG and leukotriene-mediated local and systemic symptoms (see Box 63-1).

The leukotriene pathway is also thought to contribute to the symptoms of dysmenorrhea, but leukotriene receptor antagonists have not decreased symptoms in clinical trials.[10] Finally, increased levels of vasopressin have been identified in women with dysmenorrhea, and investigators are looking at a possible role for vasopressin antagonists.[11]

## APPROACH TO THE PATIENT

The diagnosis of primary dysmenorrhea can usually be made after a complete menstrual, medical, and family history and physical examination. Box 63-5 lists questions to be included in the history and review of symptoms, and Box 63-6 lists items that favor underlying pelvic pathology. A full physical examination with an external

### Box 63-6

### *Signs and Symptoms Favoring a Diagnosis of Underlying Pelvic Pathology*

- Dysmenorrhea-like symptoms that predate or begin at menarche
- Pelvic pain not limited to menses
- Pelvic pain lasting longer than 5 days
- Noncyclic pain
- Pain unresponsive to adequate standard therapy with NSAIDs or hormonal treatments
- Other symptoms
  - Dyspareunia
  - Vaginal bleeding
  - Urinary symptoms
  - Pain with defecation
- Physical findings
  - Pelvic mass
  - Abnormal vaginal discharge
  - Pelvic tenderness on bimanual exam

genital examination is sufficient in adolescents who are not sexually active unless there is concern for pelvic pathology, when a bimanual examination should be considered. A pelvic examination, with testing for sexually transmitted infections and a bimanual examination, is advised in sexually active adolescents.

## DIFFERENTIAL DIAGNOSIS

When the history is nonclassic, positive physical findings are noted, or the pain is poorly responsive to conventional therapy, then secondary dysmenorrhea needs to be considered (see Box 63-2).

Mid-cycle pain with ovulation can be secondary to pelvic pathology, including all the etiologies that cause secondary dysmenorrhea (see Box 63-2), or it may be due to mittelschmerz. Mittelschmerz is pain that occurs with ovulation; it is typically dull or crampy, varies in duration between minutes to hours, and is thought to be caused by follicular expansion and leakage of follicular fluid or blood into the pelvic cavity.

When pelvic pathology is suspected, pelvic ultrasound is the initial diagnostic test.[12] If endometriosis is suspected, laparoscopy with biopsies is diagnostic.

### ENDOMETRIOSIS

Endometriosis, defined as "the presence of endometrial glands and stroma in aberrant locations, outside the uterine cavity," is the most common cause of secondary dysmenorrhea in adolescents. The classic clinical manifestations include the triad of pelvic pain, dyspareunia, and infertility. Genetic transmission is thought to be due to a multifactorial gene with a 6.9% incidence in first-degree relatives of women with the disease compared to controls (1%). Most young women with a positive family history are at increased risk but are still unlikely to develop the disease.[13] Chapter 61, The Uterus and Adnexa, has an in-depth discussion of endometriosis.

## MANAGEMENT OF PRIMARY DYSMENORRHEA

The principal goal in treating primary dysmenorrhea is to relieve pain and to decrease associated morbidity. It is important to educate the adolescent about the physiologic etiology of dysmenorrhea and about menstruation-associated symptoms so that treatment options make sense to the patient and parent.

### PHARMACOLOGIC THERAPY

#### Nonsteroidal Anti-Inflammatory Agents

The first-line therapies in the management of primary dysmenorrhea are NSAIDs, which alleviate symptoms by inhibiting the activity of the cyclo-oxygenase (COX) pathways and thereby reducing PG production. This leads to a decrease in the strength of uterine contractions and in menstrual flow. A Cochrane review of 63 randomized controlled trials (RCTs) confirmed that NSAIDs are the most effective treatment for dysmenorrhea, with most women experiencing pain relief compared to placebo.[14] Importantly, NSAIDs are effective both prophylactically and for immediate pain relief or "rescue" dosing. Specific guidelines for initiation, timing of treatment, and dosing schedule are provided in Box 63-7. Ibuprofen and naproxen are most frequently used, but there is no clear-cut advantage of one NSAID over another when taken at proper intervals. Mefenamic acid is a unique NSAID that inhibits PG synthesis and blocks the action of the prostaglandins that are already formed. The chosen NSAID is typically tried for 3 cycles before treatment failure is

**Box 63-7**

***NSAIDs Used in the Treatment of Dysmenorrhea***

Guidelines for use
- Start with initial loading dose (stay within daily maximum dosing)
- Medicate as early as possible
  - Optimally start 24–48 hours before anticipated menses
- Continue around-the-clock regimen for duration of cramping
- Take with food
- Maintain hydration
- Choice depends on duration, absorption, efficacy, side effects, availability, and cost

Loading and maintenance doses and scheduling (adult dosing)
- Ibuprofen (Motrin) 400–800 mg initially then 400–600 mg every 4–6 hours (3,200 mg/day max)
- Naproxen (Naprosyn) 500 mg initially then 250–500 mg every 8–12 hours (1,500 mg/day max)
- Naproxen sodium (Anaprox or Aleve) 550 mg initially then 275–550 mg every 8–12 hours (1,650 mg/day max)
- Ketoprofen (Orudis) 25–50 mg every 6–8 hours
- Mefenemic acid (Ponstel) 500 mg initially then 250 mg every 6 hours
- Diclofenac (Voltaren) 50–100 mg initially then 50 mg every 8 hours
- Celecoxib (Celebrex)[a] 400 mg initially then 200 mg every 12 hours

[a]The only COX-2 inhibitor currently available in the United States.

assumed. However, when one NSAID fails then another NSAID from a different class often is successful.

The main concerns with NSAIDs are gastrointestinal (GI) side effects and the potential for renal damage with acute or chronic use. COX is the rate-limiting enzyme in the synthesis of prostaglandins. Conventional NSAIDs inhibit COX-1 and COX-2. The newer COX-2 inhibitors effectively treat dysmenorrhea and may have fewer side effects because they selectively target COX-2, which is specific for pain and inflammation. However, concerns regarding adverse cardiovascular effects limit the availability of these medications. Celecoxib is the only COX-2 inhibitor currently available in the United States. To improve tolerance to NSAIDs, patients should take them with food and maintain good hydration to protect from GI and renal side effects, respectively. NSAIDs are contraindicated in women with a history of gastroduodenal ulcer, GI bleeding, or renal disease.

### HORMONAL TREATMENTS

Hormonal contraception is typically used to treat dysmenorrhea when NSAIDs are ineffective or contraindicated, or in young women who desire contraception or other hormonal contraceptive benefits. Combined hormonal contraceptives are well tolerated in adolescents and have many health benefits listed in Box 63-8. Chapter 52, Contraception, discusses all forms of hormonal contraception in depth. The most extensively studied combined hormonal contraceptive treatment for dysmenorrhea is the oral contraceptive pill (OCP), which works indirectly by inhibiting ovulation and directly by decreasing endometrial growth and thus reducing the amount of endometrial tissue available for PG and leukotriene production. This decrease in endometrial growth also results in less monthly bleeding.

Numerous studies with different formulations and across diverse populations support an association between OCP use and reduced dysmenorrhea. Most of these studies involved large cohorts in open epidemiologic trials, rather than RCTs, and therefore were not included in a 2001 Cochrane review of OCP use in the treatment of dysmenorrhea.[15] However, 2 recently published RCTs have confirmed the efficacy of OCPs in the treatment of primary dysmenorrhea as compared to placebo.[16,17] Other combined hormonal methods of contraception (intravaginal ring, transdermal patch) should theoretically alleviate dysmenorrhea, but have not yet been studied. The injectable long-acting progesterone-only formulation, Depo-Provera, has demonstrated efficacy in decreasing dysmenorrhea symptoms by reducing or eliminating menses.[18] There also is evidence from a number of levonorgestrel-releasing intrauterine system (LNG-IUS or Mirena) trials and observational studies that LNG-IUS effectively reduces the symptoms of dysmenorrhea.[19]

Extended OCP cycling has been used successfully to treat endometriosis and other menstrual disorders, including dysmenorrhea.[20,21] Adolescents who have exacerbation of another medical condition (see Box 63-9) during the hormone-free interval can benefit from extended cycling. Extended cycling with

#### Box 63-8

***Recognized Health Benefits of Combined Hormonal Contraceptives***

Reduced menstrual blood flow
More predictable menstrual cycles
Decreased menstrual cramps and related morbidity
Improvement in acne
Decreased catamenial headaches and other events
Decreased iron deficiency anemia
Reduced colorectal, ovarian, and endometrial cancer

#### Box 63-9

***Disorders That Can Be Exacerbated Before or During Menses***

**Affective**

Depressive disorders
Bipolar disorder
Panic disorder
Anxiety disorder
Eating disorders
Psychosocial conditions secondary to sexual or physical abuse
Schizophrenia/psychosis

**Physical**

Headaches (migraine and tension)
Asthma
Allergies
Seizures
Irritable bowel syndrome (IBS)
Inflammatory bowel disease (IBD)
Fibromyalgia
Chronic fatigue syndrome
Dermatologic problems
Pneumothorax[a]

[a]Associated with diaphragmatic endometriosis.

combined hormonal contraceptive methods, other than OCPs, should also be effective. Table 63-1 lists hormonal contraceptive methods and other pharmacologic therapies used to treat primary dysmenorrhea. Additionally, NSAIDs and hormonal contraceptives are often used together to maximize symptom relief, but clinical trials have not studied these combined regimens. Finally, depot gonadotropin releasing-hormone (GnRH) agonist (Leuprolide) has been found to be effective in the treatment of refractory cases of dysmenorrhea and endometriosis, but there are many limitations to its use, as outlined in Box 63-10.

**Box 63-10**

***Limitations to GnRH-agonist in the Treatment of Dysmenorrhea and Premenstrual Syndrome***

- Hypoestrogenic side effects
  - Vaginal dryness
  - Hot flashes
- Negative sequalae with long-term use
  - Decrease in bone mineral density
  - Osteoporosis
- Cost and limited insurance coverage
- Supplemental estrogen and periodic progesterone often required to diminish side effects[a]

[a]No established dosing regimen for adolescents.

**Table 63-1**

**Hormonal and Other Related Treatment Options for Dysmenorrhea**

| *Treatment* | *Dosing Schedule* |
|---|---|
| **Combined hormonal contraception** | |
| OCPs, all formulations | Traditional (21/7) and shorter placebo (24/4) cycling |
| Transdermal contraceptive patch | Traditional cycling (1 patch/week × 3 then 1 week off) |
| Vaginal contraceptive ring | Traditional cycling (1 ring/3 weeks then 1 week off) |
| OCPs, monophasic pills | Extended cycling[a,b] |
| Transdermal contraceptive patch | Extended cycling[a] |
| Vaginal contraceptive ring | Extended cycling[a] |
| **Progesterone-only contraceptives** | |
| Depo-Provera | 150 mg intramuscular (IM) injections every 11–12 weeks |
| Levo-norgestrel IUD (Mirena) | Uterine placement by health care provider for up to 5 years |
| Progesterone-only or "mini-pills" | One pill daily without placebo week |
| **Other pharmacologic therapies** | |
| GnRH-agonist (Depo-Lupron) | Monthly or every 3 month IM injections |
| Vasopressin antagonists[c] | 300 mg/day starting between 4 hours and 3 days before onset of pain or bleeding |
| Nitroglycerin[c,d] | 0.1–0.2 mg hourly first few days of menses |

[a]Scheduled extended cycles (predetermined number of days of hormones followed by a hormone-free interval of 7 days or less), unscheduled extended cycles (using hormones until persistent uterine bleeding occurs, at which point a hormone-free interval is initiated), or continuous cycling (using hormones continuously, without a hormone-free interval, whether or not bleeding occurs, indefinitely).

[b]More commonly used patterns for extended OCP cycling include 42/7, 84/7, 48/4.

[c]Effective in studies but not current standard practice.

[d]20% of women reported headaches as an adverse side effect.

## NONPHARMACOLOGIC AND COMPLEMENTARY AND ALTERNATIVE MEDICINES (CAM)

Most women suffering from dysmenorrhea respond to NSAIDs or hormonal therapy; however, about 10% to 20% fail these therapies.[22] There is a vast array of complementary and alternative medicines (CAM) used in the treatment of primary dysmenorrhea; however, the efficacy for each of these approaches is less well demonstrated than it is for the standard pharmacologic approaches. Table 63-2 lists CAM studied in dysmenorrhea treatment with suggested doses or mechanisms of action, efficacy, and level of evidence to support each, as available. Herbal and dietary therapies are increasingly being studied and, although easy to obtain and use, there may be concerns with dosing, quality control, and bioavailability of preparations.

**Table 63-2**

**Complementary and Alternative Medicines Studied for the Treatment of Dysmenorrhea with Doses, Efficacy, and Level of Evidence to Support Use**

| | *Dose* | *Efficacy* | *Level of Evidence[a]* |
|---|---|---|---|
| **Nutritional/supplemental Therapies** | | | |
| Omega-3-Polyunsaturated fatty acids[23] | 2 g/day fish oil or 2–3 meals/week salmon, tuna, mackerel, herring | Yes | A-B |
| Vitamin E[24] | 200 µ/day or 500 u/day for 5 days[b] | Likely | B |
| Thiamine (B1)[25] | 200 µ/day for 5 days[b] | Likely | B |
| Magnesium[25] | No standard dosing | Possible | B |
| Magnesium and B6[25] | No standard dosing | Possible | B |
| Rose tea[26] | No standard dosing | Possible | B |
| Fennel oil[27,28] | 2% extract of fennel oil 25 drops every 4 hours during first several days of menses | Possible | B |
| Toki-shakuyaku-san (TSS)[29] | Japanese herbal mix used in traditional Chinese medicine[c] | Possible | B-C[d] |
| Pyridoxine (B6)[25] | No standard dosing | Unlikely | B |
| **Traditional Chinese Medicine** | **Mechanism of Action** | **Efficacy** | **Level of Evidence** |
| Acupuncture[30] | Excites nerve fibers, which block pain impulses or alters chi | Likely | B |
| Acupressure[31] | Direct physical pressure to energy points used in acupuncture[e] | Possible | B |
| Vitamin K acupuncture[32] | Point injections on day 1 or 2 of menses | Possible | C |
| **Other Types of Therapies** | **Description** | **Efficacy** | **Level of Evidence** |
| Transcutaneous electrical nerve stimulation (TENS)[30] | Stimulates skin using currents at high frequency | Likely | B |
| Topical heat[33] | Heat pad or patch (39°C) over pelvis for 12 hours | Likely | B |
| Exercise[22] | Aerobic or muscle-strengthening | Possible | C |
| Static magnet[34] | 2,700 gauss magnet applied to pelvis 2 days before menses and continued for duration | Possible | C |
| Behavioral interventions[35] | Simple relaxation therapy, breathing exercises, stretching, muscle relaxation | Possible | C |

*(Continued)*

**Table 63-2 (Continued)**

| | Dose | Efficacy | Level of Evidence |
|---|---|---|---|
| **Other Types of Therapies** | | | |
| Spinal manipulation[36] | Techniques that move spinal vertebrae to relieve misalignment affecting sympathetic nerve supply and pelvic viscera | Unlikely | C |

[a]Level A: Large high-quality, randomized, double-blind, placebo-controlled trials, meta-analysis; Level B: lesser quality randomized trials, retrospective studies, systematic reviews; Level C: expert opinion, case series, uncontrolled studies, consensus statements.

[b]Start 2 days before menses.

[c]Requires consultation with a specialist.

[d]Difficult to grade level of evidence because study participants had a Chinese medicine diagnosis of dysmenorrhea symptoms.

[e]One study used a cotton panty brief with pads fixed over acupressure points. (Taylor D, Miaskowski C, Kohn J. A randomized clinical trial of the effectiveness of an acupressure device (relief brief) for managing symptoms of dysmenorrhea. *J Altern Compliment Med.* 2002;8:357-370.)

## PREMENSTRUAL SYNDROME AND PREMENSTRUAL DYSPHORIC DISORDER

### DEFINITION

Premenstrual syndrome (PMS) describes a constellation of recurring cyclic physical and psychological symptoms that occur in the luteal phase of the menstrual cycle, which occurs 7 to 10 days before menses. In 2000, The American College of Obstetricians and Gynecologists (ACOG) established clinical guidelines to diagnose PMS, based on a 1989 publication by Mortola et al.[37] These are detailed in Box 63-11 and include the affective and physical symptoms of PMS.[38] Premenstrual dysphoric disorder (PMDD) is a severe variant of PMS with a greater prominence of affective symptoms. The diagnosis of PMDD, as defined by the American Psychiatric Association's fourth edition revised of the *Diagnostic and Statistical Manual of Mental Disorders* (DSM IV-TR) is outlined in Box 63-12.[39]

Finally, premenstrual exacerbation (PME) of other disorders presents in a similar time frame as PMS. Exacerbations of certain diseases occur cyclically during the luteal phase or with menses, and some of these specific disorders are listed in Box 63-9. The differential diagnosis of PMS/PMDD includes all the disorders listed in Box 63-9. Importantly, women with psychiatric disorders, including schizophrenia and mood disorders, are at greater risk of exacerbation of those symptoms in the late luteal phase of their cycle.[40]

### EPIDEMIOLOGY

Premenstrual disorders occur mainly in women with ovulatory cycles, but PMS symptoms have been described in women with polycystic ovarian syndrome (PCOS), perimenopause, and those on OCPs, all of whom ovulate infrequently. Premenstrual syndrome can persist until menopause and, unlike dysmenorrhea, may become worse after childbirth.

The high prevalence of premenstrual disorders and their negative impact on a woman's quality of life are increasingly recognized. About 70% to 90% of women of reproductive age report having premenstrual symptoms at some time in their life.[41] A recent study of a large and diverse health management organization (HMO) population of 21- to 45-year-old women showed that 80% suffered from moderate to severe PMS, and 4.7% met criteria for PMDD.[42] These estimates are relatively consistent with other prospective studies, and with clinical evidence indicating that 3% to 8% of patients meet criteria for PMDD.[43,44] Premenstrual syndrome has been found to be associated with increased direct and individual medical costs in adult women, stemming from missed workdays and lower productivity.[45] Risk factors associated with PMS/PMDD are listed in Box 63-13.

### PATHOPHYSIOLOGY

The etiology of PMS and PMDD is incompletely understood. There is evidence of a connection between the

## Box 63-11

### *ACOG Diagnostic Criteria for PMS*

Patient reports at least one affective or somatic symptom highlighted in bold type below

**Affective symptoms**

**Depression**
**Angry outbursts/mood swings**
**Irritability**
**Anxiety**
**Confusion**
**Social withdrawal**
Tearfulness
Low self-esteem
Forgetfulness
Decreased concentration
Sleep disturbance
Increased appetite
Fatigue

**Physical symptoms**

**Breast tenderness**
**Abdominal bloating**
**Headache**
**Swollen extremities**
Weight gain
Myalgia
Hot flashes
Constipation
Skin problems (ie, acne)
Palpitations

---

- Symptoms occur 5 days before menses, remit within 4 days of menses onset, and do not reoccur until at least cycle day 13
- Symptoms present in the absence of any pharmacologic therapy, hormone ingestion, or drug or alcohol use
- Symptoms can occur reproducibly during 2 cycles of prospective recording
- Symptoms can cause unidentifiable dysfunction in social or economic performance

From Mortola JF, Girton L, Yen SSC. Depressive episodes in premenstrual syndrome. *Am J Obstet Gynecol.* 1989;161:1682–1687, with permission from Elsevier.

## Box 63-12

### *DSM-IV Criteria for PMDD*

Patient reports at least 5 emotional symptoms, with at least 1 of 4 specific symptoms (highlighted in bold below)

**Emotional**

**Depressed mood**
**Anxiety, tension**
**Increased sensitivity**
**Irritability, anger**
Decreased interest
Decreased concentration
Lethargy/lack of energy
Change in appetite
Insomnia or hypersomnia
Feeling overwhelmed or out of control

**Physical**

Breast tenderness or swelling
Headaches
Joint or muscle pain
Weight gain
Bloated feeling

---

- Symptoms can occur a week before menses and remit within a few days after onset of menses
- Symptoms are experienced in most of the menstrual cycles for the past year
- Symptoms are discretely related to menstrual cycle and are not merely worsening of pre-existing depression, anxiety, or personality disorder
- Symptoms occur for at least 2 consecutive menstrual cycles of prospective daily ratings
- Symptoms interfere with social, occupational, sexual, or school functioning

Modified with permission from American Psychiatric Association. *Diagnostic and Statistical Manual of Mental Disorders*, 4th ed., Text Revision. Arlington, VA: American Psychiatric Association; 2000: 774

onset of PMS/PMDD symptoms and the rise and fall of reproductive hormones associated with ovulatory cycles, as GnRH suppression relieves symptoms.[46] Women with these disorders are more sensitive to changing levels of reproductive hormones, despite normal values. The interaction between ovarian steroids and neurotransmitters plays an important role in the pathogenesis of PMS/PMDD.

Serotonin is the neurotransmitter thought to play the central role, because there is evidence that ovarian hormones affect serotonergic uptake, turnover, binding, and transport. Gamma-aminobutyric acid (GABA) and other neurotransmitters are also involved, as is the renin-angiotensin-aldosterone system (RAAS), which causes fluid retention, producing increased bloating

**Box 63-13**

***Possible Risk Factors for PMS and PMDD***

Ovulatory cycles[a]
Older age
Increased parity
History of anxiety disorder
History of depressive disorder
History of physical or sexual abuse
Family history of PMS
High stress
Smoking
Obesity

[a]Only evidence-based risk factor.

and increased breast tenderness. Progesterone inhibits and estrogen stimulates the RAAS. Women with PMS/PMDD are thought to have a different response to progesterone, but the specific pathway is poorly understood. Finally, there may be a genetic predisposition to PMS/PMDD.[47]

**Box 63-14**

***Daily Symptoms Rating Diaries***

Calendar of premenstrual experiences (COPE)

- Twenty-two symptoms that are divided into 4 factors: mood reactivity, autonomic/cognitive, appetitive, and related to fluid retention[48]

Premenstrual symptoms screening tool (PSST)

- Nineteen-item questionnaire that allows the patient to rate the severity of the symptoms used to diagnose PMDD[49]

Visual analogue scale (VAS)

- Scaled self-report of 4 core symptoms for PMDD: irritability, tension, depression, and mood swings[50]

Daily record of severity of problems (DRSP)

- Twenty-one individual items grouped into 11 distinct symptoms and 3 functional impairment items rated from 1 ("not at all") to 6 ("extreme")[a]

[a]Available at www.pmdd.factsforhealth.org/drsp/drsp_month.pdf

## APPROACH TO THE PATIENT

The established diagnostic criteria for PMS and PMDD require recording of symptoms in a prospective diary. The role of this diary is to chart progress and to differentiate PMS, PMDD, PME, and other etiologies. There are a number of daily symptom rating diaries available, which are listed in Box 63-14. Regardless of the format, it is crucial to document a symptom-free interval beginning just after the onset of menses and lasting for at least one week in order to diagnose PMS/PMDD. If symptoms are present at baseline then they should increase in intensity by greater than 30% from the follicular to the luteal phase.[39]

The prospective diary must be recorded for at least 2 months, or 2 cycles, for diagnosis and to establish a baseline. A patient history, including family history, medical comorbidities, psychologic comorbidities, drug use, sexual history, diet and exercise, and CAM use is critical. A thorough review of symptoms can rule out underlying pathology, especially hormonal disorders such as thyroid disease. A complete physical examination and mental health evaluation is advised, including a pelvic exam when indicated. Minimal, if any, laboratory work might include a complete blood cell count, thyroid-stimulating hormone, basic metabolic profile, and other tests when justified.

## MANAGEMENT

### Nonpharmacologic Medicines and Complementary and Alternative Medicines

Complementary and alternative medicine therapies are varied and suggested doses or mechanisms of action, efficacy, and level of evidence to support each as available are listed in Table 63-3. Many of these therapies are inexpensive and have an excellent safety profile, but only a few of them have been shown to significantly reduce PMS/PMDD symptoms. Because a prospective diary of at least 2 months, duration is integral to accurately diagnose PMS/PMDD, it is often practical to initiate nonpharmacologic treatment during the "diary phase."

Of all vitamin supplements studied, calcium is the best supported to decrease premenstrual symptoms with a 48% reduction in symptom score compared to placebo.[51] Calcium, vitamin D, and parathyroid hormone levels vary with menstrual cycles. Women with PMS have decreased levels of serum ionized calcium, decreased levels of 25-hydroxyvitamin D, and increased levels of parathyroid hormone. Calcium supplementation may reduce PMS symptoms and is often started in the "observational" diary phase.

**Table 63-3**

**Complementary and Alternative Medicine Used in the Treatment of PMS/PMDD**

| | *Dose* | *Efficacy* | *Level of Evidence*[a] |
|---|---|---|---|
| **Nutritional/Supplemental Therapies** | | | |
| Calcium | 400 mg/3 times/day | Yes | A |
| Magnesium | 400–800 mg/day | Likely | B |
| Chasteberry | 20 mg/day | Likely | B |
| Gingko Biloba | 80 mg twice daily | Likely | B |
| Neptune krill oil | 1 g/day with meals for a month then 8 days before and 2 days with menses | Likely | B |
| Vitamin E | 300–400 mg/day | Likely | B |
| Pyridoxine (B6)[b] | 50–100 mg/day | Possible | B |
| L-Tryptophan[c] | 6 g/day from ovulation to 3rd day of menses | Possible | B |
| St. John's wort[d] | 300 mg 3 times/day | Possible | B |
| Carbohydrate drink[e] | Increases ratio tryptophan to other large neutral amino acids | Possible | B |
| Soy isoflavones | 68 mg/day | Possible | B |
| Black cohosh | 40 mg twice daily | Possible | C |
| Kava[f] | 100–300 mg daily | Possible | C |
| Evening primrose oil | 2–3 g/day | Unlikely | B |
| **Other Therapies** | | | |
| Aerobic exercise | | Yes | B |
| Bright light therapy | | Yes | B |
| Homeopathy | | Possible | B |
| Massage | | Possible | B |
| Reflexology | | Possible | B |
| Cognitive behavioral therapy (CBT) | | Possible | B |
| Group coping skills | | Possible | B |
| Relaxation response | | Possible | B |
| Acupuncture | | Possible | B |
| Caffeine avoidance | | Possible | B |
| Biofeedback and relaxation exercises | | Possible | C |
| Guided imagery | | Possible | C |
| Yoga | | Possible | C |
| Diet high in complex carbohydrates | | Possible | C |
| Chiropractic intervention | | Unlikely | B |
| Dietary manipulation (reduce salt, alcohol) | | Unlikely | C |
| Dong Quai (Chinese herb) | | Unlikely | C |
| **No Published Studies** | | | |
| Acupressure | | | |

*(Continued)*

**Table 63-3 (Continued)**

| | Dose | Efficacy | Level of Evidence[a] |
|---|---|---|---|
| **No published studies** | | | |
| Aromatherapy | | | |
| Vaginal temperature biofeedback | | | |

[a]Level A: Large high-quality, randomized, double-blind, placebo-controlled trials, meta-analysis; Level B: lesser quality randomized trials, retrospective studies, systematic reviews; Level C: expert opinion, case series, uncontrolled studies, consensus statements.

[b]Potential toxicity with higher doses.

[c]Potential eosinophilia.

[d]Strong inducer of cytochrome p450 and may decrease levels of other drugs, including OCPs.

[e]No standard dosing.

[f]Kava use not recommended at present secondary to reports of hepatotoxicity.

Modified from Girman A, Lee R, Kligler B. An integrative medicine approach to premenstrual syndrome. *Am J Obstet Gynecol.* 2003;188:S56–S65, with permission from Elsevier.

### Pharmacologic Therapy

Pharmacologic options for managing PMS/PMDD have been more thoroughly investigated than nonpharmacologic ones. They are considered after the prospective diary confirms the diagnosis and nonpharmacologic or CAM have failed or are impractical. The strongest, evidence-based treatments for PMS/PMDD are selective serotonin reuptake inhibitors (SSRIs). Symptoms associated with PMS and PMDD overlap with those associated with decreased serotonergic neurotransmission. Any SSRI or antidepressant with sufficient serotonergic activity can help alleviate premenstrual symptoms.

SSRIs are efficacious in more than a dozen RCTs with continuous dosing and more than 8 trials with luteal phase-only dosing. A meta-analysis of 15 randomized, placebo-controlled trials showed no difference in symptom reduction between continuous- and luteal-phase administration.[52] Luteal-phase administration involves initiating medication 14 days prior to the expected onset of menstrual bleeding and discontinuing it at the onset or within several days of menses. However, luteal-phase dosing will not address untreated depression, bipolar, or anxiety disorders. Patients often prefer this intermittent dosing because there are fewer side effects, but side effects in either dosing schedule are typically mild (anxiety, nausea, insomnia, sexual dysfunction). Finally, symptom-onset dosing, recently demonstrated to be an effective treatment of PMS/PMDD in 2 small RCTs, offers the benefits of intermittent dosing with decreased medication and cost and greater patient control.[53,54]

Response rates to SSRIs are typically rapid because serotonin levels rise quickly after ingestion, and most trials show improvement in symptoms within 3 menstrual cycles. The antidepressants used to treat PMS/PMDD are listed in Table 63-4. Although most of the medications in Table 63-4 are SSRIs, other classes of antidepressants and anxiolytics are also included. Anxiolytics are sometimes added in the luteal phase for women with persistent anxiety after an adequate trial of SSRIs. Finally, spironolactone, a diuretic and aldosterone antagonist, has been shown to alleviate the physical symptoms and to improve some of the negative emotions of PMS/PMDD.[55]

### Hormonal Treatments

The more severe symptoms of PMS/PMDD typically occur at the time of declining progesterone concentrations. Progesterone has been shown to have anxiolytic properties secondary to the action of its metabolites at the GABA receptors. However, RCTs have failed to demonstrate the efficacy of progesterone supplementation. A recent meta-analysis found that progesterones were not more effective than placebo in treating PMS.[56]

PMS/PMDD does not occur in pregnancy, after oopherectomy, and is less common with anovulatory cycles, implying that hormonal inhibition of ovulation would successfully treat PMS/PMDD. However, RCTs of combined hormonal contraceptives in the treatment of PMS/PMDD found that the more traditional OCPs, containing progesterones derived from

**Table 63-4**

**Antidepressants Used in the Treatment of PMS/PMDD**

| | *Dose* |
|---|---|
| **Antidepressants** | |
| Fluoxetine (Prozac, Sarafem[a])[b] | 10–20 mg/day |
| | 90 mg/weekly |
| Paroxetine (Paxil, Paxil CR)[b,c] | 10–40 mg/day |
| Sertraline (Zoloft)[b] | 25–50 mg/day |
| Citalopram (Celexa) | 10–40 mg/day |
| Escitalopram (Lexapro)[d] | 10 mg/day |
| Fluvoxamine (Luvox) | 50 mg/day |
| Venlafaxine (Effexor) | 5-200 mg/day |
| Clomipramine (Anafranil) | 25–75 mg/day |
| Buspirone (BuSpar) | 10–30 mg/day |
| Bupropion (Wellbutrin) | 100 mg 3 times daily |
| **Anxiolytics** | |
| Alaprazolam (Xanax)[e] | 0.5–1 mg 2–4 times daily |

[a]Sold as Sarafem specifically in PMS/PMDD.

[b]FDA approved for PMDD.

[c]Contraindicated if risk for pregnancy.

[d]Citalopram isomer.

[e]Concerns for tolerance/dependence.

19-nortestosterone, were not efficacious. More recent RCTs have found that OCPs containing drospirenone, a novel progesterone, combined with varying doses of ethinyl estradiol (EE) successfully alleviate the physical and affective symptoms of PMS/PMDD.[57] Drospirenone acts as an analogue of spironolactone and has both antimineralcorticoid activity and antiandrogenic activity, increasing sodium and water excretion and potassium retention. The only OCP FDA approved for the treatment of PMDD, Yaz, contains drospirenone and EE taken for 24 days followed by 4 days of placebo. Yaz was significantly shown to decrease PMDD symptoms 62% compared to placebo (38%).[58]

GnRH-agonists have been shown to effectively treat the affective and physical symptoms of PMS/PMDD, but, as in the treatment of dysmenorrhea, there are many limitations to their use (see Box 63-11).[46] Lastly, NSAIDs are considered potentially effective in PMS/PMDD, but no studies have definitively confirmed this effect.

## CONCLUSIONS

Dysmenorrhea and PMS/PMDD are common menstrual disorders in adolescents. They can be treated with an array of well-recognized and newer therapies. These disorders cause significant morbidity and impair quality of life. Inquiry about symptoms at well adolescent and problem visits provides the opportunity to educate about the etiology and offer effective treatment options for these menstrual disorders.

## REFERENCES

1. French L. Dysmenorrhea. *Amer Fam Physician*. 2005; 71(2):285–291

2. Wilson C, Keye W. A survey of adolescent dysmenorrhea and premenstrual symptom frequency. *J Adolesc Health Care*. 1989;10:317–322

3. Banikarim C, Chacko MR, Kelder SH. Prevalence and impact of dysmenorrhea on Hispanic female adolescents. *Arch Pediatr Adolesc Med*. 2000;154:1226–1229

4. Johnson J. Level of knowledge among adolescent girls regarding effective treatment for dysmenorrhea. *J Adolesc Health*. 1988;9:398–402

5. Hillen TI, Grbavac SL, Johnston PF, et al. Primary dysmenorrhea in young western Australian women: prevalence, impact, and knowledge of treatment. *J Adolesc Health*. 1999;25:40–45

6. Campbell MA, McGrath PJ. Use of medication by adolescents for the management of menstrual discomfort. *Arch Pediatr Adolesc Med.* 1997;151:905–913

7. Campbell MA, McGrath PJ. Non-pharmacologic strategies used by adolescents for the management of menstrual discomfort. *Clin J Pain*. 1999;15:313–320

8. Weissman AM, Hartz AJ, Hansen MD, Johnson SR. The natural history of primary dysmenorrhea: a longitudinal study. *Br J Obstet Gynecol*. 2004;111:345–352

9. Chan WY, Hill JC. Determination of menstrual prostaglandin levels in nondysmenorrheic and dysmenorrheic subjects. *Prostaglandins*. 1978;15:365–375

10. Harel Z, Riggs S, Vaz R, et al. The use of the leukotriene receptor antagonist Montelukast (Singulair) in the management of dysmenorrhea in adolescents. *J Pediatr Adolesc Gynecol*. 2004;17:183–186

11. Liedman R, Skillern L, James I, et al. Validation of a test model of induced dysmenorrhea. *Acta Obstet Gynecol Scand*. 2006;85(4):451–457

12. Moore J, Copley S, Morris J, et al. A systemic review of the accuracy of ultrasound in the diagnosis of endometriosis. *Ultrasound Obstet Gynecol*. 2002;20:630–634

13. Simpson JL, Elias S, Malinak LR, et al. Heritable aspects of endometriosis (I). Genetic studies. *Am J Obstet Gynecol.* 1980;137:327-331

14. Marjoribanks J, Proctor ML, Farquhar C. Nonsteroidal anti-inflammatory drugs for primary dysmenorrhea. *Cochrane Database Systemic Review*. 2003;4:CD001751

15. Proctor ML, Roberts H, Farquhar CM. Combined oral contraceptive pill (OCP) as treatment for primary dysmenorrhea. *Cochrane Database Systemic Review*. 2001; (2):CD002120

16. Davis AR, Westhoff C, O'Connell K, Gallagher N. Oral contraceptives for dysmenorrhea in adolescent girls. *Obstet and Gynecol*. 2005;106:97-104

17. Hendrix SL, Alexander NJ. Prim dysmenorrhea treatment with a desogestrel-containing low-dose oral contraceptive. *Contraception*. 2002;66(6):393-399

18. Harel Z, Biro F, Kollar L. Depo-provera in adolescents: effects of early second injection or prior oral contraception. *J Adolesc Health*. 1995;16:379-384

19. Varma R, Sinha D, Gupta JK. Noncontraceptive uses of levonorgestrel-releasing hormone system (LNG-IUS)—a systemic enquiry. *Eur J Obstet Gynecol Reprod Bio*. 2006;125:9-28

20. Sulak PJ, Scow RD, Preece C, et al. Hormone withdrawal symptoms in oral contraceptive users. *Obstet Gynecol*. 2000;95(2):261-266

21. Vercellini P, Frontino G, De Giorgi O, et al. Continuous use of an oral contraceptive for endometriosis-associated recurrent dysmenorrhea that does not respond to a cyclic pill regimen. *Fertil Steril*. 2003;80(3):560-563

22. Proctor M, Farquhar C. Diagnosis and management of dysmenorrhea. *BMJ*. 2006;332:1134-1138

23. Harel Z, Biro F, Kottenhahn RK, Rosenthal SL. Supplementation with omega-3-polyunsaturated fatty acids in the management of dysmenorrhea in adolescents. *Obstet Gynecol*. 1996;174(4):1335-1338

24. Ziaei S, Zakeri M, Kazemnejad A. A randomized controlled trial of vitamin E in the treatment of primary dysmenorrhea. *Br J Obstet Gynecol*. 2005;112(4):466-469

25. Proctor ML, Murphy PA. Herbal and dietary therapies for primary and secondary dysmenorrhea. *Cochrane Database Syst Rev*. 2001;3:CD002124

26. Tseng YF, Chen CH, Yang YH. Rose tea for relief of primary dysmenorrhea in adolescents: a randomized controlled trial in Taiwan. *J Midwifery Womens Health*. 2005;50(5):e51-57

27. Modaress N, Asadipour M. Comparison of the effectiveness of fennel and mefenamic acid on pain intensity in dysmenorrhea. *East Mediterr Health J*. 2006;12 (3-4):423-427

28. Ostad SN, Soodi M, Shariffzadeh M, et al. The effect of fennel essential oil on uterine contraction as a model for dysmenorrhea, pharmacology and toxicology study. *J Ethnopharmacol*. 2001;76(3):299-304

29. Tanaka T. A novel anti-dysmenorrhea therapy with cyclic administration of two Japanese herbal medicines. *Clin Exp Obstet*. 2003;30(2-3):95-98

30. Proctor ML, Smith CA, Farquhar CM, Stones RW. Transcutaneous electrical nerve stimulation and acupuncture for primary dysmenorrhea. *Cochrane Database Syst Rev*. 2002;1:CD002123

31. Jun EM, Chang S, Kang DH, Kim S. Effects of acupressure on dysmenorrhea and skin temperature changes in college students: a non-randomized controlled trial. *Int J Nurs Stud*. 2007;44(6):973-981

32. Wang L, Cardini F, Zhao W, et al. Vitamin K acupuncture point injection for severe primary dysmenorrhea: an international pilot study. *MedGenMed*. 2004;6(4):45

33. Akin M, Price W, Rodriguez G Jr, Erasala G, et al. Continuous, low-level, topical heat wrap therapy as compared to acetaminophen for primary dysmenorrhea. *J Reprod Med*. 2004;49(9):739-745

34. Eccles NK. A randomized, double-blinded, placebo-controlled pilot study to investigate the effectiveness of a static magnet to relieve dysmenorrhea. *J Altern Complement Med*. 2005;11(4):681-687

35. Proctor ML, Murphy PA, Pattison HM, et al. Behavioral interventions for primary and secondary dysmenorrhea. *Cochrane Database Syst Rev*. 2007;3:CD002248

36. Proctor ML, Hing W, Johnson TC, Murphy PA. Spinal manipulation for primary and secondary dysmenorrhea. *Cochrane Database Syst Rev*. 2006;3:CD002119

37. Mortola JF, Girton L, Yen SS. Depressive episodes in premenstrual syndrome. *Am J Obstet Gynecol*. 1989;161:1682-1687

38. Mortola JF, Girton L, Beck C, Yen SSC. Diagnosis of premenstrual syndrome by a single, prospective, and reliable instrument: the calendar of premenstrual experiences. *Obstet Gynecol*. 1990;76:302

39. American Psychiatric Association. Premenstrual dysphoric disorder. In: *Diagnostic and Statistical Manual of Mental Disorders*. 4th ed., text revision. Washington, DC: American Psychiatric Association; 2000:771-774

40. Tarqum SD, Caputo KP, Ball SK. Menstrual cycle phase and psychiatric admissions. *J Affect Disord*. 1991;22 (1-2):49-53.

41. Ginsburg KA, Dinsay R. Premenstrual syndrome. In: Ransom SB, ed. *Practical Strategies in Obstetrics and Gynecology*. Philadelphia, PA: WB Saunders; 2000:684-694

42. Sternfeld B, Swindle R, Chawla A, et al. Severity of premenstrual symptoms in a health maintenance organization population. *Obstet Gynecol*. 2002;99:1014-1024

43. Freeman EW. Luteal phase administration of agents for the treatment of premenstrual dysphoric disorder. *CNS Drugs*. 2004;18 (7):453-468

44. Steiner M, Born L. Advances in the diagnosis and treatment of premenstrual dysphoria. *CNS Drugs*. 2000;13 (4):287-304

45. Borenstein J, Chiou CF, Dean B, et al. Estimating direct and indirect costs of premenstrual syndrome. *J Occup Environ Med*. 2005;47:26-33

46. Wyatt KM, Dimmock PW, Khaled MK, et al. The effectiveness of GnRHa with and without 'addback' therapy in treating

premenstrual syndrome: a meta-analysis. *BMJ Obstet Gynecol.* 2004;111(6):585-593

47. Ronchi DD, Ujkaj M, Boaron F, et al. Symptoms of depression in late luteal phase dysphoric disorder: a variant of mood disorder? *J Affect Disord.* 2005;86: 169-174

48. Feuerstein M, Shaw WS. Measurement properties of the calendar of premenstrual experience in patients with premenstrual syndrome. *J Reprod Med.* 2002;47:279-289

49. Steiner M, Macdougall M, Brown E. The premenstrual symptoms screening tool (PSST) for clinicians. *Arch Womens Ment Health.* 2003;6:203-209

50. Casper RF, Powell AM. Premenstrual syndrome: documentation by a linear analogue scale compared with two descriptive scales. *Am J Obstet Gynecol.* 1986; 155:(4) 862-867.

51. Thy-Jacobs S, Starkey P, Bernstein D, Tian J. Calcium carbonate and the premenstrual syndrome: effects on premenstrual and menstrual symptoms. Premenstrual syndrome study group. *Am J Obstet Gynecol.* 1998;179:444-452

52. Dimmock PW, Wyatt KM, Jones PW, O'Brien PM. Efficacy of SSRIs in PMS: a systemic review. *Lancet.* 2000;356:1131-1161

53. Yonkers KA, Holthausen GA, Poschman K, Howell HB. Symptom-onset treatment for women with premenstrual dysphoric disorder. *J Clin Psychopharmacol.* 2006;26 (2):198-202

54. Freeman EW, Sondheimer SJ, Sammel MD, et al. A preliminary study of luteal phase versus symptoms-onset dosing with citalopram for premenstrual dysphoric disorder. *J Clin Psychiatry.* 2005;66(6):769-773

55. Wang M, Hammarback S, Lindhe BA, Backsrom T. Treatment of premenstrual syndrome by spironolactone: a double-blind, placebo-controlled study. *Acta Obstet Gynecol Scand.* 1995;74:803-808

56. Wyatt K, Dimmick P, Jones P, Obhari M, O'Brien S. Efficacy of progesterone and progestogens in management of premenstrual syndrome: a systemic review. *BMJ.* 2001;323:776-780

57. Rapkin AJ. New treatment approaches for premenstrual disorders. *Amer J Managed Care.* 2005;11 (16):S480-S491

58. Pearlstein TB, Bachman GA, Zacur HA, Yonkers KA. Treatment of premenstrual dysphoric disorder with a new drospirenone-containing oral contraceptive formulation. *Contraception.* 2005;72:414a

# CHAPTER 64

# Abnormal Uterine Bleeding

ELBA A. IGLESIAS, MD • SUSAN M. COUPEY, MD

## INTRODUCTION

Abnormal uterine bleeding in the adolescent patient is a common complaint and reason for office visits in this age group. The normal menstrual cycle, ovulatory and anovulatory, the importance of the history and physical examination, as well as the specific etiologies of abnormal uterine bleeding will be reviewed. Many cases of irregular menses in the young adolescent population (ages 10–14) are due to immaturity of the hypothalamic/pituitary/ovarian (HPO) axis. These cases rarely lead to health problems. However, health care providers need to be aware of the spectrum of medical conditions that can contribute to abnormal uterine bleeding to appropriately evaluate, manage, and treat the underlying etiology.

## THE NORMAL OVULATORY MENSTRUAL CYCLE

In a normal ovulatory cycle, the hypothalamus secretes gonadotropin-releasing hormone (GnRH), stimulating the pituitary gland to release follicle-stimulating hormone (FSH) and stimulate the ovary to produce a follicle that secretes estrogen. The first half of the menstrual cycle, known as the proliferative phase, is dominated by the production of estrogen from the maturing follicle in the ovary, causing proliferation and thickening of the endometrial lining of the uterus. A midcycle surge of luteinizing hormone (LH), occurring usually at day 14 of the cycle, causes the follicle to release the ovum.

After ovulation, the corpus luteum remains, producing progesterone, the dominant hormone in the second half of the cycle. This is known as the secretory phase, when under the influence of progesterone the endometrial lining stops growing and stabilizes. With involution of the corpus luteum, levels of estrogen and progesterone decrease, leading to controlled shedding of the endometrial lining of the uterus, ie, menstruation.

Most normal ovulatory cycles last 28 days, counting from the first day of 1 menstrual period to the first day of the next period. Cycles that are regular, associated with premenstrual symptoms such as breast tenderness and mood changes, and those menses associated with cramps are usually ovulatory in nature.

## ANOVULATORY MENSTRUAL CYCLES

Anovulatory menstrual cycles may be seen normally in adolescents who are within 24 months postmenarche and are related to delay in maturation of the HPO axis.[1] Many of these cycles are quite regular with episodes of bleeding every 21 to 31 days, but some are irregular with missed menses. Apter and colleagues[2] looked at hormonal patterns of adolescent menstrual cycles and found that anovulatory cycles as evidenced by lack of a progesterone peak were noted in the majority of cycles in girls within 24 months of menarche. Anovulatory cycles causing irregular, infrequent menses in older adolescents who are more than 24 months postmenarche are not normal and should be investigated.

The concept of "gynecologic age" is helpful in interpreting a complaint of irregular menstrual bleeding in an adolescent. It is defined as the time in years and/or months since menarche. The gynecologic age is critical in conjunction with other factors in determining the extent of medical work-up needed in the evaluation of a menstrual complaint. For example, a 14-year-old girl would have a gynecologic age of 4 years if she began menstruating at age 10 and would be expected to have a mature HPO axis and normal regular ovulatory cycles. If this girl had irregular, infrequent menses, a work-up would be indicated. A different 14-year-old girl would have a gynecologic age of only 18 months if menarche occurred at age 12.5 years and she may still have an immature HPO axis and irregular cycles on that basis. Therefore, irregular menstrual cycles in a girl with a gynecologic age of less than 2 years, without any other contributing signs or symptoms, may simply be due to immaturity of the HPO axis, and the patient can usually be reassured and observed without anextensive work-up. The World Health Organization studied menstrual patterns in 1,472 girls aged 11 to 15 years.[1] Subjects were divided into 2 groups; those who already had menarche (802 girls) and those who experienced menarche at study onset (670 girls). The subjects kept a 2-year prospective record of their menstrual cycles. As the subjects approached a gynecologic age of 2 years, cycles became more regular, with the girls in the menarchal group approaching cycle lengths of the postmenarchal girls. When eliciting the medical history, memory prompts are helpful in determining precise gynecologic age in months with accurate time of menarche. Asking if menarche occurred in the summer, in sixth or seventh (or other) grade, near a holiday, or a birthday is helpful.

In anovulatory cycles, FSH stimulates the ovary to produce a maturing follicle. However, there is a lack of the positive feedback of estrogen in the first half of the cycle and therefore no LH surge. Ovulation does not occur, there is no corpus luteum formation, and no progesterone is produced. The endometrial lining of the uterus remains in an unstable proliferative phase. At the end of the cycle, the follicle involutes, estrogen levels fall, and a withdrawal bleed occurs. Sometimes the follicle does not involute and grows into a follicular cyst that continues to secrete estrogen leading to further proliferation of the endometrium. When this follicular cyst eventually either ruptures or involutes, a prolonged heavy bleed may occur. In young teens with anovulatory cycles due to HPO immaturity, bleeding is rarely excessive and prolonged enough to lead to complications such as anemia and/or hemodynamic instability. These complications are more commonly seen when anovulation is due to an underlying pathological condition such as polycystic ovary syndrome (PCOS).

## EXCESSIVE UTERINE BLEEDING

### DEFINITION AND EPIDEMIOLOGY

Dysfunctional uterine bleeding (DUB) is defined as irregular, painless bleeding of endometrial origin that is prolonged, excessive, and unpatterned. DUB can result from anovulatory cycles of any cause. Excessive uterine bleeding that is not unpatterned (menorrhagia) and may be painful can result from coagulopathies, medications, infections, or other illness. Box 64-1 shows the etiologies of excessive uterine bleeding.

### ETIOLOGY AND PATHOGENESIS

#### Hypothalamic Dysfunction

Hypothalamic suppression with low levels of GnRH production, resulting low LH and FSH secretion, and anovulation may lead to DUB. However, most cases of hypothalamic suppression present with primary or secondary amenorrhea. (See Chapter 62 for an in-depth discussion of amenorrhea.) Malnutrition secondary to anorexia nervosa may lead to hypothalamic dysfunction and is common in the adolescent age group. Excessive exercise may also cause hypothalamic suppression and may contribute to an underlying eating disorder. Psychosocial stressors may play a role as well. As mentioned above, DUB is not common with anovulation due to hypothalamic suppression, but it can occur.

**Box 64-1**

***Etiology of Excessive Uterine Bleeding***

**Anovulatory dysfunctional uterine bleeding:**
- Immaturity of the hypothalamic–pituitary–ovarian axis
- Hyperandrogenic chronic anovulation
  - Polycystic ovary syndrome (PCOS)
  - Adrenal disorder (congenital adrenal hyperplasia)
  - Androgen-secreting tumor
- Premature ovarian failure

**Hypothalamic dysfunction:**
- Eating disorders
- Excessive exercise
- Stress

**Blood dyscrasias:**
- von Willebrand disease
- Factor XI deficiency
- Thrombocytopenia
- Qualitative platelet disorders
- Leukemia

**Chronic illness:**
- Renal disease
- Liver disease
- Diabetes mellitus

**Complications of pregnancy:**
- Spontaneous/missed abortion
- Ectopic pregnancy

**Endocrine disorders:**
- Thyroid

**Infection**

**Trauma**

**Foreign body**

**Medications**

**Anatomical genital tract lesions:**
- Vaginal laceration
- Neoplasm
- Congenital anomalies

#### Endocrine Disorders

Endocrine disorders, most notably hyperthyroidism and hypothyroidism, commonly present in this age group with irregular menstrual bleeding that may be excessive. Patients may present with other signs and symptoms signifying a thyroid disorder, such as goiter, weight change, and/or cold or heat intolerance, but often they do not have such signs and it is always prudent to check serum levels of thyroid hormones. Another common endocrine disorder, hyperandrogenic chronic anovulation, or PCOS, can sometimes present as amenorrhea but more commonly as oligomenorrhea and is a frequent cause of DUB as well. Patients who have fewer than 6 periods a year, are overweight, or have physical signs of hyperandrogenism such as acne and/or hirsutism, should have a work-up done to investigate for PCOS.[3] Acanthosis nigricans, which is a physical sign of insulin resistance, should be looked for on physical examination.[4] Functional ovarian hyperandrogenism PCOS may be underdiagnosed in adolescent girls. It may be that some of the cases of DUB that have been attributed to immaturity of the HPO axis are, in fact, related to anovulation due to PCOS. It is important to identify these cases early so that the appropriate treatment can be implemented.[5]

Late onset 21-hydroxylase deficiency needs to be ruled out in patients with hirsutism. An adrenocorticotropic hormone (ACTH) stimulation test should be conducted if a fasting 17-hydroxyprogesterone level is elevated. Rarely, ovarian or adrenal tumors can present as hyperandrogenism with amenorrhea or oligomenorrhea, and imaging studies may be considered, especially if testosterone levels are high and/or there is rapid progression of virilization. Premature ovarian failure may initially present with anovulatory cycles and DUB. Determining FSH level is helpful as it is high with ovarian failure.

### Chronic Illness

Chronic illness such as liver disease, inflammatory bowel disease, renal failure, diabetes mellitus, and malignancies may present with excessive menstrual bleeding. Congenital or acquired coagulopathies are also associated with menorrhagia and anemia. For example, Von Willebrand disease needs to be ruled out in an adolescent girl who presents with heavy, prolonged menses and anemia at or shortly after menarche. Autoimmune hemolytic anemia, idiopathic thrombocytopenia, specific clotting factor deficiencies, and Glanzmann disease are other coagulation abnormalities that need to be considered in the differential diagnosis. Even Factor V deficiency, which is rare, should be considered and can be a diagnostic challenge.[6] Investigators from Toronto looked at diagnoses in adolescent girls admitted to their hospital for menorrhagia over a 9-year period. Of the 59 subjects, 19% had an underlying coagulopathy; in 74%, the diagnosis was DUB due to anovulation.[7] A study by Smith[8] looking at 46 adolescent admissions for menorrhagia found that a common diagnosis (33%) was hematologic disease. This included von Willebrand disease, thrombocytopenia, Fanconi's anemia, chronic idiopathic thrombocytopenic purpura, and aplastic anemia. A study done in France had similar findings. Of 41 girls presenting with anemia from excessive uterine bleeding, 12% had a coagulopathy, but most (73%) had DUB.[9] Management of patients with excessive bleeding secondary to coagulation abnormalities usually requires hormonal stabilization of the endometrium (often with combination oral contraceptives) as well as treatment of the underlying disorder.

### Infection and Pregnancy

When pain is associated with excessive uterine bleeding, etiologies other than anovulation need to be ruled out. In the adolescent, as in the adult population, infection should always be considered as a cause for painful, excessive uterine bleeding. Endometritis or salpingitis can present as heavy uterine bleeding with painful cramping. A confidential sexual history and tests for *Chlamydia trachomatis* and *Neisseria gonorrhea* should be included in the evaluation. Complications of pregnancy, such as spontaneous abortion or ectopic pregnancy, also may present with abnormal vaginal bleeding accompanied by abdominal pain. The adolescent may not be aware that she is pregnant and may not have missed a period, especially if she has a history of irregular cycles.

### Drugs

Medications such as warfarin and aspirin may cause excessive bleeding, and a complete history of all medications that the adolescent is taking is important. Use of certain contraceptives, such as depo-medroxyprogesterone acetate or levonorgestrel implants also may lead to excessive bleeding, infrequently causing anemia or hemodynamic instability. Oral contraceptive pills (OCPs) are often associated with irregular (break-through) bleeding or spotting.

### Trauma and Structural Genital Abnormalities

Structural genital abnormalities may present with abrupt bleeding that is unusual or unpatterned. This needs to be considered, especially if bleeding is not responsive to conventional treatment with OCP. A deep vaginal laceration resulting from trauma during voluntary or involuntary coitus can be associated with heavy bleeding requiring transfusion, is often difficult to diagnose, and may require examination under anesthesia and surgical repair.[10] The adolescent may be embarrassed or afraid to reveal that she has had sexual intercourse. High-pressure insufflation injuries occurring from jet ski or water ski falls, pool or spa jets, or water slides can cause vaginal tears and severe hemorrhage with no signs of external trauma. Uterine arteriovenous malformation also should be considered if bleeding occurs suddenly and is severe enough to require a blood transfusion.[11] Neoplasms of the uterus or cervix are a rare cause of menorrhagia in the adolescent. Uterine myomas (fibroids), which are more common in adults, may present as abnormal vaginal bleeding, pelvic pain, or a pelvic mass.[12] Vaginal foreign bodies usually present with purulent discharge and spotting and rarely are associated with heavy bleeding.

## CLINICAL EVALUATION, ASSESSMENT, AND DIAGNOSIS

### Taking an Adolescent Menstrual History

Obtaining an accurate menstrual history can be a challenge in the adolescent age group. Information about the period itself such as age at first menses, cycle length, duration and amount of bleeding, painful periods, and last menstrual period is basic in beginning to understand the problem. Sometimes the girl's mother tries to provide this history, but it is preferable to attempt to get as much of the information as possible from the girl herself.

The age at menarche is important because there are accepted norms for this pubertal milestone. The average girl begins menstruating at age 12.5 years, with some as early as age 9 and as late as age 14. No menarche by age 15 is unusual and therefore needs to be evaluated.[13] Determination of cycle lengths, as well as the date of last menstrual period can be difficult for some girls to recall. Using prompts, such as holidays and weekends often helps. Cycle frequency is determined by the number of days between the first day of menses and the first day of the following period. Very short cycles occurring every 2 to 3 weeks can lead to significant blood loss over time. It is especially helpful to have patients keep a prospective record of their periods. Adolescents, in their concrete thinking, may report that they had 2 periods last month. Further questioning reveals that 1 period began on January 1 and the next began on January 29, yielding a normal cycle length of 29 days. However, with a detailed review of a prospective menstrual diary a more accurate picture of the cycle is usually obtained.

It is important to specifically ask about the duration and amount of bleeding. The amount of bleeding is usually determined by inquiring about passage of blood clots and the number of times the girl changes her pad or tampon. The passing of clots is indicative of excessive bleeding. A girl who is soaking through 5 or more pads a day has excessive bleeding. It is important to ask if the bleeding is so heavy that the girl has to miss school or other activities. The duration of bleeding is also important because most normal periods last 5 to 7 days. Whether or not a pattern of heavy bleeding is new or has occurred with every menses since menarche, it can be a clue pointing to congenital coagulation disorders. Periods that are painful, depending on the nature of the pain, may point toward primary dysmenorrhea, which is associated with ovulatory cycles, or secondary dysmenorrhea which can be related to obstructive congenital anomalies, infection, pregnancy complications, or endometriosis. Prolonged menses are defined as more than 10 to 14 days of heavy bleeding. Family history is helpful because menstrual patterns tend to run in families.[14] Asking about a patient's mother and female siblings is an important part of the overall history. A patient's past medical history of chronic illness, as well as a detailed psychosocial history should be obtained. This includes asking the sexual history, in a sensitive, private, and confidential manner. Box 64-2 presents important points in eliciting a menstrual history.

> **Box 64-2**
>
> ***Menstrual History***
>
> - Age at menarche?
> - Duration of bleeding?
>   - Calculate gynecologic age
> - Amount of bleeding?
> - Passage of clots?
> - Frequency of pad or tampon change?
> - Last menstrual period?
> - Pain with bleeding?
> - Cycle length by prospective record
> - Family history of menstrual patterns

### The Physical Examination

Conducting a complete physical examination is just as important as the history. Tachycardia and orthostatic hypotension suggest rapid blood loss with severe anemia, as does pallor. Assessing height, weight, and pubertal development is especially important when evaluating menstrual disorders, because there are established norms depending on the age of the patient. Studies indicate that across the United States, girls may be developing earlier, and racial differences need to be taken into account. In a study done by Herman-Giddens,[15] secondary sex characteristics and menses were studied in 17,077 girls. Thelarche, or breast budding, is often the first sign of puberty, and black girls had earlier onset than white girls (mean of 8.87 years vs 9.96 years, respectively). On average, menarche occurred at 12.16 years in black girls versus 12.88 years in white girls. Developmental assessment via breast and genital examination for Tanner staging should be done in all patients.

Palpation of the thyroid should be done to rule out goiter or nodules as a cause of menstrual irregularity. Signs of hyperandrogenism, such as acne, hirsutism, clitoromegaly, and acanthosis nigricans need to be looked for on physical examination. Palpation of the abdomen should be performed to rule out pregnancy or masses. Careful skin examination looking for ecchymoses can be a helpful clue for coagulation disorders. Sexually active girls should have a complete pelvic examination looking for infection, pregnancy, or genital trauma. In virginal girls, a thorough external genital examination should be done, but a speculum exam may not be necessary. A rectoabdominal digital examination in the lithotomy position is usually better tolerated in a virginal girl than a vaginal bimanual examination and can provide the same information regarding pelvic masses and tenderness. Rarely, an examination under general anesthesia is warranted.

### Laboratory Testing and Studies

Initial laboratory evaluation is guided by the patient's history and physical examination. A complete blood count (CBC) to assess hematocrit, hemoglobin, and platelet count should be obtained. For girls with excessive bleeding and marked anemia, and particularly for those who must be hospitalized, coagulation abnormalities should be excluded. Chemistries, prothrombin time, activated partial thromboplastin time, fibrinogen, Factor VIII activity, Factor XI antigen, ristocetin cofactor activity, and von Willebrand factor antigen should be included in the diagnostic work-up.

In patients where PCOS is suspected, free and total testosterone, dehydroepiandrosterone sulfate (DHEAS), LH, and FSH may be included in the laboratory evaluation; blood should be drawn for these hormone tests prior to beginning estrogen or progestin therapy for management of the uterine bleeding. Women with signs of hyperandrogenism such as acne, hirsutism, and oligomenorrhea have higher levels of biologically active testosterone (free testosterone) levels than women with normal menses.[16] Other causes of hyperandrogenism may need to be excluded depending on the screening testosterone levels. An ACTH stimulation test may be helpful in evaluation of patients with hyperandrogenism and may be useful in distinguishing abnormalities of adrenal steroidogenesis if initial laboratory evaluation is abnormal.[17] Endocrinopathies including thyroid disorders need to be excluded by obtaining a free thyroxine level and thyroid-stimulating hormone (TSH) level. See Box 64-3 for laboratory evaluation.

Serum quantitative beta human chorionic gonadotropic hormone levels should be measured in all sexually active patients with abdominal pain and unusual bleeding if a urine pregnancy test is negative. In a sexually active girl with a positive pregnancy test with painful abnormal bleeding, it is critical that ectopic pregnancy be excluded by transvaginal ultrasound. Sexually transmitted infection testing also should be done in sexually active adolescents.

**Box 64-3**

***Laboratory Evaluation***

- Complete blood count: hemoglobin/hematocrit
- Platelet count
- Chemistry
- Coagulation disorders: PT/PTT, fibrinogen, von Willebrand, ristocetin, factor deficiencies
- Endocrine: LH/FSH, free and total testosterone, DHEAS, 17-OH-progesterone
- Thyroid function tests
- STI testing: GC/chlamydia
- Quantitative ßHCG

## TREATMENT AND MANAGEMENT

Treatment for excessive menstrual bleeding depends on the severity. It is helpful to divide the cases into mild, moderate, and severe. Figure 64-1 presents the management according to level of severity. Correction of any underlying pathology needs to be addressed and treated accordingly. In a patient not responding to first-line hormonal therapy, a structural or anatomical abnormality needs to be ruled out, as do other pathological causes such as neoplasms.

### Severe Hemorrhage

In severe cases with hemoglobin ≤8 gm/dL, and hemodynamic instability with orthostasis and tachycardia, the adolescent should be immediately hospitalized for aggressive management. Intravenous conjugated estrogens (Premarin) may be administered at 25 mg every 4 to 6 hours (maximum of 4 doses total) until bleeding significantly slows.[18] Oral therapy with a monophasic combination OCP every 6 hours should be started concurrently with the intravenous estrogen. Alternatively, Premarin, 2.5 mg and medroxyprogesterone acetate (Provera) 10 mg may be given by mouth.[19] An antiemetic should be administered due to the nausea that may occur from high estrogen doses. Transfusion and fluid restoration may be necessary in severe cases to correct hemodynamic instability. Examination under anesthesia for high vaginal laceration or dilatation and curettage may be necessary if an adequate response to hormonal therapy is not noted within 24 to 48 hours. The goal of treatment is to correct hemodynamic instability, stop, and prevent future episodes of excessive bleeding. Once bleeding has slowed significantly or ceased, the dose of OCPs can be tapered. Adherence is critical in management with oral hormonal regimens and needs to be addressed in particular with adolescents and their parents.

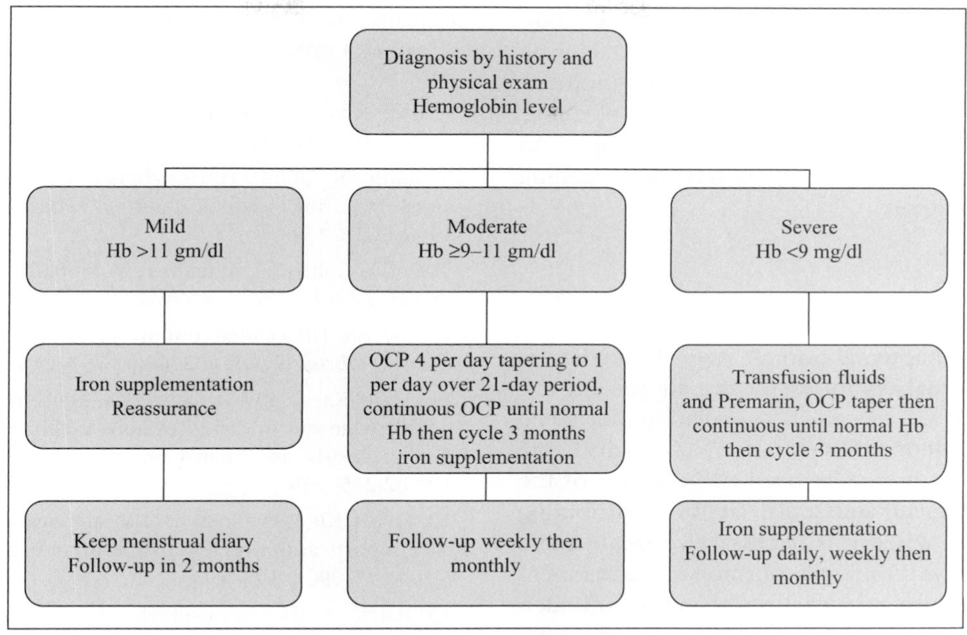


**FIGURE 64-1** Management of uterine bleeding according to severity

### Moderate Hemorrhage

In moderate cases, the anemia is not life-threatening yet significant, with hemoglobin between 9 and 11 gm/dL, and hematocrit between 25% and 35%. Monophasic combined estrogen and progestin OCP are usually adequate to control the excessive bleeding. Depending on the acuity and severity of the anemia and the rate of ongoing uterine bleeding, initial dosing of 4 OCPs per day (every 6 hours) can be started for 3 days tapering slowly to 1 pill per day. Less acute cases can start with 2 OCPs per day (every 12 hours) tapering to 1 pill per day when bleeding stops. This can be tailored to each individual case and requires close follow-up with patients and their families. In patients with very low hemoglobin levels, a withdrawal bleed should not be allowed until the hemoglobin improves. This is achieved by continuous OCP therapy. Patients should be instructed to discard the placebo pills in the 28-day pack and begin a new pack every 21 days. Alternatively, a 21-day pack may be available for some OCPs. The pharmacist must be instructed to dispense 2 packages of pills at a time as the pills will be used more quickly than with a traditional contraceptive regimen. Parents and patients should be educated about the risks and side effects of the pill. It is helpful to refer to "hormonal medication," rather than birth control or contraceptive pills because the pills are not being given for birth control but for bleeding control. Some parents are resistant to giving their daughter birth control pills for fear of this becoming an excuse to become sexually active. Again, appropriate education is sometimes needed to address these sensitive psychosocial issues.

Correction of iron stores with iron supplementation, such as ferrous gluconate, 325 mg 3 times a day is indicated. Patients should also be instructed to begin a stool softener because of constipation that often results from the iron supplement. Anticipation of this helps with patient adherence. Once the patient's hemoglobin has returned to normal, she can be cycled on a 28-day regimen of OCPs for 3 cycles while continuing to take iron and then discontinue the OCPs. If the adolescent is sexually active or if she has PCOS or a coagulopathy, she may continue taking OCPs. The levonorgestrel-releasing intrauterine system can be very helpful for girls with coagulopathies as it produces marked endometrial hypoplasia and usually amenorrhea. Because the effect of the progestin, levonorgestrel, is mainly localized to the uterus, there are few systemic side effects. In particular, the levonorgestrel-releasing intrauterine system is not associated with osteopenia and is well tolerated by nulliparous women.

### Mild Hemorrhage

Adolescents in this category may have shorter cycles and increased duration of menses; however, there is no anemia. Hemoglobin is 11 g/dL and hematocrit is 35% or more. Hormonal therapy is not required but may be given if the girl requires contraception. Reassurance, and a multivitamin pill with iron should be encouraged. Follow-up should be scheduled in 2 months for reevaluation and repeat hemoglobin level measurement. In patients with regular menses but heavy bleeding, a nonsteroidal anti-inflammatory, such as naproxen sodium, taken during the menses may reduce bleeding and improve symptoms.

## SUMMARY

As noted in this chapter, abnormal vaginal bleeding is a common menstrual complaint in the adolescent age group. Most cases are related to anovulation, but some are related to coagulopathies or other pathological conditions. Health care providers need to be aware of the physical, psychological, and social factors contributing to these disorders. When it is necessary to treat significant hemorrhage with anemia, hormonal management with OCPs is safe in this age group. Correction of underlying pathology needs to be addressed at the same time as monitoring for restoration of normal cycles.

## REFERENCES

1. World Health Organization. World Health Organization multicenter study on menstrual and ovulatory patterns in adolescent girls. *J Adolesc Health Care.* 1986;7:236–244

2. Apter D, Viinikka L, Vihko R. Hormonal patterns of adolescent menstrual cycles. *J Clin Endocrino Metab.* 1978; 47:944–954

3. Rieder J, Santoro N, Cohen HW, Marantz P, Coupey SM. Body shape and size and insulin resistance as early clinical predictors of hyperandrogenic anovulation in ethnic minority adolescent girls. *J Adolesc Health.* 2008;43:115–124

4. Barbieri RL, Ryan KJ. Hyperandrogenism, insulin resistance, and acanthosis nigricans syndrome: a common endocrinopathy with distinct pathophysiologic features. *Am J Obstet Gynecol.* 1983;147:90–101

5. Dramusic V, Goh VHH, Rajan U, et al. Clinical, endocrinologic, and ultrasonographic features of polycystic ovary syndrome in Singaporean adolescents. *J Pediatr Adolesc Gynecol.* 1997; 10:125–132

6. Bennet K, Daley ML, Pike C. Factor V deficiency and menstruation: a gynecologic challenge. *Obstet Gynecol.* 1997;839–840

7. Claessens EA, Cowell CA. Acute adolescent menorrhagia. *Am J Obstset Gynecol.* 1981;139:277–280

8. Smith YR, Quint EH, Hertzberg RB. Menorrhagia in adolescents requiring hospitalization. *J Pediatr Adolesc Gynecol.* 1998;11:13–15

9. Duflos-Cohade C, Amandruz M, Thibaud E. Pubertal metrorrhagia. *J Pediatr Adolesc Gynecol.* 1996;9:16–20

10. Merritt DF. Genital trauma in children and adolescents. *Clinical Obstet Gynecol.* 2008;51:237–248

11. Abdul-Karim RW, Badawy SZA, Adelson MD, et al. Uterine hemorrhage due to arteriovenous malformation in a teenage girl: diagnosis and management. *Adolesc Pediatr Gynecol.* 1989;2:235–239

12. Fields KR, Neinstein LS. Uterine myomas in adolescents: case reports and a review of the literature. *J Pediatr Adolesc Gynecol.* 1996;9:195–198

13. Batrinos ML, Panitsa-Faflia C, Courcoutsakis N, et al. Incidence, type, and etiology of menstrual disorders in the age group 12–19 years. *Adolesc Pediatr Gynecol.* 1990;3:149–153

14. Kantero RL, Widholm O. Correlation of menstrual traits between adolescent girls and their mothers. *Acta Obstet Gynecol Scand.* 1971;14(Suppl):30–36

15. Herman-Giddens ME, Slora EJ, Wasserman RC, et al. Secondary sexual characteristics and menses in young girls seen in office practice: a study from the pediatric research in office settings network. *Pediatrics.* 1997;99:505–512

16. Hasinski S, Telang GH, Rose LI, et al. Testosterone concentrations and oligomenorrhea in women with acne. *Int J Dermatol.* 1997;36:845–847

17. Siegel SF, Finegold DN, Murray PJ, et al. Assessment of clinical hyperandrogenism in adolescent girls. *Adolesc Pediatr Gynecol.* 1992;5:13–20

18. Iglesias EA, Coupey SM. Menstrual cycle abnormalities: diagnosis and management. *Adoles Med.* 1999;10:255–273

19. Strickland JL, Wall JF. Abnormal uterine bleeding in adolescents. *Obstet Gynecol Clin North Am.* 2003;30:321–335

# CHAPTER 65

# Hyperandrogenism

KRISTI MORGAN MULCHAHEY, MD

## INTRODUCTION

Polycystic ovarian syndrome (PCOS) and related androgen disorders are commonly encountered in the reproductive health care of the adolescent girl. Although adolescent PCOS has received more attention recently, it should be remembered that in 1980, Emans et al[1] diagnosed PCOS in 52% of adolescent females presenting with oligomenorrhea. Polycystic ovarian syndrome is increasingly recognized as a heterogeneous disorder with a variety of symptoms: ovulatory disturbances, hirsutism, skin changes such as acne or acanthosis nigricans, and obesity or metabolic disturbances with glucose intolerance and dyslipidemia. Because of these potentially serious long-term health consequences, it is imperative that those who provide medical care for adolescents recognize this endocrine disturbance early and provide appropriate diagnostic testing and treatment.

The diagnosis of PCOS is primarily clinical, without universally agreed upon diagnostic criteria. After Stein and Leventhal's[2] original description of PCOS in 1935, the World Health Organization (WHO) consensus report in 1990 defined the disorder as the presence of ovulatory disturbance and androgen excess, with no other identifiable etiology (Box 65-1). More recently, the Rotterdam criteria diagnose PCOS when 2 of the following 3 are present: clinical or laboratory hyperandrogenism, chronic anovulation, and "polycystic" ovaries by ultrasound. In Europe, clinicians stress the diagnostic importance of the "polycystic appearance" of the ovaries by ultrasound. In North America, PCOS is recognized as a functional disorder, and polycystic ovaries by ultrasound are not necessary for the diagnosis.[3,4] In fact, Behera[5] suggests replacing the term "PCOS" with "functional female hyperandrogenism" to avoid this confusion.

The diagnosis of PCOS in the adolescent is made more challenging by the complex endocrine changes of puberty. During adolescence, the accurate diagnosis of PCOS requires a clear understanding of the endocrine and ovarian changes associated with puberty and the differences between adults and adolescent menstrual function. Anovulatory cycles are common and physiologic during the first few gynecological years. (Gynecological age is chronological age minus age at menarche.) Normal ovaries often appear "polycystic" during early puberty, due to the presence of multiple small follicular cysts. Hirsutism is often subtle in the young teen due to the shorter duration of excessive androgen exposure. Serum androgen levels are different for each Tanner stage of pubarche. All of these factors add to the clinical challenge of diagnosing PCOS in the adolescent.[6–8]

Although the etiology of PCOS remains unclear, functional disturbances in the ovary, the hypothalamic-pituitary-ovarian axis, and insulin metabolism have been demonstrated.[9] This process of disordered androgen function likely begins in prenatal life. Infants who are small for gestational age are more likely to develop adolescent PCOS than appropriate for gestational age infants. Girls with premature adrenarche are at increased risk for the development of PCOS.[10,11] Apter's[12] longitudinal studies of girls from childhood through adolescence found differences in the patterns of luteinizing hormone (LH) release early in puberty in girls who later developed PCOS when compared with girls who developed normal ovulatory patterns. Although not yet fully understood, the first signs and symptoms of PCOS may present much earlier than previously appreciated.

The production of androgens is a necessary intermediate step in the process of ovarian steroidogenesis. The 2-cell model (Figure 65-1) demonstrates the conversion of cholesterol to androstenedione and testosterone in the thecal cell, followed by their conversion into estradiol

### Box 65-1

### *Definitions of PCOS*

WHO criteria: chronic hyperandrogenism (elevation of serum testosterone or other androgens) and chronic anovulation (absence of ovulation) in the absence of other specific causes of these problems.

Rotterdam criteria (of the following 3 characteristics)

1. Chronic anovulation
2. Chronic hyperandrogenism
3. Polycystic appearing ovaries (PCO) on ultrasound

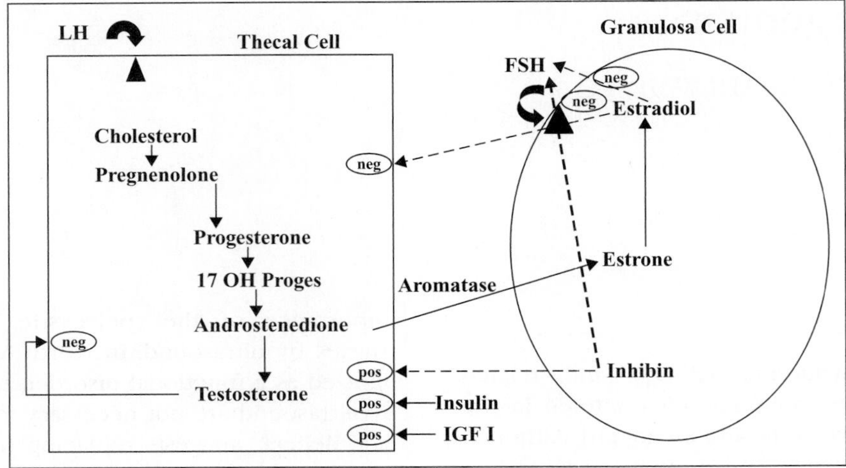


**FIGURE 65-1** Two-cell model of ovarian steroidogenesis.

in the granulosa cell. The intermediate production of ovarian androgens is also mediated by insulin and insulin like growth factor (IGF), with receptors present on the thecal cell. A theory has been proposed that a genetically based mutation in the insulin receptor results in the hyperandrogenism of PCOS. The therapeutic usefulness of insulin-sensitizing agents in the treatment of PCOS supports this theory.[13]

As research increases our understanding of pathophysiology, more light is also being shed on the natural history of PCOS. Lifelong risks of PCOS include impaired glucose tolerance, insulin resistance, gestational diabetes, and type 2 diabetes mellitus; obesity, hypertension, dyslipidemia, and coronary artery disease; fatty liver; endometrial hyperplasia and malignancy; infertility and recurrent spontaneous abortion.[9] Providers of health care for adolescents need to be aware of this common disorder and be able to diagnose and treat it effectively. Although longitudinal studies are not yet available to demonstrate improvement in long-term health from early intervention, it is hoped that improved health status may result.

## CLINICAL PRESENTATION

The clinical presentation of the adolescent girl with PCOS may be varied and is often ameliorated by the young age of the patient, a shorter duration of excess androgen exposure, and physiologic differences between adult and adolescent normal menstrual function.[14] The severity of presenting signs and symptoms may vary greatly, even within the same family. Because the diagnosis of PCOS is primarily clinical, it is critical that the clinician be very familiar with at-risk groups (Box 65-2) and varieties of presentation.

### Box 65-2

### *Identification of Girls at Risk for Polycystic Ovarian Syndrome (PCOS) and Hyperandrogenism*

**Presenting complaints**

- Menstrual dysfunction
- Primary or secondary amenorrhea
- Oligomenorrhea
- Polymenorrhea or frequent bleeding
- Weight gain
- Hirsutism
- Acne
- Family history of PCOS

**Physical assessment**

- Increased body mass index (BMI)
- Increased waist-to-hip ratio
- Hirsutism
- Acne
- Acanthosis nigricans

A careful history should begin with a neonatal and childhood history because of the recently described association between small for gestational age weight at birth and the later development of PCOS. Premature adrenarche has also been associated with an increased risk of subsequent development of PCOS.[10] Specific questions about the age of development of axillary hair, pubic hair, and the onset of body odor should be asked, because premature adrenarche may have not been diagnosed. Age of thelarche is also crucial in the assessment of menstrual function. Normal menstruation should begin within 2 to 3 years of thelarche. This milestone of thelarche is much more reliable than chronological age in evaluating the timing of menarche.

Menstrual irregularity is common among younger adolescent girls. Initially, anovulatory cycles may occur in up to 80% of healthy girls in the first gynecologic year, with the majority of girls having ovulatory cycles by the third gynecologic year. In assessing menstrual irregularities in adolescents, the gynecological age of the girl is crucial. Assessment of menstrual function should not be based on chronological age.[15]

Further studies have confirmed Emans' initial finding of a 52% incidence of PCOS among adolescent girls with menstrual disturbances. Subsequent studies have noted that these disturbances may include: primary amenorrhea, secondary amenorrhea, oligomenorrhea and polymenorrhea. Nearly any pattern of abnormal bleeding has been associated with the ovulatory disturbance of PCOS.[16] Asking teens about menstruation should involve specific questions about frequency and duration of bleeding, as well as amount of bleeding, best determined by simple questions such as "How long can you wait between changing your pad or tampon?"

Skin manifestations of PCOS are also helpful in identifying the at-risk adolescent. Excessive androgen exposure to the pilosebaceous unit may result in hirsutism and acne. In hirsutism, there is an irreversible conversion of a vellus hair into a terminal hair. This irreversible change occurs because of exposure of the androgen receptor in the hair follicle to dihydrotestosterone (DHT), created by the peripheral conversion of testosterone to DHT by 5-alpha reductase.

Hirsutism refers to terminal hair appearance on the brow, upper lip, chin, sternum, upper arm, abdomen, and bikini line. The degree of hirsutism has traditionally been measured by the Ferriman-Gallwey score, with hirsutism diagnosed by a score of 7 or more (Figure 65-2). However, the hyperandrogenic adolescent may demonstrate significant hirsutism with a score of less than 7, presumably because of the shorter duration of excess androgen exposure. The distribution and number of terminal hairs is also influenced by ethnicity. The density of hair follicles is highest in girls of Mediterranean ancestry and lowest in girls who are Asian. It is also important to distinguish between hirsutism and hypertrichosis, the excessive growth of hair. Tanner staging should also be noted.[17] On a practical note, some adolescents are very skilled at hair removal. Physical examination alone will underestimate the degree of hirsutism; it is also important to ask the teen about hair removal procedures and to estimate the degree of hirsutism before removal.

Acne is a common physical finding in adolescent girls with PCOS and a cause of great teenage angst. The increased production of sebum by the pilosebaceous unit often results in cystic acne, as well as acne on the chest and back.[18] Past and current treatment for acne should be explored, as girls may be taking oral antibiotics or isotretinoin and ongoing treatment will affect current findings.

Physical findings suggestive of insulin resistance should also be evaluated. Elevated body mass index (BMI), increased waist-to-hip ratio, and acanthosis nigricans (Figure 65-3) are often seen in PCOS. Acanthosis nigricans is the appearance of thickened, hyperpigmented skin, seen most commonly on the neck, axilla, and groin.

There are no specific findings of PCOS on pelvic examination, and a pelvic examination is not necessary for diagnostic purposes. External genital exam should include Tanner staging, assessment of acanthosis nigricans, and determination of clitoral size. Clitoromegaly, although rarely a finding in PCOS in adolescents, is a sign of virilization. Other signs of virilization, rapid progression of hirsutism, and lowering of the voice, are suggestive of an androgen-producing tumor.[19]

A history of medication use is also important. In particular, valproic acid has been documented as a cause of PCOS; fortunately, complete reversal of these changes has been achieved upon discontinuation of the medicine.[20] Especially in girls with hirsutism, the history should be evaluated for medications known to cause hypertrichosis, which can be mistaken for hirsutism.[21]

Family history also is illustrative. Keeping in mind that PCOS may have a varied presentation even within genetically related individuals,[22] it is helpful to inquire about family members with menstrual disturbance, hirsutism, infertility, and recurrent miscarriage. Families with PCOS also have an increased incidence of hypertension, type 2 diabetes mellitus, and coronary artery disease in both male and female members. Male adults may have early balding. There is also an association between PCOS and endometrial neoplasia in adult women (and occasionally older adolescents with histories of prolonged abnormal bleeding).

## LABORATORY TESTING

There are essential laboratory tests for evaluation of the girl with suspected PCOS. The diagnosis itself is primarily a clinical one, based on history and physical examination. The laboratory testing is performed to support the diagnosis by exclusion of other endocrinopathies. Studies to exclude thyroid dysfunction, hypergonadotrophic or hypogonadotrophic anovulation, and hyperprolactinemia are recommended (Box 65-3).

**Hirsutism Rating Scale***

| Patient's Name | Address | | | Date |
|---|---|---|---|---|
| Site | Grade and Definition (Enter numerical grade in box) 1 | 2 | 3 | 4 |
| **Upper Lip** | 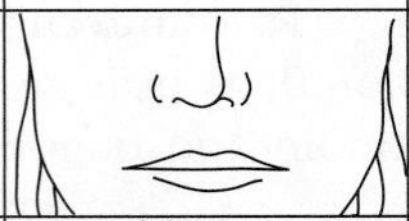 A few terminal hairs at outer margin or scattered over upper lip | A small moustache at outer margin or covering less than half of upper lip | A moustache extending halfway from outer margin or halfway up lip | A moustache extending to midline and covering most of upper lip |
| **Sideburn Area** | 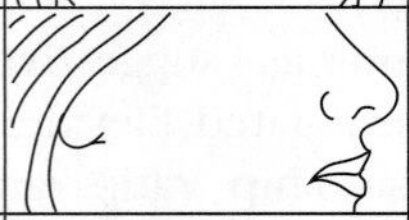 A few scattered terminal hairs | Scattered terminal hairs with small concentrations | Light coverage of entire area | Dense coverage of entire area |
| **Chin** | 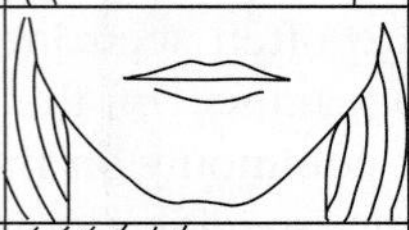 A few scattered terminal hairs | Scattered terminal hairs with small concentrations | Complete but light coverage | Complete and heavy coverage |
| **Lower Jaw and Upper Neck** | 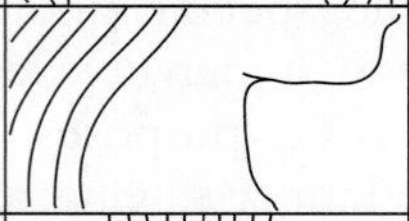 A few scattered hairs | Scattered hairs with small concentrations | Light coverage of entire area | Complete and dense coverage of entire area |
| **Upper Back** | 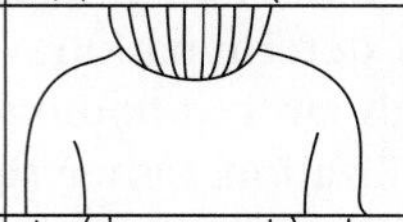 A few scattered terminal hairs | More terminal hairs, but still scattered | Complete but light coverage | Complete and dense coverage |
| **Lower Back** | 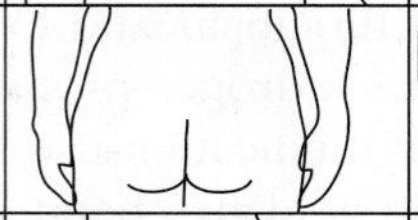 Some sacral hair (area of coverage less than 4 cm wide) | With greater lateral extension | Three-quarter coverage | Complete coverage |
| **Upper Arm** | 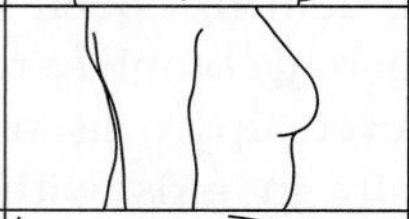 Sparse growth affecting not more than a quarter of the limb surface | More than this; coverage still incomplete | Complete but light coverage | Complete and dense coverage |
| **Thigh** | 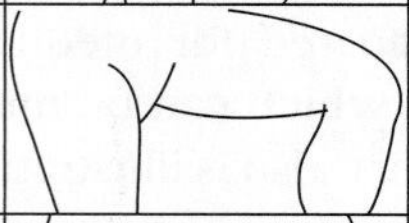 Sparse growth affecting not more than a quarter of the limb surface | More than this; coverage still incomplete | Complete but light coverage | Complete and dense coverage |
| **Chest** | 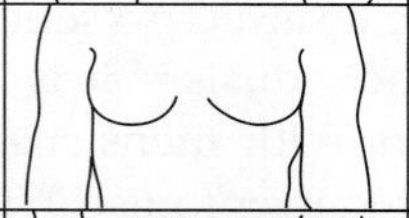 Terminal circumareolar hairs or midline hairs | Both terminal circumareolar hairs and midline hairs | Three-quarter coverage | Complete coverage |
| **Upper Abdomen** | 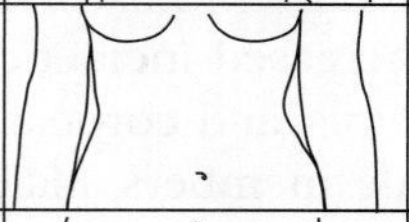 A few midline terminal hairs | More terminal hairs, still midline | Half coverage | Full coverage |
| **Lower Abdomen** | 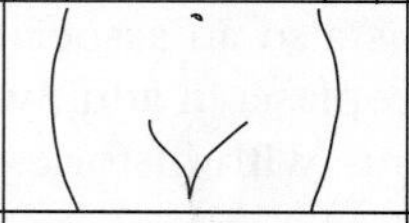 A few midline terminal hairs along linea alba | A midline streak of terminal hair | A midline band of terminal hair not more than 1/4 width of pubic hair at base | An inverted V-shaped growth 1/2 width of pubic hair at base |
| **Perineum** | 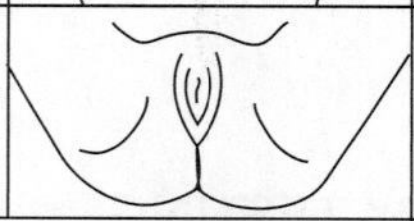 Perianal terminal hair | Lateral extension of terminal hair to edge of gluteal cleft | Three-quarter coverage of buttocks | Complete coverage of buttocks |
| Column Subtotals | | | | |

Total Score

**FIGURE 65-2** The Ferriman-Gallwey (1961) Scale for Rating Hirsutism. (Reprinted from The Practice Committee for the American Society for Reproductive Medicine. The evaluation and treatment of androgen excess. *Fertil Steril.* 2006;86:S241–S247, with permission from Elsevier.)

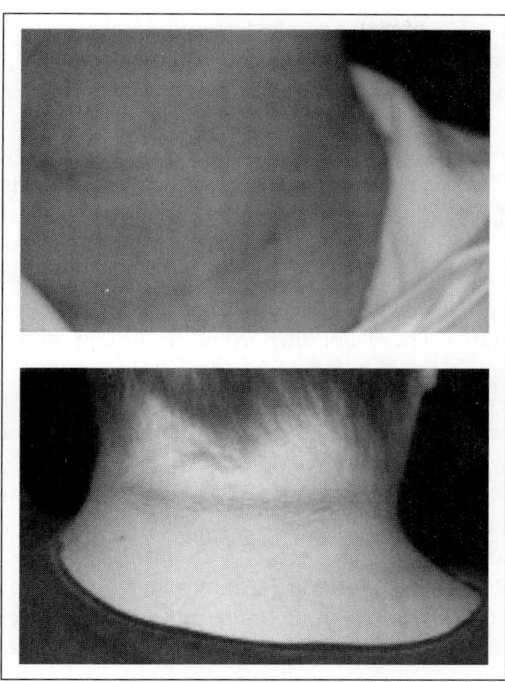

FIGURE 65-3 Acanthosis nigricans (see color insert).

### Box 65-3

#### *Essential Laboratory Testing*

- Testing for other causes of anovulation
  - Thyroid-stimulating hormone (TSH), ultrasensitive
  - Follicle-stimulating hormone (FSH)
  - Prolactin
- Testing for other causes of androgen excess
  - Dehydroepiandrosterone sulfate (DHEAS)
  - Free and total testosterone
  - 17 OH progesterone
- Testing for comorbid conditions
  - Blood sugar measurement
  - Fasting cholesterol, low-density lipoprotein (LDL), high-density lipoprotein (HDL), and triglycerides
  - Liver function testing
  - Screening for insulin resistance

Prolactin levels may be mildly elevated in females with PCOS. Although the exact etiology of this increase is unclear, it is not associated with a risk of adenoma, and minimally elevated prolactin levels may be safely followed in these patients.[23] Rising prolactin levels should be evaluated to rule out a pituitary adenoma. As a practical point, prolactin levels may be elevated in any reproductive age women when the blood sample is obtained shortly after a breast examination. The first step in evaluating minimal hyperprolactinemia is a repeat assay not preceded by a breast examination.

Traditionally, LH to stimulating hormone (FSH) ratios were performed, with LH:FSH more than 3:1 considered "suggestive" of PCOS. These ratios are not required by either the WHO or Rotterdam criteria, and there is no clear literature support for use of this ratio as a diagnostic tool.[24] In addition, LH:FSH ratios can be physiologically elevated in early puberty. It is important to avoid labeling healthy early adolescents with physiologic anovulation with a diagnosis of PCOS solely based on an elevated LH:FSH ratio.

Measurement of selected serum androgen levels is generally accepted in the evaluation of the clinically hyperandrogenic female, although it is possible for a female with PCOS to have androgen levels within the normal range. Therefore, this testing is recommended to exclude other forms of androgen excess, such as ovarian tumors, adrenal tumors, and late onset adrenal hyperplasia, sometimes called nonclassical adrenal hyperplasia (NCAH) (see Box 65-3). Dehydroepiandrosterone sulfate (DHEAS), total and free testosterone, and 17a-hydroxyprogesterone (17-HP) levels will rule out tumors and NCAH.[25] Tumor evaluation and gynecological consultation is indicated with DHEAS levels greater than 7,000 ng/dL and testosterone levels greater than 200 ng/dL.[26] Rapidly progressing evidence of androgen excess (hirsutism and acne) or virilization (clitoromegaly or lowering of the voice) are also worrisome for the possibility of a tumor and should not be ignored when androgen levels are below "tumor range," because exceptions have been noted in the literature. Imaging studies are generally not indicated in the basic evaluation of the adolescent with PCOS. However, pelvic ultrasound (Figure 65-4) is indicated with significantly elevated testosterone to rule out ovarian neoplasm; adrenal imaging by magnetic resonance imaging (MRI) or computed tomography (CT) should be obtained when DHEAS levels are in the "tumor range."

There is controversy in the literature as to whether hyperandrogenemia is necessary for the diagnosis of PCOS. As discussed in the introduction to this chapter, there is continuing debate in the literature about diagnostic criteria, and arguments may be made on both sides of this debate.[27] In adults tested by 1990 National Institutes of Health (NIH) criteria, up to 20% will meet criteria for PCOS with normal androgen levels.[28] This has several possible explanations. Testing methods are inexact and testing is best done in the follicular phase, but this may be difficult to determine in the patient with menstrual disturbances. There is also evidence

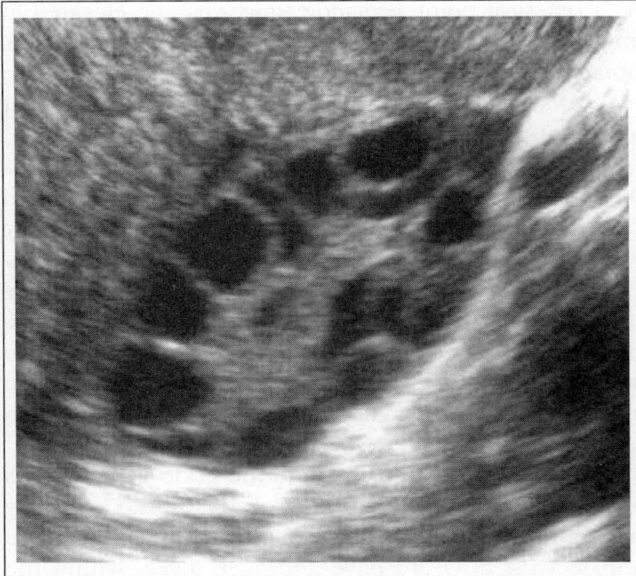

**FIGURE 65-4** Normal ultrasound of "polycystic" adolescent ovaries.

that androgen levels may decline after progestin-induced withdrawal bleeding.[29] In the evaluation of adolescents suspected of having PCOS, there are several other age-specific concerns. The levels of androgens rise through puberty and adulthood, beginning to fall in the fifth decade of life. There are normal ranges of serum androgen available by age and by Tanner stage, available from most reference labs. Should adolescent hyperandrogenemia be determined by adult or adolescent normal values? If PCOS is to be diagnosed by androgen levels, is it also important to remember that there are several other androgen levels that could be measured so which level should be used? There are a variety of assays available for serum androgens, especially with testosterone and free testosterone, and each may produce different results. What assay should be used in the adolescent? It is very clear that future research is needed to answer these questions. In the meantime, it is important to remember that serum androgens are measured in the evaluation of PCOS to "rule out" other causes of androgen excess rather than to confirm the PCOS diagnosis.

Testing to identify girls with NCAH is also important. Screening is accomplished by obtaining a serum 17a-hydroxyprogesterone during the follicular phase. In girls with menstrual disturbances, identification of the follicular phase may be difficult. Obtaining the date on the next menstrual period after the blood was drawn may indicate the laboratory studies were drawn during the luteal phase. Simultaneous measurement of progesterone with the 17a-hydroxyprogesterone will also detect laboratory studies drawn during the luteal phase.

When the follicular phase 17a-hydroxyprogesterone is elevated, definitive testing for 21 hydroxylase deficient NCAH is indicated. The adrenocorticotropic hormone (ACTH) stimulation test is performed during the follicular phase in the fasting state. Pre- and 1-hour post-ACTH stimulation levels of 17a-hydroxyprogesterone are measured and results graphed on a nomogram for interpretation. This identifies homozygous and heterozygous states. There are important treatment differences between PCOS and late-onset adrenal hyperplasia, which makes identification important. This should especially be considered in certain clinical populations, eg, Ashkenazi Jews, who are at increased risk.[30]

There is a growing body of literature confirming the increased risk of impaired glucose intolerance, insulin resistance, and type 2 diabetes mellitus in PCOS. These have also been identified in adolescent girls with PCOS and will be increasingly important with the current increasing prevalence of childhood and adolescent obesity. Dyslipidemia is also common, with unfavorable HDL:LDL ratios and elevations in triglycerides.[31–33] Modestly elevated aminotransferases, consistent with nonalcoholic fatty liver disease (NAFLD), have been recognized with both adults and adolescents with PCOS.[34,35]

When the patient has been started on oral contraceptive pills (OCPs) prior to her evaluation, several of the lab studies will be affected by the ovulation suppression of oral contraceptives. Thyroid-stimulating hormone and prolactin will be unaffected by oral contraceptives, but FSH and LH will be suppressed. Androgen levels will also be affected by OCPs. In this situation, careful history and physical exam will be essential in making a clinical diagnosis of PCOS. Screening for comorbid conditions such as type 2 diabetes, impaired glucose tolerance, insulin resistance, hyperlipidemia, and possible NAFLD may be performed in the usual manner, even if the patient is on OCPs. Therefore, diagnostic testing may be limited by the concurrent use of OCPs, but other important laboratory studies (eg, screening for comorbid conditions) can still be obtained.

## TREATMENT OPTIONS

There is no doubt that nutritional and lifestyle counseling is the most important initial step in the treatment of the adolescent with PCOS. Multiple studies have demonstrated that weight loss, accomplished through dietary changes and exercise, improves symptoms and biochemical parameters. Current nutritional guidelines suggest avoidance of simple sugars, a moderate amount of complex carbohydrates from whole grain sources, and low-fat sources of protein. Adequate calories for energy and adequate calcium for peak bone mass need to be included.

Counseling for these nutritional and lifestyle changes is challenging and is best accomplished with a multidisciplinary approach. Nutritionists with specific skills in working with adolescents and their families are extremely helpful. However, medical care providers should not completely delegate this teaching and support to their nutritionist colleagues. A team approach requires the full support of the medical portion of the team.

Counseling adolescents and their families is different than traditional weight loss counseling for adults. Teens are usually not the grocery shoppers for the family and will have less control over food choices made at home. However, when outside of the home, teens are affected by fast food easy availability and low cost, peer attitudes toward weight, food choices, body image, and school lunch programs. Nutritional counseling for the entire family is important in helping teens make better food choices. Grocery shopping, food preparation methods, and portion size need to be discussed. Highly processed convenience foods are easy but not always the best choices. Establishing a routine of family meals should be encouraged. The nutritional changes recommended for the teen will benefit the whole family, especially given the genetic tendencies for type 2 diabetes mellitus, dyslipidemia, and coronary artery disease in families with PCOS. Guidance should also include healthy food choices in snacking, fast food restaurants, school lunches as well as brown bag lunches. Internet sites that assist in tracking food intake and energy expenditure may appeal to some teens. Eating habits may be a source of conflict between the parent and teen, and this is important to address for a successful collaboration among the teen, parent, and clinician. See Chapter 79, Obesity, for a more detailed discussion of weight control in adolescents.

There are other lifestyle changes that may support better nutrition and result in desired weight loss. For example, time spent in sedentary activities, such as computer use and television watching, decreases energy expenditure and may increase caloric intake with increased snacking. Therefore, limiting these activities to a reasonable amount helps. Increased activity is important to build increased body muscle mass and decrease body fat, improving insulin utilization. Adolescents should be counseled on all forms of increased activity, not just specific sports or exercise. Organized and individual sports are excellent tools for improved physical fitness and weight loss, but less structured methods for increased energy expenditure should not be overlooked. Dancing, choosing walking or bike riding over driving for transportation, and choosing stairs over elevators are well-established lifestyle changes that support better physical fitness. Enlisting the support of the adolescent's peer group is important. Given the increasing rate of obesity in US adolescents, these strategies would benefit all groups of teens.[36-40]

Medical management of PCOS may include several different strategies. Suppressing androgen production, antagonizing androgen effect, and increasing insulin sensitivity are all medical strategies shown to benefit adult patients. More studies in adolescent patients are becoming available that have demonstrated similar benefits. In deciding the appropriate treatment, it is first helpful to determine treatment goals for each individual adolescent. The presenting complaint, whether it is acne, hirsutism, menstrual disturbance, or weight gain, should always be addressed and the patient given a realistic timetable for improvement. Need for prevention of pregnancy is also extremely important to determine in treatment planning.

Oral contraceptive pills are the most commonly prescribed treatment for PCOS. In the sexually active adolescent, OCPs offer important protection against pregnancy. Chapter 52, Contraception, provides a detailed discussion of the OCP. Menstrual cycle control is also improved with oral contraceptives. Estrogen and progestin oral contraceptives also address some of the biochemical disturbances that occur with PCOS. Oral contraceptive pills will increase sex hormone-binding globulins, decreasing the levels of free (active) testosterone. Suppression of ovarian steroidogenesis will also decrease ovarian androgen production. Adrenal androgen production may also be decreased by OCPs. They also decrease acne and hirsutism. Improvement of Ferriman-Gallwey scores have been documented. A decreased incidence of endometrial hyperplasia has also been noted among all users of OCPs.

In choosing an oral contraceptive for adolescent PCOS, it is important to remember that all oral contraceptives have antiandrogen effects, by mechanisms mentioned previously. Whether one progestin is "more antiandrogenic" than another is the subject of debate; clinically, differences are minimal. Choice of oral contraceptive should depend upon the comfort level of the clinician and medical needs of the patient. OCP For example, the choice of a 20-mcg estradiol oral contraceptive may be beneficial for the adolescent with migraine headaches. Extended cycle or continuous oral contraceptives may be helpful with menorrhagia or dysmenorrhea.

Progestin therapy has also been used in PCOS treatment. Although progestin therapy may regulate menses, treat abnormal bleeding, and protect the endometrium against the ill effects of unopposed estrogen, it does not treat the other effects of hyperandrogenemia. Specifically, acne, hirsutism, and obesity are not affected by progestin therapy and may be worsened in some patients. Protection against pregnancy is not provided. For these reasons, progestins are rarely indicated as monotherapy for PCOS. However, they may be helpful in initial treatment to induce menses in amenorrhea, control anovulatory bleeding, and treat endometrial hyperplasia.

Antiandrogen therapy with androgen receptor blockers may also be a helpful adjuvant in the medical treatment of PCOS. This is rarely indicated as monotherapy, especially because protection against pregnancy is not provided and exposure of an early pregnancy with a male fetus could be teratogenic. The most commonly used antiandrogen is aldactone, which is also a weak, potassium-sparing diuretic.[41] When combined with an oral contraceptive, additional benefits may be achieved in reduction of hirsutism and control of acne due to direct inhibition of the androgen receptor located in each hair follicle. Other androgen receptor blockers have been used in adults with treatment-resistant PCOS. None of these antiandrogen drugs are Food and Drug Administration (FDA) approved in women and there have not been adequate clinical studies in adolescent girls. Therefore, their use in routine adolescent treatment of PCOS is not recommended.

Hirsutism, especially facial, can be very distressing to the teen. Early treatment of hyperandrogenemia is important to prevent progression of hair growth, with continued conversion of the vellus hair into terminal hairs. The longer androgen levels remain elevated, the more terminal hairs will appear. Once this conversion has occurred, the terminal hair will persist unless permanently removed. It is also important to educate patients that treatment for PCOS may take 3 to 6 months before new terminal hairs stop appearing.

All measures that control hyperandrogenemia should decrease progressive hirsutism. During the 3- to 6-month time period before treatment has its full effect, temporary measures such as shaving, depilatories, and plucking are most effective. Topical eflornithine has been shown to slow regrowth of terminal hair and produce a less coarse hair. Once the progression has been stopped, permanent removal techniques such as laser or electrolysis can be offered. It is important that underlying hyperandrogenemia be corrected prior to starting any method of permanent hair removal. Laser is less painful than electrolysis with less risk of scarring; therefore, it is better tolerated by most adolescents. For adolescents of color, it is especially important that the appropriate type of laser be chosen. Referral to a dermatologist is suggested.

Insulin sensitizers have received tremendous attention in the treatment of adult PCOS, especially in treatment of infertility. Their use in the treatment of PCOS with associated insulin resistance is also becoming increasingly accepted. The use of insulin sensitizers, usually metformin, in the adolescent with PCOS is controversial, but there is a growing body of literature demonstrating benefits in this population.[42–45]

If a clinician chooses to use an insulin sensitizer in the adolescent with PCOS, it is important to have specific therapeutic goals in mind. For example, weight loss, improvement in hyperlipidemia, or normalization of increased liver function tests are specific measurable goals. If treatment does not achieve these results, it is unclear if continued insulin sensitizer treatment is beneficial. It is also unclear if insulin sensitizer therapy in the adolescent will lower the incidence of subsequent type 2 diabetes mellitus if weight loss is not achieved. It is also important to remember that the use of insulin sensitizers may result in ovulation and unintended pregnancy in a sexually active girl. It is wise to provide oral contraceptives together with metformin, unless there is a contraindication to the oral contraceptive.

## LONG-TERM MANAGEMENT ISSUES

Once the initial diagnosis and treatment plan have been established, it is important that both response to therapy as well as development of new symptoms be monitored. On subsequent visits, height, weight, BMI, and blood pressure should be assessed. If increased, BMI should fall with treatment. Elevation of blood pressure may indicate the development of hypertension associated with metabolic syndrome or as a side effect of estrogen-containing oral contraceptives. Acne should improve and hirsutism should stabilize within 3 to 6 months. If necessary, additional treatment can be initiated. Dermatologic topical treatment and oral antibiotics may be appropriate. Hair removal techniques can also be offered. Menstrual regulation will be easily achieved with oral contraceptives; insulin sensitizer treatment used alone will not regulate menses in all adolescents, and later addition of oral contraceptives may be necessary. There is no consensus among experienced physicians about monitoring of androgen levels after treatment is initiated. Some will reassess only the elevated levels; others will measure androgen levels again if clinical response is less than anticipated; and others will simply follow the patient clinically.

The patient should be screened for insulin resistance at the time of initial diagnosis, but screening needs to continue periodically. The risk of development of insulin resistance/type 2 diabetes mellitus increases as the patient ages. Periodic monitoring of blood sugar, fasting serum lipids, and liver function tests will help prompt identification.

Patients and parents will often have concerns about future fertility. While there is also abundant information available on the Internet on this topic, teens and their parents need assistance in sorting through which information is applicable in their clinical situation. The difference between "infertility" (ie, unable to conceive a pregnancy) and "subfertility" (ie, able to conceive with assistance) needs to be explained. Many women with well-controlled PCOS and appropriate treatment with insulin sensitizers and induction of ovulation, if necessary, will conceive without significant difficulty. Treatment during the first trimester of pregnancy has also been shown to decrease the risk of first trimester spontaneous pregnancy loss.

## DEVELOPMENTAL AND PSYCHOSOCIAL ISSUES

The diagnosis of any chronic illness may pose a psychological challenge, especially during the adolescent years. Symptoms such as acne, hirsutism, and weight gain can be very distressing at any age. Although a teen may be relieved to learn that there is a reason for these symptoms, she may worry about body image and appearance, the chronic nature of the disorder, and future infertility, diabetes, or hypertension. Parents may have their own concerns about future health consequences.

Limited studies have been performed addressing these issues. Dissatisfaction with body image, struggles with interpersonal trust (especially with health care providers), and increased depression have been observed among adolescents with PCOS.

The clinician should be mindful of these issues when educating the patient and her family about PCOS. It is important that the physiologic role of androgens in both men and women be explained. Often, adolescents will assume that androgens, especially testosterone, are "male hormones" not normally found in females. Most adolescents have heard the word "testosterone," sometimes offered as an explanation for the behavior of teenage boys. This assumption can lead adolescents to fearful conclusions about their future appearance, gender identity, and gender role.

Issues related to infertility and subfertility may be very troublesome for some adolescents and their families. Again, it is important to be sensitive to these issues and provide education that infertility is not a given consequence of PCOS, that therapies to induce ovulation are successful and likely to improve in the future, and that they should practice contraception if sexually active. Occasionally, the adolescent worried about infertility will assume that she cannot conceive and will not practice effective contraception. Adolescents with infertility fears have been known to intentionally try to become pregnant.

In summary, it is important that all clinicians caring for adolescent girls be very familiar with the varied presentations of PCOS. This common endocrine disorder, which usually first presents in adolescence, offers an opportunity for early intervention and significant reduction of many types of adult morbidity. This particular area is ripe for future research. Management of PCOS in the adolescent requires a thorough understanding of the normal endocrinology of adolescence and the disordered state of PCOS. Careful management requires broad knowledge of the "big picture" of PCOS effects, including cardiovascular, nutritional, reproductive, dermatological, and insulin-glucose metabolism disorders. This multidisciplinary approach with a strong emphasis on the uniqueness of the adolescent will best serve the needs of this special and important patient population.

## REFERENCES


1. Emans SJ, Grace E, Goldstein DP. Oligomenorrhea in adolescent girls. *J Pediatr.* 1980;(5):815–819

2. Stein IF, Leventhal MI. Amenorrhea associated with bilateral polycystic ovaries. *Am J Obstetr Gynecol.* 1935;29:181–191

3. Carmina E. The spectrum of androgen excess disorders. *Fertil Steril.* 2006;85(6):1582–1585

4. Ehrmann DA. Polycystic ovary syndrome. *New Eng J Med.* 2005;352:1123–1136

5. Behera M, Price T, Walner D. Estrogenic ovulatory dysfunction or functional female hyperandrogenism: an argument to discard the term polycystic ovary syndrome. *Fertil Steril.* 2006;86:1292–1295

6. Venturoli S, Porcu E, Fabbri R, et al. Longitudinal change of sonographic ovarian aspects and endocrine parameters in irregular cycles of adolescence. *Pediatr Res.* 1995;38:974–980

7. Kent SC, Legro RS. Polycystic ovary syndrome in adolescents. *Adolesc Med.* 2002;13(1):73–88

8. Rosenfeld RL, Shai K, Ehrmann DA, Barnes RB. Diagnosis of polycystic ovary syndrome in adolescence: comparison of adolescent and adult hyperandrogenism. *J Pediatr Endocrinol Metab.* 2000;13(suppl 5):1285–1289

9. Legro RS. A 27-year-old women with a diagnosis of polycystic ovary syndrome. *JAMA.* 2007;297:509–519

10. Ibanez L, de Zegher F, Potau N. Premature pubarche, ovarian hyperandrogenism, hyperinsulinism, and the polycystic ovary syndrome: from a complex constellation to a simple sequence of prenatal onset. *J Endocrinol Invest.* 1998;21:558–566

11. Porcu E, Venturoli S, Longhi M, et al. Chronobiologic evolution of luteinizing hormone secretion in adolescence: developmental patterns and speculation on the onset of polycystic ovary syndrome. *Fertil Steril.* 1997;67:842–848

12. Vihko R, Apter D. The role of androgens in adolescent cycles. *J Steroid Biochem.* 1980;12:369–373

13. Guzick DS. Polycystic ovary syndrome. *Obstet Gynecol.* 2004;103:181-193

14. Bili H, Laven J, Imani B, Eijkemans MJ, Fauser BC. Age-related differences in features associated with polycystic ovary syndrome in normogonadotropic oligo-amenorrhoeic infertile women of productive years. *Eur J Endocrinol.* 2001;145(6):749-755

15. Udoff LC, Adashi EY. Polycystic ovarian disease: current insights into an old problem. *J Pediatr Adolesc Gynecol.* 1966;9:3-8

16. Van Hooff MHA, Voorhorst FJ, Kaptein MB, Hirasing RA, Koppenaal C, Schoemaker J. Polycystic ovaries in adolescents and the relationship between menstrual cycle patterns, luteinizing hormones, androgen, and insulin. *Fertil Steril.* 2000;74:49-58

17. Azziz R. The evaluation and management of hirsutism. *Obstet Gynecol.* 2003;101:995-1007

18. Rosenfeld RL, Lucky AW. Acne, hirsutism, and alopecia in adolescent girls. *Endo Met Clinics NA.* 1993;22(3):507-532

19. Yildiz B. Diagnosis of hyperandrogenism: clinical criteria. *Best Pract Res Clin Endocrinol Metab.* 2006; 20(2):167-176

20. Luef G. Polycystic ovaries, obesity and insulin resistance in women with epilepsy. *Neurol.* 2002;249(7):835-841

21. Wendelin D. Hypertrichosis. *J Am Acad Dermatol.* 2003;48(2):161-179

22. Sanders EB, Aston CE, Ferrell RE, Witchel SF. Inter- and intrafamilial variability in premature pubarche and polycystic ovary syndrome. *Fertil Steril.* 2002;78:473-478

23. Milewicz A. Prolactin levels in the polycystic ovary syndrome. *J Reprod Med.* 1984;29:193-196

24. Taylor B, Martin KA, Anderson EG. Determinates of abnormal gonadotropin secretion in clinically defined women with polycystic ovary syndrome. *J Clin Endocrinol Metab.* 1997;82:2248-2256

25. Practice Committee of the American Society for Reproductive Medicine. The evaluation and treatment of androgen excess. *Fertil Steril.* 2004;82:s173-s180

26. Meldrum DR, Abraham GE. Peripheral and ovarian venous concentration of various steroid hormones in virilizing ovarian tumors. *Obstet Gynecol.* 1979;53:36-43

27. Lobo RA. What are the key features of importance in polycystic ovary syndrome. *Fertil Steril.* 2003;80:259-261

28. Azziz R. Androgen excess is the key element in polycystic ovary syndrome. *Fertil Steril.* 2003;80:252-254

29. Anttila L, Koskinen P, Kaihola HL, Erkkola R, Irjala K, Ruutiainen K. Serum androgen and gonadotropin levels decline after progestogen-induced withdrawal bleeding in oligomenorrheic women with or without polycystic ovaries. *Fertil Steril.* 1992;58:697-702

30. Azziz R, Hincapie LA, Knochenhauer ES, Dewailly D, Fox F, Boots LR. Screening for 21-hydroxylast-deficient nonclassic adrenal hyperplasia along hyperandrogenic women: a prospective study. *Fertil Steril.* 1999;72:915-925

31. The Rotterdam ESHREI/ASRM-Sponsored PCOS Consensus Workshop Group. Revised 2003 consensus on diagnostic criteria and long-term health risks related to polycystic ovary syndrome. *Fertil Steril.* 2004;81:19-25

32. Fernandes AR, de Sá Rosa e Silva AC, Romão GS, Pata MC, dos Reis RM. Insulin resistance in adolescents with menstrual irregularities. *J Pediatr Adolesc Gynecol.* 2005;18:269-274

33. Legro RS. Detection of insulin resistance and its treatment in adolescents with polycystic ovary syndrome. *J Pediatr Endocrinol Metab.* 2002;15:1367-1378

34. Schwimmer JB; Khorram O; Chiu V; Schwimmer WB. Abnormal aminotransferase activity in women with polycystic ovary syndrome. *Fertil Steril.* 2005;83:494-497

35. Strauss RS, Barlow SE, Deitz WH. Prevalence of abnormal serum aminotransferase values in overweight and obese adolescents. *J Pediatr.* 2000;136:727-733

36. Lefebvre P, Bringer J, Renard E, Boulet F, Clouet S, Jaffiol C. Influences of weight, body fat patterning and nutrition on the management of PCOS. *Hum Reprod.* 1997(12 suppl 1):72-81

37. Bruner B, Chad K, Chizen D. Effects of exercise and nutritional counseling in women with polycystic ovary syndrome. *Appl Physio Nutr Metab.* 2006;31(4):384-391

38. Trent M, Austin SB, Gordon CM. Overweight status of adolescent girls with polycystic ovary syndrome; body mass index as mediator of quality of life. *Ambul Pediatr.* 2005;5(2):107-111

39. Hoeger KM. Role of lifestyle modification in the management of polycystic ovary syndrome. *Best Pract Res Clin Endocrinol Metab.* 2006;20(2):293-310

40. Lewy VD, Danadian K, Witchel SF, Arslanian S. Early metabolic abnormalities in adolescent girls with polycystic ovarian syndrome. *J Pediatr.* 2001;138:38-44

41. Cumming DC, Yang JC, Rebar RW, Yen SS. Treatment of hirsutism with spironolactone. *JAMA.* 1982;247:1295-1298

42. Kolodziejczyk B, Duleba AJ, Spaczynski RZ, Pawelczyk L. Metformin therapy decreases hyperandrogenism and hyperinsulinemia in women with polycystic ovary syndrome. *Fertil Steril.* 2000;73:1149-1154

43. Ibanez L. Sensitization of insulin induces ovulation in nonobese adolescents with anovulatory hyperandrogenism. *J Clin Endocrinol Metab.* 2001;86:3595-3598

44. Gleuck CJ, Wang P, Fontaine R, Tracy T, Sieve-Smith L. Metformin to restore normal menses in oligo-amenorrheic teenage girls with polycystic ovary syndrome (PCOS). *J Adolesc Health.* 2001;29(3):160-169

45. Kay JP. Beneficial effects of metformin in normoglycemic morbidly obese adolescents. *Metabolism.* 2001;50:1457-1461

# CHAPTER 66

# Breast Disorders in the Female

YASMIN JAYASINGHE, MBBS • PATRICIA S. SIMMONS, MD

## INTRODUCTION

Adolescence is a common time for the presentation of congenital and acquired abnormalities of the breast. The relationship of breast development to adolescent self-image, the personal nature of her breasts, or anxiety may hinder an adolescent from disclosure when she has a concern about her breasts. Therefore, it is important to examine and recognize conditions of the adolescent breast and know their differential diagnosis and appropriate treatment. This chapter addresses normal development, congenital anomalies, masses, and other acquired conditions of the adolescent female breast.

## NORMAL BREAST DEVELOPMENT AND ANATOMY

The human breast is composed of a ductal and glandular system within stromal and fatty tissue. Its 15 to 20 lobules each contain many alveoli, the glandular unit of the breast. The alveoli are lined by a single layer of milk-secreting epithelial cells. The alveolar lumen drain into 10 to 100 terminal or subsegmental ducts, which drain into 20 to 40 segmental ducts, and finally into 5 to 10 primary milk ducts that are arranged radially around the nipple[1] (Figure 66-1). The ductal and glandular systems of the human breast develop in distinct phases of fetal development, early infancy, puberty, and pregnancy. Breast development begins during the 10th week of gestation, by budding of the ectoderm into the underlying mesenchyme from the primitive axilla to the primitive inguinal region to form the mammary ridge. The portion of the mammary ridge over the fourth intercostal space develops further, whereas the rest atrophies. There is a phase of breast development in early infancy, under the influence of the infant's own endocrine activity,[2] which may persist for months to years after which the breast bud remains barely palpable with a rudimentary ductal system until puberty. Under the influence of estrogen during puberty, terminal duct elongation occurs, subcutaneous adipose tissue develops, and stromal growth occurs. Progesterone promotes lobular–alveolar development, which mainly occurs after menarche. Full alveolar development normally occurs only during pregnancy. Growth hormone, glucocorticoids, insulin, thyroxine, and prolactin influence the development of breast stroma, and local growth factors also contribute to breast growth and development.

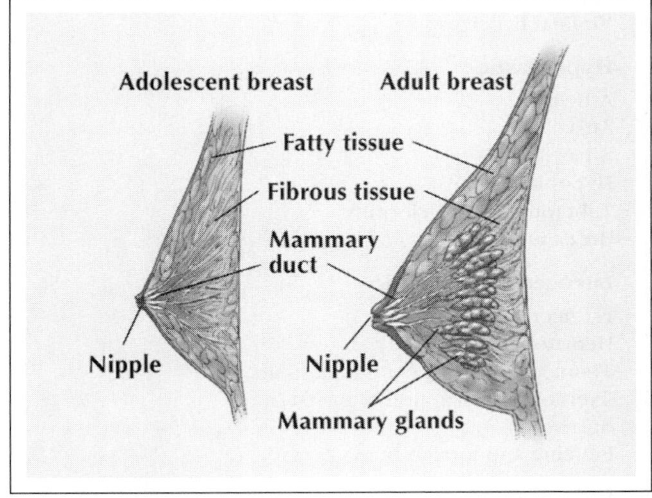


FIGURE 66-1 Anatomy of the female breast in the adolescent and adult. (By permission of Mayo Foundation for Medical Education and Research. All rights reserved.)

Normal breast development has been divided into 5 clinical stages, the Tanner stages or sexual maturity ratings (SMR).[3] Thelarche is the onset of breast development and normally occurs in girls 8 to 14 years of age. It is usually the first sign of puberty, with other secondary sexual characteristics appearing within 6 months,[4] but it may be preceded by pubic hair development. One breast bud may appear weeks or months before the other, and should not be mistaken for a breast mass, as biopsy may damage the breast bud and cause permanent breast asymmetry.

## CLASSIFICATION OF BREAST DISORDERS

Breast disorders of adolescence may be classified as developmental, traumatic, inflammatory (Box 66-1), or neoplastic (Box 66-2). Neoplastic disorders are commonly fibroepithelial and benign (Table 66-1).

**Box 66-1**

***Developmental, Traumatic, and Inflammatory Disorders of the Breast in Adolescence***[5-19]

**Hyperplastic**
Polythelia
Polymastia
Virginal hypertrophy

**Hypoplastic**
Athelia
Amazia
Amastia
Hypoplasia
Tuberous breast deformity
Breast atrophy

**Iatrogenic/Traumatic**
Fat necrosis
Hematoma
Thoracostomy or penetrating injury
Excision or disruption of breast bud
Burns
Piercing and foreign body

**Inflammatory**
Mastitis

**Miscellaneous**
Mastalgia

**Box 66-2**

***Classification of Hyperplastic and Neoplastic Disorders***

**Epithelial neoplasm**
Benign
- Juvenile papillomatosis
- Intraductal papilloma
- Papillomatosis
- Sclerosing papillomatosis
- Adenoma-tubular, nipple
- Subareolar papillomatosis

In situ carcinoma
- Lobular carcinoma in situ
- Ductal carcinoma in situ

Invasive carcinoma (stromal invasion)
- Lobular
- Ductal
- Tubular
- Mucinous
- Medullary
- Secretory/juvenile
- Papillary
- Adenoid cystic
- Metaplastic

**Mixed connective tissue and epithelial**
Benign
- Fibroadenoma
- Benign phyllodes tumor

Intermediate
- Phyllodes tumor, intermediate

Malignant
- Malignant phyllodes tumor
- Sarcoma-connective tissue

**Other**
- Soft tissue
- Skin tumors
- Lymphoid

**Metastatic**

## DEVELOPMENTAL BREAST DISORDERS

Developmental breast disorders commonly present during adolescence. They may be associated with significant embarrassment and poor self-esteem at a time when body image issues are important. It is important that providers involved with adolescent health care understand these issues and options for management.

### Hyperplastic Developmental Disorders

Hyperplastic breast disorders may be due to supernumerary nipples (polythelia) or breasts (polymastia) or hypertrophic breast tissue. Supportive care, education, and surgical excision are available treatment options.

***Polythelia (Supernumerary Nipples) and Polymastia (Supernumerary Breasts)*** Polythelia or polymastia occurs in 2% to 6% of females.[20] These lesions may appear as small pigmented macules, larger nipple-areola complexes, or accessory breasts with or without a nipple-areola complex anywhere along the mammary line, but are most commonly axillary. They result from incomplete regression of the mammary ridge, are usually sporadic but may be familial, are often bilateral, and may be mistaken for hidradenitis, lymph

**Table 66-1**

**Prevalence of Breast Disorders of Adolescence in Medical and Surgical Series**

| *Disorder* | *% Medical Series (Range)* | *% Surgical Series (Range)* |
|---|---|---|
| Fibroadenoma | 30–57% | 44–94% |
| Gynecomastia | 0–12% | 0–30% |
| Early breast bud | 0–35% | 0% |
| Fibrocystic changes (cysts, sclerosing adenosis, parenchymal fibrosis, duct ectasia) | 1.4–13% | 2–25% |
| Juvenile hypertrophy | | 13–21% |
| Phyllodes | 0–17% | 0–18.5% |
| Mastitis | 0–7% | 1–19% |
| Proliferative disease (intraductal papilloma, papillomatosis, sclerosing papillomatosis) | 0–7% | 0–7.5% |
| Polythelia/polymastia | | 0–12% |
| Soft tissue masses (keloid, neurofibroma, lipoma, hemangioma, lymphangioma, hamartoma) | 0–3% | 0–4% |
| Adenomas | 1.4–3.3% | 0–4% |
| Fat necrosis | | 0.3–3.7% |
| Malignancy | 3.3–5.4% | 0–9.5% |

nodes, or lipoma. Cyclic premenstrual tenderness of the ectopic breast tissue may occur. Though usually isolated, association with cardiovascular, skeletal, gastrointestinal, and urologic anomalies has occurred. Simple polythelia is managed conservatively with education and observation. Polymastia rarely presents before pregnancy. The ectopic tissue may undergo similar pathologic changes to pectoral breast tissue. Malignancy may develop, although the risk of this is low and rarely occurs before the fourth decade of life, therefore routine excision is not always recommended. Indications during adolescence include cosmesis, pain and tenderness, and noncyclic change in size or texture of the tissue. Postpubertal excision may necessitate wider excision due to glandular growth. Long-term follow-up is recommended, particularly in those with a glandular component, and monitoring with self-examination of the accessory breast tissue is advised.

***Juvenile Hypertrophy of the Breast*** Juvenile hypertrophy, also called virginal hypertrophy or gigantomastia, is different from macromastia (large breast size). In juvenile hypertrophy of the breast (JHB), rapid unilateral or bilateral enlargement of the breast(s) occurs during or after puberty and may occur before or after menarche. Juvenile hypertrophy involves the entire breast, and there may be minimal lobular development.[7] The condition is usually sporadic and may be due to end-organ hypersensitivity to normal levels of estrogen. Hormone levels are normal and therefore unhelpful in the diagnosis. Typically these patients otherwise exhibit normal growth and development. Women with a history of JHB are at a greater risk for gravid hypertrophy. The diagnosis of JHB is made clinically. Histopathology is benign, but not diagnostic. The clinical evaluation reveals significant breast enlargement, which may be painful or tender, and may be associated with skin hyperemia, distension of subcutaneous veins, skin necrosis, and even rupture. Patients may also experience neck, back, or shoulder pain, or poor posture. Psychological difficulties, including poor body image, poor self-esteem, and embarrassment are common, and may compromise physical activity, school attendance, and social activities. Supportive care and education are important. There is currently no medical treatment option to reduce size or retard breast growth for affected adolescents. The decision to intervene surgically and timing of any surgery must be individualized based on the clinical presentation, severity, and known substantial risk of recurrence. Complications of surgery may include cellulitis, hematoma, wound dehiscence, nipple necrosis, breast asymmetry, residual excess axillary fat tissue, and hypertrophic scarring. Preoperative weight loss in those with a body mass index (BMI) of more than 35kg/m$^2$ and cessation of smoking may reduce the risks of complications. In 1 series, reduction mammoplasty alleviated psychological distress in 90% of teenagers, and repeat operations over an average of 1.6 years were required in 17%.[21] When adequate subareolar tissue is preserved with pedicle transposition of the nipple–areola complex, breastfeeding rates comparable to the general population may be achieved. Some have recommended subcutaneous mastectomy as the procedure of choice in selected younger adolescent patients with significant gigantomastia, with a few years' delay before breast reconstruction and prosthesis. Although this approach should reduce the need for multiple surgeries, future breastfeeding is not possible.

### Hypoplastic Developmental Disorders

Hypoplastic disorders may be due to absence of development of the nipple (athelia) and/or glandular tissue (amastia, amazia), or underdevelopment of the breast tissue. Breast hypoplasia may be congenital (such as tuberous breasts) or acquired due to damage to the breast bud. Presentation may be that of breast asymmetry if the condition is unilateral.

***Athelia, Amazia, Amastia*** Athelia (absence of the nipple), amazia (absence of glandular tissue), and amastia (absence of the nipple and glandular tissue of the breast) are uncommon, but are most likely to be recognized during adolescence. Three distinct groups of patients have been identified with amastia:[22] bilateral amastia associated with ectodermal defects (involving the teeth, nails, skin, and appendages); unilateral amastia associated with Poland syndrome, which affects 1 in 20,000 to 30,000 births and is associated with other congenital abnormalities (Box 66-3); and bilateral amastia associated with palate and upper extremity abnormalities, which may be sporadic or familial. Treatment may involve a combination of chest wall reconstruction, implant insertion, and nipple reconstruction.[19]

***Breast Asymmetry*** Breast asymmetry is the most common breast condition in adolescent females, with simple difference in the size of 2 normal breasts being quite common. During pubertal development, a rapidly growing breast bud on 1 side may give the appearance of a breast mass and may account for 35% of breast presentations in young females.[16] Asymmetry usually improves once development is complete, but some visible asymmetry may persist in 25%.[23] The adolescent should be educated about variation of breast shape and size among individuals. Though less common, other causes of breast asymmetry occur and merit consideration (Box 66-4).

*Breast hypoplasia* is unilateral or bilateral underdevelopment of the breasts, and may be congenital or acquired, such as from injury to the breast bud in childhood or early adolescence. *Hypomastia* or *micromastia* refers to unilateral or bilateral small breasts, which result from a variety of causes, including breast hypoplasia (Box 66-5). Delayed puberty as a cause of hypomastia can be easily identified by absent or arrested development of secondary sexual characteristics and hormonal investigations. It differs from breast hypoplasia, as the breast still has the ability to reach full development under the influence of endogenous or exogenous sex steroids. Young women with breast hypoplasia, on the other hand, have normal ovarian function, and hormone replacement therapy is ineffective. Management of physiologic breast asymmetry may simply require augmenting the appearance of the smaller side with differential padding or a topical breast insert until catch-up growth occurs.[23] In the event of significant asymmetry, hypoplasia, or aplasia, surgery may be undertaken during puberty to avoid psychological consequences by enlarging the smaller breast over time to parallel growth of normal breast.

**Box 66-3**

***Features of Poland Syndrome***

Unilateral athelia or amastia
Absent pectoralis major/minor
Absent multiple ribs with chest wall depression
Absent axillary hair
Limited chest wall subcutaneous fat
Brachydactyly or syndactyly

**Box 66-4**

***Causes of Breast Asymmetry***

- Physiological
- Unilateral aplasia: Poland's syndrome, amastia, and athelia
- Unilateral hypoplasia: congenital (tuberous breasts) or acquired damage to the breast bud from previous surgery (thoracostomy), burns, penetrating injury, infection, radiation
- Juvenile hypertrophy
- Mastitis
- Breast mass
- Musculoskeletal abnormalities: scoliosis, chest wall condition causing pseudoasymmetry

**Box 66-5**

***Causes of Bilateral Hypomastia***

Constitutional
Delayed puberty
Breast atrophy due to:

- Weight loss
- Endocrinological: premature ovarian failure, gonadal dysgenesis, hypothyroidism, hyperandrogenism, adrenal disease
- Connective tissue disease; scleroderma

Aplasia: amastia, athelia
Hypoplasia: developmental, tuberous breasts, or acquired damage to breast bud

Revisions may be required after completion of growth. Rather than targeting a specific age or Tanner stage for surgical intervention in cases of substantial asymmetry, it is important to individualize based on the degree of asymmetry, prognosis for improvement with potential growth and development, and patient attitude.

***Tuberous Breast Anomaly*** This congenital anomaly results from a constricted breast base diameter, breast tissue herniation into the areola, a deficient skin envelope, and inframammary fold malposition. This does not improve with time. Some patients are tolerant of this anomaly, but for others it is a significant problem in terms of body image and may compromise breastfeeding. Surgical correction involves insertion of an implant and release of breast tissue herniation from the nipple–areola complex.[19]

***Iatrogenic and Traumatic Breast Disorders*** Acute injury to the breast can result in penetrating injury or hematoma and may lead to mastitis, fat necrosis, or contour deformities. Damage to the breast bud can cause hypoplastic deformities.[19] Common causes of iatrogenic injuries include tube thoracotomies, previous breast mass excision, and burns. Management may simply involve release of the fibrous tracts to allow normal breast growth, or z plasties/skin grafts for previous burns, or full reconstruction of the breast mound with implant insertion for hypoplastic deformities. The nipple–areola complex may be reconstructed after breast implant surgery with skin grafts or tattooing.

## INFLAMMATORY BREAST DISORDERS

Inflammatory problems are common in adolescents and may be related to hormonal or metaplastic factors or trauma such as nipple piercing.

### Mastitis

Mastitis accounts for up to 7% of clinical breast presentations during childhood and adolescence,[16] and mean age of presentation is around 13 years.[24] Most cases are readily diagnosed and medically treated, although presence of an abscess may necessitate surgery. In the absence of trauma and lactation, the cause of breast infection may not be apparent, but there are known risk factors (Box 66-6).

Patients present with an erythematous, warm, tender indurated area usually present for days, most often in the subareolar region. Obvious suppuration, fluctuance, or poor response to appropriate antibiotic therapy suggests abscess. Although most cases of breast infection present as mastitis without abscess formation, 1 adolescent series reported abscess formation in 38%.[25] Nipple discharge may be present. Systemic symptoms may be mild, and associated meningitis or bacteremia is rare. Breast ultrasound is indicated if abscess is suspected or if the infection does not respond to therapy. Eighty-nine percent of infections in one adolescent series were associated with breast cysts.[24] The responsible pathogen is *Staphylococcus aureus* in more than 75% of cases, with gram-negative bacilli, group A streptococcus, and enterococcus also reported. Anaerobes are more common in recurring nonpuerperal subareolar abscesses. If the patient has mastitis without systemic symptoms, she may be treated as an outpatient with oral antibiotics. An antistaphylococcus drug, such as cephalexin or amoxicillin–clavulanic acid, is appropriate first line therapy. One must always consider methicillin-resistant staphylococcus and tailor antibiotic therapy. Clindamycin may be used if there is a history of penicillin allergy or if methicillin resistance is suspected. Metronidazole may be added if anaerobic cover is indicated. The patient should be admitted for parenteral antibiotics if she has systemic symptoms or

**Box 66-6**

***Risk Factors for Adolescent Mastitis***

**Hormonal**

- Lactation causing breast engorgement with invasion of bacteria through cracked nipples

**Metaplasia of the ductal epithelium**

- Lactiferous ducts become obstructed by keratin plugs and cellular debris, causing stasis and rupture of the ducts leading to bacterial invasion of the surrounding tissue, causing subareolar infection. Risk factors for ductal metaplasia:
  - Comedomastitis
  - Congenital abnormalities of the lactiferous ducts
  - Nipple retraction
  - Vitamin A deficiency
  - Smoking (via a direct toxic effect on the ductal epithelium or promotion of secretions)
    - Ductal ectasia
    - Breast cysts
    - Breast mass
    - Trauma and hematoma
    - Repeated nipple stimulation
    - Plucking or shaving of periareolar hair
    - Nipple piercing
    - Breast implants
    - Radiotherapy
    - Hyperprolactinemia: may cause duct ectasia or increase secondary to infection

fails initial oral therapy. Incision and drainage is necessary if there is evidence of an abscess or periareolar pus. Inadequately treated infection may damage the breast bud and cause future breast hypoplasia. Success rates of more than 80% have been reported with treatment of breast abscesses with repeated needle aspiration under ultrasound guidance.[26] In adolescents, recovery from mastitis is usually complete and may take 7 to 10 days up to a few weeks. Those with bilateral breast cysts are significantly more likely to have recurrent episodes and may need longer duration of therapy. A follow-up ultrasound is recommended at 3 months to exclude underlying breast pathology not detected during the acute infection. Inflammatory breast cancer, which may mimic features of mastitis, is not a known risk in adolescents.

### Nipple Piercing

Body piercing is increasing in popularity, and prevalence of nipple piercing in adolescents and college students of up to 6% has been reported.[27] Piercings for some adolescents are a reflection of self-expression, fashion, and peer-group pressure, although in some adolescents they may serve as a marker for high-risk behaviors. There is little awareness among teens about the complications of piercing. The risk may be significant, but as yet there are no quantitative observations, only case reports (Box 66-7).[28] Until there is more data on long-term outcome, the procedure should not be encouraged, particularly in high-risk groups, and young women should be informed of possible effects on current and future health. Physicians should provide advice to the adolescent about decision making and how to proceed safely (such as awareness of infection control procedures). Subacute bacterial endocarditis prophylaxis should be provided for those at risk of endocarditis who insist on having piercing despite medical advice. Delay may occur in accessing care for complications. In the event of infection, antibiotic therapy along with foreign body removal are indicated, and if the patient has systemic symptoms or does not respond to therapy, testing for mycobacterium and diabetes as well as bacterial pathogens may be appropriate.[28]

Although nipple piercing is not recommended for anyone given the potential for negative consequences, there are certain underlying conditions that further increase the risk of complications. Patients with any of these should be further discouraged from piercing (Box 66-8).

### Mastalgia

Mastalgia (breast pain) is a common symptom and may be cyclic or noncyclic. A variety of supportive measures and empiric therapies may be used with varying success.

***Cyclic Mastalgia*** Eleven percent of the female population have moderate to severe mastalgia[29] that may disrupt physical, social, and school activity. Symptoms commonly commence up to 2 weeks prior to menstruation and are relieved with menses. Women with mastalgia are more at risk of fibrocystic disease. The etiology of cyclic mastalgia is uncertain but may represent endorphin or serotonin deficiency resulting in exaggerated response to

#### Box 66-7

#### *Complications of Nipple Piercing*

- Delayed healing up to 12 months
- Pain
- Swelling
- Allergy
- Mastitis/infection rate of up to 20%
- Granulomatous mastitis
- Keloid
- Nipple hypertrophy requiring cosmetic reduction
- Altered nipple sensation (decreased/increased)
- Metal foreign body in breast tissue
- Bacterial endocarditis, heart valve operation in those at risk
- Breast implant infection
- Psychological stress due to incorrect diagnosis of breast cancer
- Hepatitis B, C, tetanus, HIV infection
- Neurogenic hyperprolactinemia
- Theoretical problems with breast-feeding; a plastic retainer may be inserted into the piercing between feeds to maintain patency

#### Box 66-8

#### *Factors Increasing Risks from Nipple Piercing*

- Acute intoxication
- Allergy
- Coagulation disorders
- Diabetes
- Corticosteroid therapy
- Skin disease or infection
- Chronic or acute infection
- Chemotherapy
- Immunosuppression
- Past history of systemic infections or rheumatic fever
- Heart valve defects
- Breast implants

normal ovarian hormones. The condition may self-remit after months or years. Onset before the age of 20 may result in a prolonged course. Anecdotal improvement in symptoms has been reported with empiric measures, such as wearing a well-fitting brassiere, reducing caffeine, fat, and dairy intake, simple analgesics, and evening primrose oil 1 mg to 3 mg daily, although primrose has not been demonstrated to show any benefit over placebo.[30] The most effective management techniques modulate ovarian steroid function. The use of continuous, that is noncyclic, oral contraceptive pill (OCP) or depomedroxyprogesterone acetate has not been systematically studied, although anecdotally they have sometimes been of benefit. Gonadotropin-releasing hormone (GnRH) agonists are effective, but long-term use in adolescents may result in hypoestrogenism-induced osteopenia and osteoporosis as well as menopausal symptoms. Danocrine in doses of 200 to 400 mg daily is also effective, but hyperandrogenic side effects include voice changes, hirsutism, skin changes, and weight gain, so it is generally not recommended for adolescents. Luteal-phase danocrine (200 mg from day 14 to 28 of the cycle) has been demonstrated to significantly reduce premenstrual mastalgia in women older than 18 years.[31] Other treatments include neuroendocrine modulation with fluoxetine and tamoxifen. But safety and efficacy in younger women have not been established for any of these.

***Noncyclic Mastalgia*** Noncyclic mastalgia may be due to a ruptured cyst or ectatic duct, infection, tender focal nodularity, fat necrosis from trauma, stretching of the Cooper ligament, or an ill-fitting brassiere. Chest wall pain should also be excluded. Focal tenderness and localizing signs will often be elicited.

## NONNEOPLASTIC AND NEOPLASTIC BREAST DISORDERS OF ADOLESCENTS

Breast masses are common in adolescents. In 1 clinical study, 3.2% of adolescent females presenting for any reason were found on physical examination to have a breast mass.[32] Although the spectrum of etiologies that exist in adults may present during adolescence, the relative likelihood of a specific type of mass is different for the young. Masses may derive from breast parenchyma or a mass may represent nonbreast tissue that simply occurs in or near the breast. Malignancy, primary or metastatic, is rare. Therefore, the approach to evaluating a breast mass in adolescents differs from that in adults.

### Fibrocystic Changes

Fibrocystic changes are a common clinical diagnosis in young women, and that terminology is preferable to fibrocystic "disease." Fibrocystic changes confer no increased risk of breast cancer. Patients often present with diffuse symmetrical coarseness and nodularity in both breasts, for months or years, associated with cyclic mastalgia. Cystic changes (Figure 66-2) will often resolve over 1 to 2 menstrual cycles, and patients should be reassured and observed. The OCP may be used to treat cyclic mastalgia. Persistent cysts may be aspirated to relieve symptoms, and fluid may be sent for cytology if malignancy is suspected, although sensitivity of fine needle aspiration (FNA) for detection of possible malignancy due to other types of breast disease is low in adolescents. Fibrocystic changes can be focal, but when this occurs the differential diagnosis is broadened and further evaluation may be warranted to differentiate from other causes of breast mass.

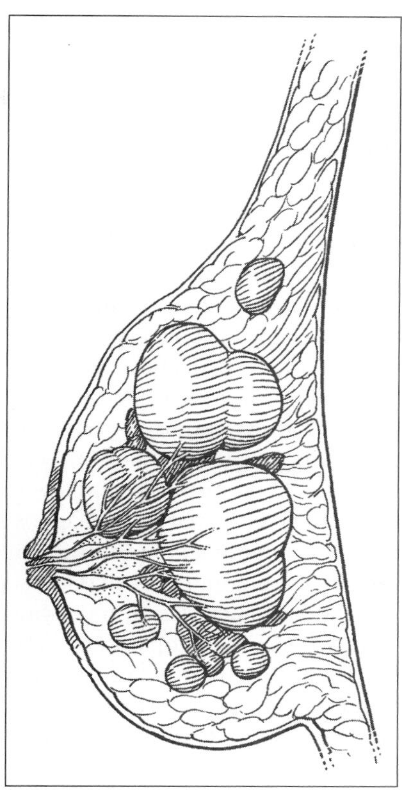

**FIGURE 66-2** Fibrocystic change. (By permission of Mayo Foundation for Medical Education and Research. All rights reserved.)

### Fibroepithelial Masses

Fibroepithelial masses encompass fibroadenomas, the most common breast mass found in adolescents, and the more rare phyllodes tumor, which may be benign, borderline, or malignant.

***Fibroadenoma*** Fibroadenomas are discrete benign tumors with connective tissue and epithelial proliferation. They are the most surgically treated or biopsied mass in adolescents.[6]

Fibroadenomas usually present after menarche, and the frequency of diagnosis increases during adolescence, with the median age of presentation 1 being around 15 years (range 11 to 16).[8] They are more common young black females than in comparably aged whites.[7] Fibroadenomas often present as a self-detected mass that may have been present for months or years. Examination reveals a rubbery smooth, mobile, well-circumscribed mass, usually in the upper outer quadrant. Although concerning signs such as immobility, nipple, and skin changes have sometimes been observed, they evoke concern for other etiologies and the need for further evaluation. Bilaterality occurs in 10% to 15% of cases. Malignant change of the epithelial component to lobular carcinoma is extremely rare, and is rarely seen in women younger than 30 years. Typing of fibroadenoma is based on histology and size (Box 66-9).[7]

Ultrasound scan is sensitive for the diagnosis of fibroadenoma, which may sometimes be indistinguishable from less common fibrous or epithelial masses, such as phyllodes tumor, mammary hamartoma, and tubular adenoma. The distinction is made on histopathological examination. A fibroadenoma smaller than 5 cm without worrisome features may reasonably be observed over 1 to 2 months for growth or regression. Regression in size allows conservative management, with clinical and as needed ultrasound follow-up. A 3- to 4-month interval is reasonable initially, with further follow-up dictated by course. The triple test (palpation, ultrasound, and core needle biopsy) is considered the gold standard for the diagnosis of breast masses in young adult women younger than 30 years. However, in adolescents a negative core biopsy may not obviate the need for surgical excisional biopsy. Large and rapidly growing masses raise concern and merit tissue diagnosis because fibroadenoma cannot be distinguished from phyllodes or other tumors clinically or by imaging. Because of the potential for tumor heterogeneity, in these instances excision is recommended over core or fine needle biopsy. Large tumors, even if benign, may distort breast architecture; therefore the patient may benefit from surgical excision. Although core needle biopsy has played an important role in evaluation of the adult woman with a breast mass, its role in the evaluation of an adolescent is not established. The primary indication for a needle biopsy in an adolescent is to establish that a mass is a manifestation of malignancy and therefore influences the patient's treatment. Although there is not a clear standard of care for surgical excision of a breast mass in the adolescent, this list is meant to provide a practical approach in deciding when surgery is indicated (Box 66-10).

### Box 66-9

#### *Variants of Fibroadenoma*

**Conventional/typical/simple fibroadenoma**

**Giant fibroadenoma:** any fibroadenoma more than 500 g or >5-10 cm, or replacing at least four-fifths of the breast. Cellular fibroadenomas are more likely to become giant fibroadenomas than simple types.

**Juvenile fibroadenoma:** rapidly growing fibroadenoma of adolescence, term is sometimes used.

**Cellular fibroadenoma:** fibroadenoma dominated by spindle cell proliferation and dense cellular appearance and/or myxoid stroma. Account for 10% of fibroadenomas in adolescence.

**Complex fibroadenoma:** have foci of sclerosing adenosis, cysts, papillary apocrine metaplasia, epithelial calcification. Not often seen in adolescence. Not premalignant, but women with complex fibroadenomas are more at risk of developing breast cancer than those with simple types.

***Phyllodes Tumor*** Phyllodes tumors are closely related to fibroadenoma but display more hypertrophy and stromal cellularity. Previously these were often called "cystosarcoma phyllodes," but that name has been replaced because of the inappropriate association with malignant sarcomas. Phyllodes tumors are uncommon in adolescence. Eight percent of these tumors occur in those younger than 20 years of age (mainly 16–19 years), and 85% in young women are benign.[33] The degree of cellularity and nuclear atypia of the stromal component determines whether it is pathologically benign, borderline, or malignant. Clinical course does not always correlate with pathologic features. Tendency to local recurrence may be largely related to incomplete excision, as microscopically the tumor lacks encapsulation and is infiltrative. Ten

### Box 66-10

#### *Indications for Surgical Excision of a Suspected Fibroadenoma*

- Rapidly growing mass
- Fibroadenoma or any mass more than 5 cm in diameter
- Mass causing distortion of breast architecture or with overlying skin changes
- Persistent mass without apparent regression
- Multiple and bilateral breast masses
- Stromal hypercellularity, cystic change on ultrasound
- Symptoms and signs worrisome for malignancy
- Presence of high-risk genetic mutation: BRCA, P53, PTEN
- Histologically complex fibroadenoma

percent of phyllodes tumors are associated with fibroadenoma, and it has been proposed that phyllodes tumors may represent fibroadenomas and may represent different ends of a disease spectrum.[34] Clinically the tumors are firm, well circumscribed, and mobile, and may be large. The overlying skin may be stretched, shiny, or ulcerated. Tumor spread is hematogenous rather than via lymphatics. Features distinguishing them from fibroadenoma are their large size, history of rapid growth, stromal cellularity, and occasionally fluid-filled spaces on ultrasound. Definitive diagnosis depends on histologic assessment. Wide local excision (with a 1-2 cm rim of surrounding tissue) is the treatment of choice for benign or malignant lesions in adolescence. Local recurrence is infrequent in adolescents with benign tumors (2%–3%), but may occur in up to 30% of malignant lesions, and usually occurs within the first 2 years. Histopathologic findings do not correlate well with clinical course, so close follow-up of all patients with phyllodes is recommended. Mastectomy is sometimes considered for biologically virulent tumors with multiple recurrence or chest wall invasion. Prognosis is good, with 5-year survival approaching 100% in adolescents, although fatalities have been reported. Phyllodes tumor may be associated with Li-Fraumeni syndrome, which manifests as multiple tumors and/or a positive family history.

### Benign Epithelial Breast Tumors in Adolescence

Epithelial breast tumors are rare in adolescence. *Tubular adenomas* are benign lesions indistinguishable from fibroadenoma clinically. Diagnosis is made histopathologically.[7] *Juvenile papillomatosis* is a distinctive clinicopathologic entity in women younger than 30 years, and 50% of cases are diagnosed by 20 years. Patients present with a discrete mass, similar to fibroadenoma. There may be a family history of breast carcinoma. Malignant potential is uncertain, although there is an association with lobular carcinoma.[7] *Papillary duct hyperplasia* (or *proliferative disease*) collectively describes *intraductal papilloma, papillomatosis*, and *sclerosing papillomatosis*, which commonly present in the fourth decade and beyond and are rare in adolescence. These conditions are considered premalignant, especially if there is a family history of breast carcinoma. Patients may present with a bloody nipple discharge. Treatment of choice is surgical excisional biopsy.[7] *Atypical ductal hyperplasia* can be seen in cellular fibroadenomas and in juvenile papillomatosis. It is unclear if it is a risk for carcinoma, as it is in adults, but caution is warranted.[7] *Breast carcinoma* in adolescents is rare.

### Malignant Breast Disease in Adolescents

Malignant breast masses are rare during adolescence, and when they do occur they are more likely to be due to metastasis or stromal malignancies rather than breast carcinoma. In a series of adolescents with surgically removed breast disease, breast malignancies were found in 1.0% to 9.5%, however only 0.02% of breast masses were due to breast carcinoma.[6–18,35]

#### Breast Carcinoma

Breast cancer in women younger than 20 years of age accounts for less than 0.2% of all breast cancers.[36] The age-specific incidence rate of breast cancer in females between 15 to 19 years is fewer than 0.5 per 100,000.[37] *Secretory carcinoma* in adolescents may present as a mobile well-circumscribed mass in the subareolar region, simulating a fibroadenoma. Prognosis is more favorable than other forms of ductal carcinoma, and breast conservation in adolescents is often the goal. *Invasive ductal carcinoma* is less common, and carcinomas in young women younger than 35 have more aggressive biological behavior and worse prognosis than breast cancer in older premenopausal women, and require more aggressive systemic therapy.[38]

***Risk Factors*** There is a growing body of evidence that risk factors present in early life influence breast cancer risk.[39] The period between puberty and first full-term pregnancy appears to be a critical time, where oncogenic risk is accumulating in the presence of vulnerable undifferentiated glandular epithelium. Risk factors include physiological hormonal factors (early menarche, late menopause, late first full-term pregnancy), perinatal factors (increased birth weight, birth length, prematurity), increased linear growth and reduced body fat in adolescence, ionizing chest radiation before the age of 10 years, and early-onset cigarette smoking. A family history of breast cancer in first-degree relatives, particularly if disease is bilateral or diagnosed before the age of 50 years, increases risk. The BRCA 1 and 2 germline mutations[40] have autosomal dominant inheritance and confer a lifetime breast cancer risk of 85%. Though the risk increases with age, the risk of premenopausal cancer also increases. Proliferative breast disease is known to be premalignant in women older than 18 years.[41] Though oncogenic risk for adolescents is not established, it is best to treat with caution. Some studies have demonstrated that OCP use in women younger than 20 years of age conferred a modest increase in the risk of premenopausal breast cancer,[42] with some risk reduction with use of lower-dose preparations containing <35 ug of ethinyl estradiol. However, over recent years, pill preparations with third-generation progestogins and lower doses of estrogen have been introduced, and breast cancer risk has not been evaluated in these preparations. Therefore, current recommendations for the use of OCPs in healthy young adolescents has not changed. A well-informed patient and a risk–benefit assessment should be part of routine care.

***Clinical Presentation of Breast Carcinoma*** Breast carcinomas in the young are associated with delayed diagnosis due to low index of suspicion by the provider resulting in delayed breast biopsy and presentation.[38,43] Clinical examination is insensitive for detection of breast carcinoma in adolescents due to normal nodularity of breast tissue and misdiagnosis of well-circumscribed carcinomas with fibroadenoma. Sensitivity of mammograms is also poor due to dense breast tissue. The triple test mentioned previously in this chapter for adult women younger than 30 has a diagnostic sensitivity of 95% for breast carcinoma.[44] Often, histologic assessment with direct surgical excisional biopsy with omission of percutaneous biopsy is performed in adolescents with a persistent solid mass due to reasons outlined previously.

### Metastatic Disease

A breast mass may be a clue to an occult primary malignancy elsewhere or the first sign of a metastasis or tumor relapse.[6,43] This is most likely to occur within the first 2 years of diagnosis of the primary. Rhabdomyosarcoma, non-Hodgkins lymphoma, and leukemia are the most common breast metastases in adolescence, but others have been reported. Symptoms and signs worrisome for malignancy include constitutional symptoms (weight loss, fever, pain, sweats, malaise, anorexia) lymphadenopathy, hepatosplenomegaly, anemia, and masses elsewhere. Breast metastases may be fixed with overlying skin changes or may be circumscribed and freely mobile. Subcutaneous or multiple masses may be important clues to their metastatic nature. If the clinical suspicion is one of metastatic disease, tissue diagnosis is needed. Fine or core needle biopsy is important, as diagnosis of metastatic disease to the breast may warrant systemic rather than surgical therapy. If the biopsy is indeterminant or negative and malignancy is suspected, further evaluation for malignancy should be pursued because the sensitivity of needle biopsy in breast masses of the young has not been established.

## BREAST HEALTH AND PREVENTIVE CARE

There is little published information available to guide physicians in the provision of appropriate preventive care in adolescents. Breast self-examination (BSE), breast screening, and genetic testing are controversial practices and currently not routinely recommended in healthy young women.

### BREAST SELF-EXAMINATION

Proponents of adolescent BSE suggest that it can promote positive behaviors when other preventive care strategies are introduced. The rationale for this practice can be questioned on the grounds of the low risk of malignancy, lack of evidence of a reduction in cancer risk or improvement in health, the possibility of increasing anxiety, the likelihood of false-positive findings leading to unnecessary intervention, and time taken away from more pressing adolescent health preventive issues. Breast self-examination is not a Bright Futures recommendation. It seems reasonable to recommend BSE to high-risk groups, however, including those at risk of metastatic disease or local recurrence because of a history of malignancy and those who have received previous chest radiotherapy. Older adolescents and young adults with familial risk because of early onset breast cancer in a first-degree relative or who are known to be BRCA 1 or 2 carriers may benefit from early introduction of BSE and regular screening. Although most of breast masses in adolescents are self-detected, most of them are benign.

### BREAST SCREENING

There is no evidence to support routine breast cancer screening in young women. Surveillance for BRCA carriers is not recommended before the age of 18 years. The medical benefits of BRCA 1 and 2 testing in adolescents is not established.[40] Referral to a genetic counselor may be appropriate in selected high-risk patients to more accurately assess the patient's cancer risk as well as the medical and psychological benefits of testing. An increased risk of OCPs has been seen in BRCA 1 but not 2 carriers, so use should be individualized with adequate education to achieve informed consent of potential users.

## EVALUATION OF A BREAST MASS IN AN ADOLESCENT

Evaluation of a breast mass in an adolescent requires a holistic and sensitive approach in accordance with principles of adolescent health care (Figure 66-3). A thorough history and physical examination pertaining to the breast mass is important. The history should include the duration of the mass, any change in size, skin changes or nipple discharge, and any history of trauma. Cyclic pain or tenderness may be indicative of fibrocystic change. A history of rapid growth after puberty may suggest a phyllodes tumor. Bloody nipple discharge may be indicative of proliferative disease. A red tender mass with or without a history of nipple trauma, nipple hair shaving, or plucking may indicate a breast abscess or infected tumor or cyst. Concerning features for malignancy include a history of constitutional symptoms (such as fever, weight loss, sweats, anorexia, and malaise), a history of prior radiation, or previous malignancy. Because young women with primary carcinoma may not have any of these symptoms, even though that diagnosis is rare in the adolescent population, patients with a breast mass should be followed. A family history of breast or ovarian carcinoma and young age of diagnosis, as well as a history of BRCA mutation should increase awareness for an epithelial neoplasm. A family or personal history of mesenchymal tumors or familial P53 mutation will increase the risk of a sarcomatous or fibroepithelial breast tumor. A history of previous breast disease may be significant. A history of OCP use, date of last use, and smoking history should be obtained.

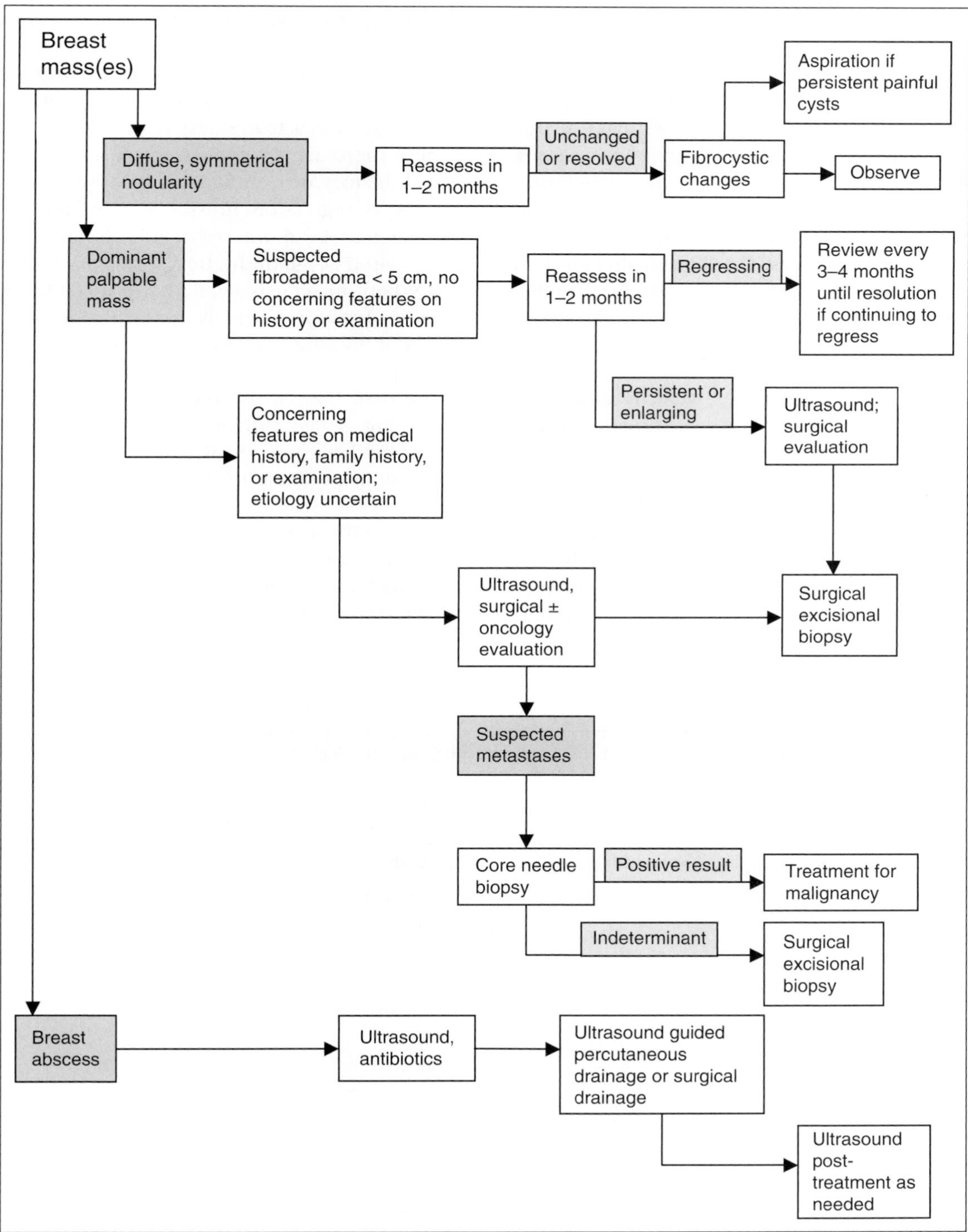


**FIGURE 66-3** Evaluation of a breast mass in an adolescent.

Physical examination should be tailored to make the young woman comfortable and confident and to look for signs of infection or systemic disease (such as fever, weight loss, anemia, systemic lymphadenopathy, hepatosplenomegaly, and masses elsewhere), because a breast mass may be the presenting sign of metastatic disease. Breast examination should begin with visual inspection for Tanner staging, inspection of the nipple–areolar complex for evidence of trauma and normal anatomy, assessment of any breast asymmetry and visible masses, documentation of skin changes such as erythema that may suggest an inflammatory mass, telangiectasia, which may indicate a hemangioma, ecchymoses, stretched shiny skin with necrosis or rupture, which may suggest a giant fibroadenoma or phyllodes, and peau d'orange and dimpling, which may suggest malignancy. The 4 quadrants of each breast should be palpated with the patient sitting up and lying down. Diffuse symmetrical nodularity is common and indicative of fibrocystic change. When a dominant mass is palpated, its location in the breast should be recorded. Most masses occur in the outer upper quadrant. A well-circumscribed, rubbery mobile mass is most likely a fibroadenoma. A warm red subareola mass is most likely a breast abscess. Concerning features for worrisome breast pathology requiring further investigation include hard masses with an irregular edge, skin tethering, and/or axillary lymphadenopathy. A feature of metastatic disease may be the presence of multiple superficial subcutaneous masses. It is important to be aware that malignant disease may not present with these concerning signs, therefore surveillance is required, even for masses clinically thought to be fibroadenoma, if managed conservatively. Pressure should be applied to the breast to assess nipple discharge, and bloody discharge may be indicative of proliferative disease or ductal carcinoma in situ. Chest wall tumors may be excluded in some by rolling the patient at 90 degrees to see if the mass is fixed or independent of the breast.

Monitored surveillance may be performed in selected adherent patients with a smooth mobile mass suggestive of fibroadenoma that is less than 5 cm in diameter and where there are no concerning features on medical or family history or examination. Review in 1 to 2 months to assess regression in size should occur. Regressing masses may be monitored clinically and by ultrasound as required at 3-month intervals.

When imaging is needed, the modality of choice is breast ultrasound, which correctly identifies different types of breast masses (such as developmental, infective, fibroepithelial, intraductal papilloma) in adolescents more than 85% of the time, although its sensitivity for detecting breast carcinoma is low (Table 66-2). Mammograms have poor sensitivity and should not be performed in adolescents because of their dense breast tissue. A breast ultrasound should be performed in any patient with a persistent mass that shows no signs of regression, or a dominant mass associated with any concerning features on history or examination, and in those where breast abscess is suspected. If metastatic disease

**Table 66-2**

**Diagnostic Modalities for Evaluation of Breast Masses in Adolescents**

| *Modality* | *Detection of a Breast Mass* | *Detection of Breast Carcinoma* | *Indication in Adolescents* | *Disadvantages* |
|---|---|---|---|---|
| **Mammography** | Insensitive | Insensitive | No indication | Radiation |
| **Ultrasound scan** | 94% sensitivity | 58% sensitivity | 1. Assessment of breast lesion<br>2. Assistance with percutaneous biopsies | Less sensitive for tumors < 2 cm<br>Difficulty distinguishing phyllodes tumor from fibroadenoma |
| **Fine needle aspiration (FNA) (cytology)** | | Insensitive | 1. Aspiration of persistent breast cysts<br>2. Suspected metastatic breast disease | May cause trauma and tumor infarction<br>Sampling errors<br>Requires expert cytopathologist |
| **Core needle biopsy (histology)** | | Sensitive for detection of malignant disease | 1. Suspected metastatic disease<br>2. Biopsy of mass that may be managed conservatively | Requires multiple samples for histological examination<br>May miss a phyllodes component in a fibroadenoma |

is suspected, core needle biopsy under ultrasound guidance is recommended to avoid the risk of operative therapy in situations where systemic therapy may be the treatment of choice. Otherwise, surgical excisional biopsy is indicated for the following:

- Patients with concerning features on medical history, family history, or examination
- Masses ≥5 cm
- Any mass that causes distortion of breast architecture
- Rapidly growing masses
- Persistent masses that have not shown any signs of regression after 3 to 4 months
- Multiple and bilateral breast masses, particularly if core biopsy is indeterminate or negative but malignancy is suspected clinically
- Bloody uniductal nipple discharge
- Concerning features on breast ultrasound scan, including cystic change, nonuniform internal echo, and irregular margin

## REFERENCES


1. Osborne MP. Breast anatomy and development. In: Harris JR, Osborne CK, Morrow M, Lippman ME, eds. *Diseases of the Breast*. Philadelphia, PA: Lippincott, Williams & Wilkins;2000: 1-13

2. McKiernan J, Coyne J, Calahane S. Histology of breast development in early life. *Arch Dis Child.* 1988;63:136-139

3. Tanner JM. *Growth in Adolescence*. 2nd ed. Oxford, England: Blackwell Scientific Publications; 1962

4. Marshall WA, Tanner JM. Variations in pattern of pubertal changes in girls. *Arch Dis Child.* 1969;44:291-303

5. Bock K, Duda VF, Hadji P, et al. Pathologic breast conditions in childhood and adolescence. Evaluation by sonographic diagnosis. *J Ultrasound Med.* 2005;24:1347-1354

6. Simmons P, Wold L. Surgically treated breast disease in adolescent females: a retrospective review of 185 cases. *Adolesc Pediatr Gynecol.* 1989;2:95-98

7. Dehner L, Hill A, Deschryver K. Pathology of the breast in children, adolescents, and young adults. *Sem Diag Pathol.* 1999;16(3):235-247

8. Cifti AO, Tanyel FC, Buyukpamukcu N, Hicsonmez A. Female breast masses during childhood: a 25-year review. *Eur J Pediatr Surg.* 1998;(8):67-70

9. Daniel W, Mathews M. Tumors of the breast in adolescent females. *Pediatrics.* 1968;41:743-749

10. Turbey W, Buntain W, Dudgeon D. The surgical management of pediatric breast masses. *Pediatrics.* 1975;56: 736-739

11. Bower R, Bell M, Ternberg J. Management of breast lesions in children and adolescents. *J Pediatr Surg.* 1976;11: 337-346

12. Stone A, Shenker I, McCarthy K. Adolescent breast masses. *Am J Surg.* 1977;134:275-277

13. Gogas J, Sechas M, Skaleas G. Surgical management of diseases of the adolescent female breast. *Am J Surg.* 1979;137: 634-637

14. Ligon R, Stevenson D, Diner W, et al. Breast masses in young women. *Am J Surg.* 1980;140:779-782

15. Goldstein D, Miler V. Breast masses in adolescent females. *Clin Pediatr.* 1982;21:17-19

16. West KW, Reseorla FJ, Schere LR, Grosfeld JL. Diagnosis and treatment of symptomatic breast masses in the pediatric population. *J Pediatr.* 1995;30:182-187

17. Elsheikh A, Keramopoulos A, Lazaris D, Ambelia C, Louvrou N, Michalas S. Breast tumors during adolescence. *Eur J Gynaec Oncol.* 2000;XXI(4):408-409

18. Vargas HI, Vargas P, Eldrageely K, et al. Outcomes of surgical and sonographic detection of breast masses in women younger than 30. *Am Surg.* 2005;71:716-719

19. Sadove AM, van Aalt JA. Congenital and acquired pediatric breast anomalies: a review of 20 years' experience. *Plast Reconstr Surg.* 2005;115:1039-1050

20. Le Savoy MA, Gomez-Garcia A, Nejdl R, Yospur G, Sylau TJ, Chang P. Axillary breast tissue: clinical presentation and surgical treatment. *Ann Plast Surg.* 1995;35:356-360

21. Aillet S, Watier E, Jarno P, Chevrier S, Pailheret JP. Hypertrophie mammaire juvenile: analyse des resultants a long-term des plasties de mammaires de reduction. *Ann Chir Plast Esthet.* 2001;46:585-594

22. Lin KY, Nguyen DB, Williams RM. Complete breast absence revisited. *Plast Reconstr Surg.* 2000;106(1): 98-101

23. Greydanus D, Matystina L, Gains M. Breast disorders in children and adolescence. *Prim Care.* 2006;33(2):455-502

24. Stricker T, Navratl F, Forster I, Hurumann R, Sennhauser F. Nonpuerperal mastitis in adolescents. *J Pediatr.* 2006;148: 278-281

25. Faden H. Mastitis in children from birth to 17 years. *Pediatr Infec Dis J.* 2005;24(12):1113

26. Christensen AF, Al-Suliman N, Nielsen KR, et al. Ultrasound guided drainage of breast abscesses: results in 151 patients. *Br J Radiol.* 2005;78:186-188

27. Armstrong ML, Roberts AE, Owen DC, Koch JR. Contemporary college students and body piercing. *J Adol Health.* 2004;35:58-61

28. Jacobs VR, Golombeck K, Jonat W, Kiechle M. Mastitis nonpuerperalis after nipple piercing: time to act. *Int J Fertil & Women's Med.* 2003;48(5):226-231

29. Ader DN, Browne MW. Prevalence and impact of cyclic mastalgia in a United States clinic-based sample. *Am J Obstet Gynecol.* 1997;177:126-132

30. Blommers J, de Lange-de Klerk ESM, Kuik DJ, Bezemer PD, Meijer S. Evening primrose oil and fish oil for severe chronic mastalgia: a randomized, double-blind, controlled trial. *Am J Obstet Gynecol.* 2002;187:1389–1394

31. O'Brien PM, Abukhalil IEH. Randomized controlled trial of the management of premenstrual syndrome and premenstrual mastalgia using luteal phase-only danazol. *Am J Obstet Gynecol.* 1999;180:18–23

32. Neinstein LS, Atkinson J, Diament M. Prevalence and longitudinal study of breast masses in adolescents. *J Adolesc Health.* 1993;14:277–281

33. Briggs R, Walters M, Rosenthal D. Cystosarcoma phylloides in adolescent female patients. *Am J Surg.* 1983;146:712–714

34. Seijo L, Sidhu J, Mizrachy B, Shafir M, Tartter P, Bleiweiss I. Malignant phyllodes tumor of the breast. *Int J Surg Pathol.* 1995;3(1):17–22

35. Ferguson CM, Powell RW. Breast masses in young women. *Arch Surg.* 1989;124:1338–1341

36. Simmons P. Breast disorders in adolescent females. *Curr Opin Obstet Gynecol.* 2001;13:459–461

37. Surveillance, Epidemiology, and End Results (SEER) Program (www.seer.cancer.gov). SEER*Stat Database: Incidence–SEER 17 Regs Public Use, Nov 2005 Sub (2000–2003), National Cancer Institute, DCCPS, Surveillance Research Program, Cancer Statistics Branch, released April 2006, based on the November 2005 submission

38. Shannon C, Smith IE. Breast cancer in adolescents and young women. *Eur J Cancer.* 2003;39:2632–2642

39. Foreman MR, Cantwell MM, Ronckers CR, Zhang Y. Through the looking glass at early-life exposures and breast cancer risk. *Cancer Invest.* 2005;23:609–624

40. Seeber B, Driscoll D. Hereditary breast and ovarian cancer syndrome: should we test adolescents. *J Pediatr Adolesc Gynecol.* 2004;17:161–167

41. Hartmann LC, Sellers TA, Frost MH, et al. Benign breast disease and the risk of breast cancer. *N Engl J Med.* 2005;353: 229–237

42. Jernstrom H, Loman N, Johannsson OT, Borg A, Olsson H. Impact of oral contraceptive use in a population-based series of early-onset breast cancer cases who have undergone BRCA mutation testing. *Eur J Cancer.* 2005;41:2312–2320

43. Corpron CA, Black CT, Singletary SE, Andrassy RJ. Breast cancer in adolescent females. *J Pediatr Surg.* 1995;30:322–324

44. Ashley S, Royle GT, Corder A, et al. Clinical, radiological, and cytological diagnosis of breast cancer in young women. *Br J Surg.* 1989;76:835–837

# CHAPTER 67

# Pubertal Gynecomastia

REUBEN D. ROHN, MD

## INTRODUCTION

Gynecomastia is defined as any visible or palpable development of breast tissue in males.[1] The tissue may be as small as 1 cm and disk-like in form or as large as that of a normal female breast (Figure 67-1). Usually, gynecomastia is noticeable only when the breast size reaches more than 2 cm in diameter. True gynecomastia represents benign proliferation of glandular tissue. It results in concentric enlargement of one or both breasts and clinically feels like a coiled rope. Many clinicians divide gynecomastia into 2 broad types characterized by the size of the tissue: <3 to 4 cm type 1, and >4 cm type 2.[2] As the size reaches that of what would be considered a typical female breast, the term macromastia or macrogynecomastia is often used to describe the degree of enlargement.

Type 1 pubertal gynecomastia is common, with an incidence of up to 70%.[3] Palpable gynecomastia may be detected once the tissue exceeds 0.5 cm in diameter. Pubertal gynecomastia usually begins between the ages of 10 to 12 years and peaks between 13 and 15 years. Gynecomastia actually correlates better with Tanner stage and is usually associated with Tanner stage 3–4. Gynecomastia usually represents a transient or possibly permanent disturbance in steroid hormone physiology. The condition originates from an imbalance in estrogen versus androgen action in the breast. Estrogen strongly stimulates breast development, whereas androgens tend to inhibit its development.

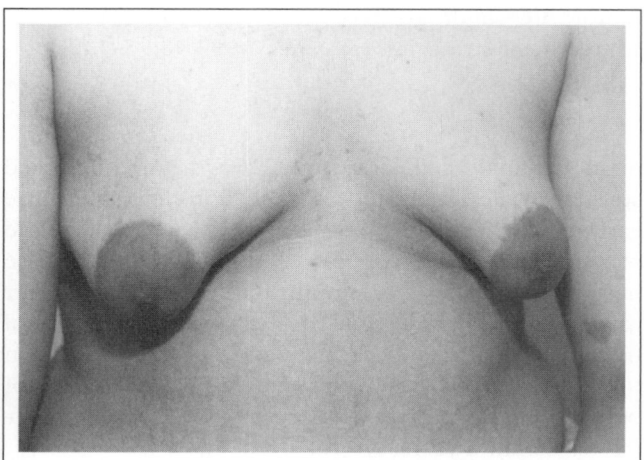

**FIGURE 67-1** Boy with type 2 gynecomastia or macromastia.

## NORMAL BREAST DEVELOPMENT

Apparently, there is no inherent difference in breast tissue between boys and girls, or in breast sensitivity to sex steroid hormones. This is well demonstrated by the fact that at birth neonates may demonstrate a 60% to 90% incidence of breast enlargement regardless of gender.[4] Estrogens from the maternal-placental-fetal unit cause a proliferation of the glandular tissue. During puberty large amounts of estrogen produced by the ovaries bring about marked proliferation of ductal and periductal tissues in girls. Progesterone production, following the development of true ovulatory menstrual cycles, leads to further differentiation of the breast tissue into terminal acini. In the adolescent male, it is the relative imbalance between estrogen and testosterone, as noted previously, that leads to the gynecomastia. Once adult androgen/estrogen ratios are achieved, then the gynecomastia usually resolves.

In boys and men the testis is the major producer of testosterone. As puberty commences, increased pituitary luteinizing hormone (LH) stimulates the testes, thus increasing testosterone output. At the same time, the testes also produce small amounts of estradiol and even smaller amounts of estrone. All 3 hormones are secreted into the circulation (Figure 67-2). Meanwhile, the adrenal glands secrete androstenedione into the circulation. Testosterone and androstenedione undergo conversion to estrogens in tissues such as liver, fat, muscle, skin, bone, and kidney through the process of aromatization—testosterone to estradiol and androstenedione to estrone.[5] Interconversion of estrone and estradiol also takes place. Most circulating estrogens in males derive from this tissue aromatization. All of these hormones circulate as free hormone or bound to sex-hormone-binding globulin (SHBG). The latter is the predominant component. The unbound hormones cross the cell membrane of the target tissue and interact, each with its specific intracellular receptor. The estrogen/

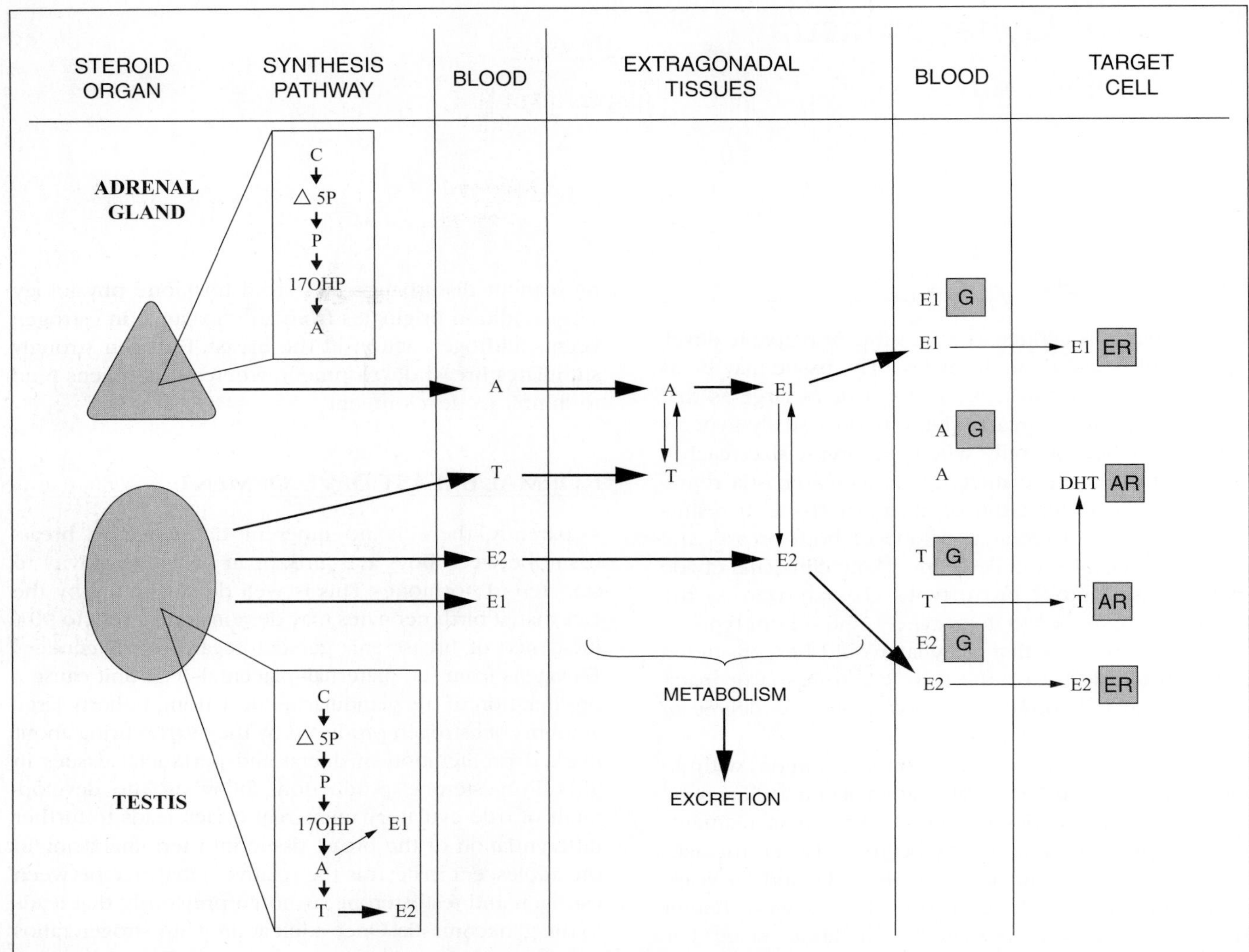


**FIGURE 67-2** Pathways of androgen and estrogen synthesis, action, and metabolism. C = cholesterol; (5P pregnenolone; P = progesterone; 17OHP = 17 hydroxyprogesterone; A = androstenedione; E2 = estradiol; E1 = estrone; G = sex hormone binding globulin; ER = estrogen receptor; AR = androgen receptor. (Modified from Mathur R, Braunstein GD. Gynecomastia: pathomechanisms and treatment strategies. *Horm Res.* 1997;48:95–102.)

receptor and androgen/receptor complexes are translocated into the nucleus where the actual hormonal action takes place.[6] The male breast is a target tissue for these hormones as noted previously.

Histopathologically, pubertal gynecomastia progresses through 3 phases: (1) Early or florid stage; (2) intermediate stage; (3) late or fibrous stage. In the florid stage, the ducts are hypoplastic with epithelial proliferation and edema of the cellular stroma associated with loose periductal connective tissue. The intermediate stage is characterized by ductal hyperplasia, stromal fibrosis, decreased cellularity, and periductal edema. The late stage is characterized by cystic dilatation of the ducts, stromal acellularity, and fibrosis with increased stromal hyalinization and inactive fibrotic tissue.[7] The early or proliferative phase lasts about 6 months, and sometimes maybe as long as 12 months. The late phase may begin as early as 12 months but certainly not longer than 2 years after the initial breast development. Medical treatment, as will be described later, is most effective in the proliferative phase. Interestingly, in 80% to 90% of boys, there is spontaneous regression of the gynecomastia within 2 years.

The exact etiology of pubertal gynecomastia is still unclear. There are 3 major hypotheses: (1) Excessive estrogen production; (2) relative rate of change in estrogen/androgen production; (3) increased sensitivity of the breast tissue to estrogens. Some researchers have reported an increase in estradiol concentration with the onset of gynecomastia either as a true increase in estradiol concentration or as an increase in the estradiol/testosterone ratio. Lee[8] found increased estradiol concentrations while LaFranchi[9] found elevated estradiol/testosterone ratios. Large and Anderson[10] found that boys with gynecomastia have an absolute increase in the 24-hour concentration of estradiol relative to testosterone. Moore et al[11] found that individuals with pubertal gynecomastia had a lower ratio of dehydroepiandrosterone (DHEA) sulfate/estrone and estradiol than those without pubertal gynecomastia at the onset of the process. It is possible that there is an actual increase of aromatization of androgen precursors in the breast itself.[12] Increased breast sensitivity to normal levels of estrogen was inferred from studies documenting that patients with protracted neonatal gynecomastia were more likely to develop pubertal gynecomastia than those who did not have excessive neonatal gynecomastia.[13] This concept has been elaborated further. In the early stages of puberty, testosterone secretion occurs only at night, whereas circulating estrogen rises throughout the 24-hour cycle. Once again, it is aromatization from testosterone and adrenal androgens that may account for this increase in circulating estrogen.[10] As mentioned previously, androgens are inhibitory of breast formation. Thus, during the daytime it may be the adrenal androgen production that inhibits breast formation. A decreased adrenal androgen/estrogen ratio in the afternoon has been found in boys with pubertal gynecomastia as opposed to those without gynecomastia.[11]

This discussion cannot be complete without mentioning that gynecomastia often is unilateral. It is thought that local tissue factors (increased aromatase activity in the affected breast) may account for this phenomenon. Unfortunately, studies of estrogen/progesterone receptors in pubertal macromastia (type 2 gynecomastia) have not been enlightening.[14]

## CLINICAL CHARACTERISTICS

Upon palpation of the breast, pubertal gynecomastia (type 1) feels like coiled rope and is subareolar in location. Adipose tissue appears less distinct, often with relative absence of subareolar tissue, making the palpation feel more like the tissue was doughnut shaped. In type 2 gynecomastia (macromastia or macrogynecomastia), the palpable characteristics become more confusing. Occasionally, one may feel central subareolar glandular-like tissue and less distinct tissue toward the periphery. In macromastia the breasts may resemble those of a female breast in stage 3 to 5 breast development (Figure 67-1). Ultrasonography may be helpful in distinguishing glandular from fatty tissue, and, hence pseudogynecomastia.[15]

Another characteristic of type 1 gynecomastia is the complaint of discomfort and true breast tenderness (mastodynia). This discomfort may be aggravated by any activity causing rubbing of the nipple or the breast against clothing. Extreme discomfort can be treated with mild analgesics or with cold compresses applied to the breast. Rarely, nipple discharge may occur as a result of attempts of a boy to reduce the gynecomastia through self-massage. The discharge is usually clear to gray in color and needs to be distinguished from galactorrhea.[16]

## PATHOLOGICAL GYNECOMASTIA

Pathological gynecomastia is defined as any breast development that occurs as a result of an underlying disorder, a disease process, or as a result of the side effect of a drug (Box 67-1).

### Box 67-1

#### *Causes of Gynecomastia*

A. Endocrine
   1. Klinefelter syndrome
   2. Hypogonadism
      a. Congenital anorchia
      b. Postnatal damage
         i. Viral orchitis
         ii. Acute lymphocytic leukemia
         iii. Radiation
   3. Defective testosterone synthesis or action
      a. Enzyme defects
      b. Partial androgen insensitivity
   4. Hermaphroditism
   5. Hyperthyroidism
   6. Adrenal disorders
      a. ACTH deficiency
      b. Congenital adrenal hyperplasia
   7. Tumors
      a. Leydig cell
      b. Sertoli cell
      c. Teratoma
      d. Choriocarcinoma

*(Continued)*

## Box 67-1 (Continued)

e. Embryonal carcinoma
f. Hepatoma, hepatocarcinoma
g. Adrenal carcinoma
h. Neurofibromatosis
i. Lipoma
j. Lymphangioma
k. Metastatic
i. Leukemia
ii. Lymphoma
iii. Rhabdomyosarcoma

B. Chronic diseases
1. Liver disorders and malnutrition
a. Cirrhosis
b. Ulcerative colitis
c. Cystic fibrosis
d. AIDS
2. Refeeding
3. Uremia
4. Nervous system

C. Familial

D. Medications/drugs

ACTH, adrenocorticotropic hormone; AIDS, acquired immune deficiency syndrome

**ENDOCRINE CAUSES**

- Klinefelter syndrome: Klinefelter syndrome is a form of hypogonadism, with increased LH levels because of lowered testosterone production in the testes. There is a relative increase in estrogen leading to an increased estrogen/androgen ratio, which promotes the gynecomastia. One must remember that Klinefelter syndrome is relatively common in males, with estimates of up to 1 in 500 males being affected. Thus, any male with gynecomastia and small testicular volume for the degree of pubertal development should undergo either gonadotrophin-level analysis or karyotyping. Rarely, 46XX males may present this way as well.
- Hypogonadism: Primary hypogonadism because of congenital anorchia or testicular damage may lead to testicular failure. Congenital anorchia most commonly results from testicular atrophy following alleged in utero testicular torsion. Postnatally, testicular damage may occur from viral orchitis, trauma, infiltrative processes (acute lymphocytic leukemia), or from radiation treatment. Gynecomastia is common in such individuals at puberty as a result of abnormal estrogen/testosterone ratios.
- Defective testosterone synthesis or action: Enzyme defects in the testosterone synthetic pathway may result in gynecomastia. These individuals are usually diagnosed before puberty because of undermasculinization of the male genitalia (eg, hypospadias) due to lack of testosterone action. Partial androgen insensitivity may also present with gynecomastia and undermasculinization of the male genitalia. Although these diagnoses would be expected to be made prior to puberty, sometimes these individuals may be diagnosed during adolescence only because of the presentation of gynecomastia and subsequent careful examination that detects undermasculinization.
- Hermaphroditism: Because of the presence of ovarian and testicular tissue, such individuals may present with breast development during puberty. The ovarian tissue component results in an increased estrogen/androgen ratio.
- Hyperthyroidism: 25% to 40% of boys with hyperthyroidism may develop gynecomastia. The mechanism of the gynecomastia results from a decrease in free testosterone secondary to increased testosterone binding. Thus, there is an increased estrogen/testosterone ratio. Moreover, hyperthyroidism causes an increased production of androstenedione. Through aromatization of androstenedione to estrogen in extraglandular sites, more estrogen is produced, further compounding the situation.
- Adrenal disorders: Rarely, isolated adrenocorticotropic hormone (ACTH) deficiency has been reported with gynecomastia secondary to increased plasma LH levels and subsequent increased estradiol levels.[17] Congenital adrenal hyperplasia, which is more common, can be accompanied by increased estrogen production as a consequence of aromatization of androstenedione into estrogen in extraglandular sites.[18]
- Tumors: Testicular tumors may secrete increased estrogen in response to chorionic gonadotropin. These tumors can be stromal cell tumors (Leydig or Sertoli cell) or germinal tumors (teratomas, choriocarcinomas, or embryonal carcinomas). Most of these tumors can be detected as unilateral masses, but occasionally ultrasound of the testes may be needed to detect smaller-sized tumors. Feminizing adrenal tumors have

been reported but are fairly rare. In all instances, the gynecomastia is secondary to secretion of large amounts of androstenedione, which are converted to estrogen by peripheral tissue aromatase.[19] Liver tumors secreting human chorionic gonadonotropin (HCG) have also been reported to present with isolated gynecomastia or feminization.[20] Other HCG-secreting tumors (brain, chest, and abdominal) may also produce gynecomastia. In the case of liver or other HCG-producing tumors, HCG increases estradiol production in the testes. Neurofibromatosis is another uncommon cause of gynecomastia. The gynecomastia may result from benign neurofibromas. Primary breast neoplasms have been the cause of unilateral breast development. These are extremely rare and various etiologies have been reported.[21]

### CHRONIC DISEASES

- Any chronic illness that can cause long-term malnutrition or liver disease may lead to gynecomastia. Specific diseases that can lead to liver problems include chronic ulcerative colitis, cystic fibrosis, AIDS, and cirrhosis. With enough damage to the hepatic cells, there is an impairment in the liver's ability to inactivate estrogen. Moreover, androstenedione extraction from circulation decreases in liver disease, resulting in more peripheral conversion of androstenedione to estrogen.
- Gynecomastia is seen in the refeeding phase of chronic malnutrition. There is transient liver impairment following starvation causing failure of estrogen degradation resulting in an increase in the estrogen/androgen ratio.[5,22–24] The gynecomastia with refeeding is usually transient because the breast enlargement regresses as liver function improves.
- Chronic uremia from renal failure results in testicular damage, leading to a mechanism similar to that of primary hypogonadism with a resultant change in estrogen/androgen ratio.[25]
- Finally, certain nervous system damage or dysfunction can also result in gynecomastia. Paraplegia secondary to trauma can result in decreased testicular function. Intercostal nerve injury during thoracoplastic surgery or herpes zoster infection leading to nerve damage have been associated with breast enlargement.[5,24] The etiology is predicated on decreased testicular function ultimately leading to a change in estrogen/androgen ratio.

### FAMILIAL GYNECOMASTIA

There is a diverse group of familial gynecomastias that seem to be transmitted as an X-linked recessive or as an autosomal-dominant trait.[21] This group of familial gynecomastia is poorly understood, and the genetic defect is hypothesized to be located in the 5'-end of the P450 aromatase gene. There is a specific form of familial gynecomastia associated with aromatase excess syndrome, which is characterized by an increase in the production and action of the CYP19 [450] aromatase. This particular enzyme is the key enzyme in estrogen biosynthesis.[26,27] These latter conditions are relatively rare, with severe breast development occurring at 10 to 11 years of age with up to a 100-fold increase in extraglandular aromatization leading to high estradiol/testosterone ratios.[21]

### DRUGS

There are many drugs that have been associated with development of gynecomastia (Table 67-1). This list is never complete because new medications causing gynecomastia are being added frequently. Estrogen or estrogen-like substances may reside in many medications, substances, or foods and may be used often without knowledge of their presence. Meat, milk, skin lotions, hair oils, embalming fluids, and delousing agents have all been implicated at 1 time or another.[21] Interestingly, androgens and anabolic steroids are listed because they may have the paradoxical effect of enhancing peripheral tissue conversion of estradiol, and thus producing gynecomastia. Illicit drug use is another common cause of gynecomastia. Boys should be questioned about androgenic steroids, which are often used to enhance physical performance. Their use has increased dramatically as evidenced by news headlines implicating more professional athletes who have been accused of using or found to have used such medications. Interestingly, marijuana as a cause of gynecomastia results from the phytoestrogens in the marijuana preparation rather than the tetrahydrocannabinol.[28] There are certain medications that are testosterone antagonists, which alter the estrogen/testosterone ratio and thus result in gynecomastia. Other drugs are noted in Table 67-1.

## DIAGNOSTIC APPROACH TO GYNECOMASTIA

Once armed with the information noted previously, the task of developing a differential diagnosis or determining the cause of the gynecomastia should be made easier. As with any other clinical condition, a thorough history and physical examination followed by the appropriate laboratory evaluation should provide the examiner with the most likely cause of the gynecomastia.

**Table 67-1**

**Drugs That Cause Gynecomastia**

| *Class* | *Drugs* |
|---|---|
| Antiandrogens/ androgen synthesis | Bicalutamide |
| | Cyproterone |
| | Finasteride |
| | Flutamide |
| | Nilutamide |
| Antibiotics/antifungal/ antituberculous | Ethionamide |
| | Isoniazid |
| | Ketoconazole (antiantrogen) |
| | Metronidazole |
| | Thiacetazone |
| Chemotherapeutic/ cancer | Busulfan |
| | Chlorambucil |
| | Cyclophosphamide |
| | Methotrexate |
| | Nitrosureas |
| | Penicillamine |
| | Procarbazine |
| | Vincristine |
| Cardiovascular/ antihypertensives | ACE inhibitors |
| | Amiodarone |
| | Calcium channel blockers |
| | Digitalis |
| | Guanabenz |
| | Hydralazine |
| | Methyldopa |
| | Propranolol |
| | Reserpine |
| Diuretics | Spironolactone (antiandrogen) |
| | Thiazide |
| Drugs of Abuse | Alcohol |
| | Amphetamines |
| | Anabolic steroids (see previous) |
| | Growth hormone (see following) |
| | Marijuana |
| | Opiates |
| Gastrointestinal | Cimetidine |
| | Omeprazole |
| | Ranitidine |

*(Continued)*

**Table 67-1 (Continued)**

| *Class* | *Drugs* |
|---|---|
| Hormones | Androgens/anabolic steroids |
| | Chorionic gonadotropin |
| | Clomiphene |
| | Estrogens |
| | Growth hormone |
| | Leuprolide |
| Psychoactive | Benzodiazepines |
| | Haloperidol |
| | Olanzepine |
| | Phenothiazines |
| | Risperidone |
| | Tricyclic antidepressants |
| Others | Atorvastatin |
| | Auranofin |
| | Diethyproprion |
| | Ergotamine |
| | Ibuprofen |
| | Metoclopramide |
| | Phenytoin |
| | Sulindac |
| | Theophylline |
| | Vitamin E |

## CLINICAL EVALUATION

A comprehensive medical history and thorough physical examination are critical to the evaluation. The history should be directed at identifying possible drug use, hormonal use, chronic illnesses, or endocrinopathies that could lead to gynecomastia. A physical examination should help differentiate between true gynecomastia and pseudogynecomastia or fatty tissue. As noted previously, true gynecomastia should be able to be differentiated on the examination. If not, ultrasonography can be helpful in questionable cases.[15]

## LABORATORY EVALUATION

Laboratory evaluation and test selection is predicated on the clinical picture. Boys who seem chronically ill may require liver, renal, and thyroid function studies. Boys with features of Klinefelter syndrome including small testes or other boys with signs of hypogonadism should have LH and follicle-stimulating hormone (FSH) levels analyzed because increased LH and FSH levels confirm the suspicion of hypogonadism. Karyotyping may also be necessary to confirm Klinefelter syndrome or hermaphroditism.

If galactorrhea is present, prolactin levels should be determined. Estrogen, testosterone, dehydroepiandrosterone sulfate (DHEAS), and HCG may also need to be obtained. Increased DHEAS levels suggest possible liver or adrenal tumors. Elevated HCG levels may signal the presence of Leydig, Sertoli, or germ cell tumors. Significant testicular asymmetry may be a clue to such tumors. Ultrasonography may be required to further investigate possible adrenal, hepatic, or testicular tumors, whereas magnetic resonance imaging of the brain, chest, or abdomen may be needed to detect certain germ cell tumors.

## TREATMENT

In boys with type 1 gynecomastia, spontaneous resolution usually occurs within 2 to 3 years. Thus, simple observation and reassurance is all that is required in most cases. Medical therapy has been attempted, but as yet none that have been approved. Various treatments aimed at altering the estrogen/androgen ratio have been tried. These remedies include dihydrotestosterone, clomiphene, tamoxifen, anastrazole, testolactone, and raloxifene. It must be remembered that for medical therapy to be effective it must be provided early in the active or proliferative phase of gynecomastia. Once the later stages of gynecomastia have been achieved, too much stromal hyalinization and fibrosis have occurred that cannot be reversed. Studies of all previously mentioned medications have shown mixed results. Dihydrotesterone cannot be converted to estrogen. Thus, it increases the androgen-to-estrogen ratio. It has been found to be effective, but dihydrotestosterone is not commercially available. Moreover, studies are limited.[29] Anastrazole and testolactone are aromatase inhibitors. In a trial, testolactone showed improvement in gynecomastia of the treated subjects, but unfortunately the study was not blinded or controlled. Plourde and associates,[30] in a well-designed (randomized, double-blind, placebo-controlled) study, demonstrated that anastrazole was ineffective in treating gynecomastia. The antiestrogens tamoxifen and raloxifene have been tried as well. Tamoxifen demonstrated effective prevention of gynecomastia in a placebo-controlled trial of 114 adult men with prostate cancer who were being treated with bicalutamide (antiandrogen; see Table 67-1).[31] Although a report in adolescent boys found that the use of tamoxifen and raloxifene was safe and effective, the study was problematic because the outcome data for the control subjects relied upon self-report of the continued presence of gynecomastia. Moreover, 5 of the 25 treated subjects had breast enlargement consistent with type I gynecomastia, which, as previously noted, resolves on its own.[32] To reemphasize, most studies have not been blinded or used controls. Hence, positive outcomes are questionable. A large multicenter, blinded, and controlled study is needed to assess the true efficacy of these medications. In boys with type 2 gynecomastia or macromastia, the only effective and proven means of treatment is surgical removal. It is often difficult to convince insurance companies that such surgery is not just cosmetic and that these boys with large breasts are often very psychologically handicapped. Surgical procedures include classic mastectomy or liposuction.[29]

## REFERENCES


1. Knorr D, Bidlingmaier G. Gynecomastia in male adolescents. *Clin Endocrinol Metab.* 1975;4:157-171

2. Schonfeld WA. Gynecomastia in adolescence: effect on body image and personality adaption. *Psychosom Med.* 1962;24:379-389

3. Carlson HE. Gynecomastia: pathogenesis and therapy. *Endocrinologist.* 1991;1:337-342

4. Schmidt-Voigt J. Brustdrüenschwellungen bei männlichen Jugendlichen des Pubertätsalter (Pubertätsmakromastie). *Z Kinderheilkd.* 1941;62:590-606

5. Wilson JD, Aiman J, MacDonald PC. The pathogenesis of gynecomastia. *Adv Intern Med.* 1980;29:1-32

6. Lazar MA. Steroid and thyroid hormone receptors. *Endocrinol Clin North Am.* 1991;20:681-695

7. Bannayan GA, Hajdu SI. Gynecomastia: clinicopathologic study of 351 cases. *Am J Clin Pathol.* 1972;57:431-437

8. Lee PA. The relationship of concentrations of serum hormones to pubertal gynecomastia. *J Pediatr.* 1975;86:212-215

9. LaFranchi SH, Parlow AF, Lippe BM, Coytupa J, Kaplan S. Pubertal gynecomastia and transient elevation of serum estradiol level. *Am J Dis Child.* 1975;129:927-931

10. Large DM, Anderson DC. Twenty-four-hour profiles of circulating androgens and estrogens in male puberty with and without gynecomastia. *Clin Endocrinol (Oxf).* 1979;11:505-521

11. Moore DC, Schlaepfer LV, Paunier L, Sizonenko PC. Hormonal changes during puberty. V. Transient pubertal gynecomastia: abnormal androgen-estrogen ratios. *J Clin Endocrinol Metab.* 1984;58:492-499

12. Bulard J, Mowszowicz I, Schaison G. Increased aromatase activity in pubic skin fibroblasts from patients with isolated gynecomastia. *J Clin Endocrinol Metab.* 1987;64:618-623

13. Hall PF. *Gynaecomastia*. Glebe: Australasian Medical Publishing; 1959

14. Lee KO, Chua DYF, Cheah JS. Estrogen and progesterone receptors in men with bilateral or unilateral pubertal macromastia. *Clin Endocrinol.* 1990;32:101

15. Garcia CJ, Espinoza A, Dinamarca V, et al. Breast US in children and adolescents. *Radiographics.* 2000;20:1605-1612

16. Rohn RD. Galactorrhea in the adolescent. *J Adolesc Health Care.* 1984;5:37–49

17. Shimatsu A, Suzuki Y, Tanaka S. Gynecomastia associated with isolated ACTH deficiency. *J Endocrinol Inv.* 1987;10:127–129

18. Zadik Z, Pertzelan A, Kaufman H, et al. Gynecomastia in two prepubertal boys with congenital and renal hyperplasia due to 11-beta hydroxylase deficiency. *Helv Pediatr Acta.* 1979;34:185–187

19. Itami RM, Amundson GM, Kaplan SA, et al. Prepubertal gynecomastia caused by an adrenal tumor in diagnostic value of ultrasound. *Am J Dis Child.* 1982;13 C:584–586

20. Kew MC, Kirschner MA, Abrahams GE. Mechanism of feminization in primary liver cancer. *N Engl J Med.* 1977;296:1084–1088

21. Mahoney CP. Adolescent gynecomastia. Differential diagnosis and management. *Pediatr Clin North Am.* 1990;37: 1389–1404

22. Braude S, Kennedy H, Hodson M,et al. Hypertrophic osteoarthropathy in cystic fibrosis. *Br Med J (ClinRes).* 1984;288:822–823

23. Couderc LJ, Claurel JP. HIV-infection-induced gynecomastia. *Ann Intern Med.* 1987;197:257

24. Leung AKC. Gynecomastia. *Am Fam Physician.* 1989;39:215–222

25. Freeman RM, Lowton RL, Fearing MO. Gynecomastia: an endocrinologic complication of hemodialysis. *Ann Intern Med.* 1968;69:67–72

26. Stratakis CA, Vottero A, Brodie A, et al. The aromatase excess syndrome is associated with feminization of both sexes and autosomal dominant transmission of aberrant P450 aromatase gene transcription. *J Clin Endocrinol Metab.* 1998;83:1348–1357

27. Bulun SE, Noble LS, Takayama K, et al. Endocrine disorders associated with inappropriately high aromatase expression. *J Steroid Biochem Mol Biol.* 1997;61:133–139

28. Sauer MA, Rifka SM, Hawks RL, Cutler GB Jr, Loriaux DL. Marijuana: interaction with the estrogen receptor. *J Pharmacol Exp Ther.* 1983;224:404–407

29. Lazala C, Saenger P. Pubertal gynecomastia. *J Pediatr Endocrinol Metab.* 2002;15:553–560

30. Plourde PV, Reiter EO, Jou HC, et al. Safety and efficacy of anastrozole for the treatment of pubertal gynecomastia: a randomized, double-blind, placebo-controlled trial. *J Clin Endocrinol Metab.* 2004;89:4428–4433

31. Boccardo F, Rubagotti A, Battaglia M, et al. Evaluation of tamoxifen and anastrozole in the prevention of gynecomastia and breast pain induced by bicalutamide monotherapy of prostate cancer. *J Clin Oncol.* 2005;23:808–815

32. Lawrence SE, Faught KA, Vethamuthu J, Lawson ML. Beneficial effects of raloxifene and tamoxifen in the treatment of pubertal gynecomastia. *J Pediatr.* 2004;145:71–76

# CHAPTER 68

## Disorders of the Male Genitalia

WILLIAM P. ADELMAN, MD • ALAIN JOFFE, MD, MPH

*The views expressed in this chapter are those of the authors and do not reflect the official policy or position of the US Army, the US Navy, the US Department of Defense, or the US government.*

The adolescent male genital examination serves to monitor sexual development, recognize common anomalies, and identify early signs of potentially serious conditions. Acute complaints in males such as abdominal, back, and flank pain, gynecomastia, supraclavicular adenopathy, and genital discomfort are potential indicators of genital disease. This chapter reviews clinically important disorders of the male genitalia.

### CRYPTORCHIDISM

Cryptorchidism refers to an undescended testis that cannot be drawn into the scrotum. The normal testicular descent occurs in the eighth month of gestation. Cryptorchidism is most commonly diagnosed in the newborn period, when the prevalence is 3.4%. The adolescent should not be presumed to have descended testes, as the prevalence of cryptorchidism in adolescent patients is 0.7%.

#### DIAGNOSIS

When a testis is not palpable in the scrotum, gentle massage should be performed along the line of descent from the anterosuperior spine, medially, and downward to the pubic tubercle. If the testis is not truly undescended, it should become palpable in the scrotum. In the young adolescent, presence of a prominent fat pad may give the false appearance of cryptorchid testes. If cryptorchidism is present, the teen should be examined for stigmata of associated disorders such as Noonan, Klinefelter, or Kallmann syndrome, or trisomy 21, or rarely, trisomy 18 or 13.

#### COMPLICATIONS

Complications of cryptorchidism include infertility and malignancy. Identification of cryptorchidism with appropriate follow-up and therapy are therefore important for optimal management of this condition. This section reviews these complications and appropriate therapy.

##### Infertility

Fertility in the cryptorchid testis may be significantly impaired. Orchiopexy is usually performed in the United States at one year of age primarily to preserve fertility. The fertility index of the descended counterparts of unilateral undescended testes may also be somewhat impaired in certain age groups. Fertility is significantly hampered in patients with bilateral cryptorchid testes if the condition is not corrected by 6 years of age.

##### Malignancy

Males who have cryptorchidism have a 10 to 40 times increased risk of testicular cancer compared with males without cryptorchidism, and 5% to 12% of men who have testicular cancer have a history of cryptorchidism. Because 1% to 5% of boys who have a history of an undescended testicle later develop germ cell tumors, any history of cryptorchidism should prompt careful long-term follow-up including teaching of testicular self-examination (TSE).

#### THERAPY

Orchiopexy of a testis located in the embryologic pathway and not in the abdomen reduces the risk of cancer in inverse relation to age. In the United Kingdom Testicular Cancer Study,[1] a significant association of testicular cancer with undescended testis (odds ratio, 3.82; 95% confidence interval, 2.24-6.52) was found. The excess risk associated with undescended testis was eliminated in men who had had an orchiopexy before the age of 10 years.

Therapy for cryptorchidism in teenagers should be corrective surgery. It is more likely that an adolescent provider will care for a male with a history of orchiopexy than to diagnose a previously unidentified case of cryptorchidism. Therefore, it is crucial to know that a testicle made palpable by surgery can be monitored better for changes. These teens should undergo yearly testicular exams by a medical provider, be aware of their increased risk of testicular cancer, and should be taught TSE.

## SCROTAL SWELLING AND MASSES

This section discusses the general approach to the adolescent with a scrotal mass or a painful scrotum.

### HISTORY

Differentiating the painless from painful scrotal complaint is a convenient way to categorize genital disease and differentiate potential surgical emergencies from less urgent conditions. The differential diagnosis for painless and painful scrotal complaints can be found in Box 68-1. A thorough history often yields the correct diagnosis, and clues to diagnosis in the history can be found in Box 68-2.

### PHYSICAL EXAMINATION

The physical examination of the male genitalia consists of inspection and palpation. The anatomy of the genitalia is straightforward and the genitalia are readily accessible for palpation. If the physical examination is difficult or uncertain, simple adjunctive tests can be used to clarify the diagnosis.

#### Inspection

In the context of a painful genital complaint, inspection can lend important information. In testicular torsion, the affected testis is often higher than on the contralateral side. With infections, such as mumps orchitis, the affected testis is often lower. In torsion, the affected testis, and often the contralateral testis, lie horizontally instead of in the usual vertical position, secondary to the congenital defect involved. In torsion, the epididymis is usually displaced anteriorly, as the testis twists on its vascular pedicle.

**Box 68-1**

***Differential Diagnosis for Painless and Painful Conditions of the Scrotum***

Painless scrotal mass or swelling

- Hydrocele
- Spermatocele
- Varicocele
- Hernia
- Testicular tumor
- Idiopathic scrotal edema

Painful scrotal mass or swelling

- Torsion of the spermatic cord
- Torsion of the appendix testis
- Epididymitis
- Orchitis
- Trauma resulting in hematoma
- Hernia—incarcerated
- Henoch-Schönlein syndrome
- Cellulitis or infected piercing
- Hymenoptera sting or insect bite
- Testicular tumor with bleeding or infarction

**Box 68-2**

***Historical Clues to Diagnosis of the Adolescent with a Scrotal Complaint***

Pain

- Abrupt onset is suggestive of torsion
- Gradual onset suggests epididymitis or orchitis
- No pain suggests tumor or cystic mass

Prior history of pain

- Torsion is often preceded by episodes of mild pain

Trauma

Recent change in testicular size or scrotum

- Reactive hydroceles are common secondary to trauma, orchitis, testicular cancer, and epididymitis
- Longstanding hydroceles are usually benign

Sexual activity

- Epididymitis in adolescence is usually sexually transmitted

#### Palpation

Understanding the anatomy of the male genitalia allows for directed diagnosis. Palpation of the testicular surfaces, the epididymis and cord (posterior structures), and the head of the epididymis (lateral structure) should be performed (Figure 68-1). Among painless findings, a mass within the testis of an adolescent or young adult is a tumor until proven otherwise. Conversely, a mass palpable separate from the testis is unlikely to be a tumor. A "bag of worms" or "squishy tube" on the left spermatic cord is a varicocele. A mass located near the head of the epididymis, above and behind the testis, is probably a spermatocele. A mass anterior to the testis or surrounding the testis is likely to be a hydrocele. A mass separate from the testis/epididymis that intensifies with straining (Valsalva) and is reducible is probably a hernia. A helpful technique on physical examination is transillumination of the scrotum. Clear transillumination of a painless mass suggests a hydrocele or a typical spermatocele. Absence of transillumination suggests a testicular tumor or, if the mass is separate from the testis/epididymis, a hernia or a large spermatocele.

In the context of a painful mass, isolated swelling and tenderness of the epididymis suggests epididymitis. A tender, pea-sized swelling at the upper pole of the

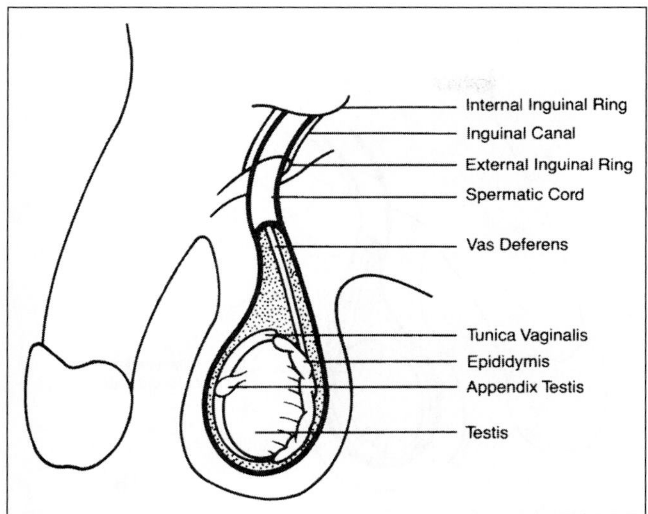


FIGURE 68-1 Anatomy of normal scrotal sac. (Kappahan C, Schlossberger N. Male reproductive health: Part 1. Painful scrotal masses. *Adolescent Health Update*. 1992;4(3):4.)

testis suggests torsion of the appendix testis. Generalized swelling and tenderness of both the testis and the epididymis can be found in either testicular torsion or epididymitis with orchitis. Presence of a cremasteric reflex makes torsion unlikely. However, it is often present in torsion of the appendix testis. Relief of pain with elevation of the testis (Prehn sign) suggests epididymitis. Lack of pain relief with elevation of the testis is not a reliable test for torsion. Nausea or vomiting with testicular pain is usually caused by torsion. Figure 68-2 illustrates scrotal disorders.

### LABORATORY EVALUATION

In cases of a painful scrotum, or dysuria, a urine dipstick test that is positive for leukocyte esterase or the presence of leukocytes on microscopy (especially if there are >20 white blood cells per high-power field) is suggestive of epididymitis rather than torsion. In cases of a painful scrotum and a history of urethritis or dysuria, a urethral gram stain is helpful. Gram-negative diplococci suggest a gonococcal epididymitis. A gram stain with white blood cells without gram-negative bacteria suggests a chlamydial epididymitis. A negative gram stain suggests an orchitis, or torsion. In cases of a painful scrotum where torsion is suspected, a Doppler ultrasound flow study, a nuclear scan, or both can be used in equivocal cases but should be obtained only after consultation with a urologist. If a reasonable suspicion of torsion exists, the primary therapy should be surgical exploration, without delaying to order diagnostic tests. In cases of torsion, the scan and Doppler study will show a decreased flow to the affected side. In the context of a painless mass, an ultrasound is a simple and noninvasive test to define anatomy and assist with diagnosis.

The next section will review painless genital masses of inguinal hernia, spermatocele, varicocele, and testicular tumor in greater detail.

## INGUINAL HERNIA

### ETIOLOGY

An inguinal hernia is a protrusion of intestine through the inguinal ring into the scrotum.

### EPIDEMIOLOGY

The incidence of hernia is less than 2% and may appear at any age. Hernia is more commonly identified in younger children than in adolescents.

### DIAGNOSIS

A hernia may resemble a hydrocele on examination but can be distinguished in the following ways: a hernia reduces when the patient is in the supine position, will not descend with traction on the testis, and may be associated with bowel sounds in the scrotum. The examiner can identify the top of a hydrocele within the scrotum but is unable to do so with a hernia. Hernias and hydroceles may coexist.

### THERAPY

The treatment for hernia is surgical correction.

## SPERMATOCELE

A spermatocele is a retention cyst of the epididymis that contains spermatozoa. Most are small (<1 cm in diameter), painless, cystic, freely movable, and will transilluminate. If it is large, the patient may present complaining of a "third testicle," and turbidity from increased spermatozoa may prevent transillumination. It is usually felt as a smooth, cystic sac located above and posterior to the testis, at the head of the epididymis. No therapy is indicated, unless it is large enough to annoy the patient, in which case a urologist may excise it.[2]

## VARICOCELE

### ETIOLOGY

A varicocele, or dilated scrotal veins, results from increased pressure and incompetent venous valves in the internal spermatic veins. Anatomical reasons explain

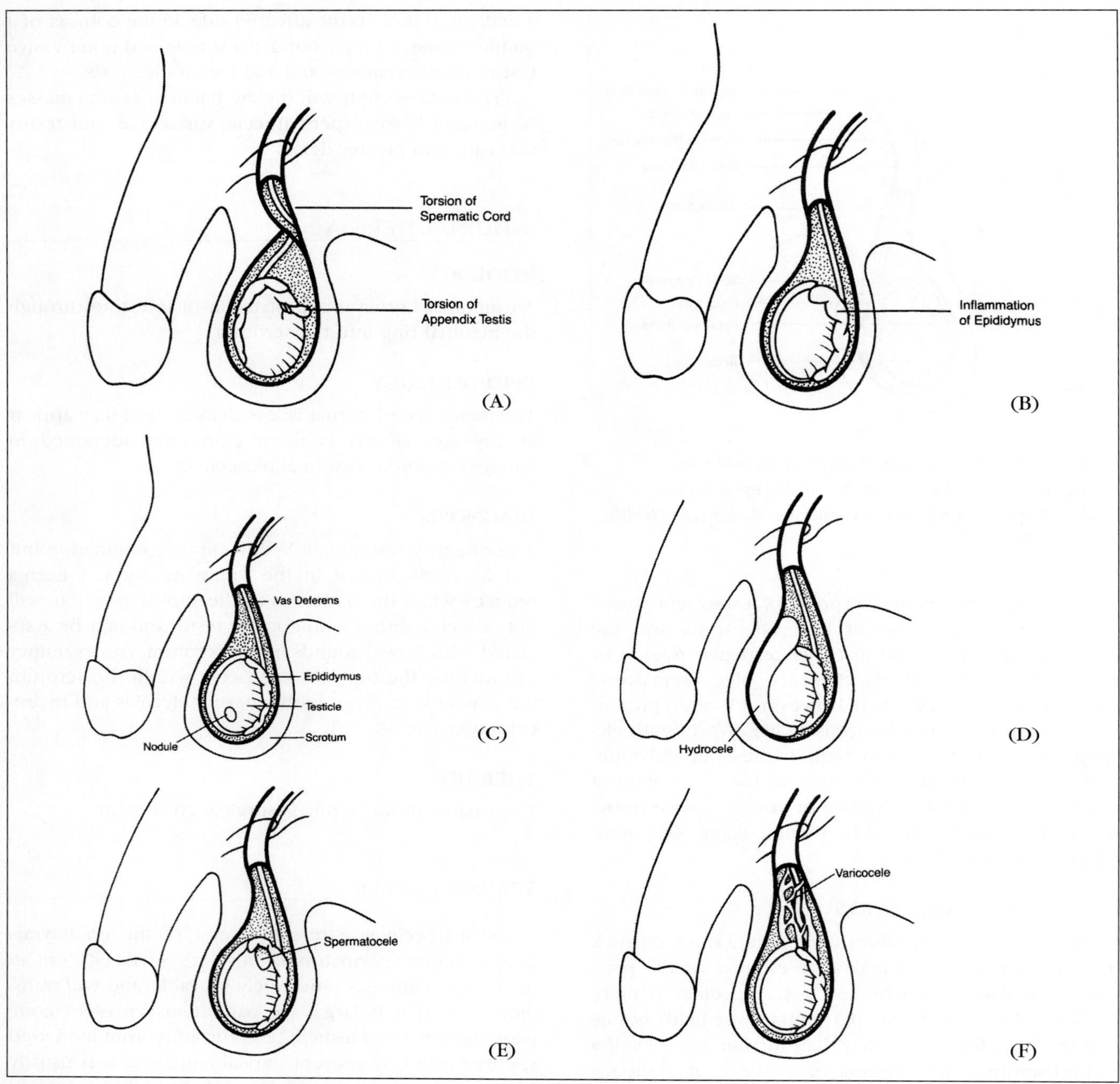


**FIGURE 68-2** Scrotal disorders. (A) Torsions; (B) Epididymitis; (C) Testis tumor; (D) Hydrocele (E) Spermatocele; (F) Varicocele [(A) and (B) from Kappahan C, Schlossberger N. Male reproductive health: Part 1. Painful scrotal masses. *Adolescent Health Update*. 1992;4(3):4; (C), (D), (E), and (F) from Kappahan C, Schlossberger N. Male reproductive health: Part 2. Painless scrotal masses. *Adolescent Health Update*. 1992;5(1):4, 7.]

why varicocele is most often noted on the left side. Recent studies suggest that the incidence of bilateral varicocele is underestimated and that percutaneous retrograde venography usually reveals bilateral disease in those with clinically evident unilateral disease.[3]

### EPIDEMIOLOGY

Varicocele is common in the 10- to 20-year age group, with a prevalence of 15%. They are rare before adolescence. Eighty-five percent of varicoceles are clinically evident on the left side, and 15% are bilateral.

### DIAGNOSIS

Varicoceles are detected in adolescents either on routine examination or secondary to a patient's discovery of a difference between 1 hemiscrotum and the other. Occasionally a patient complains of an ache or pain from the varicocele. On examination, a visible varicocele (Grade 3 or larger) has a "bag of worms" appearance and "squishy tube" feel above the testes. A varicocele that is palpable but not visible is classified as Grade 2 (moderate). More subtle varicoceles may feel like a thickened or asymmetric spermatic cord. The distension usually decreases when the patient lies down. A Grade 1 (small) varicocele is evident on Valsalva only. The benefit of identifying Grade 1 varicoceles is unknown.

### THERAPY

Multiple lines of evidence suggest that Grade 2 and Grade 3 varicoceles can have a negative effect on the growth and function of the ipsilateral testicle in up to 20% of patients with a varicocele. This may portend future problems with fertility in a subset of these patients. To assess for this possibility, it is reasonable to obtain a semen analysis, the true test of potential fertility, on willing patients once they reach Tanner stage 5. An adolescent with a normal semen analysis need not be referred for treatment of his varicocele. However, semen analysis is not often a practical test to perform on teenage boys.

Loss of testicular volume or failure of the testis to grow during puberty has been the traditional indication for surgical correction of a varicocele during adolescence. Several recommendations have been suggested as indications for varicocele repair, but definitive answers as to who should be referred and when during adolescence remain elusive.[4–7] A compilation of recommendations for varicocele repair is summarized in Box 68-3.

**Box 68-3**

***Potential Reasons to Recommend Varicocele Repair in Adolescents***[4–7]

- The results of semen analysis are abnormal.
- A testes volume difference of at least 3 mL is noted on examination.
- A difference of more than 2 mL in testicular volume is noted on serial ultrasonic examinations.
- A testicular size is smaller by 2 standard deviations when compared with normal testicular growth curves.
- The response of either luteinizing hormone (LH) or follicle-stimulating hormone (FSH) to gonadotropin-releasing hormone (GNRH) stimulation is supranormal.
- LH or FSH levels are abnormal in the absence of GNRH stimulation.
- Bilaterally palpable varicoceles are detected.
- A large, symptomatic varicocele is present.
- Varicocele is present in a patient with a single testicle.
- Scrotal pain is present.

## TESTICULAR TUMORS

### ETIOLOGY

Most testicular neoplasias are malignant and of germ-cell origin (95%). Seminomas are the most common testicular cancer of a single cell type (40% of germ cell tumors) with a peak incidence in the 25- to 45-year-old age group; nonseminoma tumors (embryonal cell, choriocarcinoma, teratoma, yolk sac, and mixed forms) peak in the 15- to 30-year-old group.

### EPIDEMIOLOGY

Testicular tumors are the most common solid tumor in males age 15 to 35 years. The incidence is 2.3 to 10 in 100,000 males. Testicular cancer is 4.5 times more common among white men than black men. The risk of a testicular tumor is increased 10 to 40 times in a teenager with a history of cryptorchidism. Testicular atrophy is also associated with cancer. Men who have a family history of testicular cancer may be at higher risk for this disease. A history of testicular cancer is associated with a higher risk of a contralateral tumor.

### DIAGNOSIS

The diagnosis of tumor should be suspected in any male with a firm, circumscribed, painless area of induration within the testis that does not transilluminate. Swelling is noted in up to 73% of cases at presentation, but is usually considered asymptomatic by the patient. Testicular pain is the presenting symptom in 18% to 46% of patients who have germ cell tumors.

### MANAGEMENT

Evaluation of a testicular mass should begin with ultrasonography, a sensitive and specific test that can discriminate between a testicular neoplasm and the nonmalignant processes included in the differential diagnosis. Even if an obvious mass is palpated on physical examination, ultrasonography should be performed on both testicles to rule out bilateral disease (2%–4%). Once a tumor is suspected, measurement of tumor serum markers such as lactate dehydrogenase, beta human chorionic gonadotropin (elevated in choriocarcinoma and seminoma), and alpha-fetoprotein (produced by yolk sac cells) is indicated. Further evaluation for staging should be performed in consultation with an oncologist and may include additional laboratory studies; computed tomography scan of the chest, abdomen, and pelvis; and other imaging as needed (eg, imaging of the brain in the case of a pure choriocarcinoma). Similarly, an appropriately trained oncologist and urologist should manage testicular cancer because treatments vary by grade and stage of tumor. Therapy involves a direct biopsy for confirmative diagnosis and cell type. All patients undergo radical orchiectomy, followed by close surveillance for certain early stage tumors or chemotherapy and radiation, usually with a positive prognosis. The most common sites of metastasis for seminoma include the contralateral testis, ipsilateral lymph nodes, pelvis, abdomen, lung, and liver.

### PROGNOSIS

Overall, the 5-year survival rate is 92%; even among those who have advanced disease at diagnosis, 5-year survival is almost 70%. Because advances in treatment have afforded an excellent prognosis, it is unknown what effect preventive measures have on mortality.

## HYDROCELE

### ETIOLOGY

A hydrocele is a collection of fluid between the parietal and visceral layers of the tunica vaginalis, which lies along the anterior surface of the testicle and is a remnant of the processus vaginalis—the embryonic sleeve through which the testes descend. If the processus vaginalis remains fully open, an inguinal hernia will result. If a small opening remains, a hydrocele will form in the scrotum. If an opening remains proximally but is closed distally before the scrotum, a hydrocele of the spermatic cord will form.

### DIAGNOSIS

A hydrocele is usually a soft, painless, fluctuant, scrotal mass that is anterior to the testis, transilluminates, and appears cystic on ultrasonography. Hydroceles often decrease in size by morning and increase in size by evening. Longstanding hydroceles are usually benign. The presence of a new hydrocele should alert the examiner to check for a possible underlying cause for a reactive hydrocele, such as a hernia, testicular tumor, trauma, or infection.

### THERAPY

Usually no therapy is required for an asymptomatic longstanding hydrocele. If a hydrocele is reactive to an underlying cause, treatment of the underlying etiology will lead to resolution of the hydrocele. Indications for treatment include a painful or tense hydrocele that might reduce circulation to the testis, a bulky mass that is uncomfortable for the teenager, or a hydrocele associated with a hernia (a communicating hydrocele). Definitive therapy involves resection of the parietal tunica vaginalis.

## PAINFUL MASSES/GENITAL COMPLAINTS

Painful genital complaints have a unique set of causes that are different from painless genital complaints. This section reviews diagnoses that present with pain as a prominent symptom.

### TESTICULAR TORSION

#### Etiology

Testicular torsion is a twisting of the testis and spermatic cord that results in venous obstruction, progressive edema, arterial compromise, and, eventually, testicular infarction. Normally the testes are covered anteriorly with a mesothelial structure, the tunica vaginalis. In some males, the tunica vaginalis is abnormally enlarged and engulfs the testes. This causes the testis to lie like a "bell clapper" in the scrotal cavity. With this deformity, a testis can twist on the spermatic cord, compromising circulation. Aside from torsion at the spermatic cord, appendages of the testes or of the epididymis can occasionally undergo torsion. Torsion can be difficult to differentiate from epididymitis (Table 68-1).

#### Epidemiology

Two-thirds of cases of testicular torsion occur in patients between 12 and 18 years of age, with incidence in the United States peaking at 15 to 16 years. The incidence of torsion is approximately 1 in 4,000, but varies according to age, geographic location, ethnicity, and other factors, and the risk of developing torsion by age 25 may be as high as 1 in 160, higher than the risk of testicular cancer.[8,9]

**Table 68-1**

**Differentiating Torsion from Epididymitis**

| *Symptoms and other findings* | *Torsion* | *Epididymitis* |
|---|---|---|
| Pain | Severe | Moderate or severe |
| Onset | Sudden/abrupt | Hours to days |
| Prior episodes | 50% of cases | Usually not |
| Nausea or vomiting | Frequent | Less frequent |
| Time to presentation | Short (<24 hours) | Longer (>24 hours) |
| Cremasteric reflex | Usually absent | Usually present |
| Epididymal abnormality | Obscured or anterior | Palpable and tender |
| Prehn sign | Absent: No relief of or increase in pain with elevation of the scrotum | Present: Pain relief with elevation of the scrotum |
| Urethral symptoms | Absent | May have dysuria, discharge |
| Urethral gram stain | Negative | May be positive for gram-negative intracellular diplococci or white cells |
| Urinalysis | Usually negative | First-catch urine positive for white blood cells and/or leukocyte esterase |

### Clinical Manifestations

The onset of testicular torsion is usually abrupt, and 50% of teenagers with torsion will report a brief prior episode of scrotal pain. Pain may be isolated to the scrotum or radiate to the abdomen, and is characteristically severe. The patient may be in extremis, and nausea and/or vomiting may occur.

Physical examination of a patient with a torsed testis reveals an exquisitely tender and swollen hemiscrotum. The affected side is often higher than the contralateral side because of the elevation from the twisted spermatic cord. The testis that undergoes torsion usually twists so that the anterior portion turns medially. In inflammatory conditions the affected side is often lower. The epididymis, if palpable, is often out of the usual posterolateral location. The affected testis and often the contralateral testis lie in a horizontal plane rather than in the normal vertical plane. The cremasteric reflex is absent. Fever and scrotal redness are not usually present.

### Diagnosis

Testicular torsion is a surgical emergency. The diagnosis of torsion should be suspected in any adolescent with a painful swelling of the scrotum. If the history (acute onset of pain, nausea, or vomiting, prior episodes of pain, lack of fever, lack of dysuria or urethral discharge) and physical examination (patient in distress, high-riding testis, horizontal position of testis, generalized swelling of the testis) are consistent with torsion, a urology consultation should be immediately obtained and decisions made for further testing or direct surgical exploration.

### Therapy

Therapy involves immediate surgery. Saving testicular function depends on early surgical intervention. If surgery is performed within 6 hours after symptoms begin, recovery is the rule; if surgery is performed between 6 and 12 hours, 62% of patients have recovery of testicular function. After 12 hours, the success rate falls to 20% to 38%, and after 24 hours, only up to 11% of testicles survive.

## TORSION OF TESTICULAR APPENDICES

Torsion of an intrascrotal appendage most often affects early adolescents, and in contrast to testicular torsion, has a good prognosis and rarely results in significant sequelae. Four intrascrotal appendages are described, but only the appendix testis and appendix epididymis are significantly prone to torsion.

Ninety-two percent of men have an appendix testis, a remnant of the Müellerian duct, located on the upper pole of the testis or in the cleft between the testis and the epididymis. It accounts for 90% of torsive appendages. Thirty-four percent of men have an appendix epididymis, a remnant of the Wolffian duct, located at the head of the epididymis. It accounts for 7% of appendage torsion. The incidence of torsion of an appendage peaks between 10 and 14 years of age, and the right and left sides are affected equally.

Usually, an early adolescent will present with subacute scrotal pain that localizes in the area of torsion. On examination, a tender mass may be palpated. The "blue dot" sign when present on examination signifies a gangrenous appendix, and may be found with transillumination or when the scrotal skin is stretched taut. Reactive hydrocele and significant erythema and edema occur as the torsion progresses, so the examination may be difficult with later presentation of disease. White blood cell count and urinalysis are unremarkable, and further studies are not required, although a testicular ultrasound may assist if the diagnosis is in doubt. Often, with urologic consultation, the affected appendage may be left to autoamputate. Some urologists advocate surgical removal. Adjunctive treatment consists of analgesics and bed rest until the pain subsides after a few days.

## EPIDIDYMITIS

### Etiology

Epididymitis is an inflammation of the epididymis caused by infection or trauma; it is primarily a problem of sexually active adolescents and is usually caused by *Chlamydia trachomatis* or *Neisseria gonorrhoeae.* Epididymitis by *Escherichia coli* or other bowel flora can be secondary to unprotected insertive anal intercourse. Uncommonly, it can be caused by urinary pathogens in males with or without genitourinary abnormalities. Nonsexually transmitted epididymitis may be caused by instrumentation, surgery, catheterization, or anatomical abnormalities. Epididymitis can be difficult to differentiate from torsion (Table 68-1).

### Diagnosis

The diagnosis is suggested by the presentation of a sexually active teenager with subacute onset of pain in the hemiscrotum, inguinal area, or abdomen with epididymal swelling and tenderness, a reactive hydrocele, urethral discharge, dysuria, and possibly fevers. Approximately two-thirds of individuals see a physician after 24 hours of pain—later than those who have testicular torsion. Swelling of the epididymis alone is more common with epididymitis than with torsion of the testes (59% vs 15%). The Centers for Disease Control and Prevention (CDC)[10] recommends one or more of the following laboratory examinations to assist with diagnosis.

- Gram staining of an endourethral swab specimen for diagnosis of urethritis and for presumptive diagnosis of gonococcal infection
- A culture of intraurethral exudates or a nucleic acid amplification test on an intraurethral swab or urine for *N gonorrhoeae* and *C trachomatis*
- Examination of first void urine for leukocytes if the urethral gram stain is negative, then sent for gram stain and culture

In addition, syphilis serology and HIV counseling and testing should be performed. In the absence of a urethral discharge, leukocytes on a gram-stained endourethral swab specimen (on microscopy) or urine dip for leukocyte esterase, or pyuria, an urgent urology consultation is called for as the likelihood of torsion increases. If any of the preceding tests shows abnormal findings and the teen has any risk factors suggesting torsion (ie, prepubertal teen, nonsexually active teen, elevated or rotated testes, history of prior pain episodes, or acute onset with rapid progression), an immediate urology consultation should be obtained and a nuclear scan or a color flow Doppler ultrasound should be considered. Orchitis can cause similar symptoms, but it usually occurs without dysuria or urethral discharge. Mumps infection is the most common cause. Mumps orchitis is usually unilateral and occasionally occurs without a history of parotitis. Other viruses (eg, adenovirus, Coxsackie virus, ECHO virus, Epstein-Barr virus) may also cause orchitis, but with less frequency.

### Therapy for Sexually Transmitted Infections

The 2010 sexually transmitted infection (STI) treatment guidelines for Sexually Transmitted Infections are available from the CDC at www.cdc.gov/std/treatment/2010/default.htm. Scrotal support, bed rest, and analgesics are an adjunct to antimicrobial therapy. Ceftriaxone, 250 mg, is given intramuscularly once, and doxycycline, 100 mg, is given orally twice a day for 10 days. If the problem is thought to be caused by enteric organisms or the patient is allergic to ceftriaxone or tetracyclines, alternative drugs are ofloxacin, 300 mg twice daily for 10 days, or levofloxacin, 500 mg orally once a day for 10 days. Failure to improve within 3 days requires re-evaluation. Sexual partners should be treated. In HIV/AIDS infection or for other immunocompromised states, therapy is the same except that fungal and mycobacterial infections are more common than in immunocompetent patients.

## PROSTATITIS

Prostatitis is an unusual condition in the adolescent. When present, the adolescent is uncharacteristically ill and complains of generalized groin or perineal pain with urinary symptoms, lower abdominal pain, and an edematous and tender prostate. Acute prostatitis in the adolescent is likely associated with an infectious process that creates an inflammatory condition in the prostate gland. Organisms may reach the prostate by means of reflux of infected urine, or by lymphogenous or hematogenic spread. Risk factors for acute prostatitis may include trauma, including cycling or horseback riding, dehydration, and sexual abstinence, but well-controlled studies are lacking. Prostatitis can also occur in patients with chronic indwelling bladder catheters and in those who perform intermittent catheterization. Although often assumed to be an STI, only minimal evidence links its etiology to *C trachomatis* or *N gonorrhoeae.* It is more likely caused by other pathogens such as *U urealyticum* and coliform bacteria such as *E coli*.

Characteristic signs of acute bacterial prostatitis may include pain in the groin, penis, scrotum, suprapubic area, perineum, or back. Pain exacerbated by ejaculation and hematospermia are consistent with this condition. Bladder symptoms such as hesitation, dribbling, increased frequency, dysuria, or even anuria may point to prostate inflammation, as may hematuria, cloudy urine, or hematospermia. Acute prostatitis often causes systemic symptoms such as fever, chills, and malaise. Although the clinical features of prostate infection can mimic urinary tract infection, isolated acute cystitis does not occur commonly in adolescent and young adult men, in whom virtually all lower urinary tract infections are caused by prostatitis or urinary instrumentation.

A typical clinical history combined with the finding of an edematous and tender prostate on physical examination should lead to a presumptive diagnosis of acute prostatitis. Empiric treatment is often successful, as antibiotic penetration of the acutely inflamed prostate gland is excellent.[11,12] Outpatient antibiotic therapy can be chosen based on urine gram stain results.

In the context of recalcitrant or chronic symptoms, a more laborious and invasive segmental culture technique may be performed that involves collection of 4 specimens: a first-void 10-mL sample, a midstream urine, prostatic secretions during prostatic massage, and a first-void 10-mL urine sample after prostatic massage. The etiology of these chronic conditions in the young adult is not well understood.

### PRIAPISM

Priapism is an unwanted painful erection. If it is prolonged, that is, lasts longer than 3 hours, it is a potential surgical emergency, requiring evaluation by a urologist. Among adolescents, priapism is most commonly encountered with sickle cell disease patients, where it may affect 6% to 40% of males with this disease, with bimodal peak frequencies in early adolescence (before age 14) and late adolescence (age 21–29).[13] It is associated with signs of increased hemolysis, decreasing the availability of nitric oxide, which then interferes with erectile function. Sickle cell disease patients who experience recurrent priapism may develop abnormal nocturnal penile tumescence and fibrotic corpora that can lead to impotence. Priapism in adolescents with normal erectile function may also occur secondary to medication abuse, specifically the widely advertised phosphodiesterase-5 inhibitors. Treatment of priapism should occur with the assistance of a urologist and is based on the classification of priapism as ischemic or nonischemic. Ischemic priapism impedes blood flow to the penis and so must be treated emergently. Options for treatment include therapeutic aspiration, intracavernous injection of sympathomimetics such as phenylephrine, epinephrine, norepinephrine or metaraminol, and surgical shunts. In addition, systemic treatment of underlying disease, such as sickle cell disease, must be undertaken. In the case of nonischemic priapism, initial observation followed by invasive arterial embolization or surgery if warranted is a reasonable approach. For individuals who have recurrent priapism, gonadotropin-releasing hormone agonists or antiandrogens may be warranted, as may intercavernosal self-injections of phenylephrine.

### URETHRITIS

Urethritis in the male adolescent is most commonly the result of STI with gonorrhea or chlamydia trachomatis. A full discussion of this condition can be found in Chapter 53, Sexually Transmitted Infections. Urinary tract infection is uncommon in adolescent males unless there is a history of instrumentation of the urethra through catheterization or surgical intervention, and in the case of congenital urogenital anomalies.

## MALE REPRODUCTIVE HEALTH CONCERNS

Male reproductive health concerns are most likely to present in the older adolescent. This section briefly reviews the topics of infertility, erectile dysfunction, and premature ejaculation.

### INFERTILITY

For providers who practice in communities where family rearing characteristically begins in late adolescence or young adulthood, concerns regarding male fertility may present regularly to the adolescent health care practitioner. Infertility may be due to problems with the male, female, or both. Twenty percent to 30% of cases of infertility may be attributed to the male alone. Another 20% of cases of infertility will have male factors in association with female factors. In addition to decreased production or function of sperm, sexual ignorance and lack of sexuality education must also be considered in the evaluation of adolescent couples. Fertility complications of varicocele are described in the previous section on varicocele.

Evaluation of an infertility complaint in the adolescent male is straightforward. A complete sexual history should be obtained to assess the couple's understanding of fertility and to determine if the type, frequency, and logistics of the sexual act are consistent with the goal of pregnancy. An adolescent couple should not be considered possibly infertile until they have been unable to achieve pregnancy after one year of unprotected intercourse. Past medical history should include history of prior fertility, cryptorchidism, childhood illnesses such as mumps or other orchitis, prior testicular torsion, childhood cancer, or trauma. Prior surgery such as inguinal hernia repair, varicocelectomy, repaired hypospadias, urologic, or renal surgery should be reviewed. Review of pubertal milestones is important. Precocious puberty may suggest the presence of an adrenal-genital syndrome, and delayed puberty may indicate hypogonadism. A complete medication history should be performed to include history of anabolic steroids, cimetidine, spironolactone, sulfasalazine, and others that may affect sperm production or motility. A history of alcohol and illicit drug use may be implicated in a decreased sperm count or hormonal abnormalities. A current history of environmental exposures should also be performed including recurrent trauma (cycling, horseback riding), excessive heat, environmental toxins, and radiation.

Physical examination should include assessment of visual fields to rule out pituitary disease, neck examination to rule out thyromegaly, and a check for gynecomastia that may suggest a feminizing state. Particular focus should be on evaluation for signs of hypogonadism (underdeveloped secondary sexual characteristics, eunuchoid body habitus, sparse axillary, pubic, and facial hair in conjunction with lack of temporal hair recession) as well as a complete genital examination looking for any abnormalities of the penis, scrotum, or epididymis, as well as to ensure fully developed testes (normal adult testes are 4.5 cm long and 2.5 cm wide with a mean volume of 20 cc).

Testing should include 2 semen analyses done 1 month apart if possible. If a low sperm count is found, or if the history or physical examination suggest signs of endocrine disease, then measurement of follicle-stimulating hormone (FSH) and testosterone are indicated. In addition, luteinizing hormone (LH) and prolactin are commonly measured. In the context of severe oligospermia (sperm counts of <5 million to 10 million per ejaculate) or nonobstructive azoospermia (absence of sperm in semen, not due to blockage), genetic testing is also indicated, as karyotype abnormalities as well as microdeletions of the Y chromosome are most commonly found in this group.

## ERECTILE DYSFUNCTION

Erectile dysfunction causes great distress in the young adult and, in this age group, it is usually psychological in nature or related to medication or substance use. The topic of erectile dysfunction is explored fully in Chapter 57, Sexual Dysfunction.

Although it is rare for an organic cause of erectile dysfunction to be present in adolescence, the possibility should not be overlooked. Physical causes of erectile dysfunction include physical injury, including prior surgery to the genital area, neurologic disease (eg, multiple sclerosis), poorly controlled diabetes, as a side effect from medications, and chronic alcohol, marijuana, heroin, or cocaine abuse. A thorough medication history is necessary in the evaluation of sexual dysfunction, as multiple medications may cause sexual adverse effects. Commonly used medications that should be asked about include: spironolactone, which inhibits testosterone, thiazide diuretics, medications that are sympathetic blockers like clonidine or methyldopa, antidepressants including selective serotonin reuptake inhibitors; ketoconazole, and cimetidine. Erectile dysfunction can be associated with multiple psychological stressors including depression, stress, generalized and sexual performance anxiety, as well as presenting as a clue to the presence of more significant problems within a relationship.

Radical prostatectomy and genital tract trauma cause a sudden loss of male sexual function. Absent history of such trauma, a patient who presents with acute onset of sexual dysfunction (ie, normal function, then sudden lack of performance) invariably is suffering from psychogenic impotence. In this setting, psychological counseling is the appropriate therapy.

A physical examination with specific attention to clues suggesting possible organic causes of dysfunction consists of the following: femoral and peripheral pulses should be evaluated, as abnormal pulses may suggest a vascular cause for impotence. A femoral bruit may indicate pelvic blood occlusion. A visual field exam should be performed to rule out defects that may be present in hypogonadal men with pituitary tumors. The presence of gynecomastia suggests Klinefelter syndrome, illicit drug use, or testicular tumor. A genital exam should look for penile strictures, testicular atrophy, asymmetry, or masses that may suggest testosterone abnormalities. A normal cremasteric reflex, elicited by stroking the inner thigh and observing for elevation of the ipsilateral testicle, assures integrity of the thoracolumbar erection center at T-11 to L-2.

If the history or physical examination suggests a possible organic cause for dysfunction, testing should include hormonal testing (serum testosterone, LH, FSH, prolactin, and thyroid function tests) as well as nocturnal penile tumescence testing. Treatment is then tailored according to the cause of dysfunction.

## PREMATURE EJACULATION

Premature ejaculation from the point of view of the adolescent is ejaculation occurring before he wishes. Clinically, premature ejaculation is defined in the context of a relationship as a failure to maintain intromission of sufficient duration to satisfy a responsive partner. Ejaculatory control is an acquired behavior that is minimal in adolescence and increases with experience. The most common reason for premature ejaculation in the adolescent is sexual inexperience that interferes with the ability to acquire the learned behavior of delaying ejaculation. In this context, the adolescent complaint of premature ejaculation is usually a normal biologic response.

Although the biology of the sexual act is straightforward, feelings of adolescent sexuality are often underexplored. Ambiguous or negative feelings toward the appropriateness of the sexual act, fear of discovery, fear of causing pregnancy, fear of contraction of a sexually transmitted disease, anxiety over performance, and depression all may contribute to premature ejaculation. It is extremely rare for a physical cause to be present, although prostatitis and genital nerve trauma or surgery, as well as medications, may be involved.

Treatment should include a history that reviews any signs of chronic illness, prior trauma, or surgery that may affect nerve pathways to the genitalia, as well as history reviewing feeling surrounding the sexual act. Usual therapy is an explanation of what causes premature ejaculation, and reassurance. Further discussion on this topic as well as treatments may be found in Chapter 57, Sexual Dysfunction.

## INTERNET RESOURCES FOR TEENS AND PARENTS

### EPIDIDYMITIS

- Medline Plus. Epididymitis. (www.nlm.nih.gov/medlineplus/ency/article/001279.htm)
- CDC. Sexually Transmitted Diseases Treatment Guidelines 2006: Epididymitis. (www.cdc.gov/std/treatment/2006/epididymitis.htm)

### TESTICULAR SELF-EXAM

- The Testicular Cancer Resource Center. How to Do a Testicular Examination. (tcrc.acor.org/tcexam.html)
- TeensHealth from Nemour. How to Perform a Testicular Self-Examination. (kidshealth.org/teen/sexual_health/guys/tse.html)

### TESTICULAR TORSION

- Rupp TJ, Zwanger M. Testicular torsion. eMedicine. (www.emedicine.com/emerg/topic573.htm)

### TESTICULAR CANCER

- National Cancer Institute. Testicular cancer. (www.cancer.gov/cancertopics/types/testicular/)

## REFERENCES


1. United Kingdom Testicular Cancer Study Group. Aetiology of testicular cancer: association with congenital abnormalities, age at puberty, infertility, and exercise. United Kingdom Testicular Cancer Study Group. *Br Med J.* 1994;308:1393–1399

2. Adelman WP, Joffe A. The adolescent male genital examination: what's normal and what's not. *Contemp Pediatr.* 1999;16:76–92

3. Gat Y, Zukerman Z, Bachar GN, et al. Adolescent varicocele: is it a unilateral disease? *Urology.* 2003;62:742–746

4. Adelman WP, Joffe A. Controversies in male adolescent health: varicocele, circumcision, and testicular self-examination. *Curr Opin Pediatr.* 2004;16:363–367

5. Kass EL, Reitelman C. Adolescent varicocele. *Urol Clin North Am.* 1995;22:151–159

6. Skoog SJ, Roberts KP, Goldstein M, et al. The adolescent varicocele: what's new with an old problem in young patients? *Pediatrics.* 1997;100:112–122

7. Guarino N, Tadini B, Bianchi M. The adolescent varicocele: the crucial role of hormonal tests in selecting patients with testicular dysfunction. *J Pediatr Surg.* 2003,38:120–123

8. Livne PM, Sivan B, Karmazyn B, Ben Meir D. Testicular torsion in the pediatric age group: diagnosis and treatment. *Pediatr Endocrinol Rev.* 2003;1 (2):128–133

9. Mansbach JM, Forbes P, Peters C. Testicular torsion and risk factors for orchiectomy. *Arch Pediatr Adolesc Med.* 2005;159:1167–1171

10. Centers for Disease Control and Prevention. Sexually transmitted diseases treatment guidelines 2010. *MMWR.* 2010;59 (No. RR-12)

11. Aagaard J, Madsen PO. Bacterial prostatitis: new methods of treatment. *Urology.* 1991;37 (suppl 3):4–8

12. Adelman WP, Joffe A. Genitourinary issues in the male college student: a case-based approach. *Pediatr Clin N Am.* 2005;52:199–216

13. Hamre MR, Harmon EP, Kirkpatrick DV, et al. Priapism as a complication of sickle cell disease. *J Urol.* 1991;145:1-5

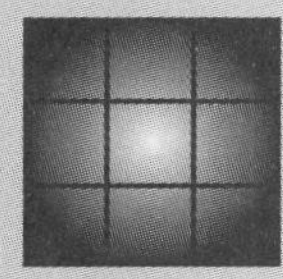

# Part 3

# Medical and Surgical Disorders

SECTION 1

# The Endocrine System

## CHAPTER 69

## Growth Disorders

GRAEME R. FRANK, MD

Multiple systemic disorders may impair linear growth and the resultant growth failure, recognized when the adolescent crosses percentiles on the growth chart, provides an important clue to an underlying abnormality. However, in the peripubertal age crossing height percentiles on the growth chart is frequently a variation of normal growth. Therefore, a clear understanding of pubertal growth and pubertal growth disorders is essential so that variations of normal growth can be readily distinguished from abnormal growth patterns that warrant a careful evaluation.

### GROWTH ASSESSMENT

Anthropomorphic measurements plotted on appropriate growth charts allow the health care provider to gain valuable insight into the adolescent's growth. Height and growth rate should be interpreted in relation to the pubertal stage of the individual, and if deemed to be abnormal a careful search is indicated for an underlying abnormality.

#### MEASUREMENTS

##### Height

Accurate height measurements are best obtained using a wall-mounted stadiometer. The subject should be standing with heels and back in contact with an upright wall. The head should be positioned in the "Frankfurt plane" (ie, an imaginary line drawn from the lower borders of the orbit to the external auditory meatus should be parallel to the ground). In the absence of a wall-mounted stadiometer, a right-angled block can be used to read a wall-mounted scale.

##### Growth Velocity

Growth velocity is expressed in centimeters per year, obtained from two readings 1 year apart. Annualized growth velocity can be calculated from two height measurements less than 1 year apart. However, because there is a seasonal variation in growth rate, with greater growth in spring and summer, a minimum of 4 to 6 months between height measurements is necessary to obtain an annualized height velocity of clinical value. Interpretation of growth rate should be done in relation to both chronological age and pubertal stage.

#### GROWTH CHARTS

The most widely available and commonly used growth charts are derived from cross-sectional growth data from the National Center for Health Statistics (NCHS). (See Chapter 9, Physical Examination and Laboratory Screening.) They are also available for free download from the Centers for Disease Control and Prevention (CDC) Web site at www.cdc.gov/growthcharts.

Although cross-sectional growth charts are useful for tracking growth during childhood (when there is little variability between the growth rates of children of similar height), one should be aware of the limitations of these charts for adolescents, in whom the timing of puberty may vary considerably. Longitudinal growth charts were therefore developed by Tanner and colleagues.[1] These allow better interpretation of growth of adolescents with varying timing of puberty.

#### BODY PROPORTIONS

##### Upper Segment/Lower Segment Ratio

To calculate the upper to lower (U/L) segment ratio, first the lower segment (symphysis pubis to floor) is measured. The upper segment is then calculated by subtracting the lower segment measurement from the standing height. In most adolescents, the U/L segment ratio is close to 1. Racial differences exist, and it should be noted that blacks are relatively long-limbed compared to Caucasians and have U/L segment ratios of approximately 0.90 after puberty.

#### Sitting Height, Subischial Leg Length, and Arm Span

Another measurement of body proportions is the sitting height (easily measured by an individual sitting on a box and then subtracting the height of the box). Subtracting the sitting height from the standing height gives the subischial leg length. Measurement of limb growth (lower segment or subischial leg length) may be more appropriate for evaluating the growth of adolescents who have undergone spinal irradiation, which impairs normal spinal growth.

Arm span is the measurement from fingertip to fingertip with the arms held at shoulder level parallel to the ground. In adolescents, the height and arm span normally are within 5 cm of each other.

Body proportion measurement may provide insight into an underlying growth disorder. Adolescents with Marfan syndrome and hypogonadal patients have increased limb length relative to the spine and therefore low U/L segment ratios (also referred to as eunuchoid proportions). Many patients with chondrodystrophies have relatively short limbs and increased U/L segment ratios.

### BONE AGE AND PREDICTED ADULT HEIGHT

An x-ray of the left hand and wrist helps determine degree of skeletal maturation. Radiographs are compared to age- and sex-matched standards to obtain the bone age.[2] The bone age can be used for the following:

- Descriptive purposes: One can plot the patient's current height according to bone age (in addition to chronologic age); the discrepancy between these measurements provides useful information regarding future growth potential.
- Predictive purposes: One can calculate the predicted adult height. In general, height prediction accuracy improves at older bone ages. It should be noted, however, that the various methods of calculating predicted adult height are based on data from normal children and are not accurate for adolescents with growth disorders.

### TARGET HEIGHT

Growth evaluation should factor in the genetic potential of the individual. Because the difference in height between men and women is approximately 13 cm, the midparental target height is determined by the equation:

- Target height in males = (height of father + [height of mother + 13 cm]) /2
- Target height in females = (height of mother + [height of father − 13 cm]) /2
- One standard deviation is ± 5 cm

## ENDOCRINE REGULATION OF GROWTH

Major hormones involved in the growth of the adolescent include growth hormone, thyroid hormone, and the sex steroids.

### GROWTH HORMONE, IGF-I, AND IGFBP3

Growth hormone (GH) is released from the pituitary in a pulsatile manner under the influence of a stimulating hormone, GH-releasing hormone (GHRH), and an inhibitory hormone, somatostatin. Ghrelin, a recently described gut hormone produced in the stomach, also stimulates GH release synergistically with GHRH.

Insulin-like growth factor-I (IGF-I), formerly known as somatomedin C, is a GH dependent protein that mediates many of the growth-promoting effects of GH. Most of the circulating GH is secreted from the liver and has classic endocrine actions. However, IGF-I is also produced by other cells (ie, chondrocytes), where it acts locally. During puberty, there is a marked rise in IGF-I levels as a result of sex steroid production, which increases the release of GH. The levels of IGF-I therefore correlate better with pubertal stage than with chronological age.

IGF-binding protein 3 (IGFBP3) is a member of the family of IGF binding proteins that modulate the action of the IGFs. Most of the IGF-I in the serum circulates in a ternary complex consisting of IGF-I, IGFBP3, and a protein called the acid-labile subunit.[3] Because IGFBP3 is also regulated by GH, IGFBP3 together with IGF-I can be used as biochemical tests to screen for GH deficiency.

### THYROID HORMONE

Thyroid hormone is critical for normal growth throughout childhood and adolescence. Thyroid hormone has direct effects on growth at the level of the growth plate. In addition, thyroid hormone is necessary for normal pituitary GH release. Untreated hypothyroidism results in profound growth failure as well as the arrest of skeletal maturation.

### SEX STEROIDS

Sex steroid production during puberty is responsible for the pubertal growth spurt that contributes approximately 18% of final adult stature. The mechanism by which the sex steroids promote growth is both direct at the level of the growth plate and indirect by increasing endogenous GH secretion. The sex steroids also promote skeletal maturation that, once complete, causes cessation of linear growth.

Recent evidence demonstrates that estrogen is essential for normal pubertal growth and epiphyseal maturation in the male as well as the female.

## SHORT STATURE AND GROWTH FAILURE

Short stature is a descriptive term generally defined as a height greater than 2 standard deviations below the mean. It follows, therefore, that 2.3% of the normal population can be defined as having short stature. Growth failure describes a subnormal growth velocity that over time results in a falling height percentile.

### CAUSES OF SHORT STATURE

#### Normal Variant Short Stature

The 2 normal variants of short stature are familial short stature and constitutional delay of growth and puberty.

***Familial Short Stature.*** There is great variation in stature among ethnic groups and also within the same ethnic group. When evaluating a child with short stature, careful attention should be paid to family background. In familial short stature, the growth velocity is normal, the bone age is not delayed, the height percentile remains stable, and the predicted adult height is appropriate for the target height.

***Constitutional Delay of Growth and Puberty (CDGP).*** In those with CDGP, there is a gradual decline in growth velocity throughout childhood, which reaches a nadir just prior to the growth acceleration that accompanies puberty. The greater the pubertal delay, the slower the growth rate will be. The increasing height discrepancy between the adolescent with pubertal delay and his or her peers becomes noticeable on the growth chart, especially when using the NCHS charts derived from cross-sectional data. It is this apparent growth failure relative to peers that frequently prompts referral for a growth evaluation. The features of CDGP are listed in Box 69-1.

**Box 69-1**

***Features of Constitutional Delay of Growth and Puberty (CDGP)***

- Short stature with a height that is ≤ 2 SD for chronological age or target height
- Growth velocity below 10th percentile for chronological age
- Delayed bone age
- No evidence of systemic illness, genetic syndrome, or endocrine disorder
- Pubertal onset at an age greater than +2 SD of average maturers (>14 years in boys and >13 years in girls)

Constitutional delay of growth and puberty is noted to be approximately 5 times more common in boys than girls. This apparent male predominance, however, may be the result of an ascertainment bias. Girls begin puberty earlier than boys, and the growth spurt in females is an early pubertal event in contrast to a late pubertal event in males. Therefore, even when a female has pubertal delay, she will not have to wait as long as a male for pubertal growth acceleration. In addition, social attitudes may result in more psychosocial problems for boys with short stature than for girls, and therefore prompt more growth consultations in males. It is also possible, however, that the frequency distribution of timing of the onset of puberty is skewed to the right in males (ie, CDGP more common) and skewed to the left in females (ie, idiopathic precocious puberty more common), which is consistent with the clinical experience reported by pediatric endocrinologists generally.

The exact etiology of CDGP is unknown. However, there is a continuum of normal GH secretion that contributes to the population variance in growth and maturation.[4] It appears that those with the lowest levels of GH secretion manifest CDGP. Many children with CDGP have been found to have subnormal levels of spontaneous GH release[5] and/or a subnormal response to provocative stimuli.[6] When spontaneous puberty occurs, GH secretion and IGF-I levels increase. Therefore, it is not surprising that GH therapy has been shown to result in an acceleration of the growth rate in CDGP.[7]

Although CDGP is a normal variant of growth, there are consequences for adult height and body proportions because of the manner in which late childhood and early pubertal growth progresses. When the pubertal growth spurt occurs in patients with CDGP, its duration and the peak height velocity achieved are both reduced; consequently, total pubertal height gain is reduced. If this were counterbalanced by an increased prepubertal height gain, final height would not be compromised. However, during late prepuberty or early puberty, height gain is mainly the result of growth in the lower segment, and spinal growth is relatively stunted. As a result, if puberty is delayed spinal growth is more compromised, so that when growth acceleration occurs, body disproportion is already recognized. During the pubertal growth spurt, spinal growth does not seem to compensate for the previous deficit. At final height, eunuchoid proportions are still present in most patients.[8–9] This likely explains the 2.3 to 6.5 cm height deficits (target height vs final height) found in adult females and males, respectively, who had CDGP during childhood and adolescence. (For the diagnosis of CDGP, see the following section on Evaluation of Short Stature, Differential Diagnosis; for treatment of CDGP, see the following section on Androgen Therapy.)

Constitutional delay of growth and puberty also has psychological consequences, as poor self-esteem and social withdrawal have been described in some patients with CDGP.[10–12] In addition, lower teacher ratings and lower scores on the Wechsler Intelligence Scales have been described in some boys with CDGP.[13] The negative impact of CDGP on self-esteem and psychosocial achievement may persist into adulthood.[10,14] It is not clear whether the psychological impact on children with CDGP results from short stature, delayed sexual development, or both.

### Endocrine Causes of Growth Failure

***Hypothyroidism.*** Thyroid hormone is essential for normal linear growth. Consequently, untreated hypothyroidism that occurs during years of active linear growth is associated with growth failure. When hypothyroidism occurs in children, there is generally a delay in bone age and in the onset of puberty; with thyroxine replacement therapy, catch-up growth occurs and adult height is normal. When hypothyroidism occurs during pubertal development, however, any delay in diagnosis may compromise final adult height because the growth failure of hypothyroidism may be associated with normal epiphyseal maturation and closure that occurs with advancing puberty. In the United States, acquired hypothyroidism that develops in adolescence generally is the result of autoimmune (Hashimoto) thyroiditis (see Chapter 72).

***Growth Hormone Deficiency.*** Growth hormone deficiency (GHD) may be congenital or acquired. In addition, GHD may be the only pituitary deficiency or may be part of multiple pituitary hormone deficiencies. Pituitary GHD has an incidence of at least 1 in 3,480 individuals.[15]

Congenital GHD may be the result of disruption of the GH axis from various congenital brain malformations. In addition, a small but significant proportion of congenital GHD has been found to be the result of genetic mutations. The anterior pituitary develops under the influence of several homeodomain transcription factors expressed at various stages of embryo development. Mutations in these transcription factors lead to a spectrum of pituitary abnormalities from selective hypopituitarism (ie, GH thyroid-stimulating hormone [TSH], and prolactin deficiency in PIT1 gene mutations)[16] to more complex disorders such as septo-optic dysplasia (optic nerve hypoplasia, absent septum pellucidum, and hypothalamic insufficiency) in HESX1 mutations.[17]

In addition, mutations in the GHRH receptor gene and the GH gene itself have been documented.[18]

Acquired GHD may be secondary to trauma, tumors, infections, cranial irradiation, or Langerhans cell histiocytosis. It may also be idiopathic (ie, no discernable cause). It is likely that in the future, a molecular basis for isolated GHD will be uncovered for many patients whose GHD is currently classified as idiopathic.

### Diagnosis of GHD

Generally, patients with GHD have subnormal linear growth for pubertal stage and delayed bone age. In severe GHD, the GH-dependent proteins (IGF-I and IGFBP3) are low. By traditional convention, the diagnosis of GHD requires failure on 2 provocative tests (eg, arginine, clonidine, levodopa, insulin, glucagon, propranolol) to optimize the specificity and predictive value.[19–20] A peak GH level of less than 10 ng/mL on two tests defines GHD. There are, however, several problems with traditional GH stimulation testing:

- There are few published age- or sex-specific normal ranges for commonly used GH tests; therefore, the upper limits used to define GHD are arbitrary.[21]
- The GH assays currently used have not been rigorously compared and can yield values that differ by up to threefold.[22]
- GH tests are not specific, that is, there is a high probability that there may be a subnormal GH test result in a hormonally normal individual. Although estrogen priming (treating the patient with estrogen for 2 to 3 days prior to the test) improves the specificity, there is no wide consensus on the use of estrogen-primed GH stimulation tests.
- GH tests are not sensitive in that they measure GH response to a nonphysiologic stimulus. There are instances where individuals do not have normal spontaneous GH secretion but are able to produce normal amounts of GH in response to a pharmacologic stimulus (neurosecretory GHD).

For the previous reasons, some have suggested that GH testing should no longer be used and that the severity of the growth impairment should guide therapy. However, the use of GH testing in combination with IGF-I and IGFBP3 levels might aid in the identification of children whose growth failure is secondary to defects downstream of GH and who may benefit from IGF-I therapy (see the following).

Given the shortcomings of GH stimulation tests, if an adolescent has a clinical picture consistent with GHD (growth failure of unknown etiology, low IGF-I and/or IGFPB3) but a normal response to provocative testing, a trial of GH therapy may be warranted.[23–24]

Whenever the diagnosis of GHD is made, imaging of the hypothalamic/pituitary region is indicated and assessment of other pituitary hormones is recommended because GHD may have an organic etiology and may be a part of multiple pituitary hormone deficiencies.

***Hypogonadism.*** Hypogonadism may be central (hypogonadotropic hypogonadism) or a result of primary gonadal failure (hypergonadotropic hypogonadism). In the absence of puberty, individuals will not have a growth spurt and therefore will have growth failure in their adolescent years. Initially, an adolescent with hypogonadism may look indistinguishable from an adolescent with CDGP.

***Cushing Syndrome.*** Supraphysiological amounts of glucocorticoid have a profound growth-stunting effect. The most common cause of Cushing syndrome in adolescents is iatrogenic, secondary to large anti-inflammatory doses of glucocorticoids used to treat a variety of inflammatory, immunologic, or rheumatologic disorders. Rarer causes of Cushing syndrome include hypersecretion of adrenocorticotropic hormone and adrenal tumors. Clinical features include truncal obesity, thin extremities due to decreased muscle mass, striae, thin skin, and growth failure. Adrenal tumors may secrete androgens that may partially obscure the growth-inhibiting effect of glucocorticoids.

***Pseudohypoparathyroidism.*** Classically, this condition is characterized by growth failure, round facies, mental retardation, truncal obesity, short fourth metacarpals, and subcutaneous ossification, along with biochemical evidence of hypoparathyroidism (low calcium and high phosphorus) despite normal or elevated levels of parathyroid hormone. It is caused by an inactivating mutation in the stimulatory G proteins involved in signal transduction.

***GH Insensitivity Syndrome.*** GH insensitivity syndrome (GHIS) encompasses a variety of conditions in which the action of GH is completely or partially absent. Primary GHIS, also known as Laron syndrome, is a hereditary defect caused by a mutation in the GH receptor. Affected patients present with marked short stature secondary to severe growth failure, physical features of severe GHD, and low serum concentrations of IGF-I despite high serum GH concentrations. Other novel mutations also may result in GH insensitivity. These include mutations in the IGF-I gene and IGF-1 receptor[18] and in the gene for signal transduction and activation of transcription-5b (STAT5b), a transcription factor involved in the GH receptor signal transduction pathway.[25]

Secondary or acquired GHIS can occur when a child with GHD caused by a deletion in the GH gene is treated with GH and develops antibodies to GH resulting in an attenuated growth response.

### Skeletal Dysplasias

Skeletal dysplasias are a heterogeneous group of a large number of inherited disorders characterized by abnormalities in cartilage and bone growth. This results in an abnormal shape and size of the skeleton and disproportion of the long bones (rhizomelia), spine, and head. These conditions were originally described by their clinical manifestations, radiographic findings, inheritance patterns, and morphology of the growth plate. More recently, the classification has been rearranged on the basis of genetics or the protein defect involved.

Achondroplasia is the most common skeletal dysplasia, occurring with a frequency of approximately 1 in 26,000. Hypochondroplasia is a milder form (short stature and rhizomelia are less prominent). Both are autosomal dominant and involve a mutation on the fibroblast growth factor receptor 3 gene. In general, management of skeletal dysplasias revolves around treatment to prevent or minimize medical complications, psychosocial support for the patients and their families, and education of the community with a view to modification of the environment where appropriate.

### Chromosomal/Genetic Abnormalities and Syndromes

Short stature is a cardinal feature of several chromosomal disorders such as Down syndrome and Turner syndrome. It is also a major feature of genetic disorders, for example, the SHOX gene mutation in the Leri-Weill syndrome. Finally, there are many syndromes associated with short stature, such as the Russell-Silver syndrome.

### Systemic Illness

***Malnutrition.*** Adequate nutrition is essential for normal linear growth. When there is significant malnutrition from starvation, malabsorption, or anorexia nervosa, a state of GH resistance develops (low IGF-I with increased GH secretion) that can result in growth failure.

***Chronic Disease.*** Several chronic disease states are associated with growth failure. The causes of growth failure may be due to malabsorption (cystic fibrosis, celiac disease, inflammatory bowel disease [IBD]), increased metabolic needs (cystic fibrosis), relative hypoxia (cyanotic congenital heart disease), the presence of inflammatory mediators (IBD, rheumatologic diseases), or medication related (chronic glucocorticoid exposure).

### Intrauterine Growth Retardation

Most children born small for gestational age as a result of intrauterine growth retardation (IUGR) exhibit catch-up growth in the first 2 years of life. However, approximately 10% of children with IUGR fail to exhibit this catch-up growth and remain very short. Growth hormone therapy has been shown to increase linear growth in these children and to result in significant improvements in final adult height.

**EVALUATION OF SHORT STATURE**

Taking a careful history of family heights, pregnancy and birth history, and a detailed past medical history (including medication history and prior growth data) are extremely important in evaluating the adolescent who presents with short stature with or without growth failure. If the growth is at a percentile inconsistent with that of siblings and parents, or if an adolescent presents with a falling height percentile, careful evaluation is warranted. It should be stressed, however, that when linear growth is followed on the NCHS growth charts, children with CDGP will appear to have significant growth failure beyond age 12 years in males and age 10 years in females. This is primarily the result of the adolescent with CDGP being compared (on the cross-sectional growth chart) to a group of adolescents who are mostly entering puberty and experiencing pubertal growth acceleration. Many conditions such as asthma, celiac disease, inflammatory bowel disease, chronic glucocorticoid use, and renal disease can mimic CDGP and should not be overlooked.[26] A careful physical examination should be performed to look for stigmata of Turner syndrome, signs of thyroid disease, visual field defects, funduscopic abnormalities, and skeletal disproportion. Pubertal status should be assessed and growth velocity calculated over a 4- to 6-month period.

The most common cause of growth failure in the adolescent is CDGP. When there is a family history of CDGP and the growth curve is characteristic, limited testing can be performed. Bone age alone (which provides an indication of residual growth potential) may be adequate. A TSH and IGF-I level (especially if considering androgen therapy) may be warranted. However, the presence of other symptoms (such as headaches), a borderline growth velocity, or incongruity in the pattern of pubertal development should raise suspicion and warrant further investigation. In addition to a bone age, other tests performed in this situation are listed in Table 69-1.

**Table 69-1**

**Evaluation of Unexplained Growth Failure/Short Stature**

| Laboratory Test | Condition |
|---|---|
| Thyroid function | Hypothyroidism |
| IGF-I and IGFBP3 | Growth hormone deficiency |
| CBC and ESR | Inflammatory bowel disease |
| Serum chemistries | Renal, metabolic, bone disease |
| Karyotype in females | Turner syndrome |
| Tissue transglutaminase and IgA | Celiac disease |

CBC, complete blood count; ESR, erythrocyte sedimentation rate

**DIFFERENTIAL DIAGNOSIS OF SHORT STATURE**

When evaluating a 14- to 15-year-old boy with short stature, pubertal delay, normal laboratory tests, and low gonadotropins, the most likely diagnosis is CDGP. However, 2 alternate conditions should be considered. First, hypogonadotropic hypogonadism might present with delayed or arrested puberty. It is extremely difficult to distinguish between CDGP and hypogonadotropic hypogonadism, and there is no single practical test that can adequately differentiate between patients with these conditions.[27] A history of micropenis, cryptorchidism, or anosmia would make the diagnosis of hypogonadotropic hypogonadism more probable and more obvious. Fortunately, the initial androgen therapy in these conditions is the same. Only in CDGP will enlargement of testicular volume and pubertal progression occur.

The second diagnostic consideration in the differential diagnosis in a short adolescent with delayed puberty is isolated GHD. Although identification of GHD before starting androgen therapy would be ideal, it appears that GHD in the setting of CDGP is frequently overdiagnosed.[28] Therefore, nonsex-steroid primed GH testing should be interpreted with caution in children with delayed puberty. This is especially true in obese subjects in whom GH secretion is reduced.[29] As a screening procedure, measurement of IGF-I and IGFBP3 might be adequate. If these levels are appropriate for Tanner stage, one might consider a short course of androgen therapy (low-dose intramuscular testosterone for 3 to 6 months). In this scenario, androgen therapy is both diagnostic and therapeutic. Doubling of the growth rate is seen in boys with CDGP but not with GHD, because much of the growth response to testosterone depends on enhanced GH secretion. Enlargement of the testicles indicates normal gonadotropin secretion. If the individual does not have a good growth response to testosterone or does not show testicular enlargement, this suggests GHD, gonadotropin deficiency, or both.[30-31] As puberty progresses in children with CDGP, there remains the normal relationship between the stages of puberty and the growth spurt. The absence of growth acceleration at a testicular volume of 10 mL would necessitate further investigation.[32]

## HORMONAL GROWTH-PROMOTING THERAPY

### Growth Hormone

***Deficiency.*** Growth hormone deficiency is the most common indication for which GH therapy is prescribed. The usual starting dose of GH is generally 0.18 to 0.3 mg/kg/week given by subcutaneous injection 6 to 7 days per week. The most robust growth response to GH therapy is in the first 2 years of treatment, and thereafter follows a progressively waning effect. Some endocrinologists keep the GH dose constant by making dose adjustments based on weight gain, whereas others use the growth rate to guide adjustments in dose. In general, GH therapy for growth promotion is discontinued when either the growth rate falls to below 2.5 cm per year or the bone age reaches 16 years in males or 14 years in females.

***GH Therapy in Non-GHD Patients.*** Recombinant human GH, which first became available in the mid-1980s, has been used for several conditions in which individuals are GH sufficient. The currently approved indications for GH therapy are listed in Box 69-2.

Use of GH therapy for idiopathic short stature (ISS) is controversial. Idiopathic short stature is a descriptive term that defines a subject who is more than 2.25 SD below the mean for age and sex or less than the 1.2 percentile, and whose final adult height is predicted to be less than 160 cm (5 feet 3 inches) in males or less than 150 cm (4 feet 11 inches) in females.

The fundamental issue underlying the controversy is uncertainty about the magnitude of effectiveness of GH for this condition. Certainly, ISS is not a specific diagnosis but rather the description of a short child with normal stimulated GH levels (>10 ng/dL) and absent comorbid conditions. Some studies investigating the efficacy of GH therapy in ISS have included normal variant short stature (familial short stature and constitutional delay of growth and puberty). Furthermore, there has been considerable variability in the doses of GH used in ISS. A meta-analysis of 10 controlled trials (434 patients) and 28 uncontrolled trials (655 patients) suggested an average gain in adult height of approximately 4 to 6 cm (range, 2.3 to 8.7 cm) with GH therapy. This gain corresponds to approximately $35,000 per inch (2.54 cm).[33]

**Box 69-2**

***Current FDA-Approved Indications for GH Therapy***

- GH deficiency or insufficiency
- Chronic renal insufficiency (pretransplant)
- Turner syndrome
- Children born short for gestational age (SGA) who fail to exhibit catch-up growth by 2 years
- Idiopathic short stature (ISS)
- Prader-Willi syndrome
- SHOX (short stature homeobox-containing gene) deficiency
- Noonan syndrome
- Adults with GH deficiency
- Adults with AIDS wasting

***Side Effects of GH Therapy.*** GH therapy is remarkably well tolerated and side effects are infrequent. Potential complications include:

- Pseudotumor cerebri (benign intracranial hypertension). Temporary discontinuation of GH therapy generally results in resolution of this condition. Thereafter, GH therapy can be restarted at a lower dose and titrated up to the original dose.
- Slipped capital femoral epiphysis (SCFE). This is particularly a concern in overweight children receiving GH therapy. Symptoms suggestive of SCFE, such as knee pain, hip pain, or unexplained limp, warrant a hip x-ray to exclude this condition. If identified, prompt referral to an orthopedic surgeon is warranted.
- Impaired glucose tolerance and diabetes. GH is a counterregulatory hormone that opposes the action of insulin. Therefore, GH therapy may cause earlier expression of impaired glucose tolerance and type 2 diabetes in susceptible individuals (eg, those who are obese and have a family history of type 2 diabetes).
- Leukemia. Although there have been some sporadic cases of leukemia reported in children receiving GH therapy, careful analysis of several worldwide databases reveals no increase in the risk of leukemia in otherwise healthy individuals (ie, those children without any risk factors such as prior malignancy, radiation therapy, chemotherapy, or premalignant conditions).

### Androgen Therapy

Androgen therapy is used relatively widely in boys with hypogonadism and also in boys with CDGP. In most cases of CDGP, the only treatment necessary is reassurance that growth and pubertal development will occur and that the final adult height will be relatively normal compared to parental heights. The knowledge that one or both of the adolescent's parents had the same pattern of growth is often reassuring. However, in some adolescents CDGP can result in significant psychological difficulties, and reassurance may not be sufficient. Androgen therapy in these cases decreases the distress caused by growth and pubertal delay.[34]

Guidelines for androgen therapy commonly used in adolescents with CDGP (age 13.5 to 14 years) is as follows:

- Testosterone is generally limited to boys whose bone age is 12 years or greater.[35] Fifty mg to 100 mg of depot-testosterone is administered monthly for 4 to 6 months. Most of the testosterone is cleared by approximately 15 days after the injection, allowing adequate time for the hypothalamic–pituitary axis to recover from any suppression induced by the testosterone. Spontaneous pubertal development, identified by enlarging testes, generally occurs within 6 months of initiating treatment.
- Oxandrolone is a nonaromatizable androgen with predominantly anabolic activity and weak androgenic activity. Because of the weak androgenic activity, oxandrolone has been used to promote growth in adolescents with CDGP. It should not be used in very young boys as this may result in both acceleration of bone age and onset of precocious puberty.[36] Adult height is not affected by oxandrolone.[37-39]
- Anticipatory treatment. Children with CDGP are frequently identified well before they have delayed puberty. Because both growth deceleration and a late spontaneous growth spurt are anticipated, some have advocated oxandrolone therapy at an earlier age to prevent the psychological difficulties associated with CDGP in the pubertal years.[40] A prolonged (approximately 1 year) course of oxandrolone given to a boy with CDGP starting at approximately age 12 allows growth acceleration to occur at the same time as his peers and achievement of a more normal height at a critical time for emotional, educational, and physical development.

### IGF-I Therapy

Recombinant IGF-I has been approved for those rare children with GHIS. IGF-I also is appropriate therapy for growth failure caused by defects in the GH-IGF-I axis downstream of the GH receptor (eg, genetic defects affecting the Janus kinase 2 [JAK2]-signal transducer and activator of transcription 5b [STAT5b])[25] and deletions or mutations of the gene for IGF-I.[41]

## TALL STATURE AND EXCESSIVE GROWTH

Tall stature is a descriptive term defined as a height greater than 2 standard deviations above the mean. It follows, therefore, that 2.3% of the normal population can be defined as having tall stature.

### CAUSES OF TALL STATURE

#### Normal Variant Tall Stature

***Familial Tall Stature.*** The diagnosis of familial tall stature is generally relatively straightforward. Although the adolescent has tall stature, the height percentile is stable and appropriate for the genetic background. In addition, the predicted adult height falls within the target height range.

***Obesity.*** Rapid weight gain is generally associated with increased growth velocity and tall stature. In addition, most children with obesity tend to have early pubertal development, which in the short term exaggerates their tall stature. However, Recombinant IGF-I has been obesity and early maturation result in advanced skeletal maturation and, as a result, final adult stature is normal.

#### Endocrine Causes of Tall Stature

***GH Excess.*** Growth hormone excess in adolescence is rare and is most commonly the result of excessive GH secretion by a pituitary adenoma. Rarely, GH excess may be secondary to excess GHRH production by a hypothalamic or other tumor. Growth hormone excess also may be part of the McCune-Albright syndrome, which is characterized by a triad of gonadotropin-independent precocious puberty, café au lait macules, and polyostotic fibrous dysplasia. The diverse features of this syndrome are the result of a somatic activating mutation in the stimulatory G proteins involved in the signal transduction of many hormone-producing cells.

Growth hormone excess in adolescence results in acceleration of linear growth and tall stature (gigantism). Facial features may become coarse, and overgrowth of hands and feet is common. Enlargement of the head, nose, and tongue, as well as separation of the teeth, may occur. Increased sweating and skin tags may also develop, and glucose intolerance and hypertension may be present. Growth hormone, IGF-I, and IGFBP3 levels are very high, and GH does not suppress following an oral glucose load.

***Thyroid Hormone Excess.*** Hyperthyroidism may be associated with rapid growth and advancement of the bone age, and should be considered in the differential diagnosis of an adolescent presenting with greater growth acceleration than expected for pubertal stage. Careful history and examination should elicit symptoms and signs of hyperthyroidism. The most common cause of hyperthyroidism in adolescence is Graves disease, and the therapeutic options include antithyroid drugs, radiation therapy, and surgery. Less commonly, a hyperfunctioning nodule may be the cause, in which case surgical removal is the treatment of choice.

***Syndromes of Estrogen Deficiency.*** Estrogen is the hormone responsible for epiphyseal maturation in both males and females. Therefore, in the absence of estrogen action linear growth continues and tall stature results. Estrogen deficiency may result from a disruptive mutation in the estrogen receptor gene[42] or as a result of a mutation in the aromatase gene,[43] which is responsible for the conversion of androgen to estrogen. These syndromes present with tall stature and continued linear growth into adulthood. They are extremely rare, inherited in an autosomal recessive manner, and should therefore be considered in the appropriate setting of continued linear growth into adulthood despite complete masculinization.

### Syndromes/Chromosomes

***Weaver Syndrome.*** This syndrome is associated with growth acceleration and advanced epiphyseal maturation, characteristic craniofacial appearance, hoarse and low-pitched cry, hypertonia, and a flexion deformity of the proximal interphalangeal joint of the little finger (camptodactyly). Other features include psychomotor delay, looseness of the skin, and hernias.

***Marfan Syndrome.*** Marfan syndrome is the connective tissue disorder that results in tall stature. Skeletal manifestations include long limbs with a decreased U/L segment ratio, arm span that exceeds the height, arachnodactyly, joint laxity, and pectus excavatum. Lung involvement may present as pneumothorax, and ectopia lentis is the common eye manifestation. The heart also is commonly affected, and mitral prolapse with regurgitation is the most common finding. Aortic root dilatation is the most serious complication that can lead to dissection and rupture. Marfan syndrome is transmitted as an autosomal dominant trait with incomplete penetrance, but in approximately 30% of cases it is the result of a new mutation. Marfan syndrome is discussed in detail in Chapter 149.

***Homocystinuria.*** Homocystinuria is an inborn error of metabolism resulting from a deficiency in cystathionine β-synthase, which results in increased urinary homocystine and methionine. Major clinical manifestations involve the skeleton, eyes, vascular system, and central nervous system. Homocystinuria shares several features with Marfan syndrome. Many of the skeletal features are the same (eg, tall stature, arachnodactyly, pectus deformity). However, unlike Marfan syndrome there is limitation of joint mobility. Affected patients also have ectopia lentis. Mental retardation and psychiatric disturbances are common. The most common cause of death is secondary to a thrombotic event.

***Klinefelter Syndrome (XXY)***

Klinefelter syndrome is a relatively common condition (frequency 1:500 to 1:1,000) that is an easily recognizable cause of tall stature. Affected individuals generally present in adolescence with small testes inconsistent with their stage of pubertal development. They generally have tall stature with a decreased U/L segment ratio and may have gynecomastia. The testes are small because of abnormal development of the seminiferous tubules (which contribute to most of the bulk of the testes). The Leydig cells are relatively normal, and therefore the testosterone level is generally in the low normal range. Serum gonadotropins are elevated.

XXYY syndrome is another chromosomal syndrome associated with tall stature and possible developmental and behavioral problems.

There are other conditions, for example, Beckwith-Wiedemann syndrome and Soto syndrome (cerebral gigantism), that cause rapid perinatal overgrowth and tall stature in early childhood. However, the period of rapid growth generally ends in mid-childhood, and these children have normal stature in adolescence and adulthood.

## EVALUATION OF TALL STATURE AND EXCESSIVE GROWTH

Obtaining a careful history of family heights, known genetic disorders, birth history, growth in infancy and early childhood, and past medical history (including prior growth data) is extremely important in evaluating an adolescent with tall stature or excessive growth. A child growing at a percentile inconsistent with that of siblings and parents, or an adolescent presenting with accelerating height percentiles, warrants careful evaluation. Examination should include determining body proportions and documenting features associated with the various overgrowth disorders.

If the predicted adult height is appropriate for the family background, the adolescent has familial tall stature. It is more common for females to be concerned about familial tall stature and, in general, reassurance is all that will be required.

If there is suspicion of GH excess, IGF-I, IGFBP3, and random GH should be measured, followed by an oral glucose tolerance test for definitive diagnosis. Failure to suppress the GH level to less than 2 ng/mL following an oral glucose load confirms the diagnosis of GH excess.

The rare syndromes of estrogen deficiency manifest with delayed bone age despite complete masculinization. The delayed skeletal maturation allows for continued linear growth in adulthood and resultant tall stature. Gonadotropins are elevated and estrogens are high in estrogen resistance, but estrogens are very low or unmeasurable in aromatase deficiency.

### MANAGEMENT OF TALL STATURE

If an endocrine cause of tall stature is discovered, the underlying condition should be treated. Therapies for GH excess include surgical removal of a pituitary tumor if well circumscribed, radiation therapy if GH hypersecretion is not normalized by surgery, and medical therapy (long-acting somatostatin analogues, dopamine agonists, GH receptor antagonists) as required. If tall stature is caused by estrogen deficiency, estrogen therapy will only be effective if the estrogen deficiency is secondary to aromatase deficiency, that is, there is a functional estrogen receptor.

High-dose estrogen therapy has been used to reduce the height of some adolescent females with familial tall stature. Certainly, with changes in cultural norms this has become much less commonly requested over the past 40 years. Several estrogen preparations can be used, with different routes of administration and different bone ages at the start of therapy. Height reductions of 2 to 10 cm have been reported.[44] There are multiple potential short-term side effects including nausea, weight gain, thrombosis, and ovarian cysts.[44] In addition, there is some concern that estrogen therapy may reduce female fertility later in life.[45] Undoubtedly, there must be careful consideration to the use of this approach in this day and age.

## REFERENCES

1. Tanner JM, Davies PS. Clinical longitudinal standards for height and height velocity for North American children. *J Pediatr.* 1985;107:317-329

2. Greulich WW, Pyle SI. *Radiographic Atlas of Skeletal Development of the Hand and Wrist.* Palo Alto, CA: Stanford University Press; 1999

3. Lewitt MS, Saunders H, Phuyal JL, Baxte RC. Complex formation by human insulin-like growth factor-binding protein-3 and human acid-labile subunit in growth hormone-deficient rats. *Endocrinol.* 1994;134:2404-2409

4. Albertsson-Wikland K, Rosberg S. Analyses of 24-hour growth hormone profiles in children: relation to growth. *J Clin Endocrinol Metab.* 1988;67:493-500

5. Bierich JR, Potthoff K. Spontaneous secretion of growth hormone in children with constitutional delay of growth and adolescence and with early normal puberty. *Monatsschr Kinderheilkd.* 1979;127:561-565

6. Gourmelen M, Pham-Huu-Trung MT, Girard F. Transient partial hGH deficiency in prepubertal children with delay of growth. *Pediatr Res.* 1979;13:221-224

7. Ivarsson SA. Can growth hormone treatment increase final height in constitutional short stature? *Acta Paediatr Scand Suppl.* 1989;362:56-60

8. Albanese A, Stanhope R. Predictive factors in the determination of final height in boys with constitutional delay of growth and puberty. *J Pediatr.* 1995;126:545-550

9. Albanese A, Stanhope R. Does constitutional delayed puberty cause segmental disproportion and short stature? *Eur J Pediatr.* 1993;152:293-296

10. Ehrhardt AA, Meyer-Bahlburg HF. Psychological correlates of abnormal pubertal development. *Clin Endocrinol Metab.* 1975;4:207-222

11. Nottelmann ED, Susman EJ, Dorn LD, et al. Developmental processes in early adolescence. Relations among chronologic age, pubertal stage, height, weight, and serum levels of gonadotropins, sex steroids, and adrenal androgens. *J Adolesc Health Care.* 1987;8:246-260

12. Lee PD, Rosenfeld RG. Psychosocial correlates of short stature and delayed puberty. *Pediatr Clin North Am.* 1987;34:851-863

13. Duke PM, Carlsmith JM, Jennings D, et al. Educational correlates of early and late sexual maturation in adolescence. *J Pediatr.* 1982;100:633-637

14. Gross RT, Duke PM. The effect of early versus late physical maturation on adolescent behavior. *Pediatr Clin North Am.* 1980;27:71-77

15. Lindsay R, Feldkamp M, Harris D, Robertson J, Rallison M. Utah Growth Study: growth standards and the prevalence of growth hormone deficiency. *J Pediatr.* 1994;125:29-35

16. Parks JS, Brown MR, Hurley DL, Phelps CJ, Wajnrajch MP. Heritable disorders of pituitary development. *J Clin Endocrinol Metab.* 1999;84:4362-4370

17. Dattani MT, Martinez-Barbera JP, Thomas PQ, et al. Mutations in the homeobox gene HESX1/Hesx1 associated with septo-optic dysplasia in human and mouse. *Nat Genet.* 1998;19:125-133

18. Lopez-Bermejo A, Buckway CK, Rosenfeld RG. Genetic defects of the growth hormone-insulin-like growth factor axis. *Trends Endocrinol Metab.* 2000;11:39-49

19. Hindmarsh PC, Swift PG. An assessment of growth hormone provocation tests. *Arch Dis Child.* 1995;72:362-367

20. Reiter EO, Martha PM Jr. Pharmacological testing of growth hormone secretion. *Horm Res.* 1990;33:121-126

21. Marin G, Domene HM, Barnes KM, Blackwell BJ, Cassorla FG, Cutler GB Jr. The effects of estrogen priming and puberty on the growth hormone response to standardized treadmill exercise and arginine-insulin in normal girls and boys. *J Clin Endocrinol Metab.* 1994;79:537-541

22. Celniker AC, Chen AB, Wert RM, Sherman BM. Variability in the quantitation of circulating growth hormone using commercial immunoassays. *J Clin Endocrinol Metab.* 1989;68:469-476

23. Consensus guidelines for the diagnosis and treatment of growth hormone (GH) deficiency in childhood and adolescence: summary statement of the GH Research Society. GH Research Society. *J Clin Endocrinol Metab.* 2000;85:3990-3993

24. Wilson TA, Rose SR, Cohen P, et al. Update of guidelines for the use of growth hormone in children: the Lawson Wilkins Pediatric Endocrinology Society Drug and Therapeutics Committee. *J Pediatr.* 2003;143:415-421

25. Kofoed EM, Hwa V, Little B, et al. Growth hormone insensitivity associated with a STAT5b mutation. *N Engl J Med.* 2003;349:1139-1147

26. Preece MA, Law CM, Davies PS. The growth of children with chronic paediatric disease. *Clin Endocrinol Metab.* 1986;15:453-477

27. Spratt DI, Carr DB, Merriam GR, Scully RE, Rao PN, Crowley WF Jr. The spectrum of abnormal patterns of gonadotropin-releasing hormone secretion in men with idiopathic hypogonadotropic hypogonadism: clinical and laboratory correlations. *J Clin Endocrinol Metab.* 1987;64:283-291

28. Adan L, Souberbielle JC, Brauner R. Management of the short stature due to pubertal delay in boys. *J Clin Endocrinol Metab.* 1994;78:478-482

29. Rosenfeld RG, Albertsson-Wikland K, Cassorla F, et al. Diagnostic controversy: the diagnosis of childhood growth hormone deficiency revisited. *J Clin Endocrinol Metab.* 1995;80:1532-1540

30. Richman RA, Kirsch LR. Testosterone treatment in adolescent boys with constitutional delay in growth and development. *N Engl J Med.* 1988;319:1563-1567

31. Kaplowitz PB. Diagnostic value of testosterone therapy in boys with delayed puberty. *Am J Dis Child.* 1989;143:116-120

32. Stanhope R, Brook CG. Clinical diagnosis of disorders of puberty. *Br J Hosp Med.* 1986;35:57-58

33. Finkelstein BS, Imperiale TF, Speroff T, Marrero U, Radcliffe DJ, Cuttler L. Effect of growth hormone therapy on height in children with idiopathic short stature: a meta-analysis. *Arch Pediatr Adolesc Med.* 2002;156:230-240

34. Houchin LD, Rogol AD. Androgen replacement in children with constitutional delay of puberty: the case for aggressive therapy. *Baillieres Clin Endocrinol Metab.* 1998;12:427-440

35. Zachmann M, Studer S, Prader A. Short-term testosterone treatment at bone age of 12 to 13 years does not reduce adult height in boys with constitutional delay of growth and adolescence. *Helv Paediatr Acta.* 1987;42:21-28

36. Doeker B, Muller-Michaels J, Andler W. Induction of early puberty in a boy after treatment with oxandrolone? *Horm Res.* 1998;50:46-48

37. Bassi F, Neri AS, Gheri RG, Cheli D, Serio M. Oxandrolone in constitutional delay of growth: analysis of the growth patterns up to final stature. *J Endocrinol Invest.* 1993;16:133-137

38. Schroor EJ, van Weissenbruch MM, Knibbe P, Delemarre-Van de Waal HA. The effect of prolonged administration of an anabolic steroid (oxandrolone) on growth in boys with constitutionally delayed growth and puberty. *Eur J Pediatr.* 1995;154:953-957

39. Joss EE, Schmidt HA, Zuppinger KA. Oxandrolone in constitutionally delayed growth, a longitudinal study up to final height. *J Clin Endocrinol Metab.* 1989;69:1109-1115

40. Papadimitriou A, Wacharasindhu S, Pearl K, Preece MA, Stanhope R. Treatment of constitutional growth delay in prepubertal boys with a prolonged course of low dose oxandrolone. *Arch Dis Child.* 1991;66:841-843

41. Woods KA, Camacho-Hubner C, Savage MO, Clark AJ. Intrauterine growth retardation and postnatal growth failure associated with deletion of the insulin-like growth factor I gene. *N Engl J Med.* 1996;335:1363-1367

42. Smith EP, Boyd J, Frank GR, et al. Estrogen resistance caused by a mutation in the estrogen-receptor gene in a man. *N Engl J Med.* 1994;331:1056-1061

43. Soliman AT, Khadir MM, Asfour M. Testosterone treatment in adolescent boys with constitutional delay of growth and development. *Metabolism.* 1995;44:1013-1015

44. Drop SL, De Waal WJ, Muinck Keizer-Schrama SM. Sex steroid treatment of constitutionally tall stature. *Endocr Rev.* 1998;19:540-558

45. Venn A, Bruinsma F, Werther G, et al. Oestrogen treatment to reduce the adult height of tall girls: long-term effects on fertility. *Lancet.* 2004;364:1513-1518

# CHAPTER 70

# Disorders of Puberty

LINDSEY ALBRECHT, MD • DENNIS M. STYNE, MD

Puberty should be considered the first stage in the continuing process of growth and development that begins during gestation and continues until the end of reproductive life. After an interval of childhood quiescence, gonadotropin-releasing hormone (GnRH) pulses increase in the peripubertal period, leading to increased secretion of pituitary gonadotropins and, subsequently, gonadal sex steroids that bring about secondary sexual development, the pubertal growth spurt, and fertility.

## PHYSICAL CHANGES ASSOCIATED WITH PUBERTY

Descriptive standards for assessing pubertal development in males and females are in wide use (sexual maturation stages or Tanner stages, as shown in Chapter 4, Physical Growth and Development). They make it possible to objectively record subtle progression of secondary sexual development.[1,2]

### FEMALE CHANGES

The first evidence that puberty is underway in females is an increase in growth velocity that heralds the beginning of the pubertal growth spurt. However, breast development is the first sign of puberty noted by most examiners. Breast development is stimulated chiefly by ovarian estrogen secretion. Breast size and shape are influenced by genetic and nutritional factors, with areolar changes in size, erectility, and color occurring in a predictable sequence. Other features reflecting estrogen action include enlargement of the labia minora and majora, dulling of the vaginal mucosa, and production of a clear or slightly whitish vaginal secretion prior to menarche. Pubic hair development is determined chiefly by adrenal and ovarian androgen secretion. Breast development and growth of pubic hair usually proceed at similar rates, but because discrepancies are possible, it is best to stage breast development separately from pubic hair progression. (See Chapter 4, for a full discussion of female breast development and pubic hair progression.) The size and shape of the uterus and ovaries also change during female pubertal development; these changes can be detected by ultrasound.

### MALE CHANGES

The first sign of normal puberty in boys is usually an increase in the size of the testes to more than 2.5 cm in the longest diameter (excluding the epididymus), which is equivalent to a testicular volume of 4 mL or greater. Pubic hair development is caused by adrenal and testicular androgen secretion and is classified separately from genital development. (See Chapter 4, for a full discussion of male genital development and pubic hair development.) The appearance of spermatozoa in early morning urinary specimens (spermarche) occurs at a mean chronologic age of 13.4 years; this usually occurs at gonadal stage 3 to 4 and pubic hair stage 2 to 4. Boys achieve reproductive maturity prior to physical maturity and certainly prior to psychologic maturity.

### AGE AT ONSET

The diagnosis of precocious puberty may be defined as secondary sexual development starting prior to age 6 years in black girls and prior to age 7 years in white girls, although these new, younger limits can only be used in the absence of findings of any condition that might predispose the girl to precocious puberty.[3,4] Although the mean age at menarche in the United States was previously stable at 12.8 years, there appears to be a recent decrease in the age of menarche by several months.[5,6] The significance of this is unclear. There is a significant concordance of age at menarche between mother-daughter pairs and within ethnic populations, demonstrating genetic effects. White girls have menarche later (12.9 years) than black girls (12.3 years), but this 6-month difference is less than the 1-year difference in the age at onset of puberty between the 2 groups.[7,8] Compensation occurs in pubertal development so that those girls who enter puberty at the earliest ages of the normal range take more time to reach menarche whereas those who enter at older ages of the normal range progress faster to menarche. In boys, 9 years is taken as the lower limit of normal pubertal development.

Many factors can alter the age at onset of puberty. Moderate obesity may be associated with an earlier onset, whereas severe obesity may delay puberty. There is much speculation that the age at onset of puberty might be decreasing in the United States, but evaluation of all major studies does not demonstrate a substantial decrease in the age at which the physical changes of puberty are seen or in the age of menarche. Increasing body mass index (BMI) may cause earlier puberty in girls; due to the epidemic of obesity in childhood, there may be an earlier age of onset of pubertal development in the future.[9]

## GROWTH SPURT

The striking increase in growth velocity in puberty is under complex endocrine control. Hypothyroidism, growth hormone deficiency, and sex hormone deficiency can decrease or eliminate the pubertal growth spurt. Estrogen indirectly stimulates insulin-like growth factor-1 (IGF-1) production by increasing the secretion of growth hormone (GH) and also directly stimulates IGF-1 production in cartilage. Estrogen is the most important factor in stimulating maturation of the chondrocytes and osteoblasts, ultimately leading to epiphysial fusion and cessation of growth. In girls, the pubertal growth spurt begins in early puberty and is mostly completed by menarche. In boys, the pubertal growth spurt occurs toward the end of puberty, at an average age 2 years older than girls. Total height attained during the growth spurt in girls is about 25 cm; in boys, it is about 28 cm. A normal growth rate does not ensure a lack of endocrine pathology, because precocious puberty may increase the growth rate sufficiently to mask the presence of coexisting GH deficiency.

## CHANGES IN BODY COMPOSITION

Prepubertal boys and girls start with equal lean body mass, skeletal mass, and body fat, but at maturity, men have approximately 1½ times the lean body mass, skeletal mass, and muscle mass of women, whereas women have twice as much body fat as men. Attainment of peak values of percentage of body fat, lean body mass, and bone mineral density is earlier by several years in girls than in boys, as is the earlier peak of height velocity and velocity of weight gain in girls. The most important phases of bone accretion occur during infancy and puberty.[10] Girls reach peak mineral acquisition velocity between 14 and 16 years of age, whereas boys reach this stage at 17.5 years; both milestones occur after peak height velocity is attained and peak bone density is reached a few years after puberty ends. Dual-energy x-ray absorptiometry (DEXA) standards exist for evaluating bone mineralization in children and adolescents; the use of young adult standards for children and adolescents that most commercial DEXA devices contain will always falsely suggest osteopenia or osteoporosis even if bone density is appropriate for age. Correct standards for age must be used.[11]

## ENDOCRINE CHANGES

Pituitary gonadotropin secretion is controlled by the hypothalamus, which releases pulses of GnRH into the pituitary-portal system to reach the anterior pituitary gland. Control of GnRH secretion is exerted by a "hypothalamic pulse generator" in the arcuate nucleus. It is sensitive to feedback control from sex steroids and inhibin, a gonadal protein, which control the frequency and amplitude of gonadotropin secretion during development in both sexes, and during progression of the menstrual cycle in females.

Episodic peaks of serum gonadotropins occur in young children until about 2 years of age; levels are lower during later years in normal childhood. The onset of puberty is heralded by an increase in amplitude of secretory events. Thus, changes in gonadotropin secretion that occur at puberty do not arise de novo, but are based on pre-existing patterns of endocrine secretion. During the peripubertal period of endocrine change prior to secondary sexual development, gonadotropin secretion becomes less sensitive to negative feedback inhibition, which partly accounts for rising gonadotropin values. An intrinsic central nervous system (CNS) inhibitory mechanism restrains puberty during childhood, but this inhibition decreases normally in the peripubertal period, or pathologically with an injury to the CNS or development of a CNS tumor of the inhibitory area.

The "switch" that triggers the onset of puberty is unknown, but several neurotransmitters are invoked in the process, including GABA (gamma amino butyric acid) and NMDA (N-methyl-D-aspartic acid). *KISS1*, a human metastasis suppressor gene that codes for metastin (or kisspeptin), a 145 AA peptide, has recently been implicated in the process. Kisspeptin is an endogenous agonist for GPR54 (G protein-coupled receptor 54) and has been shown to directly stimulate GnRH release.[12]

With the onset of puberty, serum gonadotropin secretion progressively increases from childhood levels, leading to an increase in serum gonadal steroid concentrations. Although sex steroids are secreted in a diurnal rhythm in early puberty, as are gonadotropins, sex steroids are bound to sex hormone-binding globulin (SHBG) so that the half-life of sex steroids is longer than that of gonadotropins. Thus, random daytime measurements of serum sex steroids in a sensitive and specific assay are more helpful in determining pubertal status than random measurements of serum gonadotropins.

### OVULATION AND MENARCHE

The last stage in hypothalamic–pituitary development is the onset of positive feedback, leading to ovulation and menarche. The ovary contains a paracrine system that regulates follicular development and atresia; it is only during the last stages of puberty that gonadotropins exert effects on the maturation of the follicle. After mid puberty, estrogen can either stimulate or suppress gonadotropin release, depending on estrogen level and pattern, demonstrating a biphasic effect. The frequency of pulsatile GnRH release increases during the late follicular phase of the normal menstrual cycle, the ratio of leutinizing hormone (LH) to follicle-stimulating hormone (FSH) secretion rises, and the mid cycle LH surge that causes ovulation ensues.

### ADRENARCHE

The adrenal cortex normally secretes the weak androgens dehydroepiandrosterone (DHEA), its sulfate, dehydroepiandrosterone sulfate (DHEAS), and androstenedione in increasing amounts beginning at about 6 to 7 years of age in girls, and 7 to 8 years of age in boys. A continued rise in adrenal androgen secretion persists until late puberty. Thus, adrenarche (the secretion of adrenal androgens) occurs years before gonadarche (the secretion of gonadal sex steroids). The onset of pubic hair development, or pubarche, is the result of gonadal or adrenal androgen production; premature adrenarche is the most common cause of early pubarche. The age at adrenarche does not significantly influence age at gonadarche, and suppressed gonadarche does not alter progression of adrenarche.

### MISCELLANEOUS METABOLIC CHANGES

The onset of puberty is associated with many changes in laboratory values that are either directly or indirectly caused by the rise of sex steroid concentrations. In boys, rising testosterone levels lead to a rise in hematocrit and a decline in high-density lipoprotein (HDL) concentration. In boys and girls, alkaline phosphatase rises normally during pubertal growth. Serum IGF-I concentrations rise with the growth spurt, but are even more closely correlated with sex steroid concentrations. Prostate-specific antigen (PSA) is measurable after the onset of puberty in boys and provides another biochemical indication of pubertal onset.

## DELAYED PUBERTY OR ABSENT PUBERTY

Any girl of 13 or boy of 14 years of age without signs of pubertal development falls more than 2.5 standard deviations (SD) above the mean and is considered to have delayed puberty. The examining physician must make the sometimes difficult decision about which of these patients have constitutional delay in growth and adolescence, and which have organic disease.[13] Classification of the causes of delayed puberty is presented in Box 70-1 and discussed in the following.

**Box 70-1**

***Classification of Delayed Puberty***

- **Constitutional delay in growth and adolescence**
- **Hypogonadotropic hypogonadism**
  - Central nervous system disorders
    - Tumors
    - Other acquired disorders
    - Congenital disorders of the hypothalamus or pituitary
    - Infection
    - Trauma
    - Irradiation
- **Genetic defects of the hypothalamic–pituitary axis**
  - Isolated gonadotropin deficiency
    - Kallmann syndrome
    - Gonadotropin deficiency with normal sense of smell
  - Multiple pituitary hormonal deficiencies
  - Miscellaneous disorders
    - Prader-Willi syndrome
    - Laurence-Moon, Bardet-Biedl syndromes
    - Chronic disease
    - Weight loss
    - Anorexia nervosa
    - Increased physical activity in female athletes
    - Hypothyroidism
- **Hypergonadotropic hypogonadism**
  - Males
    - Klinefelter syndrome
    - Other forms of primary testicular failure (including chemotherapy)
    - Enzymatic defects of the testes
    - Anorchia or cryptorchidism
  - Females
    - Turner syndrome
    - Other forms of primary ovarian failure (including chemotherapy)
    - Pseudo-Turner syndrome (Noonan syndrome)
    - XX and XY gonadal dysgenesis

**CONSTITUTIONAL DELAY IN GROWTH AND ADOLESCENCE**

A patient with delayed onset of secondary sexual development whose stature is shorter than that of age-matched peers but who consistently maintains a normal growth velocity for bone age and whose skeletal development is delayed more than 2 SD from the mean is likely to have constitutional delay in puberty.[14] A family history of a similar pattern of development in a parent or sibling supports the diagnosis. The subject is usually thin as well. Generally, signs of puberty will appear after the patient reaches a skeletal age of 11 years (girls) or 12 years (boys), but there is great variation. Patients with constitutional delay in adolescence will almost always manifest secondary sexual development by 18 years of chronologic age. Adrenarche is characteristically delayed—along with gonadarche—in constitutional delay of puberty.

**HYPOGONADOTROPIC HYPOGONADISM**

The absent or decreased ability of the hypothalamus to secrete GnRH, or of the pituitary gland to secrete LH and FSH leads to hypogonadotropic hypogonadism. This classification denotes an irreversible condition requiring replacement therapy. If the pituitary deficiency is limited to gonadotropins, patients are usually close to normal height for age until the age of pubertal growth spurt, in contrast to the shorter patients with constitutional delay or severely short patients with additional GH deficiency. Bone age is usually not delayed in childhood, but does not progress normally after the patient reaches the age at which sex steroid secretion ordinarily stimulates maturation of the skeleton.

**Central Nervous System Disorders**

Congenital and acquired CNS defects may lead to hypogonadotropic hypogonadism due to interruption of the normal GnRH and/or gonadotropin secretory pathways. Delayed puberty may be the only sign of a potentially life-threatening CNS disorder, such as a CNS neoplasm. All patients with delayed puberty should be carefully assessed for neurologic symptoms and neurologic deficits on physical examination.

- Tumors—A tumor involving the hypothalamus or pituitary gland can interfere with hypothalamic-pituitary-gonadal function as well as the control of GH, corticotropin (ACTH), thyrotropin (TSH), prolactin (PRL), and vasopressin secretion. Thus, delayed puberty may be a manifestation of a CNS tumor accompanied by any or all of the following: GH deficiency, secondary hypothyroidism, secondary adrenal insufficiency, hyperprolactinemia, and diabetes insipidus. The presence of an acquired (but not usually congenital) combination of anterior and posterior pituitary deficiencies should raise suspicion of a hypothalamic-pituitary tumor. Craniopharyngioma is the most common type of hypothalamic-pituitary tumor leading to delay or absence of pubertal development. This neoplasm originates in Rathke's pouch but may develop into a suprasellar tumor. Laboratory evaluation may reveal any type of anterior or posterior pituitary deficiencies. Bone age is often retarded at the time of presentation. Extrasellar tumors that involve the hypothalamus and produce sexual infantilism include germinomas, gliomas (sometimes with neurofibromatosis), and astrocytomas, although, depending upon endocrine secretory activity or location, these tumors may alternatively produce central precocious puberty.
- Other acquired CNS disorders—Langerhans cell histiocytosis may involve the hypothalamus and cause gonadotropin deficiency, although it more typically results in diabetes insipidus. Tuberculous or sarcoid granulomas, other postinfectious inflammatory lesions, vascular lesions, and trauma more rarely cause hypogonadotropic hypogonadism.
- Developmental defects—Developmental defects of the CNS may cause hypogonadotropic hypogonadism or other types of hypothalamic dysfunction. Anterior and posterior pituitary deficiencies may occur with congenital midline defects, such as cleft palate, or with other acquired defects. Early onset of such a combination suggests a congenital defect, whereas late onset more strongly indicates a neoplasm.
- Radiation therapy—CNS radiation therapy involving the hypothalamic-pituitary area can lead to hypogonadotropic hypogonadism with onset at 6 to 18 months (or longer) after treatment, although GH secretion is more frequently affected than gonadotropin secretion.

**Isolated Hormonal Deficiency**

Patients who have isolated deficiency of gonadotropins, but normal GH secretion, tend to be of normal height for age until the teenage years but will lack a pubertal growth spurt. Their skeletal development will be delayed for chronologic age during the teenage years, and they will continue to grow after an age when normal adolescents stop growing. They develop eunuchoid proportions of increased span for height, and decreased upper to lower segment ratios as adults. Kallmann syndrome 1 is the most common form of isolated gonadotropin deficiency and results from migration failure of GnRH-containing neurons during CNS development. The disorder is caused by deletions in the *KAL* gene in the region of Xp22.3, which appears to code for an adhesion molecule. Gonadotropin deficiency in these patients is associated with hypoplasia or aplasia of the olfactory lobes and hyposmia or anosmia. Ultimate height is normal, although patients are delayed in reaching adult height. Kallmann syndrome 2 is inherited in an autosomal-dominant pattern and is due to a mutation in the FGFR1 gene. Kallmann syndrome 3 exhibits an autosomal recessive pattern. Other cases of hypogonadotropic hypogonadism may occur sporadically or via an autosomal recessive pattern without anosmia due to a variety of gene defects.

### Idiopathic Hypopituitary Dwarfism

Patients with congenital GH deficiency have early onset of growth failure, in contrast to the late onset of growth failure usually seen in patients with GH deficiency due to hypothalamic tumors. Even without associated gonadotropin deficiency, untreated GH-deficient patients often have delayed onset of puberty associated with their delayed bone ages. With appropriate human growth hormone (hGH) therapy, however, onset of puberty occurs at a normal age. Patients who have combined GH and gonadotropin deficiency do not undergo puberty even when bone age reaches the pubertal stage. The syndrome of microphallus (penile length $<2$ cm at birth due to congenital gonadotropin or GH deficiency) and neonatal hypoglycemic seizures (due to congenital ACTH deficiency or GH deficiency) will not undergo spontaneous pubertal development if GnRH is also deficient. Patients with this syndrome must be diagnosed and treated early to avoid CNS damage.

### Miscellaneous Disorders

Genetic syndromes, malnutrition, and hypothyroidism can additionally lead to hypogonadotropic hypogonadism and pubertal delay. The correct diagnosis can generally be reached by assessing developmental milestones, diet, exercise frequency, and other pertinent symptoms, as well as by performing a careful physical examination to search for dysmorphic features.

- Prader-Willi syndrome—Prader-Willi syndrome is a disorder of paternal imprinting involving chromosome 15q11-q13. It occurs sporadically and is associated with fetal and infantile hypotonia, short stature, and poor feeding in infancy. After infancy, insatiable hunger leading to massive obesity, mental retardation, and a characteristic physical phenotype is typical. Delayed menarche occurs in females, and micropenis and cryptorchidism occurs in males.
- Laurence-Moon or Bardet-Biedl syndrome—These autosomal recessive conditions are characterized by obesity, short stature, mental retardation, and retinitis pigmentosa. Hypogonadotropic hypogonadism and primary hypogonadism have variously been reported in affected patients.
- Chronic disease and malnutrition—A delay in sexual maturation may be due to chronic disease or malnutrition. Weight loss to less than 80% of ideal body weight, caused by disease or voluntary dieting, may result in gonadotropin deficiency; weight gain toward the ideal usually restores gonadotropin function. Chronic disease may have effects on sexual maturation separate from nutritional state. For example, there is a high incidence of hypothalamic hypogonadism in thalassemia major even with regular transfusion and chelation therapy.
- Anorexia nervosa—Primary or secondary amenorrhea is a classic finding in patients with anorexia nervosa, and has been correlated with the degree of weight loss, although there is evidence that patients may cease to menstruate before substantial weight loss is exhibited. Additionally, weight gain to the normal range for height does not ensure immediate resumption of menses.[15]
- Increased physical activity—Girls who regularly participate in strenuous athletics may have delayed thelarche, delayed menarche, and irregular or absent menstrual periods. This effect is not always related to decreased weight but is generally attributed to insufficient nutrition relative to increased levels of activity.
- Hypothyroidism—Hypothyroidism can delay all aspects of growth and maturation, including puberty and menarche. With thyroxine therapy, catch-up growth and resumed pubertal development and menses will occur.

## HYPERGONADOTROPIC HYPOGONADISM

Primary gonadal failure is heralded by elevated gonadotropin concentrations due to the absence of negative feedback effects of gonadal sex steroids. The most common causes of hypergonadotropic hypogonadism are associated with chromosomal and somatic abnormalities, but isolated gonadal failure can also rarely present with delayed puberty without other physical findings.

### Klinefelter Syndrome

The most common form of primary testicular failure is Klinefelter syndrome (47,XXY karyotype), with an incidence of 1:1,000 males. Before puberty, patients have decreased upper segment:lower segment ratios, small testes, and an increased incidence of developmental delay and behavioral problems. Onset of puberty is not usually delayed because Leydig cell function is characteristically less affected than seminiferous tubule function, and testosterone levels are often adequate to stimulate pubertal development. After the onset of puberty, there are histologic changes of seminiferous tubule hyalinization and fibrosis, adenomatous changes of the Leydig cells, and impaired spermatogenesis. The testes become firm and are rarely larger than 3.5 cm in diameter; serum gonadotropin levels rise after the onset of puberty. Gynecomastia is common, and variable degrees of male secondary sexual development are found. Hypergonadotropic hypogonadism is found in males with mosaic sex chromosome abnormalities as well.[16]

### Other Forms of Primary Testicular Failure

Patients surviving treatment for malignant diseases form a growing category of testicular failure. Chemotherapy (primarily with alkylating agents) or radiation therapy directed to the gonads may lead to gonadal failure. Injury is more likely if treatment is given during puberty than if it occurs in the prepubertal period, but even prepubertal therapy leads to risk. Prepubertally treated boys may have normal pubertal development but have a high incidence of decreased or absent sperm counts; thus, normal development may mask significant endocrine and reproductive damage.

### Cryptorchism or Anorchia

Phenotypic males with a 46,XY karyotype but no palpable testes have either cryptorchism or anorchia. The diagnosis may be pursued by imaging studies, laparotomy or laparoscopic examination, or by endocrine evaluation (generally measurement of testosterone following hCG administration). The presence of normal basal gonadotropin levels in a prepubertal boy without palpable testes suggests the presence of testicular tissue even if the testosterone response to hCG is low, whereas the presence of elevated gonadotropin levels without any testosterone response to hCG suggests anorchia. Inhibin may be used as a clue to the presence of testicular tissue.

### Syndrome of Gonadal Dysgenesis (Turner Syndrome)

Turner syndrome (45,XO karyotype) occurs in 1:2,000 live births and is associated with sexual infantilism, short stature, and a characteristic female phenotype.[17] Patients are infertile, with "streak" gonads consisting of fibrous tissue without germ cells. Pubic hair may appear late and is usually sparse in distribution; adrenarche progresses in Turner syndrome even in the absence of gonadarche. Serum gonadotropin concentrations in Turner syndrome are extremely high between birth and age 4 years, decrease toward the normal range in prepubertal patients, and then rise again dramatically after age 10 years; this pattern is an exaggerated form of the pattern found in normal children, demonstrating the intrinsic inhibition of gonadotropin secretion that occurs even without functional gonads to produce sex steroids, which would otherwise act in a negative inhibitory feedback pattern. Patients have no pubertal growth spurt and reach a mean final height of 143 cm. Mosaicism can occur, which may attenuate the phenotype. Growth hormone function is usually normal in Turner syndrome, although GH treatment improves the growth rate and increases adult height.[17,18]

### Other Forms of Primary Ovarian Failure

Ovarian failure can occur with chemotherapy or radiation therapy. Normal gonadal function after chemotherapy does not guarantee normal function later, as late-onset gonadal failure may occur. Premature menopause has also been described in otherwise healthy girls owing to the presence of antiovarian antibodies; patients with Addison disease may have autoimmune oophoritis as well as adrenal failure. A sex steroid biosynthetic defect due to 17 alpha-hydroxylase deficiency (P450c17) is manifested as sexual infantilism and primary amenorrhea in a phenotypic female (regardless of genotype) with hypokalemia and hypertension.

### Pseudo-Turner Syndrome (Noonan Syndrome)

Individuals with Noonan syndrome have some phenotypic features that are associated with Turner syndrome and others that are not. Inheritance is autosomal dominant. Affected patients do not have intrauterine growth retardation. Characteristics of Noonan syndrome are: short stature (of postnatal onset), failure to thrive in infancy, triangular and low-set posteriorly rotated ears, nerve deafness, ptosis, hypertelorism, down-slanting palpebral fissures, epicanthal folds, myopia, blue-green irides, deeply grooved philtrum, high peaks of the upper lip vermilion border, high arched palate, micrognathia, dental malocclusion, low posterior hairline, webbed neck, cystic hygroma, congenital heart defects (usually of the right side, that include pulmonic stenosis, septal defects, and patent ductus arteriosus), shield chest, pectus carinatum superiorly and pectus excavatum inferiorly, hypogonadism and cryptorchidism, vertebral abnormalities, cubitus valgus, clinodactyly, brachydactyly, blunt fingertips, lymphedema, wooly-like consistency of hair, articulation difficulties and, in 25%, mental retardation. There may also be undescended testes and variable degrees of germinal cell and Leydig cell dysfunction.

### Primary Amenorrhea Associated with Normal Secondary Sexual Development

If a structural anomaly of the uterus or vagina interferes with the onset of menses, the patient may present with primary amenorrhea in the presence of normal breast and pubic hair development. A transverse vaginal septum or imperforate hymen may lead to retention of menstrual flow. Male pseudohermaphroditism is an alternative cause of primary amenorrhea if a patient has achieved thelarche. The syndrome of complete androgen resistance leads to female external genitalia and phenotype without axillary or pubic hair development in the presence of pubertal breast development and a 46,XY karyotype.

## DIFFERENTIAL DIAGNOSIS OF DELAYED PUBERTY

Patients who do not begin secondary sexual development by age 13 (girls) or age 14 (boys) and patients who do not progress through development on a timely basis (girls should menstruate within 5 years after development of breast buds; boys should reach stage 5 pubertal development 4½ years after onset) should be evaluated for hypogonadism. The yield of diagnosable conditions is low in children younger than these ages, but many patients and families will request evaluation well before these limits. Without significant signs or symptoms of disorders discussed previously, it is best to resist evaluation and offer support until these ages in most cases.

If the diagnosis is not obvious on the basis of physical or historical features, the differential diagnostic process begins with determining whether plasma gonadotropins are (1) elevated because of primary gonadal failure, or (2) decreased because of secondary or tertiary hypogonadism or constitutional delay of puberty.

A single ultrasensitive, third-generation determination of serum LH concentration in the pubertal range suggests that puberty is progressing. Determination of the rise in LH after administration of a GnRH or GnRH agonist (GnRHa) is helpful in the differential diagnosis; secondary sexual development usually follows within months after conversion to a pubertal LH response. A lack of LH rise after GnRH or GnRHa administration can often be seen in individuals with an abnormal hypothalamic-pituitary-gonadal axis (and can support a diagnosis of hypogonadotropic hypogonadism). Additionally, in males, a morning serum testosterone concentration more than 20 ng/dL (0.7 mmol/l) indicates the likelihood of pubertal development within 6 months. Clinical observation for signs of pubertal development and laboratory evaluation for the onset of rising levels of sex steroids may have to continue until the patient is 18 years of age before the diagnosis is definite. In most cases, if spontaneous pubertal development is not noted by 18 years of age, the diagnosis is gonadotropin deficiency. Of course, the presence of neurologic impairment or another endocrine deficiency should immediately lead to investigation for a CNS tumor or congenital defect in a patient with delayed puberty. Computed tomography (CT) or magnetic resonance image (MRI) scanning will be helpful in this situation.

## TREATMENT OF DELAYED PUBERTY

### Constitutional Delay in Growth and Adolescence

Reassurance is indicated in all cases of constitutional delay in growth and adolescence. Other forms of psychologic support, such as counseling, should be utilized on a case-by-case basis. A short course of hormonal therapy may be appropriate when additional reassurance is needed, but care must be taken to not jeopardize final adult height.

- Psychologic support—Significant psychologic problems may occur in some teenagers who are embarrassed about short stature and lack of secondary sexual development. These teens should be counseled that normal pubertal development will occur spontaneously. Although most of these patients will do well, severe depression must be treated appropriately. In some cases it helps to excuse the patient from physical education class, as the lack of development is most apparent in the locker room.
- Sex steroids—Hormonal treatment of boys or girls will elicit noticeable secondary sexual development and a slight increase in stature. The low doses recommended do not advance bone age substantially and will not significantly change final height if used for only 3 months. A short course of therapy may improve psychological outlook and allow patients to await spontaneous pubertal development with greater confidence. Continuous gonadal steroid replacement in these patients is not indicated, as it will advance bone age and lead to epiphysial fusion and a decrease in ultimate stature. After a 3- to 6-month break to observe for spontaneous development, a second course of therapy may be offered if no spontaneous pubertal progression occurs during the observation period.

### Permanent Hypogonadism

Once a patient has been diagnosed as having delayed puberty due to permanent primary or secondary hypogonadism, replacement therapy must be considered. Males with hypogonadism may be treated with testosterone gel, testosterone patches, or testosterone enanthate or cypionate given intramuscularly every month, although the gel and patch forms are not approved by the Federal Drug Administration (FDA) for this use. The dose should be gradually increased to the adult range over months to years, to mimic the normal progression of puberty and to avoid abrupt exposure to high-dose androgen and the possibility of frequent erections or priapism. Testosterone therapy may not bring about adequate pubic hair development; patients with secondary or tertiary hypogonadism may benefit, however, from human chorionic gonadotropin (hCG) administration, which will cause increased pubic hair growth resulting from endogenous testicular androgen secretion in addition to the exogenous testosterone.

Females may be treated with estradiol patches (but these are not FDA approved for use in patients younger than 16 years of age) or oral ethinyl estradiol or conjugated estrogens. Gynecologic examinations should be performed yearly for those on replacement therapy.

Hypothalamic hypogonadism may be treated with GnRH pulses by programmable pumps to achieve fertility or to promote pubertal development. Likewise, in the absence of a functional pituitary gland, hCG and menotropins (human postmenopausal gonadotropin) may be administered in pulses. These techniques are cumbersome and best reserved for the time when fertility is desired.

#### Coexisting GH Deficiency

The treatment of patients with coexisting GH deficiency requires consideration of their bone age and the amount of growth left before epiphysial fusion. If such a patient has not yet received adequate treatment with GH, sex steroid therapy may be kept at the lower dosage or even delayed to optimize final adult height. The goal is to allow appropriate pubertal changes to support psychologic development and to allow the synergistic effects of combined sex steroids and GH, but without fusing the epiphyses prematurely.[19]

#### Bone Mass

Sex steroid replacement in children with hypogonadotropic hypogonadism is helpful in increasing bone mass but has not been demonstrated to result in normal adult bone mass. Appropriate ingestion of dairy products containing calcium, as well as calcium supplementation and vitamin D, should be encouraged, at least as a commonsense measure.

## PRECOCIOUS PUBERTY (SEXUAL PRECOCITY)

All sources agree that the appearance of secondary sexual development before the age of 9 years in boys is precocious puberty. However, there remains controversy over the lower limits of normal in girls. Based on available evidence, the appearance of secondary sexual development before the age of 7 years in white girls and 6 years in black girls constitutes precocious sexual development. However, if a girl has the onset of puberty before 8 years, there must still remain a high index of suspicion for disease (particularly CNS disease).[4,20]

When the cause of precocious puberty is premature activation of the hypothalamic–pituitary axis and the condition is gonadotropin dependent, the diagnosis is central (complete or true) precocious puberty; if ectopic gonadotropin secretion occurs in boys or autonomous sex steroid secretion occurs in either sex, the condition is not gonadotropin-dependent, and the diagnosis is incomplete precocious puberty. If feminization occurs in girls, or virilization occurs in boys, the condition is isosexual precocity, but if feminization occurs in boys or virilization in girls, the condition is contrasexual precocity. In all forms of sexual precocity, there is an increase in growth velocity, somatic development, and skeletal maturation. When unchecked, this rapid epiphysial development may lead to tall stature during the early phases of the disorder but to short final stature because of early epiphysial fusion.

Classification of the causes of precocious puberty are presented in Box 70-2 and discussed in the following section.

### CENTRAL (COMPLETE OR TRUE) PRECOCIOUS PUBERTY

#### Constitutional Central (Complete or True) Precocious Puberty

Children who demonstrate isosexual precocity but no other findings and begin pubertal development near the age cutoffs noted previously may simply represent the lower reaches of the distribution curve of age at onset of puberty; often there is a familial tendency toward early puberty.[2] True precocious puberty is reported, rarely, to be due to an autosomal dominant or (in males) X-linked autosomal dominant trait.

#### Idiopathic Central (Complete or True) Isosexual Precocious Puberty

Affected children, with no familial tendency toward early development and no organic disease, may be considered to have idiopathic central isosexual precocious puberty. Electroencephalographic abnormalities or other evidence of neurologic dysfunction, such as epilepsy or developmental delay, may be found in these patients. Pubertal development may follow the normal course or may wax and wane. Serum gonadotropin and sex steroid concentrations and response to GnRH or GnRH agonists are similar to those found in normal pubertal subjects. Girls present with idiopathic central precocious

**Box 70-2**

***Classification of Precocious Puberty***

- Central (complete or true) GnRH-dependent isosexual precocious puberty
  - Constitutional
  - Idiopathic
  - Central nervous system disorders (including congenital defects)
    - Tumors
    - Infection
    - Trauma
    - Radiation
  - Following androgen exposure
- Incomplete GnRH-independent isosexual precocious puberty
  - Males
    - Gonadotropin-secreting tumors
    - Excessive androgen production
    - Testicular or adrenal tumors
    - Virilizing congenital adrenal hyperplasia
    - Premature Leydig and germinal cell maturation
  - Females
    - Ovarian cysts
    - Estrogen-secreting neoplasms
    - Severe hypothyroidism
  - Males and females
    - McCune-Albright syndrome
- Incomplete contrasexual precocity
  - Males
    - Estrogen-secreting tumor
  - Females
    - Androgen-secreting tumor
    - Virilizing congenital adrenal hyperplasia
    - Iatrogenic sexual precocity due to gonadotropin or sex steroid exposure
    - Variation in pubertal development
      - Premature thelarche
      - Premature menarche
      - Premature pubarche
      - Adolescent gynecomastia

puberty more commonly than boys. Children with precocious puberty have a tendency toward obesity with an elevated BMI in the untreated state.

### Central Nervous System Disorders

In addition to their potential to cause delayed puberty, CNS disorders may also cause precocious puberty. In many of these cases, the CNS disorder interferes with the pathways that normally inhibit GnRH secretion, leading to excessive levels of GnRH for age and untimely elevation of gonadotropins. In other instances, GnRH is secreted ectopically. Again, a high index of suspicion for neurologic disease is indicated.

- Tumors—Central nervous system tumors are a more common cause of central precocious puberty in boys than in girls, but may occur in either sex, so a high index of suspicion is essential. Tumors may cause precocious puberty by interfering with neural pathways that inhibit GnRH secretion, thus releasing the CNS restraint of gonadotropin secretion. Hamartomas of the tuber cinereum are congenital, and contain GnRH and neurosecretory cells; they may cause precocious puberty by secreting GnRH. With improved methods of imaging the CNS hamartomas are now more frequently diagnosed in patients who were previously thought to have idiopathic precocious puberty. These tumors are masses but not neoplasms and they do not enlarge; they therefore pose no increasing threat to the patient in the absence of intractable seizures, which are rare.
- Other causes of true precocious puberty—Infectious or granulomatous conditions such as encephalitis, brain abscess, postinfectious (or postsurgical or congenital) suprasellar cysts, sarcoidosis, hydrocephalus, and tuberculous granulomas of the hypothalamus can cause central precocious puberty. Brain trauma may be followed by either precocious or delayed puberty. Radiation therapy for acute lymphoblastic leukemia of the CNS or prior to bone marrow transplantation, is characteristically associated with hormonal deficiency, but an increasing number of cases of precocious puberty occurring after such therapy are being reported. Higher doses of radiation may be more likely to cause GnRH deficiency, whereas lower doses (down to 18 Grey) may lead to central precocious puberty.

### Virilizing Syndromes

Patients with long-untreated virilizing adrenal hyperplasia who have advanced bone ages may manifest precocious puberty after treatment with glucocorticoid suppression. Children with virilizing tumors or those given long-term androgen therapy may follow the same pattern when the androgen source is removed. Advanced maturation of the hypothalamic–pituitary–gonadal axis appears to occur with any condition causing excessive androgen secretion and advanced skeletal age.

## INCOMPLETE ISOSEXUAL PRECOCIOUS PUBERTY

### Boys

Males may manifest premature sexual development in the absence of hypothalamic-pituitary maturation from either of 2 causes: (1) ectopic or autonomous endogenous secretion of hCG or LH or iatrogenic exogenous administration of hCG, which can stimulate Leydig cell production of testosterone; or (2) autonomous endogenous secretion of androgens from the testes or adrenal glands or from iatrogenic exogenous administration of androgens.

1. Gonadotropin-secreting tumors—These include hepatomas or hepatoblastomas of the liver; teratomas or choriocarcinoma of the mediastinum, gonads, retroperitoneum, or pineal gland; and germinomas of the CNS. The testes are enlarged but not to the degree found in central precocious puberty.
2. Autonomous androgen secretion—Secretion of androgens can occur because of inborn errors of adrenal enzyme function, virilizing adrenal carcinomas, interstitial cell tumors of the testes, or premature Leydig and germinal cell maturation. Newly recognized forms of late-onset congenital adrenal hyperplasia, generally of the 21-hydroxylase deficiency form, may occur years after birth with no congenital or neonatal manifestations of virilization. Adrenal rest tissue may be found in the testes as a vestige of the common embryonic origin of the adrenal glands and the testes; in states of ACTH excess—primarily congenital adrenal hyperplasia—adrenal rests can enlarge (sometimes to remarkable size) and secrete adrenal androgens. In boys with familial gonadotropin-independent premature Leydig and germinal cell maturation (a sex-linked dominant condition resulting in constitutive activation of the LH receptor), plasma testosterone levels are in the pubertal range, but plasma gonadotropin levels and the LH response to exogenous GnRH are in the prepubertal range or lower because autonomous testosterone secretion suppresses endogenous GnRH release.

### Girls

Females with incomplete isosexual precocity have a source of excessive estrogens. In all cases of autonomous endogenous estrogen secretion or exogenous estrogen administration, serum LH and FSH levels are low.

1. Follicular cysts may be large enough to secrete sufficient estrogen to cause breast development and even vaginal withdrawal bleeding; some girls have recurrent cysts that lead to several episodes of vaginal bleeding.
2. Granulosa-theca cell tumors and gonadoblastomas—Granulosa cell tumors of the ovaries secrete estrogen and are palpable in 80% of cases. Gonadoblastomas found in streak gonads, lipoid tumors, cystadenomas, and ovarian carcinomas are rare ovarian sources of estrogens or androgens.
3. Exogenous estrogen administration—Ingestion of estrogen-containing substances or even cutaneous absorption of estrogen can cause feminization in children. Epidemics of gynecomastia and precocious thelarche have been attributed to ingestion of estrogen-contaminated food, estrogens in the environment, estrogenic compounds in some cosmetic products (such as certain hair creams), soy formula, or undetermined causes.

### Girls and Boys

Both males and females can be affected by disorders that do not exert their effects through the hypothalamic GnRH—pituitary gonadotropin axis, leading to incomplete isosexual precocious puberty.

1. Hypothyroidism—Severe hypothyroidism can be associated with sexual precocity and galactorrhea (Van Wyk-Grumbach syndrome), given that elevated serum TSH can act on FSH receptors, causing gonadotropic effects. Treatment with thyroxine will correct the hypothyroidism, halt the precocious puberty and galactorrhea, and lower the PRL levels.
2. McCune-Albright syndrome—McCune-Albright syndrome is classically manifested as a triad of irregular café au lait spots, fibrous dysplasia of long bones with cysts, and precocious puberty, though many other features are described as well.[21] Precocious puberty may be central or incomplete and is more common in females than in males. Some patients begin with incomplete precocious puberty and progress later to central precocious puberty.

## INCOMPLETE CONTRASEXUAL PRECOCITY IN BOYS

Estrogen may be secreted by rare adrenal tumors leading to feminization in boys. Sertoli cell tumors associated with Peutz-Jeghers syndrome are another possible etiology.

## INCOMPLETE CONTRASEXUAL PRECOCITY IN GIRLS

Excess androgen effects can be caused by premature adrenarche or by more significant pathologic conditions, such as congenital or nonclassic adrenal hyperplasia, and adrenal or ovarian tumors. Both adrenal and ovarian tumors are associated with elevation of serum testosterone, whereas adrenal tumors secrete DHEA. Thus, the source of the tumor may be difficult to differentiate if it produces only testosterone; MRI or CT scanning may be inadequate to diagnose the tumor's organ of origin, and selective venous sampling may be needed.

## VARIATIONS IN PUBERTAL DEVELOPMENT

### Premature Thelarche

The term "premature thelarche" denotes unilateral or bilateral breast enlargement without other signs of androgen or estrogen secretion of puberty. Patients are usually under 3 years of age; the breast enlargement may regress within months or remain until actual pubertal development occurs at a normal age. Areolar development and vaginal mucosal signs of estrogen effect are usually absent. Premature thelarche may be caused by brief episodes of estrogen secretion from ovarian cysts. Classically, premature thelarche is self-limited and does not lead to central precocious puberty.[22]

### Premature Menarche

In rare cases, girls may begin to menstruate at an early age without showing other signs of estrogen effect. An unproved theory suggests that they may be manifesting increased uterine sensitivity to estrogen. In most subjects, menses stop within 1 to 6 years, and normal pubertal progression occurs thereafter.

### Premature Adrenarche

The term "premature adrenarche" denotes the early appearance of pubic or axillary hair without other signs of virilization or puberty. This nonprogressive disorder is compatible with a normal age at onset of other signs of puberty. It is more common in girls than in boys and usually is found in children more than 6 years of age, sometimes overlapping with the newly suggested age limits of puberty in girls. Plasma DHEAS is elevated to stage 2 pubertal levels, which are higher than normally found in this age group. Bone and height ages may be slightly advanced for chronologic age. The presenting symptoms of late-onset adrenal hyperplasia may be similar to those of premature adrenarche, and the differential diagnosis may require ACTH stimulation testing.

### Adolescent Gynecomastia

Up to 75% of boys have transient unilateral or bilateral gynecomastia, usually beginning in stage 2 or 3 of puberty and regressing about 2 years later. Serum estrogen and testosterone concentrations are usually normal. Reassurance is usually all that is required, but some severely affected patients with extremely prominent breast development that does not regress within 2 years will require reduction mammoplasty if psychologic distress is extreme.[22] Some conditions such as Klinefelter syndrome are also associated with gynecomastia; these disorders should be clearly differentiated from the gynecomastia of normal puberty.

## DIFFERENTIAL DIAGNOSIS OF PRECOCIOUS PUBERTY

The history and physical examination should be directed toward 1 of the diagnostic possibilities discussed previously. Serum gonadotropin and sex steroid concentrations are determined in order to distinguish gonadotropin-mediated secondary sexual development (serum gonadotropin and sex steroid levels elevated) from autonomous endogenous secretion or exogenous administration of gonadal steroids (serum gonadotropin levels suppressed, sex steroid levels elevated).

If a pregnancy screening test (bhCG) is positive in a boy, the likely diagnosis is an extrapituitary hCG-secreting tumor. Luteinizing hormone values will be suppressed. Some older assays for LH cross-react with hCG; in these cases an hCG-secreting tumor may cause a falsely elevated LH level. If no abdominal or thoracic source of hCG is found, MRI of the head with particular attention to the hypothalamic–pituitary area is indicated to evaluate the possibility of a germinoma of the pineal gland. If serum sex steroid levels are high and gonadotropin levels are low, an autonomous source of gonadal steroid secretion must be assumed. If plasma gonadotropin and sex steroid levels are in the pubertal range, the most likely diagnosis is complete precocious puberty. In such patients, third-generation LH assays or the GnRH test will confirm the diagnosis. The onset of true or complete precocious puberty may indicate the presence of a hypothalamic tumor; thus, CT or MRI scanning is indicated in children with true precocious puberty. Generally, MRI is preferable to CT scan because of better resolution; the use of contrast may help evaluate possible CNS lesions.

Differentiation between premature thelarche and central precocious puberty is usually accomplished by physical examination, but determination of serum estradiol or gonadotropins may be required. The evaluation of uterine size by ultrasound may also be useful as premature thelarche causes no increase in uterine volume whereas central precocious puberty does. Ovarian size determination is a less useful method of distinguishing between the 2 possibilities, but may reveal ovarian cysts. As noted previously, some girls initially thought to have precocious thelarche progress to complete precocious puberty, but there is no way currently to distinguish girls who will progress from those who will not.

## TREATMENT OF PRECOCIOUS PUBERTY

### Central Precocious Puberty

Current treatment for precocious puberty due to idiopathic precocious puberty or a CNS lesion (over and above treatment of the lesion itself) involves the use of GnRH agonists that suppress sexual maturation and decrease growth rate and skeletal maturation. Chronic administration of highly potent and long-acting analogs of GnRH has been shown to downregulate GnRH receptors and reduce pituitary gland response to GnRH, thereby causing decreased secretion of gonadotropin and sex steroids and rapidly stopping the progression of signs of sexual precocity. Injection of these agents every 4 weeks in depot preparations has now made treatment much easier than in the past. Complete suppression of gonadotropin secretion is necessary because an incompletely suppressed patient may appear to have arrested pubertal development while actually secreting low but significant levels of sex steroids (which can advance bone age and lead to an even shorter adult stature).

Growth velocity decreases within 5 months after the start of therapy, and rapid bone age advancement decreases to a rate below the increase in chronologic age. Without therapy, final height in patients with central precocious puberty approaches 152 cm in girls and 155 to 164 cm in boys. With therapy, especially if there is early diagnosis, adult height may approach or equal normal standards.[20]

The new lower age limits of normal pubertal development in girls have led clinicians to reassess the criteria used to identify appropriate candidates for therapy. Patients without significant elevation of serum estrogen who have a predicted height appropriate for their families and who have slowly progressing variants without early menarche may achieve an appropriate final height without therapy.

Psychological support is important for patients with sexual precocity. The somatic changes and/or appearance of menses will frighten some children and may make them the object of ridicule. Thus, supportive counseling must be offered to patients and families.

### Incomplete Precocious Puberty

Treatment of the disorders discussed previously under incomplete precocious puberty is directed toward the underlying tumor or abnormality rather than toward signs of precocious puberty. If the primary cause is controlled, signs of sexual development will be halted in progression or may even regress.

Precocious thelarche or adrenarche requires no treatment, as both are self-limited benign conditions. No therapy has been reported for premature menarche, and none may be indicated. Severe, persistent cases of adolescent gynecomastia may require surgical removal of breast tissue.[22]

## REFERENCES

1. Styne DM. Puberty. In: Gardner DG, Shoback D, eds. *Greenspan's Basic and Clinical Endocrinology*. New York, NY: McGraw-Hill Companies; 2007:611-640

2. Styne DM, Grumbach MM. Puberty: ontogeny, neuroendocrinology, physiology, and disorders. In: Kronenberg HM, Melmed S, Polonsky KS, Larsen PR, eds. *Williams Textbook of Endocrinology*. Philadelphia, PA: WB Saunders; 2008:969-1166

3. Herman-Giddens ME, Slora EJ, Wasserman RC, et al. Secondary sexual characteristics and menses in young girls seen in office practice: a study from the Pediatric Research in Office Settings network. *Pediatrics.* 1997;99(4): 505-512

4. Kaplowitz PB, Oberfield SE. Reexamination of the age limit for defining when puberty is precocious in girls in the United States: implications for evaluation and treatment. Drug and Therapeutics and Executive Committees of the Lawson Wilkins Pediatric Endocrine Society. *Pediatrics.* 1999;104 (4 Pt 1):936-941

5. Euling SY, Herman-Giddens ME, Lee PA, et al. Examination of US puberty-timing data from 1940 to 1994 for secular trends: panel findings. *Pediatrics.* 2008;121:S172-S191

6. McDowell MA, Brody DJ, Hughes JP. Has age at menarche changed? Results from the National Health and Nutrition Examination Survey (NHANES) 1999-2004. *Child Adolesc Ment Health.* 2007;40(3):227-231

7. Sun SS, Schubert CM, Chumlea WC, et al. National estimates of the timing of sexual maturation and racial differences among US children. *Pediatrics.* 2002;110(5):911-919

8. Chumlea WC, Schubert CM, Roche AF, et al. Age at menarche and racial comparisons in US girls. *Pediatrics.* 2003;111(1): 110-113

9. Wattigney WA, Srinivasan SR, Chen W, Greenlund KJ, Berenson GS. Secular trend of earlier onset of menarche with increasing obesity in black and white girls: the Bogalusa Heart Study. *Ethnicity Disease.* 1999;9(2):181-189

10. Leonard MB, Zemel BS. Current concepts in pediatric bone disease. *Pediatr Clin North Am.* 2002;49(1):143-173

11. Kalkwarf HJ, Zemel BS, Gilsanz V, et al. The Bone Mineral Density in Childhood Study: bone mineral content and density according to age, sex, and race. *J Clin Endocrinol Metab.* 2007;92:2087-2099

12. Seminara SB, Messager S, Chatzidaki EE, et al. The GPR54 gene as a regulator of puberty. *N Engl J Med.* 2003;349(17): 1614-1627

13. Sedlmeyer IL, Palmert MR. Delayed puberty: analysis of a large case series from an academic center. *J Clin Endocrinol Metab.* 2002;87(4):1613-1620

14. Bertelloni S, Baroncelli GI, Ferdeghini M, Perri G, Saggase G. Normal volumetric bone mineral density and bone turnover in young men with histories of constitutional delay of puberty. *J Clin Endocrinol Metab.* 1998;83(12):4280–4283

15. Becker AE, Grinspoon SK, Kilbanski A, Herzog DB. Eating disorder. *New Engl J Med.* 1999;340(14):1092–1098

16. Acherman JC, Hughes IA. Disorders of sex development. In: Kronenberg HM, Melmed S, Polonsky KS, Larsen PR, eds. *Williams Book of Endocrinology*. Philadelphia, PA: WB Saunders; 2008:783–848

17. Frías JL, Davenport ML. Health supervision for children with Turner syndrome. *Pediatrics.* 2003;111(3):692–702

18. Bondy CA. Care of girls and women with Turner syndrome: a guideline of the Turner Syndrome Study Group. *J Clin Endocrinol Metab.* 2007;92(1):10–25

19. Ranke MB, Price DA, Albertsson-Wikland K, Maes M, Lindberg A. Factors determining pubertal growth and final height in growth hormone treatment of idiopathic growth hormone deficiency. Analysis of 195 Patients of the Kabi Pharmacia International Growth Study. *Hormone Research.* 1997;48(2)62–71

20. Kaplowitz P. Clinical characteristics of 104 children referred for evaluation of precocious puberty. *J Clin Endocrinol Metab.* 2004;89(3):3644–3650

21. Völkl TM, Dörr HG. McCune-Albright syndrome: clinical picture and natural history in children and adolescents. *J Pediatr Endocrinol.* 2006;19(suppl 2):551–559

22. Diamantopoulos S, Bao Y. Gynecomastia and premature thelarche: a guide for practitioners. *Pediatr Rev.* 2007;28(9):e57-e68

# CHAPTER 71

# Pituitary Disorders

JOAN R. DIMARTINO-NARDI, MD • BARBARA MARSHALL, MD

## PITUITARY ANATOMY

The pituitary is a pea-sized structure located at the base of the brain and attached by the hypothalamic pituitary stalk to the hypothalamus. The hypothalamus sends signals to the pituitary, which then sends signals to target tissues. The pituitary is composed of 2 portions with different embryological origins. The anterior pituitary is derived from Rathke's pouch, and the posterior pituitary arises from the infundibulum, part of the diencephalon. The location of the pituitary hormones and their functions are listed in Table 71-1.[1]

## PITUITARY IMAGING

On T1-weighted magnetic resonance imaging (MRI), the anterior pituitary appears dark and equal in intensity to the gray matter. The posterior pituitary appears white and is therefore commonly referred to as the posterior bright spot. The bright spot is typically absent in cases of hypopituitarism with diabetes insipidus (DI). The prepubertal pituitary volume increases with age to an adult size of 400 to 900 mg.[2]

## ACQUIRED PITUITARY FAILURE

Most pituitary failure that presents in adolescence is acquired. Accidents are the greatest cause of mortality in adolescents, and many of them involve traumatic brain injury (TBI). The incidence of TBI doubles between the ages of 5 and 14 years and peaks for both males and females during adolescence and early adulthood.[3] Pituitary failure may follow TBI and does not always correlate with the degree of injury. Studies show that 25% to 50% of patients have some degree of pituitary dysfunction after TBI. Growth hormone (GH) deficiency is the most common, but a complete pituitary evaluation should follow all cases of TBI.

Tumors in the hypothalamic region may cause pituitary dysfunction due to mass effects from the tumor or from treatment. Craniopharyngiomas arise from remnants of Rathke's pouch, the same tissue that forms the anterior pituitary, and are the most common tumors in this region. Although benign, they can cause pituitary damage due to compression of the pituitary structures, increased intracranial pressure, or damage to the pituitary during surgery. Head and neck radiation for tumors may also cause dose-related damage to the pituitary (Table 71-2).[4]

**Table 71-1**

**Pituitary Hormones**

| *Pituitary* | *Hormone* | *Target Organ* | *Hormone/Function* |
|---|---|---|---|
| Anterior | Growth hormone (GH) | Cartilage/liver | Insulin-like growth factor (IGF-1) |
| Anterior | Thyroid-stimulating hormone (TSH) | Thyroid gland | $T_4/T_3$ |
| Anterior | Luteinizing hormone (LH) | Ovary | Estradiol |
| | Follicle-stimulating hormone (FSH) | Testicle | Testosterone |
| Anterior | Corticotropin (ACTH) | Adrenal glands | Cortisol |
| Anterior | Prolactin (PRL) | Breast | Milk production |
| Posterior | Antidiuretic hormone (ADH) | Kidney | Urine concentration |

Adapted with permission from Geffner ME. Hypopituitarism in childhood. *Cancer Control*. 2002;9(3):212–222.

**Table 71-2**

**Radiation Dose and Associated Anterior Pituitary Hormone Deficiencies[1]**

| *Radiation Dose* | *Hormone Deficiencies* |
|---|---|
| >18 Gy (gray) | GH |
| >40 Gy (gray) | GH, FSH, LH, TSH, ACTH |
| >50 Gy (gray) | GH, FSH, LH, TSH, ACTH, hyperprolactinemia (particularly in females) |

Empty sella syndrome refers to herniation of the subarachnoid space within the sella. Primary empty sella may be due to congenital defects in the sellar diaphragm. Secondary empty sella may be caused by ische-mia, most commonly with postpartum hemorrhage (Sheehan syndrome), hemorrhage that may occur with a vascular adenoma, or infection of the pituitary. Trauma, radiotherapy, drugs, and surgery can also be causes. Global hypopituitarism is rare with empty sella syndrome, occurring if more than 90% of the pituitary is compressed or atrophied.[2] Mild hyperprolactinemia has been reported.[5]

## CONGENITAL PITUITARY FAILURE

Deficiencies in 1 or more pituitary hormones may be caused by mutations of genes involved in the development of the pituitary. The best known are mutations in pituitary transcription factors. These deficiencies may present at birth or the deficiencies may present gradually throughout young adulthood. They may or may not have associated physical malformations. Prop-1 and Pit-1 mutations are responsible for a large portion of multiple pituitary hormone deficiencies, and genetic analysis should be done for patients with familial cases (Table 71-3).[1,6]

### PIT-1

Pituitary transcription factor-1 (Pit-1, also known as Pouf-1) is responsible for pituitary development and hormone expression. It is located on chromosome 3p11. A mutation in Pit-1 leads to deficiencies of GH, prolactin (PRL), and thyroid-stimulating hormone (TSH), but ACTH (corticotropin) is intact and patients go through normal puberty. Most Pit-1 mutations are recessive, but a few dominant mutations have been described.[8]

### PROP-1

Prop-1 is expressed earlier in development than Pit-1 and is a prerequisite for Pit-1 expression. It is located on chromosome 5q.[7] Prop-1 mutations also cause deficiencies in GH, PRL, and TSH. Unlike patients with Pit-1 mutations, patients with Prop-1 mutations do not enter puberty; this is due to inadequate production of LH and FSH. Bottner et al[9] studied 9 patients with Prop-1 mutations and found that there was a progressive decline in anterior pituitary function with age, and all developed partial adrenal insufficiency that became significant in adolescence.

**Table 71-3**

**Transcription Factor Mutations and Anterior Pituitary Hormone Deficiencies[1,6]**

| *Mutation* | *Hormone Deficiency* | *Pituitary Size* | *Inheritance* | *Associated Malformations* |
|---|---|---|---|---|
| Pit-1 | GH, PRL, TSH | Small or normal | Recessive | Prominent forehead, marked midfacial hypoplasia with depressed nasal bridge, deep-set eyes, and a short nose, or no malformations[7] |
| Prop-1 | LH, FSH, GH, PRL, TSH | Small/normal or extremely large with suprasellar extension | Dominant | |
| Hesx-1 | GH, PRL, TSH, LH, FSH, ACTH | Hypoplastic or hyperplastic anterior pituitary, normal or ectopic posterior pituitary | Recessive | SOD |
| LHX-3 | GH, PRL, TSH, LH, FSH | Hypoplastic or hyperplastic anterior pituitary | | Defective neck rotation |

### HESX-1

Hesx-1 is located on chromosome 3p21.2, and its expression is earlier than Prop-1. Mutations result in deficiencies of all pituitary hormones. Hesx-1 is expressed in tissues beyond the pituitary, and mutations of Hesx-1 are responsible for some cases of septo-optic dysplasia (SOD), which involves any combination of optic nerve hypoplasia, pituitary gland hypoplasia, and midline abnormalities of the brain, including absence of the corpus callosum and septum pellucidum.[10]

### LHX3

Lhx3 is located on chromosome 9q34.3. Lhx3 persists in the adult pituitary, and the gene product may be involved in the establishment and maintenance of the differentiated phenotype of pituitary cells.[11] Lhx3 is also expressed bilaterally along the spinal cord and the hindbrain at early stages of development. In addition to deficiencies of GH, PRL, TSH, LH, and FSH, patients have limited neck rotation due to a rigid cervical spine.[12]

## DECREASED ANTERIOR PITUITARY FUNCTION

Hormones produced by the anterior pituitary include GH, TSH, ACTH, FSH, and LH. As described previously, anterior pituitary hormone production may be deficient due to congenital defects in the development of the pituitary. They may also follow pituitary insult or be iatrogenic as in the secondary adrenal insufficiency that follows long-term glucocorticoid administration. Often with GH deficiency the cause is unknown. Decreased anterior pituitary function may involve partial or complete deficiency of 1, few, or all of these. Proper testing can identify the need for hormone replacement.

### GROWTH HORMONE DEFICIENCY

Growth Hormone (GH) is the most common hormone deficiency caused by pituitary damage. It is present in approximately 45% of patients with no other pituitary hormone deficits and up to 100% of patients with multiple deficits.[13] In children and adolescents who are still growing, GH deficiency is suspected when there is a decline in the growth rate. In adults the manifestations of GH deficiency are nonspecific. Testing for GH deficiency should be done in any patient with suspicion of pituitary disease or a history of cranial irradiation. Serum IGF-1 levels that are lower than normal for age confirms the diagnosis of GH deficiency in patients with organic pituitary disease. The insulin tolerance test is the gold standard for diagnosing GH deficiency. GH levels rise above 5 μg/L in normal subjects with insulin-induced hypoglycemia. If hypoglycemia is contraindicated, then 2 stimulatory agents, such as arginine and GH releasing hormone (GHRH), may be used.[14]

### CORTICOTROPIN DEFICIENCY

ACTH is usually the last pituitary hormone lost during pituitary damage. Decreased secretion of ACTH by the pituitary results in atrophy of the adrenal glands.[15] Secondary adrenal insufficiency most commonly develops after long-term glucocorticoids are discontinued. Unlike patients with primary adrenal insufficiency, patients with decreased ACTH secretion usually have milder symptoms and do not develop hypokalemia or hyperpigmentation. They may do so, however, during a time of stress.[15] Secondary adrenal insufficiency should be suspected after brain irradiation, TBI, or when other pituitary hormone deficiencies are present.

Screening can be done by demonstrating a lack of the morning cortisol peak. Blood drawn between 6 am and 8 am should have a cortisol level >18 μg/dL, with a cortisol level <3 μg/dL indicating adrenal insufficiency.[15] If the diagnosis is not clear from the morning cortisol level, stimulation of the adrenal glands with ACTH can be used to demonstrate cortisol reserves. Inducing hypoglycemia with 0.1 u/kg of insulin tests GH secretion, as well as cortisol response to stress. Cortisol levels should be >18 μg/dL in response to a blood glucose level <40 mg/dL.[15] The insulin tolerance test requires medical supervision and is contraindicated in those prone to seizures. Intramuscular or intravenous administration of ACTH also tests the ability of the adrenals to release cortisol. The degree of adrenal atrophy depends on the duration of ACTH deficiency, and this may affect the test.[16] The high-dose test uses 250 μg of ACTH. The low-dose test uses 1 μg of ACTH, which more accurately reflects the physiologic amount of ACTH produced by the pituitary during stress.[17] A patient who cannot mount an appropriate cortisol response to the low dose of ACTH will not be able to produce adequate cortisol in a time of stress.[18]

Treatment of secondary adrenal insufficiency is with hydrocortisone 10 to 12.5 $mg/m^2/day$ divided into 3 doses.[15] Iatrogenic Cushing syndrome should be avoided by using the smallest dose that alleviates the patient's symptoms. During times of stress the steroid dose should be doubled. In addition, all patients need to be educated in the use of injected hydrocortisone and the importance of wearing a medic alert tag identifying them as having cortisol deficiency.

## HYPERPITUITARISM

Excess hormone production can be caused by pituitary tumors that oversecrete hormones or block negative feedback from the hypothalamus. Pituitary adenomas are classified as microadenomas if they are <10 mm, and macroadenomas if they are ≥10 mm. Many nonfunctioning adenomas are only discovered on autopsy, but adenomas that exceed 10 mm in size will often cause frontal headaches from distension of the diaphragmatic sella and bitemporal hemianopsia from upward distension of the optic chiasm.[19] Pituitary adenomas are also classified by the hormones they secrete (Table 71-4).[20] Pituitary carcinomas are very rare. A review of the literature by Petrossians et al[21] found only 96 cases of malignant adenomas.

### PROLACTINOMAS

Fifteen percent of the anterior pituitary is composed of lactotrophs. Prolactin is necessary for milk production during pregnancy and lactation and is under the inhibitory control of dopamine.[2] Normal baseline PRO levels are less than 20 μg/L in women and less than 10 μg/L in men. Elevated PRL levels may be caused by prolactinomas, other pituitary adenomas that compress the pituitary stalk and inhibit dopamine production, medications, or hypothyroidism. Prolactin levels greater than 200 μg/L usually indicate the presence of a prolactinoma, whereas medications rarely cause PRL levels to rise above 100 μg/L[22] (Table 71-5).[19,22]

Care must be taken when interpreting PRL values. If a patient has a macroadenoma and clinical features of hyperprolactinemia, the PRL level may be falsely low due to a "hook effect" (ie, extremely high PRL levels may saturate the assay's ability to read an accurate level, resulting in a falsely low value being reported). In this situation, samples need to be diluted 1:100 in order to obtain an accurate result.[2]

Prolactin-secreting adenomas are the most common secretory pituitary tumor. In young adults

**Table 71-4**

**Pituitary Tumors, Clinical Manifestations, and Therapy**

| *Tumor* | *Frequency* | *Primary Clinical Manifestations* | *Primary Therapy* | *Secondary Therapy* |
|---|---|---|---|---|
| Prolactinoma | 30–50% | • Females: galactorrhea, amenorrhea<br>• Males: mass effects | Dopamine agonists | Surgical resection |
| Growth hormone-producing adenoma | 20% | • Adults: acromegaly<br>• Children: gigantism | Surgical resection | Somatosatin analogue, radiation therapy |
| Corticotropin-producing adenoma | 10–15% | Cushing syndrome | Surgical resection | Radiation therapy, bilateral adrenalectomy, ketoconazole |
| Gonadotropin-producing adenoma | 10–15% | • Mass effects, hypopituitarism<br>• Females: ovarian hyperstimulation<br>• Males: increased testosterone, increased libido | Surgical resection | Radiation therapy |
| Thyrotropin-producing adenoma | 1–2.8% | Hyperthyroidism/goiter | Surgical resection | Somatostatin analogue |
| Nonfunctioning adenoma | 5–10% | Mass effect/hypopituitarism | • Microadenomas: observation<br>• Macroadenomas: surgical resection | Radiation therapy |

**Table 71-5**

**Causes of Hyperprolactinemia[22]**

| *Prolactin Level (μg/L)* | *Causes* |
|---|---|
| >200 | Prolactinoma |
| <200 | Adenoma, pituitary stalk compression |
| <100 | Medications (psychiatric, antihypertensives, estrogens), hypothyroidism, polycystic ovary syndrome |

they are more common in women, at a ratio of 10:1.[23] Prolactin hypersecretion causes menstrual irregularities, sexual dysfunction, galactorrhea, and osteopenia.[2] Decreased menstruation (oligomenorrhea or secondary amenhorrhea) is the primary symptom in up to 95% of women with prolactinomas, and 90% have galactorrhea.[19] Men usually present up to 10 years later than women, generally with larger tumors and usually with visual field defects and hypopituitarism as the first signs. Men also experience decreased libido and impotence that resolve with normalization of PRL levels.[24]

Treatment of prolactinoma is determined by the size and symptoms. Microadenomas with no symptoms from hyperprolactinemia may be observed. The risk of progression from microadenoma to macroadenoma is low, at only 7%.[25] Symptomatic microadenomas are treated with dopamine agonists. Patients with macroadenomas should be evaluated for other pituitary hormone deficiencies and visual field defects. Dopamine agonists are also the initial therapy for macroadenomas. Improvement in visual fields and hyperprolactinemia is observed in days to weeks after starting treatment, with a decrease in tumor size seen in weeks to months.[19] Bromocriptine has been used to treat prolactinomas for more than 15 years, but newer dopamine agonists, such as cabergoline, have fewer side effects and a longer half-life that allows weekly dosing with greater adherence.[14]

About 5% to 10% of patients fail to respond to medical therapy and require transphenoidal surgery.[19] Long-term normalization of PRL levels is only 59% for microadenomas and 26% for macroadenomas, so continued medical management may be necessary.[25] Radiation therapy is rarely used because only 20% to 30% of patients achieve normal PRL levels with this modality and 40% of patients develop hypopituitarism.[19]

## ACROMEGALY

Growth hormone-secreting adenomas constitute 20% of functional pituitary tumors and are the second most common pituitary adenoma.[20] Excess GH secretion causes gigantism in children and acromegaly after epiphysial fusion. Ninety-nine percent of cases of acromegaly are caused by primary pituitary adenomas that secrete GH.[26] GH-secreting adenomas tend to be large and patients present with headaches and the symptoms of space-occupying lesions. Children present with rapid linear growth. Adults have often had symptoms longer by the time they present and may complain of enlarging hands and feet, deepening of the voice, and joint pains.

Excessive IGF-1 production can also cause other endocrine abnormalities. Many patients experience GH-induced insulin resistance and glucose intolerance, but only 10% to 20% of patients become diabetic.[20] Hypertension, dyslipidemia, and diabetes, caused by insulin resistance, are reversible with normalization of IGF-1 levels.[26] Amenorrhea is common in women with pituitary adenomas, due to hypogonadism caused by compression of normal pituitary tissue or to elevated PRL levels from stalk compression.[20]

In a patient where excess GH secretion is suspected, IGF-1 is an appropriate screening test. Hypoglycemia causes an increase in GH secretion and glucose causes suppression of GH release. Failure of glucose to suppress GH secretion is the definitive test for acromegaly. In patients with acromegaly, 75 mg of oral glucose fails to suppress GH levels to <1 μg/L.[26]

Transphenoidal resection of a pituitary adenoma often results in normalization of GH levels within 1 hour of surgery, with an overall surgical remission rate of 61% to 73%.[2,19] Postoperative evaluation of the hypothalamic-pituitary-adrenal axis is necessary, because 20% of patients develop hypopituitarism postoperatively.[2,27] Medical therapy is also possible, utilizing somatostatin analogs and, more recently, GH receptor antagonists. Bromocriptine may be used, but in higher doses than used for prolactinomas.[26] Somatostatin analogs have been reported to lower GH and IGF-1 levels in 80% to 90% of patients with acromegaly and to normalize levels in 50% to 60%.[20] Newer medications include the GH-receptor antagonist pegvisomant.[28] In patients with pituitary adenomas, elevated GH levels are associated with a threefold increase in morbidity and are the most important determinant of mortality.[2] Biochemical cure is defined as a normal IGF-1, a basal-fasting GH level of less than 2.0 μg/L, and a glucose-suppressed GH level of less than 1 μg/L.[19]

## CUSHING SYNDROME

Cushing syndrome is a clinical state resulting from prolonged inappropriate exposure to excessive cortisol, characterized by loss of the normal feedback of the HPA axis and the normal circadian rhythm of cortisol production.[29] Cushing disease refers specifically to hypercortisolism caused by pituitary overproduction of ACTH.[30] Patients with Cushing syndrome are commonly described as having moon faces, central obesity, hirsutism and plethora, with weight gain and obesity being the most common presenting signs.[2] Children most commonly present with poor linear growth and development.[2] Patients may complain of weakness due to myopathy of the proximal muscles. Glucose intolerance is common, with up to one-third of patients developing overt diabetes mellitus. Although hypertension is common in patients who are overweight, patients with Cushing syndrome have a greater incidence of hypertension than those who are simply obese.[31]

Up to 85% to 90% of cases of Cushing disease are caused by a pituitary adenoma.[2] Although cortisol levels are normally higher in the morning and reach a nadir around midnight, patients with Cushing disease lose their circadian rhythm such that the morning cortisol is often normal and there is an elevated evening cortisol. For this reason a morning cortisol is not a good screening test for Cushing disease. Screening may be done with a midnight cortisol level or a 24-hour urine collection for urinary-free cortisol. If urinary-free cortisol levels are normal, it is very unlikely that the patient has Cushing syndrome.[32] Raised urinary-free cortisol levels may also be found in patients with depression and women with polycystic ovarian syndrome.[32,33] A midnight cortisol level of greater than 7 μg/dL is indicative of Cushing syndrome. The diagnosis and management of Cushing syndrome is illustrated in Figure 71-1.

Up to 85% to 90% of children and adolescents who have a pituitary adenoma have surgically identifiable microadenomas.[30] Transsphenoidal surgery has cure rates of 80% to 90% for microadenomas and 50% for macroadenomas.[2] Pituitary irradiation may be necessary for patients not cured with surgery. Bilateral adrenalectomy provides a definitive cure but requires lifelong glucocorticoid and mineralocorticoid replacement.[34]

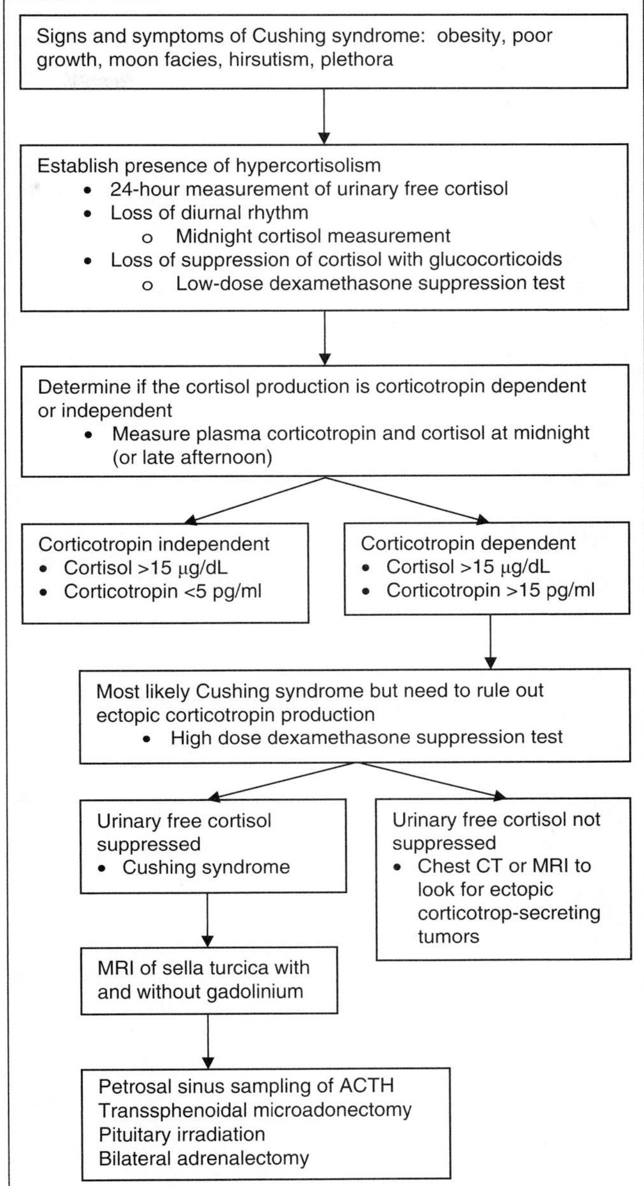


**FIGURE 71-1** Diagnosis and management of Cushing syndrome. (Modified with permission from Orth DN. Cushing syndrome. *N Engl J Med.* 1995;332(12):791–803.)

## DIABETES INSIPIDUS

Central DI is characterized by an inability to concentrate urine as a result of a deficiency of vasopressin (antidiuretic hormone; ADH) production.[35] The release of vasopressin occurs in response to volume depletion, increased plasma osmolality (from hypernatremia, hyperglycemia), nausea, pain, motion sickness, vasovagal reactions, and a number of pharmacologic agents. Normal plasma osmolality ranges between 280 and 290 mosmoles/kg/H20 (mOsm/kg). Normally, at a serum osmolality of <280 mOsm/kg, the plasma vasopressin level is ≤1 pg/mL. Above 283 mOsm/kg, the normal threshold for vasopressin release, the plasma vasopressin level rises in proportion to the plasma osmolality, up to a maximum concentration of 20 pg/ml (at a blood osmolality of 320 mOsm/kg). Peak antidiuretic effect is achieved at a vasopressin concentration of 5 pg/ml. Vasopressin secretion is inhibited by glucocorticoids. The causes of DI are listed in Box 71-1.

**Box 71-1**

***Causes of Diabetes Insipidus***

Central Diabetes Insipidus

**A. Congenital**

1. Disorders of the vasopressin gene: familial autosomal dominant DI; autosomal recessive; Wolfram syndrome (DI, diabetes mellitus, optic atrophy, deafness [DIDMOAD])
2. Congenital anatomical hypothalamic/pituitary defects: septo-optic dysplasia (SOD), holoprosencephaly, midline craniofacial defects

**B. Acquired**

1. Tumors and space-occupying lesions: germinomas, craniopharyngiomas, optic gliomas, pinealomas, hematologic malignancies (such as acute myelogenous leukemia), Langerhans cell histiocytosis, granulomatous diseases, vascular lesions
2. Empty sella syndrome
3. Basilar skull fractures and trauma
4. Inflammatory conditions: lymphocytic hypophysitis, sarcoid disease, autoimmune diseases
5. Congenital anatomic defects: SOD, agenesis of the corpus callosum
6. Neurosurgical complications
7. Drugs (ethanol, phenytoin, opiate antagonists, halothane, and α-adrenergic agents)
8. Infection: meningitis (meningococcal, cryptococcal, Listeria, toxoplasmosis), congenital cytomegalovirus (CMV), encephalitis
9. Hypotension: septic schock, postpartum hemorrhage associated with pituitary infarction (Sheehan syndrome)

In approximately 50% of children and adolescents, however, no primary etiology can be found (idiopathic, congenital defect).

## CLINICAL PRESENTATION

Diabetes insipidus causes renal loss of water, which leads to enormous urine output and acute thirst. The water loss is generally compensated for by increasing intake, so that dehydration is unusual in an awake patient. However, infants, children with altered mental status and midline brain abnormalities, and patients whose thirst centers are affected by the primary process (such as hydrocephalus or a postconcussive syndrome) are at increased risk for hypernatremic dehydration. While an infant with DI is usually irritable but eager to suck, often exhibiting a distinct preference for water over milk, the older child or adolescent presents with the abrupt onset of polyuria and polydipsia, followed by enuresis, vomiting, and constipation. Nocturia, and a preference for ice water are common. Unexplained fever and failure to thrive are other presentations. Excessive water drinking may result in a hydroureter. Central nervous system (CNS) abnormalities such as irritability, altered consciousness, increased muscle tone, convulsions, and coma can occur secondary to the hypernatremia. These findings correlate with the degree and rapidity of the rise in serum sodium.

## DIAGNOSIS AND EVALUATION

The cardinal diagnostic features of DI include a high rate of dilute urine flow (urine output >4 mL/kg/hr); clinical signs of dehydration (weight loss, hypotension), mild to marked degree of serum hypernatremia (>150 mEq/L), serum hyperosmolality (>300 mOsm/L), a low urine osmolality (<300 mOsm/kg) and a low urine specific gravity (<1.010) despite a normal or elevated serum osmolality. If the dehydration is mild, the urine osmolality is less than the serum osmolality. However, if there is severe dehydration or a low glomerular filtration rate, urine output decreases and urine osmolality increases above the serum level; this may temporarily obscure the diagnosis.

Other causes of polyuria, including psychogenic water drinking (in which nocturia is unusual), organic polydipsia (due to a hypothalamic lesion), and osmotic diuresis (due to diabetes mellitus, intravenous contrast administration, or chronic renal insufficiency), can be distinguished by the history, electrolytes, blood urea nitrogen (BUN), and creatinine. With a urinary tract infection, there will be symptoms such as urgency, frequency, and dysuria. A large urinary volume can lead to bladder distension, which can then mimic obstructive uropathy.

If DI is suspected, obtain urine for routine analysis, as well as osmolality, sodium, potassium, and culture. Obtain blood for electrolytes, calcium, BUN, creatinine, osmolality, and antidiuretic hormone (ADH) level. A serum osmolality >300mOsm/kg with urine osmolality

<300 mOsm/kg establishes the diagnosis of DI. The diagnosis is also confirmed if hypernatremia and serum hyperosmolality are documented in association with large volumes of dilute urine (specific gravity <1.005, urine osmolality < serum) that is negative for glucose. In addition, a complete neurologic examination should be performed (with evaluation of visual fields) and an MRI of the pituitary (with and without gadolinium) should be obtained. Normally, the posterior pituitary is seen as an area of enhanced brightness on T-1 weighted images following the administration of gadolinium. This "bright spot" is not present with central and nephrogenic DI—due to vasopressin defiency in the former, and due to enhanced vasopressin release in the latter. In primary polydipsia, the posterior bright spot is normal. The patient should undergo a water deprivation test if the diagnosis is uncertain or to distinguish central from nephrogenic DI.

## THERAPY

### Fluid Therapy

In infants and neonates, DI is best managed by providing fluid therapy alone. In infants, excessive fluid intake coupled with vasopressin therapy can result in water intoxication and hyponatremia.[36]

### Vasopressin and Vasopressin Analogs

In children and adolescents, antidiuretic therapy is given as vasopressin or desmopressin (DDAVP) according to the guidelines outlined in Table 71-6.

***Acute onset of DI*** Continuous Vasopressin Intravenous Infusion: Intravenous therapy with synthetic aqueous vasopressin (Pitressin) is useful in the management of central DI of acute onset or postoperatively. Aqueous vasopressin has a short half-life of 5 to 10 minutes. If continuous vasopressin is administered, fluid intake must be limited to 1 liter/m$^2$/day. One milliunit (mU) of vasopressin is equivalent to approximately 2.5 ng vasopressin. Vasopressin's effect is maximal within 2 hours of the start of infusion (vasopressin may stick to intravenous bottles and tubing). Vasopressin 1.5 mU/kg/hour results in full antidiuretic activity (See Table 71-6 for preparation and dosing of aqueous pitressin drip.)

1. Vasopressin SQ (20 units/mL): Give 0.05 to 0.1 units/kg/dose every 4 to 6 hours. Titrate the dose to the desired effect. (See Table 71-6.)
2. DDAVP (Desmopressin) Intravenous or SQ (4µg/mL): Intravenous DDAVP has a a long half-life of 8 to 12 hours. Dilute with NS (1 mL DDAVP with 9 mL NS = 0.4 µg/mL) and give 0.01 to 0.03 µg/kg/dose, every day or twice a day.

**Table 71-6**

**Medications for the Management of Central Diabetes Insipidus**

| *Medication* | *Route* | *Dose* | *Onset of Action* | *Duration* |
|---|---|---|---|---|
| Vasopressin (pitressin): 20 units/mL (0.5, 1.0, and 10 mL); conversion: 1 unit = 2.5 µg | Intramuscular/subcutaneous | 6.25–25 µg every 6–12 hours; 0.05–0.1 units/kg/dose every 4–6 hours | minutes | 2–8 hours |
| | Intravenous: dilute to 0.01 units/mL (10 mU/mL) by adding 5 units (0.25 mL) to 500 mL NS or D5 W | 0.1–1.5 mU/kg/hour (0.01–0.015 mL/kg/hour) | minutes | half-life 5–10 minutes |
| Desamino-D-arginine vasopressin (DDAVP) (desmopressin acetate) | Oral: 100, 200 µg tablets | 100–400 µg, every 12 hours | 15–30 minutes | 8–12 hours |
| | Intranasal: rhinal tube (10 µg/0.1 mL, 0.025 mL/squirt); nasal spray (10 µg/0.1 mL, 0.1 mL/spray) | 10–20 µg/dose, every 12 hours | 5–15 minutes | 8–12 hours; variable absorption with rhinitis but can be used with vomiting |
| | Intravenous or SQ: 4 µg/mL; dilute with NS (1 mL DDAVP with 9 mL NS = 0.4 µg/mL) | 0.01–0.03 µg/kg/dose, daily or twice a day | minutes | 8–12 hours |

***Chronic therapy for DI*** In the outpatient setting, treatment of central DI in older children should begin with a night-time dose of oral DDAVP of 25 µg to 300 µg. If the dose is effective but the duration is too short, the duration can be extended by increasing the dose or a second dose could be added in the morning. Patients should escape from the antidiuretic effect for about 1 hour before the administration of the second dose to avoid hyponatremia. Intranasal DDAVP can also be used. Give DDAVP 5 to 20 µg/dose daily or twice a day (start with lower dose and titrate to the desired effect).

## SYNDROME OF INAPPROPRIATE ADH (SIADH)

The syndrome of inappropriate secretion of antidiuretic hormone (SIADH), with a primary elevation in vasopressin secretion secondary to CNS pathology (meningitis, trauma) or pulmonary disease (pneumonia, tuberculosis), results in hyponatremia.[37,38] Drugs, such as nicotine, morphine, barbiturates, isoproterenol, antineoplastic agents, carbamazepine, and acetaminophen have all been implicated as antidiuretic agents. Other etiologies are hypothyroidism and water intoxication.

### CLINICAL PRESENTATION

Clinical findings are related to the serum sodium level. A rapid decrease to the 120 mEq/L to 125 mEq/L range or below may cause gastrointestinal symptoms (such as anorexia, nausea, and vomiting), agitation, headache, muscle cramps, seizures, and coma. Other neurologic signs (decreased deep tendon reflexes, pathologic reflexes, Cheyne-Stokes respiration, and pseudobulbar palsy) can be present, especially when the level is <120 mEq/L. The patient may be asymptomatic, even with a sodium <120 mEq/L, if the fall in the serum sodium occurs slowly, over days to weeks.

SIADH can occur with encephalitis, meningitis, a brain tumor, head trauma, psychiatric disease, pneumonia, AIDS, tuberculous meningitis, or secondary adrenal insufficiency. It can also occur in the postictal period after generalized seizures and after prolonged nausea.

It can also be associated with certain drugs. These include: lisinopril, carbamazepine, valproic acid, cisplatinum, vincristine, vinblastine, amantadine, haloperidol, thiroridazine, acetaminophen, clofibrate, chlorpropamide, tolbutamide, fluoxetine, sertraline, and tricyclic antidepressants.

### DIAGNOSIS AND EVALUATION

The evaluation of the patient with hyponatremia should include blood tests (electrolytes, BUN, glucose, lipids (for pseudohyponatremia), renin, aldosterone, vasopressin, uric acid, cortisol, $T_4$ and TSH) and urine tests for sodium, creatinine, and osmolality. SIADH exists when a primary elevation in vasopressin secretion results in hyponatremia, and inappropriately increased urinary osmolality (>100 mOsm/kg), normal or slightly elevated plasma volume, and a normal to high urine sodium level (because of volume-induced suppression of aldosterone and elevation of atrial natriuretic peptide). Serum uric acid is low in patients with SIADH, whereas it is high in those with hyponatremia due to systemic dehydration from other causes of decreased intravascular volume. Vasopressin is elevated in all causes of hyponatremia except for primary hypersecretion of atrial natriuretic peptide and increased water ingestion. In children and adolescents with SIADH who do not have an obvious cause, a careful search for a tumor (thymoma, glioma, bronchial carcinoid) should be considered.

### THERAPY

#### Euvolemia

Limiting the water intake to two-thirds maintenance, including all fluids (eg, intravenous medications), may be all that is required. Immediately begin treatment of the cause of the SIADH.

#### Hypervolemia

If the patient is edematous, restrict fluids to two-thirds maintenance and give furosemide (1 mg/kg IV) if there is pulmonary edema and respiratory compromise.[39]

Acute treatment of hyponatremia due to SIADH is only indicated if cerebral dysfunction is present.[40] Because patients with SIADH have volume expansion, salt administration is not very effective in raising the serum sodium level; it is rapidly excreted in the urine due to suppressed aldosterone and elevated atrial natriuretic peptide concentration.

## REFERENCES

1. Geffner ME. Hypopituitarism in childhood cancer. *Cancer Control.* 2002;9(3):212-222

2. Larsen PR, Kronenberg HM, Melmed S, Polonsky KS, Foster DW, Wilson JD. *Williams Textbook of Endocrinology*. 10th ed. Philadelphia, PA: WB Saunders; 2003:177-281

3. Baldelli R, Corneli G, Savastio S, Petri A, Bona G. Traumatic brain injury-induced hypopituitarism in adolescence. *Pituitary.* 2005;8:255-257

4. Darzy KH, Shalet SM. Hypopituitarism as a consequence of brain tumors and radiotherapy. *Pituitary.* 2005;8(3-4): 203-211

5. De Marinis L, Bonadonna S, Bianchi A, Maira G, Giustina A. Primary empty sella. *J Clin Endocr Metab.* 2005;90(9):5471-5477

6. Aarskog D, Eiken HG, Bjerknes R, Myking OL. Pituitary dwarfism in the R271WPit-1 gene mutation. *Europ J Pediatr.* 1997;156:829-834

7. Wu W, Cogan JD, Pfäffle RW, et al. Mutations in PROP1 cause familial combined pituitary hormone deficiency. *Nature Genet.* 1998;18:147-149

8. Parks JS, Brown MR, Hurley DL, Phelps CJ, Wajnrajch MP. Heritable disorders of pituitary development. *J Clin Endocr Metab.* 1999;84(12):4362-4370

9. Bottner A, Keller E, Kratzsch, Stobbe H, et al. PROP-1 mutations cause progressive deterioration of anterior pituitary function including adrenal insufficiency: a longitudinal analysis. *J Clin Endocr Metab.* 2004;89:5256-5265

10. Dattani MT, Martinez-Barbera JP, Thomas PQ, Brickman JM, et al. Mutations in homeobox gene HESX1/Hesx1 associated with septo-optic dysplasia in human and mouse. *Nature Genet.* 1998;19:125-135

11. Parks JS, Brown MR. Consequences of mutations in pituitary transcription factor genes. In: Pescovitz OH, Eugster EA, eds. *Pediatric Endocrinology: Mechanisms, Manifestations, and Management*. Philadelphia, PA: Lippincott Williams & Wilkins;2004:80-89

12. Netchine I, Sobrier ML, Krude H, et al. Mutations in LHX3 result in a new syndrome revealed by combined pituitary hormone deficiency. *Nature Genet.* 2000;25:182-186

13. Consensus guidelines for the diagnosis and treatment of adults with growth hormone deficiency: summary statement of the Growth Hormone Research Society Workshop on Adult Growth Hormone Deficiency. *J Clin Endocr Metab.* 1998;83:379-381

14. Biller BM, Samuels MH, Zagar A, et al. Sensitivity and specificity of six tests for the diagnosis of adult GH deficiency. *J Clin Endocr Metab.* 2002;87:2067-2079

15. Salvatori R. Adrenal insufficiency. *JAMA.* 2005;294(19): 2481-2488

16. Dorin RI, Qualls CR, Crapo LM. Diagnosis of adrenal insufficiency. *Ann Intern Med.* 2003;139:194-204

17. Dickstein G, Shechner C, Nicholson WE, et al. Adrenocorticotropin stimulation test: effects of basal cortisol level, time of day, and suggested new sensitive low dose test. *J Clin Endocr Metab.* 1991;72:773-778

18. Tsagarakis S, Tzanela M, Dimopoulou I. Diabetes insipidus, secondary hypoadrenalism, and hypothyroidism after traumatic brain injury: clinical implications. *Pituitary.* 2005;8:251-254

19. Pickett CA. Diagnosis and management of pituitary tumors: recent advances. *Prim Care Clin Office Pract.* 2003;30:765-789

20. Townsend CM, Beauchamp RD, Evers BM, Mattox KL, eds. *Sabiston Textbook of Surgery*. 17th ed. Philadelphia, PA: Elsevier Saunders;2004:1023-1070

21. Petrossians P, de Herder W, Kwekkeboom D, Lamberigts G, Stevenaert A, Beckers A. Malignant prolactinoma discovered by D2 receptor imaging. *J Clin Endocr Metab.* 2000;85: 398-401

22. Franks S. Polycystic ovary syndrome. *N Engl J Med.* 1995;333(13):853-861

23. Cicarelli A, Daly AF, Beckers A. The epidemiology of prolactinomas. *Pituitary.* 2005;8:3-6

24. Cicarelli A, Guerra E, DeRosa M, et al. PRL-secreting adenomas in male patients. *Pituitary.* 2005;8:39-42

25. Molitch ME. Medical treatment of prolactinomas. *Endocrinol Metab Clin North Am.* 1999;28(1):143-169

26. Sheeter RD, Wermers RA, Flinchbaugh RT, Haugo A, Ackerman JM, Shafer HI. Endocrinology. In: Rakel RE, ed. *Textbook of Family Medicine*. 7th ed. Philadelphia, PA: WB Saunders; 2007:1042-1056

27. Tindall GT, Oyesiku NM, Watts NB, Clark RV, Christy JH, Adams DA. Transsphenoidal adenomectomy for growth hormone-secreting pituitary adenomas in acromegaly: outcome analysis and determinants of failure. *J Neurosurg.* 1993;78(2):205-215

28. Trainer PJ, Drake WM, Katznelson L, et al. Treatment of acromegaly with the growth hormone-receptor antagonist pegvisomant. *N Engl J Med.* 2000;342(16):1171-1177

29. Trainer PJ, Grossman A. The diagnosis and differential diagnosis of Cushing syndrome. *Clin Endocrinol.* 1991;34:317-330

30. Sperling MA. *Pediatric Endocrinology*. 2nd ed. Philadelphia, PA: WB Saunders; 2002:385-438

31. Saruta T, Suzuki H, Handa M, Igarashi Y, Kondo K, Senba S. Multiple factors contribute to the pathogenesis of hypertension in Cushing syndrome. *J Clin Endocr Metab.* 1986;62:275-279

32. Newell-Price J, Trainer P, Besser M, Grossman A. The diagnosis and differential diagnosis of Cushing syndrome and Pseudo-Cushing state. *Endocr Rev.* 1998;19(5):647-672

33. Cizza G, Nieman LK, Doppman JL, et al. Factitious Cushing syndrome. *J Clin Endocr Metab.* 1996;81:3573-3577

34. Orth DN. Cushing syndrome. *N Engl J Med.* 1995; 332(12): 791-803

35. Maghnie M, Cosi G, Genovese E, et al. Central diabetes insipidus in children and young adults. *N Engl J Med* 2000;343:998-1007

36. McDonald JA, Martha PM Jr, Kerrigan J, Clarke WL, Rogol AD, Glizzard RM. Treatment of the young child with postoperative central diabetes insipidus. *Am J Dis Child,* 1989; 143:201-204

37. Srivatsa A, Majzoub JA. Disorders of Water Homeostasis. In: Lifshitz F, *Pediatric Endocrinology*. New York, NY: Informa Healthcare, USA, Inc; 2007: 651-692

38. Miller M. Syndromes of excess antidiuretic hormone release. *Crit Care Clin.* 2001;17:11-23

39. Decauz G. Long-term treatment of patients with inappropriate secretion of antidiuretic hormone by the vasopressin receptor antagonist conivaptan, urea, or furosemide. *Am J Med.* 2001;110(7):582-584

40. Gross P. Correction of hyponatremia. *Semin Nephrol.* 2001;21:269-272

# CHAPTER 72

## Thyroid Disorders in Adolescents

PAULA KREITZER, MD

Normal thyroid function is integral to optimal growth and pubertal development. For this reason thyroid functions are commonly evaluated in the adolescent patient. A clear understanding of thyroid function and the ability to obtain and interpret appropriate tests is, therefore, important in caring for the older child and the adolescent.

### THYROID HORMONE PRODUCTION

The 2 major products of thyroid hormone production, thyroxine ($T_4$) and triiodothyronine ($T_3$), are released into the circulation under the influence of thyroid-stimulating hormone (TSH), produced by the pituitary gland. Once released into the circulation, the hormones are largely bound to carrier proteins and transported to target tissues, where $T_3$, produced either directly by the thyroid or by peripheral deiodination of $T_4$, enters the cell and binds to nuclear receptors. The receptor-hormone complex then binds to thyroid hormone response elements, which are regulatory elements present on individual genes through which $T_3$ exerts stimulatory or inhibitory effects on gene expression, influencing the function of all bodily systems.[1]

The production of thyroid hormone is tightly regulated by the hypothalamic-pituitary-thyroid axis. $T_4$ and $T_3$ synthesis and secretion is stimulated by TSH release from the anterior pituitary. The release of TSH is in turn stimulated by the release of thyrotropin-releasing hormone (TRH) from the hypothalamus and inhibited by $T_3$ and by $T_4$, which is deiodinated in the pituitary to $T_3$. $T_4$ and $T_3$ also have a direct effect of inhibition of TRH secretion. This tightly controlled negative feedback system is the key to the interpretation of thyroid function tests. In a patient with an intact regulatory axis, high TSH indicates a lack of negative feedback and leads one to suspect hypothyroidism. Conversely, a suppressed TSH indicates excessive thyroid hormone suppression at the level of the pituitary and hypothalamus and is suggestive of hyperthyroidism.

### EVALUATION OF THYROID FUNCTION

In patients with an intact hypothalamic-pituitary-thyroid axis, the most important test for determining whether a patient has thyroid dysfunction is the measurement of TSH using a sensitive third-generation immunoassay. In a patient who is not suspected of having central nervous system dysfunction, a TSH in the normal range usually rules out thyroid dysfunction. Keeping in mind the physiology outlined above, a suppressed TSH is suggestive of hyperthyroidism, whereas an elevated TSH is usually indicative of primary hypothyroidism. However, as elevated or suppressed TSH levels may occur in euthyroid patients, a measurement of $T_4$ is often obtained along with the TSH level. Patients with an elevated TSH but a normal or low normal $T_4$ may be at the early stages of developing hypothyroidism and considered to have compensated or subclinical hypothyroidism. Conversely, patients with a suppressed TSH but normal levels of $T_4$ may be considered to have subclinical hyperthyroidism. In these cases the measurement of serum $T_3$ is useful to determine whether the patient has $T_3$ toxicosis, a condition in which the patient has symptomatic hyperthyroidism associated with elevated $T_3$ but normal $T_4$. Although the measurement of serum $T_3$ is useful in diagnosing hyperthyroidism, it is less helpful when evaluating hypothyroidism, as $T_3$ levels remain normal in many patients with primary hypothyroidism and only decrease in the more severely affected.

When there is discordance between the $T_4$ and $T_3$ levels and the level of TSH, or when the patient is known to have a condition or to take a medication that can affect levels of thyroid-binding globulin (TBG), measurement of free $T_4$ and free $T_3$ levels should be obtained. Because more than 99% of $T_4$ and $T_3$ circulate reversibly bound to protein and only the free portion is metabolically active, alterations in binding proteins can cause significant fluctuation in total thyroid hormone levels without influencing metabolic activity. In these cases, measuring free $T_4$ and free $T_3$ can be helpful in determining whether the patient has thyroid dysfunction. A potential pitfall in relying on free $T_4$ and free $T_3$ levels is that although the levels correspond well to the patient's actual thyroid function when there are mild alterations in binding proteins, severe alterations may lead to abnormal results. Some assays may also be influenced by the presence of thyroid autoantibodies.[2]

Levels of TBG can also be measured directly. Although $T_3$ is bound almost exclusively to TBG, $T_4$ is also bound to a lesser extent by transthyretin and albumin.

Therefore $T_4$ levels can be altered by alterations in binding to albumin and or transthyretin with normal TBG levels. Thyroid-binding globulin levels can be increased or decreased due to x-linked TBG deficiency or excess. Levels of TBG are elevated in acquired immune deficiency syndrome and liver disease. Of significant importance in the adolescent patient is the effect of estrogen in increasing TBG synthesis in the liver. Therefore, TBG levels are increased in pregnancy and with oral contraceptive use. Adolescents on oral contraceptives should have free $T_4$ and $T_3$ levels drawn, because total levels will be inappropriately elevated. The same goes for the pregnant adolescent. Levels of TBG are decreased in malnutrition, nephrotic syndrome, acromegaly and with the use of androgens, glucocorticoids, anabolic steroids, and l-aspariginase.[3]

Reverse $T_3$ ($rT_3$) is a major metabolite of the deiodination of $T_4$. Levels of $rT_3$ often rise in patients with acute and chronic illnesses, changing reciprocally with levels of $T_3$, which often fall in the face of illness. The pattern of a low-serum $T_3$ and an elevated $rT_3$, along with a normal level of TSH (which may rise somewhat during the recovery phase) characterizes the pattern of thyroid functions noted in nonthyroidal illness and is sometimes characterized as the "euthyroid sick syndrome."[2,4]

Thyroid ultrasonography can be helpful in estimating thyroid size as studies have shown it to be superior to palpation in children and adolescents.[5] It is also useful in the evaluation and follow-up of nodules and thyroid cancer. Radionucleotide thyroid scanning is used when it is important to determine the degree of radionucleotide uptake, such as differentiating hyperthyroidism from subacute thyroiditis.[6,7]

## SIMPLE GOITER

Not all thyroid enlargement is pathologic. Simple goiter, which is also called colloid goiter, is the most common cause of asymptomatic, diffuse thyroid enlargement in iodine-sufficient areas. This condition has also been called adolescent goiter because it is common in adolescent females. These patients present with a smooth, soft goiter. Thyroid functions are normal, and antithyroid antibodies cannot be detected, although thyroid growth-stimulating immunoglobulins may be present. This is a benign condition that does not require treatment. An ultrasound of the thyroid may be considered in those cases where there is a question of nodularity but is generally not required in the evaluation of a simple goiter. Patients with simple goiter should be followed annually. Although the goiter may regress, some patients may go on to develop positive antithyroid antibodies.[8]

## HYPOTHYROIDISM

Hypothyroidism may develop slowly over a period of time, with the patient often essentially asymptomatic. When symptoms occur they may be vague and nonspecific; therefore hypothyroidism has been said to be a "mimicker of common complaints."[9] Symptoms that may be encountered include fatigue, lethargy, weight gain, cold intolerance, constipation, dry skin, alopecia, depression, decreased appetite, and headache. In severe hypothyroidism the patient may present with nonpitting edema, bradycardia, pericardial effusion, paresthesias, and gait disturbances.[9] Symptoms particularly relevant in the adolescent patient include growth retardation, which is due to decreased growth hormone secretion, and reduced response of cartilage to insulin-like growth factor-1 (IGF-1),[10] delayed puberty, and menstrual irregularities. Hypercholesterolemia may be the initial presenting abnormality. Hyperprolactinemia may also be present and may rarely be accompanied by galactorrhea.[11]

On physical examination a goiter or enlargement of the thyroid may or may not be present. According to the World Health Organization, a thyroid gland is felt to be enlarged if the lateral lobes are larger than the distal phalanx of the thumb. Patients with significant hypothyroidism at the time of diagnosis may not have thyroid enlargement, as they are more likely to have the atrophic form of autoimmune thyroiditis.[12] Other presenting physical signs may include facial puffiness, delayed relaxation phase of deep tendon reflexes, and a yellowish tinge to the skin due to elevated carotene levels.

### AUTOIMMUNE HYPOTHYROIDISM

The thyroid gland is the most common endocrine gland to be affected by an autoimmune disease. Chronic autoimmune thyroiditis (Hashimoto thyroiditis) is the most common cause of hypothyroidism among adolescents in the iodine sufficient regions of the world.[5] In a study of healthy school children ages 11 to 18, the prevalence of autoimmune thyroiditis was found to be 1.3%.[13] In more than 90% of adult patients with chronic autoimmune thyroiditis, thyroid autoantibodies are detectable at some time in the serum; this is somewhat less predictable in younger patients.[14] Thyroid peroxidase antibody and thyroglobulin antibody are the 2 auto-antibodies most commonly associated with chronic autoimmune thyroiditis. Thyroid peroxidase antibody is the more specific indicator of thyroid disease, with thyroglobulin antibody more likely to be found in patients with no evidence of thyroid disease.[15] The antibodies are part of an inflammatory process resulting in lymphocytic infiltration of the thyroid gland. On physical examination, the classic goiter found in chronic autoimmune thyroiditis is diffusely enlarged, nontender, and firm, although as mentioned earlier, patients with the atrophic form may have severe hypothyroidism unaccompanied by a palpable goiter. The clinical presentation varies from euthyroid goiter to severe hypothyroidism. The clinical status may change over time, with patients having mild hypothyroidism or euthyroid goiter going into remission and other patients with euthyroid goiter eventually developing hypothyroidism.[13]

Adolescents at higher risk for developing autoimmune thyroid disease include children with Down syndrome, Turner syndrome, Kleinfelter syndrome,[16,17] and those with type 1 diabetes[18] and celiac disease. Autoimmune thyroiditis usually occurs as an isolated endocrinopathy but may also occur as part of an autoimmune polyendocrine syndrome.[15]

## DRUG-INDUCED HYPOTHYROIDISM

Thyroid functions can be altered by various medications. The antiepileptic drugs phenobarbital, phenytoin, and carbamazepine decrease $T_4$ levels by increasing the rate of hepatic glucuronidation of thyroid hormone; these medications also appear to blunt the hypothalamic-pituitary response to the decrease in thyroid hormone levels.[19,20] The antiarrhythmic drug amiodarone exerts its toxic effects on the thyroid both by way of a direct toxic effect on the thyroid and because of the medication's large iodine load. The effect of amiodarone is fascinating because it tends to cause hypothyroidism in iodine-sufficient areas of the world and hyperthyroidism in iodine-deficient areas. Patients with pre-existing autoimmune thyroiditis are more likely to develop amiodarone-induced hypothyroidism, and the thyroid dysfunction is more likely to be permanent, not resolving with discontinuation of the drug as in most cases without pre-existing thyroid disease.[21] Lithium administration can cause hypothyroidism at therapeutic doses by inhibition of thyroid hormone release from the gland. Patients with coexisting autoimmune thyroiditis are at higher risk. Valproic acid can also cause mild hypothyroidism with TSH elevation.[22]

## HYPOTHYROIDISM POSTCANCER TREATMENT

Because the thyroid is radiosensitive, adolescents who received mantle radiation for Hodgkin disease, cranial irradiation for brain tumors, or total body irradiation are at risk for the development of primary hypothyroidism, nodules, and thyroid cancer, necessitating lifelong follow-up. The risk of hypothyroidism is increased with higher doses of radiation and decreasing distance of the thyroid from the radiation field. Chemotherapy along with radiation may increase the risk of primary hypothyroidism. Central hypothyroidism, with a decreased $T_4$ and inappropriately low TSH, can also develop as a result of cranial irradiation.[23]

## CENTRAL HYPOTHYROIDISM

Central hypothyroidism is hypothyroidism not due to pathological processes involving the pituitary gland but hypothyroidism that is due to deficiencies of TRH or TSH or to disruption of the hypothalamic–pituitary portal circulation. The condition is rare when compared to primary hypothyroidism. Central hypothyroidism is usually associated with other pituitary and/or hypothalamic hormonal deficiencies; isolated TSH or TRH deficiency is rare, usually due to genetic defects involving TSH or TRH production or receptors.

Central hypothyroidism may be due to mass lesions, infiltrative lesions, congenital defects, trauma, or degenerative diseases affecting the pituitary or the hypothalamus. It may also be iatrogenic after surgery involving the pituitary or the pituitary stalk, or, as mentioned earlier, be the result of radiation. Central hypothyroidism has also been noted in patients with hypopituitarism secondary to defects in genes coding for pituitary-specific transcription factors such as Pit-1 and Prop-1.

In patients with central hypothyroidism, the symptoms of hypothyroidism are often masked by the symptoms of other coexisting pituitary hormone deficiencies. It can also be hard to diagnose as the TSH level, which is clearly elevated in patients with primary hypothyroidism, can be low, normal, or in up to 25% of cases, slightly elevated. Although daytime TSH secretion may be normal, patients with central hypothyroidism often have blunted nocturnal secretion of TSH. Although patients with central hypothyroidism in general have low levels of $T_4$ and free $T_4$, some patients with known central hypothyroidism have been found to have levels of $T_4$ and free $T_4$ in the lower ranges of normal.

Because central hypothyroidism is rarely isolated, patients with this diagnosis should be evaluated for other pituitary hormone deficiencies, especially adrenal insufficiency, because thyroid hormone given to a patient with untreated adrenal insufficiency may potentiate adrenal crisis. In addition, because the disorder is often associated with pituitary or hypothalamic lesions, radiographic imaging of the pituitary and the hypothalamus should be obtained.[24-27]

## TREATMENT

The treatment of hypothyroidism of any etiology is with the synthetic thyroid hormone, levothyroxine. The dose in older children and adolescents is 2 to 3 μg/kg/day.

The usual adult dose is 100 to 200 μg daily;[28] this author usually starts adolescents of normal adult size at 100 μg daily. The dose is titrated by following thyroid functions and aiming for a TSH in the normal range.

## HYPERTHYROIDISM

The symptoms of hyperthyroidism are related to an excess of thyroid hormone resulting in an increase in stimulation of cellular processes and an increase in sensitivity to catecholamines.[29] Symptoms usually develop slowly with time. Major symptoms include goiter, tachycardia and palpitations, tremor, heat intolerance, weight loss, poor sleep, diarrhea, proximal muscle weakness, systolic hypertension, headache, and fatigue.[30,31] In some adolescents hyperthyroidism may be mistaken for a primary behavioral or psychiatric disorder, because declining school performance, emotional lability, and anxiety may be the major presenting features. Various series have reported that more than 40% of children with Graves disease present with school or psychological difficulties.[30,32] Adolescent females may present with menstrual abnormalities, whereas younger adolescents may exhibit tall stature and an advanced bone age.[31]

### GRAVES DISEASE

In adolescents as well as adults, Graves disease accounts for the majority of cases of hyperthyroidism. Graves disease is an autoimmune disorder in which stimulatory autoantibodies bind to the TSH receptor, activating thyroid gland function. As in most autoimmune disorders there is a strong female predominance. Genetic factors seem to play a role in the development of Graves disease; 50% to 80% of patients have a positive family history of thyroid disease and there is a 30% concordance in monozygotic twins. The disease has been associated with human leukocyte antigen (HLA) heliotypes DR3, DQA1*0501, and B8. Studies have found racial variation, with the disease being associated with other HLA heliotypes in non-Caucasian populations. Graves disease has also been associated with certain non-HLA genes.[33] Various environmental precipitants, such as infection, stress, and hormonal changes, have been implicated in the development of Graves disease in susceptible individuals.[34] Graves, like Hashimoto thyroiditis, has an increased incidence in patients with Down syndrome and type 1 diabetes.

The diagnosis of Graves disease may be made on the basis of clinical and confirmatory laboratory findings. Aside from the clinical features of hyperthyroidism, children with Graves disease present with a goiter in more than 95% of cases.[31] A bruit may be detected over the thyroid gland, resulting from increased vascularity and blood flow. Patients with Graves disease present with positive titers of thyroid peroxidase and thyroglobulin antibodies, as well as antibodies against the TSH receptor, referred to as thyroid-stimulating antibodies or immunoglobulin (TSI). The presence of TSI can be measured by either competitive radioreceptor assay or by thyroid cell bioassay.[15] Twenty-four-hour radioactive iodine uptake is elevated in patients with hyperthyroidism due to Graves disease.[7]

Ophthalmologic findings in children and adolescents with Graves disease are usually less severe than those seen in adults, occurring in approximately one-half of patients. Patients with thyrotoxicosis from any cause may have a stare and the appearance of mild eye prominence, due to contraction of the lid muscles caused by increased sympathetic activity. True Graves ophthalmopathy results from an autoimmune process in which there is expansion of both the orbital connective tissues and the extraocular muscles due to deposition of glycosaminoglycans and increased adipose tissue. This can result in proptosis and extraocular muscle dysfunction and, in severe cases, visual loss.[34] Although children and adolescents may have resolution of findings during treatment of hyperthyroidism, patients with significant eye findings should be evaluated by an ophthalmologist for consideration of various therapies, which range from local treatment to systemic corticosteroids to surgical decompression.[35]

There remains much debate as to which is the optimum therapy for adolescents with Graves disease. The 3 main modalities of treatment are medical therapy, surgery, and radioiodine ablation. Antithyroid drugs have been in use since the 1940s. The 2 medications available in the United States, propylthiouracil (PTU) and methimazole, are thionamide drugs actively trapped by the thyroid gland. Their primary mechanisms of action are to inhibit the synthesis of $T_3$ and $T_4$ within the thyroid gland. They do not inhibit the release of thyroid hormone already synthesized by the gland. Propylthiouracil also has an effect in inhibiting extrathyroidal conversion of $T_4$ to $T_3$. Various studies have also pointed to a possible immunomodulatory effect of the drugs.[36]

Methimazole is started at a pediatric dose of 0.4 to 0.7 mg/kg/24 hours divided every 8 hours, with an adult starting dose of 15 to 30 mg divided every 8 hours. Propylthiouracil is started at 5 to 7 mg/kg/day divided every 8 hours for younger children, with older children requiring 150 to 300 mg a day divided into 3 doses and adults generally requiring 300 mg daily.[28] Larger doses may be required in some patients. Studies have shown that methimazole can be given as a once-daily dose, although PTU requires a multiple-dose regimen. Because the drugs do not inhibit release of thyroid hormone, it generally takes several weeks until patients become euthyroid. Beta blockers may be needed as adjuvant therapy in symptomatic patients until their thyroid functions normalize. Once the patient becomes hypothyroid, 2 approaches can be taken.[31] One is to lower the dose of the antithyroid drug, whereas the other approach is to add levothyroxine in addition to the antithyroid medication. Remission can be determined by the ability to decrease drug doses while maintaining euthyroidism or by the normalization of previously elevated levels of TSI.

The negative aspects of drug therapy include the need for prolonged therapy, resulting in difficulties with adherence in many patients, possible side effects, and a high rate of relapse after medication is discontinued. Side effects of the medications are more common in children. Common side effects include rash, fever, urticaria, and joint pains. If 1 of these minor side effects occurs with 1 medication, a switch to the other thioamide can be considered, although there is a risk of a similar reaction. Serious side effects include agranulocytosis, hepatitis, a lupus-like syndrome that may include renal involvement, and erythema multiforme. Patients who experience serious side effects should be taken off the medication immediately and should not be started on the other thionamide. These patients should be considered as candidates for radioiodine ablation or surgery.[29,31]

As mentioned above, drug therapy often must be long term. In a study of 63 patients ages 2 to 19 years who were followed for a period of more than 20 years, 25% of patients were found to achieve remission every 2 years, with the median time for remission 4.3 years. Duration of therapy to achieve remission, which was defined as being euthyroid 1 year after therapy was discontinued, ranged from 5 months to almost 11 years, with 1 patient not yet achieving remission after 11 ½ years.[37] Studies have indicated that patients achieving earlier remission were older than 30 and had smaller goiters and lower $T_4$ and $T_3$ levels. Therefore patients with severe thyrotoxicosis and large goiters have a poorer prognosis for early or long-term remission, as do patients with persistently elevated levels of TSI.[38]

In the United States, radioiodine is the treatment of choice for adult patients with Graves disease. For many years there was reluctance to use radioiodine in children and adolescents for fear of thyroid or other malignancies or negative effects on future offspring. In a study of 98 patients treated with radioiodine prior to age 20 and followed for a mean of 36 years, no thyroid cancer or leukemia was found and there was no increase in the rate of spontaneous abortions or congenital abnormalities in their children. Thyroid cancer has been reported in a few children who received radioiodine therapy. However, they received low doses of radioiodine in an effort to cure hyperthyroidism while preventing hypothyroidism, whereas today's practice is to give larger doses with the effect of ablating the gland.[39] Although low levels of radiation have been found to increase thyroid cancer, higher, thyroid-destructive doses do not appear to increase the thyroid cancer risk. Most patients who undergo radioiodine ablation will become euthyroid within 8 weeks, but some patients may require repeat treatment. More than 80% of treated patients will eventually develop hypothyroidism, so the need for continued monitoring must be explained to the patient. Pregnancy must be excluded prior to radioiodine therapy. Although severely hyperthyroid patients may require pretreatment with antithyroid medications, in most cases beta blockers alone are used to control the symptoms of hyperthyroidism until euthyroidism is achieved.[29,36]

Surgery is a third option for the treatment of Graves disease. The success of this therapy largely depends on the skill and experience of the surgeon, because the thyroid gland in a patient with Graves disease is vascular and friable. The 2 surgical procedures used are subtotal and total thyroidectomy. The size of the remnant of thyroid tissue left after surgery determines the likelihood of developing either hypothyroidism or recurrence. When less than 4 grams of tissue are left there is a more than 50% incidence of hypothyroidism; remnants more than 8 grams are more likely to lead to a recurrence. In children a remnant less than 3 grams is suggested, because children are more likely to relapse. Potential complications include damage to the recurrent laryngeal nerve and transient or permanent hypoparathyroidism. The patient is prepared for surgery with beta blockers. Some clinicians will treat the patient preoperatively with antithyroid drugs or iodides. One advantage of surgery is a rapid correction of the hyperthyroidism without a need for prolonged beta-blocker therapy, as is needed for radioiodine therapy. In addition, surgery may be the treatment of choice for patients with severe ophthalmopathy, as radioiodine may aggravate this condition. Patients with large glands and compressive symptoms will be helped by surgery, as will patients who are pregnant who cannot receive antithyroid medications. It is also an option for patients who cannot tolerate medications or who have failed to achieve a lasting remission and who do not desire radioiodine.[40]

## HASHITOXICOSIS

Hashitoxicosis is an uncommon but important to identify cause of hyperthyroidism in adolescents. Although Hashitoxicosis is hyperthyroidism associated with autoimmune thyroid disease, unlike Graves disease it is felt to result from unregulated secretion of stored thyroid hormone occurring during inflammation of the gland associated with Hashimoto thyroiditis. The hyperthyroidism of Hashitoxicosis usually resolves spontaneously, although patients may require beta blockers. Factors supportive of a diagnosis of Hashitoxicosis are a negative TSI titer and a low to normal uptake on a radionucleotide scan, although the features may overlap with Graves disease.[41]

### SUBACUTE THYROIDITIS

Subacute thyroiditis (de Quervain thyroiditis) is a transient, inflammatory thyroid condition in which hyperthyroidism develops due to release of thyroid hormone from an inflamed gland. There is a significant female predominance. The disorder is felt to be viral in origin and can present with symptoms of hyperthyroidism along with thyroid pain and tenderness, which may be localized or generalized. The patient may complain of pain upon movement of the neck. A high erythrocyte sedimentation rate (ESR) is found, and 24-hour uptake on a radionucleotide scan is low. Beta blockers can be used to control signs of hyperthyroidism if they are severe. Nonsteroidal anti-inflammatory medications can be used to treat mild or moderate discomfort, whereas severely affected patients may require corticosteroids. Although the initial presentation is that of hyperthyroidism, TSH elevations may be noted after resolution of the hyperthyroidism, usually within the first year. Subacute thyroiditis is usually transient; it may persist, however, in some patients who may eventually require treatment for hypothyroidism.[31,42]

### MCCUNE-ALBRIGHT SYNDROME

McCune-Albright syndrome is a rare disorder caused by an activating mutation of the gene encoding the Gs alpha membrane-associated protein, leading to activation of adenylyl cyclase and subsequent autonomous function of various endocrine glands. The classic presentation includes polyostotic fibrous dysplasia, café au lait spots, and endocrine dysfunction, most commonly pseudoprecocious puberty in females. The second most common endocrinopathy is thyroid dysfunction, caused by the autonomous activation of adenylyl cyclase at the TSH receptor, stimulating release of thyroid hormone and thyroid growth. This can lead to nodular and diffuse thyroid enlargement and hyperthyroidism, with or without goiter.[43] Rare cases of thyroid carcinoma have been associated with McCune-Albright.[44] Definitive treatment (radioiodine or surgery) is suggested for patients with hyperthyroidism secondary to McCune-Albright syndrome, as hyperthyroidism will reoccur after antithyroid medications are discontinued.[31]

### TOXIC ADENOMA

Autonomously functioning thyroid nodules are a rare cause of hyperthyroidism in children and adolescents. In general, autonomous adenomas are more common in areas of the world where there is a higher incidence of iodine deficiency. The development of these adenomas is associated with mutations in the TSH receptor or stimulating G-protein.[45] These adenomas may present with symptoms of hyperthyroidism, or if the degree of hyperthyroidism is mild the patient may come to attention because of the presence of the nodule. In general, toxic nodules tend to be large (3 cm or greater). Once the production of thyroid hormone by the adenoma exceeds that of the normal gland, the patient's TSH will be suppressed. A radionucleotide scan will show uptake in the region of the adenoma and varying degrees of suppression of the surrounding thyroid tissue. Although antithyroid medications can suppress thyroid hormone production, definitive therapy is indicated because medication will not treat the underlying adenoma. Treatment options are radioiodine ablation, surgical excision, or percutaneous injection of ethanol. Although malignancy is rare in hyperfunctioning nodules, it can occur and therefore must be ruled out.[46]

### THYROTROPIN-SECRETING PITUITARY TUMORS AND RESISTANCE TO THYROID HORMONE

Two rare conditions that can cause hyperthyroidism with inappropriately normal or elevated TSH levels are TSH-secreting pituitary adenomas and resistance to thyroid hormone. TSH-secreting pituitary tumors are rare in childhood and are usually macroadenomas when they do occur. They can also present with visual symptoms or headaches. A goiter is noted on physical examination due to chronic TSH stimulation of the thyroid. These tumors are treated by surgery, radiation therapy, or somatostatin analogues.[47] Resistance to thyroid hormone, which is due to a mutation in the THR beta gene, is present in 2 forms, generalized resistance and pituitary resistance. In generalized resistance, all tissues have variable resistance to thyroid hormone, so despite elevated levels of thyroid hormone patients may present as euthyroid or hypothyroid. This disorder has been associated with attention deficit hyperactivity disorder (ADHD), learning disabilities, poor weight gain, and auditory disorders. In pituitary resistance, the pituitary is resistant to the suppressive effects of thyroid hormone on TSH secretion whereas other tissues remain sensitive to thyroid hormone action. Euthyroid patients with resistance to thyroid hormone do not need to be treated. Hypothyroid patients with generalized resistance to thyroid hormone can be treated with high doses of thyroid hormone. Patients with pituitary resistance who are thyrotoxic may be treated with beta blockers, triodothyroacetic acid (TRIAC), or d-thyroxin, which are analogues with more potent effects on the pituitary than the periphery that have been shown to decrease TSH levels. Radioiodine therapy or thyroidectomy may be necessary, with subsequent administration of levothyroxin and careful monitoring of the pituitary for hyperplasia of thyrotropin-producing cells or adenoma formation. TSH-producing adenomas can be differentiated from resistance to thyroid hormone by the presence of a lesion on a magnetic resonance imaging (MRI) scan and high serum levels of alpha subunit. Patients with TSH-secreting tumors will also have a blunted response on a TRH stimulation test. Patients with resistance to thyroid hormone have normal levels of alpha subunit and may be noted to have a mutation in the thyroid hormone receptor β gene.[31,48,49]

#### STRUMA OVARII

Another rare cause of hyperthyroidism is struma ovarii. In this condition thyroid tissue makes up a significant component of a mature cystic teratoma. These tumors usually are benign, they can rarely undergo malignant degeneration.[50]

#### INGESTION OF LEVOTHYROXINE

Symptoms of hyperthyroidism can occur after acute ingestions of levothyroxine; usually this requires ingested doses more than 2.0 mg. Symptoms are more likely with chronic abuse. An undetectable level of thyroglobulin is consistent with chronic thyroid hormone abuse. A radionucleotide scan would also fail to show uptake in the region of the thyroid due to chronic suppression of iodine uptake. Patients with $T_4$ levels more than 25 μg/dl require follow-up. If the patient presents soon after the ingestion of 20 or more doses, activated charcoal can be used. Patients with toxic ingestions usually display few symptoms of hyperthyroidism. In patients who do become symptomatic, this may occur days after the ingestion. In these patients, thyroid hormone should be discontinued and beta blockers used if necessary for control of symptoms. Acetaminophen can be used for fever.[51]

### THYROID NODULES AND CANCER

Thyroid nodules are uncommon in the pediatric age group as compared to adults. Their prevalence has been reported to be 0.22% in 9- to 16-year-olds and 1.8% in 11- to 18-year-olds.[52] This is in contrast to 3% to 8% in adults.[53] This reported incidence in the pediatric population is likely to be an underestimation as ultrasound studies in adults have indicated the presence of nodules in 19% to 46% of the population.[54] Despite the decreased incidence in the pediatric population, thyroid nodules in children have a much higher likelihood of malignancy. Although in adults there is a 5% to 15% chance of a thyroid nodule being malignant,[53] solitary pediatric thyroid nodules have an 18% to 21% chance of malignancy.[52] The rate of malignancy in pediatric thyroid nodules has significantly decreased over time. This decrease in the rate of malignancy may be due to a decrease in the use of external radiation to treat benign conditions such as acne and tinea capitus. Radiation exposure remains the most important risk factor associated with the development of thyroid malignancy. Patients exposed to radiation prior to age 16 are twice as likely to develop subsequent thyroid dysfunction. The risk for malignancy appears to be greatest if the radiation exposure occurs prior to 10 years of age. As the latency period for developing thyroid carcinoma after radiation exposure can be as long as 40 years, those who had radiation exposure as children require lifelong surveillance. Accidental exposure to radiation also greatly increases thyroid cancer risk. The incidence of thyroid cancer in children exposed to radiation from Chernobyl increased 100 times.[52,55]

Thyroid nodules usually present as an asymptomatic mass. Concern about malignancy is increased in patients with a history of radiation, rapid growth of the nodule, symptoms of compression and pain, or a nodule that increases in size or appears while a patient is receiving levothyroxine. A nodule larger than 4 cm, firm or fixed to skin or underlying tissues, also raises concern, as does the presence of cervical adenopathy.[54] Ultrasound findings associated with malignancy are hypoechogenicity, suggestive of a solid nodule, calcifications, irregular margins, and lack of a halo sign, which indicates lack of a well-defined capsule.[53] Although these are signs suggestive of malignancy they cannot be used to either diagnose or exclude a malignancy. Like ultrasound, radionucleotide imaging can demonstrate functional properties of a nodule that may make malignancy more likely ("cold" or nonfunctional nodules are more likely to be malignant than "hot" or functioning nodules) but cannot diagnose or exclude malignancy.[52]

Fine needle aspiration (FNA) has become recognized as a safe and accurate modality in the work-up of adolescent thyroid nodules. Researchers have suggested FNA in nodules larger than 1 cm to 1.5 cm, although it has also been suggested to evaluate smaller nodules detected by ultrasound if there are risk factors. Although some authors still suggest excisional biopsy in younger children, FNA has proven useful in preventing unnecessary surgery in many adolescent cases; in highly suspicious lesions it is still most appropriate to obtain an excisional biopsy.[56] Specimens obtained by FNA are classified into 1 of 4 categories; benign, malignant, suspicious, or insufficient. If a sample is deemed insufficient, FNA should be repeated under ultrasound guidance. Suspicious lesions are often follicular or Hurthle cell neoplasms that can not be determined to be benign or malignant on the basis of FNA cytology, or lesions that show some, but not all characteristics of malignancy. Suspicious lesions need to undergo excisional biopsy. Benign nodules need to be followed up. Repeat FNA or excisional biopsy needs to be considered if clinical risk factors for malignancy are present or if the patient has had previous radiation exposure.[54,57]

Papillary thyroid carcinoma is by far the most common form of pediatric thyroid cancer, comprising 70% to 90% of all cases. Medullary carcinoma is the second most common, followed by follicular carcinoma. After papillary or follicular carcinoma is diagnosed, surgical treatment with lymph node exploration is indicated, with most centers advocating a total or near total thyroidectomy followed by levothyroxine therapy to suppress TSH.[58-60] After surgery, radioiodine ablation is used by many centers to ablate possible residual thyroid tissue, although the use in limited disease is somewhat controversial.[61] After treatment, patients are followed with radionucleotide scanning and serum thyroglobulin levels.

Medullary carcinoma, which is cancer involving the calcitonin-secreting cells of the thyroid, exists in a sporadic form and 3 hereditary forms. Familial medullary carcinoma of the thyroid and MEN2A and MEN2B are associated with mutations in the centromeric region of chromosome 10, with 95% having mutations in the RET proto-oncogene. In patients with medullary carcinoma, total thyroidectomy and lymph node dissection is the recommended treatment. Postoperative radiotherapy is controversial but can be used in patients with advanced disease.[60] As MEN2 is associated with pheochromocytoma, patients with MEN2A or B must be screened for the presence of pheochromocytoma prior to surgery. Family members should be screened for the presence of RET proto-oncogene mutations and, if present, should undergo prophylactic thyroidectomy. In patients with RET-positive MEN2B, thyroidectomy should be performed within the first few months of life.[58,59]

The overall survival rates for pediatric thyroid cancer are excellent, with long-term survival rates of more than 90% for papillary and follicular cancer. Medullary thyroid cancer has a poorer prognosis, with long-term survival rates of 65% to 90%.

## REFERENCES

1. Yen P. Genomic and nongenomic actions of thyroid hormone. In: Braverman L, Utiger RD, eds. *Werner and Ingbar's The Thyroid*. Philadelphia, PA: Lippincott Williams & Wilkins; 2005:135–150

2. Bouknight AL. Thyroid physiology and thyroid function testing. *Otolaryngol Clin North Am.* 2003;36(1):9–15

3. Langsteger W. Clinical aspects and diagnosis of thyroid hormone transport protein anomalies. *Curr Top Pathol.* 1997;91:129–161

4. Demers LM. Thyroid disease: pathophysiology and diagnosis. *Clin Lab Med.* 2004;24(1):19–28

5. Svensson J, Ericsson UB, Nilsson P, et al. Levothyroxine treatment reduces thyroid size in children and adolescents with chronic autoimmune thyroiditis. *J Clin Endocrinol Metab.* 2006;91(5):1729–1734

6. Daneman D, Daneman A. Diagnostic imaging of the thyroid and adrenal glands in childhood. *Endocrinol Metab Clin North Am.* 2005;34(3):745–768, xi

7. Meier DA, Kaplan MM. Radioiodine uptake and thyroid scintiscanning. *Endocrinol Metab Clin North Am.* 2001;30(2):291–313, viii

8. Jaruratanasirikul S, Leethanaporn K, Suchat K. The natural clinical course of children with an initial diagnosis of simple goiter: a 5-year longitudinal follow-up. *J Pediatr Endocrinol Metab.* 2000;13(8):1109–1113

9. Tews MC, Shah SM, Gossain VV. Hypothyroidism: mimicker of common complaints. *Emerg Med Clin North Am.* 2005;23(3):649–667, vii

10. Weiss RE, Refetoff S. Effect of thyroid hormone on growth. Lessons from the syndrome of resistance to thyroid hormone. *Endocrinol Metab Clin North Am.* 1996;25(3):719–730

11. Hanna CE, LaFranchi SH. Adolescent thyroid disorders. *Adolesc Med.* 2002;13(1):13–35, v

12. Matsuura N, Konishi J, Yuri K, et al. Comparison of atrophic and goitrous auto immune thyroiditis in children: clinical, laboratory, and TSH-receptor antibody studies. *Eur J Pediatr.* 1990;149(8):529–533

13. Rallison ML, Dobyns BM, Meikle AW, Bishop M, Lyon JL, Stevens W. Natural history of thyroid abnormalities: prevalence, incidence, and regression of thyroid diseases in adolescents and young adults. *Am J Med.* 1991;91(4):363–370

14. Baloch Z, Carayon P, Conte-Devolx B, et al. Laboratory medicine practice guidelines. Laboratory support for the diagnosis and monitoring of thyroid disease. *Thyroid.* 2003;13(1): 3–126

15. Devendra D, Yu L, Eisenbarth GS. Endocrine autoantibodies. *Clin Lab Med.* 2004;24(1):275–303

16. Karnis MF, Reindollar RH. Turner syndrome in adolescence. *Obstet Gynecol Clin North Am.* 2003;30(2):303–320

17. Tyler C, Edman JC. Down syndrome, Turner syndrome, and Klinefelter syndrome: primary care throughout the life span. *Prim Care.* 2004;31(3):627–648, x-xi

18. Glastras SJ, Mohsin F, Donaghue KC. Complications of diabetes mellitus in childhood. *Pediatr Clin North Am.* 2005;52(6):1735–1753

19. Miller J, Carney P. Central hypothyroidism with oxcarbazepine therapy. *Pediatr Neurol.* 2006;34(3):242–244

20. Anderson GD. Pharmacogenetics and enzyme induction/inhibition properties of antiepileptic drugs. *Neurology.* 2004;63(10Suppl 4): S3–S8

21. Basaria S, Cooper DS. Amiodarone and the thyroid. *Am J Med.* 2005;118(7):706–714

22. Correll CU, Carlson HE. Endocrine and metabolic adverse effects of psychotropic medications in children and adolescents. *J Am Acad Child Adolesc Psychiatry.* 2006;45(7): 771–791

23. Cohen LE. Endocrine late effects of cancer treatment. *Endocrinol Metab Clin North Am.* 2005;34(3):769–789, xi

24. Samuels MH, Ridgway EC. Central hypothyroidism. *Endocrinol Metab Clin North Am.* 1992;21(4):903–919

25. Alexopoulou O, Beguin C, De Nayer P, Maiter D. Clinical and hormonal characteristics of central hypothyroidism at diagnosis and during follow-up in adult patients. *Eur J Endocrinol.* 2004;150(1):1–8

26. Turton JP, Reynaud R, Mehta A, et al. Novel mutations within the POU1F1 gene associated with variable combined pituitary hormone deficiency. *J Clin Endocrinol Metab.* 2005;90(8):4762–4770

27. Borck G, Topaloglu AK, Korsch E, et al. Four new cases of congenital secondary hypothyroidism due to a splice site mutation in the thyrotropin-beta gene: phenotypic variability and founder effect. *J Clin Endocrinol Metab.* 2004;89(8): 4136–4141

28. Johns Hopkins Hospital. *The Harriet Lane Handbook.* 16th ed. Philadelphia, PA: Harcourt Health Sciences-Mosby; 2002

29. Reid JR, Wheeler SF. Hyperthyroidism: diagnosis and treatment. *Am Fam Physician.* 2005;72(4):623–630

30. Raza J, Hindmarsh PC, Brook CG. Thyrotoxicosis in children: thirty years' experience. *Acta Paediatr.* 1999;88(9): 937–941

31. Zimmerman D, Lteif AN. Thyrotoxicosis in children. *Endocrinol Metab Clin North Am.* 1998;27(1):109–126

32. O'Brien RF, Kifuji K, Summergrad P. Medical conditions with psychiatric manifestations. *Adolesc Med Clin.* 2006;17(1): 49–77

33. Pearce SHS, Kendall-Taylor P. Genetic factors in thyroid disease. In: Braverman L, Utiger RD, eds. *Werner and Ingbar's The Thyroid.* Philadelphia, PA: Lippincott William & Wilkins; 2005:407–421

34. Prabhakar BS, Bahn RS, Smith TJ. Current perspective on the pathogenesis of Graves disease and ophthalmopathy. *Endocr Rev.* 2003;24(6):802–835

35. Lee HB, Rodgers IR, Woog JJ. Evaluation and management of Graves orbitopathy. *Otolaryngol Clin North Am.* 2006;39(5):923–942, vi

36. Pearce EN, Braverman LE. Hyperthyroidism: advantages and disadvantages of medical therapy. *Surg Clin North Am.* 2004;84(3):833–847

37. Lippe BM, Landaw EM, Kaplan SA. Hyperthyroidism in children treated with long-term medical therapy: twenty-five percent remission every 2 years. *J Clin Endocrinol Metab.* 1987;64(6):1241–1245

38. Cooper DS. Antithyroid drugs for the treatment of hyperthyroidism caused by Graves disease. *Endocrinol Metab Clin North Am.* 1998;27(1):225–247

39. Read CH, Tansey MJ, Menda Y. A 36-year retrospective analysis of the efficacy and safety of radioactive iodine in treating young Graves patients. *J Clin Endocrinol Metab.* 2004;89(9):4229–4233

40. Alsanea O, Clark OH. Treatment of Graves disease: the advantages of surgery. *Endocrinol Metab Clin North Am.* 2000;29(2):321–337

41. Nabhan ZM, Kreher NC, Eugster EA. Hashitoxicosis in children: clinical features and natural history. *J Pediatr.* 2005;146(4):533–536

42. Fatourechi V, Aniszewski JP, Fatourechi GZ, Atkinson EJ, Jacobsen SJ. Clinical features and outcome of subacute thyroiditis in an incidence cohort: Olmsted County, Minnesota, study. *J Clin Endocrinol Metab.* 2003;88(5):2100–2105

43. Mastorakos G, Mitsiades NS, Doufas AG, Koutras DA. Hyperthyroidism in McCune-Albright syndrome with a review of thyroid abnormalities sixty years after the first report. *Thyroid.* 1997;7(3):433–439

44. Collins MT, Sarlis NJ, Merino MJ, et al. Thyroid carcinoma in the McCune-Albright syndrome: contributory role of activating Gs alpha mutations. *J Clin Endocrinol Metab.* 2003;88(9):4413–4417

45. Russo D, Arturi F, Wicker R, et al. Genetic alterations in thyroid hyperfunctioning adenomas. *J Clin Endocrinol Metab.* 1995;80(4):1347–1351

46. Siegel RD, Lee SL. Toxic nodular goiter. Toxic adenoma and toxic multinodular goiter. *Endocrinol Metab Clin North Am.* 1998;27(1):151–168

47. Lafferty AR, Chrousos GP. Pituitary tumors in children and adolescents. *J Clin Endocrinol Metab.* 1999;84(12):4317–4323

48. Khandwala H, Lee C. Inappropriate secretion of thyroid-stimulating hormone. *CMAJ.* 2006;175(4):351

49. McDermott MT, Ridgway EC. Central hyperthyroidism. *Endocrinol Metab Clin North Am.* 1998;27(1):187–203

50. Stepanian M, Cohn DE. Gynecologic malignancies in adolescents. *Adolesc Med Clin.* 2004;15(3):549–568

51. Tenenbein M. Thyroid hormones. In: Ford M, Delaney K, Ling L, Erickson T, eds. *Ford: Clinical Toxicology.* Philadelphia, PA: WB Saunders;2001

52. Bentley AA, Gillespie C, Malis D. Evaluation and management of a solitary thyroid nodule in a child. *Otolaryngol Clin North Am.* 2003;36(1):117–128

53. Frates MC, Benson CB, Doubilet PM, et al. Prevalence and distribution of carcinoma in patients with solitary and multiple thyroid nodules on sonography. *J Clin Endocrinol Metab.* 2006;91(9):3411-3417

54. Kim N, Lavertu P. Evaluation of a thyroid nodule. *Otolaryngol Clin North Am.* 2003;36(1):17-33

55. McClellan DR, Francis GL. Thyroid cancer in children, pregnant women, and patients with Graves disease. *Endocrinol Metab Clin North Am.* 1996;25(1):27-48

56. Corrias A, Einaudi S, Chiorboli E, et al. Accuracy of fine needle aspiration biopsy of thyroid nodules in detecting malignancy in childhood: comparison with conventional clinical, laboratory, and imaging approaches. *J Clin Endocrinol Metab.* 2001;86(10):4644-4648

57. Al Shaikh A, Ngan B, Daneman A, Daneman D. Fine-needle aspiration biopsy in the management of thyroid nodules in children and adolescents. *J Pediatr.* 2001;138(1):140-142

58. McClellan DR, Francis GL. Thyroid cancer in children, pregnant women, and patients with Graves disease. *Endocrinol Metab Clin North Am.* 1996;25(1):27-48

59. Halac I, Zimmerman D. Thyroid nodules and cancers in children. *Endocrinol Metab Clin North Am.* 2005;34(3):725-744, x

60. Vini L, Harmer C. Management of thyroid cancer. *Lancet Oncol.* 2002;3(7):407-414

61. Sawka AM, Thephamongkhol K, Brouwers M, Thabane L, Browman G, Gerstein HC. Clinical review 170: a systematic review and meta-analysis of the effectiveness of radioactive iodine remnant ablation for well-differentiated thyroid cancer. *J Clin Endocrinol Metab.* 2004;89(8):3668-3676

# CHAPTER 73

# Diabetes Mellitus

PAVEL FORT, MD

Diabetes mellitus is a leading cause of chronic illness in youth. Although insulin-dependent diabetes, also called type 1 diabetes (T1D), remains the most common type of diabetes in children, other forms of diabetes must be considered in the differential diagnosis, notably type 2 diabetes (T2D).[1-3] Thus, the diagnosis of diabetes mellitus has become a diagnostic specialty determining prognosis and appropriate treatment. Most children with diabetes mellitus are diagnosed at the beginning of adolescence, with peak incidence earlier in girls than in boys. The day-to-day management of patients with diabetes can be one of the most demanding and difficult medical problems encountered in medical practice. This is especially so in the treatment of adolescents with diabetes. Adolescents differ from younger children in their emancipation from parents, their psychosexual orientation, and their search for identity. Although adolescents with diabetes often steer a perilous course between ketosis and hyperglycemia, on the one hand, and hypoglycemic episodes on the other hand, the long-term outlook for patients with diabetes has improved significantly with intensified metabolic control of the disease. The diagnosis of diabetes represents a major challenge for the patient and family and for health professionals. Not only must the adolescent fulfill the tasks of development into adulthood, but he or she must also cope with daily and often demanding routines of proper care. Because diabetes is a chronic disease with a prognosis that is undoubtedly dependent on the degree of metabolic control, it is necessary for the patient to adhere closely to the prescribed therapeutic regimen. However, some adolescents may not readily accept recommended restrictions imposed by their parents, physicians, and diabetes educators for regulating their disease, especially when such demands interfere with their lifestyle and make them different from their peers.[4] In fact, some adolescents, knowing the importance of controlling their illness, use this as a powerful weapon in manipulating their parents. By choosing noncompliance with the prescribed therapeutic regimen or even boycotting the treatment plan to express their independence, these adolescents precipitate serious short- and long-term metabolic consequences.

## TYPES OF DIABETES MELLITUS

Most children and adolescents with diabetes mellitus have T1D. However, other types and causes of diabetes must be considered when evaluating a patient with new onset of diabetes mellitus.[5] Types of diabetes mellitus and their main characteristics encountered in the pediatric population are summarized in Table 73-1 and Box 73-1.

### TYPE 1 DIABETES MELLITUS

Most patients with T1D have an autoimmune disease whereby insulin-producing beta cells in the pancreas are destroyed by the immune system, leading to deficient or absent insulin production. Such patients require lifelong treatment with insulin. This type of diabetes is the most common entity among nonobese Caucasians, with an incidence rate (per 100,000 person-years) of

**Table 73-1**

**Major Types of Diabetes Mellitus in Adolescents and Its Main Characteristics**

| | *T1D* | | *T2D* | *MODY* |
|---|---|---|---|---|
| | *Type 1a* | *Type 1b* | | |
| Parents affected | 0–1 | 0–1 | 1–2 | 1 |
| Obesity | ± | ± | +++ | ± |
| Onset | Rapid | Rapid | Slow | Slow |
| Acanthosis nigricans | No | No | Yes | No |
| Immune markers | Yes | No | No | No |
| Environment | Yes | Yes | Yes | No |

T1D, type 1 insulin-dependent diabetes mellitus; type 1a, immune-mediated type 1 diabetes mellitus; type 1b, idiopathic (non–immune mediated) type 1 diabetes mellitus; T2D, (insulin resistance with relative insulin deficiency, previously called *non-insulin-dependent diabetes mellitus* or *adult onset diabetes mellitus*); MODY, maturity onset diabetes of the young (due to genetic defects of beta cell function).

> **Box 73-1**
>
> ***Other Types of Diabetes Mellitus***
>
> Genetic defects in insulin action and beta cell function (mitochondrial DNA)
> Diseases of exocrine pancreas
> Endocrinopathies
> Drugs and chemicals
> Infections
> Genetic syndromes
> Anti-insulin receptor antibodies
> Gestational diabetes
> Nonautoimmune diabetes of infancy

> **Box 73-2**
>
> ***Clinical Characteristics of Type 2 Diabetes in Youth***
>
> Mild incidental hyperglycemia
> Possible ketones in the urine
> Serum insulin and C-peptide levels normal to high
> Mean age at presentation, 13.5 years
> Ethnic groups (American of non-European descent)
> Females > males
> Body mass index (BMI) >85th percentile in >95% of patients
> Acanthosis nigricans in 60%–100% of patients
> Family history in 80%–100% of patients

approximately 24.3.[6] Both genetic and environmental factors play a role in the development of the disease, with a polygenic inheritance pattern. At the time of diagnosis, most patients have detectable immune markers, such as glutamic acid decarboxylase, islet cell, and autoinsulin antibodies. Such tests are readily available and are important diagnostic tools. The presence of autoantigens in relatives of a patient with T1D may help us predict the development of T1D in other family members. Environmental factors such as chemicals, milk protein, and viruses have been implicated as a trigger of an autoimmune process. Patients with T1D are at risk for other autoimmune disorders such as Hashimoto thyroiditis, Graves disease, Addison disease, celiac disease, autoimmune hepatitis, myasthenia gravis, and pernicious anemia.[7]

Idiopathic T1D is a rare type of diabetes characterized by the absence of insulin secretory reserve and autoimmune markers. Most patients are of African or Asian ancestry. Such patients may present with severe hyperglycemia and diabetic ketoacidosis (DKA). The differential diagnosis between idiopathic and immune-mediated T1D may be difficult.

## TYPE 2 DIABETES MELLITUS

Type 2 diabetes mellitus is a complex metabolic disorder that is being described with increasing frequency in children, especially adolescents.[3,6–8] The increased incidence of T2D among children has been called an epidemic. Type 2 diabetes mellitus among children was first reported as isolated cases in Native American and First Nations populations in the 1970s, and by the 1990s, physicians began to recognize T2D in black, Hispanic, Asian, and North American white children. It is estimated that 8% to 45% of children with newly diagnosed diabetes mellitus have T2D. The clinical characteristics of T2D in youth are summarized in Box 73-2. The prevalence of T2D depends on the location of a practice and its ethnic composition. Although the factors for the development of T2D are genetic and environmental, the rapidly rising incidence of obesity among children is considered the primary factor. A body mass index (BMI) >35 $kg/m^2$ is associated with 40-fold greater risk for T2D compared to a BMI <25 $kg/m^2$. The pathogenesis of T2D includes insulin resistance promoted by genetic and other risk factors, such as ethnicity, obesity, puberty, family history, polycystic ovary syndrome, and acanthosis nigricans, as well as beta cell dysfunction related to genetics, glucotoxicity, lipotoxicity, and latent autoimmunity. The hyperglycemia in T2D is due to increased insulin resistance, decreased beta cell function, and increased hepatic glucose production.

## MATURITY ONSET DIABETES OF THE YOUNG

Maturity onset diabetes of the young (MODY) usually presents as non-insulin-dependent in persons younger than 25 years who are nonobese and have a strong family history of diabetes.[9–11] It is inherited as an autosomal dominant trait in white populations, affecting approximately 1% to 2% of people with diabetes. Genetic testing is possible in 80% of MODY families. Environmental factors play little role in the pathogenesis of MODY. This type of diabetes is caused by genetic defects of beta cell function. Up to 6 genes have been identified, with glucokinase (MODY 2) and hepatic nuclear factor 1-alpha (MODY 3) being most prevalent. Patients with MODY 2 are usually asymptomatic; although they have increased fasting blood glucose, they may have a normal postprandial blood glucose value; the etiology of the disorder is due to a defect in the sensitivity of beta cells to glucose caused by reduced glucose phosphorylation. Dietary management is usually sufficient, and chronic complications of diabetes are rare. Patients with MODY 3 have abnormal regulatory gene transcription in beta cells, leading to a defect in metabolic signaling of insulin secretion, beta cell mass, or both, and up to one third of such patients will require insulin therapy. The progression of MODY 3 is variable, and the patients are at risk for chronic complication of diabetes.

### GESTATIONAL DIABETES MELLITUS

Gestational diabetes is diabetes discovered during pregnancy. Although almost any type of diabetes can present during pregnancy, the most common scenario is the unmasking of incipient T2D by the metabolic demands of pregnancy. After the child's birth, the maternal diabetes usually disappears, although such women are at increased risk for T2D later in life. Maternal diabetes is known to have profound effects on the fetus, especially when metabolic control is poor. Depending on the onset and severity of maternal diabetes, the fetus may be subjected to a metabolic insult, resulting in congenital anomalies, macrosomia, and intellectual impairment. Therefore, it is of utmost importance that gestational diabetes is recognized early so effective metabolic control can be implemented as soon as possible. If the mother is known to have diabetes, excellent metabolic control of diabetes before conception is essential. With this approach, the adverse effects of diabetes mellitus on the fetus and the mother can be minimized.[12]

### DRUG-INDUCED DIABETES MELLITUS

The list of drugs and hormones associated with abnormal glucose tolerance and diabetes mellitus is exhaustive. Some commonly used preparations causing elevated blood glucose are adrenocorticotrophic hormone, aldosterone, catecholamines, chlorpromazine, clonidine, corticosteroids, diazoxide, ethacrynic acid, furosemide, growth hormone, haloperidol, indomethacin, isoniazid, lithium carbonate, nicotinic acid, oral contraceptives, phenothiazines, phenytoin, risperidone, thiazides, and tricyclic antidepressants.

Other drugs and substances, such as ethanol, monoamine oxidase inhibitors, methimazole, probenecid, propranolol, salicylates, and sulfonamides, can cause hypoglycemia.

## DIAGNOSTIC CRITERIA OF DIABETES MELLITUS

The diagnosis of diabetes mellitus must be considered in an adolescent who presents with polyuria, polydipsia, and weight loss despite an increased calorie intake. A simple urinalysis and the measurement of blood glucose is all that is necessary to make the diagnosis of diabetes mellitus.

Fasting blood glucose ≥126 mg/dL (>7 mmol/L) and/or 2-hour postprandial blood glucose >200 mg/dL (>11.1 mmol/L) are diagnostic of diabetes mellitus.[5]

Fasting blood glucose <126 mg/dL but >100 mg/dL (<7 but >5.6 mmol/L) and 2-hour postprandial blood glucose <200 mg/dL but >140 mg/dL (<11.1 but >7.7 mmol/L) suggest impaired glucose tolerance.[13] This condition, which may or may not progress to diabetes mellitus, encompasses a variety of conditions, the scope of which is not discussed in this chapter.

## CLINICAL TESTING FOR DIABETES MELLITUS IN ADOLESCENTS

### TYPE 1 DIABETES

In asymptomatic individuals, routine testing for T1D, either by measurement of blood glucose or screening for various autoimmune markers, is not currently recommended because cut-off values for the immune marker assays have not been completely established, and there is no consensus as to what action should be taken if a child or adolescent is asymptomatic for diabetes but has the presence of antibodies.[5] The testing of healthy children for diabetes mellitus will identify only a very small number of patients (<0.5%) who at the moment may be "prediabetic." However, various experimental protocols to prevent, or at least postpone, the development of clinical diabetes have been in place.

### TYPE 2 DIABETES

Unlike patients with T1D who generally present with acute symptoms of diabetes and easily recognizable elevated blood glucose levels, many patients with T2D are frequently not diagnosed until complications of diabetes appear. Approximately one third of all people with T2D may be undiagnosed. The following criteria for testing for T2D in children older than 10 years (or at onset of puberty if puberty occurs before age 10 years) and adolescents have been established:

- Overweight (BMI >85th percentile for age and sex, weight for height >85th percentile, or weight >120% of ideal body weight for height) plus any 2 of the following risk factors:
  - Family history of T2D in first- or second-degree relative
  - Race/ethnicity (Native American, black, Latino, Asian American, Pacific Islander)
  - Signs of insulin resistance or conditions associated with insulin resistance, such as acanthosis nigricans, hypertension, dyslipidemia, or polycystic ovary syndrome
  - Maternal history of diabetes or gestational diabetes mellitus

Testing, which includes measurement of fasting and 2-hour postprandial blood glucose levels, should be done every 2 years. Measurement of glycosylated hemoglobins ($HbA_{1c}$) may be added.

## GOALS OF THERAPY AND PATIENT MANAGEMENT

The establishment of clear and reasonable goals for the treatment of diabetes mellitus is most important (Box 73-3). In the day-to-day management of patients, every attempt must be made to achieve near-normoglycemia, regardless of the philosophy of the health care professional, the resources available, and the ability of the patient and family to comply with the rigors of therapy. The presence of the classic symptoms of diabetes, such as polyuria or polydipsia or even nocturia, is not acceptable. The patient should not be allowed to develop acute complications of diabetes such as ketoacidosis or hypoglycemia. In addition, children with diabetes mellitus should exhibit normal growth and sexual maturation. In view of evidence that poor glycemic control of diabetes plays a role in the development of chronic microangiopathic complications, rigorous control of the condition must be a desirable goal.[14-17]

Ideally, blood sugar levels should be maintained in the normal nondiabetic range. However, this is difficult to achieve without imposing a great deal of limitations on the patient's lifestyle and increasing the risk of severe hypoglycemia.[18] Therefore, we and many other pediatric endocrinologists aim to reach preprandial blood sugar levels between 90 mg/dL and 130 mg/dL (5.0–7.2 mmol/L) and postprandial levels <180 mg/dL (10.0 mmol/L) in older children and adolescents. We strive to keep the urine free of ketones at all times, although ketones may be detectable during an acute illness. There has been much pressure to attain normal $HbA_{1c}$ levels the test that "does not lie." Normal $HbA_{1c}$ levels are frequently attainable during the early years of diabetes, when some residual function of endogenous insulin production remains. However, in many patients, normal $HbA_{1c}$ levels are difficult to achieve once total insulin deficiency develops. In fact, even with tight control of diabetes, such as with a continuous insulin delivery system or multiple daily injections of insulin, only 18% of patients reported by the Diabetes Control and Complications Trial study could achieve and maintain normal $HbA_{1c}$ levels.[14] Most of our patients show $HbA_{1c}$ levels between 7.0% and 8.5% (normal <6.0%) of total hemoglobin A. The goal is to keep $HbA_{1c}$ levels as close to normal as possible without risking hypoglycemia and ameliorating emotional maladaption.

A well-informed patient who has a personal, trusting relationship with the physician and other members of the health care team is ideally suited to diabetes mellitus treatment. Maladaptation for treatment, resulting in worsening of diabetes control, may occur when patients are subjected to excessive demands and to feelings of guilt associated with their difficulty in coping with care. In the management of care for adolescents with diabetes mellitus, several specific factors need to be addressed to facilitate adjustment to the disease. The location of the health center or the physician's office should be convenient to the patient. The time of appointments should be flexible, and adolescents should be reminded in writing about their next appointments. Many other factors may interfere with adherence to the therapeutic regimen, including conflicts with parents and teachers, special interests, and alcohol and drug consumption. Such issues should be well known to the medical staff who care for adolescents with diabetes mellitus. Willing and experienced medical professionals, preferably a certified diabetes educator and pediatric endocrinologist, should be the key persons providing care. They should possess up-to-date knowledge, enjoy working with teenagers, and be adept at developing a close, nonparental type of relationship with the patient. The professionals should also show flexibility and a willingness to compromise when necessary.

### Box 73-3

### *Therapy Goals for Diabetes Mellitus*

**ACHIEVABLE GOALS**

Control of symptoms
Avoidance of acute complications (eg, ketosis, hypoglycemia)
Maintenance of normal growth and maturation
Maintenance of normal blood lipids
Minimization of urinary glucose losses
Preservation of emotional well-being
Achievement of independence as mature adult

**DESIRABLE GOALS**

Normal hemoglobin A levels
Euglycemia
Prevention of long-term diabetic complications

### INSULIN THERAPY

The administration of insulin represents a mainstay of therapy for T1D and often for T2D as well.[19] Insulin is given to correct the metabolism of carbohydrates, protein, and fat, and hence to achieve as good a control of diabetes as possible. However, treatment must be individualized. Issues that need to be addressed when insulin therapy is being considered include (1) type and dosage; (2) special problems, such as inadequate insulinization, excessive insulinization, insulin resistance or sensitivity, nutrition, exercise, and stress; and (3) mode of treatment, including conventional or intensive therapy.

### Types of Insulin

The introduction of human insulin produced by DNA-recombinant techniques has expanded the availability and choice of insulin preparations. The insulin can be delivered either by subcutaneous injections or by continuous subcutaneous insulin infusion (CSII). In January 2006, the US Food and Drug Administration (FDA) approved inhaled human insulin powder (Exubera, Pfizer/Sanofi-Aventis) for adult patients with T1D and T2D. Currently available insulin preparations are shown in Table 73-2. The type of insulin used should be decided by a health care provider and should be individualized to achieve the best glycemic control possible. If one type of insulin does not provide a patient with optimal blood glucose levels, a different type of insulin must be tried. The shorter the action of insulin, the more daily injections will be required. Knowledge of the pharmacokinetics of various insulin preparations is essential for the proper management of diabetes mellitus.

**Table 73-2**

**Available Insulin Preparations on the US Market**

| *Insulin* | *Onset* | *Peak* | *Effective Duration* |
|---|---|---|---|
| **Human** | | | |
| Glulisine (Apidra) | <15 min | 0.5–1 hr | 3 hr |
| Lispro (Humalog) | <15 min | 1–2 hr | 2–4 hr |
| Aspart (Novolog) | <15 min | 1–3 hr | 3–5 hr |
| Regular | 0.5–1 hr | 2–4 hr | 3–5 hr |
| NPH | 2–4 hr | 4–10 hr | 10–16 hr |
| Lente | 3–4 hr | 4–12 hr | 12–18 hr |
| UltraLente | 6–10 hr | minimal | 18–20 hr |
| 70/30 | 0.5–1 | 2–10 hr | 10–16 hr |
| Humalog 75/25 Novolog Mix 70/30 | <15 min | 1–2 h | 10–16 hr |
| Insulin Glargine (Lantus) | 4–6 hr | NONE | 24 hr |
| Insulin Detemir (Levemir) | 3–4 hr | 50% of effect in 3–4 lasting up to 14 hours | 5.7–23 hr |



Most patients with diabetes who receive conventional insulin therapy combine a rapid and intermediate-acting insulin in the morning (before breakfast) and at night (before dinner), usually in a 1:3 ratio. Because intermediate insulin may not provide adequate coverage during the early morning hours, many patients may benefit from splitting the night time insulin such that only rapid-acting insulin is administered before dinner and intermediate-acting insulin is moved to the bedtime hours. Today, many patients with insulin-requiring diabetes use long-acting insulin, such as Lantus or Levemir, as a basal insulin given once or twice daily and short-acting insulin to cover main meals. Although a recent concern about carcinogenic activity of long-acting insulin (Lantus) has been raised,[20] there are currently no recommendations against the use of long-acting insulin in adolescents with diabetes mellitus.

### Insulin Dosages

The dosages of insulin required by patients with diabetes mellitus are fairly constant and predictable despite great variations in many factors that alter insulin action. Increased resistance to insulin is noted during puberty, in both nondiabetic and diabetic children. Under normal circumstances, insulin requirements are determined by the patient's age and the duration of diabetes.[21] Although prepubertal children with insulin-dependent diabetes mellitus usually require dosages of insulin <1 U/kg body weight per day, requirements are generally increased in adolescents, often up to 1.5 U/kg body weight daily. Higher dosages are unusual, and may worsen the control of diabetes and increase the risk of hypoglycemia. Stress, whether physical or emotional, often leads to increased insulin requirements. In contrast, exercise results in more rapid utilization of glucose with decreasing insulin requirements. However, it is important to be aware that vigorous exercise in the face of hyperglycemia may exert an opposite effect, and ketosis may result. Finally, insulin requirements are directly related to the nutritional intake of the patient. Excessive calorie consumption is associated with an increased need for insulin and an accumulation of fat, leading to undesirable weight gain.

### Inadequate Insulinization

In practical terms, an adolescent who has had insulin-requiring diabetes for several years and is receiving an insulin dose of <1 U/kg body weight per day may be having "inadequate insulinization." Regardless of what the patient claims or what is shown on the blood glucose record, it is the physician's responsibility to prove that the patient needs unusually low doses of insulin to maintain good metabolic control. It is possible that in some patients, endogenous insulin secretion is partially preserved for many years. In these patients, C-peptide levels may be measured to ascertain endogenous production of insulin. Adolescents with diabetes who receive insufficient insulin may develop complications such as peripheral neuropathy and hyperlipidemia because of an accumulation of sorbitol and decreased action of lipoprotein lipase, respectively. Moreover, chronic inadequate insulinization may contribute to the development of severe long-term complications of diabetes. When a patient seems to require small doses of insulin or when the insulin requirements decline without an apparent reason, the patient must also be checked for other autoimmune diseases. Finally, the possibility of the surreptitious use of insulin by some adolescents must be kept in mind. Such a situation generally indicates psychopathology and must be handled appropriately.

### Excessive Insulinization

The use of an insulin dose of >2 U/kg body weight per day in adolescent patients with diabetes should alert the physician to the possibility of excessive insulinization. Excessive insulinization should also be suspected when the glycemic control of the diabetes remains poor despite administration of high doses of insulin. The so-called Somogyi phenomenon denotes a situation in which blood glucose rises after insulin-induced hypoglycemia as a consequence of the sudden release of "anti-insulin hormones," causing a temporary insulin resistance.[22] The Somogyi phenomenon is often used by physicians to explain morning fasting hyperglycemia. However, others dismiss this phenomenon in many patients who have unexplained hyperglycemia.[23] Patients with T1D who exhibit hyperglycemia on awakening may be experiencing inadequate insulinization during the early morning hours without having nocturnal hypoglycemia. The Somogyi phenomenon may be suspected when the patient has frequent nightmares, has excessive perspiration during sleep, wakes up irritable, or has ketones in the urine on awakening. Body weight usually continues to increase at excessive rates. When the possibility of the Somogyi phenomenon is being considered, the insulin dose should be decreased slowly to an appropriate dosage on a per kilogram basis. This should be done despite the temptation to counteract hyperglycemia and ketonuria with extra insulin. If the Somogyi phenomenon proves to be the problem, control of diabetes is improved by decreasing the amount of insulin to the recommended level. A 10% decrease in insulin dose every few days is recommended.

Another, perhaps more common cause of early morning hyperglycemia is the so-called dawn phenomenon. This is characterized by progressively increasing blood glucose levels after 4 am and hence greater insulin requirements during that period, without preceding hypoglycemia. The exact mechanism of the dawn phenomenon has not been elucidated, although increased insulin clearance in the face of rising anti-insulin hormones, such as growth hormone and cortisol, may play a role in its development.[24] Prevention of the dawn phenomenon is best achieved by moving insulin administration to the late evening hours in patients on a conventional insulin regimen or increasing the basal rate of insulin between 4 am and 7 am in patients receiving a CSII regimen.

## HOME BLOOD GLUCOSE MONITORING

Assessment of diabetes control through home blood glucose monitoring (HBGM) is a mainstay of proper diabetes management.[25] Patients and their families must be educated about the importance of such monitoring. They must be motivated and learn how to adjust the dose of insulin according to blood glucose readings. Currently, many accurate and reliable glucose meters are on the market. Once the HBGM technique is implemented, an algorithm for multiple dosages of insulin and multiple blood glucose levels should be followed for more precise metabolic control of the diabetes. It is important to be aware that patients may falsify the HBGM records and provide the physician with unreliable data. Such a possibility should be considered whenever the clinical findings and other biochemical parameters, such as $HbA_{1c}$ levels, are in discordance with reported blood glucose values. Most patients are requested to check their blood glucose 4 times a day (before breakfast, lunch, dinner, and a bedtime snack) and, once a week, at 2 am; however, individual adjustments may be made. When blood glucose values are below or above the desired range, changes in the dose of insulin should be made. Some patients with diabetes do not adjust their insulin dosage according to blood sugar levels; such patients provide the physician with blood glucose readings, but do not use this information for better management of their illness. Obtaining a blood glucose sample is not an entirely painless procedure, even with the latest technical equipment. Some meters allow use of a blood sample from sites other than fingers, such as forearms. Various companies are presently at work on noninvasive meters, although these are currently not available for the general public. Recently, the FDA has approved an insulin pump with real-time continuous glucose monitoring (MiniMed Paradigm Real-Time System, Medtronic). The device, which takes glucose readings from interstitial fluid every 5 minutes, allows patients to view glucose trends throughout the day and night. It is hoped that this innovation could lead to the development of a closed-loop system that mimics the function of a human pancreas.

### INTENSIVE TREATMENT

Intensive insulin therapy, either in the form of multiple daily injections or as a CSII, now constitutes routine therapy for many patients with diabetes mellitus. The use of CSII among patients with T1D in the United States is estimated to be around 20%. Today, many health care providers believe that these are highly appropriate routine therapeutic modalities for patients who require insulin therapy, regardless of a patient's age, duration of diabetes, and degree of glycemic control.[26] In fact, many patients are started on intensive insulin therapy at the onset of diabetes mellitus. This attitude is based on evidence that poor metabolic control plays an important role in the pathogenesis of chronic diabetes complications.[14] Moreover, the use of multiple injections of insulin or CSII allows for a more flexible lifestyle and timing of meals, which is especially important in adolescents with diabetes mellitus. An increasing variety of ever more sophisticated and reliable CSII devices are available on the market. Because intensive insulin therapy requires close monitoring of glycemic control, it is not appropriate to start any of these therapeutic regimens unless the patient utilizes proper blood glucose surveillance and has good knowledge of carbohydrate counting. Patients undergoing such therapy need intensified overall diabetes management, covering education, nutrition, exercise, and lifestyle. Intensive treatment requires a high degree of motivation on the part of the patient and family.

Intensive therapy with multiple injections is as effective as CSII treatment. Typically, a long-acting insulin such as Lantus or Levemir is administered once daily, usually at bedtime. The main meals are then covered by a rapid-acting insulin (Humalog or Novolog), the dose of which is based on the amount of carbohydrate in a meal and the level of blood glucose. Such an approach requires, however, at least 4 daily injections of insulin, which some patients may find too demanding and thus unacceptable. With rigorous supervision, euglycemia and a near-normal $HbA_{1c}$ level can be attained on a long-term basis in many patients with diabetes mellitus.

## MAJOR COMPLICATIONS OF DIABETES MELLITUS

### DIABETIC KETOACIDOSIS

Diabetic ketoacidosis (DKA) is a major emergency in the adolescent patient.[27] It is usually defined as hyperglycemia (serum glucose concentration >250 mg/dL [13.9 mmol/L]) and metabolic acidosis (blood pH <7.30 and/or HCO <15 mEq/L). The urine is positive for glucose and ketones. Diabetic ketoacidosis results not only from an actual lack of insulin, but also from a relative deficiency of insulin, which can occur in situations marked by the presence of increased hyperglycemic hormones, such as stress, infection, and inflammation. The initial assessment, generally performed in an emergency room setting, is similar to that for any critically ill patient. Patients with DKA are always dehydrated, and the state of dehydration must be carefully assessed. Patients with DKA may continue to have a marked urinary output despite severe dehydration and impending renal shutdown. Laboratory studies consist of immediate measurement of serum glucose, electrolytes, ketones, bicarbonate, and pH, as well as serum osmolarity and a complete blood count. In the presence of fever, appropriate cultures of body fluids must be obtained. Monitoring of the serum potassium level is very important because it may fall precipitously with the initiation of therapy. Often, there is pseudohyponatremia caused by hyperglycemia and hyperlipidemia. The serum osmolarity is always elevated, but values >375 mOsm/L indicate morbid hyperosmolarity (MH), management of which is discussed later in this chapter.

*Intravenous (IV) fluid therapy* should be started immediately after the initial assessment and blood work are completed. Unless the patient presents with MH, normal saline at a rate of 20 mL/kg to 40 mL/kg body weight per hour is sufficient for initial therapy. Once the electrolyte status of the patient is known, the composition of fluids should be modified as needed to replace the severe electrolyte losses. Generally, the water and sodium replacement is given over the first 24 hours. One must be aware of ongoing urinary losses, and proper replacement of these losses must be provided. Potassium salts (half chloride and half phosphate) must be added to the IV fluids at once if there is no concomitant hyperkalemia and if the patient has good urinary output. Failure to do so may result in severe hypokalemia because both correction of acidosis and administration of insulin promote transfer of potassium into the cells.

The *acidosis of DKA* is due to a combination of mostly ketoacidosis and some lactic acidosis. Because ketoacidosis will respond to the restoration of glycolysis as the principal generator of energy by the administration of insulin, fluid therapy and insulin are the principal agents for the treatment of mild to moderate acidosis (pH >7.15). Bicarbonate administration is generally not necessary if the pH is >7.15. Marked acidosis, however, is life threatening because of its central nervous system (CNS) effects, which include respiratory depression.

The recommended treatment of marked acidosis is as follows:

- pH 7.15–7.00: correct the bicarbonate deficit slowly over 1 hour or more
- pH <7.00: 1 mEq/kg NaHCO by slow IV push
- To calculate the bicarbonate deficit: HCO deficit = (15 − serum bicarbonate) × kg body weight × 0.6.
- The sodium content of the NaHCO should be included in the calculation of total sodium maintenance and replacement. The clinician should remember that overuse of sodium bicarbonate can lead to hypernatremia. Also, as equilibration across the respiratory center of the brain is slow for bicarbonate but rapid for CO, the quick correction of metabolic acidosis will be accompanied by retention of CO and paradoxical CNS acidosis. Finally, rapid correction of acidosis may precipitate hypokalemia.

*Administration of insulin* is an essential component of therapy for DKA. Although there are many theoretical modes of insulin administration in DKA, the IV route is best in the early stages. The so-called low-dose insulin infusion has the advantage of supplying a constant steady rate of insulin administration; therefore, a steady serum level of insulin is attained. The usual dose of insulin in adolescents is regular insulin 0.1 U/kg body weight per hour. The insulin infusion rate should be governed by a reliable positive-pressure pump. Once the serum glucose falls below 250 mg/dL (13.9 mmol/L), which usually occurs before the correction of acidosis, 5% dextrose is added to the IV fluids. More glucose may be added to IV fluids as needed. A convenient method for coordinating the glucose with the insulin is to discontinue the insulin infusion, and add insulin and glucose in a fixed ratio to the hydration solution. The usual dose in adolescents is 2 units of regular insulin for every 5 g of glucose. In any given patient, the insulin/glucose ratio may vary, and proper adjustment of insulin dose and IV glucose content may be needed to maintain blood glucose levels in the 100 to 150 mg/dL range (5.6–8.3 mmol/L).

## SEVERE HYPERGLYCEMIA WITH KETONURIA

One of the important goals of therapy for T1D is to avoid acute complications such as DKA. Despite great efforts, DKA remains a real and serious complication of T1D, especially among patients with poor diabetes control. As with many diseases, the best treatment of DKA is early diagnosis and appropriate therapy. Recognition of impending DKA and institution of extra insulin administration together with vigorous oral fluid replacement, often aborts DKA, thus avoiding hospitalization. Outpatient management of severe hyperglycemia with or without ketonuria requires a reliable and cooperative patient and family, the ability to stay in close telephone contact with the physician (often on an hourly basis), and an experienced health team. The typical patient is an adolescent who is going through physical or emotional stress and presents with a blood glucose level >250 mg/dL (13.9 mmol/L) and positive urinary ketones. Often such a patient is nauseous but has not vomited. If the decision is made to treat hyperglycemia and ketonuria at home, the patient is instructed to start with a rapid-acting insulin in a dosage of 0.1 U/kg body weight subcutaneously every hour as long as the blood glucose level remains >250 mg/dL (13.9 mmol/L) and the urine shows moderate or large ketones. In conjunction with insulin administration, the patient is instructed to increase fluid intake. The amount of fluid intake recommended is based on the assumption that the patient is not more than 5% dehydrated and has had no vomiting or diarrhea. Fluid maintenance and replacement are calculated so that one half of the deficit and one third of the maintenance level are replaced in the first 8 hours. Diet (carbonated) soft drinks are a common hydration medium for patients with T1D, but these vary widely in sodium and potassium content. Resolution of ketonuria and hyperglycemia is equated with therapeutic success. Persistence of mild ketonuria with blood glucose <250 mg/dL (13.9 mmol/L) is also considered acceptable. We have found that this approach is easy for both patient and family to follow. However, the patient must be in stable condition and able to tolerate oral hydration. If there is any question about the stability of the patient's condition, he or she is instructed to go to the physician's office immediately or to an emergency facility. The details of this approach have been described by Pugliese et al.[27]

## MORBID HYPEROSMOLARITY

Morbid hyperosmolarity,[27–29] defined as serum osmolarity >375 mOsm/L and blood glucose >1,400 mg/dL (77.8 mmol/L), is a life-threatening condition with significant morbidity and mortality. It is seen in situations of near-normal insulin levels and is often precipitated by pneumonia or gram-negative sepsis. Many such patients have been receiving oral hypoglycemia agents. Drugs such as phenytoin (Dilantin), thiazides, and steroids have also been implicated as precipitating agents. The severe hyperviscosity seen in MH can lead to thromboembolic events, CNS bleeding, acute renal failure, disseminated intravascular coagulation, and shock. Rapid correction of MH, especially in young children, has been reported to result in severe cerebral edema, although the pathogenesis of cerebral edema in patients in DKA remains poorly understood. Many such patients are only mildly acidotic or not acidotic at all. Initial evaluation should quickly identify patients with MH, who should be handled in a center where various subspecialties such as neurology nephrology and hematology are available.

Management of patients with MH differs from that of typical DKA. The goals of fluid and electrolyte therapy are resuscitation of the patient from shock, maintenance of adequate perfusion of all vital organs, and a gradual reduction in serum hyperosmolarity. These goals are accomplished by carefully monitoring the interplay of arterial pressure, epidural pressure (when feasible), and urinary output. Hydration must be adequate to maintain the central venous pressure in a normal range. However, overzealous rehydration, especially with hypotonic solutions, can result in cerebral edema. If there is an increase in intracranial pressure, various methods of lowering the pressure, such as hyperventilation, barbiturate coma, and head elevation, should be employed. It is agreed that isotonic or hypertonic solutions should be used to dilute the glucose in patients with MH. In general, the fluids administered should be only 30 to 40 mOsm/L lower than serum osmolarity. Usually, this can be achieved with normal saline and potassium salts. The osmolarity of standard commercial solutions is D5W, 252 mOsm/L; normal saline, 308 mOsm/L; NaHCO, 2,000 mOsm/L; and K phosphate, 7,000 mOsm/L, or 1.7 mOsm/mEq K. As with any hypertonic dehydration, deficits should be replaced slowly over 48 to 72 hours, rather than over 24 hours, as is customary in simple DKA. Patients with MH are in need of insulin therapy. However, there has been some controversy about the dosage of insulin and the best time of administration. The general approach has been to use only half the dose of insulin (ie, 0.05 U/kg/hour) or even less if there is a precipitous decline in the blood glucose levels. The drop of serum glucose should not exceed 100 mg/dL (5.6 mmol/L)/hour, especially when the serum glucose level is approaching near-normal levels. In fact, it may be preferable to maintain serum glucose levels >250 mg/dL (13.9 mmol/L) during the first 48 hours of therapy, which can minimize the development of clinically significant cerebral edema.

## HYPOGLYCEMIA

Hypoglycemia is a common occurrence among patients receiving insulin therapy, especially because the importance of maintaining blood glucose levels as close to normal as possible to minimize long-term chronic complications of diabetes mellitus is recognized.[14] Hypoglycemia is due to the absolute or relative excess of insulin, often precipitated by a lack of food or increased exercise. Hypoglycemia can also emerge in insulin-treated patients, who develop the lack of anti-insulin hormones such as cortisol, growth hormone, epinephrine, and glucagons. Hypothyroid states, usually as a consequence of autoimmune (Hashimoto) thyroiditis or states with malabsorption (ie, celiac disease), can also be accompanied by hypoglycemia. True hypoglycemia is defined as a whole blood glucose concentration <50 mg/dL (2.8 mmol/L), although symptoms of hypoglycemia can be seen at much higher concentrations of glucose.[30] However, many patients may remain asymptomatic even at blood glucose levels <50 mg/dL (2.8 mmol/L). This has been described as the "hypoglycemia unawareness syndrome."[31]

The symptoms and signs of hypoglycemia have traditionally been divided into neuroglycopenic and adrenergic manifestations.[32] Neuroglycopenia represents a lack of the major fuel (glucose) for the CNS, which can result in cognitive dysfunction, disorientation, seizures, and death when not appropriately treated. Adrenergic symptoms result from activation of the sympathetic nervous system and are well recognized as anxiety, pallor, headaches, tremor, and increased perspiration. Although most patients can easily recognize the symptoms of hypoglycemia, repeated episodes of hypoglycemia may become asymptomatic, especially at night. It is imperative, therefore, that all patients receiving insulin therapy monitor their blood glucose several times a day and once or twice a week at 2 or 3 am. Teenagers can be at an increased risk of developing hypoglycemia because they may not comply with dietary recommendations or may experiment with alcohol intake (which aggravates hypoglycemia by blocking neoglucogenesis). Moreover, clinicians should be aware of the surreptitious administration of insulin practiced by some teenagers.[33] Treatment of documented hypoglycemia, with or without symptoms, should be prompt. When symptoms are mild, an extra 5 g to 10 g of glucose followed by a protein snack will suffice. More glucose may be needed when symptoms are more severe. If the adolescent is unconscious, 1 mg glucagon should be administered subcutaneously at once, even if a blood glucose level is not immediately available. For that reason, every family with a member having insulin-treated diabetes mellitus should have an emergency glucagon kit at their disposal and be familiar with its use. When the patient is traveling or leaves home for college, there should always be a person available who is capable of administering glucagon to the patient.

Although rare, hypoglycemia in adolescents with or without dibetes mellitus can be caused by other conditions. These include:

- missed meals
- alcohol abuse
- rapid stomach emptying (after stomach surgery)
- apart from insulin and oral hypoglycemic agents, other drugs, such as beta-adrenergic blocking agents, salicylates, certain antibiotics, and others
- severe infections

- insulin-producing tumor (such as an insulinoma)
- insulin-like substance producing tumors (such as hepatoma, mesothelioma, fibrosarcoma)
- severe liver or kidney disease
- endocrine deficiencies resulting in low levels of glucose-regulating hormones

## CHRONIC COMPLICATIONS OF DIABETES MELLITUS

Chronic complications of diabetes mellitus consist of the classic triad of retinopathy, nephropathy, and neuropathy.[34] They remain the main cause of morbidity and mortality in patients with diabetes mellitus, and once established, they are usually irreversible. Although the clinical presentation of diabetic complications usually occurs after childhood and adolescence, subclinical manifestations may be encountered at a younger age. The pathogenesis of chronic complications has not been clearly established, although several theories have been implicated. These include chronic hyperglycemia (the so-called glucotoxic theory), hemodynamic alterations (eg, hypertension), hormonal effects, and genetic and environmental factors.[35] Several animal and human studies have shown that the near-normalization of blood glucose levels reduces the frequency and severity of chronic diabetic complications.[14] However, the clustering of chronic complications among family members with diabetes mellitus points to environmental and genetic factors.[36,37]

### Diabetic Retinopathy

Visual impairment is a frequent complication of diabetes mellitus. Among adults, diabetic retinopathy is the leading cause of new cases of blindness. In addition, other eye conditions, such as glaucoma, cataracts, and corneal disease, are more likely to develop in patients with diabetes mellitus. Most patients with T1D will develop detectable eye changes after 15 years. Fortunately, new methods of treatment, such as laser photocoagulation and vitrectomy, have greatly improved the quality of life of such patients. Moreover, the availability and implementation of better metabolic control of diabetes mellitus is expected to significantly reduce all diabetic complications. It is important that all patients with diabetes mellitus receive regular ophthalmologic evaluations so that retinal changes can be detected early.[5]

### Diabetic Nephropathy

Diabetes is the most common[38–41] cause of end-stage renal disease. Diabetic nephropathy affects approximately 30% of patients with diabetes. Patients with a family history of essential hypertension or diabetic nephropathy appear to at risk for this complication. Nephropathy can be defined as the presence of clinical proteinuria (>0.5 g of protein per 24 hours). When new sensitive techniques are used, minute amounts of protein (microalbuminuria) can be detected in the urine before the appearance of clinical proteinuria. Proteinuria is associated with diabetic glomerulosclerosis, which is characterized by increased basement membrane thickness and expansion of mesangium. Renal hyperfiltration, as evidenced by an increased glomerular filtration rate, is almost always present at diagnosis. Although there is a strong association between systemic hypertension and diabetic kidney disease, it is unusual to find blood pressure measurements greater than the 97th percentile in children and adolescents with T1D. However, some normotensive patients with T1D may lack the normal night-time drop in systolic pressure and thus appear to be at risk for the development of microalbuminuria.[42]

The 2 current treatments to protect against diabetic nephropathy include tight metabolic control and the use of renin angiotensin axis blockers, such as Enalapril.

### Diabetic Neuropathy

Diabetic neuropathy, although not life threatening, is the most common and troublesome chronic complication of diabetes mellitus.[43] Fortunately, severe forms are rare among children and adolescents with diabetes mellitus, but their incidence increases with duration of disease. The most susceptible nerves are the sensory and motor fibers of the lower extremities. Diabetic neuropathy can be helped by improving glycemic control of diabetes mellitus. Autonomic neuropathy, although a difficult problem in adults with diabetes mellitus, has rarely been observed or clearly diagnosed in diabetic children and adolescents.

## OTHER COMPLICATIONS

Other, usually reversible, complications in children and adolescents with diabetes mellitus include skeletal and joint abnormalities (manifesting as thickening of skin and inability to fully extend the interphalangeal joints, and later, the larger joints), osteopenia, growth failure, and delayed sexual maturation. Diminished growth rates can be seen in poorly controlled diabetes mellitus. In the past, a common complication of insulin administration was lipoatrophy, most likely an immune-mediated phenomenon. With the introduction of more purified insulin, this condition is seen less often. However, lipohypertrophy can be observed when there are repeated injections of insulin in the same area. This can result in uneven absorption of injected insulin, leading to wide fluctuations of blood glucose levels. Another, fortunately rare condition affecting the skin of children and adolescents with diabetes mellitus is necrobiosis lipoidica diabeticorum. This usually presents as round indurated plaques over the anterior aspects of the lower legs. The lesions can become atrophic and ulcerative. The pathogenesis has not been elucidated, and treatment has been difficult.

## TREATMENT OF TYPE 2 DIABETES MELLITUS IN ADOLESCENTS

Successful treatment of adolescents with T2D should control hyperglycemia and excessive weight gain. The ultimate goal should be to decrease the risk of microvascular complications, which are similar to those with T1D. The American Diabetes Association recommendations include maintaining a fasting blood glucose between 80 and 120 mg/dL (4.4 and 6.7 mmol/L), postprandial blood glucose levels of <180 mg/dL (10.0 mmol/L), and $HbA_{1c}$ <7%.[44,45] Weight loss induced by low-calorie diet and exercise programs are the primary approaches to an obese patient with T2D. The calorie restriction improves hyperglycemia first by decreasing hepatic glucose output and later by increasing peripheral sensitivity to insulin through a reduction of adipose mass. Exercise decreases insulin resistance and is also critical for weight control. Most patients with T2D will benefit from calorie restriction and increased physical activity alone. The use of oral hypoglycemic agents (Table 73-3) should be reserved for patients who cannot control their blood glucose levels and whose $HbA_{1c}$ remains >7% despite dietary restrictions and regular physical activity. The first line of therapy in an obese adolescent patient with T2D is metformin. Some patients may also need insulin therapy to control hyperglycemia, either at the diagnosis of T2D or later in the course of the disease.

## NUTRITION

The role of proper nutrition in the management of an adolescent with diabetes mellitus cannot be overemphasized. Nutrition has been implicated as a factor in increasing the risk of T2D and contributing to the disease. Food intake can affect the presence or absence of hypoglycemia, the dosage and timing of injections and, ultimately, the patient's prognosis.[5] Because patients with T1D have lost the capacity to secrete endogenous insulin, a regular meal pattern with consistent

**Table 73-3**

**Available Hypoglycemic Agents**

| *Name* | *Indications* | *Dose* | *Side effects* |
|---|---|---|---|
| **Biguanides**—action: decreasing hepatic glucose output and peripheral insulin resistance | | | |
| Metformin | Obese with insulin resistance and hyperinsulinemia | 250–750 mg max 2,000 mg | Gastrointestinal symptoms, rare lactic acidosis |
| **Alpha-glucosidase inhibitors**—action: inhibiting absorption of carbohydrates | | | |
| Acarbose | Mild postprandial hyperglycemia | 50–300 mg | Gastrointestinal symptoms |
| Boglibose | | 0.2–0.9 mg | |
| **Sulfonylureas**—action: stimulating endogenous insulin secretion | | | |
| Tolbutamide | Nonobese or mildly obese with residual beta cell function | 250–1,500 mg | Gastrointestinal symptoms, weight gain, hypoglycemia |
| Glibenclamide | | 1.25–10 mg | |
| Gliculazide | | 40–160 mg | |
| Glimepiride | | 1–6 mg | |

Many new investigational therapeutic agents for T2D (as well as for T1D) have been studied but are generally not yet approved for the pediatric population. One promising drug is exenatide (Byetta), which received US FDA approval in April 2005 for patients with T2D whose glycemia cannot be controlled by oral hypoglycemic agents. The drug stimulates the body's production of insulin and, unlike insulin injections, can help patients to lose weight.

carbohydrate intake is important in patients with diabetes who receive conventional treatment with insulin injections. The nutritional requirements of an adolescent with diabetes mellitus are similar to those of adolescents without diabetes. In general, the term "diabetes diet" is considered improper because it connotes restriction and denial, and may induce unnecessary anxiety in patients with diabetes. Instead, terms such as "meal planning" and "nutritional requirements" are preferable for patients with diabetes.

Frequently, patients with hypoglycemia are treated with an overload of carbohydrates. This leads to hyperglycemia, which requires more insulin for treatment. As a result, a vicious cycle of hypoglycemia and hyperglycemia may ensue, leading to poor control of diabetes. The proper treatment for such patients is to avoid hypoglycemic episodes, which require extra carbohydrate intake. Another common problem is increased calorie intake and decreased calorie expenditure. Hyperglycemia may result from overeating, even in those receiving adequate insulin therapy. Some patients gain excessive weight despite marked glycosuria and hyperglycemia. Those who are gaining weight at a rate faster than that expected for height are in a positive nitrogen balance. In such patients, manipulation of insulin dosage or other methods for improving control of diabetes are bound to fail unless treatment includes nutritional rehabilitation. Rates of ketosis also appear to vary among patients with diabetes in relation to dietary factors; ketonuria may follow the ingestion of a meal with a high fat content and may not be related to insulin treatment. In addition, long-term complications of diabetes may be influenced by nutritional intake and habits. For example, when patients with diabetes having a similar degree of metabolic control are compared, patients in Japan are noted to have gangrene and coronary heart disease less frequently than their Western counterparts. Among Navajo Indians, Nigerians, and certain Pacific populations, there is a lower incidence of microvascular disease among patients with diabetes than in other populations. These differences may be related to variations in genetic factors and nutritional habits.

The key elements of sound meal planning for a person with T1D receiving conventional insulin therapy are regular timing and consistency of meals, as well as snacks that synchronize with timing of insulin doses. However, patients treated with basal insulin (CSII or long-acting insulin) have more flexibility in their meal timing because the food intake is covered by boluses of insulin. Thus, such patients do not need to follow a specific meal plan because they match insulin boluses to carbohydrate content of a meal using a carbohydrate/insulin ratio. Therefore, the learning of carbohydrate counting is essential. Nutritional recommendations for patients with T1D have been issued by the American Diabetes Association. These recommendations do not differ substantially from those for the general, or nondiabetic, population. The meal plan should be individualized and based on the usual food intake, with insulin integrated into this established eating and exercise pattern. There is no ideal, but generally 15% to 20% of calories should be provided as protein, and the remaining calories should be contributed by carbohydrates and fat. The total amount of carbohydrates consumed is more important for glycemic control than the source of carbohydrates. Fat intake should include 10% as saturated fats, less than 10% as polyunsaturated fats, and the remainder as monosaturated fats. To achieve this balance, intake of animal fats must be reduced through replacement with vegetable sources. Cholesterol intake should be reduced by limiting the intake of fatty meats, whole milk, and other dairy products. The metabolism of carbohydrates and lipids can be improved further by increased intake of dietary fiber. The protein consumed should be of high biological quality. Excess protein and fat intake may have adverse effects on both the renal and cardiovascular systems. Indeed, the deleterious effect of high protein intake on kidney function and proteinuria has been described.[38,40] As with all adolescents, adequate intake of calcium (1,300 mg/day) is important.

It has been reported that different foods exert various effects on blood glucose levels. This has led to the development of the so-called glycemic index, which compares the potential of foods containing the same carbohydrates to raise blood glucose. However, the amount of carbohydrates consumed also affects blood glucose levels, making the concept of the glycemic index less reliable. The creation of this index was considered as a possible adjunct to the construction of diets for individuals with diabetes because it identifies starchy carbohydrate foods with a low postprandial glycemic response. However, it has become increasingly apparent that the glycemic response of foods given as mixtures cannot be predicted from the values of individual foods.

Despite the many new developments in the nutritional management of patients with diabetes, much remains to be learned about optimal nutrition for this population. Moreover, even when correct recommendations are made, their adoption into an adolescent's lifestyle may not be easily accomplished.

## EXERCISE

Exercise is an integral part of the management of patients with diabetes mellitus.[46] Better physical fitness and other lifestyle modifications intended to improve the general health of the population (eg, reduced smoking) have resulted in a decline of the major risk factors associated with atherosclerosis. Regular exercise may benefit patients with diabetes in many ways, such as improved metabolic control of diabetes, better self-image, and amelioration of the chronic complications of the disease. If significant weight loss is desired, exercise must be done in conjunction with nutritional modification to achieve maximal results. Even patients who lose only a small amount of weight on an exercise regimen undergo changes in body composition, such as decreased adipose tissue mass and reduced insulin requirements, which may lead to substantial metabolic benefits. For example, it has been reported that both basement membrane thickening and pulse volume improve with better glucose control during physical training.

However, caution must be advised for patients with diabetes who are undertaking an exercise program. In patients who have had the disease for more than 15 years, ischemic heart disease may be a problem. Moreover, worsening of retinopathy has been reported in patients who have engaged in vigorous exercise. Also, more studies are needed to assess the effects of intensive exercise on microalbuminuria as postexercise proteinuria has been documented in patients with T1D who demonstrate no proteinuria at rest. Because autoimmune neuropathy may predispose a patient with T1D to orthostatic hypotension, caution must be used when these patients train in a hot environment. Also, orthopedic injuries appear to be more common in patients with T1D and diabetic patients with degenerative joint disease should avoid jogging. Meticulous attention should be given to foot care, especially in patients with peripheral vascular disease and neuropathy. Properly fitting shoes, often with orthotic aids prescribed by a podiatrist, are essential for safe exercise.

Hypoglycemia is the most frequent and dramatic complication of exercise in an individual with T1D. In healthy individuals, insulin secretion decreases during exercise, leading to increased hepatic glucose production to compensate for accelerated glucose utilization by muscles. In patients receiving exogenous insulin, such downregulation does not occur, and relative hyperinsulinism and hypoglycemia ensue. This effect occurs even in patients who are receiving an appropriate amount of insulin and whose disease is well controlled. Not only can patients develop hypoglycemia during exercise, but they also may become hypoglycemic several hours after exercise is completed. This phenomenon has been named "late onset of postexercise hypoglycemia," and it should always be kept in mind when the physician is prescribing an exercise program, especially one for the evening hours. Thus, although exercise should be a regular part of the patient's daily routine, it is best that the exercise be planned for the morning, before administration of insulin. Because it is not easy to predict the decrease in insulin requirements that may be needed during a given day's activities, we recommend that patients who have had problems with hypoglycemia take their usual insulin dose and consume an extra 15 g to 30 g of carbohydrate before and after every 30 minutes of exercise. Insulin should be administered away from sites of exercised muscle groups because increased blood flow during exercise results in increased absorption of insulin. In many instances, the abdomen may be suitable. A 10% reduction in insulin dosage may also be attempted when physical activities are planned. Under special circumstances, exercise may have an opposite effect on blood glucose. Hyperglycemia rather than hypoglycemia may be seen when blood glucose levels are already high (>250 mg/dL [13.9 mmol/L]), and vigorous exercise in this situation can lead to severe hyperglycemia and even ketosis.

## STRESS

Of all chronic diseases, diabetes mellitus probably requires the most intense and continuous involvement of the patient. The emotional effect of the unceasing demands of daily management tasks can be overwhelming under the best of circumstances, and even more so during times of stress. However, not every patient with diabetes mellitus experiences emotional disability. In fact, many patients with diabetes are emotionally stronger than their counterparts without this disease. Yet when a patient with diabetes is in poor metabolic control, an effort must be made to look for psychosocial stress. The stress may be related to the poor control, but this connection may not be apparent to the physician if the patient does not report it. The physician must explore the psychosocial and physiological aspects of the patient's condition rather than merely attempting to obliterate the consequences of stress by increasing the dose of insulin. Indeed, the role of a psychiatrist in improving control of diabetes is one of the most readily recognized successes of psychotherapy.

## EDUCATION

Diabetes self-management education is the key to achieving and maintaining the best possible metabolic control of diabetes mellitus in adolescents. Education provides adolescents and their families with skills to manage diabetes on a day-to-day basis and to incorporate diabetes into the patient's individual lifestyle. Because management of diabetes is complex, especially during the teenage years, the combined efforts of a physician (preferably a pediatric endocrinologist), a diabetes educator, a nutritionist, and an exercise physiologist are essential for designing a successful treatment plan. In other words, a comprehensive education program can be achieved only through the team approach. Diabetes education is not a one-time "fix" but a process that must continue throughout the various developmental stages of adolescence into adulthood. After the diagnosis of diabetes mellitus in an adolescent, the first and most important educational process is assessment of the adolescent and family. The assessment must include cognitive knowledge, skills necessary for care, maturity and developmental level, coping skills, and family relationships and dynamics. The adolescent's schedule, habits, and values must be taken into consideration if a successful outcome is to be expected. After completion of the initial assessment of the adolescent and family, the diabetes team must assist the family in designing initial goals that are realistic, achievable, and measurable. The overall concept is that the goals should be meaningful and the regimen kept simple: the more complex the regimen, the more likely it is to fail. Diabetes education must also be imparted. If the adolescent and the family possess incorrect or inadequate knowledge, inappropriate decisions regarding management may be made based on this lack of information.

It is important to design the educational program in such a way as to be "adolescent friendly." If there is a lack of shared philosophy between the adolescent and the diabetes team, all efforts may prove fruitless. The educational process must also be designed to impart knowledge and develop goals with the adolescent and family in a nonjudgmental atmosphere. Although this is a time when the adolescent is moving toward independence, most adolescents still want to receive approval from their parents and the treatment team and avoid confrontations. If they believe that they will be "judged," some adolescents may, for example, report false blood glucose values. The educational process should always focus on the positive, and the adolescent's self-esteem must be promoted whenever possible. Evaluation of the goals set and regimen followed must be performed with the team, adolescent, and family in order to change the regimen and adjust goals when necessary.

Adolescents should be seen at least part of the time on their own, with the parents subsequently brought in to be included in the process. Adolescents may want to address issues that they may not be comfortable discussing in front of their parents, and they should always be given that opportunity. The diabetes team must also be available at times convenient for the adolescent so that frequent follow-up can be achieved. A final factor is to encourage telephone follow-up between visits, which provides support for the family and necessary adjustments between visits. The ultimate achievement of diabetes education is to maintain healthy family dynamics while helping adolescents to develop and grow, and eventually empowering them to assess, educate, motivate, set goals for, and evaluate themselves.

## CONCLUSION

Management of diabetes mellitus in adolescents is one of the most demanding and perplexing medical problems facing health care teams today. Not only is an adolescent with diabetes prone to acute life-threatening complications, but also the unfortunate reality is that the long-term outlook remains problematic. Although a great deal of progress has been made in managing diabetes, much more needs to be done. Despite recent developments, the achievement of euglycemia on a long-term basis is difficult, if not impossible, to accomplish in many adolescents with diabetes mellitus. It seems that until implantable mechanical pancreas, isolated beta cell, or pancreatic transplantations are successful, we may not be able to achieve perfect metabolic control of diabetes.

Until better therapeutic methods have been developed, or the prevention of diabetes by specific immunosuppression or early administration of insulin has been achieved, research must continue. Our present goal for adolescents with diabetes is to provide practical, safe, and effective treatment that is best for the patient, family, and diabetes team.

## REFERENCES


1. US Department of Health and Human Services (DHHS). *Diabetes in America: Diabetes Data Compiled 1984.* Washington, DC: 1985; US Government Printing Office. DHHS Publication 85-1468 (NIH)

2. Kuller LH, Becker DJ, Cruickshanks KJ, et al. Pittsburgh Diabetes Epidemiology and Etiology Research Group: evolution of the Pittsburgh studies of the epidemiology of insulin-dependent diabetes mellitus. *Genet Epidemiol.* 1990;7:105–119

3. Fagot-Campagna A. Emergence of type 2 diabetes mellitus in children: epidemiological evidence. *J Pediatr Endocrinol Metab.* 2000;13:1395–1402

4. Drash AL, Becker DJ. Behavioral issues in patients with diabetes mellitus, with special emphasis on the child and adolescent. In: Rifkin H, Porte D, eds. *Ellenberg and Rifkin's Diabetes Mellitus: Theory and Practice.* 4th ed. New York: Elsevier; 1990:922

5. American Diabetes Association. Clinical practice recommendations. *Diabetes Care.* 2006;29(suppl 1):S43–S48

6. Dabelea D, Bell RA, Imperatore G, et al. Incidence of diabetes in youth in the United States. *JAMA.* 2007;297(24):2716–2724

7. American Diabetes Association. Standards of medical care in diabetes—2006. *Diabetes Care.* 2006;29(1 suppl):S4–S42

8. Arslanian SA. Type 2 diabetes mellitus in children: pathophysiology and risk factors. *J Pediatr Endocrinol Metab.* 2000;13:1385–1394

9. Taylor SI, Arioglu E. Genetically defined forms of diabetes in children. *J Clin Endocrinol Metab.* 1999;84:4390–4396

10. Shepherd M, Sparkes AC, Hattersley AT. Genetic testing in maturity onset diabetes of the young (MODY): a new challenge for the diabetic clinic. *Pract Diabetes Int.* 2001;18(1):16–21

11. Hattersley AT. Diagnosis of maturity-onset diabetes of the young in the pediatric diabetes clinic. *J Pediatr Endocrinol Metab.* 2000;13:1411–1417

12. American Diabetes Association. Gestational diabetes mellitus [position statement]. *Diabetes Care.* 2004;27(1):S88–S90

13. Ipp E. Impaired glucose tolerance [editorial]. *Diabetes Care.* 2000;23(5):569–570

14. The Diabetes Control and Complications Trial Research Group. The effect of intensive treatment of diabetes on the development and progression of long-term complications in insulin-dependent diabetes mellitus. *N Engl J Med.* 1993;329:977–986

15. The Diabetes Control and Complications Trial/Epidemiology of Diabetes Interventions and Complications Research Group. Retinopathy and nephropathy in patients with type 1 diabetes four years after a trial of intensive therapy. *N Engl J Med.* 2000;342:381–389

16. Drash AL. The child, the adolescent, and the Diabetes Control and Complications Trial. *Diabetes Care.* 1993;16:1515–1516

17. American Diabetes Association. Position statement. Implications of the Diabetes Control and Complications Trial. *Diabetes Care.* 1993;16:1517–1520

18. Santiago JV. Lessons from the Diabetes Control and Complications Trial. *Diabetes.* 1993;42:1549–1554

19. Bolli GB. Insulin treatment in type 1 diabetes. *Endocr Pract.* 2006;12(1):105–109

20. Weinstein D, Simon M, Yehezkel E, Laron Z, Werner H. Insulin analogues display IGF-I-like mitogenic and anti-adoptotic activities in cultured cancer cells. *Diabetes Metab Res Rev.* 2009;25:41–49

21. Drash AL, LaPorte RE, Daneman D, Fishbein H, Goldstein D, Becker D. Insulin requirements in children with diabetes mellitus: changing requirements by age and sex over the initial 5 years of therapy. In: Akerbloom H, ed. *The Remission Period: Pediatric and Adolescent Endocrinology*. Basel, Switzerland: A Krager; 1985

22. Cryer PE, Binder C, Bolli GB, et al. Hypoglycemia in IDDM. *Diabetes.* 1989;38:1193–1199

23. Tordjman KM, Havlin CE, Levandoski LA, White NH, Santiago JV, Cryer PE. Failure of nocturnal hypoglycemia to cause fasting hyperglycemia in patients with insulin-dependent diabetes mellitus. *N Engl J Med.* 1987;317:1552–1559

24. Gerich JE. Dawn phenomenon: pathophysiology, diagnosis, and treatment. *Clin Diabetes.* 1988;6(1):1–8

25. American Diabetes Association. Self-monitoring of blood glucose. *Diabetes Care.* 1994;17:81–86

26. Pickup J, Keen H. Continuous subcutaneous insulin infusion at 25 years: evidence base for the expanding use of insulin pump therapy in type 1 diabetes. *Diabetes Care.* 2002;25:593–598

27. Pugliese MT, Fort P, Lifshitz F. Treatment of diabetic ketoacidosis. In: Lifshitz F, ed. *Pediatric Endocrinology.* New York: Marcel Dekker; 1990:745

28. Glaser N. New perspectives on the pathogenesis of cerebral edema complicating diabetic ketoacidosis in children. *Pediatr Endocrinol Rev.* 2006;3(4):379–386

29. Pugliese MT, Fort P, Lifshitz F. Treatment of diabetic ketoacidosis. In: Lifshitz F, ed. *Pediatric Endocrinology.* New York: Marcel Dekker; 1990:757

30. Cryer PE, Gerich JE. Hypoglycemia in insulin-dependent diabetes mellitus: insulin excess and defective glucose counterregulation. In: Rifkin H, Porte D, eds. *Diabetes Mellitus.* 4th ed. New York: Elsevier; 1990:526

31. Veneman T, Mitrakov A, Mokan M, et al. Induction of hypoglycemia unawareness by asymptomatic nocturnal hypoglycemia. *Diabetes.* 1993;42:1233–1237

32. Kappy MS. Carbohydrate metabolism and hypoglycemia. In: Kappy MS, Blizzard RM, Migeon CJ, eds. *The Diagnosis and Treatment of Endocrine Disorders in Childhood and Adolescence*. 4th ed. Springfield, IL: Charles C.Thomas; 1994:919

33. Orr DP, Eccles T, Lawlor R, Golden M. Surreptitious insulin administration in adolescents with insulin-dependent diabetes mellitus. *JAMA.* 1986;256:3227–3230

34. Eppens MC, Craig ME, Cusumano J, et al. Prevalence of diabetes complications in adolescents with type 2 compared with type 1 diabetes. *Diabetes Care.* 2006;29:1300–1306

35. Walker JW, Viberti GC. Pathophysiology of microvascular disease: an overview. In: Pickup JC, Williams G, eds. *Textbook of Diabetes*. London: Blackwell Scientific; 1991:526

36. Becker DJ. Complications of insulin-dependent diabetes mellitus in childhood and adolescence. In: Lifshitz F, ed. *Pediatric Endocrinology*. 2nd ed. New York: Marcel Dekker; 1990:701

37. Seaquist ER, Goetz FC, Rich S, Barbosa J. Familial clustering of diabetic kidney disease. *N Engl J Med.* 1989;320:1161–1165

38. Hansen HP, Tauber-Lassen E, Jensen BR, Parving HH. Effect of dietary protein restriction on prognosis in patients with diabetic nephropathy. *Kidney Int.* 2002;62:220–228

39. Laffel LM, McGill JB, Gans DJ. The beneficial effect of angiotensin-converting enzyme inhibition with captopril on diabetic nephropathy in normotensive IDDM patients with microalbuminuria: North American Microalbuminuria Study Group. *Am J Med.* 1995;99:497–504

40. Pijls LT, de Vries H, Donker AJ, van Eijk JT. The effect of protein restriction on albuminuria in patients with type 2 diabetes mellitus: a randomized trial. *Nephrol Dial Transplant.* 1999;14:1445–1453

41. Lewis EJ, Hunsicker LG, Bain RP, Rohde RD. The effect of angiotensin-converting enzyme inhibition on diabetic nephropathy: the Collaborative Study Group. *N Engl J Med.* 1993;329:1456–1462

42. Frank GR, Pellizzari M, Speiser PW, Carey DE, Fort P, Kreitzer PM. Analysis of 24-hour ambulatory blood pressure monitoring in adolescents with type 1 diabetes: importance of defining actual sleep time. *Diabetes.* 2006;39:204A(suppl):P7

43. Vinik AI, Mehrabyan A. Diabetic neuropathies. *Med Clin North Am.* 2004;88:947–999, xi

44. Nathan DM, Buse JB, Davidson MB, et al. Management of hyperglycemia in type 2 diabetes: a consensus statement from the American Diabetes Association and the European Association for the Study of Diabetes. *Diabetes Care.* 2006;29:1963–1972

45. Urakami T. How should we treat type 2 diabetes in youth? *Pediatr Endocrinol Rev.* 2005;3(1):33–39

46. Zinman B, Ruderman N, Campaigne BN, Devlin JT, Schneider SH, American Diabetes Association. Physical activity/exercise and diabetes [position statement]. *Diabetes Care.* 2004;27 (suppl 1):S58–S62

# CHAPTER 74

# Adrenocortical Disorders

PHYLLIS W. SPEISER, MD

## INTRODUCTION

This chapter discusses the pathophysiology and treatment of adrenal diseases affecting adolescents. Adrenal cortical disease, especially adrenal insufficiency, is far more common than adrenal medullary disease and frequently goes unrecognized for extended periods. Physicians caring for adolescents should consider the diagnosis of adrenal insufficiency in any patient with unexplained fatigue, weight loss, or malaise. Such nonspecific signs and symptoms may be mistaken for, and should be differentiated from, anorexia nervosa, chronic fatigue syndrome, depression, or chronic infectious diseases.

## ANATOMY

The adrenal glands are made up of an inner medulla and an outer cortex, linked by vascular supply and hormonal influence. Within the cortex are 3 functionally distinct zones: the glomerulosa comprising about 15% of the gland; fasciculata, the largest zone, about 75% of the gland; and reticularis, about 10% at maturity.[1]

## PHYSIOLOGY

The medulla is regulated by the sympathetic nervous system and secretes catecholamines, whereas the 3 zones of the cortex secrete steroid hormones, categorized as mineralocorticoids, glucocorticoids, and sex steroids. Mineralocorticoid production, exemplified by aldosterone, is regulated principally by the renin-angiotensin axis and by ambient potassium levels.[2] Glucocorticoid and adrenal sex steroid production are regulated by pituitary corticotropin (ACTH) and hypothalamic corticotropin-releasing hormone (CRH). Cortisol is the main glucocorticoid, and dehydroepiandrosterone (DHEA) is the main adrenal sex hormone. The latter is only a weak androgen, but it may be converted via androstenedione to either estrogens or androgens.

Glucocorticoids are generally catabolic, promoting protein and lipid breakdown and inhibiting protein synthesis. The effects of cortisol counter those of insulin, increasing the concentration of glucose by stimulating gluconeogenesis and by decreasing glucose utilization in muscle. Amino acids and glycerol produced by catabolic actions of cortisol on protein and fat are used as gluconeogenic substrates. The net effect is increased production and conservation of glucose for use by essential tissues, such as the brain and red blood cells, at the expense of less essential tissues during times of stress or starvation.[3]

Cortisol also contributes to the maintenance of normal blood pressure through several mechanisms. Under normal baseline conditions, cortisol increases urine flow by stimulating glomerular filtration and decreasing water resorption. At high concentrations, cortisol acts as a mineralocorticoid agonist, causing sodium and water retention. Other vascular actions of cortisol include stimulating angiotensinogen synthesis by the liver and increasing vascular sensitivity to pressors. In the adrenal medulla, cortisol is required for the enzymatic activity of phenylethanolamine N-methyltransferase, which converts norepinephrine to epinephrine. Epinephrine stimulates cardiac output as well as hepatic glucose production. Cortisol decreases capillary permeability and also decreases the production and activity of nitrous oxide and the vasodilatory kinin and prostaglandin systems during stress, preventing life-threatening hypotension.

## PATHOLOGY

Primary adrenal disease may be associated with either hypoplasia or hyperplasia. This chapter discusses several types of adrenal pathology relevant to adolescent patients, including conditions of hypofunction and hyperfunction. The most common forms of adrenal pathology involve either deficient or excessive cortisol production.

## ADRENAL INSUFFICIENCY

### CLINICAL FEATURES

The symptoms and signs of cortisol deficiency include fatigue, weakness, dizziness, anorexia, orthostatic hypotension and tachycardia, and weight loss. These findings are nonspecific, gradual in onset, and may be mistaken for chronic fatigue syndrome, anorexia nervosa, depression, or chronic infectious diseases. In some patients gastrointestinal symptoms such as abdominal cramps, nausea, vomiting, and diarrhea are prominent. Sexual or reproductive dysfunction with decreased libido, potency, or amenorrhea may accompany either primary or secondary adrenal insufficiency. Although orthostatic hypotension is more marked in primary than secondary adrenal insufficiency because of aldosterone deficiency and hypovolemia, it can occur in the latter owing to decreased expression of vascular catecholamine receptors.[4]

The most commonly recognized sign in patients with chronic primary adrenal insufficiency is hyperpigmentation of the skin and mucosal surfaces, owing to the high plasma corticotropin and accompanying melanocyte-stimulating hormone secretion resulting from absent cortisol feedback. In contrast, patients with secondary adrenal insufficiency tend to be pale. Another specific symptom of primary adrenal insufficiency is salt craving, a result of aldosterone deficiency and resultant sodium wasting. Weight loss may also be observed. Loss of axillary or pubic hair is common among hypoadrenal patients, attributable to low levels of adrenal androgens.

Young patients with secondary adrenal insufficiency might have delayed growth and puberty, manifestations of growth hormone (GH), and gonadotropin deficiencies, in addition to ACTH deficiency. Headaches, visual disturbances, and/or polyuria and polydipsia, indicative of diabetes insipidus, may also be seen in pituitary disorders.

## PRIMARY CAUSES OF ADRENAL FAILURE

Congenital adrenal hyperplasia (CAH) is most often caused by deficiency of steroid 21-hydroxylase.[5] In classic, severe salt-wasting CAH, cortisol and aldosterone production are impaired, whereas adrenal androgen production is excessive. Owing to the lack of the vital hormones, cortisol and aldosterone, males and females are susceptible to potentially lethal adrenal insufficiency if untreated. Excess androgens cause genital ambiguity in newborn females; males affected with severe 21-hydroxylase deficiency, however, have no overt genital anomalies and therefore may not come to medical attention until they present *in extremis*. Thus, to prevent mortality from adrenal crisis, among other reasons, most states in the United States and many countries worldwide perform newborn screening for this disease.[6] Prompt treatment with glucocorticoids and mineralocorticoids is life-saving. About one-fourth of classic CAH patients produce enough aldosterone to avoid salt-wasting crises and are termed "simple virilizers."

A milder, nonclassic form of CAH not associated with genital ambiguity or adrenal insufficiency may be missed by newborn screening programs. Although nonclassic CAH is not always detected by random blood hormone measurements, it is much more prevalent at all ages than the classic forms of the disease. Because nonclassic CAH is characterized by less marked adrenal androgen excess, symptoms and signs do not often develop before middle childhood. These often include early pubic hair and/or rapid advances in height in both sexes. In many cases, these individuals either go undetected or are diagnosed in adolescent girls or women with hirsutism, oligomenorrhea, and/or acne. The mild form of CAH may be mistaken in females for polycystic ovarian syndrome.[7]

Some individuals with the typical nonclassic 21-hydroxylase deficiency profile have no symptoms. Specifically, males are much less likely to be troubled by this mild adrenal hormone imbalance. Family studies have revealed, however, that even some girls and women remain asymptomatic. Thus, adolescents with nonclassic CAH may not require treatment in all cases.

## HORMONAL DIAGNOSIS

The diagnosis of CAH rests on the clinical presentation described above and on specific hormone measurements. Deficiency of steroid 21-hydroxylase can be identified by measuring high levels of hormones that serve as enzyme substrates. The gold standard test is a corticotropin-stimulated serum 17-hydroxyprogesterone,[8] although serum or saliva levels of this hormone at 8 am may also be diagnostic. This is true because of the natural circadian pattern of endogenous ACTH secretion, which is highest between 4 am and 8 am. In endocrine specialty laboratories employing strict quality control standards, stimulated 17-hydroxyprogesterone levels are moderately elevated, exceeding 1,500 ng/dL (about 45 nmol/L) among individuals affected with nonclassic 21-hydroxylase deficiency. In contrast, both basal and stimulated 17-hydroxyprogesterone levels are markedly elevated, exceeding 10,000 ng/dL (about 300 nmol/L) in classic, simple virilizing or salt-wasting, CAH. Moreover, cortisol levels are invariably low and fail to respond robustly to stress or exogenous stimulation in classic forms of CAH. Early morning basal 17-hydroxyprogesterone measurements below 200 ng/dL (about 6 nmol/L) usually rule out even mild forms of 21-hydroxylase deficiency.[9]

## GENETICS

Phenotypic variability in CAH is attributable to allelic variation in the gene-encoding active steroid 21-hydroxylase, *CYP21A2*. The disease is inherited as an autosomal recessive trait. There are more than 100 known disease-causing mutations, but approximately 10 mutations comprise 80% to 90% of alleles in most populations.[10] The spectrum of disease ranges from severe to mild, depending on which *CYP21A2* mutations a patient carries. Genotyping can be useful in verifying an equivocal hormonal diagnosis; it is particularly valuable in prenatal diagnosis.

## TREATMENT AND LONG-TERM FOLLOW-UP

Congenital adrenal hyperplasia is treatable with oral steroid medications. In its classical form, CAH requires lifelong medical management. Salt-wasting patients require glucocorticoids and mineralocorticoids; however, with increasing age and dietary salt consumption, mineralocorticoids may be tapered, and in some cases, discontinued. Patients in tropical climates, or adolescents who engage in intense exercise with excessive sweat sodium losses, may require added sodium chloride as table salt or tablets. Poorly controlled simple virilizing patients also benefit from mineralocorticoid therapy, as it spares using high-dose glucocorticoids in some cases. Symptomatic nonclassic patients require low-dose glucocorticoid therapy only. The drug of choice for growing children or adolescents is hydrocortisone at about 10 to 15 mg/m$^2$/day.[11] The proper dose schedule is largely empiric.

There is some evidence to suggest that nighttime cortisol clearance is reduced, hence hydrocortisone dose should be weighted to the mornings.[12] Nevertheless, some clinicians prefer to treat CAH with a higher dose of cortisol or a longer-acting glucocorticoid at night in an attempt to suppress the early morning ACTH-mediated adrenal androgen production.

Once growth is nearly complete, if satisfactory control of adrenal androgens is not achieved with such a regimen, more potent glucocorticoids, such as prednisone or dexamethasone, may be used. Table 74-1 lists the approximate relative potencies of the commonly used glucocorticoids. Stress dosing is discussed below.

Dosing should be titrated to maintain the levels of adrenal androgen precursors in the normal to mildly elevated range. Levels of 17-hydroxyprogesterone, androstenedione, and testosterone should be assayed; plasma renin activity should be added to this profile in patients requiring mineralocorticoid replacement. Attempts to suppress 17-hydroxyprogesterone to the normal range usually require excessive glucocorticoid doses and have the undesirable consequence of growth suppression and iatrogenic Cushing syndrome. Measurement of ACTH is not helpful; this hormone seldom is completely suppressible in treated CAH patients. It is important to recognize that testosterone cannot be utilized as a hormonal marker of adequate therapy in adolescent boys and men, although it is quite helpful in managing prepubertal children of both sexes, as well as adolescent girls and women.

Other aspects of CAH treatment include ensuring that adolescent females with severe forms of CAH undergo gynecologic examination in anticipation of sexual activity, as vaginoplasty may be necessary, depending on whether and which genital surgical procedures may have been done in the past.[13] Psychological counseling should be provided to these young women by a professional experienced in treating this type of disorder.[14]

Adolescent boys should undergo careful testicular palpation and sonography to rule out testicular adrenal rests that can compromise fertility. Strict control of adrenal hormone levels can shrink such benign tumors in many cases.[15]

## OTHER CAUSES OF ADRENAL FAILURE

Primary adrenal insufficiency is estimated to affect about 100 per million people.[16] The syndrome, originally described by the English physician Thomas Addison, includes wasting, hyperpigmentation, and adrenal gland atrophy. In adults, more than 80% of cases are caused by autoimmune adrenal destruction,

**Table 74-1**

**Glucocorticoid Potencies**

| *Drug* | *Potency Relative to Cortisol* | *Equivalent Cortisol Dose* | *Mineralcorticoid Activity* |
|---|---|---|---|
| Cortisol (hydrocortisone) | 1 | 100 | + |
| Cortisone | 0.8 | 125 | + |
| Prednisone | 5 | 20 | – |
| Prednisolone | 5 | 20 | – |
| Methylprednisolone | 6 | 17 | – |
| Dexamethasone | 50 | 2 | – |

prevalent in women aged 25 to 45 but observed in both sexes at any age. The female-to-male ratio is about 3:1. Autoimmune adrenalitis may be isolated or found in association with other autoimmune syndromes. Autoimmune polyendocrine syndrome 1 (APS1) is associated with mucocutaneous candidiasis, Addison disease, and autoimmune hypoparathyroidism. Other systemic problems may include autoimmune pernicious anemia, hepatitis, thyroiditis, and diabetes. The onset and severity of each of these problems is variable. APS2, also termed Schmidt syndrome, is associated with Addison disease, autoimmune thyroiditis, and diabetes. Table 74-2 lists diseases associated with adrenal insufficiency, including known gene defects. Details about many of the less common diseases can be found at Online Mendelian Inheritance in Man (OMIM; www.ncbi.nlm.nih.gov/omim).

Adrenal infiltration by tuberculosis is the second most common etiology worldwide. HIV infection is another potential infectious cause of adrenalitis; both of these infectious etiologies tend to cause insidious progression to hypoadrenalism. In contrast, catastrophic adrenal hemorrhage during overwhelming bacterial sepsis causes the abrupt onset of adrenal failure.

**Table 74-2**

**Causes of Adrenal Cortical Insufficiency**

| *Disease* | *Gene* | *OMIM #* |
|---|---|---|
| **Primary** | | |
| ***Disorders associated with adrenal gland hyperplasia*** | | |
| 21-hydroxylase deficiency | CYP21A2 | 210910 |
| 3 beta-hydroxysteroid dehydrogenase deficiency | HSD3B2 | 201810 |
| Cholesterol desmolase deficiency | CYP11A | 201710, 118485 |
| Lipoid hyperplasia | STAR | 201710 |
| Glucocorticoid resistance | GCCR | 138040 |
| Wolman disease | LIPA | 278000 |
| ***Disorders associated with adrenal gland hypoplasia*** | | |
| Adrenal hypoplasia congenita | NR0B1 (DAX-1) | 300200 |
| Adrenocortical insufficiency +/- ovarian defect | NR5A1 (SF-1) | 184757 |
| Familial glucocorticoid deficiency (ACTH resistance) | MC2R/MRAP | 202200 |
| Triple A: ACTH resistance, achalasia, alacrima | AAAS | 231550 |
| IMAGe syndrome | X-linked | 300290 |
| ***Metabolic diseases*** | | |
| Adrenoleukodystrophy (X-linked) | ABCD1 | 300100 |
| Smith-Lemli-Opitz syndrome | DCHR7 | 270400 |
| Kearns-Sayre syndrome | mitochondrial DNA deletion | 530000 |
| ***Disorders associated with isolated aldosterone deficiency*** | | |
| Pseudohypoaldosteronism, type 1 (AR) | ENaC | 264350 |
| Pseudohypoaldosteronism, type 1 (AD) | MR | 177735 |
| Pseudohypoaldosteronism, type 2 (AR) | WNK4;WNK1 | 145260 |
| Corticosterone methyl oxidase deficiency I | CYP11B2 | 124080 |
| Corticosterone methyl oxidase deficiency I | CYP11B2 | 610600 |
| ***Acquired*** | | |
| Autoimmune adrenalitis, isolated | | |
| Autoimmune polyendocrine syndrome type 1 | AIRE | 240300 |

*(Continued)*

**Table 74-2 (Continued)**

| *Disease* | *Gene* | *OMIM #* |
|---|---|---|
| Autoimmune polyendocrine syndrome type 2 | MICA5.1 & HLA-DR3/DQ2 | 269200 |
| ***Hemorrhage/Infarction due to:*** | | |
| **Trauma** | | |
| Waterhouse-Friderichsen syndrome | | |
| Anticoagulation | | |
| **Drug effects** | | |
| aminoglutethimide, mitotane, ketoconazole, metyrapone, medroxyprogesterone, megestrol, tomidate, rifampin, phenytoin, barbiturates | | |
| **Infection** | | |
| viral: human immunodeficiency virus, cytomegalovirus; fungal: coccidiomycosis, histoplasmosis, blastomycosis, cryptococcosis; mycobacterial: tuberculosis; amoebic | | |
| **Infiltrative** | | |
| hemochromatosis, histiocytosis, sarcoidosis, amyloidosis; neoplasm | | |
| **Secondary** | | |
| ***Hypothalamus*** | | |
| *Congenital* | | |
| Septo-optic dysplasia | HESX1 | 182230 |
| Corticotropin-releasing hormone deficiency | CRH | 122560 |
| Maternal hypercortisolemia | | |
| *Acquired* | | |
| Inflammatory disorders | | |
| Trauma | | |
| Radiation therapy | | |
| Surgery | | |
| Tumors | | |
| Infiltrative disease (eg, sarcoidosis, histocytosis X) | | |
| Steroid withdrawal after prolonged administration | | |
| ***Pituitary*** | | |
| *Congenital* | | |
| Pituitary hormone deficiency, combined | POU1F1/PIT1, PROP-1 | 173110, 601538 |
| Pro-opiomelanocortin deficiency | POMC | 609734 |
| Proconvertase 1 | PCSK1 | 600955 |
| Isolated ACTH deficiency | TBX19/TPIT | 604614 |
| *Acquired* | | |
| Trauma | | |
| Tumor, commonly craniopharyngioma | | |
| Radiation therapy | | |
| Lymphocytic hypophysitis | | |
| Steroid withdrawal after prolonged administration | | |

Perhaps because of its rarity in children and adolescents, or because of its nonspecific symptoms, the diagnosis of adrenal insufficiency is frequently delayed or missed. If unrecognized, adrenal insufficiency may present as a life-threatening crisis with acute cardiovascular collapse. A recent survey of ambulatory adult patients with adrenal insufficiency who are members of the National Adrenal Disease Foundation reported that 60% had sought the advice of 2 or more physicians before the diagnosis was made.[17] In 5 of 16 children in Melbourne, Australia, diagnosed with primary adrenal insufficiency over a 10-year period, there was a median of 2 years delay between the onset of the first symptoms and the diagnosis.[18]

## DIAGNOSIS

Signs and symptoms of adrenal insufficiency include abdominal pain, headache, anorexia, weight loss, lethargy, postural hypotension or shock, proneness to dehydration, salt-craving, and hyperpigmentation. Patients with adrenal insufficiency with and without GH deficiency may have hypoglycemia, but this is seldom severe enough to cause seizures. Primary adrenal insufficiency can be detected on the basis of a low early morning (8 am) cortisol accompanied by elevated ACTH. If zona glomerulosa function is affected, hyponatremia and hyperkalemia will be accompanied by a high plasma renin activity and low serum aldosterone. In adrenal insufficiency due to pituitary or hypothalamic dysfunction, ACTH levels will be low. The diagnosis can be confirmed by absence of at least a twofold increment in serum cortisol 60 minutes after stimulation with intravenous cosyntropin (ACTH 1–24). If adrenal hemorrhage is suspected, this can be detected by ultrasonography or computed tomography (CT) scan.

Once the diagnosis of adrenal insufficiency is established, continuing reminders to patients, families, and medical personnel regarding the need for higher doses of glucocorticoid replacement during intercurrent illness and surgery are required. Failure to increase glucocorticoid supplementation during physical stress remains a significant cause of morbidity and mortality in these patients.

A group of investigators in Montreal recently reported their 20-year experience with primary adrenal insufficiency in children under 18 years of age.[19] The most common cause was CAH (72%), while 13% had autoimmune adrenal insufficiency, and the remaining 15% included various rare syndromes such as adrenoleukodystrophy, Wolman disease, Triple A syndrome (ACTH resistance, achalasia, alacrima), Zellweger syndrome, and unexplained adrenal insufficiency. In Melbourne,[18] where only non-CAH primary adrenal insufficiency was reported, there were 16 cases reported; 5 patients each had autoimmune adrenal insufficiency, X-linked adrenoleukodystrophy, and adrenal hypoplasia congenita, and 1 case of the IMAGe syndrome (intrauterine growth retardation, metaphyseal dysplasia, adrenal hypoplasia congenita, and genital anomalies).

## SECONDARY ADRENAL INSUFFICIENCY

Secondary causes of adrenal insufficiency are more common than primary causes. The estimated prevalence is 150 to 280 per million people.[16] Abrupt discontinuation of glucocorticoid therapy exacerbated by stress is the most common underlying cause due to the widespread use of exogenous glucocorticoids. In a survey of consultant pediatricians and adult endocrinologists in the United Kingdom, 23 children were reported to have had acute hypoglycemia following the use of inhaled glucocorticoids.[20] Most had been using more than 500 μg of inhaled fluticasone daily. Normal statural growth does not preclude the presence of adrenal suppression on inhaled glucocorticoids.[21]

Administration of steroids either orally, intramuscularly, intranasally, inhaled, transdermally, or intraorbitally may result in suppression of the hypothalamic-pituitary-adrenal (HPA) axis. In adults, as few as 2 weeks of high-dose glucocorticoid treatment may result in suppression of endogenous cortisol production for up to 1 year.[22] In children being treated for leukemia, even a short 4-week course of glucocorticoids resulted in suppression of the hypothalamic pituitary axis for up to 8 weeks after discontinuation.[23] Suppression of the axis cannot reliably be predicted by either the dose or the duration of therapy.[24]

Documentation of an intact HPA axis should be obtained before subjecting to surgery a patient who has a known history of prior high-dose, long-term glucocorticoid treatment. This may be done by documenting an 8 am plasma cortisol greater than 10 μg/dL or by performing a cosyntropin (ACTH 1–24) challenge test. If documentation cannot be obtained in time, it is safest to treat with supplemental stress steroid coverage in the perioperative period for any patient within 1 year of withdrawal of steroid therapy.[25]

Most secondary adrenal insufficiency unrelated to withdrawal of glucocorticoid therapy occurs in association with other pituitary hormone deficiencies. Panhypopituitarism, that is, deficiency of 2 or more pituitary hormones, may be either congenital or acquired. Anatomic abnormalities in the pituitary or stalk may be evident on magnetic resonance imaging (MRI). Alternatively, one may elicit a history of head trauma or cranial surgery with resulting pituitary injury.[26]

Aside from these causes of secondary adrenal insufficiency, there are several other rare syndromes. These include ACTH resistance associated with the Triple A syndrome (ACTH resistance, alacrima, and achalasia). This clinical picture is caused by mutations in the AAAS gene encoding a protein of uncertain function.[27] In contrast, an isolated form of ACTH resistance is caused by a different genetic defect in the gene encoding the ACTH receptor, MC2R. The latter syndrome is characterized by a familial form of glucocorticoid deficiency associated with hyperpigmentation and hypoglycemia without accompanying systemic abnormalities.[28] Granulomatous diseases such as sarcoid or histiocytosis can also cause pituitary failure.

The risk of adrenal crisis in adult patients with primary adrenal insufficiency is slightly higher (3.8 admissions per 100 patient years) compared to secondary adrenal insufficiency (2.5 per 100 patient years).[16] Information concerning mortality in secondary adrenal insufficiency comes primarily from recent reports regarding follow-up of individuals treated with pituitary GH. Several reports have shown up to a fourfold increase in mortality compared to the general population in children treated with pituitary GH from the 1960s and followed to the 1990s in England, Canada, and the United States.[29-31]

A substantial portion of deaths were attributed to hypoglycemia and/or secondary adrenal insufficiency. These preventable deaths were seen in individuals of all ages and were associated with a variety of causes of hypopituitarism; 74% were said to occur in individuals with known multiple pituitary hormone deficiencies. The death rate due to secondary adrenal insufficiency remained fairly constant throughout middle childhood and with advancing age (1 per 113–173 person years).

## "RELATIVE ADRENAL INSUFFICIENCY" IN THE INTENSIVE CARE UNIT

Critically ill adults in an intensive care unit with normal baseline cortisol levels (≥20 μg/dL) but inappropriately low responses of serum cortisol to acute stimulation (≤9 μg/dL increment at 30–60 minutes following 250 μg intravenous ACTH) demonstrated improved survival in one study when treated with stress doses of hydrocortisone.[32] These findings were not borne out in other centers.[33]

Among critically ill children, a low incremental cortisol response to ACTH did not predict mortality. The effect of glucocorticoid treatment was not evaluated in this study.[34]

There is still much controversy as to how to best assess for adrenal insufficiency in hospitalized pediatric and adult patients, as well as whether and when to treat.[22,33,35]

## TREATMENT OF ACUTE ADRENAL INSUFFICIENCY

Hypotension and lethargy are common presenting signs of acute adrenal insufficiency; patients and family members should be taught to recognize a change in energy level or demeanor as potential warning signs. Acute adrenal insufficiency may occur during a febrile illness, especially one accompanied by dehydration due to vomiting and/or diarrhea. Individuals who are unable to tolerate oral maintenance or stress doses during an illness require parenteral glucocorticoid administration. This may be initiated at home using intramuscular hydrocortisone sodium succinate at a dose of 50 mg/m$^2$; this will provide coverage for approximately 6–8 hours. In this situation, immediate consultation with a health care provider is recommended, because the patient will likely require emergency evaluation and treatment with intravenous hydrocortisone. Another option, provided the patient is not suffering from diarrhea, is to administer rectal hydrocortisone suppositories (25 mg in "fatty base" every 6–8 hours) until either the acute illness resolves or the patient can reach medical care for intravenous therapy.

Once the patient is seen in the emergency department, a large-bore intravenous catheter should be inserted and blood should be drawn for cortisol, electrolytes, glucose, ACTH, plasma renin activity, and aldosterone. If acute and severe adrenal insufficiency is suspected, treatment should not by delayed for diagnostic testing. Repletion of intravascular volume should begin before laboratory results are obtained; this is accomplished with isotonic solutions containing dextrose. More concentrated dextrose solutions should be administered to treat refractory hypoglycemia. Simultaneous stress doses of glucocorticoid should be given as well. Hydrocortisone is the treatment of choice due to its quick onset of action and mineralocorticoid activity (20 mg of hydrocortisone is equivalent to ~0.05 mg fludrocortisone).[16] It should be emphasized that stress dose recommendations are entirely empiric and not based on carefully controlled clinical trials. Recommended stress doses for parenteral hydrocortisone vary from 50 to 100 mg/m$^2$ initially, followed by 25 to 75 mg/m$^2$/day intravenous (divided in 4 doses), depending on the patient's size and clinical status. Hydrocortisone may be given intramuscularly or through an intraosseous line if no access exists. Rapid reversal of hypotension and lethargy should be observed following treatment with hydrocortisone.

Prednisone and dexamethasone are long-acting glucocorticoids with a slower onset of biologic action. Prednisone is not an ideal choice for treating acute adrenal crisis, as it must be converted to prednisolone to be effective. Dexamethasone administration will not immediately suppress cortisol levels or cross-react in cortisol assays if one wishes to perform a diagnostic ACTH stimulation test.

Liberal quantities of intravenous sodium chloride accompanied by large doses of hydrocortisone will usually restore normotension and correct electrolyte abnormalities, obviating mineralocorticoid treatment or pressor agents in the acute situation. As vital signs stabilize, glucocorticoids and fluid infusions are tapered over several days. Once the patient is able to eat and take oral medications, oral glucocorticoids may be substituted at physiologic replacement doses, and fludrocortisone, a synthetic oral mineralocorticoid, (0.1–0.2 mg daily) may be administered. Supplemental sodium chloride (1–2 grams daily) may be given if dietary salt intake is inadequate.

### CHRONIC REPLACEMENT THERAPY

Maintenance glucocorticoid replacement therapy is based on estimated normal cortisol secretion rates, which generally range from 5 to 7 $mg/m^2$/day without substantial variation with age or pubertal status.[36] Owing to the fact that bioavailability of orally administered hydrocortisone is reduced by gastric acids and first pass liver metabolism, a more realistic dose is 9 to 12 $mg/m^2$/day of hydrocortisone (divided in 2 or 3 doses) in primary adrenal insufficiency. Patients with partial secondary adrenal insufficiency may do well on lower doses; some patients may be able to avoid chronic replacement and reserve glucocorticoid treatment for times of illness or stress.

Glucocorticoid dosing must be individually adjusted to avert signs and symptoms of adrenal insufficiency while also avoiding the growth retardation and "Cushingoid features" that can accompany overtreatment. Once growth is complete, longer-acting glucocorticoids (eg, dexamethasone once daily) may be considered to enhance adherence. In general, lower doses of glucocorticoids are required to provide replacement therapy for patients with Addison disease compared to doses required for suppression in patients with CAH. It is not helpful to measure plasma cortisol or ACTH levels in titrating the glucocorticoid dose. Patients with low serum sodium, high potassium, or elevated plasma renin activity should receive daily oral fludrocortisone and sodium chloride supplements, adjusted to normalize these analytes.The patient's own sense of well-being, energy level, and blood pressure can help guide the adequacy of therapy. Frequent headaches, lethargy, nausea, or abdominal pain may indicate inadequate treatment. Objective signs of inadequate replacement therapy are orthostatic pulse or blood pressure changes. If skin hyperpigmentation becomes more prominent in primary adrenal insufficiency, plasma ACTH levels may be helpful.

DHEA has been considered an optional hormone supplement for older women with adrenal insufficiency and low energy or libido;[37] however, there are no data on its use in adolescents.

### STRESS DOSING

Patients with adrenal insufficiency (primary or secondary, and patients with CAH) must be informed about the need to increase their glucocorticoid dose during stress to prevent potentially lethal adrenal crisis. Prudence also dictates that all such patients wear a medical alert tag and carry an emergency medical information card to ensure that medical providers know about their underlying disorder.

Mild physical stresses, such as immunizations, uncomplicated viral illnesses, or low grade fever (<38.5°C), do not require stress doses of glucocorticoids. Athletic activity and emotional stress also do not usually require a boost in glucocorticoid dose.[11] In one study, adolescents with CAH who received an additional morning dose of hydrocortisone that resulted in a 100% increase in serum cortisol level did not have altered athletic performance. In this study, no changes were observed in blood glucose, lactate, free fatty acids, or epinephrine levels during short-term high-intensity exercise compared to placebo.[38]

More severe stresses, including illnesses accompanied by higher fever (≥38.5°C), surgery, or major trauma, should be treated by tripling the oral hydrocortisone maintenance dose to prevent the development of hypoglycemia, hypotension, and even cardiovascular collapse.

Supplemental parenteral hydrocortisone is recommended prior to general anesthesia and surgery. Again, doses are empiric and not determined by evidence-based guidelines. A commonly used preoperative dose is 50 $mg/m^2$ given 60 minutes prior to induction of anesthesia, administered either intravenously or intramuscularly. A second dose of 50 $mg/m^2$ can then be administered as a constant intravenous infusion during the procedure, followed by an intravenous bolus of 25 $mg/m^2$ every 6 hours over the following 24 hours. Intravenous or oral stress doses may be gradually tapered as the patient recovers, until the maintenance dose is resumed.

## ADRENOCORTICAL HYPERFUNCTION

The array of disorders causing adrenocortical hyperfunction is narrower than those causing hypofunction. Table 74-3 lists the possible etiologies, including the gene defect and OMIM number when appropriate.

### CUSHING SYNDROME

Cushing syndrome refers to any form of glucocorticoid excess, whereas Cushing disease refers to glucocorticoid excess due to ACTH hypersecretion. Although

**Table 74-3**

**Causes of Adrenal Cortical Hyperfunction**

| *Cause* | *Gene* | *OMIM #* |
|---|---|---|
| Iatrogenic | | |
| Glucocorticoid or mineralcorticoid treatment | | |
| ACTH treatment | | |
| Pituitary tumors | | |
| Adrenal tumors | | |
| Carcinoma | | |
| Adenoma | | |
| Nodular hyperplasia | | |
| Carney complex (AD) | PRKAR1A | 160980 |
| McCune-Albright syndrome | GNAS1 | 174800 |
| Ectopic ACTH-producing tumors | | |
| Apparent mineralocorticoid excess | HSD11B2 | 218030 |
| Glucocorticoid remediable hyperaldosteronism (AD) | chimeric CYP11B1/B2 | 103900 |

rare, Cushing disease is the most frequently identified noniatrogenic etiology for glucocorticoid excess in adolescents, about 0.5 per million persons per year.[39] Prominent clinical features of adrenocortical hyperfunction in adolescents are excess central body weight gain with stunted statural growth. It should be emphasized that most obese adolescents do not have Cushing syndrome and do not require screening, unless growth arrest or other suspicious signs are observed. Examination of annual school photographs can often be informative in revealing subtle changes in physiognomy and habitus over time. Other characteristic findings are easy bruisability, broad purplish striae, and hypertension.

Therapeutic glucocorticoids are in widespread use for a variety of inflammatory and neoplastic diseases, and exogenous administration of relatively high doses of these drugs over long periods of time cause iatrogenic Cushing syndrome. Although carefully researched studies have mainly shown the safety of alternate day oral and inhaled glucocorticoids, individual differences in drug metabolism or sensitivity may cause an apparent increase in bioavailable levels of these potent compounds, many of which have very long biologic half-lives. It is therefore important to obtain a thorough medication history. If possible, glucocorticoids should be tapered while substituting other therapeutic agents. In some patients, attenuation of the features of Cushing syndrome may take months to years.

Clinical suspicion of Cushing syndrome in the absence of exogenous glucocorticoid administration should prompt appropriate screening diagnostic studies for the presence of an ACTH-producing tumor; testing begins with measurement of midnight salivary cortisol or 24-hour urine-free cortisol. The diagnosis may be confirmed by finding a nonsuppressed morning cortisol following dexamethasone administration. The latter test has been refined by the postdexamethasone administration of CRH. An inappropriately brisk rise in plasma ACTH after CRH suggests an ACTH-producing pituitary tumor, at which point an MRI, with attention to this portion of the brain, is indicated. If the tumor cannot be localized by imaging, selective catheterization of the inferior petrosal sinuses with measurement of ACTH levels on either side may be done at a specialized center.[40] Ancillary laboratory studies frequently reveal impaired glucose tolerance and low bone density on radiographs or dual-energy x-ray absorptiometry (DXA).

Adrenal carcinomas (but not typically adenomas) will secrete cortisol as well as mineralocorticoids and androgens. If an adrenal carcinoma is suspected on the basis of an ACTH-independent cortisol excess, the patient should undergo additional hormone measurements of aldosterone and plasma renin activity, as well as DHEA-sulfate and androgens. Thin-slice CT or MRI of the abdomen including the adrenal glands should be performed. Carcinoma will often show a necrotic center and/or calcification and irregular borders, whereas benign nonfunctioning adenomas are typically more homogeneous and similar in density to normal adrenal tissue.

Treatment of Cushing syndrome varies with diagnosis. Cushing disease has traditionally been treated primarily with transsphenoidal tumor resection. Surgical success depends in large part on the skill of the surgeon and the nature of the lesion. In a review of several large series, the cure rate ranges from 60% to 80%.[41] Recent data show that directed radiotherapy, such as those employing gamma knife[42] or linear accelerator[43] techniques, can also induce gradual remission of ACTH hypersecretion. Once ACTH levels have decreased, the patient needs chronic glucocorticoid replacement therapy.

Patients with an adrenal tumor or nodular hyperplasia as the source of cortisol excess will most often undergo adrenalectomy. Another alternative for Cushing syndrome or Cushing disease is medical therapy with drugs such as ketoconazole. This can be used either short-term (eg, while waiting for radiotherapy to take effect) or long-term to reduce cortisol secretion; however, this type of treatment will not induce a permanent cure.

### PHEOCHROMOCYTOMA

Adrenal medullary disease in the adolescent is most often caused by a pheochromocytoma. This rare tumor may cause either episodic or chronic hypertension, usually accompanied by tachycardia, headaches, anxiety, sweating, or flushing. Hyperglycemia and weight loss are also sometimes present. The differential diagnosis in adolescents most saliently includes panic attacks, thyrotoxicosis, renovascular disease, and drug abuse (especially cocaine or amphetamines). The diagnosis of a pheochromocytoma is made either by measuring elevated 24-hour urine-free metanephrines (collected in an acid container), or by high-performance liquid chromatography (HPLC) tandem mass spectrometry measurement of plasma-free metanephrines.[44] Blood should be obtained from an indwelling venous catheter in a patient who has been fasting overnight and has been at rest for at least 20 to 30 minutes; the sample tube must be placed on ice and processed immediately. If possible, psychoactive drugs, especially tricyclic antidepressants, should be discontinued at least 2 weeks prior to testing. Confirmatory imaging may be done by using a metaiodobenzylguanidine (MIBG) scan,[45] which is a norepinephrine analog labeled with radioiodine that is taken up specifically by catechol-producing tumor tissue but not normal adrenal medulla. This imaging test is particularly helpful in cases where either thin-slice, contrast-enhanced CT or MRI fail to show a mass, yet biochemical tests and the clinical scenario are suspicious for the presence of a pheochromocytoma.

A careful family history should be obtained for endocrine tumors, as multiple endocrine neoplasia, type 2, may be associated with pheochromocytoma. Genotyping for the RET oncogene should be performed in the proband, and if positive, other family members should be tested. Transmission is autosomal dominant. Other syndromes that may include pheochromocytoma are von Hippel Lindau disease, neurofibromatosis type 1, and tuberous sclerosis. About 20% to 30% of patients with pheochromocytoma have one of these familial disorders; familial cases are more often bilateral.[46]

In the treatment of pheochromocytoma, calcium channel blocking drugs, such as nifedipine, are usually used to control the hypertension, because calcium is needed for catechol secretion. In preparation for surgery, the patient should be treated for at least a week with a drug with both alpha- and beta-adrenergic blocking properties (eg, labetalol). Unopposed alpha blockade would precipitate a hypotensive crisis at surgery, whereas unopposed beta blockade would exacerbate the hypertension from endogenous epinephrine, a potent vasoconstrictor. In addition, alpha-methyl-L-tyrosine (Demser) is also used to inhibit the rate-limiting step of catechol synthesis. About 10% of cases are bilateral, and thus at the time of surgery, both adrenals should be explored. If both adrenals are removed, substitution therapy will be required, as discussed above for primary adrenal insufficiency. Malignancy and recurrence may occur in about 10% to 15% of cases. Careful long-term follow-up of patients, with regular checks of blood pressure and catechol measurements, is crucial.

## REFERENCES

1. Neville AM, O'Hare MJ. Histopathology of the human adrenal cortex. *Clin Endocrinol Metab.* 1985;14(4):791-820

2. Rozansky DJ. The role of aldosterone in renal sodium transport. *Semin Nephrol.* 2006;26(2):173-181

3. Tsigos C, Chrousos GP. Physiology of the hypothalamic-pituitary-adrenal axis in health and dysregulation in psychiatric and autoimmune disorders. *Endocrinol Metab Clin North Am.* 1994;23(3):451-466

4. Walker BR, Connacher AA, Webb DJ, Edwards CR. Glucocorticoids and blood pressure: a role for the cortisol/cortisone shuttle in the control of vascular tone in man. *Clin Sci (Lond).* 1992;83(2):171-178

5. Speiser PW, White PC. Congenital adrenal hyperplasia. *N Engl J Med.* 2003;349(8):776-788

6. Therrell BL. Newborn screening for congenital adrenal hyperplasia. *Endocrinol Metab Clin North Am.* 2001;30(1):15-30

7. Azziz R, Dewailly D, Owerbach D. Clinical review 56: nonclassic adrenal hyperplasia: current concepts. *J Clin Endocrinol Metab.* 1994;78(4):810-815

8. New MI, Lorenzen F, Lerner AJ, et al. Genotyping steroid 21-hydroxylase deficiency: hormonal reference data. *J Clin Endocrinol Metab.* 1983;57(2):320–326

9. Azziz R, Hincapie LA, Knochenhauer ES, Dewailly D, Fox L, Boots LR. Screening for 21-hydroxylase-deficient nonclassic adrenal hyperplasia among hyperandrogenic women: a prospective study. *Fertil Steril.* 1999;72(5):915–925

10. Speiser PW, Dupont J, Zhu D, et al. Disease expression and molecular genotype in congenital adrenal hyperplasia due to 21-hydroxylase deficiency. *J Clin Invest.* 1992;90(2):584–595

11. Clayton PE, Miller WL, Oberfield SE, Ritzen EM, Sippell WG, Speiser PW. Consensus statement on 21-hydroxylase deficiency from the European Society for Paediatric Endocrinology and the Lawson Wilkins Pediatric Endocrine Society. *Horm Res.* 2002;58(4):188–195

12. Charmandari E, Johnston A, Brook CG, Hindmarsh PC. Bioavailability of oral hydrocortisone in patients with congenital adrenal hyperplasia due to 21-hydroxylase deficiency. *J Endocrinol.* 2001;169(1):65–70

13. Gupta DK, Shilpa S, Amini AC, et al. Congenital adrenal hyperplasia: long-term evaluation of feminizing genitoplasty and psychosocial aspects. *Pediatr Surg Int.* 2006;22(11):905–909

14. Meyer-Bahlburg HF, Dolezal C, Baker SW, Ehrhardt AA, New MI. Gender development in women with congenital adrenal hyperplasia as a function of disorder severity. *Arch Sex Behav.* 2006;35(6):667–684

15. Stikkelbroeck NM, Otten BJ, Pasic A, et al. High prevalence of testicular adrenal rest tumors, impaired spermatogenesis, and Leydig cell failure in adolescent and adult males with congenital adrenal hyperplasia. *J Clin Endocrinol Metab.* 2001;86(12):5721–5728

16. Arlt W, Allolio B. Adrenal insufficiency. *Lancet.* 2003;361(9372):1881–1893

17. Ten S, New M, Maclaren N. Clinical review 130: Addison's disease 2001. *J Clin Endocrinol Metab.* 2001;86(7):2909–2922

18. Simm PJ, McDonnell CM, Zacharin MR. Primary adrenal insufficiency in childhood and adolescence: advances in diagnosis and management. *J Paediatr Child Health.* 2004;40(11):596–599

19. Perry R, Kecha O, Paquette J, Huot C, Van Vliet G, Deal C. Primary adrenal insufficiency in children: twenty years' experience at the Sainte-Justine Hospital, Montreal. *J Clin Endocrinol Metab.* 2005;90(6):3243–3250

20. Todd GR, Acerini CL, Ross-Russell R, Zahra S, Warner JT, McCance D. Survey of adrenal crisis associated with inhaled corticosteroids in the United Kingdom. *Arch Dis Child.* 2002;87(6):457–461

21. Dunlop KA, Carson DJ, Steen HJ, McGovern V, McNaboe J, Shields MD. Monitoring growth in asthmatic children treated with high dose inhaled glucocorticoids does not predict adrenal suppression. *Arch Dis Child.* 2004;89(8):713–716

22. Lamberts SW, Bruining HA, de Jong FH. Corticosteroid therapy in severe illness. *N Engl J Med.* 1997;337(18):1285–1292

23. Felner EI, Thompson MT, Ratliff AF, White PC, Dickson BA. Time course of recovery of adrenal function in children treated for leukemia. *J Pediatr.* 2000;137(1):21–24

24. Schlaghecke R, Kornely E, Santen RT, Ridderskamp P. The effect of long-term glucocorticoid therapy on pituitary-adrenal responses to exogenous corticotropin-releasing hormone. *N Engl J Med.* 1992;326(4):226–230

25. Oelkers W. Adrenal insufficiency. *N Engl J Med.* 1996;335(16):1206–1212

26. Walvoord EC, Rosenman MB, Eugster EA. Prevalence of adrenocorticotropin deficiency in children with idiopathic growth hormone deficiency. *J Clin Endocrinol Metab.* 2004;89(10):5030–5034

27. Brooks BP, Kleta R, Stuart C, et al. Genotypic heterogeneity and clinical phenotype in triple A syndrome: a review of the NIH experience 2000–2005. *Clin Genet.* 2005;68(3):215–221

28. Clark AJ, McLoughlin L, Grossman A. Familial glucocorticoid deficiency associated with point mutation in the adrenocorticotropin receptor. *Lancet.* 1993;341(8843):461–462

29. Buchanan CR, Preece MA, Milner RD. Mortality, neoplasia, and Creutzfeldt-Jakob disease in patients treated with human pituitary growth hormone in the United Kingdom. *BMJ.* 1991;302(6780):824–828

30. Mills JL, Schonberger LB, Wysowski DK, et al. Long-term mortality in the United States cohort of pituitary-derived growth hormone recipients. *J Pediatr.* 2004;144(4):430–436

31. Taback SP, Dean HJ. Mortality in Canadian children with growth hormone (GH) deficiency receiving GH therapy 1967–1992. The Canadian Growth Hormone Advisory Committee. *J Clin Endocrinol Metab.* 1996;81(5):1693–1696

32. Annane D, Sebille V, Charpentier C, et al. Effect of treatment with low doses of hydrocortisone and fludrocortisone on mortality in patients with septic shock. *JAMA.* 2002;288(7):862–871

33. Rady MY, Johnson DJ, Patel B, Larson J, Helmers R. Cortisol levels and corticosteroid administration fail to predict mortality in critical illness: the confounding effects of organ dysfunction and sex. *Arch Surg.* 2005;140(7):661–668

34. Pizarro CF, Troster EJ, Damiani D, Carcillo JA. Absolute and relative adrenal insufficiency in children with septic shock. *Crit Care Med.* 2005;33(4):855–859

35. Menon K, Clarson C. Adrenal function in pediatric critical illness. *Pediatr Crit Care Med.* 2002;3(2):112–116

36. Kerrigan JR, Veldhuis JD, Leyo SA, Iranmanesh A, Rogol AD. Estimation of daily cortisol production and clearance rates in normal pubertal males by deconvolution analysis. *J Clin Endocrinol Metab.* 1993;76(6):1505–1510

37. Saltzman E, Guay A. Dehydroepiandrosterone therapy as female androgen replacement. *Semin Reprod Med.* 2006;24(2):97–105

38. Weise M, Drinkard B, Mehlinger SL,et al. Stress dose of hydrocortisone is not beneficial in patients with classic congenital adrenal hyperplasia undergoing short-term, high-intensity exercise. *J Clin Endocrinol Metab.* 2004;89(8):3679–3684

39. Lindholm J, Juul S, Jorgensen JO,et al. Incidence and late prognosis of Cushing syndrome: a population-based study. *J Clin Endocrinol Metab.* 2001;86(1):117–123

40. Newell-Price J, Bertagna X, Grossman AB, Nieman LK. Cushing syndrome. *Lancet.* 2006;367(9522):1605–1617

41. Oldfeld EH. Cushing disease. *J Neurosurg.* 2003;98(5):948–951

42. Jane JA Jr, Vance ML, Woodburn CJ, Laws ER Jr. Stereotactic radiosurgery for hypersecreting pituitary tumors: part of a multimodality approach. *Neurosurg Focus.* 2003;14(5):e12

43. Voges J, Kocher M, Runge M, et al. Linear accelerator radiosurgery for pituitary macroadenomas: a 7-year follow-up study. *Cancer.* 2006;107(6):1355–1364

44. Lenders JW, Pacak K, Walther MM, et al. Biochemical diagnosis of pheochromocytoma: which test is best? *JAMA.* 2002;287(11):1427–1434

45. Guller U, Turek J, Eubanks S, Delong ER, Oertli D, Feldman JM. Detecting pheochromocytoma: defining the most sensitive test. *Ann Surg.* 2006;243(1):102–107

46. Amar L, Bertherat J, Baudin E, et al. Genetic testing in pheochromocytoma or functional paraganglioma. *J Clin Oncol.* 2005;23(34):8812–8818

# CHAPTER 75

# Bone Health and Disorders

DENNIS E. CAREY, MD • NEVILLE H. GOLDEN, MD

An estimated 10 million Americans older than 50 years of age have osteoporosis and 1.5 million osteoporosis-related fractures occur each year. Fractures related to osteoporosis cost the US health care system an estimated 5 to 10 billion dollars per year.[1] In women older than 35 years, fracture incidence climbs steeply, so that rates become twice that of men.[2]

Osteoporosis is a disorder that is of concern to pediatricians and those caring for adolescents. Osteoporosis does occur in children and adolescents and may be associated with fractures and significant morbidity. In childhood the rate of fractures increases with increasing age, with a peak incidence during the pubertal growth spurt. It has been postulated that the increase in fractures is the result of rapid growth outpacing the increase in bone strength. There is increasing concern that children and adolescents who sustain fractures, especially repeatedly, may have an underlying bone problem. Perhaps more importantly, however, is the fact that the antecedents to adult osteoporosis are rooted in childhood and prevention of osteoporosis in later life is a task that must be attended to in the early stages of life.

## BONE DEVELOPMENT

An understanding of normal bone physiology and development is central to the establishment of strategies for prevention and treatment of osteoporosis. The human skeleton provides a reservoir for the important element calcium and acts as a supportive superstructure. The skeleton is an active organ, which grows dramatically in early life and continues to remodel itself after full linear growth has been achieved. The accretion of calcium, as well as phosphorus, into the fetal skeleton is initiated in earnest during the third trimester and mineral content of bone increases more than 40-fold from birth until adulthood.

From an anatomical point of view there are 2 types of bones: flat bones, such as the skull, mandible, and scapula, and long bones, such as the femur and humerus. Flat bones develop by the process of membranous bone formation while long bones develop by a combination of endochondral bone formation and membranous bone formation. Long bones consist of a hollow tube (diaphysis), which flares at the ends to form metaphyses, the regions below the growth plate, and the epiphyses, the regions above the growth plate. The diaphysis is comprised primarily of cortical bone whereas the metaphyses and epiphyses contain cancellous bone surrounded by a shell of cortical bone. About 80% of the skeleton is cortical bone and 20% is cancellous bone.

Progenitor mesenchymal cells destined to be part of the skeletal system can differentiate either into bone-forming cells (osteoblasts) or into cartilage-forming cells (chondrocytes). Differentiation into osteoblasts occurs in areas of membranous ossification including the subperiosteal bone-forming layer of the long bones. Differentiation into chondrocytes occurs in the remaining skeleton where the cartilage model develops future bone by the process of endochondral ossification. Once the skeleton is formed, it begins a continuous process of renewal that lasts throughout life. This process, termed *remodeling*, has 4 phases: activation, resorption, reversal, and formation (Figure 75-1). In the activation phase, a previously quiescent bone surface is transformed into remodeling surface. Preosteoclasts create bone-resorbing compartments juxtaposed to the organic matrix. Osteoclast formation, activation, and activity are regulated by local cytokines and systemic hormones such as parathyroid hormone (PTH), 1,25-dihydroxyvitamin D3, and calcitonin. Enzymes activated in the acidic microenvironment

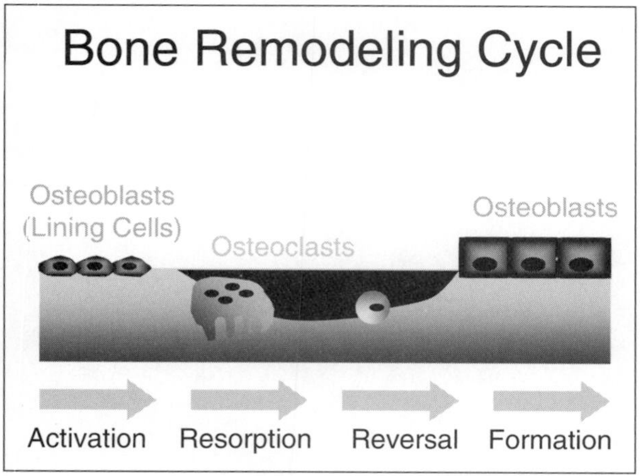


FIGURE 75-1 Bone Remodeling Cycle

dissolve and digest the mineral and organic phases of the matrix producing resorption cavities or lacunae on the surface of cancellous bone and cylindrical tunnels within the cortex. The resorption phase ends with osteoclast apoptosis and is followed by reversal. During reversal local signaling leads to recruitment of bone forming cells. The coupled process is completed when osteoblasts lead to synthesis of a new matrix and regulates its mineralization.

## PEAK BONE MASS ACQUISITION

The concept of peak bone mass suggests that bone mass reaches a zenith after which it declines. Achievement of an adequate peak bone mass is therefore a prerequisite for bone health in adulthood. Osteoporosis in adulthood is a consequence of either failure to achieve an adequate peak bone mass or accelerated loss of bone or both (Figure 75-2). Prior to achievement of peak bone mass, bone accumulates as bone formation occurs at a rate greater than bone resorption. After achievement of peak bone mass, bone resorption outpaces bone formation and bone mass declines, and if a low bone mass threshold is reached, osteoporosis is considered to be present. Implicit in the concept of peak bone mass is that osteoporosis, a disease of adulthood, has its antecedents in childhood and adolescence and therefore an understanding of the determinants of bone accumulation is an important factor in the prevention of osteoporosis.

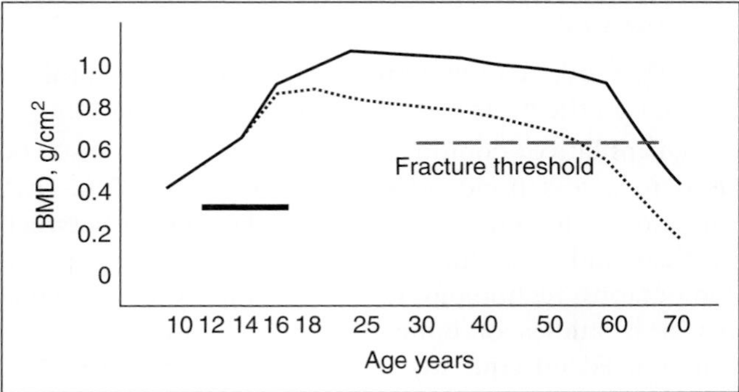


**FIGURE 75-2** Impact of a disease such as anorexia nervosa (solid bar) on achievement of peak bone mineral density (BMD). Instead of following the normal expected pattern (solid line) the patient (short dashed line) does not achieve peak bone mass and reaches the fracture threshold (long dashed line) much earlier. (Adapted from Golden NH. Osteopenia and osteoporosis in anorexia nervosa. *Adolescent Medicine: State of the Art Reviews*. 2003;14:93–108, with permission from Elsevier.)

The increase in bone mass that occurs during childhood and puberty results from a combination of growth of bone at the endplates (endochondral bone formation) and of changes in bone shape (modeling and remodeling). These processes occur at different rates and at different times at primary and secondary sites of bone formation. Longitudinal studies of total body bone mineral content (BMC) measurements show that between 40% and 60% of peak bone mass is acquired during adolescence and that up to 25% of peak bone mass is acquired during the 2-year period around peak height velocity.[3] At least 90% of net peak bone mass is acquired by age 18, and it is debatable whether any significant net gain in bone mass occurs in young adulthood.[4] The density of trabecular bone is more strongly influenced than cortical bone by the hormonal factors associated with the sexual development during late adolescence and on average bone mineral density (BMD) in the spine increases by 13% during puberty in white boys and girls. The exact role of hormones in pubertal bone mass accumulation remains to be determined but it is supposed that the increase is related to sex steroids and sex-steroid induced increases in growth hormone and insulin-like growth factor I (IGF-I).

## ASSESSMENT OF BONE HEALTH IN ADOLESCENCE

### MEASUREMENT OF BONE DENSITY

While standard skeletal radiographs are useful in diagnosing certain bone diseases such as rickets, they are unreliable for assessing bone density because reduced bone mass may be present in bones that seem normal by x-ray. Several technologies have been developed to assess bone mineral. These include dual-energy x-ray absorptiometry (DXA), quantitative computed tomography (QCT) and quantitative ultrasound (QUS). Dual Energy X-ray Absorptiometry is the most commonly utilized methodology because of its precision and minimal radiation exposure. Dual energy x-ray absorptiometry machines can measure bone mass and bone density of the whole body or in regions: lumbar spine, hip, and forearm by site-specific scanning. A DXA machine consists of a table, the scanner arm, and a dedicated computer. The spine and hip are the most commonly assessed regions. A whole body scan can assess total body BMD and can also be used to assess body composition. A scan of the spine or hip takes ~0.5 minutes and delivers an effective dose value of radiation of less than 1 microSievert (μSv). For comparison, a lateral x-ray film of the spine results in a dose of 700 μSv or more and natural background radiation is typically 2,400 μSv per year.[5]

Dual energy x-ray absorptiometry measures tissue absorption of photons emitted from an x-ray source. High-energy photons penetrate bone and soft tissue, whereas low-energy photons are able to penetrate soft tissue only. A detector quantifies photons transmitted through the body and the difference in measurement between high-energy and low-energy photons reflects photon absorption by bone.

Dual energy x-ray absorptiometry actually measures the BMC of an anatomic area. Bone mineral density is calculated by dividing BMC by the projected area in the coronal plane of the region scanned. Dual energy x-ray absorptiometry, therefore, measures areal density, expressed in grams per square centimeter. In the early 1990s, a working group of the World Health Organization, using data comparing population-based BMD to lifetime fracture risk in postmenopausal women, agreed upon a BMD threshold that used the number of standard deviations (SD) below a young adult reference mean value (at peak bone mass) of minus (–) 2.5 for the diagnosis of osteoporosis in adults.[6] The term T-score has been used to describe the SD from the mean. A T-score of 1 would be a BMD 1 SD above the young adult mean while a T-score of −1 would be a BMD 1 SD below the young adult mean. In adults, a T-score between −1 and −2.5 has been defined as osteopenia. The T-score, based on a SD value, was used rather than absolute BMD (g/cm$^2$) because the different calibrations of various manufacturers would have required device-specific BMD values. Despite these conventions, T-score discrepancy among DXA manufacturers still exists because of differences in the young-normal reference populations used by the manufacturers.

In children and adolescents, a T-score has essentially no clinical value because it compares the BMD of a child or teen to that of fully grown young adults who have a BMD that has reached its peak. Most children below a certain age or size would have a T-score for whatever bone site that was being scanned below the osteoporotic threshold of −2.5. In children and adolescents, BMD should be compared to an age-matched reference population and a Z-score registered. An increasing number of pediatric reference population databases have been developed and the manufacturers of DXA machines have incorporated these into BMD analyses. Potential inadequacy of pediatric reference data across maturational stage, ethnic group, and gender remains a limitation of DXA studies in children and adolescents. Changes in bone size and geometry in children affect measurement of BMD using DXA. Because BMD measures areal density rather than volumetric density, it may underestimate true volumetric density in small children and overestimate it in large children. Models have been developed to estimate volumetric bone density in order to reduce the influence of bone size on DXA measurement; these are frequently used in research studies.[7]

The −2.5 T-score threshold for osteoporosis was defined for post menopausal women only. To apply it to adult men or pre menopausal women and certainly children and adolescents is not appropriate. The International Society for Clinical Densitometry (ISCD) has recommended that in males and females younger than 20 years of age the terminology "low bone density for chronological age" be used if the Z-score is less than or equal to −2.0 and that the term "osteopenia" should not be used in reports on children and adolescents.[8] A Z-score of −2.5 represents the 0.6th percentile for age, −2.0, the 2.3rd percentile, and −1.0, the 16th percentile. There are no data in the pediatric population linking a given percentile to increased fracture risk during childhood or adulthood. While a very low Z-score may be found in a child or adolescent with a bone disorder, simply having a BMD Z-score of −2.0 or less does not necessarily identify the presence of abnormal bone. The ISCD Official Positions (2007) contains expanded recommendations for performing and evaluating the bone density studies in children and adolescents. The recommendations can be viewed at www.iscd.org and include the following:

- The diagnosis of osteoporosis in children and adolescents should not be made on the basis of densitometric criteria alone.
- In children with linear growth or maturational delay, spine and total body BMC and areal BMD results should be adjusted for absolute height or height age or compared to pediatric reference data that provide age, gender, and height-specific Z-scores.
- Therapeutic interventions should not be instituted on the basis of a single DXA measurement.

Quantitative computed tomography can also be used to assess bone health. In contrast to DXA, QCT measures volumetric BMD and can distinguish between cortical and trabecular bone. Quantitative computed tomography technology has been employed in several research studies of bone in children and adolescents but is used infrequently in clinical care because QCT machines are costly, not readily accessible, and the dose of radiation exposure is high (estimates vary from 30 μSv to 7000 μSv).[9] Peripheral quantitative computed tomography (pQCT) measurement of the forearm at the distal radius involves less radiation exposure and can predict hip fractures in post menopausal women. It is not yet widely available for clinical use and there are no well established reference data for children and adolescents.

Quantitative ultrasound is a non invasive method of assessing bone health by measuring speed of sound of an ultrasound wave as it is propagated along the bone.

Speed of sound propagation depends not only on BMD, but also on bone geometry and microarchitecture. Quantitative ultrasound can be performed at the calcaneus, tibia, and radius and in adults, has been shown to predict fracture risk. The use of QUS is appealing because the machine is easily portable, the test is relatively inexpensive, and the method is radiation-free. In the pediatric and adolescent population, QUS has been compared to DXA in adolescent athletes, and in patients with anorexia nervosa, celiac disease, and chronic rheumatic diseases with varying results. Reference databases are not yet available for many of the existing QUS devices for children and adolescents, but the use of QUS in pediatric populations shows promise for the future.

## MEASUREMENT OF BONE STRENGTH

An important factor determining fracture risk is the ability of the bone to resist the mechanical stresses that lead to fracture. Bone strength depends not only on BMD, but also on bone elasticity, microarchitecture, size, and shape. There is no direct measure of bone strength but assessment of section modulus provides a good estimate of bone strength. Section modulus is a mechanical engineering term used to describe bending strength of a hollow structure such as a beam, or in this case, a bone. Section modulus of the hip can be calculated from DXA scans using an interactive computer program called hip structural analysis (HSA).[10] This program measures the radius and cross-sectional area of the bone using digital images derived from the DXA scan and calculates section modulus using a mathematical formula. Section modulus of a large bone will always be greater than that of a small bone even when both bones have the same BMD. Assessment of section modulus as a measure of bone strength is primarily used for research purposes rather than for clinical care.

### BIOCHEMICAL MARKERS OF BONE METABOLISM

In recent decades, measurement of the proteins involved in bone turnover has been used to assess level of activity and the balance between bone formation and bone resorption. Table 75-1 lists the biochemical markers of bone metabolism.

Osteoblasts synthesize a number of proteins, most prominently type I collagen, but also alkaline phosphatase and osteocalcin. Alkaline phosphatase is essential for mineralization but its precise role in this process has still not been elucidated. Alkaline phosphatase levels are much higher in healthy children and adolescents than in adults and increase markedly in rachitic disorders. This enzyme also is found in the liver, intestines, spleen, placenta, and bone. Bone-specific alkaline phosphatase can be measured for research purposes, although it is not widely used in clinical practice.

Osteocalcin is considered a marker of bone formation, but since it is incorporated into the bone matrix and later released into the circulation during bone resorption, it more properly should be considered a marker of bone turnover. Like alkaline phosphatase, circulating levels of osteocalcin are higher in children and adolescents than in adults.

**Table 75-1**

**Biochemical Markers of Bone Metabolism**

| *Marker* | *Abbreviation* | *Sample Source* |
|---|---|---|
| ***Bone Formation*** | | |
| Osteocalcin | OC | Serum |
| Bone specific alkaline phosphatase | BSAP | Serum |
| Procollagen type I C-terminal peptide | PICP | Serum |
| Procollagen type I N-terminal peptide | PINP | Serum |
| ***Bone Resorption*** | | |
| Deoxypyridinoline | DPD | Urine/Serum |
| Pyridinoline | PYD | Urine |
| Cross-linked N-telopeptide | NTX | Urine/Serum |
| Cross-linked C-telopeptide | CTX | Urine/Serum |
| Type I collagen C-terminal telopeptide | ICTP | Serum |

Type I collagen is the major collagen of bone and the most abundant product of the osteoblast. Type I collagen is produced as a precursor molecule with carboxy-terminal and amino-terminal propeptides, that are cleaved prior to release into circulation. Assays have been developed to measure both the C-terminal propeptide of collagen (PICT) and the N-terminal propeptide of collagen (PINP) and, as with alkaline phosphatase and osteocalcin, levels in serum are much greater in growing children and adolescents than in adults. However, since type I collagen is not exclusive to bone, circulating levels represent total type I collagen synthesis from other tissues including skin.

Collagen degradation products can be measured as biochemical markers of bone resorption. Collagen molecules form fibrils that are joined by covalent cross-links. These consist of hydroxylysl-pyridinolines (PYD) and lysl-pyridinolines (DPD). Upon bone breakdown by osteoclasts, by-products are released into the circulation and both free and peptide-bound PYD and DPD can be measured in urine. The amino-terminal telopeptide (NTX) and the carboxy-terminal (CTX) of collagen cross-links can be measured in urine as well as in blood.

It is only recently that the use of biochemical markers has expanded out of the research field to clinical usefulness. This utility has been found in the care of osteoporosis in adults. Measurement of bone markers before and during treatment is being increasingly employed to monitor effectiveness of anti resorptive therapy. Failure to exhibit the expected reduction in bone resorptive markers can be taken to indicate therapeutic failure, improper administration, or poor compliance. It is hoped that in the future biochemical markers might prove useful to predict response to a given therapy and predict fracture risk or bone loss. In contrast to use of these markers in adults, utilization in children and adolescents remains primarily a research tool.

## FACTORS THAT AFFECT BONE MASS

Factors known to affect bone mass are listed in Box 75-1.[11] Heredity accounts for 66% to 75% of the variability in peak bone mass, but environmental factors do play an important role.[11] The fundamental issue in the field of osteoporosis with regard to genetics is the ability to identify those at risk for osteoporosis and fragility fractures so that preventive measures that optimize attainment of peak bone mass can be promoted and early treatment of developing bone loss can be instituted. Osteoporosis does run in families. Daughters of women with osteoporosis have reduced bone mass compared to controls, as do men and women with first-degree relatives who have osteoporosis.[11] However, the genotype-phenotype relationship is complex. There are likely many "osteoporosis genes" with an ever-expanding candidate list—vitamin D receptor gene, calcium-sensing receptor gene, $\alpha$-2 HS-glycoprotein gene, estrogen receptor $\alpha$ gene, calcitonin gene, PTH gene, collagen 1$\alpha$1 gene, TGF-$\beta$ genes, and others—that need to be investigated.[11]

**Box 75-1**
***Factors Affecting Bone Mass***

***Nonmodifiable***
Gender
Ethnicity
Heredity
***Modifiable***
Diet: calcium, vitamin D
Body type: body weight, body mass index
Hormonal status: estrogen, testosterone, growth hormone, cortisol
Exercise
Lifestyle choices: smoking, alcohol

Osteoporosis and fragility fractures occur more frequently in women than men. There is a four- to eight-fold higher incidence of vertebral fractures in women. The cross-sectional area of a vertebral body is 11% smaller in prepubertal girls compared with boys, and this gender discrepancy increases to 25% by the time of skeletal maturity. Bone mineral density in boys and girls is similar before puberty. Therefore, the higher fracture rate in women may be more dependent on vertebral area than actual BMD.[12] Race is a factor determining bone mass. Blacks suffer fewer fractures than whites and other racial groups. This is likely accounted for by larger bone size and greater volumetric bone density in blacks.[13] Differences in bone density among whites, Hispanics, and Asian children are essentially eliminated when corrected for height and weight.[4]

Calcium is the principal cation of bone mineral and the skeleton constitutes a reserve of calcium for bodily functions. Sustained withdrawal from this reserve, however, leads to decreases in bone mass and poses a threat to the health of the skeleton. Low calcium intake early in life is believed to predispose to fragile bones in childhood and adolescence as well as to lead to osteoporosis late in life. Calcium intake is positively correlated with bone mass at all ages. In healthy adolescents calcium supplementation has been shown to increase BMD.[14] Adequate vitamin D intake is also essential for utilization of calcium. Excessive intake of carbonated beverages is known to be associated with bone fractures in athletic adolescent girls, either because of reduced consumption of milk or because of the increased phosphorus content of soda.[15]

Adequate vitamin D intake is also essential for utilization of calcium. Vitamin D deficiency can occur in teenagers who live in northeastern climates, particularly during the winter. It is more common in blacks and in teens who keep their bodies covered for religious reasons and do not have adequate exposure to sunlight.

Body weight is a major determinant of BMD both in healthy adolescents and in those with anorexia nervosa, and weight restoration in patients with anorexia nervosa is associated with improvement in BMD.[16]

Weight-bearing exercise is protective of BMD. Immobilization is associated with reduced BMD.

Hormonal status plays an important role in maintaining bone mass. Testosterone, growth hormone, and IGF-1 all promote bone formation, while cortisol excess and hypoestrogenemia increase bone resorption leading to a reduction in net bone mass.

Smoking and alcohol are associated with reduced BMD.

## CONDITIONS ASSOCIATED WITH LOW BONE MASS

A list of conditions that are associated with low bone mass can be found in Box 75-2.

**Box 75-2**

***Low Bone Mass in Adolescence***

Primary
- Osteogenesis imperfecta
- Idiopathic juvenile osteoporosis

Secondary
- Anorexia nervosa
- Female athlete triad
- Immobilization
- Cerebral palsy
- Glucocorticoid excess
- Thyroid hormone excess
- Depot medroxyprogesterone acetate
- Anti-convulsants
- Connective tissue disorders
- Cancer
- Malabsorption
- Cystic fibrosis
- Celiac disease
- Inflammatory bowel disease
- Cushing syndrome
- Thyrotoxicosis
- Hypogonadism

### OSTEOGENESIS IMPERFECTA

Osteogenesis imperfecta (OI) is a prototypical, though rare (incidence 1:10,000), osteoporotic disorder of childhood. Sometimes referred to as "brittle bone disease," OI is a chiefly autosomal dominant genetic disorder of connective tissue, specifically type I collagen, with a wide range of clinical severity dependent on the specific type, I to IV (clinical classification of Sillence).[17] Type II OI is the most severe form and is usually lethal in the perinatal period. Fractures occur in utero. Type III and Type IV OI are intermediate in severity, with Type III patients suffering from hundreds of fractures over a lifetime, severe disability, and extreme short stature. Type IV patients generally have less disability, a lesser degree of short stature, and a decreasing rate of fractures after puberty. The diagnosis of type I, the mildest form of OI, with normal stature and little or no deformity, may be missed at an early age and present later as early onset adult osteoporosis. It should be suspected in patients with a history of fracture and low bone density who also have blue sclerae, easy bruising, or hearing loss. Screening for OI using cultured dermal fibroblasts can identify a biochemical abnormality in approximately 90% of clinically affected individuals.[18]

### IDIOPATHIC JUVENILE OSTEOPOROSIS

The other primary form of osteoporosis in childhood is idiopathic juvenile osteoporosis (IJO), which presents in pre pubertal boys and girls, typically between 8 and 12 years of age, and resolves spontaneously post puberty. There is a classical form of IJO described by Dent and Friedman[19] in 1965 but in a review on the topic, Rauch and Bishop[20] recently suggested that children with unexplained low bone mass and fractures not fitting the classical description still be considered to have "IJO in the wider sense" or what one might call non classical IJO. In their clinics IJO is approximately 10 times less common than OI. They further distinguish IJO from children in late pre-puberty and early puberty who exhibited low bone mass and fractures, mainly of the forearm, who they would consider healthy and undergoing "an adaptational bone problem." They proposed that IJO should only be diagnosed when vertebral compression fractures are present (with or without extremity fractures).

Classical IJO is characterized by metaphyseal and vertebral compression fractures with collapsed or biconcave vertebrae on lateral spine films along with radiolucent areas in the metaphyses of long bones termed "neo-osseous osteoporosis" representing new osteoporotic bone with callus formation. Unlike the thin, gracile long bones of OI, the long bones of patients with IJO have a normal diameter and cortical width. Bone histomorphometric studies indicate that in IJO there seems to be a disturbance of bone formation mainly in trabecular bone and possibly in the cortical surface adjacent to the marrow cavity. There is no biochemical marker specific for IJO.

## ANOREXIA NERVOSA AND EATING DISORDERS

Anorexia nervosa and eating disorders usually have their onset during adolescence, a time during which 40% to 60% of bone accretion is occurring. Patients with anorexia nervosa have reduced bone mass that can develop as soon as 6 months after the onset of the disease. Significant reduction in bone mass occurs in 50% to 90% of patients meeting full criteria for the condition.[21] The degree of bone mass reduction is more severe than that found in patients with other causes of hypothalamic amenorrhea, implying that, in addition to estrogen deficiency, nutritional factors play a role.[22] The reduction in bone mass in anorexia nervosa is associated with increased fracture risk and can persist for many years after recovery from the eating disorder.[23] Patients with partial eating disorders or eating disorders not otherwise specified (EDNOS) are also at risk for low bone mass, particularly if they are, or have been, at low weight. In general, patients with anorexia nervosa have the lowest BMD, followed by those with EDNOS and a prior history of low body weight. Patients with bulimia nervosa, who have never been of low weight, tend to have normal bone mass.

Factors contributing to the low bone mass in anorexia nervosa and other eating disorders include low body weight; poor dietary intake of protein, calcium, and vitamin D; hypoestrogenemia, and hypercortisolism. Studies utilizing biochemical markers of bone metabolism have demonstrated both reduced bone formation as well as increased bone resorption. The degree of bone mass reduction is directly related to the duration of amenorrhea. Many authorities suggest performing bone densitometry if a patient with anorexia nervosa has been amenorrheic for more than 6 months.

## FEMALE ATHLETE TRIAD

The female athlete triad refers to 3 interrelated conditions occurring in female athletes: disordered eating, amenorrhea, and osteoporosis. The condition is frequently not recognized and can be a cause of stress fractures. The female athlete triad is caused by an imbalance of energy intake and energy expenditure whereby energy intake is insufficient for energy requirements. As a result of the energy deficit, there is suppression of the hypothalamic-pituitary-ovarian axis resulting in amenorrhea, osteoporosis, and increased fracture risk.[24]

The female athlete triad can occur in any sport but is more likely to occur in individual sports where there is an emphasis on a lean appearance (eg, gymnastics, diving, ballet, figure skating) or in sports where it is believed that a lower weight may offer some performance advantage (eg, track, cross country, and swimming). It can also occur in sports where the athlete is required to meet a certain weight limit (eg, wrestling, rowing, and judo).

Caloric intake may be too low because the athlete is actively trying to lose weight or the athlete may be inadvertently consuming an insufficient amount of calories because of limited knowledge about the increased caloric demands of the sport. Some athletes may be using unhealthy methods to control their weight, such as self-induced vomiting or the use of laxatives, diuretics, herbal supplements, or diet pills. While some athletes with the female athlete triad may have an underlying eating disorder, many do not. They may be of normal weight and they often do not have distortion of body image. Amenorrhea in an athlete should never be considered a normal consequence of exercise but rather should be a red flag that there may be an underlying problem.

## CEREBRAL PALSY

Osteoporosis and consequent fractures are common in children with cerebral palsy (CP). Multiple factors lead to osteoporosis. Most common is the limitation to weight-bearing ambulation due to the underlying CP and temporary immobilization following orthopedic procedures. Oral-motor dysfunction with feeding difficulty can lead to poor nutrition and low calcium intake that may adversely affect bone mineralization as might concomitant anticonvulsant therapy and poor exposure to sunlight. Henderson et al[25] evaluated bone density in a population-based cohort of children and adolescents with moderate to severe CP and found a BMD Z-score at less than −2.0 in the femur in 77% of subjects. Mean Z-scores for the femur (−3.1 ± 0.2) were lower than mean Z-scores for the spine (−1.8 ± 0.1). Fractures had occurred in 26% of the children who were older than 10 years. In stepwise regression analyses, they found that the severity of neurological impairment, increasing difficulty feeding the child, use of anti-convulsants, and lower triceps skin fold Z-scores (in decreasing order of importance) all independently contribute to lower BMD Z-scores in the femur.

## CHRONIC CHILDHOOD ILLNESS

A number of chronic illnesses of childhood and adolescence such as celiac disease, inflammatory bowel disease, cystic fibrosis, juvenile rheumatoid arthritis, and childhood cancer, may predispose to low BMD either because of the underlying disorder or because of treatment of the disorder. Whether or not disease-induced low BMD in such circumstances leads to osteoporosis in adulthood remains unclear and the necessity of intervention with bone-specific therapy remains controversial.

Celiac disease is a malabsorptive disorder of the gastrointestinal tract, which has been diagnosed with increased frequency in the last decade. Low BMD has been reported in a number of studies and treatment with proper nutrition and a gluten-free diet appears to be sufficient to improve BMD. Population-based studies suggest there is not a high risk for severe fractures in patients with celiac disease.

Low BMD is reported to be common in inflammatory bowel disease and yet population studies in both Crohn disease and ulcerative colitis suggest that the risk of fractures is not elevated relative to age- and sex-matched controls.[26–27] Again, treatment of the underlying bowel disease should be both preventive and therapeutic with regard to bone health.

Certain studies have documented low BMD and fractures in pediatric and adult patients with cystic fibrosis.[28] Possible contributing factors include nutritional deficiencies, lack of exercise, hypogonadism, and various treatments. The degree of osteoporosis correlates with greater disease severity and therefore it is not unexpected that BMD is particularly reduced in patients undergoing lung transplantation. In 1 study, treatment with human growth hormone for 1 year was shown to increase total body BMC in poorly growing children with cystic fibrosis.[29] It remains to be determined if similar changes in site-specific BMD occur and if increases are sustained and are not simply a result of increased bone growth.

Low BMD and localized bone loss are seen in rheumatic disorders based on the influence of local and systemic cytokines that stimulate and support osteoclastic activity. In children with juvenile idiopathic arthritis (JIA) bone formation is also likely affected. Poor functional state, leading to decreased activity and therapeutic interventions, especially with glucocorticoids, contributes to the decrease in BMD. Vertebral compression fractures, fractures of the long bones as well as less appreciated stress fractures occur in children and adolescents with JIA resulting in considerable morbidity and cost. Although many adults with a history of JIA have a normal BMD, a subset of patients have reduced BMD for age, increasing the risk of fractures later in life.[30]

Osteoporosis and fragility fractures are part of the sequelae of childhood cancer and survival. Fractures have been reported in 25% to 30% of children with acute lymphoblastic leukemia and occur in other forms of childhood cancer, including lymphoma and solid tumors. Fractures can occur any time during and after treatment. Decreased BMD occurs as a result of multiple factors including radiotherapy, cytotoxic agents, glucocorticoids, decreased activity, impaired nutrition, and hormonal deficiencies, especially deficiency of sex steroids. Male sex and Caucasian race are factors associated with higher risk for osteoporosis in survivors of acute lymphoblastic leukemia.[31]

More research in the development and natural history of diseases associated with diminished BMD is clearly warranted. From a clinical point of view, due consideration of baseline assessment of site-specific BMD by DXA scanning in children and adolescents who develop a chronic illness should be given. Correct interpretation of BMD in chronically ill adolescents with growth failure and/or bone age delay requires analysis relative to bone age or height age in addition to chronological age.

Endocrine disorders may result in low BMD. Excess endogenous glucocorticoid secretion as in Cushing syndrome can affect the skeleton similarly to exogenous glucocorticoid excess. Thyrotoxicosis, as well as overtreatment with thyroid hormone, can cause low BMD. Growth hormone deficiency not only slows linear growth but also the accretion of bone mineral. There has been a recent move toward considering growth hormone therapy in growth hormone deficient patients beyond the closure of growth plates for the anticipated augmentation of peak bone mass. Some have recommended growth hormone therapy up to age 25 years in patients with severe growth hormone deficiency, eg, those with post-surgical growth hormone deficiency). As discussed elsewhere, achievement of optimal peak bone mass may be jeopardized by gonadal failure or even late pubertal development. Girls with anorexia nervosa are particularly at risk. In Turner syndrome, an example of congenital hypogonadism, osteoporosis has been described historically. The effect of therapy with estrogen treatment and growth hormone therapy in girls with Turner syndrome has been addressed in a recent review by Rubin.[32]

## GLUCOCORTICOID-INDUCED OSTEOPOROSIS

Pharmacologic doses of glucocorticoids are widely used in pediatric patients, especially in the treatment of inflammatory disorders such as rheumatoid arthritis, Crohn disease, and systemic lupus erythematosis. Chronic glucocorticoid therapy is one of the most common causes of osteoporosis in children. At high doses, glucocorticoids profoundly inhibit bone formation resulting in low bone mass. Glucocorticoids increase the risk of bone fractures throughout the skeleton but especially in the spine and ribs. There appears to be an "at risk population" as BMD is not lowered as much in some chronically treated patients as it is in others and it has been postulated that genetic variations in the glucocorticoid receptor account for this difference.[33]

The negative effect of glucocorticoids on bone is mainly through inhibition of osteoblastic bone formation. Bone resorption is also increased but it is a temporary phenomenon. Indirect negative effects occur through inhibition of growth factors, sex steroids, calcium absorption, and decreased mechanical strain on bone from weakened muscle.[34] Whether an individual will develop fractures as a result of glucocorticoid therapy depends on several factors, in addition to possible variations in the glucocorticoid receptor. These include the pre therapy BMD, the disease for which a glucocorticoid is being used, glucocorticoid dose, and length of treatment. A lower starting BMD, higher dose, longer administration, and more severe underlying disorder would be expected to be accompanied by higher fracture risk. A relatively short course of glucocorticoids leading to bone loss is likely to be readily reversible upon discontinuation while a longer course may reduce bone mass to a point at which recovery is not likely even after cessation of therapy and fracture risk is ongoing. Children and adolescents are more likely to recover from glucocorticoid-induced osteoporosis; however, glucocorticoid therapy could possibly prevent achievement of peak bone mass.

### DEPO-PROVERA

Depot medroxyprogesterone acetate (Depo-Provera, DMPA) is a long-acting injectable contraceptive approved for use in the United States in 1992. It is administered as a deep intramuscular injection every 12 weeks and is a very effective contraceptive because it does not rely on patient adherence. It is estimated that more than 1 million teens in the United States are being treated with DMPA annually.

Recent studies in adolescents have shown that over a period of 2 years, treatment with DMPA is associated with a 3.1% (range 1.5% to 6.0%) reduction of BMD of the lumbar spine compared with a net gain of 7.29% (range 5.9% to 9.5%) in healthy adolescent controls.[35] The mechanism of bone mass reduction is thought to be secondary to suppression of the hypothalamic-pituitary-ovarian axis, resulting in a hypoestrogenic state. Fortunately, discontinuation of DMPA use is associated with improvement in bone mass but it is not known whether subjects receiving DMPA reach the same peak bone mass they would have achieved without DMPA.[36]

In November 2004, the US Food and Drug Administration (FDA) released a black box warning informing practitioners of the risk of prolonged use of DMPA on bone mass, particularly as it relates to adolescents. Pregnancy itself can be associated with reduced bone mass and most adolescents do not continue DMPA for more than 1 year. The Society for Adolescent Health Medicine (SAHM) in its Position Paper on DMPA and BMD in Adolescents, echoing a recent statement by the World Health Organization, states that "Among adolescents, the advantages of using DMPA generally outweigh the theoretical safety concerns regarding fracture risk."[37] SAHM recommends continuing to prescribe DMPA to adolescent girls requiring contraception but to provide adequate explanation of the benefits and potential risks, including the possible risk for bone loss. SAHM recommends consideration of monitoring BMD, depending on the patient's individual risk profile for osteoporosis.

## MANAGEMENT

### PREVENTION

#### Calcium and Vitamin D

According to the American Academy of Pediatrics (AAP) report "Optimizing Bone Health and Calcium Intakes of Infants, Children, and Adolescents" provision of adequate calcium during childhood and adolescence is necessary for peak bone mass development.[38] National survey data, however, indicate that most American children older than 8 years of age fail to achieve the recommended intake of calcium, with only 10% of adolescent girls doing so. The AAP report emphasizes the critical role of the family in achieving adequate calcium intake in adolescents and the role of the pediatrician in periodically assessing calcium intake by questionnaire across the growing years. In pre adolescents and adolescents ages 9 to 18 years of age, an intake of elemental calcium of 1,300 mg/day is recommended. At intakes above this level most of the additional calcium is excreted and of no benefit. Barriers to adequate calcium intake include lactose intolerance, replacement of milk intake by soft drinks, fruit drinks, and fruit juices and avoidance of dairy products because of the misconception that they are fattening. Drinking 4 8- to 10-oz glasses of milk will provide the recommended calcium intake for adolescents. Yogurt and cheese are other good sources of calcium. Flavored milks and reduced fat milks generally contain similar amounts of calcium to regular milk. Alternate sources of calcium should be provided for adolescents who cannot drink milk. Low oxalate-containing vegetables such as broccoli and collard greens have bioavailable calcium. Bioavailability of calcium in soy foods, however, is generally low. Juices and breakfast cereals, which are fortified with calcium, are additional alternatives to dairy products. If the recommended level of calcium cannot be achieved through foodstuffs, then calcium supplements should be considered.

Per the AAP statement, optimal absorption and retention of calcium also requires intake of vitamin D. In November 2008 the AAP increased its recommendation on vitamin D intake suggesting an amount equal to 400 IU (10.0 micrograms) or 1000 ml of vitamin D-fortified milk per day.[39] Most daily multivitamins contain 400 IU vitamin D.

### Exercise and Lifestyle

Weight-bearing activity should be encouraged for all children and adolescents to optimize peak bone mass acquisition. The quantity of diet soda consumed should be limited and patients should be counseled about the effect of smoking on BMD.

In children, a 10-minute, 3 times a week, school-based exercise program conducted in 14 schools in Canada was associated with significant increases in BMD in early pubertal girls compared with a control group that did not receive the program.[40] This exercise program incorporated high impact jumping activities during regularly scheduled physical education classes. In college women randomly assigned to a weight-bearing exercise program, a resistance training program or no exercise, both weight-bearing and resistance training were associated with increases in BMD of the lumbar spine whereas in the sedentary controls there was no change in BMD.[41]

## TREATMENT

### Calcium and Vitamin D

Once reduced BMD is noted, the first step should be to ensure that the adolescent has adequate calcium and vitamin D intake as discussed in regard to prevention.

Whether additional vitamin D should be provided remains controversial. Recently the recommended amount of vitamin D supplementation in adults has been increased based on the finding that PTH levels have been shown to be elevated in the face of serum 25-OH-D levels ≤ 30 ng/ml. This 25-OH-D level is much higher than what is currently considered the lower limit of normal for children and adolescents. At the present time there is no strong evidence-based rationale for providing more than 400 IU/day of extra vitamin D in a non-deficient adolescent. In children or adolescents with reduced BMD in whom vitamin D deficiency is suspected due to certain risk factors (limited sunlight exposure, poor nutritional state, or anti convulsant therapy), laboratory tests to measure serum calcium, phosphorus, alkaline phosphatase, PTH, and 25-OH-D concentrations should be performed. If vitamin D deficiency is found to be present, standard treatment of vitamin D deficiency should be applied.

### Hormone Therapy

In general, hormone therapy is indicated only for children who have permanent hormone deficiencies, (hypogonadism, growth hormone deficiency, or hypothyroidism). Hormone replacement therapy should not be routinely prescribed to increase BMD in adolescent girls with eating disorders or for the female athlete triad because there is no evidence to support its efficacy. Despite this fact, a recent survey revealed that 78% of physicians who treat adolescents with anorexia nervosa prescribe hormone replacement therapy in an attempt to either prevent or reverse reduced BMD.[42]

In girls with hypergonadotropic hypogonadism, eg, for example, Turner syndrome, the timing of estrogen replacement must be individualized and is often delayed until final or near final height is achieved because of concern that estrogen will promote premature closure of the growth plate.

In boys who have IJO and delayed puberty, consideration of short-term, low-dose testosterone therapy may be given. Testosterone therapy should be individualized but can be introduced at low-dose and advanced slowly. Short-term, low dose testosterone therapy is often recommended for psychosocial reasons in adolescent boys with constitutional delay of growth and puberty. It was once thought that boys with delayed puberty may have reduced BMD as adults. However, recent studies assessing volumetric BMD indicate that pubertal delay does not adversely affect peak bone mass.[43]

### Bisphosphonates

In women with post menopausal osteoporosis, bisphosphonates have been the mainstay of treatment. Bisphosphonates are synthetic analogs of naturally occurring pyrophosphates. The osteoblastic enzyme alkaline phosphatase cleaves pyrophosphate preventing it from interacting with the bone matrix. Bisphosphonates are deposited in bone matrix but are resistant to cleavage by alkaline phosphastase. This results in decreased osteoclast activity, perhaps by inducing programmed osteoclast death and inhibiting the attachment of osteoclasts to the bone matrix. At very high doses bisphosphonates also inhibit bone mineralization, so only those doses that favor predominance of inhibition of bone resorption should be utilized. Bisphosphonates accumulate in bone and can remain in the bone for decades.

Bisphosphonates of greater potency continue to be developed. Zoledronate, for example, is 10,000 times more potent than the first bisphosphonate, etidronate, and 100 times more potent than the commonly used pamidronate. Bisphosphonates may be administered either parenterally or orally. Alendronate was the first bisphosphonate approved for treatment of osteoporosis.

Alendronate in a dose of 10 mg/day or 70 mg/week increases BMD, decreases bone turnover markers by 50% to 70%, decreases new fractures by approximately 50% compared to placebo, and also reduces days of decreased activity, days in bed, and use of hospital services.[44] Newer, more potent bisphosphonates have been approved recently for treatment and prevention of osteoporosis in adults and seem to have comparable safety and efficacy to alendronate.

Bisphosphonates have been much less extensively studied in children and adolescents than in adults. A 2005 position paper of the Lawson Wilkins Pediatric Endocrine Society Pharmacy and Therapeutic Committee on Bisphosphonate Treatment of Pediatric Bone Disease stated, "Because of the paucity of long-term studies among children regarding the safety and efficacy of these drugs, it is difficult to formulate strong evidence-based recommendations for their use except perhaps in children with osteogenesis imperfecta."[45]

The 2 bisphosphonates that have been investigated for use in children with osteoporosis are pamidronate, which is given intravenously, and alendronate, which is an oral preparation. Both have been evaluated in the treatment of OI, with most studies having used pamidronate, administered in cycles ranging from every 1 to 6 months. Treatment with bisphosphonates increased BMD by 50% to 120% and annualized fracture rates decreased in most patients. Other positive effects have been height gain, increased strength, increased mobility, and decreased pain. However these have not been randomized controlled studies.

There are a limited number of clinical trials of bisphosphonates in IJO and the few existing studies are hampered by the lack of a stringent definition of IJO and the natural history of spontaneous recovery. An increase in BMD and a decrease in fracture rates has been reported.[46]

In anorexia nervosa, a randomized double-blind, placebo-controlled trial compared alendronate 10 mg daily with placebo, in 32 adolescents with anorexia nervosa. Femoral neck and lumbar spine BMD increased 4.4 ± 6.4% and 3.5 ± 4.6% in the alendronate group, compared with increases of 2.3 ± 6.9% and 2.2 + 6.1% in the control group ($p = 0.41$ femoral neck, $p = 0.53$ lumbar spine). From baseline to 1 year follow-up both femoral neck and lumbar spine BMD increased significantly in the alendronate group ($p = 0.02$), but did not increase in those assigned placebo ($p = 0.22$ femoral neck, $p = 0.18$ lumbar spine).[47] Miller et al[47] administered Risedronate 5 mg daily for 9 months to 10 women with anorexia nervosa and compared the findings to those of controls followed for the same period of time. In the study group, BMD of the lumbar spine increased 4.9 + 1.0% whereas it decreased in the controls.

A double-blind, placebo-controlled trial conducted on 6 pairs of subjects with CP demonstrated that BMD increased 89% ± 21% over the 18-month study period in subjects treated with pamidronate group compared with a 9% ± 6% in the control group.[49,50]

At the present time, it is unknown how long a child and adolescent must stay on bisphosphonate therapy to maintain benefit. Recently, observations in adults have shown maintenance of benefit following discontinuation of alendronate after 5 years of therapy, suggesting that a "drug holiday" could be given in some patients. Whether such will be appropriate for children and adolescents remains to be determined.

Although it might be said that bisphosphonate usage in children and adolescents has been safe overall, bisphosphonates have been used in these age groups for little over a decade and much remains to be learned regarding their safety, especially since, in theory, bisphosphonates remain in bone and continue to be released into the circulation indefinitely. Short-term side effects relate to acute phase reactions to intravenous preparations and gastrointestinal problems with oral preparations. First or second intravenous dosing (but rarely beyond that) is often accompanied by fever and flu-like symptoms within the first 24 hours, which can generally be attenuated by prophylactic anti-pyretic therapy.

Oral bisphosphonates must be taken in the fasting state in order to ensure absorption. However, since they can cause esophageal irritation, they should be taken with 8 oz of water and the patient should remain upright until after eating, which should be delayed at least 30 minutes after ingestion of the medication. Oral bisphosphonates should be used with caution in children who cannot remain upright or who have upper gastrointestinal disorders. Similar precautions should be taken with the liquid preparation of alendronate as with the tablet form.

The potential for long-term use of bisphosphonates in children and adolescents has raised concerns regarding their effects on growth and possible reproductive toxicity. With regard to the former, linear growth has been found to be within normal limits. Animal studies using doses of pamidronate 10 times those used in humans demonstrated embryo death and poor skeletal development.[50] Little human data on bisphosphonate use during pregnancy has been published. Two women with OI who had received pamidronate prior to conception delivered infants who also had OI but were otherwise normal.[51] Kaufman et al[51] reporting in Obstetric Gynecological Survey stated, "The question remains unanswered as to when bisphosphonate therapy should be terminated before anticipated pregnancy or even if it should be administered at all to the adolescent female considering future pregnancy." The single case of osteopetrosis (marble bone disease) in a 12-year-old boy treated with 4 times the usual dose of pamidronate highlights the need to be judicious in dosing children and adolescents with bisphosphonates.[53] Poor healing following surgical osteotomy in children previously treated with bisphosphonates for OI has been reported.[54] Recently, considerable concern regarding the occurrence of osteonecrosis of the jaw (after dental procedures) has been raised in adults. However, this adverse effect has occurred mainly in patients with metastatic cancer being treated with high-dose intravenous pamidronate or zoledronic acid.[55] Transient hypocalcemia of a mild degree occurs infrequently with rapid intravenous administration. Pancreatitis, renal toxicity, and eye disorders (uveitis, conjunctivitis, scleritis) have been reported in adults.

### Recombinant Human Parathyroid Hormone

Recombinant human PTH has emerged as another treatment modality in adult osteoporosis. PTH mainly stimulates bone formation in contrast to the bisphosphonates, which mainly inhibit bone resorption. PTH has been shown to increase BMD and to decrease fracture rates and overall has a therapeutic profile at least comparable to alendronate. PTH is not likely to be used in pediatric and adolescent osteoporosis in the near future, if ever, as the FDA has prohibited its use due to an increased incidence of osteogenic sarcoma in rodents administered high-dose PTH. There have been no incidences of osteogenic sarcoma in PTH-treated humans to date.[56]

Calcitonin, a former mainstay of osteoporosis therapy, has fallen out of favor as newer modalities have proven efficacious and safe. Both injectable and nasal salmon calcitonin have a prominent analgesic effect on the bone pain of acute vertebral fracture.

## SPECIAL CIRCUMSTANCES

In most chronic illnesses accompanied by decreased BMD, treatment of the underlying disease process should be the primary intervention along with providing adequate amounts of calcium, vitamin D, and calories. Maintaining activity level, as tolerated, to prevent the added burden of immobilization-induced bone loss is important in conditions such as juvenile rheumatoid arthritis and CP. Certain conditions merit additional comment.

In girls with anorexia nervosa, weight restoration is accompanied by improved estrogen levels, resumption of menses, and some increase in BMD but levels do not return to normal. The use of hormone replacement therapy in anorexia nervosa has not been proven to increase BMD over and above standard treatment and it is not recommended for this purpose.[57,58] Furthermore, exogenously induced monthly menstrual bleeding may give a false sense of security to someone who is still of low body weight. Dehydroepiandrosterone (DHEA), a precursor of both estrogens and androgens, could theoretically inhibit bone resorption as well as increase bone formation. Gordon et al[59] studied 61 women with anorexia nervosa, randomly assigned to receive either 50 mg/d DHEA or a combination estrogen-progestin pill. Over a 1-year follow-up period, total hip BMD increased 1.7% in both groups, but after controlling for weight gain, no treatment effect was detected. In 60 adult women with anorexia nervosa and reduced bone mass, Grinspoon et al[60] compared the use of recombinant human IGF-1, a nutritionally dependent hormone that promotes bone formation, with oral contraceptives alone and in combination and found that treatment with IGF-1 alone or the oral contraceptive alone had no significant effect on BMD of the lumbar spine, but that the combination increased BMD by 1.8%. As discussed above, pilot studies have demonstrated a positive effect of bisphosphonates on BMD in anorexia nervosa, but because of the potential side effects, further study is required before clear recommendations can be made.

In female athletes with low BMD, principles of treatment include increasing caloric intake, supplementation with calcium and vitamin D, and reducing the intensity of athletic training. In adolescents who use DMPA as a means of birth control SAM suggests use of supplementation with 1,300 mg calcium plus 400 IU vitamin D.[37] Since estrogen supplementation has been shown to increase BMD in women on DMPA, consideration should also be given to estrogen supplementation in those on DMPA who have evidence of reduced bone mass.

In glucocorticoid-induced osteoporosis, the most rapid bone loss occurs in the first 6 to 12 months following commencement of high-dose glucocorticoid therapy. Sambrook[32] suggests considering 2 different therapeutic situations: (1) primary prevention and (2) treatment.[33] The minimal effective dose of glucocorticoid should be used, individual exercise programs should be established, and an appropriate diet and supplementation with calcium and vitamin D should be provided. If BMD is substantially reduced and long-term glucocorticoid therapy is anticipated, bisphosphonate therapy can be considered.

## SUMMARY

The antecedents to osteoporosis occur in adolescence, and prevention of adult osteoporosis requires that an optimal environment for the achievement of peak bone mass be established during the growing years. It is critical to the development of healthy bones that adolescents have proper nutrition with adequate calcium and vitamin D intake and that they participate in regular physical activity. Weight-bearing exercise is to be encouraged. At this time, these goals are not being achieved by most of adolescents. It is essential that those caring for adolescents educate the teens and their families how to optimize peak bone mass, and that they advocate for supportive environments in school and the community that foster development of healthy habits with regard to diet and exercise. In order to help identify the population at risk for osteoporosis, assessment of calcium intake and determination of family history of adult osteoporosis should be a routine part of adolescent health care. Adolescents with conditions associated with reduced bone mass should undergo bone densitometry early in the course of treatment and should be monitored at yearly intervals if the condition persists. Use of antiresorptive therapy in children and adolescents should be judicious. At this time, the use of bisphosphonates can only be recommended without qualification for treatment of OI. In children and adolescents with juvenile osteoporosis, CP, glucocorticoid-induced osteoporosis, or other conditions in which fractures are frequent and/or painful, bisphosphonates may provide significant relief of symptoms. In such situations, they should only be prescribed in the context of a comprehensive clinical program with specialists knowledgeable in the management of osteoporosis in children.

## REFERENCES


1. Riggs BL Melton LJ III. The worldwide problem of osteoporosis: insights afforded by epidemiology. *Bone.* 1995;17 (5 Suppl):505S-511S

2. Melton LJ III, Chrischilles EA, Cooper C, et al. Perspective. How many women have osteoporosis? *J Bone Miner Res.* 1992;7(9):1005-1010

3. Bailey DA, Faulkner RA, McKay HA. Growth, physical activity, and bone mineral acquisition. *Exerc Sport Sci Rev.* 1996;24:233-266

4. Bachrach LK. Acquisition of optimal bone mass in childhood and adolescence. *Trends Endocrinol Metab.* 2001;12(1): 22-28

5. Kalender WA. Effective dose values in bone mineral measurements by photon absorptiometry and computed tomography. *Osteoporos Int.* 1992;2(2):82-87

6. World Health Organization. *Report of a WHO Study Group: Assessment of Fracture Risk and Its Application to Screening for Postmenopausal Osteoporosis.* Geneva, Switzerland: World Health Organization; 1992

7. Leonard MB, Petit M. Research Considerations. In: Sawyer AJ, Bachrach LK, Fung EB, (eds.) *Bone Densitometry in Growing Patients. Guidelines for Clinical Practice.* Totowa, NJ: Humana Press, 2007:159-172

8. Lewiecki EM, Gordon CM, Baim S, et al. Special report on the 2007 Adult and Pediatric Position Development Conferences of the International Society for Clinical Densitometry. *Osteoporos Int.* 2008;19:1369-1378

9. Beaupré GS. Radiation exposure in bone measurements. *J Bone Min Res.* 2006;21(5):803

10. Beck TJ, Ruff CB, Warden KE, et al. Predicting femoral neck strength from bone mineral data. A structural approach. *Invest Radiol.* 1990;25(1):6-18

11. Eisman JA. Genetics of Osteoporosis. In: Favus MJ, ed. *Primer on the Metabolic Bone Diseases and Disorders of Mineral Metabolism.* Washington, DC: American Society for Bone and Mineral Research, 2006: 249-254

12. Gilsanz V, Nelson DA. Childhood and Adolescence. In: Favus MJ, ed. *Primer on the Metabolic Bone Diseases and Disorders of Mineral Metabolism.* Washington, DC: American Society for Bone and Mineral Research, 2003:71-80

13. Gilsanz V, Skaggs DL, Kovanlikaya A, et al. Differential effect of race on the axial and appendicular skeletons of children. *J Clin Endocrinol Metab.* 1998;83(5):1420-1427

14. Lloyd T, Andon MB, Rollings N, et al. Calcium supplementation and bone mineral density in adolescent girls. *JAMA.* 1993;270(7):841-844

15. Wyshak G. Teenaged girls, carbonated beverage consumption, and bone fractures. *Arch Pediatr Adolesc Med.* 2000;154(6):610-613

16. Bachrach LK, Katzman DK, Litt IF, et al. Recovery from osteopenia in adolescent girls with anorexia nervosa. *J Clin Endocrinol Metab.* 1991;72(3):602-606

17. Sillence DO, Senn A, Danks DM. Genetic heterogeneity in osteogenesis imperfecta. *J Med Genet.* 1979;16(2):101-116

18. Byers PH. Disorders of Collagen Biosynthesis and Structure, p 5241-5285. In: Scriver CR, Beaudet AL, Sly WS, et al. (eds.) *The Metabolic and Molecular Basis of Inherited Disease.* New York: McGraw-Hill, 2002: 5241-5286

19. Dent CE, Friedman M. Idiopathic juvenile osteoporosis. *QJM.* 1965; 34: 177-210

20. Rauch F, Bishop N. Juvenile Osteoporosis. In: Favus MJ, ed. *Primer on the Metabolic Bone Diseases and Disorders of Mineral Metabolism.* Washington, DC: American Society for Bone and Mineral Research, 2007: 293-302

21. Golden NH. Osteopenia and osteoporosis in anorexia nervosa. *Adolesc Med.* 2003;14(1):97-108

22. Grinspoon S, Miller K, Coyle C, et al. Severity of osteopenia in estrogen-deficient women with anorexia nervosa and hypothalamic amenorrhea. *J Clin Endocrinol Metab.* 1999;84(6):2049-2055

23. Ward A, Brown N, Treasure J. Persistent osteopenia after recovery from anorexia nervosa. *Int J Eat Disord.* 1997;22(1):71-75

24. Golden NH. A review of the female athlete triad (amenorrhea, osteoporosis, and disordered eating). *Int J Adolesc Med Health.* 2002;14(1):9-17

25. Henderson RC, Lark RK, Gurka MJ, et al. Bone density and metabolism in children and adolescents with moderate to severe cerebral palsy. *Pediatrics.* 2002;110(1: Pt 1):e5

26. Loftus EV Crowson CS, Sandborn WJ, et al. Long-term fracture risk in patients with Crohn's disease: a population-based study in Olmsted County, Minnesota. *Gastroenterol.* 2002;123(2):468–475

27. Loftus EV Jr, Achenbach SJ, Sandborn WJ, et al. Risk of fracture in ulcerative colitis: a population-based study from Olmsted County, Minnesota. *Clin Gastroenterol Hepatol.* 2003;1(6):465–473

28. Henderson RC, Madsen CD. Bone mineral content and body composition in children and young adults with cystic fibrosis. *Pediatr Pulmonol.* 1999;27(2):80–84

29. Hardin DS, Ahn C, Prestidge C, et al. Growth hormone improves bone mineral content in children with cystic fibrosis. *J Pediatr Endocrinol Metab.* 2005;18(6):589–595

30. French AR, Mason T, Nelson AM, et al. Osteopenia in adults with a history of juvenile rheumatoid arthritis. A population-based study. *J Rheumatol.* 2002;29(5):1065–1070

31. Haddy TB, Mosher RB, Reaman GH. Osteoporosis in survivors of acute lymphoblastic leukemia. *Oncologist.* 2001;6(3): 278–285

32. Rubin K. Turner syndrome and osteoporosis: mechanisms and prognosis. *Pediatrics.* 1998;102:(2: Pt 3):481–485

33. Sambrook PN. Glucocorticoid-Induced Osteoporosis. In: Favus MJ, ed. *Primer on the Metabolic Bone Diseases and Disorders of Mineral Metabolism*. Washington, DC: American Society for Bone and Mineral Research, 2006: 296–302

34. Canalis E, Bilezikian JP, Angeli A, Giustina A. Perspectives on glucocorticoid-induced osteoporosis. *Bone.* 2004;34(4):593–598

35. Cromer BA, Stager M, Bonny A, et al. Depot medroxyprogesterone acetate, oral contraceptives, and bone mineral density in a cohort of adolescent girls. *J Adolesc Health.* 2004;35(6):434–441

36. Scholes D, LaCroix AZ, Ichikawa LE, et al. Change in bone mineral density among adolescent women using and discontinuing depot medroxyprogesterone acetate contraception. *Arch Pediatr Adolesc Med.* 2005;159(2):139–144

37. Cromer BA, Scholes D, Berenson A, et al. Depot medroxyprogesterone acetate and bone mineral density in adolescents–the Black Box Warning: a Position Paper of the Society for Adolescent Medicine. *J Adolesc Health.* 2006;39(2):296–301

38. Greer FR, Krebs NF. Optimizing bone health and calcium intakes of infants, children, and adolescents. *Pediatrics.* 2006;117(2):578–585

39. Wagner CL, Greer FR, and the Section on Breastfeeding and Committee on Nutrition. Prevention of rickets and vitamin D deficiency in infants, children, and adolescents. *Pediatrics.* 2008;122(5):1142–1152

40. MacKelvie KJ, Khan KM, Petit MA, et al. A school-based exercise intervention elicits substantial bone health benefits: a 2-year randomized controlled trial in girls. *Pediatrics.* 2003;112(6 Pt 1):e447

41. Snow-Harter C, Bouxsein ML, Lewis BT, et al. Effects of resistance and endurance exercise on bone mineral status of young women: a randomized exercise intervention trial. *J Bone Miner Res.* 1992;7(7):761–769

42. Robinson E, Bachrach LK, Katzman DK. Use of hormone replacement therapy to reduce the risk of osteopenia in adolescent girls with anorexia nervosa. *J Adolesc Health.* 2000;26(5):343–348

43. Bertelloni S, Baroncelli GI, Ferdeghini M, et al. Normal volumetric bone mineral density and bone turnover in young men with histories of constitutional delay of puberty. *J Clin Endocrinol Metab.* 1998;83(12):4280–4283

44. Nevitt MC, Thompson DE, Black DM, et al. Effect of alendronate on limited-activity days and bed-disability days caused by back pain in postmenopausal women with existing vertebral fractures. Fracture Intervention Trial Research Group. *Arch Intern Med.* 2000;160(1):77–85

45. Speiser PW, Clarson CL, Eugster EA, et al. Bisphosphonate treatment of pediatric bone disease. *Pediatr Endocrinol Rev.* 2005;3(2):87–96

46. Steelman J, Zeitler P. Treatment of symptomatic pediatric osteoporosis with cyclic single-day intravenous pamidronate infusions. *J Pediatr.* 2003;142(4):417–423

47. Golden NH, Iglesias EA, Jacobson MS, et al. Alendronate for the treatment of osteopenia in anorexia nervosa: a randomized, double-blind, placebo-controlled trial. *J Clin Endocrinol Metab.* 2005;90(6):3179–3185

48. Miller KK, Grieco KA, Mulder J, et al. Effects of risedronate on bone density in anorexia nervosa. *J Clin Endocrinol Metab.* 2004;89(8):3903–3906

49. Henderson RC, Lark RK, Kecskemethy HH, et al. Bisphosphonates to treat osteopenia in children with quadriplegic cerebral palsy: a randomized, placebo-controlled clinical trial. *J Pediatr.* 2002;141(5):644–651

50. Graepel P, Bentley P, Fritz H, et al. Reproduction toxicity studies with pamidronate. *Arzneimittelforschung.* 1992;42(5): 654–667

51. Munns CF, Rauch F, Ward L, Glorieux FH. Maternal and fetal outcome after long-term pamidronate treatment before conception: a report of two cases. *J Bone Miner Res.* 2004;19(10):1742–1745

52. Kauffman RP, Overton TH, Shiflett M, Jennings JC. Osteoporosis in children and adolescent girls: case report of idiopathic juvenile osteoporosis and review of the literature. *Obstet Gynecol Surv.* 2001;56(8):492–504

53. Whyte MP, Wenkert D, Clements KL, et al. Bisphosphonate-induced osteopetrosis. *N Engl J Med.* 2003;349(5):457–463

54. Munns CF, Rauch F, Zeitlin L, et al. Delayed osteotomy but not fracture healing in pediatric osteogenesis imperfecta patients receiving pamidronate. *J Bone Miner Res.* 2004;19(11):1779–1786

55. Bilezikian JP. Osteonecrosis of the jaw—do bisphosphonates pose a risk? *N Engl J Med.* 2006;355(22):2278–2281

56. Neer RM, Arnaud CD. Effect of parathyroid hormone (1–34) on fractures and bone mineral density in postmenopausal

women with osteoporosis. *N Engl J Med.* 2001;344:1434–1441

57. Golden NH, Lanzkowsky L, Schebendach J, et al. The effect of estrogen-progestin treatment on bone mineral density in anorexia nervosa. *J Pediatr Adolesc Gynecol.* 2002;15(3):135–143

58. Strokosch GR, Friedman AJ, Shu-Chen W, Kamin M. Effects of an oral contraceptive (Norgestimate/Ethinyl Estradiol) on bone mineral density in adolescent females with anorexia nervosa: a double-blind, placebo-controlled study. *J Adolesc Health.* 2006;39:819–827

59. Gordon CM, Grace E, Emans SJ, et al. Effects of oral dehydroepiandrosterone on bone density in young women with anorexia nervosa: a randomized trial. *J Clin Endocrinol Metab.* 2002;87(11):4935–4941

60. Grinspoon S, Miller K, Herzog D, et al. Effects of recombinant human insulin-like growth factor (IGF)-I and estrogen administration on IGF-I, IGF binding protein (IGFBP)-2, and IGFBP-3 in anorexia nervosa: a randomized-controlled study. *J Clin Endocrinol Metab.* 2003;883:1142–1149

SECTION 2

# Eating Disorders

# CHAPTER 76

## Anorexia Nervosa

NEVILLE H. GOLDEN, MD • DEBRA K. KATZMAN, MD

### INTRODUCTION

Anorexia nervosa (AN) is a life-threatening disorder characterized by voluntary self-imposed starvation and cognitive distortions about body shape and weight. It usually has its onset during adolescence and is associated with significant medical and psychological morbidity. The mortality rate is reported to be the highest for any psychiatric illness. In recent years, major strides have been made in improving awareness of AN among professionals and the lay public. Primary care providers, along with families and schools, play a crucial role in early identification and treatment of this disorder.

### EPIDEMIOLOGY

#### PREVALENCE

Body dissatisfaction and dieting behavior are prevalent in industrialized societies, but relatively few patients develop full-blown AN. The lifetime prevalence of AN in the United States and Western Europe is reported to be 0.3% to 0.5%.[1] A recent study of Swedish twins found the lifetime prevalence to be 1.2% for females and 0.29% for males. Prevalence for both sexes has increased over time.[2] At the Mayo Clinic, the overall incidence of AN from 1935 to 1989 was 8.3 per 100,000 person-years, with the highest age-adjusted incidence in 15- to 19-year-old girls.[3]

#### GENDER

Anorexia nervosa primarily affects girls (90% are female). In the younger age group (<14 years of age), a greater proportion of patients are male.

#### AGE

Anorexia nervosa usually develops during adolescence. The peak age of onset is between 15 and 19 years of age, and 95% of subjects develop the disorder before the age of 25. Prepubertal AN does occur but is uncommon.

#### SOCIOECONOMIC CLASS

Though classically considered a disease of white middle-class females, AN is seen with increasing frequency in minority populations and in lower socioeconomic groups. No racial or ethnic group is immune. It is seen more frequently in industrialized countries. Epidemiological studies have shown that prevalence rates in developing countries now parallel those seen in the United States, the United Kingdom, and Europe.

#### COMORBIDITY

Major psychiatric conditions coexisting with AN are major depression or dysthymia (50%–80%); anxiety disorders (30%–65%); obsessive–compulsive disorder (OCD) (40%); and substance abuse (12%–21%). The latter usually occurs in the binge-eating purging subtype.

### ETIOLOGY

The etiology of AN is multifactorial and reflects a complex interplay among biologic, psychologic, and sociocultural factors (Figure 76-1).

There is increasing evidence supporting a genetic predisposition to development of an eating disorder. Concordance rates for AN in monozygotic twins are higher than in dizygotic twins. Women with a first-degree relative suffering from an eating disorder have a

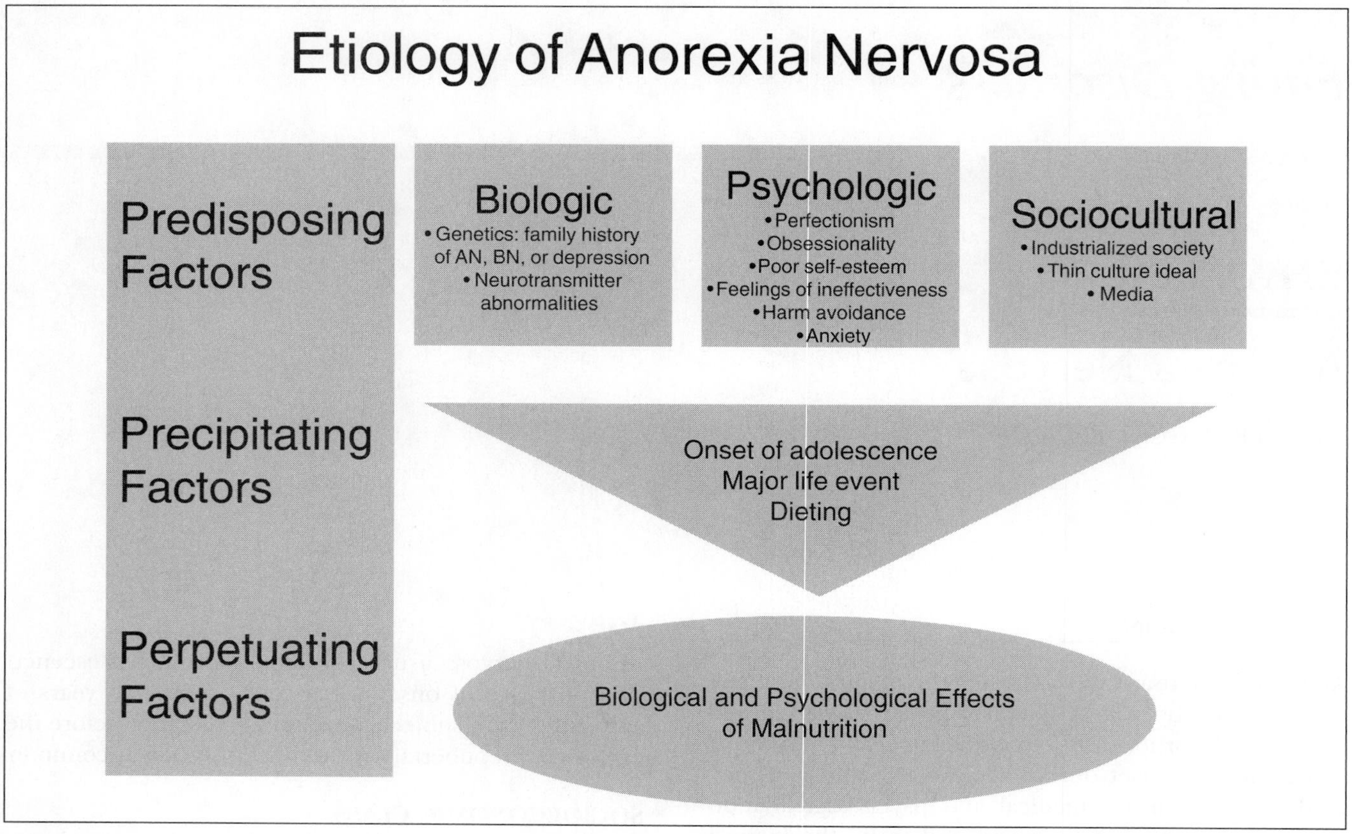

**FIGURE 76-1** The etiology of anorexia nervosa. Adapted from Allan Kaplan, MD, and based on the model of Garfinkel and Garner (Garfinkel PE, Garner DM. *Anorexia Nervosa: A Multidimensional Perspective.* New York, NY: Brunner/Mazel Publishers; 1982).

10-fold increased lifetime risk of developing an eating disorder. No single gene or group of genes has been identified, but certain areas of the human genome may harbor susceptibility genes for AN on chromosome 1.[4] Research has demonstrated an association between AN and genes coding for the serotonin system, in particular the 5-HT2a and possibly 5-HT2c receptor genes.[5]

Neurotransmitter abnormalities in serotonin, dopamine, and noradrenaline pathways have been identified in patients with AN. Some of these abnormalities resolve after weight restoration and may be secondary to malnutrition but others persist, suggesting a biological predisposition to the eating disorder. Acutely ill patients with AN have reduced levels of cerebrospinal fluid serotonin metabolites, which increase to above normal levels after weight restoration. Increased serotonin activity is thought to contribute to the core features of perfectionism, obsessionality, anxiety, and body image distortion. It has been postulated that dietary restriction reduces serum levels of tryptophan, the amino acid precursor of serotonin. Starvation-induced reduction in serotonin activity would reduce anxiety and some obsessional and perfectionistic behaviors.[6] Brain imaging with radioligands has confirmed disturbances in serotonin receptors in the ill and recovered state of AN.[7,8] Interestingly, serotonin receptors are influenced by estrogen, which may explain, in part, the female preponderance of AN and its onset during puberty. Disturbances in serotonin transmission have generated particular research interest because of the role of serotonin in the regulation of satiety, mood, and obsessional behavior, but the neurotransmitters have complex interactions and, undoubtedly, more than one neurotransmitter system is involved.

Certain personality traits such as perfectionism, obsessionality, poor self-esteem, anxiety, harm avoidance, and feelings of ineffectiveness are associated with AN. Patients with AN are usually bright, high-achieving young women but, despite their achievements, self-esteem remains low. Their perfectionistic and obsessional traits cause them to have difficulty dealing with change. The older theory of a dysfunctional family is not supported by current research. However, psychological distress in a family with a child suffering from an eating disorder is common.

Sociocultural factors most certainly play a role in the etiology of AN. The disorder occurs primarily in Western societies or in societies exposed to Western influences. In Fiji, exposure to the thin cultural ideal with the introduction of television was accompanied by increased rates of body dissatisfaction and disordered eating among adolescent girls.[9]

Anorexia nervosa usually develops during adolescence, a time of marked physical and emotional change. Young people with AN have difficulty adjusting to the changes of adolescence and struggle with mastering the psychosocial tasks of adolescence. They feel out of control and instead focus on things they can control—what they eat, how much they eat, and when they eat it. A major life event such as divorce or death in the family, childhood sexual abuse, change of school, or breakup with a partner may precipitate the onset of AN. Initially, as weight is lost the adolescent may receive approval from friends and family, but eventually the drive to lose more weight takes control. Dieting leads to further preoccupation with food and body weight, medical consequences of malnutrition, social isolation, and disturbances in mood.

In summary, genetic and biological makeup determines vulnerability to the influences of sociocultural norms. A predisposed adolescent with specific personality characteristics may feel overwhelmed and powerless. Dieting to gain control leads to further preoccupation with shape and weight and the biological and psychological effects of malnutrition.

### Box 76-1

#### *DSM-IV-TR Diagnostic Criteria for AN*

a. Refusal to maintain body weight at or above a minimal normal weight for age and height (eg, weight loss leading to maintenance of body weight less than 85% of that expected), or failure to make expected weight gain during period of growth, leading to body weight less than 85% of that expected.
b. Intense fear of gaining weight or becoming fat, even though underweight.
c. Disturbance in the way in which one's body weight or shape is experienced, undue influence of body shape and weight on self-evaluation, or denial of the seriousness of current low body weight.
d. In postmenarcheal females, amenorrhea, ie, the absence of at least three consecutive menstrual cycles. (A woman is considered to have amenorrhea if her periods occur only following hormone, eg, estrogen, administration).

*Specify Type*

Restricting type: During the current episode of AN, the person has not regularly engaged in binge-eating or purging behavior (ie, self-induced vomiting or the misuse of laxatives, diuretics, or enemas).

Binge eating/purging type: During the current episode of AN, the person has regularly engaged in binge-eating or purging behavior (ie, self-induced vomiting or the misuse of laxatives, diuretics, or enemas)

Reprinted with permission from the *Diagnostic and Statistical Manual of Mental Disorders,* 4th edition, Text Revision, Washington, DC: American Psychiatric Association; 2000: 589.

## DIAGNOSTIC CRITERIA

Anorexia nervosa constitutes part of a spectrum of eating disorders. The most widely used diagnostic criteria for AN are those published by the American Psychiatric Association in the *Diagnostic and Statistical Manual of Mental Disorders, 4th edition (DSM-IV)*[10], listed in Box 76-1. The first criterion describes weight loss or, during a period of growth, failure to make expected weight gain, leading to a body weight less than 85% of that expected. Though this criterion may seem clear, there is no consensus about whether this refers to weight loss from a premorbid weight or weight loss below an average or healthy weight for age and height. A growing adolescent could meet the first criterion even in the absence of any weight loss if there was no expected weight gain during a period of growth. Determination of expected body weight in a growing adolescent requires some clinical judgment and needs to take into account both average weight for age and height and anticipated changes in weight during growth. The patient's prior growth chart will help determine what expected height and weight would have been in the absence of the eating disorder.

The second criterion is the overriding fear of weight gain despite the patient's state of malnutrition. Despite worsening cachexia, the individual with AN continues to obsess about body weight.

The third criterion is the distortion in body image, the overemphasis of body weight in self-esteem, or the denial of the seriousness of the condition. Individuals with AN appreciate that other patients with the same condition are too thin but they see themselves, or certain parts of themselves (usually their lower abdomen, buttocks, or thighs), as being too fat.

The final criterion, amenorrhea, defined as absence of at least 3 consecutive menstrual cycles, does not apply to premenarcheal girls or to boys. The utility of amenorrhea as a diagnostic criterion has been challenged. Studies have shown that a subset of patients who menstruate have the same core psychological features as those who meet all diagnostic criteria for AN.[11,12] *DSM-IV* further divides the classification of AN into the classic restrictor and the binge-eating purging subtype.

There are problems with these diagnostic criteria particularly as they pertain to children and adolescents. The timing and rate of linear growth and weight gain during puberty are variable. The published growth curves represent smoothed curves drawn from cross-sectional data. During adolescence, a particular individual does not necessarily follow the published growth curve. An early or late maturer will not necessarily grow along the same height percentile as he or she did prior to the onset of puberty. With regard to the second and third criteria, many younger adolescents are concrete thinkers and are unable to express abstract concepts such as fear of weight gain, distortion of body image, or preoccupation with body weight and shape. They may deny these feelings, and the true fear of weight gain may only become apparent as treatment progresses. In addition, AN can delay the onset of menarche, and the expected irregularity of menstrual cycles during the first 2 years after menarche further limits the applicability of the fourth criterion. Finally, adolescents may develop pubertal delay, growth retardation, and reduced bone mineral density (BMD) at subclinical levels of an eating disorder.

In clinical practice, most patients with symptoms severe enough to warrant intervention do not meet formal criteria for AN. Under the current classification system, such patients are classified as "Eating Disorder Not Otherwise Specified" (EDNOS). Research demonstrates that in the adolescent age group, the majority of patients seeking treatment and requiring intervention fit into this category.[13,14] Eating disorder not otherwise specified includes those patients who have not yet lost enough weight to meet criteria for AN, those who purge on a regular basis to maintain a low body weight but do not binge, or those who meet all criteria for AN but have not had the absence of at least three consecutive menstrual cycles. Some individuals in the EDNOS category represent those with subthreshold AN, but others represent qualitatively distinct disorders. For example, researchers at the Great Ormond Street Hospital in London have developed a diagnostic classification that includes eating disturbances in children and young adolescents where there is no distortion in body image or preoccupation with shape or weight. Some of these conditions may be accompanied by loss of weight and growth retardation (Table 76-1).[14,15]

**Table 76-1**

**Great Ormond Street Diagnostic Criteria for Eating Disorders (Other Than Anorexia Nervosa and Bulimia Nervosa) in Children and Young Adolescents[15]**

| *Category* | *Description* |
|---|---|
| 1. Food avoidance emotional disorder | • Usually found in children 8–13 years old<br>• Food refusal for emotional reasons<br>• No distortion in body image or preoccupation with shape or weight<br>• May be accompanied by growth retardation and weight loss |
| 2. Selective eating disorder | • Narrow range of foods for at least 2 years<br>• Unwilling to try new foods<br>• No distortion in body image or preoccupation with shape and weight<br>• Weight and height are usually appropriate for age |
| 3. Functional dysphagia | • Food avoidance because of a fear of swallowing, choking, or vomiting<br>• Often a prior history of an episode of choking on a specific food<br>• No distortion in body image or fear of gaining weight |
| 4. Pervasive food refusal | • Profound refusal to eat, drink, walk, talk, or self-care<br>• Resistant to help |

## CLINICAL PRESENTATION

Adolescents with AN usually present to the physician with weight loss or amenorrhea (primary or secondary). They do not always recognize that they have a problem. The adolescent with AN usually starts by dieting or voluntarily restricting food intake leading to a preoccupation with food, intense hunger, and a distorted body image. Often a stressful life occurrence or emotional event contributes to the development of AN. The adolescent with AN, or his or her parents, can frequently identify the exact point in time and motivation for the dieting. Initially, weight loss is reinforced by positive comments from family and friends who admire the patient's self-discipline and determination. During this time, the adolescent often develops abnormal eating attitudes and behaviors. Many young people report changing their diet to a more "healthy diet." The quantity of food consumed is considerably reduced and they consistently choose low-calorie or low-fat foods. They manipulate their food, break it into small portions, separate it, mash it, eat foods of the same color, hide foods, secretly throw food away, and eat the same foods at the same time each day. Often large amounts of diet fluids are consumed to satisfy hunger or to cause diuresis (caffeine-containing beverages). Some patients purge by vomiting, using laxatives, diuretics, excessive exercise, or by using herbal remedies or complementary and alternative medicines (CAM) to lose weight. Adolescents with AN may weigh themselves daily or several times per day. The weight on the scale often determines how they feel about themselves.

Body-image distortion is a cardinal feature of AN and refers to the perception of feeling overweight when severely underweight. Young people with AN often have poor self-esteem manifested by being overly critical of themselves, being constantly worried about what others think, and feeling worthless. Furthermore, they isolate themselves from friends and family. This behavior may reflect an attempt to avoid social situations associated with food. It is not uncommon for family members to report that the adolescent has become moody or irritable. Although starvation can cause mood changes, it may also be associated with other comorbid psychiatric illnesses such as depression and obsessive compulsive disorder (OCD).

## EVALUATION

### MEDICAL HISTORY

Initial assessment of an adolescent with AN involves a thorough review of the adolescent's history, current symptoms, weight control measures, past medical history, other psychiatric issues or disorders such as depression, anxiety, or substance abuse, and physical status. The initial assessment is the first step in establishing a diagnosis and treatment plan and in evaluating medical complications.

The assessment should be completed by an interdisciplinary team of pediatric health care specialists knowledgeable about eating disorders. The team may include a pediatrician or adolescent medicine specialist, psychiatrist, psychologist, nurse, dietitian, and social worker. The pediatrician often assumes the leadership role and coordinates interdisciplinary care. The composition of the interdisciplinary team will vary depending on the availability of local expertise and the structure of the program. Communication among team members is essential to ensuring that team members' roles and responsibilities are well-defined and that their approach to the patient and family is consistent.

In most cases, the parents seek help for the adolescent with AN. Parents may notice that their child has lost a significant amount of weight, has ceased menstruating, has been avoiding friends and other social situations, or is moody and irritable. Occasionally, a teacher, coach, or family relative friend expresses concerns about changes in the adolescent. Any circumstance might cause the parents to bring the adolescent for an evaluation. Often the adolescent with AN will deny that she or he has a problem and does not understand why she or he needs medical help. At the outset of the initial interview, the adolescent and parents should meet with the physician and other members of the team. This gives an opportunity to provide an explanation of the assessment and evaluate the reason for the visit with everyone in the room together. It is important to evaluate both the adolescents' and parents' reason for coming to the evaluation. Confidential health care is particularly important for adolescents. A clear discussion of the limits of confidentiality should be reviewed with the adolescent and parents at the beginning of the assessment. Although input from parents is important, the adolescent should have an opportunity to be interviewed alone in a safe, nonjudgmental, and supportive environment. Further, when obtaining a history from an adolescent with AN, it is essential to establish a therapeutic alliance—a trusting and collaborative relationship between the health care provider and the adolescent. Such a relationship makes it possible for them to work together to accomplish treatment goals.

The first part of the interview should focus on developing an understanding of why the adolescent or the adolescent's parents have come for an assessment. The adolescent's response to this question will provide information about the patient's attitudes, motivations, and developmental stage. The next step is to obtain a complete current and past history of the problem. It is often helpful to get a detailed chronology of the events leading to the adolescent's eating attitudes and behaviors and concerns about food, weight, and shape. The physician should explore whether the adolescent has ever had a previous diagnosis (with associated investigations and hospitalizations) of an illness that can cause weight loss, disordered eating, or gastrointestinal symptoms (eg, diabetes mellitus, inflammatory bowel disease, celiac disease). Questions should be asked about the amount of weight loss, the time course of the weight loss, whether the weight loss was intentional and why, the mechanisms used to lose weight, including restricting, binging, purging, or exercise; if the patient is purging, when did it start and how often; if the patient is bingeing, when did it start, how often does it occur, and how does the patient characterize a binge; exercise, including type and quantity; substance use, including laxatives, diuretics, emetics, insulin, amphetamines and CAM products, and how often the patient uses these substances. Furthermore, questions about smoking, alcohol, and drug use or abuse should be explored.[16] A complete medication history should include the names of all medications, doses, how long the adolescent has been taking the medications (including vitamins, minerals, and supplements), and whether there are any benefits or side effects.

How adolescents feel about body weight, shape, and size should be explored, along with questions regarding their current weight and shape, how they would feel about gaining weight, whether there is anything about their body they would like to change, and at what weight they would be most comfortable.

There should be a complete nutritional history. A detailed report of food intake on a typical day should be elicited. The physician or dietitian should find out the types and quantity of foods and fluids consumed and the times of day; whether the patient counts calories or fat grams; whether there are "scary" or "forbidden" foods and are there "safe" foods; and whether there are food allergies, and if yes, how this was determined. It is not uncommon for young people with AN to be vegetarians. If this is the case, it is important to understand when the vegetarian lifestyle started and the reason for choosing it. Understanding the family's attitudes and behaviors about food (eg, does the family have meals together and who prepares the meals), weight loss, exercise, and health may provide insight into the adolescent's lifestyle and help in formulating a feasible treatment plan.

A menstrual history is critical for any assessment of the female adolescent and diagnostically important in adolescents suspected of having AN. The menstrual history should include age of menarche, mother's age of menarche, characterization of menstrual period (length of cycle, length of menstrual period, last normal menstrual period), current or past hormone replacement therapy and reason for this treatment, and past history of bone fractures. Finally, a sexual history including questions about sexual experience and sexual orientation should be sensitively reviewed with the adolescent.

The initial psychosocial assessment should include an evaluation of the patient's functioning at home, in school, and with friends. Up to two thirds of patients with eating disorders have a comorbid psychiatric disorder. Therefore, health care providers should evaluate for other psychiatric disorders, including depression, anxiety and OCD; explore whether the adolescent has been treated in other mental health care programs, and if so, the reason for the treatment and for how long; and sensitively assess the adolescent for a current or past history of self-harm, suicidality, and physical, sexual, or emotional abuse.

The adolescent should be asked about a family history of medical or psychiatric illness. This information should be reviewed and confirmed with the parents without the adolescent present because many parents are reluctant to divulge this information in front of their child or adolescent.

## PHYSICAL EXAMINATION

A thorough physical examination is essential to the assessment of an adolescent with AN. The adolescent may appear pale, tired, and wasted. She or he may wear layers of clothing to keep warm and hide the emaciation. The adolescent should be weighed in a hospital gown after voiding to get an accurate weight and to be able to assess the degree of emaciation. Weight and height should be measured. Body mass index (BMI) should be calculated (BMI = weight in kilograms divided by height in meters squared) and plotted on the Centers for Disease Control and Prevention charts. (See Chapter 9, Physical Examination and Laboratory Screening or www.cdc.gov/growthcharts.) Percentage below median weight for age and height can be determined from the National Center for Health Statistics (NCHS)[17] tables. It is important to plot previous weights and heights on the growth chart to determine whether growth arrest has occurred and to assess what the weight and height would have been without the eating disorder. Particular attention should be paid to vital signs, including oral temperature and orthostatic pulse and blood pressure. It is not uncommon for significant bradycardia, hypotension, and hypothermia to be present. Further, there may be extra heart sounds, specifically midsystolic clicks or murmurs from mitral valve prolapse. Lanugo hair may be present on the trunk, back, and arms. In those

**Table 76-2**

**Physical Findings in Adolescents with Anorexia Nervosa**

| *Organ System* | *Physical Sign* |
|---|---|
| Whole body | Weight loss, low body weight, cachexia, dehydration, hypothermia |
| Skin | Acrocyanosis, dry skin, hair loss, brittle hair and nails, lanugo hair, yellow skin, evidence of self-injurious behaviors (ie, ecchymoses, linear scratches, cuts or scars, cigarette burns) |
| Cardiac | Bradycardia, hypotension and/or orthostatic hypotension, weak and irregular pulse, extra heart sounds or murmurs, acrocyanosis, peripheral edema |
| Muscular | Muscle wasting |
| Central nervous system | Cognitive impairment, peripheral neuropathy, seizures, depressed mood, irritability, anxiety |
| Endocrine | Amenorrhea (primary or secondary), low body temperature, low energy, delay or arrested growth in height, delay or arrested pubertal growth |
| Skeletal | Bone pain, bone fractures, low BMD |
| Gastrointestinal | Abdominal distention with meals, in purging patients: parotid swelling, dental caries and gingivitis, stomatitis, glossitis |
| Hematologic | Easy bruisability, petechiae |

who purge, there may be hypertrophy of the parotid glands, dental enamel erosion, and scars or calluses on the dorsum of the hand known as Russell's sign (from contact with central incisors when using the hand to induce vomiting). Finally, determining the sexual maturity rating (breast and pubic hair for girls, genital and pubic hair for boys) is a crucial part of the examination because pubertal delay or arrest may be a consequence of malnutrition. A thorough examination of every organ system is important. Common physical signs in adolescents with AN are outlined in Table 76-2.

### LABORATORY STUDIES

Recommended laboratory tests are shown in Box 76-2. Laboratory tests are not diagnostic but they help exclude other causes of weight loss or vomiting, may help confirm the diagnosis, and may detect an occasional life-threatening situation such as hypokalemia (see following). Despite the severe degree of malnutrition, laboratory tests are usually normal.

The complete blood count (CBC) may show mild anemia, leukopenia, or thrombocytopenia, secondary to suppression of the bone marrow. The erythrocyte sedimentation rate (ESR) is usually low secondary to decreased hepatic production of fibrinogen. The

**Box 76-2**

***Recommended Laboratory and Ancillary Tests for the Evaluation of an Adolescent with Anorexia Nervosa***

- CBC
- ESR
- Urinalysis
- Chemistry profile including serum calcium, magnesium, and phosphorus levels and liver function tests
- Serum amylase—if vomiting
- Thyroid function tests
- LH, FSH, estradiol, and prolactin—if amenorrheic
- ECG
- If amenorrheic for >6 months, dual-energy x-ray absorptiometry
- MRI or CT scan of the brain for atypical presentations

CBC, complete blood count; ESR, erythrocyte sedimentation rate; LH, luteinizing hormone; FSH, follicular stimulating hormone; ECG, electrocardiogram; MRI, magnetic resonance imaging; CT, computed tomograph

presence of an elevated ESR should arouse suspicion of another diagnosis.

Electrolyte disturbances may occur with fluid restriction, self-induced vomiting, or laxative/diuretic abuse. Hypokalemia is the electrolyte abnormality most frequently seen with vomiting or laxative abuse. Hyponatremia occurs in those who are water loading to falsely elevate body weight prior to a medical visit or because of excessive water drinking to satisfy hunger urges. Serum phosphorus levels are usually normal on presentation but can drop precipitously during refeeding or episodes of bingeing. Serum transaminases are elevated in 4% to 38% of patients secondary to fatty necrosis of the liver. Serum amylase may be elevated in those who are bingeing or purging. In contrast to other forms of malnutrition, total protein and serum albumin levels are usually normal. Cholesterol levels may be high secondary to impaired lipoprotein metabolism.[18,19] Serum carotene levels are elevated in 13% to 62% of cases, probably due to a combination of increased dietary intake of pigmented vegetables (ie, carrots) and derangement of hepatic conversion of beta-carotene to vitamin A.[20,21]

The urinalysis may show ketones, mild proteinuria, and an alkaline urine. Specific gravity may be high in the presence of dehydration or low if the patient has been water loading.

Thyroid function tests may demonstrate low $T_3$ syndrome, where thyroxine ($T_4$), instead of being converted to active tri-iodothyronine ($T_3$), is preferentially converted to its metabolically inactive isomer, reverse $T_3$. Occasionally, $T_4$ levels may be low. Abnormalities in thyroid function tests, which reflect adaptive changes to malnutrition, respond to nutritional rehabilitation and should not be treated with thyroid hormone replacement. Luteinizing hormone (LH), follicle-stimulating hormone (FSH), and estradiol levels are all low, secondary to suppression of the hypothalamic-pituitary-ovarian axis.

The electrocardiogram (ECG) usually shows sinus bradycardia and low-voltage complexes, but there may be a prolonged QTc interval and nonspecific ST-segment depression or T-wave changes.[22,23] Arrythmias may occur secondary to electrolyte and acid-base imbalance due to vomiting or laxative/diuretic abuse or as part of the refeeding syndrome.

In those patients who have been amenorrheic for more than 6 months, bone densitometry of the lumbar spine and hip should be performed to evaluate for the presence of reduced bone mass. In those with atypical neurological presentations, a magnetic resonance imaging (MRI) or computed tomography (CT) scan of the brain should be performed to rule out other organic processes.

## DIFFERENTIAL DIAGNOSIS

The diagnosis of AN should be suspected in any adolescent with unexplained weight loss and food avoidance. The differential diagnosis includes both medical and psychiatric conditions.

### MEDICAL CONDITIONS

- Inflammatory bowel disease
- Malabsorption
- Endocrine conditions - hyperthyroidism, Addison disease, diabetes mellitus
- Collagen vascular disease
- Central nervous system lesions, ie, hypothalamic or pituitary tumors
- Malignancies
- Chronic infections - tuberculosis, HIV
- Immunodeficiency

### PSYCHIATRIC CONDITIONS

- Mood disorders
- Anxiety disorders
- Somatization disorder
- Substance abuse
- Psychosis

## MEDICAL COMPLICATIONS

The medical complications of AN are listed in Table 76-3. Almost every organ system can be involved.[22] Many medical complications are secondary to the effects of malnutrition. Some occur as a result of aberrant behaviors to control body weight such as self-induced vomiting or the use of laxatives, diuretics, or diet pills. Some complications, such as acute electrolyte disturbances or cardiac arrhythmias, can be life threatening, whereas others, such as growth retardation or reduced BMD may be irreversible, resulting in lifelong morbidity.

### FLUID AND ELECTROLYTES

Patients may present with dehydration and abnormal serum levels of sodium, potassium, chloride, carbon dioxide, and blood urea nitrogen. Electrolyte disturbances are more likely to be present in those who are vomiting or abusing laxatives or diuretics. The most common electrolyte disturbance is hypokalemia. Loss of hydrogen and chloride in vomitus results in compensatory reabsorption of sodium and excretion of potassium via the kidneys. Loss of electrolytes in the stool and urine in those abusing laxatives or diuretics further

**Table 76-3**

**Medical Complications of Anorexia Nervosa**

| *Organ System* | *Complication* |
|---|---|
| Fluid and electrolytes | • Increased blood urea nitrogen<br>• Hyponatremia<br>• Hypokalemia[a]<br>• Hypochloremia[a]<br>• Metabolic alkalosis[a] |
| Cardiovascular | • Bradycardia<br>• Orthostatic hypotension<br>• ECG abnormalities<br>• Cardiac arrhythmias[a]<br>• Pericardial effusion<br>• Mitral valve prolapse<br>• Emetine cardiomyopathy[a]<br>• Congestive heart failure |
| Gastrointestinal | • Constipation<br>• Delayed gastric emptying<br>• Intestinal immobility<br>• Parotid hypertrophy[a]<br>• Esophagitis[a]<br>• Erosion of dental enamel[a]<br>• Bloody diarrhea[a]<br>• Mallory-Weiss tears[a]<br>• Esophageal or gastric rupture[a]<br>• Barrett esophagus[a]<br>• Fatty necrosis of liver<br>• Acute pancreatitis<br>• Superior mesenteric artery syndrome<br>• Gallstones |
| Dermatological | • Acrocyanosis<br>• Lanugo<br>• Hypercarotinemia<br>• Calluses on dorsum of hand<br>• Edema |
| Endocrine | • Growth retardation<br>• Amenorrhea<br>• Pubertal delay<br>• Low $T_3$ syndrome<br>• Hypercortisolism |
| Skeletal | • Reduced BMD<br>• Fractures |
| Hematologic | • Anemia<br>• Thrombocytopenia<br>• Leukopenia<br>• Low ESR |
| Neurologic | • Seizures<br>• Syncope[a]<br>• Cortical atrophy |

[a]Complications secondary to self-induced vomiting or the abuse of laxatives or diuretics.

aggravates the hypokalemia. Hyponatremia can occur in those who "water load" and can lead to seizures, coma, and death. Serum phosphorus levels may be normal on presentation but can drop with refeeding. Hypophosphatemia may play a role in the development of cardiac arrhythmias and sudden unexpected death seen in the "refeeding syndrome."[24]

### CARDIOVASCULAR

Resting pulse rates may be as low as 30 to 40 beats per minute, and both systolic and diastolic blood pressures can be low. These changes reflect an adaptive response to reduced energy intake. In a population of adolescents with AN, 48% of strict dieters and 25% of those who vomited or purged had heart rates less than 40 beats per minute.[22] Within the first 4 days of hospitalization, 60% to 85% of patients were reported to have orthostatic pulse changes on standing.[25] Normalization of orthostatic pulse changes occurs after approximately 3 weeks of nutritional rehabilitation when patients reach approximately 80% of ideal body weight (IBW). Although heart size is reduced[26] and exercise capacity is diminished,[27,28] cardiac output and left ventricular function are usually preserved.[26]

Electrocardiogram abnormalities have been noted in up to 75% of hospitalized adolescents with AN and include sinus bradycardia, low-voltage complexes, a prolonged QT interval dispersion, wandering atrial pacemaker, T-wave abnormalities, ST-segment depression, first- and second-degree heart block, and various atrial and ventricular arrythmias.[22,23] A prolonged QTc interval is of particular concern because it has been reported to precede ventricular arrythmias and sudden death in patients hospitalized with AN.[29] The frequency of a prolonged QTc has been reported to be between 0% and 32% depending on the study.[22,30,31] If a prolonged QTc is found, it is a source for concern.[32]

Echocardiographic findings have demonstrated a reduced left ventricular mass and thickness with a normal left ventricular ejection fraction. A mild to moderate pericardial effusion that is clinically silent has been reported in 60% to 70% of patients with AN.[33,34] Mitral valve prolapse has been reported in patients with AN[35,36] and is thought to be the result of an apparent redundancy of the mitral valve. Emetine cardiomyopathy can occur in those using ipecac to induce vomiting. This condition is associated with necrosis of cardiac muscle and can be fatal.[37] Congestive heart failure can occur during refeeding.[38]

### GASTROINTESTINAL

Bloating and constipation are frequent complaints and reflect delayed gastric emptying and decreased intestinal motility. Liver enzymes may be elevated secondary to fatty infiltration and focal damage to the liver.[21,22,39] Weight loss can lead to the "superior mesenteric artery syndrome," a condition caused by extrinsic compression of the duodenum by the superior mesenteric artery where it originates from the aorta. Rapid weight loss can also be associated with gallstone formation.

Recurrent vomiting causes erosion of dental enamel, esophagitis, Mallory-Weiss tears and, on occasion, esophageal or gastric rupture. Prolonged recurrent vomiting causes Barrett esophagus (metaplasia of the distal esophagus), which is precancerous. Laxative abuse can be accompanied by bloody diarrhea.

### ENDOCRINE

In adolescents who develop AN prior to completing growth, growth retardation and short stature can be prominent findings. In one study, growth arrest (documented by growth curves) was observed in 15 subjects who developed AN during the prepubertal and pubertal period and who had the disease for at least 6 months.[40] Patients are shorter than expected,[41] and growth stunting may even be the presenting feature.[42,43] Growth retardation as a major feature of AN is more likely to occur in adolescent boys because boys grow, on average, 2 years longer than girls. Adolescents with AN have diminished growth hormone action resulting in decreased secretion of insulin-like growth factor-1 (IGF-1), the hormone that mediates cell proliferation and protein synthesis. Levels of growth hormone are normal or increased with low levels of growth hormone binding protein, suggesting an adaptive state of growth hormone resistance. These findings revert to normal after nutritional rehabilitation.[44] Peak height velocity is lower than expected, occurs later than expected, and menarche occurs significantly later than in healthy peers. Catch-up growth can occur with nutritional rehabilitation but, even with intervention, some adolescents may not reach their genetic height potential.[45]

Hypothalamic dysfunction is evidenced by amenorrhea as well as disturbances in satiety, difficulties with temperature regulation, and inability to concentrate urine.[46] There is activation of the hypothalamic–adrenal axis with high levels of serum cortisol. Pubertal delay is a frequent finding in those who develop AN prior to completion of puberty. One study found pubertal delay in 17% of adolescents with AN.[22] Another study found failure of breast development in 14 of 20 subjects who developed AN before menarche. Thirteen of the 20 had their first menstrual period after the age of 18.[47]

Amenorrhea in AN is associated with a disturbance in the regulation of gonadotropin-releasing hormone secretion by the hypothalamus. The cause of the amenorrhea is a combination of malnutrition, increased exercise, emotional stress, low body weight, and decreased stores of body fat. Serum LH, FSH, and estradiol levels are all low, and the uterus and ovaries revert to prepubertal size.[48] Approximately 20% to 25% of patients with AN have amenorrhea that precedes the weight loss; 50% have amenorrhea that occurs at about the same time as the weight loss; and 25% have amenorrhea only after substantial weight loss. Weight gain is usually accompanied by restoration of normal hypothalamic–pituitary–ovarian function and resumption of spontaneous menses, but in many cases amenorrhea may be prolonged.[49]

### SKELETAL

Reduced BMD is a serious and frequent complication of AN and can occur after a relatively short illness.[50] More than 90% of adolescents and young adults with AN have reduced BMD at one or more skeletal sites.[51] The etiology is multifactorial, related to a combination of poor nutrition, low body weight, estrogen deficiency, excessive exercise, and hypercortisolism. In AN there is both impaired bone formation and increased bone resorption.[52]

Adolescence is a critical time for peak bone mass attainment, achieved toward the end of the second decade of life.[48,53–55] Interference with bone mass accretion during these formative years can have long-lasting morbidity. The reduction in BMD in AN is associated with increased fracture risk many years after recovery from the eating disorder.[56–58]

### HEMATOLOGICAL

Suppression of the bone marrow leads to leukopenia (one third to two thirds of patients), anemia (approximately 30%) and thrombocytopenia (30%). The leukopenia does not appear to be associated with increased infection risk. Anemia may be secondary to bone marrow suppression but may also be due to dietary deficiency of vitamin B12, folate, or iron. All the hematologic abnormalities reverse with nutritional rehabilitation.

### NEUROLOGICAL

The major neurological complications of eating disorders are seizures (secondary to electrolyte disturbances) and cerebral atrophy noted on CT and MRI scans.[59–62] Muscle weakness and a peripheral neuropathy can also occur. In the malnourished state, the cerebral ventricles and cortical sulci are enlarged and there are volume deficits of both grey and white matter. In addition to structural brain changes, alteration in brain function has also been demonstrated. For example, evidence of reduced regional blood flow to the brain has been demonstrated in 13 of 15 children and adolescents aged 9 to 14 years.[63] Neuropsychological testing has demonstrated impairment of attention, concentration, and memory with deficits in visuospatial ability.[64] Though the ventricular enlargement and white matter changes revert to normal after weight restoration,[61,65] the grey matter volume deficits and regional blood flow disturbances persist, suggesting that these changes may even have predated the illness.[8,61,63,65] Similarly, some but not all cognitive deficits improve with weight restoration.[64]

## TREATMENT

Adolescents with AN are best treated by an interdisciplinary team of experienced health care providers. Patients can be treated in inpatient, partial hospitalization, outpatient, or residential settings. Most patients can be treated as outpatients. Some patients who are medically compromised, severely malnourished, or who failed outpatient treatment will require hospitalization. Indications for hospitalization of an adolescent with AN are listed in Box 76-3. Treatment guidelines have recently been published by the American Academy of Pediatrics, Society for Adolescent Medicine, American Psychiatric Association, and the American Dietetic Association. These guidelines provide evidence-based information and expert consensus on the diagnosis and treatment of eating disorders.[66-69]

### Box 76-3

### *Indications for Hospitalization in an Adolescent with an Eating Disorder*

1. Severe malnutrition (weight ≤75% average body weight for age, sex, and height)
2. Dehydration
3. Electrolyte disturbances (hypokalemia, hyponatremia, hypophosphatemia)
4. Cardiac dysrhythmia
5. Physiological instability
   a. Severe bradycardia (heart rate <50 beats/minute daytime; <45 beats/minute at night)
   b. Hypotension (<80/50 mmHg)
   c. Hypothermia (body temperature <96° F)
   d. Orthostatic changes in pulse (>20 beats per minute) or blood pressure (>10 mmHg)
6. Arrested growth and development
7. Failure of outpatient treatment
8. Acute food refusal
9. Uncontrollable bingeing and purging
10. Acute medical complications of malnutrition (eg, syncope, seizures, cardiac failure, pancreatitis, etc)
11. Acute psychiatric emergencies (eg, suicidal ideation, acute psychosis)
12. Comorbid diagnosis that interferes with the treatment of the eating disorder (eg, severe depression, OCD, severe family dysfunction)

Reprinted from Golden NH, Katzman DK, Kreipe RE, et al. Eating disorders in adolescents. Position paper of the Society for Adolescent Medicine. *J Adolesc Health*. 2003;33:496-503, with permission from Elsevier.

### MEDICAL TREATMENT

The aims of medical treatment are acute medical stabilization, nutritional rehabilitation, and reversal of medical complications. Dehydration and acute electrolyte disturbances can usually be corrected within 24 to 48 hours. However, hypophosphatemia and fluid shifts can continue to develop within the first 1 to 2 weeks of treatment. Weight gain is an important early goal of treatment and is accompanied by reversal of many medical complications as well as improvement in mood and cognitive functioning.

In the malnourished state, basal metabolic rate slows down as an adaptive response to malnutrition. Therefore, in the initial stages of nutritional rehabilitation, energy requirements are low. However, as nutritional rehabilitation progresses and metabolic recovery occurs, energy requirements increase rapidly, and patients may require up to 3,600 to 4,100 kcals per day for weight gain. Patients are usually started on 1,000 to 1,400 kcals per day (30–40 kcals per kg per day), and the caloric prescription is increased by 200 to 400 kcals every 24 to 48 hours. Weight gain can be achieved in outpatient, partial hospitalization, or inpatient settings. The recommended rate of weight gain for outpatients is 0.5 to 1.0 lb per week; for partial hospitalization programs, 1.o to 2.0 lb per week; and for inpatient programs, 2.0 to 3.0 lbs per week. Most patients can be refed orally. Short-term nasogastric feeding may be required in some patients failing to gain weight on oral intake alone. Nasogastric feeding should not be used as punishment.

Care should be taken to avoid the "refeeding syndrome," particularly in the severely malnourished patient (<70% of IBW). This syndrome can occur after oral, nasogastric, or parenteral feeding and is more likely to occur during the first 1 to 2 weeks of nutritional rehabilitation. The "refeeding syndrome" refers to a constellation of fluid and electrolyte shifts that occur when severely malnourished patients are refed too rapidly. In severe malnutrition, total body phosphorus is low and refeeding drives phosphorus intracellularly, leading to hypophosphatemia. Severe hypophosphatemia is associated with hemolytic anemia, cardiac failure, ventricular arrhythmias, acute delirium, seizures, coma, and sudden death. Mild to moderate hypophosphatemia has been found in more than a quarter of adolescents with AN hospitalized for their eating disorder.[70] The refeeding syndrome can be prevented by slow nutritional rehabilitation during the first 1 to 2 weeks of refeeding with careful monitoring of fluid balance, heart rate, and rhythm as well as serum phosphorus levels. Supplemental phosphorus can be administered as needed.[71]

## DETERMINING TREATMENT GOAL WEIGHT

Treatment goal weight needs to be individualized, taking into account pubertal stage, prior growth percentiles, height, and age. For adolescents, treatment goal weight is a "moving target" and should be recalculated every 3 to 6 months. Standard height and weight tables frequently used for adults are inappropriate for adolescents. The NCHS tables provide an excellent resource of normative data for height and weight of children and adolescents in the United States. These data sets provide accurate measurements of 6,768 adolescents, reliably representing data from more than 22 million United States subjects.[17] However, these tables only provide normative data and do not provide information as to what constitutes "ideal body weight."

Treatment goal weight should be the weight at which normal physical and sexual development occurs. For girls, this is the weight at which menstruation and ovulation are restored. In postmenarcheal girls, a weight approximately 90% of IBW (defined as the median weight for age and height using the NCHS percentiles) is a reasonable goal weight, as 86% of patients who achieve that weight will resume menses within 3 to 6 months.[49] For those who were previously overweight, treatment goal weight may need to be higher. In a premenarcheal girl or an adolescent boy whose growth and development are not yet complete, treatment goal weight should be 100% of IBW to maximize growth potential.

Many treatment programs provide adolescents with a weight range for their "treatment goal weight" and a clear message that this range will change with expected growth and physical development. This is done to avoid having the patient focus on one particular body weight, to acknowledge that there are daily fluctuations in body weight, and to underscore that height and weight will change with healthy pubertal development.

## MANAGEMENT OF REDUCED BMD

Weight restoration with resumption of spontaneous menses is the mainstay in the treatment of reduced bone mineral density (BMD) in AN. Dietary intake of calcium should be at least 1,300 mg per day (through diet or a calcium supplement). A multivitamin containing 400 IU of vitamin D will facilitate the absorption and utilization of calcium. Moderate weight-bearing exercise or resistance training may be helpful but should be carefully supervised. Excessive exercise that interferes with weight gain should be avoided. There is no evidence that hormone replacement therapy increases BMD in either adult[72] or adolescent[73] populations with AN, and hormone replacement therapy should not be prescribed for this purpose. The use of IGF-1, dihydroepiandrosterone (DHEA) and the bisphosphonates to treat reduced BMD in AN is being studied, but these medications are not yet recommended for routine clinical use.

## PSYCHOLOGICAL TREATMENTS

Over the past 25 years, family-based treatment (FBT) has been established as an important therapeutic approach and the treatment of choice for adolescents with AN. Almost all studies of psychological treatment in adolescents with AN have shown that younger patients can be treated quite successfully provided that parents participate in treatment.

Russell et al[74] found FBT to be superior to individual supportive therapy (IT) in adolescents who had had AN for less than 3 years. After 1 year of treatment, the FBT group had a significantly better outcome than the group treated with IT. At 5-year follow-up, 90% of the patients assigned to FBT had a good outcome compared with 36% of those in IT.[75] Recently, multifamily group treatment, in which several families are treated together in a group setting, has been demonstrated to be effective in reducing eating disorder symptoms in the adolescent while providing support for parents.[76,77] Manualization of FBT has been implemented and studied.[78] A recent study showed that a short course of FBT (6 months) was as effective as a long course of FBT (12 months) with respect to long-term follow-up (4 years) in adolescents with AN.[79]

Behavioral systems family therapy (BSFT) has been compared to ego-oriented individual treatment (EOIT).[80,81] Patients in BSFT achieved significantly greater weight gain, were more likely to have return of menses at the end of treatment, and had a more rapid treatment response compared to those in EOIT. Both treatments were similar in terms of improvements in eating attitudes, depression, and self-reported eating-related family conflict.

Finally, FBT has been compared to family group psychoeducation in adolescents with AN in an inpatient treatment setting.[82] Although both treatments were found to be equally effective, family psychoeducation was a much more cost-effective treatment modality.

This trial was uncontrolled, and therefore it is difficult to interpret the impact of these results in light of other treatments received by patients.

In summary, FBT appears to be beneficial in the treatment of adolescents with AN. However, our understanding is based on limited evidence. FBT requires further study and comparison with other psychological treatments.

### MEDICATIONS

#### *Antidepressants*

Psychopharmacology is used as an adjunct treatment strategy in adolescents with AN. Evidence for the use of antidepressants in the treatment of adolescents with AN remains quite limited. There has been much interest in the use of selective serotonin reuptake inhibitors (SSRIs) for acute treatment and relapse prevention in AN. Most of the studies have been conducted in older adolescents and young adults. Controlled trials in underweight patients have shown no benefit when medications were compared with placebo.[83,84] Other studies have explored the utility of medication after weight restoration, with differing results. In a double-blind, placebo-controlled trial, fluoxetine was found to have a significant role in preventing relapse in older adolescents and adults with AN who had attained 85% of their expected body weight.[85] However, a recent randomized, double-blind, placebo-controlled trial comparing fluoxetine to placebo in weight-restored patients with AN failed to show any benefit of fluoxetine. All subjects received individual cognitive behavioral therapy.[86] Further studies are needed to determine the effects of antidepressants in both acute treatment and relapse prevention for adolescents with AN.

The use of tricyclic antidepressants should be avoided in AN because of the risk of hypotension, cardiac conduction abnormalities, and arrythmias. Bupropion should also be avoided (especially in patients who binge and purge) because of an increased risk of seizures.

The US Food and Drug Administration has required manufacturers of antidepressant medications to include a "black box" warning label that alerts health care providers and consumers to an increased risk of suicidal thinking and behavior in adolescents being treated with the SSRI medications. As such, physicians need to inform and educate adolescents and their families about the risks and benefits of these medications. Furthermore, the use of these medications requires close monitoring for the emergence of suicidality or other unusual behaviors.[87]

Psychotropic medications such as the SSRIs (fluoxetine, sertraline, paroxetine, fluvoxamine, and citalopram) have also been used to treat comorbid depression or OCD in patients with eating disorders.

#### *Antipsychotics*

Recent case reports suggest that the atypical antipsychotic medications (such as risperidone and olanzapine) may be effective in adolescents with AN. Preliminary work has shown that these medications have helped reduce anxiety and obsessional thinking and enhanced weight gain. To date, there are no controlled studies of the use of these medications in adolescents with AN.

## OUTCOME

The long-term outcome of AN has been evaluated in more than 100 studies during the past 50 years. The outcome data vary because of differences in case definition, length of follow-up, treatment modality, type of data collected, and age range of population studied.[88] Among adolescents with AN, approximately 50% to 70% recover, 20% improve but continue to have residual symptoms such as body image disturbance, disordered eating, and other psychiatric difficulties,[89-91] and 10% to 20% develop chronic AN. Younger patients with AN who receive prompt and aggressive treatment have a much better outcome. For example, although good outcomes were observed in only 35% of 80 patients in Eisler et al's[75] 5-year follow-up study, outcomes were good in 62% of the 21 patients who had been ill for <3 years and whose illness began before age 19. In another study, 76% of adolescents had a full recovery 5 years after inpatient treatment. The time to full recovery was protracted and ranged from 57 to 79 months, and approximately 30% developed binge eating and/or purging behaviors over the course of the illness.[92]

Anorexia nervosa has the highest mortality rate among the mental disorders. According to one report, approximately 5.6% of patients diagnosed with AN die per decade of illness.[93] Females with AN are 12 times more likely to die than women of a similar age in the general population. The most common causes of death are suicide and medical complications due to starvation. The suicide rate among women with AN is up to 57 times higher than that for women of a similar age in the general population.[94]

Factors associated with a good outcome include short duration of illness, early identification and intervention, early age of onset (<14 years old), no associated comorbid psychological diagnoses, and no bingeing and purging. Factors associated with a poor outcome include lower weight at presentation, longer duration of illness, exercise compulsion, bingeing and purging, and comorbid mental illness (affective disorder, substance abuse).

## REFERENCES


1. Hoek HW, van Hoeken D. Review of the prevalence and incidence of eating disorders. *Int J Eat Disord.* 2003;34(4): 383-396

2. Bulik CM, Sullivan PF, Tozzi F, Furberg H, Lichtenstein P, Pedersen NL. Prevalence, heritability, and prospective risk factors for anorexia nervosa. *Arch Gen Psychiatry.* 2006;63(3): 305-312

3. Lucas AR, Crowson CS, O'Fallon WM, Melton LJ, III. The ups and downs of anorexia nervosa. *Int J Eat Disord.* 1999;26(4):397-405

4. Grice DE, Halmi KA, Fichter MM, et al. Evidence for a susceptibility gene for anorexia nervosa on chromosome 1. *Am J Hum Genet.* 2002;70(3):787-792

5. Klump KL, Gobrogge KL. A review and primer of molecular genetic studies of anorexia nervosa. *Int J Eat Disord.* 2005;37(suppl):S43-S48

6. Kaye WH, Barbarich NC, Putnam K, et al. Anxiolytic effects of acute tryptophan depletion in anorexia nervosa. *Int J Eat Disord.* 2003;33(3):257-267

7. Audenaert K, Van Laere K, Dumont F, et al. Decreased 5-HT2a receptor binding in patients with anorexia nervosa. *J Nucl Med.* 2003;44(2):163-169

8. Frank GK, Kaye WH, Meltzer CC, et al. Reduced 5-HT2A receptor binding after recovery from anorexia nervosa. *Biol Psychiatry.* 2002;52(9):896-906

9. Becker AE, Burwell RA, Gilman SE, Herzog DB, Hamburg P. Eating behaviours and attitudes following prolonged exposure to television among ethnic Fijian adolescent girls. *Br J Psychiatry.* 2002;180:509-514

10. American Psychiatric Association. *Diagnostic and Statistical Manual of Mental Disorders.* 4th ed. Washington, DC: APA Press; 1994

11. Garfinkel PE, Lin E, Goering P, et al. Should amenorrhoea be necessary for the diagnosis of anorexia nervosa? Evidence from a Canadian community sample. *Br J Psychiatry.* 1996;168(4):500-506

12. Watson TL, Andersen AE. A critical examination of the amenorrhea and weight criteria for diagnosing anorexia nervosa. *Acta Psychiatr Scand.* 2003;108(3):175-182

13. Fisher M, Schneider M, Burns J, Symons H, Mandel FS. Differences between adolescents and young adults at presentation to an eating disorders program. *J Adolesc Health.* 2001;28 (3):222-227

14. Nicholls D Chater R, Lask B. Children into DSM don't go: a comparison of classification systems for eating disorders in childhood and early adolescence. *Int J Eat Disord.* 2000;28(3):317-324

15. Lask B, Bryant-Waugh R. *Childhood Onset Anorexia Nervosa and Related Eating Disorders.* Melksham, Wiltshire, U: Redwood Press Limited, 1993

16. Stock SL, Goldberg E, Corbett S, Katzman DK. Substance use in female adolescents with eating disorders. *J Adolesc Health.* 2002;31(2):176-182

17. National Center for Health Statistics. *Height and Weight of Youths 12-17 Years, United States, Vital and Health Statistics. Series 11, No. 124. Health Services and Mental Health Administration.* Washington, DC: United States Government Printing Office; 1973

18. Arden MR, Weiselberg EC, Nussbaum MP, Shenker IR, Jacobson MS. Effect of weight restoration on the dyslipoproteinemia of anorexia nervosa. *J Adolesc Health Care.* 1990;11(3):199-202

19. Mehler PS, Lezotte D, Eckel R. Lipid levels in anorexia nervosa. *Int J Eat Disord.* 1998;24(2):217-221

20. Boland B, Beguin C, Zech F, Desager JP, Lambert M. Serum beta-carotene in anorexia nervosa patients: a case-control study. *Int J Eat Disord.* 2001;30(3):299-305

21. Sherman P, Leslie K, Goldberg E, Rybczynski J, St Louis P. Hypercarotenemia and transaminitis in female adolescents with eating disorders: a prospective, controlled study. *J Adolesc Health.* 1994;15(3):205-209

22. Palla B, Litt IF. Medical complications of eating disorders in adolescents. *Pediatrics.* 1988;81(5):613-623

23. Galetta F, Franzoni F, Cupisti A, Belliti D, Prattichizzo F, Rolla M. QT interval dispersion in young women with anorexia nervosa. *J Pediatr.* 2002;140(4):456-460

24. Kohn MR, Golden NH, Shenker IR. Cardiac arrest and delirium: presentations of the refeeding syndrome in severely malnourished adolescents with anorexia nervosa. *J Adolesc Health.* 1998;22(3):239-243

25. Shamim T, Golden NH, Arden M, Filiberto L, Shenker IR. Resolution of vital sign instability: an objective measure of medical stability in anorexia nervosa. *J Adolesc Health.* 2003;32(1):73-77

26. Moodie DS, Salcedo E. Cardiac function in adolescents and young adults with anorexia nervosa. *J Adolesc Health Care.* 1983;4(1):9-14

27. Nudel DB, Gootman N, Nussbaum MP, Shenker IR. Altered exercise performance and abnormal sympathetic responses to exercise in patients with anorexia nervosa. *J Pediatr.* 1984;105(1):34-37

28. Riggs S, Harel D, Biros P, Ziegler J. Cardiac impairment in adolescent girls with anorexia nervosa: what exercise stress testing reveals. *J Adolesc Health.* 2003;32(2):126

29. Isner JM, Roberts WC, Heymsfield SB, Yager J. Anorexia nervosa and sudden death. *Ann Intern Med.* 1985;102 (1):49-52

30. Lupoglazoff JM, Berkane N, Denjoy I, et al. [Cardiac consequences of adolescent anorexia nervosa.] *Arch Mal Coeur Vaiss.* 2001;94(5):494-498

31. Panagiotopoulos C, McCrindle BW, Hick K, Katzman DK. Electrocardiographic findings in adolescents with eating disorders. *Pediatrics.* 2000;105(5):1100-1105

32. Harris JP, Kreipe RE, Rossbach CN. QT prolongation by isoproterenol in anorexia nervosa. *J Adolesc Health.* 1993;14(5):390-393

33. Ramacciotti CE, Coli E, Biadi O, Dell'Osso L. Silent pericardial effusion in a sample of anorexic patients. *Eat Weight Disord.* 2003;8(1):68-71

34. Silvetti MS, Magnani M, Santill iA, et al. [The heart of anorexic adolescents]. *G Ital Cardiol.* 1998;28(2):131-139

35. Johnson GL, Humphries LL, Shirley PB, Mazzoleni A, Noonan JA. Mitral valve prolapse in patients with anorexia nervosa and bulimia. *Arch Intern Med.* 1986;146 (8): 1525-1529

36. Meyers DG, Starke H, Pearson PH, Wilken MK. Mitral valve prolapse in anorexia nervosa. *Ann Intern Med.* 1986;105(3):384-386

37. Schiff RJ, Wurzel CL, Brunson SC, Kasloff I, Nussbaum MP, Frank SD. Death due to chronic syrup of ipecac use in a patient with bulimia. *Pediatrics.* 1986;78(3):412-416

38. Powers PS. Heart failure during treatment of anorexia nervosa. *Am J Psychiatry.* 1982;139(9):1167-1170

39. Mickley D, Greenfeld D, Quinlan DM, Roloff P, Zwas F. Abnormal liver enzymes in outpatients with eating disorders. *Int J Eat Disord.* 1996;20(3):325-329

40. Danziger Y, Mukamel M, Zeharia A, Dinari G, Mimouni M. Stunting of growth in anorexia nervosa during the prepubertal and pubertal period. *Isr J Med Sci.* 1994;30 (8):581-584

41. Nussbaum M, Baird D, Sonnenblick M, Cowan K, ShenkerI R. Short stature in anorexia nervosa patients. *J Adolesc Health Care.* 1985;6(6):453-455

42. Root AW, Powers PS. Anorexia nervosa presenting as growth retardation in adolescents. *J Adolesc Health Care.* 1983;4(1):25-30

43. Modan-Moses D, Yaroslavsky A, Novikov I, et al. Stunting of growth as a major feature of anorexia nervosa in male adolescents. *Pediatrics.* 2003;111(2):270-276

44. Golden NH, Kreitzer P, Jacobson MS, et al. Disturbances in growth hormone secretion and action in adolescents with anorexia nervosa. *J Pediatr.* 1994;125(4):655-660

45. Lantzouni E, Frank GR, Golden NH, Shenker RI. Reversibility of growth stunting in early onset anorexia nervosa: a prospective study. *J Adolesc Health.* 2002;31 (2):162-165

46. Mecklenburg RS, Loriaux DL, Thompson RH, Andersen AE, Lipsett MB. Hypothalamic dysfunction in patients with anorexia nervosa. *Medicine.* 1976;53:147-157

47. Russell GF. Premenarchal anorexia nervosa and its sequelae. *J Psychiat Res.* 1985;19:363-369

48. Golden NH, Shenker IR. *Amenorrhea in Anorexia Nervosa: Etiology and Implications. Adolescent Nutrition and Eating Disorders.* Philadelphia, PA: Hanley & Belfus Inc.; 1992

49. Golden NH, Jacobson MS, Schebendach J, Solanto MV, Hertz SM, Shenker IR. Resumption of menses in anorexia nervosa. *Arch Pediatr Adolesc Med.* 1997;151(1):16-21

50. Bachrach LK, Guido D, Katzman D, Litt IF, Marcus R. Decreased bone density in adolescent girls with anorexia nervosa. *Pediatrics.* 1990;86(3):440-447

51. Golden NH. Osteopenia and osteoporosis in anorexia nervosa. *Adolesc Med.* 2003;14(1):97-108

52. Grinspoon S, Baum H, Lee K, Anderson E, Herzog D, Klibanski A. Effects of short-term recombinant human insulin-like growth factor I administration on bone turnover in osteopenic women with anorexia nervosa. *J Clin Endocrinol Metab.* 1996;81(11):3864-3870

53. Katzman DK, Bachrach LK, Carter DR, Marcus R. Clinical and anthropometric correlates of bone mineral acquisition in healthy adolescent girls. *J Clin Endocrinol Metab.* 1991;73(6):1332-1339

54. Bonjour JP, Theintz G, Buchs B, Slosman D, Rizzoli R. Critical years and stages of puberty for spinal and femoral bone mass accumulation during adolescence. *J Clin Endocrinol Metab.* 1991;73(3):555-563

55. Theintz G, Buchs B, Rizzoli R, et al. Longitudinal monitoring of bone mass accumulation in healthy adolescents: evidence for a marked reduction after 16 years of age at the levels of lumbar spine and femoral neck in female subjects. *J Clin Endocrinol Metab.* 1992;75 (4):1060-1065

56. Hartman D, Crisp A, Rooney B, Rackow C, Atkinson R, Patel S. Bone density of women who have recovered from anorexia nervosa. *Int J Eat Disord.* 2000;28 (1):107-112

57. Lucas AR, Melton LJ, III, Crowson CS, O'Fallon WM. Long-term fracture risk among women with anorexia nervosa: a population-based cohort study. *Mayo Clin Proc.* 1999;74(10): 972-977

58. Vestergaard P, Emborg C, Stoving RK, Hagen C, Mosekilde L, Brixen K. Fractures in patients with anorexia nervosa, bulimia nervosa, and other eating disorders—a nationwide register study. *Int J Eat Disord.* 2002;32 (3):301-308

59. Enzmann DR, Lane B. Cranial computed tomography findings in anorexia nervosa. *J Comput Assist Tomogr.* 1977;1(4):410-414

60. Nussbaum M, ShenkerI R, Marc J, Klein M. Cerebral atrophy in anorexia nervosa. *J Pediatr.* 1980;96(5):867-869

61. Golden NH, Ashtari M, Kohn MR, et al. Reversibility of cerebral ventricular enlargement in anorexia nervosa, demonstrated by quantitative magnetic resonance imaging. *J Pediatr.* 1996;128(2):296-301

62. Katzman DK, Lambe EK, Mikulis DJ, Ridgley JN, Goldbloom DS, Zipursky RB. Cerebral gray matter and white matter volume deficits in adolescent girls with anorexia nervosa. *J Pediatr.* 1996;129(6):794-803

63. Gordon I, Lask B, Bryant-Waugh R, Christie D, Timimi S. Childhood-onset anorexia nervosa: towards identifying a biological substrate. *Int J Eat Disord.* 1997;22 (2):159-165

64. Kingston K, Szmukler G, Andrewes D, Tress B, Desmond P. Neuropsychological and structural brain changes in anorexia nervosa before and after refeeding. *Psychol Med.* 1996;26(1): 15-28

65. Katzman DK, Zipursky RB, Lambe EK, Mikulis DJ. A longitudinal magnetic resonance imaging study of brain changes in adolescents with anorexia nervosa. *Arch Pediatr Adolesc Med.* 1997;151(8):793-797

66. American Dietetic Association. Position of the American Dietetic Association: nutrition intervention in the treatment of anorexia nervosa, bulimia nervosa, and eating disorders not otherwise specified (EDNOS). *J Am Diet Assoc.* 2001;101(7): 810-819

67. American Academy of Pediatrics Policy Statement. Identifying and treating eating disorders. *Pediatrics.* 2003;111(1): 204-211

68. Golden NH, Katzman DK, Kreipe RE, et al. Eating disorders in adolescents: position paper of the Society for Adolescent Medicine. *J Adolesc Health.* 2003;33 (6):496-503

69. American Psychiatric Association. Treatment of patients with eating disorders, third edition. *Am J Psychiatry.* 2005; 163(suppl):1-54

70. Ornstein RM, Golden NH, Jacobson MS, Shenker IR. Hypophosphatemia during nutritional rehabilitation in anorexia nervosa: implications for refeeding and monitoring. *J Adolesc Health.* 2003;32(1):83-88

71. Golden NH, Meyer W. Nutritional rehabilitation of anorexia nervosa. Goals and dangers. *Int J Adolesc Med Health.* 2004;16(2):131-144

72. Klibanski A, Biller BM, Schoenfeld DA, Herzog DB, Saxe VC. The effects of estrogen administration on trabecular bone loss in young women with anorexia nervosa. *J Clin Endocrinol Metab.* 1995;80(3):898-904

73. Golden NH, Lanzkowsky L, Schebendach J, Palestro CJ, Jacobson MS, Shenker IR. The effect of estrogen-progestin treatment on bone mineral density in anorexia nervosa. *J Pediatr Adolesc Gynecol.* 2002;15(3):135-143

74. Russell GF, Szmukler GI, Dare C, Eisler I. An evaluation of family therapy in anorexia nervosa and bulimia nervosa. *Arch Gen Psychiatry.* 1987;44(12):1047-1056

75. Eisler I, Dare C, Russell GF, Szmukler G, Le Grange D, Dodge E. Family and individual therapy in anorexia nervosa. A 5-year follow-up. *Arch Gen Psychiatry.* 1997;54 (11):1025-1030

76. Dare C, Eisler I. A multi-family group day treatment program for adolescent eating disorders. *Eur Eat Disord Rev.* 2000;8:4-18

77. Scholz M, Asen KE. Multiple family therapy with eating disordered adolescents. *Eur Eat Disord Rev.* 2001;9:33-42

78. Lock J, Le Grange D, Agra W, Dare C. *Treatment Manual for Anorexia Nervosa; a Family Based Approach.* New York, NY: Guilford Press; 2001

79. Lock J, Agras WS, Bryson S, Kraemer HC. A comparison of short- and long-term family therapy for adolescent anorexia nervosa. *J Am Acad Child Adolesc Psychiatry.* 2005;44(7): 632-639

80. Robin AL, Siegel PT, Koepke T, Moye AW, Tice S. Family therapy versus individual therapy for adolescent females with anorexia nervosa. *J Dev Behav Pediatr.* 1994;15(2):111-116

81. Robin AL, Siegel PT, Moye AW, Gilroy M, Dennis AB, Sikand A. A controlled comparison of family versus individual therapy for adolescents with anorexia nervosa. *J Am Acad Child Adolesc Psychiatry.* 1999;38(12):1482-1489

82. Geist R, Heinmaa M, Stephens D, Davis R, Katzman DK. Comparison of family therapy and family group psychoeducation in adolescents with anorexia nervosa. *Can J Psychiatry.* 2000;45(2):173-178

83. Attia E, Haiman C, Walsh BT, Flater SR. Does fluoxetine augment the inpatient treatment of anorexia nervosa? *Am J Psychiatry.* 1998;155(4):548-551

84. Zhu AJ, Walsh BT. Pharmacologic treatment of eating disorders. *Can J Psychiatry.* 2002;47(3):227-234

85. Kaye WH, Nagata T, Weltzin TE, et al. Double-blind placebo-controlled administration of fluoxetine in restricting- and restricting-purging-type anorexia nervosa. *Biol Psychiatry.* 2001;49(7):644-652

86. Walsh BT, Kaplan AS, Attia E, et al. Fluoxetine after weight restoration in anorexia nervosa: a randomized controlled trial. *JAMA.* 2006;295(22):2605-2612

87. Lock J, Walker LR, Rickert VI, Katzman DK. Suicidality in adolescents being treated with antidepressant medications and the black box label: position paper of the Society for Adolescent Medicine. *J Adolesc Health.* 2005;36(1):92-93

88. Fisher M. The course and outcome of eating disorders in adults and in adolescents: a review. *Adolesc Med.* 2003;14(1):149-158

89. Herpertz-Dahlmann B, Muller B, Herpertz S, Heussen N, Hebebrand J, Remschmidt H. Prospective 10-year follow-up in adolescent anorexia nervosa—course, outcome, psychiatric comorbidity, and psychosocial adaptation. *J Child Psychol Psychiatry.* 2001;42(5):603-612

90. Herzog DB, Nussbaum KM, Marmor AK. Co-morbidity and outcome in eating disorders. *Psychiatr Clin North Am.* 1996;19(4):843-859

91. Steinhausen HC, Boyadjieva S, Griogoroiu-Serbanescu M, Neumarker KJ. The outcome of adolescent eating disorders: findings from an international collaborative study. *Eur Child Adolesc Psychiatry.* 2003;12(Suppl 1):I91-I98

92. Strober M, Freeman R, Morrell W. The long-term course of severe anorexia nervosa in adolescents: survival analysis of recovery, relapse, and outcome predictors over 10-15 years in a prospective study. *Int J Eat Disord.* 1997;22(4):339-360

93. Sullivan PF. Mortality in anorexia nervosa. *Am J Psychiatry.* 1995;152(7):1073-1074

94. Keel PK, Dorer DJ, Eddy KT, Franko D, Charatan DL, Herzog DB. Predictors of mortality in eating disorders. *Arch Gen Psychiatry.* 2003; 60(2):179-183

# CHAPTER 77

## Bulimia Nervosa

MARK A. GOLDSTEIN, MD • DAVID B. HERZOG, MD

Bulimia nervosa is an eating disorder that is characterized by excessive eating and self-induced purging. "Bulimia" is a derivative of the Greek word for hunger. "Nervosa" is added to connect this disorder with anorexia nervosa, which is also marked by a pursuit of weight loss and fear of fatness.

For more than 2,000 years there have been references to the concept of "bulimos" as a powerful sensation of hunger; some writers, including Galen, referred to hunger followed by fainting.[1] The modern concept of bulimia nervosa developed after the middle of the 20th century. Russell[2] in 1979 described 30 patients who had an irresistible urge to overeat followed by self-induced vomiting or purging. Each had a morbid fear of becoming fat. Bulimia nervosa was added to the *DSM-III* in 1980. Patients with bulimia nervosa can be overweight, underweight, or normal weight.

### EPIDEMIOLOGY

In the past 60 years, there has been a steady increase in the numbers of adolescents with eating disorders. For adult women, the lifetime prevalence of bulimia nervosa is estimated to range from 1% to 4.2%.[3] The point prevalence for bulimia nervosa is up to 4% in a sample of adolescents from New York state.[4] About 10% to 15% of all bulimic patients are male, and about 0.2% of all adolescent and young adult males fit the criteria for bulimia nervosa.[5]

The onset of bulimia nervosa in females is generally between 15 and 18 years, whereas the onset in males is more typically between 18 and 26 years.[6] Males usually have a longer delay between the onset of bulimia nervosa and start of first treatment.

A history of sexual abuse has been reported to be common in patients with bulimia nervosa.[3] In addition, patients with bulimia nervosa have a higher likelihood of having experienced physical neglect and molestation. Homosexuality or bisexuality is reported to be common among males with bulimia nervosa.[5]

Studies have reported that up to 83% of adolescent patients with bulimia nervosa will have an additional psychiatric disorder over their lifetime.[4] These conditions include major depression (50%-75%), bipolar illness (4%-6%), anxiety disorder (13%-65%), social phobia (17%), and substance abuse (42%).[3,4,6,7]

### ETIOLOGY

Societal pressure to be thin has been shown to lead to increases in body dissatisfaction, resulting in dieting and a negative sense of self, which are risk factors for bulimia nervosa.[4] Childhood overanxious disorder and social phobia may be other risk factors for bulimia nervosa. Mothers who have experienced an eating disorder may also represent a risk factor for the adolescent.[3] In addition, compulsive exercise may precipitate bulimia nervosa; ballet dancers, gymnasts, and wrestlers may be particularly vulnerable to the onset of bulimia nervosa, although a distinction must be made between those who utilize bulimic behaviors only as a way to meet weight goals for their chosen activity and those who develop the full syndrome of bulimia nervosa.

Males with bulimia nervosa often have a significant family history of parental substance abuse, affective disorder, or parental overweight.[5] In addition, males with bulimia nervosa are more likely to have a history of premorbid obesity. Heritability estimates in twin studies range from 31% to 83% in bulimia nervosa.[4] Families of patients with bulimia nervosa display higher levels of perfectionism with an increased sense of ineffectiveness.[3]

### DIAGNOSIS

The *DSM-IV-TR* criteria for bulimia nervosa are listed in Box 77-1.[8] At least half of adolescents with eating disorders who present for specialty care do not fully meet the criteria for eating disorders and are assigned the diagnosis of Eating Disorder Not Otherwise Specified (EDNOS). Adolescents may not binge as frequently as specified in the criteria nor do some adolescents with bulimia feel as if they are eating a large amount of food. It is also difficult to quantify excessive exercise.[4] Nonetheless, adolescents with either bingeing or purging behaviors must be treated for bulimia nervosa, whether or not they meet full *DSM* criteria.

## Box 77-1

### *Diagnostic Criteria for Bulimia Nervosa*

1. Recurrent episodes of binge eating. An episode of binge eating is characterized by both of the following:
   (a) Eating within a discrete period of time (eg, within any 2-hour period) an amount of food that is definitely larger than most people would eat during a similar period of time and under similar circumstances
   (b) A sense of lack of control over eating during the episode (eg, a feeling that one cannot stop eating or control what or how much one is eating)
2. Recurrent inappropriate compensatory behavior to prevent weight gain, such as self-induced vomiting; misuse of laxatives, diuretics, enemas, or other medications; fasting; or excessive exercise
3. The binge eating and inappropriate compensatory behaviors both occur, on average, at least twice weekly for 3 months
4. Self-evaluation is unduly influenced by body shape and weight
5. The disturbance does not occur exclusively during episodes of anorexia nervosa

**Types:**

- Purging: patient regularly engages in self-induced vomiting or use of laxatives or diuretics
- Nonpurging: patient uses other inappropriate compensatory behaviors (ie, fasting or hyperexercising) without regular use of vomiting or medications to purge

Reprinted with permission from American Psychiatric Association. *Diagnostic and Statistical Manual of Mental Disorders,* Fourth Ed, Text Revision. Washington, DC: American Psychiatric Association; 2000:594

The *DSM-IV-TR* criteria for bulimia nervosa listed in Box 77-1 indicate that recurrent binge eating is a key to establishing the official diagnosis of bulimia nervosa. This may be the patient's perception of binge eating or, in fact, the actual consumption of large amounts of food. Studies have shown the amount of calories consumed during reported binges to range from as low as 200 to as high as 6,000. Patients often describe that they have no control over their eating during a binge.[4]

The second criterion, inappropriate behavior(s) performed to prevent weight gain, include purging behaviors such as the induction of vomiting or use of laxatives, diet pills, diuretics, or (rarely) ipecac. Nonpurging behaviors include excessive exercise or fasting. Two subtypes, purging and nonpurging, are described to distinguish between these behaviors. Patients who binge but do not have a mechanism for eliminating calories are classified as having a newly described *DSM* diagnosis, binge-eating disorder, which generally results in obesity and is not commonly seen in the adolescent age range.

As is the case for all patients with the official diagnosis of an eating disorder, the self-image of patients with bulimia nervosa is unduly influenced by body weight or shape. Questions formulated to elicit responses indicative of the patient's self-image are noted in Figure 77-1. This criterion may be particularly difficult to interpret because many adolescent females normatively have excessive concerns about their body shape and weight.[4]

## EVALUATION

Because the symptoms and signs of bulimia nervosa are less apparent than those of anorexia nervosa, careful screening for an eating disorder is needed. Figure 77-1 lists questions about weight history, body image, disordered thinking, exercise, and menstrual history which are important elements in eliciting information that could lead to a diagnosis of bulimia nervosa or other eating disorders.

A careful system review is important. Patients with bulimia nervosa may complain of dry skin, dental symptoms, halitosis, sore throat, excessive thirst, puffy face, broken blood vessels under the eyes, lightheadedness, and stomach pain. Menses may be irregular or absent. Despite careful questioning to screen for bulimia nervosa, adolescents may still present without any symptoms on review and many patients hide their behaviors for as long as possible.

Certain behaviors may suggest an undisclosed eating disorder, especially bulimia nervosa.[4,7] These include difficulty eating in social settings, weight fluctuations, social withdrawal, excessive exercise, and change in eating habits. Frequent trips to the bathroom after meals usually are a red flag.

Box 77-2 lists the physical signs that may be encountered in an adolescent with bulimia nervosa. Although there may be multisystem signs of bulimia nervosa, most adolescent patients present with a normal appearance and physical examination.

The differential diagnosis of an adolescent with suspected bulimia nervosa will generally encompass the differential diagnosis of eating disorders. With respect to recurrent vomiting and/or diarrhea, thought should be given to malignancy, especially those tumors that may cause increased intracranial pressure. Inflammatory bowel disease as well as celiac disease should also be considered. In regard to endocrine etiologies, review of possible pathology in the pituitary axis should be

(A) Male Lifestyle Questionnaire

Your Name: ______________________ Date: ______________________

Medical Doctor: ______________________ Nutritionist: ______________________

Mental Health Clinician(s): ______________________ ______________________

## I. Personal Health History

A. Please list any major medical problems:

______________________________________________

______________________________________________

B. Please list any medications you are currently taking:

______________________________________________

______________________________________________

C. Please list any over-the-counter medications that you are currently taking:

______________________________________________

______________________________________________

## II. Weight and Height History

A. What is your present height? __________ B. What is your present weight? __________
C. What is your highest weight? __________ D. When was your highest weight? __________
E. What is your lowest weight? __________ F. When was your lowest weight? __________
G. What was your weight at the onset of the eating disorder? __________

**Circle your answer to the following questions:**

H. Are you satisfied, dissatisfied, distressed with your current weight?
I. Are you satisfied, dissatisfied, distressed with your current body shape?
J. Have you ever thought that you were too fat or in danger of getting too fat? Yes No
K. Do you feel that way now? Yes No
L. Do you enjoy losing weight or refusing food? Yes No
M. Have you ever been concerned that you are too thin? Yes No
N. How do you feel when you lose two pounds?

______________________________________________

O. How do you feel when you gain two pounds?

______________________________________________

P. At what weight would you like to be? __________
Q. How often do you weigh yourself? __________
R. What percent of the day are your thoughts occupied with food, eating, body size, or body shape?

______________________________________________

**III. Exercise History**

A. Do you exercise regularly? Yes No B. How frequently do you exercise? ____________

C. If you exercise, what do you do? ____________________________________________

D. How long are your workouts? ______________________________________________

**IV. Diet History**

A. Do you restrict your calories? Yes No How many calories do you eat in a day? ________

B. Do you restrict certain types of foods? If so, please list: ____________________________

Do you skip meals? Yes No

C. Do you have problems controlling food intake? Yes No

D. Do you engage in any of the following behaviors (please circle)?

| | | |
|---|---|---|
| Vomiting: | Yes | No |
| Spitting: | Yes | No |
| Ruminating: | Yes | No |
| Laxative use: | Yes | No |
| Diuretic use: | Yes | No |
| Diet pill use: | Yes | No |
| Ipecac use: | Yes | No |

E. Please give a detailed description of what you ate in the past 24 hours:

______________________________________________________________________________

______________________________________________________________________________

**V. Symptom Review**

If you have experienced any of the following, please circle:

1. Thinning hair
2. Irregular heartbeat
3. Diminished sleep
4. Sensitivity to cold
5. Shrinking muscle mass
6. Muscle cramping
7. Swollen glands in cheeks
8. Puffy face
9. Broken blood vessels under eyes
10. Weakness
11. Lightheadedness
12. Excessive thirst
13. Chronic sore throat
14. Slow heartbeat
15. Rapid heartbeat
16. Fat loss
17. Diarrhea
18. Constipation
19. Stomach pain
20. Dry skin
21. Brittle nails
22. Problems with concentration
23. Depression
24. Anxiety
25. Anemia
26. Suicidal thoughts
27. Bone pain
28. Hernia

## (B) Female Lifestyle Questionnaire

Your Name: ______________________ Date: ______________________

Medical Doctor: ______________________ Nutritionist: ______________________

Mental Health Clinician(s): ______________________ ______________________

### I. Personal Health History

A. Please list any major medical problems:

______________________________________________

______________________________________________

B. Please list any medications you are currently taking:

______________________________________________

______________________________________________

C. Please list any over-the-counter medications that you are currently taking:

______________________________________________

______________________________________________

### II. Weight and Height History

A. What is your present height? ____________ B. What is your present weight? ____________
C. What is your highest weight? ____________ D. When was your highest weight? ____________
E. What is your lowest weight? ____________ F. When was your lowest weight? ____________
G. What was your weight at the onset of the eating disorder? ____________

**Circle your answer to the following questions:**

H. Are you satisfied, dissatisfied, distressed with your current weight?
I. Are you satisfied, dissatisfied, distressed with your current body shape?
J. Have you ever thought that you were too fat or in danger of getting too fat? Yes No
K. Do you feel that way now? Yes No
L. Do you enjoy losing weight or refusing food? Yes No
M. Have you ever been concerned that you are too thin? Yes No
N. How do you feel when you lose two pounds?

______________________________________________

O. How do you feel when you gain two pounds?

______________________________________________

P. At what weight would you like to be? ____________
Q. How often do you weigh yourself? ____________
R. What percent of the day are your thoughts occupied with food, eating, body size, or body shape?

______________________________________________

**III. Exercise History**

A. Do you exercise regularly? Yes No B. How frequently do you exercise? ____________

C. If you exercise, what do you do? ____________

D. How long are your workouts? ____________

**IV. Menstrual History**

A. When was your very first menstrual period? ____________

B. When was your last menstrual period? ____________

C. How many menstrual periods have you had in the past 6 months? ____________

**V. Diet History**

A. Do you restrict your calories? Yes No How many calories do you eat in a day? ________

B. Do you restrict certain types of foods? If so, please list: ____________

Do you skip meals? Yes No

C. Do you have problems controlling food intake? Yes No

D. Do you engage in any of the following behaviors (please circle)?

| | | |
|---|---|---|
| Vomiting: | Yes | No |
| Spitting: | Yes | No |
| Ruminating: | Yes | No |
| Laxative use: | Yes | No |
| Diuretic use: | Yes | No |
| Diet pill use: | Yes | No |
| Ipecac use: | Yes | No |

E. Please give a detailed description of what you ate in the past 24 hours:

____________

____________

**VI. Symptom Review**

If you have experienced any of the following, please circle:

1. Thinning hair
2. Diminished sleep
3. Sensitivity to cold
4. Shrinking muscle mass
5. Muscle cramping
6. Swollen glands in cheeks
7. Puffy face
8. Broken blood vessels under eyes
9. Weakness
10. Lightheadedness
11. Excessive thirst
12. Chronic sore throat
13. Slow heartbeat
14. Rapid heartbeat
15. Fat loss
16. Irregular heartbeat
17. Diarrhea
18. Constipation
19. Stomach pain
20. Dry skin
21. Brittle nails
22. Problems with concentration
23. Depression
24. Anxiety
25. Loss of periods
26. Painful periods
27. Heavy periods
28. Anemia
29. Suicidal thoughts
30. Bone pain

FIGURE 77-1 Lifestyle questionnaires (A) male (B) female. (Courtesy Mark A. Goldstein, MD.)

**Box 77-2**

***Physical Signs of Bulimia Nervosa***

**Vital signs:** bradycardia, hypothermia, orthostatic changes in blood pressure and/or pulse
**Skin:** periorbital petechiae, Russell's sign (calluses over the knuckles due to induction of emesis), swelling of hands and feet, dryness, lack of hair sheen
**Orofacial:** mouth sores, palatal scratches, dental caries, enamel erosion, parotid gland enlargement, submandibular adenopathy
**Gastrointestinal:** gastric dilation, abdominal fullness
**Cardiac:** arrythmia, mitral valve prolapse murmur
**Musculoskeletal:** weakness
**Metabolic:** pitting edema, poor skin turgor, Chvostek sign, Truousseau sign
**Neurological:** cognitive impairment, irritability

considered. Thyroid dysfunction, Addison disease, and pregnancy require specific attention in the differential diagnosis. Psychiatric etiologies should be considered, including major depression or obsessive-compulsive disorder. The clinician should recognize that the adolescent with bulimia nervosa may also have concurrent medical and/or psychiatric comorbidities.

Box 77-3 lists laboratory examinations that may be considered in the evaluation of an adolescent with bulimia nervosa. Clinical judgment is needed to determine the tests that should be performed for a particular patient.

Purging by vomiting or use of laxatives or diuretics can result in electrolyte disturbances.[6] Each of these modalities can cause hypokalemia. Chlorides are generally reduced in vomiting or diuretic use but may be increased or decreased in laxative abuse.[6] Sodium may be unchanged, increased, or decreased in vomiting but will be increased or normal with laxative use and decreased or normal in diuretic use.[6] The bicarbonate is usually increased in vomiting or diuretic use and decreased or increased in laxative use.[6] The serum pH is usually increased with vomiting and diuretic use and decreased or increased with laxative use.

**Box 77-3**

***Laboratory Evaluations in Bulimia Nervosa***

- Complete blood count with differential
- Electrolytes, blood urea nitrogen, glucose, creatinine, total protein, albumen, magnesium, phosphorous, calcium, liver function tests
- Urinalysis
- Electrocardiogram
- Depending on clinical status, consider ESR, estradiol, prolactin, FSH, LH, HCG, amylase, lipase, TSH, celiac panel, toxicology screen, creatine phosphokinase
- For prolonged amenorrhea, consider dual-energy x-ray absorptiometry

ESR, erythrocyte sedimentation rate; FSH, follicular stimulating hormone; LH, luteinizing hormone; HCG, human chorionic gonadotropin; TSH, thyroid stimulating hormone

Some clinicians use urine levels of electrolytes to help determine if a patient has bulimia nervosa. Table 77-1 lists the urine levels of sodium, potassium, and chloride according to the method of purging.[7] Urine pH is often increased in those who are vomiting.

In a patient with nonpurging bulimia nervosa, the urine and serum electrolytes should be normal. Some clinicians use creatine phosphokinase values to monitor patients who are suspected of excessive exercise. A serum amylase may be helpful in determining if a patient is purging by vomiting; if necessary, further testing can be used to distinguish between salivary and pancreatic causes of elevated amylase levels. Some clinicians also obtain a pancreatic lipase to help determine if an elevated amylase is due to salivary gland dysfunction

**Table 77-1**

**Urine Electrolyte Levels Associated with Purging**

| | *Urine Levels* | | |
|---|---|---|---|
| ***Method of Purging*** | ***Sodium*** | ***Potassium*** | ***Chloride*** |
| Vomiting | Decreased | Increased | Decreased |
| Laxative use | Decreased | Decreased | Normal or decreased |
| Diuretic use | Increased | Increased | Increased |

Reprinted with permission from Mehler PS. Bulimia nervosa. *N Engl J Med*. 2003;349:875–881.

in bulimia nervosa or to pancreatitis, which can also coexist with bulimia nervosa.

In adolescents with bulimia nervosa, the electrocardiogram may be normal or it may demonstrate abnormalities. Hypokalemia may cause depressed ST segments, and in severe cases it may cause widening of the QRS complex, increased P-wave amplitude and increased PR intervals.[3] Syrup of ipecac can cause muscle destruction, cardiac arrhythmias, cardiomyopathy, heart failure, and death.[4,9]

## MEDICAL COMPLICATIONS

Complications of bulimia nervosa can occur in many different organ systems. Electrolyte disturbances due to purging can cause seizures (from hyponatremia), arrhythmias (from hypokalemia), and death. Recurrent vomiting can produce esophagitis, gastrointestinal reflux, Mallory-Weiss tears, esophageal rupture, gastric rupture, and bloody diarrhea (due to laxative abuse). Laxative abuse may also lead to chronic constipation, especially when patients attempt to stop their use. Purging can cause hypovolemia and hypotension with possible syncopal episodes. Due to volume depletion from purging, secondary hyperaldosteronism may occur with loss of potassium in the urine and resultant hypokalemia. This can also lead to the development of edema on cessation of laxative or diuretic use.

Recurrent purging from vomiting has been shown to cause aspiration pneumonia, pneumothorax, and pneumomediastinum. In terms of neurological complications, there have been patients with bulimia nervosa who have abused diet pills and sustained intracranial bleeding as a sequela. Neurological complications from bulimia nervosa also include mood disorders and cognitive impairment.[3] Patients with bulimia nervosa often have irregular menstrual cycles even with normal weights, and they may have reduced levels of serum estrogen. For women with bulimia nervosa who have prolonged amenorrhea greater than 6 months, there is an increased risk for osteopenia or osteoporosis.[3] Males with bulimia nervosa have similar medical complications as do females with the disorder.[10]

## TREATMENT

Treatment of adolescents with bulimia nervosa should address the biological, psychological, and social domains of the adolescent and their illness. A long-term study[11] of women with bulimia nervosa found 74% achieving full recovery by a median of 90 months of follow-up. Another study[12] reported that earlier identification and earlier initiation of treatment for female patients with bulimia nervosa led to a higher likelihood of recovery in the study follow-up period, which was 9 years.

The goals of treatment include:[3]

- Recognizing and treating the medical complications of bulimia nervosa
- Reducing and eliminating binge eating and purging
- Enhancing the patient's motivation to restore healthy eating patterns and participate in treatment
- Providing the patient with information on healthy eating and nutrition
- Helping the patient to change core thinking, attitudes, and conflicts in regard to the bulimia
- Treating associated psychiatric conditions

An optimal way to reach these goals is to establish a multidisciplinary team comprising a physician, nutritionist, therapist, and psychiatrist, all of whom are experienced in the management of adolescent patients with eating disorders.[13] The team should be able to communicate freely. Levels of care for the treatment of bulimia nervosa include inpatient hospitalization, residential care, and outpatient care. Outpatient care may be intensive, such as a day or evening program 3 to 5 times weekly, or more standard weekly sessions in an office setting, which is the approach utilized for most patients.

The indications for inpatient hospitalization for adolescents with bulimia nervosa are listed in Box 77-4.[14] Other indications include gastrointestinal bleeding, aspiration pneumonia, and pneumomediastinum. Depending on available resources and clinical judgment, the hospitalization could be in a psychiatric facility, medical facility, or a location where both medical and mental health specialties collaborate on-site. These indications are guidelines

**Box 77-4**

***Admission Criteria for Bulimia Nervosa***

1. Syncope
2. Serum potassium concentration <3.2 mmol/L
3. Serum chlorides <88 mmol/L
4. Esophageal tears
5. Cardiac arrythmias, including prolonged QTc
6. Hypothermia
7. Suicide risk
8. Intractable vomiting
9. Hematemesis
10. Failure to respond to outpatient treatment

Source: American Academy of Pediatrics, Committee on Adolescence. Identifying and treating eating disorders. *Pediatrics.* 2003;111:204–211.

and are subject to clinical judgment. In contrast to the patient with anorexia nervosa who may require a relatively long hospitalization to accomplish significant weight gain, patients with bulimia nervosa generally have shorter hospitalizations aimed at stabilizing electrolyte values and breaking the binge–purge cycle.

The clinician responsible for the medical care of the adolescent with bulimia nervosa often assumes the role of team leader. For some patients this may be the primary care physician, or it may be a physician trained in adolescent medicine and the management of eating disorders.[15] This physician coordinates care and communicates with other treatment team members, because communication and coordination are key to the care of all adolescents with eating disorders, including those with bulimia nervosa.

Patients with bulimia nervosa may be seen weekly initially, with variations based on clinical assessment. The clinician should monitor vital signs, including sitting, supine, and standing pulse and blood pressure in order to evaluate for orthostatic signs. Hypotensive and orthostatic changes can occur in those who are having repeated and frequent purging activities, especially if there are weight fluctuations as well. If these are seen, the patient may require a hospital admission for fluid replacement.

Regular dental care is needed for adolescents with bulimia nervosa because they may develop dental erosions, caries, and complications from dental decay due to induced emesis. The adolescent with bulimia nervosa should be encouraged to brush and use a fluoride mouthwash after vomiting.[6] Sialadenosis responds to the cessation of vomiting and application of heat to the parotid area.[6]

For gastroesophageal reflux symptomatology, over-the-counter or prescription H2 blockers are indicated. Some patients may require proton pump inhibitors. Patients who purge using laxatives often encounter constipation after the laxative use is discontinued. Retraining proper bowel habits is necessary. Increased hydration and a high-fiber diet or fiber supplementation may be helpful.[10]

Patients with hypokalemia may require inpatient hospitalization to replenish body potassium. Some clinicians will treat mild hypokalemia (3.0–3.3 mmol/L) with oral supplementation of potassium chloride (20 mEq 2 times daily) until the patient is repleted, but this must be done with careful supervision. It is important that the patient also be in proper fluid balance to turn off the renin-angiotensin system. The patient should continue to be under surveillance for recurrent potassium losses. Because cardiac arrhythmia due to hypokalemia is a significant cause of mortality in those with eating disorders, it is important that careful monitoring be performed.

Patients with irregular menstrual periods, amenorrhea, or a history of anorexia nervosa may be at risk for bone loss. Oral calcium, 1,300 to 1,500 mg daily, and vitamin D, 400 IU/day, should be recommended.[13] In a clinical trial report, treatment of osteopenia with estrogen, as used in oral contraceptives, was not shown to help bone mineralization in patients with anorexia nervosa.[16] In addition, estrogen replacement did not stop progressive osteopenia in these patients. Also, false reassurances can be given to the patient if there is monthly bleeding due to oral contraception. However, there are ongoing studies in patients with anorexia nervosa and osteopenia using estrogen, testosterone, biphosphonates, and other medications to determine if bone loss can be ameliorated by these treatments.

There have been no randomized controlled studies published on the psychological treatment of adolescents with bulimia nervosa.[4] Adult-based studies have been used as the basis for psychological treatment of adolescents. Cognitive behavioral therapy (CBT) aimed at the bulimic symptoms is the psychosocial intervention that has been most extensively studied in adults. In a randomized clinical trial, CBT was noted to be more efficacious than interpersonal psychotherapy.[17] In adults, CBT has eliminated or reduced binge eating or purging in up to 50% of study subjects. However, it remains unclear whether CBT can be equally effective for adolescents, who are at various stages of cognitive development.

With rare exceptions, there have been no published, randomized controlled studies of pharmacological treatment for adolescents with bulimia nervosa, but medication has become a mainstay of treatment nonetheless.[4] In contrast to anorexia nervosa, in which selective serotonin uptake inhibitors (SSRIs) have generally not been shown to be effective, both fluoxetine and sertraline have demonstrated efficacy in the treatment of bulimia nervosa in reports of several double-blind, randomized clinical trials in adults.[18,19] These agents have been shown to reduce bingeing and purging by up to 75% in certain patients.[13] Other antidepressant medications that have been utilized include trazodone, tricyclic antidepressants such as imipramine, and several monoamine oxidase inhibitors (MAOIs), including phenelzine and isocarboxazid. These medications have been used in both adults and adolescents even though the US Food and Drug Administration (FDA) has officially approved only fluoxetine for the treatment of bulimia nervosa. Although the psychiatric member of the treatment team usually prescribes these medications, under certain circumstances the physician responsible for the medical care may be the appropriate clinician to manage this aspect of treatment. Because of a recent FDA Black Box warning regarding the development of suicidal ideation in some patients on SSRIs, care must be taken in prescribing these medications to adolescents. It is unclear whether antidepressant medication is useful for treatment of bulimia nervosa through an indirect effect on depression or a direct effect on the urge to binge or purge, but clinical experience leans toward the latter explanation.

Topiramate, an antiseizure medication, has been shown to be effective in the treatment of bulimia nervosa in a few studies. Ondansetron, which is used for nausea, decreases vagal neurotransmission and should impede vomiting. However, ondansetron is expensive, needs to be taken several times a day to be effective, and is rarely used.

The nutritionist on the treatment team needs to support the adolescent in normalizing food consumption. The nutritionist should also educate the patient in food choices, weight management, and the dangers inherent from bulimia nervosa.[15]

When possible, and based on clinical need, the mental health treatment team for adolescents may also include a family therapist. Some adolescents do well with individual therapy combined with group therapy. Intensive outpatient treatment programs may also be helpful. These may include sessions from 3 to 5 times weekly during the daytime or evening. In these settings, patients eat together as a group and also have therapeutic group sessions.

Generally, adolescents with bulimia nervosa should be treated in the least restrictive setting where effective treatment can be provided.[4] Some adolescents are admitted to residential treatment settings after having failed several trials of outpatient treatment. In these settings, patients receive intensive individual and group treatment 24 hours per day. Patients in residential facilities are "stepped down" to outpatient treatment after achieving certain goals. Because purging behaviors tend to recur in many patients with bulimia nervosa, both adolescents and adults, it is not uncommon for patients to require several modalities of treatment in various settings over time.

Overeaters Anonymous has been a helpful option for some patients in preventing relapse. There is some evidence, through a randomized clinical trial, that CBT can be administered successfully to some adults with bulimia nervosa through self-help guides or manuals while the patient receives pharmacotherapy.[20] There are no studies on the efficacy of self-help guides for adolescents.

## OUTCOME

There is considerable variability over the long-term course and prognosis of bulimia nervosa, but most adolescents recover; bulimia nervosa has a more favorable outcome than anorexia nervosa.[4,9] Bulimia nervosa that begins and is diagnosed and treated in adolescence tends to have a better outcome.[3] Early onset of treatment can be the key to improving outcomes, and 50% of patients have been reported to achieve full recovery within 2 years.[8] A history of childhood obesity[9] or obsessive-compulsive disorder[3] or low self-esteem[4] may be associated with a longer course of illness. Between 20% and 46% of adolescents with bulimia nervosa will continue to have eating disorder symptoms 6 years after diagnosis. Adolescents with bulimia nervosa have a fatality rate of approximately 0.5%.[4,9] More than 50% of adolescents with bulimia nervosa are reported to develop a mood disorder, and many will have frequent relapses after recovery.[9] There also appears to be an association between bulimia nervosa and acting-out behaviors, including substance use and promiscuity.[10] Even if the presentation of the adolescent patient does not meet all of the *DSM-IV-TR* criteria for bulimia nervosa, there will be a better outcome if treatment is started sooner.[21]

## PREVENTION

Prevention programs are needed to decrease the prevalence of bulimia nervosa in adolescents. Clinicians who give primary care to adolescents should have evidence-based questions that will help to identify adolescents who are at risk for bulimia nervosa. Conversations about healthy eating, exercise, and body mass index should occur between patient and clinician during adolescence and prior to college matriculation.[22] Research must be done on Web-based therapies, self-administered treatments, and the possible role of complementary therapies on the course of bulimia nervosa.[3]

## REFERENCES


1. Ziolko HU. Bulimia: a historical outline. *Int J Eat Disord.* 1996;20:345–358

2. Russell G. Bulimia nervosa: an ominous variant of anorexia nervosa. *Psychol Med.* 1979;9:429–448

3. Work Group on Eating Disorders. Practice guideline for the treatment of patients with eating disorders. 3rd ed. American Psychiatric Association Web site. 2006. Available at: www.psychiatryonline.com/pracGuide/pracGuideTopic_12.aspx. Accessed October 20, 2010

4. Evans DL, Foa EB, Gur RE, et al. *Treating and Preventing Adolescent Mental Health Disorders*. New York, NY: Oxford University Press; 2005

5. Carlat DJ, Camargo CA, Herzog DB. Eating disorders in males: a report on 135 patients. *Am J Psychiatry.* 1997;154:1127–1132

6. Mehler PS. Bulimia nervosa. *N Engl J Med.* 2003;349:875–881

7. Becker AE, Grinspoon SK, Klibanski A, Herzog DB. Eating disorders. *N Engl J Med.* 1999;340:1092-1098

8. American Psychiatric Association. *Diagnostic and Statistical Manual of Mental Disorders-Text Revision*. 4th ed. Washington, DC: American Psychiatric Association; 2000

9. Schiff RJ, Wurzel CL, Brunson SC, Kasloff I, Nussbaum MP, Frank SD. Death due to chronic syrup of ipecac use in a patient with bulimia. *Pediatrics.* 1986;78:412-416

10. Muise AM, Stein DG, Arbess G. Eating disorders in adolescent boys: a review of the adolescent and young adult literature. *J Adol Health.* 2003;33:427-435

11. Herzog DB, Dorer DJ, Keel PK, et al. Recovery and relapse in anorexia and bulimia nervosa: a 7.5-year follow-up study. *J Am Acad Child Adolesc Psychiatry.* 1999;38:829-837

12. Reas DL, Williamson DA, Martin CK, Zucker NL. Duration of illness predicts outcome for bulimia nervosa: a long-term follow-up study. *Int J Eat Disord.* 2000;27:428-434

13. Society for Adolescent Medicine. Eating disorders in adolescents: position paper of the Society for Adolescent Medicine. *J Adol Health.* 2003;33:496-503

14. American Academy of Pediatrics, Committee on Adolescence. Identifying and treating eating disorders. *Pediatrics.* 2003; 111:204-211

15. Rome ES, Ammerman S, Rosen D, et al. Children and adolescents with eating disorders: the state of the art. *Pediatrics.* 2003;111:e98-e108. Available at: www.pediatrics.org/cgi/content/full/111/1/e98. Accessed July 16, 2006

16. Klibanski A, Biller BM, Schoenfeld DA, Herzog DB, Saxe VC. The effects of estrogen administration on trabecular bone loss in young women with anorexia nervosa. *J Clin Endocrinol Metab.* 1995;80:898-904

17. Agras WS, Walsh T, Fairburn CG, Wilson GT, Kraemer HC. A multicenter comparison of cognitive-behavioral interventions for bulimia nervosa. *Arch Gen Psychiatry.* 2000;57:459-466

18. Romano SJ, Halmi KA, Sarkar NP, Koke SC, Lee JS. A placebo-controlled study of fluoxetine in continued treatment of bulimia nervosa after successful acute fluoxetine treatment. *Am J Psychiatry.* 2002;159:96-102

19. Milano W, Petrella C, Sabatino C, Capasso A. Treatment of bulimia nervosa with sertraline: a randomized controlled trial. *Adv Ther.* 2004;21:232-237

20. Carter JC, Olmsted MP, Kaplan AS, McCabe RE, Mills JS, Aime A. Self-help for bulimia nervosa: a randomized controlled trial. *Am J Psychiatry.* 2003;160:973-978

21. Le Grange D, Lock KL, Van Orman S, Jellar CC. Bulimia nervosa in adolescents. *Arch Pediatr Adolesc Med.* 2004;158: 478-482

22. Goldstein MA. Preparing adolescent patients for college. *Curr Opin Pediatr.* 2002;14:384-388

# CHAPTER 78

## The Female Athlete Triad

ELLEN S. ROME, MD, MPH

In 1972, the passage of Title IX marked a noteworthy shift toward inclusiveness of girls and women in competitive sports at all levels. Prior to that year, women were banned from very challenging athletic events such as marathons because officials of the Amateur Athletic Union (AAU) believed that such competition would be harmful to the female reproductive tract.[1-3] More than 30 years later, such myths appear archaic, with women's sports flourishing worldwide and much national excitement generated over women's participation in many high school and college sports.

Despite these gains, however, girls and women in the United States still get somewhat shortchanged with respect to the athletic dollar.[1,2,4] This competition for scant resources can add to the pressures placed on the female athlete. These pressures can be self-imposed, can come from a girl's parents via "achievement by proxy," or can be imposed by coaches or society. These pressures can in turn push a girl beyond the limits of healthy athleticism into the spectrum of eating disorders, which may then be accompanied by menstrual irregularities and loss of bone (or failure to deposit bone at a key age). When the behaviors reach a critical point of disordered eating, amenorrhea, and osteoporosis in combination, the constellation of findings gets labeled as the female athlete triad (which unfortunately has the acronym, the FAT). More recently, the FAT has been articulately described as low-energy availability (defined in athletes as dietary energy intake minus exercise energy expenditure) that then suppresses estradiol and certain metabolic hormones, with a resultant progressive loss of bone density.[5] The "visual" sports, where leanness has added value and performance remains heavily reliant on aesthetics (eg, ballet, gymnastics, figure skating), may put certain predisposed athletes at particular risk.[6]

In 1997, the American College of Sports Medicine published a position statement on the FAT, indicating a strong need for more epidemiological, laboratory, and clinical data to support the importance of this syndrome. This statement also documented risk for not only the elite female athlete but also for the noncompetitive, physically active girl/woman.[7] This chapter reviews the epidemiology of the triad, methodological problems in studying the triad, and practical applications for management and prevention.

### EPIDEMIOLOGY

The formal definition of the FAT was established in 1992. Although parts of the triad have been well studied since then, the prevalence of the full triad has not been well established. For instance, studies have shown that 3.4% to 66% of female athletes have amenorrhea, as compared to only 2% to 5% of the general population.[8,9] Further, 15% to 62% of female college athletes have been found to have disordered eating, in contrast with 5% to 10% in the general population.[10-12] A recent study of prevalence of the FAT among high school athletes found 18.2% of girls meeting the criteria for disordered eating, 23.5% for menstrual irregularity, and 21.8% for low bone mass, with 5.9% meeting 2 out of the 3 criteria, and 1.2% meeting criteria for all 3 components of the triad.[13] Although the percentage of girls engaging in pathogenic eating behaviors was relatively small, 24% of the girls engaging in abnormal eating behaviors used 2 or more different pathogenic behaviors in the month prior to the survey and 47% reported having engaged in pathogenic behaviors at least 4 times in the past month. Girls with oligomenorrhea or amenorrhea were more likely than eumenorrheic athletes to demonstrate abnormal eating attitudes and behaviors and were more likely to have lower bone mineral density. This study, like most others, represents a relatively finite snapshot of time; a substantial number of these young athletes might be expected to develop the full-blown triad over time without appropriate anticipatory guidance and intervention.

Researchers have tried to elucidate whether it is the elite athlete or the casual athlete who is most at risk for the FAT. In Norway, Torstveit and Sundgot-Borgen[14] surveyed 938 elite female athletes, ages 13 to 39 years, along with 900 age-matched controls. Participants were asked about diet, training, menses, oral contraceptive use, weight control methods and injuries, and completed the Body Dissatisfaction and Drive for Thinness subscales of the Eating Disorder Inventory. A total of 669 surveys completed by athletes and 607 surveys completed by controls were then analyzed, with 60.4% of athletes and 62.9% of controls classified as "at risk." Those who participated in aesthetic sports, such as ballet, dance, or figure skating were at greater risk than those who participated in athletic sports, such as soccer (66.4% vs 52.6%, $p < 0.001$).

In a related study, Torstveit and colleagues[15] also took a subgroup of elite and casual athletes to evaluate bone densitometry and perform clinical correlations. Of 186 athletes and 145 casual athletes, 8 elite athletes (4.6%) and 5 casual athletes (3.4%) met all criteria for the FAT. From these 2 studies, it has been concluded that risk for the FAT in Norwegian women is high in both elite and casual athletes. Reinking and Alexander[16] evaluated 84 college athletes and 62 nonathletes at a National Collegiate Athletic Association Division I institution in the United States. Data included questions on anthropometric measures, menstrual and exercise histories, and questions from the Eating Disorder Inventory. Results revealed no significant difference in the average body weights between the athletes and nonathletes, with 21% of both groups reporting amenorrhea or oligomenorrhea.

In a study of competitive and recreational male and female swimmers, runners, and soccer players at Stanford University, female athletes displayed disordered eating behaviors more commonly than males, with irregular periods found in 42.9% of female varsity athletes versus 13.4% of recreational female athletes.[17] Amenorrhea was found in 14.3% of varsity athletes versus 2.9% of recreational athletes.

## METHODOLOGIC PROBLEMS IN STUDYING THE FEMALE ATHLETE TRIAD

An important methodological flaw that occurs in studying the FAT is the use of cross-sectional data to describe the prevalence of each of its individual components in athletes versus nonathletes.[2] Only the Norwegian study described in the prior section evaluated simultaneous occurrence of all 3 components, resulting in the finding that the triad is rare and not significantly different among athletes and controls.[15] Several other studies have also found pieces but not all parts of the triad at one given point in time,[14,18,19] which highlights the methodological flaw of lack of longitudinal epidemiologic study; a percentage of these individuals might be expected, without appropriate intervention, to go on to the full-blown triad if studied over time.

Torsteit and Sundgot-Borgen[15,20] have been criticized for being too narrow in their definition of disordered eating, in contrast to the American College of Sports Medicine 1997 position statement, which included "inadvertently failing to balance energy expenditure with adequate energy intake" as a form of disordered eating; thus, the Norwegian data would have underestimated the prevalence of the triad.[21] Their data have also been criticized for not measuring energy intake and expenditure, for not measuring hormone levels, and for providing only a single measurement of low bone density, which is adequate in postmenopausal women but not in premenopausal women and adolescents, as epidemiological data relating bone density to the incidence of subsequent fractures are still lacking in this population.[5] Because Torsteit and Sundgot-Borgen did not measure bone density more than once, they could not document whether or not a decrease in age-matched standard deviation or Z-scores occurred. Loucks[5] argues that the lack of a dose–response relationship between the risk of triad disorders and the volume of training or level of physical activity found in their data is insufficient evidence to doubt the existence of the triad.

Other flaws include the continued reliance on self-reported data; differences between studies in the classification or definition of the 3 components; variability in study groups with regard to age, level of competition, or level of physical activity; and mixing of various terms that have very different behavioral and clinical significance, for example, disordered eating versus eating disorder.[1,2] Triad definitions have most recently been described on a continuum,[15,22] which allows for inclusiveness with respect to prevention and treatment efforts of those at risk. Thus, amenorrhea has been expanded to include menstrual cycle problems such as luteal and follicular phase dysfunctions, oligomenorrhea, and anovulation. The triad component of osteoporosis has been broadened to include osteopenia, low bone mineral density, and other measures of bone metabolism. Disordered eating can include the whole spectrum, from anorexia nervosa to bulimia nervosa to eating disorder not otherwise specified to merely "abnormal eating behaviors." From a methodologic point of view, this inclusiveness dilutes the pure "science"; it is advantageous from a clinical point of view, however, because prevention and intervention work best the earlier a problem is detected. Longitudinal data continue to be needed to clarify long-term risks.

DiPietro and Stachenfeld[1,2] have expressed concern that data related to the FAT could be misinterpreted and used as justification for setting health and social policies that may be counter to public health efforts to promote the benefits of athletic participation and an active lifestyle among children and adolescents. However, given the current public health focus on obesity, data related to the FAT are likely to help strike the right balance between combating obesity and having athletes engage in overzealous dieting in the face of intense athletics.

### INTERNATIONAL OLYMPIC COMMITTEE MEDICAL COMMISSION POSITION STAND: PRACTICAL APPLICATIONS

The International Olympic Committee (IOC) published a position statement on the FAT in 2005. According to this statement, primary amenorrhea is defined as no menarche by age 14 years in the absence of secondary sexual characteristics, or by 16 years of age with the appearance of normal growth and secondary sexual characteristics.[23] In either case, a critical time of bone deposition should occur between ages 11 and 14 years, with 40% to 60% of peak bone mass deposited in healthy girls at that time; girls with amenorrhea may be falling significantly behind in bone deposition, placing them at risk for stress fractures and osteoporosis. Secondary amenorrhea, defined as the absence of menstruation after cycles have been previously established, can vary in definition from the absence of periods for 3 to 6 consecutive months to 1 or fewer menstrual periods per year.[6] Education must continue for female athletes, their parents, and coaches on the body's need for estrogen as 1 of the 3 essential requirements for bone deposition (the other 2 being adequate calcium, or 1,200–1,500 mg per day for the young athlete, and weight-bearing exercise). Myths and misperceptions need to be addressed, for example, "She's on the pill, so we don't have to worry about periods and bones anymore," or "I've seen the Seasonale commercials, and I got periods on my own 3 times this year—January, February, and March—so I don't have to worry."

Pragmatically, few young athletes have progressed to a full definition of osteoporosis, or 2.5 standard deviations from below the mean for young adults. Osteopenia is defined strictly as bone mineral density between 1 and 2.5 standard deviations below the mean for young adults.[24] Redefining the triad to include osteopenia rather than osteoporosis allows for capturing athletes along the spectrum at risk, with more hope for reversal of bone loss with earlier detection.

Sports administrators may need to consider rule changes to discourage unhealthy weight-loss strategies, as was useful in wrestling when athletes were forbidden from dropping more than one weight category per season.[25] Recognition of any 1 of the 3 components of the FAT should provoke interventions to make sure that energy intake is in proper balance with energy expenditure without putting an athlete's mind or body at risk.

## MANAGEMENT

Side effects of extreme energy depletion include anemia, fatigue, electrolyte abnormalities, and depression; these medical complications need to be recognized and addressed (see Table 78-1). Each of these medical and psychological consequences of the FAT can impair an athlete's health and sense of well-being. The most basic treatment involves increasing energy intake while decreasing energy expenditure. Simple in premise, this task can seem insurmountable to the young athlete fixated on weight loss, or to her parent(s) who may feel they lack the knowledge and skills to change their child's behavior. Resources such as the book by Jim Lock and Daniel LeGrange, *Helping Your Teenager Beat an Eating Disorder* (New York: Guilford Press; 2005), can give concrete skills for enforcing an approach referred to as the Maudsley method, which involves placing food choices back in the hands of the parents until the teen is less brain starved and better able to perform self-care. Use of a dietitian skilled in the care of the elite athlete and versed in refeeding strategies in the face of disordered eating can be very useful. Therapists may be seen as threatening to many families; useful analogies include seeing the triad as a maladaptive coping strategy. In this analogy, the therapist can be likened to a highly skilled coach, whose skill set can make the difference between persisting problems and inability to get back to peak performance versus an expert resource to build an entirely new—and necessary—skill set. Questions that can be useful in identifying the FAT are presented in Box 78-1.

The challenge of regaining bone remains daunting. Anecdotally, a white male astronaut named Jerry Linenger, who lost 30% of his bone at age 40 years after 6 months on space station Mir, was found to regain 100% of that lost bone upon returning to earth. Granted, as an astronaut, Mr. Linenger had all the resources of NASA at his disposal, including extensive physical therapy and the support of a dietitian, allowing him to gain back his weight, strength, and bone simultaneously. However, if a white 40-year-old male astronaut can regain bone, it makes sense that young women with the FAT should be able to do the same, given proper diet, weight gain, and resistance training. Fredericson and Kent[26] provide a case study of a distance runner with the FAT followed from ages 22.9 to 30.8 years. Initially, the patient presented with primary amenorrhea at age 22.9 years with a body mass index (BMI) of 15.8 kg/m$^2$ and low bone mineral density (BMD) at the spine and hip (74% of normal, T score—2.50 and 80% of normal, T score—1.54, respectively). For the following 2 years, periods were induced with oral contraceptives but no significant

**Table 78-1**

**Medical Complications of the Female Athlete Triad**

| *Organ System* | *Complications* |
|---|---|
| Cardiovascular | Orthostatic hypotension<br>Sinus bradycardia in the face of a wasted cardiac muscle<br>Electrocardiographic abnormalities: low voltage, prolonged QTc, prominent u waves, atrial and ventricular arrhythmias, mitral valve prolapse, acrocyanosis |
| Gastrointestinal | Delayed GI motility<br>Constipation<br>Delayed gastric emptying<br>Bloating<br>Early satiety<br>Esophagitis<br>Mallory-Weiss tears<br>Esophageal rupture<br>Gastric rupture (latter four symptoms with purging)<br>Abnormal liver function tests<br>Elevated serum amylase (salivary- from vomiting) |
| Endocrine | Hypokalemia<br>Hyponatremia<br>Hypomagnesemia<br>Hypophosphatemia<br>Hypoglycemia<br>Hypothermia<br>Euthyroid sick syndrome<br>Elevated serum and urinary cortisol levels<br>Low serum estradiol levels<br>Amenorrhea<br>Oligomenorrhea<br>Delayed puberty<br>Growth failure<br>Stress fractures<br>Osteopenia/osteoporosis |
| Hematologic | Pancytopenia<br>Increased bleeding due to vitamin K deficiency |
| Renal | Decreased glomerular filtration rate<br>Renal calculi |
| Reproductive | Infertility<br>Insufficient weight gain during pregnancy<br>Low birth weight infants |
| Skin | Dry skin<br>Loss of shine/thickness and loss of hair<br>Lanugo<br>Russell's sign (calluses on the knuckles) |
| Dental | Dental caries on occlusol and lingual surfaces from vomiting |
| Neurologic | Peripheral neuropathy<br>Sciatica (from pressure)<br>Cortical atrophy |
| Fluid status | Dehydration<br>Edema<br>Electrolyte imbalances<br>Muscle cramps<br>Metabolic alkalosis<br>Fatigue |

### Box 78-1

#### *Useful Questions in Identifying the Female Athlete Triad*

What do you do for exercise? Level of intensity?
How stressed are you if you miss a workout?
What did you eat yesterday (quantity as well as quality) What foods do you avoid?
Do you count calories or fat grams? If so, how many do you allow yourself?
What is the most you ever weighed? At what height? When was that?
What is the least you ever weighed? At what height? When was that?
What do you think you should weigh? How much time/energy do you put into that?
What weight-control strategies have you tried? Have you ever tried vomiting? Diet pills? Laxatives? Diuretics? Other methods? (if yes, pursue which kinds, how much, how often)
When was your last period? The one before that? Have you missed any periods?
Have you ever had sex? If yes, what do you use for your 2 methods of contraception? Has anyone ever done anything to you sexually that made you uncomfortable?

weight gain occurred, and her bone mineral density remained essentially unchanged. At age 25.1 years, she consciously decided to gain weight and improve her nutrition; this resulted in small increases in spinal and hip BMD (+1.1% and +1.6%, respectively), and her total body bone mineral content increased by 7.6% in 4 months. By 30.8 years of age, she had reached a healthy BMI of 21.3 kg/m$^2$, with an increase in BMD of 25.5% at the spine and 19.5% at the hip (BMD now within normal, 94% at spine, 96% at hip). This case demonstrates that the answer to the FAT continues to be proper nutrition and weight gain for the significantly underweight athlete. It also demonstrates that there is no added value to hormone replacement in the FAT other than for the very low weight athlete or individual with anorexia nervosa to prevent significant ongoing loss.[27-32]

Bone formation is impaired in exercising girls and women when energy availability is reduced by more than 33%.[33] Exercise energy expenditure alone can induce reproductive dysfunction without specific disordered eating or dietary restriction.[21,34] So, if energy expenditure and/or dietary restriction occurs, the suppressive influence on bone formation outweighs the stimulatory osteogenic influence of physical activity, leaving bone at a deficit. Moreover, reproductive function and bone turnover are impaired not when physical activity is increased but when energy availability is reduced by more than 30%.[5,33,35] Amenorrheic athletes far exceed that number, having been shown to restrict their energy availability by an average of 67%.[36] The bottom line is that there is a degree of energy restriction that cannot be exceeded without impairing reproductive or bone health,[5] and those athletes (whether elite or noncompetitive) who display one or more components of the triad have exceeded that threshold. Nutritional rehabilitation, with modifications in training that can be fully accomplished, represents the cornerstone of treatment. Supportive psychological services and use of medications can help build the tools with which to enact these changes and help girls and women find strength and peace during and after the process. Finding peace of mind may be the hardest challenge for the girl or woman who is fully entrenched in an eating disorder; thus, prevention and early detection remain essential.

Hormonal therapy alone clearly does not seem to be the answer. One hypothesis is that estrogen helps to preserve bone mass in young women with anorexia nervosa by impairing osteoclast-mediated bone resoprtion.[37] In one retrospective study of young women with anorexia nervosa, oral contraceptive use was associated with a higher BMD.[38] In a small study of women with anorexia nervosa and hypothalamic amenorrhea, estrogen replacement therapy correlated with increases in bone mineral density.[39] Klibanski's[30] data on women with amenorrhea and anorexia nervosa suggested that weight gain was the main factor correlated with increases in bone mineral density, but in women of extremely low weight, oral contraceptives helped prevent further bone loss in the absence of weight gain. Other modalities, such as growth hormone and calcitonin, do not show great promise, whereas the bisphosphonates and dehydroepoandrosterone (DHEA) require further study for safety and efficacy.

## NUTRITIONAL ISSUES FOR THE ATHLETE

The necessity of gaining weight in order to improve health, so intuitive to caretakers and clinicians, is contrary to the eating-disordered part of the athlete, whether she started restrictive or insufficient eating to improve her sport, her looks, or her health. Nutritional insufficiency or disordered eating in the athlete may go undetected or overlooked until behaviors have become entrenched; early recognition and correction of nutritional imbalances is key in prevention. The nutritional insufficiency may begin unintentionally, with a failure to increase caloric intake in the face of increased energy expenditure during training.[6] Conversely, it may begin with an athlete's desire to improve performance by losing a few pounds, with the drive for weight loss or body control eventually superceding the drive for improved performance. In one study, female dance students ingested only 70% of the recommended daily allowance of energy intake to meet their needs, while professional ballerinas consumed only 80% of their needs.[40]

Disordered eating has an extremely negative effect on bone, with osteopenia best treated with weight gain accomplished by improved eating. Burrows et al[41] looked at female runners, finding that distance run per week was negatively associated with lumbar spine ($p = 0.035$) and femoral neck BMD ($p = 0.006$). Of the 52 athletes studied, 77% were eumenorrheic and 23% were oligo- or amenorrheic. There was no significant correlation between the distances run and the amount of energy/food consumed, in contrast to the logic that would suggest that longer runs should mean further energy intake. This form of disordered undereating in the face of exercise is a hallmark of the triad.

The role of leptin deserves further study. Leptin is secreted by adipocytes and has been linked with regulation of energy intake and energy expenditure.[42] Leptin inhibits the synthesis of neuropeptide Y (NPY, an appetite stimulant) after binding to a specific receptor on NPY-producing neurons in the hypothalamus.[43,44] Low leptin levels that occur during starvation suppress the reproductive access at the level of the hypothalamus, perhaps by lack of suppression of NPY.[43] Amenorrhea and disordered eating have been associated with low leptin levels,[45] and in 3 of 8 patients in one study, exogenous leptin administration was associated with a reversal of hypothalamic amenorrhea.[46] Appropriate levels of body fat used to be considered a necessary component, but Treasure and Russell[47] found one elite athlete to be eumenorrheic despite an incredibly low body fat of 4.7%, suggesting that the relationship is not so clear-cut.

## PREVENTION

As articulately outlined in the IOC Position Stand on the FAT[6] physicians, trainers, and health care providers need to provide ongoing education of athletes and coaches to recognize that weight loss does not necessarily ensure improvement in athletic performance. The position statement goes on to recommend that coaches should not be involved in decisions regarding weight or body composition but should refer athletes to health care providers to help with management of optimal weight and energy intake. Parents need to be added to this equation, as well, with education reinforcing that extreme dieting results in loss of muscle mass as well as fat, with resultant deterioration of performance.

Heightened awareness, along with a highly trained skill set, is useful for all clinicians, dietitians, psychologists, exercise physiologists, trainers, coaches, and parents working with and surrounded by female athletes. Vegan and vegetarian individuals need dietary assessment to make sure they are not intentionally or unintentionally eliminating essential foods from their diets.

Specific programs have met with some success in reducing disordered eating behaviors in athletes. The Athletes Targeting Healthy Exercise and Nutrition Alternatives (ATHENA) intervention created a scripted, coach-facilitated, peer-led, eight-session program. This program was found to reduce ongoing and new use of diet pills and to decrease female athletes' intentions to engage in disordered eating behaviors and body-shaping drug use.[48]

### FUTURE QUESTIONS

The role of heart disease in women in general, and in the female athlete in particular, remains to be clarified. Zeni Hock et al[49] looked at 20 female runners with amenorrhea or oligomenorrhea, finding that those with athletic amenorrhea displayed a reduced endothelium-dependent dilation of the brachial artery. Jorgensen et al[50] found low bone mass associated with an increased risk of echogenic calcified atherosclerotic plaques in postmenopausal women. Cause and effect remain to be clarified, but the association has ramifications for how we counsel women with the FAT, adding future heart disease to the list of problems potentially associated with the triad.

Prevention remains of paramount importance, with mounting pressure to avoid triggering eating disorders while fostering increasing athletic participation and decreasing national and international rates of obesity. Clarification on best programs to prevent both obesity and eating disorders deserves future attention. Imaging modalities such as DEXA scans involve low radiation risk but provide only 2-dimensional data; future technology may be able to give more accurate three-dimensional readings. Finally, the role of specific treatment modalities, including medications such as the anabolic steroid DHEA, currently not US Food and Drug Administration approved and under study, and the bisphosphonates, which have implications on future fetal bones and lifelong bone of young women for whom they are prescribed, requires further study.

## REFERENCES

1. DiPietro L, Stachenfeld NS. The myth of the female athlete triad. *Br J Sports Med.* 2006;40:490–493

2. DiPietro L, Stachenfeld NS. The female athlete triad myth. *Med Sci Sorts Exerc.* 2006;38(4):795

3. Macy S. *Winning Ways*. New York, NY: Henry Holt and Company; 1996

4. National Collegiate Athletic Association. *1990-2000 NCAA Gender-Equity Report.* Indianapolis, IN; 2000

5. Loucks AB. Methodological problems in studying the female athlete triad. *Med Sci Sports Exerc.* 2006;38(5):1020

6. Goodman LR, Warren MP. The female athlete and menstrual function. *Curr Opinion in Obstet Gynecol.* 2005;17(5):466-470

7. Otis CI, Drinkwater B, Johnson M, Loucks A, Wilmore J. American College of Sports Medicine position stand. The Female Athlete Triad. *Med Sci Sports Exerc.* 1997;89(3):321-325

8. Feicht CB, Johnson TS, Martin BJ, et al. Secondary amenorrhea in athletes. *Lancet.* 1978;2:1145

9. Shangold M, Rebar RW, Wentz AC, et al. Evaluation and management of menstrual dysfunction in athletes. *JAMA.* 1990;263:1665

10. Nativ A, Agostini R, Drinkwater B, Yeager KK. The female athlete triad: inter-relatedness of disordered eating, amenorrhea, and osteoporosis. *Med Clin North Amer.* 1994;78:345

11. Rosen DW, McKeag DB, Hough DO, et al. Pathogenic weight-control behavior in female athletes. *Phys Sports Med.* 1986;14:79

12. Warren BJ, Stanton AL, Blessing DL. Disordered eating patterns in competitive female athletes. *Int J Eat Disord.* 1990;9:565

13. Nichols JF, Mitchell JR, Lawson MJ, Ji M, Barkai HS. Prevalence of the female athlete triad syndrome among high school athletes. *Arch Pediatr Adolesc Med.* 2006;160:137-142

14. Torstveit MK, Sundgot-Borgen J. Participation in leanness sports but not training volume is associated with menstrual dysfunction: a national survey of 1,276 elite athletes and controls. *Br J Sports Med.* 2005;39:141-147

15. Torstveit MK, Sundgot-Borgen J. The female athlete triad: are elite athletes at increased risk? *Med Sci Sport Exerc.* 2005;37:184-193

16. Reinking MF, Alexander LE. Prevalence of disordered eating behaviors in undergraduate female collegiate athletes and nonathletes. *J Athl Train.* 2005;40:47-51

17. Hopkinson RA, Lock J. Athletics, perfectionism, and disordered eating. *Eat Weight Disord.* 2004;9(2):99-106

18. Cobb KL, Bachrach LK, Greendale G, et al. Disordered eating, menstrual irregularity, and bone mineral density in female runners. *Med Sci Sports Exerc.* 2003;35:711-719

19. Sundgot-Borgen J, Torstveit MK. Prevalence of eating disorders in elite athletes is higher than the general population. *Clin J Sport Med.* 2004;14:25-32

20. Torstveit MK, Sundgot-Borgen J. The female athlete triad exists in both elite athletes and controls. *Med Sci Sport Exerc.* 2005;37:1449-1459

21. Williams NI, De Souza MJ. Female athlete triad errors and misunderstandings. *Med Sci Sports Exerc.* 2006;38(5):1021

22. DeSouza MJ. Menstrual disturbances in athletes: a focus on luteal phase defects. *Med Sci Sports Exerc.* 2003;35(9):1553-1563

23. Sherman RT, Thompson RA. Practical use of the International Olympic Committee Medical Commission position stand on the female athlete triad: a case example. *Int J Eat Disord.* 2006;39(3):193-201

24. Khan KM, Liu-Ambrose T, Sran MM, Ashe MC, Donaldson MG, Wark JD. New criteria for female athlete triad syndrome? *Br J Sports Med.* 2002;36:10-13

25. Nattiv A, Loucks AB, Manore MM, Sanborn CF, Sundgot-Borgen J, Warren MP. American College of Sports Medicine position stand. The female athlete triad. *Med Sci Sports Exerc.* 2008;40(3):588

26. Fredericson M, Kent K. Normalization of bone density in a previously amenorrheic runner with osteoporosis. *Med Sci Sports Exerc.* 2005;37:1481-1486

27. Gibson JH, Mitchell A, Reeve J, Harries MG. Treatment of reduced bone mineral density in athletic amenorrhea: a pilot study. *Osteopor Int.* 1999;10:284-289

28. Jonnavithula S, Warren MP, Fox RP, Lazara MI. Bone density is compromised in amenorrheic women despite return of menses: a 2-year study. *Obstet Gynecol.* 1993;81:669-674

29. Keen AD, Drinkwater BL. Irreversible bone loss in former amenorrheic athletes. *Osteopors Int.* 1997;7:311-315

30. Klibanski A, Biller BM, Schoenfeld DA, Herzog DB, Sace VC. The effects of estrogen administration on trabecular bone loss in young women with anorexia nervosa. *J Clin Endocrinol Metab.* 1995;80:898-904

31. Warren MP, Brooks-Gunn J, Fox RP, Holderness CC, Hyle EP, Hamilton WG. Osteopenia in exercise-associated amenorrhea using ballet dancers as a model: a longitudinal study. *J Clin Endocrin Metab.* 2002;87:3162-3168

32. Warren MP, Brooks-Gunn J, Fox RP, et al. Persistent osteopenia in ballet dancers with amenorrhea and delayed menarche despite hormone therapy: a longitudinal study. *Fertil Steril.* 2003;80:398-404

33. Ilhe R, Loucks AB. Dose-response relationship between energy availability and bone turnover in young exercising women. *J Bone Miner Res.* 2004;19:1231-1240

34. Williams NI, Caston-Balderrama AL, Helmreich DL, Parfitt DB, Nosbisch C, Cameron JL. Longitudinal changes in reproductive hormones and menstrual cyclicity in cynomolgus monkeys during strenuous exercise training: abrupt transition to exercise-induced amenorrhea. *Endocrinology.* 2001;142:2381-2389

35. Loucks AB, Thuma JR. LH pulsatility is disrupted at a threshold of energy availability in regularly menstruating women. *J Clin Endocrinol Metabol.* 2003;88:297-301

36. Thong FS, McLean C, Graham TE. Plasma leptin in female athletes: relationship with body fat, reproductive, nutritional, and endocrine factors. *J Appl Physiol.* 2000;88:2037-2044

37. Gordon CM, Grace E, Emans SJ, et al. Effects of oral dehydroepiandrosterone on bone density in young women with anorexia nervosa: a randomized trial. *Clin Endocrinol Metab.* 2002;87(11):4935-4941

38. Seeman E, Szmukler GI, Fornica C, Tsalamandris C, Mestrovic R. Osteoporosis in anorexia nervosa: the influence

of peak bone density, bone loss, oral contraceptive use, and exercise. *J Bone Miner Res.* 1992;7(12):1467-1474

39. Hergenroeder AC, Smithe EO, Shypailo R, et al. Bone mineral changes in young women with hypothalamic amenorrhea treated with oral contraceptives, medroxyprogesterone, or placebo over 12 months. *Am J Obstet Gynecol.* 1997;176:1017

40. Loutedakis Y, Jamurtas A. The dancer as a performing athlete: physiological considerations. *Sports Med.* 2004;34(10): 651-661

41. Burrows M, Nevill AM, Bird S, Simpson D. Physiological factors associated with low bone mineral density in female endurance runners. *Br J Sport Med.* 2003;37:67-71

42. Campfield LA, Smith FJ, Burn P. The ob protein (leptin) pathway—a link between adipose tissue mass and central neural networks. *Horm Metab Res.* 1996;28:619-632

43. Stephens TW, Basinski M, Bristow PK. The role of neuropeptide Y in the anti-obesity action of the obese gene product. *Nature.* 1995;377:530-532

44. Weimann E. Gender-related differences in elite gymnasts: the female athlete triad. *J Appl Physiol.* 2002;92:2146-2152

45. Dostalova I, Kopsky V, Duskova J, et al. Leptin concentrations in the abdominal subcutaneous adipose tissue of patients with anorexia nervosa assessed by in vivo microdialysis. *Regul Pept.* 2005;128(1):63-68

46. Welt CK, Chan JL, Bullen J, et al. Recombinant human leptin in women with hypothalamic amenorrhea. *N Engl J Med.* 2004;351(10):987-997

47. Treasure JL, Russell GFM, Fogelman I, et al. Reversible bone loss in anorexia nervosa. *BMJ.* 1987;295:474

48. Elliot DL, Moe EI, Goldberg I, et al. Definition and outcome of a curriculum to prevent disordered eating and body-shaping drug use. *J School Health.* 2006;76:67-73

49. Zeni Hock A, Dempsey RI, Carrera GF, et al. Is there an association between athletic amenorrhea and endothelial cell dysfunction? *Med Sci Sports Exerc.* 2003;35:377-383

50. Jorgensen I, Joakimsen O, Rosvold-Bernsten GK, et al. Low bone mineral density is related to echogenic carotid artery plaques: a population-based study. *Amer J Epidemiol.* 2004;160:549-556

# CHAPTER 79

# Obesity

JESSICA RIEDER, MD • ALEXANDRA SALAZAR, RD

## INTRODUCTION

Obesity continues to be the most prevalent nutritional disorder of children and adolescents in the United States. Rates of overweight and obesity have been steadily climbing in the United States as well as in other developed and developing countries (Figure 79-1). Data from the combined 2003-2006 National Health and Nutrition Examination Survey (NHANES) indicated that 27.6% of US children and adolescents were obese.[1] The prevalence of overweight in female youth increased from 13.8% in 1999 to 2000 to 16.0% in 2003 to 2004 and in male youth from 14.0% to 18.2%. Overweight youth are at risk for becoming obese adults, and this risk increases with age—the probability for overweight adolescents to become overweight or obese adults may exceed 80%.[2] Although the obesity epidemic affects both genders and occurs in all age, race, and ethnic groups in the United States, prevalence rates tend to be highest among Hispanic, Native American, and black youth and in families below the poverty line when compared with families above the poverty line.[3,4]

Adolescence is a time of dramatic physical, emotional, and psychological change. Although there is a greater demand for nutrients because of the increase in physical growth and pubertal development, this period is also associated with an increased risk for the development of obesity, especially among teenage girls, where there is more deposition of fat than muscle. The greater independence and concomitant change in an adolescent's lifestyle and behavior can have an enormous impact on food choices and nutrient intake. This is a nutritionally vulnerable period of life when disordered eating and nutritional deficiencies can occur. It is increasingly important for health care providers to be educated and informed on the causes, risks, sequelae, and implications of adolescent obesity because treating overweight adolescents will become more commonplace.

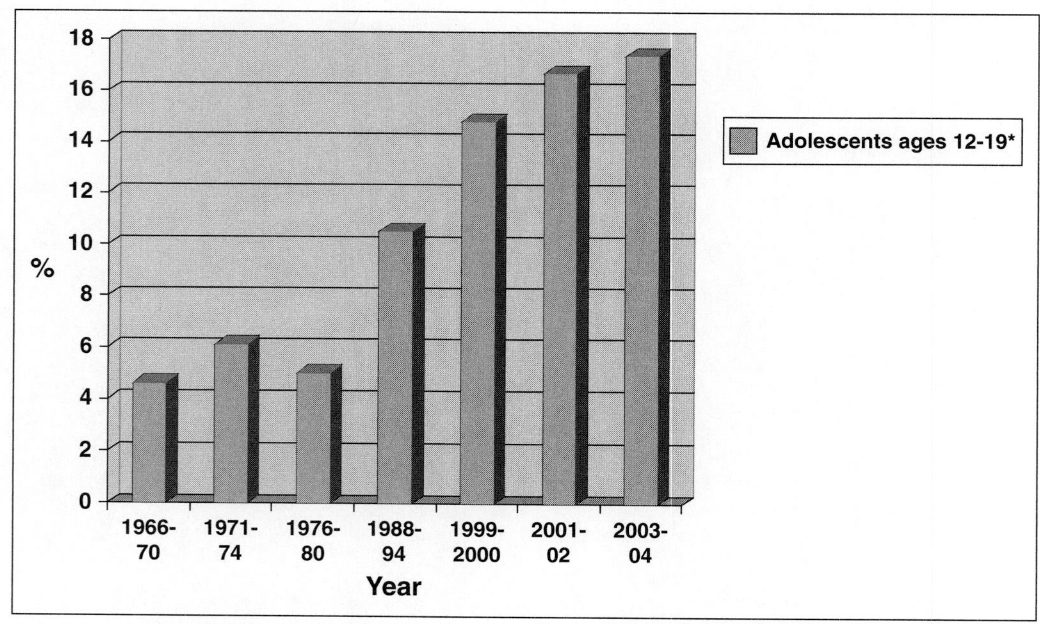


**FIGURE 79-1** Prevalence of overweight among adolescents ages 12–19 years, for selected years from NHANES 1966–1970 through 2003—2004. *Data for 1966–1970 are for adolescents 12–17 years of age, not 12–19 years. Overweight is defined as ≥ gender- and weight-specific 95th percentile from 2000 CDC growth charts. (Data from the National Center for Health Statistics.)

## DEFINITION

Obesity may be defined as a state of energy imbalance where energy expenditure does not equal energy intake and the excess is stored as fat. Assessment of overweight and obesity may be determined using weight and height measurements to calculate the body mass index (BMI) where weight in kilograms is divided by height in meters squared (kg/m$^2$).[5] In children and adolescents, the amount of body fat and height changes with age and sex and the Centers for Disease Control and Prevention (CDC) BMI-for-age growth charts take into account these differences. Recent new recommendations by the AMA Expert Committee on the Assessment, Prevention, and Treatment of Child and Adolescent Overweight and Obesity state that individuals from the ages of 2 to 18 years with a BMI >95th percentile for age and sex, or BMI exceeding 30 (whichever is smaller), should be considered obese. Individuals with BMI >85th percentile, but <95th percentile for age and sex, should be considered overweight, with this term replacing "at risk of overweight."[6]

Body mass index correlates with the amount of body fat, yet it does not directly measure body fat. It is a function of weight and height only, and when it increases in populations over time, changes in lean body mass cannot be readily distinguished from changes in body fatness mass. Further, because the BMI charts are developed from nationally representative populations and overweight youth are included in these datasets, as the population becomes heavier, the sensitivity of the measure decreases. That is, youth who were overweight using earlier BMI cutoff values may not be assessed to be overweight using updated BMI charts. Further, BMI does not take into account ethnic differences and variations in body frame. Despite these limitations, BMI is a widely used screening tool that is practical, cost-effective, and a good predictor of overweight.

Other methods of estimating body fat and body fat distribution include measurements of skinfold thickness, waist circumference, calculation of waist-to-hip circumference ratios, and techniques such as underwater weighing (hydrodensitometry), dual-energy x-ray absorptiometry, bioimpedance analysis, ultrasound, computed tomography, and magnetic resonance imaging (MRI).

## ETIOLOGY

The physiologic determinants of body weight are associated with energy intake, energy expenditure, and the division of energy stores as fat, carbohydrate, and protein. Although the basis of overweight is understood—weight gain results when energy intake exceeds energy expenditure—the etiology is not well understood. Although individuals with increased genetic susceptibility to the development of obesity are more likely than those without such susceptibility to become overweight when exposed to obesogenic environmental influences, there has been an overall societal increase in the median BMI since the 1980s and the heavier have gotten even heavier.

### GENETIC INFLUENCES

Although there are instances of single gene disorders that result in an obese human phenotype, in most overweight individuals, body fatness reflects the interaction of development and environment with genotype. The heritability of overall BMI has been estimated to be as high as 25% to 40%.[7] Further, the heritability of adipose tissue distribution (intra-abdominal vs subcutaneous fat), physical activity, resting metabolic rate, changes in energy expenditure that occur in response to overfeeding, certain aspects of feeding behavior, food preferences, and lipid metabolism are estimated to be as high as 30% to 40%.[8] Studies in twins, adoptees, and families indicate that up to 80% of the variability in BMI is genetically determined.[9] The search for candidate obesity genes focuses on those genes that play a role in mechanisms of excessive energy intake over expenditure or the preferential storage of calories as fat. To date several monogenic obesity syndromes have been identified, and most involve the leptin–melanocortin regulation pathway.[10] The obesity phenotype in the corresponding knockout mice models supports the central role of these genes in body weight regulation.

### REGULATION OF BODY WEIGHT

Body weight is thought to be regulated by complex signaling systems that provide afferent signals (including glucostatic, lipostatic, and aminostatic signals) to the central nervous system about the nutritional state of an organism, which then are translated into efferent signals that affect energy intake and expenditure.[11] The relative stability of body weight over time in most individuals despite wide variation in energy intake and expenditure, and the poor long-term results of weight-reduction efforts (90%–95% of adults and youth who lose weight regain it) suggests that attempts to maintain an altered body weight are opposed by systems of energy homeostasis that defend a highly individualized body weight or set point.[10]

### CHANGES IN THE DETERMINANTS OF ENERGY BALANCE

A number of environmental changes have affected the energy regulation of adolescents over the past decades. These changes may relate to food intake and energy expenditure and changes in the built environment, including schools and changes in parental roles.

### Changes in the Food Environment

Cross-sectional studies have established that individuals consuming fast-food meals have higher energy intake with lower nutritional values than those not consuming fast foods. Further, several studies have found that drinking sweetened beverages results in higher overall energy intake and a positive link between overweight and soft drink consumption.[11] Although youth who have higher energy intake from fast food and sweetened beverage consumption have larger weight gains than those who do not, a causal effect of fast food or sweetened beverages on overweight has not been conclusively established. Although lean and overweight adolescents consume more calories when eating fast food and drinking sweetened beverages, the lean compensate for that energy intake, whereas the overweight do not.

The positive association between fast-food and soft drink consumption and obesity may be explained by the marked increase in the overall availability and consumption of these foods and beverages over the past several decades.[12] Parallel with rising rates of soft drink consumption and consumption of soft drinks and food outside of the home, there has been an increase in the availability of tasty food at lower cost and greater convenience and a substantial increase in the portion sizes offered. Although the increase in spending for advertising soft drinks (increased by almost 50% in the latter half of the 1990s) may explain the increased rates of soft drink consumption, the evidence supporting this theory is yet to be established and the underlying reason for increased consumption of food outside the home is unclear.

### Changes in Energy Expenditure

Energy expenditure occurs through dietary thermogenesis, basal metabolic rate (BMR), and physical activity. Dietary thermogenesis relates to the energy required to digest meals, and BMR refers to the energy required to maintain the resting body's functions. Relative to non-overweight adolescents, overweight adolescents do not have a lower than average BMR that would explain a lower energy expenditure that would cause maintained obesity.[13] Although studies evaluating the link between increased physical activity and BMI have had variable results, there have been stronger links between sedentary activities, especially television viewing, and overweight and obesity. Increased television viewing may reduce time spent in physical activity and it may increase exposure to television advertising that may increase the desire for and ultimate consumption of energy-dense snack foods.[14] A reduction in children's television viewing has been associated with a drop in BMI.[15]

Although empirical studies establishing the link between physical activity and overweight are weak, it has been proposed that long-term technological and societal changes that have resulted in less physically active daily living may have resulted in changes in patterns of adolescent physical activity that promote weight gain. Urban sprawl has resulted in more travel by car and less travel by foot or by bicycle.[11] Significant changes in the school environment, including increased soft drink sales and consumption in school cafeterias and vending machines and the increased focus on academic accountability and concomitant increase in homework, have resulted in a drop in physical activity education and unstructured outdoor activity and play. A major change over the past 30 years relates to the number of children with parents (or single parent) in the labor force. Although the association of parental involvement in the labor force and obesity is not well documented, increased work time may result in less time spent preparing nutritious meals, increased consumption of convenience foods away from the home, less time to supervise active play, less time supervising walking or biking to school, or increased time unsupervised while watching television.

In summary, while there is no one critical cause in the increase in pediatric and adolescent obesity, there have been many complementary developments that have upset the crucial energy balance by simultaneously increasing energy intake and decreasing energy expenditure.

## ASSESSMENT OF THE OBESE ADOLESCENT

The evaluation of the obese adolescent should begin with a comprehensive medical and psychosocial history, a detailed assessment of nutrition, physical activity, and lifestyle behaviors, and a medical examination to evaluate the degree of obesity and its associated metabolic complications. The medical history should assess for a family history of parental obesity, type 2 diabetes, dyslipidemia, and cardiovascular disease. It should also gather information about any medication the adolescent uses, because so many common medicines, such as glucocorticoids and antipsychotic medications, promote weight gain. The goals of the assessment are to identify and treat causes of obesity that are not solely attributable to excessive caloric intake or inadequate exercise alone, that is, endogenous causes of obesity, and to identify and treat comorbid illnesses associated with obesity. Although it is imperative to assess the adolescent's readiness for change, an assessment of the adolescent's family and any other caregiver's readiness to change is also imperative for future weight loss success.

## ENDOGENOUS CAUSES OF OBESITY

Genetic and endocrinologic causes of obesity are rare. Obesity-related genetic syndromes, such as Bardet–Biedl and Cohen, typically present with dysmorphic features and developmental delay. Retinal changes and deafness may also be present. Prader-Willi usually presents in childhood with poor linear growth, dysmorphic facial features, and developmental delay. Behavior problems, especially in association with food and eating and undescended testicles in males, are other prominent features of this syndrome. Endocrinologic causes of overweight, including hypothyroidism and Cushing syndrome, characteristically present with poor linear growth. Adolescents with Cushing syndrome also typically have prominent violaceous striae as well as hypertension. These findings should prompt an evaluation with a urine free-cortisol or dexamethasone suppression test.

## COMPLICATIONS OF OBESITY

Increasing adiposity in adolescence is linked to a high prevalence of cardiovascular disease risk factors and associated cardiovascular disease as well as impaired glucose tolerance and type 2 diabetes mellitus (Table 79-1).

**Table 79-1**

**Complications of Pediatric and Adolescent Obesity**

| *System and Disorder* | *Prevalence Estimate in Obese Youth* |
|---|---|
| *Cardiovascular disease risk factors* | |
| Hypertension | 2%–40% |
| Left ventricular hypertrophy | Unknown |
| Atherosclerosis | 50% fatty streaks/8% fibrous plaques |
| *Disorders of metabolism* | |
| Insulin resistance | Unknown |
| Type 2 diabetes mellitus | 17.0 to 49.4 per 100,000 person-years[16] |
| Metabolic syndrome | 4% overall, 30% in obese |
| Dyslipidemia | 5%–10% |
| *Pulmonary complications* | |
| Asthma | 7%–9% |
| Obstructive sleep apnea | 1%–5% overall, ~ 25% in obese |
| *Gastrointestinal disorders* | |
| Nonalcoholic fatty liver disease | 3%–8% overall, ~ 50% in obese |
| Gastroesophageal reflux disease | 2%–20% |
| Cholecystitis | 50% |
| *Musculoskeletal abnormalities* | |
| Tibia vara (Blount disease) | Uncommon |
| SCFE | 1–8 per 100,000 |
| *Reproductive abnormalities* | |
| Polycystic ovary syndrome | Unknown in teens, 4%–23% in adult women |
| *Psychosocial issues* | |
| Depression | 1%–2% in children, 3%–5% in adolescents |

Source: Modified from Daniels SR. The consequences of childhood overweight and childhood obesity. *The Future of Children.* 2006;16(1):47–67. Available at: www.futureofchildren.org/futureofchildren/publications/figures-tables/figure_show.xml?fid=158. Accessed April 13, 2010. From *The Future of Children*, a collaboration of The Woodrow Wilson School of Public and International Affairs at Princeton University and The Brookings Institution.

Obese youth are also at risk for developing respiratory, gastrointestinal, orthopedic, and reproductive problems, in addition to other adverse medical and psychiatric effects. Even when the disorders do not present themselves in childhood or adolescence, these processes may be starting earlier than once thought, and the current generation of adolescents may be at risk of suffering the adverse effects of these various comorbid illnesses at younger ages than did previous generations.

### Cardiovascular Disease Risk Factors

In adults, major risk factors for future heart attack and stroke are hypertension, left ventricular hypertrophy, hypertriglyceridemia, and dyslipidemia (in particular reduced high density lipoprotein [HDL] cholesterol levels). Elevated blood pressure, left ventricular hypertrophy, hypercholesterolemia, dyslipidemia, and early development of atheromatous lesions have been associated with obesity in childhood and adolescence. In the Bogalusa Heart Study, 58% of overweight 5- to 17-year-olds had at least of the following: hypertension, hypertriglyceridemia, and reduced HDL cholesterol.[17] Early development of carotid atheromatous lesions has been demonstrated in adolescent males with obesity, increased serum cholesterol, and hypertension. Cardiovascular disease risk is identified by assessing for personal as well as family history of hypertension and dyslipidemias as well as tobacco use. Blood pressure should be measured with a cuff of an appropriate size to avoid overestimation of hypertension, and a screening lipoprotein profile will reveal dyslipidemias.

### Disorders of Metabolism

The incidence of type 2 diabetes mellitus and hyperinsulinemia in children and adolescents has also risen sharply in parallel with the rise in obesity.[18] Almost 45% of newly diagnosed cases of diabetes in youth are now type 2 diabetes.[19] Obesity in children and adolescents has been shown to be associated with decreased insulin sensitivity and increased circulating insulin, and these abnormalities persist into young adulthood.[20] The National Cholesterol Education Program has identified diabetes as a coronary artery disease risk equivalent.[19] *Acanthosis nigricans*, a condition associated with obesity, insulin resistance, and noninsulin-dependent diabetes mellitus, is characterized by hyperpigmented, velvety plaques in body folds. Fasting blood insulin and glucose, or a 2-hour oral glucose tolerance test, is indicated for insulin resistance screening.

In young people and adults the constellation of obesity, insulin resistance, inflammation, hypertriglyceridemia, reduced HDL-cholesterol, hypertension, and other risk factors that elevate the risk of atherosclerotic cardiovascular disease (ASCVD) and Type 2 Diabetes Mellitus (T2DM) is know as metabolic syndrome.[20,21] Metabolic syndrome may also be associated with other abnormalities, including fatty liver disease, polycystic ovary disease, and obstructive sleep apnea. Central obesity in overweight individuals, which can be inexpensively and accurately assessed with a waist circumference measurement, has been shown to be associated with adiposity, the metabolic syndrome, and cardiovascular disease risk.[22] Neck circumference has also been shown to be associated with the metabolic disorders related to insulin resistance.[23]

There is still no universally accepted definition of metabolic syndrome in children and adolescents for a number of reasons, including the use of adult cut points or a single set of cut points for all ages throughout childhood; the disturbances seen in the metabolic indicators in most children and adolescents are moderate; the lack of a normal range for insulin concentration across childhood; the physiologic insulin resistance of puberty changes depending on the stage of puberty; and the lack of central obesity (waist circumference) cut points linked to obesity morbidity or metabolic syndrome for children. Depending on the criteria used, the prevalence of metabolic syndrome in children and adolescents ranges from 4% to 30%.[24] With the increasing controversy related to the concept of metabolic syndrome in adolescents, and the need to understand the metabolic syndrome more fully in terms of the underlying pathophysiology and considerable variation in its manifestation related to age, sex, ethnicity, and maturation, there is a need to develop a more complex weighted scoring system that takes into account the magnitude of all the risk factors and the manner in which they interact.

### Pulmonary Complications

The prevalence and severity of childhood asthma have increased over the past 2 decades, again in parallel with the increasing prevalence and severity of childhood obesity.[25] Cross-sectional studies have demonstrated a link between overweight and asthma in children, although the link may be complicated by socioeconomic status, cigarette smoking, or other variables, and the exact mechanisms underlying the association between obesity and asthma have not yet been elucidated. OSA is a condition characterized by an abnormal collapse of the airway during sleep resulting in snoring, irregular breathing, and disrupted sleep patterns. Obstructive sleep apnea symptoms have been demonstrated in up to one-third of overweight youth, and sleep disruption can lead to excessive daytime sleepiness, poor school performance, learning disabilities, and memory defects.

Long-term complications of OSA include pulmonary artery hypertension, left ventricular hypertension, and diastolic dysfunction. A sleep study will identify sleep apnea or obesity hypoventilation syndrome, which may require continuous positive airway pressure until weight loss decreases intra-abdominal pressure, improves chest wall compliance, and restores adequate ventilation.

### Gastrointestinal Disorders

Nonalcoholic fatty liver disease is the most common form of liver disease in children and adolescents. As obesity develops, fat can be deposited in the liver, and although initially innocuous, continued fat deposition leads to steatohepatitis, which can then progress to fibrosis, cirrhosis, and even to end-stage liver disease and liver failure, ultimately requiring a liver transplant. While up to 50% of obese children may have fat deposits in their livers, some 3% of obese children have the more advanced nonalcoholic steatohepatitis. Abdominal pain or tenderness may reflect steatohepatitis, but may also indicate gall bladder disease, for which obesity is a risk factor.[26] Serum liver function evaluation and ultrasonography are indicated for the initial evaluation of these signs and symptoms.

### Musculoskeletal Abnormalities

Overweight adolescents are at risk of developing tibia vara, or Blount disease, which is a mechanical deficiency in the medial tibial growth plate that results in bowing of the tibia, which produces a bowed appearance of the lower leg and an abnormal gait. Adolescent tibia vara most often affects boys older than 9 years of age who are overweight. Slipped capital femoral epiphysis (SCFE) is a disorder of the growth plate of the hip that occurs around the age of skeletal maturity. In this disorder the femur, under mechanical stress from excess weight, is rotated externally from under the growth plate, which manifests as hip or knee pain and limited range of motion. In about one-third to one-quarter of afflicted children, both legs are affected. If radiography confirms either of these conditions, an orthopedic surgeon should evaluate the child and an appropriate weight loss intervention is needed to prevent recurrence of Blount disease or contralateral slipped epiphysis. Other obesity-related musculoskeletal deformities include flat foot, spondylolisthesis, and osteoarthritis.

### Reproductive Abnormalities

Polycystic ovary syndrome (PCOS) consists of a constellation of abnormalities, including abnormal menstrual cycles, clinical evidence of androgen excess, including acne and hirsutism, elevated serum androgen levels, and polycystic ovaries on ultrasound evaluation.[27] Obesity has been associated with PCOS, and both of these have independent effects on glucose tolerance, sex hormone binding globulin (SHBG), and androgen production. Although it is commonly acknowledged that PCOS begins at or before puberty, it can occur after puberty, particularly after excess weight gain. The syndrome is the most common cause of menstrual abnormality and hirsutism in women with prevalence estimates ranging from 4% to 23%. Women who suffer from PCOS are at risk for infertility, type 2 diabetes, and cardiovascular disease. Weight loss or pharmacologic treatment improves menstrual cycle abnormalities, insulin resistance, and often improves metabolic abnormalities. For a detailed discussion of PCOS, see Chapter 63.

### Other Adverse Health Effects

Idiopathic intracranial hypertension, or pseudotumor cerebri, is a condition in which increased intracranial pressure often results in severe headache, vision abnormalities, tinnitus, and sixth nerve paresis. Obesity is among the causes of pseudotumor cerebri, although the precise relationship between obesity and increased intracranial pressure remains unknown. Pseudotumor cerebri may be difficult to treat and may lead to loss of visual fields or visual acuity and may require aggressive weight-loss therapy, including bariatric surgery.

### Psychosocial Disorders

Underlying psychiatric disorders, including depression, anxiety, and binge eating disorder may cause or result from obesity. Depressed adolescents are at increased risk for the development of obesity during adolescence, and obese adolescents seeking weight loss treatment have more depressive symptoms than community-based obese or nonobese adolescents.[28] Binge-eating disorder, which occurs in up to 20% to 40% of obese adults and adolescents, is characterized by recurrent episodes of binge eating absent the use of the compensatory behaviors typically seen in bulimia nervosa.[29] Disturbances in self-esteem, quality of life, body image, family relations, peer relations, coping style, and self-efficacy are also associated with obesity in adolescents. Overweight adolescents who have been teased by peers or family members have been found to have increased suicidal thoughts and attempts.[30]

Overweight adolescents with underlying psychosocial or psychiatric illness require intensive psychologic evaluation and treatment. Without such treatment, a weight-control program may be ineffective. An overweight adolescent who is depressed may manifest sleep disturbance, hopelessness, sadness, and appetite changes. An adolescent with an eating disorder may report an inability to control the consumption of large amounts of food with or without the use of vomiting or laxative use to avoid weight gain.

### Economic Issues

Future health care costs associated with adolescent obesity are substantial.[31] Hospitalizations among children and adolescents (6–17 years of age) for diseases associated with obesity increased sharply between 1979 and 1999.[31] Although the indirect cost of adolescent obesity remains unknown, the indirect economic costs of adult obesity—reductions in economic opportunity or productivity—have been estimated at $23 billion a year in the United States, and the health care costs of patients with a BMI greater than 35 are approximately 44% more than those of nonobese patients.[29] Overweight individuals are often negatively stereotyped as lazy, sloppy, ugly, or stupid, and this stereotyping often affects girls more than boys. Compared to boys, obese adolescent girls become adults with less education, lower earning power, a higher likelihood of poverty, and a lower likelihood of marriage. Obese individuals have more difficulty gaining admission to college and experience more discrimination when renting apartments and houses.

## MANAGEMENT OF THE OVERWEIGHT ADOLESCENT

Although obesity is a result of energy imbalance, reversing obesity is more complex than simply restoring that balance. The societal, environmental, emotional, and physical barriers that may interfere with a patient's willingness or ability to lose weight must be taken into consideration. It is also critical to consider the developing autonomy of overweight adolescents who increasingly have more control over their time and activity when away from the family. The overarching goal of weight management is to promote healthy behaviors related to eating and physical activity.[26]

The AMA Expert Committee on the Assessment, Prevention, and Treatment of Child and Adolescent Overweight and Obesity recommends that the goal for adolescents with a BMI between the 85th and 94th percentile for age and sex is weight maintenance until the BMI is less than the 85th percentile or there is slowing of weight gain as indicated by a downward deflection in the BMI curve. The goal for adolescents with a BMI between the 95th and 98th percentile is weight loss until the BMI is less than the 85th percentile, and the weight loss should occur at no more than an average of 2 pounds per week. If greater weight loss is noted, monitor for causes of excessive weight loss. The goal for adolescents with a BMI that is >99th percentile is for weight loss not to exceed an average of 2 pounds per week.[6] If present, treatment and resolution of the medical complication is an important goal. For many with high blood pressure or high cholesterol, changes in eating and physical activity along with weight loss may improve the situation.

Management of the overweight adolescent requires a multifaceted approach that incorporates the expertise of a team of providers who can support the lifestyle and behavioral change needs of individual adolescents, their family and social supports, and the community in which they live. Although individualized medical therapies, behavior modification, and dietary and physical activity treatment modalities are focused on the overweight teen, an overall promotion of a healthy lifestyle, with support for the adolescent's family or support network, is a requisite for successful weight loss. Pharmacotherapy, bariatric surgery, treatment of underlying psychiatric disorders, and other alternative methods may be indicated in those individuals unable to respond to more conservative behavioral and lifestyle interventions. The AMA Expert Committee on the Assessment, Prevention, and Treatment of Child and Adolescent Overweight and Obesity recommends a staged approach to weight loss for youth whose BMI is above the 85th percentile (Box 79-1) and above the 95th percentile (Box 79-2).

### BEHAVIORAL TREATMENT

Behavioral treatment programs that utilize the principles of behavior change to achieve diet and physical activity modifications have shown consistent success over the short term.[32] The effective behavior therapist can help adolescents assess their readiness to change behaviors, assist in motivating to change, and teach adolescents how to change. By assisting in self-assessment and identifying small attainable goals, the behavior therapist can help the adolescent navigate and influence the environment in which he or she lives.

#### Diet

Nutrition interventions should not focus on dietary restriction; rather, they should focus on achieving an appropriate caloric intake for a growing adolescent. It is essential to identify eating patterns, the dietary content and amount of food and beverages consumed, as well as the amount and quality of snacks and the amount of juice and soft drinks consumed. The assessment will assist in identifying areas that need to be changed to facilitate the adoption of a diet that is rich in calcium, high in fiber, and with balanced macronutrients (calories from fat, carbohydrate, and protein in proportions for age as

**Box 79-1**

***The Expert Committee Recommendations for a Staged Approach to Weight Loss for Youth Whose BMI Is Above the 85th Percentile***

**Stage 1. Prevention Plus Protocol**

I. Dietary habits and physical activity
   a. 5 or more servings of fruits and vegetables per day
   b. 2 or fewer hours of screen time per day
   c. No television in the room where the child sleeps
   d. 1 hour or more of daily physical activity
   e. No sugar-sweetened beverages
II. Patients and families of the patient are to be counseled to facilitate these eating behaviors
   a. Eating a daily breakfast
   b. Limiting meals outside of the home
   c. Family meals should happen at least 5–6 times per week
   d. Allowing the child to self-regulate his or her meals
   e. Avoiding overly restrictive behaviors
III. Goal is weight maintenance with a decreasing BMI as age and height increases. Monthly follow-up
IV. Advance to Stage 2 after 3–6 months, if no improvement in BMI/weight status

**Stage 2. Structured Weight Management Protocol**

I. Dietary and physical activity behaviors
   a. Balanced macronutrient diet with low amounts of energy-dense foods
   b. Increased structured daily meals and snacks
   c. Supervised active play of at least 60 minutes per day
   d. Screen time of 1 hour or less per day
   e. Increased monitoring (eg, screen time, physical activity, dietary intake, restaurant logs) by provider, patient, and/or family
II. Goal is weight maintenance with a decreasing BMI as age and height increase
III. If no improvement in BMI/weight after 3–6 months, patient should be advanced to Stage 3

**Stage 3. Comprehensive Multidisciplinary Protocol**

I. Eating and activity goals are the same as in Stage 2
II. Activities within this category should also include
   a. Structured behavioral modification program (food and activity monitoring)
   b. Development of short-term diet and physical activity goals
   c. Behavioral training of primary caregivers/families
III. Goal is weight maintenance or gradual weight loss until BMI less than 85th percentile

Stages 1 and 2 can be implemented by the primary care physician or allied health care provider who has training in pediatric weight management/behavioral counseling. Stage 3 should be implemented by a multidisciplinary obesity care team.

Adapted from Expert Committee Recommendations on the Assessment, Prevention, and Treatment of Child and Adolescent Overweight and Obesity, January 2007. *Pediatrics*. 2007;120:S164-S192.

recommended by dietary reference intakes) and low in energy-dense foods and sweetened beverages.

### Physical Activity

As with nutrition interventions, the emphasis on physical activity behavior change should focus on gradually achieving an appropriate amount of physical activity to achieve a healthy lifestyle for the adolescent. Assessing time spent in leisure activities, light and moderate physical activity, as well as time spent in sedentary activities, provides information relating to the amount of individual baseline activity, motivation to increase activity, and barriers to increasing physical activity. The American Academy of Pediatrics recommends no more than 2 hours of quality television programming per day for children older than 2 years of age.[33] The International Consensus Conference on Physical Activity Guidelines for Adolescents recommends that "all adolescents…be

**Box 79-2**

***The Expert Committee Recommendations for Youth Whose BMI Is Above the 95th Percentile[a]***

**Stage 4. Tertiary Care Protocol**

I. Referral to pediatric tertiary weight management center with access to a multidisciplinary team with expertise in childhood obesity
II. This protocol should include continued diet and activity counseling
III. Use of meal replacement, very-low-calorie diet, medication, and surgery considered

[a]For youth BMI >95th percentile, with significant comorbidities and who have not been successful with Stages 1-3 (Box 79-1) or whose BMI is above the 99th percentile who have shown no improvement under Stage 3 (comprehensive multidisciplinary intervention).

Adapted from Expert Committee Recommendations on the Assessment, Prevention, and Treatment of Child and Adolescent Overweight and Obesity, January 2007. *Pediatrics*. 2007;120:S164-S192.

physically active daily, or nearly every day, as part of play, games, sports, work, transportation, recreation, physical education, or planned exercise, in the context of family, school, and community activities."[34] Treatment programs that include nutritional interventions in combination with exercise have higher success rates than diet modification alone.[35]

### Family Involvement

Just as the family environment can contribute to the development of obesity, in that parents and other family members share an environment that may be conducive to overeating or a sedentary lifestyle, family members may also serve as positive models that reinforce and support the acquisition and maintenance of healthy eating and exercise behaviors. Family-based interventions are needed to modify these variables in treating obese children. The involvement of at least one parent as an active participant in the weight loss process has been shown to improve short- and long-term weight regulation, and family and friend support for behavior change are related to long-term positive weight loss outcomes.[36]

### Societal Involvement

Families, physicians, allied health care, and professional organizations all have a role in advocating for increased governmental support of increasing physical activity at school through intervention programs throughout the school years and through creating school environments that support physical activity in general. There is a further role for supporting efforts to preserve and enhance parks as areas for physical activity, informing local development initiatives regarding the inclusion of walking and bicycle paths and promoting families' use of local physical activity options.

## PHARMACOTHERAPY

Pharmacotherapy may be considered as adjunctive therapy for weight loss when an adolescent with a BMI in excess of the 95th percentile for age and sex, and who may also have obesity-related comorbidities, is unresponsive to at least 6 months of a medically supervised weight loss trial. Weight loss medications assist in weight loss through several mechanisms, including increasing energy expenditure, suppressing caloric intake, limiting nutrient absorption, and by modulating the production and/or action of insulin. Clinical trials have demonstrated short-term success with weight loss medications, but unless healthy lifestyle changes are adopted and adhered to, weight loss in association with the use of medication may be reversed when the medications are discontinued. A variety of other prescription medications and over-the-counter or herbal medications, including Zonisamide, Topiramate, caffeine, green tea, bitter orange, capsaicin (chili peppers), fiber, chitosan, and chromium have been also used for weight loss. Long-term efficacy has not been determined for these agents. The American Academy of Pediatrics recommends the use of medication as adjunctive therapy for those patients who have significant weight-related health risks and who have not successfully lost weight with diet and lifestyle changes. Candidates for pharmacotherapy should be referred to a tertiary care center for evaluation and multimodal weight loss therapy, which includes modifications in behavior, diet, and physical activity.[37]

Energy expenditure may be increased through the use of stimulants, including thyroid hormone, dinitrophenol, amphetamine, fenfluramine, dexfenfluramine, phenylpropanolamine, and ephedra. At one time considered safe and effective, these stimulants have been abandoned because they are dangerous and may cause life-threatening complications.

Caloric intake may be suppressed through the use of anorectic agents. Sibutramine hydrochloride is a nonselective inhibitor of neuronal reuptake of serotonin, norepinephrine, and dopamine that has been approved by the US Food and Drug Administration (FDA) for use in adolescents older than 16 years. In combination with behavior therapy, studies in adolescents have indicated that Sibutramine produces more weight loss than behavior therapy and placebo alone when used for 6 months to 1 year. Although the adult literature shows an additional 2 kg to 10 kg weight loss reported with the use of this medication, weight regain has been demonstrated with discontinuation of the medication. Adverse events associated with the use of Sibutramine include elevations in blood pressure, tachycardia, insomnia, anxiety, headache, and depression.

Nutrient absorption may be limited through the use of Orlistat, which blocks fat absorption in the gut by inhibiting pancreatic lipase activity, thereby increasing fecal losses of incompletely hydrolyzed fat. Failure to decrease dietary fat intake while taking Orlistat results in gastrointestinal events such as borborygmi and cramps, flatus, fecal incontinence, oily spotting, and flatus, with discharge occurring at frequency rates of 15% to 30% in most studies. Orlistat has been approved by the FDA for use in adolescents older than 12 years of age. Relative to placebo, Orlistat has been shown to decrease body weight as well as total and low density lipoprotein (LDL) cholesterol levels and reduces the risk of type 2 diabetes mellitus in adults with impaired glucose tolerance. Absorption of the fat-soluble vitamins (A, D, E) may be slightly reduced and it may be advisable to give vitamin supplements to patients treated with this drug.

Metformin is a bisubstituted short-chain hydrophilic guanidine derivative that activates AMP protein kinase thereby increasing hepatic glucose uptake, decreasing gluconeogenesis, and reducing hepatic glucose production. It is the only oral antidiabetic agent FDA approved for use in pediatric patients 10 years of age or older. Relative to controls, Metformin produces weight loss, decreased fat stores (subcutaneous more than visceral fat stores), improved lipid profiles, and a reduction in conversion to type 2 diabetes mellitus among adults with impaired glucose tolerance. It is generally well tolerated, although many patients have transient abdominal discomfort, which is avoidable by taking the medication with food. An additional side effect, lactic acidosis, is extremely rare, but Metformin should not be administered to adolescents with underlying cardiac, hepatic, renal, or gastrointestinal disease.

### NONPHARMACOLOGIC TREATMENTS

Bariatric surgery may be considered a weight loss alternative for severely obese adolescents when more conservative weight loss measures fail to address the health needs of patients. Although 50% of severely obese adults maintain a weight loss of more than 50% of excess weight 5 years after surgery and this success rate far exceeds that of any other weight loss modality, the long-term success rates in adolescents have not yet been well established. Contraindications to bariatric surgery include a medically correctable cause of obesity; the presence of a substance abuse problem within the past year; a medical, psychiatric, or cognitive condition that would significantly impair the patient's ability to adhere to post-op regimens; current lactation, pregnancy, or a planned pregnancy within 2 years after surgery; and the inability or unwillingness of the patient or parents to fully comprehend the procedure and its medical consequences. Although the medical criteria for presurgical clearance have been well described for adolescents, and the safety and effectiveness of both the Roux-en-Y gastric bypass and the adjustable gastric banding (AGB) in treating and correcting obesity-related comorbidities in adolescents have been established, a comprehensive assessment of psychosocial readiness, maturity, and capacity to appreciate the risks and benefits associated with bariatric surgery have not been well detailed in the literature. Further, although improved self-esteem and socialization have been reported, the long-term metabolic, developmental, and psychosocial outcomes related to significant weight loss have not been well studied. The American Academy of Pediatrics recommends that bariatric surgery should only be performed by bariatric surgeons affiliated with a tertiary care center or pediatric hospital. Only those adolescents with a BMI >99th percentile, or a BMI of $\geq 40$ kg/m$^2$ who have comorbid conditions such as diabetes or cardiovascular disease or those adolescents with a BMI of $\geq 50$kg/m$^2$ without comorbid illnesses and who have not had significant reductions in weight through nonsurgical means over a period of a minimum of 6 months, should be considered candidates for bariatric surgery. Patients and their families are required to demonstrate an ability to follow the behavior modifications and adapt to the psychosocial adjustments that will be needed for long-term success after the bariatric surgery.[37]

## SUMMARY

Treating overweight adolescents can pose a unique challenge to health care providers. Given the magnitude and scope of the problem and the potential for significant future morbidity and mortality, the effective treatment of overweight and obesity should consist of a staged approach for weight loss with intensive behavioral, dietary, physical activity change guidance, and multifaceted treatment strategies utilizing medical, community, educational, and family resources. Only when more conservative measures fail should adjunctive measures, including pharmacotherapy and bariatric surgery, be considered.

## REFERENCES


1. Ogden CL, Carroll MD, Flegal KM. High body mass index for age among US children and adolescents, 2003-2006. *JAMA.* 2008;299:2401-2405

2. Guo SS, Wu W, Chumlea WC, Roche AF. Predicting overweight and obesity in adulthood from body mass index values in childhood and adolescence. *Am J Clin Nutr.* 2002;76(3):653-658

3. Crawford PB, Story M, Wang MC, Ritchie LD, Sabry ZI. Ethnic issues in the epidemiology of childhood obesity. *Pediatr Clin North Am.* 2001;48(4):855-878

4. Miech RA, Kumanyika SK, Stettler N, Link BG, Phelan JC, Chang VW. Trends in the association of poverty with overweight among US adolescents, 1971-2004. *JAMA.* 2006;295(20):2385-2393

5. Centers for Disease Control and Prevention. Overweight and obesity: defining overweight and obesity. Department of Health and Human Services. 2007. Available at: www.cdc.gov/nccdphp/dnpa/obesity/defining.htm. Accessed October 2, 2007

6. Barlow SE and the Expert Committee. AMA Expert Committee on the Assessment, Prevention, and Treatment of Child and Adolescent Overweight and Obesity: summary report. *Pediatrics.* 2007;120:S164-S192

7. World Health Organization. *Obesity: Preventing and Managing the Global Epidemic—Report of the WHO Consultation on Obesity*. Geneva, Switzerland: WHO Publications; 2004

8. Rosenbaum M, Leibel RL. Pathophysiology of childhood obesity. *Adv Pediatr.* 1988;35:73-137

9. Stunkard AJ, Harris JR, Pedersen NL, McClearn GE. The body-mass index of twins who have been reared apart. *N Engl J Med.* 1990;322(21):1483-1487

10. Rosenbaum M, Leibel RL. The physiology of body weight regulation: relevance to the etiology of obesity in children. *Pediatrics.* 1998;101(3 Pt 2):525-539

11. Anderson PM, Butcher KE. Childhood obesity: trends and potential causes. *Future Child.* 2006;16(1):19-45

12. Aaron DJ, Kriska AM, Dearwater SR, et al. The epidemiology of leisure physical activity in an adolescent population. *Med Sci Sports Exerc.* 1993;25(7):847-853

13. Bandini LG, Schoeller DA, Dietz WH. Energy expenditure in obese and nonobese adolescents. *Pediatr Res.* 1990;27(2):198-203

14. Dietz WH, Jr., Gortmaker SL. Do we fatten our children at the television set? Obesity and television viewing in children and adolescents. *Pediatrics.* 1985;75(5):807-812

15. Robinson TN, Killen JD, Kraemer HC, et al. Dance and reducing television viewing to prevent weight gain in African-American girls: the Stanford GEMS pilot study. *Ethn Dis.* 2003;13(1 Suppl 1):S65-S77

16. Incidence of Diabetes in Youth in the United States. The Writing Group for the SEARCH for Diabetes in Youth Study Group. *JAMA.* 2007;297:2716-2724

17. Freedman DS, Dietz WH, Srinivasan SR, Berenson GS. The relation of overweight to cardiovascular risk factors among children and adolescents: the Bogalusa Heart Study. *Pediatrics.* 1999;103(6 Pt 1):1175-1182

18. Pinhas-Hamiel O, Dolan LM, Daniels SR, Standiford D, Khoury PR, Zeitler P. Increased incidence of non-insulin-dependent diabetes mellitus among adolescents. *J Pediatr.* 1996;128(5 Pt 1):608-615

19. Type 2 diabetes in children and adolescents. American Diabetes Association. *Diabetes Care.* 2000;23(3):381-389

20. Steinberger J, Moran A, Hong CP, Jacobs DR, Jr., Sinaiko AR. Adiposity in childhood predicts obesity and insulin resistance in young adulthood. *J Pediatr.* 2001;138(4):469-473

21. Cook S, Weitzman M, Auinger P, Nguyen M, Dietz WH. Prevalence of a metabolic syndrome phenotype in adolescents: findings from the third National Health and Nutrition Examination Survey, 1988-1994. *Arch Pediatr Adolesc Med.* 2003;157(8):821-827

22. Snijder MB, Zimmet PZ, Visser M, Dekker JM, Seidell JC, Shaw JE. Independent and opposite associations of waist and hip circumferences with diabetes, hypertension, and dyslipidemia: the AusDiab Study. *Int J Obes Relat Metab Disord.* 2004;28(3):402-409

23. Laakso M, Matilainen V, Keinanen-Kiukaanniemi S. Association of neck circumference with insulin resistance-related factors. *Int J Obes Relat Metab Disord.* 2002;26(6):873-875

24. Steinberger J, Daniels SR, Eckel RH, Hayman L, Lustig RH, McCrindle B, et al. Progress and challenges in metabolic syndrome in children and adolescents: a scientific statement from the American Heart Association Atherosclerosis, Hypertension, and Obesity in the Young Committee of the Council on Cardiovascular Disease in the Young; Council on Cardiovascular Nursing; and Council on Nutrition, Physical Activity, and Metabolism. *Circulation.* 2009;119:628-647

25. Northridge ME, Meyer IH, Dunn L. Overlooked and underserved in Harlem: a population-based survey of adults with asthma. *Environ Health Perspect.* 2002;110(Suppl 2):217-220

26. Barlow SE, Dietz WH. Obesity evaluation and treatment: Expert Committee Recommendations. The Maternal and Child Health Bureau, Health Resources, and Services Administration and the Department of Health and Human Services. *Pediatrics.* 1998;102(3):E29

27. Zawadski JK, Dunaif DA. Diagnostic criteria for polycystic ovary syndrome: towards a rational approach. In: Dunaif AGJ, Haseltine F, eds. *Polycystic Ovary Syndrome*. Boston, MA: Blackwell Scientific; 1992:377-384

28. Goodman E, Whitaker RC. A prospective study of the role of depression in the development and persistence of adolescent obesity. *Pediatrics.* 2002;110(3):497-504

29. Speiser PW, Rudolf MC, Anhalt H, et al. Childhood obesity. *J Clin Endocrinol Metab.* 2005;90(3):1871-1887

30. Goodman E, Adler NE, Daniels SR, Morrison JA, Slap GB, Dolan LM. Impact of objective and subjective social status on obesity in a biracial cohort of adolescents. *Obes Res.* 2003;11(8):1018-1026

31. Wang G, Dietz WH. Economic burden of obesity in youths aged 6 to 17 years: 1979–1999. *Pediatrics.* 2002;109(5):E81

32. Epstein LH, Roemmich JN, Raynor HA. Behavioral therapy in the treatment of pediatric obesity. *Pediatr Clin North Am.* 2001;48(4):981-993

33. American Academy of Pediatrics. Children, adolescents, and television. *Pediatrics.* 2001;107(2):423–426

34. Sallis JF, Patrick K. Physical activity guidelines for adolescents: consensus statement. *Pediatr Exercise Sci.* 1994;6:302–314

35. Nemet D, Barkan S, Epstein Y, Friedland O, Kowen G, Eliakim A. Short- and long-term beneficial effects of a combined dietary-behavioral-physical activity intervention for the treatment of childhood obesity. *Pediatrics.* 2005;115(4):e443–e449

36. Epstein LH. Family-based behavioural intervention for obese children. *Int J Obes Relat Metab Disord.* 1996;20 (Suppl1):S14–S21

37. Spear BA, Barlow SE, Ervin C, et al. Recommendations for treatment of child and adolescent overweight. *Pediatrics.* 2007;120(Suppl4):S254–S288

SECTION 3

# The Cardiovascular System

# CHAPTER 80

## Chest Pain in Adolescents

ANGELA ROMANO, MD • SANAH MERCHANT, MD

### INTRODUCTION

Chest pain in the adolescent is an extremely common presenting complaint in the emergency department and in the pediatric office. It has been reported that physicians in the United States evaluate 650,000 episodes of chest pain annually in patients aged 10 to 21 years.[1] Driscoll et al[2] reported a 0.29% rate of occurrence of chest pain in a prospective study of pediatric outpatient visits; a similar rate of 0.25% was reported by Selbst et al[3] in pediatric patients presenting to the emergency department. Chest pain in adolescent patients is a source of a great deal of concern and anxiety for both the adolescents and their families. This symptom may impair the adolescent's ability to function normally in daily activities. Many may be absent from school or self-limit their extracurricular activities. Pantell and Goodman[4] reported in their study that more than 50% of the adolescents they evaluated for chest pain were fearful that cardiac disease was the cause of their pain. Many feared that they were having a "heart attack." The reality is that the overwhelming odds are against cardiac pathology in this age group. Fewer than 4% of cases presenting with chest pain can be linked to a cardiac etiology,[5] with most etiologies being idiopathic, musculoskeletal, respiratory, or psychogenic in origin. Most adolescents in whom cardiac pathology is identified, the cardiac diagnoses are not the causal link to their perceived chest pain. These asymptomatic cardiac diagnoses include bicuspid aortic (with a normal aortic root) or pulmonary valves, small atrial septal defects, and abnormalities in the electrical conduction system, such as Wolf-Parkinson-White syndrome and long QT syndrome (in the absence of tachyarrhythmias). In this chapter, a guideline to the medical assessment of the adolescent patient with chest pain, as well as a comprehensive differential diagnosis, are provided. Box 80-1 describes potential etiologies of adolescent chest pain.

**Box 80-1**

***Potential Etiologies of Adolescent Chest Pain***

**NONCARDIAC CAUSES**

- Idiopathic
- Musculoskeletal/dermatological causes
  - Trauma (accidental or abuse)
  - Chest wall syndrome (strain, bursitis)
  - Costochondritis
  - Tietze syndrome
  - Precordial catch syndrome
  - Slipping rib
  - Pleurodynia
  - Osteomyelitis
  - Primary or metastatic tumor
  - Breast tenderness
  - Cutaneous herpes zoster
- Pulmonary causes
  - Pneumonia
  - Pleurisy
  - Asthma
  - Chronic cough
  - Pneumothorax or pneumomediastinum
  - Infarction (sickle cell crisis)
  - Pulmonary embolism
  - Primary or metastatic tumor
- Gastrointestinal causes
  - Esophagitis, gastroesophageal reflux
  - Foreign body
  - Cholecystitis
  - Peptic ulcer disease
- Psychogenic causes
  - Anxiety, hyperventilation
  - Conversion symptoms
  - Somatization disorders
  - Depression

*(Continued)*

**Box 80-1 (*continued*)**

**CARDIAC CAUSES**
- Ischemic cardiac causes
  - Structural abnormalities of the heart (severe aortic stenosis or pulmonary stenosis, hypertrophic obstructive cardiomyopathies)
  - Mitral valve prolapse
  - Coronary artery abnormalities (prior Kawasaki disease, congenital anomalies, Takayasu arteritis)
  - Previous cardiac surgery in infancy or early childhood
  - Cocaine abuse
  - Familial hyperlipidemia/early coronary artery disease
- Inflammatory conditions
  - Pericarditis (viral, bacterial, or rheumatic)
  - Postpericardiotomy syndrome
  - Myocarditis
- Aortic dissection
  - Aortic dissection and aortic aneurysm (Marfan syndrome, Loeys-Dietz syndrome, Turner syndrome, and Noonan syndrome)
- Arrhythmias (palpitations)
  - Supraventricular tachycardia
  - Frequent premature ventricular contractions or ventricular tachycardia

## EVALUATION OF CHEST PAIN

Chest pain in the adolescent patient is a common problem and predominantly a benign occurrence requiring only the reassurance of the adolescent and his or her parents. However, it is important to recognize that a more serious etiology for the underlying chest pain may be possible. Although a rare event, the acute onset of severe, persistent chest pain in an adolescent constitutes a medical emergency. On presentation, these patients usually appear ill and are in significant distress (Box 80-2). Their chest pain needs to be distinguished from the more chronic, subacute, indolent, intermittent chest discomfort that besets adolescents with much greater frequency.

**Box 80-2**

***Pathology Associated with Acute, Severe Chest Pain in Adolescents***

- Aortopathies resulting in aortic dissection
- Myocardial ischemia/myocardial infarction secondary to cardiac pathology
- Myocardial/pericardial inflammation
- Persistent tachyarrhythmias
- Acute bronchospasm/reactive airway disease
- Pneumomediastinum/pneumothorax
- Esophageal rupture
- Rib fracture

During the initial encounter between the physician and the adolescent with nonacute chest pain, it is important that the physician acknowledge that the pain is a real entity and that the complaint will be taken seriously. It also is helpful to discuss at the initiation of the visit that the occurence of chest pain is extremely common in the adolescent age group. It should be pointed out that even though a comprehensive evaluation will be undertaken to investigate the cause of the pain, more often than not a definitive etiology for the chest discomfort may not be established. Rather, the purpose of the evaluation would be to eliminate serious organic pathology as an etiology. Addressing some of these issues at the onset of the visit is often helpful in assuaging the emotional fears harbored by the adolescent and the family.

### HISTORY OF THE PRESENTING COMPLAINT OF CHEST PAIN

A detailed history must be obtained and should be directed at determining the nature of the pain and associated symptoms. This history must be obtained directly from the adolescent patient. Description of the pain must include its duration, quality, location, and intensity. Chronic intermittent chest pain persisting for more than one to several months is more typically benign and less likely to be related to serious underlying pathology. Often this chest pain is short and fleeting in duration. Conversely, episodes of pain occurring for sustained periods of time with increasing frequency and intensity are more likely to be secondary to an organic cause. Precipitating occurrences such as exercise, eating, or trauma should be determined. For example, pain that worsens with deep inspiration may imply an underlying pleuritic or musculoskeletal process. Chest pain associated with dizziness, palpitations, and/or syncope may be indicative of an underlying cardiac etiology. Factors that result in relief of the pain may also aid in determining the diagnosis.

During the initial interview, it also is important to question the adolescent about his or her social situation in an attempt to elicit any relevant recent stressful life events. It may be enlightening to query adolescents as to their opinions on the cause of their chest pain.

### REVIEW OF SYSTEMS AND PAST MEDICAL HISTORY

A complete and conscientious review of systems is also crucial. Important points to establish include the presence of constitutional symptoms such as malaise, fever, and weight loss; respiratory complaints such as chronic cough, shortness of breath, and dyspnea with exertion;

cardiac symptoms of palpitations, dizziness, or syncope; gastrointestinal symptoms of vomiting or dysphagia; and visual or hearing impairments. The presence or absence of these symptoms often provides a clue to the diagnosis. For example, visual abnormalities such as high-grade myopia and subluxed lenses are associated with Marfan syndrome, and sensorineural hearing loss is found in a variant of long QT syndrome. It is important to know if the child is receiving any prescribed medications or alternative therapies. A history of any known medical conditions should be elicited at this time, including asthma, hypercholesterolemia, Marfan syndrome or Marfan-related syndromes, and pre-existing congenital or acquired heart disease (history of Kawasaki disease), as well as a history of previous cardiac surgery and rheumatologic disorders such as systemic lupus erythematosus, rheumatoid arthritis, or scleroderma. Tobacco use, as well as the use of illicit drugs, particularly cocaine, should be explored with the adolescent.

### FAMILY HISTORY

A comprehensive family history is extremely important to obtain. A family history of certain medical conditions may shed light on the etiology of the chest pain with which the adolescent is presenting. Some of these conditions include asthma, Marfan syndrome, Ehlers-Danlos syndrome, systemic lupus erythematosus, familial hypercholesterolemia, premature myocardial infarctions, hypertrophic cardiomyopathies, aortic dissections, long QT syndrome, Brugada syndrome, arrhythmias requiring pacemakers and/or defibrillators, or sudden unexplained death.

### PHYSICAL EXAMINATION

Initially, a careful general examination is necessary, including measurement of vital signs. An overall assessment of the level of acuity of illness with which the patient is presenting must be made at the onset of the encounter. If the adolescent is acutely ill and appears to be in distress (respiratory distress, hyperventilating, diaphoretic, cyanotic, tachycardic, excessively anxious, in extreme pain), then the differential diagnosis of potentially serious underlying pathology (Box 80-2) must be considered. The patient then needs to be cared for in an appropriate medical facility suited to the level of the acuity of the illness. However, it is important to reiterate that most adolescents with the presenting complaint of chest pain appear well and are in no clinical distress.

General inspection and palpation of the chest wall are crucial in the assessment of the adolescent with chest pain. Asymmetry or signs of trauma, including swelling, erythema, or bruising, should be noted. The presence of scoliosis or anterior chest wall deformities, such as pectus excavatum or carinatum, may cause musculoskeletal chest pain. One should attempt to elicit tenderness or pain on palpation of the chest wall muscles and each costochondral and chondrosternal junction. If pain is produced on palpation of the chest wall, the examiner should then question the patient whether the pain is consistent with the presenting complaint. If so, the likely etiology is musculoskeletal. If not, the finding may be incidental. It is often helpful to attempt to elicit the chest pain during the examination by having the adolescent move his or her torso and upper extremities or by performing a deep inspiration. The palpation of subcutaneous air in the neck may be indicative of asthma or a pneumothorax, pneumomediastinum, and/or pneumopericardium.

Inspection of the skin for rashes or striae may indicate an underlying disease process, such as an autoimmune disease, connective tissue disorder, or herpes zoster. Signs of trauma may be seen in areas other than the chest wall and may be a clue to the possibility of child abuse or trauma.

Careful auscultation of the lung fields for wheezing, rales, decreased breath sounds, or pleural rubs must be performed. Cardiac auscultation is focused on the detection of arrhythmias, murmurs, clicks, pericardial friction rubs, a gallop rhythm, or muffled, distant heart sounds.

On occasion, examination of the abdomen for tenderness, masses, or ascites may reveal the etiology as a cause of referred chest pain.

## POTENTIAL ETIOLOGIES OF ADOLESCENT CHEST PAIN

The various etiologies of chest pain are listed in Box 80-1. Following is a brief description of the more commonly encountered causes of chest pain.

### IDIOPATHIC CHEST PAIN

Idiopathic chest pain is the most common cause of chest pain in adolescents, accounting for 28% to 45% of cases.[6] These patients have a negative history and a negative review of systems with a normal physical examination. The typical patient presents with a long-standing history of fleeting episodes of chest pain. Recurrences may occur, but the pain usually resolves spontaneously over time. No organic or psychological factors are present to explain the underlying chest discomfort. Idiopathic chest pain is a diagnosis of exclusion.

### NONCARDIAC CAUSES

#### Musculoskeletal Chest Pain (Chest Wall Syndrome)

In 1 study, conducted by Pantell and Goodman,[4] 31% of adolescent chest pain was found to be musculoskeletal in etiology. Musculoskeletal chest pain remains the most common identifiable cause of chest pain in adolescents.

Musculoskeletal chest pain (chest wall syndrome) is most typically characterized by anterior chest wall tenderness. The pain is most often present at rest and is exacerbated by truncal movements. Chest wall strain involves the major muscles of the thorax. There often is a preceding history of zealous participation in a sport, especially a new sport. Activities commonly associated with chest wall strain include weight lifting, wrestling, and gymnastics. A previous history of trauma or vehicular accidents should be elicited. The carrying of heavy school or camping backpacks, or a recent respiratory illness characterized by excessive coughing, may also be linked to chest wall musculoskeletal strain.

Costochondritis is one of the most common causes of chest pain in adolescents. It is diagnosed by reproduction of pain with application of pressure directly over an unenlarged costochondral or costosternal junction. The pain is typically anterior in location, usually unilateral, and may be enhanced by positional changes, inspiration, or activity. Physical examination is diagnostic. The symptom may persist for weeks or months, with varying degrees of intensity; however, over time, it resolves.[7]

Tietze syndrome is a very rare disorder to be distinguished from costochondritis. In Tietze syndrome, there is a visible tender, unilateral swelling of the left second costal cartilage. Similar to costochondritis, the pain in Tietze syndrome may be exaggerated by movement, deep breathing, or pressure applied directly to the affected area. It is believed that this syndrome may be secondary to microtrauma. Tietze syndrome can have a protracted course, and recurrences are common.

Slipping rib syndrome is believed to be an unusual, rare sprain produced by trauma to the costal cartilages of the 8th, 9th, and 10th ribs.[6] These ribs do not attach directly to the sternum but join together by fibrous tissue, resulting in laxity of the joint tissues. The pain has been described as sharp, stabbing, or dull and is localized to either the abdominal upper quadrants or the inferior costal margins. Patients describe a popping or clicking sensation, followed by a dull ache in either upper abdominal quadrant. This problem is often self-limited and resolves spontaneously.

Pleurodynia is an uncommon complication of a coxsackie B viral infection. The viral process targets the chest wall intercostal muscles. It is the inflammation of these muscles that results in the occurrence of sharp chest pain. It is often accompanied by fever and malaise. Rarely does pleuritis (inflammation of the pleural lining of the lung) develop as an associated finding.

### Gynecomastia, Breast Pain, and Breast Masses

The reproduction of pain on palpation of breast tissue (either bilateral or unilateral) may occur in adolescent girls and boys. This tenderness may be secondary to benign cysts or menstrual changes, or, more likely, may be part of normal breast development in pubertal boys and girls. Heightened anxiety concerning the possibility of breast cancer is often harbored by these adolescents. Patient education and reassurance remain the therapy of choice.

### Precordial Catch Syndrome, Texidor Twinge, or "Stitch in the Side"

This is a form of intermittent, brief, left-sided chest pain of unknown etiology. The pain is typically sharp and localized. It usually occurs at rest and has a sudden onset, often taking the patient by surprise. It usually lasts a few seconds to minutes and is relieved by taking a few shallow breaths or a deep breath. Physical examination is normal, with no reproducible pain. It has been attributed by some to a slumped posture or bending position, although the origin of the pain remains unclear.

### Pulmonary Causes

Asthma is a common pediatric illness that can often cause chest pain in adolescents. Exercise, particularly in cold weather, is a frequent precipitant of asthma. Patients with exercise-induced asthma may provide a history of coughing with exercise and describe their chest pain as a tightness or a squeezing sensation. Exercise testing performed in conjunction with pulmonary function tests confirms the diagnosis. Persistent cough associated with a respiratory illness may result in chest pain, most likely secondary to strain of chest wall muscles.

Pneumonia may present with chest pain, but associated findings of fever and cough, along with physical findings on examination (tachypnea, rales, decreased breath sounds), reveal the diagnosis. A pneumothorax often presents with unrelenting, acute, severe chest pain. The patient appears ill with dyspnea, decreased breath sounds, tachycardia, and possibly cyanosis. In adolescents presenting with spontaneous pneumothoraces, the underlying diagnoses of Marfan syndrome, cystic fibrosis, or asthma should be ruled out. Chest pain can also be caused by a pneumomediastinum. The pain is usually substernal and may radiate to the neck, back, and shoulders. Palpation of crepitus in the neck and auscultation of crunching sounds over the precordium are diagnostic of this problem. The chest x-ray (CXR) is the procedure of choice for diagnosing pneumonia, pleural effusions, pneumothoraces, and pneumomediastinum. An echocardiogram performed in the presence of a pneumomediastinum or a pneumopericardium would be technically limited by the inability of sound waves to travel through air.

Pleurisy, an inflammation of the pleura, is associated with chest pain aggravated by inspiration and with respiratory distress. It may be idiopathic or may occur secondary to a viral infection, bacterial pneumonia, tuberculosis, autoimmune diseases, or pulmonary embolism.

Pulmonary embolism is a rare occurrence in pediatrics; however, it has been reported in adolescent females using oral contraceptives. Also, it may rarely occur in adolescents with a history of recent trauma to the lower limbs, necessitating a prolonged immobilization. Eliciting a family history of hypercoagulability may provide insight into the diagnosis. Affected patients may present with pleuritic chest pain, shortness of breath, cough, hemoptysis, fever, and/or hypoxia.

### Gastrointestinal Causes

More than 50% of cases of chest pain secondary to a gastrointestinal etiology involve the esophagus.[8] These include heartburn, pain on swallowing, or spontaneous esophageal spasm. Esophagitis is most likely associated with gastroesophageal reflux or hiatal hernia. These are relatively uncommon causes of chest pain in adolescents. The pain is often described as burning in nature and may be worse in the recumbent position. The pain may be related to eating certain foods, and symptoms may improve with appropriate antacid therapy or histamine H2 antagonists.

## CARDIAC CAUSES

Cardiovascular disease is identified as the cause of chest pain in fewer than 4% of children and adolescents. It is important to recognize and discern the cardiac etiologies of chest pain from the more common, benign etiologies because cardiac causes of chest pain may be life threatening. Cardiac chest pain may be caused by myocardial ischemia, aortic dissection, pericardial or myocardial inflammatory processes, and tachyarrhythmias (ventricular or supraventricular tachycardia). Ischemia is rare in children, but may occur with severe aortic stenosis or pulmonary stenosis, hypertrophic cardiomyopathies, coronary artery anomalies, cocaine abuse, pulmonary vascular occlusive disease (Eisenmenger syndrome), and possibly mitral valve prolapse. Typical anginal pain is precordial or substernal and is described as a deep, crushing pressure and choking sensation. The pain often radiates to the neck, jaws, and arms.

### Ischemic Cardiac Causes

Ischemic cardiac causes of chest pain and associated clinical findings are summarized as follows:

- **Severe aortic stenosis:** In this condition, a harsh ejection systolic murmur is heard at the upper right sternal edge with radiation to the carotids. The electrocardiogram (ECG) reveals left ventricular hypertrophy (LVH) with or without strain. The echocardiogram with Doppler evaluation is diagnostic. Patients with severe aortic stenosis may complain of chest pain with exercise. The normal physiological response to exercise includes an increase in heart rate and blood pressure, which in turn results in an increase in myocardial oxygen demands. Patients with this congenital heart disease are unable to meet their myocardial oxygen demands and may present with typical ischemic/anginal chest pain.
- **Severe pulmonic stenosis:** Physical examination reveals a loud, harsh, systolic ejection murmur at the left upper sternal border. The ECG reveals right ventricular hypertrophy with or without strain. The echocardiogram with Doppler evaluation is diagnostic.
- **Hypertrophic cardiomyopathy:** Hypertrophic cardiomyopathy is an autosomal dominant condition. The family history may be positive in approximately one-third of cases. However, spontaneous mutations do occur, and therefore, the family history may be negative. Unfortunately, a common presenting symptom in this disease is sudden death. Presence of a murmur is variable. In association with left ventricular outflow obstruction, a systolic ejection murmur may be heard. This murmur may be accentuated when the patient is standing or performing a Valsalva maneuver. The ECG may reveal LVH and/or the presence of deep Q waves. An echocardiogram is diagnostic of this condition. Hypertrophic cardiomyopathy predisposes to arrhythmias, which may also be perceived as chest pain.
- **Mitral valve prolapse:** Chest pain has been found in 18% of children and adolescents with mitral valve prolapse. In this syndrome, it is theorized that chest pain may result from papillary muscle or left ventricular endocardial ischemia; however, this is unclear. This condition often occurs in association with connective tissue disorders such as Marfan syndrome, Marfan-related syndromes, and Ehlers-Danlos syndrome. Many patients with connective tissue disorders also have thoracic skeletal anomalies (pectus excavatum, pectus carinatum, and scoliosis), which may result in chest pain. Cardiac auscultatory findings classically vary with the position of the patient because this alters the loading conditions of the heart. A mitral regurgitant murmur may be heard. The standing position results in a longer systolic murmur and an earlier systolic click. Prompt squatting from a standing position results in a delayed systolic click and a shorter systolic murmur. The ECG may be normal or may

reveal nonspecific T-wave abnormalities. Patients with mitral valve prolapse are more prone to develop tachyarrhythmias, which may present as chest pain. Also, mitral valve prolapse has been associated with psychiatric disease. These patients may complain of chest pain during an anxiety or panic attack.[9] (Mitral valve prolapse is discussed in detail in Chapter 84, Valvular Heart Diseases.)

- **Eisenmenger syndrome:** Adolescents with a history of unrepaired acyanotic congenital heart disease develop severe pulmonary hypertension secondary to fixed, irreversible pulmonary vascular disease. Physical examination is notable for cyanosis and clubbing. Precordial palpation may reveal a right ventricular impulse. Auscultation will reveal a loud second heart sound. Cardiac murmurs may often be absent. The ECG will reveal right ventricular hypertrophy. The increased myocardial oxygen demands occurring during exertion may not be met in these patients because of the underlying significant and persistent hypoxemia. Under these conditions, ischemic-like chest pain may develop.
- **Anomalous origin of the left coronary artery from the pulmonary artery (adult type):** Patients with anomalous origin of the left coronary artery from the pulmonary artery usually present with symptoms of congestive heart failure and a dilated cardiomyopathy in early infancy. In rare cases, however, extensive collateralization from the right coronary artery to the left coronary artery develops, allowing the patient to survive without symptoms until adolescence or early adulthood. These patients may then develop atypical chest pain, dyspnea, mitral regurgitation, and arrhythmias. The ECG will typically reveal abnormal Q waves in leads I and aVL consistent with an anterolateral myocardial infarction in the distribution of the left coronary artery. Surgical implantation of the anomalous coronary artery into the aortic root is the therapy of choice.
- **Anomalous origin of either the right or left coronary artery from the opposite sinus of Valsalva:** The more concerning congenital anomaly is the left coronary artery originating from the right sinus of Valsalva. Unfortunately, the most common presenting symptom of this anomaly is sudden death. Very rarely, a patient may present with chest pain consistent with myocardial ischemia secondary to this underlying coronary anomaly. The trigger for the chest pain is often intense physical exertion. During vigorous exercise, arterial vasodilation occurs, and coronary perfusion may become inadequate due to compression of the anomalous coronary artery between the aorta and the pulmonary artery and/or a relative narrowing of the anomalous coronary ostia. In an asymptomatic patient, the cardiac evaluation is normal, including a normal cardiac examination, a normal ECG, and a normal exercise stress test. The diagnosis is made on a detailed echocardiogram performed by a highly skilled echocardiographer. (See the vignette in Box 80-3 and Figure 80-1.) Unless the origin of the coronary arteries is outlined in detail on the cardiac ultrasound, this diagnosis may be inadvertently missed. More often than not, the finding of these coronary anomalies is an incidental finding on an echocardiogram performed for a different indication. Fortunately, these anomalies are rare.
- **Sequelae of Kawasaki disease:** Kawasaki disease is an acute vasculitis of unknown etiology that usually occurs in early childhood. Coronary artery aneurysms may develop during the first 4 to 6 weeks of the illness. A rare, although

## Box 80-3

### *Vignette*

A 14-year-old athletic adolescent male presented with syncope and collapse while running laps at school. He had been evaluated at an outside institution in the past for a murmur. His mother reported that his echocardiogram was "normal" at that time. In the emergency department, his initial ECG revealed marked ST depression in leads I, II, and V3–V6 and marked ST elevation in leads aVR, V1, and V2, consistent with significant myocardial ischemia (see Figure 80-1). His echocardiogram revealed poor left ventricular function and raised the suspicion of an anomalous origin of the left main coronary artery from the right aortic sinus of Valsalva. Cardiac catheterization confirmed the diagnosis of anomalous origin of the left main coronary artery. He underwent subsequent worsening in clinical status, requiring placement of an intra-aortic balloon pump and biventricular assist devices. He eventually underwent surgical repair of this anomaly with reimplantation of the left main coronary artery into the left main sinus of Valsalva. His clinical status and cardiac function improved rapidly following surgery with no significant residual sequelae. He was very fortunate to have recovered completely from what was essentially a "sudden death" episode. Appropriate emergency department management and prompt recognition of his congenital cardiac defect contributed largely to this aborted "sudden cardiac death" event.

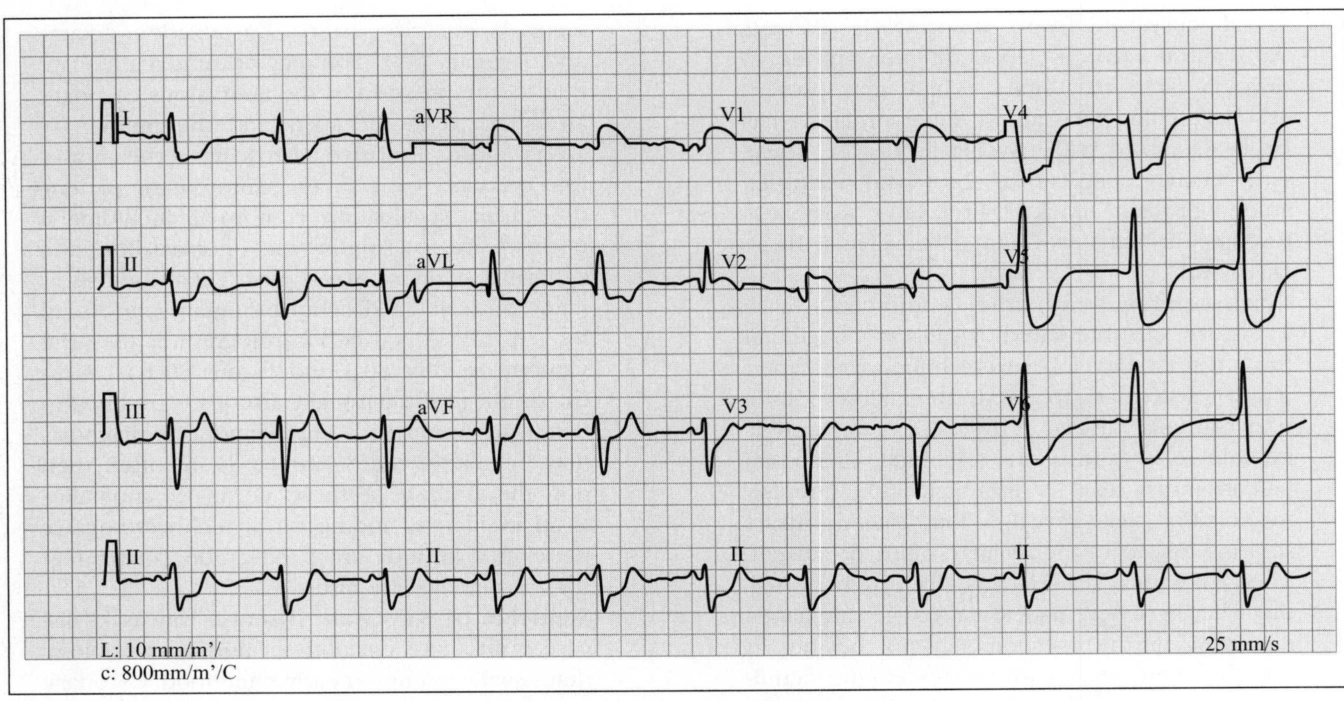


**FIGURE 80-1** Acute myocardial ischemia. Note the marked ST depression in V3–V6 and reciprocal ST elevation in V1–V2.

possible, late complication of Kawasaki disease includes coronary artery stenosis with resultant myocardial ischemia or infarction. Coronary artery insufficiency related to previous Kawasaki disease may result in anginal chest pain. In adolescents with a previous history of Kawasaki disease, chest pain must be thoroughly evaluated to rule out the possibility of myocardial ischemia or infarction.[10]

- **Takayasu arteritis:** This is a rare granulomatous vasculitis of unknown etiology that commonly affects the thoracic and abdominal aorta (see Chapter 122, Other Rheumatologic Disorders). It is an inflammatory aortitis that presents with nonspecific constitutional symptoms, such as fever, weight loss, joint pain, hypertension, and elevated markers of inflammation (erythrocyte sedimentation rate). Months later, segmental stenosis, occlusion, dilatation, and aneurysmal formation in the large and medium-size arterial vessels develop. The involvement of the ascending aorta with coronary artery narrowing, or the development of coronary artery aneurysms, may occur. These patients may then present with chest pain secondary to myocardial ischemia. Computed tomography angiography (CTA) and magnetic resonance angiography (MRA) have become valuable tools in assessing the entire arterial tree in patients with Takayasu arteritis.
- **Sequelae of previous cardiac surgery in infancy or early childhood:** An adolescent or adult who had previous open heart surgery involving the coronary arteries may present with anginal-type chest pain. Two of the surgical procedures that fall into this category are the arterial switch procedure for transposition of the great arteries and the Ross procedure, which is an autotransplantation of the patient's own pulmonary valve to replace a diseased aortic valve. The Ross procedure involves reimplantation of the coronary arteries.
- **Cocaine abuse/substance abuse:** In a recent study published by Mahle, more than 20% of their adolescent patients diagnosed with myocardial infarction also had a history of substance abuse. The abuse of both cocaine and amphetamines were associated with acute coronary syndromes.[11] Cigarette smoking may also be an additional risk factor for myocardial infarction or ischemia in adolescents. Coronary artery vasospasm resulting from cocaine abuse mimics the signs and symptoms of myocardial ischemia

or infarction. The chest pain is described as severe, crushing, and relentless. The patient appears in acute distress with tachycardia, dyspnea, and diaphoresis. Cocaine blocks the reuptake of catecholamines in the central nervous system and peripheral sympathetic nerves. An increase in the sympathetic output and circulating levels of catecholamines causes coronary vasoconstriction in the context of increased myocardial oxygen demands, thereby resulting in myocardial ischemia. The cardiac examination will likely be normal. The ECG may or may not reveal ST-segment changes consistent with ischemia. Although a history of illicit drug use may not be obtained, the diagnosis of substance abuse should be considered. Toxicology screening will confirm recent cocaine and/or amphetamine use.

### Inflammatory Causes

Inflammatory cardiac causes of chest pain include the following:

- **Pericarditis:** Inflammation of the pericardium may have a viral, bacterial, or rheumatologic (systemic lupus erythematosus, juvenile rheumatoid arthritis) etiology. Pericardial pain is usually described as sharp, stabbing, and persistent. Patients will often make an audible grunting noise with respiration, most likely secondary to pain. The pain is precordial in location and may be relieved by sitting and leaning forward. Patients with a sizable pericardial effusion are usually reluctant to lie flat. Cough, fever, and respiratory distress are often present. The CXR may reveal cardiomegaly. On examination, the heart sounds may be distant, neck veins may be distended, and a friction rub may be noted. If a large effusion is present, a friction rub may not be audible, and an exaggerated alteration in the amplitude of the pulse (pulsus paradoxus) may be noted. The ECG will reveal generalized diffuse ST elevations (Figure 80-2), and the echocardiogram may reveal a pericardial effusion. Pericarditis may occur, however, in the absence of an effusion.
- **Myocarditis/myopericarditis:** Myocarditis typically involves the pericardium and can cause a dull, persistent chest pain. The patient usually appears ill and requires immediate medical attention. Older children may complain of

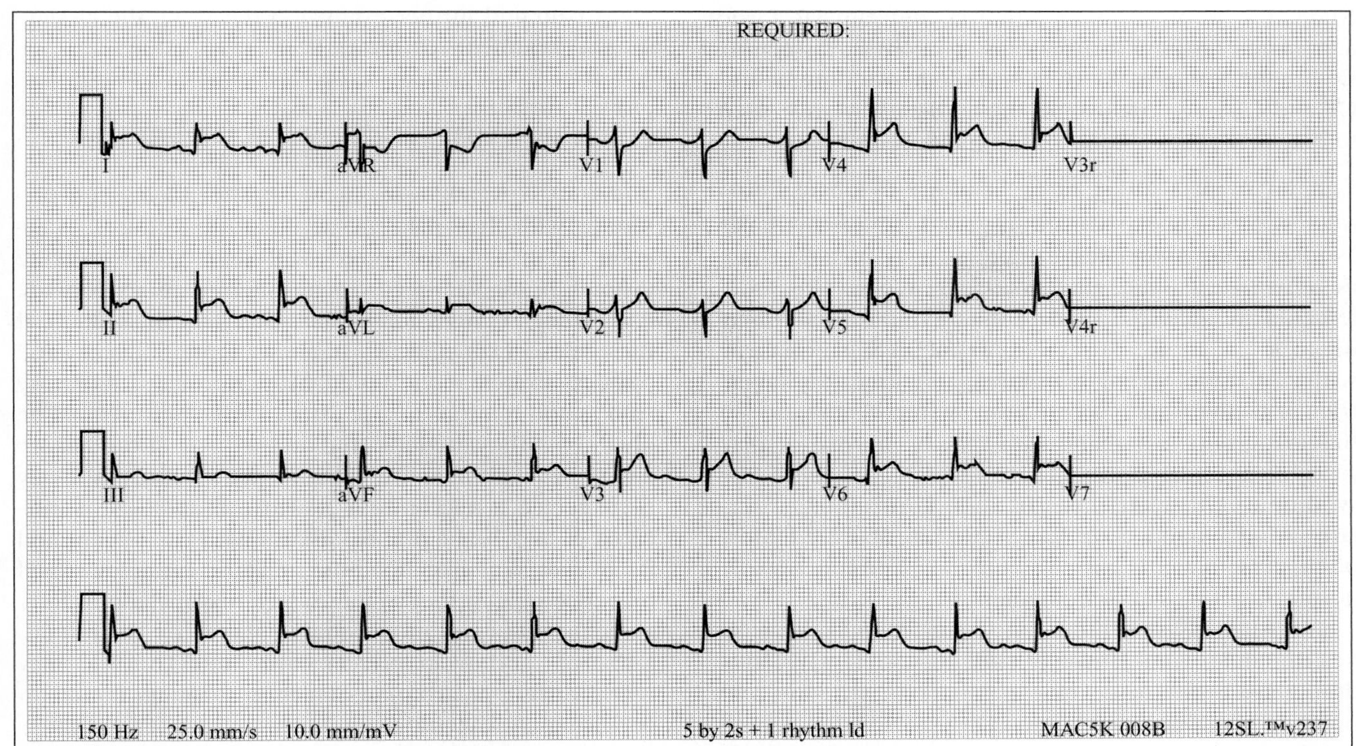


**FIGURE 80-2** Acute pericarditis. Widespread ST elevation in all leads.

abdominal/epigastric pain, most likely secondary to low cardiac output with decreased perfusion of the gut. Fever and respiratory distress may or may not be present. A prominent gallop rhythm may be noted, with or without a mitral regurgitation murmur. Viruses such as coxsackie B are the most common etiologic agent. The CXR may reveal cardiomegaly. The ECG will often reveal low QRS voltages and ST-T-wave segment abnormalities. An echocardiogram reveals decreased myocardial performance. These patients are prone to life-threatening arrhythmias.

### Trauma

Post-traumatic pericardial effusions can occur 1 to 3 months following significant blunt chest trauma. Inspection of the chest wall may not reveal any external signs of trauma such as ecchymosis or edema.

### Chest Pain Secondary to Aortic Dissection

Aortic dissection is an extremely rare occurrence in the pediatric population; however, it should be seriously considered in all patients reporting acute, sudden, and severe chest pain that is maximal in intensity at its onset. Adolescents who have a history of or a phenotype consistent with certain heritable disorders are at a higher risk for aortopathies and potential aortic dissection. Some of these disorders include Marfan syndrome, Loeys-Dietz syndrome, Turner syndrome, Ehlers-Danlos syndrome, Noonan syndrome, homocystinuria, and familial aortic aneurysms. Also, trauma may result in aortic dissection. Computed tomography (CT) scanning, including helical CT and CTA, is a highly specific and sensitive test used to diagnose aortic dissections in many institutions.

### Cardiac Arrhythmias as an Etiology of Chest Pain

Adolescents may experience sustained tachyarrhythmias as chest pain. Associated symptoms may include dizziness, nausea, fatigue, and possibly syncope. Most adolescents are able to articulate their symptoms and may describe an abrupt onset of a rapid, racing heartbeat, with an abrupt termination of the palpitations. Supraventricular tachycardia is a common rhythm disturbance in this age group. A baseline ECG may be normal or may reveal ventricular pre-excitation (Wolff-Parkinson-White syndrome). The acute onset of atrial fibrillation, particularly in adolescent boys, has also been observed. Most often, these patients have a structurally and functionally normal heart on echocardiogram.

Ventricular arrhythmias are unusual in otherwise healthy adolescents. However, patients with long QT syndrome are prone to develop palpitations, syncope, and potentially sudden death secondary to life-threatening ventricular arrhythmias. Long QT syndrome is a disorder of the electrical depolarization and repolarization of the ventricles. It is a genetic disorder and can arise from mutations in one of several genes. Often, there is a family history of sudden death. Individuals with long QT syndrome have a prolongation of the QT interval and abnormal T-wave morphology on the surface ECG.

Continued rhythm surveillance (event recorders, Holter monitors) in these patients is important to document the underlying arrhythmia and thereby appropriately diagnose and treat the arrhythmia.

### PSYCHOGENIC (FUNCTIONAL)

Adolescents often somaticize psychological stresses and may complain of chronic headaches, abdominal pain, and/or chest pain. A psychogenic etiology accounts for 9% to 20% of chest pain in adolescents and occurs more commonly in females. Anxiety and emotional stress are common in the adolescent age group and may stem from domestic conflicts, school phobias, peer problems, or other stressful life-related events such as death, divorce, or illness of a family member. A recent cardiac-related death of a family member or close friend may heighten the adolescent's fear about the health of his or her own heart and may result in functional chest pain. Sleep disturbances, depression, and anxiety disorders, often accompanied by hyperventilation and dizziness, can be associated with psychogenic chest pain. The pain is often chronic and nonspecific in nature. The physical examination is always normal. Reassurance regarding the chest pain and further evaluation regarding the anxiety are the treatments of choice in these situations.

## FURTHER EVALUATION AND MANAGEMENT

The initial overall assessment of the adolescent presenting with chest pain is crucial in formulating an evaluation and management protocol. If the patient is in acute distress, he or she needs to be referred to appropriate emergency services for further care (see Box 80-2). If the adolescent is clinically stable, a thorough history and physical examination should be performed. Laboratory studies and referrals to a pediatric cardiologist should be obtained if they are indicated on the basis of the history and physical examination (Box 80-4). If cardiac pathology is suspected, a referral to a pediatric cardiologist is indicated. It may be helpful to discuss with the patient and family that in all likelihood the pediatric cardiologist will be performing further testing, which may include an ECG, an echocardiogram, monitoring to surveil for rhythm disturbances, and/or an exercise stress test. The ECG may reveal early repolarization, which is a benign condition occurring typically in young healthy males (Figure 80-3). The T wave begins early, resulting in ST elevation predominantly in the anterior precordial leads (ie, leads

> **Box 80-4**
>
> ***When to Refer an Adolescent with Chest Pain***
>
> - Presence of acute distress
> - Significant trauma present
> - Family history of hereditary diseases associated with cardiac pathology (cardiomyopathies, Marfan syndrome, long QT syndrome)
> - Family history of sudden unexplained death or presumed seizures
> - History of underlying congenital or acquired heart disease (Kawaski disease)
> - Chest pain in the context of a previously undiagnosed pathological murmur
> - Chest pain occurring with exertion or exercise
> - Chest pain in association with dizziness, presyncope, syncope, or palpitations
> - Pleural effusion or pneumothorax
> - Serious psychological issues
> - Concern on the part of the primary caregiver of serious underlying pathology

V2–V4). Clinical correlation is extremely important when differentiating this condition from cardiac pathology. If a pulmonary condition is being considered, a CXR may be helpful to rule out pneumonia, pleural effusions, or pneumothorax. Appropriate therapy with bronchodilators or antibiotics may alleviate the chest pain. Difficult to control reactive airway disease (asthma) may benefit from a referral to a pediatric pulmonologist or allergist. Musculoskeletal chest pain is a clinical diagnosis ascertained by history and physical examination. With a history of trauma, a CXR may be necessary to rule out a rib fracture. Reassurance remains the mainstay of therapy for musculoskeletal chest pain. Analgesics, nonsteroidal anti-inflammatory medications, and rest may provide symptomatic relief. If a gastrointestinal disorder is suspected, improvement in symptoms from a trial of antacids or histamine H2 antagonists may help establish the diagnosis.

In some adolescents, chest pain may be psychogenic in origin. Adolescents experiencing psychological distress often think of themselves as sicker and tend to worry more about symptoms that most might otherwise ignore. A positive, strong bond between the patient and the primary caregiver is helpful when treating such patients. In-depth discussions focusing on the patient's fears and life stresses may ameliorate the symptoms, or enable the adolescent to cope with the pain and resume normal daily activities. Because recurrent symptoms of chest pain are common in this population, follow-up services should be routinely arranged. On occasion, a referral to a mental health provider may be indicated. Idiopathic chest pain remains a diagnosis of exclusion and is made in the context of a negative history and a normal physical examination. Reassurance remains the mainstay of therapy for these patients.

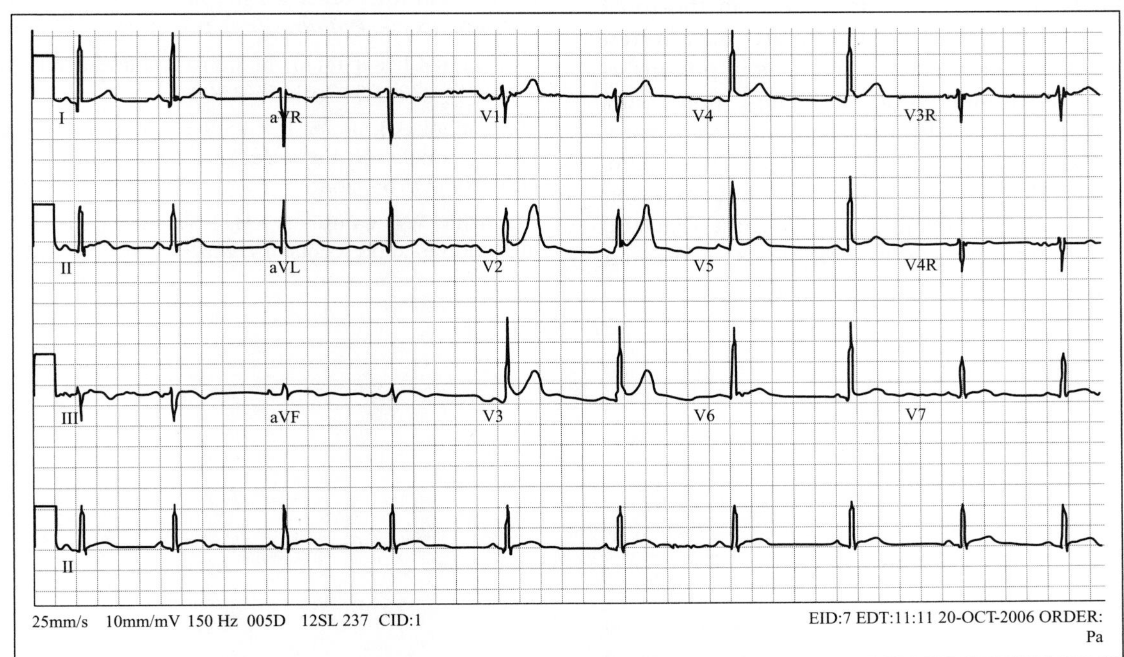


**FIGURE 80-3** Early repolarization: a benign finding.

The primary caregiver's knowledge of the family dynamics may be useful in choosing the appropriate evaluation of the adolescent with chest pain. If a low suspicion of underlying serious pathology exists, ordering additional laboratory tests may unnecessarily enhance the anxiety of the patient and family. In other families, however, laboratory testing and referrals to pediatric subspecialists may be necessary to adequately reassure the patient and family that the etiology of the chest pain is benign. (See Box 80-1.) For example, in many cases, the reassurance provided by a pediatric cardiologist that the patient has a healthy heart is therapeutic, or at least allows the adolescent to deal more effectively with the chest pain. Once the patient has been evaluated and cleared by an appropriate pediatric subspecialist and the chest pain persists, there is little reason to believe that serious cardiac or pulmonary pathology exists.[6]

## CONCLUSION

Chronic, intermittent chest pain that persists for several months is unlikely to be caused by serious organic pathology. This presenting complaint, coupled with a negative history and a normal physical examination, usually requires no further medical evaluation. The adolescent with chest pain and his or her family often manifest a heightened anxiety with respect to the possibility of serious underlying cardiac pathology. It is important to recognize that sudden cardiac death in the adolescent population is indeed a rare occurrence. Cardiomyopathies, anomalies of the coronary arteries, or an abnormal cardiac electrical conduction system are most often associated with sudden cardiac death. It is important to recognize that most adolescents with these potentially serious underlying cardiovascular conditions are asymptomatic and do not have a prodrome of chest pain. Unfortunately, sudden death is often their presenting symptom. It is also interesting to point out that the diagnosis of certain other cardiac problems such as an atrial septal defect or a bicuspid aortic valve would not be causally linked to the presenting complaint of chest pain. In general, the majority of conditions causing chest pain in adolescents are benign and self-limiting. A compassionate, thorough evaluation performed by an astute, perceptive clinician should result in the appropriate care of the adolescent with chest pain.

## REFERENCES


1. Ezzati TM. *Ambulatory Care Utilization Patterns of Children and Young Adults: National Ambulatory Medical Care Survey, United States, January-December 1975*. Vital and Health Statistics, Series 13, data from the National Health Survey. Hyattsville, MD: US Department of Health, Education, and Welfare, Public Health Office, Office of the Assistant Secretary for Health, National Center for Health Statistics; 1978. DHEW publication 39; DHEW publication (PHS) 78-1790

2. Driscoll DJ, Glicklich LB, Gallen WJ. Chest pain in children: a prospective study. *Pediatrics.* 1976;57:648-651

3. Selbst SM, Ruddy RM, Clark BJ, Henretig FM, Santulli T. Pediatric chest pain: a prospective study. *Pediatrics.* 1988;82:319-323

4. Pantell RH, Goodman BW. Adolescent chest pain: a prospective study. *Pediatrics.* 1983;71:881-887

5. Park MK. *Pediatric Cardiology for Practitioners.* 4th ed. St. Louis: Mosby; 2002:441

6. Selbst SM. Evaluation of chest pain in children. *Pediatr Rev.* 1986;8:56-62

7. Brown RT. Costochondritis in adolescents. *J Adolesc Health Care.* 1981;1:198-201

8. Feinstein RA, Daniel WA Jr. Chronic chest pain in children and adolescents. *Pediatr Annal.* 1986;15(10):685-686,691-694

9. Cava JR. Chest pain in children and adolescents. *Pediatr Clin North Am.* 2004;51(6):1553-1568

10. Madhok AB, Boxer R, Green S. An adolescent with chest pain—Sequela of Kawasaki disease. *Pediatr Emerg Care.* 2004;20(11):765-768

11. Mahle WT, Campbell RM, Favaloro-Sabatier J. Myocardial infarction in adolescents. *J Pediatrics.* 2007;151(2):150-154

# CHAPTER 81

# Hyperlipidemia and Atherosclerosis

MARC S. JACOBSON, MD

Screening for risk of atherosclerosis, whether by family history followed by cholesterol and blood pressure measurements (targeted screening) or by universal cholesterol testing, is recommended for all adolescents by the National Cholesterol Education Program Expert Panel on Blood Cholesterol in Children and Adolescents, the Committee on Nutrition of the American Academy of Pediatrics (AAP), the American Heart Association, and the American Medical Association Guidelines for Adolescent Preventive Services (AAP).[1-3] Some physicians, fearing the negative effects of low-fat diets on growth or overuse of medications, argue that no cholesterol testing should be performed until adulthood. Others consider that universal treatment with or without screening should be the standard of care and that a concerted effort should be made to lower fat and cholesterol intake, increase habitual physical activity, and prevent smoking.

Until recently, this debate took place with little scientific data available from well-designed studies. This is no longer the case. The relationship of histologic severity of atherosclerotic lesions to measurable risk factors in adolescents has been defined by the Pathobiological Determinants of Atherosclerosis in Youth study.[4] In addition, the safety and efficacy of low-cholesterol, low-fat dietary treatment has been demonstrated by the Dietary Intervention Study in Children (DISC), a prospective study of growth among early adolescents with moderate hypercholesterolemia, which demonstrated normal growth and development in both treated subjects and controls.[5] A 3-year follow-up of high-risk hyperlipidemic children and adolescents found good lipid-lowering effects and normal growth.[6] Furthermore, the powerful cholesterol-lowering effects of the statins, which are 3-hydroxy-3-methylglutaryl-coenzyme A (HMG-CoA) inhibitors, have shown clear proof of the life-saving results of cholesterol lowering in both primary and secondary prevention.[7]

Clearly, with new studies documenting the life-saving effects of cardiovascular disease prevention in adults, the safety of dietary therapy in young adolescents, and the rising prevalence of obesity and cardiovascular risk factors in adolescents, the burden of proof is now on those who state that nothing should be done for adolescents. Therefore, increasing numbers of patients with hyperlipidemia and increased atherosclerosis risk are being identified. Table 81-1 provides normative data for cholesterol, triglycerides, and lipid subfractions for US adolescents.[8] Figures 81-1 and 81-2 provide algorithms

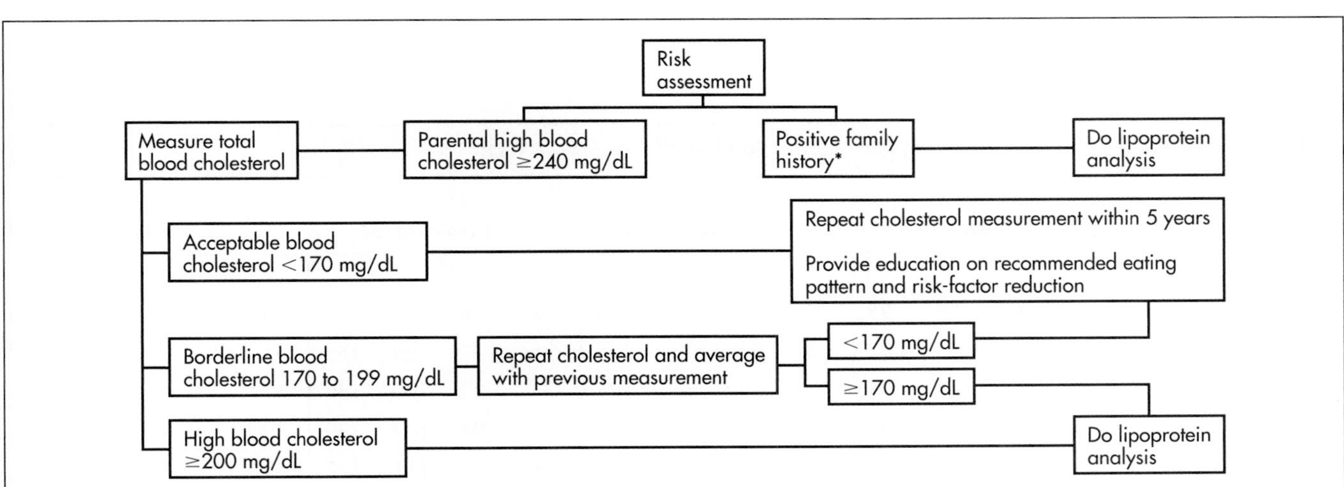


**FIGURE 81-1** Risk assessment. *Positive family history is defined as a history of premature (before age 55 in females or 60 in males) cardiovascular disease in a parent or grandparent. (Source: From US Department of Health and Human Services. *Report of the Expert Panel on Blood Cholesterol Levels in Children and Adolescents*. Bethesda, MD: US Department of Health and Human Services, Public Health Service, National Institutes of Health, National Heart, Lung, and Blood Institute, National Cholesterol Education Program; 1991. NIH publication 91-2732.)

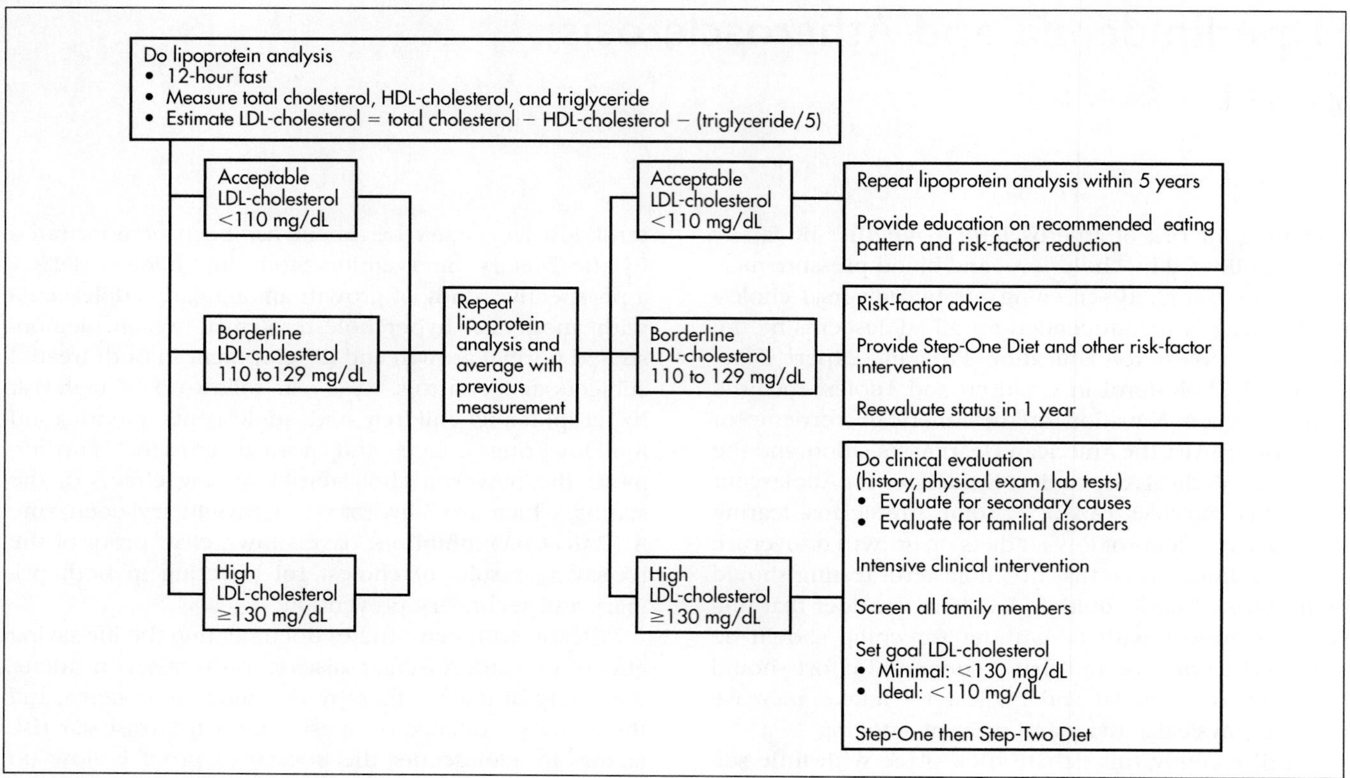


**FIGURE 81-2** Classification, education, and follow-up based on low-density lipoprotein cholesterol. (Source: From US Department of Health and Human Services. *Report of the Expert Panel on Blood Cholesterol Levels in Children and Adolescents*. Bethesda, MD: US Department of Health and Human Services, Public Health Service, National Institutes of Health, National Heart, Lung, and Blood Institute, National Cholesterol Education Program; 1991. NIH publication 91-2732.)

**Table 81-1**

## Lipid Values for Adolescent Atherosclerosis Risk Assessment

| | | *Total Cholesterol* | | | | *Triglycerides* | | | | *LDL Cholesterol* | | | | *HDL Cholesterol* | | | |
|---|---|---|---|---|---|---|---|---|---|---|---|---|---|---|---|---|---|
| ***Percentile*** | | | | | | | | | | | | | | | | | |
| *Age (yr)* | *Sex* | *5* | *50* | *75* | *95* | *5* | *50* | *75* | *95* | *5* | *50* | *75* | *95* | *5* | *50* | *75* | *95* |
| 10–14 | M | 119 | 158 | 173 | 202 | 32 | 66 | 74 | 125 | 64 | 97 | 109 | 133 | 37 | 55 | 61 | 74 |
| | F | 126 | 164 | 171 | 205 | 32 | 60 | 85 | 105 | 68 | 97 | 109 | 136 | 37 | 52 | 58 | 70 |
| 15–19 | M | 113 | 150 | 168 | 197 | 32 | 66 | 88 | 125 | 62 | 94 | 109 | 130 | 30 | 46 | 52 | 63 |
| | F | 120 | 158 | 176 | 203 | 39 | 75 | 85 | 132 | 59 | 96 | 111 | 137 | 35 | 52 | 61 | 74 |
| 20–24 | M | 118 | 159 | 179 | 197 | 44 | 78 | 107 | 165 | 66 | 101 | 118 | 147 | 30 | 45 | 51 | 63 |
| | F | 121 | 165 | 186 | 237 | 52 | 96 | 126 | 175 | 70 | 98 | 136 | 151 | 37 | 50 | 60 | 73 |

HDL, high-density lipoprotein; LDL, low-density lipoprotein.

Data from Lipid Research *Clinics Population Studies Data Book*. Pub. No. 80-1527. Bethesda, MD: National Institutes of Health; 1980.

for screening and initial evaluation of elevated cholesterol levels in adolescents.[3] Optimal treatment requires a comprehensive approach, including nutritional counseling, behavior modification, and medical therapies for the adolescent within the family context.

## DIAGNOSIS

Secondary hyperlipidemia should be ruled out in adolescents (Box 81-1). Most secondary causes can be eliminated by history and physical examination, but laboratory screening for hypothyroidism, hepatitis, nephrotic syndrome, and pregnancy should be considered. Currently used low-dose oral contraceptives have minimal effects on lipids in the average patient, but adolescents with underlying lipid abnormalities have not been studied thoroughly. Therefore, lipid screening prior to hormonal contraception initiation should be considered, if feasible. A rare form of familial hypertriglyceridemia has been reported to be exacerbated by the administration of estrogen, resulting in acute fulminating pancreatitis and death. Smoking in conjunction with the use of oral contraceptives further increases the risk of cardiovascular disease. Although lipid abnormalities are rarely contraindications to oral contraceptive use, screening and appropriate treatment should be part of a comprehensive approach to the patient.

Once secondary causes have been ruled out, hyperlipidemia can be classified as (1) familial hypercholesterolemia (FH), a dominantly inherited defect in the gene located on chromosome 19 which codes for the low-density lipoprotein (LDL) cell surface receptor; (2) familial combined hyperlipidemia (FCH), which results from a dominantly inherited excess in hepatic production of very low-density lipoprotein (VLDL) combined with abnormalities in the catabolism of VLDL cholesterol and LDL cholesterol, resulting in increased cholesterol and triglyceride levels[9]; (3) mixed environmental genetic hyperlipidemia, which may be the result of apolipoprotein phenotype abnormalities or other uncharacterized hereditary defects combined with excessive saturated fat and cholesterol dietary intake; and (4) metabolic syndrome, a combination of risk factors resulting from insulin resistance and characterized by obesity with central adiposity, hypertension, raised triglycerides, and low high-density lipoprotein (HDL) cholesterol. Table 81-2 shows typical lipid profiles for each of the four hyperlipidemias commonly seen in adolescents and for the rare homozygous FH for comparison.

Each type of hyperlipidemia may involve a family history of early myocardial infarction, stroke, and/or hypercholesterolemia. Only FH is associated with signs of peripheral lipid deposition, such as corneal arcus, xanthomas, or xanthelasmas, which are useful differentiating features. Families with FCH have some members with elevated cholesterol levels, some with elevated triglyceride levels, and some with both.[9] The homozygotes for FH present with total and LDL cholesterol levels in the 700 and 600 mg/dL range, respectively. On average, the heterozygotes for FH have a total cholesterol value of 250 to 400 mg/dL and normal triglycerides, whereas patients with FCH have average total cholesterol levels in the 200 to 250 mg/dL range, with triglycerides above 120 mg/dL. Patients with mixed environmental genetic hypercholesterolemia tend to have lower total cholesterol and triglyceride levels.[1]

### Box 81-1

### *Causes of Secondary Hyperlipidemia in Adolescents*

**Dietary**
- Excessive consumption of cholesterol, saturated fat, or calories
- Anorexia nervosa

**Endocrinologic factors**
- Diabetes mellitus
- Hypothyroidism
- Pregnancy, lactation

**Renal disease**
- Nephritis, nephrosis

**Gastrointestinal disease**
- Biliary tract obstruction, pancreatitis, hepatocellular disease

**Drugs**
- Oral contraceptives
- Corticosteroid administration
- Thiazides
- Beta-blockers
- Isotretinoin (Accutane)
- Antiretrovirals

**Other metabolic disease**
- Glycogen storage disease
- Acute intermittent porphyria
- Gout

**Connective tissue disease**
- Systemic lupus erythematosus
- Juvenile rheumatoid arthritis

**Table 81-2**

**Typical Lipid Profile Values in Adolescents with Hyperlipidemia**

| | *FH homozygous* | *FH heterozygous* | *FCH* | *Mixed Environmental Genetic* | *Metabolic Syndrome* |
|---|---|---|---|---|---|
| Total cholesterol (mg/dL) | 600–700 | 250–350 | 225–275 | 200–250 | 200–250 |
| Triglycerides (mg/dL) | 75–170 | 75–170 | 170–250 | 75–250 | 170–350 |
| LDL-C (mg/dL) | 550–650 | 160–300 | 150–200 | 150–200 | 110–160 |
| HDL-C (mg/dL) | 40–60 | 40–60 | 25–45 | 30–50 | 25–40 |

FH, Familial hypercholesterolemia; FCH, Familial combined hypercholesterolemia.

## INITIAL MANAGEMENT

Treatment of hyperlipidemia in adolescents is important. Extensive autopsy data show the acceleration of lesion formation during this age period. In addition, the direct relationship between the severity of lesions and lipid levels and smoking has been noted in recent years.[4] Treatment should begin if the adolescent's LDL cholesterol level exceeds the 95th percentile for age and sex (Table 81-1). Initial treatment for all types of hyperlipidemia consists of diet modification, weight control, and exercise. Only those with severe family histories, high levels of LDL cholesterol, and failure to respond to diet modifications require pharmacotherapy.[7,10-12] A significant adjunct to therapy for the lipid abnormality is the prevention and treatment of associated risk factors for atherosclerosis: hypertension, smoking, obesity, and sedentary lifestyle.

Dietary modification should be based on the principles of the AAP position statement on cholesterol in childhood (Box 81-2).[3] Counseling should be focused on reducing the intake of total fat and saturated fat, which is more difficult but more effective than lowering cholesterol intake per se. Generally, the clinician should attempt to modify the adolescent's baseline diet rather than attempt to construct a theoretical diet from general principles. Replacing foods that are higher in saturated fat with low saturated fat foods with similar sensory properties is the most successful approach (eg, replacing butter with olive oil in food preparation).[1,5,13,14] Adolescents with FCH may benefit from an additional emphasis on reducing refined carbohydrate intake, especially from juices and sweetened beverages. Carbohydrate intake should be principally from whole grains, fresh fruits, and vegetables. Exercise may be a useful adjunct to a comprehensive diet program because it can help maintain ideal body weight and general cardiovascular and pulmonary function.

Nutritional counseling by the physician, nurse, or registered dietitian should be followed by a repeat lipid profile no sooner than 6 to 8 weeks after diet modification. If the diet is being followed appropriately, improvement should be seen within this time. If no change or worsening occurs, further investigation of the current diet is indicated. Factors to be explored include the preparation of meals, whether school lunches are consumed, and the types and quantities of snacks and fast foods eaten. If lipids have not met targets or have not significantly improved 3 months after diet initiation, then a Step II diet (Box 81-2) and more intensive nutrition

**Box 81-2**

***Dietary Recommendations for Management of Hyperlipidemia***

**Step I**

- Cholesterol intake: 300 mg/day
- Fat intake: 20%–30% of total energy intake, averaged over several days
- Saturated fat intake: <10% of total energy intake
- Polyunsaturated fat intake: no more than 10% of total energy intake
- Monounsaturated fat intake: to make up the remainder
- Energy intake: sufficient for adequate growth achieved by eating a wide variety of foods

**Step II: For patients who do not meet LDL cholesterol target on Step I**

- Cholesterol intake: 200 mg/day
- Fat and polyunsaturated intake: as above
- Saturated fat intake: reduce to <7% of energy intake
- Monounsaturated fat intake: increase to make up the remainder

counseling is indicated. A registered dietitian with expertise in working with adolescents can be invaluable in assessing baseline nutritional status and current diet, and in providing education and counseling. Most physicians will need such support to provide comprehensive treatment for hyperlipidemia in adolescents.[1]

## PHARMACOTHERAPY

Patients who do not respond adequately to dietary intervention need pharmacotherapy in addition to diet modification. The published data on treatment with medications in the pediatric age group are based only on 1-year follow-up to this point; thus, pharmacotherapy is reserved for those at greatest risk. Medication is indicated for adolescents who have first-degree relatives who experienced early death (age 45 or younger) or disability, such as myocardial infarct or stroke, and LDL cholesterol levels persistently greater than the 95th percentile for age and sex (Table 81-1). In addition, adolescents being considered for medication should have failed to respond with 15% to 20% lowering of LDL cholesterol levels during at least 6 months of intensive diet therapy provided by a nutritionist skilled in working with adolescents with hyperlipidemia.[1]

The bile acid–binding resins—colesevelam, colestipol, and cholestyramine—have been used by many lipid specialists with good cholesterol reduction. They are generally agreed to be safe, but their effects on growth and development are just beginning to receive scientific attention. The resins are given as tablets or in a powdered form that must be mixed with water or juice. The common side effects of bile acid–binding resins, such as bloating, gas, and constipation, can be avoided by administering low doses initially, with gradual increases from 1 to 3 doses per day over the first 4 to 6 weeks. If constipation becomes a limiting side effect, the mixing of cholestyramine or colestipol with psyllium powder (Metamucil) can be helpful. Psyllium and other water-soluble fibers have their own mild cholesterol-lowering effects.[1,6]

Niacin (nicotinic acid) acts by reducing the synthesis of VLDL, the precursor of LDL, thereby lowering cholesterol and triglyceride levels and raising HDL. Dosage is in the range of 1 g to 3 g/day. The most obvious and frequent side effect of niacin is prostaglandin-mediated flushing of the skin, which may occur within a few minutes of consumption of the oral dose. Treatment with aspirin can reduce or block this side effect. More serious side effects include peptic ulcer disease, gout, and hepatic toxicity, all of which are rare.[1,7]

Statins such as simvastatin, atorvastatin, and pravastatin are now US Food and Drug Administration approved for adolescents following safety and efficacy studies.[10-12] They can be given in tablet form in a single daily dose. This simplified regimen significantly improves acceptance and compliance. The dosage is 10 mg to 40 mg/day titrated to the LDL cholesterol response. When combined with dietary therapy, statins have been shown to reduce total and LDL cholesterol levels by 25% to 40% in adolescents with hypercholesterolemia. Two rare, yet major side effects of this drug are myositis, which can progress to myolysis if untreated, and transient elevation of liver enzymes, which is reversible within 2 to 6 weeks of discontinuation of therapy. Periodic monitoring of liver enzymes and creatine kinase is indicated during statin therapy.

Gemfibrozil and fenofibrate are fibric acid derivatives that decrease VLDL levels and are useful in patients with FCH who have elevated triglyceride and LDL cholesterol levels. These agents are not indicated when cholesterol level alone is elevated, and should not be used when hepatic or renal dysfunction is present. Fibrate use is contraindicated in patients receiving anticoagulants. Fenofibrate has been used effectively in combination with statins, whereas gemfibrozil increases the risk of myosistis and should not be used with a statin. Side effects of fibrates occur in the gastrointestinal tract, nervous system, and hematologic system. Periodic monitoring of liver enzymes and complete blood cell count is advised during fibrate therapy. Fibrates and niacin have received no systematic study in adolescents. Their use should therefore be reserved for patients in whom conventional therapy has failed, and then only on an experimental basis.

## CONCLUSION

Atherosclerosis prevention is an important and rewarding aspect of adolescent medicine practice. Identification and management of risk factors such as hypercholesterolemia, hypertension, smoking, diabetes, and obesity are the keys to success. Data on therapeutic lifestyle changes, such as low saturated fat diet, decreased television time, and increased habitual physical activity, are promising.[15] Successful pharmacotherapy of lipid abnormalities has been clearly demonstrated in the short term, but long-term studies are needed.

## REFERENCES

1. Jacobson MS, ed. *Atherosclerosis Prevention: Identification and Treatment of the Child With High Cholesterol*. London: Harwood Academic; 1991

2. Elster AB, Kuznets NJ. *AMA Guidelines for Adolescent Preventive Services (GAPS): Recommendations and Rationale*. Baltimore, MD: Williams & Wilkins; 1994

3. American Academy of Pediatrics Committee on Nutrition. Cholesterol in childhood. *Pediatrics*. 1998;101:141–147

4. Pathobiological Determinants of Atherosclerosis Research Group. Relationship of atherosclerosis in young men to serum lipoprotein cholesterol concentrations and smoking: a preliminary report from the Pathobiological Determinants of Atherosclerosis Research Group. *JAMA*. 1990;264:3018–3024

5. The Dietary Intervention Study in Children Collaborative Research Group. Efficacy and safety of lowering dietary intake of fat and cholesterol in children with elevated low density cholesterol. *JAMA*. 1995;273:1429–1435

6. Jacobson MS, Tomopoulos S, Williams CL, Arden MR, Deckelbaum RJ, Starc TJ. Normal growth in high-risk hyperlipidemic children and adolescents with dietary intervention. *Prev Med*. 1998;27:775–780

7. Knopp RH. Drug treatment of lipid disorders. *N Engl J Med*. 1999;341(7):498–511

8. *Lipid Research Clinics Population Studies Data Book*. Pub. No. 80-1527. Bethesda, MD: National Institutes of Health; 1980

9. Cortner JA, Coates PM, Gallagher PR. Prevalence and expression of familial combined hyperlipidemia in childhood. *J Pediatr*. 1990;116:514–519

10. Stein EA, Illingworth DR, Kwiterovich PO Jr, et al. Efficacy and safety of lovastatin in adolescent males with heterozygous familial hypercholesterolemia: a randomized controlled trial. *JAMA*. 1999;281(2):137–144

11. McCrindle BW, Ose L, Marais AD. Efficacy and safety of atorvastatin in children and adolescents with familial hypercholesterolemia or severe hyperlipidemia: a multicenter, randomized, placebo-controlled trial. *J Pediatr*. 2003;143(1):74–80

12. de Jongh S, Ose L, Szamosi T, et al. Efficacy and safety of statin therapy in children with familial hypercholesterolemia: a randomized, double-blind, placebo-controlled trial with simvastatin. *Circulation*. 2002;106(17):2231–2237

13. Jacobson MS, Copperman N, Haas MA, Shenker IR. Adolescent obesity and cardiovascular risk: a rational approach to management. *Ann N Y Acad Sci*. 1993;699:220–229

14. Copperman N, Schebendach J, Arden M, Jacobson MS. Nutrient quality of fat- and cholesterol-modified diets of children with hyperlipidemia. *Arch Pediatr Adolesc Med*. 1995;149:333–336

15. Raitakari OT, Rönnemaa T, Järvisalo MJ, et al. Endothelial function in healthy 11-year-old children after dietary intervention with onset in infancy: the Special Turku Coronary Risk Factor Intervention Project for Children (STRIP). *Circulation*. 2005;112:3786–3794

# CHAPTER 82

# Congenital Heart Disease

MICHAEL A. LACORTE, MD

## HEART MURMUR IN HEALTHY ADOLESCENTS

It is not uncommon to detect a heart murmur for the first time during a routine examination of a healthy adolescent. Such a finding often creates anxiety on the part of the physician, the adolescent, and the family. However, most heart murmurs detected for the first time during adolescence are innocent and have no significance. Typically these functional heart murmurs are the vibratory (musical) murmur or the pulmonary ejection (flow) murmur.

Vibratory (musical) murmurs are usually heard in early infancy and childhood. This murmur can also be detected during adolescence and is believed to be caused by high-velocity, nonturbulent flow in the left ventricular outflow tract. It is typically described as vibratory or musical, is best heard at the lower left sternal border, and radiates well to the base and the apex. The quality of the murmur is typical and, once recognized, should not be confused with an organic murmur.[1]

The more important and common murmur heard in adolescence is the pulmonary flow murmur. This murmur is related to turbulence in the main pulmonary artery and seems to be commonly heard in an adolescent during the growth spurt. The pulmonary artery is anterior and close to the chest wall, so turbulence in the main pulmonary artery is easily detected with a stethoscope. These murmurs are ejection in timing, are somewhat harsh in quality, usually do not exceed grade 2 in intensity, and are well localized to the pulmonic area. They are not associated with a pulmonic ejection click, which distinguishes them from the murmur of valvar pulmonic stenosis. In addition, the second heart sound (S2) is normally split and varies with respiration, which distinguishes this murmur from the pulmonary flow murmur detected in an atrial septal defect (ASD).

These 2 types of heart murmurs are completely benign, and the adolescent and family should be reassured that they do not represent heart disease. No prophylaxis for dental work or surgery is required. Follow-up with a pediatric cardiologist is not indicated. The clinician who is comfortable with the diagnosis of an innocent murmur does not need to refer the adolescent to a cardiologist. At times, however, a patient with a pulmonary flow murmur may indeed have an atrial communication, and this should always be kept in mind when a pulmonary flow murmur is diagnosed. Therefore, in some instances echocardiography will be necessary, especially if there is concern about splitting of the S2 or interpretation of the electrocardiogram (ECG).

## EXTRA HEART SOUNDS IN THE ADOLESCENT

It is not uncommon to hear an extra heart sound during a routine cardiac examination in an adolescent. It is quite common to appreciate a third heart sound (S3) in diastole at the apex of a healthy teenager. Fourth heart sounds (S4) are less common but can also be a normal finding. A split in the first heart sound (S1) is often noted on the cardiac examination and must be differentiated from a click. Clicks have a more "snappy" quality and occur later in systole. Clicks at the base of the heart usually are secondary to thickening of the aortic valve (a fixed click at the upper right sternal border and apex) or the pulmonic valve (variable in respiration and heard at the upper left sternal border).

An important finding is a click (or clicks) at the lower left sternal border, which may be associated with a late systolic murmur, especially in the sitting or standing position. This is the hallmark of mitral valve prolapse. This condition occurs in many otherwise healthy teenagers, especially thin girls. These adolescents often have vague complaints of palpitations, atypical chest pain, and dizziness. In addition to the click and late systolic murmur found on examination, an echocardiogram will be diagnostic. An additional work-up (stress test and Holter monitor) should be performed in significantly symptomatic individuals or those with any arrhythmias (atrial or ventricular premature contractions noted on the ECG). In almost all cases, reassurance is effective in ameliorating symptoms. Uncommonly, beta blockers are required. Endocarditis prophylaxis is not needed for patients with an isolated mitral valve prolapse click but should be recommended when significant mitral insufficiency is present. As in all lesions where bacterial endocarditis prophylaxis is no longer recommended, excellent dental hygiene is paramount in preventing bacterial endocarditis. No physical restrictions are necessary and yearly follow-up is indicated.

## LESIONS COMMONLY REQUIRING THERAPY IN ADOLESCENCE

Atrial septal defects often do not come to medical attention until adolescence. There are 2 major reasons why they may go undiagnosed for many years. The first is that children and adolescents with such defects are almost always asymptomatic. The pathophysiology of an ASD is that of a volume overload of the right ventricle that is well tolerated for many years. Therefore, symptoms of heart failure, such as shortness of breath, easy fatigability, and exercise intolerance are not usually seen. The second reason is the paucity of physical findings even when there are large defects. The heart murmur of an ASD is actually a flow murmur caused by increased flow into the pulmonary artery. Thus, the murmur of an ASD is not secondary to flow across the defect itself but is essentially a functional murmur, that is, a function of increased pulmonary blood flow. Because the murmur of an ASD resembles that of a pulmonary flow murmur often heard in adolescence, it may be interpreted as an innocent murmur. The most important physical finding on cardiac examination, albeit subtle, is the fixed splitting of the S2. In healthy individuals, the S2 splits in inspiration and becomes single in expiration. The presence of an atrial communication of significant size results in the absence of the respiratory variation of S2; therefore, S2 is widely split and fixed. Primary care providers must be aware of these subtleties of the examination. The ECG can be a valuable tool in the diagnosis of an ASD. A right ventricular volume overload pattern is typical of this defect, although in some adolescents the ECG may be essentially normal. Two-dimensional echocardiography (ECHO) with color flow Doppler can be used to document the left-to-right shunt.

Although individuals with ASDs generally remain asymptomatic throughout early adult life, the consequences of the volume overload take their toll as an adult. Closure of ASD should be performed whenever they are recognized in adolescence. In certain types of ASD, that is, sinus venosus and ostium primum defects, surgery is required. However, nonsurgical closure of secundum ASDs employing an interventional approach has become the preferred corrective modality in many patients. The most commonly used device, the Amplatzer occluder, has been shown to be extremely effective in closing appropriate-sized defects (up to 3.5–4.0 cm in adults).[2] The procedure can often be performed on an outpatient basis, leaving the patient with no scar. In adolescents with a secundum ASD, which is not appropriate for interventional closure (ie, too large or in which appropriate "rim" tissue is not present), some surgeons will perform closure using a "minimally" invasive surgical technique through a right thoracotomy incision. Most surgeons, however, still prefer the median sternotomy approach, because it has been shown to be safe and effective for many decades.

Another lesion commonly undiagnosed until adolescence is subaortic stenosis, the most common form of which is a membrane beneath the aortic valve. Unlike an ASD, which clearly must be present from birth, subaortic stenosis can develop during childhood and adolescence and often does not manifest until later childhood and adolescence. The murmur of subaortic stenosis is generally a harsh systolic murmur, which is heard both at the left lower sternal border and at the right upper sternal border. The murmur is often mistaken for a small ventricular septal defect; prior to 2-dimensional ECHO, many individuals with subaortic stenosis were diagnosed as having small ventricular septal defects. Thus, it is imperative that the teenager with the clinical diagnosis of a ventricular septal defect undergo a 2-dimensional echocardiogram to make certain that a subaortic membrane is not present. Subaortic stenosis caused by a subaortic membrane is a progressive disease, and turbulence below the aortic valve will ultimately cause damage to the aortic valve and aortic insufficiency. Therefore, at the first signs of aortic insufficiency or when the gradient across the membrane is in excess of 30 mm to 40 mm, surgery should be performed. Cardiac catheterization is no longer required to treat subaortic stenosis: 2-dimensional Doppler ECHO is diagnostic, and surgery can be performed on the basis of this noninvasive technique. After recovery from surgery, the adolescent may participate in all activities as long as the pressure gradient across the subaortic region is less than 20 mm Hg. Yearly follow-up must be performed because there is an incidence of recurrence of subaortic stenosis. Endocarditis prophylaxis is lifelong in these individuals.

Congenital valvar aortic stenosis (CAS) is a lesion diagnosed early in life. However, it is not unusual for this lesion to progress during adolescence, especially in the period of rapid growth. Often, it is not until adolescence that the pressure gradient across the aortic valve becomes significant and therapy is indicated. The murmur of classic valvar aortic stenosis is a harsh systolic ejection murmur heard best in the aortic area at the right upper sternal border. A hallmark of valvar aortic stenosis is a thrill that is palpable in the suprasternal notch. A suprasternal notch thrill is present even in individuals with a relatively mild obstruction. In addition, a constant ejection click is usually audible at the apex. The adolescent with aortic stenosis is almost always asymptomatic and may want to participate in competitive sports. A pressure gradient of more than 20 mm Hg warrants restriction from competitive athletics; in individuals with pressure gradients of more than 50 mm Hg or in instances with ST-T–wave abnormalities on an exercise stress test, therapy is indicated. Balloon valvuloplasty has become an accepted mode of therapy in individuals requiring treatment for valvar aortic stenosis. The procedure is performed as part of cardiac catheterization and angiography and has proved effective as an initial stage of therapy. Valvar aortic stenosis, however, is a progressive lesion, and ultimately a valve replacement is required in many individuals with significant disease. Therefore, adolescents with valvar aortic stenosis must be counseled concerning athletic restriction and should be discouraged from participating in highly competitive athletic endeavors.[3] Endocarditis prophylaxis is no longer a requirement except in patients with a prosthetic valve.[4]

## MINOR CONGENITAL HEART DEFECTS IN ADOLESCENCE

The most common congenital heart defect, the ventricular septal defect (VAD), often persists into adolescence. This small defect does not require surgical intervention in early childhood. It would be unusual for a ventricular septal defect to be discovered for the first time during adolescence. Such defects are usually followed by a pediatric cardiologist for some time. They generally have little hemodynamic consequence other than creating a fairly harsh and loud murmur. The significance of these defects centers around the need for endocarditis prophylaxis. The adolescent with a small ventricular septal defect should be allowed full activities, with no restrictions involving athletic endeavors.

Another common minor defect followed into adolescence is valvar pulmonic stenosis (PS). Unlike aortic stenosis, which is a progressive lesion, pulmonic stenosis is usually stable from childhood to adult life. The teenager with pulmonic stenosis who has not required either surgical intervention or balloon angioplasty obviously has a minor obstruction, no more than a 30 mm to 40 mm gradient as measured by Doppler techniques. There are no restrictions, and participation in all sports is permitted. Bacterial endocarditis prophylaxis is no longer required.[4]

Minor valvular insufficiency, either secondary to congenital abnormalities of the mitral or aortic valve or secondary to a previous attack of rheumatic fever, is not uncommon in adolescents. Those with hemodynamically insignificant aortic insufficiency or mitral insufficiency need not be restricted.[3] Endocarditis prophylaxis is no longer required.[4]

## POSTOPERATIVE CONGENITAL HEART DISEASE IN ADOLESCENCE AND THE "EMERGING ADULT"

A large group of adolescents have had repair of acyanotic lesions early in life; these include ASDs, ventricular septal defects, and atrioventricular canal defects. In general, individuals who have had good hemodynamic repairs without significant residual defect lead normal lives and participate in all athletic endeavors.[5]

Although Tetralogy of Fallot (TOF) is the most common cyanotic defect in adolescence, it would be rare today to find an uncorrected "tet" in the US adolescent population. Therefore, an increasing population of adolescents has had corrective cardiac surgery performed in infancy and early childhood for Tetralogy of Fallot. After repair these children are no longer cyanotic and in most instances are asymptomatic. The teenager who has had Tetralogy of Fallot repair almost always has a residual murmur. These murmurs are usually secondary to mild residual pulmonic stenosis and pulmonic insufficiency. Murmurs of a ventricular septal defect may also be present. Endocarditis prophylaxis is mandatory in the adolescent with successful Tetralogy of Fallot repair. Individuals who have an excellent hemodynamic repair as demonstrated by clinical examination, ECHO, and exercise stress testing may participate in all activities. However, a small group of individuals, especially those in whom ventricular ectopy develops during exercise, require antiarrhythmia therapy and must have exercise limitations.

In the last decade, the operation of choice for uncomplicated transposition of the great arteries (TGA) has been the arterial switch procedure, which is performed in the first few days of life. This "anatomic" repair has superb early and late results, with approximately a 90% survival rate at 10 to 15 years and a constantly improving record. Teenagers who have had this repair lead a normal life without exercise restrictions. However, periodic evaluations with ECG and ECHO are performed. In selected patients who want to participate in strenuous athletics, nuclear stress tests are often recommended.

A growing population of adolescents have undergone a modified Fontan procedure for treatment of tricuspid atresia or other forms of complex cyanotic congenital heart disease. This procedure is in effect a form of physiologic palliative repair. Many patients who have had this operation are asymptomatic but have some degree of exercise limitation because the right ventricle is absent. The absence of the right ventricle limits cardiac output with exercise and in most instances prevents adolescents who have had this procedure from participating in more strenuous forms of competitive athletic endeavors.

## CONGENITAL HEART DISEASE AND THE PREGNANT ADOLESCENT

Corrective cardiac surgery for congenital heart disease, especially cyanotic congenital heart defects, has enabled more women with these defects to reach childbearing age. Physicians caring for the adolescent girl may be faced with a teenager who has congenital heart disease and becomes pregnant. Maternal risk of pregnancy is related to functional class (Table 82-1). Individuals with American Heart Association (AHA) class I or II have less than a 1% risk of maternal mortality. Women who have had surgery for ASD, VSD, PS, AS, TOF, or TGA repair will almost always fall into this group. In uncommon situations, pregnancy is contraindicated; these include those with severe pulmonary hypertension or hypertrophic cardiomyopathy and those with Marfan syndrome in whom the aortic root is greater than 40 mm. For those adolescents in whom it has been determined that the pregnancy can continue, a high-risk medical center, in collaboration with the pediatric cardiologist, should monitor the pregnancy.

In terms of fetal risk, this too is related to maternal clinical status. Fetuses born to mothers with class II to IV functional status will have a high risk of fetal demise, low birth weight, and prematurity. In a study by Presbitero et al,[6] 96 pregnancies were examined in 44 women with congenital heart disease. In total, only 43% of the pregnancies resulted in live births and only 26% in the birth of a full-term infant. In a review by Canobbio et al,[7] of 33 pregnancies in women who previously had a Fontan procedure for cyanotic congenital heart disease, only 45% resulted in live births, but the mean gestational age of these infants was 36.5 weeks. As the hemodynamic results of surgery for complex congenital heart disease improve, better newborn outcomes can be anticipated.

An issue often raised by the adolescent with congenital heart disease is the use of contraception. It is generally agreed that the safest available means of contraception for these adolescents are the barrier methods. Because of the risk of thromboembolism, birth control pills are generally avoided, although progestin-only pills have been used and low-dose estrogen pills are probably safe in females who are not at significant risk for thromboembolic phenomena. Intrauterine devices should not be used because of the risk of endocarditis in females with lesions such as ventricular septal defects and pulmonic or aortic stenosis.[8]

**Table 82-1**

**Classification of Functional Capacity in Patients with Cardiac Disease**

| *Class* | *Description* |
|---|---|
| Class I | Patients with cardiac disease but without resulting limitation of physical activity. Ordinary physical activity does not cause undue fatigue, palpitation, dyspnea, or anginal pain. |
| Class II | Patients with cardiac disease resulting in slight limitation of physical activity. They are comfortable at rest. Ordinary activity causes fatigue, palpitation, dyspnea, or anginal pain. |
| Class III | Patients with cardiac disease resulting in marked limitation of physical activity. They are comfortable at rest. Less than ordinary activity causes fatigue, palpitation, dyspnea, or anginal pain. |
| Class IV | Patients with cardiac disease resulting in inability to carry on any physical activity without discomfort. Symptoms of heart failure or the anginal syndrome may be present even at rest. If any physical activity is undertaken, discomfort increases. |

1994 Revisions to Classification of Functional Capacity and Objective Assessment of Patients With Diseases of the Heart.  www.americanheart.org

## REFERENCES

1. Rosenthal A. How to distinguish between innocent and pathologic murmurs in childhood. *Pediatr Clin North Am.* 1984;31:1229–1240

2. Rossi RI, de Oliveira Cardoso C, Machado PR, et al. Transcatheter closure of atrial septal defect with Amplatzer device in children aged less than 10 years old: immediate and late follow-up. *Catheterization and Cardiovasc Interv.* 2008;71(2):231–236

3. Freed MD. Recreational and sports recommendations for the child with heart disease. *Pediatr Clin North Am.* 1984;31:1307–1320

4. American Heart Association. Prevention of infective endocarditis. *Circulation.* 2007;116:1736–1754

5. Engle MA, Perloff JK. *Congenital Heart Disease after Surgery: Benefits, Residua, Sequelae.* New York, NY: Yorke Medical Books; 1983

6. Presbitero P, Somerville J, Stone S, Aruta E, Spiegelhalter D, Rabajoli F. Pregnancy in cyanotic congenital heart disease. Outcome of mother and fetus. *Circulation.* 1994;89:2673-2676

7. Canobbio MM, Mair DD, Vander Velde M, Koos BJ. Pregnancy outcomes after Fontan repair. *J Am Coll Card.* 1996;28:763-767

8. Connolly HM, Warnes CA. Pregnancy and contraception. In: Gatzoulis MA, Webb GD, Daubney PEF, eds. *Diagnosis and Management of Adults with Congenital Heart Disease.* Philadelphia, PA: Churchill Livingstone; 2003:135-144

# CHAPTER 83

# Carditis in the Adolescent

ANJI T. YETMAN, MD

Unlike in the young child, cardiac disease presenting in the adolescent is often due to an acquired rather than congenital process. Carditis, or inflammation of one or more of the cardiac structures, is the most common cardiac condition presenting in adolescence. The inflammatory process may be confined to the heart or may reflect a more widespread, systemic disorder. Inflammation of the pericardium, myocardium, or endocardium may occur in isolation or in combination.

## PERICARDITIS

The heart is surrounded by a fibroelastic sac composed of 2 layers, the parietal and visceral pericardium, between which a small amount of serous fluid is present. Inflammation of the pericardium may result in accumulation of fluid between the 2 layers known as a pericardial effusion. Although documentation of a pericardial effusion is useful in making the diagnosis of pericarditis, it is not essential.

### CLINICAL SYMPTOMS

The adolescent with pericarditis most often presents with sharp anterior chest pain of fairly acute onset. The pain is characteristically worse when the patient lies supine and relieved by sitting up and leaning forward. The pain may be aggravated by deep inspiration and may radiate to the neck or shoulder. Reportedly, pericarditis with minimal effusion is more painful than that associated with a larger effusion as the inflamed pericardial layers rub against one another. In the face of a moderate or larger effusion, dyspnea is present, but will vary in severity depending on the size of the effusion and the length of time over which it has accumulated. Dyspnea is aggravated by lying flat. A large pericardial effusion may compromise cardiac output (cardiac tamponade) and may be associated with symptoms of dizziness, presyncope, and syncope. The remaining clinical features of pericarditis are often nonspecific but may provide vital clues to the underlying disease process responsible for the inflammation. Clinical history should focus on symptoms that may favor an infectious etiology (fever, cough, coryza, gastrointestinal symptoms, conjunctivitis, jaundice) or an autoimmune etiology (arthritis, arthralgias, weight loss, rash, photosensitivity, myalgias). Past medical history of renal disease, prior cardiac surgery, or chest trauma may be relevant.[1]

### CLINICAL FINDINGS

The patient with pericarditis look often will uncomfortable. Heart rate and respiratory rate may be elevated for age. Blood pressure may be normal, or it may be diminished if there is a large effusion compromising cardiac output. Cardiac tamponade refers to a critical fall in cardiac output, which may be life threatening, and occurs when, in the face of a large effusion, intrapericardial pressure exceeds intra-atrial pressure, resulting in impaired atrial filling and subsequently impaired ventricular output. Normally, there is an increase in right heart filling with inspiration. Due to the constricting nature of a large circumferential effusion, preload returning to the right heart will limit flow into the left heart, resulting in a potentially lethal drop in stroke volume during inspiration. Pulsus paradoxus refers to a fall in systolic blood pressure of >15 mm Hg on inspiration. It is not possible to evaluate this important clinical finding with an automated blood pressure machine. Rather, a manual cuff should be used and inflated to a value above the systolic blood pressure. While allowing the cuff to slowly deflate, the presence of Korotkoff sounds should be noted. As the patient inspires, Korotkoff sounds will disappear and then reappear. If they reappear after a fall of 15 mm Hg or greater, pulsus paradoxus is present. In some instances, palpable pulsus paradoxus may be present with an appreciable decrease in peripheral pulse amplitude upon inspiration. The first and second heart sounds (S1 and S2) may be normal or may be muffled. The classic auscultatory finding of pericarditis is a pericardial friction rub. This finding, however, may be intermittent. This sound may be present during any part of the cardiac cycle and is "scratchy" in nature. It is best heard at end expiration with the patient sitting and leaning forward. Jugular venous distension will be present if the effusion is large.[1]

### ETIOLOGY

The etiology of a pericardial effusion is varied. In many instances, the cause of the effusion remains unknown. The incidence of idiopathic pericarditis will reflect the aggressiveness of the underlying clinical evaluation but has been noted to be present in up to 30% of pericardial effusions.[2] Within North America, the most common documented cause of pericarditis in the adolescent is viral pericarditis. Viruses most commonly implicated include the enteroviruses, adenovirus, and influenza. Other less common viral etiologies include hepatitis and cytomegalovirus (CMV). The most common cause of pericarditis worldwide is tuberculosis (TB), accounting for more than 50% of large pericardial effusions seen in developing countries. Within developed countries, however, tuberculous pericarditis is uncommon and accounts for 0.3% of pericardial effusions.[3] With the rise in HIV prevalence, there has been an increase in tuberculous pericarditis in all countries. Clinical history of prior TB exposure, a previous positive PPD, other opportunistic infections, and HIV status should be sought. Other infectious etiologies are rare but include Lyme disease, which may be associated with myopericarditis in up to 10% of patients, and bacterial pericarditis. Since the advent of childhood *Hemophilus* vaccination, bacterial pericarditis is rare in the immunocompetent host. Bacterial pericarditis has been reported in association with nontypeable *Hemophilus, Hemophilus influenza, Staphylococcus, Streptococcus*, and others.[1] Bacterial pericarditis most commonly occurs in the setting of widespread septicemia with secondary infection of the pericardium. A pericardial effusion is not uncommon in patients with AIDS, but true pericarditis is rare, and other infectious etiologies should be sought.[3]

## DIFFERENTIAL DIAGNOSIS

Strictly speaking, pericarditis refers to an infection of the pericardium. A pericardial effusion may occur secondary to pericarditis but may be due to a noninfectious cause.

Systemic autoimmune disorders are a common cause of pericardial effusions in the adolescent, with systemic lupus erythematosus (SLE) being the most common etiology in this category. Approximately 50% of patients with SLE will have cardiac involvement, and a pericardial effusion is the most common cardiac manifestation. A pericardial effusion may be the presenting finding in >15% of patients with SLE, thus SLE and other autoimmune disorders should be considered in the differential diagnosis of an adolescent with a pericardial effusion. Patients with SLE and an elevated creatinine, hematuria, or proteinuria, or a hemoglobin <12 g/dL have a higher incidence of cardiac complications during the course of their disease.[4] Other autoimmune conditions associated with pericardial effusion in the adolescent are much less common but include mixed connective tissue disorder (MCTD), scleroderma, juvenile rheumatoid arthritis, familial Mediterranean fever, and others.[1]

Pericardial effusions are not uncommonly seen in adolescents hospitalized and receiving treatment for malignancy. The etiology of the effusion in this instance may relate to the underlying malignancy. Pericardial effusions have been reported to occur with the leukemias, lymphomas, and other less common malignancies.[1] Other potential etiologies in this patient group are congestive heart failure related to cardiotoxic chemotherapeutic agents and volume overload in the setting of renal dysfunction.

Patients with repaired or unrepaired cardiac disease may present to medical attention with a pericardial effusion. Pericardial effusions are most commonly seen in the postoperative patient, particularly following surgical closure of an atrial septal defect. With the advent of percutaneous atrial septic defect device closures, these patients are seen less commonly. Patients may present with a pericardial effusion from days to months following surgery. Progressive dyspnea, chest pain, or increasing cardiomegaly on chest x-ray (CXR) should alert the physician to a probable postoperative pericardial effusion. Patients with elevated right heart pressures (right ventricular dysfunction, tricuspid valve disease, pulmonary valve disease, pulmonary hypertension, impaired left ventricular (LV) filling, or single ventricle physiology) may present with a pericardial effusion in association with diffuse edema.

## DIAGNOSTIC EVALUATION

In the face of suspected pericarditis or a documented pericardial effusion, each of the following tests should be ordered: 12 lead electrocardiogram (ECG), CXR, and echocardiogram. Other potentially useful diagnostic studies include: complete blood count (CBC) with differential, C-reactive protein (CRP), and erythrocyte sedimentation rate (ESR). The use of the following tests should be dictated by the presenting clinical picture: blood cultures in the febrile patient, blood urea nitrogen (BUN) and creatinine in patients suspected of having uremia or SLE, viral respiratory panel depending on local practice, hepatitis and HIV serology, and tuberculosis (TB) skin testing. If pericardiocentesis is performed (see the following), pericardial fluid should be sent for cell count with differential, gram stain and bacterial culture, and glucose, protein, and other specific analyses as dictated by the clinical picture.[1,5]

Chest x-ray may be normal or, in the case of a sizeable effusion, may reveal cardiomegaly with a globular-shaped heart. The presence of coexistent pleural effusions, a pneumonic process, and/or pulmonary edema should be noted.

Electrocardiogram typically shows diffuse ST elevation and PR-segment depression (in all leads except avR and V1) in the acute phase. Thus, the ST and PR segments change in opposite directions. Later in the course of the disease, the ECG will normalize, and subsequently diffuse T-wave inversion may be seen. ST elevation must be distinguished from early repolarization, which is a normal ECG finding in up to one-third of adolescents. Features that favor pericarditis include the presence of ST elevation in the limb leads as well as all of the precordial leads, the presence of PR-segment depression, and a ratio of ST elevation to T-wave amplitude in V6 of > 0.24 (100% positive and negative predictive values).[6]

Echocardiography may be useful in documenting the presence and size of a pericardial effusion. Compression of cardiac structures may be documented. Variation in transmitral flow velocities with respiration should be recorded. A fall of ≥20% in flow velocity indicates echocardiographic tamponade.

### NATURAL HISTORY AND TREATMENT

In most instances of viral or idiopathic pericarditis, the inflammatory process will resolve without treatment and will not recur. Treatment is directed toward symptom control and includes high-dose aspirin or nonsteroidal anti-inflammatories (NSAIDs). Long-term cardiac follow-up is not required in those patients with an uncomplicated course. Patients may resume competitive athletics once the ECG and echocardiogram have normalized.

Potential complications of pericarditis include cardiac tamponade and/or chronic recurrent pericarditis.[1,5] Cardiac tamponade occurs in 5% to 28% of cases of acute pericarditis.[5] The presence of significant respiratory distress, pulsus paradoxus, or shock all indicate cardiac tamponade and call for the immediate performance of a pericardiocentesis to evacuate the pericardial effusion. Bacterial pericarditis is associated with a purulent exudate with fibrous stranding. In addition to appropriate antibiotic therapy, surgical creation of a pericardial window is often required.[1,5]

Whereas 30% of adults with acute pericarditis will develop a recurrence, this is relatively rare in childhood. Some adolescents, however, will develop recurrent disease at varying intervals over years. Factors associated with recurrent pericarditis in the adult include initial treatment with steroids, lack of clinical response to aspirin or NSAID therapy, and inappropriate pericardiotomy or creation of a pericardial window.[5] In addition to anti-inflammatories, colchicine has been used successfully in recurrent cases.[5] Recurrent pericarditis may represent an undiagnosed systemic disorder or may reflect an autoimmune process directed at the pericardium.[2]

## MYOCARDITIS

Myocarditis is a condition resulting from inflammation of the heart muscle. The clinical spectrum is varied. Patients may be entirely asymptomatic, presenting with an incidental finding of dysfunction, longstanding symptoms due to low-grade chronic inflammation, fulminant heart failure, or sudden death. Myocarditis may be associated with transient or permanent myocellular damage.

### CLINICAL SYMPTOMS

Patients often present with a prodrome of fever, myalgia, and malaise that occurs several days prior to the onset of cardiac symptoms, which then can include dyspnea at rest, exercise intolerance, palpitations, syncope, and/or sudden death. Chest pain may be present, particularly in those patients with myopericarditis. Clinical history should be directed at determining whether the patient has acute cardiac dysfunction versus an exacerbation of previous cardiac symptomatology.

### CLINICAL FINDINGS

Patients usually have tachycardia but may have bradycardia with a finding of complete heart block if the atrioventricular node is involved in the inflammatory process. Arrhythmias are common. The patient is usually tachypneic. Blood pressure may be normal or may be severely decreased in those with poor myocardial function. Pulse pressure may be narrow. An S3 or S4 gallop may be heard; a pansystolic murmur of functional mitral or tricuspid valve regurgitation may be present; and a rub may be audible if the pericardium is involved in the inflammatory process. Hepatomegaly may be present. Perfusion may be poor.

### ETIOLOGY

The most common cause of myocarditis in the adolescent is viral infection, particularly enterovirus or adenovirus. Other viral causes include hepatitis, Epstein-Barr virus (EBV), CMV, and influenza. Other infectious causes of myocarditis in the immunocompetent host are rare.[7]

### DIFFERENTIAL DIAGNOSIS

The most common cause of new-onset heart failure in the adolescent is viral myocarditis. There are, however, other causes of LV dysfunction that need to be considered, including bacterial sepsis, cocaine usage, prior history of malignancy treated with radiation or cardiotoxic medications, neuromuscular disorders, or congenital coronary abnormalities.[8] A careful clinical history should be directed at excluding these other conditions. One of the more difficult clinical challenges in assessing the adolescent with acute heart failure is determining whether the patient has myocarditis or an underlying cardiomyopathy with a decline in clinical status due to an intercurrent infection.[7,8]

### DIAGNOSTIC EVALUATION

Initial evaluation of the patient with suspected myocarditis should include a 12 lead ECG, CXR, cardiac enzymes, and echocardiography. Other potentially useful diagnostic studies include rectal and nasopharyngeal swabs for enterovirus and adenovirus, acute and convalescent antibody titers, and arterial blood gas analysis. Cardiac catheterization with an endomyocardial biopsy and magnetic resonance imaging (MRI) of the heart may each be useful in distinguishing myocarditis from dilated cardiomyopathy secondary to another cause.

Electrocardiography may demonstrate low voltages, diffuse ST depression, or T-wave inversion. The rhythm is most commonly sinus tachycardia, but supraventricular or ventricular tachycardia may occur. It is important to rule out atrial ectopic tachycardia, as this may be the source of the myocardial dysfunction. Careful attention should be paid to determining that there is a normal p-wave axis. Complete heart block, premature ventricular contractions, and premature atrial contractions may be present.

Chest x-ray typically shows cardiomegaly with pulmonary venous congestion. Heart size, however, may be normal.

Elevated troponin levels with an increased creatine kinase MB (CK-MB) fraction may be seen and reflect myocardial necrosis. Enzyme levels may be useful in distinguishing acute myocarditis from dilated cardiomyopathy in which case troponin levels should be normal.[9]

Echocardiography is useful in quantitating and following the degree of LV systolic and diastolic dysfunction. Assessment of concomitant pericardial effusion, coronary artery abnormalities, and myocardial abnormalities, such as LV noncompaction, should also be made.

Cardiac MRI with gadolinium may show focal or diffuse subepicardial enhancement occurring in association with myocyte rupture and necrosis. This finding is in contrast to the finding of subendocardial enhancement seen with ischemia. Patients must be clinically stable to undergo such a procedure.[10]

Cardiac catheterization with myocardial biopsy is performed routinely in some centers and not in others. Perforation of the right ventricle is the most common complication,[11] but overall the risk is low. The sensitivity of the test is low, with only 50% of patients with clinically suspected disease having positive biopsy results. A positive biopsy will demonstrate lymphocyte infiltration and myocyte necrosis.[7]

### NATURAL HISTORY AND TREATMENT

Treatment protocols vary according to clinical presentation. The patient with acute myocarditis will require intensive care unit admission due to the potential for rapid hemodynamic compromise and potentially lethal arrhythmias. Treatment is supportive. Inotropic and after-load reducing agents may be required. Loss of sinus rhythm will be poorly tolerated and antiarrhythmic agents, including amiodarone or lidocaine, may be required to restore sinus rhythm. The patient with complete heart block will require placement of temporary pacing leads. The patient with hemodynamic collapse, either from refractory arrhythmias or poor cardiac output, can be supported with extracorporeal membrane oxygenation (ECMO) until myocardial recovery, or in the absence of recovery, cardiac transplantation. Immunosuppressive protocols are used in some, but not all, centers and include intravenous immunoglobulin (IVIG), corticosteroids, or other immunosuppressive agents. The one randomized trial of IVIG that exists in adult patients with myocarditis showed no benefit of therapy.[12] Retrospective data within the pediatric populations suggest some benefit of IVIG therapy,[13] but no prospective data exists. Factors associated with poor outcome include ejection fraction <30%, LV dilation, or moderate/severe mitral regurgitation on initial echocardiogram.[14] Patients may have full or partial recovery of myocardial function. Those with partial recovery may be left with a dilated cardiomyopathy necessitating chronic heart failure management with the potential of cardiac transplantation at a later date. The 5-year rate of freedom from transplantation in patients <18 years old is 81%.[8] Long-term outpatient follow-up is required. Patients should be restricted from sporting activities until LV size and function return to normal and 24-hour Holter monitoring shows no significant arrhythmias.[7]

## ENDOCARDITIS

Infective endocarditis (IE) in the adolescent patient is most commonly seen in 3 patient groups: (1) those with previously documented congenital cardiac defects, (2) patients with indwelling lines, and (3) intravenous drug users. As turbulent blood flow within the heart or great vessels occurs in the face of an underlying structural cardiac defect, or in the presence of prosthetic material, the turbulent flow traumatizes the endothelial surface, causing fibrin and platelet accumulation. Microbial invasion of the bloodstream, particularly with a highly adherent pathogen (*Streptococcus viridans, Staphylococcus*), may result in bacterial colonization and IE.[15]

### CLINICAL SYMPTOMS

There is a broad spectrum of presenting symptoms, including complete absence of cardiac symptoms in the patient presenting with fever of unknown origin, a chronic picture of low-grade fever, anemia and weight loss, or an acute presentation of fulminant heart failure.

**CLINICAL FINDINGS**

The patient may have a persistent or transient recurrent fever. He or she will often have tachycardia because anemia is common. Respiratory rate and blood pressure may be normal. Physical findings will depend on the site of involvement but may include the presence of a newly noted murmur, focal neurologic abnormalities, splenomegaly, left upper quadrant pain on palpation, or peripheral embolic phenomena (including Janeway lesions, Osler nodes, Roth spots, splinter hemorrhages, petechiae, and peripheral vascular aneurysms). Findings of a previously undiagnosed cardiac abnormality may be present. Cardiac lesions, which may escape diagnosis until adulthood and may be associated with endocarditis, include mitral valve prolapse, bicuspid aortic valve, patent ductus arteriosus, and coarctation of the aorta. Physical evidence of intravenous drug use should be sought.

**ETIOLOGY**

Mediators of bacterial adherence serve as virulence factors in the pathogenesis of IE. Highly adherent bacteria, including *Streptococci, Staphylococci*, and *Enterococci*, are the most common pathogens, with *Streptococcus viridans* being the most common in non-IV drug-using patients with native valves. Other potential organisms include the Haemophilus parainfluenzae, Haemophilus aphrophilus, Haemophilus paraphrophilus, Actinobacillus actinomycetemcomitans, Cardiobacterium hominis, Eikenella corrodens, and Kingella species (HACEK), other Gram-negative organisms, and fungi.[15]

**DIAGNOSTIC EVALUATION**

Initial evaluation in the patient suspected of having IE should include a CBC, ESR, CRP, urinalysis and urine culture, and multiple blood cultures from different sites. In the face of positive blood cultures, echocardiography is useful in assessing for the presence of vegetation or a myocardial abscess. Although a positive transthoracic echocardiogram is useful in confirming the diagnosis of IE, a negative study does not rule out the diagnosis. In the face of positive blood cultures and a clinical suspicion of IE, a transesophageal echocardiogram is required. An ECG is also required in the patient suspected of endocarditis, as a myocardial abscess at the crux of the heart may impinge on the AV node, resulting in heart block of varying degrees.[15]

**NATURAL HISTORY AND TREATMENT**

Depending on the organism involved and the site and extent of cardiac involvement, symptoms may persist for weeks to months before a diagnosis is established. The majority of patients will clear their bacteremia with appropriate antibiotic therapy. Despite this, morbidity and mortality remain high due to complications of systemic embolization and valvar destruction. Surgery during the acute bacteremic phase can be avoided unless 1 of the following conditions is present: (1) fungal infection, (2) myocardial abscess, (3) failure to clear bacteremia despite appropriate antibiotic therapy, (4) intractable heart failure, and (5) recurrent embolic phenomena. Other potential indications include the following: (1) large (>10 mm) vegetations, (2) infection with staphylococcus species, and (3) presence of a vegetation with high risk of embolization. Patients require appropriate intravenous antibiotic therapy, usually for a minimum of 6 weeks.[15] Return to physical activity is dictated by the degree of residual valvar dysfunction.

**PREVENTION**

The new American Heart Association (AHA)[16] guidelines for prevention of IE represent a marked change from prior guidelines. It is now thought that the vast majority of cases of IE result from random bacteremias occurring during daily activities rather than in association with instrumentation from dental, gastrointestinal, or genitourinary procedures. Per the new AHA guidelines, prophylaxis is recommended only in those patients at greatest risk of adverse outcome from IE, including patients with prosthetic valves or valved conduits, unrepaired cyanotic cardiac defects (including those with palliative shunts), newly repaired cardiac defects within the past 6 months, a prior history of IE, repaired congenital heart disease with residual defects at or adjacent to implanted prosthetic material, and cardiac transplant recipients with cardiac valvulopathy.[16] Amoxicillin remains the preferred choice for oral prophylaxis prior to dental procedures or instrumentation of the respiratory tract (50 mg/kg up to 2 grams 1 hour prior to the procedure). For patients who are allergic to penicillin, use of a first-generation cephalosporin, clindamycin, azithromycin, or clarithromycin is recommended, with only the latter 3 recommended in the presence of a history of anaphylaxis. Patients receiving chronic antibiotic therapy should receive a drug from a different class for IE prophylaxis. Prophylaxis is no longer recommended for body piercing, tattooing, and gastrointestinal or genitourinary procedures, including vaginal delivery.[16] Patients scheduled for elective cardiac surgery should undergo dental examination and treatment prior to surgery to lessen the risk of streptococcal bacteremia and IE in the immediate postoperative period.[16]

## PANCARDITIS

Rheumatic fever (RF) may be associated with diffuse cardiac inflammation or pancarditis. Rheumatic fever occurs as a result of a complex interaction between group A *Streptococcus* (GAS), a susceptible host, and the environment.[17] Although the incidence of RF remains high in developing countries (200–300/100,000), it had fallen in developed countries only to see a resurgence in the late 1980s.[17]

### CLINICAL SYMPTOMS

During the acute phase of RF, endocardial, myocardial, and pericardial inflammation may be present. Patients may be entirely asymptomatic; may lack cardiac symptoms but present with other features of the disease (migratory arthritis primarily affecting the large joints, chorea, erythema marginatum, subcutaneous nodules); or may present with cardiac symptoms. Pericardial effusions in RF are typically small and do not require pericardiocentesis. Myocardial dysfunction is mild. True "myocarditis" with myocyte death and lymphocyte infiltration does not occur.[17] Ventricular dysfunction may, however, be present secondary to the associated valvulitis. Endocardial inflammation results in valvar regurgitation with the mitral valve being the most commonly involved (95%). Isolated aortic insufficiency occurs in 5%. With the exception of chorea, symptoms typically occur 10 days to 5 weeks following GAS pharyngitis.[17]

### CLINICAL FINDINGS

Clinical findings of RF vary considerably depending on the extent of cardiac or other organ inflammation. Thirty percent to 70% of patients with RF will develop carditis. Clinical signs may be confined to the presence of an asymptomatic pansystolic murmur of mitral insufficiency, or less commonly a diastolic murmur of aortic insufficiency. Cardiac signs will reflect the degree of valvar regurgitation. Patients with severe mitral insufficiency will have tachycardia, tachypnea, and an active precordium. Blood pressure is usually normal. Pulmonary edema is not uncommon. Patients with severe aortic insufficiency will have, in addition to a diastolic murmur loudest at the left midsternal edge, an increase in heart rate, a widened pulse pressure with an increased systolic pressure and reduced diastolic pressure, and bounding pulses. Respiratory rate may be increased if pulmonary edema is present. The precordial impulse may be diffuse and deviated laterally.

### ETIOLOGY

The strain and virulence of the GAS organism influence the likelihood of developing RF. The M protein is thought to be an important virulence factor.[17] There is evidence to suggest that the changing demographic patterns of infection relate to a change in GAS strains.[17]

### DIAGNOSTIC EVALUATION

Diagnosis of acute RF is made in accordance with the revised Jones criteria.[17] Patients must have 2 major criteria (arthritis, carditis, chorea, subcutaneous nodules, erythema marginatum) or 1 major and 2 minor criteria (arthralgias, fever, elevated acute-phase reactants, prolonged PR interval on ECG). Exceptions to this rule include the patient with isolated chorea and the patient with a past history of RF in whom criteria are less stringent. In addition, there must be evidence of recent GAS infection as evidenced by a positive throat culture for Group A betahemolytic streptococcus, a rapid antigen test, or rising antibody titers of antistreptolysin O or anti-DNAse B. The antibody response to GAS pharyngitis peaks at 3 to 4 weeks following the infection.[17] Electrocardiography should be performed to assess for PR prolongation. Echocardiographic assessment to evaluate valvar and myocardial function, as well as to look for the presence of a pericardial effusion, is required.

### NATURAL HISTORY AND TREATMENT

Although quite variable, the duration of untreated acute RF is 0~3 months, with the outcome of patients with carditis ranging from no sequelae to intractable heart failure.[17] Treatment is largely supportive and mainly directed at preventing recurrences and the complication of chronic rheumatic heart disease. Acute treatment of patients with carditis includes activity restriction for 4 to 6 weeks and aspirin (80 to 100 mg/kg/day divided into 4 doses) for mild to moderate carditis. Steroid therapy (prednisone 2 mg/kg/day) is reserved for patients with severe carditis. Duration of therapy is guided by resolution of symptoms. Primary antibiotic prophylaxis is required, even in the presence of a negative throat culture, in order to eradicate GAS from the pharynx and prevent repetitive antigenic stimulation. A single intramuscular (IM) injection of benzathine penicillin is the most effective therapy. A 10-day oral course of therapy may also be used. Patients who are allergic to penicillin should be treated with erythromycin. Patients, especially those with carditis, remain at risk for recurrences, with the recurrence rate being as high as 40% to 60%. Recurrences result in more severe valvar dysfunction and a higher likelihood of chronic rheumatic heart disease.[17] To prevent recurrences, therefore, all patients who have had RF require secondary prophylaxis, which consists of IM or oral penicillin therapy every 3 to 4 weeks, until well into adulthood.[17]

## REFERENCES

1. Tingle LE, Molina D, Calvert CW. Acute pericarditis. *Am Fam Physician.* 2007;76(10):1509-1514

2. Pozza RD, Hartl D, Bechtold S, et al. Recurrent pericarditis in children: elevated cardiac autoantibodies. *Clin Res Cardiol.* 2007;96:168-175

3. Syed FF, Mayosi BM. A modern approach to tuberculous pericarditis. *Prog Cardiovasc Dis.* 2007;50(3):218-236

4. Yeh TT, Yang YH, Lin YT, Lu CS, Chiang BL. Cardiopulmonary involvement in pediatric systemic lupus erythematosus: a twenty-year retrospective analysis. *J Microbiol Immunol Infect.* 2007;40(6):525-531

5. Imazio M, Cecchi E, Demichelis B, et al. Indicators of poor prognosis of acute pericarditis. *Circulation.* 2007;115:2739-2744

6. Gintzen LE, Laks M. The differential diagnosis of acute pericarditis from the normal variant: new electrocardiographic criteria. *Circulation.* 1982;65:1004

7. Basso C, Carturan E, Corrado D, Thiene G. Myocarditis and dilated cardiomyopathy in athletes: diagnosis, management, and recommendations for sport activity. *Cardiol Clin.* 2007;25:423-429

8. Towbin JA, Lowe AM, Colan SD, et al. Incidence, causes, and outcomes of dilated cardiomyopathy in children. *JAMA.* 2006;296:1867-1876

9. Soongswang J, Durongpisitkul K, Ratanarapee S, et al. Cardiac troponin T: its role in the diagnosis of clinically suspected acute myocarditis and chronic dilated cardiomyopathy in children. *Pediatr Cardiol.* 2002;23:531-535

10. Laissy JP, Messin B, Varenne O, et al. MRI of acute myocarditis: a comprehensive approach based on various imaging sequences. *Chest.* 2002;122:1638-1648

11. Yoshizato T, Edwards WD, Alborliras ET, Hagler DJ, Driscoll DJ. Safety and utility of endomyocardial biopsy in infants, children and adolescents: a review of 66 procedures in 53 patients. *J Am Coll Card.* 1990;15(2):436-442

12. Robinson JL, Hartling L, Crumley E, Vandermeer B, Klassen TP. A systematic review of intravenous gamma globulin for therapy of acute myocarditis. *BMC Cardiovascular Dis.* 2005;5:12

13. Drucker NA, Colad SD, Lewis AB, et al. Gamma-globulin treatment of acute myocarditis in the pediatric population. *Circulation.* 1994;89:252-257

14. Kuhn B, Shapiro ED, Walls TA, Friedman AH. Predictors of outcome of myocarditis. *Pediatr Cardiol.* 2004;25:379-384

15. Quagliarello V. Infective endocarditis: global, regional, and future perspectives. *JAMA.* 2005;293:3061-3062

16. Wilson W, Taubert KA, Gewitz M, et al. Prevention of infective endocarditis: Guidelines from the American Heart Association. A guideline from the American Heart Association Rheumatic Fever, Endocarditis, and Kawasaki Disease Committee, Council on Cardiovascular Disease in the Young, and the Council of Clinical Cardiology, Council on Cardiovascular Surgery and Anesthesia, and the Quality of Care and Outcomes Research Interdisciplinary Working Group. *J Am Dent Assn.* 2007;138:739-760

17. Tani LY. Rheumatic fever and rheumatic heart disease. *Moss and Adams' Heart Disease in Infants, Children, and Adolescents.* Philadelphia, PA: Lippincott Williams & Wilkins; 2007:1257-1324

# CHAPTER 84

## Valvular Heart Diseases

DIPAK KHOLWADWALA, MD

### INTRODUCTION

Although most valvular heart disease in older adults is acquired, the predominant etiology in children, adolescents, and young adults is congenital. The estimated prevalence of congenital heart diseases is about 800,000 in the United States.[1] In adolescents, the congenital valvular lesions mainly comprise residual abnormalities from previous interventions performed during early childhood (balloon or surgical valvuloplasty) or uncorrected lesions that are relatively mild or awaiting interventions. Almost all acquired valvular heart diseases are rheumatic in origin. Mitral valve prolapse (MVP) is idiopathic in more than 50% of cases and is often encountered for the first time in adolescence or adulthood. It is also the most common valvular heart disease in adolescents. Despite the different causes, the pathophysiology and clinical manifestations of these valvular lesions are similar. This chapter discusses the most common valvular heart diseases seen in adolescents.

### MITRAL VALVE PROLAPSE

Mitral valve prolapse refers to abnormal displacement of mitral leaflets into the left atrial cavity. It has become the most commonly diagnosed valvular cardiac abnormality in the developed nations, occurring in 2% to 5% of the population with a 2:1 female preponderance.[2] Mitral valve prolapse is likely overdiagnosed in many patients by examiners who misidentify the auscultatory findings or overread the two-dimensional echocardiogram. There has been considerable interest and controversy regarding the diagnostic criteria of MVP and the association of MVP with arrhythmias, stroke, endocarditis, and sudden death. Despite the accumulation of considerable data, much of our knowledge remains incomplete, contradictory, and controversial.[3,4] Moreover, there is a lack of well-controlled studies and a paucity of data in children and adolescents with this abnormality.

#### PATHOPHYSIOLOGY

The mitral valve apparatus is a complex structure composed of valve leaflets, annulus, chordae tendineae, papillary muscles, and the supporting left atrial, left ventricular, and aortic walls. Primary or secondary disease processes involving any of these components can result in displacement of the mitral valve leaflet into the left atrial cavity. The normal mitral valve leaflet has three histological layers: the atrialis (facing the atrium), the fibrosa (facing the ventricular side), and the spongiosa (in the middle). In the primary form of MVP, there is myxomatous proliferation of the spongiosa tissue causing disruption of the collagen matrix in the external and internal layers. This causes reactionary fibrotic changes that result in thinning and elongation of the mitral leaflets.

Most primary forms of MVP occur as isolated cases, but MVP can also be familial and transmitted by autosomal dominant inheritance. In secondary forms of MVP, there is either (1) an underlying systemic disease of the connective tissues (ie, Marfan syndrome, Ehler-Danlos syndrome, pseudoxanthoma elasticum, osteogenesis imperfecta, Hurler syndrome) involving the mitral leaflets, chordae tendineae, and annulus; or (2) reduction in left ventricular cavity size (secondary to such entities as an atrial septal defect, anorexia nervosa, or Ebstein anomaly) that result in abnormal systolic displacement into the left atrium of an otherwise normal mitral leaflet.[5] Up to 4% of patients with MVP have Marfan syndrome, whereas almost all patients with Marfan syndrome have MVP.

#### CLINICAL MANIFESTATIONS AND DIAGNOSTIC CRITERIA

Most adolescents with MVP are asymptomatic, but a history of nonexertional chest pain, palpitations, syncope, fatigue, or anxiety may be elicited. The Framingham study found no difference in the prevalence of symptoms between those with MVP and the general population.[6] An association between MVP and panic-anxiety disorders has been suggested but never proved.[7] In 1986, Perloff et al[8] established guidelines for the clinical diagnosis of MVP similar to the Jones criteria model used for rheumatic fever (Box 84-1). The objective was to provide clinicians with a more secure basis of judgment so that the inappropriate diagnosis of healthy individuals can be avoided. The criteria for the diagnosis of MVP has been divided into three groups: (1) major

**Box 84-1**

***Diagnostic Criteria in MVP***

**Major Criteria**

- Auscultation
  - Mid to late systolic click and late systolic murmur or "whoop," alone or in combination, at the cardiac apex
- Two-dimensional echocardiogram
  - Marked superior systolic displacement of mitral valve leaflets (2 mm above annulus) with coaptation at or superior to annular plane
  - Mild to moderate superior systolic displacement of mitral valve leaflets with
    - Chordal rupture
    - Doppler mitral regurgitation
    - Annular dilation
- Echocardiogram plus auscultation
  - Mild to moderate superior systolic displacement of mitral valve leaflets with
    - Prominent mid to late systolic click at the cardiac apex
    - Apical late systolic or holosystolic murmur in the young patient
    - Late systolic "whoop"

**Minor Criteria**

- Auscultation
  - Loud S1 with an apical holosystolic murmur
- Two-dimensional echocardiogram
  - Isolated mild to moderate superior systolic displacement of the posterior mitral leaflet
  - Moderate superior systolic displacement of both mitral leaflets
- Echocardiogram plus history of
  - Mild to moderate superior systolic displacement of mitral leaflets with
    - Focal neurologic attacks or amaurosis fugax (loss of vision in one eye) in the young patient
    - First-degree relatives with major criteria

Modified from Perloff JK, Child JS, Edwards JE. New guidelines for the clinical diagnosis of mitral valve prolapse. *Am J Cardiol*. 1986;57:1124, with permission from Elsevier.

criteria, the presence of one or more of which establishes the diagnosis of MVP; (2) minor criteria, the presence of which cannot be discounted and should raise the suspicion of MVP but which by themselves are not sufficient to establish the diagnosis; and (3) other findings, which although often present in patients with MVP are nonspecific. Recognition of MVP (also known as the systolic click-late systolic murmur syndrome) is often difficult because of the extreme variability of its clinical manifestations and the diminishing auscultatory skills of physicians who may default the physical examination of the heart in lieu of noninvasive diagnostic testing.

The primary diagnostic evaluation of the patient with MVP is a careful physical examination. The principal cardiac auscultatory feature is a mid- to late systolic click that results from sudden tensing of the mitral valve apparatus as the leaflets prolapse into the left atrium during ventricular systole. The midsystolic click is frequently followed by a late systolic murmur of medium to high pitch, best heard at the apex. The presence or absence of the click or murmur, as well as its timing and intensity, can vary from one examination to the next and with various maneuvers (Figure 84-1). Mitral valve prolapse cannot be ruled out until the postural interventions necessary to elicit the click-murmur complex have been performed. In general, the click-murmur complex moves toward the first heart sound with maneuvers that decrease the volume of blood in the left ventricle (as with standing), increase contractility or decrease afterload. In contrast, any maneuver that increases the volume of blood in the left ventricle (as with squatting), reduces myocardial contractility, or increases afterload moves the click-murmur complex toward the second heart sound.

### Radiologic Examination

Radiologic examination is usually normal. The cardiac size is increased only in the presence of moderate to

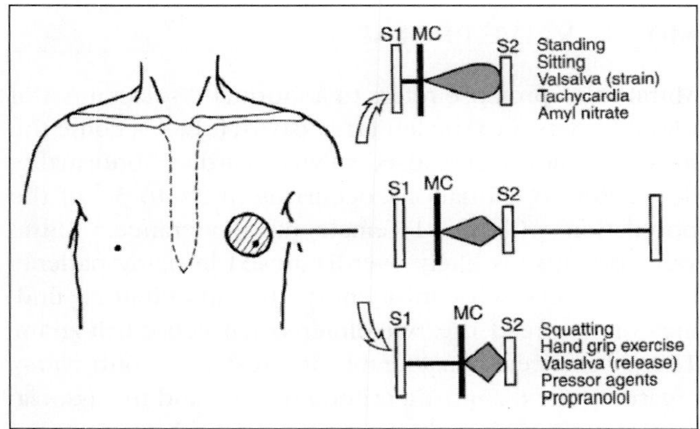


FIGURE 84-1 Auscultatory findings in mitral valve prolapse and the effect of various maneuvers on the timing of the midsystolic click (MC) and the murmur in relation to the first (S1) and second (S2) heart sounds. The maneuvers that reduce ventricular volume enhance leaflet redundancy and move the click and murmur earlier in systole. An increase in left ventricular dimension has the opposite effect. (Reprinted from Park, MK. *Pediatric Cardiology for Practitioners*. 4th ed. St. Louis, MO: Mosby; 2002, with permission from Elsevier.)

severe mitral regurgitation (MR). Coincidentally, thoracic and skeletal abnormalities such as scoliosis, pectus excavatum, and straight back syndrome may be present.

### Electrocardiogram

Most adolescents with MVP have a normal electrocardiogram (ECG). However, three types of abnormalities can be seen: abnormalities of repolarization, conduction, and rhythm. Repolarization abnormalities include prolongation of the QT interval and T-wave inversion in the inferolateral leads (II, III, aVf, V4–V6). These findings are especially intriguing due to the possible link between MVP and sudden death.[9] Although the Framingham study did not find this link, conduction and rhythm abnormalities (first-degree atrioventricular block, premature extrasystole, and reentrant tachycardia) were occasionally reported. Because these may also be found in normal subjects, the meaning remains unclear.

### Echocardiography

Echocardiography is the most useful noninvasive tool for defining MVP. Normally, the mitral valve billows slightly into the left atrium, but a "floppy valve" is regarded as an extreme form of billowing. Mitral regurgitation occurs when the leaflet edges of the valve do not coapt. Although there are M-mode criteria established, most physicians have relied on two-dimensional echocardiography for visual confirmation of the superiorly displaced mitral leaflets, along with structural changes such as leaflet thickening, redundancy, annular dilatation, and chordal elongation as additional features to establish a definitive diagnosis of MVP. Due to the "saddle-shaped" configuration of the normal mitral valve ring, a superiorly displaced appearance of the anterior mitral leaflet is seen in 30% of those in the general population. Superior displacement of the mitral valve leaflets by more than 2 mm above the plane of the annulus is an important two-dimensional echocardiographic criterion,[3,10] and systolic displacement of one or both mitral leaflets into the left atrium in the parasternal view improves the specificity of this finding (Figure 84-2). The latter criterion avoids overdiagnosis, which may occur with posterior bowing of the mitral valve on M-mode echocardiography and even in the four-chamber view on two-dimensional echocardiography.

### Natural History and Management

Most children and adolescents with MVP are asymptomatic and have a benign prognosis. Reassurance is a major part of management, with patients being encouraged to live a normal lifestyle. In adults, the age-related survival rate of both men and women with MVP is similar to that of individuals without MVP. Complications that are reported in adults, although rare in children, include infective endocarditis, progressive MR, congestive heart failure, neurological events, arrhythmias, and sudden death.

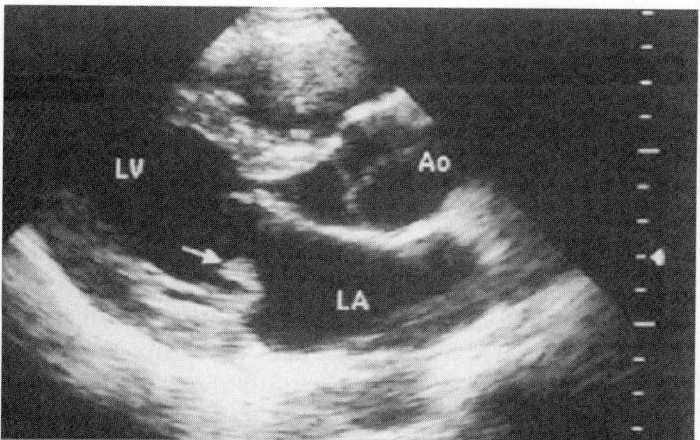


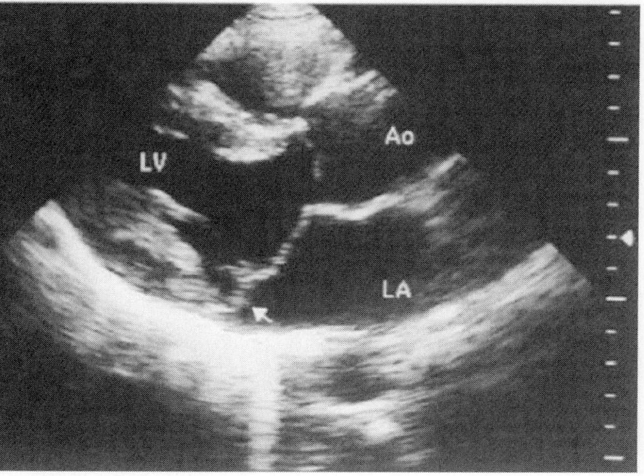


FIGURE 84-2 Parasternal long-axis view in diastole (*top*) and systole (*bottom*) in patient with MVP and myxomatous changes. In the upper panel, note the open mitral valve and the diffuse thickening of the posterior mitral valve leaflet (*arrow*). The lower panel was recorded in systole. Note that both leaflets prolapse behind the plane of the mitral valve annulus. The prolapse of the posterior leaflet is somewhat more prominent (*arrow*). Ao, aorta; LA, left atrium; LV, left ventricle. (Reprinted from Zipes DP, Libby P, Bonow RO, Braunwald E. *Braunwald's Heart Disease: A Textbook of Cardiovascular Medicine*. 7th ed. Philadelphia: WB Saunders; 2005, with permission from Elsevier.)

Infective endocarditis is a rare but serious complication that usually occurs when MR is present and mitral leaflets are thickened and redundant. According to the revised American Heart Association (AHA) guidelines,[11] antibiotic prophylaxis is no longer indicated in these individuals. The primary reasons for revision of the endocarditis prophylaxis guidelines is the lack of scientific evidence that endocarditis occurs as a result of invasive procedures, and the risk of antibiotic associated adverse events exceeds the benefit, if any. Endocarditis is much more likely to result from frequent exposure to random bacteremia associated with daily activities such as brushing or flossing teeth. It also emphasizes the importance of good oral hygiene to decrease the incidence of transient bacteremia from daily activities.

Patients with MVP who are symptomatic with increased adrenergic symptoms, as well as those with chest pain, dizziness, syncope, or anxiety, may respond to beta-blockers. However, just cessation of caffeinated products and reassurance is sufficient in most of these adolescents.

Patients who experience palpitations may undergo ambulatory Holter monitoring with or without exercise testing to detect a possible underlying cause and determine appropriate treatment. Sudden death is an extremely rare complication of MVP and almost never reported in those younger than 20 years.[4,9] In adults with MVP, sudden death seems to occur in <2% of known cases. Many cardiologists believe that this complication is so rare and has never been conclusively proven that it should not be mentioned to the patient or the family for fear of provoking undue anxiety.

Symptomatic, severe MR is rare, and indications for surgery are the same as those with other forms of nonischemic severe MR. These are shown in Table 84-1, which presents the guidelines for management of valvular heart

**Table 84-1**

**American College of Cardiology/AHA Guidelines for Management of Valvular Heart Diseases in Adolescents and Young Adults**

| *Indication* | *Class I* | *Class IIa* | *Class IIb* | *Class III* |
|---|---|---|---|---|
| Diagnostic evaluation of the adolescent or young adult with aortic stenosis[a] | 1. ECG<br>2. Echo-Doppler study | 1. Graded exercise test[b]<br>2. Cardiac catheterization for evaluation of gradient[b] | 1. Chest x-ray[a] | 1. Coronary arteriography in the absence of history suggestive of concomitant coronary artery disease |
| Aortic balloon valvotomy in the adolescent or young adult (≤21 years old) with normal cardiac output | 1. Symptoms of angina, syncope, and dyspnea on exertion, with catheterization peak gradient ≥ 50 mm Hg[c]<br>2. Catheterization peak gradient >60 mm Hg<br>3. New-onset ischemic or repolarization changes on ECG at rest or with exercise (ST depression, T-wave inversion over left precordium) with a gradient >50 mm Hg[c] | 1. Catheterization peak gradient >50 mm Hg if patient wants to play competitive sports or becomes pregnant | | 1. Catheterization gradient <50 mm Hg without symptoms or ECG changes |
| Aortic valve surgery (replacement with mechanical valve, homograft, or pulmonary autograft) in adolescent or young adult with chronic aortic regurgitation | 1. Onset of symptoms<br>2. Asymptomatic patients with LV systolic dysfunction (ejection fraction <0.50) on serial studies 1–3 months apart<br>3. Asymptomatic patients with enlargement (end-diastolic dimension >4 SD above normal) | | 1. Moderate AS (gradient >40 mm Hg) (peak-to-peak gradient at cardiac catheterization)<br>2. Onset of ischemic or repolarization abnormalities (ST depression, T-wave inversion) over left precordium at rest | |

*(Continued)*

## Table 84-1 (Continued)

| *Indication* | *Class I* | *Class IIa* | *Class IIb* | *Class III* |
|---|---|---|---|---|
| Mitral valve surgery in the adolescent or young adult with congenital, severe MR | 1. NYHA Class III or IV symptoms<br>2. Asymptomatic patients with LV systolic dysfunction (ejection fraction 0.60) | 1. NYHA Class II symptoms with preserved LV systolic function if valve repair rather than replacement is likely | 1. Asymptomatic patients with preserved LV systolic function in whom valve replacement is highly likely | |
| Mitral valve surgery in the adolescent or young adult with congenital mitral stenosis | 1. Symptomatic patients (NHYA Class III or IV) and mean mitral valve gradient >10 mm Hg on Doppler echocardiography | 1. Mildly symptomatic patients (NHYA Class II) and mean mitral valve gradient >10 mm Hg on Doppler echocardiographic survey<br>2. Systolic pulmonary artery pressure 50–60 mm Hg with a mean mitral valve gradient >10 mm Hg | 1. New-onset atrial fibrillation or multiple systemic emboli while receiving adequate anticoagulation | |
| Intervention in the adolescent or young adult with pulmonic stenosis (balloon valvotomy or surgery) | 1. Patients with exertional dyspnea, angina, syncope, or presyncope<br>2. Asymptomatic patients with normal cardiac output (estimated clinically or determined by catheterization) and right ventricular to pulmonary artery peak gradient >50 mm Hg | 1. Asymptomatic patients with normal cardiac output (estimated clinically or determined by catheterization) and right ventricular to pulmonary artery peak gradient 40–49 mm Hg | 1. Asymptomatic patients with normal cardiac output (estimated clinically or determined by catheterization) and right ventricular to pulmonary artery peak gradient 30–39 mm Hg | 1. Asymptomatic patients with normal cardiac output (estimated clinically or determined by catheterization) and right ventricular to pulmonary artery peak gradient <30 mm Hg |

ECG, electrocardiogram; LV, left ventricle; AS, aortic stenosis; SD, standard deviation; MR, mitral regurgitation; NYHA, New York Heart Association.

[a]Yearly if echo-Doppler gradient >36 mm Hg (velocity >3 m/sec); every 2 years if echo-Doppler gradient <36 mm Hg (peak velocity <3 mm Hg).

[b]If echo-Doppler gradient >36 mm Hg (velocity >3 m/sec) and patient interested in athletic participation, or if clinical findings and echo-Doppler are disparate.

[c]If gradient <50 mm Hg, other causes of symptoms should be explored.

New York Heart Association (NYHA) Classes:

Class I: conditions for which there is conflicting evidence and/or general agreement that a given procedure or treatment is useful and effective

Class II: conditions for which there is conflicting evidence and/or a divergence of opinion about the usefulness/efficacy of a procedure or treatment

Class IIa: weight of evidence/opinion is in favor of usefulness/efficacy

Class IIb: usefulness/efficacy is less well established by evidence/opinion

Class III: conditions for which there is evidence and/or general agreement that the procedure/treatment is not useful/effective, and in some cases may be harmful

Adapted from Zipes DP, Libby P, Bonow RO, Braunwald E. *Braunwald's Heart Disease: A Textbook of Cardiovascular Medicine.* 7th ed. Philadelphia: WB Saunders; 2005:1631-1632, with permission from Elsevier.

diseases in adolescents and young adults that have been developed by the AHA. The thickened, redundant mitral valve can often be repaired rather than replaced, with lower operative mortality and excellent short-term results.

Similarly, cerebrovascular complications such as stroke are a rare occurrence in children and adolescents with MVP. Management usually involves aspirin or anticoagulant therapy.

Asymptomatic adolescents with MVP and no significant MR can be clinically evaluated every 3 to 5 years to detect any changes in the physical examination. These patients need reassurance and adherence to a healthy lifestyle. The rare adolescent with MVP and MR should be seen yearly to monitor progression of the MR. A permissive approach toward competitive sports participation is warranted in most patients with MVP.

## AORTIC STENOSIS AND INSUFFICIENCY

Adolescents with congenital aortic stenosis (AS) almost always have fusion of one or more commissures resulting in a bicuspid or unicuspid valve. Although the prevalence of a bicuspid or unicuspid valve may be as high as 2% in the general population, only 1 of 50 children born with these abnormalities will actually have significant obstruction or regurgitation by adolescence.[11-13] Most adolescents with AS are asymptomatic but exertional chest pain, easy fatigability, and syncope may occur with severe AS. Balloon valvuloplasty is an effective treatment option for severe AS, resulting in good long-term function with little morbidity and a negligible risk of mortality. The indications for and timing of the intervention is usually dictated by the degree of stenosis, as estimated by a Doppler gradient of >70 mm Hg, ECG changes at rest or with exercise, and symptoms. The Doppler gradient is usually confirmed by cardiac catheterization prior to performing the balloon valvuloplasty. Guidelines for when an aortic balloon valvuloplasty should be performed in the adolescent are included in the guidelines that have been published by the AHA (Table 84-1). The guidelines recommend performing valvuloplasty in those who have a catheterization peak gradient of 50 mm Hg, along with symptoms, or a gradient of 60 mm Hg without symptoms.

Aortic insufficiency can be isolated or can be present with AS. Aortic insufficiency can also result from prior balloon or surgical interventions. The indications for surgery, as recommended by the AHA (Table 84-1), are based on symptoms, left ventricular dysfunction, or progressive dilatation of the left ventricular diastolic and systolic dimensions.

When balloon aortic valvuloplasty is ineffective or there is significant aortic insufficiency, aortic valve surgery may be necessary. Aortic valve replacement using an artificial valve or pulmonary autograft (Ross operation) is the mainstay of surgical therapy. Choice of surgical therapy is dictated by age, gender, and institutional or surgeon's preference. The Ross procedure has recently gained considerable acceptance in active young adolescents due to its advantage of not requiring anticoagulation, which can be especially important for women contemplating pregnancy.

## PULMONIC STENOSIS

In congenital valvar pulmonic stenosis (PS) the valve is thickened, with fused commissures and a domed appearance during ventricular systole. A majority of adolescents with PS are asymptomatic, even when obstruction is severe. Rarely, dyspnea and fatigue can occur due to an inability to increase cardiac output with exercise. Mild cyanosis may be seen in individuals with severe PS who have reduced right ventricular compliance when a patent foramen ovale is present, thus allowing intracardiac right-to-left shunting of blood. Sudden death is rare.

The natural history of individuals with mild PS is very benign. In 1993, the second Natural History Study of Congenital Heart Defects found that for patients with an initial transpulmonary gradient of <25 mm Hg, 96% did not require any intervention.[14,15]

Indications for intervention in the adolescent with PS are the presence of symptoms (exertional dyspnea, angina, syncope, or presyncope) or a catheterization gradient of >50 mm Hg in an asymptomatic patient. Balloon valvuloplasty (Figure 84-3) has now become the procedure of choice, with excellent long-term results. In those with severe or long-standing valvular obstruction, secondary infundibular hypertrophy may cause obstruction even after a successful valvuloplasty. This frequently regresses with time, and beta-blockers may be used as short-term therapy. Surgical repair is usually required for the dysplastic valve often seen in Noonan syndrome or an occasional failed balloon valvuloplasty due to associated annular hypoplasia.

Pulmonary insufficiency is an almost unavoidable consequence of treated PS but is usually inconsequential unless associated with distal pulmonary artery stenosis or with hypertension.

## MITRAL STENOSIS

In developed countries, mitral stenosis (MS) is almost always congenital in origin, whereas in developing countries it is almost always rheumatic in origin. Congenital MS is frequently associated with other left-sided lesions,

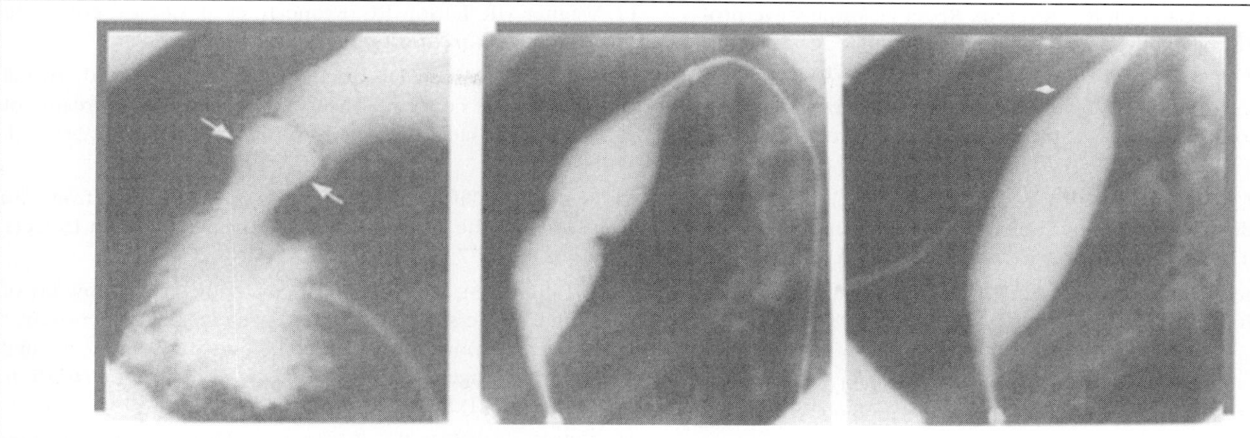

**FIGURE 84-3** Pulmonary valvuloplasty. *Left*: Right ventricular angiogram (lateral view) showing domed pulmonary valve (*arrows*). *Middle*: Balloon valvuloplasty showing appearance of a waist when the balloon is partially inflated. *Right*: Relief of valve obstruction as evidenced by complete elimination of the waist. (Reprinted with permission from Lock JE, Keane JF, Perry SB. *Diagnostic and Interventional Catheterization in Congenital Heart Disease*. 2nd ed. Netherlands: Martinus Nijhoff; 1987: 113.)

such as coarctation of the aorta or AS. Patients with mild MS are usually asymptomatic. Symptoms of dyspnea on exertion, orthopnea, or palpitations are seen with moderate to severe MS. Echocardiography is the most informative diagnostic tool for evaluating the mitral valve apparatus and papillary muscle and, at times, provides considerable insight into the feasibility of successful valve repair. Balloon valvuloplasty for congenital MS has been unsuccessful to minimally effective in the short term. This is in stark contrast to its efficacy in adolescents with rheumatic MS. According to the AHA guidelines, recommendations for mitral valve surgery in the adolescent with congenital MS are based on symptoms, pulmonary hypertension, and a mean transmitral gradient of 10 mm Hg (Table 84-1). Surgical repair or valve replacement remains the mainstay for symptomatic patients with moderate to severe MS.

## TRICUSPID VALVE DISEASE

Acquired disease of the tricuspid valve is very rare in adolescents and is usually caused by bacterial endocarditis in the presence of a small ventricular septal defect. Most cases of tricuspid valve disease are congenital, with Ebstein's anomaly being the most common cause. Some children may have severe tricuspid regurgitation (TR), whereas others have very mild abnormalities that may not be recognized until revealed by a chest x-ray. Most patients have an interatrial communication that can cause cyanosis if TR elevates the right atrial pressure, especially with exercise. One or more accessory pathways are also common, with a risk of supraventricular tachycardia of about 25%. Patients with Ebstein anomaly may be asymptomatic, with no cyanosis and no arrhythmias. More commonly, they have exercise intolerance, cyanosis, and arrhythmias. The natural history of Ebstein's anomaly varies. Predictors of poor outcome are AHA functional Class III or IV (see Chapter 82, Congenital Heart Disease), a cardiothoracic ratio of >65%, or atrial fibrillation. However, patients with Ebstein anomaly who reach late adolescence and adulthood often have an excellent outcome.[16] Surgical repair of Ebstein anomaly remains difficult. Occasionally, tricuspid valve repair is not feasible, and a bioprosthetic valve or mechanical valve is needed. In addition, if an accessory pathway is present, it can be addressed in the catheterization laboratory or during surgery.

## REFERENCES

1. Warnes CA. The adult with congenital heart disease. *J Am Coll Cardiol*. 2005;46:1-8

2. Freed LA. Benjamin EJ. Levy D, et al. Mitral valve prolapse in the general population. *J Am Coll Cardiol*. 2002;40: 1298-1304

3. Barlow JB. Pocock WA. The mitral valve prolapse enigma—two decades later. *Mod Concepts Cardiovasc Dis*. 1984;53: 13-17

4. Jersaty RM. Mitral valve prolapse: definition and implication in athletes. *J Am Coll Cardiol*. 1986;7:231-236

5. Perloff JK. Child JS. Clinical and epidemiologic issues in mitral valve prolapse: overview and perspective. *Am Heart J*. 1987;113:1324-1332

6. Savage DD, Garrison RJ, Devereux RB, et al. Mitral valve prolapse in the general population. I. Epidemiologic features: the Framingham study. *Am Heart J*. 1983;106:571–576

7. Margraf J, Ehlers A, Roth WT. Mitral valve prolapse and panic disorder: a review of their relationship. *Pyschosom Med*. 1988;50:93–113

8. Perloff JK, Child JS, Edwards JE. New guidelines for the clinical diagnosis of mitral valve prolapse. *Am J Cardiol*. 1986;57:1124–1129

9. Kliegfield P, Levy D, Devereux RB, et al. Arrhythmias and sudden death in mitral valve prolapse. *Am Heart J*. 1987;113:1298–1307

10. Otto CM. Mitral valve prolapse. In: Otto CM, ed. *Valvular Heart Disease*. 2nd ed. Philadelphia: WB Saunders; 2004:368–387

11. Wilson W, Taubert KA, Gewitz M, et al. Prevention of infective endocarditis: guidelines from the American Heart Association. *Circulation*. 2007;116:1736–1754

12. Wagner HR, Ellison RC, Keane JF, et al. Clinical course in aortic stenosis. *Circulation*. 1977;56:I-147–I-156

13. Keane JF, Driscoll DJ, Gersony WM, et al. Second natural history study of congenital heart defects: results of treatment of patient with aortic valvar stenosis. *Circulation*. 1993;87:I-16–I-27

14. Nadas AS, Ellison RC, Weidman WH, eds. Report from the Joint Study on the Natural History of Congenital Heart Defects. *Circulation*. 1977;56 (suppl I):I-1–I-87

15. O'Fallon WM, Weidman WH, eds. Long-term follow-up of congenital aortic stenosis, pulmonary stenosis, and ventricular septal defect: report from the Second Joint Study on the Natural History of Congenital Heart Defects (NHS-2). *Circulation*. 1993;87 (suppl I):I-1–I-126

16. Celermajer DS, Bull C, Till JA, et al. Ebstein's anomaly: presentation and outcome from fetus to adulthood. *J Am Coll Cardiol*. 1994;23:170–176

# CHAPTER 85

# Cardiac Dysrhythmias

CHRISTINE A. WALSH, MD

Dysrhythmias can be the cause of a variety of symptoms in the adolescent. Physicians who care for adolescents must decide whether such common complaints as "heart racing," "skipped beats," and "dizziness" are due to a significant dysrhythmia or are benign phenomena. Although dysrhythmias are a less frequent cause of syncope and sudden death in adolescents than in adults, they must be carefully considered.

## EVALUATION

The primary care practitioner is usually the first to recognize the symptoms and signs of a dysrhythmia. A thorough personal and family history and physical examination are essential in evaluating a dysrhythmia and directing diagnostic studies. Recording a suspected dysrhythmia is absolutely necessary before assuming a diagnosis and instituting therapy.

### HISTORY

#### Personal History

An adolescent with a dysrhythmia may report palpitations, which are subjective feelings of heartbeats. Paroxysms of tachycardia or single premature beats can cause palpitations or a fluttering sensation in the chest.[1] Dyspnea, chest pain, abdominal pain, nausea, or vomiting may also occur. Symptoms of congestive heart failure are much more common in infants than adolescents. Syncope and presyncope (light-headedness or "dizziness") are ominous consequences of either a tachydysrhythmia or a bradydysrhythmia. On rare occasions the presentation of a dysrhythmia is sudden death. The duration and frequency, as well as initiating events of a dysrhythmia, must be determined. Symptoms that occur with activity must be carefully evaluated because of the risk of exercise-induced ventricular tachycardia (VT). Re-entrant dysrhythmias are associated with an abrupt onset and termination, whereas automatic dysrhythmias start and stop gradually. The patient may have discovered how to terminate the dysrhythmia with a vagal maneuver, such as bearing down or drinking ice-cold water. A pulse rate taken during an episode is extremely useful.

A careful dietary history (eg, caffeine) and drug history (eg, over-the-counter cold medicines, prescription drugs) are important. The adolescent must be asked specifically about the use of alternative medicines, because they may not consider them drugs. For example, hawthorn used as a cardiac stimulant, ginkgo biloba for attention-deficit/hyperactivity disorder (ADHD), and ephedra (ma huang) as an appetite suppressant can all cause dysrhythmias. A full medical history must be taken of cardiac, neurologic (eg, neuromuscular disease), endocrinologic (eg, hyperthyroidism), and psychiatric (eg, anxiety disorder) diseases, as well as eating disorders, alcohol abuse, and illicit drug use. Intercurrent illnesses especially with fever, as well as hormonal changes and stress, can be associated with dysrhythmias. Being an athlete also puts the adolescent at higher risk.

#### Family History

A family history of sudden death, dysrhythmias, seizures (possibly due to dysrhythmias), syncope, early cardiovascular disease, or known hypertrophic cardiomyopathy, long QT syndrome (sometimes associated with congenital deafness), Wolff-Parkinson-White syndrome (WPW), Brugada syndrome (an inherited cardiac ion channelopathy, similar to long QT syndrome, which predisposes to sudden death), arrhythmogenic right ventricular dysplasia, hyperlipidemia, and Marfan syndrome are significant risk factors for dysrhythmias.

### PHYSICAL EXAMINATION

The physical examination of an adolescent with a suspected dysrhythmia may be normal, but it is important in diagnosing congenital (eg, aortic stenosis) and acquired (eg, myocarditis) heart disease, as well as exacerbating factors, such as fever, anemia, or hyperthyroidism. The adolescent with complete heart block (CHB) will have prominent pulses due to peripheral vasodilation and large stroke volume; jugular venous pulsations will occur irregularly and be prominent when the atrium contracts against a closed tricuspid valve (cannon wave). In the setting of an acute dysrhythmia, the physical examination determines the degree of hemodynamic instability, which governs therapeutic alternatives. The absence of a murmur is not reassuring because many murmurs decrease in intensity when a person is in low cardiac output, as might occur with a dysrhythmia. Similarly, flow murmurs can occur if the heart rate is fast or slow. The normal resting heart rate for an adolescent is between 60 and 100 beats per minute (see sections on Sinus Bradycardia and Sinus Tachycardia).

### ADJUNCTIVE TESTS

#### Electrocardiogram

Every patient with a suspected dysrhythmia should have a 12-lead electrocardiogram (ECG) to determine heart rate, axes (ie, P, QRS, and T), intervals (ie, PR, QRS, and QTc), AV relationships, and the presence or absence of hypertrophy and premature beats. Diagnostic abnormalities should be identified. A short PR interval, wide QRS, and a delta wave are the hallmarks of WPW. A prolonged QTc and abnormal T waves can be seen in the long QT syndrome. ST-segment changes and/or T-wave abnormalities indicate cardiac disease, electrolyte imbalance, or drug effect. However, a normal ECG does not rule out significant heart disease, such as hypertrophic cardiomyopathy, long QT syndrome, WPW, and arrhythmogenic right ventricular dysplasia/cardiomyopathy. Recording a 12-lead ECG during a dysrhythmia, especially with the onset and termination (eg, while giving adenosine), is extremely helpful in making a diagnosis.

#### Monitors

A 24-hour ambulatory ECG (Holter monitor) is useful for correlating symptoms with a dysrhythmia, which occurs at least daily, recording dysrhythmias, which a patient may not be unaware of, and quantifying dysrhythmias (eg, the number of premature ventricular contractions [PVCs] in an hour/day). On Holter monitoring, the lower limit of normal heart rate in an adolescent while asleep is 40 beats per minute,[2-5] and in an athlete, 30 beats per minute.[6]

Transtelephonic event recorders are more useful for symptoms that occur less frequently. The loop type is worn by the patient for a month and is activated by the patient or a witness by pushing a button. The ECG is recorded for a period of time before and after activation. This type is useful for dysrhythmias of short duration or if the patient's consciousness becomes altered. The nonlooping type is placed on the patient only at the time of an event. With either type the ECG is stored and transmitted telephonically later at a convenient time. Implantable loop recorders are placed in a subcutaneous pocket for up to 14 months.

#### Exercise Stress Test

Occasionally a dysrhythmia may be provoked during an exercise test, especially catecholamine-sensitive VT and AV nodal re-entry tachycardia (AVNRT). Resolution of PVCs during exercise is an indication that they are benign. Loss of delta waves as the heart rate increases is an indicator of a decreased risk of sudden death in WPW. The nature and extent of bradycardia may be evaluated with an exercise test.

#### Imaging

The echocardiogram is essential to the diagnosis of congenital and acquired heart disease, but it is important to remember that a life-threatening dysrhythmia may originate in a heart that is normal by echocardiography (eg, WPW, long QT syndrome, focal arrhythmogenic right ventricular dysplasia).

Magnetic resonance imaging (MRI) is useful in further determining if a heart is truly normal, especially in evaluating for such cardiomyopathies as arrhythmogenic right ventricular dysplasia.

#### Invasive Studies

A cardiac catheterization may be needed to diagnose coronary artery abnormalities, and a cardiac biopsy is helpful in diagnosing myocarditis.

An invasive electrophysiology study is useful for diagnosing a dysrhythmia (eg, the mechanism of a wide complex tachycardia), risk stratification (eg, determining the refractory period of an accessory pathway, such as a Kent bundle in WPW, as an indicator of risk of sudden death; inducibility of VT in a postoperative patient with tetralogy of Fallot), testing of drug efficacy, deciding if a dysrhythmia is the cause of syncope, and catheter ablation.

## CLASSIFICATION OF DYSRHYTHMIAS

A practical classification of dysrhythmias is based on auscultation of rate and regularity (Box 85-1). Is the rhythm too fast, too slow, or irregular but close to the normal rate?

### NORMAL RATE/IRREGULAR RHYTHMS

#### Sinus Arrhythmia

The most common cause of an irregular rhythm in the adolescent is sinus arrhythmia. This is a normal, physiologic rhythm in which the heart rate varies with respiration, slowing during expiration and accelerating during inspiration. Sinus rhythm requires that P waves precede each QRS complex and are of the same morphology and positive in leads I, II, and AVF (Figure 85-1). Sinus arrhythmia usually resolves with exercise and requires no treatment.

#### Wandering Atrial Pacemaker

Wandering atrial pacemaker is characterized by gradual changes in the intrinsic pacemaker of the heart from the sinus node to another part of the atrium, resulting

**Box 85-1**

***Classification of Dysrhythmias Based on Auscultation of Rate and Regularity***

I. Normal rate/Irregular
  A. Sinus arrhythmia
  B. Wandering atrial pacemaker
  C. Sinus pause
    1. Sinus arrest
    2. Sinoatrial block
  D. Premature beats
    1. Premature supraventricular contractions
      a. Premature atrial contractions (PACs)
      b. Premature junctional contractions (PJCs)
    2. Premature ventricular contractions (PVCs)
      a. Morphology (RBBB, LBBB, axis)
        i Uniform (simple)
        ii Multiform (complex)
      b. Pattern
        i Singles (simple), couplets (complex)
        ii Bigeminy, trigeminy, quadrigeminy (simple or complex)
  E. Second-degree atrioventricular (AV) block
    1. Mobitz 1 (Wenckebach)
    2. Mobitz 2
II Too slow—bradydysrhythmias
  A. Third-degree AV block
  B. Sinus bradycardia
  C. Sick sinus syndrome
  D. Ectopic atrial/junctional escape rhythm
III Too fast—tachydysrhythmias
  A. Normal QRS
    1. Sinus tachycardia
    2. Supraventricular tachycardia
      a. Re-entrant tachycardia with an accessory pathway
        i Orthodromic atrioventricular re-entrant (reciprocating) tachycardia (AVRT) (WPW)
      b. Re-entrant tachycardia without an accessory pathway
        i Atrioventricular node re-entrant (reciprocating) tachycardia (AVNRT)
      c. Ectopic (automatic) tachycardia
        i Atrial ectopic tachycardia (AET)
        ii Junctional ectopic tachycardia (JET)
        iii Chaotic atrial rhythm (multifocal atrial tachycardia)
    3. Atrial flutter/intra-atrial re-entrant tachycardia (IART)

**Box 85-1 (Continued)**

    4. Atrial fibrillation
  B. Wide QRS
    1. Ventricular tachycardia
      a. Duration
        i Sustained
        ii Nonsustained
        iii Incessant
      b. Morphology
        i Monomorphic
        ii Polymorphic
          (a) Torsade de pointes
          (b) Catecholaminergic
          (c) Bidirectional
      c. Idiopathic
        i RVOT
        ii LV fascicular re-entry
    2. Accelerated idioventricular rhythm (AIVR)
    3. Supraventricular tachycardia with aberrant conduction
    4. Antidromic atrioventricular re-entrant (reciprocating) tachycardia (AVRT) (WPW)

RBBB, right bundle branch block; LBBB, left bundle branch block

in changes in P-wave morphology (Figure 85-2). It is common and benign.

### Sinus Pause

A sinus pause is due to cessation of sinus node depolarization (sinus arrest) or exit block of the sinus node impulse to the atrium (Figure 85-3). It may be followed by an ectopic atrial, junctional, or ventricular escape rhythm. Sinus pauses are usually benign, but if frequent, prolonged (≥ 3 seconds in the adolescent), or in conjunction with a very slow escape rhythm, they may be a sign of sick sinus syndrome (see below).

### Extrasystoles

Premature beats (contractions) or extrasystoles are impulses that occur too early in the cardiac cycle and can originate from the atria, AV junction, or ventricles. Supraventricular premature contractions arise from the atria or AV junction. Premature beats usually have a fixed coupling interval to the preceding beat. When every other beat is an extrasystole, the rhythm is bigeminy (Figure 85-4). In trigeminy, there is a regular grouping of 3 impulses, 2 normal and 1 extrasystole (Figure 85-5). A couplet consists of 2 extrasystoles together; 3 or more in a row is tachycardia.

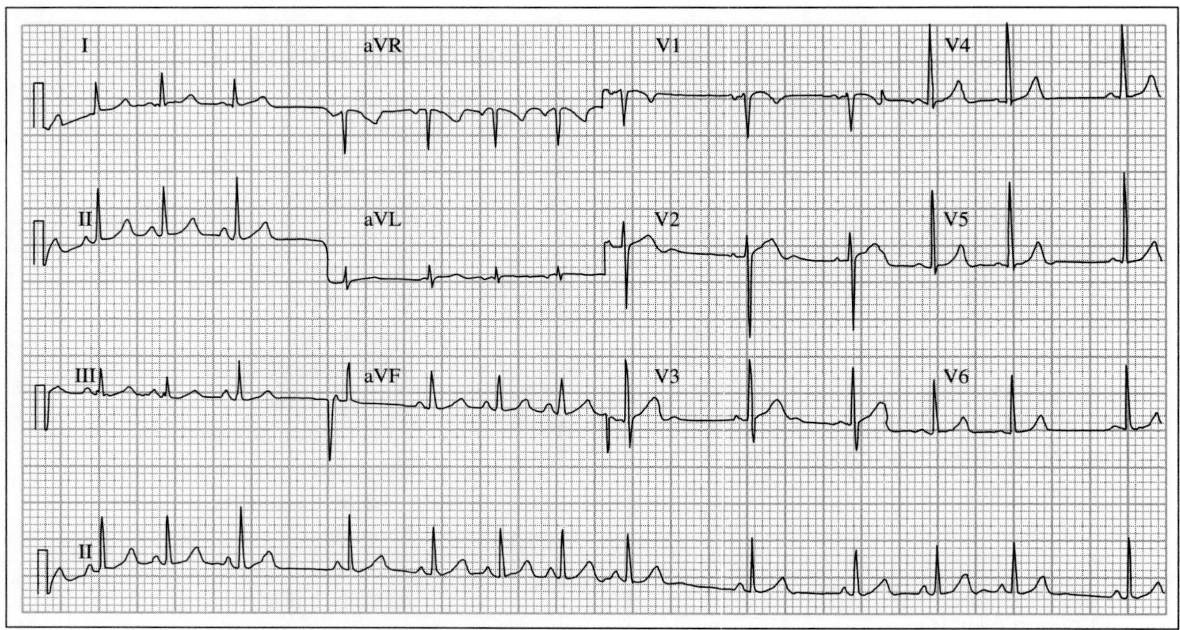


**FIGURE 85-1** ECG of sinus arrhythmia.

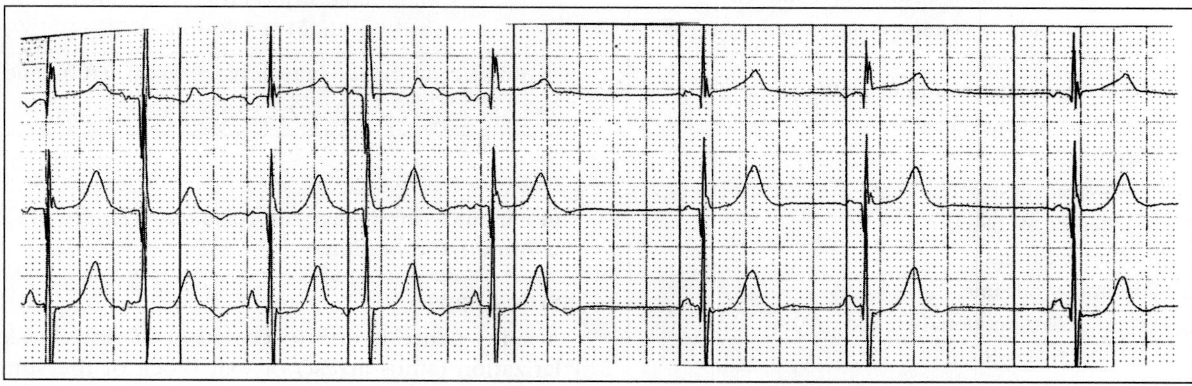

**FIGURE 85-2** ECG of wandering atrial pacemaker.

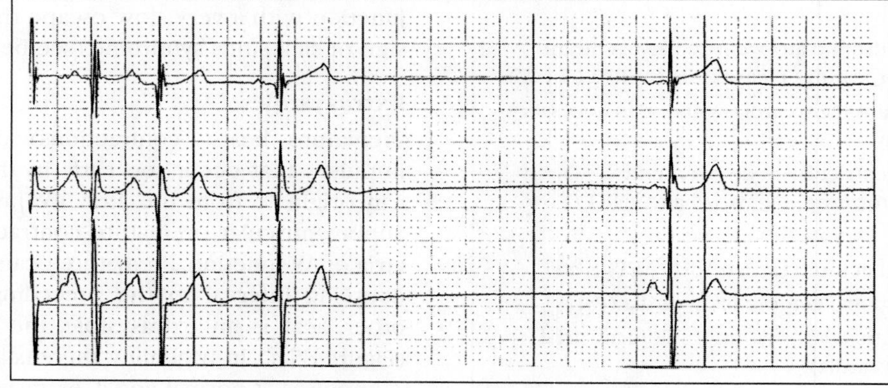

**FIGURE 85-3** ECG of sinus pause of 2.3 seconds.

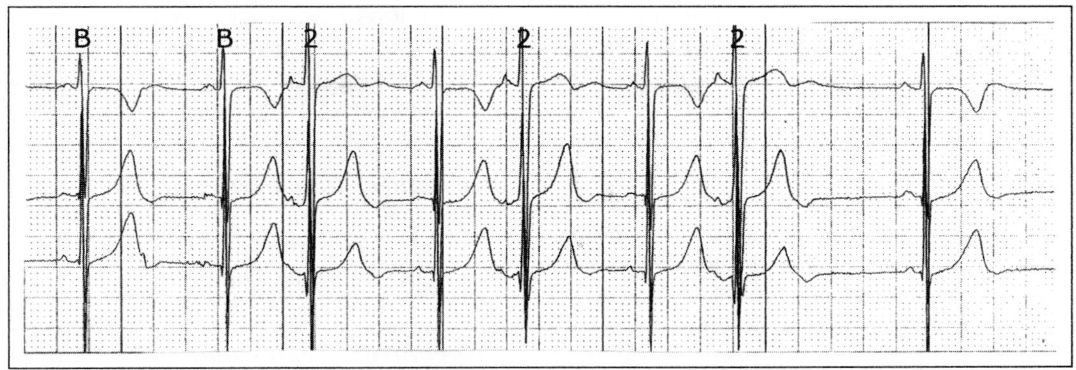


FIGURE 85-4 ECG of atrial bigeminy. Every other beat (marked 2) is a PAC.

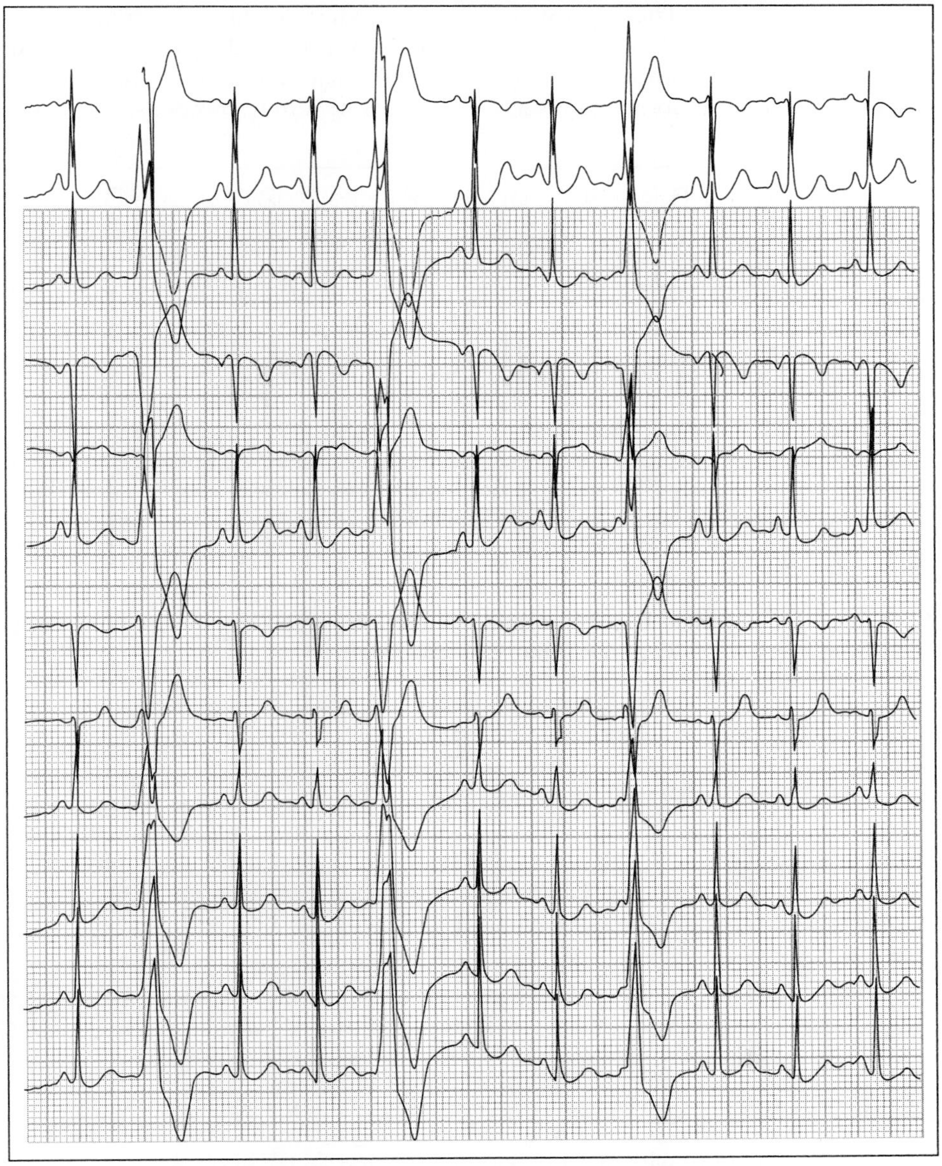

FIGURE 85-5 ECG of ventricular trigeminy. Every third beat is a PVC.

***Premature Atrial Contractions (PACs)*** In a premature atrial contraction (PAC), the P-wave morphology is usually different from the sinus P wave, but the QRS morphology is the same (narrow) (Figure 85-6). If the PAC is premature, the QRS complex may be wide (aberrant) (Figure 85-7) or absent (blocked). The preceding T wave should be examined in multiple leads for evidence of a superimposed P wave. Blocked atrial bigeminy (every other beat a blocked PAC) may be misdiagnosed as sinus bradycardia. Premature atrial contractions often reset the sinus node resulting in an incomplete compensatory pause, meaning the length of 2 cycles, including 1 premature beat, is less than the length of 2 normal cycles. However, this is not a reliable method of differentiating PACs from PVCs. Premature atrial contractions are found in 44% of normal adolescents. They are usually single and infrequent (< 1 per hour).[2–4] and Premature atrial contractions can be associated with digitalis toxicity, cardiac surgery, or with atrial abnormalities such as a tumor or an atrial septal defect. Treatment is not usually indicated, unless PACs need to be suppressed because they precipitate a tachydysrhythmia or result in significant bradycardia because of nonconduction (see treatment of SVT following).

***Premature Junctional Contractions (PJCs)*** In a premature junctional contraction (PJC), a normal QRS complex occurs prematurely, but the P wave is absent or follows the QRS complex. The clinical implications are the same as for PACs.

***Premature Ventricular Contractions (PVCs)*** Premature ventricular contractions (PVCs) are early impulses that arise from any area of the ventricles. They are characterized by a usually wide for age QRS complex, which is different from the normal QRS complex and not preceded by a P wave (Figure 85-8). Premature ventricular contractions are often, but not invariably, followed by a fully compensatory pause, that is, the length

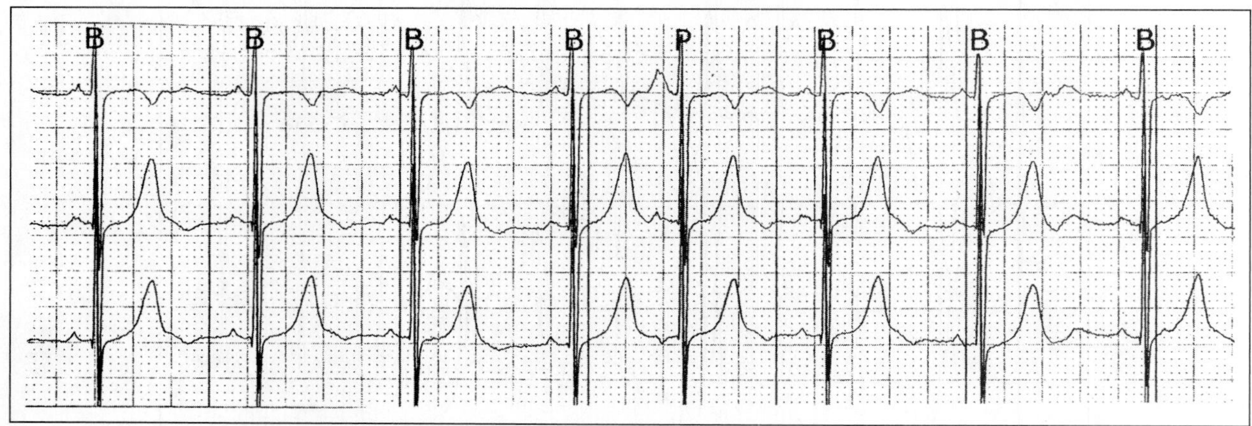


**FIGURE 85-6** ECG of PAC (Marked P) with normal conduction and an incomplete compensatory pause. The P wave differs from the sinus P wave but the QRS is the same.

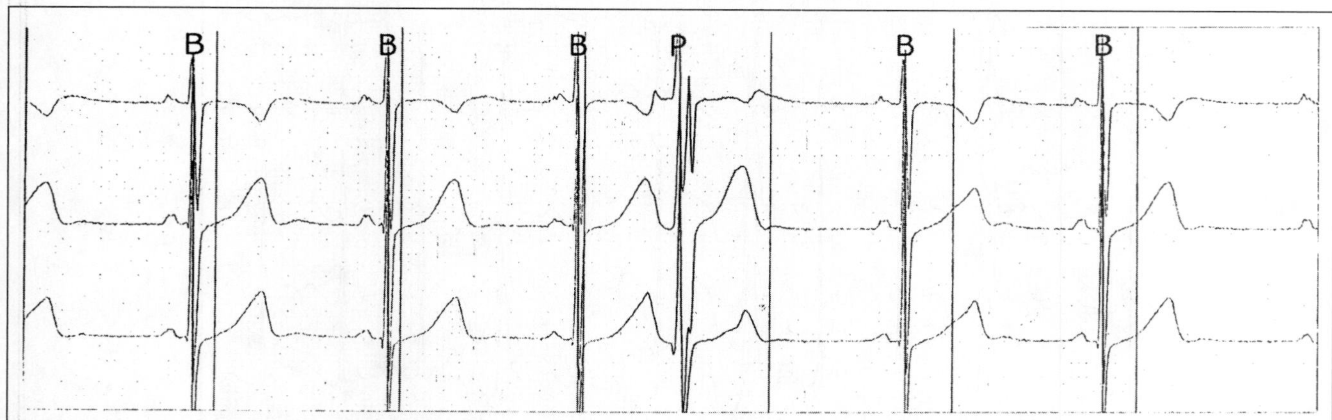


**FIGURE 85-7** ECG of PAC (Marked P) with aberrant conduction and an incomplete compensatory pause. The P and QRS differ from the sinus P and QRS.

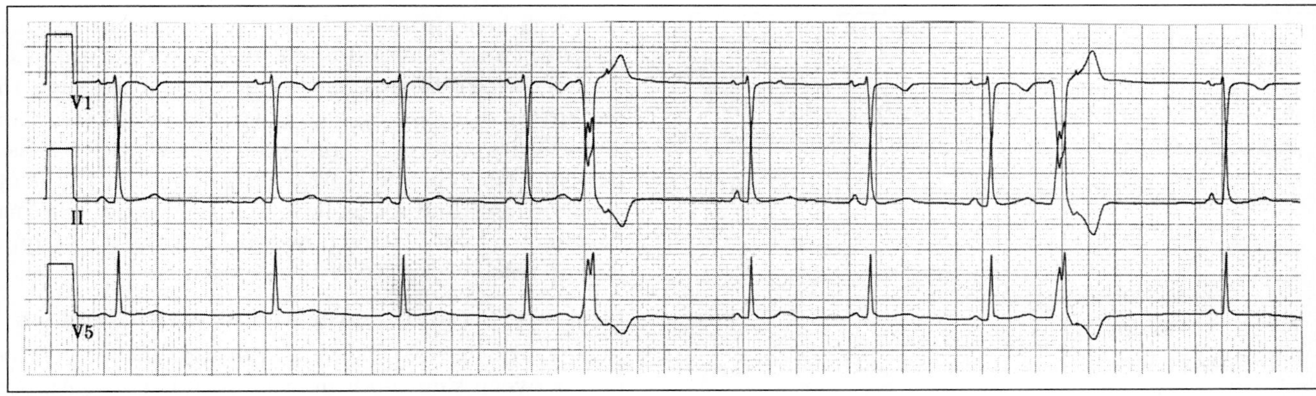


**FIGURE 85-8** ECG of uniform single PVCs.

of 2 cycles, including the premature beat, is the same as that of 2 normal cycles. The adolescent may feel the extrasystole due to the increased stroke volume of the normal beat following the compensatory pause or may be totally unaware of PVCs. Very early PVCs may not be palpable while taking a pulse.

Premature ventricular contractions with the same morphology are classified as uniform, and those with different morphologies are classified as multiform. The presence of fusion beats, with morphologic features of both the PVC and the normal sinus beat, suggests the ventricular origin of the extrasystole. Single, uniform PVCs even as bigeminy or trigeminy constitute simple ventricular ectopy. Complex ventricular ectopy consists of multiform single PVCs, uniform or multiform couplets (Figure 85-9), and VT (3 or more consecutive PVCs). During ambulatory 24-hour ECG monitoring PVCs are found in up to 41% of adolescents.[2-4] These are usually uniform and rare (< 5 per 24 hours). However, in a study of 100 healthy adolescent boys, 6 had more than 1 PVC per hour and 10 had multiform PVCs; episodes of bigeminy, trigeminy, and up to 6 beat runs of VT were

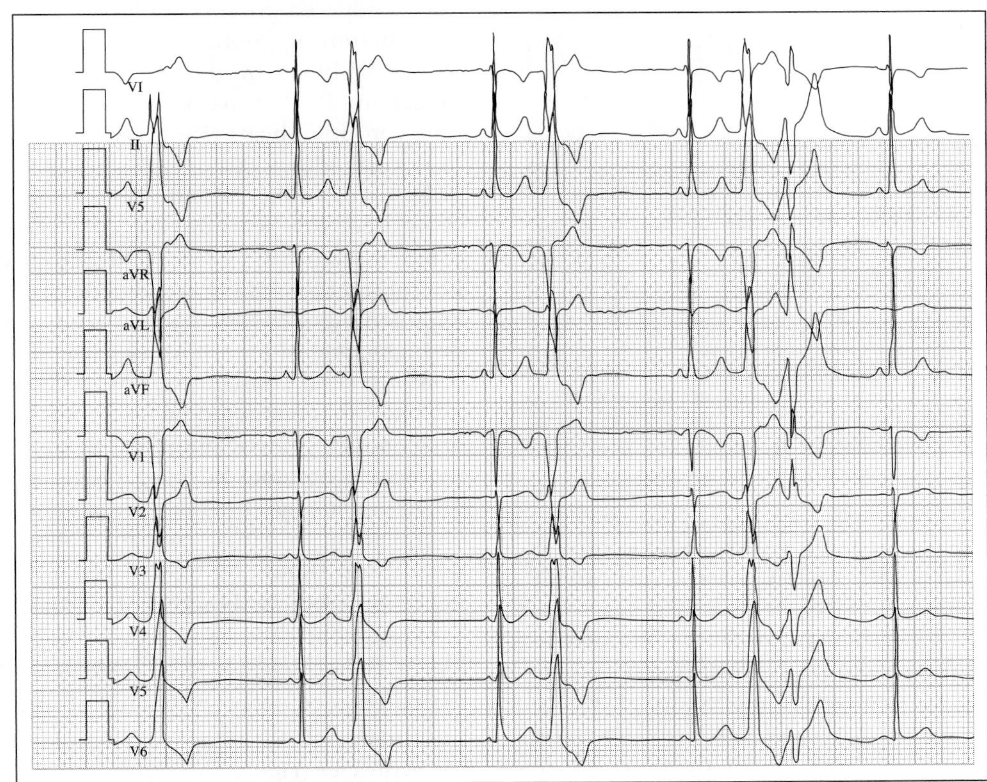


**FIGURE 85-9** ECG of ventricular bigeminy and a multiform couplet.

**Box 85-2**

***Causes of Ventricular Tachycardia and PVCs***

- Congenital heart disease
  - Unoperated
    - Aortic stenosis
    - Eisenmenger syndrome
    - Mitral valve prolapse
  - Postoperative
    - Tetralogy of Fallot
- Cardiomyopathy
  - Dilated cardiomyopathy
    - Myocarditis
  - Hypertrophic cardiomyopathy
  - Arrhythmogenic right ventricular dysplasia
- Myocardial ischemia/infarction
  - Anomalous origin of coronary artery
  - Kawasaki disease
- Cardiac tumors
- Channelopathies
  - Long QT syndrome (congenital or acquired)
  - Brugada syndrome
- Metabolic disorders
  - Hyperkalemia, hypokalemia
  - Hypoxia
  - Acidosis
- Drugs
  - Antidysrhythmic agents
  - Digitalis
  - Psychotropic agents
    - Phenothiazines
    - Tricyclic antidepressants
  - Catecholamine infusion
  - Cocaine
  - Amphetamines
- Intracardiac catheter

recorded.[5] Nevertheless, complex ventricular ectopy is more often associated with heart disease. Causes of VT are also causes of PVCs (Box 85-2).

Uniform, single PVCs that occur in the context of a normal heart and are suppressed with exercise generally do not require treatment but require investigation, which includes an echocardiogram and exercise stress test. Premature ventricular contractions in an abnormal heart and complex ventricular ectopy may be associated with a risk of sudden death and require a thorough investigation, which may include an MRI, cardiac catheterization, and/or electrophysiology study (see the following). Treatment is directed at correcting the underlying disorder (eg, electrolyte imbalance, structural abnormality) and/or suppression with drugs such as a beta blocker (eg, atenolol) or mexiletine. In the acute situation an intravenous lidocaine bolus and drip may be effective, with more powerful drugs such as amiodarone reserved for refractory ectopy.

### First- and Second-Degree Atrioventricular Block

Atrioventricular (AV) block, is a disturbance of conduction between sinus node activation and ventricular activation. There are 3 types: first-degree, second-degree, and third-degree.

In first-degree AV block, the PR interval is longer than the upper limits of normal for the patient's age and heart rate, but all atrial impulses are conducted to the ventricles (Figure 85-10). This does not cause an irregular or slow heartbeat and can occur in normal adolescents with no clinical significance. It is a minor criterion for acute rheumatic fever and can be associated with congenital heart disease such as an atrial septal defect, drugs such as digoxin, and electrolyte imbalance such as hypokalemia, hyperkalemia, hypercalcemia, hypocalcemia, and hypomagnesemia.

In second-degree AV block some atrial impulses are not conducted to the ventricles, producing an irregular rhythm. In Mobitz type I (Wenckebach) second-degree AV block, the PR interval becomes progressively longer until a P wave is not followed by a QRS complex (dropped beat) (Figure 85-11). This also can occur in normal adolescents, especially those with high vagal tone such as athletes, and needs no treatment. It can be associated with heart disease, electrolyte imbalance, and drugs. In Mobitz type II second-degree AV block, there is intermittent loss of P-wave conduction but no preceding lengthening of the PR interval (Figure 85-12). Advanced or high-grade Mobitz II AV block is the loss of conduction of several consecutive P waves. For example, in 3:1 AV block, 1 conducted atrial impulse is followed by 2 nonconducted atrial impulses. Mobitz II second-degree AV block is ominous because it is associated with Stokes-Adams attacks and sudden death and can progress to complete heart block (see the following). Any underlying cause should be treated, but a pacemaker may be necessary (see Third-Degree Atrioventricular Block).

## SLOW RHYTHMS (BRADYDYSRHYTHMIAS)

### Third-Degree Atrioventricular Block

In third-degree AV block (CHB), no atrial impulses reach the ventricles (Figure 85-13). It is a form of AV dissociation in which the ventricular rate is slower than the atrial rate. If the junctional or ventricular rate is faster than the atrial

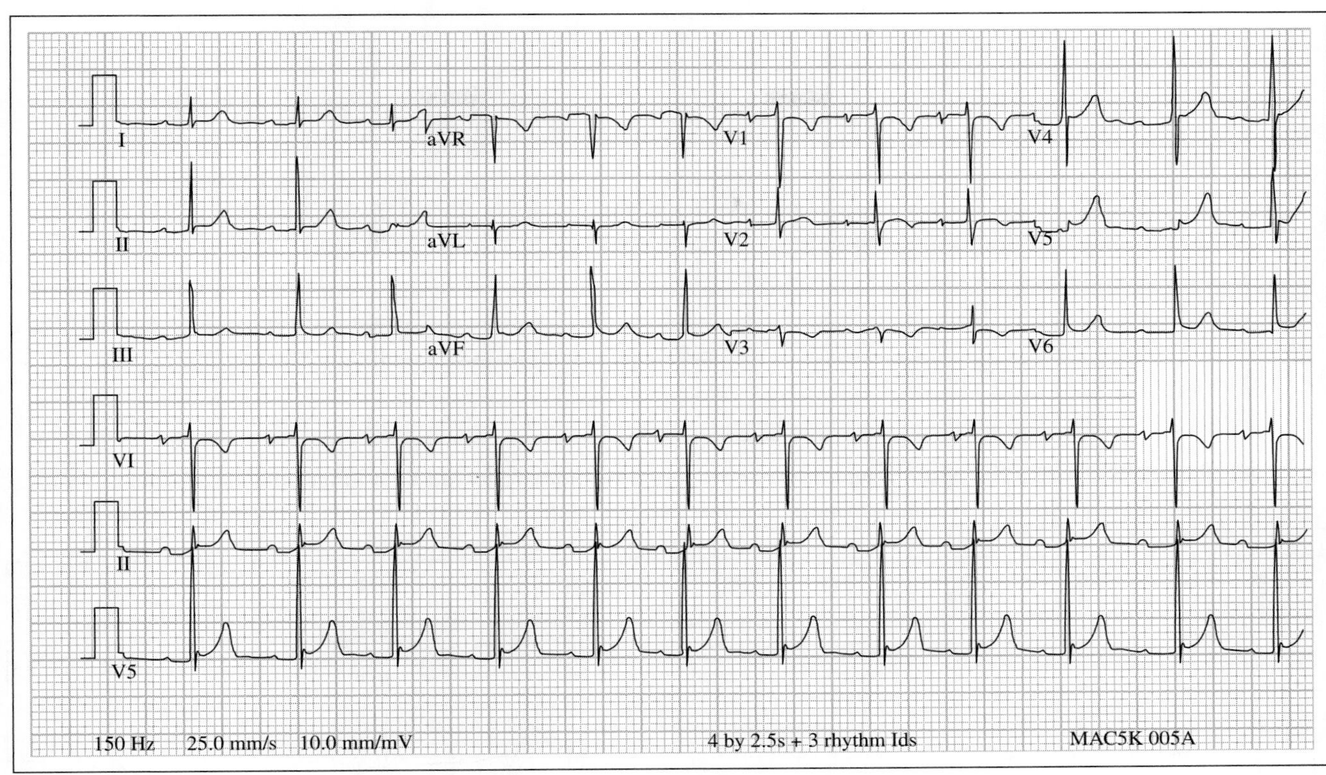


**FIGURE 85-10** ECG of first-degree AV block.

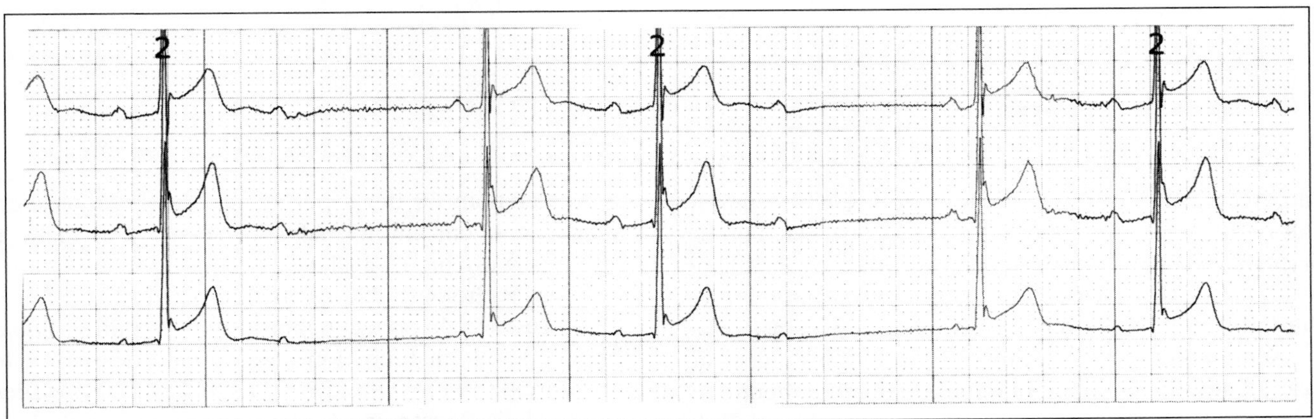


**FIGURE 85-11** ECG of Mobitz type I (Wenckebach) second-degree AV block.

rate, the AV dissociation is not due to CHB, but may be due to an accelerated junctional or ventricular rhythm or to sinus bradycardia with a junctional escape rhythm at an appropriate rate. A narrow normal QRS complex is considered more reliable because it implies a higher (junctional) origin in the conduction system.

Complete heart block is congenital or acquired. Congenital CHB can be isolated or associated with structural heart disease such as ventricular inversion or tumors or with long QT syndrome, but it is more commonly caused by autoimmune injury of the fetal conduction system by IgG antibodies (anti-SSA/Ro and anti-SSB/La) from a mother with systemic lupus erythematosus or other connective tissue disease. The adolescent with congenital CHB and a normal heart is commonly asymptomatic. However, a pacemaker is required if the

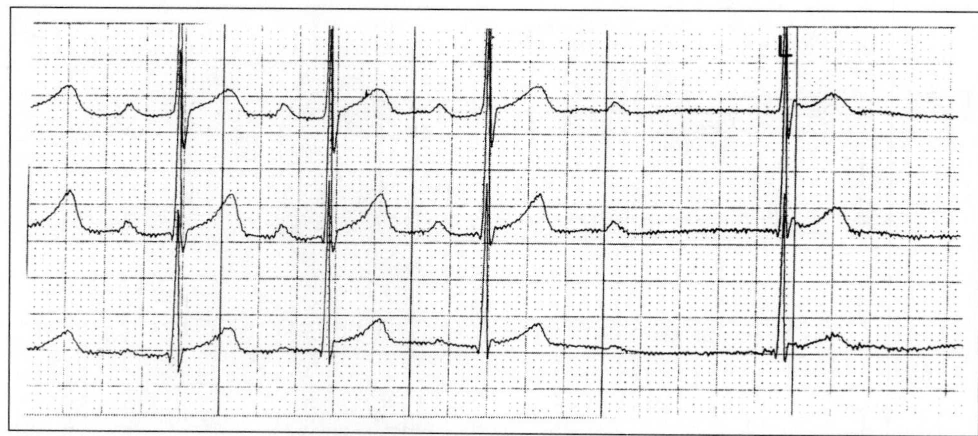

**FIGURE 85-12** ECG of Mobitz type II second-degree AV block followed by a junctional escape beat.

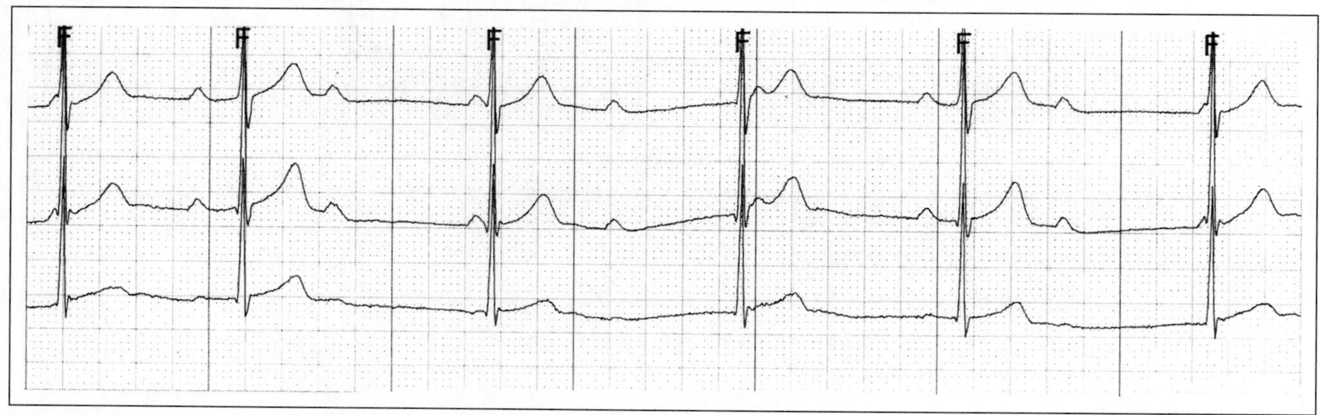

**FIGURE 85-13** ECG of third-degree AV block.

adolescent has ventricular dysfunction, a wide (unreliable) QRS escape rhythm, complex ventricular ectopy, or correlated symptoms such as syncope (Stokes-Adams attack). A patient with long QT syndrome and 2:1 or third-degree AV block most likely needs a pacemaker.[7]

Acquired CHB can be caused by infectious (eg, Lyme disease, diphtheria) or inflammatory (eg, acute rheumatic fever) myocarditis, an abscess in endocarditis, tumors in the conduction system, neuromuscular disease (eg, myotonic dystrophy, Kearns-Sayre syndrome), electrolyte imbalance, drugs (eg, tricyclic antidepressants, antidysrhythmic agents), or heart surgery (Box 85-3). Acquired CHB puts a patient at high risk for sudden death. Advanced second- or third-degree AV block that is not expected to resolve, or that persists at least 7 days after cardiac surgery is an indication for permanent pacing.[7]

## Sinus Bradycardia

The characteristics of sinus rhythm (see previous) are present in sinus bradycardia, but the awake rate is slower than 60 beats per minute in the adolescent. This can occur in normal adolescents, especially in athletes with high vagal tone, and requires no intervention. Pathologic causes include increased intracranial pressure, hypoxia, hypothermia, hypothyroidism, hyperkalemia, malnutrition (which may be secondary to anorexia nervosa) and drugs such as beta blockers (Box 85-4). Treatment is directed at the underlying cause. Sinus node dysfunction with correlation of symptoms during age-inappropriate bradycardia requires a pacemaker.[7]

## Sick Sinus Syndrome (Tachycardia-Bradycardia Syndrome)

Bradycardia alternating with episodes of atrial tachycardia, usually atrial flutter or atrial fibrillation, is often seen in patients with sinus node disease. Abrupt termination of the tachydysrhythmia can result in a prolonged pause due to overdrive suppression of the sinus node and other intrinsic pacemakers. This can result in

**Box 85-3**

***Causes of Acquired Complete Heart Block***

- Cardiac surgery
- Infection
  - Viral myocarditis
  - Bacterial endocarditis with abscess
  - Lyme disease
  - Diphtheria
  - Chagas disease
  - Typhoid
- Inflammatory/autoimmune disease
  - Acute rheumatic fever
  - Reiter syndrome
  - Guillain-Barre syndrome
  - Rheumatoid arthritis
- Neuromuscular/neurodegenerative disease
  - Kearns-Sayre syndrome
  - Myotonic dystrophy
  - Emery-Dreyfus muscular dystrophy
  - Facioscapulohumeral muscular dystrophy
- Tumors in the conduction system
- Trauma
  - Radiation therapy
  - Blunt or penetrating chest trauma
- Pharmacologic
  - Antidysrhythmic drugs
  - Tricyclic antidepressants
  - Digoxin
- Infiltrative disease
  - Amyloidosis
  - Sarcoidosis
  - Lymphoma
  - Tuberous sclerosis

syncope or sudden death. Drugs used to treat the tachydysrhythmia often exacerbate the bradydysrhythmia. Sick sinus syndrome usually results from cardiac surgery such as the atrial switch (Mustard or Senning for transposition of the great arteries) and Fontan procedures, but it can be familial. Drugs to control tachydysrhythmias may worsen sinus node and AV node function, necessitating a pacemaker.[7]

### Ectopic Atrial/Junctional Escape Rhythm

Ectopic atrial rhythms have a normal QRS complex but an abnormal P-wave axis. A negative P wave in lead I indicates that the impulse comes from the left. A negative P wave in lead AVF indicates a low atrial focus. Junctional rhythms have a normal QRS complex, but P waves that follow the QRS and are negative in AVF or are absent (Figure 85-14). Ectopic atrial or junctional rhythm may occur when the sinus node impulse fails. This may occur in normal adolescents, especially with increased vagal tone, or after cardiac surgery. No treatment is needed if the patient is asymptomatic.

**Box 85-4**

***Causes of Sinus Bradycardia***

- Normal adolescents with high vagal tone
  - Athletes
- Neurologic
  - Increased intracranial pressure
- Metabolic
  - Hypothyroidism
  - Hypothermia
  - Hyperkalemia
  - Hypoxia
  - Malnutrition (consider anorexia nervosa)
- Pharmacologic
  - Digoxin
  - Beta blockers
- Cardiac surgery
  - Mustard or Senning procedure for transposition of the great arteries

## FAST RHYTHMS (TACHYDYSRHYTHMIAS)

### Normal QRS

***Sinus Tachycardia*** The characteristics of sinus rhythm, including a normal P-wave axis (positive P wave in leads I, II, and AVF), are present but the rate is faster than the normal rate for age (Figure 85-15). The normal resting heart rate for an adolescent is between 60 and 100 beats per minute,[8] but sinus tachycardia is usually less than 220 beats per minute and varies over time. Sinus tachycardia must be differentiated from supraventricular tachycardia (SVT; Table 85-1). Anxiety, fever, pain, dehydration, shock, anemia, myocardial dysfunction, hyperthyroidism, and catecholamine excess are possible causes of sinus tachycardia (Box 85-5). Treatment is directed to the underlying etiology.

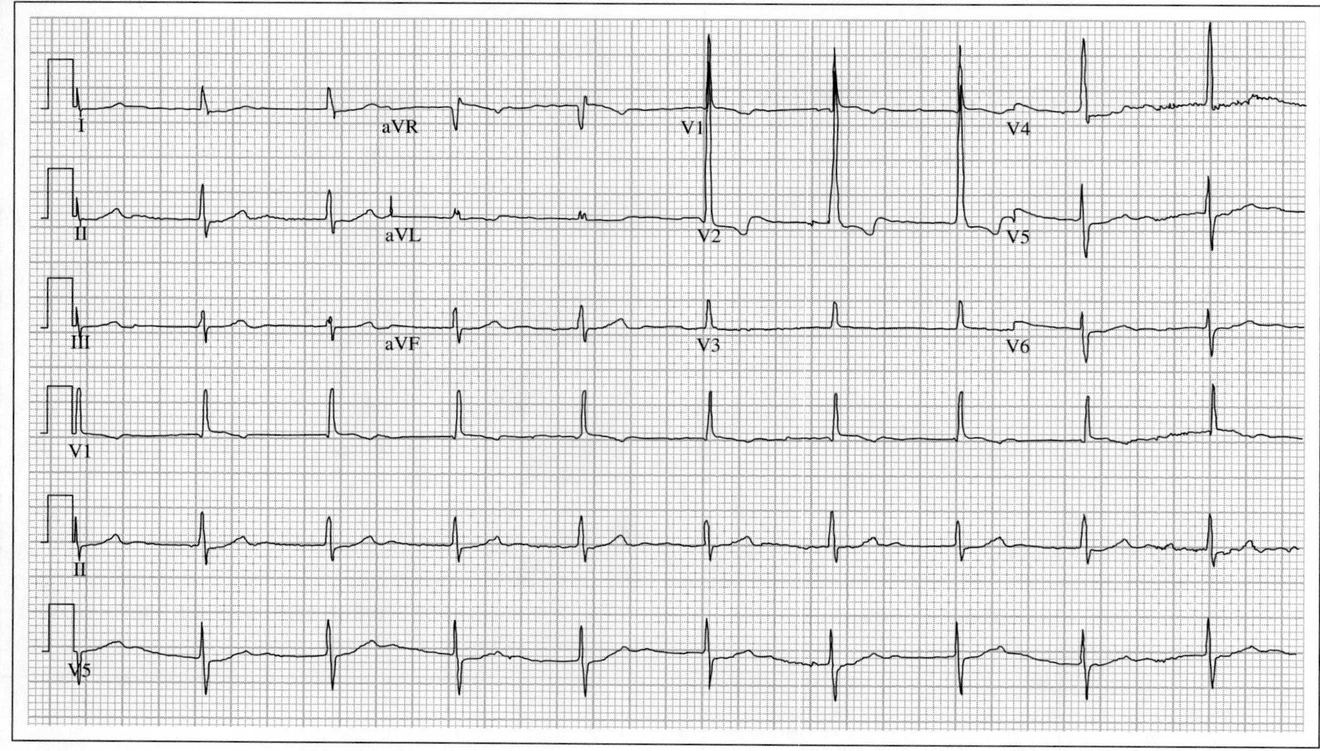


**FIGURE 85-14** ECG of junctional rhythm with absent P waves.

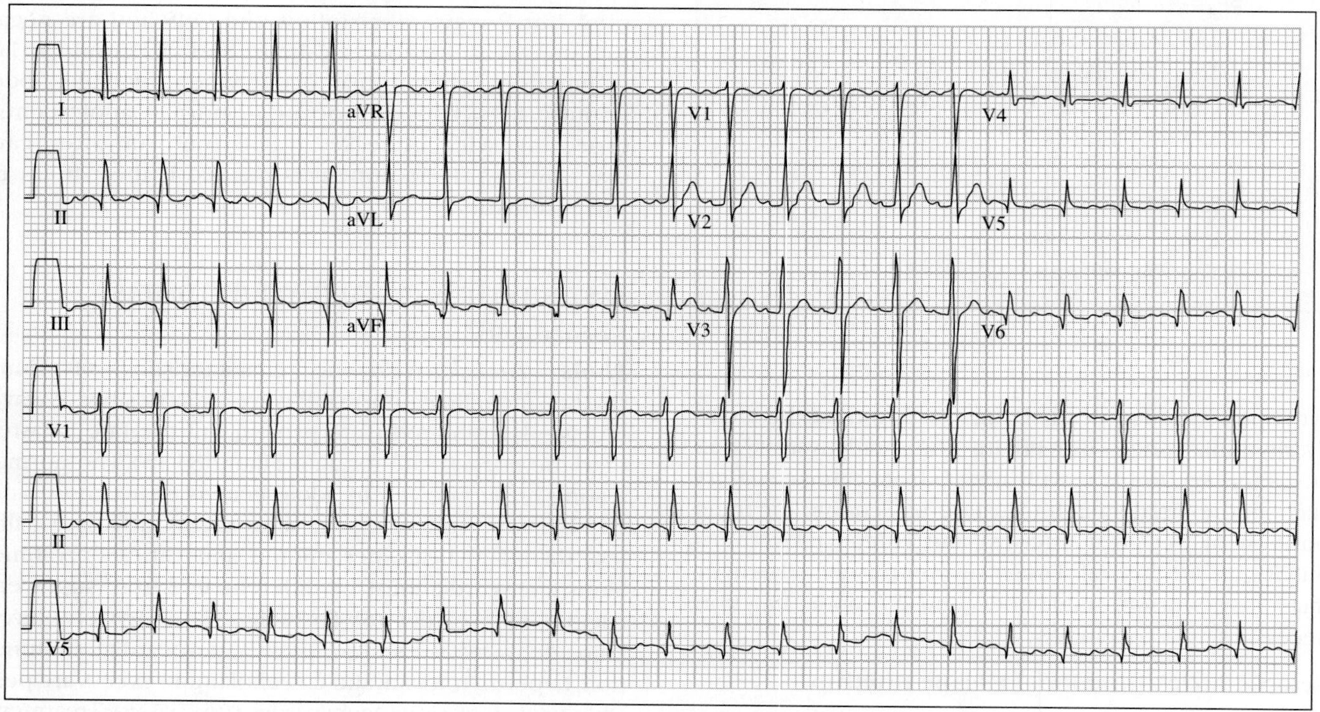


**FIGURE 85-15** ECG of sinus tachycardia in a 16-year-old boy with chest pain.

**Table 85-1**

**ECG Diagnosis of Tachydysrhythmias in the Adolescent**

| | *Sinus Tachycardia* | *SVT* | *Atrial Flutter* | *Atrial Fibrillation* | *VT* |
|---|---|---|---|---|---|
| **Rate Beats/min** | <220 | 180–240 | 250–350 | AR 400–700<br>VR 120–200 | 120–240 |
| **Regularity** | Regular (varies with time) | Regular | Regular ventricular response in multiples | Irregularly irregular | Slightly irregular |
| **QRS** | Normal | Normal 90% (aberrancy) | Normal (aberrancy) | Normal (aberrancy) | Usually wide<br>Fusion beats<br>Capture beats |
| **P** | Visible<br>Normal axis | Visible 50%<br>Abnormal axis | Flutter waves | Fibrillatory waves | Absent<br>Retrograde |
| **P-QRS** | Related | Related<br>Dissociation 3% | Varying or fixed block | Varying block | Dissociation |
| **Vagal/Adenosine** | Gradual change | Abrupt change | ↑ Block | ↑ Block | — |

***Supraventricular Tachycardia*** Supraventricular tachycardias involve the conduction system within or above the bundle of His. They can be grouped into 3 major categories: re-entrant tachycardias, which use an accessory pathway, re-entrant tachycardias without an accessory pathway, and ectopic (automatic) tachycardias. Re-entrant tachycardias are characterized by an abrupt onset and termination, whereas the onset and termination of automatic tachycardias are gradual. In SVT the QRS complex is narrow in more than 90% of cases in the pediatric population. When visible, the P-wave axis is usually abnormal (Table 85-1).

**Box 85-5**

***Causes of Sinus Tachycardia***

- Anxiety
- Pain
- Fever
- Anemia
- Myocardial dysfunction
- Hypovolemia
  - Dehydration
  - Shock
- Metabolic
  - Hyperthyroidism
- Catecholamine excess
  - Pheochromocytoma
  - Catecholamine administration

**Re-Entrant Tachycardia with an Accessory Pathway**. Atrioventricular re-entrant (reciprocating) tachycardia (AVRT) using a bypass tract occurs in 68% of patients over the age of 10 years with SVT.[9] The most common bypass tract is the Kent bundle, a muscular bridge connecting the right atrium to the right ventricle or the left atrium to the left ventricle near the AV valve ring. During sinus rhythm, the impulse is conducted down the AV node as well as down the accessory pathway, resulting in a short PR interval and a delta wave (wide QRS with slow upstroke) from pre-exciting 1 ventricle before the other (WPW syndrome) (Figure 85-16). If the bypass tract conducts only in a retrograde direction, it is called a concealed accessory pathway because the QRS complex will be normal during sinus rhythm. A PAC usually initiates the tachycardia. During *orthodromic* AVRT (Figure 85-17), the impulse from the PAC finds the accessory pathway still refractory and proceeds in an antegrade fashion down the AV node to the ventricles and up the accessory pathway, which has now recovered, to the right or left atrium, producing a narrow QRS complex

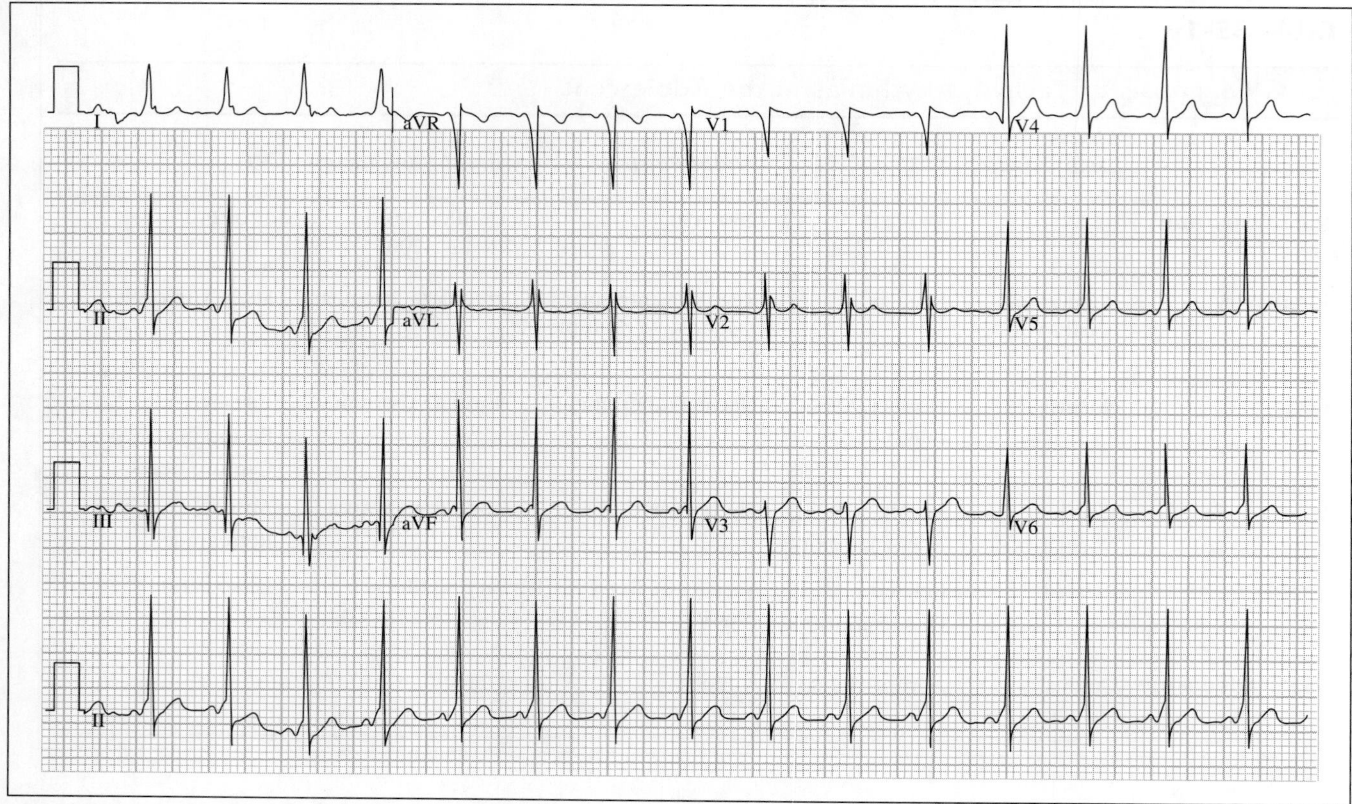


**FIGURE 85-16** ECG demonstrating a short PR interval and delta waves during sinus rhythm (WPW).

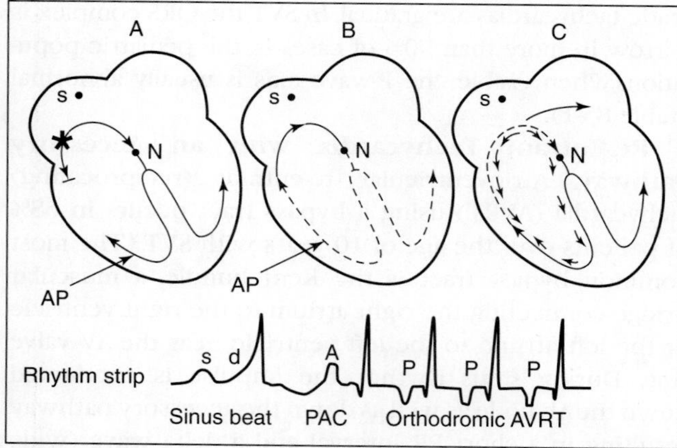


**FIGURE 85-17** Orthodromic AVRT. The ECG shows a sinus beat (S) with a short PR interval and a wide QRS due to a delta wave (d). In A the impulse from a PAC finds the accessory pathway still refractory. In B the impulse proceeds in an antegrade fashion down the AV node (N) to the ventricles, producing a normal PR interval and a normal QRS complex, and then retrogradely up the accessory pathway, which has now recovered, to the atrium, producing a negative P wave following the QRS. In C the sequence repeats itself establishing orthodromic AVRT. (Reproduced with permission from Dubin AM. Supraventricular tachycardia in children: AV reentrant tachycardia (including WPW) and AV nodal reentrant tachycardia. In: UpToDate, Basow DS (ed), UpToDate, Waltham, MA 2010. Copyright (c) 2010 UpToDate, Inc. For more information visit www.uptodate.com.)

and a negative P wave following the QRS in lead AVF (Figure 85-18). In the much less common *antidromic* AVRT (Figure 85-19), the impulse finds the AV node refractory and proceeds down the bypass tract to the right or left ventricle producing a wide QRS complex, and then travels in a retrograde direction up the now recovered AV node to the atria, again resulting in a negative P wave following the QRS complex in lead AVF (see the following).

Patients with WPW have a risk of syncope and sudden death, especially those with antidromic AVRT with a short refractory period of the bypass tract, which can lead to ventricular fibrillation especially if atrial flutter or atrial fibrillation occurs. The Wolfe-Parkinson-White syndrome can occur in adolescents with a normal heart or with a congenital heart defect such as Ebstein anomaly. As opposed to infants, WPW in adolescents is very unlikely to resolve spontaneously. A small percentage of cases of WPW are caused by mutations in the *PRKAG2* gene. This familial form is usually inherited as an autosomal-dominant trait.[10] A form of WPW associated with familial hypertrophic cardiomyopathy may be due to mutations in the *PRKAG2* gene or in the *LAMP2* gene, which is responsible for glycogen storage disease IIb (Danon disease).

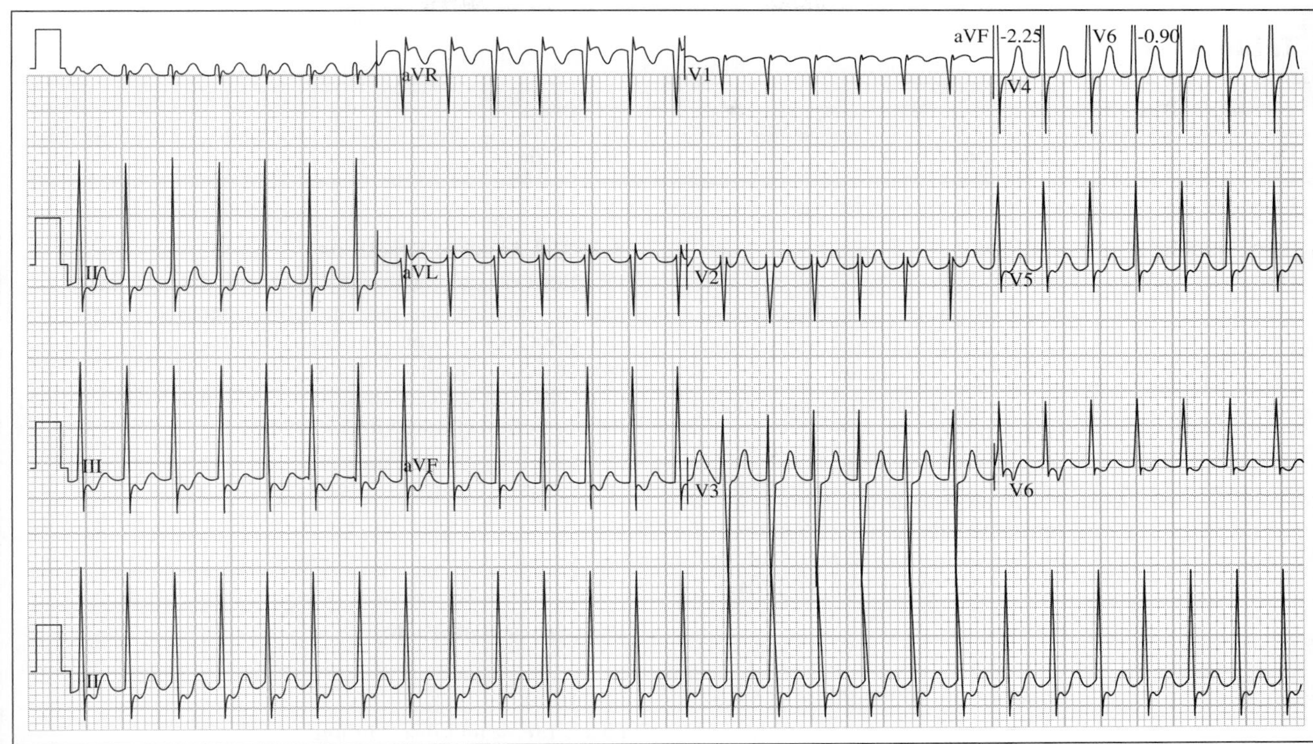


**FIGURE 85-18** ECG of orthodromic AVRT.

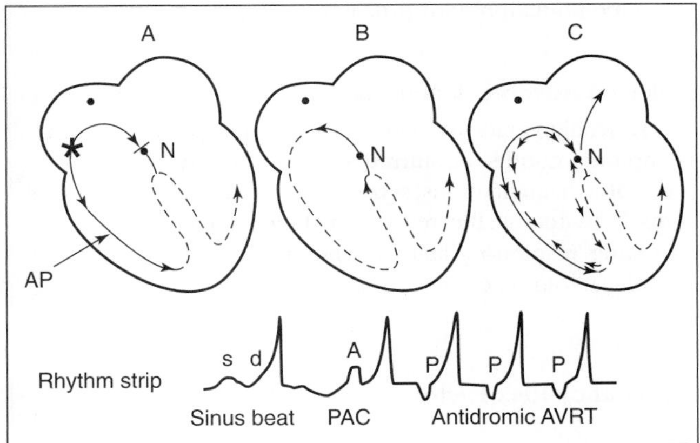


**FIGURE 85-19** Antidromic AVRT. The ECG shows a sinus beat (S) with a short PR interval and a wide QRS due to a delta wave (d). In A the impulse from a PAC finds the AV node (N) still refractory. In B the impulse proceeds down the accessory pathway, which has a short refractory period, to the ventricles, producing a wide QRS similar to the pre-excited sinus beat, and then retrogradely up the now recovered AV node to the atrium, producing a negative P wave following the QRS. In C the sequence repeats itself, establishing antidromic AVRT. (Reproduced with permission from Dubin AM. Supraventricular tachycardia in children: AV reentrant tachycardia (including WPW) and AV nodal reentrant tachycardia. In: UpToDate, Basow DS (ed), UpToDate, Waltham, MA 2010. Copyright (c) 2010 UpToDate, Inc. For more information visit www.uptodate.com.)

Acute treatment of SVT depends on the hemodynamic status of the patient.[11] If the patient is unstable without an IV, DC cardioversion at 0.5 to 1 J/kg should be performed. If ineffective the dose should be increased to 2 J/kg. Adenosine (Table 85-2) may be given to unstable patients with an IV if immediately available. Adenosine should be used with caution in patients with sinus node dysfunction because it can cause bradycardia or asystole, and in patients with asthma because it can cause bronchospasm. In addition it can precipitate atrial fibrillation, which can degenerate into ventricular fibrillation in a patient with WPW. Amiodarone or procainamide (not routinely administered together) (see Table 85-2) are used after unsuccessful cardioversion and adenosine. Digoxin and verapamil (see Table 85-2) should be avoided in a patient with suspected WPW because these drugs can potentiate conduction down the accessory pathway and precipitate ventricular fibrillation. Contributing factors (eg, hypovolemia, hypoxia, acidosis, hypokalemia, hyperkalemia, toxins) must be treated. Stable patients can be treated with adenosine and/or vagal maneuvers (eg, bearing down for 15 to 20 seconds, headstand, immersing the face in ice water).

Chronic therapy may be expectant; that is, after the first episode of SVT without ventricular dysfunction or hemodynamic instability, no antidysrhythmic agent is

**Table 85-2**

**Antidysrhythmic Agents Commonly Used in Adolescents[20-25]**

| *Drug* | *Dose and Route* | *Side Effects* |
|---|---|---|
| **Class IA** | | |
| Procainamide | **Children**:<br>IV:<br>*Loading:* 10–15 mg/kg slowly over 30–60 minutes, stop if hypotension or QRS >50% of baseline<br>*Maintenance:* 20–80 μg/kg/minute (maximum 2 g/day)<br>PO:<br>15–50 mg/kg/day, q 3–6 hours for immediate release, q 6 hours for "SR" form, or q 12 hours for "Procanbid"(maximum 4.0 g/day) | **Selected Adverse Reactions**<br>PR, QRS, QT prolongation, hypotension, dysrhythmias, nausea, vomiting, anorexia, rash, fever, agranulocytosis, thrombocytopenia, neutropenia, Coombs-positive hemolytic anemia, lupus-like syndrome, confusion, disorientation, exacerbation of periodic paralysis, hepatomegaly, elevated liver enzymes |
| | **Adults:**<br>IV:<br>*Loading:* 50–100 mg/dose, q 5–10 minutes PRN<br>*Maintenance:* 1–6 mg/minute by IV infusion<br>PO:<br>250–500 mg/dose immediate release, q 3–6 hours (usual dose 2–4 g/day) | **Pregnancy Risk Factor**<br>C<br>**Lactation**<br>Enters breast milk/use caution<br>AAP rates "compatible"<br>**Selected Drug Interactions**<br>*Antipsychotic Drugs*<br>Pimozide, thioridazine, ziprasidone-prolonged QTc—avoid combination with procainamide |
| **Class IB** | | |
| Lidocaine | **Children:**<br>IV:<br>*Loading:* 1 mg/kg bolus (maximum 100 mg/dose), second bolus of 0.5–1 mg/kg if >15 minutes delay before start of infusion<br>*Maintenance:* 20–50 μg/kg/minute (low dose with shock, hepatic disease, cardiac arrest, CHF) | **Selected Adverse Reactions**<br>Asystole, high-grade AV block, dysrhythmias, CNS symptoms, confusion, slurred speech, lethargy, anxiety, euphoria, hallucinations, seizures, coma, paresthesias, muscle twitching, blurred vision, diplopia, nausea, vomiting, respiratory failure, hypotension, rarely anaphylactoid reactions |
| | **Adults:**<br>IV:<br>*Loading:* 1–1.5 mg/kg/dose, repeat 0.5–0.75 mg/kg/dose q 5–10 minutes PRN to total of 3 mg/kg<br>*Maintenance:* 1–4 mg/minute | **Pregnancy Risk Factor**<br>B<br>**Lactation**<br>Enters breast milk (small amounts)/use caution<br>AAP rates "compatible" |
| Mexiletine | **Children:**<br>PO:<br>5–15 mg/kg/day, q 8 hours | **Selected Adverse Reactions**<br>Bradycardia, syncope, hypotension, dysrhythmias, nausea, vomiting, diarrhea, headache, dizziness, confusion, ataxia, paresthesias, tremor, rash, diplopia, tinnitus, dyspnea, hepatitis, elevated liver enzymes, positive ANA, and rarely thrombocytopenia, leukopenia, agranulocytosis |

*(Continued)*

**Table 85-2 (Continued)**

| *Drug* | *Dose and Route* | *Side Effects* |
|---|---|---|
| | **Adults:**<br>PO:<br>200 mg q 8 hours for 2–3 days, increase every 2–3 days to 300–400 mg q 8 hours (usual dose 200–300 mg q 8 hours) (maximum dose 1.2 g/day) | **Pregnancy Risk Factor**<br>C<br>**Lactation**<br>Enters breast milk/compatible<br>**Selected Drug Interactions**<br>*Selective Serotonin Reuptake Inhibitors*<br>May decrease the metabolism of mexiletine (Exception: sertraline) |
| **Class 1C** | | |
| Flecainide | **Children:**<br>PO:<br>Initial 1–3 mg/kg/day q 8 hours or q 12 hours; usual 3–6 mg/kg/day, q 8 hours or q 12 hours<br>**Adults**:100–400 mg/day, q 12 hours | **Selected Adverse Reactions**<br>Dysrhythmias, conduction disturbance, CHF, edema, dizziness, blurred vision, headache, fatigue, hypoesthesia, nervousness, paresthesia, tremor, rash, nausea, blood dyscrasias, hepatic dysfunction, dyspnea<br>**Pregnancy Risk Factor**<br>C<br>**Lactation**<br>Enters breast milk/compatible<br>**Selected Drug Interactions**<br>*Antipsychotic Drugs*<br>Pimozide, thioridazine, ziprasidone-prolonged QTc—avoid combination with flecainide |
| **Class II** | | |
| Propranolol | **Children:**<br>IV:<br>0.01–0.1 mg/kg/dose over 10 minutes (maximum 1 mg/dose in infants, 3 mg/dose in children)<br>PO:<br>1–4 mg/kg/day, q 6 hours<br>**Adults:**<br>IV:<br>1 mg/dose q 5 minutes (maximum 5 mg)<br>PO:<br>40–320 mg/day, q 6 hours or q 8 hours | **Selected Adverse Reactions**<br>Bradycardia, heart block, congestive heart failure, bronchospasm, hypoglycemia, hypotension, lethargy, weakness, depression, hypoglycemia, hyperglycemia, hyperkalemia, agranulocytosis, cold extremities, elevated liver enzymes<br>**Pregnancy Risk Factor**<br>C<br>**Lactation**<br>Enters breast milk/use caution<br>AAP rates "compatible"<br>**Selected Drug Interactions**<br>*Psychoactive Drugs*<br>Phenothiazines—may enhance the hypotensive effect and decrease the metabolism of beta blockers; beta blockers may decrease the metabolism of phenothiazines<br>Selective Serotonin Reuptake Inhibitors—may enhance the bradycardic effect of beta blockers<br>Exception: Fluvoxamine—may increase the serum concentration of propranolol<br>MAO Inhibitors—may enhance orthostatic effect |

*(Continued)*

**Table 85-2 (Continued)**

| *Drug* | *Dose and Route* | *Side Effects* |
|---|---|---|
| | | Methylphenidate—may diminish the antihypertensive effect<br>Reserpine—may enhance the hypotensive effect<br>Zolmitriptan—propranolol may increase the serum concentration |
| Atenolol | **Children:**<br>PO:<br>Initial 1 mg/kg/day, q 12 hours–q 24 hours, maximum 2 mg/kg/day<br>**Adults:**<br>PO:<br>25–50 mg daily for 1–2 weeks, may increase to 100 mg daily | **Selected Adverse Reactions**<br>Bradycardia, A-V block, CHF, chest pain, edema, Raynaud phenomenon, headache, nightmares, insomnia, depression, lethargy, postural hypotension, nausea, vomiting, diarrhea, constipation, rash, agranulocytosis, purpura, wheezing, dyspnea<br>**Pregnancy Risk Factor**<br>D<br>**Lactation**<br>Enters breast milk/use caution<br>**Selected Drug Interactions**<br>*Psychoactive drugs*<br>MAO Inhibitors—may enhance orthostatic effect<br>Methylphenidate—may diminish antihypertensive effect<br>Reserpine—may enhance hypotensive effect |
| Metoprolol | **Children:**<br>PO:<br>Initial 1–2 mg/kg/day, q 12 hours (nonsustained release), (maximum 6 mg/kg/day, ≤ 200 mg/day)<br>**Adults:**<br>PO:<br>100 mg/day, q 8 hours, q 12 hours, or q 24 hours initially, may increase to 450 mg/day, q 8 hours, or q 12 hours (usual dose 100–450 mg/day) | **Selected Adverse Reactions**<br>Bradycardia, hypotension, CHF, heart block, dizziness, depression, lethargy, bronchospasm, diarrhea, nausea, vomiting, abdominal pain, hepatic dysfunction, worsening of psoriasis, agranulocytosis, thrombocytopenia<br>**Pregnancy Risk Factor**<br>C (D if used in second or third trimester)<br>**Lactation**<br>Enters breast milk/use caution<br>AAP rates "compatible"<br>**Selected Drug Interactions**<br>*Psychoactive Drugs*<br>Phenothiazines—may enhance the hypotensive effect and decrease the metabolism of beta blockers; beta blockers may decrease the metabolism of phenothiazines<br>Selective Serotonin Reuptake Inhibitors—may enhance the bradycardic effect of beta blockers<br>Exception: Fluvoxamine<br>MAO Inhibitors—may enhance orthostatic effect<br>Methylphenidate—may diminish the antihypertensive effect<br>Reserpine—may enhance the hypotensive effect |

(*Continued*)

**Table 85-2 (Continued)**

| *Drug* | *Dose and Route* | *Side Effects* |
|---|---|---|
| Nadolol | **Children:**<br>PO:<br>Initial 0.5–1 mg/kg/day, q 12 hours or q 24 hours (maximum 2.5 mg/kg/day)<br>**Adults:**<br>PO:<br>Initial 40 mg q 24 hours; 40–80 mg q 24 hours, usual maintenance dose (maximum daily dose 640 mg) | **Selected Adverse Reactions**<br>Bradycardia, CHF, orthostatic hypotension, edema, lethargy, depression, bronchospasm, rash, Raynaud's phenomenon, GI discomfort<br>**Pregnancy Risk Factor**<br>C<br>**Lactation**<br>Enters breast milk/use caution<br>AAP rates "compatible"<br>**Selected Drug Interactions**<br>*Psychoactive drugs*<br>MAO Inhibitors—may enhance orthostatic effect<br>Methylphenidate—may diminish antihypertensive effect<br>Reserpine—may enhance hypotensive effect |
| **Class III** | | |
| Amiodarone | **Children:**<br>PO:<br>*Loading:* 10 mg/kg/day, q 12 hours for 5–14 days<br>*Maintenance:* 5 mg/kg/day, q 24 hours for several weeks<br>If effective, may reduce to 2.5 mg/kg for 5 of 7 days/week<br>IV/IO for pulseless VT or VF:<br>5 mg/kg (maximum 300 mg/dose) rapid IV bolus or IO, may repeat to a maximum total dose of 15 mg/kg/day (maximum daily dose in adolescents 2.2 g)<br>IV for perfusing tachycardia:<br>*Loading:* 5 mg/kg (maximum 300 mg/dose) over 20–60 minutes, may repeat to maximum total of 15 mg/kg/day<br>*Maintenance:* 10–15 mg/kg/day (7 μg/kg/minute) (maximum daily dose in adolescents 2.2 g) | **Selected Adverse Reactions**<br>Dysrhythmias, prolonged QT, hypotension, CHF, hypothyroidism or hyperthyroidism, hepatotoxicity, corneal microdeposits, slate blue skin, rash, angioedema, photosensitivity, pulmonary fibrosis, bronchospasm, hemoptysis, elevated triglycerides, hyperglycemia, anorexia, lack of coordination, fatigue, dizziness, headache, insomnia, nightmares, fever, behavioral changes, paresthesia, tremor, rhabdomyolysis, parkinsonian symptoms, coagulopathy, pancytopenia, hemolytic anemia, aplastic anemia, visual impairment, renal impairment |
| | **Adults:**<br>PO for ventricular dysrhythmias:<br>*Loading*: 800–1,600 mg/day for 2 weeks, then 600–800 mg/day for 1 month<br>*Maintenance:* 400 mg/day<br>IV/IO for pulseless VT or VF:<br>300 mg (in 20–30 ml $D_5W$ or NS);<br>1 supplemental dose of 150 mg for recurring VF or pulseless VT<br>IV for perfusing tachycardia:<br>150 mg over 10 minutes, may repeat to a maximum of 2.2 g/24 hours | **Pregnancy Risk Factor**<br>D<br>Lactation<br>Enters breast milk/not recommended<br>AAP rates "of concern"<br>**Selected Drug Interactions**<br>*Antipsychotic Drugs*<br>Pimozide, thioridazine, ziprasidone-prolonged QTc—avoid combination with amiodarone |

(*Continued*)

**Table 85-2 (Continued)**

| *Drug* | *Dose and Route* | *Side Effects* |
|---|---|---|
| Sotalol | **Children:**<br>PO:<br>90–180 mg/m$^2$/day, q 8 hours (maximum 160 mg/day) or 2–8 mg/kg/day, q 12 hours; 3 days between dosage increments | **Selected Adverse Reactions**<br>Dysrhythmias, prolonged QT, torsade de pointes, bradycardia, fatigue, dyspnea, orthostatic hypotension, congestive heart failure |
| | **Adults:**<br>PO for ventricular dysrhythmias:<br>80 mg once or twice daily as initial dose to 240–320 mg/day, q 12 hours (maximum total daily dose 480–640 mg for life-threatening refractory ventricular dysrhythmias) | **Pregnancy Risk Factor**<br>B<br>**Lactation**<br>Enters breast milk/use caution<br>AAP rates "compatible"<br>**Selected Drug Interactions**<br>*Psychoactive Drugs*<br>Phenothiazines—may enhance the hypotensive effect and decrease the metabolism of beta blockers; beta blockers may decrease the metabolism of phenothiazines<br>Selective Serotonin Reuptake Inhibitors—may enhance the bradycardic effect of beta blockers<br>Exception: Fluvoxamine<br>MAO Inhibitors—may enhance orthostatic effect<br>Methylphenidate—may diminish the antihypertensive effect<br>Reserpine—may enhance the hypotensive effect<br>Pimozide, thioridazine, ziprasidone-prolonged QTc—avoid combination with sotalol |
| **Class IV** | | |
| Verapamil | **Children:**<br>PO:<br>4–8 mg/kg/day, q 8 hours for standard form or q 24 hours for sustained or extended release form<br>IV:<br>0.1 mg/kg over 2 minutes, may repeat once in 30 minutes (single maximum dose 5 mg) | **Selected Adverse Reactions**<br>Bradycardia, asystole, high-grade AV block, hypotension, congestive heart failure, seizures (IV), constipation, nausea, fatigue, dizziness, headache, elevated hepatic enzymes |
| | **Adults:**<br>PO:<br>240–480 mg/day, q 8 hours for standard form or q 24 hours for sustained or extended release form<br>IV:<br>2.5–5 mg over 2 minutes; if no response in 15–30 minutes, 5–10 mg every 15–30 minutes to maximum total dose of 20 mg | **Pregnancy Risk Factor**<br>C<br>**Lactation**<br>Enters breast milk (small amounts)/not recommended<br>**Selected Drug Interactions**<br>*Psychoactive Drugs*<br>Benzodiazepines (metabolized by oxidation)—metabolism may be decreased by calcium channel blockers (nondihydropyridine)<br>Buspirone—metabolism may be decreased by calcium channel blockers (nondihydropyridine) |

(*Continued*)

**Table 85-2 (Continued)**

| *Drug* | *Dose and Route* | *Side Effects* |
|---|---|---|
| | | Lithium—the neurotoxic effect and the serum concentration may be increased by calcium channel blockers (nondihydropyridine); decreased or unaltered lithium concentrations have also been reported<br>MAO Inhibitors—may enhance hypotensive and orthostatic effects<br>Methylphenidate—may decrease antihypertensive effect<br>Resperidone—the serum concentration may be increased by verapamil |
| **Miscellaneous** | | **Selected Adverse Reactions** |
| Adenosine | **Children**:<br>IV/IO:<br>0.1 mg/kg (maximum 6 mg) rapid bolus with rapid saline flush; if not effective within 1–2 minutes, 0.2 mg/kg (maximum 12 mg) | Transient bradycardia, asystole, and tachycardia (including atrial fibrillation), transient AV block, chest pain, dyspnea, facial flushing, bronchospasm in asthmatics, headache, light-headedness, nausea, metallic taste |
| | **Adults and Adolescents ≥50 kg:**<br>IV:<br>6 mg rapid bolus, may repeat twice in 1–2 minute intervals using 12 mg bolus | **Pregnancy Risk Factor**<br>C<br>**Lactation**<br>Excretion in breast milk unknown |
| Digoxin | **Children (>10 years):**<br>PO:<br>*Total digitalizing dose:* 10–15 μg/kg, ½ total dose followed by ¼ total dose q 8–12 hours x 2<br>*Maintenance:* 2.5–5 μg/kg/day, q 24 hours<br>IV:<br>75% of PO dose | **Selected Adverse Reactions**<br>Bradycardia, AV block, PACs, PVCs, nausea, vomiting, anorexia, visual changes, headache, drowsiness, fatigue, lethargy, vertigo, disorientation |
| | **Adults:**<br>PO:<br>*Total digitalizing dose:* 0.75–1.5 mg<br>*Maintenance:* 0.125–0.5 mg/day | **Pregnancy Risk Factor**<br>C<br>**Lactation**<br>Enters breast milk (small amounts)/compatible<br>**Selected Drug Interactions**<br>*Psychoactive Drugs*<br>Milnacipran—may enhance the adverse/toxic effect of digoxin (especially IV), including postural hypotension and tachycardia<br>St John's wort—may decrease the serum concentration of cardiac glycosides |

AAP, American Academy of Pediatrics; ANA, antinuclear antibody; AV, atrioventricular block; CHF, congestive heart failure; CNS, central nervous system; GI, gastrointestinal; IO, intraosseous; IV, intravenous; MAO, monamine oxidase; PO, per os (by mouth), PRN, *pro re nata* (as needed); PVCs, premature ventricular contractions; SR, sustained release; VF, ventricular fibrillation; VT, ventricular tachycardia

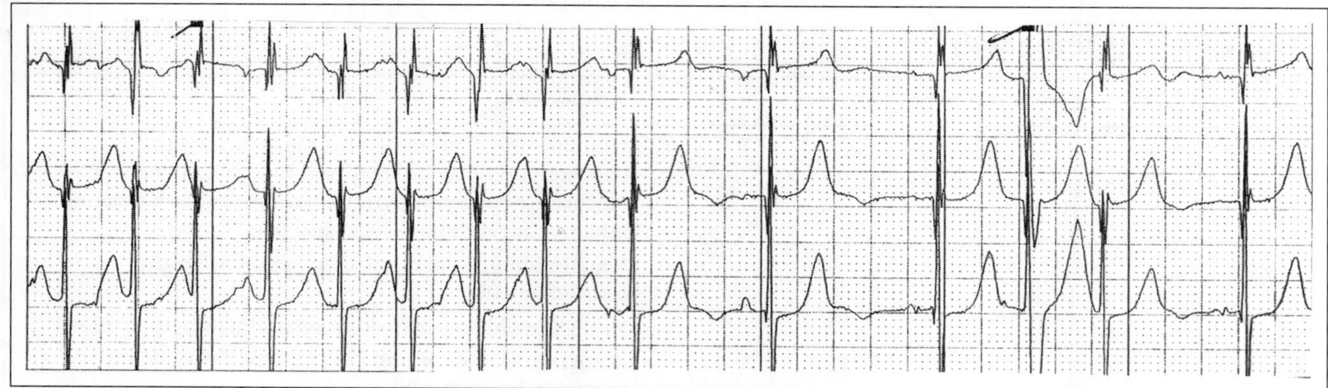

**FIGURE 85-20** ECG of multifocal atrial tachycardia.

started and the patient and parents are taught vagal maneuvers. If the episodes are frequent or produce symptoms, a long-acting beta blocker, such as atenolol or nadolol (see Table 85-2), is started. In the adolescent, the family and patient can be given the option of catheter ablation (radiofrequency ablation, cryoablation) to achieve a potential "cure." Drugs that have been effective alone or in combination include flecainide (used only in patients with a normal heart), sotalol, and amiodarone (see Table 85-2). These drugs must be started in a hospital with monitoring because of proarrhythmia. Management of the asymptomatic adolescent with WPW remains unclear.

**Re-Entrant Tachycardia without an Accessory Pathway.** Atrioventricular block node re-entrant (reciprocating) tachycardia occurs in 20% of patients with SVT over the age of 10 years, making it the second most common type in adolescents.[9] It uses dual AV nodal pathways as the re-entrant circuit. The substrate for AVNRT is much more likely to be present in adolescents than in infants or children. In the typical form, the impulse goes down the slow pathway and up the fast pathway producing a narrow QRS tachycardia with a P wave that is often invisible because it is superimposed on the QRS. During the tachycardia, palpitations are sometimes felt in the neck because of atrial contraction against a closed AV valve. In the atypical form, the impulse proceeds down the fast pathway and up the slow pathway resulting in a narrow complex tachycardia with a retrograde P wave that is negative in lead AVF and with an RP interval < 70 msec), which is shorter than with WPW. Adolescents with AVNRT may have syncope, and rarely, may have tachycardia-induced cardiomyopathy when the AVNRT is incessant. Acute therapy is similar to that for re-entrant tachycardia with an accessory pathway. It is usually amenable to digoxin, a beta blocker, or catheter ablation.

**Ectopic (Automatic) Tachycardias.** Ectopic tachycardias may be due to abnormal automaticity or triggered activity resulting from early or late afterdepolarizations. They do not respond to electrical cardioversion or adenosine.

Atrial ectopic tachycardia (AET) has a single abnormal automatic focus usually in the right atrium that produces a narrow complex tachycardia with a P wave with an abnormal axis, unless the abnormal focus is near the sinus node. Unlike re-entrant SVTs, the rate varies during the course of a day and the tachycardia has a gradual onset and termination. Atrial ectopic tachycardia can cause severe myocardial dysfunction. Patients with tachycardia-induced cardiomyopathy have been sent for cardiac transplantation with the misdiagnosis of a primary cardiomyopathy with resultant sinus tachycardia. With treatment of the AET, cardiac function improves and the cardiomyopathy may resolve. Because of the typical sensitivity of AET to adrenergic stimulation, a beta blocker may be an important part of therapy. Although many drugs have been used alone or in combination with varying success, amiodarone appears to be the most effective. If drug treatment is unsuccessful, catheter ablation should be considered because it has a greater than 90% success rate.

Junctional ectopic tachycardia (JET) is an automatic dysrhythmia characterized by a narrow complex tachycardia usually with AV dissociation with the sinus P waves marching through at a slower rate. It is most commonly seen in patients after cardiac surgery and is self-limited, but must often be treated with cooling, catecholamine reduction, and amiodarone.

Chaotic (multifocal) atrial tachycardia is rare in adolescents and usually occurs in very young children or in adults with hypoxic pulmonary disease. It is characterized by 3 or more abnormal P waves with 3 or more varying P-P intervals, frequent blocked P waves, and varying PR intervals of conducted beats (Figure 85-20). Pharmacologic therapy has included flecainide alone or in combination with digoxin or amiodarone. Catheter ablation is usually not possible.

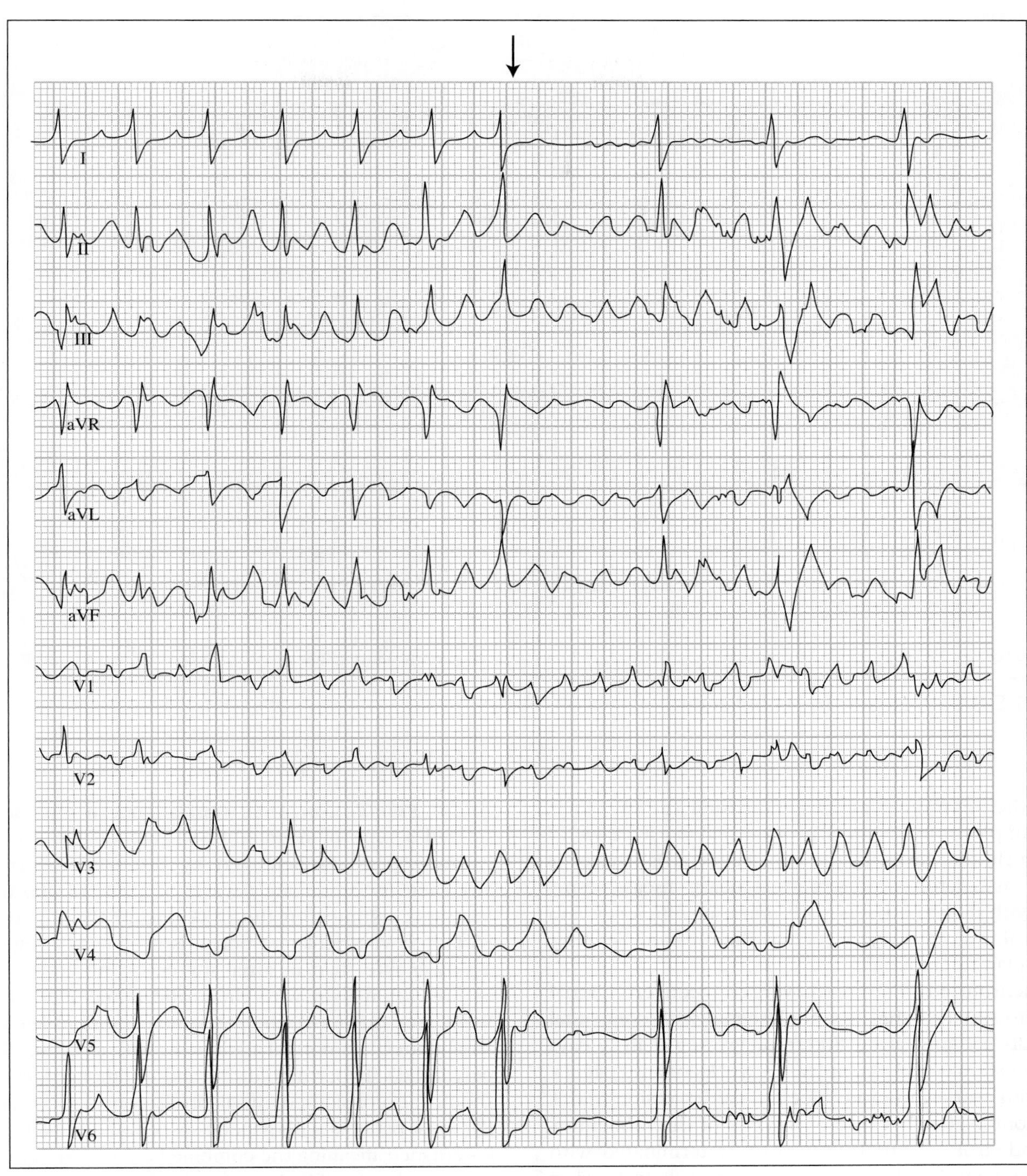


**FIGURE 85-21** ECG of atrial flutter initially with 2:1 AV block. AV block increased after adenosine was given (↓), but the rhythm did not convert to sinus.

***Atrial Flutter/Intra-Atrial Re-Entrant Tachycardia***
Atrial flutter and intra-atrial re-entrant tachycardia (IART) can be considered types of re-entrant SVT without an accessory pathway (Table 85-1). Typical atrial flutter is characterized by "sawtooth" flutter waves on the ECG at an atrial rate of about 300 beats per minute in the adolescent, usually with AV block (eg, 2:1, 3:1, 4:1), which can be variable, producing a regularly irregular rhythm, or fixed, resulting in a regular rhythm (Figure 85-21). Intra-atrial re-entrant tachycardia usually has more discrete P waves and a slower rate. The QRS complex is normal. A vagal maneuver or adenosine temporarily

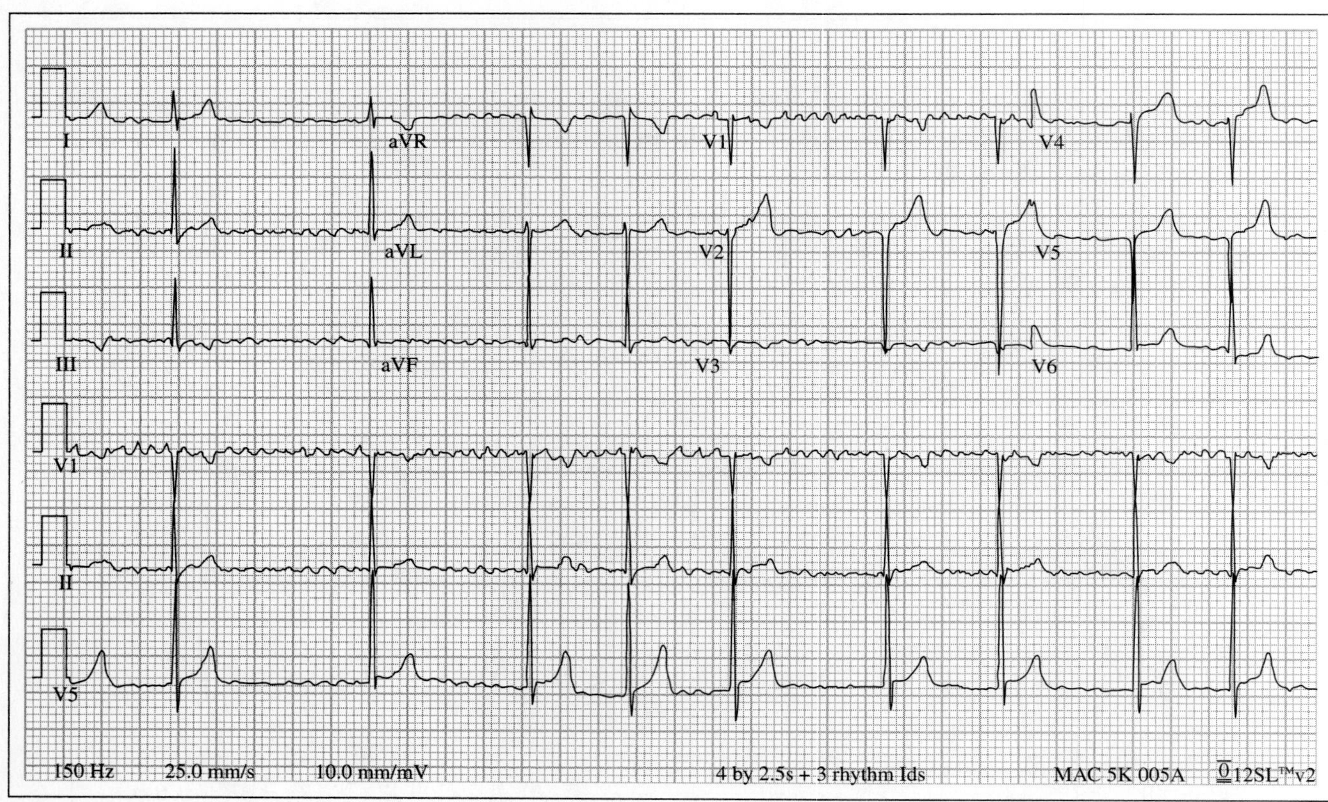


**FIGURE 85-22** ECG of atrial fibrillation.

slows the ventricular rate by increasing the AV block, for example from 2:1 to 3:1, often making it easier to discern flutter waves. In the adolescent, atrial flutter is usually associated with structural heart disease, especially with dilated atria as with mitral insufficiency, and occurs after atrial surgery such as the Mustard, Senning, and Fontan operations.

Synchronized DC cardioversion converts atrial flutter to sinus rhythm, but adolescents with congenital heart disease and atrial flutter of greater than 2 days duration should undergo at least 3 weeks of anticoagulation with warfarin before elective cardioversion and 1 to 2 months after because of the risk of thromboembolism and stroke.[12] Atrial flutter can be terminated with transesophageal atrial pacing or drugs. A beta blocker, calcium channel blocker, or digoxin is given for rate control. Procainamide or amiodarone can be used for conversion. When WPW is present, adenosine, calcium channel blockers, and digoxin must not be given.

Chronic therapy includes digoxin, diltiazem, or a beta blocker with a class IA drug such as procainamide, or a class III drug such as amiodarone or sotalol. Nonpharmacologic therapies include catheter ablation, antitachycardia pacing, and/or surgical revision.

***Atrial Fibrillation*** Atrial fibrillation can also be considered a type of re-entrant SVT without an accessory pathway. It is characterized by disorganized, irregular atrial activity producing *f* waves at a rate of 400 to 700 beats per minutes on the ECG (Figure 85-22 and Table 85-1). The ventricular response is irregularly irregular at a slower rate than in atrial flutter. In the adolescent it is most often seen with rheumatic mitral valve disease, WPW (see previous), and the same conditions seen with atrial flutter. In a normal adolescent with atrial fibrillation, pericarditis, hyperthyroidism, and pulmonary embolus should be considered. Atrial fibrillation can be familial. For most patients with genetic suscept ibility, polygenetic inheritance, meaning the combined effect of a number of genes, is responsible. However, autosomal-dominant and autosomal-recessive forms of monogenic inheritance have been identified for atrial fibrillation.[13] Vagal maneuvers or adenosine will not convert atrial fibrillation but will temporarily slow the ventricular response by increasing AV block. The same recommendations regarding anticoagulation before and after cardioversion, whether electrical or medical, hold for atrial fibrillation as well as atrial flutter. Medical therapy is similar; again when WPW is present, adenosine, calcium channel blockers, and digoxin must not be given. Catheter ablation is much less feasible for atrial fibrillation. Ablation and its surgical counterpart, the maze procedure, entail considerable morbidity.

### Wide QRS

The differential diagnosis of a tachycardia with a wide QRS complex includes VT SVT conducted aberrantly due to fixed (eg, after cardiac surgery) or rate-related bundle branch block, and pre-excited SVT.[14] Nevertheless, a wide complex tachycardia, even in a hemodynamically stable patient, should be considered VT and treated as such until proven otherwise.

***Ventricular Tachycardia*** Ventricular tachycardia is defined as 3 or more consecutive ventricular beats at a rate greater than 120 beats per minute. It must be distinguished from the benign accelerated idioventricular rhythm (AIVR), which has all the characteristics of VT but with a rate approximately the same (within 10%) as the current sinus rate and less than 120 beats per minute. Differentiating VT from SVT with aberrant conduction or pre-excited SVT (see the following) may be difficult, but the presence of AV dissociation practically makes the diagnosis of VT (see Table 85-1), although P waves may be absent or retrograde (negative in leads II, III, AVF) in VT or SVT. The presence of fusion beats or capture beats also points to VT. A fusion beat is a QRS that results from a normally conducted impulse and an ectopic ventricular impulse, and resembles both. A capture beat is a normal QRS that occurs during the wide complex tachycardia resulting from a normally conducted sinus impulse.

The QRS in VT is different from the QRS in sinus rhythm, and in adolescents it is usually wide (>0.09 second). If the QRS morphology is unchanging, the VT is termed *monomorphic* (Figure 85-23). The morphology can be a complete left bundle branch block pattern or a complete right bundle branch block pattern.[15] If the QRS complexes vary, the VT is termed *polymorphic*. *Torsade de pointes* ("twisting of points") is characterized by progressive changes in the shape and axis of the QRS complex.[16] It can self-terminate or degenerate into ventricular fibrillation. It is associated with congenital[17] or acquired long QT syndrome.[18] Catecholaminergic polymorphic VT is usually familial and occurs in the setting of physical activity or acute emotion with a normal resting ECG. In bidirectional VT, there is beat-to-beat alternating of the QRS axis. It is usually associated with hyperkalemic or hypokalemic periodic paralysis, digitalis toxicity, and catecholamine sensitivity (exercise-associated). All types of polymorphic VT are associated with significant risk of syncope and sudden death.

Ventricular tachycardia (as well as other tachydysrhythmias) may be *sustained*, lasting greater than 30 seconds, or *nonsustained*. A tachydysrhythmia is *incessant* if it lasts more than 10% of the day.[19] Incessant VT can be associated with tachycardia-induced cardiomyopathy.

Ventricular tachycardia is often associated with unoperated and postoperative congenital heart disease (eg, tetralogy of Fallot), cardiomyopathies (eg, dilated, hypertrophic, arrhythmogenic right ventricular dysplasia), myocardial tumors, metabolic abnormalities (eg, hypoxia, acidosis, hyperkalemia, hypokalemia), drug toxicity (eg, catecholamine infusion, digitalis, antidysrhythmic agents, cocaine), and channelopathies (eg, long QT syndrome, Brugada syndrome) (Box 85-2). However, VT can be idiopathic and occur in the context of a normal heart.

There are 2 types of idiopathic VT. Right ventricular outflow tract VT (repetitive monomorphic VT) has a left bundle branch block, inferior axis morphology. Its mechanism is automatic or triggered and it is catecholamine sensitive. The other type is called left ventricular fascicular re-entrant tachycardia. It has a right bundle branch

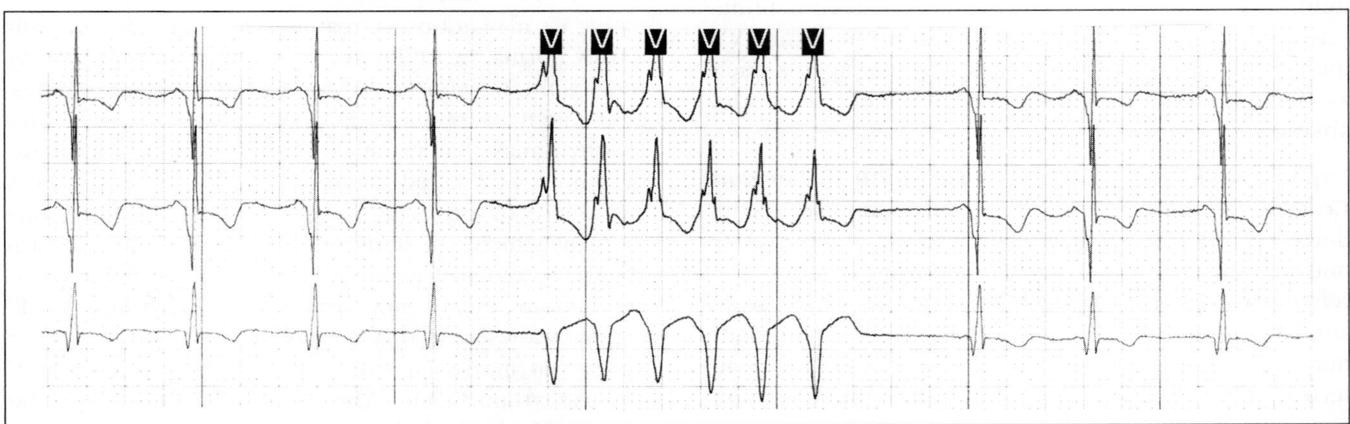


**FIGURE 85-23** ECG of nonsustained monomorphic ventricular tachycardia.

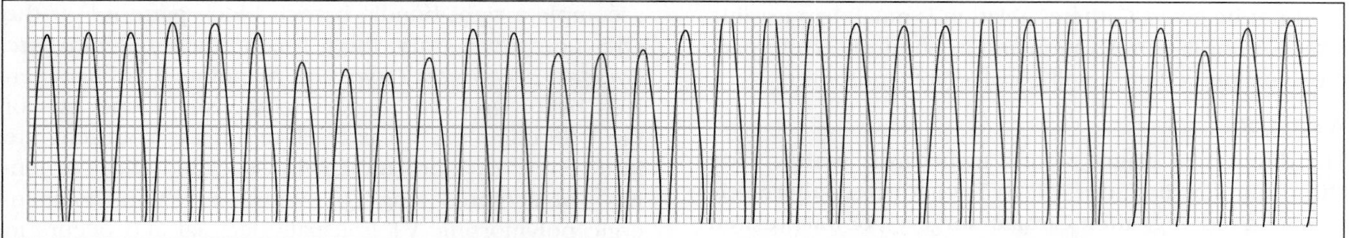

**FIGURE 85-24** ECG of AV node re-entrant tachycardia (AVNRT) with aberrant conduction.

block, left axis morphology, and a re-entrant mechanism. The prognosis is generally good.

Acute treatment of VT requires evaluation of the patient with regard to the ABCs of resuscitation.[7] Pulseless VT is treated the same as ventricular fibrillation. If the patient has pulses but poor perfusion, DC cardioversion at 0.5 to 1 J/kg should be performed. If ineffective the dose should be increased to 2 J/kg. Amiodarone or procainamide (not routinely administered together) are used after unsuccessful cardioversion. Reversible causes should be searched for and treated.

Sustained VT in the stable patient should be treated promptly with electric cardioversion or antidysrhythmic agents because of the possibility of hypotension and degeneration into ventricular fibrillation. Lidocaine (see Table 85-2) bolus and drip is usually the first line drug; other drugs include amiodarone and procainamide.

Chronic treatment requires that the underlying cause be addressed, which may necessitate a cardiac catheterization and/or electrophysiology study with possible ablation. An implantable cardioverter defibrillator may be needed in high-risk patients, especially those who have been resuscitated from sudden cardiac death. Mexiletine (see Table 85-2) may be useful if the patient responded to lidocaine. Amiodarone and procainamide are alternatives. Beta blockers are helpful in long QT syndrome and catecholamine-sensitive VT. Treatment regimens for idiopathic VT include no intervention, antidysrhythmic agents such as beta blockers or calcium channel blockers, and ablation.

***Supraventricular Tachycardia with Aberrant Conduction*** When a supraventricular impulse is conducted through the AV node and bundle of His, it may find one of the bundle branches, usually the right, still refractory (Figure 85-24). The QRS complex will be wide and have a right bundle branch block pattern if the right bundle is refractory and a left bundle branch block pattern if the left bundle is refractory. This phenomenon is very uncommon in the pediatric patient. Treatment is the same as for narrow complex SVT.

***Antidromic Atrioventricular Re-Entrant (Reciprocating) Tachycardia*** In antidromic AVRT (see previous) conduction down the bypass tract (Kent bundle) produces a wide (pre-excited) QRS complex (WPW). It is essential to avoid drugs such as digoxin and verapamil, which potentiate conduction down the accessory connection.

## MANAGEMENT

Table 85-2 lists the doses and side effects of commonly used antidysrhythmic drugs in adolescents. The doses given are for adolescents and adults. Calculating doses based on weight (kg) or body surface area ($m^2$) is recommended throughout childhood, but the maximum recommended "adult" doses should not be exceeded in full-grown adolescents and young adults. Drug interactions are common with antidysrhythmic agents. Combination drug therapy will often require reduction of doses, especially with amiodarone or digoxin.

Management of the adolescent with a dysrhythmia is determined by the severity of the dysrhythmia, symptoms, associated activity, and cardiac structure and function. In general patients with a normal heart tolerate the same dysrhythmia much better than patients with heart disease. For example, infrequent nonsustained idiopathic VT may not need treatment in an adolescent with a truly normal heart. Premature ventricular contractions that might be considered benign in a normal adolescent might be ominous in a patient with myocarditis. Dysrhythmias that produce altered level of consciousness must be treated vigorously. An adolescent who is an athlete or pregnant requires added considerations in management. In addition, adolescents have a variable psychological reaction to comparable episodes of palpitations and having to take antidysrhythmic medication. Adolescents may be taking stimulants or other drugs that may exacerbate dysrhythmias or react with antidysrhythmic agents. These complex issues should be managed by a pediatric cardiologist or pediatric electrophysiologist.

## WHO SHOULD BE REFERRED TO A PEDIATRIC CARDIOLOGIST?

A number of rhythms are benign and do not need referral, such as sinus arrhythmia. Premature atrial contractions in a normal setting and heart are benign, whereas PVCs generally need a more comprehensive cardiac evaluation with a referral to a pediatric cardiologist. Any sustained or frequently recurring dysrhythmia requires a referral. If information is obtained on personal or family history, physical examination, or testing that puts the adolescent into an "at-risk" group, he or she should be referred. Syncope that is recurrent, exercise-induced, not vasovagal (neurocardiogenic) in nature, or preceded by palpitations, may have a dysrhythmia as the etiology. Exercise-induced dysrhythmias are generally ominous.

## REFERENCES

1. Zimetbaum P, Josephson ME. Evaluation of patients with palpitations. *N Engl J Med.* 1998;338:1369-1373

2. Southall DP, Johnston F, Shinebourne EA, Johnston PGB. 24-hour electrocardiographic study of heart rate and rhythm patterns in a population of healthy children. *Br Heart J.* 1981;45:281-291

3. Brodsky M, Delon W, Denes P, et al. Arrhythmias documented by 24-hour continuous electrocardiographic monitoring in 50 male medical students without apparent heart disease. *Am J Cardiol.* 1977;39:390-395

4. Nagashima M, Matsushima M, Ogawa A, et al. Cardiac arrhythmias in healthy children revealed by 24-hour ambulatory ECG monitoring. *Pediatr Cardiol.* 1987;8:103-108

5. Dickinson DF, Scott O. Ambulatory electrocardiographic monitoring in 100 healthy teenage boys. *Br Heart J.* 1984;51:179-183

6. Vitasalo MT, Kala R, Eisalo A. Ambulatory electrocardiographic recording in endurance athletes. *Br Heart J.* 1982;47: 213-220

7. Epstein AE, DiMarco JP, Ellenbogen KA, et al. ACC/AHA/HRS 2008 guidelines for device-based therapy of cardiac rhythm abnormalities: a report of the American College of Cardiology/ American Heart Association task force on practice guidelines. *Circulation*. 2008;117:e350-e408

8. Park MK. *Pediatric Cardiology for Practitioners.* 4th ed. St. Louis, MO: Mosby; 2002:333-334

9. Ko JK, Deal BJ, Strasburger JF, Benson DW Jr. Supraventricular tachycardia mechanisms and their age distribution in pediatric patients. *Am J Cardiol.* 1992;69:1028-1032

10. Gollob MH, Green MS, Tang AS, et al. Identification of a gene responsible for familial Wolff-Parkinson-White syndrome. *N Engl J Med.* 2001;344:1823-1831

11. American Heart Association. 2005 American Heart Association guidelines for cardiopulmonary resuscitation and emergency cardiovascular care. *Circulation.* 2005;112:1 V-167-IV-187

12. Feltes TF, Friedman RA. Transesophageal echocardiographic detection of atrial thrombi in patients with nonfibrillation atrial tachyarrhythmias and congenital heart disease. *J Am Coll Cardiol.* 1994;24:1365-1370

13. Ellinor PT, Yi BA, MacRae CA. Genetics of atrial fibrillation. *Med Clin North Am.* 2008;92(1):41-51

14. Benson DW Jr, Smith WM, Dunnigan A, et al. Mechanisms of regular, wide QRS tachycardia in infants and children. *Am J Cardiol.* 1982;49:1778-1788

15. Pederson D, Zipes DP, Foster PR, Troup PS. Ventricular tachycardia and ventricular fibrillation in a young population. *Circulation.* 1979;60:988-997

16. Roden DM. A practical approach to torsade de pointes. *Clin Cardiol.* 1997;20:285-290

17. Priori SG, Schwartz PJ, Napolitano C, et al. Risk stratification in the long QT syndrome. *N Engl J Med.* 2003;348:1866-1874

18. Gutgesell H, Atkins D, Barst R, et al. Cardiovascular monitoring of children and adolescents receiving psychotropic drugs. A Statement for Healthcare Professionals from the Committee on Congenital Cardiac Defects, Counsel on Cardiovascular Diseases in the Young American Heart Association. *Circulation.* 1999;99(7):979-982

19. Fish F, Benson DW. Disorders of cardiac rhythm and conduction. In: Allen HD, Gutgesell HP, Clark EB, Driscoll DJ, eds. *Moss and Adams' Heart Disease in Infants, Children, and Adolescents.* Philadelphia, PA: Lippincott Williams & Wilkins; 2001:482-533

20. Park MK. *Pediatric Cardiology for Practitioners.* 4th ed. St Louis, MO: Mosby; 2002:489-504

21. Allen HD, Gutgesell HP, Clark EB, Driscoll DJ, eds. *Moss and Adams' Heart Disease in Infants, Children, and Adolescents.* Philadelphia, PA: Lippincott Williams & Wilkins; 2001:1462-1464

22. Dubin A. Cardiac arrhythmias. In: Behrman RE, Kliegman RM, Jenson HB, eds. *Nelson Textbook of Pediatrics*. 17th ed. Philadelphia, PA: Saunders; 2004:1554-1565

23. Walsh EP, Saul JP, Triedman JK, eds. *Cardiac Arrhythmias in Children and Young Adults with Congenital Heart Disease.* Philadelphia, PA: Lippincott Williams & Wilkins; 2001:505-507

24. Kaltman J, Shah M. Evaluation of the child with an arrhythmia. *Pediatr Clin N Am.* 2004;51:1537-1551

25. Pediatric Drug Lookup. American Academy of Pediatrics. *Pediatric Care Online.* www.pediatriccareonline.org

# CHAPTER 86

# Sudden Cardiac Death

ANDREW D. BLAUFOX, MD

## INTRODUCTION

Sudden cardiac death (SCD) is typically defined as a sudden unexpected death from a cardiovascular cause occurring within 1 hour of the onset of symptoms. An "aborted" SCD occurs when resuscitation restores spontaneous circulation. For the purposes of statistical analysis, SCD is said to occur regardless of whether it is aborted.

There are 2 general mechanisms of SCD: arrhythmic and nonarrhythmic. In arrhythmic events, there is an abrupt loss of consciousness and pulse in the absence of other conditions. This may be proven by a documented electrocardiogram (ECG) or rhythm strip during the event but is often presumed when documentation is unavailable for an event in which no structural abnormalities are found on postmortem examination. Nonarrhythmic causes occur when there is circulatory collapse in the presence of an organized rhythm, such as with an embolus or ruptured aneurysm. The overwhelming majority of SCD events in adolescents are arrhythmic.

Although SCD occurs in approximately 1/1,000 adults per year,[1] SCD is much less common in adolescents, reported to occur in approximately 1/100,000 adolescents per year.[2,3] Because most studies reporting this incidence have been limited to retrospective reviews or larger studies that rely on voluntary reporting, the true incidence may be somewhat higher. Although SCD in adolescents is rare, its effect is devastating on families and communities that experience it, particularly if it occurs in a child or adolescent with previously unknown cardiac disease. This emotional impact, as well as the advent of cases that have occurred in high-profile young athletes, have brought this problem to national attention and have made attempts to limit it a public health priority. The involvement of young athletes, both those who are prominent and highly competitive as well as those who participate for recreational purposes, has overshadowed the incidence of SCD occurring in nonathletic adolescents and has influenced efforts to concentrate on athletes. The American Board of Pediatrics recognizes the problem of SCD as being an important part of training and promotes specific learning goals related to this subject:

1. Recognize the most common causes of SCD in the adolescent.
2. Recognize that a history of exertional chest pain and syncope need further evaluation before permitting an adolescent to participate in sports.

## HIGH-RISK POPULATIONS

Sudden cardiac death is more likely to occur in individuals belonging to certain high-risk populations, regardless of whether they are athletes. Unfortunately, it may not become known that individuals belong to these populations until after SCD occurs. These populations can be divided into adolescents who have structural heart disease and those who have primary electrical disorders (Table 86-1). Although other initiating factors, such as ischemia or degeneration of a primary arrhythmia, may be involved, the common resulting mechanism of SCD in most of these individuals is ventricular fibrillation.

### STRUCTURAL HEART DISEASE

Patients with certain forms of complex congenital heart disease, such as tetralogy of Fallot, transposition of the great vessels, or severe aortic stenosis, as well as those who have had the Fontan operation, are at greater risk for SCD than the general population. However, these patients are not discussed in detail here because (1) they have generally come to medical attention by the time they reach adolescence, (2) restrictions are generally placed on their activity, and (3) SCD in these patients tends to occur in young adulthood rather than adolescence. The other forms of structural heart disease to be discussed here may be previously diagnosed but are often undiagnosed until SCD has occurred.

### HYPERTROPHIC CARDIOMYOPATHY

Hypertrophic cardiomyopathy is a familial entity that occurs in approximately 1/500 individuals, usually presents in adolescence, and is the most common cause of SCD in young athletes in the United States, representing 26% to 34% of cases.[4] Although it is sometimes difficult to distinguish from the mildly hypertrophied

**Table 86-1**

**Populations at High Risk for Sudden Cardiac Death and Recommendations for Sports Participation**

| *Abnormalities* | *Sports Participation Recommendation* |
|---|---|
| **Structural** | |
| Complex congenital heart disease | Varies depending on residual deficit |
| Hypertrophic cardiomyopathy | No competitive sports |
| Coronary artery anomalies | No competitive sports until surgically corrected |
| Marfan syndrome | No competitive sports, no isometric exercise if aorta is dilated |
| Arrhythmogenic right ventricular dysplasia | No competitive sports |
| Myocarditis/dilated cardiomyopathy | No competitive sports |
| Primary pulmonary hypertension | No competitive sports |
| **Primary Electrical** | |
| Wolff-Parkinson-White syndrome | Asymptomatic and low risk—no restriction<br>Symptomatic or high risk—ablate, then no restriction |
| Prolonged QT syndrome | No competitive sports |
| | Asymptomatic—*no data* |
| Brugada syndrome | Symptomatic—implantable cardioverter-defibrillator (ICD) and no competitive sports |
| Catecholaminergic polymorphic ventricular tachycardia | No competitive sports |
| Complete heart block | If slow escape rhythm, wide QRS escape rhythm, or concomitant ventricular ectopy, no competitive sports without pacemaker and no contact sports with pacemaker. |

For specific recommendations regarding recreational sports, see Ref. 3.

and dilated athlete's heart, hypertrophic cardiomyopathy is diagnosed if the left ventricular myocardium is excessively thickened (≥15 mm).[5] However, due to genetic variability of the causative mutations in contractile proteins, great variability may exist in phenotypic expression, including the degree of hypertrophy, which may vary greatly from massively thickened ventricles (≥30 mm) to those without obvious hypertrophy at all.

One other feature that helps support the diagnosis is asymmetric hypertrophy of the septum and left ventricular outflow obstruction. Despite occurring in a minority of cases, this asymmetry has been the reason for this entity's previous name, idiopathic hypertrophic subaortic stenosis. It is this obstruction that creates the harsh ejection murmur along the left sternal border that may be the only clue to the diagnosis on physical examination. Patients without obstruction may not have any significant physical findings. Occasionally, these patients may complain of exertional chest pain that is not musculoskeletal in description.

Histologic examination reveals that in addition to being hypertrophied, muscle cells are also in disarray. Because of the marked increase in muscle mass, these hearts are susceptible to subendocardial ischemia. This ischemia, in conjunction with the disorganized myocardial architecture, makes patients with hypertrophic cardiomyopathy vulnerable to ventricular fibrillation and SCD, which is more likely to occur with exertion as myocardial oxygen demand increases. Patients with sustained ventricular tachycardia or nonvasovagal syncope are at particular risk for SCD and may warrant placement of an implantable cardioverter-defibrillator (ICD). Other risk factors for SCD in patients with hypertrophic cardiomyopathy include (1) a family history of SCD, (2) septal thickness >30 mm, (3) nonsustained ventricular tachycardia, and (4) hypotensive response to exercise. Patients with any 2 of these other risk factors may also warrant primary prevention of SCD with ICD placement. Patients with hypertrophic cardiomyopathy should not participate in competitive sports (Table 86-1).

### CORONARY ARTERY ANOMALIES

Congenital coronary artery anomalies are the second most common nonacquired cause of SCD in the young, accounting for 16.5% of cases.[4] Of these anomalies, the most common is when the left coronary artery arises from the right sinus of Valsalva and then courses between the aorta and the pulmonary artery to perfuse the left heart. The opposite anomaly may also occur. The mechanism by which these anomalies cause SCD is disputed but possible explanations generally involve ischemia, which is often worsened by exercise and includes (1) an acute take-off of the anomalous coronary leading to kinking, (2) a small orifice of the coronary, (3) compression of the coronary as it passes between the great arteries, and (4) in some patients in whom the coronary also runs within the wall of the aorta, compression of the coronary against the aortic wall as the aorta expands during exercise. The ischemia caused by any of these mechanisms leads to ventricular fibrillation and possible SCD.

Unfortunately, these anomalies are extremely difficult to diagnose because patients are often asymptomatic and have no clinical signs of heart disease until SCD occurs, and because these anomalies are difficult to detect with noninvasive methods. Patients with syncope in the midst of exercise should be viewed with a high index of suspicion for these anomalies and may require an evaluation that includes an electrocardiogram (ECG), exercise test, echocardiogram, and possibly angiography. Patients with coronary anomalies should not participate in competitive sports. If the anomaly is amenable to surgical correction, patients may be able to participate following surgery (Table 86-1).

### MYOCARDITIS/DILATED CARDIOMYOPATHY

Myocarditis and cardiomyopathy account for approximately 7.5% of cases of SCD in the young.[4] In dilated cardiomyopathy, the left ventricle is enlarged and poorly contracts, leading to decreased cardiac output. This may be caused by prior myocarditis or inflammation of the myocardium. Myocarditis is often caused by viral infection but may be related to other etiologies such as cocaine abuse. Although patients come to medical attention because of symptoms of congestive heart failure, the degree of ventricular dysfunction can be variable, and these symptoms may be subtle. In many cases of myocarditis the disease may not progress to cardiomyopathy, and patients may be relatively asymptomatic until SCD occurs. Because of poor cardiac reserve and relative ischemia in cardiomyopathy, as well as inflammation in myocarditis, these patients are vulnerable to arrhythmias, particularly ventricular fibrillation, which leads to SCD. Patients with myocarditis or cardiomyopathy should not participate in competitive sports (Table 86-1).

### MARFAN SYNDROME

Aortic rupture or aortic dissection in patients with dilated and weakened aortic walls secondary to the connective tissue disease associated with Marfan syndrome account for approximately 3% of cases of SCD in the young.[4] Despite coming to medical attention because of their recognizable features and familial association, once aortic root dilation begins catastrophic tearing of the aorta may occur without warning, resulting in SCD. Patients with Marfan syndrome should be allowed to participate in competitive sports up until their aorta begins to dilate, after which they should be restricted from competitive sports and isometric exercise, both of which increase aorta wall stress and predispose to rupture/dissection (Table 86-1).[6]

### ARRHYTHMOGENIC RIGHT VENTRICULAR DYSPLASIA

Arrhythmogenic right ventricular dysplasia (ARVD) or cardiomyopathy is a familial condition with autosomal inheritance that usually presents in adolescence and has been reported to account for 2.8% of cases of SCD in young athletes in the United States.[4] It is the most common cause of SCD in this group in Italy.[7] Arrhythmogenic right ventricular dysplasia is characterized by replacement of myocytes with adipose and fibrous tissue, and most commonly involves the right ventricular outflow tract, resulting in right ventricular dilation and dysfunction. The left ventricle may be involved in severe cases. Although symptoms of heart failure may be present in advanced cases, the primary clinical manifestations of this disease are electrophysiologic. Patients experience palpitations or syncope from ventricular arrhythmias (premature ventricular contractions, ventricular tachycardia, or ventricular fibrillation). The likelihood of malignant ventricular arrhythmias is increased with exercise and they are the cause of syncope and SCD, either of which may be the first manifestation. Clues to this diagnosis include (1) inverted T waves through lead V3 or V4, (2) a late potential or epsilon wave at the end of the QRS, (3) left bundle branch block, (4) right ventricular dilation and dysfunction with or without evidence of aneurysm, and (5) fatty infiltration of the myocardium on magnetic resonance imaging (MRI). Family history is an important determinant of risk. Patients with ARVD should be restricted from competitive sports and may require ICD implantation (Table 86-1).

## PRIMARY ELECTRICAL DISEASES

Several diagnoses exist in which patients have structurally normal hearts but are predisposed to SCD because of electrophysiologic abnormalities that lead to malignant arrhythmias, usually ventricular fibrillation. Because these hearts are structurally normal, postmortem identification of these disorders is often difficult; thus, the relative incidence of these disorders as a cause of SCD may be higher than reported.

### WOLFF-PARKINSON-WHITE SYNDROME

Wolff-Parkinson-White syndrome (WPW) occurs in 1/1,000 infants but may spontaneously disappear by early childhood in approximately half of those affected.[8] With advances in radiofrequency ablation, the number of patients reaching adolescence with WPW is further diminished. However, because there is an overall risk of SCD of 1/1,000 per year in patients with WPW, it is still an important cause of SCD in adolescents.[9] Because it can be brought to medical attention with preexisting symptoms of palpitations due to supraventricular tachycardia, identified by the characteristic ECG findings (short PR interval, "delta" wave, and wide QRS), and because it can be cured with catheter ablation, its recognition is essential. It has been reported that 12% or more of WPW patients who experience SCD were previously asymptomatic.[10] Sudden cardiac death in WPW is due to rapid electrical conduction from the atrium to the ventricle via an accessory pathway during atrial fibrillation, resulting in a rapid and irregular ventricular rhythm that can degenerate into ventricular fibrillation. The relative risk of SCD depends on the conduction properties of this accessory pathway and may reach 6/1,000 per year in patients with a "high-risk" accessory pathway that can conduct >250 beats per minute (bpm).[10] Adolescents with WPW who are asymptomatic and have "low-risk" accessory pathways may participate in competitive sports, whereas others should undergo ablation before competing (Table 86-1).

### PROLONGED QT SYNDROME

The prolonged QT syndrome is a relatively uncommon problem that has become a paradigm for cardiovascular genetics. It may occur in as many as 1/10,000 individuals and is caused by mutations in the genes coding for the function of potassium or sodium channels of myocytes.[11] These mutations result in either delayed efflux of potassium out of the myocyte or prolonged influx of sodium into the cell, both of which result in prolongation of the action potential duration, which is manifest as prolongation of the QT interval on ECG. This prolongation predisposes individuals to the unstable ventricular arrhythmia, torsades de pointes, which may self-terminate or may degenerate into ventricular fibrillation. If the former occurs, patients may be asymptomatic or experience dizziness or syncope; if the latter occurs, patients may have SCD.

The risk of SCD from prolonged QT syndrome is highest in adolescents and young adults; it may be as high as 50% in 10 years if untreated, but may be reduced to 5% with treatment.[11] Treatment should be undertaken after ruling out transient causes of QT prolongation, such as hypocalcemia, hypomagnesemia, or hypokalemia. Treatment consists primarily of beta blockers and, in some cases, the placement of an ICD. Various diagnostic and risk-stratifying criteria have been proposed in which the risk of SCD is related to a greater length of the QT interval (after correction for heart rate), gender, ion channel mutation, the presence of symptoms, and a malignant family history.[12,13] Although there can be considerable overlap between affected and normal individuals, a good rule of thumb is that the corrected QT interval is abnormal when it is >450 msec in boys and >460 msec in girls. Importantly, individuals with genotypic prolonged QT syndrome may not manifest prolonged QT intervals until exposed to one of many drugs (www.qtdrugs.org). Patients with prolonged QT syndrome should not participate in competitive sports (Table 86-1).

### BRUGADA SYNDROME

Brugada syndrome may occur in 5/10,000 individuals and may be responsible for as many as 20% of cases of SCD occurring in individuals with structurally normal hearts.[14] Although the average age of presentation or SCD in those with Brugada syndrome is 40 years, it can also be found in adolescents. Brugada syndrome is caused by mutations to myocyte sodium channels causing a loss of function leading to dispersion of repolarization timing between the endocardium and the epicardium. This is manifest as an incomplete right bundle branch block ECG pattern with elevated ST segments in at least 2 of the 3 right precordial leads. Occasionally, infusion of sodium channel blocking agents is necessary to make the diagnosis when the ECG shows only subtle changes. The repolarization dispersion is also responsible for the initiation of a reentry-type polymorphic ventricular tachycardia that often precipitates ventricular fibrillation and causes SCD. Unlike other causes, SCD in Brugada syndrome is more likely to occur during sleep rather than exercise. Because data are lacking in asymptomatic patients with Brugada syndrome, no definitive recommendations for sports activity can be made in these patients. Symptomatic patients with Brugada syndrome should have an ICD implanted and be restricted from competitive sports (Table 86-1).

### CATECHOLAMINERGIC POLYMORPHIC VENTRICULAR TACHYCARDIA

Catecholaminergic polymorphic ventricular tachycardia (CPVT) is a rare familial disease with either autosomal dominant or recessive inheritance that is associated with malignant ventricular arrhythmias that are worsened with exercise.[15] If untreated, SCD may occur in 30% to 50% of patients. Due to compliance issues, patients treated with beta blockers are not completely free of risk; thus, ICD implantation should be strongly considered. Patients with CPVT should be restricted from competitive sports (Table 86-1).

### COMPLETE HEART BLOCK

Although most cases of pediatric complete heart block present in early childhood and are mostly related to cases of maternal systemic lupus erythematosuis (SLE), complete heart block can sometimes occur in the adolescent as a result of systemic ailments such as connective tissue disease, iatrogenic causes such as hemosiderosis from chronic transfusions, or acquired causes such as myocarditis or Lyme disease. The common link to these etiologies is scarring of the normal conduction system. Because heart block may not occur at initial presentation of these systemic diseases, careful monitoring for progressive conduction disturbances in these instances is essential; and because heart block may be the only manifestation of acquired causes, its advent may occur with an SCD event. Other symptoms associated with complete heart block are fatigue, exercise intolerance, dizziness, and syncope. Risk of SCD is related to (1) a low resting heart rate (<50 bpm), (2) a wide QRS escape rhythm, (3) frequent ventricular ectopy, (4) a prolonged QT interval, and (5) long pauses (≥3 sec). High-risk patients should not participate in competitive sports and should undergo pacemaker implantation, especially if symptomatic. After pacemaker implantation, patients should be restricted from contact sports (Table 86-1).

## CONTROVERSIAL POPULATIONS

From time to time, associations are made between foods or drugs and SCD. Before causality can be proven, public judgment, based largely on fears and lack of understanding, may be passed prematurely. It is important for health professionals to seek scientific links to events and to advise patients exposed to these agents based on scientific evidence.

### ADDERALL AND SUDDEN CARDIAC DEATH

In February 2005, the Canadian government pulled Adderall and Adderall XR from its market because of postmarketing reports of sudden unexplained death in 20 users of these drugs. Twelve of these users were children ranging in age from 7 to 16 years (mean 12.5 years), all of whom were boys. The children were using the medication for 1 day to 8 years, and total daily doses were 10 mg ($n$ = 1), 20 mg ($n$ = 5), 30 mg ($n$ = 1), 40 mg ($n$ = 1), 50 mg ($n$ = 1), and not known ($n$ = 3). In addition to Adderall, three boys were taking another prescription drug at the time of death. Considering that 30 million prescriptions were written for the medication during the same period, the risk of SCD was found to be .04/100,000 prescriptions and does not appear to be higher than the risk for the general adolescent population.

A closer look at the data reveals that (1) 3 patients had an unusual and unexplained accumulation of the drug, resulting in toxic levels; and (2) 5 patients had structural heart diseases that, in and of themselves, are conditions for which there is a higher risk of SCD. These conditions included 1 patient with an aberrant origin of the coronary artery, 1 patient with a hypertrophic cardiomyopathy, and 3 patients with possible hypertrophic cardiomyopathy. Another patient had a maternal history of ventricular tachycardia, and one patient had a bicuspid aortic valve. It is unknown whether any other children had primary electrical disorders that had not previously been diagnosed. Because of these data, the Canadian government put Adderall back on its market in August 2005. The US Food and Drug Administration (FDA) has allowed Adderall to be marketed with the following temporary recommendations: (1) the label now has a warning against abuse, and (2) the drug should not be used in individuals with known structural heart disease. In addition, in 2008, the American Heart Association (AHA) added a recommendation that all children who are to begin stimulant medication for attention deficit/hyperactivity disorder should have an initial ECG (circ.ahajournals.org/cgi/reprint/CIRCULATIONAHA.107.189473). Whether the evidence substantiates these recommendations is debatable; both the FDA and the AHA are continuing to determine whether these will remain part of the final recommendations, and the American Academy of Pediatrics issued a policy statement in 2008 recommending a targeted cardiac history, but advising against routine ECG screening in those starting on stimulant medication.[16]

### COMMOTIO CORDIS

Commotio cordis is sudden death caused by chest wall impact in individuals with a normal heart. Although the exact incidence is not known, the number of cases being reported is on the rise.[17] According to the commotio cordis registry, 78% of reported cases involved individuals younger than 18 years (median age 14 years).[17] Ninety-five percent of these adolescents are boys. The most common sports implicated are those that involve projectiles (ie, baseball, softball, hockey, football, soccer, rugby, lacrosse); however, commotio cordis can also occur in those sports that involve body blows (ie, karate, boxing).[17] Approximately half of the reported cases have occurred during baseball. Events are equally likely to occur in recreational activities as in organized activities. Regardless of the setting, the clinical outcome is devastating, with only 23% survival when resuscitation is promptly initiated within 3 minutes and 3% survival if resuscitation is delayed.[17] Neurological injury is found in many survivors.

The initial documented rhythm after commotio cordis is generally ventricular fibrillation, and this is believed to be the mechanism by which SCD occurs. Experimental models have determined that several factors are important in the generation of ventricular fibrillation from chest wall impact; these include (1) timing of impact, (2) energy of impact, (3) location of impact, and (4) hardness of impact object.[17,18] It is critical that the impact occur during cardiac repolarization when the peak of the T wave occurs.[19] Not unexpectedly, ventricular fibrillation is also more likely to occur if the impact occurs in a region over the ventricular mass.[18] Because of these findings, the athletic equipment industry has developed alternative products, such as softer balls and chest protectors, to try to minimize the detrimental effects of these impacts. Although these innovations may have helped in some cases, commotio cordis can still occur with soft baseballs or when athletes are wearing chest protectors.

## PREVENTION OF SCD

The prevention of SCD is a complicated task that involves several evolving areas: (1) screening and restrictions for sports participation, (2) patient-specific therapy for members of high-risk groups, and (3) the development of organized rescue programs. Although the first area focuses on athletes, the latter 2 are not specific to that group.

### SCREENING FOR SPORTS PARTICIPATION

The AHA recommends mandatory screening of all high school (grades 9–12) and collegiate athletes before participation in organized sports (Table 86-2).[3] This screening should be repeated every 2 years. The screening process should include a history and physical examination that is completed by a trained medical professional who is capable of detecting risk for SCD. Specific methods recommended by the AHA for preparticipation screening are listed in Table 86-2.

Although the AHA recommends national standardization of this process, it is currently regulated on the state level, and therefore many inconsistencies exist.[20] As of 1998, 1 state had no screening at all and 8 states did not have an approved standard history and physical examination questionnaire. In addition, in states with standard forms important questions were not asked: only 37 ask about syncope, 21 ask about exertional dizziness, and 28 ask about a family history of SCD.

Even if all questions are asked, it is uncertain how well screening programs can detect pathology and prevent SCD. Corrado et al[7] looked at the preparticipation screening of adolescent and young adult athletes who died suddenly and whose postmortem examinations showed ARVD ($n$ = 11), atherosclerotic coronary artery disease ($n$ = 9), or coronary artery anomaly ($n$ = 8). Factors noted on the screening included palpitations, syncope, chest pain, ST-segment or T-wave abnormalities, ventricular arrhythmias, and family history of SCD. Only in the ARVD group did most patients have

**Table 86-2**

**American Heart Association Recommendations for Preparticipation Screen**

| *Component* | *Recommendations* |
|---|---|
| Population | High school (grades 9–12) and collegiate athletes |
| Frequency | Prior to participation in organized sports and every 2 years thereafter |
| Performer | Trained health professional able to identify risks for SCD |
| History | 1. Should specifically ask about prior exertional chest pain, syncope, or excessive shortness of breath.<br>2. Inquiry should be made as to whether there is a prior history of murmur or hypertension.<br>3. A thorough family history should be documented, asking specific questions regarding sudden death or about the existence of certain familial diseases, such as prolonged QT syndrome, cardiomyopathy, Marfan syndrome, etc. |
| Physical examination | Should include blood pressure measurement, complete cardiac auscultation, assessment of the femoral pulses, and notation of any stigmata of Marfan syndrome. |

one or more of these factors: ARVD (9/11), atherosclerosis (2/9), or coronary anomaly (2/8). Unlike in Italy, where this study was conducted, ECGs are not used in screening in the United States. If the ECG findings were eliminated, the clues to the diagnosis of ARVD may have been dramatically reduced because 9 patients had ST-segment or T-wave abnormalities and 6 had ventricular arrhythmias. Likewise, 1 of the 2 coronary artery patients would not have had any positive findings on the screening. Therefore, the power to detect those at risk with the present screening system in the United States is severely limited for some conditions.

Due to the limitations with history and physical screening, many have debated whether ECGs or echocardiograms should be added to the screening process. Although each test may be beneficial for detecting different pathology (ie, ECGs for ARVD, echocardiograms for hypertrophic cardiomyopathy), instituting such a change in the screening process may also have negative effects. These other tests require additional trained pediatric personnel to perform and interpret, and the burden to accomplish this may be overwhelming. Often, these tests are inconclusive and prompt further investigation that can be invasive and that can lead to further anxiety and trauma for children and adolescents who are not at risk for SCD. Finally, although it is impossible to put a price on saving a child's life, financial limitations to funding public health initiatives demand that such initiatives have some measure of cost-effectiveness. Given the incidence of SCD, some argue that the additional costs for performing ECGs or echocardiograms make them prohibitive as parts of the screening process. Studies are currently under way in the United States to help determine the effect of these issues on SCD.

## THERAPY FOR HIGH-RISK GROUPS

Once an adolescent is diagnosed with a disease that places him or her at risk for SCD, measures can be taken to minimize the risk. Risk reducing measures can be as simple as restricting physical activity, as detailed previously in this chapter. In addition, instituting medical therapy may afford some protection as beta blockers do for patients with the prolonged QT syndrome. However, it is often the case that neither activity restriction nor pharmacotherapy prevents SCD in high-risk individuals. However, the superior effectiveness of ICDs for the prevention of SCD is widely accepted, particularly if the ICD is used as secondary prevention in patients who have experienced and survived a previous SCD. It has been shown that 75% of those who have an ICD implanted receive at least one appropriate shock for a life-threatening arrhythmia within 8 years of ICD placement.[21]

Unfortunately, it is much more difficult to determine which patients without a history of SCD would benefit from ICD implant. In hypertrophic cardiomyopathy, only 20% of patients who receive ICDs for primary prevention actually experience a life-saving shock within 8 years[21]; thus, 5 ICDs would have to be implanted for every life saved. Although some would view this as cost effective, there are other serious issues with ICD placement in children and adolescents that affect the cost-benefit calculations. First, they are bulky and come with a scar, both of which are noticeable features that may not be well tolerated in an adolescent concerned with body image. Second, significant risks are associated with repeated implantation and maintenance of vascular access that are required over the long term. Probably most important, the rate of inappropriate shocks received by pediatric patients is high, with reports of up to 40% of patients being shocked for non-life-threatening rhythms within 18 months of implant.[22] Not only are these shocks painful, they also may incur severe psychological trauma, causing some patients to be too afraid to leave their home for fear of being shocked when exerting themselves. Therefore, identification of risk does not necessarily lead to a clear understanding of the best path to take to prevent SCD.

## ORGANIZED RESCUE PROGRAMS

Despite our best efforts to identify patients at risk and institute appropriate therapies and restrictions, SCD can still occur, particularly with the unpredictability of such entities as commotio cordis. Because survival decreases exponentially with every minute of delay in resuscitation, organized rescue programs have been set up in communities to provide cardiopulmonary resuscitation (CPR) training and equipment for the prompt initiation of adequate resuscitation in the event of SCD. Although CPR alone may increase survival rates, survival is dramatically further improved when CPR is used in conjunction with defibrillation via an automatic external defibrillator (AED).[1]

There are several considerations before a community begins an organized rescue program. A decision needs to be made as to whether rescues will be performed by lay rescuers or only by first responders, such as firefighters or police officers. Important factors in making this determination include (1) the expected first responder response time, or "call to shock interval," which should be no more than 5 minutes for the best outcome; (2) the community's ability to pay for the training and equipment, which might cost more for lay rescuers because of the greater number of people and equipment needed to cover the same area covered by mobile first responders; and (3) concerns about liability, which still exist for lay rescuers

**Table 86-3**

**Core Elements of American Heart Association School Medical Emergency Response Plan**

| *Component* | *Specifics* |
|---|---|
| Effective and efficient communication | A system enabling communication across the school campus and with emergency medical professionals |
| Coordinated and practiced response plan | A plan involving the school nurse, coaches, and teachers, as well as having emergency medical service (EMS) workers visit the school to familiarize themselves with access to all areas of the campus |
| Risk reduction | Identifying students with possible medical conditions and tailoring resources to them |
| Training and equipment for first aid/CPR | Training of multiple school personnel, some of whom can act as trainers for additional school staff |
| Lay rescuer AED program | If there is a need (ie, AED has been used in past 5 years, there are students at high risk for SCD, EMS response time is >5 minutes while lay response time is expected to be <5 minutes), AED locations should be well-known and readily accessible within a few minutes of anywhere on campus |

despite legislation attempting to protect them. The AHA outlines five important additional considerations in the Medical Emergency Response Plan for Schools (www.americanheart.org/presenter.jhtml?identifier=3017969) (Table 86-3).

Although lay rescue programs offer hope to combat SCD, current analyses estimate that the cost of each life saved is $1.5 to $3.3 million.[1] Therefore, before lay rescue programs can be universally adopted, further research is required to determine how to optimize these programs and the technology they employ.

## CONCLUSION

Sudden cardiac death is a rare but devastating event in the adolescent population. Not all events occur during sports. Most of those who experience SCD have underlying heart disease, with hypertrophic cardiomyopathy and coronary anomalies being the most common. Symptoms of exertional syncope or exertional nonmusculoskeletal chest pain should be taken seriously. Commotio cordis is a preventable cause of SCD in some cases. Screening efforts fall short in the prevention of SCD. Early CPR and availability of AEDs could prevent SCD in many children.

## REFERENCES


1. Berger S, Utech L, Hazinski M. Sudden death in children and adolescents. *Pediatr Clin N Am*. 2004;51:1653–1677

2. Driscoll DJ, Edwards WD. Sudden unexplained death in children and adolescents. *J Am Coll Cardiol*. 1985;5:118B–121B

3. Maron BJ, Thompson PD, Puffer JC, et al. Cardiovascular preparticipation screening of competitive athletes. *Circulation*. 1996;94:850–856

4. Maron BJ. Sudden death in young athletes. *N Engl J Med*. 2003;349:1064–1075

5. Maron BJ. Hypertrophic cardiomyopathy. *Lancet*. 1997;350: 127–133

6. Maron BJ. Cardiovascular causes and pathology of sudden death in athletes: the American experience. In: Bayes De Luna A, Furlanello F, Maron BJ, Zipes DP, eds. *Arrhythmias and Sudden Death in Athletes*. Dordrecht, The Netherlands: Kluwer Academic;2000:31–48

7. Corrado D, Basso C, Schiavon M, Thiene G. Screening for hypertrophic cardiomyopathy in young athletes. *N Eng J Med*. 1998;339:364–369

8. Perry JC, Garson A Jr. Supraventricular tachycardia due to Wolff-Parkinson-White syndrome in children: early disappearance and late recurrence. *J Am Coll Cardiol*. 1990;16:1215–1220

9. Blaufox AD, Saul JP. Accessory pathway mediated tachycardias. In: Saul JP, Walsh E, eds. *Cardiac Arrhythmias in the Pediatric Patient: Evolving Concepts in Clinical Management*. Philadelphia: Lippincott Williams & Wilkins; 2001: 173–200

10. Klein GJ, Bashore TM, Sellers TD, Pritchett ELC, Smith WM, Gallagher JJ. Ventricular fibrillation in the Wolff-Parkinson-White syndrome. *N Engl J Med*. 1979;301:1080–1085

11. Ackerman MJ. The long QT syndrome. *Pediatr Rev*. 1998; 19:232–238

12. Priori SG, Schwartz PJ, Napolitano C, et al. Risk stratification in the long-QT syndrome. *N Engl J Med*. 2003;348:1866–1874

13. Moss AJ, Schwartz PJ, Crampton RS, Locati E, Carleen E. The long QT syndrome: a prospective international study. *Circulation*. 1985;71:17–21

14. Antzelevitch C. Brugada syndrome: overview. In: Antzelevitch C, ed. *The Brugada Syndrome: From Bench to Bedside*. Malden, MA: Blackwell; 2005;1–22

15. Francis J, Sankar V, Nair VK, Priori SG. Catecholaminergic polymorphic ventricular tachycardia. *Heart Rhythm*. 2005; 2:550–554

16. Perrin J, Friedman RA, Knilans TK, et al. Cardiovascular monitoring and stimulant drugs for attention-deficit/hyperactivity disorder. *Pediatrics.* 2008;122:451–453

17. Maron BJ, Gohman TE, Kyle SB, Estes NAM, Link MS. Clinical profile and spectrum of commotio cordis. *JAMA*. 2002;287:1142–1146

18. Maron BJ, Poliac LC, Kaplan JA, Mueller FO. Blunt impact to the chest leading to sudden death from cardiac arrest during sports activities. *N Engl J Med*. 1995;333:337–342

19. Link MS. Mechanically induced sudden death in chest wall impact (commotio cordis). *Prog Biophys Mol Biol*. 2003;82: 175–186

20. Glover DW, Maron BJ. Profile of preparticipation cardiovascular screening for high school athletes. *JAMA*. 1998; 279: 1817–1819

21. Maron BJ, Shen WK, Link MS, et al. Efficacy of implantable cardioverter-defibrillators for the prevention of sudden death in patients with hypertrophic cardiomyopathy. *N Engl J Med*. 2000;342:365–373

22. Korte T, Koditz H, Niehaus M, Paul T, Tebbenjohanns J. High incidence of appropriate and inappropriate ICD therapies in children and adolescents with implantable cardioverter defibrillator. *PACE*. 2004;27:924–932

# CHAPTER 87

# Shock in the Adolescent Patient

H. MICHAEL USHAY, MD, PhD

## INTRODUCTION

Shock is a state in which the delivery of oxygen and nutrients does not meet tissue demands.[1] Prolonged or inadequately treated shock leads to multiple organ system failure and, ultimately, death. Although most often associated with hypotension, a patient may be in shock with normal or even elevated blood pressure. Whatever the blood pressure, it is usually possible to discern signs of inadequate tissue perfusion in a patient who is in shock.

Recognition of shock is complicated by compensatory mechanisms that attempt to support oxygen delivery and thus mask its presence. These compensatory mechanisms can become exhausted, culminating in hemodynamic collapse, respiratory failure, multiple organ failure, and even death. The sometimes cryptic presentation of shock necessitates that caregivers maintain a high level of expectancy for its presence and initiate aggressive treatment as early as possible.

Etiologies of shock include sepsis, blood loss, hypovolemia, cardiac failure, and poisoning. Whatever the origin, the final common pathway of shock is failure of tissue beds to receive and use adequate amounts of oxygen, glucose, and other metabolic substrates. Tissues respond to inadequate oxygen delivery by converting from aerobic to anaerobic metabolism, which results in the production of lactic acid and development of metabolic acidosis.

When treated appropriately and in a timely manner, shock is usually reversible. An inexorable progression of untreated shock from a reversible to irreversible process emphasizes the importance of recognizing shock at its earliest manifestation and initiating appropriate and aggressive management.[2]

## EPIDEMIOLOGY OF SHOCK IN ADOLESCENT PATIENTS

Severe sepsis is the leading cause of shock in adolescent patients. The incidence of severe sepsis ranges from 0.2 per 1,000 in the 10- to 14-year-old age group to 0.4 per 1,000 in the 15- to 19-year-old age group.[3] In adolescence, the occurrence of vehicular as well as other accidental and nonaccidental trauma increases, leading to a rise in the incidence of hemorrhagic shock. Obstetric hemorrhage also enters into consideration in adolescence. Other precipitants of shock in adolescence include anaphylaxis, respiratory failure, poisoning, and decreased myocardial function secondary to myocarditis or cardiomyopathy. In the developing world, hypovolemic shock secondary to dengue, cholera, dysentery due to infectious etiologies, and severe sepsis related to pneumonia or other inadequately treated bacterial infections is common.

## PHYSIOLOGICAL ASPECTS OF SHOCK

Shock is a disorder of tissue oxygen delivery. Oxygen delivery is defined as the product of cardiac output and arterial oxygen content. Cardiac output is a function of ventricular filling (the preload), the contractile state of the myocardial muscle, and the resistance of the vasculature into which the heart chambers empty. Arterial oxygen content is a function of the hemoglobin oxygen saturation, hemoglobin concentration, and, to a much lesser extent, $PaO_2$, the blood oxygen tension.

Under circumstances of good health and normal cardiac output, about 25% of delivered oxygen is consumed in the interval between the time arterial blood leaves the left ventricle and venous blood returns to the right atrium. Therefore, venous blood is approximately 25% less saturated than arterial blood. When tissue oxygen demands increase, oxygen delivery increases by augmenting cardiac output. If cardiac output can be increased adequately, the arteriolar-venous oxygen content difference (oxygen extraction) remains constant at approximately 25%. If cardiac output cannot be increased sufficiently to meet tissue demands, then the tissue beds will extract more than 25% of the delivered oxygen, thus lowering the saturation of the venous hemoglobin and increasing the difference between arteriolar and venous oxygen contents. Thus, a decrease in mixed venous oxyhemoglobin saturation below 70% to 75% is a marker for inadequate cardiac output.[4]

Vasomotor tone, as measured by blood pressure, is required for blood volume and its cargo, oxygen, to reach all tissue beds. In some forms of shock, especially when due to septic or neurogenic etiologies, the mechanisms that regulate vascular tone are disabled and blood pressure plummets. When cardiac output is low, the body attempts to maintain perfusion by vasoconstriction, resulting in cool extremities with poorly palpable pulses.[5]

## CATEGORIES OF SHOCK

Shock may be categorized as hypovolemic, distributive, cardiogenic, obstructive, or dissociative in origin. There are general approaches to the management of shock, but definitive management requires knowing the etiology and the primary physiological disturbance.

Using physiological principles, it is possible to understand how disruptions of different components of the circulatory system can result in decreased tissue oxygen delivery. Table 87-1 summarizes the categories of shock, associated physiological disturbances, and clinical examples of each category. Although efforts are made to categorize shock, it is common for overlap to occur.

### HYPOVOLEMIC SHOCK

Hypovolemic shock results from an absolute or relative decrease in effective circulating blood volume. Decreased preload results in diminished cardiac output. In traumatic, obstetric, or gastrointestinal hemorrhage, there is an acute, absolute reduction in blood volume that results in decreased preload and decreased oxygen-carrying capacity due to a reduction in hemoglobin quantity. Excessive fluid and electrolyte losses, as occurs in diabetic ketoacidosis, diarrheal dehydration, and loss of protein-rich fluids in major burns and peritonitis, also result in a decrease in circulating blood volume, but an increase in hematocrit due to preservation of actual red cell mass. Hypovolemic shock from non blood fluid losses often develops slowly and less dramatically than hemorrhagic shock, and thus is more difficult to recognize.

**Table 87-1**

**Categories of Shock**

| *Shock Classification* | *Physiological Disturbance* | *Examples* |
|---|---|---|
| **Hypovolemic** | ↓ Preload, ↓ hemoglobin (↓ $O_2$ content) | Dehydration, hemorrhage |
| **Distributive** | ↓ Vasomotor tone, disordered tissue bed blood flow | Sepsis, toxic shock syndrome, anaphylaxis, spinal cord injury |
| **Cardiogenic** | ↓ Contractility of myocardium | Myocarditis, cardiomyopathy |
| **Obstructive** | ↓Preload, physical obstruction to blood flow | Tamponade, tension pneumothorax, pulmonary embolism |
| **Dissociative** | Disorder of $O_2$ transport or utilization | Carbon monoxide, cyanide, methemoglobinemia |

### DISTRIBUTIVE SHOCK

Distributive shock is characterized by severe alterations in peripheral vascular tone and disordered microcirculatory blood flow in tissue beds. Severe sepsis is the most important and frequent cause of distributive shock, but anaphylaxis, spinal cord trauma, and drug ingestions may present similarly. In distributive shock, regulatory mechanisms for vascular tone in large blood vessels and control of blood flow within the microcirculation of tissue beds are both disrupted.

In distributive shock due to sepsis, abnormalities in microcirculatory and tissue bed blood flow predominate, whereas, in anaphylaxis, spinal cord injury, and poisoning, loss of vasomotor tone in the macrocirculation plays a greater role. In septic shock, there is evidence for oversecretion of the intrinsic vasodilator nitric oxide, which may result in loss of large vessel tone. At the same time, alterations in the function of nitric oxide in the tissue capillary beds results in constriction, which, when combined with decreased vascular resistance in the large blood vessels, results in shunting of blood away from tissues and decreased tissue oxygen delivery.[6]

### CARDIOGENIC SHOCK

Cardiogenic shock occurs when cardiac pump failure is the principal cause of inadequate tissue oxygen delivery. The most common cause of cardiogenic shock in older adults is muscle damage from myocardial infarction. An important aspect of cardiogenic shock that distinguishes it from other forms of shock is the inability of the heart to meet the demands of an increased workload that may be required to compensate for being in shock. For example, in distributive shock, cardiac output often increases to compensate for low systemic vascular resistance, and, in hypovolemic shock, the heart rate increases and the heart pumps against increased systemic vascular resistance. Etiologies of cardiogenic shock that may occur in adolescence are listed in Box 87-1.

**Box 87-1**

***Etiologies of Cardiogenic Shock in Adolescence***

- Myocarditis
- Cardiomyopathy (dilated and restrictive)
- Arrhythmias (eg, supraventricular tachycardia or ventricular tachycardia)
- Sepsis
- Acute rheumatic fever
- Valvular heart disease
- Subacute and acute bacterial endocarditis
- Myocardial injury (eg, from trauma)
- Cardiac pump failure after cardiac surgery
- Hypoxic-ischemic injury secondary to anoxic injury
- Poisoning or drug toxicity
- Myocardial injury from myocardial infarction

Cardiogenic shock is characterized by decreased cardiac output, marked tachycardia, and peripheral vasoconstriction. The work of breathing may be increased secondary to pulmonary edema. Typically, intravascular volume is normal or increased, unless there is an intercurrent illness that results in volume depletion.

Cardiogenic shock is characterized by sequential compensatory and pathological mechanisms. However, compensatory mechanisms that maintain perfusion to the brain and heart during hypovolemic shock are deleterious in cardiogenic shock. For example, a compensatory increase in vascular tone redirects diminished blood flow from peripheral and splanchnic tissues to the heart and brain. However, increased vasomotor tone increases the afterload and, hence, the work that the ventricles must do to eject blood, and thus increases oxygen demands of the heart muscle. The heart's ejection volume decreases as afterload increases, causing further increase in heart rate in order to attempt to maintain cardiac output. Tone in the systemic and pulmonary veins increases. Antidiuretic hormone and aldosterone are secreted in order to increase fluid retention. Increased pulmonary venous pressure and volume contribute to the development of pulmonary edema.

The heart is an end organ with significant oxygen demands. Almost all shock states result in inadequate oxygen delivery to the myocardium relative to the increased demands that come from pumping against increased systemic vascular tone or from a tachycardic response to vasodilation in distributive shock. Therefore, sustained shock of any type eventually leads to impaired myocardial function (ie, patients develop cardiogenic shock in addition to a primary cause of shock). In the circumstance of a primary cardiac etiology of shock, the heart is unable to tolerate any further decline in function. Once a patient begins to develop poor myocardial function, clinical status often declines rapidly. Patients in cardiogenic shock are known to deteriorate precipitously and to be especially difficult to resuscitate.

## OBSTRUCTIVE SHOCK

Mechanical obstruction to filling or emptying of the right or left ventricle is the essence of obstructive shock. Cardiac tamponade due to pericardial effusion and tension pneumothorax are 2 causes of obstructive shock that are usually reversible when recognized and treated quickly. Cardiac tamponade occurs when blood, fluid (eg, exudates in inflammatory disorders), or air fills the pericardial space and restricts cardiac filling in diastole. Drainage of the pericardial space by pericardiocentesis can be lifesaving. In tension pneumothorax, air under pressure fills a pleural space, causing a shift of the mediastinum to the opposite side and resulting in obstruction of heart filling. A rapidly growing pleural effusion as occurs with traumatic hemothorax has the same effect. Relief of pressure in the pleural space by needle thoracostomy in tension pneumothorax or placement of a chest tube in the case of hemothorax can be effective rapidly and lifesaving. The incidence of pulmonary embolism rises in the adolescent years associated with the use of oral contraceptives in females, leg trauma in males, and hypercoagulable conditions caused by collagen vascular and oncologic diseases.[7] Massive pulmonary embolism can obstruct right ventricular outflow, resulting in a critical decrease in cardiac output and precipitating right ventricular failure due to the acute, unrelieved increase in right ventricular afterload.

## DISSOCIATIVE SHOCK

Dissociative shock results from a disorder in the transport or utilization of oxygen. Etiologies of dissociative shock include carbon monoxide (CO) and cyanide poisonings, and methemoglobinemia. In CO poisoning, the CO molecule binds to hemoglobin-occupying sites normally used for oxygen binding. In addition, CO alters the conformation of hemoglobin so as to hinder both uptake of oxygen in the lungs and offloading of oxygen in the tissues.[8] In cyanide poisoning, the cyanide ion binds to cytochrome A3, bringing oxidative phosphorylation to a halt. Oxygen that is delivered to tissue beds cannot be used to manufacture ATP.[9] In methemoglobinemia, the change in oxidation state of the iron in hemoglobin from +2 to +3 renders hemoglobin unable to bind oxygen.[10] Successful treatment of dissociative shock requires recognizing and reversing the primary defect. Carbon monoxide, cyanide, and methemoglobinemia are not usually obvious as origins of shock, and thus, a high degree of suspicion for these should be maintained when other etiologies of impaired oxygen delivery are not evident.

## CLINICAL RECOGNITION OF SHOCK

### GENERAL

Prompt recognition and institution of therapy is important to survival in all forms of shock. Many of the signs and symptoms of shock are the result of compensatory mechanisms that are activated in order to maintain oxygen delivery to the tissues. Compensatory mechanisms include tachycardia and increased vasomotor tone, strength of cardiac contraction, and venous tone. Hypovolemia triggers a number of compensatory adjustments in response to decreased organ perfusion. Decreased central venous pressure (CVP) and cardiac filling induces an increase in antidiuretic hormone release from the pituitary. Baro- and chemoreceptors in the arterial circulation sense inadequate pressure and flow, which results in an increase in sympathetic nervous system tone. Epinephrine and norepinephrine are released by the adrenals, and vasopressin is released by the pituitary gland. A decrease in renal perfusion activates the renin-angiotensin system, resulting in aldosterone secretion. Changes in the microcirculation promote movement of fluid from the interstitium into the capillaries. The result is an effort to restore, or at least maintain, blood volume by retaining sodium and water through translocation of extracellular fluid into the intravascular space at the capillary level. The increase in catecholamines induces an early increase in heart rate and contractility. In addition, the catecholamines and vasopressin cause centralization of the blood volume via venoconstriction and maintenance of systemic blood pressure via arterial vasoconstriction. Circulation to vital organs such as the brain, heart, and lungs is maintained at the expense of the peripheral tissues such as the skin, muscle, and splanchnic beds, including the kidneys.

It is important to recognize when the vital signs of heart rate, respiratory rate, and blood pressure are outside age-appropriate ranges. Abnormalities in heart rate and respirations are often present in the earliest stages of compensated shock. Although a dropping blood pressure is a sign of uncompensated shock and happens relatively late, it is the vital sign alteration that is recognized most frequently in the diagnosis of shock.

Even though vital signs exist in a wide range, there are some guidelines that can be used in assessing patients that are in shock. In adolescents, a heart rate less than 50 or greater than 130 is abnormal. A systolic blood pressure of less than 90 mm in a patient older than 10 years is hypotension. A respiratory rate greater than 30 is abnormal. Normal blood pressures for 15-year-old adolescents range from 93 to 131 systolic over 45 to 85 diastolic. An additional variable used for evaluation of adequacy of vital signs is the perfusion pressure, which is defined as the mean arterial pressure minus the CVP. A lower limit of 65 mm Hg for perfusion pressure is cited for adolescents.[1,11,12] Capillary refill should normally be brisk and less than 2 seconds. An important reason to know the normal limits of these vital signs is that they serve as targets for which to aim in the course of goal-directed resuscitation.

**Table 87-2**

**American College of Critical Care Medicine Hemodynamic Definitions of Shock**

| *Type* | *Definition* |
|---|---|
| Cold shock | Decreased perfusion manifested by altered mental status, capillary refill >2 sec, diminished peripheral pulses, mottled cool extremities, or decreased urine output <1 mL/kg/h |
| Warm shock | Decreased perfusion manifested by altered mental status, flash capillary refill, bounding peripheral pulses, or decreased urine output <1 mL/kg/h |
| Fluid refractory/ dopamine-resistant shock | Shock persists despite ≥60 mL/kg fluid resuscitation (when appropriate) and dopamine infusion to 10 mcg/kg/min |
| Catecholamine-resistant shock | Shock persists despite use of direct-acting catecholamines: epinephrine or norepinephrine |
| Refractory shock | Shock persists despite goal-directed use of inotropic agents, vasopressors, vasodilators, and maintenance of metabolic (glucose, calcium) and hormonal (thyroid, hydrocortisone, insulin) homeostasis |

Shock is described by the physical examination and response to therapeutic intervention. Table 87-2 lists the American College of Critical Care Medicine hemodynamic definitions of shock.[12] Although designed for severe sepsis and septic shock, these definitions have wide applicability in shock due to many etiologies.

## HYPOVOLEMIC SHOCK

Patients with clinical signs of early compensated hypovolemic shock are tachycardic with cool mottled extremities that show a prolonged capillary refill. Peripheral pulses are decreased in amplitude, whereas blood pressure may be within a normal range. The pulse pressure may be narrowed. Urine output is diminished and may be maximally concentrated. Neurologic status is usually normal, although mild impairment may be manifested as lethargy, irritability, or confusion. An increase in vasomotor tone may maintain perfusion to vital organs, despite a decreased blood flow. As a result, the patient's systolic blood pressure may be normal or even slightly elevated.

Failure to successfully interrupt compensated shock will result in ongoing tissue hypoperfusion and will ultimately result in worsening organ dysfunction. The heart will eventually fail, followed by rapid deterioration in pulmonary and renal function. Progressive neurologic deterioration will occur, including the autonomic centers responsible for regulation of circulation and breathing. Metabolic acidosis will become severe and intractable. Mortality becomes high in late decompensated shock.

## CARDIOGENIC SHOCK

Clinical findings in cardiogenic shock include a decrease in peripheral perfusion with cool mottled extremities and diminished pulse strength, as seen in hypovolemic shock. Clinical findings mimic cold shock (see below). It is reasonable to assume that cold shock is cardiogenic in origin, especially if it persists after volume resuscitation. In addition, there are signs of volume overload and decreased heart function, such as distended jugular veins, enlarged liver and spleen sizes, and perhaps peripheral edema. Patients in cardiogenic shock are often dyspneic and hypoxemic due to pulmonary edema. There may be crackles on lung auscultation, and these may increase with fluid administration. Gallops, murmurs, and irregular rate and rhythm may be present on cardiac examination. Central venous pressure is high as compared wtih hypovolemic shock in which the CVP is low. Cardiogenic shock may move rapidly from a compensated to an uncompensated to an irreversible state.

## DISTRIBUTIVE SHOCK

Distributive shock is characterized by inappropriate distribution of blood flow with inadequate organ and tissue perfusion as a consequence. Septic shock, anaphylactic shock, and neurogenic shock are all forms of distributive shock. Septic shock is the most prevalent and epidemiologically important of these presentations. Growing numbers of adolescents receiving immune-suppressive therapies or with primary immune deficiencies make distributive shock due to sepsis a problem of increasing importance. Distributive shock caused by sepsis is characterized by an abnormal reduction in systemic vascular tone, resulting in an abnormal distribution of blood flow. Inappropriate arterial vasodilation combined with venodilation causes pooling of blood in the venous capacitance system and relative hypovolemia. Profound inflammation in septic shock also causes increased capillary permeability, so there is loss of plasma from the vascular space, increasing the severity of the hypovolemia.

In anaphylactic shock, arterial dilation, venodilation, and increased capillary permeability combine with pulmonary vasoconstriction to reduce cardiac output due to relative hypovolemia and increased right ventricular afterload. Neurogenic shock is characterized by generalized loss of vascular tone, most often following a high cervical spinal cord injury.

Cardiac output may be increased, normal, or decreased in distributive shock. Tachycardia, increased diastolic volume, and decreased vasomotor tone combine to maintain and even increase cardiac output.[13] Tissue perfusion is compromised due to misdistribution of blood flow. Patients may present with warm extremities and bounding peripheral pulses (ie, warm shock). Patients may also present with vasoconstriction, resulting in decreased blood flow to the skin, cold extremities, and weak pulses (ie, cold shock). Cold shock is associated with severely diminished cardiac output. As distributive shock progresses unchecked, concomitant hypovolemia and myocardial dysfunction produce a fall in cardiac output. Tissues without adequate oxygen delivery generate lactic acid, leading to metabolic acidosis. In the warm phase of septic shock, unlike hypovolemic and cardiogenic shock, venous oxygen saturation may be normal or even increased. Cold septic shock is characterized by profoundly decreased venous oxygen saturation.

## SEPTIC SHOCK

Severe sepsis (acute organ dysfunction secondary to infection) and septic shock (severe sepsis plus hypotension not reversed with fluid resuscitation) affect millions of individuals around the world each year, with mortality rates ranging from 25% to 50%.[14] Outcomes from septic shock are significantly better in children and adolescents than adults.[15] The incidence of severe sepsis in all children is 0.56 per 1,000 population, with about 42,000 cases per year in the United States and an associated case fatality rate of 10.3%, and about 4,400 deaths annually. Between the ages of 10 and 19 years, the incidence ranges from 0.2 to 0.37 per 1,000 population and includes about 10,000 cases per year, with a case fatality rate of approximately 9.7%, yielding about 1,000 deaths per year in this age range.[3] Septic shock is the most common and epidemiologically important manifestation of distributive shock.

Severe sepsis is precipitated by infectious organisms (bacteria, viruses, or fungi), their by-products (eg, endotoxin or exotoxin), and the host response to these inciting triggers. The immune system's response is to secrete a mixture of proinflammatory (tumor necrosis factor, interleukin-1, and interleukin-8) and anti-inflammatory (interleukin-6, interleukin-10) cytokines. These cytokines affect neutrophil-endothelial adhesion, activation of clotting, and generation of numerous secondary inflammatory mediators, including other cytokines, prostaglandins, leukotrienes, and proteases. The anti-inflammatory cytokines may provide negative feedback to the inflammatory processes.[16]

Severe sepsis and septic shock in adolescents evolve along a continuum that begins with a systemic inflammatory response in the early stages, progressing to septic shock in the late stages. Ultimately, the failure of multiple organ systems will develop. This continuum may develop over a few hours to as long as days with a wide variety of clinical presentation and rate of progression.

In the early stages of the systemic inflammatory response, sepsis is often subtle and difficult to recognize because peripheral perfusion may appear to be good. Because sepsis is triggered by an infection or its by-products, a patient may demonstrate fever or hypothermia and an elevated or decreased white blood cell count. A patient with septic shock may have petechiae or purpura, in cases associated with meningococcemia, but any severe infection resulting in disseminated intravascular coagulopathy can have a similar presentation.

Distinct hemodynamic patterns have been observed in patients with septic shock, depending on the etiology. Fluid-resistant septic shock secondary to central venous catheter–associated infections has been found to be warm shock with a high cardiac index and a low systemic vascular resistance index. In contrast, in community-acquired sepsis, a normal or low cardiac index is predominant.[17] Younger patients tend to have greater cardiac dysfunction and hence cold shock in sepsis, thus leading to an evidence-based recommendation that dopamine be the first drug used for support of the fluid-resistant septic pediatric patient.[12] Adolescents mostly manifest the severe drop in vasomotor tone characteristic of adults but may, on occasion, have cardiovascular presentations similar to pediatric patients. The pathophysiology of the septic shock cascade includes the events in Box 87-2.[18]

### Box 87-2
### *Events of Septic Shock*

- Infectious organism or its by-products (eg, endotoxin) activate the immune system, inclu eutrophils, monocytes, and macrophages.
- These cells, or their interaction with the infecting organism, stimulate release or activation of inflammatory cytokines.
- Cytokines produce vasodilation and increased capillary permeability.
- Uncontrolled activation of inflammatory mediators can lead to organ failure, particularly cardiovascular and respiratory failure, systemic thrombosis, and adrenal dysfunction.

Vasodilatation and increased capillary permeability can produce maldistribution of blood flow, hypovolemia, and hypotension. Cardiac output may be normal or increased as a result of tachycardia and low afterload. In some patients, specific inflammatory mediators produce myocardial dysfunction that when combined with vasodilatation and capillary leak can cause low cardiac output with inadequate systemic perfusion and oxygen delivery. Absolute or relative adrenal insufficiency is often present and can contribute to cardiovascular dysfunction.[19-23]

In 2005, an international panel of experts developed consensus definitions for the clinical characteristics of pediatric sepsis,[24] based on an earlier adult consensus statement.[25] Aspects of both consensus statements are applicable to adolescent patients. There is strong emphasis on the role of the host responses to the septic insult. The continuum of host response is broken down into the systemic inflammatory response syndrome (SIRS), sepsis, severe sepsis, and septic shock.

**Systemic inflammatory response syndrome** endeavors to capture the earliest manifestations of an infectious insult that can be a harbinger of septic shock. It is defined by the presence of at least 2 of the following 4 criteria, 1 of which must be abnormal temperature or leukocyte count:

- Core temperature >101.3°F (38.5°C) or <96.8°F (36°C)
- Tachycardia (mean heart rate >2 standard deviations above normal for age) in the absence of external stimulus, chronic drugs or pain, or otherwise unexplained persistent elevation over a 0.5- to 4-hour time period

- Mean respiratory rate >2 standard deviations above normal for age or mechanical ventilation for an acute process not related to underlying neuromuscular disease or general anesthesia
- Leukocyte count elevated or depressed for age (not induced by chemotherapy) or >10% immature neutrophils

Adult SIRS criteria[10] may apply to older adolescents. Adult patients have to meet at least 3 of the following 4 criteria:

- Core temperature ≥100.4°F (38°C) or ≤96.8°F (36°C)
- Heart rate ≥90 beats/min (except in patients with medical conditions known to increase the heart rate or those receiving treatment that would prevent tachycardia)
- Respiratory rate ≥20 breaths/min or a $PaCO_2$ ≤32 mm Hg or use of mechanical ventilation for an acute respiratory process
- White blood cell count ≥12,000/mm$^3$ or ≤4,000/mm$^3$ or a differential count showing >10% immature neutrophils

**Sepsis** is defined as SIRS in the presence of, or as the result of, suspected or proven infection. **Severe sepsis** is defined as sepsis plus either cardiovascular dysfunction or acute respiratory distress syndrome or sepsis plus failure of 2 or more organs.

**Septic shock** is defined as sepsis (SIRS in the presence of, or as the result of, suspected or proven infection) and cardiovascular dysfunction, despite administration of isotonic intravenous fluid administration boluses ≥40 mL/kg in 1 hour. Cardiovascular dysfunction is characterized by the following:

- Hypotension (systolic blood pressure <5th percentile for age <2 standard deviations below normal for age) *or*
- Need for vasoactive drug to maintain blood pressure in normal range *or*
- Two of the following characteristics of inadequate organ perfusion:
  - Unexplained metabolic acidosis: base deficit >5 mEq/L
  - Increased arterial lactate greater than twice the upper limit of normal
  - Oliguria: urine output <0.5 mL/kg per hour
  - Prolonged capillary refill: >5 seconds
  - Core to peripheral temperature gap >3°C

Cardiovascular dysfunction is defined as a systolic blood pressure ≤90 mm Hg or a mean arterial pressure ≤70 mm Hg for at least one hour despite adequate fluid resuscitation, adequate intravascular volume status, or use of vasopressors in an attempt to maintain a systolic blood pressure of ≥90 mm Hg or a mean arterial pressure of ≥70 mm Hg.

Capillary permeability is increased in sepsis, and pulmonary edema may develop during volume resuscitation. The risk of pulmonary edema should not prevent adequate volume resuscitation to restore vital organ perfusion, even if mechanical ventilatory support is needed. Despite this concern, aggressive and rapid fluid resuscitation of patients with septic shock, while demonstrating improved survival and good clinical outcome, has not been associated with any increase in cardiogenic pulmonary edema or adult respiratory distress syndrome.[26,27] Vasoactive therapy is often needed to control the vasodilatation and restore adequate blood pressure. Myocardial dysfunction may develop and is an indication for inotropic support. If adrenal dysfunction is present or suspected, corticosteroid therapy is indicated.

Early recognition and treatment of septic shock are critically important determinants of outcome.[28-30] Optimally, careful evaluation of systemic perfusion and clinical signs of end-organ function will permit identification of impending shock before hypotension develops. Once sepsis is identified, there needs to be an aggressive search for and treatment of the causative organism. Management of septic shock without adequate treatment of the infectious etiology will not be successful.

## MANAGEMENT OF SHOCK

### GENERAL APPROACH

Successful outcome for a patient in shock is contingent on early implementation of aggressive measures titrated to the clinical goal of restoration of tissue perfusion and oxygenation. Current guidelines stress the importance of goal-directed resuscitation in which the restoration of threshold rates of heart rate, normal blood pressure, urine output ≥1 mL/kg/h and capillary refill ≤2 seconds are targeted. In the intensive care unit, hemodynamic support is targeted at goals of a central venous saturation of >70% and a cardiac index of 3.3 to 6 L/min/m.[12] Data show a direct relationship between the amount of time it takes to reverse shock and mortality.[28,31]

### VOLUME RESUSCITATION

Shock may result from either absolute (hypovolemic shock) or relative (distributive shock) hypovolemia. The exception to hypovolemia is cardiogenic shock in which there is usually relative hypervolemia, and fluid boluses, although sometimes necessary, must be administered very cautiously. Rapid restoration of an effective circulating blood volume is the most important first step. Isotonic crystalloids such as 0.9% sodium chloride (normal saline) or Ringer's lactate administered intravenously or by intraosseous needle are the first-line fluids. The intraosseous route of administration can be used effectively in adolescents and can be effected more rapidly than the time it takes to place a central venous catheter. In hypovolemic shock due to hemorrhage, blood should be considered if a patient remains in shock (acidosis, elevated blood lactate) after initial efforts at crystalloid resuscitation.

Evidence-based guidelines recommend boluses of 20 mL/kg of isotonic crystalloid administered up to a total volume of 60 mL/kg over a time frame of 20 minutes. The large volumes and rapidity of administration demand the presence of large-bore, secure venous access. Fluid bolus administration should be titrated to clinical and physiological end points (see previous) in order to provide adequate resuscitation and avoid complications such as pulmonary and tissue edema. Rapid bolus administration of 20 mL/kg of crystalloid or 10 mL/kg of colloid is followed by an assessment for an improvement in heart rate, blood pressure, capillary refill, strength of peripheral pulses, urinary output, and mental status. If little or no improvement occurs, a second (or third) bolus is administered.

## RESPIRATORY SUPPORT

Patients in shock often require intubation in order to ensure adequate oxygenation and ventilation. An additional advantage of intubation and mechanical ventilatory support is removal of the work of breathing. The oxygen cost of breathing can be very high in times of stress, and intubation and mechanical ventilation can take that away. The process of intubation can be hemodynamically destabilizing, however, and it is important to initiate volume and vasopressor resuscitation prior to intubation in order to minimize the cardiovascular deterioration. It is worthwhile to consider invasive monitoring of blood pressure by an arterial line in preparation for intubation in order to monitor blood pressure changes with beat-to-beat precision. The drop-in blood pressure that may occur when an inadequately resuscitated patient is placed on positive-pressure ventilation may be so severe as to cause cardiac arrest.

## MONITORING

If a patient remains in shock despite 60 mL/kg of fluid resuscitation, he or she is labeled as being in fluid refractory shock. Arterial and central venous catheters, as well as Foley urinary catheters, provide additional physiological data that can be used to guide further titration of volume infusion and institution of pharmacologic support of the circulation. Patients in advanced stages of shock with multiple organ system involvement may require placement of a pulmonary artery catheter in order to measure cardiac output and obtain a more detailed evaluation of their physiological disturbances in oxygen supply and demand. Venous saturation measuring central venous catheters, Doppler sonography, transpulmonary thermodilution, and lithium dilution are techniques developed for determining cardiac output less invasively than pulmonary artery catheters, and all have found use in monitoring patients in shock.[5]

Low CVP indicates that additional volume resuscitation is needed. A high CVP in the face of low blood pressure or compromised perfusion suggests the need for vasopressor or inotropic support. In general, a low blood pressure—especially diastolic—in the face of warm extremities (warm shock) suggests the need for a drug with primarily vasopressor qualities, such as norepinephrine or vasopressin. A patient with a low blood pressure and cool extremities and decreased pulses is presumed to be in cardiogenic shock (cold shock) and will benefit from a drug that increases the contractile properties of the heart—an inotrope. If the blood pressure is low in a patient with cardiogenic shock, then epinephrine is the drug of choice. If a patient is poorly perfused after volume resuscitation, yet has an acceptable blood pressure, then an agent such as milrinone, which strengthens the contractile properties of the heart while acting as a vasodilator, is the drug of choice. In circumstances where the picture is less clear, an agent such as dopamine, which has inotropic, pressor, and even vasodilatory properties at very low doses, is a reasonable agent with which to initiate treatment.

## METABOLIC AND ENDOCRINE RESUSCITATION

Hypocalcemia is frequently found in patients in shock. Correction of this and other biochemical abnormalities can improve hemodynamic status.

There is a role for examining the endocrinologic state of patients in shock. The use of exogenous steroids is required in the treatment of hypoadrenal states such as Addison disease and adrenal hemorrhage in Waterhouse Frederickson, and in patients who have been chronically receiving steroids as treatment for other disease processes. Contemporary studies have yielded mixed results for the use of supplemental steroids in nonsteroid-dependent patients.[15,32] It is a reasonable approach to assess baseline serum cortisol, or perhaps perform an abbreviated corticotropin stimulation test in patients who are found to be in shock states refractory to volume resuscitation and modest vasopressor and inotrope dosing in order to see if the patient is in an absolute or relative state of adrenal insufficiency. If a patient is relatively or absolutely hypoadrenal, consideration can be given to administering stress-level dosing of hydrocortisone. Similarly, examination of thyroid function can be carried out, with replacement of thyroid hormone or the active metabolite tri-iodothyronine (T3) in order to support such a patient.

Hypoglycemia and hyperglycemia are seen in shock. Hypoglycemia is corrected by administration of IV dextrose. The role of tight glucose control using insulin infusions in critically ill patients remains a topic for debate. The potential for hypoglycemia in critically ill patients without diabetes remains a concern for adolescent patients on insulin drips.[33]

## ALGORITHM FOR APPROACH TO MANAGEMENT OF SHOCK

Using evidence-based recommendations to the extent that they are available, a consensus agreement for an approach to the management of shock was designed and published under the auspices of the Society of Critical Care Medicine, the American College of Critical Care Medicine, and the Pediatric Advanced Life Support section of the American Heart Association. The algorithm was designed for septic shock specifically but has wide applicability to other forms of shock. The algorithm (Figure 87-1) stresses rapid administration of volume, careful and repetitive reassessment, and moving on to the next step as rapidly as possible when goals of normalization of vital signs are not obtained.[14]

## PHARMACOLOGIC AGENTS IN THE MANAGEMENT OF SHOCK

The use of pharmacologic agents to support the circulation is a hallmark of shock management. **Inotropic** agents improve cardiac performance by increasing myocardial contractility. **Vasoconstrictors** increase vascular tone by stimulation of α-adrenergic or vasopressin receptors. Dopamine, dobutamine, and epinephrine stimulate β-1-adrenergic receptors, resulting in increased flux of calcium into the myocardial cell, which strengthens the contractile function of the myocardium as well as increases heart rate. At higher doses, dopamine and epinephrine also stimulate α-receptors, which results in vasoconstriction in a degree proportional to the dose of the drug. These agents are administered as continuous intravenous infusions, with doses titrated to clinical and physiological end points. The onset of action for these drugs is within minutes, and they have short half-lives (minutes).[34-36]

The agents used to modulate the inotropic and vasomotor tone of the cardiovascular system are short acting and are administered by continuous infusion. Current Joint Commission guidelines recommend that these agents be prepared as fixed concentration solutions and administered at a rate that yields the desired dose of drug. Although administration of vasoconstrictors is preferably via central vein due to the risk of tissue injury from extravasation, the current recommendation is that dilute solutions of these agents may be administered by peripheral IV while central line placement is accomplished. In general, invasive arterial and CVP monitoring should be performed when these agents are used.

## SPECIFIC AGENTS

**Dopamine** is a naturally occurring catecholamine precursor of norepinephrine. Its cardiovascular effects are dose dependent. At low doses (0.5–2 μg/kg/min), the drug acts at the dopaminergic receptors of the kidney and splanchnic viscera, causing vasodilatation and increased blood flow. Although dopaminergic receptors do exist as pharmacologic entities, their role in improving splanchnic and renal blood flow has been questioned. Doses of dopamine between 2 and 12 μg/kg/min yield predominantly β-adrenergic effects that include increase in heart rate and contractility due to β1-receptor agonism. As the dose of dopamine increases, so does the degree of agonism at the α-receptor, which yields progressively increasing amounts of vasoconstriction. When the dose of dopamine approaches 12 to 15 μg/kg/min, a significant vasoconstrictor effect occurs in addition to the β-adrenergic effects already present. This mixed receptor agonism of dopamine results in significant tachycardia and increased contractility when dopamine is used predominantly as a vasoconstrictor for vasodilatory septic shock. Although dopamine continues to be the first agent for the management of shock in children and adolescents, transition to an agent with greater vasoconstrictor specificity, such as norepinephrine, should occur whenever modest doses (≤10 μg/kg/min) of dopamine do not result in acceptable clinical improvement. It is not our usual practice to administer dopamine at doses of more than 20 μg/kg/min. Prolonged use of dopamine has been associated with immune suppression due to inhibition of prolactin synthesis.[37]

**Dobutamine** is a semisynthetic derivative of isoproterenol and a β-receptor stimulator. It increases cardiac contractility with minimal to no vasoconstriction. Its action on the peripheral vasculature is to vasodilate peripheral and pulmonary arterioles. The usual dosage range is 5 to 15 μg/kg/min. It is an appropriate agent to use to support inotropy and cardiac output without increasing systemic vascular resistance. An increase in

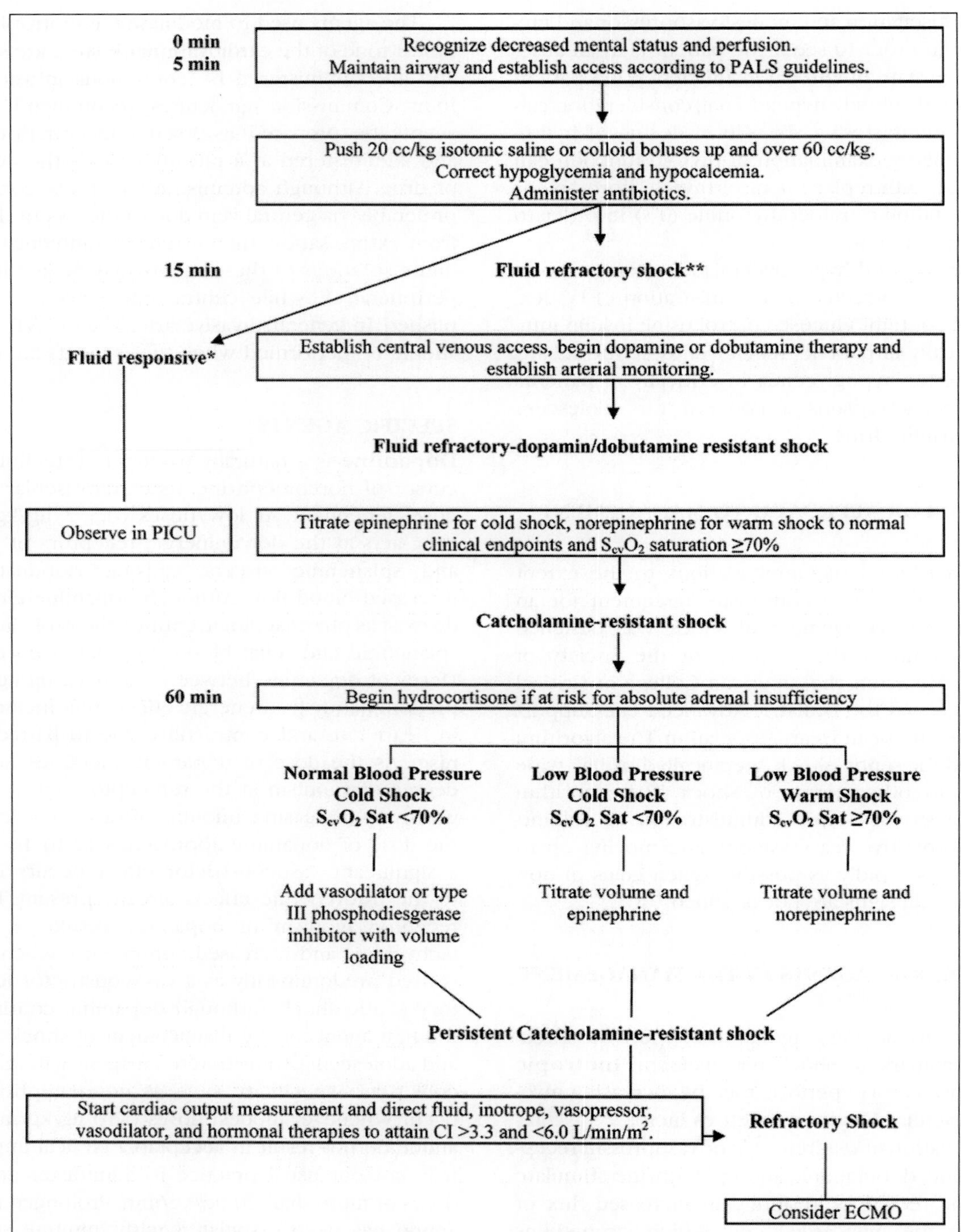


**FIGURE 87-1** Approach to pediatric shock. *Normalization of blood pressure and tissue perfusion; **hypotension, abnormal capillary refill or extremity coolness. PALS, Pediatric Advanced Life Support; PICU, pediatric intensive care unit; CI, cardiac index; ECMO, extracorporeal membrane oxygenation. (From Carcillo JA, Fields AI (task force committee members). Clinical practice parameters for hemodynamic support of pediatric and neonatal patients in septic shock. *Crit Care Med.* 2002;30:1365-1378.)

inotropy without an increase in systemic vascular resistance makes dobutamine a useful agent in the management of cardiogenic shock. In septic shock that is dominated by hypotension, dobutamine used in combination with a vasopressor, such as norepinephrine or vasopressin, serves to increase the inotropic state.

**Norepinephrine** is the major catechol neurotransmitter of the sympathetic nervous system. It has potent vasoconstrictor and inotropic effects in the dosage range of 0.1 to 1 μg/kg/min. It is particularly useful in restoring peripheral vascular tone, blood pressure, and tissue perfusion in early septic shock during the hyperdynamic "warm shock" phase. Norepinephrine is the drug of choice for warm shock in adults. As a more potent α-adrenergic agent than dopamine, norepinephrine has a greater effect on vasomotor tone and hence blood pressure at a lower dose than an agent such as dopamine.

**Epinephrine** is a potent adrenergic agent with dose-related receptor specificity. At low doses (0.05–0.2 μg/kg/min), β-1 and β-2 agonism predominate, resulting in increased heart rate, increased contractility, and peripheral and pulmonary artery vasodilatation. The systemic vascular resistance and diastolic blood pressure go down with low-dose epinephrine. This results in improved cardiac output. At higher doses (0.2–1 μg/kg/min), α-adrenergic effects occur in a dose-dependent fashion, resulting in increasing amounts of vasoconstriction. It is the drug of choice in shock with severely compromised cardiac output. High doses of epinephrine can result in severe tachycardia, a hyperdynamic contractile state, and severe vasoconstriction. Doses greater than 1 μg/kg/min are not usual. Epinephrine is the drug of choice for the management of cold shock in adolescent patients that have not responded to fluid loading and modest doses of dopamine.

**Vasopressin** is a potent endogenous noncatecholamine vasoconstrictor that can be used in situations that demand a pure vasopressor agent that does not increase myocardial oxygen demand.[38] At a dosage range beginning at 0.5 milliunit/kg/min, vasopressin has been shown to be a potent vasoconstrictor. Maximum dosages have not been established, but severe vasoconstriction may occur and must be monitored.

**Milrinone** is a phosphodiesterase-3 inhibitor and has the properties of an inodilator. Milrinone increases contractility and vasodilates the peripheral and pulmonary arterial vasculature. This vasodilatation results in decreased afterload to the right and left heart and hence increased cardiac output. Milrinone also has the unique property of being a lusitrope, which means that it improves the ability of the heart chambers to fill in diastole. This property makes it particularly helpful in diastolic heart failure. Milrinone is used in a dosage range of 0.3 to 1 μg/kg/min, with 0.5 μg/kg/min being the most typical starting dose. Due to its long half-life, a loading dose of 50 μg/kg administered over 30 minutes is usually given at the initiation of milrinone therapy. Caution should be exercised in using milrinone in patients with renal failure or worsening renal compromise in that it can accumulate, resulting in profound hypotension.

It must be emphasized that the various etiologies and stages of shock cause significant alterations in drug metabolism and response, making it necessary to titrate the dose against clinical effect.

## CONCLUSION

Early recognition of shock and aggressive resuscitation are the keys to improved outcome. Once perfusion is re-established and the patient is adequately resuscitated, a definitive diagnosis can be pursued. Appropriate cultures should be obtained and antibiotics administered to patients in septic shock. Patients in shock should be transferred to an intensive care setting where the technology and expertise exists for definitive physiological monitoring and management of the disturbances that can occur after reperfusion.

## REFERENCES


1. Ralston M, Hazinski MF, Zaritsky AL, Schexanayder AM, Kleinman ME. Recognition of shock. In: Ralston M, Hazinski MF, Zaritsky AL, Schexanayder AM, Kleinman ME, eds. *Pediatric Advanced Life Support Provider Manual*. Dallas: American Heart Association; 2005:61–80

2. Kumar A, Roberts D, Wood KE, et al. Duration of hypotension prior to initiation of effective antimicrobial therapy is the critical determinant of survival in human septic shock. *Crit Care Med.* 2006;34:1589–1596

3. Watson RS, Carcillo JA, Linde-Zwirble WT, Clermont G, Lidicker J, Angus D. The epidemiology of severe sepsis in children in the United States. *Am J Respir Crit Care Med.* 2003;167:695–701.

4. Rivers E, Nguyen JC, Havstad S, et al. Early goal-directed therapy in the treatment of severe sepsis and septic shock. *N Engl J Med.* 2001;345:1368–1377

5. Tibby SM, Murdoch IA. Measurement of cardiac output and tissue perfusion. *Curr Opin Pediatr.* 2002;14:303–309

6. Landry DW, Oliver JA. The pathogenesis of vasodilatory shock. *N Engl J Med.* 2001;345(8):588–595

7. Bernstein D, Coupey S, Schonberg SK. Pulmonary embolism in adolescents. *Am J Dis Child.* 1986;140:667–671

8. Weaver LK. Carbon monoxide poisoning. *N Engl J Med.* 2009;360:1217–1225

9. Hall AH. Cyanide and related compounds—sodium azide. In: Shannon MW, Borron SW, Burns MJ, eds. *Haddad and Winchester's Clinical Management of Poisoning and Drug Overdose*. 4th ed. Philadelphia, PA: Lippincott Wilkins & Williams;2007:1309-1316

10. Curry SC. Hematologic consequences of poisoning. In: Shannon MW, Borron SW, Burns MJ, eds. *Haddad and Winchester's Clinical Management of Poisoning and Drug Overdose*. 4th ed. Philadelphia: PA; Lippincott, Wilkins & Williams; 2007:291-295

11. Carcillo JA, Fields AI (Task Force Committee Members). Clinical practice parameters for hemodynamic support of pediatric and neonatal patients in septic shock. *Crit Care Med.* 2002;30:1365-1378

12. Brierly J, Carcillo JA, Choong K (Task Force Committee Members). Clinical practice parameters for hemodynamic support of pediatric and neonatal septic shock: 2007 update for the American College of Critical Care Medicine. *Crit Care Med.* 2009;37:666-688

13. Parker MM, Parillo, JE. Septic shock: hemodynamics and pathogenesis. *JAMA.* 1983;250:3324-3327

14. Dellinger RP, Levy MM, Carlet JM, et al. Surviving Sepsis Campaign: international guidelines for management of severe sepsis and septic shock: 2008. *Crit Care Med.* 2008;36:296-327

15. Kutko MC, Calarco MP, Flaherty MB, et al. Mortality rates in pediatric septic shock with and without multiple organ system failure. *Pediatr Crit Care.* 2003;4:333-337

16. Wheeler AP, Bernard GR. Treating patients with severe sepsis. *N Engl J Med.* 1999;340:207-214

17. Brierly J, Peter MJ. Distinct hemodynamic pattern of septic shock at presentation to pediatric intensive care. *Pediatrics.* 2008;122:752-759

18. Carcillo JA. Pediatric septic shock and multiple organ failure. *Crit Care Clin.* 2003;19:413-440

19. Annane D, Sebille V, Charpentier C,et al. Effect of treatment with low doses of hydrocortisone and fludrocortisone on mortality in patients with septic shock. *JAMA.* 2002;288:862-871

20. Pizarro CF, Troster EJ, Damiani D, Carcillo JA. Absolute and relative adrenal insufficiency in children with septic shock. *Crit Care Med.* 2005;33:855-859

21. Sarthi M, Lodha R, Vivekanandhan S, Arora NK. Adrenal status in children with septic shock using low-dose stimulation test. *Pediatr Crit Care Med.* 2007;8:23-28

22. Aneja R, Carcillo JA. What is the rationale for hydrocortisone treatment in children with infection-related adrenal insufficiency and septic shock? *Ach Dis Child.* 2007;92:165-169

23. Marik PE, Pastores SM, Annane D, et al. Recommendations for the diagnosis and management of corticosteroid insufficiency in critically ill adult patients: consensus statements from an international task force by the American College of Critical Care Medicine. *Crit Care Med.* 2008;36:1937-1949

24. Goldstein B, Giroir B, Randolph A. International Pediatric Sepsis Consensus Conference: definitions for sepsis and organ dysfunction in pediatrics. *Pediatr Crit Care Med.* 2005;6:2-8

25. Bone RC, Balk RA, Cerra FB, et al, and Members of the ACCP/SCCM Consensus Conference. Definitions for sepsis and organ failure and guidelines for the use of innovative therapies in sepsis. *Chest.* 1992;101:1644-1655 and *Crit Care Med.* 1992;20:864-874

26. Ware LB, Matthay MA. The acute respiratory distress syndrome. *N Engl J Med.* 2000;342:1334-1349

27. Carcillo JA, Davis AL, Zaritsky A. Role of early fluid resuscitation in pediatric septic shock. *JAMA.* 1991;266: 1242-1245

28. Han YY, Carcillo JA, Dragotta MA, et al. Early reversal of pediatric-neonatal septic shock by community physicians is associated with improved outcome. *Pediatrics.* 2003;112:793-799

29. Booy R, Habibi P, Nadel S, et al. Reduction in case fatality rate from meningococcal disease associated with improved healthcare delivery. *Arch Dis Child.* 2001;85:386-390

30. Ninis N, Phillips C, Bailey L, et al. The role of healthcare delivery in the outcome of meningococcal disease in children: case-control study of fatal and non-fatal cases. *BMJ.* 2005;330:1475-1480

31. Oliveira CF, de Sa Nogueira FR, Oliveira DSF, et al. Time- and fluid-sensitive resuscitation for hemodynamic support of children in septic shock: barriers to the implementation of the American College of Critical Care Medicine/Pediatric Advanced Life Support guidelines in a pediatric intensive care unit in a developing world. *Pediatr Emerg Care.* 2008;24:810-815

32. Sprung CL, Annane D, Keh D, and the Corticus Study Group. Hydrocortisone therapy for patients with septic shock. *N Engl J Med.* 2008;358:111-124

33. Vlasselaers D, Milantis I, Desmet L, et al. Intensive insulin therapy for patients in paediatric intensive care: a prospective, randomized controlled study. *Lancet.* 2009;373:547-556

34. Ushay HM, Notterman DA. Pharmacology of pediatric resuscitation. *Pediatr Clin North Am.* 1997;44:207-233

35. Zuppa AF, Barrett JS. Pharmacology. In: Nichols DG, ed. *Rogers' Textbook of Pediatric Intensive Care.* 4th ed. Philadelphia: Lippincott Williams & Wilkins; 2008:266-282

36. Ralston M, Hazinski MF, Zaritsky AL, Schexanayder AM, Kleinman ME. Pharmacology. In: Ralston M, Hazinski MF, Zaritsky AL, Schexanayder AM, Kleinman ME, eds. *Pediatric Advanced Life Support Provider Manual.* Dallas: American Heart Association; 2005:221-255

37. Van der Berghe G, de Zegher F. Anterior pituitary function during critical illness and dopamine treatment. *Crit Care Med.* 1996;24:1580-1590

38. Choong K, Kissoon N. Vasopressin in pediatric shock and cardiac arrest. *Pediatr Crit Care Med.* 2008;9:372-379

SECTION 4

# The Respiratory System

# CHAPTER 88

## Upper Respiratory Tract Infections

TSOLINE KOJAOGHLANIAN, MD

The upper respiratory tract refers to the conducting portions of the respiratory system leading to the lower respiratory tract where respiration—exchange of oxygen and carbon dioxide—occurs. The upper respiratory tract comprises the nose, pharynx, larynx, and trachea. The paranasal sinuses drain into the nose and will be included in this discussion of upper respiratory tract infections (URTI). More viral infections are acquired via the respiratory route than any other route. Many viruses, such as influenza viruses and adenoviruses, have receptors on the epithelial cells throughout the respiratory tract. Bacteria often colonize the cells of the upper airways, leading to disease and transmissibility to others. Many infectious organisms such as varicella, mumps, measles, as well as *Neisseria meningitides, and Streptococcus pneumoniae*, which subsequently spread to other organs, enter the body via the upper respiratory tract. This chapter focuses on infections that cause symptomatology in the upper airways. As in all infections, disease is a result of the balance between the characteristics of the infectious agent and the host immune response. According to the National Ambulatory Medical Care Survey,[1] URTI are responsible for the largest proportion (40%) of all infectious disease visits and a substantial proportion (10%) of all outpatient visits.

## RHINITIS

*Rhinitis* refers to inflammation of the nasal mucosa. It is the most common reason for adolescents to visit a health care provider, as well as a major cause of school absence. Rhinitis, the common cold, is caused by various viruses that infect the respiratory cells. Annual illness rates reach adult levels in adolescence, with boys tending to have slightly higher numbers of colds. Cold severity increases with smoking. Rhinitis is characterized by nasal congestion, erythema, "scratchy" throat, and sneezing. Communicability is high, and is via aerosolized droplets of various sizes, as well as from animate (from hands to mucosa) and inanimate objects (environmental surfaces) depending on the characteristics of the virus (Table 88-1).[2]

### PATHOGENESIS

Common viruses causing rhinitis include the rhinoviruses, coronaviruses, parainfluenza viruses, respiratory syncytial virus (RSV), influenza (A, B, and C) viruses, and certain adenoviruses (Ads). Recently identified viruses such as metapneumovirus and bocavirus have emerged as causes of diverse respiratory illnesses,[3] and likely many other causative viruses are yet undiscovered. Rhinoviruses cause more than half of common colds yearly. There are more than 100 serotypes and there is a lack of antibody protection against reinfection. They are stable at various temperatures and resist drying. They multiply in the nose and characteristically induce a potent innate immune system activation and inflammation, release of bradykinin, histamine, and complement, leading to the sneeze reflex. Rhinoviruses cause minimal damage, however, to the columnar epithelium of the respiratory tract. All of the previously noted characteristics contribute to their high infectivity at small inocula. The respiratory syncytial virus, which causes acute respiratory disease across all age groups, has similarly high contagion potential as rhinoviruses. Upper respiratory tract infections caused by RSV tend to last longer than those caused by other common respiratory agents. Human coronaviruses OC43 and 229E cause one-third of common colds each winter. Reinfections are possible with all of these viruses, which do not establish latency and are cleared efficiently by the host immune system. Increased crowding is the major reason for the higher prevalence of URTI in the colder months, as well as some intrinsic

**Table 88-1**

**Effect of Types of Contact and Living Conditions on the Likelihood of Contagion from Common Bacterial and Viral Respiratory Tract Pathogens**

| *Variable* | *Risk of contagion* | | | | |
|---|---|---|---|---|---|
| | **Bacteria** | ***Mycobacterium tuberculosis*** | ***Influenzavirus*** | ***Rhinovirus, RSV*** | ***Other viruses*** |
| **Type or location of contact** | | | | | |
| Casual, social contact | Low | Low | Moderate | Low | Moderate |
| School, workplace | Moderate | Moderate | High | Low | Low |
| Bar, social club | High | High | High | Low | Low |
| Travel tour | Moderate | Moderate | High | Low | Low |
| Dormitory | Moderate | High | High | Moderate | Moderate |
| Home | High | High | High | Moderate | High |
| **Special conditions** | | | | | |
| Loss of air circulation | Moderate | High | High | None | Low |

RSV, respiratory syncytial virus

Reprinted by permission from Musher DM. How contagious are common respiratory tract infections? *N Engl J Med.* 2003;**348**(13):1262.

seasonality of some viruses. Transmission of influenza viruses and Ads is even more efficient because, in addition to direct contact and large-droplet aerosolization through which the aforementioned viruses also spread, these viruses spread via microdroplets or droplet nuclei, expelled during sneezing or coughing, some of which can reach the lungs and cause pneumonia. As few as 5 influenza virus particles can initiate and transmit infection. Furthermore, the pathogenesis of influenza viruses and Ads includes significant cytolysis of columnar epithelium, the ensuing inflammation inducing the cough reflex designed to clear the airways. Thus with influenza, fever, cough, myalgias, and headaches are prominent and can last longer than the common cold. Due to the highly error-prone influenza virus RNA polymerase, there is a high rate of mutations in the influenza hemagglutinin antigen (antigenic drift) to which the host antibody is directed, such that antibodies generated during an infection only minimally protect against the newly mutated strains, thus the need for new vaccines every year. In addition, influenza A, which also infects avian species, may swap genome segments with other animal viruses such as swine as well as human influenza viruses, leading to a new virus to which the population is completely naïve. With this possibility for antigenic shift, the potential for pandemics is inevitable. The Ads elicit a good protective antibody response and thus don't have the same potential as influenza viruses to cause epidemics.[4]

## DIAGNOSIS AND TREATMENT

Testing for the specific agent is generally not sought in most common colds because of the self-limited nature of the illness. Rapid detection of the specific virus causing the infection may help in specific patient populations, such as the immunocompromised, where the few available antiviral medications may help decrease the burden of disease. Multiplex polymerase chain reaction (PCR) testing and DNA microarrays of nasopharyngeal swabs or aspirates have been developed to diagnose infections resulting from a variety of viruses.[5] Their entry into generalized use requires clinically useful sensitivity and specificity, speedy results, and low cost. Prevention remains key: hand washing and avoidance of self-inoculation; covering the mouth while coughing/sneezing; and avoiding crowded areas, especially those with poor ventilation that facilitate droplet spread are measures shown to reduce transmissibility.[6] Compared with no education, hand-hygiene education alone significantly reduced the risk for respiratory illness by 14%.[7] Influenza vaccines are highly effective and should continue to be implemented.[8] Because of the potential for severe disease with influenza viruses in immunocompromised populations, early recognition and diagnosis is essential for provision of therapy. The neuraminidase inhibitor oseltamivir has been shown to reduce the severity and duration of symptoms, the complications arising from influenza infection (pneumonia, hospitalization, antibiotic use), and mortality. Resistance to antivirals remains a concern; for example, in January 2006 the Centers for Disease Control and Prevention (CDC) recommended therapy of influenza A virus with the neuraminidase inhibitors oseltamivir or zanamivir, noting that the circulating H3N2 strains of influenza A were almost uniformly resistant to both of the first-generation drugs (amantadine and rimantadine). The prevalence of oseltamivir resistance in influenza A (H1N1) viruses was significantly increased during the early 2007–2008 influenza season. Antivirals are also useful when there is a mismatch between the vaccine and the circulating virus.

## SINUSITIS

Sinusitis is one of the most commonly diagnosed diseases in the United States. It is defined as inflammation of 1 or more of the paranasal sinuses and is categorized as acute when symptoms last less than 4 weeks, subacute when between 4 and 8 weeks' duration, and chronic if symptoms persist for longer than 8 weeks. Most often, symptoms are preceded by a viral URTI, and because the opening of the maxillary sinus meatus is upward of the drainage and stasis, there is almost always sinus involvement with any viral URTI. Sneezing increases the pressure in the nasal passages, and this back pressure leads to spreading of the virus and ensuing inflammation to the sinuses and Eustachian tubes. In a small percentage of cases (<5%–10%), there may be bacterial superinfection in the inflamed sinus, resulting in bacterial sinusitis. Symptoms of acute bacterial sinusitis are nasal congestion, purulent rhinorrhea lasting for more than 5 to 7 days, facial–dental pain, postnasal drainage, headache, and cough. On examination, the nasal mucosa may be erythematous and there may be tenderness over the sinuses with periorbital edema.

### PATHOGENESIS

Typical organisms causing acute bacterial sinusitis are *Streptococcus pneumoniae*, *Hemophilus influenzae*, and *Moraxella catarrhalis* as well as oral anaerobes, and to a lesser extent *Staphylococcus aureus*. Complications may occur and include orbital cellulitis and/or abscess manifested by periorbital swelling and/or pain, proptosis and abnormal extraocular muscle movements. The pathogenesis is secondary to the paper-thin nature of the bone, appropriately termed lamina papyracea, dividing the ethmoid sinuses from the orbit, plus the presence of valveless emissary veins through which bacteria can translocate. Frontal sinusitis, which occurs typically in adolescent boys, may lead to intracranial extension of infection resulting in subdural and epidural empyemas,[9] meningitis, or extension into the cavernous venous sinus causing thrombophlebitis manifested by abnormal neurologic signs. Headache may be the only manifestation of these complications, and thus a high index of suspicion is necessary, especially in adolescent boys. Prompt surgical intervention in addition to parenteral antibiotics are essential to avoid complications.[10]

### DIAGNOSIS AND TREATMENT

Diagnosis of sinusitis is clinical; radiologic films are not helpful. A computed tomography scan may be needed to delineate the extent of the disease and/or complications in those patients not responding to therapy or who have chronic symptoms. Nasal cultures are not helpful, but cultures from the sinuses, when available, are best. There is a higher incidence of sinusitis in patients with atopy. Guidelines put forth in 2001 by the American Academy of Pediatrics,[11] emphasize making the appropriate diagnosis in those who present with persistent or severe upper respiratory symptoms. Overdiagnosis and the resultant overuse of unnecessary antibiotics remains an active area of debate.[12,13] In adults, similar guidelines from 2005 state that for mild-to-moderate acute bacterial sinusitis, antibiotics should be avoided unless symptoms persist for at least a week and include purulent nasal discharge, maxillary pain, or tooth pain or tenderness.[14] If followed, these guidelines should lead to fewer inappropriate antibiotic prescriptions for acute respiratory infections and may aid efforts to slow the spread of antibiotic resistance. For recurrent or chronic cases of sinusitis, one should rule out an underlying predisposition such as an immunodeficiency —congenital or acquired, including human immunodeficiency virus (HIV)—or cystic fibrosis. In atopic patients, allergic fungal sinusitis may complicate the clinical picture by presenting with prolonged nasal symptoms, recurrent sinusitis, nasal polyps, and recurrent headaches. Eosinophilia and elevated IgE levels to environmental fungi aid in making the diagnosis. Surgical intervention is uniformly required and the recurrence rate is high.[15]

## PHARYNGITIS

Acute pharyngitis or "sore throat" is responsible for 1% to 2% of visits to primary care providers.[16] Most cases are caused by viruses including those causing rhinitis (Table 88-2). Clinically, pharyngitis is characterized by edema and hyperemia of the tonsils and mucous membranes.

### GROUP A *STREPTOCOCCUS*

The most important preventable complications of pharyngitis are those caused by *Streptococcus pyogenes* or group A *Streptococcus* (GAS), namely rheumatic heart

**Table 88-2**

**Microbial Causes of Acute Pharyngitis**

| *Pathogen* | *Syndrome or Disease* | *Estimated Percentage of Cases*[a] |
|---|---|---|
| **Viral** | | |
| Rhinovirus (100 types and 1 subtype) | Common cold | 20 |
| Coronavirus (3 or more types) | Common cold | ≥5 |
| Adenovirus (types 3, 4, 7, 14, and 21) | Pharyngoconjunctival fever, acute respiratory disease | 5 |
| Herpes simplex virus (types 1 and 2) | Gingivitis, stomatitis, pharyngitis | 4 |
| Parainfluenza virus (types 1–4) | Common cold, croup | 2 |
| Influenza virus (types A and B) | Influenza | 2 |
| Coxsackievirus A (types 2, 4–6, 8, and 10) | Herpangina | <1 |
| Epstein-Barr virus | Infectious mononucleosis | <1 |
| Cytomegalovirus | Infectious mononucleosis | <1 |
| Human immunodeficiency virus type 1 | Primary human immunodeficiency virus infection | <1 |
| **Bacterial** | | |
| *Streptococcus pyogenes* (group A β-hemolytic streptococci) | Pharyngitis and tonsillitis, scarlet fever | 15–30 |
| Group C β-hemolytic streptococci | Pharyngitis and tonsillitis | 5 |
| *Neisseria gonorrhoeae* | Pharyngitis | <1 |
| *Corynebacterium diptheriae* | Diphtheria | <1 |
| *Arcanobacterium haemolyticum* | Pharyngitis, scarlatiniform rash | <1 |
| **Chlamydial** | | |
| *Chlamydia pneumoniae* | Pneumonia, bronchitis, and pharyngitis | Unknown |
| **Mycoplasmal** | | |
| *Mycoplasma pneumoniae* | Pneumonia, bronchitis, and pharyngitis | <1 |

[a]Estimates are of the percentage of cases of pharyngitis in persons of all ages that are due to the indicated organism.

Adapted from Gwaltney JM, Bisno AL. Pharyngitis. In: Mandell GL, Dolan R, Bennett J, eds. *Principles and Practice of Infectious Diseases*. 5th ed. New York: Churchill Livingstone, 2000:656–662, with permission from Elsevier.

disease and glomerulonephritis, as well as suppurative complications such as peritonsillar abscess and invasive disease. Group A *Streptococcus* is disseminated through large-droplet secretions. Half of those who become colonized with GAS develop symptoms rapidly, and the disease spreads in a family soon after an index case is recognized. Group A *Streptococcus* pharyngitis is most common among school-age children and adolescents. It is difficult to make the distinction between GAS and nonstreptococcal pharyngitis on clinical grounds alone. Clinical algorithms or guidelines direct the increased probability of GAS pharyngitis to 4 clinical findings: tonsillar exudates, tender anterior cervical adenopathy, absence of cough, and history of fever. Abdominal pain can be prominent, especially in younger children. Throat culture remains the gold standard for the diagnosis of GAS pharyngitis, and negative results of rapid tests in children and adolescents should be confirmed with a conventional throat culture.[17] The differential diagnosis of exudative pharyngitis with marked pharyngeal erythema, severe pharyngeal pain, and fever in adolescents includes Epstein-Barr virus (EBV) and adenoviral pharyngitis plus bacterial infection with other beta-hemolytic streptococci, such as group C and G, and *Arcanobacterium hemolyticum*. The latter, although rarely diagnosed, has been found in higher numbers in adolescents and young adults and is frequently associated with a diffuse maculopapular skin rash. Pharyngoconjunctival fever, by adenovirus types 3 or 7, characterized by exudative pharyngitis and follicular conjunctivitis, occurs mostly in the summer. Group C *Streptococcus* has been reported as a cause of endemic pharyngitis in college students. Group C and G streptococcal infections have been linked to development of glomerulonephritis and are treated in an effort to prevent suppurative complications; non-GAS have not been shown to cause acute rheumatic fever.

## EPSTEIN-BARR VIRUS

In industrialized countries, 40% to 65% of episodes of primary EBV infection occur during early childhood and are asymptomatic. By contrast, primary infection in teenagers and young adults often causes symptomatic infectious mononucleosis (IM), which is characterized by sore throat, fever, fatigue, headache, and lymphadenopathy. The acute exudative pharyngitis is usually painful and is maximal for 5 to 7 days, with subsequent resolution within 7 to 14 days. Splenomegaly as well as atypical lymphocytosis in peripheral blood are common; heterophil agglutinins are present in up to 90% of affected adolescents. IgM antibody to viral capsid antigen can be measured for the diagnosis of acute infection. Most cases of acute IM resolve within several weeks without sequelae. Corticosteroids have been shown to reduce the upper airway obstruction caused by IM, but their efficacy for the treatment of the pain associated with the pharyngitis is unclear. Published data on EBV prevalence and IM, mainly dating from the 1970s, showed that 3% to 5% of university students in the United States and Europe develop IM annually, and this can lead to significant loss of study time. Infected patients should avoid contact sports until fully recovered and the spleen is no longer palpable. Those suspected of having IM should not be given ampicillin or amoxicillin, which cause a nonallergic morbilliform rash in a high proportion of patients with IM.[18]

## OTHER ETIOLOGIC AGENTS

There are other organisms that may manifest as acute pharyngitis, usually as part of a more generalized illness. Acute retroviral syndrome shortly after acquisition of HIV infection may manifest as febrile, nonexudative pharyngitis followed by lymphadenopathy +/– a maculopapular rash. It should be considered in adolescents in areas of the United States where HIV acquisition rates continue to be high. The antibody tests for HIV will be negative at this stage; a quantitative RNA viral load is the diagnostic test of choice. Primary HSV-1 and HSV-2 infection can also manifest as pharyngitis with mucosal ulceration and vesiculation, as do some enteroviruses, which cause herpangina characterized by palatal papules and vesicles on an erythematous base. *Neisseria gonorrhoeae* may colonize the pharyngeal mucosa and occasionally cause symptoms. Of note is Lemierre syndrome, or postanginal sepsis, generally secondary to the anaerobe *Fusobacterium necrophorum*, which, although uncommon, may be life threatening. It peaks in adolescence with a male predominance of 3:1. It is characterized by tonsillitis followed by septic thrombophlebitis of the internal jugular vein and then a septicemia with septic emboli to the lungs and other sites. Ipsilateral neck tenderness parallel to the sternocleidomastoid muscle and diffuse abdominal pain are characteristic features, if present. Some cases have been preceded by IM; EBV infection is thought to induce immunosuppression, with a transient decrease in T-cell–mediated immunity that may predispose to a bacterial superinfection. Recent evidence suggests that *Fusobacterium necrophorum* can be limited to the throat and cause persistent or recurrent tonsillitis.[19] A high index of suspicion is required for its diagnosis, and treatment includes prolonged intravenous antibiotic therapy and surgical debridement when indicated.[20] Diphtheria is rare in the United States due to successful vaccination programs; *Corynebacterium diphtheriae* forms characteristic grayish-brown fibrinous, firmly adherent, pseudomembranes on the tonsils.

## TREATMENT

As in other URTI, several factors contribute to the unnecessary use of antibiotics in many cases of pharyngitis. Up to 30% of patients with negative streptococcal test results receive antibiotic prescriptions. A recent study concluded that patients' desires for antibiotics may be based on the mistaken idea that they are the best way to alleviate pain. This raises the possibility that giving adequate analgesia may help physicians treat sore throats without antibiotics. Data also suggest that "the issue is not *which* guidelines to follow but that clinicians fail to follow *any* guideline."[21] The best approach in an adolescent would be to obtain rapid testing and if that is negative, provide a prescription to be filled only when growth of *Streptococcus* species is detected.[22] There is no harm in delaying a treatment a day or 2, and the patient is no longer contagious 24 hours after starting therapy. Group A *Streptococcus* is uniformly susceptible to penicillin, which should be the drug of choice in nonallergic patients, given orally for 10 days, or as a single injection of long-acting benzathine penicillin; erythromycin or other macrolides can be substituted in allergic patients.

## LARYNGITIS

Symptoms of laryngitis are hoarseness and a husky voice often associated with a dry cough. Students have reported laryngitis as a cause of missed sports practice more often than cough, rhinorrhea, or myalgia. The same viruses causing URTI reach laryngeal tissue, with parainfluenza and metapneumovirus playing a bigger role in young adults. Diphtheria needs to be ruled out in the developing world. In immunocompromised hosts, endemic fungi such as *Histoplasma*, *Cryptococcus,* and *Blastomyces* may invade laryngeal tissue as part of disseminated disease. A number of extraesophageal symptoms, such as chronic cough or wheezing as well as chronic laryngitis and pharyngitis, have been associated with gastroesophageal reflux disease.

## TRACHEOBRONCHITIS

Acute bronchitis refers to otherwise healthy individuals with an acute respiratory illness due to inflammation of the large airways lasting 1 to 3 weeks, with cough as the prominent feature and in whom pneumonia has been excluded.[23] The most frequent reason for visits to US ambulatory care physicians after "general medical examination" and "progress visit" is "cough." Bronchitis usually denoted as acute or "not otherwise specified," is the most frequent diagnosis given to these patients. The protracted phase of uncomplicated acute bronchitis, characterized primarily by cough, results from hypersensitivity of the tracheobronchial epithelium and airway receptors (bronchial hyperreactivity). This is often accompanied by phlegm production and wheezing and usually lasts 2 weeks. Abnormalities in pulmonary function tests peak a few weeks after infection and do not appear to be related to acute cytopathic effects of the infection or the type of infection (viral versus bacterial).

### PATHOGENESIS

#### Viral

Respiratory viruses are considered to cause most cases of uncomplicated acute bronchitis in which an agent is identified by means of culture, antibody serology, or PCR. Frequently no pathogen is isolated, probably representing viral infections for which studies did not perform appropriate analyses. The viruses most frequently associated with uncomplicated acute bronchitis are those that produce primarily lower respiratory tract disease—influenza A and B viruses, parainfluenza viruses, RSV, and Ads. Coronaviruses, rhinoviruses, and the metapneumovirus have also been implicated. The RSV URTI are more likely to be accompanied by a prolonged productive or "bronchitic" cough and are more likely to be complicated by wheezing.[24] Severe acute respiratory syndrome (SARS)-CoV, the causative agent of the SARS outbreak 5 years ago, is a coronavirus; disease in adolescents older than 12 years of age mimicked those in adults, with fever, cough, and pneumonitis. Because of the extensive cytolysis with influenza viruses, there is associated fever and a predilection for bacterial superinfection, which often complicates influenza infections and is responsible for the major morbidity and mortality generated. In recent years, severe community-acquired methicillin-resistant *Staphylococcus aureus* (CA-MRSA) pneumonia during influenza season with a fatal outcome has been reported in several states among previously healthy children and adults.[25] The short duration between any respiratory symptom onset and either death or recovery of MRSA from the patients suggested that the influenza virus and MRSA infections likely occurred concomitantly rather than in the more classically described biphasic clinical course of pneumonia after influenza illness.

#### Bacterial

When microbiological studies were performed in patients with uncomplicated acute bronchitis in non-outbreak settings, less than 10% had evidence of acute bacterial infection. To date, only *Bordetella pertussis, Mycoplasma pneumoniae*, and *Chlamydia pneumoniae* have been clearly established as causes of acute bronchitis. Pertussis, or the 100-day cough or whooping cough, was largely conquered in the United States and many Western countries by administration of whole-cell pertussis vaccines in the 1950s. Rates fell to historic lows in the 1970s, but during the 1990s the reported incidence of pertussis doubled in persons older than 10 years of age, whereas the incidence for children aged 4 months to 10 years changed little. Adolescents seem to be at particular risk for infection, and outbreaks with attack rates greater than 20% have occurred in high school settings. Attack rates as high as 100% have been reported among adult and adolescent household contacts of infected children. Sporadic cases in adults and adolescents are also quite common but are rarely diagnosed. A number of studies have described *Bordetella pertussis* as an important pathogen in adolescents and young adults, accounting for 10% to 30% of respiratory coughing illnesses of more than 2 weeks' duration, and producing symptoms that are severe and prolonged, sometimes requiring hospitalization. In adolescents, the disease may sometimes manifest solely as a protracted, nondistinctive cough. In a Canadian survey, 1 in 5 adolescents or adults with prolonged cough had laboratory evidence of pertussis, with a mean duration of cough of 8 weeks and a mean duration of violent cough of 6 weeks.[26] Forty-five percent of the subjects with pertussis experienced vomiting after their coughing episodes. The highest proportion of cough illnesses caused by *Bordetella pertussis* occurred in adolescents 12 to 19 years old. In another outbreak in a college campus investigated by the CDC, the students with laboratory evidence of pertussis (by serology in all cases) were clinically similar to those who did not meet the clinical definition of pertussis, reinforcing the difficulty facing clinicians attempting to distinguish pertussis from other causes of persistent cough, as well as the limitations of the current diagnostic methods. The largest difference was in the overall time until resolution of the cough—patients with laboratory evidence of confirmed pertussis coughed about 27 days longer than those without laboratory-confirmed pertussis.[27]

Although symptoms are not indicative of respiratory disease, of special interest in the adolescent age group is the acquisition of *Neisseria meningitidis* through the upper respiratory tract. *Neisseria meningitidis* is a gram-negative diplococcus that colonizes the nasopharynx in 5% to 10% of the population, but only a minority of strains are pathogenic, and less than 1% of carriers develop disease—a serious, rapidly progressing, and sometimes fatal disease secondary to invasion of the bacteria into the bloodstream. Worldwide, serogroups A, B, C, Y, and W-135 account for most cases, although serogroup A disease is rare in the United States. The rate for youth 11 to 19 years old (1.2–5 per 100,000) is higher than that for the general population. Risk factors for colonization and infection include household exposure, crowding, concurrent URTI, and active and passive smoking. College freshmen living in dormitories are at higher risk than college students in general. Transmission of *Neisseria meningitidis* occurs when close, "mouth-to-mouth" contact permits the exchange of salivary secretions. Although close contacts of people who are ill with meningococcal disease are at much higher risk, most people contract the bacteria from asymptomatic carriers.

## DIAGNOSIS, TREATMENT, AND PREVENTION

Culture remains the gold standard for diagnosis of Bordetella pertussis but takes at least 3 to 4 days to grow and is usually negative in late stages of the illness. Direct fluorescent antibody (DFA) testing when performed reliably can be useful. Several in-house PCR assays have been developed but have varying degrees of sensitivity, and serologic tests are only standardized and reliably used in a few states such as Massachusetts. Adolescents and young adults are thus the reservoir of the pathogen that is then transmitted to infants who are too young to have been fully vaccinated, resulting in increasing disease and mortality rates among susceptible infants. All data that have been analyzed point toward waning of vaccine-provided immunity over time. In 2006, the CDC Advisory Committee on Immunization Practices (ACIP) issued recommendations for use of a single dose of Tdap, the tetanus, diphtheria, and acellular pertussis vaccine (in a dose one-third of that given to children) to adolescents 11 to 18 years of age, instead of tetanus and diphtheria toxoids (Td) vaccine for booster immunization. The same is appropriate for those older than 18 years of age. The preferred age for Tdap immunization is 11 to 12 years old. For those at increased risk of acquiring pertussis such as child care providers and others having close contact with infants (ideally before pregnancy for mothers) as well as health care workers with direct patient contact, the CDC recommends an interval as short as 2 years from the last dose of Td.[28] Prompt antibiotic treatment of patients with pertussis is indicated to limit transmission, but (with the possible exception of therapy initiated during the first week of symptoms) there are no compelling data to support the prospect that cough will be less severe or less prolonged with antibiotic therapy. Multiplex PCR testing of nasopharyngeal swabs or aspirates is being developed to diagnose infections secondary to *B pertussis, M pneumoniae*, and *C pneumoniae*.[29]

In January 2005, the ACIP recommended routine vaccination with MCV4 (against serogroups A, C, Y, and W-135 of *Neisseria meningitides*) for children who are 11 to 12 years old, and catch-up vaccination of adolescents who have not already been vaccinated when they enter high school (at 15 years of age) or as college freshmen (living in dormitories).[30] These recommendations have now been expanded to include previously unvaccinated children who are 11 to 18 years old, and all those 2 to 55 years of age at increased risk for meningococcal disease such as patients with sickle cell disease and asplenia.[31] When Tdap and MCV4 vaccines are not administered simultaneously, the American Academy of Pediatrics suggests a minimum interval of one month between them. Persons with a history of Guillain-Barré syndrome should not receive meningococcal conjugate vaccine unless they are at substantially elevated risk for meningococcal disease.

With the development of new vaccines, some diseases in adolescents have become vaccine preventable. This provides a wonderful opportunity in which, similar to the childhood platform, immunizations draw parents and their children to routine preventive care visits at which other preventive care services can be delivered. With more vaccines targeted specifically toward 11- to 12-year-olds, the case for using vaccination to create an adolescent platform is now more compelling.

Despite the previously noted findings, the diagnosis of acute bronchitis has become synonymous with antibiotic treatment throughout the developed world. Evidence-based reviews and meta-analyses of randomized, controlled trials conclude that routine antibiotic treatment does not provide major clinical benefit in adults with acute bronchitis.[32] Noninfectious causes of acute bronchitis, such as cough-variant asthma or allergic or occupational exposures, should also be considered.

## REFERENCES

1. Armstrong GL, Pinner RW. Outpatient visits for infectious diseases in the United States, 1980 through 1996. *Arch Intern Med.* 1999;159(21):2531–2536

2. Musher DM. How contagious are common respiratory tract infections? *N Engl J Med.* 2003;348(13):1256–1266

3. Arden KE, McErlean P, Nissen MD, Sloots TP, Mackay IM. Frequent detection of human rhinoviruses, paramyxoviruses, coronaviruses, and bocavirus during acute respiratory tract infections. *J Med Virol.* 2006;78(9):1232–1240

4. Kojaoghlanian T, Flomenberg P, Horwitz MS. The impact of adenovirus infection on the immunocompromised host. *Rev Med Virol.* 2003;13(3):155–171

5. Chiu CY, Urisman A, Greenhow TL, et al. Utility of DNA microarrays for detection of viruses in acute respiratory tract infections in children. *J Pediatr.* 2008;153(1):76–83

6. Rothman RE, Hsieh YH, Yang S. Communicable respiratory threats in the ED: tuberculosis, influenza, SARS, and other aerosolized infections. *Emerg Med Clin North Am.* 2006;24(4):989–1017

7. Aiello AE, Coulborn RM, Perez V, Larson EL. Effect of hand hygiene on infectious disease risk in the community setting: a meta-analysis. *Am J Public Health.* 2008;98(8):1372–1381

8. Fiore AE, Shay DK, Broder K, et al. Prevention and control of influenza: recommendations of the Advisory Committee on Immunization Practices (ACIP), 2008. *MMWR Recomm Rep.* 2008;57(RR-7):1–60

9. Quraishi H, Zevallos JP. Subdural empyema as a complication of sinusitis in the pediatric population. *Int J Pediatr Otorhinolaryngol.* 2006;70(9):1581–1586

10. Osborn MK, Steinberg JP. Subdural empyema and other suppurative complications of paranasal sinusitis. *Lancet Infect Dis.* 2007;7(1):62–67

11. American Academy of Pediatrics. Clinical practice guideline: management of sinusitis. *Pediatrics.* 2001;108(3):798–808

12. Garbutt JM, Goldstein M, Gellman E, Shannon W, Littenberg B. A randomized, placebo-controlled trial of antimicrobial treatment for children with clinically diagnosed acute sinusitis. *Pediatrics.* 2001;107(4):619–625

13. Harris SJ, Wald ER, Senior BA, et al. The sinusitis debate. *Pediatrics.* 2002;109(1):166–167

14. Slavin RG, Spector SL, Bernstein IL, et al. The diagnosis and management of sinusitis: a practice parameter update. *J Allergy Clin Immunol.* 2005;116(6 suppl):S13–S47

15. Campbell JM, Graham M, Gray HC, Bower C, Blaiss MS, Jones SM. Allergic fungal sinusitis in children. *Ann Allergy Asthma Immunol.* 2006;96(2):286–290

16. Bisno AL. Acute pharyngitis. *N Engl J Med.* 2001;344(3): 205–211

17. Gieseker KE, Roe MH, MacKenzie T, Todd JK. Evaluating the American Academy of Pediatrics diagnostic standard for Streptococcus pyogenes pharyngitis: backup culture versus repeat rapid antigen testing. *Pediatrics.* 2003;111(6 Pt 1): e666–e670

18. American Academy of Pediatrics. Epstein-Barr virus infections. In: Pickering LK, Baker CJ, Kimberlin DW, Long SS, eds. *Red Book: 2009 Report of the Committee on Infectious Disease.* 28th ed. Elk Grove Village, IL: American Academy of Pediatrics; 2009:291

19. Batty A, Wren MW, Gal M. Fusobacterium necrophorum as the cause of recurrent sore throat: comparison of isolates from persistent sore throat syndrome and Lemierre's disease. *J Infect.* 2005;51(4):299–306

20. Riordan T. Human infection with Fusobacterium necrophorum (Necrobacillosis), with a focus on Lemierre's syndrome. *Clin Microbiol Rev.* 2007;20(4):622–659

21. Linder JA. Editorial commentary: antibiotics for treatment of acute respiratory tract infections: decreasing benefit, increasing risk, and the irrelevance of antimicrobial resistance. *Clin Infect Dis.* 2008;4(6):744–746

22. Park SY, Gerber MA, Tanz RR, et al. Clinicians' management of children and adolescents with acute pharyngitis. *Pediatrics.* 2006;117(6):1871–1878

23. Wenzel RP, Fowler AA, 3rd. Acute bronchitis. *N Engl J Med.* 2006;355(20):2125–2130

24. Hall CB. Respiratory syncytial virus and parainfluenza virus. *N Engl J Med.* 2001;344(25):1917–1928

25. Severe methicillin-resistant Staphylococcus aureus community-acquired pneumonia associated with influenza—Louisiana and Georgia, December 2006–January 2007. *MMWR Morb Mortal Wkly Rep.* 2007;56(14):325–329

26. Senzilet LD, Halperin SA, Spika JS, et al. Pertussis is a frequent cause of prolonged cough illness in adults and adolescents. *Clin Infect Dis.* 2001;32(12):1691–1697

27. Craig AS, Wright SW, Edwards KM, et al. Outbreak of pertussis on a college campus. *Am J Med.* 2007;120(4):364–368

28. Prevention of pertussis among adolescents: recommendations for use of tetanus toxoid, reduced diphtheria toxoid, and acellular pertussis (Tdap) vaccine. *Pediatrics.* 2006;117(3):965–978

29. McDonough EA, Barrozo CP, Russell KL, Metzgar D. A multiplex PCR for detection of Mycoplasma pneumoniae, Chlamydophila pneumoniae, Legionella pneumophila, and Bordetella pertussis in clinical specimens. *Mol Cell Probes.* 2005;19(5):314–322

30. Bilukha OO, Rosenstein N. Prevention and control of meningococcal disease. Recommendations of the Advisory Committee on Immunization Practices (ACIP). *MMWR Recomm Rep.* 2005;54(RR-7):1–21

31. Revised recommendations of the Advisory Committee on Immunization Practices to Vaccinate all Persons Aged 11–18 Years with Meningococcal Conjugate Vaccine. *MMWR Morb Mortal Wkly Rep.* 2007;56(31):794–795

32. Bent S, Saint S, Vittinghoff E, Grady D. Antibiotics in acute bronchitis: a meta-analysis. *Am J Med.* 1999;107(1):62–67

# CHAPTER 89

# Lower Respiratory Infections

ARTHUR ATLAS, MD

Acute respiratory infections are the most common infections in adolescents. Although most respiratory infections involve the upper respiratory tract, lower respiratory infections do occur frequently. The lower respiratory tract is defined as the respiratory system below the vocal cords that extends throughout the lungs. An infection of the lower respiratory tract can be a primary bacterial or viral infection of the lower airways, or an extension of an upper respiratory tract infection. Viral infections are the most common infections of the lower respiratory tract. Box 89-1 lists the most common viruses that infect the lower airway in adolescents.

A specific virus can cause different clinical symptoms in the same patient and different clinical syndromes in various patients. For example, parainfluenza virus type 1 is the most frequent cause of croup; however, it can also cause bronchiolitis, pneumonia, and tracheobronchitis. This phenomenon of the same organism causing different clinical syndromes also applies to bacterial infections. For example, *Mycoplasma pneumoniae* is the most common cause of bacterial pneumonia in adolescents; however, it can also cause bronchiolitis, tracheobronchitis and, less frequently, croup.

Bacterial organisms of the respiratory tract can occur as a primary infection or secondary to a viral infection.

**Box 89-1**

***Viruses Causing Acute Lower Respiratory Infections***

Adenovirus
Enterovirus
Influenza virus types A and B
Metapneumovirus
Parainfluenza virus types 1, 2, and 3
Respiratory syncytial virus
Rhinovirus
Measles virus (uncommon in United States)
Rubella virus (uncommon in United States)
Cytomegalovirus
Epstein-Barr virus
HIV
Varicella-zoster virus

**Box 89-2**

***Bacteria Associated with Acute Lower Respiratory Infections***

*Chlamydia pneumoniae*
*Mycoplasma pneumoniae*
*Haemophilus influenzae*
*Streptococcus pneumoniae*
*Staphylococcus aureus*
*Bordetella pertussis*
*Mycobacterium tuberculosis*
Anaerobes
Atypical mycobacterium

Box 89-2 lists the common bacteria causing lower respiratory tract infections. Adolescents may have increased risk for acute lower respiratory infections because of poor nutrition and inadequate sleep, which lowers their resistance. Crowded environments in college dormitories or the military increase the risk of infections due to greater exposure. Smoking, primary or secondary, and recreational drug use also increase the risk of infection by damaging cilia, which hampers the mucociliary clearance system. Intravenous drug users have a ten-fold increase in community-acquired pneumonia and are at increased risk for aspiration pneumonia. They are at risk for septic pulmonary emboli causing pneumonia and pulmonary abscesses from injected particulate matter.[1]

Acute lower respiratory infections can be divided into 4 major clinical syndromes, which are based on the predominant site of infection. The categories are laryngotracheitis, tracheobronchitis, bronchiolitis, and pneumonia. Even though this chapter discusses infections according to these classifications, the infection can be isolated to the specific anatomical site or involve numerous areas of the respiratory tract.

## HOST DEFENSE

Pulmonary defense against infection in the lung is an integrated multilayered system based on the airway epithelium as the primary interface between the host and the environment. On average, 10,000 L of air are inhaled daily, which exposes the airways and lungs to numerous pathogens, allergens, and irritants. The epithelium is involved in ciliary function and mucus production, which are the necessary components of the mucociliary transport system. The epithelium produces antimicrobial peptides, cytokines, chemokines, surfactant proteins, and proteinase inhibitors as well as stimulating adaptive and humoral immunity. These chemical mediators are also released when exposed to air pollution, cigarette smoke and, possibly, marijuana smoke, which can injure the lungs after chronic exposure. The airway epithelium functions as part of the innate system of immunity, which is activated when microorganisms are inhaled. The epithelium provides the initial protection by sensing bacterial exposure and increasing antimicrobial peptides into the airway, as well as cytokines and chemokines into the submucosa, which begins the inflammatory reaction. These mediators are capable of killing or inhibiting the growth of the microorganisms and of attracting phagocytic cells, which remove the foreign substance.[2] The particles or microorganisms not eliminated by this system are trapped in the mucus produced by the epithelial cells and are removed by the mucociliary transport system.

The mucociliary transport system is the primary system of defense for the lower airways. A thin layer of mucus on top of the ciliated epithelial cells is propelled toward the larger airways, where it can be coughed up or swallowed. Approximately 100 mL of mucus is produced and secreted daily by the goblet cells and mucous glands, which are mediated by the parasympathetic cholinergic nervous system. Atropine and various recreational and prescription drugs, such as hallucinogens, opiates, phenothiazines, and tricyclic antidepressants, can interfere with mucus secretion and impede this important clearance mechanism. Because distal airways lack ciliated epithelial cells, organisms or particles that reach this level are phagocytized by the alveolar macrophage, which either digests it or carries it to the mucociliary transport system in the larger airways. The macrophages can also move into the interstitial space and travel along the lymphatics until they reach the lymph nodes to dispose of the offending organism or particle through the lymphatics.

## LARYNGOTRACHEITIS

Laryngotracheitis is frequently termed "croup" because of the distinct sound of the cough. The clinical syndrome of hoarseness, croupy cough, and stridor result from inflammation of the distal upper and the proximal lower airway. Laryngotracheitis is an uncommon illness of adolescents and is more common in preschool-age children, with the peak incidence between 6 and 36 months. The etiology of laryngotracheitis is almost always viral, and parainfluenza is most often implicated. Parainfluenza type 1, which causes seasonal epidemics of croup, is the most frequently related infection, but parainfluenza types 2 and 3 are associated with sporadic outbreaks. Respiratory syncytial virus, influenza, rhinovirus, and measles are infrequent causes of croup. Bacterial organisms rarely cause laryngotracheitis, but *M pneumoniae* has been reported.[3]

The illness usually begins with signs and symptoms of a typical cold, including coryza, rhinorrhea, sore throat, and nasal congestion. Hoarseness, stridor, and a barky seal-like cough soon follow, frequently associated with a low-grade temperature. On physical examination, there is variability in the extent of respiratory distress. Symptoms can be mild, with minimal respiratory findings, or severe. Stridor is usually heard, either audibly or with auscultation of the upper airway. On auscultation of the chest, stridor is typically heard in the suprasternal notch but expiratory wheezes can be heard in the lower airways. There is variability in the extent of respiratory distress, occurring as isolated suprasternal retractions in mild cases and as frank respiratory failure in rare but severe cases. Lymphocytosis is seen on the complete blood count, but laboratory evaluation is nonspecific and, therefore, usually not helpful. Neck x-rays usually show subglottic narrowing, which has been called the "steeple sign" or the "pencil sign." Most cases of laryngotracheitis do not require radiographic studies. Laryngotracheitis must be differentiated from epiglottitis, which is a medical emergency and typically presents with more severe symptoms of airway inflammation, high fever, and respiratory distress.

Therapy is usually symptomatic to alleviate nasal congestion and sore throat. Racemic epinephrine improves symptoms of respiratory distress but can cause rebound symptoms within a few hours of administration. Oral steroids decrease the severity of symptoms and reduce hospitalization. High-dose inhaled steroids can decrease symptoms and length of illness.

Bacterial tracheitis is a serious, life-threatening bacterial illness that frequently develops as a complication of viral laryngotracheitis. Bacterial tracheitis has emerged as the most common cause of life-threatening large airway infection because bacterial epiglottitis and severe viral croup have almost disappeared due to widespread use of *Haemophilus influenzae* type B vaccination and corticosteroids, respectively. There has been some concern regarding the relationship of corticosteroids to the increasing prevalence of bacterial tracheitis, but there are no data supporting a cause–effect relationship. The illness is most often seen in children younger than

3 years, but there are increasing reports of bacterial tracheitis in adolescents.[4,5]

The clinical presentation of bacterial tracheitis usually begins with the typical symptoms of an upper airway infection or the flu. Fever is usually present and increases after the initial symptoms of the upper airway infection are expected to resolve. Cough, stridor, and chest wall retractions are common. Most patients appear toxic but drooling is variable.[4] *Staphylococcus aureus* is the most common bacterial organism isolated, but many patients have multiple organisms. Influenza A and B are the common viral organisms frequently identified with *S aureus*, *Streptococcus pneumoniae*, *Moraxella catarrhalis, H influenzae*, or group A streptococcus.[5] X-rays of the chest and neck reveal subglottic narrowing, with a normal-appearing epiglottis. Pneumonia can be present in the lung fields. Bronchoscopic evaluation shows an inflamed, erythematous tracheal mucosa with purulent secretions. Plaques or pseudomembranes are sometimes seen. The white blood cell count is usually elevated with a left shift, but some patients have neutropenia. Many patients develop serious and fatal complications, including acute respiratory distress syndrome (ARDS), septic and toxic shock, and multiorgan failure.[4-6] Intravenous antibiotics targeted against the common organisms and supportive care are the mainstays of therapy.

## BRONCHITIS

Acute bronchitis is a clinical entity describing symptoms of a self-limited purulent cough without pneumonia. The difficulty with using a diagnosis of bronchitis is evident from this description because many factors can lead to a self-limiting purulent cough without pneumonia. Upper respiratory tract infections, postnasal drip, smoking, sinusitis, allergy and irritant exposures, gastroesophageal reflux, and aspiration can cause similar symptoms. Therefore, for the purpose of clarity this discussion focuses on the clinical symptoms of bronchitis that are caused by inflammation of the trachea and large bronchi from infectious organisms, without the presence of pneumonia. Bronchitis is a frequently diagnosed respiratory condition in adolescence that can occur as an isolated illness or be associated with systemic conditions such as cystic fibrosis, asthma, or immune-deficiency disorders. Coughing following the onset of a typical upper respiratory tract infection (rhinorrhea, nasal congestion) is the most common clinical presentation. Coughing, which can be nonproductive but is typically productive, may be the only clinical manifestation. Vomiting associated with coughing paroxysms is more common in younger children than adolescents, but can still be observed in the older patient. The posttussive emesis often contains mucus from the lower airways or postnasal mucus in those patients with accompanying rhinosinusitis. Constitutional symptoms such as fever, malaise, and diminished appetite and activity are usually not present unless the bronchitis is secondary to a more severe systemic illness or a secondary bacterial infection.

Viruses are most commonly implicated as the cause of acute bronchitis. The yield of a specific virus is dependent on the time of year, vaccination status to influenza in the population, and presence or absence of an influenza epidemic. The viruses that have been isolated in acute bronchitis include influenza A and B, parainfluenza, respiratory syncytial virus, coronavirus, adenovirus, rhinovirus, and metapneumovirus.[7] The atypical bacteria are the most common bacterial causes of acute bronchitis; these include *Bordetella pertussis, Bordetella parapertussis, Chlamydia pneumoniae*, and *M pneumoniae*. Yeast and fungi are uncommon causes of acute bronchitis.[8] Each infectious agent damages the airway epithelium, leading to epithelial cell desquamation, denuding of the epithelial layer, and damage of the cilia. The acute airway inflammation from the infectious agents causes a lymphocytic cellular infiltration into the submucosa and increased mucus production from goblet cell hyperplasia. This infectious/inflammatory process interrupts the mucociliary clearance system and stimulates the cough receptors, resulting in increased coughing, which clears the increased mucus.

Most cases of acute bronchitis begin as an upper respiratory infection, and initial symptoms of acute bronchitis cannot be differentiated from an upper respiratory infection. However, the cough of acute bronchitis is usually present for 10 to 20 days and may persist up to 4 weeks or longer. The mean duration of coughing from all causes of acute bronchitis is 24 days.[9] In cases of more persistent cough, *B pertussis* should be considered. The duration of coughing with pertussis is between 27 and 66 days, with a median of 42 days.

A detailed history, including contacts with other coughers, smoking and drug use, and immunization history, may help identify a specific etiology. Cough is always present in acute bronchitis, but the nature of the cough is variable. Typically, the cough is initially dry and intermittent but often becomes productive and more frequent. The sputum can be thin and clear or purulent. Fever is common in viral-induced bronchitis but less common in *B pertussis*. The presence of bronchitis with fever, during an epidemic of influenza is highly predictive of influenza as the causative agent.[9] On physical examination, coryza and rhinorrhea are common and erythema of the posterior pharynx is frequent. Rhonchi and rales can be heard on auscultation of the chest, but a clear chest does not exclude the diagnosis. Wheezing can frequently be heard and may indicate the presence of either undiagnosed asthma or an exacerbation of asthma precipitated by the viral infection. In one study, asthma was diagnosed in 65% of patients with recurrent bronchitis.[10]

Laboratory evaluation is usually nonspecific and therefore unhelpful. Lymphocytosis can be seen with pertussis infections, and leucocytosis with bacterial infections. Sputum cultures are rarely helpful and commonly show no growth, or normal respiratory flora. One study evaluating the usefulness of nasopharyngeal washings, viral serologies, and sputum cultures failed to demonstrate an organism in more than two-thirds of the specimens.[11] Rapid diagnostic tests are most useful when there is a high likelihood of identifying a treatable cause of acute bronchitis or when trying to identify the etiology of a communal outbreak. Rapid influenza testing is possibly the most helpful and is becoming more widely available. Multiplex polymerase chain reaction (PCR) testing of nasopharyngeal secretions is being developed to rapidly diagnose atypical bacteria,[9] which may be helpful in the future in selecting patients for antimicrobial therapy.

Treatment of bronchitis is based on clinical symptoms and the likely underlying etiology. Generally, in adolescents who do not have fever or purulent sputum or underlying asthma most clinicians will wait 5 to 7 days (ie, the typical timing for a viral respiratory infection) before deciding if antibiotics or steroids are needed. If there is fever or purulent sputum and a negative x-ray (which is generally obtained if there is an abnormal lung exam and fever), then obtaining a sputum culture (which is usually not helpful) and starting a macrolide antibiotic (usually azithromycin) is appropriate. If there is underlying asthma using a short course of steroids is usually effective, but if symptoms persist after 5 days adding a macrolid antibiotic is appropriate at that time.

Pertussis has become more prevalent in adolescents over the past 2 decades. Initially, pertussis was a disease of infancy but since the 1940s and 1950s, when the whole-cell pertussis vaccine was introduced and came into widespread use, the overall incidence of pertussis declined dramatically. In the United States, the incidence of pertussis reached its nadir in the 1980s and has since been on the rise. However, the increased incidence of pertussis is disproportionately affecting adolescents and young adults. This change in epidemiology is probably multifactorial. The immunity from the whole-cell pertussis vaccine begins to diminish after 3 to 5 years, with lack of measurable protection by 10 to 12 years.[12] In the 1990s, because of concern of side effects from the whole-cell vaccine a less immunogenic acellular pertussis vaccine was introduced. The immunity from the acellular vaccine appears to decline after 4 to 5 years, and the duration of protection is not yet known, but it may be comparable to the whole-cell vaccine.[12] Natural infection from pertussis may offer longer immunity than the vaccine but also is not lifelong. Therefore, universal acellular pertussis vaccination for adolescents in the US is recommended.[13]

Diagnosis of pertussis is often based on clinical findings because laboratory evaluation is not always available or easy to interpret. Culture of *B pertussis* is 100% specific but has a low sensitivity because the culture is usually obtained after antibiotics have been tried or after the patient has coughed for a number of weeks, when the presence of bacteria is low. Amplification of *B pertussis* DNA through PCR increases sensitivity but decreases specificity. Immunoassay for the pertussis toxin antibody is helpful in confirming the diagnosis late in the illness. Therefore, PCR and serology are better diagnostic tests in clinical practice and are also more likely to be positive in adolescents.[12]

Chronic bronchitis in adolescents is almost always due to an underlying chronic illness or continuous exposure to a noxious environmental agent, such as cigarette or marijuana smoke. There is no consensus on the definition of chronic bronchitis or recurrent bronchitis, but "patients who have cough and sputum production on most days for at least 3 months of the year during 2 consecutive years" is frequently used.[14] Box 89-3 lists the etiologies associated with chronic bronchitis in adolescents.

**Box 89-3**

***Differential Diagnosis of Chronic and Recurrent Bronchitis in Adolescents***

Asthma
Bronchiectasis (usually secondary to prior infection)
Chronic aspiration syndromes
Cystic fibrosis
Foreign body aspiration
Heart disease (congenital)
Immunodeficiency disorders
Malignancy
Pollutants
Primary cilia dysfunction
Tracheomalacia

## PNEUMONIAS

The clinical presentation of pneumonia in the adolescent patient varies with the specific organism, extent of the disease, and competence of the patient's defense mechanisms. Cough, expectoration of sputum, fever, chest pain, and chills are common symptoms of pneumonia. Because these signs and symptoms can be present in all pneumonias, the categories of "typical" or "atypical pneumonias" have been used to differentiate the types of organisms. The typical bacterial pneumonias are caused by *S pneumoniae*, *H influenzae,* and *S aureus*. The atypical bacterial pneumonias include *M pneumoniae, C pneumoniae*, and *Legionella pneumophila*. There have been numerous attempts to differentiate etiologies of bacterial pneumonias and to differentiate bacterial from viral pneumonias, either by clinical or radiographic findings. In general, patients with typical bacterial organisms are more likely to present with higher fever, productive cough, and higher white blood cell counts. Atypical pathogens usually have a gradual onset of symptoms, with associated arthralgias, myalgias, rash, and nonproductive cough. Wheezing is frequently associated with viral infections. The term atypical pneumonia is frequently used in adolescents; however, due to a high rate of individual variability of symptoms in all types of pneumonias, clinical criteria is not a reliable predictor of specific microbial organisms.[15]

*S pneumoniae* is the most common organism to cause typical signs and symptoms of community-acquired pneumonia in adolescents but it can have a variable presentation. Even though there are more than 90 serotypes of pneumococcus, only a few account for most the cases of pneumonia. Adolescents with compromised immunity from primary or acquired immune disorders, sickle cell disease, or functional asplenia are predisposed to this organism. Transmission is from person to person, presumably from respiratory droplets. Since 2000, when the heptavalent conjugated pneumococcal vaccine (PCV7) became a routine immunization, there has been a 90% decline in infections in adolescents caused by the serotypes and related serotypes that are covered by PCV7.[16]

The classic presentation of pneumococcal pneumonia includes rapid high fever spikes, chills, and cough in the ill- or toxic-appearing patient. The sputum is frequently blood tinged and accompanied by chest pain. Milder cases can be misleading because they lack many of the classic signs. A concomitant outbreak of herpes labialis is suggestive of pneumococcal infection.[15] Diagnosis of pneumonia is usually made clinically, with radiographic confirmation. Sputum Gram stain and culture are helpful in those patients able to produce sputum. Blood cultures are usually negative and, due to the delay of obtaining a positive culture may not affect the management. Rapid testing for pneumococcal capsular antigen lacks adequate sensitivity or specificity to be of clinical value.

Penicillin, or amoxicillin, is the drug of choice in the outpatient setting. Penicillin can be used in the hospital setting in patients who are not very ill. Third-generation cephalosporins can be used in the ill-appearing patient or in those allergic to penicillin. Resistant pneumococcus is becoming more prevalent; therefore, vancomycin should be considered in the critically ill and in those with complicated pneumonias.[16] Pleural effusions, empyema, and pneumatoceles can occur as complications of pneumococcal pneumonia but are not common.

Community-acquired *S aureus* pneumonia is infrequent in adolescents, but frequency increases after influenza epidemics and with intravenous substance abuse. The pneumonia can occur by direct extension of the colonized upper airway or by hematogenous spread from another infected area. Presentation is similar to other bacterial pneumonias, but is frequently more severe. Pleural effusions and empyema develop in approximately 90% of patients, and lung abscesses are common. Spontaneous pneumothorax and pneumatoceles occur in approximately 50% of patients (Figure 89-1). *S aureus* can be rapidly progressive, with necrosis of small bronchi, which can cause pulmonary artery branch thrombosis and septic emboli to other areas of the lung. Alveolar destruction can lead to a tension pneumothorax or pneumatoceles. Pneumatoceles can enlarge, cause vascular obstruction, and possible rupture, causing a pneumothorax. *S aureus* can also be less progressive, with patchy central alveolar "bronchopneumonia" infiltrates on chest x-ray, frequently in the posterior lower lobes. The patchy areas frequently coalesce to form large consolidations, which can have central cavitations. Rapid radiographic progression is common in *S aureus* pneumonia. Even though pneumatoceles can occur with pneumonias from other bacteria including *S pneumoniae*, this complication is seen considerably more often with *Staphylococcus*. Treatment includes antistaphylococcal antibiotics; however, in the very ill or until bacterial sensitivity is available, vancomycin is used due to the emergence of methicillin-resistant *S aureus* (MRSA). Linezolid, a relatively new antibacterial agent of the oxazolidinone class, is effective against MRSA and can also be given orally. The associated pleural effusions or empyemas usually require video-assisted thoracoscopic surgery drainage or placement of a chest tube for drainage.

*Neisseria meningitidis* is another rare cause of pneumonia in adolescents. Asymptomatic colonization of the upper airway is the source of the bacteria, with person-to-person spread through respiratory droplets. Pneumonia develops from extension of the colonized upper airway or from hematogenous spread from another infected site. There are thirteen serotypes of *N meningitides* but most infections in adolescents occur from 3 serotypes, C, Y, and W135.[16] Because of overcrowding, college dormitories and military barracks are sites of outbreaks. Adolescents with immune disorders,

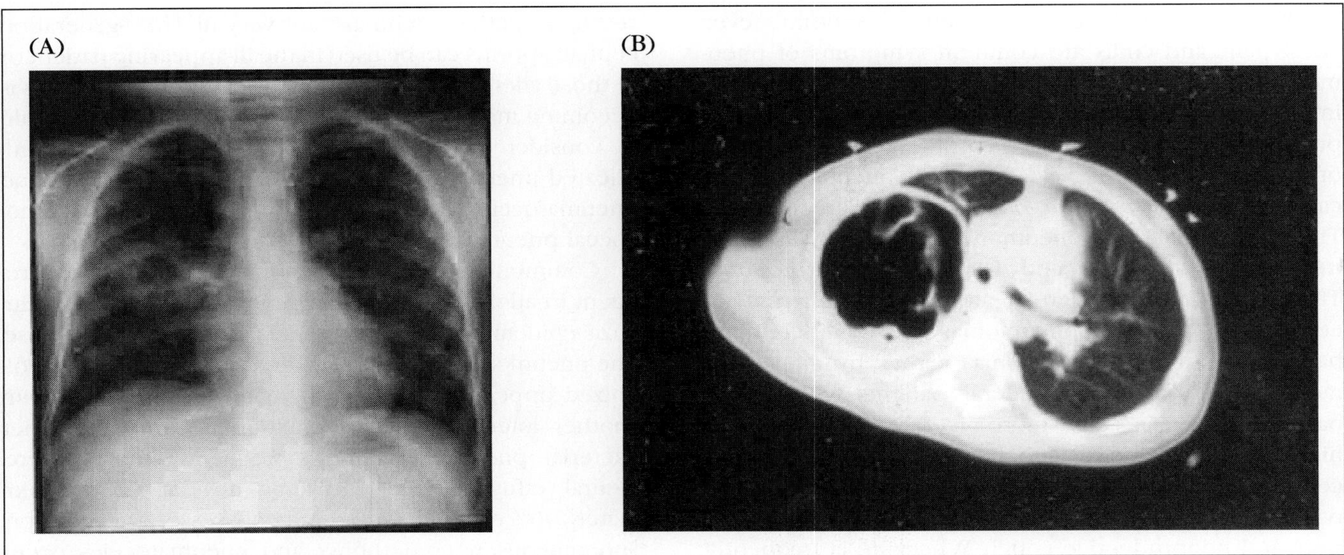

FIGURE 89-1 Complications associated with *Staphylococcus aureus* pneumonia. A: Pneumatoceles after *aureus* pneumonia. B: CT image of pneumatocele secondary to *S aureus* pneumonia.

especially complement abnormalities, and anatomical or function asplenia are at increased risk. Clinical presentation is frequently more gradual than with other bacterial pneumonias but cough, fever and crackles on examination of the chest are common. Multilobar infiltrates with pleural effusions are common but not specific for *N meningitides*. In patients with *N meningitides* septicemia or meningitis, associated pneumonia can be assumed to be from the same organism. Penicillin remains the treatment of choice in culture-proven cases.

Group A streptococci pneumonia is frequently preceded by strep pharyngitis. The onset of symptoms is usually abrupt and severe but comparable to other bacterial pneumonias, including fever, cough, and chills. Pleural effusions and pneumothorax are common complications. The antibiotic of choice is probably penicillin, but clindamycin has been shown to be superior for invasive infection.[3]

*H influenzae* has become a rare cause of pneumonia since the introduction of the Hib vaccination and the near eradication of invasive *H influenzae* type B. However, nontypeable *Haemophilus* species may cause pneumonia and can be associated with empyema, as can be seen with *Haemophilus parainfluenzae*.

## ATYPICAL PNEUMONIAS

*C pneumoniae, M pneumoniae*, and *L pneumophila* are commonly referred to as atypical pathogens, which are important causes of infection in the lower respiratory tract. Since the 1930s, atypical pneumonia has been distinguished from the classic bacterial pneumonias by its gradual onset, nonproductive cough, constitutional symptoms, lack of lobar involvement on chest radiograph, and generally benign clinical course. Another feature of atypical pneumonias was a lack of response to penicillins, which kill bacteria by damaging the cell wall, which *M pneumoniae* lacks. Atypical pneumonias (often referred to as "walking pneumonia") are the most common form of pneumonia in school-age children, adolescents, and young adults throughout the world. Of the numerous species of *Mycoplasma* to infect humans, *M pneumoniae* is the only one to cause respiratory tract infections.[17] *M pneumoniae* is the most common bacterial pathogen within the classification of atypical pneumonias, and together with *C pneumoniae*, comprises approximately 30% of community-acquired pneumonia. *C pneumoniae* is an obligate intracellular bacteria, originally known as TWAR, and recognized as a cause of respiratory tract infections in 1986.[18] Numerous viruses such as adenovirus, enterovirus, herpes viruses, measles, metapneumoviruses, non–severe acute respiratory syndrome coronavirus, respiratory syncytial virus, and rhinoviruses may cause atypical pneumonia syndromes. In the immunocompromised host, fungi such as *Cryptococcus neoformans* and protozoa such as *Pneumocystis carinii* may also be associated with atypical pneumonia presentations.

*M pneumoniae*, similar to many of the microbial pathogens listed previously, often originates in the nasal and upper airway and may be associated with a spectrum of clinical presentations that include rhinitis, laryngitis, laryngotracheitis, laryngotracheobronchitis (croup), and pneumonia. The nature of the patient's clinical presentation will depend on the inoculum, as well as the host's immune and inflammatory response. Depending on the intensity and duration of exposure, the incubation period for respiratory infections associated with *M pneumoniae* is usually 2 to 3 weeks. Initial symptoms are often comparable to a viral upper respiratory tract infection, and include acute rhinitis with rhinorrhea, sore throat, malaise, low-grade fever, and bronchitic cough. The cough may be productive or paroxysmal. If the illness progresses to pneumonia, increasing lower airway congestion accompanied by mild chest pain and dyspnea can occur. On physical examination, pharyngitis with and without exudates, otitis media or bullous myringitis, sinusitis, bronchial breath sounds, rhonchi, localized crackles, and wheezing, but rarely pleuritic chest pain, can be present. It is important to note that physical examination findings consistent with pneumonia may not correlate with chest x-ray findings. Early radiographic infiltrates, at times with small pleural effusions, may precede physical examination signs, whereas prominent physical examination findings may occur concurrently with a normal chest x-ray.

With or without antimicrobial therapy, the usual clinical course for *M pneumoniae* in the immunocompetent host is 2 to 3 weeks. Patients with sickle cell anemia, Down syndrome, and immune disorders can develop severe disease, and infections can present more like invasive bacterial infections.[3] Acute respiratory distress syndrome and acute respiratory failure have also been associated with *M pneumoniae*.

Extrapulmonary manifestations of *M pneumoniae* infections are not unusual and can occur in the previously healthy adolescent. Uveitis, erythema multiforme, Stevens-Johnson syndrome, and neurologic manifestations have been well described. These extrapulmonary conditions are usually self-limited similar to the pulmonary symptoms. Cardiomyopathy, myositis, mild arthritis, pancreatitis, and hemolytic anemia are rarely observed.[3,19]

The diagnosis of *M pneumoniae* is often elusive because sputum cultures and Gram stains are negative, and chest x-ray findings are variable. The usual radiographic appearance for a lower respiratory infection with *M pneumoniae* consists of bilateral diffuse interstitial or localized nonlobar infiltrates characteristic of bronchopneumonia. However, lobar consolidation and small pleural effusions can be observed. The diagnosis for *M pneumoniae* pneumonia is usually made by identification of elevated levels to specific antibodies during the acute and convalescent period. *M pneumoniae* PCR is a diagnostic tool being developed to identify genetic markers associated with *M pneumoniae* and other pathogens associated with atypical pneumonia.[3,15] Polymerase chain reaction may become a more readily available diagnostic tool that will assist the clinician in choosing prompt antimicrobial therapy when indicated.

Although tetracycline and doxycycline have been traditionally used to treat *M pneumoniae* and *C pneumoniae* pulmonary infections in adolescents, the macrolides, especially azithromycin, are probably more commonly used due to a more convenient dosing schedule. Fluoroquinolones are also effective in treating *M pneumoniae* and *C pneumoniae* pulmonary infections, but are more expensive. Despite appropriate antimicrobial therapy, *M pneumoniae* often can continue to be isolated from the respiratory tract.[3]

## TUBERCULOSIS

Tuberculosis (TB) is a chronic bacterial disease due to infection by the *Mycobacterium tuberculosis* complex (See Chapter 140, Mycobacterial Infections). This complex includes *M tuberculosis, Mycobacterium bovis*, and *Mycobacterium africanum*. These organisms cause similar clinical disease, but *M tuberculosis* comprises all but a small percentage of human TB. The infection is typically spread by inhalation of a single infectious aerosolized droplet, typically in an enclosed area, which penetrates into the terminal airway. For the first few weeks, the bacilli proliferate in the localized area and drain through the local lymphatics to regional lymph nodes. They then spread hematogenously to other sites in the body. The alveoli are usually the first site of infection, and the site where the alveolar macrophage ingests and then attempts to phagocytize the bacilli. Once ingested by the macrophages, the natural defenses of the tubercle can prevent the macrophage from killing it, in which case the microbe can lie dormant in the macrophage for long periods in the immunocompetent host. The contained infection is called primary TB, which is the most common type of TB in adolescents. Most adolescents remain asymptomatic throughout the process of the infection, but the dormant bacilli remain a lifelong source for endogenous reactivation. The risk of reactivation is approximately 10% over the life of those infected, and is influenced by aging, immunosuppression, and malnutrition. When the macrophages are unable to adequately contain the tubercle, clinical signs and symptoms of active infection develop. This form of TB is called progressive primary TB and is more common in the immunosuppressed, especially patients with HIV infection or AIDS. The risk of reactivation in a patient with HIV/AIDS not treated with chemoprophylaxis increases to 10% per year.[20]

Reactivation of primary TB, also called postprimary TB or chronic TB, can occur in adolescents infected as younger children due to the increased metabolic stress of rapid growth during puberty. Pregnancy also increases the risk of reactivation due to metabolic stress and possibly due to negative nitrogen balance. Active TB in adolescence can be aggressive and rapidly progressive, which has been attributed to pubertal hormonal changes as well as altered protein and calcium metabolism during periods of rapid growth. Adolescents from inner-city indigent populations, immigrants from countries with high rates of TB, intravenous drug users, and the malnourished are at greatest risk for reactivation of primary TB.[21]

Primary TB frequently occurs without symptoms but can be associated with a nonproductive cough. The clinical presentation of progressive primary TB and postprimary TB include productive cough, hemoptysis, fever, weight loss, and night sweats. The chest examination can be normal or associated with decreased breath sounds consistent with airway obstruction. Crackles are not a typical finding but wheezing can indicate airway compression from adenopathy. Increased tactile and audible fremitus and egophony can be elicited with tuberculous pleural effusions, which occur more commonly in adolescents as compared to children.[22] Radiographic findings in all stages of TB are variable and can include the presence of mediastinal lymphadenopathy, infiltrates, segmental atelectasis, cavitary lesions, pleural effusions, and a Ghon focus, which is a calcified area from primary infection usually surrounding the lobar fissure.

The Mantoux skin test is an effective method of early detection and is recommended in all high-risk adolescents. Within 2 to 10 weeks of initial infection, the Mantoux becomes positive; therefore, if there is a high level of suspicion of infection despite a negative skin test, a second Mantoux skin test should be placed at 12 weeks from the initial negative test. A positive tuberculin skin test has to be interpreted in conjunction with the patient's risk factors and clinical presentation. Less than 5 mm induration is typically considered a negative test, and greater than 15 mm induration is universally considered a positive test. Findings between 5 and 15 mm induration require individual assessment, depending on the patient's risk of infection. Chest x-rays and sputum cultures are obtained from all patients with positive skin tests. Sputum cultures for mycobacterium are the gold standard for diagnosis but have a low sensitivity. Acid-fast staining of sputum is a more rapid diagnostic tool but is frequently falsely negative, and can also be falsely positive because non-TB bacteria are ubiquitous in the environment. Two recently developed diagnostic studies, T-Spot TB and QuantiFERON-TB Gold, detect interferon gamma released by T cells in response to *M tuberculosis*-specific antigen. These methods may be better diagnostic tests than skin testing, especially in patients with HIV or AIDS. These tests will also likely be more specific for those vaccinated with bacilli Calmette-Guérin (BCG) or for those who have HIV or AIDS because delayed hypersensitivity can be affected. However, additional studies on these tests are needed.[23]

Adolescents with primary TB are rarely contagious and can continue normal activity. Treatment with isoniazid (INH) decreases the risk of reactivation later in life. It is safe to be given during pregnancy, but in the low-risk pregnant patient the medication is usually started after delivery. Chemical hepatitis is a serious complication that can occur with high-dose INH and rifampin. This risk is greatest in those with a history of hepatitis, alcohol or drug abuse, or chronic liver disease. Baseline liver function tests should be obtained in patients with these risks and in patients being treated with signs of hepatotoxicity. Pregnant and lactating teenagers and those with inadequate diets are at risk for neuropathy from INH; therefore, vitamin B6 supplementation should be considered. Adolescents with active disease, productive cough, and smear-positive sputum require respiratory isolation until the sputum becomes negative and the cough diminishes. It usually takes 2 weeks from the initiation of anti-TB therapy before respiratory isolation can be discontinued. See Box 89-4 for TB drug therapy.

### Box 89-4

### *Recommended Treatment Regimens for Drug-Susceptible Tuberculosis in Adolescents*[24]

**Positive tuberculosis (positive skin test, no disease)**

- Isoniazid (INH) once daily for 9 months. If daily therapy not possible, directly observed therapy (DOT) twice a week for 9 months
- INH resistant: Rifampin once daily for 6 months. If daily therapy not possible, DOT twice a week for 6 months
- INH rifampin resistant: Consult TB expert

**Positive skin test and hilar adenopathy**

- INH and rifampin for 6 months

**Active pulmonary disease**

- 2 months INH rifampin, and pyrazinamide daily, followed by 4 months INH and rifampin DOT

## REFERENCES

1. Gordon RJ, Lowy FD. Bacterial infections in drug users. *N Engl J Med*. 2005;353:1945-1954

2. Bals R, Hiemstra PS. Innate immunity in the lung: how epithelial cells fight against respiratory pathogens. *Eur Respir J*. 2004;23:327-333

3. Ward MA. Lower respiratory tract infections in adolescents. *Adolesc Med*. 2000;11:251-262

4. Donnelly BW, McMillan JA, Weiner LB. Bacterial tracheitis: report of eight new cases and review. *Rev Infect Dis*. 1990;12:729-735

5. Hopkins A, Lahiri T, Salerno R, Heath B. Changing epidemiology of life-threatening upper airway infections: the reemergence of bacterial tracheitis. *Pediatrics*. 2006;118:1418-1421

6. Donnelly BW, McMillan JA, Weiner LB. Bacterial tracheitis: report of eight new cases and review. *Rev Infect Dis*. 1990;12:729-735

7. Britto J, Habibi P, Walters S, Levin M, Nadel S. Systemic complications associated with bacterial tracheitis. *Arch Dis Child*. 1996;74:249-250

8. Wenzel RP, Fowler AA. Acute bronchitis. *N Engl J Med*. 2006;355(20):2125-2130

9. Knutson D, Braun C. Diagnosis and management of acute bronchitis. *Am Fam Physician*. 2002;65:1281-1282

10. Ward JL, Cherry JD, Chang SJ, et al. APERT Study Group. Efficacy of an acellular pertussis vaccine among adolescents and adults. *N Engl J Med*. 2005;353:1555-1561

11. Hallett JS, Jacobs RL. Recurrent acute bronchitis: the association with undiagnosed bronchial asthma. *Ann Allergy*. 1985;55:568-570

12. Boldy DA, Skidmore SJ, Ayres JG. Acute bronchitis in the community: clinical features, infective factors, changes in pulmonary function and bronchial reactivity to histamine. *Respir Med*. 1990;84:377-385

13. Halperin SA. The control of pertussis—2007 and beyond. *N Engl J Med*. 2007;356:110-113

14. Preventing tetanus, diphtheria, and pertussis among adolescents: use of tetanus toxoid, reduced diphtheria toxoid and acellular pertussis vaccines: recommendations of the Advisory Committee on Immunization Practices. *MMWR Recomm Rep*. 2006;55(RR-3):1-34

15. American Thoracic Society. Definition and classification of chronic bronchitis, asthma, and pulmonary emphysema. *Am Rev Respir Dis*. 1962;85:762-768

16. Gordon RC. Community-acquired pneumonias of adolescents. *Adolesc Med*. 2000;11:681-695

17. Pneumococcal infections. *Red Book: Report of the Committee on Infectious Disease*. 27th ed. Elk Grove Village, IL: American Academy of Pediatrics; 2006:525-537

18. Blasi F. Atypical pathogens and respiratory tract infections. *Eur Respir J*. 2004;24:171-181

19. Graystone JT, Kuo CC, Wang SP, Altman J. A new *Chlamydia psittaci* strain, TWAR, isolated in acute respiratory tract infections. *N Engl J Med*. 1986;315:161-168

20. Principi N, Esposito S. *Mycoplasma pneumoniae* and *Chlamydia pneumoniae* cause lower respiratory tract disease in pediatric patients. *Curr Opin Infect Dis*. 2001;15:295-300

21. American Thoracic Society/Centers for Disease Control and Prevention/Infectious Disease Society of America. Controlling tuberculosis in the United States. *Am J Respir Crit Care Med*. 2005;172:1169-1227

22. Wilcox, WD, Laufer S. Tuberculosis in adolescents. *Clin Pediatr*. 1994;33:258-262

23. Merino JM, Carpintero I, Alvarez T, Rodrigo J, Sanchez J, Coello JM. Tuberculous pleural effusion in children. *Chest*. 1999;115:26-30

24. Richeldi L. An update on the diagnosis of tuberculosis infection. *Am J Respir Crit Care Med*. 2006;174:736-742

# CHAPTER 90

# Asthma

JOSHUA P. NEEDLEMAN, MD

Asthma continues to remain one of the most significant health problems for children and adolescents. With prevalence estimates that have increased from 10% to 20% in diverse populations, asthma exacts a significant toll on teenagers and young adults. Despite advances in therapy, the impact, measured in school absences, lost days from work, emergency department visits, and reduction in health-related quality of life, is enormous. For the patients who develop acute severe exacerbations, fatal outcomes still occur with 5,000 deaths per year. Asthma is more common and more severe in minority and urban populations, increasing its affect on an already vulnerable population.[1-4]

The adolescent patient with chronic disease presents specific challenges to the clinician in terms of clinical presentation, quality of life, and other complicating medical problems. In addition, the adolescent patient will often present challenges with regard to medication adherence, communication of disease status, and the patient's evolving autonomy. The objectives of this chapter are to review the basic pathophysiology of asthma, as well as its treatment and evaluation. The issues specific to the care of the adolescent patient are emphasized.

## PATHOPHYSIOLOGY

Asthma is a complicated clinical syndrome characterized by airflow obstruction that is reversible or partially reversible, bronchial hyper reactivity, and airway inflammation. The clinical presentation can vary from episodes of severe distress with respiratory failure to a disruptive chronic cough. The elucidation of the intricate response that produces the varied asthma phenotypes continues to provide a great deal of substrate for clinical investigators.[5]

A wide variety of irritating factors have been demonstrated to provoke airway reactivity and inflammation in individuals with asthma. These include allergens, viral pathogens, *Chlamydia* and *Mycoplasma* species, and exercise.[6] When the provocative entities are inhaled into the airway, mast cells degranulate and release histamine and leukotrienes that cause constriction of smooth muscle and result in bronchoconstriction, the main element of the early phase response. The late phase response occurs 4 to 6 hours later and is a multipronged inflammatory response produced by a wide variety of inflammatory cells, including mast cells, macrophages, epithelial cells, lymphocytes, and eosinophils releasing a wide range of chemokines and cytokines.[7]

The narrowing of the airways resulting from the bronchoconstriction and inflammation affects the small airways in a heterogeneous fashion, causing an increase in airway resistance leading to breathing difficulty. The subsequent irregular distribution of ventilation throughout the lung can lead to ventilation and perfusion mismatching within the lung, resulting in hypoxemia.[8] Narrowed airways with increased secretions can trap mucus and result in plugging, atelectasis, and hypoxemia. Long standing inflammation can result in structural changes to the airway wall referred to as airway remodeling.[9]

## CLINICAL PRESENTATION AND EVALUATION

The key to successful asthma management involves careful evaluation at the time of diagnosis and assessment of therapy response at subsequent clinical contacts. Although diagnosis may seem obvious in many cases, it is incumbent on the clinician to make the diagnosis while excluding complicating factors or alternative diagnoses. As in many areas of clinical medicine, a careful history and physical examination form the cornerstone of asthma diagnosis and management.

### HISTORY

As with any other chronic illness, the history obtained from the patient and family is often the most significant piece of information in making the diagnosis of asthma and in assessing asthma control. Asthma is a disease with a highly variable clinical course. The key to evaluation is not merely to focus on the patient's current condition but on his or her clinical status throughout the preceding time period, including focusing on periods of illness and relative wellness, nighttime and daytime symptoms, and during exercise and while at rest. Because reversibility of airflow obstruction is central to the definition of asthma, clarification of the patient's response to inhaled bronchodilators is important in establishing the diagnosis.

Many patients who have asthma have been symptomatic, without a diagnosis, for years and have experienced significant impairment to their quality of life. Likewise, there are patients who carry a diagnosis of asthma who have other diagnoses that need to be clarified before they can be effectively treated. Given that the most common presenting complaints in asthma are chronic cough or recurring episodes of dyspnea or distress, complaints with broad differential diagnoses (Tables 90-1 and 90-2), care must be taken to make or exclude the diagnosis of asthma while considering all alternatives. The cough associated with asthma is often worse with upper respiratory infections, following exercise, and at night. While posterior pharyngeal irritation cough is often accentuated immediately on lying down at bedtime, the asthma cough often awakens the patient in the middle of the night.[10] Inhaled bronchodilators usually cause an improvement in cough related to asthma for several hours for a period of time.[11,12]

The complaint of wheezing can be more difficult to pursue from a historical perspective because patients and their families often refer to a wide variety of sounds and symptoms as wheezing. Patients may also report chest tightness, chest pain, pressure, tachypnea, distress, and anxiety as symptoms of asthma. Again, a key historical point to note is response to bronchodilator therapy.

When assessing the level of asthma control in a patient with a confirmed diagnosis of asthma, the history continues to play a significant role. Because patients often have trouble recalling symptoms over a period of more than 2 weeks, a symptom diary can be invaluable in quantifying severity and frequency of symptoms. A variety of checklists and other tools have been developed to assess asthma control.[13,14] A simple checklist is shown in Table 90-3. In the past, physicians caring for children and young adults with asthma focused primarily on symptoms of distress, emergency department visits, and hospital admissions. Recent research and outreach efforts have emphasized the evaluation of quality-of-life measures and the disruption that asthma can cause with symptoms that fall below the threshold of emergency or inpatient care.[15-17] A careful history should include the quality of sleep and its disruption by cough or other symptoms, school attendance, and activity levels. Patients who have previously been poorly controlled might not recognize their asthma symptoms as significant if they are part of their daily lives. The clinician must extract the information about impaired quality of life, even if the patient does not recognize it as problematic.

## PHYSICAL EXAMINATION

The physical examination of a patient with asthma can be normal or may contain important information to make the diagnosis or assess the disease state. The presence or absence of wheezing, quality of aeration and retractions, and accessory muscle use must be noted.

**Table 90-1**

**Differential Diagnosis of Chronic Cough in Adolescent Patients**

| | |
|---|---|
| Upper respiratory tract irritation | • Postnasal drip/rhinitis<br>• Sinusitis<br>• Gastroesophageal reflux disease<br>• Swallowing dysfunction |
| Infection or postinfection | • Tuberculosis<br>• Pertussis |
| Airway obstruction | • Tracheo/bronchomalacia<br>• Asthma<br>• Foreign body |
| Chronic suppurative lung disease | • Cystic fibrosis<br>• Primary ciliary dyskinesia<br>• Immunodeficiency<br>• Idiopathic bronchiectasis |
| Medication induced | • Angiotensin-converting enzyme inhibitors |
| Habit cough | • Stress/psychogenic<br>• Behavioral |

**Table 90-2**

**Causes of Recurrent or Chronic Wheezing in Adolescent Patients**

| | *Features* | *Findings on Evaluation* |
|---|---|---|
| Asthma | • Worse with exercise or respiratory infections<br>• Responds to bronchodilators<br>• Responds to steroids | • Reversible obstruction on pulmonary function tests (PFTs)<br>• Positive bronchoprovocation |
| Tracheo/ bronchomalacia | • Worse with activity<br>• Poor response to bronchodilators<br>• Poor response to steroids | • Airway collapse on fluoro<br>• Collapsible trachea or bronchus on bronchoscopy |
| Foreign body | • Sudden onset in history | • Differential breath sounds<br>• Differential hyperinflation or collapse on radiograph |
| Heart failure/ pulmonary edema | • Poor response to albuterol<br>• Poor growth | • Hepatomegaly<br>• Responds to diuresis |
| Vocal cord dysfunction | • Poor response to all therapies<br>• Severe distress reported | • PFTs: normal or with abnormal inspiratory loop<br>• Laryngoscopy: vocal cord adduction during inspiration |
| Cystic fibrosis | • History of poor growth, gastrointestinal symptoms<br>• Recurrent pneumonias | • Positive sweat test |

The response of any of these physical findings to a bronchodilator should be documented carefully. Many adolescents with airflow obstruction will breathe in a pattern of tiny breaths above their functional residual capacity, therefore masking their obstruction and appearing to have clear lungs. It is important, after examining the patient while breathing comfortably, to encourage the patient to inhale to total lung capacity and exhale forcefully. This will often reveal signs of airflow obstruction previously unappreciated.

In addition to examination of the chest, a complete physical examination is essential to exclude other

**Table 90-3**

**Asthma Control Checklist**

| | *Normal* | *Mild* | *Moderate* | *Severe* |
|---|---|---|---|---|
| **Sleep** | ☐ Undisturbed | ☐ Coughs in sleep 1–2 times per month | ☐ Coughs in sleep 1–2 times per week | ☐ Nightly symptoms |
| **Activity/exercise** | ☐ No limitations | ☐ Occasionally misses gym | ☐ Cannot take gym | ☐ Trouble on stairs<br>☐ Trouble walking long distances |
| **School absence** | ☐ None–2 days per year | ☐ Less than 1 month | ☐ 1 month | ☐ More than 1 missed school day per month |
| **Coughs** | ☐ Never–with colds for 2 days or less | ☐ Following respiratory infections, 2 weeks or more<br>☐ With heavy activity | ☐ Nightly | ☐ Daily |
| **Albuterol use** | ☐ Twice a month or less | ☐ 1–2 times per week | ☐ Daily | ☐ Multiple times per day |

complicating or alternative diagnoses. Examination of the nasal turbinates, for example, can suggest rhinitis as a complicating cause of cough and may reveal nasal polyps, which should always prompt the consideration of a diagnosis of cystic fibrosis. Specific attention should be paid to the presence of digital clubbing. Digital clubbing is not a feature of asthma and may indicate the presence of cystic fibrosis or chronic suppurative lung disease.

### DIAGNOSTIC IMAGING

Diagnostic imaging can be used judiciously in the evaluation and treatment of the patient with asthma.[18] Although not useful in the management of a patient with uncomplicated asthma, radiographs and other imaging techniques can be useful in excluding other problems in patients with a new onset of symptoms or in whom symptoms are difficult to control. A chest radiograph should be considered in an adolescent patient with a new onset of sudden and severe symptoms that respond poorly to therapy, specifically to exclude a mediastinal mass.

In the patient with asthma that is poorly controlled, a radiograph may suggest the presence of cardiac disease or suppurative lung disease. This may lead to the diagnosis of complicating or alternative diagnoses. Figures 90-1 and 90-2 are the chest radiograph and computed tomography (CT) scan of a 13-year-old patient who had been treated for years for asthma that was considered difficult to control. After the CT scan revealed bilateral apical bronchiectasis, further evaluation confirmed the diagnosis of cystic fibrosis with a rare genotype and a borderline normal sweat chloride measurement.

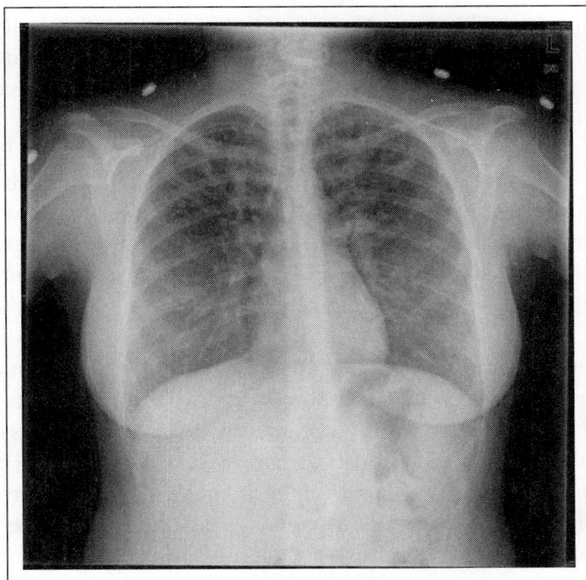

**FIGURE 90-1** Chest radiograph of 13-year-old girl treated for asthma for many years. Note chronic disease in upper lung fields.

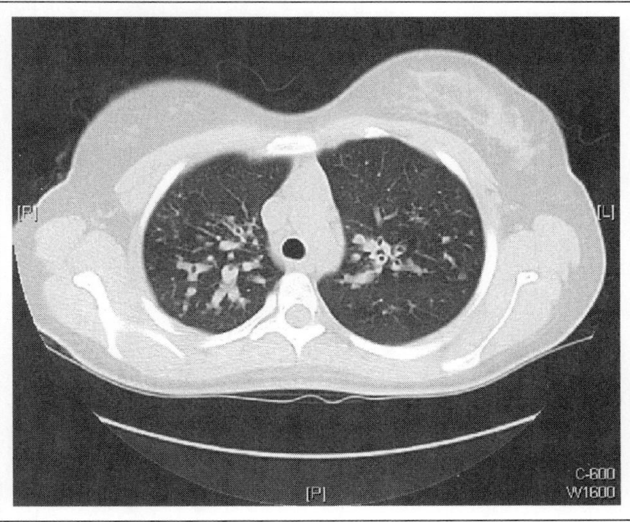


**FIGURE 90-2** Bronchiectasis on chest CT scan of patient in Figure 90-1. Patient has positive genotyping for rare cystic fibrosis mutations, confirming diagnosis.

### PULMONARY FUNCTION TESTS

Pulmonary function tests (PFTs) can be helpful in establishing the diagnosis of asthma and monitoring the course of the disease. The most commonly performed PFT is spirometry during which the patient inhales to total lung capacity and then exhales forcefully. The amount of air exhaled and the rate at which it leaves the lung is recorded. Spirometry can be used to detect obstructive lung disease and to estimate the site of obstruction, whether small or large airways. Common measurements made during spirometery include the forced vital capacity (FVC), which is the total amount of air exhaled; the forced expiratory volume in 1 second (FEV1), which is a measure of large and medium airways; and the average flow during the middle of the vital capacity [forced expiratory flow (FEF)], which is a measure of medium and small airway function. Patients with an obstructive lung disease such as asthma will have reduced FEFs. In patients with asthma, lung function can be normal or reduced, depending on the level of control and severity of disease.

Because asthma is an obstructive disease, primarily of the medium and small airways, spirometry is the test of choice. Portable spirometers are now readily available and affordable for many clinical settings, allowing measurements to be made frequently and at the time of the office visit. Figures 90-3 and 90-4 demonstrate the use of spirometry in the evaluation of 2 patients with

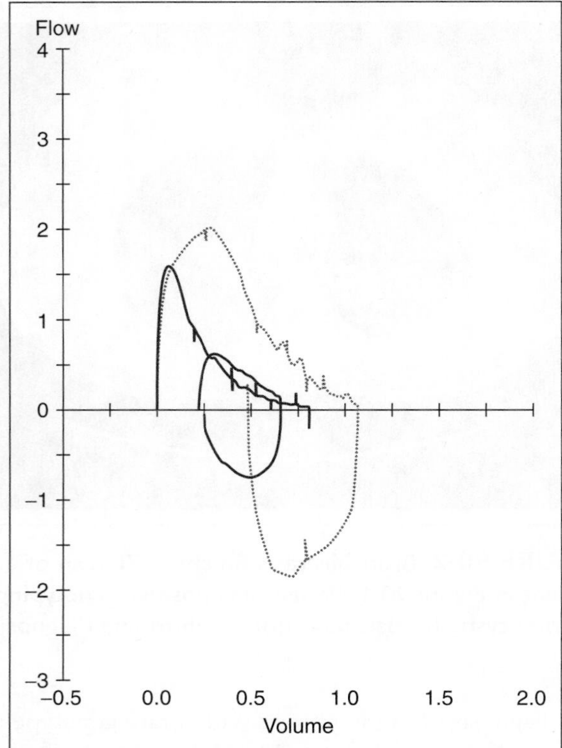


**FIGURE 90-3** Spirometry in adolescent patient with asthma who reports no symptoms. Flow is graphed as function of lung volume with expiratory flow above the baseline of 0. Solid lines represent baseline lung function, and dotted lines represent post bronchodilator administration. At baseline, the patient exhibits marked obstructive lung disease with large improvement following bronchodilator administration. Given these findings, despite a negative history by report, the patient was started on maintenance anti-inflammatory therapy, and his lung function normalized.

suspected diagnoses of asthma. Because a moderate decline in lung function can be clinically silent, regular PFT measurements can help detect disease activity that is unapparent to the patient and clinician.

In situations where asthma is suspected but physical examination and PFTs are normal, bronchial provocation could be considered. Bronchial provocation tests are used to provoke airway reactivity and aid in the diagnosis of asthma. During a bronchial provocation test, a bronchoconstrictive agent such as methacholine is administered by aerosol. Pulmonary function is measured at baseline and then after increasing doses of methacholine, while lung function is measured serially. A reduction in pulmonary function in response to the provocative agent is considered a positive sign of airway reactivity. Other agents commonly used to provoke airway reactivity include histamine, hypertonic saline, and dry cold air.

Another form of bronchial provocation that is used to evaluate exercise-induced dyspnea and suspected exercise-induced asthma is cardiopulmonary exercise testing. In a formal exercise test, the subject performs spirometry and exercises maximally on either a stationary bicycle or a treadmill. Oxygen consumption, carbon dioxide production, heart rate, oxygen saturation, and blood pressure are all measured. Following exercise, spirometry is again measured serially. A decline in FEFs following exercise is considered a positive test for exercise-induced bronchoconstriction.

The peak expiratory flow meter is an inexpensive measure of airway function that has been popular. Portable and cheap enough to be distributed to individual patients, peak flow meters became common tools for patient self-assessment and were written into many asthma action plans. The peak flow is a measurement of large airway function and is reduced during asthma exacerbations, but recent data[19] have suggested that it may be insensitive to detect the small airway dysfunction seen in early asthma exacerbations. The utility of the peak flow meter was further questioned by data[20] that demonstrated that symptom scores rose prior to a fall in peak flows during early asthma exacerbations. Comparisons of asthma plans based on symptom monitoring with plans that used peak flow failed to show any advantage to the peak flow–based plans.[21,22] Given that a peak flow meter, although inexpensive, does require some outlay of financial and time resources, and that a normal peak flow reading could give a patient with an early asthma exacerbation a false sense of security, its use should be limited to those patients who are documented to be significant over- or underperceivers of their illness.

An assessment of oxygenation is an important PFT as well. Noninvasively, pulse oximetry can be an effective, accurate measure of oxygen saturation. Patients with chronic airflow obstruction may have mild oxyhemoglobin desaturation that is clinically inapparent. A pulse oximetry measurement can be helpful both in evaluation of patients who are acutely ill and during their chronic management. An arterial blood gas (ABG) adds the measurement of acid–base status and carbon dioxide to the measurement of oxygenation. During episodes of extreme distress, an ABG can provide valuable information regarding the possibility of impending respiratory fatigue and failure. Disturbances in acid–base balance or gas exchange are often late signs during acute asthma episodes. Because patients can be severely ill but not have developed abnormal pulse oximetry or ABG findings, the clinician must be careful not to be lulled into a false sense of security by normal results from these tests.

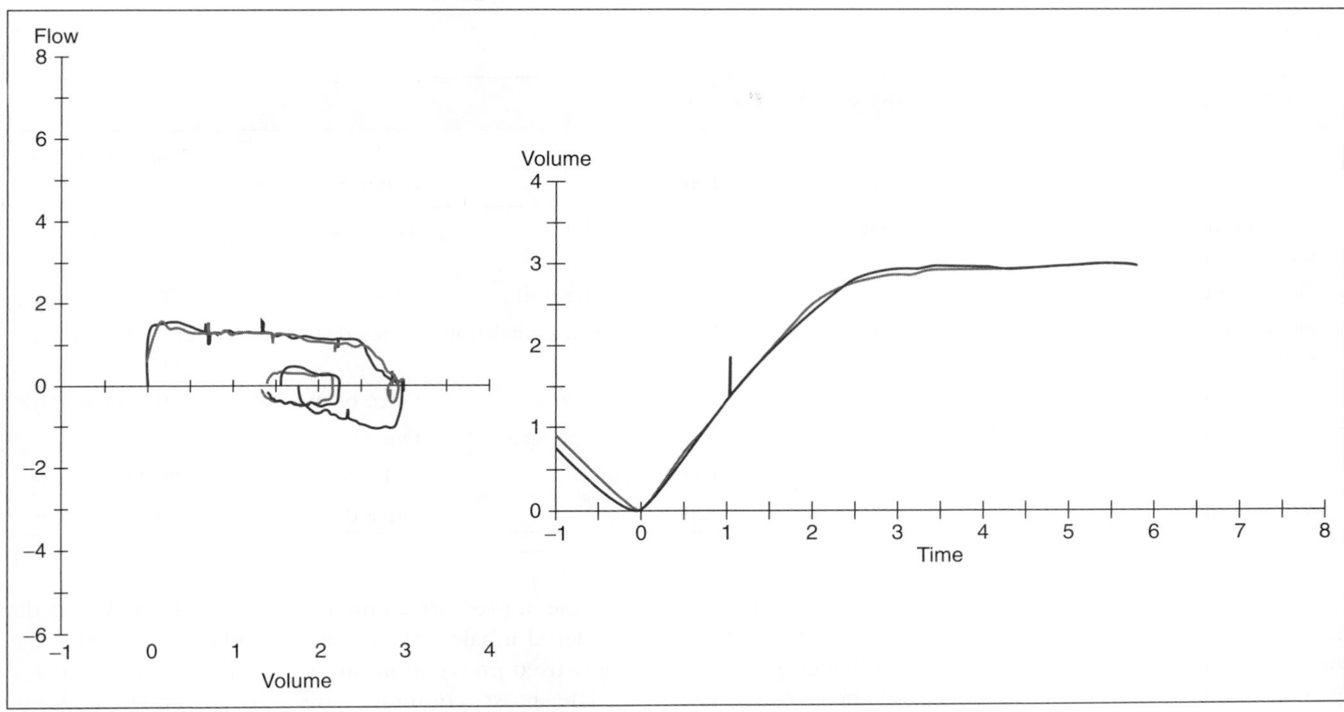


**FIGURE 90-4** A 17-year-old female with progressive dyspnea for 2 years, despite daily asthma therapy. Spirometry reveals severe obstruction with square shape that suggests large airway obstruction. There is no bronchodilator response with pre and post flow volume loops superimposed on top of each other. Airway endoscopy revealed subglottic inflammatory mass that was removed by laser excision with resolution of symptoms.

## TREATMENT

A wide range of options exist for asthma care today. There are a variety of medications available with multiple types of delivery systems. Despite this, asthma control eludes a large number of patients. In beginning to develop an asthma management plan for a particular patient, the physician and patient must first discuss and agree on the goals of therapy. In the past, asthma treatments focused on episodic care of exacerbations, and success was defined as a shortened course of illness and a rapid return to baseline clinical status. It is natural for many patients to continue to view their disease from the perspective of many, episodic illnesses. One important educational challenge is to change this perception and establish long-term goals of therapy.

Therapy is most likely to be successful if the provider and the patient agree on goals and desired outcomes. The goals must be reasonable and attainable, but allow the patient to have persistent symptoms. A typical set of goals of asthma therapy might, for example, include the following:

- Number of absences from school no greater than any other student in his or her class without asthma
- Ability to participate in gym and other sports without limitation from asthma symptoms
- No nocturnal cough
- No limitation of recreational activities due to asthma symptoms or concern about provoking asthma symptoms

If the goals and expectations are discussed from the outset, then progress can be assessed as collaboration between patient and clinician, which is significantly more likely to be successful.

A discussion of specific treatment options and therapeutic modalities for asthma in the adolescent patient follows.

### ENVIRONMENTAL CONTROLS

The reduction, or elimination, of asthma triggers, allergens, and other environmental factors in an effort to treat or reduce asthma symptoms is an attractive concept because it could, potentially, produce a clinical effect without the addition of pharmacotherapy. Although many options for environmental interventions exist, there is limited evidence for the efficacy of many of them, and the clinician must remain cognizant of their cost and effect on the patient prior to insisting on some interventions.

**Table 90-4**

**Common Inhaled Corticosteroid Preparations**

| *Name* | *Delivery Mechanism* | *Unit Doses* | *Dosing Interval* | *Common Dose Range* |
|---|---|---|---|---|
| Beclomethasone dipropionate | Metered-dose inhibitor (MDI) | 40 μg, 80 μg/puff | Twice daily | 80–320 μg/day |
| Fluticasone propionate | MDI | 44, 110, 220 μg/puff | Twice daily | 176–880 μg/day |
| Fluticasone in combination salmeterol | Dry powdered inhaler (DPI) | 100, 250, 500 μg/inhalation | Twice daily | 200–500 μg/day |
| Budesonide | DPI | 200 μg/inhalation | Once or twice daily | 400–800 μg/day |
| Budesonide | Nebulization | 0.25 mg, 0.5 mg vials | Once or twice daily | 0.5–1 mg/day |
| Triamcinolone acetonide | MDI | 100 μg/puff | 2–4 times/day | 400–800 μg/day |
| Mometasone furoate | DPI | 220 μg/puff | Once daily | 220–440 μg/day |

The creation of a smoke-free environment is an environmental approach that can be recommended strenuously without reservation. The effect of tobacco smoke, primary and environmental (secondhand), on the respiratory symptoms of patients with asthma is quite clear.[23,24] Although difficult to create, a smoke-free environment can have a positive affect on an adolescent patient with asthma. Successfully encouraging an adolescent with asthma to stop smoking can have an even greater effect. It is unlikely that smoking cessation by the patient and everyone around him or her will obviate the need for ongoing asthma treatment, but it will make the asthma easier to treat and improve daily quality of life.

The reduction of indoor allergens and irritants in an effort to reduce asthma symptoms is more difficult and has met with mixed results. The use of dust mite and allergen-impermeable mattress and pillow covers has been recommended for patients with asthma but has not been shown to be effective in reducing symptoms.[25] A significantly more aggressive approach that included air purifiers, cleaning the home regularly with a HEPA filter vacuum cleaner, mattress covers, and cockroach extermination produced a modest, yet clinically significant effect.[26] The use of air cleaners and purifiers by themselves has not been shown to be effective.[27]

## INHALED CORTICOSTEROIDS

Inhaled corticosteroids (ICSs) are the mainstay of asthma maintenance therapy. They provide effective anti-inflammatory treatment when used daily. Regular ICS use is associated with a reduced risk of fatal asthma exacerbation,[28] even in low doses. There is a wide variety of ICS products available, with multiple doses and different delivery systems. Currently, ICS preparations are available in pressurized metered-dose inhalers (MDIs), dry powdered inhalers (DPIs), and nebulizer solutions. Commonly used preparations are summarized in Table 90-4.

The most common side effects reported during the use of ICSs relate to local effects from deposition in the oropharynx. These include oral candidiasis and a hoarse voice. The incidence of both of these is reduced by routine mouth rinsing and appropriate inhalation technique.

Of more concern is the possible effect of long-term use of ICSs on bone composition and stature. This issue has been studied extensively by many methods and with many different inhaled steroids. It seems as if there is short-term fall in growth velocity when inhaled steroids are initiated, but that when they are continued consistently, catch-up growth occurs.[29] The best long-term studies available have found that the effect of chronic ICS use on final adult height is minimal and that most patients will have normal stature.[30] Untreated and uncontrolled asthma can have a negative effect on growth by delaying puberty and the associated growth spurt.[31] In summary, the effect of ICSs on growth at normal therapeutic doses is of low concern, while the withholding of ICSs can have an affect on growth and lung function. The prudent approach is to use ICSs when indicated, but to use as low a dose as possible while controlling asthma symptoms. In addition, ensuring that adolescent patients maintain adequate calcium intake seems wise, although there have been no reports of a significant effect of normal doses of ICSs on bone metabolism in adolescent patients.

## SYSTEMIC CORTICOSTEROIDS

Corticosteroids, such as prednisone, administered by mouth are effective treatments for asthma exacerbations.

In extreme cases of severe, poorly controlled asthma, they may be used chronically for maintenance. Although the side effects for a typical short course of 7 days or less are relatively low, the patient on daily oral steroids is at risk for significant untoward effects, including weight gain, hypertension, osteopenia, and myopathy. These effects are limited somewhat when steroids are reduced to every other day, and efforts should be made to place the patient on that schedule.

### SHORT-ACTING BETA AGONISTS

Short-acting beta agonist bronchodilators, such as albuterol, levalbuterol, or pirbuterol, are the basic first line asthma therapy. They are available by inhalation in MDI forms and for nebulization. They work quickly, relaxing smooth muscle surrounding the airways and reducing airflow obstruction. Although they have no protective benefit, they are most effective at improving symptoms in the short term. In addition, administration of a bronchodilator can be used diagnostically in an evaluation for asthma. A patient with obstructive lung disease and asthma should have an improvement in spirometry and physical examination following a beta agonist.

The major side effects from beta agonist use are sympathomimetic, tachycardia, and tremors. In a few patients, adverse effects will limit the use of beta agonists. For those, the single isomer beta agonist levalbuterol should be offered. Given at a lower dose, many patients will have a similar therapeutic response with less adverse effects.[32] Oral beta agonists, however, usually have side effects that many patients find intolerable.

### LONG-ACTING BETA AGONISTS

Long-acting beta agonists, such as salmeterol and formoterol, are available as single drugs or in combination with ICSs. The addition of a long-acting beta agonist to an ICS has been shown to improve asthma control and allow a reduction in inhaled steroid dose.[33] They have also been shown to have some protection in nocturnal asthma and exercise-induced asthma. These findings, coupled with the convenience of combination medication delivery systems, has led to a rapid increase in the use of long-acting beta agonists.[34]

Despite their popularity, questions regarding the appropriate role of long-acting beta agonists and their safety exist. The SMART (Salmeterol Multicenter Asthma Research Trial) study is one of several postmarketing studies that increased the level of concern regarding safety.[35] In the study, 26,355 patients were recruited before enrollment was halted prematurely. A small but significant increase in asthma-related deaths was found in the group receiving salmeterol compared to placebo (13 compared with 3). This imbalance in deaths and life-threatening experiences was highest in black patients. This study and other postmarketing data reports prompted the US Food and Drug Administration to strengthen their warnings on all drugs containing long-acting beta agonists in June 2005. The new warnings include cautions against using these drugs as first line therapy for asthma and when asthma is worsening. They also specifically state that there may be an increased risk of severe or life-threatening asthma exacerbations (www.fda.gov/Drugs/DrugSafety/PublicHealthAdvisories/ucm162678.html). Subsequent publications have continued to suggest that long-acting beta agonists may increase the risk of life-threatening asthma exacerbations or asthma-related deaths.[36]

Despite the concern regarding long-acting beta agonists, there are many patients who are using them safely with great benefit. A judicious approach must be employed in their use. Guidelines offered by this author for use of long-acting beta agonists include the following:

- Use long-acting beta agonists in patients who have poor asthma control despite MDI corticosteroid use and who demonstrate a bronchodilator response during PFTs.
- Monitor symptoms and lung function closely in patients in whom long-acting beta agonists have been started. If there is a lack of response or a decline, stop the drugs.
- Always use long-acting beta agonists with ICSs.
- Ensure the patient understands that the drugs are controller therapy and not to be increased during times of illness.
- Have direct discussions of the risks and benefits of long-acting beta agonists during the asthma education sessions.
- Do not consider long-acting beta agonists in patients who appear to have a poor understanding and perception of their disease and medication use.

### LEUKOTRIENE RECEPTOR ANTAGONISTS

Leukotriene receptor antagonists, such as zafirlukast and montelukast, block the cysteinyl leukotrienes, LTC4, LTD4, and LTE4, which are important mediators in asthma inflammation and potent bronchoconstrictors.[37] Leukotriene receptor antagonists are available in oral preparations and are used as maintenance therapy for asthma. Although some patients will be controlled by oral leukotriene receptor antagonist therapy alone, their real role seems to be as add-on therapy for patients receiving ICSs.[38] Their easy use and palatability improves adherence to therapy, especially in the adolescent patient. In addition, they have been shown to be effective in the treatment of allergic rhinitis as well, which many patients with asthma also have.

### ANTI-IgE MONOCLONAL ANTIBODIES

The development of IgE-specific antibodies is the latest addition to the asthma armamentarium. In patients who have poorly controlled asthma and elevated IgE, injecting anti-IgE antibody biweekly or monthly can reduce asthma symptoms and allow reduction of other therapies. The initial results have been encouraging, but the need for regular injections and the high cost of the medication have been barriers to patients receiving treatment.

### SELECTION OF THERAPY FOR ASTHMA MAINTENANCE

With a wide range of choices for asthma controller therapies, the clinician needs to consider the patient's needs, lifestyle, and disease status when choosing therapy. The initial decision is whether the patient needs daily controller therapy, or intermittent rescue therapy only. Most authorities agree that patients who require bronchodilator treatment, or have symptoms of asthma more that twice in a month, should be considered for daily preventative asthma therapy. Any patient who has had a hospital admission should also be considered for daily maintenance, regardless of his or her symptom frequency.

When selecting the initial therapy, the first line option should be ICSs. With a plethora of options (Table 90-4), the initial choice should be selected with consideration for patient preference. Because adherence is the major barrier to asthma control, select a medication regimen that will be readily accepted. Most MDIs should be used with a valved holding chamber spacer to maximize aerosol delivery, but many teenagers refuse to use or carry their spacers. Dry powder inhalers, such as the Pulmicort Flexhalers or the Diskus inhaler, are popular with adolescent patients due to their rapid and easy use. Some DPIs have a taste and some do not, and an adverse taste is often a reason that some adolescent patients refuse their controller regimen. Nebulizer treatments, although effective and popular, are time consuming and, therefore, difficult to use on a daily basis.

Once the initial therapy is selected, the next most important steps are education and monitoring of response. The patient must understand the regimen, the rationale, and the proper technique. Attention must be paid to inhaler technique, spacer use (if applicable), assessment of remaining medication, and importance of daily use. Written instructions are preferred. With physical examination, as well as close follow-up and monitoring of symptoms and pulmonary function, a good assessment of the success of the regimen can be obtained. If the patient is not well controlled on the initial therapy, a "step up" should be considered by increasing the inhaled steroid dose or adding an additional controller to the regimen. If the patient is well controlled while on a moderated dose of ICS, a "step down" can be considered.

### MANAGEMENT OF ASTHMA EXACERBATIONS

Even patients who are optimally controlled on their maintenance therapy will have acute deteriorations, termed "attacks" or "exacerbations," on occasion. The patient must have a plan in place for responding to these exacerbations in a rapid fashion and have the tools on hand to prevent a severe episode and to shorten the illness to as brief an interruption as possible.

The initial response to an increase of asthma symptoms is to begin administering a short-acting beta agonist. These are usually given every 3 to 4 hours as needed but can, in a situation of distress, be given in a burst of 3 treatments in an hour. If the patient is receiving regular beta agonists and is having little or partial response, the addition of oral corticosteroids is usually the next step.[39] All patients should have an emergency supply of oral steroids in their home to allow them to start, with appropriate consultation and guidance, systemic steroids early in the course of their exacerbation. Patients who have to wait for a doctor's visit and then a trip to the pharmacy before initiating oral steroids are more likely to miss school, visit the emergency department, and be admitted for hospitalization. All patients should be instructed to maintain close contact with their providers if they fail to respond to this plan.

A patient with an early asthma exacerbation who has experience and resources in the home can often be managed without an emergency department visit. This is preferable because it is less expensive and less disruptive to the patient's life. A patient who is having worsening distress or who requires bronchodilators every 2 hours or more for a prolonged time requires a physician evaluation or emergency department treatment. Any patient who seems to have a poor understanding of his or her disease and the treatment plan should also be referred for evaluation. In an emergency department setting, additional therapies such as oxygen, frequent or continuous beta agonists, inhaled anticholinergics,[40] and noninvasive ventilation[41] can be considered. A complete review of the treatment options for the severely ill acute asthmatic is beyond the scope of this chapter.

## DIFFICULT TO CONTROL ASTHMA

Most patients with persistent asthma, when identified correctly, will respond to the first or second step of maintenance therapy with a reduction in symptoms, an improvement in pulmonary function, and a reduction or elimination in the frequency and severity of exacerbations. The remaining 5% or fewer patients who fail to respond to their therapeutic interventions will consume a great deal of resources in the form of physician time, medications, and lost days of school and work.[42] These patients represent significant challenges to the clinicians, families, and the health care system as a whole.

The first step in gaining control of the patient with poorly controlled asthma is to revisit the diagnosis and ascertain its accuracy. As previously noted, there are patients who have been classified as having "recalcitrant asthma" who are having symptoms from other conditions (Tables 90-1 and 90-2). Exclusion of certain diagnoses, such as cystic fibrosis or allergic bronchopulmonary aspergillosis, can be easily achieved with several laboratory tests. Other behaviorally based diagnoses such as vocal cord dysfunction or habit cough require a high index of suspicion and can be quite difficult to confirm or exclude.

Some patients with asthma have difficulty achieving control due to complicating additional diagnoses. Common problems encountered are sinus disease, allergic rhinitis, and gastroesophageal reflux. Only when these cofactors are controlled can the patients' asthma be brought under control as well. Obesity is a complicating cofactor whose relationship to asthma is only partially understood.[43–46] It is clear, however, that patients with asthma who are obese will have fewer symptoms and improved quality of life scores when they lose weight.

When the diagnosis is secure and possible complicating factors have been addressed, the most common problem in the adolescent with poorly controlled asthma is adherence to the regimen of controller therapy. Adherence to maintenance medication is a problem for all patients with chronic illness that often escalates in the adolescent years. The emerging independence of the patient, coupled with concerns regarding body image, peer pressure, and medication use, combine to complicate the goals of asthma control. The clinician needs to confront the issue of nonadherence in a direct and nonjudgmental fashion in order to be successful. Avoid being drawn into family arguments and, if possible, validate the patient's concerns as well as the family's and physician's points of view. These situations are dealt with successfully when the patient is able to articulate his or her own barriers to medication adherence and help build strategies to improve them. Some strategies that have worked for some patients include the following:

- Designing medication schedules to help fit the patient's lifestyle
- Allowing the patient to select between several similar controller regimens to find 1 that is most acceptable, choosing 1 type of delivery system over another, for example
- Using a rubber band to attach the controller inhaler to the patient's toothbrush, toothpaste, hairbrush, or other article used on a daily basis
- Cell alarm phone reminders
- Keeping a written, weekly log that the patient signs each day after using medication; these often include some notation of symptoms and are returned to the clinician or pulmonary function laboratory or a weekly basis

The key to effective intervention in the previous examples, or in any other plan, is for the patient to be involved in selecting the system and to agree to it in advance. Success should be praised and the patient encouraged.

## SUMMARY

Asthma may be the most common chronic disease of childhood and adolescence, but it is also, frequently, controllable. Uncontrolled asthma can have an effect on an adolescent patient's health and quality of life, often in ways that are not apparent during superficial examination. With careful attention to an individual patient's needs and concerns, a personalized plan for asthma control that is effective and sustainable can be produced. Because asthma control is a goal that is only achieved through daily intervention and cooperation on the part of the patient and family, a collaborative approach that involves the patient at all times is often most successful.

## REFERENCES


1. von Mutius E. The burden of childhood asthma. *Arch Dis Child.* 2000;82(suppl II):ii2–ii5

2. Arias E, Anderson RN, Kung H-C, et al. Deaths: final data for 2001. *Nat Vital Stat Rep.* 2003;52(3). Hyattsville, MD: National Center for Health Statistics. DHHS Publication No. (PHS) 2003–1120

3. Dey AN, Schiller SJ, Tai DA. Summary health statistics for U.S. children: National health interview survey, 2002. *Vital Health Stat.* 2002;10:1–87

4. McDaniel M, Paxson C, Waldfogel J. Racial disparities in childhood asthma in the United States: evidence from the national health interview survey, 1997 to 2003. *Pediatrics.* 2006;117:868–877

5. Chu EK, Drazen JM. Asthma: one hundred years of treatment an onward. *Am J Respir Crit Care Med.* 2005;171:1202–1208

6. Lemanske RF, Busse WW. Asthma: factors underlying inception, exacerbation, and disease progression. *J Allergy Clin Immunol.* 2006;117:S456–S461

7. Busse WW, Lemanske RF. Asthma. *N Engl J Med.* 2001;344:350–361

8. McFadden ER. Acute severe asthma. *Am J Respir Crit Care Med.* 2003;168:740–759

9. Ward C, Walters H. Airway wall remodeling: the influence of corticosteroids. *Curr Opin Allergy.* 2005;5:43–48

10. Martin RJ, Banks-Schlegel S. Chronobiology of asthma. *Am J Respir Crit Care Med.* 1998;158:1002–1007

11. Schidlow DV. Cough in children. *J Asthma.* 1996;33:81–87

12. Irwin RS, Madison JM. The diagnosis and treatment of cough. *N Engl J Med.* 2000;343:1715–1721

13. Peters D, Chen C, Markson L, et al. Using an asthma control questionnaire and administrative data to predict health-care utilization. *Chest.* 2006;129:918–924

14. Vollmer WM, Markson L, O'Connor E, et al. Association of asthma control with health care utilization: a prospective evaluation. *Am J Respir Crit Care Med.* 2002;165:195–199

15. Juniper EF, Guyatt GH, Feeny DH, et al. Measuring quality of life in children with asthma. *Qual Life Res.* 1996;5:35–46

16. Juniper EF. How important is quality of life in pediatric asthma? *Pediatr Pulmonol.* 1997;15:17–21

17. Maier WC, Arrighi HM, Morray B, et al. The impact of asthma and asthma-like illness in Seattle school children. *J Clin Epidemiol.* 1998;51:557–568

18. Harty MP, Kramer SS. Recent advances in pediatric pulmonary imaging. *Curr Opin Pediatr.* 1998;10:227–235

19. Eid N, Yandell B, Howell L, et al. Can peak expiratory flow predict airflow obstruction in children with asthma? *Pediatrics.* 2000;105:354–358

20. Gibson PG, Wong BJO, Hepperle MJE, et al. A research method to induce and examine a mild exacerbation of asthma by withdrawal of inhaled corticosteroid. *Clin Experiment Allergy.* 1992;22:525–532

21. Turner MO, Taylor D, Bennett R, et al. A randomized trial comparing peak expiratory flow and symptoms self-management plans for patients with asthma attending a primary care clinic. *Am J Respir Crit Care Med.* 1998;157:540–546

22. Malo J-L, L'Archeveque J, Trudeau C, et al. Should we monitor peak expiratory flow rates or record symptoms with a simple diary in the management of asthma? *J Allergy Clin Immunol.* 1993;91:702–709

23. Dhala A, Pinsker K, Prezant DJ. Respiratory health consequences of environmental tobacco smoke. *Clin Occup Environ Med.* 2006;5:139–156

24. Chaudhuri R, Livingston E, McMahon AD, et al. Effects of smoking cessation of lung function and airway inflammation in smokers with asthma. *Am J Respir Crit Care Med.* 2006;174(2):127–133. Epub 2006 Apr 27

25. Woodcock A, Forster L, Matthews E, et al. Control of exposure to mite allergen and allergen-impermeable bedcovers for adults with asthma. *N Engl J Med.* 2003;349:225–236

26. Morgan WJ, Crain EF, Gruchalla RS, et al. Results of a home-based environmental intervention among urban children with asthma. *N Engl J Med.* 2004;351:1068–1080

27. Reisman RE. Do air cleaners make a difference in treating allergic disease in homes? *Ann Allergy Asthma Immunol.* 2001;87:41–43

28. Suissa S, Enrnst P, Benayoun S, et al. Low-dose inhaled corticosteroids and the prevention of death from asthma. *N Engl J Med.* 2000;343:332–336

29. Brand PLP. Inhaled corticosteroids reduce growth. Or do they? *Eur Respir J.* 2001;17:287–294

30. Agertoft L, Pedersen S. Effect of long-term treatment with inhaled budesonide on adult height in children with asthma. *N Engl J Med.* 2000;343:1064–1069

31. Merkus PJFM, Van-Essen Zandvliet EEM, Duiverman EJ, et al. Long-term effect of inhaled corticosteroids on growth rate in adolescents with asthma. *Pediatrics.* 1993;91:1121–1126

32. Berger WE. Levalbuterol: pharmacologic properties and use in the treatment of pediatric and adult asthma. *Ann Allergy Asthma Immunol.* 2003;90:583–592

33. Bisgaard H. Long-acting beta-2 agonists in management of childhood asthma: a critical review of the literature. *Pediatr Pulmonol.* 2000;29:221–234

34. Bisgaard H, Szefler S. Long-acting beta-2 agonists and paediatric asthma. *Lancet.* 2006;367:286–288

35. Nelson HS, Weiss ST, Bleecker ER, et al. The salmeterol multicenter asthma research trial: a comparison of usual pharmacotherapy for asthma or usual pharmacotherapy plus salmeterol. *Chest.* 2006;129:3–5

36. Salpeter SR, Buckley NS, Ormiston TM, et al. Meta-analysis: effect of long-acting beta agonists on severe asthma exacerbations and asthma-related deaths. *JAMA.* 2006;144:904–912

37. Bisgaard H. Leuokotriene modifiers in pediatric asthma management. *Pediatrics.* 2001;107:381–390

38. Simons FE, Villa JR, Lee BW, et al. Montelukast added to budesonide in children with persistent asthma: a randomized, double-blind, crossover study. *J Pediatr.* 2001;138:694–698

39. Roy SR, Milgrom H. Management of the acute exacerbation of asthma. *J Asthma.* 2003;40:593–604

40. Quershi F, Pestian J, Davis P, et al. Effect of nebulized ipratropium on the hospitalized rates of children with asthma. *N Engl J Med.* 1998;339:1030–1035

41. Needleman JP, Sykes JA, Schroeder SA, et al. Noninvasive positive pressure ventilation in the treatment of pediatric status asthmaticus. *Pediatr Asthma Allergy Immunol.* 2004;17:272-277

42. Strek ME. Difficult asthma. *Proc Am Thorac Soc.* 2006;3:116-123

43. Chen Y. Obesity and asthma in children. *J Pediatr.* 2004;144:146-147

44. Chinn S. Obesity and asthma: evidence for and against a causal relationship. *J Asthma.* 2003;40:1-16

45. Deane S, Thomson A. Obesity and the pulmonologist. *Arch Dis Child.* 2006;91:188-191

46. Li AM, Chan D, Wong E, et al. The effects of obesity on pulmonary function. *Arch Dis Child.* 2003;88:361-363

# CHAPTER 91

# Vocal Cord Dysfunction in Adolescents

MAGGIE SIFAIN, MD • EULALIA R.Y. CHENG, MD

## INTRODUCTION

Vocal cord dysfunction (VCD) is a common and often unsuspected condition in adolescents. Patients frequently present with symptoms that may not initially suggest the underlying pathology. Recognition of the clinical picture can avoid unnecessary testing and ineffective treatment. This chapter addresses the clinical presentation, pathophysiology, etiology, evaluation, and treatment of VCD.

## CLINICAL PRESENTATION

### HISTORY

Vocal cord dysfunction can occur at any age but often first occurs during childhood and adolescence.[1] Affected patients may complain of recurrent episodes of exercise-induced dyspnea.[2,3] Other chief complaints may include a sensation of throat closure, choking, stridor, wheezing, and shortness of breath.[4] Thus, the clinical picture of VCD often mimics asthma.[2,5,6] Unlike asthma, however, on detailed history, patients report dyspnea that is worse with inspiration than with expiration. Clinical severity ranges from mildly affected to severe.[6] There have been reports of adolescents presenting with significant respiratory distress and dramatic inspiratory stridor that resulted in hospitalization, intubation, and even tracheostomy.[6]

For reasons that are unclear, VCD is predominantly observed in adolescent and young adult females twice as frequently as males.[4] It is also disproportionately over-represented in young athletes, likely due to their competitive nature.

### PHYSICAL EXAMINATION

Between episodes of vocal cord adduction, the physical examination is usually normal.[7] During an acute attack, patients demonstrate harsh stridulous sounds with inspiration.[6] At times, auscultation of the lungs may reveal wheezing due to transmission of upper airways noises.[6] On comparing the regional differences in auscultation, however, the harsh breath sounds and wheezing get louder as one moves away from the lower lung up toward the upper airway. In addition, having the patient revert from mouth breathing to nasal breathing may dramatically improve the stridor and wheezing. Additional findings of rhinitis, postnasal drip, or gastroesophageal reflux disease are often present.[8,9]

## PATHOPHYSIOLOGY

During normal inspiration, the vocal cords abduct to allow the passage of inspired air from the larynx into the trachea. In patients with VCD, the vocal cords adduct or do not abduct sufficiently to allow unrestricted airflow.[6,10] This results in the turbulent passage of air into the upper trachea that leads to affected patients developing acute intermittent episodes of upper airway obstruction to airflow.

## ETIOLOGY

The underlying etiology of VCD remains unclear. Widely accepted theories suggest that altered vagal nerve outflow may alter the tone of laryngeal muscles.[9] The result is an increased sensitivity of the vocal cords to a variety of stimuli, such as chemicals, fumes, smoke, dust, and other inhalant irritants, exercise, or psychosocial conflict and stress. When exposed to these stimuli, vocal cord spasm and abnormal adduction of the vocal cords occur.

The role of gastroesophageal reflux disease and rhinitis resulting in increased sensitivity of the vocal cords has become more widely accepted.[9] There may be a higher incidence of VCD in persons with psychiatric conditions, persons working in the medical field, and obese individuals.[9] The increased prevalence of VCD among adolescent and young adult females compared to males may be related to affected females having comorbidities such as anxiety, obsessive-compulsive disorder, or depression.[9] Vocal cord dysfunction may complicate true bronchospastic asthma in a small number of patients.[6] Such cases can present challenges in management and benefit from the biopsychosocial approach, in which conventional asthma therapies may be used in combination with biofeedback techniques.

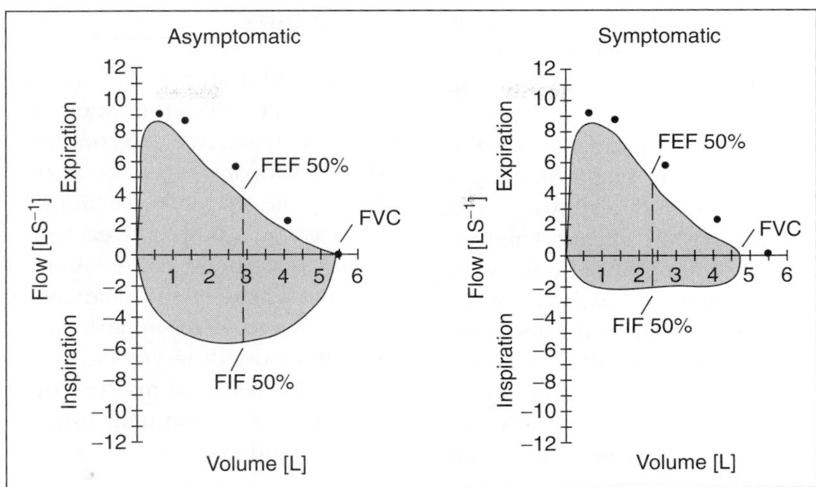


**FIGURE 91-1** Spirometry flow volume loops in vocal cord dysfunction. (A) Normal inspiratory and expiratory loops; (B) truncated inspiratory loop suggestive of variable extrathoracic large airway obstruction and normal expiratory loop. This is pathognomic of paradoxical vocal cord motion. *FVC*, forced vital capacity; *FEF 50%*, forced expiratory flow 50%; *FIF 50%*, forced inspiratory flow. (Image reprinted with permission from eMedicine.com, 2010. Available at: emedicine.medscape.com/article/137782-overview.)

## EVALUATION

History and physical examination generally suggest the diagnosis if the clinician is aware of the usual findings. Body plethysmography and diffusing capacities are usually normal.[2] Volume loops on spirometry, however, characteristically demonstrate flattening and truncation of the inspiratory flow loop (Figure 91-1).[7,8,11,12] Confirmation of the diagnosis is made by direct, flexible, fiber-optic laryngoscopy that reveals the presence of paroxysmal adduction with inspiration (Figure 91-2).[8,13] Adduction of the anterior two-thirds of the vocal cords with a posterior diamond-shaped "chink" through which air is able to flow during inspiration is also characteristic.[8,13]

A variety of laboratory studies are performed in the evaluation of an adolescent with VCD, but these will only exclude other diagnoses, which can, however, be helpful when other conditions are suspected. Chest radiographs are generally normal. Complete blood counts are usually normal, but an elevated eosinophil count may be noted in atopic adolescents. Serum IgE levels may also be normal or elevated in patients with allergies or asthma.

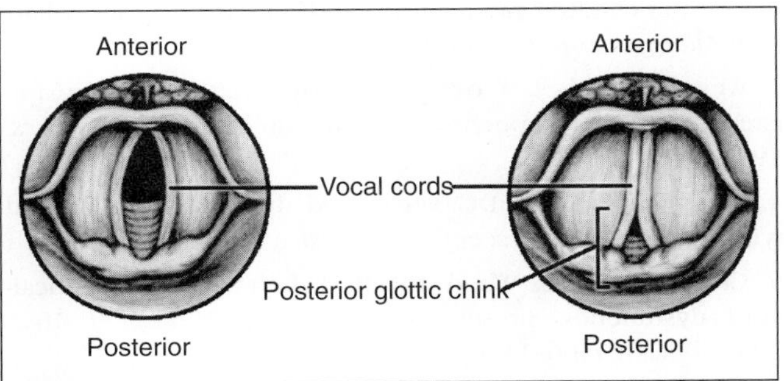


**FIGURE 91-2** Laryngoscopic appearance of vocal cord dysfunction. Note characteristic adduction of anterior vocal cords during inspiration and posterior glottic "chink." (Image reprinted with permission from eMedicine.com, 2010. Available at: emedicine.medscape.com/article/137782-overview)

### CHALLENGE TESTING

In the absence of concomitant asthma, methacholine provocation is normal. Exercise challenge testing can also be useful in further exclusion of exercise-induced asthma.[14] A *lack* of significant decline in lung function with maximal exercise supports the diagnosis of VCD.[2] Previously noted flattening of the flow-volume curves may also be observed with this study.[2,4]

## TREATMENT

A coordinated approach to the treatment of VCD starts with a definitive diagnosis. If direct laryngoscopy is not performed, characteristic history, physical examination, and volume-loop studies are sufficient. When performed, diagnostic direct laryngoscopy should include video-recording of the adduction of the vocal cords during inspiration.[6] This provides confirmation of the diagnosis and, more important, has a role in facilitating treatment.

Visually demonstrating to the patient and the family the functional changes during inspiration reinforces the location of the restricted airflow in the upper airway and also reinforces the physical nature of the condition. This is important for patients who have been treated without benefit for asthma or for whom psychological factors are considered important. The approach to patients with mental health concerns, such as anxiety, may lead the adolescent and family to believe that the symptoms of VCD are "all in the head." Reassurance and support are most easily accepted when there is a physiological explanation for the symptoms of VCD that may sometimes be triggered by stress or anxiety.

The cornerstone of the treatment of VCD is a variety of mind–body techniques that emphasize that the VCD symptoms are due to involuntary spasm of the adductor muscles of the vocal cords that may be triggered by a number of factors.[9] Awareness and avoidance of known triggers is helpful. However, it is essential for adolescent and young adult patients to realize that spasms can be brought under voluntary control, even when they are initiated involuntarily. For example, teaching patients effective breathing techniques in the form of diaphragmatic breathing and relaxation strategies provides a sense of mastery, which in itself may reduce anxiety.[6,9] This sense of mastery over a body function may be especially important for athletes.[15] Biofeedback can aid those who have difficulty focusing on such exercises by providing a target of attention related to the relaxation response.[9] These procedures are often done with the help of a speech therapist, clinical psychologist, or psychiatrist familiar with this condition.[9] They can provide extraordinary amounts of success when done properly. Instructing patients to continue to practice these techniques, even when not symptomatic, further increases the success of the procedure.

## PROGNOSIS

Vocal cord dysfunction tends to affect patients throughout their lifetimes, and symptoms that resolve in adolescence can recur later in life. In general, the prognosis is good. Patients respond well to breathing exercises and may experience complete relief of symptoms. A lack of response may indicate a concomitant pathology or a lack of compliance to therapy. These options should be thoroughly investigated in persistently symptomatic patients.

## SUMMARY

Vocal cord dysfunction is most commonly misdiagnosed as another condition, such as asthma. Because there may be associated psychological symptoms of anxiety, depression, or obsessive-compulsive disorder, the failure to respond to standard asthma treatment often results in increasingly complex treatment regimens, which when ineffective only cause more psychological distress. An awareness of the characteristic findings on history, physical examination, and spirometry can lead to confirmatory direct laryngoscopy and begin effective treatment. The sense of mastery over symptoms that occurs with effective treatment improves the quality of life in affected individuals.

## INTERNET RESOURCES

- **Allergy & Asthma Network.** Vocal Cord Dysfunction: Something to Talk About. February 19, 2009. Available at: www.aanma.org/2009/02/vocal-cord-dysfunction-something-to-talk-about/. Accessed February 19, 2010
- **American Thoracic Society.** What Is Vocal Cord Dysfunction? Patient Care Series. 2006. Available at: patients.thoracic.org/information-series/en/resources/what-is-vocal-cord-dysfunction-vcd.pdf. Accessed March 30, 2010

## REFERENCES

1. Link HW, Stillwell PC, Jensen VK, Laskowski DM. Vocal cord dysfunction in the pediatric age group. *Chest.* 1998;114 (suppl 4):255S–256S

2. Abu-Hasan M, Tannons B, Weinberger M. Exercise-induced dyspnea in children and adolescents: if not asthma then what? *Ann Allergy Asthma Immunol.* 2005;94:366–371

3. Weir M, Ehl L. Vocal cord dysfunction mimicking exercise-induced bronchospasm in adolescents. *Pediatrics.* 1997;99(6):923–924

4. Kayani S, Shannon DC. Vocal cord dysfunction associated with exercise in adolescent girls. *Chest.* 1998;113:540–542

5. Christopher KL, Wood RP II, Eckert RC, et al. Vocal-cord dysfunction presenting as asthma. *N Engl J Med.* 1983;308(26):1566–1570

6. Murray DM, Lawler PG. All that wheezes is not asthma: paradoxical vocal cord movement presenting as severe acute asthma requiring ventilatory support. *Anaesthesia.* 1998;53(10):1006–1011

7. Landwehr LP, Wood RP II, Blager FB, Milgrom H. Vocal cord dysfunction mimicking exercise-induced bronchospasm in adolescents. *Pediatrics.* 1996;98(5):971–974

8. Silvers WS, Levine JS, Poole JA, Naar E, Weber RW. Inlet patch of gastric mucosa in upper esophagus causing chronic cough and vocal cord dysfunction. *Ann Allergy Asthma Immunol.* 2006;96(1):112–115

9. Sokol W. Vocal cord dysfunction presenting as asthma. *West J Med.* 1993;158(6):614–615

10. Newman KB, Mason UG III, Schmaling KB. Clinical features of vocal cord dysfunction. *Am J Respir Crit Care Med.* 1995;152(4 pt 1):1382–1386

11. Parker JM, Mooney LD, Berg BW. Exercise tidal loops in patients with vocal cord dysfunction. *Chest.* 1998;114 (suppl 4):256S

12. Vlahakis NE, Patel AM, Maragos NE, Beck KC. Diagnosis of vocal cord dysfunction: the utility of spirometry and plethysmography. *Chest.* 2002;122(6):2246–2249

13. Brancatisano T, Collett PW, Engel LA. Respiratory movements of the vocal cords. *J Appl Physiol.* 1983;54(5): 1269–1276

14. Selner JC, Staudenmayer H, Koepke JW, et al. Vocal cord dysfunction: the importance of psychologic factors and provocation challenge testing. *J Allergy Clin Immunol.* 1987;79(5): 726–733

15. Newsham KR, Klaben BK, Miller VJ, Saunders JE. Paradoxical vocal-cord dysfunction: management in athletes. *J Athl Train.* 2002;37(3):325–328

# CHAPTER 92

# Cystic Fibrosis

KAREN Z. VOTER, MD • ANN H. MCMULLEN, CPNP • CLEMENT L. REN, MD

## INTRODUCTION

Cystic fibrosis (CF) is the most common serious genetic disease in the white population.[1] An autosomal recessive condition, CF is caused by mutations in the gene encoding the cystic fibrosis transmembrane conductance regulator (CFTR).[1] Although the genetic defect in CF was identified in 1989, the precise mechanism by which mutations in the *CFTR* gene result in the clinical manifestations of CF remain incompletely defined.[2-4] As its name suggests, CFTR is a central regulator of ion transport across epithelial cell membranes. The current leading hypothesis proposes that loss of CFTR function leads to altered ion transport, which in turn results in loss of periciliary fluid and increased viscous secretions in multiple organ systems, including the respiratory system, gastrointestinal tract, and reproductive organs.[3] However, other mechanisms, including impaired innate immunity, may also be involved.[4-6]

Cystic fibrosis was first described as a distinct clinical entity in the 1930s.[7,8] At that time, most patients did not survive past infancy. In the 1950s, the introduction of antibiotics, airway clearance therapies, and nutritional interventions resulted in significant improvements in survival.[9] Over the past 10 years, there has been a steady improvement in clinical symptoms and lung function.[10] Today, most patients with CF survive well into their fourth decade.[9] Hence, CF patients constitute a large and growing population of young adults with chronic illness.

## EPIDEMIOLOGY

The epidemiology of CF displays a distinct ethnic and racial pattern (Table 92-1).[9,11-13] Although most (94%) of patients with CF are white and of Northern European heritage, the disease can be found in people of any racial or ethnic background. The median age at diagnosis is 6 months, but the mean age of diagnosis is 3 years, indicating that there is a cohort of older individuals who are not diagnosed until later in childhood or adulthood.[9]

**Table 92-1**

**Birth Prevalence of Cystic Fibrosis in Different Racial and Ethnic Groups**

| *Racial/Ethnic Group* | *Birth Prevalence (Affected/ Number of Live Births)* |
|---|---|
| Non-Hispanic White | 1/2,500–3,500 |
| Hispanic | 1/4,000–10,000 |
| Black | 1/15,000–20,000 |
| Asian | 1/40,750 |

The prevalence rate for Asians varies depending on the specific population studied. The value listed in the table is for Asian Indians in the United States.

Although most CF patients are diagnosed in infancy or early childhood, approximately 5% are diagnosed at age 21 years or older.[9] These adolescents and young adults frequently lack the classic features of CF that would have suggested the diagnosis at a younger age. Caregivers for adolescents should therefore always remain alert to the possibility of CF in an adolescent or young adult patient presenting with the appropriate clinical history (see "Diagnosis" section).

The introduction of specific CF therapies and the development of the CF care center network has been associated with increasing improvements in survival (Figure 92-1).[9] Because the estimated median age of survival is based on deaths in the preceding year, Figure 92-2 represents a minimal expectation for survival in CF patients born today and in recent years. Analysis of survival by birth cohorts (Figure 92-2) shows that most (>80%) CF patients born in the 1980s have survived into adulthood, and the survival rate is increasing with each successive birth cohort.[9] With continued efforts in early diagnosis and intervention, the population of adolescent and adult patients with CF will continue to increase in the future.

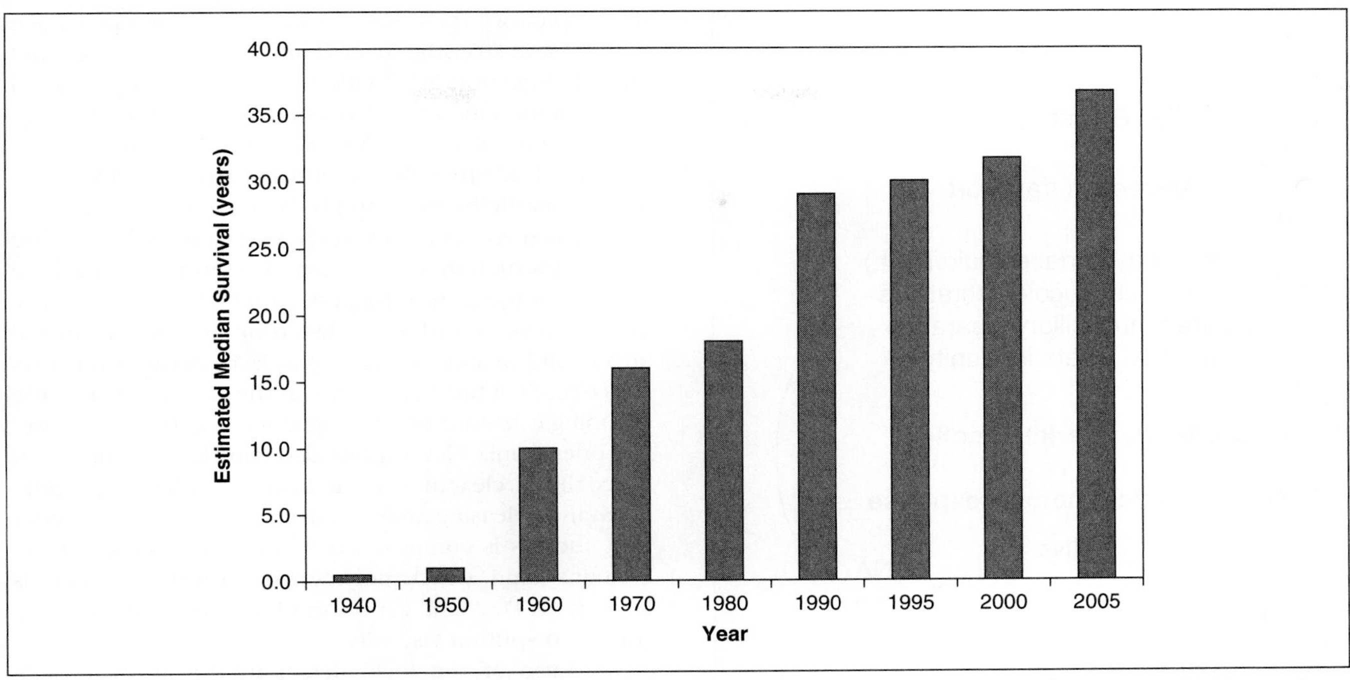


FIGURE 92-1 Estimated median survival in years for US cystic fibrosis patients. (Data are from the CF Foundation Patient Registry.)

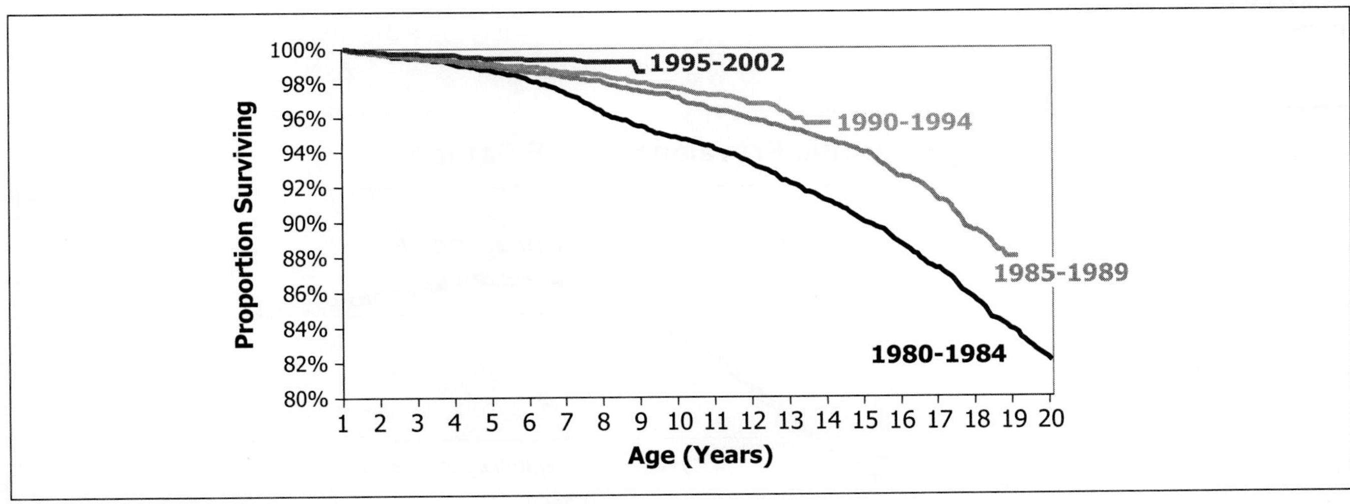


FIGURE 92-2 Proportion of US cystic fibrosis patients surviving to a given age, by 5-year birth cohort. (Data are from the CF Foundation Patient Registry.)

## CLINICAL FEATURES

Cystic fibrosis affects multiple organ systems. Respiratory disease accounts for most of the morbidity and mortality from CF, but other complications such as malabsorption, diabetes mellitus, and upper airway disease are also important.

### LUNG DISEASE

The clinical features of CF lung disease are chronic endobronchial infection and bronchiectasis.[2] Although the exact mechanism by which CF lung disease develops is still not fully understood, some of the key factors are depicted in Figure 92-3. Loss of CFTR function in

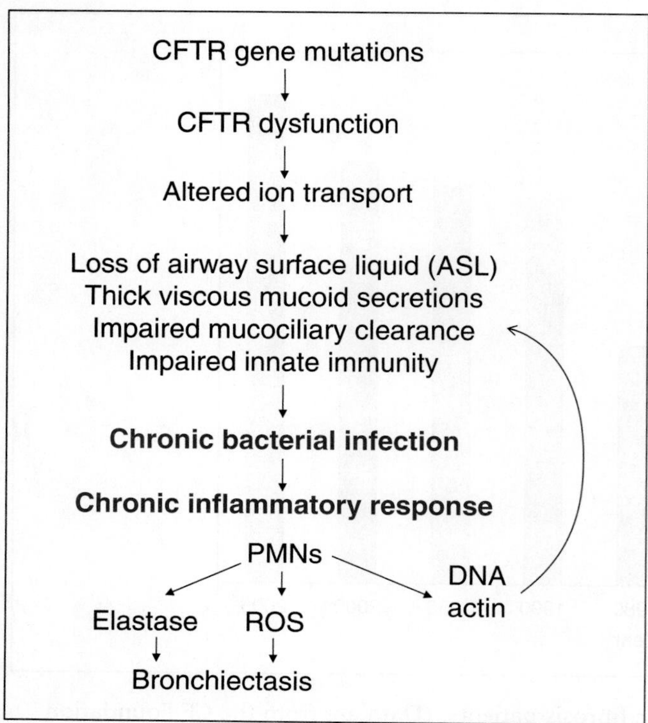


FIGURE 92-3 Pathogenesis of CF lung disease. (CFTR, cystic fibrosis transmembrane conductance regulator; PMNs, polymorphonuclear cells; ROS, reactive oxygen species)

the respiratory tract leads to loss of the airway surface liquid (ASL) layer, diminished mucociliary clearance, and chronic infection.[4,14,15] Other factors, such as impaired innate immunity, may also contribute to the development of lung disease.[5] The presence of chronic airway infection leads to a chronic inflammatory process mediated primarily by neutrophils. Neutrophil granules contain proteolytic enzymes, such as elastase, which cause tissue destruction of the airway. Chronic proteolytic damage of the airway triggers an ineffective repair process, ultimately leading to distortion and fibrosis of the airway and mucous gland hyperplasia. Because this process occurs in the airways, not in the alveolar spaces, the pathologic feature of CF lung disease is bronchiectasis, not pneumonia. Neutrophils also contribute to impaired mucociliary clearance by ultimately undergoing apoptosis and releasing their nuclear and cellular contents. The nucleus is composed of DNA, whereas the cytosol contains actin, which polymerizes to form filamentous actin. Both DNA and actin form long filaments that contribute to sputum viscosity.

Because of the local defect in the airways, once airway infection in CF is established, it can never be eradicated. Airway infection in CF is established shortly after birth, and specific pathogens vary with age (Figure 92-4).[9] Early in infancy and childhood, the most

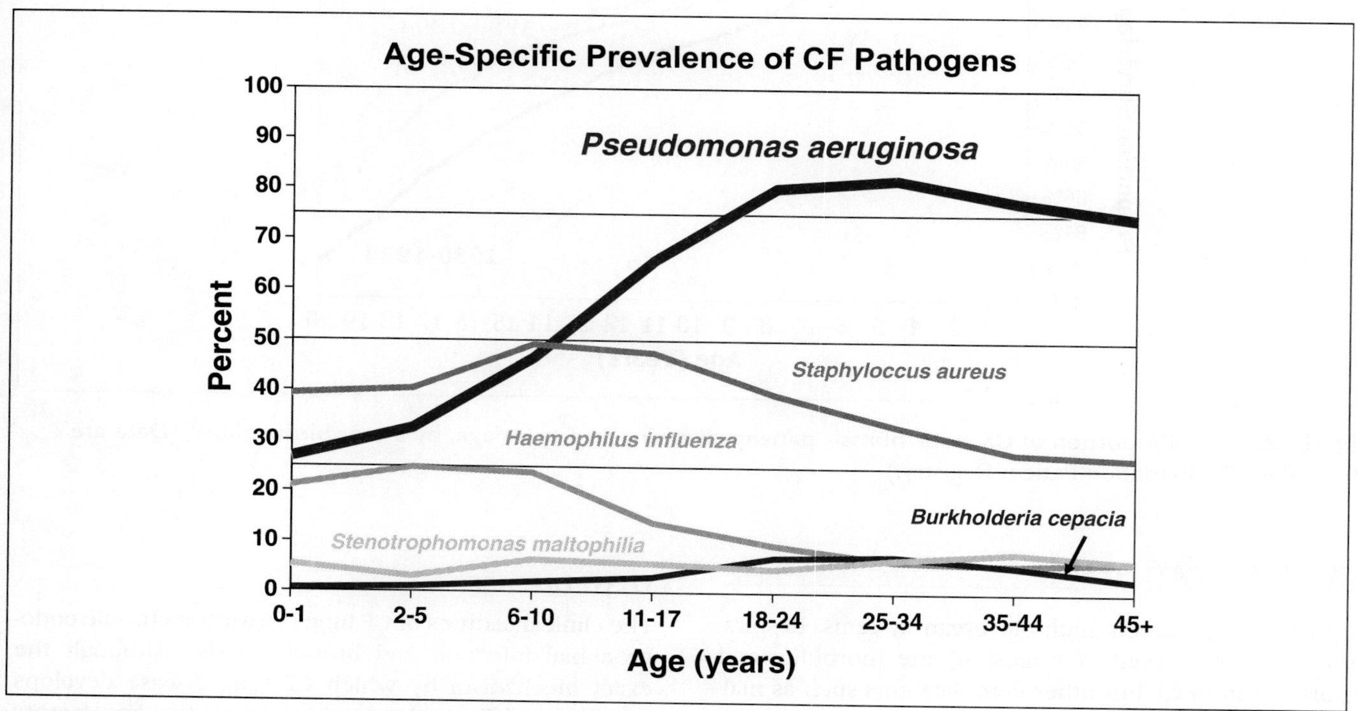


FIGURE 92-4 Age-specific prevalence of 5 CF pathogens. (Data are from the CF Foundation Patient Registry.)

common organism isolated from the respiratory tract is *Staphylococcus aureus*. However, over time the most common pathogen becomes *Pseudomonas aeruginosa* (*Pa*). Initial *Pa* infection usually has a nonmucoid phenotype, but eventually patients become infected with mucoid strains.[2,16] Once *Pa* assumes a mucoid phenotype, it cannot be eradicated. Acquisition of *Pa* is associated with a more severe clinical course, and prevention of early *Pa* infection is presently the focus of investigation.[17] Other bacteria that are less commonly recovered from CF patients include *Haemophilus influenzae*, enteric gram-negative organisms (eg, *Escherichia coli*), *Burkholderia cepacia*, and *Stenotrophomonas maltophilia*. Mirroring a general trend in *S aureus* infections, the prevalence of methicillin-resistant *S aureus* (MRSA) in CF patients has increased significantly over the past several years.[9] Some genomovars of *B cepacia* are associated with more severe disease, but the clinical impact of other organisms is not as clear.[2] Fungi such as *Aspergillus* and *Candida* are present in 25% of respiratory tract cultures in CF. Although they do not cause primary infection, the prevalence of allergic bronchopulmonary aspergillosis is increased in the CF population.[2] Mycobacterial infections usually consist of nontuberculous species.[2] Their prevalence varies depending on the geographic region, and treatment of nontuberculous mycobacterial infections can be challenging.

There is a balance in the airways of CF patients between chronic bacterial infection and the host immune response.[18] Cystic fibrosis pulmonary exacerbations arise when this equilibrium is disturbed, leading to increased bacterial density and a concomitant increase in inflammation.[19] Increased mucopurulent secretions obstruct the small and medium-size bronchioles. The clinical features of pulmonary exacerbations include increased cough, increased sputum, fatigue, weight loss, and increased airflow obstruction on pulmonary function test (PFT). Treatment with antibiotics, airway clearance therapies, and mucolytics reduces airway bacterial density and the concomitant inflammatory response, leading to a reduction in airway mucus plugging.

A higher frequency of pulmonary exacerbations is associated with decreased survival,[20] and a current goal of therapy is to prevent or reduce the number of exacerbations in CF patients. Other pulmonary complications of CF include pneumothorax, hemoptysis, and rib fractures from severe coughing.[21]

## PANCREATIC DISEASE

The original name for CF was "cystic fibrosis of the pancreas," and 85% to 90% of CF patients have loss of exocrine pancreatic function due to obstruction of the pancreatic ducts with viscous secretions.[9] Obstruction of the pancreatic ducts in utero with thick tenacious secretions results in fibrosis and atrophy of the pancreas by birth. The loss of pancreatic enzyme function leads to malabsorption and failure to thrive in infancy. Other clinical features of pancreatic insufficiency include steatorrhea and fat-soluble vitamin deficiencies.

Early in the disease, patients maintain enough pancreatic islet cell function to avoid glucose intolerance. However, over time the pancreas continues to develop fibrosis, and many adolescent and adult patients develop cystic fibrosis–related diabetes mellitus (CFRDM). The true prevalence of CFRDM is difficult to determine because of ascertainment bias. The reported prevalence in the national CF Patient Registry was 20.6% in 2007,[9] but centers that screen more aggressively for CFRDM have reported rates of 26% to 42%.[22] The incidence of CFRDM increases with age, and by age 30 years, 35% of patients will be diagnosed with this condition. Patients with CFRDM generally have more severe lung disease.[23,24] Although the psychosocial impact of CFRDM has not been formally studied, it clearly imposes an additional burden on patients already coping with a serious chronic illness.

## OTHER GASTROINTESTINAL COMPLICATIONS

Loss of CFTR function results in increased bile viscosity and biliary cirrhosis. Clinically apparent liver disease occurs in 10.8% of CF patients. Because of the likelihood that there are many more CF patients with impaired liver function who have not been formally diagnosed with liver disease,[25] patients with CF should be screened regularly for liver disease. The traditional biochemical markers, serum transaminase levels and bile canalicular proteins, are relatively insensitive at detecting liver damage, especially early in the course of disease. Likewise, although physical examination of the liver and spleen is recommended to be performed regularly, there may be no abnormalities on palpation in the early stages of CF.

Other gastrointestinal complications are common in CF.[26] Abnormal bile contributes to frequent gallbladder abnormalities in adolescents with CF. Distal ileal obstruction syndrome (DIOS) occurs in about 4% of patients with CF.[9] The pathogenesis of DIOS is believed to be inspissation of tenacious gastrointestinal mucus at the terminal ileus. The clinical features of DIOS vary, depending the severity of the episode. Mild DIOS presents simply with abdominal pain, with or without constipation, whereas severe episodes result in partial or total bowel obstruction, an emergency requiring immediate medical or surgical intervention.

Other gastrointestinal complications that occur in the CF population include pancreatitis, appendicitis, and intussusception.[26] An increased risk of gastrointestinal cancers has also been reported in CF patients, mainly in adulthood.[27]

## OTHER CLINICAL FEATURES OF CYSTIC FIBROSIS

Cystic fibrosis can affect many other organ systems, either as a primary consequence of absent CFTR function or secondary to pulmonary and gastrointestinal disease (Box 92-1). Hyponatremic dehydration resulting from loss of salt in the sweat ducts occurs most commonly in infants and young children. However, all patients should be advised to supplement their salt intake prior to vigorous physical activity or heat exposure. Azoospermia occurs in CF as a result of occlusion and involution of the vas deferens by viscous secretions. Although this renders males with CF infertile, it is important for caregivers to remind sexually active males with CF that they are still at risk for sexually transmitted infections. The fallopian tubes of females with CF can also be affected, but the overall effect on fertility seems to be minimal.

Chronic sinusitis and nasal polyps occur in about 5% of adolescents with CF, frequently requiring surgical intervention.[9] Decreased bone mineral density occurs at all ages but becomes more common and severe as patients grow older. Low bone mineral density in patients with CF occurs as a consequence of vitamin D malabsorption, overall poor nutritional status, and, possibly, chronic inflammation. Although pancreatic enzyme replacement therapy can prevent most of the nutritional deficiencies, a degree of malabsorption still exists, and kidney stones composed of calcium oxalate occur more frequently in adolescents with CF.[9]

### Box 92-1

### *Nonpulmonary Complications of Cystic Fibrosis*

- Gastrointestinal
  - Pancreatic insufficiency
  - Pancreatitis
  - Cholelithiasis/cholecystitis
  - Appendicitis
  - Intussusception
  - Meconium ileus/distal intestinal obstruction syndrome
  - Biliary cirrhosis
- Other
  - Diabetes mellitus
  - Hyponatremic dehydration
  - Chronic sinusitis
  - Nasal polyps
  - Azoospermia
  - Nephrolithiasis
  - Osteopenia

## PANCREATIC-SUFFICIENT CYSTIC FIBROSIS

Patients whose gene mutations result in a degree of residual CFTR function may not have all the classic features of CF described previously. The terms "nonclassical," "mild," and/or "atypical" have been used to describe CF in these patients. However, the CF Foundation diagnosis guidelines discourage the use of these terms[28] because they may mislead patients and families to believe that their lung disease will be less severe. These patients are usually pancreatic sufficient and their nutritional status is usually better than that of pancreatic-insufficient CF patients.[29] Because they may not have symptoms of malabsorption, these patients frequently escape diagnosis until later childhood, adolescence, or even early adulthood.[30–32]

## DIAGNOSIS

The CF Foundation consensus statement on the diagnosis of CF is summarized in Box 92-2.[28] The diagnosis is based on an appropriate clinical presentation coupled with evidence of abnormal CFTR function. Abnormal CFTR function can be demonstrated by: (1) elevated sweat chloride, (2) identification of two disease-causing mutations in the *CFTR* gene, or (3) abnormal transepithelial nasal potential difference (NPD) measurements. In recent years, newborn screening for CF has become more prevalent.[28] However, CF newborn screening is not diagnostic; a positive screen requires a diagnostic evaluation, and a negative screen does not rule out CF in a patient presenting with features suggestive of CF. In the latter case, one of the definitive diagnostic tests listed previously is needed to determine whether the patient has CF. Finally, adolescent patients may have been born

### Box 92-2

### *CF Foundation Consensus Criteria for Diagnosis of Cystic Fibrosis*

Phenotypical features of CF, or

- Positive history of CF in a sibling
- Positive CF newborn screening test result

AND evidence of abnormal CFTR function as demonstrated by ONE of the following:

- Elevated sweat chloride test
- Identification of 2 disease-causing *CFTR* gene mutations
- Abnormal nasal transepithelial ion transport

prior to implementation of CF newborn screening in their state, but develop clinically apparent signs and symptoms later in life.

Measurement of sweat chloride is the classic method of CF diagnosis.[28,33,34] Sweat chloride must be measured by quantitative pilocarpine iontophoresis (QPIT), which is generally only available at CF care centers accredited by the CF Foundation. Other methods, such as sweat conductivity, are not as accurate as QPIT and are not recommended for diagnosis. In individuals with normal CFTR function, chloride contained in sweat is reabsorbed in the sweat duct. Patients with CF lack CFTR function, fail to reabsorb chloride, and experience increased sweat chloride losses. There are very few other causes for an elevated sweat $Cl^-$ other than CF; they include Addison disease, certain glycogen storage diseases, severe peripheral edema, and hypothyroidism. Most of these conditions can be readily distinguished from CF on clinical grounds or by other appropriate laboratory studies. Therefore, a sweat $Cl^-$ ≥60 mmol/L is diagnostic for CF. Most unaffected individuals have a sweat $Cl^-$ <40 mmol/L. Beyond the newborn period, a sweat $Cl^-$ level of 40 mmol/L to 59 mmol/L is considered indeterminate. Most individuals with an intermediate sweat $Cl^-$ level do not have CF, but there are some patients with suspected CF whose sweat $Cl^-$ level is in the indeterminate range. To diagnose CF in these patients, further investigation looking for clinical features of CF and evidence of CFTR dysfunction may be necessary.

Genetic testing to identify *CFTR* gene mutations is another approach to the diagnosis of CF.[28] However, there are several limitations to using genetic testing to diagnose CF.[35] Although more than 1,500 mutations have been reported in association with patients presenting with clinical features of CF, only a few (30–40) have been definitively shown to cause loss of CFTR function. Many are missense mutations whose impact on CFTR function has been inferred but not demonstrated by either in vitro or in vivo models. Complicating the matter is the presence of numerous polymorphisms present in the *CFTR* gene. Some *CFTR* gene polymorphisms may result in altered *CFTR* function, although their clinical relevance is unclear.[35,36] In other cases, *CFTR* gene mutations only cause disease when associated with other specific polymorphisms.[28,35,37] The results of genetic testing therefore require careful interpretation by a specialist knowledgeable in CF genetics.

Genetic testing for diagnostic purposes in the clinical setting can be accomplished in 1 of 2 ways. Commercial gene mutation analysis panels screen for a number of mutations that represent the most common mutations reported to cause CF. The distribution of mutations responsible for CF may vary depending on the racial and ethnic makeup of the patient, and this affects the sensitivity of the commercial panel.[38] Complete sequencing of the coding region of the *CFTR* gene is commercially available, but even complete sequencing may not identify all mutations that lead to CF because it will not detect mutations that occur outside the coding regions or the immediate flanking exons.[39] The CF Foundation guidelines recommend *CFTR* gene mutation analysis for patients with suspected CF and an indeterminate sweat chloride level,[28] although the diagnostic yield of testing is unknown.

The knowledge gained through studying *CFTR* function can be applied to diagnostic testing through the measurements of transepithelial ion flow using NPD,[40–42] which directly assess ion transport in the nasal epithelium and represent an in vivo assessment of *CFTR* function in the respiratory tract. Performing NPD measurements is time and labor intensive, and it is available only at a few specialized research centers across the United States. Because of these limitations, NPD measurements cannot serve as a first-line diagnostic test for CF. However, they may be useful in equivocal or borderline cases. Similar to the case of genetic testing, there are no studies that have shown increased diagnostic yield when NPD measurements are added.

The diagnosis of CF depends on maintaining a high index of suspicion. Some patients do not have all the classic features, such as recurrent respiratory infections, failure to thrive, and malabsorption. This is especially common in older patients, such as adolescents, who frequently have pancreatic sufficient CF.[30–32] Because CF is a multisystem disorder patients can present with a wide spectrum of disease manifestations. Box 92-3 lists some of the indications for sweat chloride measurement, with an emphasis on symptoms presenting in adolescence. Adolescent patients with these symptoms should prompt clinicians to consider evaluation for CF.

**Box 92-3**

***Indications for Sweat Testing***

Respiratory Symptoms
- Recurrent or persistent pneumonia
- Bronchiectasis
- Chronic productive cough
- Chronic chest radiographic abnormalities
- Difficult-to-control asthma
- Pseudomonas pneumonia in an immunocompetent host
- Hemoptysis
- Chronic sinusitis
- Nasal polyps

**Box 92-3 (continued)**

Gastrointestinal Symptoms

- Failure to thrive
- Rectal prolapse
- Unexplained liver failure
- Chronic or recurrent pancreatitis
- Recurrent intussusception
- Fat-soluble vitamin loss

Other Symptoms

- Unexplained digital clubbing
- Recurrent hyponatremic dehydration
- Recurrent metabolic alkalosis
- Azoospermia
- Absence of vas deferens

## MANAGEMENT

As a multisystem disease, the management of CF requires a multidisciplinary approach that addresses the effects of disease on multiple organ systems. The treatment of CF has evolved significantly over the past 25 years, as improved survival and new drug discovery have changed CF from a fatal disease of childhood to a chronic disease of adulthood.[43] The focus of treatment today is on preserving lung function and treating late complications of the disease.

### THE CF FOUNDATION AND CF CARE CENTER NETWORK

The CF Foundation (CFF) was founded in the 1950s as a not-for-profit organization dedicated to developing the means to cure and control CF and to improving the quality of life for those with the disease. The CF Foundation accredits and funds a network of CF care centers in the United States. To be accredited by the CF Foundation, a care center must have an interdisciplinary team of physicians, nurses, nutritionists, social workers, respiratory therapist, and other specialists experienced and dedicated to the care of CF patients. It must also meet standards for respiratory care services, pulmonary function testing (PFT), microbiology, sweat testing, and other services needed for CF care.

### LUNG DISEASE

Because lung disease accounts for the overwhelming majority of morbidity and mortality in CF, a major focus of CF care is devoted to controlling chronic airway infection, poor clearance of respiratory secretions, and subsequent permanent lung damage. Similar to treatment of asthma or hypertension, treatment of CF lung disease can be viewed in terms of "controller" therapies intended to ameliorate the underlying problems in the CF airway and "reliever" therapies to be used when patients develop exacerbations (M Aitken and M Tonelli, personal communication, May 22, 2006)[43] (Box 92-4). At present, controller therapies are primarily directed at the consequences of CFTR dysfunction, but newer classes of therapies will target the underlying pathophysiology (eg, CFTR correctors or alternative channel activators).[44] The CF Foundation recently published guidelines for pulmonary therapies in CF.[45]

**Box 92-4**

***Controller and Reliever Therapies for Cystic Fibrosis Lung Disease***

**Controller Therapies**

- Mucociliary clearance
  - Airway clearance techniques
  - Inhaled beta-agonists
  - Dornase alfa
  - Hypertonic saline
- Antimicrobials
  - Oral antibiotics
  - Inhaled antibiotics
- Anti-inflammatory therapies
  - High-dose ibuprofen
  - Alternate-day prednisone
  - Low-dose azithromycin

**Reliever Therapies**

- Oral antibiotics
- Intravenous antibiotics
- Increased airway clearance therapies

### MECHANICAL THERAPIES

Improving airway clearance is one element of chronic therapy.[46] A number of therapies have been used to improve the airway clearance. These include: (1) vigorous exercise, (2) various breathing and coughing routines (Huff coughing), (3) manual postural drainage and cupping, (4) percussors, (5) devices to change exhalation (flutter, acapella, or positive expiratory pressure mask), and (6) mechanically vibrating vests. Consistency of use may be more important than the specific device used. During treatment of a pulmonary exacerbation, the frequency and duration of airway clearance therapies are usually increased.

### PHARMACOLOGIC THERAPIES

Pharmacologic therapies to improve mucus clearance include inhaled dornase alfa (recombinant human

DNase) and hypertonic saline (HS).[45] Dornase alfa reduces sputum viscosity by cleaving sputum DNA into small fragments,[47] whereas HS increases mucociliary clearance in CF patients by increasing the volume of the ASL layer, allowing the cilia to move freely.[15,48] Both therapies can improve lung function and reduce the frequency of pulmonary exacerbations.

## ANTIBIOTIC THERAPY

Antibiotics are a critical component of care for adolescents with CF.[2] Antibiotics reduce the bacterial density in the CF airway, reducing inflammation and improving airway obstruction. Antibiotic use in CF seeks to balance the beneficial effects of antibiotics with the risks of selecting resistant organisms. Although some clinicians who treat patients with CF (especially outside the US) use chronic oral antibiotics as a method to control the bacterial density in the lungs, the development of antibiotic resistance has limited this approach in general. Inhaled antibiotics provide airway drug levels without the need for intravenous (IV) therapy and with minimal systemic absorption. Chronic intermittent treatment with inhaled tobramycin for 28 days, alternating with 28 days tobramycin-free, improves lung function and reduces the frequency of pulmonary exacerbations in patients with CF without a significant increase in antibiotic resistance.[49] Other inhaled antibiotics are presently under development.

Acute use of oral or IV antibiotics is a mainstay of therapy for pulmonary exacerbations.[19] For IV therapy in patients infected with *Pa*, a combination of a beta-lactam and aminoglycoside is typically used for a treatment course of 2 to 3 weeks. The specific antibiotic choices are based on individual patient and microbiology characteristics. In the past, patients with CF receiving IV antibiotics for treatment of pulmonary exacerbation required hospitalization, which imposed a heavy burden on their quality of life. The introduction of long-term peripherally inserted central catheter lines has allowed patients to receive their therapy at home. Some studies suggest that home therapy of pulmonary exacerbations is as effective as in-hospital therapy, but each patient needs to be evaluated individually to determine his or her suitability for home IV therapy.

## ANTI-INFLAMMATORY THERAPY

Control of airway inflammation is another area of therapy in CF lung disease.[18] Alternate-day prednisone improves lung function in CF but its use is associated with unacceptable side effects, such as growth delay, cataract formation, and glucose intolerance.[50] Inhaled corticosteroids (ICS) are widely used in CF for their putative anti-inflammatory effects, but evidence supporting their efficacy is limited.[45] An epidemiologic analysis of a large observational study of CF showed that ICS therapy was associated with a significant change in lung function decline,[51] and a randomized placebo-controlled study of ICS withdrawal showed no deleterious effects of withdrawal after 6 months.[52] There have been no randomized clinical trials studying the effect of ICSs on lung function decline, and the CF Foundation pulmonary guidelines recommend against its routine use in CF patients who do not have asthma.[45] High-dose ibuprofen has been shown in prospective randomized trials to significantly slow the rate of lung function decline.[53,54] Concerns about potential side effects and the need to obtain individual pharmacokinetics have limited its use.[55] Macrolides, such as azithromycin, also have neutrophil inhibitory properties. Chronic low-dose azithromycin therapy can improve lung function and reduce the frequency of pulmonary exacerbations in patients with CF.[56] Many other anti-inflammatory therapies are under development.[18]

## SUPPLEMENTAL OXYGEN

As lung disease progresses, other complications may occur. The most common is hypoxemia, especially with exercise and at night. Supplementation with oxygen during those times may be helpful in preserving energy levels and cardiac function.

## HEMOPTYSIS TREATMENT

Hemoptysis resulting from erosion of bronchial vessels by neutrophil-derived proteases is relatively common.[21] Small amounts of bleeding may be a sign that the infection in the airways is increasing and that the patient may need a course of IV antibiotics. Clotting function may need to be evaluated because of the problem of fat-soluble vitamin K malabsorption. Massive bleeding, although less common, is an emergency and may be life threatening. This bleeding is usually from bronchial arteries. If the bleeding does not stop with rest and administration of vitamin K, tranexamic acid can be given. Often the tortuous bronchial artery will need embolization by interventional radiology.

## PNEUMOTHORAX TREATMENT

Pneumothorax should be suspected in those who present with acute severe chest pain.[21] A pneumothorax may be difficult to visualize on chest x-ray because the remainder of the lung is stiff and does not collapse. Resolution even after chest tube placement may be slow, and the risks of bed rest with its associated decreased airway clearance cannot be overestimated. Patients may benefit from surgical removal of affected cysts in the lung once a pneumothorax has occurred.

## LUNG TRANSPLANTATION

Despite appropriate therapy, patients can expect eventual progression of the lung disease. Often lung function remains relatively stable during adolescence, but some teenagers or young adults will reach the point where they will consider a lung transplant. The decision to perform lung transplantation is a difficult one that needs to be made by the patient, his or her family, and close consultation with a transplantation center. The rate of progression of lung disease, presence of other complications, history of adherence to therapies, and family support are some of the factors considered by specialized transplant centers. The decision to list a patient for transplant is generally made by applying a risk model to predict the patient's survival without transplant.[20,57] The design of these risk models for patients with CF can be controversial,[58–60] and the specific criteria used to list patients for transplantation can vary among centers.[61]

## MONITORING CF LUNG DISEASE

Just as with any other chronic illness, regular monitoring of disease severity is critical for making treatment decisions and assessing disease progression. Lung disease can be monitored by PFTs and chest radiography. Both techniques are relatively insensitive to early changes in lung function, and marked airway inflammation and structural changes can be present even in patients with normal PFTs and plain chest radiographs.[62,63] Ongoing research is helping to develop clinically useful tools for the assessment of early lung disease in CF.[64]

## GASTROINTESTINAL AND NUTRITIONAL MANAGEMENT

Pancreatic insufficiency is present in up to 90% of CF patients.[9] Although some infants with CF may have residual pancreatic function for several months, malabsorption is well established in pancreatic-insufficient patients by adolescence. Exocrine pancreatic function can be assessed by measurement of fecal elastase activity or by 3-day fecal fat collections; the former is more easily performed and less prone to measurement error.

Exogenous pancreatic enzymes taken in capsule form or sprinkled on any food or snack containing protein or fat help digestion. Generic enzyme preparations have inconsistent bioavailability compared to brand-name forms. Dosing of enzymes is usually based on clinical response, in terms of the character and number of stools and weight gain. In general, the dose is steadily increased until good clinical response is seen. Patients receiving high doses of pancreatic enzyme therapy (>10,000 lipase units/kilo/day) are at increased risk of fibrosing colonopathy, a submucosal inflammatory process that results in fibrosis of the colon.[65] If the intestinal pH is too acidic, the enzymes may not function properly; this can be remedied either by treatment with H2-blockers or by combining pancreatic enzymes with a bicarbonate capsule.

Good nutritional status is associated with better lung function and longer survival.[9,29,66] Current CF Foundation guidelines recommend that weight be maintained greater than the 10th percentile and body mass index (BMI) greater than the 25th percentile.[29] Patients with CF have increased caloric requirements due to incomplete gastrointestinal absorption (even with pancreatic enzyme replacement therapy), chronic airway infection and inflammation, and increased work of breathing as lung disease progresses. Therefore, their daily calorie needs may be 110% to 200% of the usual recommendations. Caloric requirements may increase when lung or liver disease adds to the metabolic load of the patient.

Earlier recommendations suggested that reducing the fat in the meals would decrease the steatorrhea, but this significantly limited the caloric intake. Current recommendations are for foods and beverages relatively high in fat, with enzyme supplementation to treat the malabsorption. Many adolescents, particularly when in a phase of rapid growth, will be unable to meet the requirements with food alone. They may require oral supplementation with drinks or snacks designed to provide increased calories. It is common for this to be difficult for even the most motivated adolescent, and gastrostomy placement and nighttime enteral feedings may be needed to meet the caloric needs. Maintenance of adequate caloric intake is especially important in young women during pregnancy.

Fat malabsorption is a significant problem that may affect fat-soluble vitamin levels and the ability to meet caloric needs through high-fat diets.[29] The vitamins most likely to be affected are vitamins A, D, E, and sometimes vitamin K. Vitamin supplements that are enriched in these fat-soluble vitamins should be used on a routine basis. After the newborn period, vitamin K deficiency is less of a problem because much of the vitamin K is obtained from the bacteria in the intestines; however, it should be considered if the patient has problems with bleeding. Patients with CF are particularly prone to low bone mineral density as adults. It is important to make sure that these patients get enough calcium and vitamin D during adolescence.

As previously described, individuals with malabsorption may be at risk for DIOS. This may be at the level of the rectum or at the ileocecal valve. Proper use of enzyme replacement and hydration can minimize the occurrence of this complication but may not eliminate it. Patients may get some relief by osmotic agents such as polyethylene glycol, lactulose, or enemas. In more severe cases, a gastrograffin/Tween 80 enema can be administered by a radiologist under fluoroscopy. Dietary measures such as increased fiber, good hydration, and adherence to enzymes can help prevent future episodes.

### LIVER DISEASE

In patients with CF obstruction of the biliary ducts, inspissated bile leads to biliary cirrhosis.[25] As discussed previously, early detection of CF liver disease is difficult by laboratory or physical examination. Management of CF liver disease is similar to that of other patients with hepatic disease. Ursodeoxycholic acid is frequently prescribed to patients with CF liver disease, but its impact on clinical outcomes is unknown.[25] If patients with CF progress to complete liver failure, liver transplant is indicated.

### UPPER AIRWAY DISEASE

Many adolescents with CF have recurrent problems with sinusitis or nasal polyps that may require surgical therapy.[9] An experienced otolaryngologist on the CF team can minimize the risks of surgery. This frequently requires a course of antibiotics to reduce the bacterial load prior to the surgery. The use of nasal saline lavage, nasal corticosteroids, or antibiotics may help control some of the sinus symptoms.

### DIABETES

Over time, progressive fibrosis of the pancreas leads to loss of islet cell function and the development of CFRDM.[67] The overall reported prevalence of CFRDM is 20.9%, and it increases with age.[9,22] Cystic fibrosis-related diabetes mellitus is distinct from either type 1 or type 2 diabetes mellitus (DM). In contrast to type 1 DM, patients with CFRDM retain their ability to secrete some insulin and do not develop ketoacidosis. However, they also do not have insulin resistance, a feature of type 2 DM. Rather, patients with CF are in a hypoinsulinemic state most commonly caused by low basal insulin secretion and a high demand for insulin to meet their metabolic needs. Screening for CFRDM can be done by measuring fasting blood glucose or oral glucose tolerance testing. Although some patients with CFRDM have been treated with oral hypoglycemic agents, the preferred treatment is insulin.[68] In addition to its effects on blood glucose, insulin is also anabolic. The development of CFRDM is associated with worsening lung function.[24] However, it is unclear whether CFRDM contributes directly to lung disease or merely is a marker for increased disease severity.

## PSYCHOSOCIAL ISSUES IN ADOLESCENTS WITH CYSTIC FIBROSIS

Between 1985 and 2005, there was an improvement in survival (see Figure 92-1) generally attributed to more aggressive treatment of lung disease and nutritional issues.[9] Lung function has steadily improved, whereas symptoms of disease such as chronic cough have declined.[10] However, these gains in clinical improvement and survival have come at the cost of increased treatment burden. The challenges clinicians face are in guiding adolescents to deal with current and anticipated treatment burdens as they strive to improve their quality of life and maintain lung health.

### PHYSIOLOGIC HEALTH

The prognosis of CF has dramatically improved over the past 20 years, and increasing numbers of adolescents are surviving well into adulthood. Cystic Fibrosis Patient Registry data report significant gains for adolescents during this period in nutritional health and lung function, with median BMI near the 50th percentiles and more than 60% of teens categorized as having mild lung disease.[9] Nonetheless, the progressive nature of the disease often still makes adolescence a period of greater morbidity, with 35% of 18-year-old patients categorized as having moderate to severe lung disease. Increased morbidity brings a greater focus on more arduous maintenance regimens and more frequent courses of acute therapies to treat pulmonary exacerbations. Konstan and colleagues[66] reported that 20% of adolescents with 2 or more pulmonary exacerbations per year required IV antibiotic therapy. Typically, up to 20% of adolescents[22] have CFRDM, which creates the additional burden of another chronic illness. This CF illness trajectory occurs developmentally at a time when these young people are most interested in being normal and not different from their peer group. These challenges of adolescent growth and development in the setting of individually variable disease progression pose unique and challenging issues for the clinician caring for the adolescent with CF.

#### Physical Growth and Body Image

Despite aggressive daily therapy, adolescents may still experience delayed growth and pubertal maturation that have been associated with the combined demands placed on caloric requirements by progressive lung disease, pancreatic insufficiency, and normal adolescent growth. A mean delay of 2 years in onset of puberty and menarche has been reported in females and a 1.5-year delay in puberty has been reported in males.[69] Nutritional needs are increased during pulmonary exacerbations, making the adolescent with less stable disease more vulnerable to malnutrition.[70,71] Daily treatment regimens for most adolescents are time consuming. Up to 3 hours/day may be required to complete airway clearance, nebulized therapies, and exercise. The time remaining to eat a full meal may be minimal, particularly in the morning before school. As might be anticipated similar to other adolescents, teens with CF worry about their growth and body image.[72] Developing a positive body image and sense of self in the face of increasing pulmonary and nutritional therapies can be challenging.

Good nutrition is critically important to long-term survival in persons with CF.[73] At the same time, the illness can be a formidable and relentless adversary in the arena of typical adolescent eating behaviors and the cultural emphasis on being thin. Adolescent women, in particular, may either like their thinness or regard their weight as problematic and discover how relatively easy it is for someone with CF to lose weight.[74] Adolescent boys are more likely to be concerned about poor growth and to desire weight gain.[72] However, regardless of gender these adolescents may resist recommendations for adding supplemental calories to their diet, especially if the supplementation involves initiating more invasive therapies of nighttime enteral feedings that are perceived as abnormal and that make them different from their peers. Consistent adherence to pancreatic enzyme replacement therapy may also be challenging, given adolescents' eating habits of frequent snacking and "grazing" behaviors. Teens may resist taking medication in the presence of peers, perceiving it as further labeling them as "different." Effective intervention strategies begin with increasing the adolescent's involvement in understanding the issues and in developing a plan of care to address them. For example, including the teen's favorite foods and those that can be prepared easily and independently by the teen is a helpful start to increasing the caloric intake in the diet. Also, emphasizing the potential for improved muscle strength and body image rather than weight gain may be a more acceptable approach in nutrition counseling.[29]

### Male Infertility

Adolescent males are azoospermic from bilateral absence of the vas deferens and are thus infertile. It is recommended that this diagnosis be confirmed with a semen analysis. The understanding of being infertile is often a difficult adjustment for the male adolescent and should be handled with sensitivity. In counseling, they may be reassured that infertility does not affect sexual performance. The clinician should also inform them of options for parenthood through donor sperm and, more recently, through the improvement of intracytoplasmic sperm injection techniques that allow CF men to father children.[75] Male CF patients must also be reminded that infertility does not affect their risk of acquiring or transmitting sexually transmitted diseases.

### Pregnancy

Although there may be some difficulty becoming pregnant because of the presence of thick cervical mucus, adolescent women with CF should be aware that they are capable of becoming pregnant. Recent reports on the impact of pregnancy on the mother with CF concluded that, in women who have mild lung disease, pregnancy may be not present a significant risk to their health.[76,77] However, counseling should include a discussion of pregnancy in CF being associated with increased need for therapies, more clinic visits and hospitalizations, and increased risk of developing diabetes during pregnancy that continues following childbirth.[78]

Family planning and prevention of an unwanted pregnancy is therefore critically important for adolescent women with CF. Contraception and safe sexual practices should be regularly encouraged in the young woman who is sexually active. Oral contraceptives have not been shown to have an adverse effect on CF lung disease and are routinely used in young women with CF. Oral antibiotics may decrease the effectiveness of oral contraception, so young women being treated with them should be counseled about these risks and may require higher-dose birth control pills.[79,80]

## PSYCHOLOGICAL FUNCTIONING: DEVELOPING A SENSE OF IDENTITY

Adolescence can be a time of internal turmoil with struggles for independence and a sense of identity. The addition of a chronic illness such as CF—which is progressive, associated with a shortened life expectancy and, for many, is accompanied by a significant treatment burden—can add a significant dimension to these struggles (Table 92-2).

### Socialization and Peer Relationships

Adolescents with CF are not unlike their healthy peers in their desires for socialization and development of peer relationships. However, they may have difficulty forming interpersonal relationships, exacerbated by their feelings of social isolation, delayed puberty, and misunderstandings about fertility.[81] They should have opportunities to discuss these issues with the CF team without a parent present.

As with other chronic illnesses, adolescents with CF want to meet others with CF and share illness-related concerns and ways of coping with them. It is unfortunate that these contacts and relationships are now

**Table 92-2**

**Psychosocial Challenges and Health Care for Adolescents with CF**[81,88,91]

| *Issues* | *Intervention* |
|---|---|
| • Development of sense of identity outside CF<br>• Risk-taking behavior<br>• Nonadherence to treatment<br>• Peer relationships<br>• Dating<br>• Socializing<br>• Transition to adult CF care | • Support parents in "letting go"<br>• Emphasize flexibility and honesty (not rigidity)<br>• Increased involvement of teen in own care regimen<br>• Routine discussions about sexuality (without parent)<br>• Use of newsletters and Internet to communicate with peers with CF<br>• See patient in clinic without parent<br>• Develop concrete plan for date of transfer to adult care |

discouraged because of the growing appreciation that CF pathogens can be transmitted between patients. One of these organisms, *Burkholderia cepacia*, has also been associated with rapid decline in health. As a result, support groups, camps, and social events have been curtailed and individuals with CF counseled to avoid close contact with others who have the illness. In the face of these concerns, adolescents should be encouraged to develop alternative methods of communicating with each other such as e-mail and instant messaging, telephone contact, and Internet Web sites (eg, www.hopkinscf.org/teens).

### Sexuality

Sinnema and colleagues[82] studied the effects of short stature and delayed puberty in adolescents with CF and several other chronic illnesses on a number of issues related to adolescent development, including sexuality and socialization. Adolescents with CF scored lower in these areas than controls, and the differences were deemed related to their delayed growth and sexual development. Adolescents also potentially must deal with the presence of a chronic cough, purulent sputum, malodorous breath, and general lethargy and fatigue, with impending pulmonary exacerbations. These issues may be concerning enough for the adolescent to lead to problems with socialization and sexuality.

### Adherence to Treatment Regimen

It is well documented that adherence to treatment in CF is a common problem across the age span. Adherence is known to be treatment specific, with less adherence to more arduous and time-consuming therapies and to those for which there is little immediate perceived benefit.[83,84] Adolescence can be a time of risk-taking and rebellion against authority, and CF treatments may become a potent weapon in fighting for control in the life of those with CF. Risk-taking behaviors are reported to be lower in adolescents with CF than in a nonaffected peer group; however, those risks are often more potentially damaging to their health.[85]

There are several strategies to respond to poor adherence in CF during adolescence. Overall, parents and health care providers should begin in early childhood to help the child learn about CF and to develop self-management skills that are appropriate for their age and that are designed to enhance a sense of mastery and control in the child. Education programs that promote these skills have been developed for families dealing with CF. The most widely distributed of these is the Baylor College of Medicine CF self-management program,[86] a program that features information about CF, skills development and mastery, and problem-solving skills for parents and for the child with CF during early school age, middle school age, and adolescence. Emphasis of these skills by CF clinicians using either the Baylor program or other methods can foster a collaborative patient–family/provider relationship and build disease management skills in both parents and patients.

Drotar and Lewis[87] found that adolescents with CF who were more independent in managing their illness were those who were independent in other parts of their lives. Understanding their illness and the rationale for treatments is the first priority, followed by encouragement to gradually assume more responsibility for their treatment regimen. Parents need to continue to be present and supportive to their adolescent with CF, not leaving them alone with the burden of care. Parents may struggle to walk this fine line with resulting scenarios of being described by their child as, more commonly, a nag or, less commonly, not caring about them.

In role modeling these skills for parents, the best strategy clinicians can use with adolescents is to recognize them as active and respected members of the health care team. Teens should be encouraged to participate in developing their own plan of care. Such plans should be individualized to the demands of life: school, athletics, and social needs. At the same time, the adolescent needs support and guidance in making good health care decisions as they gain a greater realization of the serious nature of their illness. Choices about their treatment should be allowed where possible in an effort to give autonomy and control. Behavioral contracts can allow the adolescent to test the need for particular therapies; however, they should be offered within the framework of a strong patient–provider relationship and close monitoring of patient outcomes. These interactions are often best developed by giving the teen an opportunity to be seen without their parents for routine clinic visits.

## TRANSITION TO ADULT CARE

With the median survival age in patients with CF now at 37 years, more than 40% of the total CF population is older than 18 years of age. As recently as 1998, only 48 of the 116 CF care centers in the United States had separate adult care programs. Historically, the issues of transition of CF specialty care have been lack of adequately trained adult CF specialists, patient and family comfort with providers they have known and trusted since diagnosis, and concerns of the pediatric CF care team about the adequacy of care for adults and the desire to remain part of patients' lives whom they have known for many years.[81,88]

Since 2000, when the CF Foundation established standards for adult care delivery, CF care centers across the United States have made significant strides in developing adult programs. Almost every accredited CF care center now has pediatric and adult programs. The emphasis in CF care centers today is (1) for pediatric and adult programs to establish a cooperative relationship and formalize a process for transition, and (2) to actively educate patients and families about CF care across the continuum from the time of diagnosis.[81,89-91]

Adolescents and their parents may find it difficult to plan for the future. Increased uncertainty about the future, lowered expectations for themselves, and the use of denial as a coping strategy may delay important planning. Discussion of education and career plans, as well as insurance issues, marriage and relationships, and building a life that incorporates CF should be part of a comprehensive plan of care.[81]

## EDUCATION CHALLENGES

Adolescents face significant challenges in the academic environment associated with absenteeism to treat the illness either at home or with hospitalizations. Their teachers also need to understand that the nature of CF is such that there will be periods of time when they are more fatigued and will be less able to function optimally in the classroom. Regular communication between faculty and students should be encouraged. A few students with more progressive disease may require an Individualized Education Plan through their school's Committee on Special Education that accommodates the need for tutorial assistance to maintain academic standing and modifications in their physical education program.

### College/Career Choices and Financial Planning

Supplemental Security Disability Insurance, Supplemental Security Income programs through the Social Security Administration, and Vocational and Educational Services for Individuals with Disabilities are available to patients with CF. Cystic fibrosis care center care teams include a social worker who is knowledgeable about resources in general and about these programs specifically, and who is able to counsel adolescents and their families about the relative benefits and limitations of these programs on individuals who are considering application. Nasr and colleagues[92] reported that counseling in the area of careers and resources for disability support was given to adolescents receiving care in a CF care center only about half the time. They concluded that periodic and regular assessment of disease severity should be done and appropriate counseling provided for adolescents and young adults.

## DEPRESSION

With advances in research, care, and treatment, hope for the future is increasingly prominent in the way adolescents and their families think about CF. Balancing hope and reality is the challenge for all patients and their families.[93] The evidence to date supports that teens with CF seem to cope well with the stress of the disease.[94] However, as the disease progresses it has a negative impact on the physical functioning aspects of quality of life. Britto and colleagues[95] found that an increasing number of pulmonary exacerbations had a detrimental effect on quality of life.

Bluebond-Langner[96] described 6 time periods specific to disease trajectory of CF, and suggested that in the later time periods of increased complications and treatment demands depression may be seen in adolescent and young adult patients. Clinicians who treat patients with CF need to be alert for the multiple kinds of support needed by adolescents with worsening disease.

This support includes pharmacologic management for pain, as well as depression and anxiety, counseling for both patient and family members in dealing with disease progression, and helping the individual maximize his or her quality of life in the face of significant progressive physical limitations.

**END-OF-LIFE ISSUES**

As young people approach the end of life, they are often not as afraid of death as they are of how to live until they die. Treatment of pain and suffering should be the highest priority in caring for the patients (see Chapter 19, Death, Dying, and Palliative Care). Two critical decisions include personal choice/advanced directives and decisions about where to die.[93] Lung transplantation has significantly altered how decisions are made regarding advanced directives. It behooves the clinician to begin these discussions at a time of relatively good health for the patient and to incorporate the reality of risks and benefits of transplantation into the discussion. Decisions about where the patient would like to die will be influenced by a number of factors, including the availability of hospice resources, the familiarity and comfort level of both patient and family with inpatient staff, and the ability of CF team members to provide in-home support.

## SUMMARY

Cystic fibrosis is a common chronic illness in children and adolescents. Although most CF patients are diagnosed in infancy, some patients, especially those with pancreatic sufficiency CF may not develop clinically apparent signs of CF until later in life. Adolescent medicine providers should consider the diagnosis of CF in patients presenting with the appropriate clinical features. Improvements in CF care over the past several decades have led to a growing adolescent population of CF patients with relatively good lung function. However, the challenges and burdens of dealing with a chronic illness remain, acting as sources of stress for patients and their families.

## REFERENCES


1. Davis PB, Drumm M, Konstan MW. Cystic fibrosis. *Am J Respir Crit Care Med.* 1996;154:1229-1256

2. Gibson RL, Burns JL, Ramsey BW. Pathophysiology and management of pulmonary infections in cystic fibrosis. *Am J Respir Crit Care Med.* 2003;168:918-951

3. Boucher RC. Airway surface dehydration in cystic fibrosis: pathogenesis and therapy. *Annu Rev Med.* 2007;58:157-170

4. Wine JJ. The genesis of cystic fibrosis lung disease. *J Clin Invest.* 1999;103:309-312

5. Bals R, Weiner DJ, Wilson JM. The innate immune system in cystic fibrosis lung disease. *J Clin Invest.* 1999;103:303-307

6. Guggino WB. Cystic fibrosis and the salt controversy. *Cell.* 1999;96:607-610

7. Fanconi G, Uehlinger E, Knauer C. Das coeliakiesyndrom bei angeborener zysticher pankreasfibromatose und bronchiectasien. *Wein Med Wchnschr.* 1936;86:753

8. Andersen D. Cystic fibrosis of the pancrease and its relation to celiac disease: a clinical and pathological study. *Am J Dis Child.* 1938;56:344-399

9. *Cystic Fibrosis Foundation Patient Registry*. Bethesda, MD: Cystic Fibrosis Foundation; 2007

10. VanDevanter DR, Rasouliyan L, Murphy TM, et al. Trends in the clinical characteristics of the US cystic fibrosis patient population from 1995 to 2005. *Pediatr Pulmonol.* 2008;43:739-744

11. Imaizumi Y. Incidence and mortality rates of cystic fibrosis in Japan, 1969-1992. *Am J Med Genet.* 1995;58:161-168

12. Mei-Zahav M, Durie P, Zielenski J, et al. The prevalence and clinical characteristics of cystic fibrosis in South Asian Canadian immigrants. *Arch Dis Child.* 2005;90:675-679

13. Wright SW, Morton NE. Genetic studies on cystic fibrosis in Hawaii. *Am J Hum Genet.* 1968;20:157-169

14. Matsui H, Grubb BR, Tarran R, et al. Evidence for periciliary liquid layer depletion, not abnormal ion composition, in the pathogenesis of cystic fibrosis airways disease. *Cell.* 1998;95:1005-1015

15. Ratjen F. Restoring airway surface liquid in cystic fibrosis. *N Engl J Med.* 2006;354:291-293

16. Li Z, Kosorok MR, Farrell PM, et al. Longitudinal development of mucoid *Pseudomonas aeruginosa* infection and lung disease progression in children with cystic fibrosis. *JAMA.* 2005;293:581-588

17. Treggiari MM, Rosenfeld M, Retsch-Bogart G, Gibson R, Ramsey B. Approach to eradication of initial *Pseudomonas aeruginosa* infection in children with cystic fibrosis. *Pediatr Pulmonol.* 2007;42:751-756

18. Chmiel JF, Berger M, Konstan MW. The role of inflammation in the pathophysiology of CF lung disease. *Clin Rev Allergy Immunol.* 2002;23:5-27

19. Ferkol T, Rosenfeld M, Milla CE. Cystic fibrosis pulmonary exacerbations. *J Pediatr.* 2006;148:259-264

20. Liou TG, Adler FR, FitzSimmons SC, Cahill BC, Hibbs JR, Marshall BC. Predictive 5-year survivorship model of cystic fibrosis. *Am J Epidemiol.* 2001;153:345-352

21. Schidlow DV, Taussig LM, Knowles MR. Cystic Fibrosis Foundation consensus conference report on pulmonary complications of cystic fibrosis. *Pediatr Pulmonol.* 1993;15:187-198

22. Moran A, Doherty L, Wang X, Thomas W. Abnormal glucose metabolism in cystic fibrosis. *J Pediatr.* 1998;133:10-17

23. Milla CE, Billings J, Moran A. Diabetes is associated with dramatically decreased survival in female but not male subjects with cystic fibrosis. *Diabetes Care.* 2005;28:2141-2144

24. Milla CE, Warwick WJ, Moran A. Trends in pulmonary function in patients with cystic fibrosis correlate with the degree of glucose intolerance at baseline. *Am J Respir Crit Care Med.* 2000;162:891–895

25. Colombo C. Liver disease in cystic fibrosis. *Curr Opin Pulm Med.* 2007;13:529–536

26. Littlewood JM. Gastrointestinal complications in cystic fibrosis. *J R Soc Med.* 1992;85 (suppl 19):13–19

27. Neglia JP, FitzSimmons SC, Maisonneuve P, et al. The risk of cancer among patients with cystic fibrosis. Cystic Fibrosis and Cancer Study Group. *N Engl J Med.* 1995;332:494–499

28. Farrell PM, Rosenstein BJ, White TB, et al. Guidelines for diagnosis of cystic fibrosis in newborns through older adults: Cystic Fibrosis Foundation consensus report. *J Pediatr.* 2008;153:S4–S14

29. Stallings VA, Stark LJ, Robinson KA, Feranchak AP, Quinton H. Evidence-based practice recommendations for nutrition-related management of children and adults with cystic fibrosis and pancreatic insufficiency: results of a systematic review. *J Am Diet Assoc.* 2008;108:832–839

30. Nick JA, Rodman DM. Manifestations of cystic fibrosis diagnosed in adulthood. *Curr Opin Pulm Med.* 2005;11:513–518

31. Rodman DM, Polis JM, Heltshe SL, et al. Late diagnosis defines a unique population of long-term survivors of cystic fibrosis. *Am J Respir Crit Care Med.* 2005;171:621–626

32. Gan KH, Geus WP, Bakker W, Lamers CB, Heijerman HG. Genetic and clinical features of patients with cystic fibrosis diagnosed after the age of 16 years. *Thorax.* 1995;50:1301–1304

33. LeGrys VA, Yankaskas JR, Quittell LM, Marshall BC, Mogayzel PJ Jr. Diagnostic sweat testing: the Cystic Fibrosis Foundation guidelines. *J Pediatr.* 2007;151:85–89

34. Gibson LE, Cooke RE. A test for concentration of electrolytes in sweat in cystic fibrosis of the pancreas utilizing pilocarpine by iontophoresis. *Pediatrics.* 1959;23:545–549

35. Grody WW, Cutting GR, Watson MS. The cystic fibrosis mutation "arms race": when less is more. *Genet Med.* 2007;9:739–744

36. Cuppens H, Lin W, Jaspers M, et al. Polyvariant mutant cystic fibrosis transmembrane conductance regulator genes: the polymorphic (Tg)m locus explains the partial penetrance of the T5 polymorphism as a disease mutation. *J Clin Invest.* 1998;101:487–496

37. Sheppard DN, Rich DP, Ostedgaard LS, Gregory RJ, Smith AE, Welsh MJ. Mutations in CFTR associated with mild-disease-form Cl- channels with altered pore properties. *Nature.* 1993;362:160–164

38. Hamosh A, FitzSimmons SC, Macek M Jr, Knowles MR, Rosenstein BJ, Cutting GR. Comparison of the clinical manifestations of cystic fibrosis in black and white patients. *J Pediatr.* 1998;132:255–259

39. Wine JJ, Kuo E, Hurlock G, Moss RB. Comprehensive mutation screening in a cystic fibrosis center. *Pediatrics.* 2001;107:280–286

40. Alton EW, Currie D, Logan-Sinclair R, Warner JO, Hodson ME, Geddes DM. Nasal potential difference: a clinical diagnostic test for cystic fibrosis. *Eur Respir J.* 1990;3:922–926

41. Boucher RC, Stutts MJ, Knowles MR, Cantley L, Gatzy JT. Na+ transport in cystic fibrosis respiratory epithelia: abnormal basal rate and response to adenylate cyclase activation. *J Clin Invest.* 1986;78:1245–1252

42. Sauder RA, Chesrown SE, Loughlin GM. Clinical application of transepithelial potential difference measurements in cystic fibrosis. *J Pediatr.* 1987;111:353–358

43. Ren CL. Cystic fibrosis: evolution from a fatal disease of infancy with a clear phenotype to a chronic disease of adulthood with diverse manifestations. *Clin Rev Allergy Immunol.* 2008;35:97–99

44. Ratjen F. New pulmonary therapies for cystic fibrosis. *Curr Opin Pulm Med.* 2007;13:541–546

45. Flume PA, O'Sullivan BP, Robinson KA, et al. Cystic fibrosis pulmonary guidelines: Chronic medications for lung health. *Am J Respir Crit Care Med.* 2007;176:957–969

46. Flume PA, Robinson KA, O'Sullivan BP, et al. Cystic fibrosis pulmonary guidelines: airway clearance therapies. *Respir Care.* 2009;54:522–537

47. Fuchs HJ, Borowitz DS, Christiansen DH, et al. Effect of aerosolized recombinant human DNase on exacerbations of respiratory symptoms and on pulmonary function in patients with cystic fibrosis. The Pulmozyme Study Group. *N Engl J Med.* 1994;331:637–642

48. Elkins MR, Robinson M, Rose BR, et al. A controlled trial of long-term inhaled hypertonic saline in patients with cystic fibrosis. *N Engl J Med.* 2006;354:229–240

49. Ramsey BW, Pepe MS, Quan JM, et al. Intermittent administration of inhaled tobramycin in patients with cystic fibrosis. Cystic Fibrosis Inhaled Tobramycin Study Group. *N Engl J Med.* 1999;340:23–30

50. Eigen H, Rosenstein BJ, FitzSimmons S, Schidlow DV. A multicenter study of alternate-day prednisone therapy in patients with cystic fibrosis. Cystic Fibrosis Foundation Prednisone Trial Group. *J Pediatr.* 1995;126:515–523

51. Ren CL, Pasta DJ, Rasouliyan L, Wagener JS, Konstan MW, Morgan WJ. Relationship between inhaled corticosteroid therapy and rate of lung function decline in children with cystic fibrosis. *J Pediatr.* 2008;153:746–751

52. Balfour-Lynn IM, Lees B, Hall P, et al. Multicenter randomized controlled trial of withdrawal of inhaled corticosteroids in cystic fibrosis. *Am J Respir Crit Care Med.* 2006;173:1356–1362

53. Konstan MW, Byard PJ, Hoppel CL, Davis PB. Effect of high-dose ibuprofen in patients with cystic fibrosis. *N Engl J Med.* 1995;332:848–854

54. Lands LC, Milner R, Cantin AM, Manson D, Corey M. High-dose ibuprofen in cystic fibrosis: Canadian safety and effectiveness trial. *J Pediatr.* 2007;151:249–254

55. Oermann CM, Sockrider MM, Konstan MW. The use of anti-inflammatory medications in cystic fibrosis: trends and physician attitudes. *Chest.* 1999;115:1053–1058

56. Saiman L, Marshall BC, Mayer-Hamblett N, et al. Azithromycin in patients with cystic fibrosis chronically infected with *Pseudomonas aeruginosa*: a randomized controlled trial. *JAMA.* 2003;290:1749-1756

57. Kerem E, Reisman J, Corey M, Canny GJ, Levison H. Prediction of mortality in patients with cystic fibrosis. *N Engl J Med.* 1992;326:1187-1191

58. Liou TG, Adler FR, Cox DR, Cahill BC. Lung transplantation and survival in children with cystic fibrosis. *N Engl J Med.* 2007;357:2143-2152

59. Aurora P, Carby M, Sweet S. Selection of cystic fibrosis patients for lung transplantation. *Curr Opin Pulm Med.* 2008;14:589-594

60. Sweet SC, Aurora P, Benden C, et al. Lung transplantation and survival in children with cystic fibrosis: solid statistics—flawed interpretation. *Pediatr Transplant.* 2008;12:129-136

61. Woo MS. Overview of lung transplantation. *Clin Rev Allergy Immunol.* 2008;35:154-163

62. Konstan MW, Hilliard KA, Norvell TM, Berger M. Bronchoalveolar lavage findings in cystic fibrosis patients with stable, clinically mild lung disease suggest ongoing infection and inflammation. *Am J Respir Crit Care Med.* 1994;150:448-454

63. Brody AS, Klein JS, Molina PL, Quan J, Bean JA, Wilmott RW. High-resolution computed tomography in young patients with cystic fibrosis: distribution of abnormalities and correlation with pulmonary function tests. *J Pediatr.* 2004;145:32-38

64. Davis SD, Brody AS, Emond MJ, Brumback LC, Rosenfeld M. Endpoints for clinical trials in young children with cystic fibrosis. *Proc Am Thorac Soc.* 2007;4:418-430

65. FitzSimmons SC, Burkhart GA, Borowitz D, et al. High-dose pancreatic-enzyme supplements and fibrosing colonopathy in children with cystic fibrosis. *N Engl J Med.* 1997;336:1283-1289

66. Konstan MW, Morgan WJ, Butler SM, et al. Risk factors for rate of decline in forced expiratory volume in one second in children and adolescents with cystic fibrosis. *J Pediatr.* 2007;151:134-139

67. Moran A. Cystic fibrosis-related diabetes: an approach to diagnosis and management. *Pediatr Diabetes.* 2000;1:41-48

68. Moran A, Hardin D, Rodman D, et al. Diagnosis, screening, and management of cystic fibrosis-related diabetes mellitus: a consensus conference report. *Diabetes Res Clin Pract.* 1999;45:61-73

69. Edenborough FP. Women with cystic fibrosis and their potential for reproduction. *Thorax.* 2001;56:649-655

70. Pencharz PB, Durie PR. Pathogenesis of malnutrition in cystic fibrosis, and its treatment. *Clin Nutr.* 2000;19:387-394

71. Steinkamp G, Wiedemann B. Relationship between nutritional status and lung function in cystic fibrosis: cross-sectional and longitudinal analyses from the German CF Quality Assurance (CFQA) project. *Thorax.* 2002;57:596-601

72. Sawyer SM, Rosier MJ, Phelan PD, Bowes G. The self-image of adolescents with cystic fibrosis. *J Adolesc Health.* 1995;16:204-208

73. Corey M, McLaughlin FJ, Williams M, Levison H. A comparison of survival, growth, and pulmonary function in patients with cystic fibrosis in Boston and Toronto. *J Clin Epidemiol.* 1988;41:583-591

74. Jelalian E, Opipari L, Carrero V, Stark L. A comparison of eating attitudes and behavior in females with cystic fibrosis and their healthy peers. *Pediatr Pulmonol.* 1996;S13:335

75. McCallum TJ, Milunsky JM, Cunningham DL, Harris DH, Maher TA, Oates RD. Fertility in men with cystic fibrosis: an update on current surgical practices and outcomes. *Chest.* 2000;118:1059-1062

76. Fitzsimmons S, Fitzpatrick S, Thompson B. A longitudinal study of the effects of pregnancy on 325 women with cystic fibrosis. *Pediatr Pulmonol.* 2009;S13:99-101

77. Goss CH, Rubenfeld GD, Otto K, Aitken ML. The effect of pregnancy on survival in women with cystic fibrosis. *Chest.* 2003;124:1460-1468

78. McMullen AH, Pasta DJ, Frederick PD, et al. Impact of pregnancy on women with cystic fibrosis. *Chest.* 2006;129:706-711

79. Sawyer SM, Phelan PD, Bowes G. Reproductive health in young women with cystic fibrosis: knowledge, behavior, and attitudes. *J Adolesc Health.* 1995;17:46-50

80. Roberts S, Green P. The sexual health of adolescents with cystic fibrosis. *J R Soc Med.* 2005;98 (suppl 45):7-16

81. Yankaskas JR, Marshall BC, Sufian B, Simon RH, Rodman D. Cystic fibrosis adult care: consensus conference report. *Chest.* 2004;125:1S-39S

82. Sinnema G, Van der Laag LH, Stoop JW. Psychological development as related to puberty, body height, and severity of illness in adolescents with cystic fibrosis. *Isr J Med Sci.* 1991;27:186-191

83. Abbott J, Dodd M, Bilton D, Webb AK. Treatment compliance in adults with cystic fibrosis. *Thorax.* 1994;49:115-120

84. Bernard RS, Cohen LL. Increasing adherence to cystic fibrosis treatment: a systematic review of behavioral techniques. *Pediatr Pulmonol.* 2004;37:8-16

85. Britto MT, Garrett JM, Dugliss MA, et al. Risky behavior in teens with cystic fibrosis or sickle cell disease: a multicenter study. *Pediatrics.* 1998;101:250-256

86. Bartholomew LK, Czyzewski DI, Parcel GS, et al. Self-management of cystic fibrosis: short-term outcomes of the Cystic Fibrosis Family Education Program. *Health Educ Behav.* 1997;24:652-666

87. Drotar D, Ievers C. Age differences in parent and child responsibilities for management of cystic fibrosis and insulin-dependent diabetes mellitus. *J Dev Behav Pediatr.* 1994;15:265-272

88. Anderson DL, Flume PA, Hardy KK, Gray S. Transition programs in cystic fibrosis centers: perceptions of patients. *Pediatr Pulmonol.* 2002;33:327-331

89. Boyle MP, Farukhi Z, Nosky ML. Strategies for improving transition to adult cystic fibrosis care, based on patient and parent views. *Pediatr Pulmonol.* 2001;32:428-436

90. Cowlard J. Cystic fibrosis: transition from paediatric to adult care. *Nurs Stand.* 2003;18:39–41

91. Flume PA, Anderson DL, Hardy KK, Gray S. Transition programs in cystic fibrosis centers: perceptions of pediatric and adult program directors. *Pediatr Pulmonol.* 2001;31:443–450

92. Nasr SZ, Welsch CC. Disability and quality of life in cystic fibrosis from early age to adulthood. *J Adolesc Health.* 1996;19:381–383

93. Markowitz M. Death and dying in cystic fibrosis. In: Bluebond-Langner M, Lask B, Angst D, eds. *Psychosocial Aspects of Cystic Fibrosis*. New York: Oxford University Press; 2001

94. Shepherd SL, Hovell MF, Harwood IR, et al. A comparative study of the psychosocial assets of adults with cystic fibrosis and their healthy peers. *Chest.* 1990;97:1310–1316

95. Britto MT, Kotagal UR, Hornung RW, Atherton HD, Tsevat J, Wilmott RW. Impact of recent pulmonary exacerbations on quality of life in patients with cystic fibrosis. *Chest.* 2002;121:64–72

96. Bluebond-Langner M. The well siblings of children with cystic fibrosis. In: Bluebond-Langner M, Lask B, Angst D, eds. *Psychosocial Aspects of Cystic Fibrosis*. New York: Oxford University Press; 2001

# CHAPTER 93

# Sleep Disorders

ASHISH R. SHAH, MD

## INTRODUCTION

Adolescents are at an increased risk for sleep problems compared with younger children. There are multiple reasons for increasing difficulty. First, adolescents need more sleep than younger children.[1] Second, there is a tendency for an increase in daytime sleepiness even when there is adequate time provided for optimal sleep.[2] Irregular sleep schedules (especially differences between weekday and weekend schedules) contribute to difficulties with initiating sleep, awakening, and fragmented or poor quality sleep. Other factors may also play a role in poor sleep, including demanding social schedules, increased schoolwork, extracurricular activities, and late night computer activities, such as online chatting and text messaging.

The consequences of sleep loss and sleep difficulties can be severe. The National Highway Traffic Safety Administration[3] identifies drowsy driving as a serious problem that contributes to thousands of automobile crashes per year. Other consequences of poor sleep include lower grades and poor school performance, negative moods (anger, sadness, fear), and an increased likelihood of stimulant use.[4]

## NORMAL SLEEP

Normal sleep consists of nonrapid eye movement (NREM) sleep and rapid eye movement (REM) sleep. Nonrapid eye movement sleep can be divided into 3 stages. Progression through these 3 stages can be characterized as a progression through deeper stages of sleep, with slow wave sleep (previously divided into stages 3 and 4 sleep) being the deepest. The electroencephalogram (EEG) pattern during NREM sleep is characterized by waveforms such as spindles (stage 2 sleep), K-complexes (stage 2 sleep), and high-voltage slow waves (which are seen in slow wave sleep). Nonrapid eye movement sleep can also be characterized as a period of minimal mental activity.

By contrast, REM sleep is defined by EEG activation, muscle atonia, and bursts of rapid eye movements. Muscle twitches and irregular cardiorespiratory activity are also seen during REM sleep. Rapid eye movement and NREM sleep alternate throughout the night at approximately 90-minute cycles. With the exception of newborns (who enter sleep in REM or active sleep), sleep begins in NREM sleep, progresses through deeper stages (from stages 1 to 2 to slow wave sleep) before the first episode of REM sleep occurs. Newborns can spend up to 50% of their sleep time in active sleep. After about the first 2 years of life, REM sleep comprises 20% to 25% of normal sleep time. Then, the percentage of REM sleep remains relatively constant through childhood, adolescence, and adulthood.

Whether an individual is awake or asleep depends on a balance between the forces that promote wakefulness and the forces that promote sleep.[5] Sleep needs vary by time of day and tend to be greatest during the early morning or early afternoon (circadian pressure). Sleepiness, in general, increases as an individual is awake for longer periods (homeostatic pressure).

Neuropeptide hormones called hypocretins promote wakefulness. Hypocretins are synthesized in the hypothalamus, and the neurons that secrete hypocretins send their projections to the ventral forebrain and brainstem. In fact, the dysregulation of hypocretins is thought to play a role in the sleep disorder of narcolepsy. By contrast, the timing of sleep is regulated by the suprachiasmatic nucleus, which is located in the hypothalamus. The suprachiasmatic nucleus receives input from the retina and regulates the timing and length of sleep. The major sleep-inducing hormone is melatonin. Melatonin is produced in the pineal gland, and melatonin levels rise just before the onset of sleep.

During adolescence, melatonin release shifts to a later time, which may play a role in the difficulty adolescents have in falling asleep at earlier times.[6] There is the development of a sleep phase delay (shift to a later bedtime) as well as an onset of increased daytime sleepiness. Adolescents also develop a pattern of midafternoon sleepiness. The change in the circadian cycle tends to occur in a relatively short period of time, and as a result adapting to these changes can have significant psychosocial effect.

There has been much controversy on whether the shift of sleep timing in adolescence is biological or behavioral. Although activities and changes in behavior such as increased schoolwork, extracurricular activities, and social pressures contribute significantly to sleep difficulties, there is also strong evidence that there is a biological explanation (a change in the function of the suprachiasmatic nucleus) to support changes in adolescents' sleep schedules and habits.[7]

The exact incidence of sleep disturbances in adolescents is difficult to determine, particularly because the term "sleep disorder" can have a broad definition. In addition, some sleep disorders may go unrecognized for years. For example, sleep-disordered breathing may not be identified in adolescents unless someone is actually observing the adolescent sleeping.

It might be fair to assume that all adolescents at one time or another will experience symptoms of either excessive daytime sleepiness or insomnia. Surveys have attempted to establish the prevalence of sleepiness in adolescents. One survey of teenagers found that up to 20% of adolescents described themselves as sleepy in the daytime and up to 25% had insomnia symptoms.[8] Studies have also shown that insomnia is not only common in adolescents, but can be a chronic condition.[9]

## CONSEQUENCES OF POOR SLEEP

The consequences of poor sleep have been well documented. Excessive sleepiness has been shown to lead to difficulties with motor and cognitive reactions, difficulties with attention and performing complex tasks, and with slowing of motor and cognitive reactions.[10] Adolescents typically have irregular sleep schedules for a number of reasons, and studies have shown that irregular sleep schedules and decreased sleep time are associated with poor school performance.[11] Sleepiness has also been implicated as a major cause of motor vehicle crashes and fatalities. In fact, people younger than the age of 25 years are the most likely to be involved in accidents caused by sleepiness.[12]

As mentioned previously, poor sleep during adolescence does not always originate from irregular schedules. *Obstructive sleep apnea syndrome* (OSAS) is a form of sleep-disordered breathing and has been associated with many neurodevelopmental consequences. There is a suggestion that individuals who only snore (but who have no associated obstructive apnea) have more attention problems, social problems, and anxious/depressive symptoms.[13] Reduced academic performance in adolescence may also be linked to snoring in early childhood. The exact cause of poor school performance from obstructive sleep apnea is not known; however, there is speculation that this may be multifactorial and related to factors such as episodic hypoxemia, sleep fragmentation and sleep deprivation, and alveolar hypoventilation.[14] There are also other more serious health consequences of sleep-disordered breathing, including an increased risk for high blood pressure, stroke, and cardiac disease. There are even indications that cardiac strain can be identified in teenagers with obstructive sleep apnea.[15]

Sleep disorders other than OSAS are also associated with daytime difficulty. *Delayed sleep phase syndrome* (DSPS) is a common sleep disorder during adolescence that involves a shift of the sleep schedule to a later bedtime. This shift in the sleep schedule coupled with early awakenings for school often leads to significant daytime sleepiness and fatigue. *Narcolepsy* is a disorder characterized by episodes of sleepiness during the day and disrupted sleep at night. Because narcolepsy and DSPS lead to significant daytime sleepiness, they have both been implicated in symptoms similar to that of attention-deficit/hyperactivity disorder (ADHD). Hyperactivity and attention difficulties have also been linked to *periodic limb movement disorder.*[16] Periodic limb movement disorder involves abnormal limb movements at night and can also lead to disrupted sleep and daytime sleepiness.

## HISTORY IN THE ADOLESCENT WITH SLEEP DISTURBANCE

Obtaining a history in an adolescent with a sleep complaint may offer some unique challenges. The complaints of excessive sleepiness and insomnia are often inseparable. The individual who complains about insomnia at night will also have daytime sleepiness. These symptoms can lead to a cycle of caffeine use, and taking daytime naps, which in turn will further magnify the insomnia complaint at night. Furthermore, sleep disorders are also not always a primary problem. Although the initial complaints may pertain to sleep, the etiology of the disorder may be neurological, pulmonary, metabolic, endocrinological, or behavioral in nature. For example, individuals with asthma may have significant respiratory symptoms while asleep, or individuals with seizure disorders may also be having seizures at night. Also, symptoms occurring at night often are misinterpreted or may go unnoticed. Therefore, obtaining an adequate history requires the examiner to have an understanding of how all systems affect sleep behavior and sleep patterns.

Interviews with the parent(s) and the adolescent (together and separately) are also essential. Parents are often unaware of the adolescent's evening and nighttime routines, and also typically do not observe the adolescent sleeping at night. In addition, the child and the parent often perceive the effect of the complaint differently. It is not unusual for the adolescent in the office to indicate that he or she does not perceive a problem at all. It may be necessary to obtain the history a second time on a subsequent office visit, after the parent has been instructed to observe the child's sleep patterns and daytime behavior.

A meaningful sleep history requires a detailed medical and social history, addressing sleep schedules and daytime activities that affect sleep hygiene. Specific questions should be asked about television and computer use prior to bedtime, daytime naps, caffeine, tobacco, alcohol, and other illicit drug use. Caffeine has a profound effect on sleep. (Even in adolescents who comment that caffeine does not prevent them from sleeping, sleep fragmentation is common.) The use of alcohol prior to bedtime can also have an adverse effect on sleep. Alcohol use leads to increased sleep fragmentation, decreased REM sleep, and may exacerbate or precipitate snoring and obstructive sleep apnea.

A common contributing factor to the adolescent's sleep difficulties is an irregular sleep schedule. The typical change in activities occurring during weekends and holidays often leads to bedtimes well past midnight. Over the long term this contributes to shifting of the schedule (DSPS). Other necessary information to be elicited includes actual bedtime, time needed to fall asleep, and frequency and duration of nighttime awakenings.

## PHYSICAL EXAMINATION AND FINDINGS ASSOCIATED WITH SLEEP DISORDERS

The physical examination of the adolescent with a sleep disorder is often normal. However, there are some particulars that should not be overlooked. For example, risk factors for obstructive sleep apnea include obesity, large tonsils and adenoids, and a large neck size. The shape and contour of the palate may also be narrowed, suggesting an increased risk for obstructive sleep apnea. Adolescents with other disorders may also have physical findings that increase the risk for obstructive sleep apnea, such as craniofacial anomalies. Cleft palate or those associated with Down syndrome, even after surgical correction, may still pose a risk for developing of sleep-disordered breathing in adolescence. Hypotonia due to underlying neuromuscular disease can increase the likelihood of upper airway collapse during sleep.

## EVALUATION AND TESTING FOR SLEEP DISORDERS

Adolescents with sleep difficulties typically have had trouble for a long time, often years prior to presenting in the office. The history obtained from a short interview at the time of the initial visit may not reflect the true extent of the difficulty. The use of a sleep log or sleep diary is essential in eliciting components of insufficient sleep, circadian rhythm disorders (such as DSPS), or poor sleep hygiene (Figure 93-1).

A sleep log should record the total sleep obtained on a daily basis and should detail the differences between schedules on school days and weekends/vacations. A list of other activities that affect sleep such as caffeine

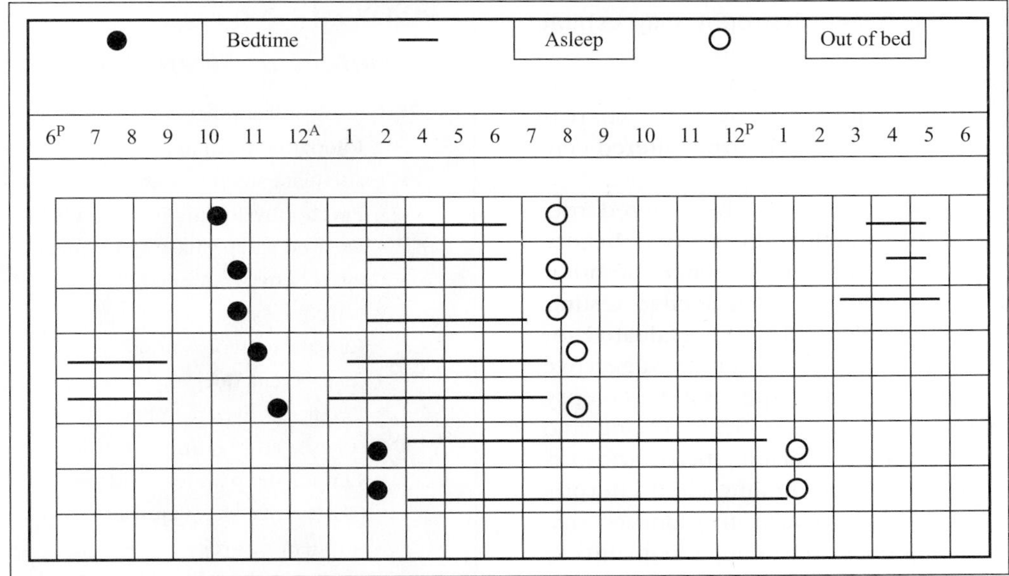


**FIGURE 93-1** Sample sleep log of an individual who has trouble falling asleep on weekdays but wakes up early for school. Naps are taken in the afternoons and evenings. On weekends, the individual stays up late, and sleep onset occurs quickly. The log shows components of delayed sleep phase and poor sleep hygiene.

intake, television, and computer/video game viewing time, and exercise during the day should also be noted. Therefore, a detailed sleep log will not only reveal the differences between total sleep actually obtained and total sleep required, but will also reveal the effects of behavior, sleep scheduling, and sleep hygiene.

When there is a concern of sleep-disordered breathing, an overnight polysomnogram (sleep study) is an essential diagnostic tool. Overnight polysomnography is considered the gold standard for the diagnosis of OSAS and other forms of sleep-disordered breathing.[17] A polysomnogram consists of monitoring multiple physiologic parameters, such as respiratory movements, oxygen saturation, sleep staging, and limb movements. Detailed respiratory monitoring includes oxygen saturation, end-tidal carbon dioxide, chest and abdominal wall motion, and airflow. Obstructive sleep apnea syndrome is diagnosed when airflow is obstructed, but abdominal and chest wall motion continues. With OSAS, a cycling of oxygen desaturation following obstructive events is often noted on the polysomnogram.

A sleep study can also identify central sleep apnea, which in contrast to OSAS can be a normal finding. However, there are circumstances where central sleep apnea is pathologic. Although not typical, cases of Arnold-Chiari malformation have been initially identified in teenagers with an initial presentation of central sleep apnea on polysomnography.[18] Central sleep apnea with oxygen desaturation may also be seen in the presence of cardiac dysfunction or congestive heart failure. Adolescents with neurological disorders such as muscular dystrophy and myotonic dystrophy may exhibit central and obstructive sleep apnea during an overnight polysomnogram. Obstructive apnea results from hypotonia and decreased upper airway tone, whereas the central apnea component may be from altered central respiratory control.

Although blood tests should not be ordered routinely as part of a sleep evaluation, a good history and physical examination or the presence of other underlying disorders should prompt selective testing. For example, an obese adolescent being evaluated for obstructive sleep apnea may have findings suggestive of thyroid dysfunction. When suspecting narcolepsy, although human leukocyte antigen (HLA) typing and cerebrospinal fluid assays are available, the diagnosis is largely based on history, clinical findings, and interpretation of polysomnography. Because drug and/or substance abuse can commonly lead to sleep complaints or exacerbate existing conditions, urine and/or blood sampling for illicit substances is often useful in the evaluation of sleep disorders.

## TREATMENT OF SLEEP DISORDERS

The differential diagnosis for complaints such as insomnia or excessive sleepiness is extensive (Box 93-1). There is frequently more than one cause or diagnosis for daytime sleepiness or insomnia. Even the adolescent with a diagnosis of obstructive sleep apnea or narcolepsy often has a behavioral component to his or her sleep problems. Poor sleep hygiene and scheduling disorders are often seen together. In fact, the institution of behavioral changes is essential to the treatment of sleep disorders. Common causes of daytime sleepiness in the adolescent include insufficient sleep, poor sleep hygiene (television or video games prior to bedtime, caffeine use, naps), and DSPS (where the bedtime is shifted toward later hours). Adolescents need 9 to 10 hours of sleep, which is equivalent to the amount of sleep that a 9- or 10-year-old typically needs.[19] However, due to school and extracurricular activities, as well as social schedules, adolescents rarely adhere to this. The typical young adult (ie, college student) will have similar sleep needs as the adolescent. Sleep patterns as a young adult also appear to remain the same, with a tendency for young adults to continue to have later bedtime hours. The shift to more usual adult bedtimes and 8 to 9 hours of sleep per night occurs gradually with age.

### Box 93-1

### *Examples of Sleep Disorders*[23]

- Causes of insomnia
  - Idiopathic insomnia
- Inadequate sleep hygiene
  - Psychophysiologic insomnia
  - Delayed sleep phase syndrome
- Causes of hypersomnia
  - Narcolepsy
  - Idiopathic hypersomnia
  - Insufficient sleep syndrome
  - Recurrent hypersomnia
- Sleep-related breathing disorders
  - Central sleep apnea syndrome
  - Obstructive sleep apnea syndrome
- Movement disorders during sleep
  - Restless legs syndrome
  - Periodic limb movement disorder

The guidelines in the list below are often quite successful when counseling an adolescent about sleep hygiene and scheduling difficulties. These guidelines can be tailored to an individual's needs based on specific information obtained from the sleep log.

- Avoid the use of electronic devices prior to bedtime (television, video games, "online" chatting)
- Sleep only in your own bed (ie, no falling asleep on the couch, television room, etc)
- Avoid naps
- Avoid use of caffeine, alcohol, tobacco products, and other illicit drugs at all times
- Engage in regular exercise

Of course, success depends on motivation and persistence. Continued follow-up for support is often necessary for success in changing sleep schedules and sleep hygiene. If there is a concern about possible associated psychiatric disorders such as anxiety or depression, professional counseling will also be helpful.

The use of medications is not necessary in cases where behavior and sleep scheduling are concerns, but selective serotonin reuptake inhibitors (SSRIs), benzodiazepines, and others may be used when there are comorbid psychiatric diagnoses. Medications to induce sleepiness and sleep onset such as melatonin, benzodiazepines, and zolpidem (Ambien) should not be considered long-term treatment for sleep disorders and may carry a risk of developing tolerance. In addition, medications may precipitate or exacerbate other sleep disorders such as obstructive sleep apnea.

The treatment for narcolepsy and obstructive sleep apnea is described in the following section. When obstructive sleep apnea is diagnosed, treatment options include a tonsillectomy/adenoidectomy or the use of continuous positive airway pressure (CPAP). Treatment for narcolepsy often involves a combination of medications along with behavioral changes.

## SPECIFIC SLEEP DISORDERS

Two specific sleep disorders are briefly discussed in the following section: narcolepsy and OSAS. Obstructive sleep apnea syndrome is a common disorder and can result in significant consequences when left untreated. There are many risk factors for OSAS, with obesity a major risk factor in adolescents and young adults. With the growing prevalence of obesity in children and adolescents, routine screening for obstructive sleep apnea will become increasingly important. Although narcolepsy is typically not diagnosed until adulthood, the symptoms of narcolepsy often present during adolescence. The diagnosis of narcolepsy should be considered in any adolescent or young adult presenting with sleepiness.

### NARCOLEPSY

Narcolepsy is a disorder characterized by a tetrad of symptoms: daytime sleepiness with sleep attacks; cataplexy (a sudden loss of muscle control in response to emotional triggers); hypnagogic hallucinations (vivid dreams at sleep onset); and sleep paralysis. Although narcolepsy is often not diagnosed until the third or fourth decades, adults often report a period of 15 years or longer between the onset of symptoms and the correct diagnosis.[20] This suggests that narcolepsy is often present but unrecognized in late childhood and adolescence.

Although little information is available as to the prevalence of narcolepsy in childhood and adolescence, its prevalence in adults in the United States has been described from 1:1,000 to 1:10,000.[21] Evidence suggests a genetic predisposition to the development of narcolepsy. Narcolepsy has been associated with the presence of histocompatibility antigens DQB1*0602 or DQA1*0102 in almost 100% of patients. In some animal models, narcolepsy has been found to be inherited in an autosomal recessive pattern. This has not been shown in humans, so it is believed that the predisposition to developing narcolepsy may be a combination of environmental factors with genetic susceptibility.[22]

Narcolepsy represents an intrusion of REM sleep into wakefulness. However, the classic tetrad of symptoms is often not present in the early stages of narcolepsy, making the diagnosis difficult in adolescents. In most cases, the presenting complaint is excessive sleepiness. Because the complaint of daytime sleepiness is nonspecific, narcolepsy is often misinterpreted by physicians, family members, and teachers. Sleepiness can also be "expressed" by behaviors such as irritability and attention difficulties, and often other diagnoses are pursued, such as psychiatric disorders and attention difficulties. The adolescent may be seen as lazy, with poor motivation, or be labeled as "difficult." The use of illicit drugs may also be suspected.

#### Diagnosis and Treatment of Narcolepsy

The differential diagnosis of excessive daytime sleepiness in an adolescent is extensive. Because the first symptom of narcolepsy is often sleepiness, the diagnosis cannot only be difficult, but it can be delayed for years. Frequent evaluation of symptoms over time is often needed to help in the assessment. The development of typical features over time may be helpful (cataplexy, sleep paralysis, hypnagogic hallucinations). The best evaluation tool for narcolepsy is overnight polysomnography followed by a multiple sleep latency test (MSLT). The overnight polysomnography may reveal typical features, such as decreased sleep latency (time to sleep onset) and decreased REM latency (time to first episode of REM sleep). The MSLT is a series of short naps undertaken the following day. In narcolepsy, the MSLT typically reveals a decreased sleep latency and sleep-onset REM. (Full diagnostic criteria can be obtained from the *International Classification of Sleep Disorders, Diagnostic and Coding Manual.*)[23] As part of the differential diagnosis of narcolepsy, exclusion of other neurologic diseases, use of an EEG, and drug screening are often helpful.

Treatment of narcolepsy should involve behavioral changes as well as medications. Good sleep habits (sleep hygiene), scheduled naps, and psychological support are essential. For daytime sleepiness, stimulants such as methylphenidate or modafinil have been used. Cataplexy can be treated with the use of tricyclic antidepressants or SSRIs.

## OBSTRUCTIVE SLEEP APNEA SYNDROME

Obstructive sleep apnea syndrome is a respiratory disorder of sleep characterized by intermittent, partial, or complete upper airway obstruction. The exact prevalence of OSAS in adolescents has not been studied, although the overall incidence of OSAS in the pediatric age group has been estimated to be anywhere from 1% to 6%. Symptoms of obstructive sleep apnea include nightly snoring (often with periods of gasps, snorts, or pauses), disturbed or restless sleep, mouth breathing, and increased respiratory effort (labored breathing) during sleep.

As mentioned previously, untreated, OSAS can lead to significant sequelae and morbidity. Cardiac evaluation, including an echocardiogram, electrocardiogram (ECG), and chest x-ray, is often helpful when moderate or severe obstructive sleep apnea is documented. Long-term follow-up to ensure improvement of obstructive apnea and its complications is essential.

### Risk Factors for OSAS

In the younger age group (ages 2–6) the most common risk factor for obstructive sleep apnea is enlarged tonsils and adenoids. Although large tonsils and adenoids are also a concern in the adolescent, obesity is also a significant risk factor for the development of obstructive sleep apnea in the adolescent. Other coexisting conditions, such as Down syndrome, craniofacial anomalies, and neuromuscular disorders, also contribute to the development of obstructive sleep apnea.

### Diagnosis of OSAS

The presence of obstructive sleep apnea is usually accompanied by some degree of snoring. Obtaining a detailed sleep history that includes screening for obstructive sleep apnea should be a part of routine health care visits. When there is a history of snoring, details about labored breathing during sleep, restless sleep, excessive daytime sleepiness, and behavioral or learning difficulties should be obtained. The physical examination in an adolescent may often be normal. However, there are nonspecific findings that may be noted, such as elevated blood pressure, adenotonsillar hypertrophy, and mouth breathing. The examiner should also take note of the size of the oropharynx, the shape of the palate, and of body habitus (obesity). Hypotonia may be noted in individuals with a history of genetic or neuromuscular disorders.

The history and physical examination for obstructive sleep apnea is useful as a screening tool to determine which individuals will need further evaluation. Even the presence of large tonsils and adenoids may not always indicate obstructive sleep apnea, as the tone of the upper airway plays a significant role in obstructive sleep apnea. Many tools have been evaluated for their usefulness in diagnosing obstructive sleep apnea; questionnaires, nocturnal saturation monitors, and home audio taping and videotaping have all been studied. All of these tools have limited usefulness and frequently have a significant degree of false-negative results. As mentioned previously, the gold standard for evaluation of obstructive sleep apnea is an overnight polysomnogram, where episodes of complete and partial airway obstruction (obstructive hypopnea) are scored and counted.

### Treatment of OSAS

Treatment for obstructive sleep apnea is pursued after underlying risk factors are considered. Because enlarged tonsils and adenoids can be a significant risk factor, a tonsillectomy and/or adenoidectomy is often the first step. However, when there are other risk factors (obesity, hypotonia, craniofacial anomalies), CPAP may be needed if obstructive sleep apnea does not resolve or if a tonsillectomy and adenoidectomy are not options. Continuous positive airway pressure is typically initiated during a second sleep study, where pressure is titrated until episodes of airway obstruction are eliminated. When obesity is present, interventions for weight loss are also essential.

## OTHER CAUSES OF DISRUPTED SLEEP

The differential diagnosis for disrupted sleep and daytime sleepiness in the adolescent is extensive, and disorders can be classified in many different ways. For example, abnormal or unusual movements during the night may be a result of periodic limb disorder, restless leg syndrome, or perhaps nocturnal seizures. Sleep-related breathing disorders may be caused or exacerbated by craniofacial anomalies, chronic lung disease, neuromuscular disorders, or cardiac disorders. Insomnia or excessive daytime sleepiness may be associated with poor sleep hygiene or circadian rhythm disorders.

In adolescents a type of circadian rhythm disorder known as DSPS is not uncommon. Delayed sleep phase syndrome occurs when sleep onset and wake times are significantly delayed beyond what would be considered appropriate or desirable. Delayed sleep phase syndrome (and circadian rhythm disorders in general) occurs when the endogenous circadian clock loses synchronization with external time cues (eg, light).

The adolescent with DSPS will often find it difficult to initiate sleep until well past midnight, leading to complaints of insomnia. Forced early awakenings on school days can lead to symptoms of excessive daytime sleepiness and irritability during the day. It is important to note that sleep times will often be normal on holidays and weekends, when the individual is allowed to sleep and wake up without other commitments. Diagnosis is often made clinically, with sleep logs and a careful history being essential. Comorbid conditions (such as depression) should also be excluded. Therapy for DSPS involves multiple approaches, such as addressing sleep hygiene and maintaining consistent schedules. Exposure to bright lights in the morning and the use of melatonin may also be effective.[24]

A clinician interested in sleep medicine is encouraged to pursue more detailed reading on the classification, physiology, and pathophysiology of the various disorders.[24,25] The diagnosis and management of most sleep disorders (obstructive sleep apnea, insomnia, scheduling disorders) can be accomplished without referral to a sleep medicine specialist. Referral to a consultant may be appropriate when less common disorders are suspected (eg, narcolepsy) or when comorbid conditions and the potential of more significant consequences exist—such as obstructive sleep apnea associated with neuromuscular disorders.

## CONCLUSION

During the adolescent years, the need for sleep does not decrease, and may be even greater than during the preadolescent years. The biological tendency for the sleep schedule to shift to a later time period, coupled with school and social schedules, becomes a barrier to obtaining an adequate amount of sleep. As a result, insomnia, disrupted sleep, and excessive daytime sleepiness are common complaints during the adolescent years. Understanding the various causes of sleep disorders and their consequences will help facilitate the evaluation and treatment of the adolescent with sleep difficulties.

## REFERENCES


1. Carskadon MA, Harvey K, Duke P, Anders TF, Litt IF, Dement WC. Pubertal changes in daytime sleepiness. *Sleep*. 1980;2: 453–460

2. Carskadon MA, Vieiri C, Acebo C. Association between puberty and delayed sleep phase preference. *Sleep*. 1993;16: 258–262

3. NCSDR/NHTSA Expert Panel of Driver Fatigue and Sleepiness. Drowsy Driving and Automobile Crashes. Available at: www.nhtsa.dot.gov/people/injury/drowsy_driving1/Drowsy.html. Accessed October 25, 2006

4. Carskadon MA. Adolescent sleepiness: increased risk in a high-risk population. *Alcohol, Drugs, and Driving*. 1990;5: 317–328

5. Saper CB, Chou TC, Scammell TE. The sleep switch: hypothalamic control of sleep and wakefulness. *Trends Neurosci*. 2001;24:726–731

6. Kotagal S, Pianosi P. Sleep disorders in children and adolescents. *BMJ*. 2006;332:828–832

7. Allen RP. Development of the human circadian cycle. In: Loughlin GM, Carroll JL, Marcus CL, eds. *Sleep and Breathing in Children: A Developmental Approach*. New York: Marcel Dekker, Inc; 2000: 313–332

8. Ohayon MM, Roberts RE, Zulley J, Smirne S, Priest RG. Prevalence and patterns of problematic sleep among older adolescents. *J Am Acad Child Adolesc Psychiatry*. 2000;39: 1549–1556

9. Johnson EO, Roth T, Schultz L, Breslau N. Epidemiology of DSM-IV insomnia in adolescence: lifetime prevalence, chronicity, and an emergent gender difference. *Pediatrics*. 2006;117:e247–e256

10. Doran SM, Van Dongen HP, Dinges DF. Sustained attention performance during sleep deprivation: evidence of state instability. *Arch Ital Biol*. 2001;139:253–267

11. Millman RP. Working Group on Sleepiness in Adolescents/Young Adults; AAP Committee on Adolescence. Excessive sleepiness in adolescents and young adults: causes, consequences, and treatment strategies. *Pediatrics*. 2005;115:1774–1786

12. Pack AI, Pack AM, Rodgman E, Cucchiara A, Dinges DF, Schwab CW. Characteristics of crashes attributed to the driver having fallen asleep. *Accid Anal Prev*. 1995;27:769–775

13. O'Brien LM, Mervis CB, Holbrook CR, et al. Neurobehavioral implications of habitual snoring in children. *Pediatrics*. 2004;114:44–49

14. Gozal D, Pope DW Jr. Snoring during early childhood and academic performance at ages 13 to 14 years. *Pediatrics*. 2001;107:1394–1399

15. Amin RS, Kimball TR, Bean JA, et al. Left ventricular hypertrophy and abnormal ventricular geometry in children and adolescents with obstructive sleep apnea. *Am J Respir Crit Care Med*. 2002;165:1395–1399

16. Chervin RD, Archbold KH, Dillon JE, et al. Associations between symptoms of inattention, hyperactivity, restless legs, and periodic leg movements. *Sleep*. 2002;25:213-218

17. Marcus CL. Section on pediatric pulmonology, subcommittee on obstructive sleep apnea syndrome. Clinical practice guidelines: diagnosis and management of childhood obstructive sleep apnea syndrome. *Pediatrics*. 2002;190:704-712

18. Zolty P, Sanders MH, Pollack IF. Chiari malformation and sleep-disordered breathing: a review of diagnostic and management issues. *Sleep*. 2000;23:637-643

19. Carskadon MA, Harvey K, Duke P, Anders TF, Litt IF, Dement WC. Pubertal changes in daytime sleepiness. *Sleep*. 1980;2:453-460

20. Hood BM, Harbord MG. Pediatric narcolepsy: complexities of diagnosis. *J Paediatric Child Health*. 2002;38:618-621

21. Kotagal S. Narcolepsy in children. *Semin Pediatr Neurol*. 1996;3:36-43

22. Guilleminault C, Heinzer R, Mignot E, Black J. Investigations into the neurologic basis of narcolepsy. *Neurology*. 1998;50(suppl 1):S8-S15

23. American Academy of Sleep Medicine. *International Classification of Sleep Disorders, Second Edition. Diagnostic and Coding Manual*. Westchester, IL: American Academy of Sleep Medicine; 2005

24. Kryger MH, Roth T, Dement WC. *Principles and Practice of Sleep Medicine*. Philadelphia, PA: Saunders Company; 2005

25. Chokroverty S. *Sleep Disorders Medicine: Basic Science, Technical Considerations, and Clinical Aspects*. Boston, MA: Butterworth-Heinemann; 1999

# CHAPTER 94

# Pneumothorax

DEBORAH LOPEZ, MD

## INTRODUCTION

Pneumothorax is an uncommon etiology of chest pain in adolescents. However, certain adolescents may be at risk and the diagnosis must be considered. This chapter discusses differences between primary and secondary pneumothorax, including diagnosis and treatment.

## PRIMARY SPONTANEOUS PNEUMOTHORAX

Primary pneumothorax is predominantly a disease of young adult males with an asthenic body habitus and a history of smoking.[1] The median age of primary pneumothorax is 16.7 years and the male-to-female ratio is 2:1.[2] The most common cause of primary pneumothorax is rupture of a subpleural bleb or bulla.[3,4] A study of chest computer tomography (CT) of 20 patients revealed various types of emphysematous lesions located predominantly in the apical fields.[5]

Symptoms are most often mild and consist of dyspnea and chest pain on the side of the pneumothorax. Contrary to the popular belief that there is an association with strenuous physical activity, primary pneumothorax frequently develops when the patient is at rest.[6] Physical examination may reveal loss of tactile fremitus, hyperresonance to percussion, and decreased breath sounds. Tension pneumothorax should be suspected if the patient has severe acute dyspnea, cyanosis, and/or a tracheal shift.

The usual radiographic findings in a patient with a pneumothorax are the demonstration of a distinct visceral pleural line with the absence of lung markings in the periphery (Figure 94-1). Chest radiographs taken during expiration or in a lateral decubitus view, with the side of the suspected pneumothorax superior, may reveal a small pneumothorax not apparent on routine chest radiograph.

Pneumothoraces that are less than 20% in a healthy adolescent may not require any treatment to re-expand the lung. It has been estimated that the rate of air reabsorption in the plural space is 1.25% per 24 hours; therefore, it can take up to 2 weeks for a 20% pneumothorax to resolve. Because of the risk of developing a trapped lung as a result of fibrotic peels being laid down on the visceral pleura, pneumothoraces that have not resolved within 2 weeks should be evacuated with either tube thoracostomy or percutaneous aspiration. Patients given 100% oxygen by face mask absorb pleural air approximately 4 times faster than those who do not receive 100% oxygen. The nitrogen gradient between the alveoli and pleural air enhances absorption.[7]

Pneumothoraces greater than 25% that are increasing in size, causing clinical deterioration, or involving a significant pleural effusion should be evacuated. Pneumothoraces can be evacuated with simple percutaneous aspiration and then monitored by serial chest radiographs. If resolution does not occur, tube thoracotomy should be considered. Method of evacuation of a pneumothorax by way of percutaneous aspiration, tube thoracotomy with underwater suction, pleurodesis, open thoracotomy with apical bullectomy, or thoracoscopy and video-assisted thoracic surgery (VATS) should be determined on a case-by-case evaluation.

## SECONDARY SPONTANEOUS PNEUMOTHORAX

The incidence of secondary pneumothorax is similar to that of primary pneumothorax. An estimated 7,500 new cases per year are diagnosed in the general population with males affected 3 times more commonly than females. Clinically, multiple disorders are associated with secondary pneumothorax (Box 94-1). Pulmonary bleb rupture is another common cause. Additionally, patients with pneumonia caused by mycoplasma, tuberculosis, and human immunodeficiency virus with underlying *Pneumocystis carinii* also are commonly affected.[8,9]

Secondary pneumothorax is a more serious condition because underlying pulmonary function is already compromised. Interpretation of the physical examination is difficult in patients with suspected secondary pneumothorax because they may have underlying hyperexpanded lungs, decreased tactile fremitus, hyperresonance to percussion, and distant breath sounds. Secondary pneumothorax should be suspected when an adolescent with an underlying pulmonary disorder, such as asthma, experiences severe acute dyspnea, tachypnea, chest pain, or cyanosis.

Once the diagnosis of a secondary pneumothorax is considered, chest radiography should be performed. Its

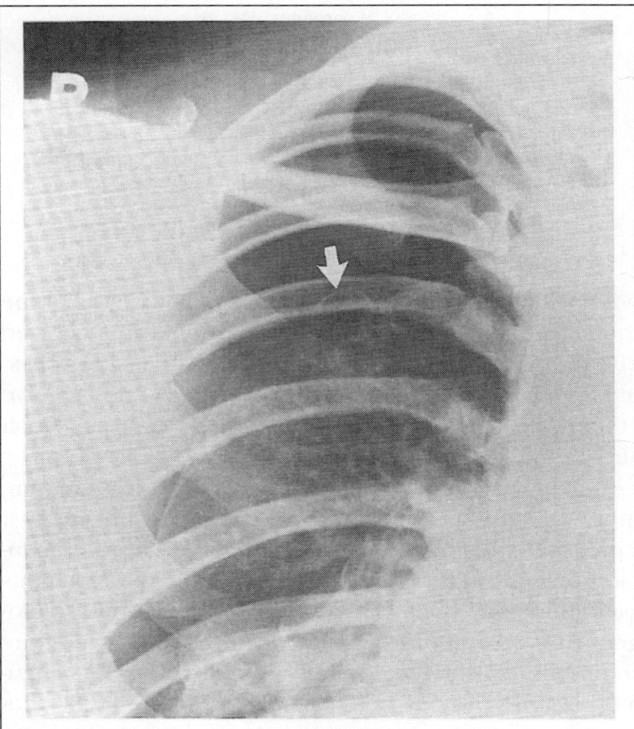

FIGURE 94-1 Primary spontaneous pneumothorax. The visceral pleural line is clearly demonstrated together with the lateral avascular space. There is a pleural bleb at the apex of the lung *(arrow)*, a common finding. Such blebs are usually not detectable when the lung re-expands. (Reprinted from Armstrong P, Wilson AG, Dee P, Hensell DM. *Imaging of Diseases of the Chest*. 2nd ed. St. Louis, MO: Mosby–Year Book;1995:696, with permission from Elsevier.)

**Box 94-1**

***Diseases Associated with Secondary Spontaneous Pneumothorax***

Asthma
Pneumonia
Cystic fibrosis
Tuberculosis
Atypical mycobacteria
Pneumocystitis carinii pneumonia
Drug abuse by inhalation
Congenital cystic lung disease
Pulmonary embolism
Collagen vascular disease
Marfan syndrome
Ehlers-Danlos syndrome
Cutis laxa (generalized elastolysis)

interpretation in patients with underlying lung disease may be difficult. Pneumothoraces as small as 5% to 10% in this population can produce severe symptoms. If the distinction between a pneumothorax and a bulla cannot be made, a CT scan should be obtained.

The main objective in treating patients with secondary pneumothorax is decreasing the possibility of a recurrence. Therapy is usually more aggressive than for primary pneumothorax because of an increased risk of pulmonary deterioration and death.

Virtually all patients with underlying pulmonary pathology require tube thoracostomy. Deterioration in respiratory status necessitating mechanical ventilation will require immediate insertion of a chest tube because of the possible continued enlargement of the pneumothorax or of the development of a tension pneumothorax. Tube thoracostomy is less effective at re-inflating the lung in secondary pneumothorax than in primary pneumothorax. The average time for lung re-expansion in secondary pneumothorax is 5 days, and patients often require multiple, prolonged use of chest tubes. Once the lung has re-expanded, it is recommended that agents such as minocycline can be instilled into the plural space to decrease the incidence of recurrence.[10] These agents produce pleuritis, with resultant adhesions between the visceral and parietal pleura. Surgical intervention should be considered in patients whose lungs remain unexpanded for more than 5 days or if an air leak persists for several days after pleurodesis.

Pneumothorax is a well-recognized complication of both inhalational and intravenous drug abuse. Drugs used for inhalation include cocaine, marijuana, nitrous oxide, and amphetamines.[11] Pneumothorax following inhalation of these agents is related to a prolonged Valsalva maneuver or other vigorous inhalation maneuvers performed by users of these substances to enhance the effects of the drug. During the Valsalva maneuver, the alveoli are overdistended and the vessels that they contact are devoid of blood. The pressure gradient created between the alveolus and the vessel leads to rupture of the alveolar wall into the perivascular adventitia, which may in turn lead to formation of a pneumothorax. Patients with pneumothorax and no underlying medical conditions should be asked about illicit drug use.

## SUMMARY

Primary pneumothorax is a relatively uncommon occurrence seen most frequently in tall, thin adolescent males with a history of smoking. Secondary pneumothorax is associated with underlying lung pathology or drug abuse. Treatment should be individualized, ranging from observation to serial chest radiographs and, in some cases, surgical intervention. The major complication associated with pneumothorax is the development of a tension pneumothorax, which should be recognized and treated promptly and aggressively.

## REFERENCES

1. Hui YW, Chan KW, Ko S, et al. Adolescent primary spontaneous pneumothorax: a hospital's experience. *HK J Paediatr. (new series).* 2006;11:128-132

2. Poenaru D, Yazbeck S, Murphy S. Primary spontaneous pneumothorax in children. *J Pediatr Surg.* 1994;29:1183-1185

3. Kjaergaard H. Spontaneous pneumothorax in the apparently healthy. *Acta Med Scand.* 1932;43(suppl):1-159

4. Brock RC. Recurrent and chronic spontaneous pneumothorax. *Thorax.* 1948;3:88-111

5. Lesur O, Delorme N, Fromaget JM, Bernadac P, Poul JM. Computed tomography in the etiologic assessment of idiopathic spontaneous pneumothorax. *Chest.* 1990;98:341-347

6. Bense L, Wiman LG, Hedenstierna G. Onset of symptoms in spontaneous pneumothorax: correlations to physical activity. *Eur J Respir Dis.* 1987;71:181-186

7. Chadha TS, Cohn MA. Non-invasive treatment of pneumothorax with oxygen inhalation. *Respiration.* 1983;44:147-152

8. Byrnes T, Brevig J, Yeoh C. Pneumothorax in patients with acquired immunodeficiency syndrome. *J Thorac Cardiovasc Surg.* 1989;98:546-550

9. Sepkowitz KA, Telzak EE, Golds JW, et al. Pneumothorax in AIDS. *Ann Intern Med.* 1991;114:455-459

10. Tanaka F, Itoh M, Esaki H, Isobe J, Ueno Y, Inoue R. Secondary spontaneous pneumothorax. *Ann Thorac Surg.* 1993;55:372-376

11. Seaman M. Barotrauma related to inhalation drug abuse. *J Emerg Med.* 1990;8:141-149

# CHAPTER 95

# Pulmonary Embolism

DIANA KING, MD • EDWARD E. CONWAY, JR, MD

## EPIDEMIOLOGY

Venous thrombosis can occur when any component of Virchow's triad is present: stasis of blood flow, injury to the vessel wall, or a hypercoagulable state. Pulmonary embolus (PE) is a potentially fatal complication of deep venous thrombosis (DVT). A clot from any location in the venous system can embolize to the pulmonary blood vessels. Both DVT and PE are discussed in this chapter, as they are components of a spectrum of disease.

Pulmonary embolism is uncommon in the adolescent. A national hospital discharge survey from 1979 through 2001 determined that 13,000 infants and children had a discharge diagnosis of PE.[1] The survey sampled 8% of hospitals, and the extrapolated rate of PE is 0.9/100,000 children/year. There is a bimodal peak in incidence in infants under 2 years and in teenagers 15 to 17 years. In the teenage group, the rate of DVT was twice as high in females, and 27% of the females were pregnant. The rate of PE was twice as high in blacks than in whites.[1] The mortality rate from PE in children and adolescents is not known. In adults, the mortality rate has dropped from 191/million in 1979 to 94/million in 1998. This is probably due to improved prevention, detection, and treatment of DVTs. The mortality rate is 50% higher in blacks than in whites and 20%–30% higher in men than women.

## RISK FACTORS

Underlying conditions associated with the risk of PE are summarized in Box 95-1. The most common predisposing conditions that lead to DVT or PE in children are central venous catheters, malignancy, congenital heart disease, trauma, infection/sepsis, nephrotic syndrome, and major surgery.[3] Venography done prior to removing implantable ports from children with cancer revealed that 50% had DVTs in the upper venous system.[4] Children with acute lymphoblastic leukemia (ALL) are at increased risk of thromboembolism because of increase in thrombin generation. Asparaginase and steroids are also known to induce a hypercoagulable state by suppression of natural coagulants.[5] Pediatric trauma patients who develop DVTs or PEs tend to be older (15 to 18 years), have higher injury severity scores, have thoracic or spinal injury, and have central venous catheters.[6] The risk of thromboembolism increases during the second and third trimesters of pregnancy, and is particularly high in teenagers (15 to 19 years). The greatest risk for DVT and PE is in the postpartum period. Fortunately, there has been a dramatic decrease in pregnancy-associated PE in recent years.[7]

**Box 95-1**

***Risk Factors for Pulmonary Embolus***

- Central venous catheters
- Malignancy
- Congenital heart disease
- Trauma
- Infection/sepsis
- Nephrotic syndrome
- Major surgery
- Pregnancy/postpartum
- Estrogen-containing contraceptives (pill, patch, ring)
- Steroids
- L-asparaginase
- Immobility
- Systemic lupus erythematosus
- Congenital prothrombotic conditions
- Ventriculatrial shunt
- Intravenous drug use
- Dehydration

Estrogen-containing contraceptives such as the birth control pill, the patch, or ring are potential causes of DVT and PE in adolescent girls. Threrefore, it is important when considering the diagonosis of DVT or PE to specifically ask the adolescent girl whether she is using any of these medications. Estrogen-containing contraceptives are contraindicated for girls with a previous history of DVT or PE.

Primary and secondary hypercoagulable states are risk factors for PE. Antithrombin III, protein C, and protein S deficiencies should be considered in a patient with recurrent thromboembolic disease, particularly if there is a family history of thrombosis. Acquired deficiencies of these proteins may occur with disseminated intravascular coagulation, liver disease, nephrotic syndrome, acute respiratory distress syndrome, pregnancy, or after surgery or L-asparaginase chemotherapy. Low protein S levels have been noted in patients infected with the human immunodeficiency virus.[8]

## PRESENTATION

Pleuritic pain is the most common symptom of PE, followed by dyspnea, cough, and hemoptysis. Fever, tachypnea, and a lower extremity DVT are other associated findings.[9] In adults, the sudden onset of dyspnea, chest pain, and syncope (singly or in combination) are the most common symptoms of PE.[10] Reproducible chest pain, generally attributed to a musculoskeletal problem, does not reliably exclude PE in adults.[11] In more than 50% of young adults 18 to 40 years of age with documented PE, there is no evidence of cardiopulmonary abnormality or DVT on physical examination.[12] Therefore, if a clinical suspicion of PE exists, diagnostic tests should be pursued, even if the patient has a healthy appearance.

## DIAGNOSIS

Clinical suspicion of PE is the crucial step in making a diagnosis. Figure 95-1 summarizes the diagnostic approach to the patient with suspected PE. The presence of risk factors and symptoms consistent with PE warrants

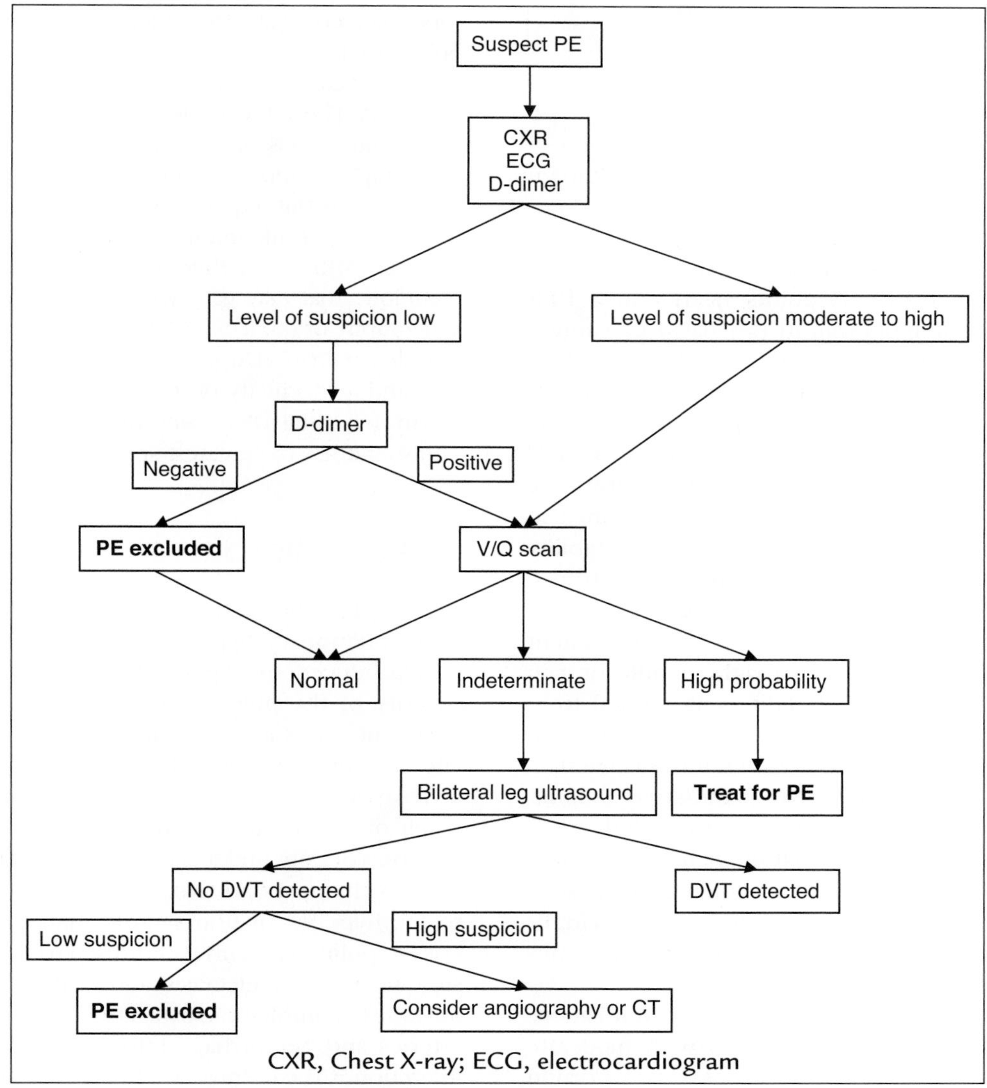


**FIGURE 95-1** Diagnostic algorithm for pulmonary embolus.

**Table 95-1**

**Wells Score**

| *Variable* | *Points* |
|---|---|
| Clinical signs/symptoms of DVT | 3.0 |
| Alternate diagnosis less likely than PE | 3.0 |
| Heart rate >100 beats per minute | 1.5 |
| Immobilization or surgery in the previous 4 weeks | 1.5 |
| Previous DVT/PE | 1.5 |
| Hemoptysis | 1.0 |
| Malignancy | 1.0 |
| ***Pretest probability determined by total of points*** | ***Total points*** |
| High | 6 |
| Moderate | 2-6 |
| Low | <2 |

further work-up. A pretest probability score, known as the Wells clinical prediction rule (see Table 95-1), is commonly used in adult patients. Points are assigned as follows: clinical symptoms of DVT = 3 points; other diagnosis less likely than PE = 3 points; heart rate > 100/min = 1.5 points; immobilization (>3 days) or surgery in past 4 weeks = 1.5 points; previous DVT or PE = 1.5 points; hemoptysis = 1 point; malignancy = 1 point. Pretest probability for PE is high if the score is >6, moderate if the score is 2 to 6, and low if the score is <2.[13] This scoring system can help guide the appropriate diagnostic strategy. Chest x-ray should be performed to exclude other processes that will lower the probability of PE, such as pneumonia or pneumothorax. Electrocardiography should be performed to exclude pericarditis or myocardial infarction. Sinus tachycardia, ST-T segment changes, right axis deviation, and right bundle branch block can be seen with PE.[14] D-dimer is formed from plasmin-mediated lysis of fibrin in a thrombus. Elevated D-dimer is seen with PE and other conditions (infection, inflammation, malignancy); a low quantitative D-dimer level (<500 ng/ml by ELISA) may help to exclude PE.[15] Normal $PaO_2$ and alveolar–arterial gradient do not help rule out PE.[16] Physical examination findings suggestive of a DVT are warmth, erythema, swelling, leg pain, or cramps. Documentation of DVT by sonography obviates the need for further tests.

The initial diagnostic test should be a ventilation/perfusion (V/Q) scan in those patients with moderate to high clinical suspicion for PE. The perfusion portion consists of an intravenous (IV) injection of technetium-labeled albumin that is distributed into the pulmonary circulation. If any perfusion defect is found, a ventilation scan should be performed.[13] Xenon gas is inhaled and its distribution recorded with a gamma camera. The perfusion scan is then compared with the ventilation scan to identify areas of mismatch. The degree of perfusion defect is then categorized as high probability, intermediate probability, low probability, or normal. A high-probability scan is diagnostic for PE and a normal scan excludes PE. Normal or high-probability scans are seen in only 25% of patients; and the remaining 75% are nondiagnostic and require further testing to confirm PE. Ventilation/perfusion scans are also difficult to interpret in adolescents with congenital heart disease. Pulmonary angiography is considered the gold standard for diagnosing PE, but it is invasive. Risks of angiography include radiation exposure, reaction to contrast medium, arrhythmia, bleeding, and infection. Sedation is often required, which imparts its own set of risk factors. Spiral computed tomography (CT) with IV contrast is being used with greater frequency as the initial examination to diagnose PE or as a follow-up to an indeterminate V/Q scan. The CT can visualize PE in the main, lobar, or segmental vessels or identify other diagnoses. Computed tomography is more cost-effective and has fewer nondiagnostic results but requires iodinated contrast and exposure to radiation. Gadolinium-enhanced Magnetic resonance imaging (MRI) is another promising, noninvasive imaging technique that may gain wider use in the future.[17] Ultrasonography of the legs may be helpful when the V/Q scan is indeterminate. Duplex ultrasound has a sensitivity of 96% and a specificity of 94% for proximal DVTs. The sensitivity for distal DVT using duplex is 71%. Compression ultrasound has the greatest specificity for DVTs (98%).[18]

## PATHOPHYSIOLOGY

After a PE, right heart failure may develop as a result of acute pulmonary hypertension. The degree of obstruction produced by the embolus is proportional to the severity of the pulmonary hypertension. Alveolar dead space increases as lung units continue to be ventilated and are not perfused. Hypoxemia and an increased alveolar–arterial oxygen gradient commonly occur as a result of V/Q mismatch, intracardiac shunt, reflex bronchoconstriction, atelectasis, or lung infarction. Proprioceptors that respond to stretch and irritation contribute to the hyperventilation seen in many patients with PE. Loss of pulmonary surfactant distal to the vascular occlusion results in atelectasis and edema. This makes the lungs less compliant. Obstruction of smaller pulmonary arteries and hemorrhage into the airways can result in infarction if the extravasated blood is not cleared.[19]

## TREATMENT

Initial care of the patient with suspected PE should focus on airway, breathing, and circulation. Supplemental oxygen should be administered for hypoxemia and patients in respiratory failure should be tracheally intubated and mechanically ventilated. If the patient is hypotensive, then a massive PE should be suspected. Judicious use of IV fluids followed by vasopressors can be utilized to treat hypotension. Empiric anticoagulant therapy should be administered when there is a high clinical suspicion for PE and considered when there is moderate or low suspicion, unless there is a contraindication. Absolute contraindications include active or potential internal or central nervous system (CNS) bleeding or a cerebrovascular accident within 2 months.[20] Heparin activates antithrombin III, which inhibits thrombin and prevents propagation of a thrombus. If heparin is used, the loading dose is 75 to 100 U/kg given intravenously (maximum adult dose is 10,000 U), followed by an infusion of 18 to 20 U/kg/hr (no maximum adult dose). Monitoring is necessary using the activated partial thromboplastin time (aPTT) or directly measuring heparin concentration. An aPTT that reflects a heparin level (by protamine titration) of 0.2 to 0.4 U/ml is considered therapeutic (2 to 2.5 times normal). Subcutaneous (SQ) low molecular weight heparin (LMWH) may be used in hemodynamically stable patients, and unfractionated heparin should be used if the patient is hypotensive. Low molecular weight heparin has high activity against factor Xa and less activity against thrombin. The dose of enoxaparin is 1 mg/kg/dose every 12 hours (adult dose is 1 mg/kg SQ q 12 hours, with no maximum). The only way of objectively monitoring LMWH is using anti-factor Xa assay, with a goal of 0.5 to 1.0 U/ml 4 to 6 hours after SQ dose. Oral vitamin K antagonists (Coumadin) reduce the plasma concentration of vitamin K-dependent factors. They are available in tablet form only and are used for long-term therapy. A dose of 0.2 mg/kg (adult dose is 5–15 mg/day) can be initiated and adjusted to maintain an international normalized ratio (INR) of 2 to 3. Heparin or LMWH should be given for 5 to 10 days and Coumadin should be initiated on day 1 to 2 of heparin. Coumadin therapy is usually continued for at least 6 months. The INR of the prothrombin time measures the degree of anticoagulation achieved by vitamin K antagonists. An INR of 2.0 to 3.0 is considered therapeutic.[21] Bleeding complications from heparin or LMWH are treated by discontinuing the heparin and giving protamine. The dose of protamine to administer is based on the amount of heparin received. Give 1 mg protamine for every 100 units of LMWH received in the last 4 hours and give 1 mg protamine for every 100 units of IV heparin received in the last 2 hours. Vitamin K can be given to reverse the effects of Coumadin. Fresh-frozen plasma should be given if significant bleeding occurs. Tissue plasminogen activator (tPA), streptokinase (SK), and urokinase (UK) are thrombolytic agents that convert plasminogen to plasmin.[22] Their use should be considered in the following situations: persistent hypotension, severe hypoxemia, or right ventricular dysfunction due to PE. An inferior vena cava filter is indicated when anticoagulation is contraindicated and when PE recurs despite therapeutic anticoagulation.[23]

## PREVENTION

Graduated-compression stockings and intermittent external pneumatic compression are routinely used in patients in the postoperative period. Heparin or LMWH prophylaxis should be considered in patients at risk for thromboembolic disease. Examples of patients at risk for thromboembolism are patients with prolonged bed rest and prolonged immobilization. See Box 95-1 for conditions associated with this risk.

## CONCLUSION

Although PE is rarely diagnosed in adolescents, it is a potentially fatal condition. The presenting signs and symptoms are nonspecific, so knowledge of conditions that predispose to PE should raise the clinician's index of suspicion. Clinical scoring systems help determine the likelihood of PE. The evolution of accessible imaging techniques should improve early detection of PE. Prompt initiation of anticoagulant therapy can be life-saving.

## REFERENCES


1. Stein PD, Kayali F, Olson RE. Incidence of venous thromboembolism in infants and children: data from the national hospital discharge survey. *J Pediatr.* 2004;145:563–565

2. Horlander KT, Mannino DM, Leeper KV. Pulmonary embolism mortality in the United States, 1979–1998: an analysis using multiple-cause mortality data. *Ann Intern Med.* 2003;163:1711–1717

3. Andrew M, David M, Adams M, et al. Venous thromboembolic complications (VTE) in children: first analyses of the Canadian Registry of VTE. *Blood.* 1994;83:1251–1257

4. Glaser DW, Medeiros D, Rollins N, Buchanan GR. Catheter-related thrombosis in children with cancer. *J Pediatr.* 2001;138:255–259

5. Athale UH, Chan AKC. Thrombosis in children with acute lymphoblastic leukemia Part II. Pathogenesis of thrombosis in children with acute lymphoblastic leukemia: effects of the disease and therapy. *Thromb Research.* 2003;111:199–212

6. Cyr C, Michon B, Petterson G, David M, Brossard J. Venous thromboembolism after severe injury in children. *Acta Haematol.* 2006;115:198-200

7. Heit JA, Kobbervig CE, James AH, Petterson TM, Bailey KR, Melton III LJ. Trends in the incidence of venous thromboembolism during pregnancy or postpartum: a 30-year population-based study. *Ann Intern Med.* 2005;143:697-706

8. Nachman RL, Silverstein R. Hypercoagulable states. *Ann Intern Med.* 1993;119:819-827

9. Bernstein D, Coupey S, Schonberg SK. Pulmonary embolism in adolescents. *Am J Dis Child.* 1986;140:667-671

10. Miniati M, Prediletto R, Formichi B, et al. Accuracy of clinical assessment in the diagnosis of pulmonary embolism. *Am J Respir Crit Care Med.* 1999;159:864-871

11. Le Gal G, Testuz A, Righini M, et al. Reproduction of chest pain by palpation: diagnostic accuracy in suspected pulmonary embolism. *BMJ.* 2005;330:452-453

12. Green RM, Meyer TJ, Drum M, Glassroth J. Pulmonary embolism in younger adults. *Chest.* 1992;101:1507-1511

13. Wells PS, Anderson DR, Rodger M, et al. Derivation of a simple clinical model to categorize patients' probability of pulmonary embolism: increasing the model utility with the SimpliRED D-dimer. *Thromb Haemost.* 2000;83:416-420

14. Crane SD, Beverley DW, Williams MJ. Massive pulmonary embolus in a 14-year-old boy. *J Accid Emerg Med.* 1999;16:289-290

15. Kearon C. Diagnosis of pulmonary embolism. *CMAJ.* 2003;168:183-194

16. Rodger MA, Carrier M, Jones GN, et al. Diagnostic value of arterial blood gas measurement in suspected pulmonary embolism. *Am J Respir Crit Care Med.* 2000;162:2105-2108

17. Babyn PS, Gahunia HK, Massicotte P. Pulmonary thromboembolism in children. *Pediatr Radiol.* 2005;35:258-274

18. Goodacre S, Sampson F, Thomas S, van Beek E, Sutton A. Systematic review and meta-analysis of the diagnostic accuracy of ultrasonography for deep vein thrombosis. *BMC Medical Imaging.* 2005;5:6-19

19. Elliott CG. Pulmonary physiology during pulmonary embolism. *Chest.* 1992;101(suppl):163S-171S

20. Evans DA, Wilmot RW. Pulmonary embolism in children. *Pediatr Clin North Am.* 1994;41:569-584

21. Hirsh J, Fuster V, Ansell J, Halperin JL. American Heart Association/American College of Cardiology Foundation Guide to Warfarin Therapy. *Circulation.* 2003;107:1692-1711

22. Monagle P, Chan A, Massicotte P, Chalmers E, Michelson AD. Antithrombotic therapy in children: the Seventh ACCP Conference on antithrombotic and thrombolytic therapy. *Chest.* 2004;126:645S-687S

23. Kucher N, Rossi E, DeRoas M, Goldhaber SZ. Massive pulmonary embolism. *Circulation.* 2006;113:577-582

# SECTION 5

# The Gastrointestinal System

## CHAPTER 96

## The Approach to Abdominal Pain

NADER N. YOUSSEF, MD

### INTRODUCTION

Abdominal pain can be a challenging complaint for both primary care and specialist physicians because it is a frequent complaint that can also herald serious acute pathology. When evaluating the complaint of abdominal pain, clinicians become responsible for trying to determine which patients can be safely observed or treated symptomatically and which require further investigation. Acute abdominal pain frequently requires urgent investigation and management. Adolescents with a suspected surgical abdomen require rapid assessment in an acute care facility where expert and urgent surgical consultation can be performed.[1] Fortunately, studies of the accuracy of history and physical examination for more dangerous causes of abdominal pain (eg, acute appendicitis, ovarian torsion), alone or in combination with focused investigations, yield good results. A partial list of diagnoses to be considered in abdominal pain emergencies is provided (Box 96-1).

Patients with less acute illness may require consultation or referral for further management following a more detailed history and initial assessment. A practical approach for further evaluation of the adolescent patient who presents with chronic abdominal pain is discussed later in the chapter.

**Box 96-1**

***Considerations in Evaluation of Abdominal Pain Emergencies***

- Enteric infection/mesenteric adenitis
- Constipation/acute fecal impaction
- Carbohydrate malabsorption/bloating
- Intestinal ileus
- Gastritis/peptic ulcer disease
- Appendicitis
- Hepatitis
- Cholelithiasis/cholecystitis
- Intussusception
- Pancreatitis
- Celiac disease
- Inflammatory bowel disease
- Vasculitis/Henoch-Schönlein purpura
- Porphyria
- Renal calculi
- Pyelonephritis
- Acute hydronephrosis
- Mononucleosis
- Nephritis
- Ovarian or testicular torsion
- Psoas abscess
- Tubo-ovarian abscess
- Ectopic pregnancy
- Pneumonia
- Sickle cell crisis
- Lymphoma
- Trauma
- Intestinal abnormalities (malrotation, volvulus, hernia, adhesions)

## APPROACH TO ABDOMINAL PAIN

The pattern and nature of the pain can vary enormously. It may be intermittent, continuous, or colicky.[2] Several illnesses, especially appendicitis, begin with vague abdominal discomfort. Respiration or movement of the patient often increases the pain, indicating generalized peritoneal inflammation and parietal peritoneal pain. Pelvic inflammation may result in painful micturition and vague lower abdominal discomfort that is occasionally relieved after defecation. Aggravating and relieving factors such as lying down and vomiting are important. The patient's activity level can aid in establishing the diagnosis. Writhing may be suggestive of colic, whereas a quiet, still patient may have peritonitis.

Night pain or pain on awakening can suggest a peptic origin, although pain that occurs in the evening or during dinner can be a feature of constipation. In addition to the complaint of heartburn, adolescents are able to articulate other features of peptic disease, including early satiety, nausea, and the supraesophageal or respiratory complications of gastroesophageal reflux. A diary that lists diet, symptoms, and associated features for 3 to 7 days is invaluable because it will indicate potential causes of the symptoms, such as exposure to lactose or the failure to have a normal bowel movement. The diary should also include any interventions initiated by the adolescent or parents.

The review of systems should focus on features that can be related to the causes of abdominal pain. These can include documented weight loss or gain, changes in linear growth, fever, joint complaints, oral sores, or rash. The presence of one or more of these signs suggests an inflammatory process such as seen in inflammatory bowel disease or celiac disease. The respiratory complications of gastroesophageal reflux, including chronic cough, reactive airway disease, or persistent laryngitis, may be more prominent than emesis or chest pain.

A careful review of recent medications may reveal potential side effects as a cause of abdominal pain; for example, antibiotics may predispose the patient to intestinal bacterial overgrowth, acne medications may induce esophagitis, and tricyclic antidepressants may cause constipation.

A family history of peptic disease, irritable or inflammatory bowel disease, pancreatitis, biliary disease, or migraine should be sought.

## DIFFERENTIAL DIAGNOSIS OF ABDOMINAL PAIN

A number of clinical features ("red flags") are commonly considered as orienting toward an organic etiology, although definitive proof for their predictive value is scant. Elements that have been classically associated with a greater likelihood of an organic condition are listed in Box 96-2. The following is an overview of common diagnoses where abdominal pain may be the key feature at presentation.

**Box 96-2**

***Alarm Features or "Red Flags" Associated with Abdominal Pain***

- Persistent right upper or right lower quadrant pain
- Dysphagia
- Persistent vomiting
- Gastrointestinal blood loss
- Nocturnal diarrhea
- Pain that awakens the patient
- Perirectal disease
- Involuntary weight loss
- Arthritis
- Deceleration of linear growth
- Delayed puberty
- Unexplained fever
- Family history of inflammatory bowel disease, celiac disease, and/or peptic ulcer disease

### Peptic Ulcer Disease

### Pancreatitis

Chronic pancreatitis is an inflammatory disease characterized by recurrent episodes of abdominal pain. In certain individuals, the recurrent bouts may result in progressive structural changes and permanent impairment of the exocrine and endocrine functions of the pancreas.[6] In one study, 1 of every 3 children and adolescents with acute pancreatitis presented with recurrences.[7] In this study, the most frequent symptom in both acute and recurrent episodes of pancreatitis was abdominal pain, followed by vomiting and ileus. Biliary stones, a family history of pancreatitis, drug ingestion, and hypercalcemia were common. Abdominal trauma and acute hepatitis A were causes in some of the patients with acute pancreatitis. Elevated triglyceride levels, pancreas divisum, and delta F508 mutation occurred in some of the patients with recurrent pancreatitis.[7]

### Inflammatory Bowel Disease

The presentation of the abdominal pain is variable in inflammatory bowel disease, depending on the site of bowel involvement. Disease of the terminal ileum and cecum in patients with Crohn disease is often associated with right lower quadrant discomfort and tenderness. In one study, a decrease in growth preceded the onset of any symptoms by at least 1 year in 24 of 50 patients with Crohn disease diagnosed in adolescence.[8]

### Celiac Disease

Adolescent patients with celiac disease rarely present with classic failure to thrive or chronic diarrhea at the time of diagnosis. Frequently, adolescents present with abdominal pain and bloating or excessive flatulence, which are common clinical manifestations of functional gastrointestinal disorders (FGIDs).[9] Any adolescent presenting with unexplained anemia and abdominal pain should be evaluated for celiac disease.[10] Some organizations have recommended that celiac disease should be added to the differential diagnosis of irritable bowel syndrome.[11] Studies in North America have shown an increased rate of diagnosis with better serological testing and subsequent histological confirmation.[12]

### Carbohydrate Intolerance

In adolescents with long-standing complaints of abdominal discomfort and increased bloating, the diagnosis of carbohydrate intolerance should also be considered. Often a dietary intervention eliminating beverages containing lactose, sorbitol, or high fructose syrup over a period of weeks to months may be both diagnostic and therapeutic. In a large series investigating nonspecific abdominal complaints using breath testing, the malabsorption rate was 34% after lactose, 61% after fructose, and 91% after the intake of a sorbitol test drink. [13] In the same study, patients themselves reported an improvement in 75% of cases with elimination of the appropriate beverages.[13]

### Genitourinary Disorders

Ureteral or pelviureteric junction obstruction may present with recurrent, cramping abdominal pain, despite a normal physical examination and urinalysis.[14] Hematuria, when present with abdominal pain, may be indicative of a urinary tract infection, abuse, trauma, Henoch-Schönlein purpura, or renal stones. Abdominal discomfort with dysuria can represent a sign of pyelonephritis, abuse, trauma, or sexually transmitted disease.[15] In adolescent females, mid-lower abdominal pain had low sensitivity but high specificity for gynecologic diseases.[16] Gynecologic pathology, such as ovarian cysts, congenital uterine abnormalities, and endometriosis, should therefore be considered in the differential diagnosis of abdominal pain. Hematocolpos due to an imperforate hymen may present with periodic lower abdominal pain, constipation, bloating, and urinary retention.[17] Clinically, endometriosis can begin as early as 3 to 4 years after menarche and may manifest by cyclic abdominal pain, nausea, vomiting, constipation, or diarrhea.[18]

### Musculoskeletal Pain

Pain related to trauma is usually well localized and sharp in nature, and may be exacerbated by movement. Pain due to costochondritis originates in the anterior chest wall, from where it may radiate to the chest, back, or abdomen. The pain of costochondritis is reproducible by palpating the affected cartilage.[19] The diagnosis of costochondritis should be considered in any adolescent complaining of chest or upper abdominal pain.

Another rarely considered cause for abdominal pain may be the abdominal wall. The abdominal wall might be considered to be an unlikely source of prolonged abdominal pain, but one study reported that in 15% of patients with prolonged, nonspecific abdominal pain, the abdominal wall was the source of the complaint.[20] Abdominal pain resulting from cutaneous nerve entrapment has been recently reported in the case of a 15-year-old girl who came to the hospital emergency department with abdominal pain of 3 months duration.[21] A comprehensive work-up had not established a specific cause for the pain. On the basis of the clinical findings, the possibility of a cutaneous nerve entrapment was suggested. After the involved cutaneous nerve was selectively blocked by subcutaneous infiltration, the pain disappeared immediately and completely. Recognition of this apparently unusual condition can lead to gratifying results.

## APPROACH TO CHRONIC ABDOMINAL PAIN

It is important to note that abdominal pain may be present on questioning of up to 75% of otherwise healthy adolescents.[1] The prevalence of abdominal pain is consistently high across diverse geographic regions and is most frequently associated with FGIDs, including dyspepsia and irritable bowel syndrome.

Chronic abdominal pain refers to a pattern that is continuous, persistent, or intermittent over a period of a few months. The pain may wax and wane, with some days being better than others.[1] On occasion, relatively short asymptomatic periods may be interposed with "painful periods," but the episodes of wellness rarely last long, generating a condition that creates profound distress in the daily life of the adolescent and the family. Many conditions can cause abdominal pain that is chronic and relapsing, but in clinical practice most adolescents presenting with this symptom have FGIDs without any evidence of organic disease. This can manifest itself as abdominal pain alone, termed "functional abdominal pain," associated with epigastric discomfort or nausea, referred to as "functional dyspepsia," or associated with alternating problems with defecation, known as "irritable bowel syndrome." Chapter 98 focuses on the most common FGIDs in adolescents.

**Table 96-1**

**ROME III Diagnostic Criteria[22]**

| *Functional Abdominal Pain** | *Functional Dyspepsia* | *Irritable Bowel Syndrome* |
|---|---|---|
| Must include *all* of the following: | Must include *all* of the following: | Must include *all* of the following: |
| Episodic or continuous abdominal pain | 1. Persistent or recurrent pain or discomfort centered in the upper abdomen (above the umbilicus)<br>2. Not relieved by defecation or associated with the onset of a change in stool frequency or stool form (ie, not IBD) | 1. Abdominal discomfort (an uncomfortable sensation not described as pain) or pain associated with *2 or more* of the following at least 25% of the time:<br>a. Improved with defecation<br>b. Onset associated with a change in frequency of stool<br>c. Onset associated with a change in form (appearance) of stool |
| No evidence of inflammatory, anatomic, metabolic, or neoplastic process | No evidence of inflammatory, anatomic, metabolic, or neoplastic process | No evidence of inflammatory, anatomic, metabolic, or neoplastic process |
| Criteria fulfilled at least *once per week for at least 2 months* before diagnosis | Criteria fulfilled at least *once per week for at least 2 months* before diagnosis | Criteria fulfilled at least *once per week for at least 2 months* before diagnosis |

*Functional abdominal pain syndrome must include functional abdominal pain *at least 25% of the time and 1 or more* of the following: some loss of daily functioning, and/or additional somatic symptoms, such as headaches, limb pain, or difficulty breathing.

## GENERAL DIAGNOSTIC EVALUATION

When needed, the exclusion of an organic condition can be accomplished using inexpensive and easily available diagnostic tests, such as a complete blood cell count, erythrocyte sedimentation rate, chemistry panel, liver and thyroid function studies, urinalysis, and stool examination for blood, ova, and parasites. The need for other diagnostic tests should be based on the history and physical examination findings. The clinician should avoid the lure of having to "rule out" an organic disease. Performing multiple tests may provide results that are often unrelated to the presenting symptom or have no clinical relevance (eg, a mildly elevated sedimentation rate). Repeating tests to confirm serendipitous findings may further increase anxiety and undermine the clinical diagnosis of functional abdominal pain.

Becoming familiar with symptom-based criteria for the FGIDs associated with chronic abdominal pain, known as the ROME III Diagnostic Criteria for Functional Gastrointestinal Disorders,[22] and using a limited diagnostic evaluation, the practitioner can work through the extensive differential diagnosis of abdominal pain without subjecting the patient to multiple testing procedures.

In patients with no alarm symptoms (Box 96-2), the ROME criteria have a positive predictive value of approximately 98%, with additional diagnostic tests providing a yield of only 2% or less.[23] The ROME criteria are symptom-based diagnostic criteria that lead to diagnoses not explained by other pathologically based disorders. The symptoms of these disorders relate to combinations of several known physiological determinants: increased gastrointestinal motor reactivity, enhanced visceral hypersensitivity, altered mucosal immune and inflammatory function (which includes changes in bacterial flora), and altered central nervous system enteric nervous system regulation (as influenced by psychosocial and sociocultural factors and exposures). Table 96-1 lists the ROME III diagnostic criteria for the 3 most common functional disorders in adolescents: functional abdominal pain, functional dyspepsia, and irritable bowel syndrome.

## SUMMARY

Adolescents with abdominal pain present a significant challenge to busy clinicians. The approach discussed in this chapter is based on clinical experience and the available data in the literature. As clinicians, we are always concerned that there may be something we are overlooking to explain the pain, and experience, vigilance, and empathy are needed to become an effective caregiver in the evaluation of abdominal pain. The treatment plan that is developed for acute abdominal pain is guided by the history, physical examination, and appropriate diagnostic testing. The evaluation of chronic abdominal pain in the adolescent heavily depends on the initial approach and first interactions with the patient. It is hoped that developing an effective relationship with the patient, using established diagnostic criteria, and having reasonable expectations for proposed treatments will lead to greater satisfaction for the patient and clinician, while also decreasing costs and improving quality of care.

## REFERENCES


1. Pollack ES. Pediatric abdominal surgical emergencies. *Pediatr Ann.* 1996;25:448–457

2. Spitz L, Kimber C. The history. *Semin Pediatr Surg.* 1997;6:58–61

3. Tsou VM, Baker R, Book L, et al. Multicenter, randomized, double-blind study comparing 20 and 40 mg of pantoprazole for symptom relief in adolescents (12 to 16 years of age) with gastroesophageal reflux disease (GERD). *Clin Pediatr.* 2006,45:741–749

4. Hirano I, Richter JE. ACG practice guidelines: esophageal reflux testing. *Am J Gastroenterol.* 2007;102:668–685

5. Bittencourt BF, Rocha GA, Penna FJ, Queiroz DM. Gastroduodenal peptic ulcer and *Helicobacter pylori* infection in children and adolescents. *J Pediatr (Rio J).* 2006;82:325–334

6. Mergener K, Baillie J. Chronic pancreatitis. *Lancet.* 1997;350:1379–1385

7. Sanchez-Ramirez CA, Larossa-Harro A, Flores-Martinez S, et al. Acute and recurrent pancreatitis in children: etiological factors. *Acta Paediatr.* 2007;96:534–537

8. Kanof ME, Lake AM, Bayless TM. Decreased height velocity in children and adolescents before the diagnosis of Crohn's disease. *Gastroenterology.* 1988;95:1523–1527

9. van de Wouden EJ, Nelis GF, Vecht J. Screening for celiac disease in patients fulfilling the Rome II criteria for irritable bowel syndrome in a secondary care hospital in The Netherlands: a prospective observational study. *Gut.* 2007;56:444–445

10. Ferrara M, Coppola L, Coppola A, Capozzi L. Iron deficiency in childhood and adolescence: retrospective review. *Hematology.* 2006;11:183–186

11. Kleibeuker JH. The Dutch College of General Practitioners' "irritable bowel syndrome" standard: reaction from the field of gastroenterology. *Ned Tijdschr Geneeskd.* 2002;146:790–791

12. Murray JA, Van Dyke C, Plevak MF, et al. Trends in the identification and clinical features of celiac disease in a North American community, 1950–2001. *Clin Gastroenterol Hepatol.* 2003;1:19–27

13. Born P, Sekatecheva M, Rosch T, Classen M. Carbohydrate malabsorption in clinical routine: a prospective observational study. *Hepatogastroenterology.* 2006;53:673–677

14. Byrne WJ, Arnold WC, Stannard MW, et al. Ureteropelvic junction obstruction presenting with recurrent abdominal pain: diagnosis by ultrasound. *Pediatrics.* 1985;76:934–937

15. McDonald JA. Abdominal pain in the adolescent female. *Clin Pediatr Emerg Med.* 2002;3:33–44

16. Yamamoto W. The relationship between abdominal pain regions and specific diseases: an epidemiologic approach to clinical practice. *J Epidemiol.* 1997;7:27–32

17. Kumar A, Mittal M, Prasad S, et al. Haematocolpos—an uncommon cause of lower abdominal pain in adolescent girls. *J Indian Med Assoc.* 2002;100:240–241

18. Tsenov D. Endometriosis in adolescence—characteristic features. *Akush Ginekol.* 2000;40:24–26

19. Brown RT. Costochondritis in adolescents. *J Adolesc Health Care.* 1981;1:198–201

20. Camilleri M. Management of patients with chronic abdominal pain in clinical practice. *Neurogastroenterol Motil.* 2006;18:499–506

21. Peleg R. Abdominal wall pain caused by cutaneous nerve entrapment in an adolescent girl taking oral contraceptive pills. *J Adolesc Health.* 1999;24:45–47

22. Rasquin A, Di Lorenzo C, Forbes D, et al. Childhood functional gastrointestinal disorders: child/adolescent. *Gastroenterology.* 2006;130:1527–1537

23. Olden KW. Diagnosis of irritable bowel syndrome. *Gastroenterology.* 2002;122:1701–1741

# CHAPTER 97

# Functional GI Disorders

NADER N. YOUSSEF, MD • STEPHANIE G. SCHUCKALO, RN, APN

## INTRODUCTION

Functional gastrointestinal disorders (FGIDs) are among the most common medical problems encountered in adolescents. In a community-based sample, 8% to 17% of middle school and high school students met the symptom-based criteria for irritable bowel syndrome (IBS).[1] In patients 12 to 19 years of age, 3% to 4% fulfilled criteria for functional dyspepsia (FD).[2] In other community-based samples, the incidence of medical presentation of abdominal pain thought to be related to FGIDs in adolescents is 3 to 7 times higher than other common episodic conditions such as asthma and migraine headaches.[3]

Functional gastrointestinal disorders have been recently defined as a variable combination of chronic or recurrent gastrointestinal symptoms not explained by structural or biochemical abnormalities. These disorders now have an accepted international criteria for symptom-based diagnosis known as Rome III.[4] A prevailing paradigm for the pathogenesis of the FGIDs is that of visceral hyperalgesia. In this concept, there has been a sensitization of primary sensory afferent fibers innervating the gut or along spinal neurons receiving input from visceral afferents. Alterations along the brain–gut axis are believed to lead to hypersensitivity to either noxious or physiologic stimuli, resulting in visceral hyperalgesia.

Recently, with innovative testing in the gastrointestinal motility laboratory, there has been a tremendous increase in the understanding of the pathophysiology of FGIDs. The early neonatal period is a time in which nocioreceptive circuits are formed. These circuits normally require use-dependent activity for appropriate development. Animal models have demonstrated a critical time during development in which the spinal cord is vulnerable to permanent structural and functional alterations in pain pathways, including those to the gastrointestinal tract.[5] Exposure to chronic antibiotic use, bacterial infections, or food allergy may all play a role at the cellular level where new insights on microscopic inflammation and immunologic dysregulation are being investigated vigorously. If these events occur early in childhood, they can lead to neuroplasticity of the enteric nervous system (ENS) and presentation of symptoms later in adolescence, theoretically through alterations in local reflex activity or via altered neural processing along the brain–gut axis.

The complex wiring system of the gastrointestinal tract that modulates its response to the internal and external environment is known as the ENS. The ENS stores more than 95% of all serotonin in the human body. An altered reflex and perceptual response within the brain–gut axis involving serotonin has emerged as a generally accepted model to explain the cardinal symptom of abdominal pain in FGIDs.[6] The 2 aspects of gut physiology most relevant to FGIDs are sensation and motility. Sustained and inappropriate gut hypersensitivity, as well as gut dysmotility, are well documented. These sensory-motor dysfunctions seem related to alterations in neural processing in the brain–gut axis and in visceral reflex pathways.[7]

## SENSORIMOTOR DYSFUNCTION

Gastrointestinal sensorimotor dysfunction has been demonstrated in several FGIDs, including IBS, functional abdominal pain (FAP), and FD. In IBS, patients reported a decreased threshold for sensation to rectal balloon distension as compared with control patients without any gastrointestinal complaints.[8] This hypersensitivity to rectal or sigmoid balloon distension can be shown in 50% to 70% of patients with IBS. Research has also revealed that site-specific hyperalgesia, rather than a generalized intestinal hypersensitivity, exists in FGID. This has been described in pediatric patients undergoing evaluation for abdominal discomfort; for instance, both a decreased sensory and motor function threshold for balloon distension in the stomach was found in patients meeting criteria for FD but not in patients with IBS.[9] Using novel, noninvasive breath testing techniques in a large number of adolescent patients, Chitkara et al[10] have confirmed that the predominant features of nausea and postprandial fullness seen in FD are the key sensorimotor dysfunctions.

The sensorimotor dysfunction that occurs in FGIDs has numerous potential causes. Enteric inflammation and immune activation have been proposed as an etiology because there is a prevalence of up to 30% of postinfectious IBS after an acute episode of bacterial gastroenteritis.[11] Alterations in enteric flora are another potential cause because bacteria can influence enteric motor activity, can modulate the host immune system development and function, and can enhance epithelial barrier function.[12]

Recently, research on disease perception and persistence of symptoms has focused on genetic alterations and early-life factors in the patient's home environment, including social learning and life experiences.[13] In addition, recent research has focused on the burden of suffering from FGIDs, providing emerging data on health care utilization, and quality of life.[14-16]

## APPROACH TO SPECIFIC FGIDS

The primary approach is to confirm a diagnosis of an FGID through an established set of symptom-based criteria. Similar to the *Diagnostic and Statistical Manual* (DSM) criteria in psychiatry, in which symptoms are described but no obvious biological markers exist, the Rome criteria, originally defined in 1999, are used for the FGIDs. The most recent Rome III criteria, established in 2006, were developed by extrapolating data from international research findings and then compiling those data into a coherent framework by committees of international experts in gastroenterology. There are more than 100 well-described FGIDs, and each FGID has specific criteria for diagnosis. For the purposes of this chapter, the description of those FGIDs that are most commonly seen in adolescents will be described. It is important to note, of course, that the underlying premise of diagnosing an FGID is that there should be no obvious evidence of an inflammatory, anatomic, metabolic, or neoplastic process that explains the adolescent's symptoms. A suggested set of laboratory investigations to aid in screening for conditions associated with inflammation, infection, and malabsorption are listed in Table 97-1. Note that one of the stool tests included in the table is for calprotectin, a protein released by neutrophils, one of the newer tests available to help distinguish between inflammatory and noninflammatory gastrointestinal disorders.

### FUNCTIONAL GASTRODUODENAL DISORDERS

A significant proportion of adolescents with FGIDs have chronic gastrointestinal symptoms that are centered around the gastroduodenal area. They include FD, belching and aerophagia, functional nausea and vomiting disorders, and rumination syndrome.

#### Functional Dyspepsia

Functional dyspepsia includes the presence of epigastric pain or burning, postprandial fullness, and early satiation.[17] Gastric hypersensitivity, delayed gastric emptying, and impaired accommodation of the proximal stomach have each been considered components of the etiology of FD. There are 2 major subtypes of FD depending on the predominant upper gastrointestinal symptom: (1) ulcer-like, in which epigastric pain is the presenting feature, and (2) dysmotility-like, which is more often associated with nausea and early satiety.

The Rome III diagnostic criteria for FD in adolescents stipulate that there is persistent or recurrent pain or discomfort centered in the upper abdomen above the umbilicus and that the pain is not relieved by defecation or associated with the onset of a change in stool frequency or form as seen with IBS.[4]

**Table 97-1**

**Suggested Laboratory and Stool Investigations to Evaluate for Inflammation, Infection, and Malabsorption**

| *Blood* | *Stool* |
|---|---|
| Complete blood count | pH |
| Comprehensive metabolic panel | Reducing substances |
| Erythrocyte sedimentation rate | Qualitative fat |
| C-reactive protein | Calprotectin |
| Amylase, lipase | Routine culture, ova, and parasites |
| Celiac serology (serum IgA, tissue transglutaminase) | *Giardia antigen, Clostridium difficile* |

Some patients may state that their symptoms began after a viral illness, often termed as postinfectious dyspepsia. It is unclear if any specific infection can be identified, but *Helicobacter pylori* infection may account for up to 5% of cases.[18,19] Several researchers have found that the pattern of symptoms of those with FD is similar in *H pylori*-positive and *H pylori* negative patients.[20,21] Therefore, patients should be aware that there is only a small chance that successful eradication of *H pylori* in those with FD will alleviate their symptoms.

In 2004, Holtmann and colleagues[22] reported an association between FD and homozygous *GNB3* 825C carrier status. The presence of this gene is also associated with depression, increased immune cell activation, and altered activation of 2 adrenoreceptors. Although this study needs to be replicated, it does illustrate a new direction in the research of the FGIDs and may explain the psychosocial comorbidities that often present with the upper FGIDs.[14,23,24]

When obtaining the history, it should be elicited whether the adolescent is experiencing early satiety, evening fullness, or vomiting of meals. An upper endoscopy is necessary if dysphagia is present or in those who have persistent symptoms despite the use of acid blocker medications or who have recurrent symptoms upon cessation of the medications.

### Aerophagia and Belching Disorders

Excessive air swallowing is usually unintentional and often associated with such conditions as anxiety or an asthma crisis in which there may be excessive use of inhaler medications. Because of concomitant abdominal distension, aerophagia is often confused with motility disorders such as chronic intestinal pseudo-obstruction or the malabsorption syndromes.

The Rome III diagnostic criteria for aerophagia stipulate that the adolescent must have at least 2 of the following: air swallowing, abdominal pain, abdominal distension because of intraluminal air, and repetitive belching or increased flatus.[4] The most important question to ask the adolescent is whether the abdominal distension decreases or resolves during sleep, which is indicative of aerophagia. A hydrogen breath test can be used to rule out carbohydrate malabsorption and/or bacterial overgrowth.[4]

This set of disorders occurs fairly commonly, can be a nuisance for adolescents and their families, and can be difficult to treat. Air swallowing during eating and drinking is a normal physiological event and so is belching of ingested air during transient relaxations of the lower esophageal sphincter. Belching should only be considered a disorder when it becomes troublesome. A detailed history and observation of air swallowing leads to the diagnosis; specific testing is usually not needed. The adolescent should be educated about avoiding gum chewing, talking during mealtimes, drinking carbonated beverages, and using a straw or pop-top bottles, all of which contribute to significant belching.

### Functional Vomiting Disorders

Vomiting is defined as the forceful oral expulsion of gastric or intestinal content associated with contraction of the abdominal and chest wall muscles. Vomiting needs to be differentiated from effortless regurgitation or rumination.

The differential diagnosis of recurrent nausea or vomiting is extensive and can include cannabinoid use, intestinal obstruction, gastroparesis, and intestinal pseudo-obstruction, as well as metabolic and central nervous system (CNS) disease. The physician must exclude gastroesophageal reflux, esophageal achalasia, gastroparesis, an eating disorder, and obstructive anatomical disorders. Psychological disturbances, including depression, anxiety, obsessive–compulsive behavior, and other disorders, are reported in up to one-third of affected individuals.[25]

It is reasonable that an initial approach may be that of referral for upper endoscopy to evaluate chronic symptoms of vomiting, especially if the vomiting is associated with dysphagia or blood in the vomitus.

### Cyclic Vomiting Syndrome

A diagnosis of cyclic vomiting syndrome (CVS) is made when the following are present: 2 or more periods of discrete, intense nausea and unremitting vomiting or retching lasting hours to days and a return to a usual state of health with complete wellness lasting weeks to months.[4]

Episodes of nausea or vomiting that occur several times a week or month are not typical of CVS. Its onset is acute and its duration is less than one week. Often what is required to distinguish chronic vomiting from CVS is a well-documented diary of symptoms over several months; the diary should include specific information such as time of day and potential triggering factors, such as foods, medications, or viral illnesses. A family history of migraine headaches is a supportive criterion for CVS, and migraine medications are often used for treatment of patients with CVS.[17]

In addition to performing a thorough history and physical examination, an upper gastrointestinal contrast series has been shown to be a cost-effective initial approach to rule out anatomical problems in patients in whom cyclic vomiting is suspected.[26] A suggested evaluation to rule out metabolic and structural abnormalities during an acute episode is provided in Table 97-2.

### Rumination Syndrome

Rumination syndrome is a condition characterized by repetitive, effortless regurgitation of recently ingested

**Table 97-2**

**Suggested Evaluation for Cyclic Vomiting Syndrome at the Time of an Acute Episode Prior to Intravenous Hydration with Dextrose**

| | |
|---|---|
| BLOOD | Complete blood count |
| | Sedimentation rate |
| | C-reactive protein |
| | Comprehensive metabolic panel (to include Na, K, Cl, $CO_2$, glucose, BUN, creatinine, ALT, AST) |
| | GGTP |
| | Amylase, lipase |
| | Carnitine |
| | Amino acids |
| | Cortisol |
| | Catecholamines |
| | Lactic acid, ammonia |
| | ACTH, ADH (vasopressin) |
| | Prostaglandin E2 |
| URINE | Urinalysis |
| | d-ALA (aminolevulinic acid) |
| | Carnitine |
| | Organic acids |
| | Porphobilinogen |
| RADIOLOGIC | Abdominal ultrasound (r/o acute hydronephrosis and uretero-pelvic obstruction) |

BUN, blood urea nitrogen; ACTH, adrenocorticotropic hormone; ADH, antidiuretic hormone; ALT, alanine transaminase; AST, aspartate aminotransferase; GGTP, gamma-glutamyl transpeptidase

food into the mouth followed by rechewing and reswallowing or expulsion.[17] Approximately 33% of affected adolescents present with nausea and vomiting, a high percentage of patients are female, and there is no relationship with cognitive abilities.[25] Significant weight loss is not a prominent feature and, when present, should prompt evaluation for underlying causes such as gastroparesis or an eating disorder. The cause of rumination is unknown but it is typically unrelated to infection or any known organic entity.

Typical of rumination is the repetitive regurgitation of gastric contents beginning within minutes of the start of a meal. This is the opposite of what occurs in those with gastroparesis, who experience vomiting in the later postprandial period. Rumination episodes generally last 1 to 2 hours, there is usually a lack of retching or nausea prior to the episode, and the regurgitant consists of partially recognizable food that has a pleasant taste according to the patient. The regurgitation is effortless or is preceded by a sensation of belching immediately before the arrival of regurgitant in the pharynx. The regurgitation may be preceded by a brisk voluntary contraction of the abdominis rectus muscle and the patient makes a conscious decision regarding what to do with the regurgitant once it is present in the oropharynx. The choice may depend on the social situation at the time. Characteristically, the patient with rumination may have up to hundreds of episodes per day without any associated epigastric or periumbilical pain.

The physician will find while obtaining the history that the symptoms rarely occur during sleep because the behavior is considered an unintentional abnormal response to drinking or eating. It most likely indicates a combination of gastric disorders including delayed gastric emptying, visceral hyperalgesia, and impaired relaxation of the proximal stomach.[27]

Treatment for rumination consists of behavioral modification, which uses habit-reversal techniques that eliminate the target behavior of rumination by the consistent use of incompatible or competing behaviors.[28] The rumination behavior is eliminated because rumination and the competing response cannot be performed at the same time. Medications and surgery, such as fundoplication, have not been useful and are not indicated as treatment. Most adolescents with rumination will have a positive outcome with behavioral treatment.[25]

### FUNCTIONAL BOWEL DISORDERS

Functional bowel disorders are FGIDs with symptoms attributable to the middle or lower gastrointestinal tract and include IBS, functional bloating, and functional constipation.

It is helpful for the adolescent suspected of having a functional bowel disorder to keep a detailed diet, symptom, and stool history for several days; this could give insight into those foods, such as lactose or "sugar-free" products (containing fructose, sorbitol, or mannitol) that may suggest a malabsorption of carbohydrates. In addition, a stool diary incorporating the Bristol Stool Form Scale (Table 97-3) is a useful method to verify stool form. The physical examination should evaluate for signs of anemia or malnutrition. An abdominal mass, particularly in the right lower quadrant of the abdomen, may suggest inflammatory bowel disease, such as Crohn's disease, and warrants further evaluation. A suggested set of laboratory investigations to aid in screening for conditions associated with inflammation and malabsorption are listed in Table 97-2. A lactose hydrogen breath test will evaluate for lactase deficiency as a cause for symptoms. Stool testing for parasites (*Giardia, Cyclospora,*

**Table 97-3**

**The Bristol Stool Form Scale**

| *Type* | *Description* |
|---|---|
| 1 | Separate hard lumps like nuts (difficult to pass) |
| 2 | Sausage shaped but lumpy |
| 3 | Like a sausage but with cracks on its surface |
| 4 | Like a sausage or snake, smooth and soft |
| 5 | Soft blobs with clear-cut edges (passed easily) |
| 6 | Fluffy pieces with ragged edges, a mushy stool |
| 7 | Watery, no solid pieces, entirely liquid |

*Isospora)* and infections (*Clostridium difficile, Salmonella, Shigella, Campylobacter jejuni)* should also be included in the work-up. Diarrhea with weight loss, blood in the stools, or suspected nutritional deficiency should prompt investigation for intestinal disease to rule out infection or mucosal pathology.

The criteria for the diagnoses described in the following are based on a certain set of well-described symptoms, as well as a detailed history, a physical examination, and limited diagnostic tests to confirm diagnoses with a high level of confidence.[29]

### Irritable Bowel Syndrome

Abdominal pain or discomfort is the predominant feature of IBS. The differentiating factor for patients with IBS compared with those with other FGIDs is that the abdominal pain in those with IBS can be often be relieved with defecation. The estimated prevalence of IBS in adolescents is approximately 15% to 20%, which indicates it is a common FGID. There is a significant female predominance in those patients who present with this condition.[4]

Visceral hypersensitivity and altered gut motility are the most common abnormalities noted in patients with IBS, whereas inflammation, disturbed CNS modulation, and psychosocial factors are implicated in its pathogenesis.[31] A study by Kellow et al[31] demonstrated that physiologic stress might be triggering motor abnormalities in patients with IBS. In their study, patients with IBS and healthy volunteers were exposed to a variety of visual and audiologic stressors; autonomic arousal in response to the stressors was measured and was compared to baseline motor characteristics for both groups. Results showed that the patients with IBS responded to the physiologic stressors with an exaggerated increase in motility. This and other studies suggest that rather than having baseline dysmotility, patients with functional bowel disorders may display an abnormal motor response to a variety of physiologic stimuli, including meals, cholecystokinin, stress, and abdominal distension.

Gastrointestinal infections may act as a triggering factor in a subgroup of patients. Physiological abnormalities of the gut in patients with postinfectious IBS include alterations in rectal sensorimotor activity, colonic transit time, and small bowel permeability.[32,33]

The Rome III criteria for IBS are defined as abdominal discomfort or pain associated with 2 or more of the following at least 25% of the time: improvement with defecation, onset associated with a change in frequency of stools, and/or onset associated with a change in form of stools.[4] Symptoms that support the IBS diagnosis include: (a) abnormal stool frequency (≥4 stools per day or ≤2 stools per week), (b) abnormal stool form (lumpy/hard or loose/watery stool), (c) abnormal passage of stool (straining, urgency, or feeling of incomplete evacuation), (d) passage of mucus, and (e) bloating or feeling of abdominal distension.[4]

Adolescents may present with constipation (IBS-C), diarrhea (IBS-D), or a mix of the two (IBS-M). Up to 75% of patients may notice a change in the subtype over time. Each subtype likely has a different pathophysiology whereby stool consistency, which can be estimated using the Bristol Stool Scale (Table 97-3), has been speculated to correlate with colonic transit time. To date, there have been no studies explaining the variations in IBS that take place in the same patient over time. There seem to be temporal fluctuations in most patients, as "flare-ups" alternate with periods of relative well-being over weeks, months, and even years.

It is important to classify whether the patient has IBS-C, IBS-D, or IBS-M because that may direct management. The diagnosis of IBS-C requires that there be >25% hard or lumpy stools and <25% loose or watery stools. There may be an overlap between IBS-C and functional constipation in terms of symptoms. The diagnosis of IBS-D requires >25% loose or watery stools and <25% hard or lumpy stools. IBS-M is defined as >25% loose or watery stools and >25% hard or lumpy stools.

### Functional Bloating

Functional bloating is a recurrent sensation of abdominal distension that may or may not be associated with measurable distension.[29] Most of the research on bloating has dealt with subjects who also have other FGIDs, because they often overlap. For example, up to 96% of patients with IBS report functional bloating. It is about twice as common in women[34] and is often associated with menses.[35] It can be distinguished from other causes of bloating by its diurnal pattern of worsening after meals and throughout the day, and improving or disappearing overnight. Epidemiologic surveys and factor analyses do not convincingly demonstrate a distinct bloating group, and physiologic studies of bloating have mainly been done on patients with IBS.[34]

Rome III diagnostic criteria include a recurrent feeling of bloating or visible distension at least 3 days/month in 3 months and insufficient criteria for a diagnosis of FD, IBS, or an other FGID. It is not related to food intolerance, abnormal gut bacterial flora, weak abdominal musculature, or abnormal retention of fluid inside and outside the gut. Studies have documented both increased intestinal gas accumulation and abnormal gas transit.

### Functional Constipation

Functional constipation presents as persistently difficult, infrequent, or seemingly incomplete defecation. Patients with functional constipation do not meet Rome III IBS criteria. The prevalence of childhood and adolescent constipation in the general population ranges widely, depending on the study, from 0.7% to 29.6%.[36] A recent long-term study suggests that childhood constipation can persist into young adulthood in about 30% of cases.[37] Abnormal defecation dynamics or pelvic dyssynergia has been reported in 63% of adolescents with chronic constipation. Progressive fecal accumulation in the rectum eventually may lead to pelvic floor muscle fatigue and theoretically to poor competence of the anal sphincter, which in turn can lead to fecal incontinence.

Slow transit constipation (STC), or "colonic inertia," is thought to have as its primary defect a slower than normal movement of contents from the proximal to the distal colon. There may be an overall paucity of motor activity in the colon, causing prolonged fecal stasis. Another cause of STC may be the presence of uncoordinated motor activity in the distal colon that offers resistance to normal transit.The 2 symptoms most suggestive of STC are reduced frequency of bowel movements and the lack of the urge to defecate.[38] A decreased urge to defecate may be the result of hyposensitivity of the rectum or acquired megarectum secondary to recurrent stool-withholding behaviors. In the presence of a much dilated rectum, there may be the need for extreme distension to provide a stimulus sufficient to trigger the urge to defecate.

Pelvic floor dysfunction (PFD) is the pathophysiologic entity considered responsible for most cases of constipation in adolescents.[39] Patients with PFD display normal or slightly delayed colonic transit overall, with a preferential storage of fecal residue for prolonged periods in the rectum. In this condition, the primary failure is an inability to adequately evacuate contents from the rectum and the characteristic symptom is a sensation of incomplete defecation. Despite the passage of stools, there often is significant straining. Paradoxical anal sphincter contraction is thought to be an essential component in the pathophysiology of this disorder. It is speculated that patients who fail to coordinate the increased intra-abdominal pressure with the relaxation of the pelvic floor will develop PFD.

The clinician should always clarify the patient's definition of constipation because there is often a lack of clarity among patients, parents, and clinicians about its nature. A detailed history should be taken; this should include questions about the time after birth of the first bowel movement, the time of onset of the problem, characteristics of stools (frequency, consistency, caliber, and volume), the presence of associated symptoms (pain at defecation, abdominal pain, blood on the stools or toilet paper, and fecal incontinence), stool-withholding behaviors, urinary problems, and neurologic deficits. A physical examination should be performed to detect any abnormalities in the perianal and anal region, such as fecal impaction, an anal stricture, rectal prolapse, a mass, or abnormal perineal descent with straining. Laboratory tests are rarely helpful; however, an abdominal x-ray can be useful in determining the presence of fecal retention in an obese adolescent or one who refuses the rectal examination.

## PSYCHOSOCIAL FEATURES OF FGIDS

Over the past 2 decades, it has been proposed that a disturbance of gastrointestinal motility in a predisposed individual with a variety of stressors, either physical or psychosocial, may contribute to persistence of symptoms in patients with FGIDs. Increasing emphasis is now being placed on the interaction among motility, sensory, and psychosocial factors as elements contributing to a variety of functional disorders in children. Psychosocial factors can enhance the patient's perception of distension of the bowel lumen and/or transient disturbances in motility through alterations in local reflex activity or via altered neural processing along the brain–gut axis.[31]

Pace et al[40] studied a group of 52 children and early adolescents with recurrent abdominal pain (RAP) of childhood or IBS and followed them for 5 to 13 years after initial diagnosis. They found that RAP in childhood can predict the later development of IBS in adulthood. They report a significant influence of an intrafamilial aggregation of symptoms, possibly through the learning of a specific illness behavior. In their study, almost one-third of subjects had IBS-like symptoms 5 to 13 years after diagnosis and they were almost 3 times more likely to have at least 1 sibling with similar symptoms compared with subjects who had no gastrointestinal complaints (40% vs 16%; $P < 0.05$). They also found a higher prevalence of extraintestinal symptoms, such as back pain, fibromyalgia, headache, fatigue, and sleep disturbances.

Although psychological and psychosocial factors can undoubtedly contribute to the clinical course of FGIDs, a causative role has not been established. German investigators[41] reviewed observational studies and found an association with anxiety and depression. For FD and IBS, it seems that severe and chronic life stress (arising from relationship difficulties, divorce, housing difficulties, etc), together with the prolonged and effortful coping required in dealing with the stress, has a significant and consistent effect on both symptom onset and exacerbations over time. In this context, it is relevant that psychological stress and other cognitive aspects have also been found to be related to sensorimotor dysfunction in FGID patients, as previously noted by Kellow et al.[31]

## TREATMENT APPROACH TO THE FGIDS

A successful approach to the treatment of FGIDs is based on an understanding of the pathophysiological mechanisms that have been proposed as the underlying causes. In patients with FGIDs, recurring symptoms of abdominal pain or discomfort are due to a combination of visceral hyperalgesia, disordered sensorimotor function of the intestinal tract, and disease perception. At the foundation of a successful approach is a strategy focused on education and an explanation of the symptoms using the Rome III criteria described in this and the previous chapter. These criteria afford the ability to offer a diagnosis of certainty rather than a diagnosis of exclusion. Confirmation of a specific diagnosis is what most patients and families are seeking when they consult multiple physicians for persistent symptoms. A successful strategy will also couple education with an effective clinician-patient-family relationship in which allocation of sufficient consultative time and availability of follow-up is encouraged. It is during this critical time of making a positive diagnosis and providing education and explanations that patient and family expectations can be set. A therapeutic plan is then installed with a focus on managing symptoms rather than curing disease.

Once these essential steps are in place, a series of goals are established to return the adolescent to a status whereby participation in expected activities can resume with minimal interruption from gastrointestinal discomfort. Despite the high prevalence of these disorders among adolescents in the community, there are few pharmacological strategies that have been evaluated with sound scientific methodology. In 1988, Klein et al[42] published a critical overview of these trials showing that most studies were flawed and that none of the drugs evaluated could reliably be regarded as an effective treatment. In addition, 2 recently approved medications for IBS, Alosetron and Tegaserod, which directly targeted serotonin receptors in the gastrointestinal tract and addressed many of the sensorimotor parameters of FGIDs, have recently been removed from the market by the US Food and Drug Administration. This was due to significant concerns about side effects, specifically reports of ischemic colitis and cardiovascular events found in postmarket analyses of patients on these selected serotonin medications. With significant limitations in available medications, other approaches need to be investigated.

Currently, therapy for the FGIDs can be divided into 2 main categories: those directed at treating the predominant symptoms (or "end organ therapy") and those that are aimed at cognitive retraining with a focus on providing patients adequate tools for modifying disease perceptions. Often an approach using both strategies is needed to reach a successful outcome in moderate to severe cases of FGID. Patients with mild symptoms may need only education and possibly diet modification if an offending food trigger can be found.

Patients with moderate symptoms may begin to experience daily impairment of function secondary to visceral hyperalgesia even while adequate nutrition is still being maintained. An example may be an infectious insult that has cleared weeks prior but there has been a resetting of the ENS with upregulation of pain receptors and now with pain being felt due to intraluminal contents such as those from food, gas, or feces. Pain intensity and persistence of symptoms may be exacerbated if underlying psychosocial issues exist. There have been some studies that have shown that patients with FGID and their family members may have associations with worry, anxiety, depression, and impaired coping mechanisms.[43,44]

### BEHAVIORAL MODIFICATION

Techniques to reduce physiologic arousal associated with chronic abdominal pain may alleviate symptoms in patients with FGIDs. There have been well-documented and designed studies, both in adults and adolescents, that have demonstrated positive effects using several techniques such as cognitive behavioral therapy (CBT), guided imagery, hypnosis, and yoga.

Cognitive behavioral therapy teaches the patient coping skills, including refraining from or modifying maladaptive thoughts such as helplessness. Studies have demonstrated effectiveness when administered to the patient and when utilized as a family intervention.[45,46] In addition, when CBT is used in combination with standard care, it appears to be more beneficial.[47] Up to 85% of ruminators will improve with behavioral therapy, and a multidisciplinary approach is associated with satisfactory recovery in most patients.[25]

Guided imagery is a form of relaxed, focused concentration similar to hypnosis. Guided imagery produces distraction from gut pain and enhances relaxation. One study showed that guided imagery was very effective in patients with treatment-refractory abdominal pain, with improvement lasting up to one year and a significant increase in quality of life.[48] In another randomized trial, Weydert et al[49] employed guided imagery effectively as first-line therapy in addition to deep breathing for symptom relief of abdominal pain in children.

Another successful mind–body technique used successfully in adolescents with IBS is yoga. In a study from Vancouver, Canada, 25 patients were randomized to yoga or to a wait-list control. There was a significant reduction in pain intensity and frequency, as well as perceived disability from pain, over a 3-month period in those who received training in yoga.[50]

### DIET

The role of diet continues to be controversial and will vary in response to the adolescent's particular FGID. Avoidance of nonsteroidal anti-inflammatory drugs and foods that aggravate symptoms (caffeine, spicy foods, fatty foods) is recommended in FD.[51] An increase in fiber could be offered as a first-line treatment method for IBS-C because it may improve bowel function by easing passage of stool.[52]

The use of peppermint oil in treating IBS has been studied with variable results. Recently, in a 4-week prospective double-blind randomized clinical trial, peppermint oil was found to significantly reduce abdominal pain complaints.[53] This beneficial effect may be due to prevention of calcium entry into intestinal smooth muscle cells leading to relaxation of the intestinal smooth muscle.

### ROLE OF PROBIOTICS

Increasing emphasis is now being placed on the interaction among motility, sensory responses, inflammation, and host gut flora in patients with IBS.[12] Recently, several studies have shown beneficial effects of utilizing lactobacillus in treatment of FGIDs in the adolescent age population.[54,55] In particular, use of probiotics appears to have a significant effect on the symptom of bloating, which is often one of the most difficult to treat.[55]

## REFERENCES


1. Hyams JS, Burke G, Davis PM, Rzepski B, Andrulonis PA. Abdominal pain and irritable bowel syndrome in adolescents: a community-based study. *J Pediatr.* 1996;129:220–226

2. De Giacomo C, Valdambrini V, Lizzoli F, et al. A population-based survey on gastrointestinal tract symptoms and *Helicobacter pylori* infection in children and adolescents. *Helicobacter.* 2002;7:356–363

3. Chitkara DK, Talley NJ, Weaver AL, et al. Incidence of presentation of common functional gastrointestinal disorders in children: a cohort study. *Clin Gastroenterol Hepatol.* 2007;5:186–191

4. Rasquin A, Di Lorenzo C, Forbes D, et al. Childhood functional gastrointestinal disorders: child/adolescent. *Gastroenterology.* 2006;130:1527–1537

5. Anand KJ, Coskun V, Thrivikraman KV. Long-term behavioral effects of repetitive pain in neonatal rat pups. *Physiol Behav.* 1999;66:627–637

6. Mayer EA, Naliboff BD, Craig AD. Neuroimaging of the brain-gut axis: from basic understanding to treatment of functional GI disorders. *Gastroenterology.* 2006;131:1925–1942

7. Kellow JE, Azpiroz F, Delvaux M, et al. Applied principles of neurogastroenterology: physiology/motility sensation. *Gastroenterology.* 2006:1412–1420

8. Van Ginkel R, Voskuijl WP, Benninga MA, Taminiau JA, Boeckxstaens GE. Alterations in rectal sensitivity and motility in childhood irritable bowel syndrome. *Gastroenterology.* 2001;120:31–38

9. Di Lorenzo C, Youssef NN. Visceral hyperalgesia in children with functional abdominal pain. *J Pediatr.* 2001;139(6):838–843

10. Chitkara DK, Camilleri M, Zinsmeister AR, et al. Gastric sensory and motor dysfunction in adolescents with functional dyspepsia. *J Pediatr.* 2005;146(4):500–505

11. Parry SD, Stansfield R, Jelley D, et al. Does bacterial gastroenteritis predispose people to functional gastrointestinal disorders? A prospective community-based, case control study. *Am J Gastroenterol.* 2003;98:1970–1975

12. O'Mahony L, McCarthy J, Kelly P, et al. Lactobacillus and Bifidobacterium in irritable bowel syndrome: symptom responses and relationship to cytokine profiles. *Gastroenterology.* 2005;128(3):541–551

13. Campo JV, Bridge J, Lucas A, et al. Physical and emotional health of mothers of youth with functional abdominal pain. *Arch Pediatr Adolesc Med.* 2007;161:131–137

14. Levy RL, Whitehead WE, Walker LS, et al. Increased somatic complaints and health-care utilization in children: effects of parent IBS status and parent response to gastrointestinal symptoms. *Am J Gastroenterol.* 2004;99:2442–2451

15. Youssef NN, Murphy TG, Langseder AL, Rosh JR. Quality of life for children with functional abdominal pain: a comparison study of patients' and parents' perceptions. *Pediatrics.* 2006;117:54–59

16. Varni JW, Lane MM, Burwinkle TM, et al. Health-related quality of life in pediatric patients with irritable bowel syndrome: a comparative analysis. *Dev Behav Pediatr.* 2006;27:451–458

17. Tack J, Talley NJ, Camilleri M, et al. Functional gastroduodenal disorders. *Gastroenterology.* 2006;130:1466–1479

18. Talley NJ, Vakil N. Practice parameters committee of the American College of Gastroenterology. Guidelines for the management of dyspepsia. *Am J Gastroenterol.* 2005;100: 2324–2337

19. Talley NJ, Silverstein MD, Agreus L, Nyren O, Sonnenberg A, Holtmann G. AGA technical review on the evaluation of dyspepsia. *Gastroenterology.* 2005;129:1756–1780

20. Sarnelli G, Cuomo R, Janssens J. Symptom patterns and pathophysiological mechanisms in dyspeptic patients with and without *Helicobacter pylori*. *Dig Dis Sci.* 2003;48(12): 2229–2236

21. Moayyedi P, Deeks J, Talley NJ, Dalaney B, Forman D. An update of the Cochrane systematic review of Helicobacter pylori eradication therapy in non-ulcer dyspepsia: resolving the discrepancy between systematic reviews. *Am J Gastroenterol.* 2003;98(12):2621–2626

22. Holtmann G, Siffert W, Haag S, et al. G-Protein β3 825CC genotype is associated with unexplained (functional) dyspepsia. *Gastroenterology.* 2004;126:971–979

23. Claar RL, Walker LS. Functional assessment of pediatric pain patients: psychometric properties of the functional disability inventory. *Pain.* 2006;121:77–84

24. Walker LS, Jones DS. Psychosocial factors: impact on symptom severity and outcomes of pediatric functional gastrointestinal disorders. *J Pediatr Gastroenterol Nutr.* 2005;41: S51–S52

25. Chial HJ, Camilleri M, Williams DE, Litzinger K, Perrault J. Rumination syndrome in children and adolescents: diagnosis, treatment, and prognosis. *Pediatrics.* 2003;111:158–162

26. Olson AD, Li B. The diagnostic evaluation of children with cyclic vomiting: a cost-effectiveness assessment. *J Pediatr.* 2002;141:724–728

27. Bredenoord AJ, Chial HJ, Camilleri M, Mullan BP, Murray JA. Gastric accommodation and emptying in evaluation of patients with upper gastrointestinal symptoms. *Clin Gastroenterol Hepatol.* 2003;1:264–272

28. Chitkara DK, van Tilburg M, Whitehead WE, Talley NJ. Teaching diaphragmatic breathing for rumination syndrome. *Am J Gastroenterol.* 2006;101:2449–2452

29. Longstreth GF, Thompson WG, Chey WD, Houghton LA, Mearin F, et al. Functional bowel disorders. *Gastroenterology.* 2006;130:1480–1491

30. Drossman DA, Camilleri M, Mayer EA, Whitehead WE. AGA technical review on irritable bowel syndrome. *Gastroenterology.* 2002;123:2108–2131

31. Kellow JE, Aspiroz F, Delvaux M, et al. Applied principles of neurogastroenterology: physiology/motility sensation. *Gastroenterology.* 2006;130:1412–1420

32. Gwee K-A, Leong Y-L, Graham C, et al. The role of psychological and biological factors in post-infective gut dysfunction. *Gut.* 1999;44:400–406

33. Spiller RC, Jenkins D, Thornley JP, et al. Increased rectal mucosal enteroendocrine cells, T lymphocytes, and increased gut permeability following acute Campylobacter enteritis and in post-dysenteric irritable bowel syndrome. *Gut.* 2000;47:804–811

34. Thompson WG, Irvine EJ, Pare P, Ferrazzi S, Rance L. Functional gastrointestinal disorders in Canada: first population-based survey using the Rome II criteria with suggestions for improving the questionnaire. *Digestive Dis Sci.* 2002;47:225–235

35. Chang L, Lee OY, Naliboff B, Schmulson M, Mayer EA. Sensation of bloating and visible abdominal distenstion in patients with irritable bowel syndrome. *Am J Gastroenterol.* 2001;96:3341–3347

36. van den Berg MM, Benninga MA, Di Lorenzo C. Epidemiology of childhood constipation: a systematic review. *Am J Gastroenterol.* 2006;101:2401–2409

37. Van Ginkel R, Reitsma JB, Buller HA, Van Wijk MP, Taminiau JA, Benninga MC. Childhood constipation: longitudinal follow-up beyond puberty. *Gastroenterology.* 2003;125:357–363

38. Youssef NN, Sanders L, Di Lorenzo C. Adolescent constipation: evaluation and management. *Adolesc Med Clin.* 2004;15:37–52

39. Chitkara DK, Bredenoord AJ, Cremonini F, et al. The role of pelvic floor dysfunction and slow colonic transit in adolescents with refractory constipation. *Am J Gastroenterol.* 2004;99:1579–1584

40. Pace F, Zuin G, DiGiacomo S, et al. Family history of irritable bowel syndrome is the major determinant of persistent abdominal complaints in young adults with a history of pediatric recurrent abdominal pain. *World J Gastroenterol.* 2006;12:3874–3877

41. Kleibeuker JH, Thijs JC. Functional dyspepsia. *Curr Opin Gastroenterol.* 2004;20:546–550

42. Klein KB. Controlled treatment trials in the irritable bowel syndrome: a critique. *Gastroenterology.* 1988;95:232–241

43. Levy RL, Langer SL, Walker LS, Feld LD, Whitehead WE. Relationship between the decision to take a child to the clinic for abdominal pain and maternal psychological distress. *Arch Pediatr Adolesc Med.* 2006;160:961–965

44. Campo JV, Bridge J, Lucas A, et al. Physical and emotional health of mothers of youth with functional abdominal pain. *Arch Pediatr Adolesc Med.* 2007;161:131–137

45. Humphreys PA, Gevirtz RN. Treatment of recurrent abdominal pain: components analysis of four treatment protocols. *J Pediatr Gastroenterol Nutr.* 2000;31:47–51

46. Robins PM, Smith SM, Glutting JJ, Bishop CT. A randomized controlled trial of a cognitive-behavioral family intervention for pediatric recurrent abdominal pain. *J Pediatr Psychol.* 2005;30:397–408

47. Heymann-Monnikes I, Arnold R, Florin I, et al. The combination of medical treatment plus multi-component behavioral therapy is superior to medical treatment alone in the therapy of irritable bowel syndrome. *Am J Gastroenterol.* 2000;95:981–994

48. Youssef NN, Rosh JR, Loughran M, et al. Treatment of functional abdominal pain in childhood with cognitive behavioral strategies. *J Pediatr Gastroenterol Nutr.* 2004;39: 192–196

49. Weydert JA, Shapiro DE, Acra SA, Monheim CJ, Chambers AS, Ball TM. Evaluation of guided imagery as treatment for recurrent abdominal pain in children: a randomized control trial. *BMC Pediatr.* 2006;6:29

50. Kuttner L, Chambers CT, Hardial J, Israel DM, Jacobson K, Evans K. A randomized trial of yoga for adolescents with irritable bowel syndrome. *Pain Res Manage.* 2006;11:217–223

51. Talley NJ. How to manage the difficult-to-treat dyspeptic patient. *Nat Clin Pract Gastroenterol Hepatol.* 2007;4: 35–42

52. Zuckerman MJ. The role of fiber in the treatment of irritable bowel syndrome: therapeutic recommendations. *J Clin Gastroenterol.* 2006;40:104–108

53. Cappello G, Spezzaferro M, Grossi L, Manzoli L, Marzio L. Peppermint oil in the treatment of irritable bowel syndrome: a prospective double-blind placebo-controlled randomized trial. *Dig Liver Dis.* 2007;39:530–536

54. Bausserman M, Michail S. The use of Lactobacillus GG in irritable bowel syndrome in children: a double-blind randomized control trial. *J Pediatr.* 2005;147:197–201

55. Gawronska A, Dziechciarz P, Horvath A, Szajewska H. A randomized double-blind placebo-controlled trial of Lactobacillus GG for abdominal pain disorders in children. *Aliment Pharmacol Ther.* 2007;25:177–184

# CHAPTER 98

# Disorders of the Esophagus

CINDY A. HALLER, MD • JAMES F. MARKOWITZ, MD

Disorders of esophageal structure and function are common in the adolescent. Although primary esophageal diseases are most common, the esophagus is also frequently the site of pathology as a consequence of systemic illness. Classically, adolescents complain of symptoms similar to those expressed by adults: dysphagia (difficulty in swallowing), odynophagia (pain on swallowing), heartburn, eructation (belching), water brash (regurgitation into the mouth), and vomiting. However, less typical complaints also appear to arise from esophageal dysfunction in the adolescent. Therefore, esophageal dysfunction should be considered in any patient who complains of nausea, especially if it is sensed in the throat rather than the abdomen, or of an ill-defined "empty" or "gnawing" sensation in the subxiphoid or upper epigastric area.

The prevalence of esophageal dysfunction during adolescence has not been determined. A sampling of any busy medical practice that involves caring for adolescents, however, will reveal that complaints suggestive of esophageal disease are frequent. Most patients with these complaints are found to have symptoms arising from gastroesophageal reflux (GER). The remainder are ultimately shown to have a variety of other gastrointestinal or biliary tract disorders. Although the other disorders of esophageal function discussed in this chapter are much less common than GER, they occur often enough to be important considerations for those who provide care for adolescent patients.

## DISORDERS OF STRUCTURE AND FUNCTION

### ANATOMIC ABNORMALITIES

Congenital esophageal lesions rarely evade detection during childhood. Occasionally, however, a congenital lesion such as esophageal stenosis from submucosal thickening of the proximal esophagus can remain undiagnosed until adolescence. Although these congenital lesions cause dysphagia from early in life, patients can compensate for their symptoms and escape diagnosis until the second or third decade of life. Other congenital lesions are recognized and treated in infancy, but the consequences of lesions such as tracheoesophageal fistula or esophageal atresia often result in ongoing problems during adolescence. Persistent dysmotility and anastomotic narrowing associated with the repair of these lesions can often lead to dysphagia or food impaction. Acquired membranous webs of the proximal esophagus associated with epidermolysis bullosa or iron deficiency anemia, and obstructing (Schatzki) rings of the distal esophagus, occasionally occur in adolescence. A traction diverticulum due to a foregut cyst also has been described in an adolescent. These esophageal lesions can cause intermittent dysphagia, food or foreign body impaction, and pain. Treatment includes dilatation, endoscopic disruption, and surgery.

### PRIMARY DYSMOTILITY

Abnormalities of esophageal motility in an otherwise healthy adolescent are unusual. However, certain disorders should be considered in an adolescent who has dysphagia or unexplained chest pain.[1]

#### Achalasia

Achalasia is characterized by incomplete relaxation of the lower esophageal sphincter (LES) after swallowing.[2,3] Frequently, LES pressure is also markedly elevated, and there is an associated absence of coordinated peristalsis in the body of the esophagus. In affected adults, 5% date the onset of their symptoms to before the age of 15 years. The cause of this condition remains unknown, although in children and adolescents achalasia has been associated with chronic intestinal pseudo-obstruction, chronic granulomatous disease, and Chagas disease. A heightened response to cholinergic agonists such as methacholine suggests denervation hypersensitivity. It is not surprising, therefore, that histopathologic studies often have demonstrated abnormalities of the enteric neurons within the esophagus. Multiple studies demonstrate loss of nonadrenergic, noncholinergic neurons that appear responsible for secreting vasoactive intestinal peptide (VIP) and nitrous oxide, 2 known mediators of smooth muscle relaxation.[4,5] Therefore, achalasia appears to be the clinical expression of unopposed contractile stimuli to the smooth muscle of the esophagus. Histologic analysis of surgical resection specimens from patients with end-stage achalasia demonstrates myenteric inflammation and progressive depletion of ganglion cells with neural fibrosis.[6] Patients with achalasia complain of intermittent but progressive, painless dysphagia. As the disease advances, the ingestion of liquids and solids is affected, and esophageal retention of ingested food occurs. Undigested food is frequently regurgitated, leading to weight loss or an aversion to eating. Chronic pulmonary aspirations result in recurrent pneumonia, chronic cough, or asthma.

The diagnosis of achalasia is suggested radiographically by an aperistaltic esophagus on barium swallow that is associated with a dilated esophageal body tapering to a narrowed distal esophagus, resulting in the typical "bird's-beak" appearance (Figure 98-1A). Retained food is also commonly identified within the esophageal lumen. Despite the apparent radiographic narrowing of the LES, the endoscope will easily pass into the stomach without resistance. Esophageal manometry (Figure 98-1B) reveals characteristic lack of LES relaxation and nonpropagated pressure waves in the distal two-thirds (smooth muscle portion) of the esophageal body. The upper esophageal sphincter (UES) and the upper third (striated muscle) of the esophageal body are usually normal. Although provocative testing with a cholinergic agonist reveals a characteristic spasm of the distal esophagus and LES, the test is painful and rarely indicated.

The optimal treatment for achalasia remains controversial. Initial treatment often consists of forceful pneumatic dilatation, which may relieve symptoms for a year or more in 60% to 80% of adolescents. Some have suggested pneumatic dilatation be used on an "on-demand" basis based on symptom recurrence. Unfortunately, about one-third of patients will develop GER, often with consequent esophagitis, within 4 years of symptomatic remission induced by pneumatic dilatation, often limiting its long-term utility.[7] Although data in adolescents are lacking, many centers prefer laparoscopic esophagomyotomy in adults as initial therapy. Although both approaches are generally effective in relieving symptoms, either can be associated with significant short- and long-term morbidity.[8] In particular, severe GER and its complications can occur after disruption of the LES barrier. Although studies in adults reveal a much lower risk of GER when the esophagomyotomy does not extend more than 5 mm into the cardia of the stomach,[9] long-term studies evaluating these patients more than 10 years after surgery reveal a progressive clinical deterioration mainly due to an increase in acid reflux disease

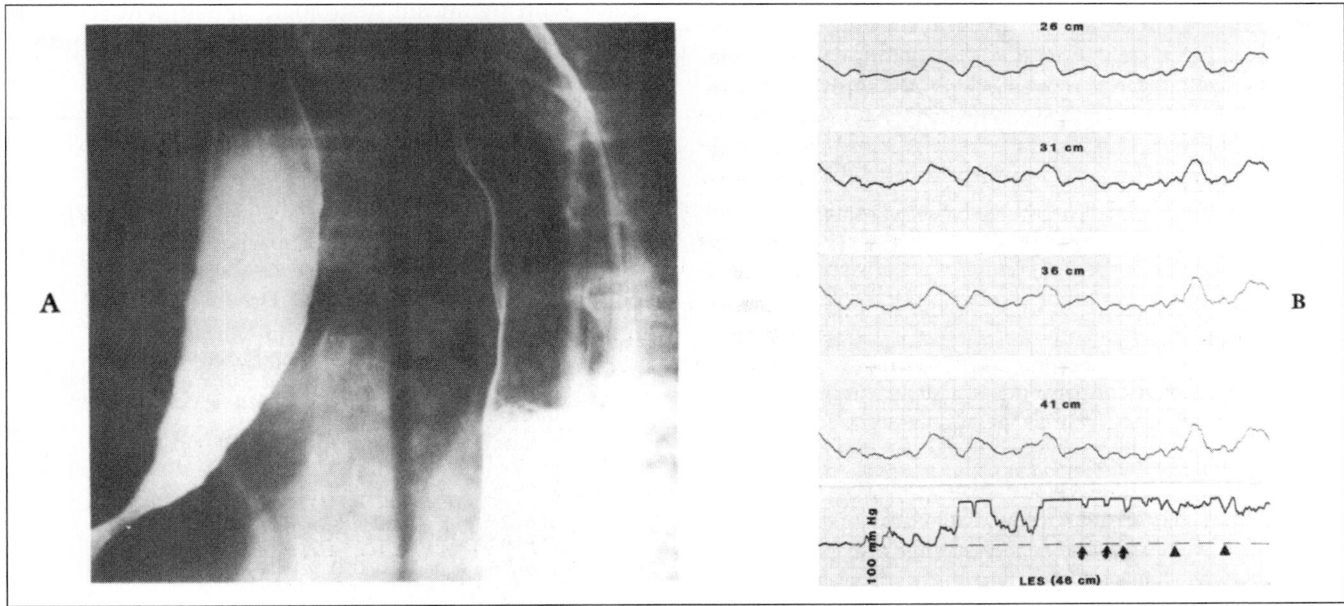


**FIGURE 98-1** (A) Barium esophagram obtained from a 16-year-old male with achalasia. Note the diffuse dilatation of the body of the esophagus with air. The barium level is depicted in the right panel. The left panel demonstrates the typical "bird's-beak" appearance of the distal esophagus. (B) Esophageal manometry in the same patient. The most distal pressure port is located in the lower esophageal sphincter (LES), 46 cm from the nares. Another four ports are located in the distal and middle esophagus at intervals of 5 cm. Total LES pressure is more than 50 mm Hg (normal = 10 to 20 mm Hg), as evidenced by the cutoff in the recorded signal in the lowermost panel (gastric baseline pressure is indicated by the dashed line). Multiple dry swallows (curved arrows) and "wet" swallows of 10 ml of water (arrowheads) do not result in relaxation of the LES to baseline gastric pressure. In the middle and distal esophagus, swallowing results in simultaneous rather than peristaltic contractions.

and the development of Barrett esophagus.[10] These are significant issues to consider in the adolescent patient population.

Pharmacologic intervention with calcium channel blockers had been advocated for patients who are not surgical candidates, but it has demonstrated only transient resolution of symptoms at best.[11] Reports have also demonstrated dramatic resolution of symptoms after endoscopic injection of botulinum toxin (botox) into the lower esophagus. The toxin directly interferes with smooth muscle contraction, resulting in reduction of LES tone that can persist for a few months. Unfortunately, as the effect of an injection wanes, repeated botox injections are necessary to provide the long-lasting relief of symptoms that patients seek. Long-term efficacy has not been established for this therapy in adults or adolescents, and subsequent esophageal fibrosis after multiple injections has been reported.[12] Although few report the use of this technique in children and adolescents, data on its use for long-term therapy in the adult population do not support its use in routine pediatric care.

### Spasm

Demonstrated manometrically by high-amplitude, usually nonperistaltic contractions of the body of the esophagus, esophageal spasm causes severe, intermittent chest pain. Patients may or may not also complain of dysphagia. Barium esophagram can reveal a "corkscrew" appearance of the lower two-thirds of the esophagus. Results of esophagoscopy are commonly normal. Treatment regimens in adolescents have not been reported extensively. Early studies in adults suggested that calcium channel blockers may be of benefit, but more recent studies have been equivocal. Dilatations and long surgical myotomies also have been of some benefit. However, symptoms may be intermittent, and a few adolescents have been reported to be either asymptomatic or having only mild, occasional symptoms 2 years after initial diagnosis despite receiving no specific therapy.[13]

### Dysfunction of the Belch Reflex

In a few young adults, incapacitating chest pain has been attributed to upper esophageal dysfunction resulting in an inability to belch.[14,15] All of these patients had symptoms dating back to adolescence. Reflux of gas from the stomach to the esophagus occurred normally, but the resultant distension of the proximal esophagus failed to trigger appropriate UES relaxation. Manometry confirmed that the tone of the UES always exceeded that of the more distal esophagus, but that the rest of the esophagus had normal manometric characteristics. Pain was relieved by lying down, which minimized gaseous GER, or by passing a nasoesophageal tube through the UES. No other specific therapies have been described.

## SECONDARY DYSMOTILITY

Abnormalities of esophageal motor function have been described as resulting from a wide variety of systemic disorders including neuromuscular disorders such as myasthenia gravis, connective tissue diseases such as scleroderma and dermatomyositis, and metabolic diseases such as diabetes mellitus (Box 98-1). In addition, toxic injuries to the esophagus—caused by radiation, chemotherapy, injection sclerotherapy, or caustic ingestion—also result in temporary or permanent disruption of normal esophageal motor function. These conditions cause abnormal motor function by different mechanisms that ultimately result in direct injury to either the esophageal smooth muscle or neural elements (Figure 98-2). Dysphagia and chest pain are common, and the diagnosis is often suggested by the patient's medical history. Treatment varies according to the nature of the underlying illness.

## GASTROESOPHAGEAL REFLUX

Gastroesophageal reflux (GER) is probably the most common disorder of the esophagus in adolescents.[16,17] Otherwise healthy patients can develop symptoms acutely or can manifest a persistence or exacerbation of symptoms present from childhood. In addition, adolescents with significant neurologic impairment represent a population at particularly high risk for the symptoms of GER and its complications.

**Box 98-1**

***Systemic Disorders Associated with Esophageal Dysfunction***

**Neurologic Disorders**
Familial dysautonomia
Static central nervous system injury secondary to cerebral palsy or cerebrovascular accidents
Multiple sclerosis
Neuropathic forms of intestinal pseudo-obstruction

**Neuromuscular Disorders**
Myasthenia gravis

**Muscular Disorders**
Muscular dystrophy
Polymyositis, dermatomyositis
Progressive systemic sclerosis
Myopathic forms of intestinal pseudo-obstruction

**Infectious Disorders**
Chagas disease

**Other Disorders**
Crohn disease
Behçet disease
Graft-versus-host disease
Chronic granulomatous disease

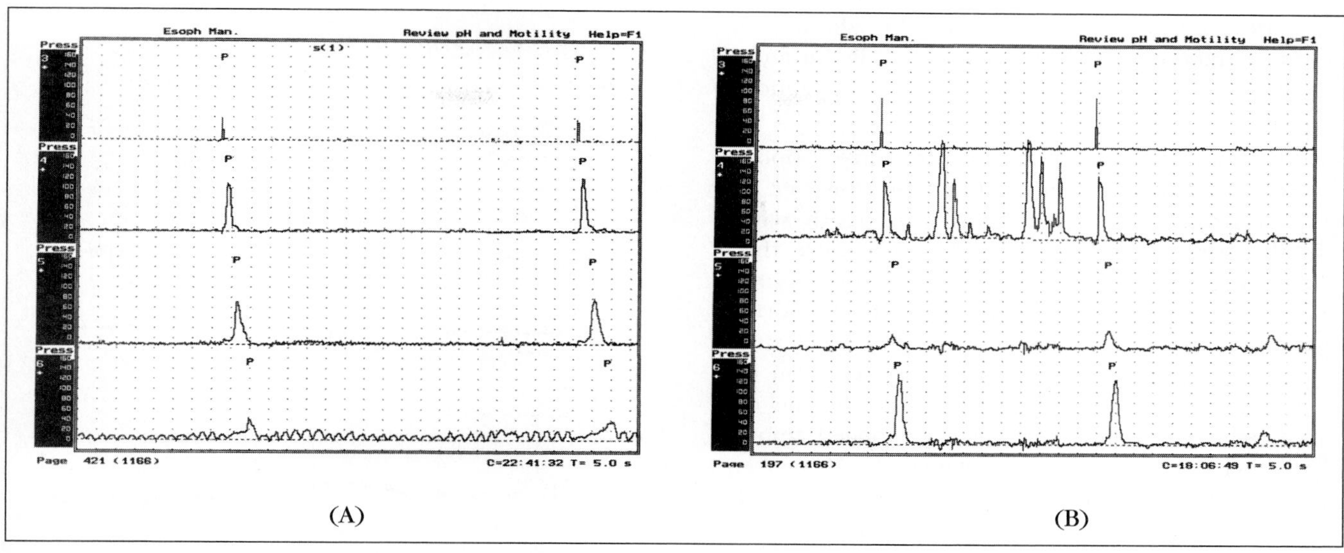


**FIGURE 98-2** (A) Normal esophageal manometry utilizing an ambulatory motility system. An esophageal catheter with four solid-state transducers 10 cm apart was situated so that the most proximal transducer (channel 3) was located in the posterior pharynx and the most distal (channel 6) in the distal esophagus. Two normal esophageal peristaltic waves progress down the esophagus in a coordinated manner, with contraction amplitudes ranging from 60 to 100 mm Hg in the midesophagus. (X axis = 5 seconds/gradation; Y axis = mm Hg). (B) Abnormal esophageal motility (localized esophageal spasm) obtained from a 17-year-old male with a neuropathic form of intestinal pseudo-obstruction. The recording device and esophageal catheter placement are identical to that described in (A). Recurrent spontaneous high-amplitude (>150mm Hg) contractions are noted only in channel 4. These contractions coincided with the subjective experience of chest pain.

### Etiology

Despite the frequency of GER, its cause remains unknown. In contrast to infants with GER who are thought to have reflux because of a relatively immature LES barrier mechanism, there is some evidence that pathologic GER in adolescents may become a lifelong condition. As in adults, only a small subset of adolescents with GER have a hypotensive LES. Instead, a transient, spontaneous, "inappropriate" relaxation of an otherwise normally functioning LES is the most commonly identified pathophysiologic event precipitating GER in the adolescent. Occasionally, patients have been identified as having GER that appears to be secondary to antropyloric dysfunction, which leads to delayed gastric emptying. The mechanisms underlying these motor disturbances remain unknown.

### Symptoms and Signs

Unlike the infant or younger child with GER whose primary presentation is usually effortless regurgitation, the adolescent with GER commonly complains of eructation, water brash, and substernal or subxiphoid pain. At times, intermittent dysphagia or odynophagia may be prominent, or hematemesis can cause the adolescent to seek medical evaluation. Occasionally, adolescent patients develop aversions to eating and lose weight, superficially mimicking patients with classic eating disorders. Adolescents with GER are also identified after evaluation of disease processes known to result as complications of GER. These include recurrent aspiration pneumonia, nocturnal asthma, chronic cough or hoarseness, chronic esophagitis, and esophageal stricture.

### Diagnosis

In the typical adolescent, a clinical diagnosis of GER can be strongly suspected on the basis of the clinical history. One or more of the following tests may be indicated, however, to differentiate between anatomic abnormalities that might be mimicking GER, to temporally relate episodes of reflux to specific symptoms, or to identify complications of GER.

- *Contrast radiography* of the esophagus and upper gastrointestinal tract delineates anatomy and to some extent function. Esophageal webs or rings, abnormalities of the gastric outlet, and intestinal malrotation can be identified, as can complications such as esophageal strictures. Careful double-contrast studies are required to delineate esophagitis. Although radiographs can reveal episodes of GER, the false-negative rate can be as high as 50%. In addition, a few uncomplicated episodes of GER during a radiographic study are not necessarily diagnostic of pathologic GER.

- *Esophageal manometry* can characterize esophageal body and LES motor function. However, in most cases LES pressure correlates poorly with the presence or severity of GER. Therefore, this procedure is not often indicated for routine clinical purposes. Manometry is useful, however, to evaluate the adolescent with dysphagia due to GER, primarily by allowing the exclusion of other motility disturbances. It can also be of benefit when performed as a prolonged ambulatory study with a simultaneous pH probe. Such a study can allow the characterization of an episodic clinical symptom such as pain and clarify the degree to which such a symptom is an "acid" as opposed to a "motor" event.
- *Radionuclide scanning* can directly demonstrate GER, but this technique generally has been more useful as a means of assessing possible pulmonary aspiration due to reflux. In addition, gastric emptying can be accurately measured with separate labels attached to the liquid and the solid components of a standardized meal.
- *Flexible esophagoscopy* allows direct visualization and biopsy of the esophageal mucosa. Anatomic lesions of the esophagus such as webs or strictures can be delineated and, at times, treated. Although endoscopy can demonstrate the consequences of GER such as esophagitis, it cannot directly demonstrate GER itself. It is important to clarify that not every patient with symptomatic GER develops esophageal mucosal lesions.
- *Intraesophageal pH monitoring* is currently the gold standard for diagnosing pathologic GER. Ambulatory 24-hour monitors and sophisticated computer analyses of the tracings are now widely available (Figure 98-3). When coupled with a careful patient diary, the pH probe is particularly valuable as a means of correlating ill-defined or atypical symptoms with episodes of GER. Recently, a wireless pH probe (Bravo) has become commercially available to allow for a more convenient and less cumbersome study in an adolescent. A recent report showed that a Bravo pH capsule placed endoscopically onto the wall of the mid- to distal esophagus in adults was safe, reliable, and well tolerated in most patients.[18]
- *Impedance/pH monitoring* has recently become commercially available. Ambulatory 24-hour monitors allow for simultaneous monitoring of acid and nonacid GER. Measurements of pH changes as well as directionality of flow and height of refluxate are determined.[19] This study is useful in the evaluation of patients on antisecretory medications, such as proton-pump inhibitors, who continue to report reflux-related symptoms. Impedance studies potentially also have a role in the evaluation of children with extraesophageal symptoms of GER such as persistent respiratory symptoms.[20]
- Reproducing a patient's symptoms by the intraesophageal perfusion of acid, or the Bernstein test, is occasionally useful in adolescents with atypical symptoms. However, the subjective nature of the test makes interpretation difficult. The Bernstein test has been supplanted almost entirely by intraesophageal pH monitoring.

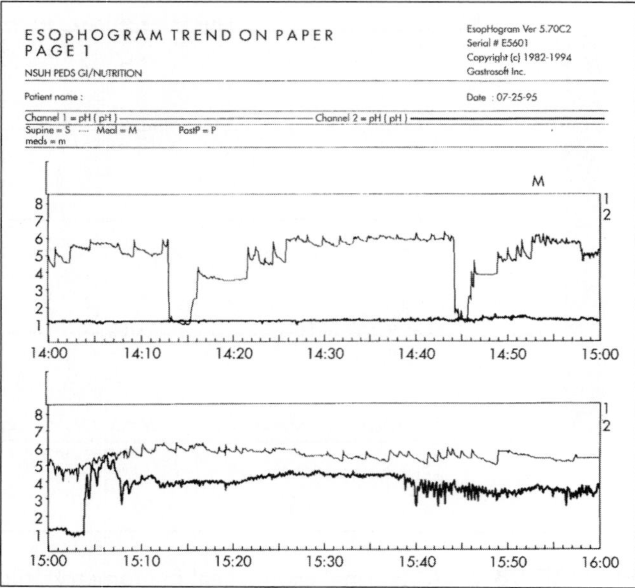


**FIGURE 98-3** Two-hour segment of a 24-hour ambulatory pH probe recording. Two probes simultaneously record the pH of the distal esophagus (channel 1, top tracing on each panel) and stomach (channel 2, bottom tracing on each panel). Intragastric contents are acid (pH = 1.2) until neutralized by the ingestion of a meal (M). In the time interval before the meal, 2 distinct, poorly cleared episodes of GER (intraesophageal pH drops to <4.0 for >5 minutes) are recorded (X axis = 1 minute/minor tick; Y axis = pH units).

### Treatment

Management of pathologic GER in the adolescent depends on the nature and severity of the symptoms. In general, most patients do well with conservative therapy directed at dietary and lifestyle changes. Patients should be counseled to eat smaller, more frequent meals. Certain foods and medications, smoking, and alcohol intake should be limited or eliminated because of their adverse effects on LES pressure or gastric emptying (see Box 98-2). Raising the head of the bed with blocks or by insertion of a foam wedge under the bedsheet is particularly helpful in patients with nocturnal GER. Coexistent constipation should be identified and treated vigorously, because significant improvement in GER symptoms often occurs as a result of such treatment. Weight loss can also be helpful in obese adolescents, as a diminished pressure gradient across the esophagogastric junction has been shown to augment GER in these patients.[21]

At times, GER does not resolve with the previously mentioned interventions, and complications develop. Gastroesophageal reflux disease (GERD) occurs when patients with GER develop sequelae such as esophagitis, and more aggressive therapy is necessary. In patients with significant pain and minimal to no esophagitis, acid neutralization with appropriate doses of antacids or H-receptor antagonists such as ranitidine, famotidine, or nizatidine is often the first line of therapy. However, frequent dosing regimens with these medications may be required to control symptoms. For severe and more chronic symptoms or esophagitis, proton-pump inhibitors such as omeprazole, lansoprazole, esomeprazole, rabeprazole, and pantoprazole, potent inhibitors of the parietal cell H,K pump, are effective, with healing of erosive esophagitis demonstrated in most patients within 4 to 8 weeks. Sucralfate, particularly the liquid preparation, may also be useful. Prokinetic agents, including metoclopramide, may help improve the abnormal esophagogastric motility underlying GER. In the past, these agents had been used as adjuncts to, or therapeutic alternatives for, acid suppression. As data support their efficacy in only about 50% of children in randomized placebo-controlled trials, and irreversible side effects, such as extrapyramidal symptoms, have been seen in children taking metoclopramide, their use should be limited. In a few patients, GER remains intractable despite aggressive medical therapy. In others, the complications of GER (eg, esophageal strictures, recurrent aspirations) make trials of medical therapy ill advised. For such patients a surgical antireflux procedure such as the Nissen fundoplication, which many centers perform laparoscopically, has been beneficial. Short-term benefits from surgery have been widely reported, but data in adults show that more than 60% are taking proton-pump inhibitors for recurrent symptoms by 7 years after antireflux surgery.[22] Therefore, further study is necessary to determine the long-term efficacy of fundoplication as an antireflux option in children and adolescents.

> **Box 98-2**
>
> ***Ingested Substances Associated with Impaired Lower Esophageal Function***
>
> **Medications**
> Anticholinergics
> Beta-adrenergic agonists
> Alpha-adrenergic antagonists
> Dopamine
> Opiates
> Calcium channel blockers
> Theophylline
>
> **Foods**
> Chocolate
> High-fat meals
> High-osmolarity meals
>
> **Miscellaneous**
> Alcohol
> Caffeine
> Cigarettes

## MUCOSAL DISORDERS

### PEPTIC ESOPHAGITIS

#### Etiology

Reflux of gastric contents through the LES exposes the esophageal mucosa to hydrochloric acid, pepsin, and (at times) bile salts and pancreatic enzymes. Because the squamous epithelium of the esophagus has a limited ability to protect itself against these noxious agents, inflammation and ulceration can result. Whether esophagitis develops depends on a number of factors, including the nature and concentration of refluxed materials, the frequency of reflux, and the efficiency of esophageal clearance. Clearance is enhanced by primary and secondary esophageal peristalsis and by the swallowing of bicarbonate-rich saliva, which directly neutralizes refluxed acid. Conversely, clearance is impaired by a hiatal hernia. Although no extensive studies in adolescents have been reported, studies in adults suggest that patients who reflux primarily at night are at greatest risk for developing peptic esophagitis. The infrequent rate of swallowing during sleep predisposes such patients to poor acid clearance and resultant prolonged episodes of acid reflux. Daytime, or so-called upright, refluxers appear to have more discomfort yet less esophagitis than do patients who reflux nocturnally. This may occur because their discomfort results in improved acid clearance through an increased frequency of swallowing saliva, food, or antacid.

Rare patients develop peptic esophagitis from ectopic gastric epithelium in the distal cervical esophagus (an "inlet patch"). This lesion secretes acid and may cause localized esophagitis adjacent to the ectopic tissue.

### Symptoms and Signs

The symptoms of peptic esophagitis are not significantly different from those of uncomplicated GER. Odynophagia and dysphagia can range from mild to severe, but patients may also be completely asymptomatic. Pain is described as burning, or crushing, or as a vague, ill-defined sensation. Food impaction or severe dysphagia is unusual unless there is a stricture. Hematemesis or occult gastrointestinal bleeding also can be present. The response to empirically prescribed antacids or dietary manipulations is variable.

### Diagnosis

Esophagitis should be suspected whenever a patient with a history of, or symptoms compatible with, GER develops hematemesis, occult gastrointestinal bleeding, or worsening dysphagia or odynophagia. Esophagoscopy is the diagnostic procedure of choice. Visualization of the esophageal mucosa may reveal hyperemia, erosions, or ulcerations with exudate that generally start at the esophagogastric junction and extend proximally for a variable distance (Figure 98-4). However, there is often poor correlation between endoscopic and histologic severity. Biopsies therefore should be obtained even when the mucosa appears normal.[23]

Barium studies of the esophagus are much less sensitive than endoscopy, but they do offer important information when symptoms suggest that a stricture might be present. However, a normal mucosal contour on a contrast study is not sufficient to rule out the possibility of even moderate degrees of esophagitis.

### Treatment

Treatment modalities have been outlined in the section on GER. Esophagitis may require vigorous therapy, not only to heal inflammatory changes but also to prevent their recurrence. Often the latter goal is far more difficult to accomplish than the former. Prolonged treatment with a combination of medications designed to suppress acid production and promote more normal esophagogastric motility may be necessary. Elimination of cigarette smoking and cessation of alcohol ingestion remain important adjuncts to therapy.

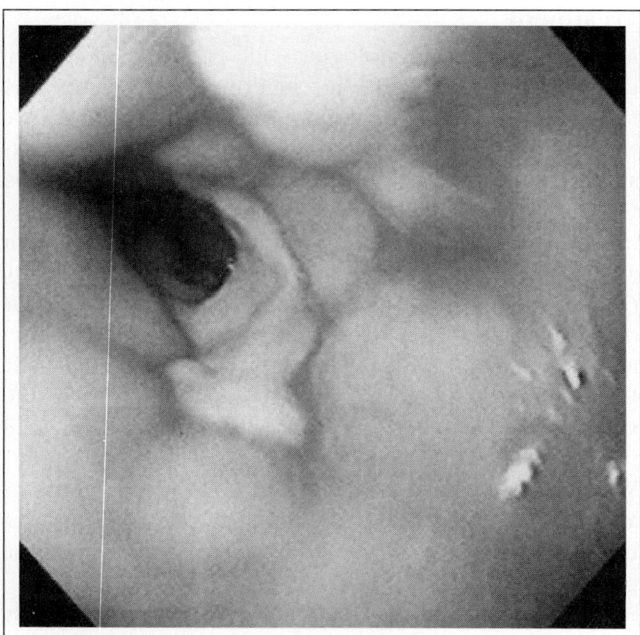

**FIGURE 98-4** Endoscopic appearance of the distal esophagus of an 18-year-old male with severe neurodevelopmental retardation. A thick membranous exudate overlies a distal esophageal ulcer. The esophageal lumen distal to the ulceration is somewhat stenotic.

### Complications

Esophageal stricture can occur as a direct result of chronic peptic esophagitis and often heralds significant morbidity. Progressive dysphagia or recurrent food impactions require multiple interventions, including recurrent esophageal dilatations. For such adolescents, nutritional intake is often compromised, and growth failure with delayed sexual maturation is not uncommon. Therefore, antireflux surgery, designed to prevent repeated GER after dilatation, is frequently indicated if chronic use of proton-pump inhibitors is unsuccessful.

Another complication of long-standing peptic esophagitis is the development of Barrett esophagus.[24,25] In this potentially premalignant lesion, the normal squamous epithelium of the esophagus is replaced by an intestinal type of columnar epithelium. It is well documented in adults that adenocarcinoma arises within the epithelium in Barrett esophagus. Adolescents with adenocarcinoma of the esophagus and Barrett esophagus changes have also been described.[23] The presence of Barrett esophagus epithelium in an adolescent is an indication for prolonged aggressive medical therapy with a proton-pump inhibitor. At times, antireflux surgery is preferable, especially in the adolescent with chronic active inflammation due to poor adherence to medical therapy. In addition, the premalignant nature of this lesion demands frequent endoscopic surveillance with careful biopsy sampling of the mucosa for the presence of dysplasia or other premalignant markers.[26]

### CAUSTIC ESOPHAGITIS

In general, ingestion of caustic agents is not seen in adolescents, except in association with suicide attempts. However, inadvertent ingestions have been reported: for example, Clinitest tablets have been ingested mistakenly. Although only mildly alkaline, these tablets generate intense heat during hydration, which can result in severe esophageal ulceration and stricture formation. Button batteries also have been inadvertently swallowed. If these objects become lodged in the esophagus, the leakage of their alkaline contents can cause necrosis, perforation, and death. Acid injuries are less common. Patients with strong alkali or acid ingestions may have burns of the oral cavity or respiratory symptoms and varying degrees of dysphagia or odynophagia. The severity of lasting injury is variable, ranging from complete healing without sequelae to intractable, long, and often occlusive esophageal strictures.

Oral medications also can cause acute esophageal damage[27] (Box 98-3). Pills can become impacted within a normal esophagus, especially if they are ingested with little or no fluid. Patients complain of the acute onset of severe odynophagia and the sensation that the pill has become stuck in the esophagus. In adolescents, oral antibiotics, such as minocycline taken for acne are common medications associated with pill-induced esophagitis. Esophagoscopy often reveals a highly localized area of ulceration that usually heals rapidly without permanent damage or specific therapy.

There are also a number of iatrogenic causes of esophageal injury in adolescent patients. Radiation and chemotherapy commonly result in esophagitis, which can be aggravated by superimposed peptic or infectious injury. Graft-versus-host disease after bone marrow transplantation also can cause severe esophageal mucosal damage. Injection sclerotherapy or band ligation for bleeding esophageal varices are other forms of treatment that can produce potentially severe mucosal and submucosal injury, ulceration, and ultimately stricture formation. In general, however, those adolescents who receive sclerotherapy or band ligation have minimal complaints, and serious strictures have not been reported.

**Box 98-3**

***Medications Associated with Caustic Esophagitis***

Tetracyclines
Potassium chloride
Theophylline
Nonsteroidal anti-inflammatory agents
Ascorbic acid
Chloral hydrate

### INFECTION

Infectious esophagitis is a cause of morbidity in both normal and immunocompromised adolescents.[28] Fungal (especially *Candida albicans*) and viral (herpes simplex and cytomegalovirus) agents are most common, but other organisms also have been seen in the immunocompromised patient. Treatment with inhaled corticosteroids, for respiratory diseases such as asthma, has also been shown to promote the development of *Candida* esophagitis. Patients complain of severe odynophagia, dysphagia, or chest pain. Diagnosis is best made by endoscopy, at which time brushings and biopsy specimens can be obtained for cytologic and histologic examination and for culture. An esophagram may suggest the diagnosis, but normal or nondiagnostic studies can be seen in 20% to 50% of patients, depending on whether double- or single-contrast studies, respectively, are performed. Treatment is determined by the specific microbiologic cause and the underlying immunocompetence of the patient.

### EOSINOPHILIC ESOPHAGITIS

#### Etiology

Eosinophilic esophagitis (EE) is a disorder that has received a considerable amount of attention over the past decade. Although initially thought to be associated with peptic or reflux esophagitis, it has been recently identified as a separate disorder.[29] Eosinophilic esophagitis is thought to occur as the result of a type IV (cell-mediated) rather than a type I (IgE immediate hypersensitivity) immunologic reaction to a food[29] or aeroallergen.[30] Consequently, patients will often have a negative reaction to skin prick or radioallergosorbent (RAST) IgE testing, with an increase in identification of allergic foods seen with a delayed reaction skin test such as skin patch testing.[31] Eosinophilic esophagitis is characterized by an extensive eosinophil infiltration of the esophagus. The eosinophilic granules are thought to release proinflammatory mediators that exert local cytotoxic effects.

#### Symptoms and Signs

Adolescents often present with vomiting, epigastric pain, or dysphagia, which may only be intermittent. Esophageal food impaction is one of the most common presentations

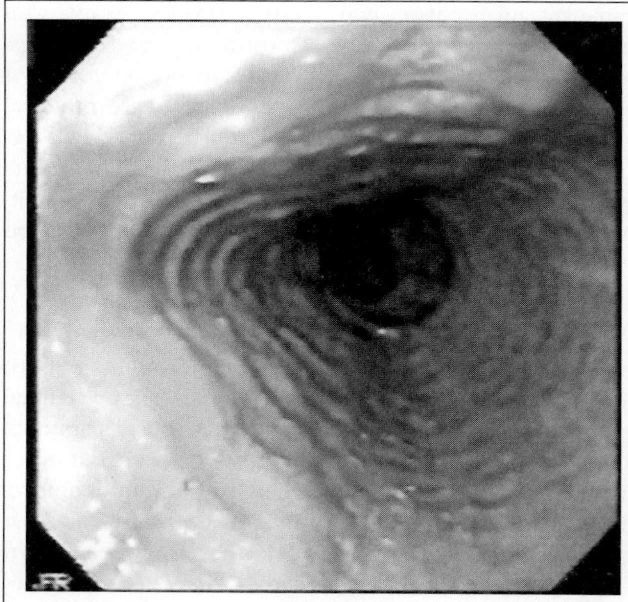


FIGURE 98-5 Endoscopic appearance of the esophagus of a 16-year-old male with eosinophilic esophagitis. Multiple circumferential rings and whitish flecks often seen in this condition are present from the mid- to distal esophagus. (See color insert.)

of EE in adolescents. Less common symptoms include water brash, globus (feeling a "lump in the throat"), and hematemesis. Patients frequently have a personal or family history of atopic disorders. Although typical symptoms may transiently improve on acid-suppressing medications such as proton-pump inhibitors, they often do not completely and consistently resolve.

### Diagnosis

A diagnosis of EE can be made in adolescents with reflux-like symptoms or dysphagia who do not respond to acid-suppressing medications, have normal or borderline normal 24-hour pH probe studies performed off medication, and have an isolated eosinophilic infiltration in the esophagus.[29] Macroscopic findings on endoscopy include white specks or concentric rings around the esophagus[32,33] (Figure 98-5). Mucosal biopsies of the esophagus, which are required to make the definitive diagnosis, reveal a more significant eosinophilic infiltration (on average >20 eosinophils per high-powered field) than that present in reflux esophagitis (5 eosinophils per high-powered field).[34] Of note, there seems to be little difference in the degree of eosinophilia in the mid-esophagus compared to the distal esophagus in EE, in contrast to peptic esophagitis, which is often more severe distally.

### Treatment

***Medications*** Although the etiology of EE is unknown, several medical therapies have been used. While systemic or topical corticosteroids were previously the mainstays of therapy, over the past 5 years other medications, including cromolyn sodium and leukotriene receptor antagonists, have been used. Proton-pump inhibitors are often useful in treating secondary acid reflux, which may accompany EE, and therefore afford some symptomatic relief.[35] Unfortunately, although symptomatic improvement may result from these therapies, they have not been shown to reverse the histologic damage. Future therapy may include biologic agents designed to specifically target proinflammatory cytokine activity in the esophagus.

***Dietary therapy*** An immunologic reaction to food allergens has been recognized as an important contributor to the inflammation seen in EE. A recent study reported an improvement in both clinical symptoms and tissue inflammation with either the temporary withdrawal of specific foods to which the patient is allergic or the removal of all foods and the use of an elemental or amino acid-based formula.[36]

Following diagnosis, patients should be evaluated by an allergist to identify IgE-mediated and non-IgE-mediated food allergies by skin prick and skin patch testing, respectively. A strict elimination diet is recommended for those foods identified by allergy testing. If after 2 months on an elimination diet symptoms and histology improve, a slow reintroduction of food is recommended. Further evaluation by endoscopy would be determined by the reappearance of symptoms and then performed at the discretion of a pediatric gastroenterologist. On the other hand, if symptoms and histology do not normalize, adherence to a strict elemental, or amino acid-based formula, is recommended.

## MISCELLANEOUS CONDITIONS

### TRAUMA

Extraluminal and intraluminal events can injure the esophagus. Penetrating wounds or the effects of externally applied blunt trauma are rare causes of esophageal injury in the adolescent, but intraluminal events are more common causes. Linear tears of the mucosa at the esophagogastric junction (Mallory-Weiss tears) are fairly common after vigorous or prolonged retching or forceful vomiting. Although bleeding can be massive, it usually ceases spontaneously, requires no specific treatment, and leaves no lasting sequelae. By contrast, spontaneous transmural rupture of the esophagus (Boerhaave syndrome), which is very rare, is associated with a high degree of morbidity and mortality.

Other mechanisms of esophageal injury result in perforations of the esophagus induced by extrinsically applied intraluminal forces. The use of instruments, such as endoscopes, dilators, and nasogastric and orogastric tubes, is the most common reason for perforation injuries, but air-pressure injuries also occur from misplaced endotracheal tubes or purposeful inhalation of materials packaged in high-pressure containers.

Most patients with esophageal perforation have pain, which may be in the neck, chest, or epigastrium, depending on the location of the injury. Dysphagia, fever, and respiratory difficulties can also occur. Subcutaneous emphysema may be palpable in the neck. Plain radiographs of the chest or neck demonstrate mediastinal or subcutaneous air, but the site of perforation is best identified by a water-soluble contrast esophagram. Esophagoscopy is rarely necessary and often ill-advised, except in the case of a suspected Mallory-Weiss tear.

Treatment depends on the site and the cause of perforation and the duration of injury before diagnosis. Surgery is often indicated, but small, noncontaminated leaks can sometimes be treated conservatively (nothing by mouth, antibiotics). Mallory-Weiss tears heal spontaneously once bleeding stops, but basic resuscitative measures applicable to all causes of upper gastrointestinal hemorrhage may be required.

### VARICES

Submucosal varices arising as a consequence of portal hypertension, in association with either liver disease or prehepatic and (occasionally) posthepatic venous obstruction, can be a cause of significant morbidity during adolescence. By one estimate, once varices develop, significant episodes of bleeding will occur in as many as 33% of patients. It is generally accepted that varices do not erode from overlying mucosal ulceration but are disrupted and perforate as a consequence of the unequal pressures that exist across the luminal wall of the varix. The current treatment trend avoids surgical intervention as a means of controlling variceal hemorrhage. Instead, endoscopic injection sclerotherapy or rubber band ligation is used to obliterate the varices, thereby preventing further episodes of bleeding.[37] Although these techniques are safe and efficacious in adolescents, sclerotherapy in particular is not without its side effects. Mucosal ulceration (occasionally accompanied by secondary massive hemorrhage), stricture formation, esophageal perforation, pneumonitis, and other less common complications have been described. In addition, these techniques deal only with the consequences of the portal hypertension rather than the cause. Given these realities, adolescents found to have varices are increasingly considered as candidates for the more definitive treatment of liver transplantation.

### SYSTEMIC DISEASES

Systemic diseases may also affect the esophagus in the adolescent by causing inflammation. These include gastrointestinal diseases, such as Crohn disease and Behcet's disease, which are associated with chronic inflammation and ulceration. These patients may present with dysphagia, chest pain, odynophagia, or vomiting. Treatment is generally disease-specific.

## REFERENCES


1. Rosen R, Nurko S. Other motor disorders. In: Walker WA, Goulet O, Kleinman RE, Sherman PM, Shneider BL, Sanderson IA, eds. *Pediatric Gastrointestinal Disease*. 4th ed. Ontario: BC Decker; 2004: 424–461

2. Illi OE, Stauffer UG. Achalasia in childhood and adolescence. *Eur J Pediatr Surg.* 1994;4:214–217

3. Myers NA, Jolley SG, Taylor R. Achalasia of the cardia in children: a worldwide survey. *J Pediatr Surg.* 1994;29:1375–1379

4. Mearin F, Mourelle M, Guarner F, et al. Patients with achalasia lack nitric oxide synthetase in the gastro-esophageal junction. *Eur J Clin Invest.* 1993;23:724–728

5. Goldblum JR, Whyte RI, Orringer MB, Appelman HD. Achalasia: a morphologic study of 42 resected specimens. *Am J Surg Pathol.* 1994;18:327–337

6. Woltman TA, Pellegrini CA, Oelschlager BK. Achalasia. *Surg Clin North Am.* 2005;85(3):483–493

7. Zerbib F. Repeated pneumatic dilations as long-term maintenance therapy for esophageal achalasia. *Am J Gastroenterol.* 2006;101(4):692–697

8. Abid S, Champion G, Richter JE, McElvein R, Slaughter RL, Koehler RE. Treatment of achalasia: best of both worlds. *Am J Gastroenterol.* 1994;87:979–985

9. Diamantis T, Pikoulis E, Felekouras E, et al. Laparoscopic esophagomyotomy for achalasia without a complementary antireflux procedure. *J Laparoendosc Adv Surg Tech.* 2006;16(4):345–349

10. Csendes A. Very late results of esophagomyotomy for patients with achalasia: clinical, endoscopic, histologic, manometric, and acid reflux studies in 67 patients for a mean follow-up of 190 months. *Ann Surg.* 2006;243(2):196–203

11. Traube M, Dubovik S, Lange RC, McCallum RW. The role of nifedipine therapy in achalasia: results of a randomized, double-blind, placebo-controlled study. *Am J Gastroenterol.* 1989;84:1259–1262

12. Pasricha PJ, Ravich WJ, Hendrix TR, Sostre S, Jones B, Kalloo AN. Intrasphincteric botulinum toxin for the treatment of achalasia. *N Engl J Med.* 1995;322:774–778

13. Milov DE, Cynamon HA, Andres JM. Chest pain and dysphagia in adolescents caused by diffuse esophageal spasm. *J Pediatr Gastroenterol Nutr.* 1989;9:450–453

14. Kahrilas PJ, Dodds WJ, Hogan WJ. Dysfunction of the belch reflex: a cause of incapacitating chest pain. *Gastroenterology.* 1987;93:818–822

15. Gignoux C, Bost R, Hostein J, et al. Role of upper esophageal reflex and belch reflux dysfunctions in non-cardiac chest pain. *Dig Dis Sci.* 1993;38:1909–1914

16. Orenstein SR. Gastroesophageal reflux. In: Hyman PE, Di Lorenzo C, eds. *Pediatric Gastrointestinal Motility Disorders*. New York, NY: Academy Professional Information Services; 1994:55–88

17. Sood MR, Rudolph CD. Gastroesophageal reflux in adolescents. *Adol Med Clinics.* 2004;15:17–36

18. Remes-Troche JM, Ibarra-Palomini J, Carmona-Sanchez RI, Valdovinos MA. Performance, tolerability, and symptoms related to prolonged pH monitoring using the Bravo system in Mexico. *Am J Gastroenterol.* 2005;100(11):2382–2386

19. Mattioli G, Pini-Prato A, Gentilino V. Esophageal impedance/pH monitoring in pediatric patients: preliminary experience with 50 cases. *Dig Dis Sci.* 2006;51:2341–2347

20. Rosen R, Nurko S. The importance of multichannel intraluminal impedance in the evaluation of children with persistent respiratory symptoms. *Am J Gastro.* 2004;99:2452–2458

21. Pandolfino JE, El-Serag HB, Zhang Q, et al. Obesity: a challenge to esophagogastric junction integrity. *Gastroenterology.* 2006;130:639–649

22. Spechler SJ, Lee E, Ahnen D, et al. Long-term outcome of medical and surgical therapies for gastroesophageal reflux disease: follow-up of a randomized controlled trial. *JAMA.* 2001;285:2331–2338

23. Dahms B. The histology of reflux esophagitis. In: Balistreri WF, Vanderhoof JA, eds. *Aspen Seminars on Pediatric Disease. Vol 4. Pediatric Gastroenterology and Nutrition.* London: Chapman & Hall; 1990:95–103

24. Hassall E. Barrett's esophagus: new definitions and approaches in children. *J Pediatr Gastroenterol Nutr.* 1993;16:345–364

25. Hassall E, Dimmick JE, Magee JF. Adenocarcinoma in childhood Barrett's esophagus: case documentation and the need for surveillance in children. *Am J Gastroenterol.* 1993;88:282–288

26. Axon ATR, Boyle P, Riddell RH, Grandjouan S, Hardcastle J, Yoshida S. Summary of a working party on the surveillance of premalignant lesions. *Am J Gastroenterol.* 1994;89:S160–S168

27. Winstead NS, Bulat R. Pill esophagitis. *Curr Treat Opt Gastro.* 2004;7:71–76

28. Thomson M. Esophagitis. In: Walker WA, Goulet O, Kleinman RE, Sherman PM, Shneider BL, Sanderson IA, eds. *Pediatric Gastrointestinal Disease.* 4th ed. Ontario: BC Decker; 2004:403–404

29. Markowitz JE, Liacouras CA. Eosinophilic esophagitis. *Gastroenterol Clin.* 2003;32(3):949–966

30. Mishra A, Hogan SP, Brandt EB, Rothenberg ME. An etiological role for aeroallergens and eosinophils in experimental esophagitis. *J Clin Invest.* 2001;107:83–90

31. Spergel JM, Beausoleil JL, Mascarenhas M, Liacouras CA. The use of skin prick and patch tests to identify causative foods in eosinophilic esophagitis. *J Allergy Clin Immunol.* 2002;109:363–368

32. Lim JR, Gupta SK, Croffie JM, et al. White specks in the esophageal mucosa: an endoscopic manifestation of non-reflux eosinophilic esophagitis in children. *Gastrointest Endosc.* 2004;59(7):835–838

33. Siafakas CG, Ryan CK, Brown MR, Miller TL. Multiple esophageal rings: an association with eosinophilic esophagitis: case report and review of the literature. *Am J Gastroenterol.* 2000;95:1572–1575

34. Ruchelli E, Wenner W, Voyek T, Brown K, Liacouras C. Severity of esophageal eosinophilia predicts response to conventional gastroesophageal reflux therapy. *Pediatric Dev Pathol.* 1999;2:15–18

35. Liacouras CA. Eosinophilic esophagitis: treatment in 2005. *Curr Opin Gastroenterol.* 2006;22:147–152

36. Liacouras CA, Spergel JM, Ruchelli E, et al. Eosinophilic esophagitis: a 10-year experience in 381 children. *Clin Gastro Hep.* 2005;3:1198–1206

37. Stiegmann GV. Endoscopic management of esophageal varices. *Adv Surg.* 1994;27:209–231

# CHAPTER 99

# Peptic Ulcers and Other Disorders of the Stomach and Duodenum

LIBIA MOY, MD • MICHAEL J. PETTEI, MD, PhD

Complaints that potentially involve disorders of the stomach or duodenum are common in adolescence. Gastroduodenal pathology can give rise to nonspecific presenting symptoms, such as pain, vomiting, nausea, or bloating, as well as those more demonstrative of an organic disorder, such as gastrointestinal (GI) bleeding or weight loss. Although the exact incidence and prevalence of gastroduodenal disorders in adolescents are not known, an understanding of these disorders, such as peptic ulcer disease and its precursor lesion gastritis, is essential when caring for adolescents with these common presenting complaints.

## MUCOSAL DISORDERS

### GASTRITIS

Gastritis is defined as microscopic evidence of inflammation affecting the gastric mucosa. Inflammation of the gastric mucosa is associated with a number of important etiologic factors. Historically, gastritis and peptic ulcer disease were divided into primary (idiopathic) and secondary causes. It is now known that most cases of "primary" gastritis are caused by gastric infection with the bacteria *Helicobacter pylori*. The most important secondary causes of gastritis/peptic ulceration are listed in Box 99-1.

**Box 99-1**

***Secondary Causes of Gastritis and Peptic Ulcer Disease in Adolescents***

**Drug related**
- NSAIDs
- KCl
- Alendronate
- Iron
- Kayexalate

**Alcohol (ethanol)**

**Severe stress**
- Burns
- Sepsis
- Shock
- Head injury
- Major surgery
- Trauma

**Bile reflux disease**

**Underlying conditions**
- Crohn disease
- Zollinger-Ellison syndrome
- Collagen vascular disease

Common causes of secondary gastritis in healthy adolescents are drug- and alcohol-induced gastritis. These should be suspected in any previously healthy adolescent with the acute onset of abdominal pain or upper GI bleeding. Stress gastritis, in contrast, should be suspected in the severely ill, hospitalized patient with upper, often painless, GI hemorrhage. Although there is a widespread perception that corticosteroid therapy is a cause for peptic ulceration, little objective evidence supports this concept. A very common cause of gastritis is use of nonsteroidal anti-inflammatory drugs (NSAIDs), the most frequently prescribed drugs in the world, which exert their effects via inhibition of the cyclo-oxygenase (COX)–catalyzed conversion of arachidonic acid to prostaglandins. Prostaglandins produced by the COX-1 pathway are largely responsible for mucosal integrity. Inhibition of COX-1 compromises mucosal protection mechanisms such as mucus and bicarbonate production, epithelial integrity and regenerative capacity, and microvascular supply. Even a single dose of a NSAID may cause petechial hemorrhages and ulceration within hours.

Stress gastropathy usually occurs within 24 hours of the onset of severe illness, such as shock, sepsis, burns, major surgery, severe trauma, multiorgan system failure, or head injury. These stressors cause reduction of gastric blood flow with subsequent mucosal ischemia[1] and breakdown of mucosal defenses.[2] Gastric acid is important in the pathogenesis of stress erosions. Stress erosions are typically asymptomatic and multiple, and do not perforate; when they are symptomatic, they produce upper GI hemorrhage. Early lesions predominate in the fundus and proximal body, later occurring in the antrum, to produce a diffuse erosive and hemorrhagic appearance. Antral involvement alone is uncommon.

Bile-induced gastritis is an uncommon condition in adolescents, notwithstanding the relatively common presence of bile seen in the stomach at upper endoscopy. It occurs mainly after surgical alteration of the gastroduodenal anatomy.

Recognizing that most "primary" or "idiopathic" cases of gastritis are caused by infection with *Helicobacter pylori* began with the isolation of spiral organisms (initially believed to be a *Campylobacter* species) from biopsies of patients with chronic gastritis or peptic ulcer disease.[3] It is now acknowledged that *H pylori* gastritis is one of the most common human bacterial infectious diseases and is causally linked with gastritis, peptic ulcer disease, gastric adenocarcinoma, and gastric B-cell lymphoma.[4] This urea-splitting, gram-negative, spiral-shaped rod thrives in the mucus layer overlying the gastric epithelium, despite the acidic milieu of the stomach, and induces inflammatory changes in the gastric (primarily antral) mucosa. In most children and adolescents, the presence of *H pylori* infection does not result in symptoms, even though it universally causes chronic active gastritis.[5]

The prevalence of infection varies depending on age and country of origin. *H pylori* is believed to infect approximately 30% to 40% of the population in the developed countries of Europe and North America, and up to 100% in many developing countries.[6] Although the overall prevalence of *H pylori* infection in the United States is relatively low, it is substantial within selected racial or ethnic groups, such as Hispanics (62%) and non-Hispanic blacks (53%).[7] The infection is usually believed to be acquired in childhood, generally before age 5 years[8]; infection may last a lifetime if untreated.[9]

Although the mechanism of transmission remains unclear, *H pylori* seems to be transmitted person to person, either by way of the oral-oral, gastric-oral, or fecal-oral route. These theories are supported by the recovery of viable *H pylori* organisms from the oropharynx, vomitus, and feces of humans.[10] Acute infection in adults is believed to result in an acute, neutrophilic gastritis with transient hypochlorhydria and a high rate of chronic infection with chronic gastritis.

*H pylori* bacteria primarily colonize the antrum of the stomach in the mucus layer overlying the epithelium and are rarely observed intracellularly, which may play some role in the evasion of antimicrobial therapy. The mechanism of gastric inflammation is unclear, but one factor that may account for the gastric damage is the large amount of urease present in *H pylori*. Urease hydrolyzes urea to ammonia and bicarbonate at the gastric mucosal surface. Ammonia can have a direct toxic effect on epithelial cells and, along with the concomitant increase in the mucosal surface pH, might interfere with gastric epithelial function, such as mucus production.[11] This enzyme is used as an indirect marker of the presence of *H pylori* in tests such as the biopsy rapid urease test and the urea breath test (URB), and as an antigen in serologic tests.

Bacterial virulence factors that may be important in the development of disease include vacuolating cytotoxin (*vacA*), cytotoxin-associated gene product E (*cagE*), adhesins such as B*abA* and S*abA*, neutrophil activating protein, and other outer membrane proteins.[12-16]

The host response to *H pylori* is now also recognized as an important factor in the pathogenesis of *H pylori* infection.[17] The best-characterized host factor is the genotype of the interleukin (IL)-1 cluster.[18] The presence of IL-1B31T and IL-IRN2 alleles has been associated with a higher risk of developing gastric cancer in those infected by *H pylori*; individuals with this genotype have an exaggerated IL-1 response. Elevated levels of IL-1 lead to more severe inflammation and to inhibition of acid production by parietal cells.

*H pylori* infection is associated with multiple clinical disorders, most of which involve the GI tract. The natural history of *H pylori* infection of the GI tract follows 2 general paths, each beginning with superficial gastritis. One path is that of a chronic-active, antral-predominant gastritis, which leads to peptic ulcer disease approximately 15% of the time.[19-22] The second, far less common path is that of an atrophic, corpus-predominant gastritis that increases the risk for gastric adenocarcinoma (<1% of infected individuals) and gastric mucosa-associated lymphoid tissue (MALT) lymphoma (approximately 0.1% of infected persons).[6,19,23,24] What dictates the pathophysiology of *H pylori*–induced gastroduodenal disease is unclear, but it seems to be a balance of bacterial factors (eg, different strains with varying virulence factors) and host responses (eg, level of acid hypersecretion, presence of duodenitis and/or gastric metaplasia).[25,26]

There have been several reports describing children and adolescents with refractory iron-deficiency anemia who have responded to treatment only after the eradication of *H pylori*.[27-30] The mechanism of *H pylori*–induced iron-deficiency anemia is unclear. Theories include *H pylori* acting as an iron-sequestering agent by means of its outer membrane receptors, which are able to capture and use iron for growth,[31] bacteria-associated changes in lactoferrin,[32] or intragastric pH changes that impair iron absorption.[33]

A diagnosis of *H pylori* infection and resulting mucosal disease can only be definitively made by upper endoscopy with biopsies. Nodularity of the antral mucosa (Figure 99-1) has been described in association with *H pylori* gastritis.[5] Histology provides information regarding the presence of *H pylori* (Figure 99-2) and the severity of gastritis. Further confirmation of infection

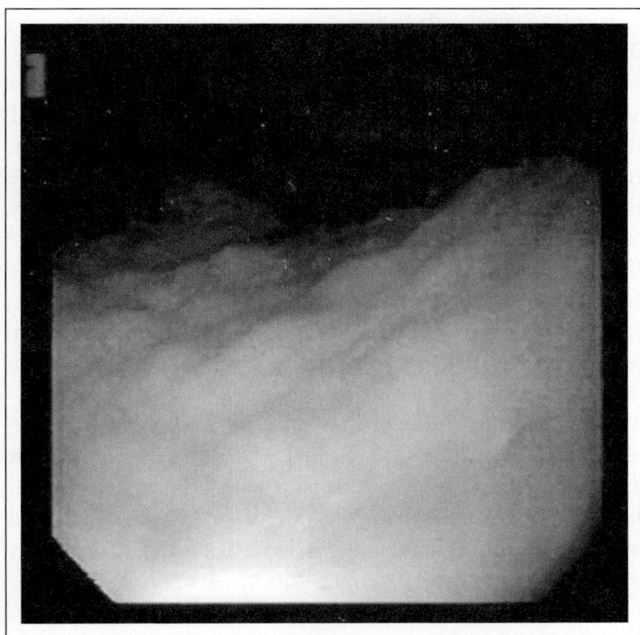

**FIGURE 99-1** Endoscopic picture of gastric antrum demonstrating nodularity often seen with *H pylori* gastritis infection. (See color insert.)

can be obtained at upper endoscopy with the use of a commercially available test based on the ability of *H pylori* organisms to produce urease. Biopsy material is placed in a chamber that contains urea and the test reagent; a color change from yellow to pink takes place within 2 hours if *H pylori* is present.

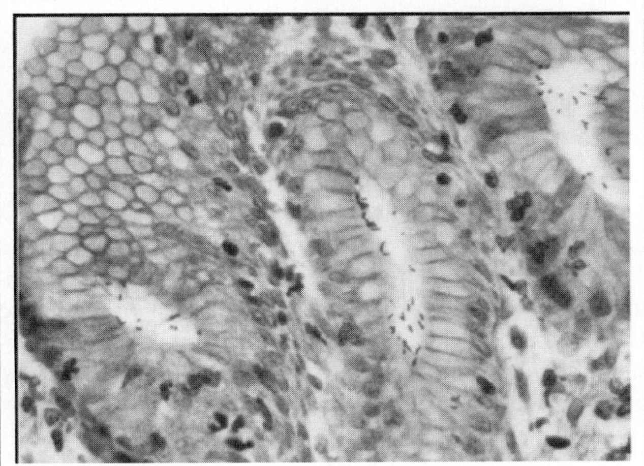

**FIGURE 99-2** Warthin-starry stain of endoscopic biopsy of gastric mucosa demonstrating *H pylori* gastritis infection (appearing as dark "dots" and "dashes" in the glandular space or surface). (See color insert.)

Although lacking the ability to define mucosal disease, a number of noninvasive, less expensive techniques, including serologic tests and URBs, have been developed to diagnose infection with *H pylori*. The presence of anti-*H pylori* serum IgG antibody titers (IgA or IgM antibodies are unreliable) has been confirmed to be an excellent measure of current or past infection in adult patients,[34] especially the third generation of this test. Unfortunately, this test is less sensitive and specific for younger patients. The carbon-13-labeled, UBT however, is a safe and noninvasive method for the diagnosis of *H pylori* infection in adults and children. Measurement of the enrichment of recovered carbon-13-labeled $CO_2$ in exhaled air by mass spectrometry following the ingestion of labeled urea indicates the presence of *H pylori* infection. The UBT has been shown to be 96% sensitive and 97% specific.[35] The detection of *H pylori* antigens in stool using polyclonal and, more recently, monoclonal antibodies provides a noninvasive method for identifying infected adults and children. One *H pylori* stool antigen test based on a polyclonal antibody is reported in adults to be 91% to 98% sensitive and 83% to 100% specific for the diagnosis of infection,[36] but it seems to be less accurate in children and adolescents.[35] The development of a monoclonal antibody has provided greater accuracy in stool antigen testing.[37]

## PEPTIC ULCER DISEASE

In contrast to erosions that are superficial, peptic ulcers are defects in the GI mucosa that extend through the muscularis mucosae. Prior to the 1980s, peptic ulcer disease was believed to be a primary or idiopathic disorder with a high rate of recurrence. It is now believed that most ulcers are related principally to *H pylori* gastritis. Studies in children have confirmed the association between *H pylori* gastritis and duodenal ulcer disease.[38,39] There are no accurate figures on the incidence of peptic ulcer disease in adolescents, but nearly three-fourths of all peptic ulcers are duodenal, and most occur within the duodenal bulb. Most gastric ulcers, in contrast, are secondary, being related to drugs, stress, and other factors. In 80% of adults[40] and almost 90% of children,[41] duodenal ulcer disease is associated with *H pylori* gastritis. Elimination of *H pylori* from the gastric mucosa results in healing of the duodenal ulcer without recurrence.[42]

The symptoms associated with peptic ulcer disease in the adolescent are variable, but more closely resemble adult rather than childhood patterns. Younger, preadolescent patients often present with atypical symptoms, such as recurrent vomiting, whereas adults and adolescents more commonly present with pain. The pain, which is often characterized as sharp or burning, is usually localized to the upper abdomen, particularly the epigastric region. The effect of eating on the pain is unpredictable, but classically symptoms are exacerbated by spicy or acidic foods. In contrast to recurrent abdominal pain (RAP), ulcer pain can often be nocturnal, awakening the adolescent from sleep. The pain of ulcers may spontaneously remit for times without any treatment. When present, vomiting is generally forceful; however, the effortless regurgitation of gastroesophageal reflux can also be mimicked. Bleeding can present as either hematemesis or melena, or it may be occult. Although life-threatening hemorrhage occurs in less than 5% of primary ulcers, it can be noted in as many as 25% to 50% of secondary peptic ulcers. Complications such as perforation or gastric outlet obstruction may occasionally be presenting symptoms, but the latter is rare in adolescents. The differential diagnosis of peptic ulceration is summarized in Box 99-2. It is divided into those presenting with abdominal pain and/or vomiting and those presenting with hematemesis.

The diagnosis of peptic ulcer or gastritis is best made endoscopically. Peptic ulcers can be visualized, and biopsy material from the duodenum and the antrum can be obtained. Biopsies are important because the ability to make the diagnosis and establish the etiology based on macroscopic appearances alone is limited.[43] There is often a poor correlation between endoscopic and histologic findings. In cases of severe hemorrhage, endoscopy offers the potential for therapeutic intervention (eg, with heater probe, bicap laser, or injection techniques) and diagnosis.

The therapy for non-*H pylori*-associated peptic ulceration in the adolescent is principally aimed at increasing gastric pH, either through suppression of acid secretion or through acid neutralization. Mucosal protective agents may also be used. The most commonly prescribed medications are listed in Box 99-3.

**Box 99-2**

***Differential Diagnosis of Peptic Ulcer Disease***

**Presentation: chronic abdominal pain/vomiting**

- Disorder of the esophagus
  - Gastroesophageal reflux
  - Esophageal stricture, membrane, web
  - Esophageal motility disorders
- Disorders affecting the stomach and duodenum
  - Antral web
  - Chronic granulomatous disease
  - Crohn disease
  - Eosinophilic gastroenteritis
  - Gastroduodenal motility disorders
  - Food bezoar
- Disorders affecting the intestine
  - Obstruction
  - Annular pancreas
  - Constipation
- Other conditions
  - Pancreatitis
  - Cholecystitis
  - Cholangitis
  - Bulimia nervosa
  - Pregnancy
  - Increased intracranial pressure

**Presentation: hematemesis**

- Swallowed blood from oropharynx or nasopharynx
- Mallory-Weiss tear
- Peptic esophagitis
- Esophageal varices
- Hemorrhagic gastritis (drug or stress induced)
- Congestive gastropathy associated with portal hypertension

**Box 99-3**

***Medical Therapy for Peptic Ulcer Disease***

**Agents that minimize intraluminal acidity**

- Acid-neutralizing agents
  - Antacids
- Antisecretory agents
  - H2-receptor antagonists: cimetidine, ranitidine, famotidine, nizatidine
  - Proton pump inhibitors: omeprazole, esomeprazole, lansoprazole
  - (Anticholinergics: pirenzepine)

**Agents that enhance mucosal protection**

- Prostaglandin analogs: misoprostil, enprostil
- Sucralfate
- Colloidal bismuth subcitrate

Patients with *H pylori*-associated peptic ulcer disease should receive treatment to eradicate the infection. There are 3, first line, triple-therapy regimens recommended by the North American Society of Pediatric Gastroenterology, Hepatology, and Nutrition, each consisting of a proton pump inhibitor and 2 antibiotics, given for 10 to 14 days (Box 99-4).[44]

## ANATOMIC OBSTRUCTION

### INTRINSIC CONGENITAL LESIONS

Most congenital anomalies of the stomach and the duodenum are noted during infancy or early childhood;

**Box 99-4**

***North American Society for Pediatric Gastroenterology, Hepatology, and Nutrition Position Statement: Recommended First Line Regimens for* Helicobacter pylori *Treatment***

Each regimen should be administered twice daily for 10–14 days:

1. PPI (1–2 mg/kg/day) + amoxicillin (50 mg/kg/day) + clarithromycin (15 mg/kg/day)
2. PPI (1–2 mg/kg/day) + amoxicillin (50 mg/kg/day) + metronidazole (20 mg/kg/day)
3. PPI (1–2 mg/kg/day) + metronidazole (20 mg/kg/day) + clarithromycin (15 mg/kg/day)

PPI, proton pump inhibitor.

Adapted from Gold BD, Coletti RB, Abbott M, et al. *Helicobacter pylori* infection in children: recommendations for diagnosis and treatment. *J Pediatr Gastroenterol Nutr*. 2000;31:490–497, with permission from Wolters Kluwer Health.

however, partially obstructing webs or membranes can remain asymptomatic until adolescence or adulthood. These rare anomalies occur primarily in the gastric antrum or the prepyloric area, and occasionally in the duodenum. Webs that are noted during adolescence can have luminal openings that vary from large to quite small central perforations. "Windsock"-shaped lesions also have been described, presumably resulting from the chronic "stretching" of a more typical membrane. Why these lesions begin to cause gastric outlet or small bowel obstructive symptoms after remaining quiescent for years has not been adequately explained. One explanation could be that inflammation and edema surrounding the central orifice result in impingement on an already limited opening. Patients may note epigastric pain, a sense of fullness, or gastroesophageal symptoms, but vomiting is most common. Antral webs may appear radiologically as a typical, contrast-absent, translucent line that sometimes creates the appearance of a "pseudopylorus." Webs may also cause markedly delayed gastric emptying or enlargement of the stomach and duodenum proximal to the obstructing lesion. Diagnostic endoscopy often reveals the nature of the lesion. Endoscopy can also be therapeutic because membranes and webs can be disrupted by "through-the-scope" balloon catheters. If surgical exploration is required, a deflated balloon catheter can be passed throughout the intestine. The balloon may then be inflated and slowly withdrawn to ensure that more distal and less obviously obstructing webs are not missed.

## EXTRINSIC CONGENITAL LESIONS

Although extrinsic obstruction of the stomach is rare, duodenal compression syndromes occasionally present during adolescence. The most common abnormality results from extrinsic fibrous bands, which may or may not be associated with malrotation. Less than 5% of all symptomatic malrotations occur after childhood; thus, adolescent cases are limited in number. When the diagnosis of extrinsic obstruction is made in an adolescent, the symptoms are usually due to intermittent partial obstruction, frequently occurring after meals. Often, however, evidence of partial obstruction is obtained unexpectedly, when an abdominal radiograph is taken for apparently unrelated reasons. Generally, the obstruction appears in the third portion of the duodenum. Similar clinical and radiographic findings have been described in adolescents and young adults with compression of the duodenum from the superior mesenteric artery or a preduodenal portal vein.

Extrinsic obstruction of the duodenum is also seen with an annular pancreas. In this situation, the obstruction is in the second portion of the duodenum and is commonly associated with underlying duodenal stenosis. Despite its congenital origin, patients with annular pancreas can initially present during adolescence; they then commonly complain of recurrent vomiting, pain, and, occasionally, hematemesis (often resulting from associated peptic disease). Pancreatitis usually does not occur. Diagnosis is aided by upper GI studies, which reveal symmetric narrowing of the second portion of the duodenum that may be associated with proximal dilation. Upper endoscopy often reveals peptic ulceration proximal to the extrinsically narrowed duodenum. Rarely, adolescents require surgery for unremitting obstructive symptoms. More commonly, vigorous therapy for the peptic ulcer disease results in marked symptomatic improvement.

## ACQUIRED LESIONS

A number of other disorders can ultimately result in obstructing lesions of the stomach or the duodenum.

Obstruction of the third portion of the duodenum from the superior mesenteric artery occurs in patients who experience marked weight loss. Adolescents with eating disorders and postoperative orthopedic patients with chronic supine positioning represent groups at high risk for this complication. Peptic ulcer disease can also produce scarring of the duodenum, pyloric channel, or antrum with resultant gastric outlet obstruction, but this particular complication is increasingly rare.

Chronic granulomatous disease (CGD) may also present with predominantly gastric/antral symptoms. It is an inherited (both X-linked and autosomal recessive) defect in the ability of phagocytes to produce superoxide and other reactive oxygen species. This results in recurrent and chronic infections with catalase-positive organisms, such as *Staphylococcus aureus*. Although the skin, lungs, and lymph nodes are the most commonly involved areas, various GI features can be present, including partial gastric outlet obstruction from granulomatous antral narrowing, as well as an enterocolitis that resembles Crohn disease. Chronic granulomatous disease should be suspected in a patient with Crohn-like findings who has recurrent infections or abscesses as seen in CGD or where the granulomas that were believed to represent Crohn disease contain foamy histiocytes that stain positive with periodic acid-Schiff (PAS). Diagnosis of CGD is confirmed by measurement of neutrophil respiratory burst activity such as performed in the traditional nitroblue tetrazolium test (NBT).

Other more common entities that can involve the stomach and duodenum are Crohn disease and eosinophilic gastroenteritis. These conditions may also occasionally delay gastric emptying anatomically by causing a marked narrowing of the gastric antrum and the proximal duodenum. Crohn disease is covered elsewhere in detail in this text (see Chapter 105, Inflammatory Bowel Disease). Findings in the gastroduodenal region can range from microscopic inflammation to granulomatous inflammation to mucosal erosions to full-blown serpiginous ulcers with heaped up margins. These latter, more severe lesions can give rise to obstructive symptoms secondary to antral or duodenal narrowing or altered gastric emptying.

Eosinophilic gastroenteritis is a clinical entity characterized by significant eosinophilic inflammation of the GI tract. Even though antral-duodenal inflammation is a known pattern, it can involve any portion of the GI tract. It is often associated with peripheral eosinophilia. Similar to what is found in patients with eosinophilic esophagitis, various food hypersensitivities may accompany the diagnosis in some cases, but many patients have no ascertainable sign of these problems. Although bearing some resemblance to childhood cow milk protein enteropathy, eosinophilic gastroenteritis, in comparison, is an uncommon finding in children, occurring with more frequency in teenagers and young adults. In the form involving the stomach, it often presents as vomiting and abdominal pain with weight loss. The antrum, in particular, is infiltrated with large numbers of eosinophils, and on a barium swallow study, a thickened antrum with consequent luminal narrowing can be observed. The differential diagnosis includes food allergy, hypereosinophilic syndrome, drug reactions, parasitic infection, *H pylori* infection, Crohn disease, connective tissue disease, CGD, celiac disease, and lymphoma or other malignancies.

## GASTRIC MOTILITY DISORDERS

The stomach, in addition to its secretory (acid, enzymes, and hormones) functions, plays a large role in digestion by virtue of its coordinated muscular contractions and relaxations. The proximal stomach functions as a reservoir, relaxing with each swallow to allow for an increase in gastric contents without acute increases in pressure. Ultimately, after a meal, the proximal stomach undergoes a sustained contraction to move contents to the antrum. The distal stomach serves to regulate the differential emptying of liquid, digestible solids, and indigestible solids into the duodenum. A 3 wave per minute cycle is generated in the distal stomach from the pacemaker region located approximately midway along the greater curvature. These contractions result in mixing of the meal, grinding of solids into particles of 1 mm size by contraction against a closed pylorus, and gastric emptying.[45] Liquids empty more rapidly than solids; digestible solids are not emptied until they are liquefied to 1 mm in size. Nondigestible solids are not emptied by this method. Instead, these solids are emptied during the fasting cycle of GI motor activity known as the migrating motor complex (MMC), specifically during the strong phase 3 contractions of the MMC accompanied by pyloric opening. Various factors (eg, meal osmolarity, fat content, acidity, amino acid content and volume) can affect the rate of gastric emptying.

Motility disorders of gastric emptying result when clinically significant alterations in these motor activities take place. Gastroparesis, delayed gastric emptying, is defined as an alteration in gastroduodenal functioning without structural or mucosal lesions present. Antral hypomotility and gastric outlet resistance due to pyloric dysfunction are possible causes. In general, signs of delayed gastric emptying in adolescents include nausea, vomiting, a sense of fullness or bloating, early satiety, and epigastric pain.[46] A wide variety of causes are associated with delayed gastric emptying, as listed in Box 99-5. The 3 most common causes are diabetes, post-GI

**Box 99-5**

***Conditions Associated with Chronic Delayed Gastric Emptying***

Anatomic (partial) obstructions
- Antral and duodenal webs
- Malrotation
- Crohn disease
- Eosinophilic gastroenteritis
- Chronic granulomatous disease

Pharmacologic agents[51]
- Opioids
- Anticholinergics
- Beta-adrenergic agonists
- Tricyclic antidepressents

Metabolic
- Hypokalemia
- Hypothyroidism
- Acidosis

Infectious
- Viral: Ebstein-Barr, herpes zoster, cytomegalovirus

Myopathic conditions
- Myopathic intestinal pseudo-obstruction (hollow viscera myopathy)
- Muscular dystrophy
- Progressive systemic sclerosis

Neuropathic conditions
- Diabetes mellitus
- Familial dysautonomia
- Multiple sclerosis
- Neuropathic intestinal pseudo-obstruction

Myoneuropathic or mixed
- Anorexia nervosa
- Gastroesophageal reflux
- Malnutrition
- Systemic lupus erythematosus

Other
- Idiopathic
- Post-GI surgery

surgery, and "idiopathic." Gastroparesis is believed to occur in 30% to 50% of those with type I diabetes mellitus, 16% to 30% of those with type II diabetes mellitus, and 20% to 40% of patients with functional dyspepsia.[47] It is always important to exclude anatomically based, obstructive causes. As noted, certain drugs are also well-known causes of emptying delay, and in the appropriate setting, metabolic/electrolyte disturbances should be investigated. Acute gastroparesis can arise from viral gastroenteritis, whereas chronic gastroparesis has been seen with herpes zoster, Epstein-Barr virus, and cytomegalovirus infections; this chronic gastroparesis can last months, usually with spontaneous recovery.[48] Chronic delayed gastric emptying also occurs secondarily in a number of systemic diseases. In adolescents, it occurs uncommonly as a result of one of the primary myopathic or neuropathic forms of chronic intestinal pseudo-obstruction. However, adolescents with anorexia nervosa frequently complain of fullness and early satiety; delayed gastric emptying that improves with treatment has been documented in those with significant weight loss.[49] Insulin-dependent diabetes mellitus is a common cause of chronic gastroparesis in adults; it can occur in adolescents as soon as 1 to 7 years after diagnosis.[50]

When (functional) delayed gastric emptying is suspected, anatomic abnormalities should first be ruled out with a radiographic contrast study and possibly esophagogastroduodenoscopy. The most commonly available measure of gastric emptying is through use of a nuclear medicine scintigraphic study. Meals are labeled with various radioisotopes, and the rate of emptying is calculated based on the disappearance of the label as determined by serial gamma-counter measurements, which are then compared to controls. Less readily available tests include electrogastrography, in which the myoelectric activity of the stomach is recorded by overlying electrodes attached to the skin, and antral duodenal manometry, in which pressure changes over time are measured by intraluminal catheters.

The outcome and treatment of adolescents with delayed gastric emptying is related to the underlying cause. When there is no underlying anatomic abnormality, surgical measures (pyloroplasty) performed to increase gastric emptying are usually not useful. Mild symptoms may respond to dietary measures, such as a low-fat and low-fiber diet and frequent small meals. Liquid or pureed meals may be better tolerated than solids. A history of constipation should be elicited, and treated if present, because resolution may favorably affect gastric emptying. Prokinetic agents, such as metoclopramide or cisapride (only available now for "compassionate use" due to reports of cardiac arrhythmias in certain clinical situations), or apparent motilin receptor stimulants, such as erythromycin, can be tried in more difficult cases. The most serious consequences of delayed gastric emptying are the adverse effects on nutritional status, with the resulting malnutrition further contributing to the gastric dysfunction. In more severe cases, enteral (usually continuous nocturnal nasogastric or gastrostomy tube) feedings are initiated, and if necessary, jejunal (nasojejunal tube, gastrojejunal tube, or jejunostomy) feedings can be used to bypass the stomach. The course and outcome for patients with delayed gastric emptying varies, ranging from rapid resolution of the dysmotility in those with acute, viral causes to potential dependence on elemental or parenteral feedings in those with primary neuropathic and myopathic intestinal motility disorders.

## REFERENCES

1. Miller TA. Mechanisms of stress-related mucosal damage. *Am J Med.* 1987;83(suppl 6A):8–14

2. Vorder Bruegge WF, Peura DA. Stress-related mucosal damage: review of drug therapy. *J Clin Gastroenterol.* 1990;12 (suppl 2):S35–S40

3. Marshall B. Unidentified curved bacilli on gastric epithelium in active chronic gastritis [letter]. *Lancet.* 1983;1:1273–1274

4. Peterson WL, Graham DY. *Helicobacter pylori*. In: Feldman M, Friedman LS, Brandt LJ, eds. *Sleisenger and Fordtran's Gastrointestinal and Liver Disease*. 6th ed. Philadelphia: WB Saunders; 1998:604

5. Drumm B. *Helicobacter pylori* in the pediatric patient. *Gastroenterol Clin North Am.* 1993;22:169–182

6. Go MF. Review article: natural history and epidemiology of *Helicobacter pylori* infection. *Aliment Pharmacol Ther.* 2002;16:3–15

7. Everhart JE, Kurszon-Moran D, Perez-Perez GI, Tralka TS, McQuillan G. Seroprevalence and ethnic differences in *Helicobacter pylori* infection among adults in the United States. *J Infect Dis.* 2000;181:1359–1363

8. Malaty HM, El-Kasabany A, Graham DY, et al. Age at acquisition of *Helicobacter pylori* infection: a follow-up study from infancy to adulthood. *Lancet.* 2002;359:931–935

9. Valle J, Kekki M, Sipponen P, et al. Long-term course and consequences of *Helicobacter pylori* gastritis: results of a 32-year follow-up study. *Scand J Gastroenterol.* 1996;31:546–550

10. Parsonnet J, Shmiely H, Haggerty T. Fecal and oral shedding of *Helicobacter pylori* from healthy infected adults. *JAMA.* 1999;282:2240–2245

11. Chemisnsky G, Blanchard S, Czinn S. *Helicobacter pylori* in children and adolescents. *Adolesc Med Clin.* 2004;15(1):53–66

12. Blaser M. *Helicobacter pylori* and the pathogenesis of gastroduodenal inflammation. *J Infect Dis.* 1990;161:626–633

13. Cover TL, Blaser MJ. Purification and characterization of the vacuolating toxin from *Helicobacter pylori*. *J Biol Chem.* 1992;267:10570–10575

14. Mahdavi J, Sonden B, Hurtig M, et al. *Helicobacter pylori* sabA adhesin in persistent infection and chronic inflammation. *Science.* 2002;297:573–578

15. Phadnis SH, Ilver D, Janzon L, et al. Pathological significance and molecular characterization of the vacuolating toxin gene of *Helicobacter pylori*. *Infect Immunol.* 1994;62:1557–1565

16. Satin B, Del Giudice G, Della Bianca V, et al. The neutrophil-activating protein (HP-NAP) of *Helicobacter pylori* is a protective antigen and a major virulence factor. *J Exp Med.* 2000;191:1467–1476

17. Ernst PB, Gold BD. The disease spectrum of *Helicobacter pylori*: the immunopathogenesis of gastroduodenal ulcer and gastric cancer. *Annu Rev Microbiol.* 2000;54:615–640

18. El-Omar EM, Carrington M, Chow WH, et al. Interleukin-1 polymorphisms associated with increased risk of gastric cancer. *Nature.* 2000;404:398–402

19. Fennerty MB. Is the only good *H pylori* a dead *H pylori*? *Gastroenterology.* 1996;111:1773–1774

20. Graham DY. *Helicobacter pylori* infection in the pathogenesis of duodenal ulcer and gastric cancer: a model. *Gastroenterology.* 1997:113:1983–1991

21. Graham DY, Yamaoka Y. Disease-specific *Helicobacter pylori* virulence factors: the unfulfilled promise. *Helicobacter.* 2000;5(suppl 1):S3–S9

22. Graham DY. *Helicobacter pylori* infection is the primary cause of gastric cancer. *J Gastroenterol.* 2000;35 (suppl 12):90–97

23. Forman D. The prevalence of *Helicobacter pylori* infection in gastric cancer. *Aliment Pharmacol Ther.* 1995;9(suppl 2):71–76

24. The EUROGAST Study Group. An international association between *Helicobacter pylori* infection and gastric cancer. *Lancet.* 1993;341:1359–1362

25. Zheng PY, Jones NL. Recent advances in *Helicobacter pylori* infection in children: from the petri dish to the playground. *Can J Gastroenterol.* 2003;17:448–454

26. Peek RM, Blaser MJ. *Helicobacter pylori* and gastrointestinal tract adenocarcinomas. *Nat Rev Cancer.* 2002;2: 28–37

27. Choe YH, Kim SK, Hong YC. The relationship between *Helicobacter pylori* infection and iron deficiency: seroprevalence study in 937 pubescent children [letter]. *Arch Dis Child.* 2003;88:178

28. Anniball B, Marignani M, Monarca B, et al. Reversal of iron deficiency anemia after *Helicobacter pylori* eradication in patients with asymptomatic gastritis. *Ann Intern Med.* 1999;131:668–672

29. Choe YH, Kwon YS, Jung MK, et al. *Helicobacter pylori*-associated iron-deficiency anemia in adolescent female athletes. *J Pediatr.* 2001;139:100–104

30. Kostaki M, Fessatou S, Karpathios T. Refractory iron-deficiency anaemia due to silent *Helicobacter pylori* gastritis in children. *Eur J Pediatr.* 2003;162:177–179

31. Barabino A. *Helicobacter pylori*-related iron deficiency anemia: a review. *Helicobacter.* 2002;7:71–75

32. Choe YH, Oh YJ, Lee NG, et al. Lactoferrin sequestration and its contribution to iron-deficiency anemia in *Helicobacter pylori*-infected gastric mucosa. *J Gastroenterol Hepatol.* 2003;18:980–985

33. Anniball B, Capurso G, Lahner E, et al. Concomitant alterations in intragastric pH and ascorbic acid concentration in patients with *Helicobacter pylori* gastritis and associated iron deficiency anaemia. *Gut.* 2003;52:496–501

34. Monterio L, de Mascarel A, Sarrasaneta AM, et al. Diagnosis of *Helicobacter pylori* infection: noninvasive methods compared to invasive methods and evaluation of two new tests. *Am J Gastroenterol.* 2001;96:353–358

35. Megraud F. Comparison of non invasive tests to detect *Helicobacter pylori* infection in children and adolescents: results of a multicenter European study. *J Pediatr.* 2005;146:198–203

36. Kabir S. Detection of *Helicobacter pylori* in faeces by culture, PCR, and enzyme immunoassay. *J Med Microbiol.* 1998;36:2772-2774

37. Suzuki N, Wakasugi M, Nakaya S, et al. Production and application of new monoclonal antibodies specific for a fecal *Helicobacter pylori* antigen. *Clin Diagn Lab Immunol.* 2002;9:75-78

38. Bourke B, Jones N, Sherman P. *Helicobacter pylori* infection and peptic ulcer disease in children. *Pediatr Infect Dis J.* 1996;15:1-13

39. Dohil R, Hassall E, Jevon G, et al. Gastritis and gastropathy of childhood. *J Pediatr Gastroenterol Nutr.* 1999;29:378-394

40. Peterson WL. *Helicobacter pylori* and peptic ulcer disease. *N Engl J Med.* 1991;324:1043-1048

41. Drumm B, Sherman P, Cutz E, Karmali M. Association of *Campylobacter pylori* on the gastric mucosa with antral gastritis in children. *N Engl J Med.* 1987;316:1557-1561

42. Goggin N, Rowland M, Imrie C, et al. Effect of *Helicobacter pylori* eradication on the natural history of duodenal ulcer disease. *Arch Dis Child.* 1998;79:502-505

43. Elta GH, Appelman HD, Behler EM, et al. A study of the correlation between endoscopic and histologic diagnoses in gastroduodenitis. *Am J Gastroenterol.* 1987;82:749-753

44. Gold BD, Coletti RB, Abbott M, et al. *Helicobacter pylori* infection in children: recommendations for diagnosis and treatment. *J Pediatr Gastroenterol Nutr.* 2000;31:490-497

45. Quigley EMM. Gastric and small intestinal motility in health and disease. *Gastoenterol Clin North Am.* 1996;25:113-145

46. Parkman H, Hasler WL, Fisher RS. American Gastroenterological Association technical review on the diagnosis and treatment of gastroparesis. *Gastroenterology.* 2004;127:1592-1622

47. Wang YR, Fisher RS, Parkman HP. Gastroparesis-related hospitalizations in the United States: trends, characteristics, and outcomes. *Am J Gastroenterol.* 2008;103:313-322

48. Sigurdsson L, Flores AF, Putman PE, et al. Postviral gastroparesis: presentation, treatment, outcome. *J Pediatr.* 1997;131:751-754

49. Rigaud D, Bedig G, Merrouche M, et al. Delayed gastric emptying in anorexia nervosa is improved by completion of a renutrition program. *Dig Dis Sci.* 1988;33:919-925

50. Reid B, DiLorenzo C, Travish, et al. Diabetic gastroparesis due to postprandial antral hypomotility in childhood. *Pediatrics.* 1992;90:43-46

51. Nimmo WS. Drugs, diseases, and altered gastric emptying. *Clin Pharmacokinet.* 1976;1:189-203

# CHAPTER 100

# Disorders of the Liver and Pancreas

HARVEY W. AIGES, MD

*This chapter was written by the late Harvey Aiges, MD, whose loss is felt by untold many. Dr. Aiges was a gifted and dedicated clinician, an inspiring and beloved teacher, and a warm and wonderful friend. He is sorely missed.*

Fortunately, the adolescent is less likely to develop serious liver disease than the neonate or the geriatric patient. However, the drug use and sexual experimentation of this age group make adolescents vulnerable to liver damage from hepatotoxic agents and at risk for developing acute and chronic hepatitis, both types B and C. In addition, adolescent girls tend to acquire autoimmune hepatitis (AH) more than any other group.

## DRUG-INDUCED HEPATOTOXICITY

Adolescents are particularly vulnerable to drug-induced hepatic damage because this physiologically and psychosocially explosive phase of life introduces many to the use of either prescribed or illicit drugs in therapeutic, recreational, or abusive ways. Recreational use of alcohol and illicit drugs at some time during the adolescent period is extremely common. These agents, even in limited amounts, by inducing the hepatic smooth endoplasmic reticulum and thus enhancing the excretion of substances requiring glucuronidation, may affect the metabolic activity of other drugs and medications. This is important to consider when prescribing medications such as anticonvulsants or estrogen-containing birth control pills because these agents may be less effective if the patient is using alcohol or illicit drugs.

Most forms of drug-induced hepatic injury spare children (acetaminophen is a good example; aspirin and valproic acid are exceptions). Adolescents are generally more vulnerable to hepatotoxicity than are children, possibly due to decreases in activity and inducibility of the hepatic mixed-function oxidase enzyme system and reductions in the glutathione content of the maturing hepatocyte in adolescents compared to children.[1]

### SUBSTANCE ABUSE

Although most illicit drugs are known to affect the central nervous and cardiovascular systems, the liver also can be damaged. Fatal hepatic necrosis in cocaine abuse has been reported, with a pattern of periportal necrosis identical to that seen in rodent models. Ischemic hepatic damage has been observed with the drug Ecstasy (methylene-dioxyamphetamine) and may be associated with specific HLA phenotypes.[2] Hepatic enzyme levels are often increased in heroin users, but this may be related to the fact that many of these individuals may show evidence of hepatitis B and exposure to HIV. Contaminants, such as talc or mannose in the diluent used to inject drugs intravenously, may cause a granulomatous hepatitis. Inhalation of halogenated hydrocarbons (carbona, carbon tetrachloride) and sniffing of airplane glue (toluene) have been associated with centrilobular necrosis that can lead to severe liver damage, hepatic coma, and even death.

Alcohol use and abuse is common among many adolescents. Ethanol is metabolized by the liver through a primary pathway that converts alcohol to acetaldehyde. This process causes an impairment of triglyceride secretion from the hepatocyte, which can cause development of a fatty liver even in the well-nourished adolescent. Other early changes associated with alcohol use may include enlargement of hepatocytes, which can lead to hepatomegaly and induction of microsomal enzymes. This change is manifested by an elevated $\gamma$-glutamyl-transferase level and mild increases in aminotransferase levels. The induction of the microsomal system may also interfere with the metabolic activity of other illicit drugs, resulting in potentiation of the effects of those drugs when combined with alcohol. More chronic or severe alcohol use can lead to alcoholic hepatitis and cirrhosis, which, fortunately, are exceedingly uncommon in adolescents. Alcoholic hepatitis, which develops in about 20% of chronic alcoholics, is associated with a high mortality rate. Alcoholic hepatitis is the intermediate step for about 75% of those who develop cirrhosis, although some alcoholics develop cirrhosis without ever manifesting overt hepatitis. The mechanisms for development of alcoholic hepatitis are still unknown.

### ANABOLIC STEROIDS AND ORAL CONTRACEPTIVES

The extremely competitive aura surrounding high school and college sports, and a desire on the part of many adolescents to enhance their appearance have fostered the abuse of anabolic steroids as a way of markedly increasing muscle mass. If such abuse occurs during the pubertal growth phase, premature closure of the epiphysis and, ultimately, shorter stature are likely. In addition, 17α-alkyl androgens—the oral form of anabolic steroids—are hepatotoxic, causing a cholestatic hepatitis in 2% to 3% of adolescents who ingest these agents. Adolescent girls who take oral contraceptives are at a slight risk (<0.01%) of developing cholestatic hepatopathy. In both cases, the abnormality is canalicular rather than parenchymal, resulting in elevations of alkaline phosphatase and bilirubin levels that are greater than elevations in transaminase levels. Patients who abuse anabolic steroids for prolonged periods also may develop hepatic adenocarcinoma later in life.

### MISCELLANEOUS DRUGS

Cyproheptadine (Periactin) is used as an appetite stimulant in thin or growth-retarded children and adolescents. Prolonged cholestasis has been reported with the use of this agent. Even after the clinical signs and symptoms of cholestatic hepatitis have disappeared in such cases, elevated levels of alkaline phosphatase and γ-glutamyltransferase may remain for up to 3 years, and liver biopsy reveals progressive portal fibrosis and decreased numbers of interlobular bile ducts. Similar findings have been reported with the use of certain psychotropic drugs, such as chlorpromazine and imipramine. Like these medications cyproheptadine has a tricyclic ring, and that structure may be involved in the hepatotoxicity of these agents. The potential hepatic damage is important in light of the recently noted tendency toward prescription of cyproheptadine, tricyclic antidepressants, and other psychotropic drugs for adolescents with psychiatric and gastrointestinal disorders. In addition, given the morbidities affecting adolescents with increasing frequency (eg, HIV, type II diabetes mellitus), it should be noted that drugs used to treat these entities can be hepatotoxic.[3]

## ACUTE HEPATITIS

In the past few years, a great deal of knowledge has been gained about the viruses that cause hepatitis. There are at least 5 such viruses, causing hepatitis A, B, C, D, and E. These are distinguished from other viruses that cause hepatic inflammation (eg, Epstein-Barr virus, herpesvirus, cytomegalovirus) by the fact that in general they cause hepatitis itself rather than a wider clinical illness that may include hepatitis. The relative prevalence of hepatitis caused by these 5 agents in American adults is hepatitis B, 50%; hepatitis A, 30%; and hepatitis C, 20%. Hepatitis D viral infection, which occurs only in conjunction with hepatitis B infection, is very infrequent in the United States; hepatitis E has been found only in Americans who have traveled to endemic areas in Asia, Africa, or Central America. Although the prevalence rate of acute hepatitis in adolescents has not been studied, it is believed to be close to adult levels. Details of the clinical features of the hepatitis viruses are presented in Table 100-1 and described in the following sections.

### HEPATITIS A VIRUS

The incidence of infection with hepatitis A virus (HAV), a RNA picornavirus, has been declining steadily in the past 20 years as sanitary conditions have improved and the introduction of universal HAV vaccination. However, the exact incidence is difficult to determine because so many cases are subclinical or anicteric and are therefore not reported. In the past, it was estimated that 30% of the adult US population show serologic evidence of previous HAV infection. The transmission of HAV is almost always by the fecal-oral route; very infrequently, transmission can occur percutaneously. The incubation period of the virus is about 25 days.

#### Diagnosis and Clinical Features

The diagnosis of HAV infection is made on serologic grounds. Liver biopsy is rarely indicated. The diagnosis is based on an immunoglobulin M (IgM) antibody that is first seen at the onset of clinical symptoms (about 5 weeks after exposure) and is evidence of acute infection. This antibody remains positive for 4 to 12 months. An anti-HAV IgG antibody develops at the end of the infection and remains positive for many years; it is evidence of previous HAV infection.

Symptoms of HAV are increasingly apparent in accordance with the age of the host. Eighty-five percent of children younger than 2 years who are infected with hepatitis A are asymptomatic (or have a viral upper respiratory illness), as are 50% of 2 to 4 year olds with the disease. Adolescents are usually symptomatic, with more than 75% of infected patients ill and 40% to 70% icteric. The symptoms of nausea, vomiting, malaise, anorexia, and cholestatic jaundice with pruritus (bilirubin >10 mg/mL) can be severe. However, almost all individuals with HAV infection, regardless of age, will recover. Fulminant hepatitis A is very rare, and chronic hepatitis A does not occur.

#### Treatment and Prevention

Because of the usually benign clinical course of acute hepatitis A, no therapy is indicated. However, immune serum globulin given before exposure or during the incubation period of HAV is protective against the clinical

**Table 100-1**

**Features of the Hepatotrophic Viruses**

| | *HAV* | *HBV* | *HCV* |
|---|---|---|---|
| Incubation | 2–6 wk | 1–6 mo | 2 wk–6 mo |
| Transmission | Fecal/oral<br>Blood/sexual (?) | Blood/sexual<br>Perinatal | Sporadic<br>Blood/sexual<br>Perinatal |
| Diagnosis | | | |
| Acute | Anti-HAV (IgM) | HBsAg<br>Anti-HBc (IgM) | Clinical |
| Chronic | N/A | HBsAg<br>Anti-HBc (total) | HCVAb<br>PCR (HCV RNA) |
| Sequelae | | | |
| Fulminant | 0.1% | <5% | <5% |
| Carrier | No | Yes | Yes |
| Chronic | No | Yes | Yes |

HAV, hepatitis A virus; HBV, hepatitis B virus; HCV, hepatitis C virus; HBsAg, hepatitis B surface antigen; Anti-HBc, antibody to hepatitis B core antigen; PCR, polymerase chain reaction.

illness. Close personal contacts and household members of patients with acute hepatitis A should receive immune serum globulin (2 mL intramuscularly) within 2 to 4 weeks of exposure. Treatment of casual contacts, such as schoolmates, is not indicated.

A vaccine against HAV is available. It can be given with immune serum globulin for postexposure prophylaxis (use at separate sites). Certainly, high-risk groups such as frequent travelers and day care workers should be vaccinated. Universal childhood HAV vaccination beginning at one year of age is now recommended as a two-dose regimen, with catch-up immunizations for adolescents recommended in higher-risk communities. Travelers previously unexposed to HAV planning to visit a developing country where hepatitis A is prevalent should receive a first dose of HAV vaccine before they travel.

### HEPATITIS B VIRUS

Hepatitis B virus (HBV) is a DNA hepadnavirus that is most often transmitted parenterally and through sexual contact. The virus has an incubation period of about 45 to 75 days. The disease has a very high prevalence rate in the Far East, Southeast Asia, and the Pacific Rim (including the Eskimo population of Alaska). The large number of people from these areas who become immigrants to the United States should make physicians aware of the possible consequences of hepatitis B (eg, in adults, cirrhosis and hepatocarcinoma; in infants, risk of perinatal exposure through a mother who is positive for the hepatitis B surface antigen [HBsAg]).

#### Diagnosis and Clinical Features

The HBV consists of an inner core (containing hepatitis B core antigen, hepatitis B e antigen, and DNA polymerase) and an outer surface shell (containing HBsAg). These antigenic markers have provided a serologic pattern to the diagnosis and various forms of the disease (Table 100-2). Routine screening for hepatitis B requires at least two serologic markers for maximal certainty. HBsAg is found in almost all patients who acquire the infection, and its rise coincides closely with the onset of symptoms. However, the surface antigen usually diminishes before the symptoms are gone so that a second marker, hepatitis B core antibody (anti-HBc), is usually needed to confirm the diagnosis. Although the hepatitis B e antigen (HBeAg) is not necessary for the diagnosis, it is an important marker, indicating viral infectivity in the patient.

**Table 100-2**

**Hepatitis B Virus: Serologic Findings**

| *Marker* | *Immunized* | *Acute* | *Recovered* | *Chronic* |
|---|---|---|---|---|
| Surface antigen (HBsAg) | – | + | – | + |
| Antibody to surface antigen (anti-HBs) | + | – | + | – |
| Antibody to core antigen (anti-HBc) | – | + | + | + |
| e Antigen (eAg) | – | + | – | ± |
| Antibody to e antigen (anti-e) | – | – | + | + |

Patients with hepatitis B are more symptomatic than those with hepatitis A. The asymptomatic patients tend to be infants and children, whereas adolescents commonly have clinically evident disease with symptoms of fever, malaise, anorexia, nausea, and vomiting. Twenty-five percent of adolescents with acute hepatitis B are icteric. In up to 10% of cases, extrahepatic (immune complex) symptoms predominate. A common presentation is a serum sickness-like illness with urticaria, arthritis (small joints), angioedema, and maculopapular rash. Other presentations include nephritis, nephrosis, myocarditis, and pancreatitis. Children may present with Gianotti-Crosti syndrome (papular acrodermatitis), an entity consisting of nonpruritic papules on the face, extremities, and buttocks associated with lymphadenopathy and anicteric hepatitis.

Fulminant, life-threatening hepatitis, although rare, can occur with hepatitis B. An asymptomatic carrier state (HBsAg positive, anti-HBs antibody negative for > 6 months) occurs in less than 0.1% of white Americans, but in 10% to 15% of Asians and Eskimos. Carriers (especially males) are at risk of developing cirrhosis and hepatocarcinoma, making hepatitis B an enormous worldwide epidemiologic problem. The chronic active form of hepatitis B can also result in cirrhosis and hepatocarcinoma.

### Treatment and Prevention

The prevention of hepatitis B is critical because of the high incidence of chronic hepatitis and the chronic carrier state with its subsequent risks. More than 90% of infants who acquire the infection perinatally become chronic carriers, as do 10% to 50% of adolescents.

Prevention can be accomplished by 2 approaches, the most important of which is hepatitis B vaccine, a recombinant DNA-synthesized vaccine that induces an antibody response to HBsAg. It is recommended for all infants as part of the routine childhood and adolescent immunization schedule, and all children who have not previously received the vaccine should be immunized by age 11 or 12 years. The safety of the recombinant vaccine and its potential for preventing this serious disease make it imperative for health care workers and others at risk to receive the vaccine before exposure may occur. There is no specific treatment for acute hepatitis B. If the infection becomes fulminant, liver transplantation is now considered a therapeutic option. Treatment of chronic hepatitis B with interferon alfa, lamivudine, and adefovir is becoming more commonplace because they have US Food and Drug Administration (FDA) approval for use in children; however, these drugs need careful monitoring when used, and this should be done by a pediatric hepatologist or physician experienced with their use.[4]

## HEPATITIS C VIRUS

In the United States, most non-A, non-B hepatitis (about 85%) is caused by hepatitis C virus (HCV). Hepatitis C is an RNA flavivirus transmitted primarily by parenteral exposure. The most important risk factors are use of intravenous drugs, transfusions, occupational exposure, and sexual exposure. Adolescents are therefore at risk of developing hepatitis C infection, with a prevalence rate in this age group estimated at about 0.4%. It is believed that the peak incidence of hepatitis C occurs between 15 and 36 years of age. About 0.5% to 1% of adults in the United States show evidence of previous hepatitis C infection. Another non-A, non-B hepatitis that has been described is hepatitis E. This RNA virus is transmitted enterally through epidemics in parts of the world where sanitary conditions are poor. In contrast to hepatitis C, hepatitis E is not a significant problem in the United States.

### Diagnosis and Clinical Features

The current diagnosis of hepatitis C infection is made by detection of an IgG anti-HCV antibody and by nucleic acid amplification testing (NAAT) to detect HCV RNA. Anti-HCV antibody is not protective. It can be positive while the virus is present.

Fifty to 70% of patients with hepatitis C develop chronic hepatitis. This is usually manifested by a fluctuating pattern of aminotransferase elevation, which occurs in approximately 80% of chronic cases. Most patients with chronic disease have a pattern of chronic active (aggressive) hepatitis, and 50% develop cirrhosis within 5 to 10 years. Primary hepatocellular carcinoma has been associated with chronic hepatitis C infection and cirrhosis.

### Treatment and Prevention

At present, there is no evidence that immunoglobulin is effective in preventing hepatitis C, and there is no vaccine currently in general use. Antiviral therapy (interferon) for acute hepatitis C is still emerging. However, the use of interferon α-2b in combination with ribavirin in patients with chronic active hepatitis C has been associated with improvement in approximately 50% of cases, although relapse is common after treatment has been discontinued. Current studies seem to indicate that very long-term or recurrent treatment may be necessary and will prove to be of greater benefit.[5-7]

## CHRONIC HEPATITIS

Chronic hepatitis is defined as an inflammatory reaction of the liver that continues for at least 6 months without resolution. This definition has been used to avoid mislabeling protracted cases of acute hepatitis, which may show evidence of biochemical and histologic aggressiveness for several months and then remit completely. The old nomenclature of chronic persistent and chronic active hepatitis based on histopathology is no longer used.

The term chronic hepatitis refers to a continuing inflammatory process of the liver that can progress to severe, irreversible destruction (cirrhosis) and death. Chronic hepatitis is associated with several etiologic agents, the most common being hepatitis C and hepatitis B infections. Autoimmune hepatitis is also seen relatively frequently in the adolescent population. Hepatitis D (delta) can evolve into chronic hepatitis. In the immunosuppressed teenager, other viral agents, such as cytomegalovirus, rubella, and Epstein-Barr virus, have been implicated in chronic hepatitis. The same histologic and clinical picture of chronic hepatitis has been described with isoniazid and methyldopa, as well as in Wilson disease and α1-antitrypsin deficiency.[8]

The mechanisms involved in the evolution and continuation of chronic hepatitis have not been totally clarified. The appearance of hepatic plasma cell infiltrates, hypergammaglobulinemia, and multiple immunogenic disturbances in patients with chronic hepatitis, and the favorable response to anti-inflammatory and immunosuppressive medications in some forms of the disease, suggest that immunologic factors are involved. It is assumed that various insults to the hepatocytes can create an antigenicity of the cells that may lead to a self-perpetuating antigen-antibody process with subsequent chronic damage. Cell-mediated immune reactions to liver cell antigens occur, and they involve sensitized lymphocytes and mononuclear cells. In vitro assays have shown that peripheral lymphocytes from patients with chronic hepatitis can destroy hepatocytes, but it is still unclear whether this is a primary or secondary event.

### AUTOIMMUNE HEPATITIS

Autoimmune hepatitis (the new nomenclature for autoimmune chronic active hepatitis) is a disease most frequently seen in adolescent and young adult females. It was first described in 1950 as an adolescent liver disease associated with acne, amenorrhea, and hyperglobulinemia. The disease has also been called lupoid hepatitis, plasma cell hepatitis, active juvenile cirrhosis, HBsAg-negative, chronic active hepatitis, and autoimmune hepatitis type 1.

#### Clinical Features

The initial clinical presentation of AH is variable, but usually falls into 1 of 3 forms: (1) prolonged typical attacks of presumed acute viral hepatitis, (2) insidious onset of malaise with or without jaundice, and (3) a finding of hepatosplenomegaly on routine physical examination. It is likely that the AH may have been present for months or years before the diagnosis is made in many patients. Amenorrhea is almost universal and should alert the physician to the possibility of chronic liver disease. Girls who are intrapubertal experience arrest of sexual development and may remain at Tanner stage 2 or 3 for a protracted time with primary amenorrhea. Girls who have reached menarche invariably develop secondary amenorrhea. The relationship between activity of liver disease and menses is so strong that physicians may use the return of menstrual flow as a marker of disease remission, especially during treatment.

Physical examination usually reveals a healthy-looking adolescent of normal size. Cutaneous vascular spiders, palmar erythema, acne, and striae may be apparent. Abdominal examination usually shows a very firm, nontender liver below the right costal margin. If the disease has progressed to cirrhosis, however, the liver may not be palpable at all. The spleen is frequently very enlarged. This splenomegaly may be secondary to reticuloendothelial hyperplasia and the spleen may shrink with therapy, or the condition may be the result of cirrhosis and portal hypertension, and therefore will persist.

### Extrahepatic Manifestations

Extrahepatic manifestations of this systemic autoimmune disease are common. Several of these are nonspecific, including fever, urticaria, erythema nodosum, generalized lymphadenopathy, and recurrent, nondeforming, migrating polyarthritis of the large joints. Specific extrahepatic disorders associated with AH include renal diseases such as nephritis, nephrosis, and renal tubular acidosis; pulmonary diseases such as pneumonitis and fibrosing alveolitis; a large variety of endocrinopathies; inflammatory bowel disease; and Coomb test–positive hemolytic anemia. These extrahepatic disorders may precede the clinical onset of AH, or they may appear during the course of the liver disease.

### Laboratory Findings

Serum aminotransferase (transaminase) levels are often elevated to 5 to 10 times the normal value. Bilirubin levels are often 2 mg/dL to 10 mg/dL, although values may be normal. The serum albumin level is usually in the low-normal range at the time of diagnosis, indicating that hepatic synthetic function has been preserved. Similarly, prothrombin and partial thromboplastin times should be normal. However, a patient occasionally presents with abnormal prothrombin and thromboplastin values; in such cases, the ability to synthesize coagulation factors is usually normal but an autoimmune circulating anticoagulant is present.

Serum globulin levels are markedly increased in AH. Serum IgG levels are almost always >2,000 mg/mL (usually this is reported as g/dL or g/L), and most often range between 2,500 and 4,500 mg/mL. The erythrocyte sedimentation rate is usually elevated. Most patients have markedly elevated titers of anti-smooth muscle antibody (SMA) or anti-nuclear antibody (ANA). A second form of AH, AH type 2, has been described (rare in North America) as being characterized by the presence of anti-liver/kidney microsomal antibodies (LKM) rather than SMA. Patients with AH type 2 are usually younger and have a more fulminant course than those with AH type 1 (SMA or ANA positive).

### Diagnosis

The diagnosis of AH is made by liver biopsy. This procedure is indicated in the presence of prolonged abnormalities of liver function; elevated IgG levels; and positive SMA, ANA, or LKM titers. The hepatic histology in this disorder is marked by the presence of an inflammatory infiltrate, usually made up of plasma cells and lymphocytes, that markedly expands the portal area. This inflammatory infiltrate extends beyond the portal area and erodes the limiting plate of the hepatocytes, causing individual hepatocellular, or piecemeal necrosis. If the cellular necrosis is more advanced, areas of necrosis are replaced by fibrosis, and "bridging" of fibrous connective tissue may be seen from portal area to portal area, or from portal area to central vein.

In view of the favorable response to medical therapy for this disease, it seems reasonable to evaluate any adolescent for AH if (1) acute hepatitis is apparent or liver function test results are abnormal, (2) serologic test results for infectious agents are negative, and (3) α-1–antitrypsin deficiency and Wilson disease have been ruled out. In these cases, if the IgG level is elevated and the SMA, ANA, or LKM is positive, a liver biopsy should be performed so that therapy can be initiated if a consistent histologic appearance is noted.

### Treatment and Prognosis

The drugs of choice for treatment of AH are prednisone (1–2 mg/kg/day), azathioprine (1–1.5 mg/kg/day), or its metabolite, 6-mercaptopurine (1–1.5 mg/kg/day). Treatment often induces biochemical, immunologic, and histologic improvement or remission, and there is no doubt that appropriate use of these agents can increase 10-year survival rates, even if cirrhosis develops.[9]

Many centers begin therapy with prednisone and continue the initial dose until a biochemical and immunologic remission is achieved. Prednisone is then tapered to a dose of <20 mg/day. Then 6-mercaptopurine is added and used as a prednisone-sparing agent, allowing a lowering of the prednisone dose to 10 mg every other day. This dose is low enough to avoid the growth-retarding and cosmetic problems associated with steroid use that are so upsetting to adolescents. Daily administration of 6-mercaptopurine and alternate-day use of steroids are continued for 2 years, at which time they are discontinued if liver function tests, serum IgG levels, and SMA, ANA, or LKM are close to or at normal levels. Experience suggests that most patients will need reinstitution of alternate-day steroids to maintain remission or stabilization of the disease.

Many adolescents with AH present with or progress to cirrhosis despite a good biochemical response to therapy. Even with cirrhosis, long-term survival is very likely, and a good quality of life possible. Some patients require liver transplantation.

## HBV CHRONIC HEPATITIS

Although most patients acutely infected with HBV have a complete recovery, 5% to 10% either become chronic carriers or develop chronic hepatitis. Infections that progress to chronic hepatitis seem to be dependent on the host's immune status and the ability of the HBV to continue replicating in the liver. It is possible that patients who contract HBV infection and have an impaired cell-mediated immune response will fail to clear the virus, and continued hepatocellular necrosis may ensue. It has also been noted in some patients that association of the delta agent (delta hepatitis) with HBV may increase the risk of development of chronic liver disease.

**Clinical Features**

Hepatitis B virus chronic hepatitis occurs predominantly in males 15 to 50 years of age, most commonly in intravenous drug abusers and homosexuals. In most cases, chronic hepatitis is not preceded by an obvious case of acute hepatitis B. However, in some patients, a mild acute hepatitis may progress to chronicity, or the patient may have chronic hepatitis at the apparent onset of the acute illness. It is interesting that patients who develop severe hepatitis B infection or survive an attack of fulminant viral hepatitis rarely develop chronic progressive disease. The condition may be recognized as unresolved acute viral hepatitis by prolonged elevation of the serum aminotransferase levels or by variable jaundice. The patient may be totally asymptomatic. However, most patients with HBV chronic hepatitis show signs of chronic liver disease, such as ascites, vascular spiders, and splenomegaly.

**Laboratory Data**

The serum aminotransferase and bilirubin levels are mildly elevated in patients with HBV chronic hepatitis. The IgG level is only moderately increased compared with the levels seen in AH. Likewise, SMA, ANA, and LKM titers are normal or minimally elevated.

HBsAg is present in the blood, and anti-HBc antibody also may be present. The diagnosis is made by the presence of HBsAg and a liver biopsy consistent with chronic hepatitis. The biopsy picture is similar to that of AH, except that HBsAg may be demonstrated as hepatic cells having a "ground-glass" appearance on orcein staining of the tissues.

**Treatment and Prognosis**

The therapeutic approach to HBV chronic hepatitis is emerging. As mentioned previously, interferon alfa, lamivudine, and adefovir are FDA approved and may have important therapeutic potential in the patient with chronic hepatitis B infection. This treatment may be associated with loss of hepatitis B DNA, seroconversion, and biochemical and histologic improvement in about one third of patients. This approach needs further evaluation.[10,11]

In most patients who do not respond to therapeutic interventions, the progression of the disease is slow and insidious. Patients with HBV chronic hepatitis may spontaneously go into remission, unlike patients with AH, who have a very high mortality rate in the first 2 years of disease if therapy has not been instituted. However, many patients with chronic hepatitis that is associated with HBV will slowly progress to cirrhosis and hepatic decompensation. A recent study has suggested that a poor prognosis may depend on the presence of e antigen. In addition, patients with HBV chronic hepatitis are at risk of developing primary hepatocarcinoma.

## OTHER LIVER DISORDERS OF ADOLESCENTS

### GILBERT SYNDROME

Gilbert syndrome is a common form of mild unconjugated hyperbilirubinemia. It is often first noticed or diagnosed in the adolescent because the jaundice may emerge during stress, illness, fasting, or menstrual periods. The serum bilirubin levels are usually less than 3 mg/dL, but occasionally may increase to as high as 7 to 8 mg/dL. The diagnosis is predicated on a mild, fluctuating indirect hyperbilirubinemia in the presence of normal liver function test results and absence of hemolysis.

In some patients, the mutation may be in the *1A1* gene. Hepatic glucuronosyltransferase activity is diminished, and there is an increased amount of monoglucuronides in the bile. These abnormalities are also seen in the neonate during the first few days of life and in patients with Crigler-Najjar syndrome type I (ie, total absence of glucuronosyltransferase leading to kernicterus). Serum bilirubin levels in Gilbert syndrome decrease with phenobarbital treatment. However, the benign nature of this entity makes therapy superfluous.

### WILSON DISEASE

Wilson disease (hepatolenticular degeneration) is a rare autosomal recessive disorder of copper metabolism first described in 1912 and considered to be a degenerative disorder of the central nervous system associated with cirrhosis. The clinical symptoms are related to excessive accumulation of copper in the liver, central nervous system, kidneys, cornea, skeletal system, and other organs. The reversal of abnormal copper metabolism in patients who receive liver transplantation strongly suggests that the primary defect for this disease is located in the liver. The abnormal gene responsible for this entity has recently been mapped and is located on chromosome 13. The specific gene defect responsible for Wilson disease seems to be *ATP7B*, which is involved in copper transport. Although the accumulation of copper in tissues begins in infancy, clinical disease rarely appears before age 6 years and more often in early adolescence. About 50% of patients develop symptoms by age 15 years.

### Clinical Manifestations

Most of the clinical manifestations of Wilson disease are related directly to copper deposition in specific organs. Most patients present with liver disease but neuropsychiatric findings are common, especially in the adolescent age group.

### Hepatic Symptoms

The hepatic symptoms, which usually appear first, can be nonspecific, mimicking a variety of acute and chronic liver diseases. In the early asymptomatic phase, or in the presence of inactive cirrhosis, liver function test results may be normal, or serum aminotransferase levels may be only minimally elevated. Wilson disease may present with clinical, biochemical, and histologic features like those of AH, which are again more common in the adolescent. It is certainly mandatory that Wilson disease be considered and evaluated in any adolescent with chronic liver disease. Occasionally, Wilson disease presents as fulminant hepatic failure, which is indistinguishable from massive hepatic necrosis and is usually rapidly fatal unless a liver transplantation can be performed.

### Neuropsychiatric Behavior

Adolescent patients with Wilson disease commonly show a significant fall off in school performance, behavioral changes that are aggressive in nature, or a psychotic disorder such as manic-depression or schizophrenia. An organic dementia can also be seen in teenagers with this disorder. The neurologic symptoms are subtle early in the course of the disease, but they progress if treatment is not begun. Lack of coordination and parkinsonian symptoms (eg, tremors, masklike facies) are most commonly seen.

### Miscellaneous Effects

Kayser-Fleischer rings (golden discoloration in the limbic region of the cornea) consist of granules of copper and are often seen in patients with Wilson disease; they are always present if there are neuropsychiatric symptoms. Acute Coomb test–negative hemolysis is the presenting symptom of Wilson disease in up to 15% of patients. The hemolysis is believed to be secondary to an oxidative injury to red blood cell membranes from excess copper. This hemolysis is usually transient and self-limiting. Renal tubular dysfunction, presenting as aminoaciduria, glycosuria, uricosuria, hyperphosphaturia, and hypercalciuria, may often be seen. The loss of calcium and phosphate may lead to bony demineralization. D-penicillamine, the primary mode of therapy, can also cause renal damage. Recently, cardiac dysfunction has been recognized in Wilson disease as a consequence of copper deposition in the myocardium, and it may present with arrhythmias, cardiomyopathy, and autonomic dysfunction.

### Diagnosis and Therapy

The diagnosis of Wilson disease is easy when the classic triad of hepatic disease, neuropsychiatric involvement, and Kayser-Fleischer rings is seen. However, in the absence of this triad the clinician must have a high index of suspicion to make the diagnosis so that therapy can be instituted immediately. No single test is diagnostic, and the work up may be frustrating. The serum ceruloplasmin level may be normal in 10% to 20% of homozygotes for Wilson disease and may be low in 10% of heterozygotes who do not have the disease. A slit-lamp examination for Kayser-Fleischer rings is necessary, but the rings may not always be present. The urinary copper level, which is usually very high (>100 μg/24 hours) in this disorder, is probably the best screening test in association with a slit-lamp examination. If the diagnosis is still unclear, a liver biopsy should be performed for a histologic study and for hepatic copper levels. Once the diagnosis has been made, the patient should be treated with D-penicillamine (a copper chelator). The usual adolescent dose is 250 mg administered orally 4 times a day. Usually there is impressive improvement in symptoms within several weeks. Patients should also receive pyridoxine 3 times a week to counteract the potential antipyridoxine effects of the chelator. In patients who have very serious side effects from penicillamine, an alternative chelating agent, trientine, has proved effective. The key to a successful outcome with either medication is early diagnosis, continuous maintenance of therapy, and a compliant patient.[12,13] In addition, a low copper diet and oral zinc therapy are necessary to decrease copper absorption from the intestines.

## UNCOMMON LIVER DISORDERS

Homozygous α1-antitrypsin deficiency is an autosomal recessive disorder associated with neonatal cholestasis and childhood liver disease and early adult-onset emphysema. The adolescent is usually not symptomatically affected by either liver or lung problems, although liver or pulmonary function test results may be abnormal. This diagnosis should be considered in any adolescent who shows biochemical or clinical evidence of chronic liver disease.[14]

An adolescent with no history of liver disease or with normal liver function test results who presents with hematemesis secondary to bleeding esophageal varices may have had silent hepatobiliary disease for many years. Cystic fibrosis, which can cause biliary cirrhosis, may be noted with signs of portal hypertension, but without evidence of liver disease. Other diseases that may manifest portal hypertension in the adolescent include congenital hepatic fibrosis/polycystic kidney disease, a heritable condition that can cause massive portal tract fibrosis with or without hepatocellular damage, and nodular regenerative hyperplasia, a noncirrhotic disease with regenerative nodules in the hepatic architecture. This entity may be an early manifestation of a collagen vascular disease.

## PANCREATIC DISEASE

Diseases of the exocrine pancreas are relatively uncommon in adolescents. Many pediatric diseases that affect the pancreas are the result of inborn errors of metabolism: for example, cystic fibrosis, Shwachman-Diamond syndrome, and exocrine enzyme deficiencies, which are most often diagnosed and treated before the patient reaches adolescence. In patients with cystic fibrosis, the pancreatic problems generally stabilize in adolescence but the hepatobiliary and pulmonary problems usually worsen. In Shwachman-Diamond syndrome, which is characterized by pancreatic insufficiency, cyclic neutropenia, and growth retardation, the steatorrhea improves when the patient reaches adolescence.[15] Pancreatitis can affect the patient during adolescence but its effects are more significant in adulthood, when alcohol abuse and hepatobiliary disease, especially cholelithiasis or choledocholithiasis, play an important role.

Most adolescents with pancreatitis develop the entity secondary to viral infections (eg, mumps, Epstein-Barr virus, coxsackie B4), *Heliobacter pylori* infection, trauma, or alcohol abuse. Other less common etiologies include hyperlipidemias, biliary tract obstructions, and drugs (eg, steroids, 6-mercaptopurine, sulfasalazine, valproate, thiazides). Signs and symptoms of acute pancreatitis include abdominal pain and tenderness, fever, and vomiting. A large amount of fluid may be lost from the vascular compartment. Laboratory evaluation usually reveals elevated serum amylase and lipase levels, as well as an increased amylase clearance. Treatment is directed at relief of pain and reduction of exocrine pancreatic secretion (nothing by mouth, nasogastric drainage, intravenous hydration), along with correction of fluid and electrolyte abnormalities. Acute pancreatitis may cause the development of a pseudocyst or a pancreatic abscess, or may lead to chronic pancreatitis or pancreatic insufficiency.[16,17]

## REFERENCES

1. Lee WM. Drug-induced hepatotoxicity. *N Engl J Med*. 1995;333:1118–1127

2. Brncic N, Kraus I, Viskovic I, et al. 3,4-Methylenedioxymethamphetamine (MDMA): an important cause of acute hepatitis. *Med Sci Monit*. 2006;12(11):107–109

3. Kress KD. Antiretroviral-associated hepatotoxicity. *Curr Infect Dis Rep*. 2005;7(2):103–107

4. Keeffe EB, Dieterich DT, Han SH, et al. A treatment algorithm for the management of chronic hepatitis B virus infection in the United States: an update. *Clin Gastroenterol Hepatol*. 2006;4:936–962

5. Zeuzem S, Buti M, Ferenci P, et al. Efficacy of 24 weeks treatment with peginterferon alfa-2b plus ribavirin in patients with chronic hepatitis C infected with genotype 1 and low pretreatment viremia. *J Hepatol*. 2006;44:97–103

6. Fried MW, Shiffman MI, Reddy KR, et al. Peginterferon alfa-2a plus ribavirin for chronic hepatitis C virus infection. *N Engl J Med*. 2002;347:975–982

7. Jonas MM. Challenges in the treatment of hepatitis C in children. *Clin Liver Dis*. 2001;5(4):128–152

8. Aiges HW. Chronic hepatitis. *Pediatr Ann*. 1985;6:439–445

9. Mieli-Vergani G. Autoimmune hepatitis in children. *Clin Liver Dis*. 2002;6(3):623–634

10. Janssen HLA, van Zonneveld M, Senturk H, et al. Pegylated interferon alfa-2b alone or in combination with lamivudine for HBeAg-positive chronic hepatitis B: a randomized trial. *Lancet*. 2005;365:123–129

11. Broderick A, Jonas MM. Management of hepatitis B in children. *Clin Liver Dis*. 2004;8(2):387–401

12. Tao TY, Gitlin JD. Hepatic copper metabolism: insights from genetic disease. *Hepatology*. 2003;37:1241–1247

13. Roberts EA, Schilsky ML. A practice guideline on Wilson disease. *Hepatology*. 2003;37:1475–1492

14. Sveger T, Erikson S. The liver in adolescents with alpha-1-antitrypsin deficiency. *Hepatology*. 1995;22:514–517

15. Aggett PJ, Cavanaugh PC, Matthew DJ, et al. Shwachman's syndrome: a review of 21 cases. *Arch Dis Child*. 1980;55:331–338

16. Trivedi CD, Pitchumoni CS. Drug-induced pancreatitis: an update. *J Clin Gastroenterol*. 2005;39(8):709–716

17. Werlin SL, Fish DL. The spectrum of valproic acid-associated pancreatitis. *Pediatrics*. 2006;118(4):1660–1663.

# CHAPTER 101

## Diseases of the Gallbladder

ERIC LAZAR, MD

Diseases of the gallbladder is relatively uncommon but not rare in the healthy adolescent. Most gallbladder disorders are a manifestation of gallstones and their sequelae. Further, most gallstones are asymptomatic. Noncalculus manifestations of gallbladder disease include acalculus cholecystitis, gallbladder dyskinesia, and polyps and should be considered in the differential diagnosis of right upper quadrant (RUQ) pain.

### ASYMPTOMATIC STONES

The incidence of asymptomatic stones is difficult to know with any certainty because such stones are found on abdominal imaging obtained to evaluate abdominal complaints. Accordingly, these stones may not be truly asymptomatic. This caveat aside, the occurrence of adolescents developing symptoms or complications from asymptomatic stones identified in childhood is low, ranging from 0% to 33%.[1,2] Therefore, asymptomatic stones may safely be observed until the onset of symptoms reasonably attributable to their presence. Such symptoms and findings might include colicky postprandial RUQ pain; constant, penetrating RUQ pain with fever and focal tenderness; or symptoms leading to an evaluation that reveals common duct obstruction or pancreatitis. In each situation, cholecystectomy will ultimately be needed to prevent recurrent symptoms or disease.

### RISK FACTORS FOR STONE FORMATION

Stone formation in adolescence may reflect stones persisting from cholestatic states in infancy and early childhood. There are a variety of factors that lead to stone formation, even in the earliest years. Total parenteral nutrition (TPN) administration for a premature infant with functional gastrointestinal failure, short gut syndrome, or ileal resection can lead to sludge or stone formation. Hemolytic states such as Rh incompatibility, hereditary anemias (sickle cell disease, spherocytosis, thalassemia), or drug-induced hemolysis produce excessive pigment that leads to the precipitation of pigment stones. Other disease states such as inflammatory bowel disease and cystic fibrosis can lead to cholestasis as a result of either the disease process or its treatment. In addition, cyclosporine used for those with renal and cardiac transplantation is a known source of gallstones. However, because cholecystectomy is routinely performed on the donor liver prior to transplant, liver transplant recipients will not develop gallstones.

Some stones are acquired later. Obesity, increasingly prevalent in adolescence, is a cholestatic state, and treatment of obesity resulting in rapid weight loss contributes to stone formation as well. As more adolescents are considered candidates for obesity surgery, we can reasonably expect to see an increase in gallstone-related disease. Pregnancy causes cholestasis, and the prevention of pregnancy using oral contraceptives has also been associated with stone formation.[3]

Other important causes of stone formation relate to the composition of bile, which may be altered in chronic hemolytic states such as sickle cell disease, hereditary spherocytosis, and thalassemia. Hypercholesterolemic states, hereditary or acquired, can unfavorably affect the composition of bile. Cholestasis and lithogenic bile separately and together can result in the precipitation of stones and resulting symptoms. These conditions often lead to symptoms necessitating cholecystectomy.

The composition of gallstones differs in the adolescent population compared to adults, in whom the most common stones are cholesterol based. As adolescents approach adulthood, their stones are more commonly cholesterol based, particularly in the obese. Younger patients tend to have black pigmented stones that are calcium bilirubinate based, but there is recent work suggesting a high incidence of calcium carbonate stones.[4] These latter stones are more common in stasis conditions, TPN use, and hemolysis, but the clinical importance of stone type in the modern era is immaterial because stone dissolution is not routinely practiced.

### PRESENTING SYMPTOMS

Presentation of the patient with gallbladder disease has some rather constant features. There may be a prodromal phase of intermittent RUQ pain that is precipitated by a fat-laden meal. This is known as biliary colic and is the mildest form of symptomatic disease. This results from intermittent obstruction of the gallbladder outlet by a stone as the gallbladder contracts to empty in response to fat in the diet. Because the gallbladder cannot empty, temporarily frustrated by the obturating stone, pressure remains high, and there is smooth muscle spasm resulting in pain. As the contraction subsides, the stone drops back into the gallbladder and relieves the obstruction. This process is mediated by the hormone cholecystokinin (CCK), which is upregulated by the presence of lipid in the antrum and duodenum, and results in gallbladder smooth muscle contraction and sphincter of Oddi relaxation.

At some point, a small stone may be propelled into the cystic duct, obstructing it without subsequent relief. The previously described scenario of colic progresses to unremitting pain. Prolonged obstruction of the gallbladder results in the emergence of an inflammatory process and fever, which marks cholecystitis. Hence, fever and persistent RUQ pain will have correlates of leukocytosis and affirmative signs on imaging.

Sometimes, a small stone passes through the cystic duct and comes to rest within the common duct, where it may reach 1 of several fates. For a time, it may lie asymptomatic, but ultimately it will enlarge in situ. It may subsequently pass through the sphincter of Oddi, which is marked by severe midepigastric pain. Pain may subside with complete passage of the stone or may persist with obstruction of the duct. Common duct obstruction can lead to biliary hypertension and stasis, which can result in life-threatening ascending cholangitis or pancreatitis.

Stone-related disease is overwhelmingly the most common pathway for the manifestation of gallbladder disease in the adolescent; however, one must always consider the possibility of persistent congenital disease that went undetected during childhood. A choledochal cyst can present in the teenager, as can Caroli disease (a rare congenital disorder of the intrahepatic bile ducts). The presence of a biliary tract tumor is extraordinarily rare in the younger patient, but can occur, particularly in the setting of longstanding inflammatory bowel disease. Increasingly, we are diagnosing dysfunctional gallbladder emptying, so-called gallbladder dyskinesia. Here, the symptoms are similar to biliary colic yet they occur in the absence of stones. Although uncommon, polyps can be formed within the gallbladder and cause symptoms that can mimic stone disease. Last, although rare, cholecystitis has followed blunt abdominal trauma, likely on the basis of vascular disruption via injury to the cystic artery.[5]

## ASSESSMENT OF THE PATIENT

The evaluation of the patient with RUQ pain always begins with a careful history and an eye toward eliciting risk factors. The physical examination is focused on the presence of fever or tachycardia, jaundice, and RUQ mass or peritonitis. Tenderness in the RUQ that is worsened on palpation during deep inspiration is the well-known Murphy sign. The initial selection of laboratory values is broad and includes assessment of aspartate, alanine, and gamma-glumatyl transaminases (AST, ALT, GGT), alkaline phosphatase, bilirubin (total and direct), and amylase/lipase. Gamma-glumatyl transaminases is proportionately higher in states of obstruction compared to the more modest elevations of ALT and AST. Very high elevations of ALT and AST must raise the suspicion of hepatitis. Elevations of amylase and lipase will raise the possibility of pancreatitis, either as an alternative primary diagnosis or as a consequence of stone disease. A leukocyte count is valuable in assessing the presence of a process escalating beyond biliary colic. Urinalysis can be helpful in confirming biliary obstruction by elevated excreted bile conjugates but is more valuable in excluding urinary tract infection. All patients with RUQ pain should have an initial hepatitis serology panel because there is significant similarity in symptom patterns, and the demonstration of gallstones does not preclude the possibility of hepatitis.

The gold standard imaging modality in gallbladder disease is the abdominal sonogram. The sonogram can detect stones or sludge in the gallbladder, as well as intrahepatic or common duct dilation resulting from stone obstruction. Gallbladder wall thickening and fluid around the gallbladder indicate cholecystitis. The examination can reproduce the pain on deep inspiration by the patient (a sonographic Murphy sign). In addition, the right kidney is assessed, which can exclude a renal source of RUQ symptoms.

Nuclear scintography (the hepatobiliary iminodiacetic acid [HIDA] scan) can yield functional information regarding the liver and gallbladder. Prompt uptake of agent by the liver and excretion in the bile demonstrates that hepatocellular function is intact. The gallbladder may fail to fill if the cystic duct is obstructed and bile cannot be concentrated within the gallbladder. The gallbladder may fill but cannot contract to empty in functional disorders or obstruction of the common duct. It is very important that the results of radionucleotide imaging of the gallbladder be interpreted in the setting of information obtained from the sonogram. Failure of the gallbladder to fill in the absence of gallstones on sonography, particularly in a critically ill patient, suggests acalculus cholecystitis. Although quite infrequent, it must be considered in a critically ill patient who experiences a clinical decline with focal RUQ pain. Similarly, the gallbladder may fill but does not empty, and the sonogram fails to demonstrate common duct stones. In this latter situation, the absence of stones in the common duct suggests the possibility of biliary (gallbladder) dyskinesia, which can be confirmed by the administration of CCK. Cholecystokinin

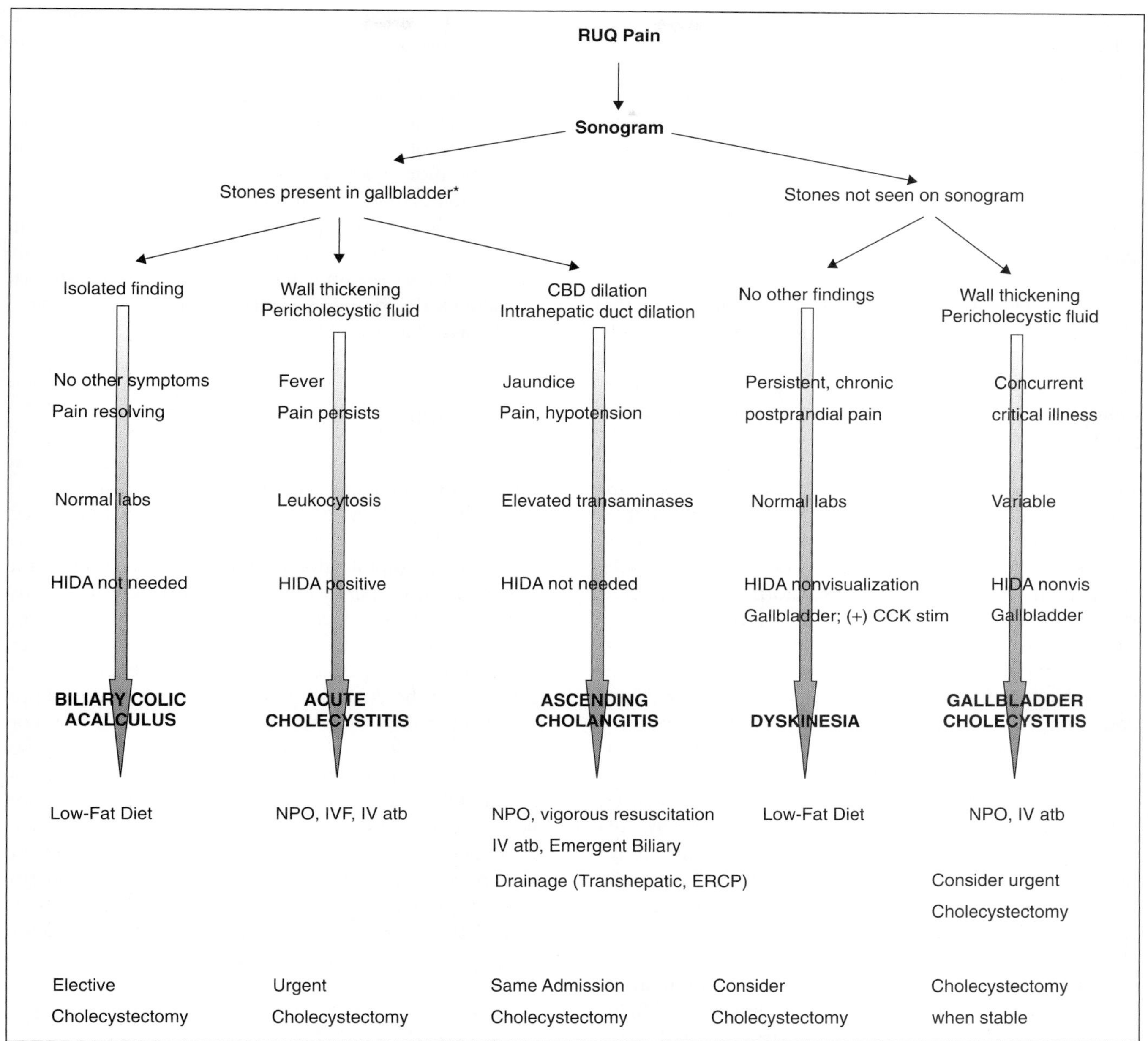


**FIGURE 101-1** Various manifestations of gallstone disease are considered in light of the presentation, clinical findings, and sonographic evaluation.*In any of these scenarios, gallstone pancreatitis may obscure the underlying gallbladder disorder and mandates some evaluation of the common duct with drainage as needed. Cholecystectomy will be required.

should reproduce the symptoms of RUQ pain and yet fail to prompt emptying of the gallbladder. An ejection fraction may be calculated, and values less than 35% ejection are consistent with the diagnosis. Figure 101-1 summarizes the evaluation of the patient with RUQ pain for the most common forms of gallbladder disease.

Computed tomography (CT) is usually unnecessary to evaluate gallbladder disease in the adolescent. Despite this, it is often obtained in the setting of abdominal pain, sometimes as a substitute for a careful assessment and methodical evaluation. Because we know that many stones are asymptomatic, the demonstration of stones on CT may be misleading to the clinician and halt other avenues of inquiry. However, the CT scan can miss smaller stones or those that are not calcified. The ionizing radiation exposure is cumulative over the life of the patient, and the test should only be ordered with specific diagnostic questions in mind after a careful clinical evaluation.

## TREATMENT

The treatment of gallbladder disease is tailored to the clinical scenario. Truly asymptomatic stones can be safely observed. Biliary colic is initially treated with a low-fat diet and non-narcotic analgesics with elective cholecystectomy planned. With the advent of laparoscopic cholecystectomy and its promise of rapid recovery, gallbladder removal is performed in preference to medical stone dissolution or lithotripsy, neither of which are part of the modern armamentarium in the treatment of gallstone disease. In the setting of cholecystitis, admission is arranged, and intravenous fluids and antibiotics are administered with cholecystectomy contemplated within the first day of admission. If the presentation of stone disease is pancreatitis, the patient is supported through the course of the pancreatitis until the pain is resolved and the laboratory values are normalized; cholecystectomy is performed at that time to prevent recurrent pancreatitis. There must be confidence that the common duct does not contain stones, either by visualizing normal ducts on sonogram and normalized laboratory values or by means of cholangiography. This can be accomplished via endoscopy (endoscopic retrograde cholangiopancreatography [ERCP]), via magnetic resonance imaging (magnetic resonance cholangiopancreatography [MRCP]), or an intraoperative cholangiogram obtained during cholecystectomy.

Ascending cholangitis, although less common, is viewed as a life-threatening emergency; intravenous fluids and antibiotics aimed at common biliary tract pathogens are rapidly instituted, and the biliary tree must be urgently decompressed. This may be accomplished by the radiologist in a transhepatic fashion or the endoscopist via the sphincter of Oddi. After drainage and stabilization, often requiring several days, cholecystectomy is planned.

Choledochal cyst is treated with excision and enterohepatic reconstruction, as dictated by the type of cyst present. Malignancy is also treated by extirpation, with survival directly related to elimination of gross disease. These latter 2 conditions are unusual and should be managed by either a pediatric surgeon or an experienced hepatobiliary surgeon. Polyps are often treated with cholecystectomy but may be observed with serial sonograms when small and unassociated with stones. Although malignant transformation has been observed in adults, this has not been shown in polyps of juvenile and adolescent onset.[6]

Some controversy exists regarding whether to treat biliary dyskinesia. Although some authors favor cholecystectomy, others are concerned that this entity may signify a more global dysmotility disorder and consider cholecystectomy unnecessary in that context. This author favors laparoscopic cholecystectomy in the absence of any other plausible cause for the symptoms when a CCK-stimulated, radionucleotide study that reproduces the patient's symptoms. Results have been excellent and affirmed by others.[7]

## OUTCOMES

Although the various forms of gallbladder disease may require different initial supportive strategies, in the end, cholecystectomy is a final common pathway. Cholecystectomy is well tolerated and when accomplished in experienced hands, complications are unusual. Nonetheless, the patient and their parents should be apprised of the possibility of common duct injury, bile leak, or unsuspected common duct obstruction. The latter problem is avoided by use of an intraoperative cholangiogram in cases where the status of the duct cannot be confidently deduced preoperatively. Conversion to open operation is uncommon and usually anticipated on the basis of pre-existing adhesions from previous operations. Patients are rapidly mobilized and fed after laporoscopic surgery, usually that same day, and discharged in 24 hours or less. Restrictive diets are unnecessary; normal amounts of fat in the diet are well tolerated. Two recent large series reporting on laparoscopic cholecystectomy in children and adolescents parallel the excellent results in adults with rare, minor complications and rapid relief of symptoms.[8,9]

## SUMMARY

Understanding gallbladder disease in adolescents essentially parallels understanding the natural history of gallstones. Asymptomatic gallstones may be safely followed in most patients; however, in patients with symptoms, cholecystectomy will be needed. The timing of surgery and the auxiliary evaluation of the common duct vary, depending on the clinical scenario. Outcomes for the vast majority of patients are excellent. Non-stone-related gallbladder disease, such as choledochal cyst, polyps, and acalculus states, are less common and generally more complex, and must be considered in the differential diagnosis, depending on the clinical presentation and patient assessment.

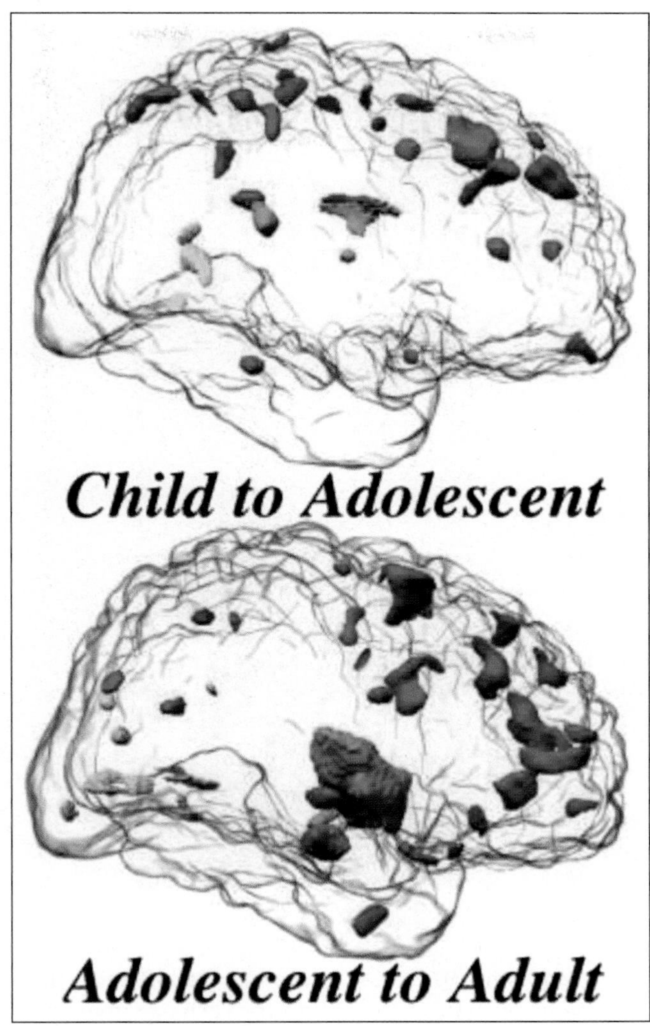


**FIGURE 5-1** Top: Child minus adolescent statistical map for the negative age effects representing gray matter density reductions observed between childhood and adolescence and Bottom: adolescence and adulthood. These maps are 3-dimensional renderings of the traditional statistical maps shown inside the transparent cortical surface rendering of one representative subject's brain. Lobes and the subcortical region were defined anatomically on the same subject's brain. Color coding is applied to each cluster based on its location within the representative brain. Clusters are shown in the frontal lobes (purple), parietal lobes (red), occipital lobes (yellow), temporal lobes (blue), and subcortical region (green). Note the increase in maturational changes in the frontal lobes between adolescence and adulthood relative to the same region in the child-to-adolescent map. (Bottom image reprinted from Sowell ER, Thompson PM, Holmes CJ, Jernigan TL, Toga AW. *In vivo* evidence for post-adolescent brain maturation in frontal and striatal regions. *Nat Neurosci.* 1999a; 2: 859–861, with permission from Macmillan Publishers, Ltd.)

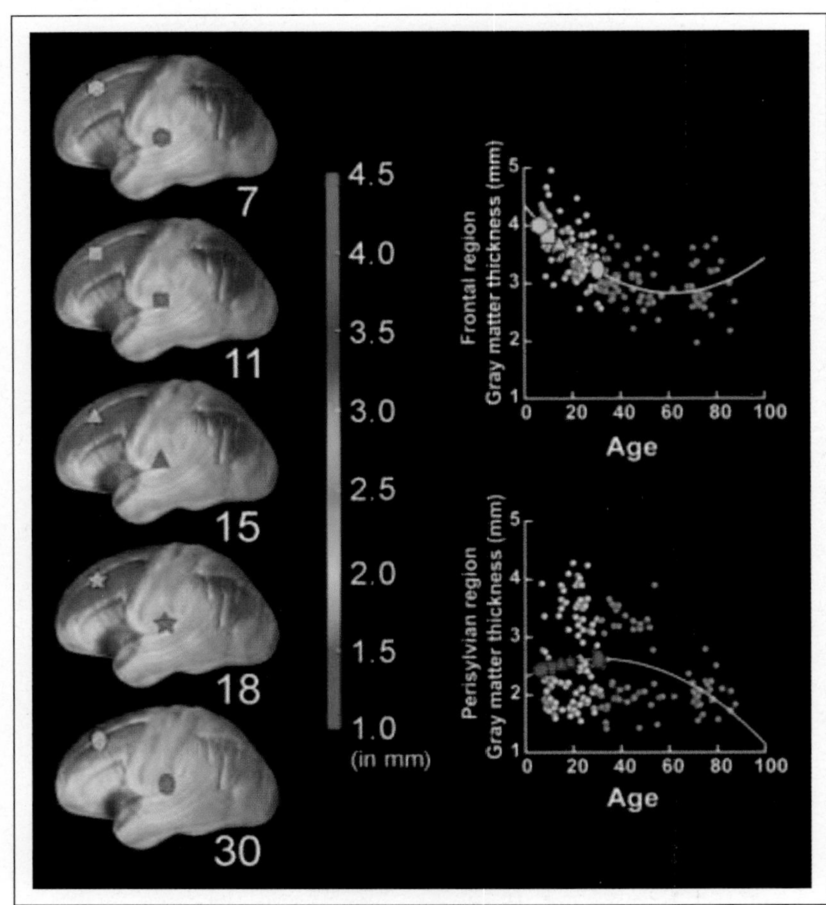


**FIGURE 5-2** Each map represents average cortical thickness in millimeters, color coded according to the color bar, for each of the represented ages between 7 and 30 years. Graphs represent the age function in each of 2 regions, dorsal frontal (top) and posterior perisylvian (bottom). Symbols for each age map shown on the left are placed in the appropriate age location on the regression line for each graph. Perisylvian thickness values are shown in red for each map in the bottom graph, and dorsal frontal thickness values are shown in yellow on the top graph. The data points in the graphs represent each subject (under age 30 represented here in white) and highlight the variability across subjects. Variability in regional patterns is also appreciated, with gray matter thickening between 7 and 30 years in perisylvian cortices and cortical thinning during the same time frame in dorsal frontal regions (based on data presented in Sowell et al, *Nat Neuroscience*. 2003; Sowell et al, *Cereb Cortex*. 2007).

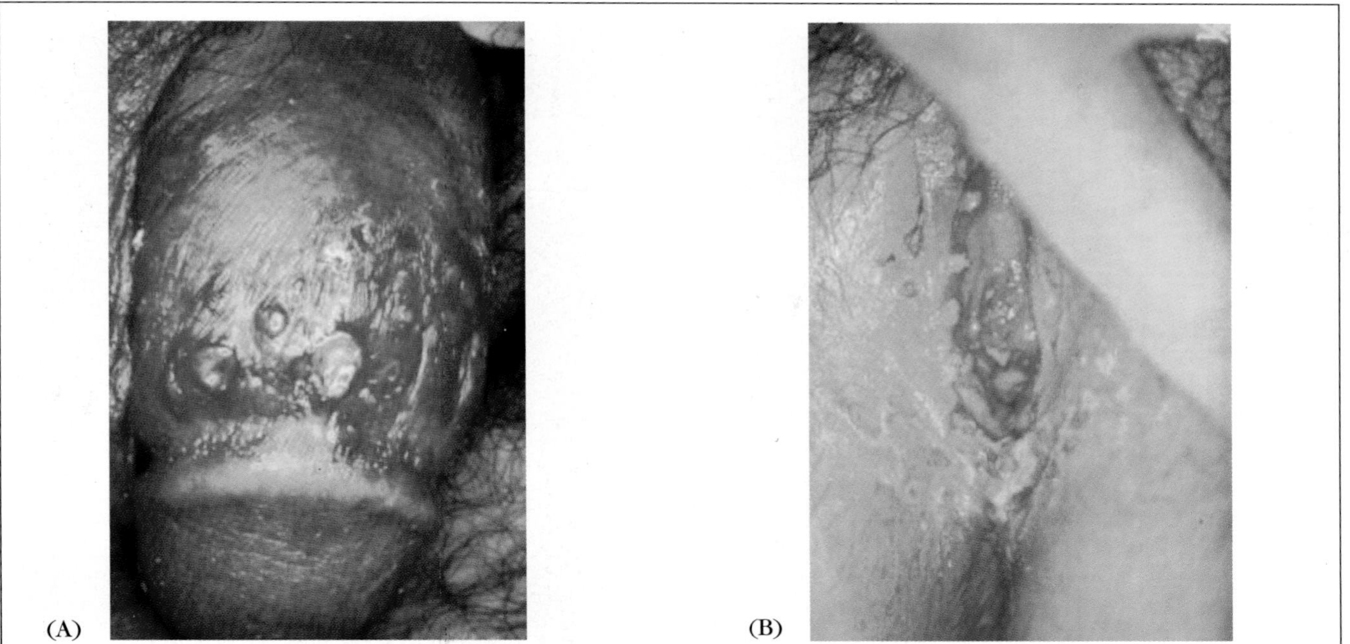


**FIGURE 53-1** Herpes Simplex Virus (HSV). (A) Primary HSV in a male patient. (B) Primary HSV in a female patient. (From Centers for Disease Control and Prevention (CDC), Training and Health Communication Branch of the Division of STD Prevention, National Center for HIV/AIDS, Viral Hepatitis, STD, and TB Prevention. Available at: www.cdc.gov/std/training/clinicalslides/slides-dl.htm.)

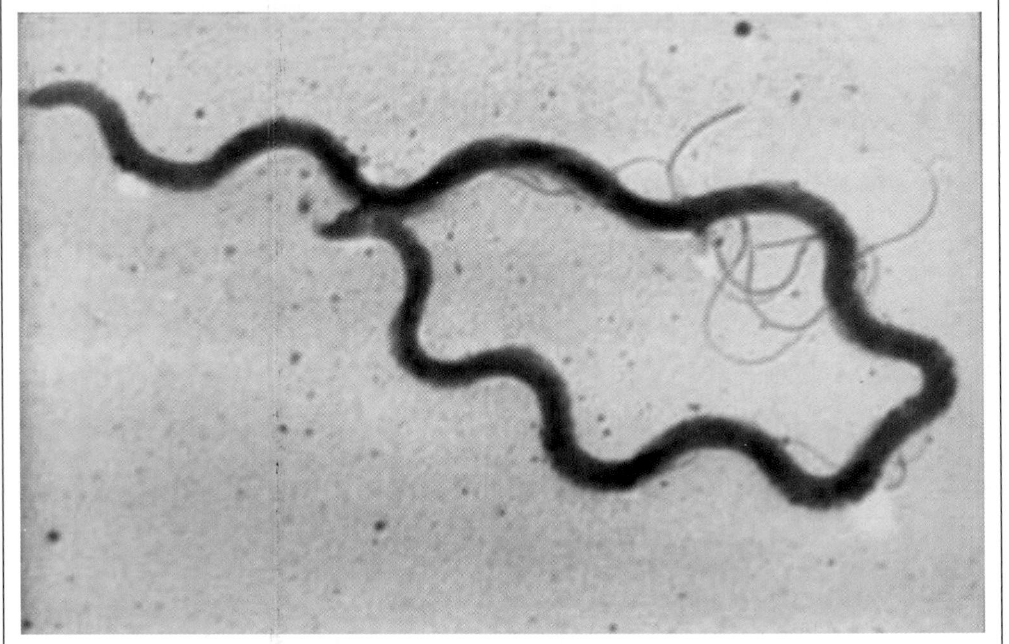

**FIGURE 53-2** Syphilis: *Treponema pallidum* organism. (From Centers for Disease Control and Prevention (CDC), Training and Health Communication Branch of the Division of STD Prevention, National Center for HIV/AIDS, Viral Hepatitis, STD, and TB Prevention. Available at: www.cdc.gov/std/training/clinicalslides/slides-dl.htm.)

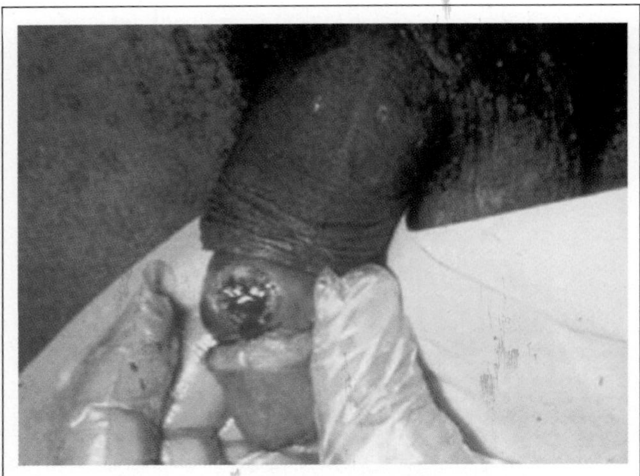

**FIGURE 53-3** Primary syphilis: Chancre on penis. Reprinted with permission of Centers for Disease Control and Prevention (CDC), Training and Health Communication Branch of the Division of STD Prevention, National Center for HIV/AIDS, Viral Hepatitis, STD, and TB Prevention. (Available at: www.cdc.gov/std/training/clinicalslides/slides-dl.htm.)

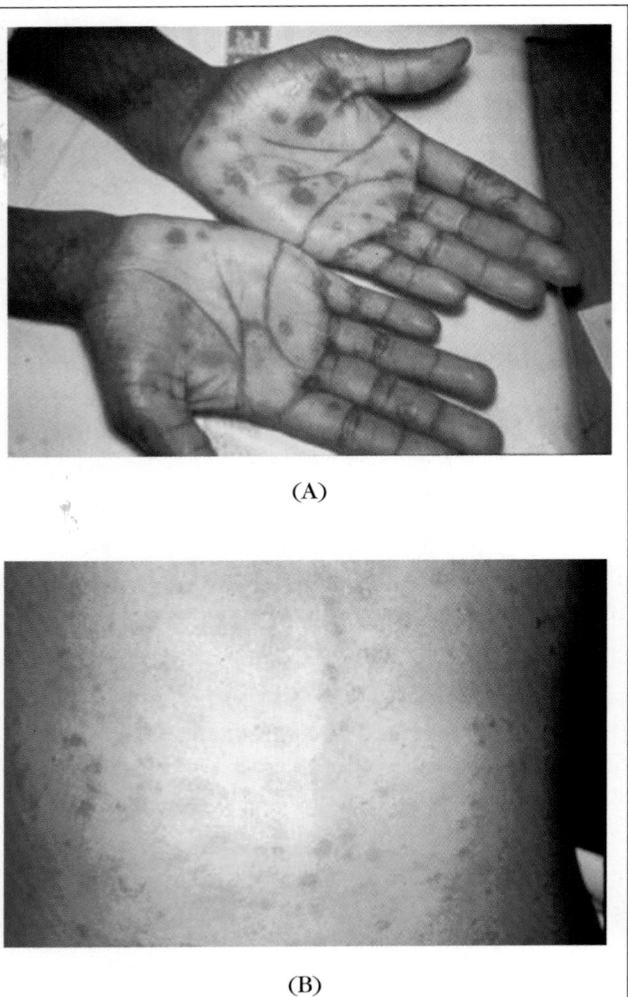

**FIGURE 53-4** Secondary syphilis. (A) Characteristic rash on palms of hands; (B) Characteristic maculopapular slightly scaly rash on the trunk. Reprinted with permission of Centers for Disease Control and Prevention (CDC), Training and Health Communication Branch of the Division of STD Prevention, National Center for HIV/AIDS, Viral Hepatitis, STD, and TB Prevention. (Available at: www.cdc.gov/std/training/clinicalslides/slides-dl.htm.)

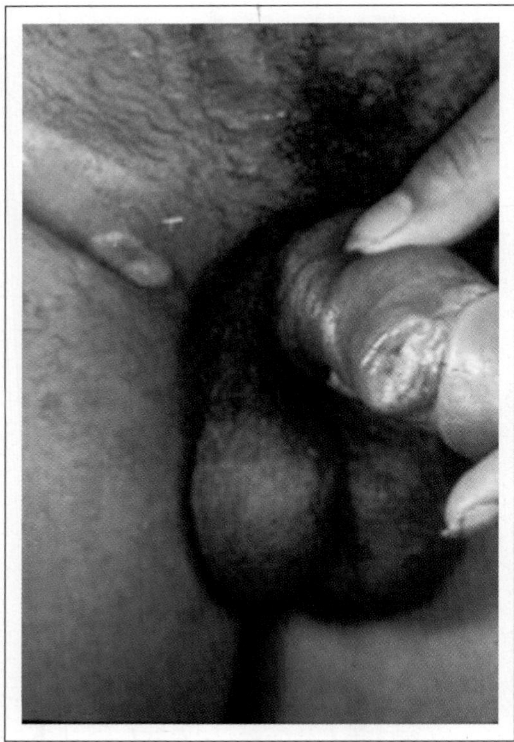

**FIGURE 53-5** Chancroid: Male with penile lesion and regional adenopathy. Reprinted with permission of Centers for Disease Control and Prevention (CDC), Training and Health Communication Branch of the Division of STD Prevention, National Center for HIV/AIDS, Viral Hepatitis, STD, and TB Prevention. (Available at: www.cdc.gov/std/training/clinicalslides/slides-dl.htm.)

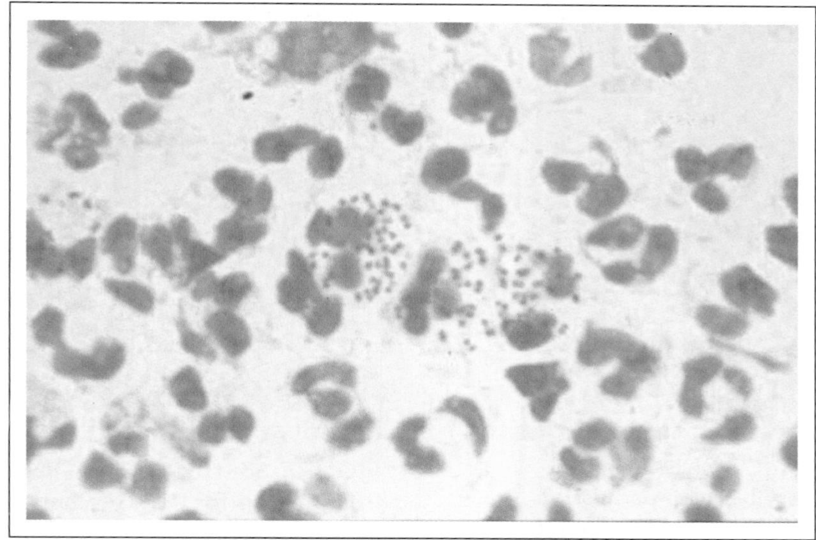

**FIGURE 53-6** Gonorrhea (GC): Gram stain of urethral discharge demonstrating Gram-negative intracellular diplococci. Reprinted with permission from Centers for Disease Control and Prevention (CDC), Training and Health Communication Branch of the Division of STD Prevention, National Center for HIV/AIDS, Viral Hepatitis, STD, and TB Prevention. (Available at: www.cdc.gov/std/training/clinicalslides/slides-dl.htm.)

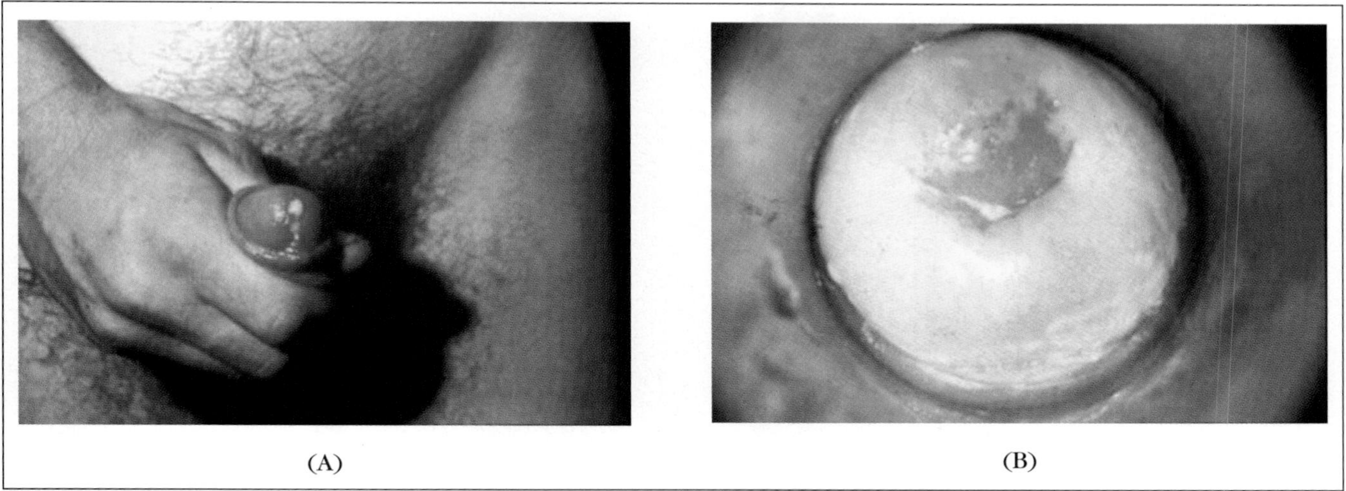


**FIGURE 53-7** Gonorrhea (GC). (A) Male with gonococcal urethritis; (B) Gonococcal cervicitis. Reprinted with permission from Centers for Disease Control and Prevention (CDC), Training and Health Communication Branch of the Division of STD Prevention, National Center for HIV/AIDS, Viral Hepatitis, STD, and TB Prevention. (Available at: www.cdc.gov/std/training/clinicalslides/slides-dl.htm.)

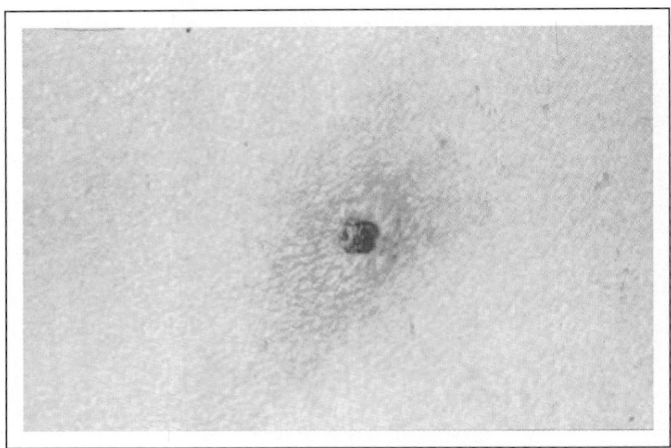

**FIGURE 53-8** Gonorrhea (GC). Disseminated gonorrhea skin lesion. Reprinted with permission from Centers for Disease Control and Prevention (CDC), Training and Health Communication Branch of the Division of STD Prevention, National Center for HIV/AIDS, Viral Hepatitis, STD, and TB Prevention. (Available at: www.cdc.gov/std/training/clinicalslides/slides-dl.htm.)

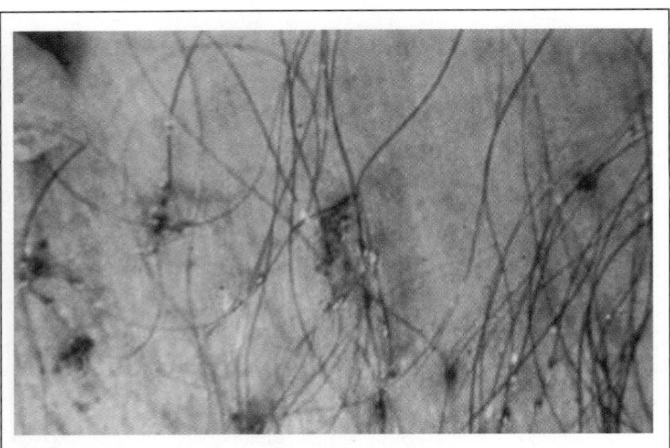

**FIGURE 53-10** Pubic lice. Reprinted with permission from Centers for Disease Control and Prevention (CDC), Training and Health Communication Branch of the Division of STD Prevention, National Center for HIV/AIDS, Viral Hepatitis, STD, and TB Prevention. (Available at: www.cdc.gov/std/training/clinicalslides/slides-dl.htm.)

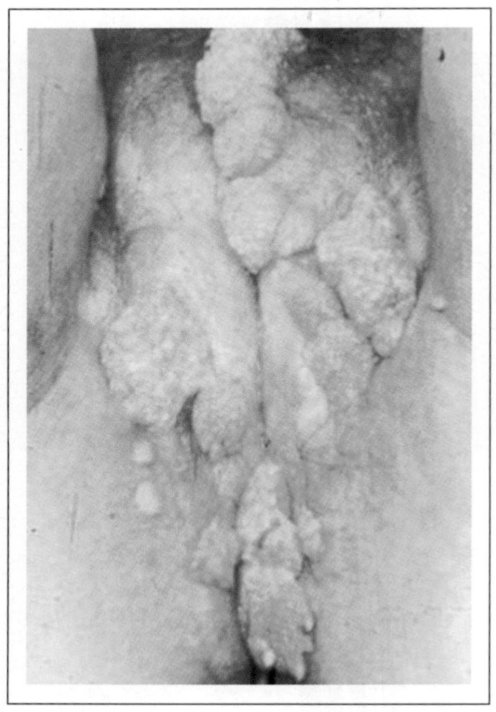

**FIGURE 53-9** Human Papillomavirus (HPV). Condyloma acuminata of vulva. Reprinted with permission from Centers for Disease Control and Prevention (CDC), Training and Health Communication Branch of the Division of STD Prevention, National Center for HIV/AIDS, Viral Hepatitis, STD, and TB Prevention. (Available at: www.cdc.gov/std/training/clinicalslides/slides-dl.htm.)

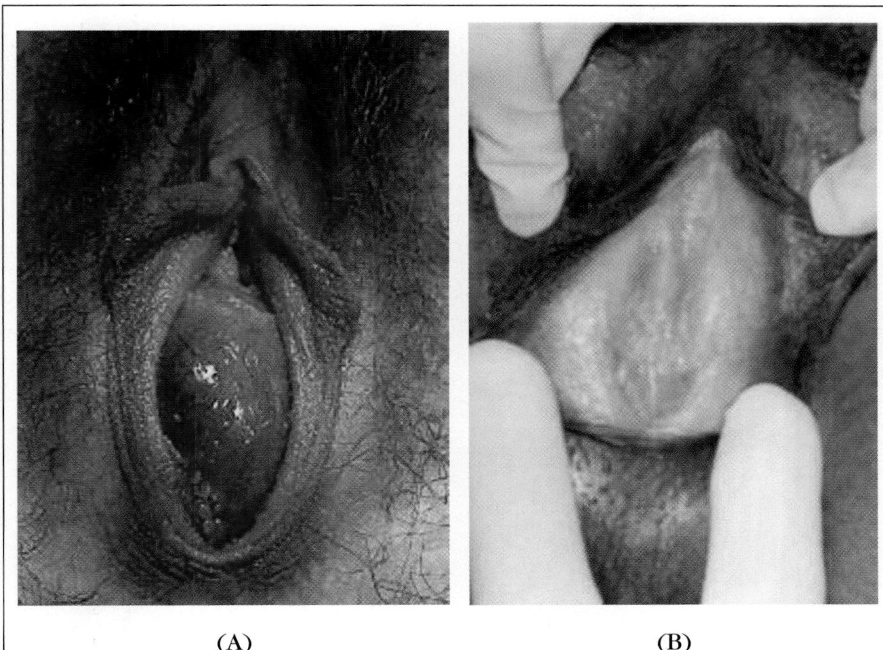


**FIGURE 59-2** Imperforate hymen vs.vaginal agenesis

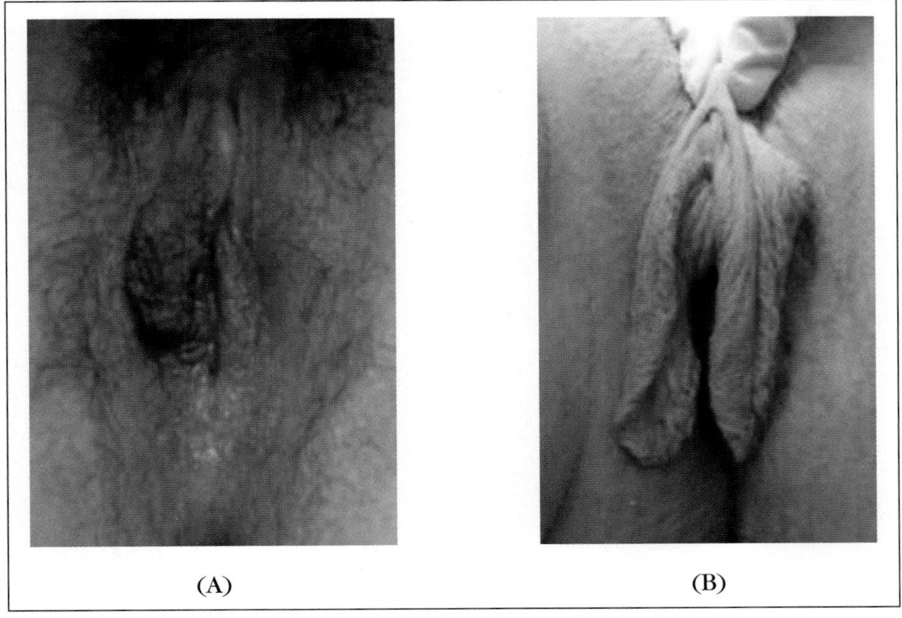


**FIGURE 59-3** Normal labial variant (asymmetry) vs. labia which required surgery

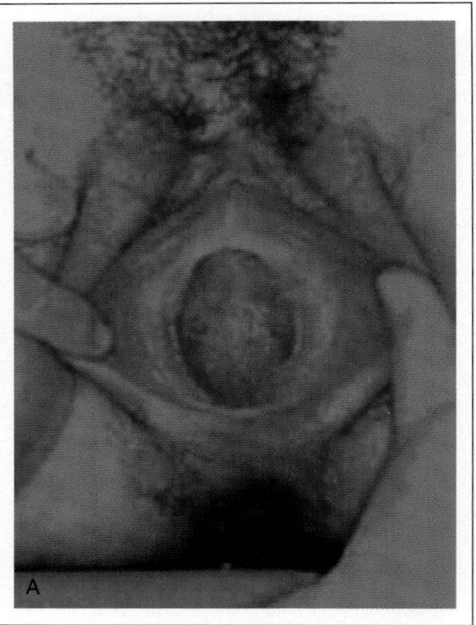


**FIGURE 62-1** Imperforate hymen. (A) Classic appearance of the bulging, blue-domed, translucent membrane. (B) Diagram of hematometra and hematocolopos with imperforate distal transverse vaginal septum. (Reprinted with permission from Judith A. Lacy, MD, clinical educator, Department of Obstetrics and Gynecologic Specialties, Pediatric and Adolescent Gynecology, Stanford University School of Medicine, and Lucile Packard Children's Hospital. Coauthor: Paula J. Adams Hillard, MD, acting professor, Department of Obstetrics and Gynecology, Stanford University Medical Center. E-Medicine Online serial available at: emedicine.medscape.com/article/269050-media)

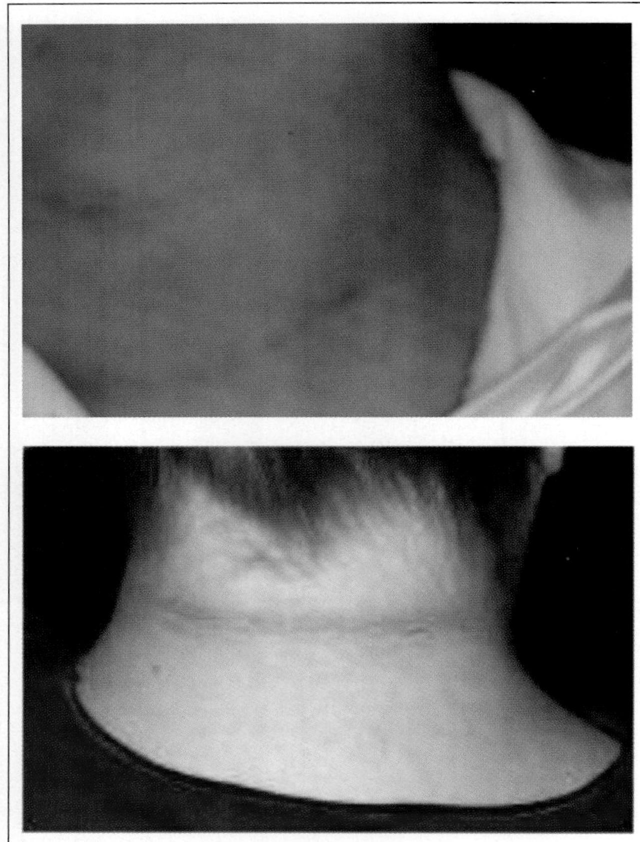

**FIGURE 65-3** Acanthosis Nigricans.

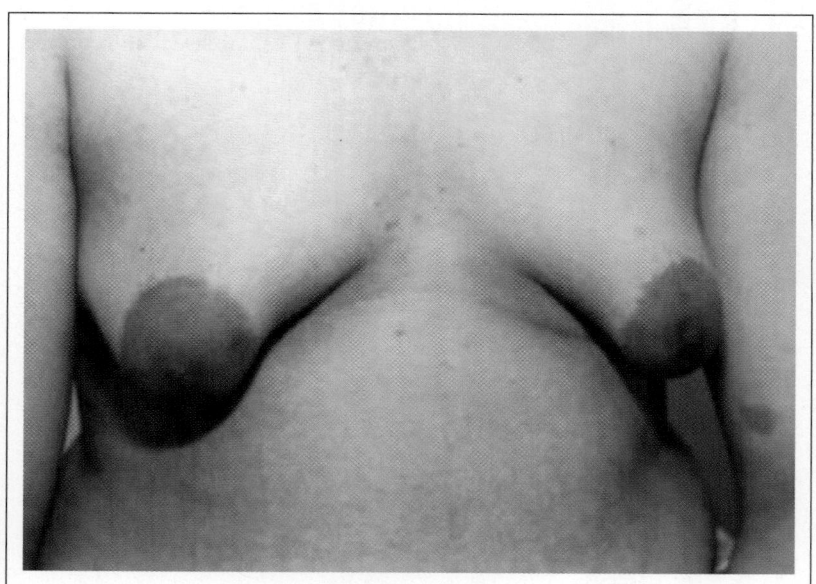

**FIGURE67-1** Boy with type 2 gynecomastia or macromastia

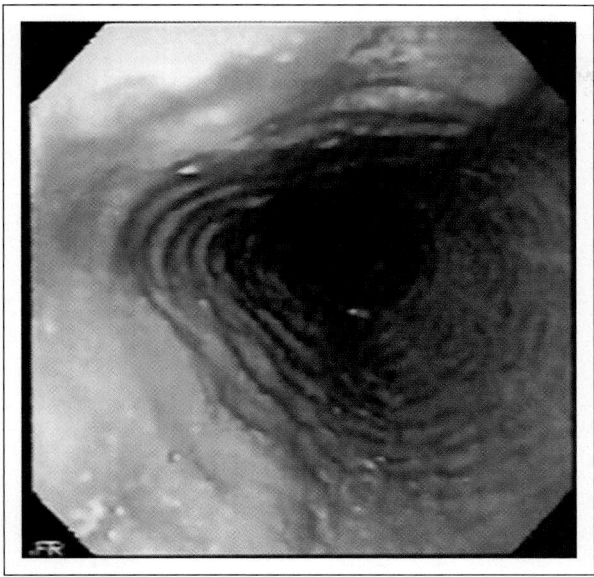


**FIGURE 98-5** Endoscopic appearance of the esophagus of a 16-year-old boy with eosinophilic esophagitis. Multiple circumferential rings and whitish flecks often seen in this condition are present from the mid- to distal esophagus.

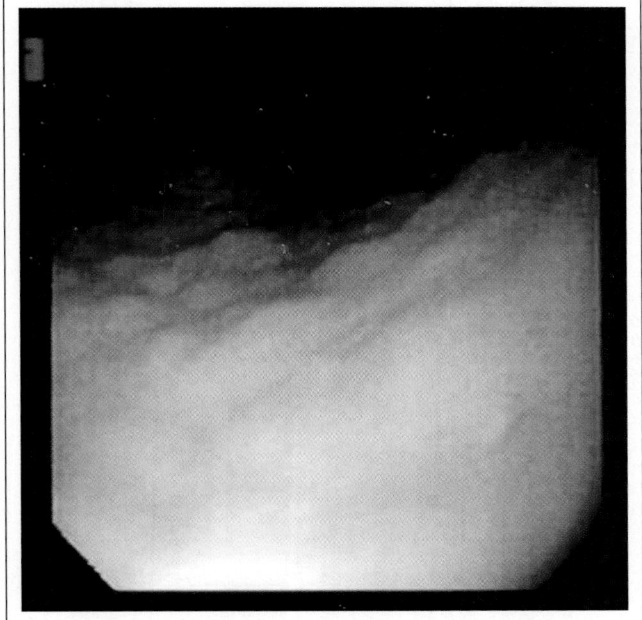

**FIGURE 99-1** Endoscopic picture of gastric antrum demonstrating nodularity often seen with *H pylori* gastritis infection.

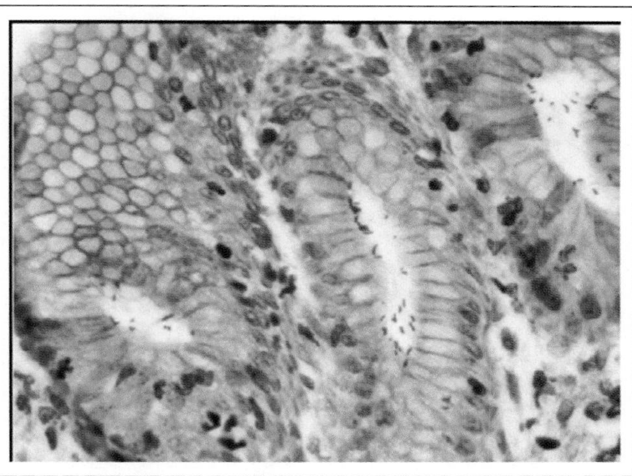

**FIGURE 99-2** Warthin-starry stain of endoscopic biopsy of gastric mucosa demonstrating *H pylori* gastritis infection (appearing as dark "dots" and "dashes" in the glandular space or surface).

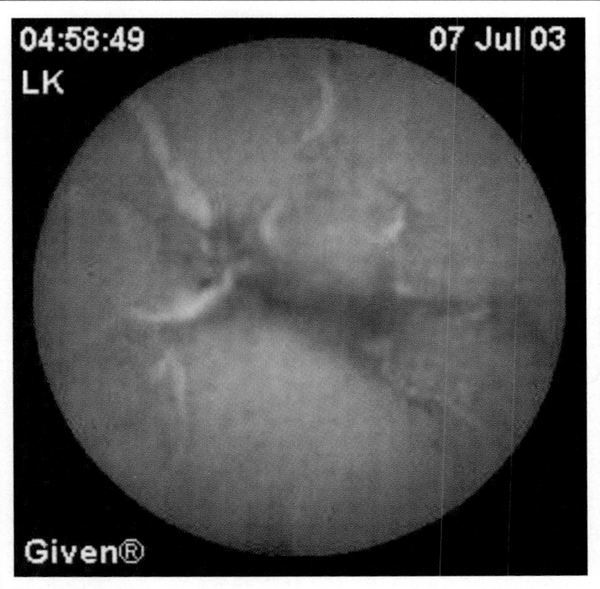


**FIGURE 104-1** Capsule endoscopy. This image from the small bowel of a patient with Crohn disease clearly shows ulceration of the mucosal lining consistent with small bowel disease.

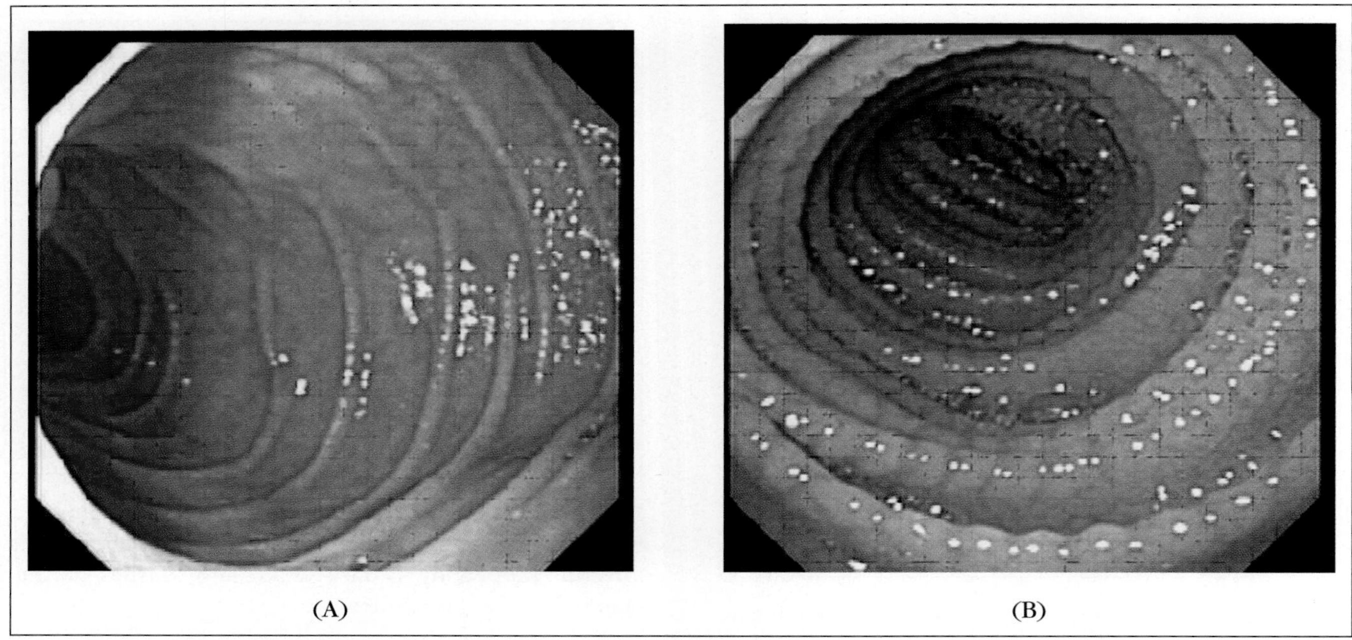


**FIGURE 105-2** (A) Normal duodenum (B) duodenal fold "scalloping" in celiac disease

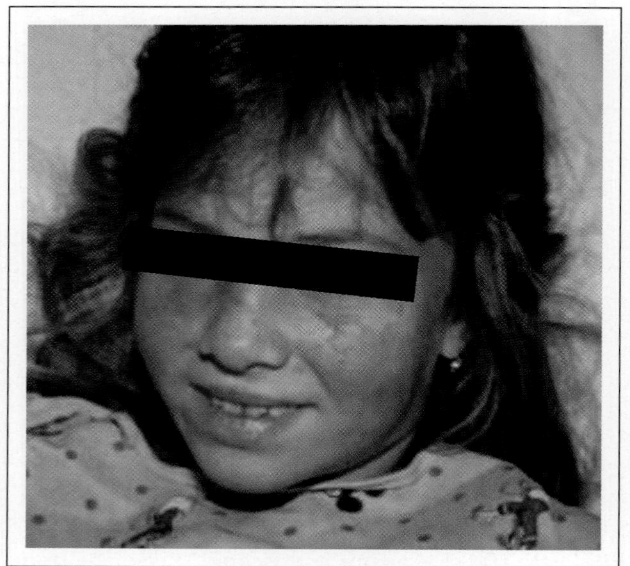

**FIGURE 120-1** Typical malar erythema in a "butterfly" distribution. Note that the erythema crosses the nasal bridge but spares the nasolabial folds.

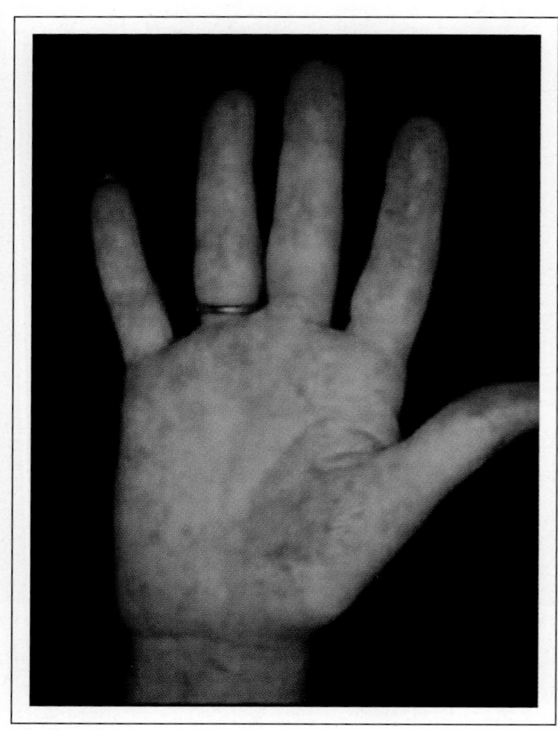

**FIGURE 120-2** Vasculitic lesions.

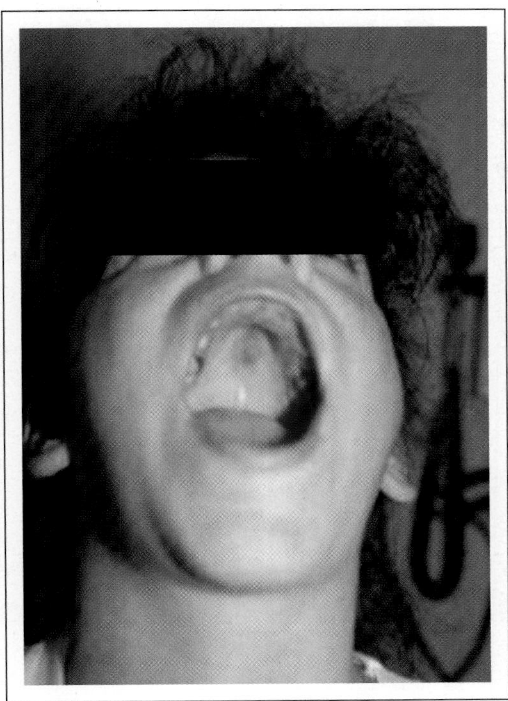

**FIGURE 120-3** Palatal erythema with a small ulceration of the hard palate.

**FIGURE 120-5** Nail-bed capillaries. Exam of the nail-bed reveals dilated loops of capillaries and areas of capillary dropout.

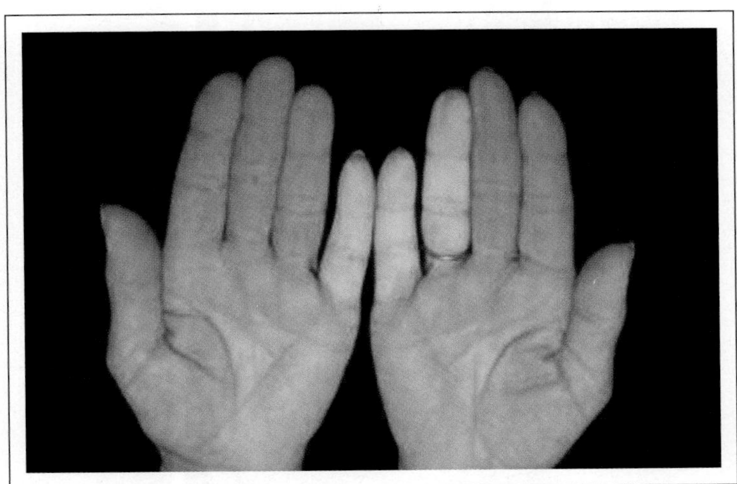

**FIGURE 120-4** Raynaud syndrome. Although all of the fingertips are usually affected, occasionally only some of the digits will show the color changes associated with the syndrome.

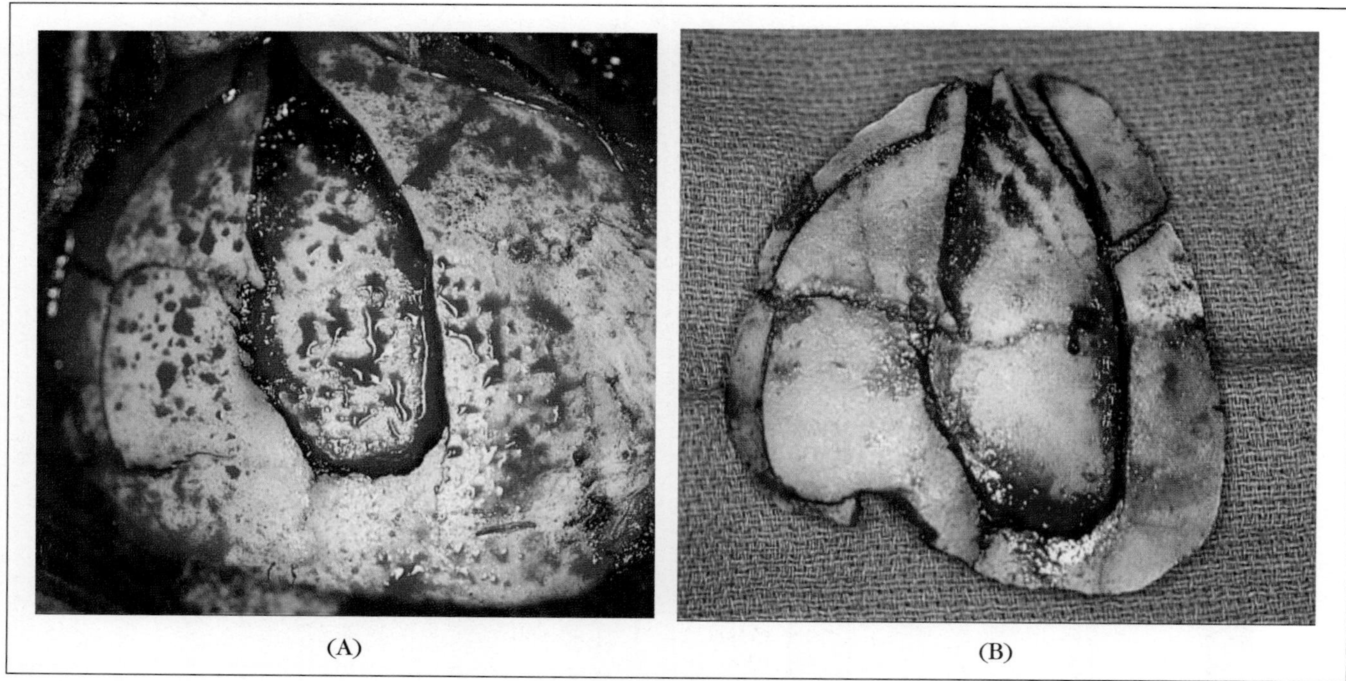

(A) (B)

**FIGURE 131-6** An adolescent female struck by a hammer over the convexity during a rape attempt. (A) A stellate fracture with multiple fracture lines. (B) After elevating of the skull fracture the multiple fractures can be easily appreciated and need to be corrected prior to placing the skull back. (Photos courtesy James Tait Goodrich.)

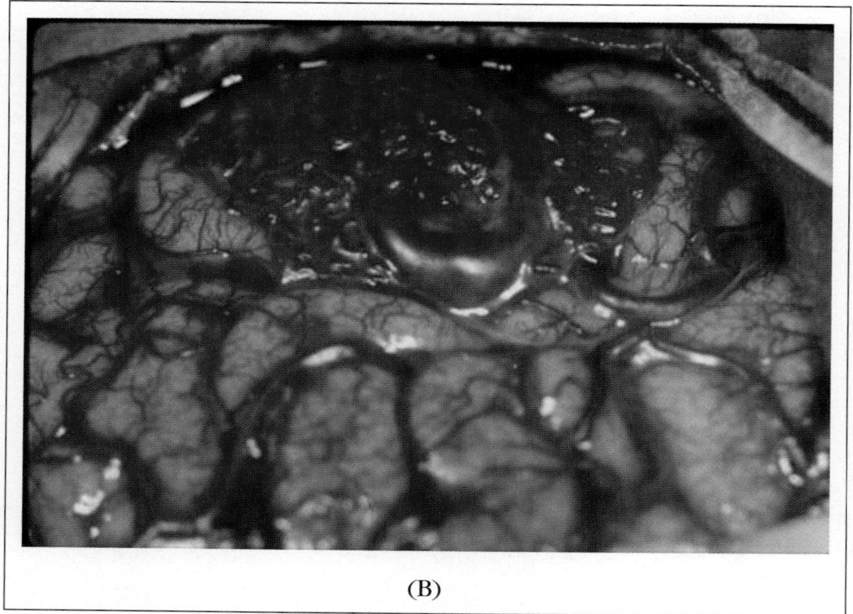

(B)

**FIGURE 132-3** (B) Intraoperative view of a cortical AVM surrounded by normal brain. The arterialized vein can be seen at the inferior margin of the AVM.

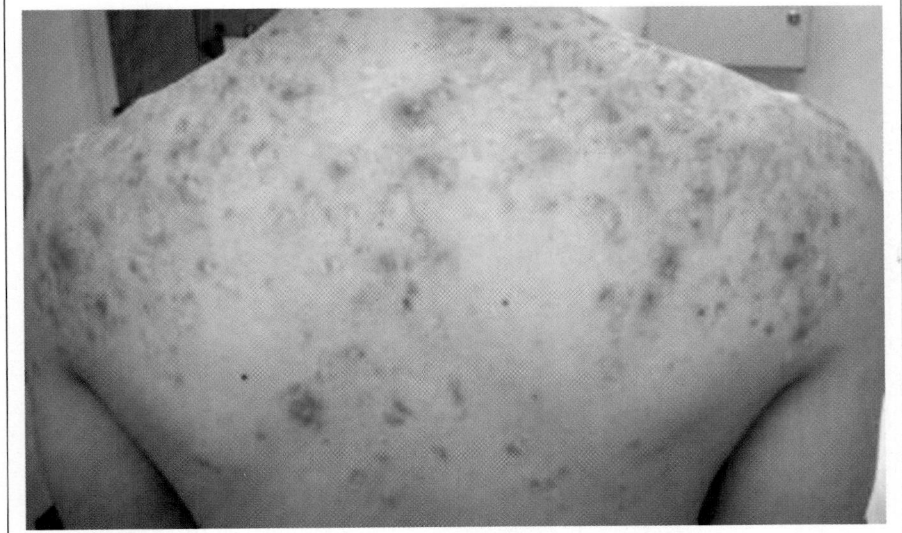

**FIGURE 144-1** Acne scarring

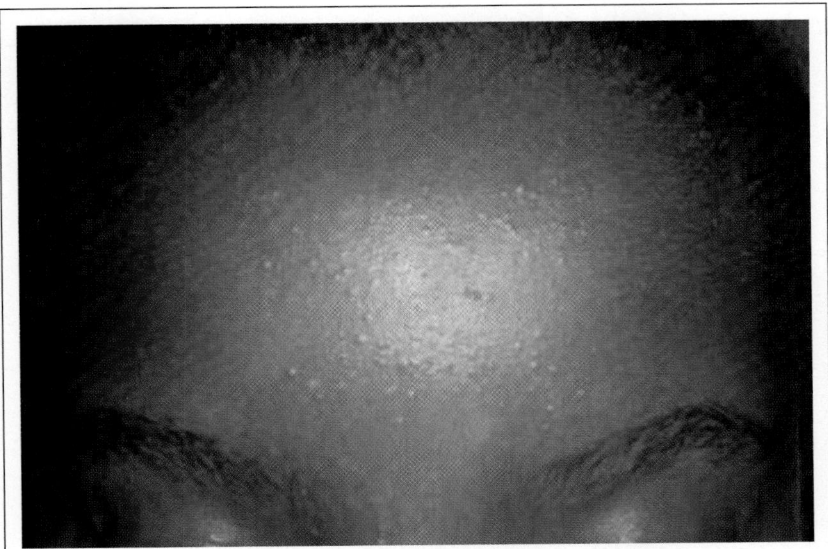

**FIGURE 144-2** Mild comedonal acne

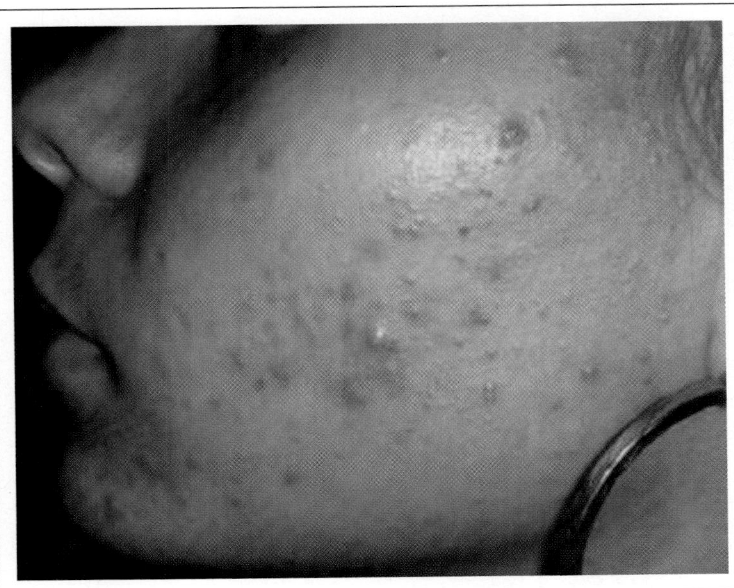

**FIGURE 144-3** Moderate papulopustular acne

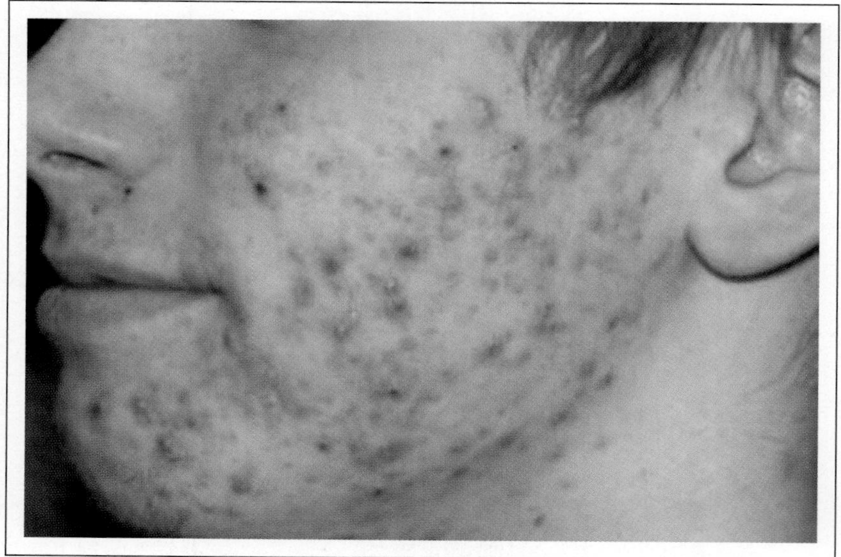

**FIGURE 144-1** Acne scarring

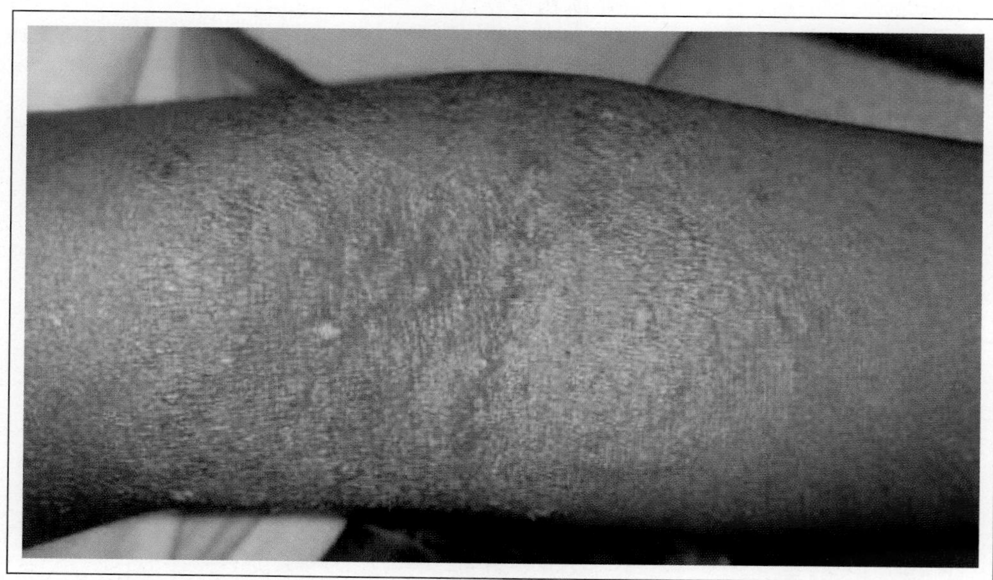

**FIGURE 145-1** Antecubital involvement in atopic dermatitis.

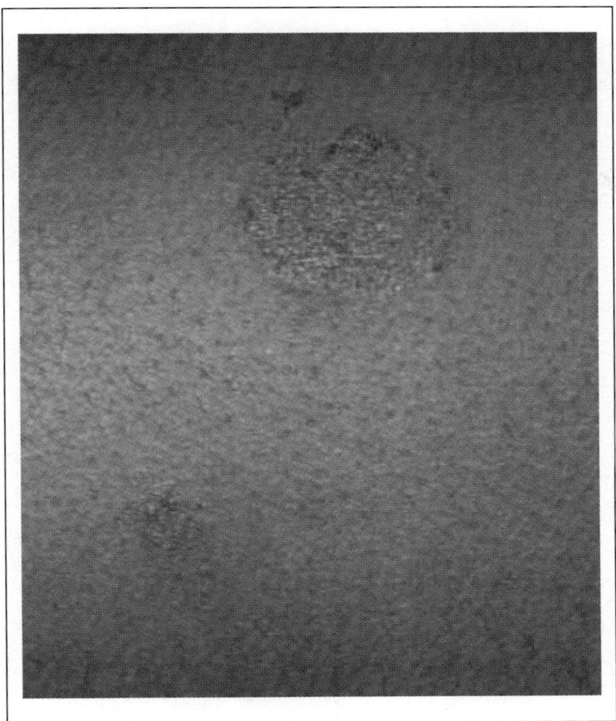

**FIGURE 145-2** Nummular eczema.

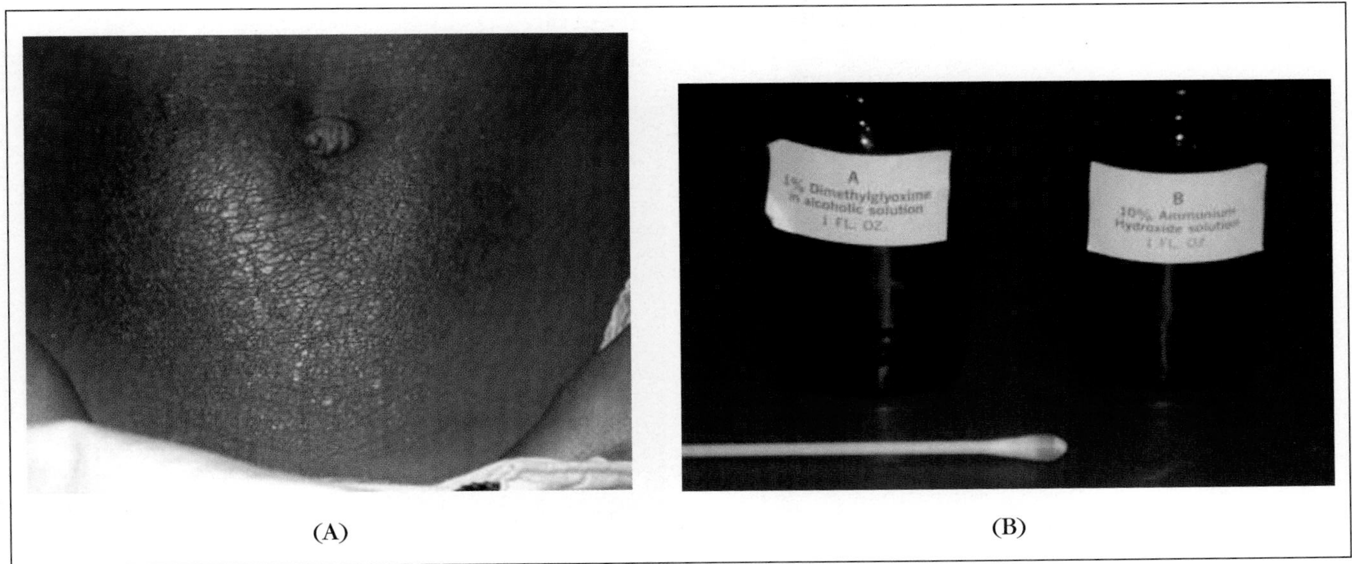


**FIGURE 145-3** Nickel dermatitis. A: Allergic contact dermatitis secondary to pant snaps made of nickel. B: Positive nickel allergy test: a cotton swab moistened with dimethylglyoxime and ammonium hydroxide was rubbed against suspected nickel-containing materials and turns pink on exposure to nickel.

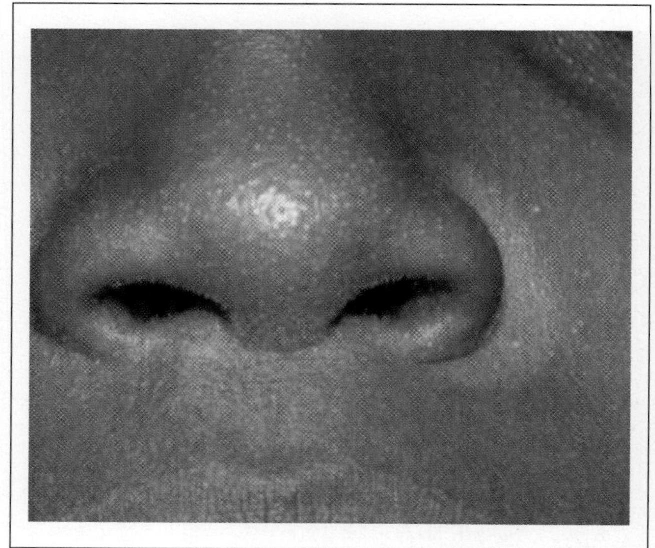

**FIGURE 145-4** Perinasal scaling in seborrheic dermatitis. Note the hypopigmentation and perinasal.

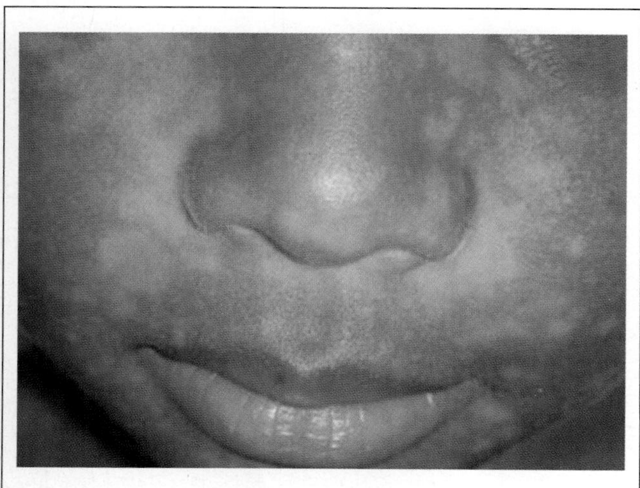

**FIGURE 145-5** Sebopsoriasis. Note the extensive hypopigmentation and scaling.

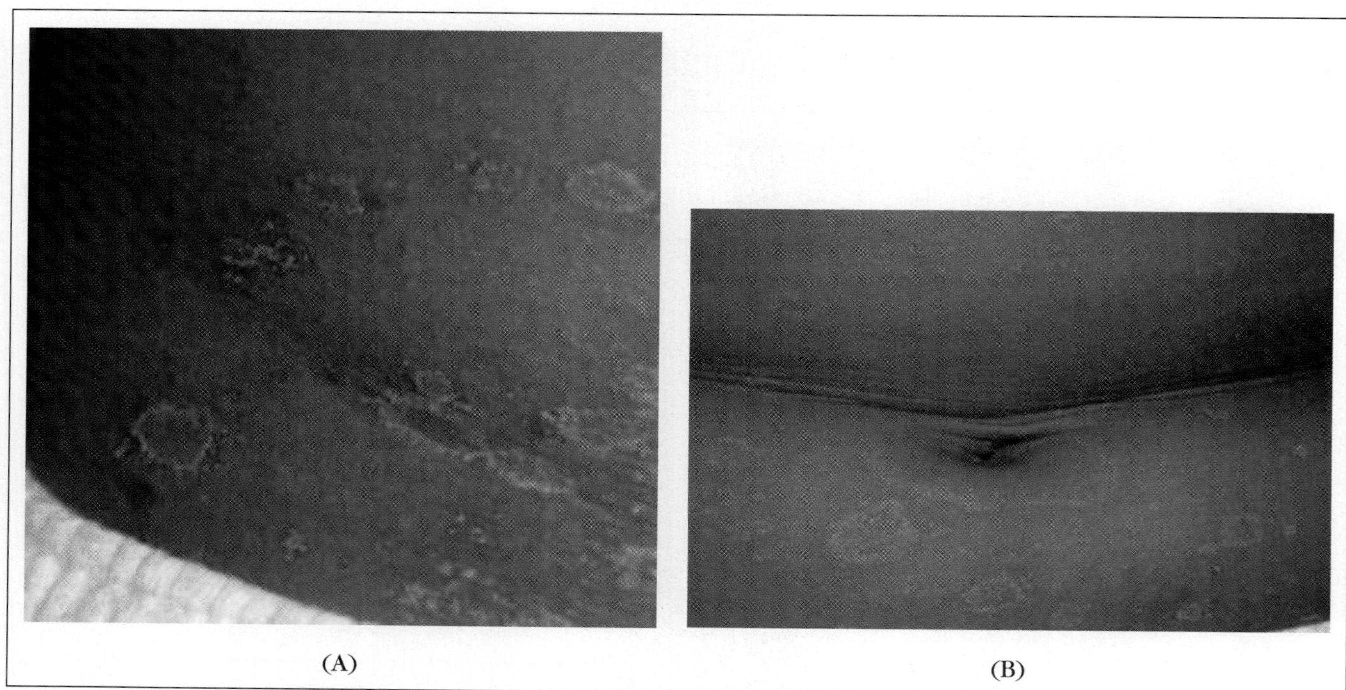


**FIGURE 145-6** Pityriasis rosea. A: Lesions possess a peripheral collarette of scale. B: Lesions follow the lines of cleavage.

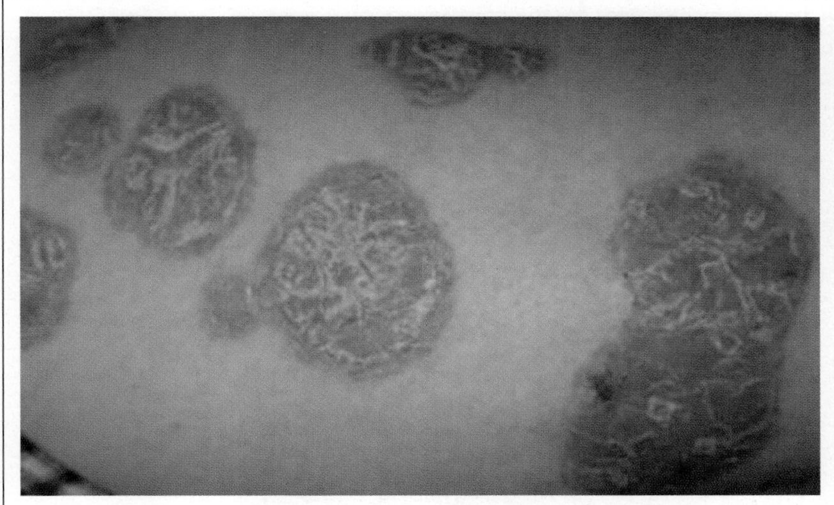

**FIGURE 145-7** Plaque psoriasis. Note the beefy red plaques and thick adherent scale.

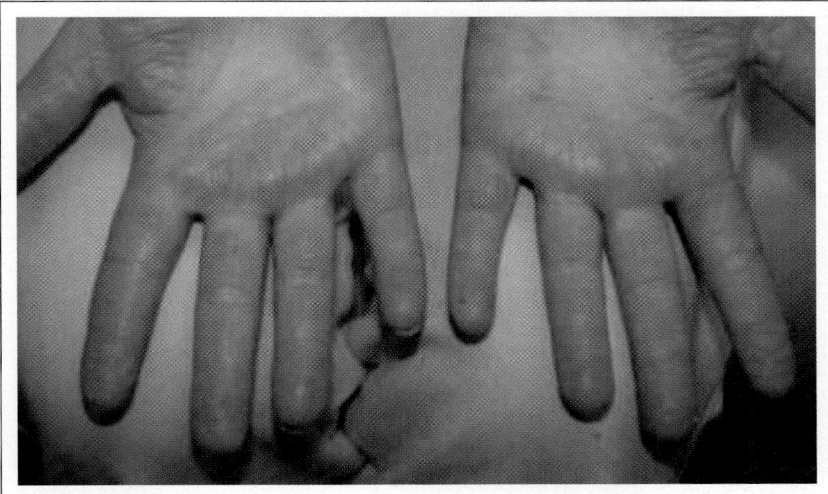

**FIGURE 145-8** Palmar psoriasis. Note the well-demarcated erythema on the palms.

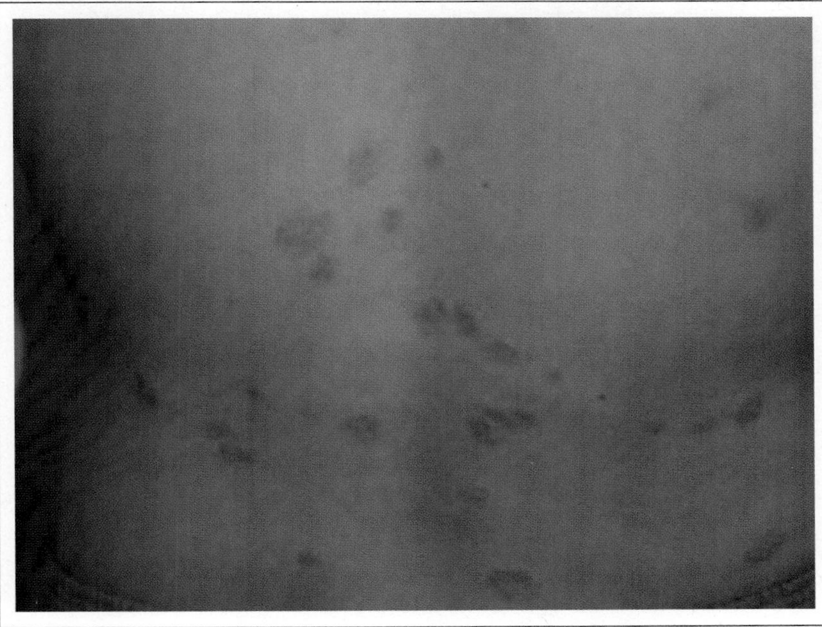

**FIGURE 145-9** Guttate psoriasis. Note the random distribution of these lesions in contrast to the distribution of lesions in pityriasis rosea.

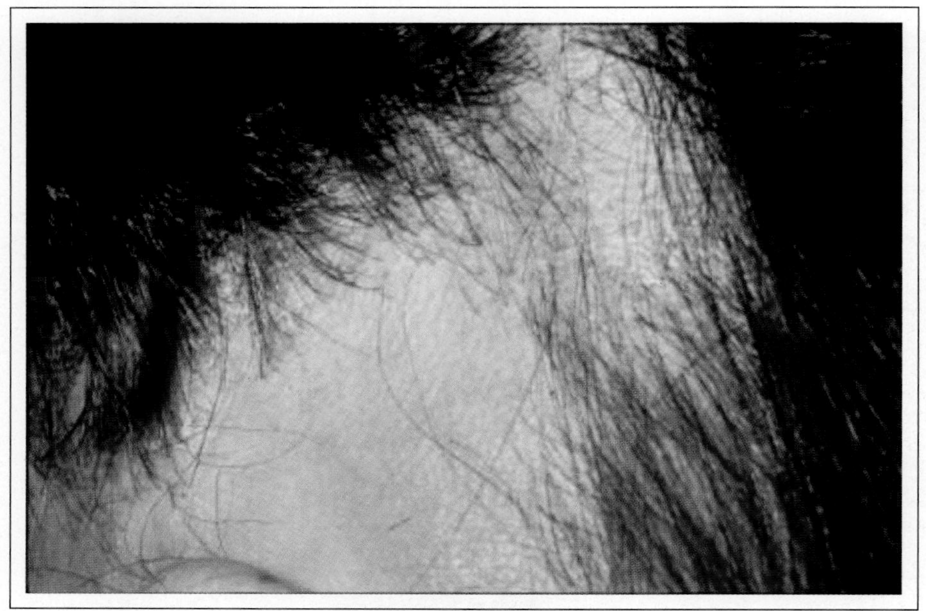

**FIGURE 146-1** Bitemporal ophiasis pattern of alopecia areata.

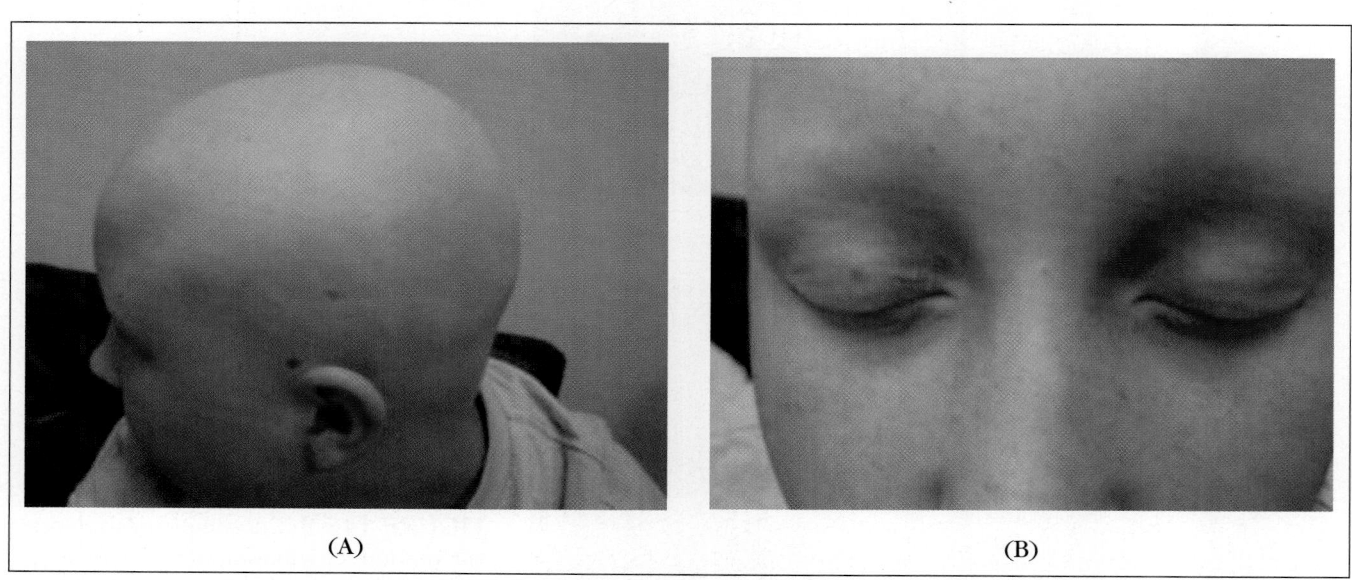

(A) (B)

**FIGURE 146-2** Alopecia universalis showing hair loss on (A) scalp and (B) eyebrows and eyelashes.

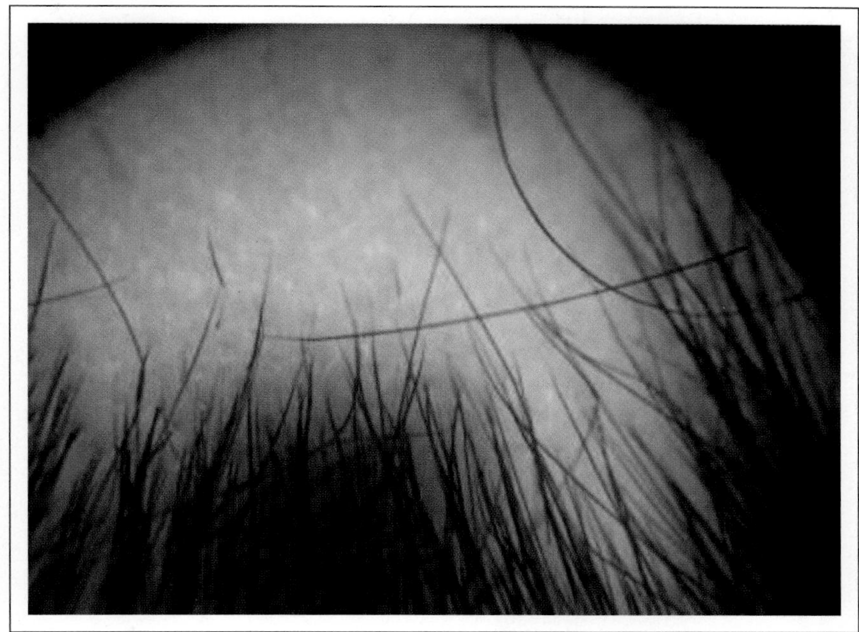

**FIGURE 146-3** Exclamation point hairs, the classic clinical finding in alopecia areata.

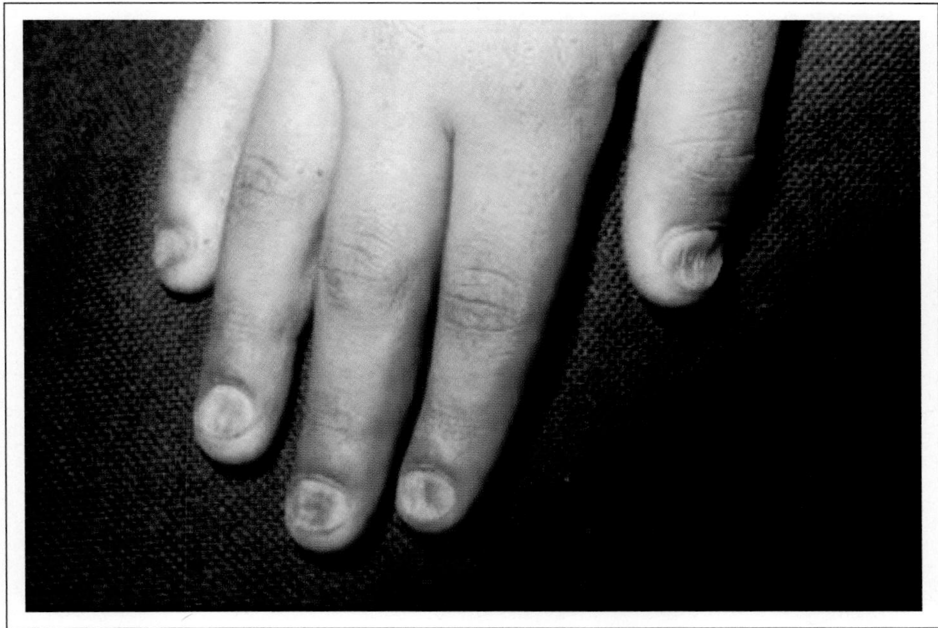

**FIGURE 146-4** Significant nail dystrophy in patient with alopecia areata.

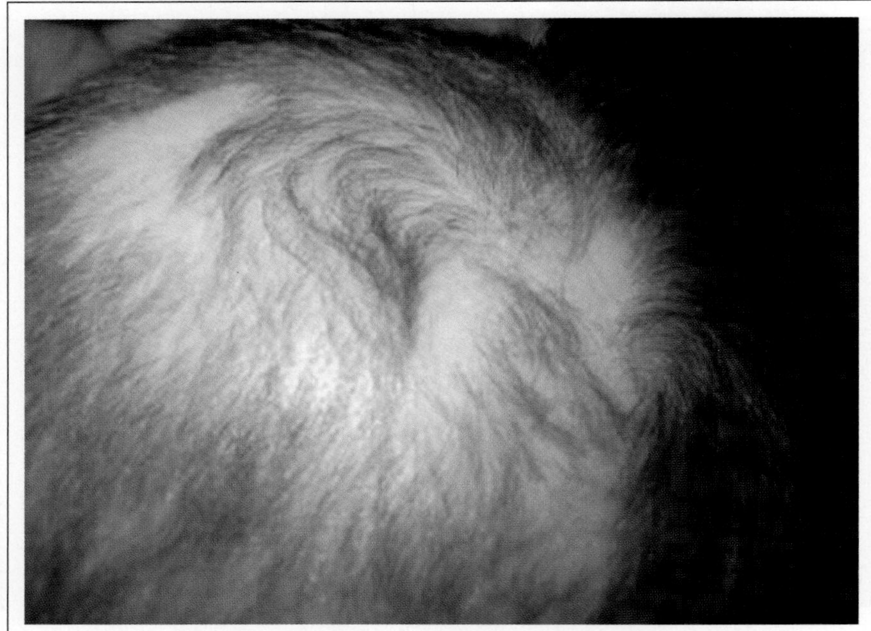

**FIGURE 146-5** Alopecia areata with evidence of hair regrowth after treatment with squaric acid.

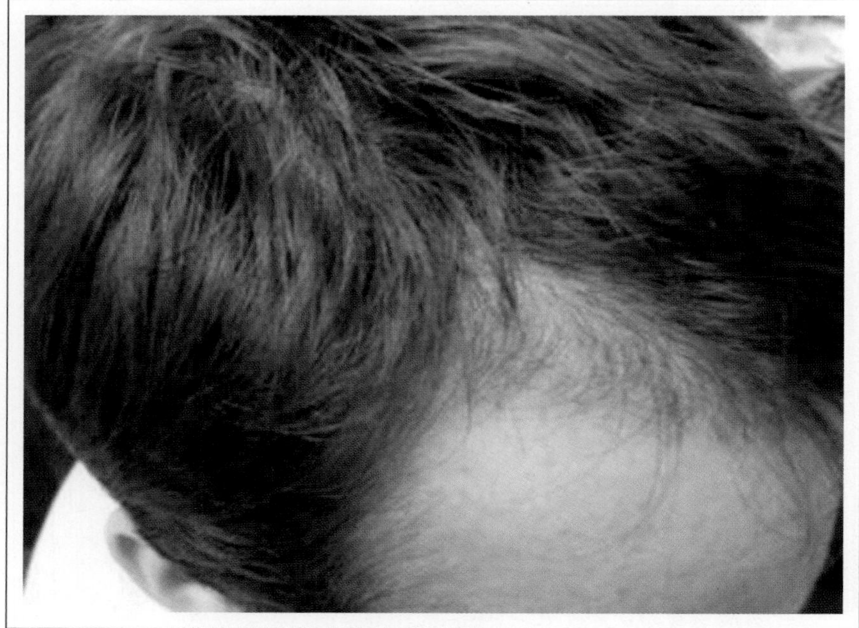

**FIGURE 146-6** Bitemporal pattern of hair loss in androgenetic alopecia.

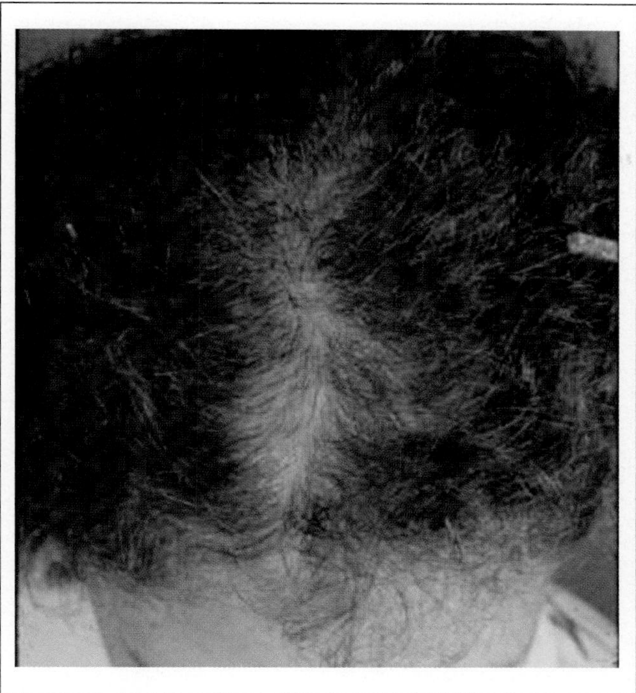

**FIGURE 146-8** Thinning of central scalp hair in female pattern hair loss.

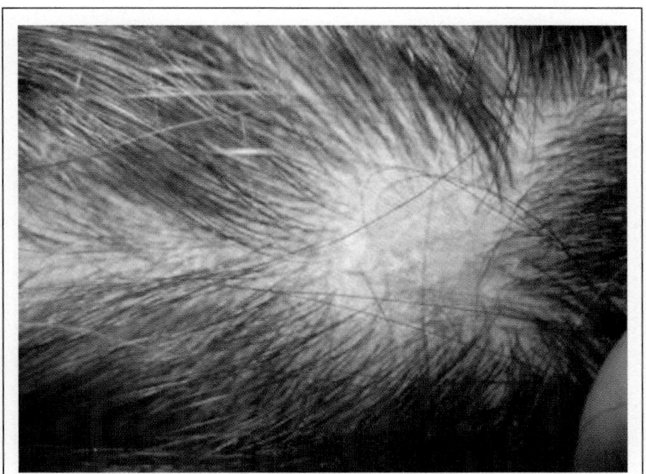

**FIGURE 146-10** Scaly erythematous plaque consistent with tinea capitis.

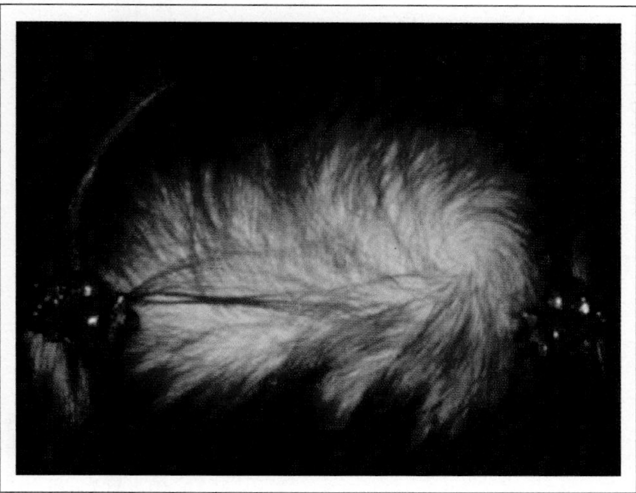

**FIGURE 146-11** Traction alopecia caused by chronic use of barrettes.

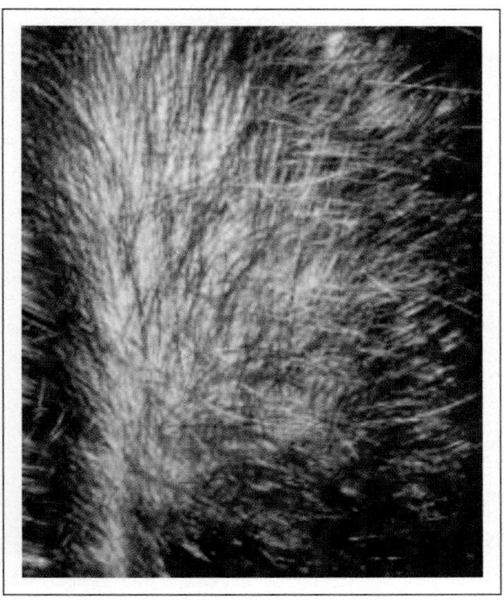

**FIGURE 146-12** Broken-off stubble commonly observed in trichotillomania.

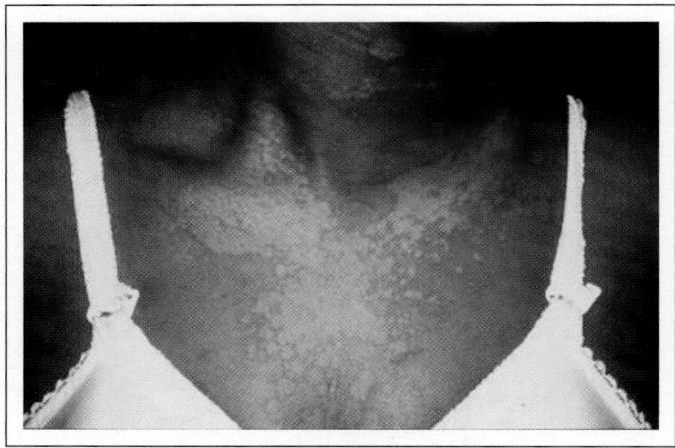

**FIGURE 147-1** Tinea versicolor.

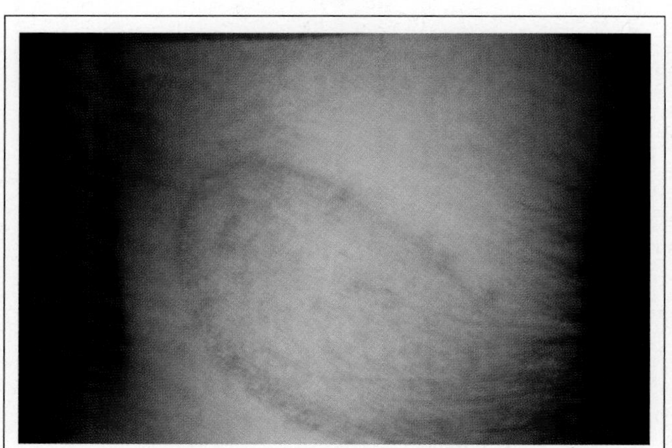

**FIGURE 147-2** Tinea corporis.

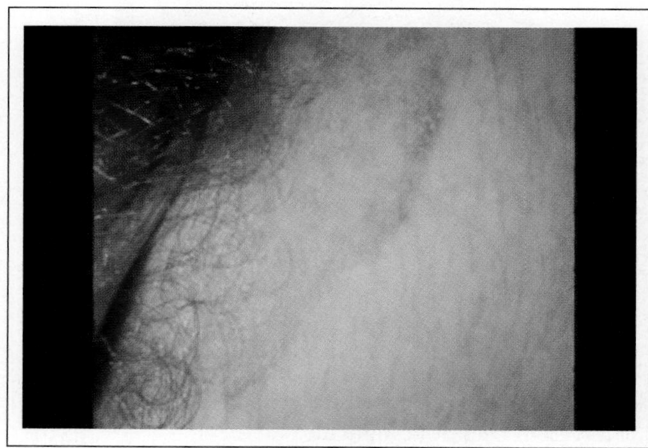

**FIGURE 147-3** Tinea cruris of the inner thigh.

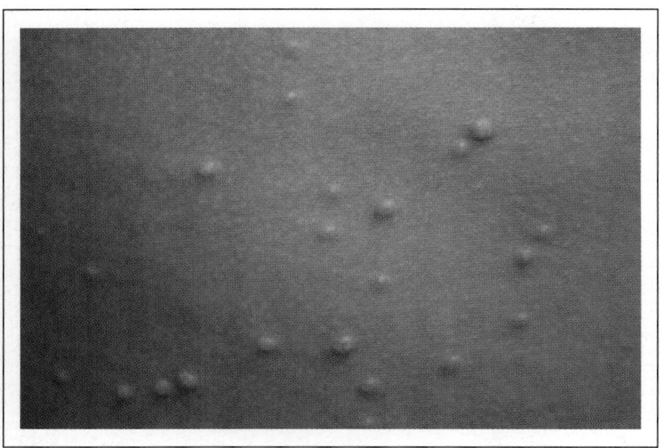

**FIGURE 147-4** Molluscum contagiosum.

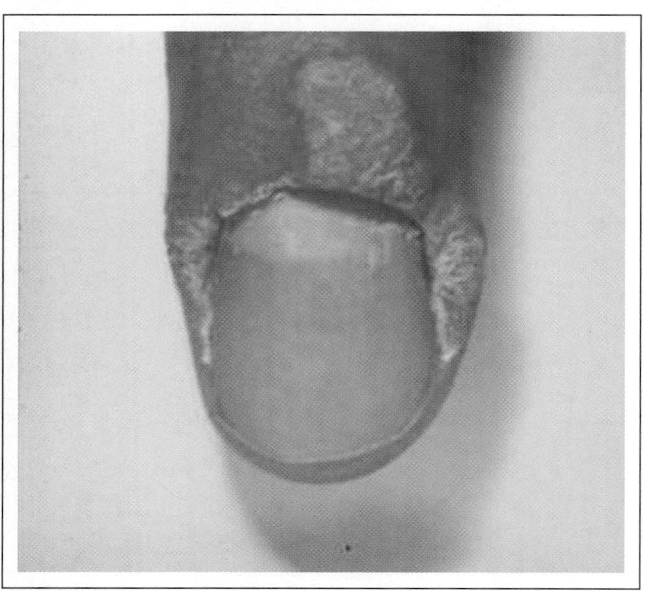

**FIGURE 147-5** Warts. (A) Periungual wart; (B) plantar wart, mosaic type.

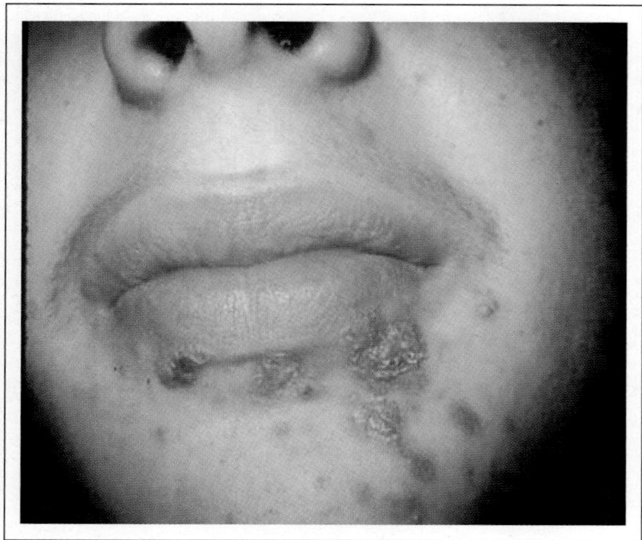

**FIGURE 147-6** Impetigo.

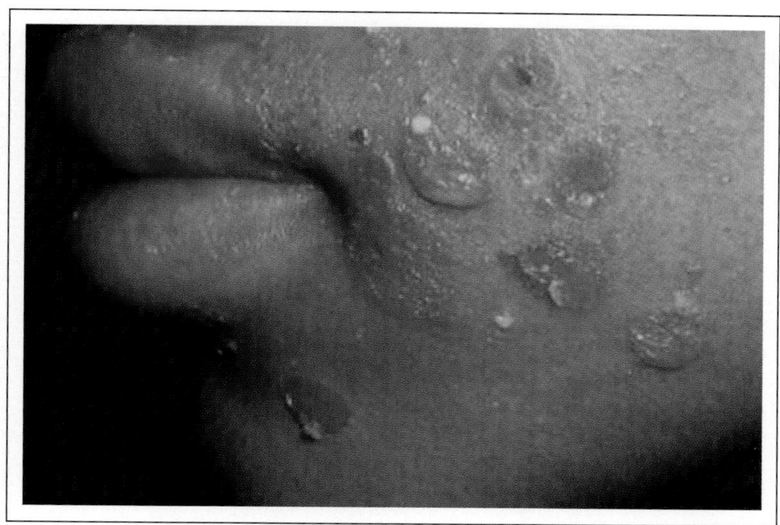

**FIGURE 147-7** Bullous impetigo.

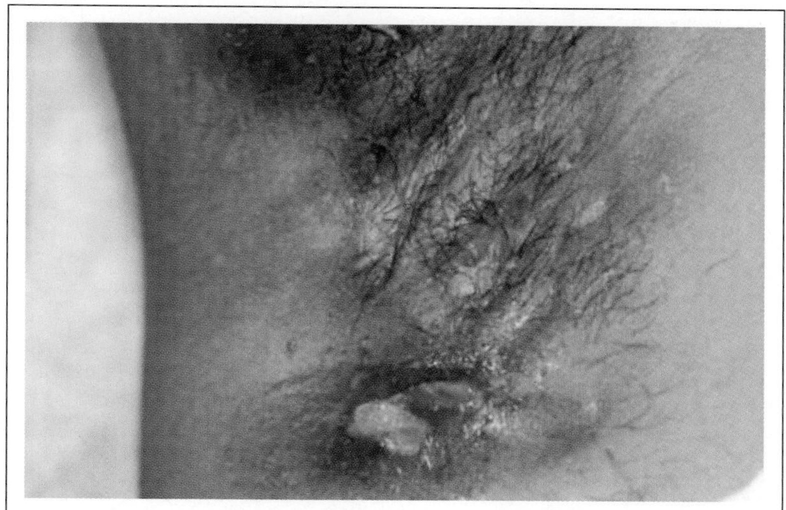

**FIGURE 147-8** Hidradenitis suppurativa.

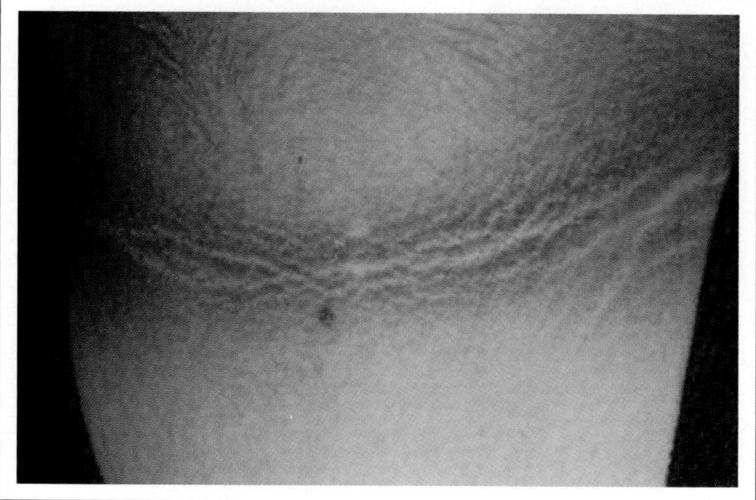

**FIGURE 147-9** Acanthosis nigricans.

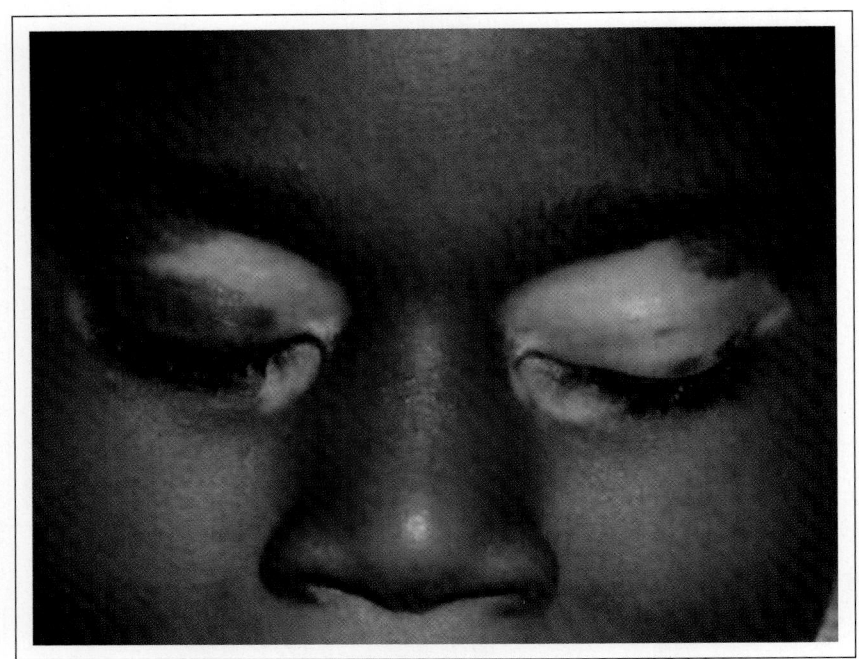

**FIGURE 147-10** Vitiligo.

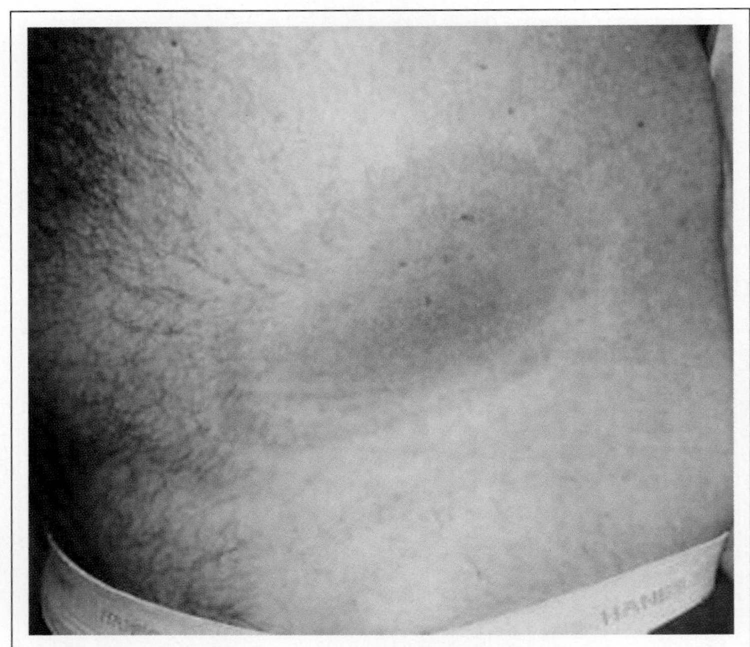

**FIGURE 147-11** Erythema migrans.

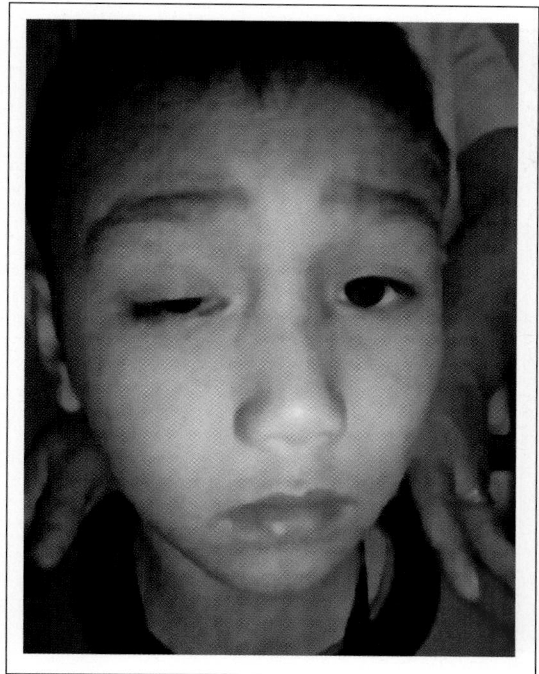

**FIGURE 154-1** Congenital ptosis of the right upper eyelid due to levator maldevelopment. Note the lack of an eyelid crease and the use of the brows to elevate the lid. (Photo courtesy of Srinivas S. Iyengar, MD.)

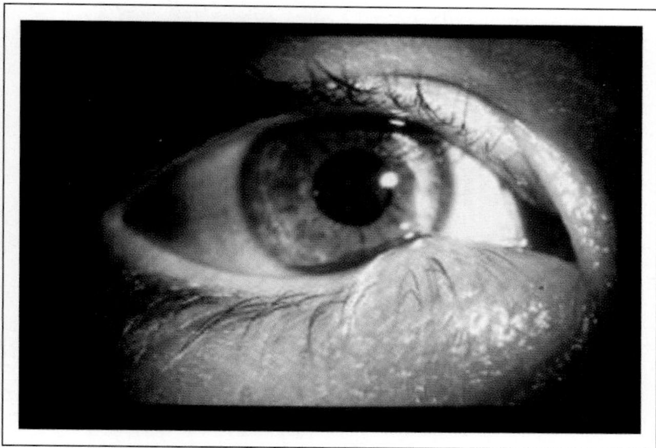

**FIGURE 154-2** Chalazion of the lower eyelid. (Photo courtesy of David Lyon, MD.)

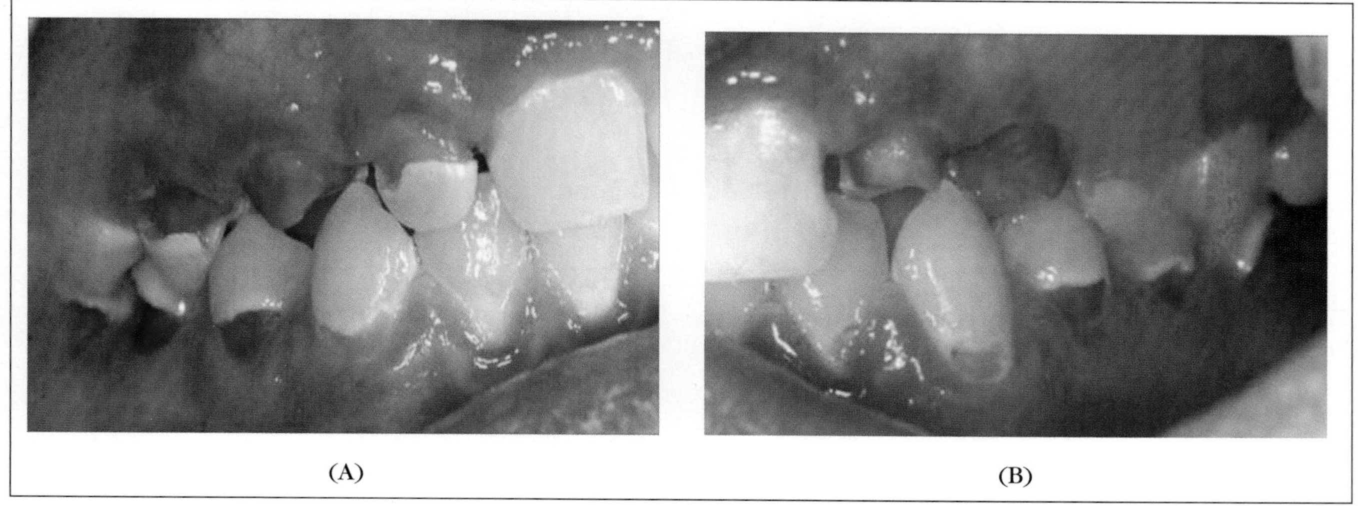

(A) (B)

**FIGURE 157-1** An adolescent patient with rampant untreated dental caries in the permanent dentition.

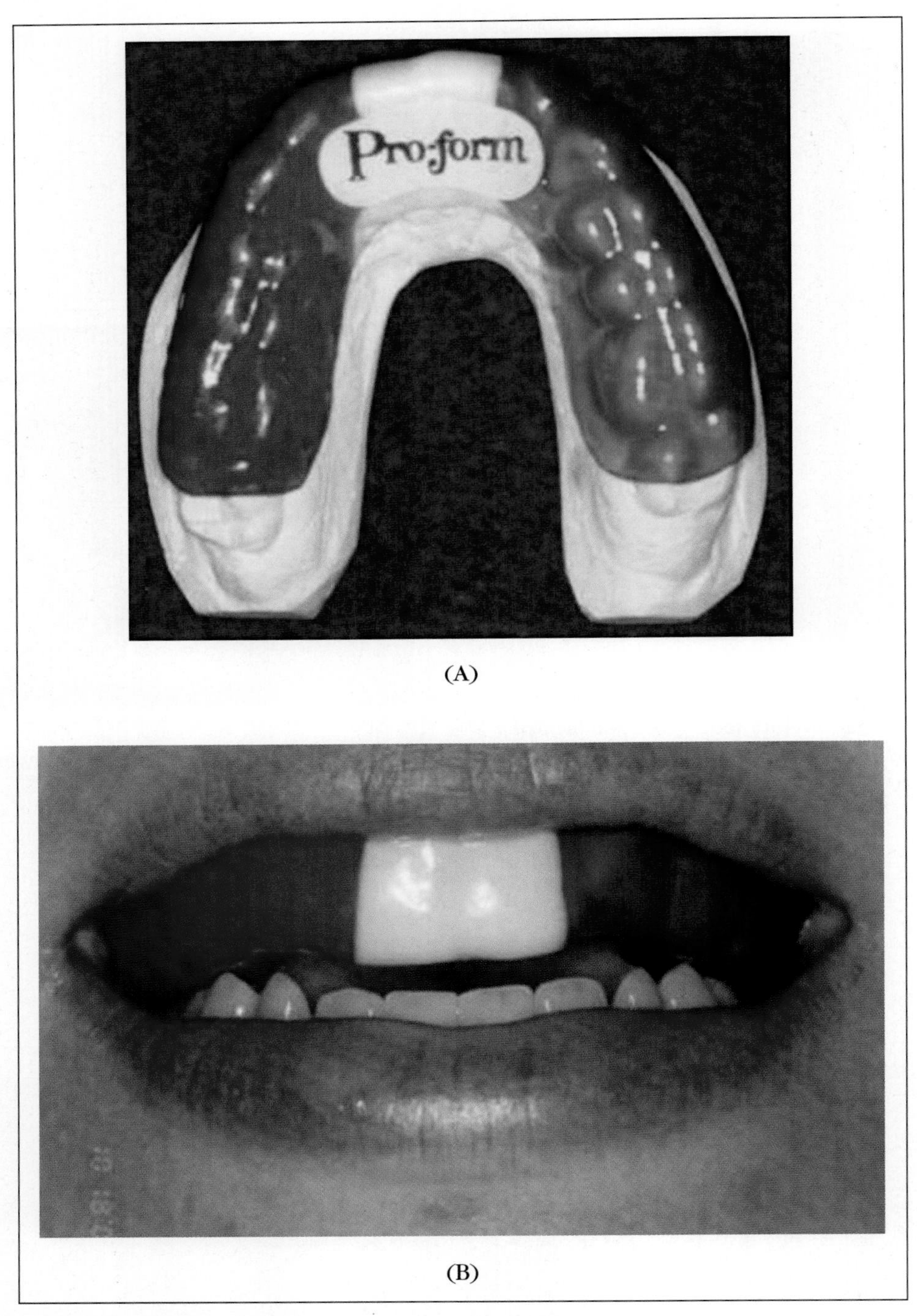


**FIGURE 157-3** (A) Custom-fabricated athletic mouthguard made over a cast of the patient's maxillary arch; (B) Properly fitted custom-fabricated mouthguard in the patient's mouth.

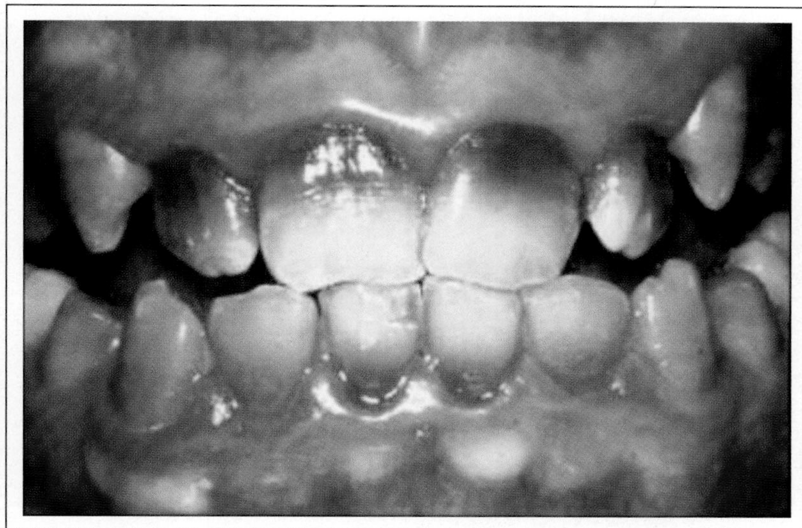

**FIGURE 157-4** Generalized moderate to severe tetracycline staining in the permanent dentition of an adolescent patient.

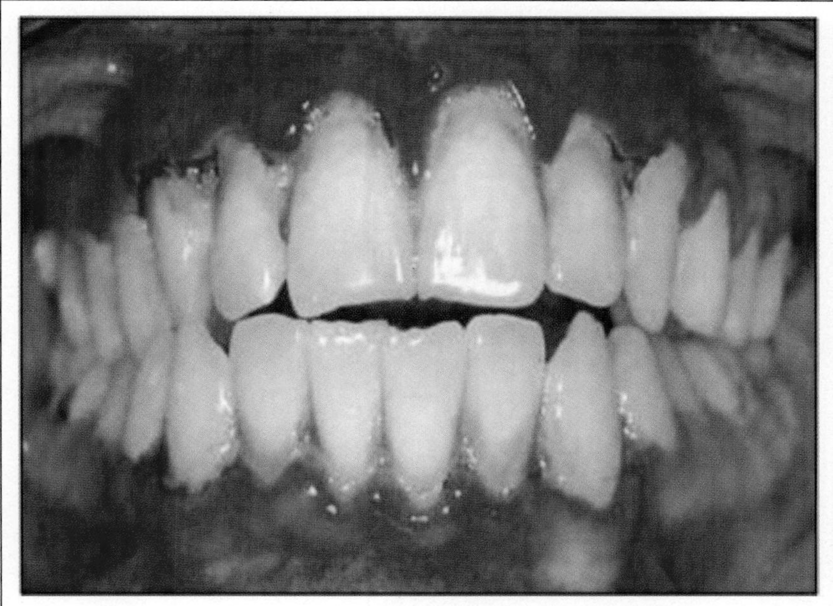

**FIGURE 157-5** Acute phase of necrotizing ulcerative gingivitis demonstrating inflammation with tissue degradation.

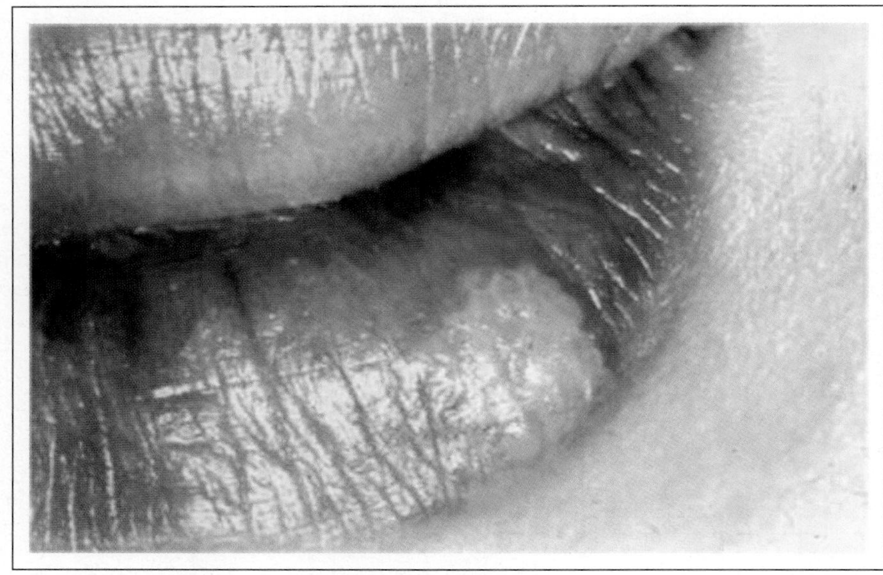

**FIGURE 157-6** Vesicular lesion of recurrent herpes labialis on the lower lip.

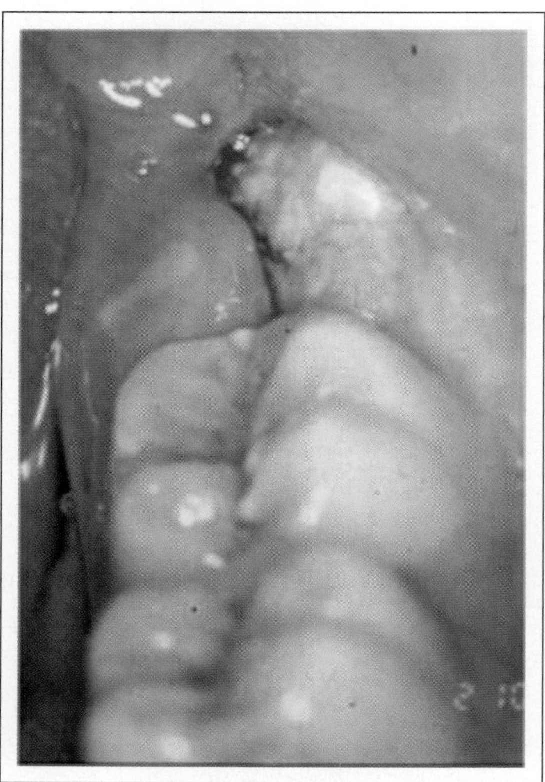

**FIGURE 157-7** Pericoronitis surrounding the crown of an erupting mandibular permanent left third molar (Tooth #17).

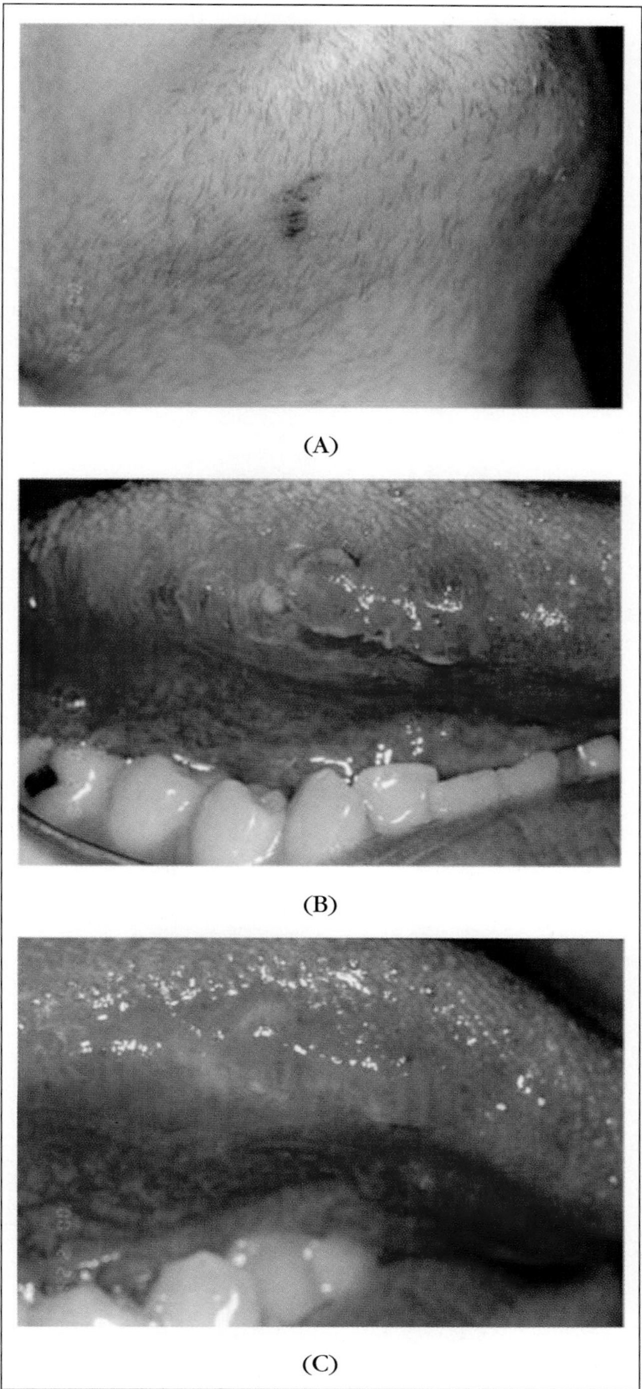

(A)

(B)

(C)

**FIGURE 157-9** (A) A 17-year-old white male wrestler received a blow to the mandible resulting in an abrasion with tissue edema; (B) The injury caused the patient to bite through the right lateral border of the tongue as demonstrated in the photo taken 2 days after the injury occurred; (C) Five days postinjury the tongue laceration healed spontaneously.

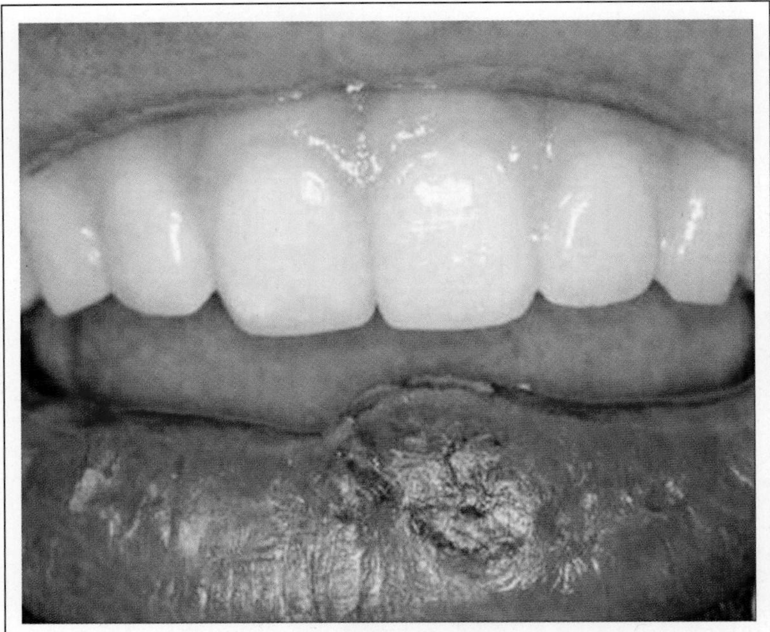

**FIGURE 157-10** Adolescent women's varsity basketball player with a self-inflicted bite wound to the lower lip that later developed into a mucocele.

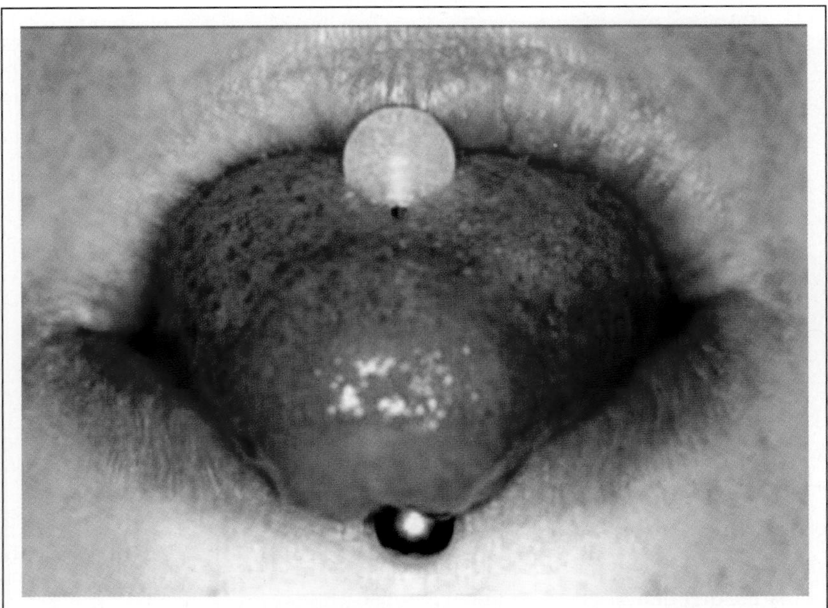

**FIGURE 157-11** Localized tissue reaction following tongue piercing and placement of jewelry.

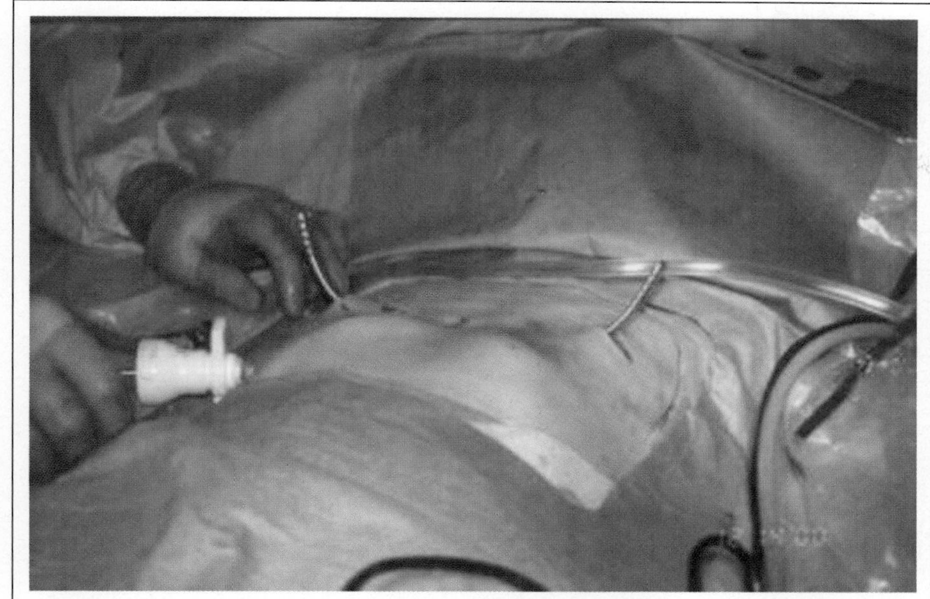

**FIGURE 163-3** Intraoperative photograph of VAPER showing convex bar in place before eversion of the sternum.

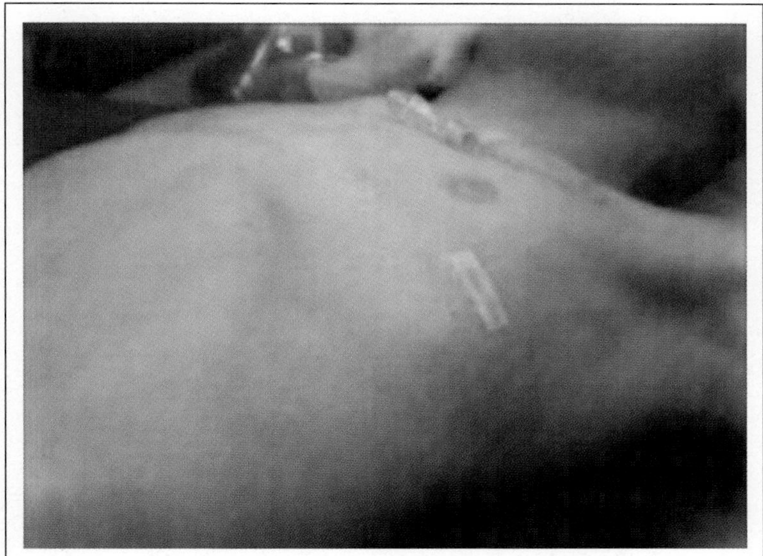

**FIGURE 163-4** Immediate postoperative photograph after eversion of sternum.

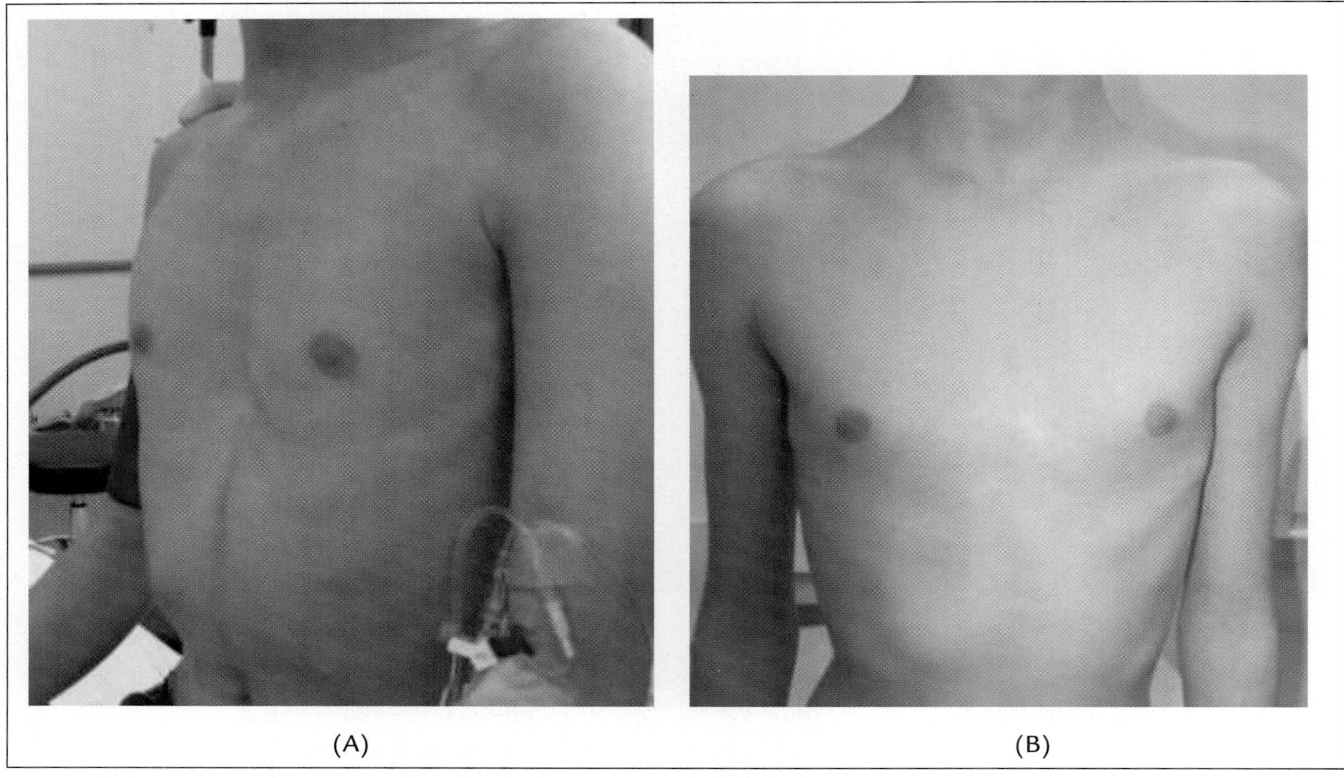


**FIGURE 163-5** PE patient (A) before and (B) after VAPER.

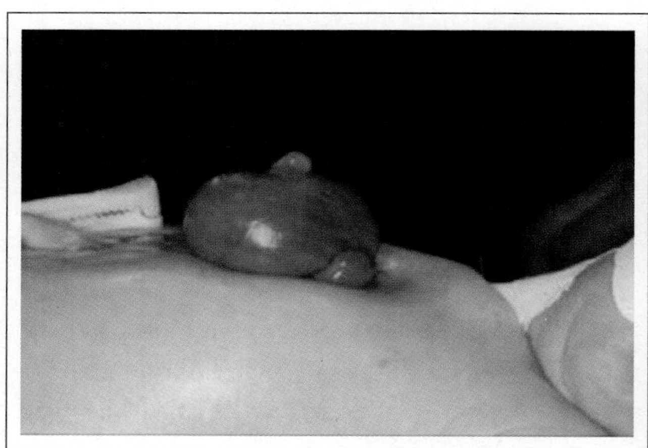

**FIGURE 163-6** Thoracic ectopia cordis.

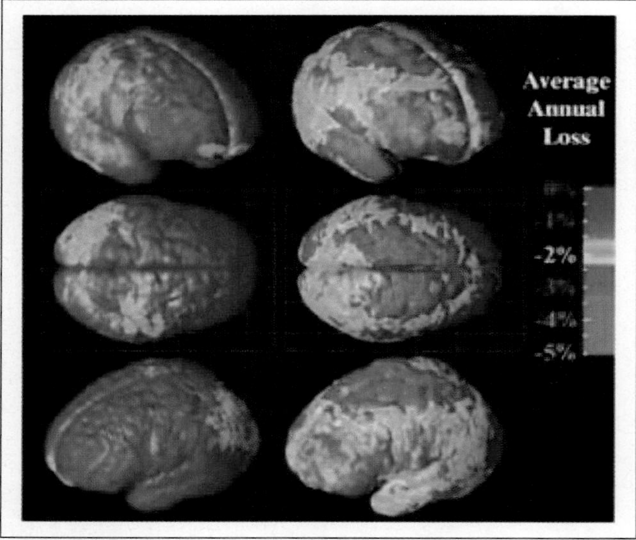


**FIGURE 188-1** Compared to gray matter loss pattern in normal adolescents (left), adolescents with schizophrenia (right) experience progressive gray matter loss in the parietal, motor, supplementary motor, and superior frontal cortices, with broad regions of the temporal cortex, including the superior temporal gyrus most severely affected. (Reprinted with permission from Thompson PM et al. Mapping adolescent brain change reveals dynamic wave of accelerated gray matter loss in very early-onset schizophrenia. *Proc Nat Acad Sci USA*. 2001;98(20):11650–11655. Copyright 2001 National Academy of Sciences, U.S.A.)

## REFERENCES

1. Bruch SW, Ein SH, Rocchi C, Kim PC. The management of non pigmented gallstones in children. *J Pediatr Surg.* 2000;35(5):729-732

2. Kumar R, Nguyen K, Shun A. Gallstones and common duct calculi in infancy and childhood. *Aust N Z J Surg.* 2000;70(3):188-191

3. Strom BL, Tamragouri RN, Morse ML, et al. Oral contraceptives and other risk factors for gallbladder disease. *Clin Pharmacol Ther.* 1986;39(3):335-341

4. Stringer MD, Soloway RD, Taylor DR, Riyad K, Toogood G. Calcium carbonate gallstones in children. *J Pediatr Surg.* 2007;42:1677-1682

5. Tanaka S, Kubota D, Oba K, et al. Gallbladder torsion-induced emphysematous cholecystitis in a 16-year-old boy. *J Hepatobiliary Pancreat Surg.* 2007;14(6):608-610

6. Beck PL, Shaffer EA, Gall DG, Sherman PM. The natural history and significance of ultrasonographically defined polypoid lesions of the gallbladder in children. *J Pediatr Surg.* 2007;42:1907-1912

7. Al-Homaidhi HS, Sukerek H, Klein M, Tolia V. Biliary dyskinesia in children. *Pediatr Surg Int.* 2002;18(5-6):357-360. Epub 2002 Apr 24

8. Holcomb GW III, Morgan WM III, Neblett WW III, et al. Laparoscopic cholecystectomy in children: lessons learned from the first 100 cases. *J Pediatr Surg.* 1999;34(8):1236-1240

9. Esposito C, Gonzalez Sabin MA, Corcione E, et al. Results and complications of laparoscopic cholecystectomy in childhood. *Surg Endosc.* 2001;15(8):890-892

# CHAPTER 102

# Appendicitis

ROBERT SAMMARTANO, PA-C • SYLVAIN KLEINHAUS, MD

The incidence of acute appendicitis is highest in adolescence and early adulthood and is the most common indication for abdominal surgery in this age group. Appreciation of the early signs and symptoms of appendicitis is of the utmost importance in diagnosing and treating the patient in an expedient manner, thus avoiding the complications associated with appendiceal perforation and peritonitis. Although the exact etiology of acute appendicitis is not always evident, obstruction of the appendiceal lumen is believed to be the cause in most cases. After obstruction, the mucosa distal to the obstruction continues to secrete mucus, and intestinal content continues to ferment in a closed system. The appendiceal lumen distends as the pressure increases, compressing the submucosal vessels and resulting in ischemia of the appendiceal wall. If this ischemia is not corrected, gangrene and necrosis will ensue, with resultant perforation, peritoneal contamination, and peritonitis. Obstruction is most commonly caused by a fecalith, which may or may not be radiopaque. Other causes such as foreign bodies, tumors, and parasitic infestation, although less frequent, are not unusual. The terminal ileum and pericecal area are rich in lymphatics (Peyer patches), especially in adolescents and lymphoid hypertrophy, which sometimes occurs during an acute viral illness, may also compress the appendiceal lumen, resulting in appendicitis.

## DIAGNOSIS

### HISTORY

Classically, the pain associated with appendicitis first presents periumbilically; this is because the appendix originates from the same dermatome as the umbilical region. Gradually, as the appendiceal inflammation and periappendiceal reaction develop, the pain shifts to the right lower quadrant. The exact location of the pain depends on the anatomic position of the appendix. If the appendix lies in the pelvis, the primary symptom may be dysuria; if it is in the cul-de-sac, tenesmus may be the most prominent sign; if the appendix lies in the right paracolic gutter, the pain may mimic cholecystitis or renal colic; if it points medially, the periumbilical pain may not shift to the right lower quadrant but remain in the midabdomen. Retrocecal appendicitis is often difficult to diagnose, because the overlying cecum can mask the evolving pathologic condition in the appendix.

The earliest symptoms are usually anorexia, nausea, and/or vomiting, which may precede or follow the onset of pain. The patient initially may be afebrile, but a low-grade fever soon develops. The patient's temperature rises as the inflammatory response to the appendicitis progresses. By the time gangrene sets in and the patient's appendix perforates, the patient's temperature has usually risen to 102°F (39°C) unless antipyretic agents have been administered.

## PHYSICAL EXAMINATION

The physical examination is the most important factor in diagnosing appendicitis. Palpation of the abdomen should be preceded by auscultation for the presence or absence of bowel sounds. In acute appendicitis the bowel sounds are usually diminished or absent, a direct result of localized or generalized peritonitis. If a perforation has occurred, intestinal motility is reduced so that the patient avoids painful stretching of the peritoneum as much as possible and therefore reduces the amount of spillage of intestinal contents. The presence of hyperactive bowel sounds should call into question the diagnosis of acute appendicitis.

The most tender area on palpation of the abdomen is usually in the right lower quadrant overlying McBurney point, which is at the junction of the lateral third and medial two-thirds of a line joining the umbilicus and anterosuperior iliac spine. As mentioned, the point of maximal tenderness also depends on the location of the appendix. As the degree of inflammation increases, so does the ability of the patient to localize the pain to a small specific area.

If the diagnosis is not made and the process is allowed to progress, perforation will eventually occur. If the perforation is localized and contained by the omentum, small bowel, cecum, and adnexa, or any combination of contiguous structures, the pain will remain localized to the right lower quadrant. If there is a free perforation, generalized peritonitis will ensue with its typical signs and symptoms. Abdominal guarding will be more generalized with rebound tenderness throughout, the abdomen will be silent, the patient will attempt to remain motionless, and paradoxically the pain will be subjectively less for a short time.

The rectal examination is most likely to be positive if the tip of the appendix lies in the posterior cul-de-sac. However, a normal rectal examination does not preclude appendicitis. The digital examination may not elicit any pain if the appendix is retrocecal or in the right pericolic gutter. If the appendix has already perforated, a pelvic abscess will often be palpable through the anterior rectal wall.

## LABORATORY TESTING

Laboratory results may also be helpful in confirming the diagnosis. Leukocytosis, which is almost always present from the onset, will progressively increase to the 12,000 to 18,000 range, with a progressive left shift as the process continues. The urinalysis may be positive, especially if the appendix overlies the ureter and/or dome of the bladder. If only the ureter is involved, a small number of white or red blood cells may be seen; if the inflammation involves the bladder wall, the cell count per high-power field may be higher. On occasion, urinary tract symptoms are so prominent in the early stages of the disease that it may even be mistaken for cystitis.

Radiographs of the chest and abdomen are helpful in diagnosing acute appendicitis. Lower lobar pneumonia, especially on the right side, may be confused with appendicitis, and recognition of a lower lobar infiltrate on a chest film can prevent the performance of an unnecessary appendectomy. On the other hand, several findings on abdominal flat films may reinforce the clinical impression of appendicitis. A localized right lower quadrant ileus and/or a mass effect in the area of the cecum are often seen in appendicitis (Figure 102-1). The presence of a fecalith is considered an absolute indication for appendectomy. Not only is obstruction of the appendiceal lumen more likely in the presence of an appendicolith, but data indicate that perforation occurs more frequently and earlier in the course of the disease in patients with calcified fecaliths than in patients without fecaliths. For this reason, we recommend elective appendectomy in the absence of symptoms in any patient with an appendicolith evident on an abdominal film (Figure 102-2).

Ultrasonography has become an important diagnostic tool in cases in which the diagnosis of appendicitis is unclear. With ultrasonography, the pelvic organs can be visualized well in most cases in females, and the presence of an unsuspected pregnancy can be excluded.

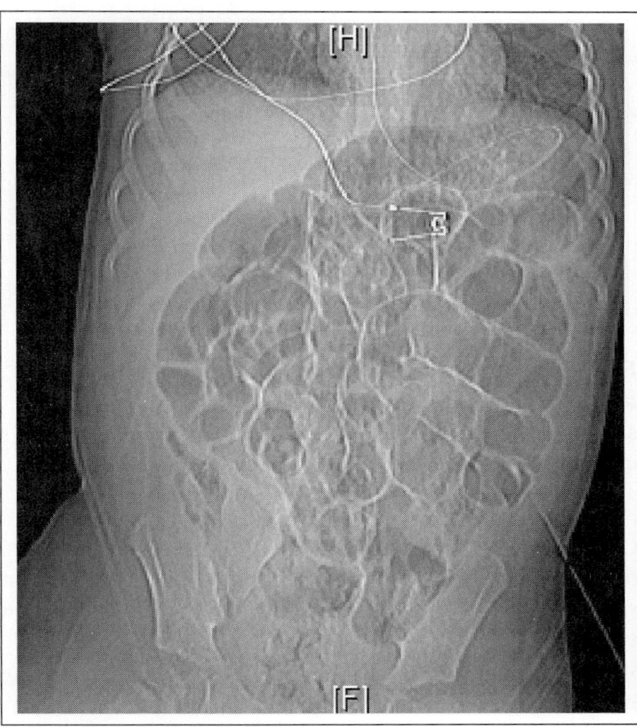


**FIGURE 102-1** Plain film of abdomen showing paucity of gas in right lower quadrant and distended small bowel loops consistent with ileus or obstruction.

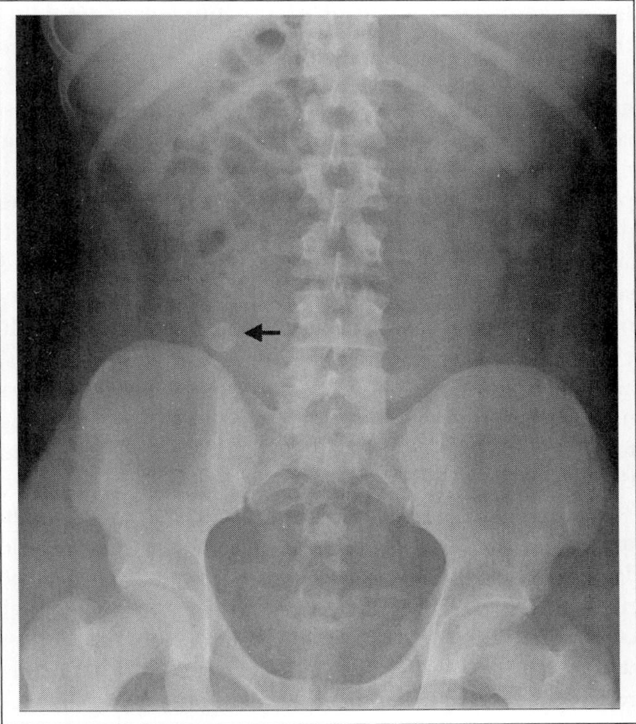

**FIGURE 102-2** Plain film of the abdomen showing large appendicolith (arrow) in right lower quadrant.

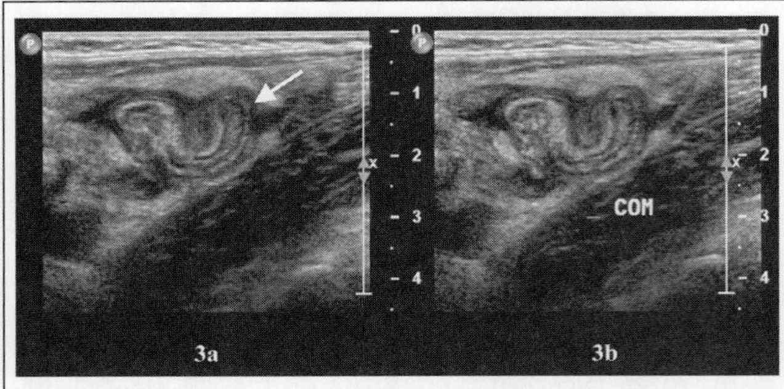


**FIGURE 102-3** (A) Ultrasound appearance of acute appendicitis showing distension, hyperemic wall, and surrounding edema of the appendix (arrow). (B) No change with compression of the abdominal wall.

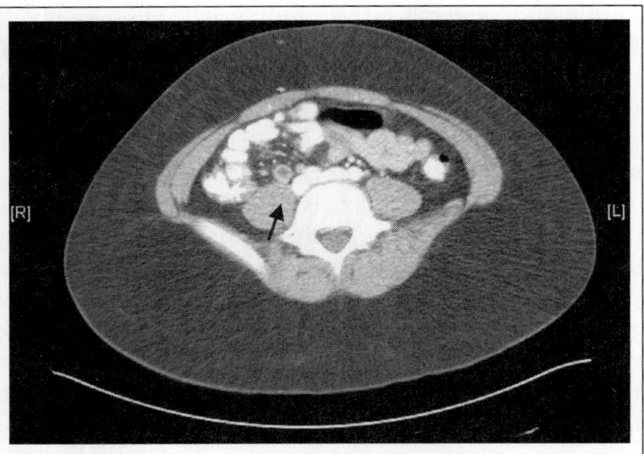


**FIGURE 102-4** CT showing acute nonperforated appendicitis with an enhancing appendiceal wall, (arrow) no free fluid.

Ovarian cysts and/or fluid in the cul-de-sac can be demonstrated, as well as adnexal abnormalities such as torsion, inflammation, and extrauterine gestation. In some cases the appendix itself can be visualized, and in some studies this finding has been used to make a presumptive radiologic diagnosis of appendicitis (Figure 102-3A and Figure 102-3B).

One of the major shortcomings of ultrasound diagnosis in general is that it is operator dependent. In other words, the ability to confirm or negate a clinical diagnosis is to a great degree dependent on the talents and determination of the individual wielding the ultrasound wand. The static images seen afterward contain only the information garnered by the radiologist who performed the study and only that radiologist is able to interpret the study accurately. If the diagnosis is clear-cut on the ultrasound screen there is no problem. However, in those cases where the ultrasound does not show a swollen, noncompressible inflamed appendix, the question always arises "did we miss something? Was the appendix obscured by bowel gas, or is another organ involved, or is this not appendicitis?" For this reason, in the last 9 years since the first article by Rao and associates appeared, many centers have substituted computed tomography (CT) scanning for ultrasound as the major auxiliary examination in those equivocal cases.

With the advent of the multidetector array CT (up to 64), a total body scan can be completed in as little as 20 seconds. The information gathered can then be reconstituted in any desired plane; coronal, sagittal, or axial. As long as the patient is relatively motionless during the procedure the CT scan will give a reliable representation of the intra-abdominal organs. The images produced contain all the information needed to formulate a diagnosis. It is the experience and knowledge of the radiologist interpreting those images that ascertains the accuracy of the diagnosis. The physician reading the study will be able to give an opinion on the state of the appendix, as well as the adjoining bowel, urinary tract, and reproductive organs.

Though not perfect, the CT scan has been found to have a high degree of accuracy and low false-positive rate (Figure 102-4). Some centers prefer the contrast material to be taken orally; others prefer a rectal route of administration. Each route has its advantages. At the authors' institution, most CT scans for appendicitis have the contrast administered orally. This has the disadvantage of having to wait for the passage of the contrast material down to the cecal area, but allows for an accurate visualization of the small bowel and terminal ileum as well as the ascending colon. The presence of a small bowel obstruction or appendiceal perforation, with or without intraperitoneal abscesses, can often be determined using the CT scan (Figure 102-5 and Figure 102-6). It also has the advantage of being able to identify gynecologic abnormalities, both structural and inflammatory, which may be the cause of the abdominal pain.

Of particular interest for patients with perforated appendicitis, Levin et al, in a study of pediatric patients evaluated by CT scan, demonstrated a ninefold increase to fail conservative management (resuscitation, antibiotics, recovery and delayed interval appendectomy) in those patients with evidence of peritonitis/absecess/ascites in more than 2 sectors of the abdominal cavity, thus necessitating surgical intervention. Those with less than 2 sectors were able in most cases to complete their non-operative therapy as planned.

Adolescent females present greater difficulties in diagnosis. Pelvic inflammatory disease and ovarian cysts

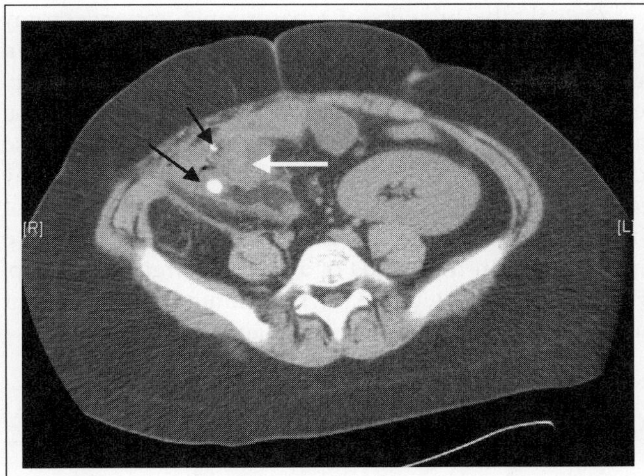


FIGURE 102-5 CT showing acute appendicitis with appendicoliths (black arrows). Phlegmon present medial to appendix (white arrow) suggests perforation.

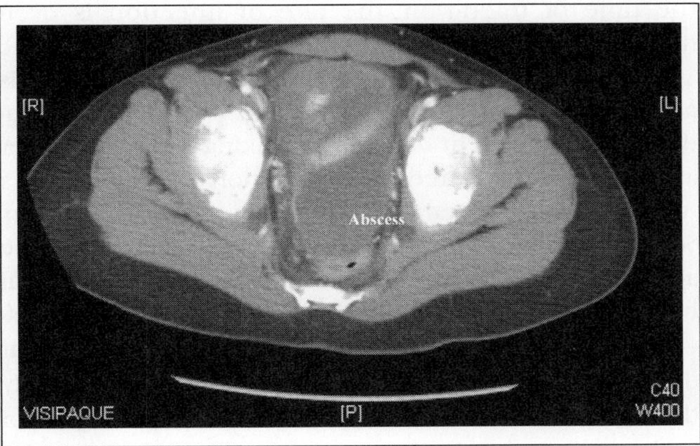


FIGURE 102-6 CT showing pelvic abscess following perforated appendicitis.

are the entities most commonly confused with appendicitis. Although pelvic inflammatory disease is associated with a history of previous sexual activity, it must be suspected even if no such history is obtained. Mittelschmerz also varies from patient to patient and from one menstrual cycle to another. Patients with pelvic inflammatory disease are most likely to present with acute abdominal pain in the immediate postmenstrual period, whereas the pain accompanying a ruptured follicular cyst occurs in midcycle. If a patient has pelvic inflammatory disease, the pelvic examination will frequently disclose a pelvic infection, and a Gram stain of any discharge may reveal intracellular diplococci. Of course, the presence of one entity does not preclude concomitant appendicitis.

## TREATMENT

The definitive treatment of appendicitis is appendectomy. Once the diagnosis is made, appendectomy should be performed as expeditiously as possible to prevent perforation. Even if there is a high degree of suspicion without clinical certainty, it is considered safer to perform an appendectomy than to delay treatment for observation. These patients are usually mildly dehydrated and require fluid resuscitation before induction of anesthesia. Serum electrolyte levels, as determined by serial serum analysis, are corrected and adequate urinary output is ensured. If there is peritonitis, the fluid requirements may be impressive. In addition, intravenous antibiotics are administered in the pre- and postoperative periods. A nasogastric tube is placed in most patients, especially those in whom an ileus has been demonstrated. Intraoperatively, the operative site should be irrigated profusely with a 0.1% kanamycin solution before closing the peritoneum, and the same solution is used to vigorously irrigate the muscle, fascia, and subcutaneous layers. In grossly contaminated cases the skin is closed over a subcutaneous Penrose drain brought out through the lateral end of the incision.

There is still a difference of opinion over surgical treatment of the perforated appendix with a periappendiceal mass or abscess. Some surgeons prefer to operate immediately, drain the abscess, and remove the appendix after proper rehydration and fluid resuscitation. Others believe that it is safer to delay the appendectomy until the patient is no longer toxic and the abdominal signs and symptoms have abated. An elective appendectomy can then be performed, usually several weeks later, without the risk of opening the contained perforation and spreading the contamination to the remainder of the peritoneal cavity. However, it is not uncommon for the patient to redevelop acute appendicitis while awaiting interval appendectomy. If the patient does not respond to nonoperative therapy, including appropriate antibiotic administration, fluid resuscitation, and nasogastric suction, the operation should be performed immediately despite the associated risks.

### LAPAROSCOPIC APPENDECTOMY

The increasing availability and variety of laparoscopic surgical instrumentation, and the large number of surgeons trained in laparoscopic operative technique for cholecystectomy, have made laparoscopic appendectomy possible at most institutions. Since laparoscopic appendectomy for acute appendicitis was first reported by Semm in 1983, numerous authors have reported randomized and nonrandomized prospective experiences comparing laparoscopic and open appendectomy.

The surgical indications in patients presenting with acute, noncomplicated appendicitis are the same for laparoscopic appendectomy and open appendectomy. For the patient whose clinical presentation suggests an intra-abdominal process that is not clearly appendicitis, laparoscopic evaluation of the abdomen is a valuable tool. This is especially so for the adolescent female patient who has reached menarche; who presents with right-sided, lower abdominal pain; and in whom the clinical investigation is equivocal for an acute abdomen. Laparoscopy allows direct visualization of the intra-abdominal and pelvic viscera and permits the surgeon to delineate the extensive differential diagnoses for the patient's symptoms. If no pelvic or abdominal pathology is found at laparoscopy, an appendectomy is performed so that if the patient presents with similar abdominal pain at a later date, a diagnosis of acute appendicitis is eliminated, sparing the patient a possible right lower quadrant laparotomy.

If the appendix is perforated, laparoscopic appendectomy affords a complete view of the abdominal viscera, as well as the ability to assess the extent of the spillage of intestinal contents into the peritoneal cavity. It also enables the surgeon to irrigate effectively those areas that are not readily accessible through a small classic open incision.

The results of treatment of acute appendicitis using an open or laparoscopic approach have been compared by various authors. Bonanni et al, reported 300 consecutive open as compared with 66 laparoscopic appendectomies, finding essentially no differences in operative complications, postoperative morbidity, pain medication requirements, or time to resumption of a regular diet. In their experience, for complicated appendicitis, laparoscopic appendectomy carried a higher postoperative rate of abscess formation. Other authors have reported an opposite experience with complicated appendicitis treated by laparoscopy or by an open operation.

Varlet et al, in a retrospective study, reported that of 403 appendectomies (200 laparoscopic and 203 open) there were definite advantages in laparoscopic appendectomy. These were noted as ease of treatment for ectopic appendix, less operative trauma, efficient peritoneal lavage, less frequent postoperative complications, and better postoperative comfort.

As for any abdominal surgery, there is an occurrence of symptomatic postoperative adhesions after open and laparoscopic appendectomy. These adhesions can present as partial or complete bowel obstruction, adnexal torsion, and also recurrent intermittent abdominal pain. Laparoscopic exploration with adhesiolysis has been used effectively to treat patients presenting with postappendectomy abdominal pain.

Overall, the benefits of laparoscopic appendectomy for noncomplicated acute appendicitis are seen in reduced length of hospital stay, decreased use of postoperative pain medications, and faster return to a normal active lifestyle. The added expense because of the use of disposable laparoscopic instrumentation noted by some authors is easily offset by the decreased length of hospital stay and the increased availability of reusable instruments. In the hands of a trained surgical staff, laparoscopic appendectomy is becoming a safe, efficient alternative to conventional open appendectomy.

## COMPLICATIONS

The complications of acute appendicitis are many despite optimal therapy. The most common is infection. Superficial wound infections occur in 6% to 15% of patients with nonsuppurative acute appendicitis, with or without perioperative antibiotic therapy. In cases in which appendicitis is more advanced at the time of operation, the rate of infection is even higher.

The second most common infectious complication is a pelvic abscess, which develops 4 to 7 days after appendectomy. The patient develops a spiking fever and lower abdominal pain; a rectal examination demonstrates a tender anterior rectal wall that bulges into the lumen. Sonography confirms the presence and extent of the abscess, as well as any other coexistent intra-abdominal collections. Many of these abscesses respond to intravenous antibiotic and symptomatic treatment without drainage. Some pelvic collections drain spontaneously through the rectum, as manifested by a transanal gush of foul-smelling mucopurulent material. Some cases require surgical drainage in the operating room; when possible, this is done transanally. In the more complicated cases, ultrasonographic guidance is used to place a catheter within the abscess cavity.

Before the availability of antibiotics, one of the most feared complications of appendicitis was pylephlebitis: infectious thrombosis of the portal vein. Fortunately, this occurrence is now rare. Inflammatory involvement of the right uterine adnexa often produces adhesions that incorporate the fimbria and may result in occlusion of the fallopian tube.

## CONCLUSION

Acute appendicitis is a common disease in the adolescent. The treatment goal is to diagnose the condition as early as possible in the disease course so that complications can be minimized. This requires appropriate pre- and postoperative care and frequent sequential examinations by the same practitioner in cases in which the diagnosis is unclear.

## BIBLIOGRAPHY


Attwood SEA, Hill ADK, Murphy PG, Thornton J, Stephens RB. A prospective randomized trial of laparoscopic versus open appendectomy. *Surgery.* 1992;112:497-501

Bagi P, Dueholm S, Karstrup S. Percutaneous drainage of appendiceal abscess: an alternative to conventional treatment. *Dis Colon Rectum.* 1987;30:532-535

Bonnani F, Reed J III, Hartzell G, et al. Laparoscopic versus conventional appendectomy. *J Am Coll Surg.* 1994;179: 273-278

Gaensler EHL, Jeffrey RB, Laing FC, Townsend RR. Sonography in patients with suspected acute appendicitis: value in establishing alternative diagnoses. *AJR.* 1989;152: 49-51

Gilchrist BF, Lobe TE, Schropp KP, et al. Is there a role for laparoscopic appendectomy in pediatric surgery? *J Pediatr Surg.* 1992;127:209-214

Heinzelmann M, Simmen HP, Cummins AS, Largiadér F. Is laparoscopic appendectomy the new "gold standard"? *Arch Surg.* 1995;130:782-785

Horrow MM, White SD, et al. Differentiation of perforated from non perforated appendicitis at CT. *Radiology.* 2003;227: 46-51

Humes DJ, Simpson J. Acute appendicitis. *BMJ.* 2006;333 (7567):530-534

Jeffrey RB Jr, Laing FC, Townsend RR. Acute appendicitis: sonographic criteria based on 250 cases. *Radiology.* 1988;167: 327-329

Jeffrey RB Jr, Laing FC, Lewis FR. Acute appendicitis: high resolution real-time US findings. *Radiology.* 1987;163:11-14

Kleinhaus S. Laparoscopic lysis of adhesions for postappendectomy pain. *Endoscopy.* 1985;30:304-305

Levin T, Whyte C, Borzykowski R, Han B, Blitman N, Harris BH. Nonoperative management of perforated appendicitis in children: can CT predict outcome? *Pediatr Radiol.* 2007;37(3):251-255

Newman K, Ponsky T, Kittle K,et al. Appendicitis 2000: variability in practice, outcomes, and resource utilization at thirty pediatric hospitals. *J Pediatr Surg.* 2003;38(3):372-379

Pulaert JBCM, Rutgers PH, et al. A prospective study of ultrasonography in the diagnosis of appendicitis. *N Engl J Med.* 1987;317:666-669

Rabau MY, Dreznik Z, et al. Indications for interval appendectomy in the management of appendicular abscess. *J Abdom Surg.* 1980;22:73-74

Rajagopalan AE, Mason JH, Kennedy M, Pawlikowski J. The value of the barium enema in the diagnosis of acute appendicitis. *Arch Surg.* 1977;112:531-533

Rao PM, Rhea JT, Novelline RA, Mostafavi AA, McCabe CJ. Effect on computed tomography of the appendix on the treatment of patients and the use of hospital resources. *N Engl J Med.* 1998;338(3):141-146

Reiertsen O, Trondsen E, et al. Prospective non-randomized study of conventional versus laparoscopic appendectomy. *World J Surg.* 1994;18:411-416

Samuelson SL, Reyes HM. Management of perforated appendicitis in children—revisited. *Arch Surg.* 1977;112:531-533

Schirmer BD, Schmieg RE, Dix J, Edge SB, Hanks JB. Laparoscopic versus traditional appendectomy for suspected appendicitis. *Am J Surg.* 1993;165:670-675

Seal A. Appendicitis: an historical review. *Can J Surg.* 1981; 24(4):427-433

Semm K. Endoscopic appendectomy. *Endoscopy.* 1983;15: 59-64

Varlet F, Tardieu D, Limonne B, Metafiot H, Chavrier Y. Laparoscopic versus open appendectomy in 403 children—comparative study. *Eur J Surg.* 1994;4:333-337

Williams MD, Miller D, Graves ED, Walsh C, Luterman A. Laparoscopic appendectomy, is it worth it? *South Med J.* 1994; 87:592-598

Whyte C, Levin T, Harris BH. Early decisions in perforated appendicitis in children: lessons learned from a study of nonoperative management. *J Pediatr Surg.* 2008;43(8):1459-63

Whyte C, Tran E, Lopez ME, Harris BH. Outpatient interval appendectomy after perforated appendicitis. *J Pediatr Surg.* 2008;43(11):1970-2

# CHAPTER 103

## Diarrhea in the Adolescent

ELIZAVETA IOFEL, MD • MICHAEL J. PETTEI, MD, PhD

The behaviors and activities often associated with adolescents place them at risk for particular patterns of diarrheal illness. Compared with younger pediatric age groups, adolescents have easier access to contaminated foods, travel more extensively, and can be sexually active. Although diarrhea may be caused by a wide variety of conditions, for adolescents most cases can be divided into 3 general categories: inflammatory, dietary, and functional gastrointestinal disorders. The most common conditions in these categories are listed in Box 103-1. Some causes of diarrhea, for example, cystic fibrosis, short bowel syndrome, and the congenital diarrheas, are not discussed because their presentation is most commonly outside the adolescent age range. The noninfectious inflammatory conditions, such as celiac disease and the idiopathic inflammatory bowel diseases, listed in Box 103-1, are described in other chapters of this text and will not be addressed here.

### INFECTIOUS CAUSES OF DIARRHEA IN ADOLESCENTS

#### VIRAL

Viruses are responsible for most cases of acute diarrhea in the United States at all ages. While rotavirus is a common cause of diarrhea in younger children, with virtually all children less than 3 years of age having had infection, noroviruses (Norwalk-like viruses), a calcivirus, are the overall most common cause of gastroenteritis, responsible for 68% to 80% of all outbreaks in industrialized countries.[1] Other viral pathogens include enteric adenoviruses and astroviruses, especially in young children. All seem to be transmitted principally via a fecal–oral route and are often food-borne. Most present with the acute onset of watery, nonbloody diarrhea with abdominal cramps, often preceded by vomiting. In immunocompetent individuals outside of infancy, symptoms are self-limited, usually lasting 1 to 2 days. The most common complication, dehydration, does not usually carry the same risk in the healthy adolescent as it does in infants or the elderly. Treatment is supportive, with attention given to replacement of oral fluids and electrolytes, with intravenous fluids rarely required.[1]

**Box 103-1**

***Common Conditions Associated with Diarrhea in Adolescence***

I. Inflammatory conditions
  A. Infectious
  B. Noninfectious
    1. Celiac disease
    2. Idiopathic inflammatory bowel disease
      a. Crohn disease
      b. Ulcerative colitis
II. Dietary agents
  A. Lactose intolerance
  B. Sugar alcohol ingestion
III. Irritable bowel syndrome

#### BACTERIAL

In developed countries, bacterial pathogens account for 2% to 10% of all cases of diarrhea.[2] *Campylobacter, Salmonella, Shigella*, and enterohemorrhagic *Escherichia coli* (EHEC) account for most cases in the United States. The presentation of bacterial gastroenteritis overlaps with viral disease, and the 2 can be indistinguishable clinically. A few features, however, are more often associated with a bacterial cause. High fevers, shaking chills, blood in the stool, and the presence of leukocytes in a stool specimen may be helpful in discriminating bacterial gastroenteritis from viral disease.[1]

##### *Shigella*

*Shigella* was discovered more than a century ago by a Japanese scientist named Shiga, for whom it is named. Humans are the natural host for *Shigella* and several different species are associated with disease. *Shigella sonnei* accounts for more than two-thirds of cases of shigellosis in the United States, while *Shigella flexneri* accounts for almost all of the rest. Other species of *Shigella* are rare in the United States although they continue to be important causes of disease in the developing world. *Shigella* is spread through the fecal–oral route. The organism is capable of surviving for up to 30 days in foods such as milk, whole eggs, oysters, shrimp, and flour.[3]

Shigellosis typically begins 1 to 4 days after exposure. Clinical features are variable, ranging from simple watery diarrhea to bloody diarrhea with severe systemic symptoms including fever and abdominal cramps. Infection usually involves the large intestine. Symptoms usually resolve in 3 to 7 days. Adolescents rarely require hospitalization while a form associated with high fevers and seizures can be seen in younger children. Rarely, toxic megacolon and intestinal perforation can be seen with severe infection. *Shigella* infection may cause a variety of extraintestinal manifestations; these most commonly include arthralgia, arthritis, the reactive arthritis previously known as Reiter syndrome (ie, arthritis, uveitis, and conjunctivitis) and hemolytic-uremic syndrome (HUS). *Shigella* infection is diagnosed by a routine stool culture.

Most infections by Shigella sonnei are self-limited and resolve without treatment, although treatment can be effective in shortening duration of diarrhea and eradicating the organisms. Therapy is recommended in those with severe disease or for those patients who have an underlying immunosuppressive condition. Because resistance to the standard medications that have been used for many years (ampicillin and trimethoprim-sulfamethoxazole) is now common, antibiotic susceptibility testing should be performed. In cases of resistant strains, a fluoroquinolone, azithromycin, or parenteral ceftriaxone may be used. Fluoroquinolones are not generally recommended for use in those under 18 years of age. The oral route of therapy is preferred, except for the cephalosporins. Antidiarrheal agents that prolong transit time may prolong the course of disease and are contraindicated.

### *Salmonella*

*Salmonella* organisms are gram-negative bacilli that belong to the *Enterobacteriaceae* family. The principal reservoirs for nontyphoidal *Salmonella* organisms are animals, including poultry, livestock, reptiles, and pets. The major mode of transmission is from foods of animal origin, including poultry, beef, fish, eggs, and dairy products.[4] Many other foods, including fruits, vegetables, and bakery products, have been implicated in outbreaks. These foods usually are contaminated by contact with an animal product or, occasionally, an infected human, or human waste. Other vehicles for transmission include ingestion of contaminated water or contact with infected reptiles.[5]

Age-specific attack rates for *Salmonella* infection are highest in people younger than 4 years of age. Rates of invasive infection and mortality are higher in infants, the elderly, and people with immunosuppressive conditions. Adolescents usually have milder cases of the disease. Most cases are sporadic, but widespread outbreaks have been reported. In 2006, *Salmonella* was reported to be the major organism causing laboratory-confirmed cases of enteric disease by the Foodborne Diseases Active Surveillance Network (FoodNet).[6]

Infection with nontyphoidal *Salmonella* causes a wide spectrum of disease, ranging from asymptomatic carriage or gastroenteritis to bacteremia, meningitis, and osteomyelitis. The most common illness associated with nontyphoidal *Salmonella* is a gastroenteritis that usually occurs 12 to 72 hours after exposure and is characterized by diarrhea, abdominal cramps, and fever. The infection usually involves the small intestine, an enteritis, but large intestinal involvement, a colitis, can occur. The illness usually lasts 4 to 7 days. Bacteremia has been reported; meningitis and osteomyelitis have been noted in 10% of patients with *Salmonella bacteremia*. Chronic fecal shedding of *Salmonella* is well known and the risk of transmission exists as long as shedding is present. Twelve weeks after infection, 5% to 45% of patients continue to shed *Salmonella*. Approximately 1% of patients shed for more than 1 year and are considered chronic carriers.[1] Diagnosis of salmonellosis is made by isolation of organisms from cultures of stool, blood, urine, or the material from the focus of infection.

Antimicrobial therapy usually is not indicated for patients with uncomplicated, noninvasive *Salmonella* gastroenteritis because therapy does not shorten the duration of disease and may prolong the duration of carriage. Although of unproven benefit, antimicrobial therapy is recommended for gastroenteritis caused by *Salmonella* species in patients with an increased risk of invasive disease or those with severe colitis.[7] Ampicillin, amoxicillin, trimethoprim-sulfamethoxazole, cefotaxime, and ceftriaxone are recommended for susceptible strains. Strains acquired in developing countries often exhibit resistance to many antimicrobial agents but usually are susceptible to ceftriaxone or cefotaxime and to fluoroquinolones.[1] Fluoroquinolones, like ciprofloxacin, are not approved for this use in those under 18 years of age.

Typhoid fever strains usually originate in developing countries and present without diarrhea as the main symptom and are thus not discussed here.

### *Escherichia Coli*

Although *E coli* is a normal component of gut flora, there are at least 5 different pathogenic strains of diarrhea-producing *E coli* that have been identified. The only *E coli* type that commonly causes diarrhea in the United States is the Shiga toxin-producing EHEC, especially *E coli* O157:H7, which is shed in the feces of cattle. Entero-hemorrhagic *E coli* can be transmitted by contaminated (undercooked) ground beef, water, raw fruits and vegetables, (unpasteurized) milk, and a wide variety of agents contaminated with bovine or infected human feces. Infections caused by *E coli* O157:H7 are detected sporadically or during outbreaks. The infectious dose is as small as 100 organisms, and person-to-person transmission is common during outbreaks.

Entero-hemorrhagic *E coli* strains are associated with diarrhea, hemorrhagic colitis, the HUS, and postdiarrhea thrombotic thrombocytopenic purpura. The incubation period is 4 to 8 days. Illness caused by EHEC often begins as nonbloody diarrhea, but usually progresses to diarrhea with visible or occult blood. Although severe abdominal pain is typical, fever occurs in less than one-third of cases. Hemolytic-uremic syndrome (HUS), defined as the triad of microangiopathic hemolytic anemia, thrombocytopenia, and acute renal dysfunction, is the most serious sequela of EHEC infection and seems to occur more frequently with *E coli* O157:H7 than other serotypes and usually in younger patients. It occurs in 8% of children with *E coli* O157:H7 diarrhea, usually developing in the 2 weeks after the onset of the diarrhea.[8] Thrombotic thrombocytopenic purpura more typically occurs in adolescents and adults and is the same disease as postdiarrhea HUS except with neurologic features.

Commensal *E coli* cannot be distinguished from diarrhea-producing *E coli* by routine culture; however, identification of *E coli* O157:H7 can be performed in most commercial laboratories. It should be ordered separately from the routine stool culture. For all patients with HUS, stool specimens should be cultured for *E coli* O157:H7 and, if results are negative, for other EHEC serotypes. When EHEC infection is considered, a stool culture and typing should be obtained as early in the illness as possible. Careful follow-up of patients with hemorrhagic colitis, including obtaining a complete blood cell count with smear, along with blood urea nitrogen and creatinine concentrations, is recommended to detect early signs of HUS. If there is no laboratory evidence of hemolysis, thrombocytopenia, or nephropathy 3 days after resolution of diarrhea, the risk of developing HUS is low.[1] A meta-analysis failed to show an increased or decreased risk of HUS in children with EHEC treated with antibiotics.[9] Most experts, however, would not treat children with *E coli* O157:H7 disease with an antimicrobial agent because no benefit has been proven, and such treatment may increase the risk of HUS.[10] Additionally, antimotility agents should not be used.

Adolescents are old enough to be educated to avoid of risk factors associated with infection with *E coli* O157:H7. Only ground beef that has been thoroughly cooked, with no pink meat and only clear juices, should be consumed. Apple juice should be pasteurized, and no raw milk products should be consumed.

### *Campylobacter*

*Campylobacter* species are motile, comma-shaped, gram-negative bacilli. *Campylobacter jejuni* and *Campylobacter coli* are the most common *Campylobacter* species responsible for diarrhea and are second only to *Salmonella* in laboratory-confirmed cases of diarrheal disease reported by the FoodNet.[6]

*Campylobacter* is found in the gastrointestinal tract of domestic and wild animals, particularly poultry. Transmission occurs by the ingestion of contaminated food or by direct contact with fecal material from infected animals or people. Typical dietary sources include improperly cooked poultry, untreated water, and unpasteurized milk. Outbreaks occur much more frequently in the summer months than in the winter.

*Campylobacter* infections present with a wide clinical spectrum.[11] Symptoms usually include diarrhea, abdominal pain, malaise, and fever. Mild infection can resemble viral gastroenteritis and last 1 to 2 days. Most patients recover in less than 1 week, but 20% relapse or have a prolonged illness.[12] Severe or persistent infection can mimic acute inflammatory bowel disease, specifically ulcerative colitis, because symptoms and the examination can be typical for a pan-colitis. Diagnosis is made by stool culture. Most cases of *Campylobacter* infection are self-limited and do not require antibiotic therapy. Treatment may be indicated in more severe cases. Erythromycin and azithromycin shorten the duration of illness and prevent relapse when given early.[7] Doxycycline for children 8 years or older is an alternative agent. If antimicrobial therapy is given, the recommended duration is 5 to 7 days. Shedding of *Campylobacter* organisms usually lasts 2 to 3 weeks in untreated cases, but only 2 to 3 days with treatment.

### *Clostridium difficile*

*C difficile* is a spore-forming, obligate anaerobic, gram-positive bacillus commonly associated with pseudomembranous colitis or antimicrobial-associated diarrhea. Disease is not related to infection by the organism per se but to the action of toxins that may be produced by this organism. Although other toxins exist, toxins A and B have been associated with human disease.

*C difficile* is commonly present in the environment, and infection is acquired from the environment or by fecal–oral transmission. Intestinal colonization rates in healthy neonates and young infants with no gastrointestinal disease can be 50%, but usually are less than 5% in children older than 2 years of age and in adults. Hospitals, nursing homes, and daycare centers are major reservoirs for *C difficile*. Risk factors for the disease include prolonged hospitalization and antimicrobial usage; antibiotics diminish the barrier effect of the normal intestinal flora, allowing *C difficile* to proliferate and elaborate toxins. Penicillins, clindamycin, and cephalosporins are the antimicrobial drugs most commonly associated with *C difficile* colitis, but colitis has been associated with almost every antimicrobial agent.[1]

Disease usually begins while the person is receiving antimicrobial therapy, but it can occur weeks after therapy is completed. Infection may occur in the setting of chronic colonic inflammation and has been seen in ulcerative colitis patients without any recent antibiotic use. Syndromes associated with infections include pseudomembranous colitis and antimicrobial-associated diarrhea. Pseudomembranous colitis is characterized by the presence of typical exudates on the colonic mucosa and clinically by diarrhea, abdominal cramps, fever, systemic toxicity, abdominal tenderness, and passage of stools containing blood and mucus. Infection also may result only in mild diarrhea or asymptomatic carriage.

Recently there have been increased numbers of severe cases of *C difficile*-associated disease documented in the United States and Canada associated with the emergence of a hypervirulent strain of *C difficile* with significantly more potent toxins.[13] The Centers for Disease Control and Prevention (CDC) has reported that this more virulent strain has caused *C difficile*-associated disease in otherwise healthy persons with little or no exposure to health care settings or antimicrobial use. Thus, in addition to causing more severe disease in high-risk populations, these strains also might cause disease in populations previously at low risk.[14]

Stool should be tested for the presence of *C difficile* toxins to diagnose *C difficile* disease. Commercially available enzyme immunoassays detect toxins A and B, or an enzyme immunoassay for toxin A may be used in conjunction with a cell culture cytotoxicity assay, the "gold standard" for toxin B detection. Sigmoidoscopic findings of pseudomembranes with erythematous, friable rectal mucosa are suggestive of pseudomembranous colitis. In patients with significant diarrhea or colitis, antimicrobial therapy should be discontinued as soon as possible. Antimicrobial therapy for *C difficile* disease is indicated for patients with severe disease or in whom diarrhea persists after antimicrobial therapy is discontinued. Metronidazole is the drug of choice for the initial treatment of most patients with *C difficile* colitis.[7] Oral vancomycin is an alternative drug and is indicated for patients who do not respond to metronidazole. Antimicrobial agents usually are administered for at least 10 days. Twenty percent to 40% of patients experience a relapse after discontinuing therapy.[1] Infection frequently responds to a second course of the same treatment. Antimotility agents should not be used. Use of intravenous immunoglobulin, colonic lavage, and probiotics, such as *Sacromyces boulardii* or *Lactobacillus GG*, have been attempted in intractable or relapsing cases.[15]

## TRAVELER'S DIARRHEA

Traveler's diarrhea affects people traveling from industrialized regions to developing countries with reduced hygiene. High-risk regions include Latin America, Africa, and southern Asia. Low-risk areas are considered to be the United States, Canada, Western Europe, Japan, Australia, and New Zealand. Intermediate risk for enteric disease is observed in travelers to the Caribbean islands, Middle East, northern Mediterranean, China, and Russia. Depending on the area of travel, risk of illness varies from 4% to 40%.[16] The most important causes of traveler's diarrhea are bacterial agents, the most common being enterotoxigenic *E coli* (ETEC). Ciprofloxacin-resistant *Campylobacter* is an important cause of illness in travelers to Thailand. Norwalk virus is a common offending agent, especially when illness is complicated by vomiting. Parasitic agents (*Giardia, Cryptosporidium, Cyclospora*) are rare, except for travelers to Nepal and Eastern Europe.

Illness typically occurs during the first week after entering the host country. It frequently is self-limited, lasting 3 to 5 days. Watery diarrhea of mild to moderate severity may be accompanied by fever and vomiting. Prevention of traveler's diarrhea should be attempted through education about high-risk foods and drinks. Cooked foods that are served steaming hot are invariably safe; temperatures over 59°C inactivate bacterial pathogens.[17] Other usually safe foods include those with minimal moisture content (ie, bread), fruits and vegetables that one peels, and items that contain a high concentration of sugar (ie, syrup, jelly, jam, and honey).[16]

In 1985, the National Institutes of Health (NIH) recommended not to use absorbed drugs as chemoprophylaxis for traveler's diarrhea due to concerns regarding systemic side effects and the potential development of antibiotic resistance. Nonantibiotic agents, such as bismuth subsalicylate (BSS) and probiotics, provide alternative possibilities for protection. The recommended adult dose of BSS is 2 tablets 3 times daily and before bedtime (263-mg BSS tablets 8 times daily). Its effectiveness has been reported to be up to 65%.[16] *Lactobacillus GG*, a probiotic, has been reported to provide protection in 12% to 45% of cases. Rifaximin, a nonabsorbable antibiotic, is the most effective in preventing traveler's diarrhea. Use of 200 mg twice daily has been reported to decrease the occurrence of symptoms in 77% of patients. Although illness is most commonly self-limited, if treatment is necessary, rifaximin (adult dose 200 mg 3 times daily for 3 days) is the first choice for presumed ETEC. It is not to be used for febrile disease. In cases of febrile dysenteric diarrhea or in cases unresponsive to rifaximin, ciprofloxacin (500 mg BID) (not approved for use under 18 years of age) or azithromycin may be considered.

## PROTOZOA

### *GIARDIA*

*Giardia intestinalis* is a flagellated protozoan that has a worldwide distribution. It is also the most common parasitic cause of diarrhea in the United States. *Giardia* exists in trophozoite and cyst forms; the infective form is the cyst. Infection is limited to the small intestine and biliary tract.

Humans are the principal reservoir of infection, but giardia can infect dogs, cats, beavers, and other animals. These animals can contaminate water with feces containing cysts that are infectious for humans. People become infected directly (by fecal–oral transfer of cysts) or indirectly (by ingestion of water or food contaminated with feces). Cyst excretion may last for many months. The disease is communicable for as long as the infected person excretes cysts.

Many people who become infected with *G intestinalis* remain asymptomatic, but infection can cause a wide spectrum of clinical manifestations. Most symptomatic patients experience a mild, watery diarrhea with abdominal cramps; however, a protracted, intermittent, often debilitating disease, characterized by the passage of foul-smelling stools associated with flatulence, abdominal distension, and anorexia, also may occur. Anorexia combined with malabsorption can lead to significant weight loss and anemia.

Identification of trophozoites or cysts in direct smear examination (ie, stool for ova and parasites) or immunofluorescent antibody testing of stool specimens or duodenal fluid is diagnostic. Direct microscopic identification of cysts or trophozoites in the stool requires 3 separate stool specimens to reach 95% sensitivity. The trophozoites can also be found on the duodenal mucosal surface by microscopy at small bowel biopsy for the evaluation of chronic malabsorption syndrome.

Metronidazole is the drug of choice for treating symptomatic giardiasis; a 5- to 7-day course of therapy has a cure rate of 80% to 95%. Tinidazole, a nitroimidazole, has a cure rate of 90% to 100% after a single dose, but limited safety and efficacy data are available in children and adolescents. Furazolidone is 72% to 100% effective when given for 7 to 10 days. A 3-day course of nitazoxanide oral suspension is as effective as metronidazole and has the advantage of treating multiple other intestinal parasites.[1] If therapy fails, a course can be repeated with the same drug. Relapses are common in immunocompromised patients, who may require prolonged treatment. Asymptomatic carriers generally do not require treatment; when there is close contact with an immunocompromised patient; however, asymptomatic carriers should be treated to prevent spread.

### *CRYPTOSPORIDIUM*

*Cryptosporidium parvum* is a spore-forming coccidian protozoan. Oocysts are excreted in feces and are the infectious form. *C parvum* has been found in a variety of hosts, including mammals, birds, and reptiles. Extensive water-borne outbreaks have been associated with contamination of municipal water and exposure to contaminated swimming pools. Transmission to humans can also occur from farm livestock and person-to-person transmission.

Infection with *C parvum* generally produces a benign, self-limited diarrhea; however, prolonged loose stools have been seen even in otherwise healthy children and adolescents. Fever and vomiting are relatively common presenting symptoms of *C parvum* in children, which often leads to a misdiagnosis of viral gastroenteritis. Infection can also be asymptomatic. Immunocompromised patients can develop chronic severe diarrhea, which may result in malnutrition, dehydration and, ultimately, death. For most, shedding of *C parvum* stops within 2 weeks, but for a few, shedding continues for 2 months.

Routine laboratory examination of stool for ova and parasites does not detect *C parvum.* Instead stool testing for *Cryptosporidium* needs to be ordered separately. The detection of oocysts on microscopic examination of the stool specimen is diagnostic. Shedding can be intermittent, thus at least 3 stool specimens collected on separate days should be examined before considering test results to be negative.

Supportive care with rehydration and adequate nutrition usually is all that is required for therapy. A 3-day course of nitazoxanide oral suspension has been licensed by the US Food and Drug Administration (FDA) for treatment of children with cryptosporidial diarrhea.[18] In immunocompromised patients with cryptosporidiosis, oral administration of human immune globulin or bovine colostrum has been beneficial. In HIV-infected patients, increasing the CD4 cell count with antiviral therapy can improve the course of cryptosporidiosis.[18]

## LACTOSE INTOLERANCE

Malabsorption of dietary lactose can result in gastrointestinal symptoms such as abdominal pain, bloating, flatus, and diarrhea. Recognition of this condition is important, because it can be easily managed by simple dietary adjustments. In its most common form, it usually presents in later childhood or adolescence.

### ETIOLOGY AND PATHOPHYSIOLOGY

Lactose malabsorption may be categorized into 3 main categories: primary, secondary, and the rare cases of congenital lactase deficiency. A genetically determined reduction of lactase activity begins soon after weaning in almost all mammals, including many human groups.[19] Lactase activity drops to about one-tenth or less of the suckling level over time, and when this situation occurs in humans it is referred to as primary lactase deficiency. It usually presents in older children and adolescents. Secondary lactase deficiency results from diseases that damage the intestinal epithelium, such as acute gastroenteritis, small bowel bacterial overgrowth, or untreated celiac disease. Lactase activity returns after the epithelium heals. Resection of a sufficient length of small bowel also can result in secondary lactase deficiency. Congenital lactase deficiency is inherited as an autosomal recessive condition and is extremely rare.[20] There have been only a few dozen documented cases in the world, most of them in Finland.

The lactase enzyme is a disaccharidase located in the brush border of the enterocyte. The enzyme hydrolyzes dietary lactose into glucose and galactose for transport across the cell membrane. If lactase is absent or deficient, the resulting osmotic activity of the unabsorbed sugar attracts fluid into the bowel lumen. This significantly increases the fluid volume of the gastrointestinal contents. In addition, unabsorbed lactose in the colon is acted upon by colonic bacteria, resulting in production of gases (methane, carbon dioxide, and hydrogen), volatile fatty acids, and monosaccharides. Monosaccharides cannot be absorbed by the colonic mucosa, thus further increasing the osmotic pressure and drawing more fluid into the bowel. All these events produce the clinical presentation of lactose intolerance: diarrhea, abdominal pain, flatulence, and bloating.[21]

## EPIDEMIOLOGY

Primary lactase deficiency is inherited through a single autosomal recessive gene,[22] which varies widely among ethnic groups. The prevalence of primary lactase deficiency is more than 50% in South America, Africa, and Asia, reaching almost 100% in some Asian countries. In the United States, the prevalence is reported to be up to 22% among those of European descent, 50% to 80% among Latinos, and 60% to 80% in blacks and Ashkenazi Jews.[23,24] A cultural-historical hypothesis has been proposed to explain the persistence of lactase after the weaning period. After the beginning of dairy farming, there would have been a survival advantage for those individuals who retained high levels of intestinal lactase postweaning. As a result, high intestinal lactase activity would have become typical in such a group. Lactase persistence is, indeed, more common in areas with long traditions of dairy farming.[19]

## CLINICAL FEATURES

Symptoms of lactose intolerance include loose stools, abdominal bloating and pain, flatulence, nausea, and borborygmi ("stomach gurgling"). The severity of the symptoms may vary according to the quantity of ingested lactose and the individual's residual lactase activity, as well as other factors not completely known. As little as 12 g of lactose (8 oz of milk) may be sufficient to cause symptoms in children and adolescents with chronic abdominal pain.[25] It has been shown, however, that the prevalence of abdominal symptoms related to lactose malabsorption documented by a hydrogen breath test varies from 2% in Finnish children to 24% in children in the southeastern United States.[26,27]

The gastric emptying rate and varying intestinal transit alter the time that lactose is exposed to intestinal lactase. After a meal, stomach contents are progressively emptied into the duodenum over a period of several hours, depending on the composition of the meal. For example, fat slows down the rate of gastric emptying. Lactose is more completely digested when consumed in milk instead of water, in a chocolate milk drink instead of plain milk, or with solid food or fiber. This is thought to be the result of differentials in gastric emptying of the above meals.[19] The temperature of a meal or drink also influences gastric emptying. Ingestion of a cold liquid at 4°C slows down the initial phase of gastric emptying for approximately 10 minutes after ingestion, compared with a control drink of 37°C.[19] Lactose in yogurt is generally better tolerated than an equivalent quantity of lactose in milk. This has been attributed to the presence of living bacteria in yogurt and the production of bacterial-derived lactases.

## DIAGNOSIS

The diagnosis of lactose intolerance can, in theory, be made on the basis of the history and response to dietary manipulations. Careful dietary history can reveal a relationship between the intake of dairy products and symptoms. A 1 to 2 week trial of elimination of all lactose-containing foods should lead to resolution of the symptoms; recurrence of symptoms with reintroduction of dairy would then be diagnostic if cow's milk protein allergy is not a consideration. In practice, any dietary modification can be difficult, especially in adolescents. Also given the frequency of lactose malabsorption in some ethnic groups and irritable bowel syndrome (IBS) in the general (adolescent) population, dietary lactose may be a contributory but not sole source of symptoms, further confusing the diagnosis.

A test demonstrating lactose malabsorption can be useful to motivate the adolescent to achieve a fair trial of dietary therapy. Measurement of breath hydrogen after ingestion of 25 g to 50 g of lactose provides evidence for lactose malabsorption. The diagnosis of lactose intolerance is a clinical diagnosis that can only be definitively established by correlating symptoms with lactose intake. The breath test is based on the principle that unabsorbed carbohydrate (lactose) that reaches the colon is metabolized by colonic bacteria that usually produce hydrogen gas. The hydrogen gas can be absorbed and pass into the colonic circulation and then be exchanged in the lungs. The breath levels of hydrogen correlate with the degree of colonic fermentation. A rise in the breath hydrogen concentration of greater than 20 parts per million (ppm) over baseline, occurring usually 1 to 3 hours after lactose ingestion, suggests lactose malabsorption. The test is positive in 90% of patients with lactose malabsorption.[28] False-negative results may be caused by the absence of bacterial flora from the recent use of oral antibiotics or the use of laxatives and enemas. Bacterial flora in some 5% to 15% of patients does not produce hydrogen in response to lactose ingestion but rather produces methane. In these cases, measurement of breath methane may establish the diagnosis.[21] Various factors can affect the baseline breath hydrogen concentration; these include inadequate fasting, a high-fiber diet, or ingestion of flatulent food the evening before the test. Small bowel overgrowth can elevate baseline levels and/or give rise to rapid elevations in breath hydrogen with carbohydrate ingestion.

## TREATMENT

Temporary avoidance of dairy for several weeks can be recommended for patients with secondary lactose intolerance. As the cause of the mucosal damage is treated or resolves, lactase deficiency resolves. In patients with primary lactose intolerance, treatment entails avoidance or a decrease in lactose intake. Given the wide variation of tolerance of lactose in those who poorly absorb lactose, the most effective correlation between symptoms and lactose intake can be made by initiation of a strict lactose-free diet for 1 to 2 weeks. If there is resolution or improvement in symptoms, then gradual liberalization of lactose intake can be tried to ascertain the individual's tolerance. Although lactose malabsorption may cause symptoms, there is no intestinal injury from isolated lactose ingestion. In a given social situation, the adolescent may reasonably choose to partake in some dietary indiscretions resulting in some discomfort.

Dairy products comprise the chief source of dietary lactose, but dairy is also the main source of calcium. Careful attention needs to be paid to calcium intake when one attempts a lactose-free or low lactose diet. Table 103-1 lists the lactose and calcium content of some common dairy products. Notably, lower fat milks contain relatively the same amount of lactose; in addition, some dairy products are rich in calcium but relatively low in lactose. There are also widely available lactose-free and lactose-reduced milks that are rich sources of calcium. Some nondairy products may serve as hidden sources of lactose and thus cause seeming failure of therapy (Box 103-2). Ingredient labels should be carefully read. Terms that may indicate lactose content that may need to be avoided include milk, milk solids, skim milk powder, butter, cream, lactose, margarine, sweet or sour cream, and milk proteins—curds, casein, caseinate, or whey.

It is important to remember that small amounts of lactose often may be tolerated without symptoms.[31] For larger lactose loads or in more severe cases, oral lactase enzyme replacement preparations may be tried. A variety of these preparations are available in pharmacies over the counter as well as in supermarkets. If

**Table 103-1**

**Lactose and Calcium Content of Common Dairy Products[23,29]**

| *Dairy Product* | *Lactose, g* | *Calcium, mg* |
|---|---|---|
| Milk, whole, 1 cup | 12.8 | 276 |
| Milk, reduced fat, 1 cup | 12.2 | 285 |
| Cottage cheese, 1 cup | 8 | 126 |
| Ice cream, ½ cup | 6 | 85 |
| Yogurt, plain, low fat, 1 cup | 5 | 415 |
| Swiss cheese, 1 ounce | 0.07 | 270 |
| Cheddar cheese, 1 ounce | 0.02 | 204 |

**Box 103-2**

***Hidden Sources of Lactose Potentially Responsible for Failure of Therapy[30]***

Bread and baked goods
Processed breakfast cereals
Mixes for pancakes, biscuits, and cookies
Breaded frozen foods
Instant potatoes, soups, and breakfast drinks
Margarines
Nonkosher luncheon meats and hot dogs
Salad dressings and commercial sauces and gravies
Some candies and other snack foods
Frostings, dessert mixes, and whipped topping

**Table 103-2**

**Calcium Content of Various Lactose-free Foods[23,29]**

| *Nondairy Products* | *Calcium Content* |
|---|---|
| Certain breakfast cereals with "complete" minerals, ¾ cup | 1,104 mg |
| Orange juice, calcium fortified, 1 cup | 300 mg |
| Spinach, frozen, boiled, 1 cup | 291 mg |
| Salmon, canned, with edible bones, 3 oz | 181 mg |
| Instant oatmeal, ¾ cup | 165 mg |
| Broccoli, frozen, 1 cup | 100 mg |
| Orange, 1 medium | 52 mg |
| Pinto beans, ½ cup | 40 mg |
| Tuna, canned, 3 oz | 12 mg |
| Lettuce greens, ½ cup | 10 mg |

avoidance of dairy products is the principal way of managing lactose intolerance in a given individual, then calcium supplementation is often necessary given the Dietary Reference Intake (DRI) for calcium in adolescents of 1,300 mg/day.[32] Alternative dietary sources of calcium other than dairy products do exist, with some listed in Table 103-2.

## INTOLERANCE OF OTHER CARBOHYDRATES

Sugar alcohols or polyols are classified by the American Dietetic Association as nutritive or nonnutritive sweeteners and used to replace sugar. They are commonly present in the diet and can cause chronic diarrhea in unsuspecting individuals. The dietary use of these substances has increased significantly over the last few years because they are utilized in many low-sugar or sugar-free products for weight management or blood glucose control as well as to promote dental health. Sorbitol and mannitol are 2 popular sugar alcohols used in dietetic foods, especially sugar-free chewing gum, candies, mints, jams/jellies, baked goods, and frozen confections. Sorbitol is present in over-the-counter medications such as liquid acetaminophen, vitamins, and cough preparations. Prescription elixirs also frequently contain sorbitol. Sorbitol and mannitol normally are poorly absorbed and thus pass into the colon. Similar to malabsorbed lactose, the colonic flora causes fermentation of these polyols. The polyols and their fermentation products result in osmotic shifts of fluid into the colon. An excessive load (eg, >50 g/day of sorbitol or >20 g/day of mannitol) frequently causes borborygmi, flatus, and diarrhea.[33] A careful dietary history is necessary to identify these substances as a cause of chronic diarrhea.

## IRRITABLE BOWEL SYNDROME

Irritable bowel syndrome is one of the most common conditions encountered in medical practice. It is generally characterized by abdominal pain and disturbed defecation—often diarrhea or periods of diarrhea alternating with periods of constipation. A formal consensus process, Rome III has created major diagnostic criteria for the definition of IBS.[34] These include at least once per week for at least 2 months of abdominal discomfort or pain, associated with 2 of 3 of the following features: abdominal pain improved with defecation, onset of pain associated with a change in the frequency of stool, and onset of pain associated with a change in the form (appearance) of stool. Absence of structural or metabolic abnormalities to explain these symptoms is, by definition, required for the diagnosis of IBS. Features supporting the diagnosis of IBS are:

- abnormal stool frequency, defined as greater than 3 bowel movements per day or less than 3 per week;
- abnormal stool form (hard or loose/watery);
- abnormal stool passage (straining, urgency, feeling of incomplete evacuation), passage of mucus, and feeling of bloating.[35]

The diagnosis of IBS is based principally on a careful history and physical examination. Symptoms that fit Rome III criteria (above), associated with the absence of red flag signs (Box 103-3), in combination with a normal physical examination and a regular growth pattern strongly suggest IBS. Screening laboratory studies are frequently performed to exclude inflammatory conditions

**Box 103-3**

***"Red Flag" Signs Suggestive of Organic Disease***

Nocturnal symptoms
Blood in the stool
Fever
Weight loss
Growth delay
Delayed puberty
Arthritis
Perirectal disease

and reassure the family and patient. They can include a complete blood count, erythrocyte sedimentation rate or C-reactive protein, and usually serologic screening for celiac disease. Stool studies for occult blood, lactoferrin, and parasites may also be warranted. Additional evaluation may be required in patients with refractory symptoms or red flag signs.

The precise pathophysiology of IBS remains elusive. IBS likely is a common clinical expression of multiple pathophysiologic factors. The most common factors contributing to IBS are thought to include genetic predisposition, dysmotility, altered visceral sensation and perception, and emotional stress. Recently a role for intestinal inflammation and enteric infection has been proposed as well.[36] Familial clustering has long been noted among patients with IBS. Levy and colleagues[37] observed that IBS is more common in monozygotic twins than in dizygotic twins. They also noted that the presence of a parent with IBS was even more predictive for the subsequent development of IBS in a child. For many years, investigators have focused on the role of abnormal motility in IBS. Patients with the predominant symptom of diarrhea seem to have accelerated whole gut and colonic transit time. Some adolescents have an abnormal contractile response to eating.[38] Whether these changes are primary or secondary to another potential etiology of IBS remains to be determined.

Sensory and motor functions of the gastrointestinal system are mediated by way of the enteric and central nervous systems. The enteric nervous system is a rich and complex system of approximately 100 million neurons. It is composed of myenteric and submucosal systems and the interstitial cells of Cajal, which primarily control motility, sensory function and gland secretion, and regulate propagation of intestinal contractions, respectively. The enteric nervous system can act autonomously or communicate with the central nervous system. Recently, serotonin (5-hydroxytryptamine) has been implicated as an important mediator of the intestinal events occurring in patients with IBS.[39] Serotonin is released by the enterochromaffin cells in response to stimulation of the enteric nerves. It then binds to multiple receptors in the enteric nervous system initiating peristalsis, smooth muscle relaxation, intestinal secretion, nausea, and vomiting. Selective serotonin agonists and antagonists have been used in attempts to treat constipation-predominant and diarrhea-predominant IBS, respectively. The central nervous system also plays a significant role in pain perception in patients with IBS. Recent work using positron emission tomography (PET) scans and functional magnetic resonance imaging (fMRI) have identified abnormalities in brain activation in patients with IBS versus controls.[40] Abnormalities have been noted consistently in activation of the anterior cingulated cortex, which likely plays a role in development of attention and an emotional response to painful stimuli. Failure of activation of this brain region has been associated with pain inhibition following noxious rectal distension.[35]

Intestinal infection frequently is reported as a precipitating event in patients with IBS. Most patients with postinfectious IBS demonstrate increased intestinal permeability, gut transit, and increased cellularity of the lamina propria and mucosa. They usually present with diarrhea-predominant IBS. Recent work by O'Mahony and colleagues[36] demonstrated improvement of IBS symptoms and normalization of a proinflammatory to anti-inflammatory cytokine ratio, IL10/IL12, after an 8-week course of a probiotic preparation of Bifidobacterium infantis 35624. This observation suggests that intestinal inflammation may play a role in a subset of patients with IBS.

Several groups have demonstrated that emotional stress alters gastrointestinal motility and sensation.[41] Anxiety, somatiform disorders, or a history of physical or sexual abuse can be identified in up to 60% of patients with IBS.[42] In particular, the presence of somatization is very common and influences the outcome in patients with IBS.

Therapeutic interventions in IBS include patient education, dietary modification, medications, and counseling. Education and reassurance are mandatory for all patients. Discussion usually includes an explanation of the brain–gut axis. The presence and severity of pain should not be disputed or minimized. Psychosocial difficulties and triggering events should be addressed even while dietary and pharmacologic interventions are instituted.[35] Dietary intervention should focus on ensuring adequate fiber intake (age + 5 = total grams of fiber per day, maximum = 25–30 g/day). Although detailed dietary manipulations may be able to achieve sufficient fiber intake, this can usually best be accomplished for adolescents through the use of any of the multiple commercially available fiber supplements (in powder, tablet, or chewable form). To avoid bloating, fiber supplementation should be started at lower doses and be increased over time. A role for lactose intolerance needs to be considered as a contributing factor to IBS; sugar alcohols should also be eliminated. Excess fructose intake may lead to carbohydrate malabsorption symptoms in some. Limitation of caffeine intake, flatulent foods, ice cold liquids, or fatty foods may also provide some symptomatic relief. For those who are interested, food diaries can be used to try to establish a relationship between symptoms and particular foods.

Antidiarrheal and antispasmodic agents are the medications most commonly prescribed in IBS patients.

Loperamide is an antidiarrheal agent that has been evaluated in prospective randomized trials.[43,44] These trials indicate that although loperamide can be effective in treating diarrhea, it does not affect abdominal pain or improve global IBS symptoms. Among antispasmodic agents, anticholinergics, such as hyoscyamine and dicyclomine, are commonly used. Studies comparing antispasmodics with placebo yield mixed results regarding improving abdominal pain;[42] however, a meta-analysis compiling 23 randomized, controlled trials found overall improvement in abdominal pain and global IBS symptoms for antispasmodics over placebo.[45] One medication, the serotonin type-3 receptor antagonist alosetron, has been shown to be an effective agent in women with severe diarrhea-predominant IBS. However, it was removed from the market in the United States due to an increased incidence of ischemic colitis in patients who had used it. Alosetron is now only available via a restricted prescribing program. The serotonin type-4 receptor agonist tegaserod is approved for women with constipation-predominant IBS. A number of other serotonin agonists and antagonists are currently under investigation.

Often, providing reassurance regarding the lack of disease, along with dietary and/or medical manipulations, is sufficient to manage the symptoms of IBS in adolescents. In those with continued problems affecting quality of life, referral to a mental health professional for antidepressant therapy, psychotherapy, or cognitive behavioral therapy may be useful. Patients with abdominal pain, diarrhea, and psychological distress may be most helped by these interventions. Although some adolescents with IBS have spontaneous improvement over time, it can be a lifelong problem.

## REFERENCES


1. Dennehey PH. Acute diarrheal disease in children: epidemiology, preventions, and treatment. *Infect Dis Clin N Am.* 2005;19:585-602

2. Koopman JS, Turkish VJ, Monto AS, et al. Patterns and etiology of diarrhea in three clinical settings. *Am J Epidemiol.* 1984;119:114-123

3. Merson MH, Goldmann DA, Boyer KM, et al. An outbreak of *Shigella sonnei* gastroenteritis on Colorado River raft trips. *Am J Epidemiol.* 1974;100:186-196

4. Daniels NA, MacKinnon L, Rowe SM, et al. Foodborne disease outbreaks in United States schools. *Pediatr Infect Dis J.* 2002;21:623-628

5. Reptile-associated salmonellosis—selected states, 1198-2002. *Morb Mortal Wkly Rep.* 2003;52:1206-1209

6. Preliminary FoodNet Data on the incidence of infection with pathogens transmitted commonly through food—10 states, 2006. *Morb Mortal Wkly Rep.* 2007;56:336-339

7. Guerrant RL, Van Gilder T, Steiner TS, et al. Practice guidelines for the management of infectious diarrhea. *Clin Infect Dis.* 2001;32:331-351

8. Rowe PC, Orrbine E, Lior H, et al. Risk of hemolytic uremic syndrome after sporadic *Escherichia coli* O157:H7 infection: results of Canadian collaborative study. *J Pediatr.* 1998;132:777-782

9. Safdar N, Said A, Gangnon RE, Maki DG. Risk of hemolytic uremic syndrome after antibiotic treatment of *Escherichia coli* O157:H7 enteritis: a meta-analysis. *JAMA.* 2002;288:996-1001

10. Tarr PI, Gordon CA, Chandler WL. Shiga-toxin-producing *Escherichia coli* and haemolytic uremic syndrome. *Lancet.* 2005;365:1073-1086

11. Blaser MJ, Wells JG, Feldman RA, et al. *Campylobacter* enteritis in the United States: a multicenter study. *Ann Int Med.* 1983;98:360-365

12. Kapperaud G, Lassen J, Ostroff SM, Aasen S. Clinical features of sporadic *Campylobacter* infection in Norway. *Scand J Infect Dis.* 1992;24:741-749

13. Muto CA, et al. A large outbreak of *Clostridium difficile*-associated disease with an unexpected proportion of deaths and colectomies at a teaching hospital following increased fluoroquinolone use. *Infection Control Hosp Epidemiol.* 2005;26:273-281

14. Centers for Disease Control and Prevention (CDC). Severe *Clostridium difficile*-associated disease in populations previously at low risk—four states. *MMWR Morb Mortal Wkly Rep.* 2005;54:1201-1205

15. Jodlowski TZ, Oehler R, Kam LW, Melnychuk I. Emerging therapies in the treatment of *Clostridium difficile*-associated disease. *Ann Pharmacother.* 2006;40(12):2164-2169

16. DuPont HL. New insights and directions in traveler's diarrhea. *Gastroenterol Clin N Am.* 2006;35:337-353

17. Bandres JC, Mathewson JJ, DuPont HL. Heat susceptibility of bacterial enteropathogens. Implications for prevention of travelers' diarrhea. *Arch Int Med.* 1988;148(10):2261-2263

18. Smith HV, Corcoran GD. New drugs and treatment of cryptosporidiosis. *Curr Opin Infect Dis.* 2004;17:557-564

19. Vesa TH. Lactose intolerance. *J Am Col Nutr.* 2000;19: 165S-175S

20. Savilahti E, Launiala K, Kuitunen P. Congenital lactase deficiency. *Arch Dis Child.* 1983;58:246-252

21. Swagerty DL. Lactose intolerance. *Am Fam Phys.* 2002;65(9):1845-1850

22. Sahi T, Launiala K. More evidence for the recessive inheritance of selective adult type lactose malabsorption. *Gastroenterology.* 1977;73:231-232

23. Scrimshaw NS, Murray EB. Prevalence of lactose maldigestion. *Am J Clin Nutr.* 1988;48(Suppl):1086-1098

24. Sahi T. Genetics and epidemiology of adult-type hypolactasia. *Scand J Gastroenterol.* 1994;29(Suppl 202):7-20

25. Gremse DA, Greer AS, Vacik J, DiPalma JA. Abdominal pain associated with lactose ingestion in children with lactose intolerance. *Clin Pediatr (Phila).* 2003;42:341-345

26. Kokkonen J, Haapalahti M, Tikkanen S, Karttunen R, Savilahti E. Gastrointestinal complaints and diagnosis in children: a population-based study. *Acta Paediatr.* 2004;93:880-886

27. Webster RB, DiPalma JA, Gremse DA. Irritable bowel syndrome and lactose maldigestion in recurrent abdominal pain in childhood. *South Med J.* 1999;92:778-781

28. Hamilton LH. *Breath Tests and Gastroenterology*. 2nd ed. Milwaukee, WI: Quin Tron Instrument Company; 1998:42

29. US Department of Agriculture. USDA National Nutrient Database for Standard Reference, Release 19. Available at: www.nal.usda.gov/fnic/foodcomp/search/. Accessed April 13, 2010.

30. US NIH National Digestive Diseases Information Clearinghouse. Lactose intolerance. Available at: digestive.niddk.nih.gov/ddiseases/pubs/lactoseintolerance/. Accessed April 13, 2010.

31. Heyman MB, for the Committee on Nutrition. Lactose intolerance in infants, children, and adolescents. *Pediatrics.* 2006;118:1279-1286

32. Food and Nutrition Board Institute of Medicine, National Academy of Science; 2004.

33. Position of the American Dietetic Association: Use of nutritive and nonnutritive sweeteners. *J Am Diet Assoc.* 2004; 104:255-275

34. Rasquin A, DiLorenzo C, Forbes D, et al. Childhood functional gastrointestinal disorders: child/adolescent. *Gastroenterology.* 2006;130:1527-1537

35. Hyams JS. Irritable bowel syndrome, functional dyspepsia, and functional abdominal pain syndrome. *Adolesc Med Clin.* 2004;15(1):1-15

36. O'Mahony L, McCarthy J, Kelly P, et al. *Lactobacillus* and *Bifidobacterium* in irritable bowel syndrome: symptom response and relationship to cytokine profiles. *Gastroenterology.* 2005;128:541-551

37. Levy RL, Jones KR, Whitehead WE, et al. Irritable bowel syndrome in twins: heredity and social learning both contribute to etiology. *Gastroenterology.* 2001;121(4):799-804

38. Van Ginkel R, Voskuijl WP, Benninga MA, et al. Alterations of rectal sensitivity and motility in childhood irritable bowel syndrome. *Gastroenterology.* 2001;120:31-38

39. Gershon MD. Roles played by 5-hydroxytryptamine in the physiology of the bowel. *Alim Pharmacol Ther.* 1999;13:15-30

40. Mertz H, Morgan V, Tanner G, et al. Regional cerebral activation in irritable bowel syndrome and control subjects with painful and nonpainful rectal distension. *Gastroenterology.* 2000;118:842-848

41. Dickhaus B, Mayer EA, Firooz N, et al. Irritable bowel syndrome patients show enhanced modulation of visceral perception by auditory stress. *Am J Gastroenterol.* 2003;98:135-143

42. Cash BD, Chey WD. Irritable bowel syndrome: a systematic review. *Clin Fam Pract.* 2004;6(3):647-669

43. Hovdenak N. Loperamide treatment of the irritable bowel syndrome. *Scand J Gastroenterol Suppl.* 1987;130:81-84

44. Efskind PS, Bernklev T, Vatn MH. A double-blind, placebo-controlled trial with loperamide in irritable bowel syndrome. *Scand J Gastroenterol.* 1996;31:463-468

45. Poynard T, Regimbeau C, Benhamou Y. Meta-analysis of smooth muscle relaxants in the treatment of irritable bowel syndrome. *Aliment Pharmacol Ther.* 2001;15:355

# CHAPTER 104

## Inflammatory Bowel Disease

MELANIE GREIFER, MD • JAMES MARKOWITZ, MD

### INTRODUCTION

The inflammatory bowel diseases (IBDs), including ulcerative colitis (UC) and Crohn disease (CD), are chronic gastrointestinal (GI) disorders that commonly affect adolescents. In this chapter, we discuss the epidemiology of IBD, current etiologic theories, clinical and pathological features, diagnosis and treatment, and the psychosocial implications associated with these lifelong conditions.

### EPIDEMIOLOGY

Inflammatory bowel disease affects more than 1 million people in the United States, and it is estimated that about 100,000 of these patients are children.[1] Age of onset demonstrates a bimodal distribution pattern, with a large peak in adolescence and a smaller, second group diagnosed in the sixth decade of life. Approximately 15% to 25% of cases are diagnosed by age 20.[2] In North America, incidence rates range from 2.2 to 14.3 cases per 100,000 person-years for UC and 3.1 to 14.6 cases per 100,000 person-years for CD.[3] These ranges are similar to other high incidence areas of the world, such as northern Europe and the United Kingdom. A prospective population-based pediatric study from Sweden, drawn from observations made between 1990 and 2001, identified high incidence rates for IBD in adolescents (15.2 per 100,000 in those aged 10–15 years) compared to younger children (5.7 per 100,000 in children aged 5–9 years and 0.9 per 100,000 in children aged 4 years and younger).[4] Similar to what has been seen in adult populations, this study demonstrated that during the period of observation, the incidence rate for UC remained relatively stable, whereas the incidence of CD increased. A population-based study from Wisconsin revealed similar incidence rates of IBD.[5] However, in contrast to previous studies, the Wisconsin study revealed an equal distribution of IBD among all racial and ethnic groups, as well as comparable rates of IBD in rural and urban environments. Data on newly diagnosed North American children with IBD compiled between 2002 and 2007 suggest that approximately 70% present with CD.

### ETIOLOGY

Although the etiology of IBD remains unknown, current research suggests that a combination of genetics, environmental factors, and immune dysregulation play a role.[6] A familial predilection for these illnesses has long been recognized, with numerous studies suggesting that 15% to 20% of all IBD patients have other first-degree relatives with IBD. Twin studies derived from population-based registries in Sweden reveal a high rate of concordance for IBD in monozygotic twins, more so in CD (58.3%) than in UC (6.3%).[7] Subsequent long-term follow-up in this same cohort of patients identified new IBD cases in previously undiagnosed twin pairs, bringing the concordance rates even higher (up to 18.8% in the UC group).[8]

The past few years have seen an explosion of new research into the genetics of IBD. As IBD genes have been identified, the potential role of the innate immune system in the etiology of IBD has become increasingly apparent. The first IBD susceptibility gene to be identified, *IBD1*, corresponds to the *NOD2/CARD15* gene located on chromosome 16.[9] Mutations in *NOD2/CARD15* predispose to the development of CD, not UC. With 2 mutated alleles, the risk of CD is increased 20 to 40 times higher than that of the general population. Heterozygotes have a two to fourfold increased risk. The gene codes for the intracellular receptor for muramyl dipeptide, a component of lipopolysaccharide (the cell wall substance of gram-negative bacteria). Mutations in this gene cause an abnormal innate immune response to luminal bacteria.[10] *NOD2/CARD15* polymorphisms appear to predispose to earlier onset of disease, with 40% of North American white pediatric patients with CD having one or more variant alleles.[11] *NOD2/CARD15* polymorphisms also appear to predispose patients to an ileal location of disease, and in some studies, fistulizing or penetrating types of the disease leading to surgery.[12] Additional genetic associations have been identified in CD, including regions of chromosome 5 (*IBD5*) and chromosome 6 (*IBD3*).

Genetics factors have not been as well established in the development of UC. Human leukocyte antigen alleles have been shown to play a role, as has a tumor necrosis factor-alpha (TNF-α) gene polymorphism—all supporting the idea of immune dysregulation because these genes are involved in control of the immune system. A multidrug resistance (*MDR1*) gene polymorphism has also been investigated as a susceptibility gene in UC. The *MDR1* gene codes for a cellular transporter that is highly expressed in intestinal epithelial cells and may function in the translocation of bacteria. It also appears to influence the outcome of corticosteroid therapy by affecting intracellular drug concentrations.[13] *MDR1* knock out mice develop spontaneous colitis in a specific pathogen-free environment, supporting the concept that the polymorphisms of this gene may contribute to the epithelial dysfunction seen in IBD.[14]

Environmental contributions to the development of IBD have also been examined. Previously, it was believed that cigarette smoking was protective against UC, but increased the risk for CD. Newer data question this protective effect with UC. Patients with CD who smoke, particularly women who are heavy smokers, are at high risk for developing more severe disease requiring surgery. Breastfeeding seems to decrease the risk of CD, whereas taking oral contraceptives potentially increases the risk, although the latter observation has been questioned, and recent reports conclude that there is no strong evidence to avoid oral contraceptive use in adolescent females at risk for developing either CD or UC. Drugs such as Accutane and nonsteroidal anti-inflammatories have been identified as possible risk factors for the development of IBD.[15,16]

The human GI tract acts as an important crossroads between the individual and the multitude of antigens and microbes that inhabit the intestinal lumen. It is the site where the interplay between an individual's genetic make up and the environment takes place. Under normal circumstances, the gut's resident immunologically active cells (including lymphocytes, plasma cells, monocytes, dendritic cells, macrophages, and epithelial cells) respond to luminally delivered antigens in a highly regulated manner characterized by immune tolerance. When IBD develops, there is immune dysregulation characterized by excessive immune responses to normal microflora. A large number of different animal models make it clear that the presence of a commensal flora is a necessary requirement for the development of IBD-like intestinal inflammation. Defects in gut epithelial barrier function may predispose to enhanced exposure of the gut immune system to the microflora. Subsequently, 1 or more different inherited genetic polymorphisms appear to result in a chronically overactive immune response. In some cases, such as in individuals with *NOD2/CARD15* mutations, the genetic variant can even result in an initially deficient immune response. In such a circumstance, it appears that the deficient response is restricted to the innate immune system. The resulting poor clearance of the initial immune stimulus subsequently results in overreactivity of the adaptive immune response. The result is an unbalanced immune response, characterized predominantly as Th-1 in CD and Th-2 in UC.[17]

## PATHOLOGY

In most patients, the 2 forms of IBD can be readily differentiated. Ulcerative colitis is confined to the colon. Characteristically, it involves the rectum and can extend proximally to affect part or all of the colon with diffuse involvement of affected areas. Inflammatory changes are restricted to the mucosa, with minimal involvement of the deeper tissues of the colon. The extent of colitis varies in different reports, with pediatric studies from France and the northeast United States compiled in the 1980s and 1990s reporting pancolitis in 32% to 41%, left-sided disease in 34% to 57%, and proctosigmoiditis in 11% to 26% of children.[18,19] A more recent report[20] from a multicenter North American consortium observed pancolitis at diagnosis in 79% of children and adolescents.

In contrast, CD can affect any portion of the GI tract from mouth to anus. At diagnosis, about 70% of children have both small and large bowel involvement, and up to 40% have identifiable inflammation in the upper GI tract. Characteristics of the disease are skip lesions, patchy inflammation, transmural involvement of affected bowel segments, and granuloma formation on biopsy. In addition, the presence of perianal fistula and abscess also characterizes CD.

Despite these differentiating characteristics, in those patients with only colonic involvement, the combination of clinical, endoscopic, radiologic, and pathological findings only characterizes 80% to 90% of adolescents into 1 of the classical IBD categories. The remaining 10% to 20% are generally diagnosed as having indeterminate colitis (IC). Over time, many IC patients can evolve to more typical CD or UC.

## CLINICAL PRESENTATION

Signs and symptoms of IBD can present suddenly or in a more chronic fashion, depending on the type and location of inflammation. Crohn disease typically presents with abdominal pain, diarrhea, weight loss, and anorexia. Although symptoms often present insidiously over a period of months or even years, about 10% of patients can present abruptly with symptoms suggestive of acute appendicitis. The location of abdominal pain is dependent on the location of disease. Patients with terminal ileal disease frequently present with right lower quadrant pain and fullness, whereas those with Crohn disease colitis often have more diffuse pain. If the colitis is predominantly left sided, bloody diarrhea may be a presenting sign. Nonbloody diarrhea can occur with right-sided colitis. Poor weight gain or weight loss, commonly with poor linear growth and delayed sexual development, may be the sole signs in a patient with small bowel disease.

Perianal disease, with the presence of chronic fissures, skin tags, fistulae, and abscesses, is another manifestation of CD and can be accompanied by other systemic symptoms or on its own. Studies have documented perianal disease in up to 49% of children and adolescents, with 13% to 16% having more complicated disease, such as fistulae or abscesses. Concurrent rectal inflammation was present in 94% of patients with fistulas and/or abscesses versus 63% of patients without perianal disease.[21]

Ulcerative colitis classically presents with the triad of diarrhea, rectal bleeding, and abdominal pain. Stooling is usually associated with frequency, urgency, and tenesmus. The severity of disease can often be determined by the frequency of stooling. One-half of children and adolescents with UC present with mild disease, having fewer than 4 stools daily, with only intermittent bloody stools and few or no other symptoms. One-third of pediatric patients present with moderate disease at diagnosis, with more than 4 stools daily, along with systemic symptoms and weight loss. Laboratory findings in these patients tend to reveal more significant anemia and elevated acute phase reactants. Fever, severe pain, profuse diarrhea, and significant anemia are present in the 10% to 15% of patients with severe disease. These patients are frequently quite sick and may require hospitalization for acute management. Some of these patients may progress to toxic megacolon, a surgical emergency requiring colectomy. Among adolescents with proctitis, the only symptoms can be minimal blood streaking of the stools or a sense of tenesmus that adolescents at times interpret as being "constipated."

Systemic findings can be present in either CD or UC, depending on severity of disease. Fever can occur in 25% to 50% of adolescents with IBD without a specific focus of infection. Temperatures can reach as high as 104°F (40°C), and fever of unknown origin can be a presenting sign of IBD. A hypochromic, microcytic anemia is common, resulting from iron deficiency due to GI blood loss, lack of incorporation of iron into erythrocytes in the bone marrow due to the effects of circulating cytokines, or both.

Anorexia can be quite profound, at times mimicking the classic adolescent eating disorder. Both UC and CD patients can suffer from significant abdominal pain, cramping, and diarrhea with meals, and frequently avoid eating to prevent the associated discomfort. Patients with CD can also have involvement of the upper GI tract, resulting in early satiety or other dyspeptic symptoms that contribute to poor food intake. Finally, increased circulating levels of cytokines such as TNF-α are believed to directly induce anorexia.

The resulting inadequate intake of nutrients is a major reason for the abnormalities of growth and development commonly seen in adolescents with IBD, especially in CD. Older data reported abnormal growth velocity in 88% of children with CD at the time of initial diagnosis.[22] Suboptimal linear growth has been described in up to 40% of children with CD and 10% of those with UC.[23] Growth curves reveal that up to 60% of adolescents with CD drop 2 standard deviations or more from their best height percentile for age during adolescence, and 19% remain 2 standard deviations below their best height percentile at maturity.[24] The cause for poor growth is multifactorial, resulting from the combination of poor caloric intake, the chronic inflammatory condition, and the side effects of treatments such as corticosteroids. Investigations into the insulin-like growth factors (IGFs I and II) and their binding proteins show that both malnutrition and chronic inflammation can cause alterations in their production, leading to a decrease in linear growth.[25]

Extraintestinal symptoms can be associated with UC and CD, and can precede, develop at diagnosis, or become apparent during the course of IBD (Box 104-1). Arthralgias are common, with nondeforming arthritis occurring less frequently. Both are associated with active intestinal disease. Aphthous ulcers in the mouth

**Box 104-1**

***Extraintestinal Manifestations of Inflammatory Bowel Disease***

- Joint disorders: arthralgia, arthritis
- Cutaneous lesions: erythema nodosum, pyoderma gangrenosum
- Ocular lesions: uveitis, episcleritis
- Mouth lesions: apthous ulcers, granulomatous cheilitis
- Autoimmune disorders: sclerosing cholangitis, autoimmune hepatitis
- Vascular disorders: venous thrombosis, vasculitis
- Cardiac disorders: myocarditis, pericarditis
- Renal disorders: nephrolithiasis
- Pulmonary disorders: pneumonitis
- Hematologic disorders: hemolytic anemia, thrombocytosis, coagulopathy

and findings such as erythema nodosum and pyoderma gangrenosum are also typically seen during flares of disease. Treatment for these extraintestinal manifestations is symptomatic, and they frequently regress as the active IBD is controlled. Other associated extraintestinal conditions, such as sclerosing cholangitis, tend to run a course that is independent of the level of intestinal inflammation. The severity of these conditions typically does not change with treatment directed at the underlying IBD.

The reports that describe the clinical features of both forms of IBD derive primarily from largely Caucasian populations with European backgrounds. Interestingly, as larger numbers of patients from other racial and ethnic groups are identified, the frequencies of many of the manifestations of IBD occur in different proportions than the literature suggests. For example, black children with CD appear to have a greater frequency of stricturing and penetrating disease than do white children.[26] Another study in adults suggests that blacks with CD are more likely than whites to have arthritis and that Hispanic patients with UC are much more likely to have a positive perinuclear antineutrophil cytoplasmic antibody (pANCA) serologic response (as discussed later in this chapter) than are whites.[27] As additional racial and ethnic populations are described, it is likely that other differences between groups will also be identified.

## EVALUATION AND DIAGNOSIS

There is a long list of disorders with similar GI signs and symptoms that are also common to IBD. Box 104-2 provides a list of possible differential diagnoses that must be investigated during the workup of an adolescent with suspected IBD.

All evaluations must start with a thorough history, reviewing all possible signs and symptoms of IBD. Questions should be focused on the presence or absence of abdominal pain, as well as its location, intensity, frequency, and association with meals or specific food ingestions. The presence of pain that awakens the adolescent from sleep is a particularly important clue to the diagnosis. Despite an adolescent's common reluctance to discuss the topic, a careful history of the defecatory pattern, including the frequency and consistency of stools and presence of gross blood in the stools, must be sought. Systemic symptoms such as fevers, night sweats, and weight loss must be reviewed. Often, a review of growth records can uncover a subtle and, at times, chronic growth decline. Family history is an important part of the evaluation because the presence of IBD in other family members increases the risk for IBD in the adolescent being evaluated.

### Box 104-2

### *Differential Diagnosis of Inflammatory Bowel Disease*

- Upper GI tract
  - Reflux esophagitis
  - Eosinophilic esophagitis
  - Acid peptic disease
  - *Helicobacter pylori* infection
  - Zollinger-Ellison syndrome
  - GI tuberculosis
- Small and large bowel
  - Celiac disease
  - Irritable bowel syndrome
  - Intestinal lymphangectasia
  - Eosinophilic gastroenteritis
  - Allergic gastroenteropathy
  - Enteric infections
  - Antibiotic-induced colitis
  - Hirschsprung disease with enterocolitis
  - Encopresis
  - Acute appendicitis
  - Neoplasms
  - Vasculitis
  - GI tuberculosis
- Other
  - Eating disorders
  - Carbohydrate intolerance

A comprehensive physical examination is also important, focusing on the systems affected by IBD. The general appearance of the patient, looking for signs of appropriate nutritional status, should be noted. A thorough skin examination should look for any lesions, as well as signs of malnutrition such as nail or hair changes. The presence of abdominal tenderness, fullness, distension, or mass must be sought. The perianal area should be inspected for any suspicious lesions, such as skin tags, fissures, fistulae, or abscess, all of which strongly suggest the presence of CD. Particular care must be taken to distinguish skin tags from hemorrhoids because the former are highly suggestive of CD and the latter only very rarely present in an adolescent. Tanner staging is also important because delay of secondary sexual characteristics is often a clue to the diagnosis.

Laboratory values are a valuable tool in uncovering IBD. Findings may be varied, depending on severity and chronicity of disease, but can frequently show anemia, leukocytosis, thrombocytosis, hypoalbuminemia, and elevation of acute phase reactants. Elevated measurements of the erythrocyte sedimentation rate or C-reactive protein can be clues to an underlying inflammatory process. Alterations in liver-related enzymes can not only occur in IBD patients as a consequence of active intestinal inflammation, but are also seen with associated sclerosing cholangitis or autoimmune hepatitis. It should be noted, however, that the laboratory assessment can be entirely normal in as many as 21% of children and adolescents with mild CD and 54% of those with mild UC at the time of initial diagnosis.[28] Stool studies must be sent to rule out enteric pathogens, parasites, and bacterial toxins such as that produced by *Clostridium difficile*. Stool markers such as lactoferrin and calprotectin can indicate intestinal inflammation, as can the identification of gross or occult blood in the stools.[29]

Serologic testing for protein markers of IBD is commercially available and can be helpful in identifying adolescents with IBD. Serologic studies can also help characterize the type of IBD in indeterminate cases. pANCAs are described in about 60% of patients with UC, and 10% of those with a "UC-like" CD.[30,31] Other microbial markers, including anti-*Saccharomyces cerevisiae* antibodies (ASCAs), anti–outer membrane porin of the cell wall of *Escherichia coli* (anti-ompC), and anti-flagellin antibodies (anti-cBir1 and anti-I2) are highly specific for CD, although sensitivity rates are not high enough for these tests to become routine tools for screening.[32,33]

Endoscopic evaluation with mucosal biopsy is still considered the gold standard in diagnosing IBD. With visual inspection and histopathological findings, extent and even type of IBD can be determined. Although upper endoscopy can help in differentiating CD and UC if granulomas are uncovered in the upper GI tract, UC patients can also have findings on upper endoscopy. Nonspecific gastritis can be present in both UC and CD patients; however, a focal, active inflammation is usually more indicative of CD. The presence of noncaseating granulomas can be found in up to 30% of patients with CD, although the absence of granulomas does not rule out CD. Colonoscopy has now virtually replaced barium enema as the method of choice for evaluating the colon because it is significantly more sensitive than the radiologic study. Continuous involvement with proximal spread from the rectum is more typical of UC, whereas skip lesions, rectal sparing, aphthous ulcers, and terminal ileal inflammation usually speaks to a Crohn disease diagnosis. Severe Crohn disease colitis, though, can look quite similar to UC. In both, the colonic mucosa can appear grossly edematous with diffuse erythema, loss of vascular markings, increased friability, ulcerations, and exudates.

An upper GI series with small bowel follow-through remains an important part of the initial diagnostic evaluation because it can uncover intestinal disease not reachable with standard endoscopic equipment (Figure 104-1). The visualization of inflammatory changes, strictures, or fistulae can support a diagnosis of CD and help direct treatment options. Computed tomography (CT) has had clearer resolution and better patient tolerance versus classical small bowel follow-through studies, but it is associated with a significantly greater radiation dose than the upper GI series.[34] Although magnetic resonance imaging (MRI) has also been used to identify areas of active intestinal inflammation or stricturing disease, it has not yet become part of the initial evaluation for most patients.

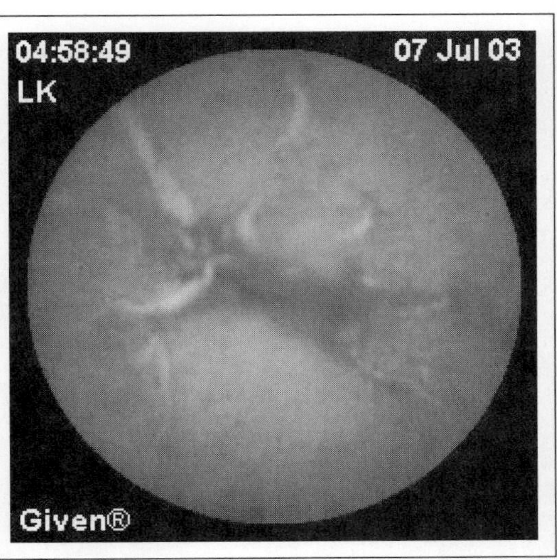


**FIGURE 104-1** Capsule endoscopy. This image from the small bowel of a patient with CD clearly shows ulceration of the mucosal lining consistent with small bowel disease.

A newer diagnostic technique, wireless capsule endoscopy, is approved for patients as young as 10 years of age and has the capability of directly visualizing the mucosa of the small bowel (Figure 104-2). The patient swallows a pill containing a camera capable of recording several hours of data. Although biopsy cannot be done, the direct visualization of the small bowel lining may identify mucosal lesions of CD not evident via traditional radiologic procedures.[35] This modality appears to be safe and well tolerated in adolescents, although there is the risk of a capsule becoming impacted in a stricture, which can prompt the need for urgent surgical intervention.[36]

## TREATMENT

The natural history of IBD is that of intermittent flares with symptoms that wax and wane over time. The type of therapy chosen is based on location and severity of

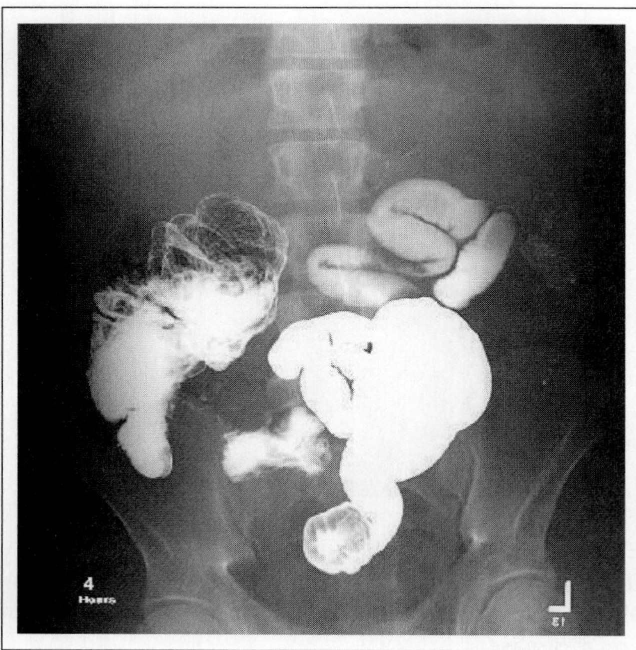


FIGURE 104-2 Upper GI and small bowel series.

disease. Possible side effects and morbidity associated with the specific treatment must be addressed, with a goal of ameliorating symptoms and preventing complications. Treatment can conceptually be divided into 2 phases: induction of remission and subsequent maintenance of remission. Some therapies can be used for both phases of treatment, whereas others are only useful as induction or maintenance agents but not both. Unfortunately, large clinical trials are often lacking in pediatric and adolescent IBD, so many therapies are extrapolated from adult studies and clinical experience.

## ANTI-INFLAMMATORY THERAPY

### 5-Aminosalicylates

This group of medications is effective in both induction and maintenance of remission in mild to moderately active UC and is also used in mild forms of CD. The 5-aminosalicylates (5-ASAs) work via multiple pathways, including inhibition of 5-lipoxygenase leading to decreased leukotriene B4, reactive oxygen metabolite scavenging, prevention of the upregulation of leukocyte adhesion molecules, and the inhibition of interleukin-1 (IL-1) synthesis.[37] These medications are available in multiple oral preparations (sulfasalazine, mesalamine, olsalazine, balsalazide) and release active 5-ASA in different locations throughout the intestine based on pH- or time-dependent delivery systems. Rectal enema and suppository preparations of mesalamine are useful to control symptoms such as tenesmus and urgency arising from inflammation of the rectosigmoid and descending colon. A combination of oral and rectal 5-ASA therapy has been superior to oral therapy alone in the treatment of UC. Sulfasalazine, the first medication to be discovered in this class, is now frequently replaced by newer agents because of its relatively common side effects, including headache, malaise, and hemolysis. Hypersensitivity reactions were also reported with rashes, fever, aplastic anemia, hepatic necrosis, pulmonary vasculitis, and neurologic complications. Pancreatitis has been reported after use of many of the 5-ASA preparations.[38] Exacerbation of colitis is also documented in adolescent patients using mesalamine preparations.[39] Megaloblastic anemia secondary to sulfasalazine can be prevented by supplementation with folic acid and is not a problem with the other 5-ASA drugs. The use of 5-ASA medications as a chemopreventative therapy against colorectal cancer in chronic colitis is controversial, although retrospective, epidemiologic studies have shown a benefit.[40]

### Corticosteroids

These preparations, in oral, parenteral, and rectal forms, are used for induction of remission in patients with moderate to severe IBD. Corticosteroids acutely decrease inflammation through a variety of mechanisms, including downregulation of proinflammatory proteins such as IL-1, 2, 3, 4, 5, 6, and 8; TNF-$\alpha$; and intracellular adhesion molecules. They also upregulate gene transcription for the production of anti-inflammatory cytokines. Although effective in obtaining clinical remission quickly, significant side effects make corticosteroid therapy difficult to use for adolescent patients. Rectal preparations, such as hydrocortisone enemas and foam-based preparations, are good options for localized left-sided disease, but still have some systemic absorption and possible side effects. A newer topically active corticosteroid, budesonide, is available in the United States as an oral preparation designed for controlled release in the ileum and right colon, and in Canada as both the oral preparation and a rectal enema. Budesonide is believed to have fewer side effects than systemic corticosteroids and has been moderately effective when used in children and adolescents with CD.[41] Parenteral corticosteroids are used in moderate to severely ill patients who have failed oral dosing or who are hospitalized.[42]

Side effects of corticosteroids include growth retardation, osteoporosis, glaucoma, cataracts, edema and weight gain, hypertension, diabetes, and avascular necrosis. The cosmetic changes of acne, hirsutism, striae, and moon facies are difficult to tolerate as adolescents deal with an already challenging time of pubertal changes. In addition, mood swings can occur, making medication compliance difficult for teenagers. Because adolescents are psychologically sensitive to changes in physical appearance, this should play a role in determining appropriate treatment regimens in these patients.

### IMMUNE MODULATORS

#### Thiopurines (6-Mercaptopurine [6-MP], Azathioprine [AZA])

By inhibiting RNA and DNA synthesis, these purine analogs ultimately downregulate cytotoxic T-cell activity and delayed hypersensitivity reactions, as well as induce T-cell apoptosis.[43] Both 6-MP and AZA are excellent maintenance treatments with significant steroid-sparing activity. The prolonged onset of action of these medications (up to 2–3 months after initiation) makes the thiopurines inappropriate agents for the induction of remission. Both observational studies and controlled clinical trials demonstrate that thiopurine use maintains remission and allows cessation of concomitant corticosteroid therapy in 60% to 80% of children and adults with CD.[44,45] Similar benefit was seen in children and adolescents with moderate-to-severe UC.

Potential toxicity is a major issue with this group of drugs.[46] Idiosyncratic reactions, including fever, malaise, rash, diarrhea, or pancreatitis, occur in 5% to 10% of patients. Potentially more serious side effects, including hepatotoxicity and bone marrow suppression, can be predicted and, to some extent, minimized by careful monitoring of routine laboratory studies and thiopurine metabolite levels.[47] Prior to starting a thiopurine, many physicians test for the activity of thiopurine S-methyltransferase (TPMT), the major inactivating enzyme for both 6-MP and AZA. Genetic polymorphisms of TPMT are common, such that 1 in 300 individuals in the general population totally lack TPMT, whereas about 11% have decreased TPMT activity. Identifying patients with TPMT deficiency can reduce, but not eliminate, the potential for severe leukopenia.[48]

#### Calcineurin Inhibitors (Cyclosporine and Tacrolimus)

These drugs inhibit T-cell activation and block transcription of proinflammatory cytokines, including IL-2 and interferon-gamma (IFN-$\gamma$), via binding to intracellular receptors. Once bound to these receptors, the complex inhibits the intracellular mediator, calcineurin, by which gene inactivation occurs. These medications have been effective inducers of remission for severe UC that is unresponsive to corticosteroids and can, at times, prevent emergency colectomy. Calcineurin inhibitors are used as a bridge to maintenance treatment with either 6-MP or AZA. Side effects are potentially serious and include nephrotoxicity, hepatotoxicity, increased risk of infection, seizures, and cortical blindness. Of note for the adolescent, hypertrichosis has also been reported.

#### Methotrexate

This drug has been used in pediatric and adult patients with CD refractory to conventional therapy. Its usage in UC is less well evaluated. Side effects include potential hepatotoxicity. Nausea is a common complaint that often limits the acceptability of this therapy. Methotrexate is prescribed as a weekly subcutaneous or intramuscular injection, or as a daily oral formulation. Controversy remains as to which mode of administration is more efficacious and better tolerated. The known teratogenicity of methotrexate complicates the use of this drug in adolescents and young adults.

### BIOLOGICAL THERAPY

#### Infliximab

This is a genetically engineered chimeric monoclonal antibody directed against TNF-$\alpha$. Its mechanism of action is believed to work through its strong binding affinity for circulating and membrane-bound TNF, as well as induction of apoptosis of activated lymphocytes. Infliximab (IFX) is given as an intravenous infusion and is approved by the US Food and Drug Administration (FDA) for induction and maintenance therapy in pediatric and adult patients with CD, and in adult patients with UC. Its success in inducing and maintaining remission in refractory patients with moderate to severe IBD has changed the face of IBD treatment. Although generally safe, this agent has a long list of potential toxicities. Because IFX is a chimeric antibody, it can induce an immunogenic response, resulting in the development of antibodies to IFX (ATI) that can increase the risk of infusion reactions and decrease the efficacy of therapy. Regularly scheduled maintenance infusions, possibly with concomitant immunomodulator therapy, have decreased the frequency of developing ATI. Other potential toxicities include immediate and delayed infusion reactions, increased risk of infection, reactivation of tuberculosis, worsening of cardiac failure, and induction of autoimmune and demyelinating diseases. In addition, recent observation raises the possibility that IFX, perhaps in conjunction with thiopurine therapy, increases the risk for lymphoma, including a rare and often fatal hepatosplenic T-cell lymphoma in adolescents and young adults.[49] The Study of Biologic and Immunomodulator Naive Patients in Crohn's Disease (SONIC) trial, an adult multicenter trial, demonstrated that monotherapy with IFX was significantly better to induce remission and mucosal healing than azathioprine alone in AZA-naive patients.[50] Other studies show that the use of concomitant IFX and AZA induce improved endoscopic healing.[51] Because the risk of lymphoma, which is often incurable, occurs in predominantly young patients, both the risks and benefits need to be weighed carefully when determining whether to use IFX along with immunomodulators in this age group.

### Other Biological Agents

New monoclonal antibodies continue to be developed. Adalimumab is a humanized anti-TNF-α monoclonal antibody, administered subcutaneously, that has recently been approved by the FDA for treatment of adults with CD. Clinical trials in adults and anecdotal reports in children and adolescents show adalimumab to be effective in the treatment of patients with CD who have developed ATI or lost responsiveness to IFX. As a humanized monoclonal antibody, adalimumab is less likely to be immunogenic than IFX. Other new biological therapies in development include agents that aim at a variety of different targets, including additional proinflammatory cytokines, intracellular adhesion molecules, growth factors, and other intracellular mediators of inflammation.

## ANTIBIOTICS

Treatment of mild to moderate inflammatory CD and perianal fistulizing CD with metronidazole and ciprofloxacin has been documented. A study of metronidazole (15–20 mg/kg/day) showed a steroid-sparing effect in adolescents with active or steroid-dependent CD. However, many of the patients with long-term use (4–11 months) developed abnormal sensory examinations with severe, but reversible, paresthesias and dysesthesias.[52] The severe abdominal pain and vomiting that arise in the patient taking metronidazole who consumes alcohol often makes the use of this antibiotic quite difficult in the adolescent. Ciprofloxacin has its own side effect profile, which includes potential growth plate damage, an important side effect in patients undergoing their pubertal growth spurts. Although studies in adolescents are lacking, a newer nonsystemic antibiotic, rifaximin, has also been effective in the treatment of adults with mild CD. There is no role for antibiotic use in UC except to treat a superimposed infection such as *Clostridium difficile*.

## PROBIOTICS, PREBIOTICS, AND SYNBIOTICS

A complex interaction between the host immune system and gut flora appears to be central to IBD expression. Animal models of IBD demonstrate that individual strains of bacteria can influence the expression and activity of GI inflammation. Probiotics are nonpathogenic bacteria that are normally found within the microflora of the GI tract. Prebiotics act as substrates for the preferential growth of probiotics. Synbiotics are preparations that include a combination of both pro- and prebiotics. Treatments incorporating the use of such preparations have decreased production of proinflammatory cytokines, interfered with bacterial adherence, and induced additional anti-inflammatory effects via increased production of anti-inflammatory cytokines such as IL-10. Pediatric studies are limited, but adult studies show some success using these products in preventing relapse in UC and "pouchitis" (see below) following colectomy for UC. Studies in CD seem less promising.

## NUTRITIONAL THERAPY

Nutritional support as an adjunctive therapy is critical in adolescents with IBD as a means of improving weight gain and preventing or reversing growth failure. However, studies also demonstrate a role for nutritional interventions as primary therapy for induction of remission in adolescents with active CD. In contrast, there appears to be no role for primary enteral therapy in the treatment of children and adolescents with UC. Studies evaluating enteral therapy describe beneficial effects from a variety of different formula types, including those that include free amino acids (elemental), peptides derived from protein hydrolysates (semielemental), and intact protein formulas.[53] Enteral therapy addresses the issues of malnutrition and nutrient deficiencies, while downregulating the inflammatory response. Enteral therapy using an elemental diet has shown similar efficacy when compared to corticosteroids and few side effects.[54] Difficulties with palatability, need for nasogastric feedings, and the inability to eat as their peers do often makes this treatment less appealing and more difficult to undertake in an adolescent with IBD.

## SURGERY

Ulcerative colitis is a condition that can be cured by a total mucosal proctocolectomy. Frequently, an ileal pouch-anal anastomosis (IPAA) is constructed at the time of colectomy to obviate the need for ileostomy. However, although these surgeries can be considered a "cure" of UC, up to 50% of children and adolescents can develop chronic inflammation of the ileal pouch ("pouchitis") that at times can require ongoing medical management.[55] Indications for elective colectomy include failure to respond to medications, significant morbidity from side effects of medications, persistent bleeding, dysplasia, and carcinoma. In UC patients, emergency surgical intervention may be needed secondary to fulminant colitis, massive bleeding, perforation, or toxic megacolon.

In contrast, CD cannot be cured by surgery. However, patients can benefit from surgery if complications of their disease occur that are unresponsive to medical therapy. Localized disease can be resected, and stricturoplasties can be performed without extensive bowel loss to alleviate strictures that lead to recurrent partial obstruction. Such interventions can result in markedly improved quality of life. Crohn disease colitis that is refractory to therapy can require total proctocolectomy and permanent ileostomy, and the risk of postoperative recurrence makes construction of an IPAA ill advised. Surgery in CD does not cure the patient of the disease, however, and recurrent disease is common. Therefore, many physicians advocate the need for continued medical treatment in the postoperative patient. Although no therapy effectively prevents recurrent CD in all patients, studies suggest a role for postoperative maintenance with metronidazole, 5-ASA, or 6-MP.[56]

Postsurgical patients, especially those with an ileostomy or IPAA, have their own set of issues and problems. In IPAA patients, "pouchitis" is common and can require continuing medication with probiotics, antibiotics, and, at times, anti-inflammatories. Possible mucosal dysplasia of the pouch, or in the remnant of colonic mucosa that remains after surgery, demands endoscopic surveillance. Quality-of-life issues such as fecal incontinence, persistent diarrhea, and even fertility are important to remember in the adolescent age group. Dietary manipulations, as well as antidiarrheal therapy, have been used to assist patients with frequent stools. In addition, for patients with permanent ileostomies, cosmetic issues and body image alteration are important concerns to be addressed.

## PSYCHOSOCIAL RAMIFICATIONS

Compared with healthy children, children with IBD are at greater risk of having difficulties in behavioral/emotional functioning.[57] Growth retardation can make athletic competition against normal-sized peers impossible. Delayed pubertal onset, the cosmetic side effects of medications, and postsurgical issues can cause significant social isolation above and beyond that of the average teenager. Recognition and appropriate management of the psychosocial impact of IBD in the adolescent population represents an important challenge to the medical team.

### PSYCHOSOCIAL FUNCTIONING

Much like those with other chronic illnesses, patients with IBD often experience psychosocial difficulties. Severe psychopathology is usually absent, but psychiatric disorders, most commonly depression and anxiety, can be identified frequently. Children with IBD tend to be more compulsive as a group than healthy controls, and have psychological styles characterized by depression, withdrawal, anxiety, and frequent somatizing.[58] When compared to healthy controls, adolescents with IBD, particularly boys, have reported significantly worse health-related quality of life.[59] In addition, significant numbers of patients report that IBD has an effect on their social lives, with 31% to 50% claiming that IBD restricts their social activities.[60] As a consequence of both the physical and social effects of these illnesses, adolescents are at risk for experiencing problems associated with low self-esteem. Addressing these issues should be a key part of managing these patients. In addition, the stress on the family in dealing with a sick sibling or child also plays a role in the care of the teenager with IBD.

### MEDICATION ADHERENCE

The treatment of the adolescent with IBD often requires multiple medications given frequently over the course of the day. As a consequence, adherence to the medically prescribed regimen becomes an important issue in managing the adolescent with IBD. In a recent review, 43% of adult patients with IBD admitted to occasionally forgetting to take their medication, but only 7.5% did it purposefully.[61] Similarly, a small study of 50 adolescents with IBD showed few patients with perfect adherence, and virtually any practitioner who treats IBD in adolescents can identify any number of patients who chose to stop their medications without their parents' or physician's knowledge.[62] Although adolescence is normally a time for acting-out behaviors, the rebellion by an IBD patient can be quite serious, especially when the outcome can lead to significant morbidity. Addressing the serious issues and complications that can occur if medication is skipped or taken incorrectly is one possible method of improving adherence and compliance. There are also electronic devices that track medication use, which can be helpful in reminding a patient to take a dose. In addition, altering the medication regimen to decrease the frequency of medication can also be helpful. Adolescents may do well with parenteral or infusional therapies that limit the need for daily dosing of medication. Newer drugs are being developed that allow for a decrease in the number and frequency of required doses.

## FERTILITY/PREGNANCY ISSUES

Many adolescent patients also need to deal with reproductive issues and the effect of IBD on fertility, pregnancy, and delivery. In general, conception is not impaired in women with IBD. Surgery, especially the creation of an ileal pouch following colectomy, however, has the potential to reduce fertility postoperatively secondary to resultant adhesions and damage to the reproductive organs.[63] It is widely recognized that, with rare exceptions, the greatest risk to the fetus during gestation is a flare of IBD that significantly comprises the mother's nutritional state. However, medication during conception and pregnancy remains an important concern. Methotrexate is a known teratogen and is contraindicated in women attempting to conceive and throughout gestation. Other immunomodulators, such as 6-MP and AZA, show increased teratogenicity in animal studies, but multiple case series of adult IBD patients during pregnancy have not shown a significant increase in congenital anomalies. However, a recently published study from Denmark identified an increased risk for premature delivery and congenital anomalies in the offspring of women with CD who received AZA during pregnancy.[64] No teratogenic risk has been demonstrated with any of the 5-ASA drugs, but sulfasalazine impairs sperm motility, making conception more difficult, and its sulfa moiety can exacerbate neonatal hyperbilirubinemia if the mother breastfeeds. Biological therapy with infliximab is believed to present a low risk to the fetus, but it is known to cross the placenta, and it is unknown whether it is safe to breastfeed while on maintenance infusions. These issues necessitate that a knowledgeable gastroenterologist and obstetrician/gynecologist work together to assure the best possible pregnancy outcome for patients with IBD.

## CANCER RISK AND SCREENING

It is now well documented that both forms of IBD increase the risk of intestinal cancer. In UC, and in CD with extensive colonic involvement, the risk of colonic adenocarcinoma increases by 0.5% to 1.0% yearly after 8 to 10 years postdiagnosis and accounts for approximately 15% of all deaths in IBD patients.[65] The primary risk factors for colon cancer include extent of disease (pancolitis > left-sided colitis > proctosigmoiditis) and duration of disease, placing pediatric and adolescent IBD patients at increased lifetime risk. Additional risk factors include concomitant primary sclerosing cholangitis, and possibly lack of treatment with 5-ASA or folic acid. Regular colonoscopic screening for dysplasia becomes a necessary part of management in these patients by 8 years after diagnosis and must be initiated during adolescence in patients who developed colitis during childhood. Other cancers cannot be overlooked, especially in light of new data showing an increased risk of lymphoma in patients on immunosuppressive medications and biological therapy.[66]

## PROGNOSIS

### CROHN DISEASE

Long-term studies in patients diagnosed as children clearly describe a pattern of waxing and waning of symptoms over the course of many years. Recurrent disease flares or the development of fistulae or strictures lead to frequent symptoms, surgeries, and multiple courses of medications.[67] Periods of growth retardation occur in up to 60% of adolescents whose disease begins before puberty, with some data illustrating permanent stunting; more recent evidence shows that once adjustments are made for parental heights, there is not always a significant difference in projected adult heights.[68] In addition, one or more operations may become necessary in many patients, especially in those who develop strictures or fistulas. These patients still have endoscopic findings post-surgery, and reoperation is common.[69] In 1 pediatric study, clinical recurrence rates were 17% at 1 year, 38% at 3 years, and 60% at 5 years, with higher rates among those with more severe disease at time of surgery.[70] In those in whom surgery is avoided, many ultimately demonstrate an increased risk of adenocarcinoma.[71]

### ULCERATIVE COLITIS

Most patients achieve remission within the first few months after diagnosis, irrespective of whether their initial attack is characterized as mild, moderate, or severe. However, 10% of those whose symptoms are characterized as moderate/severe will remain continuously symptomatic.[72] As time goes on, 55% of patients remain without symptoms, 40% suffer from chronic intermittent symptoms, and less than 10% have continuous symptoms. These data are similar to those reported in adult populations. Colectomy is a real outcome in this group, with rates increasing to about 20% by 5 years after diagnosis. The clinical outcome of children with proctitis or proctosigmoiditis appears less severe, with more than 90% without symptoms within 6 months of diagnosis and with less than 5% suffering from active disease.[73] Unfortunately, there is a strong likelihood of extension of disease that occurs over long-term follow-up in these patients. These rates of proximal extension of inflammation and colectomy appear higher than in adult populations.

## REFERENCES

1. Bousvaros A, Sylvester F, Kugathasan S, et al. Challenges in pediatric inflammatory bowel disease. *Inflamm Bowel Dis.* 2006; 12:885-913

2. Sandler RS, Eisen GM. Epidemiology of inflammatory bowel disease. In: Kirsner JB, ed. *Inflammatory Bowel Disease.* 5th ed. Philadelphia, PA: Saunders; 2000:89-112

3. Loftus EV. Clinical epidemiology of inflammatory bowel disease: incidence, prevalence, and environmental influences. *Gastroenterology.* 2004;126:1504-1517

4. Hildebrand H, Finkel Y, Grahnquist L, Lindholm J, Ekbom A, Askling J. Changing pattern of paediatric inflammatory bowel disease in northern Stockholm 1990-2001. *Gut.* 2003;52:1432-1434

5. Kugathasan S, Judd RH, Hoffmann RG, et al. Wisconsin Pediatric Inflammatory Bowel Disease Alliance. Epidemiologic and clinical characteristics of children with newly diagnosed inflammatory bowel disease in Wisconsin: a statewide population-based study. *J Pediatr.* 2003;143:525–531

6. Goyette P, Labbe C, Trinh TT, Xavier RJ, Rioux JD. Molecular pathogenesis, of inflammatory bowel disease: genotypes, phenotypes, and personalized medicine. *Ann Med.* 2007;39:177–199

7. Tysk C, Lindberg E, Jarnerot G, Floderus-Myrhed B. Ulcerative colitis and Crohn's disease in an unselected population of monozygotic and dizygotic twins: a study of heritability and the influence of smoking. *Gut.* 1988;29:990–996

8. Halfvarson J, Bodin L, Tysk C, Lindberg E, Jarnerot G. Inflammatory bowel disease in a Swedish twin cohort: a long-term follow-up of concordance and clinical characteristics. *Gastroenterology.* 2003;124:1767–1773

9. Ogura Y, Conen DK, Inohara N, et al. A frameshift mutation in *NOD2* associated with susceptibility to Crohn's disease. *Nature.* 2001;411:537–539

10. Hugot JP. *CARD15/NOD2* mutations in Crohn's disease. *Ann N Y Acad Sci.* 2006;1072:9–18

11. Cuthbert AP, Fisher SA, Mirza MM, et al. The contribution of *NOD2* gene mutation to the risk and site of disease in inflammatory bowel disease. *Gastroenterology.* 2002;122:867–874

12. Russell RK, Drummond HE, Nimmo EE, et al. Genotype-phenotype analysis in childhood-onset Crohn's disease: *NOD2/CARD15* variants consistently predict phenotypic characteristics of severe disease. *Inflamm Bowel Dis.* 2005;11:955–964

13. Annese V, Valvano MR, Palmieri O, Latiano A, Bossa F, Andriulli A. Multidrug resistance 1 gene in inflammatory bowel disease: a meta-analysis. *World J Gastroenterol.* 2006;12:3636–3644

14. Resta-Lenert S, Smitham J, Barrett KE. Epithelial dysfunction associated with the development of colitis in conventionally housed mdr1a-/- mice. *Am J Physiol Gastrointest Liver Physiol.* 2005;289:G153–G162

15. Reddy D, Siegel CA, Sands BE, Kane S. Possible association between isotretinoin and inflammatory bowel disease. *Am J Gastroenterol.* 2006;101:1569–1573

16. Guslandi M. Exacerbation of inflammatory bowel disease by nonsteroidal anti-inflammatory drugs and cyclo-oxygenase-2 inhibitors: fact or fiction? *World J Gastroenterol.* 2006;12:1509–1510

17. Strober W, Fuss I, Mannon P. The fundamental basis of inflammatory bowel disease. *J Clin Invest.* 2007;227:514–521

18. Auvin S, Molinie F, Gower-Rousseau C, et al. Incidence, clinical presentation, and location at diagnosis of pediatric inflammatory bowel disease: a prospective population-based study in northern France (1988–1999). *J Pediatr Gastroenterol Nutr.* 2005;41:49–55

19. Hyams JS, Davis P, Grancher K, Lerer T, Justinich CJ, Markowitz J.Clinical outcome of ulcerative colitis in children. *J Pediatr.* 1996;129:81–88

20. Moy LC, Markowitz J, Mack DR, et al. Clinical outcome of ulcerative colitis in children: a prospective 3-year follow-up from diagnosis (abstract T1325). Presented at: Digestive Diseases Week; May 22, 2007; San Diego, CA

21. Markowitz J, Daum F, Aiges H, et al. Perianal disease in children and adolescents with Crohn's disease. *Gastroenterology.* 1984;86:829–833

22. Kanof ME, Lake AM, Bayless TM. Decreased height velocity in children and adolescents before the diagnosis of Crohn's disease. *Gastroenterology.* 1988;95:1523–1527

23. Motil KJ, Grand RJ, Davis-Kraft L, Ferlic LL, Smith EO. Growth failure in children with inflammatory bowel disease: a prospective study. *Gastroenterology.* 2003;105:681–691

24. Markowitz J, Grancher K, Rosa J, Aiges H, Daum F. Growth failure in pediatric inflammatory bowel disease. *J Pediatr Gastroenterol Nutr.* 1993;16:373–380

25. Ballinger AB, Camacho-Hubner C, Croft NM. Growth failure and intestinal inflammation. *Q J Med.* 2001;94:121–125

26. Eidelwein AP, Thompson R, Fiorino K, et al. Disease presentation and clinical course in black and white children with inflammatory bowel disease. *J Pediatr Gastroenterol Nutr.* 2007;44:555–560

27. Basu D, Lopez I, Kulkarni A, Sellin JH. Impact of race and ethnicity on inflammatory bowel disease. *Am J Gastroenterol.* 2005;100:2254–2261

28. Mack DR, Langton C, Markowitz JM, et al. Laboratory values for children with newly diagnosed inflammatory bowel disease. *Pediatrics.* 2007;119:1113–1119

29. D'Incà R, Dal Pont E, Di Leo V, et al. Calprotectin and lactoferrin in the assessment of intestinal inflammation and organic disease. *Int J Colorectal Dis.* 2007;22:429–437

30. Sandborn WJ, Loftus EV Jr., Colombel JF, et al. Evaluation of serologic disease markers in a population-based cohort of patients with ulcerative colitis and Crohn's disease. *Inflamm Bowel Dis.* 2001;7:192–201

31. Desir B, Amre DK, Lu SE, et al. Utility of serum antibodies in determining clinical course in pediatric Crohn's disease. *Clin Gastroenterol Hepatol.* 2004;2:139–146

32. Papadakis KA, Yang H, Ippoliti A, et al. Anti-flagellin (CBir1) phenotypic and genetic Crohn's disease associations. *Inflamm Bowel Dis.* 2007;13(5):524–530

33. Ruemmele FM, Targan SR, Levy G, Dubinsky M, Braun J, Seidman EG. Diagnostic accuracy of serological assays in pediatric inflammatory bowel disease. *Gastrorenterology.* 1998;115:822–829

34. Jamieson DH, Shipman PJ, Israel DM, Jacobsen K. Comparison of multidetector CT and barium studies of the small bowel: inflammatory bowel disease in children. *Am J Radiol.* 2003;180:1211–1216

35. Seidman EG, Sant'Anna AM, Dirks MH. Potential applications of wireless capsule endoscopy in the pediatric age group. *Gastrointest Endosc Clin N Am.* 2004;14:207–217

36. Seidman EG, Dirks MH. Capsule endoscopy in the pediatric patient. *Curr Treat Options Gastroenterol.* 2006;9:416–422

37. Desreumaux P, Ghosh S. Review article: mode of action and delivery of 5-aminosalicylic acid—new evidence. *Aliment Pharmacol Ther.* 2006;24(S1):2-9

38. Fernandez J, Sals M, Panes J, Feu F, Navarro S, Teres J. Acute pancreatitis after long-term 5-aminosalicylic acid therapy. *Am J Gastroenterol.* 1997;92:2302-2303

39. Iofel E, Chawla A, Daum F, Markowitz J. Mesalamine intolerance mimics symptoms of active inflammatory bowel disease. *J Pediatr Gastroenterol Nutr.* 2002;34:73-76

40. Van Staa TP, Card T, Logan RF, Leufkens HG. 5-Aminosalicylate use and colorectal cancer risk in inflammatory bowel disease: a large epidemiological study. *Gut.* 2005;54:1573-1578

41. Escher JC. European Collaborative Research Group on Budesonide in Paediatric IBD. Budesonide versus prednisolone for the treatment of active Crohn's disease in children: a randomized, double-blind, controlled multicentre trial. *Eur J Gastroenterol Hepatol.* 2004;16:47-54

42. Steinhart AH, Ewe K, Griffiths AM, Modigliani R, Thomsen OO. Corticosteroids for maintenance of remission in Crohn's disease. *Cochrane Database Syst Rev.* 2003;(4):CD000301

43. Dubinsky MD. Azathioprine, 6-mercaptopurine in inflammatory bowel disease: pharmacology, efficacy, and safety. *Clin Gastroenterol Hepatol.* 2004;2:731-743

44. Markowitz J, Grancher K, Kohn N, Lesser M, Daum F. A multicenter trial of 6-mercaptopurine and prednisone in children with newly diagnosed Crohn's disase. *Gastroenterology.* 2000;119:895-902

45. Markowitz J, Rosa J, Grancher K, Aiges H, Daum F. Long-term 6-mercaptopurine in adolescents with Crohn's disease. *Gastroenterology.* 1990;99:1347-1351

46. Kirschner BS. Safety of azathioprine and 6-mercaptopurine in pediatric patients with inflammatory bowel disease. *Gastroenterology.* 1998;115:813-821

47. Gupta P, Gokhale R, Kirschner BS. 6-Mercaptopurine metabolite levels in children with inflammatory bowel disease. *J Pediatr Gastroenterol Nutr.* 2001;33:450-454

48. Colombel JF, Ferrari N, Debuysere H, et al. Genotypic analysis of thiopurine S-methyltransferase in patients with Crohn's disease and severe myelosuppression during azathioprine therapy. *Gastroenterology.* 2000;118:1025-1030

49. Rosh JR, Gross T, Mamula P, Griffiths A, Hyams J. Hepatosplenic T-cell lymphoma in adolescents and young adults with Crohn's disease: a cautionary tale? *Inflamm Bowel Dis.* 2007;13(8):1024-1030

50. Sandborn WJ, Rutgeerts P, Reinisch W, et al. SONIC: a randomized, double-blind, controlled trial comparing infliximab and infliximab plus azathioprine to azathioprine in patients with Crohn's disease naive to immunomodulators and biologic therapy. *Am J Gastroenterol.* 2008;103(suppl):A1117

51. D'haens G, Hommes D, Baert F, et al. A combined regimen of infliximab and azathioprine induces better endoscopic healing than classic step-up therapy in newly diagnosed Crohn's disease. *Gastroenterology.* 2006;130:A110

52. Duffy L, Daum F, Fisher SE, et al. Peripheral neuropathy in Crohn's disease patients treated with metronidazole. *Gastroenterology.* 1985;88:681-684

53. Lionetti P, Callegari ML, Ferrari S, et al. Enteral nutrition and microflora in pediatric Crohn's disease. *J Parenter Enteral Nutr.* 2005;29:S173-S175

54. Heuschkel RB, Menach CC, Megerian JT, Baird AE. Enteral nutrition and corticosteroids in the treatment of acute Crohn's disease in children. *J Pediatr Gastroenterol Nutr.* 2000;31:8-15

55. Koivusalo A, Pakarinen MP, Rintala RJ. Surgical complications in relation to functional outcomes after ileoanal anastomosis in pediatric patients with ulcerative colitis. *J Pediatr Surg.* 2007;42:290-295

56. Hanauer SB, Korelitz BI, Rutgeerts P, et al. Postoperative maintenance of Crohn's disease remission with 6-mercaptopurine, mesalamine, or placebo: a 2-year trial. *Gastroenterology.* 2004;127:723-729

57. Mackner LM, Crandall WV, Szigethy EM. Psychosocial functioning in pediatric inflammatory bowel disease. *Inflamm Bowel Dis.* 2006;3:239-244

58. Szigethy E, Levy-Warren A, Whitton S, et al. Depressive symptoms and inflammatory bowel disease in children and adolescents: a cross-sectional study. *J Pediatr Gastroenterol Nutr.* 2004;39:395-402

59. DeBoer M, Grootenhus M, Derkx B, Last B. Health-related quality of life and psychosocial functioning of adolescents with inflammatory bowel disease. *Inflamm Bowel Dis.* 2005;4:400-406

60. Moody G, Easden JA, Mayberry JF. Social implications of childhood Crohn's disease. *J Pediatr Gastroenterol Nutr.* 1999;28:43-45

61. Bernal I, Domenech E, Garcia-Planella E, et al. Medication-taking behavior in a cohort of patients with inflammatory bowel disease. *Dig Dis Sci.* 2006;51(12):2165-2169. Epub 2006 Nov 4

62. Mackner LM, Crandall WV. Oral medication adherence in pediatric inflammatory bowel disease. *Inflamm Bowel Dis.* 2005;11:1006-1012

63. Mahadevan U. Fertility and pregnancy in the patient with inflammatory bowel disease. *Gut.* 2006;55:1198-1206

64. Norgard B, Pedersen L, Christensen L, Sorenson HT. Therapeutic drug use in women with Crohn's disease and birth outcomes: a Danish nationwide cohort study. *Am J Gastroenterol.* 2007;102:1406-1413

65. Munkholm P. Review article: the incidence and prevalence of colorectal cancer in inflammatory bowel disease. *Aliment Pharmacol Ther.* 2003;18:1-5

66. Kandiel A, Fraser AG, Korelitz BI, Brensinger C, Lewis JD. Increased risk of lymphoma among inflammatory bowel disease patients treated with azathioprine and 6-mercaptopurine. *Gut.* 2005;54:1121-1125

67. Freeman HJ. Long-term prognosis of early-onset Crohn's disease diagnosed in childhood or adolescence. *Can J Gastroenterol.* 2004;18:661-665

68. Alemzadeh N, Rekers-Mombar L, Mearin M, Wit J, Lamers C, van Hogezand R. Adult height in patients with early onset of Crohn's disease. *Gut.* 2002;51:26–29

69. Rutgeerts P, Geboes K, Vantrappen G, et al. Predictability of the postoperative course of Crohn's disease. *Gastroenterology.* 1990;99:956–963

70. Baldassano RN, Han PD, Jeshion WC, et al. Pediatric Crohn's disease: risk factors for postoperative recurrence. *Am J Gastroenterol.* 2001;96:2169–2176

71. Jess T, Winther KV, Munkholm P, Langholz E, Binder V. Intestinal and extra intestinal cancer in Crohn's disease: follow-up of a population-based cohort in Copenhagen County, Denmark. *Aliment Pharmacol Ther.* 2004;19:287–293

72. Hyams JS, Davis P, Grancher K, Lerer T, Justinich CJ, Markowitz J. Clinical outcome of ulcerative colitis in children. *J Pediatr.* 1996;129:81–88

73. Hyams J, Davis P, Lerer T, et al. Clinical outcome of ulcerative proctitis in children. *J Pediatr Gastroenterol Nutr.* 1997;25:149–152

74. Ludvigsoon JF, Krantz M, Bodin L, Stenhammar L, Lindquist B. Elemental versus polymeric enteral nutrition in paediatric Crohn's disease: a multicentre randomized controlled trial. *Acta Paediatr.* 2004;93:327–335

# CHAPTER 105

# Celiac Disease

HUSAM MALLAH, MD • THOMAS M. ROSSI, MD

## INTRODUCTION

Celiac disease, also known as gluten sensitive enteropathy, is characterized by malabsorption and impaired somatic growth associated with subtotal villus atrophy of the small intestine induced by the consumption of gluten-containing grain products in susceptible individuals. Because the initial pathophysiologic link to gluten was recognized in the 1940s, these elements have been considered the essential criteria for diagnosis.[1-3] Over the last decade, however, a spectrum of pathologic changes of celiac disease has been recognized in patients who are asymptomatic or who have minimal or atypical symptoms. Furthermore, diagnostic advances, specifically the recent development of serologic diagnostic tests, have been instrumental in correlating histopathology with subtle clinical features of the disease. Through an expansion of our observations of the clinical findings associated with the condition, an unfolding of the pathophysiology has been occurring. As a result, celiac disease is now recognized as an autoimmune enteropathy of the small intestine with a broad spectrum of clinical manifestations.

Because of an increasing incidence now being reported in the United States, celiac disease has attained notoriety in recent years and has sparked public interest as a frequent topic of conversation in the community. Celiac disease has been described throughout the world, with regional differences in incidence. The disease is frequent in India and among Arabs, but is uncommon in Africans, Chinese, and Japanese populations. The prevalence of celiac disease has increased largely because of increased recognition due to the development of accurate serologic markers for the disease. For example, an older study found the incidence in Europe ranging between 12.5 and 25 per 100,000, whereas in the United States, the incidence was 12.9 per 100,000.[4] However, the diagnosis was based on a clinical presentation with classic symptoms of malabsorption. Newer sensitive and specific serologic assays for IgA antibodies to gliadin, endomysium, and tissue transglutaminase (tTG) have markedly improved detection. Data from several European countries suggest that if using endomysial antibodies (EmA) or anti-tTG as markers, the incidence may be as high as 1,000 per 100,000 in Europe, and 400 per 100,000 in the United States.[5,6] As a consequence, our awareness and understanding of the clinical spectrum of celiac disease is changing.

## PRESENTATIONS OF CELIAC DISEASE

Because celiac disease results from the injurious effects of dietary gluten on the small intestinal mucosa, abdominal symptoms and malabsorption are its classic features. Indeed, the symptoms of malabsorption were recognized for centuries before the recognition of the role of dietary gluten as the initiating factor. Because the classic features of malabsorption seen in celiac disease are shared by other malabsorptive states, one cannot rely on clinical criteria for establishing the diagnosis. The boy in Figure 105-1 presented with a vague history of progressive abdominal distension, abdominal pains, intermittent loose stools, poor appetite, and subsequent weight loss. His parents were unclear of his dietary habits, stating that they were busy working all day and would return home in the evenings and allow him to eat "junk food." On presentation he was a malnourished, edematous youth with a markedly distended abdomen. Laboratory values indicated iron deficiency anemia, hypoproteinemia,

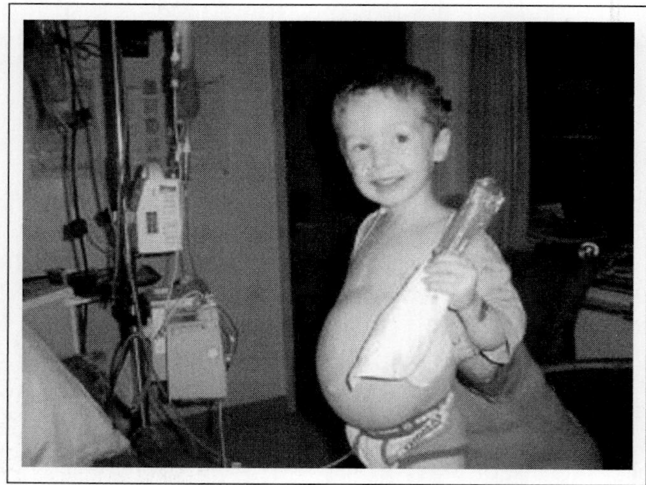

**FIGURE 105-1** Appearance of kwashiorkor in classic celiac disease

coagulopathy, and mildly elevated liver enzymes. The clinical picture was that of kwashiorkor. The differential diagnosis included protein-losing enteropathies (celiac disease, intestinal lymphangiectasia, abetalipoproteinemia, and milk/soy protein intolerance following infectious enteritis), pancreatic insufficiency from cystic fibrosis or Shwachman-Diamond syndrome, and Crohn disease. Following correction of the coagulopathy with parenteral vitamin K, a biopsy of the small intestine indicated celiac disease. This classic presentation is seen less commonly now because the diagnosis is generally made earlier in the course of the illness.

Although celiac disease may present at any age, the classic presentation described previously usually presents in infancy or early childhood (Box 105-1). As illustrated in this case, the period between the introduction of gluten and the onset of symptoms is quite variable. Although some infants are exquisitely sensitive to gluten and present with violent vomiting and diarrhea soon after the introduction of cereals into the diet, the onset is usually insidious with the progressive development of frequent, foul-smelling bowel movements, anorexia, apathy, and irritability. The abdomen becomes gradually distended and there is loss of subcutaneous fat, as well as hypotonia with muscle wasting, especially of the buttocks and proximal limbs. Stools may sometimes be bulky, suggestive of constipation, in approximately 10% of cases. Malabsorption of calcium, magnesium, iron, and the fat-soluble vitamins, as well as protein loss, may result in rickets, osseous fractures, tetany, anemia, bleeding, and pitting edema.[7]

### LATE ONSET PRESENTATION

An insidious onset of symptoms and signs is more common in preadolescents and adolescents (Box 105-2), with the chronic development of iron deficiency anemia, short stature, and delayed puberty as salient features. Adolescents may present solely with growth disturbances associated with subtle changes in stool pattern, anorexia, abdominal distension, and microcytic or macrocytic anemia. Clubbing of the fingers may also be present. Most of the adolescents who present with growth failure have a markedly delayed bone age, and some show a blunted response to hormonal stimulation, both of which are reversible with a gluten-free diet. Others might have upper intestinal tract symptoms such as nausea and gastroesophageal reflux symptoms.[7]

### ATYPICAL/EXTRAINTESTINAL PRESENTATION AND ASSOCIATED FEATURES

Celiac disease is increasingly recognized in association with many systemic symptoms and signs, as well as with other diseases. Extraintestinal manifestations may be more troublesome than the gastrointestinal symptoms, and are becoming increasingly recognized.

#### Joint Manifestations

Arthritis and arthralgias may occur either in isolation or in association with rheumatoid arthritis or systemic lupus erythematosus. A study of 200 consecutive young adults with celiac disease noted arthritis in 26%.[8]

#### Anemia

Celiac disease is associated with iron deficiency anemia. One study of 93 subjects who presented for evaluation

**Box 105-1**

***General Presenting Features of Celiac Disease***

- Diarrhea
- Weight loss
- Vomiting
- Anorexia
- Abdominal distension
- Apathy
- Constipation
- Growth failure
- Pallor
- Delayed development
- Bruising
- Rickets
- Malnutrition

**Box 105-2**

***Presenting Features of Celiac Disease in Adolescents***

- Abdominal pain, nausea, gastroesophageal reflux
- Lactose intolerance
- Anorexia
- Pubertal delay, delayed bone age, short stature
- Diarrhea
- Arthritis/arthralgia
- Clubbing of the fingers
- Anemia (micro- or macrocytic)
- Osteopenia
- Bruising
- Rickets

of iron deficiency anemia found 12% with small bowel biopsies compatible with celiac disease;[9,10] the incidence was 20% in the subgroup of non responders to supplemental iron. Megaloblastic anemia from vitamin $B_{12}$ or folate malabsorption was also reported.

### Neuropsychiatric

Mood and mental changes, depression, ataxia, epilepsy, as well as autistic behavior have all been reported with celiac disease. Autism may improve on a gluten-free diet.

### Gastrointestinal

Recurrent aphthous ulcers, anorexia, glossitis, and abdominal pain secondary to transient intussusception have also been reported. Up to 30% of patients with celiac disease have dental enamel hypoplasia.

### Musculoskeletal

Isolated short stature may be the only manifestation of the disease and may occur in up to 10% of children and adolescents undergoing testing for growth hormone deficiency. In addition, fractures of the hip, vertebrae, or upper extremities due to osteoporosis may be subtle signs of celiac disease and may occur without gastrointestinal symptoms. In one study, patients with celiac disease had significantly decreased bone mineral density (BMD) in the lumbar spine and femoral neck compared to controls.[11] The patients may have secondary hyperparathyroidism presumably due to vitamin D deficiency.[12] In a study of 30 children and adolescents maintained on a long-term gluten-free diet (average 10.7 years), BMD and serum markers of bone metabolism completely normalized.[13,14]

### Dermatologic

Celiac disease has been associated with several skin conditions. Approximately 75% of young adult patients with dermatitis herpetiformis have intestinal mucosal pathology similar to that seen in celiac disease. The enteropathy and skin lesions respond to gluten restriction. Dermatitis herpetiformis is reported to occur in 5% of celiac patients between 15 and 40 years of age. The lesions manifest as severe pruritus with erythematous blisters that are symmetrical in distribution on the face, elbows, back, buttocks, and knees. Urticaria and psoriasis have been reported in celiac disease as well.[15]

### Diabetes Mellitus

The association of celiac disease with diabetes mellitus is well established. HLA-B8 and DR3 antigens are shared by patients with celiac disease and those with diabetes. Up to 8% of patients with type 1 diabetes mellitus have characteristic changes of celiac disease on small intestinal biopsy.

### Autoimmune Disorders and Other Associated Conditions

Other clinical entities that have been associated with celiac disease include IgA deficiency, occurring in 3% of individuals, 15 times higher than in the general population. Cystic fibrosis, alpha-1-antitrypsin deficiency, Down syndrome (with a prevalence of celiac disease of 4% to 16%), autoimmune thyroid disease, inflammatory bowel disease, as well as diseases of the liver such as autoimmune hepatitis and unexplained hypertransaminasemia have all been reported in association with celiac disease.[7,16]

## ASYMPTOMATIC OR LATENT CELIAC DISEASE AND RISK OF MORBIDITY AND MORTALITY

The term asymptomatic (silent) celiac disease implies the presence of the histopathological features of celiac disease in the absence of symptoms. These individuals are usually in the group of 5% to 10% of asymptomatic family members who are screened for celiac disease. On the other hand, those patients who manifest serologic evidence of celiac disease with no histological signs are labeled "latent celiacs." The absence of histologic signs in the presence of serologic markers of celiac disease may represent biopsy sampling error, or such individuals may be ingesting a gluten-containing diet and have had prior histological lesions that have since resolved. It is known that after recovery on a gluten-free diet, some patients can tolerate a gluten-containing regular diet for years before developing a histological relapse. It is believed that some of these individuals may have had transient gluten intolerance rather than true celiac disease. Alternatively, with continued ingestion of gluten these individuals may develop overt celiac disease over time.[7]

The severity of celiac intestinal lesions does not correlate with the severity of either gastrointestinal or of atypical clinical symptoms. Celiac disease is considered a disease of the proximal small intestine, presumably on the basis of higher concentrations of gluten in this region of bowel. There is a gradient of decreasing severity of the mucosal lesion from the proximal to the distal small intestine. However, there may be a sampling error leading to a nondiffuse pattern of involvement. Although in the past subtotal villus atrophy was required for the diagnosis, the severity of the mucosal inflammation and atrophy is now recognized as being variable in celiac disease. As described in the following, the histological findings may range from a mild alteration characterized by increased intraepithelial lymphocytes to markedly abnormal, flat mucosa with total mucosal atrophy, complete loss of villi, enhanced epithelial apoptosis, and crypt hyperplasia.[7]

Persistence of the mucosal histological lesion of celiac disease may, however, have dire clinical consequences. The importance of recognizing the symptoms and establishing a diagnosis of celiac disease is emphasized because of the increased risk of malignancy, the potential presence of unsuspected nutritional deficiencies, and the association with autoimmune disorders. When unrecognized and untreated, celiac disease was associated with a high mortality rate in the past, reaching 12% in 1 retrospective study performed in 544 pediatric age patients. More recently, the death rate was reported to be twice that expected in the general population.[17] Most of the deaths are due to non-Hodgkin lymphoma, with an estimated eightfold increase in the risk of gastrointestinal malignancies and a 20- to 30-fold increase in intestinal lymphoma associated with celiac disease. The excess mortality is principally observed within 3 years after the diagnosis, and deaths are almost exclusively seen in patients who presented with severe malabsorption symptoms, rather than those diagnosed because of minor symptoms or because of antibody screening. Mortality is also higher in those who have a significant delay in diagnosis and who have poor adherence to a gluten-free diet. The risk of malignancy in patients with subclinical celiac disease is not known, although it appears to be lower than in patients who present with malabsorption symptoms. Once the disease is under remission with a gluten-free diet, the risk approaches that of the unaffected population.[18]

Other potential serious adverse effects of delays in diagnosis and treatment include permanent growth retardation and dental deformities. Some studies have found that the prevalence of autoimmune diseases may be related to the duration of undetected celiac disease and may reach more than 30% of patients diagnosed after the age of 20.[19] Delays in diagnosis will also lead to lassitude and weight loss, adversely affecting school and work performance, as well as peer and family interactions.

## DIAGNOSIS OF CELIAC DISEASE

Upper endoscopy with small intestinal biopsies remains the diagnostic gold standard for celiac disease. In addition to the histologic yield from the biopsies, visible findings such as duodenal fold "scalloping" strongly suggests celiac disease (Figure 105-2) Scalloping can also be detected by wireless capsule endoscopy.

The European Society of Pediatric Gastroenterology and Nutrition revised the criteria for the diagnosis of celiac disease in 1990. Previous criteria required at least 3 small intestinal biopsies, and the salient histological features of celiac disease were required to be present at the time of initial suspicion of the enteropathy.[20] The histological findings were expected to resolve following gluten elimination and to reappear during a gluten challenge. The success of serologic markers such as antigliadin, antireticulin, antiendomysial, and tTG antibodies has prompted revision of the criteria. Current diagnostic requirements continue to include a characteristic histological appearance of the mucosa

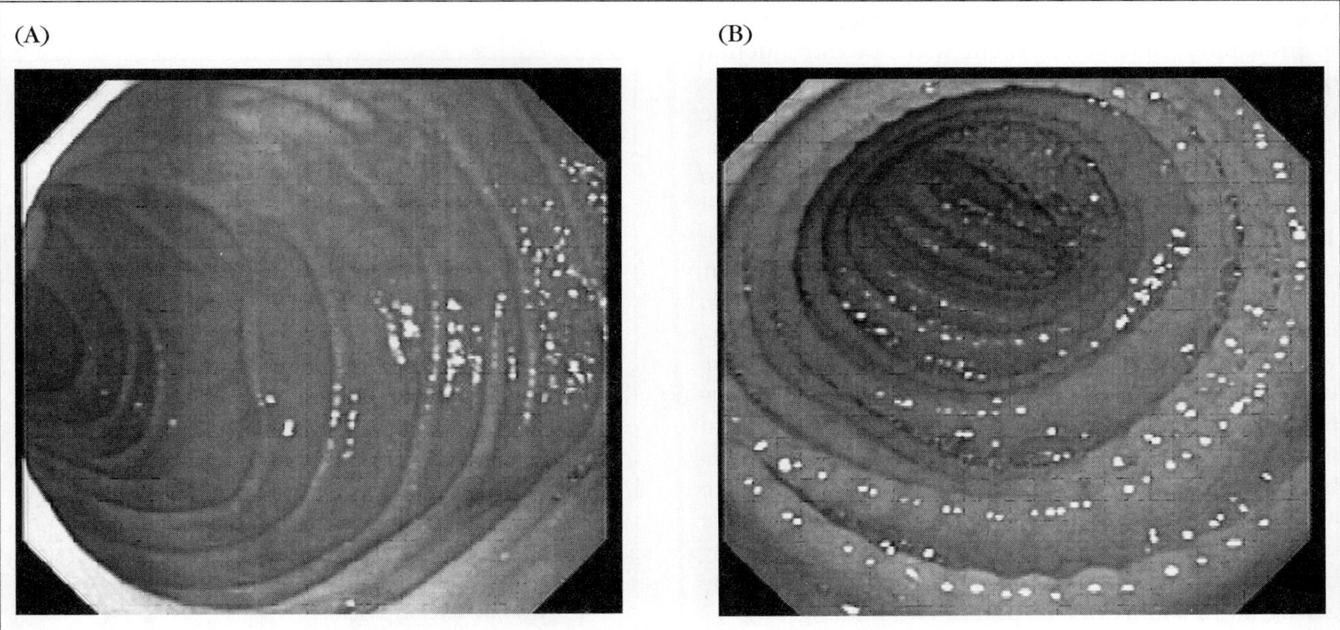


**FIGURE 105-2** (A) Normal duodenum; (B) duodenal fold "scalloping" in celiac disease (See color insert)

at presentation, with resolution of symptoms following gluten elimination. The presence of the previously mentioned circulating antibodies at time of diagnosis and disappearance following gluten withdrawal is supportive evidence of the diagnosis, especially in those who are asymptomatic. However, in certain circumstances a gluten challenge may be necessary. This is particularly true when the histological features of celiac disease are mimicked by other enteropathies such as cow milk protein sensitivity, postinfectious enteropathy, infection with *Giardia lamblia*, or regional enteritis. Additionally, a gluten challenge is indicated for patients who have been empirically started on a gluten-free diet without documentation of celiac disease, or those with noncharacteristic histology.[7] The challenge should continue for at least one year before biopsy if symptoms do not develop. Serial determinations of serologic antibody markers may be helpful. Additionally, an individual's HLA determination can be useful in ruling out celiac disease in questionable cases. Because celiac disease is almost exclusively found in HLA-DQ2- or HLA-DQ8-positive individuals, if an adolescent is negative for both of these HLA-DQ subtypes, celiac disease can be effectively ruled out. However, fewer than 1% of all DQ2 carriers have celiac disease.

## PATHOPHYSIOLOGY

The ingestion of wheat, barley, or rye is a prerequisite for the induction of celiac disease. The mucosal damage response to these grains, and to a lesser extent oats, is considered to be immune mediated through exposure to prolamins contained in them. With the introduction of peroral intestinal mucosal biopsies in the early 1950s, the histopathologic features of celiac disease in the proximal small intestine were defined. That these features were shared with adult nontropical sprue led to the conclusion that the 2 conditions were the same.[21] The mechanism and sequence of events leading to mucosal injury in celiac disease is not precisely known. Binding of gliadin peptides by the HLA-DQ molecule for antigen presentation to T cells is an important step, with the enzyme tTG considered to be a master regulator involved in both the cellular and humoral mechanisms of the disease. The tTG may modify the gliadin molecule to increase its affinity to the DQ2 peptide-binding groove by converting glutamine into glutamic acid in the gluten peptide. This results in a negative charge within the molecule that allows high affinity binding of gluten to HLA-DQ2 or DQ8 molecules, triggering an inflammatory response. The binding to DQ2 is thought to be responsible for T-cell activation and subsequent production of cytokines with resultant tissue damage. In addition, tTG cross-links with gluten and the complex can be taken up by B cells with generation of tTG-specific antibodies that are markers for the disease. Only patients with celiac disease make these antibodies, and their titers fall on gluten withdrawal. Therefore, specific immune mechanisms triggered by gluten contact may work in concert with a directly toxic effect causing remodeling of the intestinal mucosa.[22–25]

The gluten-induced enteropathy that affects the small intestinal mucosa and leads to malabsorption with associated symptoms and abnormalities is characterized by a number of histologic features, including: villus atrophy, crypt hyperplasia, and infiltration of the lamina propria with chronic inflammatory cells. The enterocytes are reduced in height and become cuboidal, and intraepithelial lymphocytes are interspersed between the enterocytes. These lymphocytes originate in the lamina propria and enter the space between the enterocytes through a break in the basal lamina of the epithelium. In untreated celiac disease, the ratio of lymphocytes to epithelial cells is typically increased to >40 lymphocytes per 100 epithelial cells. Because the histologic features of celiac disease may be interspersed with normal mucosa, it is recommended that at least 4 mucosal biopsies from different sites be obtained to ensure sufficiently representative samples to avoid sampling error.

These histologic changes, however, are not pathognomic for celiac disease. Conditions other than celiac disease may be associated with a flat or otherwise abnormal mucosa (Box 105-3). Although the cardinal

**Box 105-3**

### *Disorders Associated with Villus Atrophy*

- Celiac disease
- Viral gastroenteritis
- Cow milk or soy protein allergy
- Bacterial overgrowth
- Malnutrition
- Eosinophilic gastroenteritis
- Giardiasis
- Intestinal lymphoma
- AIDS
- Hypogammaglobulinemia
- Radiation enteritis
- Iron deficiency anemia
- Zollinger-Ellison syndrome

hallmark is villus atrophy, a spectrum of histological changes can be seen with celiac disease. Marsh and colleagues[27] have described 4 patterns of mucosal immunopathology: (1) type 0 (pre-infiltrative) no detectable changes of inflammation or changes in the crypt/villus architecture; (2) type 1 (infiltrative) with an increase in the number of intraepithelial lymphocytes; (3) type 2 (hyperplastic) with inflammation, villus blunting, and an increased crypt/villus height ratio; and (4) type 3 (destructive) with severe inflammation, flat villi, and hyperplastic crypts.

## SEROLOGICAL AUTOANTIBODY MARKERS

Current serum immunological markers for celiac disease have increased the sensitivity and specificity of diagnosis. The components of the "celiac panel" of tests are described in the following section. However, the diagnosis still relies on the small intestinal biopsy and the adolescent's clinical response to a gluten-free diet.

### ANTI-GLIADIN ANTIBODIES

Circulating anti-gliadin antibodies (AGA) are antibodies to the cereal protein gliadin, which presumably is absorbed intact across the intestinal mucosa in celiac disease. For IgA AGA, specificity ranges between 65% and 100%, whereas sensitivity ranges between 52% and 100%. For IgG AGA, specificity ranges between 50% and 100%, whereas sensitivity ranges between 82% and 100%. Because of the association of celiac disease with IgA deficiency, a negative IgG AGA can only be interpreted as a true negative if the patient is not IgA deficient. IgG AGA antibodies, however, also are found in healthy control subjects, as well as in Crohn disease and liver disease. Furthermore, IgG-AGA levels increase with age in healthy controls, making the presence of those antibodies even less specific for the purpose of diagnosing celiac disease in older persons. However, the test may be useful in screening individuals who are IgA deficient, as the screening tests described in the following are of the IgA class. In IgA-deficient patients with celiac disease, the IgG AGA should be positive. Although IgA AGA are more specific than the IgG class for celiac disease, their sensitivity can be far less than 100%, meaning that not all persons with celiac disease will have IgA AGA.[16,28]

### ANTI-RETICULIN ANTIBODIES

The specificity of IgG anti-reticulin antibodies (ARA) for celiac disease is controversial. These antibodies are also found in patients with Crohn disease and other conditions. They have a sensitivity and specificity similar to the IgA AGA. The antibodies may have the same target recognized by the EmA.[28]

### ANTI-ENDOMYSIAL ANTIBODIES

EmA are extremely sensitive and specific markers of celiac disease. These are primarily IgA antibodies directed against the intermyofibril substance of monkey esophagus smooth muscle. Unlike ARA, EmA have been demonstrated to be biologic order-specific, reacting by direct immunofluorescence only with the endomysium in the gastrointestinal tract of primates. In 1 study that compared EmA, AGA, and ARA in a group of patients with celiac disease, the specificity of EmA was 98% and the sensitivity was 97%. Anti-endomysial antibodies is a reliable serologic marker for the diagnosis of celiac disease. Anti-endomysial antibodies are diet sensitive and decline to undetectable levels by 3 to 6 months of a strict gluten-free diet.[29–31] Because EmA are IgA-class antibodies (as are IgA AGA) and because IgA deficiency occurs in approximately 3% of adolescents with celiac disease, it is necessary to measure IgA levels to interpret negative EmA results in suspected celiac disease. Thus, serum immunoglobulins should be evaluated to detect for IgA deficiency at the same time a celiac panel is obtained.

### TISSUE TRANSGLUTAMINASE ANTIBODIES

Dieterich and colleagues described that tTG is the target of the EmA characteristic for celiac disease. Screening for the presence of tTG-specific antibodies is a very specific indicator for celiac disease. The tTG IgA enzyme-linked immunosorbent assay (ELISA) test is highly sensitive and specific particularly using human recombinant tTG. In 2 studies, the sensitivity and specificity of anti-tTG IgA compared to biopsy-proven disease were 94% and 98%, respectively.[3,32] The anti-tTG IgA correlates well with the EmA and biopsy, but because it is an ELISA test, it represents an improvement over the anti-EmA IgA, which relies on indirect immunofluorescence that carries inherent human subjectivity in test interpretation.

Currently, therefore, screening of an adolescent for celiac disease should involve an assay for anti-tTG and a total serum IgA. The anti-EmA can be used as a confirmatory or prebiopsy test. The AGA determinations should be restricted to the diagnostic work-up of younger children and patients with known IgA deficiency.

## TREATMENT

Complete histologic and symptomatic resolution of the disease occurs on exclusion from the diet of the prolamins of wheat, barley, rye, and oats. Because lifelong dietary adherence is currently recommended, consultation with a nutritionist, as well as the Celiac Society of America, or the Celiac Foundation (www.celiac.org) for "hidden or unsuspected" sources of gluten is essential. Hidden sources of gluten may be found in vitamins and medications, for example. Oats remain controversial as they do not elicit the same immune response as wheat. However, the risk of contamination of oats with wheat during the process of milling is possible.[33]

Recent research addressing treatment methods alternative to the standard gluten-free diet has developed from the postulated pathogenesis of the disease. For instance, zonulin, an endogenous signaling protein that opens the tight junctions between intestinal epithelial cells, has been implicated to be overstimulated by gluten in patients with celiac disease, thereby allowing gluten to pass through the intercellular junctions to enter the mucosa and subsequently trigger the immune system. Currently zonulin receptor antagonists are under investigation to evaluate their ability to inhibit intestinal permeability of gluten in patients with celiac disease.[34] A recent in vitro study assessed the coadministration of a prolyl endoprotease, a gluten-degradating enzyme, which administered with a gluten-containing meal eliminated gluten toxicity. If further trials confirm this result, it will offer adolescents with celiac disease the possibility of loosening their strict gluten-free diet.[35]

The continuation of symptoms in adolescents with celiac disease while adhering to a gluten-free diet should prompt a search for hidden sources of gluten or other conditions (Box 105-4). Adherence to a gluten-free diet can be monitored by assays of the serological markers of celiac disease, which are elevated in the presence of gluten in the diet. If symptoms persist, other conditions within the differential diagnosis of celiac disease should be considered. Additionally, pancreatic insufficiency can be an associated feature of celiac disease, and the coexistence of celiac and Shwachman-Diamond syndrome has been reported. Immunosuppressive therapy may be required in refractory celiac disease in adolescents.

**Box 105-4**

***Potential Causes of Continued Symptoms of Treated Celiac Disease***

- Erroneous diagnosis
- Gluten ingestion
- Lactase deficiency
- Cow milk, soy, food sensitivity
- Intestinal lymphoma
- Pancreatic insufficiency

Controversy exists regarding the necessity to treat asymptomatic individuals. Adolescents who have villus atrophy on biopsy probably benefit from treatment.

## SUMMARY

Celiac disease is an autoimmune enteropathy of the small intestine with a broad spectrum of clinical manifestations that tend to be subtle if they first appear in the second decade of life. Sensitive and specific serologic assays for IgA antibodies to gliadin, endomysium, and tTG have markedly improved detection of celiac disease. Because these blood studies are still considered markers, the diagnosis rests on the remission of symptoms on a gluten-free diet combined with histologic evidence ranging from increased intraepithelial lymphocytes in mild cases to total mucosal villus atrophy, crypt hyperplasia, and infiltration of the lamina propria with chronic inflammatory cells in the small intestine in more serious cases. Alternative treatments to the standard of gluten elimination are being studied to reduce the burden of being required to avoid all wheat, barley, and rye from the diet.

## REFERENCES


1. Booth C. History of celiac disease. *BMJ.* 1999;298:527–536
2. Dicke W. Simple dietary treatment for the syndrome of GheeHerter. *Ned Tijdschr Geneeskd.* 1941;85:1715
3. Sulkanen S, Halttunen T, Laurila K, et al. Tissue transglutaminase autoantibody enzyme-linked immunosorbent assay in detecting celiac disease. *Gastroenterology.* 1998;115:1322–1328
4. Rossi TM, Albini C, Kumar V, et al. Incidence of celiac disease identified by the presence of serum endomysial antibodies in children with chronic diarrhea, short stature, or insulin-dependent diabetes mellitus. *J Pediatr Gastroenterol Nutr.* 1993;123:262–264
5. Maki M, Mustalahti K, Kokkonen J, et al. Prevalence of celiac disease among children in Finland. *NEJM.* 2003;348(25):2517–2524
6. Not T, Horvath K, Hill ID, et al. Celiac disease risk in the USA: high prevalence of antiendomysial antibodies in healthy blood donors. *Scand J Gastroenterol.* 1994;33:494–499
7. Hill ID, Bhatnagar S, Cameron DJ, et al. Celiac Disease: Working Group Report of the First World Congress of Pediatric Gastroenterology, Hepatology, and Nutrition. *J Pediatr Gastroenterol Nutr.* 2002;35(suppl 2):S78–S88
8. Lubrano E, Ciacci C, Ames PR, et al. The arthritis of coeliac disease, prevalence, and pattern in 200 adult patients. *Br J Rheumatol.* 1996;35:1314–1318
9. Ackerman Z, Eliakim R, Stalnikowicz R, Rachmilewitz D. Role of small bowel biopsy in the endoscopic evaluation

of adults with iron deficiency anemia. *Am J Gastroenterol.* 1996;91:2099-2102

10. Carroccio A, Iannitto E, Cavataio F, et al. Sideropenic anemia and celiac disease: one study, two points of view. *Dig Dis Sci.* 1998;43:673-678

11. Bottaro G, Cataldo F, Rotolo M, et al. The clinical pattern of subclinical/silent celiac disease: an analysis on 1,026 consecutive cases. *Am J Gastroenterol.* 1999;94:691-696

12. Selby PL, Davies M, Adams JE, et al. Bone loss in celiac disease is related to secondary hyperparathyroidism. *J Bone Miner Res.* 1999;14:652-657

13. Mora S, Barera G, Beccio S, et al. Bone density and bone metabolism are normal after long-term gluten-free diet in young celiac patients. *Am J Gastroenterol.* 1999;94;398-403

14. Mora S, Weber G, Barera G, et al. Effect of gluten-free diet on bone mineral content in growing patients with celiac disease. *Am J Clin Nutr.* 1993;57:224-228

15. Fry L. Dermatitis herpetitformis. *Bailliere's Clinical Gastroenterology.* 1995;9(19):371-393

16. Pietzak M, Catassi C, Drago S, Fornaroli F, Fasano A. Celiac disease: going against the grains. *Nutr Clin Pract.* 2001;16:335-344

17. Corrao G, Corazza G, Bagnardi V, et al. Mortality in patients with coeliac disease and their relatives: a cohort study. *Lancet.* 2001;358:356-361

18. Collin P, Reunala T, Pukkala E, et al. Coeliac disease-associated disorders and survival. *Gut.* 1994;35:1215-1218

19. Ventura A, Magazzu G, Greco L, et al. Duration of exposure to gluten and risk for autoimmune disorders in patients with celiac disease. *Gastroenterology.* 1999;117:297-303

20. Walker-Smith JA, Guandalini S, Schmitz J, Shmerling DH, Visakorpi JK. Revised criteria for diagnosis of coeliac disease. *Arch Dis Child.* 1990;65:909-911

21. Rubin C, Brandborg LL, Phelps PC, Taylor HC. Studies of celiac disease. I. The apparent identical and specific nature of the duodenal and proximal jejunal lesion in celiac disease and idiopathic sprue. *Gastroenterology.* 1960;38:28-38

22. Agardh D, Borulf F, Lernmark A, Ivarsson SA. Tissue transglutaminase immunoglobulin isotypes in children with untreated celiac disease. *J Pediatr Gastroenterol Nutr.* 2002;36(1): 77-82

23. McManus R. Celiac disease—the villain unmasked? *NEJM.* 2003;348(25):2573-2574

24. Mearin ML. Tissue transglutaminase: master regulator of celiac disease? *J Pediatr Gastroenterol Nutr.* 2003;36(1):10-11

25. Molberg O, McAdam SN, Körner R, Quarsten H, et al. Tissue transglutaminase selectively modifies gliadin peptides that are recognized by gut-derived T cells in celiac disease. *Nat Med.* 1998;4:713-717

26. Cellier C, Patey N, Mauvieux L et al. Abnormal intestinal intraepithelial lymphocytes in refractory sprue. *Gastroenterology.* 1998;114:471-481

27. Marsh M. Intestinal lymphoid tissue. XI. The immunopathology of cell mediated reactions in gluten sensitivity and other enteropathies. *Scanning Microscopy.* 1988;2:1663-1665

28. Paulley L. Observations on the etiology of idiopathic steatorrhoea. *Br Med J.* 1954;2:1318

29. Chan KN, Phillips AD, Mirakian R, et al. Endomysial antibody screening in children. *J Pediatr Gastroenterol Nutr.* 1994;18:316-332

30. Kumar V, Lerner A, Valeski JE. Endomysial antibodies in the diagnosis of celiac disease and the effects of gluten on antibody titers. *Immunol Invest.* 1989;18:533-544

31. Rossi TM, Kumar V, Lerner A, et al. Relationship of endomysial antibodies to jejunal mucosal pathology: specificity towards both symptomatic and asymptomatic celiacs. *J Pediatr Gastroenterol Nutr.* 1988;7:858-863

32. Dieterich W. Serum antibodies in celiac disease. *Clin Lab.* 1998;46:861-864

33. Hoffenberg EJ, Haas J, Drescher A, et al. A trial of oats in children with newly diagnosed celiac disease. *J Pediatr.* 2000;137:361-366

34. Paterson BM, Lammers KM, Arrieta MC, Fasano A, Meddings JB. The safety, tolerance, pharmacokinetic, and pharmacodynamic effects of single doses of AT-1001 in coeliac disease subjects: a proof of concept study. *Aliment Pharmacol Ther.* 2007;26(5):757-766

35. Mitea C, Havenaar R, Drijfhout JW, Edens L, Dekking L, Koning F. Efficient degradation of gluten by a prolyl endoprotease in a gastrointestinal model: implications for coeliac disease. *Gut.* 2008;57;25-32

SECTION 6

# Hematology and Oncology

# CHAPTER 106

## Disorders of the Red Blood Cells

SUJIT SHETH, MD

### INTRODUCTION

Numerous changes occur in the body of a child as development progresses through adolescence and puberty to adulthood. There are changes associated with an increase in metabolic demands as physical activity increases, hormonal changes that result in the growth spurt, and gender-specific changes in the anatomy and physiology of the adolescent as described elsewhere in this textbook. All of these factors result in an increased demand for oxygen and a corresponding increase in the total red cell mass of the body. This period of development may also be associated with the appearance of several disorders of a variety of organ systems, such as autoimmune diseases, which may manifest more commonly in the adolescent period. In addition, several changes in the psyche and habits of the individual may predispose to the development of abnormalities of red blood cell production. For all of these reasons, adolescence is a time of acute stress on erythropoiesis, and there are several factors specific to this period of development that may lead to disorders in the red blood cells that are quite different from those seen during early childhood or adulthood. It is important therefore to not only recognize the predisposition for developing anemia but also to prevent it through appropriate counseling of adolescents and their parents.

This chapter addresses the pathophysiologic approach to the problem and provide a practical guide to its management. There is an emphasis on problems that are specific to adolescents, with some discussion on the natural history of some of the congenital disorders of red blood cells during this phase of development. Most congenital disorders that present in early childhood are not discussed in detail; the reader is referred to other standard texts for a more thorough discussion of these disorders.

### DEVELOPMENTAL ASPECTS

During adolescence and the growth spurt that occurs during puberty, there is an increased demand for oxygen to the tissues, for both growth and metabolic activity. Erythropoiesis in the developing child occurs almost exclusively in the red (active) marrow of the long bones, ribs, sternum, and pelvis. In certain disease states associated with anemia, such as in myeloid metaplasia, primitive sites of red cell production, such as the liver, spleen, lymph nodes, and flat bones of the skull, may be reactivated. However, in spite of the marked increase in oxygen demand, and the increase in the total mass of erythrocytes that occurs during adolescence, the erythroid progenitors functioning in their usual marrow sites are able to produce the increased numbers of red blood cells that are required. There is an increase in the hemoglobin concentration, and in the size of the red cells, as reflected by the mean corpuscular volume (MCV), which reaches adult values by the end of puberty. Several gender-specific changes result in differences in the mean hemoglobin values between males and females. Boys have androgen production and a greater increase in muscle mass and activity, which lead to greater stimulation of erythropoietin release, resulting in a higher mean hemoglobin in boys than in girls. In addition, once girls have achieved menarche, regular monthly blood loss may contribute further to lower mean hemoglobin values. Abnormalities in the menstrual cycle may also result in excessive bleeding and the development of anemia. Nutritional deficiencies resulting in anemia are seen more often in the developing world, where food fortification is not common.

Autoimmune disorders, such as systemic lupus erythematosus (SLE), endocrine disorders, such as thyroid disease, and other conditions, such as inflammatory bowel disease, may first manifest in this period and result in anemia. Obesity and the development of type 2 diabetes may also play a role.

Adolescence is also characterized by changes in the growing child's psychological development. Some teens who develop issues with their body image may indulge in food fads or develop anorexia nervosa, predisposing them to the development of nutritional anemias. Excessive scholastic stress, strain from parent or peer relationships, and the use of recreational drugs and alcohol may also contribute to irregular eating habits or peptic ulcer disease and the development of specific nutritional deficiencies. Sexual practices resulting in the transmission of certain infections, such as human immunodeficiency virus (HIV), may also have an effect on erythroid function, both directly as well as during treatment. Exacerbation of preexisting conditions because of poor adherence with medications, which is common at this age, may also contribute to the development of anemia.

**Box 106-1**

***Causes of Anemia in Adolescence***

**Inherited disorders of the red cells**

- Disorders of erythropoiesis: thalassemia syndromes
- Disorders of the red cell membrane: hereditary spherocytosis (HS), hereditary elliptocytosis (HE)
- Disorders of hemoglobin: sickle cell syndromes
- Disorders of the enzymes: Deficiency of G6PD, pyruvate kinase deficiency, etc.

**Nutritional**

- Iron deficiency: dietary, pregnancy, chronic blood loss
- Vitamin $B_{12}$ or folic acid deficiency
- Malnutrition/malabsorption (laxative abuse)

**Chronic blood loss**

- Gastrointestinal: peptic ulcer disease, milk protein intolerance, inflammatory bowel disease
- Genitourinary: dysfunctional uterine bleeding, sexually transmitted infection, urinary tract infection
- Bleeding disorders
- Viral infections: epstein-Barr virus (EBV), cytomegalovirus (CMV), human immunodeficiency virus (HIV)

**Hemolysis**

- Immune: autoimmune hemolytic anemia

**Anemia of chronic disease (anemia of inflammation)**

- Rheumatologic disease
- Gastrointestinal disease/liver disease

**Marrow failure/replacement**

- Aplastic anemia: idiopathic, postinfectious, drug induced
- Malignancy

## ETIOLOGY AND PATHOPHYSIOLOGY OF ANEMIA DURING ADOLESCENCE

There are numerous causes of anemia in the adolescent, but in this section the discussion will be limited to those seen almost only during this period (Box 106-1). Inherited red blood cell disorders may have a somewhat different course during adolescence; as such, sickle cell anemia will be discussed individually elsewhere in this textbook (see Chapter 107, Sickle Cell Disease). It is important to remember that individuals with an underlying hemolytic process, such as sickle cell disease, or ineffective erythropoiesis, such as thalassemia, may have an increased requirement for folic acid with the increase in cellular turnover that occurs during adolescence.

### MICRONUTRIENT DEFICIENCY

Deficiencies of one or more essential nutrients remains one of the most common causes of new onset anemia in adolescents, probably second only to chronic blood loss from abnormalities in menstruation in girls. This is a particular problem in the developing world.[1] During the growth spurt that occurs at this time, the body has an increased demand for energy and certain nutrients. Several factors contribute to the development of nutritional anemia, and one or more may be present in the individual child. Teenagers who have a newfound freedom from parental influence may indulge in a variety of food fads, eating an unbalanced diet that may lack vitamins or essential elements such as iron, copper, or zinc. The absence of green vegetables or red meats in the diet may cause iron deficiency, whereas the exclusive ingestion of organic foods, fruit juices, and specific milk products that may not have been fortified may result in vitamin deficiencies. Excessive dieting, the development of eating disorders such as anorexia or bulimia nervosa (discussed in Chapters 76 and 77), binge eating, and laxative abuse may result in a more general malnutrition, which may lead to anemia simply from marrow erythroid suppression. Over the course of several weeks to months, these individuals will develop anemia typical of the specific deficiency (see differential diagnosis section) in addition to other manifestations of that deficiency.

Iron deficiency is the most common nutritional anemia worldwide and is also the most common in this age group. The prevalence of iron deficiency is common in boys and girls during adolescence.[2-5] During this time, a pregnancy may increase the iron demand still further, and, may precipitate significant iron deficiency in the teenage mother unless she takes vitamin supplements containing iron. This will have a deleterious effect first in the mother, who will become iron deficient as the developing fetus behaves as an obligate parasite. If the deficiency is severe, it may also result in iron deficiency and low birth weight in the fetus, or may result in the fetus having diminished iron stores, predisposing to iron deficiency anemia in infancy. Iron deficiency may be primary, from poor dietary intake, or secondary, due to chronic blood loss. The body has an increased demand for iron during the adolescent period to meet requirements for growth, to meet increases in muscle mass that occur especially in boys, and to compensate for menstrual blood loss in girls once they attain menarche. If they do not maintain a diet rich in iron, teens are susceptible to developing deficiency and consequently, anemia.

Although dietary deficiency of folic acid or vitamin $B_{12}$ is rare, it may occur in adolescents either because of food fads or due to overcooking of foods that causes these vitamins to be broken down. These deficiencies may also result from anatomic abnormalities (congenital or acquired) in the gastrointestinal tract, which can lead to a qualitative or quantitative defect in the absorptive intestinal mucosa. Disorders such as celiac disease, Crohn disease, and other inflammatory bowel disorders are common causes of these deficiencies. Medications such as anticonvulsants, antibiotics, or chemotherapeutic agents that interfere with folate metabolism may also cause megaloblastic anemia in this age group. Inborn errors of metabolism such as a deficiency of formiminotransferase (FIT), dihydrofolate reductase (DHFR), or methyl tetrahydrofolate reductase (MTHFR) may also be responsible, but the presentation of these disorders is usually earlier in childhood.[6-11] Some teens who abuse alcohol on a regular basis may develop folate deficiency. Strict vegetarianism, with the lack of any animal products in the diet, may result in vitamin $B_{12}$ deficiency.[12] Obese children and adolescents also tend to have lower vitamin $B_{12}$ levels.[13] Pernicious anemia, which is the most common cause of macrocytic anemia in older individuals, is relatively uncommon at a younger age but may be a rare cause of megaloblastic anemia in adolescents. It results from a defect in vitamin $B_{12}$ absorption because of a lack of intrinsic factor, which may be congenital or can occur as a result of autoimmune antibodies.[14,15] There is an association between this disorder and autoimmune thyroid disease,[16] and the diagnosis of the latter often leads to an evaluation for pernicious anemia. Folate and cyanocobalamin deficiency in pregnancy is associated with neural tube defects in the offspring.

## CHRONIC BLOOD LOSS

Any cause of chronic blood loss will result in anemia, almost always an iron deficiency anemia. The female adolescent is especially vulnerable to developing anemia around menarche because of the irregular bleeding that may occur until hormonal cycles become more regular. Older teenage girls are also prone to anemia from chronic blood loss because of dysfunctional uterine bleeding (discussed in Chapter 64, Abnormal Uterine Bleeding). Other genitourinary tract blood loss, from a sexually transmitted infection or urinary tract infection, if not treated appropriately or if recurrent, may potentially also result in chronic blood loss. Peptic ulcer disease related to *Helicobacter pylori* infection,[17] inflammatory bowel disease, and milk protein allergy (more common in younger children) are causes of chronic blood loss from the gastrointestinal tract, which may also lead to mild to moderate anemia. Bleeding disorders are discussed in more detail in Chapter 108, Hemostasis and Thrombosis.

## INFECTIONS

Acute bacterial or viral infections may cause transient anemia at any age, simply from the acute inflammatory response. Typically this anemia is not of clinical significance. Some viruses, such as cytomegalovirus (CMV) and Epstein-Barr virus (EBV), may have a more prolonged effect on the bone marrow. Teens who develop infectious mononucleosis and have a protracted course may develop significant pancytopenia from the direct effect of EBV on the marrow progenitors. Although infection with EBV is usually self-limited, an occasional patient may progress to marrow aplasia, requiring treatment. Individuals with immune deficiencies are at particular risk. Parvovirus B19, which causes fifth disease, may also cause a pure red cell aplasia, particularly in individuals with known underlying red cell disorders.

## HEMOLYSIS

Individuals with inherited hemolytic anemias do not have a distinct course in adolescence. Several of these genetic disorders have variable penetrance, and some, such as hereditary spherocytosis or mild G6PD deficiency, may not be diagnosed until the second decade of life. These individuals may have all the clinical signs of hemolysis, including episodic pallor with icterus and mild splenomegaly. Autoimmune hemolytic anemia (AIHA) may also occur at this age, either in isolation or as part of a more systemic autoimmune disorder such as SLE.[18–21] As is the case for adolescents with idiopathic thrombocytopenic purpura (ITP), the hemolytic anemia may occasionally be the very first manifestation of SLE. Most of the hemolysis is "warm antibody/agglutinin" or IgG mediated. Hemolysis occurs at normal body temperature as the antibody binds to red cells and causes extravascular hemolysis in the spleen. Many medications may cause hemolysis mediated by this mechanism. Several drugs commonly used by teens, such as antibiotics (penicillin, tetracyclines, cephalosporins, rifampin, sulfonamides), analgesics (ibuprofen, diclofenac), and psychotropic agents (doxepin), have been implicated. Some of these agents (ibuprofen, diclofenac) stimulate the production of antibodies that bind to the Rh antigen on the red cell membrane, whereas others (antibiotics, doxepin) may act as stable or unstable haptens. "Cold antibody/agglutinin" hemolysis is mediated by IgM and may be seen with CMV and mycoplasma infections. The antibody binds to red cells only when body temperature drops because of exposure to cold, and upon warming, complement, is fixed and intravascular hemolysis occurs.

### ANEMIA OF CHRONIC DISEASE (ANEMIA OF INFLAMMATION)

As at any age, this condition may develop in association with any underlying disorder that causes persistent inflammation. During adolescence, individuals may develop a variety of disorders that have a chronic, more indolent course, with persistent inflammation, such as autoimmune/rheumatologic diseases, inflammatory bowel disease, or viral infections such as HIV or hepatitis C. Anemia of inflammation is essentially a state of iron-limited erythropoiesis.[22] Erythropoietin levels may be elevated in response to the anemia, but the marrow is unable to respond by increased production of red cells. Upregulation of the recently defined iron regulatory "hormone," hepcidin, caused by the inflammatory mediators results in inhibition of iron absorption from the gut and sequestration of iron in the cells of the reticuloendothelial system, making inadequate amounts available to the erythroid progenitors in the bone marrow.

### OTHER

Hypothyroidism, primary or secondary to an autoimmune process, may also cause anemia, which is often noticed incidentally in affected adolescents and which corrects once thyroxine replacement is instituted.

## CLINICAL PRESENTATION

In most instances the adolescent will present with symptoms of the underlying disorder that is the cause of the anemia. With blood loss as the most common cause, a detailed history seeking the site, duration, frequency, and type of bleeding will most often provide the diagnosis. Some adolescent girls do not like discussing their menstrual cycles, and occasionally, a teenage girl with dysmenorrhea will simply present with symptoms of syncope. The cause of the symptoms will be clearly apparent on a routine blood count, which will show moderate to severe anemia. A detailed history is also important when nutritional causes for anemia are suspected. These will present more insidiously, developing over a period of weeks to months or years, with the onset of symptoms occurring only when the anemia is severe. Iron deficiency anemia has been shown to be associated with cognitive dysfunction in women of reproductive age,[23] with the severity of this dysfunction being correlated with the severity of anemia and the degree of iron deficiency. Individuals with pernicious anemia may present with severe anemia, or predominantly with gastrointestinal or neurologic symptoms (posterior column spinal neuropathy, peripheral neuropathy, dementia, or depression) from the $B_{12}$ deficiency.[14,15]

In cases of hemolytic anemia, the presentation may be acute, with pallor, jaundice, headache, and systemic symptoms of malaise and lethargy. A family history of anemia, gallstones, or splenectomy may point to an inherited hemolytic anemia; a medication history may provide clues for a warm-antibody, AIHA and symptoms suggestive of mononucleosis or respiratory infection with dark urine following exposure to cold may indicate a cold-agglutinin hemolytic process. A longer history, including frequent infections, bruising, or a petechial rash, and systemic symptoms may be present if the anemia is part of a more pervasive marrow process, either suppression of the marrow or infiltration by a malignant process. Symptoms of other organ system involvement or a diagnosis of a chronic inflammatory condition would point to the anemia being a result of that chronic disease.

If the underlying cause of the anemia can be found and corrected relatively quickly, there is not likely to be an effect on the continuing growth and development of the adolescent. On the other hand, a more chronic anemia may have a significant effect on the growth spurt during this period; the extent to which growth is retarded depends on the severity and duration of the anemia, as well as the nature of the underlying disease and its treatment.

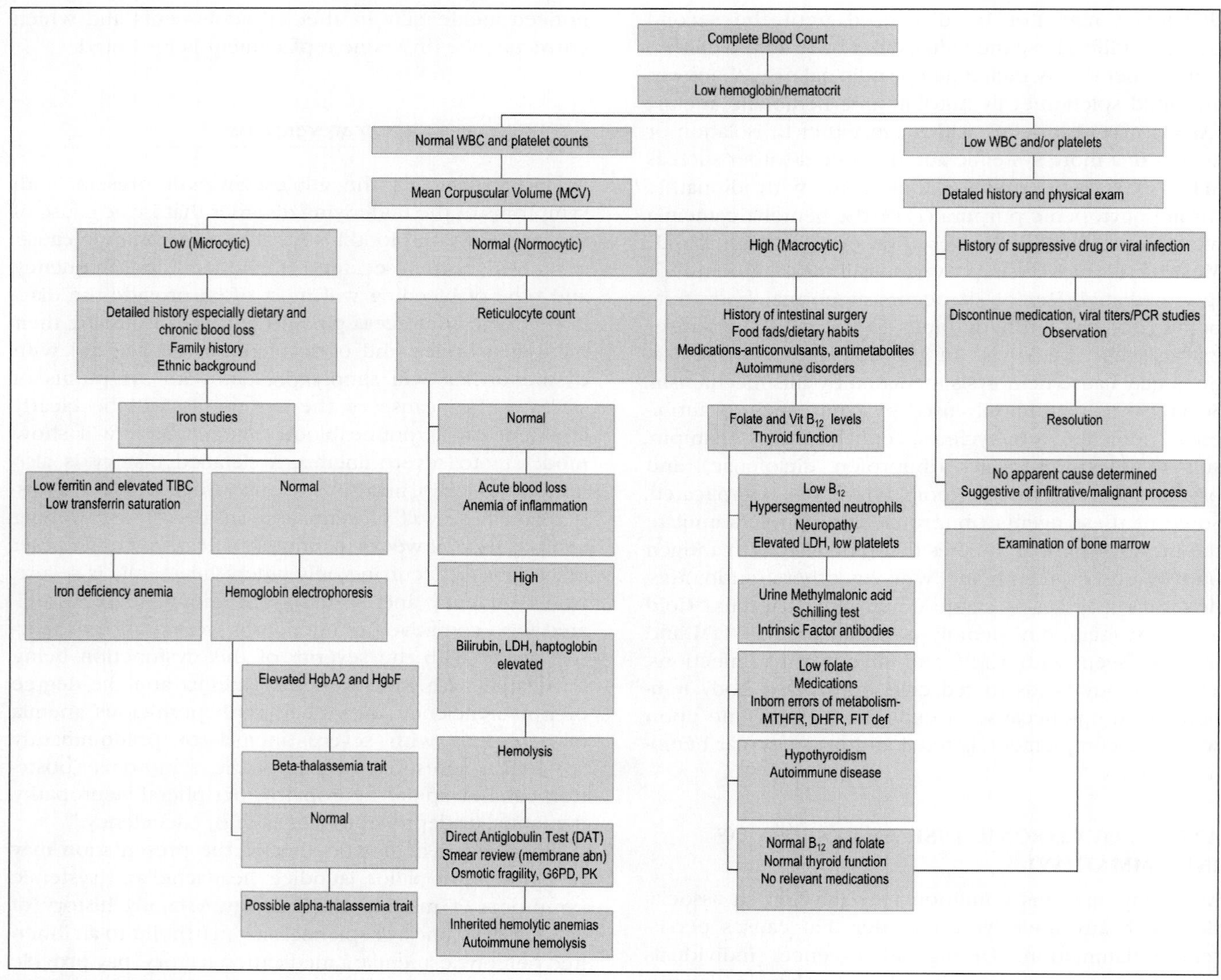


**FIGURE 106-1** Diagnostic algorithm for anemia in adolescents

The physical examination is important in determining whether the child is hemodynamically stable, in which case the diagnosis and treatment may proceed routinely, or unstable, in which case an emergent work-up may be necessary before a transfusion is administered. The degree of pallor and the presence of signs of high output cardiac failure are important in making this determination. Individuals who have petechiae or bruising, enlarged lymph nodes, or hepatosplenomegaly may warrant admission to the hospital for a more detailed evaluation of an underlying serious illness. The spleen alone may be enlarged in individuals with autoimmune hemolysis or inherited disorders such as hereditary spherocytosis.

## DIAGNOSTIC APPROACH

An algorithm outlining the diagnostic approach to the adolescent with anemia is presented in Figure 106-1. In most cases, the clinical presentation provides initial clues to the etiology of the anemia, and laboratory parameters are then used to confirm the diagnosis and to follow recovery. The complete blood count (CBC), including a reticulocyte count, may provide some or all of the necessary information required to make the diagnosis, particularly if prior normal/baseline results are available. All of the components of the CBC are useful. The hemoglobin and hematocrit are low, and the degree of anemia may be correlated with symptoms and help guide further management. The reticulocyte count will immediately indicate whether the underlying problem is one of decreased production (low reticulocyte count), or one in which there is increased destruction of red cells, either in the marrow (ineffective erythropoiesis) or in the periphery (hemolysis). The red cell indices are helpful in narrowing the differential diagnosis and guiding further testing. The MCV is one of the most useful in this regard. As children mature into adolescence, the MCV increases to reach adult levels. It is important to use age-appropriate normal ranges when using this index. A low MCV or microcytosis is usually diagnostic of iron deficiency. The red cell distribution width (RDW) may be elevated and the mean corpuscular hemoglobin (MCH) is low. It is important to remember that microcytosis is also a hallmark of the thalassemia syndromes, and the heterozygous state must be considered if the anemia is mild and the RDW is normal.

A history of blood loss or a diet poor in iron is generally enough to confirm a diagnosis of iron deficiency, and iron studies are usually not necessary in this situation. However, if there is a need to confirm the diagnosis, iron studies, including serum iron, total iron binding capacity (TIBC) and serum ferritin levels, will show a low transferrin saturation (serum iron/TIBC) and low serum ferritin. Hemoglobin electrophoresis is usually required to confirm beta-thalassemia trait, in which the hemoglobin A2 and F are elevated. Alpha-thalassemia remains a diagnosis of exclusion (if there is a mild microcytic anemia with normal iron studies and electrophoresis) unless a genetics laboratory is available to study the alpha globin genes. A macrocytic anemia (elevated MCV) is seen in vitamin $B_{12}$ or folic acid deficiency, hypothyroidism, and conditions in which there is a decrease in red cell production in the bone marrow. Further work-up includes red cell $B_{12}$ and folate levels, thyroid function tests, and if these are normal, a bone marrow aspiration or biopsy.

Most of the hemolytic anemias are also normocytic (normal MCV) and will generally have elevated reticulocyte counts, indirect bilirubin and lactic dehydrogenase (LDH) levels. If the reticulocyte count is markedly elevated, the MCV may be elevated as well, because these cells are larger than mature red cells and may shift the average. This may be seen in patients with G6PD or pyruvate kinase deficiency, hereditary spherocytosis, or an acute AIHA, after an acute hemolytic episode. Testing for these conditions includes specific assays for the enzymes, an osmotic fragility test (direct and incubated), and a direct antiglobulin test (DAT or direct Coombs') for AIHA. The latter may be specific for a warm antibody process, which will be IgG mediated and complement (C3) negative, or for a cold agglutinin process, which will be IgM mediated and C3 positive. In the latter situation, the urinalysis will show hemoglobinuria and increased urobilinogen, and EBV and mycoplasma titers may be sent to determine the responsible agent. However, most AIHA is idiopathic and a cause may not be identified. As mentioned earlier, a warm antibody process may be the first sign of an underlying autoimmune disorder, and further evaluation may be indicated.

The diagnosis of anemia related to blood loss is not complex from the hematologic standpoint. In most acute blood loss, the anemia is normocytic, the reticulocyte count may or may not have had a chance to respond, and the specific site of blood loss is evident. Appropriate evaluation for the system involved is indicated. Chronic blood loss most often results in an iron deficiency anemia, with microcytosis, elevation of the RDW, and diagnostic iron studies. Anemia of inflammation may accompany any chronic inflammatory disorder and must be considered when a normocytic anemia is present in the face of such a disorder. Iron studies characteristically show a low serum iron and TIBC, and a normal or more commonly elevated serum ferritin level, the latter being nonspecifically elevated and a marker of inflammation. If iron deficiency develops in these individuals, either from chronic blood loss or poor nutrition, the MCV may decrease and other evidence of iron deficiency may be present as well.

Macrocytic anemia has a limited list of conditions that must be considered.[24] Megaloblastic anemia as a result of vitamin $B_{12}$ or folate deficiency is rare, but the diagnosis may be made on the basis of low levels of the vitamin in the serum or, more specifically the red cell. If pernicious anemia is suspected, anti-intrinsic factor antibodies may be sent, and a Schilling test and urinary and serum methylmalonic acid levels may confirm lack of absorption of vitamin $B_{12}$. There may be mild to moderate pancytopenia, and the peripheral smear may show the typical hypersegmented neutrophils. The LDH level may also be significantly elevated. Such patients should see a neurologist and a cardiologist. If folate levels are decreased, and the diet contains adequate amounts of this vitamin, specific genetic testing for deficiencies of enzymes involved in folate metabolism may be sent. When the folate and $B_{12}$ levels are normal, hypothyroidism is likely the cause of the macrocytosis, unless there is a reason to suspect an arrest of maturation of erythroid precursors in the bone marrow because of tumor infiltration or marrow failure. In such situations, examination of the bone marrow is indicated.

The white blood cell (WBC) and platelet counts are important to pay attention to because they may be abnormal when there is a process that affects the progenitors in the bone marrow. This can be an unknown idiopathic process that could result in aplasia, or transient suppression from drugs, or viral infections such as CMV or EBV, or a complex multifactorial process as in HIV disease. In HIV disease, the virus may have a direct suppressive effect on the bone marrow or there may be autoimmune hemolysis from hypergammaglobulinemia or treatment-related marrow suppression from antiviral medications, sulfonamides, and other drugs. Many other viral infections may cause transient suppression, but this does not usually result in anemia because the red cell precursors recover rapidly before the hematocrit has a chance to drop significantly. The trimethoprim/sulfonamide combination is likely the most common cause of marrow suppression and aplasia worldwide. Most anemias related to marrow-suppressive or marrow-infiltrative processes are macrocytic because of delayed maturation of the red cell precursors.

Finally, if there is a history of significant blood loss, a more detailed past medical and family history must be obtained, with the focus of questioning being to determine if the patient should be investigated for a bleeding diathesis. Several milder conditions, such as type 1 von Willebrand disease, may not be suspected in early childhood because the only symptoms may be easy bruising. However, an adolescent girl with persistent menstrual bleeding that does not have a structural cause and does not respond to hormonal therapy may need to be referred for testing for this disorder. A detailed discussion of bleeding diatheses is presented in elsewhere in this text (Chapter 108, Hemostasis and Thrombosis).

## MANAGEMENT

Managing anemia in the adolescent is based on the underlying etiology of the condition. When the development of anemia is acute and symptoms and signs of circulatory compromise are present, such as following massive menstrual bleeding or acute hemolysis, the most prudent course would be to transfuse red blood cells. This would immediately relieve the symptoms and stabilize the patient while specific measures for treating the underlying cause are instituted.

Nutritional deficiencies are treated by supplementing the deficient element, but more importantly by providing nutritional counseling to the adolescent to prevent recurrence. Because teens are notorious for their poor eating habits, this should be a cornerstone of therapy. In addition to supplementing the deficient nutrient, as shown in Table 106-1, dietary modification for content and consistency is just as critical. In iron deficiency, 2 mg/kg/day of elemental iron for a 3-month period is generally adequate to correct the anemia, as well as to restore good iron stores. Higher doses usually result in gastrointestinal symptoms, such as diarrhea or constipation, and may further contribute to poor compliance, which is already common at this age. The same protocol may be used for iron deficiency anemia that results from chronic blood loss. In general, ferrous gluconate is better tolerated than ferrous sulfate, but the latter is still more commonly prescribed. Parenteral iron therapy is not generally recommended, except in extreme circumstances, when iron is not absorbed enterally for anatomic reasons, or if rapid replacement is desired. Iron dextran is the only form of parenteral iron available in the United States. Adolescents with anemia as a result of deficiency of vitamin $B_{12}$ and/or folate should receive supplements as described in Table 106-1. The treatment of pernicious anemia related to anti-intrinsic factor antibodies involves monthly injections of vitamin $B_{12}$ for life.

When anemia is related to blood loss, it is important to determine the site of bleeding and treat it. Most

**Table 106-1**

**Supplementation for Nutritional Deficiencies[5,9–11]**

| *Nutrient* | *Recommended Daily Intake* | *Requirement during Pregnancy or Lactation* | *Supplement Dose for Deficiency* | *Duration of Therapy* |
|---|---|---|---|---|
| Iron (elemental) | 12–15 mg | 15–30 mg | 2–3 mg/kg/day | 3 months |
| Folic acid | 800 μg | 1,200 μg | 1–5 mg/day | |
| Vitamin $B_{12}$ | 2–3 μg | 3 μg | Oral: 1–25 μg/d (200–2,000 μg/d for malabsorption) | 2–3 weeks (long term) |
| | | | IM/SQ: 30 μg/d (250–1,000 μg/d for malabsorption) | 2 weeks (Once/month long term) |

dysfunctional uterine bleeding is treated with hormonal therapy, as described in Chapter 64, Abnormal Vaginal Bleeding.

The management of inherited disorders of red cells and autoimmune processes is specific to the underlying disorder. Immune-mediated hemolysis as a result of medication is usually treated by cessation of the offending drug and providing supportive care, including a red blood cell transfusion if necessary. Acute AIHA may require red cell transfusional support, often on several occasions in the course. "Warm" agglutinin hemolysis is usually successfully treated with corticosteroids, whereas "cold" agglutinin disease does not respond to steroid therapy, but is usually self-limited, resolving when the inciting infection is controlled. In these situations, referral to a hematologist is necessary. Hemolytic anemia that is part of an underlying autoimmune disorder usually resolves as the primary condition is treated.

The management of anemia of inflammation is more complex. The primary goal is to decrease inflammation by managing the underlying systemic disorder. If the anemia persists in spite of optimizing such management, it is important to decide whether or not the severity of the anemia warrants therapy. Frequently, the anemia is mild, and therapy may be cumbersome and have little efficacy. More severe anemia, which results in impairment of normal daily activity or a poorer quality of life, may be managed by administration of erythropoietin along with iron supplementation. In the face of acute inflammatory stress, iron should be used with extreme caution, because it may cause acute decompensation in a patient with an infection. In such situations, if it is critical to correct the anemia, the best recommended course would be a transfusion of packed red blood cells.

## PREVENTION OF ANEMIA

Counseling is extremely important in the primary prevention of most causes of adolescent anemia. Two major areas include nutritional and lifestyle counseling to prevent dietary deficiencies and food fads, as well as issues related to sexual activity, pregnancy, and substance/medication abuse. It is preferable to introduce these discussions in the family setting, with a parent present, even before the child has actually entered puberty, and to continue to reinforce the message during adolescence. In the underdeveloped world, systematic food supplementation has been shown to have a positive impact on the general health of children.[25] Such programs, which have been limited to younger children, may need to be expanded to include adolescents as well.

## POLYCYTHEMIA

In addition to other secondary causes of polycythemia,[26] such as chronic lung, liver, kidney, or cardiac disease and erythropoietin or androgen-secreting tumors, there are particular causes in adolescent boys that must be considered in the differential diagnosis. Most commonly this is as a result of a very rigorous physical training program that includes either massive muscle building by nonaerobic training, such as weight training, or aerobic training for endurance activity, such as long distance bicycling or running. This may be compounded further if the training takes place at high altitudes. Other causes of polycythemia in adolescents, such as the use of anabolic steroids or erythropoietin, must be kept in mind, and referral to a hematologist may be warranted if the polycythemia is profound.

## THALASSEMIA IN ADOLESCENCE

The thalassemias are complex disorders of ineffective erythropoiesis that have a wide spectrum of severity based on underlying genetic mutations in the alpha and beta globin gene clusters. When 1 or 2 of the 4 alpha globin genes are mutated, or 1 of 2 beta globin genes is mutated, the affected individual has alpha-or beta-thalassemia trait, is usually asymptomatic, and does not require any treatment. When individuals with thalassemia trait are planning to have children, genetic counseling, and possible prenatal diagnosis if indicated, should be offered to the prospective parents. These individuals usually have a mild microcytic anemia and may receive iron supplementation, often for prolonged periods of time; however, unless there is a concomitant iron deficiency, iron supplementation will result in no improvement. The ethnic background and family history may provide clues to the diagnosis of thalassemia trait. The CBC reveals a mild microcytic anemia with a near normal red cell count, a normal RDW, and normal leukocyte and platelet counts. The Mentzer index[27] (Box 106-2) may help distinguish between thalassemia trait and iron deficiency anemia.

### Box 106-2

#### *The Mentzer Index*

Mentzer index = mean corpuscular volume (MCV)/red blood cell (RBC) count in millions

An index more than 13 is highly suggestive of iron deficiency anemia, whereas 12 or lower suggests thalassemia trait.

In beta-thalassemia trait, hemoglobin electrophoresis shows mostly HgbA, but HgbA2 and HgbF levels are usually elevated, confirming the diagnosis. In alpha-thalassemia trait, this test reveals no abnormalities, and the definitive diagnosis is made by genetic testing.

When 3 of the 4 alpha globin genes are mutated, very little alpha globin is produced, and hemoglobin H disease results. Similarly, when both beta globin genes are mutated but there is still some beta globin production, individuals are said to have beta-thalassemia intermedia. Individuals with hemoglobin H disease or beta-thalassemia intermedia have moderate to severe microcytic anemia and may require periodic transfusions, but they are not usually transfusion dependent.[28,29] However, they may have marked ineffective erythropoiesis resulting in skeletal changes from the extramedullary hematopoiesis, as well as increased iron absorption from the gut. Although the degree of iron loading is not as severe as in the regularly transfused patient, it may become significant, cause complications, and require chelation therapy. Besides the problems related to iron overload that these individuals may develop, the disfigurement that results from the extramedullary hematopoiesis may lead to serious psychological problems as well.

Although alpha-thalassemia major may be diagnosed prenatally, it may occasionally present as hydrops fetalis.[28] Likewise, beta-thalassemia major may also be diagnosed prenatally, but if it is not, it is usually manifest during infancy. Both of these disorders require either lifelong transfusion therapy or curative options such as hematopoietic stem cell transplantation or gene therapy.[29,30] Those who are treated on a regimen of regular transfusions every 2 to 4 weeks will develop significant iron overload by the age of 3 to 4 years and will require regular iron chelation therapy to prevent complications from tissue iron deposition.

Excess iron may deposit in the endocrine organs. Included are the pituitary, the gonads, the endocrine pancreas, and (somewhat less so) the thyroid and parathyroid glands. The resultant organ dysfunction can lead to growth retardation, delayed sexual maturation, infertility, type I diabetes, and osteopenia.[31] Depending on adherence with the chelation regimen, these problems may be mild or profound. Endocrine effects often become evident in adolescence when affected individuals may not have their pubertal growth spurt, may not develop secondary sexual characteristics, and/or may develop diabetes mellitus, osteopenia, and hypothyroidism. Careful monitoring for these complications is recommended.

Iron may also deposit in the myocardium, resulting in conduction abnormalities and arrhythmias, as well as progressive contractile dysfunction and eventual congestive heart failure. Regular monitoring of cardiac function by echocardiography, Holter monitoring, and myocardial magnetic resonance imaging (MRI, for measurement of iron as well as function) is recommended for early diagnosis and management. Measurement of the hepatic iron concentration (HIC) is a good indicator of the overall body iron burden and should be done regularly to assess compliance with chelation. Although there is not a good correlation between the HIC and the degree of myocardial iron loading, individuals who have always had low HIC values and are adherent with their chelation regimen are less likely to have significant myocardial loading. Other complications related to transfusion therapy, such as transmission of viral diseases (eg, HIV or hepatitis C), have become rare with the tight safety screening protocols that blood banks currently employ.

Adherence with chelation therapy has always been a major problem, especially when the chelation regimen involved subcutaneous infusions of the chelator deferoxamine. Although the situation has improved somewhat with availability of the oral chelator deferasirox, it is still not ideal. Adherence is especially difficult during adolescence when physical and psychological changes, lifestyle changes (such as moving away from home to go to college), and decreased parental supervision may result in patients either becoming irregular with their treatments or giving them up completely. Clearly, adherence is an issue with adolescents in general and is not limited to those with thalassemia, but the long-term consequences for those with thalassemia can be particularly devastating.

## REFERENCES

1. Ahmed F, Khan MR, Banu CP, Qazi MR, Akhtaruzzaman M. The coexistence of other micronutrient deficiencies in anaemic adolescent schoolgirls in rural Bangladesh. *Eur J Clin Nutr.* 2007 Feb 28; [Epub]

2. Dallman PR, Yip R, Johnson C. Prevalence and causes of anemia in the United States, 1976 to 1980. *Am J Clin Nutr.* 1984;39(3):437–445

3. Ferrara M, Coppola L, Coppola A, Capozzi L. Iron deficiency in childhood and adolescence: retrospective review. *Hematology.* 2006;11(3): 183–186

4. National Institutes of Health, Office of Dietary Supplements. Dietary supplement fact sheet: iron. Updated 2007. Available at: ods.od.nih.gov/factsheets/iron.asp. Accessed January 10, 2011

5. Centers for Disease Control and Prevention, Department of Health and Human Resources. Iron deficiency. Updated 2007. Available at: www.cdc.gov/nccdphp/dnpa/nutrition/nutrition_for_everyone/iron_deficiency/index.htm. Accessed January 10, 2011

6. Herbert V. Folic acid. In: Shils M, Olson J, Shike M, Ross AC, eds. *Nutrition in Health and Disease*. Baltimore, MD: Williams & Wilkins; 1999

7. Institute of Medicine. Food and Nutrition Board. *Dietary Reference Intakes: Thiamin, Riboflavin, Niacin, Vitamin B6, Folate, Vitamin $B_{12}$, Pantothenic Acid, Biotin, and Choline*. Washington, DC: National Academy Press; 1998

8. Kapadia CR. Vitamin $B_{12}$ in health and disease: part I—inherited disorders of function, absorption, and transport. *Gastroenterologist.* 1995;3:329-344

9. Mayo Clinic. Folic acid. Updated 2008. Available at: www.mayoclinic.com/health/folate/NS_patient-folate. Accessed January 10, 2011

10. National Institutes of Health, Office of Dietary Supplements. Dietary supplement fact sheet: folate. Updated 2005. Available at: ods.od.nih.gov/factsheets/folate.asp. Accessed January 10, 2011

11. Mayo Clinic. Vitamin $B_{12}$. Available at: www.mayoclinic.com/health/vitamin-B12/NS_patient-vitaminb12. Accessed January 10, 2011

12. Ashkenazi S, Weitz R, Varsano I, Mimouni M. Vitamin $B_{12}$ deficiency due to a strictly vegetarian diet in adolescence. *Clin Pediatr (Phila).* 1987;26(12):662-663

13. Pinhas-Hamiel O, Doron-Panush N, Reichman B, Nitzan-Kaluski D, Shalitin S, Geva-Lerner L. Obese children and adolescents: a risk group for low vitamin $B_{12}$ concentration. *Arch Pediatr Adolesc Med.* 2006;160(9):933-936

14. Toh BH, van Driel IR, Gleeson PA. Pernicious anemia. *N Engl J Med.* 1997;337(20):1441

15. Conrad ME. Pernicious anemia. Updated October 2006. Available at: emedicine.medscape.com/article/204930-overview. Accessed January 26, 2009

16. Ness-Abramof R, Nabriski DA, Braverman LE, et al. Prevalence and evaluation of $B_{12}$ deficiency in patients with autoimmune thyroid disease. *Am J Med Sci.* 2006;332(3):119-122

17. Choi JW. Association between *Helicobacter pylori* infection and iron deficiency varies according to age in healthy adolescents. *Acta Haematol.* 2007;117(4):197-199

18. Naithani R, Agrawal N, Mahapatra M, Kumar R, Pati HP, Choudhry VP. Autoimmune hemolytic anemia in children. *Pediatr Hematol Oncol.* 2007;24(4):309-315

19. Johnson ST, Fueger JT, Gottschall JL. One center's experience: the serology and drugs associated with drug-induced immune hemolytic anemia—a new paradigm. *Transfusion.* 2007;47(4):697-702

20. Schick P. Hemolytic anemia. Updated January 2007. Available at: www.emedicine.com/med/topic979.htm. Accessed January 10, 2011

21. Merck. Autoimmune hemolytic anemia. Updated 2008. Available at: www.merck.com/mmhe/sec14/ch172/ch172f.html. Accessed April 22, 2010

22. Weiss G. Pathogenesis and treatment of anaemia of chronic disease. *Blood Rev.* 2002;16(2):87-96

23. Murray-Kolb LE, Beard JL. Iron treatment normalizes cognitive functioning in young women. *Am J Clin Nutr.* 2007;85(3):778-787

24. Brigden ML. A systematic approach to macrocytosis. Sorting out the causes. *Postgrad Med.* 1995;97(5):171-172, 175-177, 181

25. Hettiarachchi M, Liyanage C, Wickremasinghe R, Hilmers DC, Abrams SA. The efficacy of micronutrient supplementation in reducing the prevalence of anaemia and deficiencies of zinc and iron among adolescents in Sri Lanka. *Eur J Clin Nutr.* 2007 May 16; [Epub]

26. Cario H. Childhood polycythemias/erythrocytoses: classification, diagnosis, clinical presentation, and treatment. *Ann Hematol.* 2005;84(3):137-145

27. Mentzer WC Jr. Differentiation of iron deficiency from thalassemia trait. *Lancet.* 1973;1(7808):882

28. Chui DH. Alpha-thalassemia: Hb H disease and Hb Barts hydrops fetalis. *Ann NY Acad Sci.* 2005;1054:25-32

29. Borgna-Pignatti C. Modern treatment of thalassemia intermedia. *Br J Haematol.* 2007;138(3):291-304

30. Urbinati F, Madigan C, Malik P. Pathophysiology and therapy for haemoglobinopathies. Part II: thalassaemias. *Expert Rev Mol Med.* 2006;8(10):1-26

31. Cunningham MJ. Update on thalassemia: clinical care and complications. *Pediatr Clin North Am.* 2008;55(2):447-460

# CHAPTER 107

# Sickle Cell Disease

BANU AYGUN, MD

## BACKGROUND

Sickle cell disease (SCD) is an inherited disorder of the red blood cells (RBCs) characterized by chronic hemolytic anemia and vascular occlusion. The clinical course of SCD is characterized by severe anemia, acute vaso-occlusive events (VOEs), acute chest syndrome (ACS), stroke, infections, and organ failure.

Adolescents with SCD have unique problems, including delayed skeletal and sexual maturation, avascular necrosis, gallstones, priapism, proteinuria, pulmonary hypertension (PH), and retinopathy (Figure 107-1). Ongoing counseling is required for issues of sexuality, drug use, birth control, and educational performance.[1] A plan should be in place for the transition of older adolescents with SCD from pediatric to adult care.

## PATHOPHYSIOLOGY

A→G nucleotide substitution in the sixth codon of the β-globin gene results in the substitution of valine for glutamic acid in the β-globin chain, leading to the formation of HbS (αβ). Hemoglobin S has reduced solubility and increased polymerization upon deoxygenation. The abnormal hemoglobin molecules form paracrystals within the RBCs, altering the cell membrane structure, leading to the typical crescent or sickle-shaped appearance and causing occlusion of the microvasculature. The anemia is due to a shortened RBC half-life. The vascular occlusion is a result of adherence of RBCs to the endothelium, increased blood viscosity, activation of adhesion molecules, and the coagulation cascade (Figure 107-2).[2] In addition, nitric oxide depletion, which results from the release of large quantities of hemoglobin and red cell arginase from the hemolyzed red cells into the plasma, has been recognized as an important contributor to the pathophysiology. The vasodilatation ordinarily caused by nitric oxide in smooth muscles is lost, resulting in unregulated vasoconstriction that promotes vaso-occlusion and contributes to tissue hypoxia and organ damage.

The vaso-occlusion that occurs in SCD can be acute, as seen in painful crises, the ACS, or stroke, or it can be insidious, as causes of such complications as splenic involution or sickle nephropathy.

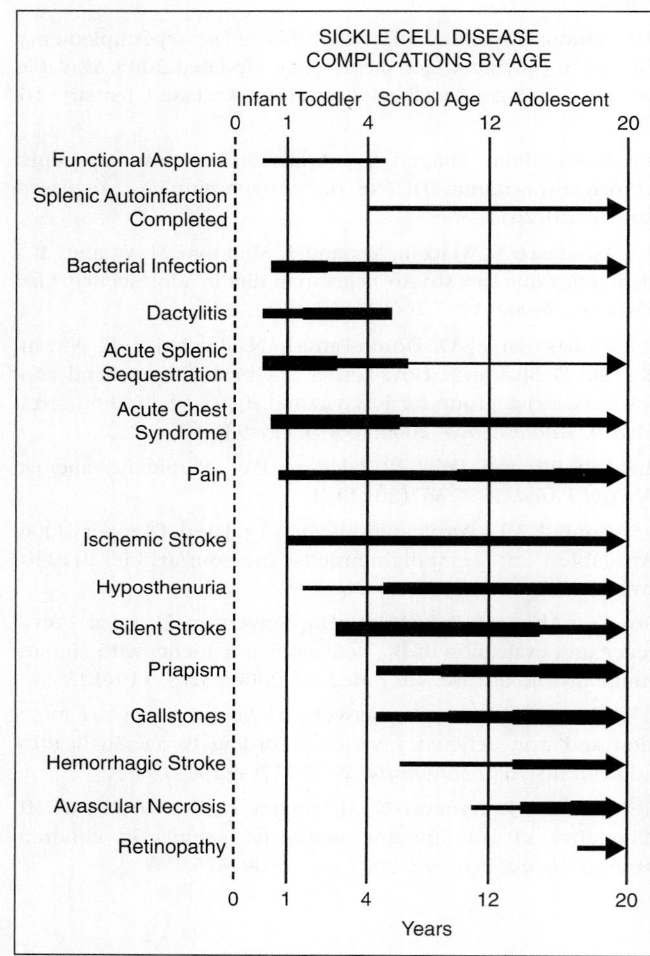


**FIGURE 107-1** Sickle cell disease complications by age. (Reprinted from Redding-Lallinger R, Knoll C. Sickle cell disease—pathophysiology and treatment. *Curr Probl Pediatr Adolesc Health Care*. 2006;36:346–376, with permission from Elsevier.)

## GENETICS

Sickle cell disease is most commonly seen in individuals whose genetic origins are in sub-Saharan Africa, southern India, and the Mediterranean. Approximately 1 in 350 blacks are born with HbSS, whereas 1 in 835 have HbSC, and 1 in 1,700 have HbSβ-thalassemia; this

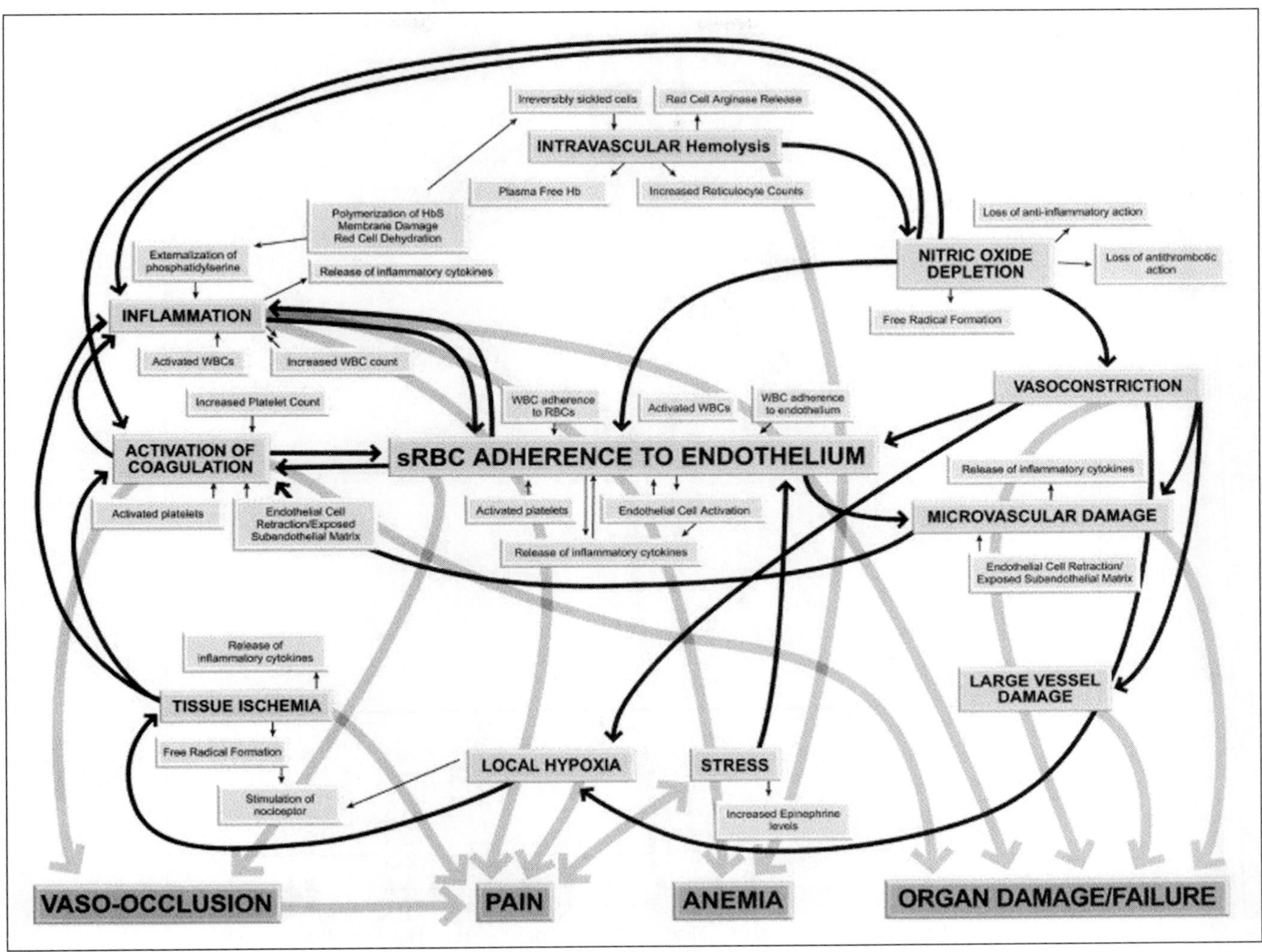


**FIGURE 107-2** Elements of the pathophysiology of sickle cell disease and their interactions. (Reprinted from Redding-Lallinger R, Knoll C. Sickle cell disease—pathophysiology and treatment. *Curr Probl Pediatr Adolesc Health Care.* 2006;36:346–376, with permission from Elsevier.)

makes SCD the most common inherited disease in the United States. The sickle cell gene protects heterozygous carriers from succumbing to endemic *Plasmodium falciparum* infection, which has been postulated to explain its persistence in the populations of endemic regions.

There are 4 globin haplotypes of the gene as determined by restriction-endonuclease-defined polymorphisms in the globin-gene cluster on chromosome 11 (Figure 107-3).[3] Three of the haplotypes, Senegal, Benin, and Bantu, are localized to 3 separate areas of Africa. The fourth haplotype, Arab-India, is seen in populations from the Arabian peninsula and India.

Sickle cell disease denotes all genotypes containing at least 1 sickle gene, in which HbS makes up at least half of the hemoglobin that is present. In addition to homozygous SCD, 4 other major sickle genotypes are linked to the disease (Table 107-1).[4] In order of frequency in the US population, they are HbSS, HbSC, HbSβ+thal, and HbSβ°thal. In order of severity, HbSS and HbSβ°thal are considered to be equivalent and more severe than HbSC, which is more severe than HbSβ+thal. Importantly, the phenotype of SCD is multigenic. There is considerable phenotypic heterogeneity among individuals who have identical alleles at the β-globin locus. Pleiotropic or secondary effector genes control other important pathological events, such as rate of destruction of sickle cells, dense cell formation, and adhesion to endothelium, and thus affect phenotypic expression.

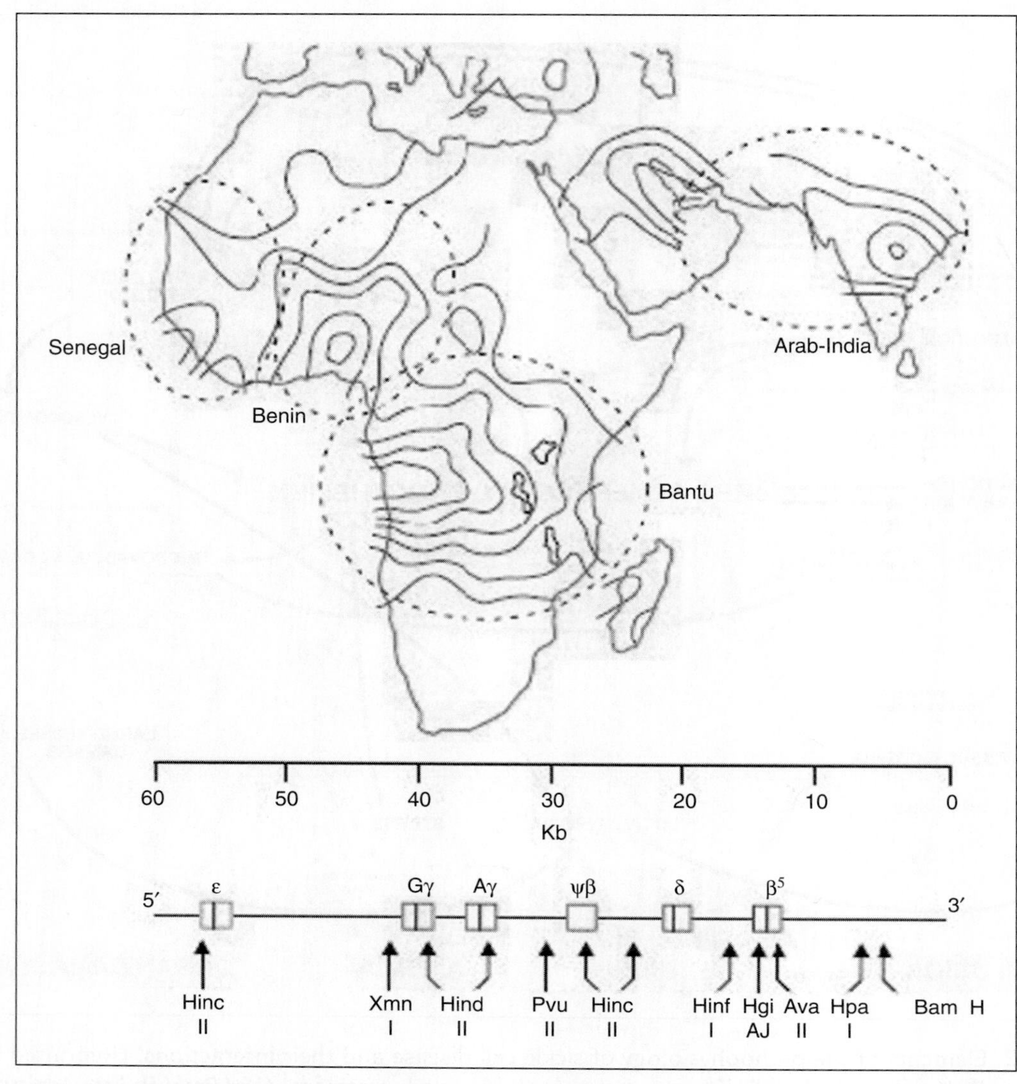


FIGURE 107-3 Geographical distribution and schematic representation of the sickle gene. (Reprinted from Stuart MJ, Nagel RL. Sickle-cell disease. *Lancet*. 2004;364:1343–1360, with permission from Elsevier.)

## CLINICAL MANIFESTATIONS

Clinical manifestations of SCD can be divided into acute and chronic manifestations. Acute problems include VOE, ACS, cerebrovascular events, infections, priapism, aplastic crises, and splenic sequestration crises. Chronic problems are related to the long-term effects of SCD on various organs.

### ACUTE PROBLEMS

#### Vaso-Occlusive Events

Vaso-occlusive events, otherwise known as painful events, are episodes of microvascular occlusion that induce local inflammation and pain. Circumstances that slow the transit of sickled RBCs through the microcirculation enhance red cell to endothelial cell adhesion, red cell dehydration, and vasomotor regulation and lead to vaso-occlusion. Microvascular occlusion occurs predominantly in localized areas of marrow, causing necrosis. Inflammatory mediators activate nociceptive afferent nerve fibers, evoking the pain response. Affected areas are the long bones, ribs, sternum, spine, and pelvis; there is often multisite involvement. Microvascular occlusion of the periosteum and cortex of bone can occasionally mimic osteomyelitis. Microvascular occlusion in the mesenteric vessels, with impaired intestinal mobility, is characteristic of the abdominal crisis that can mimic an acute abdomen. According to the Cooperative Study of Sickle Cell Disease

**Table 107-1[4]**

**Laboratory Values in Sickle Cell Syndromes Among Those Older than 5 Years**

| *Hemoglobin (HB) Variant* | *Hb[a] Electrophoresis* | *Hb (g/dL)* | *MCV[b]* | *Hb S (%)* | *Hb A (%)* | *Hb A2 (%)* | *Hb F (%)* |
|---|---|---|---|---|---|---|---|
| Hb-SS | SF | 6 to 8 | Normal or ↑[c] | >90 | 0 | <3.5 | <10 |
| Hb-S-beta° thalassemia | SF | 7 to 9 | ↓ | >80 | 0 | >3.5 | <20 |
| HB-S-beta+ thalassemia | SAF | 9 to 12 | ↓ | >60 | 5 to 30 | >3.5 | <20 |
| Hb-SC[d] | SCF | 10 to 14 | Normal or ↓ | 50 | 0 | NA[e] | <2 |
| Hb-HPFH | SF | 11 to 14 | Normal or ↓ | 60 | 0 | <2.5 | 35 to 40 |

[a]Hemoglobins are reported in order of quantity.

[b]MCV = mean cell volume.

[c]Hb-SS with coexisting alpha thalassemia may have decreased MCV and increased A.

[d]Hb C: measures ~50%.

[e]Hb A not measurable in the presence of Hb C.

HPFH, hereditary persistence of fetal hemoglobin

(CSSCD),[5] which followed 4,082 patients between October 1978 and September 1988, 39% of patients had no VOE during the 10-year period, whereas 1% had more than 6 episodes per year.

No specific form of therapy has been shown to be effective for the acute treatment of VOE. Management relies on hydration and analgesics.[6] Most VOEs are treated at home with increased oral hydration, anti-inflammatory agents, and nonopioid and opioid analgesics. Patients who fail outpatient oral treatment may benefit from several hours of intravenous hydration, parenteral anti-inflammatory agents, and analgesics in a day hospital setting or the emergency department. If there is significant improvement, patients may be discharged to home on oral analgesics. Otherwise, they are admitted to the hospital for further management.

Treatment in the hospital initially consists of round-the-clock use of analgesics, which is switched to an as-needed basis over time. Fear of drug addiction by health care providers is a common problem; however, during VOE, opioids should not be withheld for fear of addiction when the patient feels that these medications are indicated. Physicians caring for patients with VOE must be aware that different individuals have different pain thresholds. Patients who are admitted to the hospital with VOE should be monitored with pulse oximetry. They should also use incentive spirometry to prevent development of ACS. Patients with VOE may develop fever. However, because patients with SCD have increased susceptibility to bacterial infections, rigorous assessment of fever, including blood cultures, should be done and empirical antibiotic treatment should be started until culture results are available. Hydroxyurea (see following) decreases the number and duration of VOEs in HbSS patients who have frequent and severe VOEs.[7-9]

### Acute Chest Syndrome

Acute chest syndrome is the second most common cause of hospitalization and the leading cause of death in SCD. The syndrome consists of a combination of chest pain, fever, respiratory symptoms, and development of a new pulmonary infiltrate on the chest x-ray. Hypoxia is often present. The etiology is multifactorial: infection, pulmonary embolization from a distant thrombus or infarcted bone marrow, vaso-occlusion, and noncardiogenic pulmonary edema are possible mechanisms. When 671 episodes of ACS were analyzed by The National Acute Chest Syndrome Study Group,[10] a specific cause was identified in only 38% of episodes. Pulmonary fat embolism, chlamydia, mycoplasma, viruses, and bacterial infections due to coagulase-positive *Staphyloccocus aureus* and *S pneumoniae* were the most common causes. Nearly half of the patients were admitted to the hospital for a diagnosis other than ACS and developed clinical and radiographic findings within 2.5 days after admission.

In order to prevent hypoventilation induced by pain and/or analgesics, judicious use of analgesics, prophylactic incentive spirometry, and pulse oximetry monitoring should be utilized routinely during management of a VOE. Care must be given not to overload patients with fluids during intravenous hydration. Treatment of ACS is supportive, with oxygen supplementation, judicious use of intravenous fluids, broad-spectrum antibiotics (including a macrolide), and pain management. Red cell transfusions improve oxygenation. In most patients, treatment with a simple transfusion is safe and effective. However, some patients require an exchange transfusion. The use of steroids and bronchodilators has not been studied in a randomized manner, but they are used in patients who have symptoms consistent with reactive airway disease. Hydroxyurea, transfusion therapy, or bone marrow transplantation may be indicated in patients with recurrent ACS.[8]

### Central Nervous System Events

Stroke is a catastrophic complication of SCD, affecting 6% to 17% of children with SCD. Infarctive strokes occur as a result of occlusion of the major cerebral arteries and affect children from 2 to 15 years of age. Hemorrhagic stroke results from intracerebral or subarachnoid hemorrhage and affects older children and adults. Symptoms of stroke include hemiparesis, visual and language disturbances, seizures and alterations in mentation, sensation, or alertness. As soon as stroke is suspected, a prompt and thorough evaluation for therapy is recommended. Patients should receive an urgent noncontrast computed tomography (CT) of the brain to rule out hemorrhage or other nonischemic etiologies. In early ischemia (< 3 hours), the CT may be negative or show only subtle signs.

An exchange transfusion is recommended within the first few hours after the acute onset of an ischemic stroke. In a patient who has a low hemoglobin level, a simple transfusion, followed by an exchange transfusion, may be necessary. After initial stabilization and transfusion, magnetic resonance imaging (MRI) and magnetic resonance angiography (MRA) of the brain with diffusion-weighted imaging should be obtained. Strokes tend to be repetitive because of the progressive nature of the cerebral vascular disease.[11] Long-term transfusion therapy to maintain HbS levels at less than 30% slows or stops the progression of arterial abnormalities and reduces the risk of recurrent stroke from 70% to 90% to 10% to 20%. The optimal duration of chronic transfusion therapy has not been determined. Bone marrow transplantation from a histocompatible human leukocyte antigen (HLA) donor is another treatment option. Hydroxyurea is currently being studied as an alternative to transfusions for secondary stroke prophylaxis.

All children with HbSS disease between 2 and 16 years of age should have yearly transcranial Doppler (TCD) testing to assess their risk for stroke. This is a noninvasive technique that measures the flow velocity in the distal internal carotid and proximal middle and anterior cerebral arteries. Markedly increased velocities are associated with increased stenosis and an increased risk for cerebral infarction within the next 3 years. It is recommended that patients with confirmed abnormally elevated TCD velocities start chronic transfusion treatments in an attempt to prevent a primary stroke.[12]

### Infections

Children with SCD are at increased risk for invasive bacterial infections due to loss of splenic function, which occurs by 6 to 12 months of age. Common organisms are *Streptococcus pneumoniae, Staphylococcus aureus, Salmonella* species, *Haemophilus influenza* type b, *Escherichia coli*, and *Klebsiella* species. The types of infection include bacteremia, meningitis, pneumonia, and osteomyelitis.

Any fever greater than 101.3°F (38.5°C) in patients with SCD must be considered a medical emergency. Patients should be evaluated immediately with a history and physical examination, complete blood count, reticulocyte count, blood culture, urinalysis, and chest x-ray. Treatment should be started with intravenous ceftriaxone. Vancomycin should be considered in severely ill children and depending on the prevalence of penicillin-resistant pneumococcus in the community. If the patient has a toxic appearance, high fever, serious localized infection, exceptionally high or low white blood cell count, a history of invasive infection, or an unreliable social situation, he or she should be admitted to the hospital.

Penicillin prophylaxis, pneumococcal vaccines, aggressive management of the febrile child, and parental education combined to substantially lower the risk of invasive pneumococcal infections.[13] There is no advantage to continuing penicillin prophylaxis in children older than 5 years of age.[14] However, those who have had a surgical splenectomy or a previous severe pneumococcal infection, or those whose pneumococcal immunizations are not up-to-date, should continue penicillin prophylaxis until adulthood. Adolescents with SCD should receive immunization with the 13-valent and 23-valent pneumococcal polysaccharide vaccine if they have not been previously vaccinated, the meningococcal vaccine, and the hepatitis B vaccine, in addition to the influenza vaccine on an annual basis.

Osteomyelitis occurs with increased frequency at all ages in patients with SCD.[15] This may be due to infarction of the long bones during VOEs. Osteomyelitis is commonly caused by salmonella. *Staphylococcus aureus* accounts for fewer than 25% of cases in SCD.[10,11] The presenting symptoms are fever, along with pain, swelling, and tenderness over the involved area. These signs are similar to the presentation of VOE, and distinguishing between the two can be difficult. Both have similar findings on x-ray, ultrasound, and CT scan. X-ray changes are not seen until 10 to 15 days after the infection has begun. Radioisotope bone scanning cannot reliably distinguish between the two. Currently, MRI is being used most frequently for the diagnosis of osteomyelitis. Diagnosis depends on a combination of physical examination findings, MRI and bone scan results, and blood and bone cultures. If no organism is found, antibiotics that cover *Salmonella, Staphylococcus*, and gram-negative bacteria should be chosen. Treatment should continue for at least 6 weeks.

### Priapism

Priapism is an unwanted, painful erection of the penis. It is reported to occur in 5% to 45% of patients with SCD.[16] It has a bimodal age distribution. The early peak is 5 to 13 years of age and the late peak is 21 to 29 years of age. Priapism typically involves the corpora cavernosa and usually spares the corpora spongiosum and glans. It occurs in 2 general patterns: (1) prolonged, lasting 4 hours or more, and (2) stuttering, brief episodes that resolve spontaneously. The priapism in SCD is a low-flow state due to sickling and sludging of RBCs in the corpora cavernosa. After prolonged erections, blood trapped in the corpora cavernosa becomes deoxygenated, resulting in local acidosis, further sludging, and an increase in the intercavernosal pressure. When the intercavernosal pressure is increased to 80 to 120 mm Hg for 4 hours or more, the corpora cavernosa become ischemic, eliciting an inflammatory response that may result in fibrosis and impotence. Approximately half of all patients have recurrent episodes. Loss of potency is related to longer duration of the priapism and younger age at first episode. Overall, 10% to 50% of men with a history of priapism are impotent by self-report.

Most episodes of priapism occur during sleep, typically around 4 am. This may be related to the normal erections that take place during rapid eye movement sleep, as well as nocturnal acidosis and dehydration that may occur. The diagnosis is established by the finding of a tumescent phallus with a history of an unwanted painful erection lasting 30 minutes or more. When priapism lasts 4 hours or more, intervention is warranted, as there is a potential for ischemic injury. Patients report that voiding, nonsteroidal and opioid analgesics, gentle exercise, ejaculation, or taking a warm bath or shower may terminate some events. Aggressive hydration and adequate analgesia are the first steps in treatment. If there is no response within 12 to 24 hours, partial exchange transfusion may be performed. One complication of exchange transfusion is the ASPEN syndrome (SCD, priapism, exchange transfusion, and neurological events).[17] The clinical manifestations of the ASPEN syndrome range from headache to seizures to obtundation requiring ventilatory support. In one study,[18] there was rapid complete detumescence in 35 of 37 consecutive episodes of prolonged priapism in 15 patients with use of aspiration and irrigation with a dilute (1:1,000,000) epinephrine solution. Other treatment options for persistent priapism include creation of a corpora caverniosum shunt or a venous bypass. Strategies for secondary prevention of priapism include chronic red cell transfusions, vasoactive agents, pseudoephedrine, and hormonal treatments. Patients should be educated about priapism, especially the need to report recurrent events and to present for care within 4 hours of onset during a prolonged episode.

### Aplastic Crises

Aplastic crises are caused by viral infections, especially parvovirus B19, that have a direct cytotoxic effect on erythroid precursors. This results in cessation of erythropoiesis with a rapid fall in the hemoglobin. Rarely, all marrow elements may be affected. The process is self-limited. Erythropoiesis usually resumes within 10 days. Treatment is supportive with red cell transfusions as necessary.

### Splenic Sequestration

Splenic sequestration is defined as a decrease in the steady state hemoglobin concentration of at least 2 g/dL, an acutely enlarging spleen, and evidence of compensatory marrow erythropoiesis. Although it is commonly seen in children younger than 2 years of age, it can be seen in adolescents with HbSBthal or HbSC disease. Treatment is with red cell transfusions.

## CHRONIC PROBLEMS

Manifestations of chronic organ damage in SCD are listed in Table 107-2.[3]

### Delays in Skeletal and Sexual Maturation

In adolescents with SCD, pubertal increases in height and weight occur later than in the general population.[15] By adulthood, men and women with SCD reach normal or near-normal heights, but their mean weights are still lower than those of controls.

Puberty is delayed in those with SCD. Menarche occurs 2 to 3 years later than in the general population (median age, 14.0 to 15.5 years), and Tanner stage 5 is not achieved until the median ages of 17.3 years for girls and 17.6 years for boys.[19]

Physical limitations produced by SCD may prevent patients from participating in some organized sports. Decisions should be made on a case-by-case basis. Physicians should encourage their patients to participate in as many activities as possible, provided they drink fluids to avoid dehydration and rest when they become tired.

**Table 107-2**

**Chronic Organ Damage in Sickle Cell Disease**

| | *Major Clinical Manifestations* | *Underpinning Mechanisms* | *Management Issues* |
|---|---|---|---|
| Eye | Retinitis proliferans occurs with greatest frequency in HbSC disease and can lead to visual impairment. | Peripheral retinalvascular occlusion due to red-cell and leucocyte-endothelial adhesion (via surface adhesion molecules). Angiogenic factors seem crucial to seafan formation. | Periodical ophthalmologic assessment with early identification of peripheral retinal disease. |
| Kidney | Hypertrophy: occurs in all sickle genotypes, especially HbSS. Also age-dependent. | Renal enlargement is due to glomerular hypertrophy and increased renal blood volume. | |
| | Alterations in distal nephron function, resulting in hyposthenuria and nocturia. Tubular acidosis (type IV or incomplete distal acidosis) can also arise. | Hyposthenuria mainly due to hyperosmolar-induced loss of deep juxtamedullary nephrons, which also causes acidosis due to perturbation in bicarbonate reabsorption. | Hyposthenuria can lead to childhood enuresis. Urine-specific gravity is a poor index of hydration status. |
| | Tubular deficiencies in adults include increased secretion of creatinine and uric acid. Heightened reabsorption of phosphates (aldosterone-independent) leading to hyperphosphatemia can also occur. | Proximal tubular dysfunction. | Creatinine clearance might overestimate GFR. |
| | Glomerular abnormalities: increases in GFR and ERPF occur in children, preceded by microalbuminuria.<br>GFR and ERPF decline toward normal rates in adolescence, and fall to subnormal rate levels in older individuals. Proteinuria could progress to nephrotic syndrome and end-stage renal disease. HbSS patients develop renal failure earlier than those with HbSC disease (median age of onset 23 vs 50 years). | Mesangial phagocytosis of sickle cells, glomerular hypertrophy, immune-complex glomerulonephritis, and hyperfiltration-induced glomerular injury have all been implicated. NSAIDs used for pain control further impair renal function. | ACE inhibitors reduce microalbuminuria and reduce glomerular damage.<br>NSAIDs to be used with caution in patients with sickle nephropathy.<br>Transplantation is a recourse in some patients with end-stage renal insufficiency. |
| Lung | Most serious complication is PH: mean pulmonary artery pressure of >25 mm Hg, and/or a tricuspid jet velocity on echocardiograms >2–5 m/s; occurs in 5%–30% of patients, with a median survival time of 2 years. | Recurrent ACS is a predisposing factor for SCD-related PH. Chronic anemia with hypoxia, pulmonary release of inflammatory cytokines, reduction in NO synthase in small pulmonary arterioles with increases in endothelin-1, and platelet-derived factors have been implicated in pathogenesis. | Often asymptomatic in early stages. Should be suspected in those with O desaturation, syncope, or fixed dyspnea.<br>Ominous prognosis justifies experimental treatments including epoprostenol infusions, NO inhalation, oral L-arginine, or use of the endothelin antagonist bosentan. |

(*Continued*)

**Table 107-2 (Continued)**

| | *Major Clinical Manifestations* | *Underpinning Mechanisms* | *Management Issues* |
|---|---|---|---|
| Chronic leg ulcers | Usually occur over medial malleoli in chronic hemolytic anemias, including HbSS, thalassemia, and spherocytosis. | Possible incompetence of venous valves draining ankle region and a reduction in venous refilling time. Hydroxyurea treatment in SCD can cause leg ulcers. | Unra boot (gauze impregnated with zinc oxide) is effective. IV arginine butyrate also reported to cause rapid healing. Hydroxyurea to be used with caution in SCD individuals with previous history of leg ulcers. |
| Osteonecrosis | Osteonecrosis of the femoral and humeral heads occur in all sickle genotypes, most commonly in SS α-thalassemia and in HbSS individuals with a high hemoglobin concentration. | Expansion of red-cell marrow with increased pressure or end-arterialvascular occlusion of the femoral or humeral heads have been postulated. | Disease frequently asymptomatic;T1- and T2-weighted images on MRI detect early lesions not seen on radiographs. Hip coring used for early disease; surgical hip replacement indicated for more advanced lesions. |
| Spleen | Autoinfarction in patients with HbSS before age 2. Hyposplenism has slower onset in those with HbSC disease. | Distinct sinusoidal blood flow, high rates of oxygen extraction, and acidosis provide ideal conditions for HbS polymerization, leading to autoinfarction. | Elevated susceptibility to infection. Use of prophylactic penicillin and pneumococcal vaccine standard. |

ACE, angiotensin-converting enzyme; ACS, acute chest syndrome; ERPF, effective renal plasma flow; GFR, glomerular filtration rate; NO, nitric oxide; NSAIDs, nonsteroid anti-inflammatory drugs; PH, pulmonary hypertension; SCD, sickle cell disease

Reprinted from Stuart MJ, Nagel RL. Sickle-cell disease. *Lancet*. 2004;364:1343–1360, with permission from Elsevier.

### Chronic Lung Disease

As the survival of patients with SCD has increased, PH has emerged as a major cause of morbidity and mortality.[20] The normal blood pressure in the pulmonary artery is 25/15 mmHg, with a mean pulmonary artery systolic pressure (PASP) of 18 mmHg. Pulmonary hypertension in adults is defined as PASP >30 mmHg, or mean PASP >25 mmHg, or tricuspid valve regurgitant jet velocity >2.5 m/s. The pathogenesis of PH in SCD is probably multifactorial. However, intravascular hemolysis, with binding of free plasma hemoglobin to endogenous nitric oxide, is thought to play an important causative role. The development of PH in SCD carries a poor prognosis. Intensifying SCD treatment with hydroxyurea or transfusions and the use of pulmonary vasodilating and remodeling medications are currently being investigated as treatment options.

### Sickle Cell Nephropathy

Sickle cell nephropathy starts in childhood and affects the glomerulus and the tubule. Manifestations include hematuria, proteinuria, urinary-concentrating defects, type IV renal tubular acidosis (proton- and potassium-secreting defects), supernormal proximal sodium reabsorption, glomerular hyperfiltration, focal glomerulosclerosis, and papillary necrosis. The pathophysiology is not well understood. Sickle cell nephropathy is associated with renal endothelial denudation, mesangial cell expansion, basement membrane changes, impaired endothelium-dependent relaxation of blood vessels, and oxidative stress. Proteinuria, hypertension, severe anemia, and hematuria have been found to be reliable preazotemic predictors of chronic renal failure. Microalbuminuria (urinary excretion of minutely elevated amounts of albumin before the development of proteinuria) is considered to be an early marker. The prevalence of microalbuminuria is 46% in those with SCD who are between 10 and 18 years of age.[21] As many as two-thirds of patients with SCD who develop the nephrotic syndrome (proteinuria, edema, hypoalbuminemia, and hypercholesterolemia) will develop chronic renal insufficiency. Up to 18% of patients with SCD develop chronic renal insufficiency.

The median age of diagnosis of renal failure is 23.1 years.[22] Management of renal failure is the same as that for renal insufficiency due to other causes. Survival after diagnosis of renal failure in patients with SCD is only approximately 4 years.

### Gallstones

Because of the increased red cell turnover in SCD, the frequency of pigment gallstones is high. The incidence is 42% in the 15- to 18-year-old age group. Approximately 10% to 15% of patients have symptoms attributable to the biliary tract. Laparoscopic cholecystectomy has replaced open cholecystectomy in many centers due to shorter length of hospitalization, decreased postoperative pain, and other complications (see Chapter 101, Diseases of the Gall Bladder).

### Avascular Necrosis

The exact pathophysiology of avascular necrosis in SCD is unknown. The overall prevalence rate is 10%, with a rise to 50% in those older than 35 years of age.[23] There appears to be progressive occlusion of the microcirculation leading to increased intraosseous pressure and subsequent cell death. The risk factors for development of avascular necrosis include increased VOE, higher hematocrit levels, and concomitant α-thalassemia mutation. The femoral head is the most common area of bone destruction in SCD, followed by the humoral head. The initial infarct occurs in the subchondrial region, where the collateral circulation is minimal. The joint destruction almost always includes the anterior superior portion of the proximal femur, where the weight-bearing forces are the greatest. Pain may be experienced in the hip, groin, anterior or medial thigh, buttocks, knee, or lower back. Acute pain is constant and is exacerbated by weight bearing. With time, pain resolves; however, limitation of movement often remains. Plain film changes are seen only after healing of the infarct, which is late in the course of the disease. X-ray films should include antero-posterior radiographs of the pelvis and frog leg lateral views of both hips. Magnetic resonance imaging is the most accurate imaging modality, with an accuracy rate of more than 90%. Nonsurgical treatments include pain relief with nonsteroidal anti-inflammatory agents, stretching programs to improve range of motion, and strengthening exercises for stabilization and ultimately minimizing disability. Surgical treatments include core decompression, osteotomies, and total hip arthroplasty. Vertebral infarcts lead to central deterioration with preserved peripheral areas of the vertebral end-plates. This gives the typical radiographic appearance of "fish vertebrae" or "tower vertebrae." Treatment is supportive with pain medications and muscle relaxants.

### Retinopathy

The retina is especially vulnerable to vascular occlusion as it is rich in end arterioles. Vaso-occlusive changes in the retina may lead to nonproliferative and proliferative changes.[24] Nonproliferative changes consist of salmon patch hemorrhages, iridescent spots, and schisis cavities. Proliferative changes begin with the formation of arteriovenous anastomoses, followed by the development of vascular fronds resembling sea fans. Sea fans are most commonly found in the superotemporal quadrant, followed by the inferotemporal, superonasal, and inferonasal quadrants. They represent true neovascular tissue and show profuse leakage of intravascular fluorescein dye, indicating loss of the blood–retinal barrier. As sea fans grow into the vitreous cavity, traction on delicate vascular channels results in bleeding at irregular intervals for years. Treatment includes photocoagulation, cryotherapy and, in advanced cases, surgery. An additional ocular complication is hyphema. Bleeding into the anterior chamber leads to trapping of sickle cells, mechanical obstruction of the outflow apparatus, compromised circulation of the aqueous humor, and increased intraocular pressure with development of sudden blindness.

### Pregnancy, Contraception, and Genetic Counseling

Pregnancy poses potentially serious problems both for the mother and the fetus/neonate. There is an increased incidence of pyelonephritis, hematuria, and thrombophlebitis. Anemia is more severe. Infarctions of the lungs, kidneys, and brain can be seen during late pregnancy and the postpartum period. Toxemia, heart failure, and postpartum puerperal endometritis occur more commonly in women with SCD. Infants born to women with SCD are at greater risk for preterm birth, low birth weight, being small for gestational age, and neonatal jaundice.[25]

The efficacy and safety of various methods of contraception have not been studied systematically in women with SCD, and there are no controlled trials addressing the safety of oral contraceptives. However, case series have indicated that there are no detrimental effects, and it is general consensus that hormonal contraception does not increase the risk of sickling nor does there appear to be an additional risk of thrombosis in these patients compared to other groups of adolescents. Consideration has been given to use of other methods of contraception, however, and 1 study found the use of depo-medroxyprogesterone acetate decreased the number of painful episodes.

Because most of the genetic counseling efforts during childhood are directed toward the parents, most adolescents have little knowledge in this area. Adolescents should receive genetic counseling during their health care maintenance visits.

**Depression**

Depression is a common problem in patients with SCD.[1] The chronic and relapsing nature of the disease, social and economic factors, difficulty in predicting complications, and the dependence on others are factors leading to the high rate of depression. Antidepressant medications and counseling are helpful for patients with SCD who are depressed; empowering patients to assume responsibility for their illness and to be proactive and aggressive in its management is also helpful.

## TREATMENT

Due to the complexity of the illness, a comprehensive, combined-modality approach offers the best method of management for patients with SCD. Most of the treatment is supportive and preventive. There are 3 major therapeutic options:

- Red cell transfusions
- Hydroxyurea
- Hematopoietic stem cell transplantation (HSCT)

Age, antecedent history, presence of chronic organ damage, compliance, availability of an HLA-matched donor, and patient/parental choice are all factors that need to be taken into account when making treatment decisions. Advantages and disadvantages of specific treatments should be discussed with each patient/parent.

### RED CELL TRANSFUSIONS

Approximately 50% of patients with SCD receive a transfusion at some stage in their lives. The indications for transfusions are listed in Box 107-1.[26] Patients who are not on a chronic transfusion program should generally not be transfused to Hb levels above 11g/dL, because blood viscosity is markedly increased in SCD. Exchange transfusion, performed manually or by automated erythrocytapheresis, is indicated in acute stroke syndrome and ACS. In the acute setting, it has the advantage of reducing the concentration of HbS while limiting the volume administered and minimizing hyperviscosity. Chronic transfusion has been used for primary and secondary prevention of stroke as well as to ameliorate other types of end-organ damage. The most serious complications of transfusions are iron overload, allo-immunization, and transfusion-transmitted infections. Iron overload causes significant morbidity and mortality in patients with SCD who are on chronic transfusion programs. Iron overload can be minimized by limiting red cell transfusions to defined indications, by using manual or automated exchange transfusion, and by providing intensive support to enhance compliance with iron chelating treatment.

**Box 107-1**

***Indications for Red Cell Transfusion in Sickle Cell Disease***

1. Generally accepted indications
   - Acute cerebrovascular accident
   - Acute chest syndrome
   - Acute splenic sequestration
   - Aplastic crisis
   - Intrahepatic cholestasis
   - Acute blood loss
2. Possibly effective
   - Preoperative/preprocedural
   - Recurrent or persistent priapism
   - Advanced pulmonary or cardiac disease
   - Progressive renal failure
   - Unusually frequent or severe painful episodes
   - Pregnancy with exacerbation of anemia
3. Indications for chronic transfusion
   - Primary stroke prevention
   - Secondary stroke prevention
   - Recurrent acute chest syndrome and pulmonary hypertension

Reprinted from Wanko SO, Telen MJ. Transfusion management in sickle cell disease. *Hematol Oncol Clin N Am.* 2005:19:803–808, with permission from Elsevier.

### HYDROXYUREA

Hydroxyurea arrests DNA synthesis by preventing deoxyribonucleotide formation from ribonucleoside precursors. It increases the production of hemoglobin F. Additional pharmacologic effects include decreasing neutrophil count, increasing RBC volume and hydration, increasing deformability of RBCs, altering adhesion of RBCs to endothelium, and release of nitric oxide. The most common side effects are dose-dependent myelosuppression, nausea and vomiting, and skin rashes.

Potential indications for hydroxyurea treatment are delineated in Table 107-3.[4]

**Table 107-3**

**Potential Indications for Hydroxyurea Therapy in Children with Homozygous Sickle Cell Anemia**

| | | |
|---|---|---|
| Acute vaso-occlusive complications | Painful events | |
| | Dactylitis | |
| | Acute chest syndrome | |
| Laboratory markers of severity | Low hemoglobin | |
| | Low HbF | |
| | Elevated WBC | |
| | Elevated LDH | |
| Organ dysfunction | Brain | Elevated TCD velocities |
| | | Silent MRI or MRA changes |
| | | Stroke prophylaxis |
| | Lungs | Hypoxemia |
| | Kidney | Proteinuria |
| Miscellaneous | Sibling on hydroxyurea | |
| | Parental request | |

Most pediatric hematologists have accepted clinical severity with acute vaso-occlusive complications as an indication for hydroxyurea therapy, but there is little agreement about indications for children with laboratory abnormalities or organ dysfunction. Similarly, the appropriate age for hydroxyurea initiation has not been determined, although clinical trials have demonstrated safety and efficacy for infants, young children, and school-aged children with SCD.

LDH, lactate dehydrogenase; MRA, magnetic resonance angiography; MRI, magnetic resonance imaging; TCD, transcranial doppler; WBC, white blood cells

Reprinted from Heeney MM, Ware RE. Hydroxyurea for children with sickle cell disease. *Pediatr Clin North Am.* 2008;55(2):483–501, with permission from Elsevier.

Exclusion criteria are pregnancy, inability to use reliable contraception if sexually active (both men and women), and inability to comply with daily dosing and frequent monitoring.

Hydroxyurea is usually started at a daily dose of 20 mg/kg. The dose is increased by 5 mg/kg every 8 to 12 weeks to a maximum dose of 25–30 mg/kg/day or until there is evidence of toxicity. A complete blood count and reticulocyte count should be monitored every 4 weeks. Laboratory tests, including liver and kidney function tests, should be obtained every 8 weeks. Hemoglobin electrophoresis is checked periodically to assess response and adherence to treatment.

Hematologic toxicity from hydroxyurea is defined as following:

- Absolute neutrophil count <1,000/μL
- Hemoglobin <7 gm/dl with an absolute reticulocyte count <10,000/μL
- Hemoglobin <8 gm/dl with an absolute reticulocyte count <80,000/μL
- Platelet count <80,000/μL

If toxicity occurs, treatment should be stopped for at least 1 week until toxicity resolves. Hydroxyurea should then be resumed either at the same dose or a 2.5 to 5 mg/kg lower dose. If toxicity does not recur after 12 weeks on the reduced dose, the dose may then be increased by 2.5 to 5 mg/kg. In the Multicenter Study of Hydroxyurea in Sickle Cell Anemia,[27] adult patients taking hydroxyurea appeared to have reduced mortality after 9 years of follow-up. Taking hydroxyurea was associated with a 40% reduced mortality.

## HEMATOPOIETIC STEM CELL TRANSPLANTATION

Transplantation remains the only curative treatment for SCD. Indications are listed in Box 107-2. Conditioning regimens include busulfan and cyclophosphamide. Currently, antithymocyte globulin or Campath have been added to the preparatory regimen to prevent rejection. Overall survival is 92% to 94% and event-free survival is 75% to 84%. Deaths are due to acute and chronic graft-versus-host disease, intracranial hemorrhage, and sudden death. Patients with SCD have increased risk of neurological complications during or immediately after transplantation. Higher platelet transfusion threshold and rigorous control of blood pressure, with close monitoring of magnesium and cyclosporine levels prevent intracranial hemorrhage. However, a high incidence of seizures persists. Fertility is likely to be impaired. Reduced intensity, nonmyeloablative conditioning regimens may lead to stable, mixed chimerism that is sufficient to cure the disease phenotype. This also offers the potential of retaining gonadal function and fertility. However, it should only be performed in the context of a well-constructed clinical trial.

## TREATMENTS UNDER DEVELOPMENT

In addition to the developments of new drugs and therapies, combination drug therapy aimed at different

**Box 107-2**

***Indications for Hematopoietic Stem Cell Transplantation in SCD***

A. Age <16 years and HLA-matched sibling donor

B. One or more of the following:

1. Sickle cell disease-related neurological deficit, stroke, or subarachnoid hemorrhage
2. >2 episodes of acute chest syndrome and stage 1 chronic lung disease
3. Recurrent, severe debilitating pain due to vaso-occlusive crises
4. Problems relating to future medical care, ie, unavailability of adequately screened blood products
5. Sickle nephropathy with a GFR of 30%-50%
6. Bilateral proliferative retinopathy and major visual impairment
7. Osteonecrosis of multiple joints

GFR, glomerular filtration rate

Reprinted from Davies SC. Bone marrow transplant for sickle cell disease–the dilemma. *Blood Rev.* 1993;7:4-9, with permission from Elsevier.

mechanisms involved in the pathophysiology of SCD deserves further investigation.[28]

- HbF-inducing agents: Decitabine, short-chain fatty acids
- Vasodilators: Nitric oxide, arginine, sildenafil, statins
- Agents that prevent red cell dehydration: Clotrimazole, magnesium pidolate, ICA-17043 (Senicapoc)
- Others: Antiadhesive agents, Nix-0699, secretory phospholipase a2 inhibitors, antithrombotic agents
- Gene therapy

## TRANSITION FROM PEDIATRIC HEMATOLOGY TO ADULT HEMATOLOGY

One of the most difficult and traumatic events faced by adolescents with SCD is the transition from care by pediatric hematologists to care by adult hematologists. It is general consensus that there is not a specific age at which adolescents should be transferred to adult care. In practical terms, the transfer is usually coordinated around another life event, such as a birthday or graduation from high school. To prepare the patient and family, the pediatric provider should begin to discuss the transfer a year or so before it occurs. During discussions about the transfer, several issues need to be fully addressed. First, it should be emphasized that transfer is a natural phenomenon and adult providers are better trained to care for the adult patient. It is helpful to comment on the natural history of SCD, pointing out that many problems faced in childhood are acute, whereas those of the adult are more chronic. Another point of emphasis should be that the pediatric provider will still be available for questions and discussion, although not specifically involved in responsibilities of day-to-day care. Clearly, this is an issue faced by adolescents with many types of chronic illness, as discussed in Chapter 31, Adolescents with Chronic Illness.

## PROGNOSIS

Individuals with SCD have a shortened life expectancy. The CSSCD reported that the median life span of men and women who have HbSS was 42 years and 48 years, respectively.[3] An autopsy investigation of 306 patients revealed that the most common causes of death for all sickle cell variants were infection (33% to 48%), stroke (9.8%), splenic sequestration (6.6%), pulmonary thromboemboli (4.9%), renal failure (4.1%), PH (2.9%), hepatic failure (0.8%), massive hemolysis/red cell aplasia (0.4%), and left ventricular failure (0.4%). Death was sudden and unexpected in 40.8% of patients and usually occurred in the context of an acute event.[24]

The prognosis has improved in the past 2 decades, likely due to the use of prophylactic treatments, like hydroxyurea, and more comprehensive care offered by SCD centers.

## REFERENCES

1. Kinney TR, Ware RE. The adolescent with sickle cell anemia. *Hematol Oncol Clin North Am.* 1996;10:1255-1264

2. Redding-Lallinger R, Knoll C. Sickle cell disease - pathophysiology and treatment. *Curr Prob Pediatr Adolesc Health Care.* 2006;36:346-376

3. Stuart MJ, Nagel RL. Sickle-cell disease. *Lancet.* 2004;374: 1343-1360

4. Driscoll MC. Sickle cell disease. *Pediatr Rev.* 2007;28(7): 259-268

5. Platt OS, Thorington BD, Brambilla DJ, et al. Pain in sickle cell disease. Rates and risk factors. *N Engl J Med.* 1991;325:11-16

6. Rees DC, Olujohungbe AD, Parker NE, et al. Guidelines for the management of the acute painful crisis in sickle cell disease. *Br J Haematol.* 2003;120:744-752

7. Charache MD, Terrin ML, Moore RD, et al. Effect of hydroxyurea on the frequency of painful crises in sickle cell anemia. *N Engl J Med.* 1995:332:1317-1322

8. Amrolia PJ, Almeida A, Davies SC, Roberts IA. Therapeutic challenges in childhood sickle cell disease. Part 2: A problem-orientated approach. *Br J Haematol.* 2003;120:737-743

9. Heeney MM, Ware RE. Hydroxyurea for children with sickle cell disease. *Pediatr Clin North Am.* 2008;55(2):483-501

10. Vichinsky EP, Neumayr LD, Earles AN, et. Causes and outcomes of the acute chest syndrome in sickle cell disease. National Acute Chest Syndrome Study Group. *N Engl J Med.* 2000;342:1855-1865

11. Powars D, Wilson B, Imbus C, et al. The natural history of stroke in sickle cell disease. *Am J Med* 1978;65(3):461-471

12. Adams RJ, McKie VC, Hsu L, et al. Prevention of a first stroke in children with sickle cell anemia and abnormal results on transcranial Doppler ultrasonography. *N Engl J Med.* 1998;339(1):5-11

13. Gaston MH, Verter JI, Woods G, et al. Prophylaxis with oral penicillin in children with sickle cell anemia. A randomized trial. *N Engl J Med.* 1986;314(25):1593-1599

14. Falletta JM, Woods GM, Verter JI, et al. Discontinuing penicillin prophylaxis in children with sickle cell anemia. Prophylactic Penicillin Study II. *J Pediatr.* 1995;127(5):685-690

15. Almeida A, Roberts I. Bone involvement in sickle cell disease. *Br J Haematol.* 2005;129:482-490

16. Rogers ZR. Priapism in sickle cell disease. *Hematol Oncol Clin North Am.* 2005:19:917-928

17. Rackoff WR, Ohene-Frempong K, Month S, et al. Neurologic events after partial exchange transfusion for priapism in sickle cell disease. *J Pediatr.* 1992;120:882-885

18. Mantadakis E, Ewalt DH, Cavender JD, et al. Outpatient penile aspiration and epinephrine irrigation for young patients with sickle cell anemia and prolonged priapism. *Blood.* 2000;95(1):78-82

19. Serjeant GR. Physical and sexual development. In: Serjeant GR, Serjeant BE, ed. *Sickle Cell Disease*. New York: Oxford University Press;2001:393-407

20. Gladwin MT, Sachdev V, Jison ML, et al. Pulmonary hypertension as a risk factor for death in patients with sickle cell disease. *N Engl J Med.* 2004;350(9):886-895

21. Dharnidharka VR, Dabbagh S, Atiyeh B, Simpson P, Sarnaik S. Prevalence of microalbuminuria in children with sickle cell disease. *Pediatr Nephrol.* 1998;12(6):475-478

22. Powars DR, Elliott-Mills DD, Chan L, et al. Chronic renal failure in sickle cell disease: risk factors, clinical course, and mortality. *Ann Intern Med.* 1991;Oct15;115(8):614-620

23. Aguilar C, Vichinsky E, Naumayr L. Bone and joint disease in sickle cell disease. *Hematol Oncol Clin N Am.* 2005;19: 929-941

24. Emerson GG, Lutty GA. Effects of sickle cell disease on the eye: clinical features and treatment. *Hematol Oncol Clin N Am.* 2005:19:957-973

25. Serjeant GR, Loy LL, Crowther M, et al. Outcome of pregnancy in homozygous sickle cell disease. *Obstet Gynaecol.* 1994;103(6):1278-1285

26. Wanko SO, Telen MJ. Transfusion management in sickle cell disease. *Hematol Oncol Clin N Am.* 2005:19:803-808

27. Steinberg MH, Barton F, Castro O et al. Effect of hydroxyurea on mortality and morbidity in adult sickle cell anemia. *JAMA.* 2003;289(13):1645-1651

28. Hankins J, Aygun B. Pharmacotherapy in sickle cell disease - state of the art and future prospects. *Br J Haematol.* 2009;145(3):296-308

# CHAPTER 108

# Hemostasis and Thrombosis

J. NATHAN HAGSTROM, MD

This chapter focuses on the evaluation and management of the adolescent patient who may be at risk for bleeding or thrombosis. Inherited mild bleeding disorders may present during adolescence, while adolescents with existing bleeding disorders often experience a change in complications and new risks for bleeding during the adolescent years. Spontaneous deep venous thrombosis (DVT), extremely rare in children, can occur in adolescence, but more commonly, an adolescent may be found to have a prothrombotic condition because of a family history. Management of patients with bleeding and thrombotic disorders must take into account issues unique to the adolescent patient and must include the adolescent as a partner.

The goal of this chapter is to introduce the adolescent primary care provider to clinical hemostasis and thrombosis. In most cases the evaluation and management is done in partnership with a hematologist, preferably one who is associated with a hemostasis and thrombosis treatment center (also known as a hemophilia treatment center). Useful scientific data on the adolescent patient for the purpose of guiding evaluation and therapy of hemostatic and thrombotic disease are limited. Therefore one must rely on the art of medicine, using available science appropriately and judiciously, with expert interpretation and consultation when appropriate from those who have clinical experience in diagnosing and treating bleeding and thrombotic disorders. Table 108-1 lists important abbreviations used in this chapter.

**Table 108-1**

**Abbreviations**

| *Abbreviation* | *Description* |
|---|---|
| PT | Prothrombin time |
| PTT | Partial thromboplastin time |
| TT | Thromboplastin time |
| PFA-100 | Platelet function assay - 100 |
| VWF Ag | von Willebrand factor antigen |
| PAI-1 | Plasminogen activated inhibitor-1 |
| HHT | Hereditary hemorrhagic telangiectasia |
| ITP | Idiopathic thrombocytopenic purpura |
| TTP | Thrombotic thrombocytopenic purpura |
| HUS | Hemolytic uremic syndrome |
| DIC | Disseminated intravascular coagulation |
| INR | International normalized ratio |

## HEMOSTASIS

### EVALUATING THE ADOLESCENT WITH ABNORMAL BLEEDING

History is important for determining the probability that the adolescent has an identifiable bleeding disorder, or more practically speaking, is at increased risk for bleeding. Bruising is among the most unreliable symptoms. Nonetheless, spontaneous bruises that are larger than 2 to 3 centimeters and have an associated hematoma are more likely to be associated with a bleeding disorder. Bruises associated with trauma are even more difficult for determining clinical significance. Listening to the patient's level of concern can often be helpful. Epistaxis is common in bleeding disorders, but not always present, and certainly its presence is not specific for a bleeding disorder.[1] Epistaxis that requires medical attention or lasts longer than 10 minutes or occurs more frequently than once a week on average is more likely to be associated with a bleeding disorder. The examination can be helpful in validating the history. However, bruises are not always present at the time of evaluation and are not specific.

Diagnosing a bleeding disorder can be challenging for the primary care clinician.[2] Available laboratory tools lack sensitivity and specificity. The capacity for hemostasis is dynamic and there is considerable overlap between normal and abnormal. Currently available tests fail to accurately model the physiology of hemostasis and have wide ranges of normal. Mild bleeding disorders, by definition, are the result of only partial dysfunction or loss of capacity. Furthermore, the dynamic nature of the components of hemostasis exist in people with mild bleeding disorders to the same extent as those without. Normal test results do not rule out a mild bleeding disorder. In addition, abnormal test results do not always mean that the patient has a bleeding disorder or that the abnormal test result is the explanation for the abnormal bleeding. Often, repeat testing is required. In summary, because of the combination of variability introduced by physiology and inadequate testing, overlap occurs and bleeding disorders can be missed. In addition, coagulation testing is prone to inaccuracies if specimens are not collected or handled correctly, which could lead to false positives.

There is no reliable way to screen for bleeding disorders. The bleeding time lacks accuracy, precision, sensitivity, and specificity. It simply lacks the reliability necessary for clinical use, and most clinical laboratories no longer offer this test. The platelet function assay-100 (PFA-100) is an increasingly popular screening tool for defects of primary hemostasis. However, it only addresses some of the problems with the bleeding time, and therefore still lacks sensitivity and thus reliability as a screening tool.

Despite these limitations, laboratory testing still remains our primary source of data when determining the exact nature of someone's increased risk for bleeding. A laboratory evaluation starts with the complete blood count (CBC) to rule out quantitative platelet problems. The prothombin time/partial thromboplastin time (PT/PTT) and thromboplastin time (TT) are useful for ruling out a number of factor deficiencies often associated with severe bleeding. However, these simple, widely available laboratory screening tests will not detect the most common bleeding disorders, nor some rare severe bleeding disorders. Because von Willebrand disease (VWD) is so common, one must include the von Willebrand factor antigen (VWFAg) and activity as part of the initial screening. Unfortunately, the PTT is elevated in only 30% of people with mild VWD. Table 108-2 outlines the steps in laboratory testing of the adolescent with abnormal bleeding.

**Table 108-2**

**Evaluating Abnormal Bleeding**

| | *History* | *Examination* | *Labs* |
|---|---|---|---|
| Phase I | Bleeding with trauma and surgery | Bruises on the extremities | CBC |
| | Epistaxis | | PT/PTT |
| | Bruising | | TT |
| | Menorrhagia | | VWF A |
| | | | VWF activity |
| | | | Repeat VWF levels |
| Phase II | Family history of bleeding problems | | Platelet aggregation testing |
| | | | PAI-1 level |
| | | | Testing of family members for VWD, if indicated |
| | | | Factor XIII activity |
| Phase III | | | Antiplasmin level |

## EVALUATING MENORRHAGIA

A common bleeding complication in adolescent women is menorrhagia. In approximately 30% of cases, a bleeding disorder is a contributing factor.[3] Defining menorrhagia is challenging. History is important, but its sensitivity and specificity are often not sufficient. Women often think that their large amount of bleeding is normal. Objective measures of menstrual bleeding have been applied in the clinical research setting but are not practical for the everyday clinical setting. As a general rule, periods that last longer than 5 days, that include days heavy enough to use more than 6 to 8 pads a day, or that cause the adolescent to miss school because of the inability to manage the bleeding, are heavier than normal. Other features of menstrual bleeding in women with a bleeding disorder are significant dysmenorrhea, iron deficiency anemia, using both tampons and pads, and blood-soiled clothes or bed sheets. In some cases discussing how soaked the pads are when changed is helpful, but recall is often challenging and the emotional embarrassment that some adolescents experience when discussing the subject make recall even less accurate. In those patients where it is desirable to more objectively define the menorrhagia, it is possible to have the individual track blood loss using a chart, which can be scored by the practitioner. Very little exchange of words is necessary and the objectivity increases. However, the menstrual chart is a challenge to keep.

A young woman with significant menorrhagia should be evaluated for a bleeding disorder[4] with specific testing for VWD (VWFAg, VWF ristocetin cofactor activity), qualitative platelet disorders (platelet aggregation testing), factor deficiencies (PT/PTT/TT), and plasminogen activator inhibitor-1 deficiency (PAI-1). In cases where all laboratory tests are normal but the patient clinically has a significant bleeding problem, consider screening for factor XIII deficiency and alpha-2-antiplasmin deficiency (Table 108-2).

### ASSESSING SURGICAL BLEEDING RISK

The primary care practitioner is often asked to clear patients for surgery. Assessing the risk of bleeding is an important component of the evaluation. Unfortunately, there is no specific process proven sensitive in identifying an increased risk of bleeding. One can use a combination of symptoms, signs, and family history to determine a level of suspicion, followed by laboratory tests if appropriately indicated by the history or physical examination, with the intent of either increasing or decreasing that suspicion.[5]

There is no laboratory test or group of tests that have sufficient sensitivity to be considered screening tests. As noted, the bleeding time lacks accuracy and precision and most laboratories no longer even offer this test. The PT, PTT, and TT can screen for some moderate and severe bleeding disorders, but do not screen for VWD, qualitative platelet disorders, factor XIII deficiency, PAI 1 deficiency, or antiplasmin deficiency. It has been shown for tonsillectomy, 1 of the highest risk surgeries for bleeding, that the PT and PTT lack sufficient sensitivity to warrant using for routine screening.[6]

**Table 108-3**

**Assessing Surgical Risk for Bleeding**

| *Phase* | *Patient History* | *Interventions and Tests to Consider Prior to Surgery* | |
|---|---|---|---|
| Phase 1 | Have you or anyone in your immediate family had bleeding problems after surgery or dental extraction?<br>Do you bruise easily or have you ever had problems with nosebleeds or heavy periods?<br>Has anyone in your immediate family been diagnosed with a bleeding disorder? | No laboratory tests are available that have sufficient sensitivity to screen for risk of bleeding during surgery<br>If answers are not concerning for a bleeding disorder in the patient or family, then patient can be cleared for surgery as having normal risk of bleeding | |
| Phase 2a | History suggests the potential for a bleeding disorder in the family, but not in the patient. | PT/PTT<br>TT<br>CBC | VWF antigen<br>VWF activity |
| Phase 2b | History suggests the potential for a bleeding disorder in the patient. | Phase 1 testing<br>Platelet aggregation testing of Phase 1 testing normal<br>Consider repeating VWF levels if <75 with first testing | |
| Phase 3 | Patient's history very suggestive of a bleeding disorder, but Phase 2a and 2b testing normal. | Consider repeating VWF levels a third time and consider testing a potentially affected first-degree relative<br>PAI-1 level<br>Antiplasmin level<br>Factor XIII activity screen | |

If there is a personal history or a strong family history, particularly in a first-degree relative, then a laboratory evaluation needs to be carried out. Table 108-3 shows a presurgical evaluation. The importance of history cannot be underestimated as the most important clinical screening tool. However, if a patient has been challenged sufficiently to bring out a mild bleeding disorder, the history will fall short. Nosebleeds that have occurred more than once a month, and on occasion have lasted longer than 10 to 15 minutes, may be indicative. Prolonged bleeding with cuts and abrasions (eg, a cut from shaving that is still oozing an hour or 2 later) is potentially indicative. Bruises that are bigger than a quarter and associated with a hematoma, especially if they occur on places other than the distal lower and distal upper extremities, are potentially indicative. Bleeding with dental extraction or surgery is also important to note. Gum bleeding with tooth brushing is also more common in people with bleeding disorders.

## EVALUATING THE ELEVATED PTT

An elevated PTT may indicate an inherited or acquired factor deficiency, the presence of a lupus anticoagulant, a decrease in multiple clotting factors from poor production (liver disease, vitamin K deficiency) or consumption (disseminated intravascular coagulation [DIC], severe bleeding) or from lab error.[7] The first step is to repeat the test if PTT is only slightly above normal. If PTT is significantly elevated, the test is repeated with a mixing study. A mixing study is designed to separate factor deficiencies from inhibitors. The patient's plasma is mixed 1:1 with normal pooled plasma. Factor deficiencies will be corrected and the PTT will normalize. If an inhibitor is present, the PTT will either not change or will be only partially correct. Table 108-4 shows a step-wise laboratory evaluation for an elevated PTT. The author occasionally has seen the patient who has a slight elevation in the PTT, but a normal PT, who has very mild clinically insignificant vitamin K deficiency from either antibiotic therapy or a diarrheal illness. The PTT corrects after a short 3-day course of oral vitamin K at 5 mg per day.

**Table 108-4**

**Evaluating the Elevated PPT**

| *Phase* | *Test* |
|---|---|
| Phase 1 | Repeat PPT |
| | Mixing study |
| | Lupus anticoagulant screen |
| Phase 2 | Factor VIII activity |
| | Factor IX activity |
| | Factor XI activity |
| | Factor XII activity |
| Phase 3 | Prekalikrein |
| | High molecular weight kininogen |

## VON WILLEBRAND DISEASE

von Willebrand disease is the most common bleeding disorder. The precise prevalence is difficult to determine given the difficulty with making the diagnosis of mild disease. There are 3 types of VWD (Table 108-5): In Type 1, the mildest and most common, there are low levels of VWF and there may be low levels of factor VIII; in Type 2, which includes several subtypes, VWF does not work optimally; in Type 3, the most severe, there is no VWF at all and there are low levels of factor VIII. von Willebrand disease causes a defect in primary hemostasis, making bruising, epistaxis, oral bleeding, menorrhagia, and bleeding with surgeries and dental extractions common complications. Diagnosing VWD can be challenging.[8] There is no screening test that has sensitivity. The only screening tests are the tests for VWF

**Table 108-5**

**Types of von Willebrand Disease**

| *Type* | *Bleeding Complications* | *Treatment* |
|---|---|---|
| Type 1 | Bruising | Desmopressin |
| | Epistaxis | Intranasal |
| | Menorrhagia | Subcutaneously |
| | Bleeding with surgery involving mucosal surfaces (eg, dental extraction, tonsillectomy) | Intravenously<br>VWF containing factor concentrates<br>Amicar |
| Type 2 | Same as Type 1<br>Bleeding more frequent and more severe<br>Same as Type 2 | Desmopressin may be used, but effect often minimal and brief<br>VWF containing factor concentrates<br>Amicar |
| Type 3 | May have bleeding similar to hemophilia with hemarthroses | VWF containing factor concentrates |

(VWF antigen and VWF activity). von Willebrand factor activity may be tested using an enzyme-linked immunoabsorbent assay (ELISA)-based format that relies on intact Gp Ib binding function, VWF ristocetin cofactor activity, and VWF collagen binding activity. Factor VIII activity is usually done as part of the panel in the event that there is a discrepancy. A hallmark of Type 1 VWD is that a normal set of results doesn't rule out VWD. The difficulty with making the diagnosis of VWD is that VWF levels can be within normal limits at any given time in a person with deficiency, because levels rise with stress, activity, infection, and other stimuli. Only after 3 carefully collected sets of tests are done, when the patient is free of stress, can one have any certainty that VWD has been ruled out. The diagnosis of VWD needs careful evaluation of these 3 components: personal history of abnormal bleeding, laboratory tests suggestive of VWD, and a family history of abnormal bleeding (and even more helpful is a first-degree relative diagnosed with VWD).

To make a definitive diagnosis of VWD all 3 components of a strong personal history of bleeding and/or bruising, a history of VWD in a first-degree relative, and abnormal laboratory testing is required.[9] One can make a presumptive diagnosis of probable VWD if 2 of the 3 criteria are met. The typical tests done to screen for VWD are factor VIII activity, VWF antigen, and VWF activity. The activity is often measured as the VWF ristocetin cofactor activity, but can also be measured using an ELISA-based activity assay or the collagen-binding assay referred to previously.

Easy bruising, recurrent and often prolonged epistaxis, prolonged bleeding with lacerations and other similar types of tissue injury, and menorrhagia are the most common bleeding problems encountered by those with VWD.[10] Mild Type 1 VWD rarely needs specific treatment. It is advisable to use preventive therapy prior to invasive procedures such as significant dental work (eg, extractions of teeth with deep roots, deep nerve blocks) and surgical procedures. Prolonged nose bleeds and heavy periods are the most common bleeding complications requiring medical treatment. There are 2 methods used to increase VWF levels into the normal range: (1) desmopressin, given intranasally or as an injectable (subcutaneous or intravenous), and (2) VWF concentrate (eg, Humate-P).[11] Table 108-5 describes the types of VWD and their treatment options.

It is not uncommon for an adolescent to be diagnosed with a mild bleeding disorder. More severe bleeding disorders are generally diagnosed earlier in childhood. At the time of diagnosis, it is important to reassure the adolescent that this is a mild and treatable condition that doesn't lead to significant restrictions or impairments now or later in life. In fact, it is sometimes useful to point out that having a specific diagnosis is actually helpful if the adolescent has been experiencing significant problems with epistaxis or menorrhagia.

## QUALITATIVE PLATELET DISORDERS

Qualitative bleeding disorders include well-characterized severe defects, marginally defined moderate functional abnormalities, and more poorly defined, and sometimes difficult to measure, mild qualitative defects.[12] It is likely that qualitative platelet abnormalities make up the most common causes of mild bleeding problems, but that a lack of accurate and sensitive tools for diagnosing these disorders makes them second most commonly diagnosed to VWD. Platelet aggregation studies are the most common and most widely available tests for screening and diagnosing qualitative platelet disorders. However, normal testing does not necessarily rule out a defect. Additionally, platelet function testing is technically challenging and abnormal results may be falsely determined.

The mild qualitative platelet disorders are not easily characterized, but typically are of the storage pool defect type. One of the most severe is Hermansky-Pudlak syndrome. This disorder is associated with albinism. Desmopressin may assist with minor bleeding in these disorders. Aminocaproic acid is also used for recurrent, persistent, mucosal bleeding. Platelet transfusions are needed for severe bleeding and trauma and high-risk surgeries.

There are a number of rare, severe, congenital platelet disorders: Bernard-Soulier syndrome, Glanzmann thrombasthenia, and May-Hegglin anomaly to name just a few. These severe congenital platelet disorders include defects in number, function, or both. In these cases, platelet transfusions are needed for significant bleeding and for any surgical procedures.

## HEMOPHILIA

Hemophilia A and B, due to factor VIII or IX deficiency respectively, are X-linked recessive disorders, although affected females have been described, and carriers are at increased risk for bleeding. Hemophilia C, due to factor XI deficiency, is an autosomal recessive disorder and typically only homozygous patients are affected, but carriers may be at increased risk for mild bleeding, especially menorrhagia. Hemophilia (A, B, or C) can be detected using the PTT. The specific type and severity is determined using specific factor activity assays. Severe factor VIII and IX deficiencies are indistinguishable clinically, whereas severe factor XI deficiency is associated with fewer bleeding complications.

Severe hemophilia is associated with recurrent severe hemarthroses, eventually resulting in a chronic arthropathy if untreated.[13] It is also associated with a risk of intracranial hemorrhage, both spontaneous and following head trauma. In addition, severe bleeding complications can occur with trauma, even seemingly minor trauma.

Fortunately for those with hemophilia A and B, there are factor concentrates available.[14] Both plasma derived and recombinant factor concentrates are utilized, and each is safe and effective. Recombinant products have a theoretical safety advantage. The newer generation of recombinant products are manufactured without the use of animal or human proteins in the tissue culture or purification stages and do not add albumin to stabilize the factor when lyophilizing.

Prophylaxis is being increasingly used.[15] People with hemophilia are now more active and participating in a wider variety of athletic activities. A modified prophylaxis regimen is designed to be tailored to the individual, which may include the timing of infusions to certain athletic events or activities. The adolescent patient will then need to change the individualized prophylactic regimen as activities change in type or intensity. The older adolescent, who may be doing fewer activities that create a risk of trauma to the joints or head, may find himself or herself doing fewer infusions.

An issue in hemophilia care that affects young adolescents is the concept of self-infusion, which includes taking over the responsibility of hemophilia care from the parents, and performing the venous access and infusions themselves. This is a huge transition for most young adolescents. Education and encouragement from their providers is critical to success.

## PLASMINOGEN ACTIVATOR INHIBITOR-1 DEFICIENCY

Two types of PAI-1 deficiency have been described: moderately severe, autosomal recessive form, often described in isolated communities, and a milder form that may be autosomal dominant. This latter form, with unclear genetics, is considered a mild risk factor for bleeding. Mucosal bleeding is most common and is usually mild. However, menorrhagia can be significant enough to require therapeutic intervention.

## RARE BLEEDING DISORDERS

Most rare bleeding disorders are severe and diagnosed early in life.[16] Factor XIII deficiency is one example in which spontaneous bleeding and severe bruising is less common than in severe hemophilia. Prophylaxis is strongly encouraged in severe factor XIII deficiency, however, much like in severe hemophilia.

Severe factor deficiencies, such as prothrombin deficiency, factor X deficiency, factor V deficiency, afibrinogenemia and others, are also rare and have variable rates of bleeding complications. Although factor concentrates are being developed for some of these rare bleeding disorders, only severe factor VII deficiency has a US Food and Drug Administration (FDA) approved factor concentrate that can be used to replace the missing factor. In other cases, plasma (contains all factors) or cryoprecipitate (contains fibrinogen and factor XIII, as well as VWF and factor VIII) are used.

## CHRONIC MANAGEMENT FOR THE ADOLESCENT WITH A BLEEDING DISORDER

The adolescent with a bleeding disorder requires comprehensive chronic disease management much like other chronic diseases. The primary care provider is important in assisting the adolescent in transitioning from parental responsibility to self-responsibility. The primary care provider can also play a key role in reassuring adolescents that having a bleeding disorder does not mean they must consider themselves different from their peers or have less potential, and that with proper care and attention they will lead a safe and fulfilling life.

The National Hemophilia Foundation is an excellent resource for educational tools. Information about bleeding disorders and their treatment can be found on its Web site (www.nhf.org).

It is recommended that people with severe bleeding disorders receive immunizations subcutaneously.[17]

## HEREDITARY HEMORRHAGIC TELANGIECTASIA

Because hereditary hemorrhagic telangiectasia (HHT) may first present in the adolescent period, this disorder, although rare, is worth mentioning. Hereditary hemorrhagic telangiectasia is a progressive abnormal development of small blood vessels. It often presents in adolescence and early adulthood. Mucosal bleeding complications are common.[18]

## ACQUIRED BLEEDING DISORDERS

Significant bleeding of new onset is uncommon in the adolescent. Acute immune thrombocytopenic purpura (ITP) is the most common cause. Disseminated intravascular coagulation is the least common cause, but is often life threatening and challenging to manage. Acquired inhibitors of coagulation factors can occur, but are also exceedingly rare. The most common acquired inhibitor encountered in adolescents is hypothrombinemia associated with a lupus anticoagulant.[19] The lupus anticoagulant results in an elevated PTT in most cases, but the PT is usually normal. When hypoprothrombinemia is present, the PT is prolonged as well.

The lupus anticoagulant alone is not associated with bleeding; rather it can be associated with thrombosis. When hypoprothrombinemia is present, the patient is at risk for bleeding. The bleeding risk begins to increase significantly once the level falls below 20%. In cases of significant acute bleeding with a prothrombin inhibitor, recombinant factor VIIa may be used. Immunosuppressive therapy is used for more long-term management.

### THROMBOCYTOPENIA

Thrombocytopenia may be congenital or acquired. In the adolescent with new onset bruising and bleeding, acquired thrombocytopenia is more likely. Box 108-1 lists the most common causes of acquired thrombocytopenia. The initial evaluation of thrombocytopenia includes a thorough physical examination and a review of the peripheral smear and other cell lines with a repeat CBC. A bone marrow aspiration is done when bone marrow disease resulting in poor production of platelets is suspected. Consultation with a hematologist is often helpful. In cases of mild thrombocytopenia, a follow-up CBC may demonstrate quick resolution of the thrombocytopenia.

The most common cause of acquired thrombocytopenia is immune thrombocytopenic purpura (ITP).[20] In acute ITP the bruising and petechiae typically have a rapid onset, with spontaneous resolution within 3 to 6 months. Chronic ITP tends to have an insidious onset, typically does not resolve,[21] and can be associated with other autoimmune phenomena and with immunodeficiency, but usually is isolated. The treatment options for ITP are listed in Box 108-2.

**Box 108-1**
***Causes of Thrombocytopenia***

| *Causes of Acquired Thrombocytopenia* | *Causes of Congenital Thrombocytopenia* |
|---|---|
| Acute ITP | Type 2B von Willebrand disease |
| Chronic ITP | Bernard-Soulier disease |
| Viral-related suppression | May-Heglin anomaly |
| Drug related | Familial thrombocytopenia |
| TTP/HUS | |
| Aplastic anemia | |
| Bone marrow infiltrative disease | |
| DIC | |
| Hypersplenism | |

**Box 108-2**
***Treatment Options for ITP***

| *Acute ITP* | *Chronic ITP* |
|---|---|
| Observation | Observation |
| WinRho | Splenectomy |
| IVIG | Rifuximab |
| Prednisone | IVIG |
| | WinRho |
| | Dexamethasone |

## THROMBOTIC DISORDERS

Thrombosis is a rare event in children and usually occurs in the context of a combination of significant risk factors, the most important of these being a central venous catheter.[22] In adolescents, spontaneous thrombosis occurs with a higher incidence than in children, but it is still exceedingly rare. Nonetheless, it is helpful for those who treat adolescent patients to be familiar with these diseases. In addition, risk factors are commonly inherited and should be identified in asymptomatic relatives. It also is important to counsel an adolescent about signs and symptoms of thrombotic disease and acquired risk factors to avoid. Certain chronic diseases in adolescents are associated with an increased risk of thrombosis. These include sickle cell disease, systemic lupus erythematosis, inflammatory bowel disease, nephrotic syndrome, congenital heart disease, and cancer.[23]

### PROTHROMBOTIC CONDITIONS

Perhaps the most important inherited risk factor for thrombosis is having a strong family history. In most such families, an inherited risk factor for thrombosis, or a prothrombotic condition, can be identified. However, it is possible that there are genetic risk factors that have not yet been identified. As part of routine health care maintenance, it is advised that the provider inquire regarding any history of myocardial infarction, stroke, pulmonary embolism, (PE) or deep venous thrombosis at a young age in close relatives.

Unfortunately, despite an increasing scientific understanding of hemostasis and thrombosis, strong clinical tools for assessing risk are still lacking. Suffice it to say that performing a battery of tests is probably not as helpful as one would surmise.[24] This is due in large part because most of the inherited risk factors are relatively weak and the risk increases exponentially with age.[25]

**Table 108-6**

**Relative Risk (RR) of Thrombosis with an Inherited Thrombophilia and the Added Risk with Oral Contraceptive (OC) Use**

| *Risk Factor* | *Relative Risk* |
|---|---|
| Factor V Leiden | 4–5 |
| Prothrombin 20210A | 1–3 |
| Protein C deficiency | 4–5 |
| Protein S deficiency | 4–5 |
| Antithrombin deficiency | 8–12 |
| Oral contraceptives (OC) without an inherited risk factor | 2–3 |
| OC + factor V Leiden | 15–20 |
| OC + Prothrombin 20210A | 5–7 |
| OC + Protein C deficiency | 5–7 |
| OC + Protein S deficiency | 4–6 |
| OC + Antithrombin deficiency | 13–15 |

Table 108-6 lists the common inherited risk factors for thrombosis and the relative risk compared to the general population.

The most common inherited monogenetic risk factor that has clearly been linked to an increased risk of venous thrombosis across the life span is factor V Leiden.[26] Universal screening is not recommended. This is primarily because there is no specific effective primary prophylactic intervention that is sufficiently safe to use in asymptomatic individuals given the relatively low risk of thrombosis. The most common clinical scenario in which the adolescent provider will consider screening is for the adolescent girl considering oral contraceptives (OCPs).[27,28] Current cost analyses, however, fail to support screening of all women considering OCPs. A compromise is to screen those individuals with a strong family history. Given the prevalence of factor V Leiden and the prothrombin 20210 A mutations, these are the only risk factors that ought to be screened; if another specific risk factor has been identified in the family, then that specific risk factor can be tested.

Management of prothrombotic conditions in the asymptomatic individual consists primarily of counseling. As rare as thrombosis is in adolescents, it is not uncommon for adolescents to be identified as having an increased risk of thrombosis across their life span. It is helpful for adolescent practitioners to be aware of these conditions to be prepared to assist the adolescent at risk. As mentioned, primary medical prophylaxis is not done.

In general the most cost-effective and safe approach is to offer education and counseling. This includes education regarding the signs and symptoms of thromboembolic disease (including limb swelling with or without pain or discoloration, sudden chest pain with or without dyspnea, and severe headaches, neurological deficits, and partial loss of vision) and counseling regarding acquired risk factors to try to avoid (including OCPs, pregnancy, major surgery, orthopedic surgery, immobility, obesity, and smoking).

The most challenging and perhaps most common issue that the adolescent provider will face is a patient with an asymptomatic, inherited, prothrombotic condition who is considering OCPs.[28] Progesterone-only hormonal contraception is preferred over an estrogen-progesterone combination pill in these cases. The use of intrauterine systems is increasing in the adolescent population, and these may be considered in such cases. Because the risks of oral contraceptive use are still relatively low for young women (Table 108-6), this situation has not been clasified as an "absolute" contraindication but rather a "relative" one. The decision is ultimately the patient's, but careful guidance needs to be provided, and for adolescent patients, decisions regarding parental involvement need to be carefully considered. One issue included in the discussions with patients and parents is the fact that the risk of thromboembolic disease during pregnancy is higher than it is with OCPs.[29]

## DIAGNOSING THROMBOEMBOLIC DISEASE

The first step is to include thrombotic disease in the differential diagnosis when confronted with a patient complaint that could be associated with thrombosis. Because of its relative rarity, thrombosis is not often considered when an adolescent presents with limb swelling or pain, chest pain or dyspnea, or headaches. It is sometimes helpful to do a d-dimer level as a screening test. This may help increase or decrease one's suspicion, assisting in decision making about imaging.

Ultrasound is the most commonly used imaging modality and has sufficient sensitivity for ruling out a proximal lower extremity deep vein thrombosis (DVT). However, for the upper venous system, contrast venography must be considered the gold standard. Magnetic resonance (MR) venography is being used with increased frequency, but sensitivity of this method does not match that of contrast venography. Magnetic resonance imaging (MRI) is a reasonable test for dural sinus thrombosis; however, it is less reliable for cerebral vein thrombosis.

## MANAGEMENT OF THROMBOEMBOLIC DISEASE

The primary goal of antithrombotic therapy in the context of an acute DVT is to prevent death from PE. A secondary goal is to prevent extension of the thrombus, which increases the likelihood of developing localized complications, including postphlebitic syndrome. Postphlebitic syndrome is the result of chronic venous insufficiency and impedance to flow, which can result in persistent swelling, pain, and poor healing.[30]

Low molecular weight heparin (LMWH) is now the most common therapy used in the acute setting of a DVT.[31] The advantages of LMWH are much more predictable pharmacokinetics, ease of delivery (subcutaneous vs intravenous), lower risk of heparin-induced thrombocytopenia, and possibly a lower risk of bleeding complications. The dose for adolescents and adults for the treatment of acute DVT is 1 mg/kg/dose every 12 hours subcutaneously. Although not always recommended, this author uses the antifactor Xa heparin assay to follow levels, with a goal of 0.5 to 1.0 units per ml heparin activity 4 hours after an injection. When excessive bleeding occurs, protamine can be used as a reversing agent. However, its reversing effect may not be 100%, and the duration of effect may be shorter than that of the LMWH.

Standard heparin is still useful in certain settings. However, it can be a challenge to manage a heparin infusion because of all the dynamic variables that affect the therapeutic results. Heparin is especially difficult to manage in the setting of an acute-phase reaction because heparin binds to acute-phase reactant proteins.

Warfarin (eg, Coumadin) remains the standard for long-term antithrombotic therapy.[32] It is the only widely used, well-proven oral agent. Typically, Coumadin is started once heparin has been initiated and is therapeutic. The primary reason for this is that Coumadin has a long onset of action and can actually be prothrombotic when first started. The levels of protein C drop before the prothrombin levels, because of its shorter half-life. Coumadin can be started with a loading dose if the patient is anticoagulated with heparin. Once the INR has risen to >1.5, then the dose is reduced to a maintenance dose. Once the international normalized ratio (INR) has reached the therapeutic range, the heparin can be discontinued. Box 108-3 describes a common approach to managing warfarin (Coumadin); Table 108-7 lists the warfarin (Coumadin) adjustments depending on INR.

Coumadin must be carefully monitored to assure safe and therapeutic levels. The narrow therapeutic window of antithrombotic therapy reflects the many dynamic variables that affect the pharmacokinetics and actions of these medications. This is no less true for Coumadin with the many dietary, medicinal, genetic, and physiological factors that can affect the final therapeutic outcome and risk of adverse events. Because Coumadin blocks the recycling of vitamin K, anything that changes vitamin K status changes the effect of Coumadin. Vitamin K comes from certain foods, such as green leafy vegetables, broccoli and some cooking oils, and from the intestinal bacteria. Because antibiotics reduce intestinal flora, they can enhance the effect of Coumadin, increasing the INR. Genetic polymorphisms in the CYP2C9 and VKORC1 genes can also affect the response to Coumadin.[33]

The risk of bleeding with Coumadin can be minimized with careful monitoring. If the INR has risen to >5, the risk of bleeding starts to increase significantly. In some cases, rapid reversal of Coumadin may be desired. The most commonly used therapeutic intervention is to give fresh frozen plasma (FPP). Intravenous vitamin K in low doses has also been used with success.[34] Oral vitamin K can be used but is associated with difficulty

### Box 108-3

#### *Maintenance (Long-Term) Warfarin (Coumadin) Therapy*

The INR should be checked twice weekly for 1 to 2 weeks after therapeutic INR achieved following the initiation of warfarin therapy.

The INR is then checked weekly for 3 to 4 weeks, then if stable, every 2 weeks for 4 weeks, then every 3 weeks for 6 weeks, then every 4 weeks thereafter.

Five to 7 days after the start of any new medications, the INR should be checked, then follow previous sequence starting with weekly INRs.

After a dose adjustment of the warfarin, the INR should be checked in 5 to 7 days, then the previous sequence is followed, starting with weekly INRs.

### Table 108-7

#### Warfarin (Coumadin) Adjustments for Long-Term Antithrombotic Therapy

| *INR* | *Warfarin Adjustment* |
|---|---|
| 1.1–1.49 | Increase dose by 20% |
| 1.5–1.99 | Increase dose by 10% |
| 2.0–3.09 | No change |
| 3.1–3.5 | Decrease dose by 10% |
| >3.5 | Hold until INR <3.5, then restart at 20% less than previous dose (check INR every other day) |

in getting the patient to a therapeutic level once the Coumadin is restarted. In cases of severe bleeding, while awaiting FPP to arrive, some have advocated using recombinant factor VIIa.

For patients on anticoagulant therapy who need an invasive procedure, it is recommended that the anticoagulant therapy be discontinued to bring the level of anticoagulation down to a safe level. For most surgical procedures an INR of <1.5 is safe. For high-risk procedures, complete reversal to achieve a normal INR may be advisable. For most procedures, holding the Coumadin for 3 to 4 days prior to the procedure is sufficient. When using LMWH, holding 1 dose is sufficient for most procedures; for high-risk procedures, holding 2 doses is advised. Standard heparin needs to be discontinued for at least 6 hours prior to the procedure. For most procedures, the anticoagulant therapy may be restarted immediately after surgery. The decision to bridge Coumadin with heparin (standard or low molecular weight) is related to the risk of thrombosis. In most cases, bridging is not necessary. However, for some mechanical valves (eg, tricuspid valves), it is highly recommended that bridging with heparin for patients on Coumadin be used.

The duration of antithrombotic therapy depends on the risk of serious bleeding and the risk of recurrent thrombosis. Balancing these 2 risks can be challenging, but certainly need to be individualized. Those with inherited risk factors have a higher risk of recurrence, although not all risk factors are equal in this regard. For example, antithrombin deficiency is associated with a higher risk than factor V Leiden. The risk of bleeding is lower in the adolescent compared to older adults who have been included in large randomized studies investigating duration; therefore, it is somewhat unfair to extrapolate data. In addition, a spontaneous DVT in an adolescent is such a rare event that one must consider that individual to have risk factors that are inherent to that individual. The risk of bleeding is less than those patients with cancer or on multiple medications.

Interventional radiology has developed several tools over the past decade to assist in the management of acute DVT. In addition to placing caval filters, stents can be placed through venous thrombi to reduce the symptoms associated with venous obstruction; in addition catheters can be placed to deliver localized thrombolytic therapy. In some cases the clot can be mechanically removed.

The role of follow-up imaging is unclear. Some practitioners will use the rate of resolution of the thrombus or the persistence of thrombus by imaging to dictate duration of therapy or to assist the patient in determining risk of recurrence and risk of postphlebitic syndrome.

## TYPES OF THROMBOEMBOLIC DISEASE

Deep venous thrombosis most commonly occurs in the lower extremities, but can also occur in the upper venous system. In adolescents, spontaneous DVT typically occurs in the setting of acquired or inherited risk factors. In addition to the previously mentioned molecular and biochemical risk factors, there are also anatomic and mechanical risk factors. In the lower extremities, an anatomical variant in which the iliac artery passes over the vein causing compression is often found as a contributing factor in spontaneous DVT. An anatomical variant in the upper extremities may also predispose to DVT.[35]

Pulmonary embolism is a life-threatening complication of DVT and a primary reason for treating DVT with antithrombotic therapy. Significant PE typically occurs in the context of a DVT in the lower extremities, where the veins are large enough to create thrombi that will cause significant occlusion in the pulmonary arterial system.

Dural sinus thrombosis is less common in the adolescent than lower extremity DVT. It can be associated with the molecular and biochemical risk factors mentioned previously.[36] In addition, central nervous system (CNS) infections and trauma are also risk factors. Deep vein thrombosis has also been associated with OCPs, nephrotic syndrome, ulcerative colitis, and systemic lupus erythematosis.

### Hepatic and Portal Vein Thrombosis

The Budd-Chiari syndrome refers to thrombosis of the hepatic vein(s). This thrombotic event may occur in the setting of liver disease (eg, cirrhosis, liver transplant) and will present as acute hepatomegaly with pain. Portal vein thrombosis is uncommon but can occur in the setting of intra-abdominal infections or trauma, as well as liver disease, and may present with splenomegaly, abdominal pain, signs of portal hypertension, and often fever.

### Stroke

Stroke is uncommon in the adolescent. However, it can occur with carotid dissection after head or neck trauma. Stroke may also occur in systemic lupus erythematosis and/or antiphospholipid antibody syndrome. Stroke secondary to a prothrombotic condition is uncommon, but can occur, and when it does, without any other explanation, one must consider paradoxical embolism through a patent foramen ovale.[37] This is probably the most common cause of an idiopathic thromboembolic stroke in the adolescent or young adult (ie, a venous thrombus embolizing from left to right through a patent foramen ovale and then into the cerebral circulation). One can never be certain that this has been completely ruled out (or ruled in, for that matter). Nevertheless, it is advisable that a transesophageal echocardiogram be done, often with a bubble study, while the patient performs a valsalva maneuver, to rule out a setup for right to left shunting through a patent foramen ovale. If this is thought to be the cause of stroke in an adolescent or young adult, then it is advisable that the patent foramen ovale be closed.

The management of stroke depends on the underlying cause and the risk of recurrence. DVT type therapy is used in the setting of antiphospholipid antibodies and a paradoxical embolism. Antiplatelet agents are used if there is a risk of recurrence when venous thrombi or antiphospholipid antibodies are not thought to be contributing factors.

## REFERENCES


1. Sandoval C, Dong S, Visintainer PM, Ozkaynak F, Jayabose S. Clinical and laboratory features of 178 children with recurrent epistaxis. *J Pediatr Hemat/Oncol.* 2002;24:47-49

2. Favaloro EJ. Investigating people with mucocutaneous bleeding suggestive of primary hemostatic defects: a low likelihood of a definitive diagnosis? *Haematologica.* 2007;92(3):357-365

3. Bevan JA, Maloney KW, Hillery CA, Gill JC, Montgomery RR, Scott JP. Bleeding disorders: a common cause of menorrhagia in adolescents. *J Pediatr.* 2000;138:856-861

4. Matytsina LA, Zoloto EV, Sinenko LV, Greydanus DE. Dysfunctional uterine bleeding in adolescents: concepts of pathophysiology and management. *Prim Care.* 2006;33: 503-515

5. Girolami A, Luzzatto G, Varvarikis C, Pellati D, Sartori R, Girolami B. Main clinical manifestations of a bleeding diathesis: an often disregarded aspect of medical and surgical history taking. *Hemophilia.* 2005;11:193-202

6. Asaf T, Reuveni H, Yermiahu T, et al. The need for routine pre operative coagulation screening tests (Prothrombin Time PT/Partial Thromboplastin Time PTT) for healthy children undergoing elective tonsillectomy and/or adenoidectomy. *Int J Pediatr Otorhin.* 2001;61:217-222

7. Shah MD, O'Riordan MA, Alexander SW. Evaluation of prolonged APTT values in the pediatric population. *Clin Pediatr.* 2006:347-353

8. Michiels JJ, Gadisseur A, Budde U, et al. Characterization, classification, and treatment of von Willebrand diseases: a critical appraisal of the literature and personal experiences. *Sem Thromb Hemost.* 2005;31:577-601

9. Kasper CK. Von Willebrand disease. *Von Willebrand Dis.* 2005:1-57

10. Kadir RA, Chi C. Women and von Willebrand disease: controversies in diagnosis and management. *Sem Thromb Hemost.* 2006;32:605-615

11. Mannucci PM. Treatment of von Willebrand's disease. *N Engl J Med.* 2004;351(7):683-694

12. Nurden AT. Qualitative disorders of platelets and megakaryocytes. *J Thromb Haemos.* 2005;3:1773-1782

13. Manno CS. Management of bleeding disorders in children. *Hematology Am Soc Hematol Educ Program.* 2005; 416-422

14. Hoots WK, Nugent DJ. Evidence for the benefits of prophylaxis in the management of hemophilia A. *Thromb Haemost.* 2006;96(4):433-440

15. Manco-Johnson MJ, Abshire TC, Shapiro AD, et al. Prophylaxis versus episodic treatment to prevent joint disease in boys with severe hemophilia. *N Engl J Med.* 2007;357(6):535-544

16. Bolton-Maggs P. The rare coagulation disorders. *Treatment of Hemophilia.* Montréal, Québec: World Federation of Hemophilia;2006

17. Makris M, Conlon CP, Watson HG. Immunization of patients with bleeding disorders. *Haemophilia.* 2003;9:541-546

18. Sabbà C. A rare and misdiagnosed bleeding disorder: hereditary hemorrhagic telangiectasia. *J Thromb Haemost.* 2005;3(10):2201-2210

19. Harper JL, Tisdale SE, Hagstrom JN. Hypoprothrombinemia. *eMedicine Pediatrics.* 2006. Available at: www.emedicine.com/ped/topic1133.htm. Accessed October 9, 2007

20. Tarantino M. Recent advances in the treatment of childhood immune thrombocytopenic purpura. *Semin Hematol.* 2006;43(3 suppl 5):S11-S17

21. Blanchette V. Childhood chronic immune thrombocytopenic purpura (ITP). *Blood Rev.* 2002;16(1):23-26

22. Chan AK, Deveber G, Monagle P, Brooker LA, Massicotte PM. Venous thrombosis in children. *J Thromb Haemost.* 2003;1(7):1443-1455

23. Albisetti M, Moeller A, Waldvogel K, et al. Congenital prothrombotic disorders in children with peripheral venous and arterial thromboses. *Acta Haematologica.* 2006:49-155

24. Sass AE, Neufeld EJ. Risk factors for thromboembolism in teens: when should I test? *Curr Opin Pediatr.* 2002;14(4):370-378

25. Cushman M. Epidemiology and risk factors for venous thrombosis. *Semin Hematol.* 2007;44:62-69

26. Crowther MA, Keiton JG. Congenital thrombophilic states associated with venous thrombosis: a qualitative overview and proposed classification system. *Ann Intern Med.* 2003; 138:128-134

27. Straczek C, Oger E, De Jonage-Canonico MBY, et al. Prothrombotic mutations, hormone therapy, and venous thromboembolism among postmenopausal women. *Circulation* 2005;112:3495-3500

28. Blickstein D, Blickstein I. Oral contraception and thrombophilia. *Curr Opin Obstet Gynecol.* 2007;19:370-376

29. Lim W, Eikelboom JW, Ginsberg JS. Inherited thrombophilia and pregnancy-associated venous thromboembolism. *BMJ.* 2007;334:1318-1321

30. Kearon C. Natural history of venous thromboembolism. *Am Heart Assoc Circ.* 2003;107:22-29

31. Ho SH, Wu JK, Hamilton DP, Dix DB, Wadsworth LD. An assessment of published pediatric dosage guidelines for enoxaparin: a retrospective review. *Pediatr Hematol Oncol.* 2004;26(9):561–565

32. Ronghe MD, Halsey C, Goulden NJ. Anticoagulation therapy in children. *Paediatr Drugs.* 2003;5(12):803–820

33. Sconce EA, Khan TI, Wynne HA, et al. The impact of CYP2C9 and VKORC1 genetic polymorphism and patient characteristics upon warfarin dose requirements: proposal for a new dosing regimen. *Blood.* 2005;106:2329–2333

34. Mustafa S, Stein PD, Patel KC, Otten TR, Holmes R, Silbergleit A. Upper extremity deep venous thrombosis. *Chest.* 2003;123:1953–1956

35. Deveber G, Andrew M, Adams C, et al. Cerebral sinovenous thrombosis in children. *N Eng J Med.* 2001;345:417–423

36. Barnes C, Deveber G. Prothrombotic abnormalities in childhood ischaemic stroke. *Thrombosis Res.* 2006;118:67–74

37. Rigatelli G, Cardaioli P. Patent foramen ovale management: who should do what? *Eur J Neurol.* 2007;14(3):341–342

# CHAPTER 109

# White Blood Cell Disorders in Adolescents

ASHOK SHENDE, MBBS

The total white blood cell (WBC) count and differential WBC count are valuable aids in the diagnosis and treatment of various diseases. Disorders of the WBCs can be of clonal (malignant) or nonclonal origins. Clonal disorders include the acute leukemias, chronic leukemias, myelodysplastic syndromes (MDSs), and lymphomas. Nonclonal disorders include quantitative and qualitative (functional) abnormalities of the WBCs. Quantitative disorders may result from intrinsic disorders of proliferation and maturation of precursors of a specific WBC class or may result from extrinsic causes such as excessive destruction. Quantitative disorders of the WBCs are interpreted on the basis of the absolute number of a specific class of WBCs rather than its percentage in the differential count.

The normal WBC count in adolescent males and females varies between 4,500 and 13,000/mm$^3$, with an absolute neutrophil count (ANC) of 1,800 to 8,000/mm$^3$, absolute lymphocyte count of 1,500 to 6,500/mm$^3$, absolute monocyte count of 150 to 1,300/mm$^3$, absolute eosinophil count (AEC) up to 600/mm$^3$, and absolute basophil count of 20 to 120/mm$^3$.

Leukocytosis or leukopenia may occur as a result of an increase or decrease in the absolute count of 1 specific class of WBCs, or it may occur as a result of an increase or decrease in the absolute count of more than 1 class of WBCs.

## LEUKOCYTOSIS AND LEUKOPENIA

### NEUTROPENIA

Neutropenia is defined as an ANC of less than 1,500/mm$^3$; less than 500/mm$^3$ is graded as severe, 500–1,000/mm$^3$ as moderate, and 1,000 to 1,500/mm$^3$ as mild.[1] Severity, rate of decline, and duration of neutropenia correlate with susceptibility to infections.[1] Neutropenic patients are most commonly infected with their own endogenous bacterial flora that are present on the skin (eg, staphylococci), in the mouth and oropharynx (eg, anaerobic bacteria), and in the gastrointestinal tract (eg, gram-negative rods). Causes of neutropenia are shown in Box 109-1. Guidelines for the approach to the diagnosis of neutropenia are shown in Tables 109-1 and 109-2.

**Box 109-1**

***Causes of Neutropenia***

*Congenital causes*

- Benign ethnic neutropenia
- Severe congenital neutropenia
- Cyclic neutropenia
- Glycogen storage disease type 1b
- Myelokathexis syndrome
- Chronic idiopathic neutropenia
- Selective IgA deficiency
- Hyper-IgM syndrome
- Congenital bone marrow failure syndromes
  - Shwachman-Diamond syndrome
  - Dyskeratosis congenita
  - Fanconi anemia

*Acquired causes*

- Clonal diseases of bone marrow
  - Acute lymphoblastic leukemia
  - Acute myeloid leukemia
  - Myelodysplastic syndrome
- Bone marrow infiltration with neoplastic cells
  - Non-Hodgkin lymphoma
  - Rhabdomyosarcoma
  - Ewing sarcoma
- Acquired bone marrow aplasia
  - Idiopathic aplastic anemia
  - Drug-induced aplastic anemia
- Immune cytopenias
  - Rheumatic diseases
  - Autoimmune lymphoproliferative syndrome
- Hypersplenism
- Nutritional causes
  - Vitamin $B_{12}$ deficiency
  - Folic acid deficiency
  - Anorexia nervosa[2]

Patients with fever and neutropenia are treated empirically at their initial presentation with broad-spectrum antibiotics such as cefepime (a fourth-generation cephalosporin with enhanced activity against

**Table 109-1**

**Guideline for Diagnosis of Underlying Causes of Neutropenia with History and Physical Examination**

| *History and Physical Examination* | *Differential Diagnosis* |
|---|---|
| Infection: Recurrent infections (indicates chronic neutropenia) | Severe congenital neutropenia |
| | Cyclic neutropenia |
| | Myelodysplastic syndrome |
| | Congenital or acquired immune deficiency |
| Acute infection (with transient neutropenia) | Viral infections |
| | Bacterial infections |
| | Rickettsial infections |
| Absence of recurrent infections | Ethnic neutropenia |
| | Familial neutropenia |
| | Immune neutropenia |
| | Hypersplenism (eg, portal hypertension) |
| Abnormal phenotype | Faconi anemia |
| | Dyskeratosis congenita |
| | Shwachman-Diamond syndrome |
| Presence of bruises, splenomegaly, hepatomegaly, or lymphadenopathy | Acute leukemia |
| | Lymphoma |
| History of commonly used drugs | Ibuprofen |
| | Anticonvulsants |
| | Sulfonamides |
| | Penicillins |
| | Antithyroid drugs |
| | Barbiturates |
| | Benzodiazepines |
| Malnutrition | Anorexia nervosa |
| | Shwachman-Diamond syndrome |
| | Folate/B12 deficiency |

gram-positive and gram-negative aerobes) or ceftazidime (a third-generation cephalosporin) after obtaining appropriate cultures from the infected area, urine, and blood.[3] If indicated, radiologic imaging studies are also obtained. Rectal temperatures and enemas should be avoided. Antibiotic therapy is adjusted according to culture results and clinical response to therapy. After 7 days of therapy with

**Table 109-2**

**Investigations for Diagnosis of Underlying Causes of Neutropenia**

| *Investigation* | *Indication* |
|---|---|
| Complete blood counts | All patients |
| Peripheral blood smear examination | All patients |
| Identification of infectious agent | Attempted in all patients |
| Bone marrow examination | Presence of leukemic cells or dysplastic cells in peripheral blood smear |
| | Thrombocytopenia |
| | Anemia |
| | Splenomegaly, hepatomegaly, lymphadenopathy, petechiae, or bruises |
| | Abnormal phenotype |
| | Recurrent infections |
| | Chronic neutropenia |
| | Cyclic neutropenia |
| Special diagnostic studies | As indicated for suspected disease |

antibacterial antibiotics, if neutropenia persists and the cause of the fever remains unknown, then an antifungal antibiotic, such as amphotericin B, is added empirically.[3] When indicated, granulocyte colony-stimulating factor is also used.

## NEUTROPHILIA

An ANC greater than 8,000/mm$^3$ is indicative of neutrophilia. Box 109-2 shows the causes of neutrophilia.

## DISORDERS OF GRANULOCYTE FUNCTIONS

Abnormalities of granulocyte function may result from inherited or acquired defects of adhesion, chemotaxis, ingestion, degranulation, or oxidative metabolism (ie, steps that play a critical role in phagocytosis and microbial killing). Patients with these abnormalities are susceptible to the development of recurrent bacterial and fungal infections.[4]

## EOSINOPHILIA

The normal eosinophil count in the circulating blood is 400/mm$^3$ (100–600/mm$^3$).[4] Severity of eosinophilia is determined by the AEC. In mild eosinophilia, the

**Box 109-2**

***Causes of Neutrophilia***

**Acute neutrophilia**

- Acute bacterial infections
- Hypoxia
- Acute hemorrhage
- Acute hemolysis
- Exercise
- Epinephrine

**Chronic neutrophilia**

- *Clonal causes*
  - Chronic myelogenous leukemia
  - Chronic neutrophilic leukemia
- *Nonclonal causes*
  - Sickle cell disease
  - Chronic blood loss
  - Asplenia
  - Hereditary neutrophilia
  - Glucocorticoids
  - Leukocyte adhesion deficiency
  - Idiopathic

AEC range is 600 to 1,500/mm$^3$; in moderate eosinophilia, the range is 1,500–5,000/mm$^3$; and in severe eosinophilia, the count is greater than 5,000/mm$^3$. Box 109-3 shows the causes of eosinophilia, Figure 109-1 shows the diagnostic studies for the evaluation of eosinophilia, and Table 109-3 shows the treatment of eosinophilia.

### Chronic Eosinophilic Leukemia/ Hypereosinophilic Syndrome

According to World Health Organization (WHO) guidelines, the diagnosis of chronic eosinophilic leukemia (CEL) or hypereosinophilic syndrome (HES) can be made only after a number of infectious, inflammatory, and neoplastic diseases known to be associated with eosinophilia (eg, chronic myelogenous leukemia, acute myelogenous leukemia, other chronic myeloproliferative diseases, T-cell lymphoma, Hodgkin disease) have been excluded. Then, if there is no evidence of clonality, the diagnosis of HES is preferred, whereas the finding of a clonal myeloid abnormality would support the diagnosis of CEL.[5]

### Diagnostic Studies for Eosinophilia

History, physical examination, and complete blood counts, including AEC, are useful in the initial evaluation

**Box 109-3**

***Causes of Eosinophilia***

- Idiopathic hypereosinophilic syndrome
- Clonal eosinophilia
  - Eosinophilic leukemias
    - Chronic eosinophilic leukemia exclusively of eosinophilic lineage: associated with interstitial deletion of 4q12, resulting in a fusion gene *FIP1L1-PDGRFA*
    - Secondary eosinophilic clonal involvement in myeloproliferative disorders of stem cell origin
  - Eosinophilia associated with noneosinophilic clonal disorders
    - Lymphoid clonal disorders
      - Clonal CD3–, CD4+, CD8– T-cell lyphocytosis
      - T-cell non-Hodgkin lymphoma/acute lymphoblastic leukemia
      - Hodgkin disease
    - Myeloid clonal disorders: myelodysplastic syndrome/acute myelogenous leukemia
- Nonclonal or reactive causes of acute eosinophilia
  - Allergic disorders
    - Asthma
    - Hay fever
    - Urticaria
    - Eczema
    - Drug hypersensitivity
  - Skin disorders
    - Scabies
    - Dermatitis herpetiformis
    - Erythema toxicum
    - Gleich syndrome: episodic angioneurotic edema with eosinophilia and high levels of interleukin-5
  - Infections
    - Helminthic
      - *Ascaris lumbricoides*
      - Trichinosis
      - Echinococcosis
      - Toxocara
      - Hookworm
      - Strongyloides
      - Filariasis
    - Protozooal
      - Toxoplasmosis
      - Malaria
      - Pneumocystis
    - Viral
      - HIV infection
    - Fungal
      - Aspergillosis
      - Coccidiodomycosis
- Chronic eosinophilia
  - Familial eosinophilia
  - Pulmonary diseases

(*Continued*)

**Box 109-3 (Continued)**

- Chronic eosinophilic pneumonia with allergic bronchopulmonary aspergillosis
- Sarcoidosis
- Eosinophilic pneumonitis (Loeffler syndrome)

◦ Rheumatologic diseases
- Churg-Strauss vasculitis
- Eosinophilic fascitis
- Rheumatoid arthritis

◦ Gastrointestinal diseases
- Eosinophilic gastroenteritis
- Regional enteritis
- Ulcerative colitis
- Chronic active hepatitis

◦ Endocrine disorder
- Addison disease

◦ Renal conditions
- Hemodialysis
- Peritoneal dialysis

◦ Immune deficiency
- Hyper-IgE syndrome
- Organ (lung, kidney, liver) transplant rejection

From Lanzkowsky P, ed. *Manual of Pediatric Hematology and Oncology*. 4th ed. London: Elsevier Academic Press; 2005:209–249, with permission from Elsevier.

of eosinophilia. Idiopathic HES and CEL usually present with moderate to severe eosinophilia. There may be hepatosplenomegaly and evidence of other organ involvement, such as the lungs, heart, nervous system, and eyes. Bone marrow examination for microscopy, cytogenic studies, and molecular studies may reveal clonality. Patients with a dermatologic presentation may have a lymphoid clonal disorder characterized by CD3–, CD4+, and CD8– T-cell lymphocytosis.[6–8]

The autosomal dominant form of familial eosinophilia is a rare occurrence. When suspected, complete blood counts, including AEC, obtained from family members are helpful in making the diagnosis. Manifestations of Gleich syndrome include episodic angioedema, eosinophilia, and high serum levels of interleukin-5 (IL-5).

Patients with nonclonal eosinophilia usually present with a mild to moderate degree of eosinophilia. Diagnostic studies—including serology for toxocara, trichinella, strongyloides, toxoplasma, and filaria; stool examination for ova and parasites; serum immunoglobin levels; antinuclear antibody; and DNA antibody—may reveal the underlying cause, such as a parasitic infection or connective tissue disorder.

**Treatment of Eosinophilia**

Clonal eosinophilia is treated with appropriate chemotherapy for the associated malignancy. Eosinophilia with CD3–, CD4+, and CD8– T-cell lymphocytosis is treated with immunosuppressive agents such as cyclosporine A and glucocorticoids. Idiopathic HES is treated with glucocorticoids, hydroxyurea, α-interferon, vincristine, thioguanine, etoposide, or imatinib in a sequential manner according to clinical response and improvement in AEC. The myeloproliferative variant of eosinophilia (CEL), which is associated with an interstitial deletion of 4q12 with resultant *FIP1L1-PDGFRA* gene fusion, is treated with imatinib.[6–8]

Patients with parasitic infections are treated with specific therapy pertinent to the infecting parasite. Patients with HES who are refractory to imatinib treatment may be treated with nonmyeloablative allogenic bone marrow transplantation.

Interleukin 5 is a specific stimulator for eosinophilic differentiation and an eosinophilic activator. A monoclonal anti-IL-5 antibody for treatment of HES may become available in the near future.

**Surveillance Studies for Organ Damage**

Activated eosinophils release toxic granule proteins and inflammatory mediators. For this reason, patients with chronic moderate to severe eosinophilia are periodically evaluated for end-organ damage (eg, with serum troponin T levels, electrocardiogram (ECG) and echocardiogram for cardiac evaluation, chest x-ray and pulmonary function studies for lung evaluation, serology for liver function, neurologic evaluation, and eye examination).

### LYMPHOCYTOSIS, MONOCYTOSIS, AND BASOPHILIA

Boxes 109-4, 109-5, and 109-6 show causes of lymphocytosis, monocytosis, and basophilia, respectively.

## ACUTE LEUKEMIA

### EPIDEMIOLOGY

The incidence rate for acute lymphoblastic leukemia (ALL) in adolescents, aged 15 to 19 years, is 11.5 per 1 million people.[9] It is approximately twice as common in males as in females.

The majority of adolescents with ALL have precursor B-cell ALL (~75%). Approximately 25% have T-lineage ALL, and ~2% to 3% have mature B-cell ALL. The incidence of acute myelogenous leukemia (AML) in adolescents aged 15 to 19 years is 8.5 per 1 million people.[9] Its incidence rate is equal in both males and females.

### ETIOLOGY

In most pediatric patients, the underlying cause of acute leukemia is not known. However, the presence of certain conditions increases the risk for developing acute

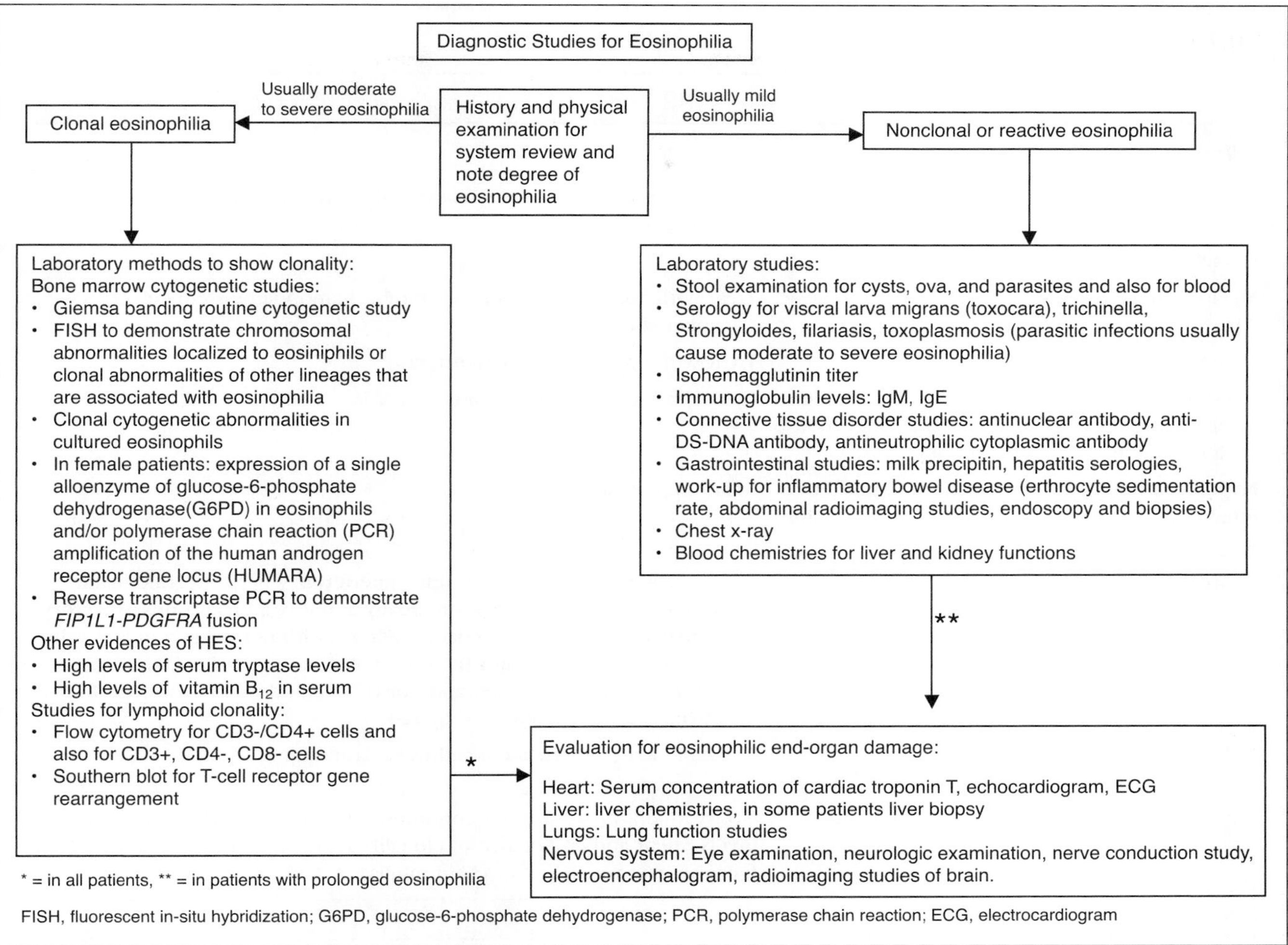


**FIGURE 109-1** Diagnostic studies for evaluation of eosinophilia. (Adapted from Shende A. Disorders of white blood cells. In: Lanzkowsky P, ed. *Manual of Pediatric Hematology and Oncology*. 4th ed. London: Elsevier Academic Press; 2005, with permission from Elsevier.)

leukemia. For ALL, the predisposing conditions include postnatal therapeutic radiation, in utero exposure to radiation, increased birth weight, Down syndrome, Bloom syndrome, ataxia telangiectasia, Shwachman-Diamond syndrome, and neurofibromatosis type I (NF-I).[10]

For AML, the predisposing factors include treatment with chemotherapeutic agents such as alkylating agents and topoisomerase II inhibitors, Down syndrome, Fanconi anemia, NF-I, Bloom syndrome, Shwachman-Diamond syndrome, familial monosomy syndrome, Kostmann granulocytopenia, familial platelet disorder with a propensity to develop AML (FPD/AML), and congenital amegakaryocytic thrombocytopenia.[10]

An in utero origin of precursor B-cell ALL with t(12;21) (TEL/AML1), as well as AML with t(8;21) (RUNX1/ETO), has been documented by the demonstration of clonotypic leukemic cells.[11,12] A long latency period before the development of overt leukemia in these patients indicates a possible role of postnatal factors as "second hit" events.

## ACUTE LYMPHOBLASTIC LEUKEMIA

### Pathogenesis

Acute lymphoblastic leukemia in children develops as a result of arrest of maturation followed by clonal expansion of a malignantly transformed lymphoid committed progenitor cell during a specific stage of its differentiation. However, in Philadelphia chromosome positive ($Ph^+$) ALL, the leukemogenic mutational events may originate in earlier stages, resulting in involvement of multiple cell lineages.[13]

**Table 109-3**

**Treatment of Conditions that Cause Eosinophilia**

| *Type* | *Treatment* |
|---|---|
| Reactive or nonclonal | Treat underlying cause (eg, treat parasitic infections with appropriate antiparasitic) |
| Clonal disease | |
| Myeloid clonal disease | Treat with appropriate chemotherapy ± hemopoietic stem cell transplantation |
| Lymphoid malignancies | Treat with appropriate chemotherapy |
| CD3–, CD4+ lymphoid clonal disease with high levels of interleukin-5 (IL-5) (usually associated with dermatologic manifestations) | Cyclosporine A, glucocorticoids, or 2CDA |
| Hypereosinophilic syndrome (HES) (caused by interstitial deletion of 4q12, resulting in a fusion gene *FIP1L1-PDGFRA*) | Imatinib mesylate |
| Idiopathic HES | Glucocorticoids, hydroxyurea, alpha-interferon, vincristine, thioguanine, or etoposide; use these agents sequentially and if response is unsatisfactory, then treat with imatinib myselate (patients with normal serum IL-5 values respond to imatinib, but not the ones with the high values); during acute, life-threatening presentation of HES, high dose of solumedrol (methylpredisolone) may be required |
| HES refractory to previously mentioned therapies | Allogenic hemopoietic stem cell transplantation |
| Idiopathic HES without organ involvement | No treatment necessary but continues periodic monitoring for organ involvement and emergence of clonality is warranted; also continue search for rare reactive causes for eosinophilia |

HES, hypereosinophilic syndrome

The following eosinophilic disorders with single organ involvement may progress into HES: eosinophilic gastroenteritis, Gleich syndrome (episodic eosinophilia with angioedema), Loeffler syndrome (eosinophilic pneumonitis), Schulman syndrome (eosinophilic fascitis), and Well syndrome (eosinophilic cellulitis). Parasitic infections with eosinophilia can also progress into HES.

(From Shende A. Disorders of white blood cells. In: Lanzkowsky P, ed. *Manual of Pediatric Hematology and Oncology.* 4th ed. London: Elsevier Academic Press; 2005, with permission from Elsevier.)

## Molecular Pathology of Acute Lymphoblastic Leukemia

Acquired genetic mutations, restricted to leukemic clones, include translocations, inversions, deletions, point mutations, and gene amplifications.[14] Translocations create leukemia-specific novel genes that make oncoproteins that act as transcription factors. Examples of such transcription factors occurring in precursor B-cell ALL include E2A-PBX in t(1;19), MLL-AF4 in t(4;11), TEL/AML1 in t(12;21), and E2A-HLF in t(17;19). E2A-HLF-positive ALL, although uncommon, is seen relatively more frequently in adolescent patients and often presents with disseminated intravascular coagulopathy (DIC) and hypercalcemia.[14] In t(9;22) precursor B-cell ALL, the BCR/ABL protein has tyrosine kinase activity that induces leukemogenesis.

Other mechanisms of leukemogenesis involve loss of tumor suppressor gene activity and loss of ability of leukemic cell to undergo apoptosis (eg, due to overexpression of antiapoptotic protein bcl-2). In T-cell or B-cell ALL, transcription factor genes, such as the *MYC* gene, are dysregulated as a result of their juxtaposition with transcriptionally active T-cell receptor genes or immunoglobulin genes.

**Box 109-4**

***Causes of Lymphocytosis***

*Clonal in origin*
- Acute lymphoblastic leukemia

*Nonclonal in origin*
- Infections
  - Infectious mononucleosis
  - Cytomegalovirus
  - Pertussis
  - Brucellosis
  - Tuberculosis
- Endocrine disorders
  - Thyrotoxicosis
  - Addison disease

**Box 109-5**

***Causes of Monocytosis***

*Clonal in origin*
- Acute monocytic leukemia

*Nonclonal in origin*
- Infectious causes
  - Tuberculosis
  - Syphilis
  - Brucellosis
  - Typhoid
- Noninfectious causes
  - Neutropenias
    - In chemotherapy-treated patients prior to recovery in absolute neutrophil count
  - Chronic inflammatory diseases
    - Juvenile rheumatoid arthritis
    - Systemic lupus erythematosus
    - Ulcerative colitis
    - Regional enteritis
    - Postsplenectomy
    - Hodgkin disease

In T-cell ALL, *HOX11, TAL1, LYL1, LMO1*, and LMO2 oncogenes are expressed abnormally, even in the absence of detectable cytogenetic abnormalities.[15] The *HOX11* mutation is associated with a favorable prognosis. Recently, gain-of-function mutations of the *NOTCH1* gene, resulting in dysregulation of the *NOTCH1* signaling pathway, have been detected in lymphoblasts of 50% of patients. *NOTCH1* signaling plays an important role in the commitment of hematopoietic stem cells to

**Box 109-6**

***Causes of Basophilia***

*Clonal in origin*
- Chronic myelogenous leukemia
- Hodgkin disease

*Nonclonal in origin*
- Hypersensitivity reactions
- Juvenile rheumatoid arthritis
- Ulcerative colitis
- Varicella

develop into T cells. Activating *NOTCH1* mutations predict a favorable prognosis in T-cell ALL.[16]

### Signs and Symptoms

Complaints of fever, lassitude, bleeding, and pallor are present in 50% to 60% of children with ALL, and bone pain is present in 25% of patients. On physical examination, lymphadenopathy, splenomegaly, and hepatomegaly are observed in 50% to 60% of patients.

The presence of a mediastinal mass with or without the superior vena cava syndrome is indicative of T-cell ALL. Usually, the peripheral blood examination shows involvement of more than 1 cell line. Anemia, thrombocytopenia, and neutropenia occur in various combinations. Anemia may manifest with pallor, tiredness, tachycardia, shortness of breath, and dizziness, and can occasionally cause congestive heart failure. Thrombocytopenia causes easy bruisability, petechiae, purpura, bleeding from mucous membranes, or internal bleeding (eg, intracranial bleeding). Neutropenia results in increased susceptibility to infections and fever. Total leukocyte counts vary from leukopenia to severe leukocytosis in the peripheral blood. Table 109-4 shows the frequency of extramedullary organ involvement, its pathogenesis, and its clinical manifestations at the initial diagnosis of ALL.

### Differential Diagnosis

***Juvenile Rheumatoid Arthritis*** Because most children with leukemia do not have blasts in the peripheral blood, a child presenting with musculoskeletal complaints such as pain or joint swelling may be misdiagnosed as having juvenile rheumatoid arthritis (JRA). In a multicenter case-control study, 3 important factors were identified that predicted a diagnosis of ALL.[17] They were low WBC count (<4,000/mm$^3$), low normal platelet count (150,000–250,000/mm$^3$), and history of nighttime pain. A positive antinuclear antibody test, presence of a skin rash, and objective signs of arthritis

**Table 109-4**

**Frequency of Extramedullary Involvement, Its Pathogenesis, and Its Clinical Manifestations at Initial Diagnosis of Acute Lymphoblastic Leukemia**

| *Extramedullary Site* | *Frequency of Involvement* | *Pathogenesis* | *Clinical Manifestation* |
|---|---|---|---|
| Lymph nodes | 50% | Leukemic infiltration | Lymphadenopathy |
| Spleen | 30%–50% | Leukemic infiltration | Splenomegaly |
| Liver | 30%–40% | Leukemic infiltration | Hepatomegaly |
| Thymus | 50% in T-cell ALL | Leukemic infiltration | Anterior mediastinal mass with or without superior vena cava syndrome |
| Central nervous system | Age: 10–14 years precursor B-cell ALL: 9%<br>T-cell ALL: 7% | Leukemic infiltration of meninges or brain parenchyma resulting in increased intracranial pressure | Headache, nausea, vomiting, convulsion, stroke |
| | Age: 15–18 years precursor B-cell ALL: 4%<br>T-cell ALL: 12% | Leukostasis, thrombosis, hemorrhage: usually associated with leukocytosis | Headache, nausea, vomiting, convulsion, stroke |
| | | Hemorrhage: thrombocytopenia, coagulopathy | Headache, nausea, vomiting, convulsion, stroke |
| Kidney | 30%–50% | Tumor lysis and uric acid nephropathy | Oliguria, uremia, renal failure, hematuria, hyperuricemia |
| | | Leukemic infiltration of kidneys | Enlarged kidneys on ultrasonography, hypertension, hematuria, uremia |
| Testis | Occult: 10%–33%<br>Overt: uncommon | Leukemic infiltration of testes: associated risk factors: T-ALL, leukocytosis, thrombocytopenia | Painless enlargement of testis |

were not helpful in differentiating between leukemia and JRA. Similarly, lactate dehydrogenase, uric acid levels in blood, fever, organomegaly, and an increased sedimentation rate have all been shown to be of limited value in differentiating leukemia from JRA.

***Benign Lymphocytosis*** An increase in immature lymphocytes, mimicking ALL, may occur in viral infections. Immunophenotyping studies on bone marrow cells are helpful in distinguishing these 2 conditions. In benign lymphocytosis, a mixture of B-lineage lymphocyte populations displaying immature (CD19+, CD20+, CD10−), early (CD19+, CD10+), and late (sIgμκ+, sIgμλ+) immunophenotypes is found, whereas in B-lineage ALL an immunophenotype at a single stage of maturation is present.[18]

***Aplastic or Hypoplastic Anemia*** Rarely, an overt phase of ALL may be preceded by the finding of an aplastic or hypoplastic bone marrow, which lasts for 1 to 4 weeks, and is then followed by a normal hematologic recovery, only to result in the development of overt ALL (CD10+, TdT+) 3 to 9 months later. This condition has been termed as the preleukemia syndrome, pre-ALL syndrome, or aplastic presentation of ALL.[18]

## LABORATORY STUDIES IN THE DIAGNOSIS OF ACUTE LYMPHOBLASTIC LEUKEMIA

### Peripheral Blood Counts

Table 109-5 shows the variability of WBC counts seen in newly diagnosed adolescents with ALL according to the subtype of ALL and the age group of the patient.[19]

Thrombocytopenia, with platelet counts less than 20,000/mm$^3$, is present in 25% of patients; these patients are at the greatest risk for severe bleeding. Platelet counts of 20,000 to 99,000/mm$^3$ are found in approximately 50% of patients. Platelet counts greater than 100,000/mm$^3$ are found in 25% of patients at the time of initial diagnosis.

**Table 109-5**

**Variability of White Blood Cell Counts in Acute Lymphoblastic Leukemia**

| *WBC Counts/mm³* | *Precursor B-Cell ALL Age (Years)* | | *Precursor T-Cell ALL Age (Years)* | |
|---|---|---|---|---|
| | *10–14* | *15–18* | *10–14* | *15–18* |
| <10,000 | 54% | 46% | 17% | 12% |
| 10,000—19,999 | 15% | 13% | 9% | 3% |
| 20,000—99,999 | 21% | 31% | 36% | 50% |
| ≥100,000 | 10% | 10% | 38% | 35% |

Low hemoglobin levels (<11 g/dL) are found in most patients. However, higher hemoglobin levels (>11 g/dL) are seen in approximately 12% of patients. A higher hemoglobin level indicates a more rapid growth rate of the leukemic cells.

### Bone Marrow Examination

Bone marrow examination shows a predominance of lymphoblasts. Morphologic classification of L1, L2, and L3 lymphoblasts, proposed by the French-American-British (FAB) Cooperative Working Group, is used widely. Generally, the FAB classification does not correlate with immunophenotypic, cytogenetic, cytochemical, or molecular features of ALL, with the exception of L3 morphology, which usually corresponds to mature B-cell ALL. Table 109-6 shows morphologic, immunophenotypic, and cytogenetic features, along with the probabilities of eventfree survival (EFS) of B-lineage ALL and T-lineage ALL in adolescent patients.

### Minimal Residual Disease

Recently, the risk of relapse has been found to correlate well with the levels of minimal residual disease (MRD) detected during induction therapy of precursor B-cell ALL and T-cell ALL. Polymerase chain reactions (PCRs) that target clonotypic leukemia-specific genes can detect 1 leukemic cell in $10^4$ to $10^5$ normal bone marrow cells. The sensitivity for detectable MRD by flow cytometry, used for leukemic cell immunophenotyping, is in the same range.

### Treatment of Acute Lymphoblastic Leukemia in Adolescents

Treatment of precursor B-ALL includes early precursor B-ALL, precursor B-ALL, and transitional precursor B-ALL. All adolescent patients with precursor B-ALL are high-risk patients and are treated on high-risk protocols. Table 109-7 shows an outline of an augmented therapy regimen for ALL patients with slow early response (SER). Adolescents with SER to induction therapy are treated with an augmented regimen during the postremission phase.[20]

Patients with rapid early response (RER) to induction therapy are treated with standard postremission therapy, which uses the same chemotherapy agents, except that interim maintenance and delayed intensification are only used once. However, patients with RER in the presence of other high-risk factors, such as t(4;11) or other *MLL* gene rearrangements, are treated with augmented regimens.

Definitions of early and late responses differ from study to study. For example, in one Children's Cancer Group (CCG) study, a slow response to induction therapy was defined as the presence of more than 25% blasts in the bone marrow on day 7.[20] Acute lymphoblastic leukemia patients with ALL with the Ph chromosome [t(9;22)] are treated with allogeneic hematopoietic stem cell transplantation (HSCT) after induction and consolidation therapy using chemotherapy and imatinib, an inhibitor of ABL-tyrosine kinase. Adolescents with T-cell ALL are also treated with intensive chemotherapy ± cranial radiation therapy. In a recent study, it was shown that improved EFS was attributable to the use of high-dose methotrexate.[21]

Adolescents with B-cell ALL are treated with an intensive protocol such as LMB89.[22] Box 109-7 shows age-specific differences in the incidence, prognostic factors, and treatment outcome of pediatric, adolescent, and adult ALL patients.

It is recommended that adolescent ALL patients between the ages of 16 and 21 years be treated with intensive pediatric treatment protocols rather than adult ALL protocols because both adult and pediatric oncologists treat patients in this age group.[23] It has been shown that the outcome is far superior when these patients are

**Table 109-6**

**Morphologic, Immunophenotypic, and Cytogenetic Features and Eventfree Survival of B- and T-Lineage Acute Lymphoblastic Leukemia (ALL) in Adolescent Patients**

| *Feature* | *B-Lineage ALL* | *T-Lineage ALL* |
|---|---|---|
| FAB (French-American-British) | L1, L2<br>L3 in mature B-ALL | L1, L2 |
| Cytochemistry | | |
| Periodic acid-Schiff | +/- | +/- |
| Tdt | + (- mature B-ALL) | + |
| Immunophenotype | **Early precursor B-ALL**<br>HLA-DR+, CD19+, CD10-, cIgμ-, sIg-, CD79a+<br>**Precursor B-ALL**<br>HLA-DR+, CD19+, CD10+, cIgμ+, sIg-<br>**B-ALL**<br>CD19+, CD10+/-, Tdt-, sIgμ+, sIgκ or λ+ | CD3+, CD7+, CD5+ |
| Some cytogenic abnormalities | **Early precursor B-ALL**<br>t(4;11), t(9;11), t(9;22), t(1;19)<br>**B-ALL**<br>t(8;14), t(2;8), t(8;22) | t(7;9), t(10;14), t(11;14), t(7;10) |
| Frequency | **Early and precursor B-ALL**<br>75%<br>**B-ALL**<br>2% | 25% |
| Eventfree survival (10-year probability) | **Early and precursor B-ALL**<br>60%<br>**B-ALL**<br>90% | 60% |

treated using pediatric-intensive protocols. As a matter of general precaution, adolescents who are to undergo chemotherapy should be advised to practice contraception if they are going to be sexually active.

### Treatment of Relapsed Acute Lymphoblastic Leukemia

Patients who relapse early in their initial treatment are treated with allogeneic HSCT after induction of remission with chemotherapy. Patients who relapse late in their treatment are treated with chemotherapy drugs not used during the initial therapy. Table 109-8 shows an outline of therapy for relapsed patients with ALL.

## ACUTE MYELOGENOUS LEUKEMIA

### Pathogenesis

The Acute myelogenous leukemia develops as a result of arrest of maturation followed by clonal expansion of a malignantly transformed early myeloid (nonlymphoid) hematopoietic cell. The leukemic stem cell in different subtypes of AML and MDS arises at various stages of differentiation.[24] Thus, the differentiation stage in which malignant transformation occurs corresponds to the subtype of AML. Box 109-8 shows the WHO classification of myeloid malignancies, which includes various subtypes of AML.

### Molecular Pathogenesis of Subtypes of Acute Myelogenous Leukemia

In acute promyelocytic leukemia (APL), the reciprocal translocation between the *PML* gene at chromosome band 15q22 and *RARα* at 17q21 results in the fusion of the *PML* gene with the *RARα* gene. This leads to aberrant recruitment of histone deacylases, which causes silencing of genes normally activated by the normal RARα nuclear hormone receptor and thus, through a

**Table 109-7**

**Augmented Therapy Regimen for Slow Early Responding Adolescents with ALL**

| *Phase* | *Therapy* |
|---|---|
| Induction (duration 4 weeks) | Vincristine<br>Prednisone<br>Daunorubicin<br>L-Asparaginase<br>Intrathecal cytarabine<br>Intrathecal methotrexate |
| Postremission therapy | |
| Augmented therapy | |
| Consolidation (duration 9 weeks) | Cyclophosphamide<br>Cytarabine<br>Mercaptopurine<br>Vincristine<br>Asparaginase<br>Intrathecal methotrexate<br>For patients with CNS disease at diagnosis: craniospinal radiation<br>Patients without CNS disease at diagnosis: cranial radiation<br>Patients with testicular disease: testicular radiation |
| Interim maintenance (course 1) (duration 8 weeks) | Vincristine<br>Methotrexate<br>Asparaginase |
| Delayed intensification (course 1) (duration 8 weeks) | Reinduction: Dexamethasone<br>Vincristine<br>Doxorubicin<br>Asparaginase<br>Reconsolidation: Vincristine<br>Cyclophosphamide<br>Thioguanine<br>Cytarabine<br>Intrathecal methotrexate<br>Asparaginase |
| Interim maintenance (course 2) (duration 8 weeks) | Same as interim maintenance course 1 |
| Delayed intensification (course 2) (duration 8 weeks) | Same as delayed intensification course 1 |
| Maintenance: 12 weeks each cycle, repeat cycles until the total duration of therapy, beginning with the first interim maintenance period, reaches 2 years in girls and 3 years in boys | Vincristine<br>Methotrexate<br>Prednisone<br>Mercaptopurine<br>Intrathecal methotrexate |

CNS, central nervous system

Reprinted with permission from Nachman JB, Sather HN, Sensel MG, et al. Augmented post-induction therapy for children with high risk acute lymphoblastic leukemia and a slow response to initial therapy. *N Engl J Med*. 1998;338:1663–1671.

**Box 109-7**

## *Age-Specific Differences According to Risk Category at Initial Diagnosis, Prognostic Factors in Context of Postremission Treatment, Cytogenetic Abnormalities and Cure Rates in Pediatric, Adolescent, and Adult Patients with Precursor B-Cell Acute Lymphoblastic Leukemia (ALL)*[15,20]

**Age-specific risk category at initial diagnosis affecting induction treatment of precursor B-cell ALL**

- Age 1–9 years and white blood cell (WBC) less than 50,000/mm$^3$: standard risk
- Age older than 10 years regardless of WBC count: high risk

**Age-specific differences in prognostic factors in the context of postremission treatment of precursor B-cell ALL**
Clinical prognostic features for precursor B-cell ALL in patients with slow response to initial therapy (ie, presence of >25% blasts in bone marrow on day 7 of induction phase of therapy)

*% 5-year eventfree survival (EFS)*

- Age 1–9 years + WBC 50,000/mm$^3$ or more: treatment with standard therapy: 42 ± 8; treatment with augmented therapy: 84 ± 5
- Age older than 10 years + WBC 50,000/mm$^3$ or more: treatment with standard therapy: 48 ± 10; treatment with augmented therapy: 67 ± 10
- Age older than 10 years + WBC less than 50,000/mm$^3$: treatment with standard therapy: 66 ± 6; treatment with augmented therapy: 73

**Age-specific differences in the context of cytogenetic abnormalities in precursor B-cell ALL**

- t(12;21) with TEL/AML1 rearrangement: less frequent in adolescents aged 15–19 years and adult patients than in children aged 1–14
- t(9;22) with BCR/ABL rearrangement: more frequent in adults than in children, including adolescents
- Hyperploidy: more common in children and adolescents than in adults

Overall cure rates

- Age group 1–14 years: 75%–85%
- Adolescent age group (15–19 years): 60%–70% (if pediatric therapy), 35%–50% (if adult therapy)
- Adult: 30%–40%

**Table 109-8**

## Outline of Therapy for Relapsed Patients with Acute Lymphoblastic Leukemia

| *Site of Relapse* | *Duration of First Remission* | *Treatment* |
|---|---|---|
| Bone marrow | Relapse occurring before completion of therapy or within 6 months of completing therapy | Allogenic HSCT |
| Isolated central nervous system | Relapse occurring before completion of 18 months of therapy | Allogenic HSCT |
| | Relapse occurring after completion of 18 months of therapy without use of cranial radiation | Chemotherapy and cranial radiation |
| | Relapse occurring after completion of 18 months of therapy with cranial radiation | Allogenic HSCT |
| Isolated testicular | Early or late relapse | Chemotherapy and radiation to both testes |

HSCT, hematopoietic stem cell transplantation

**Box 109-8**

***World Health Organization Classification of Acute Myelogenous Leukemia***

Acute myeloid leukemia with recurrent genetic abnormalities

- Acute myeloid leukemia with t(8;21)(q22;q22), (AML1/ETO)
- Acute myeloid leukemia with abnormal marrow eosinophils and inv(16)(p13;q22) or t(16;16)(p13;q22), (*CBF* β*/MYH11*)
- Acute promyelocytic leukemia with t(15;17)(q22;q12), (*PML/RAR*α), and variants
- Acute myeloid leukemia with 11q23 (MLL) abnormalities

Acute myeloid leukemia with multilineage dysplasia

- Following myelodysplastic syndrome (MDS) or MDS/myeloproliferative disorder (MPD)
- Without antecedent MDS or MPD, but with dysplasia in at least 50% of cells in 2 or more myeloid lineages
- Acute myeloid leukemia and myelodysplastic syndromes, therapy related
- Alkylating agent/radiation-related type
- Topoisomerase II inhibitor-related type (some may be lymphoid)
- Others

Acute myeloid leukemia, not otherwise categorized

- Acute myeloid leukemia, minimally differentiated
- Acute myeloid leukemia without maturation
- Acute myeloid leukemia with maturation
- Acute myelomonocytic leukemia
- Acute monoblastic/acute monocytic leukemia
- Acute erythroid leukemia (erythroid/myeloid and pure erythroleukemia)
- Acute megakaryoblastic leukemia
- Acute basophilic leukemia
- Acute panmyelosis with myelofibrosis
- Myeloid sarcoma

From Vardiman JW, Harris NL, Brunning RD. The World Health Organization (WHO) classification of the myeloid neoplasm. *Blood*. 2002;100:2292–2302. Copyright American Society of Hematology, reproduced with permission.

transcriptional repression, causes leukemogenesis. In AML with t(8;21) (q22;q22), the *AML1* gene on chromosome 21 fuses with the *ETO* gene on chromosome 8, and this fusion gene makes a protein that blocks the function of the normal core binding protein of the *AML1* gene. The *AML1* gene plays an important role in normal hematopoiesis. In AML with t(16;16) or inv(16), a fusion gene product of *CBF* β-*MYH11* causes silencing of the normal transcription factor and leukemogenesis.

### Signs and Symptoms

Signs and symptoms of AML are quite similar to those of ALL. However, chloromatous presentation of AML and a high incidence of DIC deserve special mention. Chloroma (granulocytic sarcoma, primary myeloid tumor), a mass formed by AML blasts, is a manifestation of extramedullary disease. Acute myelogenous leukemia may be present as an isolated tumor mass or may be present concurrently with the bone marrow involvement. It can occur in any anatomic site, and can also involve the spinal cord and cause paraparesis. It can also cause ptosis due to orbital involvement.[24] Bleeding due to DIC occurs with high frequency in patients with FAB morphologic subtypes M3 and M5 AML.

### Diagnosis

The presence of >20% myeloblasts in the bone marrow is required for the diagnosis of AML. There are 8 subtypes of AML. Table 109-9 lists the FAB subtypes and their cytochemical and immunophenotypic features. Auer rods are more frequently seen in the M2 and M3 subtypes of AML. Megakaryoblastic (M7) AML occurs rarely in adolescents.

### Prognostic Factors

Cytogenetic and molecular abnormalities of the AML blasts play an important role as prognostic factors. AML patients with t(15;17) (PML-RARα), t(8;21) (ETO-AML1),

**Table 109-9**

**FAB Morphologic Subtypes of Acute Myelogenous Leukemia and Their Cytochemical and Immunophenotypic Features**

| *FAB Subtype* | *Cytochemistry* *MPO* | *SBB* | *NASDA* | *Immunophenotype CD Antigen Expression* |
|---|---|---|---|---|
| M0 | –[a] | – | – | 13++, 15+, 33++, 34++, 65++, 117++, HLA-DR++ |
| M1 | + | + | – | 13++, 15+, 33++, 34++, 65++, 117++, HLA-DR++ |
| M2 | + | + | – | 13+, 15+, 33++, 34++, 65++, 117+, HLA-DR++ |
| M3 | + | + | – | 11b+, 13+, 15++, 33+++, 34+/–, 65++, HLA-DR+/–, 117+ |
| M4 | + | – | + | 11b++, 13++, 14++, 33++34+, 65++, HLA-DR+++, 117+ |
| M5 | + | + | + | 11b++, 13++, 14+, 33++, 34+/–, 65++, HLA-DR++, 117+/– |
| M6[b] | + | + | – | 13+, 33++, 65++, GPA++, 117+/– |
| M7 | – | – | + | 13+, 33++, 34+/–, 65+, 41/61++, 42++, 36++, HLA-DR+117+ |

MPO, Myeloperoxidase; SBB, Sudan Black B; NASDA, napthol-ASD chloroacetae; M0, undifferentiated leukemia; M1, acute myeloblastic leukemia without maturation; M2, acute myeloblastic leukemia with maturation; M3, acute promyelocytic leukemia; M4, acute myelomonocytic leukemia; M5, acute monocytic leukemia; M6, acute erythroleukemia; M7, acute megakaryoblstic leukemia.

[a]MPO is detected by monoclonal antibody method or by electron microscopy in M0 AML.

[b]Periodic acid-Schiff stain is positive in M6 AML. GPA; glycophorin A.

Nonmyeloid surface antigens expression in AML: T-lineage antigens: CD2 may be present on all subtypes of AML except in M6. CD7 may be expressed in all subtype of AML except in M0. CD4 may be present on M4, M5, and M7 AML. CD56 may be present on all subtypes of AML except M6. B-lineage antigens are not expressed in any subtype of AML.

Frequency of AML subtypes in children older than 2 years: M0 < 3%; M1 20%; M2 30%; M3 10%; M4 25%; M5 15%; M6 < 5%; M7 < 3%.

inv(16), or t(16;16) (MYH11-CBFB) have a favorable prognosis. Acute myelogenous leukemia with monosomy 7, –7q, t(6;9), or coplex karyotypes, evolving from MDS, therapy-induced, or with an FLT3 internal tandem duplication have an unfavorable prognosis[19,25]

### Treatment

There are several general principles of therapy for AML. Chemotherapy alone is used for patients with favorable prognostic features. Timed-sequential induction therapy was used in a study performed by the Children's Oncology Group. It demonstrated improvement in post-remission outcome (event-free survival at 3 years [42% ± 7%] for patients treated with intensive timing therapy compared with 27% ± 6% for those treated with standard timing therapy with $P = .0005$).[26] Remission is attained in 75% to 80% of AML patients, and EFS of 65% to 80% has been observed in patients with favorable prognostic features of AML. Patients presenting with isolated chloroma are also treated with the same chemotherapy. If the location of the chloroma has a potential to cause significant morbidity (eg, compression of spinal cord or loss of vision), then emergency local radiation is indicated for decompression. Matched sibling donor HSCT is indicated for AML patients with unfavorable prognostic features.

Patients with refractory or relapsed AML are treated with combinations of 2 or more drugs such as cytarabine, mitoxantrone, 2-cda, etoposide, idarubicin, or fludarabine. If AML blasts express CD33 antigen, then gemtuzumab ozogamicin (anti-CD33-calicheamicin conjugate), as a single agent or in combination with chemotherapy, is used to induce remission. Allogeneic HSCT is used as a postremission therapy. Patients with acute promyelocytic leukemia are treated with all-transretinoic acid (ATRA)-based chemotherapy. Box 109-9 shows an outline of treatments and their outcomes in newly diagnosed patients with APL.

## MYELODYSPLASTIC SYNDROMES

Myelodysplastic syndromes are clonal heterogeneous disorders of hematopoiesis that are characterized by ineffective hematopoiesis; impaired maturation of

**Box 109-9**

***Outline of Treatment for Newly Diagnosed Patients with Acute Promyelocytic Leukemia***

*Induction*

All-transretinoic acid (ATRA) daily until remission + either daunorubicin daily for 3 days or idarubicin every other day for 4 days

*Consolidation*

2–3 cycles of daunorubicin or idarubicin

Perform polymerase chain reaction (PCR) for PML-RARα.

**THEN**

- CR: 87%–97% of patients.
- PCR-negative patients: perform maintenance with ATRA daily for 15 days every 3 months + 6 MP daily and methotrexate once weekly for 2 years.
- Follow-up monitoring with PCR every 3–6 months for 2 years, and then every 6 months for 2 years. Relapse rate: 5%–10%.
- If relapse occurs, then induce remission with arsenic trioxide (CR: 85%–95% of patients) and allogeneic HSCT or molecularly negative autologous HSCT.
- Leukemiafree survival: for allogeneic HSCT: 70%; autologous HSCT: 70%.

PCR-positive patients: consider high-dose cytarabine or arsenic trioxide to induce remission, followed by allogeneic HSCT or molecularly negative autologous HSCT.

ATRA, All-transretinoic acid; PCR, polymerase chain reaction; CR, complete remission; HSCT, hematopoietic stem cell transplantation

From Lowenberg B, Griffin JD, Tallman MS. Acute myeloid leukemia and acute promyelocytic leuekemia. *Hematology Am Soc Hematol Educ Program*. 2003;82-101. Copyright American Society of Hematology, reproduced with permission.

hematopoietic cells; progressive cytopenias associated with dysplastic changes in bone marrow cells; hypercellular, normocellular or hypocellular bone marrow; and an increased risk of developing AML.[27]

## ETIOLOGY

Myelodysplastic syndromes may arise de novo; may be secondary to constitutional conditions, such as trisomy 8 mosaicism, familial MDS associated with monosomy 7 or 7q-chromosome abnormality, and Down syndrome; may occur secondary to congenital bone marrow failure syndromes; or may arise as a result of chemotherapy and/or radiation. In the adolescent age group, the incidence of de novo MDS/AML is 27 times more common than therapy-induced MDS/AML. Therapy-induced MDS represents 5% of all childhood MDS and occurs in 13% of children treated for malignancies. Alkylating agent–induced MDS has a latency period of 3 to 5 years and is associated with deletions or loss of a whole chromosome. Epipodphylltoxin-induced MDS has a latency period of 1 to 3 years and is associated with translocations involving 11q23. However, the true incidence of MDS in the adolescent age group is unknown. Table 109-10 shows the WHO classification and criteria for MDS.

## SIGNS AND SYMPTOMS

Patients with MDS usually present with similar signs and symptoms of bone marrow failure, as in acute leukemias. However, a clinical presentation with lymphadenopathy, hepatomegaly, and splenomegaly is uncommon.

## DIAGNOSIS

Dysplastic features are present in the bone marrow and peripheral blood cells. Leukemic blast cells are less than 20% in bone marrow. In de novo MDS, more than 50% of patients may have chromosomal abnormalities involving chromosomes 5, 7, 8, 9, 11, 12, 18, 19, 20, and 21. Classic chromosomal abnormalities of AML are not observed in de novo MDS. Monosomy 7 and 7q– and trisomy 8 are more common in patients with de novo MDS. Both standard Giemsa chromosome banding and fluorescent in situ hybridization (FISH) methods are used routinely for chromosomal analysis in MDS.

## TREATMENT

In refractory anemia (RA) or refractory cytopenia, the median time for RA to evolve to RA with excess blasts (RAEB) is usually 47 months. For this reason, AML chemotherapy and allogeneic HSCT are postponed until neutropenia or transfusion dependency develops. In RAEB or RAEB in transformation (RAEB-T), these patients are treated with AML chemotherapy and allogeneic HSCT. Patients with therapy-induced MDS/AML are also treated with AML chemotherapy and allogeneic HSCT.

## RESULTS OF THERAPY

In de novo MDS, 70% of patients attain remission after induction chemotherapy, and 50% of patients survive free of disease with human leukocyte antigen–matched family donor HSCT and 35% with matched unrelated donor HSCT. In therapy-induced MDS, 50% of patients attain remission after induction chemotherapy, and 20% to 30% of patients survive free of disease following allogeneic HSCT. Allogeneic HSCT is the only curative treatment for MDS.

**Table 109-10**

**World Health Organization Classification and Criteria for Myelodysplastic Syndrome**

| *Disease* | *Blood Findings* | *Bone Marrow Findings* |
|---|---|---|
| Refactory anemia (RA) | Anemia<br>No or rare blasts | Erythroid dysplasia *only*<br><5% blasts<br><15% ringed sideroblasts |
| Refactory anemia with ringed sideroblasts (RARS) | Anemia<br>No blasts | Erythroid dysplasia *only*<br><5% blasts<br><15% ringed sideroblasts |
| Refactory cytopenia with multilineage dysplasia (RCMD) | Cytopenias (bicytopenia or pancytopenia)<br>No or rare blasts<br>No Auer rods<br>$<1 \cdot 10^9$/L monocytes | Dysplasia <10% of cells in 2 or more myeloid cell lines<br><5% blasts in marrow<br><15% ringed sideroblasts<br>No Auer rods |
| Refactory cytopenia with multilineage dysplasia and ringed sideroblasts (RCMD-RS) | Cytopenias (bicytopenia or pancytopenia)<br>No or rare blasts<br>No Auer rods<br>$<1 \cdot 10^9$/L monocytes | Dysplasia <10% of cells in 2 or more myeloid cell lines<br><5% blasts<br><15% ringed sideroblasts<br>No Auer rods |
| Refractory anemia with excess blasts-1 (RAEB-1) | Cytopenias<br><5% blasts<br>No Auer rods<br>$<1 \cdot 10^9$/L monocytes | Unilineage or multilineage dysplasia<br>5%–9% blasts<br>No Auer rods |
| Refactory anemia with excess blasts-2 (RAEB-2) | Cytopenias<br>5%–19% blasts<br>Auer rods ±<br>$1 \cdot 10^9$/L monocytes | Unilineage or multilineage dysplasia<br>10%–19% blasts<br>Auer rods ± |
| Myelodysplastic syndrome, unclassified (MDS-U) | Cytopenias<br>No or rare blasts<br>No Auer rods | Unilineage dysplasia in granulocytes or megakaryocytes<br><5% blasts<br>No Auer rods |
| MDS associated with isolated del(5q) | Anemia<br><5% blasts<br>Platelets normal or increased | Normal to increased megakaryocytes with hypolobated nuclei<br><5% blasts<br>No Auer rods<br>Isolated del(5q) |

From Vardiman JW, Harris NL, Brunning RD. The World Health Organization (WHO) classification of the myeloid neoplasms. *Blood*. 2002;100(7):2292–2302. 

## CHRONIC MYELOGENOUS LEUKEMIA

In the WHO proposal, chronic myelogenous leukemia (CML) is defined specifically as a myeloproliferative disease that is characterized by the invariable presence of the Ph chromosome or the *BCR/ABL* fusion gene.[5]

### EPIDEMIOLOGY

Chronic myelogenous leukemia constitutes only 1% to 3% of leukemias in the pediatric age group. Its etiology in children is not known. Exposure to ionizing radiation is the only known environmental factor that has been implicated as a causative agent in CML. However, it is rarely the cause in pediatric CML.[28]

### SIGNS AND SYMPTOMS

Chronic myelogenous leukemia is characterized by 3 phases: the chronic phase, the accelerated phase, and the blast phase.

#### Chronic Phase

During the chronic phase, a patient may complain of nonspecific symptoms such as fever, night sweats, abdominal pain, or bone pain. Symptoms caused by hyperviscosity from extreme leukocytosis include headache, stroke, visual disturbances (due to retinal hemorrhages, papilledema), or priapism. Pallor, sternal tenderness, hepatomegaly, and splenomegaly may also be present at diagnosis.

***Laboratory Findings*** Mild normocytic, normochromic anemia and leukocytosis with a shift to the left of the neutrophilic series (characterized by a sequential orderly maturation of the myeloid series from myeloblasts to segmented neutrophils), mild eosinophilia, basophilia, and thrombocytosis are found in the peripheral blood. The bone marrow is hypercellular with a predominance of the myeloid series. Eosinophils, basophils, and megakaryocytes are increased. Cytogenetic studies by standard banding method and FISH reveal the presence of the Ph chromosome, t(9;22)(q34;q11).

### Accelerated Phase

The accelerated phase is a poorly defined phase in which a patient may experience fever, night sweats, and weight loss. Box 109-10 lists the WHO criteria for the diagnosis of the accelerated phase of CML.

### Blast Phase

During the blast phase, a patient may complain of pallor, easy bruisability, pruritus, urticaria, and bone pain. Evolution to the blast phase results from loss of ability of leukemic cells to differentiate. Clinical and laboratory features are quite similar to those in acute leukemias. Myeloid blast crisis is the most common type (80%), followed by lymphoid crisis (15%–20%) and, rarely, there may occur a multilineage, erythrocytic, or megakaryoblastic crisis. See Box 109-10 for the WHO criteria for diagnostic criteria of the blast crisis.

## BIOLOGY OF CHRONIC MYELOGENOUS LEUKEMIA

The *bcr/abl* fusion gene encodes a 210-kd tumor-specific BCR/ABL oncoprotein, which has constitutive tyrosine kinase activity and the ability to autophosphorylate by binding to ATP. This results in downstream signal transduction and activation of proteins such as RAS, PI3K, JAK-STAT, BCL-2, BCLx, and ROS, which induces cellular transformation, proliferation, inhibition of apoptosis, and altered cytoskeletal function with decreased adhesion. As a result of these molecular abnormalities, CML cells have a selective growth advantage, prolonged survival, and increased accumulation.

## TREATMENT

### Chronic Phase

Imatinib mesylate (STI 571, Gleevec) is the drug of choice to treat the chronic phase of CML in adult patients. It blocks the activity of the BCR/ABL protein by occupying the ABL-tyrosine kinase pocket and, thus, blocking ATP from binding to the site. It is more effective than the previously used regimen of α-interferon and cytarabine. Treatment with imatinib is monitored by periodically performing a cytogenetic study using both standard FISH and quantitative PCR methods.

### Blast Crisis

Myelocytic blast crisis is treated with AML-like induction phase therapy and lymphoid blast crisis with ALL-like induction phase therapy. The only curative treatment for CML is allogeneic HSCT.

### Box 109-10

***World Health Organization Criteria for Accelerated and Blast Phases of Chronic Myelogenous Leukemia (CML)***

**CML, accelerated phase (AP)**

Diagnose if 1 or more of the following is present:

- Blasts 10%–19% of peripheral white blood cells (WBCs) or bone marrow cells
- Peripheral blood basophils at least 20%
- Persistent thrombocytopenia ($<100 \cdot 10^9$/L) unrelated to therapy, or persistent
- Thrombocytosis ($>100 \cdot 10^9$/L) unresponsive to therapy
- Increasing spleen size and increasing WBC count unresponsive to therapy
- Cytogenetic evidence of clonal evolution (ie, appearance of additional genetic abnormality that was not present in initial specimen at time of chronic phase CML diagnosis)
- Megakaryocytic proliferation in sizable sheets and clusters, associated with marked reticulin or collagen fibrosis and/or severe granulocytic dysplasia, should be considered as suggestive of CML-AP. These findings have not yet been analyzed in large clinical studies, however, so it is not clear if they are independent criteria for the accelerated phase. They often occur simultaneously with 1 or more of the other features listed.

**CML, blast phase (BP)**

Diagnose if 1 or more of following is present:

- Blasts 20% or more of peripheral WBCs or bone marrow cells
- Extramedullary blast proliferation
- Large foci or clusters of blasts in bone marrow biopsy

From Vardiman JW, Harris NL, Brunning RD. The World Health Organization (WHO) classification of the myeloid neoplasms. *Blood*. 2002;100(7);2292–2302. 

## REFERENCES


1. Palmblad JEW, von dem Borne AEG Jr. Idiopathic, immune, infectious, and idiosyncratic neutropenias. *Semin Hematol.* 2002;39:113–120

2. Misra M, Aggarwal A, Miller KK, et al. Effects of anorexia nervosa on clinical, hematologic, biochemical, and bone density parameters in community-dwelling adolescent girls. *Pediatrics.* 2004;114:1574–1583

3. Walsh TJ, Roilides E, Groll AH, Gonzalez C, Pizzo PA. Infectious complications in pediatric cancer patients. In: Pizzo PA, Poplack DG, eds. *Principles and Practice of Pediatric Oncology.* 5th ed. Philadelphia, PA: Lippincott Williams & Wilkins; 2006:1269–1329

4. Dinauer MC. The phagocyte system and disorders of granulopoiesis and granulocyte function. In: Nathan DG, Orkin SH, Ginsberg D, Look TA, eds. *Hematology of Infancy and Childhood.* 6th ed. Philadelphia, PA: WB Saunders; 2003:923–1010

5. Vardiman JW, Harris NL, Brunning RD. World Health Organization (WHO) classification of the myeloid neoplasms. *Blood.* 2002;100(7):2292–2302

6. Brito-Babapulle F. The eosinophils, including the idiopathic hypereosinophilic syndrome. *Br J Haematol.* 2003;121(2):203–223

7. Shende A. Disorders of white blood cells. In: Lanzkowsky P, ed. *Manual of Pediatric Hematology and Oncology*. 4th ed. London: Elsevier Academic Press; 2005:209–249

8. Kilon AD. Recent advances in the diagnosis and treatment of hypereosinophilic syndromes. *Hematology Am Soc Hematol Educ Program.* 2005:209–214

9. Smith MA, Gloeckler Ries LA. Childhood cancer: incidence, survival, and mortality. In: Pizzo PA, Poplack DG, eds. *Principles and Practice of Pediatric Oncology.* 4th ed. Philidephia, PA: Lippincott Williams & Wilkins; 2001; 1–12

10. Spector LG, Ross JA, Robinson LL, Bhatia S. Epidemiology and etiology In: Pui CH, ed. *Childhood Leukemias.* 2nd ed. United Kingdom: Cambridge University Press; 2006: 48–66

11. Taub JW, Konrad MA, Ge Y, et al. High frequency of leukemic clones in newborn screening blood samples of children with B-precursor acute lymphoblastic leukemia. *Blood.* 2002;99:2992–2996

12. Wiemels JL, Xiao Z, Buffler PA, et al. In utero origin of t(8;21) *AML1-ETO* translocations in childhood myeloid leukemia. *Blood.* 2002;99:3801–3805

13. Margolin JF, Steuber PC, Poplack DG. Acute lymphoblastic leukemia. In: Pizzo PA, Poplack DG, eds. *Principles and Practice of Pediatric Oncology.* 5th ed. Philadelphia, PA: Lippincott Williams & Wilkins; 2006:538–590

14. Ferrando AA, Rubnitz JE, Look AT. Molecular genetics of acute lymphoblastic leukemia. In: Pui CH, ed. *Childhood Leukemias.* 2nd ed. United Kingdom: Cambridge University Press; 2006:272–297

15. DeAngelo DJ. The treatment of adolescents and young adults with acute lymphoblastic leukemia. *Hematology Am Soc Hematol Educ Program.* 2005;123–130

16. Breit S, Stanulla M, Flohr T, et al. Activating *NOTCH1* mutations predict favorable early treatment response and long-term outcome in childhood precursor T-cell lymphoblastic leukemia. *Blood.* 2006;108:1151–1157

17. Jones OY, Spencer CH, Bowyer SL, Dent PB, Gottlieb BS, Rabinovich CE. A multicenter case-control study on predictive factors distinguishing childhood leukemia from juvenile rheumatoid arthritis. *Pediatrics.* 2006;117:840–844

18. Behm FG, Campana D. Immunophenotyping. In: Pui CH, ed. *Childhood Leukemias.* United Kingdom: Cambridge University Press; 1999:111–144

19. Pui CH, Schrappe M, Ribeiro RC, Niemeyer CM. Childhood and adolescent lymphoid and myeloid leukemia. *Hematology Am Soc Hematol Educ Program.* 2004;119–145

20. Nachman JB, Sather HN, Sensel MG, et al. Augmented post-induction therapy for children with high risk acute lymphoblastic leukemia and a slow response to initial therapy. *N Engl J Med.* 1998;338:1663–1671

21. Asselin B, Shuster J, Amylon M, et al. Improved event-free survival (EFS) with high-dose methotrexate (HDM) in T-cell lymphoblastic leukemia (T-ALL) and advanced lymphoblastic lymphoma (T-NHL): a Pediatric Oncology Group (POG) study. *Proc Am Soc Clin Oncol.* 2001;20:367a (abstr 1464)

22. Patte C, Auperin A, Michon J, et al. The Societe Francaise d'Oncologie Pediatrique LMB89 protocol: highly effective multiagent chemotherapy tailored to the tumor burden and initial response in 561 unselected children with B-cell lymphomas and L3 leukemia. *Blood.* 2001;97:3370–3379

23. Boissel N, Auclerc F, Lheritier V, et al. Should adolescents with acute lymphoblastic leukemia be treated as old children or young adults? Comparison of the French FRALLE-93 and LALA-94 trials. *J Clin Oncol.* 2003;21:774–780

24. Golub TR, Arceci RJ. Acute myelogenous leukemia. In: Pizzo PA, Poplack DG, eds. *Principles and Practice of Pediatric Oncology.* 5th ed. Philadelphia, PA: Lippincott Williams & Wilkins; 2006:591–644

25. Lanzkowsky P, ed. *Manual of Pediatric Hematology and Oncology*. 4th ed. London: Elsevier Academic Press; 2005: 415–452

26. Woods WG, Kobrinsky N, Buckley JD, et al. Timed-sequential induction therapy improves postremission outcomes in acute myeloid leukemia: a report from the Children's Oncology Group. *Blood*. 1996;87:4979–4989

27. Smith FO, Woods WG. Myeloproliferative and myelodysplastic disorders. In: Pizzo PA, Poplack DG, eds. *Principles and Practice of Pediatric Oncology.* 5th ed. Philadelphia, PA: Lippincott Williams & Wilkins; 2006:673–694

28. Altman AJ, Fu C. Chronic leukemia of childhood. In: Pizzo A, Poplack DG, eds. *Principles and Practice of Pediatric Oncology.* 5th ed. Philadelphia, PA: Lippincott Williams & Wilkins; 2006:645–672

# CHAPTER 110

# Lymphadenopathy and Splenomegaly

MARK ATLAS, MD

## INTRODUCTION

The various functions of the lymph nodes and spleen, immune and otherwise, make the assessment of the adolescent patient with persistent lymphadenopathy and/or splenomegaly challenging. Lymph node enlargement occurs less frequently in adolescents than in children, but remains a common normal response to infection and other stimuli. The clinician must differentiate reactive processes, many of which require simple interventions, if any, from lymphadenopathy and splenomegaly secondary to serious or life-threatening underlying disease. Splenomegaly outside the setting of Epstein-Barr virus (EBV) infection remains uncommon in adolescence and can pose diagnostic difficulties, especially in the asymptomatic patient without concomitant lymphadenopathy. The lengthy differential diagnosis only compounds the challenge.

Normal lymph nodes are encapsulated structures of lymphoid tissue supported by reticular tissue and separated into the cortex and the medulla. The normal architecture of the cortex includes primary and secondary nodules (the latter possess a germinal center). B lymphocytes populate the outer cortex with T lymphocytes in the deep cortex, which is devoid of nodules. The medulla consists of multiple lymph sinuses that converge on the efferent lymphatic to drain the node. When presented with antigen, lymphocytes may proliferate and cause enlargement of the node. Proliferation of other intrinsic cells, including monocytes, histiocytes, and plasma cells, may also contribute to reactive hyperplasia, which is defined as a polyclonal proliferation of cells intrinsic to the lymph node. Monoclonal proliferation of dysregulated immune cells occurs in malignancies, such as leukemia and lymphoma. Infiltration by extrinsic cells, including nonhematopoietic malignant cells and storage cells, may also cause lymphadenopathy.[1]

The spleen, encapsulated with dense connective tissue from which its trabeculae emanate, consists of areas of white and red pulp. White pulp consists of lymphatic tissue in whose nodules germinal centers form in response to antigen. The red pulp contains the splenic sinuses within splenic cords of erythrocytes and white blood cells. The porous sinuses, lined by endothelial cells that do not tightly adhere to one another, allow blood cells to traverse the sinuses easily. The circulation through the sinuses is relatively slow, enabling macrophages to phagocytose damaged blood cells, which may then be easily removed from the circulation. In addition, the spleen may contain a large reserve of erythrocytes that can be mobilized into the circulation by contraction of myofibroblasts in the capsule. Similar to reactive lymphadenopathy, the spleen may enlarge secondary to polyclonal proliferation of immune cells in the white pulp, which tends to be self-limited. Splenomegaly may also occur in response to hemolysis, erythrocyte sequestration, or extramedullary hematopoiesis; in response to infiltration by malignant or storage cells; as a result of congestion secondary to hepatic disease or abnormalities of portal circulation; or as a result of primary disorders of the spleen, including vascular malformations, cysts, and hemorrhage.[1]

## CLINICAL PRESENTATION

The rapid onset of lymphadenopathy in an isolated region concurrent with symptoms of localized infection is the most common presentation (eg, strep pharyngitis). The nodes in these situations are typically firm, but not hard; relatively small (<2.5 cm); moderately tender; mobile; and nonerythematous. They may occur in any region, but true supraclavicular lymph nodes must be considered pathological until proven otherwise. Although shrinkage is reasonably rapid following resolution of infection, reactive lymph nodes may partially shrink and then persist. Such nodes typically require periodic re-evaluation by physical examination at increasing intervals. If they progressively enlarge in the absence of infection, further evaluation becomes necessary. Diffuse lymphadenopathy, with or without splenomegaly, represents a systemic process, the classic being infectious mononucleosis secondary to EBV or cytomegalovirus (CMV). Persistent enlargement for several weeks is common. However, there is typically a plateau in enlargement, so continuous growth is a cause for concern. Associated symptoms such as fever, fatigue, and minimal weight loss are common. Isolated splenomegaly is less commonly a reactive process and, if persistent, requires a thorough diagnostic evaluation.[2,3]

## DIFFERENTIAL DIAGNOSIS

The frequency with which lymphadenopathy is seen and the lack of specificity of many of the associated symptoms necessitates formulating a comprehensive differential diagnosis (Box 110-1). Isolated splenomegaly requires a similar approach (Box 110-2) and may also lead to the discovery of enlarged lymph nodes in regions too deep to palpate. The patient history must specifically focus on the numerous possible infectious etiologies. After initial broad-based questioning, specific questions regarding recent infections, wounds, medications and illegal drug use, animal bites or scratches, insect or tick bites, travel history, family history, sexual history, arthralgia, rash, fever, drenching night sweats, and weight loss (>10% without dieting) must be asked. Clearly, many of these questions should be asked or repeated without parents present.

### Box 110-1

### *Lymphadenopathy*

**Infectious Disorders**

- Bacterial infections
  - Streptococcal infection
  - Staphylococcal infection
  - *Bartonella henselae* (cat-scratch disease)
  - *Chlamydia trachomatis*
  - Diphtheria
  - Listeriosis
  - Anaerobic infection
  - *Yersinia pestis*
  - Brucellosis
  - *Salmonella typhi*
  - *Francisella tularensis*
  - *Mycobacterium tuberculosis*
  - Atypical mycobacterial tuberculosis
- Viral infections
  - Epstein-Barr virus
  - Cytomegalovirus
  - Hepatitis A, B, and C
  - Adenovirus
  - Herpes simplex virus
  - Varicella
  - Rubeola
  - Rubella
  - Mumps
  - Coxsackie virus
  - Human immunodeficiency virus (HIV)

### Box 110-1 (continued)

- Treponemal infections
  - *Treponema pallidum*
  - *Borrelia burgdorferi*
  - Leptospirosis
- Fungal infections
  - Candida
  - Aspergillus
  - Histoplasmosis
  - Coccidiomycosis
  - Blastomycosis
  - Tinea capitis
  - Cryptococcus
- Rickettsial infections
  - Rocky Mountain spotted fever (*Rickettsia rickettsii*)
  - Typhus
- Parasitic infections
  - Malaria
  - Babesiosis
  - Trypanosomiasis
  - Toxoplasmosis

**Neoplastic Disorders**

- Hodgkin disease
- Non-Hodgkin lymphoma
- Acute lymphoblastic leukemia
- Acute myelogenous leukemia
- Chronic myelogenous leukemia
- Thyroid carcinoma
- Rhabdomyosarcoma
- Nasopharyngeal carcinoma
- Parotid tumors
- Langerhans cell histiocytosis
- Hemophagocytic lymphohistiocytosis
- Malignant histiocytosis
- Macrophage activation syndrome

**Lymphoproliferative Disorders**

- Post-transplant lymphoproliferative disorder
- Castleman disease (benign "giant lymph node hyperplasia")
- Hemophagocytic lymphohistiocytosis
- Rosai-Dorfman (sinus histiocytosis with massive lymphadenopathy)
- X-linked lymphoproliferative syndrome
- Autoimmune lymphoproliferative syndrome

*(continued)*

### Box 110-1 (continued)

**Immunodeficiencies**

- Chronic granulomatous disease
- Chediak-Higashi syndrome
- Leukocyte adhesion deficiency

**Metabolic/Storage Diseases**

- Gaucher disease
- Neimann-Pick disease
- Amyloidosis
- Mucopolysaccharidoses (ie, Hunter syndrome, Hurler syndrome)

**Autoimmune Disorders**

- Erythema nodosum
- System lupus erythematosis
- Serum sickness
- Felty syndrome (rheumatoid arthritis, splenomegaly, neutropenia)
- Rheumatoid arthritis
- Sjögren syndrome
- Rheumatic fever
- Autoimmune lymphoproliferative syndrome

**Liver Diseases**

- Portal hypertension
- Budd-Chiari syndrome
- Wilson disease
- Cirrhosis
- Portal vein thrombosis
- Veno-oclusive disease of the liver

**Miscellaneous**

- Lymphatic malformation
- Splenic cyst
- Hemorrhage

### Box 110-2

### *Splenomegaly*

**Infectious Disorders**

- Bacterial infections
  - Systemic infection (acute and chronic, including sepsis)
  - Subacute bacterial endocarditis
  - Abscess
  - *Salmonella typhi*
  - *Francisella tularensis*
  - Tuberculosis

### Box 110-2 (continued)

- Viral infections
  - Epstein-Barr virus
  - Cytomegalovirus
  - Hepatitis A, B, and C
  - Human immunodeficiency virus (HIV)
- Treponemal infections
  - *Treponema pallidum*
  - *Borrelia burgdorferi*
- Fungal infections
  - Histoplasmosis
  - Coccidiomycosis
  - Blastomycosis
- Rickettsial infections
  - Rocky Mountain spotted fever (*Rickettsia rickettsii*)
  - Typhus
- Parasitic infections
  - Malaria
  - Babesiosis
  - Trypanosomiasis
  - Toxoplasmosis
  - *Toxocara canis* and *Toxocara cati*
  - Schistosomiasis
  - Leischmaniasis

**Hematologic Disorders**

- Red blood cell disorders
  - Hemoglobinopathies
    - Sickle cell syndromes: Hgb SC and S-β-thalassemia
    - β-Thalassemia major
    - Thalassemia intermedia, E-β-thalassemia, other thalassemic syndromes
    - Hemoglobin H disease
  - Hereditary spherocytosis
  - Hereditary elliptocytosis
  - Pyruvate kinase deficiency
  - G6PD deficiency
  - Erythropoietic protoporphyria
  - Autoimmune hemolytic anemia
- Thrombotic thrombocytopenic purpura
- Myeloproliferative disease (ie, polycythemia vera)
- Myelofibrosis
- Hemophagocytic lymphohistiocytosis
- Rosai-Dorfman (sinus histiocytosis)
- Mastocytosis

*(continued)*

**Box 110-2 (continued)**

**Neoplastic Disorders**

- Hodgkin disease
- Non-Hodgkin lymphoma
- Acute lymphoblastic leukemia
- Acute myelogenous leukemia
- Chronic myelogenous leukemia
- Langerhans cell histiocytosis
- Hemophagocytic lymphohistiocytosis
- Hemangioma

**Metabolic/Storage Diseases**

- Gaucher disease
- Neimann-Pick disease
- Amyloidosis
- Mucopolysaccharidoses (ie, Hunter syndrome, Hurler syndrome)

**Autoimmune Disorders**

- Erythema nodosum
- Systemic lupus erythematosis
- Serum sickness
- Felty syndrome
- Rheumatoid arthritis
- Sjögren syndrome
- Rheumatic fever
- Autoimmune lymphoproliferative syndrome

**Liver Diseases**

- Portal hypertension
- Budd-Chiari syndrome
- Wilson disease
- Cirrhosis
- Portal vein thrombosis
- Veno-oclusive disease of the liver

**Miscellaneous**

- Lymphatic malformation
- Splenic cyst
- Hemorrhage
- Familial Mediterranean fever

## EVALUATION

The physical examination should be thorough, paying particular attention to the size, location, consistency, tenderness, and mobility of lymph nodes. Particular attention to the supraclavicular region is important (assessment may be easier with hands on hips), as well as less common areas of lymphadenopathy, such as the occipital, posterior auricular, epitrochlear, and popliteal areas. Palpation of liver and spleen for size and consistency is critical, and must be performed from the pelvis superiorly to the costal margin and from the midline laterally to the anterior axillary line to avoid erroneously missing organomegaly. Measuring nodes and spleen with a tape measure greatly improves interobserver reliability. Superior vena cava (SVC) syndrome and tracheal compression are rare but critical to diagnose. Thorough examination of the skin for petechiae, ecchymoses, scratches, wounds, birthmarks, exanthema, icterus, spider angiomata, caput medusa, Osler nodes, Janeway lesions, and splinter hemorrhages must be performed. External genital examination to evaluate for sexually transmitted disease and, in males, for testicular enlargement or mass, is likewise important.

Evaluation of the history and physical examination allows formulation of a preliminary assessment of whether the lymphadenopathy or splenomegaly, alone or in combination, are acutely reactive to infection; are persistent, but temporally associated with infection and likely resolving; are scarred lymph nodes; or are nonreactive and likely secondary to an underlying disease. When lymph nodes arise in the setting of an acute febrile illness with symptoms that localize to the area (eg, strep pharyngitis) and are tender, a clinical diagnosis of reactive lymphadenopathy can readily be made. Persistent lymph nodes that are present for weeks to months may represent reactive nodes that have only partially involuted and are not pathological. Nodes that are rubbery, <2 cm in longest dimension, and mobile may be observed with serial physical examinations if basic laboratory evaluations are normal. Similarly, a minimally enlarged spleen or "spleen tip" that is relatively soft, without concerning constitutional symptoms, may be observed and will frequently recede in a few weeks. A spleen that is palpable more than 2 to 3 cm below the costal margin, especially if it has a very firm edge and feel to it, is more likely to be pathological and warrants an immediate preliminary workup. More targeted or extensive laboratory evaluation may be indicated from the specific history, signs, or symptoms. Rock hard, fixed, nonerythematous, nontender lymph nodes or massive splenomegaly are suspicious for malignancy, with or without constitutional symptoms, and demand urgent preliminary evaluation with rapid progression to biopsy unless another etiology is determined.[2] The presence of superior vena cava syndrome, respiratory distress, or evidence of pleural or pericardial effusion is a medical emergency.[4]

When a clinical diagnosis of reactive lymphadenopathy is not immediately evident, or if splenomegaly is concerning (isolated or in combination with lymphadenopathy), an initial laboratory evaluation should include the following steps:

- A complete blood count with differential, a reticulocyte count, and a review of the peripheral smear should be the starting point in most patients. Leukocytosis and leukocytopenia are frequently present and, in combination with atypical lymphocytosis, suggest viral infection. In combination with peripheral blasts, these are diagnostic of leukemia. Examination of the erythrocyte morphology may demonstrate abnormal forms consistent with hemolytic anemia; these include sickle cells, target cells, spherocytes, elliptocytes, acanthocytes, schistocytes, and cell fragments. These are evaluated in conjunction with the hemoglobin, red blood cell, and reticulocyte counts, as well as mean corpuscular hemoglobin and other indices, and may provide a preliminary diagnosis of an underlying erythrocyte disorder. Thrombocytosis is generally reactive and would typically support an infectious etiology. Thrombocytopenia with large platelets is typically a destructive process consistent with immune destruction or extravascular destruction (ie, disseminated intravascular coagulopathy or thrombotic thrombocytopenic purpura).
- The erythrocyte sedimentation rate (ESR) is relatively nonspecific when elevated, but when normal makes the diagnosis of active infection or hematologic malignancy less likely.
- Electrolytes, renal function tests, liver function tests, uric acid, and lactose dehydrogenase may give clues about viral illnesses or the tumor lysis syndrome (TLS) seen in leukemia and lymphoma. Elevation of transaminases is common in viral infections such as EBV, CMV, varicella, and hepatitis B and C, but atypical of malignancy. Elevated potassium, uric acid, phosphorus, and lactate dehydrogenase are suspicious for TLS secondary to destruction of malignant leukemia or lymphoma cells.
- Viral titers for EBV and CMV are useful because these infections are a particularly common cause of lymphadenopathy and splenomegaly in the adolescent patient.
- A chest radiograph may provide evidence of hilar lymphadenopathy, mediastinal mass, pleural effusion, or cardiomegaly. These are not specific and may be secondary to infectious, malignant, or other causes, but demonstrate acute need for further diagnosis and management.
- A tuberculin skin test, to evaluate for *Myobacterium tuberculosis*, is important because tuberculosis (Tuberculosis) can present with unilateral or bilateral cervical lymphadenopathy and hilar lymphadenopathy. (TB testing may be omitted with isolated splenomegaly if performed within the past year and a chest radiograph does not demonstrate hilar lymphadenopathy.)
- Specific tests based on the history and physical examination should be performed simultaneously, as discussed next.

In the event that any of the above examinations support the diagnosis of malignancy (eg, multiple cytopenias, presence of blasts or suspicious cells on peripheral blood smear, electrolytes suggestive of TLS, mediastinal mass or hilar lymphadenopathy with a negative tuberculin skin test), careful consideration should be given to obtaining a tissue diagnosis. If leukemia is suspected, then a bone marrow aspirate for morphology, immunophenotyping, and cytogenetics may be performed. Otherwise, if a suspicious enlarged lymph node is accessible, then an excisional lymph node biopsy should be performed. Fine-needle aspiration should be avoided because it does not reveal the lymph node architecture and, therefore, is rarely diagnostic and delays definitive diagnosis. If the lymph nodes feel malignant, then biopsy is warranted unless preliminary testing yields a definitive diagnosis. In the case of isolated splenomegaly, if the preliminary evaluation provides no answer, then further radiographic and laboratory evaluation to determine suspected conditions (Box 110-2) should be undertaken. Biopsy of the spleen is only rarely necessary to make a diagnosis, and the risk of bleeding must be considered.

Further radiographic evaluation may include the following:

- Computed tomography (CT): If lymphoma is suspected, then axial images from the Waldeyer ring in the neck through the pelvis should be obtained with intravenous and oral contrast. This provides excellent anatomic evaluation of lymphadenopathy in all major lymph node groups, as well as in the airway, lungs, liver, and spleen.
- Ultrasonography of the liver and spleen may be useful to evaluate for anatomic causes of splenomegaly, including cysts, nodular abnormalities, and vascular malformations; to serially measure spleen size; and to examine the circulation of the hepatic, portal, and splenic vasculature.

- Positron emission tomography (PET) with scans superimposed on CT images provide information on the metabolic activity of lymph nodes and organomegaly, and may be helpful in assessing the risk of malignancy in masses that are nonspecific in nature and in providing a baseline for follow-up of lymphoma to assess functional response.
- Magnetic resonance imaging (MRI) may be useful to further elucidate abnormalities, especially of the spleen and liver, that are not clear on CT scanning.
- $^{99m}$Technicium-sulfur colloid liver-spleen scanning may be useful to elucidate spleen function and size, especially in hematologic causes of splenomegaly.

Further laboratory evaluation should be guided by the history and physical examination, and may include the following:

- Specific serologic evaluation for infectious causes of lymphadenopathy (eg, *Bartonella henselae*; toxoplasmosis; HIV; hepatitis A, B, and C; Lyme disease; syphilis), a smear for malaria and babesiosis, and stool for ova and parasites.
- Evaluation for hemolytic disorders, including hemoglobin electrophoresis (hemoglobinopathy), osmotic fragility (hereditary spherocytosis), direct Coombs (autoimmune hemolytic anemia), and quantitative glucose-6-phosphate dehydrogenase levels.
- Screening for autoimmune diseases such as systemic lupus erythematosis (SLE), rheumatoid arthritis, and sarcoidosis with antinuclear antigen, anti–double-stranded DNA, C3, C4, rheumatoid factor, and angiotensin-converting enzyme levels.
- T-cell rearrangement studies to evaluate for autoimmune lymphoproliferative disorder.
- Evaluation for Gaucher disease.
- Immune function testing, including quantitative immunoglobulins, nitro blue tetrazolium (for chronic granulomatous disease), and CD 11 and 18 by flow cytometric analysis for leukocyte adhesion deficiency.

## ETIOLOGIES

### INFECTIOUS

Infectious etiologies are by far the most common causes of lymphadenopathy and splenomegaly. A thorough history and physical examination with judicious supplementary laboratory evaluation usually leads to an accurate diagnosis.

#### Viral Infections

Viral infections with EBV and CMV are the most common infectious causes of lymphadenopathy and splenomegaly in adolescents. Presentation may vary, but most commonly includes fever, fatigue (which may be severe), headache, enlarged lymph nodes in one (typically cervical) or multiple regions, mild-moderate splenomegaly, exudative pharyngitis, and malaise. History of close contact with other infected persons is common. Erythematous rash from presumptive treatment for strep pharyngitis with amoxicillin may be present. Classic hematologic findings include leukocytosis with an increased percentage of atypical lymphocytes. Neutropenia, thrombocytopenia, or autoimmune hemolytic anemia may also be present, increasing concern of hematologic malignancy. Symptoms may last for several weeks, further increasing concern, especially in the face of false-negative EBV VCA-IgM antibody and early antigen testing, which is common in the initial phase of symptomatology.[5]

Adenoviral infections commonly occur in adolescents, presenting as pharyngitis, pneumonitis, and/or conjunctivitis, among other symptoms, often with lymphadenopathy and occasionally with splenomegaly. Cytopenias may occur, increasing suspicion for underlying malignancy.

Measles and rubella are still seen periodically in adolescents because increasing numbers of families choose not to immunize children and because immunity may not occur in all vaccine recipients, hence requiring booster doses of measles in all patients. Measles characteristically presents with cough, coryza, and conjunctivitis after a prodrome of fever, anorexia, and malaise. Cervical lymphadenopathy is common, but it may be generalized. Hepatitis and mesenteric adenopathy may contribute to abdominal pain. In rubella, fever, erythematous exanthem, and suboccipital and posterior auricular lymphadenopathy are typical, often after a prodrome of anorexia, malaise, and headache. It is rarely associated with thrombocytopenic purpura.[6]

Lymphadenopathy is common in HIV infection, resulting from primary infection, secondary infection, or HIV-related lymphoma. Careful attention to history of at-risk behavior is important when evaluating the adolescent with lymphadenopathy. Frequent infection, weight loss, and persistent lymphadenopathy or hepatosplenomegaly increase concern. Adolescents presenting with B-lineage lymphomas warrant HIV testing; these are particularly challenging to treat and cure because of ongoing immunosuppression critical to surveillance for and elimination of minimal residual disease post-therapy.[7]

### Bacterial Infections

The most common bacterial infections causing lymphadenopathy are streptococcal and staphylococcal infections of the upper respiratory tract and skin, with reactive lymphadenopathy in the regional nodes associated with the site of infection, usually cervical, axillary, or inguinal.[3] Other notable infections include the following:

Brucellosis, which is usually transmitted by ingestion of infected milk or meat from farm animal reservoirs. Bacteria multiply in regional lymph nodes, and then subsequently disseminate, causing fever, chills, myalgia, anorexia, and generalized lymphadenopathy and splenomegaly.[6]

Cat-scratch disease results from inoculation of *Bartonella henselae* by a cat scratch. Regional lymph node(s) may enlarge and last for weeks to months. Mild fever and constitutional symptoms may occur. Nodes suppurate in approximately 25% of cases. Rare complications include erythema nodosum, mesenteric adenitis, and encephalitis.[8]

Lymphogranuloma venereum results in inguinal and femoral lymphadenopathy, which may be bilateral and occurs 2 to 6 weeks after infection with *Chlamydia trachomatis* via sexual contact. Lesions progress, becoming matted and painful. The overlying skin becomes adherent and erythematous, and may rupture, with drainage of pus. Fever and malaise may occur.[6]

Mycoplasma infections are common in adolescence, causing pneumonia that may be associated with hilar lymphadenopathy and sometimes cervical lymphadenopathy. Cold agglutinins are commonly positive. Autoimmune hemolytic anemia may occur. Radiographic findings vary and include diffuse infiltrates and, at times, a pleural effusion.[9]

Infection with *Francisella tularensis* causes the febrile illness tularemia, characterized by fever, chills, lymphadenopathy and splenomegaly, headache, and photophobia. The disease is rare, with exposure to wild rabbits being the most common manner of infection.[6]

*Mycobacterium tuberculosis* and atypical mycobacterial infection must be considered in adolescents, even without a history of exposure. Cervical and hilar lymphadenopathy are common in TB, often with systemic symptoms of fever, cough, and weight loss.[10] Atypical mycobacteria infections present as localized lymphadenopathy without constitutional symptoms, typically in the cervical region. Lymphadenitis may result with suppuration and sinus tract formation.[3]

### Treponemal Infections

Primary and secondary syphilis, acquired infection with *Treponema pallidum*, manifests with a painless chancre and regional lymphadenopathy during the primary phase. Systemic symptoms, including fever, myalgia, headache, malaise, rash, and generalized lymphadenopathy, especially epitrochlear lymph node enlargement, are common in secondary syphilis.[11]

### Fungal Infections

Coccidiomycosis and histoplasmosis both present typically with fever, myalgia, headache, and dry cough, with variably severe pneumonitis and hilar lymphadenopathy. The former is common in the west and southwest United States, Central and South America, and regions of Australia. Histoplasmosis is ubiquitous, but infection is more common in the Appalachian region through the Ohio, Missouri, and Mississippi River tributaries. Regional lymphadenopathy, hepatosplenomegaly, and anemia may also be present in histoplasmosis from disseminated involvement.[11]

### Parasitic Infections

Malaria should be considered in the patient with paroxysms of high fever (102.2°F–104°F [39°C–40°C]), which often occurs with chills and may be associated with myalgia, headache, and abdominal pain. Hemoglobinuria may result in anemia and jaundice. Infection with *Plasmodia* species is more common in tropical climates, but can occur in temperate climates, including parts of North America. Splenomegaly can be particularly impressive, especially in the face of anemia, where it serves as a site of hemolysis and erythrophagocytosis. Babesiosis, which is more common in North America, may mimic malaria to a certain extent, but is usually self-limited. It can be quite severe in the patient who has had a splenectomy.[6]

Trypanosomiasis (Chagas disease) is common in Central and South America and rarely presents in the southern United States. Some patients may have cutaneous erythematous nodules, but the majority of symptomatology is gastrointestinal (loss of peristalsis from smooth muscle damage) and cardiac (myocarditis that progresses). Some patients present with acute illness, including fever, generalized lymphadenopathy, hepatosplenomegaly, and malaise.[6]

## MALIGNANT

Leukemia and especially lymphoma are very common malignancies in the adolescent patient. Hodgkin disease (HD) is the most common of these, followed by the non-Hodgkin lymphomas (NHLs) (Burkitt, Burkitt-like, T- and B-lineage lymphoblastic lymphoma, diffuse large cell lymphoma [both B and T cell], and anaplastic large cell lymphoma are the most common varieties) and leukemia (both B precursor and T cell, the latter being substantially more common in adolescence than in younger children).[2,4] Patients may present with an asymptomatic single enlarged lymph node to massive diffuse lymphadenopathy with secondary effusions and hepatosplenomegaly, and severe constitutional symptoms such as fever, weight loss, night sweats, weakness, fatigue, bone pain, pain at the sites of disease, severe respiratory distress, cranial nerve palsy, and acute renal failure with electrolyte abnormalities. Hodgkin disease often presents as indolent, persistent lymphadenopathy, with the most common sites of involvement being cervical and mediastinal lymphadenopathy; splenomegaly may also occur, as can the "B symptoms" of fever, weight loss, and night sweats.[12] A history of lymphadenopathy for weeks to months is common. B-precursor cell lymphoblastic lymphoma is uncommon, but may also present with an indolent course. More often than not, bone marrow examination will demonstrate B-precursor leukemia.[7]

Other NHLs typically have a rapid aggressive onset, with doubling times of tumor mass as low as 24 hours. Burkitt lymphoma in the United States does not demonstrate the endemic phenotype of Burkitt lymphoma in Africa, which presents classically with a jaw mass. Many are nonetheless EBV related.[4] Gastrointestinal primaries are more common in the United States, at times presenting with intussusception. All may present with large mediastinal masses that may compress the airway. This is a medical emergency, and the reason all suspected lymphoma patients should have a chest radiograph urgently. Patients with airway compromise must not be sedated for any reason.[4] Patients should all have CT scans of the neck, chest, abdomen, and pelvis with oral and intravenous contrast, a PET scan, and a bone marrow aspirate. Excisional lymph node biopsy is the diagnostic method of choice, but core biopsies may provide sufficient cellular architecture to be diagnostic. Fine-needle aspirates are to be avoided because they are rarely diagnostic and do not provide sufficient tissue for immunophenotyping and cytogenetics, which are critical.[7]

Modern clinical research trials have resulted in greatly improved outcomes in leukemia and lymphoma patients. Most lymphomas are curable in 80% to 95% of patients, with the more aggressive T-cell lymphomas being the greatest exception.[13] Adolescents are, by definition, "high-risk" leukemia patients and, as a result, require more aggressive therapy, with cure rates currently in the 70% to 75% range.[14] Therapy for lymphoblastic leukemia and lymphoma consists of prolonged chemotherapy, often with cranial irradiation for central nervous system disease.[13,14] Hodgkin disease requires chemotherapy targeted to stage, with or without involved field irradiation, depending on stage, protocol, and, at times, gender. odgkin disease has a high rate of secondary malignancy, largely related to radiation. Elimination of radiation in females may decrease the high rate of secondary breast cancer. Other lymphomas are generally treated with shorter courses of very aggressive chemotherapy. Refractory disease may respond to radiation and/or autologous or allogeneic stem cell transplantation.[7]

Chronic myelogenous leukemia may present with splenomegaly and leukocytosis. More common in adolescents than in younger children, it remains a rare disease. Remission may be induced with newer targeted therapies, but the only current cure remains allogeneic stem cell transplantation.[15]

## NONMALIGNANT

### Gaucher Disease

This autosomal recessive disorder results from deficient β-glucocerebrosidase activity. It is classified based on degree of neuronal involvement in 3 categories. Type 1 is the most common and the most likely to present in adolescence. More common in Ashkenazi Jews, it exists in all populations, and presentation is variable, with splenomegaly and cytopenias being the most common signs. Type 2 disease presents in infancy, and type 3 disease in childhood.[2]

The manifestations of disease result from accumulation of glucocerebroside in macrophages of the reticuloendothelial system. Consequently, splenomegaly and hepatomegaly result from accumulation in the splenic macrophages and Kupffer cells, respectively. Secondary hypersplenism induces cytopenias, and bone marrow infiltration causes osteopenia, pathological fractures, and pain.[2]

With current enzyme replacement therapy (recombinant human glucocerebrosidase) given every 2 to 3 weeks, patients with Gaucher disease now survive into adulthood with excellent function.[7]

### Lymphoproliferative Disorders

Sinus histiocytosis with massive lymphadenopathy (Rosai-Dorfman) typically presents with impressive bilateral lymphadenopathy. The disease is benign, and there is often spontaneous regression within 12 months, but the lymphadenopathy may restrict range of motion and be cosmetically embarrassing to teenagers. Treatment with steroids or chemotherapy has variable success and is not indicated unless the patient is symptomatic.[16]

***Autoimmune lymphoproliferative syndrome*** This relatively recently described disease is characterized by one or more cytopenias, along with lymphadenopathy and splenomegaly; the adenopathy may be localized or diffuse, intermittent or persistent. There is an underlying FAS mutation that prevents normal apoptosis; lymphocytes therefore accumulate in the lymph nodes rather than dying. There are abnormalities of T-cell subsets and an increased risk of autoimmune hepatitis, uveitis, and renal disease. Patients are predisposed to certain lymphomas and other cancers.[17] Treatment of autoimmune cytopenias with immunosuppressive therapy is symptomatic. Patients tend to improve with age.[18]

***Post-transplant lymphoproliferative disorder*** Expansions of lymphoid tissue post transplant are being diagnosed with increased frequency as the number of solid organ and hematopoietic stem cell transplantations in pediatrics increases. Immunosuppression allows for EBV-induced immune dysregulation resulting in B-cell proliferation. Lymph nodes are the most commonly affected areas, but any lymphoid tissue may be affected, including the liver, spleen, and solid organs such as lungs and kidneys. Treatment of choice is to decrease or cease the use of immunosuppression. Chemotherapy may be useful in widespread or refractory disease.[19]

### Hematologic Disease

Splenomegaly is a relatively common manifestation of hemoglobinopathies. Patients with sickle cell disease may have splenic enlargement related to their chronic hemolysis because of the splenic hypertrophy that occurs with the removal of hemolyzed erythrocytes. In addition, there may be splenic sequestration that is acute or chronic, causing significant splenomegaly associated with worsening anemia, pallor, and lethargy. Transfusion of a small aliquot of packed red blood cells typically reverses sequestration. In hemoglobin SS disease, patients autoinfarct their spleens by age 6 years and should not have further splenomegaly. In hemoglobin SC, S-β-thalassemia, or other sickle genotypes, splenomegaly commonly persists throughout life. In thalassemia syndromes, the liver and spleen may serve as sites of extramedullary hematopoiesis and may be significantly enlarged. Splenectomy may decrease the rate of destruction and transfusion requirements.[20]

Other hemolytic anemias, such as hereditary spherocytosis (HS), other membrane and enzyme defects, and autoimmune hemolytic anemias, may present with splenomegaly, generally related to the removal of destroyed red blood cells. In some diseases, such as HS, splenectomy effectively cures the clinical manifestations of disease.[7]

### Congestive Splenomegaly

Splenic enlargement may occur as a result of liver disease due to increased vascular resistance and increased intravascular pressure transmitted to the splenic vessels. This may result from cirrhosis (secondary to cystic fibrosis, Wilson disease, or alpha-1-antitrypsin deficiency) or from portal hypertension or portal vein obstruction (secondary to mass, thrombosis or vascular malformation). Congestion may lead to increased collateral blood flow and formation of esophageal varices and potential bleeding complications. Hypersplenism may cause leukopenia, anemia, or thrombocytopenia.[11]

### Autoimmune Disease

Serum sickness and other autoimmune diseases may be characterized by splenomegaly and sometimes lymphadenopathy. Other findings such as rash, constitutional symptoms, arthralgia, and renal dysfunction are more likely to help lead to the appropriate diagnosis. Systemic lupus erythematosus may present with isolated splenomegaly and autoimmune cytopenias months to years before serologic evidence of SLE appears, necessitating periodic surveillance in patients with persistent symptoms.[9]

### Miscellaneous Disorders

Kikuchi disease is characterized by impressive cervical lymphadenopathy that mimics lymphoma and is most common in adolescent females. It is a benign, necrotizing histiocytic lymphadenitis that is self-limiting, generally resolving in several weeks to months. Systemic symptoms such as fever, weight loss, and night sweats may accompany the lymphadenopathy. Diagnosis is made by lymph node biopsy.[21]

Sarcoidosis typically presents with hilar lymphadenopathy and parenchymal lung involvement. Other organs affected by this inflammatory disease of unclear etiology include the eye, skin, and joints; hypercalcemia may also be present. Screening is with angiotensin-converting enzyme, but definitive diagnosis is made by biopsy demonstrating noncaseating granulomata.[9]

Cysts of the spleen may present as asymptomatic splenomegaly or with symptoms of diaphragmatic irritation such as cough and shoulder pain. They may be associated with vascular malformations, hemorrhage, inflammation, abscess, or parasitic infection. Surgical intervention is typically required for both diagnostic and therapeutic purposes.[9]

## SPLENECTOMY

Indications for splenectomy vary, depending on the underlying disease, its severity, and likelihood of spontaneous regression. Risks of splenectomy surgery are less with laparoscopic approaches, but long-term infectious risks with encapsulated organisms persist. Nonetheless, the risk–benefit ratio favors splenectomy in certain scenarios: (1) Patients with hematologic diseases, typically those with significant persistent cytopenias, will benefit from splenectomy; (2) patients with thalassemia who have increased transfusion requirements will typically require fewer transfusions annually and accumulate less iron postsplenectomy;[7] (3) patients with sickle cell disease and recurrent splenic sequestration will be cured from this life-threatening crisis by splenectomy;[22] (4) patients with refractory chronic immune thrombocytopenic purpura may benefit, although approximately 40% of patients will not respond;[23] (5) HS patients are effectively cured by splenectomy;[24] (6) massive splenomegaly prior to stem cell transplant is likewise an indication for splenectomy because the spleen may otherwise sequester some of the graft and delay or prevent engraftment.

Patients undergoing splenectomy should receive the Pneumovax and meningococcal vaccines to diminish risk from these organisms. It remains prudent for patients to receive indefinite prophylaxis with penicillin postsplenectomy.

## REFERENCES

1. Ross MH, Pawlina W. *Histology: A Text and Atlas.* Baltimore, MD: Lippincott Wiliams & Wilkins; 2006:906

2. Nathan DG, Oski FA. *Nathan and Oski's Hematology of Infancy and Childhood.* Philadelphia, PA: Saunders; 2003:1864

3. Twist CJ, Link MP. Assessment of lymphadenopathy in children. *Pediatr Clin North Am.* 2002;49(5):1009–1025

4. Pizzo PA, Poplack DG. *Principles and Practice of Pediatric Oncology.* Philadelphia, PA: Lippincott Williams & Wilkins: 2006

5. Lajo A, et al. Mononucleosis caused by Epstein-Barr virus and cytomegalovirus in children: a comparative study of 124 cases. *Pediatr Infect Dis J.* 1994;13(1):56–60

6. Feigin RD, Cherry JD. *Textbook of Pediatric Infectious Diseases.* Philadelphia, PA: Saunders; 1981:1858

7. Lanzkowsky P. *Manual of Pediatric Hematology and Oncology.* Boston, MA: Elsevier Academic Press; 2005:832

8. Windsor JJ. Cat-scratch disease: epidemiology, aetiology, and treatment. *Br J Biomed Sci.* 2001;58(2):101–110

9. Behrman RE, Kliegman R, Jenson HB. *Nelson Textbook of Pediatrics.* Philadelphia, PA: Saunders; 2004

10. Tomblin JL, Roberts FJ. Tuberculous cervical lymphadenitis. *Can Med Assoc J.* 1979;121(3):324–330

11. Avery ME, First LR. *Pediatric Medicine.* Baltimore, MD: Williams & Wilkins; 1993

12. Urba WJ, Longo DL. Hodgkin's disease. *N Engl J Med.* 1992;326(10):678–687

13. Pui CH, Evans WE. Treatment of acute lymphoblastic leukemia. *N Engl J Med.* 2006;354(2):166–178

14. Seibel NL. Treatment of acute lymphoblastic leukemia in children and adolescents: peaks and pitfalls. *Hematology Am Soc Hematol Educ Program.* 2008:374–380

15. Apperley J. CML in pregnancy and childhood. *Best Pract Res Clin Haematol.* 2009;22(3):455–474

16. Foucar E, Rosai J, Dorfman R. Sinus histiocytosis with massive lymphadenopathy (Rosai-Dorfman disease): review of the entity. *Semin Diagn Pathol.* 1990;7(1):19–73

17. Fisher GH, Rosenberg FJ, Straus SE, et al. Dominant interfering as gene mutations impair apoptosis in a human autoimmune lymphoproliferative syndrome. *Cell.* 1995;81(6): 935–946

18. Bleesing JJ, Straus SE, Fleisher TA. Autoimmune lymphoproliferative syndrome.A human disorder of abnormal lymphocyte survival. *Pediatr Clin North Am.* 2000;47(6):1291–1310

19. Garrett TJ, Drusin RE, Schulman LL, et al. Post-transplantation lymphoproliferative disorders treated with cyclophosphamide-doxorubicin-vincristine-prednisone chemotherapy. *Cancer.* 1993;72(9):2782– 2785

20. Hoffman R. *Hematology: Basic Principles and Practice.* Philadelphia, PA: Elsevier Churchill Livingstone; 2005; 2821

21. Dorfman RF. Histiocytic necrotizing lymphadenitis of Kikuchi and Fujimoto. *Arch Pathol Lab Med.* 1987;111(11):1026–1029

22. Kinney TR, Ware R, Schultz W, Filston H. Long-term management of splenic sequestration in children with sickle cell disease. *J Pediatr.* 1990;117(2 Pt 1):194–199

23. George JN, Woolf SH, Raskob GE, et al. Idiopathic thrombocytopenic purpura: a practice guideline developed by explicit methods for the American Society of Hematology. *Blood.* 1996;88(1):3–40

24. O'Brien SH. Secondary data demonstrate safety of splenectomy in spherocytosis. *Pediatr Blood Cancer.* 2009;52(7):753–754

# CHAPTER 111

# Malignant Solid Tumors

ARLENE REDNER, MD

Cancer is relatively uncommon in children and adolescents. Despite this fact, however, approximately 12,400 children and adolescents younger than age 20 are diagnosed with cancer each year in the United States, with 8,700 cases in the 0- to 14-year-old age group and 3,800 cases in the 15- to 19-year-old age group (Table 111-1). In children and adolescents younger than age 20, there is an average annual incidence rate for all cancers of 14.9 cases per 100,000 person-years. It is important to note that the likelihood of a young person reaching adulthood and having been diagnosed with cancer in childhood is 1 in 300 for males and 1 in 333 for females.

**Table 111-1**

**Age-Specific Cancer Incidence Rates (Per Million), 1986–1995**

| *Tumor Category* | *Rate per Million by Age in Years at Diagnosis* | |
|---|---|---|
| | *10–14* | *15–19* |
| All sites | 117.3 | 202.2 |
| Acute lymphoblastic leukemia | 17.8 | 12.9 |
| Acute myeloid leukemia | 5.7 | 8.5 |
| Hodgkin disease | 11.7 | 32.5 |
| Non-Hodgkin lymphoma | 10.3 | 15.3 |
| CNS tumors | 24.6 | 20.2 |
| Neuroblastoma | 0.8 | 0.5 |
| Hepatic tumors | 0.4 | 1.0 |
| Osteoscarcoma | 8.3 | 9.4 |
| Ewing sarcoma | 4.1 | 4.6 |
| Soft tissue sarcoma | 10.9 | 15.9 |
| Germ cell tumors | 6.7 | 30.8 |
| Malignant melanoma | 2.8 | 14.1 |

CNS, central nervous system.

Adapted from Ries LAG, Smith MA, Gurney JG, et al, eds. Cancer Incidence and Survival among Children and Adolescents: United States SEER Program 1975–1995. Bethesda, MD: National Cancer Institute; 1999. NIH Publication No. 99-4649.

Childhood cancer remains the leading cause of disease-related mortality (12% of all deaths) among children ages 1 to 14, with 1,400 cancer-related deaths annually in the United States in children younger than age 15. In the 15- to 19-year-old age group, cancer mortality accounts for 5% of all deaths, with 700 deaths yearly in older adolescents.

In children younger than age 15, acute leukemias, central nervous system (CNS) tumors, and lymphomas comprise most tumors. In the older adult population, carcinomas such as breast, prostate, and gastrointestinal tumors are most prevalent. In the adolescent and young adult population, musculoskeletal tumors (including osteosarcoma and Ewing sarcoma), Hodgkin disease, and germ cell tumors are most common.[1-5]

The incidence of cancer in the adolescent and young adult age group has risen faster on an annual basis than that of younger children and older adults. Also, reductions in mortality for the adolescent and young adult population are significantly less than that of younger children. It has been shown that more than 70% of patients younger than age 15 are enrolled in national clinical trials in the United States.[6] In contrast, by age 20, the percentage of patients enrolled in clinical trials is much lower. In recent years, there has been an emphasis by the Adolescent and Young Adult Committee of the Clinical Oncology Group to enroll more adolescents in clinical trials and improve the outcome for this age group. Whether the poorer outcome of this age group is due to decreased enrollment in clinical trials, less access to care and/or treatment by adult oncologists, or differences in the biology of adolescent and young adult tumors is now being investigated.[2-4]

## LYMPHOMAS

### HODGKIN DISEASE

Hodgkin disease has a bimodal age distribution that is influenced by geographic and ethnic differences. In industrialized countries, the initial peak incidence occurs in the mid to late 20s, and the second peak occurs after age 50. In contrast, in developing countries, the early peak occurs before adolescence. Epidemiologic studies have demonstrated 3 distinct forms of Hodgkin disease: a childhood form, which is seen in children and adolescents younger than age 14; a young adult form, which presents in patients between ages 15 and 34; and an older adult form, which is more commonly seen in patients ages 55 to 74.

In the childhood form, there is a predominance of males. In the adolescent form, there is an equal incidence of males and females, with older adolescents predominantly white. Interestingly, the childhood form tends to be associated with larger family size and lower socioeconomic status. The young adult form is found most commonly in industrialized countries with higher socioeconomic status. It has been postulated that delayed exposure to an infectious agent may be associated with the development of the disease in this age group. Epstein-Barr virus (EBV) infection has been implicated as a causative agent.

There are differences in the pathological subtype of Hodgkin disease in children and adolescents. The nodular sclerosis subtype occurs in 45% to 50% of childhood Hodgkin disease and 70% to 80% of adolescent and young adult Hodgkin disease. The nodular sclerosis subtype is the most common pathological subtype in adolescents. The mixed cellularity subtype is more common in the prepubertal population and is seen in 30% of pediatric cases. Mixed cellularity is most frequently associated with the presence of EBV in the tumor cells.[6]

Nodular lymphocyte-predominant Hodgkin disease occurs most commonly in childhood, with a higher predominance in males. More than 90% of patients present with peripheral adenopathy and have low-stage disease. Surgical resection as the only modality of therapy is now being studied in this group of low-stage patients with the nodular lymphocyte-predominant subtype.[7]

The lymphocyte-depleted subtype is rare in children and adolescents but predominates in older adults. It is most commonly seen associated with HIV positivity.

### Presentation

Patients usually present with painless supraclavicular or cervical adenopathy. Lymph nodes are firm and rubbery and can sometimes be sensitive to palpation. At least two-thirds of patients present with some degree of mediastinal involvement and may have a nonproductive cough or other symptoms of tracheal or bronchial compression. A chest x-ray, posteroanterior and lateral, should be performed as soon as there is suspicion of Hodgkin disease. Airway patency should be assessed before performing any surgical procedures. Primary subdiaphragmatic disease is rare, occurring in only 3% of cases. Nonspecific systemic symptoms frequently include fatigue, anorexia, and slight weight loss. Three constitutional symptoms are associated with prognosis: unexplained fever higher than 100.4°F (38°C), unexplained weight loss of more than 10% within the past 6 months, and drenching night sweats. A fourth constitutional symptom, which lacks prognostic significance, is pruritus. Interestingly, Hodgkin disease can be associated with alcohol-induced pain, whereby pain in the chest radiating to the extremities or back occurs within minutes of drinking alcohol.

Laboratory study abnormalities may include leukocytosis, eosinophilia, and anemia. Several autoimmune disorders have been associated, including nephrotic syndrome, autoimmune hemolytic anemia, autoimmune neutropenia, and immune thrombocytopenia. The erythrocyte sedimentation rate and serum copper and ferritin levels are all elevated. These tests are useful as markers of disease activity after therapy.

### Staging of Hodgkin Disease

Stages are classified into A and B, with A referring to patients who are asymptomatic and B referring to patients who have any of the following symptoms: unexplained fevers higher than 100.4°F (38°C) for longer than 3 days, unexplained weight loss of more than 10% in the previous 6 months, and/or drenching night sweats. Stage 1 involves a single lymph node region, stage 2 involves patients with 2 or more lymph node regions on the same side of the diaphragm, stage 3 involves lymph nodes above and below the diaphragm, and stage 4 involves 1 or more extralymphatic sites.

### Prognosis

Overall survival for pediatric Hodgkin disease is 90%. Significant long-term side effects are important considerations in therapy. With rare exceptions, chemotherapy is recommended for all children and adolescents. Low-dose radiation therapies with doses in the range of 15 to 25 gray (Gy) have been used in this age group. Hybrid chemotherapy regimens such as the COPP/ABV regimen, comprising cyclophosphamide, vincristine, procarbazine, and prednisone (COPP) and doxorubicin, bleomycin, and vinblastine (ABV), have been used to reduce dose-associated toxicity. Response-based therapy, with the administration of additional therapy to those patients with a slow response, has been used. Positron emission tomography (PET) scanning is now being used to help assess response to therapy.[6,7]

## NON-HODGKIN LYMPHOMA

Non-Hodgkin lymphoma (NHL) accounts for 8% to 10% of all malignancies in children and adolescents between the ages of 5 and 19. In the United States, 750 to 800 cases of NHL are diagnosed annually in those younger than age 20. Although the incidence of NHL in children and adolescents younger than age 15 has been constant over the past 2 decades, there has been an overall increase in the incidence in adolescents ages 15 to 19.

Most case of childhood and adolescent NHL involve high-grade tumors with aggressive clinical behavior. In contrast, the most adult patients with NHL have low- to intermediate-grade indolent tumors.

There are 4 major subtypes of childhood and adolescent NHL: small noncleaved cell (Burkitt and non-Burkitt), lymphoblastic, large cell lymphoma, and anaplastic large cell lymphoma.

The age-specific incidence varies according to the histological subtype. Burkitt and Burkitt-like lymphoma characteristically occur between the ages of 5 and 15. The incidence of lymphoblastic lymphoma is constant across childhood and adolescence. Diffuse large B-cell lymphoma is a disease of older adolescents, demonstrating a steady increase in incidence throughout childhood and peaking in the 15- to 19-year-old age group, where it is the dominant histological subtype. Anaplastic large cell lymphoma represents only 10% of the NHLs in these age ranges.

The etiology of NHL is unknown. Immunosuppression, either inherited or acquired, is related to the development of NHL. Inherited immunodeficiencies associated with an increased risk of NHL include Wiskott-Aldrich syndrome, severe combined immunodeficiency disease, ataxia-telangiectasia, and common variable immunodeficiency. Patients who are on immunosuppressive medications following solid organ transplantation, who are HIV positive, and who are post-allogenic bone marrow transplantation are at increased risk for development of B-cell lymphomas.

The clinical presentation of NHL depends on the histological subtype and the primary site of involvement. The most common sites at presentation are the head and neck (30%), the abdomen (30%), and the intrathoracic or mediastinal areas (25%). It commonly presents in an advanced stage in children and adolescents, with 70% presenting as stage 3 or 4 disease.

Small noncleaved NHL presents with jaw, orbital, or paraspinal masses in African Burkitt lymphoma and are associated with EBV infection. The North American and European presentation of Burkitt lymphoma includes abdominal involvement and, less commonly, head and neck or paraspinal disease. The small noncleaved cell lymphomas have a rapid doubling time, so rapid diagnosis and initiation of treatment are required.

Childhood and adolescent lymphoblastic lymphoma commonly presents with an intrathoracic or mediastinal mass. Symptoms of respiratory distress, superior vena caval syndrome, and pleural effusions may be seen.

Most large B-cell lymphomas present with abdominal disease and, to a lesser extent, with mediastinal disease.

Anaplastic large cell lymphomas present with systemic or cutaneous disease. Most anaplastic large cell lymphomas are at the advanced stages 3 or 4. In the systemic disease group, 40% to 60% have extranodal disease most commonly involving the skin, bones, and soft tissues. Primary cutaneous anaplastic large cell lymphomas are limited to the skin and occur in older adolescents.

#### Therapy

The primary modality of treatment for all types of childhood NHL is multiagent chemotherapy. Patients with newly diagnosed NHL, due to the large tumor burden and short doubling times, especially those with small noncleaved cell lymphomas, are at high risk for uric acid nephropathy and acute tumor lysis syndrome. The tumor lysis syndrome requires vigorous alkalinization, hydration, diuresis, and allopurinol or recombinant urate oxidase therapy.

Children and adolescents with localized disease (stage 1 or 2) have a more than 95% chance of survival with a short 6 to 12 weeks of combination chemotherapy without radiation therapy. Advanced stages (stage 3 or 4) have an 80% to 90% survival rate with combination therapy without radiotherapy. There are a few subtypes of NHL that have a worse prognosis, that is, in the 50% to 70% range; these include Burkitt lymphoma with bone marrow and CNS involvement, primary mediastinal diffuse lymphoblastic B-cell lymphoma, and a subgroup of patients with systemic anaplastic large cell lymphomas.[8]

## SARCOMAS

### SOFT TISSUE SARCOMAS

Traditionally, soft tissue sarcomas have been divided into 2 groups: rhabdomyosarcomas and nonrhabdomyosarcoma soft tissue sarcomas. The most common nonrhabdomyosarcoma soft tissue sarcomas are synovial sarcoma, malignant fibrous histiocytoma, malignant peripheral nerve sheath tumor, and fibromyosarcoma. Rhabdomyosarcoma is more common in children younger than age 10, whereas nonrhabdomyosarcoma soft tissue sarcomas predominate in the older adolescent age group.

#### Rhabdomyosarcoma

Two-thirds of cases of rhabdomyosarcoma develop in children younger than age 10, with 20% developing between ages 10 and 14 and 13% at older than 15 years. There is a small peak of incidence in early to middle adolescence. Extremity tumors are more commonly seen in adolescents and are more frequently of the alveolar subtype, whereas sarcomas of the extremities present with extremity swelling. Regional lymph node involvement occurs in up to half of all patients.

Genitourinary rhabdomyosarcomas are commonly embryonal in pathology. Prostate masses can occur in older male adolescents and can develop into large pelvic masses. Cervical and uterine rhabdomyosarcomas are seen in adolescent females. Paratesticular tumors produce painless unilateral scrotal or inguinal enlargement in prepubertal or postpubertal males. Retroperitoneal lymph node dissemination is present in 50% of males older than 10 years.

Principles of therapy include surgical removal, if feasible; radiation therapy for control of residual bulk or microscopic tumor; and systemic chemotherapy. Extent of disease is among the strongest predictors of long-term outcome. Treatment planning is based on clinical group (as determined by site and surgical resectability). Patients at highest risk include those with alveolar tumors and those older than 10 years with metastatic disease.[9]

### Nonrhabdomyosarcoma Soft Tissue Sarcomas

One-half of all nonrhabdomyosarcoma soft tissue sarcomas present in the extremities with a painless mass. They may also occur in the trunk, head and neck, and intrathoracic or intra-abdominal regions. These tumors are sometimes associated with the Li-Fraumeni syndrome (constitutional *p53* mutation). Patients with neurofibromatosis are at high risk for the development of malignant peripheral nerve sheath tumors, which often arise at the site of a previous neurofibroma.

The adolescent nonrhabdomyosarcomas are divided into low-, intermediate-, and high-grade tumors. Patients with high-grade tumors are at a substantially greater risk for distant metastases or recurrence. Low-risk patients include those with resectable low-grade and small high-grade tumors, and have a survival rate of more than 85%. Adolescents in the intermediate-risk category include those with large high-grade tumors and those with unresectable disease. They have about a 50% likelihood of long-term survival. Adolescents with metastatic nonrhabdomyosarcoma soft tissue sarcomas comprise the high-risk group. They have a dismal survival of approximately 6 months, and less than 10% are alive at 5 years after initial diagnosis.[10]

## BONE TUMORS

Primary bone tumors are the third most frequent neoplasm in adolescents and young adults. Osteosarcomas are exceeded only by leukemias and lymphomas.

### OSTEOGENIC SARCOMAS

Osteosarcoma is the most common malignant bone tumor of childhood, accounting for 56% of malignant bone tumors in the first 2 decades of life. Four hundred children and adolescents younger than age 20 are diagnosed with osteosarcoma each year in the United States. The peak incidence of osteosarcoma occurs in the second decade of life during the adolescent growth spurt. It has been suggested that there is a relationship between rapid bone growth during adolescence and the development of osteosarcoma. There is a genetic predisposition to osteosarcoma in patients who have hereditary retinoblastoma. The risk of developing a secondary osteosarcoma with retinoblastoma has been estimated to be between 80% and 90% at 30 years. It is believed that the retinoblastoma gene (*Rb*) is implicated in the development of osteosarcoma. The *p53* gene has also been implicated in the malignant transformation in osteosarcoma. Osteosarcoma is also seen in the Li-Fraumeni syndrome where a germ line *p53* mutation is present.

Most patients with osteosarcoma present with pain over the involved area with or without an associated soft tissue mass. The average duration of symptoms is 3 months. Osteosarcoma usually involves the long bones, especially adjacent to the knee joint. The distal femur and proximal tibia are the most frequently involved sites, followed by the proximal humerus and mid- and proximal femur. Involvement of the flat bones of the axial skeleton, especially the pelvis, occurs in 15% to 20% of cases. Approximately 15% to 20% of patients present with metastatic disease at diagnosis. Most metastatic disease involves pulmonary nodules. Bone metastasis can also be present. Multifocal sclerosing osteosarcoma, which presents with multiple simultaneous bone lesions, carries an extremely poor prognosis.

Radiographic examination of the involved bone is useful in the evaluation of the patient with a bone tumor. Plain films reveal destructive lesions with periosteal new bone formation and the formation of Codman triangle. A soft tissue mass is commonly visualized. Characteristic x-ray features, along with the clinical history and tumor location, permit the prediction of possible histological diagnosis in more than two-thirds of cases. Osteogenic sarcoma of the long bones invariably involves the metaphyseal portion of the bone. Ossification in the soft tissue, in a radial or sunburst pattern, is classic for osteosarcoma. Further radiological evaluation with computed tomography (CT) scans, magnetic resonance imaging (MRI), bone scans, and PET scans is important. Performing a CT scan of the chest is necessary to evaluate for pulmonary nodules.

Biopsy is required to make the definitive diagnosis of osteogenic sarcoma. The biopsy should be performed by an orthopedic surgeon familiar with the planning and performance of definitive limb-sparing surgery because the location of the biopsy is critical for future limb-sparing surgery options.

Patients with axial skeleton primaries have a poor prognosis because complete surgical excision with clear margins is a prerequisite for long-term disease control. Tumors that also arise in the skull and vertebrae are not amenable to curative surgery. Incomplete resection of the primary tumor is associated with a poor outcome.

Age is a prognostic indicator, with children younger than age 10 having a poorer outcome and adolescents and young adults older than age 20 having a more favorable outcome. Levels of serum lactate dehydrogenase (LDH) have had prognostic significance in patients treated with adjuvant chemotherapy.

Treatment involves the removal of the primary tumor, along with a margin of normal tissue surrounding the tumor, to prevent local recurrence. Surgical procedures involve amputation or limb salvage procedures. The selection of the definitive surgical procedure involves tumor location and size, presence of distant metastases, age, skeletal development, and lifestyle.

Adjuvant chemotherapy also is required because although surgery can control the primary tumor, more than 80% of osteogenic sarcoma patients treated with surgery alone will develop metastatic disease. Microscopic subclinical disease is present in most patients at diagnosis.

With currently available chemotherapy protocols using doxorubicin, cisplatin, and high-dose methotrexate, 60% to 70% of patients with nonmetastatic osteosarcoma of the extremity will be cured. Chemotherapy is usually begun at diagnosis, with 2 to 3 months of chemotherapy given prior to definitive surgery, followed by the definitive surgical procedure and then reinstitution of chemotherapy for up to 40 weeks. Presurgical chemotherapy has been advocated to increase the percentage of patients who are suitable for limb-sparing surgery and to provide the time to fabricate and customize an endoprosthetic device.

Patients with metastatic disease to the lung only have a 30% to 50% chance of survival. Patients with bone metastases continue to have a dismal prognosis.[9,11]

## EWING SARCOMA

Ewing sarcoma is the second most common bone tumor.[12] The annual incidence is 3 new cases per million white patients younger than 21 years in the United States. The incidence among other races is significantly less. Ewing sarcoma can arise in almost every age group, but more than half of patients are adolescents, with 15 years being the median age of diagnosis. Pain is the most common presenting symptom, sometimes accompanied by paresthesias. The pain can be intermittent and sometimes less severe at night. Pain is often mistaken for bone growth or sports injuries. A palpable mass can sometimes be present. The median time to diagnosis is 3 to 9 months. Fever and other nonspecific symptoms are seen in more advanced metastatic cases. One-third of patients present with metastatic disease.

Most Ewing sarcomas occur in bones, with the flat bones of the axial skeleton most commonly affected. In the long bones, Ewing sarcoma more frequently arises in the diaphyseal portion of the bone, whereas osteosarcoma more frequently arises in the metaphyseal portion. The most common sites are the pelvic bones, long bones of the lower extremities, and the bones of the chest wall. Metastatic disease to the lungs, bones, or bone marrow is seen in 25% of patients.

Radiological imaging reveals lytic lesions with Codman triangle and possible calcifications in soft tissue. The diaphyseal location suggests Ewing sarcoma. Magnetic resonance imaging (MRI) can delineate the extension of the bone lesions. Extent of disease evaluation includes bone and PET scans, CT scans of the lungs, and bone marrow aspirates and biopsies.

Initial surgery is usually a biopsy. The location of the biopsy site is determined by assessing the local disease and its relationship to the neurovascular bundle. The biopsy should be performed by the surgeon who will be performing the definitive resection because the biopsy tract needs to be removed in the definitive surgical procedure. The pathology reveals a small, round, blue cell tumor that is periodic acid-Schiff positive. Histochemical expression of CD 99 is seen in Ewing sarcoma. This expression is also seen in peripheral primitive neuroectodermal tumors, which are molecularly identical to Ewing sarcoma. Both have a gene rearrangement of the *EWS/FL1* gene, which is seen as a translocation of t(11, 22(q24:q12)) in 85% of cases.

### Therapy of Ewing Sarcoma

Local control by either complete surgical resection or radiation therapy, with a dose higher than 40 Gy, is needed. Chemotherapy is also required, with cyclophosphamide, vincristine, and adriamycin alternating with ifosfamide and etoposide most commonly used.

### Prognosis

Patients with nonmetastatic disease can expect a 60% to 80% long-term survival. The prognosis for adolescents and young adults with Ewing sarcoma is inferior to the outcome in pediatric patients. The older age groups frequently present with large tumors or metastatic disease. Studies show that adolescents and young adults treated on pediatric protocols have a superior outcome to those in the same age group treated using adult Ewing sarcoma protocols.[9,11]

## GENITOURINARY MALIGNANCIES

### GYNECOLOGIC MALIGNANCIES: OVARIAN AND ADNEXAL MASSES

Pediatric ovarian and adnexal masses are uncommon, accounting for 1% of all pediatric malignant neoplasms. The incidence of pediatric ovarian neoplasms is 2.6 per 100,000 girls per year. Most ovarian masses detected are benign neoplasms or functional cysts, but 10% to 30% are malignant.

Ultrasound features of an adnexal mass that suggests malignancy include large size, a complex appearance (not entirely cystic), presence of loculations within or on the surface of the tumor, and presence of measurable ascites in the posterior cul de sac.

Serum markers helpful in diagnosis include alpha fetoprotein, beta human chorionic gonadotropin (beta HCG), carcinoembryonic antigen (CEA), cancer antigen-125 (CA-125), and lactate dehydrogenase (LDH).

Germ cell tumors are the most common ovarian tumors in adolescents ages 15 to 19. These tumors originate from the primordial germ cell and express specific tumor markers that aid in preoperative detection and the response to therapy. Ovarian germ cell tumors include dysgerminomas, endodermal sinus tumors, embryonal carcinomas, and teratomas that are immature, mature, or mixed.

Mature cystic teratomas (dermoid cysts) are the most common benign ovarian neoplasms found in female adolescents. They are bilateral in 10% of cases. Fifty percent of these lesions are discovered incidentally during surgery or imaging of asymptomatic girls. Teenagers may also present with gastrointestinal symptoms, abdominal pain, or a mass. Mature cystic teratomas contain tissues from all 3 germ cell layers. The most common tissue types seen are skin, hair, teeth adipose tissue, mature brain tissue, intestinal epithelium, and cystic structures lined by squamous, cuboidal, or flattened epithelium. Approximately 2% of cases will undergo malignant degeneration. Surgical therapy should include resection of the teratoma without spillage and an attempt at ovarian preservation. Inspection of the contralateral ovary should also be performed to look for bilateral disease.

Dysgerminomas are the most common malignant ovarian germ cell tumors. The presenting symptoms include increasing abdominal girth, a palpable abdominal or pelvic mass, and pain. Symptoms are usually rapid in onset, due to rapid growth of the mass. Five percent to 10% of dysgerminomas occur in females with gonadal dysgenesis. Suspected cases should have serum markers drawn (alpha fetoprotein and beta HCG), chest x-ray or CT scan of the chest, and CT scan of the abdomen and pelvis. Surgery includes oophorectomy, biopsy of suspicious lesions and lymph nodes, omentectomy, and cytologic evaluation of peritoneal fluid. Chemotherapy includes the use of bleomycin, etoposide, and cisplatin (BEP). The overall survival rate is 85%.

Endodermal sinus tumors account for 5% of all malignant ovarian tumors. They occur at a median age of 18 years, with one-third of cases occurring in premenarchal females, making it the most common pediatric ovarian germ cell tumor. Symptoms at presentation include abdominal or pelvic pain. Ten percent of cases present with palpation of an asymptomatic pelvic mass. Tumors secrete alpha fetoprotein; are unilateral and commonly have retroperitoneal lymph nodes; and spread to the lungs, liver, peritoneum, and bowel. Treatment consists of unilateral salpingo-oophorectomy, followed by chemotherapy with BEP. Disease survival rate with chemotherapy approaches 80%.

Immature teratomas account for 48% of germ cell tumors between birth and 14 years of age, 35% in the 15- to 19-year-old age range, and 40% in the 20- to 24-year-old age range. Typical presentation is with abdominal distension, pain, and a palpable mass, with 60% of patients having an elevated alpha fetoprotein. The tumors are graded from 1 to 3 based on the proportion of primitive neuroectodermal tissue present. Surgical staging includes unilateral salpingo-oophorectomy lymph node evaluation, omentectomy, and peritoneal biopsies. All grades above 1 require chemotherapy with BEP. Survival rates range from 75% to 90%.

Embryonal carcinoma is diagnosed in 50% of patients prior to puberty. They commonly present with "pseudopuberty" due to hormonal production by the tumor. These tumors are treated using chemotherapy with BEP.

Mixed germ cell tumors have 2 or more different germ cell tumors combined. The mean age of diagnosis is 16 years. Chemotherapy with BEP is used.

Gonadoblastomas are tumors of germ cells intermixed with stromal cells. These tumors develop during adolescence, most frequently in patients with gonadal dysgenesis.[13]

### TESTICULAR TUMORS

Adolescent testicular tumors resemble adult testicular tumors. The major risk factor for the development of testicular cancers is the presence of an undescended testis. Most adolescent testicular tumors are germ cell tumors. Two-thirds of germ cell tumors are endodermal sinus tumors, and a smaller portion are teratomas. Testicular tumors present with an irregular, nontender scrotal mass. There is usually a delay of 6 to 24 months in diagnosis because of the absence of other symptoms. Metastatic tumors involve the retroperitoneal lymph nodes and chest. Surgery involves radical inguinal orchiectomy.

Teratomas occur more frequently in younger children. Embryonal carcinomas usually occur in late adolescence and young adulthood. The presenting symptoms include a scrotal mass with metastatic abdominal or mediastinal disease. Serum alpha fetoprotein or beta HCG may be elevated. Therapies may include chemotherapy with a platinum-containing agent and radiation therapy.

Mixed germ cell tumors are more common in males older than 15 years. Stage 1 disease has a 75% survival, whereas stage 4 disease portends a poor survival with conventional chemotherapy.

### MEDIASTINAL GERM CELL TUMORS

Mediastinal germ cell tumors are located in the anterior mediastinum and, in adolescents, present asymptomatically. Histological subtypes include yolk sac tumors, germinomas, choriocarcinomas, and teratomas.

## MELANOMA

Among patients younger than 15 years of age, melanoma accounts for only 0.9% of all cancers, but the incidence of melanomas rises steeply with age. It accounts for 7% of all cancers in patients ages 15 to 19, with an increase of 2.6% per year recently. The estimated annual incidence rate per million for adolescents ages 15 to 19 in the United States is 14.1.

Children with immunodeficiency have a 3 to 6 times greater risk of melanoma. Hodgkin disease survivors have an eightfold increased risk. Melanoma has been described after renal transplant or immunosuppressive therapy. Forty-four percent of melanomas that develop in people younger than age 30 arise in a small nevus, which has been present since birth or early childhood.

The most common clinical presentation of adolescent melanoma includes the increasing size of a mole, bleeding, color change, itching, palpable adenopathy, and palpable subcutaneous mass. The most common site is the trunk.

The outcome for adolescents is similar to adults, with localized disease having an excellent outcome, whereas those with nodal disease have a 10-year survival of 60% and those with distant metastasis have a 10-year survival of 25%.[14]

Early detection and surgical removal of any suspicious pigmented lesions is the mainstay of melanoma therapy in adolescents. Strategies that emphasize a decrease in sunlight exposure and early detection should be encouraged.

## MISCELLANEOUS TUMORS

Nasopharyngeal carcinoma is an uncommon tumor that has as increasing incidence in adolescence. Typical signs and symptoms are painless cervical adenopathy, nasal obstruction, sinusitis, epistaxis, chronic otitis, and headache. Cranial nerve involvement is present in 50% of affected patients. Common metastatic sites include the lungs, liver, and bones. There is a strong association with EBV infection. Therapy includes radiation and chemotherapy. The prognosis ranges from 80% survival to 25% in metastatic cases.

Hepatocellular carcinoma is the most common liver malignancy in adolescents. Predisposing conditions include long standing hepatic inflammation and hepatitis B infection. Patients treated with anabolic steroids for many years have an increased risk of developing hepatocellular carcinoma. Seventy percent of patients have unresectable disease at presentation.

Renal cell carcinoma replaces Wilms tumor as the most common primary renal tumor during adolescence. There is an increased frequency in patients with tuberous sclerosis and von Hippel-Lindau disease. In advanced disease, there is metastatic spread to nodes, the liver, the lungs, and bone. In nonmetastatic disease, wide resection offers excellent survival.

Adenocarcinoma of the colon is an uncommon malignancy in adolescence. Predisposing conditions include long standing ulcerative colitis or polyposis coli. Most adolescents with colon carcinoma have advanced disease at presentation.

## REFERENCES


1. Stiller C. Epidemiology of cancer in adolescents. *Med Pediatr Oncol.* 2002;39:149–155

2. Albritton K, Bleyer WA. The management of cancer in the older adolescent. *Eur J Cancer.* 2003;39(18):2584–2599

3. Bleyer A. The adolescent and young adult gap in cancer care and outcome. *Curr Probl Pediatr Adolesc Health Care.* 2005;35:182–217

4. Ries LAG, Smith MA, Gurney JG, et al, eds. Cancer Incidence and Survival among Children and Adolescents: United States SEER Program 1975–1996. Bethesda, MD: National Cancer Institute; 1999. NIH Publication No 99-4649

5. Bleyer A, O'Leary M, Barr R, Ries LAG, eds. Cancer Epidemiology in Older Adolescents and Young Adults 15 to 29 Years of Age, Including SEER Incidence and Survival: 1975–2000. Bethesda, MD: National Cancer Institute; 2006. NIH Publication No 06-5767

6. Schwartz CL. Special issues in pediatric Hodgkin's disease. *Eur J Haematol.* 2005;75(suppl 66):55–62

7. Herbertson R, Hancock BW. Hodgkin lymphoma in adolescents. *Cancer Treat Rev.* 2005; 31(5):339–360

8. Cairo MS, Raetz E, Lim MS, Davenport V, Perkins SL. Childhood and adolescent non-Hodgkin lymphoma: new insights in biology and critical challenges for the future. *Pediatr Blood Cancer.* 2005;45:753–769

9. Albritton KH. Sarcoma in adolescents and young adults. *Hematol Oncol Clin North Am.* 2005;19(3):527–546, vii

10. Herzog CE. Overview of sarcomas in the adolescent and young adult population. *J Pediatr Hematol Oncol.* 2005;27(4):215–218

11. Pizzo PA, Poplack DG, eds. *Principles and Practice of Pediatric Oncology*. 5th ed. Philadelphia, PA: Lippincott Williams & Wilkins; 2006

12. Kennedy JG, Frelinghuysen P, Hoang BH. Ewing sarcoma: current concepts in diagnosis and treatment. *Curr Opin Pediatr.* 2003;15(1):53–57

13. Stepanian M, Cohn DE. Gynecologic malignancies in adolescents. *Adolesc Med.* 2004;15:549–568

14. Pappo AS. Melanoma in children and adolescents. *Eur J Cancer.* 2003;39:2651–2661

# CHAPTER 112

## Brain Tumors in Adolescents

DAVID N. KORONES, MD

### INTRODUCTION

Cancer is a devastating diagnosis in an adolescent's life, but it is particularly devastating when that cancer is a brain tumor. Adolescents may present critically ill with major neurologic deficits, or with a more insidious course, characterized by declining school performance, introversion, and depression. These symptoms may initially be attributed to mood disorders or substance abuse. On diagnosis, an adolescent with a brain tumor is descended on by an army of subspecialists—neurosurgeons, neurologists, oncologists, and radiation oncologists, and an even larger support staff of nurses, nurse practitioners, physical therapists, speech therapists, and occupational therapists. At a time when autonomy is paramount, an adolescent's dependence on others is great. To complicate matters further, they may be evaluated at adult oncology centers by health care providers who are not aware of an adolescent's unique medical and psychosocial needs.

Most of the data on epidemiology, signs, and symptoms, and treatment of adolescents with brain tumors is grouped together with data on children of all ages with these tumors. Thus, adolescent-specific information on brain tumors is sorely lacking. In the following discussion, issues and data peculiar to teenagers will be highlighted whenever such information is available.

### EPIDEMIOLOGY

Brain tumors are the second most common pediatric malignancy, and the most common pediatric solid tumor. The incidence of brain tumors is highest in children younger than 5 years of age, and gradually declines from age 5 to age 19. Brain tumors account for 26% of all malignancies in adolescents 10 to 14 years old, and 11% of malignancies in 15- to 19-year-olds (Figure 112-1).[1] The incidence of brain tumors is 24.1/million/year in adolescents ages 10 to 14, and drops to 19.2/million/year for adolescents ages 15 to 19 (Table 112-1). There is a slight male predominance in adolescents. Central nervous system (CNS) tumors are significantly more common in whites (27/million/year in the 15- to 29-year-old age group) than in blacks, Hispanics, and Asians (approximately 14/million/year).

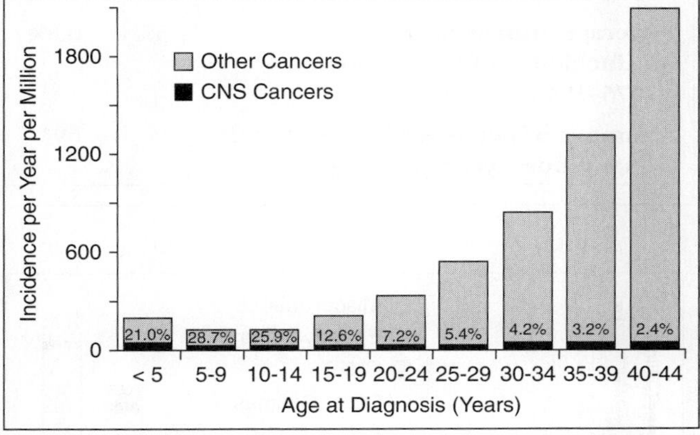


**FIGURE 112-1** Incidence of CNS tumors relative to all cancer. Central Brain Tumor Registry of the United States' Surveillance, Epidemiology, and End Results (SEER) Program 1975–2000.

There appears to be a slight increase in the incidence of brain tumors in adolescents over time. Data from the Surveillance, Epidemiology, and End Result (SEER) registry suggest an average annual increase of 0.5% to 1.0% per year from 1975 to 1998. Much of this increase occurred in the mid-1980s when magnetic resonance imaging (MRI) became available. Thus it is possible that the increase is due to increased detection of tumors and not a true increase in incidence. Astrocytoma, the most common type of brain tumor in teenagers, accounts for 64% of all brain tumors in the 15- to 29-year-old age group. Other types of gliomas, such as oligodendroglioma or oligoastrocytoma, account for 19%; primitive neuroectodermal tumors (PNET) 8%; ependymoma 6%; and miscellaneous 3%. A more detailed illustration of pediatric brain tumor types by age is shown in Figure 112-2.

### ETIOLOGY

Although there has been exhaustive evaluation of risk factors for developing brain tumors, few causes have been pinpointed. Efforts have been hampered by the

**Table 112-1**

**Incidence of Malignant CNS Neoplasms in Persons Younger than 45 Years of Age**

| *Age at diagnosis (years)* | *5* | *5–9* | *10–14* | *15–19* | *20–24* | *25–29* | *30–34* | *35–39* | *40–44* |
|---|---|---|---|---|---|---|---|---|---|
| **US population, year 2000 Census (in millions)** | 19,175 | 20,549 | 20,528 | 20,219 | 18,964 | 19,381 | 20,510 | 22,706 | 22,441 |
| **Incidence of CNS tumors, 1975–2000, per year per million** | 33.7 | 29.9 | 24.1 | 19.2 | 21.2 | 27.0 | 33.0 | 39.8 | 49.3 |
| **Average annual % change in incidence of CNS tumors, 1975–1998** | 2.5% | 0.8% | 2.1% | 0.3% | 1.1% | 1.6% | 0.8% | -0.5% | 0.2% |
| **Number of persons diagnosed with CNS tumors, year 2000, US** | 773 | 693 | 576 | 402 | 469 | 629 | 725 | 827 | 1154 |

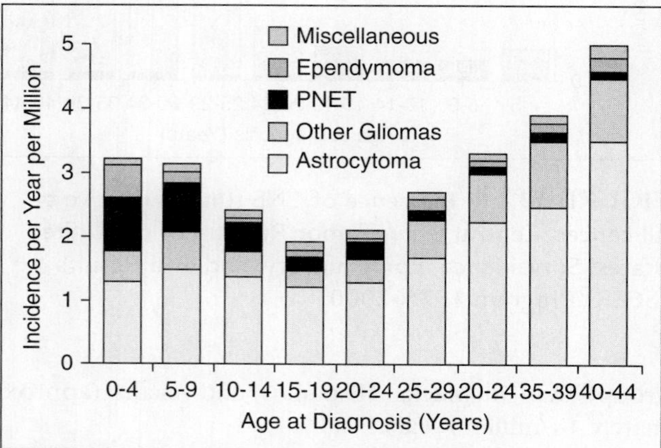


FIGURE 112-2 Age-specific incidence of childhood and adolescent primary brain and CNS tumors by selected histologies, CBTRUS' Surveillance, Epidemiology, and End Results (SEER) Program 2000–2004.

relative rarity of brain tumors in adolescents and young adults, the heterogeneity of types of brain tumors these patients develop, and the complexity of the interaction between host and environment. There are a handful of familial syndromes that predispose adolescents to developing brain tumors. Neurofibromatosis type 1 (NF) is the most common genetic condition associated with brain tumors; 15% to 20% of children with this disease develop brain tumors, most commonly optic pathway astrocytomas. Most NF-associated brain tumors are diagnosed in the preteen years, but the risk remains elevated throughout adolescence.[2] Patients with NF type 2 are prone to developing meningiomas, acoustic neuromas, and spinal cord tumors, particularly in the second decade of life.[3] Other less common syndromes predisposing patients to CNS tumors include tuberous sclerosis, as well as Von Hippel-Lindau, Li-Fraumeni, Gorlin, and Turcot syndromes. These syndromes involve the mutation of tumor suppressor genes that remove a normal check on cell growth and predispose patients to various types of malignancies.

The only firmly established environmental cause of brain tumors is external beam radiation. Children who were treated with whole brain radiation for acute lymphoblastic leukemia, and children with brain tumors who received radiation as part of their treatment regimen, are at increased risk of developing CNS tumors, particularly astrocytomas and meningiomas.[4]

## TUMOR TYPES AND LOCATION

In the United States, data regarding primary brain tumors are maintained in the Central Brain Tumor Registry of the United States (CBTRUS; Figure 112-3).[5] Data are not available on tumor location in adolescents versus younger children. The types of tumors that pediatric age patients develop varies with age. The frequency of oligodendroglioma, pituitary tumors, and CNS germinoma is significantly higher in the 15- to 19-year-old age group than in younger adolescents and children, whereas the frequency of medulloblastoma and ependymoma declines (Figure 112-4). The proportion of patients with astrocytoma remains about the same across pediatric age groups.

## SIGNS AND SYMPTOMS

The signs and symptoms of adolescents with brain tumors are highly variable. The relative rarity and heterogeneity of this disease, coupled with the many symptoms

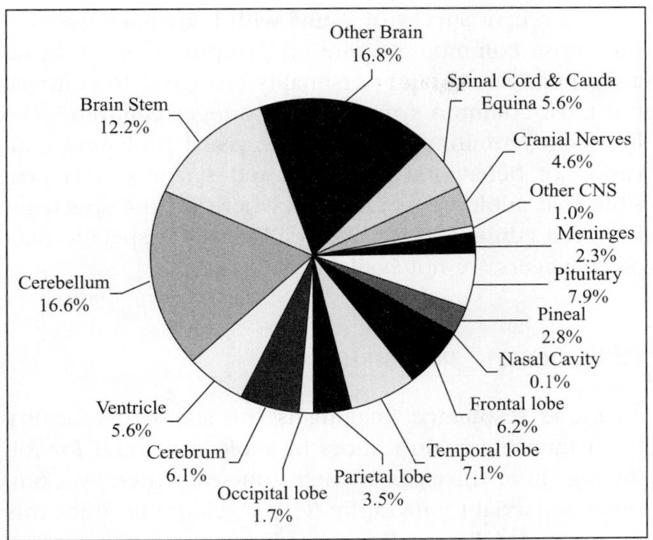


**FIGURE 112-3** Distribution of all childhood and adolescent primary brain and CNS tumors (0 to 19 years of age) by site. CBTRUS 2000–2004 (*n* = 5,873) (CBTRUS [2008]). Statistical Report: Primary Brain Tumors in the United States, 2000–2004. Published by the Central Brain Tumor Registry of the United States.

that mimic more common diagnoses, conspire to make early detection a daunting task. The challenge of diagnosing a brain tumor in the school-age or teenage child is best described by Bailey and Cushing in their original case series of children with medulloblastoma.

A preadolescent child previously in good health begins to complain of headaches or of suboccipital discomfort and to have occasional attacks of vomiting without preliminary nausea, usually on first arising in the morning. Attendance at school meanwhile may continue, but the teacher soon notices that the child is listless, inattentive, and the character of his or her work noticeably falls off. Before long, it becomes apparent that there is clumsiness in movement and awkwardness in gait. Over time it is noticed at home or in school that the adolescent's sight is impaired; or a beginning squint of one eye may be detected, even in the absence of any complaint of double vision. The physician who was previously suspecting some gastrointestinal disorder may then examine the eye grounds and find papilledema due to increased intracranial pressure. On average, 3 to 4 months elapse from the first appearance of symptoms of a brain tumor in adolescents and definitive diagnosis.[6]

In a recent study of 200 children with brain tumors, the most common presenting symptom was headache (41%), followed by vomiting (12%), unsteadiness of gait (11%), visual problems (10%), education or behavioral problems (10%), and seizures (9%).[7] The most common neurologic signs were papilledema (38%), cranial nerve deficits (49%), cerebellar abnormalities (48%), long tract signs (27%), somatosensory abnormalities (11%), and reduced level of consciousness (12%).[7] There is a paucity of data on symptoms of older children and teenagers compared to younger children. In one study, investigators examined time from onset of symptoms to time of

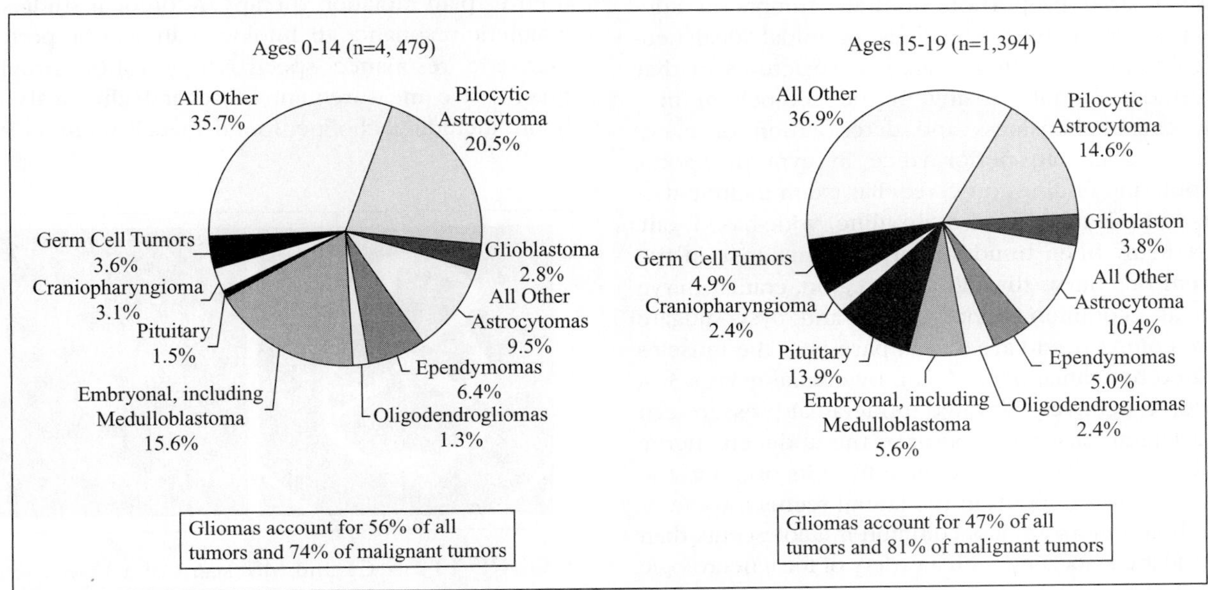


**FIGURE 112-4** Distribution of childhood and adolescent primary brain and CNS tumors by histology (CBTRUS, 2008). (Statistical Report: Primary Brain Tumors in the United States, 2000–2004. Published by the Central Brain Tumor Registry of the United States.)

diagnosis and found that the older the patient, the longer the lag time between symptom onset and diagnosis.[8] The specific signs and symptoms of brain tumors can best be categorized as nonfocal findings and focal neurologic findings as described in the following section.

### NONFOCAL SIGNS AND SYMPTOMS

Adolescents with posterior fossa and brainstem tumors frequently develop obstruction of cerebrospinal fluid (CSF) flow at the level of the aqueduct of Sylvius or foramina of Luschka or Magendie. As a consequence, their initial signs and symptoms may be due to hydrocephalus and not manifest as focal neurologic deficits. Classically these patients report headaches and morning emesis without nausea, but initially the headaches and emesis may occur intermittently and follow no discernible pattern. The patient may also suffer nonspecific changes, such as a decline in school performance, inability to concentrate, behavior changes, irritability, becoming more quiet and introverted, or depression. Some adolescents with hypothalamic/pituitary tumors have unexplained weight gain. Anorexia can also be a presenting sign of hypothalamic brain tumors, such as a Rathke pouch tumor or craniopharyngioma.[9] These nonspecific symptoms frequently are attributed to other causes. As was the case with a Cushing patient, it may take time and careful observation of patterns of behavior to establish the diagnosis.

### FOCAL SIGNS AND SYMPTOMS

Because a large proportion of brain tumors in adolescents occur in the posterior fossa, initial focal neurologic findings are often related to structures in that compartment. Tumors arising in the cerebellum may initially cause clumsiness and deterioration of handwriting or declining performance in gym or sports. Corresponding findings on cerebellar exam include dysmetria, truncal ataxia, and a shuffling, wide-based gait. Because many brain tumors in adolescents arise in the brainstem or course through that region, cranial nerve deficits are common. Facial palsies and dysconjugate gaze are common, and are due to paresis of the muscles innervated by cranial nerve 7 and by cranial nerves 3, 4, and/or 6, respectively. Elevated intracranial pressure can cause a lateral gaze palsy, because the abducens nerve (cranial nerve 6) has a long course from its origin in the brainstem to its endpoint in the lateral rectus muscle.

Cerebral tumors are less common in adolescents than adults, and are associated with a variety of focal neurologic signs and symptoms. Seizures, a common presentation for adults with brain tumors, occur in only about 10% of adolescents. Other relatively common focal findings include motor and sensory deficits and visual field compromise.[10]

In a recent survey of adults with high-grade gliomas, the most common presenting symptoms were headache, hemiparesis, and personality change.[11] In contrast, the most common symptoms in younger children were headache, vomiting, unsteadiness, visual problems, education or behavioral problems, and seizures. It is possible that adolescents fall somewhere on the spectrum between adults and younger children, but specific data on teenagers are not available.

## DIAGNOSTIC IMAGING

Magnetic resonance imaging is the standard modality for diagnosing brain tumors in adolescents and for following them throughout their course of therapy. Computerized axial tomography (CT) is seldom used for this purpose. A CT scan has the advantage of being more readily available and requiring only a few minutes to perform. A CT scan of the head may be useful to screen for hydrocephalus, bleeding, or a large mass, but if a tumor is suspected, an MRI is the imaging method of choice. Figure 112-5 illustrates the superior sensitivity and definition provided by MRI compared to CT.

Magnetic resonance imaging has many advantages over CT. Imaging can be done in 3 planes and provides much better anatomic definition of a tumor and surrounding structures. It can detect tumors that might escape notice on a CT scan. It can detect edema that often surrounds malignant lesions. In addition, the MRI can serve as a better guide for surgical planning and is used to plan radiation therapy. Additional studies using magnetic resonance technology can also be performed; magnetic resonance spectroscopy (MRS) provides a quantitative measurement of several chemicals in the brain, including choline, found in cell membranes, the

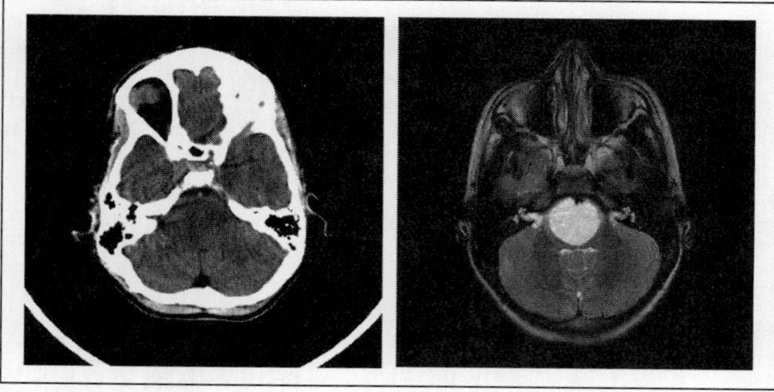

**FIGURE 112-5** CT and MRI scans of a 13-year-old boy with a brainstem tumor. What appears as an ill-defined lucency on the CT scan (left) is a well-defined lesion on a T2-weighted MRI image (right). (Images courtesy of University of Rochester Medical Center imaging archives.)

normal neural marker n-acetyl aspartate, and lactate, found in areas of necrosis. Quantitative determination of these substances assists the clinician in determining whether a lesion is due to a tumor, infection, or inflammation. Similarly, blood flow can be measured using perfusion studies and distinguish viable from nonviable tumor. Magnetic resonance angiography can often supplant intra-arterial angiography, and MR venous angiography is invaluable in detecting the presence of sagittal and transverse sinus thromboses. A newer modality, functional MRI, is now being used to pinpoint the location of important brain function, such as language, and enables the surgeon to identify and avoid these regions during tumor excision.

## TREATMENT

The treatment of brain tumors in adolescents falls into 3 broad areas: surgery, radiation, and systemic therapy that includes chemotherapy and other more targeted approaches. Progress in each of these areas has resulted in markedly improved survival and less long-term morbidity.

### SURGERY

Surgery is an essential component of treatment for adolescents with brain tumors. With the exception of a few tumor types that lie deep, or in perilous locations, such as the brainstem or optic pathways, biopsy is recommended for all other tumors to identify tumor type. Many tumors in adolescents are amenable to gross total resection, and complete removal of the tumor confers a better prognosis. For example, survival for children with gross total resection of ependymoma is approximately 70%, whereas survival for those with subtotal removal is 25% or less.[10] Gross total resection also results in significantly improved cure rates for high-grade gliomas, low-grade astrocytomas, and medulloblastoma.[10] It may be difficult to assess whether total removal of the tumor has been achieved. Assessment of the extent of tumor removal is based on the intraoperative observations and a postoperative MRI, generally performed within a few days of surgery.

Several advances in surgical techniques have enabled neurosurgeons to resect more tumor mass with less morbidity. One such advance is image-guided surgery. Preoperative digital MRI scans are transformed by computer into 3-dimensional models of the brain and tumor. Using these models intraoperatively, surgeons are aware of their exact location in the brain at any point during surgery, and thus can avoid major blood vessels and normal brain.[12] Another advance is "awake surgery." Using this approach, the skull is removed and the cortex overlying the tumor is exposed. The patient is then awakened, and various areas of the cortex are stimulated and the patient's response recorded. In so doing areas of vital function are mapped out, and the surgeon then knows critical areas to avoid during tumor resection.

The morbidity of surgery for adolescents with brain tumors can be substantial.[13] One of the more common complications of surgery is the posterior fossa syndrome, also called "cerebellar mutism," which occurs in some form in 8% to 25% of patients undergoing resection of posterior fossa tumors.[10,14] The syndrome usually develops shortly after surgery and is characterized by mutism, ataxia, behavior changes, and cranial nerve palsies. Although it usually resolves, deficits are sometimes long-lasting, and can be permanent.

### RADIATION

Radiation is a vital part of treatment for adolescents with brain tumors. It is a mainstay of therapy for medulloblastoma, incompletely resected astrocytoma and craniopharyngioma, high-grade astrocytoma, ependymoma, and CNS germinoma.[10] A major challenge of effectively delivering radiation is balancing the life-prolonging, often curative benefits of this therapy with the long-term toxicity of radiation to the developing brain.

Radiation can be delivered in a number of different ways. Standard external beam radiotherapy is reserved for large fields of radiation in which precise margins of the field are not necessary. For example, craniospinal radiation for adolescents with medulloblastoma is generally delivered in standard external beam form. When more precise margins are required, 3-dimensional conformal radiation or intensity-modulated radiation therapy (IMRT) is used. This is particularly useful for focal tumors, such as ependymoma or low-grade astrocytoma. Using 3-dimensional models of the tumor based on MRI, fields of radiation can be designed that conform to the size and shape of the tumor. In so doing, the tumor receives maximal doses of radiation, and surrounding normal brain is relatively spared. Excellent control of ependymoma and low-grade astrocytoma has been achieved using this approach in adolescents.[15,16]

There had been a great deal of enthusiasm for the use of hyperfractionated radiation for pediatric brain tumors, but data to date suggest that it is not of benefit. Hyperfractionation is an approach in which patients receive 2 smaller doses of radiation once a day instead of the standard single dose. The desired effect of delivering smaller doses more frequently was a higher cumulative dose of radiation, better control of the tumor, and less toxicity. However, the outcome is not improved and the toxicity is comparable.[17]

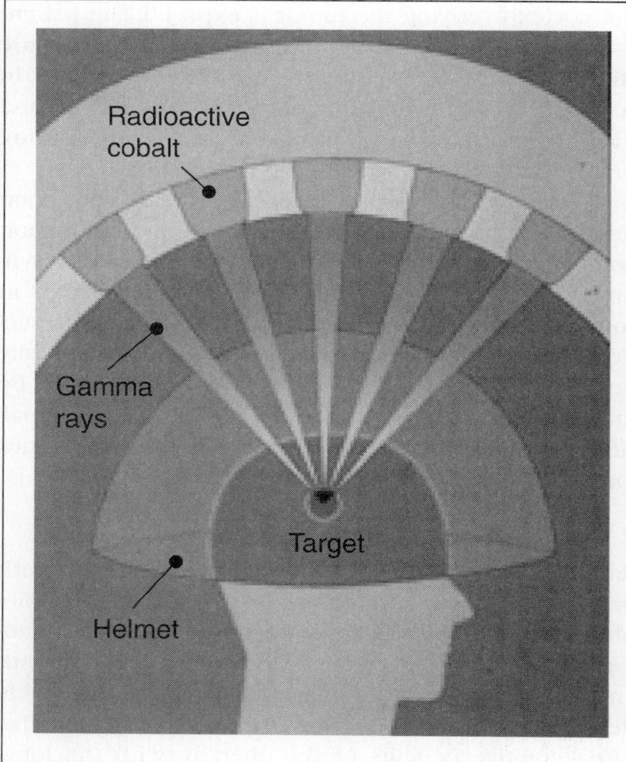


**FIGURE 112-6** Stereotactic radiosurgery. Multiple beams of gamma rays converge on the tumor. (Copyright of the Trustees of the University of Pennsylvania, www.oncolink.org)

Stereotactic radiosurgery is an even more precise means of delivering a single large dose of radiotherapy to a small tumor. Using this approach, multiple small doses of radiation are delivered from many different directions through the brain to converge at the site of the tumor, much like the spokes of a bicycle wheel converging at the axle (see Figure 112-6). In this way, the cumulative dose of radiation to the tumor is high, whereas normal brain tissue is relatively spared. This approach is most commonly used in adults with meningioma and acoustic neuroma, but it has also proved effective in small trials of younger patients with well-circumscribed low-grade astrocytomas.[18] Other less frequently used means of delivering radiotherapy include proton beam radiation and brachytherapy (surgical implantation of radioisotopes in the resection cavity).

A major limitation of radiation is long-term toxicity on the developing brain. Although such toxicity is greatest in children under the age of 5, adolescents are not immune to its effects. Cognitive deficits, growth failure, and delayed puberty are common and are discussed in detail in the following section.

## CHEMOTHERAPY

The blood-brain barrier poses a formidable obstacle to the penetration of many chemotherapeutic agents through brain vessels and into a tumor. As a result, chemotherapy historically had not been an integral part of treatment for adolescents with brain tumors. However, by the 1980s, a number of cytotoxic agents had been developed with chemical properties that enabled them to penetrate the blood-brain barrier. For example, agents that are lipophilic and low molecular weight are more likely to cross the blood-brain barrier. Furthermore, the widespread use of CT and MRI scanning enabled clinicians to more accurately assess responses to these agents. Finally, a series of carefully controlled clinical trials showed that chemotherapy improved survival for children and adolescents with selected types of brain tumors.[19,20]

Currently, chemotherapy is a standard part of therapy for teenagers with medulloblastoma, supratentorial PNET, and high-grade astrocytoma. It is being actively investigated in adolescents with CNS germinoma, ependymoma, and brainstem glioma, but it has not been shown to improve disease-free or overall survival for these patients.

Because of the limited ability of standard chemotherapeutic agents to penetrate into CNS tumors, other innovative approaches for getting chemotherapy to the tumor are being investigated. One approach is to permeabilize the blood-brain barrier to enable better penetration of the chemotherapy. Investigators have used carboplatin, which has limited blood-brain barrier penetration, in addition to RMP-7, a bradykinin analogue that permeabilizes the blood-brain barrier, but convincing activity has not been observed.[21] Another approach is high-dose chemotherapy with stem cell rescue, the rationale being that higher circulating doses of cytotoxic drugs will result in better penetration of the blood-brain barrier. This approach appears to be efficacious in patients with chemosensitive disease and small residual tumors.[22] Other approaches under investigation include intrathecal therapy, surgical placement of chemotherapy-containing "wafers" in the tumor resection cavity, and interstitial therapy (slow infusion of drug into brain parenchyma via a surgically placed catheter). These latter options have the potential not only to increase exposure of the tumor to chemotherapy, but they may also limit systemic toxicity.

## FUTURE THERAPY

Over the past 3 decades, advances in surgery, radiation, and chemotherapy have resulted in more effective targeting of the tumor, thus improving efficacy, and more effective avoidance of normal brain, thus minimizing morbidity. However, even with these advances, mortality and morbidity remain unacceptably high.

The key to improving survival and decreasing morbidity of therapy is the creation of innovative, targeted approaches based on the biology of the various brain tumors. Such therapies are being developed and tested in clinical trials. One area of active investigation is the use of antiangiogenic agents, compounds that target blood vessels supplying brain tumors, as opposed to targeting the tumor itself. Tumors can only grow if they have a blood supply. Bevacizumab is a monoclonal antibody against vascular endothelial growth factor (VEGF), a growth factor that stimulates blood vessel growth within some brain tumors. In clinical trials of adults with recurrent high-grade astrocytomas, dramatic and unprecedented responses have been observed using bevacizumab in combination with the chemotherapeutic agent irinotecan.[23] The Pediatric Brain Tumor Consortium is currently conducting a similar trial.

Another potential target is the epidermal growth factor receptor (EGFR). This growth factor receptor is mutated and constitutively activated in some tumors, and hence it may be a pivotal point of control of the growth of high-grade astrocytomas. In a recent study of adults with high-grade astrocytoma, investigators demonstrated that patients with EGFR mutations and loss of PTEN (a tumor suppressor gene) had excellent responses to gefitinib, a drug that blocks the EGF receptor.[24]

Many more mutations have been identified among the many tumor types, and treatments continue to be developed that target the specific mutations identified. As our knowledge of the molecular biology of pediatric brain tumors increases, we may eventually categorize these tumors not as they appear on the microscope, but by their molecular signature and how they respond to these more targeted therapies.

## SURVIVAL

The overall survival for adolescents with brain tumors is similar to that of younger children. As noted in Figure 112-7, the 15-year survival for 15- to 19-year-olds is more than 60%. The 5-year survival for 15- to 19-year-olds compares favorably to the 5-year survival of teens with other malignancies, having increased from 59% in the interval from 1974 to 1976 to 77% in the interval between 1995 and 2000 (Table 112-2). Overall survival data for teenagers with brain tumors are somewhat misleading because there are many different types of brain tumors, and survival is highly variable depending on the tumor type. For example, the long-term survival with CNS germinoma is approximately 90%,[10] whereas the 3-year survival for brainstem glioma is less than 10%.[25]

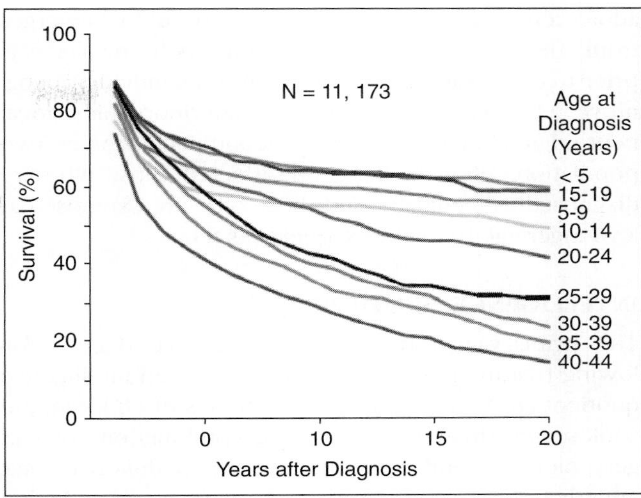


**FIGURE 112-7** Survival rates of all CNS tumors by age, SEER 1975–1998.

**Table 112-2**

**Five-Year Relative Survival Rates by Cancer Type and Time Period, Age 15–19, Surveillance Epidemiology and End Results, 1974–1976 and 1995–2000**

| *Tumor Category* | *1974–1976* | *1995–2000* |
|---|---|---|
| All sites | 64% | 80% |
| Bone and joints | 47% | 63% |
| Melanoma of the skin | 77% | 94% |
| Testis (males) | 55% | 92% |
| Brain and other nervous | 59% | 77% |
| Thyroid | 100% | 100% |
| Hodgkin lymphoma | 88% | 96% |
| Non-Hodgkin lymphoma | 41% | 72% |
| Leukemia | 22% | 54% |
| Acute lymphocytic leukemia | 21% | 60% |

Data from Ries LAG, Eisner MP, Kosary CL, et al, eds. SEER cancer statistics review, 1975–2001. Bethesda, MD: National Cancer Institute; 2004. Available at www.seer.cancer.gov/csr/1975_2001/. Accessed February 23, 2010.

## LATE EFFECTS OF THERAPY

Although the overall survival for adolescents with brain tumors continues to climb, the long-term sequelae of the tumor and the treatment can be devastating. The adolescent diagnosed with a brain tumor seldom emerges from the rigors of therapy the same as he or she was prior to diagnosis. Long-term sequelae include neurocognitive and behavioral deficits, endocrinopathies, focal neurologic deficits, and risk of second malignancies. Two populations of adolescents are affected: those who are diagnosed as teenagers, and those who are diagnosed at a younger age but suffer sequelae as teens.

### INTELLIGENCE QUOTIENT

The primary measure of neurocognitive deficits following treatment for brain tumors has been intelligence quotient (IQ). In a review of 12 studies of children and adolescents treated with varying combinations of surgery, radiation, and chemotherapy for medulloblastoma, ependymoma, or low-grade astrocytoma, most had a significant drop in IQ.[26] In addition, analysis of these studies suggests that: (1) the IQ continues to drop over time; (2) IQ drops are more pronounced for patients who receive whole brain irradiation and who are irradiated at a younger age; (3) patients receiving radiation are more affected than those treated with surgery alone; (4) factors other than radiation, such as surgery and complications of surgery, can also adversely affect IQ. In addition to the decline in IQ, survivors of pediatric brain tumors suffer from attention deficits, impaired short-term memory, and slower cognitive processing. The "real life" implications of these findings are illustrated in a large study of 341 adult survivors of pediatric and adolescent brain tumors.[27] When compared with their siblings, these survivors were less likely to be employed, married, or able to drive, and more likely to have hearing or visual deficits and emotional problems.

### ENDOCRINOLOGIC AND OTHER DEFECTS

Endocrinologic deficits are also common, due in large part to irradiation of the hypothalamic/pituitary axis and/or radiation to the full spine in a growing individual. The most common deficits are growth failure, delayed puberty, and hypothyroidism. These late effects usually can be treated effectively with hormone replacement. Hearing loss is also common in survivors of pediatric brain tumors, particularly those with medulloblastoma. Medulloblastoma is typically treated with radiation and cisplatin, an ototoxic drug, making many adolescents with this form of tumor at high risk of hearing loss.[10] Although second malignancies are uncommon in survivors of childhood brain tumors, they occur at increased frequency compared to the general population. These second tumors are associated with a prior history of radiation; the most common second tumors in adolescents are meningioma and glioma.[28]

### PSYCHOSOCIAL ISSUES

The late effects of therapy can be particularly difficult for an adolescent survivor of a childhood brain tumor. The broad spectrum of physical, psychologic, and cognitive late effects conspire to separate and isolate the teenager from his or her peers. The child successfully treated for a brain tumor may cope well as a preadolescent, but the treatment rendered in childhood may impair the rapid physical and cognitive development of normal adolescence. The increasing challenge of academic work as the adolescent enters high school can be overwhelming, and the teen may require tutoring and special classes. Growth delay and delayed puberty can physically isolate the teen, separating him or her further from peers. Social isolation can in turn cause behavior problems and depression. Current protocols for treating children with brain tumors are aimed as much at diminishing these devastating late effects of therapy as they are at improving cure rates.

## PARTICIPATION IN CLINICAL TRIALS

The field of pediatric oncology prides itself on the number of children and adolescents with cancer enrolled in clinical trials. Indeed, with 55% to 60% of eligible patients younger than 15 years of age enrolled in National Cancer Institute (NCI)-sponsored clinical trials,[29] participation in such trials is considered the standard of care in pediatric oncology. However, the proportion of participants drops in the older adolescent years, from 50% of 10- to 14-year-olds to 10% of 15- to 19-year-olds. Furthermore, the number of teens seen at institutions who are not members of NCI-cooperative groups increases from 21% in the 10- to 14-year-old group to 79% among 15- to 19-year-olds. It is likely that such older adolescents are seen at adult oncology centers or in adult private practices. Regarding older adolescents with brain tumors in England, only 30% of 15- to 19-year-olds are referred to pediatric centers and enrolled on national protocols.[30] Similar data specifically pertaining to adolescents with brain tumors in this country are not available.

## SPECIFIC BRAIN TUMORS

Management and outcome for adolescents with some of the more common brain tumors are discussed next.

### MEDULLOBLASTOMA

Medulloblastoma is one of the most common brain tumors in younger children (17.6% of children up to age 14 with brain tumors), but accounts for only 6.8%

of adolescents 15 to 19 years old with brain tumors. Although medulloblastoma is usually localized to the posterior fossa, it can disseminate throughout the CNS. Hence therapy targets the entire neuraxis. The best outcomes occur in patients who receive craniospinal radiation, followed by cisplatin-based chemotherapy. In earlier studies of medulloblastoma, survival was comparable between the older and younger age groups.[31] In a recent Children's Oncology Group[32] study of children with average-risk medulloblastoma, overall 5-year survival was 86%. Survival for 7% of the enrollees in the 15- to 19-year age group was the same as the overall group. Because patients with medulloblastoma receive whole brain radiation and cisplatin-based chemotherapy, late effects of therapy are significant (neurocognitive deficits, growth and pubertal delay, hearing loss). In the current generation of studies, investigators are examining the effect of lower-dose neuraxis radiation for these patients.

### LOW-GRADE ASTROCYTOMA

Juvenile pilocytic astrocytoma (a subtype of low-grade astrocytoma) accounts for 16% of all brain tumors in the 15- to 19-year-old age group (see Figure 112-4). When other types of low-grade astrocytomas are included along with the juvenile pilocytic astrocytomas, the proportion of older teens with low-grade astrocytoma exceeds 20%. Age-specific data on outcomes for children with this type of tumor are not available. The treatment of choice is surgery: gross total resection of low-grade astrocytomas results in at least 90% long-term survival.[10] For those in whom gross total resection is not possible, observation until the tumor grows is an acceptable approach. Radiation at the time of diagnosis or progression results in 10-year survival of 67% to 94%.[10] Chemotherapy is frequently the treatment of choice for younger children with incompletely resected astrocytomas, but its role in treating adolescents is not known.

### GERMINOMA

Central nervous system germinoma is a relatively rare type of brain tumor. However, it occurs with greatest frequency in teenagers: 6.6% of the 15- to 19-year-olds with brain tumors, compared to only 3.8% of younger children. It is far more common in boys than girls. The tumor tends to occur in the midline in the pineal or suprasellar region. Like medulloblastoma, CNS germinoma can disseminate throughout the craniospinal axis. Therefore treatment must target the entire neuroaxis. The standard therapy is craniospinal radiation. The tumor is also chemosensitive; investigators are currently examining the role of short-course chemotherapy followed by reduced-dose radiation. The long-term outcome for adolescents with this disease is excellent, with a disease-free survival rate of greater than 90%.[10]

## SUMMARY

Brain tumors are less common in adolescents than in younger children, but their effects can be devastating whether the tumor is detected in the second decade of life, or is treated in childhood with sequelae during adolescent growth and development. Most brain tumors in adolescents occur in the posterior fossa, and their presenting signs and symptoms are often related to their anatomical location. Precise definition of the location and nature of the tumor is now possible with computer-assisted 3-dimensional modeling. Depending on the tumor location and type, treatment options include surgery, radiation, and chemotherapy, alone or in combination. Although age-specific data for adolescents with brain tumors are generally lacking, involvement in clinical trials holds the best hope for determining the most effective treatment modalities over time, especially as newer treatment options develop over time.

## REFERENCES

1. Bendel A, Beaty O, Bottom K, Bunin G, Wrensch M. Central nervous system cancer. In: Bleyer A, O'Leary M, Barr R, Ries LAG, eds. *Cancer Epidemiology in Older Adolescents and Young Adults 15 to 29 Years of Age, Including SEER Incidence and Survival: 1975-2000.* National Cancer Institute, NIH Pub. No. 06-5767. Bethesda, MD; 2006

2. Listernick R, Ferner RE, Liu GT, Gutmann DH. Optic pathway gliomas in neurofibromatosis-1: controversies and recommendations. *Ann Neurol.* 2007;61:189-198

3. Ferner RE. Neurofibromatosis 1 and neurofibromatosis 2: a twenty-first century perspective. *Lancet Neurology.* 2007;6:340-351

4. Walter AW, Hancock ML, Pui CH, et al. Secondary brain tumors in children treated for acute lymphoblastic leukemia at St Jude Children's Research Hospital. *J Clin Oncol.* 1998;16:3761-3767

5. CBTRUS. *Statistical Report: Primary Brain Tumors in the United States, 2000-2004.* Central Brain Tumor Registry of the United States; 2008

6. Bailey J, Cushing H. Medulloblastoma cerebelli, common type of mid-cerebellar glioma of childhood. *Arch Neurol Psychiatry.* 1925;14:192-224

7. Wilne SH, Ferris RC, Nathwani A, Kennedy CR. The presenting features of brain tumours: a review of 200 cases. *Arch Dis Child.* 2006;91:502-506

8. Dobrovoljac M, Hengartner H, Boltshauser E, Grotzer MA. Delay in the diagnosis of paediatric brain tumours. *Eur J Pediatr.* 2002;161:663-667

9. Chipkevitch E. Brain tumors and anorexia nervosa syndrome. *Brain Development.* 1994;16:175-179

10. Blaney SM, Kun LE, Hunter J, et al. Tumors of the central nervous system. In: Pizzo PA, Poplack DG, eds. *Principles and Practice of Pediatric Oncology.* Philadelphia, PA: Lippincott Williams & Wilkins; 2006

11. Chang SM, Parney IF, Huang W, et al. Patterns of care for adults with newly diagnosed malignant glioma. *JAMA.* 2005;293:557-564

12. Barnett GH, Kormos DW, Steiner CP, et al. Use of a frameless, armless stereotactic wand for brain tumor localization with two-dimensional and three-dimensional neuroimaging. *Neurosurgery.* 1993;33:674-678

13. Cochrane DD, Gustavsson B, Poskitt KP, Steinbok P, Kestle JR. The surgical and natural morbidity of aggressive resection for posterior fossae tumors in childhood. *Pediatric Neurosurgery.* 1994;20:19-29

14. Doxey D, Bruce D, Sklar F, Swift D, Shapiro K. Posterior fossa syndrome: identifiable risk factors and irreversible complications. *Pediatric Neurosurgery.* 1999;31:131-136

15. Merchant TE, Zhu Y, Thompson SJ, Sontag MR, Heideman RL, Kun LE. Preliminary results from a Phase II trial of conformal radiation therapy for pediatric patients with localized low-grade astrocytoma and ependymoma. *Int J Radia Onc, Biol, Phys.* 2002;52(2):325-332

16. Merchant TE, Mulhern RK, Krasin MJ, et al. Preliminary results from a phase II trial of conformal radiation therapy and evaluation of radiation-related CNS effects for pediatric patients with localized ependymoma. *J Clin Onc.* 2004;22:3156-3162

17. Mandell LR, Kadota R, Freeman C, et al. There is no role for hyperfractionated radiotherapy in the management of children with newly diagnosed diffuse intrinsic brainstem tumors: results of a Pediatric Oncology Group phase III trial comparing conventional vs hyperfractionated radiotherapy. *Int J Radiat Oncol Biol Phys.* 1999;43:959-964

18. Boethius J, Ulfarsson E, Rahn T, Lippitz B. Gamma knife radiosurgery for pilocytic astrocytomas. *J Neuros.* 2002;97 (5 suppl):677-680

19. Evans AE, Jenkins RS, Sposto R, et al. The treatment of medulloblastoma. Results of a prospective randomized trial of radiation therapy with and without CCNU, vincristine, and prednisone. *J Neurosurg.* 1990;72:572-852

20. Sposto R, Ertel IJ, Jenkin RD, et al. The effectiveness of chemotherapy for treatment of high grade astrocytoma in children: results of a randomized trial. A report from the Children's Cancer Study Group. *J Neuro-oncol.* 1989;7:165-177

21. Warren K, Jakacki R, Widemann B, et al. Phase II trial of intravenous lobradimil and carboplatin in childhood brain tumors: a report from the Children's Oncology Group. *Cancer Chemotherapy Pharmacology.* 2006;58(3):343-347

22. Dunkel IJ, Boyett JM, Yates A, et al. High-dose carboplatin, thiotepa, and etoposide with autologous stem-cell rescue for patients with recurrent medulloblastoma. Children's Cancer Group. *J Clin Oncol.* 1998;16:222-228

23. Vredenburgh JJ, Desjardins A, Herndon JE II, et al. Phase II trial of Bevacizumab and Irinotecan in recurrent malignant glioma. *Clin Cancer Res.* 2007;13:1253-1259

24. Mellinghoff IK, Wang MY, Vivanco I, et al. Molecular determinants of the response of glioblastomas to EGFR kinase inhibitors. *N Eng J Med.* 2005;353:2012-2024

25. Korones DN. Treatment of newly diagnosed diffuse brainstem gliomas in children: in search of the holy grail. *Expert Review of Anticancer Therapy.* 2007;7:663-674

26. Mulhern RK, Merchant TE, Gajjar A, Reddick WE, Kun LE. Late neurocognitive sequelae in survivors of brain tumours in childhood. *Lancet Oncol.* 2004;5:399-408

27. Mostow EN, Byrne J, Connelly RR, Mulvihill JJ. Quality of life in long-term survivors of CNS tumors of childhood and adolescence. *J Clin Oncol.* 1991;9:595-599

28. Neglia JP, Robison LL, Stovall M, et al. New primary neoplasms of the central nervous system in survivors of childhood cancer: a report from the Childhood Cancer Survivor Study. *J Natl Cancer Inst.* 2006;98:1528-1537

29. Reaman GH, Bleyer WA. Infants and adolescents with cancer: special considerations. In: Pizzo PA, Poplack DG, eds. *Principles and Practice of Pediatric Oncology.* Philadelphia, PA: Lippincott Williams & Wilkins; 2006

30. Capra M, Harrave D, Bartels U, Hyder D, Huang A, Bouffet E. Central nervous system tumours in adolescents. *Eur J Cancer.* 2003;39:2643-2650

31. McNeil DE, Cote TR, Clegg L, Rorke LB. Incidence and trends in pediatric malignancies medulloblastoma/primitive neuroectodermal tumor: a SEER update. *Med Pediatr Oncol.* 2002;39:190-194

32. Packer RJ, Gajjar A, Vezina G, et al. Phase III study of craniospinal radiation therapy followed by adjuvant chemotherapy for newly diagnosed average-risk medulloblastoma. *J Clin Oncol.* 2006;24:4202-4208

# CHAPTER 113

# Hematopoietic Stem Cell (Bone Marrow) Transplantation

LAUREN BRUCKNER, MD, PhD

## INTRODUCTION

Hematopoietic stem cell transplantation (HSCT), commonly known as bone marrow transplantation, is effective in the treatment of a variety of malignant and nonmalignant conditions in adolescents. There are an estimated 4,500 HSCTs performed annually worldwide in patients younger than 20 years of age, according to 2007 data from the Center for International Blood and Marrow Transplant Research (CIBMTR).[1] The HSCT procedure involves transplanting blood and marrow stem cells into a recipient who has been pretreated with an appropriate conditioning regimen. This chapter provides an overview of HSCT including clinical indications for HSCT, sources of stem cells, types of conditioning regimens, and short- and long-term complications. Particular attention is given to those issues relevant and/or unique to adolescents. For a more in-depth review of pediatric HSCT, refer to the general references provided.[2,3]

## INDICATIONS FOR HEMATOPOIETIC STEM CELL TRANSPLANTATION

Hematopoietic stem cell transplantation can be used to treat a variety of pediatric malignancies. A limited number of hematologic as well as nonhematologic, nonmalignant conditions also respond to this modality. The fields of stem cell biology, immunology, and gene therapy are rapidly advancing, and it is anticipated that HSCT will be applied to treat many more pediatric disorders in the future than are listed in Box 113-1.

**Box 113-1**

***Clinical Indications for Hematopoietic Stem Cell Transplantation in Adolescents***

**Malignant diseases**

- Leukemia (ALL, AML, CML)
- Lymphoma (Hodgkin and non-Hodgkin)
- Myelodysplastic syndrome
- Soft tissue sarcomas (Ewing sarcoma)

**Nonmalignant hematologic or immune diseases**

- Aplastic anemia
- Fanconi anemia
- Sickle cell disease
- Thalassemia
- Immunodeficiencies (eg, DiGeorge, Wiskott-Aldrich, or severe combined immunodeficiency syndromes)

**Nonmalignant, nonhematologic diseases (usually performed in childhood)**

- Glycogen storage diseases
- Lysosomal storage disorders (lipidoses, sphingolipidoses, and leukodystrophies)
- Mucopolysaccharidoses (eg, Hurler or Hunter syndromes)
- Osteopetrosis

### MALIGNANT DISEASES

The treatment of malignant diseases is the most common clinical indication for HSCT among adolescents. It enables the use of chemotherapies and/or radiotherapies that would otherwise be limited by bone marrow toxicity. Reconstitution with hematopoietic stem cells overcomes these myelotoxic effects. There is also an immunologic basis for hematopoietic stem cells cure of malignant disease: when those cells are from a disparate individual, the transplanted immune system (the graft) can recognize the malignant cells as being nonself and promote a powerful graft-vs-tumor or graft-vs-leukemia effect.

### NONMALIGNANT DISEASES

With nonmalignant hematologic diseases, the goal is to replace defective marrow, such as in bone marrow failure syndromes, immunodeficiency disorders, or sickle cell disease. For nonmalignant, nonhematologic disorders, the introduction of hematopoietic stem cells containing a normal gene can, at least partially, alleviate the clinical symptoms related to a genetic disorder. Examples of disorders that can be treated with HSCT include mucopolysaccharidoses, leukodystrophies, glycogen storage diseases, and metabolic disorders such as X-linked adrenoleukodystrophy and osteopetrosis.

Hematopoietic stem cell transplantation for metabolic or immunodeficiency disorders is usually performed when children are younger than 12 years of age. This has long-term implications and effects on the health, development, and emotional well-being of younger patients who undergo this procedure as they progress through adolescence.

## TYPES OF HEMATOPOIETIC STEM CELL TRANSPLANTATION

To provide anticipatory guidance for an adolescent undergoing HSCT and for his or her family, the primary care provider should have a basic understanding of not only the wide spectrum of diseases that can be treated with this modality, but also the different types of procedures employed. There are several variables that affect the expected course, potential complications, and clinical outcome of transplantation, including the clinical indication, the degree of human leukocyte antigen (HLA) matching, and other variables listed in Box 113-2.

### DONOR SOURCE

#### Autologous Donor Cells

Autologous transplantation involves the removal, storage, and subsequent reinfusion of an individual's own stem cells. The major aim is to enable the use of therapies with malignant diseases (see Figure 113-1) that would otherwise be limited by bone marrow toxicity. It generally employs high-dose single- or multiagent chemotherapy with nonoverlapping toxicities that are specifically designed for complete disease eradication.

> **Box 113-2**
>
> ***Variables in Hematopoietic Stem Cell Transplantation***
>
> **Donor source**
> - Autologous
> - Allogeneic (related donor, unrelated donor)
>
> **Stem cell source**
> - Bone marrow
> - Peripheral blood
> - Cord blood
>
> **Conditioning regimen**
> - Myeloablative
> - Reduced intensity

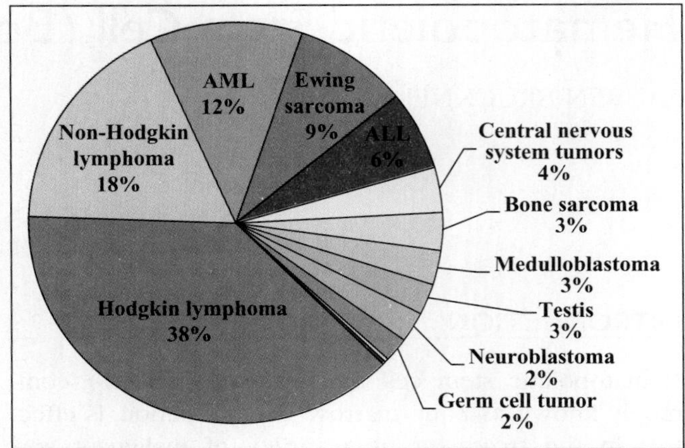


FIGURE 113-1 Indications for autologous HSCT among patients 12 to 21 years old between 1990 and 2006. Center for International Blood and Marrow Transplant Research (CIBMTR).[1] (These data are preliminary and were obtained from the Statistical Center of the Center for International Blood and Marrow Transplant Research. The analysis has not been reviewed or approved by the advisory or scientific committees of the CIBMTR.)

Thus, this type of transplantation is more accurately termed "high-dose chemotherapy with autologous stem cell rescue," and generally has less transplantation-related toxicity than allogeneic transplantation from related or unrelated donors. Hematopoietic stem cells are extracted either by peripheral apheresis or by bone marrow harvesting from the patient weeks to months prior to transplantation, frozen, and stored for future use. The stored cells are then infused 1 to 2 days after myeloablative chemotherapy has been administered. The major autologous transplantation complications are related to direct toxicities of the conditioning regimen, infections, and relapse of the underlying disease.

#### Allogeneic Donor Cells

Allogeneic transplantation involves a donor who is not genetically identical to the recipient and who may or may not be related (Figure 113-2). Hematopoietic stem cells are collected either by peripheral apheresis, bone marrow harvest, or at the time of birth from the placenta in the form of cord blood. The stem cells are then infused intravenously into the recipient, where they migrate to the bone marrow. The ideal allogeneic donor is one who is fully HLA matched and can be either from a relative, usually a sibling, or from an unrelated donor identified from volunteer registries such as the National Donor Marrow Program (NDMP). The HLA region is a series of genes arranged in 3 different clusters or classes on chromosome 6 and inherited as a genetic unit. Thus,

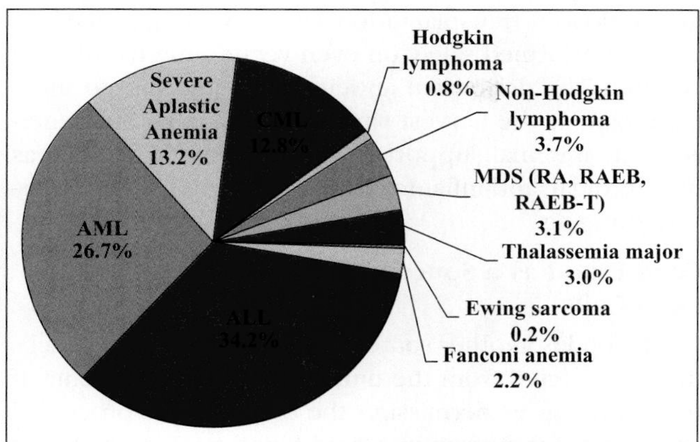


**FIGURE 113-2** Indications for allogeneic HSCT among patients 12 to 21 years old between 1990 and 2006. Center for International Blood and Marrow Transplant Research (CIBMTR).[1] (These data are preliminary and were obtained from the Statistical Center of the Center for International Blood and Marrow Transplant Research. The analysis has not been reviewed or approved by the advisory or scientific committees of the CIBMTR.)

the chance of 2 siblings having identical HLA genotypes is 25%. The time from initiation of a preliminary search to transplantation is about 3 to 4 months for an unrelated donor, but much shorter when a family member is the donor.

Human leukocyte antigen disparity directly correlates with outcome. The greater the HLA disparity, the greater the risk that donor T-lymphocytes present in the graft will recognize host tissues as foreign, resulting in graft-vs-host disease (GVHD). Graft-vs-host disease is a major allogeneic transplantation complication and a leading cause of post-HSCT morbidity and mortality. Similarly, HLA disparity increases the risk of graft rejection as host T lymphocytes recognize the donor stem cells as foreign.

When a fully HLA-matched donor is not available, partially HLA-matched family members or unrelated donors are considered. In unique circumstances, *haploidentical* HSCT are considered using the parent as the donor, as a parent will always be at least a 50% HLA match. However, these alternative transplantation types require much more aggressive immunosuppressive conditioning regimens and are associated with increased toxicity from infections and GVHD. The major obstacles in allogeneic transplantation are GVHD, organ toxicity related to the conditioning regimen, infection, and relapse of the underlying disease.

### Syngeneic Donor Cells

Identical twins have identical genotypes, and thus will be fully matched not only for HLA but for all other potential antigenic determinants, whether recognized as important in transplant immunology or not. The risk of GVHD is all but eliminated in syngeneic transplantation. However, because genetic disparity is also the basis for the desired graft-vs-tumor effect, there is a higher incidence of malignant relapse. Similarly, if a *T-cell depleted graft* is used, the risk of GVHD is less, but the risk of relapse and infections increases.

## THE HEMATOPOIETIC STEM CELL TRANSPLANTATION PROCESS

### RECIPIENT SELECTION AND EVALUATION

Preparing an adolescent as a hematopoietic stem cell transplantation recipient requires a group effort that involves a specialized transplantation unit and staff, social workers, child life specialists, transplant coordinators, stem cell processing group, insurance specialists, and clinical providers. Most adolescents considering transplantation as a treatment option will have been referred for evaluation by a hematology/oncology provider, though it is anticipated that consultations from other pediatric specialties will increase in the future as HSCT is used to treat more nonhematologic disorders.

Because of the overwhelming amount and content of information that must be absorbed by the adolescent and his or her family, the transmission of information occurs over several educational sessions and with the aid of supplemental written materials. Discussions include an explanation of the transplantation process including stem cell collection, the type of transplantation, the risk of transplant-related morbidity and mortality, and the risk of relapse of the underlying disease.

Hematopoietic stem cell transplantation is not a panacea, and the process is associated with significant morbidity. There are many circumstances where the benefits of HSCT are outweighed by the risks. The potential transplant recipient requires a thorough evaluation to determine if he or she is medically fit to proceed with transplantation. Many adolescents considering transplantation already have organ-specific toxicities related to prior treatments and/or the underlying disease, and must undergo a battery of tests to assess fitness for HSCT. These include baseline function testing of the heart, liver, kidney, and lungs, chest x-ray, neuropsychological assessment, dental assessment, audiogram, screening complete blood count (CBC) with differential, comprehensive blood chemistries, and a viral screen for herpes simplex (HSV), Epstein-Barr (EBV), cytomegalovirus (CMV), human immunodeficiency (HIV), varicella, and hepatitis viruses.

## DONOR SELECTION AND EVALUATION

Many factors are involved in choosing an appropriate donor of hematopoietic stem cells, including the recipient's disease, the type of transplantation being considered, the urgency in obtaining a donor, the size of the recipient, the age and sex of the donor/recipient pair, the parity of female donors, and ABO compatibility. The donor must be healthy and willing to undergo the stem cell collection in the required time frame. Children can safely donate hematopoietic stem cells for a sibling with parental consent and their assent. A donor evaluation includes a thorough history and physical examination, and obtaining blood work such as a CBC with differential, chemistry panel, and the viral screen performed on the recipient. Depending on the age and health of the donor, additional organ-specific evaluations may be necessary to determine whether the donor can safely undergo the stem cell collection process.

## SOURCES OF HEMATOPOIETIC STEM CELLS

There are 3 sources of hematopoietic stem cells: peripheral, cord blood, and bone marrow.

### Peripheral Blood as Source of Hematopoietic Stem Cells

Hematopoietic stem cells are primarily located in the bone marrow, with few circulating in the peripheral blood. To harvest peripheral blood stem cells, the donor is treated for several days with growth colony stimulating factor (GCSF) to mobilize these cells from the bone marrow to the peripheral blood and to improve the stem cell yield. Chemotherapy also mobilizes stem cells from the bone marrow to the peripheral blood. Therefore, when autologous transplantation is planned, cells in the peripheral blood are collected after a course of chemotherapy and GCSF. Peripheral stem cells are collected by leukopheresis using a process similar to dialysis. The donor requires placement of 2 large-bore intravenous lines, 1 to deliver blood to the apheresis machine, which centrifuges the blood and removes the leukocyte component, and the other to return the processed blood to the donor. Leukopheresis of small children can be difficult and requires specialized support services and planning.

### Bone Marrow as Source of Hematopoietic Stem Cells

Bone marrow harvesting from the posterior iliac crests is performed under sterile conditions in an operating room under general anesthesia. After filtering and processing, the final total number of nucleated cells and CD34+ cells collected is determined. Stem cells are infused into the recipient as soon as possible after being collected, but can be frozen for future use particularly for autologous transplantation. The harvesting procedure can be performed safely on even very young infants and children. The donor can anticipate having mild to moderate pain at the harvest sites for a few days, but generally only minimal supportive postoperative care such as nonsteroidal anti-inflammatory medication and a pressure dressing.

### Cord Blood as a Source of Hematopoietic Stem Cells

Cord blood is another source of hematopoietic stem cells that is collected from the umbilical cord and placenta. If the mother gives permission, the cord blood is processed and frozen for storage in a cord blood bank. Cord blood can and has been used as the source of stem cells for all the same clinical HCT indications as bone marrow. A major advantage of cord blood HSC is that the cells can be used for HSCT within 1 month compared to 2 to 3 months needed to identify and collect unrelated peripheral blood or bone marrow HSC. Additionally, cord blood improves the chance of finding an HSC donor for rarer HLA haplotypes because the HLA representation within cord blood banks is more diverse and because cord blood HSCT can tolerate a greater degree of HLA mismatch. Even units that are only matched at 4 out of 6 HLA can be successfully used because cord blood has a preponderance of naïve T-cells and thus less associated GVHD.

A major disadvantage of cord blood HSCT is that the cell doses are limited and generally small. Smaller doses of cord blood cells correlate with a greater risk of nonengraftment, delayed neutrophil engraftment, and treatment-related mortality. However, it is feasible to overcome the dose limitation by using more than one cord blood unit or by supplementing the unit with HSC from an HLA haploidentical relative. Another disadvantage of cord blood HSC is the inability to obtain additional cells from the cord blood donor should the graft fail or if donor lymphocyte infusions are needed.

## CONDITIONING REGIMENS

Many conditioning regimens are used in HSCT, including combinations of chemotherapy, total body irradiation (TBI), and biologic agents. The intensity of these regimens varies, from myeloablative regimens designed to totally eradicate malignant diseases, to reduced intensity or nonmyeloablative regimens designed to suppress the host's immune system and prevent graft rejection. The conditioning regimen varies depending on the clinical indication for the HSCT, the patient's medical condition, institutional protocols, and physician preference. Commonly used conditioning regimens include cyclophosphamide in combination with busulfan, fludarabine, or TBI with or without antithymocyte globulin (ATG).

## ACUTE POST-HSCT COMPLICATIONS

Hematopoietic stem cell transplantation can lead to potentially life-threatening toxicities and thus requires a highly specialized team of health care providers and support staff working in an appropriate environment and with the necessary pediatric-specific resources available. The primary care physician can be integral to the complex care patients receive after HSCT, and as such should be aware of the common and major post-HSCT complications.

The morbidity and mortality after HSCT is attributable to the toxicity of the conditioning regimen used (tissue injury of multiple organ systems and pancytopenia) and the HSCT-mediated effects on the immune system. Some common hematologic and nonhematologic HSCT-related complications are listed in Box 113-3. Because HSCT involves the transplantation of the immune system itself, some unique immunologic effects can occur, such as prolonged susceptibility to infection, GVHD, graft-vs-tumor/leukemia, and other morbidities that are likely multifactorial and at least in part due to immune dysregulation (hemolytic anemia, sinusoidal obstructive syndrome of the liver, hemorrhagic cystitis, and idiopathic pneumonia syndrome).

### ACUTE GRAFT-VERSUS-HOST DISEASE

Graft-versus-host disease is mediated by donor T-lymphocytes and characterized by mild to fatal skin, gastrointestinal, and/or liver injury. Even with intensive GVHD prophylaxis with immunosuppressant such as cyclosporine, tacrolimus, methotrexate, and ATG, GVHD occurs in 10% to 15% of pediatric patients receiving HLA-matched sibling hematopoietic stem cells.[4] The survival rate is 90% in grade 0–I, 60% in grade II–III, and uniformly fatal in grade IV. Risk factors for GVHD include the degree of HLA disparity, older host age, gender mismatch, CMV seropositivity, and other HSCT variables (HSCT type, conditioning regimen, stem cell source, T-cell depletion).[4] Generally, GVHD only occurs with allogeneic HCT, though GVHD with autologous HSCT can occur when post-HSCT immunomodulation is being employed to induce a graft-vs-tumor effect.

The pathophysiology of GVHD is complex and involves a combination of tissue injury and inflammation. The conditioning regimen and/or infection cause tissue injury and the subsequent release of proinflammatory cytokines, which leads to increased expression of host antigens. This in turn promotes the activation of donor T-lymphocytes and initiates a cascade of immune activation directed against antigens expressed on host tissues, leading to more tissue injury and more inflammation.[5]

Initial presentation of GVHD usually involves the skin in the form of erythema on the palms and soles that coincides with neutrophil engraftment. In severe GVHD, the maculopapular rash forms bullous lesions with toxic epidermal necrolysis. Graft-versus-host disease of the liver is characterized by elevation of the blood bilirubin and transaminase levels; Graft-versus-host disease of the GI tract can be variable in its presentation, and can include anorexia, diarrhea, abdominal pain and bloating, and malabsorption. The severity of GVHD is classified into 4 stages depending on the extent of involvement of the skin, liver, and/or GI tract.[4] Grade I GVHD is mild disease, grade II GVHD is moderate, grade III is severe, and grade IV life threatening.

Agents used to treat and/or prevent GVHD include cytotoxic agents to diminish T-lymphocyte numbers (methotrexate, pentostatin, corticosteroids), T-lymphocyte-specific inhibitors (cyclosporine, tacrolimus, sirolimus, mycophenolate mofetil), and antibody therapies to inhibit T-lymphocyte function (ATG, alemtuzumab, daclizumab). Another way to limit the number of donor T-lymphocytes infused during HSCT is to manipulate the stem cell product prior to infusion (T-cell depletion, CD34+ selection). Lastly, GVHD can be treated by extracorporeal photopheresis (ECP), in which lymphocytes are removed, exposed to ultraviolet light to inactivate the T-lymphocytes, and reinfused into the patient.[6]

> **Box 113-3**
>
> ***Acute Complications Following Hematopoietic Stem Cell Transplantation***
>
> **Hematologic:** neutropenia, anemia, thrombocytopenia
>
> **Infectious:** bacterial, fungal, viral
>
> **Immunologic:** GVHD, hemolytic anemia
>
> **Pulmonary:** pneumonia, IPS
>
> **Cardiovascular:** microangiopathy, hypertension, pericardial effusion
>
> **Genitourinary:** hemorrhagic cystitis
>
> **Gastrointestinal:** mucositis, nausea, vomiting, diarrhea, anorexia
>
> **Hepatic:** sinusoidal obstructive syndrome, hepatitis
>
> **Renal:** electrolyte wasting, renal insufficiency
>
> **Skin:** rashes, skin breakdown, radiation skin changes
>
> **Neurologic:** seizures, encephalopathies, intracranial hemorrhage
>
> **Psychological:** depression, anxiety

### INFECTION

Infection is a leading cause of morbidity and mortality during HSCT and is related to therapy-induced severe neutropenia, lymphopenia, and effects on mucosal

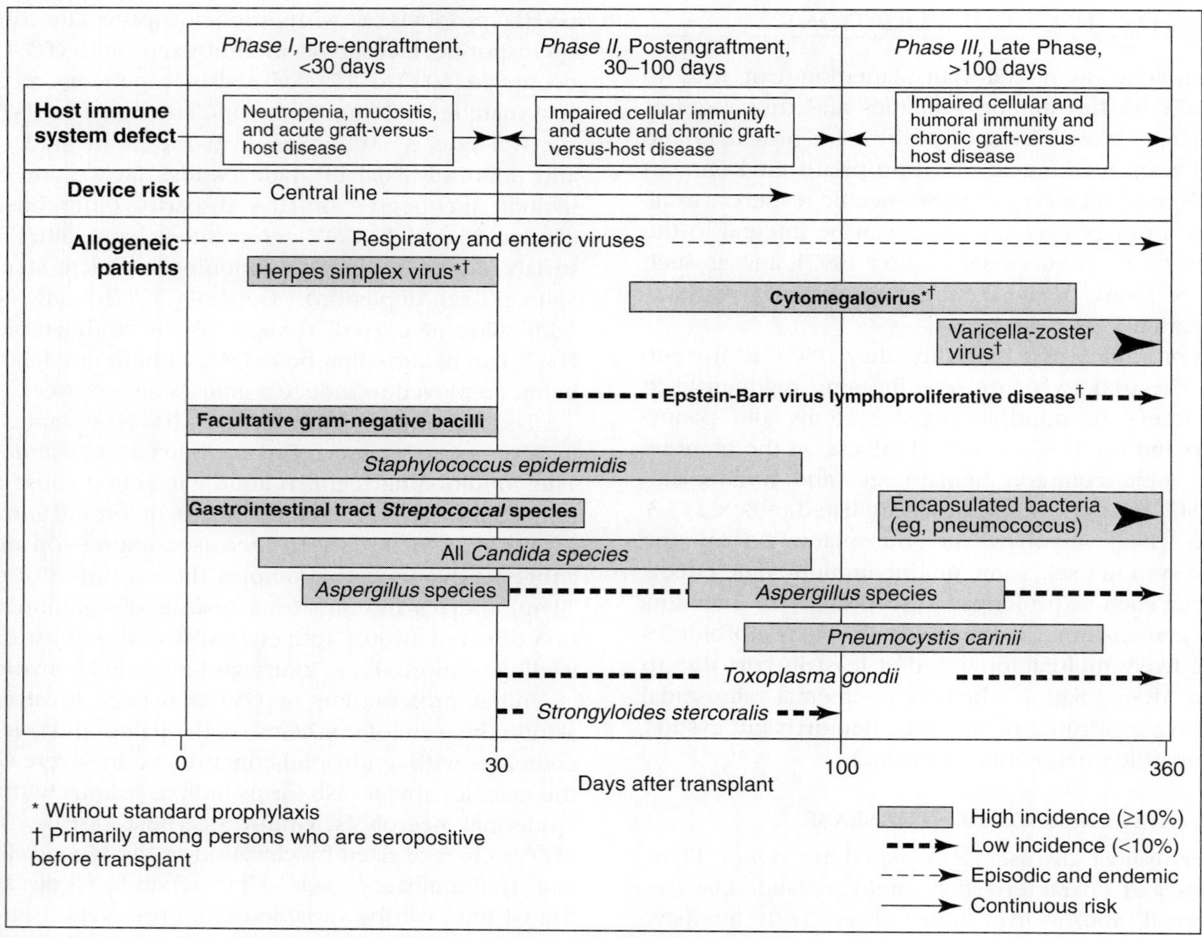


**FIGURE 113-3** Timeline of infectious risk postallogeneic HCT. (From Guidelines for preventing opportunistic infections among hematopoietic stem cell transplant recipients. *MMWR Recomm Rep*. 2000; 49 (RR-10): 1–147.)

and skin integrity. Although bacteria remain the most common cause of infection, HSCT-related deaths are more commonly attributable to fungal infections and reactivation of viruses (particularly CMV and EBV). Almost all patients will develop fever during the course of HSCT, but the risk of serious infection and potential pathogens varies as the process proceeds. The HSCT course is typically divided into 3 phases: pre-engraftment, postengraftment (through day +100) and late (after day +100).[7] Figure 113-3 shows the types of infectious risk during each of these 3 phases of HCT.

Many factors affect an adolescent's risk of infection, including the clinical state of the patient pretransplant, infectious history, mucosal and dental/oral integrity, as well as the patient's immune status, type of transplant, conditioning regimen used, and the presence of GVHD. The degree of immune system impairment is directly correlated with the risk of infection. For example, adolescents with evidence of prior CMV infection are tested weekly for CMV; if CMV reactivation is detected, therapy is started, even in the absence of symptoms. Adolescents with evidence of a prior HSV infection are started on HSV prophylaxis. Furthermore, therapies such as corticosteroids and TBI can cause further immunosuppression and also deteriorate mucosal barriers, further increasing the risk of post-transplant infection.

Almost all patients will develop febrile neutropenia in the immediate post-transplantation period. Prompt empiric initiation of antibiotics, rather than waiting for culture results, has been shown to improve overall survival.[7] Even if there is no confirmed infection, antibiotic therapy is continued until the patient is neither febrile nor neutropenic. Fevers persisting for several days without a known infectious source suggest a fungal infection and the addition of empiric antifungal coverage. Granulocyte colony-stimulating factor is frequently used to shorten the period of neutropenia and presumably reduce the risk of infection. Infusions

**Table 113-1**

**Revaccination Schedule after Hematopoietic Stem Cell Transplantation**

| *Vaccine or toxoid* | *Time after HSCT* *12 months* | *14 months* | *24 months* |
|---|---|---|---|
| **Inactivated vaccine or toxoid** | | | |
| Diphtheria, tetanus, pertussis | | | |
| Children aged <7 years | Diphtheria toxoid-tetanus toxoid-pertussis vaccine (DTP) or diphtheria toxoid-tetanus toxoid (DT) | DTP or DT | DTP or DT |
| Children aged ≥7 years | Tetanus-diphtheria toxoid (Td) | Td | Td |
| *Haemophilus influenza* type b (Hib) conjugate | Hib conjugate | Hib conjugate | Hib conjugate |
| Hepatitis B (HepB) | HepB | HepB | HepB |
| 23-valent pneumococcal polysaccharide (PPV23) | PPV23 | — | PPV23 |
| Hepatitis A | Routine administration not indicated | | |
| Influenza | Lifelong, seasonal administration, beginning before HSCT and resuming at ≥6 months after HSCT | | |
| Meningococcal | Routine administration not indicated | | |
| Inactivated polio (IPV) | IPV | IPV | IPV |
| Rabies | Routine administration not indicated | | |
| Lyme disease | Routine administration not indicated; limited data regarding safety, efficacy, or immunogenicity among HSCT recipients | | |
| **Live-attenuated vaccine** | | | |
| Measles-mumps-rubella (MMR) | — | — | MMR |
| Varicella vaccine | Contraindicated for HSCT recipients | | |
| Rotavirus vaccine | Not recommended for any person in the United States | | |

Guidelines for preventing opportunistic infections among hematopoietic stem cell transplant recipients. *MMWR Recomm Rep*. 2000;49 RR-10:84–86. See report for details and footnotes.

of IVIG are also frequently given in the post-transplant period, though generally only when the patient is hypogammaglobulinemic.

Revaccination of patients after HSCT is required because the transplantation process results in the loss of all prior immune memory. Thus, after transplantation, adolescents must be revaccinated once their new immune systems are functional, typically one year after transplant. Centers for Disease Control and Prevention guidelines regarding vaccination after transplantation are shown in Table 113-1.[8]

## PULMONARY TOXICITY

Pulmonary toxicity is the leading cause of early HSCT-related mortality and remains the major dose-limiting factor in conditioning regimens. Reported incidences of post-HSCT lung injury typically range from 40% to 60%, with associated mortality rates of up to 85%.[7] Clinical and animal studies have suggested that a noninfectious type of post-BMT lung injury, termed *idiopathic pneumonia syndrome* (IPS), results from excessive inflammation and resultant immune-mediated lung damage. The incidence of IPS among adolescents ranges from 10% to 15%, but it is associated with a significant increase in mortality (64% vs 17% overall mortality in patients with and without IPS, respectively).[9] A variety of potentially interactive lung insults have been implicated in the pathogenesis of IPS, including GVHD, occult infections, and TBI. Although the specific mechanisms remain speculative, evidence suggests the pathogenesis appears to be immune-mediated with T-lymphocytes and TNF-alpha playing key roles.[10] Clinical trials using the anti-TNF-alpha antagonist, etanercept, have shown promise in improving IPS outcomes.[11]

### SINUSOIDAL OBSTRUCTIVE SYNDROME

*Sinusoidal obstructive syndrome (SOS)* is the clinical triad of painful hepatomegaly, ascites, and hyperbilirubinemia. The conditioning regimen has direct and likely indirect cytotoxic effects on the liver endothelium. The pathogenesis of SOS involves injury to the sinusoidal endothelial cells, leading to occlusion of small vessels with fibrin deposition and disruption of hepatic function. Although generally self-limited and completely reversible, in one-quarter of pediatric patients post-transplant, SOS is severe and results in progressive endothelial damage, sinusoidal fibrosis, liver failure, and often fatal multiorgan failure.[12] Reversal of hepatic flow on Doppler is a late finding in severe SOS and portends a poor prognosis.[7] Therapy is primarily supportive and preventive including fluid restriction, pain control, and avoidance of hepatotoxic agents. One new therapy that has shown promise is the prevention and treatment of SOS is defibrotide, an anticoagulant that alters platelet activity, increases tissue plasminogen activator function, and decreases activity of tissue plasminogen activator inhibitor.[13,14]

### MUCOSITIS

*Mucositis* is a significant complication of HSCT, occurring in almost all HSCT recipients, with severe mucositis (Grade III–IV) occurring in approximately two-thirds of patients.[15,16] Mucositis causes severe pain and discomfort that results in poor nutrition and an increased risk of infection.[17] The pathophysiology involves a combination of direct cytotoxic effects of chemotherapy and/or radiation therapy, inadequate repair processes, decreased saliva production, local inflammatory responses, and changes in the normal oral flora.[7] Severe mucositis usually requires the use of narcotics and total parenteral nutrition. The mainstay of therapy continues to be supportive care and prevention of infections (such as HSV and thrush).[18] However, research is under way to develop better preventive and treatment approaches, such as the use of palifermin.[18,19]

### HEMORRHAGIC CYSTITIS

*Hemorrhagic cystitis* occurs in 10% to 50% of pediatric HSCT recipients.[20] It is usually self-limited, but can be associated with significant discomfort and can lead to urinary obstruction. In a recent retrospective study, a cohort of 163 pediatric patients with 171 HSCT was reviewed; 8.2% developed hemorrhagic cystitis at a median of 25 days post-HCT.[21] The symptoms lasted from 3 to 96 days with a median of 26 days. All symptoms eventually resolved, but 8 of the 14 affected patients died of other complications. Hemorrhagic cystitis has multiple causes, including chemotherapeutic agents such as busulfan and/or cyclophosphamide, infections such as adenovirus and BK virus, and thrombocytopenic coagulopathy.[20,22]

## LONG-TERM POST-HSCT COMPLICATIONS

The long-term effects of HSCT can be myriad and often present challenges that can significantly affect a patient's quality of life. Adolescents who have undergone HSCT can struggle with psychosocial issues such as learning disabilities, adjustment disorders, sexual and fertility difficulties, as well as growth and development impairment that can cause them to become more physically and emotionally dependent upon their parent/caregivers, interfering with the usual progression toward adulthood. Box 113-4 lists some of the long-term side effects of HSCT that can significantly affect quality of life.

For a complete list of recommended screening and preventive practices after HSCT, see the guidelines developed by a consensus panel formed by members of the CIBMTR, the European Group for Blood and Marrow Transplantation (EBMT), and the American Society for Blood and Marrow Transplantation (ASBMT).[23] The Children's Oncology Group (COG) has also developed *Long-term Follow-up Guidelines for Survivors of Childhood, Adolescent, and Young Adult Cancers* (www.survivorshipguidelines.org)[24] that is an excellent resource for primary care providers. These are risk-based, exposure-related guidelines that provide recommendations for direct follow-up care for children and young adults treated for cancer, including HSCT.

**Box 113-4**

***Potential Long-Term Complications of Hematopoietic Stem Cell Transplantation***

**Chronic graft-versus-host disease**
**Immunodeficiency**
**End-organ damage:** eye, lung, liver, bone
**Development of secondary malignancies**
**Endocrine disorders:** growth and development, gonadal dysfunction, infertility
**Neuropsychiatric functioning**
**Family and social support systems**

## QUALITY OF LIFE

A recent review of research published in the last 18 years relating to quality of life (QoL) and psychosocial sequela of pediatric patients undergoing HSCT identified older age at the time of HSCT, presence of long-term sequela, female gender, and the first 6-month period after HSCT as risk factors associated with poor QoL.[25] Although most children and adolescents experience mild to moderate psychological symptoms during the HSCT process, these adverse effects on QoL appear to be transient.[26] The studies reviewed indicated that QoL was already compromised pre-transplant and was further impaired following the conditioning regimen, but improved 4 to 12 months post-HSCT with QoL measures being comparable with, or better than, population norms at 6 months to 8 years post-HSCT.

Recently published research regarding cognitive, educational, psychosocial, and QoL outcomes of pediatric HSCT survivors compared to their siblings 2 years after transplantation found that, except for some deficits in educational outcomes and physical QoL measures, survivors' cognitive and psychological outcomes were similar to those of their siblings. Family and clinical factors were identified as critical for these outcomes.[27] The impact that pediatric HSCT has on later adult QoL was also studied in 98 disease-free survivors who were at least 18 years and 3 years post-transplant.[28] Results were compared to a control group of 58 healthy subjects of similar age. Transplant survivors, in comparison to controls, reported fewer problems regarding interpersonal relationships, sleep, depression, and leisure activities, and greater problems with physical appearance, school studies, and work possibilities.[28] Overall, the degree of family cohesion, parental adjustment, and availability of support systems appears to be among the most important variables predicting QoL outcomes. It is not clear whether interventions aimed at facilitating coping positively impact QoL, but such studies are ongoing.

## CHRONIC GVHD

*Chronic GVHD,* a significant cause of transplant-related morbidity and mortality, is an autoimmune disease similar in clinical presentation to systemic lupus erythematosus, but due to donor alloreactive T-cells reacting against antigens expressed on recipient cells.[29] The skin is the most common organ affected and can present as a lichenoid rash with pruritis, patchy erythema, scaling, and hyper- or hypopigmented papules. Some areas of cutaneous involvement can have hyperkeratotic papules and desquamation. If the disease progresses, the skin can become sclerodermatous and develop contractures. Contractures portend a more progressive and morbid disease course that is usually not reversible.[30]

Other organs that are commonly involved are the gastrointestinal tract (anorexia, diarrhea, malabsorption, cramping, and abdominal pain); respiratory tract (bronchiolitis obliterans); mucous membranes (*sicca* syndrome); liver (obstructive jaundice); eyes (ocular irritation and dryness); mouth (food sensitivity, decreased saliva production, dry and cracked lips); hair (brittle, alopecia, graying); musculoskeletal systems (fasciitis, myositis, weakness); immune system (impaired immunity due to GVHD and its treatment); and hematopoietic system (cytopenias, particularly thrombocytopenia).

The disease is classified by the degree of organ involvement as either *limited* (skin and/or liver involvement with little medical intervention necessary) or *extensive* (multiorgan system involvement). The IBMTR reported that the 3-year cumulative incidence of chronic GVHD was 15% among 2,052 pediatric patients receiving a sibling-matched HSCT. The incidence of chronic GVHD is much higher among those receiving a matched unrelated donor HSCT, with some studies reporting incidences more than 30%.[31] Factors associated with a higher incidence of chronic GVHD are patient age greater than 15 years, donor age greater than 5 years, female donor into a male recipient, use of TBI, malignant diagnosis as the indication for HSCT, and prior grade II–IV acute GVHD.[32]

Chronic GVHD is treated with immunosuppression, initially with prednisone and cyclosporine and progressing to alternative immunosuppressive regimens including thalidomide, tacrolimus, pentostatin, ECP, and oral psoralen with ultraviolet light (PUVA).[30]

## CARDIOVASCULAR COMPLICATIONS

Cardiovascular injury after HSCT can be both acute and chronic. Although cardiovascular injury can lead to significant morbidity, rarely is this injury the cause of death. Risk factors for the development of cardiac complications include the type and amount of anthracycline, radiation, and cyclophosphamide received. The injury usually manifests as congestive heart failure (shortness of breath, exercise intolerance, persistent cough, weight gain, and pulmonary edema), and increased risk of pulmonary infections. Other cardiovascular complications of HSCT include pericarditis, hypertension, and pericardial effusions.[23]

## IMMUNODEFICIENCY

Antigen-specific T- and B-cell responses are severely compromised early after HSCT and are gradually restored within the first year post-transplant. The adolescent who receives an HSCT is therefore left particularly vulnerable to viral and fungal infections. Factors that can negatively affect the recovery of the immune system include the presence of GVHD; immunosuppressive therapies necessary to treat GVHD; viral infections; lymphocyte depletion of the stem cell product; and the donor source and degree of HLA compatibility. *Pneumocystis carinii* infection prophylaxis with trimethaprim-sulfamethoxazole is given for at least the first 6 months post-transplant, longer if immune recovery is hampered. Several randomized control studies found that fluconazole prophylaxis until day +75 was effective in preventing invasive fungal infection.[33,34] Similarly, studies have shown that acyclovir was effective in preventing HSV infection and is recommended for the first 30 days post-transplant.[8]

Any adolescent with GVHD should remain on antifungal and antiviral prophylaxis, and it is recommended that antibacterial prophylaxis be initiated as well.[8] Revaccinations are started at one year post-HSCT as shown in Table 113-1. However, vaccination is not suggested for patients receiving immunosuppressive drugs and/or who have active, chronic GVHD.[8]

**ENDOCRINE**

Most childhood HSCT survivors are at risk of developing multiple endocrine complications including impaired linear and growth hormone deficiency, thyroid dysfunction, osteoporosis, and gonadal and reproductive dysfunction. The most common endocrine abnormalities are thyroid dysfunction, osteoporosis, and infertility.[6]

Several factors can impair growth in adolescents post-transplant, including growth hormone deficiency, hypothyroidism, corticosteroid use, and gonadal insufficiency. Growth hormone deficiency can develop after central nervous system (CNS) irradiation, including TBI.[35] The response to growth hormone can be dampened if there is underlying damage to bone epiphyses. Chronic corticosteroid use can also retard bone growth and result in an expected increase in height. Gonadal insufficiency can result in delayed puberty, impaired growth spurt, and shortened height. Adolescents who have delayed puberty after transplantation should be considered for sex hormone replacements, and those with growth hormone deficiency should be considered for synthetic growth hormone therapy.[36]

Depending on the specific risk, long-term post-HSCT care should include careful assessment of growth (particularly height) and development, thyroid studies and potentially thyroid replacement, periodic bone density studies, preventative measures including calcium and vitamin D supplements, smoking cessation, and weight-bearing exercises.[6]

The risk of permanent infertility after transplant depends on the specific conditioning regimen and type of HSCT (ablative versus nonablative).[36] Most adolescent HSCT survivors will have decreased fertility as adults. Females undergoing HSCT are at a high risk of ovarian failure.[37] There is a higher incidence of miscarriages among women who received TBI as part of their HSCT regimen due to radiation effects on the uterus.[38] Males are encouraged to store sperm prior to transplantation, but more strategies aimed at preventing infertility in both sexes are needed.

**SECOND MALIGNANCIES**

There are several factors that contribute to the long-term risk of developing second malignancies following HSCT. These include genetic predisposition, viruses (particularly EBV), the conditioning regimen, degree, and length of immunosuppression, and presence of chronic GVHD.[23] There are 3 general categories of second malignancies post-HSCT: *lymphoid malignancies* (B-cell post-transplant lymphoproliferative disease, T-cell lymphomas, and Hodgkin disease), *hematologic malignancies* (MDS/AML, leukemia recurrence in donor cells, new leukemia in host cells), and *solid tumors* (carcinomas, sarcomas, and CNS tumors).[23]

The risk of developing a post-transplant malignancy continues to increase even 20 years after transplant, with solid tumors developing at twice the rate expected based on that of the general population.[39] The risk reached threefold among patients followed for 15 years or more after transplantation. Most second solid cancers of the brain/CNS, thyroid, bone, and soft tissues occurred among patients younger than 17 years of age at transplantation.

In a study of 3,182 subjects specifically addressing second malignancies among children post-HSCT, 25 solid tumors and 20 post-transplant lymphoproliferative disorders (PTLDs) were observed, 45-fold higher than expected.[40] Cumulative risk of solid cancers increased to 11% at 15 years and was highest among children at ages younger than 5 years at the time of HSCT.[40]

Together, these data indicate that allogeneic transplant survivors, particularly those treated as children, have an increased risk of solid cancers and should have lifelong surveillance screening for the development of second malignancies.

## SUMMARY

Hematopoietic stem cell transplantation is an effective, potentially life-saving procedure for adolescents who have a variety of malignant and nonmalignant conditions. As scientific advances have decreased morbidity and mortality, and new indications for its use continue to emerge, primary health care providers of adolescents and young adults can expect to be faced with the challenges of caring for patients who have had a transplant, either as an adolescent or as a child. This chapter has addressed key issues that will help a primary or specialty care provider deliver health care services to these complex cases, as well as to understand the issues related to HSCT faced by affected adolescents and their families. Being aware of the indications, processes, and the acute and chronic complications of HSCT will enable health care providers to continue to work with their patients during and after transplantation.

## INTERNET RESOURCES

For professionals to obtain up-to-date information regarding HSCT

- NMDP Web site (www.marrow.org)
- CIBMTR Web site (www.cibmtr.org)
- Children's Oncology Group (www.survivorshipguidelines.org)

For adolescents and families

- National Marrow Donor Program (www.marrow.org/PATIENT/When_Child_Needs_Tx/Preparing_for_Your_Childs_Tran/Supporting_Your_Teenager_throu/index.html)
- Melissa's Living Legacy (www.teenslivingwithcancer.org/)
- 2beme (www.2bme.org/2bMe.html)

## REFERENCES


1. Pasquini M, Wang Z, and Schneider L. Summary slides of the CIBMTR. 2007. Available at: www.cibmtr.org/ReferenceCenter/SlidesReports/SummarySlides/index.html June 22, 2010

2. Kline RM. *Pediatric Hematopoietic Stem Cell Transplantation*. New York, NY: Informa Healthcare USA, Inc; 2006

3. Bishop MR. Hematopoietic Stem Cell Transplantation. New York, NY: Springer Science+Business Media, LLC; 2009

4. Jacobsohn DA. Acute graft-versus-host disease in children. *Bone Marrow Transplant.* 2008;41:215–221

5. Ferrara JL, Reddy P. Pathophysiology of graft-versus-host disease. *Semin Hematol.* 2006;43:3–10

6. Dahllof G, Hingorani SR, Sanders JE. Late effects following hematopoietic cell transplantation for children. *Biol Blood Marrow Transplant.* 2008;14:88–93

7. Afessa B, Peters SG. Major complications following hematopoietic stem cell transplantation. *Semin Respir Crit Care Med.* 2006;27:297–309

8. Guidelines for preventing opportunistic infections among hematopoietic stem cell transplant recipients. *MMWR Recomm Rep.* 2000;49 (RR-10):1–147

9. Keates-Baleeiro J, Moore P, Koyama T, et al. Incidence and outcome of idiopathic pneumonia syndrome in pediatric stem cell transplant recipients. *Bone Marrow Transplant.* 2006;38:285–289

10. Zhu KE, Hu JY, Zhang T, et al. Incidence, risks, and outcome of idiopathic pneumonia syndrome early after allogeneic hematopoietic stem cell transplantation. *Eur J Haematol.* 2008;81:461–466

11. Yanik GA, Ho VT, Levine JE, et al. The impact of soluble tumor necrosis factor receptor etanercept on the treatment of idiopathic pneumonia syndrome after allogeneic hematopoietic stem cell transplantation. *Blood.* 2008;112:3073–3081

12. Miano M, Faraci M, Dini G, Bordigoni P. Early complications following haematopoietic SCT in children. *Bone Marrow Transplant.* 2008;41(suppl 2):S39–S42

13. Behre G, Theurich S, Christopeit M, Weber T. Successful treatment of severe sinusoidal obstruction syndrome despite multiple organ failure with defibrotide after allogeneic stem cell transplantation: a case report. *J Med Case Reports.* 2009;3:69

14. Morabito F, Gentile M, Gay F, et al. Insights into defibrotide: an updated review. *Expert Opin Biol Ther.* 2009;9:763–772

15. Murphy BA. Clinical and economic consequences of mucositis induced by chemotherapy and/or radiation therapy. *J Support Oncol.* 2007;5:13–21

16. Vera-Llonch M, Oster G, Ford CM, Lu J, Sonis S. Oral mucositis and outcomes of allogeneic hematopoietic stem-cell transplantation in patients with hematologic malignancies. *Support Care Cancer.* 2007;15:491–496

17. Stiff P. Mucositis associated with stem cell transplantation: current status and innovative approaches to management. *Bone Marrow Transplant.* 2001(27 suppl 2):S3–S11

18. Mori T, Hasegawa K, Okabe A, et al. Efficacy of mouth rinse in preventing oral mucositis in patients receiving high-dose cytarabine for allogeneic hematopoietic stem cell transplantation. *Int J Hematol.* 2008;88:583–587

19. Rzepecki P, Sarosiek T, Barzal J, et al. Palifermin for prevention of oral mucositis after haematopoietic stem cell transplantation- single centre experience. *J Buon.* 2007;12:477–482

20. Decker DB, Karam JA, Wilcox DT. Pediatric hemorrhagic cystitis. *J Pediatr Urol.* 2009;5:254–264

21. Cheuk DK, Lee TL, Chiang AK, et al. Risk factors and treatment of hemorrhagic cystitis in children who underwent hematopoietic stem cell transplantation. *Transpl Int.* 2007;20:73–81

22. Gorczynska E, Turkiewicz D, Rybka K, et al. Incidence, clinical outcome, and management of virus-induced hemorrhagic cystitis in children and adolescents after allogeneic hematopoietic cell transplantation. *Biol Blood Marrow Transplant.* 2005;11:797–804

23. Rizzo JD, Wingard JR, Tichelli A, et al. Recommended screening and preventive practices for long-term survivors after hematopoietic cell transplantation: joint recommendations of the European Group for Blood and Marrow

Transplantation, the Center for International Blood and Marrow Transplant Research, and the American Society of Blood and Marrow Transplantation. *Biol Blood Marrow Transplant.* 2006;12:138-151

24. Landier W, Bhatia S, Eshelman DA, et al. Development of risk-based guidelines for pediatric cancer survivors: the Children's Oncology Group Long-Term Follow-Up Guidelines from the Children's Oncology Group Late Effects Committee and Nursing Discipline. *J Clin Oncol.* 2004;22:4979-4990

25. Tremolada M, Bonichini S, Pillon M, Messina C, Carli M. Quality of life and psychosocial sequelae in children undergoing hematopoietic stem-cell transplantation: a review. *Pediatr Transplant.* (epub ahead of print) 2009

26. McConville BJ, Steichen-Asch P, Harris R, et al. Pediatric bone marrow transplants: psychological aspects. *Can J Psychiatry.* 1990;35:769-775

27. Barrera M, Atenafu E. Cognitive, educational, psychosocial adjustment and quality of life of children who survive hematopoietic SCT and their siblings. *Bone Marrow Transplant.* 2008;42:15-21

28. Badell I, Igual L, Gomez P, et al. Quality of life in young adults having received a BMT during childhood: a GETMON study. Grupo Espanol de Trasplante de Medula Osea en el Nino. *Bone Marrow Transplant.* 1998;21(suppl 2):S68-S71

29. Tyndall A, Dazzi F. Chronic GVHD as an autoimmune disease. *Best Pract Res Clin Haematol.* 2008;21:281-289

30. Joseph RW, Couriel DR, Komanduri KV. Chronic graft-versus-host disease after allogeneic stem cell transplantation: challenges in prevention, science, and supportive care. *J Support Oncol.* 2008;6:361-372

31. Woolfrey AE, Anasetti C, Storer B, et al. Factors associated with outcome after unrelated marrow transplantation for treatment of acute lymphoblastic leukemia in children. *Blood.* 2002;99:2002-2008

32. Zecca M, Prete A, Rondelli R, et al. Chronic graft-versus-host disease in children: incidence, risk factors, and impact on outcome. *Blood.* 2002;100:1192-1200

33. Slavin MA, Osborne B, Adams R, et al. Efficacy and safety of fluconazole prophylaxis for fungal infections after marrow transplantation—a prospective, randomized, double-blind study. *J Infect Dis.* 1995;171:1545-1552

34. Goodman JL, Winston DJ, Greenfield RA, et al. A controlled trial of fluconazole to prevent fungal infections in patients undergoing bone marrow transplantation. *N Engl J Med.* 1992;326:845-851

35. Leahey AM, Teunissen H, Friedman DL, et al. Late effects of chemotherapy compared to bone marrow transplantation in the treatment of pediatric acute myeloid leukemia and myelodysplasia. *Med Pediatr Oncol.* 1999;32:163-169

36. Sanders JE. Endocrine complications of high-dose therapy with stem cell transplantation. *Pediatr Transplant.* 2004;8(suppl 5):39-50

37. Sanders JE, Buckner CD, Amos D, et al. Ovarian function following marrow transplantation for aplastic anemia or leukemia. *J Clin Oncol.* 1988;6:813-818

38. Sanders JE, Hawley J, Levy W, et al. Pregnancies following high-dose cyclophosphamide with or without high-dose busulfan or total-body irradiation and bone marrow transplantation. *Blood.* 1996;87:3045-3052

39. Rizzo JD, Curtis RE, Socie G, et al. Solid cancers after allogeneic hematopoietic cell transplantation. *Blood.* 2009;113:1175-1183

40. Socie G, Curtis RE, Deeg HJ, et al. New malignant diseases after allogeneic marrow transplantation for childhood acute leukemia. *J Clin Oncol.* 2000;18:348-357

# CHAPTER 114

# Cancer Survival Issues

JACQUELINE CASILLAS, MD, MSHS • LONNIE ZELTZER, MD

## EPIDEMIOLOGY AND DEFINITIONS

Treatment of children and adolescents with cancer is one of the major success stories in pediatrics for the 21st century. The estimated survival rate for the more than 12,000 children and adolescents diagnosed with cancer each year in the United States is now nearing 80%.[1] This translates into a prevalence of more than 300,000 childhood cancer survivors in the United States.[2] As a result of these growing numbers, more and more adolescent cancer survivors are entering general pediatric and adolescent medicine practices. It is therefore imperative for the practitioner caring for the adolescent cancer survivor to recognize that this group of patients is at risk for late effects as a result of their previous cancer therapy. A late effect is a late-occurring or chronic outcome, physical or psychosocial, which persists or develops beyond 5 years from diagnosis of cancer.[3] More than two-thirds of childhood cancer survivors develop a significant late effect, and 25% develop a life-threatening late effect.[4,5] Given these sobering statistics, the purpose of this chapter is to describe the physical and psychosocial late effects the adolescent cancer survivor may develop and thereby emphasize the importance for ongoing surveillance of this at-risk population so that future morbidity and mortality can be minimized.

## SURVEILLANCE FOR LATE EFFECTS AS A RESULT OF PREVIOUS CANCER THERAPY

Although childhood and adolescent cancer survivors comprise only 3% of the 10.7 million cancer survivors currently alive in the United States, the pediatric oncology discipline has been a leader in the field of survivorship care. Pediatric oncologists have set standards on how to define the risks that patients face as a result of their previous cancer therapy exposures through a cooperative group model. More specifically, the Children's Oncology Group (COG) has developed evidence-based guidelines to assist health care providers in providing targeted screening for physical and psychosocial late effects as a result of previous chemotherapeutic, radiation, or surgical exposures.[6] These guidelines are available online at www.survivorshipguidelines.org and are accompanied by health education materials, entitled "Health Links," so that the physician and/or patient has a "toolkit" to determine necessary long-term follow-up care. In the following sections, various physical and psychosocial late effects that may be observed in the adolescent population will be discussed in more detail.

## ORGAN SYSTEM LATE EFFECTS FROM CHEMOTHERAPY AND RADIATION

### CARDIAC

There are 2 important therapeutic risk factors for the development of cardiovascular late effects in adolescent survivors. The first important association is the risk for irreversible cardiomyopathy and congestive heart failure associated with exposure to anthracycline chemotherapeutics, including doxorubicin and daunorubicin. A high cumulative dose and concomitant exposure to radiation therapy place adolescents at greatest risk. Unfortunately, there are no studies published to date that demonstrate effective medications, such as angiotensin-converting enzyme inhibitors, to prevent long-term cardiac deterioration for childhood cancer survivors.[7] The need for monitoring of cardiac function through regularly scheduled echocardiograms therefore cannot be overemphasized.

Exposure to mediastinal radiotherapy, with or without anthracycline exposure, also places the adolescent cancer survivor at risk for cardiovascular disease. These late effects include cardiomyopathy, pericarditis, pericardial thickening, valvular heart disease, and increased risk for coronary artery disease and myocardial infarction at a young age. Recent studies demonstrate the use of cardiac stress testing to identify asymptomatic survivors at high risk for acute myocardial infarction or sudden cardiac death.[8]

Most recently, it has been found that cancer survivors are at increased risk of developing components of the metabolic syndrome (obesity, dyslipidemia, insulin resistance, hypertension). The etiology of this association is not yet known.

## ENDOCRINE

One of the most common late effects among childhood cancer survivors is the development of an endocrinopathy. There are several important therapeutic exposures that result in increased risk. Central nervous system (CNS) radiation can cause pituitary dysfunction, including deficiencies in growth hormone (GH), thyroid-stimulating hormone (TSH), luteinizing hormone (LH), follicle-stimulating hormone (FSH), gonadotropin-releasing hormone (GnRH), and corticotropin-releasing hormone (CRH). GH deficiency can result in a reduction of adult height for the adolescent survivor. Even if a survivor is not affected by short stature, GH deficiency can cause other significant chronic health problems. It has been shown in acute lymphoblastic leukemia (ALL) survivors, for instance, that those with GH deficiency have a greater risk for adverse cardiovascular events and higher diabetes risk profiles, and thus significant long-term morbidities.[9] Radiation therapy to the CNS or neck can result in hypothyroidism, which may be clinical or subclinical, and thus may only be detected by an elevation in the TSH.

Pituitary insufficiency can also result in the previously mentioned sex hormone deficiencies and, in turn, result in secondary amenorrhea or premature menopause for the adolescent female. Depending on the tumor type and associated treatment regimen, such as pelvic sarcomas requiring infradiaphragmatic radiation, both females and males may be at risk for direct gonadal damage and resultant infertility. In addition, male adolescent survivors treated for tumors in the hypothalamic–pituitary region with high-dose (24 Gy) cranial radiotherapy, as was previously used in the treatment protocols of ALL before the age of 10 years, are at risk for impaired fertility.[10,11] Furthermore, males exposed to high cumulative doses of alkylating agents, for example cyclophosphamide, are also at risk for azoospermia and infertility.[11] Given these risks for altered sex hormone production and/or spermatogenesis, it is important for the clinician to complete a careful genitourinary (GU) examination because small testicular volume may be the first clinical clue that a male adolescent is at risk for oligo- or azoospermia, which could impact future fertility status.

## GENITOURINARY

In addition to the risk for impaired fertility due to direct gonadal injury, pelvic radiation can also result in injury to the GU tract. Pelvic radiation can result in bladder fibrosis causing the bladder to become smaller in size, thus having a smaller capacity and an increased risk for recurrent urinary tract infections. Chemotherapeutic agents also place the adolescent survivor at risk for long-term GU damage. Cyclophosphamide and ifosphamide, for example, can result in hemorrhagic cystitis during chemotherapy, which can persist for months after the completion of therapy. This is particularly distressing for the adolescent male because of the often resultant urgency and pain associated with the cystitis. Ifosphamide and other nephrotoxic chemotherapeutic agents, such as cisplatin, can cause direct tubular damage and long-term electrolyte wasting of potassium, phosphorus, and magnesium. For some survivors, the electrolyte wasting may improve over time, but for others it may result in the need for long-term oral electrolyte replacement therapy. Direct glomerular damage may also occur from chemotherapy exposure, resulting in marginal renal function and placing the adolescent survivor at risk for progressive to irreversible renal failure, particularly if exposed to ongoing nephrotoxic medications, such as antibiotics.

## PULMONARY

Survivors of childhood cancer are at risk for pulmonary late effects due to chemotherapeutic agents and/or radiotherapy involving the lung fields. Bleomycin and BCNU (Carmustine), for example, place adolescent survivors at risk for pulmonary fibrosis. Similarly, radiotherapy involving the lung fields can cause paramediastinal fibrosis and interstitial fibrosis. Consequently, the adolescent survivor exposed to pulmonary toxic chemotherapy and/or pulmonary radiation who reports complaints of fatigue, decreased exercise tolerance, or inability to keep pace with peers in athletic activities should be immediately screened with pulmonary function tests to determine if there is a diffusion abnormality. Conversely, a survivor may be asymptomatic and not have respiratory complaints but may still have pulmonary sequelae from previous chemotherapy or radiation. The health care provider who obtains a history of pulmonary toxic exposure needs to complete pulmonary function testing at least once to document that there is no evidence of occult pulmonary fibrosis. A recent Medline database review to determine factors resulting in aeromedical concern for adolescent and young adults pursuing military flying careers reported a ninefold increased risk of late-occurring pulmonary fibrosis and lung cancer, with an increasing prevalence as long as 25 years following the cancer diagnosis.[12] Given this long-term risk of pulmonary disease, coupled with the association of smoking and lung cancer, targeted health education on the importance of avoidance of tobacco exposure is particularly important in providing anticipatory guidance to the adolescent cancer survivor.

## MUSCULOSKELETAL

There are various musculoskeletal late effects that adolescent cancer survivors face. These include scoliosis due to radiation exposure to the spine at a young age, phantom limb pain or pain related to poorly fitting prostheses for amputees, osteopenia or osteoporosis due to steroid and/or methotrexate exposure, avascular necrosis from steroid exposure, and peripheral neuropathy from vincristine exposure. The clinician performing sports physicals for the adolescent survivor needs to be aware of these risks so that appropriate and timely counseling and referrals can be made. For example, an adolescent complaining of inability to keep up in physical education due to increased falling when running with the group may have mild but persistent peripheral neuropathy from vincristine exposure. The adolescent may gain some improvements in strength and dexterity if referred for physical therapy. The adolescent amputee also faces challenges with properly fitting prostheses due to bony overgrowth at the stump. Appropriate referrals and advocacy for the survivor must be made by the clinician. For example, the clinician may need to advocate for insurance coverage of multiple replacement prostheses until the adolescent finally obtains a usable prosthesis that fits properly or the clinician may need to provide a doctor's note for the school administration to allow the adolescent survivor to leave classes early to allow for additional time required to walk to the next class.

### GASTROINTESTINAL

A particularly challenging late effect is the development of infectious hepatitis, such as hepatitis C, for those survivors transfused with blood products prior to July 1992, when screening was initiated.[13] The development of secondary chronic disease is particularly challenging for the teen who has undergone intensive cancer treatment at a young age and now requires ongoing, frequent evaluation by subspecialists for chronic liver disease. Counseling on safe sex practices is also another important anticipatory guidance topic, particularly for those who carry the risk of passage of infectious hepatitis.

## LATE EFFECTS ASSOCIATED WITH SURGICAL THERAPY FOR A MALIGNANCY

Hodgkin disease (HD) is a malignancy that more commonly occurs in the adolescent age group and, although it is not a disease cured by surgical intervention, it is important to recognize that surgical staging (including splenectomy) was performed in earlier treatment protocols when imaging techniques were not as sophisticated. As a result, there is a cohort of HD survivors that are asplenic and, as a result, are at risk for serious bacterial infections that can be life-threatening.[14] Providers must recognize that, similar to patients with sickle cell disease, asplenic survivors must be educated on the need to seek medical attention immediately if they have a fever so that antibiotics can be initiated promptly. In addition, clinicians must also recognize the risk for adhesions and intestinal obstruction for any adolescent survivor who has undergone abdominal surgery, either for staging or resection of the cancer.

Bone cancers, including the Ewing sarcoma family of tumors (ESFTs) and osteosarcoma (OS), are another group of malignancies that more commonly occur in the adolescent age group. Amputation and surgical resections, completed for surgical management of these diseases, can result in late effects, including cosmetic deformities and functional abnormalities. There can be functional problems associated with surgical amputations for the adolescent survivor because this is a period in which there is rapid bone growth. Prostheses can be problematic because of bony overgrowth occurring at the distal end of the surgical stump; this may result in repeated surgeries for correction of the problem. Adolescents can also be affected by chronic pain in the surgical stump or in the lower extremity, even after amputation, due to phantom limb pain, a type of pain that is a challenge to ameliorate.

Pelvic surgery with lymph node dissection, such as that which is done for germ cell tumors, can result in injury to the autonomic nervous system and impact fertility secondary to retrograde ejaculation for male adolescents. Counseling regarding fertility treatment options should be referred to urologists aware of these late effects and sensitive to the needs of adolescents with a history of cancer. There are also nonprofit organizations that can assist survivors with fertility questions and concerns by providing written educational materials, assistance in finding experienced providers, and financial assistance (eg, www.fertilehope.org).

## SECONDARY MALIGNANT NEOPLASMS

Arguably the most devastating late effect that an adolescent cancer survivor faces is the risk of developing a second malignant neoplasm (SMN) as a result of previous cancer therapy. Childhood cancer survivors have been shown to have an eightfold increased risk of death compared to age-matched controls when evaluating late mortality outcomes.[15] Using the largest national cohort of childhood cancer survivors, the Childhood Cancer Survivor Study (CCSS), Mertens found that recurrence of the primary cancer was the leading cause of death, constituting 57% of the total deaths. However, there was also a significant excess mortality rate due to subsequent malignancies. Well-known risk factors for the development of SMN include use of mantle radiation for the treatment of HD and the subsequent risk of breast cancer; use of radiotherapy and the development of skin cancer or other solid tumors in the field of radiation; and use of epipodophyllotoxins (eg, etoposide) and the development of secondary leukemias.[16,17] A recent CCSS study found additional risk factors for the development of secondary sarcomas in addition to radiation exposure to include the primary diagnosis of sarcoma, a history of other secondary neoplasms, and treatment with higher doses of anthracyclines or alkylating agents.[18]

Given this risk for excess morbidity and mortality from SMNs, the CCSS examined the self-reported cancer screening practices of more than 9,000 childhood cancer survivors and found that they were below optimal levels.[19] Thus, it is critical for the clinician to provide cancer screening, as well as education on the risk for development of future cancers, to the adolescent cancer survivor. Adolescent cancer survivors also require education on the importance of cancer prevention, such as sunscreen use, eating a diet rich in fruits and vegetables, and participation in regular exercise as integral components in maintaining a healthy lifestyle aimed at prevention of future disease. The adult survivorship community has embraced the term "teachable moment" as a result of the cancer experience that focuses on the opportunity to promote long-term health after the diagnosis of cancer.[20] The opportunity to maximize the messages of health and well-being during a "teachable moment" is also present for the clinician caring for the adolescent cancer survivor.

## NEUROCOGNITIVE LATE EFFECTS

An important lesson learned early on by pediatric oncologists regarding the late effects of cancer treatment includes the finding of the development of neurocognitive deficits associated with the use of cranial radiotherapy, particularly in children exposed prior to 3 years of age. The long-term effects can be particularly devastating for brain tumor survivors who received high doses of cranial radiation therapy as children.[21] Another risk factor for the development of neurocognitive deficits is exposure to intrathecal chemotherapy, such as methotrexate. For some adolescent survivors who have mild neurocognitive late effects, the transition from elementary school to middle and high school is when the deficits become apparent, given the higher-order functioning and multitasking that is required in higher grades. It may not be apparent to the survivor, parent, or teacher that disinterest in school or inattention to coursework may be a neurocognitive effect of cancer treatment. Therefore, it is imperative to discuss school performance during routine outpatient follow-up visits and to recognize the possible need for neuropsychological evaluation to identify cognitive deficits. Not all schools and teachers are familiar with the risks of childhood cancer treatment, so it is important for parents to advocate for their teen, for example, by requesting an Individual Education Plan should academic difficulties emerge, so that appropriate support can be provided.

## PSYCHOSOCIAL LATE EFFECTS

The scientific literature suggests that, in general, childhood cancer survivors are experiencing good psychological health years after completion of their cancer treatment. However, there have been studies suggesting that there are high-risk groups for the development of impaired mental health; one of these groups is adolescent survivors. There have also been studies that report negative psychosocial outcomes in certain populations of childhood cancer survivors. Hudson et al[22] analyzed data from the 9,535 adult survivors in the CCSS cohort compared with a randomly selected cohort of the survivors' siblings (N = 2,916). When compared with siblings, survivors in this study were significantly more likely to report adverse general health, and moderate to severe impairment in mental health, across all diagnostic groups. In this study, they found 3 diagnostic groups (survivors of HD, sarcomas, and other bone tumors) that were found to be at increased risk for continued cancer-related anxiety, and the authors specifically noted that these are 3 diagnoses that are more common in the adolescent age group.[1,2,6] They suggest that, because adolescence is the developmental period during which abstract thinking develops, adolescents diagnosed with cancer may have a better understanding of the meaning of their diagnosis and the risks of treatment, one potential reason for the findings of more severe mental health impairment compared to other groups. Similarly, studies evaluating the social impact of the cancer experience have found that there are also specific high-risk groups. These groups include those survivors who have functional (but not cosmetic) impairments, a factor that appears to increase the risk for academic and adjustment problems. Other risk factors for social and emotional problems include: older age at assessment (correlated with time since diagnosis and time since completion of therapy), history of cranial irradiation, and living in a single-parent household.[23] Given that the adolescent period is one in which peer support is critical for socialization and that childhood cancer is a rare event, it is not surprising that survivors who may be experiencing negative psychosocial sequelae may benefit from targeted psychosocial support interventions.

The brain tumor survivor population deserves special attention because it is a high-risk group for the development of diminished social functioning. Zebrack et al[24] evaluated the psychological outcomes in the brain tumor cohort (n = 1,100) within the CCSS and found that although the prevalence of psychological distress at 11% was clinically significant, no specific diagnoses or treatment-related variables were associated with distress. Instead, they found that distress was associated with diminished social functioning, which may be related to the specific diagnosis or treatment. Because there is such a great social impact on an impaired brain tumor survivor, there have been several parent-initiated, community-based organizations that provide social support for teens impacted by their brain tumor treatment, as well as for the family members who share in their experience.

## SYSTEMATIC ONGOING FOLLOW-UP OF THE ADOLESCENT CANCER SURVIVOR

It is an exciting time in the field of pediatric oncology because cure rates are reaching an all-time high and adolescent cancer survivors are increasing in such great numbers that it can now be considered an "epidemic of survivorship." It is crucial for providers caring for this population to (1) recognize the significant risk for late effects, (2) provide targeted screening for late effects of asymptomatic survivors, and (3) provide wellness counseling that will encourage healthy lifestyles and minimize future risk for the development of disease. The provider should not feel overwhelmed when evaluating the adolescent cancer survivor because there are guidelines developed by the COG at www.survivorshipguidelines.org that provide detailed recommendations on how to care for the adolescent survivor based on previous therapeutic exposure.

The first step in providing systematic, ongoing follow-up is to obtain an oncology treatment summary from the treating institution (and to not rely on parent or patient report alone). The childhood cancer experience is unique in that some adolescent survivors, given their young age at diagnosis, may not remember their cancer experience, including the specific diagnosis and the treatments that were received. After the cancer treatment summary is known, the clinician can develop a survivorship care plan using the COG guidelines. For example, one may develop a table that lists treatment exposures, associated physical late effects, and recommendations for screening (Table 114-1). Conversely, if the clinician prefers to have the adolescent survivor seen and evaluated by a late effects specialist, there are multidisciplinary, long-term follow-up programs for childhood cancer survivors across the United States to which referrals can be made to receive assistance with developing a survivorship care plan. Whether the survivorship care plan is developed by a late effects specialist or an adolescent medicine clinician, ultimately ongoing communication between the adolescent and the health care provider regarding the adolescent's risks and the need for annual screening for late effects is the cornerstone for high-quality care for this at-risk patient population.

**Table 114-1**

**Selected Physical Late Effects and Screening Recommendations**

| *Therapeutic Exposure* | *Physical Late Effect* | *Examples of Recommended Screening* |
|---|---|---|
| Anthracycline antibiotic (eg, doxorubicin) | Cardiomyopathy | Echocardiogram and electrocardiogram |
| Epipodophyllotoxins (eg, etoposide) or alkylating agents (eg, cyclophosphamide) | Second malignant neoplasm (eg, acute myelogenous leukemia [AML]) | Annual history and physical examination and complete blood count |
| Antitumor antibiotic (bleomycin) or alkylating agent (busulfan) | Pulmonary fibrosis | Pulmonary function tests |
| Heavy metal (cisplatin) | Ototoxicity/hearing loss | Brainstem auditory evoked response (BAER) or audiogram |
| Cranial/spinal irradiation | Endocrine dysfunction | Monitoring of height/weight/BMI, free $T_4$, TSH, LH, FSH, estradiol, testosterone |

## REFERENCES


1. Reis LAG, Eisner MP, Kosary CL, et al. *SEER Cancer Statistics Review, 1973-1998*. Bethesda, MD: National Cancer Institute; 2001

2. Hewitt M, Weiner SL, Simone JV. *Childhood Cancer Survivorship:Improving Care and Quality of Life*. Washington, DC:The National Academies Press; 2003

3. Bhatia S, Landier W, Casillas J, Zeltzer LK. Medical and psychosocial issues in childhood cancer survivors. In: Chang AE, Ganz PA, Hayes DF, et al, eds. *Oncology:An Evidence-Based Approach*. New York, NY: Springer Science+Business Media; 2006

4. Sklar CA. An overview of the effects of cancer therapies: the nature, scale, and breadth of the problem. *Acta Paediatr Scan Suppl.* 1999;433:1-4

5. Mertens AC. Cause-specific late mortality among 5-year survivors of childhood cancer: the Childhood Cancer Survivor Study. *J Natl Cancer Inst.* 2008;100(19):1368-1379

6. Landier W, Bhatia S, Eshelman DA, et al. Development of risk-based guidelines for pediatric cancer survivors: the Children's Oncology Group Long-Term Follow-Up Guidelines from the Children's Oncology Group Late Effects Committee and Nursing Discipline. *J Clin Oncol.* 2004;22(24):4979-4990

7. Lipshultz SE. Exposure to anthracyclines during childhood causes cardiac injury. *Semin Oncol.* 2006;33(3 Suppl 8):S8-S14; Review

8. Heidenreich PA, Schnittger I, Strauss HW, et al. Screening for coronary artery disease after mediastinal irradiation for Hodgkin's disease. *J Clin Oncol.* 2007;25(1):43-49

9. Gurney JG, Ness KK, Sibley SD, et al. Metabolic syndrome and growth hormone deficiency in adult survivors of childhood acute lymphoblastic leukemia. *Cancer.* 2006;107(6): 1303-1312

10. Byrne J, Fears TR, Mills JL, et al. Fertility of long-term male survivors of acute lymphoblastic leukemia diagnosed during childhood. *Pediatr Blood Cancer.* 2004;42(4):364-372

11. Lopez Andreu JA, Fernandez PJ, Ferris I, et al. Persistent altered spermatogenesis in long-term childhood cancer survivors. *Pediatr Hematol Oncol.* 2000;17(1):21-30

12. Landau DA, Azaria B, Fineman R, Barenboim E, Goldstein L. Long-term survivors of childhood malignancies-aeromedical dilemmas and implications. *Aviat Space Environ Med.* 2006;77(12):1266-1270

13. Castellino S, Lensing S, Riely C, et al. The epidemiology of chronic hepatitis C infection in survivors of childhood cancer: an update of the St Jude Children's Research Hospital hepatitis C seropositive cohort. *Blood.* 2004;103(7):2460-2466

14. Marina N. Long-term survivors of childhood cancer. *Pediatr Clin North Am.* 1997;44(4):1021-1042

15. Mertens AC. Cause of mortality in 5-year survivors of childhood cancer. *Pediatr Blood Cancer.* 2007 Jan 16 [Epub ahead of print]

16. Taylor AJ, Winter DL, Stiller CA, Murphy M, Hawkins MM. Risk of breast cancer in female survivors of childhood Hodgkin's disease in Britain: a population-based study. *Int J Cancer.* 2007;120(2):384-391

17. Neglia JP, Friedman DL, Yasui Y, et al. Second malignant neoplasms in five-year survivors of childhood cancer: childhood cancer survivor study. *J Natl Cancer Inst.* 2001;93(8):618-629

18. Henderson TO, Whitton J, Stovall M, et al. Secondary sarcomas in childhood cancer survivors: a report from the Childhood Cancer Survivor Study. *J Natl Cancer Inst.* 2007;99(4): 300-308

19. Yeazel MW, Oeffinger KC, Gurney JG, et al. The cancer screening practices of adult survivors of childhood cancer: a report from the Childhood Cancer Survivor Study. *Cancer.* 2004;100(3):631-640

20. Demark-Wahnefried W, Aziz NM, Rowland JH, Pinto BM. Riding the crest of the teachable moment: promoting long-term health after the diagnosis of cancer. *J Clin Oncol.* 2005;23(24):5814-5830

21. Anderson DM, Rennie KM, Ziegler RS, et al. Medical and neurocognitive late effects among survivors of childhood central nervous system tumors. *Cancer.* 2001;92:2709-2719

22. Hudson MM, Mertens AC, Yasui Y, et al. Health status of adult long-term survivors of childhood cancer. A report from the childhood cancer survivor study. *JAMA.* 2003;290

23. Mulhern R, Wasserman A, Friedman A, et al. Social competence and behavioral adjustment of children who are long-term survivors of cancer. *Pediatrics.* 1989;83:18-25

24. Zebrack BJ, Gurney JG, Oeffinger K, et al. Psychological outcomes in long-term survivors of childhood brain cancer: a report from the childhood cancer survivor study. *J Clin Oncol.* 2004;22(6):999-1006

SECTION 7

# The Urinary System

# CHAPTER 115

## Proteinuria and Hematuria

HOWARD E. COREY, MD

The clinician caring for the adolescent will at some point encounter a child with hematuria and/or proteinuria. Isolated hematuria may be difficult to diagnose, but it often carries a good prognosis. On the other hand, nonorthostatic proteinuria may be easier to diagnose, but it may be associated paradoxically with a worse outcome. There may be important age-related differences in the differential diagnosis, approach to investigation, and treatment plan of adolescents with suspected genitourinary or renal disease. Special considerations in the adolescent age group include risk behaviors (eg, use of alcohol, licit and illicit drugs, oral contraceptives, sexual activity), lifestyle issues (eg, diet, athletic participation), and adherence. These considerations argue against a "one-size-fits-all" approach to adolescents with renal disease.

### HEMATURIA

Urine with an abnormal color or appearance occurs commonly in adolescents. The differential diagnosis includes hematuria (defined as >5 red blood cells per high-power microscopic field), myoglobinuria, discolored urine due to various medications and food additives, menses, and hematospermia. In the adolescent, myoglobinuria may occur secondary to infections (eg, influenza), trauma, or drug injection (eg, opiates, Ecstasy).

Urine test reagent strips ("dipsticks"), based on the peroxidase activity of heme pigment, do not discriminate among these possibilities. Therefore, microscopic examination of the urine is the first, key step in the diagnosis.

#### PREVALENCE

In children, the prevalence of gross hematuria (visible blood in the urine), microscopic hematuria, and hematuria combined with proteinuria is estimated to be 0.15%, 1.5%, and 0.06%, respectively. Over and above the actual prevalence, hematuria in the adolescent may provoke a great deal of anxiety and concern. Because the differential diagnosis of hematuria is vast, at least some evaluation is always warranted.

Hematuria may be a solitary finding or a manifestation of a systemic disease, painless or distressful, isolated or associated with proteinuria, transient or persistent, trivial or a marker of serious illness. The urine may be yellow, tea-colored, or bright red in appearance, and may form clots or appear to be clot-free. Unraveling these possibilities always requires a disciplined approach to the differential diagnosis.

For example, the finding of microscopic hematuria in an asymptomatic adolescent without gross hematuria, proteinuria, systemic illness, hypertension, or family history of renal disease should not be a cause of great concern. On the other hand, gross hematuria (or hematuria combined with proteinuria) may indicate significant disease, and a thorough evaluation is always warranted.

#### CAUSE

Most cases of gross hematuria in children are due to genitourinary (nonglomerular) disease, most commonly viral or bacterial cystitis. Other common causes of nonglomerular hematuria include urolithiasis (renal calculi), genitourinary malformation (eg, hydronephrosis), hypercalciuria, urethritis, and trauma. Glomerular diseases that may present in the adolescent age group include

IgA nephropathy (Berger disease), Alport syndrome (AS; hereditary nephritis), and membranoproliferative glomerulonephritis (MPGN).

Of 342 children (including 122 adolescents) who presented with gross hematuria over a 10-year period, Greenfield et al[1] described 45 cases of 1 or more urogenital anomalies (including vesicoureteral reflux, ureteropelvic junction obstruction, and posterior urethral valves) and 18 cases of urolithiasis. Of the 272 males, 52 had benign urethrorrhagia (benign urethritis).

In a general pediatric emergency walk-in clinic, Ingelfinger et al[2] found that gross hematuria accounted for 158 of 128,395 (0.13%) consecutive visits. A diagnosis was made in 88 children (56%), 41 of whom had urinary tract infection (UTI) and 14 of whom had a glomerular disease. In a series of 82 children with gross hematuria, Youn et al[3] established a diagnosis in 56, including hypercalciuria ($n$ = 9), urethrorrhagia ($n$ = 8), hemorrhagic cystitis ($n$ = 7), IgA nephropathy ($n$ = 13), and AS ($n$ = 6).

Although the differential diagnosis of gross hematuria is large, these observational studies suggest that only a limited number of disorders affect most of the patients.

## DIAGNOSIS

Demographic features (age, race, and sex), genitourinary complaints, systemic (extrarenal) manifestations, family history, and urinalysis may provide important clues to the diagnosis. Once an underlying disorder is suspected, imaging studies, urine cultures, chemistries, and serologies are usually sufficient to confirm the diagnosis. In some cases, invasive procedures such as cystoscopy or renal biopsy are warranted.

## DEMOGRAPHIC FEATURES

A number of demographic features, such as age, race, country of origin, and sex, may aid in the diagnosis. For example, idiopathic hypercalciuria is relatively uncommon in black and Asian children, whereas sickle cell nephropathy is rare in whites. Some patients may originate from a "stone belt" (southeastern United States) or travel to a country that is endemic for schistosomiasis. Sex-linked disorders, such as AS, affect males disproportionately, whereas UTI and lupus nephritis are more common in adolescent girls. Wilms tumor, hemolytic uremic syndrome (HUS), Henoch-Schönlein purpura (HSP), and congenital hydronephrosis are more frequently observed in preschool-age children; acute postinfectious glomerulonephritis is most common in the school-aged population; a chronic glomerulonephritis, such as IgA nephropathy or MPGN, is seen most commonly in the adolescent.

In adults, hematuria may be an indicator of malignancy of the genitourinary tract, including renal cell carcinoma, transitional or epithelial cell carcinoma of the bladder, and tumors of the prostate. These malignancies are uncommon in children and adolescents.

## DYSFUNCTIONAL VOIDING AND ELIMINATION SYNDROMES

The voiding pattern may sometimes shed light on the likely cause of hematuria. For example, a history of recent fever (or recurring, unexplained fever), abdominal pain, dysuria, urinary frequency, incontinence, malodorous urine, hesitancy, urgency, interrupted stream, or recent enuresis suggests a past or present UTI. In young women, UTIs may be associated with recent sexual activity (referred to through the years as "honeymoon cystitis"). Sometimes, dysfunctional voiding is associated with stool withholding or constipation, and treatment with laxatives may be especially helpful. Worsening encopresis and voiding dysfunction may be due to a spinal lesion, such as a tethered cord, and should be evaluated promptly.

In boys, hematuria may be mistaken for hematospermia and in girls, with menses. Idiopathic urethritis or urethrorrhagia, the finding of blood spotting in the underwear between voids, has been associated with Cobb collar (obstruction of the bulbar urethra in males) and/or the dysfunctional elimination syndrome (DES). Treatment with behavior modification, laxatives, bowel and bladder regimens, and/or alpha blockers seems to be more effective than conventional treatment with antibiotics, urinary analgesics, and/or anticholinergics.[4] (See Chapter 119, Voiding Disorders.)

## HEMATURIA ASSOCIATED WITH PAIN OR TRAUMA

In both sexes, exercise-induced hematuria may follow vigorous athletic training, and is thought to be benign. Hematuria may result from more severe abdominal or flank trauma, especially in those with an underlying urogenital malformation (eg, hydronephrosis).

Other causes of gross hematuria associated with pain or discomfort include pyelonephritis and renal calculi. Less common causes of painful, gross hematuria include the loin pain-hematuria syndrome (LPHS) unilateral or bilateral flank pain and microscopic or macroscopic hematuria of unknown origin); chronic interstitial cystitis (CIC); and bladder endometriosis. Papillary necrosis may be seen in patients with sickle cell disease, sometimes in the setting of thrombo-occlusive crisis. In adolescents, a syndrome of flank pain and renal failure has been associated with binge (alcohol) drinking and the concomitant use of nonsteroidal anti-inflammatory drugs (NSAIDs). Renal vein thrombosis (RVT) may complicate nephrotic syndrome, hypercoagulable states (eg, oral contraceptives), and dehydration.

## RENAL AND EXTRARENAL MANIFESTATIONS

A history of recent throat, skin, or respiratory infection, periorbital or pretibial edema, weight gain, oliguria, tea-colored urine, or hypertension suggests a glomerular disease or process (eg, postinfectious glomerulonephritis, IgA nephropathy, hemolytic uremic syndrome, MPGN AS). Extrarenal complaints, including arthralgia, skin exanthem, anemia, pallor, abdominal pain, or prolonged fever suggests the possibility of an underlying vasculitis, such as HSP or Wegner granulomatosis, or a collagen-vascular disorder such as systemic lupus erythematosus (SLE).

## FAMILY HISTORY

Familial disorders that are often associated with hematuria include thin basement membrane disease ("benign familial hematuria"), AS, collagen vascular disease, urolithiasis, and polycystic kidney disease (PKD).

## PHYSICAL EXAMINATION

The physical examination should include vital signs (height, weight, pulse, respirations, blood pressure), with a notation of any new changes in these parameters. The skin should be inspected for signs of trauma, rash, or infection. The ears, nose, and throat should be examined for signs of edema (scalp, periorbital), infection (tonsils, sinus), or adenopathy. The lungs should be auscultated, and the abdomen and flank should be palpated in order to detect or elicit tenderness, organomegaly, or mass. A genitourinary examination is important to exclude local bleeding or irritation, and the extremities should be inspected for edema.

## URINALYSIS

Urine microscopy is essential to classify gross hematuria as either "glomerular" or "nonglomerular" in origin. Gross hematuria due to a nonglomerular or urological cause may be associated with dysfunctional voiding (eg, flank pain, dysuria, an abnormal voiding pattern) but not systemic illness (except fever). Visible hematuria may persist throughout micturition or appear only toward the end of micturition ("terminal hematuria"). The color of the urine may be bright red, and the urine may contain frank blood clots. The urine contains little protein, and microscopic examination reveals numerous red blood cells that are regular (concentric) in size and shape. In children with UTI, white blood cells and white blood cell casts are also present.

Gross hematuria due to a glomerular cause may be associated with systemic illness but not a dysfunctional voiding pattern. Gross hematuria persists throughout micturition. The urine is often described as tea or cola-colored, and does not form blood clots. Proteinuria is the hallmark of glomerular disease, and microscopic examination of the urine reveals irregularly shaped (dysmorphic-appearing) red blood cells. White blood cells, red blood cell casts, and granular casts may also be present. The glomerular and nonglomerular causes of both gross and microscopic hematuria are summarized in Table 115-1.

## DIAGNOSTIC TESTS OF GENITOURINARY DISORDERS

If hematuria is nonglomerular in origin, then investigations should include imaging studies (eg, renal ultrasound, abdominal computed tomography [CT] scan with and without intravenous contrast agents), and urine for bacterial or viral cultures. Also, it may be important to analyze the urine for calcium. Approximately 30% of children with isolated hematuria may have elevated urinary calcium levels (urine calcium/creatinine ratio >0.2 or urine calcium excretion >4 mg/kg/day). Children with hypercalciuria may present with renal calculi, gravel in the urine, hematuria, or voiding dysfunction (urinary frequency, urgency, dysuria). Therapy consists of hydration; a diet low in sodium and animal fat; the provision of citrate (present in orange juice and lemonade); and/or the administration of thiazide diuretics.

Rarely, cystoscopy is needed to localize the source of the bleeding (eg, harmatoma of the bladder, nephrogenic adenoma, chronic interstitial cystitis, endometriosis of the bladder, left renal vein entrapment syndrome, papillary necrosis).

## DIAGNOSTIC TESTS OF GLOMERULAR DISEASE

If a glomerular disease is suspected, the evaluation should include a complete blood count (CBC), chemistries, blood urea nitrogen (BUN), creatinine, albumin, liver function studies and serologies (antinuclear antibody test [ANA], anti-DNA, complement levels, serum IgA level, antineutrophil cytoplasmic antibodies [ANCA], antistreptolysin O [ASO] titer), and in selected cases renal biopsy. Low serum complement levels are seen in postinfectious glomerulonephritis, systemic lupus erythematosus nephritis, bacterial endocarditis, shunt nephropathy, and MPGN. Indications for a renal biopsy in adolescents with gross hematuria include impaired renal function, systemic illness (eg, systemic lupus erythematosus [SLE]), hypertension, significant proteinuria, recurring or persisting hematuria, and/or a family history of end-stage renal failure (eg, AS).

**Table 115-1**

**Causes of Hematuria in Children and Adolescents**

| | *Gross Hematuria* | *Microscopic Hematuria* |
|---|---|---|
| Glomerular | • Acute, primary (postinfectious GN, rapidly progressive GN, HUS)<br>• Chronic, primary (IgA nephropathy, Alport syndrome, MPGN)<br>• Systemic (SLE, Wegner, HSP) | Thin basement membrane disease |
| Nonglomerular | • Renal vein entrapment ("nutcracker") syndrome<br>• Papillary necrosis<br>• Hemorrhagic cystitis<br>• Nephrogenic adenoma<br>• AV malformation<br>• Harmatoma<br>• Hypercalciuria<br>• Hyperuricosuria<br>• Renal calculi<br>• Hydronephrosis<br>• Tumor<br>• Schistosomiasis<br>• Polycystic kidney disease<br>• Cobb collar<br>• Exercise induced<br>• Trauma<br>• Sickle cell<br>• Drugs/toxins (NSAIDs, anticoagulants, cyclophosphamide, ritonavir, indinavir)<br>• Coagulopathy | • Urethritis<br>• Fever<br>• Hypercalciuria |

GN, glomerulonephritis; HUS, hemolytic uremic syndrome; MPGN, membranoproliferative glomerulonephritis; NSAIDs, nonsteroidal anti-inflammatory drugs; SLE, systemic lupus erythematosis; HSP, Henoch-Schönlein purpura

Potentially serious illnesses, such as HUS, HSP, and postinfectious glomerulonephritis are important causes of hematuria in children of all ages, but are typically diseases of the school or preschool-age child. Systemic diseases, such as SLE, Wegner granulomatosis, and micropolyangitis (MPA), may be diagnosed through serological testing in consultation with a pediatric rheumatologist or nephrologist. A few glomerular diseases tend to present in the adolescent population, without evidence of systemic disease. These include IgA nephropathy, AS, and MPGN.

These 3 diseases comprise a heterogeneous group of disorders with different pathogenesis, clinical course, and outcome. Yet, patients with any of these disorders may present similarly with hematuria, proteinuria, and impaired renal function. History, laboratory investigations, and the clinical course help to distinguish these conditions, whereas the renal histology is diagnostic (Table 115-2).

### IgA Nephropathy

Berger[5] first described IgA nephropathy in 1968. Patients usually present within 48 hours after a mucosal infection with loin pain, hematuria, and proteinuria. Recurring bouts of gross hematuria are common, and vary in severity from mild and asymptomatic to severe renal failure.[6,7] IgA nephropathy is the most common primary form of glomerulonephritis in the world, accounting for almost 50% of the renal biopsies performed in Asia and Australia, almost 30% of the biopsies performed in Europe, and about 4% of biopsies performed in the United States.[8] There is a male predominance, and a higher prevalence among white patients than among black patients in the United States.[9]

Although initially thought to be a benign disease, we now know that many patients experience a slow, progressive decline in their renal function. Polymorphisms in the genes coding for the renin-angiotensin system may be important markers of disease progression.[10] Although some patients eventually remit, up to 25% of adult patients ultimately develop renal failure. Rekola et al[11] report a loss of renal function of 1 to 3 mL/minute/year, with 20% reaching end-stage after 10 years and 30% reaching end-stage after 20 years. The prognosis may be better in children.

Renal biopsy reveals IgA-containing immune complexes with proliferation of the glomerular mesangium[7] and may be the best indicator of prognosis. In a large series of children, Levy et al[12] found that none of 69 patients with minimal glomerular abnormalities, pure mesangial proliferation, or focal GN developed end-stage renal failure. However, 6 of 20 patients with a proliferative and crescentic disease eventually required dialysis or transplantation.

Although a wide variety of agents have been used to treat IgA nephropathy, few medications have been subjected to prospective clinical trials.[13] The 2 most carefully scrutinized agents have been prednisone[13] and fish oils.[14]

**Table 115-2**

**Glomerular Diseases Seen in the Adolescent Age Group**

| *Disorder* | *Incidence* | *Presentation* | *Genetics* | *Pathogenesis* | *Treatment* | *Prognosis* |
|---|---|---|---|---|---|---|
| IgA nephropathy | Common | Hematuria | ACE polymorphisms | IgA-fibronectin | Steroids<br>Fish oil | Good |
| Alport syndrome | Uncommon | Hematuria<br>Hearing loss | X-linked or autosomal | Type IV collagen | None | Poor |
| Membranoproliferative Glomerulonephritis | Uncommon | Hematuria<br>Proteinuria<br>Hypertension<br>Low C3 | Factor H deficiency | Complement activation (idiopathic, hepatitis, Hodgkin) | Alternate day steroids | Fair |

ACE, antiotensin-converting enzyme

### Alport Syndrome

In 1902, Guthrie[15] described a family in which many members had hematuria. Later, Alport[16] observed that some members of this family had developed hearing loss and that affected males died of uremia, whereas affected females survived into old age. In 1973, Spear[17] postulated that the irregular glomerular basement membrane, cochlear abnormalities, and anterior lenticonus observed in these patients may be explained by an abnormal collagen. More recent investigations indicate that AS is due to a heterogeneous genetic disorder of type IV collagen. Inheritance may be x-linked (XLAS), autosomal recessive (ARAS), or autosomal dominant (ADAS).

Iversen[18] described the characteristic course in males: "In connection with one of the infectious diseases of childhood or a common cold in early childhood or adolescence, he will suddenly begin to suffer from massive haematuria or headache, or oedema of the face. The urine shows haematuria and/or proteinuria and often also cylindruria and leukocyturia. These urinary signs may in one and the same patient vary in degree during the following months, and in some patients they may almost disappear, but they may become more pronounced again during the next infectious disease or after physical strain. There may be more or less pronounced hypertension. Most boys with this disease die from uraemia during adolescence." Extrarenal manifestations may include neurosensory deafness (about 50%), leiomyomatosis, anterior lenticonus, and other ocular lesions. See Chapter 156, Hearing Disorders and Psychosocial Development, for a further discussion of deafness in AS.

Most patients (approximately 85%) have the x-linked form of AS (XLAS).[19-21] Almost all affected males eventually develop end-stage renal disease (ESRD). However, the rate of progression varies between kindreds, and may exhibit a bimodal distribution. In families with juvenile AS, the mean age of ESRD in affected males is <31 years, whereas in adult AS the mean age of affected males is >31 years.

About 15% of female heterozygotes develop renal failure. Gross hematuria in childhood, sensorineural deafness, anterior lenticonus, and nephrotic syndrome are signs of poor prognosis. Patients with AS ARAS uniformly progress to ESRD at a young age, whereas patients with the autosomal dominant form (ADAS) seem to progress more slowly.

The diagnosis is made by renal biopsy, although immunofluorescence microscopy of skin and genetic testing may play some role. Light microscopy may reveal focal and segmental glomerulosclerosis, glomerular basement membrane (GBM) abnormalities, and interstitial foam cells. Electron microscopy is essential for the diagnosis of AS. Early in the course one observes splitting and fragmentation of the GBM. Later in the disease the GBM is thick and the lamina densa is transformed into a network of lamellae enclosing clear electron-lucent areas.

### Membranoproliferative Glomerulonephritis

First described in 1965, membranoproliferative glomerulonephritis (MPGN) is an uncommon type of glomerulonephritis. However, as patients present similarly to those with postinfectious glomerulonephritis, membranoproliferative glomerulonephritis (MPGN) is always in the differential diagnosis of adolescents with nephrotic syndrome, proteinuria, acute nephritis, or recurrent hematuria. Patients often have refractory hypertension and impaired renal function. Hypocomplementemia is present in 80%.[22-26]

Three subtypes (MPGN type I, II, and III) have been described. Patients with MPGN type I often present with the so-called nephritic-nephrotic syndrome. On the other hand, patients with MPGN type III may present insidiously with asymptomatic urinary abnormalities (see Chapter 117, Nephritis and Nephrosis).

The disorder may be either primary or secondary to hepatitis B or C, HIV, other infections, neoplasms, complement deficiency and factor H deficiency, or collagen vascular disease. Slightly more females than males develop MPGN type I. Most cases of MPGN in adults appears to be secondary to hepatitis C whereas most MPGN in children appears to be idiopathic.

Membranoproliferative glomerulonephritis is a chronic, progressive renal disease. Untreated, renal survival in adults and children at 10 years is 65%. Poor prognostic signs include nephrotic syndrome and interstitial disease. Renal survival in children with MPGN type III may be worse than those with MPGN type I.

In children, steroid therapy appears to be of benefit. In a study conducted by the International Study of Kidney Disease in Children (ISKDC),[26] 80 children with MPGN I were randomized to receive prednisone 40 mg/mm$^2$ on alternate days or placebo, with a mean duration of treatment of 130 months. At the end of the treatment period 61% of the treatment group vs 12% of the placebo group maintained stable renal function ($P < 0.05$).

**Box 115-1**

***Causes of Proteinuria***

- Transient proteinuria (fever, exercise, dehydration)
- Drugs and toxins (heavy metal poisoning, heroin nephropathy)
- Orthostatic proteinuria
- Isolated, nonorthostatic proteinuria and nephrotic syndrome
  - Minimal change nephrotic syndrome
  - Focal segmental glomerulonephritis
  - Membranous glomerulonephropathy
  - Membranoproliferative glomerulonephritis
- Congenital and acquired urinary tract abnormalities (reflux nephropathy, renal dysplasia)
- Associated with glomerulonephritis (HUS, postinfectious GN)
- Associated with hyperfiltration (surgical ablation, obesity)
- Associated with systemic disease (SLE, HSP, Wegner)

GN, glomerulonephritis; HSP, Henoch-Schönlein purpura; HUS, hemolytic uremic syndrome; SLE, systemic lupus erythematosus

## PROTEINURIA

In the adolescent, proteinuria (mostly albuminuria) may be transient or persistent, isolated or combined with hematuria, "fixed" or orthostatic, "low-grade" or "nephrotic-range." Some of the causes of proteinuria in adolescents are listed in Box 115-1.

Proteinuria is generally detected using a urinary dipstick (Albustix, Multistix), in which the concentration of protein is determined by interaction with tetrabromophenol blue. The strips react preferentially with albumin, but may give false-positive results if the urine is contaminated with bodily secretions, is very alkaline, or is very concentrated. The concentration of protein in the urine is assessed as 1+ (30 mg per dL), 2+ (100 mg per dL), 3+ (300 mg per dL), or 4+ (1,000 mg per dL). In many laboratories, a positive urinary dipstick reading is confirmed by a precipitation test with sulfosalicylic acid. A false-negative result may occur with very dilute urine.

Although 24-hour urine collections are useful in adults, they are often unhelpful in the child and adolescent because orthostatic proteinuria is quite common. Also, the finding of proteinuria on a single, random screening is common in children and adolescents, with a prevalence of up to 5% to 15% of samples. Proteinuria may be associated with fever, dehydration, or exercise. Often, the proteinuria resolves upon further testing (transient proteinuria). In the otherwise well adolescent, isolated proteinuria that is transient, orthostatic, or "low-grade" (urine protein/creatinine ratio <0.2 or <4 mg/m$^2$/h) is benign.[27,28]

However, in the patient with diabetes, collagen-vascular disease, hypertension, or recurring UTI, even a small amount of protein in the urine ("microalbuminuria," defined as 20 to 200 µg/minute/1.73 m$^2$ or 30 to 300 mg albumin/g creatinine) may warrant additional investigation and treatment.

The usual investigation for an otherwise well child with the incidental finding of proteinuria includes a first morning void for a protein/creatinine ratio. Proteinuria that is nonorthostatic and persistent, whether "low-grade" or "nephrotic range," should be investigated completely. In a study of 53 Japanese children with asymptomatic proteinuria, glomerulopathy was observed on renal biopsy in 25 patients (47%).[29] Of these, 15 had

**Table 115-3**

**Nephrotic Syndrome in Children**

| | *Minimal Change* | *MPGN* | *Focal Sclerosis* | *Membranous* |
|---|---|---|---|---|
| Hypertension | + | +++ | ++ | + |
| Hematuria | + | +++ | ++ | + |
| Hypocomplementeria | — | +++ | — | — |
| Renal failure (not due to prerenal azotemia) | — | +++ | +++ | + |
| Response to steroids | +++ | + | + | + |

—, rare; +, uncommon; ++, common; +++ very common

MPGN, membranoproliferative glomerulonephritis

focal glomerulosclerosis, 7 of whom developed renal failure.

A history of "foamy" appearing urine, oliguria, edema, UTI, sudden gain or loss of weight, exanthem, fever, photophobia, or arthralgia may aid in the diagnosis.

Non-nephrotic-range proteinuria may indicate a loss of renal mass due to congenital malformation (eg, renal dysplasia/hypoplasia), chronic pyelonephritis ("reflux nephropathy"), glomerular disease (eg, membranous nephropathy, focal segmental glomerulosclerosis), or obesity-associated hyperfiltration. Helpful diagnostic tests may include a CBC, chemistries, BUN, plasma creatinine, complement levels, ANA, hepatitis B and C profile, albumin level, liver function tests, and a renal ultrasound. In some cases a renal biopsy is indicated.

The nephrotic syndrome (proteinuria >40 mg/m$^2$/h, plasma albumin <2.5 g/dL, edema) occurs in approximately 1 to 2/100,000 children, and may be associated with a systemic illness (eg, Hodgkin disease, collagen-vascular disease, vasculitis, or a chronic infection such as hepatitis or HIV infection), a drug or toxin (eg, heroin nephropathy), or may be an isolated process. Investigations should include a chest radiograph, placement of a purified protein derivative (PPD), a varicella titer (in anticipation of steroid therapy), chemistries, albumin level, CBC, and serologies (hepatitis profile, complement levels, ANA, HIV testing). The differential diagnosis of primary nephrotic syndrome includes minimal change disease, MPGN, focal sclerosis, and membranous nephropathy.

A renal biopsy may be indicated more often in the adolescent than in the younger child because the likelihood of steroid-responsive minimal change disease decreases with age. Other indications for renal biopsy include atypical features such as persistent hematuria, renal failure, hypocomplementemia, or hypertension. Causes of primary nephrotic syndrome in children are listed in Table 115-3.

Complications of nephrotic syndrome include edema (ascites, scrotal, pleural effusion), hyponatremia, infections (including primary bacterial peritonitis), hyperlipidemia, and venous thrombosis. As the adolescent may be reluctant to report an exacerbation or worsening of disease, these complications may be especially difficult to treat.

The usual course of treatment consists of prednisone for 8 weeks (60 mg/m$^2$/day in divided doses to a maximal dose of 80 mg per day for 4 weeks, followed by 40 mg/m$^2$ every other day for an additional 4 weeks). Live-virus vaccines, sun exposure, and exposure to varicella should be avoided during and soon after treatment. In children who respond to prednisone (negative protein on dipstick), many will experience relapses or exacerbations (proteinuria 1+ or greater for 3 consecutive days), and so will receive multiple courses of treatment. As steroid therapy is associated with numerous side effects and potential complications (Cushingoid body habitus, weight gain, acne, hirsutism, hypertension, infection, thrush, striae, cataracts, osteopenia, mood swings, growth retardation), adherence may be a major issue.

Steroid-resistant patients may be treated with immunosuppressive or cytotoxic agents (eg, cyclophosphamide, cyclosporine). In addition, angiotensin-converting enzyme (ACE) inhibitors are often used as renoprotective agents, by decreasing proteinuria while preserving renal function, but they may cause fetal demise, and so are contraindicated in pregnancy. On the other hand, oral contraceptives may increase the risk of thromboembolic phenomena. As with drug use, a frank discussion about pregnancy avoidance is often important in caring for the adolescent girl with nephrosis.

## REFERENCES


1. Greenfield SP, Williot P, Kaplan D. Ross hematuria in children: a 10 year review. *Urology.* 2007;69:166–169

2. Ingelfinger JR, Davis AE, Grupe WE. Frequency and etiology of gross hematuria in a general pediatric setting. *Pediatrics.* 1977;59:557–561

3. Youn T, Trachtman H, Gauthier B. Clinical spectrum of gross hematuria in pediatric patients. *Clin Pediatr (Phila).* 2006;45:135–141

4. Herz D, Weiser A, Collette T, Reda E, Levitt S, Franco I. Dysfunctional elimination syndrome as an etiology of idiopathic urethritis in childhood. *J Urol.* 2005;173(6):2132–2137

5. Berger J, Hinglais N. Les depots intercapillaires d'IgA-IgG. *J Urol Nephrol.* 1968;74:694–695

6. D'Amico G. The commonest glomerulonephritis in the world: IgA nephropathy. *Q J Med.* 1987;64:709–727

7. Donadio JV Jr, Grande JP. Immunoglobulin A nephropathy: a clinical perspective. *J Am Soc Nephrol.* 1997;8:1324–1332

8. Julian BA, Waldo FB, Rifai A, Mestecky J. IgA nephropathy, the most common glomerulonephritis worldwide: a neglected disease in the United States? *Am J Med.* 1988;84:129–132

9. Jennette JC, Wall SD, Wilkman AS. Low incidence of IgA nephropathy in blacks. *Kidney Int.* 1985;28:944–950

10. Yoshida H, Mitarai T, Kawamura T, et al. Role of the deletion polymorphism of the angiotensin converting enzyme gene in the progression and therapeutic responsiveness of IgA nephropathy. *J Clin Invest.* 1995;96:2162–2169

11. Rekola S, Bergstrand A, Bucht H. Deterioration of GFR in IgA nephropathy as measured by 51Cr-EDTA clearance. *Kidney Int.* 1991;40:1050–1054

12. Levy M, Gonzalez-Burchard G, Broyer M, et al. Berger's disease in children. Natural history and outcome. *Medicine.* 1985;64:157–180

13. Waldo EB, Wyatt RJ, Kelly RJ, et al. Treatment of IgA nephropathy in children: efficacy of alternate-day oral prednisone. *Pediatr Nephrol.* 1993;7:529–532

14. Hogg RJ, Wyatt RJ. Scientific Planning Committee of the North American IgA Nephropathy Study: a randomized controlled trial of mycophenolate mofetil in patients with IgA nephropathy [ISRCTN62574616]. *BMC Nephrol.* 2004;255:3

15. Guthrie LB. 'Idiopathic,' or congenital, hereditary, and familial haematuria. *Lancet I.* 1902:1243–1246

16. Alport C. Hereditary familial congenital haemorrhagic nephritis. *Brit Med J.* 1927:504–506

17. Spear GS. Alport's syndrome: a consideration of pathogenesis. *Clin Nephrol.* 1973;1:336–337

18. Iversen UM. Hereditary nephropathy with hearing loss: Alport's syndrome. *Acta Paediat Scand.* 1974;245(suppl):1–23

19. Kashtan CE. Alport Syndromes: phenotypic heterogeneity of progressive hereditary nephritis. *Pediatr Nephrol.* 2000;12:502–512

20. Kashtan CE, Michael AF. Alport syndrome: from bedside to genome to bedside. *Am J Kidney Dis.* 1993;22:627–640

21. Grunfeld JP. Contemporary diagnostic approach in Alport's syndrome. *Ren Fail.* 2000;22:759–763

22. West CD. Childhood membranoproliferative glomerulonephritis: an approach to management. *Kidney Int.* 1986;29:1077–1093

23. West CD. Idiopathic membranoproliferative glomerulonephritis in childhood. *Pediatr Nephrol.* 1992;6:96–103

24. Meyers EC, Finn L, Kaplan B. Membranoproliferative glomerulonephritis type III. *Pediatr Nephrol.* 1998;12:512–522

25. West CD, McAdams AJ. The alternate pathway of C3 convertase and glomerular deposits. *Pediatr Nephrol.* 1999;12:448–453

26. Tarshish P, Bernstein J, Tobin JN, Edelmann CM Jr. Treatment of mesangiocapillary glomerulonephritis with alternate-day prednisone: a report of the International Study of Kidney Disease in Children. *Pediatr Nephrol.* 1992;6:123–130

27. Hogg RJ, Portman RJ, Milliner D, Lemley KV, Eddy A, Ingelfinger J. Evaluation and management of proteinuria and nephrotic syndrome in children: recommendations from a pediatric nephrology panel established at the National Kidney Foundation Conference on Proteinuria, Albuminuria, Risk, Assessment, Detection, and Elimination (PARADE). *Pediatrics.* 2000;105:1242–1249

28. Loghman-Adham M. Evaluating proteinuria in children. *Am Fam Physician.* 1998;58:1155–1152, 1158–1159

29. Yoshikawa N, Kitagawa K, Ohta K, Tanaka R, Nakamura H. Asymptomatic constant isolated proteinuria in children. *J Pediatr.* 1991;119:375–379

# CHAPTER 116

## Urinary Tract Infections

SUSAN MASSENGILL, MD • LEONARD G. FELD, MD, PhD

### OVERVIEW

Acute cystitis is a common problem among young adolescent females. The incidence increases during the late teen years and early adulthood, presumably due to sexual activity. Young, sexually active females have 0.5 episodes per person year, but these episodes decline by the early 30s. Urinary tract infections (UTIs) represent the fourth-leading cause of outpatient visits among adolescent females. Male patients with UTIs should be evaluated thoroughly, although such infections are uncommon in males.

### DEFINITION

Cystitis is characterized by inflammation of the mucosal surface and infection affecting the bladder. Clinical manifestations include dysuria, frequency, urgency, hesitancy, suprapubic pain, and sometimes hematuria (Figure 116-1). Pyelonephritis, on the other hand, involves an infection of the renal parenchyma. In contrast to the localized symptom complex of cystitis, upper tract infections are characterized by fever (sometimes with chills), flank pain/costovertebral tenderness or abdominal pain, and gastrointestinal symptoms such as nausea or vomiting.[1,2]

### ETIOLOGY AND PATHOGENESIS

*Escherichia coli (E coli)* is the primary uropathogen responsible for cystitis, accounting for more than 80% of all UTIs. Most other episodes are due to *Staphylococcus saprophyticus,* especially in sexually active females. Less common, gram-negative organisms include *Citrobacter, Enterobacter* species, *Klebsiella* species, and *Proteus mirabilis*. Viruses and fungi are rare causes of cystitis. Common nonbacterial pathogens include adenovirus, leading to hemorrhagic cystitis, and *Candida,* which is found in the immunocompromised patient. Indwelling catheters are a risk factor for the development of cystitis in all patients.

The ability of fecal uropathogens to adhere to and colonize the periurethral and urethral area leads to the ascent of organisms into the bladder, ureter, and renal tissue. Virulence in uropathogenic strains of *E coli* is promoted by the production of P fimbriae, which bind to glycolipid receptors on host epithelial cells, have the ability to encapsulate, produce cytolytic toxin hemolysis, sequester iron, and produce the select O-serotypes[3,4] (Table 116-1).

There are several host risk factors that predispose to development of a UTI in females. One of these is having a short urethra, which allows a closer proximity of the bladder to the warm and moist vaginal and perianal areas. Sexual intercourse is a very important risk factor for the development of cystitis.[5] Spermicidal use (with or without condom use) increases the risk of cystitis by altering the vaginal milieu, favoring colonization and enhancing adherence by uropathogenic strains. Lack of postcoital voiding or an infrequent voiding pattern have each been associated with an increased risk of cystitis. Other predisposing factors include pregnancy, a prior history of cystitis, anatomical abnormalities, vesicoureteral reflux (VUR), urolithiasis, and history of a foreign body (ie, a catheter) (Box 116-1).

The lower incidence of UTIs in males can be attributed to infrequent colonization around the urethra due to the drier periurethral environment, increased urethral length, and antibacterial substances in prostatic secretions. Given the unusual occurrence of UTIs in males, the presence of such infections warrants evaluation for structural or functional abnormalities of the urinary tract such as VUR, obstructive uropathy, or neurogenic bladder.[1] Other risk factors for males include men having sex with men, colonization of a female sexual partner, and lack of circumcision.

Host defense mechanisms exist to resist colonization by uropathogenic bacteria[4] (Box 116-2). Despite being a good culture medium for bacteria, urine contains inhibitors against growth such as an acidic environment, fluctuating osmolality, and high urea concentrations. In addition, the secretions of the epithelial surface of the urinary tract possess antibacterial properties.

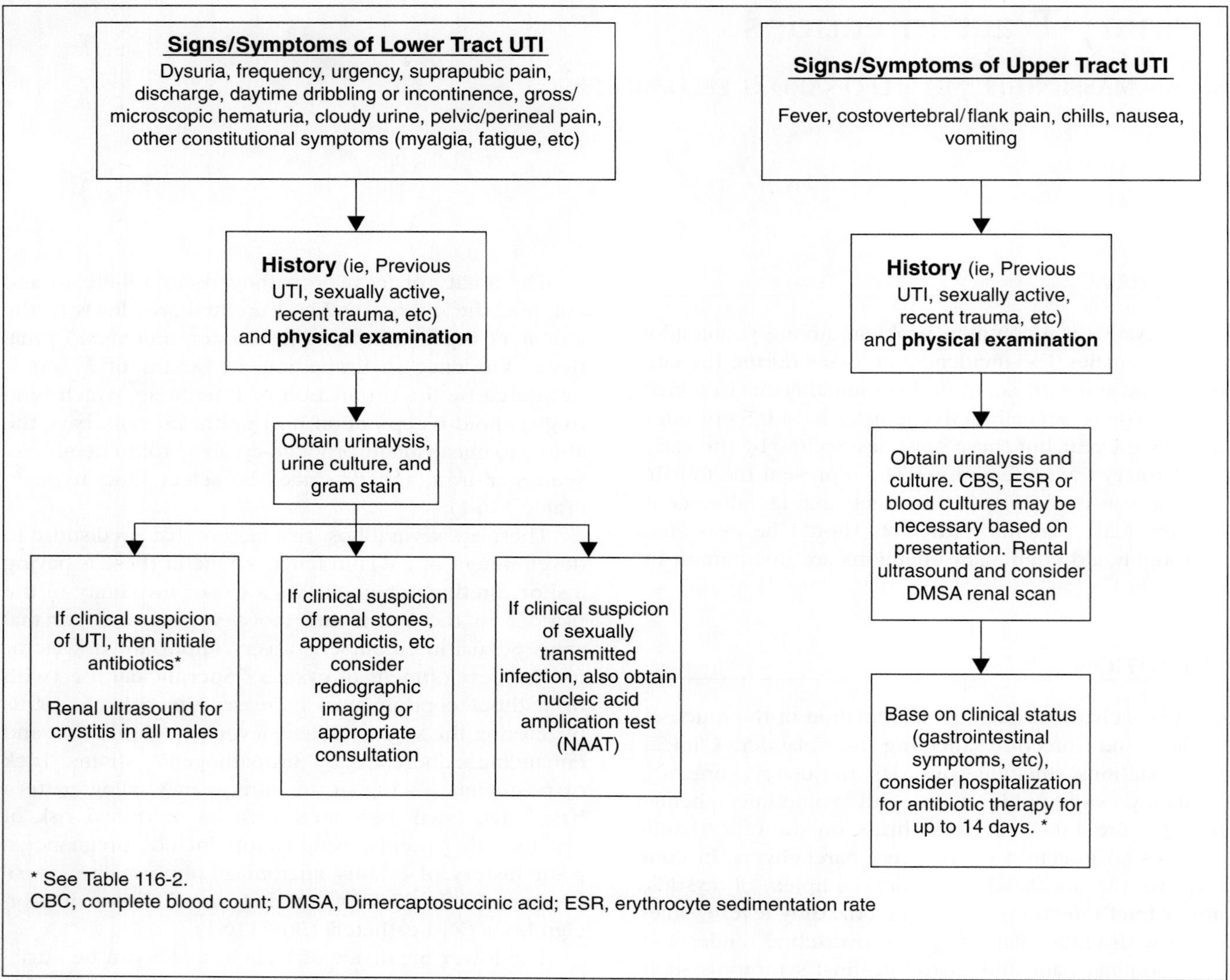


**FIGURE 116-1** Evaluation of urinary tract infection (UTI) in adolescents.

## Table 116-1

### Uropathogenic *E coli* Adhesions and Receptors

| *Adhesion* | *Receptor* | *Comments* |
|---|---|---|
| Type I fimbriae | Mannosylated proteins on epithelial cells | Binds to Tamm-Horsfall protein and sIgA |
| P fimbriae | Gal-α 1,4 (P blood group antigen) | Strongly associated with pyelonephritis and bacteremia |

Adapted from Sobel JD, Kaye D. Urinary tract infections. In: Mandell GL, Bennett JE, Dolin R (eds). *Mandell, Douglass, and Bennett's Principles and Practices of Infectious Disease*. 6th ed. Philadelphia, PA: Elsevier Churchill Livingstone;2005:875–905.

**Box 116-1**

***Host Risk Factors for Urinary Tract Infections***

| *Females* | *Males* |
|---|---|
| Sexual activity | Men having sex with men |
| Spermicide usage | Colonized female sexual partner |
| Lack of postcoital voiding | Genitourinary abnormalities |
| Prior history of UTI | Kidney stones |
| Vesicoureteral reflux | Uncircumcised |
| Pregnancy | Prior urinary catheter |
| Kidney stones | |
| Prior urinary catheter | |

**Box 116-2**

***Antibacterial Host Defenses in the Urinary Tract***

- Urine (osmolality, pH, organic acids)
- Urine flow and micturition
- Urinary tract mucosa (bactericidal activity and cytokines)
- Urinary inhibitors of bacterial adherence
- Tamm-Horsfall protein
- Bladder mucopolysaccharides
- Low-molecular-weight oligosaccharides
- Secretory immunoglobulin (sIgA)
- Lactoferrin
- Inflammatory response
- Polymorphonuclear neutrophils (PMNs)
- Cytokines
- Humoral immunity
- Cell-mediated immunity
- Prostatic secretions

Adapted from Sobel JD, Kaye D. Urinary tract infections. In: Mandell GL, Bennett JE, Dolin R (eds). *Mandell, Douglass, and Bennett's Principles and Practices of Infectious Disease.* 6th ed. Philadelphia, PA: Elsevier Churchill Livingstone, 2005:875–905.

## DIFFERENTIAL DIAGNOSIS

- **Asymptomatic bacteriuria** is the presence of a positive urine culture in an otherwise asymptomatic individual. The prevalance of bacteriuria in young, healthy, nonpregnant women is about 3% to 7%.[6] For asymptomatic females, bacteriuria is defined as 2 consecutive clean-catch voided urine specimens with isolation of the same bacterial strain in counts $\geq 10^5$ cfu/ml. For asymptomatic males, bacteriuria is defined as a single clean-catch voided urine specimen with isolation of a bacterial species in a count $\geq 10^5$ cfu/ml.[7] Asymptomatic bacteriuria in males is infrequently seen (<0.1%). In general, the same risk factors as for cystitis apply to asymptomatic bacteriuria. Conditions that predispose to asymptomatic bacteriuria include pregnancy, diabetes mellitus, VUR, renal transplantation, indwelling urinary catheter, and presence of struvite stones.
- **Cystitis** is characterized by lower urinary tract symptoms such as dysuria, hesitancy, urgency, frequency, suprapubic discomfort, and often a turbid urine due to irritation of the urethral and bladder mucosa from bacterial tissue invasion.[1,2] On occasion, the urine is grossly bloody or blood-tinged at the end of urination. Fever is not a common complaint. However, similar symptoms may be seen with other causes of lower tract inflammation, such as gonorrheal or chlamydial urethritis. Complicated cystitis is seen in individuals with special circumstances, such as male gender, pregnant women, those with a chronic illness such as diabetes mellitus or sickle cell disease, patients who are immunosuppressed (renal transplantation, systemic lupus erythematosus, etc), and those who have infection with an atypical pathogen or have had recent antimicrobial therapy or treatment of a UTI.
- **Dysuria** is defined as pain or burning with urination. Other considerations for dysuria among females include acute vaginitis/vulvovaginitis due to yeast, bacterial vaginosis, a sexually transmitted infection, localized dermatitis, subclinical pyelonephritis, or acute urethral syndrome. Among males, urethritis secondary to sexually transmitted organisms, prostatitis, and local irritation should be considered in the differential diagnosis.
- **Epididymitis** risk factors include a history of urethral manipulation, recent urinary tract surgery, catheterization, neurogenic bladder, imperforate anus, or a lower tract genitourinary anatomical abnormality such as bladder exstrophy. Clinical manifestations include dysuria, urethral discharge, and an inflamed and swollen scrotum.

In prepubertal males, cultures typically are positive for Gram negative organisms or show no growth, whereas in postpubertal males, the cause is often related to a sexually transmitted infection such as *Neisseria gonorrhoeae* or *Chlamydia trachomatis*.[8]

- **Prostatitis** (acute) tends to occur in older adolescents (>18 years of age). This is a common complaint associated with lower UTI (cystitis and epididymitis). The symptoms tend to be abrupt and include fever, chills, gastrointestinal symptoms (nausea, vomiting), dysuria, hesitancy, urgency, and frequency of urination. Some may have pain or discomfort in the suprapubic or perineal area, some have pain in the external genitalia (penis, testicles), and some have painful ejaculations.[9] Micro organisms gain entry via the urethra into the prostatic ducts (ie, unprotected intercourse—vaginal, anal) or by hematogenous or lymphatic spread.[9] Although *E coli* is the most common bacterial cause of acute prostatitis, other frequent pathogens include *Enterococci sp, Klebsiella pneumoniae, Proteus mirabilas,* and *Pseudomonas aeruginosa*. Sexually transmitted infections (STIs) such as chlamydia, gonorrhea, and trichomonas can also cause acute prostatitis. Some suggested risk factors for acute prostatitis include STIs, trauma (ie, cycling), chronic indwelling bladder catheters, and intermittent catheterization.
- **Pyelonephritis** is characterized by fever (>100.4°F [>38°C]) costovertebral angle tenderness, flank or abdominal pain, and gastrointestinal symptoms (nausea, vomiting) and may occur in the presence or absence of cystitis symptoms.[1,2] Absence of pyuria is unusual. Clinical presentation ranges from mild illness to life-threatening sepsis.
- **Urethritis** may present with dysuria in sexually active individuals; however, asymptomatic infections are common. *Neisseria gonorrhoeae* or *Chlamydia trachomatis* are often the causative organisms.[10] Symptomatic males should be treated for gonorrhea and chlamydia if gram stain microscopy is not readily available. For males and females in whom urethritis is suspected, testing for gonorrhea and chlamydia is recommended. Culture, nucleic acid amplification (NAAT), and nucleic acid hybridization tests are available. For females, a thorough pelvic examination is indicated to rule out pelvic inflammatory disease.
- **Vaginitis** may be characterized by increased vaginal secretions, odorous discharge, vulvar discomfort, dysuria, and dyspareunia.[10] Common pathogens include *Trichomonas vaginalis*, *Candida albicans,* and *Gardnerella vaginalis*. Diagnosis is dependent on a thorough history, genital examination, and collection of vaginal specimens.

## EVALUATION

### URINALYSIS

The gold standard for the diagnosis of a UTI is the urine culture. However, the incubation of 24 hours limits the immediate utility of the test. In adolescents, the urinalysis provides significant information to direct initial care for those presenting with signs or symptoms of UTI. The presence of leukocytes, with or without bacteria, is considered to be pyuria. The greatest sensitivity and specificity for the diagnosis of a UTI is the finding of 3 or more leukocytes in an unspun midstream urine specimen.[1] Although a hemocytometer may be used to quantify the number of leukocytes per microliter in urine that are indicative of a UTI, lack of routine availability makes this test impractical for most practitioners.

Recent studies have shown that perineal cleansing may not be necessary to obtain sequential specimens for sexually transmitted infection, NAAT, and urine culture.[11] Sequential testing is a 2-step procedure: the adolescent voids the first part of the urine into container #1 for NAAT, then switches cups and voids the midstream urine into container #2 for the urine culture. Because there are high rates of concurrent disease (eg, *Chlamydia trachomatis* and UTI) in sexually active adolescents, testing for both should be performed regardless of the specific urinary or vaginal symptoms.[12]

The associated finding of white cell casts would be indicative of an upper tract UTI. Leukocyte esterase detects the presence of white blood cells in the urine but false-negative test results often occur. Leukocytes are measured by a reaction of the esterases in leukocytes that catalyze the pyrrole amino acid ester to release 3-hydroxy-5-phenol pyrrole. It has a sensitivity of 75% to 96% and specificity of 94% to 98% to detect greater than 10 leukocytes per high-power field.[13] False-positive test results may occur with fecal contamination. False-negative results may occur with glucosuria, increased specific gravity, or in patients with vaginitis, urethritis, or prostatitis. A positive dipstick for urine nitrites suggests a gram-negative bacterial infection by *E coli, Klebsiella sp,* or *Proteus sp* due to the bacterial conversion of urinary nitrate to nitrite. A negative result is generally not helpful.

The presence of gross or microscopic hematuria may be found with both upper and lower tract UTIs. There are other causes of flank pain (IgA nephropathy) or suprapubic/scrotal pain with hematuria (renal stones). Microscopic hematuria may be associated with hypercalciuria, familial hematuria, or other noninfectious etiologies.[14]

### URINE CULTURE

As mentioned previously, the gold standard is the urine culture obtained by catheterization, midstream urine collection, or suprapubic aspiration. The latter is primarily used for infants and small children. Significant bacteriuria has been defined as $\geq 10^5$ colony-forming units per milliliter of voided urine. For urine specimens obtained by catheterization, values $\geq 10^2$ colony-forming units per milliliter are considered to be consistent with the presence of a UTI. Despite these standard definitions for UTI, lower colony counts may be associated with infection in *symptomatic* men and women.

### RADIOLOGICAL APPROACH TO AN ADOLESCENT WITH OR WITHOUT VESICOURETERAL REFLUX

In contrast to infants and children with either an uncomplicated or complicated UTI who undergo radiological testing with a renal ultrasound, voiding cystourethrogram (VCUG), and possibly a 99mTc DMSA nuclear medicine scan, similar testing is not routinely performed in female adolescents and young adults. This is because the chances of finding an anatomic or renal abnormality that requires attention is minimal in this patient population. In some adolescents, however, radiologic studies may be called for. In an adolescent with VUR, for example, repeat assessments to evaluate the resolution of the VUR may be performed with a radionuclide VCUG. In males, where concerns about the possible presence of anatomic abnormalities is greater, a more complete radiological evaluation is generally performed; this would include a renal ultrasound, VCUG, and possibly a renal scan (DMSA).

In many cases where radiography is required, the renal ultrasound may provide sufficient information regarding the renal architecture, renal pelvis dilatation, and bladder anatomy without the need for a VCUG. This applies especially in patients with uncomplicated cystitis or mild acute pyelonephritis. For moderate to severe acute pyelonephritis in adolescents and adults, cortical scintigraphy or spiral computed tomography (CT) should be considered to determine if there are renal parenchymal abnormalities. The use of gadolinium-enhanced magnetic resonance imaging (MRI) has been used to differentiate acute parenchymal infection from renal scarring; however, nephrogenic fibrosing dermopathy, a hardening of the skin that may progress to immobility, has been reported to occur in patients with moderate to severe chronic kidney disease. Therefore, alternative imaging should be considered in patients with compromised renal function.[15]

## TREATMENT

Therapeutic decisions, regardless of the location of the UTI, are based on clinical information. The decision to modify the choice and dosage of medication is directed by the culture and sensitivities. In many cases of lower UTIs, therapy is empirically started based on the urine dipstick (leukocyte esterase, nitrites) rather than urine culture results. The treatment of cystitis is based on the severity of the infection and whether it is uncomplicated (nontoxic appearing, no gastrointestinal symptoms such as vomiting or nausea, etc) or complicated. If a lower UTI is **uncomplicated**, a 3-day course of antimicrobial therapy with trimethoprin/sulfamethoxazole (TMP/SMX) is more reasonable than extended course regimens.[16] The 3-day course increases adherence and reduces side effects. The Infectious Diseases Society of America has provided strong evidence to support the use of TMP/SMX as the current standard of therapy. In addition, TMP alone was shown to be equivalent to TMP/SMX, and β-lactams were less effective than TMP, TMP/SMX, and the fluoroquinolones as a 3-day regimen.[16] With a high rate of resistance of *E coli* to TMP/SMX,[17] TMP/SMX should not be used as empiric therapy if the prevalence of *E coli* resistance is ≥ 20%.[17] Trimethoprin/sulfamethoxazole should also not be used if the patient is allergic to TMP/SMX, has been treated in the last 3 months with antibiotics (ie, TMP/SMX), or has been recently hospitalized. In these cases, antimicrobial treatment (ie, nitrofurantoin, third-generation cephalosporins) should be used based on identification of the pathogen and the sensitivities[18] (Table 116-2).

Even though the frequency of fluoroquinolone use for cystitis in adults has more than doubled over the past decade, ciprofloxacin is not approved by the US Food and Drug Administration (FDA) for adolescents younger than 18 years of age with uncomplicated UTI. There is also increasing concern of overuse of this class of medications. The FDA has approved ciprofloxacin for use in children 1 to 17 years of age for complicated UTI and pyelonephritis due to *E coli* (see the following). Ciprofloxacin is not a drug of first choice due to increased adverse events compared to controls, including events related to joints or surrounding tissues.

**Complicated** cystitis includes the following special circumstances: male gender, chronic conditions or

**Table 116-2**

**Suggested Treatment of Urinary Tract Infections in Adolescent Females and Males[1,9,19,20]**

| *Type of Urinary Tract Infection* | *Suggested Course of Therapy[a,b]* | *Selected Common Adverse Reactions to Therapy or Cautions (Pregnancy Risk Factor)* |
|---|---|---|
| **Cystitis**<br>Uncomplicated infection (see text) | **3-Day Oral Treatment[b]**<br>• Cefpodoxime proxetil 200 mg every 12 hours<br>• Nitrofurantoin 50–100 mg/dose every 6 hours, or macrocrystal/monohydrate 100 mg twice a day (maximum dose of 400 mg/day)<br>• TMP/SMX 160/800 mg twice a day[b]<br>• Trimethoprim 100 mg twice a day<br>• Amoxicillin 250–500 mg every 8 hours<br>• Amoxicillin-clavulanate 875/125 mg twice a day<br>• Ciprofloxacin extended release—500 mg once a day[c] | TMP/SMX (C): nausea, vomiting, anorexia, diarrhea, allergic rash, photosensitivity, dizziness, headache, lethargy<br>Ciprofloxacin[c] (C): nausea, headache, dizziness, photosensitivity, agitation, insomnia, lightheadedness, anxiety, increased risk of tendonitis and tendon rupture<br>Cephalosporins: see individual medication<br>Nitrofurantoin (B): Caution with impaired renal function, patients with G-6-PD deficiency, anemia, vitamin B deficiency, diabetes mellitus, or electrolyte abnormalities |
| Complicated/Special circumstances (see text—diabetes mellitus, sickle cell disease, prolonged symptoms, etc) | Antibiotic choices are similar to previously given for up to 7 days<br>For pregnancy, oral antibiotic choices are based on pregnancy risk factor. Based on clinical assessment, hospitalization with appropriate parenteral antibiotics may be indicated | |
| Recurrent infections including postcoital prophylaxis | For long-term prophylaxis: Half daily dose of TMP/SMX (low-dose formulation) nitrofurantoin, or ciprofloxacin[c] taken at bedtime<br>For postcoital prophylaxis: TMP/SMX (low-dose formulation), nitrofurantoin or cephalexin | |
| **Acute pyelonephritis**<br>Outpatient/ Uncomplicated (mild to moderate illness without gastrointestinal symptoms, no history of renal stones, urinary tract abnormalities, etc) | **10–14-day oral treatment (some suggest to initiate parenteral therapy for 2-3 days followed by oral therapy to complete treatment course)[b,d]**<br>• Cefixime 400 mg divided 12–24 hours<br>• Cefpodoxime proxetil 200 mg twice a day<br>• Ciprofloxacin 500 mg twice a day OR extended release—1,000 mg once a day[c]<br>• TMP/SMX 160/800 mg twice a day[b] | |

(*Continued*)

## Table 116-2 (Continued)

| *Type of Urinary Tract Infection* | *Suggested Course of Therapy*[a,b] | *Selected Common Adverse Reactions to Therapy or Cautions (Pregnancy Risk Factor)* |
|---|---|---|
| Hospitalized due to severity of symptoms | **Parenteral treatment**<br>• Cefepime 1 g every 12 hours<br>• Cefotaxime 1–2 g every 6–12 hours<br>• Ceftriaxone 1–2 g each day<br>• Gentamicin 3–6 mg/kg per day divided every 8 hours. Some studies have suggested once daily dosing. Gentamicin may be combined with ampicillin 25–50 mg/kg (maximum dose 1 g) every 6 hours<br>• Ciprofloxacin 200–400 mg every 12 hours[c]<br>• Ticarcillin/clavulanic acid and imipenem have also been given parenterally to treat urinary tract infections | |

[a]All dosages are **suggestions only** for children (>12 years of age) and adults weighing more than 40 kilograms. Some drugs require adjustment for renal disease or specific glomerular filtration rates (GFR). Use of these medications should be by physicians experienced in the treatment/management of adolescents and young adults with urinary tract infections. It is suggested that the physician should check medication dosing, maximum dosage, labeling, and safety information on all agents prior to prescribing. **For pregnant adolescents, physicians should review pregnancy risk factor categories prior to prescribing.**

[b]Local antimicrobial susceptibility should be consulted and may influence the therapeutic choice. Trimethoprim/sulfamethoxazole (TMP/SMX) should not be used as empiric therapy if the prevalence of *E coli* resistance is ≥ 20%.

[c]Ciprofloxacin is ONLY approved for patients 18 years of age or older. Recent FDA approval for ciprofloxacin has been obtained for use in children 1–17 years of age for complicated UTI and pyelonephritis due to *E coli.* Oral dosage for children is 20–30 mg/kg/day divided twice a day with a maximum dose of 1.5 g/day. **Ciprofloxacin is not a drug of first choice (due to increased adverse effects related to joints and/or surrounding tissues.**)

[d]Consider changing to oral therapy following a good clinical response, reduction in C reactive protein, and a negative urine culture to complete the treatment course. Antibiotic choice should be based on sensitivities.

immunocompromised patients (diabetes mellitus, sickle cell disease, renal transplantation), gastrointestinal symptoms, prolonged symptoms, history of urinary tract abnormalities such as VUR, atypical pathogens, recent antimicrobial use or treatment of a UTI, or a pregnant woman. In these instances, the choice of antimicrobial therapy is similar to that for uncomplicated infections, but the duration of therapy is usually at least 7 days. For pregnant adolescents and young adults, it is necessary to review the **pregnancy risk factor categories** prior to prescribing any medication.

For relief of pain, burning, and discomfort, phenazopyridine may be prescribed. The drug will turn the urine reddish-orange. Side effects, which are quite rare, include a skin rash or a skin color change to blue or blue-purple; respiratory distress, including shortness of breath, tightness in the chest, and wheezing; fever; decreased urine production; and swelling of the extremities with weight gain. The dosage for adolescents and adults is 200 mg given up to 3 times per day.

In cases of recurrent lower UTI (more than 2 documented infections in a 6-month period or more than 3 documented infections in a 12-month period), it is reasonable to prescribe a prophylactic antibiotic, at half the daily dosage, given at bedtime. TMP/SMX is used most often in children and adolescents, although nitrofurantoin and ciprofloxacin (older than 18 years of age) are also used.

In regard to asymptomatic bacteriuria, there is no apparent benefit of treatment in healthy, nonpregnant, adolescent females or in healthy males. The only populations that may benefit from screening and treatment are pregnant adolescents and young women, or patients undergoing genitourinary surgery with the potential for disruption of the mucosa and/or bleeding.

For **acute pyelonephritis** that is of mild to moderate severity, oral therapy for approximately 10 to 14 days may be appropriate (Table 116-2). Oral therapy should only be used in nontoxic-appearing and compliant patients. If patients remain symptomatic or worsen, intravenous therapy should be initiated. However, some authors suggest parenteral therapy for 2 to 3 days followed by oral therapy. In patients with **complicated pyelonephritis** (history of kidney stones or urinary tract abnormalities such as hydroureter, prune belly syndrome, posterior urethral valves) or severe cases of pyelonephritis (toxic appearing or unable to tolerate oral therapy), parenteral therapy should be started (ie, a third-generation cephalosporin or gentamicin with ampicillin). The duration of parenteral therapy will be guided by the duration of fever, clinical response to therapy/clinical status, and laboratory tests (C-reactive protein, etc). In most cases, the switch to oral therapy can occur by day 5. If parenteral therapy is required for the entire course, a peripherally inserted central catheter (PICC) line should be considered.

## SUMMARY

The evaluation and management of UTI in adolescents and young adults is different from that in infants and children. In many cases of uncomplicated cystitis and mild acute pyelonephritis in adolescents, imaging the urinary tract is not necessary. The use of empiric first line therapy with TMP/SMX is a reasonable approach unless there are high resistance rates to *E coli* in the community.

*The authors appreciate helpful suggestions from Dr. Kristin Rager.*

## REFERENCES

1. Bonny AE, Brouhard BH. Urinary tract infections among adolescents. *Adolesc Med.* 2005;16:149-161

2. Zorc JJ, Kiddoo DA, Shaw KN. Diagnosis and management of pediatric urinary tract infections. *Clinical Microbiology Reviews.* 2005;18:417-422

3. Donnenberg MS. Enterobacteriaceae. In: Mandell GL, Bennett JE, Dolin R, eds. *Mandell, Douglas, and Bennett's Principles and Practice of Infectious Diseases*. 6th ed. Philadelphia, PA: Elsevier; 2005:2567-2586

4. Sobel JD, Kaye D. Urinary tract infections. In: Mandell GL, Bennett JE, Dolin R. *Mandell, Douglas, and Bennett's Principles and Practice of Infectious Diseases.* 6th ed. Philadelphia, PA: Elsevier Churchill Livingstone; 2005:875-905

5. Hooton TM, Scholes D, Hughes JP, et al. A prospective study of risk factors for symptomatic urinary tract infection in young women. *N Eng J Med.* 1996;335:468-474

6. Hooton TM, Scholes D, Stapleton AE, et al. A prospective study of asymptomatic bacteriuria in sexually active young women. *N Eng J Med.* 2000;343:992-997

7. Nicolle LE, Bradley S, Colgan R, et al. Infectious Diseases Society of America Guidelines for the diagnosis and treatment of asymptomatic bacteriuria in adults. *Clinical Infectious Diseases.* 2005;40:643-654

8. Gearhart JP, Rink RC. *Mouriquand PDE: Pediatric Urology*. Philadelphia, PA: WB Saunders; 2001:251

9. D'Angelo LJ, Neinstein LS. Genitourinary tract disorders. In: Neinstein LS, Gordon CM, Katzman DK, Rosen DS, Woods KR, eds. *Adolescent Health Care: A Practical Guide.* 5th ed. Philadelphia, PA: Lippincott Williams and Wilkins; 2007:377- 383

10. Freeto JP, Jay MS. What's really going on down there? A practical approach to the adolescent who has gynecologic complaints. *Pediatr Clin N Am.* 2006;53:529-545

11. Blake DR, Doherty BS. Effect of perineal cleansing on contamination rate of mid stream urine culture. *J Pediatr Adolesc Gynecol.* 2006;19:31-34

12. Huppert JS, Biro FM, Lan D, et al. Urinary symptoms in adolescent females. *J Pediatr Health.* 2007;40:418-424

13. Pappas PG. Laboratory in the diagnosis and management of urinary tract infections. *Med Clin North Am.* 1991;75:313

14. Feld LG, Waz WR, Perez LM, Joseph DB. Hematuria: an integrated medical and surgical approach. *Ped Clin North America.* 1997;44:1191-1210

15. *Nephrogenic Fibrosing Dermopathy Associated with Exposure to Gadolinium-Containing Contrast Agents — St. Louis, Missouri, 2002-2006 MMWR Morb Mortal Wkly Rep.* 2007;56:137-141

16. Warren JW, Abrutyn E, Hebel JR, et al. Guidelines for antimicrobial treatment of uncomplicated acute bacterial cystitis and acute pyelonephritis in women. *Clin Infect Dis.* 1999;29:745-758

17. Gupta K. Emerging antibiotic resistance in urinary tract pathogens. *Infect Dis Clin N Am.* 2003;17:243-259

18. Hooton TM, Besser R, Foxman B, et al. Acute uncomplicated cystitis in an era of increasing antibiotic resistance: a proposed approach to empirical therapy. *Clin Infect Dis.* 2004;39:75-80

19. Hooton TM. The current management strategies for community-acquired urinary tract infections. *Infect Dis Clin N Am.* 2003;17:303-332

20. Feld LG, Cimino M, Rosenfeld WD. *Goryeb Children's Hospital Pediatric Dosing Handbook*. Lexicomp, 2005-2006 ed

# CHAPTER 117

## Nephritis and Nephrosis

ASHTON CHEN, DO • HOWARD TRACHTMAN, MD

### INTRODUCTION

Under most circumstances, glomerular disease develops as a consequence of immune-mediated injury or genetic alterations in structural proteins within the glomerular tuft that leads to disruption of filtration barrier function. In the absence of a validated classification scheme based on a specific etiology or well-characterized pathophysiological mechanisms, clinicians have been forced to rely on 2 general syndromes to categorize patients with glomerular disease, namely nephritic and nephrotic states. These terms represent relatively distinct and reproducible patterns of clinical and laboratory findings that have been used to guide the evaluation and treatment of patients with glomerulopathies. In particular, the **nephritic state** refers to the clinical picture that arises when the key feature of the illness is a reduction in glomerular filtration rate (GFR). The degree of renal dysfunction and azotemia may be mild and subclinical in degree, or it may be severe and associated with a range of other abnormalities. In contrast, the pivotal feature in patients with **nephrotic disorders** is massive proteinuria, whereas the GFR is usually well preserved. These syndromes are not mutually exclusive, have overlapping disease mechanisms, and do not definitively point to specific disease entities. Thus, the same disease often must be considered in patients with nephritic or nephrotic states. Moreover, the names of most renal diseases are frequently terms coined by nephropathologists and have no obvious connection to the cause or presentation of the illness. As a consequence, medical students, house officers, and general practitioners commonly express their utter confusion and become frustrated when confronted with a patient with new-onset glomerular disease.

This chapter attempts to provide a comprehensive diagnostic approach to patients that emphasizes that nephritic and nephrotic states are entities along a spectrum of glomerular injury. Although acknowledging the shortcomings in the state of our knowledge, it is designed to provide a rational framework for a complete and cost-effective evaluation of adolescent patients with nephritic and nephrotic disorders.

### MECHANISMS OF DISEASE

Nephritic states on the simplest level represent inflammation of the glomerulus. It can be triggered by any 1 of the following immune mediators, acting alone or in combination: (1) deposition in the kidney of preformed circulating immune complexes; (2) the formation *in situ* of immune complexes when circulating antibodies bind to endogenous or exogenous antigens present in the kidney; (3) the classical or alternative complement cascades; (4) direct antibody-mediated injury; and (5) leukocyte or mononuclear cell infiltration and damage.[1,2]

Systemic lupus erythematosus (SLE) is the paradigmatic example of a disease caused by the first mechanism, namely soluble immune complex deposition. The location and amount of immune complexes deposited in the glomerulus reflects a net effect of antibody class, molecular size and charge, and relative amount of antigen and antibody. In contrast, postinfectious nephritis probably reflects the second disease process, namely *in situ* immune complex formation provoked by alteration of native glomerular proteins and intrarenal binding of antibody to specific antibodies. Membranoproliferative glomerulonephritis (MPGN) and another form of SLE provide examples of the third type of inflammation with activation of the classical complement pathway in SLE and of the alternative complement system in MPGN. The fourth category is illustrated by Goodpasture syndrome, which results from the binding of antibodies directed against specific epitopes in the type IV collagen component of the glomerular basement membrane. In the fifth category, leukocytes or monocytes infiltrate the glomerular tuft as in postinfectious glomerulonephritis (which also belongs to the second category) and Wegener granulomatosis. These cells mediate damage to endothelial, mesangial, and glomerular epithelial cells by releasing lytic enzymes, stimulating excessive production of reactive oxygen and nitrogen molecules, and promoting the synthesis of vasoactive peptides. The mechanisms of glomerular injury in nephritic states are summarized in Table 117-1. It is worth noting that there are a handful of glomerular disorders, such as Alport syndrome, that are routinely

**Table 117-1**

**Mechanisms of Glomerular Injury in Nephritic States**

| *Category* | *Mechanism* | *Prototype Disease* |
|---|---|---|
| Preformed immune complexes | Direct injury<br>Activation of complement | Systemic lupus erythematosis (SLE) |
| *In situ* immune complexes | Podocyte injury | Postinfectious glomerulonephritis |
| Complement cascade | | |
| 1. Classical pathway | Chemotaxis | SLE |
| 2. Alternate pathway | Direct damage via membrane attack complex (MAC) | Membranoproliferative glomerulonephritis (MPGN) |
| Antibody | Injury to basement membrane | Goodpasture syndrome |
| Leukocytes | Release of proteolytic enzymes<br>Reactive oxygen molecules | Wegener granulomatosis |

included in the category of nephritic states. However, this classification is misleading because these entities do not reflect primary glomerular inflammation but rather are the consequence of genetic abnormalities in the composition of the glomerulus leading to a progressive glomerular dysfunction.

Nephrotic conditions represent an abnormal increase in the permeability of the glomerulus. They can be the consequence of either (1) loss of the negative charges normally present on the surface of endothelial and epithelial cells and the matrix components of the membrane within the glomerular barrier; or (2) an increase in the effective pore size that determines filtration of large molecular weight solutes such as albumin.[3] Although minimal change nephrotic syndrome (MCNS) results almost exclusively from loss of the net anionic charge in the glomerulus, most other causes of nephrotic syndrome represent a combination of both defects. The disturbance in glomerular barrier function can arise from genetic abnormalities in structural proteins in the podocyte, which is the terminally differentiated visceral epithelial cell that rests on the external surface of the glomerular basement membrane.[4] Alternatively, an increased permeability to protein can be caused by a variety of immune cell-derived mediators that enhance the leakage of protein without compromising GFR. Although a variety of candidate molecules have been identified, such as vascular endothelial cell growth factor, much work needs to be done to establish the immunobiology of proteinuria in nephrotic states. It is important to emphasize that, in marked contrast to nephritic states, there is minimal infiltration of the glomerulus by inflammatory cells in most cases of nephrotic syndrome.

## NEPHRITIC AND NEPHROTIC STATES: A SPECTRUM OF DISEASE

Before moving on to the discussion of the evaluation and management of specific disease states, it is worthwhile to sketch a schematic diagram that places nephritis and nephrosis, 2 interrelated glomerular disease syndromes, along a spectrum of clinical manifestations (Figure 117-1). To begin, one can draw 2 lines in opposite directions from the origin. The line extending toward the left can be labeled the nephritic axis, and it has 3 distinct positions—hematuria alone, the combination of hematuria and proteinuria with a normal GFR, and a complete nephritic syndrome with azotemia, hematuria, and proteinuria. The line extending toward the right can be labeled the nephrotic axis and it has 2 distinct positions—proteinuria and a complete nephrotic syndrome with proteinuria, edema, hypoalbuminemia, and hypercholesterolemia. The ordinate represents the percentage of patients with a given disease entity who present with 1 of the previous 5 presentations. If one then selects a specific disease, one can draw a curve with peaks of varying height that reflect the likelihood of presenting with hematuria alone, hematuria and proteinuria, acute nephritis, proteinuria alone, or nephrotic syndrome. Some diseases such as MCNS or Goodpasture syndrome, have one predominant type of presentation, nephrotic syndrome in the former and acute nephritis in the latter. The task of the nephrologist is to draw a perpendicular line through 1 of the 5 modes of presentation of nephritis, and based on the clinical history and laboratory findings, define a hierarchy of diseases in descending order of likelihood of occurrence in a given patient. This

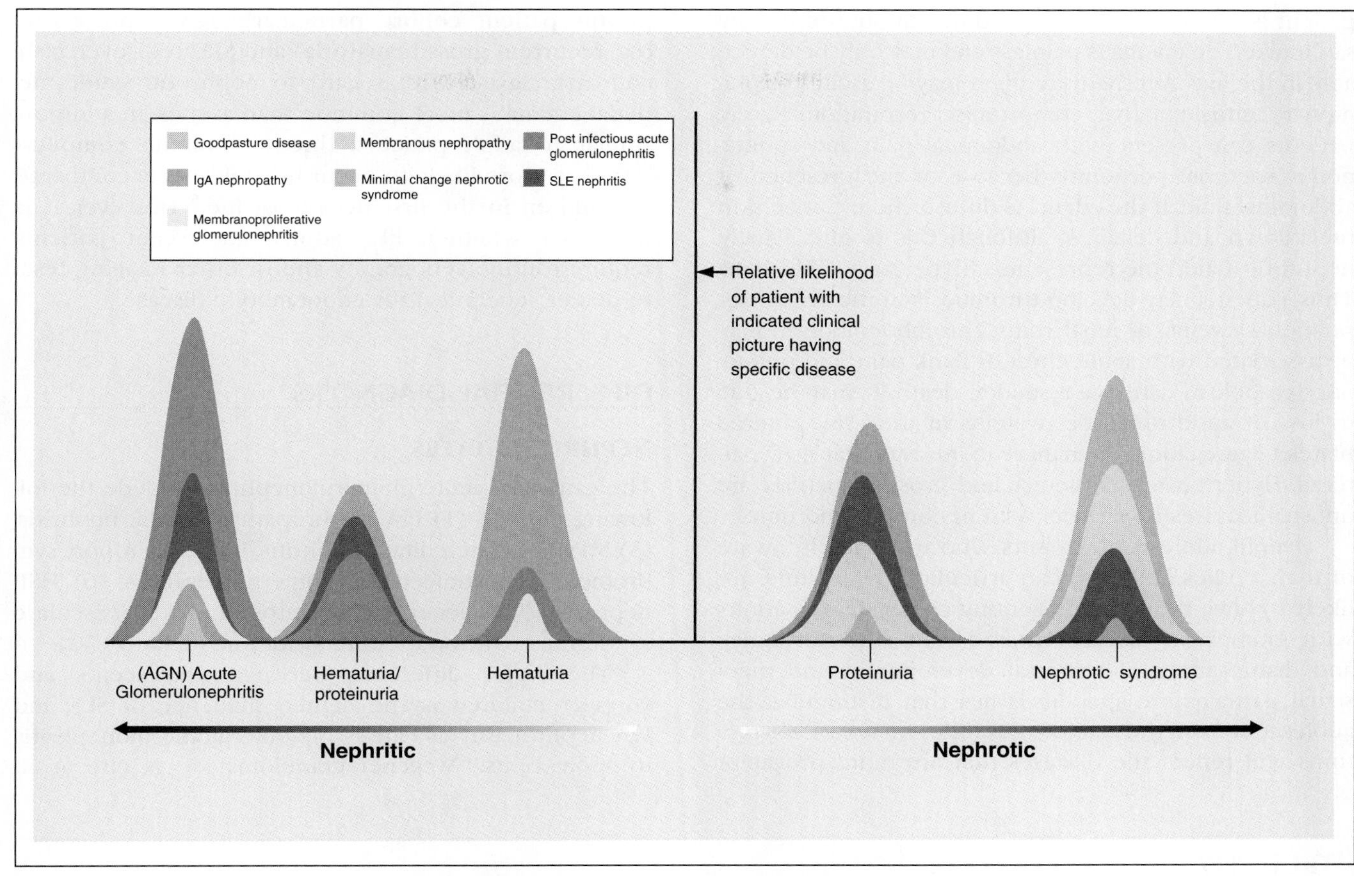


FIGURE 117-1 This illustration schematically depicts the interrelationship between nephritic and nephrotic states, the likelihood of specific clinical presentations for select entities, and the overlapping nature of glomerular diseases.

chapter delineates how this task is performed specifically for the adolescent patient and highlights where the differential diagnoses differ from infants and preadolescent patients and adults.

## CLINICAL PRESENTATION

### NEPHRITIC STATES

Acute glomerulonephritis, which is dominated by a reduction in GFR, is most commonly heralded by the sudden onset of gross hematuria. The urine is cloudy in appearance and the color can range from dark green to cola-colored, depending on the extent of chemical modification of the released hemoglobin pigment. If the urine is tea-colored but clear the likely explanation is hemoglobinuria or myoglobinuria. In glomerular hematuria, the entire stream is bloody from the onset until the completion of micturition and clots are never detected in the urine. Terminal hematuria or clots are indicative of nonglomerular hematuria. The passage of urine is usually pain free although some causes of glomerular gross hematuria such as IgA nephropathy can cause flank or loin pain. Other signs and symptoms of acute nephritis can be the result of the impaired kidney function, per se, such as lethargy, abdominal pain, anorexia, and fatigue. If the patient has acute hypertension, then there may be complaints such as headache, confusion, or seizures. Finally, the patient may display manifestations of the underlying disease process such as fever, rash, joint pains (SLE and Henoch Schönlein purpura [HSP] nephritis), melena (HSP nephritis), or hemoptysis (Goodpasture syndrome).

### NEPHROTIC STATES

Nephrotic syndrome, in which heavy proteinuria is the key feature, almost invariably presents with peripheral edema. Recognition of the cause of the edema may be delayed by inappropriate attribution to local infection or allergy. The localization and degree of swelling depends upon the interval between the onset of disease and its clinical recognition, the age of the patient, whether the patient is active or sedentary, and the amount of dietary salt intake. The edema is painless and may only be detectable in the legs. Alternatively, there may be ascites or pulmonary effusions that compromise respiration. Rarely, patients can present with abdominal pain and spontaneous bacterial peritonitis because of the presence of abdominal fluid. If the edema is diffuse, there can be skin breakdown and cellulitis, although this is rare. Finally, nephrotic syndrome represents a hypercoagulable state. Thus, patients may develop thrombosis in the arms, legs, pulmonary veins, or renal veins. Thromboembolism may be associated with acute chest or flank pain, and pulmonary embolism can cause sudden death. It may be due to loss of antithrombotic proteins in the urine, altered platelet aggregation, or changes in intravascular flow patterns. Hypertension, azotemia, and gross hematuria are unusual features in patients with nephrotic syndrome.

Overall, adolescent patients, who are generally aware of their bodies and who can articulate complaints, are likely to have the same presenting complaints as adults with glomerular disease. Altered school performance and disturbances in pubertal development and menstrual patterns are specific issues that distinguish the adolescent from the school-age child. The specific symptoms will reflect the diseases that are more prevalent in this patient cohort, particularly IgA nephropathy (eg, recurrent gross hematuria) and SLE, (eg, fever, rash, and arthralgias). With regard to nephrotic syndrome, pedal edema is more common than ascites. In addition, similar to adult patients, thromboembolic complications are more likely to occur in adolescents compared to children in the first decade of life.[5] However, it is unknown whether, like adults, adolescent patients require routine venography and/or other imaging tests to detect subclinical thromboembolic disease.

## DIFFERENTIAL DIAGNOSIS

### NEPHRITIC STATES

The causes of acute glomerulonephritis include the following entities: (1) IgA nephropathy; (2) SLE nephritis; (3) MPGN; (4) hereditary nephritis, including Alport syndrome; (5) postinfectious glomerulonephritis; (6) HSP nephritis; (7) Wegener granulomatosis and other vasculitic syndromes; (8) Goodpasture syndrome (Table 117-2).

The major difference between adolescents and younger children is the higher incidence of SLE and IgA nephropathy as causes of acute glomerulonephritis in adolescents.[6] Wegener granulomatosis is rare at all

**Table 117-2**

**Nephritic Disorders in Adolescent Patients**

| *Disease* | *Characteristic Features* |
|---|---|
| IgA nephropathy | • Male predominance<br>• Recurrent gross hematuria during upper respiratory infections |
| Systemic lupus erythematosus (SLE) | • Female predominance<br>• 5 World Health Organization (WHO) histopathological classes |
| Membranoproliferative glomerulonephritis (MPGN) | • Female predominance<br>• 3 variants, all with hypocomplementemia<br>• Initial presentation with hematuria |
| Alport syndrome/hereditary nephritis | • 85% of cases are x-linked<br>• Associated with high-tone hearing loss |
| Postinfectious glomerulonephritis | • 1-3 week latency after pharyngitis or impetigo |
| Henoch Schönlein purpura (HSP) nephritis | • No diagnostic blood test<br>• Defined by mesangial IgA deposition |
| Wegener granulomatosis/antineutrophil cytoplasmic antibody (ANCA)-associated vasculitis | • Upper respiratory/sinus infection<br>• Need for sustained immunosuppressive therapy |
| Goodpasture syndrome | • Pulmonary hemorrhage<br>• Plasmapheresis has no effect on resolution of kidney disease |

ages but is more common in the second decade of life in pediatric patients. Postinfectious glomerulonephritis is more common in the first decade of life. The other entities occur equally in children and adolescents.

### NEPHROTIC STATES

Unlike acute glomerulonephritis, nephrotic syndrome is divided into a primary or idiopathic category and a secondary category. The primary or idiopathic category includes: (1) MCNS; (2) focal segmental glomerulosclerosis (FSGS); (3) membranous nephropathy (MN); and (4) MPGN. In contrast to younger patients with primary nephrotic syndrome, in whom nearly 80% to 90% have MCNS, adolescent patients have a much higher incidence of MPGN and MN, in the range of 10% to 20% for each lesion and a corresponding decrease in the occurrence of MCNS.[7] The likelihood of FSGS has risen across the entire pediatric spectrum and accounts for approximately 20% of all cases of primary nephrotic syndrome at all ages. It is unclear whether the distribution of causes of primary nephrotic syndrome differs among various ethnic groups in adolescents (Table 117-3).

The secondary causes include: (1) SLE nephritis; (2) chronic infections, eg, HIV, hepatitis B, hepatitis C, malaria, syphilis; (3) other, namely postinfectious glomerulonephritis; HSP nephritis; medications; and malignancies (Table 117-3). One important cause of nephrotic syndrome in adult patients that is unlikely to cause clinically evident disease in pediatric patients, even in adolescents, is diabetes mellitus because of the prolonged latency between disease onset and the appearance of overt diabetic nephropathy. Hodgkin and non-Hodgkin lymphoma are rare causes of nephrotic syndrome across the entire pediatric age range.

It is worth noting that the glomerular injury caused by several glomerulopathies (eg, SLE nephritis, MPGN, postinfectious nephritis, HSP nephritis) may result in the features of an acute glomerulonephritis or the nephrotic syndrome or a combination of both. This is consistent with the previous section emphasizing the clinical nature of the classification of glomerular disease. Thus, it is not surprising that many of the disease entities under discussion appear on lists of causes both of acute glomerulonephritis and nephrotic syndrome.

**Table 117-3**

**Nephrotic Disorders in Adolescent Patients**

| *Disease* | *Characteristic Features* |
|---|---|
| *Primary* | |
| Minimal change nephrotic syndrome (MCNS) | Steroid responsive |
| Focal segmental glomerulosclerosis (FSGS) | Rising incidence<br>Proteinuria or nephrotic syndrome |
| Membranous nephropathy (MN) | Idiopathic or secondary causes such as SLE |
| Membranoproliferative glomerulonephritis (MPGN) | Persistent hypocomplementemia |
| *Secondary* | |
| Systemic lupus erythematosus (SLE) | More common presentation than nephritis |
| Chronic infections eg, HIV, hepatitis B/C, malaria | History of recent travel and exposure are key for diagnosis |
| Miscellaneous, eg, HSP, postinfectious, drugs | Nonsteroidal anti-inflammatory drugs are common cause |

## LABORATORY EVALUATION

### NEPHRITIC STATES

The key diagnostic test for a patient with acute glomerulonephritis is the urinalysis. The urine is grossly bloody in more than 80% of cases. The sample is cloudy and can be tea-colored or greenish in tint depending on the degree of oxidation of the hemoglobin pigment. Under the microscope, the erythrocytes display a dysmorphic appearance, and there are characteristic red blood cell casts. When the urine is grossly bloody, it may be easier to detect these formed elements in an unspun specimen because overlapping and clumping of the red blood cells in the urine sediment obtained after centrifugation of the sample may obscure essential features.

After obtaining a complete serum biochemical profile to assess blood urea nitrogen (BUN), serum creatinine, and potassium concentrations, and a complete blood count (CBC), the most important laboratory test is the measurement of the C3 level.[1,2] This facilitates distinguishing between hypocomplementemic forms of disease—postinfectious nephritis, SLE, and MPGN—and the normocomplementemic entities—HSP, IgA nephropathy, hereditary nephritis, vasculitis, Wegener granulomatosis, and Goodpasture syndrome. The other key diagnostic tests include antistreptolysin-O (ASLO), C4, antinuclear antibody test (ANA), double-stranded anti-DNA (dsDNA), and antineutrophil cytoplasmic antibody (ANCA) levels. Measurement of antiglomerular basement membrane is reserved for patients with concomitant hemoptysis or linear, immunofluorescence staining of the glomerular basement membrane in the renal biopsy specimen. A kidney biopsy should be performed in an adolescent with acute nephritis in whom the diagnosis is uncertain or when the disease is unusually severe or prolonged. In those cases, a tissue diagnosis and histopathological assessment is needed to define the expected response to treatment and long-term outcome.

### NEPHROTIC STATES

A dipstick examination usually is the first test used to confirm the diagnosis of nephrotic syndrome. This assessment is only semiquantitative in nature, however, and can be influenced by the urinary pH or concentration. Therefore, it is necessary to measure the protein excretion directly. Although quantitative measurement of proteinuria has traditionally been done on 24-hour urine collections, it is more physiological and convenient to measure the protein:creatinine ratio in an early-morning urine specimen.[8] This reflects urine formed in the recumbent position and prevents misclassification of orthostatic proteinuria as significant. Orthostatic proteinuria is especially prevalent in adolescents and may account for nearly 70% of patient referrals to a pediatric nephrology service for evaluation of proteinuria.[9] The urine protein:creatinine ratio is normally <0.2. A ratio that is tenfold higher, or >2.0, is regarded as nephrotic-range proteinuria.

As in acute nephritis, measurement of the C3 level is the pivotal test in determining the etiology in an adolescent with new-onset nephrotic syndrome.[1,2] Causes of nephrotic syndrome associated with hypocomplementemia include SLE, MPGN, and postinfectious nephritis. Thus, a low C3 level can help focus the diagnostic evaluation and guide therapy.

With regard to the performance of a diagnostic kidney biopsy, there are some pediatric nephrologists who recommend the procedure for all adolescent patients with new-onset nephrotic syndrome because of the relatively low likelihood of MCNS. Because steroids are usually the first line therapy in all patients and response to this treatment has such important prognostic implications, it is reasonable to give most adolescents a trial of corticosteroids. Therefore, a renal biopsy can be reserved for those patients in whom there are distinct clinical or laboratory findings that point toward a disease other then MCNS or who are resistant to a standard course of steroids.[10]

## ACUTE *VERSUS* CHRONIC DISEASE

A key question in evaluating a patient with nephrosis or nephritis is whether it is a new-onset disease or whether it represents a flare-up in activity in a previously diagnosed condition. An accurate answer to this question is important in gauging the urgency of treatment and defining the expected response to therapeutic interventions. Occasionally, patients present with manifestations of acute nephritis or the nephrotic syndrome and are found to have evidence of chronic renal insufficiency of longstanding glomerular disease, such as short stature, delayed puberty, disproportionate anemia, or x-ray findings of skeletal changes consistent with renal osteodystrophy. In these patients, there will be a marked discrepancy between the estimated GFR, which assumes that the patient is in a steady state, and the directly measured level of kidney function using radionuclide scans or a 24-hour urine collection to determine creatinine clearance.

## TREATMENT

### NEPHRITIC STATES

The treatment of the various forms of acute glomerulonephritis is far less straightforward than the management of acute nephrotic syndrome (see the following). The cornerstone is conservative medical therapy designed to prevent extracellular fluid volume overload, hypertension, and hyperkalemia. Dialysis is indicated in patients with severe refractory hypertension, respiratory distress, hyperkalemia, or symptomatic azotemia.

The therapeutic options for patients with acute nephritis include pulse intravenous methylprednisolone, 30 mg/kg per dose to a maximum of 1 gram, alkylating agents, and plasmapheresis. Pulse steroid therapy is effective in all forms of severe nephritis, provided it is initiated within 3 weeks of disease onset. However, it is usually not required in postinfectious glomerulonephritis because patients improve on their own and their long-term prognosis is favorable. Adjunctive use of alkylating agents has dramatically improved the outcome of patients with Wegener granulomatosis and systemic necrotizing vasculitis. There are numerous ongoing clinical trials to assess the efficacy and side effect profile of other immunosuppressive agents (eg, mycophenolate mofetil or rituximab) compared with cyclophosphamide. In patients with Goodpasture syndrome, plasmapheresis may prevent pulmonary hemorrhage, but does not appear to have a beneficial effect on recovery of kidney function. Recent studies suggest that adding plasmapheresis to the treatment regimen in patients with ANCA-related nephritis may improve renal function. However, this procedure does not have any beneficial effect in patients with SLE nephritis. There is an urgent need for newer, more targeted therapies for patients with acute glomerulonephritis.[11]

## NEPHROTIC STATES

The first line therapy for adolescents with new-onset primary nephrotic syndrome is an 8- to 12-week course of steroids, daily for half of the time and every other day for the remainder of the treatment period. The relative benefits of a 12- versus 8-week course are controversial and practice patterns vary.[12]

If a patient is steroid-resistant, a renal biopsy is mandatory to determine the etiology of the nephrotic syndrome, and subsequent treatment is guided by the renal histopathology. Patients with MPGN usually have persistent hypocomplementemia. They are, therefore, tentatively identified at presentation or shortly thereafter and undergo early renal biopsy. This is important because daily steroids in MPGN may greatly aggravate hypertension and provoke hypertensive encephalopathy. Steroids should not be prescribed when MPGN is suspected. Instead, on confirmation of the diagnosis, patients with MPGN should be given prolonged treatment for at least 2 years with every other day steroids until there is resolution of glomerular inflammation in a follow-up kidney biopsy. Secondary causes of nephrotic syndrome such as SLE, HSP, and hepatitis B should be treated after consultation with appropriate subspecialists. There is no proven therapy for FSGS, and the National Institutes of Health is sponsoring a multicenter randomized clinical trial comparing the efficacy of cyclosporine to the combination of mycophenolate mofetil (Cellcept) and oral pulses of dexamethasone. The treatment of MN is also highly contentious, with some nephrologists recommending supportive care alone with an angiotensin-converting enzyme inhibitor and/or an angiotensin receptor blocker, whereas others advise intensive immunosuppressive therapy with a combination of steroids and alkylating agents or cyclosporine. Because of the rarity of MN overall in pediatric patients, it is advisable to consult with an internal medicine nephrologist before embarking on a course of therapy in an adolescent with newly identified MN.

In patients with MCNS who relapse frequently or are steroid dependent and who manifest evidence of steroid toxicity, treatment options include: (1) extended administration of low-dose steroids; (2) alkylating agents; (3) calcineurin inhibitors; and (4) mycophenolate mofetil. Most adolescents are highly sensitive to the adverse cosmetic side effects of steroids and are anxious to avoid their use. Moreover, it is hard to reconcile the potential for long-term gonadal toxicity resulting from an alkylating agent to treat a disease that ultimately should resolve without permanent renal damage. Therefore, calcineurin inhibitors such as cyclosporine (Neoral) or tacrolimus (Prograf) or mycophenolate mofetil are preferred second line agents in adolescents with steroid-dependent or frequently relapsing MCNS. The calcineurin inhibitors achieve a sustained remission in 85% to 90% of patients. However, these agents do not result in permanent remission because patients invariably relapse when the drug is stopped. In addition, the drugs can cause untoward cosmetic changes (hair growth, coarsening of features, and gingival hyperplasia), hypertension, hyperkalemia, and nephrotoxicity. The latter side effect mandates regular monitoring of drug levels and the serum creatinine concentration. It is for these reasons that the use of mycophenolate mofetil is becoming more widely accepted among pediatric nephrologists. The most common side effects of this antimetabolite, which selectively inhibits lymphocyte function, include gastrointestinal upset, hepatotoxicity, and bone marrow suppression. All of these complications are reversible with reduction in dose or cessation of the drug. Although mycophenolate mofetil is less effective than the calcineurin inhibitors, it is safer, has no permanent side effects, and requires less frequent monitoring.[13] Other immunomodulatory treatments include deflazocort and levamisole, but these agents are not routinely available and this has limited their widespread use.

Immunosuppressive treatment of MCNS may require up to 3 months of therapy to achieve remission of proteinuria. Even longer periods may be required for the other causes of nephrotic syndrome. Therefore, the patient can be expected to have persistent edema, which can interfere with normal activities. Moreover, peripheral edema and ascites increase the risk of local infection and peritonitis. Strategies to alleviate edema include dietary salt restriction and diuretics. Loop diuretics are usually required to promote a diuresis, and these medications may require administration 2 to 3 times a day because of low serum albumin concentrations and shortened duration of action. Addition of metolazone (Zaroxalyn) or a thiazide diuretic (Hydrodiuril) may enhance the efficacy of furosemide and other loop diuretics. However, careful monitoring is necessary to prevent hypokalemia and metabolic alkalosis. Intravenous albumin infusions should be restricted to patients with acute renal failure, peritonitis, respiratory compromise, or disabling anasarca.

## ISSUES INVOLVED IN THE PHARMACOLOGICAL MANAGEMENT OF ADOLESCENTS

It is well known that adolescence is a time of intense psychological change, and illness can profoundly affect a patient's self-image and sense of worth. Even under the best of circumstances adolescents may rebel against parental guidance and their need for independence is exacerbated by the demands of medical treatment. Thus, nonadherence is a well-documented problem that confronts any physician responsible for treating a sick adolescent.[14] Nephrologists must recognize this as they formulate therapeutic regimens for adolescents with nephrotic syndrome or acute nephritis. There are 3 key points to remember when treating these patients.[7] First, medications such as prednisone or cyclosporine can cause cosmetic changes that may prove unacceptable to an adolescent. These include acne, altered facies, hirsutism, and weight gain. In addition, prednisone and other steroids routinely alter mood and sleep patterns, side effects that may be especially troublesome to adolescents. Failure to acknowledge this and counsel the patient is an invitation to the patient to ignore the treatment recommendations. Second, alkylating agents can cause permanent gonadal injury, a key concern to adolescents. Every effort should be made to use the lowest effective dose and consider adjunctive therapy (leutinizing hormone-releasing hormone analogues) that can ameliorate this side effect. Finally, adolescents can have chaotic schedules and spend a great deal of time outside the home. This underscores the need to design regimens that can be easily incorporated into the lifestyle of adolescents so that adherence does not mandate complete disruption of their usual day-to-day routine. If the home environment is unstable the problems may be magnified. These concerns apply to all patients, but implementation of proper treatment is even more challenging in adolescents. Success is likely to require interaction of a broad range of disciplines, including adolescent medicine, psychiatry, nutrition, nursing, and social work.

## LONG-TERM PROGNOSIS

### NEPHRITIC STATES

In general, patients with IgA nephropathy do well, although 20% to 25% may progress to end-stage renal disease over 20 to 25 years of follow-up. The outcome for SLE is determined by the World Health Organization histological category. The widespread use of intravenous cyclophosphamide has improved renal survival. Nearly 50% of patients with MPGN will develop chronic kidney failure over 10 to 15 years of treatment. Moreover, nearly 20% may have recurrent disease after renal transplantation. Boys with X-linked Alport syndrome generally reach end-stage renal disease by the end of the second decade of life. Nearly all adolescents with postinfectious nephritis recover fully and maintain normal renal function indefinitely. The prognosis in adolescents with HSP nephritis is worse in those who present with acute nephritis or nephrotic syndrome and who have a large number of glomerular crescents in their diagnostic biopsy. Wegener granulomatosis and ANCA-associated vasculitis are rare in pediatric patients and they require aggressive immunosuppressive therapy. Goodpasture syndrome is usually characterized by fulminant disease and rapid progression to end stage.

### NEPHROTIC STATES

Of the 4 forms of primary nephrotic syndrome, only MCNS has a normal long-term prognosis. Thus, even though most patients will have relapsing disease, eventually MCNS resolves and renal function is normal. Focal segmental glomerulosclerosis progresses to kidney failure in 50% of patients over 5 to 10 years of follow-up. Membranous nephropathy has a variable outcome with resolution, persistent proteinuria, or deterioration in kidney function in equal proportions of patients. Among the secondary outcomes, adequate treatment of the underlying infection or withdrawal of the causative agent can lead to resolution of the kidney disease. However, in many cases, the renal injury is too severe and irreversible, leading to end-stage kidney failure.

## CONCLUSION

Nephritis and nephrotic syndrome are relatively uncommon but important manifestations of glomerular disease in adolescent patients. The clinical presentation in the former is dominated by the reduction in GFR, whereas in the latter it is marked by massive proteinuria. The overall differential diagnosis for both entities is similar to that in younger patients; however, the ranking of diseases in order of probable occurrence in adolescents is more comparable to adult patients. The laboratory investigation should commence with a complete urinalysis with a microscopic examination of the specimen, and include a serum biochemical profile and CBC. The C3 level is a key diagnostic test in acute nephritis and nephrotic syndrome. Biopsy is reserved for unusual or severe cases in each disease category. The treatment of glomerular diseases usually commences with oral corticosteroids. The use of second line immunosuppressive medications should be guided by the specific features in each case. The management of the adolescent patient with glomerular disease should take into account the full range of side effects of all drugs prescribed to ensure acceptance and compliance with the regimen. Consultation with a pediatric nephrologist is indicated for more severe cases to define the prognosis and implement long-term treatment.

## ACKNOWLEDGMENT

*The authors want to thank Bernard Gauthier, MD, for reviewing the chapter and for his thoughtful comments and editorial suggestions, and Lois Fischman, for her skilled artwork in preparing the figure.*

## REFERENCES

1. Hricik DE, Chung-Park M, Sedor JR. Glomerulonephritis. *N Engl J Med.* 1998;339:888-899

2. Madaio MP, Harrington JT. The diagnosis of glomerular diseases: acute glomerulonephritis and nephrotic syndrome. *Arch Int Med.* 2001;161:25-34

3. Deen WM. What determines glomerular capillary permeability? *J Clin Invest.* 2004;114:1412-1414

4. Niaudet P. Genetic forms of nephrotic syndrome. *Pediatr Nephrol.* 2004;19:1313-1318

5. Crew RJ, Radhakrishnan J, Appel G. Complications of the nephrotic syndrome and their treatment. *Clin Nephrol.* 2004;62(4):245-259

6. Nair R, Walker PD. Is IgA nephropathy the commonest primary glomerulopathy among young adults in the USA? *Kidney Int.* 2006;69:1455-1458

7. Hogg RJ. Adolescents with proteinuria and/or the nephrotic syndrome. *Adolesc Med.* 2005;16:163-172

8. Houser M. Assessment of proteinuria using random samples. *J Pediatr.* 1984;104:845-848

9. Trachtman H, Bergwerk A, Gauthier BG. Isolated proteinuria in children: natural history and indications for renal biopsy. *Clin Pediatr.* 1992;33:468-472

10. Stadermann MB, Lilien MR, van de Kar NCAJ, Monnens LAH, Schroder CH. Is biopsy required prior to cyclophosphamide in steroid-sensitive nephrotic syndrome? *Clin Nephrol.* 2003;60:315-317

11. Shankland S. The podocyte's response to injury: role in proteinuria and glomerulosclerosis. *Kidney Int.* 2006;69:2131-2147

12. Tune BM, Mendoza SA. Treatment of idiopathic nephrotic syndrome: regimens and outcomes in children and adults. *J Am Soc Nephrol.* 1997;8:824-832

13. Novak I, Frank R, Vento S, Vergara M, Gauthier BG, Trachtman H. Efficacy of mycophenolate mofetil in pediatric patients with steroid-dependent nephrotic syndrome. *Pediatr Nephrol.* 2005;20:1265-1268

14. Nevins TE. "Why do they do that?" The compliance conundrum. *Pediatr Nephrol.* 2005;20:845-848

# CHAPTER 118

# Hypertension: Significance, Diagnosis, and Management

JOSEPH T. FLYNN, MD, MS

## DEFINITIONS

The approach to defining hypertension (HTN) in younger adolescents (younger than 18 years) differs significantly from the approach in older adolescents (18 years or older) and adults. In adults, large-scale studies have demonstrated the development of cardiovascular and renal disease with increasing blood pressure (BP) in a continuous fashion, with increased risk beginning at BPs >115/75 mm Hg.[1] Recognizing this relationship, *The 7th Report of the Joint National Committee on Prevention, Detection, Evaluation, and Treatment of High Blood Pressure* defined HTN in adults (18 years or older) as a BP >140/90 mm Hg on 2 or more office visits, and created a new category of "prehypertension," denoting BPs >120/80 mm Hg, to call attention to the increased risk associated with modest levels of BP elevation (Table 118-1).[1]

Children and younger adolescents, however, do not develop the cardiovascular and renal consequences of elevated BP that are seen in older adolescents and adults. The definition of HTN in the young is therefore a statistical one, based on BP percentiles derived from BPs obtained in healthy children and adolescents. Hypertension is defined as average systolic BP (SBP) and/or diastolic BP (DBP) that is ≥95th percentile for gender, age, and height on 3 or more occasions (Table 118-1).[2] Prehypertension is defined as BP levels >90th percentile, but <95th percentile. Because the 90th percentile for SBP is >120 mm Hg by age 12 years, adolescents with BP >120/80 mm Hg (but <95th percentile) should also be diagnosed with prehypertension. Normative BP values for adolescents younger than 18 years are shown in Tables 118-2 and 118-3.

For all age groups, the severity of HTN should be staged after an individual is diagnosed with HTN (Table 118-1). As discussed later in the chapter, staging the severity of HTN is helpful in guiding the subsequent evaluation and management of the patient with HTN.

## EPIDEMIOLOGY

Early screening studies, which used similar thresholds in defining HTN in children and adolescents as used for adults, demonstrated that HTN was exceedingly rare in young children, but could be seen in a small percentage of adolescents (Table 118-4). The subsequent performance of large-scale BP screening programs, typically conducted in schools, confirmed that <2% of children were hypertensive.[3-5] These screening programs also demonstrated the importance of performing repeated measures of BP before labeling a child or adolescent as

**Table 118-1**

**Classification of Hypertension in Adolescents[1,2]**

| *Blood Pressure Classification* | *Adolescents 17 Years and Younger* | *Adolescents 18 Years and Older* |
|---|---|---|
| Normal | SBP and DBP <90th percentile | SBP <120 mm Hg and DBP <80 mm Hg |
| Prehypertension | SBP or DBP 90th–95th percentile; or if BP is >120/80 mm Hg, even if <90th percentile | SBP 120–139 mm Hg or DBP 80–89 mm Hg |
| Stage 1 hypertension | SBP or DBP ≥95th–99th percentile plus 5 mm Hg | SBP 140–159 mm Hg or DBP 90–99 mm Hg |
| Stage 2 hypertension | SBP or DBP >99th percentile plus 5 mm Hg | SBP ≥160 mm Hg or DBP ≥100 mm Hg |

BP, blood pressure; DBP, diastolic blood pressure; SBP, systolic blood pressure.

**Table 118-2**

**Blood Pressure Levels for Adolescent Boys Younger Than 18 Years Based on Height Percentile**

| *Age (y)* | *BP Percentile ↓* | *Systolic BP (mm Hg) ← Height Percentile →* | | | | | | | *Diastolic BP (mm Hg) ← Height Percentile →* | | | | | | |
|---|---|---|---|---|---|---|---|---|---|---|---|---|---|---|---|
| | | *5th* | *10th* | *25th* | *50th* | *75th* | *90th* | *95th* | *5th* | *10th* | *25th* | *50th* | *75th* | *90th* | *95th* |
| 10 | 50th | 97 | 98 | 100 | 102 | 103 | 105 | 106 | 58 | 59 | 60 | 61 | 61 | 62 | 63 |
| | 90th | 111 | 112 | 114 | 115 | 118 | 119 | 119 | 73 | 73 | 74 | 75 | 76 | 77 | 78 |
| | 95th | 115 | 116 | 118 | 119 | 121 | 122 | 123 | 77 | 78 | 79 | 80 | 81 | 81 | 82 |
| | 99th | 122 | 123 | 125 | 127 | 128 | 130 | 130 | 85 | 86 | 86 | 88 | 88 | 89 | 90 |
| 11 | 50th | 99 | 100 | 102 | 104 | 105 | 107 | 107 | 59 | 59 | 60 | 61 | 62 | 63 | 63 |
| | 90th | 113 | 114 | 115 | 118 | 119 | 120 | 121 | 74 | 74 | 75 | 76 | 77 | 78 | 78 |
| | 95th | 118 | 118 | 119 | 121 | 123 | 124 | 125 | 78 | 78 | 79 | 80 | 81 | 82 | 82 |
| | 99th | 124 | 125 | 127 | 129 | 130 | 132 | 132 | 86 | 86 | 87 | 88 | 89 | 90 | 90 |
| 12 | 50th | 101 | 102 | 104 | 106 | 108 | 109 | 110 | 59 | 60 | 61 | 62 | 63 | 63 | 64 |
| | 90th | 115 | 116 | 118 | 120 | 121 | 123 | 123 | 74 | 75 | 75 | 76 | 77 | 78 | 79 |
| | 95th | 119 | 120 | 122 | 123 | 125 | 127 | 127 | 78 | 79 | 80 | 81 | 82 | 82 | 83 |
| | 99th | 126 | 127 | 129 | 131 | 133 | 134 | 135 | 86 | 87 | 88 | 89 | 90 | 90 | 91 |
| 13 | 50th | 104 | 105 | 106 | 108 | 110 | 111 | 112 | 60 | 60 | 61 | 62 | 63 | 64 | 64 |
| | 90th | 118 | 118 | 120 | 122 | 124 | 125 | 126 | 75 | 75 | 76 | 77 | 78 | 79 | 79 |
| | 95th | 121 | 122 | 124 | 126 | 128 | 129 | 130 | 79 | 79 | 80 | 81 | 82 | 83 | 83 |
| | 99th | 128 | 130 | 131 | 133 | 135 | 136 | 137 | 87 | 87 | 88 | 89 | 90 | 91 | 91 |
| 14 | 50th | 106 | 107 | 109 | 111 | 113 | 114 | 115 | 60 | 61 | 62 | 63 | 64 | 65 | 65 |
| | 90th | 120 | 121 | 123 | 125 | 126 | 128 | 128 | 75 | 76 | 77 | 78 | 79 | 79 | 80 |
| | 95th | 124 | 125 | 127 | 128 | 130 | 132 | 132 | 80 | 80 | 81 | 82 | 83 | 84 | 84 |
| | 99th | 131 | 132 | 134 | 136 | 138 | 139 | 140 | 87 | 88 | 89 | 90 | 91 | 92 | 92 |
| 15 | 50th | 109 | 110 | 112 | 113 | 115 | 118 | 118 | 61 | 62 | 63 | 64 | 65 | 66 | 66 |
| | 90th | 122 | 124 | 125 | 127 | 129 | 130 | 131 | 76 | 77 | 78 | 79 | 80 | 80 | 81 |
| | 95th | 126 | 127 | 129 | 131 | 133 | 134 | 135 | 81 | 81 | 82 | 83 | 84 | 85 | 85 |
| | 99th | 134 | 135 | 136 | 138 | 140 | 142 | 142 | 88 | 89 | 90 | 91 | 92 | 93 | 93 |
| 16 | 50th | 111 | 112 | 114 | 116 | 118 | 119 | 120 | 63 | 63 | 64 | 65 | 66 | 67 | 67 |
| | 90th | 125 | 126 | 128 | 130 | 131 | 133 | 134 | 78 | 78 | 79 | 80 | 81 | 82 | 82 |
| | 95th | 129 | 130 | 132 | 134 | 135 | 137 | 137 | 82 | 83 | 83 | 84 | 85 | 86 | 87 |
| | 99th | 136 | 137 | 139 | 141 | 143 | 144 | 145 | 90 | 90 | 91 | 92 | 93 | 94 | 94 |
| 17 | 50th | 114 | 115 | 116 | 118 | 120 | 121 | 122 | 65 | 66 | 66 | 67 | 68 | 69 | 70 |
| | 90th | 127 | 128 | 130 | 132 | 134 | 135 | 136 | 80 | 80 | 81 | 82 | 83 | 84 | 84 |
| | 95th | 131 | 132 | 134 | 136 | 138 | 139 | 140 | 84 | 85 | 86 | 87 | 87 | 88 | 89 |
| | 99th | 139 | 140 | 141 | 143 | 145 | 146 | 147 | 92 | 93 | 93 | 94 | 95 | 96 | 97 |

BP, blood pressure.

Source: National High Blood Pressure Education Program Working Group on High Blood Pressure in Children and Adolescents. *The Fourth Report on the Diagnosis, Evaluation, and Treatment of High Blood Pressure in Children and Adolescents*. Bethesda, MD: National Institutes of Health, National Heart, Lung, and Blood Institute; 2005. NIH publication 05-5267.

**Table 118-3**

**Blood Pressure Levels for Adolescent Girls Younger Than 18 Years Based on Height Percentile**

| *Age (y)* | *BP Percentile* ↓ | *Systolic BP (mm Hg) ← Height Percentile →* | | | | | | | *Diastolic BP (mm Hg) ← Height Percentile →* | | | | | | |
|---|---|---|---|---|---|---|---|---|---|---|---|---|---|---|---|
| | | *5th* | *10th* | *25th* | *50th* | *75th* | *90th* | *95th* | *5th* | *10th* | *25th* | *50th* | *75th* | *90th* | *95th* |
| 10 | 50th | 98 | 99 | 100 | 102 | 103 | 104 | 105 | 59 | 59 | 59 | 60 | 61 | 62 | 62 |
| | 90th | 112 | 112 | 114 | 115 | 116 | 118 | 118 | 73 | 73 | 73 | 74 | 75 | 76 | 76 |
| | 95th | 116 | 116 | 118 | 119 | 120 | 121 | 122 | 77 | 77 | 77 | 78 | 79 | 80 | 80 |
| | 99th | 123 | 123 | 125 | 126 | 127 | 129 | 129 | 84 | 84 | 85 | 86 | 86 | 87 | 88 |
| 11 | 50th | 100 | 101 | 102 | 103 | 105 | 106 | 107 | 60 | 60 | 60 | 61 | 62 | 63 | 63 |
| | 90th | 114 | 114 | 116 | 118 | 118 | 119 | 120 | 74 | 74 | 74 | 75 | 76 | 77 | 77 |
| | 95th | 118 | 118 | 119 | 121 | 122 | 123 | 124 | 78 | 78 | 78 | 79 | 80 | 81 | 81 |
| | 99th | 125 | 125 | 126 | 128 | 129 | 130 | 131 | 85 | 85 | 86 | 87 | 87 | 88 | 89 |
| 12 | 50th | 102 | 103 | 104 | 105 | 107 | 108 | 109 | 61 | 61 | 61 | 62 | 63 | 64 | 64 |
| | 90th | 116 | 116 | 118 | 119 | 120 | 121 | 122 | 75 | 75 | 75 | 76 | 77 | 78 | 78 |
| | 95th | 119 | 120 | 121 | 123 | 124 | 125 | 126 | 79 | 79 | 79 | 80 | 81 | 82 | 82 |
| | 99th | 127 | 127 | 128 | 130 | 131 | 132 | 133 | 86 | 86 | 87 | 88 | 88 | 89 | 90 |
| 13 | 50th | 104 | 105 | 106 | 107 | 109 | 110 | 110 | 62 | 62 | 62 | 63 | 64 | 65 | 65 |
| | 90th | 118 | 118 | 119 | 121 | 122 | 123 | 124 | 76 | 76 | 76 | 77 | 78 | 79 | 79 |
| | 95th | 121 | 122 | 123 | 124 | 126 | 127 | 128 | 80 | 80 | 80 | 81 | 82 | 83 | 83 |
| | 99th | 128 | 129 | 130 | 132 | 133 | 134 | 135 | 87 | 87 | 88 | 89 | 89 | 90 | 91 |
| 14 | 50th | 106 | 106 | 107 | 109 | 110 | 111 | 112 | 63 | 63 | 63 | 64 | 65 | 66 | 66 |
| | 90th | 119 | 120 | 121 | 122 | 124 | 125 | 125 | 77 | 77 | 77 | 78 | 79 | 80 | 80 |
| | 95th | 123 | 123 | 125 | 126 | 127 | 129 | 129 | 81 | 81 | 81 | 82 | 83 | 84 | 84 |
| | 99th | 130 | 131 | 132 | 133 | 135 | 136 | 136 | 88 | 88 | 89 | 90 | 90 | 91 | 92 |
| 15 | 50th | 107 | 108 | 109 | 110 | 111 | 113 | 113 | 64 | 64 | 64 | 65 | 66 | 67 | 67 |
| | 90th | 120 | 121 | 122 | 123 | 125 | 126 | 127 | 78 | 78 | 78 | 79 | 80 | 81 | 81 |
| | 95th | 124 | 125 | 126 | 127 | 129 | 130 | 131 | 82 | 82 | 82 | 83 | 84 | 85 | 85 |
| | 99th | 131 | 132 | 133 | 134 | 136 | 137 | 138 | 89 | 89 | 90 | 91 | 91 | 92 | 93 |
| 16 | 50th | 108 | 108 | 110 | 111 | 112 | 114 | 114 | 64 | 64 | 65 | 66 | 66 | 67 | 68 |
| | 90th | 121 | 122 | 123 | 124 | 126 | 127 | 128 | 78 | 78 | 79 | 80 | 81 | 81 | 82 |
| | 95th | 125 | 126 | 127 | 128 | 130 | 131 | 132 | 82 | 82 | 83 | 84 | 85 | 85 | 86 |
| | 99th | 132 | 133 | 134 | 135 | 137 | 138 | 139 | 90 | 90 | 90 | 91 | 92 | 93 | 93 |
| 17 | 50th | 108 | 109 | 110 | 111 | 113 | 114 | 115 | 64 | 65 | 65 | 66 | 67 | 67 | 68 |
| | 90th | 122 | 122 | 123 | 125 | 126 | 127 | 128 | 78 | 79 | 79 | 80 | 81 | 81 | 82 |
| | 95th | 125 | 126 | 127 | 129 | 130 | 131 | 132 | 82 | 83 | 83 | 84 | 85 | 85 | 86 |
| | 99th | 133 | 133 | 134 | 136 | 137 | 138 | 139 | 90 | 90 | 91 | 91 | 92 | 93 | 93 |

BP, blood pressure.

Source: National High Blood Pressure Education Program Working Group on High Blood Pressure in Children and Adolescents. *The Fourth Report on the Diagnosis, Evaluation, and Treatment of High Blood Pressure in Children and Adolescents*. Bethesda, MD: National Institutes of Health, National Heart, Lung, and Blood Institute; 2005. NIH publication 05-5267.

**Table 118-4**

**Prevalence of Hypertension in Children and Adolescents**

| *Study Location* | *Number screened* | *Ages (y)* | *Number of Screenings* | *Normative Criteria* | *Prevalence* | *Ref* |
|---|---|---|---|---|---|---|
| Muscatine, IA, United States | 1,301 | 14–18 | 1 | 140/90 mm Hg | 8.9% SHTN, 12.2% DHTN | 3 |
| Edmonton, Canada | 15,594 | 15–20 | 1 | 150/95 mm Hg | 2.2% | 4 |
| Dallas, TX, United States | 10,641 | 14 | 3 | 95th percentile | 1.2% SHTN, 0.4% DHTN | 5 |
| Minneapolis, MN, United States | 14,686 | 10–15 | 1 | 1987 TF | 4.2% | 6 |
| Tulsa, OK, United States | 5,537 | 14–19 | 1 | 1987 TF | 6.0% | 7 |
| Buraidah, Saudi Arabia | 3,299 | 3–18 | 1 | 1996 WG | 10.6% | 8 |
| Minneapolis, MN, United States | 14,686 | 10–15 | 2 | 1996 WG | 0.8% SHTN, 0.4% DHTN | 9 |
| Houston, TX, United States | 5,102 | 12–16 | 3 | 1996 WG | 4.5% | 10 |

DHTN, diastolic hypertension; SHTN, systolic hypertension; TF, Second Task Force Report[11]; WG, Working Group Report[12].

hypertensive; studies that used a single BP determination demonstrated significantly higher "prevalences" of HTN than studies in which repeated screenings were performed.[3-10]

More recent studies have generally confirmed a low prevalence of HTN in children and adolescents. However, data from the Houston Screening Project[10] have demonstrated that the childhood obesity epidemic has resulted in an increased prevalence of HTN. In this study, more than 5,000 primarily minority Houston public school children underwent BP and obesity screening. The prevalence of HTN among these children after 3 screenings was 4.5%, significantly higher than in prior studies. Among children whose body mass index (BMI) was ≥95th percentile, 11% had HTN, compared to 1% to 3% of those whose BMI was at or less than the 75th percentile.

The influence of the obesity epidemic on the epidemiology of HTN in children and adolescents cannot be underestimated. As illustrated in Figure 118-1, the prevalence of obesity in children and adolescents has increased from <5% in 1963 to nearly 20% in 2004.[13] Among the many health sequelae of obesity, elevated BP is one of the more common. Luepker et al,[14] for example, obtained anthropometric measurements and BPs in 18,000 Minneapolis school children in 1986 and 1996. Between 1986 and 1996, a significant increase of BMI occurred in both boys and girls, and this increase in BMI was associated with an increase in SBP. These findings have recently been confirmed with data from the National Health and Nutrition Examination Survey (NHANES),[15] which demonstrated that mean SBP among children and adolescents in the United States was 1.4 mm Hg higher and DBP 3.3 mm Hg higher in 1999 to 2000 compared with 1988 to 1994. Twenty-nine percent of the increase in SBP and 12% of the increase in DBP was explained by the increase in BMI seen over the same time period.

Given these statistics, it is no surprise that among published studies of children and adolescents with HTN, obesity is an increasingly common finding. Among 70 children and adolescents with primary HTN seen at the University of Michigan, the mean BMI was 27 ± 7.5 kg/m$^2$, and 34 (48.5%) were classified as obese (BMI ≥95th percentile).[16] In another series from Texas Children's Hospital, the mean BMI among 139 children and adolescents with primary HTN was 30 ± 7.9 kg/m$^2$, and the mean BMI percentile was 88 ± 14.[17] Hypertension has become a significant problem in obese children and adolescents with important potential public health ramifications.[18]

## ETIOLOGY

In infants and preadolescent children, secondary causes of HTN predominate, and primary HTN is rare. Renal and cardiac disorders are the most common identifiable

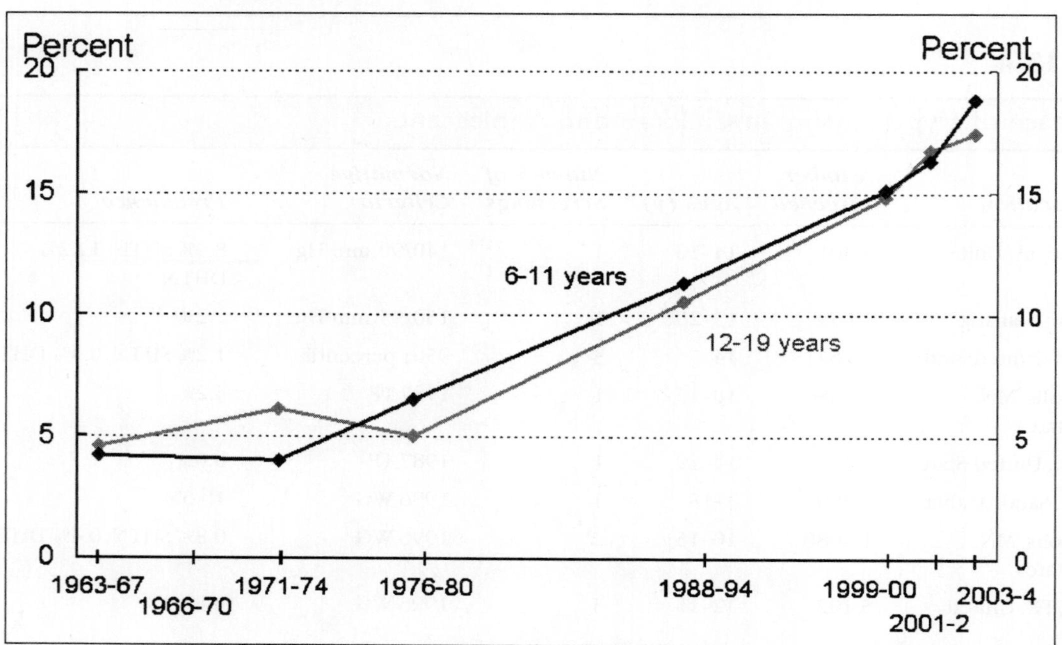


**FIGURE 118-1** Percentage of children and adolescents classified as overweight, 1963–2004. (*Source:* Data from Centers for Disease Control and Prevention. Trends in child and adolescent overweight. Available at: www.cdc.gov/nchs/products/pubs/pubd/hestats/overweight/HealthEstat1206.gif. Accessed October 5, 2009.)

causes in these age groups. The reader who is interested in a more detailed discussion of the differential diagnosis and evaluation of HTN in infants and young children should consult one of the recent comprehensive texts on pediatric HTN.[19,20]

In adolescents, however, it has been increasingly recognized that primary HTN accounts for the majority of cases. This was clearly seen in a 1992 study by Wyszynska et al[21] of 1,025 children referred to a Polish children's hospital for evaluation of HTN (defined as BP persistently >95th percentile). Overall, 45% of their study population had primary HTN, and 55% had secondary HTN. Among adolescents (aged 15–18 years), who comprised 60% of those studied, 75% had primary HTN. Causes of secondary HTN in the adolescents studied included many of the conditions listed in Box 118-1, especially renal causes. Similarly, in the University of Michigan series mentioned previously,[16] of 92 adolescents with confirmed HTN, 64% had no identifiable underlying cause for their HTN, whereas the rest had secondary causes.

Certain factors increase the likelihood of primary HTN in adolescence, including a family history of HTN and obesity, which has already been discussed. Offspring of hypertensive parents have higher BPs and an increased prevalence of other cardiovascular risk factors.[22–25] The prevalence of a positive family history of HTN in children and adolescents with primary HTN has recently been reported to be more than of 80%.[16] Thus, a family history of HTN (or other cardiovascular disease such as stroke) increases the likelihood of a diagnosis of primary HTN, especially when the results of initial diagnostic studies are normal.

## ASSOCIATED CARDIOVASCULAR RISK FACTORS

Several characteristics of adult cardiovascular disease, such as systolic HTN, dyslipidemia, and impaired glucose tolerance, occur commonly in hypertensive adolescents. Isolated systolic HTN, a major risk factor for cardiovascular morbidity and mortality in adults,[26] is now commonly seen in hypertensive children and adolescents. Data from a multicenter trial of an antihypertensive medication in children showed that among the 140 subjects in the trial, 37% had isolated systolic HTN, with this finding occurring significantly more often in obese subjects (50% vs 30% of nonobese subjects, $P = .02$).[27,28] In the school-based screening study conducted by Sorof et al,[27] the prevalence of isolated systolic HTN among adolescents who were obese and

**Box 118-1**

***Differential Diagnosis of Secondary Hypertension in Adolescents***

***Renal***

- Obstructive lesions (UPJ, UVJ)
- Glomerulonephritis (acute or chronic)
- Other acquired renal parenchymal disease (pyelonephritis, reflux nephropathy, infarction)
- Renovascular disease
- Intrinsic: fibromuscular hyperplasia, arterial or venous thrombosis
- Extrinsic: compression
- Congenital defects (hypoplasia/dysplasia, autosomal dominant or recessive PKD)
- Hemolytic uremic syndrome

***Vascular***

- Thoracic aortic coarctation
- Midaortic syndrome
- Vasculitis (Takayasu arteritis, polyarteritis nodosa)

***Neurologic***

- Increased intracranial pressure
- Guillain-Barré syndrome
- Cervical and leg traction
- Pain

***Endocrine***

- Diabetes (type 1 or type 2)
- Cushing syndrome
- Primary aldosteronism
- Hyperparathyroidism
- Congenital adrenal hyperplasia
- Genetic
- Turner syndrome
- Williams syndrome
- Neurofibromatosis
- Tuberous sclerosis
- Single gene defects (Liddle syndrome, AME, GRA)

***Neoplastic***

- Renal tumors (renal cell carcinoma, Wilms tumor)
- Pheochromocytoma
- Neuroblastoma

***Miscellaneous***

- Drug induced (Box 118-2)
- Stress
- Organ transplantation

AME, apparent mineralocorticoid excess; GRA, glucocorticoid-remediable aldosternonism; PKD, polycystic kidney disease; UPJ, ureteropelvic junction; UVJ, ureterovesical junction.

had BP >95th percentile on a single set of measurements was 94%. Given the frequency of development of hypertensive target-organ damage in hypertensive adolescents, it is clear that isolated systolic HTN is not as benign as previously thought.

It is well-known that dyslipidemia occurs commonly in children with elevated BP,[29] and several more recent studies confirm this association.[16,30] The typical pattern is normal to slightly elevated total cholesterol with low high-density lipoprotein (HDL) cholesterol and elevated triglycerides. This pattern is similar to that which occurs in type 2 diabetes, most likely reflecting underlying insulin resistance, even in nonobese hypertensive patients. Impaired glucose tolerance also occurs frequently in obese hypertensive children, typically as part of the metabolic syndrome.[31] Other studies have demonstrated that these cardiovascular risk factors may be associated with the early development of atherosclerosis in the young.[32] It is therefore reasonable, as recommended by *The Fourth Report*,[2] to screen for these risk factors/comorbidities when evaluating hypertensive children and adolescents. Identification of multiple cardiovascular risk factors at an early age may, in turn, permit institution of measures aimed at prevention of adult cardiovascular disease.

## CONSEQUENCES IN ADOLESCENCE AND BEYOND

As noted previously, the long-term cardiovascular sequelae of HTN seen in adults, such as stroke and myocardial infarction, do not occur in children. However, a large body of evidence has accumulated over the years, documenting that persistent BP elevation in children and adolescents can produce other target-organ effects that may be important to consider, especially when making treatment decisions.

Left ventricular hypertrophy (LVH) is probably the most common and most easily identified target-organ effect of HTN in children and adolescents. More recent studies have established a prevalence of LVH in hypertensive children and adolescents as high as 40%.[33] Although the adverse effects of LVH, such as sudden cardiac death,[34] seen in adults have not been proven to occur in hypertensive children, LVH is still considered an important cardiovascular risk factor in hypertensive children, and treatment recommendations from consensus organizations have emphasized that if LVH is present, the adolescent should be aggressively treated with antihypertensive medications.[2]

Other vascular effects of HTN have also been demonstrated in hypertensive youth, including retinal changes and increased carotid intimal-medial thickness (cIMT). Retinal changes, when systematically looked for, occur in a large number of hypertensive children and adolescents,[35] and in one study appeared more often in those with higher DBP.[36] Increased cIMT, which is well established as a correlate of atherosclerosis and increased cardiovascular risk in adults,[37,38] has recently been found to also occur in hypertensive children and adolescents.[39,40] As in hypertensive adults, increased cIMT in the young is correlated with obesity and LVH.[39] Although more studies are needed,[41] it may soon be possible to use cIMT as a marker of increased cardiovascular risk in hypertensive children and adolescents.

The other major target organ in HTN is the kidney. In adults, HTN is one of the most common causes of chronic kidney disease (CKD). According to the *2004 US Renal Data Systems (USRDS) Annual Data Report*, HTN was the second leading cause of end-stage renal disease (ESRD) in adults in 2002, affecting approximately 125,000 individuals, or 24.4% of the entire ESRD population.[42] In children, however, it is not clear whether HTN alone may result in ESRD. The North American Pediatric Renal Trials and Collaborative Studies (NAPRTCS) dialysis, transplant, and chronic renal insufficiency (CRI) registries do not list HTN among the causes of CKD/ESRD in children.[43] However, close analysis of the USRDS data reveals that HTN was reported as the cause of ESRD in more than 150 children in 2002.[42] Hypertension was reported less often than other forms of kidney disease, and was primarily reported as a cause of ESRD in children ≥10 years of age. Reconciling these 2 databases is difficult because they are derived from significantly different sources. Because HTN was reported as a cause of ESRD mostly in adolescents, it is tempting to speculate that perhaps long-standing HTN may indeed lead to CKD/ESRD in adolescents, adding further weight to recent recommendations advocating earlier use of antihypertensive medications in some children and adolescents.

It is possible that HTN may also impair mental function. In adults, long-standing BP elevation may cause impaired performance on neuropsychological testing,[44] with at least one study demonstrating an inverse relationship between BP level and measures of attention and memory.[45] In a pediatric study, Lande et al[46] examined data from NHANES III, which included information on BP as well as results of standardized neuropsychological testing (including tests of short-term memory, attention, concentration, and constructional skills). They found that children with BP >90th percentile had decreased performance on the neuropsychological tests compared to controls with normal BP. These findings are especially provocative given that only a single BP measurement was obtained in the NHANES III. Further studies are clearly needed to examine the effects of sustained BP elevation on mental function in the young, as well as the potential effects of treatment on neuropsychological function in hypertensive children and adolescents.

The final and perhaps most intriguing consequence of elevated child and adolescent BP is that it likely predicts the development of adult HTN. This phenomenon, known as BP "tracking," has been the subject of much study, with the overall conclusion in the literature being that BP does indeed track into adulthood,[47] especially in children with BPs in the prehypertensive range. Perhaps the most convincing of the available studies is the Muscatine Study,[48] which enrolled school children and adolescents aged 7 to 18 years in Muscatine, Iowa, between 1971 and 1978. A subgroup (the "longitudinal cohort") was then recalled as young adults (aged 23–28 years). Subjects with SBP in childhood >90th percentile were 3.9 times more likely than expected to develop HTN as adults, and those with DBP in childhood >90th percentile were 1.9 times more likely than expected to develop adult HTN. The likelihood of developing adult HTN increased with readings >90th percentile for SBP and DBP. In addition, the absence of abnormal readings in childhood was associated with a reduced risk of developing adult HTN. A meta-analysis of tracking studies[49] has confirmed this relationship, highlighting the importance of early detection and treatment of HTN in the young.

## DIAGNOSTIC EVALUATION

Evaluation of the hypertensive adolescent should begin with a comprehensive medical history and physical examination. Although some laboratory testing will always be needed, the extent of this should be decided after the history and physical examination have been completed, so that only the necessary tests are obtained.

The history should begin with asking whether any symptoms suggestive of HTN are present, such as headaches, dizziness, diplopia, vomiting, or epistaxis. The interview should then focus on uncovering symptoms of other underlying disorders, including symptoms of possible renal disease, heart disease, or diseases affecting other organ systems (Table 118-5). The past medical history should include questions about recent and chronic illnesses, prior hospitalizations or episodes of trauma, recurrent urinary tract infections or unexplained fevers, and neonatal history. Family history of HTN, diabetes, renal disease, and other cardiovascular disease (hyperlipidemia, myocardial infarction at an early age) should be elicited. Finally, it is important to ask about over-the-counter, prescription, and illicit drug use because many substances can either cause or exacerbate HTN (Box 118-2).

Physical examination begins by obtaining the patient's weight and height so that growth percentiles can be plotted and BMI calculated. Blood pressures should be obtained in both upper extremities in the seated position, and in at least one arm and one leg in the supine position. If initial BPs are obtained using an automated oscillometric device, they should be confirmed by auscultation using an aneroid sphygmomanometer. Cuff sizes should be chosen in accordance with the recommendations of the National High Blood Pressure Education Program (NHBPEP) Task Force.[2] Consideration should be given to performing ambulatory BP monitoring (ABPM) to confirm the diagnosis of HTN. Ambulatory BP monitoring can detect white coat HTN and masked HTN,[50] correlate with the presence of hypertensive target-organ damage,[51] and be used to help differentiate between primary and secondary HTN.[52,53] Increased use of ABPM is supported by research studies and has been endorsed by the NHBPEP Task Force.[2] However, it may not be widely available, especially in the primary care setting, and there are still issues related to interpretation of ABPM in children and adolescents that need to be resolved[50] before it can be considered standard of care.

As with the history, the rest of the physical examination should focus on uncovering signs of specific underlying disorders that may be causing the adolescent's HTN (Table 118-5). In obese adolescents, there may be signs of insulin resistance such as acanthosis nigricans, or in females, findings may be suggestive of polycystic ovarian syndrome (PCOS) such as hirsutism. The physical examination may also provide clues as to the severity/chronicity of the patient's HTN, such as LVH (signified by an apical heave) or hypertensive retinopathy.

Patients with confirmed HTN should then undergo diagnostic testing to follow up on findings from the history and physical examination, and to assess for other coexisting cardiovascular risk factors.[2] It is typical to obtain a basic set of screening studies in all patients, including a urinalysis, serum chemistries, fasting lipid panel, and fasting glucose. Plasma renin activity and aldosterone are sometimes also included in this initial

**Table 118-5**

**History and Physical Examination Findings Suggestive of Secondary Hypertension**

| *Present in history* | *Suggests* |
|---|---|
| Known UTI or UTI symptoms | Reflux nephropathy |
| Joint pains, rash, fever | Vasculitis, SLE |
| Acute onset of gross hematuria | Glomerulonephritis, renal venous thrombosis |
| Renal trauma | Renal infarct, RAS |
| Abdominal radiation | Radiation nephritis, RAS |
| Renal transplant | Transplant RAS |
| Precocious puberty | Adrenal disorder |
| Muscle cramping, constipation | Hyperaldosteronism |
| Excessive sweating, headache, pallor and/or flushing | Pheochromocytoma |
| Illicit drug use | Drug-induced hypertension |
| ***Present on examination*** | ***Suggests*** |
| BP >140/100 mm Hg at any age | Secondary hypertension |
| Leg BP < arm BP | Aortic coarctation |
| Poor growth, pallor | Chronic renal disease |
| Turner syndrome | Aortic coarctation |
| Café-au-lait spots | Renal artery stenosis |
| Delayed leg pulses | Aortic coarctation |
| Precocious puberty | Adrenal disorder |
| Bruits over upper abdomen | Renal artery stenosis |
| Edema | Renal disease |
| Excessive sweating | Pheochromocytoma |
| Excessive pigmentation | Adrenal disorder |
| Striae in males | Drug-induced HTN |

BP, blood pressure; HTN, hypertension; RAS, renal artery stenosis; SLE, systemic lupus erythematosus; UTI, urinary tract infection.

**Box 118-2**

***Substances that May Elevate Blood Pressure in Adolescents***

***Prescription Medications***

- Calcineurin inhibitors (cyclosporine, tacrolimus)
- COX-2 inhibitors (rofecoxib, others)
- Erythropoietin
- Glucocorticoids
- Migraine medications (ergotamine, sumatriptan)
- Oral contraceptives
- Phenylpropanolamine
- Pseudoephedrine
- Stimulant medications[a] (dexedrine, methylphenidate, amphetamine derivatives, atomoxetine)
- Tricyclic antidepressants[a]

***Nonprescription Medications***

- Caffeine
- Ephedrine
- Nonsteroidal antiinflammatory drugs[a]
- Pseudoephedrine

***Others***

- Cocaine
- DHEA (dehydroepiandosterone)
- Ethanol
- Heavy metals (lead, mercury)
- Herbal preparations (ephedra, glycyrrhiza)
- MDMA ("ecstasy")
- Tobacco

[a]These cause elevated BP relatively infrequently compared with the other agents in the table.

set of studies, especially when the patient's HTN is severe, or if systolic and diastolic HTN are present.

Renal ultrasound, which should be routinely obtained in all hypertensive preadolescent patients, may be omitted in adolescents with stage 1 HTN if the screening studies are normal, and if other features of primary HTN are present, including obesity, a positive family history, and isolated systolic HTN. Those with stage 2 HTN, abnormal screening studies, or diastolic HTN should get an ultrasound. As recommended by consensus organizations,[2] additional imaging studies, including renal angiography, nuclear renal scans, and voiding cystourethrograms, should only be obtained as indicated based on the results of the history, physical examination, and initial diagnostic studies.

Given the high prevalence of LVH in hypertensive adolescents, two-dimensional (2D) and m-mode echocardiography should be obtained to assess for the presence of hypertensive target-organ damage.[2] Left ventricular mass should be indexed to height to correct for the effect of obesity. Ophthalmologic examinations should be obtained, but should be performed by an experienced pediatric ophthalmologist because hypertensive retinal changes are likely to be subtle in adolescents. At some point in the future, carotid imaging and urine microalbumin testing may also find roles in the assessment of hypertensive adolescents, but more data are needed before these studies should be obtained routinely.

## APPROACH TO THERAPY

Treatment of the hypertensive adolescent includes 3 components: nonpharmacologic measures, antihypertensive medications when indicated, and long-term assessment of the success of treatment and monitoring for the development of other cardiovascular risk factors. Given the frequency of primary HTN in adolescents, those caring for adolescents should be familiar with initiating these measures, especially in teens with uncomplicated HTN.

### NONPHARMACOLOGIC APPROACHES

Weight loss, aerobic exercise, and dietary modifications have all been shown to successfully reduce BP in children and adolescents, and are therefore considered primary treatment, especially in those with obesity-related HTN. Studies in obese adolescents have demonstrated that modest weight loss not only decreases BP, but also improves other cardiovascular risk factors such as dyslipidemia and insulin resistance.[54-56] In studies where a reduction in BMI of about 10% was achieved, short-term reductions in BP were in the range of 8 to 12 mm Hg. Unfortunately, weight loss is difficult and frequently unsuccessful. In addition, even intensive efforts at weight loss in childhood may be followed by recidivism and an increased prevalence of adverse consequences of obesity in adulthood.[57] However, identifying a medical complication of obesity such as HTN can perhaps provide the necessary motivation for patients and families to make appropriate lifestyle changes.

Similarly, exercise training over 3 to 6 months has been shown to result in a reduction of 6 to 12 mm Hg for systolic BP and 3 to 5 mm Hg for diastolic BP.[58] However, cessation of regular exercise is generally promptly followed by a rise in BP to preexercise levels. Aerobic exercise activities such as running, walking, or cycling are usually preferred to static forms of exercise. Many adolescents may already be participating in one or more appropriate activities and may only need to increase the frequency and/or intensity of these activities. At the very least, the amount of time spent in sedentary activities such as television viewing should be restricted to less than <2 hours/day.[59] Increasing physical activity may not only reduce BP, but can help with weight loss and/or maintenance and may also forestall the development of type 2 diabetes.[60] Exercise should be combined with dietary changes such as those discussed later in the chapter for best results in terms of BP reduction[61] and weight control. The combination of dietary changes and exercise training may also improve vascular function in addition to reducing BP.[62]

Dietary modification in the management of HTN in children and adolescents has received a great deal of attention. Nutrients that have been examined include the obvious, such as sodium, potassium, and calcium, as well as folate, caffeine, and other substances. Manipulation of sodium intake has received extensive study.[63] Many authors have noted that the typical dietary sodium intakes of children and adolescents, at least in the United States, far exceed any nutritional requirement for sodium. Trials of dietary sodium restriction in hypertensive children and adolescents have had mixed results, with some studies showing no benefit, and others showing a modest BP reduction in obese adolescents but not lean adolescents.[64] This suggests that dietary sodium restriction may have an important role in treatment of overweight hypertensive adolescents, a substantial proportion of whom are likely to be salt sensitive.

Other nutrients that have been examined in hypertensive patients include potassium and calcium, both of which have been shown to have antihypertensive effects. A 2-year trial of potassium and calcium supplementation in hypertensive, salt-sensitive Chinese children demonstrated that this combination significantly reduced SBP.[65] Therefore, a diet that is low in sodium and enriched in potassium and calcium may be more effective in treatment of HTN than a diet that restricts sodium only.

An example of such a diet is the so-called DASH (Dietary Approaches to Stop Hypertension) diet, developed by the National Institutes of Health and National Heart, Lung, and Blood Institute, which has an antihypertensive effect in adults with HTN, even in those receiving antihypertensive medication.[66,67] The DASH diet also incorporates higher intake of such micronutrients as folate, which may have an antihypertensive effect, as well as measures designed to reduce dietary fat intake, an important strategy given the frequent presence of dyslipidemia in hypertensive adolescents. The basic elements of the DASH eating plan are logical to apply to the treatment of hypertensive adolescents, especially if accompanied by counseling from a pediatric dietitian, and its antihypertensive efficacy in adolescents has recently been confirmed.[68]

## USE OF ANTIHYPERTENSIVE MEDICATIONS

Despite weight loss, exercise, and dietary changes, antihypertensive medications will be needed in some hypertensive adolescents in order to achieve the desired BP. Although there are potential theoretical benefits of initiation of drug therapy early in life, it is important to recognize that the long-term consequences of untreated HTN in the young remain unknown. Similarly, there is a lack of data on the benefits of drug therapy in the pediatric age group, which adds further uncertainty to the decision to initiate drug treatment.

For these reasons, consensus statements[2] have emphasized that a definite indication for initiating pharmacologic therapy should be ascertained before antihypertensive medication is prescribed in an adolescent. These are generally self-explanatory:

- Stage 2 HTN
- Symptomatic HTN
- Secondary HTN
- Hypertensive target-organ damage
- Diabetes (types 1 and 2)
- Persistent HTN despite nonpharmacologic measures

Only the final indication is somewhat unclear because the length of time needed to see an effect of lifestyle changes may vary significantly from patient to patient. At the very least, hypertensive adolescents who either do not adhere with or do not respond to a reasonable (6 - to 12-month) trial of nonpharmacologic measures should probably be prescribed antihypertensive medications due to the likely risk of development of hypertensive target-organ damage in these patients.

The choice of drug class for the initial antihypertensive agent in adolescents is controversial. In adults, studies such as the Antihypertensive and Lipid-Lowering Treatment to Prevent Heart Attack Trial (ALLHAT)[69] have provided evidence that a diuretic should be the first choice of medication due to their demonstrated benefit in reducing cardiovascular endpoints such as myocardial infarction. This evidence base is lacking for pediatric patients because studies comparing different classes of antihypertensive agents have not been conducted in the young. Until data are available to differentiate the advantages and disadvantages of different classes of antihypertensive medications in adolescents, it is advisable to consider several classes of agents, including diuretics, beta-blocking agents, angiotensin-converting enzyme (ACE) inhibitors, ARB agents, and calcium channel blockers, as acceptable first-line agents.[2]

Some authors have advocated a pathophysiologic approach to the choice of initial agent, at least in adults. One such approach is based on measurement of plasma rennin activity (PRA).[70] Those with elevated PRA would be classified as having HTN on the basis of renin-mediated vasoconstriction and should therefore be prescribed an antirenin agent such as an ACE inhibitor, whereas those with low PRA would be believed to have volume overload HTN and should be prescribed a diuretic. Although this approach has not been studied in children and adolescents, it might be reasonable to consider, especially given the higher renin values seen in hypertensive children, particularly in obese adolescents.[16] The well-known activation of the renin-angiotensin system in obesity[71] would provide additional rationale for the use of ACE inhibitors as initial therapy in obese hypertensive adolescents.

There are some clinical situations in which specific classes of antihypertensive agents should be chosen preferentially. The best example of this would be patients with underlying CKD, in whom ACE inhibitors or angiotensin receptor blockers (ARB) are preferred due to their beneficial effects on slowing progression.[72] Similarly, in hypertensive adolescents with the metabolic syndrome, the effect of the antihypertensive drug on glucose metabolism needs to be considered.[73] In adults, this so-called compelling indications approach centers on data from numerous large-scale clinical trials that have demonstrated significant reductions in morbidity and mortality based on treatment with specific classes of antihypertensive medications.[1] In children and adolescents, such data are lacking, so these decisions need to be made empirically.

Adherence to prescribed therapy is another important issue that should be considered in the treatment of HTN because most patients have so few symptoms. In adolescents, this is particularly difficult because they often fail to remember to take their medications and do not like to be perceived as different from their peers. If BP control can be achieved with a single, once-daily agent, this will improve the likelihood of adherence to the medication and should be taken into consideration when the initial agent is chosen. Adverse effects of the chosen agent should also be considered. Some classes of antihypertensive agents, particularly newer ones such as ACE inhibitors and ARBs, have a lower incidence of adverse effects[74] and may be preferable when compliance is a concern. There are also combination preparations available that can improve adherence when more than one agent is needed to achieve the desired goal BP.[75]

A "stepped-care" approach to the use of antihypertensive medications in children and adolescents has been recommended by the NHBPEP since *The Second Task Force Report* and was recently reendorsed in *The Fourth Report*.[2] In this approach (Figure 118-2), initial treatment consists of adding a single antihypertensive agent to nonpharmacologic measures, beginning with a low dose of the drug chosen. Increases in the dose of the initial medication should then be made as necessary to achieve BP control. Efficacy and adverse effects should be monitored during titration; if significant adverse effects appear, the dose should be reduced or another drug chosen. If BP control is not achieved, proceed to combination treatment by adding another drug with a different mechanism of action. In many patients, the second agent will be a diuretic, given the complementary effects that diuretics have when used in combination with other classes of antihypertensive medications. If BP control is still not achieved, a third antihypertensive drug can be added, or the patient should be referred to a pediatric HTN specialist. Poor adherence should always be considered throughout this process if the desired BP goal is not attained.

Recent clinical trials of antihypertensive agents in children and adolescents have greatly expanded the available information on dosing, efficacy, and safety of these medications in the young,[76] enabling practitioners to prescribe these medications with greater confidence than in the past. Because these trials have resulted in US Food and Drug Adminstration (FDA)-approved pediatric labeling for many antihypertensive agents, primary care practitioners should only prescribe agents that are labeled for use in children or adolescents younger than 18 years. Suggested initial and maximum doses of various antihypertensive agents are given in Table 118-6. More comprehensive references, especially the results of pediatric trials (if available), should be consulted for detailed discussion of the specific adverse effects of these medications.

Recommended treatment goals for hypertensive children and adolescents have varied widely in the past.

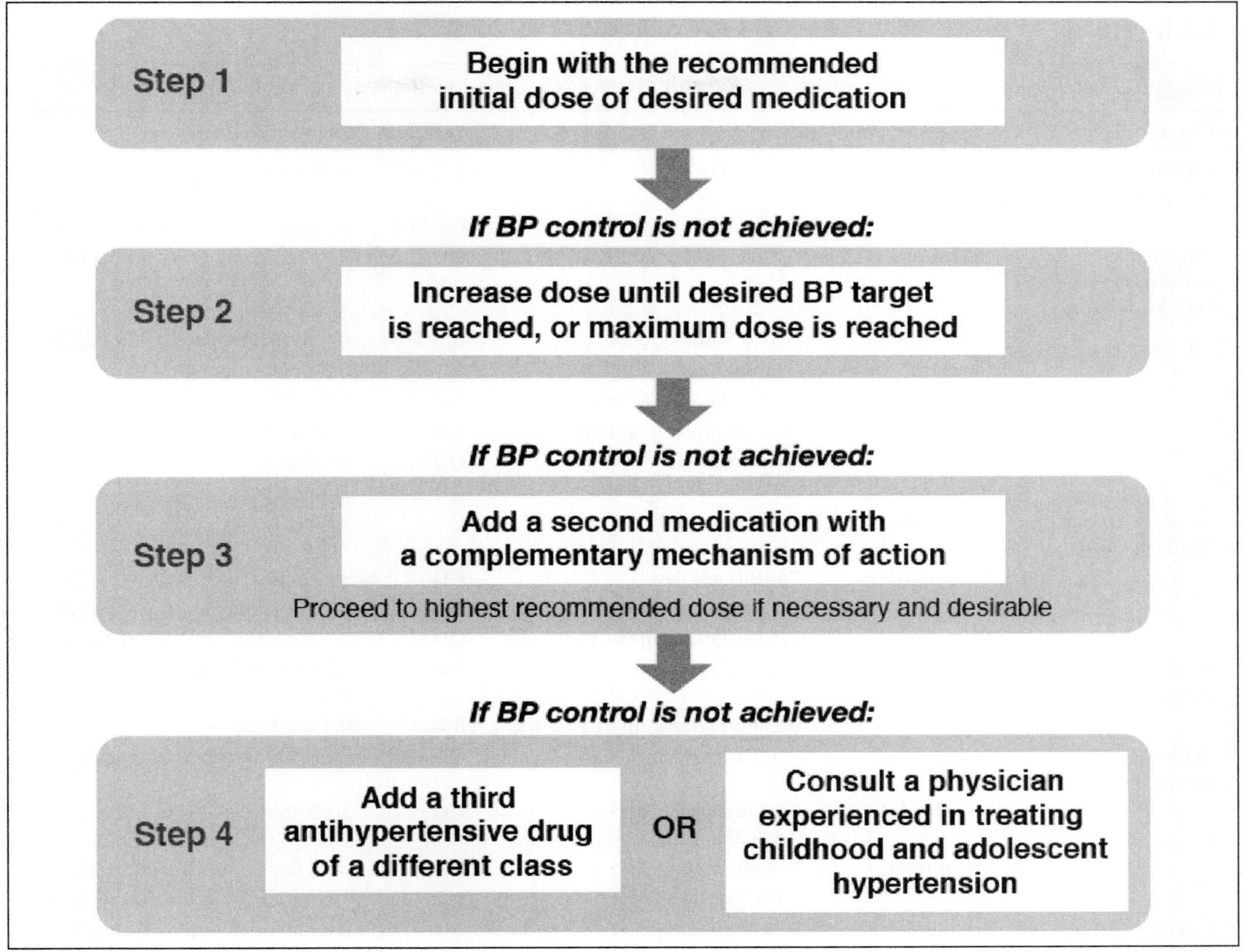


**FIGURE 118-2** Stepped-care approach to pharmacologic management of HTN in adolescents.

The NHBPEP has attempted to rectify this situation in *The Fourth Report*.[2] For patients with uncomplicated primary HTN and no hypertensive target-organ damage, goal BP should be <95th percentile for age, gender, and height, whereas for those with secondary HTN, diabetes, or hypertensive target-organ damage, goal BP should be <90th percentile for age, gender, and height. These goals are consistent with current recommendations for therapy of HTN in adults that recommend treatment to a lower BP goal in patients with complicated HTN, such as those with diabetes or renal disease.[1] In such patients, it is recommended to reduce BP to <130/80 mm Hg, a goal that would also be reasonable for hypertensive adolescents aged ≥18 years with similar conditions.

Finally, it must be emphasized that treatment of HTN does not end when medications are prescribed. Adolescents with hypertension should be seen at regular intervals to assess compliance with therapy and to monitor for medication-related adverse effects. They should be encouraged to monitor their BP at home using an over-the-counter automated sphygmomanometer. This will increase their involvement in treatment and hopefully improve compliance. Similarly, continued nonpharmacologic measures should be encouraged because these may help improve BP control. Laboratory studies should be repeated periodically, especially fasting lipids and glucose in obese adolescents, and electrolytes in those treated with diuretics, ACE inhibitors, or ARBs. Female patients receiving ACE inhibitors or ARBs should be counseled to use effective contraception due to the risks of ACE inhibitor fetopathy, which has recently been described to occur even in fetuses exposed early in pregnancy.[77]

**Table 118-6**

## Suggested Doses of Antihypertensive Medications for Use in Adolescents

| *Class* | *Drug* | *Starting Dose* | *Interval* | *Maximum Dose* |
|---|---|---|---|---|
| Aldosterone receptor antagonists | Eplerenone | 25 mg/day | QD-BID | 100 mg/day |
| | Sprionolactone | 1 mg/kg/day | QD-BID | 3.3 mg/kg/day up to 100 mg/day |
| Angiotensin-converting enzyme (ACE) inhibitors | Benazepril | 0.2 mg/kg/day up to 10 mg/day | QD | 0.6 mg/kg/day up to 40 mg qd |
| | Captopril | 0.3- 0.5 mg/kg/dose | BID-TID | 0 6 mg/kg/day up to 450 mg/day |
| | Enalapril | 0.08 mg/kg/day | QD | 0.6 mg/kg/day up to 40 mg/day |
| | Fosinopril | 0.1 mg/kg/day up to 10 mg/day | QD | 0.6 mg/kg/day up to 40 mg/day |
| | Lisinopril | 0.07 mg/kg/day up to 5 mg/day | QD | 0.6 mg/kg/day up to 40 mg/day |
| | Quinapril | 5–10 mg/day | QD | 80 mg/day |
| | Ramipril | 2.5 mg/day | QD | 20 mg/day |
| Angiotensin receptor blockers (ARB) | Candesartan | 4 mg/day | QD | 32 mg |
| | Irbesartan | 75–150 mg/day | QD | 300 mg/day |
| | Losartan | 0.75 mg/kg/day up to 50 mg/day | QD | 1.4 mg/kg/day up to 100 mg/day |
| | Valsartan | 1.3 mg/kg/day up to 40 mg/day | QD | 2.7 mg/kg/day up to 160 mg/day |
| α- and β-Adrenergic antagonists | Labetalol | 2–3 mg/kg/day | BID | 10–12 mg/kg/day up to 1.2 g/day |
| | Carvedilol | 0.1 mg/kg/dose up to 12.5 mg | BID | 0.5 mg/kg/dose up to 25 mg |
| β-Adrenergic antagonists | Atenolol | 0.5–1 mg/kg/day | QD-BID | 2 mg/kg/day up to 100 mg/day |
| | Bisoprolol/ HCTZ | 0.04 mg/kg/day up to 2.5/6.25 mg/day | QD | 10/6.25 mg |
| | Metoprolol | 1–2 mg/kg/day | BID | 6 mg/kg/day up to 200 mg/day |
| | Propranolol | 1 mg/kg/day | BID-TID | 16 mg/kg/day up to 640 mg/day |
| Calcium channel blockers | Amlodipine | 0.06 mg/kg/day up to 5 mg/day | QD | 0.6 mg/kg/day up to 10 mg/day |
| | Felodipine | 2.5 mg/day | QD | 10 mg/day |
| | Isradipine | 0.05–0.15 mg/kg/dose | TID-QID | 0.8 mg/kg/day up to 20 mg/day |
| | Extended-release nifedipine | 0.25–0.5 mg/kg/day | QD-BID | 3 mg/kg/day up to 120 mg/day |
| Central α-agonists | Clonidine | 5–10 mcg/kg/day | BID-TID | 25 mcg/kg/day up to 0.9 mg/day |
| | Methyldopa | 5 mg/kg/day | BID-QID | 40 mg/kg/day up to 3 g/day |
| Diuretics | Amiloride | 5–10 mg/day | QD | 20 mg/day |
| | Chlorothiazide | 10 mg/kg/day | BID | 20 mg/kg/day up to 1 g/day |
| | Chlorthalidone | 0.3 mg/kg/day | QD | 2 mg/kg/day up to 50 mg/day |
| | Furosemide | 0.5–2.0 mg/kg/dose | QD-BID | 6 mg/kg/day |
| | HCTZ | 0.5–1 mg/kg/day | QD | 3 mg/kg/day up to 50 mg/day |
| | Triamterene | 1–2 mg/kg/day | BID | 3–4 mg/kg/day up to 300 mg/day |
| Peripheral α-antagonists | Doxazosin | 1 mg/day | QD | 4 mg/day |
| | Prazosin | 0.05–0.1 mg/kg/day | TID | 0.5 mg/kg/day |
| | Terazosin | 1 mg/day | QD | 20 mg/day |
| Vasodilators | Hydralazine | 0.25 mg/kg/dose | TID-QID | 7.5 mg/kg/day up to 200 mg/day |
| | Minoxidil | 0.1- 0.2 mg/kg/day | BID-TID | 1 mg/kg/day up to 50 mg/day |

BID, twice daily; QD, once daily; QID, 4 times daily; TID, 3 times daily.

**Table 118-7**

## Antihypertensive Drugs for Management of Severe Hypertension

| *Drug* | *Class* | *Dose* | *Route* | *Comments* |
|---|---|---|---|---|
| Clonidine | Central α-agonist | 0.05–0.2 mg/dose, may be repeated hourly up to 0.8 mg total dose | PO | Side effects include dry mouth and sedation. |
| Enalaprilat | ACE inhibitor | 0.05–0.10 mg/kg/dose up to 1.25 mg/dose | IV bolus | May cause prolonged hypotension and acute renal failure, especially in patients with high-renin hypertension. |
| Esmolol | ß-Blocker | 100–500 mcg/kg/min | IV infusion | Very short-acting—constant infusion preferred. May cause profound bradycardia. |
| Fenoldopam | Dopamine receptor agonist | 0.2–0.8 mcg/kg/min | IV infusion | Produced modest reductions in BP in a pediatric clinical trial in patients up to 12 years. |
| Hydralazine | Vasodilator | 0.2–0.6 mg/kg/dose | IV, IM | Should be given q 4 h when given IV bolus. |
| Isradipine | Calcium channel blocker | 0.05–0.1 mg/kg/dose up to 10 mg/dose | PO | Stable suspension can be compounded. |
| Labetalol | α- and ß-Blocker | Bolus: 0.20–1.0 mg/kg/dose—up to 40 mg/dose<br>Infusion: 0.25–3.0 mg/kg/h | IV bolus or infusion | Asthma and overt heart failure are relative contraindications. |
| Minoxidil | Vasodilator | 0.1–0.2 mg/kg/dose up to 5 mg/dose | PO | Most potent oral vasodilator; long acting. |
| Nicardipine | Calcium channel blocker | Bolus: 30 mcg/kg up to 2 mg/dose<br>Infusion: 0.5–4.0 mcg/kg/min | IV bolus or infusion | May cause reflex tachycardia. |
| Sodium nitroprusside | Vasodilator | 0.5–10 mcg/kg/min | IV infusion | Monitor cyanide levels with prolonged (>72 h) use or in renal failure; or coadminister with sodium thiosulfate. |

ACE, angiotensin-converting enzyme; IM, intramuscular; IV, intravenous; PO, oral.

Source: National High Blood Pressure Education Program Working Group on High Blood Pressure in Children and Adolescents. *The Fourth Report on the Diagnosis, Evaluation, and Treatment of High Blood Pressure in Children and Adolescents*. Bethesda, MD: National Institutes of Health, National Heart, Lung, and Blood Institute; 2005. NIH publication 05-5267.

## HYPERTENSIVE EMERGENCIES

A detailed discussion of the pathophysiology of severe HTN in adolescents is beyond the scope of this chapter. The interested reader should consult one of the available reviews for this information.[78–80]

Severe HTN has traditionally been divided into hypertensive emergencies and hypertensive urgencies, the former denoting severe HTN associated with life-threatening symptoms (congestive heart failure, seizures), and the latter denoting severe HTN with less severe symptoms (headache, vomiting). However, it is more important clinically to recognize that patients with severe, symptomatic HTN require prompt, careful management in order to either ameliorate or prevent the adverse effects of HTN on other organs such as the heart and brain.

Most adolescents with severe HTN will have underlying renal parenchymal disease, either previously known or newly diagnosed. Other causes may include renal artery stenosis, pheochromocytoma, and medication nonadherence in a patient with known HTN. Whatever the cause, it is important to highlight that hypertensive encephalopathy occurs frequently in adolescents with severe HTN, although perhaps somewhat less often than in younger children. Blood pressure reduction in such patients should be performed in a slow, controlled fashion to prevent ischemic strokes and other complications related to rapid BP reduction in the face of loss of normal autoregulatory processes.[78,81]

The usual goal in treatment of a hypertensive emergency is to reduce the BP by no more than 25% during the first 8 hours, with a gradual return to normal/goal BP during the next 24 to 48 hours.[79] Given the need for controlled BP reduction, treatment of hypertensive emergencies should be initiated with a continuous infusion of an intravenous antihypertensive, with nicardipine and labetalol finding the greatest popularity in most centers.[80,82] The dopamine receptor agonist fenoldopam has also been reported effective,[83] although it may not be as potent as nicardipine or other agents.[84] Sodium nitroprusside has fallen out of favor in most centers due to the possibility of thiocyanate accumulation with prolonged use.[80]

For less severe degrees of BP elevation, or if the patient's symptoms permit, oral antihypertensive agents can be used. Many choices are available; the practitioner should familiarize themselves with one or two agents and make them easily available in patient care settings where they may be needed. A list of recommended doses for drugs used to treat severe HTN in adolescents is found in Table 118-7.

## REFERENCES


1. Chobanian AV, Bakris GL, Black HR, et al. The 7th report of the Joint National Committee on prevention, detection, evaluation, and treatment of high blood pressure: the JNC 7 report. *JAMA.* 2003;289:2560-2572

2. National High Blood Pressure Education Program Working Group on High Blood Pressure in Children and Adolescents. *The Fourth Report on the Diagnosis, Evaluation, and Treatment of High Blood Pressure in Children and Adolescents.* Bethesda, MD: National Institutes of Health, National Heart, Lung, and Blood Institute; 2005. NIH publication 05-5267

3. Lauer RM, Connor WE, Leaverton PE, et al. Coronary heart disease risk factors in school children: the Muscatine Study. *J Pediatr.* 1975;86:697-706

4. Silverberg DS, Nostrand CV, Juchli B, et al. Screening for hypertension in a high school population. *Can Med Assoc J.* 1975;113:103-108

5. Fixler DE, Laird WP, Fitzgerald V, et al. Hypertension screening in schools: results of the Dallas Study. *Pediatrics.* 1979; 63:32-36

6. Sinaiko AR, Gomez-Marin O, Prineas RJ. Prevalence of "significant" hypertension in junior high school-aged children: the Children and Adolescent Blood Pressure Program. *J Pediatr.* 1989;114(4 pt 1):664-669

7. O'Quin M, Sharma BB, Miller KA, Tomsovic JP. Adolescent blood pressure survey: Tulsa, Oklahoma, 1987 to 1989. *South Med J.* 1992;85:487-490

8. Soyannwo MAO, Gadallah M, Kurashi NY, et al. Studies on preventative nephrology: systemic hypertension in the pediatric and adolescent population of Gassim, Saudi Arabia. *Ann Saudi Med.* 1997;17:47-52

9. Adrogue HE, Sinaiko AR. Prevalence of hypertension in junior high school-aged children: effect of new recommendations in the 1996 updated Task Force report. *Am J Hypertens.* 2001;14(5 Pt 1):412-414

10. Sorof JM, Lai D, Turner J, et al. Overweight, ethnicity, and the prevalence of hypertension in school-aged children. *Pediatrics.* 2004;113:475-482

11. Task Force on Blood Pressure Control in Children. Report of the second task force on blood pressure control in children—1987. *Pediatrics.* 1987;79(1):1-25

12. National High Blood Pressure Education Program Working Group on Hypertension Control in Children and Adolescents. Update on the 1987 task force report on high blood pressure in children and adolescents: a working group report from the National High Blood Pressure Education Program. *Pediatrics.* 1996;98:649-658

13. Centers for Disease Control and Prevention. Trends in child hood obesity. www.cdc.gov/obesity/childhood/trends.html. Accessed November 1, 2010

14. Luepker RV, Jacobs DR, Prineas RJ, Sinaiko AR. Secular trends of blood pressure and body size in a multi-ethnic adolescent population: 1986 to 1996. *J Pediatr.* 1999;134: 668-674

15. Muntner P, He J, Cutler JA, et al. Trends in blood pressure among children and adolescents. *JAMA.* 2004;291:2107-2113

16. Flynn JT, Alderman MH. Characteristics of children with primary hypertension seen at a referral center. *Pediatr Nephrol.* 2005;20:961-966

17. Croix B, Feig DI. Childhood hypertension is not a silent disease. *Pediatr Nephrol.* 2006;21:527-532

18. Sorof J, Daniels S. Obesity hypertension in children: a problem of epidemic proportions. *Hypertension.* 2002;40:441-447.

19. Feld LG, ed. *Hypertension in Children A Practical Approach.* Boston: Butterworth-Heinemann; 1997

20. Portman RJ, Sorof JM, Ingelfinger JR, eds. *Pediatric Hypertension.* Totowa, NJ: Humana Press; 2004

21. Wyszynska T, Cichocka E, Wieteska-Klimczak A, et al. A single center experience with 1,025 children with hypertension. *Acta Padiatrica.* 1992;81:244-246

22. Kellogg FR, Marks A, Cohen MI. Influence of familial hypertension on blood pressure during adolescence. *Am J Dis Child.* 1981;135:1047-1049

23. Munger RG, Prineas RJ, Gomez-Marin O. Persistent elevation of blood pressure among children with a family history of hypertension: the Minneapolis Children's Blood Pressure Study. *J Hypertens.* 1988;6:647-653

24. Buonomo E, Pasquarella A, Palombi L. Blood pressure and anthropometry in parents and children of a southern Italian village. *J Hum Hypertens.* 1996;10(suppl 3):S77-S79

25. Diaz Martin JJ, Malaga Dieguez I, Arguelles Luis J, et al. Clustering of cardiovascular risk factors in obese offspring of parents with essential hypertension. *An Pediatr (Barc).* 2005;63:238-243

26. Izzo JLJ, Levy D, Black HR. Importance of systolic blood pressure in older Americans. *Hypertension.* 2000;35:1021-1024

27. Sorof JM, Urbina EM, Cunningham RJ, et al. Screening for eligibility in the study of antihypertensive medication in children: experience from the Ziac Pediatric Hypertension Study. *Am J Hypertens.* 2001;14:783-787

28. Sorof JM, Poffenbarger T, Franco K, et al. Isolated systolic hypertension, obesity, and hyperkinetic hemodynamic states in children. *J Pediatr.* 2002;140:660-666

29. Gidding SS. Relationships between blood pressure and lipids in childhood. *Pediatr Clin North Am.* 1993;40:41-49

30. Boyd GS, Koenigsberg J, Falkner B, et al. Effect of obesity and high blood pressure on plasma lipid levels in children and adolescents. *Pediatrics.* 2005;116:442-446

31. Weiss R, Dziura J, Burgert TS, et al. Obesity and the metabolic syndrome in children and adolescents. *N Engl J Med.* 2004;350:2362-2374

32. Berenson GS, Srinivasan SR, Bao W, et al. Association between multiple cardiovascular risk factors and atherosclerosis in children and young adults. *N Engl J Med.* 1998;338:1650-1656

33. Brady TM, Fivush B, Flynn JT, Parekh R. Ability of blood pressure parameters to predict left ventricular hypertrophy in children with primary hypertension. *J Pediatr.* 2008;152:73-78, 78e1

34. Koren MJ, Devereux RB. Mechanism, effects, and reversal of left ventricular hypertrophy in hypertension. *Curr Opin Nephrol Hypertens.* 1993;2:87-95

35. Daniels SR, Lipman MJ, Burke MJ, Loggie JM. Determinants of retinal vascular abnormalities in children and adolescents with essential hypertension. *J Hum Hypertens.* 1993;7:223-228

36. Daniels SR, Lipman MJ, Burke MJ, Loggie JM. The prevalence of retinal vascular abnormalities in children and adolescents with essential hypertension. *Am J Ophthalmol.* 1991;111:205-208

37. Chambless LE, Heiss G, Folsom AR, et al. Association of coronary heart disease incidence with carotid arterial wall thickness and major risk factors: the Atherosclerosis Risk in Communities (ARIC) Study, 1987-1993. *Am J Epidemiol.* 1997;146:483-494

38. Cuspidi C, Mancia G, Ambrosioni E, et al. Left ventricular and carotid structure in untreated, uncomplicated essential hypertension: results from the Assessment Prognostic Risk Observational Survey (APROS). *J Hum Hypertens.* 2004;18:891-896

39. Sorof JM, Alexandrov AV, Cardwell G, Portman RJ. Carotid artery intimal-medial thickness and left ventricular hypertrophy in children with elevated blood pressure. *Pediatrics.* 2003;111:61-66

40. Lande MB, Carson NL, Roy J, Meagher CC. The effects of childhood primary hypertension on carotid intima-media thickness: a matched controlled study. *Hypertension.* 2006;48:1-5

41. Flynn JT. What is the significance of increased carotid intima-media thickness in hypertensive adolescents? *Hypertension.* 2006;14:23-24

42. US Renal Data System. *2002 USRDS Annual Data Report: Atlas of End-Stage Renal Disease in the United States.* Bethesda, MD: National Institutes of Health, National Institute of Diabetes and Digestive and Kidney Diseases; 2002

43. North American Pediatric Renal Transplant Cooperative Study. *2004 Annual Report.* Potomac, MD: Emmes Corporation; 2005

44. Mazzucchi A, Mutti A, Poletti A, et al. Neuropsychological deficits in arterial hypertension. *Acta Neurol Scand.* 1986;73:619-627

45. Elias ME, Wolf PA, D'Agostino RB, et al. Untreated blood pressure level is inversely related to cognitive functioning: the Framingham Study. *Am J Epidemiol.* 1993;138:353-364

46. Lande MB, Kaczorowski JM, Auinger P, et al. Elevated blood pressure and decreased cognitive function among school-age children and adolescents in the United States. *J Pediatr.* 2003;143:720-724

47. Lever AF, Harrap SB. Essential hypertension: a disorder of growth with origins in childhood? *J Hypertens.* 1992;10:101-120

48. Lauer RM, Clarke WR. Childhood risk factors for adult blood pressure: the Muscatine Study. *Pediatrics.* 1989;84:633-641

49. Chen X, Wang Y. Tracking of blood pressure from childhood to adulthood: a systematic review and meta-regression analysis. *Circulation.* 2008;117:3171-3180

50. Lurbe E, Sorof JM, Daniels SR. Clinical and research aspects of ambulatory blood pressure monitoring in children. *J Pediatr.* 2004;144:7-16

51. Sorof JM, Cardwell G, Franco K, Portman RJ. Ambulatory blood pressure and left ventricular mass index in hypertensive children. *Hypertension.* 2002;39:903-908

52. Flynn JT. Differentiation between primary and secondary hypertension in children using ambulatory blood pressure monitoring. *Pediatrics.* 2002;110:89-93

53. Seeman T, Palyzova D, Dusek J, Janda J. Reduced nocturnal blood pressure dip and sustained nighttime hypertension are specific markers of secondary hypertension. *J Pediatr.* 2005;147:366-371

54. Rocchini AP, Katch V, Anderson J, et al. Blood pressure in obese adolescents: effect of weight loss. *Pediatrics.* 1988;82:16–23

55. Williams CL, Hayman LL, Daniels SR, et al. Cardiovascular health in childhood: a statement for health professionals from the Committee on Atherosclerosis, Hypertension, and Obesity in the Young (AHOY) of the Council on Cardiovascular Disease in the Young, American Heart Association. *Circulation.* 2002;106:143–160

56. Reinehr T, Andler W. Changes in the atherogenic risk factor profile according to degree of weight loss. *Arch Dis Child.* 2004;89:419–422

57. Togashi K, Masuda H, Rankinen T, et al. A 12-year follow-up study of treated obese children in Japan. *Int J Obes Relat Metab Disord.* 2002;26:770–777

58. Alpert BS. Exercise as a therapy to control hypertension in children. *Int J Sports Med.* 2000;21 (suppl 2):S94–S96

59. Daniels SR, Arnett DK, Eckel RH, et al. Overweight in children and adolescents: pathophysiology, consequences, prevention, and treatment. *Circulation.* 2005;111:1999–2012

60. Diabetes Prevention Program Research Group. Reduction in the incidence of type 2 diabetes with lifestyle modification or metformin. *N Engl J Med.* 2002;346:393–403

61. Watts K, Jones TW, Davis EA, Green D. Exercise training in obese children and adolescents: current concepts. *Sports Med.* 2005;35:375–392

62. Ribeiro MM, Silva AG, Santos NS, et al. Diet and exercise training restore blood pressure and vasodilatory responses during physiological maneuvers in obese children. *Circulation.* 2005;111:1915–1923

63. Falkner B, Michel S. Blood pressure response to sodium in children and adolescents. *Am J Clin Nutr.* 1997;65(2 suppl):618S–621S

64. Rocchini AP, Key J, Bondie D, et al. The effect of weight loss on the sensitivity of blood pressure to sodium in obese adolescents. *N Engl J Med.* 1989;321:580–585

65. Mu JJ, Liu ZQ, Liu WM, et al. Reduction of blood pressure with calcium and potassium supplementation in children with salt sensitivity: a 2-year double-blinded placebo-controlled trial. *J Hum Hypertens.* 2005;19:479–483

66. Appel LJ, Moore TJ, Obarzanek E, et al. A clinical trial of the effects of dietary patterns on blood pressure. *N Engl J Med.* 1997;336:1118–1124

67. Appel L, Brands, M, Daniels SR, et al. Dietary approaches to prevent and treat hypertension: a scientific statement from the American Heart Association. *Hypertension.* 2006;47:296–308

68. Couch SC, Saelens BE, Levin L, et al. The efficacy of a clinic-based behavioral nutrition intervention emphasizing a DASH-type diet for adolescents with elevated blood pressure. *J Pediatr.* 2008;152:494–501

69. ALLHAT Officers and Coordinators for the ALLHAT Collaborative Research Group. Major outcomes in high-risk hypertensive patients randomized to angiotensin-converting enzyme inhibitor or calcium channel blocker vs diuretic: The Antihypertensive and Lipid-Lowering Treatment to Prevent Heart Attack Trial (ALLHAT). *JAMA.* 2002;288:2981–2997

70. Laragh JH. Abstract, closing summary, and table of contents for Laragh's 25 lessons in pathophysiology and 12 clinical pearls for treating hypertension. *Am J Hypertens.* 2001;14:1183–1187

71. Hall JE. The kidney, hypertension, and obesity. *Hypertension.* 2003;41:625–633

72. Puri M, Flynn JT. Management of hypertension in children and adolescents with the metabolic syndrome. *J Cardiometab Syndr.* 2006;1:259–268

73. Shatat IF, Flynn JT. Hypertension in children with chronic kidney disease. *Adv Chronic Kidney Dis.* 2005;12:378–384

74. Anonymous. After the diagnosis: adherence and persistence with hypertension therapy. *Am J Manag Care.* 2005;11(13 suppl):S395–S399

75. Wells T, Stowe C. An approach to the use of antihypertensive drugs in children and adolescents. *Curr Ther Res Clin Exp.* 2001;62:329

76. Flynn JT, Daniels SR. Pharmacologic management of hypertension in children and adolescents. *J Pediatr.* 2006;149(6):746–754

77. Cooper WO, Hernandez-Diaz S, Arbogast PG, et al. Major congenital malformations after first-trimester exposure to ACE inhibitors. *N Engl J Med.* 2006;354:2443–2451

78. Vaughan CJ, Delanty N. Hypertensive emergencies. *Lancet.* 2000;356:411–417

79. Adelman RD. Management of hypertensive emergencies. In: Portman R, Sorof J, Ingelfinger J, eds. *Pediatric Hypertension.* Totowa, NJ: Humana Press; 2004:457–469

80. Patel HP, Mitsnefnes M. Advances in the pathogenesis and management of hypertensive crisis. *Curr Opin Pediatr.* 2005;17:210–214

81. Schwartz RB. Hyperperfusion encephalopathies: hypertensive encephalopathy and related conditions. *The Neurologist.* 2002;8:22–34

82. Flynn JT, Mottes TA, Brophy PB, et al. Intravenous nicardipine for treatment of severe hypertension in children. *J Pediatr.* 2001;139:38–43

83. Strauser LM, Pruitt RD, Tobias JD. Initial experience with fenoldopam in children. *Am J Ther.* 1999;6:283–288

84. Murphy MB, Murray C, Shorten GD. Fenoldopam: a selective peripheral dopamine-receptor agonist for the treatment of severe hypertension. *N Engl J Med.* 2001;345:1548–1557

# CHAPTER 119

# Voiding Disorders

MANJU CHANDRA, MD

## INTRODUCTION

In higher vertebrates, Mother Nature interposed the urinary bladder between the kidneys and the external environment to allow continence. The urinary bladder has been entrusted 2 major functions: storage of urine without leakage and efficient emptying at appropriate intervals. Normal bladder function bestows humans with the dual skills of storing urine until the time and place is convenient and appropriate for bladder emptying, and passing urine at will, even when the bladder is not full.

An efficient voiding mechanism depends on a normal anatomy of the lower urinary tract and coordination of the various events of the micturition reflex by the central nervous system. The storage of urine is achieved by maintenance of low pressure in the bladder despite continued distension, a good urethral closure mechanism, and a gradual increase in the tone of the external urethral sphincter and pelvic floor during bladder filling. No leakage of urine occurs despite bursts of high intra-abdominal pressure from coughing or sneezing as long as the urethral closure pressure remains higher than the intravesical pressure. The usual bladder capacity ranges from 200 mL to 400 mL in adults, whereas most individuals with an average fluid intake void 4 to 8 times in 24 hours.

Bladder emptying results from a neurally induced detrusor (bladder muscle) contraction coordinated with widening of the bladder neck and opening up of the urethra from pelvic floor relaxation. The bladder is able to empty at low pressure because widening of the urethra provides a low resistance channel for urine flow. The bladder may or may not empty completely but the postvoid residual rarely exceeds 20 mL. The synergy between pelvic floor relaxation and detrusor contraction is mediated in the brain stem micturition center located in the pons, whereas the widening of the bladder neck depends on the pulling action of a strong detrusor contraction.

Human beings are able to sense varying degrees of bladder fullness and can plan bladder emptying rather than respond to the urgent calls of the bladder. Most people can hold urine, even after an urge to void has been felt, by centrally relaxing the detrusor. Central postponement of micturition becomes increasingly difficult as the bladder fills beyond the usual capacity; most people will then hold urine by voluntarily tightening the pelvic floor musculature, because this maneuver reflexively inhibits detrusor contractions.

## MATURATION OF BLADDER CONTROL

The bladder manifests changes in storage and emptying patterns from infancy through the toddler stage, reaching a mature pattern during early childhood. During infancy, the bladder empties reflexively when it fills to functional capacity, hence involuntary passage of urine is normal in infants and toddlers. With growth, a series of maturational processes, hormonal, neural, and structural, result in diurnal and nocturnal urinary continence by age 5 in most children. These maturational processes lead to all of the following: increased functional bladder capacity, perception of bladder fullness and impending detrusor contraction, ability to void voluntarily even when the bladder is not full, ability to hold urine despite a full bladder (by inhibition of reflex detrusor contractions by the cerebral cortex), decrease in nocturnal urine volume, and improvement in arousal from sleep in response to bladder fullness. Maturational delay or pathological alteration in one or more of these processes can result in primary diurnal or nocturnal enuresis (NE), or secondary onset of enuresis.

## CLASSIFICATION OF VOIDING DISORDERS

Voiding disorders can be classified as disorders of storage and disorders of emptying. A storage problem, such as urinary incontinence, can result from low urethral resistance or high intravesical pressure, either from reflex detrusor contractions or poor detrusor compliance. Emptying problems, such as a weak or intermittent urinary stream or urinary retention, can result from impaired detrusor contractility or an inability to lower urethral resistance due to a functional or mechanical urethral obstruction.

**Box 119-1**

***Voiding Disorders in Adolescents***

**Disorders of Storage**

- Urinary frequency: Voiding every 2 hours or more often
- Infrequent voiding: Voiding 3 times or less in 24 hours or not voiding for 12 hours overnight
- Urinary urgency: Short latency between the urge and imperative need to void
- Incontinence: Involuntary urine leakage
- Intermittent diurnal urge incontinence, nocturnal enuresis
- Continuous ectopic ureter, iatrogenic damage to the external urinary sphincter
- Diurnal urge syndrome: Combination of urinary frequency, urgency, urge incontinence, and pelvic withholding maneuvers to postpone voiding
- Postvoid dribble

**Disorders of Emptying**

- Hesitancy of urination: difficulty in initiating a void
- Straining or manual compression of the bladder to initiate or continue voiding
- Slow or interrupted urinary stream
- Urinary retention
- Feeling of incomplete bladder emptying
- Dysuria and strangury (slow, painful urination)

Box 119-1 lists common voiding disorders encountered in adolescents. The 3 most commonly encountered voiding disorders in adolescents are discussed here.

## PATHOPHYSIOLOGY AND MANAGEMENT OF COMMON VOIDING DISORDERS

### OVERACTIVE BLADDER

Acute urinary frequency and urgency can result from bladder and urethral mucosal inflammation or irritation from a urinary tract infection (UTI), crystalluria, stone formation, or foreign bodies. In the absence of the previously mentioned problems, urinary frequency, urgency, and urge incontinence in adolescents are generally related to an overactive bladder (OAB), that is, a bladder prone to reflex detrusor contractions that occur at less than full bladder capacity and are not inhibited by the cerebral cortex.

The prevalence of OAB is estimated to be 15% in adolescents, although not all adolescents will have readily apparent symptoms. The OAB in some adolescents may be of primary onset, that is, present since the toddler years as a result of delayed maturation of cerebral inhibitory control over the bladder, whereas in others the diurnal urinary urgency and urge incontinence is of secondary onset, occurring after at least a 6-month period of normal diurnal voiding control. The etiology of OAB comprises reflex detrusor contractions from neurogenic and nonneurogenic causes. The former include inadequate cortical inhibition of the micturition reflex, cerebral or spinal cord lesions, and degenerative neuropathies. Nonneurogenic causes include bladder outlet obstruction, stool retention in the rectosigmoid, and chronic bladder mucosal irritation from infection, stones, or a tumor. Overactive bladder is common in patients with cerebral palsy and in those with learning delays and attention-deficit/hyperactivity disorder (ADHD), although the vast majority of adolescents presenting with OAB do not manifest these problems.

The response to sudden unannounced detrusor contractions may vary in different adolescents at different times. For many it may include a mad rush to the toilet, total urge incontinence, or attempts to postpone voiding and minimize urine leakage by tightening of the pelvic floor muscles (because the latter reflexively inhibits and aborts a detrusor contraction). Some patients with OAB learn to restrict fluid intake as a method for increasing voiding intervals and minimizing leakage. Patients who manifest urinary urgency and pelvic withholding maneuvers are labeled as having the "diurnal urge syndrome."

Some patients with OAB use pelvic withholding maneuvers repeatedly to postpone voiding to a more opportune time and to prevent socially embarrassing urine leakage. The pelvic withholding maneuvers in some adolescents change from a volitional act intended to prevent urine leakage to a conditioned behavior; these adolescents may habitually contract their pelvic floor during voiding, causing functional urethral obstruction that in turn manifests as a weak or interrupted urinary stream. This dysfunctional pattern of voiding results in high intravesical pressures, detrusor hypertrophy, and incomplete bladder emptying. Patients with these behaviors are at risk for development of recurrent UTI, secondary vesicoureteral reflux, a decompensated detrusor with decreased contractility, and stool retention.[1,2] Patients with dysfunctional voiding often suffer from psychological comorbidity or behavioral problems. These include outwardly directed visible behaviors, such as conduct disorder or ADHD or internalizing, emotional disorders, such as social anxiety, sibling rivalry, or depressive disorders. The patient's voiding problems may additionally elicit punitive behavior from the parents, which may compound the underlying psychosocial disturbances.

### Evaluation of Patients with Overactive Bladder

All patients with urinary frequency, urgency, or urge incontinence should have a urinalysis to rule out the presence of a UTI, glucosuria from diabetes mellitus, and urolithiasis-related crystalluria. Polyuria secondary to a urinary concentrating defect can be excluded by documenting a urine-specific gravity of 1.016 or higher in a random urine, or a urine collected after fluid deprivation. Patients with dysuria or leukocyturia should have a urine culture.

An underlying neurogenic or organic cause of voiding dysfunction should be ruled out in all patients by obtaining a detailed history of voiding patterns and performing a directed physical examination. Evaluation utilizing structured questionnaires, a voiding pattern chart (bladder diary), and observation of voiding all yield important information.[3] Renal and bladder ultrasonography is indicated in those with a UTI and severe voiding dysfunction to rule out an underlying structural abnormality. Additional tests, such as noninvasive uroflowmetry, pelvic floor electromyography, and measurement of the postvoid residual, are helpful in assessing lower urinary tract function and determining which patients will require more invasive urodynamic investigations.

### Treatment of Overactive Bladder

The treatment of OAB is aimed at preventing reflex detrusor contractions and retraining the patient with dysfunctional voiding to relax his or her pelvic floor during voiding. Patients are educated about normal functioning of the lower urinary tract, in what way their voiding habits deviate from normal, proper voiding posture, and treatment measures that can help achieve normal voiding habits and avoid pelvic withholding maneuvers.

***Behavioral and Motivational Therapy*** Patients with OAB are taught bladder control by following a regimen of frequent voluntary voiding that is timed to occur before the bladder has a chance to fill to its functional capacity and contract reflexively. The frequent voluntary voidings help break the pattern of reflex detrusor contractions and train the bladder to respond to the patient's commands instead of the patient having to respond to the unwanted detrusor contractions. In order to focus his or her attention on the problem, the patient is asked to maintain a voiding diary with planned voids, urgent voids, and incontinence episodes.[4] Positive feedback is provided to reinforce patient behavior. Voiding intervals are gradually increased from every 2 to every 3 to 4 hours if the patient demonstrates the ability to hold urine comfortably without urgency or pelvic withholding maneuvers.

***Pharmacological Therapy of Overactive Bladder*** Anticholinergic drugs are extremely useful as an adjunct to behavioral treatment. These agents increase the threshold for reflex detrusor contractions and decrease their amplitude and frequency. With anticholinergic agents, a balance between efficacy and tolerability should be considered because systemic side effects related to blockade of cholinergic receptors at sites other than the detrusor muscle may preclude use of the higher doses needed to combat detrusor overactivity. The older anticholinergic agents, including propantheline and short-acting oxybutynin hydrochloride, had significant side effects of dry mouth, dryness of the skin, and blurred vision. However, newer agents are more specific for M3-type muscarinic receptors in the bladder and have slow-release formulations, and some have additional direct antispasmodic activity on the detrusor muscle. These medications include oxybutynin extended-release tablets, tolterodine tartrate short- and long-acting capsules, trospium chloride tablets, darifenacin extended release tablets, and solifenacin tablets.[4] Whichever anticholinergic medication is used, the dose should be increased to the maximum tolerable level if there is not sufficient improvement in voiding symptoms despite motivated efforts on the part of the patient. Medication is continued daily until the patient is able to comfortably hold urine for 3 to 4 hours without intervening urinary urgency or urge incontinence for 4 weeks; medication is then either discontinued or titrated to the lowest dose required to maintain a normal voiding pattern.

***Pelvic Floor Relaxation Training*** Patients with incomplete bladder and rectal emptying related to inadequate pelvic floor relaxation, as well as those with hesitancy of urination and hesitancy of bowel elimination, will benefit from efforts directed at teaching pelvic floor relaxation using slow and deep breathing. This can also be done by having the patient perceive and observe in a mirror the movement of the pelvic floor while using a pelvic withholding maneuver. The patient then tries to achieve the opposite, that is, pelvic floor relaxation and descent. Optimal posture during voiding and defecation is emphasized.

In the setting of a urodynamics laboratory, biofeedback training can be provided with visual or audio demonstration of the child's pelvic floor electromyogram activity obtained with sticky patch electrodes placed around the anus while the patient's urine flow curve is monitored simultaneously. Intermittent urine flow and lack of suppression of pelvic floor electromyographic activity can thus be demonstrated to the patient in a graphic manner and compared over several voids.

***Treatment of Comorbidities*** Addressing the accompanying psychological and behavioral problems is important in the management of those with OAB; for example, treatment of associated ADHD will help the child focus better on his or her voiding problem.[5,6]

It is important to treat associated constipation or stool retention because stool retention predisposes to OAB and sets up a vicious cycle that may negatively affect the patient socially and psychologically.[2] The treatment of constipation or stool retention includes patient education about the biologic basis of the problem, institution of dietary modifications and laxatives, and gentle persuasion to attempt 1 or 2 bowel movements per day with the goal of keeping the rectum empty. Several effective treatment regimens for constipation are available.

***Unconventional Therapies*** For patients with OAB resistant to standard therapy and continued severe voiding problems, other nonevidence-based interventions have included periodic intravesical instillation of capsaicin or resiniferatoxin (neurotoxins that desensitize the C-fiber afferent neurons), electrical stimulation of sacral nerve roots, and injection of botulinum toxin into the detrusor muscle.[7]

## NOCTURNAL ENURESIS

### Prevalence

Nocturnal enuresis is noted in 1% of 18-year-olds and 0.5% of adults. Although NE occurs in 6% to 10% of 7-year-olds, its prevalence goes down with age. However, not everyone outgrows bed-wetting. The estimated risk for a patient who has had persistent NE from the toddler years to continue with NE for the rest of his or her life is 3% if the NE is not treated in childhood.[7]

### Pathophysiology

Nocturnal enuresis results when the amount of urine produced at night exceeds the nocturnal bladder capacity and the patient is unable to awaken to the stimulus of a full bladder. Nocturnal enuresis is a heterogeneous disorder that reflects an interplay of decreased nocturnal bladder capacity, nocturnal polyuria, and difficult sleep arousal.[8,9] Whether NE has always been present, or develops after a minimum of 6 months of dryness is an important question because the pathophysiology may be different in those with primary versus secondary onset of NE.[10] Psychosocial problems often result in the secondary onset of NE.[5,10] Some adolescents manifest NE as the only voiding problem and have a perfectly normal daytime voiding pattern; they are labeled as having monosymptomatic NE. Many others manifest bed-wetting in association with diurnal symptoms related to OAB.

Whereas the healthy nonenuretic individuals can hold 1.6 to 2.1 times more urine during sleep than awake, decreased nocturnal functional bladder capacity possibly related to OAB has been noted in many patients with NE.[11,12] Diurnal urinary frequency, urgency, and urge incontinence coexist with NE in 50% of affected boys and 75% of affected girls.[10] Patients with monosymptomatic NE have normal bladder capacity in the day whereas those with NE associated with diurnal frequency and urgency have low functional bladder capacity both during the day and during sleep.

Nocturnal polyuria has been noted in many children and adolescents with NE. Most people develop a circadian rhythm of urine production in early childhood, with nocturnal urine production approximating half of daytime levels.[9,12] Lower nocturnal urine volume results from decreased free water and solute excretion. Factors that may affect nocturnal urine production include: blood levels of arginine vasopressin, angiotensin II, and atrial natriuretic peptide; renal production of various prostaglandins; aquaporin dysfunction; hypercalciuria; and obstructed breathing. Lack of a normal nocturnal surge in arginine vasopressin secretion has been noted in some patients with NE, and this deficiency seems to correlate with nocturnal polyuria as well as improvement in NE with use of the vasopressin analogue DDAVP.[9] The urine output in those with NE, however, varies considerably from night to night, and nocturnal urine volume appears to be much larger on wet nights compared to dry nights.

Obstructed breathing during sleep has been found to be associated with an increased prevalence of NE which may in part be related to nocturnal polyuria due to an increased release of atrial and brain natriuretic peptides and impaired sleep arousal. In a recent community-based survey of 5- to 7-year-old children, NE was reported in 26.9% of 53 habitual snoring children compared to 11.6% in 15,670 nonsnoring children.[13]

Regardless of the cause of the mismatch between nocturnal bladder capacity and nocturnal polyuria, NE only occurs when the patient is unable to wake up before voiding is initiated. This has caused many to conclude that an abnormal sleep pattern and deep sleep contribute to bed-wetting. However, recent studies suggest that the problem is with sleep arousal rather than with the depth of sleep. Difficult arousal from sleep has been noted in patients with NE, based on parental beliefs as well as on objective assessments of arousal from sleep by a questionnaire-based scoring system, auditory stimulation, and simultaneous sleep EEG and sleep urodynamic studies.[14] Our own studies have noted difficult arousal from sleep in 59% of patients with NE and 20%

of controls, but only in 5% of patients who were dry at night despite daytime symptoms of urinary frequency and urgency.[10]

Bed-wetters do not awaken to void as often as their peers. We have found in our studies that only 6% of bed-wetters awakened to void at least twice a month whereas one-third of controls and one-third of patients with isolated daytime bladder overactivity did so.[10] The frequency of nocturia was 11-fold lower in those with NE than in those with isolated diurnal urge syndrome.

There is a significant difference in sleep arousal among subgroups of patients with NE. Patients with monosymptomatic NE and those with primary onset of NE have a higher prevalence of difficult sleep arousal than those with secondary onset of NE or NE associated with diurnal voiding symptoms. It appears that difficult sleep arousal is an important pathogenic factor for primary monosymptomatic NE but plays a lesser role in patients with secondary onset of NE associated with diurnal voiding problems.[10] The variability in sleep arousal can explain why some patients awaken after bed-wetting and change into dry clothes whereas others continue to sleep, remaining unaware of their being wet.

Sleep stage and arousal response may affect nocturnal urine production and reflex detrusor contraction, thereby modifying the ability of the bladder to hold urine overnight. The brainstem nuclei that control arousal and that inhibit detrusor contractions are in close proximity to the pontine micturition center.[6] Therefore, lower arousal can result in decreased inhibition of the micturition reflex during sleep.

Familial clustering of NE has long been known. Genetic factors are paramount in the etiology of NE whereas environmental factors, both somatic and psychosocial, exert modulatory effects on the phenotype. Empirical family studies have demonstrated a high rate of relatives affected by enuresis; 22% to 39% of fathers, 23% to 24% of mothers, 46% of parents,17% of siblings, and 63% of relatives.[7] The risk of a child being affected by NE is 40% if 1 parent and 70% if both parents had bed-wetting. Genetic linkage studies have identified different "loci" for susceptibility to NE. There is, however, no clear association of any of the identified loci with any particular type of NE.

The rate of clinically relevant behavioral disorders in children and adolescents with NE is between 12% (ICD-10 criteria) and 14.3% (*DSM-IV-TR*) criteria.[7] Children with monosymptomatic NE, however, have a much lower incidence of behavioral problems than those with NE associated with diurnal urge syndrome. In a study[10] we performed in 2004, only 2% of patients with monosymptomatic NE manifested psychosocial/learning problems compared to 21% of those with NE and the diurnal urge syndrome. Although none of the children with primary onset of monosymptomatic NE had any psychosocial problems, 10% of those who had secondary onset of monosymptomatic NE did so.

Several adverse factors operative during the critical years of maturation of the central nervous system's control over voiding may result in primary or secondary onset of NE and the coexistence of diurnal urge syndrome with the NE. The stressors that may impair bladder control include: OAB, large urine volume during sleep related to a urine concentrating defect or solute diuresis, obstructed breathing, immature sleep arousal mechanism, a nonnurturing environment, emotional stress, UTI, and stool retention. Monosymptomatic NE represents impaired inhibitory control of the cerebral cortex over the bladder selectively during sleep and appears to be related to the first 3 stressors only. Most other stressors lead to both NE and diurnal voiding symptoms or to diurnal voiding symptoms only.

### Evaluation of Patients with Nocturnal Enuresis

An important role for the physician in managing the adolescent with NE is to rule out structural or neurogenic lower urinary tract dysfunction and to identify additional daytime voiding symptoms. This can be done with a detailed history of voiding and bowel elimination patterns and a good physical examination. A urinalysis is needed in all children with enuresis to rule out polyuria secondary to glucosuria, or a urinary concentrating defect. A urine-specific gravity of 1.016 or more in a random or first morning urine sample rules out a concentrating defect. Monosymptomatic NE rarely, if ever, is the only symptom of structural or neurogenic urinary tract disease; hence imaging studies of the urinary tract are not indicated in children with monosymptomatic NE.

A careful voiding and sleeping pattern history, preferably with the use of a structured questionnaire, is crucial to discovering the predominant underlying pathophysiological mechanisms operative in a particular patient: nocturnal polyuria, OAB and difficult sleep arousal.[11] Sleep arousal can be assessed with the use of a previously validated and standardized questionnaire-based scoring system.[10]

The suspicion that there is an associated diurnal urge syndrome should be high in all girls with NE because it coexists with NE in 75% of affected girls. The suspicion for coexistent diurnal urge syndrome should also be high in any patient with a history of a UTI, encopresis, psychosocial/learning problems, or a family history of UTI, because patients with OAB are prone to UTI, stool retention, and psychological and behavioral comorbidity.[10] Moreover, the tendency to have OAB runs in families. Patients with such a history should be further questioned for the presence of daytime voiding symptoms, even if those symptoms were not volunteered, because patients with OAB from early childhood who leak only a few drops may be unaware that their daytime voiding pattern is abnormal. Moreover, parents of subjects with diurnal urge incontinence often blame it on the patient's laziness and waiting until the last minute to void.

Certain clinical pearls are worth noting. The timing and frequency of wetting at night, as well as the amount of wetness, may reflect nocturnal functional bladder capacity and the nocturnal urine volume. Patients who wet after several hours of sleep are likely to have a larger bladder capacity than those who wet soon after falling asleep, unless they drank a large amount of fluid prior to sleep. Patients with small functional bladder capacity may leak small amounts of urine more than once each night. Patients with polyuria usually wet large amounts. A history of obstructed breathing should raise suspicion for nocturnal polyuria. A patient manifesting nocturia or awakening after wetting has easy sleep arousal and is therefore likely to have either low bladder capacity or nocturnal polyuria as the cause of the NE. Patients with constipation and encopresis are prone to OAB hence low bladder capacity, as the cause of the NE.

### Treatment of Nocturnal Enuresis

The treatment of NE is directed at the major pathophysiologic mechanisms of NE at work in a particular patient, that is, nocturnal polyuria, OAB at night, or difficult sleep arousal. Patients should be labeled as having monosymptomatic NE only when additional diurnal voiding symptoms are ruled out with a careful voiding history. In patients with NE and diurnal urge syndrome, the daytime voiding habits first need to be normalized, with use of anticholinergic agents and frequent timed voluntary voiding, as described in the previous section.

The treatment of monosymptomatic NE includes general measures, including patient education, motivation, and fluid restriction, as well as specific therapy with either a moisture alarm, vasopressin analogue, or tricyclic antidepressants. The efficacy and mode of action of these treatments have recently been reviewed. In those with obstructed breathing, alleviation of the respiratory tract obstruction by removal of the adenoids or application of positive airway pressure often improves or cures the NE. Monosymptomatic NE has no adverse medical consequences. It is, however, a treatable condition and treatment does offer psychosocial benefits and improved self-image. The goal of treatment is complete dryness at night for at least 6 consecutive weeks and not just a reduction of wetting frequency.

***Patient Education and General Measures*** Education of the patient and family about the pathogenic factors for monosymptomatic NE is an important part of treatment and well worth the time invested at the initial visit. The patient should be advised, in lay language and with the use of Venn diagrams, of the interaction of difficult sleep arousal, nocturnal polyuria, and low bladder capacity in the causation of NE. The patient and family should be advised about the actions and side effects of different therapeutic agents, to help them decide which treatment option best suits their lifestyle. The therapeutic agent is described as the "coach" and the patient as the "player." The player has the pivotal role in achieving the goal, whereas the coach just helps and guides.

To minimize the possibility of nocturnal polyuria, the patient is counseled to restrict fluid intake to 8 ounces in the 3 to 3½ hours prior to bedtime, to avoid any fluid intake thereafter and to empty the bladder just before retiring to bed. The patient is encouraged to have a bedtime resolution to stay dry and to keep a chart of wet and dry nights; both of these activities serve to focus the patient's attention on the problem. The patient is provided positive feedback for dry nights and effort in the form of words of praise, a pat on the back, or a more substantial reward. Any punitive reaction to the patient's bed-wetting is discouraged. The combination of a motivated patient and a cooperative family is a good predictor of positive outcome.

***Conditioning with a Moisture Alarm*** The moisture alarm works on the principle that urine leakage will complete an electrical circuit and sound an alarm. The recommended alarm system consists of a small sponge pad, worn in the pajamas, to which an electric sensor is clipped. The wire from the sensor reaches a small alarm box that can be strapped to the shoulder by Velcro or a pin. The alarm serves as a conditioning device. The child initially responds to the noise by awakening just after a voiding detrusor contraction. After several nights of alarm use, the patient will learn to avoid the noise stimulus by not leaking at night. Dryness may result either from the patient awakening to void or because of increased nocturnal bladder capacity.

About two-thirds of patients with monosymptomatic NE are deep sleepers and unlikely to awaken with the noise of the alarm; in those cases, parents or guardians should take the responsibility of awakening the adolescent when they hear the alarm and assist him or her to the bathroom to finish voiding. After several nights of alarm use, many of these adolescents will learn to either awaken to the noise of the alarm, or leak less, or not leak. As patients manifest improvement with alarm use, the time of wetting moves from early in the night to the early hours of the morning and the amount of wetness decreases. After achieving 28 consecutive dry nights, fluid intake after supper should be liberalized. It is wise to discontinue alarm use only after the patient demonstrates continued dryness for another 2 weeks despite normal fluid intake. This overconditioning improves the long-term success rate. In the event of a relapse of NE, the alarm use should be reinitiated and continued until 28 consecutive dry nights are achieved.

Many families discontinue alarm use in frustration if the alarm continues to go off most nights, not realizing the subtle improvement in bladder capacity and sleep arousal manifesting as wetting later at night with less wetness each time.

The long-term cure rate of bed-wetting with alarm use has been variable, but can be as high as 83%. The alarm is most effective in children with frequent wet nights per week and more than one episode of wetness per night. Close follow-up every 2 weeks is important to sustain motivation and monitor results. The commercial alarms presently available are fairly safe and free of side effects. The alarms that have a vibrator but no sound are not likely to awaken patients with difficult sleep arousal and are therefore not useful for this subgroup of patients.

Awakening of the adolescent to void at a time convenient to the parents or with an alarm clock is often helpful in achieving some dry nights but does not achieve the long-term cure that the moisture alarm therapy does, because awakening with the latter is conditioned to the stimulus of a full bladder and voiding detrusor contraction.

***Treatment with Tricyclic Antidepressants*** Tricyclic antidepressants help patients with monosymptomatic NE either by enhancing their arousal from sleep in response to a full bladder or due to their anticholinergic effect. Imipramine works better than other tricyclic antidepressants.

Imipramine works best in patients with frequent wet nights and difficult sleep arousal and is a better alternative to alarm treatment when parents do not wish to be bothered at night by the noise of the moisture alarm. Imipramine use may result in dry nights from the first dose or after a few weeks. It is generally given as a single dose of 1.5 to 2 mg/kg body weight about 1½ to 2 hours prior to bedtime with a maximum dose of 75 mg, or 2.5 mg/kg. Imipramine is prescribed nightly until 21 consecutive dry nights are achieved (a minimum of 4 weeks daily if the adolescent was dry from the first day of its use) and then the dose is reduced to every other night for 2 weeks in association with liberalization of fluid intake in the evening. If the patient continues to stay dry, the medication is stopped. For patients who relapse after discontinuation of medication, the nightly dosage is reintroduced until at least 6 weeks of dryness is achieved before the dose is tapered to every other night.

Imipramine has about a 6% incidence of side effects, including decreased concentration at work or in school, sleep disturbance, mood alteration, and decrease in appetite. Imipramine can induce serious cardiac arrhythmias with overdosage or when used in concert with other antipsychotic agents. Thus, patients should be screened for risk factors for cardiac arrhythmia before use, and the family should be cautioned about not exceeding the prescribed dose. The medication has to be kept out of reach of other children to prevent inadvertent overdose.

***Treatment with DDAVP*** DDAVP decreases urine volume because of its antidiuretic effect and is usually started at a dose of 20 μg of nasal spray or 2 mg orally, 1 to 2 hours prior to bedtime, along with general measures to help the bed-wetting. The dose can be increased to 40 μg of nasal spray or 6 mg orally per night if the response is inadequate. The medication is continued until 28 consecutive dry nights have been achieved, at which point it can be tapered gradually over 3 to 4 weeks. DDAVP has been shown to reduce the number of wet nights by approximately 50% and provides a long-term cure of bed-wetting in about 25% of patients. It is most effective in patients with a low frequency of wet nights, only one wet episode per night, and a large amount of wetness per night, suggestive of nocturnal polyuria. It is not effective in patients with low daytime bladder capacity. The relapse rate is high on discontinuance of the medication, presumably because it does not improve nocturnal bladder capacity. If patients repeatedly relapse on discontinuing DDAVP, it can still be used nightly as symptomatic therapy or as needed for sleep-away nights. History of OAB and stool retention should be repeatedly sought in patients felt to have monosymptomatic NE who do not improve with DDAVP therapy.

DDAVP therapy can result in headaches and seizures from water intoxication if fluid intake is not curtailed. Hence, patients should be advised to limit their fluid intake 3½ hours prior to bedtime.

***Combination Therapy*** When one form of therapy (alarm, DDAVP, or imipramine) fails or results in an inadequate response, another can be substituted.[15]

## INFREQUENT BLADDER EMPTYING

Although most adolescents void 4 to 6 times a day, some have a lower bladder capacity and have to void more frequently, whereas others have a larger bladder capacity and void infrequently. The former have a tendency for OAB, whereas the latter have a tendency for bladder inertia or an underactive bladder. Patients who habitually void 3 times or less in 24 hours, or hold urine for 12 hours or more overnight, are considered infrequent voiders. Although 7% of elementary school children are infrequent voiders, the percentage of adolescents with infrequent bladder emptying is probably higher than that.[16] The pattern of infrequent voiding starts in infancy in some, although others acquire this habit once they are confronted with unpleasant public bathrooms or a job that does not allow them to empty the bladder as often as they need to. These individuals are able to hold urine comfortably for a long time without using any pelvic withholding maneuver, have a normal urinary stream, and can empty their bladder completely. An overstretched bladder, however, can lose its elasticity and over time lose its ability to empty completely.

Adolescents with infrequent bladder emptying are at risk for UTIs because of infrequent washout of bacteria. Urinary infections in these adolescents generally do not present with urinary urgency or urge incontinence but with dysuria, back pain, lower abdominal pain, or fever. Infrequent bowel emptying because of colonic inertia often coexists with bladder inertia. However, stool withholding and encopresis are distinctly rare in this group.

Adolescents who void infrequently need to be encouraged to reset their voiding pattern by emptying their bladders 5 to 6 times a day. These individuals are often quite stubborn and require gentle coaxing along with a reward incentive. In those with coexistent colonic inertia, more frequent bowel emptying can be facilitated with the use of laxatives.

There is a small group of infrequent voiders whose detrusor contractions are suppressed because of high basal pelvic floor tone. Their pelvic floor spasticity is often a consequence of repeated conditioned pelvic tightening maneuvers related to having an OAB [1,2] The treatment in these patients is directed to the OAB and pelvic floor relaxation training.

## RELATION OF UTI TO VOIDING DISORDERS

Most UTIs in humans are ascending infections. Voiding disorders are the major predisposing factors for the development of UTIs in children and adolescents. Despite colonization of the distal urethra by bacteria, the bladder is able to defend itself against bacterial colonization and invasion. Bladder defense mechanisms include mechanical clearance of organisms by frequent and complete washout of its contents, antibacterial chemical constituents of the urine, presence of microbe-binding proteins like Tamm-Horsfall protein in the urine, inducible production of antimicrobial peptides like B-defensins and cathelicidins by the uroepithelial cells, and shedding of colonized uroepithelial cells.[17] Bacterial adhesion to their corresponding receptors on the uroepithelial cells is prevented by a layer of mucus that shields the epithelial receptors. Bacterial invasion of the bladder wall is prevented by intact mucosal integrity, the influx and phagocytosis of invading bacteria by neutrophils, and by adaptive immunity, that is, bactericidal antibodies and effector immune cells.

UTIs generally occur with the following abnormalities in voiding mechanics: infrequent and incomplete bladder emptying, distension of the bladder beyond capacity, infravesical obstruction, and high intravesical pressure. Infrequent voiding and large residual urine result in inadequate washout of invading bacteria. Bladder overdistension and high intravesical pressure result in increased mucosal permeability to bacteria due to mucosal disruption and impaired vesical blood flow. Infravesical obstruction, either structural or functional, results in turbulent urine flow and retrograde passage of bacteria from the urethra into the bladder, as well as a high voiding pressure.

In several surveys, the incidence and prevalence of voiding dysfunction was found to be significantly higher in patients with a history of UTI than in those without UTI.[1,4,10] This association not only reflects the predisposition to UTI in those with voiding dysfunction, but also the ability of UTI to trigger and aggravate the voiding dysfunction.

Detection and correction of the underlying voiding disorder, either infrequent bladder emptying or the diurnal urge syndrome, is the key to the prevention of an initial UTI, as well as its recurrence. This is especially important in sexually active adolescents where an acute alteration of the vaginal flora, either from the use of a spermicidal jelly or flora acquired from a sexual partner, can predispose to development of a UTI. In patients with a UTI and associated diurnal urge syndrome, the rate of resolution of the UTI is much higher in patients who are treated for their voiding dysfunction with anticholinergic agents or cognitive bladder training than in those provided antibacterial prophylaxis alone; cessation of UTI development can be correlated with achievement of normal voiding patterns in these patients.

## REFERENCES

1. Chandra M. Reflux nephropathy, urinary tract infection, and voiding disorders. *Curr Opin Pediatr.* 1995;164–170

2. Koff S, Wagner T, Jayanthi V. The relationship among dysfunctional elimination syndromes, primary vesicoureteric reflux, and urinary tract infection in children. *Jour Urol.* 1998;160:1019–1022

3. Starkman JS, Dmochowski RR. Urgency assessment in the evaluation of overactive bladder (OAB). *Neurourol Urodyn.* 2008;27:13-21

4. Chandra M. Enuresis and voiding dysfunction. In: Burg F, Ingelfinger J, Polin R, Gershon A, eds. *Current Pediatric Therapy.* Vol 9. Philadelphia, PA: Saunders Elsevier; 2006: 588-594

5. von Gontard A, Mauer-Mucke K, Pluck J, et al. Clinical behavioral problems in day-and-night-wetting children. *Pediatric Nephrol.* 1999;13:662-667

6. Rickenbacher E, Baez MA, Hale L, Leiser SC, Zderic SA, Valentino RJ. Impact of overactive bladder on the brain: central sequelae of a visceral pathology. *Proc Natl Acad Sci USA.* 2008;105(30):10589-10594

7. Hjalmas K, Arnold T, Bower W, et al. Nocturnal enuresis: an international evidence-based management strategy. *J Urol.* 2004;71:2545-2561

8. Neveus T, Lackgren G, Tuvemo T, et al. Enuresis—background and treatment. *Scand J Urol Nephrol.* 2006:2000(suppl):1-44

9. Rittig S, Knudsen UB, Norgaard JP, et al. Abnormal diurnal rhythm of plasma vasopressin and urinary output in patients with enuresis. *Am J Physiol.* 1989;256:F664- F671

10. Chandra M, Saharia R, Hill V, Shi Q. Prevalence of diurnal voiding symptoms and difficult arousal from sleep in children with nocturnal enuresis. *J Urol.* 2004;72:311-316

11. Abrams P, Klevmark B. Frequency volume charts: an indispensable part of lower urinary tract assessment. *Scand J Urol Nephrol.* 1996;179:47-53

12. Kawauchi A, Yamao Y, Nakanishi H, et al. Relationships among nocturnal urinary volume, bladder capacity, and nocturia with and without water load in nonenuretic children. *Urology.* 2002;59(3):433-437

13. Sans Capdevila O, Crabtree VM, Kheirandish-Gozal L, Gozal D. Increased morning brain natriuretic peptide levels in children with nocturnal enuresis and sleep-disordered breathing: a community-based study. *Pediatrics.* 2008;121:e1208-e1214

14. Watanabe H, Kawauchi A, Kitamori T, et al. Treatment system for nocturnal enuresis according to an original classification system. *Eur Urol.* 1994;25:43

15. Kruse S, Hellstrom AL, Hjalmas K. Daytime bladder dysfunction in therapy-resistant nocturnal enuresis. A pilot study in urotherapy. *Scand J Urol Nephrol.* 1999;33:49

16. Chandra M. Voiding and its disorders in children. In: Trachtman H, Gauthier B, eds. *Monographs in Clinical Pediatrics*. Chur, Switzerland: Harwood Academic Publishers; 1998:217-229

17. Zasloff M. Antimicrobial peptides, innate immunity, and the normally sterile urinary tract. *J Am Soc Nephrol.* 2007; 18:2810-2816

SECTION 8 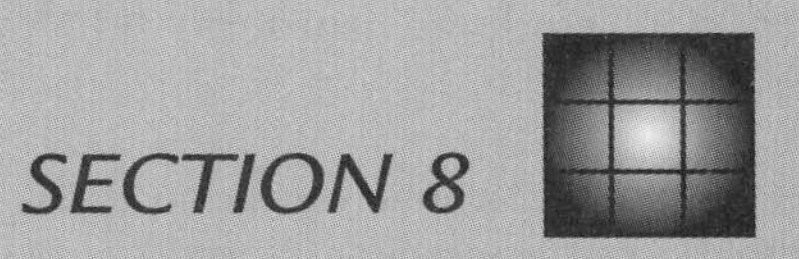

# Connective Tissue Disease, CFS, Fibromyalgia

## CHAPTER 120

# Systemic Lupus Erythematosus

BETH S. GOTTLIEB, MD

## INTRODUCTION

Systemic lupus erythematosus (SLE, or "lupus") is a chronic, multisystem autoimmune disease characterized by the presence of antinuclear antibodies. The clinical manifestations of this disease are determined by the target of the autoantibodies produced. The severity of SLE can range from very mild to a severe, life-threatening disease. The disease is episodic and characteristically has episodes of flares and remissions. Persistent unexplained symptoms in a preteen or teenager should prompt consideration of this diagnosis.

## EPIDEMIOLOGY

The diagnosis of SLE is rare in children younger than age 5. Most cases diagnosed in pediatric patients occur in adolescents. Overall, approximately 20% of SLE patients are diagnosed during childhood. Systemic lupus erythematosus is predominately a disease found in females. Prior to puberty the female to male ratio is 3:1, whereas after the onset of puberty that ratio changes to 9:1. Ethnicity also plays a role in the differences observed in the disease course of SLE. Most susceptible are Native Americans, followed by blacks, Hispanics, Chinese, and Filipinos. Blacks and Hispanics tend to have more severe disease.

The etiology of lupus remains unknown, although it is likely multifactorial and may involve dysregulation of the immune system, hormonal abnormalities, and environmental factors, such as infectious agents or ultraviolet radiation in an individual with a genetic predisposition. Immune system dysfunction may play an important role in SLE. Multiple manifestations of SLE are linked to antibody production and immune complex formation, such as the hematologic manifestations of cytopenia (ie, hemolytic anemia) and lupus nephritis. Altered T-cell function may result in reduced suppression of B cells, which may lead to autoimmune phenomena. Ultraviolet light has been linked to flares of lupus in up to 70% of SLE patients. Infections have long been thought to trigger lupus, possibly through molecular mimicry or immune dysregulation. Some medications have been found to induce a lupus-like syndrome. This is discussed later in this chapter.

Family history reveals that between 10% and 16% of patients with SLE have a first- or second-degree relative with lupus.[1] In monozygotic twins there is more than a 20% concordance rate, and in dizygotic twins and siblings a 5% concordance rate.[2] This suggests a genetic component to the etiology of lupus. Complement deficiencies likely predispose to SLE because they result in defective processing and clearance of immune complexes. Such deficiencies include C1q, C1r, and C1s, which have been associated with lupus nephritis and the presence of anti-double stranded DNA (anti-dsDNA) antibodies.[3] C1q deficiency is found especially in lupus patients who experienced disease onset as a child. C2, C3, and C4 deficiencies have also been associated with lupus.

Antigens of the major histocompatibility complex (MHC) have also been studied in relation to lupus. HLA-DR2 and DR3 are found to increase the risk of SLE in white patients. HLA-DR3 has in particular been associated with the production of autoantibodies and lupus.[4] HLA-DR2 and DR7 are common in those with SLE. Multiple other factors will likely be found as new knowledge and testing capabilities become available.

Currently, studies examining the multigenic nature of SLE are also assessing polymorphisms in tumor necrosis factor alleles, Fc and T-cell receptors, interleukins, and a variety of enzymes.[5] The greater the understanding of the potential genetic predisposition to lupus, the greater the realization that the disease is complex and that multiple risk genes may be required in any one individual patient.

## CLINICAL MANIFESTATIONS

Most adolescents who develop SLE present with a history of persistent fevers, weight loss, and alopecia and are found on examination to have mucositis, rash, and arthritis. Routine laboratory tests frequently reveal cytopenias that may include leukopenia, anemia, or thrombocytopenia, and an elevated sedimentation rate. Findings such as these should prompt further serologic testing, which will reveal a positive antinuclear antibody (ANA) titer in addition to other positive serologic tests for lupus.

### CONSTITUTIONAL

Fever, malaise, and weight loss are frequent symptoms at the onset of SLE in adolescents. These symptoms are frequently experienced during disease flares as well. Fever occurred at initial presentation in 58% of pediatric patients with SLE in a recent study.[6]

### MUCOCUTANEOUS

Mucocutaneous manifestations are common at the onset of lupus, as well as during the course of the disease. The classic butterfly rash is often an early feature of SLE (Figure 120-1). This rash is a photosensitive erythematous rash that appears over the cheeks and across the bridge of the nose but spares the nasolabial folds. Although this rash is the hallmark of SLE, it may also occur in dermatomyositis. Rosacea may be confused with the butterfly rash of lupus, but this common facial rash has pustular and papular lesions and may include some areas of telangiectasia.

Many other photosensitive rashes are also found frequently in lupus. Discoid lesions on the scalp or extremities are most often photosensitive. These lesions have clearly demarcated borders and appear in an asymmetric distribution. Discoid lesions heal, leaving behind a scarred area of atrophic skin. Subacute cutaneous lesions and bullous lesions are uncommon in children and adolescents. When they occur, subacute lesions appear as papulosquamous, erythematous lesions on the trunk and limbs. Additionally, vasculitic rashes occur and may take on different forms, including nodules, palpable purpura, petechial lesions, or ulcerations. Vasculitic lesions often occur on the palms and result in generalized palmar erythema (Figure 120-2). Unlike other lupus lesions, vasculitic lesions may be painful. Livedo reticularis is a lacey erythematous rash over the extremities that is commonly seen in SLE.

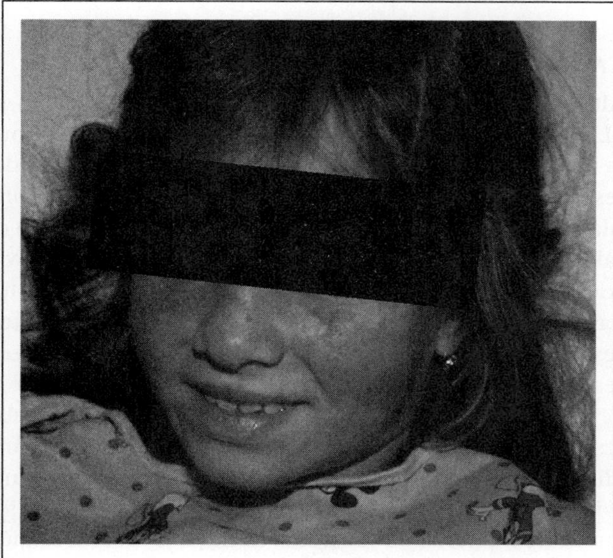

**FIGURE 120-1** Typical malar erythema in a "butterfly" distribution. Note that the erythema crosses the nasal bridge but spares the nasolabial folds. (See color insert.)

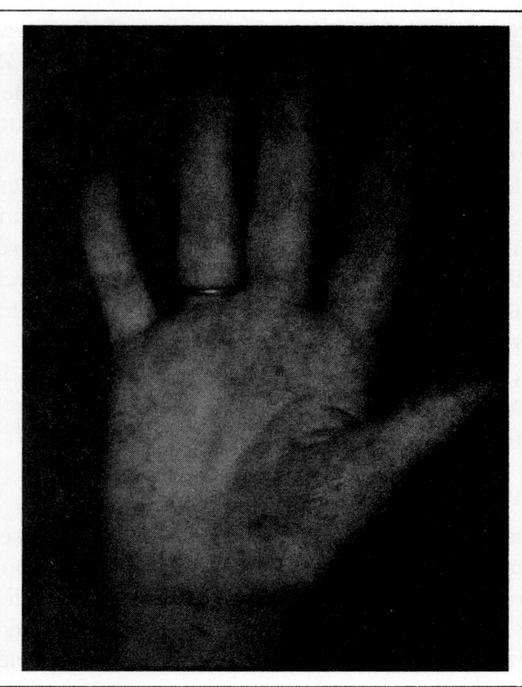

**FIGURE 120-2** Vasculitic lesions. (See color insert.)

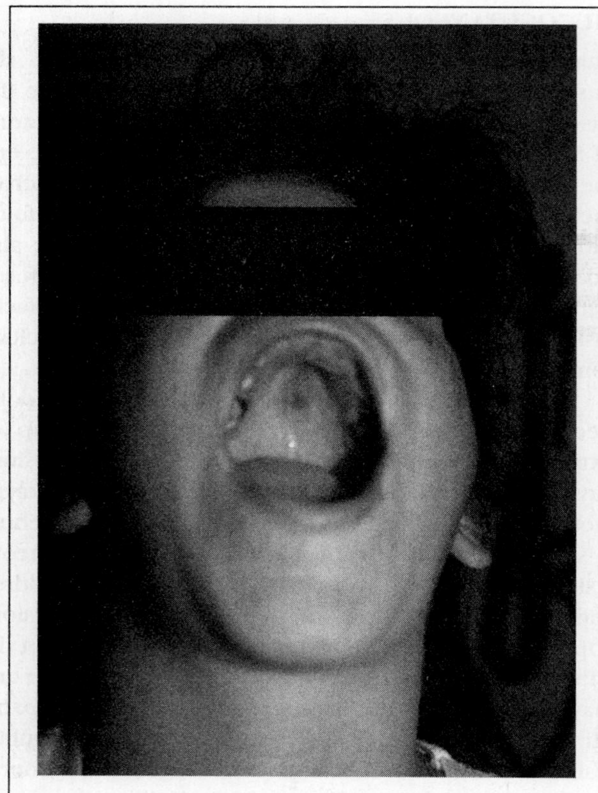

**FIGURE 120-3** Palatal erythema with a small ulceration of the hard palate. (See color insert.)

Mucous membrane involvement generally manifests as erythema over the hard palate, but shallow painless ulcerations may also be observed (Figure 120-3). The nasal mucosa may become similarly involved. Because patients are not aware of these ulcers, they may only be realized as a result of careful physical examination.

Alopecia is a difficult cosmetic issue for adolescents with SLE. (See Chapter 146, Alopecia, for photos and further information.) It generally begins in the frontal regions and then becomes diffuse over the scalp. Alopecia frequently accompanies active disease. Fortunately, alopecia resolves as the disease is treated, except in the rare cases when discoid lesions occur in the scalp.Because discoid lesions result in scarring, ensuing areas of alopecia are permanent and occur in patches over the scalp.

## NERVOUS SYSTEM

Central nervous system (CNS) involvement is the second-leading cause of morbidity and mortality in lupus and the most difficult to diagnose.The CNS manifestations of lupus are frequently vague and are varied. Generally these symptoms occur within the first year of the disease; only 25% of children and adolescents develop CNS symptoms later in the course of their illness.[7] Neuropsychiatric symptoms may include depression, cognitive impairment (such as difficulty with concentration or memory), and psychosis. Headaches that are refractory to usual treatment modalities are common in CNS lupus. Multiple causes for headaches are possible, including CNS vasculitis, pseudotumor cerebri, CNS infection, and cerebral vein thrombosis. Because these common CNS symptoms occur frequently, even without lupus, and may be attributed to multiple factors, such as treatment (corticosteroids may cause mood swings, psychosis, etc) or the psychological effects of a teenager coping with chronic illness and the effects of its treatment, it can be very difficult to determine the etiology of these symptoms. Seizures, which are usually generalized and tonic-clonic, may be the first manifestation of SLE in some adolescents. Although chorea, neuropathies, and transverse myelitis occur less frequently in SLE, when they do occur they can be more easily attributed to the disease itself. Infection must always be considered in the differential diagnosis of CNS manifestations in patients with SLE, especially in those receiving immunosuppressive therapy.

Evaluation of CNS lupus depends on the specific manifestations but may include examination of the cerebral spinal fluid to assess opening pressure, protein content, cell count, and fluid for culture. Imaging studies, an electroencephalogram, and neurocognitive testing may also be considered. Antiribosomal P antibodies are sometimes found in lupus patients with CNS symptoms, especially those with neuropsychiatric manifestations. Anticardiolipin antibodies are almost always detected in patients with chorea and usually in those with thrombotic events.

## CARDIOVASCULAR

Although all structures of the heart may be involved in SLE, the most common cardiac manifestation of lupus is pericarditis, with approximately 15% to 25% of adolescent patients developing pericardial effusion.[8] Complaints of chest pain exacerbated by lying down or taking a deep breath, especially when accompanied by a friction rub, should prompt a chest x-ray, to evaluate for cardiomegaly, and an echocardiogram. Myocarditis, manifesting as congestive heart failure or arrhythmia, occurs less commonly in SLE.

Libman-Sachs endocarditis is the classic valvular lesion of SLE. This sterile, verrucous vegetation is subclinical and may be present in up to 50% of patients with SLE. Because these lesions place patients at risk for subacute bacterial endocarditis (SBE), it is recommended that all patients with SLE receive SBE prophylaxis prior to dental, upper respiratory, or genitourinary procedures. Prolonged fever without an obvious cause, or a new or changing heart murmur, should prompt investigation for SBE, including performance of a transesophageal echocardiogram when necessary. Antiphospholipid antibodies may also promote the occurrence of Libman-Sachs endocarditis.

Premature atherosclerotic disease is becoming an important cause of morbidity in patients with SLE, including adolescent patients. Multiple factors contribute to atherosclerotic disease in SLE. Factors inherent to the disease, such as ongoing inflammation, nephritis, elevated homocysteine levels and dyslipoproteinemia, increased expression of adhesion molecules by endothelial and inflammatory cells, as well as presence of antiphospholipid antibodies, all play a role in the development of premature atherosclerosis. Hypercholesterolemia secondary to the nephrotic syndrome also contributes to this problem in some patients. The dyslipoproteinemia of SLE is characterized by elevated very low density lipoprotein (VLDL) cholesterol and triglycerides and decreased high density lipoprotein (HDL) cholesterol and apoprotein A-I.[9] In addition to disease-related factors, treatment with glucocorticoids results in accelerated atherosclerosis due to increased total cholesterol, VLDL cholesterol, and triglyceride levels. Prevention of these complications should begin in the pediatric age group. It is important to monitor fasting lipid profiles in teens with SLE, as well as other factors that may compound the risk of heart disease, such as hypertension. Adolescents should be counseled on proper nutrition and exercise. Fish oil capsules may be added in order to improve lipid profiles. Some patients will require treatment with statins if these other measures fail to result in sufficient improvement.

Raynaud syndrome, which describes the 3 phases of color change of the digits commonly seen in adolescents, usually in response to cold exposure (Figure 120-4), may occur in patients with SLE. The digits first become pale, which is followed by a cyanotic phase and, finally, erythema occurs with rewarming. In most cases, Raynaud syndrome is primary, and investigations do not demonstrate any evidence of rheumatologic disease. However, Raynaud syndrome may occur secondary to SLE or other connective tissue diseases. Examination of the nail bed capillaries often provides a clue to distinguishing between primary and secondary Raynaud syndrome. Visibly dilated, corkscrew-shaped nail bed capillaries or areas of dropout (a large gap between capillaries) are suggestive of vasculopathy and, therefore, secondary Raynaud syndrome (Figure 120-5). Aside from cold exposure, emotional stress, caffeine, and cigarette smoke may also precipitate or exacerbate these symptoms. Counseling patients to dress warmly in multiple layers and to limit prolonged exposure to the cold is very important. Patients who experience frequent or prolonged episodes of cyanotic changes in their digits are at risk for infarction of the digits. These patients may require treatment with a vasodilator (such as nifedipine), particularly during the winter months.

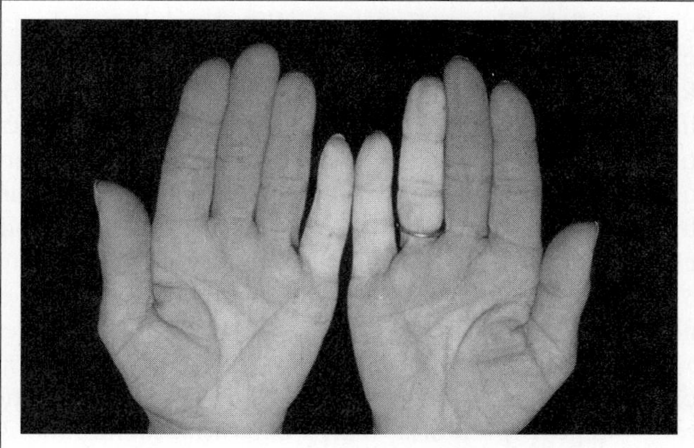

**FIGURE 120-4** Raynaud syndrome. Although all of the fingertips are usually affected, occasionally only some of the digits will show the color changes associated with the syndrome. (See color insert.)

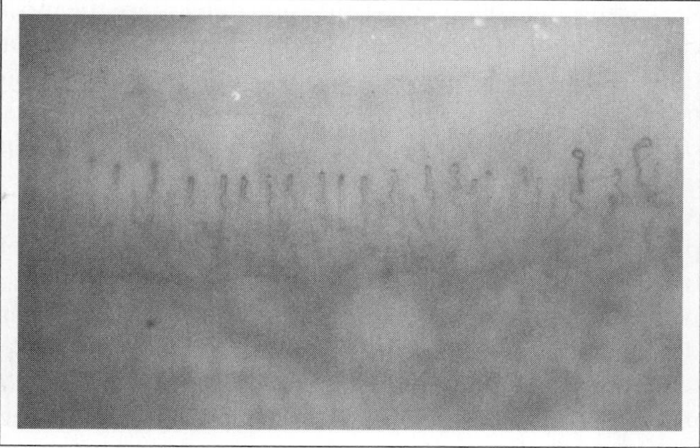

**FIGURE 120-5** Nail-bed capillaries. Examination of the nail bed reveals dilated loops of capillaries and areas of capillary dropout. (See color insert.)

### PULMONARY

Pleuropulmonary disease is a frequent manifestation of SLE in adolescents. Pleuritis is the most common pulmonary manifestation of lupus and it may occur together with pericarditis or alone. Patients with pleuritis typically complain of chest pain that is worse with inspiration. This may be a presenting sign of lupus. The pleuritis may be unilateral or bilateral. Effusions are generally exudative and are present in low volumes.

Approximately 60% of adolescent patients with SLE have subclinical pulmonary disease with abnormal pulmonary function tests in the absence of symptoms.[10]

Restrictive lung disease and diffusion defects are the most common abnormalities. These findings may worsen over time. "Shrinking lung syndrome," a relatively uncommon manifestation of lupus in both adolescents and adults, occurs from dysfunction of the diaphragm resulting in its elevation and subsequent loss of lung volume. A chest x-ray is required to make the diagnosis. Lupus pneumonitis, manifesting as dyspnea with a finding of basilar rales on auscultation, occurs in 13% of pediatric patients with lupus according to 1 study.[10] Radiographs demonstrate infiltrates and atelectasis. Pulmonary hemorrhage, although uncommon in children, does occur more often in adolescents with SLE and may be severe and life threatening. Hemoptysis may occur at the onset. Pallor, dyspnea, tachycardia, and the finding of a falling hemoglobin with pulmonary infiltrates should raise the possibility of pulmonary hemorrhage. Pulmonary embolism may also occur, especially in patients with antiphospholipid antibodies.

Infection should always be considered a possible cause for pulmonary distress in adolescents with SLE. It is important to rule out infections prior to initiating immunosuppressive therapy.

### GASTROINTESTINAL

Peritonitis, mesenteric vasculitis, and hepatitis may all occur in lupus. Abdominal pain radiating to the shoulder that may be accompanied by nausea and vomiting should prompt testing of amylase and lipase levels for the evaluation of pancreatitis. Gastrointestinal symptoms that occur in an adolescent with lupus may also be the result of an adverse effect of treatment or may be due to an etiology completely unrelated to the disease.

### RENAL

Approximately 75% of children who have SLE develop renal involvement, most often within the first 2 years of onset of the disease.[11] Renal disease is a major cause of morbidity in SLE. Microscopic hematuria and proteinuria provides evidence of early renal disease and, when persistent, may prompt renal biopsy. Patients also may have hypertension, a decreased glomerular filtration rate, and elevated blood urea nitrogen (BUN) and creatinine concentrations. Renal biopsy provides useful information that defines the specific type of nephritis and helps determine proper treatment. Lupus nephritis has been classified by the World Health Organization based on light microscopy. An updated version is presented in Box 120-1. Mesangial proliferation (class II) is relatively mild in most cases and generally has a better long-term prognosis than other subtypes. However, in 20% to 30% of patients this lesion may progress to class III or IV lupus nephritis over time. Focal segmental (class III) and diffuse proliferative glomerulonephritis (class IV) lupus nephritis are the most severe forms. Patients with these types of nephritis frequently have hypertension and may have impaired renal function. Urinalysis reveals proteinuria, hematuria, and often urinary casts. Laboratory evaluation typically reveals hypoalbuminemia, decreased levels of C3 and C4, and elevated anti-dsDNA antibody levels. In approximately 35% of patients with focal segmental disease, the nephritis will progress to diffuse proliferative disease. Membranous nephritis (class V) occurs in 10% to 20% of patients with lupus nephritis. This results in nephrotic range proteinuria with hematuria. Membranous lupus nephritis may be seen in combination with the other types of nephritis as well. Glomerulosclerosis represents advanced lupus nephritis where more than 90% of glomeruli observed in a biopsy specimen demonstrate global sclerosis.

**Box 120-1**

***Lupus Nephritis***

- Class I: Normal
  1. Normal by all techniques
  2. Normal by light microscopy but deposits by electron microscopy or immunofluorescence
- Class II: Mesangial nephritis
  1. Mesangial widening and/or hypercellularity
  2. Moderate hypercellularity
- Class III: Focal segmental glomerulonephritis
  1. With active necrotizing lesions
  2. With active lesions and sclerosing lesions
  3. With sclerosing lesions
- Class IV: Diffuse proliferative glomerulonephritis
  1. Without segmental lesions
  2. With active necrotizing lesions
  3. With active and sclerosing lesions
  4. With sclerosing lesions
- Class V: Membranous glomerulonephritis
  1. Pure membranous lesions
  2. Also with lesions of class II
  3. Also with lesions of class III
  4. Also with lesions of class IV
- Class VI: Glomerulosclerosis

Adapted from Churg J, Sobin LH. *Renal Disease: Classification and Atlas of Glomerular Disease*. Tokyo: Igaku-Shoin; 1982.

Histopathology also is helpful in determining the acuity or chronicity of inflammation, which determines responsiveness to treatment. Electron microscopy and immunofluorescence provide details about the location of immune complex deposits, which affects prognosis.

**MUSCULOSKELETAL**

Arthralgias or arthritis are very common in adolescents with SLE and are present at onset in more than 60% of pediatric patients.[6] Arthritis in SLE is typically a symmetric polyarthritis that is nonerosive and nondeforming, and involves small and large joints. In some cases, arthritis may cause Jaccoud arthropathy, a nonerosive but deforming arthritis that results from joint subluxation secondary to tenosynovitis. Myalgias and proximal muscle weakness may develop in patients who have SLE. Myositis occurs more often in an overlap syndrome such as mixed connective tissue disease. Steroid-induced myositis must also be considered in patients with SLE treated with prolonged high-dose glucocorticoids. In this case muscle enzymes are within normal limits.

**HEMATOLOGIC**

Hematologic manifestations represented the most common initial findings of lupus in childhood in 1 study,[6] occurring in 72% of children diagnosed with SLE. All cell lines may be affected. Leukopenia may result from either neutropenia or lymphopenia. Anemia occurs in approximately 50% of patients and most often is a normocytic, normochromic anemia consistent with that of chronic disease. However, in some cases, the anemia is an autoimmune hemolytic anemia and is found to be Coombs positive. Immune-mediated thrombocytopenia also may occur. SLE should be considered in adolescent girls who have chronic idiopathic thrombocytopenic purpura or Evans syndrome (thrombocytopenic purpura and hemolytic anemia).

## DIAGNOSIS

There is no specific symptom or diagnostic test for lupus; rather the diagnosis is based on clinical manifestations and abnormal laboratory and serologic tests. The diagnosis of SLE should be considered in an adolescent with unexplained multisystem disease and the presence of autoantibodies. There are classification criteria for SLE that are helpful when considering the diagnosis of lupus; however, they are not strictly diagnostic criteria (Box 120-2). Because lupus is such a diverse disease there are many instances where a patient may be diagnosed with SLE even though he or she does not meet the classification criteria. Furthermore, these criteria have not been validated in children and adolescents.

### Box 120-2

### *1997 Classification Criteria for SLE*

- Malar rash ("butterfly rash")
- Discoid rash
- Photosensitivity
- Oral or nasal mucosal ulcers
- Nonerosive arthritis
- Serositis: pleuritis or pericarditis
- Renal manifestations: persistent proteinuria (>0.5 g/dl) or cellular casts
- Neurologic manifestations: seizure or psychosis
- Hematologic manifestations: hemolytic anemia, leukopenia (<4,000/mm$^3$), lymphopenia (<1,500/mm$^3$), thrombocytopenia (<100,000/mm$^3$)
- Immunologic manifestations: positive anti-dsDNA Ab or anti-Sm Ab or evidence of antiphospholipid antibodies (elevated anticardiolipin immunoglobulin IgG or IgM Ab or positive lupus anticoagulant test or false-positive serologic test for syphilis for ≥6 months)
- Antinuclear antibody elevation

Ab, antibodies

Adapted with permission from Hochberg M. Updating the American College of Rheumatology revised criteria for the classification of systemic lupus erythematosus. *Arthritis Rheum.* 1997;40(9):1725.

Laboratory assessment is important for establishing the diagnosis of SLE and for monitoring the disease course. ANA is the best screening test for SLE because it is positive in almost all patients who have active disease. It is important to know, however, that although the ANA is a sensitive test for SLE, it is not specific and may be positive in up to 33% of the general healthy population.[12] In 1 study,[13] 71% of patients referred to a pediatric rheumatology center for a positive ANA did not have any rheumatic disease. This study showed that there was no increase in the frequency of rheumatologic disease diagnosed at ANA titers below 1:1280. Several autoimmune diseases are associated with elevated ANA titers aside from SLE, including juvenile idiopathic arthritis, dermatomyositis, scleroderma, and thyroid disease. Positive ANA titers may also result from recent infectious illnesses.

Antibodies to double-stranded DNA (anti-dsDNA) are more specific for SLE because they are rarely positive in healthy individuals or in other rheumatologic diseases. These antibodies are helpful in monitoring disease activity because they tend to be present at high

**Table 120-1**

**Antibodies Found In SLE**

| | |
|---|---|
| Anti-dsDNA antibodies | Positive in 73% of patients with SLE, very specific for SLE, often correlates with active lupus glomerulonephritis |
| Anti-SSA (Ro) antibodies | Positive in 40% of patients with SLE, most strongly associated with neonatal lupus phenomenon, often correlates with cutaneous manifestations, Sjögrens syndrome, renal and pulmonary disease |
| Anti-SSB (La) antibodies | Positive in 10% of patients with SLE, usually present when anti-SSA is positive, often correlates with neonatal lupus, Sjögrens syndrome |
| Anti-Sm antibodies | Positive in 20% to 30% of patients with SLE, very specific for SLE |
| Anti-RNP antibodies | Positive in 15% of patients with SLE, in low-titer correlates with SLE, in high-titer correlates with mixed connective tissue disease |
| Anticardiolipin antibodies | Positive in 37% of patients with SLE |

Data from: Peng SL, Craft J. Antinuclear antibodies. In: Ruddy S, Harris ED, Sledge CB, eds. *Kelly's Textbook of Rheumatology*. 6th ed. Philadelphia, PA: WB Saunders Co; 2001:165; Edworthy SM. Clinical manifestations of systemic lupus erythematosus. In: Ruddy S, Harris ED, Sledge CB, eds. *Kelly's Textbook of Rheumatology*. 6th ed. Philadelphia, PA: Saunders Co; 2001:1110; Gedalia A, Molina JF, Garcia CO, et al. Anti-cardiolipin antibodies in childhood rheumatic diseases. *Lupus*. 1998;7:551.

titers when the disease is active. They also may be predictive of disease flares, commonly increasing prior to an exacerbation of symptoms. Other specific antibodies for SLE include the extractable nuclear antigens anti-Sm (Smith) and anti-RNP (ribonucleoprotein), anti-Ro (also called SSA), and anti-La (also called SS-B) (Table 120-1). High titers of anti-RNP are suggestive of mixed connective tissue disease. Both anti-Ro and anti-La may be positive in Sjögren syndrome. Anti-Ro antibodies are most well known for their association with neonatal lupus erythematosus and the development of congenital heart block. Levels of serum complement components 3 and 4 may provide information of active disease, as C3 and C4 levels are typically diminished in active lupus nephritis. Rising levels of anti-dsDNA antibodies are also suggestive of active renal disease. Routine monitoring of C3 and C4 levels and anti-dsDNA titers are therefore important as they may indicate a need for more aggressive therapy, especially in patients who have class III or IV nephritis. Testing for antiphospholipid antibodies and results of a complete blood count, electrolytes, BUN, creatinine, hepatic enzymes, acute-phase reactants (such as erythrocyte sedimentation rate or C-reactive protein), and urinalysis are helpful in the routine monitoring of affected patients.

### DRUG-INDUCED LUPUS

Many drugs are known to result in a transient syndrome of lupus or "drug-induced lupus" (Box 120-3). The most common presentation consists of fever, fatigue, arthritis, serositis, and a positive ANA. Renal disease and CNS involvement are rare in drug-induced lupus. Anti-dsDNA antibodies are notably negative and C3 and C4 levels are normal. Symptoms resolve with discontinuation of the drug and do not recur. The same medications that may cause drug-induced lupus are not implicated in precipitating flares of the disease and are therefore not contraindicated for patients with SLE.

**Box 120-3**

***Medications Associated with Drug-Induced Lupus***

Proven association
- Hydralazine
- Isoniazid
- Methyldopa
- Phenytoin
- Procainamide

Possible association
- Beta blockers (atenolol, labetalol, propranolol, etc)
- Captopril
- Carbamazepine
- Cimetidine
- Ethosuximide
- Minocycline
- Penicillamine
- Quinidine

**ANTIPHOSPHOLIPID ANTIBODY SYNDROME**

Antiphospholipid antibody syndrome (APLS) may occur as a primary disease or may be secondary when associated with SLE or other diseases. Antiphospholipid antibodies include many antibodies against a family of negatively charged phospholipid proteins and areas of lipid-protein complexes. Diseases other than SLE that may cause APLS include other autoimmune diseases, malignancies, and human immunodeficiency virus (HIV) infection. Antiphospholipid antibody syndrome may also occur transiently after other viral infections. Lupus anticoagulant (LAC) and anticardiolipin (aCL) antibodies place patients at risk for both arterial and venous thrombosis, recurrent fetal loss, hemolytic anemia, thrombocytopenia, neurologic symptoms (ie, chorea, transverse myelitis), Libman-Sachs endocarditis, livedo reticularis, and Raynaud syndrome.

Laboratory features of this syndrome include the presence of anticardiolipin antibodies, prolonged phospholipid-dependent coagulation tests (such as the partial thromboplastin time and the dilute Russell viper-venom time, or DRVVT), and circulating lupus anticoagulants, as documented by a failure to correct the prolonged coagulation time with mixing studies. One study revealed that 66% of pediatric patients who had SLE had positive anticardiolipin antibodies, 62% had lupus anticoagulants, and 39% had a false-positive Venereal Disease Research Laboratory (VDRL) test, which is also a phospholipid-dependent test.[14] In 12% of the patients, only 1 of these tests was positive. Therefore, no single test can be relied on for the diagnosis. The DRVVT is reported to be the most sensitive test for APLS, with positive results in 73.8%.[15] This still emphasizes the need for multiple tests in order to diagnosis this syndrome as accurately as possible.

## TREATMENT

The treatment of SLE must be tailored carefully to each patient. The choice of medications depends on the extent of organ system involvement. Although the disease itself may result in significant morbidity and mortality, much of the emerging morbidity in SLE today results from medications used to control the disease. This morbidity includes infections and osteoporosis. Thus, therapy must be monitored closely, and decreased whenever possible to diminish iatrogenic sequelae. All patients with lupus are advised to use sunscreen for ultraviolet A and ultraviolet B protection for all skin exposed to the light (indoor lighting or sunlight) year-round to prevent exacerbation of skin disease and internal organ disease. Due to the risk of Libman-Sachs endocarditis, all patients with lupus should receive SBE prophylaxis.

Nonsteroidal anti-inflammatory drugs are useful in treating fevers and arthritis. Methotrexate is efficacious for more extensive arthritis. Hydroxychloroquine is used to reduce fatigue, mucocutaneous lesions and alopecia. Due to potential retinal toxicity associated with this medication, patients must have routine ophthalmologic examinations. Glucocorticoids are reserved to treat exacerbations of internal organ system disease, especially CNS, renal, and hematologic disease.

Glucocorticoids have the advantage of a rapid onset of action and control of symptoms. However, glucocorticoids are associated with multiple toxicities including cushingoid features, cataracts, glaucoma, osteoporosis, hypertension, glucose intolerance, aseptic necrosis of the femoral head, immune suppression, abnormal lipid handling, and myopathy. Therefore, although high doses are initially required for treatment (often divided into multiple doses during the day), patients must be closely monitored so that steroid doses can be reduced as quickly as possible once clinical improvement allows. Toxicity-sparing strategies include consolidating the dose into a single morning dose, alternate-day dosing, or intravenous "pulse" doses of methylprednisolone.

Intravenous immunoglobulin may be helpful, primarily for the treatment of chorea and thrombocytopenia. Immunosuppressive therapy has 2 important roles: as steroid-sparing agents and in the treatment of steroid-resistant disease. Cyclophosphamide has been considered the therapy of choice for serious organ involvement in SLE. This medication is used especially for focal segmental and diffuse proliferative glomerulonephritis and for CNS disease. Cyclophosphamide has substantial potential toxicity, including infection, bone marrow suppression, nausea, vomiting, alopecia, hemorrhagic cystitis, and bladder malignancy. Administering this drug as monthly intravenous pulse doses instead of daily oral doses may diminish some of the toxicity. Azathioprine and cyclosporine are also used to treat some manifestations of SLE. Newer therapies aim to target the processes believed to be important in the pathogenesis of lupus. Mycophenolate mofetil (MMF) inhibits purine synthesis, lymphocyte proliferation, and T-cell-dependent antibody responses. Studies suggest that MMF may be useful in the treatment of some forms of lupus nephritis (such as class V) with less toxicity. Mycophenolate mofetil is currently being studied to determine if it can be used in place of cyclophosphamide for induction treatment for diffuse proliferative glomerulonephritis. Mycophenolate mofetil is also being used for maintenance therapy after a course of intravenous cyclophosphamide.

Many biologic agents are currently being tested for the treatment of SLE. These target specific cytokines (eg, anti-interleukin-10 monoclonal antibody) and costimulatory molecules (eg, anti-CD40 ligand) and/or attempt to enhance B-cell tolerance (eg, LJP 394). Rituximab is a chimeric monoclonal antibody against the CD20 receptor found on B lymphocytes. This anti-CD20 therapy has been used for the treatment of non-Hodgkin B-cell lymphoma and is now being used to treat SLE that is refractory to cyclophosphamide. Rituximab is being studied further to fully understand its efficacy and potential toxicities in the treatment of lupus. Autologous stem cell transplant is being investigated as a treatment for severe SLE refractory to available treatments.

## OUTCOME AND PROGNOSIS

The long-term prognosis of patients who have SLE has improved in recent years, which may be attributed to better monitoring and treatments. Morbidity in adolescents with lupus is related mainly to infection, renal disease, and CNS manifestations. Five-year survival rates for Class IV lupus nephritis range from 88% to 93%, with an overall 10-year survival rate of 85%.[16]

A recent study found the 5-year survival rate of pediatric SLE to be almost 100%; the 10-year survival rate is nearly 90%. Although the life-span has been improved, cumulative organ damage is unfortunately still significant, with 50% to 60% of pediatric lupus patients developing organ damage over time.[17] This study also found that teens with lupus have poorer health-related quality of life and lower socioeconomic achievements than those without SLE.

It is important that a multidisciplinary team approach be used in the care of adolescents with SLE. A pediatric rheumatologist, nurse, and when necessary physical/occupational therapist, psychologist, and social worker, should all be available. The teen must be involved in his/her own treatment and viewed as a partner in the monitoring and treatment of the disease. As new treatments are found for SLE, attention will be focused on minimizing toxicity and improving quality of life.

## REFERENCES


1. Ruddy S, Harris ED, Sledge CB, eds. *Kelly's Textbook of Rheumatology.* 6th ed. Philadelphia, PA: W.B. Saunders; 2001:1089–1152

2. Deapen D, Escalante A, Weinrib L, et al. A revised estimate of twin concordance in systemic lupus erythematosus. *Arthritis Rheum.* 1992;35(3):311–318

3. Bowness P, Davies KA, Norsworthy PJ, et al. Hereditary C1q deficiency and systemic lupus erythematosus. *Q J Med.* 1994;87(8):455–464

4. Kelly JA, Moser KL, Harley JB. The genetics of systemic lupus erythematosus: putting the pieces together. *Genes Immun.* 2002;3(suppl 1):S71–S85

5. Sestak AL, Shaver TS, Moser KL, et al. Familial aggregation of lupus and autoimmunity in an unusual multiplex pedigree. *J Rheumatol.* 1999;26(7):1495–1499

6. Bader-Meunier B, Armengaud JB, Haddad E, et al. Initial presentation of childhood-onset systemic lupus erythematosus:a French multicenter study. *J Pediatr.* 2005;146(5):648–653

7. Steinlin MI, Blaser SI, Gilday DL, et al. Neurologic manifestations of pediatric systemic lupus erythematosus. *Pediatr Neurol.* 1995;13:191–197

8. Guevara JP, Clark BJ, Athreya BH. Point prevalence of cardiac abnormalities in children with systemic lupus erythematosus *J Rheumatol.* 2001;28:854–859

9. Ilowite NT, Samuel P, Ginzler E, Jacobson MS. Dyslipoproteinemia in pediatric systemic lupus erythematosus. *Arthritis Rheum.* 1988;31(7):859–863

10. Delgado EA, Malleson PN, Pirie GE, Petty RE. The pulmonary manifestations of childhood onset systemic lupus erythematosus. *Semin Arthritis Rheum.* 1990;19:285–293

11. Cameron JS. Lupus nephritis in childhood and adolescence. *Pediatr Nephrol.* 1994;8:230–249

12. Egner W. The use of laboratory tests in the diagnosis of SLE. *J Clin Pathol.* 2000;53:424–432

13. Malleson PN, Sailer M, Mackinnon MJ. Usefulness of antinuclear antibody testing to screen for rheumatic diseases. *Arch Dis Child.* 1997;77:299–304

14. Seaman DE, Londino V, Kwoh C, Medsger TA Jr, Manzi S. Antiphospholipid antibodies in pediatric systemic lupus erythematosus. *Pediatrics.* 1995;96:1040–1045

15. Proven A, Bartlett RP, Moder KG, et al. Clinical importance of positive test results for lupus anticoagulant and anticardiolipin antibodies. *Mayo Clin Proc.* 2004;79:467–475

16. Hagelberg S, Lee Y, Bargman J, et al. Longterm follow-up of childhood lupus nephritis. *J Rheumatol.* 2002;29:2635–2642

17. Ravelli A, Nicolino R, Martini A. Outcome in juvenile onset systemic lupus erythematosus. *Curr Opin Rheumatol.* 2005;17(5):568–573

# CHAPTER 121

# Juvenile Idiopathic Arthritis

PATRICIA IRIGOYEN, MD • NORMAN T. ILOWITE, MD

Juvenile idiopathic arthritis (JIA) is among the most common chronic conditions of childhood and adolescence. Occurring in about 1 of 1,000 children, JIA is more common than diabetes mellitus. Juvenile idiopathic arthritis is the term now used to encompass a heterogenous group of related disorders presenting in children who are younger than 16 years of age. All types of JIA share an inflammatory arthritis of apparently autoimmune etiology. Although the terms are somewhat different, JIA can also be referred to as juvenile rheumatoid arthritis and as juvenile chronic arthritis (JCA). The terms rheumatoid arthritis (RA) and spondyloarthropathy are reserved for adolescents and adults who develop chronic inflammatory arthritis disease at or after age 16.

In 2001, the International League of Associations for Rheumatology (ILAR) published an updated set of classification criteria for the different subtypes of JIA. Although debate still exists regarding the best mode of classification, we will refer to the ILAR criteria in this chapter for the sake of simplicity.[1] The diagnostic criteria for adult RA remain the 1987 American College of Rheumatology (ACR) criteria.[2]

Juvenile idiopathic arthritis is a chronic, potentially debilitating disease. The course of JIA can be highly variable, from monophasic disease with lifelong remission to persistent erosive disease causing complete disability or requiring joint replacement. In a large case series of patients who developed JIA, a third were in remission 10 years after diagnosis, a third had a mild chronic course, and a third had severe functional limitations.[3] The prognosis varied by subtype of disease. For example, in patients with polyarticular and systemic disease, the remission rate was as low as 1 in 5, and some patients had developed joint erosions. Oligoarticular JIA patients had a high risk of developing impaired vision due to chronic uveitis.[4] In another large series, 10% of all patients were severely impaired in activities of daily living after 16 years of follow-up.[5] The advent of newer medications, particularly the "biologics," has the potential for improving outlook.

Juvenile idiopathic arthritis can cause not only physical disability but emotional and social difficulties as well. Even more than 20 years after disease onset, patients with JIA report significantly greater pain and lower physical functioning, health perception, and vitality than case control subjects.[6] An interdisciplinary approach to this chronic disease can best provide an optimal medical and psychological outcome. Those who care for adolescents need to be familiar not only with the presentation of JIA during the teenage years but also with the continued care of children who present at a younger age.

## ETIOLOGY AND PATHOPHYSIOLOGY

The etiology of JIA is not known; however, it is considered to be a disease of autoimmunity. Often, the patient with JIA will have laboratory abnormalities consistent with a high degree of inflammation. Commonly seen are an elevated erythrocyte sedimentation rate (ESR) and C-reactive protein (CRP), elevated white blood cell (WBC) and platelet count, and an anemia of chronic disease. A positive antinuclear antibody (ANA) can be found in about 40% of children with JIA and a positive rheumatoid factor (RF) in about 10%.[7] Histopathology reveals synovial lining layer hyperplasia and pronounced inflammatory cell infiltration.[8] Overall, these laboratory and pathological findings support an autoimmune etiology for JIA.

This autoimmune process occurs in individuals who have a genetic predisposition. In these patients, JIA is triggered by an unknown environmental factor, possibly a viral infection. In contrast to diseases with single genetic defects, such as cystic fibrosis, JIA seems to be a complex genetic trait with risk alleles differing by subtype. There is now supportive evidence that points to specific genetic markers in individuals with JIA. Most notably, HLA class I and class II alleles have been implicated as JIA risk genes.

Different subtypes of JIA have been associated with different genetic risk alleles. For example, oligoarticular JIA is associated with HLA DRB1*08 and *11, DQA1*04 and 05. RF-negative polyarticular JIA is associated with HLA-DRB1*08, and systemic JIA with HLA-DRB1*11. Similar to the adult diseases, HLAB27 is associated with enthesitis-related arthritis (ERA) and juvenile psoriatic arthritis (JPsA), and HLA DRB1*04 is associated with RF-positive polyarticular JIA.[9]

## DIFFERENTIAL DIAGNOSIS

Although the most common presentation of JIA is joint stiffness and functional limitation, the most common referrals to the rheumatologist are due to joint pain. Musculoskeletal pain, however, is a common childhood complaint, particularly in adolescents. A detailed description of the pain is very important in making the diagnosis. Inflammatory pain—such as in JIA—is associated with morning stiffness and alleviated by movement. In contrast, pain due to mechanical causes generally improves with rest and is exacerbated by activity. Particularly concerning signs include nighttime pain and functional disability, because these may also point to a diagnosis of leukemia.[10] The diagnosis of JIA also requires prolonged arthritis of at least 6 weeks' duration. More common causes of joint pain in adolescents include viral infections, orthopedic conditions (including overuse syndromes), and reactive arthritis. Potentially concerning causes include bacterial infections, malignancies, and musculoskeletal injuries. These conditions must be excluded to make the diagnosis of JIA.

## CLINICAL EVALUATION

In the evaluation of adolescent joint pain, it is important to obtain a complete clinical history. Nonjoint complaints should be thoroughly assessed, because they can provide critical clues to diagnosis. For example, inflammatory symptoms such as fever, night sweats, and weight loss are concerning and may point to a diagnosis of infection, rheumatic disease, or malignancy.[10] Abdominal involvement must be evaluated, because inflammatory bowel disease (IBD) can be a concomitant illness. Rashes may also accompany specific diseases such as systemic lupus erythematosus or Henoch-Schönlein purpura, which commonly have joint involvement. In JIA, 2 subtypes are associated with rashes: systemic JIA and psoriatic JIA.

Physical evaluation should include a thorough evaluation of the joints, as well as a complete physical examination. Concerning signs include joint redness, swelling, and heat (rubor, tumor, calor). In addition, range of motion should be assessed to look for limitation or hypermobility. Particular attention should be paid to gait analysis (antalgic, Trendelenburg), eyes (cataracts, irregular pupils, band keratopathy), and skin (rash or change in temperature). Lymphadenopathy and hepatosplenomegaly can point to either inflammatory disease or malignancy. Focal tenderness at the insertion of the tendon into bone suggests enthesitis, which may be associated with JIA. If localized to a particular joint, such tenderness may indicate an overuse syndrome.

Laboratory evaluation can be helpful in making the diagnosis, but there is no one test that can make the diagnosis of JIA. A complete blood count is essential to evaluate for hematologic malignancy. Laboratory abnormalities more often seen in patients with leukemia who present with joint pain include decreased WBC count, relative thrombocytopenia (low to normal platelets in the setting of an elevated inflammatory marker, such as ESR), low hemoglobin, and high uric acid. Generally, elevated markers of inflammation, such as ESR or CRP, can be suggestive of JIA. However, many subtypes present with normal inflammatory indices. HLA-B27 and RF are helpful prognostic indicators once the diagnosis is made; however, neither is specific for rheumatic disease. An ANA should be performed only when there is clinical suspicion for JIA or systemic lupus erythematosus, because the test is helpful only with a high pretest probability for disease.[11]

Imaging is helpful to exclude other diagnoses, particularly trauma or malignancy. A plain radiograph can show the destructive changes of longstanding, erosive JIA.[12] Magnetic resonance imaging (MRI) and ultrasound are more specific for detecting joint effusions. Currently, however, the expense of such studies precludes their general use. An initial plain radiograph is indicated if a specific joint is a concern and an MRI is warranted if subtle trauma is considered. For example, an MRI of the knee may reveal a torn patellar tendon, meniscal tear, or other soft tissue abnormalities. The axial skeleton is best imaged with either computed tomography (CT) or MRI scanning.

## SINGLE JOINT INVOLVEMENT: DIFFERENTIAL DIAGNOSIS

In the patient with monoarticular arthritis, the most critical entity to exclude is a septic joint. Septic arthritis generally presents with acute onset of one red, swollen, painful joint with associated fever. Any patient with this clinical presentation requires arthrocentesis to exclude this diagnosis. In culture-positive septic arthritis, the most common causative organism is *Staphylococcus aureus*. In a significant minority of patients, however, the synovial culture will remain negative. If there is a strong clinical suspicion, these patients are treated presumptively with a full course of antibiotic therapy to prevent the permanent joint damage that can occur in this condition. Helpful laboratory tests include an elevated WBC count, elevated ESR or CRP, and a positive blood culture. A small proportion of patients with septic arthritis, approximately 5%, can have involvement of multiple joints. In addition, associated osteomyelitis can be seen and a bone scan should be included in the evaluation. Of note, infectious sacroiliitis and diskitis may be more indolent in nature.

Musculoskeletal pain in adolescents is frequently of mechanical origin. Overuse syndromes, such as the patellofemoral syndrome, are common in young athletes, particularly females. Osgood-Schlatter disease and osteochondrosis may be seen in young adolescents and can be diagnosed with the classic tenderness and swelling at the tibial tuberosity. Similar overuse syndromes affect the patella (Sinding-Larsen-Johansson) and heel (Sever), and may be difficult to differentiate from enthesopathy. These diagnoses should be considered if the patient does not have evidence of joint swelling. Trauma to the joint structures—such as the meniscus or ligament in the knee—should be considered as well. Generally these are associated with a history of acute injury or repetitive trauma.

Lyme disease must also be considered in the differential diagnosis of monoarthritis in children. Most typically, the arthritis caused by *Borrelia burgdorferi* presents as a large knee effusion that develops weeks to months after a tick bite. Erythema migrans can be present, but is not required for the diagnosis. Frequently, the patient cannot recall a history of a tick bite. Because there is a wide range of presentations in this disease, Lyme titers are recommended for all children and adolescents with arthritis who have traveled to endemic areas.

Reactive arthritis is an acute, sterile autoinflammatory arthritis that can occur following either a viral or bacterial infection. It is believed to be mediated by "molecular mimicry" caused by T- or B-cell-mediated cross-reactivity to similar antigens. One form comprises a classic triad of urethritis, conjunctivitis, and arthritis following bacterial infections. However, reactive arthritis can occur in isolation. Common predisposing organisms include *Chlamydia, Yersinia, Shigella, Salmonella,* and *Campylobacter*. Like viral arthritis, this type of inflammatory arthritis is self-limited and generally does not have future sequelae. It is more commonly seen in HLA-B27-positive patients. Isolated reactive arthritis following a Group A streptococcal pharyngitis is termed poststreptococcal arthritis. This entity is believed to be on a spectrum with acute rheumatic fever (ARF), and patients receive penicillin prophylaxis accordingly. ARF is diagnosed by fulfilling the modified Jones criteria. Major manifestations include carditis, arthritis, chorea, erythema marginatum, and subcutaneous nodules. Minor criteria are fever, arthralgia, elevated acute phase reactants, and a prolonged P-R interval on the electrocardiogram (ECG). In addition, there must be evidence of an antecedent streptococcal infection such as a positive throat culture or positive antibody titer for Group A streptococcus. The arthritis associated with ARF is classically migratory and sensitive to salicylate therapy. Although manifestations such as chorea can linger, the arthritis of ARF generally does not last longer than one week. Poststreptococcal arthritis, on the other hand, can occur in the absence of other manifestations and is often associated with a longer course.

An underlying malignancy should always be considered in the patient with arthritis, bone pain, or bone tenderness. A discrepancy between the blood counts and sedimentation rate (ie, relative thrombocytopenia) may be a clue to diagnosis, as should nighttime pain and low-grade fever.[10] This is particularly relevant when considering the diagnosis of systemic JIA in a patient with persistent fever and joint pain.

## MULTIPLE JOINT INVOLVEMENT: DIFFERENTIAL DIAGNOSIS

Viral arthritis can be seen with multiple viruses including Epstein-Barr virus (EBV), cytomegalovirus (CMV), rubella, and parvovirus infection. Viral arthritis generally involves multiple joints and is frequently associated with fatigue and morning stiffness. Viral arthritis may initially appear to be JIA, but resolves spontaneously. It does not cause erosions or joint damage. This condition is self-limited, lasting up to 6 to 8 weeks, and has no future implications for the patient. It is because of the frequency of viral arthritis that more than 6 weeks of persistent disease are required for the diagnosis of JIA.

One infection that must be considered in the adolescent with joint pain is disseminated *Neisseria gonorrhoeae*. Signs and symptoms include fever, rash on the hands, wrists, and feet, tenosynovitis of the hands or feet, and asymmetric polyarthritis. Culture of joint fluid is usually negative, although blood culture may be positive. Urethral, pharyngeal, or rectal cultures are helpful in making the diagnosis.

Chronic pain syndromes, such as fibromyalgia or complex regional pain syndrome, will often have their onset during adolescence. Seen more often in females, fibromyalgia typically manifests as multiple diffuse aches and pains accompanied by fatigue. Symptoms of headaches and abdominal pain are also quite frequent. Because changes in sleep patterns have been found in these patients, it is felt that the disorder begins with some insult or stress to the body, which results in poor quality of sleep, which in turn results in the patient feeling ill with multiple muscle aches. The patient tends to focus on the pain, which then leads to a more disturbed sleep pattern, and so on. Examination of these patients shows consistently reproducible tender points with an otherwise normal examination and laboratory findings (See Chapter 123 for further information on fibromyalgia syndrome.)

## DEFINITION AND CLASSIFICATION OF JIA

As per the ILAR criteria, JIA is an arthritis of unknown etiology that begins before age 16 years and persists for at least 6 weeks in which other known conditions are excluded.[1] Arthritis is defined as a swollen joint (excluding bony swelling) or a joint that exhibits limitation of movement accompanied by pain or tenderness of the joint.

The major JIA classifications are based on onset type. Prognosis for the disease is influenced by the type of JIA at onset, but also by the course of the disease. Over time, types of JIA may overlap because of evolving symptomatology. For instance, systemic-onset JIA can eventually become indistinguishable from polyarticular JIA.[7] Patients with this pattern of onset and disease course may be particularly difficult to treat.

Prognosis varies among the disease types. Overall, the following are indicators for poor long-term outcome: active systemic disease at 6 months, polyarticular onset or disease course, female gender, RF, persistent morning stiffness, tenosynovitis, subcutaneous nodules, ANAs, early involvement of small joints of the hands and feet, rapid appearance of erosions, and extended pauciarticular disease course.[6]

### SYSTEMIC ARTHRITIS

Systemic arthritis is arthritis in 1 or more joints with or preceded by fever of at least 2 weeks' duration, that is documented to be daily ("quotidian") for at least 3 days, and accompanied by 1 or more of the following:[1]

1. Evanescent (nonfixed) erythematous rash
2. Generalized lymph node enlargement
3. Hepatomegaly and/or splenomegaly
4. Serositis

Systemic JIA comprises 10% to 20% of all patients with JIA.[7] The most dramatic form of childhood arthritis, systemic JIA, often presents as a prolonged fever with associated rash. In many cases, the appearance of arthritis lags and can occur months after the onset of illness. Systemic JIA, therefore, is often a diagnosis of exclusion in the evaluation of a patient with fever of unknown origin. The classic fever curve is 1 of high spiking quotidian or double quotidian fever (1 or 2 daily spikes are seen, with rapid return to baseline or below baseline). The fever is generally accompanied by the classic rash that is comprised of small, evanescent, salmon-colored macules that often have central clearing and perilesional pallor. The rash is generally worse when fever is present and can be elicited with gentle stroking of the skin (known as the Koebner phenomenon). Occasionally pruritic, it is generally seen on the trunk and extremities but can be seen on the face, palms, and soles.

Clinical features of systemic JIA are often nonspecific. Generalized lymphadenopathy and hepatosplenomegaly are often present. Typically, the patient with systemic JIA will have laboratory abnormalities consistent with a high degree of inflammation. Commonly seen are an elevated ESR and CRP, elevated WBC and platelet count, and an anemia of chronic disease. Patients with systemic JIA can have associated serositis, including pericarditis, peritonitis, and pleuritis. Uveitis is not generally seen with systemic JIA. However, unless the characteristic rash and/or arthritis are present, other etiologies must be ruled out before the diagnosis can be made. Generally, this will involve an infectious work-up for sepsis, viral syndromes including EBV, CMV, and parvovirus, or other infectious etiologies. In addition, a bone marrow biopsy may be required to rule out hematologic malignancies. This is particularly important when the use of corticosteroids is being considered in a patient without a definitive diagnosis.

The prognosis of systemic JIA depends largely on the course during the first 6 months. Poor prognostic indicators at 6 months include persistence of systemic symptoms, elevated inflammatory markers, and polyarthritis. In most patients, the systemic symptoms resolve within a few years, but they can persist in some cases. Approximately half of all patients who present with systemic JIA will go on to develop a severe, persistent polyarthritis.[6]

Macrophage activation syndrome (MAS) is a rare but severe complication of systemic JIA. More correctly called a secondary hemophagocytic lymphohistiocytosis, MAS is fatal in up to 22% of cases. Typically seen in patients with unremitting systemic symptoms, MAS is characterized by fever, elevated transaminases, and a disseminated intravascular coagulation (DIC)-type picture in a toxic-appearing patient. Complications can include encephalopathy, bleeding, hepatic failure, renal failure, and death. Laboratory findings include an elevated ferritin, elevated aspartate aminotransferase (AST) and alanine aminotransferase (ALT), elevated triglycerides, and a paradoxically low ESR. The ESR is decreased due to the hypofibrinogenemia caused by the consumptive coagulopathy. Evidence of increased macrophage activity is present, with elevated cytokines such as interferon-gamma and tumor necrosis factor (TNF) alpha. Definitive diagnosis requires a biopsy specimen showing macrophages engulfing erythrocytes. This is typically found in the bone marrow, although a liver biopsy may show abnormalities earlier in the disease. Other indicators include a very elevated ferritin level (generally above 5,000), decreased fibrinogen, and low platelet count.[13] The treatment for MAS must be rapid and aggressive, and typically consists of high-dose intravenous corticosteroids. Subsequent therapy generally includes cyclosporine, although TNF alpha antagonists have been used with some success.

## OLIGOARTHRITIS

Oligoarthritis is arthritis affecting 1 to 4 joints during the first 6 months of disease. Two subcategories are recognized:[1]

1. Persistent oligoarthritis: Affecting not more than 4 joints throughout the disease course
2. Extended oligoarthritis: Affecting a total of more than 4 joints after the first 6 months of disease

Oligoarthritis is the most common subtype, seen in 50% to 60% of children with JIA.[7] Oligoarthritis, particularly when ANA positive, is frequently associated with uveitis. An oligoarticular JIA patient who is ANA positive has a 50% risk of developing uveitis.[6] Although most of these patients present before adolescence, it is important to recognize the chronic nature of this illness. Even if arthritis has resolved, persistent morbidity, such as leg length discrepancy requiring shoe lifts, may be seen.

Patients with oligoarticular JIA typically have asymmetric involvement of the large joints, such as the knees and ankles. Monoarthritis involving the knee is seen in approximately half of these patients. Often, patients complain more of morning stiffness than pain and are functionally intact. Patients are often younger and present with a subtle limp. Common physical findings include a leg length discrepancy and atrophy of associated muscles, indicating chronicity. Patients who follow a persistent oligoarticular course have a generally good outcome, with a remission rate of 75%. The 50% of patients who develop arthritis in more than 4 joints after 6 months have a worse prognosis, with an overall remission rate of only 12%.[5]

## POLYARTHRITIS (RHEUMATOID FACTOR NEGATIVE)

Polyarthritis (RF negative) is arthritis affecting 5 or more joints during the first 6 months of disease; a test for RF is negative.[1]

A quarter (20% to 30%) of all JIA patients will fall into the category of polyarthritis at presentation. This percentage includes RF-positive and RF-negative subtypes. Usually presenting in early childhood, RF-negative polyarthritis has a variable prognosis. It is likely that this group encompasses several disorders that cannot be differentiated clinically. However, many patients will have arthritis that persists into adolescence.[5]

In addition, patients with polyarticular disease may have involvement of the temporomandibular (TMJ) joints, as well as involvement of the cervical spine. Even in patients with remission, instability of the cervical spine from prior disease may result in cervical fracture.[14] RF-negative polyarticular JIA is associated with HLA-DRB1*08.[9]

## POLYARTHRITIS (RHEUMATOID FACTOR POSITIVE)

Polyarthritis (RF positive) is arthritis affecting 5 or more joints during the first 6 months of disease; 2 or more tests for RF at least 3 months apart during the first 6 months of disease are positive.[1]

This subtype is believed to be an early expression of RA as seen in adults. Like RA, RF-positive polyarticular JIA is associated with HLA DRB1*04, and has a poor prognosis, with a high likelihood of erosive disease. As in adult RA, anticyclic citrullinated peptide (CCP) antibodies may be seen. This type of arthritis occurs in approximately 10% of children with JIA.[5] The arthritis usually involves the large and small joints of the hands and feet. The axial skeleton, including the cervical spine and TMJ joints, may also be involved. Boutonniere deformities (proximal interphalangeal [PIP] joint flexion and distal interphalangeal joint [DIP] hyperextension) and swan neck deformities (PIP hyperextension and DIP flexion) are common. Chronic uveitis is less frequently seen. Like adult RA, remissions are rare in this subtype.[14]

## PSORIATIC ARTHRITIS

Psoriatic arthritis consists of arthritis and psoriasis, or arthritis and at least 2 of the following:[1]

1. Dactylitis (inflammation/swelling of the digits)
2. Nail pitting or onycholysis (separation of the nail from the nail bed)
3. Psoriasis in a first-degree relative

Juvenile psoriatic arthritis is a difficult diagnosis to make, as the arthritis may precede the cutaneous manifestations by several years. It has a peak age of onset in mid-childhood, and typically presents as an asymmetric arthritis that often affects the knees, ankles, and small joints of the hands and feet. PIPs, DIPs, and the tendon sheath are often inflamed, resulting in diffuse swelling of the digit, referred to as dactylitis, or a "sausage digit."

Extra-articular manifestations include rash, nail changes (including pitting, onycholysis, oil drop sign), and uveitis. One-third of these patients develop the rash by 15 years of age. This subtype is also frequently associated with asymptomatic anterior uveitis, which may be found in up to 17% of patients.[15]

## ENTHESITIS-RELATED ARTHRITIS

Enthesitis-related arthritis (ERA) includes either arthritis and enthesitis, or arthritis or enthesitis, with at least 2 of the following:[1]

1. Presence of or history of sacroiliac joint tenderness and/or inflammatory lumbosacral pain
2. Presence of HLA-B27 antigen
3. Onset of arthritis in a male older than 6 years of age
4. Acute (symptomatic) anterior uveitis
5. History of ankylosing spondylitis (AS), ERA, sacroiliitis with IBD, reactive arthritis, or acute anterior uveitis in a first-degree relative

This subtype includes patients with juvenile ankylosing spondylitis (JAS) and arthritis associated with IBD. It is similar to adult spondyloarthropathy. Both have an asymmetric polyarthritis that usually involves the axial skeleton and the large joints of the lower extremities. Inflammatory back pain may be seen, which can lead to eventual loss of mobility of the back. Peripheral arthritis generally precedes arthritis of the axial skeleton, which can take years to develop. Over time, sacroiliitis will produce radiographic changes including joint space narrowing, erosions, sclerosis, osteoporosis of the pelvis, and fusion. As in adults, this type of arthritis is strongly associated with HLA-B27.

Acute anterior uveitis is seen in about a quarter of patients. Unlike the asymptomatic uveitis associated with other subtypes, this presents as a red, painful, photophobic eye. Extra-articular manifestations can also include aortic insufficiency, aortitis, muscle weakness, and low-grade fever. Elevated inflammatory markers, such as the ESR, may be found. Two forms may be seen: an acute polyarticular type that mirrors the activity of the bowel disease, and another type that is more like ERA with the course of arthritis independent of bowel disease.

In addition, this type of arthritis may precede the onset of the IBD. Because the arthritis may present before the development of abdominal symptoms, the diagnosis of IBD must always be considered in patient follow-up.

## UNDIFFERENTIATED ARTHRITIS

Undifferentiated arthritis is arthritis that fulfills criteria in no category or in 2 or more of the previous categories.

These are patients who cannot be grouped in any of the previous criteria. A heterogenous group, they need to be further studied in order to determine where they belong in the classification system.

## RHEUMATOID ARTHRITIS

In an adolescent who develops polyarticular disease after age 16 years, the appropriate diagnosis is RA. Symptoms include morning stiffness, arthritis of 3 or more joints, arthritis of hand joints, symmetric arthritis, rheumatoid nodules, serum RA positive, and radiographic changes consistent with RA. The prognosis and treatment is similar to RF-positive polyarticular JIA.

RA is often associated with HLA-DR4. A positive RF may be seen but is not required for diagnosis. Anticyclic CCP antibodies can also be found. Very specific for RA, these antibodies imply a worse prognosis. Both RF and anti-CCP antibodies are associated with erosive disease. The treatment of RA is similar to polyarticular JIA.

RA is generally a chronic disease, with few spontaneous remissions. It tends to be erosive and can cause significant morbidity over time. Extra-articular manifestations, such as vasculitis, pericarditis, and interstitial lung disease, can be seen in RA. Commonly, patients will develop rheumatoid nodules. Uveitis is not generally associated with RA, but patients can develop associated rheumatologic diseases, such as secondary Sjögren syndrome.

## SPONDYLOARTHROPATHY

The term spondyloarthropathy encompasses a spectrum of diseases that includes AS, psoriatic arthritis, reactive arthritis, and arthritis associated with IBD. The diseases, seen most commonly in young men, comprise a group of disorders that symmetrically affect the large joints, particularly in the lower extremities. They commonly are accompanied by enthesitis and strongly associated with the HLA-B27 allele. Like ERA, spondyloarthropathies are associated with an acute, symptomatic form of uveitis. This is the appropriate diagnosis for an adolescent who presents with symptoms after age 16 years.

Ankylosing spondylitis generally begins with inflammatory pain of the back. This is typically a dull, low back pain that is worse with rest and relieved by exercise. The diagnosis of AS formally requires limitation of lumbrosacral mobility along with radiologic evidence of sacroiliitis. However, these are late findings, and many patients must be categorized as "probable" AS early in the course of disease. Similar to ERA, large joints of the lower extremities and enthesitis are often seen. Enthesitis-related arthritis may, in fact, be a juvenile form of AS. A similar type of arthritis may be associated with IBD and psoriasis, as in children. Psoriatic arthritis can include dactylitis ("sausage joint") as described in the pediatric form.

## NONARTICULAR MANIFESTATIONS

Although JIA is predominantly a disease of the joints, it can have systemic effects. In fact, the largest percentage of morbidity in the disease is due to uveitis.[4] These other manifestations must be considered in the diagnosis and care of children with JIA.

### UVEITIS

Chronic, anterior, nongranulomatous uveitis (iridocyclitis) develops in up to 30% of patients with oligoarticular JIA and 10% with polyarticular JIA. It is most common in young girls with oligoarticular disease and a positive ANA titer. The uveitis is usually asymptomatic, but may also present as headache, conjunctivitis, unequal pupils, or eye pain. It can occur before, during, or well after the onset of JIA. Visual loss occurs in a significant minority and can occur before diagnosis. In 85% of affected children, uveitis is bilateral. The recommendation is that patients with JIA receive a baseline ophthalmology evaluation at onset, and then throughout their course, as indicated in Table 121-1.

Complications of uveitis include posterior synechiae, cataracts, band keratopathy, and/or glaucoma in up to 64% of patients. Eighteen percent of children with JIA-associated uveitis have been reported to have significantly impaired visual acuity of 20/200 or worse. Overall, it seems that time to diagnosis is the most important factor in determining outcome for JIA-associated uveitis.[4]

Initial treatment of uveitis includes topical corticosteroids to treat inflammation and mydriatics to prevent posterior synechiae. In patients who do not respond to topical therapy, oral or intravenous corticosteroids may be used. Corticosteroids may also be applied locally via subtenon injection. In persistent uveitis, methotrexate, cyclosporine, and infliximab may be used.

### GROWTH DISTURBANCE

Generalized growth retardation and delayed puberty can be seen in children with JIA. This is particularly true of patients with systemic and polyarticular JIA, who are at higher risk for diminished growth. The causes are multifactorial and include malnutrition, increased catabolic demands, inflammation, and corticosteroid therapy. Maximizing nutrition, particularly in patients who have significant TMJ involvement and difficulty chewing, is critical. Using alternate-day dosing, when corticosteroids are required, can help minimize the growth effects. In addition, growth hormone may be effective in selected patients.

Localized growth disturbances can occur in any JIA subtype. These can be seen in up to 1 in 4 patients. They can result from several etiologies such as destruction of a growth center (which can cause micrognathia), accelerated bone maturation (which can lead to leg length discrepancy), or premature closure of the physis (which can result in brachydactyly). These disturbances occur primarily in children with disease onset after 9 years of age. However, these abnormalities persist throughout life and cause significant morbidity, even if JIA is quiescent.[5,6]

### OSTEOPOROSIS

Patients with JIA have interference with the acquisition of bone mass in adolescence. In fact, osteoporosis has been noted in 46% of patients by 32 years of age.[14] For this reason, JIA patients should be prescribed calcium and vitamin D. They should also be instructed about the value of exercise and advised to avoid smoking.[14]

### PSYCHOSOCIAL EFFECTS

Psychosocial consequences are also associated with JIA. Half of all adults with a history of JIA report adverse

**Table 121-1**

**Recommended Screening Intervals for Uveitis in JIA, Stratified by ANA Status**

| *Subtype of JIA* | *Type of Uveitis* | *Onset <7 Years* | *Onset >7 Years* |
|---|---|---|---|
| Oligo: ANA+ | Asymptomatic, common | 3–4 months | 6 months |
| Oligo: ANA– | Asymptomatic | 6 months | 6 months |
| Poly: ANA+ | Asymptomatic | 3–4 months | 6 months |
| Poly: ANA– | Asymptomatic | 6 months | 6 months |
| Systemic | Rare | 12 months | 12 months |
| ERA | Symptomatic | 6 months | 6 months |

ANA, antinuclear antibody; ERA, Enthesitis-related arthritis

affects on body image and the ability to interact socially. An increase in unemployment is seen in up to 35% to 40% of adults with JIA. Up to 20% of patients with JIA may experience a period of depression, typically in late adolescence or early adulthood. It has also been noted that adolescents with a history of JIA cope with their illness differently than those with adult-onset disease. Typically they are more passive about seeking therapy and more commonly alter personal goals to accommodate their disease. This trait can be difficult when managing the transition from pediatric to adult care, as many patients can "fall through the cracks."[6,14]

## TREATMENT OF JIA

For all patients, the goals of therapy are to decrease chronic joint pain, suppress the inflammatory process, and maintain function. Accomplishing these goals leads not only to improved short-term and long-term function but also to normal growth and development. The toxicities associated with therapeutic agents pose a significant problem in effective treatment. For instance, agents that work by general immunosuppression may be associated with increased susceptibility to infection, interference with vaccine administration, or increased oncogenic risk. The distinction between symptom control and prevention of erosive disease must also be recognized. Many of the agents that are most effective at pain and symptom control, including corticosteroids and nonsteroidal anti-inflammatory drugs (NSAIDs), have no effect on erosive disease.

### JOINT INJECTION

Local corticosteroid injections often are the first line of treatment in JIA, particularly in oligoarticular disease. By performing an intra-articular injection, generally with a triamcinolone hexacetonide, the local inflammation is often well controlled without the need for systemic medication. It has been shown that aggressive use of joint injections prevents morbidity, such as leg length discrepancies.[16] On average, the injected joint will remain symptom free for about 9 months. However, injections can be performed up to every 3 months as necessary. Arthrocentesis, or joint aspiration, is not commonly performed in pediatric rheumatology unless infection is suspected. This is due to the very low incidence of crystal-induced arthropathy in children and adolescents.

Side effects to intra-articular joint injections are minimal. Most commonly seen are the development of periarticular atrophy at the site of injection or intra-articular calcification. A very uncommon potential adverse event is the development of septic arthritis. This can be largely prevented with the use of sterile techniques.

### NONSTEROIDAL ANTI-INFLAMMATORY DRUGS

If intra-articular injection is insufficient to control all symptoms, as is the case in polyarticular JIA, NSAIDs are used. Conventional NSAIDs inhibit both the cyclo-oxygenase (COX)-1 constitutive form of the enzyme, which releases prostaglandins that protect the stomach and kidneys, and the COX-2 inducible form, which produces prostaglandins involved in the inflammatory process. Only a handful of NSAIDs have been approved by the US Food and Drug Administration (FDA) for use in JRA: ibuprofen, naproxen, tolmetin, and choline magnesium trisalicylate. Celecoxib (Celebrex), a selective COX-2 inhibitor, has also been approved for use in children. Although cardiovascular events in children on selective COX-2 inhibitors have not been reported, as in adults, this issue still needs to be fully studied. Many other NSAIDs are also commonly used for JRA, including indomethacin and diclofenac.

The most commonly used agents include ibuprofen and naproxen, both available over the counter. Naproxen is often preferred due to its longer half-life and easier dosing regimen. However, particularly in fair-skinned younger children, this drug can produce a pseudo-porphyria rash that can be scarring. It is suggested that children on naproxen limit their exposure to the sun, as this is a photosensitive reaction.

### TRADITIONAL DMARDS

The term "disease-modifying antirheumatic drugs" (DMARD) is limited to agents that retard radiologic progression of disease. Only 3 DMARDs have been proved to be effective in controlling disease activity in double-blind, placebo-controlled studies of children with JRA: methotrexate, sulfasalazine, and etanercept.

The most commonly used second line therapy for JIA is methotrexate. This agent, demonstrated to be effective in polyarticular JIA, has been used to treat juvenile arthritis for more than 10 years. Highest response rates to methotrexate are obtained in children with oligoarticular onset, particularly those with extended polyarticular disease. Patients with systemic onset may respond less frequently. Overall, between 60% and 80% of JIA patients who are treated with methotrexate experience some clinical improvement.[17] Given once weekly, either orally or subcutaneously, methotrexate is well tolerated in the pediatric population.

The most common adverse events associated with methotrexate use in children with JIA are gastrointestinal symptoms, which occur in approximately 13% of patients.[18] Other common side effects include fatigue for a day following the dose, and oral ulcers. These can be ameliorated with the use of folic acid or folinic acid (leucovorin) supplementation. Although hepatic fibrosis has been seen in adults on rheumatologic doses of methotrexate, this does not appear to be a concern in the pediatric population. Serum transaminase and albumin levels are monitored every 4 to 8 weeks. Significant liver damage seems to be rare, probably in part because comorbid hepatotoxic risk factors are absent in most pediatric patients. In a study of 14 JIA patients who were treated with methotrexate for a mean of 6.3 years, needle biopsies failed to detect signs of significant liver fibrosis in any of the patients, although some histologic abnormalities were noted.[19] Likewise, pulmonary toxicity is rare in children.

Despite the widespread use of methotrexate, data on immunosuppressive, teratogenic, or oncogenic risks associated with long-term methotrexate therapy in JIA patients are lacking. Current recommendations are not to administer live virus vaccines to patients who are taking methotrexate. In addition, patients are generally cautioned about increased susceptibility to infection. In adolescent females, the teratogenic risk of this medication must be emphasized.

Other second line agents include sulfasalazine and leflunomide. In a double-blind, placebo-controlled, multicenter study of patients with JCA, sulfasalazine was significantly more effective than placebo in suppressing disease activity, as indicated by decreases in overall articular severity scores, all global assessments, and laboratory parameters.[20] However, drug toxicity is a problem. Elevated liver transaminases, leukopenia, hypoimmunoglobulinemia, and gastrointestinal problems contributed to a 30% withdrawal rate in this trial. The manufacturer recommendations are to check blood counts and transaminase levels before treatment every other week for the first 3 months, monthly for the next 3 months, then every 3 months.

Leflunomide, an immunosuppressive agent that acts as a reversible inhibitor of de novo pyrimidine synthesis, has been shown to be significantly superior to placebo and comparable to sulfasalazine and methotrexate in controlling measures of disease activity in patients with adult RA.[21] The ability of these agents to retard radiographic progression is also similar. The most common adverse effects associated with leflunomide are diarrhea, elevated liver enzymes, alopecia, and rash. In particular, the teratogenic potential of this agent may be a concern when treating pediatric patients, especially adolescent females.

Systemic JIA, once diagnosed, is initially treated with NSAIDs. Indomethacin is often used to control the systemic symptoms. Unlike other forms of JIA, corticosteroids are a mainstay of treatment for severe unresponsive systemic features. They are not typically used in children with isolated arthritis. Therapy is used to induce clinical remission and tapered as tolerated. Second line agents include methotrexate and the biologics (as below). In addition, immune suppressive agents, such as azathioprine, cyclosporine, intravenous immunoglobulin (IVIG), cyclophosphamid, and thalidomide, have been used with varying levels of success.[22]

## BIOLOGICS

Currently, methotrexate continues to be the first line DMARD. Until more clinical experience is gained, biologics, which are created by recombinant technology and work by modulating the immune system, should be reserved until after methotrexate failure because long-term study data of biological therapy in JIA are not yet available. Nevertheless, due to the significant proportion of incomplete responders or nonresponders to methotrexate, biological therapies will be a valuable addition to JIA treatment options.

Etanercept is a biologic agent approved by the FDA for use in reducing signs and symptoms and delaying structural damage in patients with moderately to severely active adult RA, and for reducing signs and symptoms of moderately to severely active polyarticular-course JIA that is refractory to 1 or more DMARDs. This agent consists of 2 soluble p75 TNF receptors fused to the Fc portion of immunoglobulin G. Etanercept is a potent inhibitor of TNF alpha, which is a key proinflammatory cytokine found in the synovial tissue of patients with JIA and is believed to play an important role in proinflammatory signaling.[23]

Etanercept is generally well tolerated in pediatric patients. The most common adverse events are injection site reactions, headaches, and upper respiratory infections of mild to moderate severity. Although not observed in the placebo-controlled phase of the study, concern exists regarding increased susceptibility to infection. No increased rates of infection have been observed, however, in long-term, controlled trials of etanercept versus placebo. This agent is well tolerated by both adults and children, and data from long-term studies have not revealed any cumulative toxicity. However, infections, neoplastic complications, hematologic complications, and multiple sclerosis-like neurologic disease have been identified in small numbers of patients during postmarketing surveillance, and concerns regarding these events exist because long-term experience is still limited.[24]

Another TNF-neutralizing agent, infliximab (also known as cA2), is a chimeric human–mouse monoclonal antibody to TNF.[25] Given as an intravenous infusion, infliximab has become widely used in the treatment of adult RA, as well as Crohn disease patients of any age. In addition, infliximab is being used more and more often to control uveitis that is unresponsive to current first and second line therapy. A risk with this therapy is the development of infusion reactions, particularly because of the murine components of the antibody. Adalimumab, a humanized monoclonal antibody to TNF-a, is now also available. Its efficacy appears similar to infliximab, but biweekly subcutaneous injections performed at home make it easier to use.[26]

International studies show that TNF alpha inhibition renders the tuberculosis (TB)-exposed patient at high risk for disseminated TB. Due to this concern, all patients placed on anti-TNF therapy are screened with a purified protein derivative (PPD) test. If the PPD is positive, anti-TNF therapy should not be given until appropriate antimicrobial therapy has been instituted. It also is recommended that pediatric patients be brought up to date with all immunizations before receiving these agents. Because of cases of aseptic meningitis with varicella zoster infection, immunization with varicella in susceptible children, and administration of varicella zoster immune globulin in exposed individuals, have been recommended. However, live vaccines should not be given concurrently with etanercept.[27] Ideally, approximately 3 months should be allowed to elapse between live virus vaccination and initiation of biologic therapy. Pediatric patients with significant exposure to varicella should temporarily discontinue their anti-TNF agent.

TNF alpha antagonists such as etanercept, infliximab, and adalimumab have been shown to be less useful in systemic JIA than the other subtypes. Other biologic agents, particularly therapy targeting interleukin-1 (IL-1) or interleukin-6 (IL-6), appear to be more promising in the treatment of this subtype of arthritis. Currently, the only available IL-1 blocker is anakinra, a soluble IL-1 receptor. This medication is delivered as a daily subcutaneous injection and results in frequent injection reactions.[28] In open label trials, and one placebo-controlled, double-blind study, anti-IL-6 receptor antibody IV infusions appear to be effective in treating systemic JIA. However, this medication is currently not approved for use in the United States.[29]

Two new biologic agents that have demonstrated efficacy in adult RA may also be helpful in JIA. Rituximab, an anti-CD20 B-cell antibody, has been used for more than 10 years to treat B-cell lymphoma. Currently, rituximab has been approved for use in adult RA but there are no current data regarding rituximab use in JIA. The newest available biologic is abatacept, which is an antibody to CD28, a T-cell costimulator. Like rituximab, this drug has been approved for use in adult RA. Preliminary studies suggest efficacy and relative short-term safety.

## SYSTEMIC CORTICOSTEROIDS AND OTHER IMMUNOSUPPRESSIVE AGENTS

Corticosteroids are seldom used in the treatment of JIA. They are most often required in the treatment of systemic JIA with refractory systemic symptoms. Occasionally they are used in the other forms of JIA as a "bridging" medication to provide relief until other treatments take effect.

In refractory JIA, or refractory uveitis, several immunosuppressive drugs may be used to attempt to control the disease. These include cyclosporine, tacrolimus, thalidomide, and mycophenolate mofetil. There are no double-blind, case-control studies of these medications in JIA. There are, however, conflicting case reports as to their efficacy. Certain patients may benefit from these alternative medications, and a trial is warranted in severe, refractory disease. However, hydroxychloroquine, D-penicillamine, oral gold, and azathioprine, which have been used in the past, seem to be ineffective.

Systemic JIA appears to have a different response to immune suppressants than the other drugs. Thalidomide, in particular, may be effective in refractory systemic JIA.[22] In addition, IVIG and cyclophosphamide are occasionally used in the patient with systemic JIA who has severe systemic symptoms. In the most ill patients, bone marrow transplant has been performed. However, there continues to be a high rate of mortality with this treatment.

## PAIN MANAGEMENT

It is clear that children with JIA experience chronic pain. In 1 study, 76% of children reported feeling pain on most days. Most reported mild or moderate pain, but up to 25% reported more intense pain. However, disease activity correlated poorly with reported pain. Instead, more successful models to predict JIA pain have taken into account multiple factors, including disease status, demographics, psychological issues, and environmental factors. Older children, including adolescents, appear to report increased levels of pain. In a study[30] that used thermography as an objective measure of joint inflammation, it was noted that the amount of pain reported by adolescents did not correlate with the degree of joint inflammation.

The first step in treating pain in JIA is the use of anti-inflammatory therapy. By treating the underlying disease, pain can be improved acutely and painful deformities can be avoided. In particular, corticosteroids can provide rapid symptomatic relief. However, chronic use is associated with significant morbidity. In patients with longstanding disease, such as adolescents or adults, pain is common despite clinical remission.[14] This is due to inflammation in the immature joint causing cartilage loss and bone erosion. Also, limb length discrepancies cause biomechanical pain. Opioids are used in the most severe cases, where they are required to allow increased mobility. If a patient reports sleep disturbances, tricyclic antidepressants can be helpful. Studies have suggested that cognitive behavioral therapy, as well as improvement in sleep patterns, can help alleviate the pain of JIA.[31]

Surgical management is used in extreme cases of pain or functional limitation. This can include synovectomy, soft tissue release, joint fusions, and arthroplasty. Generally, it is preferable to wait until the growth plates have fused.[31] In a large series of adult patients with persistent JIA, joint replacement had been required in half. Adults with a history of JIA may have, for example, small femoral heads and poorly formed acetabuli. Custom joint replacements may be required because of abnormal bone morphology, osteopenia, and contractures.[14]

## REFERENCES


1. Petty RE, Southwood TR, Manners P, et al. International League of Associations for Rheumatology classification of juvenile idiopathic arthritis: second revision, Edmonton, 2001. *J Rheum.* 2004;31:390-392

2. Arnett FC, Edworthy SM, Bloch DA, McShane DJ, Fries JF, Cooper NS, et al. The American Rheumatism Association 1987 revised criteria for the classification of rheumatoid arthritis. *Arthritis Rheum.* 1988; 31(3):315-324

3. Fantini F, Gerloni V, Gattinara M, Cimaz R, Arnoldi C, Lupi E. Remission in juvenile chronic arthritis: a cohort study of 683 consecutive cases with a mean 10 year follow-up. *J Rheumatol.* 2003;30(3):579-584

4. Kump LI, Castaneda RA, Androudi SN, Reed GF, Foster CS. Visual outcomes in children with juvenile idiopathic arthritis-associated uveitis. *Ophthalmology.* 2006;113(10):1874-1877

5. Minden K, Niewerth M, Listing J, et al. Long-term outcome in patients with juvenile idiopathic arthritis. *Arthritis Rheum.* 2002;46:2392-2401

6. Packham JC, Hall MA. Long-term follow-up of 246 adults with juvenile idiopathic arthritis: functional outcome. *Rheumatology (Oxford).* 2002;41(12):1428-1435

7. Cassidy JT, Levinson JE, Bass JC, et al. A study of classification criteria for a diagnosis of juvenile rheumatoid arthritis. *Arthritis Rheum.* 1986;29(2):274-281

8. Kruitof E, Van Den Bossche V, De Rycke L,et al. Distinct synovial immunopathological characteristics of juvenile onset spondylarthritis and other forms of juvenile idiopathic arthritis. *Arthritis Rheum.* 2006;54:2594-2604

9. Thomson W, Barrett JH, Donn R, et al. Juvenile idiopathic arthritis classified by the ILAR criteria: HLA associations in UK patients. *Rheum.* 2002;41:1183-1189

10. Jones OY, Spencer CH, Bowyer SL, Dent PD, Bottlieb BS, Rabinovich CE. A multicenter case-control study on predictive factors distinguishing childhood leukemia from juvenile rheumatoid arthritis. *Pediatrics.* 2006;117:840-844

11. Malleson PN, Sailer M, Mackinnon MJ. Usefulness of antinuclear antibody testing to screen for rheumatic diseases. *Arch Dis Child.* 1997;77(4):299-304

12. Graham TB. Imaging in juvenile arthritis. *Curr Opin Rheumatol.* 2005;17(5):574-578

13. Ravelli A, Magni-Manzoni S, Pistorio A, et al. Preliminary diagnostic guidelines for macrophage activation syndrome complicating systemic juvenile idiopathic arthritis. *J Ped.* 2004;12:598-604

14. Nigrovic PA, White PH. Care of adult with juvenile rheumatoid arthritis. *Arthritis Rheum.* 2006;55:208-216

15. Southwood TR, Petty RE, Malleson PN, et al. Psoriatic arthritis in children. *Arthritis Rheum.* 1989;32(8):1007-1013

16. Sherry DD, Stein LD, Reed AM, Schanberg LE, Kredich DW. Prevention of leg length discrepancy in young children with pauciarticular juvenile rheumatoid arthritis by treatment with intra-articular steroids. *Arthritis Rheum.* 1999;42(11):2330-2334

17. Giannini EH, Brewer EJ, Kuzmina N, et al. Methotrexate in resistant juvenile rheumatoid arthritis. Results of the USA-USSR double-blind, placebo-controlled trial. The Pediatric Rheumatology Collaborative Study Group and The Cooperative Children's Study Group. *N Engl J Med.* 1992;326(16):1043-1049

18. Giannini EH, Cassidy JT. Methotrexate in juvenile rheumatoid arthritis. Do the benefits outweigh the risks? *Drug Saf.* 1993;9(5):325-339

19. Hashkes PJ, Balistreri WF, Bove KE, Ballard ET, Passo MH. The long-term effect of methotrexate therapy on the liver in patients with juvenile rheumatoid arthritis. *Arthritis Rheum.* 1997;40(12):2226-2234

20. Van Rossum MA, Fiselier TJ, Franssen MJ, et al. Sulfasalazine in the treatment of juvenile chronic arthritis: a randomized, double-blind, placebo-controlled, multicenter study. Dutch Juvenile Chronic Arthritis Study Group. *Arthritis Rheum.* 1998;41(5):808-816

21. Silverman E, Mouy R, Spiegel L, et al. Leflunomide in Juvenile Rheumatoid Arthritis (JRA) Investigator Group. Leflunomide or methotrexate for juvenile rheumatoid arthritis. *N Engl J Med.* 2005;352(16):1655-1666

22. Lehman TJ, Schechter SJ, Sundel RP, Oliveira SK, Huttenlocher A, Onel KB. Thalidomide for severe systemic onset juvenile rheumatoid arthritis: a multicenter study. *J Pediatr.* 2004;14(6):856-857

23. Grom AA, Murray KJ, Luyrink L, et al. Patterns of expression of tumor necrosis factor alpha, tumor necrosis factor beta, and their receptors in synovia of patients with juvenile rheumatoid arthritis and juvenile spondylarthropathy. *Arthritis Rheum.* 1996;39(10):1703-1710

24. Lovell DJ, Reiff A, Jones OY, et al. Pediatric Rheumatology Study Group. Long-term safety and efficacy of etanercept in children with polyarticular-course juvenile rheumatoid arthritis. *Arthritis Rheum.* 2006;54(6):1987-1994

25. Scallon B, Cai A, Solowski N, et al. Chimeric anti-TNF-alpha monoclonal antibody cA2 binds recombinant transmembrane TNF-alpha and activates immune effector functions. *Cytokine.* 1995;7(3):251-259

26. Biester S, Deuter C, Michels H, et al. Adalimumab in the therapy of uveitis in childhood. *Br J Ophthalmol.* 2007;91(3): 319–324. Epub 2006 October 11

27. Milojevic DS, Ilowite NT. Treatment of rheumatic diseases in children: special considerations. *Rheum Dis Clin North Am.* 2002;28(3):461–482

28. Pascual V, Allantaz F, Arce E, Punaro M, Banchereau J. Role of interleukin-1 (IL-1) in the pathogenesis of systemic onset juvenile idiopathic arthritis and clinical response to IL-1 blockade. *J Exp Med.* 2005;201(9):1479–1486

29. Woo P, Wilkinson N, Prieur AM, et al. Open label phase II trial of single, ascending doses of MRA in Caucasian children with severe systemic juvenile idiopathic arthritis: proof of principle of the efficacy of IL-6 receptor blockade in this type of arthritis and demonstration of prolonged clinical improvement. *Arthritis Res Ther.* 2005;7(6):R1281–R1288

30. Ilowite NT, Walco GA, Pochaczevsky R. Assessment of pain in patients with juvenile rheumatoid arthritis: relation between pain intensity and degree of joint inflammation. *Ann Rheum Dis.* 1992;51(3):343–346

31. Anthony KK, Schanberg LE. Pediatric pain syndromes and management of pain in children and adolescents with rheumatic disease. *Pediatr Clin North Am.* 2005;52(2):611–639

# CHAPTER 122

# Vasculitis and Associated Illnesses

BARBARA ANNE EBERHARD, MD

## INTRODUCTION

Chronic vasculitides are rare in the adolescent population and many may not be seen in a lifetime of treating children with rheumatic diseases. The presentation of the vasculitides can be vague and therefore a challenge to diagnose. Developing multiorgan involvement, occurring over sometimes weeks but more often months, may be an early clue. Although there may be no diagnostic tests to definitively confirm clinical suspicion of a vasculitis, there are invariably signs of inflammation, such as an elevated erythrocyte sedimentation rate (ESR) or C-reactive protein (CRP), along with evidence of a vasculitis, such as a rash, mucositis, neurologic and renal involvement, and possibly arthritis.

## RAYNAUD DISEASE

It is estimated that approximately 10% of adolescent girls have symptoms consistent with Raynaud disease.[1] The disorder is characterized by a triple-phase color change of the hands and feet in response to cold temperatures or emotional stress. This triple color change of the extremities was described by Raynaud and is called Raynaud phenomenon. The hands/feet turn blue due to arterio-vasoconstriction and resultant venous stasis, then white due to a further decrease in cutaneous blood flow, and finally red secondary to reflex vasodilation. These changes can be seen in one fingertip or a whole hand. There may also be similar color changes on the tips of the ears and nose. Often, idiopathic (primary) Raynaud disease is familial and seen mainly in the females of the family. The episodes are often more of a nuisance and the patient is instructed to avoid cold exposure, to wear a coat, hat, scarf, and mittens and, if necessary, hand warmers in the cold weather. Vasodilators have been used in more persistent cases, nifedipine being the drug of choice. Medication does not prevent the episodes but can make them shorter and less severe. Raynaud disease should be separated from acrocyanosis, a benign condition often seen in thin adolescents whose hands are always cold and blue.

Raynaud phenomenon can occur in association with a connective tissue disease, such as systemic sclerosis or systemic lupus erythematosus.[1-3] Here, spasm of the vessels is accompanied by inflammation within the blood vessels, which can lead to fingertip infarction. A distinction is made between the benign form of Raynaud and the more severe form by presence of a positive antinuclear antibody (ANA) and abnormal nail-bed capillaries.[1-4] The combination of the 2 confers a 90% risk of developing a connective tissue disease. In patients with secondary Raynaud phenomenon, aggressive treatment is needed with vasodilators, including nifedipine; in those with severe disease, sildenafil and bosentan can be considered.

## DERMATOMYOSITIS/POLYMYOSITIS

Diagnostic criteria for adult dermatomyositis were developed by Bohan and Peters[5] and can be applied equally well to any age group. The diagnosis is based on finding at least 4 of the following 5 criteria: (1) progressive, symmetric weakness of the proximal limb girdle, anterior neck flexors, and abdominal muscles; (2) a classic rash over the eyelids (heliotrope) or papules over the metacarpal and interphalangeal joints, elbows, knees, and medial malleoli (Grotton papules); (3) elevated muscle enzymes: CPK, AST, ALT, aldolase or LDH (Box 122-1); (4) electromyograph (EMG) evidence of myopathy and denervation; and (5) a biopsy demonstrating inflammatory myositis characterized by necrosis and inflammation. Newer tools may in the future make EMG and muscle biopsy unnecessary. A T2 fat-suppressed magnetic resonance imaging (MRI) of the proximal quadriceps and the pelvic musculature provides excellent information on both the presence and extent of muscle inflammation, whereas dilated nail-bed capillaries, present in most patients with dermatomyositis, are a useful adjunct in making the diagnosis (Box 122-1).[6,7]

In adolescence, the presentation of dermatomyositis peaks between the ages of 10 and 14 years. Although the classic presentation of rash and proximal muscle weakness allows the diagnosis to be made relatively easily, when the rash is absent (polymyositis), other etiologies need to be excluded, and in this instance a muscle biopsy may prove diagnostic (Box 122-2). In adolescents, muscular dystrophy, myotonia congenita, and periodic paralysis are important considerations in the differential diagnosis.[8]

**Box 122-1**

***Work-up for a Patient with Suspected Dermatomyositis***

- ***Laboratory work***
  - Muscle enzymes: Creatinine kinase (CK), lactate dehydrogenase (LD), aldolase, aspartate transaminase (AST), alanine transaminase (ALT). *Should be elevation of at least 1 muscle enzyme*
  - Measures of inflammation: ESR, CRP *Generally normal in inherited muscle dystrophies*
  - Markers of endothelial damage: Factor VIII-related antigen (von Willebrand factor) *may be elevated in active dermatomyositis*
  - Autoantibodies: Antinuclear antibody *can be positive but is not diagnostic.* Muscle-specific antibodies such as Jo-1, anti-Mi-2 *may be seen, if the ANA is positive, in a small number of patients*
- ***Other diagnostic tests***
  - EMG: *not absolutely necessary but can be useful if diagnosis in doubt*
  - Fat-suppressed T2-weighted MRI of quadriceps and pelvic musculature: *diagnosis strongly suggested by muscle edema*
  - Muscle biopsy: of either the deltoid or quadriceps muscle. *Perifascicular muscle atrophy, vasculitis*

**Box 122-2**

***Differential Diagnosis of Proximal Muscle Weakness in Adolescence***

Dermatomyositis
Muscular dystrophy
Central core and nemaline myopathy (mitochondrial myopathies)
Congenital hypotonia
Glycogen storage disease
Myoadenalate deaminase deficiency
Endocrine myopathy (thyroid, Cushing disease)
Amyloidosis
Proximal familial muscular disorders
Steroid myopathy

Although the etiology is unknown in this disease, in the past various infectious agents have been implicated. Coxsackie virus B and influenza A and B can cause a transient myositis. Toxoplasma invasion of muscle may present in a similar fashion to dermatomyositis and should be excluded either through serological testing or on muscle biopsy.

Weakness and fatigue are the prime complaints in dermatomyositis. The most noticeable muscle groups affected are the proximal limb-girdle muscles, the anterior neck flexors, and the trunk muscles. Functionally, activities such as climbing stairs, getting out of a chair or bed, brushing hair, and reaching for objects overhead can be difficult. Occasionally there will be pain associated with the weakness. The more worrying muscle weakness occurs in the bulbar musculature. Weakness in these muscles can present with swallowing difficulties, nasal speech, and nasal regurgitation of liquids. These are concerning signs and signal impending aspiration. Any patient with these complaints should be observed in the hospital.

The classic rash of dermatomyositis is the well-known heliotrope rash over the upper eyelids. This can be associated with malar erythema, which can involve the nasolabial folds, hence distinguishing this from a lupus rash. Gottron papules are wartlike in appearance and appear over the metacarpal and proximal phalangeal joints of the fingers. The papules may be erythematous or violaceous in color, over the elbows and knees. The rash can be scaly and look suspiciously like psoriasis. The rash in dermatomyositis, like the rash in lupus, is photosensitive, and flares of the disease can occur after prolonged sun exposure. A rash can also appear in sun-exposed areas such as the upper chest, neck, and upper back. Recently, visualization of nail-fold capillaries has aided diagnosis.[6] The changes that are seen can be extensive and include capillary dropout accompanied by dilated capillary loops. Capillary repair, along with improving muscle strength, provides a means of monitoring improvement in disease activity.

There are 2 unique features that can be seen in dermatomyositis. One is the development of cutaneous calcinosis[9] and the other is the appearance of lipodystrophy.[10] Both seem to be related to poorly controlled disease. Cutaneous calcification can present at any time during the course of dermatomyositis; a postulated mechanism could be via the release of calcium from the mitochondria of damaged muscles with the free calcium accumulating under the skin. Symptoms are dependent on where the calcinosis appears and the amount of calcinosis that develops. If it occurs around a joint, it can lead to joint contractures; if it appears in areas of frequent trauma, it can result in pain or even ulceration.

Lipodystrophy in active dermatomyositis may be accompanied by metabolic abnormalities including acanthosis nigricans, abnormal oral glucose tolerance testing (OGTT), and hypertriglyceridemia. An impaired OGTT or abnormal fasting glucose/insulin ratio suggestive of insulin resistance, with or without hypertriglyceridemia, can be seen in many patients with dermatomyositis even without lipodystrophy.[10]

Treatment has been debated for many years between lower-dose (1 mg/kg) and higher-dose (2 mg/kg) therapy of prednisone (max 80 mg/day). In general, patients do better long term on the higher dose of prednisone and improvement may be more rapid if the dose is divided throughout the day. Unfortunately, long-term prednisone has significant and often irreversible side effects. Therefore, to minimize its use other agents have been tried. The most commonly used steroid-sparing agent in dermatomyositis is methotrexate, given in a standard dose of 10 to 15 mg/m$^2$ and up to a maximum dose of 25 mg. It is given once per week, either by mouth or subcutaneously. It may take many weeks for its full effect to be seen, and for that reason is often started shortly after diagnosis rather than waiting for a flare on weaning the steroids.[11] Another treatment that may be effective is intravenous gammaglobulin (IVIG), given every month. This is not used as an initial therapy but rather as an adjunct when it is difficult to wean steroids. In severe disease, with aggressive vasculitis of major organ systems, such as the skin, central nervous system (CNS), lungs, and gastrointestinal tract, cyclophosphamide can be used.

Overall the outcome is excellent, and in most patients the disease will go into remission over months to years.[12,13] Provided there are no significant complications from prolonged steroid therapy, patients will return to a normal lifestyle without any restrictions. However, the minority who follow a chronic continuous course often have significant functional impairment, especially if there is significant loss of muscle mass.[13]

## VASCULITIS

These are a group of rare conditions united by the presence of inflammation in the blood vessels. The classification of these conditions is confusing, and pathogenesis remains unknown. The most widely used classification is based on blood vessel size—small, medium, and large. There is blurring between the small and medium blood vessel category (Box 122-3), with most illness in either category having some crossover into the other category. An outline of the work-up for a patient with vasculitis is outlined in Box 122-4. One blood test that may be helpful in these conditions is the antineutrophil cytoplasmic antibody (ANCA). The vasculitis most frequently encountered in adolescent patients is Henoch–Schonlein purpura (HSP).

**Box 122-3**

***Classification of Vasculitis Seen in Adolescence***

**Large vessel**
Takayasu arteritis

**Medium-sized vessel**
Polyarteritis

**Small-vessel vasculitis**
*ANCA positive*
Microscopic polyangiitis
Wegener granulomatosus
Churg–Strauss
*Immune complex vasculitis*
Henoch–Schonlein purpura
Behçet disease
Serum sickness

**Box 122-4**

***Work-up of a Patient with Vasculitis***

**Laboratory tests**
CBC/ESR/CRP *eosinophilia (Churg–Strauss)*
BUN/Creatinine
Complement C3 and C4 *will be low in immune complex disease*
Urine analysis, urine microscopy *hematuria/proteinuria*
Metabolic panel *may see abnormalities in liver function tests*
Antinuclear antibody *(ANA)*, antineutrophil cytoplasmic antibody *(ANCA)*
ASCA and ANCA testing *(rule out IBD)*
ASO, Hepatitis B

**Radiology**
CXR *infiltrates, hemorrhage, nodules*
Sinus x-ray
High-resolution chest CT scan

**Other tests**
Pulmonary function tests *restrictive/obstructive disease*
Diffusing capacity of oxygen (DCO) *may be raised if pulmonary hemorrhage*
Doppler tests for blood flow

### HENOCH–SCHÖNLEIN PURPURA

Henoch-Schönlein is the most prevalent primary vasculitis. It is an IgA-mediated, immune complex, small-vessel, leukocytoclastic vasculitis. The term leukocytoclastic refers to the presence of polymorphoneutrophils (PMNs) within a necrosed vessel wall. The diagnosis of HSP is based on the presence of palpable purpura (skin vasculitis), abdominal pain (intestinal vasculitis/bowel angina), arthritis, and glomerulonephritis.[14] Henoch-Schönlein purpura occurs infrequently in adolescence and rarely in adulthood.[15,16] Because infections can trigger HSP, especially Group A Streptococcus infections, it is presumed that the decreasing incidence in older age groups is due to decreased exposure to infections or a possible decrease in vaccinations, another potential trigger. For unknown reasons, there is a higher incidence of renal involvement in adolescents than in children, with some cases presenting as a nephritic or nephrotic syndrome and resultant renal failure.[17] Although there are no diagnostic tests for HSP, the studies outlined in Box 122-5 can be helpful in making the diagnosis or excluding other less common vasculitides that can mimic HSP (Box 122-6).

In general, pharmacologic treatment is not needed unless there is significant rash, renal disease, or gastrointestinal symptoms. Despite the liberal use of corticosteroids in this condition, there are few studies that have proven them to be beneficial.[18] When used, the initial dose should be 2 mg/kg/day (maximum: 80 mg/day) given orally; tapering the dose depends on the response to therapy. For severe renal disease, other immunosuppressive agents have been used, including azathioprine or cyclophosphamide.

**Box 122-5**

***Work-up for Patient with Henoch–Schönlein Purpura***

**Laboratory examination**

Blood urea nitrogen (BUN), creatinine
Complete blood count (CBC) with platelet count (rule out thrombocytopenia), leukocytosis
Urinary abnormalities: hematuria, proteinuria
Complement levels: normal C4, low C3
ASO (antistreptolysin antibody)
ANCA (may occasionally be positive; usually done to rule out other vasculitis)

**Skin biopsy**

Leukocytoclastic vasculitis with IgA and C3 deposition

**Box 122-6**

***Differential Diagnosis of Henoch–Schönlein Purpura***

Idiopathic thrombocytopenic purpura
Poststreptococcal glomerulonephritis
Systemic lupus erythematosus
Septicemia
Disseminated intravascular coagulation
Hemolytic uremic syndrome

## POLYARTERITIS NODOSA

Polyarteritis nodosa (PAN) is a rare vasculitis that is characterized by necrosis in medium and small vessels accompanied by aneurysm formation. Clinical presentation varies depending on the vessels involved. Polyarteritis nodosa has a predilection for the nervous system and the gastrointestinal tract. There are 2 types of PAN. Cutaneous PAN is generally limited to the skin, with the classic livedo reticularis rash, although other skin manifestations may include panniculitis and nonspecific skin edema. There may also be arthritis, mainly of the large joints. There seems to be an association with streptococcal infections in cutaneous PAN, and recurrent streptococcal infections can be a cause of disease flares. Treatment of cutaneous PAN is with anti-inflammatory medications, including corticosteroids and nonsteroid anti-inflammatories. This type of PAN usually resolves, although a few cases can develop into systemic PAN.

Systemic PAN is a more severe disease, which can result in major organ failure. It too can be associated with infection, particularly hepatitis B and C. The presentation in this illness is protean, and this is reflected in the diagnostic criteria (Box 122-7). The diagnosis rests on identifying the characteristic aneurysm formation in the involved blood vessels. There are no diagnostic laboratory criteria, although signs of ongoing inflammation such as raised ESR and acute-phase reactants are present. Antineutrophil cytoplasm antibodies (ANCAs) are not diagnostic in this condition.[19] Aggressive

**Box 122-7**

***American College of Rheumatology 1990 Criteria for the Classification of Polyarteritis Nodosa***

*Requires 3 or more criteria to make the diagnosis*
Unexplained weight loss of 4 kg or more
Livedo reticularis
Testicular pain
Myalgia in the absence of muscle weakness
Mono or polyneuropathy
Diastolic B/P >90
BUN >40 mg/dl or creatinine >1.5 mg/dl
Hepatitis B surface antigen
Unexplained aneurysms or vessel occlusion on arteriography
Vasculitis in a medium- or small-sized artery on biopsy

Adapted with permission from Lightfoot RW Jr, Michel BA, Bloch DA, et al. The American College of Rheumatology 1990 criteria for the classification of polyarteritis nodosa. *Arthritis Rheum.* 1990; 33:1088.

treatment is needed to prevent end organ damage; high dose cortico steroids, combined with a stronger immunosuppressive agent such as cyclophosphamide, is generally required.[20]

### TAKAYASU ARTERITIS

Takayasu arteritis is a granulomatous vasculitis of unknown origin that affects the aorta and its branches.[21,22] Its other (and better known) name is "pulseless disease." Although uncommon in North America, Takayasu arteritis is the third most common vasculitis worldwide. There has been a vague association with tuberculosis in countries such as Mexico and India, where both illnesses are more common. The clinical presentation is dependent on where in the aorta or its branches the vasculitis occurs. For example, involvement of the renal arteries occurs from hypertension; abdominal pain can result from celiac axis involvement; intermittent claudication occurs from narrowing in the descending aorta; and strokes or headache may result from carotid or vertebral artery involvement. In an attempt to aid diagnosis, the American College of Rheumatology has developed diagnostic criteria (Box 122-8). The findings in Takayasu arteritis are based on longstanding inflammation in the arteries, with resultant stenosis, and are irreversible.

The initial phase of the illness has a nonspecific prodrome of fever, arthralgia, weight loss, and fatigue, without apparent vascular abnormalities. Theoretically, if the illness can be diagnosed early, then stenosis of the arteries may be prevented; however, the lack of a diagnostic test makes this scenario unlikely. Antiendothelial antibodies may be helpful in this endeavor but are still only a research tool. Diagnosis requires vessel imaging, initially Doppler ultrasound, with confirmation by arteriography or a magnetic resonance arteriogram. Treatment is directed at preventing ongoing inflammatory damage with the hope that a surgical repair of the vascular lesions is possible. High-dose steroids are used until the ESR and CRP have returned to normal, then a steroid-sparing agent, such as methotrexate or cyclophosphamide, is added.[23] Hypertension needs aggressive treatment.[24] Low-dose aspirin has been used to prevent thrombus formation within the poststenotic, dilated portion of the artery. Prognosis is dependent on several factors, including the location of the vessel involved and the degree of reversibility of the lesion. The illness itself runs a relapsing and remitting course, which can make timing of surgical repair challenging, but most patients do go into remission.

**Box 122-8**

***Classification Criteria for Takayasu Arteritis***

Subclavian or aortic bruit
Age <740 at diagnosis
Decreased brachial artery pressure
Blood pressure difference of >10 mm Hg between arms
Claudication of extremities
Arteriographic evidence of narrowing or occlusion of the aorta and/or its branches

Adapted with permission from Arend WP, Michel BA, Bloch DA. The American College of Rheumatology (1990) criteria for the classification of Takayasu's arteritis. *Arthritis Rheum.* 1990; 33;1129.

### BEHÇET DISEASE

Behçet disease has a particular relevance in adolescence as it is included in the differential diagnosis of recurrent genital ulceration. As originally described by Dr Behçet, this illness is a triad of genital ulceration, apthous stomatitis (oral ulceration), and uveitis. However, over the years the illness has expanded to include complete and incomplete forms, and the involvement of other organ systems, but recurrent apthous ulceration is a necessity, no matter whose definition of the disease is used (Box 122-9).[25]

**Box 122-9**

***Diagnostic Criteria for Behçet Disease***

**Major criteria**

Recurrent oral ulceration with at least 3 episodes over a 12-month period
Recurrent genital ulceration
Uveitis either anterior or posterior
Skin lesions, eg, erythema nodosum, acneiform nodules, pseudofolliculitis
Pathergy (skin reaction to a needle prick)

**Minor**

Gastrointestinal lesions
Thrombophlebitis
Cardiovascular lesions
Arthritis
Central nervous system lesions
Family history

Requires at least 3 major or 2 major criteria and 3 minor criteria; recurrent oral ulceration must be 1 of the major criteria.

Reproduced from Mason RM, Barnes CG. Behçet's syndrome with arthritis. *Ann Rheum Dis.* 1969;28:95, with permission from BMJ Publishing Group, Ltd.

In Europe, where the disease is more prevalent, HLA-B51 confers an increased risk of developing the disease. There does not appear to be a similar finding in North America. The cause for the illness is unknown; infectious etiologies have been considered, particularly herpesvirus-1 (HSV-1), but not proven.

This illness evolves over time. Most patients develop bouts of apthous stomatitis, lasting up to 2 weeks, that heal, usually without scarring. Recurrent, painful ulcerations of the genital area in either sex occurs, usually starting after the oral ulcerations. Eye involvement can be severe.[26] Patients can develop a pan-uveitis, which if left untreated can progress to blindness. All patients therefore need to be followed regularly by an ophthalmologist. The following organ systems can be involved in decreasing frequency: (1) Musculoskeletal: arthritis occurs in 50% to 75% of cases, mainly in the large joints, such as the knees and ankles, and occasionally with sacro-iliac joint involvement; (2) vascular: 5% to 15% of patients have venous thromboses and, rarely, aneurysm formation; and (3) CNS: 5% to 15% have CNS involvement, the most common being encephalomyelitis or aseptic meningitis. The most important illness to consider in the differential diagnosis of Behçet disease is inflammatory bowel disease, in particular Crohn disease, where aphthous ulcers, arthritis, and erythema nodosum are also seen.

Treatment is directed by the severity of organ system involvement. Patients with primarily oral and genital involvement can generally be managed with daily colchicine. More serious involvement such as CNS and eye disease warrant corticosteroid therapy. Current therapies adequately treat the symptoms but do not put the disease into remission, meaning that disease recurrence during the lifetime of the patient is common.

## WEGENER GRANULOMATOSIS

This is a granulomatous vasculitis involving predominantly the upper and lower respiratory tract and the kidneys and is an important cause of the pulmonary-renal syndrome. Two types of Wegener granulomatosis have been described: the first is limited to the upper respiratory tract without any evidence of kidney involvement and is called localized Wegener granulomatosis. The second is the classic form of Wegener granulomatosis, which presents with nasal or oral inflammation, nodules or infiltrates on chest x-ray (CXR), the presence of glomerulonephritis on examination of the urine sediment, and evidence of granulomas on biopsy.[27-29]

Most patients present with an aggressive, recurrent sinusitis, often associated with epistaxis secondary to nasal mucosal ulcerations. The classic saddle nose deformity is the end result of vasculitis affecting the nasal cartilage. Less frequent manifestations include hoarseness secondary to subglottic stenosis and persistent nasal discharge secondary to chronic sinusitis. Although there are often nodules or pulmonary infiltrates on CXR, pulmonary symptoms such as pleuritis or cough are uncommon. The classic lesion in the kidneys is that of a rapidly progressive glomerulonephritis, and renal failure can occur in the course of a few days. Less frequent findings include a vasculitic rash virtually indistinguishable from HSP, ocular findings (in particular scleritis or episcleritis), and nonspecific complaints that include weight loss and fever.[28-30]

Findings of the typical granulomas on biopsy will confirm the clinical suspicion of Wegener granulomatosis. Other granulomatous vasculitides associated with infections, such as tuberculosis, fungal infections, or a helminth infestation, are part of the differential diagnosis but are generally easy to exclude. Other vasculitides, especially polyarteritis, could be considered, but granulomas should be absent and the ANCA, which is a diagnostic antibody test in Wegener, is negative.[30-32]

Over the past decade, the diagnosis of Wegener has been confirmed by ANCAs. There are several different types of these antibodies directed against different antigens. In Wegener granulomatosis, the cANCA is positive in up to 90% of cases. This antibody is directed against the PR3 antigen and appears to be highly specific for Wegener granulomatosis. In some patients ANCAs can be used to monitor the disease; a raised level may indicate a flare of the illness, whereas a negative ANCA may indicate that the disease is in remission.

Aggressive treatment for active Wegener granulomatosis is needed; the combination of oral cyclophosphamide and corticosteroids will induce a remission, but with significant morbidity.[33] Recently, treatment has become similar to cancer chemotherapy, with an induction phase consisting of a combination of corticosteroids (IV or oral) and cyclophosphamide (oral or IV) and a consolidation phase utilizing other agents, such as methotrexate or even a tumor necrosis factor (TNF-$\alpha$) inhibitor (Remicade). As infection can precipitate the illness, trimethoprim–sulfamethoxazole has been used with some success. It is often used as sole treatment for the localized form of the disease.

Previously this illness was uniformly fatal, but with the current forms of treatment it has now become a chronic illness, with relapses occurring in more than 50% of patients. Morbidity as a consequence of both the illness and the treatment is high, particularly due to the occurrence of serious infections and pulmonary hemorrhage. Renal failure is seen in about one-third of patients despite treatment.

**MICROSCOPIC POLYANGIITIS**

Another cause of the pulmonary-renal syndrome, microscopic polyangiitis, is a necrotizing vasculitis involving the small vessels of the kidney and lung. Antineutrophil cytoplasm antibodies are often positive in this condition, but unlike in Wegener granulomatosis, the pANCA, with reactivity to the myeloperoxidase (MPO) antigen, is positive. Treatment is very similar to Wegener granulomatosis and involves a combination of corticosteroids and cyclophosphamide.[34]

**CHURG–STRAUSS SYNDROME**

Churg-Strauss syndrome is an extremely uncommon vasculitis in children and adolescents. There is always a history of asthma, often difficult to control, with associated eosinophilia and pulmonary infiltrates on CXR. Vasculitis is a later finding, and can be accompanied by systemic features such as fever, fatigue, and weight loss. Diagnosis is confirmed both by a positive cANCA and/or pANCA and a biopsy showing granuloma formation with perivascular infiltration by eosinophils.[35] Treatment tends to be empiric and dependent on the patient's organ system involvement; response to corticosteroids determines whether other agents such as cyclophosphamide need to be introduced.

## REFERENCES


1. Nigrovic PA, Fuhlbrigge RC, Sundel RP. Raynaud's phenomenon in children: a retrospective review of 123 patients. *Pediatrics.* 2003;11(4 Pt 1):715–721

2. Dolezalova P, Young SP, Bacon PA, Southwood TR. Nailfold capillary microscopy in healthy children and in childhood rheumatic diseases: a prospective single-blind observational study. *Ann Rheum Dis.* 2003;62(5):444–449

3. Meli M, Gitzelmann G, Koppensteiner R, Amann-Vesti BR. Predictive value of nail-fold capillaroscopy in patients with Raynaud's phenomenon. *Clin Rheumatol.* 2006;25(2):153–158

4. Luggen M, Belhorn L, Evans T, Fitzgerald O, Spencer-Green G. The evolution of Raynaud's phenomenon: a long-term prospective study. *J Rheumatol.* 1995;22(12):2226–2232

5. Bohan A, Peter JB. Polymyositis and dermatomyositis. *N Engl J Med.* 1975;292:344

6. Nascif AK, Terreri MT, Len CA, Andrade LE, Hilário MO. Inflammatory myopathies in childhood: correlation between nail-fold capillaroscopy findings and clinical and laboratory data. *J Pediatr.* 2006;82(1):40–45

7. Reed AM, Mason T. Recent advances in juvenile dermatomyositis. *Curr Rheumatol Rep.* 2005;7(2):94–98

8. Compeyrot-Lacassagne S, Feldman BM. Inflammatory myopathies in children. *Pediatr Clin North Am.* 2005;52(2):493–520

9. Pachman LM, Veis A, Stock S, et al. Composition of calcifications in children with juvenile dermatomyositis: association with chronic cutaneous inflammation. *Arthritis Rheum.* 2006;54(10):3345–5330

10. Huemer C, Kitson H, Malleson PN, et al. Lipodystrophy in patients with juvenile dermatomyositis—evaluation of clinical and metabolic abnormalities. *J Rheumatol.* 2001;28(3):610–615

11. Ramanan AV, Campbell-Webster N, Ota S, et al. The effectiveness of treating juvenile dermatomyositis with methotrexate and aggressively tapered corticosteroids. *Arthritis Rheum.* 2005;52(11):3570–3578

12. Huber A, Feldman BM. Long-term outcomes in juvenile dermatomyositis: how did we get here and where are we going? *Curr Rheumatol Rep.* 2005;7(6):441–446

13. Pachman LM, Abbott K, Sinacore JM, et al. Duration of illness is an important variable for untreated children with juvenile dermatomyositis. *J Pediatr.* 2006;148(2):247–253

14. Trapani S, Micheli A, Grisolia F, et al. Henoch-Schönlein purpura in childhood: epidemiological and clinical analysis of 150 cases over a 5-year period and review of literature. *Semin Arthritis Rheum.* 2005;35(3):143–153

15. Yang YH, Hung CF, Hsu CR, et al. A nationwide survey on epidemiological characteristics of childhood Henoch-Schonlein purpura in Taiwan. *Rheumatology (Oxford).* 2005;44(5):618–622

16. Blanco R, Martinez-Taboada VM, Rodriguez-Valverde V, Garcia-Fuentes M, Gonzalez-Gay MA. Henoch-Schönlein purpura in adulthood and childhood: two different expressions of the same syndrome. *Arthritis Rheum.* 1997;40(5):859–864

17. Chang WL, Yang YH, Wang LC, Lin YT, Chiang BL. Renal manifestations in Henoch-Schönlein purpura: a 10-year clinical study. *Pediatr Nephrol.* 2005;20(9):1269–1272

18. Huber AM, King J, McLaine P, Klassen T, Pothos M. A randomized, placebo-controlled trial of prednisone in early Henoch-Schönlein Purpura. *BMC Med.* 2004;2(2):7

19. Bakkaloglu A, Ozen S, Baskin E, et al. The significance of antineutrophil cytoplasmic antibody in microscopic polyangitis and classic polyarteritis nodosa. *Arch Dis Child.* 2001;85(5):427–430

20. Feinstein J, Arroyo R. Successful treatment of childhood onset refractory polyarteritis nodosa with tumor necrosis factor alpha blockade. *J Clin Rheumatol.* 2005;11(4):219–222

21. Eke F, Balfe JW, Hardy BE. Three patients with arteritis. *Arch Dis Child.* 1984;59(9):877–883

22. Martini A. Behçet's disease and Takayasu's disease in children. *Curr Opin Rheumatol.* 1995;7(5):449–454

23. D'Souza SJ, Tsai WS, Silver MM, et al. Diagnosis and management of stenotic aorto-arteriopathy in childhood. *J Pediatr.* 1998;132(6):1016–1022

24. Milner LS, Jacobs DW, Thomson PD, et al. Management of severe hypertension in childhood Takayasu's arteritis. *Pediatr Nephrol.* 1991;5(1):38–41

25. On behalf of Turkish Pediatric Vasculitis Study Group; Ozen S, Bakkaloglu A, Dusunsel R, et al. Childhood vasculitides in Turkey: a nationwide survey. *Clin Rheumatol.* 2006;2196–2200

26. Pivetti-Pezzi P, Accorinti M, Abdulaziz MA, La Cava M, Torella M, Riso D. Behçets disease in children. *Jpn J Ophthalmol.* 1995;39(3):309–314

27. Roberti I, Reisman L, Churg J. Vasculitis in childhood. *Pediatr Nephrol.* 1993;7(4):479–489

28. Belostotsky VM, Shah V, Dillon MJ. Clinical features in 17 paediatric patients with Wegener granulomatosis. *Pediatr Nephrol.* 2002;17(9):754–776

29. Ozen S, Ruperto N, Dillon MJ, et al. EULAR/PReS endorsed consensus criteria for the classification of childhood vasculitides. *Ann Rheum Dis.* 2006;65(7):936–941

30. Frosch M, Foell D. Wegener granulomatosis in childhood and adolescence. *Eur J Pediatr.* 2004;163(8):425–434

31. Dillon MJ. Systemic vasculitis. *Clin Exp Rheumatol.* 1993;11(Suppl 9):S1–S21

32. Watts RA, Scott DG. Epidemiology of the vasculitides. *Semin Respir Crit Care Med.* 2004;25(5):455–464

33. Rottem M, Fauci AS, Hallahan CW, et al. Wegener granulomatosis in children and adolescents: clinical presentation and outcome. *J Pediatr.* 1993;122(1):26–31

34. Peco-Antic A, Bonaci-Nikolic B, Basta-Jovanovic G, et al. Childhood microscopic polyangiitis associated with MPO-ANCA. *Pediatr Nephrol.* 2006;21(1):46–53

35. Boyer D, Vargas SO, Slattery D, Rivera-Sanchez YM, Colin AA. Churg-Strauss syndrome in children: a clinical and pathologic review. *Pediatrics.* 2006;118(3):e914–e920

# CHAPTER 123

# Fibromyalgia Syndrome in Adolescents

DAVID M. SIEGEL, MD, MPH

## INTRODUCTION

Fibromyalgia syndrome (FS) is characterized by widespread pain, fatigue, poor sleep, and some or all of a variety of other complaints, including arthralgia, stiffness, recurrent headache, irritable bowel syndrome, dysmenorrhea, irritable bladder syndrome, Raynaud phenomenon, paresthesias, and depression. The prevalence of FS in a general population of adults has been estimated at 3.4% in women and 0.5% in men,[1] whereas in adolescents the figure is likely to be less.[2] In a North America Pediatric Rheumatology registry, 7.65% of newly referred diagnoses were FS.[3] Establishing the presence of FS can be challenging for the clinician, and a significant number of patients will have had prolonged pain, fatigue, and other symptoms prior to diagnosis. Thus, patients with FS have often accrued a meaningful degree of disability. In the teenager, this can manifest as increasing school absence, withdrawal from usual activities, and decline in school performance. Because the entity of FS has received increasing attention in the lay media, it is common for patients with varied somatic symptoms to incorrectly self-diagnose and somewhat insistently query their provider as to whether FS is present. It is therefore important for the clinician to have a working understanding of the diagnostic approach to FS in order to correctly identify those who do and do not have the condition. Once FS is properly identified, it is equally important that an appropriate treatment strategy be implemented, which should result in a decrease in symptoms and return to and maintenance of a normal level of functioning and quality of life.

Descriptions of patients with widespread pain, tender points, and fatigue, in the absence of an alternative biomedical or psychiatric diagnosis, have appeared in the literature since the 1800s. These early reports used terms such as "neurasthenia," "muscular rheumatism," or "soft tissue rheumatism" as diagnostic labels for patients, many of whom we would now identify as having FS. The term "fibrositis" appeared in a paper by Gowers in 1904[4] and persisted until the 1980s, when it was replaced by "fibromyalgia," which was deemed more accurate given the lack of objective evidence for inflammation in the disorder. Concurrent with this evolution in nomenclature was the landmark observation reported by Smythe and Moldofsky in 1978 characterizing the sleep disturbance in FS.[5]

To standardize the diagnosis of FS, a multicenter study was undertaken in which 558 adult patients (293 with FS, 265 controls) seen in rheumatology centers were enrolled, and various elements of the history, physical examination, and laboratory studies were analyzed as to their predictive and discriminating value in diagnosing FS. Published in 1990, this American College of Rheumatology collaborative study[6] identified 2 major diagnostic criteria: widespread (defined as above and below the waist and on both sides of the body) pain for at least 3 months, and a minimum of 11 out of 18 tender points on the physical examination. The latter used an agreed-on template of 18 defined points (9 symmetrically arrayed on each side of the body; Figure 123-1), which were digitally palpated with 4 kg of pressure. Control points were incorporated into the examination to eliminate the potentially confounding factor of patients who might have an exaggerated and generalized hyperalgesia. In adolescents, the author and others contend that if clinical and laboratory findings support the diagnosis, observing less than 11 tender points does not preclude identification of FS.

## PRESENTATION AND DIAGNOSIS

The adolescent with FS describes the gradual onset of diffuse achiness in the periarticular soft tissue or in the joints themselves. There is no redness or warmth, but patients frequently describe muscle or joint swelling that is not apparent to the physician or other provider. Although a precipitating event (eg, trauma or acute infection) can be reported, more commonly, the onset is insidious. A high percentage of patients report fatigue with everyday activity, and a progressive decrease in exercise tolerance, which is aggravated by the decline in aerobic activity that usually occurs. Numerous associated somatic complaints include recurrent headache, abdominal pain with cramping, and alternating diarrhea and constipation (irritable bowel syndrome), dysmenorrhea, joint stiffness, intermittent subjective swelling of hands and feet, Raynaud phenomenon, mood disturbance, and

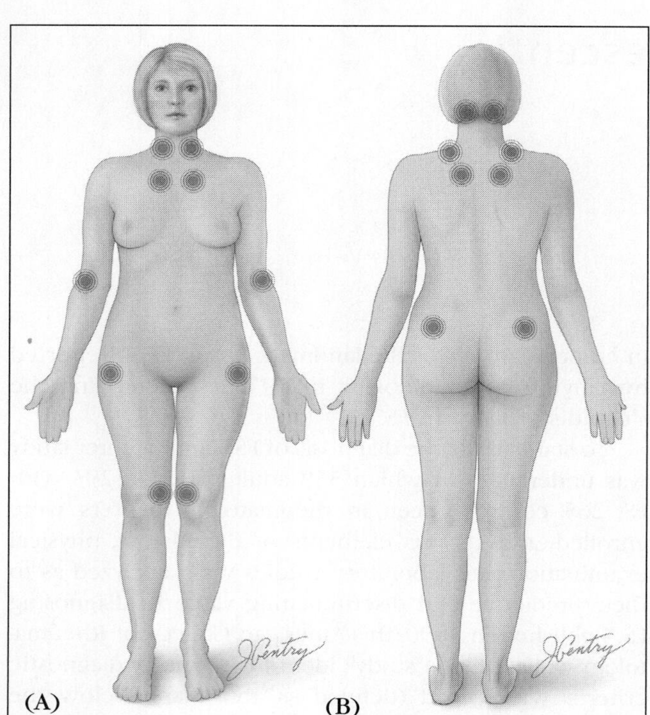


FIGURE 123-1 Fibromyalgia tender points. (From head to toe) (A) Anterior: low cervical (C6); 2nd rib costochondral junction; lateral epicondyle; posterior to greater trochanter; knee medial fat pad; (B) Posterior: suboccipital; mid-trapezius; supraspinatus insertion; upper outer buttocks.

difficulty with concentration. A study has found familial clustering of FS.[7] This is consistent with mothers presenting to our clinic with their daughters and stating that the child has the same disease they have (ie, FS). Of course, the parent's diagnosis of the daughter is not always borne out by the physician's evaluation.

Although the previously associated symptoms are often enumerated by the patient and parent(s), a key area that merits careful questioning and discussion by the provider is the quality of sleep and whether the adolescent is fatigued much of the time. Having trouble falling asleep may be a problem, but more typical is nocturnal restlessness and lack of energy in the morning. Furthermore, if asked "How many hours of sleep do you need in order to feel rested and refreshed?", the adolescent with FS will have difficulty answering. "No matter how many hours of sleep I seem to get, I am always tired. Even if I nap during the day (*which many of these patients do*) I am never able to feel refreshed and ready to go." In our study, this nonrestorative sleep was found in 98% of adolescents with FS.[8] Further questioning will find that the patient is quite restless during the night, with multiple awakenings and descriptions of bed covers significantly disheveled, or even entirely off the bed, in the middle of the night or morning. As found by Smythe and Moldofsky[5] and others,[9] this restless, nonrestorative sleep pattern represents inadequate delta wave, or stage IV, sleep due to the intrusion of lighter alpha wave sleep. Eliciting a careful sleep description in an achy, tired teen is an essential part of the history.

Not found in adolescents with FS are fever; weight loss; oral lesions; or joints with swelling, warmth, erythema, or limited motion. In addition to the usual elements of the physical examination, a diagnostic consideration of FS should incorporate systematic palpation of each of the 18 tender points and some control points. When establishing the presence of tender points, the examiner should apply 4 kg of pressure using the thumb or another finger. The physician can standardize his or her examination pressure by using a pinch strength meter to gauge one's technique.[10] The proper force results in some degree of discomfort, even in patients without the diagnosis. However, in those with FS, the examination experience is much more unpleasant and characterized by marked grimacing and withdrawal. Typically, the patient is resistant to undergoing a repeat examination because of the magnitude of pain. Other parts of the physical examination in FS are normal.

No diagnostic testing is absolutely confirmatory of FS, and laboratory and imaging studies in FS are consistently normal. In an adolescent with persistent symptoms suggestive of FS, and nothing found in the history or physical examination to suggest a competing condition, a complete blood count with differential, an erythrocyte sedimentation rate (and/or C-reactive protein), and, perhaps, thyroid function studies should be sufficient. If the clinician ascertains that depression is likely, a standardized metric such as the Beck Depression Inventory might be used to gauge severity and the possible need for formal mental health consultation.

## TREATMENT

Management of the adolescent with FS should focus on sleep quality, pain, exercise, and, if present, depression. The poor, nonrestorative sleep pattern in FS is often at the root of the pain and fatigue. Thus, the first priority is to establish proper sleep hygiene. This includes a consistent bedtime and morning wake-up time throughout the week. Variation in when the adolescent goes to bed at night and gets up in the morning should be no more than 1.5 hours, regardless of the day of the week. We strongly encourage avoidance of napping, as well as eliminating intake of alcohol, caffeine, nicotine, or other stimulants. Although sleep hygiene is necessary, it is not usually sufficient in the initial management of FS. Most patients will also require medication, the effect of which is to facilitate stage IV sleep. The most commonly used preparations are tricyclic antidepressants (TCAs) given in low doses 1 to 1.5 hours prior to bedtime. Specifically, cyclobenzaprine (which is not an antidepressant, but shares the same tricyclic chemical structure as TCAs) at a dose of 10 to 20 mg nightly is often very effective, although some adolescents may require higher doses. In a meta-analysis of adults with FS, those taking cyclobenzaprine were 3 times as likely to report overall improvement and enhanced sleep as compared to subjects treated with other medications.[11] The first signs of improvement are less nighttime awakening and decreased disruption of bed covers. Usually, after 2 to 3 weeks of quieter, more restful sleep, an increase in energy and a decrease in pain begin to occur. If the quality of sleep is not changing within a few weeks, then increasing the medication dose by 5- to 10-mg increments is appropriate. Excessive morning grogginess can be a sign that the dose is too high or the medication should be taken earlier in the evening.

If there is no clinical response to cyclobenzaprine, or if adverse effects (eg, morning sleepiness) occur, alternative medications should be tried. Examples of alternative medications include nortriptyline or doxepin. Other classes of drugs have shown response to treatment are selective serotonin reuptake inhibitors[12] and serotonin/norepinephrine reuptake inhibitors.[13] Although tramadol (a weak μ-opioid receptor) and sedative hypnotics (eg, zolpidem tartrate) have been shown to be beneficial in FS, we discourage their use in adolescents because of the potential long-term complication of dependency. A combination of tramadol and acetaminophen (Ultracet) is effective in adults with FS and may be safer than tramadol alone because of the lower dose.[14] Although nonsteroidal anti-inflammatory drugs and acetaminophen are not consistently helpful, for the individual teen these analgesics might offer some interim relief while more definitive therapy takes hold.

The first US Food and Drug Administration (FDA)–approved treatment for fibromyalgia is pregabalin, which attained this status in June 2007.[15] Although the approval is for adult use, it is an appropriate therapeutic option in those adolescents with fibromyalgia who have not responded adequately to other forms of treatment. Pregabalin has anticonvulsant, analgesic, and anxiolytic properties. With regard to its effect on decreasing pain, the mechanism of action is believed to be mediated through reducing the synaptic release of glutamate, noradrenalin, and substance P.[16] In 2005, Crofford et al[17] published results of an 8-week, double-blind, placebo-controlled trial in which doses of 300 mg/day and 450 mg/day were observed to be effective in reducing pain as well as fatigue and disrupted sleep.

Based on these findings, a more extensive trial was undertaken by Arnold et al[18] to explore longer-term efficacy, additional dose response characteristics, and expanded quantification of outcome parameters, including not only pain but also sleep disturbance, fatigue, quality of life, anxiety, and depressive symptoms. Not only did these investigators use a double-blind, placebo-controlled experimental design, but they also stipulated that with the exception of as-needed acetaminophen, pregabalin was the only treatment that study subjects received. Using the American College of Rheumatology definition of fibromyalgia,[6] 750 patients were enrolled and randomized to 4 conditions: placebo, or pregabalin at 300 mg/day, 450 mg/day, or 600 mg/day, respectively. The dosing interval was twice daily and subjects were followed for 14 weeks.

The initial primary outcome measure was patient daily pain diaries. For those who recorded significant decreases in pain as compared to the placebo group, other standardized instruments including the Patient Global Impression of Change and the Fibromyalgia Impact Questionnaire (FIQ) were administered, as were metrics of sleep quality, anxiety, and depression. The authors found that pain and sleep improved significantly for all 3 doses of pregabalin, as compared to placebo, whereas only those with the 2 higher doses (450 mg/day and 600 mg/day) demonstrated improvements in the more global assessment represented by the FIQ. It was also observed that adverse effects of dizziness and somnolence were more common among the 2 higher-dose groups, but only 3% to 4% reported that these effects were sufficiently severe to necessitate withdrawal from the drug. Although the literature on pregabalin efficacy in fibromyalgia (and subsequent FDA approval of the medication in this disorder) does not warrant making pregabalin the treatment of first resort for adolescents with fibromyalgia, it does make for a meaningful addition to the therapeutic armamentarium. Its success as monotherapy in the condition is certainly appealing as well.

Along with these strategies to address the nonrestorative sleep, regular moderate exercise has also been shown to improve the status of patients with FS, in terms of physical and psychological outcomes.[19] Brisk walking for 20 to 30 minutes, 3 times per week, is an example of an appropriate, low-intensity physical activity that can be incorporated into a treatment plan for FS. Referral to a physical therapist, or to a gym and trainer, may be necessary for those who are unable to initiate this level of activity on their own. In such instances, a more careful and graded exercise routine must be created. For the competitive athlete, or the adolescent who desires regular participation in high-intensity exercise, it is important to design a schedule of *gradual* return to this more strenuous activity. Abruptly taking on a demanding regimen of physical exertion in the patient with FS who has not yet established consistently restful sleep and restoration of aerobic capacity and muscle endurance can very well result in clinical deterioration and regression. The physician may need to counsel the adolescent to hold back on aggressive exercise until it is clear that improved sleep, decreased pain, and restoration of adequate aerobic capacity have occurred.

In addition to these physical and pharmacologic interventions, many of those with FS will benefit from psychological support and intervention. Obviously, if overt depression is present, appropriate mental health referral and treatment should take place. However, for some patients, clinical depression is not the issue as much as is distress and feeling discouraged and frustrated with the persistent fatigue and pain. This may be complicated by deterioration in school performance and/or disruption of peer relationships. In many families, the presence of a teen with FS also introduces stress on siblings and parents. With all of the latter in mind, attention to the emotional and psychological burden of FS is an important priority. The adolescent medicine provider, pediatrician, or family physician can certainly assess the emotional dimension of the problem and undertake initial counseling for the patient and family as appropriate for his or her training background and level of expertise. Cognitive behavioral therapy has been studied in FS and found to be a useful adjunct to treatment.[20] For some of these patients, formal mental health consultation will be necessary to fully address the psychological morbidity of the illness.

## PROGNOSIS

Overall, the adolescent with FS responds reasonably well to the previous approach and, over a period of weeks following initiation of treatment, will become increasingly less symptomatic with regard to pain and fatigue, although restoring complete exercise tolerance may take longer than correction of fatigue and pain, depending on the duration of symptoms and degree of deconditioning at the onset of therapy. If recovery does not proceed, then reformulation of the treatment plan should be undertaken and/or consultation with a pediatric rheumatologist should be considered. If new symptoms or signs appear that introduce the possibility of alternative diagnoses, then the clinician should readdress the correctness of the FS label and undertake further evaluation as needed. Whereas some of the popular information available concerning adults with FS might suggest a gloomy outcome, we emphasize with teens that early and prompt diagnosis, coupled with appropriate treatment, is an effective means to prevent chronic, pathological behavioral and physical maladaptations. Most adolescents with FS should be able to return to their previous premorbid status.[8,21]

## INTERNET RESOURCES

- National Institute of Arthritis and Musculoskeletal and Skin Diseases fact sheet on fibromyalgia: www.niams.nih.gov/Health_Info/Fibromyalgia/fibromyalgia_ff.asp
- Patient handout from American Academy of Family Physicians on fibromyalgia and exercise: www.familydoctor.org/handouts/061.html
- The American Fibromyalgia Syndrome Association, Inc: www.afsafund.org/
- Fibromyalgia Network: www.fmnetnews.com
- American College of Rheumatology: www.rheumatology.org

## REFERENCES


1. Wolfe F, Ross K, Anderson J. The prevalence and characteristics of fibromyalgia in the general population. *Arthritis Rheum.* 1995;38:19

2. Buskila D, Press J, Gedalia A, et al. Assessment of nonarticular tenderness and prevalence of fibromyalgia in children. *J Rheumatol.* 1993;20:368

3. Bowyer S, Roettcher P. Pediatric rheumatology clinic populations in the United States: results of a 3-year survey. Pediatric Rheumatology Database Research Group. *J Rheumatol.* 1996;23:1968

4. Gowers WR. Lumbago: its lessons and analogues. *BMJ.* 1904;1:117

5. Smythe HA, Moldofsky H. Two contributions to understanding the "fibrositis" syndrome. *Bull Rheum Dis.* 1978;26:928

6. Wolfe F, Smythe HA, Yunus MB, et al. The American College of Rheumatology 1990 criteria for the classification of fibromyalgia. *Arthritis Rheum.* 1990;33:160

7. Arnold LM, Hudson JI, Hess EV, et al. Family study of fibromyalgia. *Arthritis Rheum.* 2004;50:944

8. Siegel DM, Janeway D, Baum J. Fibromyalgia syndrome in children and adolescents: clinical features at presentation and status at follow-up. *Pediatrics.* 1998;101:377

9. Moldofsky H. Management of sleep disorders in fibromyalgia. *Rheum Dis Clin North Am.* 2002;28:353

10. Baum J. Use of the pinch strength meter in tender point examination. *Arthritis Rheum.* 1991;34:128

11. Tofferi JK, Jackson JL, O'Malley PG. Treatment of fibromyalgia with cyclobenzaprine: A meta-analysis. *Arthritis Rheum.* 2004;51:9

12. Arnold LM, Hess EV, Hudson JI, et al. A randomized, placebo-controlled, double-blind, flexible-dose study of fluoxetine

in the treatment of women with fibromyalgia. *Am J Med.* 2002;15:191

13. Sayar K, Aksu G, Ak I, Tosun M. Venlafaxine treatment of fibromyalgia. *Ann Pharmacother.* 2003;37:1561

14. Bennett RM, Schein J, Kosinski MR, et al. Impact of fibromyalgia pain on health-related quality of life before and after treatment with tramadol/acetaminophen. *Arthritis Rheum.* 2005;53:519

15. Pzifer, Inc. Lyrica (pregabalin) Package Insert. New York: Pfizer, Inc; June 2007

16. Field MJ, Cox PJ, Stott E, et al. Identification of the α-δ-1 subunit of voltage-dependent calcium channels as a molecular target for pain mediating the analgesic actions of pregabalin. *PNAS.* 2006;103:17537-17542

17. Crofford LJ, Rowbotham MC, Mease PJ, et al. Pregabalin for the treatment of fibromyalgia syndrome: results of a randomized, double-blind, placebo-controlled trial. *Arthritis Rheum.* 2005;52:1264-1273

18. Arnold LM, Russell J, Diri EW, et al. A 14-week, randomized, double-blinded, placebo-controlled monotherapy trial of pregabalin in patients with fibromyalgia. *J Pain.* 2008;9:792-805

19. Mannerkorpi K, Iversen MD. Physical exercise in fibromyalgia and related syndromes. *Best Pract Res Clin Rheumatol.* 2003;17:629

20. Williams DA. Psychological and behaviorial therapies in fibromyalgia and related syndromes. *Best Pract Res Clin Rheumatol.* 2003;17:649

21. Buskila D, Neumann L, Hershman E, et al. Fibromyalgia syndrome in children—an outcome study. *J Rheumat.* 1995;22:525

# CHAPTER 124

# Chronic Fatigue Syndrome

MARTIN FISHER, MD

It has been approximately 20 years since a difficult-to-define illness, marked by ongoing fatigue and a series of other symptoms, was first identified in several cohorts of adults in the United States, England, and Australia. Originally considered to be chronic mononucleosis or a chronic Epstein-Barr virus (EBV) infection, later called "chronic fatigue immunodeficiency syndrome," and for the past 10 to 15 years referred to as "chronic fatigue syndrome (CFS)," the illness has also been seen in small but distinct groups of adolescents. It remains difficult to define, there are no definitive explanations for its etiology, and there are no treatment approaches that have shown significant effectiveness. Yet much has been learned during these 20 years about the definition, epidemiology, and presentation of CFS in adults and adolescents; possible etiologies and the most appropriate approaches to evaluation and management; and the clinical course and outcome of the syndrome. These are reviewed in this chapter.

## DEFINITION AND EPIDEMIOLOGY

In the late 1980s and early 1990s, diagnostic criteria for CFS were developed in the United States, England, and Australia. Each definition, which varied somewhat in its approach, emphasized that the illness is *chronic* (lasting at least several months), includes debilitating *fatigue* (affecting the individual's lifestyle), and can be categorized as a *syndrome* (including symptoms other than the fatigue). In 1994, the Centers for Disease Control and Prevention (CDC) updated the original definition developed in 1988, and it is this definition (Box 124-1) that continues to be used to date.[1] The criteria indicate that for an illness to be defined as CFS, it must last at least 6 months, cause a decrease in activity of at least 50%, not be due to other discernible causes, and include at least 4 other symptoms, as listed in Box 124-1.

These criteria have functioned well to define CFS as it is seen in adults. Studies have shown that as many as 1 in 300 adults in the United States can be considered to have CFS and that most adults who have CFS have had symptoms for at least 6 to 12 months, and sometimes several years, before a diagnosis is made.[2,3] Approximately 85% of adults with CFS have an abrupt onset of symptoms, and 75% are bedridden or unable to work during the course of their illness. Approximately two-thirds of adults with CFS are female, the median age of diagnosis is 36 to 41 years, and most adults with CFS remain ill for many years, if not indefinitely.

### Box 124-1
### *Chronic Fatigue Syndrome: A Working Definition*

**Fatigue**

Lasts at least 6 months
Limits the person to ≤50% of premorbid activity
May be persistent or recurrent

**Additional symptoms (4 or more)**

Impaired memory or concentration
Pharyngitis
Tender lymph nodes (cervical or axillary)
Low-grade fever (or sensation of fever/chills)
Muscle pain (myalgia)
Multiple joint aches (arthralgia)
New onset headaches
Sleep disturbance (hypersomnia or insomnia)
Postexertion fatigue

**Exclusion**

Another cause of, or diagnosis, that accounts for the person's fatigue and symptoms

From Fukuda K, Straus SE, Hickie I, et al. The chronic fatigue syndrome: a comprehensive approach to its definition and study. *Ann Intern Med*. 1994;121: 953–959

The criteria do not work quite as well in defining the syndrome as seen in adolescents. Although some adolescents meet the full criteria in Box 124-1, others may have a milder form of the condition or are diagnosed before having symptoms for 6 months. Many adolescents who otherwise meet all other criteria for CFS do not quite have a 50% decline in activities (because they are able to attend school and participate in other activities, although with difficulty), whereas others are not yet ill for 6 months when presenting for a diagnosis (because parents are likely to bring their adolescents for evaluation earlier than adults may choose to go on their own).[4] There is some controversy as to whether CFS is an adolescent illness at all, and certainly whether these milder forms can be considered CFS.[5] Accordingly, some clinicians have chosen to refer to the earlier or milder cases seen in adolescents as "postviral fatigue," reserving the diagnosis of CFS for those who have been ill for at least 6 months and meet full CDC criteria. There is evidence in the literature that adolescents who present before 6 months of illness have a better prognosis than those who present later and that adolescents in general have a better prognosis than adults.

Studies of adolescents with CFS indicate that approximately 70% are female and most are white and middle class, which is not different than that seen in adults; half are 10 to 14 years of age and half are 15 to 19 years of age, indicating that younger and older adolescents are equally affected, with only rare cases seen in children; the mean time to diagnosis is 6 to 12 months, less than that seen in adults; and 75% have an abrupt onset of illness, with the other 25% having had other symptoms, such as headaches, abdominal pains, or milder forms of fatigue, interfering with functioning prior to the onset of the CFS.[6] Adolescents reported to have CFS in the United States have sometimes been part of miniepidemics along with adults (eg, as reported from a suburb of Buffalo, New York, in the early 1990s),[7] but most cases have been sporadic, as reported in case series from several parts of the country (Seattle, Washington; Hartford, Connecticut; Lexington, Kentucky; Long Island, New York) by specialists treating adolescent CFS throughout the 1990s.[6,8-10] These case series have reported remarkably similar findings, regardless of location, and it is estimated that less than 1 in 1,000 adolescents suffer from CFS, a much lower prevalence than that reported in adults.

## PRESENTATION

It is certainly not unusual for adolescents to present to their primary care provider with the complaint of fatigue, but it is the rare adolescent among this group who will be determined to have CFS. Only those who have debilitating fatigue along with other symptoms lasting for at least 6 months and no other reason for the fatigue can be considered within the CFS spectrum. Most adolescents who present with the symptom of fatigue do not have CFS; the differential diagnosis for the cause of their fatigue must be determined outside the CFS spectrum.

The CDC criteria in Box 124-1 lists the symptoms seen in patients with CFS. These symptoms include recurrent sore throat and adenopathy, joint and muscle pains, new onset headaches and changes in concentration and/or memory, low-grade fever or a feeling of "fever" or chills, and 2 symptoms that describe aspects of the fatigue (ie, nonrefreshing sleep and fatigue on exertion). By definition, all patients with CFS, including all adolescents, have some, but not necessarily all, of these symptoms. In addition, however, many patients with CFS, especially adolescents, have other symptoms as well. Table 124-1 lists the symptoms found in a series of 58 adolescents diagnosed with CFS.[6] Three things should be noted about this list: (1) most of the adolescents had many more symptoms than those listed in the CDC criteria; (2) pediatric-type symptoms, such as abdominal pain, are reported more frequently by adolescents with CFS than adults; and (3) a very prominent symptom not included in the CDC criteria, but reported by many adolescents and adults with CFS, is orthostatic hypotension.

### Table 124-1

### Symptoms of 58 Children and Adolescents with Chronic Fatigue Syndrome

| *Symptom* | *Number (%)* |
|---|---|
| Fatigue | 58 (100%) |
| Headache | 43 (74%) |
| Sore throat | 34 (59%) |
| Abdominal pain | 28 (48%) |
| Fever | 21 (36%) |
| Impaired cognition | 19 (33%) |
| Myalgia | 18 (31%) |
| Diarrhea | 17 (29%) |
| Adenopathy | 17 (29%) |
| Anorexia | 16 (28%) |
| Nausea or vomiting | 5 (26%) |
| Dizziness | 10 (17%) |
| Arthralgia | 10 (17%) |
| Sweats | 5 (9%) |
| Chills | 4 (7%) |
| Depression | 4 (7%) |

Krilov L, Fisher M, Friedman S, et al. Course and outcome of chronic fatigue in children and adolescents. *Pediatrics*. 1998;102(2):360–366.

In most cases, the story of an adolescent with CFS involves a well teenager who develops the relatively sudden onset of fatigue and other symptoms, often starting in conjunction with a viral illness, and the continuation of the fatigue and accompanying symptoms despite resolution of the initial illness. Some patients may have a more insidious onset of the fatigue, but almost all adolescents with CFS can describe a time when they made a transition from having no more than mild fatigue and no other symptoms to a time when they developed debilitating fatigue and accompanying symptoms. Some patients describe ups and downs in their symptoms, varying by days or weeks, whereas others feel the same day after day. In patients with CFS, the sense that something has changed significantly in their lives is a prominent feature.

In determining the approach for those who present with a possible diagnosis of CFS, it is useful to divide patients into 3 categories: (1) those who meet full criteria for CFS and whose histories fit the expected profile; (2) those who do not fully meet CDC criteria or whose histories do not fully match the expected profile, but whose symptoms clearly overlap with what is seen in CFS; and (3) patients who have fatigue, but whose histories and symptoms do not fit into the CFS spectrum. Thus, a first step in the evaluation and management of the adolescent who presents with fatigue is to determine whether the patient does have CFS or a milder variant. If the adolescent does have CFS, then a series of steps will follow, as described later in this chapter, which will include looking for possible alternate or underlying explanations for the fatigue. If the adolescent does not have CFS, then the general differential diagnosis of fatigue in adolescents must be considered as described in the next section.

## DIFFERENTIAL DIAGNOSIS OF FATIGUE

The differential diagnosis of fatigue in adolescents can be divided into 4 categories (Box 124-2). Most adolescents who complain of fatigue have neither a medical nor a psychological condition to account for the fatigue. A recent study indicated that as many as 20% of girls and 6% of boys report severe fatigue of at least 1 month's duration.[11] Most of these adolescents with fatigue are merely feeling tired because of a combination of too little sleep or a busy schedule. However, it is important to distinguish a second category from this group, those who have a psychological cause (most often depression) for their fatigue. A search for the signs and symptoms of depression (see Chapter 184, Disorders of Mood) should be included in the evaluation of any adolescent presenting with fatigue.

### Box 124-2
### *Differential Diagnosis of Fatigue and Chronic Fatigue Syndrome*

1. Lifestyle causes
   - Too little sleep
   - Busy schedule
2. Psychological causes
   - Depression
   - Anxiety
   - Stress
   - Psychiatric disorders
3. Organic causes
   - Medications
     - Antihistamines, sedatives
     - Alcohol, drug use
     - Other medications
     - Heavy metal intoxication
   - Infectious diseases
     - Mononucleosis, other viral infections
     - HIV, lyme, brucellosis, tuberculosis
     - Bacterial infections, bacterial endocarditis
   - Endocrine disorders
     - Hypothyroidism, hyperthyroidism
     - Diabetes mellitus, hypoglycemia
     - Addison disease, Cushing syndrome
     - Hypopituitarism, hypoparathyroidism
   - Systemic illnesses
     - Anemia, neoplasms
     - Allergies, connective tissue diseases
     - Congenital heart disease, asthma
     - Inflammatory bowel disease, celiac disease
     - Renal failure, liver failure
   - Sleep disorders
     - Delayed sleep phase syndrome
     - Obstructive sleep apnea
     - Narcolepsy
     - Restless leg syndrome

A third category, medical illness, is an uncommon cause of fatigue in adolescents, especially if it is not accompanied by other symptoms. Although the differential diagnosis of fatigue can theoretically include almost every illness and every organ system (Box 124-2), caution must be used in creating a balance between searching for the occasional medical diagnosis as a cause of fatigue and performing an extensive evaluation for all possible causes. It seems most prudent, in the evaluation of those adolescents who do not have obvious scheduling or psychological causes for their fatigue, to perform a complete review of systems and basic laboratory testing (looking for such diagnoses as anemia or hypothyroidism) and to pursue further testing in those with other findings on their history, physical examination, or laboratory screening.

A fourth category in the differential diagnosis of fatigue is sleep disorders. Although considered extremely rare in adolescents, sleep disorders as a cause of fatigue is receiving increasing attention of late. Two disorders in particular may be more common than previously realized: the delayed sleep phase syndrome (DSPS) and obstructive sleep apnea [also referred to as sleep disordered breathing (SDB)].[12] Delayed sleep phase syndrome is a circadian rhythm abnormality in which the individual's internal clock is not synchronized with external time. It represents an exaggeration of the tendency of adolescents to sleep at odd hours and is reported to occur in up to 7% of adolescents. Sleep disordered breathing, which involves recurrent collapse of the pharynx during sleep, may occur in up to 3% of adolescents. It is marked by loud snoring during sleep and may be caused by enlarged tonsils and adenoids, retrognathia, or nasal obstruction. Other entities, such as narcolepsy and restless leg syndrome, are still considered to be rare in adolescents and more common with aging. With the greater use of sleep studies, it is expected that the diagnosis of sleep disorders in all age groups, including adolescents, will rise in the coming years.

In general, although the differential diagnosis of CFS in adolescents is shown in Box 124-2, the approach is different. By definition, the adolescent with CFS has more than just too little sleep and a busy schedule, the most common cause in those without CFS, although appropriate scheduling can be an important factor in managing patients with CFS. Instead, in those with CFS, the psychological, medical, and sleep problems listed in Box 124-2 must be considered as a possible differential diagnosis (ie, another cause of fatigue masquerading as CFS) and/or as an underlying cause (ie, the reason for the CFS). Patients with CFS may ultimately have another diagnosis, although this is uncommon in clinical practice and the medical literature. Alternately, some patients with CFS may have an underlying cause of their syndrome, as discussed in the next section. Also, there are some syndromes (eg, fibromyalgia or lyme disease) whose symptoms overlap with CFS (see Chapter 123, Fibromyalgia, and Chapter 140, Tick-Borne Diseases).

## ETIOLOGY: THEORIES AND EVIDENCE

The etiology of CFS is yet to be determined. Many theories have been proposed, many possibilities tested, and many controversies engendered during the past 20 years.[13] At first, an infectious etiology was most suspected. Over time, immunologic and endocrine possibilities have been considered. Of late, cardiovascular abnormalities and sleep disorders have received the most attention. Throughout the 20 years, psychological underpinnings have been apparent, with some people arguing that CFS is nothing more than depression in another guise. At this point, however, the most prevalent thinking is that the etiology is multifactorial, involving the interplay of an initial infection that precipitates ongoing symptoms in an individual who has an underlying physiological vulnerability and is also psychologically primed. According to this theory, it may be possible for any infection to serve as the precipitating agent, the physiological vulnerability may not need to be the same in all individuals, and the relative importance of physiological and psychological factors may vary between individuals. At this time, the search for a single cause of CFS has waned, but the study of factors that may play a role continues. The factors that have been, and continue to be, under consideration are listed in the following sections.

### INFECTIOUS DISEASES

In the mid- and late 1980s, when CFS first began to be reported, the illness was considered to be due to mononucleosis; hence, the earliest names of chronic mononucleosis and chronic EBV infection. In fact, many individuals with mononucleosis report ongoing fatigue for up to one year after the onset of the illness (see Chapter 137, Infectious Mononucleosis and Mononucleosis-Like Syndromes), but an initial finding that patients with CFS have an abnormal and persistently elevated antibody (early antigen-EA) was found to be incorrect on a repeat study. At this point, it is believed that EBV may be one of many viral illnesses that can serve as the precipitant for CFS, and many people with CFS, especially adolescents, are able to point to a bout of mononucleosis that initiated the syndrome, but it is not currently considered that CFS represents an ongoing case of mononucleosis. Errors in interpreting the antibody responses to EBV infection, in which the IgG and EBNA (Epstein-Barr nuclear antigen) antibodies remain elevated lifelong, continue to lead some to a false impression of ongoing infection, but this has not been an accepted explanation for CFS for more than 15 years.

Other infections have also been considered. These have included coxsackie virus, studied extensively in England in the early 1990s; brucella, leading to consideration of a diagnosis of "chronic brucellosis"; an unnamed "spongy virus," found once on electron microscope studies, but never replicated; and lyme disease, whose chronic manifestations may overlap with those seen in CFS. As noted previously, it is now believed that any infection can play a role in the initiation of CFS and that it is unlikely any single agent will turn out to be responsible for the syndrome.

### PSYCHOLOGICAL FACTORS

It is clear that psychological symptoms play a prominent role in adults and adolescents with CFS, and, accordingly, the role of psychological factors in the etiology of the syndrome has been strongly considered. Studies in adults have shown that those with CFS have a much higher incidence of previously diagnosed depression than do controls, and many adolescents and adults exhibit depression during the course of their illness. Hence, the relationship between depression and CFS has been extensively studied. Several possibilities exist: (1) CFS may be an alternate manifestation of depression, as some believe; (2) an underlying tendency toward depression may be a necessary precursor for the development of CFS; (3) depression may be a reaction to the debilitation caused by CFS; or (4) depression may be one of the physiological consequences, as are concentration and memory difficulties, of CFS. Other psychological possibilities have also been considered, including separation anxiety and conversion reaction, and it has been shown that adolescents with CFS have greater psychological difficulties than those with other chronic illnesses, but the true role of psychological factors in the etiology of CFS remains unknown.

### IMMUNOLOGIC CONSIDERATIONS

There was an early suspicion that CFS was a manifestation of an immunologic disorder that caused the body to either under- or overreact to infection, thus leading to ongoing symptoms. One of the names used to describe the disorder in the late 1980s, "chronic fatigue immunodeficiency syndrome," reflected this thinking. Over time, studies have shown some minor immunologic abnormalities in patients with CFS, but these have never been replicated from study to study, they have never been correlated with the severity of illness, and opportunistic infections have not been found.[14] At this point, it is considered that immunologic abnormalities may play some role in the underlying mechanism of CFS, but neither an immunodeficiency nor an inflammatory reaction are believed to be components of the etiology. Of interest, however, has been a clinical finding that patients with CFS frequently have significant allergy and asthma histories, more so than the general population. It is possible that these atopic illnesses may serve as a marker for unknown immunologic abnormalities; it is also possible that these allergic conditions may predispose patients to sinus inflammation and infection, which can either exacerbate CFS or cause symptoms similar to those seen in CFS.

### ENDOCRINE ABNORMALITIES

Thyroid function has never been found to be abnormal in patients with CFS. Abnormalities in the hypothalamic-pituitary-adrenal axis have been more seriously considered, with one study of steroid administration showing minimal effects,[15] but endocrine disorders are not currently considered a major factor in the etiology of CFS. Computed tomography (CT) scans and magnetic resonance imaging (MRIs) of the brain have not been found to be abnormal in CFS.

### CARDIOVASCULAR ABNORMALITIES

Cardiovascular abnormalities in patients with CFS have been extensively evaluated for the past 10 years because initial studies showed abnormalities on tilt table testing in adults and adolescents with CFS.[16-29] Although there is some controversy about the accuracy of tilt table testing, and patients with CFS do not usually show abnormalities on standard orthostatic (lying-sitting-standing) blood pressure measurements, it is known clinically that patients with CFS do complain of orthostatic symptoms and often come from families with histories of low blood pressures. At this time, it is believed that cardiovascular instability may be one of the physiological abnormalities that make an individual vulnerable to CFS.

### SLEEP DISORDERS

In more recent years, the possibility that sleep abnormalities may underlie CFS has been increasingly considered. As more patients, including adolescents, with CFS are being evaluated by overnight sleep studies, abnormalities such as sleep apnea are being discovered in some patients. It may be that sleep abnormalities will be found to be one of the physiological abnormalities that can predispose an individual to the development of CFS, in which case sleep studies will become an important part of the evaluation of the patient who presents with CFS.

## EVALUATION

Obtaining a history from the patient and parents of an adolescent who presents for evaluation of presumed CFS can be a complicated process. The details of the story generally involve multiple symptoms, a varying course over a relatively long period of time, and frequent disagreements between patients and parents regarding the severity, sequence, and importance of the various details. The goals of the history are to determine whether the adolescent does or does not have CFS; whether there may be other medical and/or psychological conditions that are part of, causing, or an alternate to the CFS; and which aspects of the disorder in a particular individual are amenable to treatment. In most cases, it is the adolescent's primary care provider who sees the evolution of the syndrome in its early stages, usually in discrete visits over several weeks and months. Most patients then see several specialists to evaluate specific complaints (eg, headaches or joint/muscle aches) that may predominate. Eventually, a specialist may then be called on to put the whole picture together.

In so doing, it is necessary to obtain a comprehensive history, which may take longer than an hour to complete, to perform a physical examination and appropriate screening tests, and to proceed from there. The history should be obtained in 5 sections:

1. Chronological order—The patient and parents should be asked to present the history in the order that it occurred. Emphasis is placed on how the syndrome began; the course over time; and variations in symptoms by days, weeks, and seasons. Specific questions are asked about sleep patterns, including hours of sleep at night, naps during the day, difficulties falling asleep and/or awakening, degree of fatigue (using a 1–10 scale can be helpful), whether sleep is refreshing, and how exertion affects the fatigue.
2. Review of systems—Even though many symptoms will have been mentioned in the chronological history, a specific accounting of each organ system should be undertaken. Presence or absence of all symptoms should be noted, and details of all positive symptoms, especially variability over time, should be explored.
3. Health care providers seen and tests done—Reports have shown that patients with CFS often see multiple medical specialists and sometimes see alternative care providers as well.[6] It is important to determine who has been seen, tests that have been done, and what has been said. Families should be asked to bring as many test results as possible (ie, laboratory tests, imaging studies, consultation letters) to the initial visit.
4. Family history—In addition to general questions about family history, emphasis should be placed on whether anyone else in the family has had CFS or other difficult-to-understand syndromes; whether there is a history in the family of orthostatic symptoms, sleep difficulties (including snoring), or migraine headaches; and whether there are any psychiatric disorders in the family.
5. Psychological/psychosocial Issues—In this section of questioning, issues explored include school attendance; current and past psychological symptoms (especially depression, but also including anxiety disorders, separation issues, and psychosomatic problems); changes in activity levels; interactions with friends and family; and goals/expectations for the future.

Obtaining the history in the manner described allows for all details to be covered in a way that minimizes confusion and limits the amount of "jumping around" and debate that might otherwise occur among patients and parents. It also serves as a first step in modeling for families the ways to look at and understand the illness, making connections that will ultimately be important in management.

Physical examination of the adolescent with CFS is almost always normal. Findings of fever or weight loss should be a cause for concern. Despite orthostatic symptoms, pulse and blood pressure readings are generally normal. Mild pharyngeal redness and/or adenopathy may be seen, but even these are unusual without the presence of an intercurrent viral illness. Examination of the lungs, heart, and abdomen are usually normal; if hepatomegaly and/or splenomegaly are noted, these should prompt a search for an underlying cause. Any neurological findings should also be considered a cause for concern.

Laboratory tests performed in the evaluation of CFS in adolescents fall into 2 categories. Tests performed in almost all patients with CFS include a complete blood count and complete metabolic panel, thyroid function tests ($T_4$ and thyroid-stimulating hormone), and an erythrocyte sedimentation rate. These tests serve as a general screen for underlying or alternative diagnoses that may explain the patients' symptoms and are usually performed by the primary care physician early in the course of the illness. Additional laboratory tests may be performed if called for by specific symptoms, if there are abnormalities on initial screening, or if needed to help explain the initiation of the CFS. These can include tests in the realms of endocrinology (ie, cortisol levels), rheumatology (ie, antinuclear antibody and rheumatoid factor), or infectious diseases (eg, titers for EBV, lyme, cytomegalovirus, parvovirus, or toxoplasmosis). Caution must be used when interpreting the results of these tests because it is rare for either abnormal cortisol levels or elevated ANA or RF to be responsible for the symptoms, and it is common for EBV and lyme titers to be falsely considered positive.

Imaging studies that are often performed in patients with CFS include (1) MRI or CT of the brain in those with severe headaches; (2) x-rays or CT of the sinuses in those with recurrent sinus symptoms; (3) chest x-ray in those with pulmonary symptoms or a positive purified protein derivative; or (4) x-rays of joints in those with specific joint symptoms. As is the case for laboratory testing, it is rare to find abnormal imaging studies in adolescents with CFS.

Of late, 2 additional studies have been performed in patients with CFS. As mentioned previously, these are tilt table testing and sleep studies. In contrast to the laboratory testing and imaging studies listed previously, which are generally performed to look for alternative diagnoses that may be causing the fatigue or other symptoms, tilt table testing and sleep studies are performed to evaluate for abnormalities that may be causes of CFS symptoms that are amenable to therapy.

Whether and when to refer patients with CFS to a specialist is an important part of the evaluation of adolescents with CFS. Because patients with CFS usually have multiple symptoms, it is possible but not always reasonable to refer each patient to multiple specialists. In fact, studies have shown that most adolescent patients with CFS do tend to see several specialists. As a rule, referral to specialists depends on a combination of severity of the symptoms, anxiety of the family, and style of the clinician. Specialists most often seen by patients with CFS include neurologists and rheumatologists (to rule out underlying conditions such as migraine headaches or brain tumors and inflammatory diseases or fibromyalgia); ear, nose, and throat and infectious disease (ID) specialists (to evaluate the possibility of sinusitis and rule out infectious causes); and cardiology and sleep specialists (to consider the possibilities of tilt testing and sleep studies).

Psychological evaluation is also an important component of the evaluation. It is the rare adolescent who does not have psychological issues as a cause or effect (or both) of CFS. Therefore, evaluation for depression, anxiety, and more severe psychological symptoms should be undertaken; detailed evaluation of the effects of CFS on the adolescent's lifestyle should be determined; and reactions of family, friends, and school personnel should be explored. In some specialty settings, a social worker or psychologist may see each patient as part of the initial evaluation (either with the clinician or on a separate visit), whereas in other settings the psychological evaluation may be less formal and some patients are referred for psychiatric evaluations as needed.

## MANAGEMENT

There is no definitive treatment for CFS. Although multiple medications and approaches have been tried, and some have been reported in the lay press to be useful, controlled studies showing any approaches that have been at all beneficial are rare. The only 2 approaches to be shown to have any beneficial effects on randomized controlled studies are cognitive behavioral therapy and a graded exercise program, and these are only mildly beneficial for a relatively small subset of patients.[20] Therefore, those who treat CFS in adolescents are generally careful to let patients and parents know that they should not expect a "cure," but that there are management principles that can help alleviate the symptoms and effects of the illness. In the course of an initial visit with a patient with CFS, these principles are generally discussed as categorized here.

### EVALUATION AND EXPLANATION

It is important for parents and patients to have the diagnosis of CFS confirmed, to have underlying pathology excluded, and to have psychological status evaluated. This is followed by a detailed explanation of CFS, the meaning of the laboratory tests that have been performed, and the relationships of physical symptoms and psychological status. Most important, reassurance is given that the symptoms are real, that the adolescents is neither "crazy" nor "lazy," and that adolescents with CFS get better over time. Families and patients are encouraged to avoid doctor shopping, the use of unnecessary testing, and an ongoing search for unproven therapies. A goal of this part of treatment is to prevent secondary problems, family strain, and secondary gain. Families are advised to consider the CFS to be a temporary situation that will ultimately improve with time, and adolescents are advised on how to maximize their performance of adolescent activities, both academic and social, within the constraints of the illness. Patients and families are counseled to look at CFS as a temporary setback during adolescence that will not interfere with adult functioning if handled correctly. When all is said and done, because there is no cure for the illness, it is this approach to CFS that ultimately leads to the most positive course and outcome.

### MEDICATION MANAGEMENT

The use of medications in the treatment of adolescents with CFS includes those that are used for the management of specific symptoms of the illness, which have shown varying degrees of success, and those that have been proposed for management of the illness as a whole, which have generally not shown any success in changing the severity or course of the illness.[21]

Specific medications for symptom control include the anti-inflammatory medications that are used for control of the aches and pains (headaches, muscle aches, joint pains) that are often part of the illness. Medications such as ibuprofen and acetaminophen may be helpful for some patients, but there are others whose symptoms are refractory to use of these medications. In some cases, medications such as amitriptyline, which is sometimes used in pain syndromes, can be useful in CFS patients.

Various medications have been used for management of the sleep difficulties, especially nighttime insomnia, associated with CFS. Some clinicians prescribe sleep medications (eg, zolpidem) to adolescents with CFS, although psychoactive substances must be prescribed cautiously in adolescents. More recently, melatonin and modafinil have been used, but there are no studies evaluating their effects in adolescents, and recent reports about Stevens-Johnson syndrome have been raised regarding modafinil.

Antidepressant medications, especially in the selective serotonin reuptake inhibitor class, have been prescribed for many adults and adolescents with CFS. Some patients, especially those with more apparent depression, have shown benefit from this approach, but there are no studies demonstrating a definitive effect on the course or severity of CFS.

Several medications have been used in adolescents to try to alleviate the symptoms of orthostatic intolerance experienced by many patients with CFS. These include fludrocortisone (usually given along with an increase in salt and water intake), atenolol (a beta blocker), and midodrine (an alpha-agonist). Although many patients have reported anecdotally that they feel better symptomatically with these medications, neither controlled studies nor clinical experience have indicated any change in the course of the illness.[22,23] Some cardiologists have also used methylphenidate for its ability to elevate blood pressure; clinical experience with this approach has shown that patients report an improvement in their concentration, not unlike that seen in attention-deficit/hyperactivity disorder, but not other CFS symptoms.

Other medications that have been studied include cortisone and galantamine, an acetyl cholinesterase inhibitor.[15,24] Neither has shown positive effects. Experimental approaches to immunoregulation and infection control (including use of immunoglobulins, acyclovir, and Ampligen) have also been tried, also without effect. Many patients try various vitamins (including B and folate), herbs (such as valerian and ginkgo biloba), nutritional supplements (NADH and Co-Enzyme Q10), hormones (DHEA and 5HTP) and other complementary/alternative medications and approaches, sometimes with anecdotal improvement, but rarely any effects in controlled studies.[25,26]

In general, the approach to use of medications in adolescents with CFS involves a combination of family preference and physician style. Some families and/or clinicians prefer to try multiple medications and approaches, expecting to achieve symptom control at the least, and hoping to also affect the severity and course of the illness. Other families and/or clinicians prefer to use medications sparingly, concentrating instead on educational, lifestyle, psychological, and behavioral approaches to improvement of the illness.

## EDUCATIONAL AND LIFESTYLE ISSUES

How well the adolescent with CFS functions during the course of the illness ultimately depends on how the adolescent and his or her family manage the day-to-day educational and lifestyle issues that arise. Guiding families through these issues becomes one of the most important components of managing CFS.

The ability of adolescents with CFS to attend school varies greatly among adolescents. Some adolescents attend school regularly and participate in outside activities while complaining of fatigue; some attend school regularly but refrain from any out-of-school or extracurricular activities; some cannot attend school full-time but are able to participate in a partial program; others do not attend school at all but keep up with their work via a home tutoring program; and those with the most severe illness cannot even do that. Adolescents with CFS may switch back and forth between these levels as their illness gets better or worse, whereas some seem to be using the illness for secondary gain; it is seldom useful to try to distinguish between those who cannot do more and those who will not do more. School districts also vary greatly in their ability and/or willingness to make accommodations for adolescents with CFS. Working with school districts often becomes one of the roles served by the clinician treating adolescents with CFS.[27] Of interest, patients with CFS often find college to be easier than high school because of the flexibility allowed in schedules, and almost all adolescents do better during the summer when there are no schedules at all.

Although it would be logical to expect that nutrition would play a role in CFS, this does not appear to be the case. It is the rare adolescent with CFS who has either a change in appetite or weight, despite their multiple other symptoms, and there have been only rare hints of a possible relationship (as cause or effect) between CFS and eating disorders.[28] In contrast, exercise does seem to play a major role in the management of CFS. There are some thoughts that part of the exertional fatigue in patients with CFS may be due to a deconditioning effect, and there are studies showing that a graduated exercise program may be beneficial for some patients, including adolescents, with CFS. Clinical experience shows that although many adolescents are "too tired" to attempt an exercise program, those who are willing to give it a try may find benefit from such an approach.[29,30]

Similarly, some adolescents are able to participate in activities with friends, whereas others are not, and some adolescents try to continue their outside activities, sometimes at the expense of their school performance. In general, the approach to educational and lifestyle issues includes creating realistic expectations and schedules while also encouraging as much activity (in school, extracurricular activities, with friends) as possible. Experience has shown that adolescents who "overdo it" suffer the short-term consequences of increased fatigue for several days but do not have any lingering effects over the following weeks.

**PSYCHOLOGICAL AND BEHAVIORAL APPROACHES**

Management of issues such as depression and family stress may be handled by the primary care clinician, a social worker or psychologist, or occasionally a psychiatrist. Some patients may benefit from individual therapy and/or medication (as described previously). The network of self-help groups that are beneficial for many adults with CFS are discouraged for adolescents, in whom the goal is to not develop an identity as a patient with CFS but to get back to school and other activities as quickly as possible. In line with that, some studies have shown benefits to a cognitive behavioral approach in adolescents.[20] As with the benefits of a gradual exercise program, the only other approach to demonstrate a benefit in controlled studies, clinical experience shows it is only some adolescents who are willing and able to use this approach.

**FOLLOW-UP MANAGEMENT**

Establishing an ongoing plan of follow-up serves several important purposes. Changes in clinical status are monitored, with additional testing or referrals called for if a particular symptom develops or becomes more prominent. Ongoing guidance on educational and lifestyle issues is provided, including working with schools as needed. Psychological status and reactions are monitored, with guidance and referrals provided as required. It is also during follow-up that continued reassurance regarding the generally positive outcome that can be expected for adolescents with CFS can be reinforced.

## COURSE AND OUTCOME

As the name implies, patients with CFS have a long course to their illness. However, one hopeful finding is that adolescents with CFS most frequently have a shorter course than that reported in adults. Although most adults with CFS remain ill for many years, most adolescents improve over time and become well within a few years of the onset of the illness. As noted, this information is used as an important part of guiding adolescents with CFS in managing the illness.

The course of the illness follows a fairly similar pattern, with variability in timing and severity, for most adolescents with CFS. Adolescents are generally most ill during the first few months of illness, with some adolescents sleeping up to 18 hours per day during that time, and many complaining of other symptoms as well. During the next few months, there is usually some decrease in fatigue and lessening of symptoms, but the adolescent is still not well enough to resume usual activities. As the months proceed, most adolescents will have an "up-and-down" course, feeling better on some days than others, having some weeks that are better than others, and even having variability by month. During this time, most adolescents, but not all, will have a general improvement such that the number of better days or weeks increases, they feel better than previously on the bad days, and the interval between bad days or weeks increases. Several factors play a role in the variability: adolescents with CFS generally feel better when they have lighter schedules and worse when they attempt to be more active or when they have of an intercurrent illness. In general, when adolescents in the improvement phase get set back several days by increased exertion, or several weeks by illness, they get progressively less debilitated with each episode, and episodes become less prolonged over time.

Studies of outcomes for adolescents with CFS have reported that approximately three-fourths of adolescents return to their normal status after 2 to 3 years.[6,9,31] We found that about half are feeling much better by the year after their consultation, two-thirds are much better by the second year, three-fourths by the third year, and seven-eighths by the fourth year. It is the rare adolescent in our experience who remains ill for many years, the way most adults do. Ultimately, it is this information that should guide the clinician, family, and adolescent in the management of the illness and provide the hope that is needed to most successfully proceed through the ups and downs of CFS during adolescence.

## INTERNET RESOURCES

- The Centers for Disease Control and Prevention's Chronic Fatigue Web site "aims to provide evidence-based information concerning the illness, its manifestations, and treatment": www.cdc.gov/ncidod/diseases/cfs/index.htm
- The CFIDS (chronic fatigue immunodeficiency syndrome) Association of America "serves the CFIDS community through patient education, public awareness, public policy, and research": www.cfids.org

## REFERENCES

1. Fukuda K, Straus SE, Hickie I, et al. The chronic fatigue syndrome: a comprehensive approach to its definition and study. *Ann Intern Med.* 1994;121:953–959

2. Reyes M, Nisenbaum R, Hoaglin D, et al. Prevalence and incidence of chronic fatigue syndrome in Wichita, Kansas. *Arch Intern Med.* 2003;163:1530–1536

3. Jason L, Richman J, Rademaker A, et al. A community-based study of chronic fatigue syndrome. *Arch Intern Med.* 1999;159:2129–2137

4. Krilov LR, Fisher M. Chronic fatigue syndrome in youth: maybe not so chronic after all. *Contemp Pediatr.* 2002;19:61

5. Smith MS. Adolescent chronic fatigue syndrome. *Arch Pediatr Adolesc Med.* 2004;158:207–208

6. Krilov L, Fisher M, Friedman SB, Reitman D, Mandel FS. Course and outcome of chronic fatigue in children and adolescents. *Pediatrics.* 1998;102:360–366

7. Bell DS, Jordan K, Robinson M. Thirteen-year follow-up of children with chronic fatigue syndrome. *Pediatrics.* 2001;107:994–998

8. Smith MS, Mitchell J, Corey L, et al. Chronic fatigue in adolescents. *Pediatrics.* 1991;88:195–202

9. Feder HM, Dworkin PH, Orkin C. Outcome of 48 pediatric patients with chronic fatigue: a clinical experience. *Arch Fam Med.* 1994;3:1049–1055

10. Carter BD, Edwards JF, Kronenberger WG, et al. Case control study of chronic fatigue in pediatric patients. *Pediatrics.* 1995;95:179–186

11. Wolbeek M, van Doornen L, Kavelaars A, Heijnen C. Severe fatigue in adolescents: a common phenomenon? *Pediatrics.* 2006;117:e1078–e1086

12. Millman RP, Working Group on Sleepiness in Adolescents/Young Adults, American Academy of Pediatrics Committee on Adolescence. Excessive sleepiness in adolescents and young adults: causes, consequences, and treatment strategies. *Pediatrics.* 2005;115:1774–1186

13. Natelson BH. Chronic fatigue syndrome. *JAMA.* 2001; 285:2557–2559

14. Lyall M, Peakman M, Wessely S. A systematic review and critical evaluation of the immunology of chronic fatigue syndrome. *J Psychosom Res.* 2003;55(2):79–90

15. McKenzie R, O'Fallen A, Dale J, et al. Low-dose hydrocortisone for treatment of chronic fatigue syndrome. *JAMA.* 1998;280:1062–1066

16. Rowe PC, Bou-Holaigah I, Kan JS, et al. Is neurally mediated hypotension an unrecognized cause of chronic fatigue? *Lancet.* 1995;345:623–624

17. Rowe PC. Orthostatic intolerance and chronic fatigue syndrome: new light on an old problem. *J Pediatr.* 2002;140: 387–389

18. Stewart J, Gewtiz M, Weldon A, et al. Orthostatic intolerance in adolescent chronic fatigue syndrome. *Pediatrics.* 1999;103(1):116–121

19. Stewart J, Gewtiz M, Weldon A, et al. Patterns of orthostatic intolerance: the orthostatic tachycardia syndrome and adolescent chronic fatigue. *J Pediatr.* 1999;135(2 pt 1):218–225

20. Tovey D, ed. Chronic fatigue syndrome. In: *Clinical Evidence: Concise.* London: BMJ; 2005:358

21. Whiting P, Bagnall A-M, Sowden AJ, et al. Interventions for the treatment and management of chronic fatigue syndrome: a systematic review. *JAMA.* 2001;286:1360–1368

22. Peterson PK, Pheley A, Schroeppel J, et al. A preliminary placebo-controlled crossover trial of fludrocortisone for chronic fatigue syndrome. *Arch Intern Med.* 1998;158(8):908–914

23. Rowe PC, Calkins H, DeBusk K, et al. Fludrocortisone acetate to treat neurally mediated hypotension in chronic fatigue syndrome. *JAMA.* 2001;285:52–59

24. Blacker CVR, Greenwood DT, Wesnes KA, et al. Effect of galantamine hydrobromide in chronic fatigue syndrome: a randomized controlled trial. *JAMA.* 2004;292:1195–1204

25. Forsyth LM, Preuss HG, MacDowell AL, et al. Therapeutic effects of oral NADH on the symptoms of patients with chronic fatigue syndrome. *Ann Allergy Asthma Immunol.* 1999;82:185–191

26. Werbach M. Nutritional strategies for treating chronic fatigue syndrome. *Altern Med Rev.* 2000;5(2):93–108

27. Tillet A, Glass S, Reeve A, et al. Provision of health and education services in school children with chronic fatigue syndrome. *Ambul Child Health.* 2000;6(2):83–89

28. Fisher M, Krilov L, Ovadia M. Chronic fatigue syndrome and eating disorders: concurrence or coincidence? *Int J Adolesc Med Health.* 2002;14:307–316

29. Viner R, Gregorowski A, Wine C, et al. Outpatient rehabilitation treatment of chronic fatigue syndrome. *Arch Dis Child.* 2004;89:615–619

30. Powell P, Bentall RP, Nye FJ, et al. Randomized controlled trial of patient education to encourage graded exercise in chronic fatigue syndrome. *BMJ.* 2001;322:387

31. Gill AC, Dosen A, Ziegler JB. Chronic fatigue syndrome in adolescents: a follow-up study. *Arch Pediatr Adolesc Med.* 2004;158(3):225–229

SECTION 9

# Central Nervous System

## CHAPTER 125

# Central Nervous System Infections

TINA Q. TAN, MD

Meningitis is an important and serious infection that may occur at any age. It is defined as an inflammation of the leptomeninges (dura, arachnoid, and pia mater) surrounding the brain and spinal cord. It is caused by a number of etiologic agents (both infectious and noninfectious) and identified by an increased number of white blood cells (WBCs) in cerebrospinal fluid (CSF). Bacterial meningitis is caused by bacterial organisms; aseptic meningitis lacks evidence of a bacterial organism detectable in the CSF by routine laboratory techniques (eg, gram stain, culture) and most commonly is attributed to a viral etiology.

## BACTERIAL MENINGITIS

### EPIDEMIOLOGY AND ETIOLOGIC AGENTS

The microbiologic causes of meningitis vary depending on the age of the patient.[1] In all age groups, including adolescents, boys are affected more frequently than girls. Bacterial meningitis has a peak incidence during the late fall and winter months. The most common bacterial organisms that cause meningitis in the adolescent age group are *Neisseria meningitidis* and *Streptococcus pneumoniae*. *Mycoplasma pneumoniae* can also be a cause of severe meningitis and meningoencephalitis in this age group but is not commonly seen.

In the adolescent population, the overall incidence of meningitis due to *S pneumoniae* is 0.5/100,000[2] and for *N meningitidis* the incidence is 1.5 to 2.2/100,000.[3]

Patients with certain underlying conditions are predisposed to the development of bacterial meningitis. Deficiencies in the terminal components of complement lead to an increased risk for meningococcemia and meningococcal meningitis. Patients with CSF leaks, basilar skull fractures, cribriform plate fractures, cochlear implants, anatomic or functional asplenia, hemoglobinopathies, malignancy, and human immunodeficiency virus (HIV) infection have an increased risk for pneumococcal meningitis and other invasive pneumococcal diseases. *Listeria* meningitis may be seen in those with cellular immune defects, whereas nontypeable *Haemophilus influenzae* meningitis has been associated with immunoglobulin deficiencies. Persons with a dermal sinus or abnormality of the neuroenteric canal, or recent penetrating head trauma, neurosurgery, or ventriculoperitoneal shunt placement are at increased risk for development of meningitis caused by streptococci, staphylococcal species, and gram-negative enteric bacilli, especially *Klebsiella* species, *Escherichia coli*, and *Pseudomonas aeruginosa*. In the immunocompromised host with meningitis, in addition to the usual pathogens, consideration must also be given to more unusual pathogens, such as *Cryptococcus, Toxoplasma*, fungi, tuberculosis, and HIV as the cause of the meningitis.

The most common bacterial meningeal pathogens share a similar multistep route of pathogenesis. The first step involves attachment of the organism to the nasopharyngeal mucosa, leading to colonization and infection of the upper respiratory tract. These pathogens all have polysaccharide capsules that contribute to their invasiveness by aiding them in evading local host defenses. This allows the organism to invade between or through the respiratory epithelial cells into the subepithelial tissues where they can enter the bloodstream, the second step in the pathogenesis. The presence of a preceding viral upper respiratory infection seems to further to aid this process. The third step involves the replication of the organism in the bloodstream, establishing bacteremia that leads to the seeding of the meninges through the cerebral capillaries and the choroid plexus. In this protected environment, the organism can quickly multiply and spread throughout the CSF. Bacterial products (eg, endotoxins, peptidoglycans, teichoic acid) stimulate the release of proinflammatory cytokines (eg, tumor necrosis factor-α, interleukin-1) from endothelial cells and macrophages, leading to inflammation of the meninges and brain. Each of these cytokines in turn can stimulate the production of other inflammatory mediators (eg, interleukin-6, platelet-activating factor, interferons, other interleukins), activate and attract leukocytes, and activate the coagulation cascade. The end result is increased permeability of the blood-brain barrier, thrombosis of vessels and decreased cerebral blood flow, and, finally, cerebral edema with increased intracranial pressure. The administration of antibiotics can further augment the inflammatory response and elevate intracranial pressure because of rapid bacterial lysis resulting in the release of bacterial cell wall and membrane fragments.[4]

## CLINICAL FINDINGS

Patients with meningitis may experience a wide range of presenting signs and symptoms. Presentation may have a gradual onset of symptoms, beginning as nonspecific upper respiratory manifestations that progress over a period of several days until the disease becomes obvious. Alternatively, the course may be fulminant and result in death less than 24 hours after the onset of symptoms; the risk for this type of presentation is increased in adolescents with meningococcal disease. Despite appropriate antibiotic therapy and intensive medical care, a significant level of morbidity and mortality remains.

Fever and severe headache may be the initial presenting symptoms of meningitis in the adolescent. As the disease progresses, malaise and anorexia increase with respiratory distress and photophobia often developing. As the meningeal inflammation increases, back pain, stiff neck, hearing loss, difficulty with balance, and Kernig (when patient lies on the back and the thigh is flexed to a right angle with the axis of the torso, extension of the leg is not possible) or Brudzinski (when neck is passively flexed, flexion of the legs occurs) signs may be present; at the time of initial evaluation, 90% of adolescents will have a stiff neck. As intracranial pressure begins to increase, nausea and vomiting develop. The increase in intracranial pressure ultimately may produce papilledema, confusion, and mental status changes. Seizures can occur at any time during the disease, but focal seizures or cranial nerve findings suggest central nervous system (CNS) injury. In approximately 12% of patients with bacterial meningitis, seizures occur before hospital admission, with another 26% having seizures within the first 48 hours after hospital admission. Eventually, lethargy, sommolence, and shock may ensue. Petechiae, purpura, and end-organ dysfunction may develop; these findings are seen in more than 50% of adults with meningitis.[1,5]

## DIAGNOSIS AND TREATMENT

Early and accurate diagnosis of bacterial meningitis is a major factor in the successful treatment of the infection. Prompt initiation of therapy with intravenous fluids and antibiotics can minimize the severity of the illness, the development of complications, and the emergence of sequelae. If there is suspicion of bacterial meningitis in an adolescent with the appropriate signs and symptoms, lumbar puncture (LP) must be performed immediately to obtain CSF for analysis and culture. Every effort should be made to perform an LP prior to the administration of antibiotic therapy; however, if there is a delay in LP (eg, difficult LP access, computed tomography (CT) scan, or unstable patient), antibiotic administration should ***not*** be delayed until the LP is completed. The LP should be performed as soon as possible thereafter, even though the culture results will be altered.

The typical CSF WBC count in bacterial meningitis is more than 1,000 cells/mm$^3$ (range several hundred to tens of thousands); however, WBCs may be few to none in the early stages of infection. Most of the WBCs are polymorphonuclear leukocytes (PMNs), with the presence of immature PMNs being highly suggestive of a bacterial process. In addition, the CSF glucose concentration usually is depressed to <30 mg/dL or less than two-thirds of the concurrent serum glucose, whereas the protein concentration usually is elevated (>100 mg/dL). Gram stain of the CSF specimen may be positive in 80% to 90% of patients with untreated meningitis. Detection of polysaccharide antigen in the CSF by latex agglutination may be used to aid in the determination of the etiology of meningitis (*N meningitidis, S pneumoniae*), especially in patients who have abnormal CSF parameters with a negative gram stain and culture. Antigen detection testing also may be helpful in the setting of partially treated bacterial meningitis where the organisms are no longer viable but can be detected by antigen methods. However, a positive CSF culture still remains the gold standard in confirming the diagnosis.

For adolescents with possible or proven bacterial meningitis, empiric therapy is guided by the knowledge of the most likely pathogens and their current antimicrobial susceptibilities. Empiric therapy for bacterial meningitis consists of a parenteral third-generation cephalosporin, either cefotaxime (300 mg/kg/day divided every 6 hours; maximum daily dose 12 grams) or ceftriaxone (100 mg/kg/day divided every 12 hours; maximum daily dose 4 grams), plus vancomycin (60 mg/kg/day divided every 6 hours). The initial empiric regimen provides coverage for antibiotic-resistant organisms, especially penicillin-resistant *S pneumoniae*. Once an organism has been identified and the antimicrobial susceptibilities are known, the antimicrobial regimen can be tailored.

For susceptible organisms, aqueous penicillin G can be used to complete therapy for meningococcal and pneumococcal meningitis. For pneumococcal isolates that are penicillin resistant but susceptible to the extended-spectrum third-generation cephalosporins, vancomycin can be discontinued and these agents used to complete therapy. If a patient is found to have a pneumococcal isolate that is highly resistant to penicillin and extended-spectrum third-generation cephalosporins, vancomycin and a third-generation cephalosporin are continued and rifampin should be added. However, if the patient does not clinically improve, imipenem or meropenem may be used as alternative agents. The duration of antibiotic therapy varies by the organism isolated and the patient's clinical response. Meningitis due to *S pneumoniae* is treated for 10 to 14 days and meningitis due to *N meningitidis* for 5 to 7 days.[5,6]

The use of dexamethasone adjunctive therapy in the treatment of meningitis remains controversial. Studies have shown that for patients with meningitis caused by *H influenzae* type b (Hib), adjunctive therapy with dexamethasone significantly improvesd outcomes, especially neurosensory hearing loss. However, with the virtual disappearance of meningitis caused by Hib in the United States, the value of dexamethasone adjunctive therapy with meningitis caused by *S pneumoniae* remains unclear. Several studies have shown that its use in pneumococcal meningitis may negatively influence clinical outcome. It also may reduce the penetration of vancomycin into the CSF, resulting in significantly decreased levels. In contrast, a study of adults with bacterial meningitis demonstrated that early treatment with dexamethasone was associated with a reduction in mortality, although there was no difference in morbidity noted.[7] There are no data to support its use in meningococcal meningitis, viral meningitis, or other infectious causes of aseptic meningitis. If dexamethasone is used, all potential benefits and possible risks need to be carefully considered. For it to have any potential benefit, it must be given ***before or simultaneously with*** initial antibiotic therapy.[5,6]

### COMPLICATIONS

The morbidity and mortality associated with meningitis is considerable, even with early diagnosis and appropriate therapeutic intervention. The most common complications include subdural effusions, subdural empyemas, and seizures.[5] Typically they are associated with persistent fever and may cause increased intracranial pressure due to a mass effect. Drainage usually is not necessary unless the patient has neurologic symptoms due to this mass effect. In that setting, drainage is needed to relieve pressure. Subdural empyema occurs in approximately 1% of patients with bacterial meningitis and clinically presents with persistent fever, irritability, and other meningeal signs. This complication requires drainage and prolonged antibiotic therapy. Persistent seizures are a problem that usually requires long-term antiepileptic therapy and follow-up evaluations.

Neurologic sequelae have been detected in 25% to 56% of survivors, and death can be expected in 5% to 15% of cases. The most common neurologic sequela is neurosensory hearing loss. This is seen in approximately 30% of patients after pneumococcal meningitis and in up to 10% of patients after meningitis due to *N meningitidis*. Varying degrees of impairment of motor functions and intellectual processes may occur. In more severe cases, hydrocephalus, infarction of brain or spinal cord, or neurologic devastation may result.[5]

### PREVENTION

There are vaccines available that protect against Hib, some serogroups of *N meningitidis*, and many types of *S pneumoniae*. The Advisory Committee on Immunization Practices recommends routine vaccination of all persons 11 to 18 years of age with 1 dose of meningococcal conjugate vaccine.

## VIRAL MENINGITIS

### EPIDEMIOLOGY AND ETIOLOGIC AGENTS

Viral or aseptic meningitis is an inflammation of the leptomeninges caused by infection with multiple different viruses. Viral meningitis is the most common form of meningitis in adolescents. It occurs most frequently during the summer and fall seasons, but may be seen year round. In all age groups, disease occurs more commonly in males than in females, with a ratio of 1.5:1 or greater.[8] Infection rates are also higher among persons of lower socioeconomic status and in areas of crowding.[9] The most common etiologic agents of viral meningitis include: the enteroviruses, which account for 85% of cases, and include disease caused by the polioviruses, coxsackieviruses, echoviruses, and nonpolio enteroviruses; the herpesviruses (eg, herpes simplex virus-2 [HSV-2], adenoviruses, and *human herpesvirus* 6 [HHV-6]); and the arboviruses (eg, West Nile, St Louis, Eastern equine, Western equine, California-LaCrosse strain).[9,10] Other, less common causes of viral meningitis in this age group include Epstein-Barr virus, lymphocytic choriomeningitis virus, rabies virus, and influenza A and B viruses. The most common mode of transmission is from person to person through the fecal–oral route (eg, enteroviruses) or from mosquitoes (eg, West Nile, St Louis) and ticks (eg, Colorado tick fever). Retrograde neuronal spread is common in cases of HSV and rabies.[9] Hematogenous spread of the virus occurs after replication at the site of entry or in regional lymph nodes, with the virus reaching the CNS after passive transport across the blood–brain barrier. The severity of the disease depends on viral virulence, viral replication rate, and extent of brain involvement.

### CLINICAL FINDINGS

The clinical manifestations of viral meningitis are often initially nonspecific and do not correspond to a particular agent. Onset of symptoms is usually sudden and acute but may be preceded by a nonspecific acute febrile illness of several days duration. The most common clinical findings in the adolescent age group include: headache (92%), fever (76%), nuchal rigidity (67%), photophobia, nausea, vomiting, pharyngitis, and general malaise. Upper respiratory tract symptoms and the development of a rash may or may not be present.[9,11]

### DIAGNOSIS AND TREATMENT

Obtaining a careful history is an important step in making the diagnosis and identifying a potential etiologic agent in patients with viral meningitis. Evaluation for exposure to ill contacts, mosquitos, ticks, animals and history of recent travel are important pieces of information to obtain. An LP should be performed so that CSF can be examined. Usually the CSF is colorless or mildly turbid. The CSF WBC count usually is <500 cells/mm$^2$ (but may be as high as several thousand), with most of the cells being lymphocytes or mononuclear cells; early in the illness, a PMN predominance may be present. The CSF glucose concentration is usually normal and the protein concentration is normal or slightly elevated. The gram stain and latex agglutination tests are negative.

Three methods are available to aid in the detection of the etiologic agents that cause viral meningitis: viral culture, serology, and nucleic acid amplification. CSF viral cultures are infrequently positive (<25%), whereas nasopharyngeal and rectal viral cultures are more often positive and can help in reaching a specific diagnosis. However, some of the agents that cause viral meningitis cannot be cultured. So even though tissue culture has been the mainstay of diagnosis, it has limitations as a diagnostic modality with a sensitivity of only 65% to 75% in the detection of enteroviruses. Also, because on average it takes 3 to 8 days for viruses to grow in tissue culture, it may not be cost-effective or efficient enough to have an impact on patient care.[12] Serologic testing for the etiologic agents of viral meningitis is of limited value clinically because it usually requires acute and convalescent samples; serology is really useful only in the event of an outbreak. For detection of the arboviruses, paired serology may be an effective retrospective diagnostic method. However, the diagnosis of the arboviruses as a cause of viral meninigitis is usually made by the performance of an immunoglobulin M (IgM) antibody capture enzyme-linked immunosorbent assay (ELISA) on CSF and serum specimens.[13] Polymerase chain reaction (PCR) is the most promising alternative to viral culture for diagnosis of viral meningitis.[14] It is available for the detection of various viruses in the CSF, including HSV and the enteroviruses, and has several features that make it ideal as a diagnostic modality: it requires small amounts of clinical material; it is rapid, sensitive, and specific; and it is available in most areas of the United States.

For most viral meningitis cases, only supportive therapy (eg, fluids, pain medications) is needed. Patients with seizures should receive anticonvulant medication. Currently there are no antiviral agents available for treatment of this condition.

### COMPLICATIONS

Complications of viral meningitis occur rarely and have little long-term sequelae. The most commonly reported complications include: seizures, severe lethargy, muscle weakness, increased intracranial pressure, and coma. The risk of developing bacterial meningitis when someone has viral meningitis is extremely small.

## VIRAL ENCEPHALITIS

### EPIDEMIOLOGY AND ETIOLOGIC AGENTS

Encephalitis is defined as an inflammation of the cerebral cortex and meningoencephalitis is an inflammation of the cerebral cortex accompanied by the presence of meningitis. Acute viral encephalitis refers to the direct infection of neural cells by a variety of viral agents that manifests pathologically as perivascular inflammation, neuronal destruction, neuronophagia, and tissue necrosis. The reported incidence of acute encephalitis

**Table 125-1**

**Common Viruses That Cause Acute Viral Encephalitis**

| *Virus* | *Comments on encephalitis* |
|---|---|
| Arboviruses | 1% to 50% of cases may be fatal |
| Cytomegalovirus | May cause encephalitis with infectious mononucleosis |
| Epstein-Barr virus | May cause encephalitis with infectious mononucleosis |
| Enteroviruses | May cause fatal encephalitis in neonates; most common cause of viral encephalitis |
| Herpes simplex viruses | More than 75% of cases are fatal if untreated |
| HIV | May cause acute encephalitis at time of primary infection |
| Human herpesvirus 6 | Causes mild encephalitis |
| Lymphocytic choriomeningitis viruses | Causes mild encephalitis |
| Mumps virus | Causes mild encephalitis |
| Rabies virus | More than 99% of cases are fatal |

is between 3.5 and 7.4 cases per 100,000 patient-years. The Centers for Disease Control and Prevention suggest that approximately 20,000 cases of encephalitis occur in the United States each year, with most being mild.[15-17] More than 100 different agents have been associated with encephalitis, with the most important life-threatening causes are HSV and arthropod-borne viruses (arboviruses, eg, West Nile, St Louis, California, Eastern equine, etc). Other viruses that more commonly cause encephalitis include: the enteroviruses, adenoviruses, HHV-6, mumps virus, lymphocytic choriomeningitis virus, and rabies virus.[17] Shown in Table 125-1 are the more common viruses that cause acute viral encephalitis.

Encephalitis due to HSV can occur year round and is the most common cause of severe sporadic fatal encephalitis accounting for between 10% and 20% of cases of viral encephalitis in the United States. In adolescents, HSV encephalitis is caused primarily by HSV type 1 and has a biphasic age predilection with the first peak occurring in patients between 5 and 30 years of age and the second peak in those more than 50 years of age. In children and adolescents, HSV encephalitis is different from neonatal disease in that it usually has an acute onset and a fulminant course. This can lead rapidly to coma and death, which may occur in up to 75% of untreated patients.

In the United States, arboviral infections occur most commonly during the summer months and are the cause of sporadic and epidemic CNS viral infections. There are 5 arboviruses that account for most of the cases in the United States: West Nile virus, California encephalitis (LaCrosse strain), St. Louis encephalitis, Western equine encephalitis, and Eastern equine encephalitis.[18]

West Nile virus infection has a peak incidence from July through September and an incubation period ranging from 2 days to 2 weeks. Most persons infected have an asymptomatic illness, with only 1 in 5 persons developing West Nile fever and 1 in 150 developing more severe neurologic disease, which includes meningitis, encephalitis, or a polio-like illness. The disease is recognized much less frequently in children and adolescents, in part because it commonly presents as an aseptic meningitis or encephalitis that is clinically indistinguishable from other causes of aseptic meningitis and encephalitis. It has been seen in children as young as one year of age, and older teenagers have a course similar to that seen in adults.[19] Mortality rate is around 12%.

Disease caused by the California encephalitis viruses (LaCrosse strain) occurs most commonly in the Midwestern states. Children, adolescents, and adults are infected, but 90% of clinical disease occurs in children and adolescents 15 years of age or younger. St Louis encephalitis virus causes clinical disease in both children and adults with the amount of disease varying greatly from year to year. Disease caused by Western equine encephalitis occurs in adults and children and is seen in areas west of the Mississippi River, whereas Eastern equine encephalitis virus is restricted largely to the Atlantic and gulf coasts. This virus is associated with the most severe disease. It has a mortality rate of more than 50%, with 70% of pediatric survivors suffering severe sequelae.[18]

### CLINICAL FINDINGS

The hallmark of viral encephalitis is the acute onset of a febrile illness. The clinical findings common to most viral encephalitides include: fever, headache, altered mental status or level of consciousness, disorientation, and behavioral and speech disturbances. Focal neurologic signs may be present but more commonly are diffuse and include findings such as hemiparesis or seizures. The clinical findings reflect disease progression and the cells of the CNS that are infected.

Other hallmark symptoms that may be seen with West Nile virus, meningitis, and encephalitis are severe muscle weakness, abdominal pain, nausea, vomiting, diarrhea, and cranial nerve abnormalities. Ten percent of patients will develop complete flaccid paralysis of one or more body parts, which is indicative of West Nile poliomyelitis.[19]

For HSV encephalitis, in addition to the symptoms mentioned previously, because of the predisposition for HSV to have a tropism for the temporal lobes, other clinical findings may include: aphasia, anosmia, superior quadrant visual field defects, paresthesias, temporal lobe seizures, personality changes (which may dominate the clinical presentation for up to one week before other signs evolve), hemiparesis, and focal neurologic findings.[16,18]

### DIAGNOSIS AND TREATMENT

In patients with viral encephalitis, evaluation of CSF parameters usually demonstrates an increase in pressure (if measured) and several hundred WBCs (most of which are mononuclear cells); however, early in the illness, up to 20% of CSF specimens may be acellular or the CSF may have a PMN leukocyte predominance. The protein concentration in the CSF is elevated, but the glucose concentration is usually normal or only slightly lowered. Red blood cells (RBCs) may be present; however, an increased number is not clearly indicative of herpetic encephalitis (increased RBCs seen in only about 50% of patients), nor does the absence of RBCs exclude it. Neurodiagnostic tests, including electroencephalography (EEG), CT, and magnetic resonance imaging (MRI), all can provide useful information in the evaluation of patients with viral encephalitis.

EEG usually shows diffuse slowing of the brain waves; however, in patients with HSV encephalitis, the classic EEG finding is the presence of periodic lateralized epileptiform discharges, which are periodic high-voltage spike waves emanating from the temporal region coupled with slow-wave complexes at 2- to 3-second intervals. In patients with HSV disease, CT abnormalities appear later in the disease and the classic finding is a low-density abnormality in one or both temporal lobes. MRI demonstrates lesions earlier and also shows abnormalities in the temporal lobe region.

The diagnostic method of choice for HSV, CMV, HHV-6, and enterovirus infections is PCR analysis of the CSF. The specificity of PCR is 99%, and the sensitivity is 90% to 98%. Rapid diagnosis of arbovirus encephalitis is done by antibody-capture ELISA testing for virus-specific IgM on CSF (95% sensitivity) and serum (90% sensitivity). For most of the agents, antibody is usually present at the time of medical presentation. Viral cultures usually are of low yield and, in general, are not recommended unless for epidemiologic purposes. Brain biopsy may also be helpful in diagnosis (eg, HSV, rabies), however, it is seldom performed.

Treatment of viral encephalitis (including that caused by arboviruses) is primarily supportive with fluid restriction, anticonvulsant administration if seizures occur, and artificial ventilation for respiratory failure. Corticosteroids are not generally indicated. Most patients empirically are started on a course of high-dose IV acyclovir (30 mg/kg/day divided every 8 hours) until the results of various tests for HSV (eg, PCR, IgM, EEG, and/or MRI) are found to be negative. If a patient is found to have HSV encephalitis, IV acyclovir therapy is continued for a 21-day course. For encephalitis caused by West Nile virus, alpha interferon and IV ribavirin have been shown to have some activity against this virus in vitro and have been used empirically in some patients, but these drugs have not been studied in a controlled trial.

### COMPLICATIONS

Two percent to 5% of patients with viral encephalitis die from their disease, and patients who present with lethargy, loss of consciousness, or disorientation have a poor prognosis. Prognosis also depends on the age of the patient and the etiologic agent causing the encephalitis (eg, HSV, rabies). Severe neurologic sequelae include mental retardation, spasticity, paralysis, and seizures. For patients who survive herpetic encephalitis, severe, permanent, debilitating sequelae may occur and include major motor and sensory deficits, aphasia, and an amnestic syndrome.

For patients with encephalitis caused by West Nile virus, the overall morbidity is substantial, with 50% of those infected not returning to baseline functioning by hospital discharge and two-thirds not being ambulatory. Persistent headaches, memory loss, and focal neurologic deficits may persist for a long time, with more than 50% of those infected continuing to have symptoms 1 year after the illness.

## MISCELLANEOUS AGENTS OF MENINGITIS

### *M TUBERCULOSIS* MENINGITIS

The incidence of tuberculosis has increased in recent years in the United States, especially in the HIV-infected population, blacks, and immigrants from countries where tuberculosis is endemic. This increase has also resulted in an increase in the number of cases of tuberculous meningitis. About 0.5% of children, and a lower percentage of adolescents with active, systemic *M tuberculosis* disease will develop tuberculous meningitis as a complication of untreated primary tuberculosis. The meningitis develops as a result of rupture of a caseous lesion in the cerebral cortex or meninges into the subarachnoid space.

### Clinical Signs and Symptoms

The onset of symptoms may be rapid or gradual. The most common symptoms include: fever, headache, irritability, and increased sleepiness, which may progress to meningeal signs, seizures, hypertonia, vomiting, cranial nerve palsies (especially of cranial nerves III, VI, VII), coma, hemi- or paraplegia, and ultimately death.[20,21]

### Diagnosis and Treatment

Tuberculin skin test results are initially negative in up to 40% of cases but will convert on repeat testing, and miliary tuberculosis may be present on physical examination and on chest radiograph up to 50% of the time. Typical CSF leukocyte counts range from 10 to 500 cells/μL; PMN cells may be the major cell type early on, but a lymphocytic pleocytosis is most common. The CSF glucose level varies but is usually depressed (≤30 mg/dL), and protein concentrations are usually elevated. The diagnosis is confirmed by smear, biopsy, and cultures obtained from extraneural sites and CSF. Acid fast bacilli are seen on CSF smear of patients with tuberculous meningitis in about 10% to 22% of cases; however, yield may be increased by obtaining a large volume of CSF (5 ml-10 ml), which is centrifuged and the sediment carefully examined. Cerebrospinal fluid cultures are positive in 30% to 75% of cases; cultures of gastric aspirates or sputum will increase the diagnostic yield.[20,21] Rapid antigen and antibody detection tests are also available to aid in the diagnosis. The detection of tuberculostearic acid in CSF is both specific and sensitive for *M tuberculosis*.[22,23] Polymerase chain reaction to detect mycobacterial DNA in CSF is also available; the specificity is very high at 95% to 100%; however, sensitivity varies widely ranging from 27% to 85%.[24,25] Adenosine deaminase CSF levels have been found to be elevated in patients with tuberculosis meningitis but not in viral or bacterial meningitis.[26]

Treatment consists of a regimen of 4 antituberculous drugs: isoniazid, rifampin, pyrazinamide, and ethambutol for the first 2 months of therapy and the adjunctive use of corticosteroids (1-2 mg/kg/day of prednisone [maximum 60 mg/day]) or its equivalent, which are tapered over a 6- to 8-week period. After 2 months, therapy is tailored to isoniazid and rifampin to complete a total of 12 months of therapy.[27]

### Complications

Prognosis is influenced by a number of factors including age, duration of symptoms, and neurologic deficits. Neurologic sequelae include focal neurologic deficits, hydrocephalus, paraplegia, or hemiplegia. Mortality is greatest in patients in whom illness has been present for more than 2 months (80%) and in those younger than one year or older than 50 years of age.

## TRANSMISSIBLE SPONGIFORM ENCEPHALOPATHY

Prion disease, or transmissible spongiform encephalopathy, is caused by infectious agents whose nature has not been delineated. There are 3 main hypotheses about the nature of these infectious agents. The first is that the diseases are caused by a protein known as PrP that replicates second is that the agent is a small virus;[29] and the third is that the agent is a virion that is a small informational molecule (probably a nucleic acid) associated with a host protein (possibly PrP).[30] The newest form of the disease is a variant, Creutzfeldt-Jakob disease, which was first reported in 1995. This disease is thought to be caused by an agent that is similar to the agent that causes bovine spongiform encephalopathy. This disease differs from sporadic Creutzfeldt-Jakob disease in that it occurs in young, healthy patients, median age 29 years (range 16-41 years), and its presenting features and EEG pattern are different. Also the time between the onset of symptoms and death ranges from 7.5 to 22.4 months (median 12 months), which is longer than in most patients with spontaneous Creutzfeldt-Jakob disease.[31] An identifiable risk factor for patients with this disease has not been identified, although acquisition of this disease has been possibly linked to the consumption of tissues from cows with bovine spongiform encephalopathy. Minimal incubation period is probably somewhere between 5 and 10 years.[31]

### Clinical Symptoms, Diagnosis, and Treatment

The presenting features of the new variant Creutzfeldt-Jakob disease are often behavioral changes, ataxia, and peripheral sensory disturbances followed by progressive dementia, rather than changes in mentation as seen in spontaneous Creutzfeldt-Jakob disease. Brain biopsy is the method of choice for diagnosis. The neuropathological findings demonstrate extensive plaques resembling those seen in kuru, which are different from the spongiform changes, astrocytosis, and neuronal loss seen in spontaneous Creutzfeldt-Jakob. Therapy is supportive as there is no known treatment.[31]

### Complications

This disease is uniformly fatal, with the time between the onset of symptoms and death, as noted, ranging from 7.5 to 22.4 months (median 12 months).[31]

**AMEBIC DISEASE**

Small free-living amebae of the genera *Naegleria*, *Acanthamoeba*, and *Balamuthia* cause severe CNS infections in humans characterized by few distinguishing symptoms and an almost uniformly poor prognosis with few reports of survival. Free-living amebae cause primary amebic meningoencephalitis and granulomatous amebic meningoencephalitis.[32] Primary amebic meningoencephalitis caused by *Naegleria fowleri* is an acute fulminant illness affecting healthy children and young adults, which usually results in death within a week of presentation. In contrast, granulomatous amebic encephalitis caused by *Acanthamoeba* spp. or *Balamuthia mandrillaris* is an insidious, subacute, and protracted illness affecting primarily, but not exclusively, immunocompromised or debilitated patients, which leads to death in weeks to months. Most cases occur during the summer months. Boys are affected more commonly than girls, with a ratio of 12:1. Cases are typically associated with a history of swimming, diving, or playing in bodies of warm fresh water, man-made lakes, hot springs, and streams. The incubation period in natural infection is several months after exposure.[33]

**Clinical Symptoms, Diagnosis, and Treatment**

Patients with primary amebic meningoencephalitis caused by *N fowleri* present with symptoms similar to the clinical picture of a fulminant bacterial meningitis. Commonly there is the abrupt onset of severe headache, fever, nausea and vomiting, malaise, rhinitis, meningeal signs, and mental status changes. A history of abnormalities in taste and smell have also been reported. There is rapid progression from the onset of fever to the development of meningoencephalitis. The development of seizures is common and coma is present at or soon after hospital admission.[33]

For patients with granulomatous amebic meningoencephalitis cuased by *Acanthamoeba* spp and *B mandrillaris*, the clinical course is usually prolonged and the clinical picture resembles that of a bacterial brain abscess or brain tumor. Patients develop chronic severe headache, intermittent low-grade fever, nausea, vomiting, symptoms of increased intracranial pressure, and altered mental status. Depending on the area of the brain that is affected, patients may also have focal neurologic signs, hemiparesis, drowsiness, aphasia, personality changes, and seizures. The progression from focal neurologic signs to diffuse meningoencephalitis occurs over a period of weeks to months.[34]

CSF parameters in patients with primary amebic meningoencephalitis are abnormal but nonspecific with increased pressure, elevated protein, and low to normal glucose concentrations and a modest PMN pleocytosis. Gram stain and cultures are negative. In patients with granulomatous amebic meningoencephalitis, CSF parameters are also nonspecific with elevated protein and low glucose concentrations and a mononuclear pleocytosis. Gram stain and cultures are also negative.

If the diagnosis of primary amebic meningoencephalitis caused by *Naegleria* spp is suspected, a wet mount of fresh CSF should be examined for the presence of motile amebae. *Naegleria, Acanthamoeba* spp, and *Balamuthia* may all be seen in fixed sections of brain tissue biopsy or autopsy specimens. Immunofluorescent stains using monoclonal and polyclonal anti-*Acanthamoeba* and *Balamuthia* antibodies, immunoperoxidase staining, and electron microscopy of tissue sections have all been used to confirm the diagnosis. *Naegleria*, *Acanthamoeba* spp, and *Balamuthia* can be cultured from CSF and brain tissue; however, *Balamuthia* cultures take a long time to grow.[32,35,36]

Mortality among patients with primary and granulomatous amoebic encephalitis is more than 95%. Early diagnosis and treatment are major factors that influence outcome. Treatment regimens are difficult because no single drug is effective against all free-living amoebae. Amphotericin is the drug of choice for infection due to *Naegleria* but is not effective against *Acanthamoeba* and *Balamuthia*. Empiric therapy that has been suggested includes a combination of agents such as: amphotericin and flucytosine or voriconazole and miltefosine. Adjunctive corticosteroid therapy seems to exacerbate the amebic infection and should be avoided.[37]

## REFERENCES


1. Wubbel L, McCracken GH. Management of bacterial meningitis: 1998. *Pediatr Rev.* 1998;19:78–84

2. Zangwell KM, Vadheim CM, Vannier AM, et al. Epidemiology of invasive pneumococcal disease in Southern California: implications for the design and conduct of a pneumococcal conjugate vaccine efficacy trial. *J Infect Dis.* 1996;174: 752–759

3. Rosenstein NE, Perkins BA, Stephens DS, et al. The changing epidemiology of meningococcal disease in the United States, 1992–1996. *J Infect Dis.* 1999;180:1894–1901

4. Saez-Llorens X, Ramilo O, Mustafa MM, et al. Molecular pathophysiology of bacterial meningitis: current concepts and therapeutic implications. *J Pediatr.* 1990;116: 671–684

5. Kaplan SL. Clinical presentation, diagnosis, and prognostic factors of bacterial meningitis. *Infect Dis Clin North Am.* 1999;13:579–594

6. Quagliarello VJ, Scheld WM. Treatment of bacterial meningitis. *N Engl J Med.* 1997;336:708–716

7. de Gans J, van de Beek D. Dexamethasone in adults with bacterial meningitis. *N Engl J Med.* 2002;347:1549–1556

8. Nicolosi A, Hauser WA, Beghi E, et al. Epidemiology of central nervous system infections in Olmstead County, Minnesota, 1950–1981. *J Infect Dis.* 1986;154:399–408

9. Rotbart HA. Viral meningitis. *Semin Neurol.* 2000;20: 277-292

10. Sawyer MH. Enterovirus infections: diagnosis and treatment. *Curr Opin Pediatr.* 2001;13:65-69

11. Rotbart HA, Brennan PJ, Fife KH, et al. Enterovirus meningitis in adults. *Clin Infect Dis.* 1998;27:896-898

12. Chonmaitree T, Baldwin CD, Lucia HL. Role of the virology laboratory in diagnosis and management of patients with central nervous system disease. *Clin Microbiol Rev.* 1989;2:1-14

13. Tsai TF. Arboviruses. In: Murray PR, Baron EJ, Pfaller MA, et al, eds. *Manual of Clinical Microbiology*. Washington, DC: ASM Press; 1999:1107-1124

14. Rotbart HA, Sawyer MH, Fast S, et al. Diagnosis of enteroviral meningitis using the polymerase chain reaction with a colorimetric microwell detection assay. *J Clin Microbiol.* 1994;32:2590-2592

15. Nicolosi A, Hauser WAS, Beghi E, et al. Epidemiology of central nervous system infections in Olmstead County, Minnesota, 1950-1981. *J Infect Dis.* 1986;154:399-408

16. Whitley RJ, Kimberlin DW. Viral encephalitis. *Pediatr Rev.* 1999;20:192-198

17. Johnson RT. Acute encephalitis. *Clin Infect Dis.* 1996; 23:219-226

18. Calisher CH. Medically important arboviruses of the United States and Canada. *Clin Microbiol Rev.* 1994;7:89-116

19. Hayes EB, O'Leary DR. West Nile virus infection: a pediatric perspective. *Pediatrics.* 2004;113:1375-1381

20. Waecker NJ Jr, Connor JD. Central nervous system tuberculosis in children: a review of 30 cases. *Pediatr Infect Dis J.* 1990;9:539-543

21. Kent SJ, Crowe SM, Yung A, et al. Tuberculous meningitis: a thirty-year review. *Clin Infect Dis.* 1993;17:987-994

22. Brooks JB, Daneshvar MI, Haberberger RL, et al. Rapid diagnosis of tuberculous meningitis by frequency-pulsed-electron-capture gas liquid chromatography detection of carboxylic acids in cerebrospinal fluid. *J Clin Microbiol.* 1990; 28:989-997

23. Daniel TM. New approaches to the rapid diagnosis of tuberculous meningitis. *J Infect Dis.* 1987;155:603-607

24. Kox LFF, Sjoukje Kuijper I, Kolk AHJ. Early diagnosis of tuberculous meningitis by polymerase chain reaction. *Neurology.* 1995;45:2228-2232

25. Bonington A, Strang JIG, Klapper PE, et al. Use of Roche AMPLICOR *Mycobacterium tuberculosis* PCR in early diagnosis of tuberculous meningitis. *J Clin Microbiol.* 1998;36: 1251-1254

26. Petterson T, Klockars M, Weber TH, et al. Diagnostic value of cerebrospinal fluid adenosine deaminase determination. *Scand J Infect Dis.* 1991;23:97-100

27. American Academy of Pediatrics. Tuberculosis. In: Pickering LK, ed. *Red Book: 2009 Report of the Committee on Infectious Diseases*. 28th ed. Elk Grove Village, IL: American Academy of Pediatrics; 2009

28. Prusiner SB. Molecular biology and pathogenesis of prion diseases. *Trends Biochem Sci.* 1996;21:482-487

29. Manuelidis L. Dementias, neurodegeneration, and viral mechanisms of disease from the perspective of human transmissible encephalopathies. *Ann NY Acad Sci.* 1994;724:259-281

30. Dickinson AG, Outram GW. Genetic aspects of unconventional virus infections: the basis of the virino hypothesis. *Ciba Found Symp.* 1988;135:63-83

31. Haywood AM. Transmissible spongiform encephalopathies. *N Eng J Med.* 1997;25:1821-1828

32. Ma P, Visvesvara GS, Martinez AJ, et al. *Naegleria* and *Acanthoamoeba* infection. *Rev Infect Dis.* 1990;12:490-513

33. McKee T, Davis L, Blake P, et al. Primary amebic meningoencephalitis-Georgia, 2002. *MMWR.* 2003; 52:962-964

34. Gavin PJ, Tan TQ. Naegleria, Acanthamoeba, and Balamuthia. In: Feigin RD, Cherry J, Demmler-Harrison GJ, Kaplan SL (eds.) *Feigin and Cherry's Textbook of Pediatric Infectious Diseases*. 6th ed. Philadelphia, PA: Saunders; 2009: 2942-2953

35. Marciano-Cabral F, Cabral G. *Acanthamoeba* spp as agents of disease in humans. *Clin Microbiol Rev.* 2003;16:273-307

36. Martinez AJ, Visvesvara GS. Laboratory diagnosis of pathogenic free-living amoebas: *Naegleria, Acanthamoeba,* and *Leptomyxid. Clin Lab Med.* 1991;11:861-872

37. Schuster FL, Guglielmo BJ, Visvesvara GS. In-vitro activity of miltefosine and voriconazole on clinical isolates of free-living amoebas: *Balamuthia mandrillaris, Acanthoamoeba* spp, and *Naegleria fowleri*. *J Eukaryot Microbiol.* 2006;53:121-126

# CHAPTER 126

# Headaches

ZHICHENG LI, MD • SHLOMO SHINNAR, MD, PhD

Headaches are among the most common complaints in adolescents. By age 15 as many as 15% of teenagers will have recurrent headaches.[1] Chronic headaches constitute 1 of the most common reasons for referral to a pediatric neurology practice. Most headaches are not associated with intracranial structural lesions. Diagnosis can usually be made by careful history-taking and physical examination, and laboratory investigations are rarely required. Most headaches can be managed with simple analgesics. For more severe cases, particularly of migraine, effective pharmacologic agents are available.

**Box 126-1**

***Primary Headaches***

- Migraine with aura
- Migraine without aura
- Tension-type headache
- Cluster headache
- Paroxysmal hemicrania
- Episodic paroxysmal hemicrania
- Chronic paroxysmal hemicrania
- Short-lasting unilateral neuralgiform headache attacks with conjunctival injection and tearing (SUNCT)
- Other primary headaches
  - Primary stabbing headache
  - Primary exertional headache
  - Primary cough headache
  - Primary headache associated with sexual activity
  - Hypnic headache
  - Primary thunderclap headache
  - Hemicrania continua
  - New daily-persistent headache

## TYPES OF HEADACHE

Headaches may be classified as primary or secondary. The primary headache disorders (migraine, tension-type, and cluster headaches) represent illnesses in which the headache itself is the problem (Box 126-1). In contrast, the term "secondary headaches" implies that headache is a manifestation of some underlying pathology such as a brain tumor, an infection, or some other systemic illness. Most headaches seen in clinical practice are primary, but headaches from secondary causes must always be excluded (Box 126-2). An accurate diagnosis can usually be made on the basis of the history and physical examination.[2]

## PRIMARY HEADACHE DISORDERS

### MIGRAINE

Migraine headaches affect all age groups, although the clinical manifestations may differ. Children are less likely than adults to complain of severe headache and may therefore be less likely to have their headaches correctly diagnosed. There is an equal gender incidence before puberty, but in adolescents migraine occurs more frequently in girls. A first- or second-degree relative also has migraine in 70% to 80% of cases. Migraine headaches are typically unilateral, throbbing, and associated with nausea and vomiting. They occur at any time of day, last from 30 minutes to 2 or 3 days, and are often relieved by vomiting or sleep. Precipitating factors include stress, fatigue, exertion, head trauma, illness, and dietary factors.[4,5] In 2004 the International Headache Society (IHS)[3] proposed new criteria for the diagnosis of migraine and other headaches. Common migraine is now known as ***migraine without aura,*** and the term classical migraine has been replaced by ***migraine with aura.*** The IHS classification of migraine may be found in Box 126-3. The IHS criteria are quite restrictive and best reserved for research purposes. In clinical practice it is useful to divide migraine into 4 phases:

1. *Prodrome.* Many people with migraine experience premonitory symptoms that precede the aura or headache phase. These symptoms, which may occur hours to days before the headache, are in 30% to 80% of patients with migraines. The most common prodromal symptoms are

**Box 126-2**

### *Suggestions for Secondary Etiology in Adolescent Headache*

1. New headache <6 months history
2. Sudden onset and maximally intense immediately
3. Headache does not respect sleep—waking up in the middle of the night; headache on awakening, headache not relieved by sleeping
4. Radical change or progressive worsening in established headaches
5. Headache with new deficit, facial pain/tenderness, stiff neck/neck pain, vomiting, papilledema, altered mental status or seizure, motor/sensory/cranial nerve/cerebellar deficit
6. Headache triggered or worsened by increasing intracranial pressure maneuvers—cough, squatting, Valsalva maneuver, exertion, et al
7. Headache with a fever that is otherwise unexplained
8. Headache in immunocompromised, cancer, ventriculo peritoneal shunt patients
9. Headache with exclusive and persistent unilaterality
10. Headache without a familial history

From Winner P, Hershey AD, Li Z. Headaches in Children. In: Silberstein SD, Lipton RB, Dodick DW (eds.) *Wolff's Headache and Other Head Pain*. New York: Oxford University Press;2008, with permission.

**Box 126-3**

### *Migraine Classification*

- Migraine without aura
  1. At least 5 attacks fulfilling criteria B–D
  2. Headache attacks lasting 1–72 hours (untreated or unsuccessfully treated)
  3. Headache has at least 2 of the following characteristics:
     1. unilateral location
     2. pulsating quality
     3. moderate or severe pain intensity
     4. aggravation by or causing avoidance of routine physical activity (eg, walking or climbing stairs)
  4. During headache at least 1 of the following:
     1. nausea and/or vomiting
     2. photophobia and phonophobia

*(continued)*

**Box 126-3 (continued)**

  5. Not attributed to another disorder
- Migraine with aura
  1. At least 2 attacks fulfilling criterion B
  2. Migraine aura fulfilling criteria B–C for 1 of the following subforms
  3. Not attributed to another disorder
- **Typical aura with migraine headache**
  1. At least 2 attacks fulfilling criteria B–D
  2. Aura consisting of at least 1 of the following, but no motor weakness:
     1. fully reversible visual symptoms including positive features (eg, flickering lights, spots, or lines) and/or negative features (ie, loss of vision)
     2. fully reversible sensory symptoms including positive features (ie, pins and needles) and/or negative features (ie, numbness)
     3. fully reversible dysphasic speech disturbance
  3. At least 1 of the following:
     1. homonymous visual symptoms and/or unilateral sensory symptoms
     2. at least 1 aura symptom develops gradually over ≥ 5 minutes and/or different aura symptoms occur in succession over ≥ 5 minutes
     3. each symptom lasts ≥ 5 and ≤ 60 minutes
     4. Headache fulfilling criteria B–D for 1. 1 *Migraine without aura* begins during the aura or follows aura within 60 minutes
     5. Not attributed to another disorder
- **Typical aura without headache**
  1. *As typical aura with migraine headache*
  2. Aura consisting of at least 1 of the following, with or without speech disturbance but no motor weakness:
     1. fully reversible visual symptoms including positive features (eg, flickering lights, spots, or lines) and/or negative features (ie, loss of vision)
     2. fully reversible sensory symptoms including positive features (ie, pins and needles) and/or negative features (ie, numbness)
     3. Headache does not occur during aura nor follow aura within 60 minutes

From Headache Classification Subcommittee of the International Headache Society. The international classification of headache disorders. *Cephalalgia*. 2004; 24 (suppl): 1–160, with permission.

irritability, sluggishness, depression, excessive energy, increased yawning, impaired concentration, increased urination, fluid retention, hunger, food cravings, photophobia, phonophobia, and osmophobia.

2. *Aura.* Only 20% of migraine sufferers experience auras, and although their presence is not necessary to establish the diagnosis, many sufferers are misdiagnosed because of their absence. Auras are transient neurologic disturbances that last 5 to 60 minutes and then spontaneously resolve. They are believed to occur more commonly in adults than in children, although some studies have reported visual auras in up to 50% of childhood migraine sufferers.[1] The most common auras consist of visual disturbances such as scotomas, blurred vision, flashing lights, and hemianopsias. Other aura phenomena include paresthesias, hemiparesis, vertigo, aphasias, and visual hallucinations.
3. *Headache phase.* The headache is considered the hallmark of migraine. Typically, the pain is described as throbbing or pounding, is worsened with movement or exertion, and usually involves the temple, orbital, and frontal regions. Migraine headache tends to be hemicranial, although attacks demonstrate side-shift (ie, they alternate sides during subsequent bouts). The headache may not be hemicranial in children; instead, children complain of generalized or bifrontal headaches more frequently than of hemicranial pain. Hemicranial headaches occur in only 22% to 31% of childhood migraine.[1,6,7] Headaches may be associated with nausea, vomiting, photophobia, phonophobia, osmophobia, and tenderness of the scalp and pericranial muscles. During attacks, patients prefer to sleep or lie quietly in a dark room. Attacks last from 1 to 72 hours, although episodes tend to be shorter in children than in adults.
4. *Postdrome.* After the headache, many adolescents with migraines experience a period of decreased concentration, fatigue, and limited food tolerance for up to 24 hours.

Migraines with prolonged aura or complicated migraines have been abandoned in ICHD-II.[3,5,8,9] These disorders consist of migraine subtypes with transient neurologic deficits or alterations in state of consciousness. The aura symptoms last more than 60 minutes but less than one week. The deficits are presumably due to prolonged vasoconstriction and ischemia to the affected cerebral areas. The onset of the deficit usually precedes the headache. The symptoms are extremely diverse and depend on the vascular territory involved. The natural course of complex migraine is usually benign and most patients later go on to develop typical migraine. It is important to differentiate migraine syndromes from more serious intracranial pathology. In general, adolescents with complex migraine should be referred to a neurologist for evaluation. The more common complex migraine syndromes are listed in Box 126-4.

**Box 126-4**

***Common Complex Migraine Syndromes***

- Familial hemiplegic migraine
- Sporadic hemiplegic migraine
- Basilar-type migraine
- Childhood periodic syndromes that are commonly precursors of migraine
- Cyclical vomiting
- Abdominal migraine
- Benign paroxysmal vertigo of childhood
- Retinal migraine
- Complications of migraine
- Chronic migraine
- Status migrainous
- Persistent aura without infarction
- Migrainous infarction
- Migraine-triggered seizures

## CLUSTER HEADACHE

Cluster headache is a rare and distinct entity in children, although it is somewhat more common in late adolescence.[10] Cluster attacks are characterized by intense (the most severe pain), nonthrobbing periorbital pain that may then generalize to the entire hemicranium. The headaches are often associated with unilateral conjunctival injection, ptosis, lacrimation, and rhinorrhea ipsilateral to the headache. The attacks are brief, not preceded by an aura, last 15 to 180 minutes, and occur in groups of one headache every other day to 8 attacks daily for a period of 6 to 12 weeks. The cluster of headaches is followed by prolonged periods of remission lasting months to years.[9] Cluster headaches are usually refractory to simple analgesic therapy and generally require treatment with preventive agents. Patients with cluster headaches should be referred to a neurologist for treatment, as these headaches tend to have a less favorable prognosis than migraine and do not respond well to the standard treatments for migraine and tension headaches.[10]

### TENSION-TYPE HEADACHE

Tension-type headaches are the most common form of headache in adolescents, but they are less common in children. They were once called tension or muscle contraction headache because they were believed to arise secondarily to increased contraction of the muscles of the head and neck. Recent evidence suggests this is not the case, and these headaches may in some way have pathophysiologic mechanisms similar to those of migraine. Tension-type headaches may be subdivided into episodic and chronic varieties. In chronic tension-type headache, sufferers report more than 15 headaches per month or more than 180 headache days per year.[3] Adolescents with tension-type headaches typically describe a sensation of tightness or pressure in a bandlike distribution around the head. Physical examination may reveal tenderness or tightness of the muscles in the occipital scalp or posterior cervical region. They are often quite frequent and may last all day if untreated. The episodic variety usually does not interrupt regular daily activities and often responds well to mild analgesics such as acetaminophen or ibuprofen. Tension-type headaches differ from migraine headaches by the absence of vomiting and associated autonomic symptoms and by the ability of patients to continue their daily activities during the attack.

## SECONDARY HEADACHES

### POST-TRAUMATIC HEADACHES

The existence of a post-traumatic headache is controversial, but in the authors' experience it is a real entity. The headaches are often self-limited and usually resolve after a few weeks. They can, however, persist for months to years even after relatively minor trauma. Other symptoms of post-traumatic syndrome, such as sleep disturbances and behavior changes, are often present.[11] The headache may be migraine or tension-type in character.

### HEADACHES AND CHILDHOOD DEPRESSION

A serious and often unrecognized cause of chronic headache is depression.[12] The patient usually complains of a dull, constant headache that may be generalized or localized to the occipital region. Other symptoms can often be elicited, such as significant mood changes, withdrawal, increasingly poor school performance, school problems, sleep disturbances, aggressive behavior, lack of energy, weight loss, anorexia, and other somatic complaints. Appropriate treatment depends on recognition of the underlying depression. Headaches as a primary manifestation of depression are relatively uncommon and must be distinguished from tension-type or migraine headaches, whose frequency and severity are often increased by stress.[4]

### NONMIGRAINOUS VASCULAR HEADACHES

#### Convulsive States

Headache may occur as a postictal symptom but is rarely the sole manifestation of a seizure.[13] On occasions, patients with nocturnal seizures may awaken afterward with a postictal vascular headache. Migraine and epilepsy are distinct syndromes that can usually be differentiated on clinical grounds.[2,14] Some cases of complex migraine that may involve altered states of consciousness and transient neurologic deficits may be difficult to distinguish from complex partial seizures.

#### Traction Headache

A traction headache is caused by traction on the intracranial pain-sensitive structures. The traction may be exerted by a mass lesion such as a brain tumor, an abscess, or a subdural hematoma; by the weight of the brain after removal of cerebrospinal fluid by lumbar puncture; or by distortion of intracranial structures from increased intracranial pressure, as in hydrocephalus or pseudotumor cerebri. Although a relatively uncommon form of headache, it is often associated with serious intracranial pathology.

Brain tumors are an extremely rare cause of headache in adolescence. Several characteristics help to distinguish brain tumor headaches from more benign varieties. Headaches associated with brain tumors are usually chronic and progressive, present in the morning on first arising, and exacerbated by changes in position, coughing, or a Valsalva maneuver. In a 1993 review, however, the classic triad of headache, sleep disturbance, and vomiting was present in only one-third of patients with brain tumors.[15] Localization of the headache is also of limited value, because a mass lesion may cause distortion of distant pain-sensitive structures. Associated symptoms such as vomiting, diplopia, weakness, ataxia, and personality changes are usually present within a few weeks of the onset of headache.[16] Physical examination often reveals papilledema, nuchal rigidity, irritability, focal neurologic deficits such as a field cut, or a hemiparesis. As a general rule, the child with headaches of more than 6 months' duration who still has normal neurologic examination results is exceedingly unlikely to have a brain tumor.

### Pseudotumor Cerebri

This syndrome is characterized by the clinical manifestations of increased intracranial pressure in the absence of hydrocephalus or a mass lesion. It occurs most frequently in obese young women.[17] Headache is the most common presenting complaint and is frequently associated with nausea and vomiting. Visual symptoms such as diplopia are not uncommon, and are often present between headaches. Imaging studies are typically normal. However, on examination papilledema is almost invariably present. Prompt treatment is necessary to prevent visual loss.

### HEADACHE ASSOCIATED WITH OTHER HEAD OR NECK STRUCTURES

Refractive errors and eye muscle imbalance are common but rarely cause frank headaches. Instead, they may cause dull pain localized to the periorbital or frontal area and are clearly related to prolonged eye strain. Correction of the visual deficit will lead to prompt resolution of the headache. Headache from ear disease is usually associated with acute otitis externa, acute otitis media, or serous otitis media. The associated ear pain and physical examination should make the diagnosis clear. Dental disease can also cause headache in association with severe local pain. However, in the absence of local pain, temporomandibular joint dysfunction is rarely a cause of headaches. Sinus disease can cause a chronic headache, with pain and tenderness to percussion over the forehead and maxillary regions. There is usually a history of chronic sinus disease or recurrent upper respiratory tract infection. On close inspection, most patients diagnosed with sinus headaches usually meet the criteria for migraine or tension-type headaches.

## DIAGNOSIS

The foremost important task for diagnosis is the differentiation of primary and secondary headache.

**History** is the key for diagnosis. A detailed history should be obtained from the patient and parent(s), including information regarding the character of the headache, its frequency and severity, and associated symptoms (Box 126-5).[18,19–23] History-taking can be conducted in an orderly manner, as outlined next to facilitate differential diagnosis and to avoid misdiagnosis. A detailed investigation of the triggering events and the events surrounding the first attack may provide a clue not only to the diagnosis but also to treatment. An aura may point to the diagnosis of migraine or temporal lobe seizures. Associated deficits between headaches, such as weakness, ataxia, personality change, and visual disturbances should make one suspicious of a mass lesion. The type and number of medications used in the past are an indication of the perceived magnitude of the problem. Prolonged use of multiple medications should alert the physician to the potential of drug dependence or abuse. A therapeutic response to a previously used agent may be of diagnostic as well as therapeutic significance. At the end of the interview the physician should have a good idea as to the type of headache present.

### Box 126-5

### *Questions to Ask for Differentiating a Headache*

**Temporal Nature of the Headache**

***History***
When was your first and last headache (HA)?

***Onset***
Is it a sudden onset, thunderclap HA, or more like a gradually building-up type of HA? Is it a cluster of HA? How long does it take to achieve maximal intensity?

***Duration***
How long does it last (seconds, minutes, hours, days)?

***Frequency***
How often is it? How many days per week/month?

***Timing***
What time of the day? Morning or evening? Before or after school? Does it only happen on weekdays, or weekends, or evenly distributed? Does it happen in the morning right after getting up? Does it wake you up in the middle of the night?

***Variability***
Is it stable over time? Is it getting progressively or suddenly worse in any aspect? Is it getting better? Is this a persistent headache or does it come and go with HA-free interval?

***Termination***
How does it stop? Does sleep get rid of it?

**Physical Nature of the Headache**

***Aura***
Can you tell if a headache is coming? Do you have any of the prodomal symptoms listed below? If so, how long do they last? Do they go away afterward? How soon after the aura does the headache start?

- Blurry vision or loss of vision?
- Flashing light?
- Difficulty talking or any speech problems?
- Numbness, pain, or pin-and-needle sensation?

*(continued)*

## Box 126-5 (continued)

***Motor Deficit***
Any focal weakness/heaviness to 1 side of the body/face?

***Severity***
Rate the pain on a scale of 0 to 10: Missed school? Hospitalized? Suicidal ideation?

***Location***
Is it in front, back, vertex, or temporal, or behind the eyes/ears, above or below the eyes or all over the place? Is it unilateral or bilateral? Is the face involved? Indicate where it hurts the most.

***Quality***
Is it a pounding, throbbing, pulsating? Or a dull pain like squeezing, or a sharp pain like pin pricking, "ice-pick" jabs or stabbing, band-like or something else? Can you draw a picture?

**Association of Nausea and/or Vomiting—How Often?**

- Photophobia and phonophobia?
- Does walking or climbing upstairs make it worse?
- Brainstem deficit
    - Dysarthria
    - Dysphagia
    - Vertigo; ataxia
    - Tinnitus; hypacusia; hyperacusis
    - Diplopia
    - Syncope
    - Decreased consciousness
    - Simultaneously bilateral paresthesias
    - Perioral numbness
- Abdominal pain? Leg pain?
- Seizure?

***Influential Factors***
What triggers it? What makes it better or worse?

***Variety***
One kind of headache or more? Describe them all.

### EXAMINATION

A complete general and neurologic examination is essential for diagnosis, as well as to rule out organic disease. Temperature, respiration rate, heart rate, and blood pressure should be determined. Disturbances in growth parameters such as weight and height, and their change over a period of time, may indicate chronic disease or the presence of a pituitary tumor. Particular attention should be given to the structure of the head and neck.

Neurologically, a thorough funduscopic examination, visual acuity, visual fields, and assessment of extraocular movements are essential. Abnormalities of other cranial nerve or cerebellar functions may indicate a posterior fossa mass. Gait disturbances and asymmetric motor findings also point to possible structural abnormalities. When a properly performed general and neurologic examination fails to reveal any significant abnormalities and the history is reassuring, the physician can usually rule out an intracranial structural lesion and make a clinical diagnosis without laboratory testing.

### ACCESSORY TESTS

The use of accessory tests serves to confirm a clinical suspicion or guide treatment options. Different investigation modalities have different indications, contraindications, advantages, and disadvantages.

Neuroimaging is not indicated in children who have recurrent headache with a normal neurological examination.[24] The American Academy of Neurology (AAN) and Child Neurology Society (CNS)[24] recommend neuroimaging in children with abnormal neurologic examination, or with historical features such as severe headache of recent onset, change of headache type or pattern, or neurological dysfunction. In practice, neuroimaging may be considered if the history or examination suggests secondary etiology (Box 126-2).

In those patients for whom neuroimaging is indicated, magnetic resonance imaging (MRI) and computed tomography (CT) scanning of the head offer relatively safe, sensitive imaging for detecting a variety of structural lesions of the central nervous system. Magnetic resonance imaging is superior to CT in offering detailed anatomical and pathologic information of the brain and soft tissue, but it is time-consuming and may require sedation in young or agitated patients. Computed tomography is better than MRI at providing information about an acute bleed, bony lesion, or calcification, but less so for tumors. It takes only minutes to complete and is much more readily available in many medical facilities.

Magnetic resonance angiogram (MRA) is a noninvasive, 3-dimensional digital graphic reconstruction of the brain arterial system. It is indicated when there is a clinical suspicion of aneurysm, vascular malformation/dissection, or vasculitis. A conventional angiogram may be needed as a golden standard when MRA evidence is equivocal or clinical suspicion of a vascular lesion is strong, such as in the instance of an aneurysm less than 5 mm in diameter.

Magnetic resonance venogram (MRV) demonstrates the anatomical integrity of the venous and sinus drainage system of the brain. It is indicated when cephalic sinus thrombosis or venous malformation is suspected as an etiology of a headache.

Contrast material for either CT or MRI is indicated when a disruption of the blood-brain barrier or abnormal vasculature is suspected. Tumor, infection, and vascular malformation are regular indications for contrast enhancement imaging studies.

The electroencephalogram (EEG) is not recommended in the routine evaluation of pediatric headaches.[25,24] However, EEG remains an important diagnostic test in children when the differential diagnosis includes migraine and seizures.

Lyme disease is a cause of chronic daily headaches.[26-28] Lyme antibodies should be obtained for patients from endemic areas such as the northeast United States, in particular New York, New Jersey, and Connecticut.

Thyroid function tests should be considered in patients with chronic headaches.[29,30]

Substance abuse is of particular importance in the adolescent population. A toxicology screen should be carried out in suspected patients.

## TREATMENT

The goal of headache treatment is to stop an ongoing headache, and/or to prevent a headache from happening. The emphasis should be placed on reassurance, removal of precipitating factors, adequate sleep and hydration, a headache diary to track pain, and treating a headache early rather than later with simple analgesics.

### NONPHARMACOLOGIC THERAPY

A large number of external and constitutional factors play a role in triggering and exacerbating migraine and tension headaches in adolescents. Although these factors often cannot be completely eliminated, their identification and reduction will reduce the frequency and severity of the symptoms. Foremost among precipitating factors are the emotional stress of school, peer relations, and family tensions. In adolescents the stresses of maturation, puberty, and the struggle toward independence are additional factors. The irregular lifestyle of many adolescents also contributes to their headaches, particularly in those with migraines. Fasting or missing meals, sleeping late, or lack of sleep have all been implicated in triggering headache attacks. Contrary to popular belief, dietary factors have not been conclusively implicated in studies of large numbers of people with migraines. However, in selected patients, when there is a clear history of headaches after the ingestion of specific foods, dietary manipulation may be beneficial. In adolescent girls, both migraine and tension headaches are often associated with menstruation, and oral contraceptives may exacerbate their headaches.

Biofeedback and relaxation techniques are nonpharmacologic tools that are achieving an increasingly accepted role in the management of chronic headaches. They are particularly effective in tension-type headaches, but are also proving effective for migraine.[31,32] The safety of these techniques, and their avoidance of the potential pitfalls of drug dependency and abuse, make them attractive for use in adolescents with chronic headaches of all causes. Biofeedback and relaxation techniques work best when provided in the context of a comprehensive stress management approach.

General management includes resting in a cool, dark, and quiet room, which provides a conducive healing environment for migraine. Hydration, either intravenously or orally with attention to imbalance of electrolytes secondary to vomiting or poor intake, should be instituted upon early encounter patients with a migraine. Once a thorough and focused history and examination is taken and a secondary etiology is ruled out, induction of sleep is helpful for acute migraine. Pharmacologic treatment should be part of a comprehensive management. Such integrated multidisciplinary strategy constitutes the cornerstone of any successful treatment plan.

### PHARMACOLOGICAL THERAPY

Pharmacological therapies for headache are divided into 3 classes: abortive, symptomatic, and prophylactic. Abortive medications are taken at the onset of an attack to eliminate pain. The usage of any acute headache medication should be limited to no more than 2 days per week to avoid rebound headache. Symptomatic medications are prescribed to treat the accompanying symptoms, such as nausea and vomiting. These agents are also useful in treating an attack that has already begun (such as during sleep) in which abortive agents would be of no help. Prophylaxis is used to prevent headache.

The following are evidence-based, adolescent-specific headache treatments; however, they are limited by the paucity of clinical trials.

#### Abortive Treatment

Several medications have been proven to be efficacious in treating migraine in adolescents.

##### *Nonsteroidal Anti-inflammatory Agents*

**Ibuprofen** at 7. 5 to 10 mg/kg PO dose has been shown to be superior to placebo in treating acute migraine headache in adolescents.[33,34] **Ketorolac** at 0. 5 mg/kg (maximum 30 mg) can be given intravenously for acute migraine treatment in adolescents.[35] In addition, **Naproxen** at 750 to 825 mg PO was shown to be effective in reducing migraine pain, shortening the duration of attack, and improving nausea, vomiting, photophobia, and phonophobia in adult populations.[36–38] No significant side effects were observed. Given its efficacy in adults, many neurologists use naproxen 500 mg (lower dosage) for migraine attack in adolescents as well.

### Triptans

Triptans are tryptamines chemically similar to serotonin. They act as agonists for $5\text{-}HT_{1B}$ and $5\text{-}HT_{1D}$ receptors and constrict mainly cranial blood vessels.

**Sumatriptan** 25 mg, 50 mg, and 100 mg are effective in relieving migraine headaches at 3 and 4 hours after dosing in adolescents with moderate or severe pain. Another formulation, sumatriptan NS 20 mg significantly improves headache at 30 minutes, 1 hour, and 2 hours after application in an adolescent patient with moderate to severe migraine headache.[39,40,41–43] Side effects are mild in general, with taste disturbance in nasal spray as an exception.

### Rizatriptan

Rizatriptan at 5 mg produced pain relief at 66% of 12 to 17 year old patients at 2 hours postdosing. Of these, 32% were headache-free.[44] No serious side effects were reported.

**Zolmitriptan** at 2.5 mg or 5 mg tablets has been shown to relieve headaches in 70% and 88% of adolescent patients, respectively.[45] Its nasal spray form has also been used, but to a lesser degree of efficacy.[46]

**Eletriptan** 40 mg is not superior to placebo in reducing migraine in adolescents.[47]

**Almotriptan** at 12. 5 mg is effective in reducing the migraine headache in 71% of adolescent patients. It also reduces photophobia, phonophobia, and nausea.[48]

Triptans in general can be given a second dose in approximately 2 hours if the first dose does not resolve the headache. However, it should not be given more than twice a day. Triptans should not be combined.

Triptans should not be used in patients who have a history of stroke or vascular diseases due to its weak vasoactive property. They have not been tested in patients with basilar migraine, hemiplegic migraine, nor migraine with prolonged aura. More recently, the Food and Drug Administration (FDA) issued a Black Box warning regarding the possible serotonin syndrome occurring in patients who take triptans or certain classes of antidepressants. This warning should be mentioned to patients who are at risk, but its practical risk is remote.

**Other: Acetaminophen** at 15 mg/kg is also effective.[33,49]

**Isometheptene mucate** (Midrin) is a useful abortive agent in adults as well as older children and adolescents. In children older than 8 years the adult dosage is given: 2 capsules at headache onset, and then 1 every hour as needed. The maximal daily dose is 5 capsules.[29]

### Ergotamine Compounds

In adults with migraine, ergot compounds were the mainstay of therapy in the past.[9] The usual dose is 1mg to 2 mg orally at the onset of the aura, and an additional 1 mg 30 to 60 minutes afterward if necessary, for a maximum of 12 mg/week. Ergotamine compounds are contraindicated in patients with complicated migraine, as they may theoretically prolong the ischemic phase. Ergotamine preparations should not be used in young children.

Intravenous dihydroergotamine (DHE) has been used to treat headaches in adults and adolescents.[18] It causes severe nausea and vomiting and has adverse cardiovascular effects. It should be reserved for inpatients only, under the supervision of a headache specialist.

### Symptomatic Relief

**Prochlorperazine** at 0.15 mg/kg single dose intravenously (maximal 10 mg) can be used to terminate an ongoing headache.[35] It is also a good symptomatic medicine for migraine-associated nausea and vomiting. If side effects, such as dystonia occur, diphenhydramine 25 mg intravenously or orally can be used.

### Migraine Prophylaxis

No guideline exists for the indication of migraine prevention. However, several clinical criteria can be used to determine if a patient needs prophylaxis. These include patients who have at least 4 headaches per month,[29] patients who have lost 1 day of school per month for 2 months, patients who have been in the emergency department (ED) or admitted to a hospital for headache treatment or whose acute headache medication is contraindicated or not tolerated. In short, if headaches interfere with a patient's life or schooling in a consistent manner, then pharmacologic prevention is probably needed.

All headache prevention drugs were invented for nonheadache purposes initially. Four of them (propranolol, timolol, topiramate, divalproex sodium) are approved by the FDA for headache prophylaxis. They can be used at lower doses in headache prevention than their original indication. However, it usually takes 3 to 4 weeks to achieve therapeutic efficacy.

***Beta Blockers*** **Propranolol** is an excellent agent for migraine prophylaxis and has been studied in children and adolescents in well-designed clinical trials.[50,51] It is well tolerated by most adolescents. The most common side effects include nausea and easy fatigability on exertion. It is contraindicated in patients with bronchial asthma, sinus bradycardia, and congestive heart failure. It is relatively contraindicated in patients with major affective disorders because it can exacerbate the disorder. Propranolol is effective for the various types of migraine in all age groups. The starting dose in adolescents is 40 to 80 mg orally daily; this may need to be increased. However, propranolol is only partially effective in tension-type headaches and rarely effective in cluster headaches.

**Nadolol** is also well tolerated and tends to produce fewer behavioral side effects.

### Anticonvulsants

These are a heterogeneous group of medications used to treat seizures. Topiramate and valproic acid are approved for headache prophylaxis by the FDA. Although the dosages for headache prevention are generally lower than those for epilepsy, side effects are still common. Therefore they should not be used as first line medication.

**Topiramate** at a dose of 100 mg daily significantly reduces headache frequency, headache days, and usage of headache acute medication in adolescent patients.[52-57] Higher dosages cause more frequent side effects and lower dosages do not deliver as many benefits. It should be slowly titrated from 25 mg PO QHS over 4 to 6 weeks to 50 mg PO BID.

Topiramate is a weak diuretic and carbonic anhydrase inhibitor. It causes hypokalemia and metabolic acidosis. Patients may develop generalized fatigue, paresthesias, anorexia, and kidney stones (long-term usage). The hypokalemia and acidosis can be helped by prescribing potassium-rich food such as bananas and oranges, adequate hydration, and abalanced diet.

Topiramate's more concerning adverse effects include psychomotor slowing, poor concentration, and memory deficits, which can be disturbing for adolescents who attend school. Although slow titration may reduce the occurrences, the authors do not use it as first line therapy due to these cognitive side effects. Another common side effect includes weight loss; oligohidrosis and hyperthermia may also occur. A patient who is on oral contraceptive pills should be told that it might lower the efficacy. Rarely, acute myopia and secondary angle closure glaucoma may occur.

**Valproic acid** has been found to be efficacious in blinded, randomized, controlled clinical trials for migraines in adults and children.[58-60] Dosage range from 500 mg to 1,000 mg per day. It is a drug of long clinical history with well-established therapeutic and side effects profile.

Common side effects include weight gain, tremor, and hair loss. It can also cause thrombocytopenia, which tends to occur in a dose-dependent fashion and can be dose limiting. Rare but serious side effects include pancreatitis and liver failure, although the latter mostly occurs in young children rather than adolescents. A major concern regarding valproate use is teratogenicity. It causes neural tube defects in 1% to 3% of pregnancies and it is unclear if folic acid prevents this, although folic acid is indicated in all women of childbearing age on valproate. In addition, recent studies suggest that infants exposed in utero to valproate may have a lower IQs.[61] Therefore, valproate should be used with caution in young women of childbearing age. As migraine is most common in young women, this side effect profile limits its usage as the first line preventive medication in adolescents.

Lately, **levetiracetam** (20 mg or 40 mg/kg) has been implied (a chart review and open-label study) to reduce migraine frequency and improve dysfunction in children.[62,63] This drug has a relatively benign side effect profile (mild behavior change), however, concrete evidence is needed.

### Tricyclic Antidepressants

The headache prophylaxis effect is independent of the antidepressant activity.[64] These agents are the drugs of choice for adolescents with migraine, severe and frequent tension-type headaches, and post-traumatic headaches. Therapy must be instituted gradually, and a therapeutic effect may require 3 to 4 weeks. Two drugs have clinical evidence to support their efficacy.

***Amitriptyline.*** Two open-label, nonrandomized trials in children implied the efficacy for pediatric migraine prophylaxis.[64,66,67] The targeted dose is 1 mg/kg daily after a 2-month titration. A lower dose may work. Side effects are minimal. Amitriptyline was implied in the reduction in migraine/headache frequency, duration, severity, and missed school days. One case series implies its usefulness in cyclic vomiting syndrome in adolescents.[68]

***Nortriptyline.*** A second-generation tricyclic, it has fewer side effects than amitriptyline. It is often used for headache prevention despite the lack of clinical trial data. The dose is 1 mg/kg after titration.

The side effects of tricyclics must be discussed with patients and their parents. The anticholinergic effects such as constipation, dry mucosa, and orthostatic hypotension are frequent. Cardiac arrhythmia is rare. Drowsiness, fatigue, and weight gain can occur.

***Desyrel (trazodone)*** A randomized, double-blinded, placebo-controlled crossover trial in children and adolescents showed that trazodone (1 mg/kg divided into 3 doses daily) can reduce migraine frequency and duration compared to placebo.[65] Subjects reported no serious side effects. Specifically, no mood, school performance, or sleep/wake pattern changes were reported.

### Calcium Channel Blockers

**Nimodipine** is effective in the prophylaxis of migraine headaches in adolescents.[69] It can be used in asthmatic children when beta blockers, such as propranolol, are contraindicated. We have found that calcium channel blockers are relatively well tolerated in older adolescents, in whom they are often first line drugs. These agents are the drugs of choice in the treatment of basilar migraine, hemiplegic migraine, and migraine with prolonged auras. Nimodipine at 10 to 20 mg PO TID can significantly reduce migraine frequency and duration. Flunarizine[70] is also effective but, is unavailable in the United States.

### Other Prophylactic Agents

**Cyproheptadine** (Periactin) is an antihistaminergic, antiserotonergic, and anticholinergic medication with weak calcium channel blocker property. It has been shown in 2 randomized blinded placebo-controlled trials involving adolescents (15 or 16 years old and older) to be efficacious.[71,72] The usual dose is 2 or 4 mg twice daily. Side effects, including drowsiness, increased appetite, and weight gain, often limit its usefulness in treating adolescents. The authors find it of limited use in this population.

**Methysergide** (Sansert) is rarely used now due to its many side effects, including hallucinations, muscle cramping, and ischemic and gastrointestinal symptoms. It is a treatment of last resort and should only be used by a headache specialist after other treatment options have failed.

## WEANING OFF PROPHYLAXIS

There is no evidence-based guideline for stopping preventive medications. The termination of a medication should be accorded the same rationale for starting one, which is weighing the benefits and the risks. When prophylaxis is no longer indicated, medication withdrawal over a period of a month can be attempted after at least 6 months (due to a high rate of spontaneous remission). Even if complete remission has not occurred, the symptoms may have improved sufficiently to warrant discontinuation of daily medication.

## LONG-TERM MANAGEMENT

Headache medication is only one facet of the management of this multifactorial disease. Adolescents who are placed on prophylactic medication should also be instructed in proper sleep hygiene, biofeedback, and stress management techniques. Medication will not be efficacious if these other factors are not managed well. Conversely, medications may be only needed initially, and nonpharmacologic techniques alone may be sufficient, or may reduce the need for chronic medications later.

Emphasis on nonpharmacologic techniques and on prophylaxis of headaches, rather than seeking acute pharmacologic relief will help prevent some of the pharmacologic overtreatment commonly found in the management of patients with chronic headaches.

## REFERENCES


1. Bille B. Migraine in school children. *Acta Paediatr Scand.* 1962;51(suppl 136):1–151

2. Shinnar S, D'Souza BJ. The diagnosis and management of headaches in childhood. *Pediatr Clin North Am.* 1982;29:79–94

3. Headache Classification Subcommittee of the International Headache Society. The international classification of headache disorders. *Cephalalgia.* 2004;24(suppl):1–160

4. Cooper PJ, Bowden HN, Camfield PR, Camfield CS. Anxiety and life events in childhood migraine. *Pediatrics.* 1987;79:999–1004

5. Shinnar S. Headaches in children. In: Kaufman DM, Solomon G, Pfeffer M, eds. *Pediatric Neurology for Psychiatrists.* Baltimore, MD: Williams & Wilkins; 1991:158–168

6. Congdon PJ, Forsythe WI. Migraine in childhood: a study of 300 children. *Dev Med Child Neurol.* 1979;21:209–216

7. Prensky AL, Sommer D. Diagnosis and treatment of migraine in children. *Neurology.* 1979;29:506–510

8. Barlow CF. *Headaches and Migraine in Childhood.* Clinics in Developmental Medicine No. 91. London: Spastics International Medical Publications; 1984

9. Dalessio DJ, Silberstein SD. *Wolff's Headache and Other Head Pain.* 6th ed. New York, NY: Oxford University Press; 1993

10. Maytal J, Lipton RB, Solomon S, Shinnar S. Childhood onset cluster headaches. *Headache.* 1992;32:275–279

11. Levin HS, Eisenberg HM, Benton AL, eds. *Mild Head Injury.* New York, NY: Oxford University Press; 1983

12. Ling W, Oftedal G, Weinberg W. Depressive illness in childhood presenting as severe headache. *Am J Dis Child.* 1970;120:122–124

13. Swaiman KF, Frank Y. Seizure headaches in children. *Dev Med Child Neurol.* 1978;20:580–585

14. Andermann F, Lugaresi E, eds. *Migraine and Epilepsy.* Boston, MA: Butterworths; 1987

15. Forsyth PA, Posner JB. Headaches in patients with brain tumors: a study of 111 patients. *Neurology.* 1993;43:1678–1683

16. Honig PJ, Charney EB. Children with brain tumor headaches: distinguishing features. *Am J Dis Child.* 1982;136:121–124

17. Weisberg LA, Chutorian AM. Pseudotumor cerebri of childhood. *Am J Dis Child.* 1977;131:1243–1248

18. Silberstein SD. Twenty questions about headache in children and adolescents. *Neurology.* 1991;41:786–793

19. Lapkin ML, Golden GS. Basilar artery migraine: a review of 30 cases. *Am J Dis Child.* 1978;132:278–281

20. Brown JK. Migraine and migraine equivalents in children. *Dev Med Child Neurol.* 1977;19:683–692

21. Illingworth RS. *Common Symptoms of Disease in Children*. 5th ed. Oxford:Blackwell Scientific Publications; 1975:98

22. Prensky AL. Migraine and migrainous variants in pediatric patients. *Pediatr Clin North Am.* 1979;23:461–471

23. Vahlquist BO. Migraine in children. *Int Arch Allergy.* 1955;7:348–355

24. Lewis DW, Ashwal S, Dahl G, et al. Practice parameter: evaluation of children and adolescents with recurrent headaches: report of the Quality Standards Subcommittee of the American Academy of Neurology and the Practice Committee of the Child Neurology Society. *Neurology.* 2002;59:490–498

25. Millichap JC. Recurrent headaches in 100 children: electroencephalographic abnormalities and response to phenytoin (Dilantin). *Childs Brain.* 1978;4:95–105

26. Bingham PM, Galetta SL, Athreya B, Sladky J. Neurologic manifestations in children with Lyme disease. *Pediatrics.* 1995;96:1053–1056

27. Belman AL, Iyer M, Coyle PK, et al. Neurologic manifestations in children with North American Lyme disease. *Neurology.* 1993;43:2609–2614

28. Moses JM, Riseberg RS, Mansbach JM. Lyme disease presenting with persistent headache. *Pediatrics.* 2003;112: e477–e479

29. Bigal ME, Sheftell FD, Rapoport AM, et al. Chronic daily headache: identification of factors associated with induction and transformation. *Headache.* 2002;42:575–581

30. Fenichel NM. Chronic headache due to masked hypothyroidism. *Ann Int Med.* 1948;29:456–460

31. Adler CS, Adler SM. Biofeedback psychotherapy for the treatment of headaches: a 5-year follow-up. *Headache.* 1976;16:189–191

32. Diamond S. Biofeedback and headache. *Headache.* 1979;19:180–184

33. Hamalainen ML, Hoppu K, Valkeila E, Santavuori P. Ibuprofen or acetaminophen for the acute treatment of migraine in children: a double-blind, randomized, placebo-controlled, crossover study. *Neurology.* 1997;48:103–107

34. Lewis DW, Kellstein D, Dahl G, et al. Children's ibuprofen suspension for the acute treatment of pediatric migraine. *Headache.* 2002;42:780–786

35. Brousseau DC, Duffy SJ, Anderson AC, Linakis JG. Treatment of pediatric migraine headaches: a randomized, double-blind trial of prochlorperazine versus ketorolac. *Ann Emerg Med.* 2004;43:256–262

36. Johnson ES, Ratcliffe DM, Wilkinson M. Naproxen sodium in the treatment of migraine. *Cephalalgia.* 1985;5:5–10

37. Pradalier A, Rancure IG, Dordain S, Verdure L, Rasco lA, Dry J. Acute migraine attack therapy: comparison of naproxen sodium and an ergotamine tartrate compound. *Cephalalgia.* 1985;5:107–113

38. Nestvold K, Kloster R, Partinen M, Sulkava R. Treatment of acute migraine attack: naproxen and placebo compared. *Cephalalgia.* 1985;5:115–119

39. Korsgaard AG. The tolerability, safety, and efficacy of oral sumatriptan 50 mg and 100 mg for the acute treatment of migraine in adolescents. *Cephalalgia.* 1995;15(suppl 16):99

40. Linder SL. Subcutaneous sumatriptan in the clinical setting: the first fifty consecutive patients with acute migraine in a pediatric neurology office practice. *Cephalalgia.* 1995;15(suppl 16):98

41. Winner P, Prensky A, Linder S. *Efficacy and safety of oral sumatriptan in adolescent migraines.* Presented at: American Association for the Study of Headache; 1996; Chicago, IL

42. Winner P, Rothner AD, Wooten J, Webster B, Ames M. Randomized, double-blind, placebo-controlled study of sumatriptan nasal spray in adolescent migraineurs. *Neurology.* 2004;62:A182

43. Winner P, Rothner A, Webster C, Ames M. Overall efficacy of sumatriptan nasal spray in adolescent migraineurs: pooled results from US placebo-controlled trials. *Headache.* 2004;44:465

44. Winner P, Lewis D, Visser WH, Jiang K, Ahrens S, Evans JK. Rizatriptan Adolescent Study Group. Rizatriptan 5 mg for the acute treatment of migraine in adolescents: a randomized, double-blind, placebo-controlled study. *Headache.* 2002;42(1):49–55

45. Linder SL, Dowson AJ. Zolmitriptan provides effective migraine relief in adolescents. *Int J Clin Pract.* 2000;54(7):466–469

46. Lewis D, Winner P, Hershey AD, Wasiewski W. Efficacy of zolmitriptan nasal spray in adolescent migraine. *Pediatrics.* 2007;120(2):390–396

47. Winner P, Linder SL, Lipton RB, Almas M, Parsons B, Pitman V. Eletriptan for the acute treatment of migraine in adolescents: results of a double-blind, placebo-controlled trial. *Headache.* 2007;47(4):511–518

48. Charles JA. Almotriptan in the acute treatment of migraine in patients 11–17 years old: an open-label pilot study of efficacy and safety. *J Headache Pain.* 2006;7:95–97

49. Soriani S, Battistella PA, Naccarella C, Tozzi E, Fiumana E, Fanaro S. Nimesulide and acetaminophen for the treatment of juvenile migraine: a study for comparison of efficacy, safety, and tolerability. *Headache Q.* 2001;12:233–236

50. Bille B, Ludvigsson J, Sanner G. Prophylaxis of migraine in children. *Headache.* 1977;17:61–63

51. Ludvigsson J. Propranolol used in prophylaxis of migraine in children. *Acta Neurol Scand.* 1974;50:109–115

52. Brandes JL, Saper JR, Diamond M, et al. Topiramate for migraine prevention: a randomized controlled trial. *JAMA.* 2004;291:965–973

53. Diener HC, Tfelt-Hansen P, Dahlof C, et al. Topiramate in migraine prophylaxis—results from a placebo-controlled trial with propranolol as an active control. *J Neurol.* 2004;251: 943–950

54. Silberstein SD, Neto W, Schmitt J, Jacobs D. Topiramate in migraine prevention: results of a large controlled trial. *Arch Neurol.* 2004;61:490–495

55. Winner P, Gendolla A, Stayer C, et al. Topiramate for migraine prevention in adolescents: a pooled analysis of efficacy and safety. *Headache.* 2006;46:1503–1510

56. Winner P, Pearlman EM, Linder SL, et al. Topiramate for migraine prevention in children: a randomized, double-blind, placebo-controlled trial. *Headache.* 2005;45:1304–1312

57. Campistol J, Campos J, Casas C, Herranz JL. Topiramate in the prophylactic treatment of migraine in children. *J Child Neurol.* 2005;20:251–253

58. Hering R, Kuritzky A. Sodium valproate in the prophylactic treatment of migraine: a double-blind study vs placebo. *Cephalalgia.* 1992;12:81–84

59. Silberstein SD, Saper J, Mathew NT, et al. The safety and efficacy of divalproex sodium in the prophylaxis of migraine headache: a multicenter, double-blind, placebo-controlled trial. *Headache.* 1993;33:264–265

60. Ashrafi MR, Shabanian R, Zamani GR, Mahfelati F. Sodium valproate versus propranolol in paediatric migraine prophylaxis. *Eur J Paediatr Neurol.* 2005;9:333–338

61. Adab N, Kini U, Vinten J, et al. The longer term outcome of children born to mothers with epilepsy. *J Neurol Neurosurg Psychiatry.* 2004;25:1575–1583

62. Miller GS. Efficacy and safety of levetiracetam in pediatric migraine. *Headache.* 2004;44:238–243

63. Pakalnis A, Kring D, Meier L. Levetiracetam prophylaxis in pediatric migraine—an open-label study. *Headache.* 2007;47:427–430

64. Couch JR, Hassanein RS. Amitriptyline in migraine prophylaxis. *Arch Neurol.* 1979;36:695–699

65. Battistella PA, Ruffilli R, Cernetti R, et al. A placebo-controlled crossover trial using Trazodone in pediatric migraine. *Headache.* 1993;33(1):36–39.

66. Sorge F, Barone P, Steardo L, Romano MR. Amitriptyline as a prophylactic for migraine in children. *Acta Neurol (Napoli).* 1982;4:362–367

67. Hershey AD, Powers SW, Bentti AL, Degrauw TJ. Effectiveness of amitriptyline in the prophylactic management of childhood headaches. *Headache.* 2000;40:539–549

68. Andersen JM, Sugerman KS, Lockhart JR, Weinberg WA. Effective prophylactic therapy for cyclic vomiting syndrome in children using amitriptyline or cyproheptadine. *Pediatrics.* 1997;100:977–981

69. Battistella PA, Ruffilli R, Moro R, et al. A placebo-controlled crossover trial of nimodipine in pediatric migraine. *Headache.* 1990;30:264–268

70. Sorge F, Marano E. Flunarizine v. placebo in childhood migraine. A double-blind study. *Cephalalgia.* 1985;5 (suppl 2):145–148

71. Rao BS, Das DG, Taraknath VR, Sarma Y. A double-blind controlled study of propranolol and cyproheptadine in migraine prophylaxis. *Neurol India.* 2000;48(3):223–226

72. Mehvari J, Rafieian-kopaei M. Recommendations for the management of migraine in paediatric patients. *Iran J Med Sci.* 2005;30(2):84–87

# CHAPTER 127

# Seizures in Adolescents

SHLOMO SHINNAR, MD, PhD • HENRY HASSON, MD

## INTRODUCTION

Epilepsy, one of the most common chronic neurologic disorders affecting adolescents, is defined as "recurrent seizures without immediate provocation."[1] Most cases of epilepsy begin in childhood and adolescence. The prevalence of epilepsy in the 10- to 19-year-old group has been conservatively estimated at 4.1 per 1,000 population.[1-3] Using less strict criteria and including single convulsions, prevalence rates as high as 20 to 30 per 1,000 population have been reported.[2] Recent advances in the development of new antiepileptic drugs (AEDs) and improved understanding of their proper use have had a major effect on our ability to treat adolescents with epilepsy. The rational use of these drugs can result in complete seizure control in many cases. Surgery is an increasingly available option for those with intractable partial seizures. Recognizing psychosocial issues is also important because many adolescents are hampered more by their fears than by their seizures. Proper management of the adolescent with epilepsy will help ensure a transition to life as an independent adult.

## CLASSIFICATION OF SEIZURES IN ADOLESCENTS

The internationally accepted classification currently being used is the one established by the International League Against Epilepsy (ILAE). The classification of epileptic seizures was adopted in 1981, and the revised Classification of Epilepsies and Epileptic Syndromes was adopted in 1989. The 1981 classification replaced the often confusing older classification.[4] A simplified summary of the classification is shown in Table 127-1. The basic distinction in this classification is between those seizures with focal onset, which are referred to as partial seizures whether or not they generalize, and those seizures generalized from the onset. The old "psychomotor" seizure is now referred to as a complex partial seizure, which is defined as a partial seizure with impaired consciousness. The new term recognizes that many complex partial seizures do not have motor phenomena. This classification has a rational basis in terms of common electrophysiologic features of the various seizure types and the spectrum of drugs that are effective in their treatment.

**Table 127-1**

**Classification of Seizures in Adolescents**

| *Classification* | *Examples* |
|---|---|
| Generalized | Absence |
| | Atypical absence |
| | Myoclonic |
| | Tonic |
| | Tonic-Clonic |
| | Atonic |
| Partial | Simple partial |
| | Complex partial |
| | Partial with secondary generalization |

Adapted with permission from Commission on Classification and Terminology of the International League against Epilepsy. Proposal for revised clinical and electroencephalographic classification of epileptic seizures. *Epilepsia*. 1981;22:489–501.

## EPILEPTIC SYNDROMES

The major contribution of the 1989 classification[5] was that it recognized not only seizure types, but epileptic syndromes. An epileptic syndrome is defined based on seizure type(s), characteristics of the electroencephalogram (EEG), age of onset, and other features. Selected epileptic syndromes with special relevance to adolescents are discussed in the following. Although primary generalized and partial epilepsies can have their onset in adolescence, most adolescent onset seizures are of partial origin. This is different from childhood onset seizures, most of which are generalized. Almost three-quarters of adolescents and adults with onset of seizures above age 15 have a partial epilepsy.[1-3] This explains why neuroimaging studies, which are not usually necessary in children with a generalized tonic-clonic seizure, are routinely performed in adolescents with a new onset of seizures.

### PARTIAL EPILEPSIES

Most adolescent onset epilepsies are partial, even if the patients present with what appears to be a generalized tonic–clonic seizure and a normal EEG. The temporal lobe is the most common site of onset for partial seizures, with the frontal lobe being next most common. Adolescent onset partial seizures have the same clinical characteristics and prognosis as adult onset epilepsy and represent part of the same spectrum.

One specific epileptic syndrome that should be mentioned is benign rolandic epilepsy. Benign rolandic epilepsy is the best described benign focal epilepsy of childhood.[3,5-7] It is thought to be an autosomal dominant disorder with incomplete penetrance. Onset is in children between 4 and 10 years of age. Seizures tend to occur at night and can be generalized tonic–clonic or partial. When partial, they often involve the mouth and face. The EEG shows characteristic centro-temporal stereotyped spikes, with a horizontal dipole, which are often bilateral and increase with drowsiness and sleep. The seizures remit in early adolescence and the EEG abnormality generally disappears a few years later. The physician caring for the adolescent with this disorder must be aware that this epilepsy almost always remits in adolescence. Therefore it is often decided not to treat these patients because the risks associated with treatment may not outweigh the benefit of stopping the seizures. If medication is started, patients should be taken off medications at the appropriate time so they may enter adult life off medications. The other benign focal epilepsies of childhood are less well understood and have far more variable prognoses.[3,5-7]

### PRIMARY GENERALIZED EPILEPSIES

Primary generalized epilepsies comprise a spectrum of disorders with a presumed genetic basis. They all share the EEG marker of generalized spike and wave.[3,5,6] The most common are childhood absence, juvenile absence, and juvenile myoclonic epilepsy (JME). Childhood absence has a typical age of onset of 3 to 12 years, with a peak at 6 to 7 years of age. Affected children have multiple brief episodes of classical absences, usually easily provoked by hyperventilation. Most of these cases go into remission during adolescence with disappearance of both the seizures and the EEG trait.

Adolescents with a new onset of absence seizures more commonly have a diagnosis of juvenile absence epilepsy. Juvenile absence has a typical age of onset of 8 to 17 years.[3,5-7] Although the age of onset and clinical characteristics overlap with childhood absence, these children have somewhat fewer seizures. More importantly, however, they have a far worse prognosis in terms of eventually outgrowing the need for medications. As patients with juvenile absence get older, the absence seizures often disappear even if the EEG trait and the generalized tonic–clonic seizures persist.

Juvenile myoclonic epilepsy (JME) is characterized by myoclonic jerks that most often occur on awakening.[3,5-8] Most patients have at least occasional generalized tonic–clonic seizures, which is what typically brings them to medical attention. The history of "morning jerks" must be specifically elicited or it is likely overlooked. Approximately 30% of patients with JME will have absence seizures. Age of onset is in the second and third decades of life. Although JME in most of these patients is well controlled with AEDs, spontaneous remission of the underlying epileptic trait is rare.[6] The need for continued medications, as well as the underlying EEG abnormality, usually persists at least into the fifth decade of life. Relatives of patients with JME have an increased incidence of seizures, but the affected relatives do not necessarily have JME.

## EVALUATION OF THE ADOLESCENT WITH NEW ONSET SEIZURES

All adolescents who present with an initial seizure require a comprehensive medical and neurological evaluation. The evaluation should include a careful history, including potential precipitating factors and a description of the ictal event and postictal state, looking especially for any focal components.[9,10]

Additionally, one must ascertain that this is truly the first seizure, not merely the first convulsive event. After careful questioning, many adolescents who present with a first convulsion will in fact have a history of previous nonconvulsive ictal events such as absence, myoclonic, or complex partial seizures. Indeed, in a prospective study of first seizures at our institution, approximately one-third of children and adolescents who were referred with the diagnosis of a first seizure were found, after taking a careful history, to have had prior seizures.[11]

Laboratory studies in the emergency department should be performed in a systematic fashion looking for specific abnormalities.[3,9,10] Routine electrolytes and hematologic studies are rarely helpful in the afebrile patient. A lumbar puncture should be reserved for those cases where a central nervous infection, such as encephalitis or meningitis, is suspected. In the afebrile patient with normal mental status and no focal deficits, a lumbar puncture is rarely helpful. In contrast, a toxicology screen is very important in adolescents with a first seizure. Several popular drugs of abuse, most notably cocaine, can present with seizures following even occasional use. The author has seen a number of teenagers with recurrent seizures who experienced seizures each time they abused cocaine and never had any other seizures. A detailed history should include any medications or supplements the patient may be taking as well.

An EEG should be performed on all adolescents who present with new onset seizures.[9,10] The EEG is not only an important predictor of seizure recurrence but may also identify patients with those specific epileptic syndromes in which the long-term prognosis is known. If possible, an EEG in the awake and sleep states should be performed. As most adolescent onset seizures are of partial origin, a neuroimaging study usually is indicated, even in patients without obvious focal features.[9,10] Magnetic resonance imaging (MRI) is the study of choice due to its superior abilities to detect low-grade gliomas, vascular malformations, mesial temporal sclerosis, and heterotopias.[3,9] With current state-of-the-art neuroimaging, an increasing number of lesions are being detected. With the exception of those patients known to have a primary generalized epilepsy, performance of an MRI should be considered for any adolescent who has longstanding epilepsy that is not in remission. In most cases, both the EEG and MRI can be performed electively.

## PRINCIPLES OF ANTIEPILEPTIC DRUG THERAPY

The basic principle of AED therapy is to select the drug most likely to be effective for the individual patient's seizure type. The drug is then administered in a sufficient quantity to control seizures fully without undue toxicity. If the initial dose is inadequate, the drug is gradually increased until complete control of seizures is achieved or the patient experiences clinical toxicity. When several drugs with a similar spectrum of activity are available, one should select the drug with the least objectionable toxicities for the given patient. When a patient has 2 or more seizure types, one should select, whenever possible, a single drug that will be effective against all the seizure types, rather than a different drug for each seizure type. Given the range of AEDs now available, initial therapy with a single agent is almost always possible.

Over the past 15 years, a large number of new AEDs have been approved in the United States and Europe.[12,13] Although pediatric experience remains somewhat limited, the trials did include adolescents and there is sufficient experience with adolescents to justify their use when appropriate. As with all new drugs, they were first tried as add-on therapy in refractory patients. However, by now sufficient experience has been accumulated on many of these agents to justify their use even as first line agents in some cases.[12] The new drugs include felbamate, gabapentin, lamotrigine, leviteracetam, pregabalin, tiagabine, topiramate, and zonisamide.

As a group, the new AEDs are not necessarily more effective than the older drugs because it is hard to find more effective drugs than carbamezpine or phenobarbital for partial seizures, and valproate for generalized seizures. However, many of them do have a more favorable side effect profile, including relative lack of enzyme induction and drug-drug interactions, including less effect on oral contraceptives, and less harmful effect on bone health, which is an increasingly recognized adverse effect of chronic AED therapy. A few of them, specifically lamotrigine and leviteracetam, have achieved first line status due to their efficacy and adverse event profile.[7,12-15]

Cryptogenic epilepsy in most adolescents can be controlled fully with a single drug. This is particularly true of primary generalized seizures. If the first drug is ineffective, a second drug is added, and the dosage is gradually increased. If the second drug is effective, the physician should consider whether the original AED is still necessary. In principle, one should always try to use monotherapy because of decreased toxicity, but some adolescents will require treatment with more than one agent. If complete seizure control without toxicity is not achieved with 2 drugs, the patient should be referred to a neurologist specializing in epilepsy. Complete seizure control is attainable in only 70% to 80% of adolescents with epilepsy. However, because there is a major difference in quality of life between having complete control without toxicity versus having an occasional seizure or toxicity, every adolescent should have an attempt at complete control. Also, adolescents with refractory epilepsy may be candidates for surgery, as discussed in the following.

The older and newer AEDs are briefly described in the following in alphabetical order. In adolescents, for partial seizures the authors' current first line choices in alphabetical order include carbamazepine/oxcarbazepine, lamotrigine, and leviteracetam. For generalized seizures they are lamotrigine, leviteracetam, and valproate.

### OLDER AEDS

**Carbamazepine** remains a first line agent for the treatment of partial seizures and along with **oxcarbazepine** is considered the most commonly used first line therapy for partial seizures.[7,12,14,15] It is effective against both generalized tonic-clonic seizures and focal seizures. Oxcarbazepine, which is one of the newer AEDs, is discussed here because it is a structural analog of carbamazepine.[7,12,14,15] Its indications and side effects are similar to carbamazepine, but it less commonly causes rash. Although oxycarbazepine was initially thought to be just the prodrug, it is now clear that some patients have different responses to the 2 drugs, but the indications for using them are the same. Both should be considered enzyme inducers of the hepatic cytochrome P450 system, though oxcarbazepine may be less inducing.

Initial rare reports of aplastic anemia associated with use of carbamazepine, and the possible need for frequent blood monitoring, created some concern about use of this drug. However, as increased experience accumulates with its use, many epileptologists have questioned the need for frequent hematologic monitoring, which now seems to have a purely medicolegal basis.[7,16] In using carbamazepine, one must start with a low dose and gradually titrate to a full maintenance dose. This is due to the unusual pharmacokinetic properties of the drug, which specifically autoinduces its own metabolism.

The relative lack of cosmetic and cognitive side effects, and proven efficiency and safety, make carbamazepine and oxcarbazepine, in the opinion of the author, first line drugs in treating most adolescents with secondarily generalized tonic–clonic or focal seizures. However, in women the possible teratogenic effects must be considered as well.[17,18]

**Clonazepam** is a benzodiazepine AED. It has a similar clinical spectrum to valproic acid, although it is usually not as effective. Clonazepam is rarely used as a first line drug for any seizure type because of its sedative side effects. These side effects are also present with the other more recently introduced AEDs in the benzodiazepine class, such as **lorazepam** and **nitrazepam**.

**Ethosuximide** remains the drug of choice for treatment of typical absence seizures. However, classic petit mal epilepsy rarely has its onset in adolescence. For this reason, ethosuximide would rarely be used in adolescents with new-onset seizures. It remains, however, a valuable and relatively safe drug for selected patients.

**Phenobarbital** is the oldest AED still in common use. It is effective against both generalized tonic–clonic and partial seizures. **Primidone**, also a barbiturate, is metabolized to phenobarbital, but in addition it has anticonvulsant properties of its own. It is primarily used in treating refractory partial seizures. As with phenobarbital, primidone has been shown to be less effective and less well tolerated than phenytoin or carbamazepine.[19] This medication has limited use in the adolescent patient due to side effects such as cognitive[20] and behavioral changes, sedation, depression, and suicidal ideation.[21] In general, although phenobarbital remains a useful drug in selected cases, it is not currently the initial or even the second drug in the management of most adolescents with epilepsy.

**Phenytoin** is an effective AED for the treatment of both generalized tonic–clonic and focal seizures. Phenytoin's advantages are that it is inexpensive and can often be given on a once-a-day schedule, which may improve adherence. It is available in intravenous formulation (often used as fosphenytoin, which is the prodrug and more soluble) and it can be given with a full loading with only minor side effects, making it most effective in cases where a therapeutic level must be reached quickly. For this reason, it is the drug of choice in the emergency department setting and in situations where short courses of therapy are indicated. The major drawbacks of phenytoin are its chronic toxicities, including gingival hyperplasia, coarsening of the facial features, and hirsutism, each of which can occur even with therapeutic doses. Although less severe and less frequent in adolescents than in younger children, the side effects can still be a significant problem, particularly in young females. Phenytoin is also an enzyme-inducing agent. Therefore although widely used in emergency settings, it is infrequently used for chronic AED therapy in adolescents.

**Valproic acid** is a very effective drug in the treatment of generalized seizures of all types, including generalized tonic–clonic, absence, myoclonic, and akinetic seizures. Its structure and clinical spectrum of activity are quite different from the AEDs discussed previously. Valproate is a first line drug of choice in the treatment of myoclonic and akinetic seizures and of photoconvulsive epilepsy.[14,15] An intravenous formulation is available. In a clinical trial it was the most effective drug for the secondarily generalized epilepsies.[14,15,22] Some authors consider valproic acid the drug of choice for all primary generalized epilepsies.[6,15] The major advantages of valproic acid are its broad spectrum of activity against all types of generalized seizures and its relative lack of cognitive side effects.[20] The disadvantages are its potential toxicities, the most common of which is nausea. Less common side effects include weight gain, alopecia (usually transient), tremor, and hyperammonemia. The latter, which is often asymptomatic, may occur in the presence of otherwise normal liver-function tests. Significance of this finding in the asymptomatic patient is unclear.

Of more concern is the occurrence of a rare idiosyncratic, fatal hepatotoxicity. At particular risk are children who are younger than 2 years of age, who have neurological handicaps, and who are taking multiple drugs. However, it has also been reported in adolescents.[23] Also of concern are the teratogenic effects of valproate, which includes a high incidence of fetal malformations (including spina bifida) and cognitive deficits in infants born to women receiving valproic acid. Valproate appears to have a significantly worse profile in terms of teratogenicity than the other commonly used AEDs.[17,18]

### NEW AEDS

**Felbamate**, although a very effective drug for partial and generalized seizures, is being used only for intractable cases due to concerns about its hepatic and hematopoietic toxicity. It should only be used by experienced epileptologists when other options have failed.[7,12,13]

**Gabapentin**[7,12,13] has been shown to be effective in adults with partial seizures. It is ineffective against absence seizures and may make them worse. Its main advantages are that it is not appreciably metabolized in humans and is excreted unchanged by the kidney. It does not alter the levels of other AEDs or comedications and does not induce the microsomal liver system. It should therefore not affect the metabolism and efficacy of oral contraceptives. Most of its usage today is in the management of pain rather than of epilepsy, but it remains a useful drug in selected patients.

**Pregabalin**,[7,12,13] which is the prodrug for gabapentin and appears to be more potent, is approved by the Food and Drug Administration (FDA) for adjunctive treatment in patients with partial seizures and of pain. It has a similar efficacy profile to gabapentin with the most frequently reported side effects being dizziness and somnolence. Other reported adverse effects include ataxia, peripheral edema, headache, and weight gain.

**Lamotrigine**[7,12,13] has been shown to be effective as add-on therapy in adults with partial seizures and generalized seizures. The most notable side effect is the occurrence of a rash that can progress to full-blown Stevens-Johnson syndrome. Children are more susceptible. The rash is unusual because it can occur even after several months of therapy if the dose is increased. For this reason titration is very slow. The adverse effect profile is otherwise favorable, including lack of enzyme induction and a relatively favorable teratogenicity profile.[7] In randomized trials lamotrigine was superior to carbamazepine on a combined efficacy tolerability measure.[24] It is considered first line therapy for partial and generalized seizures, especially in women of childbearing potential. Lamotrigine is strongly affected by other AEDs. The usual dose in monotherapy in adults and adolescents is 300 mg to 400 mg per day. That dose is often doubled in the presence of an enzyme-inducing AED and is halved if also taking valproate. In addition, although lamotrigine does not alter the metabolism of oral contraceptives, its metabolism is affected by them. This aspect of lamotrigine use in adolescent girls is important to consider.[18] Although it does require slow titration and careful attention to what other medications are being used, its favorable efficacy and adverse event profile have made it a first line drug for the treatment of partial seizures as well as of generalized seizures.[12-15,24]

**Levetiracetam**[7,12,13] is effective in the treatment of partial seizures, as well as generalized tonic–clonic seizures, and myoclonic seizures (specifically with JME) in adults and children older than 4 years. It is a relatively safe drug with no known drug interactions. Although it may have mood and behavioral side effects such as agitation, anger, anxiety, and depression, particularly at high doses, its side effect profile is favorable. It has the benefit of not being metabolized in the liver like other seizure medications, is not an enzyme inducer, and has no known significant drug–drug interactions (including with oral contraceptives). An intravenous formulation is available, allowing for rapid loading and titration in cases where it is desirable to achieve a therapeutic dose rapidly. There is insufficient experience with pregnancy outcomes, but to date the reports have been reassuring.[18] For these reasons, it is often being used in adolescent women who are entering their childbearing years.

**Tiagabine**[7] is effective in treating partial seizures. Similar to other gamma-aminobutyric acid agonists, it exacerbates absence seizures. The use of tiagabine is limited due to an unfavorable adverse event profile that includes potential exacerbation of seizures. It should only be used by experienced epileptologists when other treatments have failed.

**Topiramate**[7,12,13] is effective in treating partial and primary generalized tonic–clonic seizures. It is also effective in treating myoclonic seizures, and atonic seizures associated with the Lennox-Gastaut syndrome. The major side effect of concern is cognitive slowing, with specific effect on memory and language. Another consideration when prescribing topiramate to teenagers is its side effect of decreasing appetite, leading to weight loss. This can be either a beneficial or adverse reaction depending on the specific circumstances. Other side effects include nephrolithiasis, open angle glaucoma, and metabolic acidosis, which can adversely affect bone health. Although an effective drug, topiramate has not become a first line agent due to its unfavorable cognitive side effect profile.

**Zonisamide**[7,12,13] is a broad spectrum drug that has been used to treat partial, primary generalized tonic–clonic, absence, atonic, and myoclonic seizures. Although zonisamide has some interactions with other medications, it does not have any interactions with oral contraceptives. Another benefit of zonisamide, specifically for adolescents, is the once-daily dosing. It should be noted that zonisamide is a sulfonamide and should not be administered to patients with known hypersensitivity to this drug class. Some of the side effects of this drug include somnolence, dizziness, weight loss, headache, nausea, and irritability. It is not considered a first line agent but can be a useful agent in adjunctive therapy.

## THERAPEUTIC DOSAGE RANGE AND DRUG MONITORING

The ability to measure serum drug levels has led to a greater understanding of the pharmacokinetics of

AEDs and has permitted correlations between serum levels and both clinical efficacy and toxicity. Although the availability of serum drug levels is important, it should be understood that the therapeutic range is a statistical concept based on studies of small populations of patients with epilepsy. Thus, many patients will be fully controlled on a dose that produces a "subtherapeutic" level. Conversely, some adolescents may become toxic with serum levels in the therapeutic range. As a general rule, any adolescent patient on a single drug who is having no seizures and experiencing no clinical toxicity has a serum level that is therapeutic for that individual regardless of the numeric value. It should also be noted that the "therapeutic range" is calibrated for morning trough levels, whereas random levels obtained in the office or clinic are generally closer to peak levels. This is particularly important to consider when dealing with drugs such as valproate, which, because of their short serum half-life, will have large differences between peak and trough levels. It should also be noted that the correlation between serum levels and a therapeutic response is not well established for most of the newer AEDs and that the utility of monitoring levels in these drugs is not clear.

Despite previous caveats, drug monitoring is a useful tool in the management of adolescents with epilepsy.[25] When initiating therapy, the concept of a therapeutic range enables one to choose a drug dosage that will result in full control without undue toxicity most of the time. If one achieves control of seizures with a given drug dosage, obtaining a baseline level is useful, particularly in the growing adolescent, in whom changes in metabolism and body weight over time may lead to significant changes in the serum drug level achieved by a given dose. Last, but not least, serum drug levels are a useful, though very imperfect, way of monitoring adherence, which is a major problem in adolescents. Adherence is a particularly difficult problem with AEDs because they must be taken daily for years, often have unwanted side effects (hirsutism, sedation, etc), and have a social stigma associated with their use. In addition, there are medicolegal issues that require monitoring the adolescent with epilepsy who wishes to drive. Adolescence is a time of profound metabolic changes. The therapeutic level ranges are the same as for adults. However, the dosage requirements change throughout adolescence because of changes in body weight and composition as well as pharmacokinetic changes in the drug's half-life.

## DRUG–DRUG INTERACTIONS

Antiepileptic drugs, especially the older ones, which were enzyme inducers and protein bound, had many drug–drug interactions. Comprehensive reviews are available[7] but are beyond the scope of this chapter. A few general principles are worth noting. The most common drug interactions are due to competition for protein binding and induction of the hepatic microsomal enzyme system, especially cytochrome P450. Many AEDs are protein bound, some heavily. The presence of another protein-bound drug will alter the protein-bound fraction of both drugs. This will in turn affect the clearance, as well as the toxicity, both of which depend on the free fraction of the drugs. Antiepileptic drugs, particularly phenobarbital, but also phenytoin and carbamazepine, induce the hepatic microsomal enzyme system. This induction causes increased biotransformation of all liver-metabolized drugs, including other AEDs, theophylline, steroids, and oral contraceptives. The latter is of particular importance to the physician treating adolescents, as there have been several reports of failure of oral contraception in women also taking AEDs.[7,17,26,27] The interaction with theophylline is also of importance, as it is a drug with a very narrow therapeutic window that can be altered by initiating or stopping AED therapy. Enzyme-inducing agents can also have adverse effects on bone health even in children and adolescents.[28,29] One of the main advantages of the newer AEDs is the relative lack of both protein binding and enzyme induction in many of them that reduces the risk of drug–drug interactions and thus makes them particularly useful for use in populations with comorbid medical conditions that require medications or in women who may be using oral contraceptives.

## BONE HEALTH

Recently, it has been found that many AEDs have adverse effects on bone health, with lower bone density and an increased rate of osteopenia and even osteoporosis diagnosed in adults who have been on chronic therapy for many years. Of particular concern are the enzyme-inducing AEDs including carbamazepine, oxcarbazepine, phenobarbital, phenytoin, and primidone. There is evidence that they may reduce bone density by increased metabolism of vitamin D. However, valproate may also reduce bone density, and there is concern about topiramate and zonisamide because acidosis increases bone resorption. There is now reason to be concerned even in adolescents. A recent study of ambulatory children ages 6 to 18 years with epilepsy demonstrated significant bone mineral density deficits compared to controls during the initial 1 to 5 years of treatment, which progressively worsened thereafter.[28,29] Therefore bone health should be added to the list of concerns in managing the adolescent with epilepsy. It influences choice of initial therapy as well as suggests the need for monitoring bone density in adolescents on chronic AED therapy.[28-30]

## EPILEPSY SURGERY

A major development in the treatment of intractable epilepsy has been the increased availability of epilepsy surgery.[3,7,31] Recent advances in our ability to localize the epileptic focus has made this procedure, which had been sparingly used for more than 40 years, an increasingly used option in comprehensive epilepsy centers. Even though there is some controversy regarding the use of epilepsy surgery in young children, in adolescents the indications for epilepsy surgery are the same as for adults. Epilepsy surgery is particularly valuable in those with temporal lobe epilepsy, where the success rates in properly selected patients is 70% to 80%.[31]

Candidates for epilepsy surgery must meet specific eligibility criteria, including the exclusion of nonepileptic events, failure to achieve control with optimal pharmacologic management, consistent localization to a single focus in a surgically accessible area, localization to an area that is not neuropsychologically vital, and a high likelihood of substantial improvement in function or quality of life if seizure control is improved.

The protocol for evaluation of these surgical candidates requires recording, through videotape and EEG monitoring, of a sufficient number of seizures to electrographically localize the single source of origin. This is particularly important in patients who have more than 1 clinically distinguishable seizure type.

Initially, all patients receive an extensive outpatient evaluation, that may include an EEG, computed tomography (CT), MRI, single photon emission computed tomography (SPECT), or positron emission tomography (PET) scan, and neuropsychological testing. These tests are designed to yield as much information as possible for the epileptologist. In patients previously followed in a community setting, an effort is made to manage their seizures with medications. Patients who are felt to be candidates for surgery after this initial screening will then have prolonged video and EEG monitoring to record the precise location of their seizure onset. To record a sufficient number of seizures, it is often necessary to reduce the antiepileptic medications. This then requires inpatient monitoring, as patients are at significant risk of having many or prolonged seizures. The monitoring data are then analyzed. If prolonged EEG monitoring (Phase I) supports eligibility for surgery but does not adequately localize the focus, recording electrodes may then be surgically placed via a craniotomy, either onto the surface of the brain or within it, using depth electrodes or a subdural grid (Phase II). This allows more precise localization of the epileptic focus but requires an invasive procedure.

As part of the presurgical assessment, detailed neuropsychological evaluation also is required. This testing assists localization by defining specific areas of cognitive defect, as well as areas necessary for vital functions such as speech and memory. It also helps to assess the patient's baseline level of functioning for comparison with the patient's abilities after surgery and subsequent alterations in the pharmacological regimen.

Patients who are deemed appropriate surgical candidates undergo focal resection. The ideal candidate is an adolescent or young adult who has no other neurological deficits and has normal intelligence, no motor deficits, and a single consistent EEG focus.[7,31] An abnormal MRI or CT with a focal abnormality in the same area is also a favorable prognostic sign, presumably because it increases the probability that the area being resected is in fact the site of origin of the seizures. The success rate in the best group is greater than 80%, with success being defined as complete or almost complete seizure control on AEDs. Excellent results are also achieved in patients with temporal lobe foci even when no mass lesions are present, particularly in the presence of mesial temporal sclerosis. Special coronal views with thin cuts are often needed to detect mesial temporal sclerosis, which can be missed on routine MRI. The field is rapidly evolving, with ever-improving neuroimaging modalities and EEG localization techniques. At this time, surgery should be seriously considered for any adolescent with intractable partial seizures, particularly if they have no other neurological deficits and a single EEG focus.

## SINGLE SEIZURE

Recent prospective studies have shown that the risk of seizure recurrence following a first unprovoked seizure in adolescents is 30% to 40%.[11,32-35] Risk factors for recurrence include a remote symptomatic etiology and an abnormal EEG. However, even adolescents with positive risk factors have recurrence risks of 60% to 70%. Treatment with AEDs lowers the risk of having a second seizure but does not alter long-term prognosis.[34-38] For this reason, as well as the morbidity associated with drug therapy, many neurologists and pediatricians now feel that therapy is usually not indicated in the adolescent with a first seizure.[35-37] This is particularly true in females who are entering their childbearing years and in adolescents who are about to start driving. In both settings, waiting until at least a second seizure occurs will avoid committing the adolescent to long-term medications until it is sure they are needed. However, it is important to note that an adolescent with JME who has been having myoclonus, and presents with his or her first generalized tonic-clonic seizure may not be treated as a first-time seizure patient, as the myoclonic seizures are seizures as well.

Similarly, many adolescents seek medical attention for a tonic–clonic seizure, often after sleep deprivation, but on careful history have a history of complex partial seizures for several months.[9,37]

Whatever the decision, it must be made jointly by the physician, the adolescent, and the family after careful discussion, including not only an assessment of the risks and benefits of treatment but also a review of measures to be taken in the event of a recurrence. Even adolescents with good prognostic factors may experience a recurrence. Informed decision making will allow the adolescent and the family to select the risks with which they are most comfortable. It is the author's experience that, when adolescents and families are informed of the risks of another seizure and its potential consequences, as well as the morbidity and consequences of AED therapy, they rarely opt to initiate or continue drug therapy after a single seizure.

## PROGNOSIS OF SEIZURES

Although studies based on tertiary care centers specializing in refractory epilepsy have shown a low rate of remission, population-based studies show exactly the opposite.[3] The best available data on seizure remission come from longitudinal studies of the population of Rochester, Minnesota.[2,39] Within 6 years of the diagnosis of epilepsy, 42% of patients had been seizure-free for 5 years either on or off medication. By 20 years, 70% had been seizure-free for 5 years, and 50% were seizure-free off medications. The probability of attaining remission was highest in those with idiopathic epilepsy and onset of seizures prior to age 10. The probability of being at least 5 years seizure-free 10 years after diagnosis was 75% in those with onset of seizures prior to 10 years of age, 68% in those with onset between 10 and 19 years of age, and only 63% for those with onset above 20 years of age. The group with the worst outcomes were those with neurologic dysfunction since birth. However, even those patients had a 46% probability of being seizure-free for 5 years or more within 20 years of the onset of their epilepsy. More recently, a population-based study from Finland of childhood onset seizures reported similar results.[40] The favorable prognosis of a younger age of onset presumably reflects the capacity of the immature central nervous system to "outgrow" seizures as it matures.

## PUBERTY AND SEIZURES

A variety of disorders, both neurological (epilepsy, migraine) and nonneurological (asthma), tend to either remit or have their onset in adolescence. It would seem logical to conclude that, in addition to central nervous system development and maturation, systemic maturation may also be an important variable in the onset and remission of seizures. Therefore, one would assume that neurological factors associated with puberty most likely play a role. Nevertheless, at present, a definitive link between seizure onset or remission and puberty has not been shown.[3,39-41] In fact, a variety of epidemiologic studies, as well as studies on the remission of childhood seizures and on withdrawing AEDs in children[37,39-44] do not show a reproducible pattern that correlates with puberty. Studies of the long-term prognosis of seizures suggest that the probability of attaining remission is more a function of the age of onset and the duration of the seizure disorder rather than puberty, per se. However, studies of the relationship between puberty and seizure disorders have been less than satisfying due to the inadequate definition of puberty. Few investigators have even used Tanner staging and none has used endocrine markers of puberty.

## WITHDRAWING ANTIEPILEPTIC DRUGS

The available data suggest that adolescents who are seizure-free on medication for 2 or more years have a very high likelihood of remaining in remission after medications are withdrawn.[37,42-44] The clinician must decide how long to maintain an adolescent on medications before attempting to discontinue them. This decision will be influenced by a variety of factors, including the probability of remaining seizure-free after withdrawal in a given patient, the potential risk of injury from a seizure recurrence, and the potential adverse effects of continued AED therapy.

A large number of prospective and retrospective studies involving more than 4,000 children and adolescents have been done over the past 20 years and have been analyzed.[37,44] The overall results have been very similar.[37,42-45] Between 60% and 90% of children with epilepsy who have been seizure-free for more than 2 years on medications remain seizure-free when AEDs are withdrawn. Furthermore, the majority of recurrences occur shortly after medication withdrawal, with almost half the relapses occurring within 6 months of medication withdrawal, and 60% to 80% within one year.

Recent studies indicate that there are no major differences between stopping after a 2-year seizure-free period compared with a 4-year period. Favorable risk factors for withdrawing medications include cryptogenic epilepsy, a normal EEG prior to discontinuing medications, and age of onset under 12 years.[37,42-45] Puberty has no effect on the success rate.[37,42,43] One should remember that the adolescent usually still lives in a relatively supervised environment. It is often far safer to attempt discontinuation of AEDs while adolescents are still living at home and before they start driving or become pregnant. The authors[37] recommend attempting to discontinue AEDs in adolescents with reasonable risk factors as long as the patient and the family understand the risks involved. The authors are even more aggressive in trying to withdraw adolescent females from AEDs due to the teratogenicity of the drugs, and the need to determine whether they are necessary before pregnancy occurs. When planning to discontinue AEDs one should also take into account other factors such as the adolescent beginning to drive a car or going away to college.

When discontinuing AEDs, one must consider not only the half-life of the drug but also the potentially lower seizure threshold of the patient with epilepsy, even after a 2-year seizure-free interval. On the other hand, once the decision to withdraw medications has been made, there is no justification for tapering them over years. A recent randomized study found no difference in recurrence rates between children whose AEDs were tapered over 6 weeks and those tapered over 9 months.[45] The author, in general, tapers each drug over a 1- to 3-month period, depending on the dosage, the serum level, and the type of medication.

## EPILEPSY AND PREGNANCY

In treating a pregnant adolescent with seizures, the physician must try to maintain the patient in a seizure-free state while minimizing drug toxicity and the possible teratogenic effects on the fetus.[17,18,26,27] Pregnant women often require higher doses of their regular AEDs because of alterations of drug clearance (both volume of distribution and metabolism) in pregnancy. In addition, there is a much higher incidence of nonadherence, secondary to concerns about teratogenicity. Less commonly, the underlying seizure disorder is exacerbated by pregnancy.

Most of the teratogenic effects of AEDs occur in the first 6 to 8 weeks of gestation. Because adolescent pregnancies often are unplanned, this implies that by the time the pregnancy is confirmed, these effects have generally already occurred and underscores the importance of the adolescent girl using reliable contraception if she is sexually active. Therefore it is usually too late to consider changing to other AEDs with lower teratogenicity. In general, major changes in the AED regimen during pregnancy are not recommended because the risks of uncontrolled seizures during the changeover period that can cause damage to the fetus (due to direct injury or metabolic factors such as maternal hypotension) outweigh the possible benefits to the mother and fetus.[17,26,27]

Recent evidence suggests that valproate has a particularly high rate of adverse effects on the fetus including fetal malformations and in particular spina bifida, but also decreased cognitive levels in children exposed to valproate in utero.[17,18,26,27] There is now a growing consensus that when possible, it is a drug to be avoided during pregnancy. It has also been recommended that pregnant women receiving valproic acid therapy undergo prenatal diagnosis with amniocentesis and ultrasonography.[17,26] More recently, carbamazepine has also been linked with neural tube defects[17,18] although the magnitude of the risk is not yet clear. In general, supplementation with folic acid (1 mg to 2 mg daily) is recommended for all females of childbearing age on AEDs to help reduce the risk of neural tube defects.[26,27]

It should be emphasized that these issues affect the choice of therapy of adolescent women who will often be on AEDs for many years. But pregnancy is not the time to switch AEDs. By the time a woman knows she is pregnant most of the teratogenic effects will have occurred. Switching drugs at that point exposes the woman and the fetus to the risks of seizures and to potential effects of the new agent, though probably too late to avoid the adverse effects of the original AED. Furthermore, although some AEDs have a worse profile than others, seizures also have an adverse impact on pregnancy outcomes, and their effect was as significant as that of any AED including valproate. Therefore efficacy of the AED is also a key factor, and even valproate is a rational choice for some women if it is the drug that controls seizures where others have failed.

## SPORTS

In recent years, pediatricians and neurologists alike have recognized that with proper medical management, good seizure control, and proper supervision, adolescents with epilepsy may participate in most competitive sports. The AAP now recommends that epilepsy per se should not be considered a sufficient reason to exclude a child from contact sports, and that each case be evaluated on its own merits.[46] Certain activities such as competitive underwater swimming, high diving, and rope climbing, where the occurrence of a seizure could be unusually dangerous, should be avoided. The new policy recognizes that sports and athletic activities are important for the physical and emotional well-being of children and adolescents and undue limitations to "be on the safe side" do more harm than good.

## DRIVING

Patients with epilepsy whose seizures are fully controlled on medications are legally allowed to drive in every state in the United States and in almost all developed countries. The precise reporting and certification requirements as well as the required seizure-free period vary tremendously among different jurisdictions. In the United States, specific information on the requirements in any particular jurisdiction can be obtained through the Epilepsy Foundation of America (www.epilepsyfoundation.org) or through the American Epilepsy Society (www.aesnet.org) Adolescents with epilepsy often view driving as an important issue.The ability to drive validates to them that they can indeed lead a relatively unrestricted life. The author will, in general, permit adolescents whose seizures are well controlled to drive as long as there is a reasonable expectation of adherence. However, it should be noted that accident rates in patients with epilepsy, particularly in young males, are somewhat higher than in the general population.[47] It must be understood that driving is a privilege, not a right, and that in return for the privilege, adherence to a medication regimen is expected. Because most adolescents who are seizure-free for more than a year will remain so and become candidates for medication withdrawal, it is often reasonable to delay driving by a few years so that an attempt at medication withdrawal can be made first.

## PSYCHOSOCIAL ADAPTATION

In treating the adolescent with epilepsy, the physician must recognize that controlling seizures with AEDs is not enough. Psychosocial problems in patients with epilepsy are frequent and are often more debilitating than the seizures themselves.[3,48-50] It is not uncommon to see an adolescent with relatively mild, well-controlled epilepsy whose emotional development and growth have been severely hampered by the family's inability to deal with the fear of a seizure.The psychosocial problems noted in these patients are due to several factors, including the presence of chronic illness,[3,7,48-51] the patient's fears about epilepsy, and the social stigma associated with epilepsy.[3,7,48-51] Although only a few studies have investigated the specific psychosocial problems of adolescents[3,50,51] these confirm the wide extent of psychosocial problems encountered in adolescents with epilepsy. Additional studies are needed to evaluate the differences between psychosocial problems encountered in adolescents and adults, and whether appropriate early interventions in adolescence may prevent some of the problems encountered in adult life.

## REFERENCES

1. Hauser WA, Annegers JF, Kurland LT. Incidence of epilepsy and unprovoked seizures in Rochester, Minnesota 1935 through 1984. *Epilepsia.* 1993;34:453–468

2. Hauser WA, Hesdorffer DC. *Epilepsy: Frequency, Causes, and Consequences*. New York, NY: Demos Medical Publishing; 1990

3. Shinnar S, Amir N, Branski D, eds. *Childhood Seizures.* Basel, Switzerland: S Karger; 1995

4. Commission on Classification and Terminology of the International League against Epilepsy. Proposal for revised clinical and electroencephalographic classification of epileptic seizures. *Epilepsia.* 1981;22:489–501

5. Roger J, Dreifuss FE, Martinez-Lage M, et al. Proposal for revised classification of epilepsies and epileptic syndromes. *Epilepsia.* 1989;30:389–399

6. Roger J, Bureau M, Dravet C, Genton P, Tassinari CA, Wolf P, eds. *Epileptic Syndromes in Infancy, Childhood, and Adolescence with Video*. 4th ed with video. London: John-Libbey Eurotext; 2006

7. Pellock JM, Bourgeois BFD, Dodson WE, eds. *Pediatric Epilepsy: Diagnosis and Therapy*. 3rd ed. New York, NY: Demos; 2008

8. Greenberg DA, Durner M, Resor S, Rosenbaum D, Shinnar S. The genetics of idiopathic generalized epilepsies of adolescent onset: differences between juvenile myoclonic epilepsy and epilepsy with random grand mal and with awakening grand mal. *Neurology.* 1995;45:942–946

9. Hirtz D, Ashwal S, Berg A, et al. Practice parameter: evaluating a first nonfebrile seizure in children: Report of the Quality Standards Subcommittee of the American Academy of Neurology, the Child Neurology Society, and the American Epilepsy Society. *Neurology.* 2000;55:616–623

10. Krumholz A, Wiebe S, Gronseth G, et al. Quality Standards Subcommittee of the American Academy of Neurology; American Epilepsy Society. Practice parameter: evaluating an apparent unprovoked first seizure in adults (an evidence-based review): Report of the Quality Standards Subcommittee of the American Academy of Neurology and the American Epilepsy Society. *Neurology.* 2007;69:1996–2007

11. Shinnar S, Berg AT, Moshe SL, et al. The risk of seizure recurrence following a first unprovoked afebrile seizure in childhood: an extended follow-up. *Pediatrics.* 1996;98:216–225

12. French JA, Kanner AM, Bautista J, et al. Efficacy and tolerability of the new antiepileptic drugs I: Treatment of new onset epilepsy: Report of the Therapeutics and Technology Assessment Subcommittee and Quality Standards Subcommittee of the American Academy of Neurology and the American Epilepsy Society. *Neurology.* 2004;62:1252–1260

13. French JA, Kanner AM, Bautista J, et al. Efficacy and tolerability of the new antiepileptic drugs II: Treatment of refractory epilepsy: Report of the Therapeutics and Technology Assessment Subcommittee and Quality Standards

Subcommittee of the American Academy of Neurology and the American Epilepsy Society. *Neurology.* 2004;62:1261–1273

14. Karceski S, Morrell MJ, Carpenter D. Treatment of epilepsy in adults: expert opinion, 2005. *Epilepsy Behav.* 2005;7(suppl 1):S1–S64

15. Wheless JW, Clarke DF, Arzimanoglou A, Carpenter D. Treatment of pediatric epilepsy: European expert opinion, 2007. *Epileptic Disord.* 2007;9:353–412

16. Camfield CS, Camfield PR, Smith E, Tibbles JAR. Asymptomatic children with epilepsy: little benefit from screening for anticonvulsant-induced liver, blood, and renal damage. *Neurology.* 1986;36:838–841

17. Commission on Genetics, Pregnancy, and the Child, International League Against Epilepsy. Guidelines for the care of women of childbearing age with epilepsy. *Epilepsia.* 1993;34:588–589

18. Meador K, Reynolds MW, Crean S, Fahrbach K, Probst C. Pregnancy outcomes in women with epilepsy: a systematic review and meta-analysis of published pregnancy registries and cohorts. *Epilepsy Res.* 2008;81:1–13

19. Mattson RH, Cramer JA, Collins JF, et al. Comparison of carbamazepine, phenobarbital, phenytoin, and primidone in partial and secondarily generalized tonic-clonic seizures. *N Engl J Med.* 1985;313:145–151

20. Vining EPG, Mellits ED, Dorsen MM, et al. Psychologic and behavioral effects of antiepileptic drugs in children: a double-blind comparison between phenobarbital and valproic acid. *Pediatrics.* 1987;80:165–174

21. Brent DA, Crumrine PK, Varma RR, Allan M, Allman C. Phenobarbital treatment and major depressive disorder in children with epilepsy. *Pediatrics.* 1987;80:909–917

22. Marson AG, Al-Kharusi AM, Alwaidh M, et al. The SANAD study of effectiveness of valproate, lamotrigine, or topiramate for generalised and unclassifiable epilepsy: an unblinded randomised controlled trial. *Lancet.* 2007;369(9566):1016–1026

23. Scheffner D, St. Konig J, Rauterberg-Ruland I, Kochen W, Hoffman WJ, St. Unkelbach. Fatal liver failure in 16 children with valproate therapy. *Epilepsia.* 1988;29:530–542

24. Marson AG, Al-Kharusi AM, Alwaidh M, et al. The SANAD study of effectiveness of carbamazepine, gabapentin, lamotrigine, oxcarbazepine, or topiramate for treatment of partial epilepsy: an unblinded randomised controlled trial. *Lancet.* 2007;369(9566):1000–1015

25. Commission on Antiepileptic Drugs, International League Against Epilepsy. Guidelines for therapeutic monitoring on antiepileptic drugs. *Epilepsia.* 1993;34:585–587

26. Morrell MJ. Guidelines for the care of women with epilepsy. *Neurology.* 1998;51(5 suppl 4):S21–27

27. Zahn CA, Morrell MJ, Collins SD, Labiner DM, Yerby MS. Management issues for women with epilepsy: a review of the literature. *Neurology.* 1998;51(4):949–956

28. Sheth RD, Binkley N, Hermann BP. Progressive bone deficit in epilepsy. *Neurology.* 2008;70(3):170–176

29. Abou-Khalil BW. Why should clinicians worry about bone density for patients with epilepsy? *Epilepsy Currents.* 2008;8:148–149

30. Petty SJ, O'Brien TJ, Wark JD. Anti-epileptic medication and bone health. *Osteoporos Int.* 2007;18(2): 129–142

31. Engel J Jr, Wiebe S, French J, et al. Practice parameter: temporal lobe and localized neocortical resections for epilepsy: Report of the Quality Standards Subcommittee of the American Academy of Neurology, in Association with the American Epilepsy Society and the American Association of Neurological Surgeons. *Neurology.* 2003;60:538–547

32. Hauser WA, Anderson VE, Loewenson RB, McRoberts SM. Seizure recurrence after a first unprovoked seizure. *N Engl J Med.* 1982;307:522–528

33. Berg AT, Shinnar S. The risk of seizure recurrence following a first unprovoked seizure: a quantitative review. *Neurology.* 1991;41:965–972

34. First Seizure Trial Group. Randomized clinical trial on the efficacy of antiepileptic drugs in reducing the risk of relapse after a first unprovoked tonic–clonic seizure. *Neurology.* 1993;43:478–483

35. Hirtz D, Berg A, Bettis D et al. Practice parameter: treatment of the child with a first unprovoked seizure. Report of the QSS of the AAN and the Practice Committee of the CNS. *Neurology.* 2003;60:166–175

36. Musicco M, Beghi E, Solari A, and the First Seizure Trial Group. Effect of antiepileptic treatment initiated after the first unprovoked seizure on the long-term prognosis of epilepsy. *Neurology.* 1994;44(suppl 2):A337–A338

37. O'Dell C, Shinnar S. Initiation and discontinuation of antiepileptic drugs. *Neurologic Clinics.* 2001;19:289–311

38. Shinnar S, Berg AT. Does antiepileptic drug therapy alter the prognosis of childhood seizures and prevent the development of chronic epilepsy? *Seminars in Pediatric Neurology* 1994;1:111–117

39. Annegers JF, Hauser WA, Elveback LR. Remission of seizures and relapse in patients with epilepsy. *Epilepsia.* 1979;20:729–737

40. Sillanpaa M, Jalava M, Kaleva O, Shinnar S. Long-term prognosis of seizures with onset in childhood. *N Engl J Med.* 1998;338:1715–1722

41. Diamantopoulos N, Crumrine PK. The effect of puberty on the course of epilepsy. *Arch Neurol.* 1986;43:873–876

42. Holowach-Thurston J, Thurston DL, Hixon BB, Keller AJ. Prognosis in childhood epilepsy: additional follow-up of 148 children 15 to 23 years after withdrawal of anticonvulsant therapy. *N Engl J Med.* 1982;306:831–836

43. Shinnar S, Berg AT, Moshe SL, et al. Discontinuing antiepileptic drugs in children with epilepsy: a prospective study. *Ann Neurol.* 1994;35:534–545

44. Berg AT, Shinnar S. Relapse following discontinuation of antiepileptic drugs: a meta-analysis. *Neurology.* 1994; 44:601–608

45. Tennison M, Greenwood R, Lewis D, Thorn M. Discontinuing antiepileptic drugs in children with epilepsy: a comparison of a six-week and nine-month taper period. *N Engl J Med.* 1994;330:1407–1410

46. American Academy of Pediatrics. Committee on Children with Handicaps and Committee on Sports Medicine. Sports and the child with epilepsy. *Pediatrics.* 1983;72:884–885

47. Hansotia P, Broste SK. The effect of epilepsy or diabetes mellitus on the risk of automobile accidents. *N Engl J Med.* 1991;324:22–26

48. Dodrill CB, Breyer DN, Diamond MB, Dubinsky BL, Geary BB. Psychosocial problems among adults with epilepsy. *Epilepsia.* 1984; 25:168–175

49. Hoare P. Does illness foster dependency: a study of epileptic and diabetic children. *Dev Med Child Neurol.* 1984;26:20–24

50. Ziegler RG. Impairments of control and competence in epileptic children and their families. *Epilepsia.* 1981;22:339–346

51. Westbrook LE, Silver EJ, Coupey SM, Shinnar S. Social characteristics of adolescents with idiopathic epilepsy: a comparison to chronically ill and non chronically ill peers. *J Epilepsy.* 1991;4:87–94

# CHAPTER 128

# Motor Unit Disorders

ALFRED J. SPIRO, MD

Motor unit disorders are those that affect the anterior horn cells of the spinal cord, portions of the peripheral nerve, the myoneural junction, and/or the muscle cells. Although many of the more common disorders of the motor unit, such as spinal muscular atrophy (SMA types 2 and 3) and Duchenne muscular dystrophy (DMD), are clinically apparent in infancy or childhood, several motor unit disorders characteristically become apparent or have their major effect on the patient and family during the adolescent years.

## APPROACH TO THE PATIENT

The cardinal symptoms of a motor unit disorder are muscle weakness and/or sensory complaints such as numbness or tingling. Weakness may be manifested by difficulty in walking, running, rope climbing, and raising the arms above the head or a decrease in athletic abilities. To determine whether facial muscle weakness is present, for example, as in facioscapulohumeral muscular dystrophy (FSHMD), patients should be asked whether they can whistle normally or whether their eyelids are open during sleep. Appropriate questioning will reveal whether patients have been toe walkers in childhood, as in Becker' muscular dystrophy (BMD) or in SMA (type 3), or whether they trip easily while walking, which suggests weakness of the anterior tibialis muscles, as noted in peripheral neuropathies. Inquiries should be made about abnormal functional capacity of the hands, as seen in peripheral neuropathy or myotonic dystrophy—for example, by asking about difficulty in opening jars, using a screwdriver, or writing. Patients should be asked whether they have difficulty letting go of objects, a symptom common in myotonic dystrophy. Although it occasionally is difficult to ascertain when symptoms were originally noted, every effort should be made to obtain this information, because the duration of illness can be important in establishing a definitive diagnosis. Old photographs or videotapes of the patient sometimes may provide useful information. Inquiries also should be made concerning the presence of muscle pain or pigmented urine, as evidenced in some inflammatory or metabolic myopathies. In addition, patients should be asked whether they have been paralyzed in the past, even for a brief period, a clue that would suggest a periodic paralysis. They also should be questioned about easy fatigability, double vision, and dysphagia, and about the variability of these symptoms, as observed in myasthenia gravis (MG). Because many motor unit disorders are inherited, a careful genetic history should be undertaken. At times, examination of other family members for preclinical involvement is indicated.

Certain details of the physical examination should be stressed. These include assessment of gait, ability to walk on the heels and toes and to climb stairs, scoliosis, highly arched feet, increase in lumbar lordosis, and muscle enlargement or wasting; manual muscle testing; testing for deep tendon reflexes and sensory abnormalities and extraocular muscle weakness; and tests for shoulder, neck, and facial muscle weakness.

Genetic and other studies can be helpful in arriving at a correct diagnosis when correlated to clinical data. Electromyography (EMG), performed with needle electrodes, records electrical activity from the muscle itself. Determination of nerve conduction velocities (NCV), sensory and motor, is a test done with surface electrodes. The physician ordering the tests must remember that they are uncomfortable, sometimes painful, and expensive. For ancillary studies to be useful, they should be performed by a physician who has an understanding of the information sought. Serum muscle enzyme determinations, particularly creatine kinase (CK) levels, can be useful in searching for a primary muscular disorder. However, in some muscle disorders seen in adolescents, for example, in FSHMD, the CK level may be normal. In selected instances a muscle biopsy can provide a definitive diagnosis, provided that appropriate morphologic, histochemical, biochemical, and any other necessary studies are performed. A muscle biopsy should not be taken unless state-of-the-art studies can be obtained.[1]

There are many clinics supported by the Muscular Dystrophy Association to which a patient with a motor unit disorder can be referred for diagnosis and multidisciplinary management.

## ANTERIOR HORN CELL DISEASE

Since the virtual eradication of poliomyelitis, with the exception of West Nile disease, the most common disorder of anterior horn cells observed in adolescents is SMA type 3.[2] This is a genetically determined disorder in which the primary lesion is degeneration of the anterior horn cells, resulting in wasting of the skeletal musculature. The inheritance pattern is generally autosomal recessive, but autosomal dominant types (in late onset SMA) or, rarely, X-linked recessive forms are known. The recessive form has been mapped to the long arm of chromosome 5, and prenatal diagnosis is possible in selected informative families.

The clinical characteristics of SMA type 3 include painless proximal symmetric muscle weakness and atrophy, with manifestations more pronounced in the legs than in the arms. Initial symptoms usually consist of difficulty in running, climbing stairs, or arising from a chair; toe walking, enlarged calves, and a waddling gait may be prominent. Intellectual function is generally normal, as are the muscles supplied by the cranial nerves. An increase in the normal lumbar lordosis may be apparent, and scoliosis and joint contractures may develop. Muscle fasciculations are present in only a few patients. Deep tendon reflexes are reduced or absent, and toe responses and sensations are normal. A mild irregular tremulousness (minipolymyoclonus) of the outstretched hands may be apparent. Spinal muscular atrophy type 3 is usually static or slowly progressive; however, in some patients it can lead to wheelchair status.

The diagnosis of SMA type 3 is established when the clinical picture is coupled with (1) normal serum muscle enzymes (although the CK level can be moderately elevated), (2) neuropathic EMG with normal NCV (although in some instances an element of myopathic dysfunction may be present), and (3) DNA confirmation. DNA studies are available in several commercial laboratories. Similar patterns of weakness may be observed in BMD, limb-girdle muscular dystrophy (LGMD), and some metabolic muscle disorders, but these can usually be distinguished through the studies already noted.

Management is symptomatic, because there is no specific therapeutic agent that will alter the course of the disease; at the time of this writing there are experimental therapeutic trials with various drugs. Physical therapy should be provided for the patient.

A disorder that may be related to SMA type 3 has been termed "juvenile type of distal and segmental muscular atrophy of the upper extremities."[3] In this disorder, commonly seen in Japan but less commonly in the United States, the onset in approximately 90% of cases occurs in the age range from 18 to 22 years. Males are affected more frequently than females. The distribution of muscular atrophy is initially limited to the hand and forearm. Deep tendon reflexes in the affected limb are hypoactive or absent, but no sensory abnormalities are noted. Rapid progression of the disease takes place during the initial 2 to 3 years after onset, with a slowly progressive course thereafter. No abnormal laboratory findings are noted, except for the results of EMG studies and structural changes on muscle biopsy that indicate neurogenic atrophy of the muscles. Although the cause of this disorder is unknown (and there does not seem to be a genetic pattern), the site of the lesion is thought to range from the fifth cervical to the first thoracic spinal segments, with intramedullary involvement. No specific therapeutic modality has been identified.

## BRACHIAL PLEXUS AND PERIPHERAL NERVES

### BRACHIAL PLEXUS NEUROPATHY

Brachial plexus neuropathy[4] is observed in adolescents and adults. Although many patients with this disorder describe an antecedent illness (sometimes trivial) suggesting an autoimmune etiology, or an injection, the pathogenesis of this disorder is otherwise unknown.

The major symptom of brachial plexus neuropathy is pain in one or both shoulders. This pain may be severe and can last from a few hours to several weeks before it abates. Lessening or cessation of pain is accompanied or followed by varying degrees of weakness and atrophy of the arm muscles. Sensory loss is also extremely variable, but most patients do not exhibit weakness and/or sensory abnormalities of the entire arm, indicating incomplete or diffuse involvement of the brachial plexus. Electrodiagnostic studies may be helpful in substantiating the diagnosis of brachial plexus neuropathy.

Physical therapy, consisting of active exercise (when possible) and passive movement, should be prescribed, as well as measures to lessen pain. The prognosis for recovery is excellent, but full restitution of function may take place over a prolonged period.

### GUILLAIN-BARRÉ SYNDROME

Guillain-Barré syndrome (GBS)[5] has an incidence of 0.4 to 2 per 100,000 population. The incidence is moderately higher in females, and somewhat lower in adolescents than in older individuals. Uncertainty still exists about the exact cause of the resultant polyradiculoneuropathy, but GBS is often associated with a preceding viral infection, and there is evidence for an autoimmune mechanism.

Characteristically, but not necessarily, GBS begins approximately 1 to 2 weeks after a viral infection or other illness, surgery, or inoculation. At the onset of illness, the patient is usually afebrile. Symmetric weakness generally develops acutely or subacutely, and its degree may vary from mild to severe, with paralysis of the facial, trunk, and bulbar muscles. The extraocular muscles also may become paralyzed; in fact, in some variants (Miller-Fisher syndrome) of the disorder may begin with muscle weakness.

Areflexia is the rule in GBS, but sensory symptoms and signs are generally mild, although significant pain can be a major complaint. Autonomic dysfunction, characterized by fluctuations in blood pressure and heart rate and postural hypotension, is common. Progression of weakness generally stops approximately 3 weeks after onset of the illness. Recovery usually begins a few weeks after the cessation of the progression. Although most patients recover fully, improvement may be delayed and may take place over several months. A few patients are left with some residual weakness and joint contractures.

Diagnosis can be made on the basis of the clinical pattern coupled with the results of cerebrospinal fluid (CSF) examination and electrodiagnostic studies. The CSF protein is usually increased after the first week of symptoms, and there are generally less than 10 mononuclear cells per cubic millimeter. Electrodiagnostic tests can provide diagnostic and prognostic information early in the disease. Possible infection with *Mycoplasma*, *Campylobacter*, Epstein-Barr virus, and Lyme disease should be investigated. Other conditions, including poliomyelitis, paralysis resulting from a conversion reaction, botulism, toxic neuropathies (eg, addictive glue sniffing), acute intermittent porphyria, tick paralysis, and hypokalemic periodic paralysis, occasionally may resemble GBS, but these possibilities can be readily excluded by appropriate assessments. In addition, a GBS-like syndrome has been described in adults with acquired immunodeficiency syndrome (AIDS).

Patients diagnosed with GBS should spend the first few weeks in an intensive care unit with very careful monitoring of vital signs and respiratory function, because autonomic dysfunction and respiratory failure are important causes of complications and possible death. The immediate availability of respiratory assistance is mandatory. Intravenous administration of high doses of gamma globulin[6] has been documented to shorten the course and lessen the severity of GBS; this should be begun as early as possible and may sometimes obviate the need for respiratory assistance. Physical therapy also should be begun early in the course of the disease to prevent joint contractures.

## PERIPHERAL NEUROPATHIES

Peripheral neuropathies[7] are disorders of various causes—hereditary, toxic, traumatic, metabolic, idiopathic—that affect the function and/or structure of the peripheral nervous system. They occur in all age groups, and the manifestations can be recognized in adolescents, in whom hereditary causes are common. Sensory or motor symptoms may predominate but frequently coexist. The manifestations depend on the degree of involvement of large myelinated, small myelinated, or nonmyelinated fibers and on which portion of the peripheral nerve is involved. A peripheral neuropathy may occur with certain central nervous system (CNS) degenerative disorders in adolescents.

Symptoms include numbness, burning, or paresthesias (primarily in the hands or feet); insecurity of gait; and weakness in the fingers and/or dorsiflexors or plantiflexors of the feet. Weakness may be identified by functional muscle testing (eg, by asking patients to walk on their heels or toes, which may be difficult or impossible) and by manual muscle testing. Sensation for pain, touch, or vibration may be reduced, and deep tendon reflexes, usually ankle jerks, are absent.

Electrodiagnostic studies are extremely useful for assessing patients in whom peripheral neuropathies are suspected. A demyelinating neuropathy results in a marked decrease in motor nerve conduction velocity. In neuropathies in which axonal degeneration is the primary pathologic alteration, there is either no change or only a minor decrease in nerve conduction velocity; however, there is EMG evidence of denervation. Sensory nerve action potentials also may be assessed in conventional electrodiagnostic studies; and these may be useful in confirming the diagnosis of peripheral neuropathy.

Peripheral nerve trauma in adolescents is generally no different from trauma in other individuals. As in children and adults, there are certain vulnerabilities, such as injury to the radial nerve in the spiral groove, associated with fractures of the humerus, and trauma to the long thoracic nerve in backpackers, resulting in winging of the scapula. A problem encountered in adolescents who ride bicycles for long distances is compression neuropathy of the ulnar nerve at the wrist. This is related to riding with the hands in an extended position and the wrists pressing on the handlebars. This problem is found more commonly in the dominant hand. It is characterized by pain and tingling in the 2 ulnar fingers, with sensory abnormalities noted in the ulnar half of the ring finger; associated weakness of the muscles innervated by the ulnar nerve is sometimes also seen. A change in bicycle riding habits usually results in alleviation of symptoms.

Diabetic peripheral neuropathy is less frequently a problem in adolescents than in adults. Manifestations include numbness and paresthesias, sometimes painful, of the toes and feet, and, to a lesser extent, the fingers and hands. Loss of pain, touch, and vibratory perception are found in a glove-stocking distribution; this sign is associated with depressed deep tendon reflexes, especially ankle jerks. Abnormalities can be documented by determinations of nerve conduction velocity. Rigorous control of the diabetes may delay the onset of peripheral neuropathy or lessen the severity when it exists. Relief of symptoms sometimes can be obtained with carbamazepine. Additional drugs such as imipramine may be needed to provide symptomatic relief.

Uremic neuropathy may be observed in adolescents with chronic renal disease. Such patients develop a chronic, symmetric, and predominantly sensory neuropathy in which the major complaints are burning paresthesias, restless legs, and numbness spreading upward from the feet, and occasionally present in the hands. Motor problems, such as foot drop, also may be present. The severity of the involvement is not necessarily related to the degree of uremia. Nerve conduction velocity determinations can be used to substantiate the diagnosis. Renal dialysis may prevent the progression of the neuropathy or provide some degree of recovery when it exists. Renal transplantation, when indicated, also results in a good response.

Toxic neuropathy may be noted in adolescents who might be exposed to a wide variety of agents that potentially damage the peripheral nervous system. These include heavy metals, many industrial solvents and organic compounds, and nitrous oxide. In addition to the usual symptoms and signs of this disorder, toxic neuropathies are frequently associated with pain and weight loss. In any adolescent who has a peripheral neuropathy of unclear origin, a careful search for toxins should be undertaken.

Hereditary sensory motor neuropathies (HSMN) or Charcot-Marie-Tooth disease[8] include several disorders in which various pathologic changes in peripheral nerves play a central role. Hereditary sensory motor neuropathy type I, in which demyelination is the major alteration, and HSMN type II, in which axonal degeneration is the major pathologic condition, are the most common. Both types may become clinically apparent in the adolescent years as motor and/or sensory problems, but it is often difficult to ascribe a date of onset because the symptoms are often insidious. Hereditary sensory motor neuropathies disorders are often inherited in an autosomal-dominant pattern, but individual differences in severity of symptoms occasionally make diagnosis in the parents or a sibling of the patient difficult when an affected relative is only subclinically involved. Elucidation of the hereditary pattern often necessitates careful neurologic and electrophysiologic studies of close relatives if possible because X-linked and autosomal forms are well recognized.

Motor and sensory signs and symptoms are highly variable, but they generally involve the feet more than the hands. The initial complaints may be slowly evolving equinovarus deformity, generally symmetric, which may result in increasing tripping and difficulty in walking; this deformity also may be associated with increased fatigability after routine activities. The rate of progression is variable but usually slow. Wasting of the calf muscles may become apparent. Weakness of the hand muscles also can become a problem, as can wasting of the intrinsic muscles of the hands. Weakness, wasting, and difficulty in walking on the heels and/or toes usually can be detected at the time of examination. Sensory loss in a stocking or (less commonly) glove distribution, with diminished or absent ankle jerks, also may be noted at this time. Loss of vibratory perception is usually the most easily detected sensory abnormality. In some patients, the ability to walk independently can be lost after many years.

The diagnosis can be confirmed by electrophysiologic studies, which also can be used to characterize the defect in the peripheral nerves as axonal or demyelinating. There is no specific medical treatment; however, physical therapy, prudent bracing with acceptable orthoses, and surgery, if needed, can be helpful. Genetic counseling should be provided; DNA studies can be useful in selected cases.

Chronic (or relapsing) inflammatory demyelinating polyradiculoneuropathy (CIDP)[9] can have its onset in adolescence, although it is more commonly observed in older individuals. The pathogenesis is not fully understood but is probably related to an abnormal immune response.

The onset of symptoms is subacute. Proximal and distal symmetric muscle weakness, associated with sensory loss and diminished to absent deep tendon reflexes (especially ankle jerks), is the cardinal characteristic. Facial muscle weakness may also be present. A relapsing course is commonly observed.

Diagnosis of CIDP is substantiated when the characteristic clinical pattern is coupled with slowed NCV, usually with conduction block; an elevated CSF protein level; and a nerve biopsy specimen with characteristic features. Most patients with CIDP respond to prednisone therapy. Initially, high single daily doses of prednisone are commonly used for 2 to 4 weeks. Subsequently, single-dose, alternate-day therapy can be given until clinical improvement is achieved. Some patients with CIDP require azathioprine; others respond very quickly to high-dose intravenous gamma globulin administration. After improvement, this therapy can be maintained, with courses given when needed.

## DISORDERS OF THE MYONEURAL JUNCTION

### MYASTHENIA GRAVIS

Myasthenia gravis (MG),[10] an acquired autoimmune disorder affecting the myoneural junction, is not uncommon in adolescents. In this age group, MG is noted more frequently in females than in males.

The most common initial symptoms of MG are ptosis and/or diplopia because of selective vulnerability of the extraocular muscles. These symptoms may be variable in severity. They may not be present in the morning or if the patient is not fatigued, and therefore the diagnosis is sometimes missed. Spontaneous remission of symptoms may occur. Other clinically more severe forms of MG may occur; in these types, bulbar involvement with rapid development and progression of severe generalized weakness, and resultant ventilatory failure, are present. Because of muscle weakness, the patient may experience problems in speaking full sentences, chewing, and holding up the head. Deep tendon reflexes are characteristically preserved. No sensory abnormalities are noted.

Diagnosis can be established with edrophonium (Tensilon), an anticholinesterase drug that acts rapidly and briefly to provide prompt relief of myasthenic weakness. A test dose of 2 mg is given intravenously to determine whether the patient has any abnormal sensitivity to the drug or a beneficial response. If there are no untoward reactions, the edrophonium can be given in further small increments up to a total of 10 mg. After each dose, the response of the patient is determined by assessing changes in a specifically defined endpoint, such as the size of the palpebral fissure or the range of motility of the extraocular muscles.

Specialized electrodiagnostic studies are sometimes of great assistance in establishing the diagnosis. Antibodies against acetylcholine receptor sites, present in approximately 80% of patients with MG, also can be assessed as a definitive diagnostic measure. In seronegative individuals suspected of having MG, muscle-specific antibodies (MUSK) can be assessed. Because thymic enlargement or tumors are associated with MG, careful assessment of the thymus should be done with computed tomography or magnetic resonance imaging. Because of the association of dysthyroid states and MG, thyroid function should be assessed. In some cases of very mild ocular MG, therapy may consist of eye-patching alone if diplopia is mild. Some patients experience spontaneous remission during the first 2 years of the disease. Most patients with ocular MG need anticholinesterase drugs, the most useful of which is pyridostigmine bromide (Mestinon), for relief of symptoms. The dosage needs to be titrated to the patient's activities and response. Single-dose, alternate-day administration of prednisone is frequently required in mildly to moderately severe generalized MG.

In adolescents with MG, thymectomy may be indicated to provide long-term beneficial results, even if thymic enlargement is not demonstrated on imaging. The procedure can be done either through a sternal splitting operation or through a mediastinoscope. Each technique has its own advantages and disadvantages. Immunosuppression with azathioprine can prove useful as therapy in some cases; although this drug is usually well tolerated, its effects may not be noted for several months. When the patient experiences an acute exacerbation of severe or generalized weakness, plasmapheresis can be performed as part of the treatment. Administration of high doses of intravenous gamma globulin can be equally effective. In patients with MG in whom ventilatory failure is imminent, treatment in an intensive care unit is necessary, and intubation with respiratory assistance is frequently indicated. Patients with MG and their caretakers should be provided with a list of contraindicated drugs.[11]

### BOTULISM

Botulism[12] is another disorder of the myoneural junction in which symptoms appear within hours after ingestion of contaminated food and often are manifested in several members of the same family. Diplopia and ptosis appear rapidly, with spreading of the paralysis to produce respiratory failure. Therefore, immediate respiratory support must be provided for the patient. There are no sensory abnormalities. Repetitive nerve stimulation demonstrates the defect of the myoneural junction. Bacterial testing may be used to confirm the diagnosis.

## MYOPATHIES

### BECKER MUSCULAR DYSTROPHY AND DUCHENNE MUSCULAR DYSTROPHY

Becker muscular dystrophy and DMD[13] are X-linked recessive disorders of muscle, the major features of which are progressive muscular weakness and wasting. The prevalence of DMD is about 3 in 100,000; that of BMD is approximately one-tenth of that figure. The defective gene in both of these disorders has been isolated and is on the short arm of the X chromosome. Dystrophin, the protein product of the gene, has been identified; it is found to be absent in DMD and variably reduced or altered in BMD skeletal muscle. There is a positive relationship between the amount of dystrophin present and the severity and onset of weakness. Because virtually all boys with DMD use a wheelchair before the age of 12, are all severely affected by the time they reach adolescence but may survive for an additional decade or more. In contrast, patients with BMD generally become symptomatic at school age and frequently during adolescence or even adulthood. Adolescent boys with DMD often have scholastic learning difficulties that had been identified earlier; in addition, scoliosis must be identified and treated, as well as cardiac and pulmonary involvement. Cardiac problems, due to absence of dystrophin in cardiac muscle, can be treated with digoxin, angiotensin-converting enzyme (ACT) inhibitors, and diuretics. Pulmonary involvement can be treated with ventilatory support. Physical therapy and psychological support should be continued.

Generally, painless weakness in BMD is noted initially in the proximal muscles of the legs, although a tendency to walk on the toes may be noted earlier, along with markedly enlarged calf muscles. Manifestations include difficulty with running, climbing stairs, and riding a bicycle, and a waddling gait. Weakness and wasting of the proximal arm muscles are seen later. Progression of weakness may be slow, and patients with BMD may lead a relatively normal life for several decades. As in DMD, mental subnormality may coexist. The deep tendon reflexes are usually diminished or absent, with the exception of the ankle jerks, which are maintained indefinitely. No sensory abnormalities are present. Diagnosis of BMD is made when the characteristic clinical pattern is seen in association with high serum levels of muscle enzymes, especially CK. Elevations of CK are noted at birth, long before weakness is clinically apparent. Results of EMG studies are consistent with a myopathy; muscle biopsy is characteristic, but quantitative or qualitative abnormalities of dystrophin can substantiate the diagnosis and aid in providing a prognosis. Sequencing of the dystrophin gene is commercially available. An in-frame deletion can document the diagnosis, eliminating the necessity for a muscle biopsy. Differential diagnosis includes other syndromes in which limb-girdle weakness is present. Differentiation can be based on the changes noted in genetic studies on blood, or muscle biopsies when required. Elevated CK values can be observed in McLeod syndrome, in which acanthocytes are seen; muscle weakness is absent.

There is no specific medical management; however, appropriate physical therapy, including unlimited exercise, and genetic counseling should be provided. Daughters of affected patients are obligate carriers of the gene, but sons are uninvolved. Sisters more than 15 years of age should be checked for cardiomyopathy, which may be present in the absence of skeletal muscle weakness.

## LIMB-GIRDLE MUSCULAR DYSTROPHY

Limb-girdle muscular dystrophy[14] represents a group of disorders of either autosomal recessive or autosomal dominant inheritance in which symptoms of proximal muscle weakness may begin at virtually any age, but commonly during the second decade of life and in adolescence. Proximal muscles in the legs are generally more involved than the proximal muscles of the arms, resulting in the gait difficulties that are usually the first symptoms. Weakness may be manifested by difficulty climbing stairs or running, and it can be documented by manual and functional testing. Deep tendon reflexes are usually reduced; however, the ankle jerks may be preserved. Sensory examination results are normal. Cardiac muscle involvement is exceptionally rare.

Creatine kinase values are variable but generally elevated. Electromyogram studies can be used to document the myopathic basis, and a muscle biopsy usually helps to delineate the myopathic nature of the disorder. However, for several of the many types of LGMD, genetic studies from blood samples can confirm the diagnosis.

Treatment is symptomatic. In general, physical therapy should be aimed at preserving muscle function as long as possible and aborting joint contractures. The course of LGMD is extremely variable, but it may be severe enough to result in wheelchair status and/or dependence on a ventilator for respiration. Prenatal diagnosis is possible in selected cases.

## FACIOSCAPULOHUMERAL MUSCULAR DYSTROPHY

Facioscapulohumeral muscular dystrophy[15] is transmitted as an autosomal dominant trait. The onset may occur anytime from childhood until adulthood, but onset in adolescence is common. Facial musculature is involved initially, but there is a great potential for subsequent involvement of the shoulder-girdle musculature and of the leg muscles. Because of the limited involvement seen initially in this disorder, the patient may be described as being round-shouldered or having poor posture; diagnosis is considered when weakness in the typical distribution is detected through manual muscle testing. The diagnosis is substantiated when other members of the family are found to be similarly affected, even if muscle weakness is limited to the face and no other symptoms are present. A history of inability to whistle in the usual manner (with pursed lips), to blow up a balloon, or to puff up the cheeks frequently is noted but not volunteered by the patient. Winging of the scapulae is common. The CK values, although sometimes elevated, may be normal. Results of electrodiagnostic studies and muscle biopsies, when performed, may be extremely variable and should be correlated with the clinical findings. DNA testing can be used to confirm a clinical suspicion of FSHMD.

Treatment of this type of muscular dystrophy is symptomatic, and physical therapy is aimed at preserving muscle function. Genetic counseling should be provided. The defective gene in FSHMD has been localized to chromosome 4; prenatal diagnosis is available.

## MYOTONIC DYSTROPHY

Myotonic dystrophy type 1 (MyD),[16] an autosomal dominant disorder with a prevalence of approximately 7 in 100,000 population, often has its symptomatic onset in adolescence or the school-age years. The gene responsible for MyD is located on the long arm of chromosome 19; an abnormal expansion of a CTG sequence repeat is present. Although myotonia, or difficulty in relaxing after muscular contraction, is the characteristic feature, MyD is a multisystemic disorder. It is often associated with distal muscle weakness and wasting, frontal baldness, presenile cataracts, cardiac conduction defects, testicular atrophy, and subnormal intelligence.

The clinical picture of MyD is extremely variable and the diagnosis is frequently overlooked. In some adolescents, myotonia is recognized only when it is actively sought: for example, in mothers of "floppy babies" in whom infantile MyD is considered in the differential diagnosis. In other patients with mental retardation or hypernasality of speech, which are common features of MyD, the diagnosis is made only if percussion or reflex myotonia is sought specifically, because patients often do not complain of difficulty in relaxing muscles. Percussion myotonia is noted when the muscles of the thenar eminence are struck briskly with a reflex hammer; there is contraction of the muscle with markedly delayed relaxation. In reflex, or action, myotonia, the patient has difficulty opening the hand after grasping an object. Ptosis and an expressionless face are also common signs. Wasting of the muscles of mastication and smallness of the sternocleidomastoid muscles are typical. Wasting and weakness of the distal muscles of the limbs, sometimes leading to foot drop, may be seen. Lenticular cataracts are frequently identified on slit-lamp examination in the adolescent age group.

Electrocardiographic (ECG) abnormalities are often observed. The course of MyD is variable; in some cases there is a slow deterioration, usually over 15 to 20 years. There is an increased risk of complications during general anesthesia.

Diagnosis is verified by DNA testing. Severity correlates with the numbers of expanded repeats. Electromyography findings are characteristic but not necessary in typical cases. Serum muscle enzyme levels are generally normal or only slightly elevated. There is usually no need for a muscle biopsy.

Treatment is symptomatic, but the patient should be provided with physical therapy and genetic counseling. However, because of the mental subnormalities so common in this disorder, these modes of therapy are not always useful. Prenatal diagnosis is readily available and extremely accurate. The judicious use of phenytoin or imipramine may be helpful; however, as in other disorders in which mental subnormality is present, drugs should be administered with a great deal of caution.

## INFLAMMATORY MYOPATHIES

Polymyositis and, more commonly, dermatomyositis,[17] occur in virtually all age groups, including adolescence. These disorders probably result from an alteration of normal immune mechanisms and are not genetically determined.

Onset of symptoms is generally subacute or subchronic, lasting over weeks or a few months, although rarely, onset can be acute. Muscular weakness, generally proximal and more severe in the legs than in the arms, is the most common presenting complaint. Neck flexor muscles are often weak, but extraocular and facial muscles are spared. Variably intense muscular pain is present infrequently in adolescence. Muscular atrophy or muscular enlargement, as seen in BMD or JPSMA, is not seen early in inflammatory myopathies. In dermatomyositis, skin manifestations are present in the periorbital and malar regions and on the extensor surfaces of the limbs; the skin over the metacarpophalangeal and interphalangeal joints also may be reddened. Arthralgias are present in about one-quarter of patients. The course of the disease is variable: it may be limited, polycyclic, or continuous. Some patients may exhibit features of other connective tissue disorders.

Diagnosis can be established when the clinical pattern is correlated with appropriate biochemical, electrodiagnostic, and pathologic studies. Values of serum CK are generally elevated, but they may be normal in rare cases. Electrodiagnostic studies are useful in verifying the diagnosis. These studies should be limited to one side of the body, to enable subsequent performance of a muscle biopsy in a muscle that has not been tested with a needle. A muscle biopsy, when done properly, can be diagnostic in that an inflammatory exudate and/or perifascicular atrophy is confirmatory. The erythrocyte sedimentation rate is abnormal in approximately one-third of patients.

The differential diagnosis includes genetically determined or metabolic myopathies, anterior horn-cell disease, and sporadically occurring disorders; also included are acute viral myositis, "growing pains," conversion reactions, and toxic myopathies. In adolescents with an eating disorder, an ipecac (emetine)-induced myopathy can produce a pattern of muscle weakness similar to that seen in polymyositis. Careful analysis of the history in correlation with the clinical examination, negative genetic history, serum muscle enzyme values, results of electrodiagnostic tests, and muscle biopsy results generally provide the correct diagnosis.

Prednisone is considered the preferential agent in the treatment of inflammatory myopathies. Treatment is usually begun with a daily, single-morning, high-dose regimen. After a period this may be switched to an alternate-date, single-morning, high-dose schedule to reduce the possibility of side effects. High-dose intravenous steroid administration has also been used successfully. If patients do not experience a beneficial response after a reasonable period of prednisone therapy, or if they experience intolerable side effects, immunosuppressive agents (eg, azathioprine, methotrexate, or cyclosporine) may be added or substituted. High doses of intravenous gamma globulin have proved very effective. Physical therapy is generally part of the treatment plan.

With treatment the prognosis is generally good, although complications, which may be related to the disease itself or to the therapy, can be significant. These include severe respiratory involvement and dysphagia, gastrointestinal bleeding, subcutaneous calcifications, recurrence, and death. The relationship of polymyositis or dermatomyositis with malignancy, as noted in older patients, does not exist in adolescents, with rare exceptions.

## MISCELLANEOUS MYOPATHIES

*Hypokalemic periodic paralysis,*[18] a rare autosomal dominant disorder, frequently first appears in adolescence. This disorder is manifested by an acute quadriplegia with areflexia, most commonly occurring in the early morning hours. Results of an ECG may suggest hypokalemia, which is confirmed by a very low serum potassium determination. Treatment with potassium can overcome the paralysis, and diuretics can be used prophylactically to lessen the frequency and intensity of the attacks. Hyperkalemic periodic paralysis, also autosomal dominant, usually has its onset in early childhood, and by adolescence, treatment, also with diuretics, must be initiated and continued.

*Carnitine palmityl transferase deficiency*[19] may be manifested in adolescent males through sudden onset of severe weakness and myoglobinuria, frequently occurring after a fast. Respiratory difficulty is occasionally present during an attack. Serum muscle enzyme levels are elevated, and the diagnosis can be confirmed by specialized morphologic and biochemical studies of a muscle biopsy. In the presence of episodic myoglobinuria and weakness, other rare metabolic disorders of skeletal muscle that frequently have initial manifestations in adolescence, such as McArdle disease (phosphorylase deficiency) and phosphofructokinase deficiency, should be considered in the differential diagnosis.

Specialized studies of muscle biopsies can help confirm the diagnosis in these disorders. Serum muscle enzyme levels, especially CK, are generally elevated in these myopathies and in myoadenylate deaminase deficiency of muscle, in which muscle pain and myoglobinuria may be present.

*Intramuscular pentazocine (Talwin)* or *meperidine (Demerol) abuse* in adolescents can result in induration and contracture of the muscles injected, with associated fibrosis. This effect may be severe and may produce a woodlike sensation to palpation of the muscles. Patients may complain of weakness, but diagnosis is frequently difficult because of their denial of drug abuse.

*Ipecac abuse*[20] in adolescents with an eating disorder also can result in damage in both skeletal and cardiac muscles because of the toxic effect of emetine. This results in a generalized myopathy, with manifestations of proximal muscle weakness. Prognosis is guarded but generally good when the ipecac abuse is stopped.

In hyperthyroidism, *hyperthyroid myopathy*[21] may occur, frequently before the onset of symptoms of the underlying thyroid disorder. Proximal muscle weakness, which is the rule, is frequently associated with fatigability out of proportion to the degree of weakness. In addition, hyperthyroidism is occasionally associated with MG. The deep tendon reflexes are normal. Electromyography may be helpful in confirming the presence of an underlying myopathy, but the diagnosis is established on confirmation of the hyperthyroid state. Treatment of the underlying disorder is generally successful.

*Malignant hyperpyrexia,*[22] which can be encountered in all age groups (including adolescence), is triggered by succinylcholine, halothane, and other anesthetic agents during the induction of anesthesia or shortly thereafter. The exact pathogenesis is unclear, but it is associated with a rapidly evolving metabolic acidosis with lacticacidemia, rapid rise in body temperature, muscle rigidity, hyperkalemia, extremely elevated CK levels, myoglobinuria, hypocalcemia, and other changes. Prompt termination of anesthesia and immediate administration of intravenous dantrolene, coupled with body cooling, rehydration, administration of sodium bicarbonate, and associated ventilatory assistance, have proved effective.

## INTERNET RESOURCES

- Muscular Dystrophy Association: www.mda.org
- Online Mendelian Inheritance in Man: www.ncbi.nlm.nih.gov/omim
- Charcot-Marie-Tooth Association: www.charcot-marie-tooth.org/index.php
- Families of Spinal Muscular Atrophy: www.fsma.org

## REFERENCES


1. Dubowitz V. *Muscle Biopsy: A Practical Approach,* 3rd ed. London: WB Saunders; 2007

2. Han JJ, McDonald CM. Diagnosis and clinical management of spinal muscular atrophy. *Phys Med Rehabil Clin N Am.* 2008;19:661

3. Kikuchi S, Tashiro K. Juvenile muscular atrophy of distal upper extremity (Hirayama's disease). In: Jones HR Jr, DeVivo DC, Darras BT. *Neuromuscular Disorders of Infancy, Childhood, and Adolescence.* Amsterdam: Butterworth Heinemann; 2003:167-181

4. Beghi E, Kurland LT, Mulder DW, Nicolosi A. Brachial plexus neuropathy in the population of Rochester, Minnesota, 1970-1981. *Ann Neurol.* 1985;18:320-323

5. Nagasawa K, Kuwabara S, Misawa S, et al. Electrophysiological subtypes and prognosis of childhood Guillain-Barre syndrome in Japan. *Muscle Nerve.* 2006;33: 766-770

6. Alshekhlee A, Hussain Z, Sultan B, Katirit B. Immunotherapy for Guillain-Barre syndrome in the US hospitals. *J Clin Neuromusc Dis.* 2008;10:4-10

7. Ouvrier RA. *Peripheral Neuropathies in Childhood.* 2nd ed. New York, NY: Raven Press; 1999

8. Ouvrier R. Correlation between the histopathologic, genotypic, and phenotypic features of hereditary peripheral neuropathies in childhood. *J Child Neurol.* 1996;11:133-146

9. Ryan MM, Grattan-Smith PJ, Procopis PG, et al. Childhood chronic inflammatory demyelination polyneuropathy: clinical course and long-term outcome. *Neuromuscul Disord.* 2000;10:398-406

10. Osserman KE, Genkions G. Studies in myasthenia gravis: review of a twenty-year experience in over 1,200 patients. *Mt Sinai J Med.* 1971;38:497

11. Howard JF. Guidelines for the pharmacist. In: Howard JF, ed. *Myasthenia Gravis: A Manual for the Health Care Provider*. St. Paul, MN: Myasthenia Gravis Foundation of America; 2008. Available at: www.myasthenia.org/docs/MGFA_ProfessionalManual.pdf. Accessed January 13, 2010

12. Sasser H, Nussbaum M, Beuhler M, Ford M. Classification tree methods for development of decision rules for botulism and cyanide poisoning. *J Med Toxicol.* 2008;4:77-83

13. Bushby KM, Gardner-Medwin D. The clinical, genetic, and dystrophin characteristics of Becker muscular dystrophy. I. natural history. *J Neurol.* 1993;240:98-104

14. Bushby KM, Beckmann JS. The limb girdle muscular dystrophies—proposal for a new nomenclature. *Neuromuscul Disord.* 1995;4:337-343

15. Padberg GW, Frants RR, Brouwer OF, et al. Facioscapulohumeral muscular dystrophy in the Dutch population. *Muscle Nerve.* 1995;2:S81-S84

16. Harper PS. *Myotonic Dystrophy.* 3rd ed. London: WB Saunders; 2001

17. Pachman LM, Hayford JR, Chung A, et al. Juvenile dermatomyositis at diagnosis: clinical characteristics of 79 children. *J Rheumatol.* 1998;25:1198-1204

18. Venance SL, Cannon SC, Fialho D, et al. The primary periodic paralyses: diagnosis, pathogenesis, and treatment. *Brain.* 2006;129:8-17

19. Van Adel BA, Tarnopolsky MA. Metabolic myopathies: update 2009. *J Clin Neuromusc Dis.* 2009;10:97-121

20. Bennett HS, Spiro AJ, Pollack MA, Zucker P. Ipecac-induced myopathy simulating dermatomyositis. *Neurology.* 1982;32:91-94

21. Ruff RL, Weissman J. Endocrine myopathies. *Neurol Clin.* 1988;6:575

22. Larew RE. Malignant hyperthermia: quick recognition and treatment to avoid death. *Postgrad Med.* 1989;85:117

# CHAPTER 129

## Movement Disorders and Ataxia

REBECCA K. LEHMAN, MD • JONATHAN W. MINK, MD, PhD

### OVERVIEW OF MOVEMENT DISORDERS

Movement disorders are defined as abnormalities of movement that are not due to weakness or abnormal muscle tone. They can be classified as *either hyperkinetic* disorders (dyskinesias), which are characterized by abnormal, repetitive, involuntary movements, or *hypokinetic* disorders (akinetic/rigid disorders), which are characterized by slow voluntary movements, reduction of spontaneous movements, and rigidity. Most childhood onset movement disorders are hyperkinetic in nature, including tics, chorea/ballismus, dystonia, myoclonus, stereotypies, and tremor (Table 129-1). Abnormalities of coordination, such as ataxia, are typically not included under the umbrella of movement disorders. However, ataxia is covered in this chapter.

Smooth, coordinated movement requires communication among several components of the nervous system—basal ganglia (caudate, putamen, globus pallidus, subthalamic nucleus, substantia nigra), frontal cortex, thalamus, cerebellum, spinal cord, peripheral nerve, and muscle. A detailed description of the precise neural pathways involved is beyond the scope of this chapter, but it is important to recognize that dysfunction in any of these regions can result in a movement disorder.

When approaching an adolescent with a movement disorder, several key questions need to be answered (Box 129-1). Although the patient's and parents' answers to these questions provide useful information, accurate diagnosis relies on the clinician seeing the movements. If the movements are not apparent during the examination, it is often helpful to have the parents videotape the movements at home. Most movement disorders are recognized by the spatial and temporal features of the movements.

The clinical features and treatments of movement disorders depend entirely on the specific disorder. In the following sections, the important movement disorders occurring during adolescence are discussed. These include tics, chorea, dystonia, myoclonus, stereotypy, tremor, parkinsonism, and ataxia.

### TICS

Tics are the most common movement disorder occurring during childhood and adolescence.[1,2] Tics are defined as intermittent, discrete, repetitive, stereotyped movements or vocalizations that occur many times a day, nearly every day. Older children may report a

**Table 129-1**

**Classification of Movement Disorders**

| *Movement Disorder* | *Brief Description* |
|---|---|
| Tics | Intermittent, discrete, repetitive, stereotyped, nonrhythmic movements, most frequently involving head and upper body. |
| Chorea/ballismus | Rapid, chaotic, purposeless movements with "dance-like" quality. High-amplitude, proximal choreic limb movements are referred to as ballismus. |
| Dystonia | Repetitive, sustained, abnormal postures and movements. Abnormal postures typically have twisting quality. |
| Myoclonus | Sudden, brief, shock-like movements that may be repetitive or rhythmic. |
| Stereotypy | Patterned, episodic, repetitive, purposeless, rhythmic movements. |
| Tremor | Rhythmic, oscillatory movement around central point/plane. |
| Parkinsonism | Hypokinetic syndrome characterized by rest tremor, slow movement (bradykinesia), rigidity, and postural instability. |

Schlaggar BL, Mink JW. Movement disorders in children. *Pediatr Rev*. 2003;24(2):39–51.

**Box 129-1**

***Key Historical Questions for Diagnosing Movement Disorders***

1. Are the adolescent's movements excessive (hyperkinetic) or diminished (hypokinetic)?
2. If hyperkinetic, do the individual movements appear normal or abnormal?
3. Is the movement paroxysmal (sudden onset and offset), continual (repeated again and again), or continuous (without stop)?
4. What is the developmental stage of the adolescent, and has the development been normal?
5. How does voluntary movement affect the movement disorder?
6. Are the symptoms and signs present at rest (body part supported against gravity), with maintained posture, with action, with approach to a target (intention), or a combination thereof?
7. Has the movement disorder changed over time?
8. Is the adolescent aware of the movements?
9. Can the movements be suppressed voluntarily?
10. Does the movement disorder abate with sleep?
11. Is there a family history of a similar or related condition?

premonitory sensation,[2] such as an itchy feeling that precedes the need to blink repeatedly, which often results in their movements being misattributed to allergy symptoms. Other characteristic features of tics are that they change in anatomic location, frequency, type, complexity, and severity over time. They may be suggestible (ie, tics can be precipitated by talking about or demonstrating the tic) and are suppressible for brief periods of time. Tics typically disappear with sleep, but in some individuals they may persist in all stages of sleep.[3]

Tics typically start in childhood, peak in severity between 10 and 13 years of age, and then become less severe during the later teenage years and early adulthood.[4] However, tics may worsen during the teenage years for some individuals. Furthermore, tics may be more disabling for adolescents due to their social ramifications. Many patients also have comorbid obsessive-compulsive disorder (OCD), attention-deficit/hyperactivity disorder (ADHD), anxiety, depression, learning disorders, and/or oppositional behavior/conduct disorder, all of which may be more impairing than the tics themselves.[1,2]

Primary tic disorders can be classified into 5 different groups: transient tic disorder, chronic motor tic disorder, chronic vocal tic disorder, Tourette syndrome, and tic disorder not otherwise specified (NOS) (Table 129-2). Although most patients fall into 1 of these 5 categories, secondary tic disorders exist (Table 129-3). However, when tics are secondary to another neurologic or psychiatric disorder, other signs or symptoms are usually present. Patients who have tics in conjunction with other developmental or neurologic abnormalities should be further evaluated by a neurologist.

Once a tic disorder has been diagnosed, it is critical to provide anticipatory guidance. Specifically, it is important to talk about the fact that tics wax and wane over time and tend to worsen with anxiety, depression, fatigue, illness, and stress (including "good stress," such

**Table 129-2**

**Classification of Tic Disorders (Based on *DSM-IV-TR*)**

| *Disorder* | *Age of Onset* | *Duration* | *Description of Tics* |
|---|---|---|---|
| Transient tic disorder | Younger than 18 years | 4 weeks but <12 months | Single or multiple motor and/or vocal tics |
| Chronic motor tic disorder | Younger than 18 years | 1 year without ever having tic-free period longer than 3 months | Motor only |
| Chronic vocal tic disorder | Younger than 18 years | 1 year without ever having tic-free period longer than 3 months | Vocal only |
| Tourette syndrome | Younger than 18 years | 1 year without ever having tic-free period longer than 3 months | Motor and vocal |
| Tic disorder NOS | May include patients older than 18 years | May include tics lasting <4 weeks | May include rare patient with 1 motor and 1 vocal tic |

NOS, not otherwise specified

American Psychiatric Association. *Diagnostic and Statistical Manual of Mental Disorders.* 4th ed. Text Revision. Washington, DC: American Psychiatric Association; 2000.

**Table 129-3**

**Selected Causes of Secondary Tic Disorders**

| *General Cause* | *Specific Cause* |
|---|---|
| **Heredodegenerative disorders** | Huntington disease |
| | Neuroacanthocytosis |
| | PKAN |
| | Wilson disease |
| **Infectious** | Encephalitis (measles, herpes virus) |
| | *Mycoplasma pneumoniae* |
| **Postinfectious** | Sydenham chorea |
| | PANDAS |
| **Developmental** | Cerebral palsy |
| | Mental retardation syndromes (eg, Down syndrome, fragile X) |
| | Autism spectrum disorders |
| | Fetal alcohol syndrome |
| **Metabolic** | Lesch-Nyhan syndrome |
| | Phenylketonuria |
| | Citrullinemia |
| **Other genetic/ chromosomal disorders** | Klinefelter syndrome |
| | Congenital adrenal hyperplasia |
| **Drugs** | Stimulants (cocaine, amphetamines) |
| | Antiepileptic drugs (carbamazepine, phenytoin, phenobarbital, lamotrigine) |
| | Levodopa |
| | Dopamine-blocking drugs (tardive tourettism) |
| **Toxins** | Carbon monoxide |
| | Wasp venom |
| | Mercury |
| **Psychiatric** | Conversion disorder |
| | Schizophrenia |
| **Other** | Head trauma |
| | Stroke |
| | Malignancy |
| | Neurocutaneous syndromes |

PANDAS, pediatric autoimmune neuropsychiatric disorder associated with streptococcal infection; PKAN, pantothenate kinase-associated neurodegeneration (also known as neuronal brain iron accumulation type 1)

Jankovic J. Tics in other neurologic disorders. In: Kurlan RM, ed. *Handbook of Tourette's Syndrome and Related Tic and Behavioral Disorders*. New York: Marcel Dekker; 1992:167–182.

as anticipation of holidays, birthdays, etc). Patients often worry that they will involuntarily swear (coprolalia) or perform obscene gestures (copropraxia), but they should be reassured that these symptoms are present in a small minority of patients. Another frequent concern is that tics will interfere with driving, which they typically do not.

The decision to treat tics is based on whether they are causing morbidity. If treatment is initiated, it is important to establish the goal of suppressing tics to a tolerable level, rather than eliminating them altogether. Patients with tics frequently benefit from an α2-agonist, such as clonidine or guanfacine. Second line agents include typical neuroleptics (eg, haloperidol, pimozide) and atypical neuroleptics (eg, risperidone, zprasidone). For some patients, their tics may be less problematic than their comorbidities, in which case pharmacotherapy should target the most troublesome issues first. Cognitive behavioral therapy should be considered in patients with comorbid obsessive-compulsive behaviors or anxiety.

Historically, methylphenidate has been contraindicated in patients with a personal or family history of tics. This was initially based on single case reports. Subsequently, it has become recognized that nearly half of patients with chronic tics, including Tourette syndrome, have comorbid ADHD and that ADHD symptoms typically begin at least one year before tics appear.[1] A more recent randomized, placebo-controlled, double-blinded study found that methylphenidate and clonidine, particularly in combination, were effective for treating ADHD in children with comorbid chronic tics. Significantly, patients in all 3 treatment groups had decreased tic severity when compared to placebo.[5] Thus, there is no overall worsening, and there may even be improvement, of tics when ADHD is treated with methylphenidate.

## PEDIATRIC AUTOIMMUNE NEUROPSYCHIATRIC DISORDER ASSOCIATED WITH STREPTOCOCCAL INFECTIONS

Pediatric autoimmune neuropsychiatric disorder associated with streptococcal infections (PANDAS) refers to a subset of patients whose tics or OCD symptoms started in the setting of, or were exacerbated by, a streptococcal infection, presumably via an immune-mediated mechanism involving molecular mimicry.[6] Proposed diagnostic criteria include (1) the presence of OCD and/or tic disorder; (2) prepubertal age of onset; (3) sudden, "explosive" onset of symptoms and a course of sudden exacerbations and remissions; (4) temporal relationship between symptom onset/exacerbations and group A beta-hemolytic streptococcus infection; and (5) the presence of neurologic abnormalities, including tics, hyperactivity, and choreiform movements during exacerbations.[6] Although there has been significant interest in this area, it remains unclear whether pediatric autoimmune neuropsychiatric disorder associated with streptococcal infection (PANDAS) is a distinct disease entity.[7] Regardless, there are no convincing data to indicate that tics should be treated differently regardless of whether there is an apparent link to a preceding strep infection. Because antistreptolysin (ASO) titers do not reliably reflect the existence of a recent strep infection, we do not recommend measuring ASO in children with tics. Furthermore, we do not recommend treatment of tic exacerbations with antibiotics in the absence of a proven strep infection.

## CHOREA

Chorea describes rapid, chaotic, purposeless movements that often have a dance-like quality. These movements may coexist with dystonia or athetosis (slow, nonrhythmic, writhing movements), in which case some apply the term "choreoatheosis." High-amplitude, proximal choreic limb movements are referred to as "ballismus." Finally, some use the term "choreiform" to describe the minimal twitching or "piano-playing" movements that are seen in many neurologically normal children when they are asked to extend their arms.

Chorea is associated with motor impersistence (eg, patients have difficulty keeping the tongue protruded or maintaining grip, so-called milkmaid's grip). It tends to occur both at rest and with action, resulting in a fidgety appearance. Patients may try to incorporate these fidgety movements into more purposeful movements, a phenomenon known as parakinesis. Chorea disappears with sleep but may worsen with drowsiness.

In most cases, chorea in adolescents occurs secondary to an identifiable disorder. Such "secondary" chorea can result from myriad metabolic, infectious, immune-mediated, vascular, and heredodegenerative disorders (Table 129-4). In addition, many commonly used drugs can precipitate chorea either during treatment or as a tardive symptom, particularly in individuals with pre-existing basal ganglia dysfunction.

### SYDENHAM CHOREA

Sydenham chorea (St Vitus' dance) is the most common cause of secondary chorea in children and adolescents. It is a symptom of acute rheumatic fever, typically beginning weeks to months following a group A β-hemolytic streptococcus infection.[8] Thomas Sydenham, MD, originally described the disorder as follows: "*Chorea Sancti Viti*, is a form of Convulsion, which chiefly invades

**Table 129-4**

**Selected Causes of Secondary Chorea**

| *General Cause* | *Specific Cause* |
|---|---|
| **Metabolic** | • Hypo/hypernatremia<br>• Hypo/hyperglycemia<br>• Hypocalcemia<br>• Hyperthyroidism |
| **Infectious/ parainfectious** | • Epstein-Barr virus<br>• HIV<br>• Rheumatic fever (Sydenham chorea)<br>• Viral encephalitis |
| **Immune mediated** | • Lupus<br>• Antiphospholipid antibody syndrome<br>• Paraneoplastic syndrome |
| **Vascular** | • Stroke<br>• Moya-moya syndrome<br>• Global hypoxia |
| **Structural** | • Cerebral palsy<br>• Trauma |
| **Heredodegenerative disease** | • Niemann-Pick type C<br>• Gangliosidoses<br>• Lesch-Nyhan disease<br>• Wilson disease<br>• PKAN<br>• Ataxia telangectasia |
| **Drugs/toxins** | • Anticholinergics (eg, trihexyphenidyl)<br>• Antihistamines<br>• Tricyclic antidepressants<br>• Neuroleptics, including antiemetics<br>• Antiepiletics (eg, carbamazepine, phenytoin, valproate, phenobarbital)<br>• Stimulants (eg, bronchodilators, cocaine)<br>• Oral contraceptives<br>• Manganese<br>• Methanol<br>• Carbon monoxide |
| **Pregnancy (chorea gravidarum)** | |
| **Psychogenic** | |

PKAN, pantothenate kinase-associated neurodegeneration

Schlaggar BL, Mink JW. Movement disorders in children. *Pediatr Rev*. 2003;24(2):39–51.

Boys and Girls, from ten Years of Age to Puberty: First, it shows itself by a certain Lameness, or rather Instability of one of the Legs, which the Patient drags after him like a Fool; afterwards it appears in the Hand of the same side; which he that is affected with this Disease, can by no means keep in the same Posture for one Moment, if it be brought to the Breast, or any other Part, but it will be distorted to another Position or Place by a certain Convulsion, let the Patient do what he can."[9]

Although the mechanism for Sydenham chorea is still not fully understood, it is generally believed that there is molecular mimicry between streptococcal surface antigens and basal ganglia peptides, with resultant immune-modulated damage to the basal ganglia. The diagnosis of Sydenham chorea is a clinical one, but a combination of acute *and* convalescent serum ASO O titers help confirm an acute infection. Negative titers do not exclude the diagnosis. All patients with suspected Sydenham chorea should be evaluated for carditis.

If there is evidence of an acute streptococcal infection, the patient should receive antibiotics. All patients should receive long-term antibiotic prophylaxis because this has been shown to decrease the risk of developing rheumatic heart disease.[10] There is no agreement about the best way to administer penicillin; we advocate giving penicillin G benzathine 1.2 million units IM every 2–3 weeks to ensure adherence.[10] If the chorea is impairing, treatment options include valproate, carbamazepine, and/or dopamine receptor antagonists. There is insufficient evidence to recommend routine use of corticosteroids or intravenous immunoglobulin in Sydenham chorea.

Sydenham chorea usually persists for weeks to months, but almost always resolves spontaneously within 6 months. Rarely, chorea can recur in the setting of future streptococcal infections, pregnancy (chorea gravidarum), or oral contraceptive use.

## DYSTONIA

Dystonia is characterized by repetitive, sustained muscle contractions that cause abnormal postures and movements, often with a twisting quality, along the long axis of a limb. It is usually triggered or exacerbated by voluntary movement. In some cases, the trigger may be task specific (ie, posturing occurs while performing a specific task, but not while performing other tasks that require the same muscles). The muscle contractions abate during sleep. Many individuals with dystonia find that touching the involved body part or assuming a particular position will alleviate their dystonia; this phenomenon is referred to as a sensory trick or *geste antagoniste*.

Dystonias can be classified according to age of onset (childhood vs adult), anatomic distribution (Table 129-5), or etiology (primary vs secondary). Dystonia can also be subclassified by whether it occurs at rest (fixed), with particular tasks (task specific), with movement of the involved region (action), or with movement of an

**Table 129-5**

**Dystonia by Anatomic Distribution**

| *Anatomic Distribution* | *Definition* | *Examples* |
|---|---|---|
| Focal | Involving single body part, such as limb, neck, or face | Writer's cramp<br>Focal hand or foot dystonia<br>Torticollis<br>Blepharospasm (eyelids)<br>Oromandibular dystonia<br>Spasmodic dysphonia (vocal cords) |
| Segmental | Involving muscles of 2 contiguous body parts | Cranial segmental dystonia (face and neck)<br>Axial dystonia (neck and trunk)<br>Brachial dystonia (arm and trunk)<br>Crural dystonia [leg(s) and trunk] |
| Multifocal | Involving 2 or more noncontiguous body parts | |
| Hemidystonia | Involving most or all muscles on 1 side of body | |
| Generalized | Involving multiple limbs on both sides of body, including at least 1 leg | |

uninvolved region (overflow), or by whether it improves with talking or other voluntary movements (paradoxical). Primary dystonias are those in which dystonia is the predominant or only clinical feature, and in which the cause is either a specific genetic mutation or is unknown. Conversely, secondary dystonias are those in which the dystonia is due to another identifiable cause, such as cerebral palsy (CP), trauma, stroke, or degenerative disease. The 2 most important primary dystonias in adolescents are idiopathic torsion dystonia and dopa-responsive dystonia.

### IDIOPATHIC GENERALIZED TORSION DYSTONIA

Symptoms of childhood onset idiopathic generalized torsion dystonia (DYT1 dystonia, dystonia musculorum deformans) usually begin in the legs, with a mean age of onset of 12.5 years of age (typical range 6–28 years). In some cases, the arms are affected first. Typically, the symptoms become generalized within 5 years of disease onset.[11] Childhood onset idiopathic torsion dystonia is caused by a *GAG* deletion at the DYT1 locus on chromosome 9 and is inherited in an autosomal dominant fashion with 30% penetrance. Genetic testing is commercially available for this disorder.

Any child with prominent dystonia should receive a trial of levodopa for the possibility of dopa-responsive dystonia (DRD).[12] Commonly used therapies for primary dystonia include the anticholinergic medication trihexyphenidyl, baclofen (alone or in combination with trihexyphenidyl), and benzodiazepines.[13,14] Botulinum toxin may be beneficial for patients whose impairment is attributable to a few muscle groups. Patients with generalized dystonia may benefit from deep brain stimulation of the globus pallidus.[15]

### DOPA-RESPONSIVE DYSTONIA

Dopa-responsive dystonia (DYT5 dystonia) typically begins between 1 and 12 years of age (median 6.5 years), most often with progressive foot dystonia and resultant gait abnormality. In adolescence, most patients develop diurnal variation in their symptoms.[12] Patients may have associated findings, including hyperreflexia, extensor plantar responses, and parkinsonism, which may result in DRD being misdiagnosed as spastic diplegia CP, hereditary spastic paraplegia, intractable epilepsy, or a neurodegenerative disorder.[16] Untreated, DRD is a progressive disorder; however, it is highly responsive to low-dose levodopa.

The most common type of DRD is caused by mutations in the guanosine triphosphate cyclohydrolase 1 gene on chromosome 14q22.1–2.[8] Inheritance is autosomal dominant with incomplete penetrance. Mutations in the tyrosine hydroxylase gene on chromosome 11p15.5 can yield a similar clinical picture but with earlier onset and a more severe course. Inheritance is autosomal recessive with full penetrance.

**Table 129-6**

**Causes of Secondary Dystonia[1,8]**

| *General Cause* | *Specific Cause* |
|---|---|
| **Heredodegenerative disorders** | • Gangliosidoses<br>• Niemann-Pick type C<br>• Huntington disease (particularly, Westphal variant)<br>• Lesch-Nyhan syndrome<br>• PKAN<br>• Wilson disease<br>• Metachromatic leukodystrophy<br>• Ataxia telangiectasia<br>• SCAs; particularly, Machado-Joseph disease/SCA3 |
| **Metabolic** | • Glutaric aciduria<br>• Methylmalonic acidemia<br>• Mitochondrial disorders |
| **Structural brain lesions** | • Perinatal hypoxia-ischemia/cerebral palsy<br>• Infection (eg, varicella)<br>• Acute disseminated encephalomyelitis<br>• Basal ganglia stroke<br>• Tumor<br>• Head trauma |
| **Paroxysmal** | • Complex migraine<br>• Paroxysmal dyskinesias |
| **Drugs/toxins** | • Neuroleptics (haloperidol, chlorpromazine, risperidone)<br>• Antiemetics (metoclopromide, prochlorperazine)<br>• Anticonvulsants (carbamazepine, phenytoin)<br>• Manganese<br>• Carbon monoxide |
| **Psychogenic** | • Coping mechanism |

PKAN, pantothenate kinase–associated neurodegeneration (neuronal brain iron accumulation type 1); SCAs, spinocerebellar ataxias

### SECONDARY DYSTONIA

Among the many causes of secondary dystonia (Table 129-6), CP is by far the most common due to its high prevalence.[8] Dyskinetic CP represents 6% to 15% of all CP cases, and dystonia tends to be the primary feature. Although, by definition, CP is a static encephalopathy, the dystonia in CP may worsen over time. Moreover, the onset of dystonia may occur several years after the initial injury. Patients with dystonic CP should receive a trial of levodopa because some patients may have functional benefit from this medication.[17]

## MYOCLONUS

Myoclonus is described as a sudden, brief, shock-like movement. Positive myoclonic jerks are caused by rapid contraction of a muscle or group of muscles, whereas negative myoclonus (asterixis) is caused by a brief interruption of sustained, voluntary muscle contraction, often followed by a compensatory jerk. Myoclonus can be classified by whether it occurs at rest, in response to a sensory stimulus (reflex myoclonus), or with volitional movement (action myoclonus).

Distal myoclonus may be difficult to differentiate from chorea, but it does not have the same "flowing" quality, nor is it associated with motor impersistence. Unlike tics, myoclonus cannot be suppressed. Unlike dystonia, chorea, and tremor, myoclonus may persist during sleep.

Myoclonus can be generated at almost every level of the neuraxis, including the motor cortex, subcortical reflex centers, spinal cord, and peripheral nerve, although the motor cortex is the most common source. Cortical myoclonus predominantly affects the face and hands because these areas have large cortical representations.[18]

There are several physiological forms of myoclonus that occur in healthy adolescents, including hypnic jerks and hiccups. When myoclonus is pathological, it can be either an epileptic (eg, juvenile myoclonic epilepsy) or nonepileptic phenomenon (Box 129-2).

The best treatment for myoclonus is treatment of the underlying disorder; however, this is not possible in most cases. Many medications have been used for the symptomatic treatment of myoclonus, generally with suboptimal results. Cortical myoclonus may respond to high doses of sodium valproate, clonazepam, piracetam, or levetiracetam.[18] Zonisamide may be helpful in some cases. Many patients eventually require multiple medications. Posthypoxic myoclonus seems to be particularly responsive to serotonergic medications, including selective serotonin reuptake inhibitors (SSRIs). Baclofen has been used, but the mechanism of action is not clear. Phenytoin and carbamazepine can make central myoclonus worse.

### Box 129-2

### *Selected Etiologies of Myoclonus in Adolescents*

1. **Physiological**
   a. Hiccups
   b. Hypnic jerks (sleep starts)
   c. Nocturnal (sleep) myoclonus
2. **Essential (primary symptom, nonprogressive course)**
   a. Hereditary
   b. Sporadic
3. **Epileptic**
4. **Symptomatic**
   a. Storage diseases
      i. Juvenile Gaucher (type III)
      ii. Sialidosis (type 1)
      iii. GM-1 gangliosidosis
      iv. Neuronal ceroid lipofuscinosis (late infantile > juvenile)
   b. Degenerative conditions
      i. DRPLA
      ii. Huntington disease
      iii. Progressive myoclonus ataxia
      iv. Ramsay-Hunt syndrome
      v. Wilson disease
      vi. PKAN
   c. Dementias
      i. Bovine spongiform encephalopathy
      ii. Creutzfeldt-Jakob disease
      iii. Rett syndrome
   d. Infectious and postinfectious
      i. Meningitis (viral or bacterial)
      ii. Encephalitis
      iii. Epstein-Barr virus
      iv. Coxsackie
      v. Influenza
      vi. HIV
      vii. Lyme disease
      v. Acute disseminated encephalomyelitis
   e. Metabolic
      i. Uremia
      ii. Hepatic failure
      iii. Electrolyte disturbances
      iv. Hypo- or hyperglycemia
      v. Metabolic alkalosis
      vi. Hyperthyroidism
      vii. Vitamin E deficiency
      viii. Aminoacidurias
      iv. Organic acidurias
      v. Urea cycle disorders
      vii. Mitochondrial disorders (MERRF, MELAS)
   f. Toxic
      i. Psychotropic medications (tricyclics, lithium, SSRIs, MAOIs, neuroleptics)

(*Continued*)

**Box 129-2 (*Continued*)**

- ii. Antibiotics (penicillin, cephalosporins, quinolones)
- iii. Antiepileptics (phenytoin, carbamazepine, lamotrigine, gabapentin, vigabatrin)
- iv. Opioids
- v. General anesthetics
- vi. Antineoplastic drugs
- vii. Strychnine, toluene, lead, carbon monoxide, mercury

g. Hypoxia (Lance-Adams syndrome)
h. Paraneoplastic
i. Opsoclonus-myoclonus syndrome

**5. Focal lesions**

a. Stroke
b. Tumor
b. Trauma (central or peripheral nervous system)

**6. Psychogenic**

DRPLA, dentatorubral-pallidoluysian atrophy; MAOI, monoamine oxidase inhibitor; MELAS, mitochondrial myopathy, encephalopathy, lactic acidosis, and stroke-like episodes; MERRF, myoclonic epilepsy and ragged red fiber; PKAN, pantothenate kinase–associated neurodegeneration; SSRI, selective serotonin reuptake inhibitor.

## STEREOTYPY

Stereotypies are patterned, episodic, repetitive, purposeless, rhythmic movements. Examples include head banging, body rocking, leg shaking, arm flapping, and hand waving. Unlike tics, stereotypies are not preceded by a premonitory urge, and they do not change over time. Stereotypies are usually suppressed by distraction. Although stereotypies are more common in adolescents with autism, mental retardation, sensory deprivation, and neurodegenerative disorders, they can also be seen in many healthy, developmentally normal children.[19]

In general, stereotypies do not require treatment; however, treatment may be warranted if the movements are extremely severe or are causing psychosocial distress. Many medications have been used to treat stereotypies, including benzodiazepines, α-adrenergic agonists, opiate antagonists, beta blockers, antiepileptic drugs, antipsychotic agents, and SSRIs, with variable effects.[20] The combination of habit reversal therapy and differential reinforcement of other behaviors may also be beneficial in reducing motor stereotypies.[21]

## TREMOR

Tremor is defined as a rhythmic, oscillatory movement around a central point or plane. Tremor can affect the extremities, head, trunk, or voice and can be classified as rest, postural, action, or intention tremor, according to the position in which the tremor is most pronounced. Rest tremor is maximal when the affected body part is inactive and supported against gravity. Postural tremor is most notable when the patient sustains a position against gravity, whereas action tremor is precipitated by movement. Intention tremor, which is defined as tremor that worsens as the patient's limb approaches a target, is associated with cerebellar disease. Tremor can also be characterized by its frequency. For example, parkinsonian tremor is 4 to 6 Hz, and essential tremor (ET) is 5 to 8 Hz. Physiological tremor has 2 components: 1 each at 8 to 12 Hz and at 20 to 25 Hz.[8]

Some of the more common etiologies of tremor in adolescents are listed in Table 129-7. A detailed discussion of the various causes of secondary tremor is beyond the scope of this chapter; however, it is important to exclude Wilson disease, which has a characteristic "wing-beating" tremor, because this is a treatable condition in adolescents.

### ESSENTIAL TREMOR

Although often thought of as a disease of the elderly, 4.6% of cases of ET begin during childhood.[22] Essential tremor is primarily postural, but may be worsened by actions, such as trying to pour water from cup to cup. Tremor with handwriting is a common complaint, and affected patients typically have difficulty reproducing an Archimedes spiral. In 1 study of 39 children with ET, the mean age of onset was 8.8 ± 5.0 years; however, the mean age of evaluation was 20.3 ± 14.4 years.[23] Approximately three-fourths of the affected patients were male. A family history of tremor was noted in 79.5% of patients, consistent with the putative autosomal dominant inheritance with variable penetrance. Treatment of ET is symptomatic with strong evidence for propranolol and primidone and good evidence for sotalol, atenolol, gabapentin, topiramate, and alprazolam.[24] Botulinum toxin A may be effective for treating limb tremor, although it causes nonpermanent, dose-dependent limb weakness.[24] Surgical treatments, which include deep brain stimulation of the thalamus and unilateral thalamotomy, are generally reserved for adults.

## PARKINSONISM

Parkinsonism is characterized by bradykinesia (slowness of movement), rigidity (nonvelocity-dependent resistance to passive movement), postural instability, and rest tremor, although the latter feature is less common in children. Patients may also have hypokinesia, typified by hypophonia (soft speech), micrographia (small handwriting), and decreased amplitude of movement.

**Table 129-7**

**Selected Causes of Tremor in Adolescents**

| *General Cause* | *Specific Cause* |
|---|---|
| Physiological | Enhanced physiological tremor |
| Static injury/structural | Stroke (particularly in midbrain or cerebellum), MS |
| Hereditary/degenerative | Familial essential tremor, Wilson disease, Huntington disease, juvenile parkinsonism (tremor is rare), pallidonigral degeneration |
| Metabolic | Hyperthyroidism, hyperadrenergic state (including pheochromocytoma and neuroblastoma), hypomagnesemia, hypocalcemia, hypoglycemia, hepatic encephalopathy, vitamin B12 deficiency |
| Drugs/toxins | Valproate, lithium, tricyclic antidepressants, stimulants (cocaine, amphetamine, caffeine, thyroxine, bronchodilators), neuroleptics, cyclosporin, toluene, mercury, thallium, amiodarone, nicotine, lead, manganese, arsenic, cyanide, naphthalene, ethanol, lindane, SSRIs |
| Other causes of tremor | Peripheral neuropathy, cerebellar disease or malformation, anxiety, psychogenic tremor |

MS, multiple sclerosis; SSRIs, selective serotonin reuptake inhibitors

**Table 129-8**

**Causes of Parkinsonism[8]**

| *General Cause* | *Specific Causes* |
|---|---|
| Static injury/structural | Basal ganglia infarcts, brain tumor, hydrocephalus |
| Hereditary/degenerative | Juvenile Parkinson disease, SCA, Huntington disease (Westphal variant), PKAN, Rett syndrome, Pelizaeus-Merzbacher disease, Machado-Joseph disease (SCA3) |
| Metabolic | Dopa-responsive dystonia, tyrosine hydroxylase deficiency and other abnormalities of bioamine metabolism, abnormalities of folate metabolism, Wilson disease, basal ganglia calcification (Fahr disease, hypoparathyroidism) |
| Infectious/parainfectious | Encephalitis lethargica (von Economo disease), viral encephalitis, acute demyelinating encephalomyelitis |
| Drugs/toxins | MPTP poisoning, rotenone, tetrabenazine, reserpine, methyldopa, sedatives, neuroleptics, antiemetics, calcium channel blockers, isoniazid, SSRIs (sertraline, fluoxetine), meperidine |
| Disorders that mimic Parkinsonism | Catatonia, spasticity, hypothyroidism, depression, PKAN |

PKAN, pantothenate kinase–associated neurodegeneration; MPTP, methy-phenyl-tetrahydropyridine; SCA, spinocerebellar ataxi; SSRI, selective serotonin reuptake inhibitors,

In adolescents, most cases of parkinsonism are secondary (Table 129-8). Treatment consists of levodopa/carbidopa 1 mg/kg (or 50–100 mg total) every morning for 3 or 4 days. If this dose is tolerated, levodopa/carbidopa can be administered 3 times per day and then titrated to effect (maximum dose 10–15 mg/kg/day).[8] Dopamine-sparing strategies, using dopamine-agonists or dopamine breakdown inhibitors, have not been studied in adolescents.

## JUVENILE PARKINSON DISEASE

Juvenile Parkinson disease is a rare disorder that typically presents with leg dystonia in younger children and with bradykinesia and rigidity in adolescents. Many cases are due to mutations in the *PARK-2* gene on chromosome 6q25.2–27, which is inherited in an autosomal recessive fashion.[8] Juvenile Parkinson disease responds to levodopa and dopamine-sparing medications; however, escalating doses are required, and patients ultimately develop dyskinesias.

## DRUG-INDUCED MOVEMENT DISORDERS

Drugs, particularly high-potency neuroleptics, are a relatively common cause of movement disorders in adolescents. Acute drug reactions include acute dystonic reactions, parkinsonism, and neuroleptic malignant syndrome. An acute dystonic reaction typically involves involuntary gaze deviation (oculogyric crisis), severe back arching (opisthotonos), torticollis, and uncontrollable tongue movements.[1] Such reactions respond to anticholinergic medications, such as diphenhydramine (1 mg/kg/dose IV every 6 hours) or benztropine (0.5-2 mg daily to BID). Neuroleptic malignant syndrome is a life-threatening condition characterized by rigidity, hyperthermia, autonomic instability, and encephalopathy. Treatment consists of discontinuing the offending agent, fever control, correction of electrolyte disturbances, and dantrolene to decrease the excessive muscle contractions.

In addition to the acute drug reactions, neuroleptic medications can cause a variety of tardive syndromes, including tardive dyskinesia, tardive dystonia, and tardive chorea. Although the word "tardive" means late onset, these syndromes can actually occur anytime from shortly after starting the medication to months or years later. In some cases, the symptoms become apparent as the medication is discontinued. Treatment involves rapid withdrawal of the causative medication, although symptoms do not always resolve once the medication is discontinued. Patients with tardive syndromes should not be rechallenged with neuroleptics in the future.

## PSYCHOGENIC MOVEMENT DISORDERS/ CONVERSION DISORDER

Many adolescents have abnormal movements without any identifiable neurologic basis. Most often, these patients are labeled as having conversion disorder—a condition in which there are symptoms affecting voluntary motor or sensory function that suggest a neurologic or general medical condition but are not fully explained by that condition. Rather, the symptoms are associated with psychological factors. Other defining features of conversion disorder are that the symptoms cause impairment and are not produced intentionally.

The incidence of conversion disorder varies considerably depending on the population surveyed, ranging from 33% in some outpatient psychiatric populations to 1% among neurology service admissions.[25] The typical age of onset is during adolescence.

Psychogenic movement disorders can mimic almost any organic movement disorder, although tremor, dystonia, and myoclonus are the most common manifestations. Several historical and clinical features help distinguish psychogenic disorders from organic disorders (Box 129-3). Even so, it is often necessary to perform diagnostic testing to exclude organic etiologies.

When delivering the diagnosis, it is often helpful to explain the patient's symptoms in terms of a "mind-body imbalance," while stressing that patient is not "crazy" or "faking it." In adolescents, symptoms of conversion disorder typically resolve within 3 months.[25] Treatments such as psychotherapy, physiotherapy, and biofeedback provide insight into the psychological underpinnings of conversion disorder and may expedite recovery.

### Box 129-3

### *Clues to Diagnosis of Psychogenic Movement Disorders*[25]

Historical clues
- Abrupt onset
- Static course
- Spontaneous remission or inconsistency over time
- Obvious psychiatric disturbance
- Multiple somatizations
- Pending litigation or compensation
- Presence of secondary gain

Clinical clues
- Inconsistent character of movement (amplitude, frequency, distribution, selective disability)
- Paroxysmal movement disorder
- Movements increase with attention to movement and/or decrease with distraction
- Ability to trigger or relieve abnormal movements with unusual or nonphysiological interventions (eg, body trigger points)
- False ("give-way") weakness
- False sensory findings
- Self-inflicted injuries
- Deliberate slowness of movements
- Functional disability out of proportion to examination findings
- Prominent pain out of proportion to movements

Therapeutic responses
- Unresponsiveness to appropriate medications
- Response to placebos
- Remission with psychotherapy

## ATAXIA

Ataxia refers to a disturbance in the smooth performance of voluntary motor acts and is usually the result of primary or secondary cerebellar dysfunction.[26] There are myriad causes of ataxia, but most either present prior to adolescence or have associated findings that point to a specific etiology (Table 129-9). Given that the list of potential etiologies for ataxia is quite long, it is helpful to first determine whether the symptoms are acute or chronic. Acute symptoms suggest an infectious/postinfectious, endocrinologic, toxic, traumatic, vascular, or psychogenic process, whereas more chronic symptoms suggest a metabolic, neoplastic, or degenerative process.

Treatment depends on the underlying etiology but generally involves supportive care and physiotherapy. Pharmacologic treatment is largely ineffective.

**Table 129-9**

**Selected Causes of Ataxia[26]**

| *General Cause* | *Specific Causes* |
|---|---|
| Congenital | • Agenesis, aplasia, or dysplasia of cerebellum<br>• Chiari malformation<br>• Dandy-Walker malformation<br>• Progressive hydrocephalus |
| Degenerative/genetic | • Ataxia-telangiectasia<br>• Friedreich ataxia<br>• Spinocerebellar ataxia |
| Infectious/parainfectious | • Coxsackievirus<br>• Epstein-Barr virus<br>• Mycoplasma pneumonia<br>• Rubeola<br>• Acute disseminated encephalomyelitis |
| Metabolic | • Hypoglycemia<br>• Hypothyroidism |
| Neoplastic | • Frontal lobe, cerebellar, pontine, or spinal cord tumors |
| Psychogenic | • Conversion reaction |
| Toxic | • Alcohol<br>• Benzodiazepines<br>• Antiepileptics (eg, carbamazepine, phenytoin, phenobarbital)<br>• Lead encephalopathy |
| Traumatic | • Acute frontal lobe injury/edema<br>• Acute cerebellar injury/edema |
| Vascular | • Cerebellar stroke<br>• Vasculitis<br>• Basilar migraine |

## SUMMARY

The characteristic features of tics, chorea, dystonia, myoclonus, stereotypy, tremor, parkinsonism, and ataxia have been described as movement disorders seen in adolescents. As is true of most clinical symptoms, the diagnosis depends on a detailed history and comprehensive assessment, including a complete physical examination with emphasis on the neurologic and mental health aspects. Treatment options vary by the diagnosis, as described previously.

## REFERENCES


1. Schlaggar BL, Mink JW. Movement disorders in children. *Pediatr Rev.* 2003;24(2):39–51

2. Kurlan R, ed. *Handbook of Tourette's Syndrome and Related Tic and Behavioral Disorders.* 2nd ed. New York: Marcel Dekker; 2005

3. Leckman J, Walker D, Cohen D. Premonitory urges in Tourette's syndrome. *Am J Psychiatry.* 1993;150:98–102

4. Leckman J, Zhang H, Vitale A, et al. Course of tic severity in Tourette syndrome: the first two decades. *Pediatrics.* 1998;102:14–19

5. Tourette Syndrome Study Group. Treatment of ADHD in children with tics: a randomized controlled trial. *Neurology.* 2002;58:527–536

6. Swedo SE, Leonard HL, Garvey M, et al. Pediatric autoimmune neuropsychiatric disorders associated with streptococcal infections: clinical description of the first 50 cases. *Am J Psychiatry.* 1998;155:264–271

7. Kurlan R, Kaplan EL. The pediatric autoimmune neuropsychiatric disorders associated with streptococcal infection (PANDAS) etiology for tics and obsessive-compulsive symptoms: hypothesis or entity? Practical considerations for the clinician. *Pediatrics.* 2004;113:883–886

8. Sanger T, Mink J. Movement disorders. In: Swaiman K, Ashwal S, Ferriero DM, eds. *Pediatric Neurology Principles and Practice.* 4th ed. Philadelphia: Mosby; 2006:1271–1303

9. Pechey J, trans. *The Whole Works of That Excellent Practical Physician, Dr. Thomas Sydenham: Wherein Not Only the History and Cures of Acute Diseases Are Treated of, after a New and Accurate Method; But Also the Shortest and Safest Way of Curing Most Chronical Diseases.* London:

R. Ware; R. and B. Wellington; J. Brindley; C. Corbett; and R. New; 1740

10. Manyemba J, Mayosi BM, The Cochrane Heart Group. Penicillin for secondary prevention of rheumatic fever. *Cochrane Database Syst Rev.* 2007;4

11. Bressman SB, de Leon D, Kramer PL, et al. Dystonia in Ashkenazi Jews: clinical characterization of a founder mutation. *Ann Neurol.* 1994;36(5):771-777

12. Mink JW. Dopa-responsive dystonia in children. *Curr Treat Options Neurol.* 2003;5:279-282

13. Fahn S. High dosage anticholinergic therapy in dystonia. *Neurology.* 1983;33:1255-1261

14. Mink JW. Dystonia (DRD, primary, secondary). In: Singer HS, Kossoff EH, Hartman AL, Crawford TO, eds. *Treatment of Pediatric Neurologic Disorders.* Boca Raton, FL: Taylor & Francis; 2005:139-144

15. Vidailhet M, Vercueil L, Houeto JL, et al. Bilateral deep-brain stimulation of the globus pallidus in primary generalized dystonia. *N Engl J Med.* 2005;352(5):459-467

16. Jan MMS. Misdiagnosis in children with dopa-responsive dystonia. *Pediatr Neurol.* 2004;31:298-303

17. Brunstrom JE, Bastian AJ, Wong M, Mink JW. Motor benefit from levodopa in spastic quadriplegic cerebral palsy. *Ann Neurol.* 2000;47(5):662-665

18. Caviness JN, Brown P. Myoclonus: current concepts and recent advances. *Lancet Neurol.* 2004;3(10):598-607

19. Mahone EM, Bridges D, Prahme C, Singer HS. Repetitive arm and hand movements (complex motor stereotypies) in children. *J Pediatr.* 2004;145:391-395

20. Mink JW, Mandelbaum DE. Stereotypies and repetitive behaviors: clinical assessment and brain basis. In: Tuchman R, Rapin I, eds. *Autism: A Neurological Disorder of Early Brain Development.* London: Mac Keith Press; 2006:68-78

21. Miller JM, Singer HS, Bridges DD, Waranch R. Behavioral therapy for treatment of stereotypic movements in nonautistic children. *J Child Neurol.* 2006;21:119-125

22. Louis ED, Dure LS, Pullman S. Essential tremor in childhood: a series of nineteen cases. *Mov Disord.* 2001;16(5):921-923

23. Jankovic J, Madisetty J, Vuong KD. Essential tremor among children. *Pediatrics.* 2004;114(5):1203-1205

24. Zesiewicz TA, Elble R, Louis ED, et al. Practice parameter: therapies for essential tremor: report of the Quality Standards Subcommittee of the American Academy of Neurology. *Neurology.* 2005;64(12):2008-2020

25. Kirsch DB, Mink JW. Psychogenic movement disorders in children. *Pediatr Neurol.* 2004;30(1):1-6

26. Maricich SM, Zoghbi HY. The cerebellum and the hereditary ataxias. In: Swaiman K, Ashwal S, Ferriero DM, eds. *Pediatric Neurology Principles and Practice.* Vol 2. 4th ed. Philadelphia: Mosby; 2006:1242-1269

# CHAPTER 130

# Demyelinating Diseases

MITCHELL STEINSCHNEIDER, MD, PhD

## OVERVIEW

The hallmark of demyelinating diseases is their disruption of myelin sheaths that encase axons in the white matter of the brain and spinal cord, leading to an interruption of normal nervous impulses. Because white matter lesions can occur anywhere in the central nervous system (CNS), signs and symptoms also vary widely. Demyelination is most effectively identified by magnetic resonance imaging (MRI), and the observed lesion patterns frequently serve as keys for accurate diagnosis. Infectious, parainfectious, metabolic, and idiopathic etiologies, the latter exemplified by multiple sclerosis (MS), are the main causes of CNS demyelination in the adolescent (Box 130-1). Treatments can be given for most demyelinating disorders, necessitating their accurate and rapid diagnosis (Box 130-2). As a group, demyelinating diseases are relatively common in this age group, and a pediatric neurology practice, clinic, or children's hospital can expect to see new cases regularly.

### Box 130-1

***Selective Adolescent-Onset Demyelinating Disorders***

- **Infectious**[1-8]
  - HIV
  - HTLV-I
  - Cytomegalovirus (CMV)
  - Polyomavirus
  - JC (progressive multifocal leukoencephalopathy)
  - Lyme disease
  - *Mycoplasma pneumoniae*
  - Influenza[9]
  - West Nile virus[10]
- **Parainfectious (acute disseminated encephalomyelitis)**[11-12]
  - Measles
  - Mumps
  - Rubella
  - Varicella

### Box 130-1 (Continued)

  - Herpes simplex
  - Epstein-Barr
  - Coronavirus
  - Influenza
  - Coxsackie
  - Enterovirus
  - Hepatitis (A and C)
  - *Mycoplasma pneumoniae*
  - *Streptococcus pyogenes*
  - Vaccinations
- **Optic neuritis**
- **Transverse myelitis**
- **Neuromyelitis optica**
- **Multiple sclerosis**
- **Systemic autoimmune disorders**
  - Systemic lupus erythematosus (SLE)
  - Sjögren syndrome
  - Behçet disease
- **Posterior leukoencephalopathy**
- **Metabolic**
  - Adrenoleukodystrophy/adrenomyelopathy
  - Mitochondrial disorders

## INFECTIOUS CAUSES OF DEMYELINATION

Central nervous system demyelination frequently results from infectious illnesses. Although demyelination usually is caused by a parainfectious, autoimmune response directed against white matter elements, it can also be caused directly by the infectious agent (Table 130-1). Retroviruses are important direct causes of CNS demyelination. White matter in the brain and spinal cord is disrupted by HIV-1 infection.[1,2] Spinal cord involvement is generally restricted to the corticospinal tracts in children and adolescents. White matter changes in the brain typically occur in the centrum semiovale and periventricular areas, and may mimic the appearance of MS. Atrophy, basal ganglia calcifications, and ventricular

## Box 130-2

### *Selective Treatments of Demyelinating Diseases*

**Acute disseminated encephalomyelitis (ADEM):**

A. Weight >30 kg: IV methylprednisolone 250 mg every 6 hours for 3-5 days, followed by 1 mg/kg/day of oral prednisone for 10 days, and then a slow taper over 3-6 weeks. The slow taper is recommended to limit the risk of relapse, which can occur in up to one-third of patients.[11]

B. Weight <30 kg: IV methylprednisolone 10–30 mg/kg/day to maximum dose of 1 g/day, then follow previous protocol.[12-13]

C. Intravenous immunoglobulin (IVIG) 0.4 g/kg/day for 5 days or plasmapheresis may also be of benefit.[11]

**Optic neuritis:**

A. Weight >30 kg: IV methylprednisolone 250 mg every 6 hours for 3 days, followed by 1 mg/kg/day of oral prednisone for 11 days, and then taper over 4 days.[14]

B. Weight <30 kg: consider ADEM dosing for initial treatment.[12,15]

**Transverse myelitis, neuromyelitis optica:**

A. Consider previously stated steroid therapies for acute treatment.[16]

B. If no improvement consider plasmapheresis, 7 exchanges delivered every other day at 55 ml/kg per exchange.[17]

**Multiple sclerosis:**

A. Acute therapy: see therapies used for optic neuritis.[18] Consider intravenous gamma globulin (IVGG) or plasmapheresis.[19]

B. Chronic therapy:[18]

- Interferon beta-1 a (Avonex): 30 mcg IM once weekly.
- Interferon beta-1 a (Rebif): 22–44 mcg SC 3 times weekly. Lower and higher doses have been tested in adolescents.[20]
- Interferon beta-1b (Betaseron): 0.25 mg SC every other day. This dose has been tested in adolescents.[21]
- Glatiramer acetate (copaxone): 20 mg SC once daily.

enlargement also are observed. Opportunistic infections associated with HIV and other immunocompromised states may also produce white matter abnormalities, including cytomegalovirus (CMV) and progressive multifocal leukoencephalopathy, a potentially lethal and progressive demyelinating disease caused by reactivation of the polyomavirus JC.[2,3] Another retrovirus, human T-lymphotropic virus (HTLV-1), produces demyelination of the spinal cord (HTLV-1 myelopathy/tropical spastic paraparesis).[4,5] The disorder is endemic to the Caribbean, southern Japan, and central Africa, and population mobility has increased the frequency of it in more temperate locations. Disease progression usually is insidious with progressive back and leg pain, weakness and spasticity of the legs, and bowel/bladder dysfunction. Diagnosis is made by demonstrating increased HTLV-1 titers in serum and cerebrospinal fluid (CSF).

Demyelinating lesions of the brain also are caused by Lyme disease.[6,7] Focal, multifocal, and more expansive lesions have all been described. Serological evidence of Lyme disease will be present in the CSF, and the white matter lesions generally resolve with antibiotic therapy. These lesions may be associated with multiple neurological complications including Bell's palsy, other cranial neuropathies, meningitis, encephalitis, optic neuritis, pseudotumor cerebri, headache, and behavioral changes. Similarly, demyelinating lesions caused by *Mycoplasma pneumoniae* infections also are associated with a host of CNS presentations, including a diffuse or focal encephalitis, stroke, optic neuritis and other cranial neuropathies, and transverse myelitis.[8] A more in-depth discussion of Lyme disease can be found in Chapter 140, Tick-Borne Disases.

## PARAINFECTIOUS CAUSES OF DEMYELINATION

Central nervous system demyelination frequently is caused by immunological reactions to infections, and less commonly by vaccinations. The disorder, acute disseminated encephalomyelitis (ADEM) (see Box 130-2), accounts for 15% of childhood-onset (prepubertal) encephalitis[11,12] and also is common in adolescence. Incidence ranges from 0.4 to 0.8 per 100,000. As a primary response to infection, an inflammatory reaction in the CNS ensues, with resultant leakage of myelin antigens into the systemic circulation, development of autoantibodies, and subsequent attack by activated immune cells through a compromised blood–brain barrier. As a secondary response, homology between pathogen antigens and constituents of myelin produces demyelination when the activated immune cells enter the CNS. Pathologically, ADEM is characterized by perivascular infiltration with lymphocytes and macrophages, vasculitis, demyelination, and brain edema. Acute hemorrhagic leukoencephalitis (AHL), a more fulminant form of ADEM, is characterized by a necrotizing vasculitis and hemorrhage.

Clinical presentation classically begins 1 to 2 weeks after an infection, most commonly upper respiratory, or vaccination.[11,12] Historically, measles is the most common precipitating agent of ADEM worldwide, complicating 1 in every 1,000 cases with a severe form of the disorder that has a 25% mortality rate. *Mycoplasma pneumoniae* is another common precipitant of ADEM. Other causes of ADEM include a wide variety of viruses, other infectious agents, and immunizations, and are listed in Box 130-1. However, in 25% to 50% of cases, a precipitating cause cannot be identified.

Patients usually present with signs of encephalitis that include fever, headache, focal neurological deficits, altered mental status, and seizures.[11,12] Ataxia, hemiparesis, and cranial nerve dysfunction are the most frequent focal deficits. Focal-onset seizures are observed in about one-third and may progress to focal status epilepticus. More discrete disorders such as optic neuritis (usually bilateral and classically associated with varicella) and transverse myelitis can frequently be considered variants of ADEM.

Diagnosis is facilitated by serological evidence of a recent systemic illness, exclusion of other disorders, analysis of CSF, and neuroimaging.[11,12] Cerebrospinal fluid usually reveals a lymphocytic infiltration with mild to moderately increased protein, normal glucose, occasionally elevated pressure, and negative cultures. Increased CSF IgG and oligoclonal bands, indicative of an intrathecal immunological response, may be transiently present in about one-third. Magnetic resonance imaging most commonly reveals widespread, multiple small lesions in the white matter, though large confluent areas may occur and take on a tumor-like appearance. Edema and ring-like enhancement of lesions with gadolinium may be observed. Less commonly, thalamus and basal ganglia may be affected, the latter often appearing when the ADEM initiates a movement disorder. Hemorrhage is present in AHL. Rarely, brain biopsy may be required for diagnosis.

Occasionally, it is unclear whether a patient is presenting with ADEM or an infective encephalitis.[22] Patients with ADEM are more likely to have had a prodromal illness; have visual acuity loss in one or both eyes, signs and symptoms referable to the spinal cord, and more extensive white matter lesions. Viral cultures and DNA evidence of viral infection may also be helpful. Other disorders may present with white matter lesions that mimic ADEM and usually require evaluation.[11] The most common dilemma with regard to the differential diagnosis of ADEM is whether the attack constitutes a first episode of MS. Several criteria can be used to help differentiate these 2 disorders (Table 130-1).[11,13]

Although controlled evidence is lacking, standard of care treatment generally involves use of intravenous (IV) high-dose steroids (Box 130-2).[11-13] Intravenous gamma globulin and plasmapheresis may also be of benefit.[11] Clinical outcome of patients is generally favorable, although a prolonged recovery period may be necessary.[12] Despite modern therapies, ADEM still carries a 5% mortality rate, and higher if associated with measles. In one long-term follow-up study of ADEM, 89% of patients were either normal or had mild residual deficits without significant disability.[12] Most favorable outcomes occurred in patients with small lesions on MRI, although even patients with large or thalamic lesions had 80% favorable results.

**Table 130-1**

**Differentiation between ADEM and MS[11,13]**

| | *ADEM* | *MS* |
|---|---|---|
| Age | Usually younger children | Usually adolescents |
| Presentation | Many signs and symptoms | Few signs and symptoms |
| MRI lesions | Gray/white matter junction | Periventricular |
| | Deep gray matter | Corpus callosum |
| Repeat MRI | Lesion resolution | New lesions |
| CSF | Transient oligoclonal bands | Persistent oligoclonal bands |

**OPTIC NEURITIS**

Optic neuritis is an inflammation of the optic nerves that manifests as a subacute loss of visual function.[13,14] Visual deficits, which can be severe, are most often unilateral, though in children almost half develop bilateral dysfunction. Ocular pain exacerbated by eye movements and more generalized headaches are very common symptoms. Onset follows a prodromal viral illness in about 30%. Visual loss is maximal centrally and color vision is affected. Examination reveals an afferent papillary defect if visual loss is unilateral. Swelling of the optic disc (papillitis) is commonly observed in adolescents, contrasting to normal funduscopy indicative of a retrobulbar inflammation that is more common in older patients. Magnetic resonance imaging shows swelling of the optic nerve and enhancement with gadolinium. Cerebrospinal fluid may show a lymphocytosis, an elevated protein, and oligoclonal bands. Additional symptoms and more diffuse MRI abnormalities indicate that the optic neuritis is a component of ADEM. In this case, the optic neuritis is usually bilateral. Other

**Box 130-3**

***Differential Diagnosis of Optic Neuritis***[14]

Retinal detachment
Compressive optic neuropathy
Ischemic optic neuropathy
Leber hereditary optic neuropathy
Autoimmune disorders (eg, SLE)
Sarcoidosis
Infection: Lyme disease, cat scratch neuroretinitis produced by *Bartonella henselae*, syphilis, cryptococcal infection, and viral illnesses such as HIV, CMV, and varicella

disorders that should be considered in the differential diagnosis are listed in Box 130-3.

Optic neuritis may be a harbinger of MS.[13-23] Multiple series have reported a 10% to 40% risk of developing MS after a first episode of optic neuritis, with risk increasing when patient follow-up is extended over decades. Factors increasing risk include: (1) presence of additional neurological symptoms, (2) optic neuritis recurrence, (3) presence of demyelinating lesions in the brain, and (4) increased cells or oligoclonal bands in the CSF.

Optic neuritis therapy has become standardized in adults (Box 130-2).[14] Therapy hastens recovery of visual functions, diminishes pain, and decreases the probability that MS will develop within the subsequent 2 years. Recovery from an attack of optic neuritis usually occurs within a month, though subtle visual deficits may persist.

### TRANSVERSE MYELITIS

Transverse myelitis is an acute or subacute inflammatory process of the spinal cord.[24,25] Signs and symptoms include back pain, weakness, diminished sensation, and bowel/bladder dysfunction. Inflammation is usually greatest within the thoracic spinal cord, leading to weakness that is maximal in the legs. Paralysis may ensue, and a sensory level can usually be identified. Both idiopathic forms and those caused by defined entities occur. These entities are essentially identical to those associated with other demyelinating disorders such as ADEM (Box 130-1), with the caveat that transverse myelitis may be a component of neuromyelitis optica (see the following). Infectious and parainfectious etiologies are the most common causes of transverse myelitis in adolescents.

A compressive etiology must be rapidly excluded at patient presentation.[24] If an acute surgical lesion is not identified, a lumbar puncture should be performed to search for additional signs of inflammation and to exclude noninflammatory causes of myelopathy (eg, spinal cord infarction). A negative MRI of the brain and orbits suggests the diagnosis of acute transverse myelitis. Positive findings point toward the diagnosis of MS, ADEM, or neuromyelitis optica, though in either case other disease causes need to be excluded. Therapy of transverse myelitis is similar to those for ADEM (Box 130-2).[24]

### NEUROMYELITIS OPTICA (DEVIC DISEASE)

Neuromyelitis optica is a severe disorder characterized by optic neuritis and transverse myelitis.[17-25] Episodes do not have to occur in close temporal proximity. Clinical and MRI evidence of demyelination within the brain may occur in patients with an otherwise typical presentation. Relapses frequently occur, and the misdiagnosis of MS is often made. Newly modified criteria for clinically definite neuromyelitis optica include the requirements that patients have optic neuritis, acute myelitis, and 2 of 3 additional findings: (1) contiguous spinal cord lesions that extend across at least 3 vertebrae, (2) brain MRIs that do not meet criteria for MS, and (3) NMO-IgG seropositivity. NMO-IgG is a serological marker with high specificity and good sensitivity that binds near the blood–brain barrier to small blood vessels and astrocytic foot processes via aquaporin-4, a major water channel involved in CNS fluid homeostasis. In the younger patient, extensive spinal cord lesions consistent with neuromyelitis optica are seen in more routine cases of transverse myelitis. Although high-dose steroid therapy is used for acute exacerbations, plasmapheresis may bring better initial relief. Preventive therapy against relapses generally includes a combination of an immunosuppressive agent and prednisone.

## MULTIPLE SCLEROSIS

The clinical hallmarks of MS are multiple episodes of neurological dysfunction produced by more than one demyelinating lesion in the CNS (dissemination in space and time).[18-26] Although MS is generally a disease of young adults, 2% to 5% of cases begin in childhood, most in the teenage years. Girls are more likely to be affected than boys by a ratio of 2:1. Multiple sclerosis is common, with a prevalence of 0.5/1,000 in northern latitudes. Thus, although only a small percentage of MS occurs in children, its high overall prevalence makes it a relatively frequent pediatric neurological disorder. Although the etiology of MS is unknown, 2 main hypotheses are dominant. In the first, systemic T cells reactive to myelin enter the CNS and initiate an inflammatory cascade. In the second, processes initiated in the CNS, such as a persistent infection, cause myelin antigens to be released into the systemic circulation with resultant antibody formation, CNS attack, and damage. In either case, the complex inflammatory cascade that initiates, maintains, and transforms the disorder into a chronic, treatment-resistant entity is being heavily investigated, resulting in novel and ever-evolving treatment options.[19]

White matter plaques with a predilection for periventricular and corpus callosal locations are the pathological hallmark of MS. Plaques are inflammatory regions containing T cells, B cells, and macrophages that cause demyelination. Although variable degrees of remyelination occur, chronic disease ultimately leads to loss of oligodendrocytes, progressive axonal damage, and gliosis. This latter stage, which represents a transition from a relapsing/remitting pattern to chronic progressive MS, occurs in most patients and is associated with significant clinical disabilities.

Multiple sclerosis most commonly begins with a clinically isolated syndrome, including optic neuritis (generally unilateral in MS) and transverse myelitis. Because demyelination can occur at any white matter site, the symptoms and signs of MS are protean. Sensory disturbances, ataxia, limb weakness, and bowel/bladder symptoms are common initial problems in children and adults, whereas headache, seizures, and encephalopathy are more common in children.[27] The clinical course is characterized by periods of relapses and remissions in most adolescents,[28] with the first relapse averaging 10 months after initial presentation.[27] Initial remissions are usually associated with return to normal function, but further relapses tend to produce permanent residual deficits. Cognitive deficits maximal in language and attentional functions commonly accrue in children and adolescents.[29] Clinical outcome is variable and ranges from no long-term disabilities to progressive acquisition of multiple permanent deficits.

Definitive diagnosis rests on demonstrating multiple CNS lesions that produce clinical evidence of CNS dysfunction separated in time (Box 130-4).[26] However, the advent of disease-modifying therapies has made the need for early diagnosis more critical. Laboratory-supported criteria allow CSF abnormalities and the number, distribution, and enhancement characteristics of lesions identified on MRI at initial presentation, in association with documentation of new white matter lesions on MRI, to take the place of a second clinical episode for making a diagnosis of clinically definite MS (Box 130-4).[26] Thus, it is recommended that a follow-up MRI with gadolinium contrast be obtained 3 months after initial presentation.[18] More lenient criteria may be required for early diagnosis in children.[27] Evoked potentials may occasionally reveal lesions unseen on MRI and hasten diagnosis.[30]

### Box 130-4

### *Diagnostic Criteria for Clinically Definite Multiple Sclerosis*[26]

**Poser criteria:**

1. Two or more attacks AND clinical evidence of at least 2 separate CNS lesions.
2. Two or more attacks, clinical evidence of 1 lesion, AND laboratory evidence (MRI, evoked potentials) of at least 1 other.

**McDonald criteria also allow:**

1. One attack with 2 lesions on examination AND evidence of a new MRI lesion (new T2 lesion or gadolinium-enhancing lesion) at least 3 months after the clinical attack.
2. One attack with 1 lesion on examination AND MRI at time of attack demonstrating dissemination in space (see following) OR at least 2 MRI lesions with abnormal CSF (elevated IgG or demonstration of CSF oligoclonal bands) AND a new MRI lesion at least 3 months after the clinical attack.

**MRI criteria for dissemination in space (need 3 of 4):**

1. At least 1 gadolinium-enhancing lesion or at least 9 T2 lesions.
2. At least 1 infratentorial lesion.
3. At least 1 lesion at the junction of the gray/white matter.
4. At least 3 periventricular lesions.

Note: One spinal cord lesion can replace 1 brain lesion.

**Other relevant disorders must always be excluded.**[18,26]

In general, patients presenting with optic neuritis or isolated sensory symptoms and a normal initial brain MRI have the best prognosis for not developing MS, whereas presenting with multifocal signs and symptoms, motor system involvement, and a large lesion load on the initial MRI carries the worst prognosis.[23]

Alternative diagnoses must always be excluded. Analysis of CSF is especially important to rule out other etiologies, especially infection.[18] Cerebrospinal fluid cell count may show a mild mononuclear pleocytosis in MS, and protein content is usually elevated slightly. An increase in CSF IgG levels and ratio of CSF IgG to total protein is often present. Oligoclonal bands are found in the CSF of most patients. Positive findings, although supportive of MS, are also found in many other chronic inflammatory disorders. Therefore, clinical judgment must always be the deciding factor for making the diagnosis of MS.

Management must be tailored to the individual patient. There is no cure for MS, but multiple new therapies exist that can significantly ameliorate symptoms, reduce exacerbations of the disease, and retard disease progression (Box 130-2). The duration of acute exacerbations can be shortened by high-dose steroid therapy, although the clinical outcome is unaffected.[18] Three different preparations of interferon beta therapy and glatiramer acetate decrease the number of clinical relapses by about 33%, diminish the formation of new MRI lesions by 50% to 80%, and improve cognitive functions and quality of life parameters.[18,19] Initiating therapy early in the course of the disease is more beneficial than using conservative measures alone, because those compounds are better able to prevent new lesion formation than heal old lesions.[18] Interferon beta-1b and SQ beta-1 a may be somewhat more efficacious than IM beta-1 a, though the latter requires administration only once weekly.[31] Principal side effects of interferon therapy include local injection site reactions, flu-like symptoms, and usually mild anemia, thrombocytopenia, and elevated liver transaminases.[18] Development of neutralizing antibodies directed against the interferons may reduce their efficacy and necessitate changing therapy to glatiramer acetate. Interferons have a safety and tolerability profile in adolescents similar to adults, though controlled trials of efficacy are lacking.[21,20] Adjunct therapies are crucial components in the care of patients with MS.[18,32] Physical, psychological, and urological therapies play major roles, as do medications to counter the effects of fatigue, depression, dizziness, tremor, pain, spasticity, and bladder/bowel dysfunction.

## AUTOIMMUNE DISORDERS

Multiple autoimmune diseases, most commonly systemic lupus erythematosus (SLE) antiphospholipid antibody syndrome, Sjögren syndrome, and Behçet disease, can mimic demyelinating disorders both clinically and radiographically.[33] Neurologic dysfunction may precede the classic systemic symptoms of each disorder. Thus, appropriate diagnostic studies should be obtained at patient presentation. Diagnostic confusion may occur from the false-positive presence of antinuclear antibodies in some patients with MS.

## POSTERIOR LEUKOENCEPHALOPATHY

Multiple etiologies, most commonly severe, acute hypertension, can produce this disorder with the characteristic radiographic appearance of edema maximal in the white matter of the posterior parietal and occipital lobes (Box 130-5).[34,35] Patients present with seizures, headache, nausea and vomiting, altered mental status, and visual loss. Diagnosis often requires excluding stroke, venous thrombosis, encephalitis, and other demyelinating disorders.[34] Treatment beyond symptomatic therapies requires amelioration of the underlying causative condition. In the case of hypertensive encephalopathy, IV antihypertensive medications should be used to gently lower blood pressure over a period of several hours.[35] Prompt and appropriate therapy causes reversal of the clinical symptoms and the white matter edema.

### Box 130-5
### *Selected Causes of Posterior Leukoencephalopathy*[34,35]

Hypertensive encephalopathy
Severe renal disease
Eclampsia immunosuppressive drugs
Cytotoxic drugs
Erythropoietin
Autoimmune disorders
Thrombotic-thrombocytopenic purpura
Organ transplantation

## METABOLIC DISORDERS

Inborn errors of metabolism are important causes of CNS demyelination in older children. The most common are adrenoleukodystrophy and mitochondrial disorders.

### ADRENOLEUKODYSTROPHY/ ADRENOMYELONEUROPATHY

Adrenoleukodystrophy (ALD) is an X-linked disorder with an incidence in males of 1:17,000 that is associated with serum elevations and impaired ß-oxidation within peroxisomes of very long chain fatty acids (VLCFA), saturated fatty acids with carbon chain lengths of 24 to 30).[36,37] The genetic defect mutates a membrane protein involved in the transport into the peroxisome of the enzyme VLCFA acyl CoA synthetase, which catalyzes the formation of the CoA derivative of the VLCFA. Multiple phenotypic expressions of the disorder exist.

Classic ALD is characterized by a severe white matter demyelination that is most prominent in the parieto-occipital region. Onset generally begins at 3 to 10 years of age, though adolescent-onset ALD occurs in 4% to 7% of patients. Initial neurological symptoms usually include behavioral problems that may resemble attention-deficit disorder with hyperactivity. Seizures, hearing and visual loss, dementia, and progressive spastic motor disturbances are also common. Adrenal cortical insufficiency (Addison disease) occurs in most patients and may be the only clinical manifestation of ALD, which is slowly progressive, leading to a vegetative state and subsequent death within several years.

Another common phenotypic expression of the disorder is adrenomyeloneuropathy (AMN) which generally begins in the second to third decade. It is characterized by neurologic dysfunction of the spinal cord and peripheral nerves, leading to a progressive spastic paraparesis, sphincter dysfunction, and sensory loss. Adrenal cortical insufficiency is common. Many patients who present with this phenotype develop cerebral involvement.

Diagnosis is confirmed by demonstrating elevated serum levels of VLCFAs. Adrenal dysfunction should be treated with steroid replacement. Dietary treatments that reduce serum levels of VLCFAs (Lorenzo's oil) have been disappointing in reversing the rate of disease progression in symptomatic patients, but may be useful in delaying disease onset in presymptomatic individuals. Bone marrow transplantation may be the treatment of choice for patients with early neurological involvement.

### MITOCHONDRIAL DISORDERS

Mitochondrial diseases are a remarkably diverse and common group of disorders (prevalence of 1-1.5:10,000) produced by genetic mutations in both nuclear and mitochondrial DNA.[38] Almost all organs can be affected, though those with high energy requirements (eg, brain) are particularly susceptible to damage. Symptoms can occur at any age, placing mitochondrial disease in the differential diagnosis of a host of degenerative disorders. White matter lesions of the brain are commonly observed.[39,40] Leukoencephalopathy with small cystic components, concurrent cerebral and cerebellar white matter involvement, and additional basal ganglia lesions are especially characteristic of mitochondrial disease. Diagnosis may require determinations of plasma and CSF lactate and pyruvate, DNA analysis, muscle biopsy, and enzyme assays.[38-40]

A mitochondrial disease, Leber hereditary optic neuropathy, deserves special comment as it often presents in the teen years and enters into the differential diagnosis of optic neuritis.[14] It is a maternally inherited disorder predominantly seen in males and is characterized by severe, acute, or subacute visual loss that occurs sequentially in both eyes.[14,39] Additional neurological deficits and diffuse or periventricular white matter lesions may coexist, mimicking ADEM and MS.

## REFERENCES

1. Belman AL. Central nervous system involvement in pediatric HIV-1 infection. *Int Pediatr.* 1992;7:126–135

2. Offiah CE, Turnbull IW. The imaging appearances of intracranial CNS infections in adult HIV and AIDS patients. *Clinical Radiology.* 2006;61:393–401

3. Koralnik IJ. New insights into progressive multifocal leukoencephalopathy. *Curr Opin Neurol.* 2004;17:365–370

4. Bagnato F, Butman JA, Mora CA, et al. Conventional magnetic resonance imaging features in patients with tropical spastic paraparesis. *J Neurovirology.* 2005;11:525–534

5. Primo JRL, Brites C, de Oliveira M de FSP, Moreno-Carvalho O, Machado M, Bittencourt AL. Infective dermatitis and human T-cell lymphotropic virus type 1-associated myelopathy/tropical spastic paraparesis in childhood and adolescence. *Clinical Infectious Diseases.* 2005;41:535–541

6. Belman AL, Coyle PK, Roque C, Cantos E. MRI findings in children infected by *Borrelia burgdorferi. Pediatr Neurol.* 1992;8:428–431

7. Stanek G, Strle F. Lyme borreliosis. *Lancet.* 2003;362:1639–1647

8. Tsiodrasa S, Kelesidisa I, Kelesidisa T, Stamboulisb E, Giamarelloua H. Central nervous system manifestations of *Mycoplasma pneumoniae* infections. *J Infection.* 2005;51:343–354

9. Maricich SM, Neul JL, Lotze TE, et al. Neurologic complications associated with influenza A in children during the 2003–2004 influenza season in Houston, Texas. *Pediatrics.* 2004;114:e626–e633

10. Jeha LE, Sila CA, Lederman RJ, Prayson RA, Isada CM, Gordon SM. West Nile virus infection: a new acute paralytic illness. *Neurology.* 2003;61:55–59

11. Menge T, Hemmer B, Nessler S, et al. Acute disseminated encephalomyelitis: an update. *Arch Neurol.* 2005;62:1673–1680

12. Tenembaum S, Chamoles N, Fejerman N. Acute disseminated encephalomyelitis: a long-term follow-up study of 84 pediatric patients. *Neurology.* 2002;59:1224–1231

13. Dale RC, Branson JA. Acute disseminated encephalomyelitis or multiple sclerosis: can the initial presentation help in establishing a correct diagnosis? *Arch Dis Child.* 2005;90:636–639

14. Balcer LJ. Optic neuritis. *New Engl J Med.* 2006;54:1273–1280

15. Wilejto M, Shroff M, Buncic JR, Kennedy J, Goia C, Banwell B. The clinical features, MRI findings, and outcome of optic neuritis in children. *Neurology.* 2006;67:258–262

16. Wingerchuk DM. Neuromyelitis optica. *The International MS J.* 2006;13:42–50

17. Wingerchuk DM, Lennon VA, Pittock SJ, Lucchinetti CF, Weinshenker BG. Revised diagnostic criteria for neuromyelitis optica. *Neurology.* 2006;66:1485–1489

18. Calabresi PA. Diagnosis and management of multiple sclerosis. *Am Fam Phys.* 2004;70:1935-1944

19. Frohman EM, Racke MK, Raine CS. Multiple sclerosis—the plaque and its pathogenesis. *New Engl J Med.* 2006;354:942-955

20. Pohl D, Rostasy K, Gärtner J, Hanefeld F. Treatment of early onset multiple sclerosis with subcutaneous interferon beta-1a. *Neurology.* 2005;64:888-890

21. Banwell B, Reder AT, Krupp L, et al. Safety and tolerability of interferon beta-1b in pediatric multiple sclerosis. *Neurology.* 2006;66:472-476

22. Kennedy PGE. Viral encephalitis: causes, differential diagnosis, and management. *J Neurol Neurosurg Psychiatry.* 2004;75(suppl 1):i10-i15

23. Miller D, Barkhof F, Montalban X, Thompson A, Filippi M. Clinically isolated syndromes suggestive of multiple sclerosis, part I: natural history, pathogenesis, diagnosis, and prognosis. *Lancet Neurology.* 2005;4:281-288

24. Kerr DA, Ayetey H. Immunopathogenesis of acute transverse myelitis. *Curr Opin Neurol.* 2002;15:339-347

25. Pittock SJ, Lucchinetti CF. Inflammatory transverse myelitis: evolving concepts. *Curr Opin Neurol.* 2006;19:362-368

26. Frohman EM, Goodin DS, Calabresi PA, et al. Report of the Therapeutics and Technology Assessment Subcommittee of the American Academy of Neurology. The utility of MRI in suspected MS. *Neurology.* 2003;61:602-611

27. Hahn CD, Shroff MM, Blaser SI, Banwell BL. MRI criteria for multiple sclerosis: evaluation in a pediatric cohort. *Neurology.* 2004;62:806-808

28. Banwell B, Tremlett H. The use of immunomodulatory therapy in children with multiple sclerosis. *Neurology.* 2005;64:778-779

29. MacAllister WS, Belman AL, Milazzo M, et al. Cognitive functioning in children and adolescents with multiple sclerosis. *Neurology.* 2005;64:1422-1425

30. Pohl D, Rostasy K, Treiber-Held S, Brockmann K, Gärtner J, Hanefeld F. Pediatric multiple sclerosis: detection of clinically silent lesions by multimodal evoked potentials. *J Pediatrics.* 2006;149:125-127

31. Goodin DS. Treatment of multiple sclerosis with human beta interferon. *The International MS J.* 2005;12:96-108

32. Henze T. Managing specific symptoms in people with multiple sclerosis. *The International MS J.* 2005;12:60-68

33. Theodoridou A, Settas L. Demyelination in rheumatic diseases. *J Neurol Neurosurg Psych.* 2006;77:290-295

34. Garg RK. Posterior leukoencephalopathy syndrome. *Postgrad Med J.* 2001;77:24-28

35. Stott VL, Hurrell MA, Anderson TJ. Reversible posterior leukoencephalopathy syndrome: a misnomer reviewed. *Internal Medicine J.* 2005;35:83-90

36. Moser HW, Raymond GV, Dubey P. Adrenoleukodystrophy: new approaches to a neurodegenerative disease. *JAMA.* 2005;294:3131-3134

37. Loes DJ, Fatemi A, Melhem ER, et al. Analysis of MRI patterns aids prediction of progression in X-linked adrenoleukodystrophy. *Neurology.* 2003;61:369-374

38. DiMauro S, Schon EA. Mitochondrial respiratory-chain diseases. *New Engl J Med.* 2003;348:2656-2668

39. Lerman-Sagie T, Leshinsky-Silvera E, Watemberga N, Luckman Y, Lev D. White matter involvement in mitochondrial diseases. *Mol Genet Metab.* 2005;84:127-136

40. Moroni I, Bugiani M, Bizzi A, Castelli G, Lamantea E, Uziel G. Cerebral white matter involvement in children with mitochondrial encephalopathies. *Neuropediatrics.* 2002;33:79-85

# CHAPTER 131

# CNS Trauma

BRIAN J. SNYDER, MD • JAMES TAIT GOODRICH, MD, PhD, DSci (*HON*)

Head injury remains among the leading causes of significant morbidity and mortality in the adolescent population. Most injuries result from motor vehicle accidents, but in urban areas, missile injuries (eg, gun shot wounds), stabbings, and injuries with blunt objects (such as baseball bats) predominate. Because 50% to 60% of deaths in these cases occur within the first 24 hours after injury, this time frame is the window within which aggressive management must occur if long-term morbidity and mortality are to be reduced.[1]

## INITIAL NEUROLOGIC EVALUATION

On arrival in the emergency department (ED) a patient who has sustained a serious head injury requires a thorough evaluation. The evaluation is similar to the standard emergency department trauma examination and is performed in a methodical step-wise fashion[2] (Box 131-1).

### PROVISIONS FOR ADEQUATE AIRWAY AND VENTILATION

Patients with severe head injury tend to be obtunded, with altered mental status; a seizure may have resulted from the initial injury. Vomiting with aspiration is not an uncommon sequela to head injury (particularly closed blunt injury). Injury to the brainstem can significantly alter breathing regulation. For these reasons an open and secured airway must be established and maintained. A low threshold for intubation should exist in all patients with altered mental status, as there is potential for a sudden precipitous further decline in the patient's neurologic examination. There may be a short-term benefit to hyperventilation in a patient with progressive intracranial hypertension (see section on hyperventilation).[3]

**Box 131-1**

***Emergency Department Evaluation for the Head Injured***

- Provision of an adequate airway and ventilation
- Volume—evaluate for blood loss and potential hypovolemia
- Vital signs and evaluate for associated injuries (rule out cervical spine injuries)
- Scalp hemorrhage
- Glasgow Coma Scale (GCS)
- Focal neurological examination
- History of trauma (mechanism of injury, loss of consciousness, progression of symptoms, history of alcohol and drug use, blood screening) should be obtained

### OBSERVATION OF VITAL SIGNS

The vital signs must be documented, monitored closely, and recorded frequently. By doing so the physician can detect trends and try to predict and avoid impending catastrophe. The well-known Cushing phenomenon—systemic hypertension with bradycardia—occurs when intracranial pressure (ICP) is significantly increased. Cushing phenomenon is an ominous sign and an indication for immediate efforts to reduce increased ICP. Blood loss due to scalp injury and lacerations can be significant if not life threatening. The scalp is well perfused and can bleed extensively in the field, so early evaluation of hematocrit can be important.

### DETERMINATION OF STATE OF CONSCIOUSNESS

The patient's level or state of consciousness must be documented to provide a baseline for measuring changes. Chapter 134, Altered States of Consciousness, has an in-depth discussion of the evaluation and treatment of such patients. If the patient is brought in by family members or paramedics it is critical to question them about the mental status of the patient before arrival, as well as any new changes, and to document this information. The Glasgow Coma Scale (GCS)[4] is most commonly used for this purpose. Drug and alcohol use is prevalent in the adolescent population; therefore the emergency evaluation should also include a drug and alcohol screening profile, especially in a patient with altered mental status.

### NEUROLOGIC EXAMINATION

The neurologic examination need not be a thorough and complete examination of all 12 cranial nerves and all motor groups. Rather it should document the level of consciousness and the function of the third, fifth, sixth, seventh, and tenth cranial nerves. The physician must determine and document the pupillary responses and extraocular function (Are the pupils reactive? Is the pupillary response symmetric?). The corneal reflex can be quite sensitive; its loss is a grave prognostic sign. Is there facial symmetry? Does the patient have an intact gag response? Motor and sensory function is evaluated simply: Does the patient follow commands? Is the examination symmetric? If not, does the patient withdraw from pain and is it symmetric? Decorticate or decerebrate posturing is a clinical sign of injury to the brainstem or severe compression of the neural axis. The presence of either of these signs may be associated with Cushing phenomenon and is an ominous prognostic indicator.

### HISTORY OF TRAUMA

It is distressing to know how often the history of trauma is not obtained in the ED. In most cases the history can be obtained from a family member, the police, or the ambulance crew. This information is extremely important, because it determines how the neurosurgical team will treat the patient, eg, a history of blunt trauma can require a surgical protocol entirely different from that for a penetrating injury.

### GLASGOW COMA SCALE

Determining the GCS has become the standard of practice in most EDs. Over the years, trauma services have correlated this score with eventual neurologic outcome. As a result, it is a useful grading system, not only for the evaluation but also for the neurosurgical team's determination of long-term prognosis. The score is standardized and should be available to all physicians.[4]

Typically, a patient who arrives with a GCS of 15 will do well unless there is an acute change. However, a patient with a GCS of 8 has a severe neurologic injury, and the injury may become permanent if not managed promptly and appropriately. A patient who arrives in the ED with a GCS of 3 to 5 is severely injured and carries an extremely poor prognosis.

**Table 131-1**

**Glasgow Coma Scale**

| *Findings* | *Score* |
|---|---|
| **Eyes** | |
| Open spontaneously | 4 |
| Open to verbal command | 3 |
| Open to pain | 2 |
| No response | 1 |
| **Best Motor Response** | |
| *To verbal command* | 6 |
| Obeys | |
| *To painful stimuli* | 5 |
| Localizes pain | |
| Flexion—withdrawal | 4 |
| Flexion—abnormal | 3 |
| Extension | 2 |
| No response | 1 |
| **Best Verbal Response** | |
| Oriented and converses | 5 |
| Disoriented and converses | 4 |
| Inappropriate words | 3 |
| Incomprehensible sounds | 2 |
| No response | 1 |

## MANAGEMENT OF ELEVATED INTRACRANIAL PRESSURE

Because elevated ICP is found in more than half of all head injuries, any patient who arrives in the ED must be evaluated for this condition. In a number of studies it has been found that in patients with an ICP greater than 20 mm Hg that remains uncontrolled the mortality rate exceeds 80%. Early recognition and treatment are therefore critical.

The management of patients with increased ICP has undergone significant changes over the last 10 to 15 years. The earlier emphasis was on the management of increased ICP rather than assessing cerebral perfusion pressure (CPP). To do this the patient was routinely hyperventilated, dehydrated with agents like mannitol, and in severe cases placed in a barbiturate coma. In recent years, and due to rigorous literature reviews and case studies, the methods of recommended treatment have changed. The introduction of the "Management of the Severe Head Injury by the American Association of Neurological Surgeons" led to these changes.[2] As a result of these guidelines, the management of the patient with a head injury depends on a key principle: maintenance of CPP rather than the previously held concept of management of ICP. The CPP is the difference between the mean arterial blood pressure (MABP) and the ICP. If CPP falls below the acceptable range oxygenation of brain tissue is compromised and permanent brain injury will result.[5,6] The concept now is to manage brain injury

**Box 131-2**

***Formula Showing the Relationship of ICP to CPP***

CPP = MABP − ICP
ICP = increased intracranial pressure
CPP = cerebral perfusion pressure
MABP = mean arterial blood pressure

**Table 131-2**

**Intracranial Pressure Levels[a]**

| *Pressure* | *Range* |
|---|---|
| Normal | 1–10 mm Hg |
| Slightly increased | 11–20 mm Hg |
| Moderately increased | 21–40 mm Hg |
| Severely increased | 21–40 mm Hg |

[a]Patients with ICP >20 need immediate and aggressive management to lower ICP and increase CPP.

by maintaining or increasing perfusion rather than just focusing on the reduction of ICP (Box 131-2 and Table 131-2).

**MANNITOL**

Before the introduction of the new guidelines[2] a patient with a severe head injury was routinely placed on a dehydrating agent such as mannitol. The thought was that mannitol would reduce overall blood volume and reduce ICP, a situation that often did occur. However, the use of mannitol also reduced significantly the CPP, causing an undesired effect of reduced perfusion. As a result of these findings the guidelines have changed in the use of dehydrating agents. In cases where there is acute evidence of a severely elevated ICP or clinical signs of herniation its use is indicated. Mannitol's effects are twofold. Immediately upon administration of mannitol (typical dose, 0.25 to 1.0 mg/kg) there is a hemodilutent effect that causes a reduction in hematocrit, reduces blood viscosity, and improves the delivery of oxygen to the brain. This positive rheological effect is the cause of the reversal of signs of herniation, if immediately observed, and is best accomplished via bolus administration. The second method by which mannitol works is through its osmotic effect on the brain, thereby dehydrating it. This is not observed until approximately 15 to 30 minutes following administration. Mannitol does have a number of side effects that must be considered. It can cause a change in fluid balance, altered serum electrolytes, a rebound rise in ICP (more frequently seen when mannitol is administrated as a continuous infusion), and seizures. Patients being treated with mannitol should have frequent laboratory tests, and serum osmolarity should be maintained at or below 320 mOsm to reduce the potential risk of renal injury. Furthermore, hypotension from dehydration should be carefully treated with fluid to prevent its occurrence.[7,8] The older practice of a continuous infusion of mannitol or other dehydration agents in the management of head injury is no longer routinely recommended.

**HYPERTONIC SALINE**

Although the experience with and use of hypertonic saline to treat intracranial hypertension remains small, several studies have supported its use in adolescents as well as adults. Hypertonic saline acts in a similar fashion to mannitol to promote positive rheologic properties and enhance delivery of blood to the brain as well as act as a hyperosmolar agent. Hypertonic saline may also aid restoration of cell membrane potential, inhibit inflammation, stimulate the release of atrial natriuretic potential (ANP), and enhance cardiac output. There are several potential side effects of hypertonic saline and these include rebound increases in ICP, central pontine myelinolysis, and subarachnoid hemorrhage. Hypertonic saline should be given using a sliding scale continuous dose infusion ranging from 0.1 to 1.0 mL/kg. The minimum dose needed to control the ICP should be used.[7]

**BARBITURATES**

Approximately 10% to 15% of patients and 21% to 42% with severe head injury will develop refractory intracranial hypertension. High doses of barbiturates have been known to reduce ICP. Enthusiasm for their use has been hampered by the significant morbidity associated with its use, especially cardiovascular suppression and hemodynamic instability. Nonetheless, barbiturates have been found to be effective in lowering ICP and decreasing mortality in patients refractory to any other treatment. Studies of barbiturates have not, however, evaluated long-term neurological outcome. Patients given barbiturates for ICP control necessitate close hemodynamic monitoring with invasive lines.[9]

**STEROIDS**

Glucocorticoids are used in the treatment of many neurologic diseases and were noted to be of benefit in reducing edema associated with brain tumors. This led to their use in head-injured patients. Sufficient evidence exists that demonstrates no benefit to the use of steroids in traumatic brain injury (TBI), and they are not recommended for use in that setting.[10]

### HYPERVENTILATION

The use of hyperventilation was historically a first line treatment of choice in severe head injury and ICP. With the recent rigorous review of the literature by the American Association of Neurological Surgeons, the guidelines have changed significantly in its use. Hyperventilation through an endotracheal tube, can lead to a rapid decrease in ICP. The reduction in a patient's $PCO_2$ level from a normal level of 40 mm Hg to 20 mm Hg results in an immediate 50% drop in ICP. It is due to this fact that aggressive hyperventilation has been utilized in the management of head injury. However, the method of reduction in ICP is due to cerebral vasoconstriction leading to an undesired result of decreased perfusion pressure. Research has demonstrated a pre-existing decrease in cerebral blood flow (CBF) in the acute periods following TBI. A prospective randomized study found improved outcomes in patients at 3 and 6 months when *prophylactic* hyperventilation was *not* utilized. Chronic hyperventilation to $PaCO_2 \leq 25$ should now be avoided in patients with TBI especially within the first 24 hours. The recent guidelines recommend keeping the patient eucarbic with ventilations of $PaCO_2$ in the range of 35 to 40. However, hyperventilation may be implemented as a short treatment in patients with acute neurologic decline or with intracranial hypertension refractory to other therapy.[11]

### TEMPERATURE CONTROL

There is little clinical data on temperature control and the effects on outcome in adolescents with TBI. Data in adult animal models have shown that hypothermia increases the degree of posttraumatic damage by furthering the pathophysiologic response to injury. Clinical data in adults have also demonstrated a poorer outcome with hypothermia. Due to these 2 factors, the avoidance of hypothermia in severe head-injured adolescents should be considered.[12] The converse of hyperthermia should also be avoided as the hypermetabolism that occurs decreases oxygenation to the brain.

## INDICATIONS FOR MONITORING OF INTRACRANIAL PRESSURE

Only 3% of patients with mild head injury (GCS 14–15) and 10% to 20% of patients with moderate head injury (GCS 9–13) deteriorate into coma and are reclassified as severe head injury patients. Therefore, routine ICP monitoring in these 2 groups is not felt to be warranted.

Due to the association between elevated ICP and poor outcome in severe head injury patients, ICP monitoring is felt to be appropriate in patients with a GCS of 3 to 8 with evidence of an abnormal head computed tomography (CT) scan (defined as the presence of hematoma, contusions, edema, or compressed basal cisterns). Patients with severe head injury but a normal head CT may still be considered appropriate for monitoring if they have 2 of the following risk factors: age >40 years, unilateral or bilateral motor posturing, and/or a systolic blood pressure (SBP) of <90 mm Hg.[13] The monitoring of ICP has several criteria associated with it, and we have outlined those in Box 131-3.

**Box 131-3**

***Monitoring ICP—Ideal Criteria***

1. Little or no trauma to intracranial structures
2. Risk of infection should be minimal
3. No leakage of CSF fluid from the system
4. Length of time of monitoring should not interfere with patient comfort
5. Continuous recordings possible despite changes of position and diagnostic procedures
6. Easily used by the nursing and house staff

CSF, cerebrospinal fluid

## MONITORING INTRACRANIAL PRESSURE

### INTRAVENTRICULAR CATHETER

The most common means of monitoring ICP is the intraventricular catheter. It is placed within the ventricular system by means of a frontal burr hole and coupled to an external strain gauge transducer. It is the least expensive and most accurate method for measuring ICP. In addition, the ventricular catheter offers the advantage of therapeutic drainage of cerebrospinal fluid (CSF), which is not offered by any other ICP-measuring device. The catheter may be readily placed in an intensive care unit. The procedure usually requires less than 10 minutes with either a burr hole or twist drill technique. The main disadvantages of a ventricular catheter are the risk of infection and the risk of hemorrhage associated with insertion (average incidence of hemorrhage 1.1%). To minimize the infectious risk, the catheter is typically tunneled in the subcutaneous tissues prior to externalization. The ventricular catheter must be placed within the ventricle to function properly and may occasionally become plugged with particulate material, necessitating reinsertion/revision.[14]

### INTRAPARENCHYMAL MONITORS

The intraparenchymal monitor with a pressure transducer tip is currently felt to be the second best option for ICP monitoring in head trauma. The monitor is a wire that is placed into the substance of the patient's brain by means of a burr hole or twist drill. The advantage of this type of monitoring is the lower risk of infection as well as the ease in placement. This should be considered when ventricular catheterization has failed or is obstructed. The disadvantage is that it may have a tendency to drift due to an inability to recalibrate the device upon insertion and it does not have the ability to withdraw cerebrospinal fluid (CSF) associated with it.[14]

### SUBARACHNOID, SUBDURAL, AND EPIDURAL MONITORS

Monitors exist that can be placed in all 3 of these spaces within the brain. They are currently felt to be less optimal for ICP measurement in the head trauma patient. The advantages of these 3 systems are that they do not enter the brain parenchyma. However, all 3 systems are considered to be less accurate than the use of ventricular catheters or the intraparenchymal device, and none offers the ability to remove CSF if the pressure increases.[14]

## INTRACRANIAL HEMORRHAGE IN HEAD TRAUMA

There is a high incidence of intracranial hemorrhage in severe head injury. Knowledge and recognition of the types of hemorrhage are critical for optimal management. Essentially, 4 types of intracranial hemorrhages are seen in adolescents: (1) subdural, (2) intraparenchymal, (3) epidural, and (4) traumatic subarachnoid. Chapter 134, Altered States of Consciousness, discusses evaluation and management of contusions and concussions in adolescent patients.

### ACUTE SUBDURAL HEMATOMA

Subdural hematoma (Figure 131-1) is a common injury in the adolescent population and carries a poor prognosis. It occurs when direct injury to the brain results in a torn bridging vein or artery or direct injury to a pial vessel. Greater force is required to cause injuries of this type in adolescents because most of them do not have brain atrophy and therefore the subdural space is less generous and the bridging vessels exist in less of a state of stretch. It is essential to recognize this injury early, because it is a surgical emergency requiring urgent evacuation of the clot.

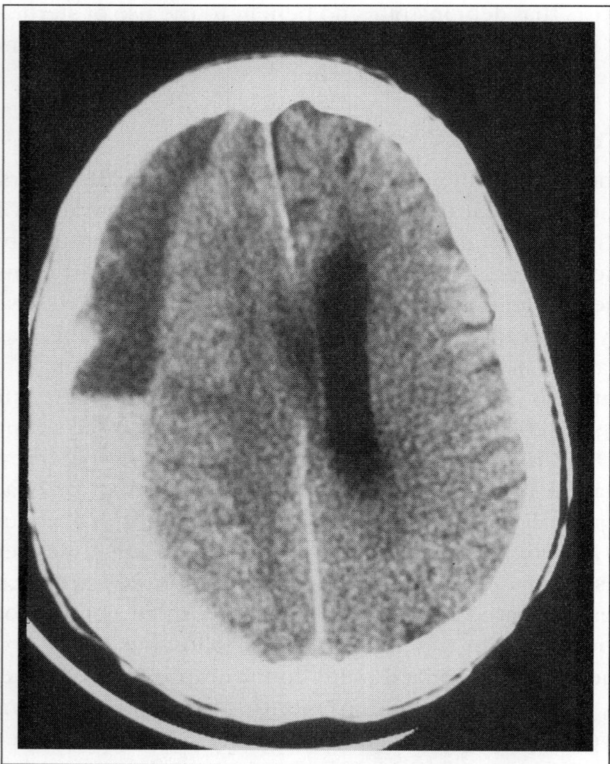

**FIGURE 131-1** Computed tomography (CT) scan showing a mixed chronic and acute subdural hematoma (SDH) over the right hemisphere. Fresh blood is evident as seen in the starkly white blood, which has layered out in the chronic component. There is shift and mass effect from the SDH evidenced by the midline shift of the ventricles and obliteration of the right lateral ventricle. (Photo courtesy of James Tait Goodrich.)

### ACUTE INTRAPARENCHYMAL HEMATOMA

The most common sites of intraparenchymal injury are the frontal and temporal lobe tips (Figure 131-2). This most commonly occurs as a result of a motor vehicle injury where the victim is thrown forward. The sites of injury are the points at which the brain comes into contact with the decelerated skull. The other common cause of intraparenchymal trauma is penetrating injury, such as a gunshot wound (Figure 131-3). These grave injuries almost always carry a long-term morbidity. In most cases of penetrating intraparenchymal hematoma, craniotomy is required for removal of the intraparenchymal clot and debridement of surrounding devitalized tissue.

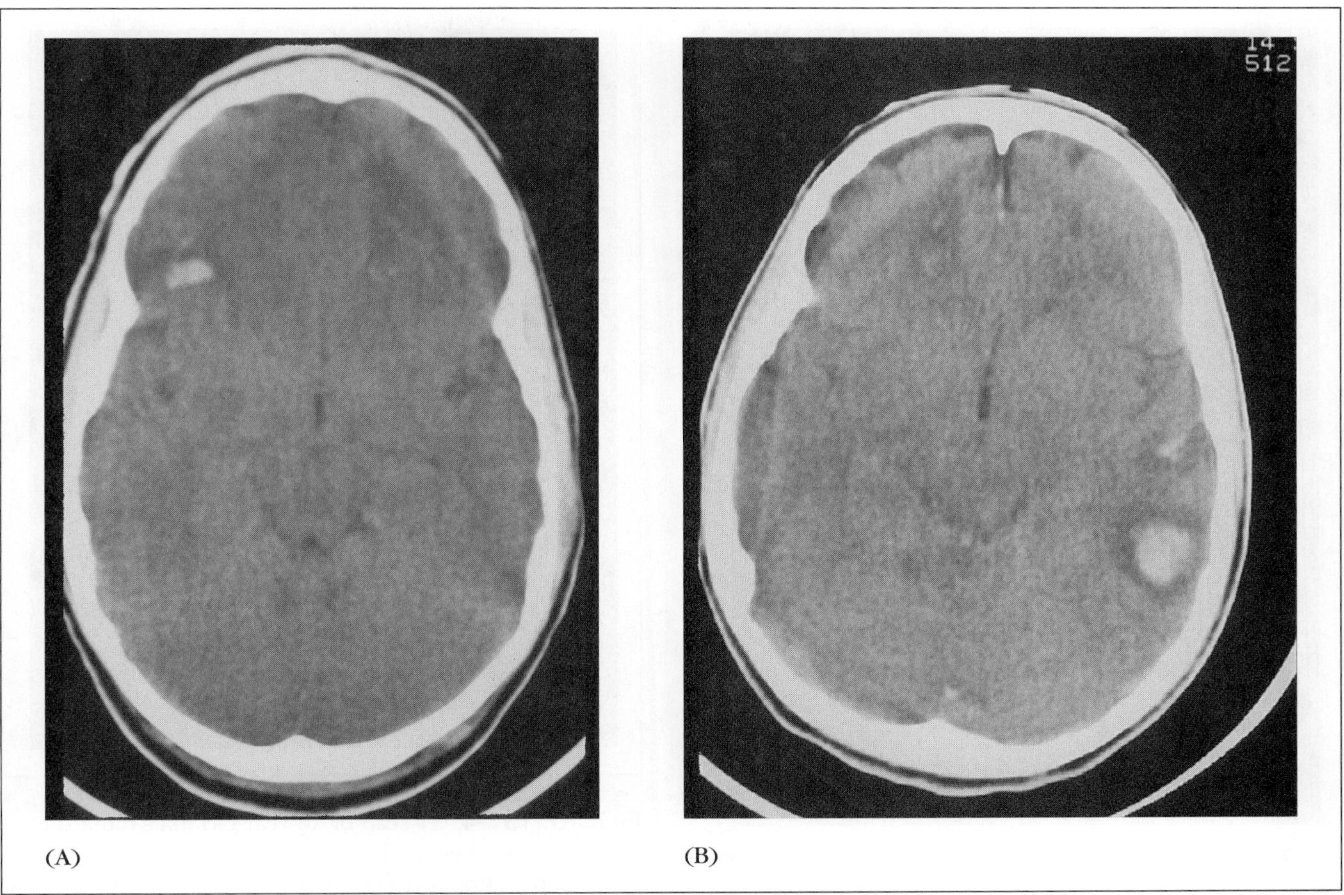


**FIGURE 131-2** (A) CT scan showing an acute intraparenchymal hemorrhage of the right frontal lobe occurring as a result of a fight and a blow to the head. The hemorrhage is acute as seen in the bright white signal. There is surrounding brain edema suggesting a more diffuse brain injury. (B) CT scan showing 2 acute fresh intraparenchymal bleeds in the left temporal–parietal region; there are also several small bleeds throughout the brain—blunt head trauma from a motor vehicle accident: an 18-year-old unbelted male thrown into the windshield. (Photos courtesy of James Tait Goodrich.)

## ACUTE EPIDURAL HEMATOMA

This injury results from hemorrhage into the potential space between the dura and skull (Figure 131-4). Often injury to the middle meningeal artery causes an acute epidural hematoma. In our experience, this lesion is the most common type overlooked in the emergency department. Typically, the patient suffers some sort of head blow, in many cases a mild one. In the emergency department the patient walks, talks, and seems fine and is sent home, only to be brought back obtunded with a fixed and dilated pupil. What is observed in the emergency department is the so-called lucid interval. Because the hematoma expands slowly, a period of minutes to hours can elapse during which the patient appears well. Only when the hematoma expands to a critical mass does the patient become obtunded and exhibit altered mental status. If these injuries are recognized early and surgically treated the long-term morbidity is low. Because the brain is only compressed, prompt removal of the blood clot is sufficient to ensure a good prognosis.

## TRAUMATIC SUBARACHNOID HEMORRHAGE

Trauma is the most common cause of subarachnoid hemorrhage. This results from tearing of veins and arteries along the skull base or in the subarachnoid space. Traumatic subarachnoid hemorrhage is found in a high proportion of severe head injury patients. Its presence also correlates with a worsened outcome in retrospective studies (Figure 131-4 and Figure 131-5).

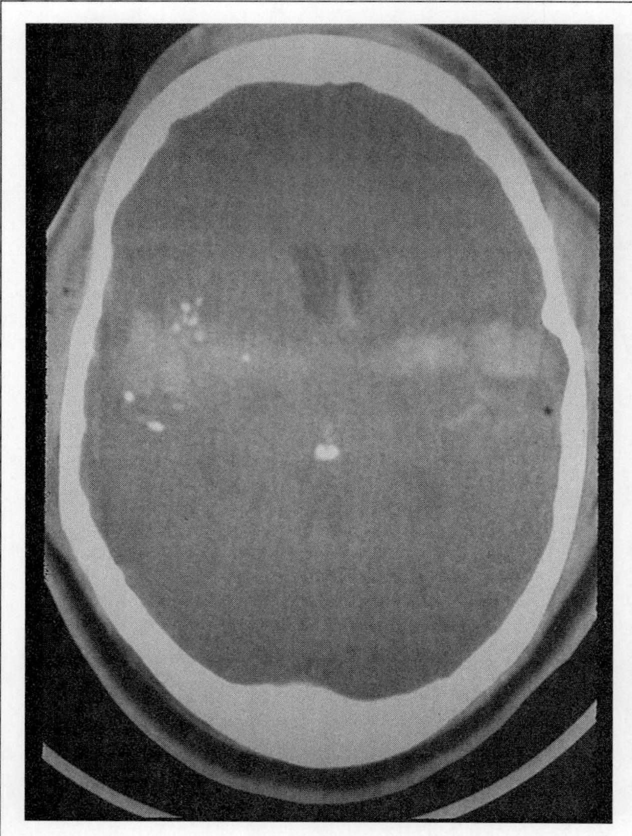

FIGURE 131-3 CT scan of a 16-year-old male who committed suicide by placing a large caliber gun to his temporal region. The CT shows a devastating through-and-through gunshot wound. Injuries of this type are ominous and survival is rare. (Photo courtesy of James Tait Goodrich.)

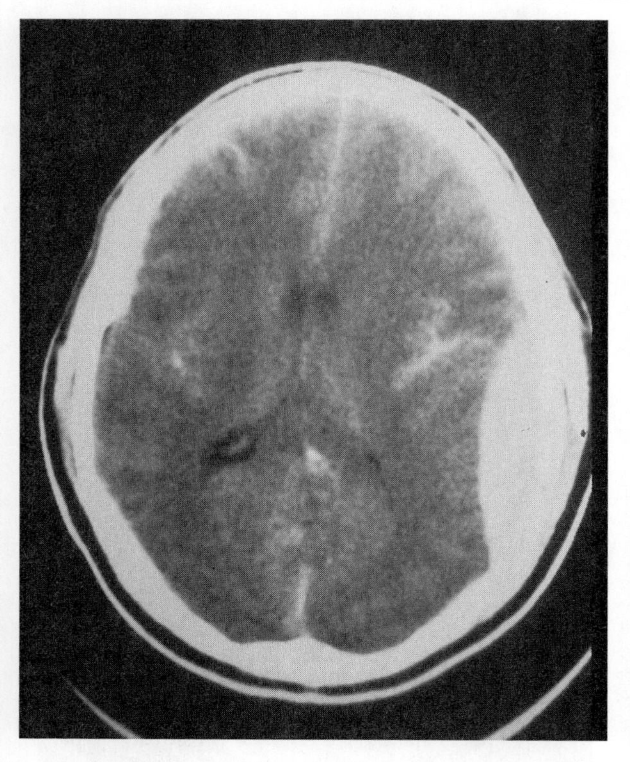

FIGURE 131-4 CT scan of 14-year-old male hit in the side of the head with a baseball. The crescentic shape epidural hematoma (EPH) seen in the left temporal region is a classic finding. The smooth edge of the clot against the brain is what distinguishes this type of bleed, EPH, from an SDH. There is, in addition, a picture of diffuse subarachnoid bleeding, seen in the high white signal in the subarachnoid spaces. (Photo courtesy of James Tait Goodrich.)

## BRAIN HERNIATION

Brain herniation is defined as the movement of a portion of the brain from its normal position to an adjacent compartment, caused by the presence of a pathological mass lesion or by focal or generalized brain edema. No matter what its cause, it is an ominous finding and needs to be aggressively treated. Herniation causes a stretching or compression of vascular or neural structures against bone and dural edges. Interestingly, brain herniation does not necessarily imply elevated ICP, because some brains can compensate for the presence of sizable pathological masses by reduction in CSF volume. In head trauma, brain herniation is most frequently caused by hematoma (epidural, subdural, intracerebral) or the resultant diffuse brain edema that follows. A useful diagnostic sign on CT is loss or obliteration of the ambient cisterns, the CSF cisterns that surround the mesencephalon. As a result of the uncal herniation that occurs, these cistern become obliterated—an ominous early sign in head trauma. An example of a normal versus obliterated cistern is shown in Figure 131-5.

## SKULL FRACTURES AND MANAGEMENT

One of the most common head injuries seen in adolescents is a fracture of the skull. Some skull fractures require surgery, whereas others can be managed conservatively. The types of skull fractures and guidelines for managing them are discussed in the following (Box 131-4 and Box 131-5).

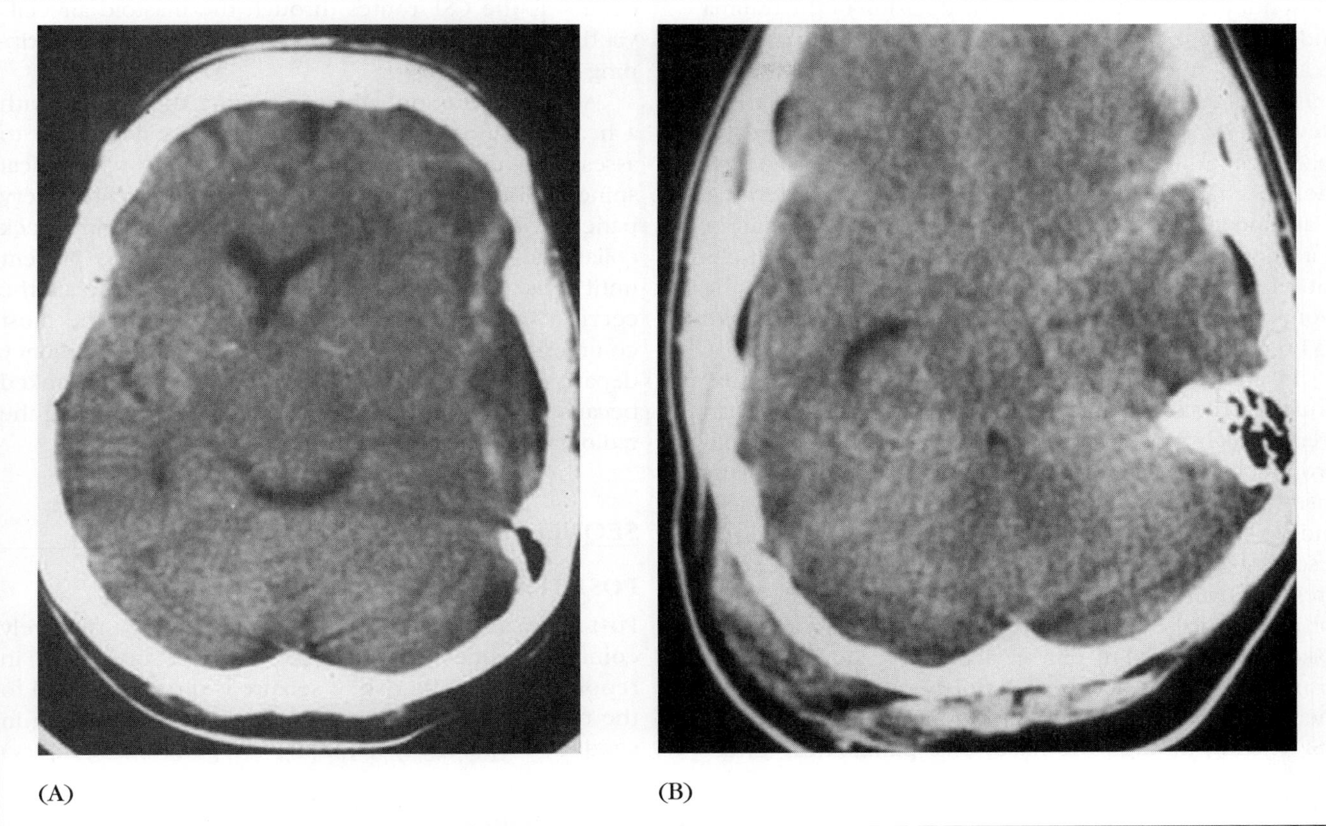


**FIGURE 131-5** (A) An axial CT scan reveals a large right chronic subdural hematoma with some left to right shift of the ventricles. The ambient cistern, a space around the mesencephalon, is open and not at all compressed. (B) An axial CT scan of a severe head injury with completely obliterated ambient cisterns plus diffuse subarachnoid bleeding, seen as the white haze throughout the CT. (Photos courtesy of James Tait Goodrich.)

**Box 131-4**

***Types of Skull Fractures***

- Linear: 2 bone edges of fracture not displaced
- Stellate: multiple fractures in "stellate" fashion (see Figure 131-6A)
- Comminuted: open (overlying scalp laceration) and depressed fracture
- Depressed: 1 edge of fracture is below the other (see Figure 131-7 A)
- Basilar: fracture involved anywhere along the skull base; most common sites are subfrontal and cribriform plate, temporal bone, and mastoid sinuses
- Compound

**Box 131-5**

***Criteria to Consider in Skull Fracture Evaluation/Elevation***

- Bone fragments driven into brain
- Depressed skull fracture >1 cm
- Underlying hematoma (with potential brain compression)
- Neurological deficit
- CSF leak
- Presence of air in subarachnoid space
- Fracture over paranasal or mastoid sinuses
- Basilar skull fracture with persistent CSF leak

CSF, cerebrospinal fluid

A number of criteria guide the decision of the trauma and neurosurgical teams to operate on a skull fracture. In any skull fracture with bone fragments driven into the brain, the fractures and the bone fragments need to be elevated. Typically any depressed skull fracture greater than 1 cm in diameter in which the outer table is below the inner table as detected on CT needs to be elevated. If an underlying hematoma is compressing the brain or if a neurologic deficit is suspected, exploration and elevation are indicated. If CSF is seen issuing through the wound, there is an increased risk of meningitis (Figure 131-6 and Figure 131-7).

In adolescents there is a high incidence of basilar skull fractures, usually manifested by Battle sign, an area of ecchymoses behind the ear around the mastoid prominences. There is a cerebral spinal leak in many cases, but fortunately most leaks resolve spontaneously and do not require surgery. In the 5% or so that do not resolve, placement of lumbar spinal drain with negative pressure over a 7-day period usually suffices. The need for intracranial exploration is rare, occurring in less than 2% of cases treated by our service. Also it should be kept in mind that a paradoxical rhinorrhea can occur when the fracture is in the mastoid/temporal region with CSF leaking through the nose. This "paradoxical" effect occurs as the CSF routes through the mastoid air cells via the Eustachian tube to the nose, leading to CSF dripping from the nares.

As a final caution, when managing the patient with a head injury, the emergency team must not forget to assess the cervical region. The incidence of cervical spine injuries is high in this population. Therefore every patient with a head injury should be stabilized in a neck collar and treated as though a spine injury is present until it is proved otherwise. It is critical that all the cervical vertebrae down to C7 be evaluated. The most commonly missed cervical injury in the emergency department is the C7-T1 injury, which is overlooked because of failure to pull the shoulders down during the radiographic examination (Figure 131-8).

## SEQUELAE OF HEAD TRAUMA

### POST-TRAUMATIC EPILEPSY

Post-traumatic epilepsy in the adolescent is a relatively common sequelae with a 2.5% to 9% incidence in reported series. The risk of seizure is directly related to the type and mechanism of injury. Injuries resulting in subdural or parenchymal injury (ie, penetrating injury)

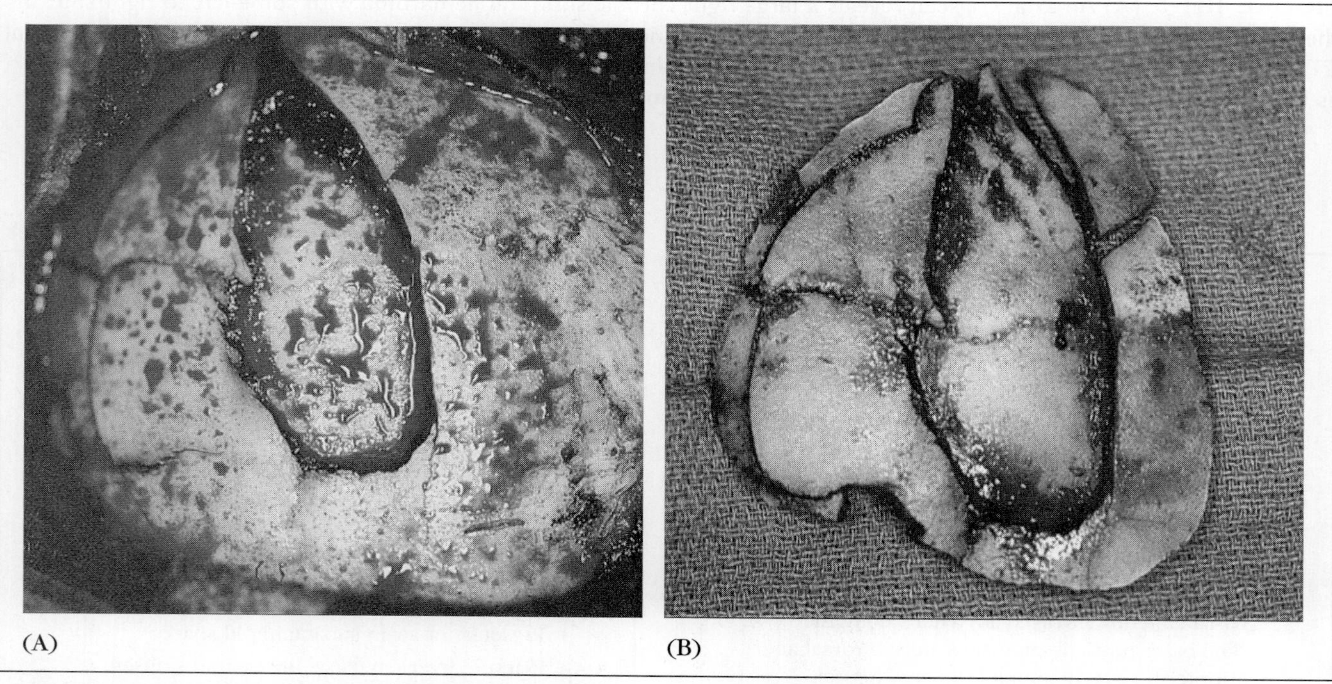

**FIGURE 131-6** An adolescent female struck by a hammer over the convexity during a rape attempt. (A) A stellate fracture with multiple fracture lines. (B) After elevating of the skull fracture the multiple fractures can be easily appreciated and need to be corrected prior to placing the skull back. (Photos courtesy of James Tait Goodrich.) (See color insert.)

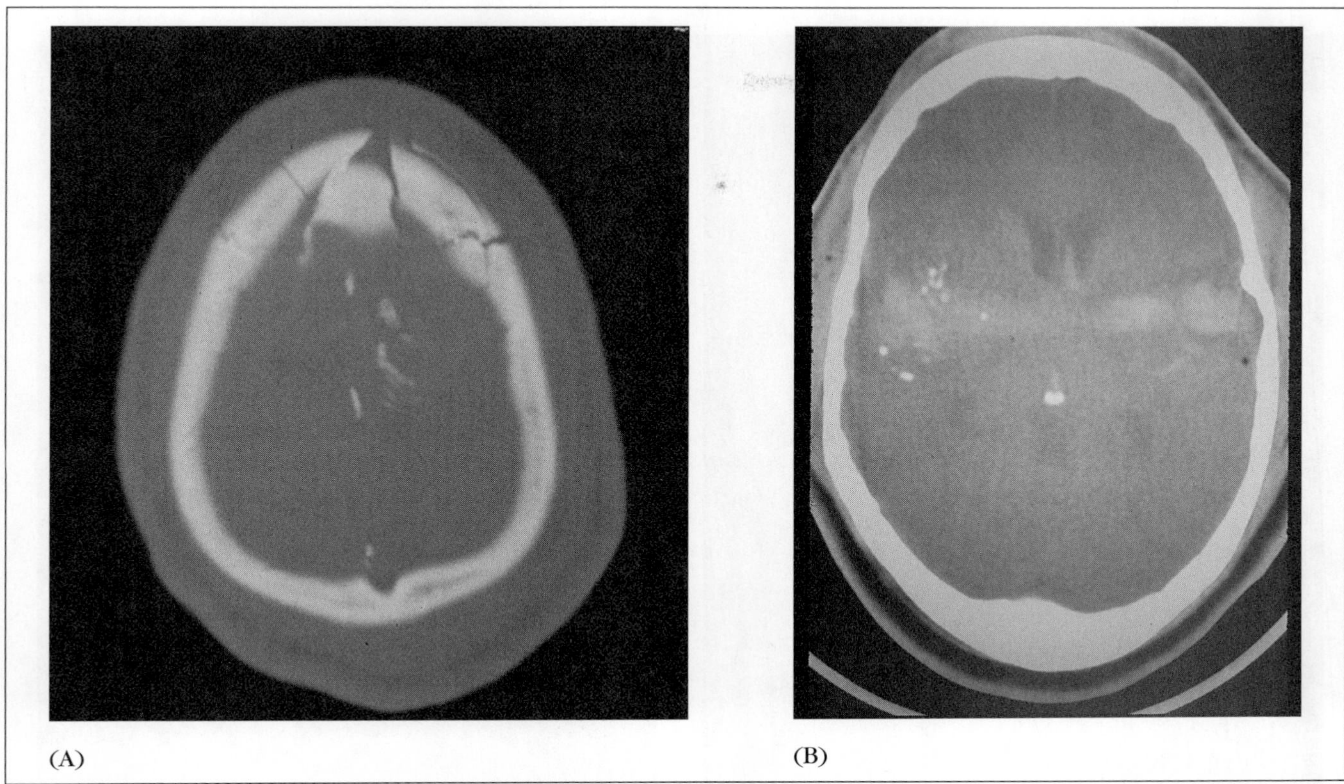

**FIGURE 131-7** (A) CT scan using bone windows showing a large left frontal depressed skull fracture within driven bone fragments. Due to significant depression and compression of the brain plus in driven fragments this fracture needs to be elevated. (B) CT with axial view showing a 15-year-old who committed suicide with a gun; a temporal through-and-through track can be seen. In our experience this is an ominous injury with rare survivors. (Photos courtesy of James Tait Goodrich.)

have the highest risk of seizures: 30% to 36%. Epidural hematomas and skull fractures have a rate of 9% to 13%, and even with minor head injury without neurological sequelae there is a reported incidence of 1% to 2%. Post-traumatic seizures can be divided into those that are early (within 1 week) and those that are late (more than 1 week from the traumatic event). There is no evidence to suggest that *prophylactic* antibiotics have any effect on the prevention of late seizures. Studies in the adult literature have shown that prophylactic anticonvulsants do decrease the rate of early seizure occurrence without having an effect on outcome. If late post-traumatic seizures do occur in a patient with only closed head trauma they can be followed to see what pattern (ie, frequency) develops. In patients with penetrating injury, particularly those who develop focal neurological symptoms, there is a higher risk of permanent epilepsy that may necessitate medications.[15]

## LONG-TERM MANAGEMENT

Late post-traumatic seizures greatly affect adolescents in learning and development and need to be aggressively managed. In adults, it has been shown that late seizures greatly lessen the chance of gainful employment after treatment. The single most ignored factors in the adolescent who has sustained a head injury are the psychologic sequelae. After a head injury has occurred, particularly in an assault case, the adolescent can become fearful, with retrograde amnesia, and a loss of learning skills is not uncommon. If these conditions are recognized and treated the outcome will be much improved.

## POST-TRAUMATIC SYNDROME

General sequelae following a head injury may include the following:

1. Headache (mild to excruciating) typically in the occipital region, which can often persist for up to 6 to 12 months after the injury
2. Irritability, which often affects social interactions and school performance
3. Forgetfulness: retrograde amnesia is common, and school performance can be affected in that these patients have difficulty acquiring new knowledge

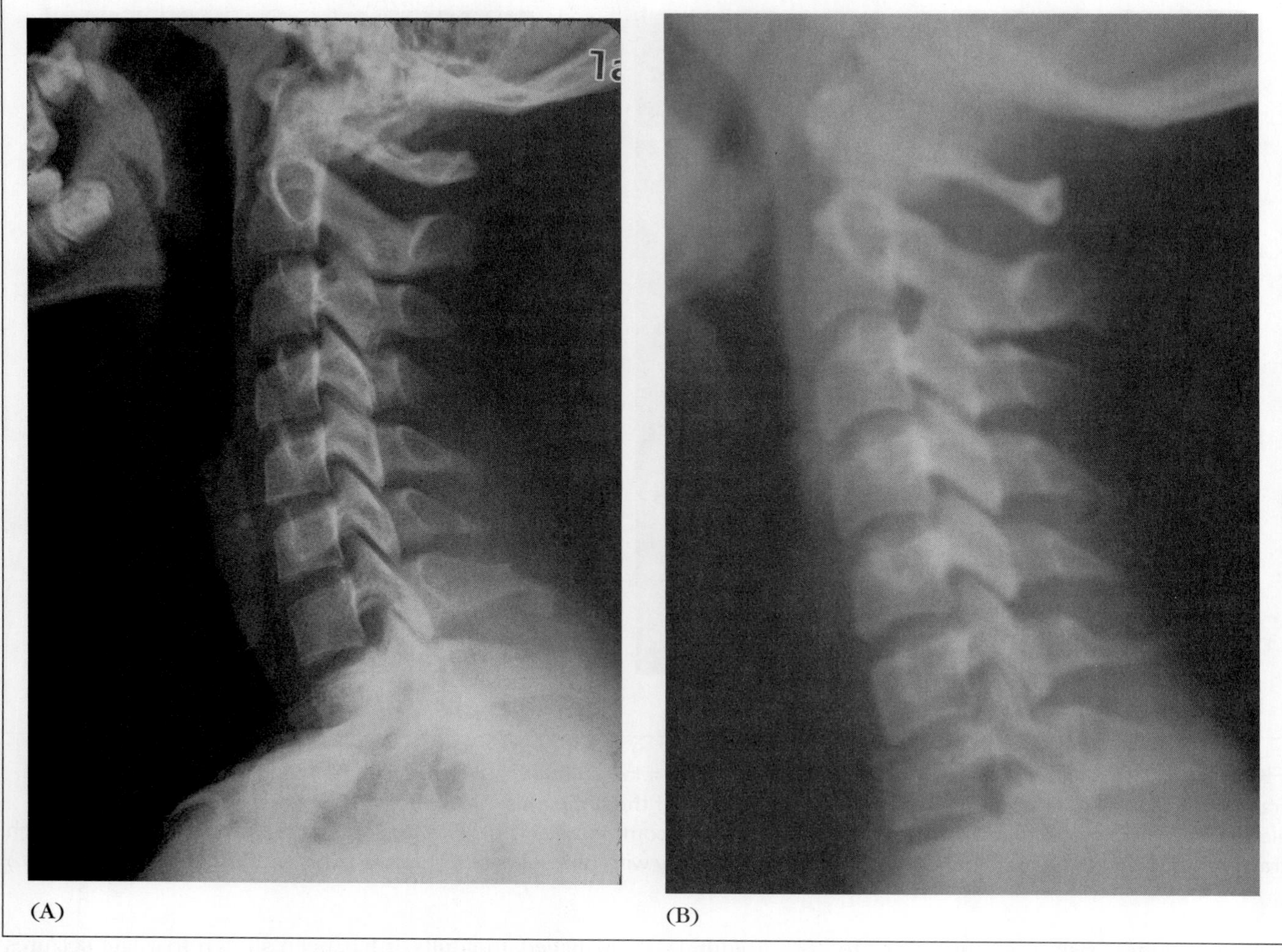

**FIGURE 131-8** (A) A lateral cervical spine radiograph showing a C7 spinous process "teardrop" fracture. The fracture was initially missed because of the patient's large shoulders. The repeat radiograph with the shoulders pulled down clearly showed the fracture. (B) Lateral spine x-ray revealing a C6-C7 subluxation from a football injury in a 16-year-old male. Additionally there is an abnormal straightening of the spine. (Photos courtesy of James Tait Goodrich.)

4. Postural vertigo (dizziness)
5. Enuresis
6. Disturbances in sleep patterns
7. Episodic aggressive behavior, particularly in adolescent males
8. Decline in school performance; teachers typically note impaired concentration skills

It should also be borne in mind that whenever there is a medicolegal coincident situation, patients may not do well until the legal matter is resolved.

The post-traumatic syndrome is one of the most ignored sequelae in the adolescent population. This is particularly the case in adolescent males, in whom a bravado attitude tends to lead the family and school to ignore the problem. In adolescent females, particularly those who are victims of assault, the psychological sequelae can be devastating and need to be closely monitored. Typically the earliest subtle signs in females and males are changes in school performance. Fortunately, a persistent post-traumatic syndrome is uncommon in adolescents and almost always resolves with time. This does not negate the fact that these patients need close monitoring in the first 6 months after injury.

## CONCLUSION

Head injury remains an all too common cause of mortality and morbidity in the adolescent population. Through early and aggressive management of the patient with head injury outcomes can be improved. Recognizing, and understanding the new guidelines in the management of adolescents with head injury is key to treatment and a better outcome.

## REFERENCES


1. Alberico AM, Ward JD, Choi SC, Marmarou A, Young HF. Outcome after severe head injury. Relationship to mass lesions, diffuse injury, and ICP course in pediatric and adult patients. *J Neurosurg.* 1987;67(5):648-656

2. The Brain Trauma Foundation. The American Association of Neurological Surgeons. The Joint Section on Neurotrauma and Critical Care. Initial management. *J Neurotrauma.* 2000;17 (6-7):463-469

3. Adelson PD, Bratton SL, Carney NA, et al. Guidelines for the acute medical management of severe traumatic brain injury in infants, children, and adolescents. Chapter 4. Resuscitation of blood pressure and oxygenation and prehospital brain-specific therapies for the severe pediatric traumatic brain injury patient. *Pediatr Crit Care Med.* 2003;4(3 suppl):S12-S18

4. The Brain Trauma Foundation. The American Association of Neurological Surgeons. The Joint Section on Neurotrauma and Critical Care. Glasgow Coma Scale score. *J Neurotrauma.* 2000;17(6-7):563-571

5. Adelson PD, Bratton SL, Carney NA, et al. Guidelines for the acute medical management of severe traumatic brain injury in infants, children, and adolescents. Chapter 8. Cerebral perfusion pressure. *Pediatr Crit Care Med.* 2003;4(3 suppl):S31-S33

6. Adelson PD, Bratton SL, Carney NA, et al. Guidelines for the acute medical management of severe traumatic brain injury in infants, children, and adolescents. Chapter 6. Threshold for treatment of intracranial hypertension. *Pediatr Crit Care Med.* 2003;4(3 suppl):S25-S27

7. Adelson PD, Bratton SL, Carney NA, et al. Guidelines for the acute medical management of severe traumatic brain injury in infants, children, and adolescents. Chapter 11. Use of hyperosmolar therapy in the management of severe pediatric traumatic brain injury. *Pediatr Crit Care Med.* 2003;4(3 suppl):S40-S44

8. The Brain Trauma Foundation. The American Association of Neurological Surgeons. The Joint Section on Neurotrauma and Critical Care. Use of mannitol. *J Neurotrauma.* 2000;17 (6-7):521-525

9. Adelson PD, Bratton SL, Carney NA, et al. Guidelines for the acute medical management of severe traumatic brain injury in infants, children, and adolescents. Chapter 13. The use of barbiturates in the control of intracranial hypertension in severe pediatric traumatic brain injury. *Pediatr Crit Care Med.* 2003;4(3 suppl):S49-S52

10. Adelson PD, Bratton SL, Carney NA, et al. Guidelines for the acute medical management of severe traumatic brain injury in infants, children, and adolescents. Chapter 16. The use of corticosteroids in the treatment of severe pediatric traumatic brain injury. *Pediatr Crit Care Med.* 2003;4(3 suppl):S60-S64

11. Adelson PD, Bratton SL, Carney NA, et al. Guidelines for the acute medical management of severe traumatic brain injury in infants, children, and adolescents. Chapter 12. Use of hyperventilation in the acute management of severe pediatric traumatic brain injury. *Pediatr Crit Care Med.* 2003;4(3 suppl):S45-S48

12. Selden PD, Bratton SL, Carney NA, et al. Guidelines for the acute medical management of severe traumatic brain injury in infants, children, and adolescents. Chapter 14. The role of temperature control following severe pediatric traumatic brain injury. *Pediatr Crit Care Med.* 2003;4(3 suppl):S53-S55

13. Adelson PD, Bratton SL, Carney NA, et al. Guidelines for the acute medical management of severe traumatic brain injury in infants, children, and adolescents. Chapter 5. Indications for intracranial pressure monitoring in pediatric patients with severe traumatic brain injury. *Pediatr Crit Care Med.* 2003;4(3 suppl):S19-S24

14. Adelson PD, Bratton SL, Carney NA, et al. Guidelines for the acute medical management of severe traumatic brain injury in infants, children, and adolescents. Chapter 7. Intracranial pressure monitoring technology. *Pediatr Crit Care Med.* 2003;4(3 suppl):S28-S30

15. Adelson PD, Bratton SL, Carney NA, et al. Guidelines for the acute medical management of severe traumatic brain injury in infants, children, and adolescents. Chapter 19. The role of antiseizure prophylaxis following severe pediatric traumatic brain injury. *Pediatr Crit Care Med.* 2003;4(3 suppl):S72-S75

# CHAPTER 132

# Intracranial Vascular Malformations

DAVID GORDON, MD • JAMES TAIT GOODRICH, MD, PhD, DSci (*HON*)

## INTRODUCTION

Few lesions of the brain have a more devastating impact than hemorrhage from an intracranial vascular malformation. Some vascular malformations present with warning signs, allowing an alert physician to make an early diagnosis. The most common vascular malformations in adolescents that lead to brain injury are arteriovenous malformations (AVMs), aneurysms, and cavernous malformations.

## ARTERIOVENOUS MALFORMATIONS

Arteriovenous malformations are pathologic collections of vessels within brain parenchyma consisting of abnormal arteries and veins with no intervening capillary beds. Histologically, there is no functional brain tissue within the center, or nidus, of the AVM. They are thought to be congenital lesions; however, they do have dynamic tendencies and may change in morphology and size over time.

### EPIDEMIOLOGY

They are the most common abnormality of the intracranial circulation in the pediatric and adolescent populations. Autopsy data suggests an overall prevalence of 0.14%, with a range as high as 1.5% to 4% in these younger age groups. Patients with Rendu-Osler-Weber syndrome have a cerebral AVM prevalence of 5% to 10%.[1] Although patients most often present in the third and fourth decades of life, presentation in adolescence is common.

### CLINICAL PRESENTATION

#### Hemorrhage

Due to direct arteriovenous shunting, AVMs tend to be high-flow lesions that present most commonly with rupture and intracerebral hemorrhage (ICH). The rate of presentation with hemorrhage is generally considered to be higher in the pediatric age group (60% to 85%) than in adults (40% to 65%), although Stapf et al[2] found increasing age to correlate with higher rates of hemorrhage in a prospective cohort of 542 patients (Figure 132-1).

There is a 2% to 4% annual incidence of hemorrhage from previously unruptured lesions.[3,4] Certain risk factors predispose to higher rates of ICH. Using a multivariate model in 622 patients, a recent study found a higher risk of ICH as the initial presentation in patients with AVMs having the following characteristics: small size, deep location (ie, basal ganglia, thalamus, brainstem), deep venous drainage, and the presence of an associated aneurysm. Multivariate predictors of recurrent hemorrhage following the initial presentation included older age, initial hemorrhagic presentation, deep AVM location, and deep venous drainage. The strongest predictor of a subsequent hemorrhage was hemorrhage at initial presentation[5] (Table 132-1).

#### Seizure

Up to one-third of patients present with seizure.[5-7] Seizure types include simple partial, complex partial, and secondarily generalized activity. Turjman et al[5] found an increased risk of seizure presentation with several AVM characteristics, including cortical location, the presence of middle cerebral artery (MCA) supply, the absence of an associated aneurysm (which predisposes to rupture), the presence of varices, and larger size.[8]

#### Other

A small but significant minority of patients will present with nonspecific neurological complaints such as headache. With the liberalization of indications for computed tomography (CT) and magnetic resonance imaging (MRI), an increasing number of lesions are being discovered incidentally. Patients may also present with progressive neurological deficits as a result of vascular steal phenomena. The proposed mechanism for such a process is the shunting of blood through an arteriovenous fistula away from normal brain parenchyma, thus resulting in focal areas of relative hypoperfusion leading to focal ischemia and possible stroke.[9]

#### Imaging

The first imaging study performed in the initial evaluation of patients with AVMs often is CT, due to the fact that most patients present with an ictus of sudden onset headache with accompanying focal neurological deficit.

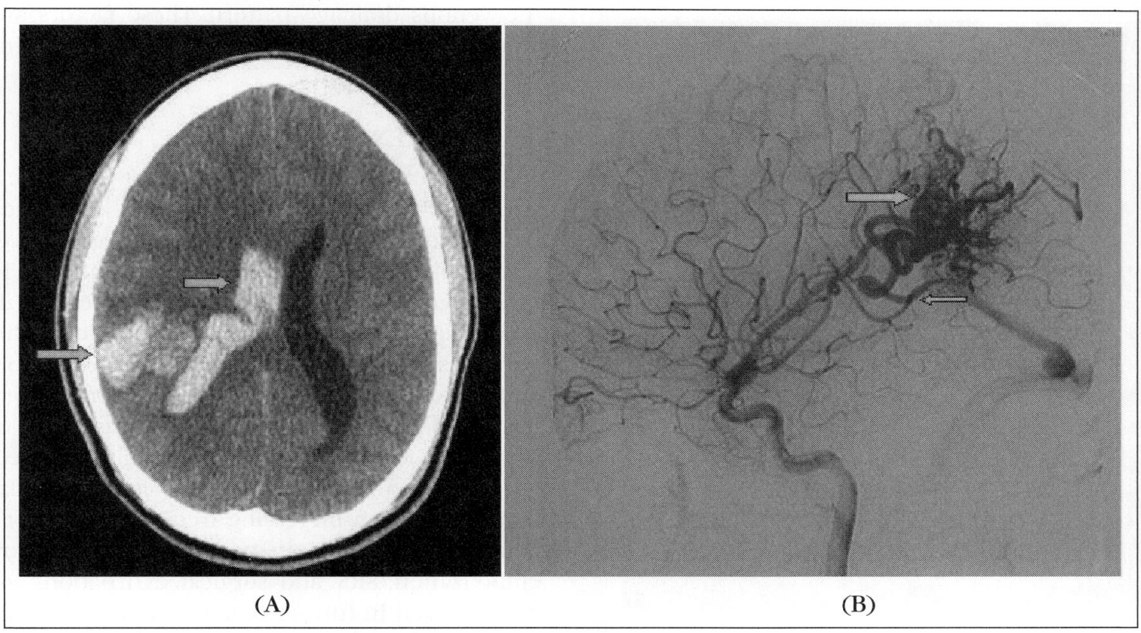


**FIGURE 132-1** (A) A CT scan of an 18-year-old male who presented with a severe headache, lethargy, and left-sided weakness. This noncontrast axial scan reveals an acute intracerebral hemorrhage with extension into the right lateral ventricle. (B) A lateral cerebral angiogram demonstrating a right parietal AVM in the same patient. The large feeding arterial vessels are seen arising from the middle cerebral artery. The nidus of the AVM is seen with a large caliber vein draining into the straight sinus. (Photos courtesy of James Tait Goodrich.)

The lesion itself is usually seen as a region of mixed hyperdensity that often has areas of calcification. However, it is not uncommon to find the AVM to be obscured by the uniform hyperdensity of an acute hemorrhage (Figure 132-2 and Figure 132-3).

**Table 132-1**

**Vascular Malformations of the Central Nervous System: Aneurysm, Arteriovenous Malformation, Cavernous Angioma**

| | |
|---|---|
| Clinical presentation | • Headache - sudden and explosive<br>• "Worst headache of my life"<br>• Followed by brief to prolonged loss of consciousness<br>• Photophobia<br>• Meningimus (stiff neck) |
| Diagnostic work-up | • Lumbar puncture ("bloody tap")<br>• CT for subarachnoid hemorrhage<br>• MRI for signal void<br>• Angiogram/Angiogram (CTA) definitive test |

On T2-weighted MRI, AVMs show heterogeneous signal intensity with focal hypointense regions representing flow voids in the abnormal vessels. The

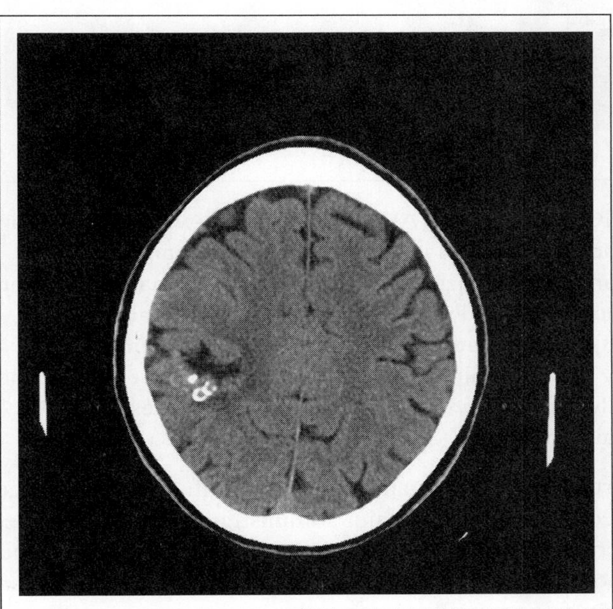

**FIGURE 132-2** A CT scan showing the presence of an AVM without rupture; areas of calcification are evident. (Photo courtesy of James Tait Goodrich.)

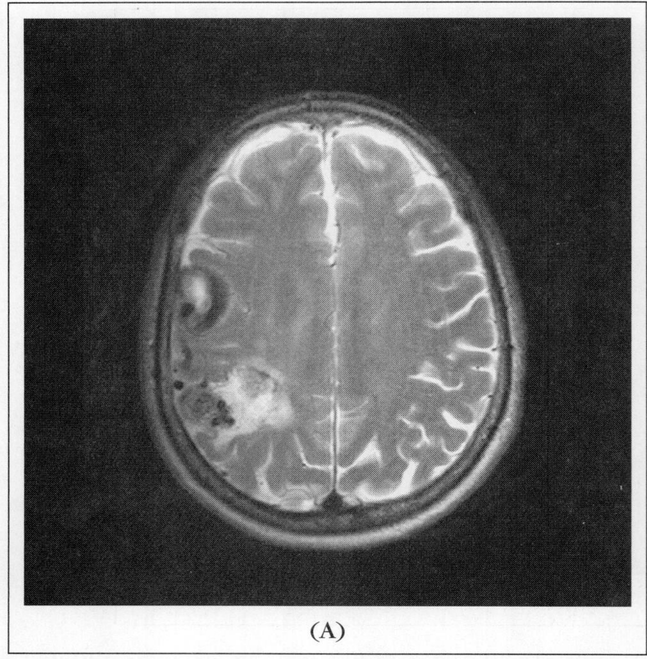

(A)

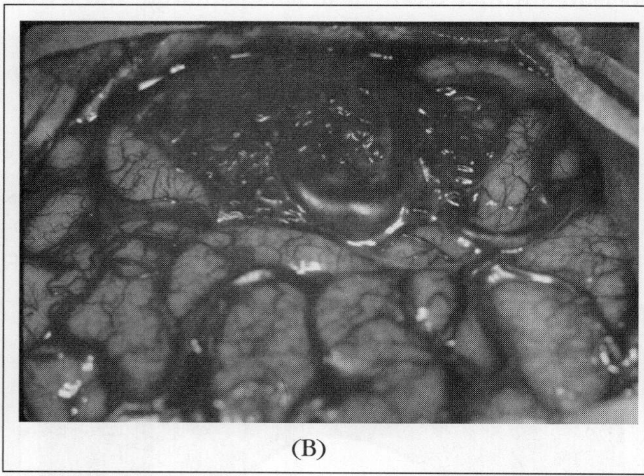

(B)

**FIGURE 132-3** (A) An MRI with T2-weighted imaging showing an AVM in the right posterior parietal area; surrounding edema is evident. A large signal void is seen more temporally consistent with a large draining vein. (B) Intraoperative view of a cortical AVM surrounded by normal brain. The arterialized vein can be seen at the inferior margin of the AVM. (Photos courtesy of James Tait Goodrich.) (See color insert.)

Arteriovenous malformations enhance heterogeneously with gadolinium administration on T1-weighted sequences. The study of choice for localizing the exact intraparenchymal location of the AVM and its relationship to potentially eloquent brain structures is MRI.

Digital subtraction angiography (DSA) is critical for the complete evaluation of an AVM. It defines the exact size, the anatomy of the nidus, the arterial supply, and the venous drainage pattern. These factors are crucial in planning an individualized management strategy for each patient.

## MANAGEMENT

The primary goal of AVM treatment is to decrease the risk of subsequent hemorrhage and its attendant morbidity and mortality. Treatment also has been geared to decreasing morbidity related to intractable epilepsy and neurological dysfunction. Surgical resection has long been the mainstay of treatment. However, technological advances in the fields of interventional neuroradiology and stereotactic radiosurgery (SRS) have significantly improved the success rate and decreased the treatment morbidity for patients with difficult and deep-seated lesions.[10] As a result, combined treatment modalities are being used with increasing frequency in most comprehensive centers. These modalities include intra-arterial embolization, SRS, and surgical extirpation, which will be discussed in further detail. Due to the fact that AVM treatment is largely a preventative measure, the risks of treatment must always be weighed against the natural history of the disease process.

### Surgery

*If an adventurous young surgeon cuts into the body of a tumour of tortuous veins and arteries, he has vessels throwing out their blood over both his shoulders. But if he keeps wide of the diseased mass, he perhaps cuts across one artery which throws out its blood with no uncommon velocity.* (Sir Charles Bell, London, 1812)

As Sir Charles Bell so clearly pointed out in 1812, few surgical lesions present such a daunting task as AVMs. Their locations, a propensity for significant blood loss, and identifying normal from abnormal tissue are all issues that make for enormous challenges to the surgical team. The Spetzler-Martin grading scale stratifies patients into surgical risk categories based on a combination of AVM location, size, and venous drainage pattern[11] (Table 132-2). Patients with low-grade lesions (Spetzler-Martin Grade I–II) may undergo craniotomy for resection with acceptably low morbidity and mortality rates. Patients with high-grade lesions (ie, Spetzler-Martin Grade IV–V) are most often advised against surgical treatment due to the prohibitive risk involved.[12] Patients with Grade III lesions[13] will often undergo preoperative embolization to decrease surgical morbidity (Table 132-2).

Surgical outcome tends to be better in younger patients. In a recent comparison of 32 patients younger than 18 years of age with 192 adults treated surgically, Sanchez-Mejia et al[14] found that the younger cohort was 78% less likely to have poor outcome and 86% less likely to have further neurological deterioration. These authors

**Table 132-2**

**Spetzler-Martin Grading System**

| *Feature* | *Points* |
|---|---|
| SIZE | |
| Small (<3 cm) | 1 |
| Medium (3-6 cm) | 2 |
| Large (>6 cm) | 3 |
| ELOQUENCE OF ADJACENT BRAIN | |
| Noneloquent | 0 |
| Eloquent | 1 |
| VENOUS DRAINAGE PATTERN | |
| Superficial only | 0 |
| Deep | 1 |

Reprinted with permission from Spetzler RF, Martin NA. A proposed grading system for arteriovenous malformations. *J Neurosurg*. 1986;65(4):476-483.

hypothesize that a greater capacity for neural plasticity in the younger patient affords this benefit.[14]

### Embolization

Endovascular embolization involves selective catheterization of feeding vessels with the goal of partial or complete nidus occlusion. Embolization may be used for cure, as an adjunct to more definitive treatment, or for palliation. Complete cure is rare with interventional techniques alone,[15] and thus the main utility of embolization in current practice is to decrease the morbidity and enhance the success rate of surgery, SRS, or, in some instances, both.

Embolization is not without risk. Haw et al[15] reported a permanent disability/mortality rate of 3.9%. Overall morbidity/mortality approached 7.5%. The authors[15] caution that risk is additive with combined modalities and must be balanced with the risk of no treatment. Kim et al[16] noted a periprocedural morbidity of 11.8% with long-term morbidity/mortality of 8.6%. Greater than 3 embolized branches per patient predicted significant morbidity.[16]

### Stereotactic Radiosurgery

Stereotactic radiosurgery targets high-energy radiation to a lesion while minimizing exposure to surrounding normal tissue. It is most often performed in a single setting, although centers have recently begun to stage the procedure for larger lesions.[17] A growing body of data exists in support of SRS as a primary treatment option, particularly for small, deep AVMs whose surgical risk precludes that method of treatment.[6,7,17-23] Obliteration rates in recent series range from 35% to 95%,[6,17-19,21-25] and seizure-free status has been achieved in up to 51% of selected patients presenting with intractable epilepsy.[7] In a series of 100 patients aged 4 to 19 years, predictors of obliteration included age less than 12, nidus less than 2 cm in diameter, and 3.8 $cm^3$ in volume, and Spetzler-Martin Grade III or less.[24] A radiosurgery-based AVM score[26] based on AVM volume, AVM location, and age of patient has been found to better predict outcome than the Spetzler-Martin grade[21] and has recently been validated in a series of 38 patients younger than 18 years of age.[18] Other predictors include radiation dose,[6,19,24] number of draining veins,[26] and location.[24,26]

The complication rates of SRS are not insignificant. Vasculopathy, radiation necrosis, and cerebral edema may develop with resultant neurological morbidity. The greatest risk, however, is related to the fact that a latency period exists between treatment and obliteration that may last for greater than 3 years. During this time, the patient remains at risk for ICH. Annual rates of new ICH during the latency period range from 1.5% to 4.7% in series that combine pediatric and adolescent patients.[6,19,24] One study even reports an annual ICH risk of 0.3% in SRS-treated patients with obliteration confirmed by angiography.[20] These factors must be considered when individualizing treatment plans, especially in patients at high annual risk of hemorrhage.

### PROGNOSIS

Prognosis varies and is predominantly based on the occurrence and severity of ICH. Again younger patients tend to fare better in their long-term outcomes.[14] Parenchymal hemorrhage predicts unfavorable outcome[27] and results in 30% to 50% morbidity and approximately 10% mortality per hemorrhage. Due to the age of the adolescent patient, overall favorable outcome with treatment, and relative high incidence of hemorrhage, strong consideration must be given to aggressive treatment of these potentially devastating lesions. All treatment options should be considered, including surgery, embolization, SRS, and a combination of modalities in order to effect cure.

## ANEURYSMS

Intracerebral aneurysms are potentially life-threatening lesions of the cerebral vasculature. Their etiology is controversial, although a congenital defect in the musculature of the arterial media has been postulated as a predisposing factor to their development. Most aneurysms occur at branch points of major cerebral arteries in the direction of blood flow. Their propensity to

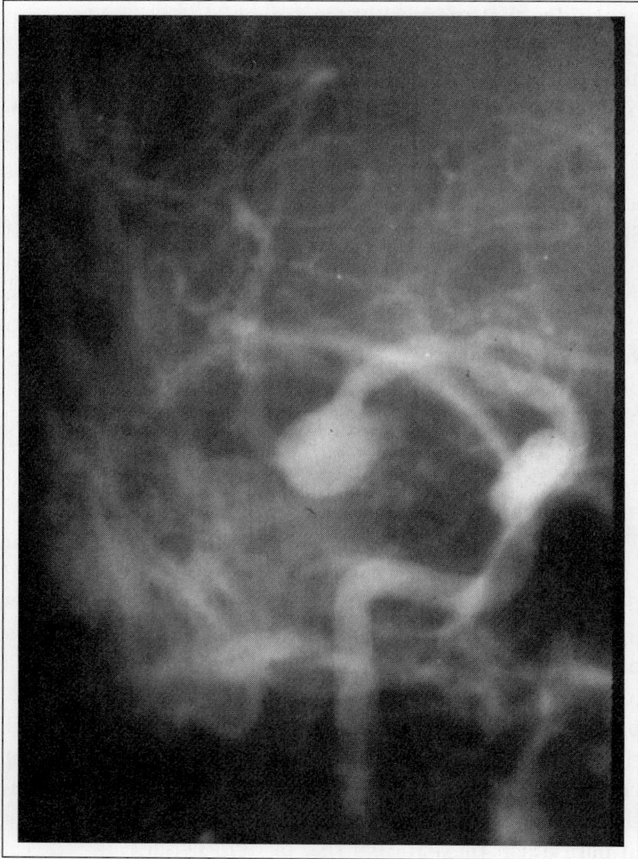

FIGURE 132-4 Cerebral angiogram showing an aneurysm of the middle cerebral artery. The large dome of the aneurysm is clearly seen. (Photo courtesy of James Tait Goodrich.)

rupture with attendant high morbidity and mortality drives aggressive treatment plans (Figure 132-4).

Acquired aneurysms may also result from bacterial endocarditis. These "mycotic" aneurysms tend to occur in more distal locations, and are managed primarily with appropriate, aggressive antibiotic therapy, although surgery may become necessary. Patients with rheumatic heart disease, intracardiac shunts, prosthetic heart valves, and intravenous drug users are particularly at risk.

Penetrating trauma is an important environmental cause of intracerebral aneurysms. A cerebral angiogram should be considered following any penetrating injury (eg, knife, nails, gunshot wounds) of the brain that may have compromised the cerebral vasculature (Figure 132-5).

## EPIDEMIOLOGY

Aneurysms in adolescence differ significantly from those in adults. The most frequent site of occurrence is the internal carotid artery (ICA) bifurcation, as compared to the anterior communicating artery in adults.[28-30] Patients younger than 18 years old represent approximately 1% to 2% of patients who present with aneurysmal subarachnoid hemorrhage (SAH) and approximately 0.17% to 4.6% of patients who undergo surgical clip ligation of aneurysms.[29-38] There tends to be a male predominance in this age group[31,38,39] and an increased incidence of giant aneurysms (>2.5 cm in diameter).[28,39] Multiplicity of aneurysms, occurring in 15% to 25% of adult patients, is rare in adolescence. Patients with coarctation of the aorta, polycystic kidney disease, connective tissue disorders (eg, Ehlers-Danlos syndrome), and fibromuscular dysplasia are known to be at higher risk for the development of aneurysms.

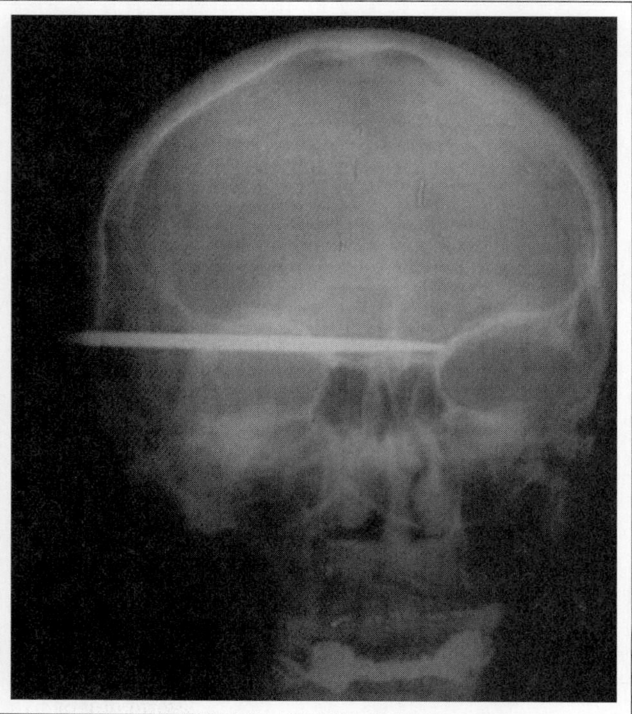

FIGURE 132-5 Skull x-ray of a severely depressed 15-year-old female who attempted suicide by driving a large nail into her skull. Due to the location of the nail in relation to the Circle of Willis, an angiogram would be helpful here in the surgical work-up to rule out any potential aneurysm. (Photo courtesy of James Tait Goodrich.)

## CLINICAL PRESENTATION

Patients most often present with signs and symptoms of SAH. Classically, an awake patient will describe the sudden onset of the "worst headache of my life." Associated nausea, vomiting, photophobia, and changes in mental status are common. Headache is the presenting symptom in up to 97% of patients with aneurysmal SAH.

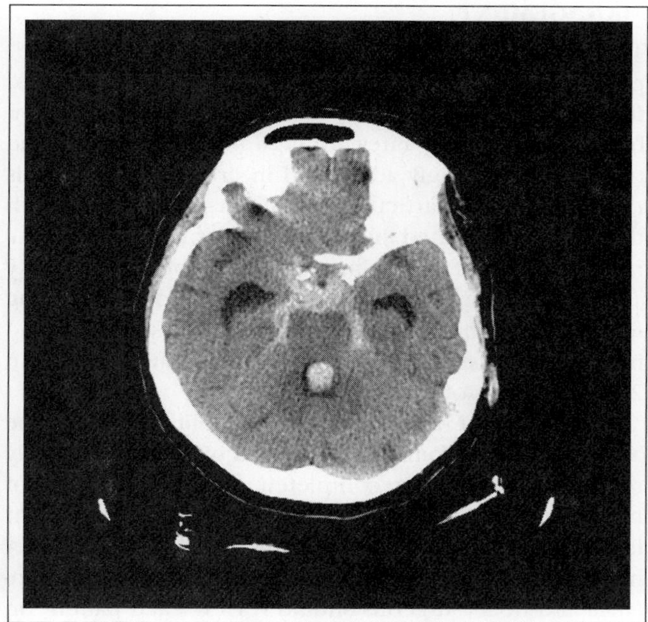

**FIGURE 132-6** CT scan showing a diffuse subarachnoid hemorrhage, seen as a diffuse white haze throughout the basilar cisterns subarachnoid spaces. Of further concern is the dilation of the temporal horns, a finding consistent with acute hydrocephalus, not uncommonly seen with these conditions. (Photo courtesy of James Tait Goodrich.)

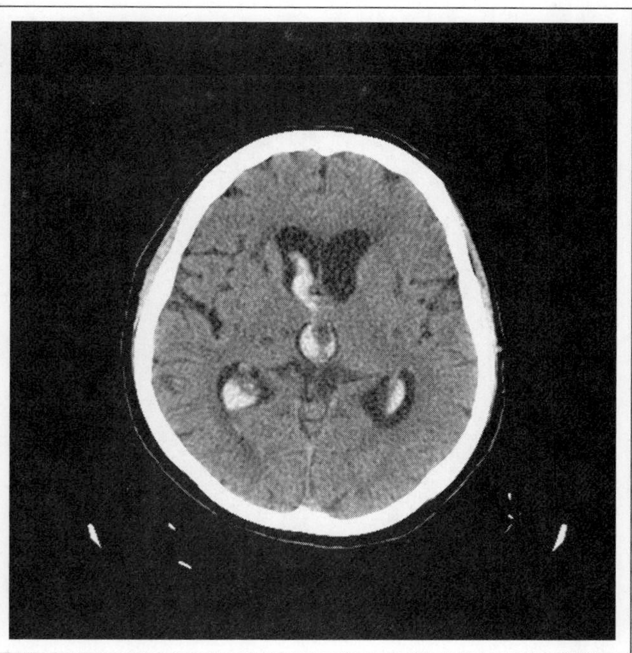

**FIGURE 132-7** CT scan with a diffuse intraventricular bleed, with blood seen as the white material in the right lateral ventricle, the third ventricle, and both atria. This proved to be a hemorrhage from an anterior communicating artery aneurysm. (Photo courtesy of James Tait Goodrich.)

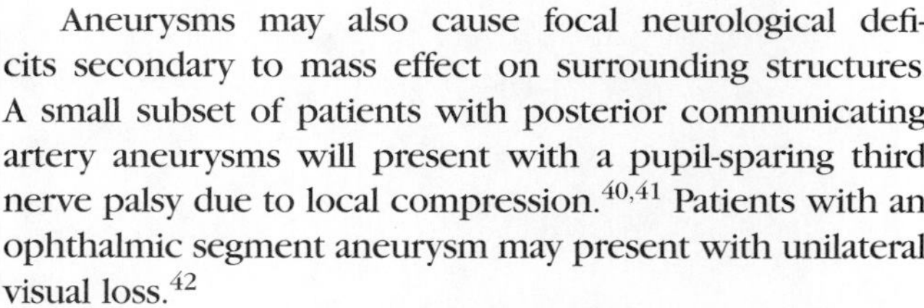

Aneurysms may also cause focal neurological deficits secondary to mass effect on surrounding structures. A small subset of patients with posterior communicating artery aneurysms will present with a pupil-sparing third nerve palsy due to local compression.[40,41] Patients with an ophthalmic segment aneurysm may present with unilateral visual loss.[42]

Due to advances in neuroimaging, an increasing number of aneurysms are being discovered incidentally after presentation with more protean symptomatology (Figure 132-6 and Figure 132-7).

## DIAGNOSIS

As in AVMs, CT is often the first study obtained in the evaluation of a patient with a suspected aneurysm. Following rupture, diffuse hyperdensity may be seen in the subarachnoid space, including the Sylvian fissures, the interhemispheric fissure, and the basal cisterns. Intraventricular hemorrhage is common,[43] particularly with aneurysms that abut the ventricular system (eg, anterior communicating artery, distal basilar artery, posterior inferior cerebellar artery). Focal ICH may also occur, most often in the context of a ruptured MCA aneurysm.

Vascular anatomic detail with CT angiography (CTA) and MR angiography (MRA) has improved substantially over the last decade. Because of their noninvasive nature, CTA and MRA are frequently used to evaluate patients with suspected aneurysms, particularly in the absence of SAH.[44]

Despite advances in alternative imaging modalities, DSA remains the standard diagnostic tool. It allows for a dynamic, albeit qualitative, assessment of cerebral blood flow. Three-dimensional reconstructions of rotational acquisitions now allow a remarkably accurate assessment of aneurysm morphology and its relationship to the normal vasculature. In patients whose aneurysms are amenable to coil embolization (discussed in the following section), DSA provides a single examination to both diagnostic and therapeutic ends (Figure 132-8).

Lumbar puncture is used less frequently because of the accuracy of current imaging. However, cerebrospinal fluid (CSF) studies may provide essential information in patients for whom there is high clinical suspicion for aneurysmal rupture without radiographic confirmation. The presence of xanthochromia in CSF is highly indicative of SAH.

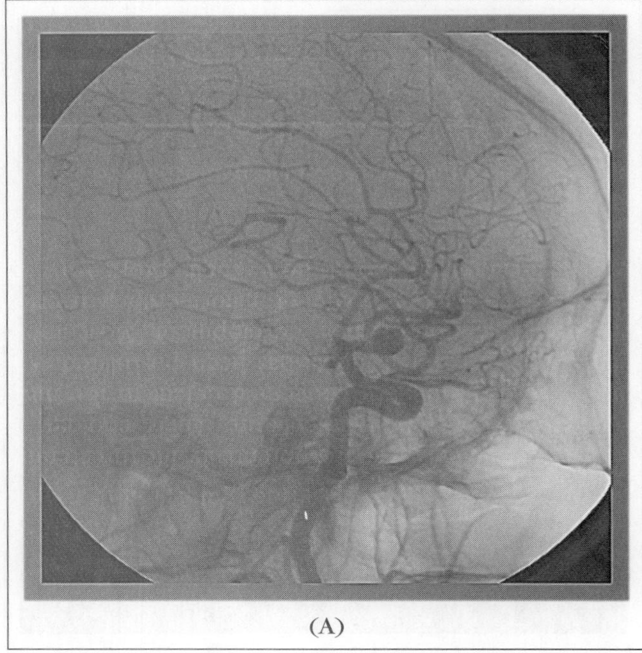

(A)

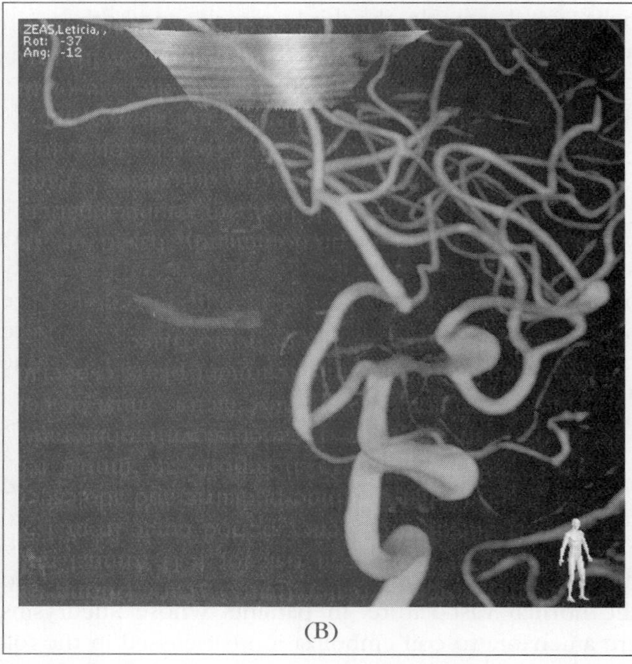


(B)

**FIGURE 132-8** (A) A digital subtraction angiogram (DSA) demonstrating a large fusiform aneurysm arising from the communicating artery. (B) A 3-dimensional reconstruction of a conventional angiogram showing the same communicating artery aneurysms seen in (A). Due to its less invasive nature, CT angiograms will become the diagnostic treatment of choice in the future. (Photos courtesy of James Tait Goodrich.)

## MANAGEMENT

The risk of an aneurysm rupture approximates 1% to 2% per year, although 1 large prospective study estimated this risk at 0.05% per year for small aneurysms.[45] Morbidity and mortality rates are high for each rupture, and treatment is strongly advocated in order to obviate this risk. This holds particularly true for adolescents with their long anticipated life expectancy. For ruptured aneurysms, the risk of rebleeding with its attendant morbidity and mortality are highest in the first 48 hours following the initial hemorrhage. Therefore most surgeons and interventionalists advocate definitive treatment within 24 to 48 hours of the ictus.

The goal of any treatment is obliteration of the aneurysmal sac from the parent circulation. This greatly reduces, but does not completely eliminate, the risk of hemorrhage and allows for aggressive medical treatment in the aftermath of SAH for patients who have bled. A multidisciplinary team consisting of neurointerventionalists and neurosurgeons should review each patient on an individual basis and come to a consensus regarding the most effective means of achieving this common goal (Figure 132-9).

### Surgery

Microsurgical treatment of aneurysms most often involves the placement of a spring-loaded metal clip around the neck of the aneurysm, effectively isolating

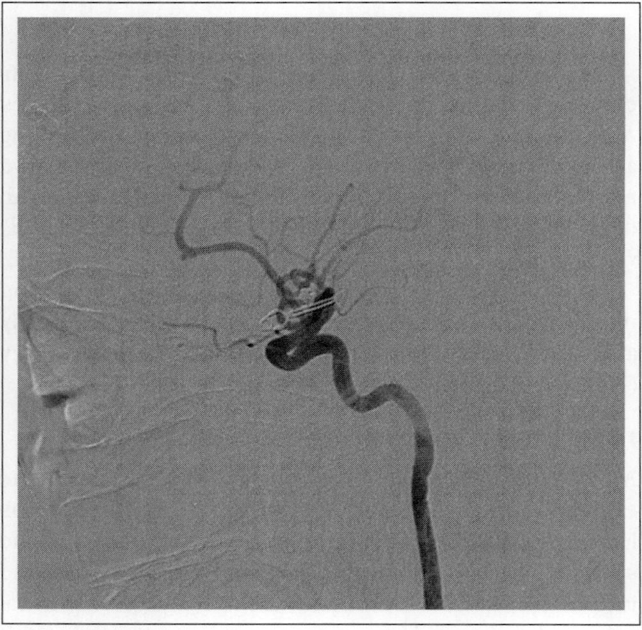

**FIGURE 132-9** Postoperative angiogram of a clipped aneurysm showing the spring-loaded clip on the neck of the aneurysm with complete occlusion of the aneurysm. (Photo courtesy of James Tait Goodrich.)

the aneurysm from its feeding vessel while reconstituting normal distal blood flow patterns. Saphenous vein and radial artery bypass grafts may be used in the setting of large or dysplastic aneurysms that are not amenable to direct clip ligation or coil embolization. Following bypass, the vessel segment that gives rise to the aneurysm may then be sacrificed via either surgical or endovascular means. Various approaches to the cranial base have been employed for exposure and treatment of aneurysms in difficult to reach locations, such as the basilar and ophthalmic arteries. More recently, surgery and coil embolization have been used in concert with each other for the treatment of more complex lesions.

### Embolization

Coil embolization involves the intraluminal detachment of malleable platinum coils into the sac of an aneurysm under fluoroscopic guidance during cerebral arteriography. The coils reduce blood flow into the aneurysm and are thought to then induce thrombosis, thus eliminating the aneurysm from the circulation. In approximately 15 years, coil embolization has gone from an experimental treatment to the procedure of choice for many aneurysms. The multicenter International Subarachnoid Aneurysm Trial (ISAT) enrolled 2,143 patients with ruptured ICAs who were felt to be suitable for both treatments, and who were then randomized to either surgical clipping or endovascular coiling.[46,47] The authors found that the risk of death or dependence at one year was significantly less in patients who underwent endovascular coiling. The absolute and relative risk reductions were 7.4% and 23.9%, respectively[47] (Figure 132-10).

However, the incidence of rebleeding is higher in coil embolization, ranging from 0.11% to 1.4% per year.[47,49] The incidence of recanalization of the aneurysm secondary to coil compaction is also higher, approaching as much as 21% in some series.[48-53] The occurrence of recanalization on follow-up angiography necessitates retreatment in a significant number of patients over time, with rates ranging from 4.7% to 18.9% in the recent literature.[48-50,52] The need for retreatment following clip ligation is substantially lower.[48] Because of these data, patients who undergo coiling procedures must have long-term follow-up to ensure complete aneurysm obliteration and to minimize the risk of rerupture.

At this time, some aneurysms continue to be unsuitable for coil embolization due to unacceptable occlusion rates. Aneurysms that have small necks and higher dome-to-neck size ratio have better occlusion rates and improved outcome.[52-54] Occlusion rates for MCA aneurysms have traditionally been poor.[55] However, as technology advances and patient selection criteria are refined, these rates are beginning to improve as well.[56]

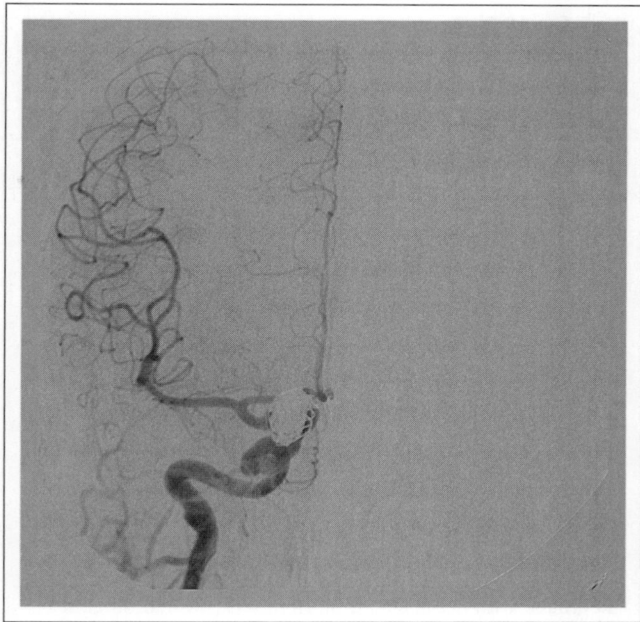

**FIGURE 132-10** An anterior posterior view of an angiogram of the right carotid artery plus the middle and anterior artery circulation. At the level of the ophthalmic segment of the internal carotid artery, there is a large aneurysm that has been treated using a series of platinum coils. The coiled aneurysm is seen in outline with the coils clearly evident. (Photo courtesy of James Tait Goodrich.)

Newer interventional techniques are continuously being developed and refined to minimize recanalization rates, achieve higher complete occlusion rates, and decrease the incidence of rehemorrhage and its associated morbidity. As such, indications for coil embolization as first-line therapy continue to broaden. Stenting technology and balloon-remodeling techniques are now widely used to improve angiographic occlusion. Promising areas of research include the use of coated coils that increase thrombogenicity and packing ratios, liquid embolic agents, and biological manipulation of traditional coils to promote thrombus organization, collagen formation, and endothelialization of the aneurysm neck.[57-59]

## PROGNOSIS

It is important to note that the mortality for aneurysmal SAH is approximately 50% at 30 days, with 10% to 15% of patients dying before they reach the hospital. Approximately 50% of survivors have major neurological disability.[29,30,35-37] The 2 predominant causes of long-term morbidity are rehemorrhage and post-SAH vasospasm. Because of these ominous numbers, with rare exception, treatment is recommended in adolescents who are found to have aneurysms. This concept holds true regardless of rupture status (Table 132-3).

**Table 132-3**

**Hunt and Hess Classification of Subarachnoid Hemorrhage[60]**

| *Grade* | *Description* |
|---|---|
| 1 | Asymptomatic, or mild headache and slight nuchal rigidity |
| 2 | Cranial nerve palsy, moderate/severe headache, nuchal rigidity |
| 3 | Mild focal deficit, lethargy, or confusion |
| 4 | Stupor, moderate/severe hemiparesis, early decerebrate rigidity |
| 5 | Deep coma, decerebrate rigidity, moribund appearance |

Hunt-Hess classification has proven to be a useful predictor of outcome and in surgical design making. The lower the grade, the better the prognosis and long-term outcome.

Reprinted with permission from Hunt WE, Hess RM. Surgical risk as related to time of intervention in the repair of intracranial aneurysms. *J Neurosurg*. 1968; 28 (1): 14–20.

## CAVERNOUS MALFORMATIONS

Cavernous malformations are congenital vascular lesions composed of thin-walled sinusoidal channels lined with a single layer of epithelium. Intervening neural tissue, feeding arteries, and draining veins are lacking, distinguishing them from other vascular malformations.[61] Surrounding parenchyma shows evidence of prior hemorrhage with hemosiderin deposition. Calcification, cystic degeneration, and cholesterol deposition may be seen pathologically.[62] Cavernous malformations tend to have a more benign clinical course than aneurysms and AVMs, and treatment strategies are therefore more controversial.

### EPIDEMIOLOGY

The estimated prevalence of cavernous malformations ranges from 0.02% to 0.53%,[62] distributed equally between males and females in most series. They tend to present in the third and fourth decades, and are rare in adolescents, representing only 5% to 13% of all clinically detected vascular malformations.[62,63] Males tend to present earlier than females,[64] and there has been a suggestion of a higher incidence in the Hispanic population.[65] The presence of multiple lesions is common and is significantly higher in those with familial inheritance patterns.

Most lesions occur in the supratentorial space. Lesions in the pons and cerebellum, however, are not uncommon, and can pose difficult management problems.

### CLINICAL PRESENTATION

Seizure is the most common presentation for patients with cavernous malformations, occurring in an average of approximately 60% of patients in representative series.[62] Epilepsy is much more common in patients with cavernous malformations than in those with other vascular malformations, and therefore a larger percentage of treatment strategies are aimed at seizure control as the primary outcome measure.[66]

Overt ICH occurs in approximately one-third of patients[67] and tends to be more common in younger patients.[68] The annual risk of hemorrhage is estimated at approximately 0.7% to 1.1% per year,[62,64,69,70] with hemorrhages having a more benign course than those associated with AVMs and aneurysms. Morbidity is location dependent, with long-term neurological sequelae being more common and more profound when hemorrhage occurs in eloquent areas such as the brainstem.

A minority of patients (15%-45%)[62] will present with either focal or progressive neurological deficit without overt ICH. These occurrences are thought to be related to intralesional hemorrhages resulting in local mass effect on surrounding eloquent brain structures. Females are more likely to present in this manner.[62]

### IMAGING

Magnetic resonance imaging findings are quite characteristic and extremely sensitive for cavernous angioma. Cavernous malformations are usually discrete lesions with heterogeneous signal intensity on both T1- and T2-weighted imaging. There is a characteristic hypointense ring on T2 and gradient echo sequences that represents hemosiderin deposition sometimes referred to as a "halo-ring" appearance[71,72] (Figure 132-11).

Computed tomography has relatively high sensitivity but low specificity for the detection of cavernous malformations. Hyperdense calcifications (Figure 132-12) and blood products and hypodense cystic components may be seen. Overt hemorrhage will be easily detected but may obscure the underlying lesion.

Cavernous malformations are rarely seen on cerebral angiography. The absence of a lesion on angiography in concert with characteristic MRI findings lends support to the diagnosis.

### MANAGEMENT

Surgical excision is the treatment of choice for symptomatic lesions in surgically accessible locations. Surgery is also advocated by most surgeons for patients with progressive neurological deterioration, regardless of location.[73] Intractable epilepsy also can serve as an indication for lesionectomy, and long-term seizure control may be improved if concomitant resection of

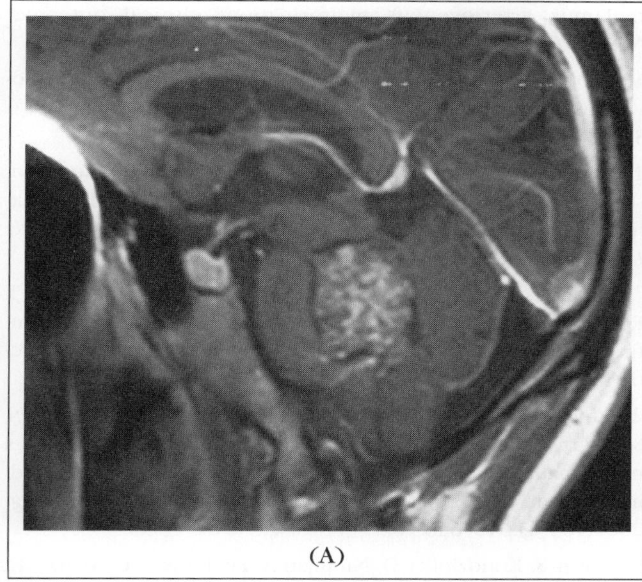

(A)

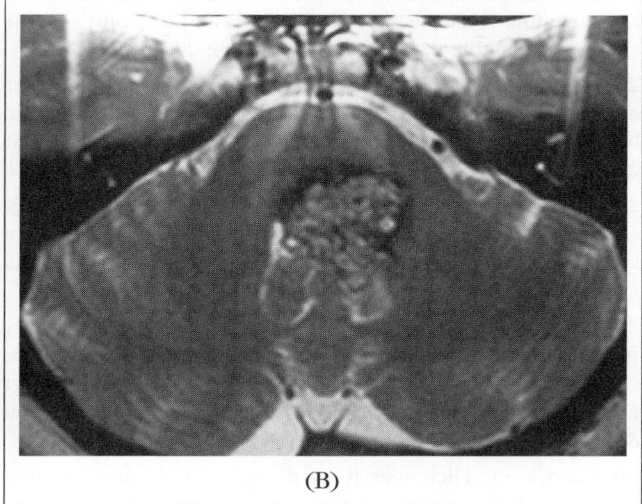

(B)

**FIGURE 132-11** (A) Sagittal MR T1-weighted showing findings consistent with a cavernous angioma of the brainstem, deeply invading the pons. This patient is a 16-year-old female with progressive gait ataxia, and sixth nerve palsy. The lesion has evidence of several small microhemorrhages. (B) Axial MR of same patient showing again multiple areas of small hemorrhages and invasion of the brainstem. (Photos courtesy of James Tait Goodrich.)

surrounding hemosiderin-laden brain is performed.[66,74] As in AVMs and aneurysms, the long life expectancy of adolescents lends support to the argument for early intervention in the context of acceptable treatment morbidity.

Stereotactic radiosurgery has emerged as a potential treatment option for patients with deep-seated lesions or residual lesion following craniotomy. Although treatment morbidity and rehemorrhage rates appear acceptably low, long-term obliteration rates are variable.[75,76] As more long-term data become available, indications for SRS will likely become more defined.[75-77]

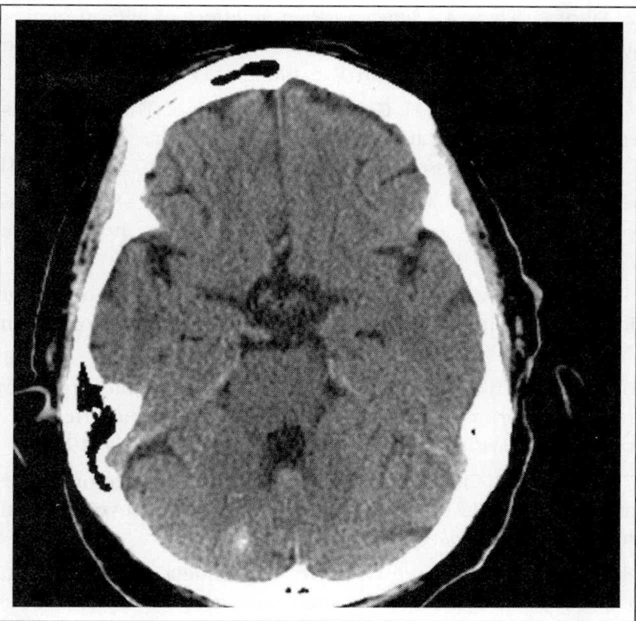

**FIGURE 132-12** CT scan showing a discrete cavernous angioma of the right cerebellum; the whitish haze represents calcifications in the cavernous angioma. (Photo courtesy of James Tait Goodrich.)

As in the other pathologies discussed in this chapter, the natural history of the disease process must be considered when determining a treatment strategy that is largely prophylactic in nature.

## PROGNOSIS

The prognosis for patients with cavernous malformations is favorable compared with other intracranial vascular malformations. Location of the lesion is of primary importance in determining outcome from both hemorrhage and intervention, with eloquent and infratentorial locations carrying greater risk of morbidity. Seizure-free survival following resection of epileptogenic lesions and surrounding abnormal brain is excellent, and surgery should be considered strongly for these patients.

## REFERENCES

1. Mei-Zahav M, Letarte M, Faughnan ME, Abdalla SA, Cymerman U, MacLusky IB. Symptomatic children with hereditary hemorrhagic telangiectasia: a pediatric center experience. *Arch Pediatr Adolesc Med.* 2006;160(6):596–601

2. Stapf C, Khaw AV, Sciacca RR, et al. Effect of age on clinical and morphological characteristics in patients with brain arteriovenous malformation. *Stroke.* 2003;34(11):2664–2669

3. Ondra SL, Troupp H, George ED, Schwab K. The natural history of symptomatic arteriovenous malformations of the brain: a 24-year follow-up assessment. *J Neurosurg.* 1990;73(3):387–391

4. Kondziolka D, McLaughlin MR, Kestle JR. Simple risk predictions for arteriovenous malformation hemorrhage. *Neurosurgery.* 1995;37(5):851–855

5. Stapf C, Mast H, Sciacca RR, et al. Predictors of hemorrhage in patients with untreated brain arteriovenous malformation. *Neurology.* 2006;66(9):1350–1355

6. Nataf F, Schlienger M, Lefkopoulos D, et al. Radiosurgery of cerebral arteriovenous malformations in children: a series of 57 cases. *Int J Radiat Oncol Biol Phys.* 2003;57(1):184–195

7. Schäuble B, Cascino GD, Pollock BE, et al. Seizure outcomes after stereotactic radiosurgery for cerebral arteriovenous malformations. *Neurology.* 2004;63(4):683–687

8. Turjman F, Massoud TF, Sayre JW, Viñuela F, Guglielmi G, Duckwiler G. Epilepsy associated with cerebral arteriovenous malformations: a multivariate analysis of angioarchitectural characteristics. *AJNR Am J Neuroradiol.* 1995;16(2):345–350

9. Sheth RD, Bodensteiner JB. Progressive neurologic impairment from an arteriovenous malformation vascular steal. *Pediatr Neurol.* 1995;13(4):352–354

10. Bristol RE, Albuquerque FC, Spetzler RF, Rekate HL, McDougall CG, Zabramski JM. Surgical management of arteriovenous malformations in children. *J Neurosurg.* 2006;105(2):88–93

11. Spetzler RF, Martin NA. A proposed grading system for arteriovenous malformations. *J Neurosurg.* 1986;65(4):476–483

12. Han PP, Ponce FA, Spetzler RF. Intention-to-treat analysis of Spetzler-Martin grades IV and V arteriovenous malformations: natural history and treatment paradigm. *J Neurosurg.* 2003;98(1):3–7

13. Lawton MT. UCSF Brain Arteriovenous Malformation Study Project. Spetzler-Martin Grade III arteriovenous malformations: surgical results and a modification of the grading scale. *Neurosurgery.* 2003;52(4):740–748; discussion 748–749

14. Sanchez-Mejia RO, Chennupati SK, Gupta N, Fullerton H, Young WL, Lawton MT. Superior outcomes in children compared with adults after microsurgical resection of brain arteriovenous malformations. *J Neurosurg.* 2006;105(2):82–87

15. Haw CS, terBrugge K, Willinsky R, Tomlinson G. Complications of embolization of arteriovenous malformations of the brain. *J Neurosurg.* 2006;104(2):226–232

16. Kim LJ, Albuquerque FC, Spetzler RF, McDougall CG. Postembolization neurological deficits in cerebral arteriovenous malformations: stratification by arteriovenous malformation grade. *Neurosurgery.* 2006;59(1):53–59; discussion 53–59

17. Andrade-Souza YM, Zadeh G, Scora D, Tsao MN, Schwartz ML. Radiosurgery for basal ganglia, internal capsule, and thalamus arteriovenous malformation: clinical outcome. *Neurosurgery.* 2005;56(1):56–63; discussion 63–64

18. Cohen-Gadol AA, Pollock BE. Radiosurgery for arteriovenous malformations in children. *J Neurosurg.* 2006;104(6 Suppl):388–391

19. Smyth MD, Sneed PK, Ciricillo SF, et al. Stereotactic radiosurgery for pediatric intracranial arteriovenous malformations: the University of California at San Francisco experience. *J Neurosurg.* 2002;97(1):48–55

20. Shin M, Kawahara N, Maruyama K, Tago M, Ueki K, Kirino T. Risk of hemorrhage from an arteriovenous malformation confirmed to have been obliterated on angiography after stereotactic radiosurgery. *J Neurosurg.* 2005;102(5):842–846

21. Andrade-Souza YM, Zadeh G, Ramani M, Scora D, Tsao MN, Schwartz ML. Testing the radiosurgery-based arteriovenous malformation score and the modified Spetzler-Martin grading system to predict radiosurgical outcome. *J Neurosurg.* 2005;103(4):642–648

22. Sirin S, Kondziolka D, Niranjan A, Flickinger JC, Maitz AH, Lunsford LD. Prospective staged volume radiosurgery for large arteriovenous malformations: indications and outcomes in otherwise untreatable patients. *Neurosurgery.* 2006;58(1):17–27

23. Maity A, Shu HK, Tan JE, et al. Treatment of pediatric intracranial arteriovenous malformations with linear-accelerator-based stereotactic radiosurgery: the University of Pennsylvania experience. *Pediatr Neurosurg.* 2004;40(5):207–214

24. Shin M, Kawamoto S, Kurita H, et al. Retrospective analysis of a 10-year experience of stereotactic radio surgery for arteriovenous malformations in children and adolescents. *J Neurosurg.* 2002;97(4):779–784

25. Steiner L, Lindquist C, Steiner M. Stereotactic radiosurgery, part 1: radiosurgery with focused gamma-beam irradiation in children. In: Edwards MSB, Hoffman HJ, eds. *Cerebral Vascular Disease in Children and Adolescents.* Baltimore, MD: Williams & Wilkins; 1989:367–388

26. Pollock BE, Flickinger JC. A proposed radiosurgery-based grading system for arteriovenous malformations. *J Neurosurg.* 2002;96(1):79–85

27. Choi JH, Mast H, Sciacca RR, et al. Clinical outcome after first and recurrent hemorrhage in patients with untreated brain arteriovenous malformation. *Stroke.* 2006;37(5):1243–1247

28. Krishna H, Wani AA, Behari S, Banerji D, Chhabra DK, Jain VK. Intracranial aneurysms in patients 18 years of age or under, are they different from aneurysms in adult population? *Acta Neurochir (Wien).* 2005;147(5):469–476; discussion 476

29. Meyer FB, Reeves AL. Pediatric and adolescent aneurysms. *Contemp Neurosurg.* 1990;12:1–6

30. Amacher A. Subarachnoid hemorrhage in children and adolescents. *Contemp Neurosurg.* 1984;6:1–6

31. Meyer FB, Sundt TM Jr, Fode NC, Morgan MK, Forbes GS, Mellinger JF. Cerebral aneurysms in childhood and adolescence. *J Neurosurg.* 1989;70(3):420–425

32. Norris J, Wallace MC. Pediatric intracranial aneurysms. *Neurosurg Clin N Am.* 1998;9(3):557–563

33. Ostergaard JR, Voldby B. Intracranial arterial aneurysms in children and adolescents. *J Neurosurg.* 1983;58(6):832–837

34. Patel AN, Richardson AE. Ruptured intracranial aneurysms in the first two decades of life. A study of 58 patients. *J Neurosurg.* 1971;35(5):571–576

35. Amacher AL, Drake CG. The results of operating upon cerebral aneurysms and angiomas in children and adolescents. I. Cerebral aneurysms. *Childs Brain.* 1979;5(3):151–165

36. Heiskanen O. Ruptured intracranial arterial aneurysms of children and adolescents. Surgical and total management results. *Childs Nerv Syst.* 1989;5(2):66–70

37. Humphreys RP. Intracranial arterial aneurysms. In: Edwards M, Hoffman HJ, eds. *Cerebral Vascular Disease in Children and Adolescents.* Baltimore, MD: Williams & Wilkins; 1989:247–254

38. Storrs BB, Humphreys RP, Hendrick EB, Hoffman HJ. Intracranial aneurysms in the pediatric age-group. *Childs Brain.* 1982;9(5):358–361

39. Lustgarten L, John T, Lopez R, et al. Paediatric intracranial aneurysms: results of a surgical series and literature review of Guglielmi detachable coil embolization. *J Clin Neurosci.* 1999;2:133–137

40. Branley MG, Wright KW, Borchert MS. Third nerve palsy due to cerebral artery aneurysm in a child. *Aust N Z J Ophthalmol.* 1992;20(2):137–140

41. Preechawat P, Sukawatcharin P, Poonyathalang A, Lekskul A. Aneurysmal third nerve palsy. *J Med Assoc Thai.* 2004;87(11):1332–1335

42. Day AL. Aneurysms of the ophthalmic segment. A clinical and anatomical analysis. *J Neurosurg.* 1990;72(5):677–691

43. Mohr G, Ferguson G, Khan M, et al. Intraventricular hemorrhage from ruptured aneurysm. Retrospective analysis of 91 cases. *J Neurosurg.* 1983;58(4):482–487

44. Wong GK, Boet R, Poon WS, Yu S, Lam JM. A review of isolated third nerve palsy without subarachnoid hemorrhage using computed tomographic angiography as the first line of investigation. *Clin Neurol Neurosurg.* 2004;107(1):27–31

45. Unruptured intracranial aneurysms—risk of rupture and risks of surgical intervention. International Study of Unruptured Intracranial Aneurysms Investigators. *N Engl J Med.* 1998;339(24):1725–1733

46. Molyneux A, Kerr R, Stratton I, et al. International subarachnoid aneurysm trial (ISAT) of neurosurgical clipping versus endovascular coiling in 2143 patients with ruptured intracranial aneurysms: a randomised trial. *Lancet.* 2002;360(9342): 1267–1274

47. Molyneux AJ, Kerr RS, Yu LM, et al. International subarachnoid aneurysm trial (ISAT) of neurosurgical clipping versus endovascular coiling in 2143 patients with ruptured intracranial aneurysms: a randomised comparison of effects on survival, dependency, seizures, rebleeding, subgroups, and aneurysm occlusion. *Lancet.* 2005;366(9488):809–817

48. CARAT Investigators. Rates of delayed rebleeding from intracranial aneurysms are low after surgical and endovascular treatment. *Stroke.* 2006;37(6):1437–1442

49. Kole MK, Pelz DM, Kalapos P, Lee DH, Gulka IB, Lownie SP. Endovascular coil embolization of intracranial aneurysms: important factors related to rates and outcomes of incomplete occlusion. *J Neurosurg.* 2005;102(4):607–615

50. Henkes H, Fischer S, Mariushi W, et al. Angiographic and clinical results in 316 coil-treated basilar artery bifurcation aneurysms. *J Neurosurg.* 2005;103(6):990–999

51. Ross IB, Dhillon GS. Complications of endovascular treatment of cerebral aneurysms. *Surg Neurol.* 2005;64(1):12–18; discussion 18–19

52. Gallas S, Pasco A, Cottier JP, et al. A multicenter study of 705 ruptured intracranial aneurysms treated with Guglielmi detachable coils. *AJNR Am J Neuroradiol.* 2005;26(7): 1723–1731

53. Li MH, Gao BL, Fang C, et al. Angiographic follow-up of cerebral aneurysms treated with Guglielmi detachable coils: an analysis of 162 cases with 173 aneurysms. *AJNR Am J Neuroradiol.* 2006;27(5):1107–1112

54. Debrun GM, Aletich VA, Kehrli P, Misra M, Ausman JI, Charbel F. Selection of cerebral aneurysms for treatment using Guglielmi detachable coils: the preliminary University of Illinois at Chicago experience. *Neurosurgery.* 1998;43(6):1281–1295; discussion 1296–1297

55. Regli L, Uske A, de Tribolet N. Endovascular coil placement compared with surgical clipping for the treatment of unruptured middle cerebral artery aneurysms: a consecutive series. *J Neurosurg.* 1999;90(6):1025–1030

56. Doerfler A, Wanke I, Goericke SL, et al. Endovascular treatment of middle cerebral artery aneurysms with electrolytically detachable coils. *AJNR Am J Neuroradiol.* 2006;27(3):513–520

57. Lanzino G, Kanaan Y, Perrini P, Dayoub H, Fraser K. Emerging concepts in the treatment of intracranial aneurysms: stents, coated coils, and liquid embolic agents. *Neurosurgery.* 2005;57(3):449–459; discussion 449–459

58. Gaba RC, Ansari SA, Roy SS, Marden FA, Viana MA, Malisch TW. Embolization of intracranial aneurysms with hydrogel-coated coils versus inert platinum coils: effects on packing density, coil length and quantity, procedure performance, cost, length of hospital stay, and durability of therapy. *Stroke.* 2006;37(6):1443–1450

59. Niimi Y, Song J, Madrid M, Berenstein A. Endosaccular treatment of intracranial aneurysms using matrix coils: early experience and midterm follow-up. *Stroke.* 2006;37(4):1028–1032

60. Hunt WE, Hess RM. Surgical risk as related to time of intervention in the repair of intracranial aneurysms. *J Neurosurg.* 1968;28(1):14–20

61. New PF, Ojemann RG, Davis KR, et al. MR and CT of occult vascular malformations of the brain. *AJR Am J Roentgenol.* 1986;147(5):985–993

62. Maraire J, Awad IA. Intracranial cavernous malformations: lesion behavior and management strategies. *Neurosurgery.* 1995;37(4):591–605

63. McCormick W. The pathology of angiomas. In: Fein J, Flamm ES, eds. *Cerebrovascular Surgery.* New York, NY: Springer-Verlag; 1985:1073–1095

64. Robinson JR, Awad IA, Little JR. Natural history of the cavernous angioma. *J Neurosurg.* 1991; 75(5):709–714

65. Mason I, Aase JM, Orrison WW, Wicks JD, Seigel RS, Bicknell JM. Familial cavernous angiomas of the brain in an Hispanic family. *Neurology.* 1988;38(2):324–326

66. Baumann CR, Schuknecht B, Lo Russo G, et al. Seizure outcome after resection of cavernous malformations is better when surrounding hemosiderin-stained brain also is removed. *Epilepsia.* 2006;47(3):563–566

67. Tagle P, Huete I, Méndez J, del Villar S. Intracranial cavernous angioma: presentation and management. *J Neurosurg.* 1986;64(5):720–723

68. Scott RM, Barnes P, Kupsky W, Adelman LS. Cavernous angiomas of the central nervous system in children. *J Neurosurg.* 1992;76(1):38–46

69. Del Curling O Jr, Kelly DL Jr, Elster AD, Craven TE. An analysis of the natural history of cavernous angiomas. *J Neurosurg.* 1991;75(5):702–708

70. Zabramski JM, Wascher TM, Spetzler RF, et al. The natural history of familial cavernous malformations: results of an ongoing study. *J Neurosurg.* 1994;80(3):422–432

71. Rigamonti D, Drayer BP, Johnson PC, Hadley MN, Zabramski J, Spetzler RF. The MRI appearance of cavernous malformations (angiomas). *J Neurosurg.* 1987;67(4):518–524

72. Tomlinson FH, Houser OW, Scheithauer BW, Sundt TM Jr, Okazaki H, Parisi JE. Angiographically occult vascular malformations: a correlative study of features on magnetic resonance imaging and histological examination. *Neurosurgery.* 1994;34(5):792–799; discussion 799–800

73. Ferroli P, Sinisi M, Franzini A, Giombini S, Solero CL, Broggi G. Brainstem cavernomas: long-term results of microsurgical resection in 52 patients. *Neurosurgery.* 2005;56(6):1203–1212; discussion 1212–1214

74. Awad IA, Robinson J. Cavernous malformation and epilepsy. In: Awad IA, Barrow DL, eds. *Cavernous Malformations*. Park Ridge, IL: AANS; 1993:49–63

75. Liscák R, Vladyka V, Simonová G, Vymazal J, Novotny J Jr. Gamma knife surgery of brain cavernous hemangiomas. *J Neurosurg.* 2005;102 Suppl:207–213

76. Hasegawa T, McInerney J, Kondziolka D, Lee JY, Flickinger JC, Lunsford LD. Long-term results after stereotactic radiosurgery for patients with cavernous malformations. *Neurosurgery.* 2002;50(6):1190–1197; discussion 1197–1198

77. Pollock BE, Garces YI, Stafford SL, Foote RL, Schomberg PJ, Link MJ. Stereotactic radiosurgery for cavernous malformations. *J Neurosurg.* 2000;93(6):987–991

# CHAPTER 133

# Myelomeningocele

ROBERT W. MARION, MD

*"Things are going pretty well for me, at least for the top half of my body. Sometimes, I wish I could cut off my lower half and start over. Things would be a lot better for me...."*

—Jose L, 15-Year-old Patient at Einstein/Montefiore Spina Bifida Center

## INTRODUCTION

Due to the development of new technology such as the ventriculoperitoneal (VP) shunt, and following the introduction of multidisciplinary management in the 1960s, the natural history of spina bifida has undergone a revolution. In 1960, in most affected infants, myelomeningocele (MMC) (which is used interchangeably in this chapter with the term "spina bifida") was a lethal congenital defect. In 1989, writing in *The Birth Defects Encyclopedia,* Louis Bartoshesky, MD,[1] noted that "of 13,600 American children born with Spina Bifida between 1980 and 1987, an estimated 9,800 were still alive in 1987,"[1] suggesting that the mortality rate in the first 7 years of life was as high as 28%. Between 1987 and 2007, the Einstein/Montefiore Spina Bifida Center (SBC), in the Bronx (NY), reported that 12 patients out of 211 with spina bifida had died, a 10-year death rate of less than 5%.

The result of this striking improvement in survival is that more infants and children with spina bifida are surviving into adolescence and adulthood. As they age, individuals with spina bifida develop medical, psychological, and emotional problems, presenting management issues that alter the way that care must be provided. The quote from Jose L, a patient at the Einstein/Montefiore SBC, just scratches the surface of the psychological burden that this disorder has on affected adolescents. Consequently, it is important that the practitioner providing primary care to adolescents has a good understanding of these issues. In this chapter, we review the etiology of spina bifida, the medical and surgical problems that occur in affected individuals, and the special problems that occur in adolescents and young adults. In addition, we discuss information regarding the prevention of neural tube defects (NTDs) and methods of diagnosing them.

## SPINA BIFIDA DEFINITIONS AND ETIOLOGY

In this chapter, the term "spina bifida" is used as a synonym for MMC. Myelomeningocele is the most common of NTDs, a group of disorders that includes rachischisis totalis, anencephaly, and meningocele. Spina bifida occulta, a common variant of normal in which a fusion defect of one or more vertebrae occurs, is not considered an open NTD and thus is not discussed in this chapter.

The neural tube, the embryonic structure that forms the spine and skull, develops early in the first trimester of gestation. At approximately 18 days after conception, neuroectodermal cells form the neural plate (Figure 133-1). By day 21, the neural plate invaginates, leading to the formation of the neural groove, the structure that ultimately becomes the central portion of the neural tube. Eventually, the 2 edges of the neural plate come together, meeting at a point that will ultimately become the cervical spine; from this point, the tube forms through a "zipping closed" caudadly (to form the lower spine) and cephaladly (to form the skull). By day 24, closure of the cranial end of the tube is complete; the caudal end's closure is finished by 26 days after conception.

Neural tube defects result from either a primary failure or a secondary reopening of the neural tube. In 1980, approximately 1 in 1,000 liveborn children in the United States had an NTD, with a total of about 2,000 affected children born that year. The prevalence significantly decreased, however, following 1998, when the American diet began to be fortified with folic acid. In 2007, the prevalence of NTDs in liveborn children in the United States was approximately 1 in 4,000, and only about 500 children with NTDs were born each year. Thus, folic acid supplementation has been one of the most effective public health initiatives since the introduction of the Salk polio vaccine in the 1950s.

Neural tube defects are multifactorial disorders caused by the interplay of genetic and environmental factors. Evidence pointing to this multifactorial inheritance includes the following facts:

- Once a couple has had a child with an NTD, the recurrence risk for subsequent pregnancies is between 2% and 4%, significantly greater than the risk in the general population (suggesting a genetic etiology).
- They are more common in individuals from the British Isles than they are in other parts of the world (suggesting a genetic etiology).

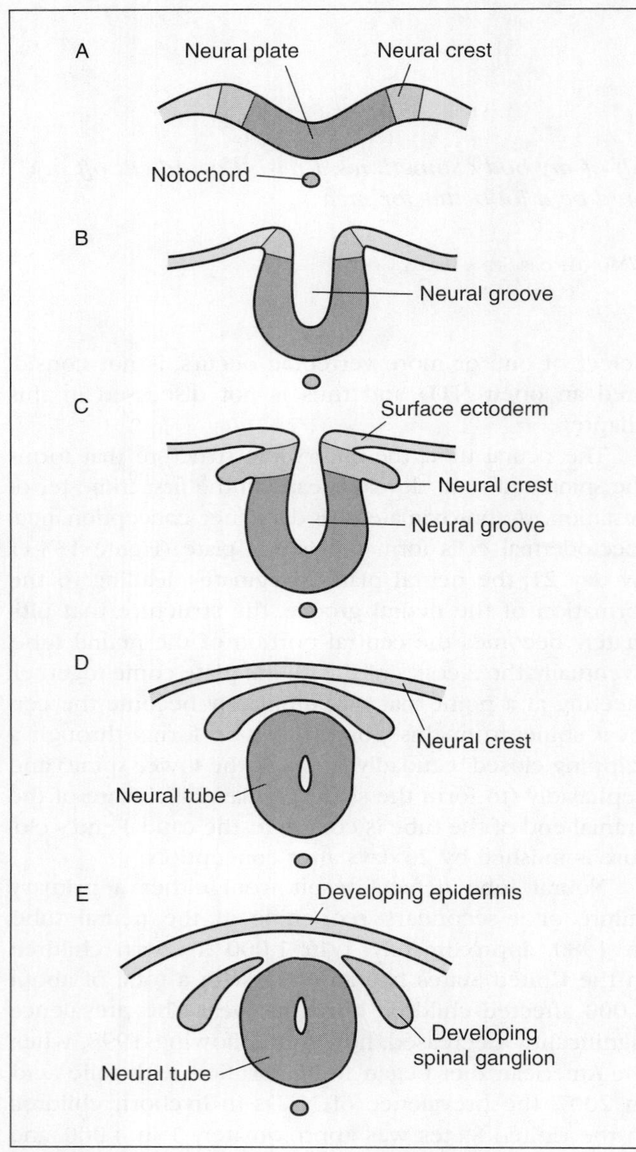


**FIGURE 133-1** A-E, Embryonic process of neural tube closure.

- Individuals from the British Isles who emigrate to other parts of the world have a lower risk of having a child with an NTD than do their relatives back home (suggesting an environmental etiology).
- In the northern hemisphere, infants with NTDs are more likely to be born in late fall and early winter than at other times of the year (ie, their neural tubes would have been closing in early spring, suggesting an environmental etiology).

It was the latter observation that ultimately led to the discovery that maternal dietary factors, specifically, folic acid, played a role in the etiology of NTDs. As a result of these observations and studies performed by multiple groups in Europe and the United States in the 1980s and 1990s, the important preventive role of pre- and periconceptual folic acid supplementation was definitively demonstrated. This is discussed in more detail later in the chapter.

As seen in Figures 133-2 and 133-3, an infant with spina bifida presents with a glistening sac herniating through the midline of the back. The covering of the sac is formed from the meninges, and the contents of the sac consist of cerebrospinal fluid and a portion of the spinal cord. In most cases, the spinal cord present in the sac and the portion of the cord caudal to that section are unable to perform normal functioning. As a result, individuals with MMC are paralyzed from the level of the lesion downward.

All problems—medical, cognitive, psychological, and emotional—that occur in individuals with spina bifida are caused, either directly or indirectly, by this disruption of the functioning of the spinal cord. Individuals who have low lesions (ie, in the sacral spine) generally have a better prognosis; those whose lesions are high (ie, in the thoracic spine) suffer from more severe consequences. As such, at the time of birth or following prenatal diagnosis, a general assessment of an individual's prognosis can be made with some certainty.

All adolescents with spina bifida need to be cared for by a team of providers from an array of specialties. Studies have shown that prognosis of these patients is improved if the specialists providing care work together in a team. Thus, over the last quarter of the 20th century, multidisciplinary clinics such as the Einstein/Montefiore SBC have developed. These clinics must provide the

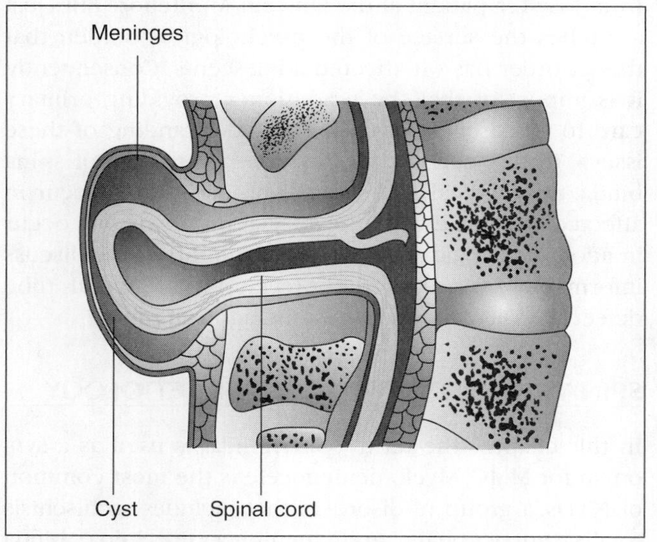


**FIGURE 133-2** Schematic view of myelomeningocele.

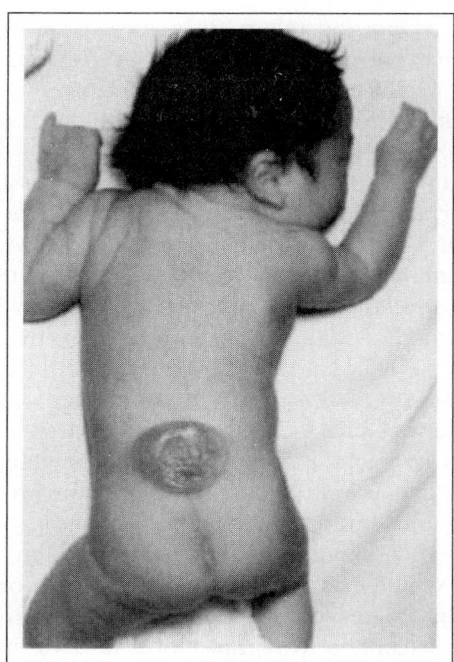

FIGURE 133-3 Newborn with myelomeningocele.

following services: neurosurgery, orthopaedic surgery, physiatry, urology, gastroenterology, and general medicine. In addition, representatives from nursing, social work, orthotic manufacture, radiology, genetic counseling, developmental medicine, and psychiatry should be available for consultation.

As infants and children with spina bifida grow into adolescence and adulthood, additional problems can be anticipated. Adolescents with spina bifida are often scorned or ignored by their contemporaries; their ambulatory impairments often prevent them from participating in typical activities; and due to neurogenic bowel and bladder, they require clean intermittent catheterization every 4 hours and often use diapers. They need assistance from adults, usually their parents, a situation that serves to infantilize them at a time when they should be gaining independence. They learn to live with chronic pain, and they have difficulty finding housing, jobs, and sexual partners (a problem compounded in men by the fact that their allergy to latex, believed to be universal in individuals with spina bifida, prevents them from being able to use standard condoms; they must instead use lambskin condoms, which are not as optimal for prevention of pregnancy and sexually transmitted infections). These and other issues cause an additional psychological and emotional burden in adolescents and young adults with this condition, a situation that must be explored and addressed by their health care provider.

The medical and surgical problems of the adolescent with spina bifida are discussed in the next section.

## MEDICAL AND SURGICAL PROBLEMS OF THE ADOLESCENT WITH SPINA BIFIDA

### NEUROSURGERY

For most patients with spina bifida, the neurosurgeon is the first member of their treatment team they meet. In the newborn period, because the meninges-covered spinal defect represents a portal through which bacteria can have easy access, it is necessary for the surgeon to close the back within the first few days after birth. In addition, due to Arnold-Chiari malformation, type II, a herniation of the hindbrain through the foramen magnum that occurs in every child with spina bifida and that, in many, leads to a disruption in the flow of spinal fluid, hydrocephalus is seen in 70% to 90% of affected individuals. As such, most newborns with spina bifida will require the placement of a VP shunt before they leave the hospital.

Even after the child has left the hospital, the neurosurgeon must continue to be closely involved with the patient. Following closure of the spinal defect and placement of the VP shunt, the neurosurgeon must monitor the functioning of the shunt, and be alert to serious consequences of spina bifida, including symptomatic Arnold-Chiari malformation and tethering of the spinal cord. In the former, the blood supply to the herniated portion of the hindbrain is compromised, leading to infarction of the critically important elements located in that region. During the first year of life, children with symptomatic Arnold-Chiari malformation usually present with hoarseness of their voice, inspiratory stridor, apnea, or sudden death. The presence of any of these findings in a child with spina bifida represents a true medical emergency: if the obstruction of blood flow to the hindbrain is not relieved within 6 hours, the child will be left with serious, permanent neurologic deficits. Most children with symptomatic Arnold-Chiari malformation whose obstruction is not acutely relieved die within 24 months of their initial event. Any child with spina bifida who displays any of these symptoms or signs should have an emergency computed tomography (CT) scan or magnetic resonance imaging (MRI), and the neurosurgeon should be immediately consulted.

In children with spina bifida, tethering of the spinal cord, a phenomenon seen in 10% to 20% of patients, occurs as a direct result of growth and the initial closure of the spinal defect. Following this initial surgery, scar tissue forms between the spinal cord and the spine. Normally, as the child grows, the spine grows more rapidly than the spinal cord, changing the relationship between the lower portion of these 2 structures. When scarring is present, the growing spine pulls and stretches the lower portion of the spinal cord, causing it to thin and progressively interfering with its function.

Spina bifida is a static lesion. The neurologic status of an affected individual should remain stable throughout life. Tethering of the spinal cord should be considered in children or adolescents exhibiting any changes in neurologic functioning. Such changes include the following:

- Alterations in gait (especially the appearance of a previously absent limp)
- Alterations in the appearance or posture of the foot
- Rapidly worsening scoliosis
- Changes in bowel or bladder habits
- Increased number of urinary tract infections

Any child or adolescent exhibiting one or more of these symptoms and signs should be referred to the neurosurgeon and undergo MRI.

Tethering of the spinal cord is a problem all adolescent care providers should know about. Because of its relationship to growth of the spine, the problem is often seen during the adolescent growth spurt. If left untreated, the neurologic deterioration will continue, leading to worsening functioning, and early surgical treatment is warranted. During surgery, the neurosurgeon lyses the scar tissue, a procedure that results in the spinal cord "springing" upward into its normal position. It is important to note, as well as to point out to the adolescent and his or her family, that recovery of lost neurologic function following an untethering procedure may not occur for as long as 6 months to 2 years. In fact, immediately following the procedure, due to edema and manipulation, deterioration of function is often seen, an occurrence for which the patient requires anticipatory guidance and reassurance.

## ORTHOPAEDIC SURGERY AND PHYSIATRY

The goal of orthopaedic management of the individual with spina bifida is to make and keep the patient as ambulatory as possible. Children with low spinal lesions will be able to walk without encumbrance, requiring little or no assistance from the orthopaedist and physiatrist. Those with thoracic lesions may never be able to ambulate; in these cases, making the patient as comfortable as possible in a wheelchair or other device is the main task of the orthopaedist and the physiatrist. In between these 2 extremes, the orthopaedist and physiatrists may use surgical intervention, bracing, canes, walkers, and other devices to achieve the desired outcome.

There is controversy among groups who care for adolescents and young adults with spina bifida about how aggressive to be in encouraging patients to ambulate. On the one hand, the argument is made that because muscle strength in the lower extremities does not increase proportionately with body size, it is inevitable that individuals who are ambulatory early in life will become wheelchair bound as they get older. This group argues, therefore, that forcing young children with spina bifida to work hard to maintain their tenuous ability to walk and performing surgical procedures to assist in this endeavor actually serve to deceive the patient. On the other hand, an argument is made that not giving those able to ambulate the opportunity to walk will ultimately result in a self-fulfilling prophecy. Because they have not been pushed to walk, they will never have the strength to walk.

At the SBC, we agree with the latter philosophy. Our experience has been that most children who were ambulatory in childhood continue to be able to walk in adolescence and adulthood. Our team provides all services and equipment necessary to get patients to become and remain ambulatory. In addition, because obesity, which has reached epidemic proportions in the United States, can be doubly disabling in ambulatory adolescents with spina bifida, it is essential that consultation with a nutritionist be available.

Due to their spinal lesions and the limitation of motion caused by the cord's disruption intrauterinely, newborns with spina bifida can have clubfeet, contractures of ankles and knees, and dislocated hips; due to the spinal defect, older children and adolescents can develop scoliosis. Thus, ongoing surveillance by an orthopaedic surgeon and physiatrist, with intervention as necessary, is an important component of care for adolescents with spina bifida.

Ongoing physical therapy also is important. Although, as noted previously, spina bifida is a static neurologic lesion; over time, children with the condition are liable to develop progressive joint limitation and contractures below the level of their lesion. Such contractures can limit their mobility, make it difficult for those who are wheelchair bound to maintain a comfortable sitting position, and, due to osteopenia and osteoporosis (discussed later in the chapter), cause them to be more prone to developing long bone fractures. It is essential that these children continue to receive physical therapy to maintain range of motion of all joints in the lower extremities throughout childhood and adolescence and into adulthood. It is the role of the physiatrist to assess these needs and write appropriate prescriptions.

In recent years, a growing problem of osteopenia and osteoporosis has become appreciated in adolescents and young adults. This is especially important in individuals who are paraplegic and who, due to lack of strength, are not able to bear weight on their legs. In this nonambulatory population, fractures can occur while the patient is transferring to and from a wheelchair and while toileting. In many cases, due to a lack of pain sensation, fractures may go undiagnosed until severe swelling is seen. For these reasons, it is important for the adolescent care provider to carefully examine the lower limbs of patients with spina bifida, searching for signs of recent fractures. Also, adolescents and young adults should be screened with periodic bone densitometry, and when osteoporosis is identified, appropriate treatment should be offered.

## UROLOGY

The bladder is controlled by nerves emanating from the lower sacral spine. Because approximately 90% of individuals with spina bifida have a lesion at S4 or above, most patients will have a partial or complete neurogenic bladder, a condition that will cause them to remain incontinent and prone to develop recurrent urinary tract infections. Improvement in bladder management has been the main reason for the markedly improved survival of individuals with spina bifida over the past 40 years. Prior to the 1970s, when clean intermittent bladder catheterization became the accepted form of treatment in children with neurogenic bladders, vesicoureteral reflux and recurrent urinary tract infections led to recurrent episodes of pyelonephritis that, in turn, contributed to the development of chronic renal failure. Today, through the use of bladder catheterization and scrupulous urologic management, these individuals can expect to maintain normal renal function throughout their lives.

The goals of urologic management in individuals with neurogenic bladder are twofold. The first goal is to ensure the healthy maintenance of the urinary tract, and the second is to attempt to keep patients dry and "accident free," so that they can attend school without requiring the use of diapers. To accomplish these 2 goals, it is essential that children and adolescents with a neurogenic bladder receive regular follow-up with a urologist, and routine testing to assess bladder function. Patient management should include the following:

- Yearly sonography of the kidneys and bladder, looking for changes in appearance, and searching for calculi.
- Periodic urodynamic studies to assess bladder capacity and functioning.
- Use of anticholinergic medications, such as oxybutynin, to increase bladder tone.
- Use of prophylactic antibiotics, such as sulfamethoxazole and trimethoprim, to prevent the development of urinary tract infections.
- Surgical interventions, such as bladder augmentation, which increase bladder capacity, and the Mitrofanoff procedure, which establishes a channel connecting the bladder and the abdominal wall, to facilitate an easier and less frequent need for catheterization. As discussed below, combining the Mitrofanoff procedure with one that will establish bowel continence has become an important part of the management of older children and adolescents.

Finally, the urologist plays an important role in the management of males with spina bifida, that is, in the determination of their ability to produce viable sperm. Depending on the level of the spinal lesion and because of the neurologic deficit, at least half of all males with spina bifida will not be able to either initiate or maintain an erection. In those who are able to maintain an erection, at least half will have ejaculatory difficulties, including retrograde ejaculation. Thus, between 80% and 90% of males with spina bifida will be unable to complete sexual intercourse. In such adolescents and young adults, the urologist performs tests to assess fertility and, in cases in which fertility is compromised, may perform surgery or offer other options that will enhance the chances that these men will be able to father children (fertility in females with spina bifida is normal).

## GASTROENTEROLOGY

As is the case with bladder function, the bowel depends on innervation from as far down the spinal cord as the fourth sacral spine for normal functioning. Because, as already stated, 90% of individuals with spina bifida will have a lesion at or above S4, most of these children and adolescents will also suffer from neurogenic bowel.

The consequences of a neurogenic bowel can be overwhelming for adolescents and young adults. Because they have no control over function, they are prone to having bowel movements at any time. As a result, affected individuals wear diapers; they often smell; and, as a result, are shunned by their classmates, have difficulty making friends, develop low self-esteem, and are often embarrassed about initiating sexual encounters.

Adolescents and young adults with spina bifida will go to great lengths to avoid embarrassment. For instance, at the SBC, some of our patients have told us that, in order to make sure they don't "have an accident," they will not eat for 8 hours prior to going out in public. Many of our patients use laxatives and enemas in an attempt to "clean out" their bowels or to develop more "normal" bowel function. However, in many cases, these strategies also fail, again leading to overwhelming embarrassment, worsening self-esteem and depression, and a sense of isolation.

Thus, the gastroenterologist plays a significant role in the management of these patients. Similar to that noted previously in the Urology section, the goal of gastroenterologic management is to allow the patient to go to school without needing to wear diapers. This goal can be accomplished by eliminating or significantly decreasing the chance of fecal soiling. Working with the urologist, the gastroenterologist assesses bowel function through such tests as urodynamics. Management of neurogenic bowel starts with emptying the bowel. In most cases, these children and adolescents will suffer from severe constipation, and no manipulation of the bowel will be successful until the bowel has been appropriately emptied. Thus, fecal impaction should be relieved via manual manipulation, the rigorous use of enemas and suppositories, and the use of oral laxatives.

Once fecal impaction has been resolved, children and adolescents with spina bifida should be maintained on a regular bowel protocol. This might include the administration of a colonic stimulant, such as bisacodyl; a bulking agent, such as psyllium; or a stool softener, such as docusate sodium, at night. In the morning, the patient is advised to "sit on the toilet" for a given period of time, accompanied by digital rectal stimulation, in an attempt to establish a routine. Although this plan is often successful, it is far from foolproof.

In some cases, biofeedback and behavioral training may be of benefit. Such techniques may improve sensory and motor awareness in children and adolescents who do not have complete absence of innervation, but instead have incomplete neurogenic bowel lesions.

In recent years, a new operation that combines the Mitrofanoff procedure, described previously in the Urology section, with an intervention that provides fecal continence has been developed. Called the Malone antegrade continence enema (MACE), this procedure uses the appendix as a conduit between the skin and cecum. Following establishment of this conduit, enema fluid can be introduced using a catheter, resulting in the ability to flush the retrograde bowel. Patients are instructed to perform the enema in the morning, ensuring that the bowel will remain empty throughout the school day. This procedure has met with great success; however, it is not appropriate for every patient. Because the fistulae must be carefully and scrupulously maintained, MACE should only be offered to children and adolescents who are highly motivated and of high enough intelligence to perform self-care.

## MEDICAL ISSUES

Thus far, this discussion has focused on the role that surgical subspecialists play in the treatment of individuals with spina bifida. However, the primary care provider plays a larger role than any one of these individuals. In addition to the complicated problems already described, adolescents with spina bifida also have a series of serious and sometimes life-threatening medical issues not addressed or addressable by these subspecialists. For instance, in recent years, as more children with spina bifida have survived into adolescence, the problems of latex allergy, skin breakdown, osteoporosis, chronic pain, and obesity have surfaced. In addition, there are issues of fertility in males, self-image, and psychological and emotional factors that require ongoing attention. It is the role of the primary care provider to address these issues, and they are discussed in some depth here.

In addition to managing these problems alluded to previously in this chapter, it is also the role of the primary care provider to serve as a guide and advisor to the adolescent and his or her family. In many cases, the adolescent with spina bifida will need assistance in making decisions: should he or she undergo a MACE procedure? Is scoliosis surgery really necessary, or do other options exist? Can I get by without wearing my ankle-foot orthoses, which are ugly and stigmatizing? These and many other questions may be asked. To assist the patient, it is essential that the primary care provider communicate regularly with the spina bifida team.

At the Einstein/Montefiore SBC, the medical director sends summaries of each patient's visits to the primary care provider. Although this system works well, other centers may not have developed effective systems of communications. Thus, it is essential that the primary care provider develop some relationship with the clinic's coordinator, so that a free and easy exchange of information can take place.

### Allergy

The observation that latex allergy is ubiquitous in individuals with spina bifida is recent, and its etiology remains mysterious. In 1980, allergy to latex was not considered a problem in these patients, whereas 7 years later, approximately 10% of patients attending the Einstein/Montefiore SBC reported having had some reaction, usually development of a rash, after coming into contact with latex. In 1997, a survey revealed that 70% of these patients had developed a rash or other reaction after exposure to latex, and, in that year, a 10-year-old boy died of anaphylaxis after inadvertent exposure to an oxygen mask in the recovery room following successful scoliosis surgery.

It is now believed that every child with spina bifida will, at some point during his or her life, develop an allergy to latex. As a result, the Spina Bifida Association (SBA) has made the following recommendations:

1. All individuals with spina bifida should be considered at high risk for having an allergic reaction to natural rubber (not synthetic rubber) and should avoid contact with latex products in all settings from birth. Alternative products made

of silicone, plastic, nitrile, or vinyl can usually be safely substituted.

2. Individuals who have had an allergic reaction to latex should
   - Wear a MedicAlert bracelet or necklace.
   - Carry autoinjectable epinephrine.
   - Carry sterile nonlatex gloves and other necessary nonlatex equipment for emergency use.
3. Latex allergy and latex avoidance should be discussed with all health care and community providers, including school, day care, camp, and visitors bringing gifts to the child.
4. Consultation with health care providers familiar with the latex allergy is recommended before hospitalization or surgery to prevent inadvertent exposure and to plan for latex-safe care.

Unfortunately, latex is ubiquitous, found in many products, both medically related and those that are not medically related. The SBA lists the following items that contain latex:

- **Health care items:** gloves, catheters, tourniquets, elastic bandages, ace bandages, intravenous tubing injection ports, medication vial stoppers, adhesive tape, dental dams, bandages.
- **Home/community items:** balloons, pacifiers, rubber bands, elastic in clothing, beach toys, Koosh balls, baby bottle nipples, condoms, diaphragms, diapers, art supplies.

A more complete list of latex-containing products is maintained by the SBA and can be accessed via their Web site (www.sbaa.org). It should be remembered that most condoms are made of latex. This presents a significant problem for adolescents and young adults with spina bifida because both males and females can have reactions. All adolescents with spina bifida should be instructed to avoid latex-containing condoms, using instead those made of silicone, which offer protection against both pregnancy and the spread of sexually transmitted diseases. Also, cross-reactivity exists between latex and a group of tropical fruits, including bananas and mangoes; thus, some individuals with spina bifida who are allergic to latex may also have reactions to those fruits.

It is the role of the primary care provider to educate the patient and his or her family about the danger of latex, communicate this danger to all health care providers who will come in contact with the patient, and provide the patient and his family with a list of items that should be avoided, as well as a prescription for autoinjectable epinephrine and instructions for its use. The author finds it useful to provide 3 EpiPens: 1 to be kept in a known location at home, 1 to be kept in the nurse's office at school (or in an identifiable location in the workplace), and 1 to travel with the patient. In this way, in case of emergency, a treatment option will always be accessible.

### Dermatology

Perhaps the greatest medical problem encountered by our team in the SBC in older individuals is the development of decubitus ulcers. Although less commonly a problem in younger children, stubborn and unrelenting decubiti cause distress; infection; and serious, life-threatening complications. The reasons for the increase in the number of ulcers are multiple and include the following:

1. Patients are insensate below the level of the lesion; thus, they cannot respond to pain.
2. Sitting in a wheelchair, especially if there is a disturbance in seating posture (as might occur with scoliosis or dislocation of the hip), leads to the development of "pressure points," locations on the perineum or leg that are at special risk for breaking down.
3. Because of the neurogenic bladder, the perineum is often damp with acidic urine.
4. The growing problem of obesity makes it difficult for patients to adequately clean at-risk sites.

The care provider should try at all costs to prevent decubiti from occurring. This can be accomplished through education; careful and frequent surveillance of at-risk skin locations by the patient, the family, and all care providers; and the avoidance of certain activities (eg, crawling across carpeted floors) by the patient. However, even under the best of circumstances, decubiti will occur. Medical management should be attempted first; if this is unsuccessful, surgical management via a skin flap may be necessary.

After a decubitus ulcer has appeared, it must be carefully examined and assessed. How large is the lesion? How deep is it? Are there any signs of infection? If possible, it should be photographed, so that comparisons can be made to assess whether the lesion is improving or worsening over time. Initial and subsequent management of the lesion will depend on answers to these questions.

Decubiti should be classified into 1 of 4 stages, using a classification system developed by Barczak et al[2]:

- Stage 1—The skin is intact but reddened for longer than 1 hour after relief of pressure
- Stage 2—Blister or other break in dermis with or without infection

- Stage 3—Subcutaneous destruction into muscle with or without infection
- Stage 4—Involvement of bone or joint with or without infection

In adolescents with spina bifida, most decubiti will initially be in 1 of the first 3 stages. In these cases, medical management, including local wound care using antimicrobial creams such as silver sulfadiazine, debridement of necrotic tissue, release of pressure by keeping the patient off the pressure point as much as possible, and cleanliness, should be attempted first. If available, hydrotherapy may also be a useful adjunct. The wound should be frequently re-evaluated to make sure it is improving.

Infection of the decubitus should be treated with both topical and, if necessary, oral antibiotics. The most common organisms found in pressure sores include *Staphylococcus aureus, Proteus mirabilis,* and *Streptococcus* species.

If the decubitus is stage 3 or 4, surgical intervention may be necessary. A plastic surgeon should be involved, and a flap reconstruction performed. Prior to surgery, it is essential that any infection be cleared. Sometimes, especially in individuals who are nutritionally compromised, the placement of soft tissue expanders prior to the flap surgery may be necessary.

### Bone Density

As mentioned previously, an emerging problem in adolescents and young adults with spina bifida is osteoporosis. Although decreased bone density is a known problem in older individuals who are wheelchair bound, the problem in the spina bifida population involves both those who are ambulatory and those who are more sedentary.

In 2006, Valtonen et al[3] reported that of 21 adult subjects (mean age 30 years) with spina bifida who had undergone densitometry studies, 7 (33%) had osteoporosis in at least 1 of the measured sites, and an additional 3 had osteopenia. Among the 15 subjects whose bone mineral density (BMD) of the hip region could be reliably measured, 7 (47%) had osteoporosis in the femoral neck or trochanteric region of the hip. The experience of our center is similar to that of the Valtonen group, suggesting that this is a widespread problem in affected adolescents and adults. Due to the risk of fracture in patients with spina bifida who are wheelchair bound and suffer from osteoporosis, especially those who self-transfer and self-toilet, this is a major concern, one that the primary care provider must evaluate and, when appropriate, treat.

Our policy is that all patients with spina bifida should undergo a densitometry study during early adolescence. Those who have normal BMD should be re-evaluated every 2 years, whereas those with values that place them in the osteopenic group should begin taking calcium supplementation with vitamin D and receive yearly follow-up. Those who are osteoporotic should also be given calcium with vitamin D, but treatment with a bisphosphonate should also be considered. Follow-up densitometry in this latter group should be performed 6 months after the start of therapy to assess the efficacy of the treatment, and therapy should be adjusted based on the results of that follow-up study.

### Obesity

According to the SBA, obesity, which has reached epidemic proportions in the United States, is an even greater health problem for people with spina bifida. By the age of 6 years, approximately 50% of children with MMC will be greater than 95th percentile for weight. Because it limits mobility, obesity in affected individuals causes a cyclical gain of weight, which further limits mobility. As already noted, obesity increases the problem of skin breakdown and, in individuals with osteoporosis, increases the likelihood of fracture. In addition, obesity further damages self-image, contributing to depression and the further eating of unhealthy food. For these reasons, it is essential for the health and well-being of adolescents and young adults that primary care providers assist them in managing their weight.

For adolescents and young adults with spina bifida, the prevention of obesity must begin early in life and remain a lifelong task. The regimen must focus on education, an attempt to teach the individual about "good foods" and "bad foods," on cutting calories in the diet, and on identifying ways of increasing physical activities so that more calories are burned. It is important to include consultation and periodic follow-up with a nutritionist in this plan.

The SBA Web site (www.sbaa.org) provides important advice on how to increase physical activity. The SBA notes that it is important to help children who have spina bifida enjoy exercise because physical activity has 2 benefits: it burns more calories, and it decreases hunger. Most physical activities can be adapted for children who have mobility impairments, and wheelchair sports such as basketball and track are lifelong activities that families can enjoy together.

### Development

Through the years, it has become appreciated that most children, adolescents, and young adults with spina bifida have learning disabilities and that developmental disabilities, including mental retardation, occur in approximately 25%. Because they tend to have strengths in the area of personal social functioning, causing them to appear to have higher cognitive skills, the diagnosis of a developmental disability can be more challenging; thus, it is essential that formal developmental testing be carried out in all children and adolescents with spina bifida.

In discussions in the literature of cognitive functioning in children and adolescents with spina bifida, a distinction has been made between those who have hydrocephalus (representing between 70% and 90% of the population) and those who do not. Our own experience and that of many published studies have confirmed that the following observations about the majority of individuals with spina bifida with hydrocephalus are true:

- Most of these children have average IQs, often with significantly higher verbal than nonverbal scores, a phenomenon that results in their having greater reading skills and poorer math skills.
- Most have diminished perceptual-motor abilities, a phenomenon that causes poor hand-eye coordination, leading to problems with penmanship and other fine motor activities.
- There is a direct relationship between the number of shunt malfunctions that have occurred and the severity of the neurocognitive impairment (the more shunt malfunctions, the worse the prognosis).
- Children with seizures have a worse prognosis that those who do not.
- There is a correlation between the level of the spinal lesion and the severity of the neurocognitive disability: those with higher lesions are more severely affected than those with lower lesions.
- Most individuals with spina bifida and hydrocephalus often have problems with higher executive functioning, including memory, comprehension, and attention. This must be taken into account when assigning a school placement.

Attention-deficit/hyperactivity disorder (ADHD) occurs in a majority of adolescents with spina bifida. Because of its frequency in this population, it is essential for the primary care provider to assess the patient for this problem and, when found, offer treatment. There is no contraindication to the use of stimulants or other medications commonly used to treat ADHD.

### Behavioral

In early childhood, individuals with spina bifida exhibit a characteristic personality. As noted in the following anecdote, they tend to be outgoing and friendly, as well as loquacious and happy, and to smile in the face of terrible adversity.

At age 15, Cecil suffered a VP shunt malfunction that led to increased intracranial pressure and chronic papilledema. Unfortunately, before the problem was identified, the latter had caused permanent loss of vision due to irreversible damage to the optic nerves. When told that his vision loss was permanent, Cecil responded cheerfully, "Oh, don't worry about me, Dr Marion. I've been through a lot of bad stuff in my life and I've done okay. Besides, seeing is overrated!"

The characteristic personality is similar to that seen in children with Williams syndrome, who are described as having a "cocktail party" personality because of their happy chatter.

Much of this behavior changes, however, in later adolescence and early adulthood. As they reach the end of high school, these children become isolated. They have no place to go in the morning, and due to ambulatory limitations and the lack of transportation available to them, they often become shut-ins, cut off from friends and contemporaries. Their lack of mobility, coupled with their developmental issues and their lack of work skills, all conspire to make it difficult for them to obtain employment. Their dependence on parents and other family members for basic care, including the need for assistance with toileting and bladder catheterization and with transferring to and from a wheelchair, cause them to never be able to leave home alone, a problem that is worsened by the fact that few residences are available to wheelchair-bound individuals who require assistance with bladder catheterization. As a consequence, once they finish high school, many individuals with spina bifida become depressed and isolated; develop anxiety; and lose the joyful, outgoing personality that was a characteristic feature earlier in life.

The problem of dependence is especially troubling. Most adolescents and young adults with spina bifida yearn to be independent, live on their own, handle their own finances, and make important decisions about their future without input from their families. However, due to their constant need for assistance from their parents, who, since infancy, have bathed them, changed their diapers, helped with bladder catheterization, and made all decisions of consequence, they have become infantilized, reduced to dependent children. In inner-city areas, this problem may be magnified by financial interests: in order to survive, families come to rely on the government support checks that these individuals receive every month. In some cases, achieving independence may be nearly impossible.

As in other adolescents, the problems of depression and anxiety can be overwhelming and life altering. With accurate diagnosis, complete evaluation and appropriate treatment, these consequences may be avoidable. It is essential that the primary care provider periodically screen the adolescent with spina bifida for symptoms and signs of depression and anxiety. As in other adolescents in whom depression is being considered, the care provider should inquire about changes in appetite and sleep patterns, as well as ability to concentrate in class and function as usual. In the spina bifida clinic, however, additional information can be gleaned from inquiring about self-care skills. Depressed adolescents with spina bifida often cease catheterizing themselves, choosing instead to remain wet through most of the day, endangering their health. They may also stop changing diapers. Furthermore, it is necessary to assess whether activities that were once appealing are no longer interesting.

As in other adolescents with depression, symptoms to look for include weight loss or gain, insomnia and daytime somnolence, agitation, hand wringing, restlessness, or oppositional behavior. Changes in speech pattern, such as slowed speech, should also be assessed.

In dealing with the depressed or anxious adolescent with spina bifida, in addition to providing routine medical care, the physician needs to serve as a friend (a "shoulder to cry on") and an advocate for the patient. Discussions about the problem alone are often helpful; in an attempt to get the parents and siblings to understand the issues facing the patient, the care provider can serve as an intermediary between the patient and his or her family. As they transition from high school, referral to vocational training or college programs and assistance with housing can go a long way toward improving patients' states of mind. When depression and anxiety persist, referral for ongoing psychological and psychiatric services is essential.

It should be noted that the role of exercise in alleviating depression and anxiety in individuals with spina bifida is well known. Providing improved body image and the ability to increase social contacts can have profound effects on depression.

In adolescents with spina bifida and intractable depression, medications and counseling may be crucial, especially if the patients have low self-esteem. A short course of selective serotonin reuptake inhibitors (SSRIs) may be effective in improving symptoms and signs of depression, but medication alone should not be the answer. Rather, use of medication should be coupled with counseling and advocacy, while attempts to improve the living conditions of the patient are continued.

## PREVENTING SPINA BIFIDA: WHAT THE ADOLESCENT PRIMARY CARE PROVIDER SHOULD KNOW

Although the focus of this chapter has been on the role the primary care provider plays in the medical management of the adolescent with spina bifida, care providers also need to know about the prevention of NTDs in their female patients who are either contemplating a pregnancy or who are pregnant. In this section, information about the prevention, both primary and secondary, of spina bifida is presented.

### PRIMARY PREVENTION OF SPINA BIFIDA: PERICONCEPTUAL FOLIC ACID SUPPLEMENTATION

As alluded to in the previous section on etiology, in the past 20 years, a significant change in the epidemiology of NTDs has occurred. Spina bifida, a condition that was found in 1 in 1,000 liveborn children in the United States in 1987,[1] now occurs in 1 in 4,000. This change, seen in all ethnic and racial groups and in all parts of the country, is reflected in our experience at the Einstein/Montefiore SBC: prior to 1998, an average of 9.3 infants with spina bifida entered our clinic each year; since 1998, that number has shrunk to 2.5, a decrease of nearly 75%. This marked reduction in cases, seen in a poor, underserved, inner-city population, is the result of the introduction of folic acid fortification of the food supply.

The story of how folic acid came to be found as an agent that prevented spina bifida goes back to detective work that was begun in the 1930s. As noted previously, NTDs are multifactorially inherited conditions, caused by the interplay between genetic and environmental factors. Although their identities were unknown, evidence of the environmental influences that played a role in the etiology of NTDs were obvious: children with spina bifida were more likely to be born in the late fall and early winter in places such as the British Isles. Because neural tube closure is completed during the first month after conception, in babies born in the late fall or early winter, this event occurs in the early spring. As a result, investigations focused on factors known to be present during this time of the year, including infectious agents and maternal dietary deficiencies.

Between 1930 and the 1950s, multiple studies in animals showed that maternal vitamin deficiencies could result in congenital malformations in offspring. In 1980, Elwood and Elwood[4] speculated that the naturally occurring decrease in the prevalence of NTDs that had occurred in the 40 years since 1940 was the result of improved maternal nutrition.

The earliest studies focused on the recurrence risk of NTDs in offspring of women who had previously given birth to infants affected with these disorders, a risk that, as noted previously, was predicted to be between 2% and 4%. In 1980, Smithells et al[5] reported a 70% reduction in that rate in children born to women who had taken multivitamin supplementation beginning at least 2 months prior to conception. A year later, Laurence et al[6] demonstrated that folic acid was the important agent in those multivitamins: they noted that periconceptual folic acid supplementation alone decreased the recurrence risk of NTDs by this amount. In the years following this seminal article, multiple international studies confirmed the findings of Laurence et al. Simply providing folic acid to women who had previously borne a child with an NTD 3 months prior to the time of conception decreased the risk of recurrence of an NTD[6] in that next child by up to 70%.

But what of women who had not previously borne an affected child? In 1992, studying a Hungarian population, Czeizel and Dudás[7] demonstrated that periconceptual folic acid supplementation also decreased first time occurrence of NTDs by approximately 70%. It was the results of this study that led the US Public Health Service to issue a recommendation that "all women of childbearing age in the United States who are capable of becoming pregnant should consume 0.4 mg of folic acid a day." In women who had had a previous child with an NTD, the recommended dose was 4 mg per day.

Although these recommendations were somewhat effective, it was not until January 1, 1998, that the major public health initiative that forever altered the epidemiology of NTDs occurred. On that day, fortification of the food supply in the United States with folic acid was begun. Because of fortification of bread, cereal, orange juice, and other dietary staples, an individual who consumes a regular diet would obtain a dose of folic acid that may have been enough to reduce the risk of NTDs. Although some controversy still exists about whether the amount of folic acid is enough, the fact is that, following the start of this new program, the prevalence of NTDs throughout the United States dropped dramatically.

Today, these recommendations remain in place. Because the supplementation must begin at least 2 months prior to conception, all adolescent women capable of becoming pregnant should receive 0.4 mg of folic acid per day. In women who are not eating a regular diet, supplementation with folic acid should be encouraged. For women who have spina bifida or who are the first-degree relative of an individual with an NTD (ie, a previous child, a parent, or a sibling), the dose should be raised to 4 mg per day.

This higher dose should also be offered to women who are taking medications, such as valproic acid and tegretol, with known teratogenic potential whose consequences include development of NTDs in the fetus (of course, as noted in Chapter 148, Genetic Disorders, if possible, efforts should be made prior to conception to change these women to medications with lower or, preferentially, no teratogenic potential). All women in this higher-risk group should also be offered referral for prenatal diagnosis (described in more detail later in the chapter).

## SECONDARY PREVENTION OF SPINA BIFIDA: PRENATAL DIAGNOSIS AND COUNSELING

A detailed review of prenatal diagnosis of genetic disorders is presented in Chapter 148, Genetic Disorders. In this section, we review only the information pertinent to the prenatal diagnosis of NTDs.

As noted in Chapter 149, Genetic Predisposition to Common Disorders, it is important that those providing care for pregnant adolescent women, as well as partners of adolescent men who have genetic disorders, have an understanding of prenatal diagnostic techniques so that appropriate referrals can be made in a timely fashion. As described previously, women with spina bifida and those who are taking drugs, such as valproic acid and tegretol, known to have teratogenic potential, are at increased risk for having a child with an NTD. Such women should be offered the opportunity to have their pregnancy monitored for these anomalies; all deserve sensitive, accurate risk counseling, performed either by their primary care provider or by a genetic counselor.

There are currently 3 main modalities that are helpful in the prenatal diagnosis of NTDs: maternal serum biochemical screening, sonography, and amniocentesis.

### Maternal Serum Biochemical Screening

As noted in Chapter 148, Genetic Disorders, alpha-fetoprotein (AFP), a normal component of fetal serum, "leaks" in low concentration into the amniotic fluid and subsequently into the maternal blood. When defects exist in the fetal skin, such as occurs in NTDs, excess leakage of AFP into the maternal serum occurs. Alpha-fetoprotein screening is thus useful as an indicator of fetal NTDs. In the 1970s, screening maternal serum for levels of AFP became a routine part of prenatal care in the United States. Although screening for other biochemical markers such as unconjugated estriols, human chorionic gonadotropin, and inhibin A has been added to the AFP testing due to their relevance as a screening tool in the prenatal diagnosis of fetal chromosomal abnormalities, maternal serum AFP (MSAFP) is still the gold standard screening test for NTDs.

Ideally, MSAFP testing is performed between 15 and 18 weeks' gestation, but may be performed as early as 14 weeks or as late as 22 weeks. Because it is used only as a screening test, an abnormal MSAFP screen must be followed up with further testing (amniocentesis and ultrasonography). Prior to testing, it is important to point out to patients that in most cases, abnormal levels of AFP are not associated with any fetal abnormality; similarly, a normal result does not completely rule out the possibility that a defect will be found in the newborn. However, because of both the low risk and the low cost of testing, maternal serum biochemical screening is a valuable initial step in the evaluation of women at risk for having a child with an NTD.

### Sonography

At present, most women receiving prenatal care in the United States have at least one ultrasonographic examination during pregnancy. The examination is relatively inexpensive and can be performed at any time; however, for the detection of NTDs, it is best done after 16 weeks' gestation. When an abnormal MSAFP screen is found, a first step should be a sonogram to "date" the pregnancy; because acceptable AFP levels change throughout the first 2 trimesters of pregnancy, if the dates are incorrect and the fetus is either "older" or "younger" than suspected, an apparently abnormal MSAFP may actually be normal.

If the initial sonogram reveals that the dates are accurate and that, in fact, the MSAFP is truly elevated, a careful, targeted sonogram should be performed in an attempt to detect NTDs and other fetal anomalies. Numerous studies have shown that success in identifying abnormalities is dependent on the experience of the sonographer; as such, a more experienced radiologist should be called on to perform this anatomy scan.

Often, sonography alone may be sufficient to identify the presence of an NTD in a fetus. However, in more subtle cases, amniocentesis may be used as an adjunct to these other modalities.

### Amniocentesis

As with maternal biochemical serum screening and sonography, amniocentesis is discussed in more detail in Chapter 148, Genetic Disorders. For purposes of this discussion, this procedure is performed after the finding of an elevated MSAFP in order to confirm the presence of an NTD in the fetus.

The test is done for 3 reasons: (1) to determine the level of AFP in the amniotic fluid (AFAFP); (2) to check for the presence of acetylcholinesterase, a specific marker for NTDs; and (3) to determine the fetal karyotype (although usually an isolated defect, an NTD may be part of a more serious genetic or chromosomal abnormality, such as trisomy 18 or trisomy 13; thus, before counseling the client, it is important to know "the whole story").

Although the risk incurred from amniocentesis has traditionally been cited as approximately 1 in 300, which is believed to be the frequency with which fetal loss, either through introduction of infection or from other complications, is actually caused by the procedure, more recent evidence suggests that the risk is much lower than this, in the range of 1 in 1,000 or less. The reliability of information obtained through amniocentesis is extremely high, and incorrect information, caused by sampling and growing maternal cells rather than those from the fetus, failure of cells to grown in culture, or laboratory error, occurs much less than 1% of the time.

After detection of an NTD, 2 options are available. The pregnant woman may choose to continue the pregnancy, knowing that her baby will be affected with a specific disorder, or she can choose to terminate it. The role of the primary care provider and the genetic counselor is to provide the client and her partner with enough information to make an appropriate decision, and then, after a decision has been made, to support the couple through the rest of the pregnancy.

### Chorionic Villus Sampling

Although in many cases chorionic villus sampling (CVS) offers some real advantages over amniocentesis, it is unfortunately not a useful technique in evaluating pregnancies for NTDs. As such, CVS has no role in the evaluation of individuals at risk for these malformations.

## REFERENCES

1. Bartoshesky L. Myelomeningocele. In: Buyse ML, ed. *The Birth Defects Encyclopedia.* Boston: Blackwell Sciences;1990

2. Barczak CA, Barnett RI, Childs EJ, Bosley LM. Fourth National Pressure Ulcer Prevalence Survey. *Adv Wound Care.* 1997;10(4):18-26

3. Valtonen KM, Goksor LA, Jonsson O, et al.Osteoporosis in adults with meningomyelocele: an unrecognized problem at rehabilitation clinics. *Arch Phys Med Rehabil.* 2006,87(3): 376-382

4. Elwood JM, Elwood JH. *Epidemiology of Anencephalus and Spina Bifida.* New York: Oxford University Press; 1980:85-119

5. Smithells RW, Shephard S, Schorah CH, et al. Possible prevention of neural-tube defects by periconceptional vitamin supplementation. *Lancet.* 1980;1(8164):339-340

6. Laurence KM, James N, Miller M, et al. Double-blind randomized controlled trial of folate treatment before conception to prevent recurrence of neural-tube defects. *Br Med J* 1981;282:1509-1511

7. Czeizel AE, Dudás I. Prevention of the first occurrence of neural-tube defects by periconceptional vitamin supplementation. *N Engl J Med.* 1992;327(26):1832-1835

# CHAPTER 134

# Altered States of Consciousness

EDWARD E. CONWAY, JR, MD, MS

Adolescent patients may present with alterations in behavior or an impaired level of consciousness. Consciousness and coma appear to be the extremes of mental alertness; however, there is a spectrum of impaired mental states that may include lethargy, confusion, delirium, obtundation, stupor, and coma. *Lethargy* is a state in which one is easily distracted and misjudges sensory perceptions but retains the ability to communicate. *Confusion* is the loss of clear thinking. *Delirium* is characterized by disorientation, fear, irritability, and visual hallucinations. *Obtundation* is a state of mental blunting with a decreased interest in the environment. *Stupor* is a state of deep sleep from which the patient can be aroused for short periods only by vigorous and repeated stimuli. There is much confusion and disagreement about which terms should be used to describe these clinical states because there is a lack of uniformity in the literature as to how these states are defined. There is, however, a consensus definition on *coma*. It is manifested with absence of awareness of one's self and one's environment. It is a state of unarousable unresponsiveness in which the patient lies without spontaneous movement with his or her eyes closed.[1]

These states of impaired consciousness represent a severe derangement in cerebral function that may be structural or nonstructural in origin. Most patients who present with either coma or a depressed level of consciousness have an underlying metabolic or systemic disease rather than a structural lesion. Such patients present the clinician with a simultaneous diagnostic and management challenge requiring a rapid, organized evaluation and management plan. It is important to remember that although the underlying pathophysiologic processes may be life threatening, they are also potentially reversible. A change in the level of consciousness may be caused either by a diffuse toxic/metabolic/infectious state (approximately 80% of coma cases in adolescent and adult patients) or by structural damage (ie, trauma, hemorrhage, tumor) to the central nervous system (CNS). Alterations in consciousness may be transient (concussion, seizure, or syncope) or may be longer in duration, such as those following severe intracranial catastrophies (ie, head trauma, hemorrhage, drowning, hypoxic-ischemic insult following cardiac arrest).

## PATHOPHYSIOLOGY

Consciousness may be seen as the product of 2 closely related cerebral functions: wakefulness (ie, arousal, vigilance, alertness) and awareness of the self or the environment (content of consciousness).[2] The content of consciousness encompasses several other brain functions including attention, sensation and perception, explicit memory, executive function, and motivation.[2] Wakefulness is linked to the ascending reticular activating system (ARAS), a network of neurons originating in the tegmentum of the pons and midbrain and projecting to diencephalic and cortical structures.[3] Consciousness is maintained by the interaction of *both* cerebral cortices and the ARAS located within the brainstem (Figure 134-1). This interaction relates wakefulness (arousal, alertness, and awareness of one's environment) with consciousness. To affect consciousness, lesions of

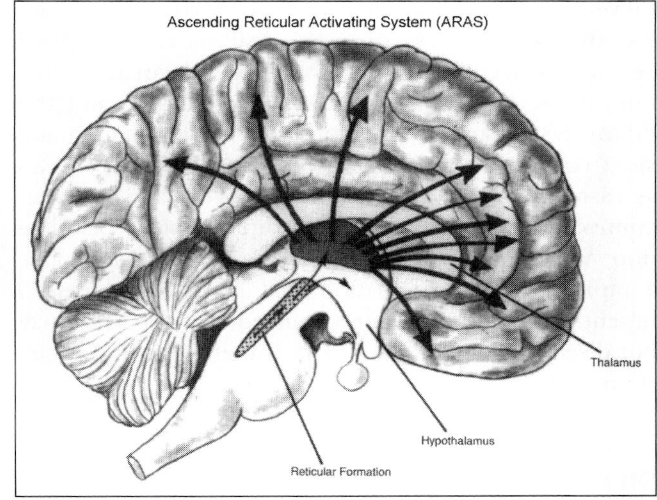


**FIGURE 134-1** The ARAS shown as a network beginning in the rostral brainstem and projecting to the thalamus and then to the cerebral cortex. (Reprinted with permission from Young GB. Consciousness. In: Young GB, Ropper AH, Bolton CF, eds. *Coma and Impaired Consciousness: A Clinical Perspective.* New York, NY: McGraw-Hill; 1998:7.)

the cerebral cortex must involve both hemispheres or must be unilateral lesions large enough to cause displacement or shift of midline structures.[4] Brainstem and diencephalic lesions resulting in coma may be comparatively small; however, they must also involve bilateral structures. A compartmental shift of sufficient magnitude will disrupt the ARAS and its projections resulting also in coma. Normal consciousness requires the interaction of neurons at the cellular level with specific CNS structures at the gross anatomic level.[1] CNS function may be disrupted at the cellular level secondary to a disruption in delivery of substrate (hypoglycemia, hypoxia, electrolyte abnormalities), alterations in neuronal excitability and signaling (seizures, acidosis, drug toxicity), or changes in brain volume (hypernatremia, hyponatremia, diabetic ketoacidosis [DKA]). The degree of neurologic impairment is related to the time course of the underlying cerebral pathology. An adolescent with a massive interhemispheric bleed following the rupture of an arteriovenous malformation with mass effect may have depressed consciousness whereas a patient with a slow growing tumor in the same anatomic region may be asymptomatic.

Coma is best assessed and described using the Glasgow Coma Scale (GCS)[5] (Table 134-1). The GCS rates the patient's performance in 3 major areas: (1) eye opening, which relates to arousal and alertness; (2) verbal ability, which relates to content and mentation; and (3) motor ability, which reflects mentation as well as the functional integrity of the major CNS pathways. A fully alert patient is given a score of 15, whereas a score less than 8 indicates coma. The scale is easily applied and reproduced. The ability to speak is a cortical function, eyelid opening is a brainstem function, and the motor responses require both the cortical and brainstem pathways to be intact. The GCS therefore allows assessment of the integrity of the cortex and its interconnections on the basis of a simple clinical examination. A decrease of more than 2 in the GCS indicates a rapidly changing situation that must be addressed urgently. It must also be recognized that the GCS may not discern subtle alterations in wakefulness and brainstem findings.

**Table 134-1**

**Glasgow Coma Scale**

| *Test* | *Finding* | *Score* |
|---|---|---|
| Eye opening | Spontaneously | 4 |
| | Response to voice | 3 |
| | Response to pain | 2 |
| | No response | 1 |
| Verbal response | Oriented and appropriate | 5 |
| | Disoriented conversation | 4 |
| | Inappropriate words | 3 |
| | Incomprehensible sounds | 2 |
| | No response | 1 |
| Motor response | Obeys commands | 6 |
| | Localizes pain | 5 |
| | Flexion withdrawal | 4 |
| | Decorticate posturing | 3 |
| | Decerebrate posturing | 2 |
| | No response | 1 |
| Maximal total score | | 15 |

## DIFFERENTIAL DIAGNOSIS

The differential diagnosis of coma is extensive. The mnemonic AEIOU THIPS can help classify the causes of coma (Box 134-1). A major consideration is whether the coma is the result of a correctable toxic/metabolic etiology (ie, ingestion or electrolyte abnormality) or of a structural lesion (ie, CNS hemorrhage, trauma, or tumor).

**Box 134-1**

***Etiologies of Coma***

- A Alcohol/abuse/anoxia
- E Encephalopathy/endocrinopathy/electrolytes/epilepsy
- I Ingestions/insulin
- O Opiates/overdose
- U Uremia
- T Trauma
- H Hypo/hypertension/hyper/hypothermia/hypoglycemia
- I Infection
- P Psychogenic
- S Structural lesions/seizures/syncope

**INFECTION**

Most infections of the CNS are life threatening, and there must be a high index of suspicion. Fever, photophobia, headache, vomiting, and a change in mental status suggest CNS infection. Kernig and Brudzinski signs may be absent in patients in deep coma. Cerebrospinal fluid (CSF) studies should be performed in all patients with symptoms suggesting CNS infection; however, in patients with papilledema or focal neurologic findings a head computed tomography (CT) scan should be performed to rule out a mass lesion. An opening pressure should be determined and CSF obtained for cell counts, chemistries (glucose and protein), and bacterial and viral cultures. Cryptococcal antigen determination should be performed in all immunocompromised patients.

If there is a strong consideration that a CNS infection is present, antibiotics should be started empirically, with the major bacterial organisms to consider in adolescent meningitis being *Streptococcus pneumoniae* and *Neisseria meningitidis.* Complications associated with meningitis that may lead to coma include seizures, subdural effusions, subdural empyema, cerebral abscess, cerebral venous infarcts, the syndrome of inappropriate antidiuretic hormone (SIADH), hyponatremia and both communicating and obstructive hydrocephalus.[6,7]

**ENCEPHALITIS**

Encephalitis is an unusual complication of common viral infections. These usually involve the meninges, as in aseptic meningitis, or cause a mild clinical syndrome of meningoencephalitis.[8,9] They present with the acute onset of fever; headache; altered mental status; disorientation; behavioral and speech disturbances; and neurologic signs, sometimes focal, but generally diffuse, such as hemiparesis or seizures. There is no evidence of bacteria, fungi, spirochetes, or parasites in the CSF, but there is usually a mild elevation in the cell count, usually lymphocytes, with normal chemistries. The differential diagnosis includes parameningeal infections and carcinomatous meningitis.

The most common viral cause of sporadic acute focal encephalitis is herpes simplex. In the absence of therapy, mortality exceeds 70%, and only about 2.5% of persons affected regain normal function. There is an associated classic electroencephalographic picture called PLEDs (periodic lateralized epileptiform discharges) that shows periodic focal spikes from the temporal area where the virus localizes. Treatment should be instituted with acyclovir as soon as a herpes infection is suspected.

Lastly, patients with AIDS may present with chronic encephalitis. The virus itself may cause damage to deep cortical structures, and these patients may have unusual opportunistic infections of the CNS. Unusual primary and secondary malignancies have also been noted.[10]

**INGESTIONS/ALCOHOL/OPIATES/ABUSE**

Drugs that are commonly ingested and lead to changes in mental status and coma include barbiturates, opiates, psychedelics, amphetamines, cocaine, ethanol, atropine, tricyclic antidepressants, phenothiazines, methaqualone, benzodiazepines, anticonvulsants, and antihistamines. Some agents have a direct effect on the CNS (barbiturates, opiates, ethanol, and benzodiazepines). Others induce seizures or other physiologic changes that produce a coma (hyper/hypotension, hyperthermia). Drug withdrawal (opioids and benzodiazepines) produces neurologic findings including confusion, hallucinations, myoclonus, seizures, hyperthermia, and pupillary constriction. Many of the above cited ingestions may be suggested by a toxidrome, which is a group of clinical signs and symptoms associated with a particular group of pharmacologic agents summarized in Table 134-2. Section 2 Substance Abuse, discusses common ingestions and their management.

Ethanol appears to be 1 of the more frequently cited drugs that may alter the level of consciousness. Ethanol is a weak sedative in that much greater doses of ethanol are required than benzodiazepines or barbiturates to obtain the same depressant effect. It appears that ethanol causes gamma-aminobutyric acid-like effects (GABA, which is an inhibitory neurotransmitter) on neurons in a similar manner to benzodiazepines via a chloride channel leading to hyperpolarization (inability to fire) of the cell. Ethanol has also been shown to decrease the activity of excitatory neurotransmitters such as N-methyl-D-aspartate (NMDA) in certain areas of the brain. Receptors are located in large concentrations in the hippocampus, and thus a proposed mechanism for the cognitive and blackout effects of ethanol may be explained by NMDA receptor blockade.

**METABOLIC/ELECTROLYTE/ENDOCRINE ABNORMALITIES**

Metabolic etiologies of coma commonly include hypoglycemia and hypoxia. Both globally disrupt neuronal function at the cellular level and produce a change in consciousness. Hypoglycemia is defined as a blood concentration less than 40 mg/dL (2.5 mmol/L) in an adult patient; a glucose determination should be one of the first investigations in a comatose patient. If it is not possible to obtain an immediate serum glucose level, 50 ml of D50 W should be administered intravenously.

Hypoglycemia has 3 important effects on the CNS: (1) it invokes a stress response, (2) it causes cerebral bloodflow disturbances, and (3) it alters cerebral metabolism, ultimately leading to permanent neurologic damage.[11] Common causes include fasting, liver

**Table 134-2**

**Toxidromes**

| Toxidrome | Mental Status | Pupils | Vital Signs | Other Manifestations | Examples of Toxic Agents |
|---|---|---|---|---|---|
| Sympathomimetic | • Hyperalert<br>• Agitation<br>• Hallucinations<br>• Paranoia | Mydriasis | • Hyperthermia<br>• Tachycardia<br>• Hypertension<br>• Widened pulse pressure<br>• Tachypnea<br>• Hyperpnea | • Diaphoresis<br>• Tremors<br>• Hyperflexia<br>• Seizures | • Cocaine<br>• Amphetamines<br>• Ephedrine<br>• Pseudoephedrine<br>• Phenylpropanolamine<br>• Theophyline<br>• Caffeine |
| Anticholinergic | • Hypervigilance<br>• Agitation<br>• Delirium with mumbling speech<br>• Coma | Mydriasis | • Hyperthermia<br>• Tachycardia<br>• Hypertension<br>• Tachycardia | • Dry, flushed skin<br>• Dry mucous membranes<br>• Decreased bowel sounds<br>• Urinary retention<br>• Myoclamus<br>• Choreoathosis<br>• Picking behavior<br>• Seizures (rare) | • Antihistamines<br>• Tricyclic antidepressants<br>• Cyclobenzaprine<br>• Orphenadrine agents<br>• Antispasmodics<br>• Phenothiazines<br>• Atropine<br>• Scopolamine<br>• Belladonna alkaloids (eg, Jimson weed) |
| Hallucinogenic | • Hallucinations<br>• Perceptual distortions<br>• Depersonalization<br>• Agitation | Mydriasis (usually) | • Hyperthermia<br>• Tachycardia<br>• Hypertension<br>• Tachypnea | • Nystagmus | • Phencyclidine<br>• LSD<br>• Mescaline<br>• Psilocybin<br>• Designer amphetamines (eg, MCMA, MDEA) |
| Opioid | • CNS depression<br>• Coma | Miosis | • Hypothermia<br>• Bradycardia<br>• Hypotension<br>• Hypopnea<br>• Bradypnea | • Hyporeflexia<br>• Pulmonary edema<br>• Needle marks | • Opiates (eg, heroin, morphine, methadone, oxycodone, hydromorphone)<br>• Diphenoxylate |
| Sedative-hypnotic | • CNS depression<br>• Confusion<br>• Stupor<br>• Coma | Miosis | • Hypothermia<br>• Bradycardia<br>• Hypotension<br>• Hypopnea<br>• Bradypnea | • Hyporeflexia | • Benzodiazepines<br>• Barbiturates<br>• Carisoprodol<br>• Meprocarnate<br>• Glutethimide<br>• Alcohols<br>• Zolpidem |

*(Continued)*

**Table 134-2 (Continued)**

| *Toxidrome* | *Mental Status* | *Pupils* | *Vital Signs* | *Other Manifestations* | *Examples of Toxic Agents* |
|---|---|---|---|---|---|
| Cholinergic | • Confusion<br>• Coma | Miosis | • Bradycardia<br>• Hypertension<br>• Hypotension<br>• Tachypnea or bradypnea | • Salivation<br>• Urinary and fecal incontinence<br>• Diarrhea<br>• Emesis<br>• Diaphoresis<br>• Lacrimation<br>• GI cramps<br>• Bronchoconstriction<br>• Muscle fasciculation and weakness<br>• Seizures | • Organophosphate and carbamate insecticides<br>• Nerve agents<br>• Nicotine<br>• Pilocarpine<br>• Physostigmine<br>• Edrophonium<br>• Bethanechol<br>• Urecholine |
| Serotonin syndrome | • Confusion<br>• Agitation<br>• Coma | Mydriasis | • Hyperthermia<br>• Tachycardia<br>• Hypertension<br>• Tachypnea | • Tremor<br>• Myoclonus<br>• Hyperreflexia<br>• Clonus<br>• Diaphoresis<br>• Flushing<br>• Trismus<br>• Rigidity<br>• Diarrhea | • MAOIs alone or with SSRIs, meperidine, dextromethorphan, TCAs, or L-tryptophan |
| Tricyclic antidepressant | • Confusion<br>• Agitation<br>• Coma | Mydriasis | • Hyperthermia<br>• Tachycardia<br>• Hypertension then hypotension<br>• Hypopnea | • Seizures<br>• Myoclonus<br>• Choreoathetosis<br>• Cardiac arrhythmias and conduction disturbances | • Amitriptyline<br>• Nortriptyline<br>• Imipramine<br>• Compromise<br>• Desipramine<br>• Doxepin |

CNS, central nervous system; GI, gastrointestinal; MAOI, monoamine oxidase inhibitor; SSRI, selective serotonin reuptake inhibitor; TCA, tricyclic antidepressant

and renal disease, excess insulin, glucocorticoid deficiency, sepsis, malnutrition, heart failure, and drugs (oral hypoglycemics, ethanol, salicylates, propranolol).

The effects of hypoxia are different for different cell types, but brain cells can be permanently damaged after only 4 to 6 minutes of hypoxia.[12] Neuronal dysfunction is caused by the development of cellular acidosis, generation of free radicals, an increase in the concentration of metabolic products, and degradation of membrane phospholipids. Central nervous system anoxia is most commonly seen after cardiopulmonary arrest. In the United States, there are more than 1,000 cardiac arrests daily; 80% of persons successfully resuscitated are unconscious at 1 hour, and 39% of victims never regain consciousness.[13]

Extremes of temperature may cause neuronal dysfunction. Hyperthermia is directly toxic to neurons and it produces renal and hepatic failure that contribute to neuronal dysfunction. Electrolyte abnormalities that cause a change in consciousness include hyponatremia, hypercalcemia, hypermagnesemia, and hypernatremia. Extreme changes in serum osmolarity (seen in DKA, diabetes insipidus, and SIADH) also contribute to cellular dysfunction. Toxic metabolites may accumulate in patients with renal and hepatic failure and cause neuronal depression. Endocrinopathies that produce a change in mental status include DKA, hypo- or hyperthyroidism, and adrenal disease. Extremes of acid-base disturbance produce cellular neuronal dysfunction.

**STRUCTURAL PROCESSES**

Structural processes cause focal disruption or destruction of either the cerebral cortices or the ARAS. Central nervous system lesions may be subdivided as occurring in either the supra- or subtentorial regions. The supratentorial compartment mainly contains the cortex, thalamus, and other structures above the midbrain. Trauma resulting in an epidural, subdural, or intracerebral hematoma or diffuse cerebral swelling is the leading cause of supratentorial lesions. Cerebrovascular accidents (in sickle cell disease and systemic lupus erythematosus patients), venous thrombosis, subdural empyema, or intracerebral tumor may also produce supratentorial lesions. These lesions may produce focal destruction in one hemisphere, which in turn may cause cerebral swelling or pressure on the other hemisphere or on the brainstem and, ultimately, coma.

The subtentorial compartment is the area under the tentorium and contains most of the brainstem, the cerebellum and the cranial nerves (CN), and CSF foramina that allow the egress of CSF to bathe the spinal column. Subtentorial (posterior fossa) lesions result from tumors, trauma, and primary hemorrhage into the brainstem. These directly affect/compress the ARAS and thus depress consciousness.

Subarachnoid hemorrhage (SAH), although a focal lesion, may cause global dysfunction because the blood released is transported by way of the CSF to the entire CNS. Approximately one-third of patients with SAH present in a comatose state. The most common causes are a ruptured aneurysm or an arteriovenous malformation.

**TRAUMA**

Head injury accounts for almost 25,000 deaths per year in pediatric patients. Younger patients with severe head injury (GCS score of <8) have better outcomes than adults and approximately one-half the mortality rate. Alcohol and drugs play an increased role in head injury in adolescent patients. Also as patients enter adolescence, the etiologies of head trauma change from being predominantly falls to now include motor vehicle accidents (both as pedestrian and driver), assaults, and sports injuries. Traumatic brain injury is classified by using the GCS: 13 to 15 is considered minor, 9 to 12 moderate, and below or equal to 8 is severe. Head injuries are classified as primary (that occur at the moment of impact) and secondary, as those that occur as the result of injury or death of brain cells that initially survived the traumatic event and then succumbed to either worsening damage from the primary injury or complications of other simultaneous injuries. Primary brain injury is usually the result of an impact blow or an acceleration–deceleration force. Secondary injury results from hypoxia, hypercarbia, and hypotension (ischemia). The goal of treating any patient with head injury is to minimize or prevent secondary injury. Recovery from severe head injury depends on the severity of injury, rapid initiation of medical treatment, and rehabilitation.

Chapter 131, CNS Trauma, contains a full discussion of the evaluation and treatment of the adolescent patient with CNS trauma resulting in intracranial injury and bleeding, including epidural hematoma, subdural hematoma, and intracerebral bleeds. Another type of injury that may occur is a contusion. Contusions are a bruising or tearing of brain tissue. They result from coup-countercoup injuries and occur when the brain impacts against the bony prominences of the skull, and they may also be seen under fracture sites. The most commonly affected area of the brain are the temporal lobes and the subfrontal regions over the cortex. Symptoms may include unconsciousness, disturbance in strength, changes in visual awareness, and seizures.

The most common type of head injury seen is defined as minor; however, these can have significant long-term implications for adolescent patients. The term concussion has been used interchangeably with mild head injury (MHI) or mild traumatic brain injury (mTBI). A concussion is defined as a trauma-induced alteration in mental status that may or may not involve a loss of consciousness.[14] Immediate signs and symptoms include a change in playing ability, vacant stare, loss of consciousness, confusion, slowing, memory loss, increased emotionality, incoordination, headache, dizziness, and vomiting. Most children and teenagers recover fully from a single, uncomplicated mTBI. It is important to realize that recovery does take time and in the days, weeks, and months after injury a number of neurobehavioral problems can be seen.[15] Postconcussive symptoms have been divided into somatic (headaches, fatigue, sleep disturbance, nausea, tinnitus, dizziness, balance problems, sensitivity to light and noise), emotional (lowered frustration, irritability, depression, anxiety, clinginess, personality changes), and cognitive (slowed thinking, mental fogginess, poor concentration, distractibility, memory problems, disorganization). The World Health Organization (WHO) has published criteria for the diagnosis of postconcussive syndrome[16] (Table 134-3).

The pathophysiologic changes seen in concussion include abrupt neuronal depolarization, release of excitatory neurotransmitters, ionic shifts, altered glucose metabolism, altered cerebral blood flow, and impaired axonal function. These changes result following a rapid deceleration that causes a mild form of diffuse axonal injury. A controversial entity called "second-impact syndrome" seems to exist and results from a second

**Table 134-3**

**Guidelines for the Management of Sport-Related Concussion[a]**

| *Symptoms* | *First Concussion* | *Second Concussion* |
|---|---|---|
| Grade 1: no loss of consciousness, transient confusion, resolution of symptoms and mental abnormalities in <15 minutes[b] | Remove from play<br>Examine at 5-minute intervals<br>May return to play if symptoms disappear and results of mental-function examination return to normal within 15 minutes | Allow return to play after 1 week if there are no symptoms at rest or with exertion |
| Grade 2: as above, but with mental symptoms for >15 minutes | Remove from play and disallow play for rest of day<br>Examine for signs of intracranial lesion at sidelines and obtain further examination by a trained person on same day<br>Allow return to play after 1 week if neurologic examination is normal | Allow return to play after 2-week period of no symptoms at rest or with exertion<br>Remove from play for season if imaging shows abnormality |
| Grade 3: any loss of consciousness | Perform thorough neurologic examination in hospital and obtain imaging studies when indicated<br>Assess neurologic status daily until postconcussive symptoms resolve or stabilize<br>Remove from play for 1 week if loss of consciousness lasts seconds; for 2 weeks if it lasts minutes; must be asymptomatic at rest and with exertion to return to play | Withhold from play until symptoms have been absent for at least 1 month |

[a]These guidelines reflect consensus opinion, are not evidence-based, and are under revision. Adapted from the American Academy of Neurology guidelines.[19]

[b]Testing includes orientation, repetition of digit strings, recall of word list at 0 and 5 minutes, recall of recent game events, recall of current events, pupillary symmetry, finger-to-nose and tandem-gate tests, Romberg test, and provocative testing for symptoms with a 4-yard (3.5-meter) sprint, 5 push-ups, 5 sit-ups, and 5 knee bends.



concussion while the adolescent is still symptomatic from a prior concussion. It is thought that there is a disruption of the autoregulation of cerebral blood flow and this may lead to vascular engorgement, cerebral edema, and increased intracranial pressure (ICP) and death.[17]

As mentioned earlier, most athletes will recover within the first hours, days, or weeks after an mTBI; however, no 2 injuries are exactly alike.[15] Although there is a lack of consensus regarding the management of concussion there are several published guidelines to date that describe the grading of a concussion and a suggested clinical pathway as to when or if the athlete should be allowed to compete again[18] (Box 134-3). The most important point is not to let an athlete back to practice until he or she has become totally symptom and complaint free.[19]

## SEIZURES

A seizure is a paroxysmal disorder of the CNS (gray matter) characterized by an abnormal neuronal discharge associated with a change in function of the patient. Chapter 126 discusses seizure disorders in adolescents. Patients may present in a postictal state after a protracted seizure that may not have been witnessed. Certain factors are known to provoke seizures; these include fever, hyponatremia, hypoglycemia, hypocalcemia, hyperglycemia, meningitis, head trauma, toxin exposure, ethanol, and many clinically used medications. The mnemonic *GRANDMALS* will help the reader recall the common cause of seizures (Box 134-3). One must be vigilant in following the postictal patient because approximately 15% of patients who have their seizures pharmacologically controlled may develop nonconvulsive status epilepticus (NCSE).[20] NCSE is an entity in which patients have a persistent altered mental status after their clinical seizure appears to be controlled. This entity can present in very subtle ways (ie, a slight finger twitch), and thus if a patient is not waking up in a reasonable time period (60 minutes) following a seizure, NCSE should be considered. The diagnosis is made electrographically using an electroencephalogram (EEG).

### Box 134-2

### *International Classification of Diseases, 10th Revision, Criteria for Postconcussion Syndrome (Code 310-2)*

Interval between head trauma with loss of consciousness and development of symptoms, ≤4 weeks

Symptoms in at least 3 of the following categories:
- Headache, dizziness, fatigue, noise intolerance
- Irritability, depression, anxiety, emotional lability
- Subjective concentration, memory, or intellectual difficulties without neuropsychological evidence of marked impairment
- Insomnia
- Reduced alcohol tolerance
- Preoccupation with above symptoms and fear of brain damage, with hypochondriacal concern and adoption of sick role

### Box 134-3

### *Seizure Mnemonic*

- **G**lucose
- **R**ising blood pressure
- **A**lcohol/anatomic
- **N**eoplasms/neuroinfections
- **D**rugs
- **M**etabolic
- **A**rterial disease
- e**L**ectrolytes
- **S**DH/SAH/ICH (subdural hematoma, subarachnoid hemorrhage, intracranial hemorrhage)

### PSYCHIATRIC SYNDROMES

Several psychiatric syndromes are associated with a depressed mental state, including akinetic mutism, psychogenic unresponsiveness, conversion disorder, and catatonia. Catatonic stupor is characterized by either acute or subacute development of stupor with waxy flexibility of limbs and sometimes echolalia and echo-praxia. Catatonia is an uncommon manifestation of schizophrenia, but a similar state that may be seen is severe depression. These syndromes are not life threatening but must be differentiated from other potentially reversible causes of coma.

### CONDITIONS THAT MAY MIMIC COMA

The clinician must be astute to always consider the "locked-in syndrome" where the patient may present with total paralysis of the limbs and most CN, with preserved mentation and some afferent input. Patients with brainstem stroke, critical illness polyneuropathy (CIPN, seen occasionally in those who have received protracted courses of steroids and neuromuscular blockers in the intensive care unit [ICU]) and Guillain-Barré syndrome may present in this manner. Jean Dominique Bauby is a famous brainstem stroke survivor who wrote an entire book by using eyelid signals to a stenographer to publish *The Diving Bell and the Butterfly.*

## MANAGEMENT

The patient who presents in a comatose state represents a true diagnostic dilemma for the physician. The goal of therapy is to prevent further CNS injury and to stabilize the patient quickly. Rapid identification and reversal of toxic or metabolic causes of coma may be life-saving. Once the patient's airway is secure and he or she is hemodynamically stable, one may then consider the AEIOUTHIPS approach to further elucidate the possible cause of the coma. An organized approach is presented in Figure 134-2.

The initial assessment of adolescents with a change in mental status may have begun in the field. Such patients are usually administered dextrose, thiamine, and a trial of naloxone, a narcotic antagonist. The routine empiric naloxone dose is intravenous administration of 0.8 mg to 2.0 mg. It may also be administered endotracheally, intramuscularly, or subcutaneously or injected intralingually.[21] The half-life of naloxone is 40 to 90 minutes, a much shorter time course than that of most opioids being reversed.[22] A continuous infusion should be considered if the initial dose is successful. Naloxone should be administered to patients with a respiratory rate less than 8 to 10 breaths per minute, those with pinpoint pupils, and those with circumstantial evidence of opioid abuse (drug paraphernalia, needle tracks, bystander corroboration). Flumazenil, a benzodiazepine antagonist, has been administered to patients with multiple drug ingestions, but its use has precipitated seizures in patients who have ingested both tricyclic antidepressants and benzodiazepines. It is a reversal agent that should be viewed with great caution in pediatric patients.[23]

The initial (or continued, if instituted in the field) assessment should consist of the ABCDs: airway, breathing, circulation, and disability. The physician must identify conditions that are rapidly correctable (hypoxemia, hypotension, hypoglycemia) and be able to identify a deteriorating

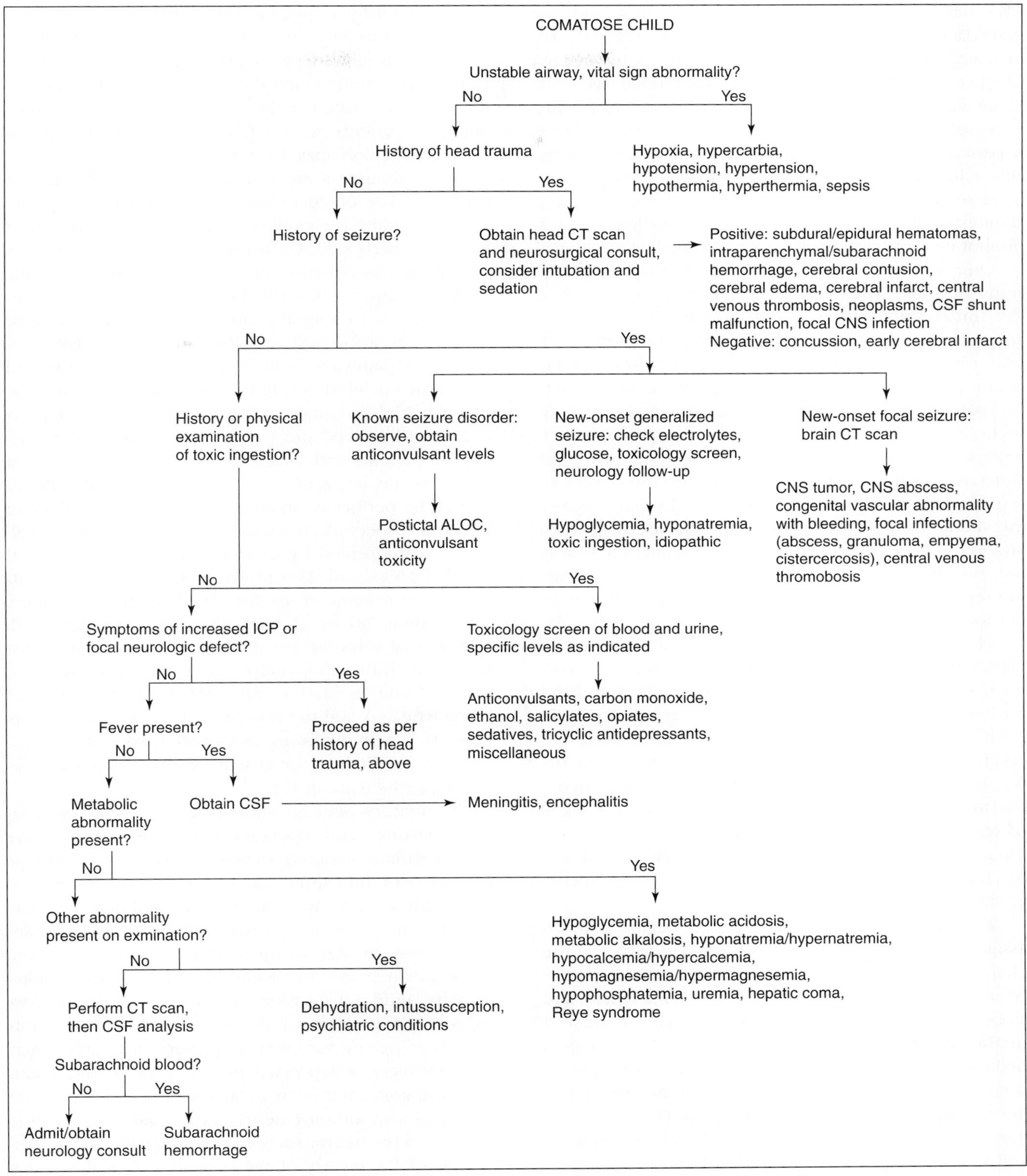


**FIGURE 134-2** Diagnostic algorithm for the assessment of the comatose patient. (Modified with permission from Nelson D. Coma and altered level of consciousness. In: Fleischer GR, Ludwig S, Henretig FM, eds. *Textbook of Pediatric Emergency Medicine.* 5th ed. Philadelphia, PA: Lippincott, Williams & Wilkins 2006:207.)

CNS status. After the ABCD assessment, it should be immediately determined whether there are any signs of increased or if the patient is at risk for cerebral herniation. Chapter 131, CNS Trauma, also outlines the management of increased ICP. Symptoms include vomiting, headache, a decrease in GCS score, papilledema (a late finding), hypertension, bradycardia, apneustic breathing, posturing, and unilateral dilation of a pupil. If there is a suggestion of increased ICP, the patient should be hyperventilated, administration of 1 g/kg of mannitol considered, and a prompt neurosurgical consultation obtained.

One must carefully assess for focal neurologic signs that may suggest a structural CNS lesion. After the initial stabilization of the patient, history-taking and a careful physical examination must be performed. The history may have to be obtained from emergency personnel, bystanders, or someone other than the patient. Specific items to evaluate in the history include chronic underlying diseases (pulmonary, renal, hepatic, immunodeficiency), ingestion of any drugs or substances (including over-the-counter medications), trauma, seizures, previous episodes, thyroid disease, metabolic disease, malignancy, psychosocial history, and possible exposure to any environmental toxins (carbon monoxide).[24] The time course of the change in mental status and focal findings may also suggest an etiology.

The physical examination includes evaluation of the vital signs: heart rate, blood pressure, respiratory pattern, and temperature. The neck should be stabilized until a C-spine fracture can be safely excluded. Abnormalities of vital signs suggest a possible etiology or result in a worsening of the patient's mental status (ie, hypotension, hypertension, hyperthermia, hypothermia). The patient should be examined for signs of trauma and the scalp palpated for possible hematomas or the presence of a ventriculoperitoneal shunt. Nuchal rigidity may not be present in the deeply comatose patient.

A detailed neurologic examination begins with an assignment of the GCS score, as discussed earlier in the chapter. The neurological examination in the comatose patient focuses on examination of the brainstem and associated reflexes. The ARAS courses from the medulla to the thalamus. The ARAS's location overlaps several brainstem reflex pathways, particularly those responsible for the pupillary light reflex and the reflex eye movements that allow conjugate gaze. Thus preservation of these reflexes suggests that the ARAS is normal and that the altered mental status is due to cerebral dysfunction, whereas conversely if there is pupillary asymmetry or dysconjugate gaze, then the ARAS is the site of the problem.[25] Focal or lateralizing neurologic findings may help with the diagnosis. If everything can be explained by a specific lesion, this points the clinician in the direction of a structural cause. Examination of the pupils may suggest a possible cause of the coma. In toxic/metabolic coma the pupils are small but react symmetrically, whereas there may be dilation or asymmetry in patients with a CNS lesion. Thus the pupillary examination may be the most important sign to help differentiate a medical from a structural cause of the coma. The oculocephalic (doll's eye) reflex is elicited by holding the eyelids open and turning the head briskly to each side. A normal response is for the eyes to shift in the direction opposite to the head turning, so for example when the head is turned abruptly to the left the eyes normally move to the right to attempt to return to a forward gaze. This reflex is mediated by brainstem pathways originating in the labyrinths and vestibular nuclei involving the high spinal cord and the medulla. It also requires integrity of the midbrain, pons and CN III and IV, and the medial longitudinal fasciculus. In patients with brainstem lesions the eyes remain fixed and do not return to midline. This reflex should NEVER be performed in any patient in whom a C-spine injury is suspected. The oculovestibular reflex (cold calorics) is performed by elevating the head of the bed to 30 degrees, and then inserting a small catheter into the external auditory meatus, holding the eyes open, and flushing 30 cc of cold water into the ear canal. The normal response in an unconscious patient is nystagmus with the slow component toward the ear being irrigated and the fast component away from the ear being irrigated, and the reverse being true in conscious patients.[26] A funduscopic examination should evaluate signs of papilledema or absent venous pulsations suggesting an increase in ICP.

Respiratory patterns should be observed. The position, posture, and spontaneous movements of the patient should be noted. Decorticate positioning (flexor posturing of the upper extremities) is usually associated with a CNS injury above the midbrain, whereas decerebrate positioning (extensor posturing) is associated with damage to the midbrain or diencephalon. These postures may be produced by a variety of lesions in many different locations and do not of themselves suggest the location of the lesion. Babinski sign (an extensor upgoing toe) may be present bilaterally when consciousness is depressed from any cause, but a unilateral upgoing toe is an indicator of a CNS structural lesion.[4] An important clue to a structural CNS lesion is focality on the neurologic examination. Table 134-4 presents a brief summary of the expected clinical findings associated with a specific anatomic lesion.

The choice of laboratory studies should be guided by the history. All patients must undergo an immediate determination of serum glucose levels and arterial

**Table 134-4**

**Clinical Findings Correlated with Level of Central Nervous System Injury**

| *Anatomic Dysfunction* | *Response to Noxious Stimuli* | *Pupils* | *Eye Position and Movements* | *Breathing* | *Motor Findings for Structural Lesions* |
|---|---|---|---|---|---|
| Both cortices | Withdrawal | Small, reactive | Extraocular movements can be elicited | Post-hyperventilation apnea or Cheyne-Stokes respiration | |
| Thalamus | Decorticate posturing | Equal and small unless the optic tract is damaged | Eyes deviated down and toward the side of the lesion | Same as above | Contralateral hemiparesis |
| Midbrain | Decorticate or decerebrate posturing | Midposition, fixed to light | Nystagmus may be present; loss of ability to adduct; both eyes may be deviated laterally and down in CN III damage | Usually same as above; potential for central reflex hyperpnea | Hemiplegia with contralateral CN III palsy |
| Pons | Decerebrate posturing | Bilateral pinpoint pupils, reactive to light | Ocular bobbing; absent conjugate horizontal movements with retained vertical movements and accommodations; often eyes are deviated medially; CN VII damage | Central reflex hyperpnea; cluster (Biot) breathing or apneustic breathing | Hemiplegia with contralateral CN VI and VII palsy |
| Medulla | Weak or no leg flexion | Nonreactive, normal size | Usually no effect on spontaneous eye movements | Rarely, ataxic respiration; apnea if respiratory center is involved | Flaccid weakness with difficulty swallowing, phonating, and incoordination |
| Spinal cord | None | Normal reaction, abnormal response if brainstem is affected | Normal response | Normal | Flaccid weakness; loss of bowel and bladder control |

CN, cranial nerve

Reproduced from Pearson-Shaver AL, Mehta R. Coma and depressed sensorium. In: Fuhrman BP, Zimmerman JJ, eds. *Pediatric Critical Care*. 3rd ed. Philadelphia, PA: Mosby Elsevier; 2006:859, with permission from Elsevier.

blood gases to ascertain their acid-base status. Serum electrolytes to be evaluated include sodium, calcium, bicarbonate, urea nitrogen, and creatinine. If the history and physical examination suggest an infectious cause, appropriate cultures should be obtained along with a complete blood count. A spinal tap should be performed unless contraindicated. Serum and urine toxicologies should be guided by the most likely substance ingested, keeping in mind the possibility of administering an antidote. Although the decision to perform head CT will be guided by the patient's presentation and physical examination, it is strongly recommended that a CT be performed in any patient with an acute loss of consciousness.

## OUTCOME

In general the prognosis of coma is much better in the adolescent patient than in the adult. The outcomes that may be seen include death, vegetative state (VS), various degrees of neurologic disability, and full neurologic recovery.[4] Patients with toxic/metabolic etiologies have a better outcome than those patients with a structural lesion. Signs that correlate with poor prognosis include the length of time the patient was comatose, brainstem damage, and the GCS. Brain death represents a complete and irreversible loss of brain and brainstem function. It is recognized by the abolition of consciousness, CN activity, motor reflexes, and spontaneous breathing.[26] In contrast to comatose patients in whom there is an absence of arousal and awareness, patients in a VS present with a global impairment in consciousness, in which awareness of self or the environment is absent, but signs of arousal may be retained. These patients may spontaneously open their eyes but do not react in a meaningful way to environmental clues. They are not able to follow visually nor can they fixate on specific objects or people. Vegetative state usually results following severe head injury or a significant hypoxic-ischemic event such as cardiac arrest. The VS results from extensive damage to the cerebral cortex with sparing of the brainstem.[2]

Adolescent patients presenting with an altered level of consciousness often present a diagnostic and management challenge for the clinician. One must maintain a high degree of concern in these patients and follow a systematic approach in assessing their clinical situation to ensure an optimal outcome. Most adolescent patients who present with altered mental status or coma will have a toxic/metabolic etiology and the clinician must remember that many of these are reversible when recognized early.

## REFERENCES

1. Plum F, Posner JB. *The Diagnosis of Stupor and Coma.* 3rd ed. Philadelphia, PA: FA Davis; 1980

2. Stevens RD, Nyquist PA. Coma, delirium, and cognitive dysfunction in critical illness. *Crit Care Clin.* 2007;22:787–804

3. Parvizi J, Damasio AR. Neuroanatomical correlates of brainstem coma. *Brain.* 2003;126:1524–1536

4. Stevens RD, Bhardwaj A. Approach to the comatose patient. *Crit Care Med.* 2006;34(1):31–40

5. Teasdale G, Jennett B. Assessment of coma and impaired consciousness. *Lancet.* 1974;2:81–84

6. Saez-Llorens X, McCracken GH. Bacterial meningitis in children. *Lancet.* 2003;361:2139–2148

7. El Bashir H, Laundy M, Booy R. Diagnosis and treatment of bacterial meningitis. *Arch Dis Child.* 2003;88:615–620

8. Silvia MT, Licht DJ. Pediatric central nervous system infections and inflammatory white matter disease. *Pediatr Clin N Am.* 2005;52(4):1107–1126, ix

9. Lewis P, Glaser CA. Encephalitis. *Pediatr Rev.* 2005;26(10):353–358

10. Burchett SK, Pizzo PA. HIV infection in infants, children, and adolescents. *Pediatr Rev.* 2003;24(6):186–194

11. Sieber FE, Traystman RJ. Special issues: glucose and the brain. *Crit Care Med.* 1992;20:104–114

12. Gutierrez G. Cellular energy metabolism during hypoxia. *Crit Care Med.* 1991;19:619–626

13. Shewmon DA, De Giorgio CM. Early prognosis in anoxic coma: reliability and rationale. *Neurol Clin.* 1989;7:823–843

14. Collins MW, Lovell MR, McKeag DB. Current issues in managing sports-related concussion. *JAMA.* 1999;282(24):2283–2285

15. Kirkwood MW, Yeates KO, Wilson PE. Pediatric sport-related concussion: a review of the clinical management of oft-neglected population. *Pediatrics.* 2006;117(4):1359–1367

16. World Health Organization. *International Statistical Classification of Diseases and Related Health Problems.* 10th ed. Geneva, Switzerland: World Health Organization; 1992

17. McCrory PR, Berkovic SF. Second impact syndrome. *Neurology.* 1998;50:667–683

18. Quality Standards Subcommittee, American Academy of Neurology. Practice parameter: the management of concussion in sports (summary statement). *Neurology.* 1997;48(3):581–585

19. Ropper AH, Gorson KC. Concussion. *N Engl J Med.* 2007;356(2):166–172

20. Delorenzo RJ, Waterhouse EJ, Towne AR. Persistent nonconvulsive status epilepticus after the control of convulsive status epilepticus. *Epilepsia.* 1998;39:833–840

21. Zimmerman JL. Poisonings and overdoses in the intensive care unit: general and specific management issues. *Crit Care Med.* 2003;31(12):2794–2803

22. Mokhlesi B, Leiken JB, Murray P, Corobridge TC. Adult toxicology in critical care. Part I: General approach to the intoxicated patient. *Chest.* 2003;123:577–592

23. Mokhlesi B, Leiken JB, Murray P, Corobridge TC. Adult toxicology in critical care. Part II: Specific poisonings. *Chest.* 2003;123:897–922

24. Bazakis AM, Kunzler C. Altered mental status due to metabolic or endocrine disorders. *Emerg Med Clin N Am.* 2005;23:901–908

25. Avner JR. Altered states of consciousness. *Pediatr Rev.* 2006;27(9):331–337

26. King D, Avner JR. Altered mental status. *Clin Ped Emerg.* 2003;4:171–178

# CHAPTER 135

## Fever of Unknown Origin

LORRY G. RUBIN, MD

Fever is a common symptom of illness and usually signifies the presence of an infection. As for a patient of any age, the most common cause of fever in an adolescent is viral infection. A viral infection typically presents with concomitant symptoms of an upper respiratory infection or acute gastroenteritis but may occur in the absence of localizing symptoms. Fever represents the host response to a number of stimuli, and occasionally an illness other than an infection initiates the cascade of biologic processes that results in fever. This chapter focuses on the approach to the adolescent with persistent fever (fever of unknown origin, or FUO) and the approach to the febrile adolescent who appears seriously ill.

### PATHOGENESIS OF FEVER

Pathogens and their components or products may serve as exogenous pyrogens. For example, the lipopolysaccharide of *Escherichia coli* is a pyrogen. Fever and other signs of systemic illness are induced by intravenous injection into experimental animals of live *E coli* and killed *E coli* or lipopolysaccharide purified from the cell wall of *E coli*. Endotoxin from the lipopolysaccharide of *E coli* or other gram-negative bacteria, lipoteichoic acid of gram-positive bacteria, and certain other microbial products serve as exogenous or indirect pyrogens by stimulating host cells to produce and secrete cytokines termed endogenous pyrogens, the direct mediators of fever. Interleukin-1 (IL-1) and tumor necrosis factor (TNF) along with interferons and interleukin-6 (IL-6) are cytokines that function as endogenous pyrogens. These polypeptides, produced mainly in cells of macrophage/monocyte lineage, enter the circulation and act on the thermoregulatory center of the anterior hypothalamus, resulting in a rise in the thermostat set point. In addition, microbial product interaction with the toll-like receptor of the innate immune system adjacent to the vascular network supplying the thermoregulatory center in the anterior hypothalamus provides an additional mechanism for the genesis of fever independent of endogenous pyrogens as intermediary molecules.[1] The change in the thermostat set point, mediated by cyclo-oxygenase activity and prostaglandin E, causes neural stimulation that activates peripheral mechanisms including vasoconstriction (that results in heat conservation) and muscle contraction (that results in heat generation). Nonmicrobial stimuli, including trauma and burns that result in production and secretion of endogenous cytokine pyrogens, can also cause fever.[2]

### FEVER OF UNKNOWN ORIGIN

Fever of unknown origin has not been studied specifically in adolescents but has been defined in the pediatric and adolescent age groups as fever without a diagnosis persisting for 21 days,[3,4] or a daily fever for a minimum of 14 days,[5] despite multiple examinations and screening laboratory testing. Although in some cases the fever is self-limited and a diagnosis is not established or the patient is classified as having a presumed viral infection, patients who fulfill these criteria warrant investigation because in many cases the patient will not recover without a specific diagnosis and therapy. Infections comprise most cases. It is more common for FUO to be caused by an atypical presentation of a common infection than a rare condition. When fever persists for 4 weeks or more without a diagnosis, the likelihood of an infectious etiology is lower and the likelihood of a noninfectious diagnosis such as a connective tissue disease or malignancy is higher.

Anatomically, infections of the upper or lower respiratory tracts, particularly occult infection of a paranasal sinus (especially the sphenoid sinus[6]) or occult pneumonia, including pneumonia due to tuberculosis, are important causes. Pyelonephritis, particularly in a patient who has received antimicrobial therapy that temporarily results in a nondiagnostic urinalysis or urine culture, is a relatively common cause especially in female adolescents. Osteomyelitis of the axial skeleton (ie, vertebral body, disk space, sacroiliac joint or pelvis) or infection in contiguous muscles may be clinically occult or may result in nonspecific symptoms and present as FUO. Occult dental abscess, meningitis, and endocarditis are occasional causes of FUO.[7]

The pathogen most often responsible for FUO in adolescents is the Epstein-Barr virus (EBV), the most commonly identified cause of infectious mononucleosis, but primary infection with other viruses, particularly an enterovirus, cytomegalovirus (CMV), or human immunodeficiency virus (HIV), may cause FUO. Primary HIV in the adolescent is generally sexually acquired and may be accompanied by other sexually transmitted infections. Although infection may occur without initial symptoms, approximately 50% of adolescents develop symptoms 3 to 6 weeks after primary infection and present with symptoms suggestive of infectious mononucleosis including fever, fatigue, pharyngitis, myalgia, and cervical lymphadenopathy.[8] An opportunistic infection, such as disseminated *Mycobacterium avium-intracellulare* infection in an adolescent with previously unrecognized HIV infection with severe immune deficiency, may present with FUO. Among bacterial pathogens, recent studies have emphasized the importance of infection with *Bartonella henselae*, the etiologic agent of cat scratch disease, as a cause of FUO in children and adolescents.[5] Typically, patients with cat scratch disease do not have clinically evident lymphadenitis but may present with fever and may sometimes have occult intra-abdominal or retroperitoneal lymphadenopathy, with or without multiple small abscesses in the liver and/or spleen that are only detectable by performing imaging studies.[5] Other bacterial pathogens that may cause FUO include enteric fever due to extraintestinal infection with *Salmonella typhi* (typhoid fever, foreign travel) or a non-*S typhi* salmonella species (most commonly acquired from food, especially poultry or egg- or milk-containing products), *Brucella* spp (brucellosis), *Francisella tularensis* (tularemia), and rarely *Borrelia burgdorferi* (Lyme disease). Rat bite fever due to *Streptobacillus moniliformis* may cause fever lasting several weeks and is associated with rodent contact and clinical signs of rash and arthritis.[9] The tick-borne infections babesisos and ehrlichiosis may cause fever without a focus, but in healthy adolescents these infections usually resolve without specific therapy in less than 2 weeks.

Immune-mediated diseases may be triggered by an infection that has resolved by the time the patient presents with fever. Acute rheumatic fever following a *Streptococcus pyogenes* throat infection is most commonly recognized by the presence of fever in association with major criteria of carditis and/or migratory polyarthritis. The life-threatening hemophagocytic syndrome (also called macrophage activation syndrome or hemophagocytic lymphohistiocytosis), characterized by fever, cytopenia of two or three blood cell lines, hypertriglyceridemia and hemophagocytosis, often occurs after an antecedent infection with one of a variety of pathogens, including EBV or adenovirus.[10]

The etiology of fever may be unrelated to an infection.[7] Autoimmune diseases, including systemic lupus erythematosus (with the presence of one or more of a variety of clinical findings including rash, arthritis, and nephritis in the presence of antinuclear antibodies or autoantibodies to Rho and La antigens, polyarteritis nodosa (fever, hypertension, renal involvement), and Wegener granulomatosis (fever, renal and respiratory tract involvement, and classic antineutrophil cytoplasmic antibody serology-positive), often present with fever as a predominant feature. Although systemic onset juvenile idiopathic arthritis (JIA) often presents with persistent fever, this form of JIA is relatively uncommon in the adolescent age group. Sarcoidosis may present with fever, often in the presence of pulmonary or ophthalmologic symptoms. Malignancy, particularly leukemia and lymphoma, inflammatory bowel disease, especially Crohn disease, and drug fever[3] are additional causes of prolonged fever. Factitious fever, including Munchausen syndrome (self-induced or feigned infections) and Munchausen syndrome by proxy (induced by a parent), occurs in adolescents and may require observation in an inpatient setting to document the absence of fever or the mechanism of feigned or induced fever. Factitious or pseudofever should be suspected in a patient with a normal pulse rate and results of laboratory testing that indicate the absence of signs of an acute-phase response, that is, normal erythrocyte sedimentation rate (ESR) and C-reactive protein concentration, absence of anemia, and a normal rather than elevated platelet count.

An approach to the history, physical examination, diagnostic testing, and management of the adolescent with FUO is delineated in Box 135-1. Suggested diagnostic tests have been divided into initial tests that should be performed in all patients and subsequent tests that are appropriate if a diagnosis has not been established despite repeated elicitation of history and physical examinations and review of the results of initial tests. In every case it is appropriate to aggressively

## Box 135-1

### *Approach to the Adolescent with Persistent Fever*

1. Detailed history to include:
   a. Travel outside the United States (at risk for malaria, tuberculosis, typhoid fever, dengue) and prophylactic measures taken (eg, use of insect repellent, malaria chemoprophylaxis, typhoid vaccine)
   b. Travel or residence within the United States, for example, Midwest: histoplasmosis; Southwest: coccidiomycosis
   c. Sexual history: relevant to primary HIV infection; disseminated gonococcal infection; syphilis
   d. Animal or animal product exposure: kitten contact in cat scratch disease; livestock contact in brucellosis; rodent contact in leptospirosis and rat bite fever; reptile contact in *Salmonella*
   e. Tick bite: relevant to babesiosis, tularemia, Lyme disease, ehrlichia and anaplasma infection, Rocky Mountain spotted fever
   f. Fever pattern: once daily in malaria
   g. Means of documentation of fever: possibility of pseudofever or factitious fever; measured versus tactile, tympanic often less accurate than oral or rectal
   h. Antimicrobial therapy, including self-prescribed microbials
   i. Other medications that might cause drug fever, for example, anticonvulsants
2. Physical examination
   a. Document fever
   b. Flank tenderness: urinary tract infection
   c. Spine or pelvic tenderness: axial skeleton osteomyelitis
   d. Lymphadenopathy, hepatosplenomegaly: EBV, CMV, HIV, cat scratch, lymphoma, leukemia, extrapulmonary tuberculosis, Kikuchi disease (histiocytic necrotizing lymphadenitis)
   e. Tenderness overlying the paranasal sinuses, posterior pharyngeal wall with mucus or cobblestone pattern: sinusitis
   f. Skin rash
3. Diagnostic testing
   a. Initial tests: complete blood count (CBC) with differential, erythrocyte sedimentation rate (ESR) or C-reactive protein (CRP) (normal values suggest pseudo-fever), blood culture (two-bottle system for aerobic and anaerobic cultures), hepatic profile including albumin and total protein, urinalysis, serum creatinine and blood urea nitrogen (BUN), chest radiograph
   b. Subsequent tests if diagnosis is not established and fever has not resolved; consider gallium scan, FDG-PET scan, or indium-labeled leukocyte scan; note that indium scan is not helpful for osteomyelitis of axial skeleton; bone marrow aspiration if presence of neutropenia or thrombocytopenia or suspicion of leukemia or lymphoma; culture bone marrow aspirate, including inoculation of media designed for culture of blood
      i. General additional tests: repeat blood culture (at least 2 days after discontinuation of antimicrobial therapy), urine culture, serology for EBV and CMV, radiograph or CT scan of paranasal sinuses, stool for occult blood (screening test for inflammatory bowel disease), bacterial culture of stool (*Salmonella*), tuberculin skin test (extrapulmonary tuberculosis), ultrasound of abdomen (urinary tract abnormalities, lesions in the liver or spleen) and subsequent CT scan of abdomen (occult abscess such as due to ruptured appendicitis, inflammatory bowel disease)
      ii. Tests to perform if history or physical examination findings are supportive: *Bartonella* (cat scratch) serology; serology for HIV if sexually active; serology for *Anaplasma* (ehrlichiosis; if epidemiology is suggestive), MRI, or CT of pelvis or spine (if osteomyelitis or adjacent soft tissue infection is suspected based upon history or physical examination); antinuclear antibody, c-ANCA
4. Management
   a. Discontinue antimicrobial therapy in absence of a diagnosis
   b. Discontinue or replace other medications that may be causing drug fever
   c. Minimize antipyretic therapy
   d. Have patient record temperature twice daily and when perception of fever and record associated symptoms
   e. Repeat history and physical examination to include measurement of body temperature and body mass at frequent intervals

follow clues from the history and physical examination. For example, if focal abdominal tenderness is present, an ultrasound or computed tomography (CT) scan of the abdomen should be performed; if there is focal tenderness of the spine or pelvis, a CT or magnetic resonance imaging (MRI) of these areas should be performed. For imaging the paranasal sinuses, CT may be preferable to MRI because of the high rate of false-positive findings on

MRI. Nuclear medicine scans are occasionally helpful.[11] An indium-labeled leukocyte scan or a gallium scan are most often considered. [$^{18}$F]fluoro-deoxyglucose positron emission tomography (FDG-PET), of established value in diagnosis of malignant diseases, is a newer technique for diagnosing infection and studying patients with FUO but may eventually replace gallium scanning because it may be more accurate and is completed more rapidly.[12] Nuclear scans have limited specificity, and there is almost always a need to follow up a positive finding with additional testing to establish a specific diagnosis.

## SYSTEMIC INFLAMMATORY RESPONSE SYNDROME

The invasion of a pathogen or tissue injury unrelated to an infectious agent triggers a localized inflammatory response resulting in migration of components of the immune system to the injury site. However, if an infectious agent gains access to the systemic circulation in response to a variety of traumatic, surgical, immunologic, or drug-induced insults, there is activation of a number of host responses, collectively called the systemic inflammatory response syndrome (SIRS),[10–13] which can be triggered by the lipopolysaccharide of gram-negative bacteria, cell wall products of gram-positive bacteria, enterotoxins, and by viral or fungal components. The most important cytokine in the genesis of this syndrome is TNF, although many other mediators, including IL-1, IL-6, IL-8, colony-stimulating factors, and platelet-activating factor, are also involved. These mediators stimulate production of leukotrienes, thromboxane A2 and prostaglandins from arachidonic acid that affect the vascular endothelium, which then undergoes an increase in permeability and synthesizes a variety of mediators of inflammation, including additional IL-1. Stimulation of vascular endothelium and leukocytes results in changes in expression of ligands and receptors and promotes transmigration of leukocytes across endothelial surfaces. Degranulation of neutrophils occurs and results in release of proteolytic enzymes and toxic oxygen radicals that contribute to increased vascular permeability. The coagulation and complement systems are activated with resultant disseminated intravascular coagulation, vascular abnormalities, and neutrophil activation. Together, these processes cause vascular injury and increase capillary permeability. Also, there is participation of anti-inflammatory cytokines and other molecules that attenuate the potentially autodestructive effects of the proinflammatory substances.

The clinical definition of SIRS in the adolescent age group requires 2 or more of the following criteria (one of which must be fever/hypothermia or an elevated/depressed leukocyte count): (1) fever or hypothermia, (2) tachycardia (>110 beats/minute), (3) elevated respiratory rate (>14 breaths/minute), and (4) elevated or depressed leukocyte count ($>11 \times 10^3$ or $<4.5 \times 10^3$).[14] Sepsis is defined as SIRS in the presence of an infection. Severe sepsis is defined as sepsis plus cardiovascular organ dysfunction, acute respiratory distress syndrome (ARDS), or 2 or more other organ dysfunctions. Septic shock is defined as sepsis plus cardiovascular organ dysfunction.

## THE ACUTELY ILL FEBRILE ADOLESCENT

As noted previously, the presence of shock with multiorgan dysfunction due to SIRS may be caused by a wide variety of infectious agents as well as tissue injury unrelated to infection. The differential diagnosis of a febrile adolescent patient who appears acutely ill is broad but includes life-threatening infections that constitute medical emergencies (Table 135-1). A rapid but thorough history and physical examination is critical for formulating and initiating a rational, empiric antimicrobial regimen. The empiric antimicrobial regimen should provide coverage for the potential bacterial pathogens and should be administered expeditiously. Clues that suggest an etiologic agent should broaden rather than limit empiric antimicrobial coverage while awaiting the results of blood cultures and other diagnostic tests. One suggested empiric antimicrobial regimen for community-acquired sepsis syndrome without a definable focus of infection or etiological agent is combination therapy with ceftriaxone (provides treatment of meningococcus, *E coli*-causing urosepsis, disseminated gonococcal infection, and Lemierre syndrome) vancomycin for treatment of methicillin-resistant *Staphylococcus aureus* (MRSA) and enterococcal urosepsis, and clindamycin for coverage of *Streptococcus pyogenes* causing toxic-shock syndrome, necrotizing fasciitis or other soft tissue infection, many strains of MRSA, and Lemierre's syndrome. If Rocky Mountain spotted fever is suspected (see discussion following and Table 135-1), doxycycline should be added. If intra-abdominal sepsis is suspected, the empiric antimicrobial regimen should include antimicrobials with activity against aerobic gram-negative bacilli including *E coli*, the anaerobic gram-negative bacillus *Bacteroides fragilis*, and enterococci; either piperacillin/tazobactam (Zosyn) or ticarcillin/clavulanate (Timentin) is an excellent choice for this purpose.

Meningococcemia is the prototype bacterial infection that presents acutely in a previously healthy adolescent, may progress rapidly to septic shock, and may have a fatal outcome (Table 135-1).[15] This infection, caused

**Table 135-1**

**Infectious Causes of Illness in Acutely Ill Febrile Adolescents**

| *Infectious Disease* | *Pathogen* | *Presentation (in Addition to Fever)* | *Physical Findings* | *Diagnostic Tests* | *Antimicrobial Therapy* | *Comments* |
|---|---|---|---|---|---|---|
| Disseminated gonococcal infection (arthritis-dermatitis syndrome) | *Neisseria gonorrhoeae* | Onset just after menstrual period; joint and tendon pain; discrete skin lesions | Tenosynovitis, arthritis, right upper quadrant tenderness; purulent cervicitis usually not present | Blood culture; cervical swab or culture for *N gonorrhea*; DNA detection | Ceftriaxone (cefotaxime) | Predominantly in females who are sexually active. Caused by particular serum-resistant strains of *N gonorrhoeae* |
| Intra-abdominal sepsis | Mixed aerobic/anaerobic infection: *E coli* or other gram-negative bacilli including *Pseudomonas* spp, *Bacteroides fragilis*, often enterococcus | Abdominal pain, vomiting; if appendicitis—right lower quadrant pain | Abdominal tenderness with rebound tenderness, diminished bowel sounds | Surgical evaluation and laparotomy or laparoscopy. If imaging is needed, perform ultrasound or CT scan | Piperacillin/tazobactam (Zosyn) or ticarcillin/clavulanate (Timentin) | Acute appendicitis is most common. In sexually active females, salpingitis (pelvic inflammatory disease) can present as intra-abdominal sepsis. Differential diagnosis includes pancreatitis, primary peritonitis, intra-abdominal abscesses. Ruptured ovarian cyst or torsion or ruptured ectopic pregnancy can present in a similar fashion |
| Lemierre syndrome (suppurative jugular vein thrombophlebitis) | *Fusobacterium necrophorum* (or other oral anaerobic bacterial species) | Neck pain and stiffness, headache, or other neurological symptoms; cough/chest pain | Pain anterior to sternocleidomastoid muscle, torticollis, pulmonary findings consistent with pneumonia or pulmonary embolus | Anaerobic blood culture, CT scan with IV contrast demonstrating thrombosed internal jugular vein | Clindamycin or metroniadazole or cetriaxone (cefotaxime) | Septic phlebitis of jugular vein originating from pharyngitis. Can result in septic pulmonary emboli or cephalad extension with cerebral venous sinus thrombosis |
| Meningococcemia | *Neisseria meningitidis* | Acute onset (within hours), vomiting, headache, rash | Shock, petechial and/or purpuric rash | Blood culture, CSF culture, gram stain, and culture of petechial lesion scraping) | Penicillin G | There may be accompanying meningitis. Most cases are vaccine preventable. Antimicrobial prophylaxis of household contacts is indicated |
| Necrotizing fasciitis | *Staphylococcus aureus*, *Streptococcus pyogenes*, gram-negative bacilli | Localized severe pain in extremity, back, or perineal areas | Toxic appearance, localized extreme tenderness out of proportion to local findings; local findings of inflammation may include bullae | MRI of affected area; biopsy with frozen section; culture of blood and tissue specimen | Piperacillin/tazobactam (or another broad spectrum regimen) ± vancomycin | Surgical and medical emergency. Obtain urgent surgical consultation. Extensive debridement is often required |

*(Continued)*

**Table 135-1 (Continued)**

| *Infectious Disease* | *Pathogen* | *Presentation (in Addition to Fever)* | *Physical Findings* | *Diagnostic Tests* | *Antimicrobial Therapy* | *Comments* |
|---|---|---|---|---|---|---|
| Rocky Mountain spotted fever | *Rickettsia rickettsii* | Tick bite history or exposure; fever, severe headache, and myalgia precedes maculopapular rash that starts on wrists and ankles; petechial rash follows | Conjunctival injection, tender muscles, diffuse maculopapular or petechial rash with rash on palm and soles | Serology, acute and convalescent for *R rickettsii* | Doxycycline | Diagnosis is made clinically and empiric treatment is started with doxycycline. Differential diagnosis includes Kawasaki syndrome and ehrlichiosis |
| Staphylococcal septicemia | *Staphylococcus aureus* | Possible skin lesions or extremity pain, cough, tachypnea | Evidence of pneumonia, cellulitis, or deep soft tissue infection | Blood culture, culture of infected site | Vancomycin plus nafcillin ± gentamicin; D/C vancomycin or nafcillin when susceptibility test results are known | Can have no focus or have associated soft tissue infection, pneumonia, and/or osteoarticular infection, at times multifocal. May be caused by community-associated MRSA |
| Toxic shock syndrome | *S aureus, Streptococcus pyogenes* | Dizziness, erythematous skin rash, diarrhea, decreased urine output, at times pain in soft tissue or evidence of infection at wound site | Multiorgan system involvement including rash | • *S pyogenes:* blood culture, throat culture (antistreptolysin O titer)<br>• *S aureus*: culture of sites of clinical infection; culture of skin, vagina, nares (reference lab to test for toxin gene or production) | • Staphylococcal toxic shock syndrome (TSS): vancomycin plus nafcillin; D/C vancomycin or nafcillin based upon results of susceptibility tests<br>• Streptococcal TSS: clindamycin plus penicillin G | Frequently, a large volume of intravenous fluids is required for resuscitation. Administration of intravenous immune globulin may be helpful. In TSS due to *S aureus*, blood culture is negative, whereas in TSS due to *S pyogenes* blood culture is frequently positive |
| Urosepsis | *Escherichia coli;* other gram-negative bacilli, enterococcus, *Staphylococcus saprophyticus* | Back pain, abdominal pain, vomiting, often dysuria | Abdominal tenderness, flank tenderness | Urine culture, blood culture | Ceftriaxone (cefotaxime) plus ampicillin if gram-positive cocci on gram stain of urine | Urinalysis with pyuria. Cystitis symptoms of dysuria or urinary frequency are not reliably present |

by the gram-negative bacterium *Neisseria meningitides,* presents acutely with fever, vomiting, and headache and often progresses to shock within hours of presentation. Adolescents with invasive meningococcal disease have a case-fatality rate of 23%.[16] The most useful clinical sign is a petechial and at times purpuric skin rash, a finding suggestive but not specific for this pathogen. In fact, the majority of episodes of fever with a petechial skin rash is caused by a virus, particularly an enterovirus. A polysaccharide-protein conjugate vaccine for serogroups A, C, W135, and Y was licensed in the United States in 2005 and 2010, and is recommended for all early adolescents at age 11 or 12 years, with a booster dose at age 16 years as well as older adolescents who have not received a dose.[16] This vaccine has no activity against serogroup B strains that comprise approximately 20% of cases of invasive disease in the adolescent age group.

Sepsis caused by *S aureus* may present with petechiae or purpura, but in contrast to patients with meningococcemia who rarely present with a focal infection, most cases of *S aureus* sepsis are associated with a focal infection of the skin/soft tissue, bone, joints, lung, or heart.[17,18] Increasingly, episodes of *S aureus* sepsis in adolescents are caused by community-associated MRSA that not only contains genes encoding an altered penicillin-binding protein resulting in methicillin resistance but also genes encoding additional virulence factors such as the Panton-Valentine leukocidin.[19] Therefore, empiric therapy for suspected *S aureus* septicemia must include an antimicrobial with activity against MRSA such as vancomycin. Similar to patients with meningococcemia, adolescents with the tick-borne rickettsial infection Rocky Mountain spotted fever may develop a petechial skin rash and shock but are distinguishable because the onset of illness occurs several days prior to the development of petechiae and shock. Early symptoms of illness include fever, headache, myalgia, and a nonpetechial rash that first appears on the wrists and ankles. Other characteristic features are occurrence during the summer months and, in most patients, a history of a tick bite.

Toxic shock syndrome (Table 135-1) is the term used for a shock syndrome with SIRS and multiple organ system involvement due to *S pyogenes* or *S aureus* infection in which the major clinical manifestations are caused by bacterial exotoxins, specifically a streptococcal pyrogenic exotoxin or a staphylococcal toxic shock syndrome toxin (enterotoxin), respectively.[20] In cases of *S pyogenes* TSS, there may be no evident focus of infection, or a focus such as cellulitis or necrotizing fasciitis may be present. In cases of *S aureus* TSS, cases are most commonly associated with menses and the use of tampons or with the presence of a wound, particularly a wound with packing. In both cases, *S aureus* multiplies locally and elaborates exotoxin that results in systemic symptoms and signs. The case definition of streptococcal TSS requires hypotension or shock plus isolation of *S pyogenes* from a sterile (definite case) or nonsterile (probable case) site plus multiorgan system involvement with two or more of the following: renal impairment, adult respiratory distress syndrome, scarlet fever rash, soft tissue necrosis, hepatic abnormalities, or disseminated intravascular coagulation. The case definition of staphylococcal TSS requires fulfillment of all 3 of the following criteria: (1) fever, hypotension, and a macular erythroderma rash, (2) evidence of organ dysfunction of 3 or more of the following organs: mucous membrane inflammation such as conjunctivitis or pharyngitis, vomiting and/or diarrhea, muscle abnormalities as evidenced by myalgia and/or elevated creatine kinase level, central nervous system symptoms such as confusion, obtundation, or coma, hepatic abnormalities such as elevated bilirubin or transaminase concentrations, or a decreased platelet count, and (3) absence of another explanation and a negative blood culture (other than growth of *S aureus*). In some cases *S aureus* septicemia is difficult to differentiate from staphylococcal TSS. Generally, patients with *S aureus* septicemia have a positive blood culture, and in many cases there is a focus for infection such as cellulitis or soft tissue abscess, osteomyelitis, pneumonia, or less commonly, endocarditis. Adolescent girls with tampon-associated TSS should avoid tampon use or at a minimum replace the tampons frequently.

Another infectious syndrome that presents in an acutely ill adolescent is Lemierre syndrome (Table 135-1).[21] Lemierre syndrome, or suppurative thrombophlebitis of the internal jugular vein, is a life-threatening septicemic infection that occurs in previously healthy adolescents or young adults. This syndrome is caused by infection with the anaerobic bacterium *Fusobacterium necrophorum* or on occasion another anaerobic bacterial species that is a constituent of the normal flora in the oral cavity. Infection originates in the oropharynx, and typical initial symptoms are sore throat and fever. Tissue invasion results in unilateral suppurative thrombophlebitis of the internal jugular vein and bacteremia accompanied by systemic toxicity. In some cases, there is neck stiffness and swelling in the anterior cervical area. Patients may develop cerebral venous sinus or cavernous sinus thrombosis with headache and other neurological symptoms or septic pulmonary emboli with chest pain and respiratory distress. The diagnosis is proven by demonstration of thrombosis of the jugular vein on imaging and recovery of the bacterium in a blood culture. Inoculation of an anaerobic bottle, a routine component of the 2-bottle blood culture system used in adults, is imperative. An adult blood culture system should be used routinely for blood cultures obtained from adolescents rather than the single-bottle blood culture used for infants and young children that does not support the growth of obligate anaerobic bacteria. Intravenous metronidazole, clindamycin, or ceftriaxone is effective. The role of anticoagulant therapy is controversial but should be considered, particularly in cases with extensive thrombosis. Adjunctive surgery of the jugular vein is occasionally needed.

## REFERENCES


1. Dinarello CA. Infection, fever, and exogenous and endogenous pyrogens: some concepts have changed. *J Endotoxin Res.* 2004;10:201–222

2. Matsuda N, Hattori Y. Systemic inflammatory response syndrome (SIRS): molecular pathophysiology and gene therapy. *J Pharmacol Sci.* 2006;101:189–198

3. Steele RW, Jones SM, Lowe BA, Glasier GM. Usefulness of scanning procedures for diagnosis of fever of unknown origin in children. *J Pediatr.* 1991;119:526–530

4. Lohr JA, Hendley JO. Prolonged fever of unknown origin. A record of experiences with 54 childhood patients. *Clin Pediatr.* 1977;16:768–773

5. Jacobs RF, Schutze GE. *Bartonella henselae* as a cause of prolonged fever and fever of unknown origin. *Clin Infect Dis.* 1998;26:80–84

6. Marseglia GL, Pagella F, Licari A, et al. Acute isolated sphenoid sinusitis in children. *Int J Pediatr Otorhinolaryngol.* 2006;70:2027–2031

7. Long SS, Edwards KM. Prolonged, recurrent, and periodic fever syndromes. In: Long S, ed. *Principles and Practice of Pediatric Infectious Diseases.* 3rd ed. Philadelphia, PA: Churchill Livingstone; 2008:126–135

8. Vanhems P, Routy JP, Hirschel B, et al. Clinical features of acute retroviral syndrome differ by route of infection but not by gender and age. *J Acquir Immune Defic Syndr.* 2002; 31:318–321

9. Rubin LG. *Streptobacillus moniliformis* (Rat Bite Fever). In: Long S, ed. *Principles and Practice of Pediatric Infectious Diseases.* 3rd ed. Philadelphia, PA: Churchill Livingstone; 2008:927–928

10. Palazzi DL, McClain KL, Kaplan SL. Hemophagocytic syndrome in children: an important diagnostic consideration in fever of unknown origin. *Clin Infect Dis.* 2003;36:306–312

11. Mourad O, Palda V, Detsky A. A comprehensive evidence-based approach to fever of unknown origin. *Arch Intern Med.* 2003;163:545–551

12. Blockmans D, Knockaert D, Maes A, et al. Clinical value of [$^{18}$F] fluoro-deoxyglucose positron emission tomography for patients with fever of unknown origin. *Clin Infect Dis.* 2001;32:191–196

13. Robertson CM, Coopersmith CM. The systemic inflammatory response syndrome. *Microbes Infect.* 2006;8:1382–1389

14. Goldstein B, Giroir B, Randolph A. Members of the International Consensus Conference on Pediatric Sepsis. *International pediatric septic consensus conference: definitions for sepsis and organ dysfunction in pediatrics. Pediatr Crit Care Med.* 2005;6:2–8

15. Centers for Disease Control and Prevention. Prevention and Control of Meningococcal Disease. Recommendations of the Advisory Committee on Immunization Practices (ACIP). *Morb Mort Weekly Report. Recommendations and Reports.* 2005;54(RR07):1–21

16. American Academy of Pediatrics. Prevention and control of meningococcal disease: recommendations for use of meningococcal vaccines in pediatric patients. *Pediatrics.* 2005;116:496–505

17. Francis JS, Doherty MC, Lopatin U, et al. Severe community-onset pneumonia in healthy adults caused by methicillin-resistant *Staphylococcus aureus* carrying the Panton-Valentine leukocidin genes. *Clin Infect Dis.* 2005;40:100–107

18. Gonzalez BE, Hulten KG, Dishop MK, et al. Pulmonary manifestations in children with invasive community-acquired *Staphylococcus aureus* infection. *Clin Infect Dis.* 2005;41:583–590

19. Etienne J. Panton-Valentine leukocidin: a marker of severity for *Staphylococcus aureus* infection? *Clin Infect Dis.* 2005;412:591–593

20. Stevens DL. Streptococcal toxic shock syndrome associated with necrotizing fasciitis. *Annu Rev Med.* 2000;51:271–288

21. Chirinos JA, Lichtstein DM, Garcia J, Tamariz LJ. The evolution of Lemierre syndrome: report of 2 cases and review of the literature. *Medicine (Baltimore).* 2002;81:458–465

# CHAPTER 136

# Common Viral Infections in Adolescents

SUJATHA RAJAN, MD • CHRISTY BENERI, DO

## INTRODUCTION

Adolescents experience a wide range of viral infections. Clinical presentation can vary significantly, reflecting the underlying viral predilection for a particular organ system, the immune status of the patient, and the importance of early recognition of disease in certain instances. A baseline understanding of these viruses will enable one to recognize the disease entity and appropriately manage patients. Although most viral infections resolve without treatment or sequelae, there are instances when viral infections have a significant effect and morbidity. Examples of such instances include a pregnant adolescent who was not vaccinated for rubella and then delivers a child with congenital rubella syndrome, a sexually active adolescent who acquires genital herpes and then must manage outbreaks, or a healthy adolescent who becomes ill with influenza and acquires a secondary bacterial infection as has been seen in past influenza pandemics.

This chapter reviews some of the most common viral infections encountered in adolescents. Traditionally, viruses have been divided into RNA and DNA viruses. For easier review, this chapter is divided according to the organ systems that the virus affects or other similar groupings. The sections are as follows: respiratory infections, gastrointestinal infections, vaccine-preventable diseases, herpes infections, and other (to include Parvovirus and Enterovirus). Other common viruses, such as Epstein-Barr virus (EBV), the hepatitis viruses, and human papillomavirus (HPV), are discussed in other chapters in this textbook.

## RESPIRATORY INFECTIONS

### INFLUENZA

Influenza is an important cause of acute, febrile respiratory illness that occurs annually worldwide. In temperate climates, infection with influenza generally occurs in the late autumn and winter months. There are 3 different antigenic types of influenza virus (ie, influenza A, B, and C), with the former 2 mainly responsible for outbreaks and epidemics worldwide. Influenza type C infections cause a mild respiratory illness and are not thought to cause epidemics. In the United States, 5% to 20% of the general population becomes infected with influenza each year, resulting in more than 200,000 hospitalizations and 36,000 deaths.[1] Those most at risk are the young (<2 years of age) and the elderly (>65 years of age).

#### Microbiology

Influenza is a negative-sense, single-stranded RNA virus of the *Orthomyxoviridae* family. Influenza A and B viruses contain 8 segmented genomes that code for proteins. The viral envelope consists of 2 glycoproteins: hemagglutination (HA), which enables the virus to attach to the host cell, and neuraminidase (NA), which releases new viral particles from cells. There are 16 different hemagglutinin subtypes and 9 different NA subtypes. Variable combinations of these proteins allow influenza A viruses to be divided into several subtypes.

#### Nomenclature

The name of each viral strain is based on the World Health Organization (WHO) naming system. This system identifies each virus type (A, B, C), geographical origin, isolate strain number, year of isolation, and virus subtype (HA subtype and NA subtype). The vaccine is produced each year based on strains most likely to be circulating during the upcoming season. An example of the WHO naming system is as follows: during the 2007–2008 season an influenza strain identified as type A, originally isolated in Wisconsin as isolate number 67, was named A/Wisconsin/67/2005 (H3N2).

#### Epidemiology

Influenza epidemics are associated with high morbidity and mortality, mostly in the form of pneumonia, influenza-associated hospitalizations, and deaths. Mortality is generally highest among older adults, although infants and young children have significant morbidity due to influenza-related hospitalizations and secondary complications such as otitis media and pneumonia. Groups at increased risk for complications due to influenza are (1) children <5 years of age, (2) pregnant women, (3) persons ≥65 years of age, (4) residents of nursing homes and chronic care facilities, and (5) adults and children with chronic respiratory conditions (such as asthma and cystic fibrosis), sickle cell disease and other hemoglobinopathies, immunosuppressive disorders or therapies, human immunodeficiency virus (HIV), hemodynamically significant cardiac disease, chronic metabolic conditions such as diabetes mellitus, chronic renal dysfunction, neurologic conditions that can compromise respiratory function or handling of respiratory secretions, and patients on long-term aspirin therapy.

Influenza occurs worldwide. In tropical regions it is prevalent year round; in temperate climates epidemics occur almost exclusively in the winter. In the United States, the season is generally between late November and early March. Changes in the antigenic subtypes of the virus cause variations in epidemiologic patterns. This antigenic variation occurs by 2 processes: antigenic drift and antigenic shift. Antigenic drift is due to point mutations in the HA and NA glycoproteins and occurs in both influenza A and B. Antigenic shift occurs only in influenza A and is due to a novel and significantly different subtype of HA or NA that circulates in an animal reservoir and enters a human population without pre-existing immunity. These changes in the antigenic subtypes cause different epidemiologic patterns in the community. Antigenic drifts are associated with localized outbreaks, whereas antigenic shifts are associated with epidemics and pandemics of influenza A. The 3 most infamous outbreaks were the 1918 Spanish influenza, the 1957 Asian influenza, and the 1968 Hong Kong influenza.

### Transmission/Pathophysiology

Transmission is likely person-to-person by small-particle aerosols (<10 μm mass median diameter) via sneezing, coughing, or talking. The primary site of infection is the tracheal epithelium; the virus then spreads to the upper respiratory tract or lungs. The incubation period is 24 to 72 hours; levels of virus peak within 24 hours of onset of replication and then slowly decrease over 4 to 5 days.

### Clinical Findings

Disease severity varies from uncomplicated cases to those that are severe and life threatening. Uncomplicated, or classic, influenza begins with the abrupt onset of symptoms after a 1- to 2-day incubation period. Patients have fever, chills, headache, myalgia, malaise, anorexia, arthralgia, and dry cough. Respiratory symptoms such as rhinorrhea, nasal congestion, and sore throat are present but are generally overshadowed by the systemic symptoms during the first 3 days of illness. The cough is initially dry and hacking and changes to a productive cough later in the illness. Pain in eye muscles with lateral gaze, tearing, burning, and photophobia may also occur. Fever and systemic symptoms usually last 3 to 4 days. Fever is the most important sign and may be as high as 104°F (40°C) within 12 hours of onset and is usually continuous. A clear nasal discharge, hyperemia of the throat, and a normal chest examination are usually observed. Transient rhonchi or localized rales are sometimes auscultated. Influenza B is thought to be milder than influenza A. Influenza C, when it occurs, causes an afebrile "common cold."

Complications of influenza include more severe pulmonary disease, either directly from influenza or related to a secondary bacterial infection. Organisms most commonly implicated are *Staphylococcus aureus*, *Streptococcus pneumoniae*, *Streptococcus pyogenes*, and *Haemophilus influenzae*.[2] Nonpulmonary complications include:

- Myositis—myoglobinuria and elevated creatine phosphokinase (CPK)
- Cardiac—myocarditis and pericarditis
- Toxic shock syndrome—viral infection changes colonization and replication of toxin-producing *Staphylococcus aureus or Group A Streptococcus*
- Central nervous system (CNS)—Guillain-Barré syndrome, transverse myelitis, encephalitis
- Reye syndrome—mental status changes due to encephalopathy; seen in children given aspirin as an antipyretic

In April 2009, a new influenza virus (initially called "swine flu") was detected in an outbreak in Mexico, with subsequent spread to the United States and other countries in the world, prompting the WHO to call this outbreak a pandemic. This novel swine-origin influenza A (H1N1) virus represented a quadruple reassortment of 2 swine strains, 1 human strain, and 1 avian strain of influenza. Based on ongoing data from the WHO, transmissibility and the secondary attack rate of this strain seemed to be higher than for seasonal influenza. The incubation period ranged from 1 to 7 days with an average of 4 days. The signs and symptoms of influenza caused by novel H1N1 are similar to those of seasonal influenza. Symptoms consist of fever, cough, sore throat, malaise, and headache. Vomiting and diarrhea were also common, which are unusual features of seasonal influenza.

Most cases in the United States have been mild, although some patients required hospitalization and some deaths occurred. Data from the Centers for Disease Control and Prevention (CDC) show that the 2009 novel H1N1 flu caused greater disease burden in people younger than 25 years of age, rather than an older population as seen during seasonal influenza. This was thought to be due to pre-existing immunity among those older than 60 years against antigenically similar influenza viruses that have circulated in the past. Complications of novel H1N1 viral infection were similar to seasonal influenza. Laboratory confirmation was made by real-time (reverse transcriptase—polymerase chain reaction [RT-PCR]) on nasal aspirates or nasopharyngeal swabs. Based on limited data, the sensitivity of rapid antigen testing for detection of H1N1 was probably similar to or lower than that for seasonal influenza. Treatment is reserved for those who were hospitalized and those with high-risk medical conditions. A new H1N1 vaccine was manufactured, becoming available to the public in the fall of 2009. This, likely along with the natural progression of the epidemic, resulted in a dimunition of cases by the end of 2009. Current information and updated recommendations regarding the novel H1N1 virus remain available at the CDC Web site (www.cdc.gov/h1n1flu/).

Avian influenza virus refers to influenza A virus found chiefly in birds, but infections with these viruses have occurred in humans. The pandemics of 1957 and 1969 were due to new viruses that contained components of human and avian genomes. More recently, an avian influenza A H5N1 virus subtype has been responsible for infections in birds (poultry) and has caused more than 400 cases of infections in humans since 2004. Most of these cases have been reported from Asia and Europe and have occurred in those who have close contact with H5N1-infected poultry or H5N1-contaminated surfaces. Human-to-human spread has been limited and inefficient but has occurred rarely. However, there is concern that this virus can mutate and one day cause more efficient transmission and result in a pandemic. Symptoms of avian influenza in humans have ranged from typical human influenza-like illness (fever, cough, sore throat, muscle aches) to eye infections, pneumonia, and severe respiratory distress.

### Treatment

The Advisory Committee on Immunization Practices (ACIP) of the CDC states that the most effective way of preventing influenza is through annual vaccination. Each year the vaccine is reformulated and strains are derived from the H3N2, H1N1, and B strains most likely to circulate in the upcoming season.

Two types of vaccine are available in the United States: the trivalent inactivated vaccine (TIV) and the live attenuated influenza vaccine (LAIV). Trivalent inactivated vaccine is a noninfectious, semipurified split of viral proteins given intramuscularly. Live attenuated influenza vaccine is a live, attenuated viral vaccine administered intranasally. It has the same trivalent antigenic composition of TIV but is cold adapted. It is designed to replicate in the cooler nasopharynx and is approved for healthy, nonpregnant persons ages 2 to 49.

The newest **recommendations** for annual seasonal influenza vaccination are vaccination of (1) all children aged 6 months to 18 years of age, (2) household contacts and out-of-home caregivers of children 0 to 59 months of age and adults 50 years of age or older, (3) household contacts and caregivers of those with underlying medical conditions that place them at increased risk for influenza complications, (4) people 19 to 49 years of age with chronic medical conditions who are at increased risk of severe complications, (5) persons ≥65 years of age, (6) residents of nursing homes and chronic care facilities, (7) pregnant women, (8) siblings of high-risk patients of any age and children 0 to 59 months of age, and (9) children who are members of households with high-risk adults.[3] A recent change for health care professionals in contact with patients in the hospital, outpatient care settings, or chronic care facilities will be a yearly influenza vaccination requirement. More information on the influenza vaccine and annual updates are available at the CDC Web site: www.cdc.gov/flu.

There are 2 classes of medication to prevent or treat influenza. The first class of drugs are the M2 channel inhibitors, which are active only against influenza A. The 2 drugs in this class are amantadine and rimantidine. However, recent reports of resistance have limited their use.[4] The other class of drugs are the neuramidase inhibitors, which are active against influenza A and B. The 2 drugs in this class are oseltamivir and zanamivir. This is the class of drugs currently being recommended, although resistance has been reported now for this class of therapy as well, particularly oseltamivir resistance for seasonal influenza A (H1N1).[5,6] Use of oseltamivir for treatment of influenza A (H3N2) or influenza B is recommended, but combination therapy is needed if the decision to treat is made for influenza A (H1N1). The CDC Web site contains more details and regular updates on medication use. Oseltamivir (Tamiflu) is an oral medication approved for children >1 year and adults. Zanamivir (Relenza) is an intranasal medication approved for healthy adolescents and adults (see Table 136-2 for dosing).

## RHINOVIRUS AND CORONAVIRUS

Rhinovirus and coronavirus are the most common viruses implicated in the "common cold."

### Microbiology

Rhinovirus is a single-stranded RNA virus belonging to the Picornavirus family. There are more than 100 different serotypes. Rhinovirus derives from the Latin word "rhino" meaning nose. Coronavirus is an enveloped, non-segmented, single-stranded, positive-sense RNA virus. There are a number of serogroups; the most common serogroups causing clinical diseases are serogroups OC43, NL63, HKU1, and 229E. Coronavirus gets its name from its "corona" or crown-like surface spike proteins.

### Epidemiology/Transmission

Rhinoviruses are found throughout the year and worldwide, peaking with children's return to school in September.[7] Coronaviruses occur throughout the year, but epidemics are seen in the winter and spring months.[8-10]

Infection in both viruses is generally limited to the respiratory tract epithelium of the nose and pharynx, but rhinovirus can also infect the lower respiratory tract. In addition, like with respiratory syncytial virus (RSV), rhinovirus has been associated with asthma exacerbations.[11]

Rhinovirus transmission is person-to-person with self-inoculation of nasal mucosa or conjunctiva with infected secretions on hands; aerosol spread may occur, but sneezing and coughing are generally inefficient means of transmission. Coronavirus transmission is similar, with person-to-person or infected fomite contact followed by self-inoculation.

### Clinical Manifestations

Rhinovirus causes nasal congestion or rhinorrhea, pharyngitis, and cough. On physical examination there may be mild erythema of the nasal mucosa and pharynx. Inflammatory mediators like cytokines and chemokines contribute to symptomatology but are also responsible for limiting viral replication. The course of illness generally lasts 5 to 7 days in adults and 10 to 14 days in children. Rhinovirus has also been implicated in lower respiratory tract illness, especially in immunocompromised individuals.

Coronavirus infection is generally a respiratory illness, although in more than 50% of cases, people are asymptomatic. There has been debate over coronavirus as a cause of gastroenteritis. In older children and adults, coronavirus-like agents have been found in stools of both asymptomatic patients and those with diarrhea.[12] Coronavirus has also been identified as the cause of severe acute respiratory syndrome (SARS), recognized first in China in 2002. Severe acute respiratory syndrome is characterized by fever, headache, malaise, and myalgia, but upper respiratory symptoms do not occur. Twenty-five percent of patients have diarrhea. About a quarter of patients go on to develop severe disease that progresses to acute respiratory distress syndrome (ARDS). Although SARS spread worldwide in 2002, the WHO response program that was instituted helped lead to cessation of transmission by June 2003. Control measures and treatment are being studied should another epidemic occur.

### Treatment

Treatment of rhinovirus and coronavirus infections is supportive.

## PARAINFLUENZA VIRUSES

### Microbiology

Parainfluenza virus (PIV) is a pleomorphic-enveloped, single-stranded, negative-sense RNA virus with nonsegmented genomes coated with nucleocapsid protein. Parainfluenza virus belongs to the family Paramyxoviridae. There are 4 serotypes (1-4; with 2 antigenic subtypes of PIV 4, 4A, and 4B).

### Epidemiology/Transmission

There is seasonal variability for the 4 serotypes: parainfluenza 1—autumn; 2—variable; 3—spring and summer but can extend into autumn; 4—sporadic. Reinfections are common and most people have been infected with types 1-3 universally by age 5.

The incubation period is 2 to 6 days. Infection occurs by contamination of hands with secretions followed by autoinoculation. Infection starts in the nasal mucosa and upper respiratory tract but may infect the lower tract.

### Clinical Manifestations

There are a variety of respiratory illnesses. Most of the infections are manifested as upper respiratory tract infections. Symptoms include rhinorrhea, sneezing, pharyngitis, laryngitis, and occasionally cough. Pneumonia is uncommon in those without HIV. Risk factors for progressive infection include a bone marrow transplant within the previous 100 days, substantial myelosuppression, or relapse of a malignancy.[13] Otitis media is a common complication.[14] Rare cases of myopericarditis, encephalitis, and aseptic meningitis have been reported due to PIV.[15-17]

### Treatment

Treatment is supportive, and most infections are self-limited in healthy individuals. No antiviral treatment is approved for immunocompromised patients, but aerosolized ribavarin has been used with some success. See treatment of adenovirus in the following for more details on ribavarin.

## ADENOVIRUSES

### Microbiology

Adenovirus is a small, nonenveloped DNA virus in the family Adenoviridae (adenos is the Greek word for "gland," as the virus was first isolated from adenoid tissue). There are 51 serotypes characterized into 6 subgroups, A-F, based on different patterns of HA. The virus readily infects human epithelial cell lines with a characteristic cytopathic effect.

### Epidemiology/Transmission

The virus has been reported worldwide and infections occur throughout the year. It has a high prevalence and is associated with outbreaks in day care centers, summer camps, military barracks, and swimming pools. Nosocomial infection can occur. Transmission occurs via aerosol droplets, the fecal-oral route from person-to-person, and by contaminated fomites. Development of serotype-specific neutralizing antibodies protects against each specific serotype, but no cross-reactivity occurs.

### Clinical Features

Infection in the adolescent age group is generally manifested as a respiratory infection (upper respiratory infection [URI] or bronchitis) or an ocular infection (viral conjunctivitis). Infections in general manifest as follows:

- Respiratory and ocular infections. Respiratory tract infections can be of the upper or lower tract. Upper respiratory infections include symptoms of fever, coryza, and pharyngitis/tonsillitis. Lower respiratory infections include symptoms of fever and cough, clinically evident as bronchiolitis, bronchitis, laryngotracheobronchitis, or pneumonia. In addition, adenovirus can mimic pertussis with a paroxysmal cough, fever, and vomiting. Ocular infections include acute hemorrhagic conjunctivitis marked by subconjunctival hemorrhage, chemosis, fever, and periauricular lymphadenopathy. Epidemic keratoconjunctivitis can be another manifestation with keratitis, headache, pharyngitis, periauricular lymphadenopathy, and fever. Most common is pharyngoconjunctival fever, presenting with fever, coryza, conjunctivitis, adenopathy, headache, pharyngitis (which may be exudative), and sometimes a rash.
- Gastrointestinal and genitourinary infections. Gastroenteritis with vomiting and diarrhea can be caused by adenoviral serotypes 3, 5, 7, 31, 40, or 41. Abdominal pain can be significant and may mimic appendicitis or cause a mesenteric adenitis or intussusception. Cystitis (usually hemorrhagic), nephritis, urethritis, orchitis, cervicitis, and ulcerative genital lesions may occur. Stool and urine can be sent for adenovirus antigen.
- Cardiac and neurologic infections. Cardiac disease can include myocarditis and pericarditis. Central nervous system infections include meningitis, encephalitis, and Reye syndrome.
- Infections in immunocompromised hosts. Respiratory disease can be severe and life threatening in immunocompromised patients. Hepatitis, hemorrhagic enterocolitis, cystitis, and severe disseminated disease can occur.

### Treatment

Most infections will resolve in healthy individuals. In immunocompromised patients, antiviral agents may be helpful. Two antiviral medications have been used with some success: ribavirin and cidofovir.

Ribavirin is a synthetic nucleoside analogue that interferes with viral messenger RNA. It has activity against many viruses including paramyxoviruses and adenoviruses. Aerosolized ribavirin has been used with success in immunocompetent patients with adenovirus, parainfluenza, and RSV (see below), but cost and concern about toxicity to health care providers has limited its use. Ribavirin may be considered, however, in immunocompromised patients, particularly those undergoing bone marrow or solid-organ transplant. Cidofovir is a nucleotide that in its active diphosphate form serves as a competitive inhibitor of DNA polymerase. It has been used in severe adenoviral infections and is given with probenicid to reduce renal toxicity. Adenoviral immunization is only available in military settings.

## RESPIRATORY SYNCYTIAL VIRUS

Respiratory syncytial virus is the most commonly identified respiratory viral infection and mostly presents as bronchiolitis or pneumonia in young infants. By 24 months of age, most children have been infected. Infection in adolescents is uncommon.

### Microbiology

The name of the virus is derived from its ability to form syncytia in tissue culture and its predilection for the respiratory tract. It belongs to the family Paramyxoviridae and the genus Pneumovirus. It has a single-stranded RNA genome and encodes at least 10 proteins. Fusion (F) and attachment (G) glycosylated surface proteins are targets for host immune response. There are 2 subgroups, A and B.

### Epidemiology/Transmission

Respiratory syncytial virus infections occur in the winter and early spring. Though most children are infected at a young age, repeated infections are common and can occur in adulthood. Most infections are symptomatic, usually with URI symptoms. Risk factors for infection include exposure to cigarette smoke, larger number of siblings, lower socioeconomic status, day care attendance, family history of asthma, certain ethnic groups, and absence of breastfeeding.[18] Exposure occurs through contact with infected children or adults. Direct spread occurs via contact with contaminated surfaces, as demonstrated in a study by Hall et al.[19] The incubation period is 5 days; viral shedding lasts about 1 week, but can be longer in immunocompromised patients. Nosocomial infections have been reported.

### Clinical Manifestations

In infancy, infections are manifested as bronchiolitis, pneumonia, upper respiratory infections (URI), croup, apnea, and otitis media. In older children and adults, URI, bronchitis, and pneumonia (especially in the elderly) are commonly seen. Older children and adults may have rhinorrhea, pharyngitis, cough, and congestion lasting 7 to 10 days. The virus has rarely been associated with meningitis, encephalitis, cardiac dysfunction, or exanthems. There is a high mortality from RSV infection in infants with congenital heart disease or chronic lung disease, premature infants, and immunocompromised patients. It is unclear whether an RSV infection early in life leads to repeated wheezing and residual abnormalities in pulmonary function later in life.

### Treatment

Treatment is supportive. Aerosolized ribavarin (which is approved by the Food and Drug Administration [FDA] for treatment of RSV) has been used with some success in immunocompromised patients. Used alone, or in combination with palivizumab (Synagis), ribavirin has shown promise in recent trials.[20] Palivizumab is a humanized mouse monoclonal antibody that is currently given as a monthly intramuscular injection for high-risk infants and children as immunoprophylaxis.

## HUMAN METAPNEUMOVIRUS

Like RSV, human metapneumovirus (hMPV) is more common in infants and the elderly. Human metapneumovirus is a more recently recognized virus that causes respiratory disease.[21]

### Microbiology

Human metapneumovirus is a negative-sense single-stranded RNA virus of the Paramyxoviridae family, subfamily pneumovirus. It seems infection is limited to the respiratory tract, where viral replication occurs.

### Epidemiology/Transmission

Infection occurs in late winter and early spring in temperate climates,[22] which overlaps with RSV and influenza. Human metapneumovirus is most common in children younger than 2 years of age.[23] There have also been reports of hMPV in adults, particularly the elderly.[24] Transmission is believed to be similar to that of RSV, via respiratory droplets. The incubation period is 3 to 5 days.

### Clinical Manifestations

Human metapneumovirus may cause both upper and lower respiratory tract disease. Upper respiratory infections are marked by rhinorrhea, fever, and cough. Lower respiratory infections include bronchiolitis, croup, bronchitis, and pneumonia. Some patients may also have symptoms of rash, vomiting, and diarrhea. Some may develop otitis media. Symptomatic infection in young adults has been reported in 2.9 to 9.1% of cases.[25]

### Treatment

Treatment is supportive.

## DIAGNOSIS OF VIRAL RESPIRATORY INFECTIONS

Several methods are used to detect viruses to aid in the diagnosis of respiratory tract infections. The gold standard for viral detection is to obtain a culture of the virus from the respiratory tract. However, this method is time-consuming and has varying sensitivity, but good specificity. Generally, sensitivity is greatest early in the course of an acute illness. Several newer methods have evolved that utilize the presence of viral antigens or nucleic acid in respiratory secretions. Methods used to detect these antigens include various assays, such as enzyme immunoassay, direct fluorescent antigen assay (DFA—detects viral antigens on cell surfaces by using a fluorescent tagged monoclonal antibody), and latex agglutination tests. These tests are rapid and results are generally available within 24 hours. Some of these tests are commercially available to be used in office settings (ie, flu kit). Molecular techniques detect viral nucleic acids by nucleic acid amplification using PCR technology; these tests are more sensitive than culture but are very labor intensive and technically demanding. Although serologies are available for most of the viruses, they do not play a role in the acute setting and are generally not recommended. Seroconversion and a fourfold rise in titers are needed to establish a diagnosis.

Specimens for laboratory detection are generally obtained by either swabbing or washing the nasopharynx, swabbing the pharynx, or obtaining washes from the bronchus or trachea. Rarely, tissue from a lung biopsy can be used as a specimen. The methods available for the laboratory diagnosis of the common viral respiratory infections are summarized in Table 136-1.

**Table 136-1**

**Viral Diagnostic Methods**

| *Virus* | *DFA or EIA* | *Culture* | *PCR* | *Type of Specimen* |
|---|---|---|---|---|
| Influenza | + | + | + | NP, BAL |
| Rhinovirus | | | + | NP, BAL |
| Coronavirus | | | + | NP, BAL |
| Parainfluenza | + | + | + | NP, BAL |
| Adenovirus | + | + | + | NP, BAL, stool (antigen detection only) |
| RSV | + | + | + | NP, BAL |
| hMPV | + | | + | NP, BAL |

BAL, bronchoalveolar lavage; DFA, direct fluorescent antigen; EIA, enzyme immunoassay; hMPV, human metapneumovirus; NP, nasopharyngeal; PCR, polymerase chain reaction; RSV, respiratory syncytial virus

**Table 136-2**

**Antiviral Medications for Influenza Virus Infection**

| *Medication* | *Class of Drug* | *Coverage* | *Treatment Dose* | *Prophylactic Dose* |
|---|---|---|---|---|
| Amantadine (Symmetrel)[a] | M2 inhibitor | Type A only | 5mg/kg/day div BID for 3–5 days (ages 1–9) (max 150 mg) 100 mg BID for 3–5 days (ages ≥10 years) | Same as treatment but for 10 days |
| Rimantadine (Flumadine)[a] | M2 inhibitor | Type A only | Same as amantadine (only ≥18 years) | Same as amantadine, including age breakdown |
| Oseltamivir (Tamiflu) | Neuramidase inhibitor | Types A and B | ≥1 year:<br><15 kg: 30 mg BID<br>>15–23 kg: 45 mg BID<br>>23–40 kg: 60 mg BID<br>>40 kg: 75 mg BID<br>≥13 year: 75 mg BID<br>Total 5 days | Dosing as per treatment but only once daily for 10 days<br>*Household* setting (≥5 years and older): same dose as treatment but once daily for 10 days |
| Zanamivir (Relenza) | Neuramidase inhibitor | Types A and B | 2 inhalations (5 mg/inhalation) BID for 5 days (age ≥7 year)<br>Administer within 2 days of onset and on day 1 give 2 doses at least 2 hours apart | *Household* setting (≥5 years and older): same dose as treatment but once daily for 10 days<br>*Community* setting (adolescent age and older): same dose as treatment but once daily for 28 days |

[a] Should not be used in the United States secondary to resistance as per the Centers for Disease Control and Prevention; possible consideration in pandemic setting as combination therapy.

### TREATMENT OF VIRAL RESPIRATORY INFECTIONS

For most viral respiratory infections, treatment is supportive and the illness is usually self-limited. See the discussion of each individual virus for specific treatment options. Good hand washing and proper infection-control measures are the keys to prevention.

Table 136-3 summarizes the characteristics of respiratory viral pathogens.

## GASTROINTESTINAL INFECTIONS

Gastroenteritis is most commonly caused by 3 viral pathogens, caliciviruses (including Norwalk virus), rotavirus, and adenovirus.

### CALICIVIRUSES

#### Microbiology

Caliciviruses are nonenveloped, single-stranded RNA viruses. They are divided into 4 genera. The relevant human viruses are the Norwalk-like and Sapporo-like viruses. Caliciviruses were first recognized during an outbreak in school children in Norwalk, Ohio, in 1972.[26]

#### Epidemiology

Viral distribution is worldwide. Disease occurs in all age groups, and outbreaks have been associated with contaminated seafood or water. Norwalk virus has been the cause of gastrointestinal outbreaks on many cruise ships.[27] Outbreaks have also occurred in child care centers.[28] Transmission is person-to-person and by the fecal–oral route. Illness begins within hours to days and may last up to a week.

#### Clinical Manifestations

Fever, vomiting, diarrhea (often explosive), and abdominal cramping are features of the illness. Stools are generally loose or watery, usually without blood or mucous.

#### Diagnosis/Treatment

Stool samples generally lack leukocytes. Diagnosis could be suspected if associated with an outbreak. Most routine laboratories do not have methods to detect the virus.

**Table 136-3**

## Summary of Respiratory Viral Pathogens

| Virus | DNA vs RNA Virus | Serotypes | Incubation Period | Isolation | Common Clinical Manifestations | Diagnosis | Treatment |
|---|---|---|---|---|---|---|---|
| Adenovirus | DNA virus | 1–4 | Respiratory tract infection: 2–14 days | CONTACT and DROPLET precautions | Common cold, pharyngitis, tonsillitis, otitis media, pharyngo conjunctival fever | DFA<br>Culture<br>PCR<br>Serology | Supportive |
| Coronavirus | RNA virus | OC43229E NL63 | 2–5 days<br>SARS: 2–7 days | STANDARD precaution<br>SARS: AIRBORNE, DROPLET, and CONTACT precautions | Common cold; SARS-CoV: fever, malaise, myalgia, then cough, +/- URI symptoms | Not available; culture in research labs; PCR in future | Supportive |
| Human metapneumovirus | RNA virus | | 3–5 days | CONTACT precaution | Bronchiolitis, croup, pneumonia | DFA<br>PCR | Supportive |
| Influenza virus | RNA virus | A, B, C | 1–4 days | DROPLET precautions | URI (rhinitis, sore throat, nasal congestion), cough, fever, headache, myalgia, malaise<br>Rare: vomiting and diarrhea | Rapid test<br>DFA<br>Culture<br>PCR | Supportive<br>Neuramidase inhibitors (oseltamivir, zanamivir): see dosing table<br>Prevent with vaccination (TIV or LAIV) |
| Parainfluenza virus | RNA virus | 1–4 | 2–6 days | CONTACT precautions (isolate immunocompromised patients with PIV-3) | Croup, URI, pneumonia, bronchiolitis<br>Rare: parotitis, aseptic meningitis, encephalitis | DFA<br>Culture<br>PCR | Supportive |
| Respiratory syncytial virus | RNA virus | A and B | 2–8 days | CONTACT precautions | Bronchiolitis, pneumonia in young infants and children<br>URI in older patients<br>LRI in elderly and immunocompromised patients<br>RAD exacerbations | Rapid test<br>DFA<br>Culture<br>PCR | Supportive<br>Ribavirin for immunocompromised patients<br>Palivizumab for high-risk infants (consult ID specialist) |
| Rhinovirus | RNA virus | | 2–3 days (up to 7 days) | STANDARD precautions and CONTACT precautions for hospitalized patients | Common cold, pharyngitis, OM, bronchiolitis, bronchitis, pneumonia, RAD exacerbation | Culture<br>PCR | Supportive |

DFA, direct fluorescent assay; LAIV, live attenuated influenza vaccine; LRI, lower respiratory infection; OM, otitis media; PCR, polymerase chain reaction; RAD, reactive airway disease; SARS, severe acute respiratory syndrome; TIV, trivalent inactive influenza vaccine; URI, upper respiratory infection

Diagnostic methods available at research labs include ELISA to detect viral antigen and RT-PCR to detect viral DNA in stool. Treatment is supportive.

### ADENOVIRUSES

Adenovirus can cause many clinical syndromes, including gastrointestinal disease. This is more common in infants. Transmission occurs from person-to-person by the fecal-oral route. Clinical signs and symptoms include fever, nausea, vomiting, diarrhea, and a mild respiratory viral illness. The most frequent serotypes are 3, 5, 7, 31, 40, and 41. Because children may shed the virus in the stool for months, it may still be detected despite resolution of symptoms. Adenovirus has been associated with appendicitis, mesenteric lymphadenitis, and intussusception. Hepatitis has been seen in patients with disseminated disease and in immunocompromised patients, for whom the disease may be fatal.[29-31]

To diagnose adenoviral enteric infections, stool can be sent for antigen detection for serotypes previously mentioned. Rapid diagnostic kits are available. Treatment is supportive. Antiviral therapy is not routine. The use of aerosolized ribavarin or intravenous cidofovir has been used in severely ill patients with underlying immunosuppression with limited success.[32]

### ROTAVIRUS

#### Microbiology

Rotavirus is a nonenveloped RNA virus with a double-stranded genome of the Rotaviridae family. The virus has the appearance of a hubbed wheel (*rota* in Latin) under electron microscopy, from which it gets its name. There are 7 antigenic groups (A–G). A, B, and C are associated with disease in humans. The virus is classified by serotype. This is based on 2 outer capsid proteins, VP4 protease-cleaved HA (P), and VP7 glycoprotein (G). P1A, P1B, and G types 1–4 are most common.

#### Epidemiology

Illness is most common in young children and most children are seropositive by age 4. Reinfection is common. Outbreaks occur in child care centers, and rotavirus is one of the most common nosocomial infections in children's hospitals. Peak incidence is in the winter. The epidemiology of the G types is complex, although G1, 2, 3, and 4 have been recovered in more than 90% of infections. The incubation period is 2 to 4 days, and infection lasts approximately 4 to 8 days.

#### Clinical Manifestations

Illness is associated with fever, vomiting, diarrhea, and respiratory tract disease, and can cause severe dehydration. Stools are generally soft to watery and usually lack blood or mucus.

#### Diagnosis

Fecal leukocytes are generally absent. Commercial assays for antigen detection in the stool are widely available. Most assays detect group A-specific antigens (mainly VP6 on the inner capsid, which is the major group-specific antigen). Rotavirus can also be detected by electron microsopy, nucleic acid techniques, or tissue culture.

#### Treatment

Care is supportive with special attention to maintaining proper hydration. A vaccine is currently available for infants (Rotateq, Rotarix).

Table 136-4 summarizes the characteristics of the gastrointestinal viral infections.

## VACCINE PREVENTABLE VIRAL INFECTIONS

### MEASLES

#### Microbiology and Pathogenesis

Measles is in the Morbillivirus genus of the Paramyxoviridae family with one serotype. It is also known as rubeola virus and contains a single-stranded, negative-sense, linear RNA genome. It is most infective during the prodromal period (7–10 days after exposure) through the fourth day after the rash appears. The virus enters via the nasopharynx, invades the respiratory epithelium, and then spreads to regional lymphatics. Cell-associated viremia occurs a few days after exposure. Approximately one week after infection a second viremia occurs and shortly thereafter disease is manifested as URI, fever, and rash. As humoral and cell-mediated immunity is activated after exposure, further viral replication and clinical illness resolves.

#### Epidemiology/Transmission

Measles is endemic worldwide and humans are the only natural host. Prior to the availability of vaccination, epidemic cycles occurred every 2 to 3 years in the United States, most often in late winter and early spring, and most frequently in crowded, urban areas. In developing countries, measles accounts for approximately one million deaths per year.[33,34] In the United States, vaccination programs have resulted in a significant decrease in reported cases since the vaccine was licensed in 1963. As a result of these successful vaccination programs, the United States was declared measles free in 2000.[35] Outbreaks continue to occur in unvaccinated patients; most of these are associated with importation.[36] The number of cases in the United States doubled (to 131 cases) between January and July of 2008 as compared with the prior 7 years.[37] Among these, 17 (13%) cases were importations whereas an additional 99 (76%) cases were linked epidemiologically or virologically to importation. Most of

## Table 136-4

### Summary of Gastrointestinal Viral Infections

| *Virus* | *DNA vs RNA Virus* | *Serotype* | *Incubation Period* | *Exposure and Isolation* | *Common Clinical Manifestations* | *Diagnosis* | *Treatment* |
|---|---|---|---|---|---|---|---|
| Adenovirus | DNA | 40, 41, 31 | Gastrointestinal infection: 3–10 days | Enteric strains by fecal–oral route<br>CONTACT and DROPLET precautions | Gastroenteritis | Specific antigen detection from stool | Supportive |
| Caliviruses (includes Norwalk virus) | RNA | | 12 hours–4 days | Fecal–oral route, contamination of seafood and water<br>STANDARD precautions | Gastroenteritis (vomiting, explosive diarrhea, abdominal cramps), respiratory symptoms in one-third of patients | Based on outbreak with a common source, commercial assays not available | Supportive |
| Rotavirus | RNA | Seven distinct antigenic groups (A–G; A, B, C in humans) | 2–4 days | Direct or indirect contact with infected patients<br>STANDARD and CONTACT precautions | Vomiting, nonbloody diarrhea | Enzyme immunoassay or latex agglutination for group A antigen | Supportive |

these cases occurred in those <20 years of age who were unvaccinated or partially vaccinated.

Measles is transmitted by aerosolized particles from respiratory secretions of infected patients. The measles virus is highly contagious. Patients are contagious from 3 to 5 days before the rash and for 4 days after; therefore, airborne precautions should be in place until 4 days after the appearance of the rash.

### Clinical Manifestations

Measles is classically characterized by the three "Cs": **cough** (hacking or brassy), **coryza**, and nonpurulent **conjunctivitis**, which develop after an 8- to 12-day incubation period. Koplik spots develop within 2 to 3 days; they are typically located opposite the lower premolars, have been described as appearing like "grains of salt," and present for 12 to 72 hours. At the height of respiratory symptoms (generally 2 weeks after exposure and 2 to 3 days after appearance of the Koplik spots) the rash appears. It is an erythematous and initially macular or maculopapular rash that starts on the forehead or posterior occipital area and then spreads to the trunk and extremities within 3 days, becomes confluent, and eventually fades with fine desquamation. Disease severity is proportional to the extent and degree of rash confluence.[38] High fever, pharyngitis, and cervical adenopathy can occur; in developing countries, diarrhea also occurs. Leukopenia and marked lymphopenia are sometimes seen.

Measles can be mild, with a variable degree of symptoms of the classic presentation in those with some degree of passive immunity (such as babies with maternal antibodies to measles virus or individuals who received immune globulin). In the 2008 outbreak, 76% of cases were in children and adolescents; most presented with fever and a rash, and 91% of those infected were unvaccinated or had unknown vaccine status.[39] Adults, those who are malnourished, and immunocompromised patients can have more severe manifestations, including a higher incidence of complications such as bacterial superinfections and pneumonitis.

### Immunization

The vaccine currently licensed in the United States is the Moraten strain of live-attenuated measles. It was originally given as one dose. However, in 1990 there was a measles outbreak partly due to the fact that there is primary immunization failure in some adolescents. This prompted institution of a 2-dose regimen. The first dose is given at 12 to 15 months of age and the second dose is given between the ages of 4 to 6 years. Adolescents who have not received both doses require catch-up doses.

Measles vaccine is not recommended for pregnant women or those considering pregnancy within 3 months. It is contraindicated in immunocompromised patients, except those with asymptomatic HIV or those with symptomatic HIV who are not severely immunocompromised. Adverse reactions to measles vaccine include high fever in up to 15% of patients and transient rash in up to 5% of patients. The fever generally occurs 6 to 12 days after vaccination and usually persists for 1 to 2 days.

For those who are receiving the measles vaccine and a Mantoux test, the 2 should be placed at the same visit or the Mantoux test should be delayed at least 4 weeks. If a measles vaccine is given prior to the placement of the Mantoux test, the vaccine may inhibit the immune response to the Mantoux test and a false-negative result may occur.

### Diagnosis

Serologic tests help confirm the diagnosis. A fourfold rise or greater in antibody titer from paired sera or a single elevated immunoglobin M (IgM) is indicative of recent infection. The IgM antibody is detectable 1 to 2 days after onset of rash and lasts for 30 to 60 days. Measles can be isolated from blood, urine, and nasopharyngeal secretions.

### Treatment

Treatment is generally supportive. Ribavarin can be used in severely affected immunocompromised patients with pneumonia or encephalitis, but there are no controlled clinical trials and it is not approved by the FDA for those purposes. Vitamin A is given in developing countries to decrease complications such as diarrhea and pneumonia, in which the vitamin may act as an immunomodulator.[40–42] In the United States, vitamin A is given to children aged 6 months to 2 years of age who are hospitalized with measles and have complications and to those older than 6 months of age with immunodeficiency, Vitamin A deficiency, malnutrition, malabsorption, or recent immigration. The dose is 200,000 IU intramuscularly as a 1-time dose (100,000 IU for children 6 months–1 year); for those with ophthalmologic evidence of vitamin A deficiency, a repeat dose is given 24 hours later and at 4 weeks.

### Complications

Deaths from measles usually occur from encephalitis or pneumonia. The most common complication is otitis media (7%–9% of cases). Bacterial superinfection of the lower respiratory tract occurs in 1% to 6% of cases and accounts for significant morbidity and mortality.[43–45] Uncommon complications include thrombocytopenia, hepatitis, appendicitis, ileocolitis, pericarditis, myocarditis, glomerulonephritis, hypocalcemia, Stevens Johnson syndrome and toxic shock syndrome. In developing countries, mastoiditis, pneumonia, and diarrhea are the most common life-threatening complications. In developed countries, with the exception of encephalitis, most complications resolve without sequelae.

Measles can infect the CNS and may result in acute encephalitis, subacute sclerosing panencephalitis (SSPE), and subacute encephalitis in immunocompromised hosts. Acute encephalitis is generally mild and self-limited in most children. About one-fourth of survivors have long-term sequelae (seizures, hearing loss, developmental delay, and paralysis). Subacute encephalitis is a rare, slowly progressive disease that results in fatal neurologic deterioration. It manifests in the first decade of life usually between 4 to 8 years after measles infection; death occurs within 6 to 9 months after onset of symptoms.

### Prevention

Vaccine may provide protection if given within 72 hours of exposure. Those exposed need respiratory isolation from 5 to 21 days after exposure. Immunocompetent patients should be isolated until 5 days after onset of rash and immunocompromised patients should be isolated during the entire illness.

Immunoglobulin has been used to prevent or modify disease in susceptible contacts at high risk for complications (ie, infants <12 months of age, pregnant women, immunocompromised patients); it must be given within 6 days of exposure. The dose is 0.25 ml/kg IM (immunocompromised patients 0.5 ml/kg; max dose 15 ml).

Vaccine should be deferred if a patient receives immunoglobulin, depending on the indication for therapy.

## MUMPS

### Microbiology and Pathogenesis

Mumps virus is a member of the genus Rubulavirus in the Paramyxoviridae family. It is an enveloped negative-stranded RNA virus with an irregular spherical shape. Illness classically presents as unilateral or bilateral parotid swelling. Contact with infected respiratory secretions causes replication in the nasopharynx and regional lymph nodes. Primary viremia ensues and infection spreads to multiple organs.

### Epidemiology/Transmission

Infection occurs most commonly in the winter and early spring. Males and females are infected equally but males are more likely to have complications. The incubation period is 16 to 18 days (range 12–25 days). The most infectious period is 1 to 2 days prior to the onset of parotid swelling to 5 days thereafter; the virus is isolated from saliva 7 days before symptoms to 9 days after parotid swelling. Clinical and subclinical infection provides lifelong immunity; reinfection is rare. Mumps outbreaks continue to occur, with the largest reported in 2006, despite a high coverage rate with 2 doses of mumps-containing vaccine. Although the exact cause of this outbreak is unclear, failure of the 2-dose vaccine or a change in the virus have been postulated.[46]

### Clinical Manifestations

Subclinical or mild respiratory disease occurs in one-third of patients. The most common finding is parotid swelling, which can begin as unilateral and then become bilateral. Prodromal symptoms include headache, abdominal pain, and decreased appetite. Parotid swelling often blunts the angle of the mandible and lasts 7 to 10 days. The opening of the Stensen duct is swollen and erythematous. Trismus can occur.

Other salivary glands can be involved. In addition, a morbilliform rash may develop. Fevers last 3 to 5 days. Adults and adolescents have worse disease than young children.

Other entities that can result in parotitis and should be included in the differential diagnosis include: bacterial (supprative) parotitis, parotid duct stone, drug reaction, parotid tumor, Sjogren syndrome, and infection with other viruses, including coxsackievirus A, echovirus, parainfluenza virus 1 and 3, and HIV.

In the 2006 outbreak, parotitis was the most common clinical manifestation (92% of cases). Complications were reported in 5% of patients and 2% were hospitalized. Complications were more common in males and were mostly related to orchitis.[46]

### Complications

Mumps is a neurotropic virus. Somewhat fewer than 50% of patients have parotitis, and some patients have clinical evidence of meningitis or encephalitis.[47] Central nervous system involvement is more often diagnosed in males, with meningitis being more common than encephalitis. Systemic CNS symptoms usually occur 3 to 10 days after onset of parotitis and include headache, fever, lethargy, nuchal rigidity, delirium, and vomiting; seizures occur in 20% of patients.[48] The cerebrospinal fluid (CSF) profile demonstrates an increased white blood cell count with a lymphocytic predominance; protein is normal or elevated; glucose may be decreased in some patients; the pleocytosis can persist for prolonged periods. Disease is usually self-limited without sequelae, although behavioral problems, aqueductal stenosis with hydrocephalus, sensorineural hearing loss, paralysis, and retrobulbar neuritis can occur. Death occurs rarely in encephalitis cases.

Orchitis occurs in up to a third of males; the highest incidence occurs between 15 to 29 years of age, and it is uncommon in prepubertal males. Symptoms begin 4 to 8 days after the onset of parotid swelling; the orchitis is usually unilateral with associated epididymitis in most cases. Symptoms include fever, malaise, headache, vomiting, lower abdominal pain, and testicular pain. Treatment is supportive with bed rest, scrotal support, ice packs, and anti-inflammatory agents. Fifty percent recover completely and 50% have some testicular atrophy. Infertility occurs rarely, although decreases in sperm amount and motility have been described.

Other complications include glomerulonephritis, which is usually self-limited; reports of renal failure are rare. Arthralgia, polyarticular migratory arthritis, and monoarticular arthritis, with an onset 1 to 3 weeks after parotitis, can occur; joint symptoms are more common in males and usually involve the large joints. Myocarditis can occur in a small number of patients, more often adults, and resolves in 2 to 4 weeks. Mumps pancreatitis is poorly defined and a possible role in insulin-dependent diabetes is yet unclear.

### Diagnosis

Mumps should be suspected in any patient with parotid swelling for more than 2 days without an apparent cause. An increased serum amylase can be detected in the first week, with a low or normal white blood cell count, generally demonstrating a lymphocytosis. A definitive diagnosis depends on isolation of the virus, a rise in specific antibodies, viral antigen detection, or a positive PCR. Suitable specimens include a swab of the pharynx or the area near the duct of Stenson, CSF, and urine. A rise in IgG between the acute and convalescent titers or a positive IgM antibody test also can confirm the diagnosis.

### Treatment and Prevention

Treatment is supportive. Infected individuals are considered noninfectious 9 days after the onset of the parotid swelling. Droplet precautions are necessary for hospitalized patients. Neither vaccine nor immunoglobulin are beneficial as postexposure prophylaxis.

### Mumps Vaccine

Mumps vaccine is a live, attenuated virus of the Jeryl Lynn strain. It was first licensed in 1967. Universal vaccination began in 1977. Neutralizing antibodies develop in >90% of recipients. There are lower neutralizing antibodies after vaccine versus natural infection, but vaccine-induced immunity is long-lasting. Outbreaks in highly vaccinated populations are thought to be due to primary vaccine failure or, less commonly, waning immunity. Protective efficacy of the vaccine is 91%. A multistate outbreak of mumps that occurred among college students in 2006 prompted changes in the guidelines for college entry, requiring documentation of 2 doses of measles-mumps-rubella (MMR) vaccination.[49]

The vaccine is a 2-dose series given subcutaneously to children at 12 months of age and again at 4 to 6 years of age. Adverse reactions secondary to gelatin or the neomycin component are uncommon; anaphylaxis is rare. A temporal association with fever, febrile seizures, meningitis, encephalitis, orchitis, and parotitis is extremely rare. There are theoretical risks to a fetus, so pregnant women should not be immunized and conception should be avoided up to 3 months after vaccination. The vaccine can be given to children whose mothers are pregnant. Most children with egg allergy can be immunized. Immunoglobulin interferes with the serologic response to live-attenuated vaccines; hence, the mumps vaccine should be given either 2 weeks before or 3 months after receipt of immunoglobulin or a blood transfusion, and longer for those who received higher doses of immunoglobulin. Immunization should not be given to those with most immunodeficiency diseases, or those on immunosuppressive therapy. A patient can receive the vaccine if off immunosuppressive therapy for 3 months and the underlying disease is in remission. It can be given to patients with HIV, unless the patient is severely immunocompromised. The next dose should be given as early as 4 weeks later to induce seroconversion as early as possible. Contacts of immunocompromised patients can be vaccinated, as vaccine recipients do not transmit attenuated virus.

## RUBELLA

### Microbiology

Rubella virus is the only member of the Rubivirus genus of the Togavirus family. It is a spherical virus with a single-stranded positive-sense RNA genome. In general, rubella is a benign, self-limited viral illness. It is classically characterized by an exanthem and lymphadenopathy, although it frequently can be asymptomatic. Congenital rubella syndrome is a more devastating illness, however, characterized by growth retardation, deafness, congenital heart disease, and mental retardation.

### Epidemiology

Infection generally occurs in late winter and throughout the spring. Rubella is endemic worldwide; general epidemics occur in 2- to 4-year cycles, with larger pandemics occuring in 6- to 9-year cycles. The pandemics that occurred in 1941 and 1963 increased knowledge about the virus worldwide, and rubella became a reportable illness in the United States in 1966. Vaccine licensure in the United States occurred in 1969.

Attack rates are 75% to 90% in close quarters, approaching 100% in household contacts. Prevalence has decreased dramatically since the introduction of vaccination, with an estimated current incidence of 0.06 to 0.09 per 100,000. In the prevaccine era, the highest attack rate was in children 3 to 9 years of age. Outbreaks now occur in susceptible groups that refuse vaccine, immigrants, or communities with large adolescent and young adult populations. Fortunately, because of vaccination, congenital rubella in the United States is now extremely rare. Only 4 cases were reported between 2001 to 2004.[50]

### Pathogenesis of Acquired Infection

The virus is likely transmitted by aerosolized particles from respiratory tract secretions of infected patients. Viral shedding begins 3 to 8 days after exposure and lasts about 11 to 14 days; those with rash are infectious from 5 days before until 6 days after the onset of the rash.

The virus attaches to and invades respiratory epithelium and spreads hematogenously to regional lymphatics, then to the rest of the reticuloendothelial system, followed by a second viremic phase. Within 8 to 14 days after exposure active replication occurs in the body. This is the maximum time of viral shedding; clinical symptoms appear with the development of a humoral immune response. Antibodies to viral antigens then develop.

### Pathogenesis of Congenital Infection

Placental and fetal infection occur after maternal infection in the first trimester at rates of 90% to 100%; the fetal infection rate drops to 20% by 16 weeks, but rises to 60% after 30 weeks and above. The rubella virus induces a generalized, progressive, necrotizing vasculitis, which leads to parenchymal hypoplasia and then the characteristic clinical findings. Other pathologic effects are focal inflammation, edema, and granulomatous changes. There is a varied clinical spectrum, with later disease including more focal defects in the eyes and auditory system.

### Clinical Manifestations of Acquired Infection

The incubation period from the onset of exposure to the exanthem is 14 to 21 days. There is a nonspecific prodromal period of 1 to 5 days before the exanthem appears, which is manifested as fever, eye pain, sore throat, arthralgia, and gastrointestinal complaints. Characteristic clinical findings are rash and suboccipital adenopathy; the rash usually begins on the face, spreads in a cephalocaudal manner within 24 hours, and then fades over 2 to 3 days. The rash is usually maculopapular but can be scarlitiniform, morbilliform, or macular; in adolescents it can sometimes be confused with acne.

Lymphadenopathy always occurs with rubella and lasts up to one week from the onset of the exanthem; the posterior auricular and suboccipital nodes are generally involved. Reinfection is uncommon.

### Clinical Manifestation of Congenital Infection

Congenital rubella infection is a chronic, progressive disease. Infection in the first 8 weeks leads to miscarriage in 20% of cases; among live births, the severity of the defects is inversely related to the gestational age at the time of maternal infection. Congenital defects occur in more than 80% of infants whose mothers were infected during the first trimester. These defects include sensorineural hearing loss, cardiac defects, retinopathy, cataracts, microphthalmia, psychomotor retardation, cryptorchidism and some delayed features including mental retardation, central language defects, immune complex disease, and hypogammaglobulinemia.

### Complications of Acquired Infections

The most common complication is arthropathy; it occurs in 20% of children and 75% of adults older than 30 years of age. Arthritis and arthralgia of multiple joints can occur 1 to 6 days after the onset of the rash, and can persist for a mean of 9 days. There is an association with rheumatoid arthritis. Acute encephalitis occurs in 0.02% of cases and is usually seen within 4 days of the onset of the rash; lumbar puncture shows mild pleocytosis ($<300/mm^3$ and $>50\%$ lymphocytes), a normal or slightly increased protein, and a normal glucose. Symptoms of peripheral neuritis are reported commonly. Rare, though reported, is SSPE as seen in measles. Thrombocytopenia with purpura occurs in 0.03% of cases, more often in girls; it is usually self-limited but can last months. Other rare complications include myocarditis, pericarditis, follicular conjunctivitis, hemolytic anemia, and hepatitis.

### Diagnosis of Acquired Infection

Commonly seen are leukopenia and a relative neutropenia. A fourfold or higher rise in antibody titer, or a single elevated IgM, indicates active infection. Hemagglutinin antibodies or the more sensitive enzyme immunoassays that detect rubella-specific IgA, IgM, and IgG, can be used. Rubella can be cultured from nasopharyngeal secretions and urine. Polymerase chain reaction detection has also been described.

### Diagnosis of Congenital Infection

There should be suspicion for congenital infection if a neonate has microcephaly, hepatosplenomegaly, ocular abnormalities, and thrombocytopenia (with or without the "blueberry muffin" rash of purpura and petechiae). The diagnosis of congential infection requires virologic or serologic confirmation. Rubella virus may be isolated for up to one year from the nasopharynx, the buffy coat of blood, the spinal fluid, and the urine of congenitally infected infants. Rubella-specific IgM can be measured in cord blood or neonatal serum. However, false positives can occur in the presence of rheumatoid factor or maternal IgG and false-negative reactions can occur if maternal infection occurred late in the pregnancy, so serial measurements are necessary. Blood should be drawn at 3 and 6 months and tested in parallel; the presence of rubella-specific HA inhibition antibodies or enzyme immunoassay antibodies is considered diagnostic.

### Treatment

No specific treatment is available. If congenital rubella syndrome is suspected, ophthalmologic, auditory, cardiac, and neurodevelopmental assessments are required. Children with acquired rubella should be excluded from school until 7 days after the onset of the rash; infants with congenital rubella are contagious for up to 1 year, unless viral studies are negative at or after 3 months of age.

### Rubella Vaccine

Universal vaccination of infants eliminates congenital rubella in subsequent generations. The first dose is given at 12 to 15 months of age and the second dose at 4 to 6 years of age; any adolescent who has not received 2 doses requires immediate catch-up (or serologic testing). Rubella vaccine is given as part of the MMR. The RA 27/3 strain of the live-attenuated rubella virus is immunogenic in 98% of recipients and probably confers lifelong immunity for up to 90% of vaccinees. It produces a mild, noncommunicable disease. Adverse reactions include rash, fever, and lymphadenopathy in up to 15% of recipients; joint pains occur in fewer than 1% of children, but as many as 25% of postpubertal women have arthritis and arthralgia after vaccination. Arthropathy can occur 1 to 3 weeks after vaccination and is transient. Rarely, thrombocytopenia, a transient neuropathy, and other CNS manifestations have been described. The vaccine should not be given to pregnant women or those considering pregnancy within 3 months. It should not be given to immunocompromised patients, but can be given safely to patients with HIV.

## HERPES INFECTIONS

The Herpesviridae family is divided into 3 subfamilies: Alpha-herpesviridae, Beta-herpesviridae, and Gamma-herpesviridae. They cause the clinical syndromes associated with herpes simplex virus (HSV) infection, human herpesvirus (HHV) infection, varicella zoster virus (VZV) infection, cytomegalovirus (CMV) infection, and EBV infection. These infections are divided as follows:

- Alpha-herpesviridae, genus simplex virus: HSV-1, HSV-2, HHV-8; genus Varicellovirus: VZV
- Beta-herpesviridae, genus Cytomegalovirus: CMV; genus Roseolovirus: HHV-6, HHV-7
- Gamma-herpesviridae, genus Lymphocryptovirus: EBV

This chapter will concentrate on HSV-1, HSV-2, and VZV.

## HSV-1 AND HSV-2

### Microbiology

In general, members of the Herpesviridae are linear double-stranded DNA viruses; replication occurs in the nucleus, latency follows primary infection, and potential for reactivation exists.

There are 2 types of HSV, types 1 and 2. They each can become latent after primary infection. The HSV-1 initially infects the oral mucosa in most cases and then establishes latency in the trigeminal nerve; HSV-2 initially infects the genital region in most cases and then establishes latency in the sacral ganglia.

### Epidemiology

Infections occur worldwide, and humans are the only reservoir. It is often difficult to determine the epidemiology because many infections are asymptomatic. However, primary HSV-1 infection tends to occur in infancy or childhood and primary HSV-2 infection tends to occur in adolescence or adulthood (in relation to sexual activity). Neonatal infections are not discussed in this chapter. Exposure consists of contact with infected mucocutaneous surfaces and secretions from a person with primary infection or a reactivation. Risk factors include socioeconomic status, age, race and geographic location.[51] Individuals of lower socioeconomic status have been found to have a higher incidence of disease by age 5 (⅓ versus ¼ in the middle class), which increases to three-fourths by adolescence.

Although HSV-1 causes oral infections most commonly, 15% to 30% of primary genital infections and 2%–3% of recurrent genital infections are caused by HSV-1.[52] Most HSV-2 infections are asymptomatic and account for the most shedding, and thus the greatest exposure, during these periods.[53]

### Pathophysiology and Immunity

Infection occurs when the virus enters through abraded skin or mucosal surfaces. Replication occurs at the site of inoculation and then likely along the sensory ganglia. Visible lesions occur with subsequent destruction of the epithelial cells. Inflammatory cells are recruited to the site and then healing slowly occurs. Disseminated disease can occur if the host is immunocompromised and viral replication is not controlled. In all individuals, the virus remains dormant in the dorsal root ganglia after control of the illness and the genome remains repressed unless the host's immune system is challenged by another infection, stress, hormonal changes, damage to the ganglia, and, in some cases, sun (ultraviolet light) exposure. Table 136-5 lists the clinical manifestations of HSV-1 and HSV-2 infections.

### Diagnosis

Obtaining a viral culture of the herpes virus is the most sensitive and specific means of diagnosis. Lesions can be unroofed and the base scraped with a cotton swab or mucosal lesions can be swabbed at the base with a cotton applicator; the material is then placed in a viral transport medium. The virus can grow in 24 hours if there is a high inoculum; growth will take longer if viral concentrations are low. For rapid diagnosis, a direct fluorescent antigen (DFA) can be performed using monoclonal HSV-specific antibodies. The DFA is 80% to 90% sensitive compared to culture.[54,55] A serologic diagnosis can be made using monoclonal antibodies to the glycoprotein G of HSV-2; it is more specific than DFA and is available commercially, but its utility in clinical practice is unclear.[56]

Herpes simplex virus detection by DNA PCR is an important diagnostic modality in cases of encephalitis, in addition to the electroencephalogram (EEG) and neuroimaging studies. The EEG may show temporal lobe spikes or characteristic paroxysmal lateralizing epileptiform discharges (PLEDs). Neuroimaging may be normal early in the disease process but later is marked by edema, focal disease, or hemorrhagic necrosis. Cerebral spinal fluid reveals pleocytosis with lymphocyte predominance. Elevated red blood cells may also be seen. Protein may initially be normal but increases later in the course of the infection.

### Treatment

Treatment is based on type of infection (primary versus recurrent) and location (mucocutaneous versus CNS). Refer to the following table for appropriate management. Medication can be used safely in pregnancy. Table 136-6 lists antiviral therapy for herpes infections.

## VARICELLA ZOSTER VIRUS

Varicella, more commonly known as chickenpox, is the primary infection caused by VZV. The infection becomes latent in the dorsal root ganglia and can reactivate, causing herpes zoster (shingles).

As with HSV-1 and HSV-2, infections occur worldwide and humans are the only reservoir. Prior to vaccination in the United States, 90% to 95% of children had VZV.

**Table 136-5**

**Herpes Clinical Manifestations**

| *Location* | *Primary* | *Reactivation* |
|---|---|---|
| Orolabial | **HSV-1** most common<br>Incubation: 3–4 days<br>Younger children: high fever, submandibular lymphadenopathy, vesiculo-ulcerative lesions on an erythematous base located on the palate, gingiva, tongue, lip, and face<br>Adolescents/Adults: fever, cervical lymphadenopathy, and pharyngitis with erythema, exudates, or ulcerative lesions in the posterior pharynx<br>**HSV-2** also possible in sexually active adolescents | Generally asymptomatic shedding<br>About one-third have recurrent disease<br>Usually milder<br>Related to trigger |
| Genital | **HSV-2** most common<br>Incubation: 7 days<br>Viral shedding: average of 11 days<br>Prodrome with headache, myalgias, and backache<br>Local burning pain, itching 1–2 days prior to outbreak<br>Lesions are vesicular, pustular, or ulcerative on labia, mons pubis, vaginal mucosa, or cervix (females) or shaft of penis (males)<br>Females can experience vaginal discharge and dysuria<br>Inguinal lymphadenopathy<br>Complications: aseptic meningitis, pharyngitis, visceral dissemination | Most asymptomatic<br>Usually mild<br>Generally few, localized lesions<br>Viral shedding shorter (4 days)<br>Less systemic symptoms |
| Cutaneous | **HSV-1:** *herpetic whitlow*, finger contamination from oral or genital secretions<br>Tingling, burning pain, erythema, and edema<br>Small vesicles and pustules that coalesce<br>Surgical intervention can make worse<br>**HSV-1:** *Herpes gladiatorum* in wrestlers or "scrum-pox" in rugby players related to close contact of abraded skin with infected oral secretions | Rare |
| Ocular | Keratoconjunctivitis: follicular conjunctivitis<br>Pain, photophobia, blurred vision, tearing, chemosis, periorbital edema, and preauricular lymphadenopathy<br>Skin involvement around eye<br>Corneal ulcers<br>**HSV-1** more common after neonatal period | About one-third of patients have recurrences over following 5 years<br>Can be severe and result in blindness<br>Unlikely |
| CNS | Encephalitis: fever, change in mental status, focal neurologic signs<br>Accounts for 10%–20% of viral encephalitis cases<br>Occurs more likely with reactivation than primary disease<br>Affects 5–30-year-olds and those >50 years old<br>Sequelae: seizures, cognitive impairments, behavioral disorders<br>Other: Bell palsy, trigeminal neuralgia, vestibular neuritis, temporal lobe epilepsy<br>Unusual: recurrent aseptic meningitis, brainstem encephalitis, acute disseminated encephalomyelitis (ADEM) | |

Epidemics occur during late winter and early spring. The transmission rate is high in households, 90%, versus 12% to 33% in classrooms or hospitals.[57] Herpes zoster in adults is a potential source of infection for those still susceptible. Transmission of VZV is by aerosol or contact with skin lesions, so isolation involves airborne and contact precautions. The incubation period is 14 to 16 days (range 10–21 days). It may be as long as 28 days

**Table 136-6**

## Antiviral Therapy for Herpes Infections

| *Type of Infection* | *Medication* | *Dose* | *Doses/Day* | *Route* | *Length of Therapy (Days)* |
|---|---|---|---|---|---|
| Orolabial | Acyclovir | 5 mg/kg | 3 | IV | 7 |
| | | 15 mg/kg (max 400 mg) | 4 | po | 5–7 |
| | Valacyclovir | 2,000 mg | 2 | po | 1 |
| | Famciclovir | 500 mg | 2 | po | 7 |
| Immunocompromised (Orolabial or genital) | Acyclovir | 400 mg | 5 | po | 14–21 |
| | | 5 mg/kg | 3 | IV | 7 |
| (HIV patients) | Famciclovir | 500 mg | 2 | po | 7 |
| (HIV patients); can also use for chronic suppressive treatment | Valacyclovir | 500 mg | 2 | po | 5–10 |
| Genital, primary | Acyclovir | 400 mg | 3 | po | 7–10 |
| | Valacyclovir | 1,000 mg | 2 | po | 7–10 |
| | Famciclovir | 250 mg | 3 | po | 7–10 |
| Genital, recurrent | Acyclovir | 800 mg or | 3 | po | 2 |
| | | 400 mg | 3 | | 5 |
| | Valacyclovir | 500 mg or | 2 | po | 3 |
| | | 1,000 mg | 1 | | 5 |
| | Famciclovir | 1,000 mg or | 2 | po | 1 |
| | | 125 mg | 2 | | 5 |
| Cutaneous | Acyclovir | 400 mg | 3 | po | 10 |
| Ocular | Trifluridine or Virdarabine ophthalmic drops | Refer patient to ophthalmologist | | | |
| Encephalitis | Acyclovir | 10 mg/kg | 3 | IV | 14–21 |

IV, intravenous; PO, *per os* (by mouth)

in patients who have received VariZIG or intravenous immune globulin. Herpes zoster has no seasonal predilection, as infection is due to individual reactivation; it is uncommon in children younger than 10 years old. There has been a dramatic decrease in the incidence of varicella because of licensure and use of the varicella vaccine in the United States. However, breakthrough cases of varicella have continued to occur at an average rate of 21.7 cases/1,000 person-years over an 8-year follow-up period.

Infection occurs when VZV infects the respiratory epithelial cells and then spreads to the lymphoid tissues that comprise Waldeyer rings. Primary viremia causes infection of reticuloendothelial organs, such as the liver and spleen, followed by secondary viremia that disseminates infection to the skin and other organs. During primary infection the virus reaches neurons in the sensory ganglia and establishes latency. IgA, IgM, and IgG antibodies are made in response to infection. T lymphocytes also play a critical role in fighting the infection, as those with cellular immunodeficiencies have more severe disease.[58]

Primary infection results in chickenpox. The rash is a generalized, pruritic, vesicular rash consisting of 250 to 500 lesions, appearing first on the face, scalp, or trunk. A distinguishing feature is that the lesions are at varying stages of development and healing. Patients may also develop fever, malaise, headache, and abdominal pain. Complications include bacterial superinfection, particularly by *Streptococcus pyogenes*, pneumonia, and CNS infection (aseptic meningitis, encephalitis, and acute cerebellar ataxia). Rarely, other complications can include hepatitis, nephritis, and arthritis. Reye syndrome was also seen in patients with chickenpox in relation to the use of salycilates, although that became less of a problem as the use of aspirin in children as a fever reducer was discontinued. Varicella is more severe in adolescents and adults. Varicella zoster virus pneumonia appears a few days after the rash; it usually resolves quickly but can result in interstitial pneumonitis and ultimately respiratory failure. Most breakthrough cases of chickenpox after vacination are mild, usually with fewer than 50 lesions. Herpes zoster is a vesicular eruption presenting in a dermatomal pattern. Usually the rash is preceded by tingling, burning sensation, or hyperesthesias. Complications include eye involvement and facial nerve palsies if the cranial nerves are involved. Postherpetic neuralgia is uncommon in children.

Prior to immunization, when chickenpox was seen more commonly, the diagnosis was generally made clinically. In healthy children, further work-up is seldom needed. In immunocompromised hosts, in which the diagnosis affects treatment and exposure decisions, a more definitive diagnosis may be required. Culture of VZV is the most definitive way to make the diagnosis, although it can be difficult to make a culture diagnosis and it can take 3 to 7 days to isolate the virus. Rapid diagnosis can be made by DFA detection using monoclonal antibodies. Polymerase chain reaction is used on CSF in the setting of CNS disease. Cerebrospinal fluid often reveals a mild pleocytosis (<100 cells/mm$^3$) and a slight elevation of protein with a normal glucose.[59] Use of serology, specifically IgM, to make a diagnosis can be challenging because of high rates of false-positive and false-negative results. IgG serology may be useful to establish previous immunity; however, these can be negative despite documented infection or vaccination.[60,61]

For those who require it, acyclovir is the treatment for varicella and herpes zoster. In adolescents and adults, oral agents like valacyclovir and famciclovir have been used in chickenpox and zoster.[62] Intravenous acyclovir is indicated for patients with immunodeficiencies (malignancy, bone marrow transplant, high-dose steroid therapy, congenital T-lymphocyte deficiencies, HIV), neonates in whom the mother had varicella within 5 days before and 2 days after delivery, and in patients with pneumonia or encephalitis. Treatment should begin within 24 hours. Dosing is based on underlying disease and age, as listed in Box 136-1.

Other alternative agents are listed in Table 136-7.

Varicella vaccine should be given to children and adults who are considered susceptible. Children age 1 to 13 years should get 2 doses at a minimal interval of 3 months between doses, whereas for those older than 13 years of age the minimal interval is 4 to 8 weeks. Vaccine is contraindicated in (1) those with a malignancy before chemotherapy has been discontinued for at least 3 months, (2) patients with symptomatic HIV, (3) those with congenital or acquired immunodeficiency, (4) patients on systemic immunosuppressive therapy, (5) patients with a blood dyscrasia, (6) those on high-dose steroids (≥2 mg/kg/day or 20 mg daily of prednisone for >1 month), (7) pregnant patients, (8) and anyone who has had anaphylaxis to any of the vaccine components. For further information please refer to the CDC Web site.

Passive antibody postexposure prophylaxis is available for those at high risk using VariZIG, a VZV immunoglobulin that is available through a research protocol. VariZIG is indicated after exposure for any pregnant woman or immunocompromised patient who does not have a history of varicella or varicella immunization; any newborn whose mother had varicella 5 days prior or 2 days after delivery; hospitalized preterm infants <28 weeks gestation or <1,000 grams, regardless of maternal history; and hospitalized preterm infants ≥28 weeks in whom the mother lacks a reliable history of disease or lacks antibodies to VZV. The dose is 1 vial (125 units/10 kg body weight; max 5 vials) given intramuscularly within 96 hours of exposure. Antiviral prophylaxis with acyclovir has been used but is generally not recommended.

Table 136-8 summarizes the characteristics of the herpes viruses.

## Box 136-1

### *Acyclovir Dosing*

Immunocompromised patients, neonates, and those with complicating pneumonia or encephalitis:

- <1 year: 30 mg/kg/day divided every 8 hours
- >1 year: 1.5 gm/m$^2$/day divided every 8 hours
- Given for 7 days or 48 hours after no new lesions appear

Healthy children, especially those >12 years, those with chronic skin conditions (ie, eczema), those with chronic conditions that may be exacerbated by VZV (ie, cystic fibrosis, other pulmonary diseases, diabetes, chronic salicylate therapy): 80 mg/kg/day divided every 6 hours for 5 days

Oral acyclovir can also be used for herpes zoster in healthy and immunocompromised hosts. For those at risk of dissemination dosing is 1.5 gm/m$^2$/day or 30 mg/kg/day divided every 8 hours intravenously usually for 7 days or 48 hours after new lesions appear

**Table 136-7**

**Treatment for Varicella Zoster**

| *Type of Infection* | *Host Status* | *Medication* | *Dose* | *Dose/Day* | *Route* | *Length of Therapy (Days)* |
|---|---|---|---|---|---|---|
| VZV | Normal host | Acyclovir | 20 mg/kg (2–12 years) | 4 | po | 5 |
| | | | 800 mg | 5 | po | 5–7 |
| | | Valacyclovir | 1,000 mg | 3 | po | 5 |
| | | Famciclovir | 500 mg | 3 | po | 5 |
| | Pneumonia or third trimester of pregnancy | Acyclovir | 800 mg | 5 | po | 5 |
| | | | 10 mg/kg | 3 | IV | 5 |
| | Immunocompromised | Acyclovir | 10–12 mg/kg | 3 | IV | 7 |
| Shingles | Normal host | Acyclovir | 800 mg | 5 | po | 7–10 |
| | | Valacyclovir | 1,000 mg | 3 | po | 7 |
| | | Famciclovir | 500 mg | 3 | po | 7 |
| | Immunocompromised host (not severe) | Acyclovir | 800 mg | 3 | po | 7 |
| | Not severe | Valacyclovir | 1,000 mg | 3 | po | 7 |
| | Not severe | Famciclovir | 500 mg | 2 | po | 7 |
| | Severe | Ayclovir | 10–12 mg/kg | 3 | IV | 7–14 |

IV, intravenous; PO, *per os* (by mouth)

## OTHER VIRAL INFECTIONS

### PARVOVIRUS B19

#### Microbiology

Parvovirus is a nonenveloped, isohedral, single-stranded DNA virus. Parvovirus is from the family Parvoviridae and a member of the Erythrovirus genus, as its replication occurs only in human erythroid progenitor cells. B19 is the only human antigenic type described.

Viremia occurs about a week after exposure, at which time patients have a nonspecific febrile illness. In those who are immunocompetent, IgM and IgG are produced as the viremia resolves. A second immune-mediated phase occurs 2 to 3 weeks after infection, at which time the typical rash, and an arthralgia or arthritis, may occur. Cytotoxicity results in decreased reticulocyte production and a subsequent decrease in the red blood cell count. This can be particularly problematic, resulting in aplastic anemia, in patients who have increased erythropoeisis due to hemolysis (such as those with sickle cell disease), those with blood loss and chronic anemia, and immunocompromised hosts who are unable to clear the infection.

#### Epidemiology/Transmission

Parvovirus B19, also known as fifth disease, is a common childhood illness. By age 15, approximately 50% of individuals have been infected, as evidenced by positive IgG titers.[63] Secondary attack rates are as high as 50% in household contacts. Transmission is by the respiratory route, probably by droplet spread, and highest at the time of viremia.

#### Clinical Manifestations

Most infections are asymptomatic or mild. The most common childhood form of the disease, fifth disease, also known as erythema infectiosum, is marked by mild fever and a rash. The rash has a lacy, reticular pattern and the classic "slapped cheek" appearance; it occurs when the viremia resolves. Another presentation of parvovirus infection, which occurs less commonly, is development of a rash known as the papular-pupuric gloves and stocking syndrome (PPGSS). This presentation is characterized by swelling and petechiae of the hands and feet with a mild fever and oral lesions.

Polyarthropathy syndrome, another possible presentation of parvovirus infection, is more common in

**Table 136-8**

**Summary of Herpes Viruses**

| *Virus* | *DNA vs RNA Virus* | *Incubation Period* | *Exposure and Isolation* | *Common Clinical Manifestations* | *Diagnosis* | *Treatment* |
|---|---|---|---|---|---|---|
| Herpes simplex virus-1 | DNA virus | 2 days–2 weeks | Mucocutaneous secretions and direct contact<br>STANDARD precautions | Most asymptomatic, gingivostomatitis, genital, eczema herpeticum, conjunctivitis, or keratitis, encephalitis<br>Recurrent cold sores, conjunctivitis, or keratitis, encephalitis | DFA<br>Culture<br>PCR<br>Serology | Supportive<br>Acyclovir<br>Valacyclovir<br>Famciclovir |
| Herpes simplex virus-2 | DNA virus | 2 days–2 weeks | Mucocutaneous secretions and direct contact<br>STANDARD precautions | Genital, oral, encephalitis | DFA<br>Culture<br>PCR<br>Serology | Supportive<br>Acyclovir<br>Valacyclovir<br>Famciclovir |
| Varicella zoster virus | DNA virus | 3–5 days | Highly contagious<br>Direct person-to-person contact, by contact with vesicular fluid or contact with lesions, or airborne by respiratory secretions<br>AIRBORNE and CONTACT precautions | Chickenpox; complications: pneumonia, acute cerebellar ataxia, encephalitis, bacterial superinfection of skin lesions<br>Reactivation: zoster ("shingles") | DFA<br>Culture<br>PCR<br>Serology | Supportive<br>Acyclovir if within 48–72 hours of symptoms<br>Pulmonary involvement<br>VariZIG<br>Prevent with vaccination |
| Epstein-Barr virus | DNA virus | 30–50 days | Close personal contact; occasionally by blood transfusion<br>STANDARD precautions | Fever, pharyngitis, lymphadenopathy, hepatosplenomegaly, rash if given ampicillin<br>Associated with other lymphoproliferative disorders and cancers | Heterophil antibody<br>Serology<br>PCR | Supportive |

(*Continued*)

**Table 136-8 (Continued)**

| *Virus* | *DNA vs RNA Virus* | *Incubation Period* | *Exposure and Isolation* | *Common Clinical Manifestations* | *Diagnosis* | *Treatment* |
|---|---|---|---|---|---|---|
| CMV | DNA virus | Horizontal transmission unknown<br>3–12 weeks after blood transfusion<br>1–4 months after tissue transplantation | Horizontal (direct person–person contact), vertically, or via transfusions<br>STANDARD precautions | Most asymptomatic, mono-like illness with fever and mild hepatitis<br>Pneumonia, colitis, & retinitis in immunocompromised patients<br>Congenital infection | Culture<br>PCR<br>Blood antigenemia | Supportive<br>Ganciclovir in immunocompromised patients |
| Human herpes virus-6 (HHV-6) | DNA virus; Serotypes A & B | ?, 10 days | Unclear, perhaps asymptomatic shedding from secretions<br>STANDARD precautions | Roseola<br>Mono-like illness, meningitis/encephalitis, seizures | PCR<br>Serology | Supportive |
| Human herpes virus-7 | DNA virus | 2–3 days (up to 7 days) | Unclear, perhaps asymptomatic shedding from secretions<br>STANDARD precautions | Similar to HHV-6 | PCR<br>Serology | Supportive |
| Human herpes virus-8 | DNA virus | | Sexual transmission via semen or saliva in United States, vertical, or possible nonsexual horizontal transmission | Usually asymptomatic<br>Manifestations of disease from reactivation:<br>Kaposi sarcoma (often HIV-associated) | PCR<br>Serology | For Kaposi sarcoma: irradiation, surgery, or chemotherapy<br>Reconstitution of immune system |

DFC, direct flourescent assay; PCR, polymerase chain reaction

adolescents and adults, with a female predominance. The joint distribution in this presentation is symmetrical, with arthralgia or arthritis affecting the small joints of the hands, ankles, knees, and wrists. Resolution generally takes a few weeks, but the joint symptoms can sometimes last on and off for years.

Transient aplastic anemia can occur in some patients, particularly those with hematologic disorders (ie, hereditary sperocytosis), hemoglobinopathies (ie, sickle cell disease, thalessemia), red cell enzymopathies (glucose-6-phosphate dehydrogenase deficiency, pyruvate kinase deficiency), and autoimmune hemolytic anemias. Pure red cell aplasia has been reported in immunocompromised patients. Temporary cessation of immunosuppressive therapies may be necessary for clearance of infection. Parvovirus can also cause transient neutropenia and thrombocytopenia and has been associated with the hemophagocytic syndrome. Idiopathic thrombocytopenia and Henoch-Schönlein pupura have been reported in rare cases after parvovirus B19 infection.

### Diagnosis

Culture is difficult so detection of the virus is usually done by molecular means (PCR) in addition to serology. IgM antibodies can be detected at the time of the rash or a few days into the aplastic crisis. IgG is usually present by the seventh day.

### Treatment

Treatment consists of supportive management. There are no antiviral treatments. Blood transfusion and IVIG have been used in immunocompromised patients with severe illness.

## ENTEROVIRUS

### Microbiology and Pathogenesis

Enteroviruses belong to the Picornaviridae family. The genus Enterovirus is subdivided into different classes and serotypes. The major subgroups are poliovirus serotypes 1-3, coxsackievirus A serotypes 1-24, coxsackievirus B serotypes 1-6, echovirus serotypes 1-34, and enterovirus serotypes 68-72. These viruses are single-stranded RNA viruses.

Infection with this virus occurs by the fecal–oral route or by secretions from the upper respiratory tract. The virus replicates in the upper respiratory tract or the small intestine. Virus is shed from the upper respiratory tract for 1 to 3 weeks after infection and from the feces for up to 8 weeks. Viral replication occurs in submucosal lymphoid tissues, resulting in a viremia with spread to other reticuloendothelial tissues. With continued replication, there is further dissemination to other organs, such as the heart, brain, and skin. The initial viremia is usually asymptomatic, but patients become symptomatic with dissemination to other organs and the subsequent inflammatory response of the immune system. The incubation period is 3 to 5 days for most enterovirus illnesses, but CNS manifestations of poliovirus may occur as long as 9 to 12 days after exposure.

Immunity is serotype specific. Neutralizing humoral antibodies represent past infection. Secretory IgA antibodies can be detected at mucosal sites of viral replication and appear 2 to 4 weeks after infection. These antibodies can also be found in the breast milk of immune mothers.

### Epidemiology

Enteroviruses result in 5 to 10 million infections yearly in the United States. Infections occur throughout the year but generally are most common in the summer and fall in temperate climates.[64] Infection occurs in all age groups but is most common in younger children.

### Clinical Manifestations

Most infections are asymptomatic. When symptoms occur, they vary based on the different serotypes. In general, presentation in the adolescent age group includes a nonspecific rash and aseptic meningitis.

Nonpolio enteroviruses are a common cause of nonspecific febrile illnesses, especially in children younger than 3 months of age. In young infants, the presentation of the illness may include lethargy, poor feeding, rash, vomiting, diarrhea, or an upper respiratory tract infection. Infants have an aseptic meningitis in about half of the cases. The illness generally resolves in 2 to 10 days without sequelae.

The enteroviruses can cause a broad range of different rashes. The rash may resemble that of measles, rubella, or roseola, and may be vesicular, petechial, purpuric, or urticarial. Echovirus is most commonly associated with rash. Hand-foot-and-mouth disease is an enteroviral illness characterized by a vesicular stomatitis (on the buccal mucosa and tongue) and a macular, papular or vesicular-like rash on the distal extremities (most commonly the hands and feet). The illness is most commonly caused by coxsackievirus A16 and enterovirus 71 and generally lasts about 7 days. Herpangina, an enanthem characterized by painful vesicular oral lesions, often accompanied by fever, headache, and sore throat, is another distinct illness caused by a variety of enteroviruses.

Enteroviruses are a common cause of aseptic meningitis, particularly in the summer and early fall. Group B coxsackievirus and the echoviruses cause most cases. Symptoms vary widely in adolescents and adults. The onset can be gradual or abrupt and is marked by fever, headache, and meningismus. Kernig and Brudzinski signs are present in only one-third of these cases. Generally the illness is uncomplicated, although a small percentage of

**Table 136-9**

**Summary of Other Viral Infections – Parvovirus and Enterovirus**

| *Virus* | *DNA vs RNA Virus* | *Serotypes* | *Incubation Period* | *Exposure and Isolation* | *Common Clinical Manifestations* | *Diagnosis* | *Treatment* |
|---|---|---|---|---|---|---|---|
| Parvovirus | DNA | | 4–14 days (up to 21 days)<br>Rash and joint symptoms occur 2–3 weeks after infection | Contact with respiratory secretions, percutaneous exposure to blood and blood products, vertical transmission<br>STANDARD precautions; DROPLET precautions for hospitalized children with aplastic anemia, PPGSS, or immunocompromised patients | Erythema infectiosum (fifth disease)<br>Asymptomatic infection<br>Papular-purpuric gloves and socks syndrome (PPGSS)<br>Polyarthropathy syndrome<br>Aplastic anemia | Serology<br>PCR | Supportive |
| Enterovirus | RNA | Group A and B coxsackie viruses, echoviruses, other enteroviruses | 3–6 days<br>24–72 hours for acute hemorrhagic conjunctivitis | Fecal–oral and respiratory routes, fomites, vertical<br>STANDARD and CONTACT precautions | Most common: nonspecific febrile illness or<br>1. Respiratory: cold, pharyngitis, herpangina, stomatitis, pneumonia, pleurodynia<br>2. Skin: exantham<br>3. Neurologic: aseptic meningitis, encephalitis paralysis<br>4. GI: vomiting, diarrhea, abdominal pain, hepatitis<br>5. Eye: acute hemorrhagic conjunctivitis<br>6. Heart: myopericarditis | Culture<br>PCR<br>Serology | Supportive |

PCR, polymerase chain reaction

hospitalized children may experience seizures, obtundation, or increased intracranial pressure.[65,66]

Encephalitis is caused by enterovirus in 10% to 20% of those cases proven to be viral in origin. In particular, patients with x-linked agammaglobulinemia can develop a chronic meningoencephalitis. Group A coxsackieviruses are most commonly isolated from infants and children with focal disease. A poliomyelitis-like syndrome is seen uncommonly but is characterized by acute weakness and paralysis that is clinically and pathologically indistinguishable from poliomyelitis. Other neurologic illnesses have been associated with enteroviruses, including Guillain-Barré syndrome and acute transverse myelitis.

Pleurodynia, an acute disease characterized by fever and sharp, spastic pain involving the intercostal and abdominal muscles, can occur with enteroviral infections. Pain or swelling of the affected areas may be noted. It usually lasts 4 to 6 days and analgesics may give patients some relief. Myositis can also occur, and can be focal or generalized. Myoglobinuria, myoglobinemia, and elevated CPK can be found. It is more common in adults.

Myopericarditis can also be caused by enteroviruses, particularly group B coxsackieviruses. Signs and symptoms may be that of pericarditis or myocarditis. It can occur in all age groups. Disease may result in congestive heart failure or cardiac arrhythmias. Fatalities are rare. Intravenous immunoglobulin and corticosteroids have been used with some proven benefit, but there have been no randomized control trials.

Enterovirus 70 and coxsackievirus A24 can cause hemorrhagic conjunctivitis, which is highly contagious and presents with eye pain, eyelid swelling, and subconjunctival hemorrhage. Infection may be accompanied by fever and headache. Conjunctival edema, follicle formation, punctuate epithelial keratitis, and preauricular lymphadenopathy are common. The signs and symptoms generally last a few days and resolve without residual eye problems.

Hepatitis and pancreatitis have been reported but are rare. Acute parotitis has also been reported.

### Diagnosis

The gold standard for diagnosis of the enteroviral infections is cell culture. The virus can be isolated from throat and rectal swabs, CSF, tissue, pericardial fluid, or blood.

Detection of enterovirus by PCR from CSF is more sensitive and rapid, and can also be used to detect virus in respiratory secretions, blood, urine, and cardiac tissue.

Serologic diagnosis is generally not used and often not well standardized.

### Treatment

Intravenous immunoglobulin has been used in myocarditis with some success. Pleconaril, an antiviral in the oxazoline class, has shown some benefit in the treatment of aseptic meningitis by decreasing the duration and severity of symptoms and shortening the duration of viral shedding,[67–69] but given the self-limited nature of the disease, it is not routinely used. Current trials are ongoing for use in enteroviral sepsis in infants. Good hand washing is prudent to avoid spread of infection.

Table 136-9 summarizes details of parvovirus and enterovirus infections.

## INTERNET AND PRINT RESOURCES

- *Principles and Practice of Pediatric Infectious Diseases* (2009) by Sarah Long, Larry Pickering, and Charles Prober
- *Textbook of Pediatric Infectious Diseases* (2009) by Ralph Feign and James Cherry
- *Red Book* by the American Academy of Pediatrics, updated every 3 years
- *Principles and Practice of Infectious Diseases* (2004) by Gerald Mandell, John Bennett, and Raphael Dolin
- Centers for Disease Control and Prevention: www.cdc.gov
- Infectious Disease Society of America: www.idsociety.org
- American Academy of Pediatrics: www.aap.org

## REFERENCES

1. Centers for Disease Control and Prevention. Flu activity and surveillance. Available at: www.cdc.gov/flu/weekly/fluactivity.htm. Accessed October 21, 2009

2. Bhat N, Wright JG, Broder KR, et al. Influenza-associated deaths among children in the United States, 2003–2004. *NEJM.* 2005;353:2559–2567

3. Fiore AE, Shay DK, Broder K, et al. Prevention and control of influenza. *MMWR.* 2008;57:1–60

4. Sato M, Hosoya M, Kato K, et al. Viral shedding in children with influenza virus infections treated with neuraminidase inhibitors. *Pediatr Infect Dis J.* 2005;24:931–932

5. Dharan NJ, Gubareva LV, Meyer JJ, et al. Infections with oseltamivir-resistant influenza A (H1N1) in the United States. *JAMA.* 2009;301:1034–1041

6. Centers for Disease Control and Prevention. Seasonal influenza. Available at: www.cdc.gov/flu. Accessed October 21, 2009

7. Gwaltney JM Jr, Hendley JO, Simon G, et al. Rhinovirus infections in an industrial population. I: The occurrence of illness. *N Engl J Med.* 1966;375:1261–1268

8. Kaye HS, Marsh HB, Dowdle WR. Seroepidemiologic survey of coronavirus (strain OC 43) related infections in a children's population. *Am J Epidemiol.* 1971;94:43–49

9. Kaye HS, Dowdle WR. Seroepidemiologic survey of coronavirus (strain 229E) infections in a population of children. *Am J Epidemiol.* 1975;101:238–244

10. Monto AS, Lim SK. The Tecumseh study of respiratory illness. VI: Frequency and relationship between outbreaks of coronavirus infection. *J Infect Dis.* 1974;129:271–276

11. Gern JE, Busse WW. Association of rhinovirus infections in asthma. *Clin Microbiol Rev.* 1119;12:9–18

12. Monroe SS, Glass RI, Noah N, et al. Electron microscopic reporting of gastrointestinal viruses in the United Kingdom, 1985–1987. *J Med Virol.* 1991;33:193–198

13. Englund JA, Piedra PA, Whimbley E. Prevention and treatment of respiratory syncytial virus and parainfluenza virus in immunocompromised patients. *Am J Med.* 1997;102(3A):61–70, discussion 75–76

14. Henderson FW, Collier AM, Sanyal MA, et al. A longitudinal study of respiratory viruses and bacteria of acute otitis media and effusion. *N Engl J Med.* 1982;306:1377–1383

15. Wilkes D, Burns SM. Myopericarditis associated with parainfluenza virus type 3 infection. *Eur J Clin Microbiol Infect Dis.* 1998;17:363–365

16. Arisoy ES, Demmler GJ, Thakers S, et al. Meningitis due to parainfluenza virus type 3: report of two cases and review. *CID.* 1993;17:995–997

17. Jantausch BA, Weidermann BL, Jeffries B. Parainfluenza virus type 2 meningitis and parotitis. *South Med J.* 1995; 88:230–231

18. Weisman LE. Populations at risk for developing respiratory syncytial virus and risk factors for respiratory syncytial virus severity: infants with predisposing conditions. *Pediatr Infect Dis J.* 2003;22:S33–S39

19. Hall C, Douglas RJ. Modes of transmission of respiratory syncytial virus. *J Pediatr.* 1981;99:100–103

20. Chavez-Bueno S, Meijas A, Merryman RA, et al. Intravenous palivizumab and ribavarin combination for RSV disease in high-risk pediatric patients. *Pediatr Infect Dis J.* 2007;26: 1089–1093

21. Van Den Hoogan BG, DeLong JC, Groen J, et al. A newly discovered human pneumovirus isolated from young children with respiratory tract disease. *Nature Medicine.* 2001;7: 719–724

22. Crowe JE. Human metapneumovirus as a major cause of human respiratory tract disease. *Pediatr Infect Dis J.* 2004;23:S215–S221

23. McAdam AJ, Hasenbein ME, Feldman HA, et al. Human metapneumovirus in children tested at a tertiary-care hospital. *JID.* 2004;190:20–26

24. Boivin G, De Serres G, Hamelin M-E, et al. An outbreak of severe respiratory tract infection due to human metapneumovirus in a long-term care facility. *CID.* 2007;44:1152–1159

25. Falsey AR, Erdman D, Anderson LJ, Walsh EE. Human metapneumovirus in young and elderly adults. *J Infect Dis.* 2003;187:785–790

26. Kapikian AZ, Wyatt RG, Dolin R, et al. Visualization by immune electron microscopy of a 27-nm particle associated with acute infectious nonbacterial gastroenteritis. *J Virol.* 1972;10:1075–1081

27. Isakbaeva ET, Widdowson M-A, Beard RS, et al. Norovirus transmission on cruise ship. *EID.* 2005;11:154–157

28. Matson DO, Estes MK, Glass RI, et al. Human calicivirus-associated diarrhea in children attending day care centers. *JID.* 1989;159:71–78

29. Bertheau P, Parquet N, Ferchal F, et al. Fulminant adenovirus hepatitis after allogeneic bone marrow transplantation. *Bone Marrow Transplant.* 1996;17:295–298

30. Somervaille TC, Kirk S, Dogan A, et al. Fulminant hepatic failure caused by adenovirus infection following bone marrow transplantation for Hodgkin's disease. *Bone Marrow Transplant.* 1999;24:99–101

31. Chakrabarti S, Collingham KE, Fegan C, et al. Fulminant adenovirus hepatitis following unrelated bone marrow transplantation: failure of intravenous ribavirin therapy. *Bone Marrow Transplant.* 1999;11:1209–1211

32. Munoz FM, Piedra PA, Demmler GJ. Disseminated adenovirus disease in immunocompromised and immunocompetent children. *Clin Infect Dis.* 1998;27:1194–2000

33. Centers for Disease Control and Prevention. Advances in global measles control and elimination: summary of the 1997 international meeting. *MMWR.* 1998;47(RR-11):1–23

34. Sabin AB. My last will and testament on rapid elimination and ultimate global eradication of poliomyelitis and measles. *Pediatrics.* 1992;90:162–169

35. Orenstein WA, Papania MJ, Wharton ME. Measles elimination in the United States. *J Infect Dis.* 2004;189(suppl 1): S1–S3

36. Centers for Disease Control and Prevention. Measles—United States 2004. *MMWR.* 2005;54:1229–1231

37. Centers for Disease Control and Prevention. Update: measles: United States—January-July 2008. *MMWR.* 2008;57:893–896

38. Maldonado YA, Lawrence EC, DeHovitz R, et al. Early loss of passive measles antibody in infants of mothers with vaccine-induced immunity. *Pediatrics.* 1995;96:447–450

39. Grigg MA, Brzezny AL, Dawson I, et al. Update measles—United States, January-July 2008. *MMWR.* 2008;57:893–896

40. Sommer A. Vitamin A, infectious disease, and childhood mortality: a 2 cent solution? *J Infect Dis.* 1993;167:1003–1007

41. Cantorna MT, Nashold FE, Hayes CE. In vitamin A deficiency multiple mechanisms establish a regulatory T helper cell imbalance with excess Th1 and insufficiency Th2 function. *J Immunol.* 1994;152:1515–1522

42. Rumore MM. Vitamin A as an immunomodulating agent. *Clin Pharm.* 1993;12:506–513

43. Makhene MK, Diaz PS. Clinical presentations and complications of suspected measles in hospitalized children. *Pediatr Infect Dis J.* 1993;12:836–840

44. Mason WH, Ross LA, Lanson J, et al. Epidemic measles in the postvaccine era: evaluation of epidemiology, clinical presentation, and complications during an urban outbreak. *Pediatr Infect Dis J.* 1993;12:42–48

45. Gremillian DH, Crawford GE. Measles pneumonia in young adults. An analysis of 106 cases. *Am J Med.* 1981;71: 539–542

46. Dayan GH, Quinlisk MP, Parker AA, et al. Recent resurgence of mumps in the United States. *NEJM.* 2008;308: 1580–1589

47. Bang HA, Bang J. Involvement of the central nervous system in mumps. *Acta Med Scand.* 1943;113:487

48. Azimi PH, Cramblett HG, Haynes RE. Mumps meningoencephalitis in children. *JAMA.* 1969;207:509

49. Centers for Disease Control and Prevention. Update: multistate outbreak of mumps—United States, January 1-May 2, 2006. *MMWR.* 2006;55(Dispatch):1-5

50. Centers for Disease Control and Prevention. Achievements in public health: elimination of rubella and congenital rubella syndrome—United States, 1969-2004. *MMWR.* 2005;54:279-282

51. Whitley RJ, Roizman B. Herpes simplex virus infections. *Lancet.* 2001;357:1513

52. Lafferty WE, Downey L, Celum C, et al. Herpes simplex virus type 1 as a cause of genital herpes: impact on surveillance and prevention. *J Infect Dis.* 2000;181:1454

53. Koutsky LA, Stevens CE, Holmes KK, et al. Underdiagnosis of genital herpes by current clinical and viral-isolation procedures. *N Engl J Med.* 1992;326:1533

54. Goldstein LC, Corey L, McDougall JK, et al. Monoclonal antibodies to herpes simplex viruses: use in antigenic typing and rapid diagnosis. *J Infect Dis.* 1983;147:829

55. Pouletty P, Chomel JJ, Thouvenot D, et al. Detection of herpes simplex virus in direct specimens by immunofluorescence assay using a monoclonal antibody. *J Clin Microbiol.* 1987;25:958

56. Ashley RL, Wald A. Genital herpes: review of the epidemic and potential use of type-specific serology. *Clinical Microbiol Rev.* 1999;12:1

57. Arvin AM. Varicella-zoster virus. In: Long S, Pickering L, Prober C, eds. *Principles and Practice of Pediatric Infectious Diseases,* 3rd ed. Philadelphia, PA: Churchill Livingstone; 2008

58. Cohen J, Straus S, Arvin A. Varicella-zoster virus. In: Fields BN, Knipe DM, Chanock R, et al, eds. *Virology,* 5th ed. Philadelphia, PA: Lippincott-Raven; 2007:2774-2806

59. Johnson R, Milbourne PE. Central nervous system manifestations of chickenpox. *Can Med Assoc J.* 1970;102:831-834

60. Gershon AA, LaRussa P, Hardy I, et al. Varicella vaccine: the American experience. *J Infect Dis.* 1992;166(suppl 1):S63-S68

61. Lieu TA, Black SB, Takahashi H, et al. Varicella serology among school-age children with a negative or uncertain history of chickenpox. *Pediatr Infect Dis J.* 1998;17:120-125

62. Balfour HH Jr, Rotbart HA, Feldman S, et al. Acyclovir treatment of varicella in otherwise healthy adolescents. The Collaborative Acyclovir Varicella Study Group. *J Pediatr.* 1992;120:627-633

63. Centers for Disease Control and Prevention. Risks associated with human parvovirus B19 infection. *MMWR.* 1989;38:81-97

64. Strikas RA, Anderson LJ, Parker RA. Temperate and geographic pattern of isolates of nonpolio enteroviruses in the United States. *J Infect Dis.* 1986;153:346-351

65. Rorabaugh ML, Berlin LE, Heldrich F, et al. Aseptic meningitis among infants less than two years of age. Acute illness and neurologic complications. *Pediatrics.* 1993;92:206-211

66. Lepow ML, Coryne N, Thompson LB, et al. A clinical, epidemiologic, and laboratory investigation of aseptic meningitis during the four-year period, 1955-1958. II. The clinical disease and its sequelae. *N Engl J Med.* 1962;266:1188-1193

67. Sawyer M, Holland D, Aintablian N, et al. Diagnosis of enteroviral central nervous system infection by polymerase chain reaction during a large community outbreak. *Pediatr Infect Dis J.* 1994;13:177-182

68. Pozo F, Casas I, Tenorio A, et al. Evaluation of a commercially available reverse transcription-PCR assay for diagnosis of enteroviral infection in archival and prospectively collected cerebrospinal fluid specimens. *J Clin Microbiol.* 1998;36:1741-1745

69. Verboon-Maciolek MA, Nijhuis M, van Loon AM, et al. Diagnosis of enterovirus infection in the first 2 months of life by real-time polymerase chain reaction. *Clin Infect Dis.* 2003:37:1-6

# CHAPTER 137

# Infectious Mononucleosis and Mononucleosis-Like Syndromes

SUJATHA RAJAN, MD

## INFECTIOUS MONONUCLEOSIS

Infectious mononucleosis (IM) is one of the most frequently encountered infections in adolescence. It was initially described in 1921 in 6 otherwise healthy adolescents who had fever, lymphadenopathy, and absolute lymphocytosis with atypical mononuclear cells in the peripheral blood smear.[1,2]

The clinical syndrome of IM is caused by the Epstein-Barr virus (EBV), a double-stranded DNA virus that belongs to the *Herpesviridae* family. Although the clinical syndrome was described much earlier, the virus was not discovered until 1964, when it was isolated from continuous cell lines derived from African Burkitt lymphoma tissue.[3] The etiologic link between EBV and IM was made when a laboratory technician working with the virus became ill and developed EBV-specific antibodies. In addition, at about the same time, several large population studies confirmed the relationship between the clinical syndrome of IM and the development of EBV-specific antibodies.[4,5]

### EPIDEMIOLOGY

Humans are the only source of EBV. Close personal contact, such as kissing or sharing of food, is usually required for transmission. The virus is shed in saliva and respiratory tract secretions and can last for many months following primary infection. Hence, the period of communicability is prolonged and indeterminate. Epstein-Barr virus affects all age groups, with the highest incidence in those aged 15 to 25 years. The age of initial infection varies in different cultural and socioeconomic settings, with 80% to 100% of children being seropositive by 3 to 6 years of age in developing countries. In developed countries, primary infection generally occurs later in life, most often between the ages of 10 and 30. More than 95% of adults have acquired the disease by age 35 in all settings.[6]

### PATHOGENESIS

Studies indicate that EBV infects B lymphocytes present in the lymphoid-rich areas of the oropharynx, after an initial round of lytic replication in the oral and tonsillar epithelium. This is followed by dissemination of infection via B lymphocytes in the peripheral blood and throughout the lymphoreticular system, including the liver and spleen. This then invokes a host immune response that primarily consists of activated cytotoxic-supressor (CD8+) T lymphocytes. The atypical lymphocytes seen in the peripheral blood of patients with IM are primarily CD8+ cells. This surge in CD8+ cells is responsible for reducing the number of EBV-infected B lymphocytes. Clinical manifestations of lymphadenopathy and hepatosplenomegaly in IM are believed to be due to this immunopathological response, rather than direct tissue destruction, as seen in other viruses.[7]

Similar to other herpes viruses, EBV establishes a latent infection after the primary infection. The viral genome is maintained as a plasmid or episome within the nucleus of host B lymphocytes. Only a few viral gene proteins, such as Epstein-Barr nuclear antigen (EBNA) and latent membrane protein, are expressed during this latent phase. These, in turn, activate a number of complex host cellular responses that are responsible for maintaining latency. About 1 to 50 B cells per million remain quiescently infected and serve as the reservoir for lifelong infection of the individual.[8] Latent EBV virus has been associated with a number of benign (hemophagocytic syndrome, pulmonary interstitial pneumonitis) and malignant (Burkitt lymphoma) proliferative disorders.[9]

### INCUBATION PERIOD

The onset of clinical symptoms after exposure is usually prolonged and varies from 10 to 45 days. A prodromal period characterized by fatigue, generalized malaise, myalgias, and headache often precedes the onset of IM and lasts 7 to 14 days.[10]

### CLINICAL FEATURES

Epstein-Barr virus infects all age groups, and the presentation is variable. It is often asymptomatic or associated with mild nonspecific symptoms such as fever, malaise, and anorexia in infants and children. Even in adolescents and young adults, a significant number of infections can be subclinical. In one group of about 110 children prospectively studied with serologic evidence of primary EBV, 50% were diagnosed as upper respiratory tract infection, otitis media, pharyngitis, and/or nonspecific febrile illness, with or without lymphadenopathy.[11,12]

Classic IM symptoms are seen in most adults and adolescents (>50%) and usually start with low-grade fever, headache, and malaise. The classic clinical triad consists of tonsillitis, cervical lymphadenopathy, and moderate to high fever (also referred to as the "anginose").[13] Fever ranges between 102.2°F and 104°F (39°C and 40°C) and lasts from 1 to 3 weeks. Pharyngitis, which is usually most severe during the first 3 to 5 days of illness, is associated with enlarged tonsils that are coated with thick, white-gray-green exudates (30% of cases); the tonsils may sometimes appear necrotic. Red macules and petechiae may be seen at the junction of the hard and soft palate. This finding is indistinguishable from group A streptococcal (GAS) pharyngitis. Lymphadenopathy primarily involves the posterior cervical area. Anterior cervical, axillary, and inguinal groups can be enlarged, and involvement of these other lymph nodes distinguishes the illness from GAS pharyngitis. The lymph nodes in IM are symmetric, discrete, and tender but not fixed, and commonly appear in the first week of illness, with gradual resolution over the next 2 to 3 weeks.

Hepatomegaly is seen in 50% of cases. Splenomegaly is seen in 75% of cases and is most prominent in the second and third week of illness. If present, care should be taken to avoid repeated palpation because this may increase the risk of splenic rupture.[6,14,15] Approximately 10% of individuals have a rash that can range from erythematous, maculopapular, morbilliform, or urticarial to erythema multiforme. Almost all patients who are inadvertently given beta-lactam antibiotics will develop a drug eruption, typically within 24 to 72 hours, but sometimes as late as 5 to 9 days after receiving the antibiotics. This is believed to be an immune-mediated rash and resolves without specific treatment.[16,17] Other common symptoms include malaise, headache, myalgias, sweats, and anorexia. Palpebral or periorbital edema is sometimes seen early in the disease and is believed to be due to lymphatic obstruction.[15]

## ATYPICAL PRESENTATIONS

Apart from the classic presentation of IM, other presentations are (1) a typhoidal form of IM characterized by prolonged high fever with insignificant pharyngitis and a delay in appearance of lymphadenopathy; and (2) a glandular form of IM in which there is marked lymphadenopathy, mild pharyngitis, and low-grade fever.[13]

Other unusual manifestations may occur in older patients with primary EBV, who tend to present with prolonged fever, fatigue, myalgia, malaise, and liver function abnormalities. Pharyngitis and lymphadenopathy are relatively rare in these patients. Hence, IM should be considered as part of the differential diagnosis of any prolonged febrile illness. Sometimes complications of EBV can be the initial presentation of an EBV infection without any of the classic signs and symptoms of IM.[18,19]

## LABORATORY ABNORMALITIES

The white cell count ranges from 12,000 to 20,000, with more than 50% lymphocytes and at least 10% atypical lymphocytes (also called Downey cells) on the peripheral smear. They appear larger than mature lymphocytes and have a vacuolated, basophilic cytoplasm, with a lobulated and eccentrically placed nucleus.[15] A lymphocyte-to-white cell count ratio higher than 0.35 in those with tonsillitis is a quick screening tool to detect patients with IM; this tool showed a sensitivity and specificity of >90% in a recent study.[20] However, atypical lymphocytes in the peripheral blood are not pathognomonic for IM and can be associated with infection by cytomegalovirus (CMV), adenovirus, rubella, herpes simplex virus, *Toxoplasma gondii*, and other viral infections.[6] Thrombocytopenia (<140,000/mm$^3$) may occur in half of the cases of IM due to increased destruction by an enlarged spleen or antiplatelet antibodies.

Abnormal liver function tests are seen in 80% of cases during the second and third weeks of illness. Two- to threefold elevations are seen in transaminases and alkaline phophatase. Bilirubin is usually only mildly elevated, although clinical jaundice can occur in rare cases.[15]

## DIAGNOSIS

A presumptive diagnosis can be based on the presence of typical clinical signs (ie, fever, sore throat, lymphadenopathy [posterior cervical, axillary, or inguinal], splenomegaly, and palatal petechiae). The sensitivity of these signs and symptoms varies between 20% to 60%, with a relatively good specificity of 80% to 99%.[21]

Serologic tests available for confirmation are the rapid heterophile antibody and EBV-specific antibodies.

### Rapid Heterophile Antibody Test

This test was first described by Paul and Bunnel. Heterophile antibodies are an IgM response due to polyclonal activation of the B-cell system and are so called because they agglutinate red blood cells from unrelated species (ie, sheep or horses).[22] The heterophile antibodies are detectable at variable levels, depending on the duration of illness: 40% by week 1, 60% by week 2, and 80% to 90% by week 3. These antibodies are transient and usually last up to 3 months in most patients, but can last up to 6 to 12 months in some cases. The most widely used method is the qualitative rapid slide test in which the test serum is initially absorbed by guinea pig kidney cells (increases specificity) before addition of either sheep or horse erythrocytes. Agglutination of the red cells is

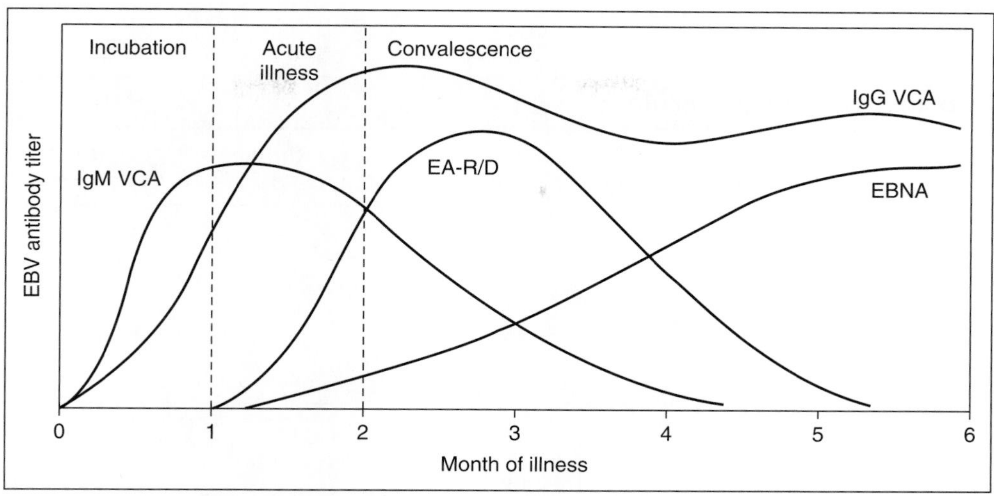


**FIGURE 137-1** Infectious mononucleosis. Antibody response to Epstein-Barr virus. (Adapted with permission from Johnson DH, Cunha BA. Epstein-Barr virus serology. *Infect Dis Pract.* 1995;19:26–27.)

regarded as positive. A quantitative microtiter agglutination assay is also available. Titers can remain elevated for 3 to 6 months and occasionally up to 1 year.[23] A recent study comparing several "monospot" kits showed a sensitivity ranging from 63% to 84% and a specificity of 84% to 100%.[24]

Patients with classic IM symptoms, atypical lymphocytosis, and a positive heterophile test do not require further testing.

False-negative tests usually occur in children younger than 6 years of age, or if performed in the first week of illness.[25] Other causes of false-negative tests are due to IM-like illnesses that are not due to EBV. False-positive heterophile tests are uncommon (<10%) and are usually due to erroneous interpretation. Other causes of false-positive tests are viral hepatitis, rubella, malaria, connective tissue diseases, and lymphoma.[26]

### Epstein-Barr Virus–Specific Antibody Response

Obtaining specific EBV serologies is the definitive diagnostic study for EBV infection. It is usually reserved for those with an IM-like illness who have a negative heterophile test or those who have atypical features of IM. Antibody responses to several EBV antigens, namely, viral capsid antigen (VCA), early antigen (EA), and EBNA, are used to help make a serologic diagnosis in these situations.

In the acute phase, there is an initial IgM response to VCA, followed by an IgG response. The IgM anti-VCA response is transient and can last from 4 to 12 weeks. The IgG anti-VCA response peaks a little later than the IgM response and lasts for life. Antibodies to EBNA are the last to develop; these take several weeks to months (6–12 weeks) to become positive and persist for life. Presence of anti-EBNA antibodies excludes an active primary infection (Figure 137-1). For practical purposes, antibodies to VCA and EBNA are sufficient to differentiate acute from past infections (Table 137-1). However, some laboratories also report antibodies to EA, and these are sometimes useful. There are 2 types of IgG anti-EAs based on the region of cell staining. The anti-D EA has diffuse staining in the nucleus and cytoplasm, whereas the anti-R EA has staining restricted to the cytoplasm. The IgG anti-D EA response usually peaks by 3 to 4 weeks after the onset of IM symptoms and persists for about 3 to 6 months. They are present in only 70% of infected patients. Levels are also elevated in patients with nasopharyngeal carcinoma or chronic active EBV infection. Early antigen-restricted (EA-R) antibodies are only occasionally detected in patients with IM, but are often found at elevated titers in patients with African Burkitt lymphoma or chronic active EBV infection.[6,15]

A recent study compared several commercial kits for EBV-specific antibodies in patients with recent primary EBV infection. The average sensitivity was 97% (95%–99%), and average specificity was 94% (86%–100%).[27] Several different methods, including indirect immunofluorescence assay, enzyme immunoassays, and immunoblot techniques, are used to detect EBV-specific antibodies.

### Other Methods

Epstein-Barr virus can be cultured from oropharyngeal secretions or lymphocytes of patients by infecting specialized cell lines and allowing for immortalization to occur. However, this process takes 6 to 8 weeks and is not routinely available.

**Table 137-1**

**Patterns of Epstein-Barr Virus Serology**

| *Type of Infection* | *Heterophil Antibody* | *Viral Capsid Antigen (VCA)-IgM* | *VCA-IgG* | *Early Antigen (EA)D-EA* | *R-EA* | *Epstein-Barr Nuclear Antigen (EBNA)* |
|---|---|---|---|---|---|---|
| Acute primary infection | + | + | + | +/− | − | − |
| Recent infection | − | +/− | + | +/− | − | +/− |
| Past infection | − | − | + | +/− | − | + |

Polymerase chain reaction (PCR) technology can be used to detect the DNA of EBV in serum, plasma, and tissue specimens. This test is available commercially and is useful in patients with post-transplantation lymphoproliferative disease and other patients who are immunocompromised.

## COMPLICATIONS

Most patients with IM have a benign clinical course and recover completely within 3 weeks. However, complications can occur, including upper airway obstruction, immune-mediated phenomena, rash associated with beta-lactam antibiotic administration, and splenic rupture. Almost all organ systems can be affected by IM, as listed in Box 137-1.

**Box 137-1**

***Complications of Epstein-Barr Virus***

- Respiratory: upper airway obstruction, pneumonitis
- Liver: clinical jaundice (5%), subclinical hepatitis (80%–90%), liver failure (rare)
- Spleen: rupture
- Neurologic: aseptic meningitis or meningoecephalitis, cerebellar ataxia, Guillain-Barré syndrome, cranial nerve palsies, transverse myelitis
- Cardiac: myocarditis, pericarditis, arrhythmias
- Dermatology: rash related to drug administration
- Hematology: hemolytic anemia, thrombocytopenia, neutropenia, hemophagocytic syndrome
- Renal: glomerulonephritis

### Upper Airway Obstruction

This potentially dangerous complication ccurs in 0.1% to 1% of cases of IM and is due to lymphoid hypertrophy of the Waldeyer ring and surrounding edema. Onset can be acute or insidious. Impending obstruction can sometimes be prevented with administration of steroids.

### Hematologic Complications

Hemolytic anemia of the Coombs positive type occurs in 1% to 3% of cases and is mediated by IgM cold-agglutinin antibodies directed at the I antigen of the red cell. Patients can present clinically with hemolytic anemia, usually during the second or third week of illness and without the classic IM findings. Aplastic anemia is another rare complication. Mild thrombocytopenia ($<140{,}000/mm^3$) occurs in more than half of IM cases, and profound thrombocytopenia has been reported. Neutropenia is seen commonly but is usually mild and self limited.[15]

### Splenic Rupture

Splenic rupture is rare but is the most feared and well-remembered complication. The risk is estimated to be about 0.1% to 0.2% and almost always occurs between 4 and 21 days after the onset of illness.[28] The longest interval of rupture to be documented has been at 7 weeks after illness. Rupture is believed to occur due to lymphocytic infiltration of the trabeculae and capsule, causing distortion of the normal anatomy and increased splenic fragility. Signs and symptoms of splenic rupture include left upper quadrant abdominal pain, with or without radiation to the left shoulder (Kehr sign). Other findings include hypotension, anemia, and increased polymorphonuclear leukocytes in the peripheral smear. Splenic rupture during IM has occurred either spontaneously or after trauma, and is almost always associated with splenomegaly.[29]

Based on the previous observations, the general consensus is for patients to avoid sports activity for at least 3 to 4 weeks after the onset of the illness. Return to sports based on resolution of splenomegaly is controversial. It is well known that documentation of splenomegaly by the physical examination is insensitive and may be particularly challenging in an athlete with well-developed abdominal muscles. Some authorities advocate the use of ultrasound to document spleen size, especially in high-risk athletes involved in contact sports (ie, football, gymnastics, lacrosse, basketball, hockey, diving, karate, judo) and repeating it in 1 to 2 weeks if still enlarged.[30–32] Yet, there is wide variability in the normal spleen size, especially with single measurements, and 3% of healthy college students have splenomegaly. Because imaging is unreliable in the absence of a baseline measurement, it is most prudent that the return-to-play decision be based on clinical judgment of each case.[33] The most recent preparticipation physical examination monograph suggests return to light activities in asymptomatic individuals after a 3-week recovery period from onset of symptoms and full participation the following week if all goes well.[34,35] It is understood, however, that there is no definitive way to be sure that there is no splenomegaly; thus, patients and parents need to know that the safest approach is to avoid contact sports for as long as possible and that there is some risk, although probably minimal, even after waiting a full 4 weeks from the onset of symptoms.[34,35]

### Neurologic Complications

Neurologic symptoms usually tend to present 2 to 3 weeks after the initial onset of symptoms, but sometimes can present in the absence of the classic triad. Meningits and encephalitis are the most common neurologic manifestations of IM. Other reported complications are Guillain-Barré syndrome, mononeuritis, cerebellar dysfunction, and transverse myelitis.

### Other Complications

A rash related to ampicillin or amoxicillin occurs in 50% to 100% of patients with IM. The rash is erythematous and maculopapular, and it is believed to be immune related rather than a true allergy to penicillins. Other reported complications include hepatitis, myositis, myopericarditis, pneumonitis, pancreatitis, and postanginal sepsis resulting from phlebitis of the jugular veins. Glomerulonephritis and genital ulcerations have also been described.[13,15]

## THERAPY

Supportive care is the mainstay of uncomplicated IM and consists of nonsteroidal anti-inflammatory agents, adequate nutritional and fluid intake, and bed rest.

Acyclovir and ganciclovir have been shown to inhibit EBV in vitro. Acyclovir is a nucleoside analog that blocks EBV replication through inhibition of viral DNA polymerase, present only during the lytic stage of the infection. However, a meta-analysis of several randomized controlled trials indicated that although patients who took acyclovir had less oropharyngeal shedding at the end of therapy, these patients demonstrated no significant clinical benefit from treatment.[6,36]

### Steroids

Studies have indicated that a short course of steroids can either shorten (or have no effect on) the duration of symptoms of IM (ie, fever, sore throat). Steroids, however, are generally not recommended in uncomplicated cases.[37] The main indications for steroid use in IM are severe toxic exudative tonsillitis and pharyngeal or laryngeal edema with impending or early airway obstruction. Other indications are acute hemolytic anemia, severe thrombocytopenia, and severe neurologic or cardiac disease.

A short course of prednisone, 1 mg/kg per day orally (maximum 20–40 mg/day), can be administered for 7 to 10 days. Once there is a good clinical response, the dose can be rapidly tapered.[15]

## PROGNOSIS

Most EBV infections are self limited, and symptoms usually last 2 to 4 weeks. About one-third of patients have symptoms (usually fatigue) that can last for 6 to 12 months. However, most recover completely, and the prognosis is generally excellent.

## OTHER CLINICAL CONDITIONS ASSOCIATED WITH EPSTEIN-BARR VIRUS

### Chronic Active Epstein-Barr Virus Infection

Chronic active Epstein-Barr virus infection (CAEBV) is a rare disorder characterized by the following key features:

- Severe illness of more than 6 months' duration that begins as a primary EBV infection
- Histologic evidence of organ disease, such as pneumonitis, hepatitis, bone marrow hypoplasia, or uveitis
- Demonstration of EBV antigens or EBV DNA in tissue
- Absence of an alternative explanation for the disease process[38]

Clinical features include intermittent or prolonged fever, lymphadenopathy, and hepatosplenomegaly. Other symptoms include complaints of sore throat, fatigue, myalgia, and arthralgia. The EBV serologic pattern is similar to that of acute IM, but with extreme elevations of VCA IgG, EA IgG, and very low or absent levels of anti-EBNA. In addition, these patients have high serum EBV viral loads.[39] This syndrome has been reported mainly in Asians. The disease is associated with a high mortality and morbidity, and most of these patients are believed to be in the process of developing either hemophagocytic lymphohistiocytosis or other EBV-related neoplasms. There is no effective treatment, although ganciclovir, intravenous immunoglobulin, bone marrow transplantation, and adoptive immunotherapy have been used.

### X-Linked Lymphoproliferative Syndrome

This is a rare familial condition that affects young boys following primary EBV infection. It is believed to be due to dysregulation in the polyclonal expansion of EBV-infected B cells and the CD8+ cytotoxic T-cell response. The disease is characterized by rapid and progressive involvement of various organs, leading to fulminant hepatic and bone marrow failure. Ninety percent of patients with X-linked lymphoproliferative syndrome (XLPS) have evidence of hemophagocytosis. The *XLP* gene has recently been cloned and is responsible for a product called signal lymphocyte activation molecule–associated protein (SAP), a small protein involved in lymphocyte signaling.[40] A SAP deficiency is believed to be caused by an abnormal interaction between T and B cells, resulting in proliferation of EBV-infected B cells.[9] Most patients with this gene defect are clinically and immunologically well until they get primary EBV; approximately 50% of patients die after getting IM or go on to develop hypogammaglobulinemia or malignant lymphomas.

### Epstein-Barr Virus–Associated Malignancies

Epstein-Barr virus is associated with several malignancies that include Burkitt lymphoma, nasopharyngeal carcinoma, and Hodgkin lymphoma. In patients with severe cellular immunodeficiency or those who have had a solid organ or bone marrow transplantation, an uncontrolled proliferation of EBV-infected B lymphocytes can occur due to lack of effective immune surveillance. This leads to a disorder referred to as lymphoproliferative disease or as post-transplant lymphoproliferative disease (PTLD) when it occurs after a transplant. Patients who are EBV naive prior to a transplant are at particularly high risk, especially if they receive an organ from an EBV-positive donor. Patients with PTLD develop a mononucleosis-like illness from which they recover or to which they succumb, and those who recover can go on to develop solid tumors. The diagnosis is established by the presence of a primary or reactivated EBV serologic response and/or decreasing EBNA titers, as well as the presence of viral genome and antigens within lesions. Treatment is difficult, including mainly a decrease in immunosuppression and the use of antiviral agents.[6,15]

### Chronic Fatigue Syndrome

Adolescents with nonspecific complaints of malaise or fatigue are sometimes labeled as having a chronic EBV infection or chronic fatigue syndrome (CFS) because they have persistent EBV titers or slight changes in the titers of specific EBV antibodies. While CAEBV infection is a rare disorder with specific criteria, as detailed previously, many studies have shown that EBV is not the cause of CFS. Instead, CFS is a syndrome that can follow any flu-like illness, with multiple symptoms that then last for several months to years. Although many patients with CFS are seropositive for EBV, this does not mean that EBV is the cause of the CFS. Specific criteria have been established to provide better guidelines to diagnose CFS; these are reviewed in detail in Chaper 124, Chronic Fatigue Syndrome.[41]

## MONONUCLEOSIS-LIKE SYNDROMES

There are a number of infections that closely mimic EBV-induced IM; these infections are often referred to as mononucleosis-like syndromes (MLSs). These IM-like syndromes are characterized by some or all of the following features of IM: fever, malaise, pharyngitis, adenopathy, hepatomegaly, and splenomegaly. Peripheral lymphocytosis with atypical lymphocytes can be seen in most of them. However, the heterophile antibody response is negative. The most common causes of IM-like syndromes are CMV, toxoplasmosis, and primary HIV. Other less common causes are human herpesvirus (HHV)-6, rubella, and viral hepatitis. It is important to remember these conditions in order to avoid misdiagnosis and unnecessary diagnostic and invasive procedures during the evaluation of a mononucleosis-like illnesses. Table 137-2 lists the causes of heterophile-negative IM with some important differentiating features. The more common causes are discussed in the next sections.

## CYTOMEGALOVIRUS MONONUCLEOSIS

Cytomegalovirus is a member of the herpesvirus group and is the leading cause of heterophile-negative IM-like syndrome. Like other herpes viruses, it exists in a latent state and can reactivate at a later time.

Infection can be acquired via various routes:

1. Horizontal transmission by direct person-to-person contact with virus-containing secretions from saliva, urine, the cervix, semen (sexual contact), stool, or tears. The 2 main routes of transmission seem to be through oral and sexual secretions.
2. Vertical transmission occurs from mother to child either in utero via transplacental passage of

**Table 137-2**

**Clinical and Laboratory Features of Mononucleosis-Like Syndromes**

| *Syndrome* | *Distinguishing Features when Compared to Infectious Mononucleosis due to Epstein-Barr Virus* | *Diagnostic Tests for Acute Infection* |
|---|---|---|
| Cytomegalovirus (CMV) | Prolonged fever and malaise<br>Absent or mild sore throat<br>Mild cervical lymphadenopathy<br>Splenomegaly may be slightly more prominent than EBV<br>Atypical lymphocytes less prominent<br>Increased liver function tests (LFTs)<br>Fever<br>Posterior cervical lymphadenopathy | Positive CMV IgM<br>CMV polymerase chain reaction (PCR)<br>CMV p65 antigen |
| Toxoplasmosis | Pharyngitis not prominent<br>Mild lymphocytosis<br>Normal LFTs<br>Fever<br>Pharyngitis | Anti-toxoplasma IgM<br>Anti-toxoplasma IgG<br>Avidity assay |
| Human Immunodeficiency Virus (HIV) | Lymphadenopathy<br>Maculopapular rash and mucocutanenous ulceration<br>Leukopenia and thrombocytopenia, fever and malaise<br>No pharyngitis | HIV ELISA<br>HIV Western blot<br>HIV-1 plasma viral load |
| Viral hepatitis | No lymphadenopathy<br>Transaminase enzymes are elevated >10 times normal level Less common in adults | Serologies for hepatitis A, B, and C |
| Human herpesvirus (HHV)-6 | Fever with mild bilateral anterior and posterior cervical lymphadenopathy<br>Mild liver function abnormalities and atypical lymphocytosis<br>Fever | Anti-HHV-6 IgM and IgG<br>HHV-6 PCR |
| Rubella | Postauricular and suboccipital adenopathy, a characteristic exanthem, and a shorter course than classic IM | Not done routinely |
| Group A streptococcus pharyngitis | Abrupt onset of sore throat<br>Tonsillopharyngeal erythema with or without exudates<br>Tender enlarged anterior cervical lymphadenopathy | Rapid streptococcal antigen detection test<br>Positive throat culture |
| Adenovirus | Absence of hepatosplenomegaly<br>Fever with pharyngitis and coryza, with or without conjunctivitis<br>Exudates on pharynx<br>Fever | Nasopharyngeal swab or wash for direct fluorescent antigen (DFA) testing or viral isolation |
| Herpes simplex virus type 1 | Pharyngitis with or without exudates or ulcerations<br>Cervical lymphadenopathy | Pharyngeal swab for viral isolation or DFA |

the virus, at birth by passage through an infected birth canal, or postnatally by ingestion of CMV-positive human milk.

3. Transfusion of blood, platelets, or white blood cells from previously infected people is another potential source of infection, but use of filters and CMV-negative blood has greatly decreased this route of transmission. Cytomegalovirus mononucleosis infection can also follow organ transplantation.[42]

The incidence of infection with CMV depends on such factors as socioeconomic status, child care attendance, and sexual behaviors. Primary infection often occurs in children attending child care who then bring it to their homes and infect parents and older siblings. The infection can vary from a subclinical illness to a full-blown mononucleosis-like illness. As many as 5% to 10% of all cases of "mononucleosis" may be due to CMV infection.[43] Patients have fever, malaise, hepatitis, splenomegaly, and lymphocytosis with atypical lymphocytes, as in classic IM. However, the degree of pharyngitis, cervical adenitis, and splenomegaly is less with CMV than with EBV. Fever is seen in more than 90% of symptomatic cases and can last for more than 2 weeks.[44,45]

In patients with immunocompromising conditions (ie, HIV, transplants), CMV can cause disease in any organ, and patients can present with retinitis (common in HIV), pneumonitis (common in bone marrow transplant), hepatitis, central nervous system (CNS) disease, colitis, and fever of unknown origin. The infection may represent either primary infection through the acquisition of CMV-positive donor tissue or reactivation of a latent infection.[46]

### Diagnosis

Diagnosis is usually made via serologic tests. The heterophile or Monospot test is negative. Assays for anti-CMV IgM antibodies are positive during the acute infection. The IgM assay is neither very sensitive nor specific, and caution should be used in interpretation of results. Care should be taken to elute out the IgG while looking for the IgM in order to avoid false-positive IgM results. Either the presence of IgM or a fourfold rise in IgG helps in making the diagnosis.

Cytomegalovirus can be isolated from the throat, urine, or blood; however, presence of the virus in these fluids does not unequivocally indicate a direct causal relationship between CMV and current symptoms. Other newer diagnostic methods that have become available are detection of CMV by PCR in the blood and other body fluids, and antigenemia assays that detect a component of the virus nucleoprotein in CMV-infected cells or tissue. These methods have been well established in immunocompromised patients and may have a role in immunocompetent patients as well.[46]

### Treatment

Treatment is generally supportive for the immunocompetent patient.

Several antiviral agents (ie, ganciclovir, foscarnet, cidofovir) have in vitro and in vivo activity against CMV, but are reserved for immunocompromised patients.[46]

## TOXOPLASMOSIS

*Toxoplasma gondii* is probably the second leading cause of the heterophile-negative IM syndrome. *T gondii* is a protozoan found in many species of warm-blooded animals throughout the world, although the definitive host is the domestic cat. The parasite undergoes the sexual phase of reproduction in the intestines of the cat, and the oocysts that are produced are shed in cat feces and deposited in soil. The oocysts are ingested by intermediate hosts, including wild animals, cattle, and humans. In humans, the oocysts transform into freely motile tachyzoites that invade the gut epithelium and disseminate. The tissue cysts persist in a viable latent form in the host for life, retaining the potential for reactivation at any time.

Humans acquire infection by various routes. These include ingestion of oocysts from handling cat feces or contaminated dirt, or ingestion of raw or undercooked meat of another intermediate host that contains cysts (ie, chicken, beef, pork).

Acute acquired infection in the immunocompetent host can vary from subclinical infection to a MLS with fever, malaise, and lymphocytosis. Adenopathy usually involves the posterior cervical nodes or may be generalized. Pharyngitis and hepatosplenomegaly are not prominent features. Rash is sometimes seen. Liver function tests are normal.[47–49]

Acute infection in pregnancy can result in congenital toxoplasmosis of the fetus, the presentation of which is variable, depending on the stage of gestation. Congenital toxoplasmosis can present with chorioretinitis, various CNS manifestations (hydrocephalus, microcephaly, intracranial calcification, developmental delay), hepatosplenomegaly, and jaundice.[48] Ocular toxoplasmosis generally results from the reactivation of the cysts previously deposited in or near the retina during a congenital or primary infection, but can also occur during a primary infection.

Manifestations of toxoplasmosis in the immunocompetent host most commonly involves the CNS (encephalitis), but can involve any organ system (ie, lungs or eyes).[50]

### Diagnosis

The diagnosis of infection in pregnancy is particularly important because toxoplasmosis can potentially cause congenital infection. Antitoxoplasma IgM and IgG antibodies are routinely used in the diagnosis. Antitoxoplasma IgM antibodies can persist for years after infection; hence, their presence alone cannot be used to diagnose primary infection. Acute versus chronic infection may be distinguished by IgG "avidity" testing. Weaker binding of IgG in an avidity assay is suggestive of more recent infection. Chronic exposure to the organism results in antitoxoplasma IgG antibodies with progressively stronger binding to toxoplasma antigens. Diagnosis can also be made by isolating the organism from body fluids and tissues (amniotic fluid, cerebrospinal fluid, placenta) by mouse or tissue culture inoculation. Organisms can also be identified histologically from tissue and body fluid specimens. Currently, PCR amplification of *T gondii* DNA in body fluids and tissues is used to diagnose infection in pregnant and immunocompromised patients.

### Treatment

Specific treatment is not necessary for most immunocompetent patients with toxoplasmosis. Indications for treatment include active chorioretinitis, infections in immunocompromised and pregnant patients, and congenital toxoplasmosis. Therapeutic regimens include use of sulfadiazine or clindamycin, in combination with pyrimethamine. Pyrimethamine is considered to be the most effective antitoxoplasma agent; it is a folic acid antagonist and hence should always be given with folinic acid. Several other drugs (azithromycin, clarithromycin, atovaquone, dapsone, and trimethoprim-sulfamethoxazole) have activity against toxoplasma and have been used as alternatives. Spiramycin is the drug of choice used in pregnancy to reduce transmission to the fetus.[47,48]

## ACUTE PRIMARY HIV INFECTION

Also known as acute retroviral syndrome (ARS), this syndrome is the earliest clinical manifestation of HIV infection and represents the initial stage of disease that immediately follows viral entry into the body. Most infected patients (40%–90%) experience this syndrome, and symptoms typically occur 2 to 6 weeks after exposure to the virus. Symptoms include fever, fatigue, pharyngitis, weight loss, night sweats, lymphadenopathy (usually generalized), myalgias, headache, nausea, and diarrhea. Leukopenia, thrombocytopenia, and/or mild transaminitis are seen. About one-fourth of patients have a truncal maculopapular rash or urticarial rash that occurs on the trunk and palms and soles. Neurologic manifestations can include aseptic meningitis, peripheral neuropathy, and Guillain-Barré syndrome. A combination of mucosal ulcerations, rash, lymphadenopathy, and neurologic signs are important clues to the acquisition of a primary HIV infection, especially in individuals with risk factors for the illness. It is important to have a high index of suspicion in patients who present with a mononucleosis-like illness, especially in those who have risk factors. The symptoms of the primary infection usually last 2 weeks but can persist for up to 10 weeks. Early identification of patients with primary infection allows for interventions to prevent further transmission and the opportunity to provide early treatment.

### Diagnosis

Antibodies may not have yet been formed at the time of ARS; hence, routine serologic assays for HIV (HIV enzyme immunoassay antibody assay and Western blot) may be negative or indeterminant. Diagnosis is established by the presence of viral RNA levels in the plasma.[50,51]

### Treatment

Adolescents with ARS should be referred to and managed by specialists who have expertise in this disease. Treatment of ARS is considered optional; details are available at www.aidsinfo.nih.gov. Because treatment remains controversial, enrollment into available clinical trials should be encouraged to provide more information about outcomes of early intervention. Information about trials for children and adolescents is found at www.clinicaltrials.gov or by contacting the AIDS Clinical Trials Information Service.

## STREPTOCOCCAL PHARYNGITIS

Because most patients with IM have pharyngitis, a routine throat culture for GAS is often performed by clinicians in these patients. Studies indicate about 3% to 30% of patients with IM have a positive throat culture for GAS. This could be due to either colonization or true coinfection. Distinguishing between IM and GAS can be difficult to determine clinically. Presence of axillary or inguinal lymph nodes and splenomegaly makes IM the more likely diagnosis. Conversely, normal hepatic enzymes make the diagnosis of IM less likely. Distinguishing between colonization and coinfection in those with IM who have a positive throat culture for GAS can also be difficult. Serologic tests for recent infection with GAS may help make this distinction but are usually not available immediately. Two studies compared throat cultures of patients with confirmed IM and healthy controls and found the carriage rate of GAS to be 4% in each, and in one study there was not the expected fourfold rise in antistreptococcal antibodies among the patients with IM, implying that they had colonization and not coinfection. For that reason, routine testing for GAS in those with confirmed IM is not warranted. However, for those with IM who do have a positive GAS culture, most experts would recommend treatment with antibiotics (but not with a beta-lactam antibiotic that can cause a rash in the presence of IM) because of the risk of poststreptococcal complications.[6,52,53]

## VIRAL HEPATITIS

Early viral hepatitis may resemble the prodrome of EBV with fever and malaise. Pharyngitis and lymphadenopathy are not seen. Lymphocytosis and atypical lymphocytes are of lesser magnitude when compared with EBV. Liver enzymes in viral hepatitis are markedly elevated (at least 10 times more than normal limits) with disproportionately higher alkaline phosphatase levels.

**RUBELLA VIRUS**

Although rarely seen at this time because of vaccination, rubella can manifest as a mild illness with fever, sore throat, and lymphadenopathy. Atypical lymphocytosis is mild. Appearance of the characteristic rash generally helps in making the diagnosis of rubella.

**HUMAN HERPESVIRUS TYPE 6**

Human herpesvirus type 6 typically causes roseola infantum (exanthema subitum or sixth disease) in children. Eighty percent of children acquire infection by age 3. Several cases have been reported in the literature of a mononucleosis-like illness that presents with mild fever, sore throat, lymphadenopathy, and rash in older children, adolescents, and adults. Laboratory evaluation shows elevated liver enzymes and a mild atypical lymphocytosis. Some patients may also have evidence of aseptic meningitis. Diagnosis is usually established by serologic conversion (ie, a fourfold rise in IgG titers) or detection of viral DNA in peripheral blood or involved tissue.[54-56]

## REFERENCES

1. Sprunt TP, Evans FA. Mononucleosis in reaction to acute infections (infectious mononucleosis). *Johns Hopkins Bull.* 1920;31:410

2. Evans AS. The history of infectious mononucleosis. *Am J Med Sci.* 1974;267:189

3. Henle G, Henle W, Diehl V. Relation of Burkitt's tumor associated herpes type virus to infectious mononucleosis. *Proc Natl Acad Sci USA.* 1968;59:94

4. Niederman JC, McCollum RW, Henle G, et al. Infectious mononucleosis: clinical manifestations in relation to EB virus antibodies. *JAMA.* 1968;203:205

5. Evans AS, Niederman JC, McCollum RW. Seroepidemiologic studies of infectious mononucleosis with EB virus. *N Engl J Med.* 1968;279:1121

6. Johannsen EC, Schooley RT, Kaye KM. Epstein-Barr virus (infectious mononucleosis). In: Mandell GL, Bennett JE, Dolin R, eds. *Principles and Practice of Infectious Diseases.* 6th ed. Philadelphia: Churchill Livingstone; 2005

7. Rickinson AB, Kieff E. Epstein-Barr virus. In: Knipe DM, Howley PM, Griffin DE et al, eds. *Fields Virology.* 5th ed. Philadelphia: Lippincott Williams & Wilkins; 2006: 2656–2700

8. Williams H, Crawford DH. Epstein-Barr virus: the impact of scientific advances on clinical practice. *Blood.* 2006;107: 862–868

9. Cohen JI. Epstein-Barr virus infection. *N Eng J Med.* 2000;343:481–492

10. Hoagland RJ. The incubation period of infectious mononucleosis. *Am J Public Health.* 1984;54:1699–1705

11. Sumaya CV, Ench Y. Epstein-Barr virus infectious mononucleosis in children. I. Clinical and general laboratory findings. *Pediatrics.* 1985;75:1003

12. Hoagland RJ. The clinical manifestations of infectious mononucleosis: a report of 200 cases. *Am J Med Sci.* 1960;240:55

13. Hickey SM, Strasburger VC. What every pediatrician should know about infectious mononucleosis in adolescents. *Pediatr Clin North Am.* 1997;44:1541–1556

14. Rea TD, Russo JE, Kaon W, Ashley RL. Prospective study of the natural history of infectious mononucleosis caused by Epstein-Barr virus. *J Am Board Fam Pract.* 2001;14:234

15. Katz BZ. Epstein-Barr virus infections (mononucleosis and lymphoproliferative disorders). In: Long S, Pickering L, Prober C, eds. *Principles and Practice of Pediatric Infectious Diseases.* 3rd ed.

16. Renn CN, Straff W, Dorfmuller A, et al. Amoxicillin-induced exanthema in young adults with infectious mononucleosis: demonstration of drug-specific lymphocyte reactivity. *Br J Dermatol.* 2002;147:1166

17. Haverkos HW, Amsel Z, Drotman DP. Adverse virus–drug interactions. *Rev Infect Dis.* 1991;13:697

18. Auwaerter PG. Infectious mononucleosis in middle age. *JAMA.* 1999;281:454–459

19. Axelrod P, Finestone AJ. Infectious mononucleosis in older adults. *Am Fam Physician.* 1990;42:1599–1606

20. Wolf DM, Friedrichs I, Toma AG. Lymphocyte-white blood cell count ratio: a quickly available screening tool to differentiate acute purulent tonsillitis from glandular fever. *Arch Otolaryngol Head Neck Surg.* 2007;133:61–64

21. Ebell MH. Epstein-Barr virus infectious mononucleosis. *Am Fam Physician.* 2004;70:1279–1287

22. Paul JR, Bunnell WW. Classics in infectious diseases: the presence of heterophile antibodies in infectious mononucleosis. *Rev Infect Dis.* 1982;4:1062–1068

23. Aronson MD, Komaroff AL, Pass TM, Erwin CT, Branch WT. Heterophil antibody in adults with sore throat: frequency and clinical presentation. *Ann Intern Med.* 1982;96: 505–508

24. Linderholm M, Boman J, Juto P, Linde A. Comparative evaluation of nine kits for rapid diagnosis of infectious mononucleosis and Epstein-Barr virus specific serology. *J Clin Microbiol.* 1994;32:259–261

25. Sumaya CV, Ench Y. Epstein-Barr virus infectious mononucleosis in children: II. Heterophil antibody and viral-specific responses. *Pediatrics.* 1985;75:1011–1019

26. Schumacher HR, Austin RM, Stass SA. False-positive serology in infectious mononucleosis. *Lancet.* 1979;1:722

27. Bruu AL, Hjetland R, Holter E, et al. Evaluation of 12 commercially available tests for detection of Epstein-Barr virus specific and heterophile antibodies. *Clin Diag Lab Immunol.* 2000;7:451–456

28. Farley DR, Zietlow SP, Bannon MP, Farnell MB. Spontaneous rupture of the spleen due to infectious mononucleosis. *Mayo Clin Proc.* 1992;67:846-853

29. Maki DG, Reich RM. Infectious mononucleosis in the athlete: diagnosis, complications, and management. *Am J Sports Med.* 1982;10:162-173

30. Burroughs KE. Athletes resuming activity after infectious mononucleosis. *Arch Fam Med.* 2000;9:1122-1123

31. Sevier TL. Infectious disease in athletes. *Med Clin North Am.* 1994;78:389-412

32. Waninger KN, Harcke HT. Determination of safe return to play for athletes recovering from infectious mononucleosis: a review of the literature. *Clin J Sport Med.* 2005;15:410

33. Hosey RG, Rodenberg RE. Infectious disease and the collegiate athlete. *Clin Sports Med.* 2007;26:449-471

34. Putukian M, O'Connor FG, Stricker PR, et al. Mononucleosis and athletic participation: an evidence-based subject review. *Clin J Sport Med.* 2008;18:309-315

35. Bernhardt DT, Roberts WO (eds). *Preparticipation Physical Evaluation.* Fourth Edition. Elk Grove Village, IL: American Academy of Pediatrics; 2010

36. Torre D, Tambini R. Acyclovir for treatment of infectious mononucleosis: a meta-analysis. *Scand J Infect Dis.* 1999;31:543-547

37. Tynell E, Aurelius E, Brandell A, et al. Acyclovir and prednisolone treatment of acute infectious mononucleosis: a multicenter, double-blind, placebo-controlled study. *J Infect Dis.* 1996;174:324-331

38. Macsween KF, Crawford DH. Epstein-Barr virus—recent advances. *Lancet Infect Dis.* 2003;3:131-140

39. Kimura H, Hoshino Y, Kanagane H, et al. Clinical and virologic characteristics of chronic active Epstein-Barr virus infection. *Blood.* 2001;982:280-296

40. Grierson H, Purtilo DT. Epstein-Barr virus infections in males with the X-linked lymphoproliferative syndrome. *Ann Intern Med.* 1987;106:538-545

41. Fukuda K, Strauss SE, Hickie I, et al. The chronic fatigue syndrome: a comprehensive approach to its definition and study. *Ann Intern Med.* 1994;121:953-959

42. Pass RF. Cytomegalovirus. In: Long S, Pickering L, Prober C, eds. *Principles and Practice of Pediatric Infectious Diseases.* 3rd ed. New York, NY: Churchill Livingstone; 2008: 1029-1036

43. Klemola E, von Essen R, Henle G, et al. Infectious-mononucleosis-like disease with negative heterophil agglutination test: clinical features in relation to Epstein-Barr virus and cytomegalovirus and antibodies. *J Infect Dis.* 1970;121:608-614

44. Wreghitt TG, Teare EL, Sule O, et al. Cytomegalovirus infection in immunocompetent patients. *Clin Infect Dis.* 2003;37: 1603-1606

45. Betts RF. *Mononucleosis Syndromes in Williams Hematology.* 7th ed. New York, NY: McGraw-Hill; 2006

46. Crumpacker CS, Wadhwa S. *Cytomegalovirus.* In: Mandell GL, Bennett JE, Dolin R, eds. *Principles and Practice of Infectious Diseases.* 6th ed. Philadelphia: Churchill Livingstone; 2005

47. Montoya JG, Kovacs JA, Remington JS. *Toxoplasma gondii.* In: Mandell GL, Bennett JE, Dolin R, eds. *Principles and Practice of Infectious Diseases.* 6th ed. Philadelphia: Churchill Livingstone; 2005: 947-1091

48. Boyer KM, Marcinak JF, McLeod RL. *Toxoplasma gondii* (toxoplasmosis). In: Long S, Pickering L, Prober C, eds. *Principles and Practice of Pediatric Infectious Diseases.* 3rd ed. New York, NY: Churchill Livingstone; 2008

49. McCabe RE, Brooks RG, Dorfman RF, et al. Clinical spectrum in 107 cases of toxoplasmic lymphadenopathy. *Rev Infect Dis.* 1987;9:754-774

50. Kahn JO, Walder BD. Acute human immunodeficiency virus type I infection. *N Engl J Med.* 1998;339:33-39

51. Kassutto S, Rosenberg ES. Primary HIV type I infection. *Clin Infect Dis.* 2004;15(38):1447-1453

52. Merriam SC, Keeling RP. Beta-hemolytic streptococcal pharyngitis: uncommon in infectious mononucleosis. *South Med J.* 1983;76:575-576

53. Collins M, Fleisher GR, Fager SS. Incidence of beta hemolytic streptococcal pharyngitis in adolescent with infectious mononucleosis. *J Adolesc Health Care.* 1984;5:96-100

54. Steeper TA, Horwitz CA, Ablashi DV, et al. The spectrum of clinical and laboratory findings resulting from human herpesvirus-6 (HHV-6) in patients with mononucleosis-like illness not resulting from Epstein-Barr virus or cytomegalovirus. *Am J Clin Pathol.* 1990;93:776

55. Akashi K, Eizur Y, Sumiyoshi Y, et al. Severe infectious mononucleosis-like syndrome and primary human herpes virus-6 infection in an adult. *N Engl J Med.* 1993;329:168-171

56. Maric I, Bryant R, Abu-Asab M, et al. Human herpesvirus-6–associated acute lymphadenitis in immunocompetent adults. *Mol Pathol.* 2004;17:1427-1433

# CHAPTER 138

# HIV and AIDS in Adolescents

DONNA C. FUTTERMAN, MD

## EPIDEMIOLOGY OF HIV AND SEXUALLY TRANSMITTED INFECTIONS IN YOUTH

International and domestic data demonstrate that the acquired immune deficiency syndrome (AIDS) pandemic continues to evolve in adolescents. Worldwide, a third of the 2.5 million infections in 2007 occurred among youth between the ages of 15 to 24, with some 2,300 young people per day acquiring human immunodeficiency virus (HIV).[1] Based on reported cases in 45 states and 5 territories, the Centers for Disease Control and Prevention (CDC) calculates that as of December 2006, young Americans aged 13 to 24 made up about 16% of the national population with a diagnosis of HIV.[2]

The CDC figure probably undercounts the number of young people with HIV because most HIV infections in this age group were recently acquired. Young people with HIV have had a relatively brief time in which to be diagnosed. Adolescence is defined by the American Academy of Pediatrics (AAP) to include young people aged 13 to 21 years, but the CDC breaks down HIV/AIDS data for youth into 3 different age groups: 13- to 14-, 15- to 19-, and 20- to 24-year-olds.

Adolescent HIV incidence and prevalence figures therefore are incomplete, whereas the census of AIDS diagnoses is more precise. The AIDS cases in teenagers and young adults represent the rapid progressors who did not receive HIV treatment, so they are only a small sample of the entire US adolescent HIV population. The major exception is the small but growing numbers of perinatally infected youth who are now surviving into their teenage years. These include nearly all the 711 13- to 14-year-olds with AIDS who entered the US adolescent population in 2006.

There were 478 new AIDS diagnoses among 13- to 19-year-olds in 2006 and another 1,669 in 20- to 24-year-olds.[3] The CDC surveillance figures indicate that although total new AIDS diagnoses declined by 4% between 2000 and 2006, AIDS rose by 21% among 13- to 24-year-olds.

Blacks are more disproportionately represented among HIV-positive youth than among adults. They made up 60% of the 2005 incident AIDS cases in the 13-to-24 age bracket[4] while accounting for approximately 15% of the US population in that age group. Young women also represent a higher proportion of incident HIV and AIDS among teens and young adults as compared to older adults. In 2005, females comprised 43% of incident AIDS cases in 13- to 19-year-olds compared to 26% among older persons with AIDS. From 2001 to 2005, about three-fourths of all 13- to 24-year-old women with AIDS were infected through heterosexual contact. Injection drug use accounted for a smaller percentage of transmission (16%) than among older women (28%).

The exposure categories for cases of AIDS among young males differ somewhat in the 2 adolescent age groups.[4] Sex with other men is the leading cumulative transmission category—57% of transmission in 13- to 19-year-old males and 69% in males aged 20 to 24. Injection drug use is the probable route of transmission in 10% of cumulative young male AIDS cases and heterosexual contact in 14%.

One of the more rigorous surveys of HIV in young people was the CDC's Young Men's Survey.[5] From 1994 to 1998, investigators recruited 3,448 men in 6 US cities who have sex with men and were aged 15 to 22. They found an overall HIV prevalence of 5.6% in 15- to 19-year-olds and 8.6% in 20- to 22-year-olds. Particularly alarming were the HIV rates in young black men: This subgroup had a total prevalence of 16%.[6] Nearly all (93%) were unaware of their infection. Of those with unrecognized infection, 71% thought that it was unlikely or impossible that they were infected. Yet 57% had had unprotected anal intercourse.

Men for this study were recruited at various homosexually oriented social venues, such as clubs and video arcades, many of them sites for anonymous sex. This might have biased the cohort toward young men most at risk for HIV. The National Longitudinal Study of Adolescent Health[7] found that young blacks as a whole have safer patterns of sexual and drug behavior than white youth. Yet even the blacks with the most conservative behavior (few sexual partners, low alcohol and drug use) had 7 times the combined prevalence of HIV and sexually transmitted infections (STIs) than their white counterparts. For the men who reported sex with other men, the whites had a combined HIV-STI prevalence of 6.7% whereas the comparable prevalence in blacks was 33.7%

The reasons for blacks' heightened population risk remains controversial. Discussion centers around a variety of environmental, or "structural," factors as well as individual ones.[8] Among these factors are blacks' segregated sexual networks, unstable housing leading to lack of family and community cohesion, poor health care, black men's high incarceration rates and low educational attainment, and the special isolation and double stigma weighing on black men who have sex with men.[9]

## RISK FOR HIV INFECTION AND SEXUALLY TRANSMITTED INFECTIONS

In 1996, the Institute of Medicine[10] released a report highlighting the interaction of behavioral, biological, and socioeconomic pathways that increase adolescent susceptibility (particularly young women's risk) to sexually transmitted diseases, including HIV infection.

The inflammation arising from STIs is known to increase susceptibility to HIV, and adolescents have relatively high rates of these diseases. Of the 12 million cases of STIs reported in the United States each year, 25% occur among teenagers.[11] In women, chlamydia and gonorrhea rates are highest among 15- to 19-year-olds, and in men second only to the 20- to 24-year-old age group.[12]

### Behavioral Factors

Many normative behaviors of adolescents intersect with risk-taking behaviors. Sexual activity is usually initiated during adolescence. More than half of young Americans have had sexual intercourse by the time they reach 17 years of age, a figure that does not differ markedly from most countries in the world.[13] A 2001 CDC[14] survey found that a third of US high school students were sexually active in the prior 3 months and that 14% reported having had more than 4 partners. About 58% of these teens reported using condoms during their last sexual intercourse.

There are subpopulations of youth who are at particularly high risk. Youth who are gay, bisexual, and transgender, homeless or runaway, injection drug users, incarcerated, in the foster care system, mentally ill, or sexually or physically abused are all at increased risk for exposure to HIV infection. These vulnerable youth experience higher rates of health and social problems in general than other youth.[15,16,17]

Young males who have sex with males are particularly vulnerable to HIV, as their social networks are more likely to include many HIV-infected persons.[18] The difference between behavior and sexual identity is an important distinction in youth. Development of sexual identity is a process that unfolds over several years. Same-sex experimentation is more common than ultimate gay or bisexual identity. Because some youth infected in male–male encounters do not consider themselves gay or bisexual, they may not view the limited safe sex messages targeted to gay males as personally relevant. For those youth who are gay, support and age-appropriate social outlets during the process of "coming out" can be life saving.[19]

Experimentation with alcohol and other drugs is frequent during adolescence and may impede the development of psychosocial skills. Substance use is also associated with increased risk-taking activities, including sexual activity and violence. Some 30% of high school students report drinking 5 or more alcoholic beverages at least once in the month prior to the CDC survey, and 4.2% had used heroin more than once in the month before the survey.[14] Heroin use among teens has doubled since 1991 to 3.1%, and 2.3% reported having ever injected drugs in the 2001 CDC survey. Adolescents are less likely to recognize their use as problematic. They rarely initiate drug treatment on their own, and if they do enter treatment it is often under the guidance of their schools, parents, or the criminal justice system as opposed to the medical system.

One of the most representative samples of HIV-positive youth was the 13-city REACH cohort (Reaching for Excellence in Adolescent Care and Health) funded by the National Institutes of Health (NIH).[20] It consisted of 325 HIV-positive adolescents (75% females) and 171 uninfected individuals. The cohort was recruited at 15 adolescent medical centers throughout the United States, where teens receive comprehensive health care and counseling. Nonetheless, risk behaviors remained disturbingly high among the HIV-positive members of the cohort.[21] About two-thirds were sexually active, with only half saying they had used a condom during their latest sexual intercourse. (Condom use increased to 60% by the end of the study.) Self-reported frequent alcohol use (15%) and frequent marijuana use (33%) were common, though both declined by half as the study progressed. Unprotected sex was significantly associated with depression, as was frequent alcohol use. Frequent marijuana use was associated with health anxiety.

These results were echoed by findings in the CDC Young Men's Survey[22] among men who kept their homosexual relations secret. These men (11% of the total and 18% of the blacks) were distinguished by greater feelings of isolation as well as societal and self-disapproval due to their sexual orientation. They had more frequent unsafe sex with men and women than those who were public about their sexuality. They also were more likely to have sex in public settings.

### Biological Factors

Biological factors contributing to the heightened infection rate among young women include: (1) During puberty, the single-layer columnar cells on the exocervix are progressively replaced by multilayer squamous cells, which are less susceptible to HIV, chlamydia, and gonorrhea; (2) Sexually transmitted infections are transmitted with greater efficiency from males to females due to the mechanics of sexual intercourse and the larger surface area of the female genital tract; (3) Sexually transmitted infections that enhance susceptibility to HIV are more likely to remain asymptomatic in women, and hence unnoticed and untreated, for a longer period of time.

### Socioeconomic Factors

Socioeconomic factors that heighten vulnerability to HIV are poverty and lack of access to health care, education, and prevention skills. Youth are the least insured sector of the population—35% of youth ages 18 to 24 have no, or partial, health insurance, and youth in this age group were 3 times more likely to be uninsured than youth ages 12 to 17 years.[23] They also face other barriers to accessing care, including mistrust of the health system, fear of inappropriate disclosure, and lack of understanding of their rights to confidentiality in the provider–client relationship.

Young people often use walk-in facilities and hospital emergency rooms for their acute health care needs. Providers in these settings tend to be unable to adequately communicate risk-reduction messages. Adolescence is a formative period in regard to behavioral patterns and decision-making ability in general and in regard to health care in particular. Teenagers' experiences with health care providers form the basis for future provider–client relationships and help-seeking patterns.

### Youth of HIV-Positive Parents

Tens of thousands of US children and teenagers have lost a parent to AIDS. In addition to the emotional devastation of this loss, parental illness and death from AIDS may raise youths' vulnerability to HIV and risk behaviors. This arises from the great disruption that occurs in families where a parent is sick. Children of HIV-positive parents are also frequently living in the same high seroprevalence communities as their parents, which increases their risk for acquiring infection. The percentage of these "affected" youth who are themselves HIV-positive is unknown. A review of 81 sexually infected teens followed at the Bronx-based Montefiore Medical Center Adolescent AIDS Program[24] found that 21% reported having at least 1 HIV-positive parent. Further research into the ways in which parental HIV infection mediates sexual risk behaviors and subsequent HIV infection in children would help elucidate the reasons for this risk factor. However, it is important to counsel and test the adolescent children of HIV-positive parents in a more systematic way.

## ADOLESCENT HIV DISEASE COURSE

Although the clinical course of HIV infection for most adolescents follows that seen in adults, there may be features that distinguish them from adults and children. The previously mentioned REACH study was undertaken by the Adolescent Medicine HIV/AIDS Research Network (AMHARN) to provide more definitive information on the clinical course of adolescents with sexually or injection-acquired HIV infection. It is the first prospective observational study of this nature.

In order to conduct comparative studies, REACH enrolled 325 HIV-positive youth 12 to 18 years old and 171 HIV-negative youth matched for age, sex, ethnicity, and risk behavior. (Adolescents with perinatally acquired HIV were excluded from the study.) Between 1996 and 2000, REACH examined unique features of HIV disease progression and manifestations, pubertal changes, the interaction of HIV and sexually transmitted disease as well as social and mental health correlates of disease progression in adolescents.

One of REACH's features was the preponderance of females in the cohort (373 out of 496 total study participants).[25] A major early finding concerned human papilloma virus (HPV) infection. REACH found high HPV prevalence among the HIV-positive (77.4%) and HIV-negative girls (54.5%), though the rate in the HIV-positive cohort was significantly higher. More striking was that the types of HPV infecting the HIV-positive girls were more likely to be those that confer high risk of cervical dysplasia (the type 16 and 18 groups). Only 29.9% of the girls with both HIV and HPV had normal cervical cytology, compared to 70% of the girls with only HPV. Overall, the relative risk for HPV in the HIV-positive cohort was 3.3 (95% CI, 1.6–6.7), and for squamous interepithelial lesions (SIL) it was 4.7 (95% CI, 1.8–14.8). The presence of HIV was significantly associated with HPV and SIL, but there was no correlation with a higher viral load or lower CD4 count, at least not in this group with relatively early HIV disease. This result suggests that HIV itself may somehow directly stimulate HPV, making the high-risk HPV harder for the immune system to clear.

### CLINICAL STATUS OF HIV-POSITIVE ADOLESCENTS IN CARE

Descriptive studies of HIV-positive adolescents in care consistently show that most youth enter care with significant immune dysfunction[26,27] and that clinical status varies markedly by transmission category.[28] Most youth have acquired their infection sexually during adolescence and enter care asymptomatic but with moderate immune dysfunction (median CD4 count: 410 cells/mm$^3$ for males and 464 cells/mm$^3$ for females).[27] In the REACH cohort, 49% of the HIV-positive females and

66% of the HIV-positive males had a CD4 count below 500 cells/mm$^3$ at study entry.[29] Viral loads were higher in the males (9% of the girls had viral loads above 50,000 copies/mL at study entry, compared with 23% of the boys), yet a similar percentage of each group were in treatment (45% and 41%, respectively). Among the females, 16% had AIDS at study entry whereas 18% of the males did. The higher lab values in the girls, coupled with a similar proportion with AIDS, gives an adolescent perspective to the debate over whether and why women might progress to AIDS at lower viral loads and higher CD4 counts.

In contrast, youth with perinatally acquired HIV have a different clinical course reflecting long-term infection. Of note, one pre-HAART (highly active antiretroviral therapy) study[30] reported that among such children surviving to adolescence, about one-fifth remained asymptomatic or with CD4 counts above 500 cells/mm. With the introduction of HAART, the subpopulation of HIV-positive adolescents with perinatal infection will grow steadily in number.[31] These youth are confronted with their own physical disability, isolation, and stigma, as well as the illness and death of their parent(s). At the same time, they are challenged by the tasks of adolescence. Some are first told of their infection only after they reach puberty.[32] Clinicians need to be aware of the possibility that perinatally infected, slowly progressing children will not be diagnosed until adolescence. Teenage children of HIV-positive parents need HIV testing if their infection status has not been confirmed previously.

## CLINICAL CARE

### ADOLESCENT-CENTERED CARE

Adolescents prefer health care settings that are oriented to their age group and providers who are attuned to their many needs.[33] The state of the art for adolescent care is a "1-stop shopping" multidisciplinary model that integrates primary and gynecological care with HIV, mental health, prevention, and case management services.[34] Many programs are not able to create adolescent programs separate from those for children or adults, but it may at least be possible to create a provider "team" that understands and wants to work with adolescents. Availability of flexible appointments that do not conflict with school or work, attention to payment barriers, and walk-in capacity for youth (who may not plan ahead) can facilitate adolescents' participation in health services. In 2007, the Health Resources and Services Administration (HRSA) launched a new Web site (www.hivcareforyouth.org), which covered clinical and mental health care as well as prevention and transition issues for HIV-infected youth.

### LEGAL ISSUES

All states have laws that allow minors to access, without their parents' consent, specific health services including emergency care, STI treatment, reproductive health support, and substance abuse therapy, but not all providers are aware of minors' right to consent on their own.[34,35] This right exists because adolescents might avoid needed care if they have to first turn to their parents.[36] In the case of HIV, providers must make a careful assessment of an adolescent's ability to understand HIV-related information and try to involve a supportive adult in his or her care while recognizing that this disclosure might take months. Additionally, the possibility of neglect and abuse of minor adolescents necessitates awareness of local child protection services and regulations.

### PHYSICAL EXAMINATION

Privacy is an important feature of the adolescent physical examination as adolescents often have a high level of modesty (due to anxiety about physical changes and a lack of understanding of their anatomy). Pubertal assessment using the Tanner staging system (which characterizes breasts, genitalia, and pubic hair) is helpful in interpreting normative blood values and choosing appropriate drug doses. The rest of the physical examination follows guidelines for adults.

### LABORATORY STUDIES, SEXUALLY TRANSMITTED INFECTION SCREENING, AND IMMUNIZATIONS

The high prevalence of STIs in this age group warrants integrating gynecological care and providing routine screening for HPV, chlamydia, gonorrhea, syphilis, herpes simplex virus (HSV), and hepatitis B[26,34,37,38] (see Box 138-1). Tuberculosis screening should also be done according to guidelines for HIV-positive adults. Utilizing community-based resources such as a mobile-medical van, school-based clinic, or youth recreation center can increase the rate of completion of tuberculosis testing.[39] The number of immunizations is greater for HIV-positive adolescents than for adults (see Box 138-2). Because immunizations transiently increase viral load, immunizations should not be scheduled in the few weeks before viral load tests.

### HIV TREATMENT

#### Dosing

Adolescents have not been extensively studied in the clinical trial system, and thus there is little direct data on them at present. Based on expert opinion, the Department of Health and Human Services (DHHS)[40–42] combined postpubertal adolescent treatment guidelines with those for adults. Because the pharmacokinetics

**Box 138-1**

***Baseline Laboratory Testing***

Confirmatory HIV serology (confirmation is recommended for adolescents, based on anecdotal reports of HIV-negative youth presenting for HIV care)
CD4-cell count (absolute and %)
Viral load
Complete blood count
G6PD level
Liver function tests
Serum BUN and creatinine
Urinalysis
Serology

- Hepatitis (A,B,C) – use HBcAb for prevaccination and HBsAb for postvaccination 1 month after completion of series
- Toxoplasmosis, CMV, and varicella (if no history of chickenpox)
- Pregnancy testing if needed
- Syphilis serology (RPR or VDRL)

Sexually transmitted diseases

- Gonorrhea/chlamydia (cervix or urethra via DNA-based method)
- Gonorrhea at oropharynx and anus (use culture media as DNA assays not reliable at these sites)

---

Papanicolaou smears of cervix for sexually experienced female patients. (As per HIV-negative adolescents, with colposcopy for follow-up of any abnormalities. The utility of HPV typing and anal Pap smears in both men and women is still under investigation.)

BUN, blood urea nitrogen; CMV, cytomegalovirus; G6PD, glucose-6 phosphate dehydrogenase; RPR, rapid plasma reagin; VDRL, Venereal Disease Research Laboratory

of some medications change during adolescence due especially to alterations in hepatic enzyme activity and plasma protein binding, care must be taken with medication dosing during pregnancy. See Chapter 20, Pharmacologic Considerations, for a more in-depth discussion of pharmacokinetics in adolescents. Researchers have yet to demonstrate any clinical effect on nucleoside analogs resulting from these changes. Less information is available for nonnucleoside reverse transcriptase inhibitors (NNRTIs) and protease inhibitors. At present, dosing is based on Tanner staging of pubertal development and not age.[40] Pediatric dosing should be used for adolescents who have not yet initiated puberty or are early in puberty (Tanner I/II). Dosing for adolescents who are in the middle of puberty (Tanner III/IV) should be based on whether they have completed their growth spurt.

**Box 138-2**

***Immunizations for Adolescents***

- Tetanus, diphtheria (TdaP), influenza, hepatitis B, and pneumococcal polysaccharide vaccines
- Pneumococcus: revaccinate once after 5 years or more have elapsed since initial vaccination, and vaccinate as close to diagnosis as possible when CD4 cell counts are highest
- For persons with medical/exposure indications including MSM and HIV infection: hepatitis A
- Catch-up on childhood vaccinations: measles mumps rubella (MMR) (Withhold MMR or other measles-containing vaccines from HIV-infected persons with evidence of severe immunosuppression.)
- Annual influenza vaccine (intranasal vaccine is contraindicated)
- Human papilloma virus vaccine
- Varicella vaccine is contraindicated

---

MSM, men who have sex with men

CDC. Recommended adult immunization schedule—United States, 2002–2003. *MMWR Morb Mortal Wkly Rep*. 2002;Oct 11;51(40):904–908.

Adolescents who have completed puberty (Tanner V) should be given adult doses.

### Drug Interactions

It is important to note that several key medications commonly prescribed to adolescent patients have significant interactions with antiretroviral medications.[40] For instance, ritonavir and indinavir increase levels of clarithromycin and possibly azithromycin (prescribed for uncomplicated cervicitis or urethritis) as well as metronidazole (employed for treating bacterial vaginosis and trichomoniasis). Because ritonavir and nevirapine decrease estradiol levels, concurrent use with combined oral contraceptive pills (OCPs) may reduce contraceptive efficacy. Clinicians should consider switching to injectable Depo-Provera or progestin-only formulations of OCPs for better contraception efficacy. Ritonavir and nevirapine as well as efavirenz reduce methadone levels. An increase in methadone dose may be required to prevent withdrawal symptoms. These warnings also apply to the protease inhibitor lopinavir/ritonavir (Kaletra), which contains ritonavir, though not at full dose.

Drug interactions become very complicated. Efavirenz usually reduces the drug levels of coadministered drugs, but it should not be given with astemizole, midazolam, triazolam, cisapride, and ergot derivatives, whose increased levels might lead to life-threatening toxicities. Indeed, alcohol and any psychoactive drug should be taken with caution by persons receiving efavirenz. These agents can reinforce each other's effects on the central nervous system (CNS).

### Treatment Strategy

The timing of treatment initiation has been the subject of continuing debate. It is difficult to determine the optimum balance between protecting patients from immune decline and clinical disease while minimizing side effects and the development of drug-resistant HIV. The playing field is constantly evolving along with the introduction of more effective antiretroviral agents and improved management of toxicities.[43-46]

According to the latest federal guidelines, antiretroviral therapy of postpubertal adolescents should start when a patient's CD4 count falls below 350 cells/mm$^3$.[40] Therapy initiation is also indicated by the presence of AIDS-defining illnesses, HIV-associated nephropathy, or advanced hepatitis B requiring treatment. If patients with CD4 counts above 350 cells/mm$^3$ lack these signs, physicians may still wish to commence therapy when considering their patients' various comorbidities and general prognosis. (See Table 138-1 for the

## Table 138-1

**Department of Health and Human Services Panel on Antiretroviral Guidelines for Adults and Adolescents (Recommended Antiretroviral Therapies for Treatment-Naïve Patients)**

| *Select 1 Component from Column A and 1 from Column B* | *Column A (NNRTI or PI Options)* | *Column B (Dual-NRTI Options)* |
|---|---|---|
| **Preferred components** | *NNRTI:* efavirenz[a]<br>or *PI:*<br>atazanavir + ritonavir<br>fosamprenavir + ritonavir (2x/day)<br>lopinavir/ritonavir[b] (2x/day) (coformulated) | abacavir/lamivudine[c] (for patients who test negative for HLAB*5701) (coformulated)[d]<br>tenofovir/emtricitabine[c] (coformulated) (AII) |
| **Alternative to preferred components** | *NNRTI:* nevirapine[e]<br>or *PI:*<br>atazanavir[f]<br>fosamprenavir<br>fosamprenavir + ritonavir (1x/day)<br>lopinavir/ritonavir (1x/day) (coformulated)<br>saquinavir + ritonavir | zidovudine/lamivudine[c] (coformulated)<br>didanosine + (emtricitabine or lamivudine) |

[a]Efavirenz is not recommended for use in the first trimester of pregnancy or in sexually active women with childbearing potential who are not using effective contraception.

[b]The pivotal study that led to the recommendation of lopinavir/ritonavir as a preferred PI component was based on twice-daily dosing. A smaller study has shown similar efficacy with once-daily dosing but also showed a higher incidence of moderate to severe diarrhea with the once-daily regimen (16% vs 5%). In addition, once-daily dosing may be insufficient for those with viral loads > 100,000 copies/mL.

[c]Emtricitabine may be used in place of lamivudine and vice versa.

[d]Please refer to "DHHS Adults and Adolescents Antiretroviral Treatment Guidelines Panel's Communication Regarding Abacavir – April 4, 2008" at: www.aidsinfo.nih.gov/guidelines.

[e]Nevirapine should not be initiated to the following treatment-naïve patients: women with CD4 count > 250 cells/mm$^3$ or in men with CD4 count > 400 cells/mm$^3$ because of increased risk for symptomatic hepatic events in these patients.

[f]Atazanavir must be boosted with ritonavir if used in combination with efavirenz or tenofovir.

Panel on Antiretroviral Guidelines for Adults and Adolescents. Guidelines for the use of antiretroviral agents in HIV-1-infected adults and adolescents. Department of Health and Human Services. January 29, 2008; 63 (Table 6). Available at: www.aidsinfo.nih.gov/ContentFiles/AdultandAdolescentGL.pdf. Accessed April 20, 2008.

These guidelines change frequently. The most recent version is viewable at: aidsinfo.nih.gov/guidelines.

NNRTI, non-nucleoside reverse transcriptase inhibitors; NRTI, nucleoside reverse transcriptase inhibitors; PI, protease inhibitor

recommended antiretroviral regimens in treatment-naïve patients.)

Several key features mark a steady stream of treatment innovations that support the guidelines' move toward earlier treatment. The first is the gradual replacement of zidovudine and stavudine by more benign nucleoside analogs less likely to promote limb fat loss (lipoatrophy). For example, the combination of tenofovir and emtricitabine plus efavirenz was found superior to zidovudine and lamivudine plus efavirenz in terms of virologic suppression and adverse events.[47,48] After nearly 3 years (144 weeks), initially treatment-naïve patients receiving tenofovir-emtricitabine had significantly more limb fat (7.9 kg compared to 5.4 kg in zidovudine/lamivudine recipients) and fewer had use discontinued due to adverse events (5% vs 11%, respectively). Concerns persist, however, about the association between tenofovir use and gradual renal impairment.[40]

Another important innovation has been the widespread adoption of ritonavir-enhanced protease inhibitor therapy.[49-51] Low, subtherapeutic doses of ritonavir slow down the hepatic metabolism of other HIV protease inhibitors, stabilizing their plasma levels for longer periods. Ritonavir also flattens out the intra- and interpersonal variations in protease inhibitor metabolism, reducing the proportion of patients with marginal drug levels on any given day. Protease inhibitors combined with ritonavir attain more consistent viral suppression with reduced emergence of drug-resistant HIV.[49,52] Such therapy is also more likely to achieve virologic suppression in patients who have acquired HIV with partial protease inhibitor resistance, whether during HIV transmission or previous therapy. The major disadvantage to these ritonavir-including regimens is that ritonavir markedly increases blood lipid levels.

Still more striking are the introduction of new drugs, including agents either less susceptible to HIV drug resistance mutations (the protease inhibitor darunavir[53] and the NNRTI etravirine)[54] or utilizing novel mechanisms of action (the integrase inhibitor raltegravir[55] and the entry inhibitor maraviroc).[56] These have greatly widened the possibilities for HIV suppression after failure of initial regimens. In large trials of patients with broadly drug-resistant HIV, the proportion exhibiting week 24 virologic suppression (plasma viral load below 50 copies/mL) were 60% (etravirine plus darunavir/ritonavir), 63% (raltegravir), and 45% (maraviroc). (All patients also received additional antiviral drugs in the form of optimized background therapy, which took into account their virus' drug resistance profile. Virologic suppression in patients who received the background therapy without the investigational agent or agents was much lower in the trials—40%, 33%, and 22%, respectively).

Comparative trials currently are evaluating these new agents in treatment-naïve patients. Preliminary results have indicated that they perform comparably to such established agents as lopinavir or efavirenz.[40] In the maraviroc trial, the results were slightly better for the efavirenz arm, and the difference was just large enough that noninferiority could not be concluded under the trial protocol's statistical standards. Existing antiretroviral therapies are highly suppressive in treatment-naïve patients. It will be difficult to prove that the new agents represent an improvement, except over the long run or in terms of tolerability. As it stands now, these agents give greater confidence when offering earlier initial therapy. They can provide adequate back-up therapy when first regimens fail.

The REACH cohort[19] reported that 45% of the females and 41% of the males were receiving antiretroviral therapy at study entry. But as noted previously, REACH did not include perinatally infected youth, and participants were at a relatively early disease stage. Half of the HIV-positive females had entry CD4 counts above 500 cells/mm$^3$. The proportion was lower among the males—only 34%.

A REACH immunology study[57] indicated that thymic function in HIV-positive teenagers was stable throughout adolescence rather than declining as had been thought previously. Investigators found evidence of active lymphocyte regeneration in perinatally infected teens as well as those with more recent infection. The capability for immune restoration is high in young people and remains until late in HIV disease progression. When effective antiretroviral therapy is administered, CD4 counts are able to rebound at older ages and with more years of living with HIV infection than had been previously thought.

### Treatment Adherence

HIV medications require strict adherence to prevent the emergence of resistant HIV. Unfortunately, incomplete adherence remains an active problem among HIV-positive youth. Common reasons for missing doses are side effects, the inconvenience of taking so many pills, forgetfulness, and feeling that medications continually reinforce the reality of being HIV infected. Adolescents often blame the complications of daily life for their inability to follow dosing schedules.[58] In the REACH study,[59] only 41% claimed good adherence. Eighteen percent had never taken their prescribed antiretroviral drugs. Depression and higher pill burdens were associated with decreased adherence. Poor adherence was frequent even though strictly following dosing schedules correlated with undetectable viral loads and high CD4 counts.

As with any successful effort to provide teens with comprehensive care, the first step to ensuring adherence is establishing a therapeutic alliance between patients and health care staff. The Montefiore Adolescent AIDS Program systematically addresses adherence issues using

> **Box 138-3**
>
> ***Adherence: Using Your EARS***
>
> **ENGAGE**
>
> - Establish therapeutic alliance and build trust; goal is active participation by adolescent in all aspects of treatment
> - Address immediate needs (health, housing, insurance, family, partners)
> - Educate about HIV infection: transmission, disease course, and HAART
>
> **ASSESS**
>
> - Stage HIV infection
> - Assess mental health and cognitive abilities
> - Assess physical ability to take medicines
> - Assess support systems and disclosure issues: family and friends
> - Assess readiness to begin medications (using stages of change model)
>
> **READINESS**
>
> - Decide with adolescent on regimen that integrates clinical needs with lifestyle—show different pills/combinations
> - Solidify support systems: family and/or treatment buddy
> - Practice chosen regimen with surrogate vitamins; distribute medications into a weekly medication planner, program 1-day pill timer with the adolescent
> - Address adherence barriers discovered in vitamin practice run
>
> **SUPPORT**
>
> - Provide ongoing support with frequent clinic visits and phone contact
> - Acknowledge and address side effects
> - Develop strategies to ensure tolerability and regularity
> - Facilitate interactions with other youth taking medications
>
> HAART, highly active antiretroviral therapy

the acronym EARS (Engage, Assess, Readiness/Regimens, Support) (see Box 138-3).

Doctors have historically prescribed twice-daily medication regimens, but now a more convenient once-daily schedule is available for a number of antiretrovirals. Notably, a single once-daily tablet is available that provides a complete antiretroviral regimen of tenofovir, emtricitabine, and efavirenz. In addition, ritonavir enhancement has lengthened dosing periods for protease inhibitors. Once-daily schedules are feasible for treatment-naïve patients with low viral loads (and atazanavir is always once daily).[40] Serum half-lives still do not approach those of efavirenz or other NNRTIs, however. Many providers prefer a protease inhibitor-sparing regimen for the initial regimen because adherence tends to be more critical with protease inhibitors and side effects more difficult to manage.[60]

An adult AIDS Clinical Trials Group (ACTG) study[60] found that Trizivir, a coformulation of abacavir, AZT, and 3TC, was less effective than a combination of efavirenz plus either Trizivir or Combivir (AZT-3TC coformulation). The NNRTI-containing regimens are the only good alternatives to protease inhibitors for initial therapy,[40] at least until raltegravir or maraviroc are established as protease inhibitor replacements in this situation. Efavirenz (Category D) has the potential to cause birth defects. It is not recommended for women who may become pregnant. Another major NNRTI, nevirapine, can cause severe liver impairment that seems more frequent in women. Also, maraviroc is only effective in patients whose HIV uses only the CCR5 coreceptor when entering CD4+ cells. Some 80% to 90% of treatment-naïve patients and 50% to 55% of treatment-experienced patients test positive for this exclusively R5-tropic HIV.[61]

## PSYCHOSOCIAL ISSUES

An understanding of adolescent development is crucial for viewing the adolescent as a health care client and participant in treatment. In addition to the physical changes in puberty, adolescence consists of a series of cognitive and psychosocial development phases. The Montefiore Adolescent AIDS Program[34] has observed 5 key stages for HIV-positive adolescents coping with their changing health status.

### Stages of Coping with HIV

***Being Informed of HIV Status*** In helping youth cope with their HIV infection, it is simultaneously necessary to instill hope and provide support for the challenging years that lie ahead. Many adolescents are still concrete thinkers. They have a hard time comprehending the concept of disease latency and asymptomatic infection. Young people without apparent symptoms must learn to strike a balance between healthy denial of their condition and morbid preoccupation.

The complexities inherent for all adolescents in the process of integrating sexuality into self-identity are compounded for HIV-positive youth. For substance-abusing youth, learning one's status may be a powerful motivator for entering substance abuse treatment or conversely may make drug treatment less likely. Some youth may need psychotropic medications for premorbid psychiatric problems or newly occurring symptoms such as anxiety and depression. We have found individual and peer group interventions with psychosocial providers to be very effective.

Since 2003, with the approval of "point of care" rapid HIV testing (negative and preliminary reactive results are known within 20 minutes), the experience of learning one's results will increasingly take place the day of testing, heightening the need for immediately available support and referral resources. Most clinicians have found that youth prefer getting their results immediately, and this has also greatly increased the percentage of those tested who get their results.

***Disclosure and Partner Notification*** A major initial hurdle confronting HIV-positive teenagers is deciding when, and to whom, they should disclose their status.[61] Although the involvement of a supportive adult (preferably a parent) is ideal, many youth fear losing the love of their parent or hurting them. The need to rely on adults because of illness is often in sharp contrast to the developmental need to establish independence and identify with one's peer group. For gay or substance-abusing youth, disclosure to a parent is especially threatening as they may have to simultaneously reveal their HIV status, sexuality, or drug use at the same time. That could lead to rejection, harassment, and even violence.[19]

Disclosure becomes a particularly salient issue with advancing disease because it is difficult to conceal medications from the people with whom one lives. Adolescence is one of the most "observed" times of life. Young people often do not have much space to call their own. Privacy is especially compromised for adolescents living in crowded homes or residential programs. Even in school, institutional bathrooms provide no seclusion for taking medication.

Disclosure to sexual partners is ethically compelling and complicated. Of course, HIV-positive teens should inform any sexual partners and always engage in safe sex. But youth face several unique issues when disclosing their HIV status: In the first place, the adolescent's social world is smaller and more intense than that of adults, so confidentiality is more easily compromised. Providers must be aware that young people in earlier stages of sexual behavior have had fewer partners than adults and that the notified sex partner might figure out the source of the exposure. If 1 person knows, soon everyone in the group might know. Adolescents greatly fear that their current partner will reject them if they disclose. Disclosure and partner notification should be well planned. Providers can help the adolescent to "play out the scenario" and offer to participate in the disclosure process, as well as make available the health department partner notification program. The prevention plan of the CDC currently places an increased emphasis on "prevention with positives" highlighting the importance of this phase of clinical work. Increasingly, adolescent programs are partnering with local departments of health to facilitate the identification and testing of sexual partners, and to identify sexual networks with heightened rates of transmission utilizing the long experience of partner notification for STIs.

***Learning about Viral Load and CD4 Marker Changes*** Given the prognostic significance of these markers, adolescents need to understand how viral load and CD4 counts relate to the course of their HIV disease. Viral load and CD4 counts vary widely and even when they do change significantly, a satisfying and productive life remains possible. This too may be difficult to comprehend for youth who still think in concrete terms.

***Becoming Symptomatic*** The presence of HIV-related symptoms is often anxiety-inducing. Developing concrete symptoms can pierce denial in those who have only superficially grasped their infection. For some youth, the appearance of symptoms increases their determination to fight HIV and makes them willing to consider treatment. When symptoms occur, it is important to explore their meaning, correct any misconceptions, and ensure that adequate services and supports are in place.

***Death and Dying*** Many adolescents have naïve notions about death and dying, like adults. They often avoid the topic. If the end of life becomes a real prospect, providers can assist by exploring the perceptions of dying and helping a young person plan for that time. Discussions should include options for dying in the hospital or at home, funeral, or memorial services. For HIV-positive adolescents who are parents themselves, a critical consideration is child custody or permanency planning, including creation of "memories" for offspring. Resolving relationships with family, close friends, and others is another important task. Introducing the topics of living wills and health care proxies are practical ways to initiate such discussion at a time when the adolescent patient has advanced disease but is not imminently dying.

### Mental Illness and Substance Use

Mental illness and substance abuse are important comorbidities for HIV-positive adolescents, as they increase an adolescent's vulnerability to HIV. Failure to identify and address these issues will hobble a patient's ability to cope with his or her disease. Adherence to antiretroviral treatment will be problematic.

Several case series indicate a high prevalence of depression, bipolar disorder, and anxiety in HIV-positive adolescents.[62] Similarly, researchers have also found a frequent history of sexual abuse among HIV-positive adolescents. A New York City study cohort[26] reported that 30% of the males and 35% of the females described childhood sexual abuse. In the REACH study,[20] 6% of the girls and 17% of the boys reported using illicit drugs beyond marijuana in that period. Mental health practitioners should ideally be part of the clinical team. They should intervene as needed with such therapies as medication and individual and peer group support.

### Age Transitions

As medical care continues to improve, a considerable number of HIV-positive adolescents will be healthy enough to "graduate" from pediatric to adolescent and finally adult care programs. Emerging adults require programs that address their developmental needs. They face the concurrent challenges of health care maintenance, medication adherence, and illness within the context of maturing sexuality and establishing an independent life. The concept of transition from pediatric and adolescent to adult health care settings has been described in the literature for other chronic illnesses.[63-65] Little has been written about introducing HIV-positive adolescents to adult health care systems. Even a recent consensus statement on health care transition, signed by 3 major US medical associations, did not mention HIV.[66]

Young people can be quite reluctant to leave their established providers. In response, many adolescent HIV programs have expanded their upper age limit from ages 21 to 24 years. But inevitably, there comes a time when transfer to adult care is appropriate. Adolescent HIV programs frequently begin addressing transition months before it takes place. Patients and program staff conduct an intensive effort to formulate the patient's life and treatment goals, and the patients have a chance to consult with their future providers before the move.

The other group facing transition is perinatally infected youth. New medications now allow survival into their teens and beyond. These emerging adolescents face the usual struggle to achieve independence, but for them rebellion often includes a self-destructive decline in treatment adherence. Also, young HIV-positive teenagers develop sexually just as other adolescents do. They need particular training on communicating with sex partners and risk-reduction strategies. Their health care providers should either expand the scope of their services or collaborate with adolescent health specialists. Alternatively, they can work to transfer their maturing patients to adolescent HIV programs.

## HIV COUNSELING AND TESTING, PREVENTION, AND OUTREACH

The promise of new advances in HIV care, in the context of continued HIV transmission among adolescents, heightens the need for routine HIV testing among youth in more settings than just prenatal care. Adolescents engaging in high-risk behaviors often do not believe that they are at risk, but it is a myth that adolescents refuse HIV testing or that they do not want providers to ask personal questions. In fact, many youth prefer that the clinician initiate such discussions.[67,68]

HIV-testing programs must be accessible to youth to have any chance of success. In addition to primary care sites, venues that should consider offering routine HIV counseling and testing include mobile units, school-based health clinics, drug treatment, and family planning programs. Services need to be youth-friendly, flexible, free or low cost, and help overcome barriers such as transportation. Youth need special help with the implications of partner notification requirements. They should be made aware of the availability of anonymous HIV testing, although the patient–provider relationship, which is confidential but not anonymous, establishes a stronger clinical bond. It establishes the momentum for youth-sensitive follow-up, including treatment and counseling.

In addition to providing basic HIV information and obtaining consent during the pretest counseling visit, the health provider can also promote preventive healthy behaviors and assess substance use or family planning issues. The counseling session is an invaluable teaching opportunity to educate teens about condom use and safer sex, whether or not testing occurs. Providers should be aware that the prevention benefits of HIV testing have been established for HIV-positive patients (who reduce their risk behaviors by up to 50% after finding out they are HIV-positive) but unfortunately not as clearly for HIV-negative patients. HIV counseling for adolescents should be culturally sensitive and tailored to the developmental needs of adolescents. Youth considered potentially self-destructive or impulsive require careful assessment prior to testing. Special measures to preserve confidentiality should be taken in settings such as foster care, residential institutions, or detention facilities.[69] All states currently require confidential reporting of names of those testing HIV-positive to their local department of health.

The continued unacceptably high level of HIV transmission in the United States—40,000 new cases per year with half to one-fourth among 13- to 24-year-olds—has increased concerns that the epidemic is not being brought under control. It is quite shocking that 25 years into the epidemic, fully 25% of those who are HIV-positive do not know they are infected. Beyond the traditional gay neighborhoods and IV drug-using populations, a number of poor communities have reached HIV prevalences of 1% or greater. This is a disturbing level that indicates a high concentration of HIV risk in the community and the chance for a runaway epidemic. To help counter the threat, the CDC[70] now recommends making HIV testing a "routine" part of health care in such communities.

A survey conducted by Montefiore Medical Center[71] found that Bronx clinics screened only one-third as many patients for HIV as for other STIs (10% vs 30%). Yet 1% of these clinics' patients are already known to have HIV. Making HIV testing part of a standard medical work-up poses great challenges for health care staff. The traditional HIV counseling, testing, and referral process involves 2 sessions totaling about an hour and requires staff with specific training. Counseling adolescents poses particular challenges: Special sensitivity is required to address their level of sexual and emotional development. Even to have teens return for follow-up visits where they receive test results calls for special effort, like telephone reminders.

To ease the burden and extend HIV testing, Montefiore's Adolescent AIDS Program has created a streamlined testing protocol called ACTS, for Advise, Consent, Test, and Support (www.ACTSHIVtest.org).[70] This 4-step protocol (see Figure 138-1) assigns only about 1 to 5 minutes to counseling and relies heavily on referrals for any further services, especially for those who test positive. ACTS provides a practical, "reality-based" response to the demands of testing many people in clinics with limited resources. It is quite suitable for the new rapid HIV test, which can deliver results in as little as 20 minutes. It helps ease the organizational restructuring that this test requires.

Ideally, broad-based education and skills-building to form healthy behavioral patterns occurs before teens become sexually active. Providers should carefully evaluate the resources to which they refer their patients. A number of key elements mark successful adolescent programs. Beyond providing basic information, such programs incorporate interventions to increase self-esteem, individual competence, and social skills. They incorporate a peer-support model and take advantage of adolescents' inherent psychosocial development to diffuse skills they acquire into the community at-large.

## PREVENTION

A comprehensive prevention strategy requires multiple levels that target youths' various psychosocial and health care needs. These levels include primary care encounters, education in schools, open discussions in religious and community organizations, and public service announcements.

Comprehensive programs that teach sexual decision making (including declining to have sex [abstinence] and condom use) are desperately needed. But as long as sex education remains a cultural battleground, with "abstinence-only" programs congressionally mandated, the lack of adequate programs will lead to new cases of HIV. "Abstinence-only" messages or delay of sexual behaviors are validating for many youth but not effective for youth who are already sexually active. The range of prevention can be briefly summarized as ABC—Abstain, Be Faithful, and Condomize. Although each of these steps is important, none of them stands alone or is perfect.

The AIDS Risk Reduction Model[72] (ARRM) has been the most widely applied approach to primary prevention programs for high-risk youth and secondary prevention to deter transmission and reinfection of those who are HIV-positive.[73] The ARRM maintains that to change behavior, one must first label that behavior as risky, then make a commitment to change or reduce the behavior, and, lastly, take action to perform the desired change. Fear, anxiety, and social norms influence movement between these stages.

All adolescent care facilities should make condoms available for sexually active youth and provide education on proper condom use using anatomical models. Young people have difficulty incorporating condom use into their sexual encounters for a number of reasons. Among these are: (1) lack of knowledge on using condoms properly, (2) lack of communication and social skills, (3) lack of available condoms at the time of sexual activity, and (4) impulsive behavior exacerbated by drug or alcohol use. Because condoms are used by men, gender and power imbalances in relationships contribute to greater vulnerability of adolescent females and gay males. These imbalances are heightened when the male partner is older. Encouraging youth to develop their personal values and social skills adds to self-esteem and enhances their ability to fend off pressures to engage in sexual risk behaviors.

### School and Community-Based Programs

Schools are logical venues for health education, and school-based health clinics could provide immediate health care for youth with sexually acquired infections and pregnancy-related needs. The most comprehensive meta-analysis of school-based programs was conducted by Kirby.[74,75] He found that the elements of successful programs included (1) a narrow and specific focus, (2) instruction on social influences and pressures, (3) age- and experience-appropriate reinforcement of values and norms against unprotected sex, and (4) skill-building activities. Schools' refusal to take up "healthy sexuality" or to include condom demonstrations undermines the effectiveness of their curricula for all students.[29] The implementation of supportive safe sex programs for gay and bisexual youth is even more constrained, denying health-enhancing information to the most vulnerable youth.

The most vulnerable adolescents are those most likely to be outside systems that could provide prevention,

# ACTS

ADVISE
CONSENT
TEST
SUPPORT

## A Rapid System for HIV Counseling and Testing

### ADVISE Routine HIV testing is for all patients.

- ▷ HIV is the virus that causes AIDS, only an HIV test can detect infection
- ▷ Testing benefits HIV+ patient's health and improves prevention for all
- ▷ HIV can be transmitted sexually, via needle-sharing or perinatally

### CONSENT Use NYS DOH (Part B) form.

- ▷ Testing is voluntary and can be confidential or anonymous
- ▷ For patients who test HIV+, NY protects confidentiality and requires partner notification and name reporting
- ▷ Obtain signature on consent form

### TEST Use rapid or conventional test with blood or oral fluid.

- ▷ Rapid tests: have patient wait for results
- ▷ Conventional tests: verify contact information and make plans to deliver results later, as done with other test results

### SUPPORT Give results and allow time to process.

- ▷ HIV-negative:
  - Explain the test by itself is not prevention and discuss staying negative
  - Encourage partner testing and annual testing; retest sooner if new risk: pregnancy, unsafe sex, STD, new partner, IV drug use or acutely ill
  - Clarify if client needs to retest in three months (window period)
- ▷ HIV-positive:
  - Coping: Ask about/respond to patient's concerns, call counselor if needed
  - Treatment: Link patient to care, emphasize benefits of treatment, support
  - Prevention: Discuss prevention and partner disclosure
  - Review DOH reporting, partner notification and domestic violence laws

ACTSHIVTest.org

**FIGURE 138-1** ACTS pocket card. Reprinted with permission from Adolescent AIDS Program, Montefiore Medical Center. Available at: www.actshivtest.org.

counseling and testing, and treatment services. School-based programs cannot link up with youth who are drug users, juvenile offenders, truants, runaways, homeless, or migrants, as these youth are most often not in school.

**Parents**

Frank discussions between parents and their adolescents about condoms can lead teens to adopt behaviors that will protect them from STIs. Recent results from a large school-based survey of 12,118 youth in grades 7 to 12 (the National Longitudinal Study on Adolescent Health)[76] point to the importance of family and school influences as well as that of individual characteristics on healthy behaviors in adolescents. A multisite study[77] of 372 sexually active adolescents 14 to 17 years old conducted in New York, Alabama, and Puerto Rico found that condom use increased 3 times among teens whose mothers talked to them before their first sexual encounter. Further, teens who used condoms during their first intercourse were 20 times more likely to use condoms on subsequent occasions.

## OUTREACH

Community outreach is critical to programs focusing on HIV in youth. It is essential to point out HIV care and prevention services to at-risk youth and their providers. Given that most HIV-infected teenagers are unaware of their infection, linkages with agencies serving high-risk youth are crucial for clinics. But these connections are not by themselves sufficient to identify HIV-positive youth and bring them into care. Social marketing campaigns that span the continuum from HIV prevention through testing and care can make a major contribution.[78] One example—"HIV. Live with it. Get Tested."—uses youthful sex slang, like "Knockin' Boots" or "Gettin' Busy," to talk about the links between unprotected sex, HIV risk, and the importance of HIV testing. Designed in collaboration with an ad agency, a medical communications company and, most importantly, young people themselves, the campaign promoted testing and care services backed up by a citywide coalition of adolescent HIV programs and community-based youth agencies. It combined media placements with community outreach and services at places frequented by at-risk youth.[79]

## VACCINES AND OTHER FORMS OF MEDICAL PREVENTION

The ultimate AIDS prevention strategy would be an HIV vaccine, but such a development presents formidable biologic and social hurdles not encountered in other diseases.

The virus envelope is coated with protective layers of carbohydrate and host cell membrane. It also quickly mutates to escape immune pressure. Worse yet, HIV is highly toxic to the very lymphocytes that form the main immune defense against it. Probably for these reasons, the immune system has proven ineffective in controlling HIV infection. Stimulating antibodies appears at first glance to be the most effective vaccine strategy, 1 that works in other diseases, but the HIV-infected slow progressors and the few persons who seem resistant to contracting HIV are not distinguished by their antibody production but by high levels of cytotoxic lymphocytes that kill HIV-infected cells.[80] Probably, vaccines should trigger some combination of cellular and antibody responses, but against what targets on HIV exactly? Conserved viral regions that would be vulnerable to effective immune attack have not yet been found.[81]

In the absence of a vaccine, microbicides represent an alternative approach to medical prevention. Prior to sexual intercourse, users would apply these topical agents to the vagina or rectum to inhibit HIV transmission. Microbicides' main advantage is that they give receptive sexual partners a nonintrusive way to reduce their relatively high HIV risk without having to negotiate condom use with potentially unwilling and intimidating males. (Microbicidal penile gels and wipes are also under investigation.[82]) Most of the microbicides in advanced trials are polyanionic surfactants, or detergents, that disrupt viral coatings. The rest are simple buffering agents that increase vaginal acidity during sex. Trials to date have failed to show any benefit for vaginal gels and have even observed higher HIV rates in the active microbicide users compared with those assigned to a neutral placebo gel.[83–85] (Previously unappreciated vaginal irritation may be an issue here.) Microbicide development is shifting to agents with specific antiretroviral activity, and hopefully, less potential for local toxicity. Among these products are gels containing tenofovir or daprivirine, which block the action of HIV reverse transcriptase. Entry inhibitors such as maraviroc do not need to penetrate cells to have a protective effect. They are another strong possibility.

It is noteworthy that the major success in medical prevention research is a one-time intervention that required no further commitment by trial participants. This measure is male circumcision. Circumcision eliminates a site in men that is highly susceptible to HIV, the mucosal surface under the foreskin. In contrast to the microbicide studies described here, 3 male circumcision trials in South Africa, Kenya, and Uganda involving 11,000 men ended prematurely because circumcision proved so successful.[86–88] Men circumcised at the start of these trials experienced 60% less new HIV infection than their uncircumcised peers in the trials' control arms.

Testing vaccines in adolescents is especially important for successful vaccines. It will be necessary to demonstrate the extent of a vaccine's protection in this population because young people's immune patterns could well be different than adults. Immune cytokines in the genital track are influenced by the presence of other STIs,[89] of which HIV-vulnerable teens have a plentitude. But even in normal times, the genital tract of adolescents, especially adolescent girls, may differ from that of adults. For example, a recent small study[90] found that teens experience a greater drop in vaginal immunoglobulin during the follicular phase before ovulation.

A warning of the confusion that comes from leaving adolescents out of vaccine testing comes from a small REACH substudy[37] of responses to the hepatitis B vaccine. REACH participants who received the vaccine before entering the study (ie, at a younger age) had a differential response according to HIV status. Seventy percent of those who were HIV-negative responded, which is already rather low, versus 41.1% of those who were HIV-positive. Study participants who were vaccinated during the course of REACH (median age of 17) had a similar response rate regardless of HIV status—37%. One immediate issue is that all these teenagers received the pediatric vaccine dose. Another is the confounding factor that stems from the high levels of STIs in this teenage cohort. The high frequency of STIs may have dampened immune responses even in the HIV-negative study participants.

Testing vaccines in a high-risk young population should be attractive to vaccine developers because it provides quicker answers on a vaccine's effectiveness. However, there are unique community and ethical issues in conducting vaccine trials in youth. A vital issue is the counseling that would accompany any trial. It is crucial that trial participants do not assume that a vaccine is protective and abandon condom use and other safe sex strategies. Such an increase in risk-taking might overwhelm the benefits of a vaccine that turns out to be only partially protective, to the grief of trial participants and investigators. Counseling teenagers, with their special psychosocial needs, would be qualitatively different from adults. This educational process would have to teach the tenuous promise offered by an experimental vaccine, the chance of being randomly assigned to the placebo arm, and the need to conscientiously return for scheduled visits even though the vaccine is doing no apparent good. Beyond that, the necessary safe sex section would be more basic and more controversial than for adults. Then there are the legal and ethical issues in obtaining informed consent and assent from minors, who also need parental approval.

Once a vaccine is on the market, administration to teenagers will be a central part of vaccine distribution. There may be little point to immunizing children years before their sexual debut if that gives immunity against HIV a chance to decline before it is needed. Childhood vaccination, the only effective system we have, is enforced by school entry requirements. Current controversies over immunizing school students with the new HPV vaccine presages what is in store for an HIV vaccine. Both viruses are sexually transmitted, and the HIV vaccine, like the HPV vaccine, will be expensive. Despite strong trial data, public questioning of the HPV vaccine's effectiveness continues. HIV vaccines, especially the initial versions, probably will not have as strong supporting data. And HIV is much less prevalent than HPV.

HIV vaccine distribution may need to focus on high-risk populations, at least at first. Considering the past failures of targeted hepatitis B vaccine programs, the HIV effort will have to develop innovative motivational techniques and delivery channels. These programs should include careful discussion of the continuing contribution of other prevention methods to healthy sexuality. That is an abstract concept that adolescents may well find hard to grasp—as will many adults.

## CONCLUSION

HIV infection in adolescents continues to challenge health providers, policy makers, and advocates for youth. There will be no relief from its complexities in the foreseeable future. Primary care providers are in a unique position to utilize effective HIV prevention and care interventions. Successful programs move beyond moralism to realism. They show a willingness to engage young people and their families in a sensitive dialogue on the needs of youthful sexual development. Youth at high risk for HIV should be identified and referred to comprehensive care and counseling as soon as possible. HIV-positive youth need intensive individual and group interventions to keep themselves healthy and reduce transmission to others. To protect their patient populations, health care providers have to commit time and effort to making adolescent services visible, flexible, affordable, confidential, culturally appropriate, and universally available.

## REFERENCES

1. UNAIDS/World Health Organization. Coreslides: global-summary of the HIV and AIDS epidemic. November 2007. Available at: data.unaids.org/pub/EPISlides/2007/2007_epidupdate_core_en.ppt. Accessed April 16, 2008

2. Centers for Disease Control and Prevention. HIV/AIDS surveillance—epidemiology of HIV infection (through 2006). March 2008. Available at: www.cdc.gov/hiv/topics/surveillance/resources/slides/general/index.htm. Accessed April 18, 2008

3. CDC. HIV/AIDS surveillance report, 2006. Vol 18. March 2008

4. CDC. HIV/AIDS surveillance in adolescents and young adults (through 2005). June 2007. Available at: www.cdc.gov/hiv/topics/surveillance/resources/slides/adolescents/index.htm. Accessed April 19, 2008

5. CDC. HIV incidence among young men who have sex with men—7 US cities, 1994-2000. *MMWR Morb Mortal Wkly Rep.* 2001; Jun 1;50(21):440–444

6. CDC. Unrecognized HIV infection, risk behaviors, and perceptions of risk among young black men who have sex with men—6 US cities, 1994–1998. *MMWR Morb Mortal Wkly Rep.* 2002; Aug 23;51(33):733–736

7. Hallfors DD, Iritani BJ, Miller WC, Bauer DJ. Sexual and drug behavior patterns and HIV and STD racial disparities: the need for new directions. *Am J Public Health.* 2007;97(1):125–132

8. Fullilove RE. *Africa Americans, Health Disparities, and HIV/AIDS*. Washington, DC: National Minority AIDS Council; November 2006

9. Millett GA, Flores SA, Peterson JP, Bakeman R. Explaining disparities in HIV infection among black and white men who have sex with men: a meta-analysis of HIV risk behaviors. *AIDS.* 2007;21(15):2083–2091

10. Institute of Medicine. *The Hidden Epidemic: Confronting Sexually Transmitted Diseases*. Washington, DC: National Academy Press; 1997

11. Centers for Disease Control and Prevention. *Tracking Hidden Epidemics. Trends in STDs in the United States, 2000.* Centers for Disease Control and Prevention; April 2001

12. Centers for Disease Control and Prevention. *Sexually Transmitted Disease Surveillance, 2001*. Atlanta, GA: US Department of Health and Human Services; September 2002

13. Singh S, Wulf D, Samara R, Cuca YP. Gender differences in the timing of first intercourse: data from 14 countries. *Int Fam Plann Perspect.* 2000;(1):21–28, 43

14. Grunbaum JA, Kann L, Kinchen SA, et al. Youth risk behavior surveillance—United States, 2001. *MMWR Surveill Summ.* 2002;51(4):1–62

15. D'Angelo LJ, Getson PR, Luban NL, Gayle HD. Human immunodeficiency virus infection in urban adolescents: can we predict who is at risk? *Pediatrics.* 1991;88(5):982–986

16. Rotheram-Borus M, Koopman C, Ehrhardt AA. Homeless youth and HIV infection. *Am Psychol.* 1991;46(11):1188–1197

17. Morris R, Baker C, Huscroft S. Incarcerated youth at risk for HIV infection. In: DiClemente RJ, ed. *Adolescents and AIDS: A Generation in Jeopardy.* Newbury Park, CA: Sage; 1992: 52–70

18. Katz MH, McFarland W, Guillin V, et al. Continuing high prevalence of HIV and risk behaviors among young men who have sex with men: The Young Men's Survey in the San Francisco Bay Area in 1992 to 1993 and in 1994 to 1995. *J Acquir Immune Defic Syndr Hum Retrovirol.* 1998;19(2):178–181

19. Ryan C, Futterman D. *Lesbian and Gay Youth: Care and Counseling*. New York, NY: Columbia University Press; 1998

20. Wilson CM, Houser J, Partlow C, Rudy BJ, Futterman DC, Friedman LB. The REACH (Reaching for Excellence in Adolescent Care and Health) Project: study design, methods, and population profile. *J Adolesc Health.* 2001; 29(3suppl):8–18

21. Murphy DA, Durako SJ, Moscicki AB, et al. No change in health-risk behavior over time among HIV-infected adolescents in care: role of psychological distress. *J Adolesc Health.* 2001;29(3S):57–63

22. CDC. HIV/STD risks in young men who have sex with men who do not disclose their sexual orientation - 6 US cities, 1994-2000. *MMWR Morb Mortal Wkly Rep.* 2003;52(5):81–86

23. National Adolescent Health Information Center. 2008 fact sheet on health care access and utilization: adolescents and young adults. Available at: nahic.ucsf.edu//downloads/HCAU2008.pdf. Accessed October 5, 2010

24. Chabon B, Futterman D, Hoffman ND. HIV infection in parents of youths with behaviorally acquired HIV. *Am J Public Health.* 2001;91(4):649–650

25. Moscicki AB, Ellenberg JH, Vermund SH, et al. Prevalence of and risks for cervical human papillomavirus infection and squamous intraepithelial lesions in adolescent girls: impact of infection with human immunodeficiency virus. *Arch Pediatr Adolesc Med.* 2000;154(2):127–134

26. Futterman D, Hein K, Reuben N, Dell R, Shaffer N. Human immunodeficiency virus-infected adolescents: the first 50 patients in a New York City program. *Pediatrics.* 1993;91(4):730–735

27. Rogers AS, Futterman D, Levin L, D'Angelo L. A profile of human immunodeficiency virus-infected adolescents receiving health care services at selected sites in the United States. *J Adolesc Health.* 1996;19(6):401–408

28. Futterman D, Rogers A, D'Angelo L, et al. Transmission dynamics and clinical status of youth. *J Adolesc Health.* 1995;16:134

29. Dryfoos JG. *Adolescents at Risk: Prevalence and Prevention*. New York, NY: Oxford University Press; 1990

30. Grubman S, Gross E, Lerner-Weiss N, et al. Older children and adolescents living with perinatally acquired human immunodeficiency virus infection. *Pediatrics.* 1995;95(5):657–663

31. Gortmaker SL, Hughes M, Cervia J, et al. Effect of combination therapy including protease inhibitors on mortality among children and adolescents infected with HIV-1. *N Engl J Med.* 2001;345(21):1522–1528

32. Committee on Pediatrics AIDS, American Academy of Pediatrics. Disclosure of illness status to children and adolescents with HIV infection. *Pediatrics.* 1999;103(1):164–166

33. Resnick M, Blum RW, Hedin D. The appropriateness of health services for adolescents: youth's opinions and attitudes. *J Adolesc Health Care.* 1980;1(2):137–141

34. Kunins H, Hein K, Futterman D, Tapley E, Elliot AS. Guide to adolescent HIV/AIDS program development. *J Adolesc Health.* 1993;14(5suppl):1S-140S

35. English A. Expanding access to HIV services for adolescents: legal and ethical issues in adolescents and AIDS. In: DiClemente R, ed. *A Generation in Jeopardy*. New York, NY: Sage; 1992:262-283

36. Cheng TL, Savageau JA, Sattler AL, DeWitt TG. Confidentiality in health care. A survey of knowledge, perceptions, and attitudes among high school students. *JAMA.* 1993;269(11): 1404-1407

37. Wilson CM, Ellenberg JH, Sawyer MK, et al. Serologic response to hepatitis B vaccine in HIV infected and high-risk HIV uninfected adolescents in the REACH cohort. *Reaching for Excellence in Adolescent Care and Health. J Adolesc Health.* 2001;29(3suppl):123-129

38. CDC. Sexually transmitted diseases treatment guidelines 2002. Centers for Disease Control and Prevention. *MMWR Recomm Rep.* 2002;10;51(RR-6):1-78

39. Hoffman ND, Kelly C, Futterman D. Tuberculosis infection in human immunodeficiency virus-positive adolescents and young adults: a New York City cohort. *Pediatrics.* 1996;97(2):198-203

40. Panelon Clinical Practices for Treatment of HIV Infection. *Guidelines for the Use of Antiretroviral Agents in HIV-Infected Adults and Adolescents.* Washington, DC: Department of Health and Human Services; 2008

41. SPHS/IDSA. Prevention of Opportunistic Infections Working Group. *2001 USPHS/IDSA Guidelines for the Prevention of Opportunistic Infections in Persons Infected with Human Immunodeficiency Virus*. Washington, DC: Department of Health and Human Services; 2001

42. Working Group on Antiretroviral Therapy and Medical Management of HIV-Infected Children. *Guidelines for the Use of Antiretroviral Agents in Pediatric HIV Infection*. Washington, DC: Department of Health and Human Services; 2003

43. Gallant JE. Should antiretroviral therapy be started earlier? *Curr HIV/AIDS Rep.* 2007;4(2):53-59

44. Holmberg SD, Palella FJ Jr, Lichtenstein KA, Havlir DV. The case for earlier treatment of HIV infection. *Clin Infect Dis.* 2004;Dec 1;39(11):1699-1704

45. Lichtenstein KA, Armon C, Buchacz K, et al. Initiation of antiretroviral therapy at CD4 cell counts >/=350 cells/mm$^3$ does not increase incidence or risk of peripheral neuropathy, anemia, or renal insufficiency. *J Acquir Immune Defic Syndr.* 2008;Jan1;47(1):27-35

46. Nguyen A, Calmy A, Schiffer V, et al. Lipodystrophy and weight changes: data from the Swiss HIV Cohort Study, 2000-2006. *HIV Med.* 2008;Mar;9(3):142-150

47. Arribas JR, Pozniak AL, Gallant JE, et al. Tenofovir disoproxil fumarate, emtricitabine, and efavirenz compared with zidovudine/lamivudine and efavirenz in treatment-naïve patients: 144-week analysis. *J Acquir Immune Defic Syndr.* 2008;Jan1;47(1):74-78

48. Gallant JE, DeJesus E, Arribas JR, et al. Tenofovir DF, emtricitabine, and efavirenz vs zidovudine, lamivudine, and efavirenzfor HIV. *N Engl J Med.* 2006; Jan19;354(3): 251-260

49. Johnson M, Grinsztejn B, Rodriguez C, et al. Atazanavir plus ritonavir or saquinavir, and lopinavir/ritonavir in patients experiencing multiple virological failures. *AIDS.* 2005; 19(7):685-694

50. Gathe JC Jr, Ive P, Wood R, et al. SOLO: 48-week efficacy and safety comparison of once-daily fosamprenavir/ritonavir versus twice-daily nelfinavir in naïve HIV-1-infected patients. *AIDS.* 2004;18(11):1529-1537

51. Murphy RL, daSilva BA, Hicks CB, et al. Seven-year efficacy of a lopinavir/ritonavir-based regimen in antiretroviral-naïve HIV-1-infected patients. *HIV Clin Trials.* 2008;9(1): 1-10

52. Cohen C, Nieto-Cisneros L, Zala C, et al. Comparison of atazanavir with lopinavir/ritonavir in patients with prior protease inhibitor failure: a randomized multinational trial. *Curr Med Res Opin.* 2005;21(10):1683-1692

53. Prezista Product Monograph [package insert]. Tibotec Therapeutics. Raritan, NJ. February 2008

54. Intelence Product Monograph [package insert]. Tibotec Therapeutics. Raritan, NJ. January 2008

55. Isentress Product Monograph [package insert]. Merck & Co. Whitehouse Station, NJ. October 2007

56. Selzentry Product Monograph [package insert]. Pfizer. New York, NY. August 2007

57. Pham T, Belzer M, Church JA, et al. Assessment of thymic activity in human immunodeficiency virus-negative and-positive adolescents by real-time PCR quantitation of T-cell receptor rearrangement excision circles. *Clin Diagn Lab Immunol.* 2003;10(2):323-328

58. Murphy DA, Sarr M, Durako SJ, Moscicki AB, Wilson CM, Muenz LR. Barriersto HAART adherence among human immunodeficiency virus-infected adolescents. *Arch Pediatr Adolesc Med.* 2003;157(3):249-255

59. Murphy DA, Wilson CM, Durako SJ, Muenz LR, Belzer M; Adolescent Medicine HIV/AIDS Research Network. Antiretroviral medication adherence among the REACH HIV-infected adolescent cohort in the USA. *AIDSCare.* 2001; Feb;13(1):27-40

60. Gulick RM, Ribaudo HJ, Shikuma CM, et al. ACTG 5095: a comparative study of 3 protease inhibitor-sparing antiretroviral regimens for the initial treatment of HIV infection [abstract 41]. In: Program and Abstracts of the 2nd IAS Conference on HIV Pathogenesis and Treatment. *Antiviral Therapy.* 2003;8(suppl 1):S194-S195

61. Hoffmann C. The epidemiology of HIV coreceptor tropism. *Eur J Med Res.* 2007;Oct15;12(9):385-390

62. Henderson R, Colgrove J, Lusk H. A survey of the mental health care needs of HIV+ adolescents and young adults [abstract 24230]. In: *Program and Abstracts of the 12th World AIDS Conference*. Geneva; 1998:485

63. Blum RW, Garell D, Hodgman CH, et al. Transition from child-centered to adult health-care systems for adolescents with chronic conditions. A position paper of the Society for Adolescent Medicine. *J Adolesc Health.* 1993;14(7):570-576

64. Johnson CP. Transition into adulthood. *Pediatr Ann.* 1995;24(5):268-273

65. Telfair J, Myers J, Drezner S. Transfer as a component of the transition of adolescents with sickle cell disease to adult care: adolescent, adult, and parent perspectives. *J Adolesc Health.* 1994;15(7):558-565

66. American Academy of Pediatrics; American Academy of Family Physicians; American College of Physicians-American Society of Internal Medicine. A consensus statement on health care transitions for young adults with pecial health care needs. *Pediatrics.* 2002;110(6 Pt 2):1304-1306

67. Rawitscher LA, Saitz R, Friedman LS. Adolescents' preferences regarding human immunodeficiency virus (HIV)-related physician counseling and HIV testing. *Pediatrics.* 1995;96(1Pt1):52-58

68. Goodman E, Tipton AC, Hecht L, Chesney MA. Perseverance pays off: health care providers' impact on HIV testing decisions by adolescent females. *Pediatrics.* 1994; 94(6Pt1):878-882

69. Chabon B, Futterman D, Jones C. Adolescent HIV counseling and testing protocol. In: Ryan C, Futterman D, eds. *Lesbian and Gay Youth: Care and Counseling.* New York, NY: Columbia University Press; 1998

70. Technical Expert Panel Review of CDC HIV Counseling, Testing, and Referral Guidelines. Revised guidelines for HIV counseling, testing, and referral. *MMWR.* 2001;50(RR19):1-58

71. Futterman D, Stafford SR, Madhava V. To test or not to test is no longer a question: time to ACTS (assess, consent, test, support)...a rapid new paradigm. 2003 [abstract M2-C0803. In: Proceedings and Abstracts of the 2003 National HIV Prevention Conference. Atlanta, GA; 2003

72. Catania JA, Kegeles SM, Coates TJ. Towards an understanding of risk behavior: an AIDS risk reduction model (ARRM). *Health Educ Q.* 1990; 17(1):53-72

73. Rotheram-Borus MJ, Miller S. Secondary prevention for youths living with HIV. *AIDS Care.* 1998;10(1):17-34

74. Kirby D, Short L, Collins J, et al. School-based programs to reduce sexual risk behaviors: are view of effectiveness. *Public Health Rep.* 1994;109(3):339-360

75. Kirby BD. Understanding what works and what doesn't in reducing adolescent sexual risk-taking. *Fam Plann Perspect.* 2001;33(6):276-281

76. Resnick MD, Bearman PS, Blum RW, et al. Protecting adolescents from harm. Findings from the National Longitudinal Study on Adolescent Health. *JAMA.* 1997;278(10):823-832

77. Miller KS, Levin ML, Whitaker DJ, Xu X. Patterns of condom use among adolescents: the impact of mother-adolescent communication. *Am J Public Health.* 1998;88(10):1542-1544

79. Futterman DC, Rudy BJ, Peralta L, Wolfson S, Guttmacher S, Rogers AS, and the ACCESS Project Team. The ACCESS project (adolescents connected to counseling, evaluation, and special services): social marketing to promote HIV testing to adolescents, method and first-year results from a six-city campaign. *J Adolesc Health.* 2001;29(3S):19-29

78. Futterman DC, Stafford SR, Marrero L, Tobkes C, Harriet Jackson P. Hittin' the zips: utilizing social marketing and targeted community-based HIV testing to improve HIV case finding and prevention in HIV vulnerable neighborhoods [abstract T1-C2004]. In: *Proceedings and Abstracts of the 2003 National HIV Prevention Conference.* Atlanta, GA; 2003

80. Kaur A, Johnson RP. HIV pathogenesis and vaccine development. *Top HIV Med.* 2003;11(3):76-85

81. McMichael AJ, Hanke T. HIV vaccines 1983-2003. *Nat Med.* 2003;9(7):874-880

82. National Institute of Allergy and Infectious Diseases. 62% and 15% ethanol in emollient gel as topical male microbicides. January 2008. Available at: clinicaltrials.gov/ct2/show/NCT00469547?term=15%25+ethanol+emollient+gel&rank=1. Accessed April 21, 2008

83. Van Damme L, Govinden R, Mirembe F, et al. Lack of effectiveness of cellulose sulfate gel for the prevention of vaginal HIV transmission. *N Engl J Med.* 2008;359(5):463-72

84. Halpern V, Wang L, Obunge O, et al. Effectiveness of cellulose sulfate gel for prevention of HIV: results of the phase III trial in Nigeria. 4th IAS Conference on HIV Pathogenesis, Treatment, and Prevention. Sydney. July 22-25, 2007. Abstract WESS302

85. Family Health International. FHI letter regarding further analysis of Savvy results [public letter]. Research Triangle Park, NC. September 18, 2007

86. Auvert B, Taljaard D, Lagarde E, et al. Randomized, controlled intervention trial of male circumcision for reduction of HIV infection risk: the ANRS 1265 Trial. *PLoS Med.* 2005; Nov;2(11):e298

87. Bailey RC, Moses S, Parker CB, et al. Male circumcision for HIV prevention in young men in Kisumu, Kenya: a randomised controlled trial. *Lancet.* 2007;Feb24;369(9562):643-656

88. Gray RH, Kigozi G, Serwadda D, et al. Male circumcision for HIV prevention in men in Rakai, Uganda: a randomised trial. *Lancet.* 2007;Feb24;369(9562):657-666

89. Rudy BJ, Crowley-Nowick PA, Douglas SD. Immunology and the REACH study: HIV immunology and preliminary findings. *Reaching for Excellence in Adolescent Care and Health. J Adolesc Health.* 2001;29(3 suppl):39-48

90. Shrier LA, Bowman FP, Lin M, Crowley-Nowick PA. Mucosal immunity of the adolescent female genital tract. *J Adolesc Health.* 2003;32(3):183-186

# CHAPTER 139

## Bacterial Infections

LORRY G. RUBIN, MD

This chapter describes the infections caused by bacterial pathogens that commonly and uncommonly affect adolescents. *Streptococcus pyogenes* and *Staphylococcus aureus*, including the highly prevalent community-associated, methicillin-resistant *S aureus* (MRSA) strains, are the most important pathogens and cause a variety of localized infections of the skin (*S pyogenes* and *S aureus*) and upper respiratory tract (*S pyogenes* only). These pathogens are also responsible for more serious invasive infections, including sepsis, deep soft tissue and osteoarticular infections, and complicated pneumonias. The adolescent and young adult age groups are most commonly affected by toxic shock syndrome (TSS) caused by these pathogens. *Escherichia coli* is the most important pathogen of urinary tract infections and causes gastrointestinal infection by a number of mechanisms. The features of infections from less commonly encountered bacterial pathogens that affect adolescents are summarized in the table and described briefly in the text.

### *STREPTOCOCCUS PYOGENES* (GROUP A BETA-HEMOLYTIC STREPTOCOCCUS)

#### THE PATHOGEN

*Streptococcus pyogenes* is a gram-positive coccus that grows well on nutrient agar media containing sheep erythrocytes (blood agar) under anaerobic or aerobic conditions. Colonies of *S pyogenes* exhibit beta-hemolysis, that is, complete lysis of erythrocytes in the vicinity of the colony with clearing of the media, and are inhibited by bacitracin disk, findings that are a presumptive test for this bacterial species. *S pyogenes* is also known as Group A beta-hemolytic streptococcus because of the group-specific carbohydrate antigen on the cell surface that forms the basis for immunologic tests to type beta-hemolytic streptococci and differentiate *S pyogenes* from other beta-hemolytic streptococci such as *Streptococcus agalactiae* (Group B streptococcus). M protein is a surface-exposed protein important in virulence because it facilitates evasion of phagocytosis. Although anti-M protein antibodies provide immunity against infection with the homologous M type, the greater than 120 M types explain why repeated infection with *S pyogenes* occurs.[1] *S pyogenes* produces a capsule composed of hyaluronic acid, exotoxins, and enzymes that contribute to pathogenesis of infection. Streptococcal pyrogenic exotoxins are a family of bacterial superantigens that mediate the rash of scarlet fever and streptococcal TSS.[1] Other biologically active extracellular enzymes include the streptolysin hemolysin O, antibody to which is measured in the antistreptolysin O titer ([ASLO titer]) and indicative of recent *S pyogenes* infection, streptokinases, hyaluronidase and DNAses.[1]

*S pyogenes* may be found asymptomatically in the oropharynx, a state known as carriage or colonization. The most common symptomatic infection is pharyngitis ("strep throat"), and *S pyogenes* is the most common bacterial etiology of pharyngitis in adolescents (although most episodes of pharyngitis are viral in etiology). Other respiratory tract infections caused by this pathogen are peritonsillar abscess, sinusitis, mastoiditis, suppurative lymphadenitis, and pneumonia. *S pyogenes* is also an important cause of cellulitis and other skin and soft tissue infections and also causes invasive infections including septicemia, necrotizing fasciitis, and osteoarticular infection. TSS and scarlet fever are toxin-mediated manifestations of *S pyogenes* infections. Nonsuppurative, immune-mediated sequelae of *S pyogenes* infection are acute rheumatic fever, acute glomerulonephritis, and reactive arthritis. A syndrome of pediatric autoimmune neuropsychiatric disorders associated with streptococcal infections (PANDAS) has been associated with this pathogen.[2]

#### PHARYNGITIS

The cardinal symptoms of *S pyogenes* pharyngitis are sore throat, headache, fever, and abdominal pain. The presence of rhinorrhea, cough, laryngitis, or conjunctivitis make a viral etiology of pharyngitis more likely than *S pyogenes*. On physical examination, findings that increase the likelihood of *S pyogenes* infection are tonsillar exudates, soft palatal petechiae, tender anterior cervical lymph nodes, and a diffuse erythematous blanching rash with a sandpaper consistency (ie, scarlet fever rash). A diagnosis of Group A streptococcal pharyngitis based solely on clinical grounds is neither sensitive nor specific, so the diagnosis should be confirmed by testing a throat swab using a test to directly detect the Group A carbohydrate antigen or nucleic acid or by culturing the swab on a blood agar plate. Culture is more sensitive than direct detection tests such that if a direct detection test is negative, a culture should be performed. The clinical symptoms of streptococcal pharyngitis resolve without antimicrobial therapy. However, all patients with streptococcal pharyngitis should be treated because symptoms resolve at least 1 day more rapidly with antimicrobial therapy, contagion is terminated within 24 hours of the start of antimicrobial therapy, and (of most importance) treatment prevents suppurative complications such as peritonsillar abscess and most cases of acute rheumatic fever.

In patients with pharyngitis where there is high suspicion that *S pyogenes* is the etiology, treatment can be started empirically while awaiting the results of diagnostic testing; alternatively, antimicrobial therapy can be delayed until a positive diagnostic test result is obtained. Penicillin, given orally as penicillin V 500 mg twice daily for a 10-day course or as a single intramuscular injection of 1.2 million units of benzathine penicillin G (or a benzathine/procaine penicillin G combination), is the drug of choice for treatment. A 10-day course of amoxicillin given once daily at a dose of 750 to 1,000 mg is an alternative.[3] Although occasionally a clinical treatment failure occur, and failure to eradicate Group A beta-streptococcus from the pharynx is noted in as many as 25% of patients treated with oral penicillin, no isolate has been described that exhibits resistance to penicillin in vitro. Some experts prefer to treat with a cephalosporin antibiotic because of an apparently higher bacteriologic cure rate. For penicillin-allergic patients, erythromycin, clarithromycin, or azithromycin are indicated unless erythromycin-resistant Group A beta streptococci are prevalent in the particular community. A first-generation cephalosporin may be used unless the patient has a type I hypersensitivity to penicillin. Penicillin is not reliably effective for eradication of carriage of *S pyogenes* in asymptomatic carriers, but a 10-day course of clindamycin[4] or a 10-day course of penicillin with addition of rifampin for the last 4 days of treatment are often effective.

### SOFT TISSUE INFECTIONS

*S pyogenes* and *S aureus*, either alone or in combination, are the etiologic agents of impetigo, a common localized superficial skin infection that tends to blister and crust. Erysipeles is a form of superficial Group A streptococcal cellulitis characterized by tender erythema with a rapidly advancing border and is often accompanied by fever. Necrotizing fasciitis ("flesh-eating disease") is a life-threatening, deep soft tissue infection most commonly caused by *S pyogenes* that presents with fever and severe localized pain, at times with overlying edema, erythema, and bullae, but at times with no cutaneous findings.[5] Magnetic resonance imaging (MRI) may be useful, especially in excluding the diagnosis. Management of necrotizing fasciitis due to *S pyogenes* includes intravenous antimicrobial therapy with penicillin and clindamycin and urgent surgical consultation for biopsy, culture, and debridement of infected tissue.[5]

### SEPTICEMIA

*S pyogenes* can cause septicemia, invading the bloodstream from a soft tissue focus of infection (eg, superinfected varicella skin lesions) or via the lung or upper respiratory tract. Alternatively, *S pyogenes* can cause TSS a multiorgan systemic syndrome with hypotension or shock accompanied by at least 2 of the following clinical features: erythroderma/scarlet fever rash, renal dysfunction, hepatic abnormalities, acute respiratory distress syndrome, disseminated intravascular coagulation and soft tissue necrosis; and isolation of Group A beta streptococcus from the blood or another sterile site (definite case) or from a nonsterile site such as the pharynx (probable case). The syndrome is mediated by the action of *S pyogenes* pyrogenic exotoxin. Differentiation of Group A streptococcal TSS from *S aureus* TSS may be difficult, particularly at presentation. Patients should receive antimicrobials directed at both *S aureus* and *S pyogenes*. Also, clindamycin should always be prescribed because in addition to its antimicrobial activity, it inhibits toxin production (by inhibiting bacterial protein synthesis) and thereby may act rapidly and improve outcome.[6] Adjunctive therapy with intravenous gammaglobulin can be considered.[6]

## *STAPHYLOCOCCUS AUREUS*

*S aureus* is a gram-positive coccus that grows well on most agar media under anaerobic or aerobic conditions. Colonies of *S aureus* generally exhibit beta-hemolysis (complete lysis of erythrocytes) due to production and action of a hemolysin exotoxin. Other extracellular products such as additional hemolysins and leukocidins, hyaluronidase, and DNAse (locally destructive to host tissue), TSS toxin, exfoliative toxin (scalded skin syndrome, bullous impetigo), enterotoxins (food poisoning), and scarlet fever toxin contribute to the pathogenesis of infection. A hemolysin termed the Panton-Valentine leukocidin (PVL) is associated with skin infections and hemorrhagic pneumonia in children, adolescents, and young adults. Community-associated strains of methicillin-resistant *S aureus* (CA-MRSA) are increasingly prevalent and may exhibit enhanced virulence due to the presence of PVL or other virulence factors.[7] Other bacterial factors that contribute to virulence include an antiphagocytic polysaccharide capsule; surface adhesins that allow binding to immunoglobulin, fibrinogen, collagen, or fibronectin; and lipoteichoic acid involved in induction of host inflammation by triggering release of cytokines such as tumor necrosis factor.

Staphylococci that do not produce coagulase are termed coagulase-negative staphylococci (CoNS). *Staphylococcus epidermidis* is the most commonly isolated CoNS, which have a lower intrinsic virulence than *S aureus* and regularly colonize the skin. In the absence of a foreign body such as an intravascular catheter, ventriculoperitoneal shunt, or prosthetic cardiac valve, the recovery of CoNS from an adolescent patient is generally the result of colonization or contamination. *Staphylococcus saprophyticus* is a CoNS that is an important cause of pyelonephritis in adolescent and young adult women.

Asymptomatic carriage of *S aureus* with colonization of the anterior nares, skin, and at times the stool, is common; there is a prevalence of 25% in the adolescent age group. Skin is the most common site of *S aureus* infection. Localized skin lesions tend to form pus. Impetigo reflects infection of the epidermis, and if there is elaboration of exfoliative toxin there is blister formation, an entity known as bullous impetigo. Folliculitis is an infection of the superficial dermis, whereas furuncles, carbuncles, and hidradenitis are infections of the deep dermis. Erisipelas, cellulitis, and fasciitis are examples of deeper tissue infections. This bacterial species also causes invasive or systemic infections including osteomyelitis, septic arthritis, endocarditis, necrotizing pneumonia, septic shock, and TSS. In the adolescent age group, *S aureus* is the most common etiology of septic arthritis, osteomyelitis, myositis, and other deep soft tissue infections. Systemic *S aureus* infection such as pneumonia and osteomyelitis may result in infection in more than one site.[7]

Almost all *S aureus* isolates elaborate beta-lactamase and are penicillin-resistant. The semisynthetic penicillins for intravenous administration, nafcillin or oxacillin, or oral administration, dicloxacillin or cloxacillin, are the drugs of choice for methicillin-susceptible strains. In addition, most cephalosporin antibiotics, including all first-generation cephalosporin antibiotics (eg, cefazolin, cephalexin), exhibit excellent activity. However, most *S aureus* that cause health care-associated infections and an increasing proportion of isolates that cause community-acquired infections are methicillin-resistant.[7] Such strains are resistant to all penicillin and cephalosporin antibiotics. Vancomycin is the parenteral drug of choice for suspected or proven serious infection with MRSA, although patients with pneumonia or patients who are bacteremic with strains that have a minimum inhibitory concentration at the upper end of the concentrations considered susceptible (2 μg/mL) may have a delayed response to therapy.[8] Potential alternative antimicrobials include linezolid, daptomycin, tigecycline, and quinupristin/dalfopristin.[9] Localized superficial cutaneous infections can be treated with topical mupirocin and should be drained if appropriate. Most CA-MRSA strains exhibit in vitro susceptibility to trimethoprim-sulfamethoxazole (Bactrim, Septra), and many are susceptible to clindamycin and doxycycline/minocycline.[9] For patients with recurrent cutaneous infections, eradication of colonization may be attempted; however, treatment of an infection with any of the intravenous or oral antimicrobials listed previously does not reliably eradicate carriage. Nasal mupirocin, alone or in combination with body washes using chlorhexidene and/or oral rifampin, plus a second antimicrobial such as trimethoprim-sulfamethoxazole or doxycycline, may be used to eradicate carriage to prevent additional episodes of infection.[10]

## *ESCHERICHIA COLI*

*E coli*, an aerobic gram-negative bacillus and normal resident of the flora of the colon, is the etiology of most urinary tract infections (UTIs). Most strains, including the majority of strains causing community-acquired urinary tract infection, are resistant to both amoxicillin (due to beta-lactamase production) and trimethoprim-sulfamethoxazole, and neither antibiotic is recommended for empiric treatment of a UTI. Acceptable oral antimicrobials include a cephalosporin or amoxicillin-clavulanate (also active against enterococci). A fluoroquinolone antibiotic such as ciprofloxacin is also effective but is not approved for use by the US Food and Drug Administration (FDA) for adolescents younger than 18 years of age unless they have a complicated UTI.

*E coli* strains that elaborate particular virulence factors cause gastroenteritis by one of several mechanisms (see Chapter 103, Diarrhea in the Adolescent). Enterohemorrhagic *E coli* most commonly serotype O157H7 strains, cause bloody diarrhea; some infected patients develop hemolytic-uremic syndrome (HUS). Antimicrobial therapy is not indicated because there is no data on effectiveness, and some data suggest antimicrobial therapy may increase the risk of HUS.[11] Enterotoxigenic *E coli* is the most common etiology of travelers' diarrhea; treatment with a fluoroquinolone antibiotic such as ciprofloxacin or levofloxacin is effective, as is azithromycin.

## LESS COMMON BACTERIAL PATHOGENS

Table 139-1 lists the less common pathogens of bacterial infections. A discussion of each follows.

**Table 139-1**

**Pathogens of Bacterial Infections**

| Bacterial Species | Disease Name | Bacterial Forms | Incubation Period | Epidemiology & Risk Factors | Common Clinical Manifestations | Diagnosis | Antimicrobial Treatment |
|---|---|---|---|---|---|---|---|
| *Bacillus anthracis* | Anthrax | Gram-positive spore-forming bacilli | 1-7 days; rarely up to 60 days | Contact with infected animal, animal hide, or soil; bioterrorism-inhalation of spores | Painless cutaneous ulcer with black eschar with regional lymphadenopathy ± fever; inhalation severe pneumonia, fever, septicemia | Culture and gram stain of skin lesion; blood culture; serology; rapid tests at state health department | Cutaneous: penicillin, doxycycline, or ciprofloxacin for 7–10 days. Pneumonia or systemic infection: 2 to 4 drugs, doxycycline or ciprofloxacin plus rifampin, vancomycin, imipenem, and/or clindamycin |
| *Bartonella henselae* | Cat scratch disease | Fastidious, slow-growing gram-negative bacilli (after culture on media) | 7–10 days for skin lesion at inoculation site | Cat (kitten) scratch, bite, or contact | Localized, tender lymphadenitis, ± fever, ± initial papule 1–2 weeks prior to onset of lymphadenopathy | Clinical diagnosis; confirmed by serology | Supportive care or azithromycin, TMP-SMX, or ciprofloxacin, ± rifampin |
| *Brucella abortus, B melitensis, B suis* | Brucellosis | Gram-negative coccobacilli | 1–4 weeks | Contact with infected animal (cattle, goat, swine) or animal product, unpasteurized milk | Fever, sometimes prolonged, malaise, arthalgia; lymphadenopathy, hepatosplenomegaly, occasional osteomyelitis | Serology; blood culture with prolonged incubation | Doxycycline + rifampin × 4–8 wks (alt: TMP-SMX + rifampin) |
| *Capnocytophaga carimorsus* | | Gram-negative bacilli | 1–8 days | Dog (or cat) bite or scratch; asplenia, corticosteroid therapy | Septicemia; meningitis, cellulitis | Blood culture | Penicillin if pathogen has been recovered (or amoxicillin-clavulanate if etiology of infection unknown and oral therapy is appropriate). Prophylactic amoxicillin-clavulanate (see text) should be considered in asplenic adolescents after a dog bite |
| *Francisella tularensis* | Tularemia | Gram-negative pleomorphic coccobacillus | 2–10 days | Tick bite, contact with sick rabbit | Regional lymphadenitis ± cutaneous papule/ulcer, fever, septicemia | Serology; culture on special media | Gentamicin for at least 7–10 days; alternative: ciprofloxacin |

*(Continued)*

**Table 139-1 (Continued)**

| *Bacterial Species* | *Disease Name* | *Bacterial Forms* | *Incubation Period* | *Epidemiology & Risk Factors* | *Common Clinical Manifestations* | *Diagnosis* | *Antimicrobial Treatment* |
|---|---|---|---|---|---|---|---|
| *Fusobacterium necrophorum* | Lemierre syndrome | Anaerobic gram-negative bacillus | | Adolescent or young adult | Pharyngitis, neck pain, thrombophlebitis, neurologic symptoms, pulmonary symptoms | Anaerobic blood culture | Clindamycin, ceftriaxone (cefotaxime) |
| *Haemophilus influenzae, nontypable* | | Gram-negative coccobacillus | | - | Acute otitis media, sinusitis; bronchitis in patients with underlying lung disease | Culture | Amoxicillin; amoxicillin-clavulanate |
| *Legionella pneumophila; other Legionella spp.* | Legionnaire disease | Gram-negative bacillus (after culture on media) | 1–21 days | Residence near cooling tower; depressed cellular immunity; hospital-associated pneumonia | Pneumonia, at times with neurologic or gastrointestinal symptoms | Urine antigen detection, sputum culture, or direct fluorescent antibody test | Intravenous azithromycin, levofloxacin; addition of rifampin for severe infections |
| *Pasteurella multocida* | | Gram-negative (cocco) bacillus | Less than 24 hours | Animal bite, especially dog or cat; cat scratch | Cellulitis | Culture of drainage | Amoxicillin-clavulanate (also effective against *S aureus*, another common pathogen of animal bites). Prophylactic administration should be considered in high-risk situations (see text) |
| *Streptobacillus moniliformis* | Rat bite fever; Haverhill disease | Gram-negative filamentous | 2–10 days; up to 3 weeks | Rat bite or contact | Fever with maculopapular or petechial rash, polyarthritis; occasionally septicemia | Culture of blood or joint fluid on special media | Penicillin |
| *Yersinia enterocolytica* | Yersiniosis | Gram-negative bacillus | Usually 4–6 days; range 1–14 days | Pig or other animal (cow, rabbit) contact; consumption of chitterlings | Diarrhea, mesenteric adenitis ("pseudoappendicitis"); bacteremia in patients with iron overload | Culture; stool on selective media (cold enrichment) | No treatment for enterocolitis; TMP-SMX or fluorquinolone for immunocompromised host or invasive syndrome |

### *BACILLUS ANTHRACIS* (ANTHRAX)

*Bacillus anthracis* is the cause of anthrax, a zoonotic infection spread to humans after contact with wild or domestic infected animals or their products, including hides, wool, and imported dolls and toys made from animal materials. The most common presentation of anthrax is cutaneous infection with an initial papule that is painless and evolves to a vesicular lesion and eventually an eschar with painful regional lymphadenopathy (Table 139-1).[12] Antibiotic therapy prevents progression to systemic infection with a possibly fatal outcome.[12] Inhalation anthrax results from inhalation of aerosolized spores and is the anthrax form associated with bioterrorism that occurred in the United States in 2001 with 22 cases of mail-associated anthrax.[13,14] Antimicrobial therapy with a single antimicrobial agent for 7 to 10 days is recommended for cutaneous anthrax without systemic symptoms, but intravenous therapy with at least 2 antimicrobial agents is recommended for inhalation or systemic infection. When disease occurs from aerosol exposure, antimicrobial therapy should be continued for 60 days.

### *BARTONELLA HENSELAE*

Cat scratch disease is a zoonotic infection that occurs after a scratch or bite by a cat with inoculation of the zoonotic bacterium *Bartonella henselae*.[15] The hallmark of this infection is the development of tender regional lymphadenitis in the axillary, cervical, or submandibular areas; there may be an antecedent erythematous papule at the inoculation site. Some patients have fever and other constitutional symptoms. Patients may present with fever of unknown origin with 1 to 3 weeks of fever, at times with abdominal pain associated with abdominal lymphadenopathy and/or hepatosplenomegaly, or with encephalopathy. Immunocompromised patients with HIV infection develop bacillary angiomatosis with cutaneous lesions and fever. Although the lymphadenitis is self-limited in immunocompetent patients and treatment is supportive, resolution takes 4 to 6 weeks or more, and antimicrobial therapy (Table 139-1) may offer clinical benefit.

### *BRUCELLA* SPP (BRUCELLOSIS)

Brucellosis is a zoonosis with humans as accidental hosts who acquire infection by contact with infected animals such as cattle or goats, their carcasses, or milk. Most cases are acquired outside the United States, or via imported foods such as goat's milk or cheese. The clinical presentation can be acute or insidious and includes fever and nonspecific findings such as malaise, lethargy, anorexia, arthralgia, and headache. Physical findings are often scant, with the occasional occurrence of hepatomegaly or arthritis. Antimicrobial treatment consists of a long course (minimum of 4 weeks) with 2 drugs to reduce the risk of relapse (Table 139-1).[16]

### *CAPNOCYTOPHAGA CANIMORSUS*

*Capnocytophaga canimorsus* is a fastidious, slow-growing gram-negative bacillus that exists as normal oral flora in dogs and cats but causes infection in humans after a dog bite or exposure. The most common clinical manifestations are septicemia, at times fulminant, and meningitis with or without an associated cellulitis.[17,18] This occurs more commonly in asplenic patients. Isolated cellulitis at the site of a bite is more commonly caused by *Pasteurella multocida*, which also exists as normal oral flora in dogs and cats, or *S aureus*. Penicillin is the drug of choice. However, for asplenic adolescents who sustain a dog bite, prophylaxis with amoxicillin-clavulanate should be considered because of the increased risk of sepsis.[19] Other potential indications for antimicrobial prophylaxis are described in the paragraph on *P multocida* following.

### *FRANCISELLA TULARENSIS* (TULAREMIA)

Tularemia, caused by *Francisella tularensis*, is a zoonotic infection with humans as accidental hosts. Infection is most commonly acquired through the skin by contact with infected wild rabbits or transmission by ticks.[20] Most cases present with one or more enlarged, inflamed lymph nodes, often with a swollen painful papule at the inoculation site proximal to the lymph node that evolves to an ulcer ("ulceroglandular" presentation).[20,21] Enlarged lymph nodes may be seen in more than one location, and most patients have fever or other systemic symptoms. Tularemia pneumonia occurs following inhalation of organisms by landscape workers or through bioterrorism with intentional aerosolization of *F tularensis*. The microbiology laboratory should be notified when specimens are submitted for culture because culture of *F tularensis* requires special medium and there is a potential biohazard for infection of laboratory personnel. The diagnosis of tularemia is most commonly confirmed by serology. A 7-day course of gentamicin is the treatment of choice, with ciprofloxacin or another fluoroquinolone antibiotic as an alternative.[22] If tetracycline is used for treatment, relapse occurs commonly.

### *HAEMOPHILUS INFLUENZAE*

*Haemophilus influenzae* is a fastidious gram-negative coccobacillus that may express one of 6 polysaccharide capsules (designated with the letters a-f) or may be unencapsulated. Prior to routine immunization of infants, serotype b strains were an important cause of meningitis and other invasive infections in children younger than age 5 years. Nontypable, unencapsulated *H influenzae* commonly and asymptomatically colonize the nasopharynx and are important pathogens for acute and chronic sinusitis, acute otitis media, and in adolescents with chronic lung disease, bronchitis, or pneumonia. Up to 40% of isolates are ampicillin-resistant, most commonly due to production of beta-lactamase. Thus, although amoxicillin remains a first-line treatment for sinusitis and acute otitis media, in part because of its activity against *Streptococcus pneumoniae*, amoxicillin-clavulanate, a beta-lactamase stable oral or parenteral second- or third-generation cephalosporin antibiotic (a requirement that excludes cefaclor or cefprozil) or trimethoprim-sulfamethoxazole, will be active against a higher proportion of strains.

### *LEGIONELLA PNEUMOPHILA*

*Legionella pneumophila* is often grouped with *Mycoplasma pneumoniae* and *Chlamydophila (Chlamydia) pneumoniae* as the trio of atypical bacterial pathogens causing community-acquired pneumonia in adolescents. However, in adolescents pneumonia due to *Legionella* is much less common than pneumonia due to *M pneumoniae* or *C pneumoniae*. Most cases have occurred in patients with impairment of cell-mediated immunity caused by therapy with high doses of corticosteroids or cancer chemotherapy.[23] The clinical presentation of *Legionella* pneumonia, fever, and cough, at times accompanied by chest pain, is not distinctive. Chest radiographs usually show a unilateral, focal alveolar infiltrate that can progress to bilateral disease.[24] *Legionella* can also cause outbreaks of a self-limited, nonpneumonic, influenza-like illness with fever, malaise, myalgia, and cough, which is known as Pontiac fever. Intravenous azithromycin or a fluoroquinolone antibiotic (eg, levofloxacin) is the drug of choice for treatment of *Legionella* pneumonia. Beta-lactam antibiotics and clindamycin are ineffective.

### *PASTEURELLA MULTOCIDA*

*Pasteurella multocida* is a gram-negative pleiomorphic coccobacillus that, like *Capnocytophaga canimorsus,* exists as normal flora in the mouths of cats and dogs. This bacterial species is the most common cause of wound infection following the bite of a cat or dog but does not commonly cause septicemia. Typically, the onset of a wound infection due to *P multocida* occurs 12 to 24 hours after the injury and may be accompanied by regional lymphadenopathy and fever. Amoxicillin-clavulanate is recommended for initial therapy of wound infections following a cat or dog bite because it has activity against both *P multocida* and *S aureus*, both of which are important pathogens in this setting. Trimethoprim-sulfamethoxazole or azithromycin can be considered for penicillin-allergic patients. Antimicrobial prophylaxis with amoxicillin-clavulanate may be indicated in situations where the risk of infection or the morbidity of infection is high, such as for cat bites, bites on the hands, feet, or genital areas, or bites in patients with an immunocompromising condition such as asplenia.

### *STREPTOBACILLUS MONILIFORMIS*

*Streptobacillus moniliformis*, a fastidious, pleomorphic, and often filamentous gram-negative bacillus that exists as normal flora in the mouth of rodents, is the main etiologic agent of rat bite fever.[25] Infection occurs most commonly after a rat bite, with an abrupt onset of fever, chills, headache, vomiting, myalgia, and a maculopapular and sometimes petechial rash most prominent on the extremities including the palms and soles. Migratory polyarthritis or polyarthralgia occurs in half of patients and generalized lymphadenopathy is common.[26] Untreated rat bite fever will undergo a relapsing course for several weeks. Haverhill fever is an *S moniliformis* infection acquired through ingestion of the organism via milk or water contaminated with rat excreta and may present in epidemic form. Penicillin is the drug of choice for treatment.[27] Following a rat bite, the risk of rat bite fever is approximately 10%; therefore, postexposure prophylaxis with penicillin should be considered.

### *YERSINIA ENTEROCOLYTICA*

*Yersinia enterocolytica* is a gram-negative aerobic bacterium that is a member of the family *Enterobacteriaceae*. Like *Salmonella* and *Campylobacter*, bacterial gastrointestinal pathogens, *Y enterocolytica* is a common infection of animals. Pigs are the most important animal reservoir. These organisms proliferate at refrigerator temperatures, so milk and other dairy products may be a source of infection. Human infections are more common in cooler climates and in the winter months. The most common clinical syndrome is enterocolitis with fever, abdominal pain, vomiting, and diarrhea, usually without mucus or blood (see Chapter 103, Diarrhea in the Adolescent). Mesenteric adenitis (pseudoappendicitis), or less commonly terminal ileitis, may occur and may present with fever and abdominal pain, as occurs in patients with acute appendicitis. Bacteremia may occur in adolescents with iron overload, for example, those who receive frequent red blood cell transfusion due to beta-thalassemia (including those patients undergoing chelation therapy), patients with cirrhosis or who are on hemodialysis, or those receiving oral iron supplementation. These patients present with fever, often with enteritis or a pseudoappendicitis syndrome, and may have a palpable abdominal mass. Infection with *Y enterocolytica* may be associated with erythema nodosum, uveitis, and reactive arthritis.

## REFERENCES

1. Bisno AL, Brito MO, Collins CM. Molecular basis of group A streptococcal virulence. *Lancet Infect Dis.* 2003;3:191-200

2. Shulman ST. Pediatric autoimmune neuropsychiatric disorders associated with streptococci (PANDAS). *Pediatr Infect Dis J.* 1999;18:281-282

3. Clegg HW, Ryan AG, Dallas SD, et al. Treatment of streptococcal pharyngitis with once-daily compared with twice-daily amoxicillin: a noninferiority trial. *Pediatr Infect Dis J.* 2006;25:761-767

4. Tanz RR, Poncher JR, Corydon KE, Kabat K, Yogev R, Shulman ST. Clindamycin treatment of chronic pharyngeal carriage of group A streptococci. *J Pediatr.* 1991;119:123-128

5. Anaya DA, Dellinger EP. Necrotizing soft-tissue infection: diagnosis and management. *Clin Infect Dis.* 2007;44:705-710

6. Stevens DL. Streptococcal toxic shock syndrome associated with necrotizing fasciitis. *Annu Rev Med.* 2000;51:271-288

7. Gonzalez BE, Hulten KG, Dishop MK, et al. Pulmonary manifestations in children with invasive community-acquired Staphylococcus aureus infection. *Clin Infect Dis.* 2005;41:583-590

8. Deresinski S. Vancomycin: does it still have a role as an antistaphylococcal agent? *Expert Rev Anti Infect Ther.* 2007;5:393-401

9. Sakol KE, Echevarria KL, Lewis JS II. Community-associated methicillin-resistant Staphylococcus aureus: new bug, old drugs. *Ann Pharmacother.* 2006;40:1125-1133

10. Laupland KB, Conly JM. Treatment of Staphylococcus aureus colonization and prophylaxis for infection with topical intranasal mupirocin: an evidence-based review. *Clin Infect Dis.* 2003;37:933-938

11. Tarr PI, Gordon CA, Chandler WL. Shiga-toxin-producing Escherichia coli and haemolytic uraemic syndrome. *Lancet.* 2005;365:1073-1086

12. Dixon TC, Meselson M, Guillemin J, Hanna PC. Anthrax. *New Engl J Med.* 1999;341:815-826

13. Bartlett JG, Inglesby TV Jr, Borio L. Management of anthrax. *Clin Infect Dis.* 2002;35:851-858

14. Jernigan DB, Raghunathan PL, Bell BP, et al. Investigation of bioterrorism-related anthrax, United States, 2001: epidemiologic findings. *Emerging Infect Dis.* 2001;8:1019-1028

15. English R. Cat-scratch disease. *Pediatr Rev.* 2006; 27:123-128

16. Pappas G, Akritidis N, Bosilkovski M, Tsianos E. Brucellosis. *N Engl J Med.* 2005;352:2325-2336

17. Pers C, Gahrn-Hansen B, Frederiksen W. *Capnocytophaga canimorsus* septicemia in Denmark, 1982-1985: review of 39 cases. *Clin Infect Dis.* 1996;23:71-75

18. Campbell JR, Edwards M. *Capnocytophaga* species infections in children. *Pediatr Infect Dis J.* 1991;10:944-948

19. Rubin LG. *Capnocytophaga* species. In: Long S, ed. *Principles and Practice of Pediatric Infectious Diseases.* 3rd ed. Philadelphia, PA: Churchill Livingstone; 2008: 874-875

20. Rubin LG. *Francisella tularensis* (tularemia). In: Long S, ed. *Principles and Practice of Pediatric Infectious Diseases.* 3rd ed. Philadelphia, PA: Churchill Livingstone; 2008:891-892

21. Jacobs RF, Condrey YM, Yamauchi T. Tularemia in adults and children: a changing presentation. *Pediatrics.* 1985;76:818-822

22. Jacobs RF. Tularemia. *Adv Pediatr Infect Dis.* 1997; 12:55-69

23. Rubin LG. *Legionella* species. In: Long S, ed. *Principles and Practice of Pediatric Infectious Diseases.* 3rd ed. Philadelphia, PA: Churchill Livingstone; 2008: 912-915

24. Edelstein PH. Legionnaires' disease. *Clin Infect Dis.* 1993;16:741-747

25. Rubin LG. *Streptobacillus moniliformis* (rat bite fever). In: Long S, ed. *Principles and Practice of Pediatric Infectious Diseases.* 3rd ed. Philadelphia, PA: Churchill Livingstone; 2008:927-928

26. Roughgarden JW. Antimicrobial therapy of rat bite fever. *Arch Intern Med.* 1965;116:39-54

27. Dendle C, Woolley IJ, Korman TM. Rat-bite fever septic arthritis: illustrative case and literature review. *Eur J Clin Microbiol Infect Dis.* 2006;25:791-797

# CHAPTER 140

# Tick-Borne Diseases

SUNIL K. SOOD, MD

The recreational and occupational activities of adolescents put them at risk for tick bites. Worldwide, there are more than 30 known tick-transmitted species of viruses, rickettsiae, ehrlichiae, spirochetes, and piroplasms. Also included as tick-borne diseases are tick paralysis and the gram-negative bacillary infection tularemia. This chapter emphasizes the well-characterized tick-borne human infections on the North American continent. Many tick-borne infections acquired on other continents are closely related to those encountered in North America; those that are different will not be covered in this chapter.

## LYME BORRELIOSIS

### ETIOLOGY AND EPIDEMIOLOGY

Lyme disease is caused by the spirochete *Borrelia burgdorferi* sensu lato. The term "sensu lato" means "in a broad sense" and is used to indicate that other genospecies of the organism are included in the name. The genospecies *B afzelii* and *B garinii* cause Lyme disease in Europe, whereas Lyme disease in North America is caused only by the genospecies *B burgdorferi* "sensu stricto" ("in a narrow sense"). Lyme disease is more common in children than in adults, with about a quarter of all reported cases occurring in children younger than 14 years of age.

The spirochetes are transmitted by hard-bodied ticks of the *Ixodes persulcatus* complex in temperate zones of North America, Europe, and Asia (Figure 140-1A). In the United States, the disease occurs primarily in the northeastern and north central regions where *I scapularis*, the deer tick, is the vector (Figure 140-1B). The only other endemic area in the United States is on the West Coast, primarily in northern California. Therefore, reported cases from other parts of the country in all probability represent misdiagnosis or travel-associated acquisition.

Lyme borreliosis has been called a disease of place.[1] The incidence of reported cases in the United States ranges from 0 in several states to 76.6/100,000 in Delaware.[2] The states with the highest incidence are in northeastern and northern midwestern regions—Connecticut, Delaware, Rhode Island, New York, New Hampshire, New Jersey, Pennsylvania, Maryland, Massachusetts, Wisconsin, and Minnesota; these states account for more than 90% of cases on the continent. Underreporting, to the extent of 10- to 12-fold, has been shown in some studies, and 1 estimate gives an overall national case rate of about 20/100,000 to 30/100,000.[2]

The difference in epidemiology in different regions is related to variations in animal reservoirs needed to sustain the life cycle, as well as to ambient temperatures. For example, the ubiquitous white-footed mouse is the most common reservoir for *Borrelia burgdorferi* in the northern United States, and this is coupled with high populations of white-tailed deer. A lower incidence on the West Coast is attributed to a relatively incompetent host for *Borrelia*, the western fence lizard.

Longitudinal studies have demonstrated that there is an increasing incidence of cases in focal suburban and rural residential areas in the northeastern United States. The main reasons for the increased outbreaks in this region are greatly increasing deer populations and the migration of people into rural and wooded areas where opportunities for tick exposure are greatest.

### CLINICAL MANIFESTATIONS

The clinical presentations of Lyme borreliosis are well defined. The original investigations in the United States, and several subsequent North American and European studies, have included children predominantly.[3] In a large pediatric, practice-based community study, patients presented with a single erythema migrans (EM) skin lesion (66%), multiple EM lesions (23%), arthritis (7%), facial palsy (3%), aseptic meningitis (1%), or carditis (0.5%).[4] In Europe, as compared to the United States and especially in the pediatric age group, nervous system involvement is more common as a proportion of all manifestations, with Bannwarth polyradiculoneuritis (as described in the following) being particularly common. In general, neurologic manifestations are significantly more common in children (17%–38% of cases) than in adults.

In a study in Slovenia, a presentation of multiple EM lesions accounted for 40% of children who had EM, which may be due to a higher prevalence of

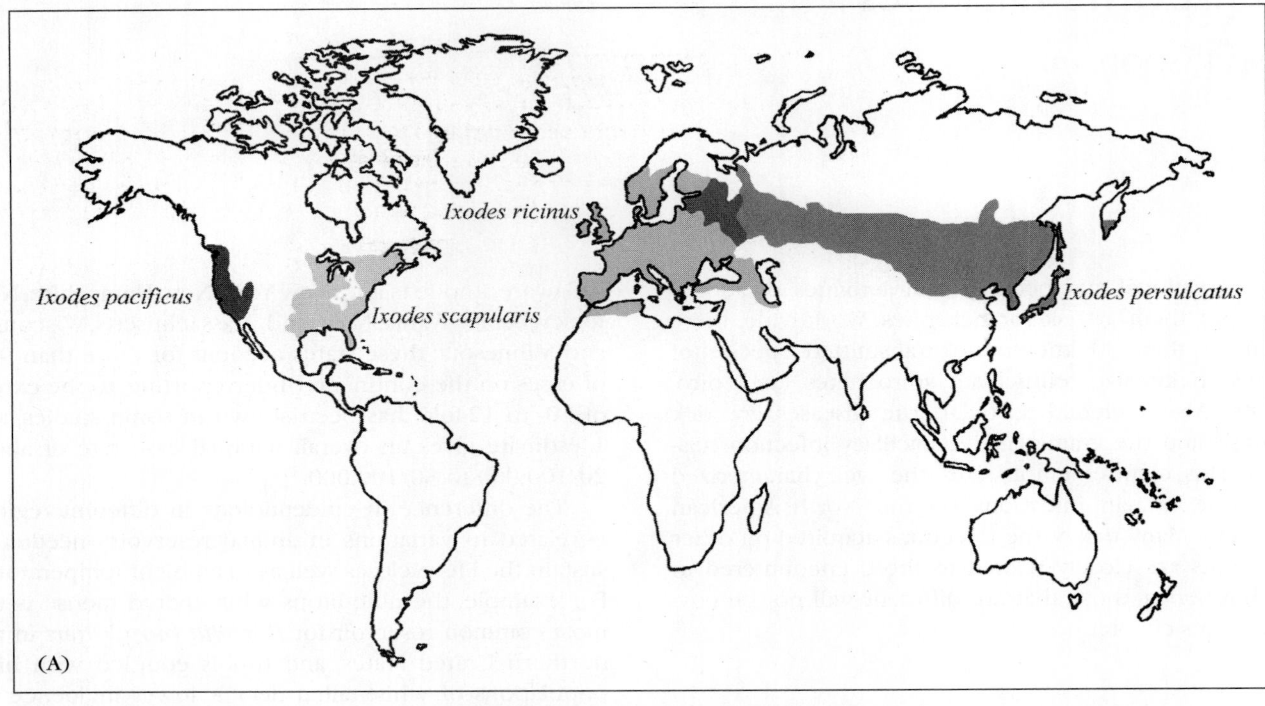


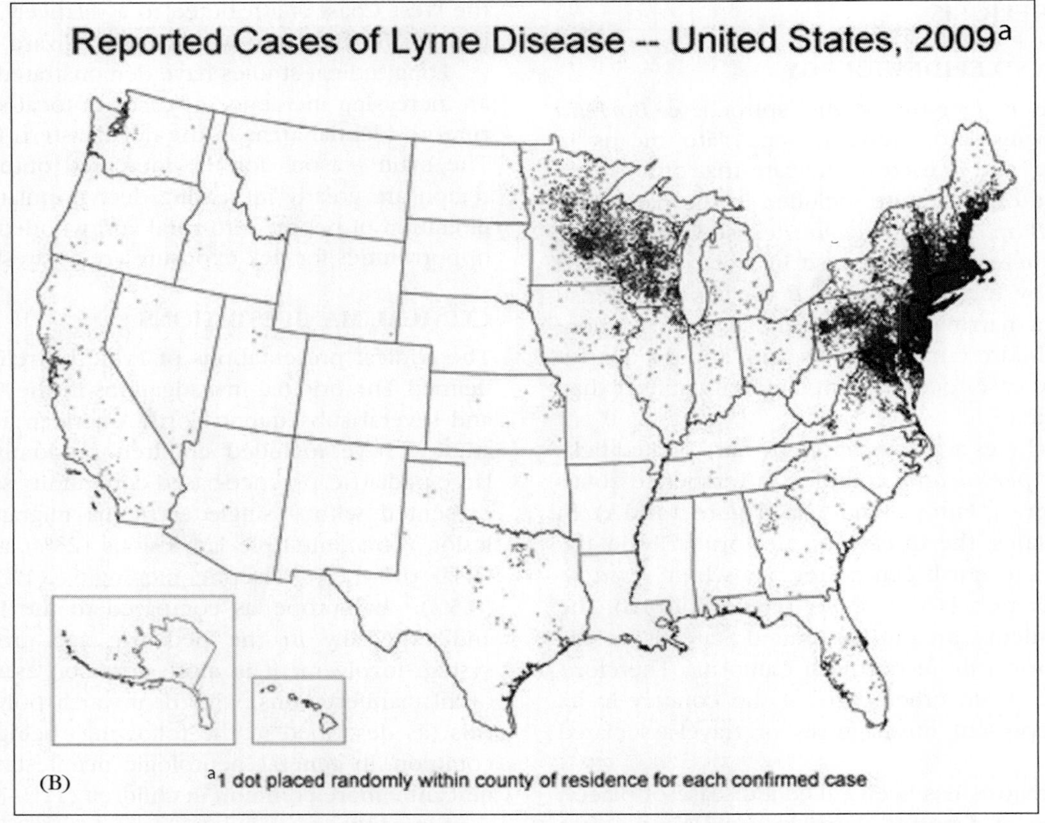


**FIGURE 140-1** (A) The contiguous and overlapping distributions of the 4 principal tick vectors of *Borrelia burgdorferi* around the world. (J. Piesman, CDC); (B) Reported cases of Lyme disease, United States, 2009. Available at: www.cdc.gov/ncidod/dvbid/lyme/ld_statistics.htm.

*Borrelia afzelii*.[5] Two additional forms of the disease, borrelial lymphocytoma and acrodermatitis chronica atrophicans (ACA), are seen exclusively in Europe, where borrelial lymphocytoma comprised 7% of pediatric borreliosis in 1 study.[6] Although localized EM is the most common manifestation in all locations, the spirochete can disseminate shortly after the tick bite. Therefore, the clinical manifestations have been classified as early (early-localized or early-disseminated) or late. Although there is no clear temporal demarcation between early and late Lyme disease, the onset of early Lyme disease usually occurs within 8 weeks of the tick bite.

### Early-Localized Disease

***Erythema Migrans*** Early-localized Lyme disease manifests as a single EM lesion at the site of inoculation (Figure 140-2A and B). The mean incubation period to appearance of EM is 10 days (range 1–27). Mild systemic symptoms may accompany the rash, chiefly arthralgia, headache, and fatigue. The erythema migrans begins as a red macule or papule at the tick bite site, which develops into a circular erythematous flat rash that then expands concentrically for days. In about two-thirds of cases there is no central clearing, as shown in a study of culture-proven lesions.[7] Clearing tends to appear if the rash is present for several days. Erythema migrans is usually not accompanied by pain, but a mild stinging sensation may occur. The diagnosis of EM can be made if the rash attains a diameter of at least 5 cm to 6 cm; a ring lesion smaller than this is more likely to be an insect bite reaction or a reaction to tick saliva that will fade without expansion as it is monitored over several days. Variants of the EM lesion, such as vesiculation, urticaria, mild scaling, a purpuric appearance, and even noncircular linear shapes can be seen.

Several patients with rashes morphologically resembling EM were reported in 1997 in Missouri and North Carolina.[8,9] The nomenclature of these illnesses has not been generally accepted as Lyme disease to date. There is an apparent association with lone star, not deer tick, bites in these cases. There is evidence that a novel species of *Borrelia*, provisionally named *B lonestari*, is present in southern lone star ticks, but a causal link for spirochetes with what has been called "southern tick-associated rash illness" (STARI) has not been definitively established.

Bloodstream dissemination (spirochetemia) can result in multiple EM lesions (Figure 140-2C). Multiple EM is the most common type of early-disseminated Lyme disease. An important differential diagnosis is erythema multiforme. Although the latter is a hypersensitivity reaction in which the skin lesions vary in morphology, with some being urticarial, all of the lesions in multiple

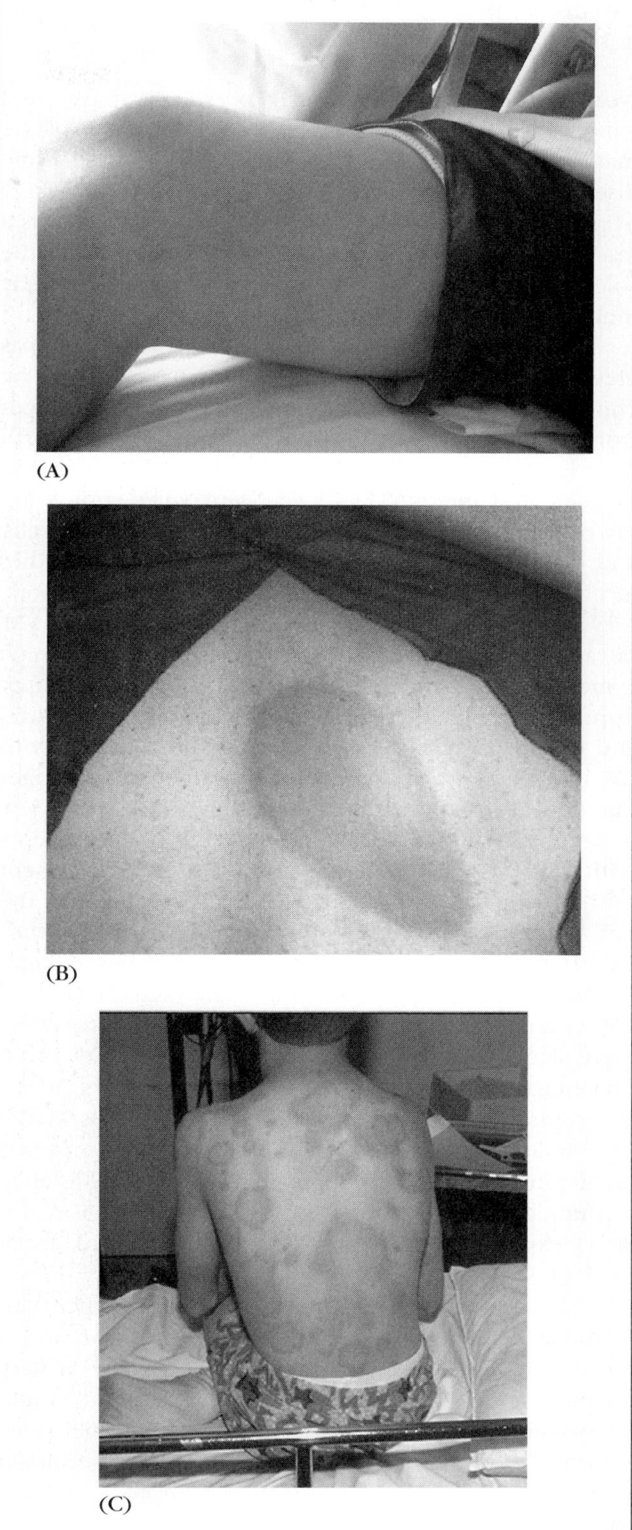
(A)
(B)
(C)

**FIGURE 140-2** Erythema migrans. (A) and (B) Single lesions at site of innoculation; (C) Multiple erythema migrans lesions. (See color insert.)

EM are morphologically similar despite their variations in size.

***Neurologic Infection*** Cranial nerve VII palsy and lymphocytic meningitis are the common neurologic manifestations of early-disseminated Lyme disease. Lyme disease should especially be considered in the etiology of peripheral facial palsy in an endemic area, and it is a leading cause of bilateral palsy. Facial palsy can be the sole manifestation of Lyme disease, and it is clinically indistinguishable from Bell palsy.

The meningitis of Lyme disease is lymphocytic, has elevated cerebrospinal fluid (CSF) protein, and may be complicated by pseudotumor cerebri.[10] Some differences from viral meningitis (VM) have been noted in North America. Kernig and Brudzinski signs are less common in Lyme meningitis (LM);[11] CSF leukocyte counts are lower, with a greater percentage of mononuclear cells; and papilledema is more common.[12] Several studies in children have identified clinical features and laboratory parameters that can help differentiate LM from VM, because both are common diseases in areas in which Lyme disease is endemic, at least in the United States. Eppes et al[11] analyzed features of children age 2 years and older, 12 with LM and 10 with VM. Children with LM had significantly lower temperatures and a longer duration of symptoms at presentation. Papilledema, EM, or cranial neuropathy was present in all of the patients with LM (with the exception of 1 patient) but absent in the patients with VM. Fewer white blood cells in the CSF were observed in LM than in VM (mean, 80/mm$^3$ vs 301/mm$^3$) as were significantly greater percentages of mononuclear cells. Shah et al[12] analyzed 24 LM and 151 enteroviral meningitis cases in children. Parameters with significant differences are listed in Table 140-1. The negative predictive value for LM was 99% when neutrophils constituted more than 10% of cells in the CSF. Similarly, a study of LM (14 children) versus aseptic meningitis (16 children) in Belgium[13] found a difference in duration of symptoms before admission (15 vs 1.6 days), except when the LM was associated with facial palsy (1.3 days).

Cranial and peripheral mononeuropathies other than a cranial nerve VII palsy have been reported in adults but are rare in children. Bannwarth syndrome is very uncommon in North American Lyme disease, but should be suspected if a child has evidence of a spinal polyneuropathy in association with either EM or serologic evidence of *B burgdorferi* infection. Symptoms include any combination of motor weakness, neuralgia, sensory impairment, or paresthesia, especially in the cervical and thoracic dermatomes. Other neurologic manifestations have also been reported in association with a positive serologic test, although these have not always been confirmed by immunoblot assay. These include optic neuritis, Guillain-Barré-like syndrome, and acute meningoencephalitis.[14] Immunoblot confirmation is essential before an atypical manifestation is ascribed to *B burgdorferi* infection.

**Table 140-1**

**Lyme Meningitis vs Enteroviral Meningitis at the Children's Hospital of Philadelphia**

| *Category* | *Incidence of Lyme Meningitis vs Enteroviral Meningitis* |
|---|---|
| Median age (yr) | 10.5 vs 5.5 |
| Median symptom duration (d) | 12 vs 1 |
| Median headache duration (d) | 7.5 vs 2 |
| Cranial neuropathy | 17 (71%) vs 0/151 |
| Papilledema | 6/13 (46%) vs 0/21 |

Modified from Shah SS, Zaoutis TE, Turnquist J, Hodinka RL, Coffin SE. Early differentiation of Lyme from enteroviral meningitis. *Pediatr Infect Dis J*. 2005;24(6):542–545, with permission from Wolters Kluwer.

The acute neurologic manifestations of Lyme disease, including meningitis, are generally self-limited. Facial palsy usually resolves in 2 to 8 weeks with or without treatment. A long-term study[15] (mean follow-up 17 years) of untreated facial palsy in Swedish children, including some with CSF pleocytosis, revealed no long-term sequelae. Still, it is important to assess the need for lumbar puncture clinically, for example, when neck stiffness or headache accompanies the palsy, as the presence of pleocytosis will change the treatment of choice to an intravenous antibiotic.

A rare but ominous complication of neuroborreliosis is transient or permanent impairment of vision. This was highlighted in a report by Rothermel et al.[16] They described impairment of vision in 4 children. Visual loss associated with increased intracranial pressure (ICP) occurred early in the course in one patient. Visual loss in 2 patients manifested weeks to months after treatment, due to optic neuritis (as a sole manifestation in 1 and following arthritis in the other). Loss of sight resulted in permanent bilateral blindness as a consequence of persistent raised ICP or optic neuritis in one patient. Unequivocal meningitis was present in only one patient. Among 6 previously reported cases in the United States, Rothermal et al[16] identified a report of a 10-year-old with permanent visual loss in 1 eye. An antecedent of the visual loss is raised ICP in most cases. Headaches are an important sign of raised ICP in Lyme disease, as underscored by reports of 9- and 13-year-old females with waxing and waning headaches and blurred optic discs.

***Other Manifestations of Early-Disseminated Disease*** Migratory and recurrent arthralgia and periarticular pain without swelling can develop within weeks of the tick bite. Frank arthritis with effusion may also occur early. Cardiac involvement consists of a first-, second-, or third-degree atrioventricular conduction block or a bundle branch block. Rare complications are myocarditis and congestive heart failure. Because cardiac conduction abnormalities are often asymptomatic, an electrocardiogram (ECG) should be done in an adolescent with disseminated Lyme disease.

### Late-Disseminated Disease

***Arthritis*** Among 90 children in Connecticut, arthritis developed a mean of 4 months after the initial manifestation of early Lyme disease, mostly in children who did not receive appropriate treatment, although the range of onset was wide (2 days to 20 months).[17] A single joint is involved in about 66% of cases, fewer than 4 joints are involved in all cases, and the knee is involved in 90% of cases. It is common to have a preceding period of migratory arthralgias and periarticular inflammation. The involved joint is swollen and painful, with swelling and stiffness being out of proportion to the pain, which tends to be mild to moderate. There is a neutrophil-predominant pleocytosis in the synovial fluid and an elevated erythrocyte sedimentation rate (ESR). As in reactive arthritis, the fluid tends to reaccumulate rapidly after arthrocentesis. Severity of arthritis increases with age; the median duration of active inflammation for an episode was 1 month in 2- to 4-year-olds but 22 weeks in teenagers.[18]

***Late Neurologic Disease*** Findings of sensorineural peripheral neuropathy and low-grade encephalopathy with cognitive deficits occur as late sequelae of Lyme disease in adults, but late neurologic disease is rarely encountered in children and adolescents. Patients with these syndromes present a diagnostic challenge because it is difficult to prove an etiologic link with earlier *B burgdorferi* infection at this chronic stage of the illness. Culture of the CSF is negative and DNA antibody or antigen detection tests have poor specificity and sensitivity. Manifestations in adolescents sometimes attributed to Lyme borreliosis include behavioral and sleep changes; auditory or visual sequential processing deficits revealed by a battery of neuropsychologic tests; focal or large patchy high signal areas in the white matter on magnetic resonance brain imaging; and periventricular focal necrosis. There is a marked paucity of evidence to confirm that these are consequences of *B burgdorferi* infection.

A common concern, and an area of much controversy, is whether chronic CNS Lyme disease could be the explanation for cognitive disturbances such as emotional lability, memory loss, sleep disorders, and even diminished academic performance. It has been demonstrated that the long-term neuropsychologic outcome in children who have had documented Lyme disease is excellent. Neuropsychologic or emotional problems are therefore more likely to be pre-existing conditions rather than related to previous Lyme disease. Positive serology may also reflect past, resolved infection unrelated to present complaints.

***Other Manifestations***

- **Asymptomatic Seroconversion.** The development of an antibody response to *B burgdorferi* in the absence of a recognized illness, termed asymptomatic seroconversion, is well documented. In a prospective study in an endemic area, the ratio of asymptomatic to symptomatic disease was 4:10.[19] It is likely that asymptomatic seroconversion represents successful elimination of the spirochete rather than latent infection. There is no evidence that treatment is necessary.
- **Acute Constitutional Illness without Focal Manifestations.** Because previous studies had suggested that 8% to 17% of patients with well-documented Lyme borreliosis, including a patient with a positive blood culture, have only a "flu-like illness" without EM, Feder et al[20] studied 24 untreated children older than 4 years of age with "undefined flu-like illness." These patients developed self-limited fever and fatigue that resolved spontaneously in 5 to 21 days; had 1 or more symptoms of arthralgias or myalgias, headache or neck pain, and fatigue; and were confirmed by immunoblot (paired acute and convalescent serology) to be infected with *B burgdorferi*. The authors concluded that a "flu-like illness without EM" was a form of early Lyme disease. The proportion of children with *B burgdorferi* infection who develop this form, better termed acute constitutional or viral-type illness, is unclear. The term "flu-like" illness is not accurate for this presentation, and the presence of respiratory or gastrointestinal symptoms suggest that the patient does not have *B burgdorferi* infection. The diagnosis can only be made if seroconversion is demonstrated, and antibiotic treatment should not be prescribed without such evidence. Other tick-borne illnesses should

also be considered for a clinical presentation such as this in endemic areas.

- **Borrelial Lymphocytoma and Acrodermatitis Chronica Atrophicans.** Borrelia lymphocytoma is a localized manifestation of disseminated Lyme disease seen in Europe. It mimics a benign tumor of the skin, usually on the ear lobes or breast areolae.[14] Acrodermatitis chronica atrophicans (ACA), a chronic *Borrelia* infection of the skin, is rarely encountered in children and adolescents, as it takes many years to manifest. It consists of painful bluish-red, discolored areas of swelling on the extremities, usually accompanied by a sensory peripheral neuropathy.
- **Coinfections with Other Deer Tick-Borne Pathogens.** Human granulocytic anaplasmosis (HGA) and babesiosis are deer tick-borne diseases that are occasionally co-transmitted with *B burgdorferi*. Coinfection with either agent may increase the severity of Lyme disease. Diagnostic testing and treatment should be expanded accordingly.

## DIAGNOSIS

*B burgdorferi* is a fastidious organism; the culture yield is high from skin aspirates in EM and from blood in early-disseminated Lyme disease, very low from CSF, and almost negligible from synovial fluid. The culture medium is expensive to purchase and the procedure and controls laborious to maintain. Confirming the diagnosis by culture, therefore, is not feasible in practice settings. Instead, the diagnosis of Lyme borreliosis, except for EM, is confirmed by serologic assays. A diagnosis of EM should be made clinically, because patients are frequently seronegative at this early stage of the infection and the rash, when typical, is pathognomonic for Lyme disease. If the rash is atypical and the patient is not treated, and the initial serology is negative or equivocal, a second specimen should be obtained within 2 to 4 weeks.[21]

A diagnosis of Lyme disease should never be made solely on the basis of a laboratory test. Serologic testing is often ordered indiscriminately, at great economic and emotional cost, in patients with nonspecific symptoms and even in asymptomatic individuals. This leads to overdiagnosis based on false-positive results, especially in areas with low prevalence, where the predictive value of a positive test is very low. Consequences include patient anxiety, unnecessary antibiotic treatment, and missing other diagnoses.[22] Indiscriminately ordered screening tests to "rule out" Lyme disease are prevalent and should be discouraged. Serology should be ordered only in the clinical situation of a patient with an objective sign that can be a manifestation of Lyme disease, and at least a reasonable possibility of exposure to ticks.

The commonly available serologic screening tests are enzyme immunoassays (EIA), in which false-positives are common, but the "2-step" approach has been widely adopted and has markedly improved the specificity of diagnosis.[23] It is recommended that the laboratory automatically follow through with the second step test, an immunoblot (Western blot) on any serum sample that yields a positive or equivocal result. Antibodies to *B burgdorferi* appear as bands on an immunoblot that represent antibodies to different polypeptides of *B burgdorferi*, their molecular weight expressed in kilodaltons (kD or K). IgM and IgG blots are run separately. As in most infectious diseases, IgM antibodies appear early and there is a more gradual rise in IgG antibodies. False-positives are commonly observed. Moreover, results of an IgM immunoblot are invalid after the first 4 weeks of the illness because IgM antibodies can persist beyond the early stage.[24] Seroconfirmation is obtained by the IgG assay and repeated 1 to 3 weeks later if initially negative. Antibodies persist after antibiotic treatment, so a positive serologic assay does not imply persistent infection and cannot be used to monitor the effectiveness of treatment. Serologic testing should not be repeated following treatment.

Tests to detect antigens of *B burgdorferi* in urine are not Food and Drug Administration (FDA)-approved, and they have no current role in the diagnosis or management of Lyme disease.

## TREATMENT

The drugs of choice for treatment of Lyme borreliosis in adolescents are oral doxycycline or amoxicillin, and parenteral ceftriaxone or cefotaxime (Table 140-2). In addition, cefuroxime axetil is approved for treatment of early Lyme disease in children 12 years and older. Doxycycline is the preferred drug for adolescents in most clinical situations. Its advantages include central nervous system (CNS) penetration and the opportunity to treat *Anaplasma* or *Ehrlichia* coinfection. Macrolides have inferior efficacy. Anti-inflammatory drugs are used to treat musculoskeletal symptoms that persist after successful treatment of Lyme arthritis. Hydroxychloroquine therapy, intra-articular steroids, and synovectomy are measures considered by the rheumatologist to alleviate symptoms in the small subset of children with chronic arthritis.

Intravenous antibiotic therapy is indicated for treatment of meningitis and can be considered for recurrences of arthritis. There is no evidence that prolonged

## Table 140-2

### Treatment of Lyme Borreliosis

| *Manifestation* | *First Line Drugs* | *Equivalent Alternate Drugs* | *Second Line Drugs* |
|---|---|---|---|
| **Early localized EM** | **Amoxicillin** PO 10–**21** days or doxycycline PO 10–**21** days | Cefuroxime axetil PO[a] 10–**21** days | Erythromycin PO 10–**21** days or **clarithromycin** 10–**21** days |
| Early disseminated | | | |
| Multiple EM | Amoxicillin PO 21–**28** days or **doxycycline** PO 21–**28** days | **Cefuroxime axetil** PO[a] 21–**28** days or **ceftriaxone** IV 14 days or cefotaxime IV 14 days | Erythromycin PO 21–**28** days or **clarithromycin** PO 21–**28** days |
| Facial palsy | Amoxicillin PO 21–**28** days or **doxycycline** PO 21–**28** days | **Ceftriaxone** IV **14**–28 days or cefotaxime IV 14–**28** days | Erythromycin PO 21–**28** days or **clarithromycin** PO 21–**28** days |
| Meningitis/Facial palsy with meningitis/polyneuropathy | **Ceftriaxone** IV **14**–28 days or cefotaxime IV 14–**28** days | Doxycycline PO 28 days | Penicillin IV **14**–28 days |
| Cardiac[b] | Amoxicillin PO 21 days or **doxycycline** PO 21 days OR **ceftriaxone** IV 14 days or cefotaxime IV 14 days | | Erythromycin PO 21 days or **clarithromycin** PO 21 days or penicillin IV 14 days |
| **Late** | | | |
| Arthritis | **Amoxicillin** PO **28** days or **doxycycline** PO **28** days | **Ceftriaxone**[c] IV 14–28 days or cefotaxime[c] IV 14–**28** days | Penicillin IV 14–**28** days |
| Neurologic | **Ceftriaxone** IV 14–**28** days or cefotaxime IV 14–**28** days | Doxycycline PO **28** days | Penicillin IV 14–**28** days |
| **Other** | | | |
| Asymptomatic seroconversion<br>Viral-type illness | Amoxicillin PO 21–**28** days or **doxycycline** PO 21–28 days | Cefuroxime axetil PO[a] 21–28 days | Erythromycin PO 21–**28** days or **clarithromycin** PO 21–**28** days |
| **Prophylaxis for engorged deer tick bite** | **Amoxicillin** PO 10 days or doxycycline PO 10 days | Cefuroxime axetil PO[a] 10 days | Erythromycin PO 10 days or **clarithromycin** PO 10 days |

[a]Cefuroxime axetil was tested in children 12 and older

[b]First-degree block with PR interval <0.3 sec, PO therapy; PR >0.3 sec or higher grade, IV initially, then PO if responds rapidly

[c]For oral therapy failures only

**Doses:**
- Doxycycline PO 2–4 mg/kg/day divided into 2 doses, up to adult dose of 100 mg bid
- Amoxicillin PO 40–50 mg/kg/day divided into 3 doses, up to adult dose of 2 g/day
- Cefuroxime axetil PO 30 mg/kg/day divided into 2 doses, up to adult dose of 500 mg bid
- Erythromycin PO 30–40 mg/kg/day divided into 4 doses, up to adult dose of 250 qid
- Clarithromycin PO 15 mg/kg/day divided into 2 doses, up to adult dose of 500 bid
- Ceftriaxone IV 100 mg/kg/day once daily, up to adult dose of 2 g once daily
- Cefotaxime IV 180 mg/kg/day, up to adult dose of 2 g every 8 hours
- Penicillin IV 200,000–400,000 units/kg/day, divided into 4 doses, up to adult dose of 24 million units/day

**Duration: The author's preferences are indicated in bold type.**

bid, twice a day; EM, erythema migrans; qid, 4 times a day

courses of treatment that exceed a month are efficacious for adults with ongoing symptoms of post-Lyme disease syndrome, and this knowledge can be extrapolated to children. It is inappropriate to prescribe an antibiotic for a child who has positive serology in the absence of accompanying or recent specific clinical manifestations.

### PROGNOSIS

Early-localized EM responds rapidly to treatment, irrespective of the duration of rash. Recurrent episodes of arthritis can occur after treatment for the first episode of Lyme arthritis. Musculoskeletal symptoms persist for several weeks in some children, and ongoing knee pain is often from patellofemoral joint disease rather than true knee arthritis. The long-term prognosis of treated arthritis is excellent in children. Of children ages 1.8 to 16 years at the time of diagnosis, in a telephone follow-up study 2 to 12 years after the onset of arthritis, 4 of 90 children had ongoing musculoskeletal complaints, but none had evidence of active arthritis.[25] The same authors' review of previous studies suggested that the success rate of treatment in children is about 95%. Of 55 children in Germany (ages 2–16), in 27 the arthritis was either chronic at onset or became chronic during treatment or follow-up. One year after antibiotic treatment, 12 (24%) of 51 evaluable children still had arthralgia or frank arthritis.[26] In 8 children, synovectomy was used as part of treatment. Factors associated with a poorer outcome were older age and female gender.[27] The long-term prognosis of children with treated neurologic infection is excellent. Because of concern that infection of the nervous system in Lyme disease could have adverse neuropsychological consequences in the long term, Adams et al[28] conducted a prospective controlled study in an endemic area. The 41 children consisted of 25 with proven Lyme disease and 16 healthy sibling controls. At 2- and 4-year follow-up, none had impairment of cognitive functioning. In a New England endemic area, children with prior Lyme disease did not have a higher prevalence of musculoskeletal or neurological symptoms, an abnormal ECG, or behavioral difficulties a mean of 3.2 years from the initial manifestation, compared to children with no history of Lyme disease. Behavioral difficulties were assessed by a battery of questions designed to assess a wide range of behavioral and emotional problems. These data contrast with those in adults, who have significantly more arthritic, neurologic, and global health impairment than controls.[29]

Infection with *B burgdorferi* does not confer lasting immunity, for unknown reasons. The incidence of reinfection was 3% in a prospective pediatric study.[4]

## ROCKY MOUNTAIN SPOTTED FEVER

### ETIOLOGY AND EPIDEMIOLOGY

*Rickettsia rickettsii* infection is common in the United States, and has increasingly been recognized in Mexico, Canada, Central America, and a few countries in South America.[30] It has emerged in urban parks in New York City and recently in the southwest, in the latter outbreak being transmitted by a new tick vector for this organism. Rocky Mountain spotted fever (RMSF) is somewhat misleading as a name for the disease, as most cases occur outside the Rocky Mountain states. It owes its name to the initial recognition in Idaho as the "black measles." The current highest prevalence is in North Carolina and Arkansas. Definitive characterization of the organism was achieved by Dr. Howard Ricketts at the Rocky Mountain laboratory of the National Institutes of Health (NIH) in Hamilton, Montana.[31] *Rickettsia rickettsii* is a tick-transmitted obligate intracellular pathogen. There are 3 proven vectors, which vary in their predominant geographic distribution: the American dog tick (*Dermacentor variabilis*) in the northeastern and eastern endemic areas, the wood tick (*D andersoni*), also known sometimes as the Rocky Mountain wood tick, in the Rocky Mountain states, and the brown dog tick (*Rhipicephalus sanguineus*) in the southwest and south.

Most cases occur in children younger than 15 years of age. April through September is the period associated with the highest incidence, but RMSF can occur in any month of the year. The incubation period after the tick bite is between 2 days and 2 weeks, but the bite may go unnoticed.

### CLINICAL MANIFESTATIONS

Rocky Mountain spotted fever is a systemic infection that results in vasculitic phenomena.[30] In endemic areas, the possibility of RMSF should be considered in any patient who presents with an acute febrile constitutional illness during the spring and summer months. Certain combinations of signs and symptoms suggest RMSF in the appropriate epidemiologic setting, but adherence to "classic triad" rules of thumb may be misleading, especially because different triads have been described. More importantly, in an adolescent with fever, myalgia, malaise, and headache, the appearance of a characteristic rash has a much better predictive value. The rash begins as a blanching and nonpruritic erythematous macular rash, which may be difficult to appreciate, then progresses to petechial and purpuric lesions, and in some patients to frank skin hemorrhages and larger areas of skin necrosis or even gangrene. The rash usually makes its initial appearance on the distal extremities. There are several caveats regarding the rash.[32] It may be delayed until the sixth day of illness, and about 10% of patients never develop it. Involvement of the palms and soles may be absent or only appear in the later phases of illness. Centripetal progression has been emphasized but only occurs in a minority of patients with RMSF.[33]

The illness may last as long as 3 weeks and may be severe, with progression to disseminated intravascular coagulation (DIC), as well as CNS, gastrointestinal, and renal involvement, and shock leading to death. Complications observed in RMSF include edema, hypovolemia, hypoalbuminemia, azotemia, hypotension, cardiac dysrhythmia, respiratory involvement (8% require mechanical ventilation), meningoencephalitis, and occasionally purpura fulminans.[34] Mortality is higher in males and in those for whom recognition and initiation of antirickettsial treatment is delayed.

### DIAGNOSIS

Certain laboratory findings serve as criteria that support a diagnosis of RMSF: elevated polymorphonuclear (PMN) band forms in association with normal white blood counts or leukopenia; thrombocytopenia; hyponatremia; elevated hepatic transaminases; and elevated creatine kinase. Because similar laboratory findings are observed in other rickettsial illnesses and babesiosis, and because the symptoms can be similar in the absence of a characteristic rash, the diagnostic work-up should include these illnesses.[35]

An indirect immunofluorescence antibody assay (IFA) is the most widely available serologic test. A probable diagnosis can be established by a single serum titer of 1:64 or greater by IFA, but only a fourfold or greater rise in titer on convalescent serum confirms the diagnosis. *R rickettsii* can be identified by immunohistochemical (immunofluorescence or immunoperoxidase) staining of tissue (biopsy or autopsy) obtained at the site of the rash. This method is highly specific, but not sensitive, and not practical in today's laboratory settings. The nonspecific and insensitive Weil-Felix serologic test (*Proteus vulgaris* OX-19 and OX-2 agglutination) is not recommended. Polymerase chain reaction assay for detection of *R rickettsii* during the acute phase may confirm the diagnosis, but this test is not universally available.

### TREATMENT

Adolescents who are able to maintain adequate oral intake and are stable hemodynamically do not have to be hospitalized for treatment. Supportive care is essential for those with severe symptoms, often in the intensive care unit (ICU) setting. Prophylactic antibiotic therapy after a tick bite is not recommended, as it potentially can delay the diagnosis by partially masking the symptoms. Treatment should be started promptly based upon clinical suspicion and should not await confirmation of the diagnosis. Doxycycline is the drug of choice. The dose is 3 mg/kg to 5 mg/kg per day in 2 divided doses, maximum dose 100 mg twice daily. Duration of therapy is 5 to 7 days or 2 days after defervescence of symptoms.

## HUMAN EHRLICHIOSES

At least 5 related species of obligate intracellular bacteria that are classified as ehrlichiae, which are rickettsia-like organisms, are known to be tick-borne pathogens of humans.[36] Three of these have well-characterized and overlapping clinical manifestations: *Anaplasma phagocytophilum, Ehrlichia chaffeensis, and Ehrlichia ewingii.* The hallmark of these pathogens is infection of leukocytes, which enables early diagnosis in many instances.[36] *Anaplasma phagocytophilum* causes HGA, previously called human granulocytic ehrlichiosis (HGE). *Ehrlichia ewingii* also infects granulocytes and the illness is termed human *ewingii* ehrlichiosis. *Ehrlichia chaffeensis* is the agent of human monocytic ehrlichiosis (HME), where the target is monocytes.

### ETIOLOGY AND EPIDEMIOLOGY

#### Human Granulocytic Anaplasmosis

*Anaplasma phagocytophilum* is transmitted by the same vector ticks that transmit *B burgdorferi:Ixodes scapularis* in the northeastern and upper midwest of the United States, *I pacificus* in the northern Pacific coastal region, and *I persulcatus* group ticks in Eurasian regions. Up to a quarter of adult deer ticks have been found to be coinfected with *B burgdorferi* and the HGE agent in Westchester County, New York, and cotransmission with *B burgdorferi* has caused dual infection in several instances.[37,38] Babesia spp. and, in Europe, tick-borne encephalitis virus are also transmitted by *Ixodes* ticks. Coinfection with another tick-borne pathogen in HGA-infected individuals may be as high as 10%.[36] Because of its relatively nonspecific clinical syndrome (see the following), it is likely that most cases go unrecognized. Further evidence of this is inferred from the seroprevalence rates found in endemic areas, ranging from 9% to 36%. Vertical transmission from a mother to her baby, and percutaneous, mucosal, aerosol, or transfusion-mediated exposures, have also been suspected.[39]

#### Human Monocytic Ehrlichiosis

Human monocytic ehrlichiosis is prevalent in the southern and mid-Atlantic regions of the United States, where the lone star tick (*Amblyomma americanum*) is prevalent along with high populations of white-tailed deer. The American dog tick (*Dermacentor variabilis*) has a role in the natural history of the HME agent but has not been proven to be a vector for humans.

### Human Ewingii Ehrlichiosis

Human ewingii ehrlichiosis is restricted to the United States and is transmitted by *Amblyomma americanum*, the lone star tick. Its epidemiology is not as well defined as for the other ehrlichiosis infections.

### CLINICAL MANIFESTATIONS

The syndrome caused by these pathogens consists of fever (almost universally); constitutional symptoms such as myalgia, malaise, arthralgias, headache, and gastrointestinal symptoms; and varying occurrence of other constitutional symptoms such as malaise, nausea, leukopenia and/or thrombocytopenia, and hepatic inflammation detectable by elevated serum transaminases.[37] In general, HME is the most severe illness among the human ehrlichiosis infections, with renal failure and fulminant illness occurring at higher rates.

As there is no pathognomonic clinical sign for these infections, the diagnosis will frequently be missed in the absence of a high index of suspicion. In those patients who report a known tick bite, the incubation period is most often between 1 and 2 weeks. A rash is reported in 2% to 16% of published HGA cases, most often erythematous and maculopapular. Rashes are significantly more common in HME, noted in 31% in a meta-analysis.[38] They are distributed on the trunk or extremities and can be macular, maculopapular, petechial, or a combination thereof. The spectrum of severity of HGA ranges from asymptomatic to fatal infection. There is a 50% hospitalization rate and a 17% ICU admission rate, with complications that include shock, opportunistic infections, respiratory failure due to adult respiratory distress syndrome (ARDS), renal failure, brachial plexopathy, and demyelinating neuropathy.[39] Another complication of note for HGA in an immunocompromised patient is serious and fatal infections from viral and fungal opportunistic pathogens.

### DIAGNOSIS

The laboratory hallmarks of human ehrlichial infections are leukopenia, thrombocytopenia (more commonly than leukopenia, about 75% of cases), and elevation of hepatic transaminases. One or more of these abnormalities are present in the majority of patients. In HGA, a pronounced left shift of the differential white blood cell count has been noted. Spontaneous resolution of these abnormal laboratory findings may begin during the second week of the illness.

The confirmatory tests for the human ehrlichial infections are visualization of morulae (intraleukocytic mulberry-shaped inclusions) on Wright or Giemsa stained blood smears; PCR or culture evidence of the organism from blood; or seroconversion by assay-specific antibodies detected by IFA testing. Although the presence of IgM antibodies is supportive of the diagnosis, a fourfold rise in IgG titers is needed for confirmation.

A diagnostic testing approach based on time intervals is recommended.[37] Within the first week of illness onset, evaluation of blood smears for morulae is a specific, though relatively insensitive test, with 25% to 75% of HGA but fewer than 10% of HME patients yielding a positive finding. The polymerase chain reaction assay on a blood specimen is 60% to 90% sensitive, whereas IgM and IgG serologic assays are positive in 25% to 50% of cases at this stage. During the second week, smear and PCR should still be ordered but serology is on average 68% sensitive for HME and 91% sensitive for HGA, whereas after the third week both HME and HGA can be confirmed by serology more than 90% of the time. Culture is confirmatory at any stage but not routinely available, and the organisms may take weeks to grow. Testing for *E ewingii* should be arranged in collaboration with a research laboratory.

### TREATMENT

Because of the limitations involved in early diagnostic confirmation, and because an ehrlichial illness can rapidly worsen and result in fatality, treatment should be initiated based on clinical suspicion using the following minimal presumptive diagnostic criteria: unexplained fever, constitutional symptoms, and suggestive lab findings on the complete blood count (CBC) and chemistry panel. The antibiotic of choice is doxycycline.[40] In most cases, complete resolution of the illness is achieved in 24 to 48 hours. Some patients, mostly in the adult age group, are ill enough to be hospitalized and require supportive care; hemodynamic and renal functions need to be monitored in these patients.

## TICK-BORNE RELAPSING FEVER

### ETIOLOGY AND EPIDEMIOLOGY

Tick-borne relapsing fever (TBRF) is a variety of relapsing fever illness that is widespread on many continents. In the United States it occurs west of the Mississippi River, primarily in western and southern states.[41,42] In Canada it is endemic in British Columbia. Three related species of *Ornithodoros* soft ticks (*B hermsii*, *turicata,* and, rarely, *parkeri*) transmit 3 respectively eponymous species of *Borrelia* (*B hermsii, turicatae*, and, *parkeri*).[43] *B hermsii* infections are mostly observed in the western states, with *B turicatae* infections mostly in the lower elevation and desert terrain of the southern and southwestern states. The tick bites are usually acquired in lake or mountain cabins in the former instance and in caves in the latter instance. The most common epidemiologic setting is a previously rodent-infected seasonal cabin where ticks seek out a human host, being present in coats and bedding.

### CLINICAL MANIFESTATIONS

The blood meal is rapid and the bite usually asymptomatic, and the incubation period of the febrile illness is 4 to more than 18 days (mean 7 days). Following an initial brief febrile illness of up to 106.7°F (41.5°C) that lasts about 3 days, the fever ends abruptly in a "crisis." During the crisis there are chills, higher fever, profuse diaphoresis, tachycardia, and hypotension, which is life threatening. The illness relapses about a week later. Untreated, relapsing fever can continue for several weeks, with 4- to 14-day intervals, during which the person feels well or has malaise. The relapsing course is attributed to the ability of these *Borrelia* species to change the antigenic composition of their outer surface proteins rapidly, thus evading the immune response. The most common accompanying symptoms are headache, myalgia, and chills, present in about 90% of patients. Gastrointestinal symptoms, especially nausea, vomiting, and abdominal pain, are present in about 75% of patients, as are arthralgias. Altered sensorium may be part of the presentation. A minority of patients will also have eye pain or photophobia, neck pain, or overt signs of meningitis. Some patients present with jaundice or hepatosplenomegaly. A rare but significant complication is ARDS, but the overall mortality is very low. Neurologic complications, especially cranial and other neuropathies, are more common in *B turicatae* infection than in other North American infections.

Because of the wide variability in illness severity, TBRF should be in the differential diagnosis of any summertime febrile illness. In particular, there are a number of domestically acquired zoonotic illnesses that can present with a relapsing or at least biphasic course, including Colorado (viral) tick fever, brucellosis, bartonellosis, leptospirosis, rat bite fever, and lymphocytic choriomeningitis. A history of foreign travel would add malaria, yellow fever, and dengue and other hemorrhagic fevers to the list.

### DIAGNOSIS

It is possible to obtain early confirmation of a diagnosis of TBRF by visualization of organisms on blood smears (Wright or Giemsa stain examined under oil immersion, or wet mount examined by dark or bright field microscopy). Examination of a buffy coat further enhances the sensitivity. The highest yield is on a blood specimen drawn as the fever begins to rise, as the spirochete density diminishes rapidly after the fever has peaked.[43] Isolation of the bacteria on culture is not practical in the clinical laboratory, as a modified cell culture medium (Kelly) must be used. In practice, confirmation is achieved by demonstration of a fourfold titer rise between acute and convalescent sera, typically by ELISA, using whole cell preparations of the organism. Serologic assays have not yet been rigorously evaluated or standardized, and a more specific immunoassay that uses the GlpQ protein is in development.

### TREATMENT

Because diagnostic confirmation may be delayed, empiric treatment with antibiotics is indicated if it is determined on history that exposure to an *Ornithodoros* tick is likely. In most cases, oral treatment as an outpatient is adequate. Adolescents and adults should receive a 7- or 10-day course of doxycycline (100 mg every 12 hours), with erythromycin as an alternative. In hospitalized patients, the same antibiotics can be administered parenterally, if necessary, with intramuscular procaine penicillin G as an additional option; intravenous penicillin G or ceftriaxone are preferred in cases with suspected neurologic involvement. In contrast to other tick-borne infections discussed in this chapter, there is a high incidence of the Jarisch-Herxheimer reaction occurring with treatment of TBRF (54% in 1 review of North American cases).[44] This results in a worsening of the patient's signs and symptoms, similar to the aforementioned crisis, secondary to massive release of cytokines as the spirochetes are killed and phagocytosed. Because fatal cardiovascular collapse can ensue, patients should be closely monitored for at least 4 hours after the first dose of antibiotic is administered. This precaution is particularly pertinent to treatment in the outpatient setting. The use of meptazinol, an opioid antagonist, has been shown to ameliorate the reaction.

### PROPHYLAXIS

In a placebo-controlled trial in Israel where subjects were exposed or suspected to be exposed to other species of *Borrelia* that cause relapsing fever, postexposure treatment with a single dose of doxycycline was efficacious in preventing TBRF.[44] This option should be considered in exposed persons, given the approximately 50% transmission rate, and the unproven effectiveness of repellents, considering that most persons are bitten while asleep.

## BABESIOSIS

### ETIOLOGY AND EPIDEMIOLOGY

Babesiosis is a tick-borne infection of red blood cells caused by piroplasms ("pear-shaped" unicellular tick-borne organisms) belonging to several species of the genus *Babesia*.[45] The species prevalent in the northeastern and Great Lakes regions of the United States is *B microti*, transmitted by the hard-bodied tick *I scapularis*, which is also a vector for *B burgdorferi* and *Anaplasma phagocytophilum*. One of the most endemic foci is on the southern New England coast of Massachusetts, Rhode Island, and Connecticut and in New York (especially Long Island). The distribution is more focal than that of Lyme disease, but in this region the main mammalian reservoir, *Peromyscus leucopus*, is the same as that for *B burgdorferi*. *B burgdorferi* and *Babesia* spp have been concurrently recovered from 18.6% of nymphal *Ixodes* ticks from Nantucket Island and concurrent human infection occurs.[46] Infections from related species have been identified in California and Washington (*B duncani* WA1) and Missouri, Kentucky, and Washington (*B divergens*-like). In Europe, babesiosis is primarily caused by *B divergens* and is a more fulminant disease, with *B microti* and a novel species, EU1, identified recently. Cases of babesiosis have also been reported from the Asian, African, and South American continents. Rarely, transfusion-acquired and transplacental transmissions have been reported.[47,48]

### CLINICAL MANIFESTATIONS

The clinical presentations of babesiosis vary widely, the spectrum of illness ranging from asymptomatic infection to fulminant disease resembling blackwater fever of malaria with fever, hemolysis, and hemoglobinuria. In a recent compilation of outpatients and inpatients, 85% presented with fever, most with chills or rigors, and 79% presented with fatigue; about a third had headache and myalgia, and other constitutional symptoms occurred, but less often. Acute respiratory failure is the most common complication of babesiosis, followed by disseminated intravascular coagulation (DIC), heart failure, and coma. A 5% mortality rate was noted in a retrospective survey of 136 patients on Long Island.[49] The disease is usually mild in children, but the uncommon scenario of fatal infection in asplenic or immunocompromised patients is an important consideration.[27] Babesiosis should be in the differential diagnosis of an adolescent with fever of uncertain origin with anemia and/or thrombocytopenia. Persistent infection for up to 2 years, with clinical recrudescence, has been described.[28]

### DIAGNOSIS

The diagnosis of babesiosis should be considered in any patient with fever of uncertain origin in an endemic area year round, but especially during the transmission season (May to October). The incubation period is estimated to vary from 1 to 6 weeks, but the tick bite is often unnoticed. The optimal method of diagnosis is examination of a blood smear for intraerythrocytic forms, typically seen in less than 1% of erythrocytes. The ring form is seen most commonly and can be mistaken for malarial parasites by an inexperienced microscopist. Visualization of the less common "Maltese cross" tetrad form is pathognomonic. The current serologic test of choice is an indirect IFA for IgM and IgG antibodies. Titers of 1:1,024 or greater signify active or recent infection. Other confirmatory tests are small animal inoculation and PCR for babesial DNA, the latter now being increasingly available in commercial laboratories. Testing for coinfection with Lyme borreliosis and HGA should be emphasized whenever the clinical suspicion of babesiosis is high.

### TREATMENT

Treatment regimens for babesiosis are matched to clinical severity (Table 140-3). The standard regimen of clindamycin and quinine is associated with a high incidence of side effects. Quinine is poorly tolerated in about half of treated patients, who experience hearing loss, tinnitus, gastrointestinal symptoms, and occasionally, hypotension. As more experience is gained, combination treatment with azithromycin and atovaquone may become the therapy of choice.

## TULAREMIA

### ETIOLOGY AND EPIDEMIOLOGY

Tularemia is a bacterial infection caused by the gram-negative bacillus *Francisella tularensis.* Its synonyms have included rabbit fever, deerfly fever, Pahvant Valley plague, Ohara disease, Francis disease, and lemming fever. The name is derived from the original description in the United States a century ago of a plague-like disease of ground squirrels in Tulare County, California. Tularemia has been reported in all states in the United States except Hawaii. Over the past half-century or so, about half of reported US cases in which the source of exposure could be determined have been due to tick exposure,[50,51] most commonly *Dermacentor* species (dog or wood ticks) and less commonly *Amblyomma americanum* (lone star tick).[52] The highest incidence of tick-borne tularemia is in Arkansas, Missouri, and Oklahoma, where both *Dermacentor* and *Amblyomma* ticks are prevalent.[53]

In Europe and Asia most tularemia is not tick-borne, despite isolation of *F tularensis* from several species of ticks. This has been attributed to the absence of *Dermacentor variabilis* and *andersoni* ticks outside of North America. Other modes of transmission include "mechanical" transmission from deerfly, horsefly, and mosquito

**Table 140-3**

**Treatment of Babesiosis**

| *Severity* | *Agents* | *Dosing* | *Comments* |
|---|---|---|---|
| Asymptomatic | No treatment, unless persistent parasitemia ≥3 months or immunocompromised (see the following) | | |
| Mild-to-moderate | Atovaquone PO+<br>Azithromycin PO | 20 mg/kg up to 750 mg 12 hourly for 7–10 days<br>10 mg/kg up to 500 mg once 15 mg/kg daily up to 250 mg for 7–20 days | About a third of patients will not be able to continue the medications due to tinnitus, GI disturbances, or other adverse reactions |
| Severe | Clindamycin IV + quinine PO partial or complete exchange transfusion | 7–10 mg/kg up to 600 mg/dose every 6–8 hours<br>8 mg/kg up to 650 mg/dose every 6–8 hours | *B divergens* infection always treated as severe |
| Immunocompromised | Either of previously noted combination regimens. Atovaquone + azithromycin for 6 weeks followed by 2 weeks after smear negative has been associated with cure | Consider following with lower doses for longer durations | Repeat smears every 2–3 months until clear |

bites, as well as inhalation, ingestion, and handling of infected animals. *F tularensis* is a zoonotic organism that has been identified in more than 100 species, but the primary reservoirs are rodents, lagomorphs, domestic cats, and captive primates, which differ in the subspecies they typically harbor (Table 140-4). *F tularensis* has 2 main subspecies: A (also known as subspecies *tularensis*) and B (also known as subspecies *holarctica*).[54] Tick transmission is strongly linked to type A organisms, which are considered more pathogenic than type B. The A subspecies is subdivided into A1 and A2 clades. There are distinct geographic distributions for A1, A2, and B that correlate with tick species distributions (Figure 140-3). Further molecular subtyping of A types into A1a, A1b, A2a, and A2b genotypes has demonstrated significant differences in human mortality for infection with A1b (24%) compared with A1a (4%), A2 (0%), and B (7%).[54]

**Table 140-4**

***F Tularensis* Isolates, by Subspecies and Animal Source Groups**

| *Source* | *Type A (n = 97)* | *Type B (n = 87)* | *Total (n = 184)* |
|---|---|---|---|
| Domestic cats | 41 | 3 | 44 |
| Lagomorphs | 52 | 6 | 58 |
| Primates | 2 | 27 | 29 |
| Rodents | 2 | 46 | 48 |
| Other (dog, bird, weasel) | 0 | 5 | 5 |

Adapted from Kugeler KJ, Mead PS, Janusz AM, et al. Molecular epidemiology of *Francisella tularensis* in the United States. *Clin Infect Dis*. 2009;1;48(7):863–870 by permission of the University of Chicago Press.

## CLINICAL MANIFESTATIONS

Tularemia can present in many clinical forms including fever without localizing signs (typhoidal), oropharyngeal, pneumonic, oculoglandular and a typhoid-like syndrome, and lymphadenitis with or without cutaneous lesions. The latter, termed glandular or ulceroglandular tularemia, is the most common presentation. The incubation period is usually less than 2 weeks. The tick-acquired illness has sudden onset with fever and chills, headache, myalgia, gastrointestinal, and several other constitutional symptoms. Various rashes, including erythema nodosum and erythema multiforme, have been observed, and complications include

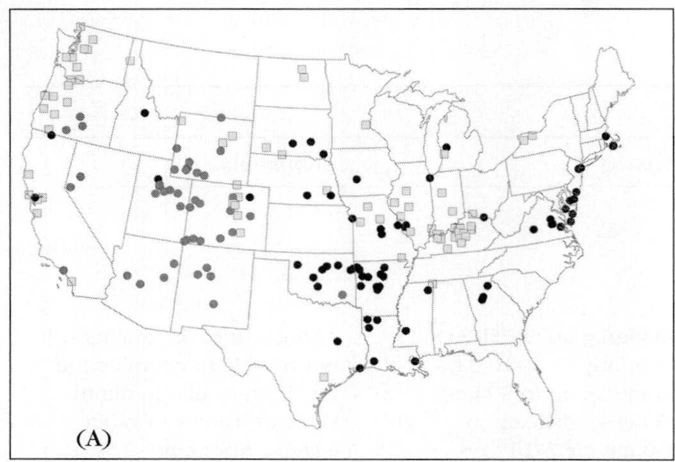


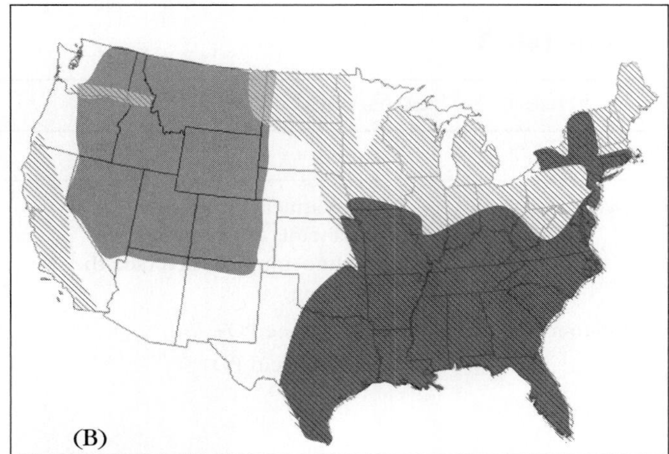


**FIGURE 140-3** Map of *F tularensis* strains and their vector ticks in the United States. (A) The distribution of human infections caused by *F tularensis* subsp holarctica (type B) (light gray squares) and subsp tularensis clades A1 (black circles) and A2 (gray circles) in the USA. (Human infection data is from Staples JE, Kubota KA, Chalcraft LG, Mead PS, Petersen JM. Epidemiologic and molecular analysis of human tularemia, United States, 1964–2004. *Emerg Infect Dis*. 2006;12(7):1113–1118.) Cases are plotted randomly with the county of infection. Infections represent all routes of exposure (arthropod, animal contact, inhalation, etc). (B) Approximate geographic distributions of tick species associated with human tularemia in the USA, *D variabilis* (light gray diagonal striped shading), *A americanum* (black shading) and *D andersoni* (gray shading). (Reprinted with permission from Petersen JM, Mead PS, Schriefer ME. *Francisella tularensis*: an arthropod-borne pathogen. *Vet Res*. 2009;40:7. Available at www.vetres.org/index.php?option=com_article&access=standard&Itemid=129&url=/articles/vetres/full_html/2009/02/v09004/v09004.html; tick distributions are from Brown RN, Lane RS, Dennis DT. Geographic distribution of tick-borne diseases and their vectors. In: Goodman JL, Dennis DT, Sonenshine DE, eds. *Tick-Borne Diseases of Humans*. Washington, DC: ASM Press; 2005:363–391.)

meningitis, septic arthritis, endocarditis, and pericarditis. With antibiotic treatment, mortality is about 2%.

### DIAGNOSIS

A hemagglutination assay to detect antibodies to the causative bacterium is available from most commercial laboratory services and is a sensitive means of detecting evidence of recent or current infection. Typically, IgM and IgG titers of hemagglutinating antibody are markedly elevated. Because a single elevated IgG titer could be from past infection, a fourfold or greater rise on a 2-week convalescent sample is diagnostic. Tissue samples can be used for direct detection of the organism by culture, PCR, and direct fluorescent antibody or slide agglutination tests, but they entail a hazard for laboratory personnel. Importantly, *F tularensis* is an agent of bioterrorism, and culture is to be undertaken only in biosafety level 3 laboratories. The organism can survive in harsh conditions, including freezing at −15°C, in carcasses and hides of animals, and on fomites.

### TREATMENT

Mild cases, especially those presenting with unifocal lymphadenitis, are self-limited. Severe disease is treated with antibiotics. Streptomycin is the most effective antibiotic, but the most practical alternative is intramuscular gentamicin, with oral ciprofloxacin or doxycycline as alternatives.

## POWASSAN ENCEPHALITIS

A "tick-borne encephalitis complex" of flaviviruses is important in the causation of encephalitis. The only well-characterized viral lineage of this group in North America is the Powassan viruses, which encompass the deer tick virus. These viruses have been isolated from several species of *Ixodes* ticks and from *Dermacentor* species. Prototypic Powassan virus strains have caused encephalitis chiefly in Ontario and New York state, whereas deer tick virus may be prevalent in all the states endemic for Lyme borreliosis because its enzootic cycle relies on the white-footed mouse and *I scapularis*.[55] Symptomatic disease from these viruses appears to be rare, but this may be a consequence of lack of testing. Most patients with Powassan encephalitis reported in the literature suffered short- or long-term neurologic sequelae, or died. It is important to suspect tick-borne flaviviruses in the etiology of encephalitis of unknown origin.[56] Serologic assays to detect specific antibodies in serum or CSF should be sought in consultation with the state health department or the Centers for Disease

Control and Prevention (CDC). There is no specific treatment, and standard supportive measures are used.

## COLORADO TICK FEVER

Another virus transmitted by a tick in the United States is a reovirus (genus *Coltivirus*), an acronymous name for Colorado tick fever. *D andersoni* is the identified vector for humans, and the prevalence of the disease correlates with the geographic distribution of this tick.[55] Colorado tick fever is fairly common, as up to 400 cases are reported in the United States every year, and mild disease probably goes unreported. There is a wide clinical spectrum that spans constitutional, musculoskeletal, and gastrointestinal symptoms, rashes, meningoencephalitis, and rarely the involvement of other organ systems. Rashes can be maculopapular or petechial and occur in 5% to 15% of patients. The onset is abrupt, heralded by fever and chills along with constitutional symptoms, as seen in arboviral and enteroviral illnesses. A biphasic illness with a 1- to 2-day reprieve of fever occurs in about 50% of patients, earning it the name "saddleback fever."

On laboratory testing, the presence of combinations of leukopenia, neutropenia, and thrombocytopenia is common, as is a lymphocytic pleocytosis in the meningitic form. Confirmatory testing can be accomplished in consultation with the CDC, which offers PCR, viral culture, and specific serology. There is no specific therapy. Fortunately, the encephalitic presentation is rarely severe, and mortality from Colorado tick fever is rare.

## PREVENTION AND MANAGEMENT OF TICK BITES

As has been detailed previously, tick-borne diseases are a common problem. Nevertheless, most clinicians, even in endemic areas, are not familiar enough with recommendations for prevention and management of tick bites. This discussion is divided into prevention of tick bites and prevention of infection after a tick bite. Many of the measures discussed are also useful for the reduction of risk from mosquito bites.

### PREVENTION OF TICK BITES

#### Avoidance

An obvious piece of advice is to avoid infected areas, but because recreational, occupational, and even residential habits make exposure inevitable for most people in endemic areas, other preventive measures need to be implemented.[57] Visitors to public parks and nature preserves in endemic areas are usually aware of the need to minimize contact with brush, bushes, and heavily wooded areas. However, ticks can attach during even minimal or passing exposure and can be present on grassy areas and in leaf litter. An additional protective measure is wearing long-sleeved clothing and light-colored clothing that would enable crawling ticks to be seen more readily, but most adolescents would be unlikely to comply. Tucking socks into long pants and even taping them will prevent tick attachment, but this measure is likely to be more effective in conjunction with repellents.[58]

#### Repellents

Of the variety of topical repellents available commercially, DEET (N, N-diethyl-m-toluamide, or N-N-diethyl-3-methylbenzamide) is the most effective.[59] The more concentrated the preparation, the longer lasting the protection, with formulations of 10%–30% DEET adequate in most circumstances. Because a 30% formulation provides about 6 hours of protection, the use of even higher concentrations may be superfluous and has been phased out in Canada.

Concerns about potential toxicity from transcutaneous absorption of DEET has resulted in underutilization of this very effective modality.[60] Only a very small proportion of DEET is absorbed after topical application, and its metabolism and elimination are rapid. The use of combination DEET-sunscreen preparations is not recommended, as certain DEET-sunscreen combinations and topical retinoids can enhance the absorption of DEET. DEET decreases the effectiveness of sunscreen,[61-63] so sunscreen should be applied before DEET.

Permethrin is an insecticide, acaricide, and repellent that is not approved for use as a repellent because neurotoxic effects are reported with exposure to high doses. However, it is highly effective at killing ticks on contact when applied to clothing, shoes, and fomites. It is used on clothing by professional groups at high risk of tick exposure, such as military personnel, hunters, and forestry workers.

The role of garlic, other plant-based natural products, and the synthetic compound picaridin (KBR 3023) in repelling *Ixodes* ticks remains tentative.[63-66] Although several repellents are marketed under the Skin-So-Soft brand, preparations containing di-isopropyl adipate and benzophenone demonstrate poor effectiveness, even as an *Aedes aegypti* mosquito repellent, whereas IR3535 and picaridin are not yet proven as tick repellents.[67]

#### Tick Checks

Adolescents should perform tick checks under a bright light at the end of each day of exposure. The use of a washcloth may help dislodge recently attached ticks, and special attention should be paid to the armpit, groin, back, and scalp. In studies in the United States, early removal of an *Ixodes* tick minimized the risk of acquiring *B burgdorferi* infection from the bite.[68] There is a small risk that ticks on clothing can survive washing, so killing the ticks by subjecting them to heat in a dryer for an hour should be considered.[58]

## PREVENTING INFECTION AFTER A TICK BITE

In most cases, Lyme borreliosis can be readily diagnosed and easily treated. Still, the apprehension associated with a tick bite, and the confusion among physicians regarding the preferred course of action, warrants an evidence-based approach. This will allay anxiety, decrease the indiscriminate use of antibiotics, and prevent some cases of *B burgdorferi* infection.

### Tick Removal

Tick removal is achieved using an ordinary pair of thin-tipped tweezers or forceps by grasping the tick by its mouth-end, if discernible, and gently pulling straight up until detached. There is no evidence that embedded mouth parts that remain increase the risk of transmission or that crushing the tick enhances transmission.[69] Methods that use petroleum jelly, lidocaine, isopropyl alcohol, volatile substances such as nail polish and gasoline, lighted matches, or heated nails are ineffective, dangerous, and not recommended.[70]

### Tick Identification

An important component of education about tick bites is to remind patients not to discard the suspected tick, but to save it in any dry container. Even in an endemic area, almost a third of suspected deer ticks in one report were either other ticks or not a tick at all.[68] The non-ticks included beetles, lice and their nits, and artifacts that included scabs and eraser bits. For this reason, the practitioner should attempt to identify the tick. With a little practice, it should be possible in the office to distinguish an insect (6-legged) from a nymphal or adult tick (8-legged), differentiate a dog tick and a lone star tick from a deer tick, and identify a nymphal tick because of its small size. The availability of tick images on the Internet has made this simple office task much easier.[71] The only tools needed are a magnifying glass and a pair of tweezers to handle the tick. Alternatively, commercial laboratories perform tick identification, and in endemic counties in the United States it is usually done free of charge at health departments.

### Tick Analysis for Spirochete

The most common request from the patient is to have the tick sent for "testing for Lyme disease." Polymerase chain reaction testing for *B burgdorferi* DNA is offered in many commercial laboratories. This is unreliable and has no utility. A variable percentage of *Ixodes* ticks will harbor *B burgdorferi* in an endemic area, but a positive PCR does not correlate with transmission.

### Assessment of the Risk of Lyme Borreliosis from an Ixodes Tick Bite

The incidence of *B burgdorferi* infection following an *Ixodes* tick bite is low, even in endemic areas, in the range of 1.2% to 4.4% in US studies. However, inordinate anxiety on the part of patients, parents, and clinicians leads to many unnecessary prescriptions for antibiotics.[72] A decision to treat prophylactically needs to be

**Table 140-5**

**Clinical Scenarios of Tick-Borne Illness in Which Empiric Therapy Should Be Strongly Considered**

| *Clinical Scenario* | *Tick-Borne Diseases to Consider* |
|---|---|
| Fever with rash (maculopapular, petechial, or hemorrhagic), ± headache or neurologic findings | Rickettsial |
| | Ehrlichial (including *Anaplasma*) |
| | Tick-borne relapsing fever (TBRF) |
| Fever with eschar | Rickettsial |
| | Typhus |
| | Tularemia |
| Relapsing fever paroxysms | TBRF |
| Fever with leukopenia and thrombocytopenia | Ehrlichial (including *Anaplasma*) |
| Fever with anemia and thrombocytopenia | Babesiosis |
| Erythema migrans-like rash, especially if no pain or purulence | Lyme borreliosis |
| Ulcerative skin lesion with lymphadenopathy ± fever | Tularemia |
| Fever with unexplained sepsis syndrome or hypotension ± rash | Rickettsial |
| | Ehrlichial (including *Anaplasma*) |
| | Tularemia |

Content adapted from Goodman JL. Clinical approach to the patient with a possible tick-borne illness. In: Goodman JL, Dennis DT, Sonenshine DE, eds. *Tick-Borne Diseases of Humans*. Washington, DC: American Society for Microbiology; 2005:87–101.

balanced against the incidence of adverse effects from use of an antibiotic, which has been shown to be as high as 30% in an efficacy study.[73] The best decision can be made if all of the variables that influence the risk of infection are taken into consideration. The main factors are the developmental stage and duration of attachment of the tick. Most cases of human infection result from the nymphal stage.[73] This reinforces the importance of tick identification.

### Duration of Attachment

Duration of attachment is a key factor influencing infection risk, but it has been proven only for Lyme borreliosis. The history is generally unreliable as most patients are usually only able to report a broad window of time in which they could have been bitten, for example, a long weekend spent outdoors.

Because the spirochetes reside and replicate in the midgut of the tick, there is a delay between the onset of feeding and the appearance of spirochetes in the saliva. In a prospective study of tick bites conducted in the New York tri-state metropolitan area, which includes several hyperendemic foci of Lyme borreliosis, the incidence of human infection was 20% from ticks attached for 72 hours or more and 1.1% from ticks attached for fewer than 72 hours (odds ratio, 23.3).[68] This study demonstrated that tick identification and a measurement of engorgement could be used to identify a small, high-risk subset of persons who may benefit from antibiotic prophylaxis. This subset consisted of roughly 1 of every 8 persons for whom the tick's duration of attachment could be determined.

### Antibiotic Prophylaxis after an Ixodes Tick Bite

In a placebo-controlled antibiotic prophylaxis study conducted in the hyperendemic county of Westchester, New York, persons 12 years of age and older were enrolled if an *I scapularis* tick was brought in within 72 hours of the tick bite.[73] In this study as well, a duration of attachment of 72 hours, as measured objectively by

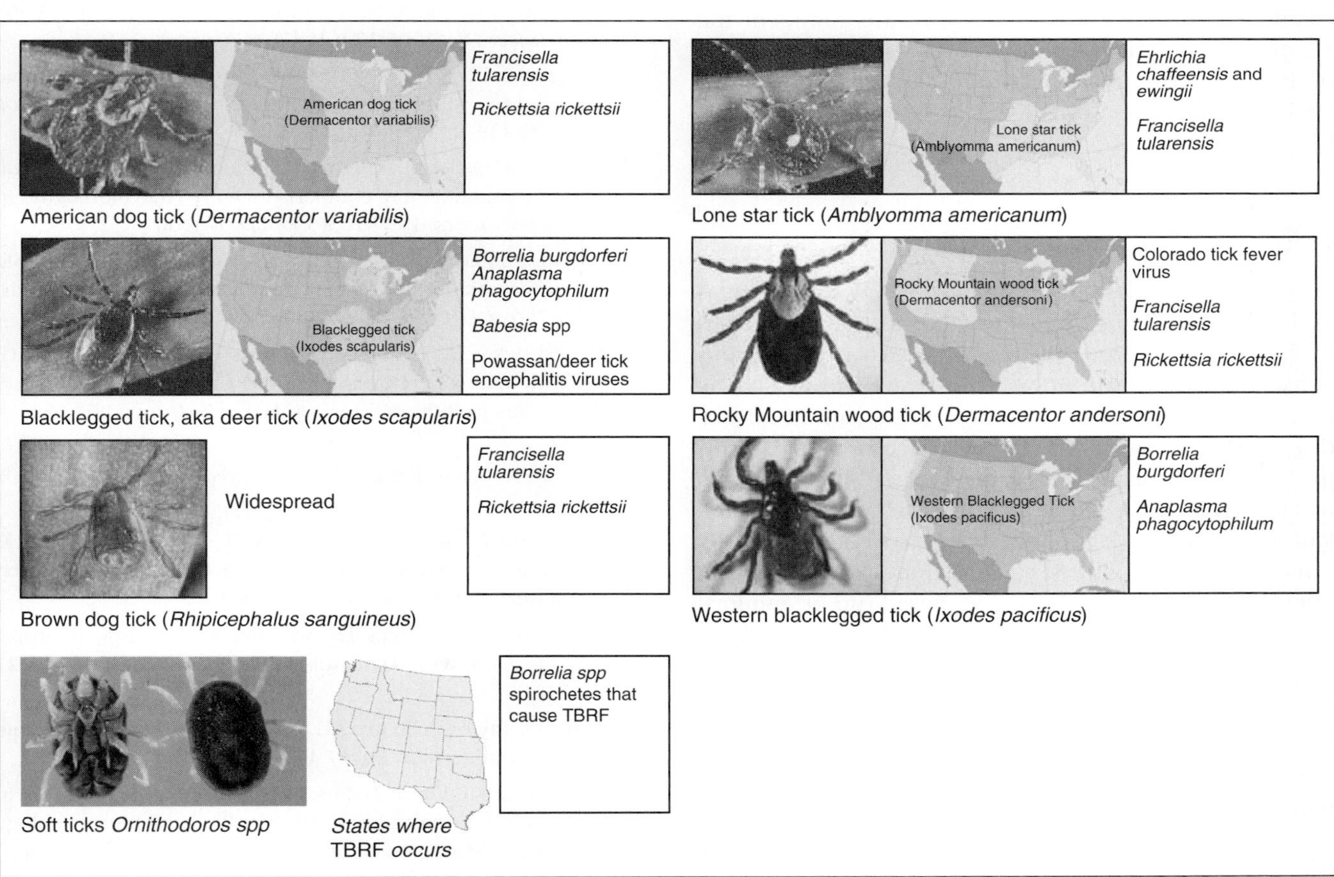


FIGURE 140-4 Common ticks that transmit infections to humans in the United States: Identification, geographic distribution, and infections transmitted. (CDC. Ticks: geographical distribution. Available at www.cdc.gov/ticks/geographic_distribution.html Accessed August 3, 2010; Goodman JL, Dennis DT, Sonenshine DE, eds. *Tick-Borne Diseases of Humans*. Washington DC: ASM Press; 2005).

the scutal index method, was found to be the cutoff for a significant increase in risk of acquiring *B burgdorferi* infection (and developing EM). A single 200-mg dose of doxycycline was 87% effective in prevention of Lyme borreliosis, but adverse effects occurred in 30% of doxycycline recipients. Identification of persons at higher risk of acquiring infection is possible with the help of stage identification (nymph) and assessment of duration of attachment (>72 hours in North American studies). In all other cases a "wait and watch" approach is completely acceptable given the low risk of Lyme borreliosis following a tick bite, and this is the approach favored in Europe.[74] The value of acute-and-convalescent paired serum testing for antibodies to *B burgdorferi* in this setting has not been demonstrated. Therefore, the use of serologic testing to aid in management decisions after a tick bite, still commonly considered by physicians in the United States, is not recommended. Adolescent patients who are treated with antibiotics need to be cautioned to screen themselves from sun exposure because tetracyclines can induce photosensitivity reactions. They should also not lie down before they are confident the doxycycline capsule has entered the stomach because of the propensity to cause esophageal ulceration. A practical tip is to "chase down" the capsule with adequate food or water.

## CONCLUSIONS

Tick-borne infections are common. Their incidence is underreported because acute constitutional illnesses may go unrecognized, but they can also cause serious consequences; a proportion of many of the tick-borne illnesses can progress to become fulminant. Moreover, the geographic range of many tick species is expanding, probably secondary to climate changes such as rising mean night time temperatures in previously uninfected latitudes. Specific laboratory tests are not sufficiently sensitive in early illness, so initiation of empiric antimicrobial treatment should be based upon minimal presumptive criteria[35] (Table 140-5). A pictorial reference for the common tick vectors in North America, along with their geographic distribution, is presented in Figure 140-4.

## REFERENCES

1. Brown RN, Lane RS, Dennis DT. Geographic distributions of tick-borne diseases and their vectors. In: Goodman JL, Dennis DT, Sonenshine DE, eds. *Tick-Borne Diseases of Humans.* Washington, DC: American Society for Microbiology; 2005:363-392

2. Lyme disease—United States, 2003-2005. *MMWR Morb Mortal Wkly Rep.* 2007;56(23):573-576

3. Sood SK. What we have learned about Lyme borreliosis from studies in children. *Wien Klin Wochenschr.* 2006;118(21-22):638-642

4. Gerber MA, Shapiro ED, Burke GS, Parcells VJ, Bell GL. Lyme disease in children in southeastern Connecticut. Pediatric Lyme Disease Study Group. *N Engl J Med.* 1996;335(17):1270-1274

5. Arnez M, Pleterski-Rigler D, Ahcan J, Ruzic-Sabljic E, Strle F. Demographic features, clinical characteristics and laboratory findings in children with multiple erythema migrans in Slovenia. *Wien Klin Wochenschr.* 2001;113(3-4):98-101

6. Berglund J, Eitrem R, Norrby SR. Long-term study of Lyme borreliosis in a highly endemic area in Sweden. *Scand J Infect Dis.* 1996;28(5):473-478

7. Nadelman RB, Nowakowski J, Forseter G, et al. The clinical spectrum of early Lyme borreliosis in patients with culture-confirmed erythema migrans. *Am J Med.* 1996;100(5):502-508

8. Kirkland KB, Klimko TB, Meriwether RA, et al. Erythema migrans-like rash illness at a camp in North Carolina: a new tick-borne disease? *Arch Intern Med.* 1997;157(22):2635-2641

9. Campbell GL, Paul WS, Schriefer ME, Craven RB, Robbins KE, Dennis DT. Epidemiologic and diagnostic studies of patients with suspected early Lyme disease, Missouri, 1990-1993. *J Infect Dis.* 1995;172(2):470-480

10. Kan L, Sood SK, Maytal J. Pseudotumor cerebri in Lyme disease: a case report and literature review. *Pediatr Neurol.* 1998;18(5):439-441

11. Eppes SC, Nelson DK, Lewis LL, Klein JD. Characterization of Lyme meningitis and comparison with viral meningitis in children. *Pediatrics.* 1999;103(5 Pt 1):957-960

12. Shah SS, Zaoutis TE, Turnquist J, Hodinka RL, Coffin SE. Early differentiation of Lyme from enteroviral meningitis. *Pediatr Infect Dis J.* 2005;24(6):542-545

13. Tuerlinckx D, Bodart E, Garrino MG, de Bilderling G. Clinical data and cerebrospinal fluid findings in Lyme meningitis versus aseptic meningitis. *Eur J Pediatr.* 2003;162(3):150-153

14. Sood SK. Lyme disease. *Pediatr Infect Dis J.* 1999;18(10):913-925

15. Berglund J, Stjernberg L, Ornstein K, Tykesson-Joelsson K, Walter H. 5-year follow-up study of patients with neuroborreliosis. *Scand J Infect Dis.* 2002;34(6):421-425

16. Rothermel H, Hedges TR 3rd, Steere AC. Optic neuropathy in children with Lyme disease. *Pediatrics.* 2001;108(2):477-481

17. Szer IS, Taylor E, Steere AC. The long-term course of Lyme arthritis in children. *N Engl J Med.* 1991;325(3):159-163

18. Huppertz HI, Karch H, Suschke HJ, et al. Lyme arthritis in European children and adolescents. The Pediatric Rheumatology Collaborative Group. *Arthritis Rheum.* 1995;38(3):361-368

19. Steere AC, Sikand VK, Schoen RT, Nowakowski J. Asymptomatic infection with Borrelia burgdorferi. *Clin Infect Dis.* 2003 15;37(4):528-532

20. Feder HM Jr, Gerber MA, Krause PJ, Ryan R, Shapiro ED. Early Lyme disease: a flu-like illness without erythema migrans. *Pediatrics.* 1993;91(2):456-459

21. Aguero-Rosenfeld ME, Nowakowski J, McKenna DF, Carbonaro CA, Wormser GP. Serodiagnosis in early Lyme disease. *J Clin Microbiol.* 1993;31(12):3090–3095

22. Feder HM Jr, Johnson BJ, O'Connell S, et al. A critical appraisal of "chronic Lyme disease." *N Engl J Med.* 2007; 357(14):1422–1430

23. Aguero-Rosenfeld ME, Wang G, Schwartz I, Wormser GP. Diagnosis of lyme borreliosis. *Clin Microbiol Rev.* 2005;18(3):484–509

24. Hilton E, Tramontano A, DeVoti J, Sood SK. Temporal study of immunoglobin M seroreactivity to Borrelia burgdorferi in patients treated for Lyme borreliosis. *J Clin Microbiol.* 1997;35(3):774–776

25. Gerber MA, Zemel LS, Shapiro ED. Lyme arthritis in children: clinical epidemiology and long-term outcomes. *Pediatrics.* 1998;102(4 Pt 1):905–908

26. Bentas W, Karch H, Huppertz HI. Lyme arthritis in children and adolescents: outcome 12 months after initiation of antibiotic therapy. *J Rheumatol.* 2000;27(8):2025–2030

27. Sood SK, Ilowite NT. Lyme arthritis in children: is chronic arthritis a common complication? *J Rheumatol.* 2000;27(8):1836–1838

28. Adams WV, Rose CD, Eppes SC, Klein JD. Cognitive effects of Lyme disease in children: a 4-year follow-up study. *J Rheumatol.* 1999;26(5):1190–1194

29. Steere AC. Lyme borreliosis in 2005, 30 years after initial observations in Lyme, Connecticut. *Wien Klin Wochenschr.* 2006;118(21–22):625–633

30. Chen LF, Sexton DJ. What's new in Rocky Mountain spotted fever? *Infect Dis Clin North Am.* 2008;22(3): 415–432,vii–viii

31. Ricketts H. The study of "Rocky Mountain spotted fever" (tick fever?) by means of animal inoculations. A preliminary communication. *JAMA.* 1906;47:33–36

32. Helmick CG, Bernard KW, D'Angelo LJ. Rocky Mountain spotted fever: clinical, laboratory, and epidemiological features of 262 cases. *J Infect Dis.* 1984;150(4):480–488

33. Buckingham SC, Marshall GS, Schutze GE, et al. Clinical and laboratory features, hospital course, and outcome of Rocky Mountain spotted fever in children. *J Pediatr.* 2007; 150(2):180–184

34. Dantas-Torres F. Rocky Mountain spotted fever. *Lancet Infect Dis.* 2007;7(11):724–732

35. Goodman JL, Dennis DT, Sonenshine DE. *Tick-Borne Diseases of Humans.* Washington, DC: American Society for Microbiology; 2005

36. Dumler JS, Choi KS, Garcia-Garcia JC, et al. Human granulocytic anaplasmosis and Anaplasma phagocytophilum. *Emerg Infect Dis.* 2005;11(12):1828–1834

37. Dumler JS, Madigan JE, Pusterla N, Bakken JS. Ehrlichioses in humans: epidemiology, clinical presentation, diagnosis, and treatment. *Clin Infect Dis.* 2007;45(suppl 1):S45–S51

38. Bakken JS, Dumler JS. Human granulocytic ehrlichiosis. *Clin Infect Dis.* 2000;31(2):554–560

39. Bakken JS, Dumler S. Human granulocytic anaplasmosis. *Infect Dis Clin North Am.* 2008;22(3):433–448,viii

40. Thomas RJ, Dumler JS, Carlyon JA. Current management of human granulocytic anaplasmosis, human monocytic ehrlichiosis, and Ehrlichia ewingii ehrlichiosis. *Expert Rev Anti Infect Ther.* 2009;7(6):709–722

41. CDC. Reported cases of tick-borne relapsing fever by county, United States, 1990–2002; 2008

42. Dworkin MS, Anderson DE Jr, Schwan TG, et al. Tick-borne relapsing fever in the northwestern United States and southwestern Canada. *Clin Infect Dis.* 1998;26(1):122–131

43. Dworkin MS, Schwan TG, Anderson DE Jr, Borchardt SM. Tick-borne relapsing fever. *Infect Dis Clin North Am.* 2008;22(3):449–468, viii

44. Hasin T, Davidovitch N, Cohen R, et al. Postexposure treatment with doxycycline for the prevention of tick-borne relapsing fever. *N Engl J Med.* 2006;355(2):148–155

45. Perkins ME. Rhoptry organelles of apicomplexan parasites. *Parasitol Today.* 1992;8(1):28–32

46. Krause PJ, Telford SR 3rd, Spielman A, et al. Concurrent Lyme disease and babesiosis. Evidence for increased severity and duration of illness. *JAMA.* 1996;275(21):1657–1660

47. Esernio-Jenssen D, Scimeca PG, Benach JL, Tenenbaum MJ. Transplacental/perinatal babesiosis. *J Pediatr.* 1987; 110(4):570–572

48. Leiby DA. Babesiosis and blood transfusion: flying under the radar. *Vox Sang.* 2006;90(3):157–165

49. Meldrum SC, Birkhead GS, White DJ, Benach JL, Morse DL. Human babesiosis in New York State: an epidemiological description of 136 cases. *Clin Infect Dis.* 1992;15(6):1019–1023

50. Staples JE, Kubota KA, Chalcraft LG, Mead PS, Petersen JM. Epidemiologic and molecular analysis of human tularemia, United States, 1964–2004. *Emerg Infect Dis.* 2006;12(7):1113–1118

51. Goethert HK, Telford SR, 3rd. Nonrandom distribution of vector ticks (Dermacentor variabilis) infected by *Francisella tularensis*. *PLoS Pathog.* 2009;5(2):e1000319

52. Petersen JM, Mead PS, Schriefer ME. *Francisella tularensis*: an arthropod-borne pathogen. *Vet Res.* 2009;40(2):7

53. Nigrovic LE, Wingerter SL. Tularemia. *Infect Dis Clin North Am.* 2008;22(3):489–504, ix

54. Kugeler KJ, Mead PS, Janusz AM, et al. Molecular epidemiology of *Francisella tularensis* in the United States. *Clin Infect Dis.* 2009;48(7):863–870

55. Romero JR, Simonsen KA. Powassan encephalitis and Colorado tick fever. *Infect Dis Clin North Am.* 2008; 22(3):545–559, x

56. Deibel R, Srihongse S, Woodall JP. Arboviruses in New York State: an attempt to determine the role of arboviruses in patients with viral encephalitis and meningitis. *Am J Trop Med Hyg.* 1979;28(3):577–582

57. Hayes EB, Piesman J. How can we prevent Lyme disease? *N Engl J Med.* 2003;348(24):2424–2430

58. Stafford KC, 3rd. Tick management handbook. In: Station TCAE, ed. *The Connecticut Agricultural Experiment Station New Haven: The Connecticut Agricultural Experiment Station;* 2007:1-80

59. Fradin MS, Day JF. Comparative efficacy of insect repellents against mosquito bites. *N Engl J Med.* 2002;347(1):13-18

60. Goodyer L, Behrens RH. Short report: the safety and toxicity of insect repellents. *Am J Trop Med Hyg.* 1998;59(2): 323-324

61. Ross EA, Savage KA, Utley LJ, Tebbett IR. Insect repellent interactions: sunscreens enhance DEET (N,N-diethyl-m-toluamide) absorption. *Drug Metab Dispos.* 2004;32(8): 783-785

62. Montemarano AD, Gupta RK, Burge JR, Klein K. Insect repellents and the efficacy of sunscreens. *Lancet.* 1997;349(9066):1670-1671

63. Katz TM, Miller JH, Hebert AA. Insect repellents: historical perspectives and new developments. *J Am Acad Dermatol.* 2008;58(5):865-871

64. Pretorius AM, Jensenius M, Clarke F, Ringertz SH. Repellent efficacy of DEET and KBR 3023 against Amblyomma hebraeum (Acari: Ixodidae). *J Med Entomol.* 2003;40(2): 245-248

65. Jaenson TG, Palsson K, Borg-Karlson AK. Evaluation of extracts and oils of tick-repellent plants from Sweden. *Med Vet Entomol.* 2005;19(4):345-352

66. Carroll JF, Klun JA, Debboun M. Repellency of DEET and SS220 applied to skin involves olfactory sensing by 2 species of ticks. *Med Vet Entomol.* 2005;19(1):101-106

67. Chou JT, Rossignol PA, Ayres JW. Evaluation of commercial insect repellents on human skin against Aedes aegypti (Diptera: Culicidae). *J Med Entomol.* 1997;34(6):624-630

68. Sood SK, Salzman MB, Johnson BJ, et al. Duration of tick attachment as a predictor of the risk of Lyme disease in an area in which Lyme disease is endemic. *J Infect Dis.* 1997;175(4):996-999

69. Piesman J, Dolan MC. Protection against lyme disease spirochete transmission provided by prompt removal of nymphal Ixodes scapularis (Acari: Ixodidae). *J Med Entomol.* 2002;39(3):509-512

70. Needham GR. Evaluation of 5 popular methods for tick removal. *Pediatrics.* 1985;75(6):997-1002

71. Sood SK. Effective retrieval of Lyme disease information on the Web. *Clin Infect Dis.* 2002;35(4):451-464

72. Murray T, Feder HM Jr. Management of tick bites and early Lyme disease: a survey of Connecticut physicians. *Pediatrics.* 2001;108(6):1367-1370

73. Nadelman RB, Nowakowski J, Fish D, et al. Prophylaxis with single-dose doxycycline for the prevention of Lyme disease after an Ixodes scapularis tick bite. *N Engl J Med.* 2001;345(2):79-84

74. Stanek G, Kahl O. Chemoprophylaxis for Lyme borreliosis? *Zentralbl Bakteriol.* 1999;289(5-7):655-665

# CHAPTER 141

# Mycobacterial

MARGUERITE M. MAYERS, MD

Tuberculosis (TB) has been a significant cause of morbidity and mortality since the days of Hippocrates. Over the centuries, although amplified in populations by crowding, malnutrition, and concurrent disease, it has not respected wealth or position. The World Health Organization (WHO) estimates that 2 billion people are infected worldwide, most with latent disease, and in 2007 there were 9.4 million new cases and 1.32 million deaths.[1] The burden of disease in the United States is less. It is estimated between 9.6 million and 14.9 million persons have latent disease.[2] Active TB is at an all-time low in the United States, with 13,299 cases (4.4 cases/100,000 persons) reported in adults in 2007.[3] The prevalence of active TB in adolescents is difficult to determine nationally except in high-incidence areas where the number of cases encourages more exact statistics. In 2007, New York City reported a 22% increase (from 37 to 45) in the number of TB cases in children between the ages of 10 and 19 years compared with the preceding year.

## ETIOLOGY

Mycobacterium is a genus of aerobic, nonmotile bacteria designated *acid-fast bacilli* (AFB) because of their ability to absorb Ziehl-Neelsen (carbolfuchsin) stain when heated and to then resist decolorization by acid alcohol. In this genus, *M tuberculosis* is the most common cause of TB in the United States and worldwide. *M bovis*, an organism able to cause disease in both man and cattle, continues to be seen in parts of the world where bovine TB has not been eradicated and unpasteurized milk is the norm. Atypical mycobacteria, *M scrofulaceum*, *M kansasii, M marinum, M fortuitum*, *M abscessus*, and *M chelonei*, are also pathogenic but usually cause a mild or self-limited infection of lymph nodes or skin. *M avium-intracellulare* complex is a significant pathogen for individuals deficient in cell-mediated immunity (CMI), such as those infected with human immunodeficiency virus (HIV).

## PATHOPHYSIOLOGY

Tuberculosis is usually acquired through the respiratory tract, although gastrointestinal and cutaneous acquisition has been reported. *M tuberculosis* is an airborne pathogen found in air-droplet nuclei that when inhaled initiates infection in lung alveoli, usually in the lower lobes. Alveolar macrophages phagocytize the bacilli, killing some and releasing the still viable remainder as the macrophages die. These bacilli and cell products then attract circulating macrophages that ingest the bacilli and carry them to the regional lymph nodes. They enter the systemic circulation and are spread throughout the body. The most vascular organs receive the greatest number of organisms, with the lungs, liver, bone marrow, spleen, kidneys, adrenals, central nervous system (CNS), bones, and joints all affected. This bacillemia occurs silently and unchecked in all individuals in the first few weeks of their infection. At this time, clusters of epithelioid cells called tubercles are formed. They consist of viable organisms surrounded by the host's cellular response, forming a granuloma. Within 6 to 8 weeks, CMI is stimulated, and the macrophages are activated to kill instead of containing the ingested bacilli. Central caseating necrosis is produced. This host immune response halts the progression of disease, eliminates most of the bacilli, and contains the remainder in a latent condition.

## CLINICAL PRESENTATION OF ACTIVE DISEASE

In 90% of all infected individuals, the acquisition and containment of the mycobacteria is entirely asymptomatic, although there exists a lifetime risk of reactivation. In the other 10%, a symptomatic illness develops. Adolescents are particularly susceptible to clinical illness or significant reactivation disease both because of their relatively recent acquisition of infection and the metabolic stress associated with their recent accelerated growth. Clinical manifestations are usually nonspecific, consisting of fever, malaise, anorexia, weight loss or poor weight gain, and/or night sweats. Headache, abdominal pain, and chronic fatigue have been seen, and occasionally symptoms are directly referable to the affected organ. Pulmonary disease is the most common form of symptomatic TB and can present with a chronic nonproductive cough. When progressive primary TB occurs, a pleural effusion develops causing pleuritic chest pain and respiratory distress. Adolescents with reactivation upper lobe disease or a cavity formation have adult-type pulmonary TB, with a productive cough or hemoptysis. Those with miliary or disseminated pulmonary TB have only nonspecific signs and symptoms, which get progressively worse. Extrapulmonary TB, either primary or reactivation, is less common. Tuberculous meningitis presents insidiously. Initially there is fever, headache, and vomiting, followed by signs of increased intracranial pressure, focal neurologic signs, seizures, coma, and finally death over 1 to 3 weeks. Tuberculomas of the CNS present as space-occupying lesions, with increased intracranial pressure and/or focal neurologic signs. Tuberculous lymphadenitis is most commonly seen in the cervical and axillary nodes. Other sites of TB are bone, the peritoneum, the kidney, the adrenal or the genital-urinary system. In these instances, pain, swelling, or organ dysfunction indicates the site of the infection.

## DIAGNOSIS OF ACTIVE DISEASE

All patients with suspected active TB should be hospitalized to obtain an organism for culture and sensitivity before the initiation of therapy or concurrent with the start of empiric therapy in life-threatening situations. The evaluation should include the following steps.

### MICROBIOLOGY

Body fluid and tissue specimens should be smeared and examined by Ziehl-Neelsen or auramine O stain and blue-light fluoroscopy for the presence of AFB. Nucleic acid amplification has been used on positive specimens to identify the presence of *M tuberculosis*.[2] This result has immediate implications for infection control and supports the initiation of therapy. Traditional solid culture methods take weeks to months for definitive results. Modern automated methods use liquid culture media with a carbon-labeled substrate specific for mycobacteria and can yield positive cultures in 2 weeks and sensitivities in 3 weeks. Early growth detected in this media can be rapidly identified by DNA probe. Sputum for smear and culture can be obtained by expectoration or saline induction. Morning gastric aspirate specimens of at least 50 mL can only be obtained from the cooperative patient. Bronchoscopy can yield results from either the lavage fluid or from postbronchoscopic bronchorrhea. A large volume first morning urine specimen can be sent from the patient with sterile pyuria. Blood cultures can be positive when TB is disseminated. Cerebral spinal fluid (CSF) in patients with meningitis will show a lymphocytic pleocytosis with a low glucose and an elevated protein. Cerebrospinal fluid should be centrifuged and the pellicle stained and examined for AFB. Smear and culture are positive only when organisms are present in the CSF. A parameningeal tuberculoma, which has not ruptured into the cerebral spinal space, can cause a CSF pleocytosis yet have negative smears and cultures.

### PATHOLOGY

Lymph node, liver, and bone marrow biopsies, and surgical specimens from any involved site are diagnostic when caseating granulomas are found.

### IMAGING

The chest x-ray (CXR) in primary TB can have a variety of abnormalities: an infiltrate alone, a Ghon complex (an infiltrate and hilar adenopathy), an infiltrate and pleural effusion (a progressive primary), or a diffuse miliary (or snow storm-like) pattern. In pulmonary reactivation disease, apical abnormalities or a cavity are seen. Old healed TB is manifested by fibrotic scars or calcifications. The CXR is negative in most patients with extrapulmonary disease even though the pathophysiology of acquisition supports an initial respiratory infection. A chest computed tomography scan (CT) can reveal adenopathy or cavity formation that is not seen on routine films. X-rays of bones and joints can show destruction. In the spine, the destruction of 2 adjacent vertebral bodies with anterior collapse and loss of the intervening disc space correlates with a prominent posterior kyphosis or gibbous deformity on physical exam. The head CT in patients with meningitis shows hydrocephalus and basilar enhancement. The magnetic resonance imaging (MRI) in patients with tuberculomas shows rim enhancement and perhaps calcifications.

### GENETIC FINGERPRINTING

In clinical settings with a strong research component, organisms are now being evaluated by restriction fragment length polymorphism (RFLP) to identify the infecting species. This molecular genotype or fingerprint can then be used to determine the geographic clustering of strains to delineate the epidemiology of transmission and to differentiate reinfection from reactivation disease.[5]

### TUBERCULIN SKIN TESTS

The Mantoux test has been used to identify individuals with both active and latent TB infection. It measures in vivo the delayed-type hypersensitivity (DTH) response of the host. Reproducible results, with high sensitivity and specificity, are obtained when 0.1 mL of 5 tuberculin units of purified protein derivative (PPD) is injected intradermally on the volar forearm, forming a visible wheal of 6 to 10 mm at the site of the injection. This area is then inspected at 48 to 72 hours and induration, not erythema, is measured transversely to the long axis of the forearm. Trained personnel should administer and read the test as there are significant personal and public health implications of a positive test.[6] Table 141-1 defines positive results for this PPD test.[6] If it is suspected that an adolescent is so recently infected that CMI has not yet developed, that individual should be retested in 8 to 10 weeks.[7] If it is suspected that immunity may have waned over time, a second PPD should be placed 1 to 2 weeks after the first and its result considered the true baseline against which all subsequent tests are compared. This *2-step testing* boosts the immune system, triggering an amnestic response and recalling the cell-mediated response to PPD that may have diminished with time. Repeated tuberculin skin test (TST) testing in the noninfected individual does not sensitize a person to PPD and will not cause a positive response in an uninfected individual. Repeated testing, however, in those infected with nontuberculous mycobacteria or those vaccinated with bacillus Calmette-Guerin (BCG) can boost the response to PPD. Boosting appears to be a nonspecific response to any prior mycobacterial exposure.[8]

## IMMUNODIAGNOSTIC TESTS

Several immunodiagnostic tests, interferon gamma release assays (IGRA), which measure in vitro interferon

**Table 141-1**

**Positive TST Reaction Supporting the Diagnosis of TB**

| *Induration* | *Clinical History* |
|---|---|
| ≥5 mm | • Persons who have had recent contact with an active TB case<br>• Persons whose chest x-ray shows findings of active or old TB<br>• Persons infected with HIV<br>• Persons immunosuppressed due to disease or medication |
| ≥10 mm | • Persons born in high TB prevalence areas, especially those who have emigrated within the past 5 years<br>• Persons who travel to high TB prevalence areas or who have frequent visitors from those areas<br>• Persons who themselves or their frequent contacts are homeless, incarcerated, reside in an institution or shelter, are migrant workers, or are drug users<br>• Persons who have certain chronic illnesses: uncontrolled type 1 diabetes, renal failure, gastrectomy or jejuno-ileal bypass, or lymphoma<br>• Persons with malnutrition |
| ≥15 mm | All others without risk factors |

Stratification of induration creates cutoffs based on the sensitivity and specificity of the TST and the prevalence of TB in the population being tested. Therefore, a positive test is not 1 absolute size but varies with the likelihood that an individual has both been exposed to *M tuberculosis* and has become infected. A positive test does not differentiate between those with active or latent infection and its size does not predict who will develop active disease. A positive response can also be seen in those infected with atypical mycobacteria and in some individuals vaccinated with a Bacille Calmette-Guèrin vaccine (BCG). The current public health recommendation is to evaluate the response to PPD as if BCG had not been given. A negative response does not always indicate the absence of infection, as those with recent infection may not yet have had time to develop CMI. False-negative tests are seen in those with overwhelming disease, immunosuppression, infection in the distant past, and concurrent viral infections such as measles, varicella, and influenza. These individuals are said to manifest anergy, that is, a lack of DTH response in 1 truly infected. A variety of technical problems may also cause false-negative results.

Modified from American Academy of Pediatrics. Tuberculosis. In: Pickering LK, Baker CJ, Kimberlin DW, Long SS, eds. *Red Book: 2009 Report of the Committee on Infectious Diseases*, 28th ed. Elk Grove Village, IL: American Academy of Pediatrics; 680–701.

released by T cells sensitized by *M tuberculosis*, are available. These tests offer a new 1-visit approach to assess both active and latent TB infection, and their results are not confounded by either infection with atypical mycobacteria or BCG vaccination. The ELISPOT is licensed in Europe. The T-spot, the Quantiferon TB Gold (QFT), and the Gold In Tube, all enzyme-linked immunosorbent assays (ELISA) are approved by the FDA for individuals age 17 years and older to be used in all circumstances in place of a Mantoux test.[9] Experts suggest that IGRAs can be used in place of a TST to evaluate an immunocompetent child >5 years. A positive test should be indicative of TB, but a negative or indeterminant test cannot necessarily be interpreted as the absence of infection.[6]

## DIFFERENTIAL DIAGNOSIS OF ACTIVE DISEASE

Signs and symptoms of active TB are similar to diseases caused by bacterial, viral, and fungal infections, autoimmune disease, sarcoid, and cancers. The diagnosis of TB is supported by the history of exposure and risk factors, TST or immunodiagnostic tests, imaging studies, tissue examination, and culture results. It is important to remember that TB can be found concurrently with any condition that causes immunosuppression.

## ISOLATION AND INFECTION CONTROL

Adolescents with primary pulmonary TB without a productive cough are rarely contagious and need not be isolated in the hospital or at home. Those with positive sputum, a productive cough, or a cavity must be isolated for airborne infectivity, preferably in a negative pressure room until effective therapy has been started, 3 sputum smears are AFB-negative, and the patient's cough is diminished. This process can take 2 to 4 weeks. When the adolescent is no longer contagious, a rapid return to school and normal activities is encouraged.[2] Extrapulmonary TB, whether it is found in the lymph node, the bone, or the CNS, does not require isolation unless there is drainage from the infected site. A draining site should be covered, gloves should be used for dressing changes, and all dressings disposed of as potentially infectious. Urine from patients with renal or genital-urinary TB should also be considered infectious. Adult contacts should be evaluated for active disease before being allowed to visit in the hospital because they can unknowingly be a source of infection for other patients and staff.

## TREATMENT OF ACTIVE DISEASE

All cases of suspected active TB should be hospitalized to obtain an organism for culture and sensitivity; to initiate a contact investigation in conjunction with the local department of health (DOH); to assess the degree of infectivity of the index case; to start therapy in a controlled environment assessing tolerability and adverse events; to evaluate behavioral/social conditions that might affect the treatment plan; and to enroll the patient in a supervised therapy program, directly observed therapy (DOT). Current chemotherapy is based on the biology of the organism in vivo, its drug susceptibility in the context of drug resistance and tissue penetration, and the immunity of the host. A long duration of treatment is required because the bacilli are killed by most agents only when they are actively growing. Combination therapy is required to minimize the emergence of drug-resistant organisms. Individuals with *immune dysfunction* due to HIV, malnutrition, chronic illness, or receiving immune-modulating agents may have particular difficulty in being treated for TB. Their immune dysfunction and the resistance pattern of their infecting organism can restrict their options for therapy. Additionally, drug interaction is of concern in those individuals requiring simultaneous administration of both anti-TB therapy (TB-Rx) and antiretroviral therapy (ART). Table 141-2 lists the first line drugs, their dosages, and side effects. Box 141-1 further describes the available medication. Table 141-3 displays the guidelines of the American Thoracic Society (ATS) for empiric treatment of active TB.[10]

ATS recommends that 4 drugs be started initially to sterilize the tuberculous lesion as rapidly as possible. For *pulmonary* TB, including *hilar adenopathy*, intensive, short course, supervised therapy encompassing 6 months of treatment is the standard of care. For *miliary or disseminated* TB, *meningitis*, or *bone or joint* TB, more prolonged supervised therapy is generally recommended. These presentations of TB may be life threatening or have a greater burden of disease than that seen in pulmonary infection and thus require a longer treatment. In addition, for CNS TB it is essential that the chemotherapeutic agents used cross the blood–brain barrier and reach therapeutic concentrations in the CSF. *M bovis* infections need to be treated for 9 to 12 months due to innate pyrazinamide (PZA)resistance.[6] For those individuals with HIV, the number of drugs and the duration of therapy are based on the infecting organism, the site of the infection, and the response to therapy, not their immune status. Rifabutin should be used instead of rifampin (RIF) if protease inhibitors are also being administered. However, if the patient does not require ART, RIF can be used. When multi-drug resistant

**Table 141-2**

**Commonly Used Drugs for the Treatment of Tuberculosis**

| | *Dosage* | | | |
|---|---|---|---|---|
| | *Daily* | *2x/Week* | *Route* | *Major Side Effects* |
| **Bactericidal Drugs** | | | | |
| Isoniazid (INH) | 10–15 mg/kg (300 mg max) | 20–30 mg/kg (900 mg max) | Oral/IM/IV | • Hepatitis<br>• Peripheral neuropathy<br>• Hypersensitivity |
| Rifampin (RIF) | 10–20 mg/kg (600 mg max) | 10–20 mg/kg (600 mg max) | Oral/IV | • Hepatitis<br>• Thrombocytopenia<br>• Flu-like reaction |
| Rifabutin | 5 mg/kg (300 mg max) | 5 mg/kg (300 mg max) | Oral | • Leucopenia<br>• Rash, hepatitis<br>• Arthralgia, uveitis |
| Pyrazinamide (PZA) | 20–40 mg/kg (2 g max) | 50 mg/kg (4 g max) | Oral | • Hepatitis<br>• Rash, arthralgia<br>• Increased uric acid |
| Streptomycin (SM) | 20–40 mg/kg (1 g max) | N/A | IM/IV | • Ototoxicity<br>• Nephrotoxicity<br>• Rash |
| **Bacteriostatic Drugs** | | | | |
| Ethambutol (EMB) | 15–25 mg/kg (2.5 g max) | 50 mg/kg | Oral | • Optic neuritis<br>• Decreased color vision<br>• Decreased visual acuity |
| Ethionamide (ETH) | 15–20 mg/kg (1 g max) | N/A | Oral | • Hepatitis<br>• Hypersensitivity<br>• GI intolerance |
| Para-aminosalicylic acid (PAS) | 200 mg/kg tid (12 g max) | N/A | Oral | • Hepatitis<br>• GI intolerance |

Bactericidal drugs kill without the help of the host immune system. Bacteriostatic drugs assist the intact host immune system to eradicate the organisms. Second line drugs include the oral agents levofloxacin and cycloserine; and the parenteral agents capreomycin, kanamycin, and amikacin.

IM, intramuscular; IV, intravenous; tid, 3 times a day

tuberculosis (MDR-TB) is suspected, the initial regimen should include 5 drugs of which at least 3 should be active for suppression of resistance. This number can be reduced or modified once sensitivities are known. The available agents are usually second line drugs, with less efficacy and/or greater side effects, and they must be given up to 24 months. Recent reports have defined a new highly resistant strain of TB termed extremely drug-resistant TB (XDR-TB), found to be resistant to the first line isoniazid (INH) and RIF, and also certain second line agents, 1 of the fluoroquinolones and 1 of the 3 parenteral medications: capreomycin, kanamycin, or amikacin. This strain has been identified in a small number of African patients with acquired immunodeficiency syndrome and has had a high mortality because its drug resistance makes eradication almost impossible.[11]

## ADJUVANT THERAPY

In addition to chemotherapeutic agents, surgery and corticosteroids also have a place in the treatment of TB. Biopsy has been used to obtain a specimen from extrapulmonary sites. Incision and drainage has been used to relieve

**Table 141-3**

**Empiric Therapy for Presumed Susceptible Tuberculosis[10]**

| *Clinical* | *Initial Phase* | *Continuation Phase* |
|---|---|---|
| Pulmonary<br>Extrapulmonary | INH, RIF, PZA, EMB daily or 5 days/week DOT for 2 months (#doses 56–40) | INH, RIF daily or 5 days/week DOT for 4 months (#doses 126–190) or 2x a week (#doses 36) |
| Bone and joint | INH, RIF, PZA, EMB daily or 5 days/week DOT for 2 months (#doses 56–40) | INH, RIF daily or 5 days/week DOT for 7 months (#doses 217–155) or 2x a week (#doses 62) |
| Meningitis | INH, RIF, PZA, SM, or ETH daily DOT for 2 months (#doses 56) | INH, RIF daily or 5 days/week DOT for 10 months (#doses 308–220) or 2x a week (#doses 88) |
| HIV coinfection with protease inhibitors as part of ART | INH, rifabutin, PZA, EMB daily or 5x/week DOT for 2 months (#doses 56–40) | INH, rifabutin daily or 5 days/week DOT for 4, 7, or 10 months depending on clinical diagnosis |

These recommendations have the strongest evidence-based support for pulmonary TB and have been generalized to other forms of the disease.

Drugs are given in an *initial* phase for early and rapid sterilization of all or most lesions. If a clinical and bacteriologic response is seen at 2 months, and the patient is AFB smear negative, a reduction of the number of drugs occurs in the *continuation* phase. For those individuals with pulmonary TB still AFB smear positive at 2 months, therapy is extended to 9 months total. Using DOT, alternative schedules for better compliance include: 4 drugs 3× a week for 6 months; or 14 days of daily therapy followed by 2× a week for 6 months.

The American Academy of Pediatrics 2009 Red Book Committee (AAP) recommends the same therapy as the ATS. However, a 3-drug initial regimen can be used in those children with pulmonary TB where the index case has a pansensitive organism isolated. The *continuation* phase is still 2 drugs for 4 months.[6]

pressure or debulk large areas of infected material for improved drug penetration; and corticosteroids have been used to decrease intracranial pressure in CNS disease[12] to reduce obstruction from large hilar nodes, and to reduce inflammation and postinflammatory fibrosis in pericarditis.

## OUTPATIENT MANAGEMENT

There has been a shift in the responsibility for treatment of TB from the patient to the health care system and the provider because of the public health implications of failure to cure an infected individual. A therapeutic alliance should be developed between the adolescent, the family, the provider of medical supervision, and the physician. At the time of hospitalization the DOH is notified for contact investigation and to provide DOT in the outpatient setting. This involvement of all concerned parties facilitates the monitoring of patient adherence and response to therapy and proactively addresses the effect of incomplete therapy on the individual and society. A physician must still prescribe the medication, counsel the adolescent concerning side effects, follow clinical and bacteriologic parameters, and accept responsibility for the overall health of the adolescent. Monthly appointments should be the norm with more frequent visits as needed to address intercurrent problems. Transportation and incentives may also be provided. Microbiologic specimens from body sites that originally yielded positive cultures should be recultured. X-rays and scans that originally showed disease should be repeated until there is improvement or resolution of the abnormality. Pregnant or lactating adolescents, those with HIV, and any teenager whose diet is deficient in meat or milk should be prescribed pyridoxine (vitamin $B_6$) to prevent INH-related peripheral neuropathy. Adolescents at risk for preexisting liver disease because of a history of hepatitis or drug or alcohol abuse should have baseline liver function tests (LFTs). Pregnant teenagers and those taking hepatotoxic agents should also have baseline tests. All others are presumed to have normal liver function and can be monitored only for symptomatic illness. Hepatitis is the most serious side effect of all TB medications. The earliest signs are malaise, anorexia, and a flu-like illness, which if ignored can lead to clinical jaundice and acute liver failure. This occurs most frequently in patients

## Box 141-1

### *Important Characteristics of Selected Drugs*

- Isoniazid (INH) has some activity in the macrophage and the caseating granuloma, but it is most active in the cavity where organisms are actively replicating. It is well absorbed from the gastrointestinal tract, penetrates all body fluids, including the CNS, is metabolized in the liver, and excreted through the kidneys.
- Rifampin (RIF) is the most active agent at all sites, especially against intermittently replicating organisms in the caseating lesions. It is actively absorbed when taken orally, penetrates all body fluids including the CNS when inflammation is present, and is metabolized in the liver. It is excreted in the bile, urine, tears, and sweat with an orange pigment.
- Rifabutin, a related rifamycin with a similar profile to RIF, is better suited for use in individuals being treated with protease inhibitors for HIV infection. Both drugs can interfere with the efficacy of oral contraceptives.
- Pyrazinamide (PZA) is active mainly in the acidic PH of the macrophage with particular usefulness during the first few months of therapy. It is well absorbed, penetrates body fluids, and achieves detectable levels in the CNS. It is metabolized by the liver. It cannot be used against *M bovis*, as all strains are intrinsically resistant to this drug.
- Streptomycin (SM), the first anti-TB drug to be developed, is effective against extracellular organisms only. It is an intramuscular injection that must be given daily and has poor CNS penetration except when inflammation is present.
- Ethambutol (EMB) diffuses well into most tissues except the CNS. At high doses, 25 mg/kg, it becomes bactericidal, but reversible and irreversible optic neuritis is more commonly seen at this dose than at lower doses. It should not be used in children where visual acuity and color vision cannot be reliably tested.
- Ethionamide (ETH) is well tolerated in children, although less so in adults, and it achieves CSF levels.
- Para-aminosalicylic acid (PAS) is poorly tolerated because of severe gastric irritation, and when included in a regimen it is significantly associated with interruptions of therapy.
- Rifamate (INH and RIF) and Rifater (INH, RIF, and PZA) are fixed drug combinations that have been used when DOT is not available to minimize inadvertent monotherapy and subsequent selection for resistance. They reduce the number of pills, but must be taken daily, not intermittently. They are formulated in proportions compatible with most but not all daily treatment regimens.
- Levofloxacin, cycloserine, capreomycin, kanamycin, and amikacin all have been used for the treatment of multidrug-resistant TB (MDR-TB), defined as an organism that is resistant to both INH and RIF.

taking both INH and RIF, especially in high doses, and in patients with pre-existing liver disease. When the adolescent is symptomatic, all medication should be immediately discontinued and LFTs should be checked. If the transaminase AST is more than 3 times normal, all TB-Rx should be stopped and only reinstituted in consultation with a specialist. If the LFTs are normal, another etiology is the cause of the symptoms, and TB-Rx can be restarted. In the asymptomatic patient, if AST is found to be more than 5 times normal the TB-Rx should be stopped and drugs should be restarted judiciously only when the AST returns to less than 2 times normal. Rifampin is restarted first, followed in 1 week by INH. If the patient tolerates this regimen and the hepatitis was severe, PZA can be presumed to be the cause and can be dropped, extending the duration of therapy to 9 months. Consultation with an infectious diseases specialist may be needed to plan a different regimen if LFT abnormalities are persistent.

Latent tuberculosis infection (LTBI) is found in individuals infected with *M tuberculosis* but not clinically symptomatic and without radiographic or bacteriologic evidence of disease. These adolescents remain at risk for developing active disease throughout their lifetime. In the immune-competent host, the risk is greatest immediately after the acquisition of infection, peaking at 2 years and diminishing after 5 years, but persisting at a low level approaching a cumulative lifetime incidence of 10%.[2,13] In individuals coinfected with HIV, those with other chronic illnesses with defective immunity, or those taking immunosuppressant drugs, this risk may approach up to 10% per year. Targeted testing has replaced routine screening to identify those at high risk of having LTBI and of developing active illness.[14,15] TST has been the standard, but the immunodiagnostic tests are becoming an acceptable alternative in the immunocompetent host. In the adolescent with a history of BCG they are the test of choice because of their greater specificity. See Box 141-2 for those at high risk for LTBI, the same groups most at risk for active TB. Adolescents with LTBI should be treated because they are likely to be recently infected, their adolescent growth spurt puts

### Box 141-2

### *Recommendations for TB Screening in Adolescents*

Adolescents for whom targeted tuberculin skin test (TST) or interferon gamma release assays (IGRA) are indicated:

1. Those exposed to a person with active disease
2. Those found to have an abnormal chest x-ray consistent with active or healed TB
3. Those immigrating from countries where TB is endemic, especially within the last 5 years
4. Those with frequent visitors from countries where TB is endemic
5. Those traveling to endemic areas and residing there for more than 1 month should be tested 8–10 weeks after their return provided they remain well in the interim
6. Those found to be HIV positive
7. Those who live or work in an institutional setting, eg, prison, hospital, shelter, or who have frequent contact with others who live or work in these areas
8. Those individuals about to start prolonged therapy with immunosuppressive or immune-modulating drugs
9. Those who use illicit injection drugs or who have frequent contact with those who do
10. Migrant farm workers

Adolescents for whom an annual TST or IGRA is indicated:

1. Those who are HIV infected
2. Those who are incarcerated

Modified from American Academy of Pediatrics. Tuberculosis. In: Pickering LK, Baker CJ, Kimberlin DW, Long SS, eds. *Red Book: 2009 Report of the Committee on Infectious Diseases,* 28th ed. Elk Grove Village, IL: American Academy of Pediatrics; 680–701.

them at risk for progression of disease, and they have a lifetime to reactivate their infection. Most DOT programs do not accept individuals with LTBI, so the burden of convincing a teenager that a course of medication is in their best interest falls on their physician or health provider. See Box 141-3 for the recommended therapy and its duration.[13]

## SPECIAL CLINICAL SITUATIONS

### INTERRUPTIONS IN THERAPY

Interruptions in therapy do occur even in the best DOT program. The ATS (see Box 141-4) has addressed this

### Box 141-3

### *Treatment for Individuals with LTBI*[10]

1. Nine months of daily INH (10 mg/kg, 300 mg max) for those who have been exposed to an INH-sensitive organism or an unknown contact. Total: #270 doses within 12 months
2. Nine months of 2x a week INH (20–30 mg/kg, 900 mg max) under directly observed therapy (DOT) for those who have been exposed to a known INH sensitive organism or an unknown contact. Total: #76 doses within 12 months
3. Four months (adults) or 6 months (children) of daily RIF (10–20 mg/kg, 600 mg max) for those who have been exposed to a known INH-resistant and RIF-sensitive organism. Total: #120 doses. This regimen can also be used for those who cannot tolerate INH or for those who will not be able to complete the 9-month course of INH
4. Rifabutin daily (5 mg/kg, 300 mg max) can be given instead of RIF to those with HIV and exposed to an INH-resistant organism
5. Those with known contact with MDR-TB should either be observed and treated only if they develop symptomatic disease or should receive treatment in consultation with a specialist

It is for the group that is infected with an INH-sensitive strain that there is the strongest evidence for risk reduction with therapy. Even patients who complete only 6 months of therapy, and have received 180 doses on the daily schedule and 52 doses on the 2x/week schedule, have reduced their lifetime risk of reactivation by 65%, and if adherence is a major problem, this duration of therapy is acceptable.[16] Interrupted treatment should be managed according to the recommendations for active disease, ie, the shorter the course of TB-Rx, and the longer the interruption, the more likely that treatment should be restarted from the beginning. If more than 2 months has passed since therapy was interrupted, the patient should be re-examined for active TB. Patients with HIV and exposed to active TB should be treated for 9 months even if PPD negative.

Adolescents with LTBI also represent a point source for contact testing.

Positive TST are reportable in some areas, and there the DOH can be mobilized to pursue contact tracing. Most areas, however, rely on the provider to encourage or provide household and close contact testing to this group. Before starting therapy, the individual should have a nutritional assessment, a determination of the need for baseline LFTs, and an HIV test if risks are present. After contracting with the adolescent to complete the required therapy, there should be monthly follow-up visits to ensure adherence and to assess for complications.

## Box 141-4

### *Management of Treatment Interruption*

Interruption during initial treatment phase

- If interval is ≥14 days, restart from beginning
- If interval is <14 days, continue therapy

Interruption during the continuation phase

- If ≥80% of doses have been given and cultures before start of therapy are negative:
  - Stop further therapy and manage the patient with a total of 4 months of therapy for culture-negative TB
  - If ≥80% of doses have been given and cultures were initially positive:
  - Re-evaluate the patient, as more therapy may be required
- If <80% of doses have been given and <3 months have elapsed:
  - Continue therapy as appropriate for this phase
  - If <80% of doses have been given and ≥3 months have elapsed:
  - Restart therapy from the beginning, returning to the original initial regimen, unless clinical deterioration or symptomatic disease supports a more drug-resistant infection

In general, the earlier in treatment or the longer the duration that the interruption has occurred, the more likely that therapy has to start over from the beginning. At the time of return to therapy the patient should be re-evaluated by physical exam, culture, and x-ray. If therapy is to be resumed, the number of doses required should dictate the duration of therapy. The major concern for the patient and for public health is that the interruption has occurred at a point in therapy when all sensitive organisms have been eliminated, leaving the relatively resistant bacilli to cause a clinical relapse.

issue and recommends that treatment be individualized for each patient.[10]

### HUMAN IMMUNODEFICIENCY VIRUS

Human immunodeficiency virus requires a baseline assessment of the individual's immune status before initiation of TB-Rx. Tuberculosis can be cured in those coinfected with HIV, but severe immunodeficiency and concomitant ART can be associated with drug interactions. Those already being treated with ART should have their TB-Rx initiated as appropriate for their clinical illness. Rifabutin is the rifamycin that should be used because it has fewer drug interactions and is as effective as rifampin in most situations. Dosage adjustment may be required as rifabutin induces cytochrome P450 enzymes in the liver. The American Academy of Pediatrics (AAP) recommends 9 months of therapy for adolescents with active TB and coinfected with HIV.[9] The ATS recommends 9 months of therapy for LTBI for those with HIV infection who are exposed to active TB, even if their PPD is negative.

### THE IMMUNE RECONSTITUTION SYNDROME

The immune reconstitution syndrome (IRIS) is a paradoxical exacerbation of clinical illness that can occur in an HIV-infected individual who starts TB-Rx, and ART is added either simultaneously or within 4 to 8 weeks. Symptoms include fever, generalized lymphadenopathy, pleural effusion, CNS dysfunction, and a worsening of infiltrates on CXR. These reactions are the result of host defenses, restored by ART, being mobilized against the TB infection. If treatment failure and other causes of clinical deterioration have been excluded, patients can be treated symptomatically with nonsteroidal anti-inflammatory drugs or with a tapering short course of corticosteroids. In most individuals, TB-Rx should be started first and ART delayed for at least 2 months, and in some instances, the total course of TB-Rx can be completed before the initiation of ART.

### PREGNANCY

Pregnant adolescents with active TB should be treated appropriately for their clinical disease. Drugs that have been used without teratogenic effect include INH, RIF, and EMB. Streptomycin has been associated with congenital deafness, and the other aminoglycosides presumably have this same toxicity. There is a paucity of information on PZA and its effect on the developing fetus, but the WHO recommends its use in pregnancy. Women at high risk for MDR-TB require a broader spectrum of drugs, many of which have not had extensive use in pregnancy. The effects of these drugs on the mother and fetus are unknown. This information must be disclosed and the woman counseled concerning the risk/benefit of treatment because untreated or inadequately treated TB poses a significant risk to both. Those exposed to active TB should be evaluated by TST and shielded CXR, and if they are found to have active disease should have their therapeutic options discussed as previously. Women suspected of having LTBI, and not active disease, can have their evaluation and treatment deferred until postpartum or can begin appropriate therapy after their first trimester. Breastfeeding is not contraindicated for women who are being treated with first line agents. The small amount of drug found in breast milk has not been found to be toxic; however, it is insufficient to treat an infant with congenital TB.

## BACILLE CALMETTE-GUÈRIN VACCINE

Bacille Calmette-Guerin (BCG), a live vaccine prepared from attenuated strains of *M bovis*, is given in many countries to protect infants and children from disseminated or life-threatening TB. The available strains have variable efficacy and do not confer a lifelong protection. Many adolescents we evaluate have emigrated from countries that routinely employ this vaccine as a public health strategy. When these teenagers are given a TST, the history of BCG administration should be ignored and the cutaneous response interpreted in the same manner as for individuals who have not had the vaccine. Chest x-rays should be obtained in all individuals with a positive TST. Interferon gamma release assays are the preferred diagnostic test for this population as they have a similar sensitivity for TB but greater specificity with no cross-reaction with BCG exposure.

## INTERNET AND PRINT RESOURCES

- Centers for Disease Control and Prevention. Tuberculosis. Available at: www.cdc.gov/tb/. Accessed May 13, 2010
- World Health Organization. Tuberculosis. Available at: www.who.int/tb/en/. Accessed September 21, 2009
- Francis J. Curry National Tuberculosis Center. Available at: www.nationaltbcenter.edu/index.cfm. Accessed September 21, 2009
- American Thoracic Society, CDC, Infectious Disease Society of America. Diagnostic standards and classification of tuberculosis in adults and children. *Am J Respir Crit Care Med.* 2000; 161(4 Pt 1):1376–1395

## REFERENCES

1. World Health Organization. WHO Report 2009 Global Tuberculosis Control—Epidemiology, Strategy, Financing. Available at: www.who.int/tb/publications/global_report/2009/en. Accessed June 29, 2009

2. Centers for Disease Control and Prevention. Controlling tuberculosis in the United States: recommendations from the American Thoracic Society, CDC, and the Infectious Disease Society of America. *MMWR.* 2005;54(No. RR-12):1–81

3. CDC. *Reported Tuberculosis in the United States.* Atlanta, GA: US Department of Health and Human Services, CDC; 2007

4. *TB Annual Summary, 2007.* New York, NY: New York City Department of Health and Mental Hygiene; 2008

5. Barnes PF, Cave MD. Molecular epidemiology of tuberculosis. *N Engl J Med.* 2003;349:1149–1156

6. American Academy of Pediatrics. Tuberculosis. In: Pickering LK, Baker CJ, Kimberlin DW, Long SS, eds. *Red Book: 2009 Report of the Committee on Infectious Diseases.* 28th ed. Elk Grove Village, IL: American Academy of Pediatrics; 2009;680–701

7. Centers for Disease Control and Prevention. Guidelines for the investigation of contacts of persons with infectious tuberculosis; recommendations from the National Tuberculosis Controllers Association and CDC. *MMWR.* 2005;54(No. RR-15):1–47

8. Menzies D. Interpretation of repeated tuberculin tests: boosting, conversion, and reversion. *Am J Respir Crit Care Med.* 1999;159:15–21

9. Centers for Disease Control and Prevention. Guidelines for using the QuantiFERON® TB Gold test for detecting *Mycobacterium tuberculosis* infection, United States. *MMWR.* 2005;54(No. RR-15):49–55

10. American Thoracic Society, CDC, Infectious Diseases Society of America. Treatment of tuberculosis. *Am J Respir Crit Care Med.* 2003;167:603–662

11. Raviglione MC, Smith MB. XDR tuberculosis—implications for global public health. *N Engl J Med.* 2007;356:656–659

12. Thwaites GE, Nguyen DB, Nguyen HD, et al. Dexamethasone for the treatment of tuberculous meningitis in adolescents and adults. *N Engl J Med.* 2004;351: 1741–1751

13. American Thoracic Society, CDC. Targeted tuberculin testing and treatment of latent tuberculosis infection. *Am J Respir Crit Care Med.* 2000;161(4):S221–S247

14. Pediatric Tuberculosis Collaborative Group. Targeted tuberculin skin testing and treatment of latent tuberculosis infections in children and adolescents. *Pediatrics.* 2004;114:1175–1201

15. Munsiff S, Nilsen D, Dworkin F. *Guidelines for testing and treatment of latent tuberculosis infection.* NYC Department of Health and Mental Hygiene, Bureau of Tuberculosis Control. October 2005;1–25

16. Comstock GW. How much Isoniazid is needed for prevention of tuberculosis among immunocompetent adults. *Int J Tuberc Lung Dis.* 1999;3:847–850

# CHAPTER 142

## Parasitic Infections

PETER J. HOTEZ, MD, PhD • SIMON BROOKER, DPhil • DONALD A.P. BUNDY

### GENERAL COMMENTS ON HELMINTH INFECTIONS IN ADOLESCENTS

Parasitic worms (helminths) rank among the most common infectious agents of humans. An estimated 807 million, 604 million, and 576 million people are infected with the soil-transmitted helminths (STHs), *Ascaris lumbricoides, Trichuris trichiura*, and the hookworms (*Necator americanus* and *Ancylostoma duodenale*), respectively,[1] whereas 200 million people are infected with schistosomes,[2] and 120 million with filarial worms.[3] Most of these infections are found in the developing regions of sub-Saharan Africa, Asia, and the Americas, where they occur primarily in individuals living in extreme poverty.

Adolescents who live in impoverished conditions in the developing world are at high risk for severe morbidity from helminth infections. To understand why, it is important to introduce the concept of infection intensity. The STHs, schistosomes, and filariae do not replicate within the human host, and it has been observed that the amount of host morbidity they cause is roughly proportional to their numbers. Therefore, the epidemiology and control of human helminth infections relies significantly on identifying the populations at risk for acquiring moderate and heavy helminth burdens, ie, high-intensity infections, as opposed to light infections.[4] Studies conducted in Africa (where the prevalence of schistosomiasis is highest) have determined that populations between the ages of 10 and 14, on average, harbor the highest burden of schistosomes, particularly for the urinary schistosome *Schistosoma haematobium*[5] whereas human hookworm burdens are highest in both adolescents and adults.[6,7] This concept is sometimes surprising to clinicians who think of parasitic worm infections as pediatric problems, which exclusively affect younger children. However, cross-sectional studies conducted in many developing countries indicate that among the most prevalent helminthiases, the 3 major STH infections, schistosomiasis, and lymphatic filariasis (LF), only ascariasis and trichuriasis exhibit their highest intensity in young children and adolescents (Figure 142-1).[4,8]

The basis by which adolescents exhibit high-intensity schistosome and hookworm infections compared with other age groups is not known. Of interest is the observation made recently in the Philippines that following treatment with the drug praziquantel, the intensity of post-treatment reacquisition of schistosomiasis (caused by *Schistosoma japonicum*) inversely correlated with levels of the hormone dehydroepiandrosterone sulfate (DHEA-S).[13] These data suggest that an intrinsic property of host pubertal development may mediate the apparent resistance to infection observed in some older individuals.[13] Alternatively, it has been suggested that some aspects of exposure to the infective stages of these parasites or host immunity following repeated parasite invasion may mediate susceptibility or resistance to helminth infections.[1,7]

Although adolescents might exhibit higher-intensity schistosome and hookworm infections compared with other groups, within the adolescent population there is typically a wide variation in infection intensities. Parasitic worm infections are said to be aggregated, such that across a given age group most individuals in an endemic region (usually 70%–80%) will harbor light infections, whereas a minority (usually 20%–30%) will harbor moderate and heavy infections.[6-8] The higher mean intensity of schistosomiasis and hookworm infection observed in adolescents is therefore accounted for by a relatively high percentage of this age group harboring moderate and heavy infections. Such populations are at the highest risk for long-term chronic sequelae of hookworm and schistosomiasis.

One of the most important clinical consequences of chronic heavy infections with hookworm and schistosomiasis in adolescence is anemia.[7,14-16] As Crompton points out, "teenage girls grow against a background of iron stress in developing countries where vegetarian diets are the norm and food containing stores of haem iron are unavailable or prohibitively expensive."[14] For such teenagers, additional iron stress arises because of increased demands that result from pubertal growth and menstruation, which typically requires an added dietary iron intake of between 2 and 3 mg daily.[14,17] Pregnancy creates additional iron stress. Therefore teenage girls, both pregnant and nonpregnant, have lower underlying iron reserves compared to other populations and are particularly susceptible to anemia resulting from the

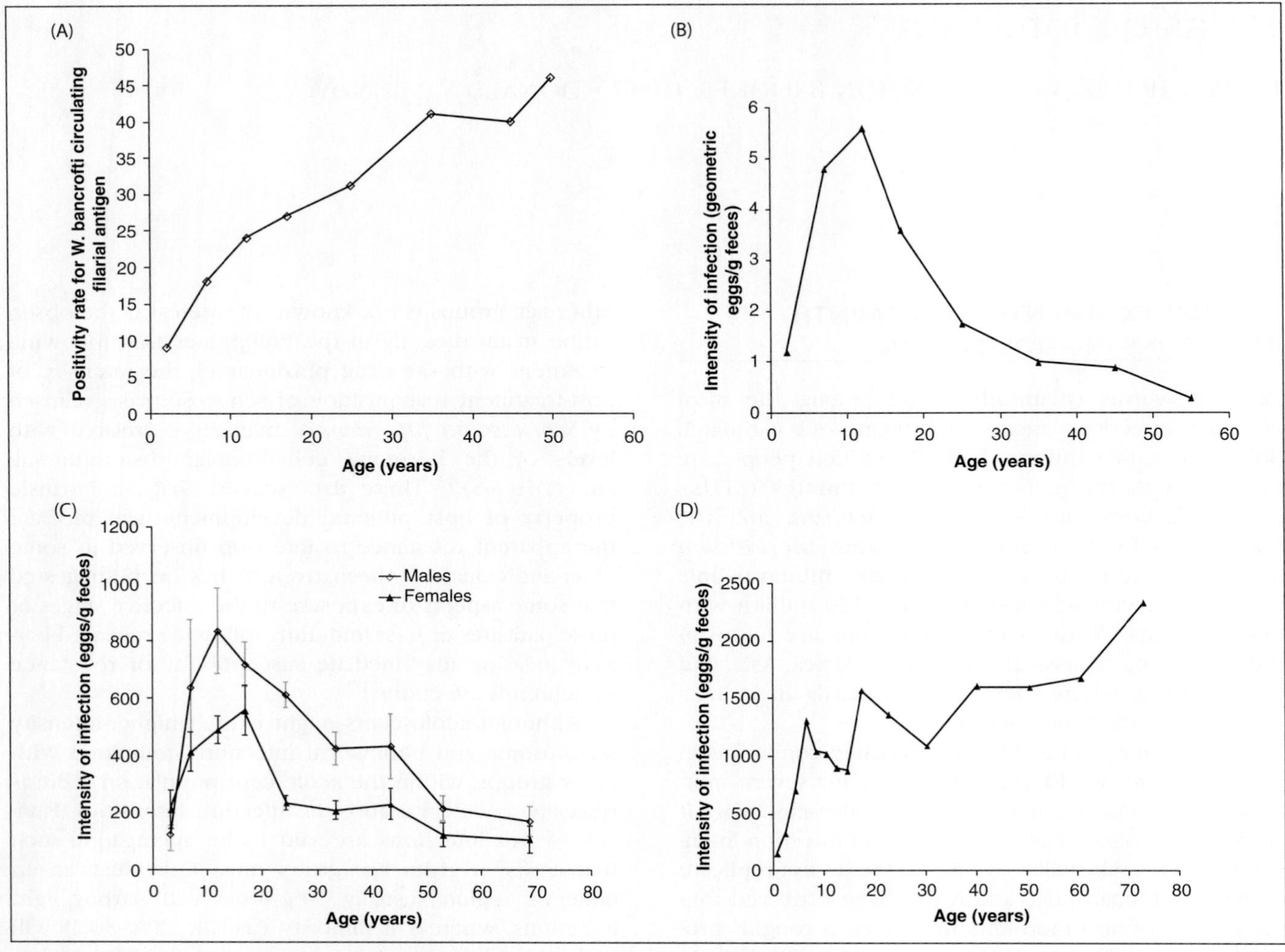


**FIGURE 142-1** (A) Age-specific positivity for *W bancroft* circulating filarial antigen in a Uganda village;[9] (B) age-specific intensity of *S haematobium* infection among individuals in Zimbabwe;[10] (C) age-specific intensity of *S mansoni* infection among males and females in Uganda;[11] and (D) age-specific hookworm intensity of infection among individuals in Brazil.[12]

added iron losses from chronic hookworm infection and schistosomiasis.

Iron deficiency in human hookworm infection results from intestinal blood loss, with moderate hookworm infection causing losses of between 1.1 mg (*N americanus* infection) and 2.3 mg (*A duodenale* infection) of iron loss daily.[18] Anemia results when blood losses exceed the low underlying iron reserves of hookworm-infected adolescents,[16] such that among Zanzibari nonpregnant women hookworm accounts for 19% of iron deficiency anemia and 56% of moderate to severe anemia.[18] Similarly, iron deficiency in schistosomiasis also results primarily from blood loss, which includes intestinal blood loss from *S mansoni* and *S japonicum* infections and urinary tract blood loss from *S haematobium* infection.[19] Severe *S haematobium* infection results in 2.1 mg of daily iron loss.[18] This largely explains the association between schistosomiasis and anemia and the observation made in Kenya that girls heavily infected with *S mansoni* were twice as likely to be anemic as uninfected or lightly infected girls.[20] However, other mechanisms may also add to the anemia of schistosomiasis, including splenomegaly and red blood cell sequestration, autoimmune hemolysis, and anemia of inflammation.[15] Moreover, in Africa and Brazil, coinfections with hookworm and schistosomiasis are not uncommon.[21,22] In many cases, the anemia resulting from helminth coinfections among teenagers is likely to be additive. The long-term consequences of iron-deficiency anemia among adolescents include impaired physical growth and development, as well as impaired cognition and school performance. Worldwide, irondeficiency anemia accounts for approximately 841,000 deaths and 35 million disability adjusted-life years lost, with the developing regions of sub-Saharan Africa and Asia bearing the brunt of the disease burden.[23] The potential for frequent and periodic antihelminthic drug administration ("deworming") to improve iron status provides an important rationale for targeting adolescents with either albendazole or mebendazole for hookworm and other STH infections and/or praziquantel for schistosomiasis.[24]

In addition to its effect on adolescent growth and development, severe anemia resulting from hookworm and schistosomiasis is being increasingly recognized as an important public health threat among pregnant women, including pregnant teenagers. Anemia is the major contributory cause of death in 20%–40% of the 500,000 maternal deaths that occur every year, with 16%–20% of those maternal deaths resulting from iron deficiency anemia.[25] This observation has stimulated several studies looking at the effect of prenatal anthelminthic therapy on pregnancy outcome, with the results so far pointing to significant effects both in terms of improved maternal morbidity and mortality and increased neonatal birth weight.[25,26] World Health Organization (WHO), United Nations' Children's Fund (UNICEF), and International Nutritional Anemia Consultive Group (INACG) currently recommend inclusion of anthelminthic treatment with either albendazole or mebendazole in prenatal programs in areas where prevalence of hookworm exceeds 20%–30%.[25] Treatment is only recommended for the second or third trimester.[24,27] Studies to evaluate the safety and efficacy of praziquantel during pregnancy are in progress.[28]

## SPECIFIC HELMINTH INFECTIONS

The major helminth infections of adolescents include schistosomiasis, and the STH infections, especially hookworm infection and toxocariasis. Emphasis here will be given to clinical aspects of the major helminth infections, which are of particular importance in adolescence.

### LYMPHATIC FILARIASIS

The largest numbers of cases of LF occur in India (45.5 million) and sub-Saharan Africa (40 million), with the highest prevalence occurring in the Pacific Islands of Papua New Guinea and the Republic of Tonga.[29] Most of the cases worldwide are caused by *Wuchereria bancrofti*. In endemic regions, LF has been traditionally considered an infection of adults, and in most endemic regions the highest prevalence occurs in individuals over the age of 20 (Figure 142-1A). Over the last decade, however, there has been increasing appreciation of LF as an important public health problem among children and adolescents, with evidence indicating that infection is first acquired during the first decade of life.[29] This observation has come about through improved diagnostic techniques including filarial-specific antigen assays and ultrasound of the lymphatics, which have improved the sensitivity of detecting cases of LF.[29] These efforts have also revealed an important adolescent component to the burden of filarial disease.[30] In areas of high transmission and endemicity, it is estimated that the prevalence of LF among adolescent populations is approximately 69% of the corresponding adult population.[30] It is believed that the acute (eg, adenolymphangitis and filarial fevers) and chronic (eg, hydrocele and lymphoedema) manifestations found commonly in adults can also be detected in adolescents, although usually at an earlier stage of progression.[30]

Subclinical or asymptomatic lesions are common in adolescents living in endemic areas. These cases can be identified by ultrasound of the proximal lower extremities and the inguinal region, primarily as nests of living worms in the lymphatics (sometimes known as the "filarial dance sign") together with surrounding lymphangiectasia.[29] Such adolescents are frequently microfilaremic. The acute manifestations of LF are common in adolescents and manifest as acute filarial fevers, which are typically recurrent and associated with either lymphangitis or lymphadenitis (adenolymphangitis), with inflammation occurring most commonly in the inguinal, axillary, and epitrochlear regions.[29] This condition must be differentiated from other causes of lymphadenitis, such as tuberculosis, as well as neoplasms or inguinal hernias.[30] The chronic manifestations of LF occur approximately 10 to 15 years after initial infection, and therefore in a substantial number of adolescents.[29] When lymphoedema occurs in this population it is usually at either the Grade 1 (pitting edema reversible on limb elevation) or 2 (nonreversible pitting/nonpitting edema with normal skin) stages.[30]

Detection and early treatment of clinical cases with diethylcarbamazine (DEC) are important for potentially reversing some of the long-term consequences of filarial infection. With increasing recognition of the importance of LF among children and adolescents, it is expected that these populations will be incorporated into mass drug administration efforts using either DEC and albendazole or ivermectin and albendazole. Current WHO preventive chemotherapy guidelines recommend these drugs for children more than 90 cm (15 kg).[31] The WHO dose recommendations can be found at the following Web site: whqlibdoc.who.int/publications/2006/9241547103_eng.pdf.

### SCHISTOSOMIASIS

In terms of their global disease burden, the 2 most important forms of human schistosome infection are urinary schistosomiasis caused by *S haematobium* and intestinal/biliary schistosomiasis caused by *S mansoni*.

Approximately 112 million cases of *S haematobium* occur worldwide with almost all of the cases occurring in sub-Saharan Africa. Global morbidity estimates indicate that urinary schistosomiasis results in 70 million cases of hematuria, 18 million cases of major bladder wall pathology, and almost 10 million cases of major hydronephrosis.[32] Adolescents are at high risk for these chronic sequelae because of their higher-intensity infection compared to other age groups. Peak intensity typically occurs among 10- to 14-year-olds[5] (Figure 142-1B), and women under the age of 20 are considered at particular risk for heavy infection.[33]

Most of the morbidity of *S haematobium* infection results from the tissue deposition of terminal-spine-shaped eggs that cause direct damage and host inflammation. The resulting granulomas cause major bladder wall pathology leading to urinary tract obstruction and hydronephrosis. Another important sequela is anemia, which is especially prominent among teenage girls.[19] The anemia results from blood loss caused by tissue invasion by the eggs in the bladder mucosa and submucosa, as well as from longstanding host inflammatory responses.[15]

Of particular importance to female adolescent populations is the observation that up to 75% of women with *S haematobium* infection develop female genital schistosomiasis (FGS), associated with ulcerations in the vulva, vagina, and cervix.[34] This has been largely a neglected problem[35] despite efforts by the WHO Tropical Disease Programme to highlight this condition through a task force on gender.[36] The condition is typically diagnosed by gynecological inspection and colposcopy,[37,38] which reveal the presence of either sandy patches or evidence of neovascularization.[39] Upper genital tract lesions can also occur, although these are less easily discernible and require diagnosis by laparascopy and ultrasound.[37,38] It is associated with genital bleeding, abdominal pain and pain on sexual intercourse, and infertility.

Newer data from Zimbabwe and elsewhere indicate that FGS significantly increases the risk of HIV transmission,[34,35,40] possibly as much as threefold.[34] Increased risk of HIV infection occurs because the ulceration of the vaginal and cervical mucosa that results from FGS erodes a critical first line of defense for young women exposed to HIV infection[34,2] and the inflammatory cells associated with these lesions, which include CD4+ cells, macrophages, and dendritic cells, also provide a reservoir for cellular invasion by the human immunodeficiency virus.[41] There is also evidence that *S haematobium* infection in men results in elevated numbers of CD4+ T cells and cytokines associated with HIV infection, and this may result in higher concentrations of virus and virus-infected cells in semen.[42]

*S mansoni* infection is a significant cause of intestinal and liver disease in Africa (with approximately 54 million cases[32]) and it is the only cause of schistosomiasis in the Americas. Like *S haematobium* infection, the disease of *S mansoni* infection results from the invasion of eggs (which have a lateral spine instead of a terminal spine) in the tissues and a host inflammatory response, but primarily in the intestine and liver. It is associated with bloody diarrhea and fibrosis of the liver. FGS can also occur in *S mansoni* infection.[43] *S japonicum* and *S mekongi* are the predominant schistosomes occurring in Asia, with intestinal/biliary infection occurring in less than 1 million people. The greatest numbers of cases occur along the Yangtze and Mekong rivers in China and Southeast Asia, respectively, as well as the Philippines. Age-specific infection patterns are typically similar to those for *S haematobium* (Figure 142-1C). Chronic infection with all 4 major schistosomes is an important cause of impaired child growth and cognition as well as anemia, chronic pain, exercise intolerance, and undernutrition.[44,45]

Praziquantel is the treatment of choice for both forms of schistosomiasis. For *S haematobium* and *S mansoni* infections, praziquantel should be administered PO at 40 mg/kg in 2 divided doses (1 day only), whereas for *S japonicum* infection it should be administered PO at 60 mg/kg in 3 divided doses (1 day only). However, in resource-poor settings the WHO recommends administration of praziquantel according to size through the use of a height pole (whqlibdoc.who.int/publications/2006/9241547103_eng.pdf).[27] Some of the urinary, intestinal, and liver pathology is reversible following treatment, although not the lesions associated with FGS. Therefore, it is critical to prevent the lesions of FGS from developing through regular preventive chemotherapy with praziquantel.[34,39] When started in childhood, preventive chemotherapy with praziquantel has an important positive effect on physical growth and development, as well as improved cognition, school performance, and school attendance.[24] Based on newer data on the risk associated with HIV infection, preventive chemotherapy with praziquantel may 1 day be shown to represent an important new tool in the fight to improve women's reproductive health and to combat HIV/AIDS.

## HOOKWORM AND OTHER SOIL-TRANSMITTED HELMINTH INFECTIONS

The STH infections are almost ubiquitous throughout impoverished rural areas of sub-Saharan Africa, Asia, and the Americas. Although ascariasis and trichuriasis occur frequently in adolescents, hookworm is considered the most important infection in this population because of the high worm burdens that can occur in adolescents and the resulting intestinal blood loss and anemia (Figure 142-1D).[6,7] Adolescent girls and women of reproductive age are particularly vulnerable to hookworm infection because of their impaired iron status.[16,18] It is estimated that approximately 32 adult *N americanus* worms (corresponding to 1,000 eggs per gram of feces) produce 1.3 to 2.2 ml of blood loss per day or 0.45 to 0.65 mg of daily iron loss (corresponding to 1,000 eggs per gram of feces).[14] For many teenage girls on the verge of iron deficiency because they cannot keep up their high body iron requirements resulting from growth and menstruation, such hookworm-associated blood losses quickly throw them into negative iron balance and iron deficiency anemia.[16] For that reason, the WHO currently recommends regular and periodic deworming of adolescent populations with either mebendazole or albendazole.[27] Both drugs are well tolerated and considered safe, although because of their embryotoxic and teratogenic effects in laboratory animals, they need to be used with caution in pregnancy. However, an estimated 44 million pregnant women globally and 7 million in sub-Saharan Africa alone are infected with hookworm,[46] which represents an important cause of anemia in pregnancy,[47] particularly among multigravidae.[48] Therefore, the WHO has proposed prenatal deworming in the second or third trimester emerging as an important reproductive health strategy (whqlibdoc.who.int/publications/2006/9241547103_eng.pdf),[24,27,31] which improves neonatal birth weight and child survival and reduces maternal morbidity and mortality.[25,26] Added iron supplementation may also be an important adjunct therapy during pregnancy.[25,26]

In both industrialized and developing countries the canine zoonosis, toxocariasis, is an important cause of ocular larval migrans and impaired vision in adolescent populations.[49] Unlike visceral larval migrans, which is primarily a condition of young children, ocular larva migrans has its peak incidence among school-aged children, recently estimated at 9.7 per 100,000 persons.[49]

## REFERENCES


1. Bethony J, Brooker S, Albonico M, et al. Soil-transmitted helminth infections: ascariasis, trichuriasis, and hookworm. *Lancet.* 2006;367:1521–1532

2. Chitsulo L, Engels D, Montresor A, Savioli L. The global status of schistosomiasis and its control. *Acta Tropica.* 2000;77:41–51

3. Michael E, Bundy DA, Grenfell BT. Reassessing the global prevalence and distribution of lymphatic filariasis. *Parasitology.* 1996;112:409–428

4. Bundy DA. Control of intestinal nematode infections by chemotherapy: mass treatment versus diagnostic treatment. *Trans R Soc Trop Med Hyg.* 1990;84:622–625

5. Kojima S, MacDonald AS. Schistosomes:general (Chapter 28). In: Cox FEG, Wakelin D, Gillespie SH, Despommier DD, eds. *Topley Wilson Microbiology Microbial Infection.* 10th ed. Hoboken, NJ: Wiley-Blackwell; 2006:600–609

6. Bundy DAP. Is the hookworm just another geohelminth? In: Schad GA, Warren KS, eds. *Hookworm Disease Current Status and New Directions.* London: Taylor and Francis; 1990:147–164

7. Brooker S, Bethony J, Hotez PJ. Human hookworm infection in the 21st century. *Adv Parasitol.* 2004;58:197–288

8. Anderson RM, May RM. Helminth infections of humans: mathematical models, population dynamics, and control. *Adv Parasitol.* 1985;24:1–101

9. Onapa AW, Simonsen PE, Pedersen EM, Okello DO. Lymphatic filariasis in Uganda: baseline investigations in Lira, Soroti, and Katakwi districts. *Trans R Soc Trop Med Hyg.* 2001;95:161–167

10. Woolhouse ME, Watts CH, Chandiwana SK. Heterogeneities in transmission rates and the epidemiology of schistosome infection. *Proc Biol Sci.* 1991;245:109–114

11. Kabatereine NB, Brooker S, Tukahebwa EM, Kazibwe F, Onapa A. Epidemiology and geography of *Schistosoma mansoni* in Uganda: implications for planning control. *Trop Med Int Hlth.* 2004;9:372–380

12. Fleming F, Brooker S, Geiger SM, et al. Synergistic associations between hookworm and other helminth species in a rural community in Brazil. *Trop Med Int Hlth.* 2006;11:56–64

13. Kurtis JD, Friedman JF, Leenstra T, et al. Pubertal development predicts resistance to infection and reinfection with Schistosoma japonicum. *Clin Infect Dis.* 2006;42:1692–1698

14. Crompton DWT. The public health importance of hookworm disease. *Parasitology.* 2000;S39–S50

15. Friedman JF, Kanzaria HK, McGarvey ST. Human schistosomiasis and anemia: the relationship and potential mechanisms. *Trend Parasitol.* 2005;21:386–392

16. Hotez PJ, Brooker S, Bethony JM, et al. Hookworm infection. *N Engl J Med.* 2004;351:799–807

17. Viteri FE. The consequences of iron deficiency and anaemia in pregnancy on maternal health, the foetus and the infant. *SCN News.* 1994;11:14–8

18. Stoltzfus RJ, Dreyfuss ML, Chwaya HM, Albonico M. Hookworm control as a strategy to prevent iron deficiency. *Nutr Rev.* 1997;55:223–232

19. Stephenson LS. The impact of schistosomiasis on human nutrition. *Parasitology.* 1993;107:S107–S123

20. Leenstra T, Kariuki SK, Kurtis JD, Ojoo AJ, Kager PA, ter Kuile FO. Prevalence and severity of anemia and iron deficiency, cross-sectional studies in adolescent school girls in western Kenya. *Eur J Clin Nutr.* 2004;58:681–691

21. Raso G, Vounatsou P, Singer BH, N'Goran EK, Tanner M, Utzinger J. An integrated approach for risk-profiling and spatial prediction of Schistosoma mansoni-hookworm coinfection. *Proc Natl Acad Sci USA.* 2006;103:6934–6939

22. Brooker S, Alexander N, Geiger S, et al. Contrasting patterns in the small-scale heterogeneity of human helminth infections in urban and rural environments in Brazil. *Int J Parasitol.* 2006;36:1143–1151

23. Stoltzfus RJ. Iron deficiency: global prevalence and consequences. *Food Nutr Bull.* 2003;24(4 Suppl):S99–S103

24. WHO (World Health Organization). *Deworming for Health and Development: Report of the Third Global Meeting of the Partners for Parasite Control.* Geneva: World Health Organization; 2005

25. Larocque R, Casapia M, Gotuzzo E, Gyorkos TW. Relationship between intensity of soil-transmitted helminth infections and anemia during pregnancy. *Am J Trop Med Hyg.* 2005;73:783–789

26. Christian P, Khatry SK, West KP. Antenatal antihelmintic treatment, birthweight, and infant survival in rural Nepal. *Lancet.* 2004;364:981–983

27. WHO (World Health Organization). *Prevention and Control of Schistosomiasis and Soil-Transmitted Helminthiasis. Report of a WHO Expert Committee.* Geneva: World Health Organization. WHO Technical Report Series #912; 2002

28. Ndibazza J, Muhangi L, Akishule D, Kiggundu M, Ameke C, Oweka J, et al. Effects of deworming during pregnancy on maternal and perinatal outcomes in Entebbe, Uganda: a randomized controlled trial. *Clin Infect Dis.* 2010;50:531–540

29. Babu S, Nutman TB. Lymphatic filariasis (Chapter 38). In: Cox FEG, Wakelin D, Gillespie SH, Despommier DD, eds. *Topley Wilson Microbiology Microbial Infection,* 10th ed. Hoboken, NJ: Wiley-Blackwell; 2006:769–780

30. Witt C, Ottesen EA. Lymphatic filariasis: an infection of childhood. *Trop Med Int Health.* 2001;6:582–606

31. WHO (World Health Organization). *Preventive Chemotherapy in Human Helminthiasis.* Geneva: World Health Organization; 2006. Available at: whqlibdoc.who.int/publications/2006/9241547103_eng.pdf. Accessed January 24, 2009

32. Van Der Werf MJ, de Vlas SJ, Brooker S, et al. Quantification of clinical morbidity associated with schistosome infection in sub-Saharan Africa. *Acta Tropica.* 2003;86:125–139

33. Ndhlovu PD, Mduluza T, Kjetland EF, et al. Prevalence of urinary schistosomiasis and HIV in females living in a rural community of Zimbabwe: does age matter? *Trans R Soc Trop Med Hyg.* 2007; 101:433–438.

34. Kjetland EF, Ndhlovu PD, Gomo E, et al. Association between genital schistosomiasis and HIV in rural Zimbabwean women. *AIDS.* 2006;20:593–600

35. Feldmeier H, Krantz I, Poggensee G. Female genital schistosomiasis. A neglected risk factor for the transmission of HIV? *Trans R Soc Trop Med Hyg.* 1995;89:237

36. Vlassoff C. The gender and tropical diseases task force of TDR: achievements and challenges. *Acta Tropica.* 1997;67:173–180

37. Helling-Giese G, Kjetland EF, Gundersen SG, et al. Schistosomiasis in women: manifestations in the upper reproductive tract. *Acta Tropica.* 1996 a;62:225–238

38. Helling-Giese G, Sjaastad A, Poggensee G, et al. Female genital schistosomiasis (FGS): relationship between gynecological and histopathological findings. *Acta Tropica.* 1996b;62:257–267

39. Kjetland EF, Ndhlovu PD, Mduluza T, et al. Simple clinical manifestations of genital Schistosoma haematobium infection in rural Zimbabwean women. *Am J Trop Med Hyg.* 2005;72:311–319

40. Poggensee G, Kiwelu I, Saria M, Richter J, Krantz I, Feldmeier H. Schistosomiasis of the lower reproductive tract without egg excretion in urine. *Am J Trop Med Hyg.* 1998;59:782–783

41. Poggensee G, Feldmeier H, Krantz I. Schistosomiasis of the female genital tract: public health aspects. *Parasitol Today.* 1999;15:378–381

42. Leutscher PDC, Pedersen M, Raharisolo C, et al. Increased prevalence of leukocytes and elevated cytokine levels in semen from Schistosoma haematobium-infected individuals. *J Infect Dis.* 2005;191:1639–1647

43. Feldmeier H, Correia Daccal R, Martins MJ, Soares V, Martins R. Genital manifestations of schistosomiasis mansoni in women: important but neglected. *Mem Inst Oswaldo Cruz.* 1998;93:127–133

44. King CH, Dickman K, Tisch DJ. Reassessment of the cost of chronic helminth infection: meta-analysis of disability-related outcomes in endemic schistosomiasis. *Lancet.* 2005;365:1561–1569

45. Ajanga A, Lwambo NJ, Blair L, Nyandindi U, Fenwick A, Brooker S. Schistosoma mansoni in pregnancy and associations with anaemia in northwest Tanzania. *Trans R Soc Trop Med Hyg.* 2006;100:59–63

46. Bundy DA, Chan MS, Savioli L. Hookworm infection in pregnancy. *Trans R Soc Trop Med Hyg.* 1995;89:521–522

47. Brooker S, Hotez PJ, Bundy DAP. Hookworm-related anaemia among pregnant women: a systematic review. *PLoS Negl Trop Dis* 2. 2008;(9):e291

48. Guyatt HL, Brooker S, Peshu N, Shulman CE. Hookworm and anaemia prevalence. *Lancet.* 2000;356:2101

49. Good B, Holland CV, Taylor MRH, Larragy J, Moriarty P, O'Regan M. Ocular toxocariasis in schoolchildren. *Clin Infect Dis.* 2004;39:173–178

# CHAPTER 143

# Prevention of Travel-Related Infections

SUNIL K. SOOD, MD

*There is no unhappiness like the misery of sighting land (and work) again after a cheerful, careless voyage.*

—MARK TWAIN

American adolescents are traveling abroad in increasing numbers as travel opportunities are made possible by shorter air travel times, more elaborate school trips, and increasingly popular college semester or year abroad programs. Adolescents and young adults are engaging in both distant travel and adventure travel. Moreover, many pediatric and adolescent practices in the United States today take care of immigrant families, who frequently travel back and forth between their countries of origin. For these reasons, it is important that those who care for adolescents be familiar with "travel medicine."

There are some basic considerations in the practice of travel medicine. For example, whether to stock vaccines that may be used infrequently or whether to instead make referrals to a travel medicine center is ultimately a business decision. Giving travel advice also means that the physician should be familiar with world geography, have ready access to online resources, and be willing to perform background research prior to the patient's visit. Depending on the volume of "travel" visits, a subscription to a travel medicine reference service may be worth the investment. This chapter reviews prevention of travel-related infectious diseases, including vaccine-preventable diseases, traveler's diarrhea, and malaria. Other prophylaxis measures are beyond the scope of this chapter. A recent study on mountain sickness in adolescents was published.[1]

## VACCINE-PREVENTABLE DISEASES

Vaccination is the first step in prevention of travel-related infectious diseases in adolescents. Because travel vaccines are not typically covered by insurance, the out-of-pocket expenses required may deter some parents. Advice to vaccinate could go unheeded, or parents may request that the bare minimum be prescribed. With experience, the clinician can become knowledgeable in weighing the risks versus the costs for each patient's circumstances.

The so-called "3 Rs" of immunization for travel are the administration of *routine, required*, and *recommended* vaccines. The status of the adolescent's *routine* immunizations should be reviewed well in advance of the departure date. Important examples of vaccines that should be up to date include measles (2 doses), hepatitis A (HAV), hepatitis B (HBV), and polio (a booster administered by age 18 years if traveling to pockets of persistent endemicity in south Asia and Africa). Patients should be reminded that infectious diseases such as diphtheria and measles, although now seen very infrequently in the United States, are still prevalent in the world at large.[2]

At the present time, only yellow fever vaccine is legally *required* to cross international borders. Meningococcal vaccine, however, is *required* for all pilgrims traveling to the Hajj. Saudi Arabia is also currently enforcing 2009 H1N1 (swine-origin) influenza vaccination for Hajj pilgrims. All other immunizations that would be used in a travel medicine context fall under the *recommended* category.

Considerations include whether the adolescent is embarking on adventure travel or on a "sanitized" tour, whether rural areas will be visited, and, most important, what provinces he or she is visiting in endemic countries. These are especially important for protection against yellow fever, Japanese encephalitis, and drug-resistant malaria.

### HEPATITIS A

Acute hepatitis A virus (HAV) infection is often a debilitating disease in adolescents, presenting with jaundice, anorexia, and prolonged convalescence, with the rare occurrence of fulminant hepatitis.

#### Geographic Distribution

The hepatitis A virus vaccine should always be recommended because the risk of hepatitis A is not limited to developing nations. An intermediate to low risk exists throughout the rest of the world.[3] In fact, domestic risk has been the rationale for the recent introduction of catch-up hepatitis A immunization for all children in the United States. For the adolescent who is likely to travel abroad more than once, completion of the 2-dose regimen, which confers long-term immunity, obviates the need for revaccination.

### Vaccines

Two manufacturers (GlaxoSmithKline and Merck & Co) currently market hepatitis A vaccines in the United States. Both are formalin-inactivated whole virus vaccines that cause only mild side effects and have excellent immunogenicity: 97% to 100% of adolescents develop protective levels of antibody 1 month after receiving 1 dose, and a second dose administered 6 to 12 months later ensures long-term protection. GlaxoSmithKline also markets a combination vaccine of HAV and hepatitis B virus (HBV).

### Recommendations for Immunization of Traveling Adolescents

Other than a severe allergic reaction to a vaccine component or documented immunity (IgG antibody to HAV), there are no exceptions to the HAV recommendation for travelers.[4] If there is not enough time before the start of the trip, theadolescent can be assured that a single dose provides protection for up to 3 months; arrangements should then be made to return for the second dose 6 to 12 months after the first dose.

## RABIES

Human rabies results from intimate contact with the saliva of an infected mammal, usually from a bite. For adolescents, consideration of pre-exposure prophylaxis for this almost universally lethal viral infection is one of the most important travel precautions.

### Geographic Distribution

Very few countries, and in the United States only the state of Hawaii, are considered rabies free. A list of rabies-endemic countries and reasonably up-to-date, country-specific information and maps from the World Health Organization (WHO) are easily accessible on the Internet at www.who.int/rabies/rabies_maps/en/index.html.

### Vaccines

The current cell culture–derived vaccines are much safer than the old neural tissue–derived vaccines, are more immunogenic, and require fewer doses.[2,5] Human rabies immune globulin, used for passive, immediate prophylaxis also has an excellent safety profile. Both vaccines are filtration- and ultracentrifugation-purified, inactivated virus vaccines (Table 143-1). Human diploid cell vaccine (HDCV) and purified chick embryo cell culture vaccine (PCECV) are grown on MRC-5 human diploid cell and chicken fibroblast cultures, respectively. They are recommended for use as an intramuscular injection in the deltoid for optimal immunogenicity.

Physicians should be aware that cell culture–derived vaccines are not always available abroad, and patients may incur a higher risk of adverse reactions from vaccines prepared by older technology. If immunization is initiated abroad, the titer of neutralizing antibody should be checked on return and immunization completed with a cell culture–derived vaccine, if necessary.

**Table 143-1**

**Rabies Vaccines in the United States**

| *Type* | *Name* | *Route* | *Indications* |
|---|---|---|---|
| Human diploid cell vaccine (HDCV) | Imovax rabies | Intramuscular | Pre- or post-exposure |
| Purified chick embryo cell vaccine (PCECV) | RabAvert | Intramuscular | Pre- or post-exposure |

Centers for Disease Control and Prevention (CDC), Preexposure Vaccinations. Available at: www.cdc.gov/rabies/specific_groups/travelers/pre-exposure_vaccinations.html. Accessed September 9, 2010.

### Recommendations for Immunization of Traveling Adolescents

Rabies prophylaxis should be strongly considered for those who have even a small risk of contact with rabid animals. This includes travel to rural areas or farms, and those who are camping. The most common exposure will be from stray dogs, which can be encountered in many cities in the developing world. Advance planning is essential because all vaccines in the United States are administered in a 3-dose regimen (days 0, 7, and 21–28). Because concern about side effects of rabies vaccines can be a deterrent to acceptance of pre-exposure prophylaxis, it is helpful to be familiar with the data. Local reactions occur in 30% to 74% of recipients,[6] and systemic side effects such as headache, malaise, fever, or nausea occur in up to one-half of all recipients. In a recent study in the United States that compared 83 subjects who received PCECV and 82 who received HDCV,[7] none of the adverse events were serious, and almost all events were of mild or moderate intensity. It is strongly recommended that adolescents experiencing side effects after 1 or 2 doses should complete the immunization course with the help of anti-inflammatory medications. A relative contraindication to immunization with a rabies vaccine is severe hypersensitivity to previous rabies immunization.

## ENTERIC FEVER

Enteric fever, also known as typhoid fever and caused by the exclusively human pathogens *Salmonella typhi* and *Salmonella paratyphi*, is a severe and debilitating infection. It is a bacteremic illness that may be accompanied by severe toxicity, prostration, diarrhea or constipation, and life-threatening complications, mainly, intestinal perforation or hemorrhage and encephalopathy. Acquisition of infection is by the feco-oral route, usually by ingestion of contaminated food or water while traveling in the developing world. However, the infection can also be acquired by contact with carriers in the household, and thus a history of travel is not universal in patients with typhoid fever.

### Geographic Distribution

The highest current incidence is in south and Southeast Asia, with an estimated 100 or more cases per 100,000 population per year, but a medium level of risk (10–100/100,000) exists throughout Asia, Eastern Europe, Africa, and Latin America.[8] The risk to travelers has been estimated to be 1 in 3,000 people per month for travelers to India, northern and western Africa, and Peru, and 10-fold lower in other developing countries.[9] The risk of acquiring multidrug-resistant infection is highest for travelers to south Asia, which makes it very important to immunize before travel to India, Pakistan, and Bangladesh, as well as their neighboring, smaller countries. Just 6 countries account for 76% of travel-associated cases (India, Pakistan, Mexico, Bangladesh, the Philippines, and Haiti).[10]

### Vaccines

Although enteric fever in travelers is caused by *S typhi*, as well as by at least 3 strains of *S paratyphi*, the only recommended vaccines contain whole (live-attenuated) *S typhi* or *S typhi* subunit antigens (capsular polysaccharide). Two vaccines are currently available in the United States (Table 143-2). The oral live-attenuated vaccine (Vivotif Berna) is manufactured from the *S typhi* Ty21a strain; the intramuscular polysaccharide vaccine (Typhim Vi) consists of purified cell surface Vi polysaccharide extracted from the *S typhi* Ty2 strain. The former is administered as enteric-coated capsules containing lyophilized bacteria. An impediment is the need to take 4 doses over 8 days, so adherence may be an issue. In addition, capsules need to be refrigerated at 35.6°F to 46.4°F (2°C–8°C) and all 4 doses should be completed at least 1 week before travel. Antibiotics cannot be coadministered nor should the person ingest hot fluids or alcohol within a few hours of the vaccine capsules. Typhim Vi is a more convenient, albeit less efficacious, vaccine that is administered as a single intramuscular dose. The live-attenuated vaccine provides some cross-protection against *S paratyphi,* whereas the Vi polysaccharide vaccine does not. Both vaccines have a very favorable safety profile.

**Table 143-2**

**Typhoid Vaccines in the United States**

| *Vaccine* | *Fever* | *Headache* | *Local Reactions* |
|---|---|---|---|
| Ty21a[a] | 0%–5% | 0%–5% | Not applicable |
| Vi capsular polysaccharide | 0%–1% | 16%–20% | 7% Erythema or induration 1 cm |

[a]The side effects of Ty21a are rare and mainly consist of abdominal discomfort, nausea, vomiting, and rash or urticaria. The incidence did not exceed that in placebo recipients.

Centers for Disease Control and Prevention (CDC). The pre-travel consultation: Travel-related vaccine-preventable diseases. In: Yellow Book. Available at. wwwnc.cdc.gov/travel/yellowbook/2010/chapter-2/typhoid-paratyphoid-fever.aspx. Accessed September 9, 2010.

### Recommendations for Immunization of Traveling Adolescents

Immunization is recommended even for short travel periods to high-risk areas, such as the Indian subcontinent, because 1 in 7 US cases occurs after trips lasting less than 2 weeks.[9] Typhoid fever was the most common vaccine-preventable infection in a study of 24,920 travelers returning to North America.[11]

Because of the limited efficacy of typhoid vaccines, immunized adolescents must pay careful attention to food and water precautions in the prevention of typhoid fever. In particular, milk products can harbor large inocula of *Salmonella*, so ice cream and other cold milk products should be avoided. Booster doses are recommended every 5 years for the oral Ty21a vaccine and every 2 to 3 years for the capsular polysaccharide vaccine.[12]

## YELLOW FEVER

Yellow fever is an infection caused by a virus from the flaviviral group (Latin: *flavus*, "yellow"), transmitted most commonly by the mosquito *Aedes aegypti*. Although most patients experience a mild to moderate illness, and only 15% experience an icteric illness, there is no specific treatment, and yellow fever is occasionally a fulminant and fatal disease.

### Geographic Distribution

Yellow fever is restricted to the South American and African continents, with the most endemic countries currently being Peru, Brazil, Bolivia, and Colombia in South America, and several countries in western, central, and eastern Africa (Figure 143-1). An increase in yellow fever epidemics over the past 2 decades or so has correlated

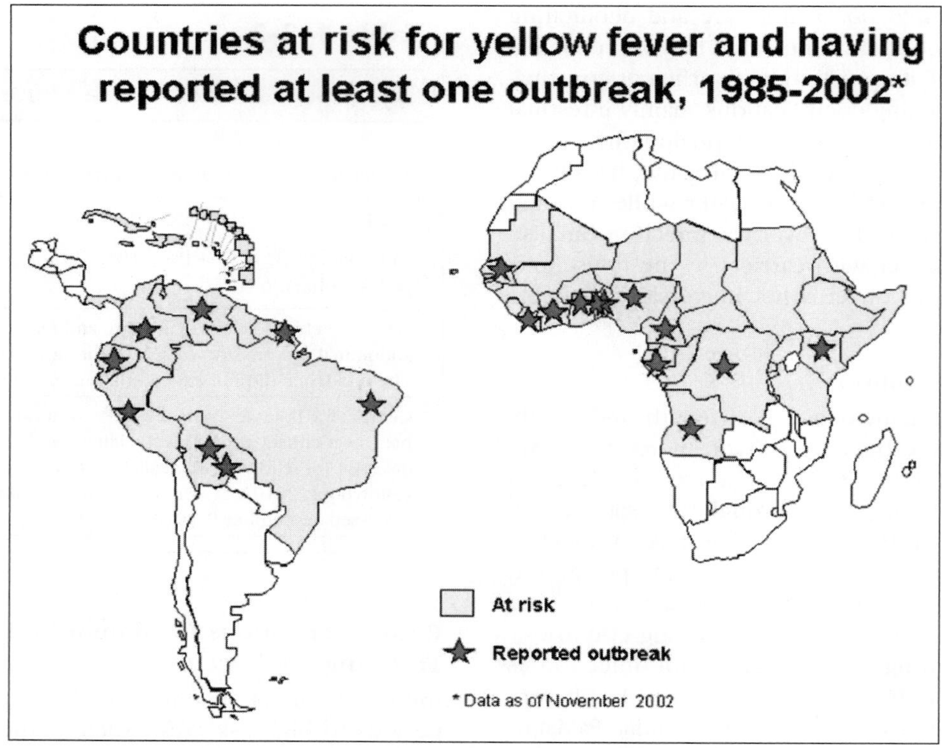


**FIGURE 143-1** Maps of the Americas and Africa that illustrate countries at risk and those that have reported outbreaks in recent years within the endemic zones on these continents. (Reprinted with permission from WHO. Yellow fever: Global vaccination control strategies and vaccine safety overview. Available at: www.who.int/vacine_safety/topics/yellow_fever/yellowfever_dec03.pdf)

with changes in the environment such as deforestation and urbanization, which result in the expansion of mosquito habitats. Widespread international travel and large unvaccinated and susceptible populations could also be playing a role.

The overall risk for an unvaccinated traveler staying 1 week in an African country that has yellow fever is estimated at 1 in 4,200 and is 10-fold less in South America.

About 10 cases have been reported in US travelers over the past quarter century or so, and most were usually fatal.

### Vaccines

Currently, only 1 formulation is available in the United States, a live-attenuated viral vaccine strain 17D (YF-VAX, Sanofi-aventis, Swiftwater, PA). Immunity lasts for more than 10 years, although international guidelines require revaccination after 10 years have lapsed. The Advisory Committee on Immunization Practices (ACIP) of the Centers for Disease Control and Prevention (CDC) recommends immunization for travelers at risk and states that the vaccine is "considered to be one of the safest and most effective live virus vaccines ever developed."[13] The vaccine is generally well tolerated. The vaccinated adolescent should be counseled about mild headache or myalgias that may occur 5 to 10 days after vaccination. More severe reactions are extremely rare. Contraindications for use of 17D vaccine are pregnancy, allergy to egg products, and conditions that compromise the immune system.

### Recommendations for Immunization of Traveling Adolescents

A vaccination regimen should be based on 2 considerations—any requirements of the destination country and recommended prophylaxis based on known risk in the areas being visited. This can be confusing because not all countries in the so-called yellow fever zones, and not all areas within endemic countries, are "infected" (ie, have had recent cases). For the purposes of *recommending* a vaccine, a working and current knowledge of the prevalence of yellow fever in specific areas is needed. This information is best available via subscription to reporting services such as Travax (Shoreland), but it may be necessary to consult with a travel immunization center. Those countries *requiring* a vaccine as a condition of entry are listed on the CDC Web site in a convenient tabular form.

To prevent reintroduction of virus where the competent mosquito vector is present, some countries have required vaccine despite the fact that the WHO does not consider it necessary. The WHO has now issued new regulations, with the expectation that all countries will comply. Under the 2005 International Health Regulations (IHR), the terms "infected" and "endemic" are obsolete, and vaccination decisions should be made based on whether the destination falls under "areas/countries with risk of yellow fever transmission." Nevertheless, some countries may continue to impose requirements and reserve the right to quarantine an unvaccinated traveler. A stamped and completed valid International Certificate of Vaccination ("Yellow Card") must be completed, and the traveler should be reminded to carry this with his or her passport. To administer yellow fever vaccine, the medical facility needs to obtain permission to be an approved yellow fever vaccination facility.

### MENINGOCOCCAL DISEASE

Infectious syndromes caused by *Neisseria meningitidis* infection result in severe disease, and meningococcemia is often fatal.[14] Certain destinations entail an increased risk of acquiring meningococcal disease.

#### Geographic Distribution

In addition to sporadic cases and periodic, unpredictable outbreaks anywhere in the world, outbreaks of serogroup A meningococcal disease regularly occur in the sub-Saharan African region known as the "meningitis belt." The seasonality of these outbreaks allows the physician to specifically recommend meningococcal vaccine for travel during the dry season, which is December through June, in that geographic area. In addition, travel as a Hajj pilgrim to Saudi Arabia involves an increased risk of meningococcal infection, notably from serogroup W-135. In fact, Saudi Arabia requires that pilgrims show proof of vaccination with tetravalent (A, C, Y, W-135) meningococcal vaccine on entry. Fortunately, both the serogroup A and W-135 antigens are components of each of the 2 available meningococcal quadrivalent vaccines.

#### Vaccines

The 3 currently marketed vaccines in the United States are quadrivalent A, C, Y, W-135 meningococcal polysaccharide vaccine for subcutaneous injection (MPSV4, Menomune, Sanofi-aventis), quadrivalent A, C, Y, W-135 meningococcal polysaccharide vaccine conjugated to diphtheria toxoid for intramuscular injection (MCV4, Menactra, Sanofi-aventis), and quadrivalent A, C, Y, W135 meningococcal polysaccharide vaccine conjugated to $CRM_{197}$ (Menveo, Novartis).

#### Recommendations for Immunization of Traveling Adolescents

Despite ACIP and American Academy of Pediatrics (AAP) recommendations in effect for immunization of adolescents beginning at 11 years of age, adolescents who are traveling may not be up to date with meningococcal vaccination. However, college students would most likely have received a vaccine as a requirement before enrollment. A single dose of meningococcal conjugate vaccine is recommended, whereas a recipient of polysaccharide vaccine should be revaccinated, with conjugate vaccine, if 3 or more years have elapsed since vaccination.[15]

### JAPANESE ENCEPHALITIS

Japanese encephalitis (JE) is an arboviral infection caused by a flavivirus related to the yellow fever and dengue viruses, and is transmitted by the bite of *Culex* mosquitoes. Most bites occur around dusk and can be avoided by staying indoors after dark. Illness can range from a simple febrile illness with headache to aseptic meningitis or severe encephalitis.

#### Geographic Distribution

Japanese encephalitis is endemic to Asia, chiefly in rural agricultural areas where flooding irrigation is practiced. Very few cases now occur in Japan.[16]

#### Vaccines

The previously licensed vaccine in the United States, JE-VAX (Biken, Japan/distributed by Sanofi-Aventis USA), a mouse brain-derived inactivated virus vaccine, has been discontinued. In its place, "IC51," a killed, cell culture–based vaccine, is now available.[17] The brand name is Ixiaro, manufactured by Intercell (Vienna, Austria). It was approved by the US Food and Drug Administration (FDA) in early 2009 and is distributed by Novartis. It is formulated as a ready-to-use liquid formulation in prefilled syringes. Ixiaro is indicated for active immunization against JE virus for persons 17 years of age and older, administered in 2 doses, 28 days apart.

#### Recommendations for Immunization of Traveling Adolescents

Although the reported incidence of JE among visitors to Asia is less than 1 case per 1 million travelers, the vaccine is recommended if the person plans to stay 1 month or longer in endemic areas during the transmission season. This includes those who will be based in urban areas but will visit endemic rural or agricultural areas during that period. The season differs for temperate and subtropical or tropical areas, and can be determined by referring to authoritative sources.[18] The ACIP issued provisional recommendations in July 2009.[19]

## TRAVELER'S DIARRHEA

The cornerstone of prevention of traveler's diarrhea is meticulous avoidance of potentially contaminated food and water, but physicians often neglect to

**Box 143-1**

***Etiology of Traveler's Diarrhea in Cases with Identifiable Pathogens***

**Bacterial**
Enterotoxigenic *Escherichia coli*
Enteroaggregative *E coli*
Enteroinvasive *E coli*
*Campylobacter jejuni*
*Salmonella* spp
*Shigella* spp
*Aeromonas* spp
*Plesiomonas shigelloides*
*Vibrio* spp (*cholerae, parahemolyticus)*

**Viral**
Norovirus
Rotavirus

**Protozoal**
*Giardia intestinalis*
*Entamoeba histolytica*
*Cryptosporidium parvum*
*Cyclospora cayetanensis*

**Noninfectious**
Fish, mushroom, toxin, and chemical food poisonings

provide advice on the many effective self-treatment options. Most cases are caused by the organisms and chemical agents listed in Box 143-1. It is inevitable that adolescent travelers, like all travelers, will ingest contaminated sources containing one or more of these agents, either inadvertently or from indiscretion.[20] Preventive counseling includes instruction on rehydration, a recommendation to purchase over-the-counter (OTC) loperamide, and prescribing one of the antibiotic agents listed in Table 143-3.[21] Initial self-treatment consists of rehydration and loperamide. If the diarrhea worsens or persists, either a single dose or 3-day course of antibiotics (as listed in Table 143-3) should be initiated. The patient is to be warned that life-threatening diarrhea can rapidly ensue with *Vibrio cholerae* infection, for which treatment at a hospital is imperative.

## MALARIA

Several species of the *Plasmodium* parasite cause malaria, but prophylaxis efforts are directed primarily at preventing *Plasmodium falciparum* infection, which causes the most severe morbidity and can result in death. The choice of chemoprophylaxis is based on the epidemiology of chloroquine resistance (Figure 143-2).

**Table 143-3**

**Self-Treatment Options for Traveler's Diarrhea**

| *Drug* | *Recommended Doses* | *Adverse Effects* |
|---|---|---|
| Loperamide | 4 mg STAT, then 2 mg after each loose stool; max, 16 mg/day | Abdominal cramping, rarely dizziness, dry mouth, skin rash; do not use with high fever or bloody stools or for longer than 48 hours |
| Ciprofloxacin | 500 mg bid × 1–3 days | Infrequently gastrointestinal (GI) disturbance, central nervous system (CNS) effects, skin rash |
| Levofloxacin | 500 mg qd × 1–3 days | Infrequently GI disturbance, CNS effects, skin rash |
| Azithromycin | 500 mg qd × 3 days | GI disturbance, drug interactions |
| Rifaximin | 200 mg tid × 3 days or 400 mg bid × 3 days | GI disturbance, headache |

STAT, immediately; bid, twice a day; qd, once a day; tid, 3 times a day.

Modified from Diemert DJ. Prevention and self-treatment of traveler's diarrhea. *Clin Microbiol Rev*. 2006;19: 583–594, with permission from American Society for Microbiology

The drug of choice is determined as follows: if the area has chloroquine-susceptible malaria, use chloroquine; if chloroquine resistant, use mefloquine, doxycycline, or atovaquone/proguanil; if mefloquine resistant, use atovaquone/proguanil or doxycycline.

Despite proven safety and efficacy, the use of mefloquine for prophylaxis in adults has fallen out of favor.[22] It is contraindicated in persons with a history of seizures or manic-depressive illness because patients with these conditions are at an increased risk of developing neurologic and psychiatric adverse events. Atovaquone/proguanil (Malarone), a relatively new addition to the drugs available for prophylaxis, is well tolerated. The disadvantage of daily administration (versus weekly for mefloquine) is balanced by the need to continue it for 1 week after return (versus 4 weeks for mefloquine).

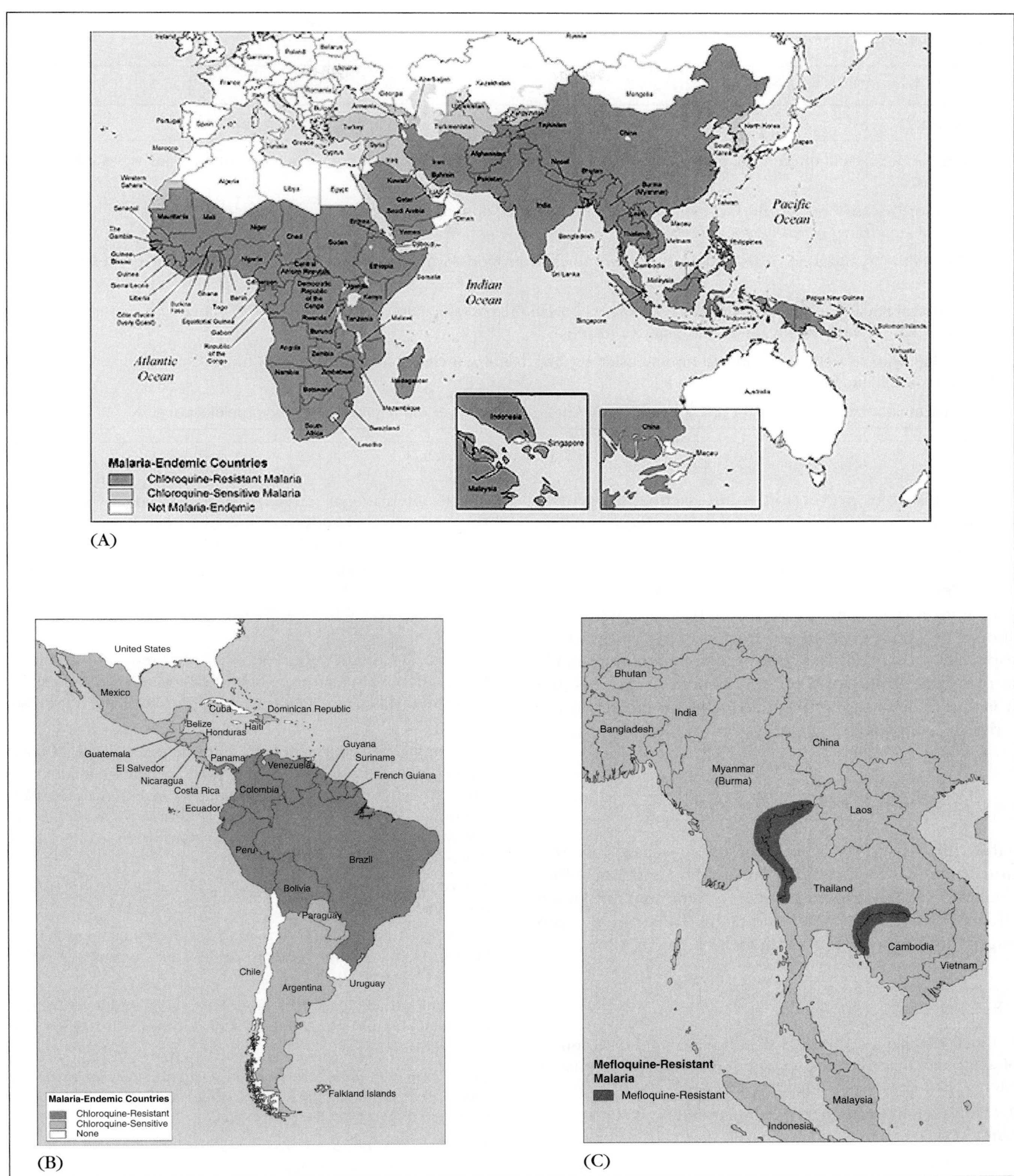


**FIGURE 143-2** Malaria-endemic countries with depiction of chloroquine- and mefloquine-resistant *falciparum* species. (A) Africa and Asia. (B) North and South America. (C) Detail of south Asia. Available at: wwwnc.cdc.gov/travel/yellowbook/2010/chapter-2/malaria.aspx#978

**Table 143-4**

**Travel Medicine Resource Examples**

| *Resource* | *Web Address* |
|---|---|
| Patient. He or she will often bring recommendations from his or her travel agent or own research. | www.tripprep.com, www.cdc.gov |
| Centers for Disease Control and Prevention (CDC). Also order or download latest version of *Health Information for International Travel (The Yellow Book)*. | www.cdc.gov/travel |
| World Health Organization (WHO). Most useful for rabies, arthropod-borne disease outbreaks. | www.who.int/ith/en/index.html |
| International Society of Travel Medicine (ISTM). Inexpensive membership-based resource that provides handy guide and practice materials. | www.ISTM.org |
| Travax EnCompass from Shoreland. Comprehensive service that also includes news and literature highlights by e-mail. | www.travax.com |
| US Department of State. Postings of disease outbreak alerts and country-specific regulations. | www.travel.state.gov |

Mosquito bite prevention is an essential preventive health measure for travel because of the large number of arthropod-borne infections besides malaria to which a traveler could be exposed. These include West Nile virus, dengue, yellow fever, JE, and Rift Valley fever. A preparation that contains between 10% and 30% DEET should be considered an essential part of the travel kit, especially because it may not be conveniently available in many countries. An additional benefit of DEET is that it is an effective tick repellent. Tickborne infections are a risk in many locations worldwide.

## LAY AND PROFESSIONAL RESOURCES

Table 143-4 lists key resources for up-to-date information, some of which can be consulted by patients before their vaccination appointment. At a minimum, the office should consult the CDC and State Department Web pages for appropriate travel advice.

## REFERENCES

1. Bloch J, Duplain H, Rimoldi SF. Prevalence and time course of acute mountain sickness in older children and adolescents after rapid ascent to 3,450 meters. *Pediatrics.* 2009;123:1–5

2. Sood SK. Immunization for children traveling abroad. *Pediatr Clin North Am.* 2000;47:435–448, viii

3. Steffen R, Kane MA, Shapiro CN, Billo N, Schoellhorn KJ, van Damme P. Epidemiology and prevention of hepatitis A in travelers. *JAMA.* 1994;272:885–889

4. Centers for Disease Control and Prevention. Update: prevention of hepatitis A after exposure to hepatitis A virus and in international travelers. Updated recommendations of the Advisory Committee on Immunization Practices (ACIP). *MMWR Morb Mortal Wkly Rep.* 2007;56:1080–1084

5. Wiktor TJ, Plotkin SA, Koprowski H. Development and clinical trials of the new human rabies vaccine of tissue culture (human diploid cell) origin. *Dev Biol Stand.* 1978; 40:3–9

6. Noah DL, Smith MG, Gotthardt JC, Krebs JW, Green D, Childs JE. Mass human exposure to rabies in New Hampshire: exposures, treatment, and cost. *Am J Public Health.* 1996;86: 1149–1151

7. Manning SE, Rupprecht CE, Fishbein D, et al. Human rabies prevention–United States, 2008: recommendations of the Advisory Committee on Immunization Practices. MMWR Recomm Rep. 2008 May 23;57(RR-3):1-28. Available at: www.cdc.gov/mmwr/preview/mmwrhtml/rr57e507a1.htm. Accessed September 15, 2010

8. Crump JA, Luby SP, Mintz ED. The global burden of typhoid fever. *Bull World Health Organ.* 2004;82:346–353

9. Steffen R, Rickenbach M, Wilhelm U, Helminger A, Schar M. Health problems after travel to developing countries. *J Infect Dis.* 1987; 156:84–91

10. Steinberg EB, Bishop R, Haber P, et al. Typhoid fever in travelers: who should be targeted for prevention? *Clin Infect Dis.* 2004;39:186–191

11. Wilson ME, Weld LH, Boggild A, et al. Fever in returned travelers: results from the GeoSentinel Surveillance Network. *Clin Infect Dis.* 2007;44:1560–1568

12. Keitel WA, Bond NL, Zahradnik JM, Cramton TA, Robbins JB. Clinical and serological responses following primary and booster immunization with *Salmonella typhi* Vi capsular polysaccharide vaccines. *Vaccine.* 1994;12:195–199

13. Cetron MS, Marfin AA, Julian KG, et al. Yellow fever vaccine. Recommendations of the Advisory Committee on

Immunization Practices (ACIP), 2002. *MMWR Recomm Rep.* 2002; 51:1-11; quiz CE1-4

14. Salzman MB, Rubin LG. Meningococcemia. *Infect Dis Clin North Am.* 1996;10:709-725

15. Centers for Disease Control and Prevention. Revised recommendations of the Advisory Committee on Immunization Practices to vaccinate all persons aged 11-18 years with meningococcal conjugate vaccine. *MMWR Morb Mortal Wkly Rep.* 2007;56:794-795

16. Arai S, Matsunaga Y, Takasaki T, et al. Japanese encephalitis: surveillance and elimination effort in Japan from 1982 to 2004. *Jpn J Infect Dis.* 2008;61:333-338

17. Tauber E, Kollaritsch H, von Sonnenburg F, et al. Randomized, double-blind, placebo-controlled phase 3 trial of the safety and tolerability of IC51, an inactivated Japanese encephalitis vaccine. *J Infect Dis.* 2008;198:493-499

18. Fischer M, Griggs A, Erin Staples J. The Pre-Travel Consultation/Travel-Related Vaccine-Preventable Diseases/ Japanese encephalitis (JE). The Yellow Book [serial on the Internet]. 2009. Available at: www.cdc.gov/travel/yellowbook/2010/chapter-2/japanese-encephalitis.aspx. Accessed February 22, 2010

19. Centers for Disease Control and Prevention. ACIP Provisional Recommendations for the Use of Japanese Encephalitis Vaccine. *MMWR.* 2010;59(RR01):1-27. Available at: www.cdc.gov/mmwr/preview/mmwrhtml/rr5901a1.htm

20. Ang JY. Traveler's diarrhea: updates for pediatricians. *Pediatr Ann.* 2008;37:814-820

21. Diemert DJ. Prevention and self-treatment of traveler's diarrhea. *Clin Microbiol Rev.* 2006;19:583-594

22. Wells TS, Smith TC, Smith B, et al. Mefloquine use and hospitalizations among US service members, 2002-2004. *Am J Trop Med Hyg.* 2006;74:744-749

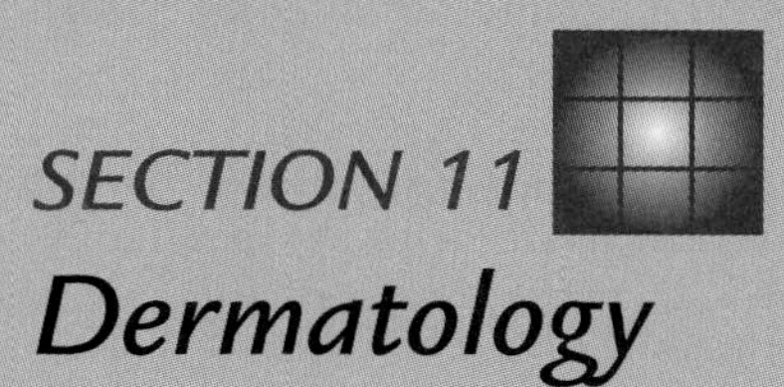

SECTION 11

# Dermatology

## CHAPTER 144

## Acne

RICHARD ANTAYA, MD • SEVERINE CHAVEL, MD

### INTRODUCTION

Acne vulgaris is a common skin disorder that usually peaks during adolescence but can be seen in children and adults. Approximately 40 to 50 million Americans between the age of 12 and 24 years have acne. The effect of acne on adolescent quality of life is not trivial. Quality of life measurements have revealed that acne patients report similar levels of psychosocial impairments as patients with diabetes, asthma, arthritis, and epilepsy.[1] These psychological and emotional issues include problems with body image, self-esteem, social withdrawal, embarrassment, anxiety, and depression. Even patients with mild to moderate acne may have significant mental health sequelae.[2] Acne scarring may have a lifelong effect on self-esteem.

### PATHOGENESIS OF ACNE

Acne vulgaris is a multifactorial disease of the sebaceous follicle, which is composed of large multilobulated sebaceous glands, a hair shaft, and a follicular canal lined by keratinized epithelium. These specialized pilosebaceous units are located primarily on the face, chest, and back. Although the exact pathogenesis of acne is still unknown, increased sebum production, follicular hyperkeratinization, *Propionibacterium acnes* colonization, and inflammation all seem to play a role in the development of acne lesions.

The current understanding of acne begins with the formation of the microcomedo, through the combination of hyperproliferation, abnormal differentiation, and altered desquamation of the corneocytes in the follicle. Obstruction of the follicular opening results from accumulation of cells in the pilosebaceous duct. The increasing pressure causes the comedo wall to rupture and spill its content into the surrounding tissue, resulting in foreign body-like inflammation.

Bacteria in the sebaceous follicle also play a role in the development of acne. *Propionibacterium acnes* are anaerobic gram-positive rods that reside deep within the sebaceous follicle and are found in increasing numbers during puberty in normal individuals and, in at least some studies, even higher numbers in acne-prone patients. During puberty, *P acnes* proliferate in the sebum-enriched environment of the sebaceous follicle and are thought to contribute to the inflammation of acne lesions through their release, directly and indirectly, of proinflammatory factors.

Sebum production is controlled by androgens, mainly testosterone, and peaks during adolescence. Although androgens are produced mainly by the gonads and the adrenal glands, androgen-metabolizing enzymes also are found in the pilosebaceous units of the skin. At the onset of adrenarche, the adrenal glands begin to release increasing levels of dehydroepiandrosterone sulfate (DHEAS), the precursor to more potent androgens, with a subsequent increase in sebum production. However, despite the appearance of comedonal acne at the onset of puberty, most patients with acne have normal hormone levels.

### CLINICAL PRESENTATION

Acne lesions are divided into noninflammatory (ie, comedones) and inflammatory lesions (ie, papules, pustules, nodules, and cysts). Microcomedones are too small to be seen clinically but become visible in the form of open or closed comedones as they enlarge. Closed comedones, or whiteheads, are approximately 1 mm skin-colored to white papules with no apparent follicular opening. They are best appreciated with palpation, gentle stretching of the skin, or observed with side lighting. On the other

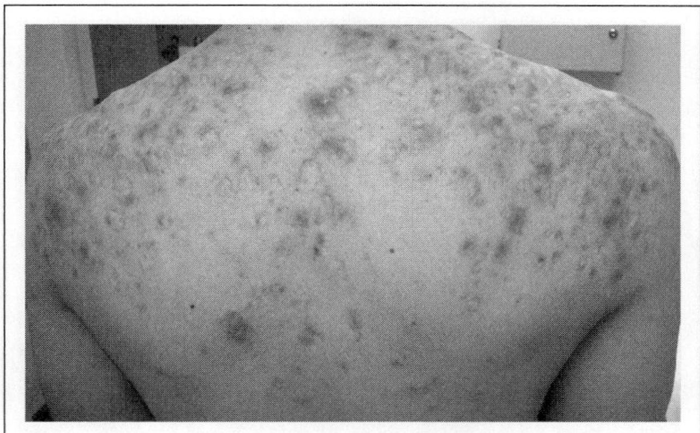

FIGURE 144-1 Acne scarring. (See color insert.)

hand, open comedones, or blackheads, are 1 mm to 2 mm lesions that are dilated follicular openings filled with packed keratin. Oxidation of melanin within the keratin debris, not dirt, causes the black discoloration seen at the opening.

The inflammatory lesions of acne are papules, pustules, nodules, and cysts, in order of increasing severity. Papules and pustules are small, erythematous, superficial lesions. Once the follicular wall ruptures in the dermis, the papules enlarge to form deeper nodules and can become increasingly tender. In severe cases, pus can occur within the nodule to form deep pustules, which have been incorrectly called "cysts" as they have no lining. Scarring may result if acne is not treated, and although it is usually seen with severe nodulocystic acne, it can also result from papulopustular acne. The types of scars usually seen are either atrophic scars (eg, depressed or ice-pick) or hypertrophic scars (Figure 144-1).

### ACNE VARIANTS

#### Acne Fulminans

Acne fulminans is a rare acne presentation characterized by the sudden onset of severe suppurative and often ulcerating acne accompanied by systemic manifestations, including fever, malaise, myalgias, and arthralgias. It usually presents in young males with a history of mild to moderate acne who abruptly develop microcomedones, followed by coalescing inflamed papules and plaques with serosanguineous crust. Of note, initiation of oral isotretinoin therapy can rarely trigger acne fulminans, whereas acute inflammatory flares without systemic symptoms are common.

#### Acne Conglobata

Acne conglobata is an uncommon severe form of acne characterized by suppurative nodulocystic acne on the face, chest, back, shoulders, upper arms, thighs, and buttocks that form sinuses and abscesses without systemic manifestations. The resulting scarring can sometimes be disfiguring.

#### Acne Excoriée

Acne excoriée is a condition seen more commonly in young women characterized by neurotic manipulation of comedonal and inflammatory acne lesions, which results in excoriations, erosions, and scarring. History-taking should include psychiatric history to look for any underlying disorders such as anxiety disorder, personality disorder, or obsessive-compulsive disorder.

#### Drug-Induced Acne

Numerous medications can cause acneiform eruptions, including corticosteroids, anabolic steroids, lithium, iodides, bromides (found in over-the-counter cold remedies), and phenytoin. Drug-induced acne is characterized by abrupt onset of monomorphous inflammatory papules or pustules on the face, back, and/or chest.

#### Acne Mechanica

Acne mechanica is acne resulting from or exacerbated by repetitive friction, pressure, and heat of the pilosebaceous unit. It is usually localized and may be linear or geometrically distributed. It may be sports-related such as acne developing under helmets, pads, straps, or headbands. Acne mechanica can also be seen on the neck of violin players.

## EVALUATION AND WORK-UP

History-taking is an important part of the evaluation of acne. Specific questions relevant to the patient with acne are outlined in Box 144-1. The physical examination should include the face, neck, upper arms, chest, and back. Assessing the acne type and severity is crucial for developing an effective treatment plan. Is the acne mainly comedonal or inflammatory? Is it mild, moderate, or severe? (See Figure 144-2, Figure 144-3, and Figure 144-4.) If mild, who is more concerned about the acne, the parent or the patient? Is there scarring? An approximate lesion count may be helpful to assess the acne severity and to measure responsiveness to treatment.

Laboratory tests such as serum androgens are not routinely ordered unless signs of hyperandrogenism, such as hirsutism, deepening of the voice in females, irregular menstrual cycles, acanthosis nigricans, androgenetic alopecia, or obesity are detected in the history or on physical examination. Other indicators of possible endocrine abnormalities are sudden onset of acne and treatment-resistant acne. If an endocrine abnormality

**Box 144-1**

***Acne-Relevant History-Taking***

- How motivated is the patient to treat the acne?
- How much does the acne affect the patient's quality of life?
- Which over-the-counter or prescription medications for acne has the patient used in the past?
- What is the patient's current skin care routine?
- Does the patient have sensitive skin?
- Does the patient use cosmetics and/or hair products?
- Does the patient have other medical problems?
- Is the patient taking any medications (specifically, oral contraceptives, corticosteroids, anabolic steroids, lithium, halogen-containing medication)?
- What are the patient's hobbies and occupational activities, including sports? Does he/she wear a helmet, hat, or chin strap?

Female specific:

- Does the patient's acne worsen premenstrually?
- Is the patient using oral contraception?
- Is there any history of irregular menstrual cycles, hirsutism, or deepening of the voice?

is suspected, serum levels of free testosterone, total testosterone, DHEAS, and luteinizing hormone (LH) and follicule-stimulating hormone (FSH) ratio can be useful in determining the source of androgens. Of note, oral contraceptives should be discontinued 4 to 6 weeks before the endocrine evaluation because they can mask underlying hyperandrogenism.[3]

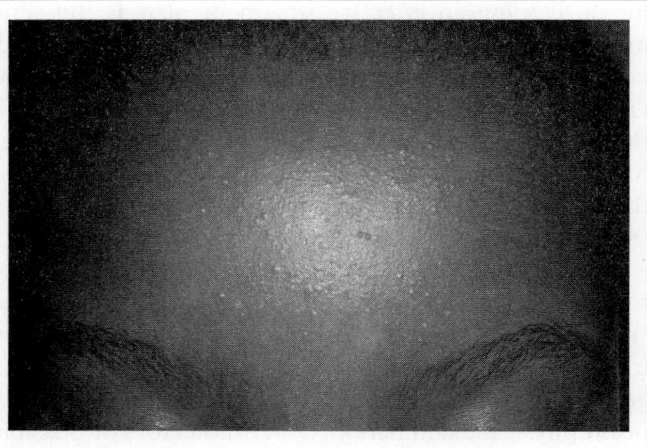

FIGURE 144-2 Mild comedonal acne. (See color insert.)

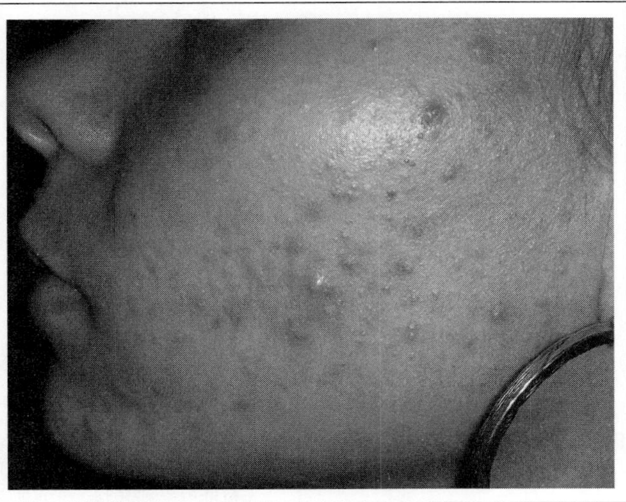

FIGURE 144-3 Moderate papulopustular acne. (See color insert.)

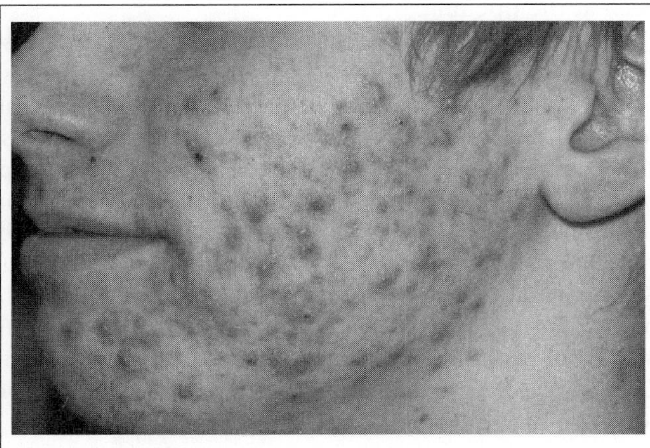

FIGURE 144-4 Severe papulopustular/nodular acne. (See color insert.)

## DIFFERENTIAL DIAGNOSIS OF ACNE

The differential diagnosis of comedonal acne includes milia, keratosis pilaris, and nevus comedonicus. The inflammatory lesions of acne need to be differentiated from folliculitis (staphylococcal, gram-negative, or eosinophilic), keratosis pilaris, perioral dermatitis, neurotic excoriations, angiofibromas (as seen with tuberous sclerosis), and scars. A medication history and physical examination can help distinguish between acne vulgaris and acne caused by systemic corticosteroids or anabolic steroids.

## TREATMENT

### APPROACH TO TREATMENT

An approach to treatment depending on the severity of the patient's acne is shown in Figure 144-5. Mild acne should be treated with topical therapy whereas moderate to severe acne warrants a combination of topical and oral therapy. The common topical and oral treatments used for acne vulgaris, their dosage, preparations, and side effects are outlined in Table 144-1. Patients should return in approximately 3 months to assess the success or failure of therapy, or earlier if side effects or worsening of acne occurs (unless expected, as in worsening of acne after initiation of topical retinoids).

### PATIENT EDUCATION

The successful treatment of acne relies considerably on the motivation and adherence of the patient. It is therefore important when treating adolescents with acne to explain in simple terms the causes of acne and the different roles of medications used to treat acne. Adherence might be improved if the patient understands the reasoning behind the treatment. The physician also needs to set appropriate expectations by explaining the length of treatment, the side effects of the different medications, and the importance of adherence to see results. The patient should be counseled on behaviors that may exacerbate acne. The use of cosmetics, sunscreen, and moisturizers should be limited to noncomedogenic,

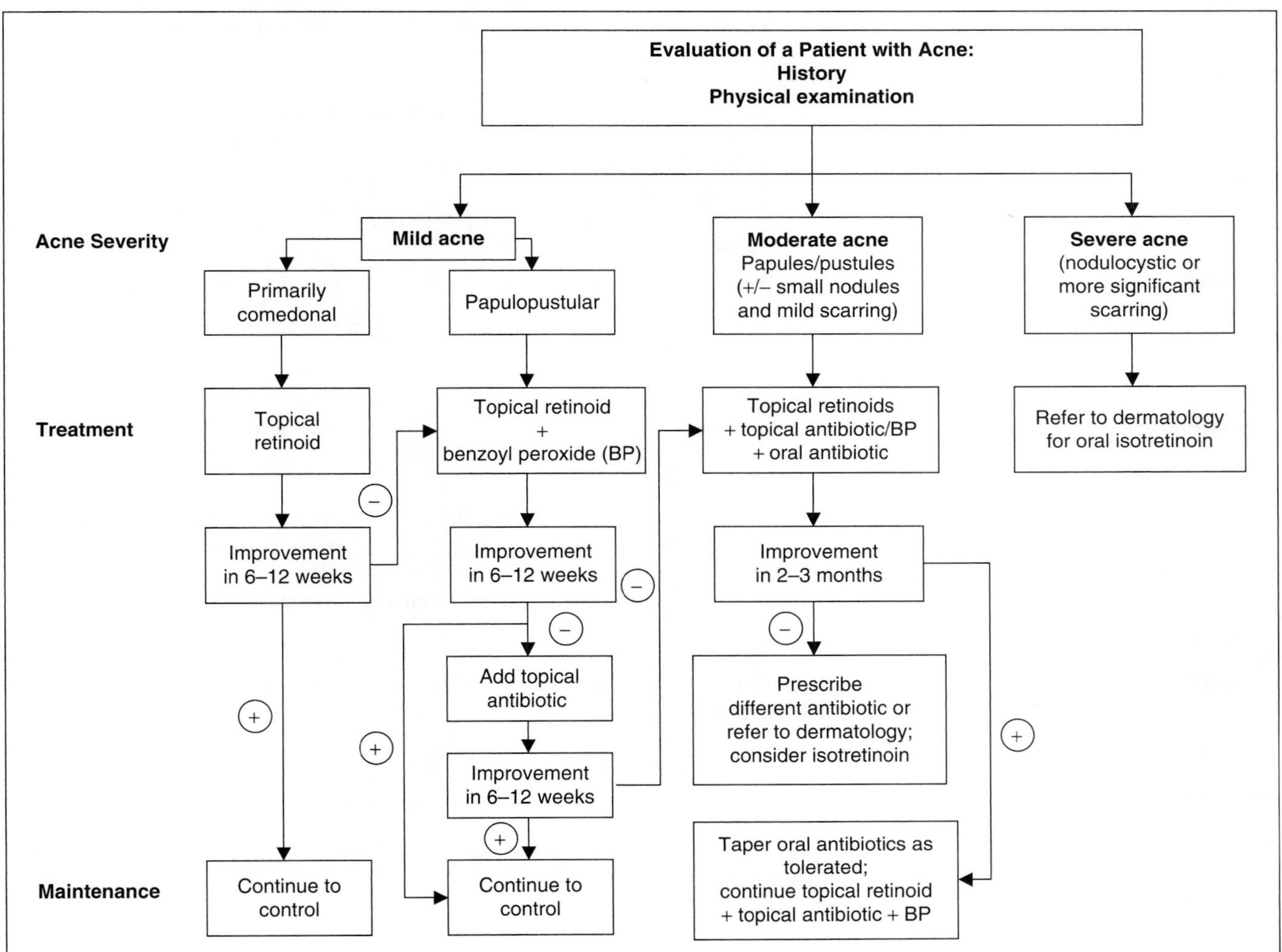


FIGURE 144-5 Treatment algorithm for acne.

**Table 144-1**

**Topical Treatments for Acne**

| *Topical Agent* | *Dose* | *Preparation* | *Concentration (%)* | *Side Effects/Considerations* |
|---|---|---|---|---|
| **Retinoids** | | | | |
| Tretinoin | qhs | Cream,<br>gel,<br>solution,<br>gel/microsponge | 0.02, 0.025, 0.05, 0.1%<br>0.01, 0.025%<br>0.05%<br>0.04, 0.1% | Erythema and dryness, increased sunburn and wind burn, inactivated by sunlight |
| Adapalene | qam or qpm | Gel,<br>solution, cream,<br>swab | All 0.1% | Erythema, scaling, increased sunburn and wind burn, bleaching of clothing and bedding |
| Adapalene/ benzoyl peroxide | qd | Gel | 0.1%/2.5% | Increased sunburn and wind burn, bleaching of clothing and bedding |
| Tazarotene | qhs | Gel,<br>cream | 0.05, 0.1%<br>0.05, 0.1% | Erythema, scaling, increased sunburn and wind burn |
| **Antimicrobials** | | | | |
| Benzoyl peroxide | qd or bid | Gel,<br>cream,<br>lotion,<br>shaving cream,<br>pad,<br>cleanser | 2.5, 3, 4, 5, 6, 7, 8, 9, 10%<br>2.5, 5, 10%<br>2.5, 4, 5, 5.5, 8, 10%<br>5, 10%<br>3, 4.5, 6, 6.5, 8.5, 9, 10%<br>4, 5, 8, 10% | Bleaching of clothing and bedding, dryness and erythema |
| Clindamycin | qd or bid | Solution,<br>foam,<br>gel,<br>lotion,<br>pad | All 1% | May develop resistance |
| Erythromycin | qd or bid | Solution,<br>gel,<br>swab | All 2% | May develop resistance |
| Benzoyl peroxide (BP)/ clindamycin or BP/erythromycin | qd or bid<br>qd | Gel | 2.5% or 5% BP/1% clindamycin<br>5% BP/3% erythromycin | Found to be more effective than antibiotics alone, decreased development of resistance |
| **Other** | | | | |
| Azelaic acid | qd or bid | Gel,<br>cream | 15%<br>20% | Well tolerated |

(*Continued*)

**Table 144-1 (Continued)**

| *Topical Agent* | *Dose* | *Preparation* | *Concentration (%)* | *Side Effects/Considerations* |
|---|---|---|---|---|
| **Other** | | | | |
| Sulfur/sodium sulfacetamide | qd or bid | Cream, lotion | 5%/10% | Well tolerated |
| Salicylic acid | qd or bid | Cream,<br>solution,<br>gel,<br>lotion,<br>foam,<br>patch,<br>stick | 0.5, 2, 2.5, 6%<br>2%<br>2, 3, 5, 6, 17%<br>0.5, 0.6, 1.5, 2, 3, 6%<br>2%<br>0.5, 1, 2%<br>1.25, 2% | Well tolerated |
| Dapsone | bid | Gel | 5% | Oiliness/peeling, erythema, dryness |

bid, twice a day; qam, every morning; qd, daily; qhs, at bedtime; qpm every evening

oil-free products. Picking and squeezing acne lesions should be discouraged to avoid causing inflammation, infection, and scar formation. Identifying possible environmental or occupational factors, such as the use of helmets in sports or after-school jobs with exposures to greases or oils (ie, fast-food restaurants or gas stations) can direct changes in behavior.

## TOPICAL THERAPY

The commonly used topical treatments for acne include topical retinoids, benzoyl peroxide, topical antibiotics, and azelaic acid (Table 144-1).

### Topical Retinoids

Topical retinoids should be used as first-line therapy for mild to moderate acne because they target the microcomedo—the precursor of comedonal and inflammatory acne.They have been shown to correct the abnormalities in follicular keratinization, expulse existing comedones, and prevent new comedo formation. The available topical retinoids in the United States are tretinoin, adapalene, and tazarotene (Table 144-1).

Tretinoin was the first topical retinoid to be used in the treatment of acne and was shown to reduce the number of comedones and inflammatory lesions. The original formulation of tretinoin is associated with moderate irritation of the skin, which can be decreased by initiating treatment at a low concentration and decreasing the frequency of application. The patient should be instructed to start applying the topical retinoid every other night or third night initially and then increase the frequency as tolerated over 2 to 3 weeks. Newer formulations of tretinoin have been developed to decrease skin irritation, including tretinoin microsphere (Retin-A micro) and 0.025% tretinoin cream containing polyolprepolymer-2 (Avita).[4] Topical tretinoin degrades with sunlight and oxidation; therefore, nighttime application is preferred. Benzoyl peroxide should be applied in the morning if both treatments are used concurrently. Photosensitivity may result from irritation of the skin and thinning of the stratum corneum, and patients should use sunscreen during the day. To ensure adherence, patients should be warned that initial worsening of the acne 2 to 4 weeks after initiation of tretinoin may occur before improvements are seen.

Although studies have not shown an increased risk of birth defects in children born to women using topical tretinoin during the first trimester of pregnancy, its similarity to isotretinoin raises concerns about potential teratogenicity and its use is discouraged in pregnancy. It is listed as a pregnancy category D drug.

Adapalene (Differin) is a naphthoic acid derivative that possesses retinoid-like activities, which has been shown to have equivalent efficacy as tretinoin with improved skin tolerability.[5] Because of its improved cutaneous irritation profile compared to tretinoin, it may be more suited for individuals with dark skin who are more likely to experience hyperpigmentation after inflammation. Unlike tretinoin, adapalene is photostable and does not oxidize with benzoyl peroxide. Adapalene is listed as a pregnancy category C drug.

Tazarotene is a receptor-specific retinoid. Once daily and short contact applications (3–5 minute application and rinse off) of topical tazarotene have been shown to be safe and effective for comedonal and inflammatory acne. Similar to all retinoids, the main side effect is skin irritation. Contraceptive counseling in women of child-bearing age is necessary with topical tazarotene, as it has been labeled a pregnancy category X drug.

### Benzoyl Peroxide

Benzoyl peroxide is a bactericidal agent that reduces the number of *P acnes* through the release of free oxygen radicals in the sebaceous follicle. It is used in acne for its anti-inflammatory property. Benzoyl peroxide alone or with clindamycin or erythromycin has been shown to be as effective as oral tetracycline or minocycline in treating mild to moderate facial acne.[6] Contrary to topical antibiotics, benzoyl peroxide has not been associated with bacterial resistance. Over-the-counter and prescription-strength formulations are available in multiple concentrations and vehicles (see Table 144-1). Patients should be warned about the bleaching effect of benzoyl peroxide on clothing and bedding. Its major side effect is irritation, presenting as redness and scaling, which can be improved by decreasing the frequency and/or concentration of the product and/or choosing a water-based instead of alcohol-based product. Allergic contact dermatitis to benzoyl peroxide has been reported.

### Topical Antibiotics

Topical antibiotics, mainly erythromycin and clindamycin, are commonly used in the treatment of mild to moderate acne, alone or with benzoyl peroxide. The different preparations and concentrations are found in Table 144-1. They are generally well tolerated without significant side effects. The rising incidence of antibiotic resistant *P acnes* is an important problem in acne treatment. The use of benzoyl peroxide with topical antibiotics such as erythromycin has been shown to reduce the pattern of bacterial resistance to topical antibiotics.[7] The addition of benzoyl peroxide in combination therapy is thought to reduce the number of resistant organisms as well as counteract the selection of erythromycin-resistant strains.[8] Some studies have shown improved efficacy when a combination of topical benzoyl peroxide and clindamycin gels were used compared with benzoyl peroxide or clindamycin gel alone.[9,10]

### Second-Line Topical Therapy

Salicylic acid, azelaic acid, and sodium sulfacetamide/sulfur preparations are used as alternative topical treatments for acne.

Salicylic acid, a β-hydroxyacid, has mild keratolytic and anti-inflammatory properties and is found in over-the-counter preparations to treat mild comedonal acne. No side effects are reported. Azelaic acid is a dicarboxylic acid with antikeratinizing and antibacterial properties. It is therefore useful for comedonal and inflammatory acne. One study found that 20% azelaic acid cream had comparable efficacy in treating comedonal acne as 0.05% tretinoin cream and caused less irritation.[11] Azelaic acid may also be helpful in reducing the postinflammatory hyperpigmentation seen in some acne patients.[12] Sodium sulfacetamide is a topical antibiotic used alone or in combination with sulfur to limit the growth of *P acnes*.

## ORAL THERAPY

The indications for systemic therapy are outlined in Box 144-2. Oral treatments for acne vulgaris include oral antibiotics, hormonal therapy, and oral retinoids. As expected, systemic acne therapies have more side effects than topical treatments. Counseling patients on possible adverse reactions with oral acne medications should be done before initiating therapy.

### Oral Antibiotics

Oral antibiotics are usually prescribed for moderate to severe inflammatory acne. Erythromycin and tetracycline, and the derivatives doxycycline and minocycline, suppress *P acnes* growth and therefore have anti-inflammatory properties in the treatment of acne. Erythromycin is currently used less frequently than tetracycline and its derivatives due to the higher rate of *P acnes* resistance.[13] The dose, duration, and adverse effects of oral antibiotics prescribed for acne are summarized in Table 144-2.

Tetracycline, and its lipophilic derivatives doxycycline and minocycline, prevent *P acnes* growth by binding to the 30S ribosomal subunit and subsequently block bacterial protein synthesis. Tetracycline is usually prescribed as 500 mg twice a day (adult doses) and should be taken 1 hour before or 2 hours after eating, and its absorption may be decreased by polyvalent cations (eg, iron, zinc, calcium). This constraint may compromise adherence in adolescent patients. Tetracycline may cause gastrointestinal upset and vaginal yeast infections in women. It

**Box 144-2**

***Indications for Systemic Therapy***

- Moderate to severe acne
- Scarring
- Postinflammatory hyperpigmentation
- Widespread distribution (back, chest, shoulders)
- Significant effect on quality of life
- Failure of topical medications

**Table 144-2**

**Oral Antibiotics for Acne**

| *Antibiotic* | *Dosage* | *Duration* | *Adverse Effects* | *Comments* |
|---|---|---|---|---|
| Tetracycline | 250–500 mg twice a day | 3–4 months | Gastrointestinal upset<br>Vaginal candidiasis<br>Photosensitivity | Need to take on empty stomach<br>Resistance<br>Inexpensive<br>Cannot be used in pregnant girls |
| Doxycycline | 50–100 mg twice a day | 3–4 months | Photosensitivity<br>Gastrointestinal upset<br>Esophageal ulceration | Can take with food<br>Certain preparations less irritating to gastrointestinal tract<br>Cannot be used in pregnant girls |
| Minocycline | 50–100 mg once or twice a day | 3–4 months | Dizziness, vertigo<br>Hyperpigmentation of skin/ oral mucosa/teeth<br>Pseudotumor cerebri<br>Drug-induced lupus<br>Autoimmune hepatitis | Can take with food<br>Expensive<br>Certain preparations irritate GI tract less<br>Cannot be used in pregnant girls |
| Erythromycin | 250–500 mg 2-4 times a day | 3–4 months | Gastrointestinal upset<br>Vaginal candidiasis | Inexpensive<br>Take on empty stomach<br>Resistance |
| Trimethoprim-sulfamethoxazole | One dose twice a day (160 mg/ 800 mg) | 3–4 months | Allergic eruption<br>Toxic epidermal necrolysis/ Stevens-Johnson syndrome<br>Pancytopenia | Inexpensive |
| Trimethoprim | 300 mg twice a day | 3–4 months | Allergic eruption | Inexpensive |

should not be prescribed to pregnant women or children younger than 9 years old to avoid delayed bone growth and tooth discoloration in the fetus or child.

Doxycycline and minocycline are usually prescribed as 50 mg to 100 mg twice a day. They can be taken with food, which may increase adherence. Photosensitivity can be seen with all the tetracyclines, but is more commonly associated with doxycycline. Minocycline is thought to have the least *P acnes* resistance of the tetracyclines. However, minocycline has a greater tendency than tetracycline or doxycycline to cause rare side effects, such as pseudotumor cerebri, hypersensitivity reaction, serum sickness-like reaction, dizziness, and vertigo. Unlike the other tetracyclines, rarely minocycline can also cause drug-induced lupus and hyperpigmentation of the skin over time. A Cochrane system database review[14] in 2000 on the clinical efficacy of minocycline in the treatment of inflammatory acne vulgaris could not reliably determine its efficacy relative to other acne therapies due to the lack of randomized controlled trials.

Alternatives to tetracycline and its derivatives are erythromycin and trimethoprim with or without sulfamethoxazole. Erythromycin, a macrolide antibiotic, is a bacteriostatic inhibitor of bacterial protein synthesis. The most common adverse effect is gastrointestinal upset, which can be improved by taking the medications with food, but may compromise absorption. Erythromycin is usually prescribed as 500 mg twice a day. It is currently used less frequently in the United States because of *P acnes* resistance. Trimethoprim with or without sulfamethoxazole can also be used as a second line agent. The most common adverse effect is drug eruption.

The need for a second form of contraception in women using oral contraceptives (OCs) and oral antibiotics is still controversial. A conservative approach is recommended.

### Hormonal Therapy

Hormonal therapy can be useful to treat acne in women with hyperandrogenism, but also in women with normal serum androgen levels. Three OCs are currently approved by the Food and Drug Administration (FDA) for the treatment of acne: norgestimate-ethinyl-estradiol (Ortho-Tri-cyclen), norethindrone acetate-ethinyl estradiol (Estrostep), and drospirenone-ethinyl estradiol (Yaz). Oral contraceptives contain estrogen (usually ethinyl estradiol) and progestin. Estrogen in OCs is thought to improve acne by decreasing the circulating androgen levels. It causes an increase in levels of sex hormone-binding globulin, which in turn decrease circulating free testosterone levels and indirectly decrease sebum production. The progestin drospirenone has antiandrogenic activity similar to that of spironolactone. The hormones in OCs also prevent ovulation by suppressing luteinizing hormone and follicular stimulating hormone secretions by the anterior pituitary through negative feedback. The lack of ovulation decreases androgen levels and subsequently sebum production.

Adolescents found to have severe acne exacerbated by endocrine abnormalities will generally be treated with hormonal therapy. Ovarian androgen blockers, such as oral contraceptives, are one of many options to choose. Androgen receptor blockers (eg, spironolactone), glucocorticoids, and gonadotropin-releasing agonists are other types of hormonal therapies that might be indicated. Management of patients with endocrine abnormalities will usually be shared by endocrinologists and gynecologists.

### Isotretinoin

Isotretinoin, or 13-*cis* retinoic acid, was approved by the FDA in 1983 for the treatment of severe recalcitrant nodular acne that is unresponsive to conventional therapy, including systemic antibiotics. Indications for use of oral isotretinoin are outlined in Box 144-3. Isotretinoin causes sebaceous gland atrophy and reduction of sebum production by up to 90%. Dosing is usually 0.5 to 2.0 mg/kg/day for 15 to 20 weeks. It is better absorbed if taken with a fatty meal. The main side effects of isotretinoin are outlined in Box 144-4, the most common being dry skin and cheilitis. Due to its association with teratogenicity and possible lipid and liver abnormalities, patients need close monitoring while on the medication. Furthermore, the FDA issued a warning in 1998 about a possible increased risk for depression, suicidal ideation, and psychosis while on isotretinoin. No conclusive evidence has been found to date. Since March 2006, all wholesalers, prescribers, pharmacies, and patients involved with isotretinoin need to register in the iPLEDGE program, which came about to minimize the number of pregnancy exposures to isotretinoin.

**Box 144-4**

***Side Effects of Oral Isotretinoin***

Common:

- Dry skin, cheilitis, retinoid dermatitis (red, scaly patches mostly on extremities)
- Myalgia, arthralgia, back pain
- Epistaxis
- Dry eyes, conjunctivitis
- Clinically insignificant increase in serum triglyceride and occasionally cholesterol levels

Less common:

- Decreased night vision
- Mild mood changes
- Clinically significant increase in serum triglyceride levels

Rare:

- Pseudotumor cerebri
- Depression, violent behavior
- Severe, symptomatic elevation in serum triglyceride levels
- Pancreatitis
- Hair loss

Very rare:

- Hepatotoxicity
- Anaphylaxis
- Hearing impairment or tinnitus
- Inflammatory bowel disease
- Neutropenia

**Box 144-3**

***Indications for Use of Oral Isotretinoin***

- Severe nodulocystic acne
- Acne associated with scarring
- Acne unresponsive to appropriate combined oral antibiotic and topical treatment

## SURGICAL TREATMENTS

Comedo extraction has been used in conjunction with a topical retinoid or other comedolytic agent to aid in treatment. Reports of treatment with light electrocautery and electrofulguration can be found in the literature. Intralesional injection of corticosteroid can be used for deep, inflamed nodules and cysts to improve cosmetic appearance and accelerate healing. Low-concentration chemical peels may help reduce the number of comedones. A few small studies have shown that diode laser and photodynamic therapy might be efficacious treatments for otherwise resistant inflammatory acne.[15,16]

**WHEN TO REFER TO DERMATOLOGY**

Adolescents with mild to moderate acne can first be managed by their primary care physician using the simple guidelines outlined in this chapter. A referral to a dermatologist should be initiated for refractory acne that does not respond to treatment, severe acne, such as nodulocystic acne, or any form of acne that is causing significant scarring. Patients who might require oral isotretinoin should be referred to a dermatologist as early as possible.

## REFERENCES


1. Mallon E, Newton JN, Klassen A, Stewart-Brown SL, Ryan TJ, Finlay AY. The quality of life in acne: a comparison with general medical conditions using generic questionnaires. *Br J Dermatol.* 1999;140:672–676

2. Gupta MA, Gupta AK. Depression and suicidal ideation in dermatology patients with acne, alopecia areata, atopic dermatitis and psoriasis. *Br J Dermatol.* 1998;139:846–850

3. Thiboutot DM. Endocrinological evaluation and hormonal therapy for women with difficult acne. *J Eur Acad Dermatol Venereol.* 2001;15:57–61

4. Lucky AW, Cullen SI, Funicella T, Jarratt MT, Jones T, Reddick ME. Double-blind, vehicle-controlled, multicenter comparison of 2 0.025% tretinoin creams in patients with acne vulgaris. *J Am Acad Dermatol.* 1998;38:S24–S30

5. Cunliffe WJ, Poncet M, Loesche C, Verschoore M. A comparison of the efficacy and tolerability of adapalene 0.1% gel versus tretinoin 0.025% gel in patients with acne vulgaris: a meta-analysis of five randomized trials. *Br J Dermatol.* 1998;139:48–56

6. Ozolins M, Eady EA, Avery AJ, et al. Comparison of five antimicrobial regimens for treatment of mild to moderate inflammatory facial acne vulgaris in the community: randomised controlled trial. *Lancet.* 2004;364:2188–2195

7. Harkaway KS, McGinley KJ, Foglia AN, et al. Antibiotic resistance patterns in coagulase-negative staphylococci after treatment with topical erythromycin, benzoyl peroxide, and combination therapy. *Br J Dermatol.* 1992;126:586–590

8. Eady EA, Farmery MR, Ross JI, Cove JH, Cunliffe WJ. Effects of benzoyl peroxide and erythromycin alone and in combination against antibiotic-sensitive and -resistant skin bacteria from acne patients. *Br J Dermatol.* 1994;131:331–336

9. Leyden JJ, Hickman JG, Jarratt MT, Stewart DM, Levy SF. The efficacy and safety of a combination benzoyl peroxide/clindamycin topical gel compared with benzoyl peroxide alone and a benzoyl peroxide/erythromycin combination product. *J Cutan Med Surg.* 2001;5:37–42

10. Lookingbill DP, Chalker DK, Lindholm JS, et al. Treatment of acne with a combination clindamycin/benzoyl peroxide gel compared with clindamycin gel, benzoyl peroxide gel and vehicle gel: combined results of 2 double-blind investigations. *J Am Acad Dermatol.* 1997;37:590–595

11. Katsambas A, Graupe K, Stratigos J. Clinical studies of 20% azelaic acid cream in the treatment of acne vulgaris. Comparison with vehicle and topical tretinoin. *Acta Derm Venereol Suppl.* 1989;143:35–39

12. Shemer A, Weiss G, Amichai B, Kaplan B, Trau H. Azelaic acid (20%) cream in the treatment of acne vulgaris. *J Eur Acad Dermatol Venereol.* 2002;16:178–179

13. Coates P, Vyakrnam S, Eady EA, Jones CE, Cove JH, Cunliffe WJ. Prevalence of antibiotic-resistant propionibacteria on the skin of acne patients: 10-year surveillance data and snapshot distribution study. *Br J Dermatol.* 2002;146:840–848

14. Garner SE, Eady EA, Popescu C, Newton J, Li WA. Minocycline for acne vulgaris: efficacy and safety. *Cochrane Database Syst Rev.* 2003;(1):CD002086. Review

15. Friedman PM, Jih MH, Kimyai-Asadi A, Goldberg LH. Treatment of inflammatory facial acne vulgaris with the 1450-nm diode laser: a pilot study. *Dermatol Surg.* 2004;30:147–151

16. Wiegell SR, Wulf HC. Photodynamic therapy of acne vulgaris using methyl aminolaevulinate: a blind, randomized, controlled trial. *Br J Dermatol.* 2006;154:969–976

# CHAPTER 145

# Dermatitis and Papulosquamous Diseases

ALBERT C. YAN, MD • DIONNE LOUIS, MD

## INTRODUCTION

The terms *eczema* and *dermatitis* are often used synonymously to signify a skin rash that is characterized by various degrees of erythema, the presence of macules and papules, lichenification, scaling, and exudate. Pruritus may or may not be present. This chapter focuses on the more common and important forms of dermatitis that affect adolescents, including atopic dermatitis (AD), contact dermatitis (CD), and seborrheic dermatitis. Papulosquamous disorders such as pityriasis rosea (PR) and psoriasis are also reviewed as part of this section.

## ATOPIC DERMATITIS

Atopic dermatitis is a common inflammatory skin disorder characterized by pruritus, a typical morphology and distribution, and a chronic and relapsing course that remits in the majority of patients. Many patients also suffer from related atopic disorders, such as asthma and allergic rhinitis. Those affected often exhibit a predisposition to secondary skin infections, sleep disturbances, impaired social interactions, and, in more severe cases, alterations in normal growth and development. Although 75% to 90% of children see marked improvement in severity by age 10 to 14 years, a sizable minority of patients continue to suffer into adolescence and adulthood, and a proportion of those who had experienced childhood remission may suffer occasional relapses as teenagers or adults, particularly on acral sites.[1,2]

The etiology of AD is multifactorial, and involves interactions between an abnormal skin barrier, dysregulation of the immune response, genetic factors, and exposure to environmental agents. Skin barrier dysfunction appears to play a critical role in the pathogenesis of AD. Homozygous null mutations in the gene encoding filaggrin, a key protein in the stratum corneum, have been strongly associated with ichthyosis vulgaris, AD, and asthma.[3] Likewise, mutations in the gene encoding collagen XXIX have been linked to AD.[4] Presumably, an impaired skin barrier provides entry of environmental allergens into the systemic circulation that may then sensitize and predispose to development of bronchiolar hyperreactivity and allergic rhinitis as part of the so-called atopic march.[5] This "outside-in" conceptualization notwithstanding, it is clear that intrinsic immunologic abnormalities may also trigger cutaneous manifestations in understanding AD as an "inside-out" phenomenon. Abnormalities in immune regulation, particularly of Th2 and Th1 cells; disturbed phosphodiesterase activity and fatty acid metabolism; and suppression of antimicrobial peptide production also play key roles in the pathogenesis of AD.

Foods have also been implicated as relevant triggering factors in AD in 5% to 30% of children and are more common among severe atopics.[6] The most common food allergens are egg, soy, milk, wheat, fish, shellfish, and peanut, which together account for 90% of food-induced cases of AD in double-blind placebo-controlled food challenges. Fortunately, many food allergies remit after children reach 1 year of age, eliminating the need for long-term restrictive diets. Radioallergosorbent (RAST) testing and skin prick testing can be performed to evaluate patients for food allergies relevant to AD. Although these may frequently produce false-positive results, the negative predictive value of these studies is excellent.

Patients with AD share pruritus as a common complaint that is often more severe at night. This symptom typically precedes the skin manifestations, hence the popular attribution "the itch that rashes." Along with pruritus, patients with AD show early onset of their disease, a typical age-dependent distribution and morphology, a positive family history of other atopic disorders, and other supportive clinical manifestations.[7] In infancy, AD is often widespread, with an exudative erythema with scaling located on the face and extremities, as well as the neck, torso, and scalp. Characteristic sparing of the nose, perinasal folds, and diaper area is classic. By later childhood and adolescence, the dermatitis often subsides and localizes to flexural creases—antecubital, popliteal, posterior thighs, wrist, ankle, neck—as well as to the hands (Figure 145-1). Previously spared due to the occlusive nature of the diaper, the buttocks are frequently involved as well. Some patients present with a nummular variant of AD in which coin-shaped areas of erythema, scaling, and lichenification predominate (Figure 145-2).

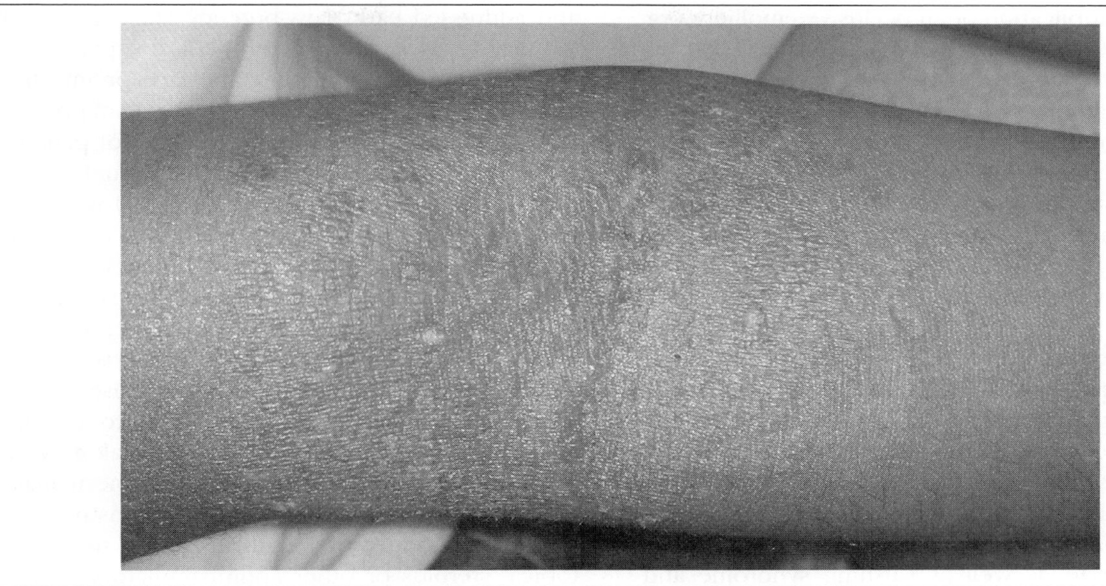

**FIGURE 145-1** Antecubital involvement in atopic dermatitis. (See color insert.)

**FIGURE 145-2** Nummular eczema. (See color insert.)

Patients with AD have a predilection for colonization and infection by both bacterial and viral organisms, especially *Staphylococcus aureus*, herpes simplex virus, and molluscum contagiosum virus. The propensity for microbial colonization within AD patients is likely multifactorial, a combination of impaired skin integrity permitting a favorable environment for adherence of organisms and a disease-associated suppression in the production of antimicrobial skin peptides. Certain bacterial superantigens are known to bind glucocorticoid receptors, and as a result, patients with significant bacterial colonization may exhibit steroid resistance or tachyphylaxis.[8]

Most patients with AD are successfully managed in the outpatient setting, although severe acute flares associated with superinfection may require hospitalization. Treatment goals include optimizing atopic skin care, controlling pruritus and cutaneous inflammation, avoiding exacerbating factors, and addressing secondary infection.

Controversy exists regarding the optimal frequency for bathing. Although some physicians advocate increased frequency and duration of baths to reduce exposure to environmental allergens and hydrate the skin ("the wet school"), others have argued that increased bathing alters normal skin pH and reduces the presence of natural skin proteins (eg, ceramides) that help maintain skin hydration status ("the dry school"). The choice of a wet versus dry approach depends on the clinician's individual expertise and experience, as well as on the motivation of the individual patient and family. Most teenagers are unwilling to avoid bathing every day, so informing them that shorter lukewarm showers are preferable to long, hot baths will help. Following use of a mild soap (eg, Tone) or syndet (eg, Aveeno, Caress, Cetaphil, Dove, Oil of Olay), the skin should be lightly patted to remove excess moisture, and then followed by the immediate application of an occlusive emollient (eg, Absorbase, Acid Mantle Cream, Aquaphor, Aveeno cream, Cerave cream, Cetaphil cream, Eucerin cream, petrolatum) over the entire skin surface.

Antihistamines are widely used as a therapeutic adjunct in patients with AD to treat pruritus, although the evidence supporting their use is relatively weak. However, when used, sedating antihistamines such as hydroxyzine, diphenhydramine, and doxepin appear to be more effective at moderating itch than less sedating antihistamines.

Topical corticosteroids (TCS) are the mainstay of treatment of AD. These medications reduce inflammation and pruritus primarily by inhibiting the transcriptional activity of various proinflammatory genes. The selection of the TCS should be based on the age of the patient, anatomic site being treated, and severity of disease. Steroid-related adverse effects include cutaneous atrophy and striae, as well as Cushing syndrome and hypothalamic-pituitary-adrenal axis suppression. Fortunately, most adverse effects are reversible if identified and addressed early. Low-potency TCS (classes VII and VI) may be used safely under medical supervision on all areas of the body, including the face or intertriginous areas for short periods of time. Medium-potency TCS (classes V, IV, and III) may be necessary for patients with more active disease. These agents should be avoided on the face and intertriginous areas and warrant closer medical supervision. Nummular eczema lesions often require treatment with medium-potency TCS because lower-potency agents are often ineffective for this variant of eczema. High-potency TCS (classes II and I) may be considered for short-term supervised use on the hands and feet for more recalcitrant disease on these acral surfaces. The use of *systemic* steroids should be avoided in patients who suffer from AD alone whenever possible. If steroids are necessary for the management of other comorbid conditions such as asthma, the steroids should be tapered gradually over 7 to 14 days, and topical steroids or other antiinflammatory agents instituted as part of the regimen to minimize the potential rebound flares (Table 145-1).

**Table 145-1**

**Atopic Dermatitis Topical Therapies**

| *Type* | *Examples* |
|---|---|
| **Topical Corticosteroids** | |
| Low potency (Classes VI and VII) | Alclometasone 0.05% cream, ointment<br>Desonide 0.05% cream, foam, hydrogel, ointment<br>Fluocinolone 0.01% oil, shampoo, solution<br>Hydrocortisone 1%, 2.5% cream, ointment |
| Medium potency (Classes IV and V) | Fluocinolone 0.025% cream, ointment<br>Fluticasone 0.05% cream, lotion<br>Hydrocortisone valerate 0.2%, butyrate 0.1% cream, ointment<br>Mometasone 0.1% cream<br>Prednicarbate cream, ointment<br>Triamcinolone 0.025% cream, ointment |
| High potency (Classes II and III) | Betamethasone valerate 0.1% cream, lotion, ointment<br>Fluticasone 0.005% ointment<br>Mometasone 0.1% ointment<br>Triamcinolone 0.1% cream, ointment |
| Ultrahigh potency (Classes I and II) | Betamethasone diproprionate cream, ointment<br>Clobetasol 0.05% cream, lotion, ointment, shampoo, solution<br>Desoximetasone 0.05% cream, ointment<br>Fluocinonide 0.05%, 0.1% cream, ointment |
| **Topical Calcineurin Inhibitors** | Pimecrolimus 1% cream<br>Tacrolimus 0.03%, 0.1% ointment |
| **Barrier Repair Products** | MAS063DP (glycerrhetinic acid, hyaluronic acid, telmestine, and others in hydrolipidic cream—Atopiclair)<br>Palmitimide MEA (MimyX)<br>Ceramide-dominant barrier creams (TriCeram, EpiCeram) |

The topical calcineurin inhibitors Protopic (tacrolimus) and Elidel (pimecrolimus) are effective in the treatment of AD. These macrolide immunosuppressive agents act by binding to cytoplasmic macrophilin receptors, thereby reducing inflammation by decreasing the production of proinflammatory cytokines. These agents are nonsteroidal and therefore do not cause skin atrophy. For this reason, they may be particularly useful on the face, eyelids, neck, skin folds, and perineal areas. Both topical preparations are approved by the US Food and Drug Administration (FDA) for use in children older than 2 years in immunocompetent patients.[9] Pimecrolimus is indicated for mild-to-moderate AD and is currently available as a 1% cream. Tacrolimus is indicated for moderate-to-severe AD and is currently available as an ointment in both 0.03% and 0.1% formulations (Table 145-1).

Several nonsteroidal barrier repair agents have recently been cleared by the FDA for the treatment of AD. MAS063DP (glycerrhetinic acid, hyaluronic acid, telmestine, and others in hydrolipidic cream), palmitimide MEA (MimyX), and ceramide-dominant barrier creams all focus on improving skin barrier function in AD patients (Table 145-1).

Severe, recalcitrant AD may require therapy with systemic immunosuppressive or immunomodulating medications, including ultraviolet light phototherapy, cyclosporine, methotrexate, interferon-$\gamma$, oral mycophenolate mofetil, omalizumab, efalizumab, and etanercept, but these treatments have little data available to accurately evaluate their efficacy.

Any associated infection should also be appropriately treated. With more severe staphylococcal bacterial infections, and especially in communities where methicillin resistance is high, clindamycin, cotrimoxazole, or vancomycin should be used. For those with recurrent problems with staphylococcal infection, use of a diluted formulation of chlorine bleach may help provide broad-spectrum reduction in bacterial skin colonization.[10] Typically, 0.5 to 1 capful per gallon of water or approximately 0.25 to 0.5 cup of bleach per bathtub of water may be used once or twice a week for 5 to 10 minutes as a bath soak. It should be noted that patients may experience stinging or burning with fissured skin, and white towels are recommended for the patient because colored towel fabrics may become bleached. Kaposi varicelliform eruption should be suspected if vesicles are present or if no improvement is observed with oral antibiotics. The most common virus is herpes simplex, although cases of coxsackievirus and vaccinia can occur. Appropriate antiviral therapy should be instituted where possible in these cases.

Most patients with AD can be successfully managed by the primary care clinician. Consider consultation with an allergist, dermatologist, immunologist, infectious disease specialist, or ophthalmologist for the following conditions: severe AD, disease refractory to conventional therapy, infectious complications, ocular complications, identification of triggers and allergens, AD requiring hospitalization, dependency on systemic steroid, or when the diagnosis is uncertain.

## CONTACT DERMATITIS

Contact dermatitis refers to a group of heterogeneous cutaneous disorders that is elicited by exposure to an external agent, and includes irritant contact dermatitis (ICD), allergic contact dermatitis (ACD), phototoxic contact dermatitis (PTCD), photoallergic contact dermatitis (PACD), and contact urticaria (CU) (Box 145-1).

### Box 145-1

#### *Clinical Forms of Contact Dermatitis*

Irritant contact dermatitis
Allergic contact dermatitis
Phototoxic contact dermatitis
Photoallergic contact dermatitis
Contact urticaria

Irritant contact dermatitis describes a nonspecific inflammatory reaction in the skin that is dose dependent and occurs in response to direct cumulative toxicity of an agent against epidermal cells. For example, children who wash their hands with harsh soaps throughout the day may develop an irritant contact hand dermatitis.

Allergic contact dermatitis in contrast, indicates an inflammatory skin disorder that is caused by an allergen-specific delayed-type hypersensitivity reaction that can occur even with exposure to small quantities of an allergen (Box 145-2). The prototypical forms of ACD encountered in children include reactions to poison ivy and nickel. Nickel dermatitis frequently manifests with nummular areas of lichenification located on common areas of nickel contact—lower abdomen (pant snaps and belt buckles), ear lobes (earrings), sides of the neck (necklaces and chains), and wrists (watches and bracelets) (Figure 145-3A). Adolescents with nickel dermatitis can use a portable nickel test kit to detect nickel in jewelry and clothing before purchasing. The test uses dimethylglyoxime and ammonium hydroxide that turns the cotton swab pink in the presence of nickel (Figure 145-3B). The test carries high specificity but relatively lower sensitivity.

## Box 145-2
### *Common Causes of Allergic Contact Dermatitis*

Plants in the genus Rhus such as Poison Ivy or Sumac
Nickel
Topical medications
- antibiotics: neomycin, bacitracin
- antihistamines and related compounds:
  - diphenhydramine, ethylenediamine
- anesthetics: benzocaine
- steroids

Adhesives: PTBP resin
Chromates
Colophony
Disperse dye
Formaldehyde-related compounds
- Quaternium-15
- Imidazolidinyl urea, diazolidinyl urea
- DMDM hydantoin

Fragrances
Preservatives
Rubber-related compounds (IPPD, mercaptobenzathiazole, mercapto mix, thiurams)

Light exposure can be an eliciting factor for some forms of CD. Phototoxic contact dermatitis as exemplified by phytophotodermatitis, is an inflammatory skin disorder that occurs when a photosensitizing agent such as lime juice is applied to the skin and exposed to sunlight.[11] A PACD, in contrast, arises in response to a specific allergen like ACD, but is only elicited in response to light exposure. The presence of photosensitivity in a teenager should also raise the suspicion for collagen vascular disorders and other photosensitive disorders.

Finally, CU refers to an immediate-type hypersensitivity that results in urticaria on contact with an allergen. Latex allergy, for instance, can manifest as CU when sensitized patients wear latex gloves.[12] Foods, and even insects such as caterpillars, have been associated with urticaria. Patients with this type of reaction may be at risk for anaphylaxis and should be counseled accordingly.

The physical findings of CD are classically characterized by linear or geometric patterns elicited by contact with an external allergen. ICD, ACD, PTCD, and PACD may present with erythema, papules, and vesicles in these unusual configurations. As might be expected, CU manifests as urticaria and at times angioedema. Pruritus can be seen with most forms of CD, although patients with PTCD may also note burning discomfort and residual postinflammatory hyperpigmentation.

Evaluation of these heterogeneous disorders starts with a detailed history of potential exposures that might pinpoint a particular etiologic allergen. Patch testing and, where appropriate, photopatch testing should be obtained to identify or confirm the identity of underlying allergens.

Acute management involves the use of topical steroids—low potency for the face and intertriginous areas; medium or high potency for other affected areas on the

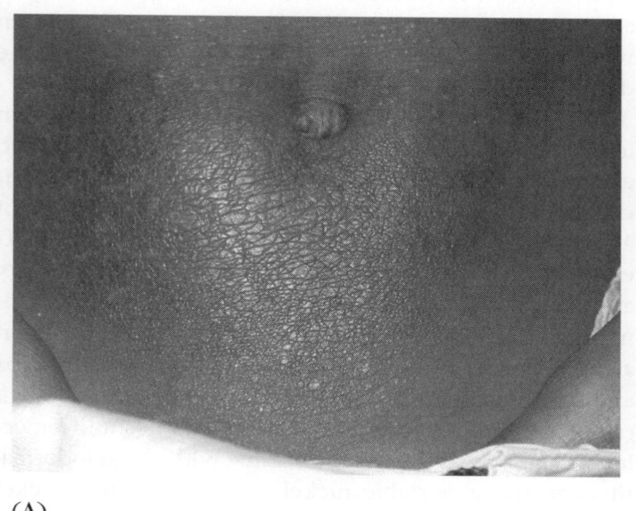

(A)

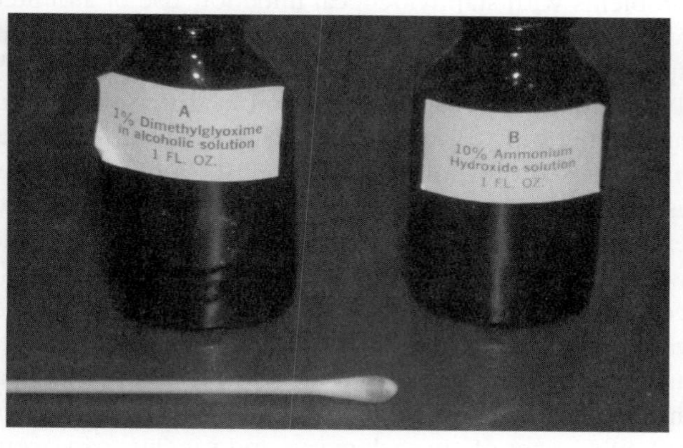


(B)

FIGURE 145-3 Nickel dermatitis. A: Allergic contact dermatitis secondary to pant snaps made of nickel. B: Positive nickel allergy test: a cotton swab moistened with dimethylglyoxime and ammonium hydroxide was rubbed against suspected nickel-containing materials and turns pink on exposure to nickel. (See color insert.)

body; antihistamines to moderate pruritus; and, in severe cases, systemic corticosteroids may be indicated. However, identification and avoidance of potential allergens is perhaps the most effective therapy.

## SEBORRHEIC DERMATITIS

Seborrheic dermatitis is a superficial, inflammatory process affecting the sebum-rich (seborrheic) areas of the scalp, face, and trunk. The occurrence of seborrheic dermatitis parallels the increased sebaceous gland activity that occurs in infancy and during puberty. This condition has been associated with proliferation of *Malassezia furfur*, immunologic abnormalities (eg, HIV), and the activation of complement. Commonly aggravated by emotional stress, trauma, changes in humidity, and climate, activity is intermittent and seasonal, with worsening in winter and early spring.

Clinical severity varies widely from a mild dandruff to a widespread exfoliative erythroderma. Although rare, generalized seborrheic erythroderma is most often encountered in association with AIDS, congestive heart failure, Parkinson's disease, and the relative immunosuppression observed in premature infants.[13] A seborrheic-like dermatitis may also be observed as part of riboflavin, biotin, and pyridoxine micronutrient deficiencies.

Dandruff of the scalp represents the mildest form of seborrheic dermatitis. The patches and plaques of seborrheic dermatitis are characterized by greasy scaling over erythematous, inflamed skin. Distribution follows the oily and hair-bearing areas of the head and the neck (ie, scalp, forehead, eyebrows, lash line, periauricular and nasolabial folds), midchest, and intertriginous areas (ie, axillae, groin, gluteal crease, and inframammary folds). In contrast to AD, pruritus is mild when present. The concomitant presence of oozing and crusting may indicate secondary infection.

After infancy, the incidence of "cradle cap" seborrheic dermatitis wanes until puberty when the condition once again becomes more common, presumably as sebum production increases. In adolescents and adults, seborrheic dermatitis usually starts as mild, greasy scaling of the scalp, with erythema and scaling of the nasolabial folds or the postauricular skin (Figure 145-4). The scaling is often concurrent with an oily complexion and appears in areas of increased sebaceous gland activity (eg, auricles, beard area, eyebrows, trunk, flexure, inframammary areas). Otitis externa, coexistent acne vulgaris, or pityriasis versicolor may also be evident. Some patients may also exhibit features that at some anatomic sites resemble seborrheic dermatitis, whereas in others appears more consistent with psoriasis. This hybrid condition may be referred to as sebopsoriasis (Figure 145-5).

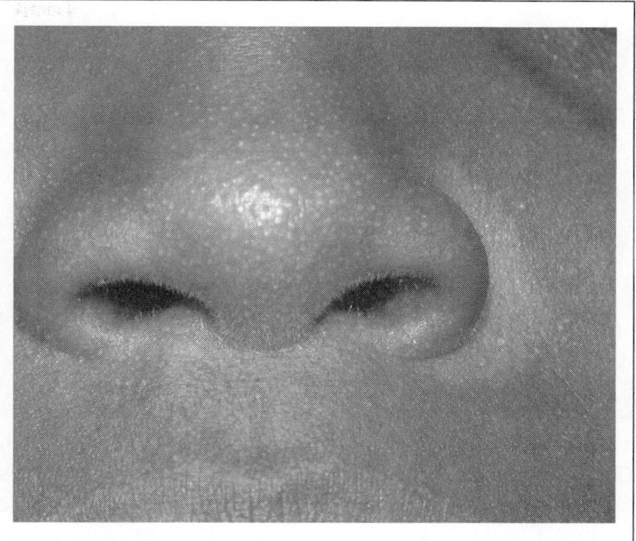

**FIGURE 145-4** Perinasal scaling in seborrheic dermatitis. Note the hypopigmentation and perinasal. (See color insert.)

A diagnosis of seborrheic dermatitis is made by clinical examination and rarely requires skin biopsy for confirmation. Evaluation of the adolescent patient with seborrheic dermatitis will often document a history of waxing and waning severity, as well as observation of a characteristic morphology and distribution of involvement.

The differential diagnosis of seborrheic dermatitis can be formulated based on the distribution of anatomic site involved (Box 145-3). With prominent scalp involvement, tinea capitis, psoriasis, AD, and folliculitis should be considered. On the face, perioral dermatitis, rosacea,

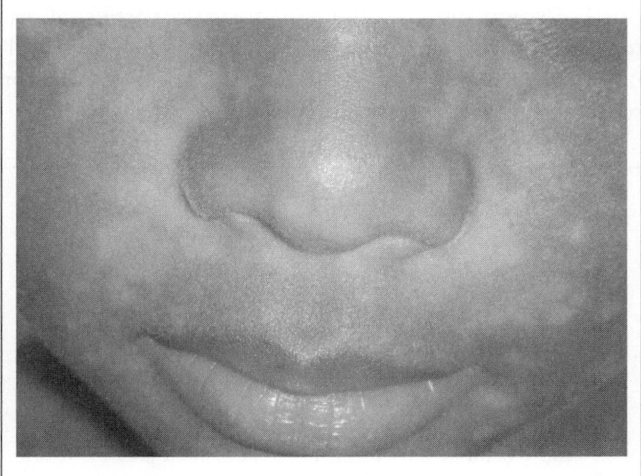

**FIGURE 145-5** Sebopsoriasis. Note the extensive hypopigmentation and scaling. (See color insert.)

### Box 145-3

#### *Differential Diagnosis of Seborrheic Dermatitis*

- Severe seborrheic dermatitis: consider HIV or other underlying immunocompromised state
- Seborrheic-like dermatitis
  - Face: perioral dermatitis, rosacea, nutritional deficiency (B complex), contact dermatitis
  - Scalp: tinea capitis, psoriasis, Langerhans cell histiocytosis
  - Body areas: tinea (pityriasis) versicolor, pityriasis rosea

CD, and psoriasis might resemble seborrheic dermatitis. On the trunk, pityriasis (tinea) versicolor and PR should be considered. Fever, petechiae, and failure of standard therapy should raise suspicion of Langerhans cell histiocytosis. Seborrheic dermatitis is common in HIV infection and can be a presenting finding.[14] It is clinically atypical, however, with often greater severity (often with a more sebopsoriatic appearance) and characteristically distinct histologic findings. Before the introduction of effective antiretroviral therapies, up to 40% of HIV-seropositive individuals and 80% of those with AIDS demonstrated evidence of seborrheic dermatitis.

Intermittent treatment of the scalp and other hair-bearing areas using antiproliferative, antimicrobial, and antiinflammatory shampoos or scalp treatments can assist in controlling scaling and pruritus by removing excess sebum and scaling (Box 145-4). Tar-based shampoos, those containing selenium sulfide (1%, 2.5%) and zinc pyrithione, help decrease scaling and pruritus.[15] Topical antifungal shampoos—ketoconazole (1%, 2%) and ciclopirox—target *Malassezia* species, but may possess some mild antiinflammatory properties. Short-term use of topical steroid preparations such as fluocinolone 0.01% (solution or oil) provide good efficacy for reducing pruritus and erythema.

### Box 145-4

#### *Treatment of Seborrheic Dermatitis*

***Topical Agents***

Low-potency topical corticosteroids: hydrocortisone 1% or 2.5%, fluocinolone 0.01%

Topical calcineurin inhibitors: pimecrolimus 1%, tacrolimus 0.03%, 0.1%

Shampoos: tar-based compounds, salicylic acid products, antifungal agents (selenium sulfide, zinc pyrithione, ketoconazole, ciclopirox)

More severe, recalcitrant cases may benefit from intermittent therapy with an oral antifungal agent. Once-weekly doses of an oral agent such as fluconazole, for instance, can significantly reduce the clinical features of sebopsoriasis.

As with hair-bearing sites, TCS, antifungals, or combinations of the two are the standard treatments for seborrheic dermatitis. Low-potency TCS (class VI or VII) are used daily for 1 to 2 weeks until improvement is seen and then tapered. Selection of an appropriate vehicle is important to patient compliance. Where ointments may be tolerated by infants, adolescents, and young adults often prefer creams or lotions for facial use and solutions or foams for hair-bearing areas. Patients often respond rapidly and appreciate prompt resolution of erythema and scaling.

Useful topical and systemic antifungal agents include clotrimazole (cream), ketoconazole (shampoo, cream, oral), ciclopirox (shampoo, cream, lotion, solution), terbinafine (cream, oral), and fluconazole (oral). Shampoo products may be used not only on the scalp, but also on the face or other affected sites while in the shower. Therapy can be prescribed daily for 1 to 2 weeks and then tapered to twice weekly as needed. These topical products are well tolerated and can be used up to twice daily for as long as needed. Patients who require oral antifungal therapy need to be followed closely for potential adverse effects.

Topical calcineurin inhibitors (eg, tacrolimus ointment, pimecrolimus cream [Elidel]) possess antiinflammatory and limited fungicidal properties without the long-term risks attendant to TCS therapy. As a result, calcineurin inhibitors offer a long-term noncontinuous and steroid-sparing alternative when the face and ears are affected.

## PITYRIASIS ROSEA

Pityriasis rosea (PR) is an acute, self-limited inflammatory exanthem of uncertain origin. PR is most commonly diagnosed in children and young adults, with a peak incidence in persons between 15 and 29 years of age. Although there is no consistent gender predilection, a seasonal variation is noted, with most cases occurring during spring and fall months. Pityriasis rosea is a self-limited disease, and treatment is usually not necessary.

A prodrome of headache, malaise, and pharyngitis may occur in a small number of cases. With the exception of itching, the condition is usually asymptomatic. Individual lesions are oval or round and characterized by a central, wrinkled, salmon-colored area with a collarette of scale just proximal to the margin. The eruption frequently announces itself with a herald patch—actually a larger solitary stereotypical plaque—that may persist for a week or more before multiple, smaller macules and papules start to appear. The herald patch ranges from 2 to 10 cm and is usually located on the trunk, but can also be seen on the neck or extremities. Involvement is maximal over the torso and abdomen. The smaller secondary lesions of PR follow Langer's lines or lines of skin cleavage. When the lesions occur on the back, they often align in a typical "Christmas tree" or "fir tree" pattern (Figure 145-6). Oral lesions consisting of erythematous plaques, hemorrhagic puncta, and ulcers have also been reported.

In children and in patients with more darkly pigmented skin, the distribution and morphology of the lesions is often atypical. These patients may have PR involving the scalp and face; it may be completely "inverse," affecting the face and distal extremities, while sparing the trunk. Individual lesions may be folliculopapular, vesicular, pustular, urticarial, or purpuric.

Although PR is a self-limited eruption and generally heals without scarring, some patients may observe areas of postinflammatory hyperpigmentation at sites of previous involvement that may take weeks or months to spontaneously improve.

The etiology of PR is unclear, although a variety of viruses and other microbial pathogens have been associated with PR, including HHV-7, HHV-6, *Chlamydia pneumoniae, Legionella pneumophila,* and *Mycoplasma pneumoniae.*

Drugs such as bismuth, barbiturates, captopril, gold, organic mercurials, methoxypromazine, metronidazole, D-penicillamine, isotretinoin, omeprazole, terbinafine, and naproxen have been implicated in causing drug-induced PR-like reactions and should be considered when patients are taking medications. The eruption does not represent a hypersensitivity to the drug; rather, the response is dose related and can be managed safely by reduction in dose size and frequency of administration.

The diagnosis of PR is often straightforward. If the eruption is atypical, especially if the palms and soles are affected and the patient is sexually active, the clinician should consider the possibility of secondary syphilis, the clinical manifestations of which closely resemble those of PR. Other clinically similar conditions include nummular eczema, tinea corporis, pityriasis lichenoides, guttate psoriasis, lichen planus, medication reactions, and various viral exanthems. With atypical presentations, a rapid plasma reagin or VDRL should be obtained, and a skin biopsy considered.

The rash of PR typically lasts about 5 weeks and resolves by 8 weeks in more than 80% of patients. Although PR is generally a one-time infection, recurrences are estimated in approximately 2% of cases.

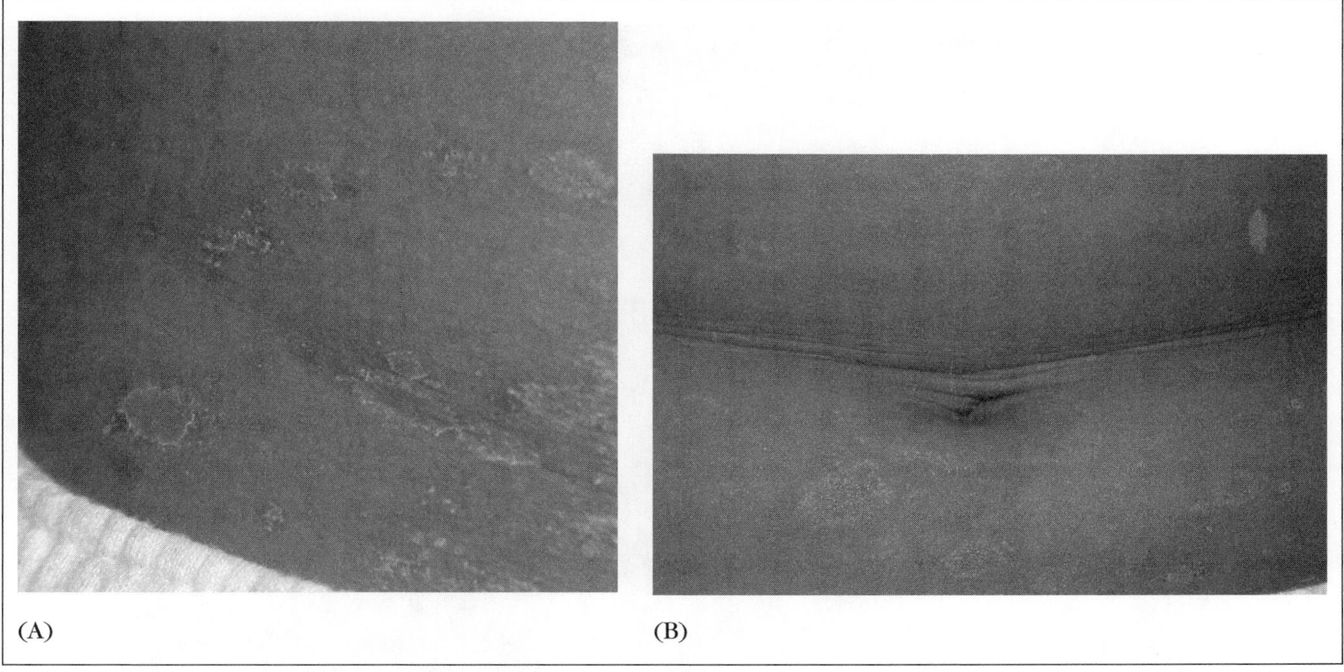


**FIGURE 145-6** Pityriasis rosea. A: Lesions possess a peripheral collarette of scale. B: Lesions follow the lines of cleavage. (See color insert.)

Pruritus can be managed with oral antihistamines, TCS, topical antipruritics (eg, pramoxine), and topical preparations (eg, calamine lotion).

Most cases are managed expectantly. However, a trial of erythromycin may be useful in selected cases of PR.[16] One well-controlled study of 90 patients found that erythromycin taken orally (250 mg QID for 14 days) was effective in reducing both the duration and the severity of the disease. The therapeutic positive effect of erythromycin may stem more from antiinflammatory and immune-modulating effects rather than direct antimicrobial effects. A nonrandomized single-blind trial suggested that high-dose acyclovir (800 mg 5 times daily for 7 days) may be beneficial.[17] Patients treated with acyclovir had more rapid resolution of lesions (mean time to clearance 19 vs 38 days), and fewer new lesions after 1 week of therapy. Additional study with blinded evaluation is needed before it can be determined whether acyclovir actually shortens the duration of PR. Ultraviolet B light therapy has been shown to accelerate resolution of lesions, but may be associated with postinflammatory hyperpigmentation. Consultation with a dermatologist for phototherapy may be considered in patients who have severe itching and extensive disease, and who are unable to make time for natural sunlight exposure.

## PSORIASIS

Psoriasis is a common papulosquamous disorder that manifests as beefy red papules and plaques, and superficial silvery scales. Classic plaque psoriasis peaks in onset during late adolescence and during middle age (50s–60s), and although characterized as a skin disorder, a significant minority (10%–20%) suffer from associated psoriatic arthritis. The disorder is now understood to represent an immunological disorder mediated by activation of T cells and release of cytokines, such as tumor necrosis factor, which result in skin inflammation and hyperproliferation. Several different clinical forms of psoriasis are recognized on the basis of morphology and distribution of the lesions: plaque, guttate, inverse, pustular, and erythrodermic forms.

Plaque psoriasis as suggested by its name involves round, circular, or nummular plaques of varying sizes associated with erythema and scale (Figure 145-7). This form of psoriasis classically involves the scalp (especially the occipital scalp), symmetric areas on the extensor surfaces of the extremities, and, in some patients, the palms and soles (Figure 145-8). Not infrequently, the genital areas are also affected.

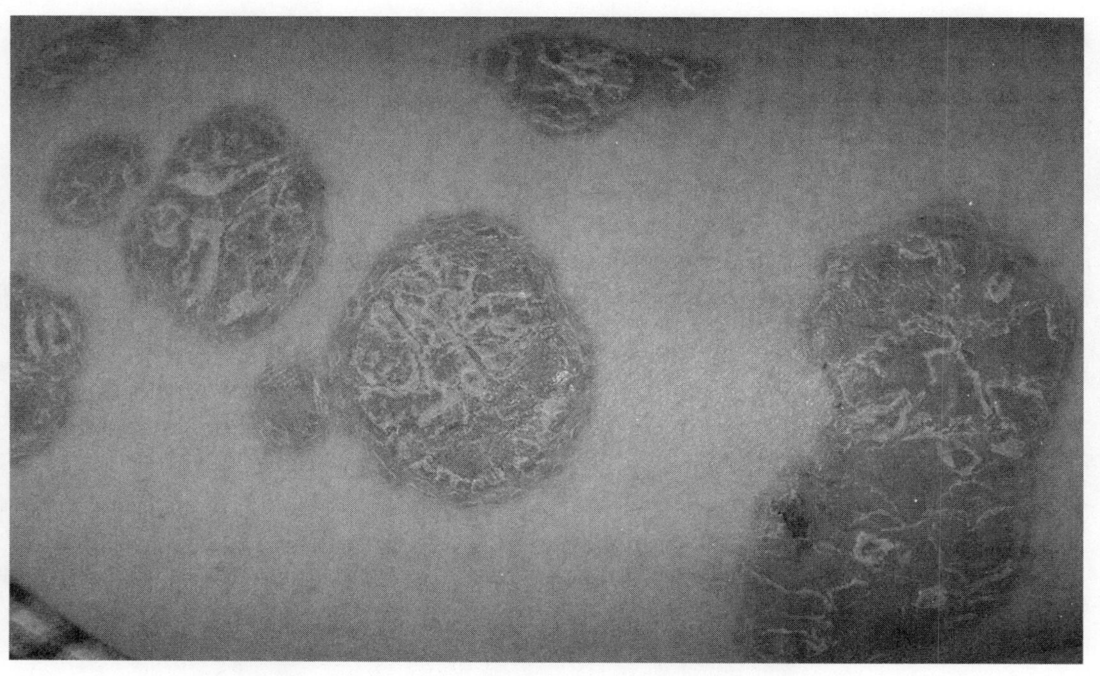

**FIGURE 145-7** Plaque psoriasis. Note the beefy red plaques and thick adherent scale. (See color insert.)

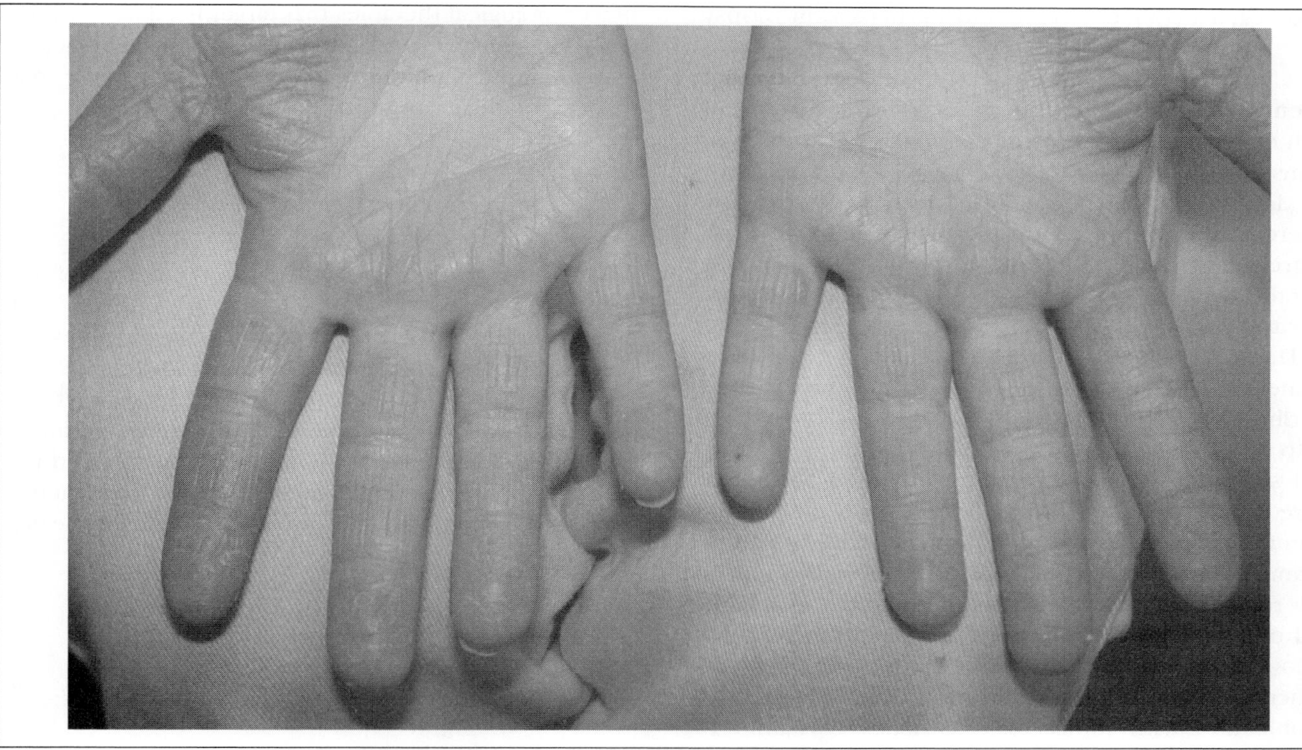

FIGURE 145-8 Palmar psoriasis. Note the well-demarcated erythema on the palms. (See color insert.)

Guttate psoriasis manifests as small drop-like areas of psoriasis that can be generalized (Figure 145-9). This form of psoriasis occurs more commonly in children and can be triggered by group A streptococcal infections. In some patients, antibiotic treatment of the underlying streptococcal infection may induce the guttate flare to remit temporarily.

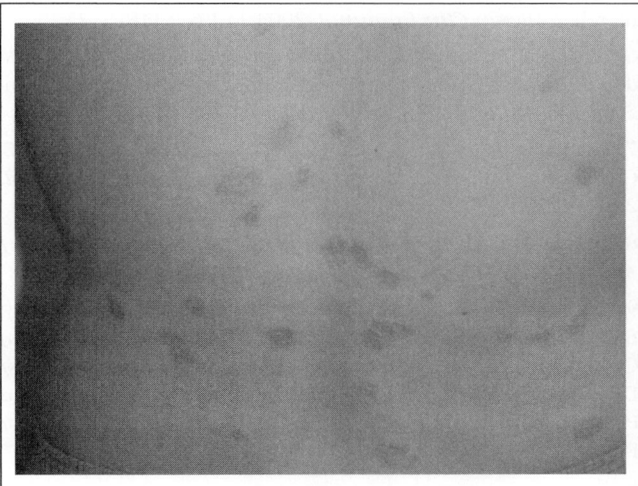

FIGURE 145-9 Guttate psoriasis. Note the random distribution of these lesions in contrast to the distribution of lesions in pityriasis rosea. (See color insert.)

Patients with inverse psoriasis present with disease in intertriginous zones, such as the axillary and inguinal folds. However, in contrast to the papules and plaques of plaque-type and guttate psoriasis, lesions of inverse psoriasis appear as macerated areas of erythema at intertriginous sites.

Pustular psoriasis is a more severe form of psoriasis. Affected patients develop localized areas of erythema that are at times painful or tender and become studded with lakes of coalescent pustules. These may rupture, leaving collarettes of scale. Pustular flares may result from use of systemic corticosteroids in psoriatic patients, particularly as the steroid is tapered.

Erythrodermic psoriasis, by definition, describes generalized erythema and scaling involving more than 90% of the body surface area. Because of the widespread disruption in the normal skin barrier, patients with this form of psoriasis are at risk of hypothermia, increased insensible water loss and electrolyte abnormalities, and sepsis.

Patients with psoriasis also present with characteristic nail changes, such as nail pits and onycholysis manifesting as tan or brown "oil spots."

The diagnosis of psoriasis is made on clinical grounds, although a skin biopsy can be helpful in situations where the diagnosis is unclear. Guttate psoriasis may be confused with PR or pityriasis lichenoides chronica; a detailed history and perhaps skin biopsy will help with diagnosis. Palmoplantar psoriasis must be distinguished from dyshidrotic or hand-foot eczema. Although nail pitting may be a feature of both conditions, palmoplantar psoriasis tends to favor palms and soles, whereas eczematous disorders favor the dorsal hands and feet. Scalp psoriasis should be differentiated from tinea capitis; where scalp psoriasis is rarely associated with frank alopecia, tinea capitis is characterized by prominent features of hair loss and pruritus.

The selection of therapeutic agents for the management of psoriasis will depend in large part on the distribution and the severity of disease (Box 145-5). Scalp areas, for instance, can be managed using salicylic acid shampoos to reduce scaling, tar-based shampoos to reduce the hyperproliferation and thereby reduce scaling, or topical steroid solutions or foams to reduce inflammation. Areas on the face or intertriginous areas may respond most safely to lower-potency topical steroid or calcineurin inhibitor creams or ointments. Psoriatic areas on the body respond better to medium- or higher-potency topical steroids that may be used in combination with topical calcipotriene (a vitamin D analog) or the retinoid tazarotene (a vitamin A analog), both of which help reduce the hyperproliferation and inflammation in psoriatic lesions.

More severe cases will benefit from consultation with a dermatologist and may require ultraviolet light phototherapy (290–320 nm), which targets skin-resident T cells. Although traditional systemic chemotherapeutic agents such as methotrexate, oral retinoids (acitretin and isotretinoin), and cyclosporine remain useful, newer biological therapies that target T-cell activation or trafficking, or that help reduce production of associated cytokines, offer a more directed approach to the treatment of moderate to severe psoriasis.

**Box 145-5**

***Common Treatments for Psoriasis***

**Topical Agents**

Corticosteroids
Calcipotriene
Calcineurin inhibitors (pimecrolimus, tacrolimus)
Retinoids (tazarotene, tretinoin, adapalene)
Tar compounds
Keratolytics (urea, ammonium lactate, salicylic acid)

**Systemic Agents**

Ultraviolet light phototherapy
Oral retinoids (acitretin, isotretinoin)
Methotrexate
Cyclosporine
Biological agents (etanercept, infliximab, efalizumab, alefacept, adalimumab)

## CONCLUSION

Adolescents may be predisposed to a number of skin conditions, including several forms of dermatitis (AD, CD, seborrheic dermatitis) and papulosquamous disorders (PR and psoriasis). These heterogeneous skin conditions have characteristic clinical findings that help differentiate them from each other. An understanding of the underlying pathophysiology helps the clinician provide an appropriate and timely diagnosis, and thereby select safe and effective therapeutic options for the adolescent patient.

## REFERENCES

1. Vickers CFH. The natural history of atopic eczema. *Acta Derm Venereol Suppl (Stockh).* 1980;92:113–115

2. Williams HC, Wüthrich B. The natural history of atopic dermatitis. In: Williams HC, ed. *Atopic Dermatitis.* Cambridge: Cambridge University Press; 2000:41–59

3. Palmer CAN, Irvine AD, Terron-Kwiatkowski A, et al. Common loss-of-function variants of the epidermal barrier protein filaggrin are a major predisposing factor for atopic dermatitis. *Nat Genet.* 2006;38:441–446

4. Söderhall C, Marenholz I, Kerscher T, et al. Variants in a novel epidermal collagen gene (*COL29A1*) are associated with atopic dermatitis. *PLoS Biol.* 2007;5(9):1952–1961

5. Spergel JM, Paller AS. Atopic dermatitis and the atopic march. *J Allergy Clin Immunol.* 2003;112(6):S118–S127

6. Sicherer SH, Sampson HA. Food hypersensitivity and atopic dermatitis: pathophysiology, epidemiology, diagnosis, and management. *J Allergy Clin Immunol.* 1999;104 (suppl):114–122

7. Eichenfield LF, Hanifin JM, Luger TA, Stevens SR, Pride HB. Consensus conference on pediatric AD. *J Am Acad Dermatol.* 2003;49:1088–1095

8. Leung D. Update on glucocorticoid action and resistance. *J Allergy Clinical Immunol.* 2003;111(1):3–22

9. US Food and Drug Administration. Public Health Advisory: Elidel (pimecrolimus) Cream and Protopic (tacrolimus) Ointment. February 15, 2005. Available at: www.fda.gov/Drugs/DrugSafety/PostmarketDrugSafetyInformationforPatientsandProviders/DrugSafetyInformationforHeathcareProfessionals/PublicHealthAdvisories/UCM051760. Accessed November 17, 2010

10. Winter J, Ilbert M, Graf PCF, et al. Bleach activates a redox-regulated chaperone by oxidative protein unfolding. *Cell.* 2008;135:691–701

11. Goskowicz MO, Friedlander SF, Eichenfield LF. Endemic "lime" disease: phytophotodermatitis in San Diego County. *Pediatrics.* 1994;93(5):828-830

12. Guillet MH, Guillet G. Contact urticaria to natural rubber latex in childhood and associated atopic symptoms: a study of 27 patients aged under 15 years. *Ann Dermatol Venereol.* 2004;131(1 Pt 1):35-37

13. Vega ML, Vega J, Vega JM. Moneo I, Sanchez E, Miranda A. Cutaneous reactions to pine processionary caterpillar. *Pediatr Allergy Immunol.* 2003;14(6):482-486

14. Dunic I, Vesic S, Jevtovic DJ. Oral candidiasis and seborrheic dermatitis in HIV-infected patients on highly active antiretroviral therapy. *HIV Med.* 2004;5:50-54

15. Danby FW, Maddin WS, Margewwon L, Rosenthal D. A randomized, double-blind, placebo-controlled trial of ketoconazole 2% shampoo versus selenium sulfide 2.5% shampoo in the treatment of moderate to severe dandruff. *J Am Acad Dermatol.* 1993;29(6):1008-1012

16. Sharma PK, Yadav TP, Gautam RK, Taneja N, Satyanarayana L. Erythromycin in pityriasis rosea: a double-blind, placebo-controlled clinical trial. *J Am Acad Dermatol.* 2000;42:241-244

17. Drago F, Vecchio F, Rebora A. Use of high-dose acyclovir in pityriasis rosea. *J Am Acad Dermatol*. 2006;54 (1):82-85

# CHAPTER 146

# Alopecia

BROOK E. TLOUGAN, MD • JUDITH O'HAVER, PhD, RN, CPNP • RONALD C. HANSEN, MD

## INTRODUCTION

The importance of hair may be affected by social and cultural norms.[1] Hair often is associated with beauty, attraction, and virility.[2] Hair loss in teenagers may be an isolated finding or may be indicative of an underlying disorder.[1] Disorders of the hair in the adolescent may be a source of concern for teens and parents. Accurate diagnosis of hair disorders is necessary for effective counseling and treatment.

## GROWTH CYCLE OF HUMAN HAIR

Hair follicles are present at birth and are capable of producing 3 types of hair: lanugo, vellus, and terminal hair. Lanugo is normally found in the neonatal period as nonpigmented, soft, fine hair; however, it can also be acquired later in life in disorders such as anorexia nervosa or occult malignancy. Vellus hairs are short, fine, and lightly pigmented, and are present over most of the adult body. Terminal hair is long, thick, and strongly pigmented. It is found in areas such as the scalp, eyebrows, and in postpubertal children and adults, in both the axilla and pubic area, as well as on the chest and face of mature males.[1]

Hair growth follows a cyclic pattern. Each human scalp hair grows over a period of 1 to 6 years at about 1 cm per month. This is called the anagen phase.[3] The duration of the anagen phase is usually fixed by adolescence.[1] Once the growth period is complete, the hair undergoes an involution stage known as the catagen phase that lasts about 3 weeks. Finally, the telogen phase occurs over a period of 3 months. Hair shedding occurs normally in the telogen phase. This period is followed by regrowth and return to the anagen phase. Most individuals shed between 50 and 100 hairs each day. At any given time, approximately 85% to 90% of scalp hair is in the anagen/growth phase, 1% is in catagen, and 10% to 15% is in telogen. Normal growth may be interrupted when a larger portion of anagen hairs progress to the telogen phase.[3]

## COMMON CAUSES OF ADOLESCENT ALOPECIA

### TELOGEN EFFLUVIUM

Telogen effluvium is characterized by an increase in the shedding of normal hair due to physiological stress. The 10% of hair normally in the telogen phase increases to 30%. Thinning hair may not be observable to the naked eye until more than 50% of hairs are lost. Telogen effluvium may occur at any age and is induced by factors that affect follicle growth; examples include pregnancy, significant weight loss, or significant medical illness, especially if associated with high fevers or significant emotional stress.[4] Medications such as lithium, angiotensin-converting enzyme inhibitors, beta blockers, and oral contraceptives also may cause telogen effluvium.[3] Acute telogen effluvium usually occurs about 3 months after the triggering event, so history can be an important aspect of this diagnosis. There is usually an appearance of overall decreased hair density. The shedding is transient and often resolves in 3 to 6 months, returning the hair to normal density.[1,3]

Diagnosis is suggested by a positive hair pull test. Firm traction on hair results in more than 6 hairs lost in each pull[3] and the bulbs of the plucked hair are "club hairs" typical of the telogen phase. Management of telogen effluvium includes identifying the underlying cause and avoiding the trigger. Reassurance is important as improvement is anticipated. Vigorous manipulation of hair must be avoided until regrowth occurs.[1,3]

### ALOPECIA AREATA

Alopecia areata is a condition in which well-circumscribed patchy hair loss may occur on any part of the body. More dramatic variants of alopecia areata include the bitemporal bandlike ophiasis pattern alopecia areata (Figure 146-1); alopecia totalis, where the patient's scalp is bald; and alopecia universalis, which involves the total loss of body hair (Figure 146-2). Common alopecia areata is usually characterized by sharply defined oval or circular patches of hair loss. The incidence is about

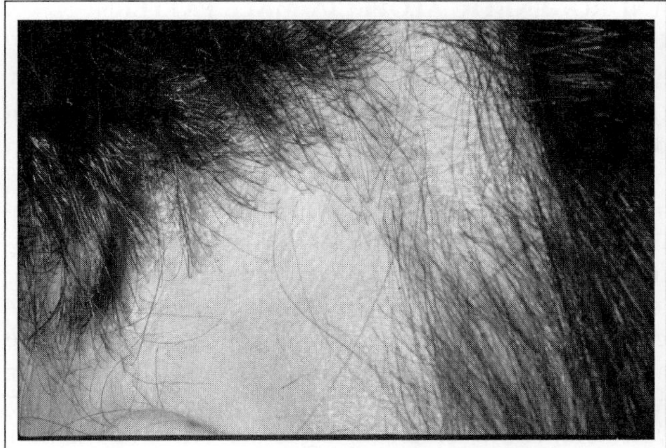

**FIGURE 146-1** Bitemporal ophiasis pattern of alopecia areata. (See color insert.)

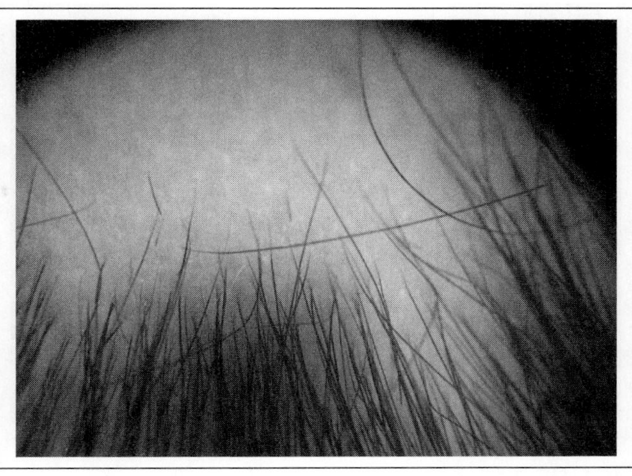

**FIGURE 146-3** Exclamation point hairs, the classic clinical finding in alopecia areata. (See color insert.)

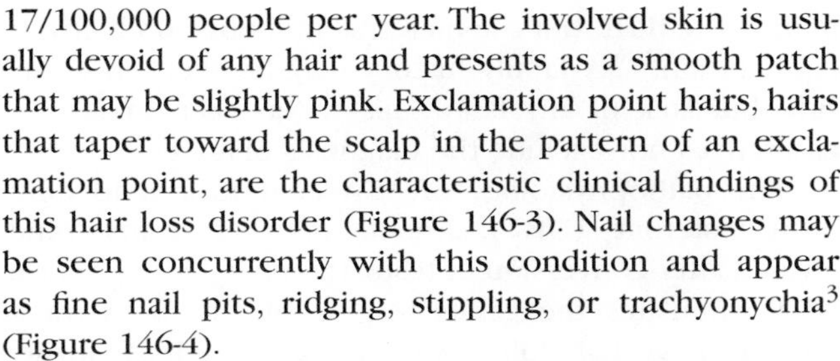

17/100,000 people per year. The involved skin is usually devoid of any hair and presents as a smooth patch that may be slightly pink. Exclamation point hairs, hairs that taper toward the scalp in the pattern of an exclamation point, are the characteristic clinical findings of this hair loss disorder (Figure 146-3). Nail changes may be seen concurrently with this condition and appear as fine nail pits, ridging, stippling, or trachyonychia[3] (Figure 146-4).

Alopecia areata is usually a chronic inflammatory condition associated with T-cell infiltration around the hair bulb, classically referred to as a "swarm of bees" on histopathology. The hair pull test in newer patches of the areas bordering the alopecia reveals increased numbers of telogen and dystrophic hairs.[5] Later in the course, more of the hairs will be in the anagen phase of hair growth.[3] A poorer prognosis is associated with this alopecia if it occurs prior to puberty, is prolonged, or occurs in other family members.[5] There is no permanent tissue destruction associated with this condition, and the alopecia is usually nonscarring as a result.[1]

The course of alopecia areata is variable. Local treatments may help control the problem, but there is currently no cure. In some children, alopecia areata will resolve spontaneously within the year, and the option to not treat is a valid consideration.[3] A variety of treatments have been tried with variable success. These include topical corticosteroids; intralesional corticosteroids; oral corticosteroids; and topical agents, such as

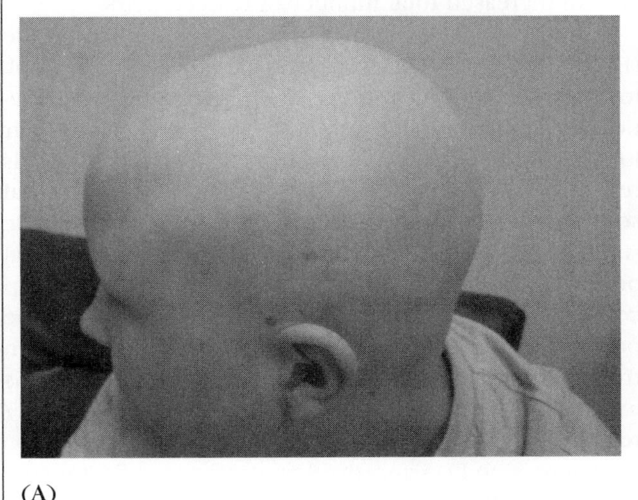

(A)

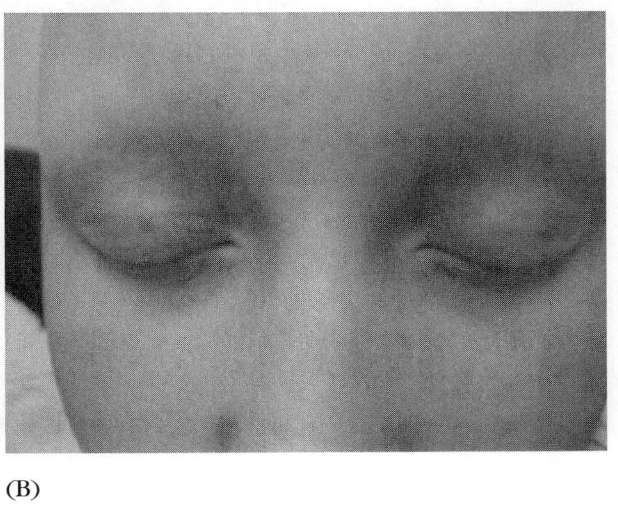

(B)

**FIGURE 146-2** Alopecia universalis showing hair loss on (A) scalp and (B) eyebrows and eyelashes. (See color insert.)

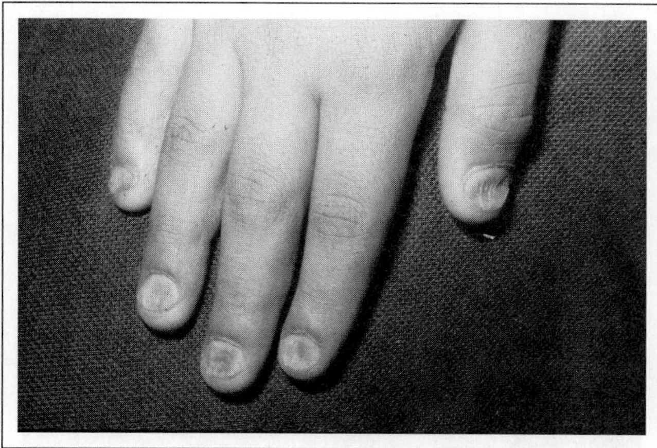

**FIGURE 146-4** Significant nail dystrophy in patient with alopecia areata. (See color insert.)

anthralin, minoxidil, and topical immunotherapy with multiple contact sensitizers. The contact sensitizers that have been used are squaric acid dibutylester and diphenylcyclopropenone. Figure 146-5 demonstrates alopecia areata with some hair regrowth following contact sensitization. Dinitrochlorobenzene is no longer used, and diphencyprone is not licensed for use in the United States. Systemic psoralen used with psoralen ultraviolet type A, cryosurgery, azathioprine, and cyclosporin have also been tried, but are not recommended for use in children. Cosmetic solutions, such as wigs and altered hairstyles, should be considered to address the emotional distress and anxiety associated with this hair loss condition in adolescents.[1]

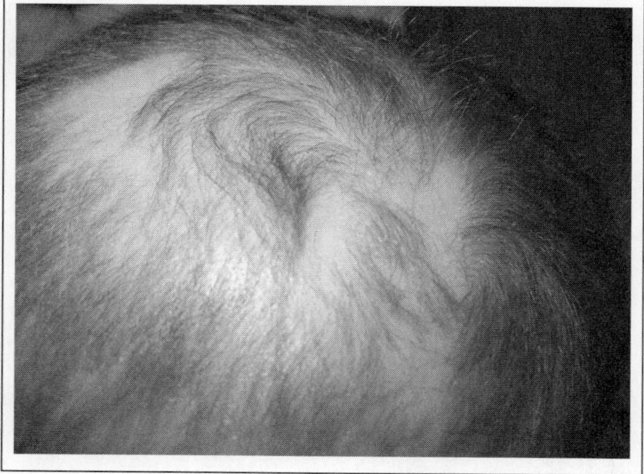

**FIGURE 146-5** Alopecia areata with evidence of hair regrowth after treatment with squaric acid. (See color insert.)

## ANDROGENETIC ALOPECIA/MALE PATTERN HAIR LOSS

Androgenetic alopecia (AGA) or male pattern hair loss (MPHL) is a common, but often psychosocially harmful disorder for the adolescent patient. In males, it can occur any time after the onset of puberty and is clearly androgen dependent. In fact, as demonstrated by Hamilton's studies in the 1940s, AGA is absent in males castrated before the onset of puberty.[6] In addition, there is a higher incidence of this disorder in girls with polycystic ovarian syndrome, an androgenizing disorder. The average onset of MPHL occurs in the mid 20s; however, approximately 14% to 15% of healthy teenagers (15–17 years old) show some early signs of AGA.[7,8] In addition, there seems to be a racial predilection whereby whites, in general, have more extensive hair loss than other ethnicities.[7,8] The genetics of MPHL are not precisely defined, but are polygenetic with variable penetrance. An increased frequency of AGA is observed in sons of men with MPHL, but the maternal influence on hair loss is uncertain.[7-9] A family history may be seen on either side, but lack of any family history, as seen in 20% of cases, does not exclude the diagnosis of AGA.[7,8]

The pathophysiology of AGA centers around dihydrotestosterone (DHT), a metabolite of testosterone, formed after conversion of testosterone by 5α-reductase. DHT stimulates the genes responsible for both transforming large hair follicles (terminal hair) into smaller follicles (vellus hair) and shortening the cycle of hair growth. It is important to note that there is no actual loss of hair follicles in AGA; instead, progressive miniaturization of the terminal hair follicles occurs, and the shorter, finer, nonpigmented vellus hair is produced. The normal ratio of terminal to vellus hairs in the scalp is 7:1, but in AGA, the ratio is reduced to 2:1. There is also an increased total number of telogen hairs.

Clinically, AGA is a simple diagnosis to make (Figure 146-6). The history of progressive hair loss following a frontal, bitemporal, and vertex scalp distribution as outlined by the Hamilton-Norwood scale of hair loss (Figure 146-7) is diagnostic. The occipital scalp is relatively spared because the follicles in the occipital scalp are largely androgen independent; embryologic studies have demonstrated a cephalic mesodermal origin of these follicles, whereas the rest of the scalp comes from neural crest cells.[10] A hair pull test may be positive in early disease, but is usually negative when the hair loss is long-standing.[8] The differential diagnosis includes acute or chronic telogen effluvium and diffuse/reverse ophiasis alopecia areata.[8]

There is no FDA-approved treatment for AGA for adolescents younger than age 18, but minoxidil and finasteride, used as monotherapy or in combination, have proven quite useful for men with MPHL. Minoxidil is a

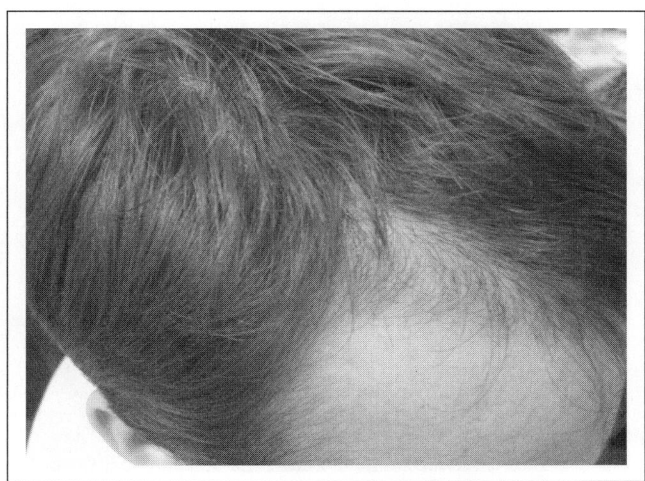

**FIGURE 146-6** Bitemporal pattern of hair loss in androgenetic alopecia. (See color insert.)

potassium channel opener; it seems to increase the duration of the anagen phase and reverse miniaturization of the terminal hair follicles. It is marketed in both 2% and 5% topical formulations (solution and foam), with studies showing greater hair regrowth with the 5% over the 2% solution (57% vs 40%).[7,11] For maximum efficacy, the hair should remain dry for an hour after applying the medication. Finasteride, given in a 1-mg dose for AGA, inhibits the activity of the type 2 isoenzyme of 5α-reductase, which converts testosterone to DHT at the level of the hair follicle (specifically in the dermal papilla and the outer root sheath). It has been shown to reverse miniaturization, as well as increase hair density, growth rate, and thickness over placebo.[7,8,10] Neither medication reverses complete baldness nor restores all hair loss, but both medications seem to stop hair loss and stimulate some regrowth.[8] It is important to note, however, that baldness will progress with discontinuation of treatment. In severe disease, hair transplantation, scalp reduction, and cosmetic aids, such as wigs, are additional options; however, none of these treatments address the underlying pathophysiology of the condition.[7]

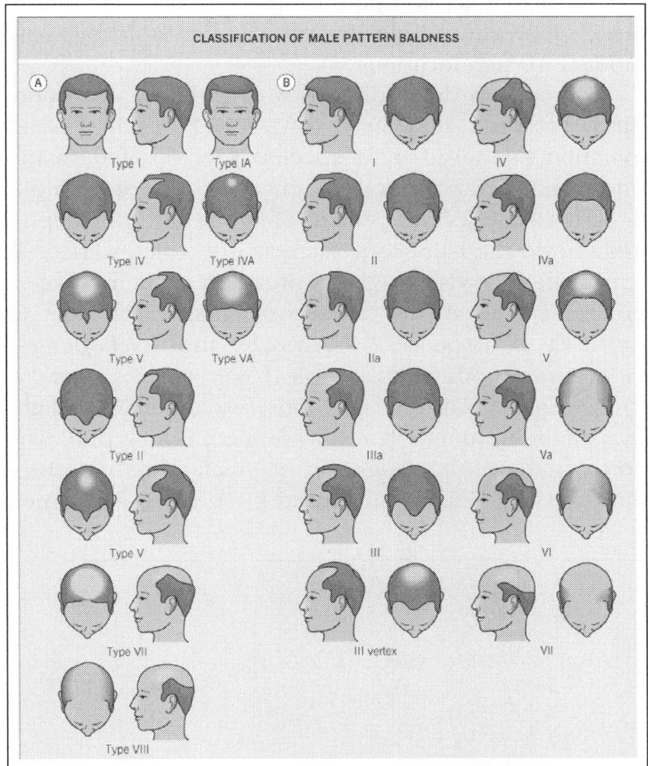


**FIGURE 146-7** Hamilton-Norwood Scale for classification of male pattern hair loss. (Reprinted from Bolognia JL, Jorizzo JL, Rapini RP. *Dermatology*. London: Mosby; 2003:1046, with permission from Elsevier.)

## FEMALE PATTERN HAIR LOSS

Much less is known about hair loss in females, and because the role of androgens is less certain, the term female pattern hair loss (FPHL) is used. Studies show that adolescent females with hair loss have an even lower sense of psychosocial well-being than males.[9] FPHL can be seen in the mid-teenage years as well; however, unlike MPHL, FPHL tends toward 2 other unique patterns: (1) diffuse thinning of the crown and central scalp or (2) frontal accentuation (Christmas tree pattern) (Figure 146-8).[8] Depending on the severity, Ludwig's classification system is used to divide FPHL into 3 stages, as seen in Figure 146-9.[12,13] In females, screening blood work is usually recommended to include thyroid-stimulating hormone (TSH) and iron studies because both hypothyroidism and iron deficiency may cause telogen effluvium, a diagnosis included on the differential for FPHL.[8] Minoxidil is effective in FPHL, but finasteride is only advised in females who demonstrate symptoms suggesting hyperandrogenism. Other medications with occasional efficacy include oral contraceptive pills, spironolactone, flutamide, and cyproterone acetate. Patients should also be counseled to avoid excessive use of hair care products that cause additional damage to the scalp.[8]

## TINEA CAPITIS

Tinea capitis (scalp ringworm) is the most common dermatophyte infection of childhood (Figure 146-10).[14] It generally affects urban school-age children, but is occasionally observed in adolescents as well. Males are more widely affected than females and black children are more widely inflicted than whites. Three different

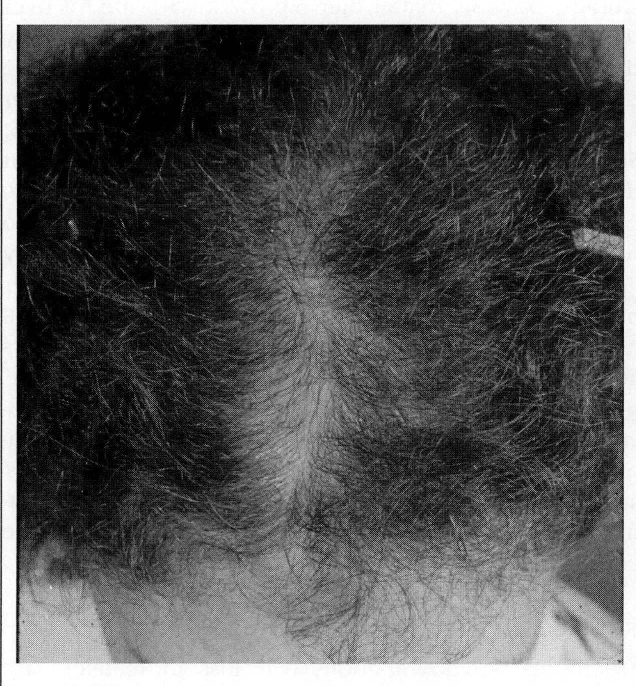

FIGURE 146-8 Thinning of central scalp hair in female pattern hair loss. (See color insert.)

genera of dermatophyte cause this invasion of the scalp hair; these include *Microsporum*, *Trichophyton*, and *Epidermophyton*. There are 3 different types of reservoirs for these fungi: (1) zoophilic (acquired from animals), (2) anthropophilic (infections from close human contact), and (3) geophilic (soil-originating infections).[1] In the United States and the United Kingdom, *Trichophyton tonsurans*, an anthropophilic dermatophyte causing mild scaling and alopecia, is the most prevalent species.[14,15] In addition, there are data to support a 5% to 15% asymptomatic carrier rate

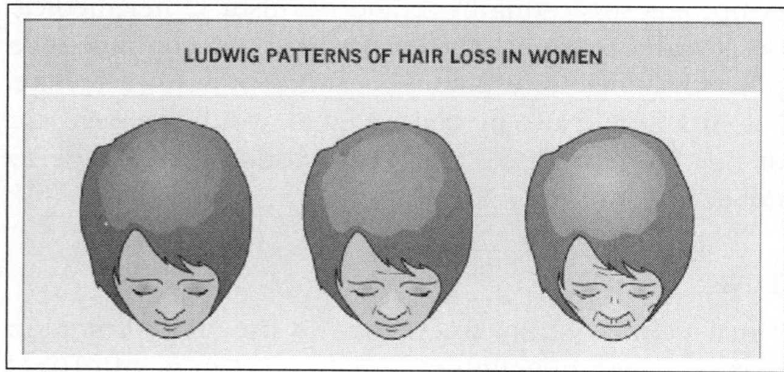


FIGURE 146-9 Ludwig classification of female pattern hair loss. (Reprinted from Bolognia JL, Jorizzo JL, Rapini RP. *Dermatology*. London: Mosby; 2003:1047, with permission from Elsevier.)

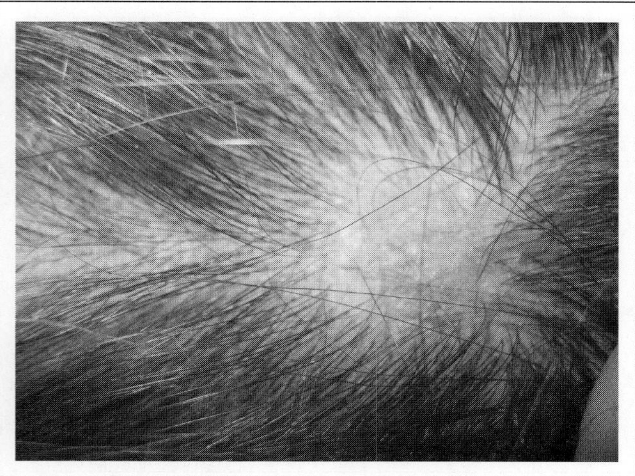

FIGURE 146-10 Scaly erythematous plaque consistent with tinea capitis. (See color insert.)

for *T tonsurans*. In central Europe, the pet-carrying *Microsporum canis* is the predominant organism causing disease.[14] Dermatophytes have a short incubation period, which varies widely depending on the species (2 days–3 weeks). Fomite spread is not uncommon because infectious fungal matter can be viable for many months in such locations.[14]

There are 3 different modes of hair invasion: endothrix, ectothrix, and favus (Box 146-1). Each type of infection is caused by a specific species of dermatophyte, and each presents different clinically. For example, in endothrix infections, chains of large spores are deposited within the hair shaft, whereas the cuticle surface is left intact. Likewise, the hairs break off at their weakest points, leaving an appearance of small black dots in the area of alopecia. *T tonsurans* and *Trichophyton violaceum* produce this clinical pattern of "black-dot ringworm," which does not fluoresce under Wood light examination. Nonetheless, a Wood light is a helpful diagnostic tool in the diagnosis of small-spore ectothrix infections, such as those caused by *M canis*. The green

**Box 146-1**

***Presentations of Tinea***[3,14]

Gray patch type
Diffuse scale type
Black dot type
Favus
Kerion
Diffuse follicular pustular type
Scale with or without hair loss

fluorescence is observed when a dermatophyte invades the hair keratin.[1] Another noninflammatory clinical pattern of hair loss usually caused by *T tonsurans* is the "gray patch type," where one sees multiple circular patches of minimal hair loss and abundant scaling.[14] In general, the anthropophilic infections cause less inflammation than either the zoophilic or geophilic infections. Zoophilic and geophilic organisms may produce either kerion or favus that can lead to extensive and permanent scarring alopecia. Favus is characterized by red scaly plaques with hyperkeratotic honeycomb-yellow crusts (scutula) and a central hair shaft. The infection is usually caused by *Trichophyton schoenleinii*, and a mouselike odor is distinctive.[14] Kerion is an extremely inflammatory and painful form of tinea capitis. Any hairs still present in the boggy mass are easily pulled out, and scarring may occur. Adolescents with a kerion may also present with constitutional symptoms, including fever, malaise, and lymphadenopathy.

In addition to the Wood light, obtaining a direct sample of the fungus is paramount to making the diagnosis. The chosen area should be cleaned with 70% rubbing alcohol to minimize contamination and scraped with a blunt scalpel. Scale and hair debris are placed in a single layer on a glass microscope slide, and 10% to 30% potassium hydroxide is added before covering the material with a coverslip.[14] To definitively identify the fungal source, a culture is performed, most commonly with Sabouraud's agar as the growth medium. Unfortunately, culture results may take up to 4 weeks to grow an organism.

Griseofulvin is, at present, the only FDA-approved treatment of tinea capitis in patients younger than age 18. The medication is fungistatic in vitro, interfering with cell wall synthesis by altering microtubule function. Absorption is augmented by administration of griseofulvin with fatty foods.[14] Treatment with griseofulvin can be variable and depends on the formulation (microcrystalline vs ultramicrocrystalline). In adolescents, the typical doses would include 750 mg daily for the microcrystalline and 250 mg twice a day for the ultramicrosized. Other options for treatment, though not FDA-approved, include itraconazole, fluconazole, and terbinafine. Griseofulvin and the azole drugs are contraindicated in pregnancy; terbinafine, although a pregnancy category B medication, is also not recommended during pregnancy as adequate controlled studies have not been performed in humans. Some authors suggest 2 negative fungal cultures before systemic therapy is considered to be effective.[14] Others treat until the clinical cure is noted, usually at least 6 weeks on griseofulvin. The use of selenium sulfide, povidone iodine, and ketoconazole shampoos can help reduce transmission and infectivity to others, but do not provide a cure.[14] It has also been shown that hair conditioner proffers a protective effect against tinea capitis infections.[16]

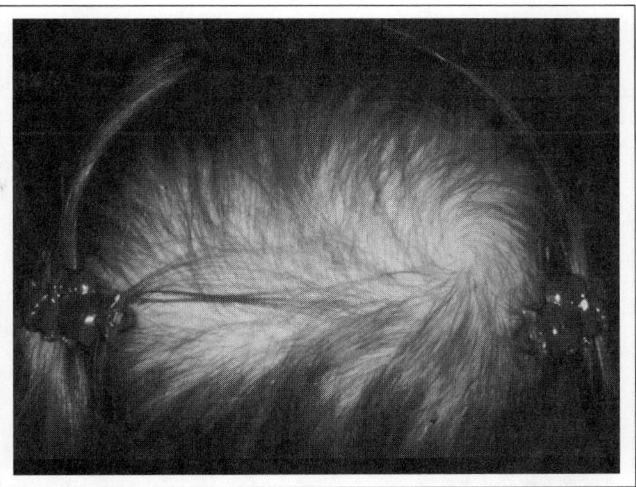

**FIGURE 146-11** Traction alopecia caused by chronic use of barrettes. (See color insert.)

## TRACTION ALOPECIA

Traction alopecia is a reversible condition if the causative factors are corrected early in the course of the alopecia. It is more common in females on the frontal or parietal scalp, and it is caused by the constant tension applied to the hair by certain styling techniques such as tight braids, corn rows, or ponytails (Figure 146-11). Prolonged traction may cause scarring with resulting little regrowth, even when the traction is discontinued.[1,3] Although there is an absence of terminal hair in the area of alopecia, numerous fine vellus hair may be apparent on close inspection.[3] Recognition of the causative factors of the problem is essential to treating the patient because the patient and his or her family must be convinced that a change of hairstyle is important to prevent permanent hair loss.

## TRICHOTILLOMANIA

Trichotillomania is a form of traction alopecia. It is classified as an impulse control disorder in which there is a compulsion or habit to pull or pluck the hair.[1] Adolescent patients with trichotillomania have reported an irresistible impulse associated with anxiety that causes them to pull out the hair.[2] The scalp and eyebrows are the most common sites affected; however, other sites may also be involved. The affected area is usually without scarring unless the same area is plucked consistently enough to cause permanent hair loss.[1]

The condition most often begins with irregular geometric pattern of hair loss appearing on the contralateral side of the patient's dominant hand. The broken-off

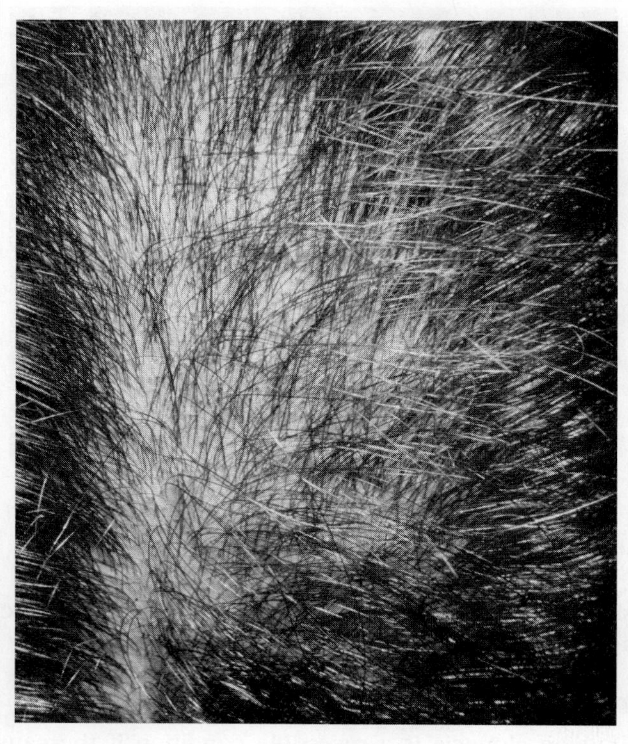

FIGURE 146-12 Broken-off stubble commonly observed in trichotillomania. (See color insert.)

**Box 146-2**

***Diagnostic Criteria for DSM-IV-TR 312.39 Trichotillomania***

1. Recurrent pulling out of one's hair resulting in noticeable hair loss
2. An increasing sense of tension immediately before pulling out the hair or when attempting to resist the behavior
3. Pleasure, gratification, or relief when pulling out the hair
4. The disturbance is not better accounted for by another mental disorder and is not due to a general medical condition (eg, a dermatological condition)
5. The disturbance causes clinically significant distress or impairment in social, occupational, or other important areas of functioning

*Source:* Reprinted with permission from American Psychiatric Association. *Diagnostic and Statistical Manual of Mental Disorders, Fourth Edition, Text Revision*. Washington, DC: American Psychiatric Association; 2002:677.

hair is firmly rooted in the scalp and is classically varied in length (Figure 146-12). Examination with the fingertip demonstrates an easily palpable stubble. There is an absence of scale, but focal perifollicular erythema with hemorrhagic excoriations may be noted.[3] This plucking of the hair may fracture the hair above or within the follicle, and the result is a fractured end unlike the fine tapered silkiness usually associated with new anagen hair.[2] Examination of the hair under magnification shows stable broken-off hair of normal caliber.

Trichotillomania may be diagnosed when hair is found in the patient's bed, or there is observation of the habit by a caregiver.[3] In adolescents, the behavior may occur in secret, and the patient may deny the manipulation.[1] Parents may be unaware of the habit, and the diagnosis may be resisted (Box 146-2).[17] Histopathological examination of a scalp biopsy in the affected areas often revealed melanin pigment in the follicular canals, known as pigmented hair casts.The condition may be episodic; however, it can also become chronic and difficult to treat.[2] An interdisciplinary approach to the management of trichotillomania can be quite helpful.[18] Psychiatric evaluation may be necessary to identify comorbidities, and counseling and adjunctive pharmacotherapy (chlormipramine, selective serotonin reuptake inhibitors) might be required to assist in the modification of the behavior.[2,3,18]

## MEDICAL CONDITIONS PRESENTING AS ALOPECIA

Diffuse and chronic telogen shedding (longer than 3 months) in the adolescent patient may warrant investigation of a secondary cause of hair loss.The most common systemic disease manifesting with hair loss is iron deficiency. Another disorder of particular importance in the adolescent patient is anorexia nervosa.[10] Additional causes of alopecia in teenagers from systemic sources include thyroid disease (hyperthyroidism and hypothyroidism), secondary syphilis, systemic lupus erythematosus, zinc deficiency, fatty acid deficiency, protein malnutrition, drug-induced hair loss, and chronic renal failure.

### IRON DEFICIENCY

Iron deficiency is an occasional finding during an investigation of chronic hair loss in the teenage patient. A positive history of anemia, heavy menses, or vegetarianism can be helpful to suggest this diagnosis.[10] Symptoms may include pallor, easy fatigability, and lethargy.[19] Many dermatologists believe that iron deficiency with or without anemia is a cause of diffuse alopecia.

Nonetheless, this has recently become more controversial. There is no firm evidence to establish the relationship between low serum ferritin or serum iron and hair loss.[10,20,21] Previously, it was believed that oral iron supplementation was necessary to treat this alopecia until ferritin or iron levels returned to normal, but presently the role of iron supplementation therapy in the management of hair loss and the utility of serum ferritin in the investigation of patients with chronic diffuse telogen alopecia is unclear.[20,21] Some authors have observed, however, that treatment of hair loss is enhanced when iron deficiency is also treated.[21]

### ANOREXIA NERVOSA AND NUTRITIONAL DISORDERS

An increasingly common diagnosis in the adolescent patient population, especially in females, is anorexia nervosa. A history of weight loss or crash dieting can facilitate diagnosis.[10] Symptoms of anorexia nervosa are mostly attributable to starvation, including amenorrhea, constipation, abdominal pain, cold intolerance, lethargy, emaciation, hypotension, bradycardia, and skin dryness. Some individuals develop lanugo, a fine downy body hair, on their trunks along with the scalp alopecia.

Another disorder involving chronic starvation, marasmus, results in dry, straight, sparse hair that is easily plucked.[19] Essential fatty acid deficiency and kwashiorkor produce much telogen hair loss with a lightening of hair color.[19] Alopecia may also be an important clue to the diagnoses of either zinc or B deficiencies.[19]

### THYROID DISEASE

Diffuse scalp alopecia occurs in patients with either hypothyroidism or hyperthyroidism. When a patient is profoundly hypothyroid, in addition to the barrage of classic symptoms and loss of the outer third of the eyebrows, patients may have significant hair loss.[19] Hypothyroidism inhibits cell division in skin appendages, thereby inducing catagen and delayed reentry to the anagen phase.[19] Interestingly, telogen effluvium-like alopecia occurs in severe hyperthyroidism, although the mechanism is not well understood. If thyroid disease is suspected, TSH, T3, and T4 should be evaluated.[10] With treatment, hair loss usually rapidly reenters the anagen phase in hypothyroid patients; hair loss usually ceases within 3 months of becoming euthyroid in hyperthyroid patients.[19]

### SECONDARY SYPHILIS AND CONNECTIVE TISSUE DISORDERS

With the increasing sexual activity of adolescents and the resurgence of syphilis in recent years, secondary syphilis is a consideration in a teenage patient presenting with patchy alopecia. The incidence of hair loss in secondary syphilis is 3% to 7%, and is most classically observed as patchy "moth-eaten" alopecia.[19,22] In addition to the scalp, hair loss may occur in the eyebrows, beard, and pubic area.[22] Traction alopecia, alopecia areata, and trichotillomania may present in a similar pattern to secondary syphilis.[22] When associated with a skin rash or lymphadenopathy, confirmation should be sought using serologic testing. Incidentally, the treatment of syphilis has also been shown to cause alopecia. As part of the Herxheimer reaction, sudden alopecia may result with the injection of penicillin.[22] Connective tissue disorders, most notably lupus erythematosus and dermatomyositis, can frequently present with a nonscarring diffuse alopecia.[14]

### METABOLIC DISORDERS AND DRUG-INDUCED ALOPECIA

Metabolic disorders such as chronic renal failure and chronic liver failure may present with alopecia, although these conditions are somewhat uncommon in the adolescent patient. Drug-induced anagen or telogen hair loss, however, is exceptionally common, especially in patients undergoing chemotherapy. Many medications and drugs have been implicated in alopecia (Box 146-3). Cessation of the drug in question is advised, but may be inappropriate with the necessary treatment of an underlying malignancy or other disorder.[19]

**Box 146-3**

***Common Drugs That Cause Alopecia in Adolescents***[3,19]

Phenytoin
Valproic acid
Amphetamines
Propanolol
Cimetidine
Lithium
Oral contraceptives
Retinoids
Vitamin A
Allopurinol
Interferon
Sulfasalazine
Propylthiouracil
Thyroxine
Anabolic steroids
Chemotherapeutic agents

## CONCLUSION

The origin of hair loss in adolescents is multifactorial. It may be an isolated finding leading to a specific diagnosis, or it may be indicative of an underlying metabolic, nutritional, or psychiatric disorder. Teens often seek treatment due to the major psychosocial implications that accompany alopecia. Successful treatment of hair loss in adolescents is dependent on identifying and treating underlying factors. Support of the teenage patient during the entire process is an essential component of treatment.

## REFERENCES


1. Harrison S, Sinclair R. Optimal management of hair loss (alopecia) in children. *Am J Clin Dermatol.* 2003;4(11):757–770

2. Hautmann G, Hercogova J, Lotti T. Trichotillomania. *J Am Acad Dermatol.* 2002;46(6):807–821

3. Rogers M, Tay Y. Hair disorders. In: Schachner LA, Hansen RC, eds. *Pediatric Dermatology*. 3rd ed. Edinburgh: Mosby; 2003

4. Fitzpatrick T, Johnson RA, Wolff K, Suurmond D. *Color Atlas and Synopsis of Clinical Dermatology*. 4th ed. New York: McGraw-Hill; 2001

5. Mandt N, Vogt A, Blume-Peytavi U. Differential diagnosis of hair loss in children. *J Deutschen Dermatologischen Gesellschaft.* 2004;2:399–411

6. Hamilton JB. Male hormone stimulation is prerequisite and an incitant in common baldness. *Am J Anat.* 1942;71:451–480

7. Stough D, Stenn K, Haber R, et al. Psychological effect, pathophysiology, and management of androgenetic alopecia in men. *Mayo Clin Proc.* 2005;80(10):1316–1322

8. Olsen EA, Messenger AG, Shapiro J, et al. Evaluation and treatment of male and female pattern hair loss. *J Am Acad Dermatol.* 2005;52(2):301–311

9. Price VH. Androgenetic alopecia in adolescents. *Cutis.* 2003;71(2):115–121

10. Chartier MB, Hoss DM, Grant-Kels JM. Approach to the adult female patient with diffuse nonscarring alopecia. *J Am Acad Dermatol.* 2002;47(6):809–818

11. Olsen EA, Dunlap FE, Funicella T, et al. A randomized clinical trial of 5% topical minoxidil versus 2% topical minoxidil and placebo in the treatment of androgenetic alopecia in men. *J Am Acad Dermatol.* 2002;47(3):377–385

12. Price VH, Menefee E, Sanchez M, Kaufman KD. Changes in hair weight in men with androgenetic alopecia after treatment with finasteride (1 mg daily): 3 and 4-year results. *J Am Acad Dermatol.* 2006;55(1):71–74

13. Bolognia JL, Jorizzo JL, Rapini RP. *Dermatology*. St Louis, MO: Mosby; 2003

14. Mohrenschlager M, Seidl HP, Ring J, Abeck D. Pediatric tinea capitis: recognition and management. *Am J Clin Dermatol.* 2005;6(4):203–213

15. Trovato MJ, Schwartz RA, Janniger CK. Tinea capitis: current concepts in clinical practice. *Cutis.* 2006;77(2):93–99

16. Sharma V, Silverberg NB, Howard R, Tran CT, Laude TA, Frieden IJ. Do hair care practices affect the acquisition of tinea capitis? A case-control study. *Arch Pediatr Adolesc Med.* 2001;155(7):818–821

17. American Psychiatric Association. *Diagnostic and Statistical Manual of Mental Disorders, Fourth Edition, Text Revision*. Washington, DC: American Psychiatric Association; 2002

18. Tay YK, Levy ML, Metry DW. Trichotillomania in childhood: case series and review. *Pediatrics.* 2004;113(5):e494–e498

19. Sinclair R. Diffuse hair loss. *Int J Dermatol.* 1999;38 (suppl 1):8–18

20. Sinclair R. There is no clear association between low serum ferritin and chronic diffuse telogen hair loss. *Br J Dermatol.* 2002;147(5):982–984

21. Trost LB, Bergfeld WF, Calogeras E. The diagnosis and treatment of iron deficiency and its potential relationship to hair loss. *J Am Acad Dermatol.* 2006;54(5):824–844

22. Vafaie J, Weinberg JM, Smith B, Mizuguchi RS. Alopecia in association with sexually transmitted disease: a review. *Cutis.* 2005;76(6):361–366

# CHAPTER 147

# Miscellaneous Dermatologic Disorders in Adolescence

LEONARD KRISTAL, MD • ELENA C. HALIASOS, MD

## INTRODUCTION

Although acne is the most common skin condition seen in adolescents, there are other skin conditions that occur with increased frequency. Among the more common conditions are infection and infestations. Primary skin conditions such as vitiligo and hidradenitis suppurativa, although uncommon, can have significant psychosocial effect on the adolescent patient. Adolescent behaviors such as tanning, tattooing, and body piercing are associated with short- and long-term potential health risks.

## FUNGAL INFECTIONS

### TINEA VERSICOLOR

Tinea versicolor is an asymptomatic, superficial fungal infection caused by overgrowth of *Malassezia furfur*, an organism normally found on the skin of almost all adolescents. There is an equal incidence in males and females and it is seen equally in all races. Warm, humid climates and sweating predispose to infection by this organism. Other predisposing factors include genetic predisposition, immunosuppression, malnutrition, and Cushing syndrome.

Tinea versicolor typically presents as hypo- or hyperpigmented scaly, tan, brown, or reddish-brown macules favoring the upper trunk and arms, although the neck, abdomen, and antecubital fossae are commonly involved. The individual lesions are round or oval, and coalescence into larger lesions is common. During the summer months, if a tan is present the lesions may appear hypopigmented. In darker-skinned individuals the lesions are usually hypopigmented but may be hyperpigmented (Figure 147-1). All lesions tend to be the same color in the individual patient. Scaling associated with the macules may be subtle but is more evident when the lesions are slightly scraped. Examination with a Wood light will reveal a mustard yellow fluorescence. The diagnosis of tinea versicolor can be confirmed by microscopic potassium hydroxide (KOH) examination of scale revealing the yeast and hyphal forms of *M furfur*, giving a "spaghetti and meatballs" appearance. Box 147-1 lists the differential diagnosis of tinea versicolor, which includes vitiligo, where scaling is not seen, and pityriasis rosea and seborrheic dermatitis, where lesions are more inflammatory than tinea versicolor.

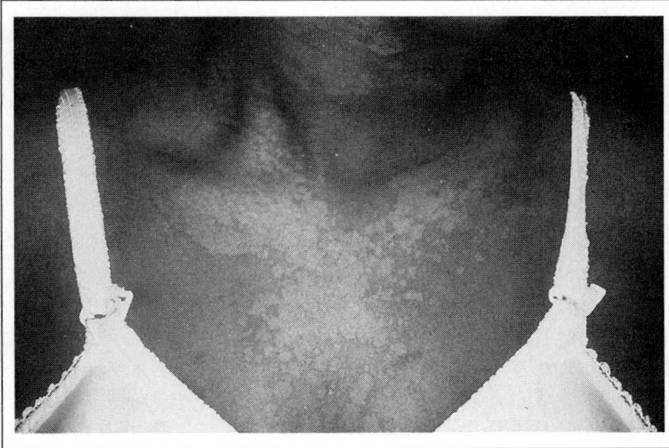

FIGURE 147-1 Tinea versicolor. (See color insert.)

When treating adolescents with tinea versicolor it is important to explain that the hypo- or hyperpigmentation can take months to resolve, and the rash can recur in the future. Most patients can be treated topically. Selenium sulfide 2.5% suspension applied daily and washed off after 10 minutes, over a 2-week period, is an effective treatment. Selenium sulfide 2.5% suspension also may be applied to the skin at night and washed off in the morning, but this may cause some irritation. One or 2 applications should be beneficial. Selenium sulfide can be used prophylactically for a few minutes in the shower once to twice monthly. Ketoconazole shampoo is an

**Box 147-1**

***Differential Diagnosis of Tinea Versicolor***

- Vitiligo
- Pityriasis alba
- Pityriasis rosea
- Seborrheic dermatitis

alternative to selenium sulfide. Shampoos are more economical for use over large areas.

Topical antifungal medications such as azoles and allylamines applied once daily for 2 weeks also are effective. For severe cases, or those where topical treatments have not provided the desired effect, systemic antifungal agents may be used. Oral fluconazole taken as a single 400-mg dose or itraconazole 200-mg daily for 5 days is effective. Oral ketoconazole can be given as a 400-mg single dose followed by activity leading to sweating, or as a 200 to 400 mg daily dose for 3 to 5 days. Oral antifungal medications do not prevent recurrence. It is important to discuss potential risks associated with oral antifungal therapy.[1-3]

### TINEA CORPORIS

Tinea corporis is a superficial dermatophyte infection occurring on the skin of the body not involving the scalp, groin, palms, or soles. *Trichophyton rubrum* infections are most common, although infections, with *Trichophyton tonsurans* and *Microsporum canis* are also seen. Adolescent males and females may be infected by coming in contact with others who are infected, or by exposure to infected animals. Two unique presentations include tinea gladiatorum, a superficial fungal infection spread by skin contact among wrestlers, and Majocchi granuloma, an infection of hair follicles leading to granuloma formation that occurs often in females who shave their legs.

The typical lesion in tinea corporis is an annular or ring-like plaque, with a peripheral scaly border and central clearing (Figure 147-2). The lesions expand centrifugally. The peripheral border may have scale, crusts, papules, pustules, or vesicles. Infections are often unilateral, although multiple lesions may occur. Tinea gladiatorum typically presents on the head, neck, and arms corresponding to areas of most skin-to-skin contact in wrestlers.

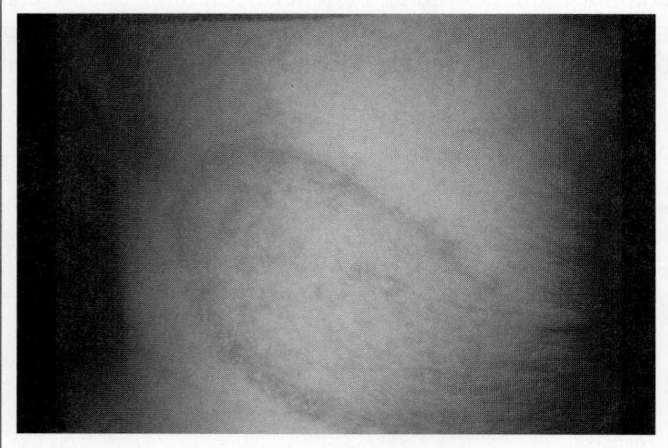

**FIGURE 147-2** Tinea corporis. (See color insert.)

**Box 147-2**

***Differential Diagnosis of Tinea Corporis***

- Nummular dermatitis
- Candidiasis
- Psoriasis
- Pityriasis rosea (especially the herald patch)
- Tinea versicolor
- Granuloma annulare
- Systemic lupus erythematosus (especially subacute cutaneous lupus)

The diagnosis of tinea corporis infections can be made easily and quickly by performing a KOH microscopic examination on scale obtained from scraping the border of a lesion. The KOH will dissolve the keratin in the scale making it possible to visualize hyphae within the scale. A fungal culture is a useful adjunct, especially in those cases where clinical suspicion is high but a KOH is negative. Box 147-2 lists the differential diagnosis of tinea corporis.

Topical antifungal preparations are effective in treating tinea corporis and should be applied once or twice daily for 1 week after clinical resolution. The cream should be applied 1 cm to 2 cm beyond the clinically visible area of involvement. Inflammatory lesions may be treated with a mild topical corticosteroid such as 1% hydrocortisone, but the use of potent topical steroids and steroid/antifungal combinations should be avoided as this may prolong the infection and cause local side effects, including unsightly striae.

### TINEA PEDIS

Tinea pedis, also known as athlete's foot, is most commonly caused by *Trichophyton rubrum*. This superficial dermatophyte infection occurs more commonly in males and tends to develop in most cases after puberty. Risk factors include swimming, sweating associated with prolonged use of occlusive shoes, and hot, humid environments. The interdigital type, the most common, presents with erythema, maceration, scaling, and fissures, typically starting in the fourth toe web space. Itching is common, and the rash may spread to the toes or the plantar portion of the foot. A second type, called moccasin tinea pedis, presents with fine dry scaling and erythema, or at times thickened hyperkeratotic areas located on the

**Box 147-3**

***Differential Diagnosis of Tinea Pedis***

- *Candida* infection
- Erythrasma
- Dyshidrotic eczema
- Contact dermatitis
- Eczematous dermatitis
- Psoriasis

plantar aspect of the foot. A third type associated with vesicles and bullae most often found on the instep or anterior portion of the plantar portion of the foot tends to be pruritic. Box 147-3 lists the differential diagnosis of tinea pedis.

Diagnosis can be made by a KOH examination of skin scrapings or from a fungal culture.

Most cases of tinea pedis can be treated topically, although oral antifungal therapy may be required. In addition to medications, measures should be taken to try to prevent reinfection by wearing less occlusive footwear or protective footwear around swimming pools or common bathing areas. Topical antifungal creams include azoles, allylamines, and pyridones. Over-the-counter preparations may be tried initially and, if not effective, a prescription antifungal can be used. As with any treatment, adherence is important for the medication to be effective. Interdigital tinea pedis requires treatment for 2 to 4 weeks. The dry, scaly, moccasin-type of tinea pedis may require longer durations of treatment and at times require oral antifungal therapy. The vesicular type may also require oral antifungal therapy especially if the infection is extensive, although initial therapy with a topical antifungal agent may be effective.

### TINEA CRURIS

Tinea cruris is a superficial fungal infection of the groin area commonly seen in adolescent males and most frequently caused by *Trichophyton rubrum*. Predisposing factors include the wearing of tight-fitting clothes or wet garments. In adolescents this infection may be seen in those using communal bathing areas or living in close quarters where the fungus has been found on clothing, towels, and bedding. The rash presents as erythema and scaling that is typically sharply demarcated, sometimes with central hyperpigmentation, located on the groin and inner thighs, sometimes spreading to the perianal area and buttocks, and typically sparing the penis and scrotum (Figure 147-3). In acute cases the eruption may be moist and macerated. Pruritus is a frequent complaint. Box 147-4 lists the differential diagnosis of tinea cruris.

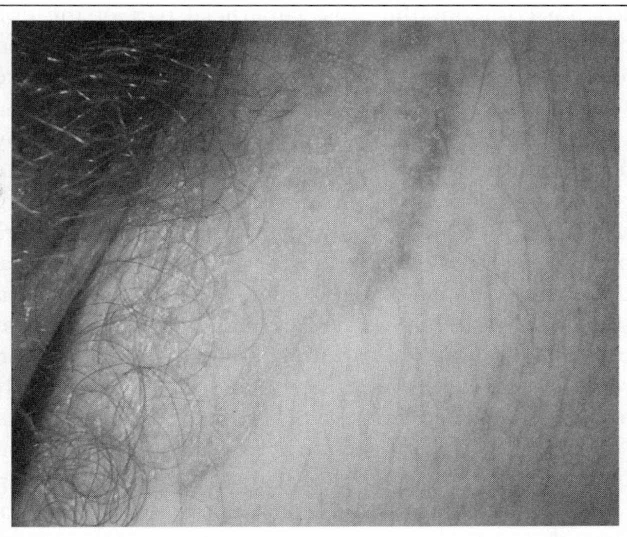

**FIGURE 147-3** Tinea cruris of the inner thigh. (See color insert.)

**Box 147-4**

***Differential Diagnosis of Tinea Cruris***

- Intertrigo
- Psoriasis
- Seborrheic dermatitis
- *Candida* infection
- Erythrasma
- Irritant contact dermatitis

Potassium hydroxide examination and fungal culture can confirm the diagnosis of tinea cruris. Topical treatment would be similar to treatments mentioned in the section on tinea pedis.

## INFESTATIONS

### SCABIES

Scabies is an infestation caused by the *Sarcoptes scabiei* var *hominis* mite. It is common worldwide and is seen in all age groups. The infestation is transmitted primarily by close physical contact with an infested person and is not uncommon in adolescents, especially those sharing close quarters on college campuses. After contact with an infested person, the mite burrows into the stratum corneum, the most superficial part of the epidermis. There it begins a cycle of growth, reproduction leading to new larvae development, and finally more scabies mites. In addition, the mites burrow through the stratum corneum, depositing feces, as well as eggs by female mites. After about a month, the body's immune response leads to a very pruritic eruption. The scratching that occurs secondary to the pruritus limits the numbers of mites in the skin but does not eradicate the infestation. Some patients may have moderate itching without significant rash, whereas others will have a significant papular eruption. Typical physical findings include burrows, erythematous papules, nodules found particularly in the axillae and groin, and vesiculopustular lesions. Lesions may be found anywhere on the body, but in older children, adolescents, and adults the face and scalp tend to be uninvolved. Numerous scattered excoriations and at times secondary eczematous changes may lead one to think of a nonspecific dermatitis. Patients may also develop a secondary bacterial infection due to scratching.

Scabies burrows are very small, thin, serpiginous tracts that are not inflammatory. Burrows are generally few in number and are more commonly found on the wrists or finger webs, although they may be found on the feet, axillae, penis, and breasts. Erythematous papules reflecting the inflammatory reaction to the presence of the infestation are far more common and when scraped will not yield a diagnosis. Box 147-5 lists the differential diagnosis of scabies.

Confirmation of the diagnosis can be made by scraping the end of a burrow with a No. 15 scalpel blade, placing it on a microscope slide with mineral oil, and then examining for the mite, eggs, or fecal material called scybala.

Secondarily infected patients may be improperly diagnosed as having a primary diagnosis of impetigo. A high level of suspicion should lead one to think of scabies in a patient with a nonspecific, pruritic eruption. It is important to ask about unexplained pruritus, rash, or even treated scabies in other family members or close contacts. Many times, when only the index case, and not all close contacts are treated, the infestation can continue to spread. Some affected individuals may just have itching on their fingers, breasts, or genitalia.

**Box 147-5**

***Differential Diagnosis of Scabies***

- Atopic dermatitis
- Contact dermatitis
- Insect bites
- Papular urticaria

Treatment of scabies is aimed at treating the mite infestation with a topical scabeticide as well as treating secondary eczematous or infectious processes. Topical permethrin 5% cream is the treatment of choice for most cases of scabies. The medication should be applied from the neck down, covering all body surfaces including the tips of nails, and be left on for about 12 hours. The treatment should be repeated in one week. Lindane is generally not recommended at this time due to the small risk of neurotoxicity. Topical crotamiton 10% is much less effective than permethrin, and precipitated sulfur 6% in petrolatum is an option for pregnant women or those who have hypersensitivities to the other scabeticides. Oral ivermectin has also been found to be effective in adolescent populations but is generally not accepted as first-line treatment.[4] All household members and close contacts should be treated. All clothing, towels, and bedding used within the past week should be washed in hot water. Clothing that cannot be washed in hot water should be dry-cleaned or placed in a plastic bag for one week. Itching can be treated with oral antihistamines or menthol/camphor lotions. Eczematous rashes will benefit from topical steroid application. Secondary bacterial infections should be treated with antibiotics that cover both streptococcal and staphylococcal organisms. Symptoms resolve within 1 to 3 weeks after appropriate treatment, although nodular lesions may persist for months.

## PEDICULOSIS PUBIS

Pubic or crab lice, *Phthirus pubis*, cause pediculosis pubis. The infestation is spread by close physical or sexual contact, although it may be transmitted from contaminated clothing, towels, or bedding.[5] The louse has a short, broad body with large claws in the front giving it the appearance of a crab. The large claws enable it to cling to pubic hair as well as hair in the axillae, beard, and at times, eyelashes, eyebrows, and body hair.

The predominant symptom in patients with pediculosis pubis is pruritus, whereas on physical examination excoriations may be noted. On close inspection, a louse may be found grasping the hair close to the skin. Some patients present with maculae ceruleae, bluish macules caused by bites on the skin by the pubic louse. Patients should be checked for another sexually transmitted disease when they are found to have pubic lice, as the incidence is increased.

Treatment of pubic lice is similar to head lice. The most effective treatment is the overnight application of 5% permethrin cream to all affected hairy areas with a repeat application 1 week later. All sexual contacts should be treated. Other treatments include 1% permethrin or synergized pyrethrin shampoos.[5]

## VIRAL INFECTIONS

### MOLLUSCUM CONTAGIOSUM

Molluscum contagiosum is a cutaneous viral infection caused by a DNA poxvirus that affects children, adolescents, and adults, with an incubation period ranging from 2 weeks to 6 months. Molluscum contagiosum can be transmitted by sexual contact and close physical contact including sports, such as wrestling. Infection can occur secondary to contact with fomites such as sharing towels and sports equipment in gyms. Spread may also occur among children who share baths and swimming pools. The prevalence is increased in those with immune deficiency, especially patients infected with HIV.

Molluscum contagiosum present as skin-colored to pearly white, dome-shaped papules with a central white umbilication (Figure 147-4). Lesions range in size from 1 mm to 5 mm, although larger lesions up to 15 mm may occur. Molluscum may appear anywhere on the body, although the neck, axillae, trunk, and thighs are common areas of involvement. Genital involvement is not unusual, especially in adolescents. Lesions in the intergluteal cleft may appear like skin tags or even resemble warts. About 10% of patients will develop an eczematous dermatitis around the molluscum, which sometimes may not clear until the molluscum are gone.

Molluscum contagiosum is a self-limited eruption that resolves within a few months to a few years if left untreated. When the patient exhibits immunity to the virus the lesions may become inflamed, sometimes appearing infected. Molluscum, even untreated, can heal with atrophic scarring.

There is no distinct cure for molluscum, although there are many treatment strategies. Destructive modalities such as the topical application of cantharidin, cryotherapy, or curettage are effective at treating individual lesions. Topical medications such as tretinoin cream 0.025% to 0.1%, imiquimod 5% cream, salicylic acid, and podophyllotoxin have all been used with some degree of success, although irritation may be associated with these treatments.

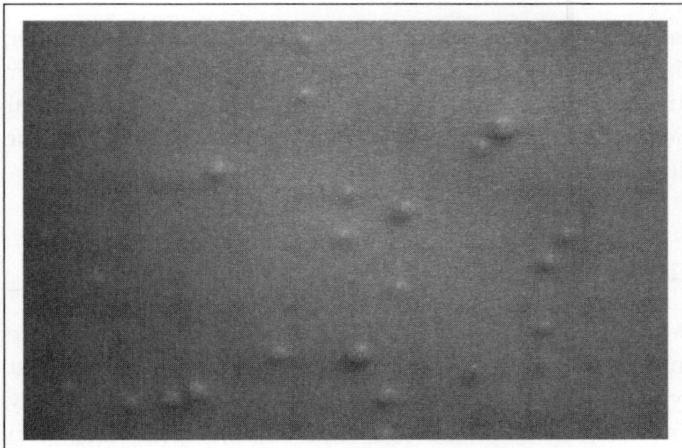

FIGURE 147-4 Molluscum contagiosum. (See color insert.)

### WARTS

Warts are infections caused by the human papillomavirus (HPV), of which there are more than 100 types. Warts can occur on the skin and mucosal surfaces. Cutaneous warts in adolescents include common warts, palmar and plantar warts, flat warts, and genital warts. Common warts, known as verruca vulgaris, may occur anywhere, but areas of predilection include the fingers, dorsal hands, elbows, and knees (Figure 147-5). They present

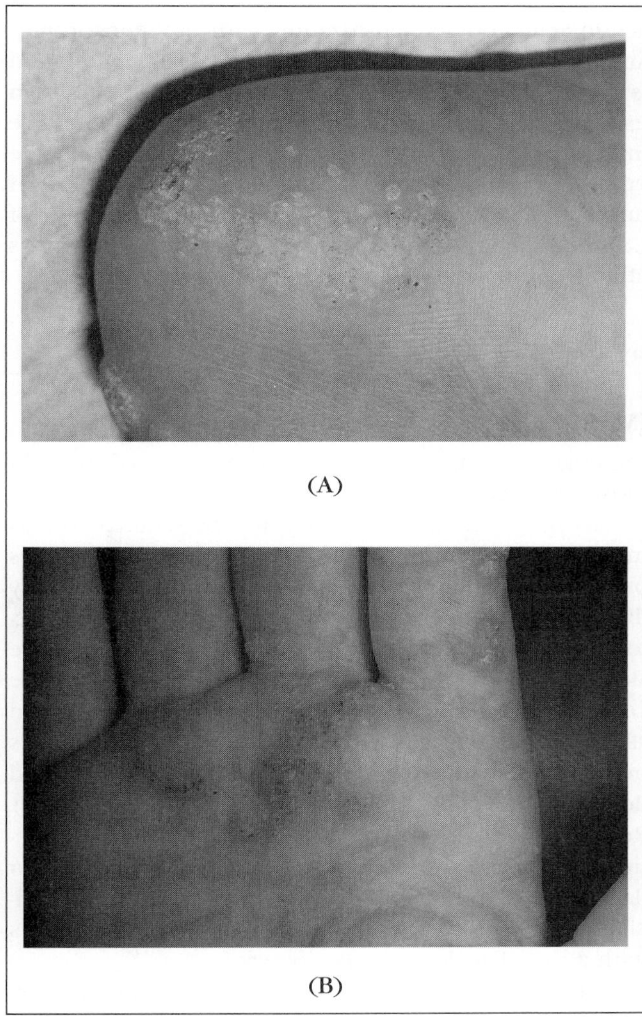

(A)

(B)

FIGURE 147-5 Warts. (A) Plantar wart, mosaic type. (B) Palmar warts. (See color insert.)

as exophytic, hyperkeratotic, cauliflower-like growths. Plantar warts grow down within the epidermis and may coalesce into large plaques called mosaic warts. Plantar warts may cause pain when walking. Flat warts are skin colored or pink, flat-topped papules with a smooth surface most commonly seen on the face, dorsal hands, or arms. Anogenital warts, also known as *condyloma acuminata*, are often found on the external genitalia and perineum, but may also be seen in the pubic area and inguinal folds. See Chapter 53, Sexually Transmitted Infections, for an in-depth discussion of anogenital warts.

There is no true cure for warts, but there are many treatment modalities available. About two-thirds of warts will go away within 2 years if left untreated. Treatments range from noninvasive topical therapies to destructive modalities.[6] Topical therapy includes the use of salicylic acid available over the counter as a 17% preparation in a base of flexible collodion or as a 40% salicylic acid plaster patch. Other topical treatments include trichloroacetic acid, contact sensitization with diphencyprone,[7] and imiquimod cream, although the use of imiquimod is more effective for the treatment of genital warts than extragenital warts. Topical tretinoin is often effective in treating flat warts.[8] Destructive modalities include cryotherapy, electrosurgery, and laser therapy. A form of immunotherapy involving the intralesional injection of *Candida*, mumps, or *Trichophyton* skin test antigens is effective in patients with recalcitrant warts.[9,10]

## BACTERIAL INFECTIONS

### IMPETIGO

Impetigo is a superficial bacterial infection of the skin most often caused by *Staphylococcal aureus*. *Streptococcus pyogenes* infections may also be seen, as well as mixed infections with staphylococcus and streptococcus organisms. This highly contagious infection is spread by direct person-to-person contact, with predisposing factors including warm, humid climate and trauma to the skin. Clinically, the nonbullous presentation is more common than the bullous type. Lesions typically begin as small erythematous macules that evolve into vesicles or pustules, in turn becoming superficially eroded and developing a yellow honey-colored crust (Figure 147-6). Regional lymphadenopathy may be seen. Bullous impetigo presents with small vesicles that rapidly enlarge into flaccid, transparent bullae (Figure 147-7). These superficial bullae rupture, leaving a superficial erosion, at times with a rim of scale at the periphery.

Treatment of impetigo includes antibiotic therapy and local wound care, such as cleansing and soaks to remove the crusts. Localized infections without systemic symptoms may be treated topically with either mupirocin or retapamulin. Widespread infections or those in which constitutional symptoms or deeper infections are present should be treated with an oral *B*-lactamase-resistant antibiotic such as dicloxacillin or cephalexin.

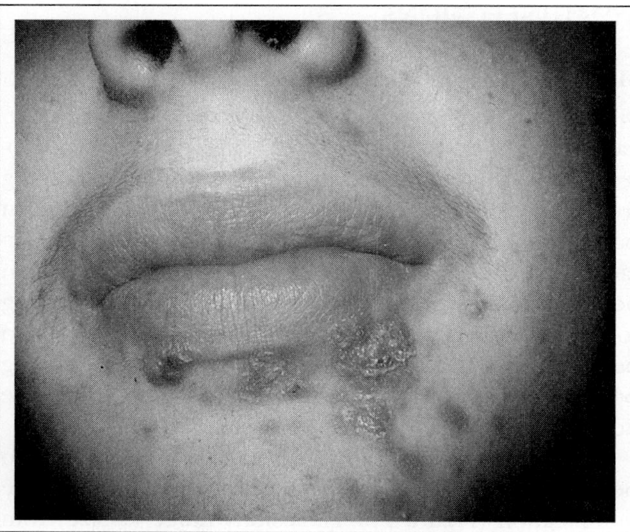

**FIGURE 147-6** Impetigo. (See color insert.)

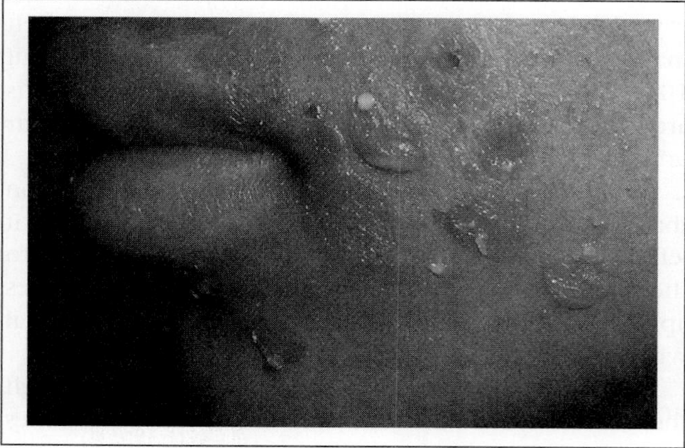

**FIGURE 147-7** Bullous impetigo. (See color insert.)

## GONORRHEA

Patients with a disseminated *Neisseria gonorrhoeae* infection can present with fever, arthritis, and a rash that typically involves the extremities. Chapter 53, Sexually Transmitted Infections, contains an in-depth discussion of the genital manifestations of infection with *Neisseria gonorrhoeae*. The rash consists of erythematous papules that develop a central vesicle or pustule with a hemorrhagic base. The center of the lesion may become hemorrhagic or necrotic. Skin lesions tend to be painless. It is important to recognize these skin lesions in the context of other symptoms that an adolescent patient presents with because this is a disseminated infection that requires systemic antibiotic treatment.

## OTHER DERMATOLOGIC HAZARDS AND CONDITIONS

### SUN EXPOSURE

Current cultural trends advocate tan bodies. A survey conducted on 10,079 boys and girls ages 12 to 18 reported that 10% had used a tanning bed in the previous year.[11]

These data were also replicated in another study showing that, between 1998 and 2004, the incidence of tanning among adolescents aged 11 to 18 years was 10%.[12]

Ultraviolet light has been documented to cause increased numbers of nevi in children,[13] increased risk of skin cancers including melanomas,[14] in addition to promoting signs of skin aging. Exposure to natural sunlight is a combination of ultraviolet A and B light, with the strongest exposure being between the hours of 10 am and 4 pm. Although not a common entity in adolescents, incidence of melanomas is rising in this age group.[15-17] Early detection of melanoma enables better outcomes.

Tanning beds have become popular among adolescents and are perceived to be safer than actual sun exposure. Tanning beds are programmed to release ultraviolet A light; however, depending on the quality of the bulbs, ultraviolet B light is also released to a certain degree. Because there currently are no national regulations to monitor the amount of ultraviolet B light being emitted, individuals who expose themselves to tanning beds place themselves in precarious positions.[18] The American Academy of Pediatrics[18] recommends that sun protection counseling for teenagers include warnings about using sunbeds and sunlamps.

Many states have implemented measures that either prohibit tanning salon use or mandate parental permission for minors to attend tanning salons.[19] Such public health measures are instrumental in decreasing the morbidity and mortality from skin cancer. Further concerns are being raised as to the addictive behavior of habitual tanners. Recent studies suggest an opioid-type mechanism in those who receive ultraviolet light and their desire to return for more sessions.[20]

Preventive measures include discontinuation of any tanning practices, sun avoidance between 10 am and 4 pm, regular sunscreen use, hat use when outdoors, and regular skin examinations. The use of artificial tanners may be an alternative to tanning beds for those who desire darker skin tones, but adolescents must be aware that they are not alternatives for sunscreen. It is important that a dermatologist evaluate patients with numerous nevi, especially with a family history of atypical nevi or melanoma, or patients who develop a new, unusual nevus or have an older nevus that has changed.

### HIDRADENITIS SUPPURATIVA

Hidradenitis suppurativa is a chronic inflammatory disease affecting areas bearing apocrine glands, especially the axillae and anogenital regions. Although the exact etiology remains unknown, current theories speculate that shortly after puberty the apocrine glands become occluded in predisposed individuals. This occlusion results in rupture of the apocrine-follicular unit releasing the keratin contents into the dermis, eliciting an inflammatory response.[21] Hidradenitis suppurativa is more common in blacks and women, with an onset after puberty.

Clinical findings of hidradenitis suppurativa include comedones behind the ears, double comedones, and deep nodules and draining abscesses in the axilla, inframammary, groin, or perianal areas (Figure 147-8). As the lesions resolve, scarring results, often with palpable subcutaneous cord-like structures or a honeycombed appearance. The deep lesions are characteristically sterile upon culture; however, secondary infection may be present, and treatment will then be dictated by culture results. Long-term sequelae include scarring, fistulae to the urethra, bladder, peritoneum, and rectum, hypoproteinemia, anemia, and squamous cell carcinoma at scarred sites.[21]

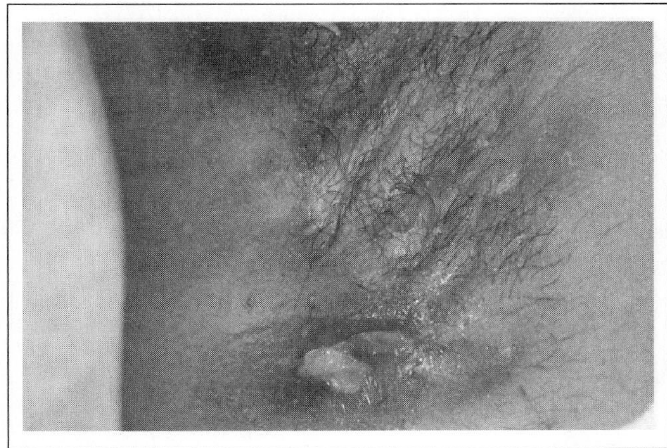

**FIGURE 147-8** Hidradenitis suppurativa. (See color insert.)

Treatment is difficult, as few have been successful in remitting the disease. Topical measures include antiseptic soaps and benzoyl peroxide washes to minimize bacterial superinfection. Topical clindamycin has benefited patients with *Staphylococcus aureus* secondary infection, and oral antibiotics may be necessary depending on abscess culture results. Although incision and drainage relieves symptoms temporarily, scarring and chronic sinus formation may result. Other adjuvant therapies include weight loss, wearing loose-fitting clothing, and absorbent powders or drying solutions.

Oral treatments with corticosteroids, hormonal therapy, isotretinoin, ametidine, and finasteride have led to temporary improvements but are not curative.[21] Biologic agents such as infliximab have recently been reported as successful in certain patients, but there are limited case reports so far.[22,23] Surgical excision and grafting, or $CO_2$ laser ablation, have also shown promising results.[24] It is important not to discount the psychological effect this chronic disease has on adolescents.

## ACANTHOSIS NIGRICANS

Acanthosis nigricans presents as a symmetric, velvety, thickening of the skin with hyperpigmentation (Figure 147-9). Usual sites of involvement are the axilla, groin, posterior neck, knuckles, thighs, areola, and umbilicus; however, acanthosis nigricans can become generalized and include mucosal involvement.[25] Acanthosis nigricans is associated with insulin resistance and fibroblast growth factor receptor defect syndromes. Acanthosis nigricans has been found in several clinical settings with paraneoplastic, endocrine, congenital, familial, and pharmacologic associations. The most common cause, however, is hyperinsulinemia associated with obesity. (See Chapter 79, Obesity.) Polycystic ovary syndrome is also associated with acanthosis nigricans and insulin resistance. Chapter 65 discusses the association of acanthosis nigricans and polycystic ovarian syndrome.

In blacks, acanthosis nigricans is strongly associated with obesity and insulin resistance, and has been suggested to be a marker for increased risk of noninsulin-dependent diabetes mellitus. It is possible that increased insulin levels lead to acanthosis nigricans by the activation of the insulin-like growth factor-1 (IGF-1) pathway.[26]

Adolescents with acanthosis nigricans should be evaluated for insulin resistance. It is important to try to improve the underlying disease process. There is no effective treatment for acanthosis nigricans, although weight loss may minimize the signs of acanthosis nigricans, as do topical retinoids and lactic acid- or salicylic acid-containing emollients.[26]

## VITILIGO

Vitiligo is an acquired disorder of skin pigmentation, possibly autoimmune in nature, resulting in the destruction of melanocytes in the skin. Although this disorder usually manifests on its own, it has been associated with autoimmune endocrinopathies such as thyroid disease and occurs slightly more frequently in individuals with a family history of autoimmune disease. Half of patients manifest the disease by 20 years of age.[27]

The lesions of vitiligo appear as white, depigmented macules with discrete borders (Figure 147-10). Vitiligo commonly appears in a generalized form where the depigmented macules are bilaterally symmetric, typically

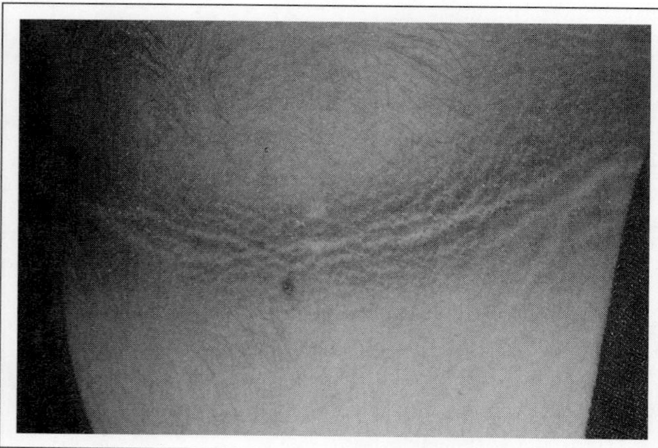

FIGURE 147-9 Acanthosis nigricans. (See color insert.)

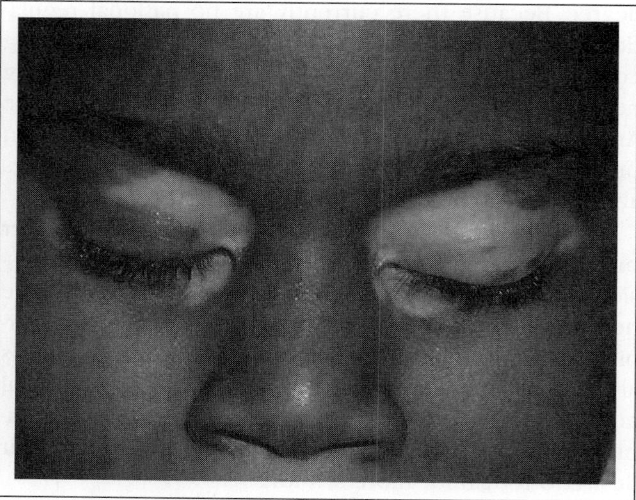

FIGURE 147-10 Vitiligo. (See color insert.)

**Box 147-6**

***Differential Diagnosis of Vitiligo***

- Postinflammatory hypopigmentation
- Nevus depigmentosus
- Tinea versicolor
- Hypopigmented macules of tuberous sclerosus
- Pityriasis alba

involving the upper eyelids, perioral area, fingers, wrists, elbows, axillae, groin area, knees, shins, dorsal ankles, and toes. Vitiligo may also occur in a localized or segmental distribution. There may also be depigmentation of the hairs in involved areas. On Wood lamp examination these lesions enhance with a bright white hue. This contrasts with hypopigmentation, which also accentuates on Wood lamp but lacks the characteristic bright white appearance. Box 147-6 lists the differential diagnosis of vitiligo.

Disorders of hypopigmentation include postinflammatory hypopigmentation commonly seen after eczematous skin conditions, nevus depigmentosus, tinea versicolor, and the hypopigmented macules of tuberous sclerosis.

Spontaneous resolution of vitiligo is rare. When repigmentation does occur it begins as 2 to 3 mm tan macules originating at hair follicles. Poor rates of repigmentation occur at sites where hair follicles are minimal, such as the dorsal fingers and wrists. Topical corticosteroids, calcineurin inhibitors, laser and ultraviolet phototherapy approaches to repigmentation have been attempted with variable success rates.[28]

Given the fact that vitiligo is very difficult to treat, the adolescent with vitiligo will seek some type of intervention to improve the cosmetic appearance of these lesions. Cosmetic cover-ups such as Dermablend and Covermark can help conceal bothersome areas. It is important to stress the importance of sun protection to adolescents with vitiligo, as the affected areas are more prone to sunburn. Artificial tanners may make the skin look more pigmented but do not offer photoprotection.

## ERYTHEMA MIGRANS

Erythema migrans represents the first sign of Lyme disease. Lyme disease is a multistage, multisystem disease caused by infection with *Borrelia burgdorferi*. The spirochete is acquired through the bite of an *Ixodes* species tick. Chapter 140, Tick-Borne Infections, contains an in-depth discussion of Lyme disease.

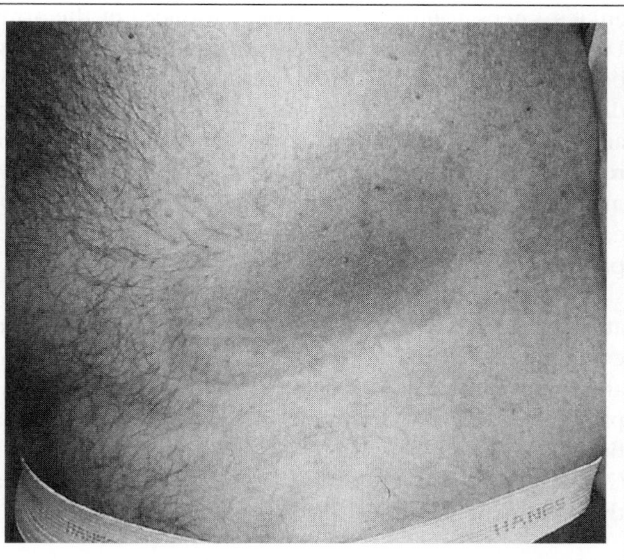


**FIGURE 147-11** Erythema migrans. (See color insert.)

Erythema migrans develops typically within 1 to 2 weeks after the tick bite. It begins as a red papule at the site of the bite and progresses to an annular, expanding erythematous patch (Figure 147-11). At this stage, the spirochete infection is limited to the skin. Multiple annular patches would insinuate disseminated disease with the spirochete. Erythema migrans will resolve after a few weeks. Failure to treat patients at this stage risks dissemination of the infection.

Treatment of early Lyme disease in adolescents consists of a 14- to 21-day course of doxycycline 100 mg every 12 hours. Alternative treatments include amoxicillin 500 mg every 8 hours for 14 to 21 days, or cefuroxime axetil 500 mg every 12 hours for 14 to 21 days.[29] Tick avoidance by wearing long-sleeve clothing in endemic areas, and permethrin or DEET (N,N-diethyl-3-methylbenzamide) repellent is recommended.

## ERYTHEMA NODOSUM

Erythema nodosum is a cutaneous hypersensitivity reaction. Despite the many causes associated with this cutaneous reaction, in up to as many as half of the cases there is no etiology found. β-hemolytic streptococcal infection is the most common identifiable cause; however, others include infections such as mycoplasma, tuberculosis, inflammatory bowel disease, and sarcoidosis; medications such as oral contraceptives, sulfonamides, and penicillins; and medical conditions such as pregnancy.

The diagnosis is often made clinically with characteristic tender erythematous nodules symmetrically located over pretibial surfaces. Other sites of involvement include ankles, knees, thighs, and extensor surfaces of the arms. Lesions on the trunk, face, and neck are rare. There may be associated arthritis, arthralgia, or fever. After a few days the lesions may take on a bruise-like appearance and resolve within a few days to weeks. The lesions resolve without scarring. As many as one-third of cases may recur.[30] Although the diagnosis may be made clinically, a biopsy will show diagnostic features of a septal panniculitis.

Treatment for erythema nodosum begins with attempts to determine the underlying cause. A streptococcus culture test, antistreptolysin O titers, chest x-ray, and tuberculin testing along with a complete history and physical examination may reveal the etiology. Leg elevation, bed rest, and nonsteroidal anti-inflammatory drugs (NSAIDs) help with the discomfort of the lesions. Alternative treatments include salicylates and potassium iodide.

## DRUG-ASSOCIATED RASH

Skin reactions to medications manifest in various ways. The spectrum ranges from transient urticaria, fixed drug eruptions, maculopapular or morbilliform eruptions, serum sickness-like reactions, drug hypersensitivity syndrome, Stevens-Johnson syndrome, (SJS) and toxic epidermal necrolysis (TEN). The reader is referred to *Litt's Drug Eruption Reference Manual* for a comprehensive guide on medications and drug eruptions.[31]

Pruritic exanthematous or maculopapular eruptions develop 7 to 14 days after ingestion of a medication and are the most common types of cutaneous drug reactions. The lesions typically begin on the chest and progress caudally. The hands and feet may exhibit lesions, but the mucous membranes are spared. The lesions may desquamate upon resolution of the eruption. Administration of ampicillin in the presence of Epstein-Barr virus infection often elicits this type of exanthem. Penicillins, sulfonamides, cephalosporins, and anticonvulsants are commonly associated with this type of drug reaction. The morphology of these drug eruptions may be identical to viral exanthems. Discontinuation of the offending agent and supportive care are treatments for this type of eruption.

Urticaria is a type I, IgE-mediated hypersensitivity reaction to a particular protein. Penicillin and penicillin derivatives are the most common medications that cause urticaria. The lesions have a characteristic edematous center with an erythematous border. Individual lesions by definition resolve within 24 hours. The treatment of urticaria is primarily through antihistamines, with subcutaneous epinephrine and systemic corticosteroids administered to those with severe urticaria or angioedema.

Serum sickness-like reactions present with fever, urticarial or erythema multiforme-like skin lesions, arthralgias or arthritis, lymphadenopathy, and eosinophilia developing 2 to 3 weeks after the ingestion of a medication. Cefaclor is most commonly associated with this eruption, although other medications including cefprozil, penicillins, and minocycline have been implicated. Unlike serum sickness, circulating immune complexes resulting in vasculitis and renal disease are not present. Serum sickness-like reactions resolve within 2 to 3 weeks after discontinuation of the medication. Antihistamines and corticosteroids may be used to treat severe symptoms.[32]

Stevens-Johnson syndrome is on the moderate end of the spectrum of drug reactions, characterized by at least 2 sites of mucosal erosions, targetoid dusky red lesions with less than 10% of epidermal detachment, and constitutional symptoms. Toxic epidermal necrolysis is at the more severe end of the spectrum, with more than 30% of body surface area epidermal detachment and less mucosal involvement. The most common triggers of SJS and TEN are sulfonamides, phenytoin, penicillin, NSAIDs, lamotrigine, carbamazepine, barbiturates, and allopurinol. Individuals with HIV are at a slightly higher risk for the reaction than the immunocompetent. Infections, neoplasia, autoimmune disorders, and vaccination have also been associated with this cutaneous eruption.[32]

Stevens-Johnson syndrome and TEN are potentially life-threatening disorders with mortality rates of 25% to 50%. Admission to burn units may decrease morbidity and mortality in these patients.[33] Meticulous wound care, hydration, nutrition, and pain management are required for successful outcomes. Consultation with ophthalmology is also vital to avoiding ocular sequelae. Although controversy exists as to the proper management of SJS-TEN, intravenous immunoglobulin (IVIG) at 2.5 to 3 mg/kg/day for 2 to 3 days has recently shown success in reducing progression of the reaction. Further studies are needed to assess the usefulness of IVIG. The use of systemic corticosteroids also remains controversial.

## TATTOOING AND BODY PIERCING

Tattooing and body piercing are becoming increasingly popular in adolescents. These practices may lead to scarring, bacterial infections, and viral infections such as hepatitis B, hepatitis C, and HIV/AIDS. Body piercing can cause site-specific side effects such as tooth fractures, gingival recession, or speech impediments in patients who get tongue and lip piercings.[34] Tattoos and body piercings may be associated with risk-taking behaviors in adolescents, and health care professionals should probe about potential high-risk behaviors in adolescents with tattoos and piercings.[35]

## REFERENCES


1. Kose O, Bulent Tastan H, Riza Gur A, Kurumlu Z. Comparison of a single 400-mg dose versus a 7-day 200 mg daily dose of itraconazole in the treatment of tinea versicolor. *J Derm Treatment.* 2002;13:77–79

2. Gupta AK, Bluhm R, Summerbell R. Pityriasis versicolor. *J Eur Acad Dermatol Venereol.* 2002;16:19–33

3. Friedlander SF, Rueda M, Chen BK, Caceres-Rios HW. Fungal, protozoal, and helminthic infections. In: Schachner LA, Hansen RC, eds. *Pediatric Dermatology.* 3rd ed. St. Louis, MO: Mosby; 2003:1106–1109

4. del Mar Saez-De-Ocariz M, McKinster CD, Orozco-Covarrubias L, Tamayo-Sanchez L, Ruiz-Maldonado R. Treatment of 18 children with scabies or cutaneous larva migrans using ivermectin. *Clin Exp Dermatol.* 2002;27:264–267

5. Meinking TL, Burkhart CN, Burkhart CG, Elgart G. Infestations. In: Bolognia JL, Jorizzo JL, Parini RP, eds. *Dermatology.* Vol 1. St Louis, MO: Mosby; 2008:1297–1298

6. Allen AL, Siegfried EC. Management of warts and molluscum in adolescents. *Adol Med.* 2000;12:229–242

7. Upitis JA, Krol A. The use of diphenylcyclopropenone in the treatment of recalcitrant warts. *J Cutan Med Surg.* 2002;6: 214–217

8. Bodemer C. Human papillomavirus. In: Schachner LA, Hansen RC, eds. *Pediatric Dermatology.* 3rd ed. St Louis, MO: Mosby; 2003:1088

9. Horn TD, Johnson SM, Helm RM, Roberson PK. Intralesional immunotherapy of warts with mumps, Candida, and Trichophyton skin test antigens: a single-blinded, randomized, and controlled trial. *Arch Dermatol.* 2005;141:589–594

10. Maronn M, Salm C, Lyon V, Galbraith S. One-year experience with candida antigen immunotherapy for warts and molluscum. *Pediatr Dermatol.* 2008.25:189–192

11. Geller AC, Colditz G, Oliveria S, et al. Use of sunscreen, sunburning rates, and tanning bed use among more than 10,000 US children and adolescents. *Pediatrics.* 2002;109(6): 1009–1014

12. Cokkinedes V, Weinstock M, Lazovich D, Ward E, Thun M. Indoor tanning use among adolescents in the US, 1998 to 2004. *Cancer.* 2009;115:190–198

13. English DR, Milne E, Simpson JA. Sun protection and the development of melanocytic nevi in children. *Cancer Epidemiol Biomarkers Prev.* 2005;14:2873–2876

14. Rivers JK, Wang B, Marcoux D. Ultraviolet radiation exposure: public health concerns. *J Cutan Med Surg.* 2006;10(suppl):8–13

15. Karlsson P, Boeryd B, Sander B, Westermark P, Rosdahl I. Increasing incidence of cutaneous malignant melanoma in children and adolescents 12–19 years of age in Sweden 1973–1992. *Acta Derm Venereol.* 1998;78:289–292

16. Downard CD, Rapkin LB, Gow KW. Melanoma in children and adolescents. *Surg Oncol.* 2007;16:215–220

17. Silverberg NB. Update on malignant melanoma in children. *Cutis.* 2001;67:393–396

18. American Academy of Pediatrics Committee on Environmental Health. Ultraviolet light: a hazard to children. *Pediatrics.* 1999;104:328–333

19. Dellavalle RP, Parker ER, Cersonsky N,et al. Youth access laws: in the dark at the parlor. *Arch Dermatol.* 2003:139:443–448

20. Kaur M, Liguori A, Lang W, et al. Induction of withdrawal-like symptoms in a small, randomized controlled trial of opioid blockade of frequent tanners. *J Am Acad Dermatol.* 2006;54:709–711

21. McMichael A, Guzman Sanchez D, Kelly P. Folliculitis and the follicular occlusion tetrad. In: Bolognia JL, Jorizzo JL, Parini RP, eds. *Dermatology.* Vol 1. St Louis, MO: Mosby; 2008:528–529

22. Moul DK, Korman NJ. The cutting edge. Severe hidradenitis suppurativa treated with adalimumab. *Arch Dermatol.* 2006;142:1110–1112

23. Giamarellos-Bourboulis EJ, Pelekanou E, Antonopoulou A, et al. An open-label phase II study of the safety and efficacy of etanercept for the therapy of hidradenitis suppurativa. *Br J Dermatol.* 2008;158:567–572.

24. Madan V, Hindle E, Hussain W, August PJ. Outcomes of treatment of nine cases of recalcitrant severe hidradenitis suppurativa with carbon dioxide laser. *Br J Dermatol.* 2008;159:1309–1314

25. Schwartz RA. Acanthosis nigricans. *J Am Acad Dermatol.* 1994;31:1–19

26. Higgins SP, Freemar M, Prose NS. Acanthosis nigricans: a practical approach to evaluation and management. *Dermatol Online J.* 2008;14(9):2

27. Morelli J. Vitiligo. In: Schachner LA, Hansen RC, eds. *Pediatr Dermatol.* 3rd ed. St Louis, MO: Mosby; 2003:513–515

28. Ortonne JP. Vitiligo and other disorders of hypopigmentation. In: Bolognia JL, Jorizzo JL, Parini RP, eds. *Dermatology.* Vol 1. St Louis, MO: Mosby; 2008:913–920

29. Wormser GP, Dattwyler RJ, Shapiro ED,et al. The clinical assessment, treatment, and prevention of lyme disease, human granulocytic anaplasmosis, and babesiosis: clinical practice guidelines by the Infectious Diseases Society of America. *Clin Infect Dis.* 2006;43:1089–1134

30. Mert A, Ozaras R, Tabak F, Pekmezci S, Demirkesen C, Ozturk R. Erythema nodosum: an experience of 10 years. *Scand J Infect Dis.* 2004;36:424–427

31. Litt J. *Litt's Drug Eruption Reference Manual.* 13th ed. New York, NY: Informa Healthcare; 2007

32. Knowles SR, Shapiro LE, Shear NH. Drug eruptions. In: Schachner LA, Hansen RC, eds. *Pediatric Dermatology.* 3rd ed. St Louis, MO: Mosby; 2003:1267–1276

33. Pereira F, Mudgil AV, Rosmarin DM. Toxic epidermal necrolysis. *J Am Acad Dermatol.* 2007;56(2):181–200

34. De Moor RJ, De Witte AM, Delme KI, De Bruyne MA, Hommez GM, Goyvaerts D. Dental and oral complications of lip and tongue piercings. *Br Dent J.* 2005;199:506–509

35. Carroll ST, Riffenburgh FH, Roberts TA, Myhre EB. Tattoos and body piercings as indicators of adolescent risk-taking behaviors. *Pediatrics.* 2002;109:1021–1027

SECTION 12

# Genetic Disorders

## CHAPTER 148

## Genetic Disorders

ROBERT W. MARION, MD • MARCIE B. SCHNEIDER, MD

In recent years, the field of medical genetics has undergone a revolution. Because of changes in prevailing ethical views and improved and more aggressive medical and surgical care delivered during infancy and childhood, increasing numbers of children born with congenital malformations and genetic syndromes are living longer. They are "aging out" of the pediatric population and appearing in increasing numbers in the waiting rooms of physicians who provide care to adolescents and adults. Better, more sophisticated diagnostic techniques, such as microarray comparative genomic hybridization (array CGH) and recombinant DNA technology have allowed earlier diagnosis of inherited and chromosomal disorders and have led to intervention at a younger age and the elucidation of the natural history of a number of these disorders from infancy into adulthood. Because of this, it has become increasingly important for professionals caring for adolescents to have a working knowledge of genetic disorders so that correct, sensitive counseling can be offered, medical problems such as hypothyroidism in individuals with Down syndrome (DS) can be anticipated and treated in an early stage, and referral for prenatal and preimplantation genetic testing can be offered early enough to provide the pregnant client with a choice.

Providers generally encounter a patient with or at risk for a genetic disorder in 1 of 3 ways. First, and most common, is when a diagnosis has already been established and the adolescent comes for assessment or management of a specific complaint. Most children with congenital or genetic disorders will have had their conditions diagnosed well before entering adolescence. Although this group represents only a small percentage of adolescents, they are often overrepresented in adolescent clinics and inpatient services; it is estimated that individuals with congenital or genetic disorders account for between 20% and 35% of all inpatient pediatric admissions.[1]

The second situation occurs when an individual whose condition has not been previously diagnosed seeks evaluation. Confirmation of the diagnosis of disorders such as Turner syndrome (TS) in females or Klinefelter syndrome (KS) in males must await the development of characteristic phenotypic changes that may become apparent only around or after puberty. Therefore, it is essential that those caring for adolescents are able to recognize the signs and symptoms so that the diagnosis will not be missed.

Finally, because they may be providing care for young women during pregnancy, it is important for clinicians to have knowledge of techniques for prenatal diagnosis of genetic disorders, such as amniocentesis, and to know when to refer for appropriate testing. Also, an understanding of teratogenesis is important in order to know what should be done to monitor the pregnant woman whose embryo or fetus has been exposed to a potential teratogen.

This chapter offers a simple approach to the adolescent affected with, or at risk for, genetic disorders. After a review of the categories of genetic diseases and standard prenatal diagnostic techniques, the natural history of specific disorders will be discussed and guidelines regarding management of these disorders offered.

## CATEGORIES OF GENETIC DISORDERS

When evaluating a patient with an apparent syndrome, the clinical geneticist attempts to classify the disorder into 1 of 4 categories: (1) chromosomal abnormalities, (2) single gene mutations, (3) multifactorially inherited disorders, and (4) teratogenically induced syndromes.

Chromosomal abnormalities account for approximately 7% of all congenital anomalies in the newborn period. Although individuals with some of the more common chromosomal disorders, such as trisomy 13 and trisomy 18, may be unlikely to survive infancy, patients with other aberrations, such as Down (trisomy 21), Turner (monosomy X), and Klinefelter (XXY) syndromes, most often do survive to adulthood.

Single gene mutations, which account for approximately 7.5% of all congenital malformations and illustrate mendelian inheritance patterns, include 4 major subcategories. In autosomal-dominant inheritance, a single copy of a nonworking gene is sufficient to cause symptoms. As such, these disorders are usually passed vertically, from affected parent to affected child, and each child of an affected parent has a 50% chance of also being affected. In autosomal-recessive inheritance, 2 copies of a nonworking gene are necessary to produce symptoms. Thus, parents who carry 1 copy of the nonworking gene are usually themselves healthy, and each child born to 2 such carrier parents has a 25% chance of being affected. X-linked recessive inheritance is marked by male preponderance of affected individuals. In this form of inheritance, a nonworking gene causing disease is carried on the X chromosome. Females, who have 2 copies of the X chromosome, do not usually manifest symptoms; males who carry the nonworking gene, however, because of their hemizygous state (that is, having only 1 copy of the gene), suffer the full consequences of the disorder. Thus, male offspring of a woman known to be carrying an X-linked recessive trait have a 50% chance of being affected. Female children of such women are not at risk but have a 50% chance of being a carrier, like their mother. Finally, in X-linked-dominant inheritance, a single dose of a nonworking gene that is carried on the X chromosome is sufficient to cause symptoms. In X-linked-dominant inheritance, males and females are affected in equal numbers, but male-to-male transmission, a hallmark of autosomal-dominant inheritance, does not occur.

In multifactorial inheritance, abnormalities result from an interplay of many factors, genetic and environmental. This form of inheritance accounts for 20% of all congenital malformations, including such common conditions as meningomyelocele, which will be discussed in a subsequent chapter, and nonsyndromic cleft lip and palate, as well as a great number of chronic disorders of childhood and later life, such as asthma, allergies, atherosclerotic heart disease, and many forms of cancer.

Teratogen-induced disorders, such as fetal alcohol syndrome (FAS), result from the adverse effects of drugs, chemicals, and other environmental agents on the developing embryo and fetus. Teratogens account for approximately 7% of all congenital malformations.

Nearly half of all congenital disorders do not fit into any of these 4 categories. Presumably, as more information about the human genome becomes available, these disorders will ultimately be classified into the known categories.

## CHROMOSOMAL ABNORMALITIES

### DOWN SYNDROME

Down syndrome (DS), which occurs in 1 in 700 newborns, is caused by an extra copy of chromosome 21 in every cell of the body. Trisomy 21, caused by nondisjunction, is present in more than 94% of affected individuals; the remaining cases are due to chromosomal translocation (in 3.3%) and mosaicism (in 2.4%).

#### Medical Problems

The management of adolescents with DS must reflect current knowledge of the medical problems that occur in patients with this disorder.

***Central Nervous System*** Every individual with DS has some degree of intellectual disability, ranging from mild (low normal or borderline range) to profound retardation. Most patients fall in the mild to moderately retarded range, with IQs in the 50s. Because of this intellectual disability, adolescents and adults with DS typically are unable to live independently; most live with their families or in supervised group homes and hold jobs in sheltered settings.

Young adults with DS are at increased risk for developing presenile dementia. This condition, which rarely begins before the age of 20, is seen with some frequency during the third decade of life. It resembles Alzheimer disease both clinically and pathologically.

***Craniofacial Features*** The facial phenotype, a hallmark of DS in infancy, becomes less striking with advancing age so that by adolescence some of the typical features may be lacking. With age the nasal bridge becomes more prominent and the epicanthal folds may vanish. Dental disease is common in older patients because of a predilection for infections and poor oral hygiene. Therefore, regular dental follow-up is essential in the management of these patients.

Controversy has developed over the issue of performing facial plastic surgery in people with DS in an effort to mask some of the dysmorphic features. Requests for such surgery often come from parents who are disturbed by their child's "stigmatized" appearance. Because subjecting a child or young adult to surgery for his or her parents' sake seems inappropriate, it is our opinion that such procedures should be offered only when patients themselves request them; thus, these operations would be reserved for higher-functioning individuals.

***Cardiovascular System*** Between 33% and 50% of newborns with DS have congenital heart disease, most commonly because of endocardial cushion defects, including especially atrioventricular canals, and ventricular or atrial septal defects. Because most of these anomalies are now repaired surgically, the cardiovascular complications in adolescents and adults with DS do not differ from those in older patients who have survived congenital cardiac disorders.

***Endocrinologic Features*** Abnormalities of thyroid function are common in young adults with DS. By the age of 18, 20% have hypothyroidism and 3% have hyperthyroidism. These figures increase through adult life. In nearly all cases the thyroid disease represents an autoimmune defect. Pathologically, the thyroid tissue resembles that seen in Hashimoto thyroiditis. Because the number affected increases with age, it is essential that thyroid function testing be performed frequently in all adolescents and adults with DS.

Obesity is another significant problem in young adults with DS. In some cases a marked increase in weight may herald the onset of hypothyroidism. Often, however, no thyroid dysfunction can be uncovered. In these individuals, weight gain is caused by a combination of complicated factors, including a sedentary lifestyle and excessive caloric intake. In addition, early in life behavior-modification techniques that involve food as a reward are often used in children with DS. This clearly can contribute to the later obesity and make it more difficult to use other types of rewards in adolescence. It is essential that the care provider aid these families by helping them devise appropriate, nutritious diets; encouraging increased physical activity; and using rewards other than food in behavior modification efforts.

Sexual development in the adolescent with DS is usually less complete than in typical patients. Females are fertile, however, and there have been many reports of affected women bearing children. As expected, the incidence of trisomy 21 in progeny of women with DS is markedly increased over the general population. Birth control counseling is indicated but is made difficult by the developmental disability that occurs with DS, a fact that makes barrier methods of birth control unreliable. Methods of birth control applicable in women with DS therefore are limited to medroxyprogesterone (Depo-Provera), levonorgestrel (Norplant), and birth control pills. The issue of birth control raises a major ethical concern: Who should make the decision regarding use of birth control in women with DS? The answer to this complex question is beyond the scope of this chapter.

There have been no proven cases of paternity in men with DS. Although testicular histology appears to be normal, the semen produced by affected men contains no viable sperm. This may be due to a postmeiotic maturational defect or to some other as yet unidentified endocrinologic abnormality.

***Skeletal System*** Adult height is significantly shorter than that seen in the general population; mean height is 154 cm for males and 144 cm for females. Growth hormone has been found to be normal in these patients. It is important that the clinician monitoring a young adolescent's growth use the specific growth chart for DS. Such charts are available online at www.growthcharts.com/charts/DS/charts.htm.

Atlantoaxial instability, related to an increased distance between the first and second cervical vertebrae, occurs in 10% of individuals with DS, and is believed to predispose to spinal cord compression. It has been recommended that lateral radiographs of the cervical spine in full flexion, extension, and neutral positions be performed in children with DS at 3 years of age, and that participation in contact sports be restricted if the atlantoaxial distance is greater than 4.5 mm. It has further been recommended that these radiographs be repeated again at least once on completion of puberty. In adults in whom atlantoaxial instability was present in childhood, osteoarthritis of the cervical spine has been reported. Therefore, radiographs of the spine should be taken in adolescents and young adults complaining of neck pain. Individuals with abnormalities should be referred to appropriate specialists.

***Eyes and Ears*** Strabismus, common in childhood, continues to be a problem in adults with DS. Conductive hearing loss, related to recurrent otitis media in childhood, is significantly increased in the adult population.

***Hematologic Features*** Individuals with DS have a markedly higher risk for developing leukemia during their lives compared with the general population. Other forms of cancer are believed to be more common, but there are no figures available to support this. The reason for this predilection is not certain but probably relates to errors in basic cellular regulatory mechanisms caused by the chromosomal aneuploidy that exists in these individuals.

***Gastrointestinal System*** Since the 1990s, clinicians have appreciated that individuals with DS are at a substantially increased risk of developing celiac disease compared with the general public. Various studies have shown that between 5% and 10% of children with DS in the United States are affected. Because of this high frequency, it is recommended that adolescents with DS be screened with appropriate blood tests (the so-called celiac panel) and that, if positive, they be referred to a gastroenterologist for management.

### Clinical Management

The management of adolescents with DS must be geared toward the medical problems just noted.[2] The first visit should include the following:

1. Full history and physical examination, with height and weight plotted on the DS growth curve (available online at www.growthcharts.com/charts/DS/charts.htm).
2. Hearing and vision testing, with referral to otolaryngologist if abnormalities are found.
3. Blood work to include a complete blood count, thyroid function tests, and a celiac panel.
4. Lateral radiographs of the neck in neutral, flexion, and extension positions, to rule out atlantoaxial instability. These radiographs should be performed during childhood, during adolescence, and after age 30.
5. Check of school placement to confirm that it is appropriate.
6. Confirmation that vocational and long-term living arrangement planning is ongoing.
7. Reinforcement of genetic counseling for the family and the beginning of birth control counseling, if the patient is female.

For subsequent visits:

1. Continue to plot height and weight.
2. Annually check thyroid function, and perform ophthalmologic examination to rule out keratoconus and cataracts.
3. If obesity is present, help with dietary advice and behavioral modification.
4. Continue to monitor educational placement, vocational and social situation.

## TURNER SYNDROME

Although Turner's description of 7 adolescent and adult women with short stature, "sexual infantilism," webbed neck, and cubitus valgus appeared in 1938, the chromosomal basis of Turner syndrome (TS) was not discovered until 1959, when a single copy of an X chromosome was identified in the cells of a girl with clinical features of this condition. Since that time, it has become evident that the phenotype of TS, which occurs in 0.4 per 1,000 live-born females, represents the mildest expression of the 45,X genotype; more than 95% of 45,X conceptuses are lost during early gestation. Furthermore, 40% of females with clinical TS have karyotypes other than 45,X, including partial monosomy X caused by structural anomalies of the X chromosome (in 20%) and monosomy X mosaicism (in 20%). This observation suggests that such aberrations may produce a milder phenotype. Studies of women with deletions of portions of the X chromosome have produced a "phenotypic map," short stature being associated with monosomy of the short arm of the chromosome (del Xp) and failure of sexual development associated with deletions of the long arm (del Xq).

### Medical Problems

Clinically, TS is variable. The classic neonatal features, including lymphedema of the extremities, redundant skinfolds, and webbing of the neck, occur in less than 25% of affected girls. The diagnosis is more commonly made later in childhood or adolescence, during an evaluation for either growth failure, delayed thelarche or puberty, or primary amenorrhea. Because many affected girls are diagnosed after infancy, it is essential that the clinician not only understand the natural history of TS, but be able to recognize the clinical features of the disorder so that appropriate chromosomal testing can be performed.[3]

***Endocrinologic Features*** Three major endocrinologic problems occur commonly in women with TS: (1) hypogonadism, (2) growth failure, and (3) Hashimoto thyroiditis, as well as other forms of autoimmune endocrinopathies. Careful evaluation of each of these is vital in the management of patients with TS. Ovarian dysgenesis, with hypoplasia to absence of germinal elements, occurs in more than 90% of women with a 45,X karyotype and less commonly in women with TS who have other X chromosome anomalies. This pathologic finding, resulting in ovarian failure and lack of estrogen production at adolescence, leads to failure of development of the clinical signs of puberty.

It is stressed that in women with TS the timing and extent of ovarian failure varies. Approximately 10% of patients have sufficient estrogen production to enter thelarche spontaneously. A smaller percentage may initiate menarche, but the continuation of regular menses throughout adolescence is rare. Finally, there are multiple reports of successful conceptions and pregnancies in women with both 45,X and variant karyotypes, but they account for far less than 1% of all affected females.

The second major endocrinologic problem in women with TS is growth failure. Short stature, the cause of which is as yet unidentified, is the single most common clinical finding, occurring in 100% of females with 45,X karyotypes and a significant percentage of those with structural variants or mosaicism. Children with TS tend to deviate progressively from the normal height percentages until 14 years of age when, because of delayed closure of the epiphyses, growth approaches more closely the normal percentile chart. Adult stature, not usually reached until the early 20s, ranges from 142 to 147 cm. The growth chart for females with TS is available online at www.kidsgrowth.com/resources/articledetail.cfm?id=521.

The final group of endocrinologic disorders occurring commonly in TS are autoimmune endocrinopathies, Hashimoto thyroiditis being the most frequent. Although thyroid autoantibodies are found in 30% to 50% of women with TS, only 10% manifest clinical hypothyroidism. In addition to Hashimoto disease, other autoimmune phenomena, including Graves disease, Addison disease, vitiligo, and type 2 diabetes mellitus, may be seen. The clinical approach and management of these endocrinologic problems are covered in the chapters on endocrinology (Chapters 69 to 75).

***Cardiovascular Problems*** Cardiovascular anomalies occur in approximately 30% of girls with TS. The major malformations, in descending order of frequency, include bicuspid aortic valve, coarctation of the aorta, mitral valve prolapse, and dissecting aortic aneurysm resulting from median cystic necrosis. Although some of these anomalies may be diagnosed in infancy or childhood, others, such as mitral valve prolapse, may not be detected until adolescence or adulthood. Therefore, it is essential that every woman with TS undergo a cardiac evaluation at some time during childhood or adolescence.

***Renal Features*** Abnormalities of the kidneys have been found in 25% to 70% of women with TS. Most anomalies, including horseshoe and pelvic kidneys and partial or complete duplication of the collecting system, can remain clinically silent. Occasionally, however, urinary tract obstruction may occur and result in hydroureter, hydronephrosis, and recurrent infections. Because of the high frequency of anomalies, a renal ultrasound examination should be performed as part of the initial evaluation of affected females.

***Skeletal System*** A large number of skeletal anomalies have been reported in females with TS, including disproportionately short legs, leading to an increased upper- to lower-segment ratio; a "shieldlike" chest; hypoplasia of the cervical vertebrae; short fourth and fifth metacarpals; and genu valgum. These features, although helpful in establishing the diagnosis, do not cause medical problems. Nevertheless, they should be sought whenever the diagnosis of TS is being considered.

***Neurodevelopmental Problems*** Although most women with TS have normal intelligence, their performance on tests of mathematical ability, visual-motor coordination, and spatial-temporal processing may be below average. However, with appropriate remedial assistance and counseling, individuals with TS can succeed, often attending college and graduate school.

### Clinical Management

When, because of the presence of 1 or more of the clinical features, a diagnosis of TS is suspected in an adolescent female, chromosomal studies should be performed. For diagnostic purposes, karyotype analysis should always be carried out on lymphocytes cultured from peripheral blood. Analysis of Barr bodies, obtained from smears of buccal mucosa, is unreliable and should never be used for primary confirmation of the diagnosis.

The informing interview after cytogenetic confirmation of the diagnosis must be conducted in a respectful and sensitive manner. The diagnosis, unsuspected by the adolescent and her parents, often comes as a blow. Virtually assured that she will be infertile, with no possibility of bearing children without advanced technological assistance, and learning that she will be strikingly shorter than most of her friends, the adolescent may react angrily or violently to the care provider delivering the news. In some instances, it may prove valuable for the information to come from the geneticist, who may not be involved in providing ongoing medical care. On the other hand, hearing the news from the primary care provider, who has been offering care and support for the patient and her family, may soften the blow. The decision should be made by the primary care provider on a case-by-case basis.

After the informing interview, a comprehensive work-up should be performed in all patients and generally includes the following:

1. *Endocrinologic evaluation.* First, thyroid function and growth hormone secretion should be tested. More specific testing for other associated endocrinologic abnormalities that occur in TS should be performed only if the patient is symptomatic.

2. *Renal evaluation.* Because of the association of urinary tract anomalies, a renal ultrasound examination and voiding cystourethrography should be performed.

3. *Cardiovascular evaluation.* As previously stated, cardiovascular anomalies occur in 30% of females with TS, and some may not be detected until adulthood. A full evaluation, including chest radiography, electrocardiography, and echocardiography,

should be performed in all patients in whom TS has been confirmed.

4. *Other.* Radiographic examination of the skeletal system should be considered in any woman who has symptoms such as bone or joint pain. Special consideration is given to other anomalies, as mentioned previously. In addition, hearing loss, both sensorineural and conductive, occurs in affected women. For this reason, an audiographic evaluation should be performed.

After completion of this evaluation, the adolescent should be monitored on a routine basis. Because the diagnosis may lead to a great deal of emotional distress, it may be propitious for the primary caretaker to see the patient at least once a month to reinforce the counseling and to check on the patient and her family's understanding and acceptance of the diagnosis. In addition to helping support the patient through these emotionally difficult times, it will also allow the primary caretaker, by checking on the woman's adherence with subspecialty appointments and medications, to coordinate and monitor the patient's medical progress.

The use of growth hormone to increase the adult height of women with TS has been advocated by many endocrinologists in recent years. Also, estrogen replacement therapy, to produce secondary sexual characteristics, has been helpful in normalizing the lives of many women with TS. For these reasons, a good rapport and long-term follow-up with an endocrinologist is essential in the management of women with TS.

In recent years, advances in *in vitro fertilization* techniques have been instrumental in helping women with TS bear children. In these cases, eggs obtained from a donor and fertilized in vitro have been implanted in those women who have been hormonally primed. This breakthrough offers significant hope to young women with this disorder who previously had no possibility of bearing children. However, more recent evidence suggests that pregnancy in a woman with TS may significantly worsen underlying cardiac disease; between 6% and 20% of such women will develop dissection of a poststenotic aortic aneurysm. As such, it is imperative that women with TS be carefully monitored by a cardiologist during pregnancy.

## KLINEFELTER SYNDROME

In the first half of the 20th century, Harry Klinefelter described males with gynecomastia, testicular atrophy with azoospermia but without atrophy of Leydig cells, and increased excretion of follicle-stimulating hormone. It was not until 1959, however, that a 47,XXY karyotype was demonstrated in affected males. Because virtually none of the clinical findings are expressed in infancy or childhood, nearly all cases of Klinefleter syndrome (KS) not picked up during prenatal testing are diagnosed in adolescence.[4] Because of this and because of its relatively high frequency (1 to 2 per 1,000 males), it is essential that the adolescent care provider be able to recognize the phenotype of KS and respond appropriately.

### Medical Problems

***Endocrinologic Problems*** Commonly, gynecomastia is the initial sign of KS, a finding that occurs in one-third of affected patients. The breast enlargement, which may be present by 12 years of age, is of moderate volume and is not associated with hyperpigmentation; although it may be strikingly asymmetric at the outset, symmetry is usually present by adulthood.

Gynecomastia also occurs commonly in males who do not have KS during early to middle adolescence. This syndrome should be suspected only when additional phenotypic features (listed in the following) are present or when the gynecomastia persists into later adolescence.

Testicular atrophy, the only constant feature, is usually the second sign noted. The testes are small, measuring less than 5 cc, and are soft to the touch; this is in sharp contrast to apparent normal development of the penis and relatively normal pubertal development. Although puberty is usually normal, clinical manifestations related to testicular dysfunction include the absence of beard and body hair, a high-pitched voice, decreased libido, and lack of muscular development.

Histologically, at puberty, the seminiferous tubules are sclerotic and atrophic, containing almost nothing but Sertoli cells. Although elements of germinal maturation are present, mature sperm are almost never seen.

***Skeletal Problems*** The typical KS phenotype includes a tall, long-limbed, and somewhat eunuchoid body habitus, but these features are extremely variable. The absence of the typical skeletal pattern in a male with small testes and normal pubertal development should not impede the evaluation process.

***Neurodevelopmental Problems*** Although most men with KS have normal intelligence, the incidences of psychiatric disturbances and developmental delay are higher than in the general population. The literature is replete with anecdotal reports of men with KS who have immature emotional development. However, the frequency of this finding in the KS population is not known.

### Clinical Management

The initial management of patients suspected of having KS is similar to that of those with TS. Chromosome analysis of peripheral blood lymphocytes should be performed in any male in whom micro-orchia is found during adolescence. Again, analysis of buccal mucosal cells for the presence of Barr bodies is unreliable and should never be used to confirm this diagnosis. As in TS, the professional informing the patient and his family of the diagnosis must be sensitive and respectful. Once the diagnosis is explained, the patient must begin to deal with its consequences, most importantly the infertility that is virtually always a feature. After the informing interview, frequent visits to the primary care provider should be encouraged to assess and reinforce acceptance of the diagnosis and adherence with the medical regimen. After confirmation of the diagnosis, testosterone production should be evaluated and testosterone replacement therapy offered.

In recent years, through assisted reproductive techniques, men with KS have been able to father children. When biopsied, testicular tissue discloses occasional mature spermatozoa. These can be selected with a syringe and needle and injected into an ovum (through a technique known as intracytoplasmic sperm injection or ICSI); following implantation of the fertilized ovum in the uterus of the female, successful pregnancies have ensued. The offspring of these pregnancies have all been normal.

## PRADER-WILLI SYNDROME

Although Prader-Willi syndrome (PWS) is not a commonly encountered disorder, it is important for the practitioner caring for adolescents to recognize its features because, as in KS and TS, this diagnosis is often made during adolescence. Prader-Willi syndrome has been classified here as a chromosomal disorder because, during the past 2 decades, evidence has pointed to the fact that a small deletion of the long arm of chromosome 15 (del 15q11–13) is associated with the phenotype in most cases. For this reason, for purposes of diagnosis and genetic counseling of the patient and other family members, a fluorescent in situ hybridization (FISH) study, with a probe specific for this region of chromosome 15, should be performed as a first step in every individual in whom the diagnosis of PWS is being considered (as discussed in the following, mechanisms other than a deletion can give rise to this disorder).

### Medical Problems

The clinical features of PWS are variable and change as the affected individual grows older. In infancy the hallmark of the disorder is hypotonia, with failure to thrive because of the inability to suck and swallow. During early childhood, the hypotonia resolves and the course is marked by the development of an unusual eating pattern: affected individuals develop a seemingly insatiable appetite, often eating anything available to them. As a result, pica is a common feature. Obtaining food becomes a major activity for these children, and affected individuals have been known to steal or beg for food on the streets and eat garbage. As a result of the insatiable appetite, obesity usually is present by 3 or 4 years of age and becomes progressively more striking. In the older child, adolescent, and young adult, this obesity leads to serious, ongoing medical problems such as type 2 diabetes mellitus and coronary artery disease.

Intellectual disability is often not severe in adolescence. Adolescents typically have outgoing, cheerful personalities. Because of their loquaciousness, the examiner may conclude that these patients can function at a level higher than that indicated by schoolwork or IQ tests. However, behavioral problems, such as stubbornness, tantrums, and rage-type outbursts (frequently centered around issues of obtaining food), tend to be common in adolescence and young adulthood, making management of affected individuals a real challenge.

Hypogonadotropic hypogonadism is an important feature of PWS. In males, this may be manifested early in life by the finding of micropenis and cryptorchidism. In females, however, the hypogonadism may become apparent only when the changes of puberty or menarche do not occur at an appropriate age. It is for this reason, especially in females with PWS, that the diagnosis may first be considered by the adolescent care provider.

### Clinical Management

As mentioned previously, when the diagnosis of PWS is suspected, a sample of blood for FISH studies should be obtained. But even if this test reveals no identifiable deletion, the diagnosis should still be pursued.

Prader-Willi syndrome is caused by deficiency of the product of the *SNRPN* gene. Located in the PWS critical region on chromosome 15, *SNRPN* is expressed only in the chromosome 15 inherited from the father; for reasons that are still unknown, maternal *SNRPN* is methylated, preventing transcription of the gene. As such, PWS results whenever no paternal chromosome 15 is present. In 60% of cases, this is related to a deletion of the region, an abnormality that is identifiable via FISH analysis. In the remaining cases, the absence of the paternal chromosome 15 is related to maternal uniparental disomy, the phenomenon in which both copies of chromosome 15 have been inherited from the mother. When PWS is suspected and FISH analysis is negative, methylation studies to check for maternal uniparental disomy are indicated.

As in Turner and Klinefelter syndrome, counseling of the adolescent and his or her family must be sensitive and respectful. Because of the intellectual problems in the affected individual, more time than might be expected may have to be allotted before the information is clearly understood. Therapy for the adolescent with PWS must be aimed at 3 major problems: weight reduction and control, treatment of hypogonadism, and management of the behavioral and psychological sequelae of the disorder.[5]

***Weight Reduction and Control*** Because weight gain is directly caused by the eating disorder that occurs in PWS, weight control must be attempted through correction of the eating disorder. This is not a simple task. By the time their child is an adolescent, most parents of children with PWS have placed a padlock on their refrigerators and cabinets. This is rarely successful. Because of their compulsive need for food, the patients usually solve this dilemma quickly by obtaining food from a neighbor's kitchen or through some other source. In fact, the only method that has enjoyed any success in controlling food intake is behavior modification. Surgical intervention to reduce stomach capacity should be avoided. Surgery fails to get at the cause of the problem, and thus such procedures are rarely, if ever, successful.

In addition to trying to reduce weight and control the eating compulsion, the care provider must be vigilant for signs of obesity-related disease. Periodic testing for glycosuria, with appropriate follow-up of glycohemoglobin ($HbA_{1C}$) and serum cholesterol levels, must be done.

***Treatment of Hypogonadism*** Because these patients have hypogonadotropic hypogonadism and are therefore deficient in either estrogen or testosterone, they may never spontaneously enter puberty. As a result, replacement therapy should be attempted during adolescence. This may be especially important in an attempt to prevent osteoporosis, a problem that becomes increasingly important in older individuals with this condition.

***Management of Behavioral and Psychological Sequelae*** Dealing with the psychologic aspects of PWS often goes hand in hand with management of the compulsive eating disorder. As a result, the clinician supervising the patient's behavior modification should also address this issue.

## SINGLE GENE MUTATIONS

Disorders caused by a single gene mutation demonstrate 1 of 4 mendelian inheritance patterns: autosomal-dominant and recessive patterns, and X-linked dominant and recessive patterns. Because few disorders result from X-linked dominant inheritance, this discussion includes only entities falling into the other 3 categories.

### AUTOSOMAL DOMINANTLY INHERITED DISORDERS

#### Marfan Syndrome

Because the features of Marfan syndrome (MS) involving the skeletal, ophthalmologic, and cardiovascular systems are related to the fact that aberrations in connective tissue lead to the pathologic findings, research efforts have focused on the composition of the extracellular matrix. Within the last 2 decades, 2 breakthroughs have occurred in MS research: (1) demonstration of abnormalities in the myofibrillar array in the connective tissue of some patients with MS, coupled with a defect in the production of fibrillin, a major constituent of these myofibrils; and (2) linkage of at least one gene responsible for MS (*FBN1*) to the long arm of chromosome 15. These findings have allowed the beginning of an understanding of the molecular pathogenesis of MS and, in turn, breakthroughs in its treatment. The diagnosis is best made on clinical grounds, using the diagnostic criteria system adopted in 1996.[6] Marfan syndrome is an autosomal dominantly inherited disorder; thus, each offspring of an affected individual has a 50% chance of also being affected. Although it might be expected that one of the parents of an affected individual would be similarly affected, the fact is that in 25% of cases no such history is available. This phenomenon is explainable in 1 of 2 ways: either because of variability of expression of the gene, the features are so subtle in the affected parent that a diagnosis has not been made; or the disorder may have arisen as the result of a spontaneous mutation in the affected individual. Before it is concluded that the latter is the case, it is essential that both parents be examined carefully for features of the disorder.

***Medical Problems*** Perhaps the best known of the abnormalities that occur in MS are those of the skeletal system: dolichostenomelia (a tall, thin body habitus) with distal lengthening of the extremities (on examination, the upper- to lower-segment ratio is often greater than 2 standard deviations below the mean, and the arm span is greater than the height); and arachnodactyly, with long, "spidery" fingers and excessive and disproportionately long hand measurements. Additional manifestations include progressive scoliosis and lumbar lordosis, joint laxity, pes planus (flat feet), and abnormalities of the sternum, most commonly pectus excavatum.

In addition to skeletal abnormalities, weakness in the wall of the aorta (caused by abnormalities in the protein fibrillin) leads to the most dramatic and life threatening of the clinical features of MS: aneurysmal dilatation of the ascending aorta with dissection. The natural history of this catastrophic event is now well known. Individuals with MS show progressive dilatation of the aortic root, often beginning in infancy, frequently accompanied by aortic regurgitation. Eventually, the wall weakens and dissection occurs. Prior to recently developed therapies, which are detailed in the following, the average age at death in individuals affected with MS was approximately 45. Dilatation and dissection of other parts of the aorta (the thoracic and abdominal segments), as well as of other vessels (the pulmonary artery and the ductus arteriosus), have also been known to occur.

Ophthalmologic problems may also occur. Subluxation of the lens (ectopia lentis) caused by a defect in the lens' suspensory ligament, is a common feature of MS. The subluxation often occurs in an upward and outward direction. In addition, myopia is a nearly constant feature, and the sclerae often have a bluish tinge.

***Diagnosis*** The initial step in managing the patient with MS is to confirm the diagnosis. Marfan syndrome is often diagnosed in childhood, but it is not unusual for patients to reach puberty without the diagnosis having been made. The gold standard for diagnosis of MS relies on fulfilling diagnostic criteria established in 1996,[6] which involves the presence of physical findings and a positive family history. In our experience, the diagnosis should be made only in individuals who demonstrate 2 or more of the following: (1) involvement of the cardiovascular system, including aortic root dilatation or aortic valve insufficiency; (2) skeletal manifestations, including dolichostenomelia, with an aberrant upper- to lower-segment ratio, abnormally long total hand and foot lengths, and evidence of pectus excavatum or carinatum; (3) ophthalmologic abnormalities (ectopia lentis and/or "high" myopia); and (4) a history of MS, diagnosed by these criteria, in a first-degree relative. Thus, an individual with only a dolichostenomelic body habitus does not have MS.

***Clinical Management***

- **Cardiovascular system.** Until recently, the use of beta-adrenergic blocking drugs, such as atenolol, have been advocated in the treatment of all patients with MS. Theoretically, the decrease in cardiac preload induced by these medications serves to decrease the pressure with which cardiac output reaches the proximal aorta, thus cutting down on the "wear and tear" affecting this vulnerable vessel. In addition, echocardiograms are performed at least every 6 months to monitor the size of the aortic root. Because the risk of dissection increases significantly in individuals whose aortic root diameter exceeds 6 cm, replacement of the ascending aorta with a composite graft (replacing the aorta and valve) is performed electively in such patients. The need for a decrease in physical activity and for the daily taking of medication represents a marked change in lifestyle for many patients with MS. In 2005, Yetman and colleagues[6] suggested that use of angiotensin-converting enzyme (ACE) inhibitors, such as losartin, may be more beneficial in the protection from progressive aortic enlargement in individuals with MS than beta blockers. Trials to examine the long-term effects of this regimen are ongoing.
- **Ophthalmologic management.** Careful ophthalmologic follow-up is a necessity because of the risk of blindness, from either untreated ectopia lentis or vitreo-retinal degeneration (secondary to high myopia).
- **Skeletal system.** Orthopedic care must be directed toward 2 complications: the progressive scoliosis, which may be treatable with bracing but often requires surgery; and pectus excavatum, which can be a confounding factor in the cardiac surgery described earlier and may lead to respiratory compromise. For these reasons, orthopedic surgery is not unusual in patients with MS, and close follow-up is necessary.
- **Genetic counseling.** The risk of MS occurring in each child born to an affected individual is 50%. Recently, molecular diagnostic testing has become available, and in some families, direct DNA-based prenatal testing is possible; however, in most families, a definitive prenatal diagnosis cannot be offered. Although some infants with MS are symptomatic and the diagnosis has been reported by sonographic demonstration of disproportionately long arms and legs in some fetuses, this has generally been unreliable. Therefore, affected adults must currently make a decision about reproduction based only on risk estimates. In addition, in some women with MS, pregnancy has accelerated aortic dilatation, leading to dissection during the third trimester. Further, because of the risk of teratogenic effects, ACE inhibitors are contraindicated during pregnancy. As such, before becoming pregnant, women with MS must have careful consultations with their health care providers. However, most affected women remain relatively stable throughout the pregnancy. Because the risk of pregnancy may be considerable and affected teenagers may be sexually active, the issue of family planning needs to be addressed early in adolescence. Furthermore, birth control pills are not contraindicated in this disorder; they can be safely prescribed for women with MS, even those in whom cardiovascular disease has been diagnosed.
- **Psychologic concerns.** Marfan syndrome is a disorder that is not infrequently diagnosed during adolescence. Suddenly, the "normal" adolescent must come to grips with the fact that he or she is not "perfect"; in addition, the teenager must begin taking cardiac medications,

limit physical activity, and face difficult reproductive decisions. Because of the risk of aortic dissection, adherence with the medical regimen may be crucial. Thus, the primary caretaker must encourage adherence, facilitate understanding and acceptance of the disorder, and monitor the psychosocial development of these adolescents.

### The Neurofibromatoses

In recent years a great deal of progress has been made in the delineation of the neurofibromatoses.[7] Table 148-1 shows the chromosomal map positions of neurofibromatosis (NF) types 1 and 2, the most important of the 8 currently accepted types of NF.

***Neurofibromatosis-1*** Formerly called von Recklinghausen disease, NF-1 is an autosomal dominantly inherited condition that occurs in 1 in 4,000 people. The disease, characterized by a large number of seemingly unrelated clinical findings, is caused by a mutation in the *NF1* gene, which codes for the protein neurofibromin.

The diagnosis of NF-1 is confirmed by fulfilling the criteria developed by the National Institutes of Health (NIH) Consensus Conference. The clinical criteria, summarized in Box 148-1, include cafe au lait spots (pigmented nevi 5 mm or more in diameter that increase in number throughout childhood), axillary or inguinal freckling (clusters of small, 1- to 3-mm macules, similar in color to cafe au lait spots), and neurofibromas (benign tumors of the Schwann cells and fibroblasts that can arise virtually anywhere and, because of their presence, cause a large variety of complications). Rarely present in the newborn, neurofibromas gradually increase in number and size through life. During puberty, they may grow rapidly or become apparent for the first time. Optic gliomas (neurofibromas of the optic nerve, which have the potential to cause blindness), Lisch nodules (melanocytic hamartomas of the iris, identifiable through slit-lamp examination, which cause no symptoms but are a unique, pathognomonic hallmark of NF-1), skeletal defects (including scoliosis, a serious problem in adolescents with NF-1), and sphenoid wing dysplasia are other cardinal features of NF-1. In addition to these features, growth (the average height in adolescents with NF-1 is at the 33rd percentile on the normal growth curve), development (attention-deficit/hyperactivity disorder, learning disabilities, and, less commonly, mental retardation), neurologic function (headaches, seizures), and emotional status are often affected by NF-1. Finally, individuals with NF-1 are at increased risk for the development of many types of malignancies, including soft tissue sarcomas and astrocytomas.

**Table 148-1**

**Neurofibromatoses**

| *NF-Type* | *Alternate Name* | *Chromosome Localization* |
|---|---|---|
| NF-1 | von Recklinghausen disease | 17q11.2 |
| NF-2 | Central or bilateral acoustic neurofibromatosis | 22q11.21-q13.1 |
| | Schwannomatosis | 22q.12.2 |

**Box 148-1**

***NF-1: Major Diagnostic Criteria***

Two or more of the following features must be present to confirm a diagnosis of NF-1:

1. Cafe au lait spots
   A. Prepubertal: 5 or more of at least 0.5 cm in diameter
   B. Postpubertal: 6 or more of at least 1.5 cm in diameter
2. Axillary or inguinal freckling
3. Neurofibromas: 2 or more of any type or 1 plexiform
4. Optic glioma (neurofibromas of the optic nerve)
5. Lisch nodules (melanotic hamartomas of the iris)
6. Skeletal defects: include scoliosis, pseudarthrosis, and sphenoid wing dysplasia
7. Family history of first-degree relative with NF-1, diagnosed by these criteria

- **Clinical management.** As in MS, the initial step in managing the adolescent with NF-1 is to confirm the diagnosis. The individual in whom NF-1 is suspected must have at least 2 of the 7 features listed in Box 148-1. Thus, a patient with multiple cafe au lait spots and no other symptoms, signs, or family history does not have NF-1 and is not at risk for any of the other disorders that occur in this disease. Most individuals with NF-1 have nothing more than cafe au lait spots, axillary and/or inguinal freckling, Lisch nodules, and subcutaneous neurofibromas. For this reason, the care provider should help the patient maintain a positive attitude while providing careful surveillance for signs of more serious symptoms. In 10% to 20% of affected individuals, more severe complications occur. Once the diagnosis of NF-1 has been confirmed, possible courses of action include surgery, surveillance, and genetic counseling.
- **Surgery.** In most cases, surgery to remove subcutaneous neurofibromas is inappropriate or unnecessary and should be discouraged. The

reasons for this include medical factors (tumor regrowth is likely) and psychologic factors (the patient must come to grips with the fact that removal of all neurofibromas would be impossible in most cases). With this in mind, there are several clear indications for removal of neurofibromas: (1) when the size becomes excessive, (2) when pain becomes significant, (3) when the tumor causes disfigurement, and (4) when a tumor interferes with normal function.

- **Surveillance.** The care provider must maintain a constant search to identify any of the serious complications that may accompany NF-1. At the time the diagnosis is made, we recommend initial magnetic resonance imaging (MRI) of the head and orbits (to search for hamartomas in the basal ganglia, common concomitants to NF-1 that in most cases are associated with no symptoms) and of the spine (to search for paraspinal NFs), yearly ophthalmologic examinations (to check for Lisch nodules and to evaluate the development of optic gliomas), and vision and hearing tests every 6 to 12 months. Because of risk of hypertension, blood pressure should be checked at least annually. Any complaint made by the patient should be seriously evaluated, as should any change in the physical examination. Because of the increased risk of malignancy in NF-1 patients, some authors have recommended a regular series of radiographic studies such as a periodic skeletal survey, along with computed tomographic scans of the brain, orbits, cervical and thoracic spine, abdomen, and pelvis. In our opinion, these tests should not be routinely performed unless specific symptoms occur.
- **Genetic counseling.** Because the gene for NF-1 has been identified and clinical genetic testing is now widely available, direct prenatal diagnosis, through amniocentesis or chorionic villus sampling (CVS), is currently available. Because each child born to an affected individual has a 50% chance of being affected, such testing should be offered. However, because of the marked variability of clinical features in NF-1, the decision concerning abortion of an affected fetus will undoubtedly be a difficult and troubling one.

***Neurofibromatosis-2*** Although characterized by some skin hyperpigmentation and peripheral neurofibromas, NF-2 presents a markedly different clinical picture from that of NF-1. The hallmark of NF-2, the presence of bilateral acoustic neuromas and other central nervous system (CNS) tumors, is a serious, life-threatening complication. After confirmation of this diagnosis, all efforts must be focused on identifying small neuromas at a point at which they can be surgically removed and function can be preserved.

Like NF-1, NF-2 has an autosomal-dominant inheritance pattern, but it is genetically distinct. The gene responsible, *NF2*, which has been mapped to the long arm of chromosome 22, is responsible for production of the protein, merlin, which may coordinate the processes of growth-factor receptor signaling and cell adhesion. The position of this gene is adjacent to a gene responsible for familial meningiomas, and these CNS tumors also occur commonly in individuals with NF-2.

In 50% of cases, individuals with NF-2 have a history of an affected parent. In the other 50% of cases, the condition arises presumably due to a spontaneous mutation in the *NF2* gene. An autosomal dominantly inherited condition, the offspring of an individual with NF-2 has a 50% chance of also being affected.

Clinically, the adolescent with NF-2 has fewer cafe au lait spots than does the patient with NF-1. At the time of diagnosis, the individuals with NF-2 should have the following tests:

- Head MRI
- Hearing evaluation, including brainstem auditory evoked response (BAER)
- Ophthalmologic evaluation
- Cutaneous examination

Surveillance MRI scans to determine the presence of CNS tumors should be performed every year, and affected individuals should be monitored by a neurosurgeon, with an eye toward early detection and removal of acoustic neuromas and other tumors.

### Achondroplasia

The most common bone dysplasia in humans, achondroplasia is a condition that affects 1 in 10,000 newborns. A disorder of endochondral bone, it causes rhizomelic ("root of the limb") shortening of the extremities, as well as many other clinical signs and symptoms.[8] Achondroplasia is an autosomal dominantly inherited condition, with 80% presumably arising secondarily to spontaneous mutations. Caused by a mutation in the gene *FGFR3*, which codes for fibroblast growth factor receptor type 3, a protein expressed in early bone development, achondroplasia is diagnosed on the basis of clinical and radiographic findings and can be confirmed by molecular genetic testing.

#### *Medical Problems*

- **Orthopedic problems.** The most striking feature in individuals with achondroplasia is the disproportionate shortening of stature. The mean adult height (131.5 cm in males, 123.4 cm in females) renders affected individuals immediately obvious and carries with it the potential for significant psychologic and orthopedic dysfunction. The growth chart for individuals with achondroplasia is available at: aappolicy.aappublications.org/cgi/content/full/pediatrics;116/3/771. In adolescence, knee pain becomes a common complaint. Associated with obesity and progressive genu varum (related to unequal growth of the tibia and fibula), the pain is caused by strain on the lateral collateral ligaments and is difficult to treat. In addition, spinal disorders are common orthopedic problems in young adults with achondroplasia, occurring in 70%. Exaggerated lumbar lordosis is seen first, and spinal stenosis is common later in life, leading to a spectrum of problems. If spinal surgery is indicated in these individuals, the use of instrumentation, such as rods, should be avoided, because these devices have been known to leave the patient with permanent neurologic sequelae.

- **Neurologic problems.** Complaints referable to neurologic dysfunction occur in 70% of young adults with achondroplasia. Early in life, hydrocephalus and other problems related to dysplasia of the cranial base and upper cervical spine may occur. Later, spinal deformities causing nerve root compression may lead to diverse symptoms (central apnea, paraplegia, claudication, numbness).
- **Respiratory problems.** Hypoventilation and apnea, caused by cord compression, can occur at any age. It has also been our experience that obstructive apnea, resulting from a combination of factors, including an acute cranial base angle and obesity, may become a significant problem in early adolescence. Changes in school performance, daytime somnolence, and alterations in sleeping patterns should lead to a careful evaluation of the airway in such patients.
- **Obstetrics/family planning.** Both males and females with achondroplasia have normal genitalia and endocrine functioning. Pregnancies are not significantly different from those of unaffected women during the first 2 trimesters. However, because of a markedly increased risk of stillborn infants when delivered vaginally (because of abnormalities in the size and shape of the pelvis), elective cesarean section is indicated in women with achondroplasia. Like children with NF and MS, children born to men or women with achondroplasia have a 50% chance of also being affected. However, as a result of involvement with social organizations such as Little People of America, patients with achondroplasia frequently meet and mate with other affected individuals. In such matings, although each offspring still has a 50% chance of having heterozygous achondroplasia, there is a 25% risk that the child will inherit both abnormal genes and have homozygous achondroplasia, an almost universally lethal disorder. Because of this and the need for cesarean section, the decision to bear children is a significant one. As noted previously, because of the recent discovery that achondroplasia is caused by a mutation in *FGFR3*, prenatal diagnosis through amniocentesis or CVS is now available to many affected individuals. This is especially important in matings between individuals with achondroplasia, because the diagnosis of the homozygous condition can be accomplished.
- **Psychosocial problems.** Nearly all people with achondroplasia have normal intelligence. Because of the short, disproportionate size of adolescents with achondroplasia, many in society react to them with curiosity, surprise, fear, and concern. Affected adolescents, faced with the frequent disruptions of their lives caused by people's reactions, adopt 1 of 4 defense mechanisms: (1) withdrawal and isolation (a combination that may contribute to obesity); (2) denial (a defense that is likely to last for only a short time); (3) accepting the role of "mascot" (which leads to poor body image and serious psychologic problems); and (4) finally, realizing the effect their size has on other people and helping society cope with their abnormality by learning methods of putting people at ease. According to Little People of America, the last named is the most effective and healthy mechanism. School and employment present special problems for people with achondroplasia. At school, special tools, such as a step stool at the toilet and a second set of books, so that heavy books need not be carried, may be necessary. Traditionally, people with achondroplasia have been forced to find work in the entertainment field and have often had a difficult time finding white-collar jobs. Finally, because of the rarity of achondroplasia and other bone dysplasias, it is not uncommon for some affected adolescents never to have seen another person with achondroplasia. As a result, organizations such as Little People of America and the Human Growth Foundation have served an important role in the social development

of young adults with achondroplasia. Through local functions and annual national conventions, people with achondroplasia have an opportunity to meet others with bone dysplasias. In addition, these groups deal with such day-to-day problems as the inability to buy life or health insurance, the need to purchase appropriate clothing, and discrimination in the workplace.

***Clinical Management*** The diagnosis of achondroplasia is always made in infancy or early childhood. By the time of adolescence, the psychologic and physical effects of achondroplasia have already been felt.

- **Growth.** At present, no consistently effective treatment is available for the disproportionate short stature that occurs in achondroplasia. Growth hormone therapy currently has little place in the management of these patients. Leg-lengthening procedures, performed surgically, have been successful in some cases; however, these procedures take an extremely long time, require a great deal of dedication and adherence on the part of patient and family, are expensive, and are fraught with complications. These procedures should therefore be offered only to highly motivated individuals on whom the shortened stature is having the most serious effects.
- **Orthopaedic surgery.** Surgery to repair the genu varum is important and should be performed in early adolescence. Surgical correction of the spinal malalignment may be needed later in life. For these reasons, it is important that patients with achondroplasia be monitored by an orthopedist.
- **Respiratory management.** As noted previously, there is a significant risk for the development of obstructive apnea. The care provider must be ever-vigilant for symptoms and signs of airway obstruction. If such symptoms are evident, the practitioner should (1) conduct a sleep study to confirm the presence of apnea, (2) evaluate the airways (through endoscopy) to find any causes of obstruction, and (3) select a treatment aimed at specific causes (some patients may require continuous positive airway pressure, others a tracheostomy).
- **Genetic counseling.** Careful counseling is imperative in adolescence. Patients need to know their risks of having an affected child, or an unaffected child, which may prove more of a burden. As already discussed, prenatal diagnosis through amniocentesis or CVS is possible. Ultrasonographic and radiologic prenatal diagnosis can also be accomplished.

## AUTOSOMAL RECESSIVELY INHERITED DISORDERS

The 2 most common autosomal recessively inherited disorders, sickle cell disease and cystic fibrosis, are discussed in depth in Chapters 107 and 92, respectively. This section focuses only on genetic counseling.

### Sickle Cell Anemia

More information about the molecular genetics of sickle cell anemia (SCA) is known than about nearly any other genetic disorder. All clinical signs and symptoms in this disease are caused by a single base change in the gene coding for the beta-globin chain, which has been mapped to the short arm of chromosome 11. This minute change, leading to a substitution of the amino acid valine for glutamine at the sixth position from the protein's amino terminal end, affects the conformation of the hemoglobin molecule and leads to its sickled shape when oxygen saturation is low.

Because so much about the molecular genetics of SCA is known, definitive prenatal diagnosis, through amniocentesis, CVS, or preimplantation genetic diagnosis (PGD) is possible. However, only women at risk of having an affected child should be referred for testing. Therefore, one of the following criteria should be met: (1) both parents have previously had a child with SCA either together or separately; (2) both parents have been tested and found to be heterozygotes (have the sickle cell trait); or (3) one parent has had a child with SCA and the other has tested positive. Each child born to a couple in which any of these criteria have been fulfilled has a 25% chance of having SCA and a 50% chance of inheriting the sickle cell trait. Children born to couples in which one parent is affected with SCA and the other has a trait each have a 50% chance of being affected with the disease. If both parents are affected, all offspring will have SCA.

In counseling couples that fulfill these criteria, it is important to emphasize that SCA is clinically variable; some affected individuals are chronically ill and others only mildly symptomatic. The decision to undergo prenatal diagnosis and then to continue or end the pregnancy must be made by the couple.

### Cystic Fibrosis

Caused by mutations in the *CFTR* gene, cystic fibrosis (CF) is the most common single gene disorder in the US population, occurring in 1 in 3,200 live births. Responsible for producing cystic fibrosis transmembrane conductance regulator, mutations in *CFTR* are responsible for causing an array of clinical features that affect the respiratory, gastrointestinal, endocrine, and reproductive systems. Hundreds of mutations of this gene have been identified and there is a clear correlation between severity of disease and mutation present. Cystic fibrosis exists as a spectrum: classical CF stands at one of the spectrum, whereas at the other is congenital absence of the vas deferens, presenting as infertility in the male with no other phenotypic anomalies.

Cystic fibrosis is an autosomal-recessive disorder; in order to be affected, the individual must have inherited 2 copies of nonworking genes, 1 from each parent. Parents who are both carriers have a recurrence risk in future pregnancies of 1 in 4. Males who are affected are infertile; affected females, however, can reproduce. Their offspring would all be expected to be heterozygotes (carriers); if the spouse of an affected female is a heterozygote, each offspring has a risk of 50% of also having CF.

Because the genetic defect in CF is known, prenatal diagnosis via amniocentesis, CVS, or PGD is available.

### X-LINKED RECESSIVELY INHERITED DISORDERS

The 2 most common disorders in this group are Duchenne muscular dystrophy (DMD) and hemophilia. Again, both have been covered in detail elsewhere in this text: the former in Chapter 128, Motor Unit Disorders, and the latter in Chapter 108, Hemostasis and Thrombosis, respectively. As a result, only the genetics of these disorders will be discussed here.

#### Duchenne Muscular Dystrophy

Although DMD has long been known to be linked to the X chromosome, characterization of the gene responsible for this disorder was accomplished only in the 1980s. The gene, termed *DMD,* is responsible for production of the protein dystrophin, an important component of muscle cells that is deficient in men with this and some other forms of muscular dystrophy, including the milder Becker muscular dystrophy and *DMD*-related dilated cardiomyopathy (now known collectively as "the dystrophinopathies"). The characterization of dystrophin has led to major advances in the diagnosis and potential treatment of DMD.

Because DMD shows an X-linked recessive inheritance pattern, most affected patients are male, and the disorder occurs in 1 in 5,500 boys. Mothers and sisters of affected males may or may not be carriers of the abnormal gene. In the past, counseling was offered on the basis of statistical probabilities: the chances that a first-degree female relative of a male affected with DMD carried the abnormal gene depended on the number of other affected males in the family and the level of creatine kinase in the woman's blood. Furthermore, in women believed to be carriers, fetal sex determination was the only possible method of prenatal diagnosis. Because of the identification of the actual gene defect responsible for DMD, however, counseling with certainty can now be offered after testing of affected relatives. In addition, once a female has been identified as a carrier, direct prenatal diagnosis can now be offered through amniocentesis, CVS, or PGD.

Recently, it has become clear that heterozygote females are at risk for developing *DMD*-related cardiomyopathy, a life-threatening condition that also affects hemizygous males. In affected males, the heart involvement usually begins in the teens and 20s, with rapid progression. In carrier females, involvement of the cardiac muscle usually does not begin until the fourth or fifth decade of life, and is more slowly progressive.

Because of the inheritance pattern, those men with DMD who reproduce cannot have children who are affected. Rather, all daughters born to such men will be obligate carriers, whereas sons, having received their father's Y chromosome, will be free of the disease. Because of the risk of carrier status in first-degree female relatives of men with DMD, all such women should be offered definitive testing, and if testing reveals them to be heterozygous, genetic counseling and evaluation by a cardiologist should be carried out. Because such testing should ideally be performed before childbearing has begun, much of this testing will take place in adolescence.

#### Hemophilia

Appropriate genetic counseling in hemophilia is nearly identical to that for DMD. Similarly, the gene responsible for producing the clotting factors deficient in hemophilia A and B, as well as for some of the other inherited bleeding diatheses, has been characterized, and direct DNA diagnosis is possible. As in DMD, children of males affected with hemophilia cannot be themselves affected; however, daughters will all be carriers and should be offered prenatal diagnosis. First-degree relatives of affected males (ie, mothers and sisters) should routinely be offered the opportunity to be tested and, if found to be carriers, be referred for prenatal diagnosis by CVS, amniocentesis, or PGD.

## MULTIFACTORIALLY INHERITED DISORDERS

Multifactorially inherited traits result from a combination of many factors, genetic and nongenetic, each of which makes a significant contribution to the overall picture. These disorders tend to cluster in families, but the inheritance does not conform to simple mendelian patterns. Approximately 20% of all congenital malformations are multifactorially inherited; included in this group are neural tube defects, congenital heart disease, nonsyndromic cleft lip and palate, and hypospadias. In addition, many diseases of childhood and adult life, including asthma, autism, diabetes mellitus, alcoholism, atherosclerotic heart disease, and some forms of cancer, are determined by the interplay between genetic background and environmental exposures. One of the multifactorially inherited disorders faced commonly by those providing care to adolescents, meningomyelocele, will be discussed in detail in Chapter 133.

## ENVIRONMENTALLY INDUCED CONGENITAL MALFORMATION SYNDROMES

A "teratogen" is defined as any chemical or environmental agent that has the potential to damage embryonic tissue primordia, ultimately resulting in one or more congenital malformations. Since the early 1960s, when it became apparent that the drug thalidomide, a tranquilizer often prescribed during pregnancy, caused phocomelia (limb reduction defects) and a series of other life-threatening congenital malformations, information has been collected for a large series of drugs and chemical agents that, when administered during pregnancy, appear to induce birth defects. Today, teratogens are responsible for approximately 6.5% of all malformations recognized in the newborn period.

There are 3 major reasons why those providing care to adolescents need to understand teratogenesis. First, within the patient population being served, some individuals are bound to be affected with such entities as fetal alcohol and congenital rubella syndromes. To provide optimal care to such individuals, the care provider must understand the natural history of these disorders. Second, because of the growing number of women who become pregnant during adolescence, the care provider should question the patient about use of such agents as crack cocaine, alcohol, and other teratogenic agents. Finally, the care provider, in treating the pregnant adolescent, may wish to prescribe drugs, such as *cis*-retinoic acid, hydantoin, or tetracycline, all of which have been implicated in causing birth defects. For these reasons, the concepts of when and how teratogens cause their adverse effects, the work-up after a teratogen exposure, and the natural history of some resulting syndromes will be covered in this section.

### TERATOGENESIS

Before specific teratogenic agents are discussed, 3 concepts need elucidation. First, teratogens often have different effects when administered at different periods during gestation. The 3 important periods during fetal life are (1) the preimplantation phase, from conception until 10 days after conception, when implantation is completed; (2) the organogenic phase, from implantation to approximately 8 weeks after conception, when formation of all major organ systems has been completed; and (3) the fetal phase, from 9 weeks after conception until birth. When a teratogen is administered during the preimplantation phase, either it will cause such severe damage to the blastocyst that the conceptus will be lost and a spontaneous abortion will occur (at a time when the woman may be completely unaware that she is pregnant), or no harmful effects will occur and normal implantation will take place. This latter phase has been referred to as the safe period; although this is technically inaccurate, it is understood that if pregnancy does ensue, no significant harm has been done to the embryo. The same teratogen administered during the organogenic phase may cause serious harm to many developing structures, but if it is administered after the completion of organogenesis, it is possible that no harmful effects will occur. Alcohol, described later in greater detail, provides a good example of this phenomenon. If a woman drinks alcohol heavily during the preimplantation phase and then stops, any surviving offspring will be unharmed; if she drinks in the organogenic phase, her child may be affected with FAS; if she abstains from alcohol until the second trimester of pregnancy, her infant will appear morphologically normal but is at risk for serious intellectual abnormalities. Alcohol is therefore considered both a structural (capable of causing congenital malformations) and a behavioral (capable of inducing behavioral alterations) teratogen.

A second important concept of teratogenesis is that of tissue specificity. Some agents known to be teratogenic exert harmful effects on only 1 or 2 tissue types. The antibiotic tetracycline is a good example; it is harmful only to developing bone and teeth. If it is administered during the early first trimester, before this tissue has begun to develop, no harmful effects will result. If it is administered later, in the second and third trimester, tooth defects (hypoplasia of enamel) and diminished growth of long bones may result.

A third concept that should be understood is that of facilitation. In the context of teratogenesis, facilitation refers to the enhancement or alteration of an agent's effect by the presence of a second agent or factor. For example, the anticonvulsant hydantoin causes different effects on the embryo and fetus when the mother who uses the drug is free of seizures than it does when seizures occur. Therefore, facilitation may have a confounding effect on epidemiologic analysis and may affect the type of counseling offered to the mother.

## TERATOGENS

### Maternal Factors

***Maternal Infections*** Table 148-2 lists some of the more common infectious agents that produce harmful effects and the consequences of infection on the conceptus. The effect of each of these infectious agents on the developing embryo or fetus is related to the timing of infection. Generally, the earlier the infection, the more devastating the effects.

***Noninfectious Maternal Illness*** The fetus is sensitive to a number of maternal metabolic disturbances. In most cases, strict control of the underlying metabolic abnormality in the mother will serve to protect the fetus.

Infants of mothers with diabetes are at significantly greater risk for congenital malformation than are infants whose mothers do not have diabetes. It is estimated that between 6% and 10% of these infants have an abnormality in form or function that is detectable in the neonatal period.[9] Malformations that occur more commonly in this group include the caudal regression sequence (a severe defect in the development of the posterior blastema, in which absence of the sacrum, defects of the lower limb, imperforate anus, and abnormalities of the genitourinary tract combine); and the VACTERL association (association of vertebral anomalies, anal stenosis, cardiac anomalies, tracheo-esophageal fistula, and renal and limb malformations). The presence and severity of anomalies appear to be directly related to the degree of glycemic control during the first trimester of pregnancy.

In addition to these congenital malformations, infants of mothers with diabetes are at greater risk for nonmalformation-related disorders at the time of birth. Macrosomia, cardiomyopathy, hypoglycemia, polycythemia, and hyperbilirubinemia are all known neonatal sequelae of gestational diabetes.

Through the use of neonatal screening and the institution of special diets low in phenylalanine, phenylketonuria (an inborn error of metabolism caused by a deficiency of phenylalanine hydroxylase) has become a relatively innocuous disease since the 1960s. The tendency in the past has been to limit intake of phenylalanine in affected individuals until late childhood, when liberalization of the diet has occurred. However, Mabry et al,[10] in 1966, were the first to note that offspring of women with phenylketonuria are at significant risk for mental retardation, microcephaly, and congenital heart disease.[10] In the late 1980s, suggestions were made that women in the childbearing years be returned to a low phenylalanine diet; it has been shown that, if this diet is instituted before the start of pregnancy, the fetus is at little or no increased risk for these anomalies.

**Table 148-2**

**Selected Infectious Teratogens**

| | Congenital Malformation | | | | |
|---|---|---|---|---|---|
| *Agent* | *Central Nervous System* | *Eye* | *Ear* | *Heart* | *Other* |
| Rubella virus | MR, microcephaly | Cataract, glaucoma, other | Deafness | VSD, ASD, PDA | Growth deficiency, bone dysplasia, other |
| Cytomegalovirus | Microcephaly, calcifications, MR | Microphthalmia, blindness | Deafness | | Miscarriage |
| *Toxoplasma gondii* | Microcephaly, calcifications, MR | Microphthalmia, chorioretinitis | | | Miscarriage |
| Herpes simplex virus | Microcephaly, MR | Microphthalmia, retinal dysplasia | | | |
| Varicella | Microcephaly, MR | Cataracts, microphthalmia | | | Limb deficiency, cicatricial skin lesions |
| Human immunodeficiency virus | Microcephaly, calcifications, MR | Prominent eyes, blue sclerae | | | Characteristic facies, immunodeficiency |

ASD, atrial septal defect; MR, mental retardation; PDA, patent ductus arteriosus: VSD, ventricular septal defect.

### Drugs and Chemicals as Teratogens

This category of teratogenic agents has special significance because, to some extent, their use by pregnant women is determined by the physician, whose prescription and advice can cause these agents to be used or avoided. Therefore, it is essential for the physician to have a clear understanding of drugs and chemicals that can cause birth defects.

***Nonprescription Drugs*** Alcohol, cocaine, marijuana, and heroin are all nonprescription drugs with teratogenic potential. Also considered as part of this group are caffeine and nicotine, but these agents are believed to have no teratogenic potential. In 1973, Jones et al[11] described a recognizable pattern of malformations in infants born to chronic alcoholic women and named the condition fetal alcohol syndrome. Features of FAS include prenatal and postnatal growth deficiency; microcephaly with intellectual delay; various skeletal defects, such as radioulnar synostosis and atlantoaxial instability; cardiac anomalies, including ventricular and atrial septal defects; and a characteristic facial appearance, including short palpebral fissures, ptosis, a hypoplastic malar region, a flat philtrum, and a thin upper vermilion border of the lip. The full-blown syndrome occurs in 3 to 5 per 1,000 newborns, making FAS the most common teratogenic syndrome encountered in humans.[12] Medical problems that occur in the adolescent with FAS include growth retardation, serious intellectual defects and mental retardation, and seizure disorders. Adolescents and adults with FAS are fertile; if affected women refrain from drinking alcohol during their pregnancies, their offspring are at no increased risk for congenital defects.

More recently, the term fetal alcohol spectrum disorder (FASD) has been used to describe the range of effects that occur in individuals who were exposed to alcohol during gestation. The more subtle effects of FASD include physical, mental, behavioral, and/or learning disabilities with possible lifelong implications. Individuals with FASD frequently have attention-deficit/hyperactivity disorder, learning disabilities, mild mental retardation, memory disturbances and subtle physical findings, including slow growth, and mild facial dysmorphic features. Fetal alcohol spectrum disorder is far more common than full-blown FAS, and should be suspected in any individual with a known history of exposure to alcohol during gestation.

Over the past 2 decades, cocaine has remained a common and popular drug of abuse. A spectrum of anomalies has been observed in some offspring of women using these substances. Malformations, including intracranial hemorrhages leading to intellectual disabilities and microcephaly, intestinal atresias, limb reduction defects, and striking urinary tract anomalies such as the prune-belly syndrome, have been reported.[13] The cause of these anomalies appears to be related to vascular disruption. Thus, the vasoconstrictive effects of the drug occurring at critical times of gestation lead to this pattern of anomalies.

Although this pattern of malformations has been seen repeatedly in infants of cocaine-using women, the overall incidence of congenital malformations in this group of infants does not exceed the 3% expected in all populations. This suggests that some exposed embryos and fetuses are lost as spontaneous abortions, and that cocaine effects can be seen in only a small minority of exposed conceptuses who survive to term.

More troubling is the recent evidence that offspring of women who used cocaine during pregnancy are at significant risk for the development of behavioral and psychologic disturbances during childhood and later in life. Although the pathogenetic mechanism for this association has not yet been firmly established, it appears that these neurodevelopmental aberrations are direct sequelae of exposure to cocaine during gestation, and thus represent behavioral teratogenic effects.

***Prescription Drugs*** Thalidomide was the first prescription drug known to cause malformations. The effects of 2 other drugs are described in the following.

A vitamin A congener, *cis*-retinoic acid is an effective agent in the treatment of cystic acne, which is common in adolescence. In the early 1980s, this drug, marketed in the United States as Accutane, was also found to be a potent teratogen. Up to 70% of the fetuses exposed to Accutane during the first trimester were found to be abnormal. Some of the pregnancies ended in spontaneous abortion. Others resulted in the birth of a child with what has become known as Accutane embryopathy, a pattern of anomalies including severe craniofacial disorders (abnormalities of the skull, ears, eyes, nose, and palate), cardiac defects, and DiGeorge syndrome (hypoparathyroidism and T-cell deficiency). Because of the clear cause-and-effect relationship, *cis*-retinoic acid, as well as all other vitamin A congeners, should never be prescribed, recommended, or used during pregnancy.[14]

Hydantoin is another drug known to cause malformations. Convincing epidemiologic evidence of an association between the anticonvulsant hydantoin and congenital anomalies was provided by Fedrick.[15] In 1975, Hanson and Smith[18] described a recognizable pattern of malformations in offspring of women using hydantoin to control seizures during pregnancy. Features of the fetal hydantoin syndrome include a characteristic facies (ocular hypertelorism, a broad depressed nasal bridge, low-set ears with abnormal pinnae, cleft lip and palate); occasional mild mental retardation; and hypoplasia of the distal phalanges of the fingers and toes, with tiny or absent nails, a striking characteristic of the disorder. In recent years, the pathogenetic mechanism responsible for the malformations has been described. The risk of the syndrome is low; less than 10% of exposed embryos prove to have features of the disorder. Therefore, recommended counseling at this time is as follows: if a woman is already pregnant and taking hydantoin, she should continue taking the medication; if she is not pregnant, she should be switched to an anticonvulsant that has not been shown to be teratogenic.

#### Environmental Agents as Teratogens

This category of teratogens represents a group apart from those mentioned previously because, in contrast to prescription and street drugs, exposure to chemicals and agents in the environment is not easily controllable. One agent and some "nonagents" are described here.

***Radiation*** From the experience in the Japanese cities of Hiroshima and Nagasaki at the conclusion of World War II, it became clear that radiation exposure during fetal life can have lethal or devastating consequences. In addition to a significantly higher rate of spontaneous abortion, pregnant women exposed to high doses of radiation from the atomic bomb explosions (ie, those close to "ground zero") gave birth to a higher number of children with microcephaly, mental retardation, and skeletal malformations. However, the dose of radiation needed to induce these defects is greater than 5 rad and probably closer to 25 rad. The radiation dose used in diagnostic radiology is extremely low, with most exposure in the range of a few millirad. The literature offers no good evidence that a single (or even multiple) chest radiograph, upper gastrointestinal tract series, or other commonly performed radiologic study can harm the developing fetus.

***Nonteratogenic Environmental Agents*** Contrary to some media reports, there is no convincing evidence that exposure to video display terminals, electromagnetic fields, or caffeine causes malformations. Finally, although the active inhalation of cigarette smoke can cause a decrease in birthweight, there is no evidence that the smoking of cigarettes induces malformations in exposed fetuses.

#### Evaluation of Embryo/Fetus with Potential Teratogen Exposure

Women who have been exposed to potential teratogens often seek advice from their physician. To serve the best interests of both mother and baby, a careful evaluation must be carried out, as follows:

1. Obtain a complete history of the agent, including the dates, type, and length of exposure. The woman should bring any information about the agent (eg, package insert, label information) in her possession.
2. Obtain a complete history of the pregnancy, including last menstrual period, last normal menstrual period before the last menstrual period (to ascertain the length of the menstrual cycle), date when the pregnancy test became positive, and any symptoms of pregnancy noted. It is essential to make sure that the putative exposure actually occurred during the pregnancy and after the "safe period," as defined earlier, before proceeding with the evaluation.
3. Perform a literature search to investigate previously reported teratogenic effects of the agent. Because it does not give sufficiently helpful or specific information, the *Physicians' Desk Reference* should never be used for purposes of teratogen counseling. Rather, use appropriate online computer services and textbooks,[16,17] or refer to specific articles that cite large retrospective or prospective studies.
4. Armed with the information obtained from the literature, counsel the woman regarding the risks. She may then opt to terminate the pregnancy. If she decides to continue the pregnancy, proceed to the next step.
5. Plan an evaluation using prenatal diagnostic modalities (see earlier discussion), looking for anomalies previously reported after agent exposure.
6. Provide the information necessary so that an intelligent decision can be made about the pregnancy, and support the woman in any decision she has made.

## PRENATAL DIAGNOSIS OF GENETIC DISORDERS

It is essential that those providing care for pregnant adolescent women, as well as partners of adolescent men who have genetic disorders, have an understanding of prenatal diagnostic techniques so that appropriate referrals can be made in a timely fashion. Some women affected with congenital disorders, such as meningomyelocele, are themselves at increased risk for having a child with a similar condition.[18] Others, like those who have had multiple spontaneous abortions of unknown cause or who have a brother with muscular dystrophy, may, by virtue of their medical or family history, be at increased risk for having a child with a specific problem. Finally, some women are exposed to drugs or chemicals, such as *cis*-retinoic acid (Accutane), that are known teratogens during early embryogenesis. All of these women should be offered the opportunity to have their pregnancy appropriately monitored for specific anomalies; all deserve sensitive, accurate risk counseling, performed either by their primary care provider or by a genetic counselor.

Prenatal diagnosis originated in the 1960s with the first midtrimester amniocentesis performed for detection of fetal chromosomal abnormalities. Since that time, the field has blossomed and other diagnostic modalities, including ultrasonography, CVS, biochemical screening (quad screen), and percutaneous umbilical blood sampling have been developed. As a result of these new techniques, a greater number of congenital anomalies can now be safely detected at a relatively early stage of pregnancy.

## MATERNAL SERUM BIOCHEMICAL SCREENING

In 1984, an association between low levels of alpha-fetoprotein (AFP) and chromosomal trisomies, such as DS, was reported. This association has led to the use of AFP as a screening test for chromosomal disorders. Subsequently, levels of 3 other biochemical markers, unconjugated estriols (uE, produced by the fetus and the placenta), human chorionic gonadotropin (hCG, a hormone produced by the placenta), and inhibin A (a protein produced by the placenta and ovaries), have been found to be useful additions to the AFP screen. Using all 4 of these tests, commonly referred to as the quad screen, coupled with information regarding maternal age and underlying medical conditions, a risk profile for a fetal chromosomal abnormality can be developed for every pregnancy.

Maternal serum biochemical testing is ideally performed between 15 and 18 weeks of gestation. Because it is used only as a screening test, an abnormal quad screen must be followed up with further testing (amniocentesis and/or ultrasonography). In most cases, abnormal levels of AFP, uE, hCG, and Inhibin A are not associated with any fetal abnormality; similarly, a normal result does not completely rule out the possibility that a defect will be found in the newborn. However, because of the low risk and the low cost of testing, maternal serum biochemical screening is a valuable initial step in the evaluation of women at risk for having a child with a neural tube defect or chromosomal abnormality.

In recent years, earlier screening for fetal chromosomal abnormalities has emerged as an option for women. Performed between 11 and 13 weeks of gestation, first-trimester screening combines sonographic measurement of the fetal nuchal translucency (see the following) with measurement of levels of pregnancy-associated plasma protein A (PAPP-A) and free beta hCG in the maternal serum. Using this technique, approximately 85% of fetuses with DS and 97% of fetuses with trisomy 18 can be detected. As with second-trimester biochemical screening, an abnormal result of the combined screen requires confirmation via amniocentesis. Further, because this test does not evaluate levels of AFP, women require further testing to rule out the possibility that their fetus is affected with an open neural tube defect or abdominal wall defect later in pregnancy.

## SONOGRAPHY

Currently the most commonly used form of indirect fetal imaging, in addition to being used for assessment of fetal age, evaluation of gestational bleeding, and evaluation of intrauterine growth retardation, sonography can also be helpful in the diagnosis of a growing number of structural congenital malformations and as an adjunct to other forms of prenatal diagnosis (eg, amniocentesis, AFP screening, and CVS). As noted previously, it is also an essential component of the first-trimester screening protocol, in which the width of the nuchal translucency is assessed at 11 to 13 weeks. At levels used for diagnosis, sonography does not have any harmful effect on the fetus.

At present, most women receiving prenatal care in the United States have at least one ultrasonographic examination during pregnancy. The examination is relatively inexpensive and can be performed at any time, but for the detection of fetal malformations it is best done after 16 weeks of gestation.

## AMNIOCENTESIS

Traditionally, amniocentesis has been the cornerstone of prenatal diagnosis. When used for detection of fetal genetic disorders, it usually is performed between 14 and 18 weeks of gestation. The procedure is carried out under sonographic guidance to assess fetal age, rule out gross structural anomalies, and choose a suitable site for insertion of the needle. Approximately 30 ml of amniotic fluid is aspirated, and aliquots of this fluid are placed in a culture medium (to allow growth of fetal cells so that chromosomal or DNA analysis can be performed) and are also used to determine the AFP level. If the latter is significantly elevated, a study of acetylcholinesterase, a specific marker for neural tube defects, is also performed.

The principal use of amniocentesis today is for detection of chromosomal abnormalities in women at increased risk for having a child with one of these anomalies. As such, the applicability of amniocentesis in adolescent women is limited to those who have a family history of a chromosomal aberration in a first-degree relative (eg, a sibling or child), or who have had an abnormal quad or first-trimester screen. In addition to detection of chromosomal abnormalities, however, amniocentesis is used when the fetus is at increased risk for (1) neural tube defects (eg, when the mother or a first-degree relative has meningomyelocele, or when the fetus has been exposed to teratogens known to cause such defects, such as valproic acid); (2) specific X-linked disorders (eg, when the mother carries the gene for DMD or hemophilia); (3) inborn errors of metabolism in which an enzyme defect (eg, Tay-Sachs disease) or an abnormal metabolite (eg, congenital erythropoietic porphyria) can be detected; or (4) any single gene defect that can be diagnosed through analysis of DNA (eg, CF).

Recent studies have demonstrated that amniocentesis is a low-risk procedure, with the risk of fetal loss in the range of 1 in 1,000 or less. The reliability of information obtained through amniocentesis is extremely high; incorrect information, caused by sampling and growing maternal cells rather than those from the fetus, failure of growth of the cells in culture, or laboratory error, occurs much less than 1% of the time.

After detection of an abnormality through amniocentesis, 2 options are available. The pregnant woman may choose to continue the pregnancy, knowing that her baby will be affected with a specific disorder, or she can choose to terminate it. By the time the diagnosis is relayed to the woman, the pregnancy is relatively far advanced, often between weeks 18 and 21, and the abortion techniques available are psychologically and medically more complicated than those performed during the first trimester. As a result of these problems, prenatal diagnosis through CVS has been developed.

### CHORIONIC VILLUS SAMPLING

This modality has been developed in response to the need for a safe, accurate test that will provide information about anomalous pregnancies during the first trimester. The technique employs sampling of the chorionic villi, structures derived from fetal mesenchymal tissue that eventually form the cytotrophoblast and the placenta.

Removing a small number of villi is relatively easily accomplished between 9 and 11 weeks of gestation. The cells of the villi, embryonic in origin, are actively dividing, and analysis of the karyotype and isolation of DNA can be rapidly performed. As a result, these investigations can be completed within a week after the procedure, allowing detection of chromosomal defects and single-gene mutations within the first trimester, a marked advantage over amniocentesis.

At present, CVS is performed through a transcervical or transabdominal approach. The procedure is preceded by sonographic examination to assess fetal viability. Data concerning the risks for transcervical CVS indicate that the fetal loss rate is only 0.8%, suggesting that it is a safe and effective technique for the early prenatal diagnosis of cytogenetic abnormalities, but that it entails a slightly higher risk of procedure failure and fetal loss than amniocentesis. Also, as in amniocentesis, analysis of cells obtained from CVS is not always guaranteed. Cells may fail to grow in the culture, and occasionally inadvertent inclusion of maternal cells may occur. In CVS, however, an additional problem has occasionally been seen, that of chromosomal mosaicism; experience has shown that detection of an abnormal karyotype during CVS does not always reflect an underlying fetal anomaly. Some aberrations, such as tetraploidy, trisomy 16, and monosomy X, may be found in direct chorionic villus preparations but not in the embryonic tissue.

Chorionic villus sampling is useful for diagnosing many of the same conditions detected by amniocentesis, such as chromosomal anomalies, certain inborn errors of metabolism, and single-gene mutations in which DNA defects are known. Detection of neural tube defects through AFP determination cannot be accomplished by CVS, however.

### PREIMPLANTATION GENETIC DIAGNOSIS

Relatively new to the armamentarium of prenatal genetic diagnosis, preimplantation genetic diagnosis (PGD) uses in vitro fertilization technology to allow detection of the presence of single-gene disorders and chromosomal abnormalities in a fertilized ovum prior to implantation in the uterus.

Preimplantation genetic diagnosis begins with routine in vitro fertilization. Following hormonal stimulation to cause hyperovulation, mature ova are harvested from the woman using a laparoscope. Ova are evaluated and placed in a culture medium and fertilized using spermatozoa from the woman's partner. After fertilization, the cells begin to divide.

Soon after cell division has begun, as early as at the 16- or 32-cell stage, a single cell is sampled using a micropipette. Using either PCR to amplify a specific region of the genome, or FISH to identify a number of copies of chromosomes, the cell's DNA is analyzed, searching for the presence of a particular single-gene mutation or an abnormality in the number of chromosomes. Cell division progresses; at the time that implantation takes place, only pre-embryos found to be free of the particular genetic disorder of concern are used, ensuring that the resulting embryo, fetus, and child will be free of that condition.

Because only nonaffected pre-embryos are implanted, the couple using this technique will not have to face the prospect of terminating an affected fetus later in the pregnancy (as occur in both amniocentesis and CVS). Preimplantation genetic diagnosis is most useful for families in which single-gene disorders, such as CF or SCA, are segregating, or in couples in whom one partner carries a balanced chromosomal translocation that may lead to an unbalanced trisomy or monosomy in his or her offspring.

Unfortunately, PGD is expensive, limiting its usefulness in most families. Also, because the mutation present must be identified before use, it is further limited to only those disorders in which the molecular basis has been found.

### PERCUTANEOUS UMBILICAL BLOOD SAMPLING

Occasionally, rapid and accurate assessment of a fetus's karyotype is necessary in the second and third trimesters of pregnancy. Chorionic villus sampling is not possible at this stage, and diagnosis through amniocentesis may require more time than is available. In these instances, direct sampling of fetal blood and culturing of lymphocytes is an appropriate technique. In this procedure a catheter equipped with a small needle and a syringe allows sampling of a small aliquot of blood from an umbilical cord vessel, which can be used for appropriate testing.

The applicability of percutaneous umbilical blood sampling is limited to those instances in which an immediate obstetric or neonatal decision must be made. For instance, percutaneous umbilical blood sampling can be helpful when significant intrauterine growth retardation is found or in a fetus noted to have congenital malformations on routine ultrasonography.

## SUMMARY

Although each genetic disorder encountered by the adolescent health care provider may be rare, taken together they compose a significant portion of the burden of chronic disease in the young adult population. Because of this, it is essential that care providers working with this population have knowledge of genetics. Although much more information is available about each of the conditions listed previously, this chapter was intended to serve as an outline, a beginning for this understanding.

## REFERENCES

1. Hall JG, Powers EK, McIlvaine RT, Ean VH. The frequency and financial burden of genetic disorders in a pediatric hospital. *Am J Med Genet.* 1978;1(4):417–436

2. Down syndrome preventive medicine check list. *Down Syndrome Papers and Abstracts for Professionals.* 1989;12:2

3. Rosenfeld RG. *Turner Syndrome: A Guide for Physicians.* Los Angeles, CA: Mason Medical Communications; 1989:1–23

4. Caldwell PD, Smith DW. The XXY syndrome in childhood: detection and treatment. *J Pediatr.* 1972;80(2):250–258

5. Butler MG, Meaney FJ, Palmer CG. Clinical and cytogenetic survey of 39 individuals with Prader-Labhert-Willi syndrome. *Am J Med Genet.* 1986;23(3):793–809

6. Dietz HC. Marfan syndrome. In *Gene Clinics.* Available at: www.ncbi.nlm.nih.gov/bookshelf/br.fcgi?book=gene&part=marfan. Accessed November 17, 2010

7. Riccardi VE, Eichner JE. *Neurofibromatosis: Phenotype, Natural History, and Pathogenesis.* Baltimore, MD: Johns Hopkins University Press; 1986

8. Jones KL. *Smith's Recognizable Patterns of Human Malformations.* 4th ed. Philadelphia, PA: WB Saunders; 1988:298

9. Merlob P, Reisner SH. Fetal effects from maternal diabetes. In: Buyse ML, ed. *Birth Defects Encyclopedia.* Cambridge, MA: Blackwell Scientific Publications; 1990:700

10. Mabry CC, Denniston JC, Coldwell JG. Mental retardation in children of phenylketonuric mothers. *N Engl J Med.* 1966;275(24):1331–1336

11. Jones KL, Smith DW, Ulleland CN, Streissguth AP. Pattern of malformations in offspring of chronic alcoholic women. *Lancet.* 1973;1:1267–1271

12. Jones KL. Fetal alcohol syndrome. *Pediatr in Rev.* 1986;8(4):122–126

13. Bingol N, Fuchs M, Diaz V, Stone RK, Gromisch DS. Teratogenicity of cocaine in humans. *J Pediatrics.* 1987;110(1):93–96

14. Lammer EJ, Chen DT, Hoar RM, et al. Retinoic acid embryopathy. *N Engl J Med.* 1985;313(14):837–841

15. Fedrick J. Epilepsy and pregnancy: a report from the Oxford Record linkage study. *Br Med J.* 1973;2:442–448

16. Shepard TH. *Catalog of Teratogenic Agents.* 6th ed. Baltimore, MD: Johns Hopkins University Press; 1989

17. Briggs GG, Freeman RK, Yaffe SJ. *Drugs in Pregnancy and Lactation.* 2nd ed. Baltimore, MD: Williams & Wilkins; 1986

18. Marion RW, Chambers P, Schendel LF. Myelomeningocele. In: Johnson RT, ed. *Current Therapy in Neurologic Disease-3.* St Louis, MO: Mosby-Year Book; 1990:85

19. Hanson JW, Buehler BA. Fetal hydantoin syndrome: current status. *J Pediatr.* 1982;101(5):816–818

# CHAPTER 149

# Genetic Predisposition to Common Disorders

DEANNE MRAZ ROBINSON, MD • CHIN-TO FONG, MD

## INTRODUCTION

Genes contribute, at some level, to the etiology of almost every human disease. Such contributions can vary from a single gene causing a recognized disorder in mendelian fashion to a combination of genes conferring a mild to moderate increase in risk for a disease, whereas environmental, lifestyle, or life history factors make more significant contributions in a multifactorial fashion. Most traits or disorders can be categorized into a well-defined genetic syndrome, a likely syndrome that has not been well defined, or an isolated finding that is nonsyndromic. Within each category, traits or disorders can be further subcategorized into whether it is familial or sporadic, or genetic or nongenetic, and if genetic whether it is mendelian ("simple") or multifactorial ("complex").

This chapter addresses common patterns of predisposition to genetic diseases in adolescents, including the contributions of complex phenotypes and genotypes, as well as environmental and random influences and gene–environment interactions that can each play a role. With obesity as a model of a common condition affecting adolescents, the contribution of familial versus sporadic, genetic versus nongenetic, and mendelian versus multifactorial influences are explored. With the completion of the sequencing of the human genome and advances in genetics technology, a number of means are available to identify human disorders associated with adolescent obesity, including gene and linkage mapping, genetic associations, and linkage disequilibrium (LD). In addition to helping future understanding of monogenic, oligogenic, and multifactorial nonsyndromic conditions, these techniques will also be invaluable in expanding our knowledge about a variety of other conditions affecting adolescents.

## PATTERNS OF PREDISPOSITIONS TO GENETIC DISEASES IN ADOLESCENTS

Most common diseases or disorders in adolescent health care follow a multifactorial pattern of inheritance. Often referred to as "common complex traits," the word "complex" denotes the unknown manner in which genetic and environmental factors interact to cause many of these diseases or disorders. In the medical genetic literature, the term "complex diseases" is operationally defined as those conditions whose genetic contributions are not easily traced through traditional methods of genetic dissection, which were constructed based primarily on a mendelian genetic framework.

### COMPLEX GENETIC CONDITIONS

There are several ways for a condition in an adolescent to be genetically "complex," including the influence of (1) phenotype, (2) genotype, (3) environment, (4) random events, and (5) risk. In addition, it may be difficult to differentiate between affected and unaffected adolescents. Each trait is detailed in the following sections.

#### Complex Phenotypes

Many adolescent disease phenotypes or traits are complex, including a plethora of behavioral or mental health traits, ranging from psychiatric diseases, such as schizophrenia or bipolar disorders, to addiction, risk-taking behavior, sexual orientation, and, perhaps, intelligence. This partly reflects the true complexity of the traits, but mostly reflects our inability to properly define and subclassify them. For example, the kind of intelligence needed to become a chess master differs from that to be a race car driver.

#### Complex Genotypes

Some disease phenotypes and traits have multiple genetic etiologies. For example, although most patients with Alzheimer disease do not follow a mendelian pattern of inheritance, there are subsets of patients with Alzheimer disease who do. At least 4 different genes have been identified that account for the mendelian forms of Alzheimer disease. Variants of one or more of these genes may contribute to the common forms for Alzheimer disease, but the combinations of variants may vary from individual to individual.

This is an example of *genetic heterogeneity*. There are 2 kinds of genetic heterogeneity: *locus heterogeneity* and *allelic heterogeneity*. Locus heterogeneity refers to more than one gene, or combination of genes, causing the same phenotype. Allelic heterogeneity, in contrast, refers to different alleles of a given gene at a given locus resulting in a different manifestation of the total phenotypic spectrum of a disease. Locus heterogeneity and allelic heterogeneity are not mutually exclusive.

In addition to genetic heterogeneity, complex diseases generally require contributions from a few to many genes. Thus, the contribution from an individual gene may be difficult to discern, making the identification of candidate genes particularly challenging. Furthermore, genes that do not cause a phenotype may modify phenotypic expression. These *modifier genes* are the focus of increasing attention because they provide important clues to the treatment of the diseases for which they modify phenotypic expression. Modifier genes are also believed to be responsible for such genetic phenomena as *incomplete penetrance* and *variable expressivity*.

### Environmental Influences

Environmental factors are important in the manifestation, progression, treatment response, morbidity, and mortality of complex genetic diseases. Common environmental factors include physical, chemical, and biological exposures; diet, lifestyle, and other physiological life processes, such as pregnancy or aging. In the genetic analysis of complex diseases, nongenetic factors are considered "environmental," even if no specific environmental agent has been identified. In addition, effects of environmental agents are often mediated through "epigenetic" processes that change the phenotype without changing the genotype, mostly through altering gene expression profiles.

### Random (Stochastic) Events

Some traits may require additional random events to occur before they become manifested. Examples include somatic mutation(s) on specific cell or tissue types, skewed X inactivation, or uneven segregation of abnormal mitochondria among mitotic daughter cells. In these circumstances, an adolescent's genotype may result in a decreased ability to "remedy" such events, as occurs in DNA repair disorders. Although the cause of the event itself may be environmental, the occurrence of the actual event is governed by rules of probability following a Poisson distribution and, as such, may influence the penetrance and variability of the trait.

### Risk of Being Affected by a Condition

When considering a complex disease, the demarcation between an affected and unaffected status becomes blurred. In simplistic classification, an adolescent showing the signs and symptoms of a disease is "affected," and one who is not showing the same signs and symptoms is "unaffected." However, this classification scheme is unsatisfactory because many individuals in the general population may be *presymptomatic* and not develop signs and symptoms until later in life. Thus, for complex diseases, it is more important to consider the risk of an adolescent developing a certain disease than to focus solely on the presence or absence of disease manifestations. This implies that every adolescent has the potential of developing a complex disease, but some individuals are far more *predisposed* to do so than others as a result of their genetic makeup and environmental exposure.

Although nongenetic factors generally exert their effects over time, genetic factors are inherited and present at birth. Thus, prior to the manifestation of a disease or disorder, predisposed adolescents possessing the requisite genetic factors that will make them vulnerable to nongenetic triggers can most effectively delay or minimize their adverse genetic factors by altering their environmental exposure or lifestyle. This is a keystone of preventive medicine in the era of modern genetics that makes the exploration of genetic contributions to diseases and disorders so essential.

## GENES AND ENVIRONMENT IN COMPLEX DISORDERS

Among many clinicians, there is significant skepticism about the investment of resources to study the genetic contribution of common complex disorders when it seems obvious that environmental factors, and hence lifestyle interventions, appear to be the key to address problems at a public health level. For example, as obesity trends started to emerge in the late 1980s and early 1990s, a common aphorism was "the cause of increasing rates and levels of obesity cannot be accounted for by genetics because the gene pool does not change in one generation." This was prior to advances in the understanding of environmental influences on gene expression. The conclusion was that because the trend in obesity in developed countries could be accounted for almost exclusively by changes in environment and lifestyle (diet and physical activity), investing in the study of the genetics of obesity was considered ill advised because resources could be more effectively allocated to public education and health systems alterations to combat these changes.

There are at least 2 counterpoints to this position. First, taking a Darwinian view of our genome, there is consensus among many evolutionary geneticists that the human genome and the manner in which it is expressed had been "optimized" through natural selection to cope with the environment or lifestyle of the stage of human history when large-scale evolution began to slow due to the advent of cultural intervention, perhaps at the hunter-gatherer stage. From this viewpoint, many "mismatches" between our genome and our modern society are manifested in many diseases of our time, such as obesity or coronary heart

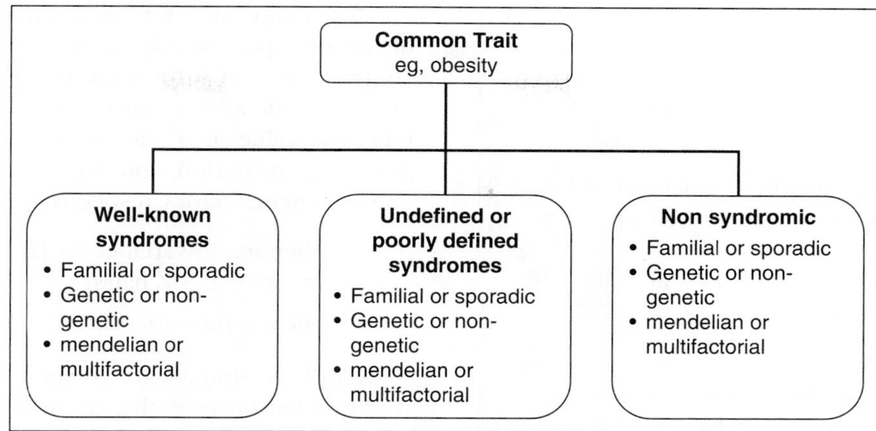


**FIGURE 149-1** Categorization of common traits in terms of genetic etiology.

disease. It is unlikely that even with the most comprehensive personal education or public health intervention that the environment and lifestyle of modern humans will return to that of the hunter-gatherer stage. Hence, understanding where our genome has fallen short of adapting to the modern environment will help bridge the gap of "maladaptation."

Second, the understanding of genetic and metabolic pathways has the potential of helping with the development of pharmacologic interventions. For example, the genetic and metabolic underpinnings of statin therapy were elucidated in patients affected by the rare genetic trait familial hypercholesterolemia. The knowledge from the study of patients with this rare genetic disorder has had a profound effect on innumerable patients within more common forms of hypercholesterolemia. Foregoing study of genetic contributions to hypercholesterolemia in favor of public health interventions exclusively might have prevented the discovery of statins.

Numerous common complex traits affect the adolescent population, including, but not limited to, obesity, hypertension, asthma, and mental health disorders. Obesity serves as an example to illustrate the overall approach to elucidating the genetic predisposition to any common complex genetic disorders,[1,2] following the schema depicted in Figure 149-1.

## ADOLESCENT OBESITY: A COMMON COMPLEX TRAIT

In the United States, the prevalence of obesity has increased from 5.0% to 17.6% from 1980 to 2006 in adolescents 12 to 19 years of age.[3] This increase is paralleled by associated comorbidities. For example, from 1981 to 1999, the percentage of discharges in children and adolescents due to gallbladder disease tripled, and those due to sleep apnea increased fivefold.[4] The rising prevalence of obesity, in part, can be explained by changes in our environment; there is an abundance of calorie-rich foods, increased sedentary time in front of televisions and computers, and less time spent engaging in physical activity. However, an "obesogenic" environment is only one component of the multifactorial disorder of obesity, and much evidence exists for the contribution of genetic factors. Other factors include familial or sporadic traits and genetic and nongenetic traits.

### FAMILIAL VERSUS SPORADIC TRAITS: RELATIVE RISK RATIO

To demonstrate the genetic contribution(s) of a trait or disease, it is useful to first demonstrate familial aggregation, or *familiality*. A convenient measure of the familial aggregation of a disease is the relative risk ratio, or $\lambda$. The relative risk ratio is the ratio of the prevalence of a trait/disease in a relative of an affected individual to the prevalence of the same trait/disease in the general population.

$$\lambda_R = \frac{\text{prevalence of disease in relative "R" of affected individual}}{\text{prevalence of disease in general population}}$$

For example, $\lambda_R$ for obesity among siblings ($\lambda_s$, where s = siblings) is the prevalence of obesity among siblings of an obese individual compared with the general population incidence of obesity. Because $\lambda$ is a ratio, any statistically significant value greater than one is evidence of familiality. It is a versatile parameter because the relative category can be parents, mothers, fathers, offspring, first-degree relatives, or second-degree relatives (with the relative ratio designated as $\lambda_p$, $\lambda_m$, $\lambda_f$, $\lambda_o$, $\lambda_1$, and $\lambda_2$, respectively). Traits caused by strong mendelian genetic factors, such as cystic fibrosis, tend to have higher $\lambda_s$,

**Box 149-1**

***Classic Examples of Relative Risk Ratio***

Nonsyndromic cleft lip and palate (a multifactorial trait)

- Recurrence risk among siblings is about 3% (3 in 100)
- General population risk is about 1 in 1,000
- $\lambda_s = (3/100)/(1/1{,}000) = 30$

Cystic fibrosis (a mendelian trait)

- Recurrence risk among siblings is 25% (1 in 4)
- General population risk (among whites) is 1 in 2,500
- $\lambda_s = (1/4)/(1/2{,}500) = 625$

whereas polygenic or multifactorial traits tend to have somewhat lower $\lambda_s$.

Relative risk ratio (Box 149-1) estimates for obesity based on body mass index (BMI) data from family studies suggests $\lambda_R$ of 3 to 6 for BMI exceeding the 95th percentile, and the risk of obesity is 2 to 3 times higher for an individual with a positive family history for obesity.[5] Similarly, family studies conducted by Whitaker et al[6] found that parental obesity more than doubled the risk of obesity in obese and nonobese children younger than 10 years. The results of these investigations point clearly to a familial aggregation of obesity.

## GENETIC VERSUS NONGENETIC: TWIN STUDIES AND HERITABILITY

Familiality of a trait can be attributed to the sharing of genetic or environmental risk factors among family members, such as diet and amount of time spent watching television; alone, it does not provide proof of genetic causation. To address genetic causality, twin studies are often used. Twin studies are based on a comparison of disease concordance in monozygotic (MZ) and dizygotic (DZ) twin pairs. If the causation of the disease is purely genetic, MZ twins, who share essentially 100% of their genes, will display absolute concordance of their trait status. Less than 100% trait concordance in MZ twins is evidence of environmental and/or stochastic factors. Because DZ twins share on average only 50% of their genes, a greater disease concordance rate among MZ compared to DZ twins is consistent with a genetic etiology for the disease. In addition, for traits that can be measured in quantitative terms, such as weight or BMI, observation of the phenotypic variance in MZ and DZ twin pairs allows for a reliable computation of *heritability* ($h^2$).

Heritability of a trait is defined as the proportion of the total phenotypic variance that is due to genetic contribution and is the measure of the sum total effect of the genetic alleles that may contribute to the phenotype. The value of $h^2$ varies from 0 to 1, indicating no genetic contribution, and the variance observed being due to genetic factors, respectively.

$$h^2 = \frac{\text{phenotypic variance in DZ pairs} - \text{phenotypic variance in MZ pairs}}{\text{phenotypic variance in DZ pairs}}$$

Adoption studies are a special category of twin studies that provide the most powerful evidence of heritability because a shared postnatal environment is no longer a confounding variable. For example, MZ twins adopted by different families at birth and raised separately can be assessed for trait concordance. Loos et al[7] reviewed a large number of twin, adoption, and family studies conducted in obesity research and concluded that the heritability of human adiposity ranged from 30% to 70%. The highest heritability values were obtained from studies of MZ and DZ twins, indicating a clear familial and genetic component to obesity.

## MENDELIAN VERSUS MULTIFACTORIAL: SEGREGATION ANALYSIS

To establish the mode of inheritance for human traits or disorders, it is necessary to observe their segregation among family members of individuals with the trait. The proportion of affected individuals in a class of relatives such as parents, offspring, or siblings, is used to determine the mode of inheritance that best fits the observed data in a hypothesis testing statistical approach. For example, assuming 100% penetrance, a parent with an autosomal dominant trait is expected to pass the trait on to 50% of his or her children. Similarly, 25% of the siblings of an individual with an autosomal recessive trait are expected to have the trait as well. Comparing observed to expected family data provides support for various modes of inheritance. This procedure is termed *segregation analysis*.

For example, in 1954, Neel and Schull[8] studied the dental condition opalescent dentine. They suspected that opalescent dentine followed an autosomal dominant mode of inheritance. They identified a large number of families in which one parent was affected with the trait, but the other parent was not affected. Among 112 offspring, 52 were affected, and 60 were unaffected. The segregation data, when analyzed by the simple chi-square statistical analysis, were consistent with the opalescent dentine trait being transmitted by an autosomal dominant mode of inheritance.

However, most segregation analyses are not this straightforward and require the best fit of collective family data of a complex trait against a number of possible patterns of inheritance. Using a statistical method called maximum likelihood estimate (MLE), a procedure called *complex segregation analysis* can aid in the determination of likely transmission patterns. With MLE, other unknown variables can be incorporated in the analysis, such as the frequency of the mutant allele in the general population (allelic frequency), the penetrance of the trait, and possible environmental influences. Precaution and statistical adjustment of ascertainment bias are essential in such studies.

## IDENTIFYING HUMAN DISEASE GENES

A number of elements are involved in the identification of genes predisposing adolescents to be affected by various conditions. In the following section, adolescent obesity provides a framework to explore the processes involved.

### GENETIC MAPPING

The identification of human disease genes generally follows a number of steps. It usually begins with *genetic mapping* of chromosomes to define the location of a hypothesized gene that is believed to correspond to a specific trait locus. Elements of genetic mapping include the following:

- Formulating a genetic model that explains a trait, including demonstrating a genetic contribution to the trait, and defining the most likely mode of inheritance by pedigree studies, segregation analysis, and epidemiologic studies.
- Identifying the chromosomal location of the putative gene, including the region, band, and sub-band location. This approach is often serendipitous and depends on a chance encounter with patients with a trait who also have chromosomal abnormalities.
- Defining the location of a putative gene by its relative distance to other known genes or genetic markers by *linkage mapping*. If the linkage mapping depends on specific parameters of a genetic model, it is called *parametric* (or *model-based*) *linkage analysis*. *Nonparametric* (or *model-free*) *linkage analysis* refers to linkage mapping performed without a genetic model.
- Locating the putative gene by detailed molecular examination of a chromosomal region where the gene is believed to reside, a process called *physical mapping*. This is followed by definitively identifying and cloning the gene(s); sequencing of the gene(s) responsible for the trait has largely already been accomplished in the human genome sequence.
- Searching the human genome sequence database for genes that may contribute to the trait or disease using the map location information as a road map; the process requires bioinformatics tools and genomic databases.
- Verifying the causal relationship between the putative genes and the disease by identifying and characterizing mutations within the gene(s) in affected individual.

### LINKAGE MAPPING

The goal of linkage mapping is to identify genes that cosegregate with the disease of interest. The more closely a gene cosegregates with the disease in affected families, the more likely the gene is the causative gene (pending further verification on DNA sequencing). Because such a gene is not known a priori, a "trial-and-error" approach is often taken by querying whether there is cosegregation between the disease and a "candidate gene" with known function or a large number of genetic loci "markers" with known positions in the genome. In the candidate gene approach, the test locus is a gene speculated to contribute to the disease based on what is known about its function (eg, the insulin receptor gene for diabetes mellitus). In the genome scan approach, however, the test loci represent carefully chosen "random" genetic markers that are evenly distributed throughout the genome at a high density. Cosegregation of any of these test loci with the disease is taken as evidence that the disease gene resides in the location in the genome that is in the vicinity of the cosegregating test locus. In other words, the disease is considered "mapped" to the genetic location where the locus resides.

Traditional linkage mapping requires specification of parameters such as pattern of inheritance, allelic frequencies, penetrance, and genetic heterogeneity. For common complex traits, these variables are largely unknown but can be estimated using maximum likelihood approaches as part of complex segregation analysis. However, the power of the linkage analysis decreases dramatically with each additional estimated parameter. Moreover, the power to detect linkage with any given gene is also diminished in the setting of common diseases due to the contribution of multiple genetic and environmental factors. Utilization of a nonparametric linkage analysis addresses these issues and greatly aids the mapping of common complex traits.

One example of a nonparametric linkage mapping method is *sib-pair analysis*. The affected sib-pair analysis (ASP) method examines large numbers of sib-pairs that are similarly affected with a disease. In this approach, the genotypes at the locus under consideration are obtained for both members of each sib-pair. Because siblings share an average of half of their alleles that are identical by descent (IBD) at each locus (because an allele from each parent has a 50% chance of passing it on to each member in a sibship), observation of significant increase more than 50% of IBD allele sharing among ASPs is an indication of linkage between the locus and the disease. As in parametric linkage analysis, both candidate gene and genomic scan approach can be used in sib-pair analysis.

## GENETIC ASSOCIATION STUDIES

Another versatile nonparametric gene mapping approach takes advantage of the concept of genetic association that has seen increasing application in the mapping of common complex disorders. When 2 events occur together more often than expected from the combined probabilities of occurrence of the individual events, there is an *association* of these 2 events. If one of the "events" is the occurrence of a specific allele and the other "event" is the occurrence of a disease (or trait) under question, there is a *genetic association*.

The *case-control study* is a method to establish a genetic association. In this method, the genotypes at any locus under consideration are determined for a large number of affected cases and unaffected control individuals. A significant increase of allelic frequency in the cases over that of the controls establishes a genetic association.

A pitfall of case-control studies is *population stratification*, in which populations are nonhomogeneous because they contain hidden subgroups, or strata, of genotypes and other characteristics, including environmental exposure and socioeconomic status. If cases and controls come from different population strata, observed genetic associations may be erroneous. This problem can be circumvented by studying a large number of unrelated loci to demonstrate that the cases and the controls are genetically similar with respect to loci that do not contribute to the disease.

An alternative to case-control study that avoids the need for unaffected controls is the *transmission disequilibrium test* (TDT). The TDT uses families with one or more affected offspring, in which at least one of the parents is heterozygous for a genetic allele, the test locus, hypothesized to be associated with the trait. The offspring and parents from a large number of such affected families are genotyped at the test locus, and the frequencies of the test allele among the transmitted and untransmitted alleles are determined. Any transmission significantly in excess of 50% to the affected offspring is a demonstration of positive genetic association. Because the TDT employs no unrelated unaffected controls, it eliminates the population stratification problem entirely. However, a larger number of individuals need to be genotyped (requiring a parent-affected offspring triad compared to a case-control pair in case-control studies), TDT are generally less cost efficient when compared to case-control studies. Similar to other gene mapping studies, the TDT can employ the candidate gene or genome scan approach.

## LINKAGE DISEQUILIBRIUM AND GENOMEWIDE ASSOCIATION STUDIES

Linkage describes the relationship between 2 loci in close proximity to each other in the same chromosomal region; linked alleles tend to "travel" together during meiosis because of this proximity. Within a family, transmission of specific combinations of alleles across linked loci, haplotypes, can be predicted. However, the relationship between specific alleles cannot be extended to unrelated families. In the general population, linkage does not presume a "preference" of specific alleles at one locus for specific alleles at the linked locus. However, when a specific allele at one locus is "preferentially" associated with a specific allele at a linked locus, there is *linkage disequilibrium*. If one of the alleles is a disease-causing allele and the other is a test allele in a genetic association study, one can easily see why LD may be a cause for genetic association. In mapping complex diseases, the most common reason for LD is a *recent mutation* event. The study of a large number of test alleles at loci representing the entire genome is referred to as a genomewide association study (GWAS). A GWAS is increasingly being used in the mapping of common complex disorders.

Thus, observation of LD between a disease trait and an allele is a changing phenomenon in a population. In generations subsequent to the mutation event, even absolute LD will progressively dissipate due to recombination between chromosomes during meiosis, with the rate of dissipation dependent on the distance between the linked loci. The phenomenon of LD dissipation can be used to map causative genes for mendelian disorders in a relatively inbred population.

## MONOGENIC OBESITY

Most cases of obesity are multifactorial in nature, caused by the interplay of genetics, environment, and lifestyle, without a mendelian pattern of inheritance. However, there are a number of rare forms of obesity caused by mutations in a single gene, the study of which can provide important knowledge. As depicted, monogenic obesity can be divided into those associated with specific genetic syndromes in which obesity is a prominent feature along with other physical or developmental characteristics, and nonsyndromic cases in which obesity appears to be an isolated finding.

There are approximately 30 mendelian syndromic forms of obesity,[9] a sample of which is summarized in Tables 149-1 and 149-2.

The most well-known syndromic cause of obesity in adolescents is the Prader-Willi syndrome (PWS). Various epidemiologic studies report a prevalence of 1 in 25,000, resulting in 350,000 to 400,000 individuals affected worldwide.[10] Prader-Willi syndrome is characterized by decreased fetal movement, neonatal hypotonia, short stature, hypothalamic hypogonadism, mental retardation, and characteristic facial features, including narrow bitemporal diameter and almond-shaped eyes. Voracious hyperphagia develops in childhood, and by adolescence, obesity is generally advanced. The obesity is centrally distributed with relative sparing of the distal extremities and is the major cause of morbidity and mortality in affected individuals.[11]

Prader-Willi syndrome was also the first identified human disorder of *genetic imprinting*, which refers to certain genes or groups of adjacent genes being expressed differently, depending on the gender of the parent from which they were inherited. Approximately 75% of affected individuals with PWS have a deletion of the region of the long arm of *paternal* chromosome 15, the Prader-Willi critical region (PWCR) (15q11–q13).

**Table 149-1**

**Human Obesity Syndromes**

| *OMIM No.* | *Syndrome* | *Additional Clinical Features* | *Locus* |
|---|---|---|---|
| *Autosomal recessive* | | | |
| 209900 | Bardet-Biedl syndrome | Mental retardation, postaxial polydactyly, retinal dystrophy/ pigmentary retinopathy, hypogonadism, structural abnormalities of the kidney, or functional renal impairment | 11q13 (BBS1); 16q21(BBS2); 3p12-q13 (BBS3); 15q22.3 (BBS4); 2q31 (BBS5); 20p12 (BBS6); 4q27 (BBS7); 14q32.11 (BBS8); 7p14 (BBS9); 12q (BBS10); 9q33.1 (BBS11); 4q27 (BBS12) |
| 203800 | Alstrom syndrome | Retinal dystrophy, neurosensory deafness, diabetes | 2p13 |
| 216550 | Cohen syndrome | Prominent central incisors, ophthalmopathy, microcephaly | 8q22 |
| *Autosomal dominant* | | | |
| 181450 | Ulnar-mammary syndrome | Ulnar defects, delayed puberty, hypoplastic nipples | 12q24.1 |
| 176270 | Prader-Willi syndrome | Hypotonia, mental retardation, short stature, hypogonadotropic hypogonadism, small hands and feet | Lack of paternal segment of 15q11.2–q12 |
| 103580 | Albright hereditary osteodystrophy | Short stature, skeletal defects, impaired olfaction | 20q13.2 |
| *X-linked* | | | |
| 301900 | Borjeson-Forssman-Lehmann syndrome | Mental retardation, hypogonadism, large ears | Xq26.3 |
| 300148 | Mehmo syndrome | Mental retardation, epilepsy, hypogonadism, microcephaly | Xp22.13–p21.1 |
| 309585 | Wilson-Turner syndrome | Mental retardation, tapering fingers, gynecomastia | Xp21.2–qq22 |

ACTH, adrenocorticotropic hormone; OMIM, Online Mendelian Inheritance in Man (www.ncbi.nlm.nih.gov/sites/entrez?db=omim.).

**Table 149-2**

**Human Monogenic Nonsyndromic Obesity Disorders**

| OMIM No. | Disorder | Clinical Features | Locus |
|---|---|---|---|
| 164160 | Leptin deficiency | Severe early onset obesity, hyperphagia, hypogonadotrophic hypogonadism, central hypothyroidism | 7q31.3 |
| 601007 | Leptin receptor deficiency | Severe early onset obesity, hyperphagia, hypogonadotrophic hypogonadism, central hypothyroidism, mild growth retardation | 1p31 |
| 155541 | Melanocortin 4 receptor deficiency | Severe early onset obesity, hyperphagia, increase in lean body mass and bone density, increased linear growth through childhood, severe hyperinsulinemia | 18q22 |
| 609734 | Pro-opiomelanocortin deficiency | Severe early onset obesity, ACTH deficiency leading to adrenal insufficiency, red hair and pale skin, hyperphagia | 2p23.3 |
| 600955 | Proprotein convertase 1 deficiency | Severe early onset obesity, abnormal glucose homeostasis, hypoinsulinemia with elevated plasma proinsulin, hypogonadotrophic hypogonadism, elevated plasma POMC, hyperphagia | 15q15–q21 |
| 600456 | Neurotrophic tyrosine kinase receptor type 2 deficiency | Obesity, severe hyperphagia, delayed speech and language development, impaired short-term memory, loss of nociception | 9q22.1 |

ACTH, adrenocorticotropic hormone; OMIM, Online Mendelian Inheritance in Man (www.ncbi.nlm.nih.gov/sites/entrez?db=omim).

Most remaining affected individuals exhibit maternal *uniparental disomy*, in which they possess 2 copies of the maternal PWCR. In both instances, there is absence of the normally active paternally inherited genes in the PWCR.

The PWCR contains several interesting genes, the expression of some of which have been shown to be absent in the brains of patients with PWS. Two such genes include *necdin* (*NDN*) and small nuclear ribonucleoprotein polypeptide N (*SNRPN*). Other nonexpressed genes include the *Ring Zinc finger 127-polypeptide* gene, the *MAGE-like 2* gene, and the *PWCR1* gene. The exact functions of these genes and how they result in the phenotype of PWS remain to be elucidated.

Many nonsyndromic monogenetic obesity disorders have been studied. These single gene mutations all cause severe childhood-onset obesity. Table 149-2 shows a subset of the known nonsyndromic monogenic causes of obesity, including those involving the genes for leptin or its receptor. Leptin is an endocrine hormone produced by adipocytes, the gut, and placenta. Its key role is to communicate with the brain regarding the quantity of fat stored. Obesity due to congenital leptin deficiency was first described in 2 severely obese cousins from a highly consanguineous family. They had undetectable levels of leptin despite florid obesity, and were homozygous for a frameshift mutation that resulted in a truncated and nonsecreted form of leptin.[12,13] The children were profoundly obese and severely hyperphagic from a young age, a presentation similar to 3 adults and one child from a highly consanguineous family found to be homozygous for a missense mutation in the leptin gene.[14] In addition, one family has been identified with a leptin receptor mutation and exhibited a similar phenotype to those individuals with leptin gene mutations.[15] Leptin therapy has been demonstrated to be beneficial for these patients.

## OLIGOGENIC OBESITY

The Bardet-Biedl syndrome (BBS) is an interesting paradigm in genetic obesity. Clinically, it is characterized by retinal cone-rod dystrophy, postaxial polydactyly, truncal obesity, cognitive impairment and learning disability, hypogonadotropic hypogonadism, renal abnormalities, or nephropathy. This syndrome is genetically heterogeneous, and to date, mutations in 12 genes have been identified that are causally related to the syndrome. Most BBS cases follow the autosomal recessive pattern of inheritance. Under this model, siblings of an affected individual have a 25% chance of being similarly affected. However, in about 10% of BBS cases, another mutation in 1 of the 12 BBS genes is required, called *triallelic inheritance*.

Because mutations in more than one gene are involved, the inheritance pattern is referred to as *oligogenic inheritance*. Bardet-Biedel syndrome bridges the gap in transitioning from monogenic obesity disorders to those of multifactorial obesity.

### MULTIFACTORIAL NONSYNDROMIC OBESITY

Individuals with mendelian syndromic or nonsyndromic obesity represent the minority of those with the obesity phenotype. They clearly do not account for the current obesity epidemic. Rather, obesity is a complex multifactorial phenotype resulting from polygenetic factors, environment, and lifestyle. Human studies using linkage analysis and association studies, as described previously, have been conducted in efforts to map the specific genes involved in common obesity.

The last update of the Human Obesity Gene Map[16] cited 253 quantitative trait loci (QTLs) for obesity-related phenotypes that have been localized from 61 genome-wide linkage studies in humans (Table 149-3).

In total, QTLs in 52 genomic regions have been substantiated. Twenty-two genes were found to be supported in at least 5 positive association studies[17] (Table 149-4).

**Table 149-3**

**Evidence for Presence of Linkage with Body Mass Index**

| *DNA Marker* | *Chromosomal Location* | *Study Sample* | *LOD Score*[a] |
|---|---|---|---|
| D2S1788 | 2p22.3 | 66 white families (349 subjects) | 3.08 |
| D2S347 | 2q14.3 | 1,249 white European-origin sibling pairs | 4.44 |
| D2S347 | 2q14.3 | 53 white families (758 subjects) | 3.42 |
| | 2q37 | 451 white families (4,247 subjects) | 3.34 |
| D3S1764 | 3q22.3 | 1,055 pairs (white, black, Mexican American, and Asian) | 3.45 (black) |
| D3S2427 | 3q26.33 | 507 white families (2,209 subjects) | 3.3 |
| D3S2427 | 3q26.33 | 128 black families (545 subjects) | 4.3 |
| D3S2427 | 3q26.33 | 1,055 pairs (white, black, Mexican American) | 3.4 |
| D3S3676 | 3q26.33 | 128 black families (545 subjects) | 4.3 |
| D4S1627 | 4p13 | 37 Utah families (994 subjects) | 3.4 |
| D4S3350 | 4p15.1 | 37 Utah families (994 subjects) | 9.2 |
| D4S2632 | 4p15.1 | 37 Utah families (994 subjects) | 6.1 |
| D6S403 | 6q23.3 | 27 Mexican-American families (261 subjects) | 4.2 |
| D6S1003 | 6q24.1 | 27 Mexican-American families (261 subjects) | 4.2 |
| D7S817 | 7p14.3 | 182 African families (769 subjects) | 3.83 |
| D7S1804 | 7q32.3 | 401 American families (3,027 subjects) | 4.9 |
| D8S1121 | 8p11.23 | 10 Mexican-American families (470 subjects) | 3.2 |
| D10S212 | 10q26.3 | 18 Dutch families (198 subjects) | 3.3 |
| Chr. 10 region | 10q26.3 | 279 white families (1,848 non-Hispanic subjects) | 3.2 |
| D11S2000 | 11q22.3 | 182 African families (769 subjects) | 3.35 |
| D11S912 | 11q24.3 | 264 Pima Indian and American families (1,766 pairs) | 3.6 |
| D12S1052 | 12q21.1 | 66 white families (349 subjects) | 3.41 |
| D12S1064 | 12q21.33 | 66 white families (349 subjects) | 3.41 |
| D12S2070 | 12q24.21 | 260 European-American families (1,297 subjects) | 3.57 |

*(Continued)*

## Table 149-3 (Continued)

| DNA Marker | Chromosomal Location | Study Sample | LOD Score[a] |
|---|---|---|---|
| | 12q24 | 933 Australian families (2,053 subjects) | 3.02 |
| D13S257 | 13q14.2 | 401 American families (3,027 subjects) | 3.2 |
| D13S175 | 13q12.11 | 580 Finnish families | 3.3 |
| D13S221 | 13q12.13 | 580 Finnish families | 3.3 |
| D13S1493 | 13q13.2 | 1,124 American families (3,383 subjects) | 3.2 |
| D19S571 | 19q | 109 French white families (447 subjects) | 3.8 |
| D20S149 | 20q13.31-qter | 92 American families (513 subjects, 423 pairs) | 3.2 |
| D20S476 | 20q13 | 92 American families (513 subjects, 423 pairs) | 3.06 |
| D20S438 | 20q12 | 103 Utah families (1,711 subjects) | 3.5 |
| D20S107 | 20q12 | 92 American families (513 subjects, 423 pairs) | 3.2 |
| D20S211 | 20q13.2 | 92 American families (513 subjects, 423 pairs) | 3.2 |

[a]LOD, logarithm of the odds to the base 10. An LOD of 33 generally indicates that 2 gene loci are near each other on a chromosome.

Reprinted from Yang W, Kelly T, He J. Genetic epidemiology of obesity. *Epidemiol Rev*. 2007; 29: 49–61, with permission from Oxford University Press.

## Table 149-4

### Genes with 5 or More Associations with Obesity or Obesity-Related Phenotypes

| Gene Symbol | Full Name | Chromosomal Location | No. of Studies | *p* Value |
|---|---|---|---|---|
| *ACE* | Angiotensin I-converting enzyme (peptidyl-dipeptidase A) 1 | 17q24.1 | 6 | 0.05–0.0023 |
| *ADIPOQ* | Adiponectin, C1Q and collagen domain containing | 3q27 | 11 | 0.05–0.001 |
| *ADRB2* | Adrenergic, beta-2-, receptor, surface | 5q31–q32 | 20 | 0.05–0.0001 |
| *ADRB3* | Adrenergic, beta-3-, receptor | 8p12–p11.2 | 29 | 0.05–0.001 |
| *DRD2* | Dopamine receptor D2 | 11q23.2 | 5 | 0.03–0.002 |
| *GNB3* | Guanine nucleotide binding protein (G protein), beta polypeptide 3 | 12p13.31 | 14 | 0.05–0.001 |
| *HTR2 C* | 5-Hydroxytryptamine (serotonin) receptor 2C | Xq24 | 10 | 0.05–0.0001 |
| *IL6* | Interleukin 6 (interferon, beta 2) | 7p21 | 6 | 0.03–0.003 |
| *INS* | Insulin | 11p15.5 | 7 | 0.05–0.0002 |
| *LDLR* | Low density lipoprotein receptor (familial hypercholesterolaemia) | 19p13.2 | 5 | 0.04–0.001 |
| *LEP* | Leptin (obesity homologue, mouse) | 7q31.3 | 10 | 0.05–0.003 |
| *LEPR* | Leptin receptor | 1p31 | 16 | 0.04–0.0001 |
| *LIPE* | Lipase, hormone sensitive | 19q13.2 | 5 | 0.05–0.002 |
| *MC4R* | Melanocortin 4 receptor | 18q22 | 8 | 0.04–0.002 |
| *NR3C1* | Nuclear receptor subfamily 3, group C, member 1 (glucocorticoid receptor) | 5q31 | 10 | 0.05–0.001 |
| *PLIN* | Perilipin | 15q26 | 5 | 0.05–0.0008 |

*(Continued)*

**Table 149-4 (Continued)**

| *Gene Symbol* | *Full Name* | *Chromosomal Location* | *No. of Studies* | *p Value* |
|---|---|---|---|---|
| *PPARG* | Peroxisome proliferative activated receptor, gamma | 3p25 | 30 | 0.05–0.001 |
| *RETN* | Resistin | 19p13.2 | 5 | 0.048–0.001 |
| *TNF* | Tumor necrosis factor (TNF superfamily, member 2) | 6p21.3 | 9 | 0.05–0.004 |
| *UCP1* | Uncoupling protein 1 (mitochondrial, proton carrier) | 4q28–q31 | 10 | 0.05–0.001 |
| *UCP2* | Uncoupling protein 2 (mitochondrial, proton carrier) | 11q13.3 | 11 | 0.05–0.001 |
| *UCP3* | Uncoupling protein 3 (mitochondrial, proton carrier) | 11q13 | 12 | 0.049–0.0005 |

## SUMMARY

The sequencing of the human genome and advances in genetics technology facilitates the understanding of the genetic predisposition of adolescents to a variety of conditions. The key elements related to patterns of predisposition, including the contributions of complex phenotypes and genotypes, as well as environmental and random influences and gene-environment interactions, can each play a role. With adolescent obesity as a model of a common condition affecting adolescents, the contribution of familial versus sporadic, genetic versus nongenetic, and mendelian versus multifactorial influences must be considered. A number of means to identify human disorders associated with adolescent obesity, including gene and linkage mapping, genetic associations, and LD will help with the future understanding of monogenic, oligogenic, and multifactorial nonsyndromic conditions. In addition, these same techniques will be invaluable in expanding our knowledge about a variety of other conditions affecting adolescents.

## REFERENCES

1. Haines JL, Pericak-Vance MA. *Genetic Analysis of Complex Disease.* 2nd ed. New York: Wiley-Liss; 2006

2. Rao DC, Province MA. *Genetic Dissection of Complex Traits.* New York: Academic Press; 2001

3. Centers for Disease Control and Prevention. NHANES Surveys (1976–1980 and 2003–2006). November 17, 2009. Available at: www.cdc.gov/nchs/nhanes.htm Accessed March 8, 2010

4. Wang G, Dietz WH. Economic burden of obesity in youths aged 6 to 17 years: 1979–1999. *Pediatrics.* 2002;109:e8

5. Allison DB, Kaprio J, Korkeila M, Koskenvuo M, Neale MC, Hayakawa K. The heritability of body mass index among an international sample of monozygotic twins reared apart. *Int J Obes Relat Metab Disord.* 1996;20:990–999

6. Whitaker RC, Wright JA, Pepe MS, Seidel KD, Dietz WH. Predicting obesity in young adulthood from childhood and parental obesity. *N Engl J Med.* 1997;337:869–873

7. Loos RJF, Bouchard C. Obesity—is it a genetic disorder? *J Intern Med.* 2003;254(5):401–425

8. Neel JV, Schull WJ. *Human Heredity.* Chicago: The University of Chicago Press; 1954

9. Beales PL, Farooqi IS, O'Rahilly S. *Genetics of Obesity Syndromes.* New York: Oxford University Press; 2009

10. Butler MG, Hanchett JM, Thompson T. Clinical findings and natural history of Prader-Willi syndrome. In: Butler MG, Lee PDK, Whitman BY, eds. *Management of Prader-Willi Syndrome.* New York: Springer;2006 (1) 3–48

11. Chen C, Visootsak J, Dills S, Graham JM Jr. Prader-Willi syndrome: an update and review for the primary pediatrician. *Clin Pediatr (Phila).* 2007;46:580–591

12. Montague CT, Farooqi IS, Whitehead JP, et al. Congenital leptin deficiency is associated with severe early-onset obesity in humans. *Nature.* 1997;387:903–908

13. Rau H, Reaves BJ, O'Rahilly S, Whitehead JP. Truncated human leptin (delta133) associated with extreme obesity undergoes proteasomal degradation after defective intracellular transport. *Endocrinology.* 1999;140:1718–1723

14. Strobel A, Issad T, Camoin L, Ozata M, Strosberg AD. A leptin missense mutation associated with hypogonadism and morbid obesity. *Nat Genet.* 1998;18:213–215

15. Clement K, Vaisse C, Lahlou N, et al. A mutation in the human leptin receptor gene causes obesity and pituitary dysfunction. *Nature.* 1998;392:398–401

16. Rankinen T, Zuberi A, Chagnon YC, et al. The human obesity gene map: the 2005 update. *Obesity.* 2006;14(4): 529–644

17. Yang W, Kelly T, He J. Genetic epidemiology of obesity. *Epidemiol Rev.* 2007;29:49–61

# CHAPTER 150

# Special Issues of Genetic Testing in Adolescent Patients

AMY MAYHEW, MD • CHIN-TO FONG, MD

## BACKGROUND

The past few decades have witnessed tremendous transformations in the field of medical genetics related to the expansion in understanding the important role of genes in illness and health. Prior to successful sequencing of the human genome, human genetic research and its clinical applications had focused mainly on disorders caused by mutations in single (mendelian) genes, such as cystic fibrosis or Huntington disease. In the post-genomic era, research and clinical emphases have changed rapidly. For mendelian disorders with known gene mutations, research has shifted to examining efficient diagnostic testing (including genetic screening); searching for "modifier genes" that may determine the course and prognosis of the disease; and developing novel interventions, such as targeted molecular medicine and gene therapy. For common complex disorders (see Chapter 149, Genetic Predisposition to Common Disorders) research focuses on elucidating their genetic contributions through a combined genetic and epidemiological approach. This chapter focuses on important considerations in genetic testing of adolescents. Following a description of definitions of genetic testing and types of genetic variations, the purposes of genetic testing in adolescents are examined. The dimensions of clinical and genetic information are then explored in the context of available technology in genetic testing. Pre- and post-testing issues for adolescents and their families are then detailed. The chapter closes with brief discussions of "recreational" genetic testing and costs.

## CONTRIBUTION OF RECENT GENETICS RESEARCH

Based on human genome sequence data, there are an estimated 20,000 genes in the human genome. The clinical consequence of mutations in most of these genes, however, is unknown. The rapid pace of discovery of disease-associated genes is paralleled by a proliferation of genetic tests. As a result, well-recognized genetic disorders increasingly can be diagnosed by genetic testing long before the onset of symptoms. In addition, the wider application of genetic testing is leading to a greater array of new medical diagnoses, many of which were not recognized previously as genetic. Genetic parameters in medical nosology now provide a comprehensive framework with which to understand progress in disease processes, prognosis, and treatment, such as in cancer pathogenesis and staging. Also, genetic epidemiology research promises to bring about a better understanding of the interaction among gene–gene and gene–environment interactions that contribute to the cause of common disorders that affect a much larger percentage of the population.[1]

Using genetic risk factors to guide presymptomatic risk reduction by lifestyle modification and medical prophylaxis will likely become a routine component of preventive medicine. Because adolescence is a critical period for the establishment of lifelong health habits, it is reasonable to assume that genetic testing in adolescents will become increasingly important, and, as such, will have profound implications for transitioning an adolescent into a healthy adult.

## IMPORTANT FACTORS TO CONSIDER IN GENETIC TESTING OF ADOLESCENTS

Genetic testing is not without complications. An adolescent's genetics status concerns not only the individual being tested (due to permanence and lifelong implications) but may hold implications for other family members (parents as gene donors and siblings as potential carriers or affected individuals). Thus, genetic testing is unlike simple clinical testing of blood for electrolytes or even for HIV status because it requires careful deliberations and thorough counseling prior to testing.

The issues related to genetic testing of adolescent patients include:

- Definition of a genetic test
- Understanding of the concept of genetic variations
- Purpose(s) of genetic testing in adolescents
- Clinical and genetic definition of the disorder being tested and the technical aspects of the

test itself related to test sensitivity and specificity (see Chapter 13, Screening)

- Proper anticipatory interpretation of the genetic test based on such factors as the nature of the test result, family history, disease penetrance, and ethnicity or geographic ancestry
- Pretesting consent and assent processes as well as counseling related to the capacity of the adolescent being tested to understand key issues related to testing as well as the psychosocial dynamic between parents and the adolescent
- Post-testing understanding of test results, privacy, confidentiality, and the long-term psychological burden
- Increasing trend of direct-to-consumer genetic testing and the use of genetic testing in "recreational" contexts
- Cost and access to genetic testing

These issues will be discussed in order, using common genetic disorders as illustrative examples. For more thorough coverage, refer to the excellent reviews by other authors.[2–6]

## DEFINITION(S) OF GENETIC TESTING

The definition of a genetic test is complex. One definition is "a test that involves analysis of genes." This definition emphasizes the technical aspects of the testing process and includes any DNA testing, both at the molecular and cellular level. However, it does not discriminate between the detection of constitutional and somatic genetic variations, even though somatic mutations are usually not familial or heritable.

Another definition of a genetic test is one that "determines the genetic status of an individual with respect to a certain trait." This definition focuses on the purpose of the test performed, rather than the actual technique employed. This definition can be overly inclusive in that many commonly used non-DNA-based tests can be used to determine status, such as a sweat chloride determination for cystic fibrosis, or a lipid profile for an individual from a family with familial hypercholesterolemia.

Some states determine the definition of a genetic test. For example, the New York State Civil Rights Law (section 79-l and amendment)[7] defines a "genetic test" as any laboratory test of "DNA, chromosomes, genes, or gene products to diagnose the presence of a genetic variation linked to a *predisposition* to a genetic disease or disability in the individual or the individual's offspring; such a term shall also include DNA profile analysis." It does provide exclusions: genetic tests do not include "any test of blood or other medically prescribed test in routine use that has been or may be hereafter found to be associated with a genetic variation, unless conducted purposely to identify such genetic variation." Although the exclusion is ambiguous regarding what "purposely" means, it is a reasonable compromise, given the complexity of the issues. As more diseases are found to have a genetic contribution, it will become increasingly difficult to define what a "genetic disease or disability" is. However, this chapter will focus on the type of genetic testing that is DNA-based and directed at the detection of constitutional genetic variations that cause disease or predispose to disabilities.

## GENETIC VARIATIONS

Genetic variations include genetic mutations and genetic polymorphisms. Understanding these concepts is essential to understanding genetic conditions in adolescents.

### Genetic Mutations

Genetic mutations fall into 2 broad categories. A *molecular* genetic mutation is present in all of the cells of an adolescent, which means that it was present within the fertilized egg that eventually gave rise to the individual. These genetic mutations are considered constitutional (or germline) and are generally inherited from one or both parents, who likewise carry the genetic alteration in a germline fashion. Occasionally germline mutations are the consequence of new mutational events limited to an egg or sperm and in such cases may not be familial. Regardless of the origin, germ-line genetic alterations can be passed on to the next generation in a predictable fashion. Sometimes genetic alterations are only present in certain cells, tissues, or organs of an individual, and not in most the body cells. These confined genetic mutations are called *somatic* mutations. Affected adolescents are most often born with a normal constitution, with the genetic mutation taking place some time after the fertilized egg begins to divide. Somatic genetic mutations are not inherited and are likewise not generally passed onto the next generation.

Molecular and somatic genetic mutations are not mutually exclusive categories. For example, an individual may inherit a constitutional mutation that predisposes him or her to a somatic mutation. This is the basis for many familial cancer predisposition syndromes. Alternatively, somatic mutations may take place in the gonads of an individual, such that these mutations may be passed on to the next generation through the egg or sperm.

### Genetic Polymorphisms

Genetic polymorphisms represent naturally occurring variations in DNA, RNA, or protein sequences found throughout a population that are part of an adolescent's genetic makeup. A good example of genetic polymorphism is ABO blood group differences among individuals. These polymorphisms are generally not thought to be directly disease-causing. However, much of the current human genetic research on common complex disorders seeks to establish associations between specific genetic polymorphisms and *predisposition* to disease states. A good example of this is the association of *ApoE4* polymorphism with an increased risk of Alzheimer disease. Other genetic polymorphisms are believed to modify an individual's *resistance* to known pathogens, highlighting the genetic–environmental interaction of many common diseases, such as the association of mutations in the chemokine gene *CCR5* and resistance to HIV infection. Genetic polymorphisms are part of an individual's genetic constitution, and as such are passed on to their offspring following rules of inheritance. Although they have enormous potential, they provide a particular challenge in determining risks and benefits in clinical and research settings.

## PURPOSE(S) OF GENETIC TESTING IN ADOLESCENTS

There are many reasons for performing genetic testing in an adolescent. These purposes are generally regarded as potential benefits in the consent process and may include any of the following 5 reasons for genetic testing for an adolescent:

- Confirming a diagnosis to inform the workup, prevention, treatment, or management of a condition, including genetic counseling. This diagnostic testing should be offered at the earliest age when health benefits might be realized. Examples of conditions in which early diagnosis improves outcomes is multiple endocrine neoplasia or familial adenomatosis polyposis.[4]
- Determining a molecular abnormality that accounts for an established diagnosis. This can benefit other family members who are presymptomatic or demonstrating mild or otherwise ambiguous signs and symptoms by receiving genetic counseling. In addition, it can be valuable in the obstetric and perinatal management of a pregnant adolescent with a genetic condition, such as neurofibromatosis type 1 or 2.
- Searching for a scientific cause related to a clinical diagnosis. Such genetic information may provide some families with the feeling of closure, catharsis, and/or decrease in parental guilt (though the opposite can happen as well). Angelman syndrome is a good example of a condition in which genetic information can explain symptoms in an adolescent, whereas the condition itself is generally not familial.
- Contributing to the scientific understanding of a disease or disability that may benefit other adolescents in the future. Such altruism is surprisingly common among families in difficult or tragic situations that seek to find a higher purpose or meaning for their own suffering.
- Determining the genetic risk of a condition occurring for family planning purposes. This is especially pertinent when the risk is deemed to be significantly higher than the general population. There are few conditions in adolescents for which this is relevant. When this is requested by a parent on a minor offspring, it can present ethical problems and may reflect some measure of parental coercion, such as identification of the carrier status for an adolescent who has a sibling with cystic fibrosis or fragile X syndrome.

## CLINICAL AND GENETIC DEFINITIONS IN CONTEXT OF TECHNOLOGY

The definition of a "disorder" is an important consideration in genetic testing. For example, cystic fibrosis as characterized by chronic pulmonary disease, pancreatic insufficiency, absent of the vas deferens males. Elevated sweat chloride has long been the *sine qua non* of this diagnosis and is considered a requirement for the diagnosis. Most patients satisfying the clinical diagnostic criteria of cystic fibrosis will have 2 mutations in the cystic fibrosis transmembrane conductance regulator (*CFTR*) gene (Chapter 92, Cystic Fibrosis), as expected from the autosomal recessive nature of the disorder. In these patients, the clinical and genetic findings are concordant with each other.

There are, however, adolescents in whom clinical findings, including sweat chloride studies, are discordant with genetic testing results. Although there are many reasons for this discordance, the definition of cystic fibrosis should be rooted in clinical criteria and not in the presence of *CFTR* gene mutations. Thus, patients with isolated congenital absence of vas deferens and no pulmonary or pancreatic disease and normal sweat chloride do not have cystic fibrosis, even if they have mutations in the *CFTR* gene. Likewise, although most adolescents with Marfan syndrome have a single mutation in the gene that codes for the protein fibrillin-1 (*FBN1*), the presence of the *FBN1* mutation helps establish, but does not define, Marfan syndrome. There are a number of genetic syndromes distinct from Marfan syndrome—albeit having overlapping clinical features—that are also caused by mutations in *FBN1*. Once a clinical diagnosis of Marfan syndrome is made in a family, the presence of an *FBN1* mutation in the index case is helpful in the presymptomatic diagnosis of other family members. Amid this complex interplay of clinical and genetic diagnoses, when a clinical diagnosis should be sufficient and when a genetic test should be utilized is described next.

### Genetic Testing Techniques and Applications

Advances in molecular genetics have spawned a diverse array of techniques for detecting mutations. Each of these techniques has advantages and disadvantages in terms of cost, efficiency, resolution, and the kind of mutations best detected. Standard chromosome analysis by G-banding is light microscope-based and has a resolution of 10 megabase ($10^7$ base pairs) of DNA. Chromosomal deletions under this size limit will not be detected. G-banding chromosome study can also detect such abnormalities as aneuploidies such as trisomies and monosomies, as well as translocations or other gross rearrangements. On the other hand, DNA sequencing based on polymerase chain reaction (PCR) of a targeted gene region is very sensitive in detecting small-scale genetic alterations down to the base pair level, but is not easily adaptable to detect large-scale chromosomal alterations. The resolutions of these 2 genetic techniques to detect mutations differ by several orders of magnitude.

Because the capability of modern genetics technology tends to be inflated in the mass media, patients and families often have the common misconception that genetic testing has a high degree of sensitivity and specificity. This is most often not the case. With very few exceptions, such as sickle cell disease, genetic testing almost never achieves 100% sensitivity or specificity, and often much less than that. Moreover, the sensitivity in genetic testing—the percentage of patients with a given diagnosis who test positive for mutation(s) in the causative gene—can be elusive. For some genetic disorders where the diagnostic criteria are clear, this concept is less ambiguous. For other disorders, such as rare syndromes for which diagnostic criteria are yet to be established, the denominator on which the sensitivity could be estimated is too small to be meaningful.

In some diseases, such as cystic fibrosis, a common mutation accounts for most of the patients with the disease, but the remaining patients have a diverse number of other mutations. For adolescents who are at low risk of having a condition, it is reasonable to use a test for the prevalent mutation, which will have a lower sensitivity in identifying all adolescents with the condition. In higher-risk situations, such as adolescents who have a strong family history of the disease, more comprehensive (and expensive) tests with higher sensitivity would be appropriate.

For other disorders, there may not be highly prevalent or common mutations. When the range and number of mutations associated with a condition are diverse, focusing on a subset of mutations is not reasonable. The sensitivity of the genetic test is then determined by the power of the molecular techniques being used and the range of possible mutations for that disorder. To increase the sensitivity of individual techniques, a laboratory offering testing for a certain disorder may employ a series of techniques, beginning with more cost-efficient ones and advancing to more sophisticated techniques when a less sensitive test fails to reveal a mutation. For example, the genetic testing of neurofibromatosis type 1 (*NF1*) may require a panel of techniques such as protein truncation assay, DNA sequencing, fluorescence *in situ* hybridization (FISH), multiplex ligation-dependent probe amplification (MLPA) analysis, and cytogenetic studies.

Although the diagnosis of Prader-Willi syndrome (PWS) has long been based on clinical features, the current mainstay of diagnosis is based on the absence of paternal contribution of genes from within a region of the long arm of chromosome 15 (15q11.2-q13), called the Prader-Willi critical region (PWCR). Genes from the PWCR demonstrate the phenomenon of genomic imprinting: in a normal individual, only paternally inherited genes from the PWCR are active, whereas the maternally inherited genes are silenced; lack of paternal contribution of these genes renders an individual without any gene expression from the PWCR, resulting in the phenotype of PWS. The silencing of maternal genes from the PWCR is mediated by DNA methylation. Thus, 99% of adolescents with PWS have an abnormality on methylation pattern studies on the PWCR. More than two-thirds of patients with PWS have an abnormal methylation pattern due to deletion of the paternal PWCR. In others, this deleted paternal copy is replaced by a second maternal copy that is also inactive (ie, maternal uniparental disomy or UPD). Fluorescence in situ hybridization study of the PWCR will detect abnormalities in adolescents who have a deletion, but not in those with UPD, even though both groups of patients will show an abnormal methylation pattern. Thus, when interpreting a genetic testing report on a PWS, it is critical to take into account the technique employed. The sensitivity of a methylation test (99%) is much higher than that of a FISH test (70%) due to the higher percentage of mutations the former can detect, and should be the first test employed.

Another cause of decreased test sensitivity is due to the same condition being caused by mutations in different genes. For example, both familial breast cancer and tuberous sclerosis are caused by germline mutations in 1 of 2 possible genes (*BRCA1* and *BRCA2*, and *TSC1* and *TSC2*, respectively). Testing for only 1 of the 2 causative genes for each disorder will be associated with a significant decrease in test sensitivity. To compensate for this, testing laboratories are increasingly using an optional paneled testing approach, including the option of testing for a single gene or for all genes that can cause the disorder. Noonan syndrome, for example, is associated with 4 potential causative genes: *PTPN11* (50% sensitivity), *SOS1* (11% sensitivity), *RAF1* (10% sensitivity), and *KRAS* (4% sensitivity). The panel of 4 tests will only have a combined sensitivity of 85%, partly due to the inadequacy of the techniques employed in mutation detection of these 4 genes, but partly due to the possibility that more causative genes are yet to be discovered for Noonan syndrome.

Compounding these complex factors of test sensitivity is that some genetic disorders show different mutation patterns among individuals of different geographic or ethnic ancestry. For example, 3 common mutations in the *BRCA1* and *BRCA2* genes account for about 90% of all mutations in these genes among individuals of Ashkenazi descent, whereas the same 3 mutations account for only a small fraction of mutations in similarly affected individuals from other ethnic backgrounds.

The concept of genetic testing specificity has been briefly discussed earlier in the discussion of *FBN1* mutations that can cause Marfan syndrome or a number of other overlapping clinical entities, such as familial isolated aortic root dilatation, familial isolated lenticular dislocation, Marfanoid hypermobility syndrome, MASS (mitral valve, aorta, skeleton, skin) syndrome. An ever-increasing number of such examples are found each year, promising increasing complexity to challenge medical nosology in the future. The lack of 1-to-1 correspondence between clinical diagnoses and molecular genetic abnormalities—manifesting as decreased sensitivity and specificity—provides a significant pretesting burden to the ordering medical provider, as well as to the individual or family undergoing the testing, that needs to be addressed during the process of informed consent, discussed in the following.

## ANTICIPATORY INTERPRETATION OF GENETIC TESTS DURING PRETESTING GENETIC COUNSELING

In addition to exploring with the adolescent and family the purpose of genetic testing, the nature of the genetic tests being offered, and the strategy of testing, one of the most important elements in pretesting genetic counseling is to describe the possible outcomes of the testing and anticipate their interpretation prior to testing.

In general, test results will be either positive (ie, the test demonstrates the presence of a deleterious mutation) or negative (ie, the test does not demonstrate the presence of a deleterious mutation). Negative test results can be further separated into 2 different categories: (1) the test result is identical to that obtained from testing a predominant proportion of unaffected individuals in the general population; or (2) the test result is different from that obtained from testing a predominant proportion of unaffected individuals in the general population, but current data have demonstrated this difference to be of no significant clinical consequence. This represents a benign genetic polymorphism until evidence to the contrary emerges in the future.

In anticipating a *positive* test result, one should distinguish between the adolescent who is symptomatic and one who is presymptomatic. With symptomatic adolescents, counseling should focus on diagnostic certainty and how a positive test result will help predict prognosis or guide management. With presymptomatic adolescents, the discussion before testing should focus on the likelihood that the patient will manifest symptoms (ie, the penetrance of the disease) and the likely severity or approximate age of onset (ie, the variability of the disease), as well as surveillance and management options.

The anticipatory discussion of a *negative* test result is more complicated. If the testing is done for presymptomatic diagnosis when a gene mutation has already been identified in the family (ie, there is an index mutation in an affected family member, the index case), a negative test result is often considered a "true negative." This means that the adolescent being tested has neither the mutation nor the disease with which it is associated. If, however, no such mutation has been identified in the family, this presymptomatic testing will have lower interpretive value because a negative test result, although decreasing the overall likelihood that the adolescent will develop the disease, does not prove the absence of the condition, unless the test has 100% sensitivity. It is best, therefore, to have the index case tested before making a decision about presymptomatic testing on other family members. This reasoning, however, does not apply when there is no other affected family member, or if the patient is already manifesting signs and symptoms of the disease. A negative result in these situations either reflects an incorrect clinical diagnosis or imperfect test sensitivity.

For many genetic tests, a troublesome third category of results, "variant of unknown significance," occurs when the test result identifies a genetic difference between the adolescent compared with unaffected individuals in the general population, but the clinical significance of this difference is unknown (neither a deleterious mutation, nor a benign polymorphism). This category may have devastating psychological consequences because of the uncertainty or perceived risk status that would not have occurred if the test were not performed. Because of this potential for harm, this outcome is often considered a "complication" of genetic testing and needs to be adequately explored with the patient and family in the consent process prior to genetic testing.

Because the need for testing other family members can arise, another potential complication of genetic testing is that occasionally the test result may reveal false biological parental or sibling identity, most commonly false paternity. This possibility needs to be skillfully articulated prior to any family genetic testing.

### PRETESTING PARENTAL CONSENT AND ADOLESCENT'S ASSENT IN PRETESTING COUNSELING

Since 1979, the Belmont Report has served as a "constitutional document" in guiding the conduct of research involving human subjects. Its 3 major ethical pillars—respect for persons, beneficence, and justice—are so broadly applicable that they have also become the guiding principles for medical providers in many clinical situations. The principle of respect for persons leads one to acknowledge the adolescent as the unit of autonomy. The principle of beneficence necessitates one to maximize benefits and minimize risks. The principle of justice further dictates that there should be fairness in the distribution of benefits and risks at the individual and social level.

Because of the potential for psychological harm, genetic testing is almost universally regarded as a process requiring an individual's explicit consent. In this context, the conceptual framework outlined in the Belmont Report is often invoked in approaching genetic testing. Despite some decision-making ability, an adolescent patient is still considered psychosocially and legally vulnerable, and requires additional protection in all clinical decision-making processes, the need for which can be further compounded by the pre-existing psychosocial burden of the disease status that had necessitated the consideration of genetic testing.

The complexity of the issues concerning genetic testing can make the consent process arduous and consent documents difficult to comprehend even for a well-educated adult. Adolescents may lack the ability to understand the underpinning and purpose of genetic testing and may not be able to have an adult perception of present and future psychosocial risks of the testing. In consenting adolescent patients, priority is generally given to beneficence over that of autonomy, and this is particularly true for genetic testing. Thus, the consent of parents (or other health care proxies) is generally sought, and the consent process is based on criteria of disclosure, understanding, voluntariness, and competence. However, the principle of respect for persons would insist that anyone capable of autonomous activity, albeit limited as in children, should be treated as autonomous. This reasoning leads to the important consideration of assent or dissent by minors that should parallel the consent process by the health care proxy.

A large number of publications have addressed the issue of assent by pediatric subject in the research arena.[8–14] The considerable disagreement about the age when a minor becomes competent for assent or dissent is reflected in the wide variability among institutions' requirements for documentation of assent for ages between 6 and 15.[15] In 1977, the National Commission for the Protection of Human Subjects of Biomedical and Behavioral Research recommended that active affirmation be required for all patients over age 7, and the objection of a patient over 7 should be binding. However, if there is the prospect of a significant direct benefit to the patient's health or well-being, the objection may be overridden. This age of assent was endorsed by the American Academy of Pediatrics,[16] but some have argued that assent of such young children is inappropriate and propose that the age of assent should be raised to as high as 14 years.[17] Others invoke religious traditions in determining the ripe age of competency, such as the age of confirmation, adult baptism, and bar or bat mitzvah.[5]

Although there are such guiding standards for judging competency—such as the abilities to show voluntariness[18] and make rational choices in terms of individual and family social and cultural situation and lifestyle; to evaluate risks, benefits, and tangible alternatives—complex family dynamics often confound the decision making of an adolescent. Thus, it is often difficult to judge the voluntariness of an adolescent who often experiences an external locus of control, sensing other people or external events are controlling them. Studies of 14- and 15-year-olds asked to make hypothetical medical decisions suggest that adolescents generally defer to perceived parental wishes.

This consideration of competency is made more difficult by the lack of strict correspondence between chronological age and measures of competency and maturity in decision-making processes. Paul[11] pointed out that just as in adults, competence is not simply present or absent, but depends on age, cognitive capacity of child, level of competence required, and conditions under which the question is asked. In the case of emancipated minors, ambiguities are common concerning whether the emancipated adolescent is considered competent to make decisions for her offspring and/or for herself. Some states recognize that "mature" minors are able to make decisions about health care without meeting emancipation criteria.[2]

In light of this complexity, health care providers of adolescent patients considering genetic testing should individualize their approach in seeking assent. At the beginning of the assent process, competence should neither be assumed nor rejected without evidence. The adolescent should be presented with information that parallels the consent process for the parent, albeit in an age-adjusted level of sophistication. Furthermore, the health care provider should provide a fair opportunity for the adolescent to voice his or her opinions and to take such opinions seriously and thoughtfully. If a final decision for genetic testing is made contrary to the wish of the adolescent, the reasoning for the decision should be thoroughly explained using the framework of beneficence.

Traditionally, parents are assumed to be best suited to make decisions for adolescents regarding genetic testing. Likewise, society recognizes a sphere of privacy for family life and the need to protect family relationships from outside interference.[3] However, there can occasionally be conflict of interest between the parent and the adolescent patient being considered for genetic testing. For example, an adolescent who has a paternal grandparent affected by familial adenomatous polyposis could be tested for the autosomal dominant *APC* gene. If positive, an early management plan can be initiated. However, if the test is positive, his father could also carry the gene. This "double jeopardy" in genetic testing is not uncommon, and should the intervening family member (in this case the father) not desire to know his own genetic status, he may veto testing for the adolescent to protect his own self-interest.

A different example of conflict of interest concerns parental coercion in situations when the genetic information sought on the affected adolescent will not alter the management plan or provide benefit for the future, but there is a perceived benefit for other unaffected siblings. The patient may feel coerced to be tested, and such feelings need to be explored.

Because of the content conveyed in the pretesting consent process, some have advocated that formal genetic counseling be offered to subjects before or during the consent process. In some states, such an offer is an explicit legal requirement prior to genetic testing. However, there is no generally agreed upon definition of who is qualified to give genetic counseling; a "professional" can be interpreted to include not only medical geneticists and genetic counselors, but all physicians, health care providers, research investigators, or support personnel. Clearly, the quality of such counseling varies widely.

Some states have attempted to codify consent form requirements for genetic testing. For example, the New York State Civil Rights Law 79-1 states that the "written informed consent to a genetic test shall consist of written authorization that is dated and signed and includes at least the following":[7]

- General description of the test
- Statement of the purpose of the test
- Statement indicating that the individual may wish to obtain professional genetic counseling prior to signing the informed consent
- Statement that a positive test result is an indication that the individual may be predisposed to or have the specific disease or condition tested for and may wish to consider further independent testing, consult their physician or pursue genetic counseling
- General description of each specific disease or condition tested for
- Level of certainty that a positive test result for that disease or condition serves as a predictor of such disease. If no level of certainty has been established, this may be disregarded
- Name of the person or categories of persons or organizations to whom the test results may be disclosed
- Statement that no tests other than those authorized shall be performed on the biological sample and that the sample shall be destroyed at the end of the testing process or not more than 60 days after the sample was taken, unless a longer period of retention is expressly authorized in the consent
- Signature of the individual subject of the test or, if that individual lacks the capacity to consent, the signature of the person authorized to consent for such individual

Despite this rather exhaustive list of consent form requirements, the law does not mandate any requirement in discussing risks and benefits, perhaps presuming that this would be subsumed under the broad category of "genetic counseling," highlighting that often laws do not mandate an established ethical standard of practice. Simply put, what is legally sound practice may not be ethically adequate in caring for individuals who are medically and psychosocially vulnerable. Discussion about risks and benefits should be routine practice in medicine and an integral part of any pretesting counseling.

In respecting the principle of beneficence, one would have to consider whether there are current or future medical or psychosocial benefits to genetic testing. If one has established some degree of current or future benefit, the next step is to address what each of these may mean to the patient and family. For example, a potential future benefit of being able to be more expeditiously enrolled in a treatment trial may mean more or less to a family depending on the family's interest in such research endeavors. Certainly any discussion of potential benefits has to be balanced against potential risks.

For most genetic tests, the physical risk to individuals is minimal, often involving no more than a blood draw, cheek scraping, or use of biological tissues obtained in the course of clinical care.

Far more insidious, however, are the psychosocial or financial risks. Genetic testing intended to clarify the risk for one disease may inadvertently reveal the risk for another disorder for which the adolescent and family did not seek information. A well-known example is that of testing of the *APOE* gene to assess risk for coronary heart disease. Although having 1 copy of the *APOE4* allele predicts a higher risk for coronary heart disease, an individual having 2 copies of the *APOE4* may also have a greatly increased risk for developing Alzheimer' disease. Because many patients do not expect nor desire this information, if inadvertently discovered, such test results represent a significant psychosocial risk of the testing. Such possibilities should be anticipated prior to testing and explained to the patient and family undergoing testing. However, to other individuals, this collateral discovery may represent a benefit because it may lead to early attention, preventive care, and knowledge about future genetic risk to patients and their families. In such case, the potential benefit for the collateral testing, or lack thereof, should also be adequately discussed. As genetic testing increases in scale and scope, this possibility of collateral harm and benefit will surely increase. Other potential risks relating to a positive or negative test result can be categorized into those imparted by external or internal factors.

### Potential Pretesting Risks due to External Factors

- Positive results confirming a diagnosis with a well-known prognosis may accentuate parental guilt, affect parent–adolescent bonding, and/or negatively modify parental expectations, which may reallocate family resources away from the adolescent with a diagnosis.
- Potential for leading to a variation of the vulnerable child syndrome due to parental overcompensation. This may result in decreased socialization for the patient. Such risks may also extend beyond the affected child to all unaffected siblings because such overly protective parents have a tendency to limit opportunities to healthy siblings because they do not want the affected sibling to feel isolated because of lack of opportunity due to disease status.
- Discrimination against the patient from adolescence into adulthood in terms of medical and life insurance or job opportunities. The recent passage of the federal Genetic Information Non-Discrimination Act (GINA)[19] should greatly mitigate against this concern, although the act does not change life insurance policies, which have traditionally been premised upon individualized risk assessment.
- Misunderstanding of test results by others may lead to misconceptions about carrier status and reproductive risks that can affect current or future romantic relationships.
- Negative test result may lead to a sense of futility in parents, who may lose hope in future diagnostic work-ups.

### Potential Pretesting Risks due to Internal Factors

- Positive test results may adversely affect self-esteem and enforce latent feelings of unworthiness and self-blame for illness. All of these can interfere with peer integration.
- Worries about disease or carrier status may lead to fear of intimacy and interpersonal relationships.
- Overemphasis on genetic determinism may result in the feeling of loss of control about one's life.
- Confirmation of genetic status may challenge religious beliefs in the context of suffering and divine intention.
- Patients and family may develop a sense of guilt if they belong to a religious tradition that believes that humans should not interfere with divine providence, and that genetic testing is not compatible with their beliefs.[4]
- Negative test result in a presymptomatic diagnosis setting may disrupt normal family relations due to "survivor guilt."

The sensitivity surrounding genetic testing heightens the concern for privacy and confidentiality issues. Although this needs to be addressed during pretesting counseling, we defer this discussion to the following section when we explore post-testing counseling issues.

Finally, in approaching the discussion patients and parents should be advised not to treat the testing as a risk in which all their expectations are focused on one possible test outcome (positive or negative), and the test serves only to prove their expectations. This is a potentially dangerous approach because when the final result does not fit their prior expectations, the likelihood for unintended psychosocial harm increases. Adolescents and families should be encouraged to treat the testing as a means to acquire useful information concerning their health, which should empower them to take better control of current and future risk. With this attitude, even if the test result fails to meet their expectation, they have gained useful knowledge.

The intent of the consent process is based on the notion that consenting is more than just providing an affirmative signature on a form, and such consent should be given only after there is demonstration of a clear understanding of all the issues previously outlined. Despite genuine efforts toward that end, this full understanding is rarely achieved or assured. Right or wrong, trust between patient/proxy and the health care provider often substitutes for a full understanding. In these instances, the health care provider serves as an implicit proxy for the patient and family. This further emphasizes the high ethical standard that health care providers have to adhere to when it comes to offering genetic testing. To limit the potential for harm in situations when there is significant psychological stress that could potentially be exacerbated by the consideration of genetic testing or by the outcome of test results, the health care provider can request psychological counseling prior to genetic testing. The most effective counseling should be directed at the family as a whole and not only focused on the affected individual. The ideal genetic testing process will strengthen the family unit while respecting the individuality of the adolescent.

## POST-TESTING COUNSELING, PRIVACY, CONFIDENTIALITY, AND PSYCHOLOGICAL CONSEQUENCES

Once the results are available, the health care provider will be faced with the task of informing the adolescent and the parents of the test results. This is not a trivial process due to the potential implications of the test results and the unpredictably of how it may be received. Telephone, electronic, mail, or indirect communication is generally not the best medium, and a direct face-to-face session should always be considered. Because there is no easy way to justify an *ad hoc* appointment for result disclosure without providing some information, in situations when the testing is associated with a high degree of anxiety or sensitivity, scheduling a result–disclosure meeting well in advance of the availability of the test result is prudent.

Other than providing the test results along with a thorough discussion of the technical limitations and implication for the adolescent and the family, including current and future reproductive implications, it is good to revisit many of the elements of the consent process, including how to further take advantage of the benefit the result is now providing and how to avoid the risks that may be anticipated. With the results of the test known, questions and discussion are more specific and concrete in post-testing counseling. One of the most common questions that patient and family may have concerns the issues of privacy and confidentiality. At the most basic level, genetic information is considered part of an individual's medical information and as such is protected by rules and regulations pertaining to the confidentiality of medical records, such as the Health Insurance Portability and Accountability Act (HIPAA). However, several unique features of genetic information deserve further attention.

Another important consideration is whether the genetic test result belongs to the individual or to the family from which the individual comes. The prevailing Western view of autonomy assigns such ownership to the individual on whom the testing is done. In the case of the adolescent patient, the test results are also available to the parents or the health care proxy. Because parents often treat the family unit as a single unit of autonomy, it is not uncommon for such genetic information to find its way into their own medical records or into the medical records of other siblings. This is especially true if follow-up testing is being considered in other immediate family members. An explicit consent for release of medical records is rarely asked of the adolescent. When the adolescent becomes an adult, such prior sharing of private genetic records may come as a surprise.

On the other hand, over the course of a genetic work-up, critical and sensitive parental information (eg, biological parentage, history of past pregnancy exposures, or termination of pregnancies) will often become part of the adolescent's permanent medical record. Upon attaining adulthood the adolescent will have access to this information, which the parents may have had no intention of sharing. These issues require vigilance and proactive thinking during the entire genetic work-up process. With nontraditional family structures and electronic records, it is increasingly difficult to compartmentalize or selectively suppress medical information; these issues challenge health care providers to minimize such risks during the entire genetic work-up process in years to come.

In general, it is difficult to maintain confidentiality of genetic testing results among family members participating in genetic testing as a group. Sometimes, the genetic testing results of one individual may lead one to draw certain conclusions about the results for another individual. There can be significant coercion concerning sharing of testing results in an extended family. Health care providers need to be sensitive to these issues. In addition, the complex and sometimes unpredictable relationship among family members makes it important to protect against disclosure of genetic testing information through legal proceedings.

Counterbalancing the need for privacy and confidentiality is the judicious disclosure of genetic test results to benefit the adolescent and the family from information obtained with genetic testing. Although special education and services should be made available on an as-needed basis, often the limitation in resources available to educational and social agencies lead them to adopt diagnosis-based criteria in disbursing services. In these situations, disclosure of genetic testing results confirming a "medical diagnosis" often result in the availability of critical services. The responsibility of the health care provider performing the genetic testing to inform at-risk family members needs to be recognized, and it is often most appropriate if the parent of the tested individual is the "messenger" for the rest of the family. However, family dynamics vary such that such information is often not communicated, or not communicated accurately. Thus, the ethical and legal responsibility for disclosing genetic information to other at-risk family members against the adolescent's will is a thorny issue. Legal precedent and the National Society of Genetic Counselors has supported that individuals are responsible for the dissemination of their medical information; however, other legal cases suggest that physicians are liable to warn at-risk individuals. The American Society of Human Genetics takes the position that information should be disclosed in situations in which serious and foreseeable harm is likely to occur and/or if the disease is preventable or treatable. Although this is contrary to the spirit of HIPAA, and there are clear logistic difficulties in how to adequately inform family members, this issue should be discussed during the result-disclosure meeting.

A common question asked by parents receiving a positive test result for their adolescent son or daughter is whether, when, and how to discuss the test results with the patient. This is particularly true when the adolescent has limited capacity to understand the result and its implications, or has behavioral or psychological concerns that preclude the adolescent from participating in the result-disclosure meeting. In general, parents should be guided toward full disclosure of such information and should share their feelings with the patient. These discussions should be tailored to the developmental stage and competence of the adolescent patient. Whenever possible, the adolescent should be included in the initial result-disclosure meeting.

Depending on the nature of the results and their implications, health care providers should be prepared to counsel the patient and family on such issues as grief, anger, guilt, change in self-esteem, feeling of lack of control, alteration in family and peer relationships, and long-term psychological burdens and their emotional consequences. It should also be emphasized to the adolescent and the family that these issues often re-surface recurrently in the future. Health care providers should use the post-testing counseling meeting for such anticipatory counseling, and to lay out management plans that will help minimize these adverse possibilities.

## DIRECT-TO-CONSUMER GENETIC TESTING AND "RECREATIONAL" GENOMICS

Increased media coverage of the development in the genetic technology and its application has resulted in changes in public perception and attitude toward genetics, both positively and negatively. Among the positive changes is an increasing curiosity about how the new technology may be applied to them as individuals. Some of this curiosity is channeled toward identifying health-related vulnerabilities in one's genome, but others are directed at questions of a non medical nature, which may range from mate choice decisions, to enhancing a hobby. The latter category of pursuits has been referred to as "recreational genomics."

At the heart of the issues is marketing by some commercial genetic testing companies directly to target consumers. Some traditional genetic testing laboratories, in an effort to widen their market, are increasingly marketing to non-genetic specialists and primary care physicians. In many of these situations, it is unclear whether there had been adequate pretesting and post-testing counseling, as the testing companies generally do not provide direct genetic counseling to the patients, but consult with the practitioners in helping them interpret testing results.

In the past few years, there has been increasing expectation that genome-wide association studies (GWAS) will identify a large number of genes to predict an array of health risks and personal traits, including behavioral characteristics. Most of these GWAS are sponsored by federal research funds, and the data generated are required to be in the public domain. Recognizing the commercial value of these datasets, a number of newer companies have taken advantage of the vast amount of GWAS data that have accumulated—and will continue to accumulate—and are offering to do genome-wide testing of individuals in the general population. In these ventures, the general public is their consumer target. Individuals may send their own biological samples to the testing laboratories, along with the requisite fee, and in return will get a detailed listing of the estimates of their risks for a large number of common complex disorders. Many professional organizations point out that this form of direct-to-consumer marketing is risky because it provides no safety net for any potential misunderstanding or psychosocial trauma that may be incurred as a consequence of these tests. It is likely that when confronted with questions about the test results, individuals will turn to their own health care providers who are ill-equipped to handle such complex information. On the other hand, some consumer advocates believe that this is a good development that will over time decrease medical costs and make genetic data more widely applicable to the common person. They argue that many medical tests went through this phase in their evolution and that public demand for quality in a competitive market will eventually lead to increasing quality of such products (eg, home-based pregnancy tests).

A further example of consumer-driven genomics is a group of commercially available genetic tests that are not of direct medical significance. For example, paternity testing is now available without a medical indication. One can envision that genome-based data with implications for health-related or nonhealth-related traits will be added to sperm and egg donor portfolio in the future. Other applications with an increasingly recreational flavor include genetic testing to aid genealogical studies—a fast-growing hobby—and potentially those that can be applied to help in dating services or mate choice. Although there is no current evidence to suggest that adolescents are engaged in these kinds of recreational genomics, being open-minded and easy targets for new vogue consumer technologies, they could conceivably become the consumer targets for future commercial genetic testing ventures.

### COST AND ACCESS TO GENETIC TESTING

Genetic testing is expensive. Many factors contribute to the absolute cost of the tests, including the specific laboratory technique(s) used, the size and number of genes being examined, the demand for the particular test(s), and the level of details needed to define a mutation in the gene(s) tested. In addition, as technology improves over time, retesting using more current methodology further adds to the costs of genetic testing. Thus genetic testing for an individual can range from a few hundred dollars to thousands of dollars. Because of this, genetic testing requested by health care providers not accustomed to the nuances of the procedure can quickly become problematic not only from the counseling, interpretative, or psychosocial perspectives, but also from the financial and logistical perspectives.

In addition to the health care disparity due to socioeconomic factors, many adolescents may face access barriers for genetic testing especially if the testing is deemed to not result in change in medical management. Yet, for many adolescent patients who are in the process of transitioning into an adult care system, there is often time pressure to complete genetic testing before their insurance as a dependent child expires, or before they move away from home in pursuit of higher education. Sometimes, when a disabled adolescent's continued education and social support into adulthood are being threatened because of the lack of medical diagnosis, the parents may desire a genetic diagnosis to use as evidence to justify to the service agencies that the patient needs continued services. All these factors complicate the financial environment for genetic testing of adolescents.

## SUMMARY

Genetic testing in adolescents raises a number of issues not relevant to young children or young adults. This chapter addressed key concepts related to genetic testing, including areas of concern in the future as advances in technology provide new challenges to clinicians caring for adolescents with conditions not previously recognized as genetic, as well as adolescents who have diseases recognized as genetic. The principles contained in this chapter should remain applicable regardless of future advances in genetic testing.

## REFERENCES

1. Patenaude AF, Guttmacher AE, Collins FS. Genetic testing and psychology: new roles and responsibilities. *Am Psychol.* 2002;57:271-282

2. Wertz DC, Fanos JH, Reilly PR. Genetic testing for children and adolescents: who decides? *JAMA.* 1994;272:875-881

3. Ross LF, Moon MR. Ethical issues in genetic testing of children. *Arch Pediatr Adolesc Med.* 2000;154:873-879

4. Kodish E. Informed consent for pediatric research: is it really possible? *J Pediatr.* 2003;142:89-90

5. Ensenauer RE, Michels VV, Reinke SS. Genetic testing: practical, ethical, and counseling considerations. *Mayo Clin Proc.* 2005;80:63-73

6. Twomey JG. Issues in genetic testing of children. *MCN Am J Matern Child Nurs.* 2006;31:156-163

7. New York State Legislature. Section 79-I of the New York State Civil Rights Law. Available at: www.wadsworth.org/labcert/regaffairs/clinical/79-l_1_2002.pdf. Accessed June 22, 2009

8. Department of Health and Human Services, National Institutes of Health. Policy and guidelines on the inclusion of children as participants in research involving human subjects. Available at: grants.nih.gov/grants/guide/notice-files/not98-024.html. Accessed June 22, 2009

9. Society for Adolescent Medicine. Guidelines for adolescent health research. *J Adolesc Health.* 2003;33:410-415

10. American Academy of Pediatrics Committee on Bioethics. Informed consent, parental permission, and assent in pediatric practice. *Pediatrics.* 1995;95:314-317

11. Paul M. Informed consent in medical research: children from the age of 5 should be presumed competent. *BMJ.* 1997;314:1480

12. Burns JP. Research in children. *Crit Care Med.* 2003;31(3)(suppl):S131-S136

13. Fisher CB. Informed consent and clinical research involving children and adolescents: implications of the revised APA ethics code and HIPAA. *J Clin Child and Adolesc Psychol.* 2004;33:832-839

14. Kon A. Assent in pediatric research. *Pediatrics.* 2006;117:1806-1810

15. Kimberly MB, Hoehn KS, Feudtner C, Nelson RM, Schreiner M. Variation in standards of research compensation and child assent practices: a comparison of 69 institutional review board-approved informed permission and assent forms for 3 multicenter pediatric clinical trials. *Pediatrics.* 2006;117:1706-1711

16. American Academy of Pediatrics, Committee on Drugs. Guidelines for the ethical conduct of studies to evaluate drugs in pediatric populations. *Pediatrics.* 1995;95:286-294

17. Miller VA, Drotar D, Kodish E. Children's competence for assent and consent: a review of empirical findings. *Ethics Behav.* 2004;14:255-295

18. Roberts LW. Informed consent and the capacity for voluntarism. *Am J Psychiatry.* 2002;159:705-712

19. Department of Health and Human Services, National Institutes of Health. National Human Genome Research Project. Genetic Information Non-discrimination Act of 2008. Available at: www.genome.gov/Pages/PolicyEthics/GeneticDiscrimination/GINAInfoDoc.pdf. Accessed June 22, 2009

# SECTION 13

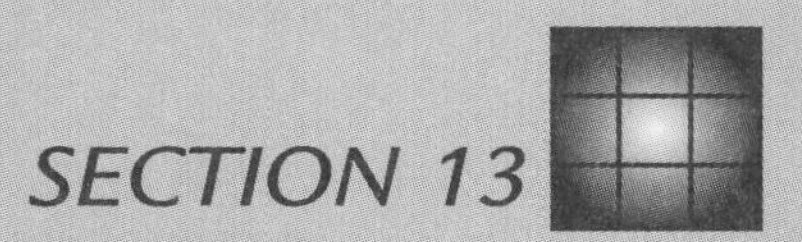

# Allergies and Immunologic Disorders

## CHAPTER 151

## Environmental Allergies

PETER M. G. DEANE, MD

### ALLERGY AND ATOPY

*Allergy* refers to a clinically significant immunologic hypersensitivity reaction that occurs when a patient is re-exposed to the sensitizing antigen (*allergen*). *Atopy* is the genetic predisposition to develop symptomatic IgE-mediated hypersensitivity to extrinsic allergens. This hypersensitivity manifests as extrinsic atopic dermatitis (EAD; atopic eczema), allergic rhinoconjunctivitis (AR), extrinsic asthma (EA), or some combination of these. An abrupt, systemic IgE-mediated reaction is *anaphylaxis*; insect venom hypersensitivity is an example. Diffuse urticaria, if due to an allergic reaction, is mild anaphylaxis. *Anaphylactoid* reactions are caused by agents that directly and systemically trigger mast cell activation, such as opioids, some radiocontrast media and, uncommonly in adolescents, cyclo-oxygenase inhibitors.[1]

Atopy has a characteristic natural history, the atopic march. Atopic dermatitis (AD) is the first step; its incidence peaks in infancy. Over the next few years AD recedes and may clear, while AR develops. A few years after that, asthma declares itself. The prevalence of asthma continues to increase through the second decade of life. More severe AD and higher total IgE levels are risk factors for the development of AR and asthma. Over these same years, hypersensitivity to aeroallergens increases in prevalence, to 36% in 1 study. Figures vary among studies (and locations) but typically range between 10% and 40% for each of the 3 ailments at peak prevalence.[2] Total serum IgE levels normally increase to 10 to 15 years of age then slowly decline. A value of >333 IU/mL is strongly associated with atopic disorders, but there is also a wide overlap between atopic and nonatopic populations, enough so that tests for total IgE have poor sensitivity and specificity in the diagnosis of atopic disorders.[3]

The prevalence of atopy has increased over the past several decades for reasons not known. One explanation has been termed "the hygiene hypothesis." Greatly simplified, this posits that more septic living conditions in infancy prevent the development of atopy. Infections with wild-type viruses and higher airborne endotoxin levels seem to be protective. These agents drive naïve T-helper cells (Th0) to develop into cells that drive cell-mediated immunity and secrete interferon gamma (IFN-γ) and interleukin 12 (IL-12), known as Th1 cells. In more aseptic, immunization-ridden, developed-world conditions, Th0 cells tend to become Th2 cells, which secrete IL-4, -5, -6, and -13. These cytokines promote B-cell antibody secretion and class switching, from IgM to IgE and, to a lesser extent, IgG. Th1 and Th2 cytokines suppress each other, so that 1 type of response predominates.[4]

### ALLERGY TESTS

Two useful methods to test for hypersensitivity to environmental allergens are available: skin and in vitro radioallergosorbent (RAST) tests. Skin tests are preferred because they are faster, more specific, less costly per test, and provide the patient with visual proof of hypersensitivity. In the usual method, drops of solutions, each containing one allergen, are placed upon the skin of the patient's arm, and a slight abrasion of the skin is made through the drop with a sterile pronged device. If a wheal and flare of significant size has formed at the site 20 minutes later, this is read as positive. Controls—histamine for positive and diluent for negative—are also placed. In general, a reaction to allergen at least comparable in size to the reaction to histamine is considered positive. If the scratch test is negative, intradermal (ID) tests may be done for allergens strongly associated with symptoms. Usually, about 0.2 ml of allergen solution is placed with a 27-gauge needle and read compared to the same controls 15 to 20 minutes later. Radioallergosorbent tests are preferred if the patient cannot tolerate skin tests, has dermatographism (positive reaction to diluent) or no reaction to histamine, or has a rash affecting the skin needed for tests. The patient needs to be free of antihistamines for 3 to 7 days (depending on the half-life in circulation of the particular antihistamine) prior to skin testing for the tests to work properly. Radioallergosorbent tests are not affected by antihistamine therapy.

A variety of other tests are offered to patients by alternative medicine practitioners, such as the "pulse test." They are unproven and inaccurate.[5]

## ALLERGENS AND AVOIDANCE

One difference between the atopic and many other immunologic diseases is that the antigens driving atopic response have been defined. Allergens have traditionally been divided into seasonal (pollens) and perennial (all others). Pollens come from trees, grasses, and weeds. Prevalence varies by biome, and in the United States timely local pollen counts are available from the National Allergy Bureau.[6] The most important perennial allergens are from house dust mites, pets (especially cats and dogs), cockroaches, and molds (fungal spores).[7,8] With knowledge of the specific antigens (allergens) involved, allergen-specific treatments have been devised. The most basic treatment is avoidance.

Environmental controls have been proven to help control symptoms of atopic diseases. Dust mite controls are the best studied and are listed in Box 151-1.[7] They have been shown to benefit AR, EA, and EAD if the patients are allergic to dust mites.[8,9] Pet allergen control by means of removing the pet from the home has been shown to be helpful for pet-allergic asthma due to cats, dogs, ferrets, and hamsters.[10] Washing pets does not help. Air filters can improve dog (but not cat) allergic asthma.[11] Box 151-2 lists helpful measures.

### Box 151-1

### *Environmental Controls for House Dust Mite Allergy*

*Minimum to be effective:*

- Use impermeable encasements for mattress, box spring, and all pillows
- Wash all bedding outside encasements in water >130°F (>55°C)

*Also helpful:*

- Maintain household humidity <50%
- Remove all carpeting
- Vacuum with high-efficiency particulate air (HEPA) filter bags
- Freeze or expose rugs (beaten outdoors) and bed toys to the sun

*Possibly helpful:*

- Use acaricide or a denaturant on furniture and carpets

### Box 151-2

### *Environmental Controls for Pet Allergens*

- Keep the pet out of the patient's bedroom
- Keep the bedroom door closed
- Run a HEPA filter in the room
- Keep the room windows closed
- Place vent filters on ducts bringing air into the room

## SPECIFIC IMMUNOTHERAPY

Specific immunotherapy (SIT) involves the induction of clinical tolerance to clinically significant allergens. This has been shown to be helpful in hypersensitivity to allergens from dust mites, cats, the perennial molds *Alternaria* and *Cladosporium*, tree, grass, and ragweed pollens, among others. It affects the response to those antigens only, and therefore is true immunomodulation. Immunotherapy is the only disease-modifying therapy available, that is, it can alter the natural course of these diseases.[12] Although SIT has been used for decades, how it works is not fully known. In part, SIT converts the immune response against allergens from a Th2 to Th1 type. So, the response shifts from intensely humoral to more cellular in nature.[13] One consequence is shown in Figure 151-1. IgE levels increase promptly but no longer change with exposure (eg, increase in pollen season). Within 60 days, IgG titers can be found to increase. They continue to do so for a few years, then decline.[14,15] This decline is not seen in clinical response (and in general the IgG response correlates weakly with clinical response), so the response must be due at least in part to nonhumoral changes. The IgG decline seems to be due to the development of tolerance at the T-cell level, which may be SIT's most important effect. T cells that secrete

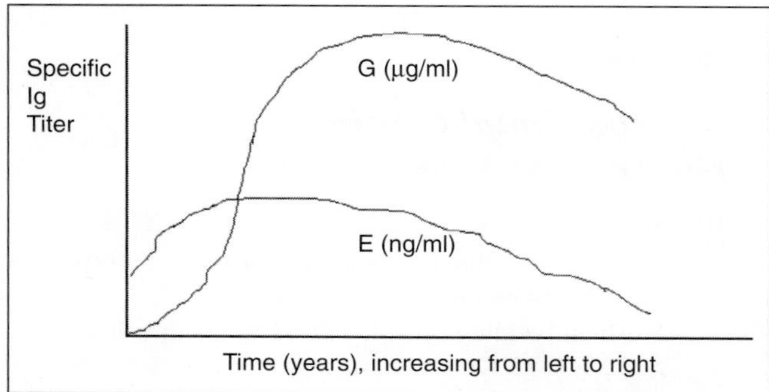


FIGURE 151-1 Typical course of specific antibody response to specific immunotherapy.

Il-10 (Th3 cells) in response to allergen are present by 2 years of immunotherapy. Il-10 is profoundly inhibitory of both Th1 and Th2 responses. The Th3 response is long-lived and may account for SIT's prolonged effects after discontinuation.[16]

Specific immunotherapy typically is administered weekly at first. The dose of allergen increases in small increments until the maintenance dose is reached. Maintenance doses are given at intervals gradually increased up to every 4 weeks. The usual therapeutic dose of inhalant allergens is in the range of 5 to 20 mcg per injection (2,000 to 4,000 allergy units). Clinical benefit is a slow onset; more than a year can elapse before patients note symptomatic improvement.[14] If continued for 3 to 5 years, benefit is maintained for at least 3 years afterward. For this reason, one long-term effect of SIT is reduced cost of care.[12] A major limit on its usefulness are systemic (anaphylactic) reactions, which can occur in 5% to 10% of patients, with severe reactions occurring in 1% to 3%.[17]

It has been shown to be effective for AR related to dust mites, cats, dogs, common molds and tree, grass, and ragweed pollens.[12] It also has been shown to be associated with two-thirds reductions in medication use and symptom scores, and to be cost-effective because it reduces long-term medication use.[17]

## ALLERGIC RHINITIS

Some patients have developed AR prior to adolescence, but the most common time of onset is between 12 and 15 years of age. Most AR patients have symptoms by 20 years of age.[18] Parents often hope that their child will "outgrow" their allergies; perhaps a third will, while others worsen.[19]

Environmental controls should be the first line of treatment. If that is unsuccessful, then medications may be prescribed, usually H1 blockers. Different classes of antihistamines are summarized in Table 151-1. First-generation products are sedating and drying but may be more effective at full therapeutic doses and are most often taken at bedtime.[20] The second-generation antihistamines have little or no sedation or drug interactions and are generally used at adult dosages from 12 years of age and older. Decongestants may be added or used by themselves. They reduce total nasal symptom and congestion scores and provide added benefit in combination with antihistamines. As alpha-adrenergic agonists, they can also act as stimulants, and this may be problematic. Over-the-counter topical decongestants/vasoconstrictors, whether for nasal or eye symptoms, can induce tolerance with subsequent rebound after as few as 4 days of regular use. They should be avoided in the treatment of chronic symptoms. Prescription eyedrops for allergic conjunctivitis are described in Table 151-2. Two of the ophthalmic antihistamines, azelastine and olopatadine, are also used as nasal sprays. Antihistamines may be more effective as nasal spray than in the oral form, as they work directly on the site of the symptoms.[17] Their bitter taste often limits acceptance by adolescents. Table 151-3 lists nasal sprays for rhinitis.

### Table 151-1

**Antihistamines for Rhinitis**

| *Medication* | *Dose* |
|---|---|
| **Second generation** | |
| Cetirizine[a,b] | 10 mg daily |
| Levocetirizine[b] | 5 mg daily |
| Fexofenadine | 180 mg daily |
| Loratidine[a] | 10 mg daily |
| Desloratidine | 5 mg daily |
| **First generation** | |
| Carbinoxamine | 4–8 mg up to 4 times daily or 10 mg 2 times daily |
| Chlorpheniramine[a] | 4 mg up to 4 times daily or 12 mg 2 times daily |
| Clemastine[a] | 1–2 mg up to 3 times daily |
| Cyproheptadine | 4 mg up to 3 times daily |
| Diphenhydramine[a] | 25–50 mg up to 4 times daily |

[a]Available without prescription.

[b]Can be mildly sedating and is often taken at bedtime.

Note: These medications are often used for urticaria at similar doses.

**Table 151-2**

**Eyedrops for Allergic Conjunctivitis**

| *Medication* | *Dose* |
|---|---|
| **Antihistamines** | |
| Azelastine | 1 drop twice daily |
| Epinastine | 1 drop twice daily |
| Ketotifen[a] | 1 drop twice daily |
| Olopatadine | 1 drop twice daily |
| **Mast cell stabilizers** | |
| Cromolyn | 1 drop up to every 4 hours |
| Lodoxamide | 1 drop up to 4 times daily |
| Nedocromil | 1 drop up to 4 times daily |

[a]Available without prescription.

**Table 151-3**

**Nasal Sprays for Allergic Rhinitis**

| *Medication* | *Dose* |
|---|---|
| **Steroids** | |
| Budesonide | 1–2 puffs per nostril daily |
| Ciclesonide | 2 puffs per nostril daily |
| Fluticasone furoate | 2 puffs per nostril daily |
| Fluticasone propionate | 2 puffs per nostril daily |
| Mometasone furoate | 2 puffs per nostril daily |
| Triamcinolone acetonide | 2 puffs per nostril daily |
| **Antihistamines** | |
| Azelastine | 2 puffs per nostril 2 times daily |
| Olopatadine | 2 puffs per nostril 2 times daily |
| **Mast cell stabilizers** | |
| Cromolyn[a] | 2 puffs per nostril 4 times daily |

[a]Available without prescription.

For more severe rhinitis, topical nasal steroids are the preferred therapy. They are more effective than oral antihistamines. The available agents are all aqueous and comparable in efficacy and side effects, the most significant of which is epistaxis. Adolescents may prefer the unscented and lower-volume products. Growth retardation has not been a major issue among adolescents. Combination treatments with oral antihistamines have not been shown to be better than nasal steroids alone.[17]

Compared with other agents, cromolyn, in any topical form, requires frequent and regular dosing and takes weeks to reach full effect, so it is often not useful. Antileukotriene agents are equivalent in effect to second-generation antihistamines and have usually not shown added benefit for rhinitis when combined with them.[17]

Not all rhinitis is allergic, just as not all asthma is extrinsic (ie, allergic). For intrinsic (nonallergic) forms of rhinitis and asthma, medication therapy is used the same way as for extrinsic forms.

## EXTRINSIC ASTHMA

From 1980 to 1996 the prevalence of asthma among people younger than 18 years of age increased by about 4% annually, from 3.2% to 6.2%. Between 1996 and 2000 its prevalence leveled off.[21] However, if one considers adolescents with undiagnosed frequent wheezes, prevalence in that age group about doubles.[22] Chapter 90 has a more in-depth discussion of asthma.

About half of those under 18 years of age with asthma have AR, and about half with AR have asthma. Treatment of AR has been shown to improve asthma control, with reduced symptoms and emergency care use. Nasal steroids are more effective than nasal cromolyn, with the effect of antihistamines inconsistent.[23,24] Sinusitis and nasal polyposis are also associated with asthma, and treatment of sinusitis and polyposis improves associated asthma.[25]

Environmental controls, not only for pets but also for dust mites, are helpful for EA. Benefits include fewer symptoms and hospitalizations.[10,24]

The role of SIT in asthma has been controversial. On balance, SIT has been shown to be helpful for asthma related to dust mites, cats, several pollens, and common molds. Benefits include reduced symptom burden, medication use, and bronchial hyperresponsiveness, but not lung function measures.

## EXTRINSIC ATOPIC DERMATITIS

Acute lesions of AD show a predominance of Th2-type inflammation as seen in AR and EA. But unlike the airway conditions, persistent areas of involvement—chronic lesions—evolve to a Th1-predominant response. Adolescents with AD typically have markedly elevated

IgE levels (>150 IU/mL, sometimes >10,000 IU/mL), associated with sensitization to aeroallergens. (Food allergy seems not to play a significant role in adolescent AD.)[9] Lesions are intensely itchy, and the consequent scratching grossly traumatizes the epithelial barrier. *Staphylococcus aureus* colonizes 93% of lesions.[2] IgE then develops against superantigens from *S aureus* and also to antigens from common skin-colonizing fungi.[26]

Patients with AD have not only an immunologic disorder but also a disordered immune system. Th1 function is impaired and cutaneous anergy is common. Patients with AD are at high risk for cutaneous dissemination of certain viral infections: molluscum, herpes simplex (eczema herpeticum), and vaccinia (eczema vaccinatum). The smallpox vaccine should not be given to teens with AD.[2]

Adequate moisturization is crucial in treating AD. It helps restore the skin's barrier function and relieves pruritus. Lotions are convenient but may be harmful; by definition, a lotion is oil in water kept in solution with alcohols. Alcohols dry and irritate skin. Remember: *Lotions are the enemy.* Creams are water in oil and are tolerable and efficacious. They should be applied liberally, at least twice daily. Ointments are oils; they work, but are messy.

Dust mite controls are helpful in sensitized patients if done rigorously. Controls for pet allergy are likewise recommended, but their benefit is not well proven. Specific immunotherapy has not been shown helpful for AD.[9,26]

## INSECT VENOM HYPERSENSITIVITY

Bee and wasp stings are parenteral exposure to allergenic toxins. Some people get only mild local inflammation, primarily a toxic effect. Others have larger local reactions due to IgG and IgE produced after prior stings. A *local* reaction is defined as a reaction limited to the stung extremity. Venom sensitivity tests are often positive among these patients, but the natural history is that 90% will continue to have only localized sting reactions; evaluation with testing is not indicated because SIT will not be helpful with local reactions. Treatment, if necessary, consists of 2 or 3 days of prednisone (eg, 60 mg then 40 mg), and an antihistamine if desired.

Systemic reactions are a different matter. A systemic sting reaction is an allergic reaction to a sting that extends beyond the stung extremity (ie, anaphylaxis). Adolescents should be considered as adults in this setting. Most systemic reactions occur in those younger than 20 years of age. About 60% of those with 1 systemic reaction will have such reactions subsequently; the more severe the reaction, the more likely the recurrence. Recurrence risk falls with time but never normalizes.[27,28]

The treatment for acute anaphylaxis, due to insect sting or not, is epinephrine. Patients should have an epinephrine auto-injector handy at all times. Antihistamines help only cutaneous manifestations, and corticosteroids take hours to work.

Venom SIT is remarkably effective in preventing systemic venom reactions in up to 98% of patients. After an adequate 3- to 5-year course, 80% of patients will remain desensitized permanently. How to predict the other 20% is not yet known. In general, the more severe the last reaction, the more likely the recommendation to continue beyond 5 years.[27,28]

## REFERENCES

1. Task Force on Allergic Disorders. *The Allergy Report: Volume 1: Overview of Allergic Diseases.* Milwaukee, WI: American Academy of Allergy, Asthma, and Immunology; 2000

2. Spergel JM, Paller AS. Atopic dermatitis and the atopic march. *J Allergy Clin Immunol.* 2003;112:S118–S127

3. Hamilton RG, Adkinson NF Jr. Clinical laboratory assessment of IgE-dependent hypersensitivity. *J Allergy Clin Immunol.* 2003;111:S687–S701

4. McGeady SJ. Immunocompetence and allergy. *Pediatrics.* 2004;113:1107–1113

5. Terr AI. Controversial and unproven diagnostic tests for allergic and immunologic diseases. *Clin Allergy Immunol.* 2000;15:307–320

6. National Allergy Bureau Web Site. Available at: www.aaaai.org/nab. Accessed February 6, 2009

7. Platts-Mills TAE, Vervloet D, Thomas WR, et al. Indoor allergens and asthma: report of the third international workshop. *J Allergy Clin Immunol.* 1997;100:S1–S24

8. Platts-Mills TAE. Allergen avoidance in the treatment of asthma and rhinitis. *N Engl J Med.* 2003;349:207–208

9. Akdis CA, Akdis M, Bieber T, et al. Diagnosis and treatment of atopic dermatitis in children and adults. *J Allergy Clin Immunol.* 2006;118:152–169

10. Shirai T, Matsui T, Suzuki K, Chida K. Effect of pet removal on pet allergic asthma. *Chest.* 2005;127:1565–1571

11. Chapman MD, Wood RA. The role and remediation of animal allergens in allergic diseases. *J Allergy Clin Immunol.* 2001;107:S414–S421

12. Bousquet J, Lockey R, Malling H. Allergen immunotherapy: a WHO position paper. *J Allergy Clin Immunol.* 1998; 102:558–562

13. Till SJ, Francis JN, Nouri-Aria K, Durham SR. Mechanisms of immunotherapy. *J Allergy Clin Immunol.* 2004;113: 1025–1034

14. Creticos PS. Immunotherapy with allergens. *JAMA.* 1992;268:2834–2839

15. Mosbech H, Frew HJ. The immunologic response to hymenoptera venoms. In: Levine MI, Lockey RF, eds. *Monograph on Insect Allergy.* 4th ed. Milwaukee WI: American Academy of Allergy, Asthma, and Immunology; 2003:75-81

16. Norman PS. Immunotherapy: 1999-2004. *J Allergy Clin Immunol.* 2004;113:1013-1023

17. Plaut M, Valentine MD. Allergic rhinitis. *N Engl J Med.* 2005;353:1934-1944

18. Hagy GW, Settipane GA. Bronchial asthma, allergic rhinitis, and allergy skin tests among college students. *J Allergy Clin Immunol.* 1969;44:323

19. McKnee WD. The incidence and familial occurrence of allergy. *J Allergy.* 1966;38:226

20. Simons FER. Advances in H1-antihistamines. *N Engl J Med.* 2004;354:2203-2217

21. Akinbami LJ, Schoendorf KC. Trends in childhood asthma. *Pediatrics.* 2002;110:315-322

22. Yeatts K, Davis KJ, Sotir M, et al. Who gets diagnosed with asthma? *Pediatrics.* 2003;111:1046-1054

23. Thomas M, Kocevar VS, Zhang Q, et al. Asthma-related health care resource among asthmatic children with and without allergic rhinitis. *Pediatrics.* 2005;115:129-134

24. Bousquet J, van Cauwenberge P, Khaltaev N, ARIA Working Group. Allergic rhinitis and its impact on asthma. *J Allergy Clin Immunol.* 2001:108(suppl):146 S-344 S

25. Bachaert C, Patou J, van Cauwenberge P. The role of sinus disease in asthma. *Curr Opin Allergy Immunol.* 2006;6:29-36

26. Boguniewicz M, Schmid-Grendelmeier P, Leung DYM. Atopic dermatitis. *J Allergy Clin Immunol.* 2006;118:40-43

27. Golden DBK. Insect sting allergy and venom immunotherapy. *J Allergy Clin Immunol.* 2005;115:439-447

28. Reisman RE. Clinical aspects of hymenoptera allergy. In: Levine MI, Lockey RF, eds. *Monograph on Insect Allergy.* 4th ed. Milwaukee WI: American Academy of Allergy, Asthma, and Immunology; 2003:55-61

# CHAPTER 152

# Food Allergies

SCOTT H. SICHERER, MD

A *food allergy* is the result of an adverse immune response directed toward food proteins. Food allergies can be broadly categorized by immunopathology, among those that are or are not associated with detectable food-specific IgE antibodies.[1] Disorders with an acute onset of symptoms following ingestion, such as anaphylaxis, are typically mediated by IgE antibodies. Food-specific IgE antibodies arm tissue mast cells and blood basophils, a state termed *sensitization*. Upon re-exposure, the causal food proteins bind to the IgE antibodies specific for them and may trigger the release of mediators, including histamine, causing symptoms that may affect the skin, gastrointestinal tract, respiratory tract, and cardiovascular system. Atopic dermatitis and allergic gastrointestinal disorders characterized by eosinophilic inflammation, are variably associated with food allergy and are often associated with detectable IgE antibodies, although not always (mixed IgE associated/cell-mediated disorders). Nonimmune adverse reactions to foods must also be considered in the differential diagnosis of a food-related adverse reaction. Examples of adverse reactions to foods that may affect adolescents are shown in Box 152-1. Behavioral problems, arthritis, and headache have not been convincingly or commonly linked to food allergy.

**Box 152-1**

***Examples of Adverse Reactions to Foods***

- Intolerance (nonallergic hypersensitivity)
  - Lactose intolerance (lactase deficiency)
  - Alcohol
  - Caffeine (jitteriness)
  - Tyramine in aged cheeses (migraine)
- Toxins
  - Bacterial food poisoning
  - Scombroid (in dark-meat fish, may mimic allergy)
- Food allergy (immune responses, see Table 152-2)
- IgE-mediated
  - Not IgE-associated
  - Mixed IgE/non-IgE (eosinophilic gastrointestinal disease, atopic dermatitis)
- Neurologic and psychological/psychiatric
  - Auriculotemporal syndrome (facial flush with salivation)
  - Gustatory rhinitis (rhinitis from hot or spicy foods)
  - Anorexia nervosa and food aversions

## EPIDEMIOLOGY

Prevalence data for the adolescent age group support an observation noted in other age groups, that perceived food allergies often lead to avoidance of foods not verified to cause a reaction when physician-supervised oral food challenges are undertaken. A cohort study on the Isle of Wight, United Kingdom, evaluated 11- ($n$ = 757) and 15-year-old ($n$ = 775) children.[2] Food avoidance rates were 16% and 19% for the 11- and 15-year-olds, respectively. By means of objective assessment, 2.3% of both 11- and 15-year-old children had food allergy. However, estimated rates of food allergy, and the specific causal foods, vary by age and geographic region. It is estimated that 6% of young children and 3.7% of adults in the United States have a food allergy.[3] In young children, the most common causal foods are cow's milk, egg, peanut, wheat, soy, tree nuts such as walnut and cashew, fish, and shellfish. Adolescence is an age when certain childhood food allergies have resolved (eg, egg, milk, wheat, soy), but allergy to peanuts, tree nuts, fish, and shellfish may persist or develop. Adults, and presumably adolescents, rarely (<0.3%) have allergies to milk, egg, soy, or wheat and are more commonly allergic to shellfish (2%), peanut (0.6%), tree nuts (0.5%), and fish (0.4%).[3] Reactions to fruits and vegetables also are common (~5%), but usually not severe. Severe reactions to seeds (eg, sesame, poppy) are being increasingly reported.[3] Allergy to additives and preservatives are uncommon (<1%). Studies in the United States and United Kingdom have indicated at least a doubling in the rate of peanut allergy in young children within the past decade, which may indicate that more teenagers will be affected by food allergies in the coming years.[4,5] Genetic risk factors for food allergy include a family or personal history of atopic disorders (asthma, atopic dermatitis, allergic rhinitis, food allergy).

## CLINICAL MANIFESTATIONS

The clinical manifestations of food allergy are determined by the underlying immune mechanisms and their affect on particular target organs.[3,6,7] Specific disorders are listed in Table 152-1 according to their immunopathologic basis.

### DISORDERS AFFECTING THE SKIN

Although there are many causes of *acute urticaria* and *angioedema*, food allergy accounts for up to 20% of episodes. Lesions usually occur within an hour of ingestion or skin contact (termed *contact urticaria*) with the causal food. In contrast, chronic urticaria, characterized by periods of hives that continue to occur over 6 weeks, is rarely associated with a food allergy. *Atopic dermatitis* (AD) is a chronic, pruritic, and relapsing rash that often develops in infancy. The flexural creases are typically affected in adolescents. One-third of children with moderate to severe AD have food allergy;[8] however, AD is rarely associated with food allergy in adults, and presumably is not a common trigger for teenagers. Chapter 146, Papulosquamus Diseases, has an in-depth discussion of AD.

### DISORDERS AFFECTING THE GASTROINTESTINAL TRACT

A number of food hypersensitivity disorders affect primarily the gastrointestinal tract.[7] *Immediate gastrointestinal hypersensitivity* is characterized by acute gastrointestinal symptoms following the ingestion of a triggering food protein. Considered here as a distinct syndrome, it is more commonly associated with reactions in other organ systems, eg, during anaphylaxis. *Pollen-food related syndrome (oral allergy syndrome)* is characterized by oral pruritus and possibly angioedema of the lips, tongue, and palate occurring from certain raw fruits and vegetables. The reaction occurs primarily in

**Table 152-1**

**Food-Allergic Disorders**

| *Immunopathology/Disorder* | *Comments* |
|---|---|
| **IgE antibody associated** | Acute onset, detectable food-specific IgE |
| Urticaria/angioedema | Most common manifestation of food allergy |
| Immediate gastrointestinal reaction (GI anaphylaxis) | Usually associated with systemic reactions |
| Oral allergy syndrome (pollen-related) | Usually mild oral pruritus |
| Rhinitis | Not a frequent sole manifestation of food allergy |
| Asthma | Not a frequent sole manifestation of food allergy<br>Inhalation of food-borne allergen (cooking, occupational exposure) may trigger exacerbation |
| Anaphylaxis | Adolescent age group at risk for fatal food-induced anaphylaxis<br>Common triggers: peanut, tree nuts, fish, shellfish |
| Food-associated, exercise-induced anaphylaxis | Often associated with wheat |
| **IgE antibody associated/cell mediated, chronic** | Variable relationship to foods; IgE tests variably associated with specific food triggers |
| Atopic dermatitis | Food may be a trigger in a subset |
| Eosinophilic gastroenteropathies | Elimination diets are typically effective; symptoms vary by site and degree of inflammation |
| **Non-IgE associated** | |
| Dietary protein enterocolitis, proctitis, and enteropathy | Usually resolve in infancy/early childhood |
| Celiac disease | See Chapter 105 |
| Dermatitis herpetiformis | Papulovesicular eruption associated with gluten hypersensitivity |
| Contact dermatitis | Usually associated with occupational food exposure |
| Pulmonary hemosiderosis | Typically isolated to infancy |

persons with pollen allergy sensitized to cross-reacting proteins in particular fruits and vegetables. Persons allergic to birch pollen may experience symptoms from pitted fruits such as apple, peach, and plum, and persons with ragweed pollen allergy may develop symptoms with melons. The proteins in these foods are labile; therefore, cooked forms such as applesauce generally do not induce symptoms. About 1% to 2% of the time, more severe symptoms may occur. Several gastrointestinal disorders are characterized by eosinophilic inflammation of the gastrointestinal tract and may be food-responsive. The disorders are named according to the site(s) of inflammation. *Allergic eosinophilic esophagitis* (AEE) may present with symptoms of severe reflux disease, and typically with dysphagia. The diagnosis requires a biopsy showing eosinophilic infiltration. Treatment may include dietary restriction and medications including corticosteroids.[9]

#### DISORDERS AFFECTING THE RESPIRATORY TRACT

*Allergic rhinitis*, or hay fever, symptoms may accompany a systemic food-allergic reaction but are rarely an isolated manifestation of food allergy.[10] Similarly, *asthma* can occur during a systemic allergic reaction but is not commonly a sole manifestation of food allergy.

#### ANAPHYLAXIS

*Food-induced anaphylaxis* is a serious systemic allergic reaction that is rapid in onset and may cause death.[11] Symptoms can vary and may affect any of a combination of organ systems among the skin, respiratory tract, gastrointestinal tract, and cardiovascular system. Symptoms may also include an aura of "impending doom," and uterine contractions. Life-threatening symptoms include laryngeal edema, severe asthma, and cardiovascular compromise. Food is the most common cause of out-of-hospital anaphylaxis. Additional triggers for anaphylaxis, such as insect stings, medications, exercise, and others, and masqueraders of anaphylaxis, such as anxiety, vasovagal syncope, choking, and others, must be considered in the differential diagnosis. Case series of fatal, food-allergic reactions indicate that the adolescent age group is at increased risk.[12] In a registry of 32 fatalities, 69% were between 12 and 21 years of age.[13] Characteristics of fatal reactions are listed in Table 152-2. It has been presumed that teenagers are at higher risk because they are more likely to take risks in eating unsafe foods, may not carry emergency medications, and are less likely to treat themselves promptly in the event of a reaction.[14] *Food-associated, exercise-induced anaphylaxis* is an uncommon disorder in which patients are able to ingest a particular food or exercise without a reaction but the combination of exercise following the ingestion of a particular food results in anaphylaxis.

## PATHOPHYSIOLOGY

Immune responses to foods are a normal phenomenon leading to a state of oral tolerance.[3] Approximately 2% of ingested food enters the bloodstream in an immunologically intact form but causes no symptoms in the

**Table 152-2**

**Risk Factors for Fatal Food-Induced Anaphylaxis**

| *Risk Factor* | *Comments* |
|---|---|
| Allergies to peanut, tree nuts, fish, and shellfish | Other foods are potential, but less common, causes |
| Delay in treatment with epinephrine | Barriers to prompt treatment include: lack of autoinjector, hesitation to use, failure to recognize symptoms, expectation of resolution using asthma inhalers |
| Teenagers and young adults | Presumably because of risky eating practices and denial of symptoms leading to treatment delay |
| Asthma | Including well-controlled asthma |
| Lack of skin rash during a reaction | Fatal reaction may not include skin symptoms (or, lack of skin symptoms may delay recognition/treatment) |
| Reactions to trace amounts | Increased sensitivity to allergen |
| Previous severe reactions | Fatal reactions have occurred to a first known ingestion, but more typically to a known allergen. Reactions are not automatically more severe with each exposure, but prior severe reactions may identify a future risk |

normal individual. When a protein enters the intestine, antigen-presenting cells (APCs) process the protein and present a small portion to T cells, and may direct an allergic immune response. Th-2 types of T cells may direct the generation of a food-specific IgE antibody from B lymphocytes. In addition to immediate responses, chronic disease attributed to food allergy may result from proinflammatory cytokines elaborated by T cells leading to chronic allergic inflammation (eg, eosinophilic esophagitis).

The most common food allergens to cause severe reactions are heat and acid stable. Although many botanically related proteins or animal proteins from similar species share regions of homology and may show cross-reactivity on allergy testing, clinical evidence of cross-reactivity is not as common.[15] For example, most persons (95%) with peanut allergy (a legume) tolerate other beans and most persons with a wheat allergy (80%) tolerate other grains. However, it is common (>50%) for persons allergic to 1 type of finned fish or 1 type of shellfish to be allergic to other types. Virtually every food or derivative (eg, gelatin, spices, colors, or flavors) from meats, fruits, vegetables, grains, seeds, etc, has been described to at least rarely cause a food allergic reaction.[6] Chemical additives are not likely to cause IgE-associated allergic reactions, but some may have drug effects that can rarely cause adverse reactions.

## DIAGNOSIS

A *history and physical examination* is performed to consider nonimmunologic adverse reactions to foods or to consider other allergic (ie, environmental trigger) or nonallergic causes for symptoms.[1,6] The history should focus on the symptoms attributed to food ingestion, food(s) involved, consistency of reactions, quantity of food-eliciting symptoms, timing between ingestion and onset of symptoms, and associated factors (ie, exercise, aspirin, or alcohol ingestion that may enhance reactions). If the symptoms being evaluated are typical of an IgE-mediated reaction, and if the symptoms follow soon after a food ingestion, that history may clearly implicate a particular food, and a positive test for the specific IgE antibody, discussed in the following, would be confirmatory. If the ingestion was of mixed foods, the history may help eliminate some of the foods—those frequently ingested without symptoms—and specific tests for IgE may further narrow the possibilities. In chronic disorders, such as AD and eosinophilic gastroenteritis, trial elimination diets and supervised oral food challenges may be necessary.

For IgE-mediated food allergy, specific tests can help identify, or exclude, responsible foods. One method to determine the presence of specific IgE antibody is *prick-puncture skin testing* performed by allergists. While the patient is off antihistamines, a probe is used to puncture the skin through a glycerinated extract of a food and appropriate positive (histamine) and negative (saline) controls. A local wheal and flare response indicates the presence of food-specific IgE antibody. *Serum tests for food-specific IgE antibodies* are commercially available to the general practitioner and are not influenced by antihistamines. These tests are often called RAST (radio-allergosorbent test) although the modern tests do not use radioactivity.

The food-specific IgE antibody tests are most valuable when they are negative because the negative predictive value of the tests is very high (more than 85%).[6] Unfortunately, the positive predictive value is on the order of only 50%. Various factors regarding diagnosis using these tests are summarized in Table 152-3. Based on studies in young children, the stronger an individual's food-specific IgE antibody response, indicated by increasingly higher food-specific IgE antibody concentrations or larger skin test wheal size, the more likely it is that there would be an allergic reaction to the tested food.[16,17] However, comprehensive studies to correlate test results with clinical outcomes have not been reported for teenagers or adults. The degree of IgE response does not generally correlate with the severity of an allergic reaction. Tests for IgE antibodies do not help in diagnosing food allergies that are not necessarily associated with IgE. Studies are underway for improved tests for non-IgE mediated disorders, including the use of a skin patch test where an area of skin is exposed to food protein for 24 to 48 hours and the area is examined for the development of a rash in the ensuing days.[18] Tests such as measurement of IgG4 antibody, provocation–neutralization, cytotoxicity, and applied kinesiology (muscle strength tests) among others, are considered unproved methods.[6]

As an adjunct to testing, a first step to determine a cause and effect relationship with a particular chronic illness and food allergy is to show resolution of symptoms with *elimination* of the suspected food(s). If symptoms persist, the eliminated food(s) is (are) excluded as a cause of symptoms. Elimination diets may target suspected foods, based upon history, epidemiology, and test results, or may be comprised of nutritionally complete elemental formula (elemental diet). To establish whether there is a food allergy when the history and test results are otherwise inconclusive, an allergist may perform a physician-supervised *oral food challenge* by gradually feeding the patient the suspected food under observation. Food challenges may elicit severe reactions and are therefore conducted under medical supervision with emergency medications to treat anaphylaxis immediately available. The "gold standard" of oral challenge

**Table 152-3**

**Key Factors in Diagnosis**

| *Factor* | *Examples/Implications* |
|---|---|
| The history is paramount to provide prior probability assessments | • To determine which foods to test<br>• To assess whether the reaction is likely IgE-associated<br>• A convincing history may be "confirmed" with a positive test to the implicated food<br>• It is more likely that a food that is not commonly eaten is the cause of a reaction, compared to a new allergy to a routinely tolerated food |
| Epidemiologic factors influence test selection/interpretation | • Peanuts, tree nuts, fish, and shellfish are more likely to cause severe reactions (anaphylaxis)<br>• Egg, milk, wheat, soy, peanut, tree nuts, fish, shellfish, and seeds account for most significant food-allergic reactions<br>• Foods with similar proteins may "test positive," but true clinical cross-reactivity is variable (eg, peanut and other beans) |
| Tests for IgE antibodies have limited sensitivity and specificity | • In the event of a convincing reaction, a negative test should not be relied upon to exclude allergy; additional testing and physician-supervised oral food challenges may be needed<br>• Testing of large "panels" of foods without regard to patient history or epidemiology of allergic diseases is often misleading because sensitization (positive tests for IgE) may occur without clinical consequence. It is not generally recommended to test for "panels" of foods. |

feedings is the double-blind, placebo-controlled challenge (DBPCFCs) where a placebo feeding is included and neither the patient nor the physician knows which challenges contain the food being tested.

## MANAGEMENT

Treatment for food allergy requires dietary elimination of the offending food, which is not a simple task. Improved food allergen labeling under the Food Allergen Labeling and Consumer Protection Act of 2004 (FALCPA) came into effect January 2006. The law requires that the 8 major allergens or allergenic food groups—milk, egg, fish, crustacean shellfish, tree nuts, wheat, peanut, and soy—be declared on ingredient labels using plain English words. The plain English words used to identify the foods may be placed within the ingredient list or as a separate statement "contains." The law does not exclude using scientific terms for food allergens, for example casein or whey, as long as the label indicates, in some location, the plain English term for the food. Limitations of the law include that foods other than the "major" allergens, eg, sesame, garlic, etc, may not be disclosed individually. The law does not govern the use of "may contain" labels. The law applies to all types of packaged foods except for meat, egg, and poultry products, and raw agricultural foods such as fruits and vegetables. The specific requirements of the law may change, and updates are available at the Web site of the Center for Food Safety and Applied Nutrition, www.cfsan.fda.gov.

Teenagers and parents must also be made aware that the food protein, as opposed to sugar or fat, is the ingredient being eliminated. For example, lactose-free cow's milk contains cow's milk protein. Patients and families undertaking an avoidance diet must also be taught about avoidance in a variety of settings, such as in obtaining restaurant meals where issues of cross-contact (shared utensils, grills, pans, etc) during food preparation may pose dangers. Having the teenager partner with his or her parents from an early age to learn how to order safe meals and to read ingredient labels is suggested. When multiple foods are eliminated, it is prudent to enlist the help of a dietitian in formulating a nutritionally balanced diet. Lay organizations such as The Food Allergy & Anaphylaxis Network (FAAN; 800-929-4040; www.foodallergy.org) assist in the difficult task of dietary elimination. For example, "Chef cards" listing the allergenic foods and issues of cross-contact may be used to improve safety in acquiring restaurant meals. Plans for allergen avoidance must extend to school, camp, trips, sporting activities, and college. Program materials and a Web site specifically for teenagers are available through FAAN.

For life-threatening food allergies, a physician-directed emergency plan must be in place to treat reactions caused by accidental ingestions and periodically reviewed (examples available at www.foodallergy.org). Antihistamines may be required to reduce itching/rash. However, for patients experiencing more severe symptoms of anaphylaxis with respiratory and/or cardiovascular symptoms, or progression of symptoms, or for a known ingestion of an allergen that previously triggered a severe reaction, prompt injection of epinephrine is required. Self-injectable epinephrine should be readily available and administered without delay to treat severe reactions. Teenagers and their caregivers must be familiarized with indications for the use and method of administration of these medications.[19] It is essential to periodically review the indications and the technique of administration of self-injectable epinephrine because mistakes are common. Following the administration of

**Table 152-4**

**Management Issues for Food-Allergic Adolescents**

| *Concerns* | *Suggested Actions* |
|---|---|
| May misperceive need for self-treatment with epinephrine | • Teach symptoms of anaphylaxis, not just word "anaphylaxis"<br>• Educate about treatment circumstances, review self-injector technique and actions to take (inform others, call 911, etc) for an allergic reaction<br>• Review that antihistamines and asthma inhalers cannot replace epinephrine in treatment of anaphylaxis |
| Rates of carrying self-injecting epinephrine vary by social circumstances, perceived risks, and convenience (eg, lower if sports, activities with friends, tight clothing, small purse) | • Impress need for consistency even when not expecting to eat<br>• Reminders to carry, especially for social activities (parties, dances, etc)<br>• Offer carrying alternatives (larger purse, holster, belt clip)<br>• Have back-up medication on site when appropriate (eg, coach for sporting activities) |
| Ignoring risks: eating items that "may contain allergen," neglecting to read ingredient labels, not asking questions when dining out, testing foods for safety by taste, kissing after a partner may have ingested an allergen, etc | • Review risks of exposures and discourage risky behavior<br>• Encourage practice in obtaining safe foods under supervision early to instill good habits<br>• Encourage peer education<br>• Review risks |
| Feeling "different" or "less concerned" are emotional markers for those who take risks | • Address issues of social isolation associated with food allergies<br>• Encourage peer education<br>• Address bullying<br>• Review teenagers' thoughts about their allergy/risks<br>• Refer to Web site for food-allergic teenagers (www.faanteens.org) |
| Quality-of-life easements | • Increase safe food choices<br>• "Point person" for safe meals at school, camp, college |
| Poor communication of allergy to friends may enhance social isolation, increase risk-taking | • Third-party education about allergy directed to friends (eg, FAAN's "PAL-Protect A Life" program) |

the medications, prompt (ie, ambulance) transportation to an emergency facility for advanced care (intravenous fluids, oxygen, corticosteroids, respiratory and cardiovascular support, etc) should be sought with prolonged observations (>4 hours) because recurrence of severe symptoms is possible.[11,13] Patients should obtain medical emergency bracelets identifying their allergy and be reminded to update their epinephrine prescriptions. An important component of the school and camp management of food allergy is to have a clear emergency plan in place, medications readily available, and personnel trained in recognizing and treating reactions. A study of coping strategies of food-allergic teenagers revealed significant deficiencies in self-care.[14] These findings and suggested solutions to improve safety for food-allergic adolescents are shown in Table 152-4. Although studies are under way for improved therapy, current treatment requires education about avoidance and emergency management to protect adolescents at risk for severe or fatal anaphylactic reactions to foods.

## REFERENCES

1. Sicherer SH. Food allergy. *Lancet.* 2002;360(9334):701–710

2. Pereira B, Venter C, Grundy J, Clayton CB, Arshad SH, Dean T. Prevalence of sensitization to food allergens, reported adverse reaction to foods, food avoidance, and food hypersensitivity among teenagers. *J Allergy Clin Immunol.* 2005;116(4):884–892

3. Sicherer SH, Sampson HA. Food allergy. *J Allergy Clin Immunol.* 2006;117 (2 Suppl Mini-Primer):S470–S475

4. Grundy J, Matthews S, Bateman B, Dean T, Arshad SH. Rising prevalence of allergy to peanut in children: data from 2 sequential cohorts. *J Allergy Clin Immunol.* 2002;110(5): 784–789

5. Sicherer SH, Muñoz-Furlong A, Sampson HA. Prevalence of peanut and tree nut allergy in the United States determined by means of a random digit dial telephone survey: a 5-year follow-up study. *J Allergy Clin Immunol.* 2003;112(6):1203–1207

6. American College of Allergy, Asthma, and Immunology. Food allergy: a practice parameter. *Ann Allergy Asthma Immunol.* 2006;96(3 Suppl 2):S1–S68

7. Sampson HA, Sicherer SH, Birnbaum AH. AGA technical review on the evaluation of food allergy in gastrointestinal disorders. *Gastroenterol.* 2001;120(4):1026–1040

8. Eigenmann PA, Sicherer SH, Borkowski TA, Cohen BA, Sampson HA. Prevalence of IgE-mediated food allergy among children with atopic dermatitis. *Pediatrics.* 1998;101:E8. Available at: pediatrics.aappublications.org/cgi/content/full/101/3/e8. Accessed October 18, 2007

9. Liacouras CA, Spergel JM, Ruchelli E, et al. Eosinophilic esophagitis: a 10-year experience in 381 children. *Clin Gastroenterol Hepatol.* 2005;3(12):1198–1206

10. Sicherer SH, Sampson HA. The role of food allergy in childhood asthma. *Immunol Allergy Clinics NA.* 1998;18:49–60

11. Sampson HA, Muñoz-Furlong A, Campbell RL, et al. Second symposium on the definition and management of anaphylaxis: Summary report—Second National Institute of Allergy and Infectious Disease/Food Allergy and Anaphylaxis Network symposium. *J Allergy Clin Immunol.* 2006;117(2):391–397

12. Sampson HA, Mendelson LM, Rosen JP. Fatal and near-fatal anaphylactic reactions to food in children and adolescents. *N Engl J Med.* 1992;327:380–384

13. Bock SA, Muñoz-Furlong A, Sampson HA. Fatalities due to anaphylactic reactions to foods. *J Allergy Clin Immunol.* 2001;107(1):191–193

14. Sampson MA, Muñoz-Furlong A, Sicherer SH. Risk-taking and coping strategies of adolescents and young adults with food allergy. *J Allergy Clin Immunol.* 2006;117(6): 1440–1445.

15. Sicherer SH. Clinical implications of cross-reactive food allergens. *J Allergy Clin Immunol.* 2001;108(6):881–890

16. Roberts G, Lack G. Diagnosing peanut allergy with skin prick and specific IgE testing. *J Allergy Clin Immunol.* 2005;115(6):1291–1296

17. Sampson HA. Utility of food-specific IgE concentrations in predicting symptomatic food allergy. *J Allergy Clin Immunol.* 2001;107(5):891–896

18. Spergel JM, Beausoleil JL, Mascarenhas M, Liacouras CA. The use of skin prick tests and patch tests to identify causative foods in eosinophilic esophagitis. *J Allergy Clin Immunol.* 2002;109(2 Pt 1):363–368

19. Sicherer SH, Simons FE. Quandaries in prescribing an emergency action plan and self-injectable epinephrine for first-aid management of anaphylaxis in the community. *J Allergy Clin Immunol.* 2005;115(3):575–583

# CHAPTER 153

# Immunodeficiencies

MAHESH C. PATEL, MD • SIMA S. TOUSSI, MD • HARRIS GOLDSTEIN, MD

The general adolescent practitioner is often confronted with patients who have recurrent infections. Although most recurrent infections are not due to any identifiable host immune defect, complete formulation of a differential diagnosis requires consideration of whether the recurrent infection is due to an underlying immunodeficiency. In addition, the life expectancy for patients with primary immunodeficiencies has increased as a consequence of improved medical management, resulting in many such patients surviving well into adolescence and young adulthood. Therefore, it is important for those who care for adolescents to have an understanding of the diagnosis and management of patients with a possible immunodeficiency. This chapter is not meant to be an exhaustive list of primary immunodeficiencies that may be encountered in adolescence, but rather to enable the practitioner to identify the most common immunological causes for recurrent infections and to provide a general overview of the diagnosis and treatment of the more commonly encountered primary immunodeficiencies in the adolescent population.

## APPROACH TO THE ADOLESCENT PATIENT WITH RECURRENT INFECTIONS

As a general rule, the more severe the underlying immunodeficiency, the younger the affected individual will be when he or she presents with recurrent infections. Therefore, the most severe congenital immunodeficiencies will have been diagnosed before the adolescent years. Consequently, the initial presentation of congenital immunodeficiencies in adolescence is uncommon and most adolescent patients who present with recurrent infections are unlikely to have a detectable abnormality of the immune system.

The cause of immunodeficiency in adolescents who present with recurrent infections is likely either an acquired or a mild congenital deficiency. A full discussion of AIDS is given in Chapter 138, HIV and AIDS. If a primary immunodeficiency is suspected, various laboratory tests can be performed that will assist in identifying a possible etiology for the patient's presentation (Table 153-1).

**Table 153-1**

**Laboratory and Screening Tests for Suspected Primary Immunodeficiencies[1-3]**

| *Laboratory Test* | *Associated Disorders* |
|---|---|
| Chest radiograph to assess thymus size and lung fields | DiGeorge syndrome, hyper-IgE syndrome, others |
| White blood cell count with differential and quantification of B-cell and T-cell lymphocyte count | T-cell, B-cell, and mixed disorders (for a definitive diagnosis, B- and T-cell levels can be obtained) |
| Delayed-type hypersensitivity skin test | T-cell disorders |
| Total and individual serum immunoglobin levels | Humoral immunodeficiencies, hyper-IgE syndrome |
| Measurement of specific antibody levels to protein and polysaccharide antigens | Humoral immunodeficiencies |
| Nitroblue tetrazolium test | Chronic granulomatous disease |
| Total hemolytic complement assay (CH) | Phagocyte disorders |

Identification of the underlying immune defect can frequently be deduced from the microbiology, anatomic site affected, and patterns of infection. For instance, recurrent sinus, otic, or pulmonary infections, as well as bacteremia or meningitis with encapsulated bacteria, are most often seen in patients with immunoglobulin or complement defects. As a specific example, recurrent *Neisseria* infection is classically seen in patients with late complement component deficiency. In fact, HIV-infected patients (who have a diminished number of T helper cells) are frequently infected with organisms in these categories. Patients with phagocytic defects frequently have recurrent skin infections, especially with abscess formation. Cell-mediated immunity defects predispose the host to infections with viruses, fungi, mycobacteria, and intracellular pathogens[1] (Table 153-2).

**Table 153-2**

**Disease History, Associated Pathogens, and Subgroups of Primary Immunodeficiency Disorders[2,3]**

| *Characteristic Immunodeficiency* | *History and Features* | *Host Defense Affected* | *Pathogen* |
|---|---|---|---|
| • Severe combined immunodeficiency<br>• Hyper-IgE syndrome | • Disseminated infections<br>• Opportunistic infections<br>• Eczema<br>• Pulmonary and cutaneous infections<br>• Mucocutaneous candidiasis | T-cell defects and combined B- and T-cell defects | • *Pneumocystis jirovecii*<br>• *Cryptococcus neoformans*<br>• Herpes viruses<br>• *Candida* spp<br>• Enteroviruses<br>• Mycobacteria<br>• *Staphylococcus aureus*<br>• *Streptococcus pneumoniae*<br>• *Haemophilus influenzae* |
| • Common variable immunodeficiency<br>• X-linked agammaglobulinemia | • Recurrent sinopulmonary infections with encapsulated organisms<br>• Chronic gastrointestinal malabsorption<br>• Postvaccination paralytic polio | Pure B-cell | • *H influenzae*<br>• *S pneumoniae*<br>• *Streptococcus* spp<br>• *Giardia lamblia*<br>• Enteroviruses<br>• *Campylobacter* spp<br>• *Cryptosporidium* spp |
| • Late complement component deficiency | • Recurrent meningitis and bacteremia<br>• Rheumatoid disorders<br>• SLE-like syndrome | Complement | • *Neisseria meningitidis* and *Neisseria gonorhoeae* |
| • Chronic granulomatous disease<br>• Chediak-Higashi syndrome<br>• Leukocyte adhesion deficiency<br>• Systemic lupus erythematosus | • Recurrent, severe infections with typical and common pathogens<br>• Granuloma formation<br>• Recurrent skin infections and abscess formation<br>• Gingivitis and aphthous ulcers | Phagocytes | • *S aureus*<br>• *Pseudomonas* spp<br>• *Serratia* spp<br>• *Klebsiella* spp<br>• *Candida* spp<br>• *Nocardia* spp<br>• *Aspergillus* spp |

Further assisting the diagnosis of immunodeficiencies is a careful family history because most primary immunodeficiencies are inherited in an autosomal recessive or X-linked manner[2] (Table 153-3). Because congenital immunodeficiencies are rarely newly diagnosed in the teenage years, we also discuss alternative etiologies for serious recurrent infections presenting during adolescence. We have grouped the discussion into the following 3 categories based on their most common presentations: (1) recurrent skin, (2) recurrent sinopulmonary, and (3) central nervous system or disseminated infections.

**Table 153-3**

**Primary Immunodeficiency Disorders and Genetic Inheritance Patterns**

| *Disorder* | *Genetic Inheritance Pattern*[a] |
|---|---|
| **B-Cell Differentiation and Antibody Production** | |
| Common variable immunodeficiency | Not determined |
| Selective IgA deficiency | AR |
| IgG subclass deficiencies | Not determined |
| **T-Cell Defects and Combined B- and T-Cell Defects** | |
| DiGeorge syndrome | AD or spontaneous |
| Ataxia-telangiectasia | AR |
| X-linked hyper-IgM syndrome | X linked |
| **Phagocytic** | |
| Chronic granulomatous disease | X linked or AR |
| Chediak-Higashi syndrome | AR |
| LAD types 1 and 2 | AR |
| Myeloperoxidase deficiency | AR |
| Hyper-IgE syndrome (Job syndrome) | Sporadic, AD, rarely AR |
| Interferon gamma receptor deficiency | AR |
| G-6-PD deficiency | X linked |
| **Complement** | |
| Complement deficiencies | Generally AR |

[a]AD, autosomal dominant; AR, autosomal recessive; LAD, leukocyte adhesion deficiency

## RECURRENT SKIN AND SOFT TISSUE INFECTIONS

The most common cause of recurrent cellulitis is nasal carriage of *Staphylococcus aureus*. Treatment of patients without an underlying immunodeficiency who have recurrent soft tissue infections due to *S aureus* should include decolonization of *S aureus* nasal carriage with intranasal mupirocin, as well as the use of antimicrobial skin cleansers and washes. Whether the addition of suppressive oral antibiotics is superior to mupirocin and cleansers alone in promoting long-term decolonization and therefore fewer infections remains to be seen.[3]

Patients with lymphatic stasis, compromise of the normal dermal barrier as a consequence of trauma, or coexisting skin infections such as eczema can also be predisposed to developing recurrent cellulitis. The most common organisms involved in recurrent soft tissue infections are *S aureus* and *Streptococcal pyogenes* in the normal host. Recurrent abscess formation is usually associated with anatomic abnormalities such as pilonidal cysts, branchial cleft cysts, or a foreign body.[1] However, if the recurrent abscess formation occurs in unusual anatomical sites, or if the infection is due to an unusual organism, this should prompt an immunological evaluation, especially for chronic mucocutaneous candidiasis (CMC), hyper IgE syndrome, phagocyte defects, or granulocytopenia.

## CHRONIC MUCOCUTANEOUS CANDIDIASIS

### Background, Epidemiology, and Pathogenesis

Although CMC can be secondary to inhaled steroid therapy, HIV infection, or the use of dentures, this section focuses on CMC as a primary immune deficiency. Patients with CMC are unable to effectively clear fungal infections of the genus *Candida*, namely, *Candida albicans*. This leads to persistent and recurrent infections of the skin, nails, and mucous membranes with yeasts. Studies have described various defects that likely predispose these individuals to candidiasis, but the precise mechanism remains unknown.[4] Patients with CMC can have abnormal lymphoproliferative responses and cytokine production to Candida antigens. Some may lack delayed-type hypersensitivity responses to Candida antigens.

Three clinical syndromes of CMC that present in early childhood are familial CMC, chronic localized candidiasis, and autoimmune polyendocrinopathy-candidiasis-ectodermal dystrophy (APECED).[5] The CMC with thymoma usually presents in adults and is not reviewed here. Candidiasis in the setting of hyper-IgE syndrome is discussed in the next section. Chronic mucocutaneous candidiasis may be the only manifestation in affected patients, or it may be associated with endocrine, immune, or inflammatory disorders. Patients affected with APECED are predisposed to autoimmune disorders.

### Clinical Manifestations and Diagnosis

Individuals with familial CMC have chronic and recurrent oral candidiasis, and less commonly, cutaneous and ungual candidal infection.[5] Males and females are affected equally and are often symptomatic by age 2 years. Patients with chronic localized candidiasis (candida granuloma) present by the age of 5 years with thick, crusty lesions at the scalp, face, and mouth, and do not develop endocrinopathies. Patients with APECED have extensive oral and cutaneous candidiasis, and may present with recurrent oral and diaper candidiasis that progresses to involve the scalp, extremities, and nails. Later in adulthood, they can develop autoimmune disorders and endocrinopathies such as hypoparathyroidism, hypoadrenalism, and ovarian failure.[6] Other disorders commonly found in patients with APECED include alopecia, keratoconjunctivitis, enamel dysplasia, nail dystrophy, malabsorption, and autoimmune hepatitis.

Although *C albicans* is the main pathogen infecting CMC patients, they may also be infected with other fungi, viruses, and bacteria. Most CMC patients have normal numbers of T cells and serum immunoglobulins, as well as normal responses to vaccines.[5] However, patients with CMC can have a wide range of immunological abnormalities, which may explain their susceptibility to Candida and significant infections with bacteria, viruses, and other fungi.

#### Management

Patients with CMC rarely develop disseminated candidiasis. The mainstay of therapy is oral antifungals, such as fluconazole for oral, vaginal, and cutaneous candidiasis. Topical antifungal creams or oral nystatin solutions are typically ineffective alone, but can be given in addition to oral azoles to enhance response. Treatment duration may need to be prolonged in these patients. For patients with more severe recurrent oral or cutaneous candidiasis who may be at risk of developing APECED, there should be careful monitoring for the development of endocrinopathies and autoimmunity. Regular monitoring, in addition to appropriate treatment of candidiasis and other infectious complications, should allow for a reasonably good quality of life.

## HYPER-IgE SYNDROME

### Background, Epidemiology, and Pathogenesis

Hyper-IgE syndrome, or Job syndrome, is a rare disorder affecting the immune system, connective tissue, skeletal system, and dentition. Hyper-IgE patients have extremely elevated IgE levels, and many have eosinophilia in blood and sputum, defective neutrophil chemotaxis, deficient cytokine production, and poor antibody responses to immunizations and antigens. Most cases of hyper-IgE syndrome are sporadic, but inheritance can be autosomal dominant or autosomal recessive. Although chromosome 4 has been implicated in some families, a common molecular defect has not been consistently identified in affected patients.

### Clinical Manifestations and Diagnosis

Hyper-IgE syndrome usually presents with the classic triad of abscesses, pneumonia, and elevated IgE levels (>2,000 IU/mL), but these may not always be present. In a review of 30 patients with hyper-IgE syndrome, other common features included CMC (83%), recurrent long bone fractures after minor trauma (57%), hyperextensible joints (68%), and delayed shedding of primary teeth (72%).[7] By adolescence, individuals develop coarse facial features, a broad nasal bridge, and frontal bossing.

Other infections seen include sinusitis, otitis, and bone infections. *S aureus* is the most common pathogen in respiratory and skin infections. Other important pathogens are *Haemophilus influenzae*, *Pseudomonas aeruginosa*, and invasive fungal infections with *Aspergillus fumigatus* and *Cryptococcus neoformans*. Skin manifestations begin in infancy, where an atypical neonatal rash may be seen. Children and adolescents have an eczematous rash, which on biopsy displays an eosinophilic infiltrate. They are prone to recurrent skin infections, including furuncles, cold abscesses, and cellulitis. A hallmark of the syndrome is the development of cold abscesses, large soft tissue infections that lack warmth and are not associated with fever or pain. Pneumonias are often severe and complicated by empyemas, pneumatoceles, or effusions; they may lead to subsequent pulmonary damage, including bronchiectasis and bronchopleural fistulas.

Patients with hyper-IgE syndrome have extremely elevated levels of serum peripheral IgE and usually peripheral eosinophilia 2 standard deviations above normal. IgE levels can fluctuate over time, but do not correlate with disease severity. Levels of IgA, IgM, and IgG are usually normal but can be elevated.

#### Management

Skin care with adequate hydration and emollients, and possibly steroids, is critical for effective management of the eczematous dermatitis and to prevent superinfection. Infection can be prevented by treatment with prophylactic antibiotics that cover *S aureus*, such as bactrim. When they occur, infections should be treated promptly with appropriate antibiotics or antifungals. Deep-seated abscesses and complicated pneumonias may need surgical intervention. There are cases reporting treatment with cimetidine, cyclosporine, intravenous immunoglobulin (IVIG), and interferon in hyper-IgE patients with varying levels of success, but none were evaluated in randomized controlled trials and thus cannot be recommended at this time.

## PHAGOCYTE DISORDERS/DEFECTS

Neutrophils and monocytes are the primary phagocytic cells; they play an important role in microbial killing. Adolescents who suffer from these defects develop repeated infections at sites on the body that are exposed to the environment and present with infections that form minimally purulent abscesses and granulomas, skin infections, furuncles, organ abscesses, and lymphadenitis.

### Chronic Granulomatous Disease

***Background, Epidemiology, and Pathogenesis*** The prototypical syndrome due to phagocyte cell dysfunction is chronic granulomatous disease (CGD). It is estimated that CGD in the United States occurs in upward of 1 per 200,000 live births and is characterized by mutations in genes responsible for the ability of phagocytes to generate reactive oxygen intermediates from molecular oxygen. Specifically, CGD is caused by defects in the reduced nicotinamide adenine dinucleotide phosphate (NADPH) oxidase, the enzyme that assists in the generation of superoxide, which in turn activates granule proteins inside the phagocytic vacuole, which are necessary to kill microbes. Mutations in any of the 4 structural genes of NADPH oxidase can result in a person being affected with Chronic granulomatous disease CGD, which is found in both X-linked and autosomal recessive forms. Approximately 65% to 70% of all cases arise from mutations in the gene encoding gp91phox and are inherited in an X-linked recessive manner; the remainder are due to mutations in the autosomally encoded p22phox, p47phox, and p67phox subunits and are inherited in an autosomal recessive form.

***Clinical Manifestations and Diagnosis*** Patients with CGD are generally diagnosed as toddlers or young children, although milder forms have been described with onset in the teenage or early adult years. The primary clinical manifestations include recurrent, life-threatening infections with catalase-positive bacteria and fungi, as well as granulomatous inflammation that can affect any organ in the body. Most of these infections are due to *S aureus*, *Serratia marcescans*, *Burkholderia cepacia*, *Nocardia* spp, and *Aspergillus* spp, especially *Aspergillus fumigatus*. Granulomas form as a compensatory response by lymphoid cells due to the ineffective destruction of phagocytized microbes. Infections that occur in affected individuals include pneumonia, abscesses, suppurative adenitis, osteomyelitis, bacteremia/fungemia, and superficial skin infections, such as cellulitis or impetigo. Isolation of the previous organisms in patients with particularly severe or recurrent infections should prompt an investigation for CGD. Patients with CGD often pose a diagnostic dilemma because they frequently have little signs or symptoms of clinical infection. Other noninfectious manifestations seen include granuloma formation, chorioretinitis, lupus syndromes, and significant gastrointestinal involvement. Patients with CGD have an increased risk of developing inflammatory bowel disease, especially Crohn disease.

Patients with CGD have normal neutrophil counts, and the chemotactic, adherence, and phagocytic functions of these cells are preserved. The diagnosis of CGD is made by demonstrating that the patient's neutrophils are unable to generate superoxide ions detected by nitroblue tetrazolium (NBT) dye reduction, measurement of chemiluminescence, or quantitative determination of phagocyte reactive oxygen production using flow cytometry (the dihydrorhodamine assay); the latter method can distinguish the X-linked from the autosomal form of CGD.[8]

***Management*** Chemoprophylaxis with antibiotics, especially trimethoprim-sulfamethoxasole, and antifungals has helped reduce the frequency of serious infections in affected patients. However, despite effective prophylaxis, the incidence of fungal infections, particularly with *Aspergillus* spp, is increasing. The mainstay for treatment of *Aspergillus* infections is voriconazole or amphotericin B with alternate-day normal granulocyte transfusions. Antifungal prophylaxis with itraconazole has decreased the incidence of fungal infections in patients with CGD. Subcutaneous IFN-gamma injections have also been shown to reduce the number of serious infections in select patients with CGD and has been used successfully for long-term prophylaxis.[9] Finally, bone marrow transplantation is the treatment of choice and has been performed on some patients with limited success.

### Leukocyte Adhesion Deficiencies

***Background, Epidemiology, and Pathogenesis*** The ability of leukocytes to adhere to the epithelium, other leukocytes, and bacteria is necessary for leukocytes to communicate, travel, and fight infection. Any defect in these processes leads to poor recruitment of neutrophils to sites of inflammation or infection. Leukocyte adhesion deficiency is an inherited syndrome that consists of 2 different disorders that are characterized by recurrent skin, mucous membrane, and subcutaneous infections.

Leukocyte adhesion deficiency type 1 (LAD-1) is an autosomal recessive disorder that is due to a mutation in the B2 integrin family, CD18. This molecule, along with others, makes up the leukocyte function-associated antigen 1 (LFA-1). Leukocyte function-associated antigen 1 mediates adhesion of leukocytes to endothelial cells, and without it, leukocytes would not be able to reach sites of infection. Leukocyte adhesion deficiency type 2 (LAD-2) is due to the absence of the carbohydrate structure sialyl-Lewis X on the outer surface of neutrophils.

The absence of this molecule prevents leukocytes from initiating attachment to vascular endothelium. The incidence of LAD-1 is rare, affecting one in a million individuals. Other forms of the LAD complex are even rarer with only a few case reports and, therefore, are not discussed in this chapter.

***Clinical Manifestations and Diagnosis*** Patients with severe LAD-1 have persistent leukocytosis, delayed umbilical stump separation, omphalitis, and severe destructive gingivitis with alveolar bone resorption. Therefore, they are usually diagnosed early in life and likely will not be encountered by the adolescent practitioner due to early death of those with the severe phenotype. Recurrent infections of the skin and gastrointestinal and respiratory tracts are common, and patients usually have minimal inflammation or neutrophilic infiltration at the sites of infection. Those with the moderate form of LAD-1 typically have milder disease and, therefore, may be diagnosed later in life. Clinically, these patients have normal umbilical cord separation, fewer infections, and a much longer life expectancy. Periodontal disease, poor wound healing, and leukocytosis are still, as is the case with the severe phenotype, the hallmark of this disease.[8] Diagnosis of LAD-1 is typically made by flow cytometric analysis of blood from affected individuals. CD18 and its associated molecules (CD11a, CD11b, and CD11c) are reduced or absent (depending on the severity of the phenotype) on the surface of neutrophils and other leukocytes in patients with LAD. Functional assays are typically carried out in conjunction with flow cytometric analysis.

Patients with LAD-2 are characterized by having severe mental retardation; short stature; abnormal facies; and the traditional immunologic features of LAD, which include the risk of increased infection, poor pus formation, and leukocytosis. Needless to say, it is an extremely rare disorder and likely will not be encountered by the general adolescent practitioner. Diagnosis is made by flow cytometry to identify surface expression of CD15 s or sialyl-Lewis X.

***Management*** Affected patients are usually treated for the underlying infectious process. Initiation of appropriate antibiotics targeted toward the more common isolates, such as *S aureus* and gram-negative bacilli, is the mainstay of treatment. Given the penchant for these infections to cause ulceration and necrosis, aggressive medical and surgical management with debridement and grafting is necessary in many cases. Chronic granulomatous disease. Management also includes antimicrobial prophylaxis with trimethoprim-sulfamethoxasole and bone marrow transplantation, if possible.[10]

### Neutrophil Granule Defects

***Background, Epidemiology, and Pathogenesis*** Patients with disorders in neutrophil granule function have varied presentations ranging from being asymptomatic to having an increased susceptibility to infection. The abnormalities are either inherited or acquired and can be divided into 3 distinct categories, which include myeloperoxidase (MPO) deficiency, Chediak-Higashi syndrome (CHS), and specific granule deficiency. The latter has only 5 described cases and is not discussed in further detail.

The myeloperoxidase deficiency is characterized by a dysfunctional peroxidase in neutrophils and monocyte azurophilic granules. The gene has been located on chromosome 17q22–23. The MPO itself is necessary for the chlorination and iodination of microbes that are ingested by neutrophils. It occurs in about 1 in 4,000 persons in the United States.[10]

Chediak-Higashi syndrome is a rare autosomal recessive disorder characterized by a mutation on chromosome 1 at position q42–43 that affects the lysosomal transport protein LYST. The classic feature is giant lysosomal granules. These abnormal lysosomes are unable to fuse with phagosomes (to form a phagolysosome) and thus are unable to lyse ingested bacteria.

***Clinical Manifestations and Diagnosis*** Although the majority of patients with MPO deficiency have no increased risk of infection and are clinically asymptomatic, patients may occasionally have disseminated candidiasis. Myeloperoxidase deficiency is also acquired and can be seen in patients with acute myelogenous leukemia and in myelodysplastic syndromes. Patients are easily diagnosed by testing leukocytes for MPO content, and because automated differential white blood cell counters identify granulocytes by their MPO content, they would be able to readily identify routine samples of affected individuals.[11]

Patients with CHS have a unique phenotypic appearance characterized by partial oculocutaneous albinism and photophobia. Patients suffer from recurrent infections caused by fungi and gram-positive and gram-negative bacteria. The most common organisms are *S aureus* and beta-hemolytic streptococci. Patients also suffer from motor or sensory neuropathy, typically beginning in the adolescent years. Individuals with CHS have mild neutropenia and platelet dysfunction (with normal counts), but immunoglobulin and antibody production is normal. The diagnosis is largely clinical, with findings of large inclusions in nucleated blood cells and characteristic giant cytoplasmic granules on peripheral blood smear. Many patients develop a lymphoproliferative disorder characterized by high fever, pancytopenia, and lymphohistiocytic infiltration of the lymphatic organs. This lymphocytic proliferation results in recurrent viral and bacterial infections, which ultimately lead to death.

***Management*** Patients with MPO deficiency are largely asymptomatic, so these individuals do not require therapy.

Patients with disseminated candidiasis, often associated with diabetes mellitus, should be treated with appropriate antifungals and should have their diabetes better controlled.

Some CHS patients have improved with ascorbic acid therapy (500–2,000 mg daily). After patients develop the lymphoproliferative disorder, they can be treated with bone marrow transplantation. Corticosteroids and splenectomy have been used in some patients in the accelerated phase of lymphoproliferation with limited success.[10]

### GLUCOSE-6-PHOSPHATE DEHYDROGENASE DEFICIENCY

Although typically thought of as a disease that causes acute and chronic hemolytic anemia, patients with glucose-6-phosphate dehydrogenase deficiency (G6PDD) have diminished peroxide production, which results in decreased intracellular bactericidal activity. This X-linked enzyme deficiency is very common and affects more than 200 million people worldwide. Individuals with G6PDD commonly inherit abnormal alleles of the gene responsible for the synthesis of G6PD, and patients with G6PDD activity reduced by more than 95% are more severely affected.[12] The diminished levels of cellular NADH and NADPH in the presence of normal NADPH oxidase activity results in a microbicidal defect that is similar to those in patients with CGD.[2] Diagnosis is made by demonstrating the reduced level of G6PDD in red blood cells. Treatment is directed toward appropriate therapy for infections, supportive care, and prevention of hemolysis.

### OTHER DISORDERS RESULTING IN PHAGOCYTE DEFECTS

There are many other diseases that effectively result in phagocyte deficiencies or dysfunction, most of which are acquired. Although disorders causing congenital neutropenia such as Kostmann and Shwachman-Diamond syndromes are exceedingly uncommon, one should be aware of other causes of neutropenia such as cyclic neutropenia. Cyclic neutropenia can present in children or adults, and the underlying defect in the childhood form is a mutation in the neutrophil elastase gene. This leads to cycles where patients can have marked neutropenia that typically lasts 3 to 7 days per cycle. During that time, they may present with fever, aphthous ulcers, and soft tissue infections due to the neutropenia. However, they can rarely present with severe infections. Treatment is supportive, and for those with recurrent, severe disease, GC-SCF may be warranted. Acquired neutropenias are seen more commonly in the teenage years than primary neutropenias and include drug-induced, autoimmune, infection-induced, and marrow-infiltrating neutropenias. Furthermore, syndromes may overlap to affect several different arms of the immune system and phagocyte function; these are discussed in other sections in this chapter and include hyper-IgE syndrome, immune complex disease, and complement deficiencies. Finally, compromised splenic function, as seen in patients following splenic removal or vascular occlusion of the spleen, results in impaired function of splenic macrophages and increased susceptibility to infections with encapsulated bacteria.

## RECURRENT SINOPULMONARY INFECTIONS

Given the high incidence of sinopulmonary infections, complaints of recurrent sinopulmonary disease often pose a challenge to the general adolescent provider. The overwhelming majority of patients with recurrent sinusitis and otitis media infections, especially in the absence of lower respiratory tract disease, have no host defense defects. These infections can be attributable to such factors as poor antibiotic selection or use, anatomic abnormalities, and allergic disorders. Careful physical examination; appropriate use of decongestants, antihistamines, and antimicrobials; and possible referral to an otolaryngologist will help these patients enormously. Similarly, patients with recurrent pharyngitis often have persistence of the same isolate, instead of recurrent infections with multiple isolates; these patients may, in fact, be simply colonized with group A beta-hemolytic streptococci.[13] Finally, patients with recurrent pneumonias, especially if they are in the same anatomic location, often have structural abnormalities such as tracheal deviation, retained foreign body, tracheobronchial fistulae, bronchial sequestration, or neoplasm. Widespread pulmonary infection should prompt evaluation for cystic fibrosis, immotile cilia syndrome, neurologic dysfunction (as a cause for recurrent aspiration), and/or esophageal dysfunction (as seen with gastroesophageal reflux).[1] Finally, noninfectious causes such as vasculitis and other collagen-vascular disorders should be entertained. Careful physical examination, limited laboratory studies, enhanced radiologic imaging, and pulmonary bronchoscopy will typically identify individuals with these processes. If careful evaluation has ruled out most of these possibilities, then attention should be directed toward immunological etiologies such as granulocyte disorders, hypogammaglobulinemia, combined primary immunodeficiencies, and complement disorders. Some of the more commonly encountered illnesses in these categories are discussed next.

## DIGEORGE SYNDROME

### Background, Epidemiology, and Pathogenesis

DiGeorge syndrome describes individuals presenting with hypocalcemia, cardiac disease, abnormal facies, hypoplastic thymus and parathyroid glands, and T-cell immunodeficiency.The most common cause is a deletion at chromosome 22q11.2, which occurs in nearly 1 out of 4,000 births. The clinical manifestations resulting from this deletion are broad, and similar manifestations occur in patients with velocardiofacial syndrome and conotruncal anomaly face syndrome, and sometimes these patients are categorized as having CATCH (Cardiac, Abnormal facies, Thymic hypoplasia, Cleft palate, and Hypocalemia) 22 syndrome. The immunodeficiency in patients with DiGeorge syndrome is due to decreased levels of circulating T cells; however, T cells that are produced function normally. Thus, the varying degrees of immunodeficiency seen in DiGeorge syndrome depends on the levels of T cells produced, with individuals having an aplastic thymus (complete DiGeorge syndrome) presenting with severe immunodeficiency comparable to children with severe combined immunodeficiency.[14]

### Clinical Manifestations and Diagnosis

The most common clinical findings in patients with DiGeorge syndrome are cardiac anomalies, renal anomalies, developmental delay, speech delay, and cleft palate or velopharyngeal insufficiency.[15] Most are diagnosed in infancy during evaluation of hypocalcemia or cardiac anomalies. Interestingly, there are rare case reports of adults diagnosed with DiGeorge syndrome after presenting with hypocalcemia.[16] The most common infections seen in patients with DiGeorge syndrome are otitis media, sinusitis, and pneumonia.

More than 90% of patients with DiGeorge syndrome have a hemizygous deletion of chromosome 22q11.2, which can be demonstrated by cytogenetic analysis using fluorescent in situ hybridization (FISH) or by polymerase chain reaction (PCR). The reduction in peripheral T-cell counts can vary depending on the degree of thymic hypoplasia, ranging from almost complete deficiency to moderately decreased T-cell levels. Most DiGeorge syndrome patients have milder T-cell deficiencies and seldom develop opportunistic or life-threatening infections. Immunoglobulin levels are usually normal, but selective IgA deficiency may occur in up to 10% of patients.

### Management

Children with complete DiGeorge syndrome have severe T-cell deficiency and will need prompt and prolonged treatment of infections. Although Pneumocystis carinii pneumonia (PCP) is a rare opportunistic infection in this population, children with severe immunodeficiency should be started on prophylaxis with trimethoprim-sulfamethoxazole. Live-attenuated vaccines should be avoided in these patients. Patients with complete DiGeorge syndrome will need to undergo either sibling-matched hematopoietic stem cell transplant or thymic tissue transplant to survive beyond infancy.

Most children with DiGeorge syndrome have a milder degree of immunodeficiency. For patients whose CD4 T-cell counts are below 25%, bactrim prophylaxis should be considered. These patients often require a multidisciplinary approach, including an immunologist, cardiologist, and additional attention for possible impaired cognitive development and growth. Patients with DiGeorge syndrome are also predisposed to developing autoimmune diseases such as juvenile rheumatoid arthritis and hematologic autoimmune diseases. Therefore, an adolescent provider should monitor T-cell counts annually and be aware of these secondary disorders.

## IgA DEFICIENCY

### Background, Epidemiology, and Pathogenesis

Selective IgA deficiency is the most common primary immunodeficiency with an incidence affecting 1 in 300 to 1 in 700 whites. More than 90% of IgA-deficient individuals are asymptomatic. The fraction of individuals who are symptomatic are at increased risk of developing recurrent upper respiratory tract infections, otitis media, autoimmune disorders, allergic symptoms, and gastrointestinal infections. IgA deficiency may occur in isolation, or it may be associated with other immunodeficiencies, such as IgG subclass deficiency. Some may later progress to common variable immunodeficiency (CVID).

There are many case reports where IgA deficiency is associated with immune disorders such as myasthenia gravis, systemic lupus erythematosus (SLE), juvenile rheumatoid arthritis (JRA), Hashimoto thyroiditis, dermatomyositis, and idiopathic thrombocytopenia. One study evaluated 65 children with IgA deficiency and diagnosed 7.7% of them with celiac disease.[17] Despite familial clustering of IgA deficiency and its association with other immunodeficiencies, the genetics of IgA deficiency remains unknown.

### Clinical Manifestations and Diagnosis

Adolescents with IgA deficiency are often identified after evaluation of recurrent sinopulmonary infections or allergic symptoms. One study found that of the 67 children evaluated for recurrent infections at an immunology clinic who did not have combined or acquired immunodeficiency, 31% had IgA deficiency.[18] A more recent study found that IgA and IgG subclass deficiencies were more prevalent in children with recurrent respiratory infections, and these children may be at greater risk of chronic pulmonary damage.[19]

The diagnosis of IgA deficiency in adolescents relies on an extremely low IgA concentration (<7 mg/dL), with normal serum levels of IgG and IgM. If the diagnosis was made prior to age 5 years, IgA levels should be rechecked because it may have been a transient form of IgA deficiency. If the patient is on any medication that may induce IgA deficiency, attempts should be made to make a reasonable substitute and re-evaluate IgA levels. IgA-deficient patients who are symptomatic should have B cells evaluated and complete quantification of immunoglobulins, including IgG subclasses. Some would also recommend evaluating antibody responses to polysaccharides and protein antigens.

#### Management

Patients with selective IgA deficiency and IgG subclass deficiencies that have recurrent infections may benefit from prophylactic antibiotics. If antibiotics are not helpful in preventing recurrent infections, intravenous immunoglobulin (IVIG) may need to be administered. This may be necessary in patients with chronic asthma and recurrent pulmonary infections to prevent long-term lung damage. If IVIG is to be given, the patient should be screened for IgE anti-IgA antibodies. If positive, the risk of anaphylaxis should be minimized by choosing an IVIG preparation with the least IgA content. If symptoms are consistent, patients may also need to be screened for celiac disease. Patients with isolated IgA deficiency who do not develop other disorders, such as CVID, have a very good prognosis.

## IgG SUBCLASS DEFICIENCY

### Background, Epidemiology, and Pathogenesis

Individuals with IgG subclass deficiency have normal levels of total IgG but are deficient in 1 or more of the 4 subclasses. In general, each of these subclass deficiencies may be seen concomitantly with another subclass deficiency, IgA deficiency, or another primary immune disorder such as CMC. Patients with IgG subclass deficiency are predisposed to recurrent otitis, sinusitis, and respiratory infections. IgG subclass deficiency is a common finding in children being evaluated for recurrent infections, severe asthma, and atopic diseases.

### Clinical Manifestations and Diagnosis

In children and adolescents, selective deficiency of IgG2 is often associated with respiratory tract infections, sinusitis, and otitis, and less frequently with more severe infections. Because IgG2 is responsible for the antibody response against polysaccharide capsular antigens, IgG2-deficient patients are at increased risk for *S pneumoniae*, *H influenzae* type b, and *Neisseria meningitides* infections. Some of these patients also have IgA and/or IgG4 deficiency. IgG2 deficiency has been associated with other immunodeficiencies such as ataxia-telangiectasia.

IgG1 and IgG3 are important in antibody responses to protein and viral antigens. Selective IgG3 subclass deficiency has been associated with asthma, gastrointestinal infections, and meningitis. IgG1 deficiency can be seen in younger children, but likely represents transient hypogammaglobulinemia of infancy. Adults with IgG1 deficiency may progress to hypogammaglobulinemia and, subsequently, CVID. IgG4 deficiency may occur alone or in combination with IgG2 and/or IgA deficiencies. Most patients with isolated IgG4 deficiency are asymptomatic.

The diagnosis of IgG subclass deficiency is made when the particular subclass is more than 2 standard deviations below what is expected for age. Because of the difficulty in measuring IgG subclass levels and standardizing normal ranges in children, if abnormal, the IgG subclass levels should be repeated and confirmed. Patients with IgG subclass deficiency who are symptomatic should also be tested to determine their capacity to mount an antigen-specific IgG subclass response. Antibody responses to protein antigens can be assessed by measuring tetanus and diphtheria titers, while responses to pathogens can be evaluated by testing a patient's response to challenge with a vaccine such as pneumococcal vaccine.

#### Management

Patients with IgG subclass deficiency who are symptomatic are at risk of developing chronic pulmonary disease following repeated infections. Prompt treatment with antibiotics is critical to prevent this outcome, and some may need prophylactic antibiotics if infections are frequent or severe. Many patients with IgG subclass deficiencies who have recurrent infections, severe asthma, and even chronic rhinosinusitis with nasal polyps, or who are refractory to standard treatment, have responded well to IVIG therapy.

Patients who have not responded to polysaccharide vaccines may need immunization with the conjugate vaccines. Because IgG subclass deficiency may evolve into CVID, these patients should have immunoglobulin levels reassessed annually.

## COMMON VARIABLE IMMUNODEFICIENCY

### Background, Epidemiology, and Pathogenesis

Common variable immunodeficiency has an incidence ranging from 1 in 25,000 to 1 in 66,000. Common variable immunodeficiency is usually sporadic, although autosomal dominant transmission has been described in some families. It can present at any age, and the diagnosis is often made in the second or third decade of life. Common variable immunodeficiency is characterized by hypogammaglobulinemia, poor antibody responses, and recurrent bacterial infections. A failure of B-cell differentiation results in low immunoglobulin levels and poor antibody response.

Common variable immunodeficiency patients also have T-cell abnormalities, including reduced CD4 levels, decreased cytokine production, and decreased T-cell proliferation and activation in response to mitogens and antigens. Macrophage defects have also been described frequently, as has increased tumor necrosis factor production, which may lead to inflammatory manifestations. Several genetic defects underlying CVID have been identified that affect ICOS, TACI, BAFF-R, or CD19. These defects together account for about 10% of the cases because they are not found in most patients.

### Clinical Manifestations and Diagnosis

Most CVID patients become symptomatic after puberty and present with recurrent sinopulmonary infections. The most common infections are sinusitis, otitis, pneumonia, and gastroenteritis. Organisms usually implicated are *S pneumoniae* and *H influenzae*. Patients who progress to chronic lung disease may also require treatment for *S aureus*, *P aeruginosa*, and *Pneumocystis jiroveci*. Physical examination of patients may demonstrate weight loss, clubbing, lymphadenopathy, and hepatosplenomegaly. Inflammatory gastrointestinal disease is common in this disorder, and patients may have diarrhea and malabsorption. A study that evaluated 248 patients with CVID found an increased risk in other disorders: 8% with non-Hodgkin lymphoma, 22% with autoimmune diseases such as idiopathic thrombocytopenic purpura and autoimmune hemolytic anemia, and 8% developed granulomatous disease.[20] Women with CVID had a far greater risk of developing malignancy and autoimmune disorders.

Common variable immunodeficiency patients have reduced levels of IgG, IgA, and often IgM. To diagnose CVID in a patient who presents with recurrent infections and hypogammaglobulinemia, other diseases that overlap may need to be excluded. These include X-linked agammaglobulinemia (XLA) in young boys, lymphoproliferative disorder, hyper-IgM syndrome, and immunodeficiency secondary to medications.

### Management

Patients will likely require monthly IVIG. The 20-year survival after the diagnosis of CVID is estimated to be 64% for men and 67% for women compared to an expected 92% to 94% survival for similar ages in the general population. The major causes of death are lymphoma and chronic pulmonary disease.

In 1 study of 24 patients, monthly IVIG therapy helped reduce the incidence of bacterial infections and prevented progression of chronic pulmonary disease as determined by pulmonary function tests and high-resolution computed tomography (CT).[21] Patients with diarrhea should also be evaluated for the presence of *Giardia lamblia*. For patients who develop autoimmune disease and require immunosuppressive therapy, it should be used with caution and given only for short periods of time.

## ATAXIA-TELANGIECTASIA

### Background, Epidemiology, and Pathogenesis

Ataxia-telangiectasia is an autosomal recessive disorder characterized by immune deficiency, progressive cerebellar ataxia, oculocutaneous telangiectasia, chromosome instability, predisposition to malignancy, and premature aging. Patients with ataxia-telangiectasia have a single gene mutation on chromosome 11 (ataxia-telangiectasia, mutated [*ATM*]). The prevalence is about 1 in 40,000. The ATM protein is involved in mitogenic signal transduction, intracellular protein transport, and cell cycle control. In the absence of functional ATM, the cell cycle does not stop for repair of double-stranded DNA breaks, such as those caused by V(D)J recombination of immunoglobulin and T-cell receptor genes, interfering with appropriate B- and T-lymphocyte maturation.

There are variable degrees of immune deficiency secondary to ATM deficiency that involves both the humoral and cellular compartments. Although the most common deficiencies of cell-mediated immune function are lymphopenia with diminished numbers of CD4 T cells and impaired lymphoproliferative responses to mitogens and antigens, there is often a defect in B-cell maturation in some patients, which leads to hypogammaglobulinemia.

### Clinical Manifestations and Diagnosis

Neurologic sequela are the most dramatic manifestation, with most affected patients displaying deterioration of fine and gross motor skills by age 7 years. Most are confined to wheelchairs by the second decade of life. Recurrent otitis media, sinusitis, bronchitis, and pneumonia are common infections in patients with ataxia-telangiectasia, and the incidence of lower respiratory tract infections increases with age as the risk for aspiration increases due to the progression of chewing and swallowing difficulties over time. Clinical findings can include clubbing of the digits and bronchiectasis in patients with chronic pulmonary damage. The major cause of death in patients is bacterial pneumonia and chronic lung disease, followed by cancer, most commonly non-Hodgkin lymphoma.

In a study evaluating immunodeficiency in 100 patients with ataxia-telangiectasia, immunoglobulin deficiencies and lymphopenia were common.[22] Many patients had low or absent levels of IgA, IgE, or IgG subclasses, particularly IgG2 and IgG4. Some had elevated serum immunoglobulin levels; IgM was elevated in 26%, IgG in 13%, and IgA in 7%. Lymphopenia was found in

71% of patients, with reduced B lymphocytes in 75%, CD4 T lymphocytes in 69%, and CD8 T lymphocytes in 51%. Despite the wide-ranging immune deficiencies seen in patients with ataxia-telangiectasia, it is uncommon for them to develop sepsis, severe viral infections, or opportunistic infections.

### Management

Immune function needs to be carefully evaluated and monitored. As with most other disorders, prompt treatment of infections and supportive care are the mainstays of therapy. Intravenous immunoglobulin has been used in patients with hypogammaglobulinemia and antibody deficiency. Unfortunately, most patients die in the second or third decade of life either due to pneumonia or malignancy.

## COMPLEMENT PROTEIN DEFICIENCIES

The complement system has been traditionally divided into the classical pathway (so named because it was the first pathway discovered) and the alternative pathway. In general, patients with a complement defect can be stratified into 1 of 4 different categories: (1) those with defects in factors involved in the early steps of the pathway usually present with a lupus-like or vasculitic process; (2) those patients with defects in factors involved in the late steps of the pathway typically present with recurrent or disseminated *Neisseria* infection; (3) those with a specific deficiency in mannose-binding lectin are prone to lupus and recurrent infections in childhood and infancy; and (4) those with a specific C3 deficiency have an increased incidence of both infections and collagen vascular disorders. Although these defects are typically congenital (or primary), they can also be acquired (or secondary) and contribute to about 2% of the overall number of primary immunodeficiency disorders.

### Primary Complement Deficiencies

Primary complement deficiencies are inherited and present with either lupus-like disease, recurrent or disseminated *Neisseria* infections, or features of both. Defects in the early classical pathway components includes factors C1, C2, and C4 of the classical pathway and factors B, D, and P of the alternative pathway. Depending on which complement component is defective, patients can develop lupus-like diseases ranging from typical SLE to an ANA-negative SLE-like illness to true SLE without systemic manifestations. Deficiencies in the late complement components, C5–C9, typically present with infections caused by *Neisseria* spp, such as gonococcal arthritis, recurrent meningococcal meningitis, or gonococcemia. Several studies have shown that about 15% of patients with systemic meningococcal disease have deficiencies of C5–C9 complements.[23] Because patients with selective C9 deficiency retain some complement titers, these patients are less susceptible to infections with *Neisseria* spp. Deficiencies in the mannose-binding lectin pathway are not discussed in detail because the infectious complications primarily occur in the preadolescent years. Finally, deficiency in C3 tends to result in collagen vascular disease and susceptibility to recurrent infections. This is due to the dual role of C3 as a facilitator of the clearance of immune complexes in the blood and as an opsonin, critical in the activation of the membrane attack complex, a complex that is ultimately required for bacteriolysis in the classical and alternative pathways.[2]

Hereditary angioedema is an autosomal dominant disorder due to the absence of C1 inhibitor (C1 INH). Interestingly, it is not associated with a lupus-like syndrome or an increased incidence of infections. The majority of patients with this disorder have decreased levels of C1 INH, with a subgroup of patients having a normal level of a nonfunctional C1 INH. In the absence of C1 INH, uncontrolled C1 activity leads to catabolism of C4 and C2, as well as the consequent release of a vasoactive peptide called "kinin" that causes episodic swelling of the hands, abdomen, or other body parts. Swelling is usually not associated with pruritus, erythema, or urticaria. Episodes typically last 1–3 days and may be precipitated by trauma, menses, or emotional stress. Although episodes may initially occur early in life, they tend to increase in severity in the teenage years. Diagnosis is made by measuring a diminished or absent level of nonfunctional C1 INH, although as discussed previously, a minority of patients (~15%–20%) may have a normal or elevated level of C1 INH. The latter group may have an abnormally functioning C1 INH, which can be determined by a functional assay.

### Acquired Complement Deficiencies

Many diseases that are encountered by the adolescent practitioner can cause an acquired complement disorder. Membranoproliferative glomerulonephritis results in the production of nephritic factor, which can activate the alternative pathway and lead to increased consumption of C3. Patients with anorexia nervosa or malnutrition often have significantly decreased activity of complement, not only due to decreased synthesis of complement factors, but also as a consequence of increased depletion. Patients with liver cirrhosis may have decreased synthesis of C3. Furthermore, disorders associated with immune complex formation such as endocarditis, infectious mononucleosis, malaria, and acute hepatitis B have been known to cause a consumption of complement components. Unidentified defects in the alternative pathway have been described in about 10% of patients who are asplenic or have beta-thalassemia.[23] Finally, individuals with nephrotic syndrome have been shown to have decreased serum opsonizing activity. Although most cases of C1 INH deficiency are hereditary, acquired forms have been seen in patients with SLE, glomerulonephritis, autoantibodies to C1 INH, and B-cell cancers.[23]

***Diagnosis*** Patients with any of the previous suspected disorders, those who have had severe or recurrent encapsulated bacterial or gonococcal infections, or those with lupus-like illness/immune complex disease should have their serum total hemolytic complement activity (CH50) measured. If this is normal, measurement of the alternative pathway activity can be assessed with an AH50. If either the CH50 or AH50 are abnormal, analysis of the concentration of specific complement components should be performed.

***Management*** Treatment for the primary disorders is limited, and care should be directed toward prevention. In addition to the avoidance of precipitating factors, hereditary angioedema has been treated effectively with a C1 INH concentrate, which has shown to be helpful in aborting acute attacks and as a means for long-term prophylaxis.[2] Although other primary disorders have no true therapy, emphasis on prevention strategies and heightened awareness of disease processes (ie, infections and vasculitis) can greatly benefit the patient. Patients, as well as their family members, should be strongly encouraged to be vaccinated against *H influenzae*, *N meningitidis*, and *S pneumoniae*. A greater awareness by both patients and their practitioners for the increased susceptibility toward infections and collagen vascular diseases can increase the vigilance for the development of these processes during times of illness or hospitalization.

**Box 153-1**

***Primary Immunodeficiency Resources***

**Immune Deficiency Foundation**
40 West Chesapeake Avenue, Suite 308
Towson, MD 21204
(800) 296-4433
www.primaryimmune.org

**National Institute of Allergies and Infectious Diseases (NIAID)**
NIAID Office of Communications and Government Relations
6610 Rockledge Drive, MSC 6612
Bethesda, MD 20892-6612
(301) 496-5717
www.niaid.nih.gov

**International Patient Organisation for Primary Immunodeficiencies (located in the UK)**
(+44) 01503 250 668
www.ipopi.org

**Jeffrey Modell Foundation**
747 Third Avenue
New York, New York 10017
(212) 819-0200/(800) JEFF-844
www.jmfworld. com

## RECURRENT CENTRAL NERVOUS SYSTEM OR DISSEMINATED INFECTIONS

Although uncommon, clinicians may encounter a patient with recurrent meningitis, typically viral or bacterial. The most common etiology of recurrent bacterial meningitis is *S pneumoniae*, followed by *N meningitides*. Recurrent bacterial meningitis is often due to a congenital defect in the bony or meningeal architecture surrounding the brain. Many patients may have a history of head trauma and subsequent development of a cerebrospinal fluid leak. Some patients may have a parameningeal focus that predisposes them to recurrent meningitis. This includes an infected intraventricular shunt, sinusitis, mastoiditis, or an infected dermoid sinus. Anatomic or structural abnormalities are also seen in patients with recurrent brain abscesses.[1] Patients should have a head CT scan and consultation with a neurosurgeon to better identify and correct these causes.

Primary immunological defects that increase a patient's risk of recurrent bacterial meningitis include complement deficiencies, hypogammaglobulinemia, and congenital asplenia. As discussed previously, deficiency in terminal complement factors is classically associated with recurrent meningococcal meningitis, and immunoglobulin deficiency predisposes the individual to infection with encapsulated organisms. HIV and malignancies are secondary immunodeficiencies that can similarly predispose patients to recurrent meningitis.

Finally, recurrent viral meningitis is seen in patients with Mollaret meningitis and in those with XLA. Mollaret meningitis, classically presenting in the adolescent years, is a viral meningitis typically due to recurrent genital herpes simplex virus infection. Immunocompetent patients with this disorder have rapid recovery and resolution without significant sequelae. Consideration should be given to prophylaxis with antiviral agents if recurrence is frequent. X-linked agammaglobulinemia is a rare antibody deficiency syndrome that usually presents by infancy with recurrent sinopulmonary infections and invasive disease such as bacteremia and meningitis. Although most of the infections in these patients are due to encapsulated bacteria, they commonly have severe and chronic meningoencephalitis secondary to enterovirus. Patients are treated regularly with IVIG to maintain adequate IgG levels, and they may need higher doses in the setting of chronic enteroviral meningoencephalitis.

In general, the adolescent with recurrent infection rarely has an identifiable immune defect. More commonly, recurrent infections in this age group are due to anatomical defects or are acquired immunodeficiencies. However, a working knowledge of the previously listed most commonly encountered primary immunodeficiencies in adolescents can help the practitioner arrive at a timely diagnosis so that specialty referral and treatment, if needed, can be started as soon as possible. Furthermore, knowledge of some of the immunodeficiencies that present earlier in life will be necessary for the practitioner so that he or she can help manage and care for these patients in adolescence and beyond. For practitioners, their patients, and families, a brief listing of available resources is provided in Box 153-1.

## REFERENCES

1. Avery RK, Pasternack MS. Approach to the adult patient with recurrent infections. *Cleve Clin J Med.* 1997;64(5):249–257

2. O'Neil KM, Ballow M. Approach to the patient with recurrent infections. In: Adkinson NF, Yunginger JW, Busse WW, Bochner BS, Holgate, ST, Simons FE, eds. *Middleton's Allergy Principles and Practice.* Saint Louis, MO: Mosby; 2003

3. Simor AE, Phillips E, McGeer A. Randomized controlled trial of chlorhexidine gluconate for washing, intranasal mupirocin, and rifampin and doxycyline versus no treatment for the eradication of methicillin-resistant *Staphylococcus aureus* colonization. *Clin Infect Dis.* 2007;44:178–185

4. Antachopoulos C, Walsh TJ, Roilides E. Fungal infections in primary immunodeficiencies. *Eur J Pediatr.* 2007;166:1099–1117

5. Kirkpatrick CH. Chronic mucocutaneous candidiasis. *Pediatr Infect Dis J.* 2001;20:197–206

6. Ahonen P, Myllarniemi S, Sipila I, Perheentupa J. Clinical variation of autoimmune polyendocrinopathy-candidiasis-ectodermal dystrophy (APECED) in a series of 68 patients. *N Engl J Med.* 1990;322:1829–1836

7. Grimbacher B, Holland SM, Gallin JI, et al. Hyper-IgE syndrome with recurrent infections—an autosomal dominant multisystem disorder. *N Engl J Med.* 1999;340:692–702

8. Rosenzweig SD, Holland SM. Phagocyte immunodeficiencies and their infections. *J Allergy Clin Immunol.* 2004;113:620–626

9. Marciano BE, Wesley R, De Carlo ES, et al. Long-term interferon-gamma therapy for patients with chronic granulomatous disease. *Clin Infect Dis.* 2004;39:692–699

10. Boxer LA. The immunologic system and disorders: disorders of phagocyte function. In: Behrman RE, Kliegman RM, Jenson HB, eds. *Nelson Textbook of Pediatrics.* Philadelphia: WB Saunders; 2004

11. Parry MF, Root RK, Metcalf JA, Delaney KK, Kaplow LS, Richar WJ. Myeloperoxidase deficiency and other enzymatic WBC defects causing immunodeficiency. *Ann Intern Med.* 1981;95(3):293–301

12. Segal GB. Diseases of the blood: enzymatic defects. In: Behrman RE, Kliegman RM, Jenson HB, eds. *Nelson Textbook of Pediatrics.* Philadelphia: WB Saunders; 2004

13. Pichichero M. Streptococcal pharyngitis: sore throat after sore throat after sore throat. Are you asking the critical questions? *Postgrad Med.* 1997;101:205–206, 209–212, 215–218

14. Stiehm ER, Ochs HD, Winkelstein JA. *Immunologic Disorders in Infants and Children.* 5th ed. Philadelphia: Elsevier Saunders; 2004

15. Sullivan KE. Chromosome 22q11.2 deletion syndrome: DiGeorge syndrome/velocardiofacial syndrome. *Immunol Allergy Clin North Am.* 2008;28:353–366

16. Kar PS, Poole R, Meeking D. DiGeorge syndrome presenting with hypocalcaemia in adulthood: two case reports and a review. *J Clin Pathol.* 2005;58:655–657

17. Meini A, Pillan NM, Villanacci V, Monafo V, Ugazio AG, Plebani A. Prevalence and diagnosis of celiac disease in IgA-deficient children. *Ann Allergy Asthma Immunol.* 1996;77:333–336

18. Finocchi A, Angelini F, Chini L, et al. Evaluation of the relevance of humoral immunodeficiencies in a pediatric population affected by recurrent infections. *Pediatr Allergy Immunol.* 2002;13:443–447

19. Ozkan H, Atlihan F, Genel F, Targan S, Gunvar T. IgA and/or IgG subclass deficiency in children with recurrent respiratory infections and its relationship with chronic pulmonary damage. *J Investig Allergol Clin Immunol.* 2005;15:69–74

20. Cunningham-Rundle C, Bodian C. Common variable immunodeficiency: clinical and immunological features of 248 patients. *Clin Immunol.* 1999;92:34–48

21. de Gracia J, Vendrell M, Alvarez A, et al. Immunoglobulin therapy to control lung damage in patients with common variable immunodeficiency. *Int Immunopharmacol.* 2004;4:745–753

22. Nowak-Wegryzyn A, Crawford TO, Winkelstein JA, Carson KA, Lederman HM. Immunodeficiency and infections in ataxia-telangiectasia. *J Pediatr.* 2004;144:505–511

23. Johnston RB Jr. The immunologic system and disorders: disorders of the complement system. In: Behrman RE, Kliegman RM, Jenson HB, eds. *Nelson Textbook of Pediatrics.* Philadelphia: WB Saunders; 2004

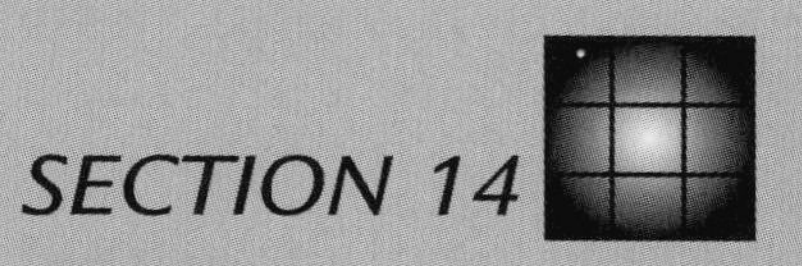

SECTION 14

# Disorders of the Eyes, Ears, Nose, and Throat

## CHAPTER 154

## Eye Disorders

DENISE HUG, MD • SCOTT E. OLITSKY, MD • LAURA PLUMMER, MD

### THE BASIC EYE EXAMINATION

The basic eye examination, whether done by the primary physician or an ophthalmologist, generally includes a measurement of visual acuity, evaluation of the visual field, assessment of the pupils, ocular motility and alignment, general external eye examination, and ophthalmoscopic examination of the fundi.

#### VISUAL ACUITY

The visual acuity should be checked as a routine part of any eye examination. Each eye should be tested separately. When evaluating an eye that has been injured, measurement of the visual acuity is important regardless of the severity of the injury. If the patient is unable to see a chart, the ability to count fingers, see the movement of a hand, or perceive light should be noted.

#### VISUAL FIELD ASSESSMENT

Using a confrontational visual field, a gross measurement of the visual field can be obtained and can detect diagnostically significant changes such as the bitemporal hemianopia of a chiasmal lesion or the homonymous hemianopia of a cerebral lesion.

#### PUPILLARY EXAMINATION

The size and symmetry of the pupils are noted. The pupils should be examined for direct and consensual reaction to light. The swinging flashlight test is an important objective test that is useful for detecting unilateral or asymmetric optic nerve defects (Marcus Gunn pupil).

#### OCULAR MOTILITY

Alignment of the eyes and the movements of each eye individually (ductions) and of the 2 eyes together (versions and vergences) should be assessed. The corneal light reflex test is a rapid and easy method to evaluate ocular alignment. The examiner projects a light source onto the cornea of both eyes simultaneously as the patient is asked to look directly at the light. Comparison is then made of the placement of the corneal light reflex in each eye. If the eyes are straight, the light reflection appears symmetric. If strabismus is present, the reflected light is asymmetric and appears off-center in one eye.

#### EXTERNAL EXAMINATION

The external examination starts with general inspection of the eye and its surrounding anatomy. The examiner notes the size, shape, and symmetry of the orbits, position and movement of the eyelids, and the position and symmetry of the globes. The lids and conjunctiva are examined for signs of inflammation. The anterior segment of the eye is evaluated making note of the luster and clarity of the cornea, the depth and clarity of the anterior chamber, and features of the iris. Fluorescein dye can be instilled onto the surface of the eye to help in diagnosing abrasions, ulcerations, and foreign bodies. Biomicroscopy (slit lamp examination) provides a highly magnified view of the structures of the eye. It also provides a cross-sectional view through the cornea, aqueous humor, lens, and vitreous. Lesions can be identified and localized according to their depth within each of the structures.

### FUNDUS EXAMINATION

The fundus examination (ophthalmoscopy) is best done with the pupil dilated. The posterior landmarks, the disc and macula, as well as retinal arteries and veins are examined.

## ABNORMALITIES OF REFRACTION

Emmetropia is the ideal refractive state. This occurs when parallel rays of light travel through the cornea and lens and come to focus on the retina when the eye is not accommodating. Although emmetropia occurs in a large number of people, a less than ideal refractive state (ametropia) frequently occurs. Three principal types of refractive errors occur: hyperopia (farsightedness), myopia (nearsightedness), and astigmatism. Most children are born slightly hyperopic. Their hyperopia decreases as the axial length of the eye grows through childhood. If the eye continues to grow, myopia may develop and is common in teenagers.

Measurement of the refractive state of the eye (refraction) can be accomplished objectively and subjectively. The objective method involves using a beam of light from a retinoscope and focusing it on the patient's retina with lenses of various powers. This method can be carried out at any age. In most adolescents, a subjective refraction can be performed. This involves placing various lenses in front of the eye and having the patient report which lenses provide the clearest vision.

### HYPEROPIA

If parallel rays of light come to focus posterior to the retina, hyperopia exists. This may occur if the anterior–posterior diameter of the eye is too short or if the refractive power of the cornea or lens is less than normal. Patients who are hyperopic use accommodation (focusing) to bring objects into focus when viewing distance and near objects. Low levels of hyperopia do not require treatment. With high degrees of hyperopia, greater accommodative effort is needed and the patient may complain of blurred vision or eyestrain. Glasses or contact lenses may be prescribed when indicated.

### MYOPIA

When parallel rays of light are brought to focus anterior to the retina, myopia is present. This most commonly occurs secondary to the anterior–posterior diameter of the eye being too long. It can also occur if the refractive power of the cornea or lens is greater than normal. The most common symptom of myopia is blurred vision for distant objects. The far point of clear vision varies inversely with the degree of myopia. Myopia generally starts to increase after 6 to 7 years of age and continues to increase throughout the teenage years as the posterior segment of the eye grows. Although a few medications have shown some efficacy in slowing the progression of myopia, none have gained widespread use. As the myopia increases, the far point of clear vision moves closer to the patient. Squinting is common and improves the vision by allowing fewer rays of light to enter the eye requiring focusing. The effect is similar to that achieved by closing down the aperture of the diaphragm of a camera. When the level of myopia is high enough to warrant treatment, glasses or contact lenses are prescribed. Contact lenses may be used at almost any age. Most ophthalmologists suggest that they are most appropriate for the treatment of myopia when the child begins to express an interest in them and when they can properly care for them. For most children, this occurs in the early teen years. Refractive surgery may also be an option for some patients. Because refractive surgery does not prevent further growth of the eye, it is usually only considered when the refractive error has stabilized and no further growth is expected. This generally takes place during the late teen years. The age varies for each person but often occurs between the ages of 16 and 18. Refractive surgery is currently Food and Drug Administration (FDA) approved for patients over the age of 18.

### ASTIGMATISM

In astigmatism, the refractive power of the eye varies in different meridians. Most cases are caused by an irregularity in the curvature of the cornea, although some cases may occur due to changes in the lens. Significant levels of astigmatism can cause blurring of vision at near and far distances. Astigmatism may be corrected with glasses and contact lenses.

## DISORDERS OF VISION

### AMBLYOPIA

Amblyopia is a decrease in visual acuity, unilateral or bilateral, that develops in visually immature children as a result of a lack of a clear image falling upon the retina. Although uncommon in adolescents, amblyopia may develop secondary to a deviated eye, an unequal need for vision correction between the eyes, an abnormally high refractive error in both eyes, or a media opacity within the visual axis. Amblyopia develops during the first decade of life and is generally treated by forcing the poorer seeing eye to be used with either a patch or drops.[1] Recent studies have shown that treatment can be successful in teenagers who may have developed amblyopia as young children but were never treated for it.[2]

### DIPLOPIA

Diplopia, double vision, is most often a result of a misalignment of the eyes (binocular diplopia). Cases of monocular diplopia are caused by an optical defect such as a cataract or uncorrected refractive error. Occluding one eye eliminates the diplopia and affected patients may close one eye to relieve the bothersome symptom of seeing double. Diplopia that does not disappear by closing either eye (monocular diplopia) is not due to a misalignment of the eyes. Monocular diplopia may be caused by astigmatism, disorders of the pupil, or changes in the lens such as dislocation or cataract.

### AMAUROSIS

Amaurosis is partial or total loss of vision. It is used to describe profound visual impairment, blindness, or near blindness. Amaurosis that develops in an adolescent who once had useful vision may have serious implications. In the absence of obvious ocular disease (cataract, uveitis, retinal disorders), consideration should include many neurologic and systemic disorders that can affect the visual pathway. If the amaurosis develops rapidly, it may indicate encephalopathy, demyelinating disease, vasculitis, migraine, toxins, or trauma. A more slowly progressive loss of vision suggests a tumor or neurodegenerative disorder. Amaurosis should prompt a thorough ophthalmic evaluation and further diagnostic work-up as needed.

### FUNCTIONAL VISION LOSS

In functional vision loss, conversion reactions and willful feigning are frequently encountered. The usual presentation is a complaint of reduced vision in one or both eyes. In most cases discrepancies between the symptoms and the findings during a thorough examination raise the suspicion of the examiner. Using various techniques, it is generally possible to document a visual acuity that is better than that which was first claimed. Most patients fare well with reassurance and positive suggestion. If the functional vision loss persists, psychologic consultation may be helpful.

## STRABISMUS

Strabismus, a misalignment of the eyes, occurs in many children and may persist or present during the teenage years. For diagnostic and therapeutic reasons, strabismus can be divided into comitant and incomitant forms. In comitant strabismus, the deviation of the eyes remains the same regardless of the position of gaze. In incomitant strabismus, the deviation changes as the position of the eyes change. Patients may be able to place their eyes into a position of alignment to eliminate their diplopia, causing an abnormal head posture to develop.

### NONPARALYTIC STRABISMUS

#### Esotropia

Esotropia is a convergent strabismus ("cross eye") that typically develops early in life. Congenital esotropia describes the form of esotropia that develops within the first 6 months of life and requires surgical correction. Many children with congenital esotropia display unstable ocular alignment and may require additional surgeries throughout their life. Accommodative esotropia is a convergent deviation associated with activation of the accommodative (focusing) reflex. It generally occurs in children with high levels of hyperopia who cross their eyes because of the effort needed to see well. Glasses or contact lenses eliminate the need to accommodate and are used to maintain normal alignment. Hyperopia begins to decrease after the age of 7 and will continue to lessen during the teenage years. If a child is only moderately hyperopic, he or she may lose enough farsightedness to no longer need to focus to see well and will therefore outgrow the need for corrective lenses.

#### Exotropia

Exotropia is a divergent form of strabismus ("walleye") that commonly occurs in teenagers. Intermittent exotropia is the most common type of exotropia. It is characterized by an outward drifting of one eye. Early in the disease process, the drifting usually occurs when the patient is tired. With time, the deviation becomes more frequent and may eventually become constant if not treated. Surgery is usually required once the deviation begins to worsen.

### PARALYTIC STRABISMUS

Paralytic strabismus represents an important type of incomitant strabismus. A paralytic strabismus will demonstrate a deviation that is greatest when the patient is asked to look into the field of gaze of the affected muscle(s). Paralytic strabismus may be congenital or acquired due to trauma, systemic disease, or neurologic abnormalities such as a brain tumor.

#### Third Nerve Palsy

In a third nerve palsy, only the lateral rectus and superior oblique muscles continue to function. This results in an exotropia and an associated downward deviation of the eye along with an inability to adduct, elevate, or depress the eye. There may also be a complete or partial ptosis of the upper eyelid. If the internal branch of the third nerve is involved, the pupil may be dilated. A newly acquired third nerve palsy should be considered a neurologic emergency and be referred for further evaluation and treatment of a possible brain tumor or aneurysm.

**Fourth Nerve Palsy**

This type of palsy can be congenital or acquired. Closed head trauma is the most common cause for an acquired palsy. A weakness of the fourth nerve results in an upward deviation of the eye, which may be controlled with a compensatory head posture that includes a head tilt and face turn away from the affected eye.

**Sixth Nerve Palsy**

A sixth nerve palsy produces markedly crossed eyes with limited ability to move the affected eye(s) laterally. Patients may present with their head turned toward the palsied muscle. An acquired sixth nerve palsy is often an ominous sign because the sixth nerve is susceptible to increased intracranial pressure associated with intracranial tumors. Patients presenting with a new onset sixth nerve palsy should undergo neurologic evaluation promptly.

## DISORDERS OF THE EYELIDS

The eyelids can be affected by congenital and acquired abnormalities including infections, inflammatory conditions, positional changes, neoplastic processes, and trauma.

Congenital eyelid anomalies present early in life and thus are not diagnosed in adolescence but persist into the teen years. Ptosis refers to inferodisplacement of any anatomic structure. Blepharoptosis specifically refers to inferodisplacement of the upper eyelid and may be congenital or acquired (Figure 154-1). If congenital, there is a longstanding history of eyelid drooping, and vision may be reduced secondary to amblyopia. Congenital ptosis is most often due to levator maldevelopment but may be secondary to congenital third nerve palsy, or congenital Horner syndrome. Acquired ptosis may be due to various processes including neuromuscular dysfunction, neurologic defect, a mechanical reason, or trauma (Box 154-1). Ptosis treatment is most often surgical.

Additional eyelid anomalies include entropion (inversion of the eyelid) and ectropion (eversion of the eyelid). Entropion may be congenital or acquired secondary to spasticity or scarring because of ocular irritation or trauma. Ectropion may also be congenital as seen with blepharophimosis and ichthyosis or acquired due to paralytic, mechanical (mass or lesion), or traumatic causes. Severe ectropion results in exposure keratitis (corneal disease) and constant epiphora (tearing flowing down the face).

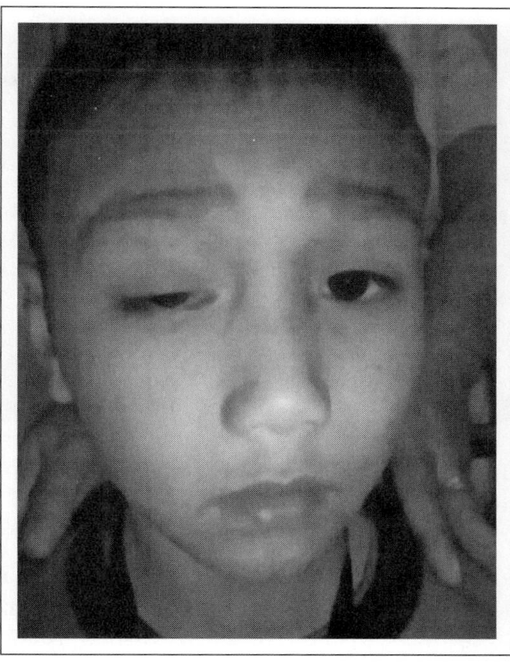

FIGURE 154-1 Congenital ptosis of the right upper eyelid due to levator maldevelopment. Note the lack of an eyelid crease and the use of the brows to elevate the lid. (Photo courtesy of Srinivas S. Iyengar, MD.) (See color insert.)

### Box 154-1

*Differential Diagnosis of Ptosis*

**Congenital ptosis**

- Levator muscle maldevelopment
- Horner syndrome
- Cranial nerve 3 palsy

**Acquired ptosis**

- Myogenic: muscular dystrophy, myasthenia gravis, progressive external ophthalmoplegia
- Neurogenic: cranial nerve 3 palsy, Horner syndrome, Marcus Gunn jaw wink
- Mechanical: neoplasm
- Traumatic: disinsertion of levator muscle

**Pseudoptosis**

- Enophthalmia
- Micro-/Anophthalmia
- Contralateral eyelid retraction

Common acquired eyelid abnormalities are chalazia and styes. A chalazion is a focal inflammatory process due to obstruction of the meibomian glands in the eyelid. (Figure 154-2) Treatment initially consists of

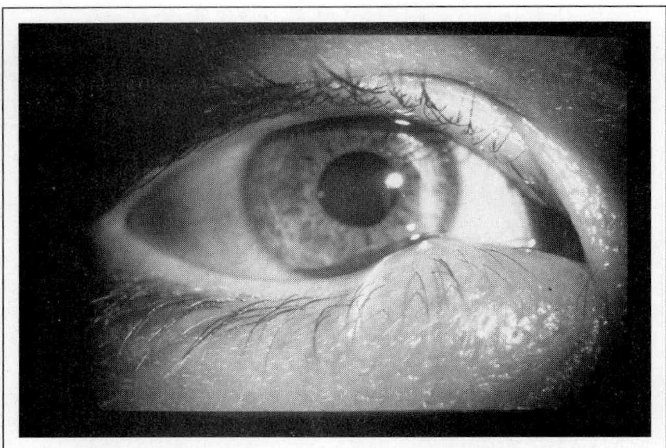

**FIGURE 154-2** Chalazion of the lower eyelid. (Photo courtesy of David Lyon, MD.) (See color insert.)

warm compresses and lid scrubs using baby shampoo diluted with 50% water. Some cases may require systemic doxycycline for suppression or if secondary bacterial infection is suspected. Chalazia that do not respond to lid hygiene therapy may require surgical intervention. Styes, involving either meibomian or the sebaceous glands of Zeis, are due to an infectious process, most often staphylococcal in origin. Spontaneous resolution is common but warm compresses and topical antibiotic therapy may also be used, such as topical bacitracin or erythromycin ointment. A stye may progress to cellulitis or an abscess requiring systemic antibiotics covering for staphylococcal organisms.

Trichiasis refers to misdirection of the eyelashes with treatment directed at removal of the offending lashes. Distichiasis refers to extra eyelashes that arise from the meibomian glands. This process may be congenital or due to chronic irritation and trauma. Treatment is only indicated if ocular surface irritation occurs.

Eyelid edema may be secondary to inflammation as with insect bites or allergic reactions, infection, trauma, or due to certain systemic disorders including renal disease Graves disease, and collagen vascular diseases. Blepharochalasis is a rare form of angioneurotic edema. It presents with recurrent idiopathic inflammation of the eyelids. It is most common in young females and results in thin, wrinkled eyelid skin due to the recurrent episodes.

Eyelid neoplasms that occur in adolescence include papillomas, benign epithelial cysts, nevi, basal cell carcinoma (especially in susceptible persons having Gorlin syndrome or xeroderma pigmentosum), and melanoma. Gorlin syndrome also is known as nevoid basal cell carcinoma syndrome, an autosomal-dominant disorder with basal cell carcinomas, broad facies, rib anomalies, among other abnormalities.

## DISORDERS OF THE CONJUNCTIVA

The conjunctiva is a thin tissue composed of connective tissue and blood vessels that covers the front of the eye.

Conjunctivitis is the term used when the eye appears red secondary to inflammation of the conjunctiva, regardless of the cause. The differential diagnosis of conjunctivitis in adolescents is extensive (Box 154-2). The etiology of conjunctivitis can be divided into infectious and noninfectious. The most common infectious causes of conjunctivitis are bacterial, viral, and chlamydia.

### BACTERIAL CONJUNCTIVAL INFECTIONS

Most bacterial conjunctival infections present in an acute manner with a sudden onset of a red eye and mucopurulent discharge. Common causative agents are: *Staphylococcus, Streptococcus, Haemophilus, Moraxella,* and *Neisseria* (Box 154-3). Diagnosis is by clinical presentation and appearance. Bacterial conjunctivitis is often self-limited but a course of broad- spectrum topical antibiotic drops is appropriate to shorten the course and decrease the severity of the conjunctivitis. Examples of topical antibiotics that can be used include gentamicin, polymyxin/trimethoprim, and moxifloxacin. A

**Box 154-2**

***Differential Diagnosis of the Red Eye***

Bacterial conjunctivitis
Viral conjunctivitis
Allergic conjunctivitis
Ocular surface foreign body
Toxic keratoconjunctivitis
Keratitis
Blepharitis
Uveitis: anterior/posterior
Scleritis
Endophthalmitis
Orbital cellulitis

**Box 154-3**

***Etiology of Bacterial Conjunctivitis***

*Streptococcus*: viridans, pneumonia
*Haemophilus* influenza
*Staphylococcus*: aureus, coagulase negative
*Moraxella* species
*Neisseria*: gonorrheae, meningitis
*Pseudomonas*

special mention of *N gonorrhea* should be made. The presentation is often hyperacute with eyelid swelling, conjunctival chemosis (swelling), and copious amount of purulent discharge. Preauricular lymphadenopathy is often present. This type of infection can rapidly progress to involve the cornea and in fact can penetrate the cornea leading to loss of the eye. Treatment should be done in conjunction with an ophthalmologist and involves topical as well as systemic modalities.

### VIRAL CONJUNCTIVITIS

Diagnosis of viral conjunctivitis is again based on clinical presentation. Signs and symptoms include: burning, tearing, foreign body sensation, red eye, conjunctival follicles, red/swollen eyelids, preauricular lymphadenopathy, and history of recent upper respiratory infection. Many different viruses cause conjunctivitis (Box 154-4), but adenovirus is a very common cause of acute conjunctivitis in the adolescent population. Clinically there are 2 main presentations: epidemic keratoconjunctivitis (EKC) and pharyngoconjunctival fever (PCF). Epidemic keratoconjunctivitis is highly contagious and tends to occur in epidemics, most commonly in fall and winter months. Clinical course involves unilateral onset of conjunctival hyperemia, preauricular lymphadenopathy, watery discharge, and foreign body sensation. The fellow eye often becomes involved within 5 days. Peak intensity of the conjunctivitis is 5 to 7 days. Clinical course usually lasts 2 to 3 weeks but may last longer in severe cases. Treatment is palliative. Because transmission is through direct and indirect contact with the infected individual, the patient should minimize personal contact for 2 weeks. Careful hygiene measures must be observed. Pharyngonconjunctival fever has a similar ocular course as EKC but is unilateral in almost all cases. The conjunctivitis is accompanied by fever and pharyngitis.

**Box 154-4**

***Etiology of Viral Conjunctivitis***

- Adenovirus
  - Epidemic keratoconjunctivitis
  - Pharyngoconjunctival fever
- Herpes virus
  - Herpes simplex virus
  - Herpes zoster virus
  - Epstein-Barr virus
- Paramyxovirus
  - Measles
  - Mumps
- Picornavirus
  - Enterovirus 70
  - Coxsackie A/B

#### Chlamydia

Unlike other infectious etiologies of conjunctivitis, chlamydia usually presents in a chronic manner with symptoms of redness, irritation, and stringy mucous discharge. Chlamydia is sexually transmitted by direct contact. In developing countries, chlamydia ocular infection is usually present in the form of trachoma. It is prevalent in areas with poor sanitation and overcrowding. Treatment with topical antibiotics is recommended, but systemic treatment with azithromycin or doxycycline is also necessary. Topical erythromycin ophthalmic ointment 3 times per day for 7 days in addition to azithromycin 1 g in a single dose or doxycycline orally twice per day for 7 days often is recommended. The sexual partners of the patient must also be treated.

### ALLERGIC CONJUNCTIVITIS

Allergic conjunctivitis usually presents with itching, watery discharge, and conjunctival hyperemia and often occurs with systemic allergic symptoms. Treatment includes: cool compresses, artificial tears, and topical antihistamine with mast cell stabilizer preparations (olopatadine, ketotifen). The patient may benefit from systemic antihistamines in severe cases.

### OTHER DISORDERS OF CONJUNCTIVA

#### Subconjunctival Hemorrhage

Subconjunctival hemorrhage manifests as a red area on the sclera. It can be very small to quite large, with larger hemorrhages often having a dark red, swollen appearance. No treatment needs to occur other than trying to establish the etiology. Most are idiopathic, traumatic, or related to Valsalva maneuver. If traumatic, mechanism of injury and presence of associated injury must be determined. More uncommonly, hemorrhages may be caused by hypertension or bleeding disorders.

#### Conjunctival Nevus

Conjunctival nevus often develops in childhood and adolescence. They are variable in size, location, and elevation. They are often pigmented but may be nonpigmented and appear pinkish. Growth of previously stable nevi may occur during adolescence. Conjunctival nevus should be followed because malignant transformation has been reported.

## DISORDERS OF THE CORNEA

The cornea is the clear window of the eye, and many issues including infections, injury, degeneration, and dystrophy may have a significant effect on the cornea. The best way to examine the cornea is with a biomicroscope, but an ophthalmoscope or Wood lamp also can be used. Fluorescein dye is very useful in examining the integrity of the corneal epithelium. A fluorescein strip should be moistened with sterile saline and gently applied to the internal surface of the lid. After instillation, the cornea should be inspected with the blue filter on the direct ophthalmoscope or with a Wood lamp. Abnormalities in the corneal surface will appear green against the blue background.

### HERPES SIMPLEX KERATITIS

Herpes simplex keratitis can cause serious, permanent decrease in vision. Clinical presentation includes unilateral photophobia, pain, tearing, conjunctival hyperemia, and corneal epithelial dendrite. A history of oral or genital ulceration is often present but not necessary. Treatment is with topical antiviral medication.[3] Recurrence of ocular herpes simplex virus (HSV) keratitis is common.[4]

### BACTERIAL CORNEAL ULCERS

Bacterial corneal ulcers threaten vision as well as the eye (Box 154-5). Clinical presentation includes unilateral red eye, pain, photophobia, and decreased vision with focal opacity in the cornea. Surrounding corneal edema (haziness) and hypopion (layered white blood cells in the anterior chamber) may be present. Contact lens wear, especially overnight wear, is a known risk factor for development of corneal ulcers. If a contact lens is present, removal is necessary followed by urgent referral to an ophthalmologist. Treatment includes corneal scraping for culture followed by intensive antibiotic treatment sometimes requiring hospitalization. The antibiotic used depends on the location, size, depth, and whether the infection is related to contact lens wear. If not deemed to be immediately vision threatening, moxifloxacin may be used every 1 to 2 hours with tobramycin ophthalmic ointment 4 times per day. If the infection is more serious, fortified ceftazidime and fortified vancomycin hourly is required. As always, antibiotics are guided by Gram stain and culture.

**Box 154-5**

***Etiology of Corneal Ulcer***

Bacterial: *Staphylococcus, Streptococcus, Pseudomonas, Serratia, Haemophilus, Moraxella*
Viral: HSV, HZV
Acanthamoeba
Fungal: fusarium, aspergillus candida
Neurotrophic
Exposure
Autoimmune: rheumatoid arthritis, Mooren

HSV, herpes simplex virus; HSZ, herpes zoster virus

### KERATOCONUS

Keratoconus is a bilateral, central thinning of the cornea. Onset or progression often occurs during the adolescent years. Patients present with the complaint of blurred vision secondary to the large amount astigmatism and myopia that is caused by the corneal thinning. Initial treatment is with glasses. Patients will progress to needing gas-permeable contact lenses when vision is not improved with glasses. In severe cases, corneal transplant is required.

Corneal manifestations of systemic disease are many and varied (Table 154-1).

## DISORDERS OF THE UVEAL TRACT

The uveal tract lines the inside of the eye and consists of the iris, ciliary body, and choroid. Uveitis is inflammation of the uveal tract. Uveitis is often divided into anterior, involving the iris and/or ciliary body, and posterior, involving the choroid, or panuveitis, involving all uveal structures.

**Table 154-1**

**Corneal Manifestations of Systemic Disease**

| *Disorder* | *Corneal Findings* |
|---|---|
| Tyrosinemia type II | Crystalline deposits |
| Alkaptunuria | Yellow-brown pigmentation at limbus |
| Cystinosis | Refractile corneal crystals |
| Hyperlipoproteinemia type II and III | Arcus (white ring at lumbus) |
| Hyperlipoproteinemia | Diffuse corneal clouding |
| MPS I-H, I-S, I-HS, II-B, IV | Diffuse corneal clouding |
| Mucolipidosis IV | Diffuse corneal clouding |
| Fabry | White-golden brown whorl opacities |
| GM, gangliosidosis type 1 | Mild, diffuse, corneal cloudy |
| Wilson | Brown ring at lumbus (Kayser-Fleischer ring) |
| Hypercalcemia | Band keratopathy |

MPS, mucopolysaccharidosis

### ACUTE ANTERIOR UVEITIS

Acute anterior uveitis presents with conjunctival hyperemia, photophobia, pain, and decreased vision. With a slit lamp examination, cells are seen in the anterior chamber, and inflammatory deposits might be seen on the corneal endothelium.[5] The etiology of anterior uveitis is extensive (Box 154-6), but the most common causes are trauma and idiopathic. Infectious and systemic causes must always be considered. Adolescents with juvenile rheumatoid arthritis can have significant asymptomatic iritis and require routine surveillance. Untreated or delayed treatment of inflammation can cause significant damage including: glaucoma, synechia, cataracts, band keratopathy, and phthisis. This in turn can lead to significant loss of vision. Treatment of the underlying etiology is necessary in addition to topical steroidal anti-inflammatories and cycloplegics. In some cases, systemic immunosuppression is required.

### POSTERIOR UVEITIS

Posterior uveitis presents with decreased vision. Floaters, redness, photophobia, and pain may be present. The etiology of posterior uveitis is again extensive (Box 154-7). The clinical course, treatment, and visual prognosis depends on the underlying etiology.

**Box 154-6**

***Etiology of Anterior Uveitis***

**Infections**
Herpes simplex virus
Herpes zoster virus
Lyme disease
Tuberculosis
Syphilis

**Inflammatory**
HLA-B27
Juvenile rheumatoid arthritis
Ankylosing spondylitis
Inflammatory bowel disease
Reiter syndrome
Psoriatic arthritis
Behçet disease
Kawasaki disease
Sarcoid

**Masquerading Syndromes**
Leukemia
Lymphoma
Intraocular tumor

**Trauma**
**Idiopathic**
**Medications**

**Box 154-7**

***Etiology of Posterior Uveitis***

**Infections**
- Toxoplasmosis
- Syphilis
- Ocular histoplasmosis
- CMV
- HSV
- Lyme disease
- Toxocara
- TB

**Inflammatory**
- Sarcoid
- Pars planitis (idiopathic inflammation in the area anterior to the retina)
- Behçet disease
- Vogt-Koyanagi-Harada syndrome (systemic disease including uveitis, alopecia, poliosis, hearing loss, headache, and seizure)

**Masquerading Syndromes**
- Leukemia
- Lymphoma
- Intraocular foreign body
- Intraocular tumor
- Retinal detachment

CMV, cytomegalovirus; HSV, herpes simplex virus; TB, tuberculosis

## DISORDERS OF THE LENS

The crystalline lens of the eye is a clear structure suspended just posterior to the iris.

### CATARACT

A cataract is any opacification of the lens. The opacification often leads to visual disturbance. The cause of cataracts in the adolescent population is extensive (Box 154-8). Trauma is a common etiology and can be secondary to a penetrating injury as well as a blunt injury. Sporadic and autosomal dominant are the most common inheritance patterns. Onset of presentation is quite variable from congenital to adolescence. The patient will present complaining of decreased vision. On examination of the red reflex with the direct ophthalmoscope, a dark spot, a white spot, or distortion will be noted in the pupil. Treatment should occur if there is a significant reduction in vision. Treatment requires surgical removal of the lens material to clear the visual axis. The resulting refractive error must be corrected.

**Box 154-8**

***Etiology of Adolescent Cataracts***

**Hereditary**
- Autosomal dominant
- Autosomal recessive
- X-linked
- Sporadic

**Metabolic**
- Diabetic mellitus
- Fabry disease
- Hypoglycemia
- Wilson disease
- Hypocalcemia

**Systemic Syndrome/Disease**
- Trisomy 21
- Alport syndrome
- Myotonic dystrophy
- Neurofibromatosis 2
- Intercontinental pigmenta
- Atopic dermatitis
- Cockayne syndrome
- Smith-Lemli-Opitz

**Ocular**
- Posterior lenticonus
- Uveitis
- Retinitis pigmentosa
- Aniridia
- Intraocular tumor

Intraocular lens implantation is the most common method of visual rehabilitation, but contact lenses or glasses may be used. Visual prognosis in adolescent cataracts is usually quite good. In the case of traumatic cataract, the prognosis depends on the accompanying injury.

### LENS DISLOCATION

Lens dislocation is the term used when the lens is not in its normal anatomic position. As mentioned, the lens is suspended behind the iris by the zonules from the ciliary body. When the zonules are disrupted, regardless of cause, the lens may move out of its normal anatomic position (subluxated). The patient presents with a complaint of blurred vision. Because of the shape of the natural lens, horizontal subluxation results in large amounts of myopia and astigmatism. In terms of etiology (Box 154-9), most conditions, except trauma, are bilateral, although the amount of subluxation may be asymmetric. Treatment initially involves optical correction with glasses or contact lenses. In some cases the dislocated lens causes vision-threatening complications such as glaucoma. If this occurs, prompt surgical removal of the lens is necessary. In addition, some patients require surgical removal of the lens for visual rehabilitation.

**Box 154-9**

***Etiology of Dislocated Lens***

**Inherited**
- Ectopia lentis
- Ectopia lentis et pupillae

**Systemic Disorder**
- Marfan syndrome
- Homocystinuria
- Weill-Marchesani syndrome
- Ehlers-Danlos syndrome

**Ocular Disorder**
- Aniridia
- Congenital glaucoma
- Microspherophakia

**Trauma**

## DISORDERS OF THE RETINA

Various metabolic disorders may cause retinal diseases that appear at or shortly after birth. Retinitis pigmentosa (RP) is a group of hereditary disorders affecting retinal function, leading to progressive night blindness, visual field loss, and loss of central visual acuity. Retinitis pigmentosa may be isolated or associated with systemic abnormalities. Congenital retinal disorders will typically limit vision early in life with a possible secondary nystagmus. Those progressing in adolescence will be associated with complaints of vision loss or night vision problems.

Acquired retinal disorders affecting adolescents include retinal vascular diseases such as diabetic, hypertensive, and sickle cell retinopathies. Adolescents with these systemic diseases require at least yearly dilated eye examinations combined with good systemic control in an effort to provide the best visual outcome possible.[6] In addition, hereditary retinal and choroidal dystrophies may lead to reduced vision. Symptomatic onset varies with the disorder.

## DISORDERS OF THE OPTIC NERVE

### PAPILLEDEMA

Papilledema is, by definition, optic nerve elevation and swelling secondary to increased intracranial

**Box 154-10**

***Differential Diagnosis of Optic Nerve Elevation***

Papilledema
Optic neuritis
Diabetic papillitis
Malignant hypertension
Infiltrative optic neuropathy
Leber optic neuropathy
Ischemic optic neuropathy

pressure (Box 154-10). Presenting symptoms include transient episodes of visual loss often related to postural change, headache, nausea, vomiting, and diplopia. When a patient has increased intracranial pressure without intracranial mass or hydrocephalus, the patient is classified as having pseudotumor cerebri. The etiology of pseudotumor cerebri may be idiopathic or secondary (Box 154-11). Idiopathic intracranial hypertension in pubescent and postpubescent children tends to have a female preponderance and be related to obesity. If papilledema is suspected a complete history, physical, and ocular examination must be performed. Urgent neuroimaging should be obtained followed by lumbar puncture with opening pressure, if no mass is present. Treatment is dictated by underlying etiology. If pseudotumor cerebri is present, treatment may include: weight loss, acetazolamide, systemic steroids, optic nerve sheath decompression, or lumboperitoneal shunt. The patient must be monitored carefully by an ophthalmologist to try to prevent permanent vision loss.

**Box 154-11**

***Etiology of Pseudotumor Cerebri***

**Idiopathic**
**Secondary**

- Dural sinus thrombosis
- Medications: oral contraceptives, tetracyclines, nalidixic acid, cyclosporine, vitamin A, somatotropin, and systemic steroid withdrawal
- Malnutrition
- Anemia
- Addison disease
- Meningitis

## OPTIC NEURITIS

Optic neuritis is caused by inflammation of the optic nerve. The signs and symptoms involve decrease in vision, orbital pain, pain with eye movement, and decreased color vision. Optic neuritis is usually unilateral but may be bilateral. The typical course of optic neuritis is that of rapid loss of vision followed by a slow visual recovery.[7,8] The etiology is variable (Box 154-12) but in the adolescent population, the greatest concern is that of multiple sclerosis. Chapter 130, Demyelinating Diseases, discusses multiple sclerosis in depth. Magnetic resonance imaging (MRI) is recommended to look for periventricular plaques. If at least one area of brain demyelination is present, pulse intravenous steroids followed by oral steroids is recommended.[6,9] With a normal MRI the same treatment may be recommended in an attempt to hasten visual recovery.[7]

## OPTIC ATROPHY

Optic atrophy refers to the death of the retinal ganglion cells that come together to form the optic nerve. This causes a painless, permanent loss of vision that may be unilateral or bilateral depending on the etiology. Initially, the optic nerve may appear swollen or normal. With time, the optic nerve becomes pale. The main inherited forms of optic atrophy are dominant optic atrophy and Leber optic neuropathy. Leber optic neuropathy is transmitted by mitochondrial DNA so it usually affects adolescent to young adult males. Because the disease is transmitted by mitochondrial DNA, it is passed by mothers to all offspring. Fifty percent to 70% of sons and 10% to 15% of daughters manifest the disease. Daughters are carriers, yet sons

**Box 154-12**

***Etiology of Optic Neuritis***

Idiopathic
Multiple sclerosis
Infectious/postinfectious
- Measles
- Mumps
- Chicken pox
- Lyme disease
- Infectious mononucleosis
- Cat scratch disease

Inflammatory
- Sarcoidosis
- Systemic lupus

cannot transmit the disease. Rapid loss of vision occurs in one eye followed by the second eye, usually within days. Toxic/nutritional optic neuropathies are also usually bilateral. The causative agents include: thiamine deficiency, $B_{12}$ deficiency, methanol, ethambutol, isoniazid, chloroquine, lead, and radiation. Treatment involves exploring for pernicious anemia, malabsorption disorders, eating disorders, and alcoholism. Compressive optic neuropathies can be bilateral or unilateral depending on the location of the compression. The loss of vision is usually gradual. Two of the more common compressive lesions in adolescents are visual pathway glioma and craniopharyngioma. A full discussion of craniopharyngioma may be found in Chapter 70, Disorders of Puberty. One of the most common causes of optic atrophy in adolescents is traumatic optic neuropathy. This can be caused by penetrating or blunt trauma to the periorbital area. Treatment is controversial, but many practitioners use high-dose steroids within 24 hours of injury.

## DISORDERS OF THE ORBIT

When evaluating orbital processes it is important to distinguish between a true orbital and a periorbital disorder. Important history and physical items are type of onset, duration of symptoms, presence of systemic illness or sinus disease, and associated trauma.

Congenital orbital anomalies are apparent very early in life and may persist into adolescence. Anophthalmos is the absence of the eye or often the presence of a small ocular remnant. Orbital expansion conformers are used early in life to promote orbital growth and prevent asymmetric orbits. Microphthalmos is the presence of a small, disorganized eye. The size of the eye may vary, with the same secondary hypoplastic orbit possible. Craniofacial clefting syndromes that affect the orbit and eyelids include midline clefting abnormalities, mandibulofacial dysostosis (Treacher Collins-Franceschetti syndrome), and oculoauricular dysplasia (Goldenhar syndrome). In addition, craniosynostosis syndromes, such as the Crouzon and Apert syndromes result in orbital abnormalities including shallow orbits and exorbitism (lateral displacement of the lateral orbital walls). Amblyopia and strabismus are important ocular consequences of these syndromes observed into adolescence.

Proptosis refers to the forward displacement of any anatomical structure and is used to describe protrusion of the eye. The many causes of proptosis vary in frequency according to age (Box 154-13).

### Box 154-13

#### *Differential Diagnosis of Proptosis*

- Graves disease (thyroid ophthalmopathy)
- Lymphoma/leukemia
- Idiopathic orbital inflammatory disease (orbital pseudotumor)
- Vasculitis
- Solid tumor
- Orbital cellulitis
- Fibrous dysplasia
- Pseudoproptosis

Orbital cellulitis is a bacterial infection of the orbital and periorbital regions, most commonly resulting from direct extension from an adjacent sinusitis. It may also occur via direct infection or trauma and even from distant spread such as from otitis media or pneumonia. Distinction between orbital and preseptal cellulitis is clinically important. Preseptal refers to infection of the periorbital and eyelid region anterior to the orbital septum. If no direct site of infection is noted on exam, investigation is indicated with a computed tomographic (CT) scan of the orbit and sinuses. Preseptal cellulitis in adolescents typically results from a superficial source and responds well to oral antibiotics. Orbital cellulitis often results from chronic bacterial sinusitis. Orbital cellulitis is generally treated with intravenous antibiotics covering gram-positive, gram-negative, and anaerobic organisms. The specific choice of therapy should be based on the most likely pathogen present in the patient until results from nasal, nasopharyngeal, or blood cultures are known. Close follow-up is essential, examining for clinical improvement. Clinical features suggesting orbital rather than preseptal cellulitis include: proptosis, limited ocular motility, chemosis (swollen conjunctiva), pain with eye movement, and fever. Prompt action is recommended to prevent posterior spread of the infection. Computed tomography scans may be beneficial to determine if an orbital abscess requiring drainage is present, especially if minimal clinical improvement is noted on therapy.

Orbital inflammatory conditions include thyroid ophthalmopathy, idiopathic orbital inflammation, and vasculitis. Thyroid eye disease (Graves ophthalmopathy) is an autoimmune inflammatory disorder characterized by proptosis, eyelid retraction, conjunctival injection, extraocular muscle restriction, and optic neuropathy. These symptoms are often associated with hyperthyroidism but can also occur with hypothyroidism or even a euthyroid state. The ophthalmologic course may run independent of both the thyroid gland abnormalities and treatment. Idiopathic orbital inflammation may present as a diffuse or localized process. Typically the onset is abrupt with orbital pain, restricted motility, proptosis, conjunctival injection, chemosis, and eyelid erythema. Formally referred to as orbital pseudotumor, this is a self-limited but variable disorder and responds quickly to systemic steroid therapy. Additional inflammatory conditions affecting the orbit include sarcoidosis, the vasculitides, and Wegener granulomatosis.

Orbital neoplasms may be congenital, such as choristomas, including dermoid cysts and lipodermoids, and hamartomas, including capillary hemangiomas. Neoplasms presenting later include lymphangiomas, which may present with sudden proptosis and spontaneous hemorrhage, optic nerve gliomas, which can be associated with neurofibromatosis, rhabdomyosarcoma, lymphoproliferative disorders, and metastatic tumors. Urgent work-up is indicated with imaging and biopsy.

## TRAUMA

Eyelid trauma occurs via blunt and penetrating mechanisms. Eyelid injuries should be accompanied by a thorough ocular examination and appropriate imaging studies. Blunt eyelid trauma may result in ecchymosis, edema, and eyelid laceration. Penetrating eyelid injuries may appear minimal despite significant damage to the eyelid, orbit, and/or the eye itself. The canaliculi of the tear duct system may be disrupted in medial eyelid lacerations. Proper primary wound closure is important in the repair of eyelid laceration as improperly sutured injuries may lead to significant scarring and possible tear duct abnormalities requiring reconstruction.

Orbital injuries include fractures, orbital foreign bodies, and intraorbital hemorrhage. Orbital fractures may involve any of the orbital walls, roof, or floor. A CT scan of the orbits with axial and coronal views is beneficial for complete evaluation, as is a complete motility examination. Most orbital fractures do not require urgent repair. Fractures with entrapment of orbital soft tissue, especially an extraocular muscle, suggest urgent attention. A blowout fracture is typically a floor fracture but may extend to or involve only the medial wall and not involve the orbital rim. Suspicion for a blowout fracture is warranted for any patient sustaining a blunt periorbital injury resulting in ecchymosis. Additional signs include diplopia, limited motility in upgaze or downgaze, enophthalmos (sinking of the eye), hypoesthesia involving the maxillary division of cranial nerve 5, and emphysema of the orbit or lids on CT scan. Intraorbital foreign bodies are suggested by the history. Imaging is recommended, typically CT, as MRI should be avoided if the possible foreign body is ferromagnetic. Intraorbital hemorrhage may result from trauma or eye surgery. The hemorrhage is typically only drained if optic nerve function is compromised.

Ocular trauma may be secondary to chemical, thermal, blunt force, or penetrating damage. Chemical injuries require immediate and generous irrigation of the eye. Alkali burns especially can result in rapid corneal damage leading to permanent scarring. Thus, irrigation should be continued until the pH normalizes. Thermal burns result from items such as cigarettes and curling irons. Typically, the injury is similar to a corneal abrasion (loss of epithelium) and therefore should be treated similarly with antibiotic drops or ointment and ophthalmologic follow-up. Blunt trauma may result in subconjunctival hemorrhage and corneal abrasions as well as intraocular injuries such as traumatic iritis (inflammation in the anterior chamber), hyphema (blood in the anterior chamber), traumatic cataract (opacity of the lens), and/or retinal hemorrhage or edema. The management of hyphema is aimed at preventing a rebleed, maintaining normal intraocular pressure, decreasing associated inflammation, and ensuring proper drainage of the blood in the anterior chamber. An important consideration with hyphema is the presence of sickle cell trait or disease. These patients can have dramatic intraocular pressure elevations even with small hypemas that do not fill the anterior chamber due to sickling of the red blood cells, which slows the resorption of blood and blocking the drainage system of the eye. Hyphema management options include topical steroids, cycloplegics, and pressure medications, as well as systemic medications and surgical evacuation depending on the specific case. Ocular penetrating injuries enter the eye and perforating injuries enter and exit the eye. Both may lead to devastating, permanent vision loss. The injury may be quite obvious, secondary to a large laceration, or hidden by dense hemorrhage. Any penetrating or perforating injury requires urgent ophthalmologic evaluation and treatment. If an ocular foreign body is suspected, a CT scan should be performed.

## REFERENCES


1. Pediatric Eye Disease Investigator Group. A randomized trial of atropine vs patching for treatment of moderate amblyopia in children. *Arch Ophthalmol.* 2002;120:268–278

2. Scheiman MM, Hertle RW, Beck RW, et al. Randomized trial of treatment of amblyopia in children aged 7 to 17 years. *Arch Ophthalmol.* 2005;123:437–447

3. Barron BA, Gee L, Hauck WW, et al. Herpetic Eye Disease Study. A controlled trial of oral acyclovir for herpes simplex stromal keratitis. *Ophthalmology.* 1994:101:1871–1882

4. The Herpetic Eye Disease Study Group. Acyclovir for the prevention of recurrent herpes simplex virus eye disease. *N Engl J Med.* 1998;300:300–306

5. Jabs DA, Nussenblatt RB, Rosenbaum JT, Standardization of Uveitis Nomenclature (SUN) Working Group. Standardization of uveitis nomenclature for reporting clinical data. Results of the First International Workshop. *Am J Ophthalmol.* 2005;140(3):509–516

6. Optic Neuritis Study Group. The clinical profile of optic neuritis: experience of the optic neuritis treatment trial. *Arch Ophthalmol.* 1991;109:1673–1678

7. Optic Neuritis Study Group. Visual function more than 10 years after optic neuritis: experience of the optic neuritis treatment trial. *Am J Ophthalmol.* 2004;137(1):77–83

8. Optic Neuritis Study Group. High- and low-risk profiles for the development of multiple sclerosis within 10 years after optic neuritis: experience of the optic neuritis treatment trial. *Arch Ophthalmol.* 2003;121(7):944–949

9. Early Treatment Diabetic Retinopathy Study Research Group. Early photocoagulation for diabetic retinopathy. ETDRS report 9. *Ophthalmology.* 1991;98:766–785

# CHAPTER 155

# ENT Disorders

MARK N. GOLDSTEIN, MD

The onset of adolescence causes a shift in the focus of head and neck health care problems. The childhood diseases of otitis media and upper respiratory infections are replaced in adolescence by illnesses resulting from nasal obstruction, sinusitis, and sinus-related headache. These maladies are attributed to the growth and development of the anatomic structures, as well as to reactions of the nasal and paranasal mucosa to inflammation due to allergies and/or infection.

In the adolescent, the eustachian tube has matured anatomically and functionally, and the middle ear function has improved. There is a regression of the adenotonsillar tissue, and tonsillitis becomes less of a problem except in a small percentage of adolescents. Voice strain or improper voice projection techniques result in laryngeal problems presenting as hoarseness, which is secondary to inflammation, and occasionally in the form of nodules.

Obesity in adolescents predisposes them to obstructive sleep apnea with nighttime symptoms affecting daytime activities.[1]

## EXAMINATION OF THE HEAD AND NECK

Beginning with the external aspect of the nose, the clinician should note whether a horizontal crease appears in the lower portion, indicating constant wiping of the nose. A persistent discharge from the nose frequently causes erythema and crusting around the nares. The internal nose is examined for congestion, edema, and erythema of the mucosa. The mucosal lining in patients with allergies that affect the nose appears gray or bluish in color. The position and appearance of the nasal septum and turbinates should be noted to determine whether a deviated septum or enlarged turbinates are causing obstruction. Enlarged boggy turbinates are consistent with allergic rhinitis. Enlarged turbinates with a clear discharge are consistent with pregnancy. Discharge near the turbinates, either clear or purulent, unilateral or bilateral, also should be examined to determine whether there is an infection in the paranasal sinuses. A vasoconstricting agent should be placed on the mucosa and allowed to absorb for several minutes so that the mucosal lining will contract. Subsequent examination will reveal the degree of mucosal congestion and underlying bony hypertrophy. In addition, the repeat examination may enable visualization of the posterior aspect of the nasal cavity to detect anatomic deformities or purulent discharge. Posterior rhinoscopy may be performed either with a flexible endoscope through the anterior nares or by a mirror examination looking at the nasopharynx from the oropharynx. In addition, nasal polyps, a posterior spur of the septum, or adenoidal hypertrophy may be diagnosed by rhinoscopy.

During otologic examination, the color and thickness of the external canal skin should be noted. Tenderness on pulling the pinna implies otitis externa; tenderness on palpation of the tragus and the anterior canal wall implies temporomandibular joint syndrome. Wax should normally be present in the lateral, hair-bearing aspect of the external auditory canal, and the tympanic membrane should be examined to detect any discoloration, scarring, retractions, or loss of mobility. Pneumatic otoscopy is performed to assess the movement of the tympanic membrane, while tuning forks (256 and 512 Hz) are used to assess the patient's hearing status. The extraocular motions of both eyes are noted to rule out nystagmus, which is rhythmically repetitive movement of the eyes.

The oral cavity and oropharynx are examined for signs of infection involving the mucosa, teeth, or opening of the salivary ducts. Tonsillar size and symmetry and the presence of erythema, exudate, and inspissated food are recorded as abnormalities. Tenderness of the pterygoid muscles is frequently associated with temporomandibular joint pain.

The hypopharynx and larynx are examined by indirect laryngoscopy or by further advancing the flexible endoscope from the nose through the oropharynx and hypopharynx. The larynx is examined for mobility, color, and thickness of the vocal cords, as well as for abnormalities such as nodules or polyps. The posterior portion of the larynx, the arytenoids, is examined to see if any erythema or edema exists. The neck is palpated for enlarged lymph nodes, the size and location of which are noted, and the major salivary glands and the temporomandibular joint are palpated. Thyroid position and size are noted. Palpation of the carotid vessels, including the bifurcation, and the larynx complete the initial examination.

## NASAL OBSTRUCTION

The primary functions of the nose include humidification, filtration, heat exchange, olfaction, and speech. Except for olfaction and speech, the autonomic nervous system controls most of the functions of the nose. The nasal cavities process approximately 10,000 L of air per day, and they normally contribute 30% of the airflow resistance to the lungs. The specific resistance of each side of the nose varies, owing to the alternating swelling and constriction of the mucosa over the nasal turbinates. This variation in resistance is cyclic, occurring every 45 to 90 minutes, and is known as the nasal cycle. Rhinologic obstruction can be the result of the nasal cavity anatomy itself. Whereas the external nose is formed of an upper portion consisting of bone and a lower portion of cartilage, the internal nose is divided in the midline by the cartilaginous septum anteriorly and bony septum posteriorly. Inferior and middle turbinates form the lateral wall of the internal nose, and the superior turbinate forms the posterior aspect. Deviation of the septum becomes more pronounced as the child grows, and the turbinates may hypertrophy, causing unilateral or bilateral obstruction.

Patients presenting with nasal obstruction frequently complain of airway "stuffiness," which may be seasonal, acute, or chronic. This sensation may be unilateral or bilateral, and it is important to determine changes with the nasal cycle. These patients also complain of a dry mouth and frequently have recurrent sore throats as a result of mouth breathing. Headaches develop from referred pain to other areas in the paranasal region, and sleep disturbance may be secondary to the nasal obstruction. A careful history must be obtained to rule out antecedent trauma. Allergy symptoms, including rhinorrhea, postnasal discharge, sneezing, headaches, and itching, should be thoroughly investigated. Exposure to specific irritants, such as fumes or smoke, and the use of medications or illegal drugs should be determined. During history-taking, the patient should be specifically questioned about excessive use of nasal sprays, which is a common cause of nasal obstruction.

Physiologic causes of nasal obstruction include the nasal cycle, the nasopulmonary reflex, paradoxical obstruction, and hormonal alterations. The nasopulmonary reflex occurs when increased nasal resistance produces increased pulmonary resistance and decreased pulmonary compliance, causing abnormal blood gases. This phenomenon may explain why an active upper respiratory infection causes breathlessness. Paradoxic nasal obstruction results from a longstanding anatomic deformity such as septal deviation. The normally patent side of the nose intermittently obstructs, leading to complaints of difficulty in breathing from the patent side. Puberty causes changes in the mucosal lining of the nasal cavity, which are mediated by increases in the estrogen hormone levels in both sexes. Intermittent nasal obstruction may be secondary to hormonal changes during menses. Normal vasomotor reaction to external stimuli, such as temperature, humidity, dust, and smog, frequently causes nasal obstruction. However, the most common cause of acute nasal obstruction is the common cold. Persistent acute rhinitis (for longer than 7 to 10 days) associated with significant nasal or nasopharyngeal discharge suggests sinusitis. Table 155-1 summarizes the more common causes of rhinitis.

After a thorough physical examination, appropriate laboratory tests should be performed and should include cultures of any thickened secretions or purulent material. Nasal cytology showing greater than 1 neutrophil per high-power field correlates with an 80% chance of a radiographic diagnosis of sinusitis. The presence of eosinophils on a nasal smear suggests allergy. With nasal cytology there is a false-negative incidence of 11%, which should be considered when basing therapeutic decisions on the results.

Rhinomanometry is used to calculate airway resistance by measuring airflow and pressure differences across the nasal cavity. This technique is useful in documenting the amount of obstruction and recording the changes of resistance with the use of vasoconstrictors. The testing of olfaction has now been standardized by a scratch-and-sniff technique that forces the patient to choose 1 of 4 answers. It documents the degree of olfactory loss and is effective in unmasking malingerers.

Inflammation of the nose is the most common cause of nasal obstruction and is produced by bacterial, viral, allergic, or toxic agents. Adenoidal hypertrophy, an anatomic problem, is exacerbated by any inflammatory reaction. Metabolic abnormalities that cause obstruction include cystic fibrosis, diabetes mellitus, thyroid disease, and immune deficiency disease. In adolescent men the most common neoplasm causing obstruction is juvenile angiofibroma.

## SINUSITIS

Sinusitis may complicate the treatment of nasal obstruction by causing inflammation of the adjacent nasal mucosa. This diagnosis should be considered when a patient fails to respond to medical management of nasal obstruction. The clinical manifestations of sinusitis in

**Table 155-1**

**Rhinitis**

| *Etiologies* | *Comments* | *Management* |
|---|---|---|
| **Infectious** | | |
| Viral | URI<br>HIV | Decongestants<br>Saline irrigations |
| Bacterial | | Antibiotics |
| Fungal | Asthmatics | Antifungals |
| | Immunocompromised | Drainage |
| | | Debridement |
| **Allergic** | | |
| Polyps | | Steroids/oral, nasal antibiotics<br>Excision |
| Fungal | | Antifungals |
| **Rhinitis Medicamentosum** | | |
| Irritants | | Oral steroids<br>Saline irrigations |
| **Medication** | | |
| Oral contraceptive pills | | Adjust medicine |
| Antihypertensives | | |
| **Pregnancy** | | Saline irrigations |
| **Drugs** | | |
| Smoking | | Saline irrigations |
| Cocaine | Perforation/necrosis | |
| **Inherited** | | |
| Cystic fibrosis | | Antibiotics, irrigations |
| Immotile cilia | | |
| Immune deficiency | | |

URI, upper respiratory infection

adolescents are different from those in children.[2] By adolescence, most of the sinuses are developed. Malodorous breath and a persistent cough, as well as headache in the periorbital area, facial pain, and dental pain, may indicate sinusitis. In evaluation of patients with headache of possible sinus origin, it should be noted that 4% of patients have aplasia of the frontal sinuses and 16% have hypoplasia of the frontal sinuses. The complication of periorbital swelling is a common manifestation of sinusitis and may be the initial presenting symptom of a sinus infection. Tenderness to palpation of the face is a more reliable symptom of sinusitis in adolescents than in children.

Transillumination does not add significantly to the diagnosis, but radiographic films are generally used. Standard radiographs include the Waters view for the maxillary sinus, the Caldwell view for the frontal and ethmoid sinus, and the submental vertex and lateral views for the sphenoid sinuses. The lateral view also assists in visualizing the ethmoid and frontal sinuses. When the sinus radiographs are reviewed, an air-fluid level, complete opacification, or mucosal thickening of 4 mm or more is correlated with pus in the sinus. Computed tomography (CT) and magnetic resonance imaging (MRI) have been used more frequently than routine radiographs to diagnose and monitor sinusitis. When plain films are compared with CT scans, there is up to an 84% discrepancy in findings. The plain films are useful in monitoring acute disease using the criteria of opacification, air–fluid levels, or mucosal thickening. Computed tomography scans are superior for monitoring chronic disease (infection of 4 weeks or longer) in which the ethmoid sinuses are most frequently involved. A CT provides a significant amount of detail, particularly when performed in the coronal plane, because on CT the osteomeatal complex of the sinuses is better defined. This superior definition on CT is especially important for determining the cause of recurrent sinusitis. Orbital complications are clearly demonstrated when the 2 planes of the CT view are compared. The scans are also used in preparation for endoscopic sinus surgery involving the osteomeatal complex and the ethmoid sinuses, in which diseased mucosa is removed using telescopic lenses and instruments. An Magnetic resonance imaging is useful for noting the inflammatory process and areas of opacification, but bony detail is better visualized by CT. Chronic rhinosinusitis is a clinical diagnosis and the decision to perform a CT scan of the sinuses and the interpretation of the scan should include the clinical context. Follow-up scans, usually after 6 weeks, depend on the patient's clinical course.

It is important to recognize the relationship between nasal obstruction, sinusitis, and asthma, and to obtain the appropriate diagnostic studies. Medical and/or surgical treatment of sinus infection frequently helps to manage asthma. Effective treatment of sinusitis in asthmatic adolescents improves pulmonary function and frequently permits reduction of asthma medications.

Cystic fibrosis is another special case in which extensive sinusitis is involved. Nasal polyposis occurs in 6% to 9% of children with cystic fibrosis and is more common in adolescents with this disease than in younger children. A sweat chloride test should be obtained for all children who have nasal polyps before surgery to remove the polyps is contemplated. Excision of the polyps and appropriate drainage of the involved sinuses lead to a significant disease-free interval, with less nasal obstruction and/or sinusitis. Appropriate cultures are taken from the area of the polyps and antibiotic therapy directed by the culture results. *Pseudomonas aeruginosa* is a common pathogen in this population.

Treatment of nasal or sinus infection consists of the administration of antibiotics; topical and systemic decongestants; and, when allergy is a possible underlying etiology, antihistamines, intranasal, and/or oral steroids. The most common bacterial organisms are *Streptococcus pneumoniae, Haemophilus influenzae,* and *Branhamella catarrhalis.* Anaerobic organisms account for approximately 40% of the bacteria isolated. The initial oral antibiotic therapy should involve either amoxicillin, amoxicillin-clavulanate, trimethoprim-sulfamethoxazole, or erythromycin-sulfazoxisol. Intranasal and/or oral decongestants reduce mucosal swelling and aid sinus drainage. Antihistamines reduce mucosal reactivity to environmental factors. Steroids can be used in severe inflammatory states, but antibiotic administration is necessary if there is any possibility of an infection. The possibility of fungal infections, although rare, should be considered in patients with longstanding sinus infections (ie, asthmatics) or those who have compromised immune function. The treatment regimen of antibiotics and decongestants usually takes 10 days, with several weeks of treatment necessary in some cases.

The patient usually responds within the first 2 to 3 days of medical treatment. Intranasal lavage of the sinus is recommended for patients with persistent symptoms, documented radiographic findings, or therapeutic failure. Lavage clears disease from the sinus, and an accurate culture of the infected sinus can be obtained. Hospitalization with administration of intravenous antibiotics is recommended for patients who fail to respond to medical management, suffer recurrent episodes of sinusitis, or develop a complication. Orbital complications are the most common, intracranial complications being the second most common (Box 155-1 and Box 155-2).

**Box 155-1**

***Orbital Complications from Sinusitis***

Periorbital inflammatory edema
Orbital cellulites
Subperiosteal abscess
Orbital abscess
Cavernous sinus thrombosis

**Box 155-2**

***Intracranial Complications from Sinusitis***

Meningitis
Epidural abscess
Subdural abscess
Venous sinus thrombosis
Brain abscess

Once the patient has been treated for an acute nasal or paranasal sinus condition, a full evaluation, with special attention to the possibility of allergic rhinitis or anatomic deformities should be performed. If the patient has medical problems, including allergic rhinitis, desensitization, or the use of oral or intranasal medications to control the disease is appropriate. Surgical intervention is used acutely to drain an infected sinus and adjacent area if a complication has developed. Surgical management is also used to correct nasal obstruction due to a deviated septum or enlarged turbinates. These procedures are usually performed on an outpatient basis. Postoperative visits to the clinician are necessary to clear the nasal cavity of crusts until the mucosa has healed. The patient also may undergo sinus drainage as an outpatient procedure. The removal of any anatomic abnormalities and the opening of the sinus ostia permit appropriate drainage from the sinuses to the nasal cavity. Patients require follow-up care for the next few weeks to remove crusts from the surgical sites. Occasionally, the endonasal procedures fail owing to blockage of the ostia or recurrent infection, and external procedures are necessary. These external procedures generally require hospitalization for several days and a subsequent recuperative period at home for an equal amount of time.[3]

## EPISTAXIS

Evaluation of epistaxis should always include the history of whether the bleeding is unilateral or bilateral, the amount of bleeding (eg, the patient stained a tissue, filled a cup), the time and duration, and whether it was a posterior bleed (went down the back of the throat while the patient was sitting up) or an anterior bleed (all blood comes anteriorly). Systemic problems relating to blood loss should be recorded (diaphoresis, tachycardia, orthostatic hypotension, perfusion of the skin, petechiae).

Most epistaxis is from the anterior septum, and only 10% is thought to be from the posterior septum or nasal cavity. The patient should sit up and lean forward to clear the airway, and blood should be collected in a basin to estimate the amount of blood lost. If blood goes down the back of the throat, this is believed to indicate a posterior bleed requiring hospital evaluation and management. Vital signs indicate the amount of blood lost. Tachycardia can result from blood loss or the patient's anxiety. Normal blood pressure indicates less than 10% blood loss; postural hypotension indicates more than 10% blood loss. If the blood pressure is low and the pulse rapid, the loss of blood is causing impending shock. Elevated blood pressure may be a contributing factor or may be related to the patient's mental status.

Treatment consists of packing the nose with cotton to which Neo-Synephrine 0.5% or Afrin Nasal spray has been applied. Hold the nostrils closed for several minutes. If bleeding continues or is profuse, pack the nose with expandable packing or gauze and call for consultation. Transferring the patient to the hospital is appropriate so that an intravenous line can be started and blood samples obtained for complete blood count, type, and cross-match, as well as coagulation screening.

If the bleeding subsides, replace the cotton with the constricting agent with cotton soaked in 4% lidocaine. Remove this cotton after several minutes and cauterize the bleeding area with silver nitrate applicators. Place a third cotton, this time mixed with antibiotic ointment, in the nose after the cauterization and keep it in place for several hours. The patient should refrain from hot foods for 2 or 3 days. No excessive activity should be allowed for 5 days, although the patient may go to school. Antibiotic ointment should be applied to the nose twice daily to cover the cauterized area for 5 to 7 days.

Bleeding that is severe, necessitating admission to the hospital, requires team management to monitor the need for blood or blood products. A posterior pack may be necessary, and sinus radiographs or a CT scan should be obtained, when this type of pack is placed, to examine the anatomy. Antibiotics are given because of the possibility of sinusitis. Supplemental oxygen is given via a mask. If the bleeding is controlled, the packing is advanced after 48 hours and removed shortly thereafter. If the bleeding continues, the patient is evaluated for either angiographic embolization or surgical ligation of the appropriate arteries.

## TONSILLITIS

The incidence of all upper respiratory infections diminishes in adolescence. However, recurrent tonsillitis remains a significant problem in a small portion of this population and is frequently associated with adenoiditis.[4] At puberty the tonsils and adenoid regress further, having previously been reduced in size between the ages of 6 and 8 years. Persistence of large tonsils and adenoids causes problems with the upper airway, such as mouth breathing, snoring, occasional snorting, and some difficulty eating, because the mouth cannot be closed to chew properly. Poor sleeping may lead to morning tiredness with excessive daytime sleepiness and poor attention span in school. These symptoms may indicate obstructive sleep apnea, especially in the obese patient. Occasionally, an adolescent presents for evaluation because of halitosis that does not respond to antibiotics. The patient may have cryptic tonsils that trap food and lead to malodorous breath. Other causes of bad breath include chronic adenoiditis and sinusitis.

In the adolescent who has recurrent problems with tonsils and the adenoid, a careful examination of both nasal cavities must be performed to rule out purulent discharge, intranasal pathologic conditions, or sinusitis. The adenoids are visualized by flexible endoscopy to observe the size, degree of erythema, and presence of any purulent exudate on their surface. The oropharynx and hypopharynx are examined endoscopically to see whether the hypertrophied tonsils are impinging on the airway. The larynx is examined to ensure that the lingual tonsils are not part of the obstructing complex. Oropharyngeal examination is performed to determine the exact relationship between the tonsils and the palate. The palate is palpated for the presence of a submucous cleft. The neck is palpated for persistent cervical adenopathy.

Serous otitis media is a frequent presentation of adenoidal hypertrophy. Cervical adenopathy associated with adenotonsillar hypertrophy points to an infectious etiology. Laboratory evaluation for Epstein-Barr virus and, if suspected, human immunodeficiency virus, should be included. Surgery for drainage of serous fluid or for adenotonsillar hyperplasia is deferred if the patient has an acute viral infection (Box 155-3). Infection of the tonsils occurs frequently during upper respiratory infections. In addition to pain, patients have erythema, possibly exudate, and cervical adenopathy. Fever may be present. It is important to take a throat culture to rule out group A beta-hemolytic streptococci. Asymmetry of the tonsils may indicate a peritonsillar abscess; this is associated with trismus, voice changes ("hot potato voice") with fullness, and erythema of one tonsillar pillar more than the other.

Infectious mononucleosis mimics tonsillitis but is frequently more severe with both tonsils enlarged with exudate and the characteristic posterior cervical adenopathy. Therapy is directed at reducing the upper airway obstruction with the use of steroids and antibiotics (ampicillin is not used because this is associated with a rash in a high percentage of patients). Owing to airway obstruction, it may be necessary either to provide a nasopharyngeal airway or to intubate the patient.

**Box 155-3**

***Tonsil and Adenoid Surgery: Indications***

OBSTRUCTION

- Hypertrophy of tonsils or adenoids
- Obligate mouth breathing not attributed to other causes
- Sleep apnea
- Speech abnormalities
- Chronic otitis media with effusion
- Recurrent or chronic otitis media with perforation
- Chronic or recurrent nasopharyngitis

INFECTION

- Recurrent tonsillitis despite adequate medical therapy
- Peritonsillar abscess
- Recurrent tonsillitis with cardiac disease
- Recurrent tonsillitis with persistent streptococcal carrier state
- Halitosis

**Box 155-4**

***Sleep Apnea***

**Nighttime Symptoms**
Mouth breathing
Snoring
Snorting
Apnea
Restless sleep
Diaphoresis
Enuresis

**Daytime Symptoms**
Morning headache
Morning tiredness
Daytime sleepiness
Learning problems
Behavioral problems
Attention-deficit/hyperactivity disorder

**Signs**
Obesity
Hypertension
Pulmonary hypertension

Obstructive sleep apnea should be considered in any child with adenotonsillar hypertrophy and/or obesity with a history of snoring, respiratory pauses during sleep, morning tiredness, or headache (Box 155-4).[1]

If intervention is indicated, treatment is generally surgical. If an abscess is suspected, local anesthesia is administered to the anterior pillar of the tonsil. The tonsillar pillar is aspirated; if this is unsuccessful the pillar is incised with a No. 15 blade through the mucosa, and the area of the tonsillar capsule is exposed, the incision being enlarged with a tonsil clamp.

Tonsillectomy is performed as ambulatory surgery in an outpatient setting of a hospital or ambulatory surgical facility. In older patients, recuperation takes 7 to 14 days. The lengthy recuperative time is due to the large surface area at the site of excision. Postoperative pain, frequently referred to the ears, is controlled with analgesics. A healing white eschar fills the tonsillar fossae and is often considered to represent infections. The eschar separates after one week, occasionally causing some bleeding. By the seventh postoperative day the patient generally returns to school, with athletics permitted on the 17th to 21st postoperative day. The complication of bleeding generally occurs in less than 1% of patients, so blood typing is usually not performed preoperatively.

## ORAL CAVITY LESIONS

The most common types of nontraumatic ulcerative lesion in the oral cavity are aphthous ulcers. Immunologic factors have been implicated in the etiology. The lesions may be minor, major, or herpetiform. There is usually a tingling or burning sensation before the eruption of the ulcer. Over-the-counter medications can provide good control of the disease, and prescription medications are not usually necessary. Topical or systemic steroids are occasionally used for severe cases.

Gonorrhea also presents with multiple ulcerations, but more commonly there is a general erythema with the ulcers, along with cervical adenopathy. After appropriate cultures, antibiotics are prescribed.

Smokeless tobacco presents as white lesions in the oral mucosa where the tobacco is usually kept. The mucosa has a granular, irregular appearance. The lesions are painless and asymptomatic initially. Cessation of tobacco use leads to regression. If the lesion persists or becomes larger or more ulcerative, malignancy should be suspected and appropriate referral and biopsy recommended.

## OTOLOGIC PROBLEMS

Otologic problems that occur during adolescence are usually either a progression of ear disease that presented during infancy or a manifestation related to noise exposure. The child who has recurrent ear infections with frequent perforations, or who has had the tympanic membrane surgically manipulated, may develop softening of the tympanic membrane with a retraction of the membrane toward the medial aspect of the middle ear space or onto the ossicular chain. Frequently this condition progresses, causing potential ossicular disruption with hearing loss. If hearing loss exists, amplification to improve the hearing level or surgical treatment is recommended. Surgery is planned to repair the tympanic membrane and/or repair the ossicular chain. Overnight hospitalization is usually not necessary, with return to school or work within a week.

For the ear that continues to be infected, the infectious process should first be controlled medically or surgically before any reconstructive procedures are performed. Cholesteatoma is a possibility that should be considered with all ongoing infections that do not clear within a 4- to 6-week period. A discharge from the ear associated with otitis externa may represent a chronic infection of the middle ear. The outer ear must be treated first to permit good visualization of the tympanic membrane. Preoperative radiographic evaluation consists of a CT scan to visualize any bony abnormalities of the mastoid and to determine the extent of the disease.

Otitis externa tends to be extremely painful and is common during the summer months. The use of expandable wicks has reduced the difficulty in treating this disease. Spongelike wicks are inserted into the swollen ear canal with little difficulty, and the topical drops then cause the wick to expand, reducing the edema, minimizing the pain of the ear canal, and ensuring that the medication stays in contact with the skin surface. The wick is usually removed in 24 to 48 hours and the ear canal cleansed thoroughly, enabling visualization of the tympanic membrane. To avoid otitis externa, the patient can use most commercial preparations of acetic acid and alcohol to dry the ear and prevent infections. This solution is used regularly at the end of the day, with cotton placed on the outside for 15 to 20 minutes.

Ear piercing is common and is mentioned because of the possibility of infection (see Chapter 147, Miscellaneous Dermatologic Disorders in Adolescence). The patient should have the piercing removed and treatment started to cover *Pseudomonas aeruginosa*, not just normal skin pathogens.

Sensorineural hearing loss noted in adolescence may be related to noise exposure or a sequela of persistent otitis media of childhood. Loud music, even when listened to through headphones, has been known to cause unsafe levels of sound. It is especially advisable for adolescents who use headphones to keep the volume level low to avoid causing hearing problems. Frequently, the first sign of hearing loss is a temporary threshold shift after exposure to loud noises. If exposure occurs regularly, a permanent threshold shift will be experienced.

All patients who have ear complaints should undergo a complete audiological evaluation, including the testing of acoustic reflexes, to determine whether hearing loss exists and the type and degree of loss. The audiogram should include pure tone testing from 250 to 8000 Hz. Air and bone conduction should be examined to determine whether conductive loss, as opposed to sensorineural loss, has occurred. The normal hearing range is 0 to 25 dB; above 25 dB, one may experience hearing difficulties. The audiogram also examines word recognition—the ability to understand phonetically balanced words (think, pink, sink) at a given decibel level. Tympanometry is used to measure tympanic membrane mobility. Acoustic reflexes test the integrity of the cochlear nerve to elicit a stapedial reflex (governed by cranial nerves VII and VIII) when a loud noise is present. The reflex is both ipsilateral and contralateral. At high frequency (above 4000 Hz), audiometry can identify unsuspected hearing loss not apparent during routine screenings. If unilateral hearing loss exists, further evaluation should include vestibular function tests and specialized audiometric tests to rule out retrocochlear pathologic conditions such as a tumor. Magnetic resonance imaging is extremely useful in identifying the cochleovestibular complex to visualize any pathologic conditions in this area.

Sensorineural hearing loss due to noise exposure is often in the upper frequencies, corresponding to the basal turn of the cochlea near the oval window where sound enters. Acute sensorineural hearing loss usually affects many frequencies. Because of the emergent nature of this loss, treatment is directed at possible causes, including inflammation (bacterial, viral) and poor circulation to the inner ear (sludging of blood or vasoconstriction). Treatment with antibiotics, oral steroids, vasodilating agents, and anticoagulants (aspirin, dipyridamole [Persantine]) is common. The results of treatment depend on the degree of the patient's pre-existing hearing loss before acute loss occurred. If a hearing loss existed previously, the prognosis is less favorable.

Tinnitus is frequently associated with hearing loss.[5] Causes of tinnitus in adolescents also include eustachian tube dysfunction, temporomandibular joint disease, allergy, and metabolic problems. Using the tones available from the audiometer, one can try to match the tinnitus tone that the patient senses. There is no specific treatment, but a thorough understanding of the problem helps the patient. Specific psychosocial stress factors associated with adolescence should be identified. Helpful suggestions include the use of competing noise as the child attempts to go to sleep, and the avoidance of any loud noises that may aggravate the tinnitus or hearing problems. Treatment of underlying medical problems should help. Biofeedback has been used with some success.

Vertigo is relatively uncommon in adolescents and is usually related to an inner ear infection or trauma to the head, causing an inner ear problem. It is important to distinguish vertigo from dizziness. The patient should be questioned specifically concerning aural symptoms; if there is no associated hearing loss, it is unlikely that there is end-organ (vestibular) disease. A thorough head and neck examination should be performed, including pneumatic otoscopy, which may unmask a fistula of the inner ear. A full neurologic test is also important, including cerebellar testing. Having the patient hyperventilate for 30 seconds frequently produces the symptom complex and identifies hyperventilation as the etiology. A full audiological evaluation is necessary. Should any of the initial clinical tests prove abnormal, an electronystagmogram, and possibly CT or MRI, should be performed. If no specific cause is found and the examination is clinically normal, Cawthorne exercises, designed specifically to strengthen balance function, can be used by the patient to compensate for the sensation of imbalance. These exercises are done twice daily for approximately 15 minutes. The patient is re-evaluated at 2-week intervals to check on progress. Laboratory tests, including hematologic evaluation with tests for infectious and metabolic abnormalities, should be performed.

## LARYNGEAL PROBLEMS

Laryngeal problems in the adolescent are usually related to either acute infections affecting the vocal cords or vocal abuse, which leads to persisting hoarseness. The acute infections are frequently viral in origin, causing edema of the cords, and hoarseness. The patient is usually treated with decongestants, humidification, and voice rest with good resolution. Persistence of the hoarseness or an attempt to use the voice during the acute episode frequently leads to irritation of the vocal cords at the junction of the anterior and middle thirds of the vocal cord. Persistent irritation or vocal abuse can lead to the development of small nodules at this location. The nodularity can also develop from chronic vocal abuse, shouting, or use of poor technique in an attempt to project the voice to large audiences. Any hoarseness that persists for more than 4 to 6 weeks should be evaluated by a specialist, and if vocal cord nodules are present, voice rest and instruction on the proper use of the voice should be the primary therapy. Evaluation by a speech pathologist is generally indicated to diagnose the specific problems patients are having with their voice, and therapy is usually performed once or twice a week. Occasionally adolescents who use their voice in a professional manner, as in singing or acting, may need instruction from a voice coach on a regular basis. Once they have improved speech habits, persistent nodules may be excised in an outpatient procedure under microscopic control to avoid damage to the delicate surrounding structures. Postoperatively, 4 to 6 weeks of voice rest are required, with continued speech therapy to solidify gains the patient made during the initial treatment. Surgical intervention is not indicated as the primary treatment because poor vocal habits cause recurrence of the nodules. With good speech therapy, surgical intervention can frequently be avoided.

Gastroesophageal reflux can present with symptoms of persistent hoarseness. Associated symptoms include a globus sensation (feeling a lump in the throat) and/or chronic cough. Heartburn and chest pain are usually absent. On examination the larynx will frequently have erythema of the arytenoids located in the posterior aspect of the larynx, near the cricopharyngeus muscle and the upper esophageal sphincter. The area may also be edematous. Dietary changes, weight loss, cessation of smoking and reflux precautions are the initial treatment. If unsuccessful, then 3 months of antireflux therapy is recommended. Failure to respond requires further diagnostic evaluation.[6]

## REFERENCES

1. Marcus CL, Chapman D, Davidson Ward S, McColley SA. Clinical practice guideline: diagnosis and management of childhood obstructive sleep apnea syndrome. *Pediatrics.* 2002:109(4);704–712

2. Wald ER, Clayton Bordley W, Darrow DH, et al. Clinical practice guideline: management of sinusitis. *Pediatrics.* 2001;108(3):798–808

3. Graney DO. Paranasal sinuses, anatomy. In: Cummings CW, Fredrickson JM, Harker LA, et al, eds. *Otolaryngology—Head and Neck Surgery.* St Louis, MO: Mosby-Year Book; 1986:845

4. Hibbert J. Tonsils and adenoids. In: Mackay IS, Bull TR, eds. *Scott-Brown's Otolaryngology. Vol 6.* London: Butterworth; 1987:368

5. Leonard G, Owen Black F, Schramm VL. Tinnitus in children. In: Bluestone CD, Stool SE, eds. *Pediatric Otolaryngology. Vol 1.* Philadelphia, PA: WB Saunders; 1983:271

6. Rudolph CD, Mazur LJ, Liptak GS, Baker RD. Clinical practice guidelines: pediatric GE reflux. *J Pediatr Gastroenterol Nutr.* 2001;32(S2):1–31

# CHAPTER 156

## Medical and Psychosocial Considerations for the Deaf Adolescent

ERIC C. WEISELBERG, MD • IRENE W. LEIGH, PhD

Historically, medical interest in deafness has been one of diagnosis and intervention, including the prevention of intermarriage among Deaf people (Box 156-1), postmortem dissection, and crude attempts at hearing augmentation. Now, newborn screening, gene mapping, and cochlear implantation are the focus. A milestone occurred in 1990 with the passage of the Americans with Disabilities Act (ADA), which, in part, mandates accessibility to health care. The D/deaf adolescent, however, may not always reap the benefits of these advances. Newborn screening is obviously for the newborn. Cochlear implantation, approved for use in children 1 year of age and older, has been shown to have the best results when done as early as possible. Although Deaf adults may be offered sign language interpreters, adolescents may have a more difficult time negotiating the health system to obtain equal services. The challenge for the practitioner is to provide the D/deaf adolescent the full range of health services, including anticipatory guidance, education, risk assessment, evaluation, and management as would be provided for the hearing adolescent, as well as to assess psychosocial development and provide any medical treatment specifically related to the deafness.

**Box 156-1**

***Distinction between "Deaf" and "deaf"***

"Deaf" refers to deaf people as a cultural group, whereas "deaf" denotes the audiological condition of severe to profound hearing loss. The term "Deaf" (with an uppercase D) is used here to denote those who identify as culturally Deaf. It indicates a cultural significance to those who identify as culturally Deaf. When the lowercase D is used, it indicates a technical or medical sense of hearing loss. "D/d" is sometimes used to indicate both categories. It may indicate that an individual is deaf but may not necessarily identify as culturally Deaf.

### ETIOLOGY

The incidence of congenital deafness is approximately 1 in 1,000 births, with another 1 in 1,000 children becoming deaf prior to adulthood. Although the incidence has remained fairly constant, our understanding of the causes of deafness, as well as the individual etiologies, has changed markedly secondary to advances in medicine. In the 19th century, a common cause of acquired deafness was catarrhal deafness, that is, blockage from inflamed adenoids and nasal passages, which, once adenoidectomies were perfected, has become obsolete. Other reported causes of that era included scarlet fever, scrofula (tuberculosis), worms, bathing, lightning, and fright.[1] The introduction of antibiotics in the 20th century decreased the incidence of some infectious causes, while increasing the incidence secondary to ototoxicity. Prior to Mendel's work on patterns of inheritance in 1865, the cause of a second deaf child born in a family was considered a result of "sad mental impressions" in the expectant mother.[2] However, early reports of deaf children among intermarriage of near relations were also appearing in the literature. During the mid-19th century, deaf children began to attend residential educational institutions, which gave them the opportunity to meet, develop a community and culture, and marry. In the early 20th century, interest in genetics, along with the observation that Deaf couples were having children with a slightly increased rate of deafness compared with hearing couples, led to failed attempts to try to legislate the prevention of marriage among Deaf people.

The rubella epidemic of the 1960s left thousands of newborns with deafness, blindness, and other serious medical complications. Subsequent licensure of the rubella vaccine in 1969 has virtually eliminated the disease as an etiologic cause of deafness in the United States. The incidence of meningitis, once the leading cause of acquired deafness, has also been declining since the conjugate *Haemophilus influenzae* vaccine was issued in 1987. Advances in perinatal medicine have led to the increased incidence of hearing loss seen in extremely low birth weight babies and those neonates receiving extracorporeal membrane oxygenation (ECMO) and prolonged ventilation.[3]

To date, more than 400 genetic syndromes involving deafness have been described[4] and more than 75 genes identified (Hereditary Hearing Loss home page: webh01.ua.ac.be/hhh). Although in-depth discussion can be found elsewhere, highlighted in the following are several genetic causes and one nongenetic cause (rubella) of deafness with specific importance for the Deaf adolescent.

### CONGENITAL RUBELLA SYNDROME

First described in Australia in 1941, congenital rubella syndrome (CRS) has virtually been eliminated in the United States.[5] The 1960s rubella epidemic in the United States left thousands of individuals with multisystem teratogenic effects of rubella. For the present-day practitioner, CRS is considered a syndrome "of the past." However, for those caring for adults or immigrant Deaf children and adolescents, CRS remains a relevant nongenetic etiology. The World Health Organization (WHO) estimates more than 100,000 cases of CRS worldwide, and therefore schools serving deaf students that have immigrant populations should expect to see individuals with CRS.

Newborns with CRS may present with sensorineural deafness, although at times the hearing loss develops over months to years, and classically with cataracts and congenital heart disease (patent ductus arteriosis being the most common) depending on when during gestation the rubella was contracted. Of utmost concern for those caring for adolescents, CRS is not a static disease, but has late manifestations often presenting in the second and third decades of life. Delayed onset disease includes diabetes mellitus type 1 (12% to 20%; another 20% have pancreatic islet cell cytotoxic antibodies suggesting future development of diabetes), diabetes mellitus type 2, glaucoma, thyroid disease (19%), early menopause (73%), osteoporosis (13%), cardiac disease (pulmonary stenosis, peripheral pulmonary stenosis), growth retardation,[6] and progressive subacute panencephalopathy.

Providers need to maintain a high index of suspicion for CRS, especially regarding patients born in countries where rubella vaccine is not mandated or offered. History of gestational rash, small for gestational age, congenital heart disease, congenital cataracts, and continued short stature and microcephaly into adolescence may provide clues to the diagnosis. Hypo- and hyperpigmentation of the retina (salt and pepper retinopathy) are sometimes seen. After diagnosis, recommendations include screening for late manifestations and educating the individual and family about these concerns.

### CONNEXIN 26

Most congenital deafness is genetic in nature, and most genetic deafness is nonsyndromic, having no other associated medical findings. Approximately half of all nonsyndromic deafness is caused by mutations in Connexin 26 (GJB2).[7] Connexin 26 is a gap junction protein felt to be involved in ion transport, specifically in recycling potassium within the cochlea that allows proper functioning of the cochlear hair cells. More than 40% of genetic deafness appears to be secondary to Connexin 26. Diagnosis by genetic analysis for the Connexin 26 gene is available, which can aid in early diagnosis and management and ensure that other causes, such as Jervell and Lange-Nielsen or Usher syndrome (US; see the following) are not present.

### WAARDENBURG SYNDROME

A common form of autosomal-dominant deafness is Waardenburg syndrome (WS), first defined in 1948 and responsible for 3% to 6% of congenital deafness.[8,9] It has marked variable penetrance, and therefore a detailed family history may be needed to see a more complete presentation. There are 4 described types: WS type 1 features deafness (25% of cases), dystopia canthorum (lateral displacement of the inner canthi), isochromic pale blue irides or heterochromic irides, white forelock (poliosis), various degrees of hypopigmentation (piebaldism, vitiligo), premature graying, medial fusion of the eyebrows (synophrys), and hypoplastic alae nasi. Waardenburg syndrome type 2 is similar to type 1, but without dystopia canthorum, and 50% of patients are deaf. Waardenburg syndrome type 3, also known as Klein-Waardenburg, is similar to type 1, with limb anomalies. Waardenburg syndrome type 4, also known as Shah-Waardenburg, has features similar to type 2 but is associated with Hirschsprung disease and has autosomal-recessive inheritance. Several genetic mutations have been described and mutation analysis is available.

### USHER SYNDROME

First described by Von Graefe in 1858, but named after the ophthalmologist who noted its pattern of inheritance, Usher syndrome significantly affects adolescent development. Usher syndrome (US) involves sensorineural hearing loss and retinitis pigmentosa (RP) and is responsible for 3% to 6% of congenital deafness, making it the leading cause of deafblindness.[10] Transmission is autosomal-recessive and there are 3 types described. Usher syndrome type 1: profound deafness at birth, early onset of RP, and vestibular dysfunction; US type 2: moderate to severe hearing loss at birth, later and slower onset of RP, and no vestibular dysfunction; US type 3: normal to mild hearing loss at birth that progresses in childhood, variable later onset of RP, and no vestibular dysfunction. There may also be a fourth type that has x-linked inheritance.

The challenges people with US face are quite different depending on the type. Those with type 1 often communicate visually with sign language, and those with type 2 often, though not always, use spoken language and speechread with the assistance of auditory amplification. When each of these groups is met with progressive vision loss, the challenges in interacting with the world around them can be great. Those with US type 1 are congenitally deaf; they therefore often communicate using sign language, which is dependent on vision, and identify with Deaf peers and Deaf culture.

The early signs of US often go unrecognized. The vestibular dysfunction may manifest as delayed acquisition of motor milestones, specifically walking, and babies may use a 5-point (head used as a prop) crawl. The night vision loss seen in infancy and childhood may be passed off as behavior problems that present as night terrors and enuresis. Usually by 10 to 12 years of age, as the child enters early adolescence, the cone cells begin to deteriorate and blind spots (scotomas) develop. The child may not realize at this stage that his/her vision is different than that of peers. As these blind spots coalesce into full-ringed scotomas, the individual may experience significant visual field loss. The vision loss often becomes prominent during mid-adolescence, at a time when the adolescent is asserting his/her independence and looking to peers to establish a "sense of normal" and an identity as a member of the Deaf community. Communication is hindered as the adolescent may miss conversation off to the side. The teen is considered clumsy and often made fun of for tripping over large objects, walking into doorways, or bumping into people in the hall. Sports may prove difficult as it becomes increasingly hard to track a moving object, such as a ball, or an opponent running or to see contrast, such as a white ball, in the sky. Also faced with difficulties seeing at night, the adolescent may begin to socially withdraw and isolate, without even understanding the cause of these feelings.[11]

Diagnosis is made by establishing a negative (extinguished) response by electroretinogram (ERG). Findings on funduscopy of retinal pigmentation and vessel attenuation can often be seen by the skilled clinician or ophthalmologist. Relaying the diagnosis to the adolescent and family should be done by people knowledgeable in US. The term "blind" or "Deafblind" should be minimized as individuals with US can have useful, albeit deteriorating, vision for decades. As the diagnosis is often devastating for both the adolescent and family, appropriate psychological support services should be provided. Giving adolescents an opportunity to meet other adolescents and young adults with US through local organizations or the Helen Keller National Center can help with the fear and isolation many of these adolescents face. Once a diagnosis is made, visual field testing should be performed to "map out" the scotomas and areas of useful vision. These tests are useful in establishing class seat assignments, sports participation clearance, and addressing concerns regarding activities of daily living, and should be repeated as needed (yearly or biannually) to discern changes. Orientation and mobility assessment should be provided to ascertain the need for any visually related education or independence skills services. Gene testing might allow individuals to be diagnosed as early as possible, prevent injuries, such as pedestrian–motor vehicle accidents, and allow intervention before symptoms are apparent.

Often seen as a rite of passage into adulthood, a specific concern is the ability to drive. Because most states do not require peripheral field screening to obtain a driver's license, it is quite possible that individuals with US do drive. However, at least one study has shown that there is a significant correlation of motor vehicle crashes with visual field loss in those with RP.[12] Adolescents should be encouraged to obtain a nondriving license and through orientation and mobility services gain independence by alternative means of transportation.

## JERVELL AND LANGE-NIELSEN SYNDROME

An infrequent but potentially lethal disorder is Jervell and Lange-Nielsen syndrome (JLN), first described in 1957 in a family of 4 children with congenital deafness, 3 of whom died suddenly.[13] The syndrome is one of congenital deafness and long QT that can lead to sudden death, and it has autosomal-recessive inheritance. The incidence has been reported to be at 0.17% of all congenital deafness.

Jervell and Lange-Nielsen syndrome is heterogenetic, with several genetic mutations described, giving rise to several subtypes and presentations. Type 1 presents with cardiac events that occur with physical exertion; type 2 with events that occur with emotional stress; type 3 has events that occur during rest or sleep. Cardiac presentations include syncope, atypical seizure-like episodes, and cardiac arrest from torsades de pointe and ventricular fibrillation. The significance of early recognition and management of this syndrome is highlighted by the high rate of sudden death (up to 30% to 40%) at time of first cardiac event, as well as a 10-year mortality rate of 50% to 70% in untreated individuals.

Management is aimed at preventing a malignant ventricular tachyarrhythmia with the use of beta blockers as a first line of defense. Implantable cardioverter defibrillators are recommended for those who are resistant to standard treatment, are nonadherent with treatment, or whose presenting event was a rescued cardiac arrest. Future treatments will focus on gene-based therapy targeting ion channels. For the adolescent with JLN, the challenge is to promptly diagnose, help ensure compliance, limit physical exercise and stressful stimuli, and help foster normal adolescent development.

### ALPORT SYNDROME

Alport syndrome (AS) represents a genetically heterogeneous disease that primarily manifests as renal impairment, along with eye and cochlear disease.[14] Alport syndrome is present in approximately 3% of all children with end-stage renal disease (ESRD) in the United States. Eighty percent of the pedigrees show x-linked-recessive inheritance; however heterogeneous females can show some symptoms of the disease as well. Another 15% show autosomal-recessive inheritance, with males and females equally affected, and the remainder consists of autosomal-dominant forms.

The genetic mutations are varied and usually unique to individual family lines. Clinically affected males (x-linked-recessive) present with microscopic hematuria in the first decade of life, with further development of proteinuria and hypertension with age. The progression to ESRD, although inevitable, varies in its timing in accordance with the family line. The juvenile form of x-linked AS presents with ESRD before age 30, whereas the adult form is after 30. The hearing loss is progressive in nature, usually starting in the first or second decade of life and invariably accompanied by renal disease. Profound deafness may occur by adolescence or young adulthood, depending on family genetics. The ocular manifestations primarily include anterior lenticonus. The treatment for AS is renal transplantation.

### PENDRED SYNDROME

Vaughn Pendred[15] first recognized the association between deafness and goiter in 1896. Pendred syndrome (PS) is considered one of the most common causes of syndromic congenital deafness, responsible for up to 7.5% of cases. It is an autosomal-recessive disorder characterized by bilateral sensorineural hearing loss (often secondary to Modini malformation of the cochlea) and goiter, with occasional vestibular dysfunction. The appearance of the goiter is quite variable; it usually presents in adolescence or early adulthood but can be absent in up to 40% of individuals. Testing shows an abnormal perchlorate discharge test, which evaluates iodine uptake by the thyroid gland and is classically positive in PS, although most individuals are chemically and clinically euthyroid. Several mutations of the Pendred gene (PDS) have been localized and shown to code for pendrin, an ion transport protein. Treatment for the goiter consists usually of thyroxin, and less often surgery.

## PSYCHOSOCIAL CONSIDERATIONS

### EARLY INTERVENTION AND FAMILY VARIABLES

To understand the deaf adolescent, an awareness of antecedent issues is critical. Universal infant hearing screening has facilitated earlier diagnosis of deafness, although progressive hearing loss or a later central nervous system etiology can delay diagnosis.[16] Pending parent adjustment to the diagnosis, caregiver participation in quality early intervention programs will minimize childhood developmental delays and facilitate cognitive, linguistic, and social development, taking into account developmental differences based on factors such as individual characteristics, cultural contexts, parenting styles, emotional and social resources, use of hearing technology, exposure to auditory/visual language, and ability to adapt to the needs of the deaf child.[17,18] Participation in such programs is less frequent and less satisfactory for families of lower socioeconomic status and those with minority/racial/ethnic identification.[19] In immigrant families, adjustment to a new culture and language creates additional burdens, with the deaf adolescent having to confront limited linguistic access to information and emotional stress.[20] Approximately 5% of deaf parents will have deaf children; these children typically demonstrate higher academic achievement and self-concept based in part on accessible communication in the home and parental awareness of the needs of their deaf children.[21]

In dealing with deaf adolescents, communication factors are paramount. One of the earliest decisions that parents or caregivers have to make is how to provide language access for their deaf child. Such decisions may be heavily dependent on available local programs and their communication philosophy, that is, spoken language, bicultural–bilingual (use of American Sign Language [ASL] and English separately), signed English (spoken English accompanied by signs), cued speech (sign system on the face to illustrate spoken phonemes simultaneously).[22] For any approach, parents/caregivers have to decide on hearing aids or cochlear implantation (see later discussion), adjust to the technology, and orient their children to the meaning of sound or to visual linguistic input. Early intervention will facilitate the effectiveness of family communication, which has critical bearing on the deaf adolescent's social and emotional adjustment.

### EDUCATIONAL TRENDS

Deaf individuals are educated in a variety of settings, depending on educational philosophy, local availability, and individual needs. The historical reliance on specialized schools for deaf children is no longer the main option; approximately three-fourths of deaf children and youth are educated in the mainstream.[23] Mainstream educational options include full-time resource room placement, placement in both regular nonacademic classes and specialized academic classes, or full inclusion in standard classrooms with or without support services such as FM systems, sign language interpreters, and itinerant teachers.[24] Despite numerous success stories, adolescents frequently are not fully integrated into the academic and social processes of the school setting due to limited communication access and subpar academic achievement, even if they have moderate to severe, rather than severe to profound, hearing losses. Complex classroom discussions create communication barriers not easily overcome, even with support services.

Specialized schools are often preferred by Deaf parents of Deaf students because of communication ease through the use of ASL and Deaf culture exposure, though there are some settings exclusively based on spoken language. However, specialized schools have increasingly become a resource for deaf students with additional disabilities who have difficulty in mainstream education. There seems to be a recent trend of deaf mainstreamed adolescents gravitating back to specialized schools for socialization with deaf peers and ease in accessing classroom instruction, although more research is needed to confirm this.[25]

### PSYCHOSOCIAL IMPLICATIONS FOR DEAF ADOLESCENTS

Deaf adolescents are not immune to the usual adolescent issues predominant in the United States. Secure emotional attachment and effective parent–child communication facilitate confident adolescent exploration beyond the family.[26] Success depends on the adolescent's social and communication capabilities.

Adolescents require skill in matching group norms for expressive and receptive communication, keeping in mind that optimal receptive communication with hearing peers is not always readily achievable, either because of limitations in using vision or speech reading, or because of noisy situations. Inadequately understood speech is often an issue. Consequently, mainstreamed adolescents are often prone to social neglect by hearing peers, potentially leading to adjustment difficulties. When critical masses of deaf adolescents are available, there tends to be greater emotional security with deaf friendships as opposed to hearing friendships.

Adolescence is a critical time for self-esteem and identity development, which are influenced by messages from family and peers. Depending on the social context, the deaf adolescent may develop a hearing-based identity (mirroring the ways hearing people behave and viewing deafness as a disability to be surmounted), a Deaf identity (connecting with the Deaf community as a positive identifier rather than adopting a stance that denies deafness as a normal variation of the diversity spectrum), a bicultural identity (reflecting comfort in both Deaf and hearing environments), or a marginal identity (rootless in either environment).[27]

Social neglect, implying as it does the stigmatizing aspect of being deaf in a mainstream hearing setting, is a breeding ground for feelings of marginality. Positive exposure to Deaf culture, which is rooted in ASL, may result in improved self-esteem. Various studies indicate that having Deaf or bicultural identities is more strongly associated with positive self-esteem in contrast to hearing identity, presumably due to stress in maintaining positive interactive communication with hearing peers. The emotionally healthy deaf adolescent is supported by parents, peers, and appropriate educational interventions based on strengths and needs. Lacking these, the risk for psychopathology increases.

## HEALTH CARE ACCESS

Access to private and confidential health care is a right for all adolescents. There is limited information in the literature regarding the health risks of D/deaf adolescents. It is clear, however, that these adolescents face similar health concerns as do hearing adolescents but are often faced with barriers that may impede access to appropriate information and services. Reports indicate that D/deaf adolescents are involved in high-risk behaviors, with more than 50% of Deaf youth becoming sexually active by age 18, only one-third using condoms at last sexual encounter,[28] and many exhibiting limited knowledge regarding AIDS.[29] Ninety-six percent of deaf offspring have hearing parents, and health care professionals are more comfortable communicating with the parents. A pilot study suggested that at the most recent medical visit, the parents were kept in the room in 60% of cases, and in only 7% was there a sign language interpreter present.[30]

The ADA Title III (Public Accommodations) legislates that ancillary services, including qualified sign language interpreters, be provided as needed by doctors' offices and hospitals. Adolescents are often dependent on parents to arrange their medical appointments. This can place them at a disadvantage in trying to navigate the medical system and negotiate interpreter services to ensure confidentiality. It should therefore also become the responsibility of the health care provider to ensure access for Deaf adolescent patients and arrange for sign language interpreter services as needed. Certainly, parents or family members should never be used to obtain confidential information from a Deaf adolescent. One may also need to provide interpreter services for patients with cochlear implants (CIs) or those who are mainstreamed, as many of those adolescents also use sign language.

## COCHLEAR IMPLANTS

The earliest descriptions of hearing loss and its treatments can be found in the ancient Egyptian papyri dating to before 1500 BC. In the 17th and 18th centuries various "speaking trumpets" and horns were used to amplify sound. Treatments such as repetitive noise exposure for auditory re-education and electrical stimulation can also be found in 19th-century literature. The first wearable carbon hearing aid was introduced in 1902 for mild hearing loss. For more severe hearing loss, electronic vacuum tube hearing aids appeared in the 1920s, with wearable versions becoming available in the 1930s. After World War II, the return of many veterans with noise-induced hearing loss led to an increased interest in developing audiometers to better fit hearing aids. The 1950s transistor behind-the-ear hearing aid has evolved into the digital hearing aids of the 1980s. The most significant effect on auditory rehabilitation has been the CI, first licensed by the Food and Drug Administration (FDA) in 1984 and approved for use in children in 1990.[31] Whereas conventional hearing aids amplify sound and rely on working cochlear hair cells, the CI bypasses the hair cells to directly stimulate the auditory nerve. The CI consists of an external microphone, speech processor and transmitter, an internal receiver and stimulator placed in a shallow well in the parietal bone, and an electrode that is surgically introduced through a mastoidectomy into the cochlear canal.

Studies have shown that the earlier implantation can be done after an acquired hearing loss, the better result for speech recognition, leading to implantations being approved by the FDA for congenital deafness in children 12 months of age and older. Candidates for CIs undergo extensive screening, including imaging studies and otologic and psychosocial evaluations. For adolescents with congenital deafness considering implantation, careful screening regarding appropriate expectations and motivation of both the adolescent and the parents, as well as previous experience with auditory amplification, must be included. Although further long-term studies are needed to document real-world outcomes, CIs have been shown to provide the possibility of understandable speech in many recipients with early implantation and to be an adjunct to speech reading in others. Investigations are being done regarding implanting children younger than 12 months of age, the use of bilateral CIs to help localize sound, fully implantable CIs, and bone-conductive devices for those who are not candidates for CIs. Most of the educational research on users of CIs focuses on children rather than adolescents. The general consensus is that with implantation before age 3 and appropriate intensive habilitation, the likelihood of improved language and speech, and in turn greater academic competency, is greater compared with earlier generations, but not necessarily equivalent with hearing peers.[32,33] Individual variation, including cognitive skills and consistency of habilitation, complicates the research picture insofar as educational achievement is concerned.

Surgical complications are considered to be minimal and consist primarily of skin flap infections, facial nerve weakness, cerebrospinal fluid leak, perilymphatic fistulae, and tinnitus. More serious complications, including facial nerve stimulation, skin flap necrosis, and electrode extrusion, are infrequent. In 2002, a 30 times increased rate of bacterial meningitis, especially secondary to *Streptococcus pneumoniae*, was reported in children who received CIs.[34] Many, but not all, of these cases were felt to be secondary to the use of a positioner that holds the electrode against the wall of the cochlear. Since July 2002 the model that used a positioner (Advanced Bionics) has been removed from the market, although there is no recommendation that those who currently have this model have it surgically removed. Although the risk of meningitis decreases over time after surgery, there remains an ongoing increased risk of meningitis beyond at least 2 years postimplantation.[35] All children who are to undergo cochlear implantation or who have CIs should receive appropriate immunization prophylaxis.

Because of the possible relationship with otitis media and the development of meningitis in some of these patients, prompt diagnosis and management of otitis media is necessary. Further studies are needed to assess the actual role of otitis media in these patients and the appropriate course of antibiotics. Because there is a magnet placed under the scalp to hold the external transmitter in place, patients with CIs are often unable to undergo magnetic resonance imaging (MRI) or need to have the magnet removed prior to the study, depending on the nature of the technology. Other considerations include participation in certain athletics where there may be a possibility of damaging the implant, for example boxing and wrestling. Participation in these sports, including football, hockey, and rugby, needs to be discussed with the surgeon. In other contact/collision sports, the player should wear a protective helmet. Various modes of communication should be discussed, even for those able to understand speech using the CI, for times when the CI is not being worn, for example, during swimming, certain sports activities, or at night.

From a psychosocial perspective, it is imperative to recognize that CIs do not make deaf individuals "hearing." The sounds produced by this device differ drastically from normal sounds, and deaf children must learn to identify these through intensive training. Deaf culture adherents have feared potential psychological maladjustment based on being forced into "hearing molds." A review of psychosocial research on adolescents[32] indicates that factors other than the CIs per se, including personality, social support, and communication access, will affect psychosocial adjustment. Communication access and interaction with hearing peers can be facilitated by the effective use of CIs. However, difficulties with background noise and individual variation in the ability to identify meaningful sounds affect the ability to interact in one-on-one and group situations. Evidence of adolescents with CIs who continue to sign when in Deaf environments has allayed concerns that getting a CI automatically implies rejection of Deaf culture.

## REFERENCES


1. Fay EA. Reports of American institutions for the deaf and dumb. *Am Ann Deaf.* 1875;20(4):252–271

2. Turner WW. Causes of deafness. *Am Ann Deaf.* 1847;1(1):25–32

3. Roizen NJ. Etiology of hearing loss in children, nongenetic causes. *Pediatr Clin North Am.* 1999;46:49–64

4. Gorlin RJ, Toriello HV, Cohen MM, eds. *Hereditary Hearing Loss and Its Syndromes.* New York, NY: Oxford University Press; 1995

5. Banatvala JE, Brown DWG. Rubella. *Lancet.* 2004;363:1127–1137

6. Chiriboga-Klein S, Oberfield S, Casullo AM, et al. Growth in congenital rubella syndrome and correlation with clinical manifestations. *J Pediatr.* 1989;115:251–255

7. Marlin S, Feldmann D, Blons H, et al. GJB2 and GJB6 mutations. *Arch Otolaryn Head Neck Surg.* 2005;131:481–487

8. Nayak C, Isaacson G. Worldwide distribution of Waardenburg syndrome. *Ann Otol Rhinol Larygol.* 2003;112:817–820

9. Jones KL, ed. Waardenburg syndrome, types I and II. *Smith's Recognizable Patterns of Human Malformation.* 6th ed. Philadelphia, PA: Elsevier Saunders; 2006:278–279

10. *Usher Syndrome. National Institute on Deafness and Other Communication Disorders.* NIH publication No. 98–429; 2003

11. Miner I. The impact on Usher syndrome, type 1, on adolescent development. *J Vocational Rehab.* 1996;6:159–166

12. Szlyk JP, Alexander KR, Severing K, Fishman G. Assessment of driving performance in patients with retinitis pigmentosa. *Arch Ophthal.* 1992;110:1709–1713

13. Chian CE, Roden D. The long QT syndromes: genetic basis and clinical implications. *J Am Coll Cardio.* 2000;36:1–12

14. Kashtan C. Alport syndrome—an inherited disorder of renal, ocular, and cochlear basement membranes. *Medicine.* 1999;78(5):338–360

15. Reardon W, Coffey R, Chowdhury T, et al. Prevalence, age of onset, and natural history of thyroid disease in Pendred syndrome. *J Med Genetics.* 1999;36:595–598

16. NCHAM. Early Hearing Detection and Intervention. National Center for Hearing Assessment and Management Web site. Available at: www.infanthearing.org/earlychildhood/index.html. Accessed March 16, 2010

17. Sass-Lehrer M, Bodner-Johnson B. Early intervention. In: Marschark M, Spencer P, eds. *Oxford Handbook of Deaf Studies, Language, and Education.* New York, NY: Oxford University Press; 2003:65–81

18. Traci M, Koester LS. Parent-infant interactions. In: Marschark M, Spencer P, eds. *Oxford Handbook of Deaf Studies, Language, and Education.* New York, NY: Oxford University Press; 2003:190–202

19. Moores DF, Jatho J, Dunn C. Families with deaf members: American Annals of the Deaf, 1996–2000. *Am Ann Deaf.* 2001;146:245–250

20. Akamatsu CT, Cole E. Immigrant and refugee children who are deaf: crisis equals danger plus opportunity. In: Christensen K, ed. *Deaf Plus: A Multicultural Perspective.* San Diego, CA: DawnSign Press; 2000:93–120

21. Mitchell R, Karchmer M. When parents are deaf versus hard of hearing. *J Deaf Studies Deaf Edu.* 2004;9:133–152

22. Marschark M, Lang HG, Albertini JA. *Educating Deaf Students.* New York, NY: Oxford University Press; 2002

23. Karchmer M, Mitchell R. Demographic and achievement characteristics of deaf and hard-of-hearing students: In: Marschark M, Spencer P, eds. *Oxford Handbook of Deaf Studies, Language, and Education.* New York, NY: Oxford University Press; 2003:21–37

24. Stinson M, Antia S. Considerations in educating deaf and hard-of-hearing students in inclusive settings. *J Deaf Studies Deaf Edu.* 1999;4:165–175

25. Holden-Pitt L. A look at residential school placement patterns for students from deaf- and hearing-parented families: a ten-year perspective. *Am Ann Deaf.* 1997;142:108–114

26. Sheridan M. *Deaf Adolescents: Inner Lives.* Washington, DC: Gallaudet University Press; 2008

27. Glickman N. The development of culturally Deaf identities. In: Glickman N, Harvey M, eds. *Culturally Affirmative Psychotherapy with Deaf Persons.* Mahwah, NJ: Lawrence Erlbaum Associates; 1996:115–153

28. Joseph J, Sawyer R, Desmond S. Sexual knowledge, behavior, and sources of information among deaf and hard of hearing college students. *Am Ann Deaf.* 1995;140:338–345

29. Baker-Duncan N, Dancer J, Gentry B, Highly P, Gibson B. Deaf adolescents' knowledge of AIDS. *Am Ann Deaf.* 1997;142:368–372

30. Weiselberg EC, Sondike S, Jacobson M. Deaf adolescents' attitudes in seeking health care information. *Amb Child Health.* 1997;3

31. Papsin BC, Gordon KA. Cochlear implants for children with severe-to-profound hearing loss. *New Eng J Med.* 2007;357:2380–2387

32. Spencer P, Marschark M. Cochlear implants. In: Marschark M, Spencer P, eds. *Oxford Handbook of Deaf Studies, Language, and Education.* New York, NY: Oxford; 2003: 434–448

33. Marschark M, Rhoten C, Fabich M. Effects of cochlear implants on children's reading and academic achievement. *J Deaf Studies Deaf Edu.* 2007;12:269–282

34. Reefhuis J, Honein MA, Whitney CG, et al. Risk of bacterial meningitis in children with cochlear implants. *New Eng J Med.* 2003;349:435–445

35. Biernath KR, Reefhuis J, Whitney CG, et al. Bacterial meningitis among children with cochlear implants beyond 24 months after implantation. *Pediatrics.* 2006;117:284–289

# CHAPTER 157

# Adolescent Oral Health

DEBORAH STUDEN-PAVLOVICH, DMD • DENNIS N. RANALLI, DDS, MDS

Adolescent oral health is a topic of current relevance and is being recognized with increasing emphasis within the dental and medical communities. The complexity of the adolescent period provides an opportunity for interdisciplinary collaboration among various health care professionals to enhance the quality of integrated comprehensive care to the adolescent patients we treat.

The American Academy of Pediatrics[1] is keenly aware of the importance of adolescent oral health and in conjunction with the American Academy of Pediatric Dentistry has initiated programs such as Protecting All Children's Teeth (PACT): A Pediatric Oral Health Training Program. The aims of PACT are to educate pediatricians about the role of oral health in the overall health of infants, children, and adolescents. And further, to enable pediatricians to more comfortably provide oral health guidance and preventive measures in collaboration with their dental colleagues.

Adolescence is accompanied by physical, psychological, and social transitions, as well as being a time of transition in dentition. Maintaining good oral health is an essential component to the overall health and well-being of the adolescent as a gateway to adulthood. It is important to note that lifestyles and habits, healthful and harmful, that are formed during adolescence are more likely to continue into adulthood.

It is the intent of this chapter to provide an overview of common oral and dental conditions encountered in the clinical practice of adolescent dentistry with particular reference to the oral changes and dental needs that occur during this period.

The cornerstone of pediatric dentistry is prevention. A total prevention program for adolescents should include strategies that address the hard and soft tissues of the orofacial complex. Although some of these disease processes are reversible, such as gingivitis, others may be irreversible, such as dental caries once cavitation has occurred.

## HARD TISSUE

### DENTAL CARIES

Despite the numerous techniques and products aimed at preventing dental caries, it remains the single most common chronic disease of childhood and adolescence. During adolescence, caries risks and clinical patterns transition from those encountered during middle childhood. For example, pit and fissure caries are more common among early school-age children; a shift occurs to increased frequency of interproximal decay among teenagers. In fact, by 17 years of age, 78% of adolescents have experienced at least 1 irreversible carious lesion.[2]

One potential negative aspect of adolescent independence is related to the selection of food. Increased snacking patterns, the consumption of sugar-containing beverages, and carbohydrate overloading all contribute to dental decay.[3] Further, adolescents of lower socioeconomic status have been identified as having higher rates of caries (Figure 157-1).

On the other hand, this same characteristic of adolescent independence and assimilation of information to make informed decisions can be used as an entree to the prevention of dental caries in this age group. An exciting opportunity in working with individual adolescents is their maturing cognitive capabilities to understand cause-and-effect relationships that promote general and oral health.[4]

In terms of primary prevention, identifying healthful food choices should be emphasized. Comprehensive nutrition and dietary counseling not only enhances the prevention of dental caries but also contributes to positive measures for weight control among adolescents in general, but perhaps more importantly for adolescents with disordered eating patterns.[5] The relationship between good oral health and good systemic health is an important foundation for the adolescent to assimilate into health-enhancing behaviors.

In addition to healthful food choices, intensified efforts on establishing a proper oral home care routine including thorough and regular tooth brushing with fluoridated toothpaste, interproximal flossing, and fluoride mouth rinses, if necessary, are critical to caries prevention. If brushing is not possible after eating, swishing with water will dilute and clear food debris from the mouth. Chewing xylitol-containing gum is effective as a plaque-inhibiting agent as are chlorhexidine gluconate mouth rinses for bacterial clearance.[6] Although most community water supplies are fluoridated, in nonfluoridated

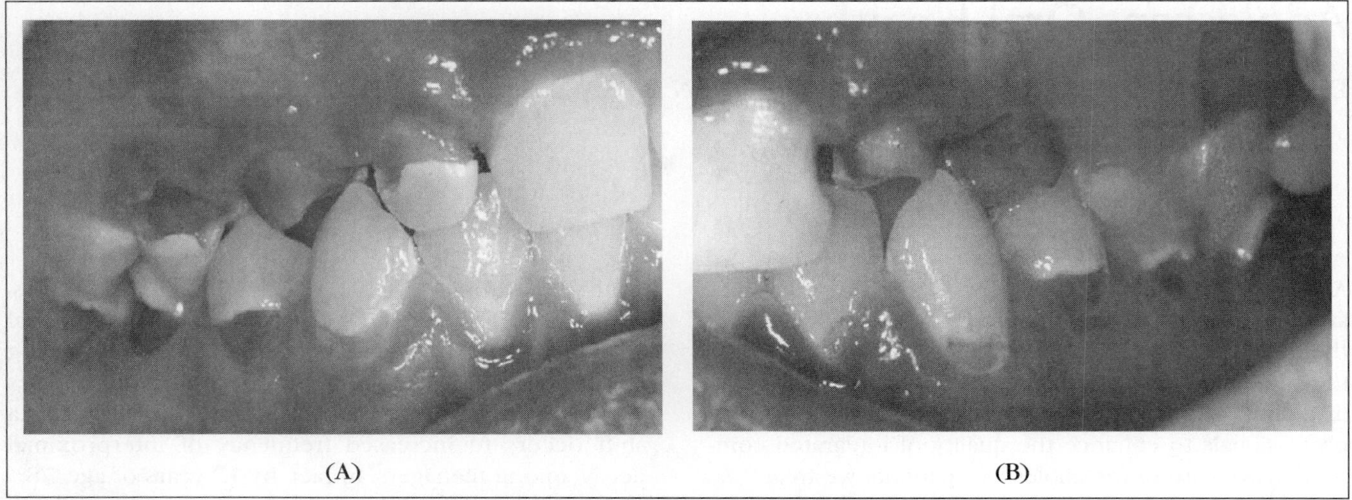

FIGURE 157-1 An adolescent patient with rampant untreated dental caries in the permanent dentition. (See color insert.)

areas fluoride supplementation should be continued until the adolescent has reached the age of 16.

Another aspect of primary prevention is the use of pit and fissure sealants. They have been proven to be effective in preventing dental caries on the occlusal surfaces of newly erupted posterior permanent teeth.[7] Because sealants cannot be placed on the tooth's interproximal surfaces, these areas are more vulnerable to the development of dental caries during adolescence.

In terms of secondary prevention, the restoration of teeth and regular 6-month recall examinations, including radiographs as necessary, are critical to the maintenance of adolescent oral health and the developing occlusion.

One area of increasing concern among dental practitioners is the rampant tooth decay associated with the use of the illicit drug methamphetamine. The term "meth mouth" includes devastating dental caries that progress rapidly.[8] The teeth literally crumble as they become nonrestorable and require extraction. Several causal factors may contribute to the inception of "meth mouth" including the acidity of the drug; the 12-hour duration of the drug; xerostomia; cravings for highly caloric, carbonated beverages; clenching and grinding of the teeth; and lack of attention to oral hygiene. Health care professionals who treat adolescents should be alert to physical signs of malnutrition along with unaccounted for and accelerated tooth decay.[9]

Thus, an essential component of an effective caries prevention program is an individualized approach for each adolescent patient because dental caries is an infectious process that can be interrupted before cavitation.

## DENTAL INJURIES

The epidemiology and etiology of traumatic dental injuries vary among age groups. For children in primary dentition, the most common injury is intrusive luxation of the maxillary incisors, often associated with the development of motor skills. In the adolescent population, traumatic dental injuries are frequent occurrences often associated with high-risk behaviors. The most prevalent type of injury is a crown fracture of the maxillary permanent incisors.

High-risk behaviors among adolescents may include participation in sports and recreational activities without the use of adequate protective equipment, altercations with peers, motor vehicle crashes, substance abuse by the adolescent or within the family, and oral piercings, among others.[10] Studies have demonstrated that adolescent males experience a higher frequency of dental injuries when compared with their female counterparts. However, when comparing male to female athletes, the occurrence of dental trauma is similar.[11]

Traumatic dental injuries of the hard tissue may be categorized as crown fractures, root fractures, luxations, or combinations of these. Evaluation of the severity and extent of oral trauma is essential for proper triage to the appropriate health care provider. It is important to note that any traumatic injury to the orofacial complex should alert the pediatrician to evaluate the patient for possible signs of mild traumatic brain injury (concussion).[12]

Enamel-only tooth fractures may go unnoticed by the patient and the physician, and such fractures do not constitute a true dental emergency, whereas fractures that extend through the enamel and dentin into the underlying vital tooth pulp will be evident and painful for the patient. Such injuries require immediate referral for definitive dental treatment. Often the prognosis for such injuries is dependent upon the time interval between the injury and the initiation of intervention.[13]

On the other hand, because most horizontal root fractures are not visible and occur subgingivally within the alveolar socket, they may be less readily recognized clinically and without the use of dental radiographs may go undetected (Figure 157-2). One indication of a displaced root fracture is that the tooth is not aligned with the contralateral tooth in the arch. These injuries should be referred immediately to the adolescent's dental practitioner for thorough evaluation, segmental repositioning, and placement of a semirigid splint.[14,15] During transport to the dentist, the pediatrician may instruct the patient to bite on a gauze pad to prevent further displacement and to absorb possible hemorrhage or oral fluids.

A traumatic force to a tooth that does not result in either a crown fracture or a root fracture may exhibit luxation ranging from subluxation to exarticulation (avulsed tooth).[16,17] Regardless of the extent of the luxation injury, the patient should be referred for definitive diagnosis, repositioning, and splinting of the tooth as required. In addition, for teeth that have been exarticulated, the tooth should be replanted as soon as possible on site to maximize the prognosis for successful reattachment. It should be emphasized that during the process the tooth should be handled by the crown only, that any debris should be gently rinsed from the tooth using saline solution, and positioning should be verified by comparison to the contralateral tooth. For instances in which this procedure is not feasible, the tooth should be placed in a liquid transport medium to preserve the periodontal ligament cells that remain on the root surface. Hank's balanced saline solution is the preferred transport medium.[18] An alternative is to place the tooth in a container of milk, preferably skim milk. Moreover, most neutral liquids are preferable to placing the tooth in a dry paper towel or gauze. Dry transport will result in desiccation and necrosis of the periodontal ligament cells, and reattachment failure with subsequent tooth loss. The replacement of lost anterior teeth during adolescence is confounded by the continuation of jaw growth and tooth eruption until the completion of craniofacial growth. These injuries often require extended and costly dental management into adulthood.

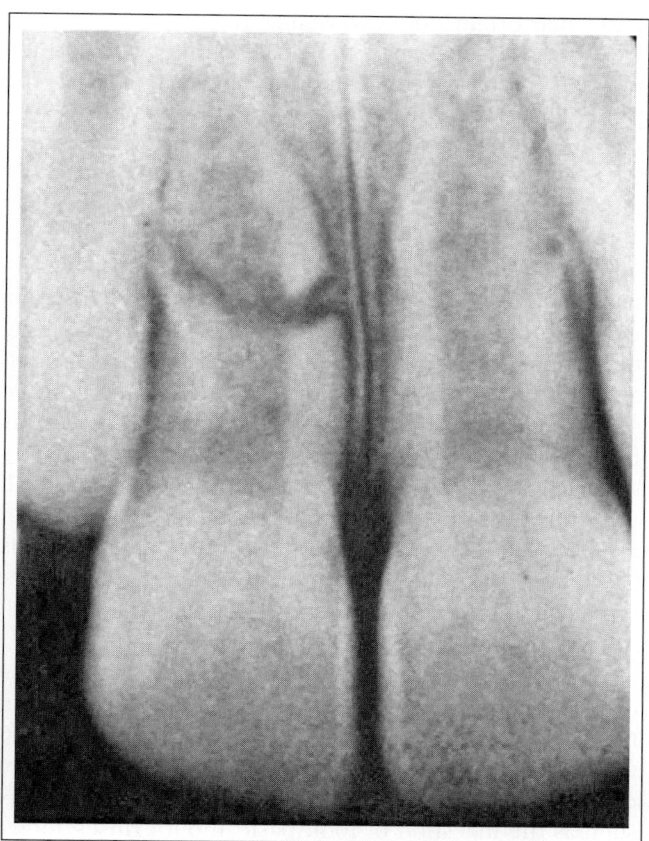

**FIGURE 157-2** A periapical radiograph illustrating a midroot fracture of the maxillary permanent right central incisor (Tooth #8).

In many instances of dental trauma the use of protective equipment has been demonstrated to be effective in preventing such injuries. Such equipment may include seat belts, helmets, face masks, and athletic mouthguards.[19] As part of the pediatrician's adolescent evaluation, inquiries should be made to determine the adolescent's participation in recreational activities or competitive sports. The use of a properly fitted custom mouthguard should be the recommendation of choice for all adolescent athletes (Figure 157-3).

## TOOTH DISCOLORATION

Because of an increased focus on aesthetics during adolescence, the presence of an unsightly dentition can be used as another motivational factor for improving oral hygiene. Discolored teeth may result from a variety of local and/or systemic conditions. Permanent teeth that are discolored may be classified into 2 broad categories: extrinsic (exogenous) staining or intrinsic (endogenous) staining.[20]

Localized extrinsic staining is commonly associated with bacteria and discoloring agents. The most commonly observed tooth staining is green and is associated with *Bacillus pyocyaneus*, *Aspergillis*.[21] Orange staining is associated with chromogenic bacteria such as *Serratia marcescens* and *Flavobacterium lutescens*, poor oral hygiene, and doxycycline, a commonly used prescription among teenagers to treat acne.[22]

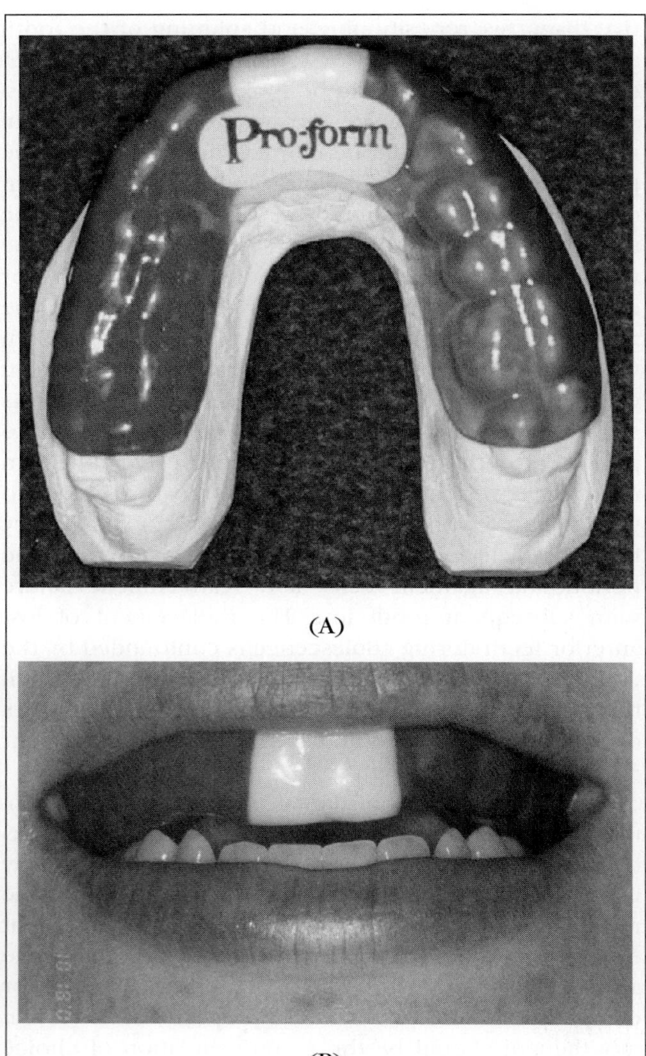


(A)

(B)

FIGURE 157-3 (A) Custom-fabricated athletic mouthguard made over a cast of the patient's maxillary arch; (B) Properly fitted custom-fabricated mouthguard in the patient's mouth. (See color insert.)

In addition to chromogenic bacteria, food pigments may cause brown stains due to the deposition of tannins found in tea and coffee, and coloring agents in cola drinks. Other foods and beverages that may result in staining include red wine, berries, and betel nuts. A more tenacious dark brown to black staining is associated with tobacco use in the form of pigments contained in chewing tobacco and the tars deposited by smoking cigarettes. Marijuana smoking has been associated with a gray-green stain from the oils, resins, and pigments in cannabis.

Many drugs and therapeutic agents may cause tooth staining. Black stains are associated with extrinsic metallic compounds such as iron sulfide and silver nitrate. Extended use of chlorhexidine gluconate rinses may also cause brown staining after several weeks of use, particularly on aesthetic tooth-colored restorations.

Another type of staining that may be present in the adolescent dentition is intrinsic staining. Intrinsic stains are endogenous and may be the result of pigments, drugs, and disorders.[20]

Blood-borne pigments may be a cause of intrinsic staining that is reflected by differences in the coloration of the teeth. For example, individuals with porphyria may demonstrate purplish-brown intrinsic staining whereas those with bile duct defects may present with green staining of the teeth. In addition, adolescents with various forms of anemia may demonstrate gray staining from hemosiderin deposition. It should be noted that although extrinsic staining is usually confined to the outer surfaces of the enamel covering the teeth, intrinsic stains are located in the deeper layers of the enamel and into the dentin. Thus, intrinsic stains are derived from the pulpal bloodstream within the tooth; extrinsic stains have their origin from external factors.

Drugs that may cause intrinsic staining include tetracycline and systemic fluoride ingested during the period of tooth development.[23,24] This staining is permanent and results in varying degrees of discoloration. Even when taken by the mother during pregnancy, tetracycline may stain the developing teeth of the child. Tetracycline can cross the placental barrier and also may pass into human milk. Thus, the effects of maternal use of tetracycline may appear years later in the permanent dentition of the adolescent. In addition, prescribing tetracycline between the fifth month *in utero* through age 8 of the offspring should be avoided. The degree of staining is related to the dosage and duration as well as the type of tetracycline compound used (Figure 157-4). The yellow discoloration caused by tetracycline will transition to brown by slow oxidation when the teeth are exposed to ultraviolet light. The threshold dosage is 21 to 26 mg/kg/day in a brief period, such as 3 days; tetracycline hydrochloride results in more staining than oxytetracycline.[23]

Repeated ingestion of low dosages of systemic fluoride over time may result in dental fluorosis, varying from opaque white spots to mottled enamel with diffuse brown striations. The critical issue is the additive effects of fluoride (halo effect) from multiple sources such as the ingestion of toothpaste, mouth rinses, foods, beverages, and water.

Determination of the fluoride content in the community water supply is essential in formulating an appropriate fluoride regimen. The fluoride concentration of

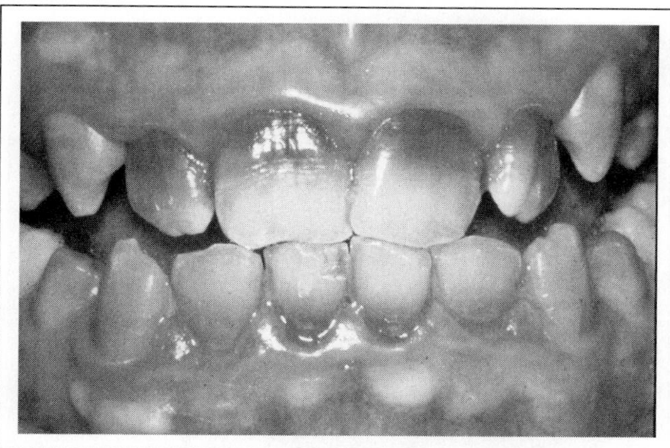

FIGURE 157-4 Generalized moderate to severe tetracycline staining in the permanent dentition of an adolescent patient. (See color insert.)

commercial products such as bottled water is often not taken into consideration when prescribing additional fluoride. Indiscriminant supplementation, especially with the use of fluoride-containing vitamins when other fluoride sources are unknown, may result in fluorosis. Despite the nonaesthetic appearance of teeth affected by dental fluorosis, these teeth are more resistant to dental decay.

Extrinsic tooth stains in the enamel are more easily removed than intrinsic staining that affects the deeper layers of enamel and extends into the dentin. For extrinsic stains a wide range of clinical treatment options is available such as mechanical scaling and prophylaxis with abrasive pumice or calcium carbonate; ultrasonic cleaning, air abrasion, or tooth-whitening agents in dentifrices, strips, or vital bleaching. For more penetrating intrinsic stains, professional bleaching, microabrasion, veneers, or crowns may be required to enhance the aesthetic results and self-image of the adolescent.[25]

## TOOTH WEAR

Posteruption tooth wear during adolescence is a noncarious pathologic loss of tooth structure that can be classified into 3 groups based on etiology: abrasion, attrition, and erosion. All 3 categories involve irreversible structural wear to the dentition that often requires dental restorations for patient comfort, aesthetics, and function.

Abrasion is the physiologic wearing away of tooth structure from tooth-to-tooth contact. This type of structural wear is often related to bruxism and affects the chewing surfaces of the teeth. Attrition is the wearing away of tooth structure by repeated use of an object. This type of structural wear is commonly associated with overzealous use of the toothbrush in the cervical portion of the crown. Erosive tooth wear involves chemical dissolution of tooth enamel caused by acid. Unlike dental caries, erosive tooth wear is without a bacterial component. It may affect all surfaces of the teeth, particularly the facial, occlusal, or lingual.

Of the 3 types of posteruption tooth wear, the effects of abrasion and attrition become evident later in life than erosion, which is the most prevalent type encountered during adolescence. Almost 46% of 13- to 19-year-olds sampled in the United States were found to have at least one tooth with erosive tooth wear.[26] Erosion may be categorized either as extrinsic or intrinsic.

Extrinsic erosion is associated with factors such as high intake of candy, soda, or acidic foods. Recent research indicates that high intake of candy, particularly the sour versions, is more erosive and less likely to be neutralized by saliva.[27] In addition, tooth erosion can be drug-induced with either prescription medications such as albuterol or illicit drugs such as methamphetamine, as described previously. For asthmatic adolescents following the use of an albuterol inhaler, drinking a glass of water to clear the medication from the teeth and to reduce its xerostomic effects is recommended.

In contrast, intrinsic erosion is often associated with acid reflux from gastrointestinal disorders or from purging related to eating disorders. Perioral and intraoral findings in patients with eating disorders involving self-induced vomiting may include enlargement of the parotid glands, xerostomia, and perimylolysis. The specific type of enamel erosion termed perimylolysis is the result of chemical effects caused by regurgitation of gastric contents and mechanical effects activated by the movement of the tongue. Typically, perimylolysis is seen on the lingual surfaces of the maxillary teeth. In addition, the incisal edges of the anterior teeth may become chipped and rough, and existing amalgam restorations in the posterior teeth may appear to be raised due to the surrounding enamel destruction. Continued loss of tooth structure on the chewing surfaces of the posterior teeth ultimately results in premature loss of vertical dimension. Because of the complexity of such eating disorders, a multidisciplinary approach is essential to address not only the oral and dental manifestations, but more importantly the underlying behavioral, psychosocial, and medical issues among affected adolescents.[28]

The key factor in the successful dental management of tooth wear such as erosion must include identifying and eliminating the underlying cause. Without control of these factors, dental therapeutic interventions are likely to be ineffective. Once the underlying causes have been addressed, dental interventions may proceed and include meticulous oral hygiene, dietary modifications, the use of topical fluoride rinses, and placement of aesthetic tooth-colored restorations. In extreme cases, full-mouth rehabilitation may be necessary.

## SOFT TISSUE

### PERIODONTAL DISEASES

The transition from childhood to adolescence is often accompanied by the development of and increased prevalence for periodontal diseases. The combined effects of genetics, hormonal fluctuations, medications, diet, and lack of proper oral hygiene all contribute to the spectrum of periodontal diseases during the adolescent period.[29] Pediatricians should be aware of the various oral manifestations of adolescent periodontal diseases as well as the increasing research evidence that supports the linkage between oral health and systemic health.

### GINGIVITIS

The most common reversible periodontal disease of adolescence is gingivitis. The underlying factors for the development of this inflammatory condition include the accumulation of plaque around the teeth due to inattention to brushing and flossing, sex hormone changes, host-parasite interactions, increased blood vessel permeability, and exaggerated responses to micro-organisms.[30] Effective interventions consist of regular professional prophylaxis and intensified educational efforts to improve self-care dental practices. The adolescent's need for peer acceptance and vanity may be used advantageously as motivational factors to stimulate positive behavioral changes.

### NECROTIZING ULCERATIVE GINGIVITIS

Compared to gingivitis, necrotizing ulcerative gingivitis (NUG) is a painful periodontal disease that often occurs in adolescent patients. This reversible condition has as its basis 2 components: altered host resistance and stress. The 2 primary causal bacteria are *Borelia vincentii* and *Prevotella intermedia*.[31] Stress among adolescents is often related to factors such as peer pressure, athletic events, school examinations, or lack of sufficient sleep, all of which may alter host resistance and bacterial proliferation. The clinical course of the disease begins initially with interproximal tissue necrosis of the gingivae. As the soft tissue begins to desquamate from the necrosis, patients experience the rapid onset of pain, metallic-tasting saliva, and fetid breath.[29] The tissue degradation results in a "punched-out" appearance of the gingival tissues (Figure 157-5). Dental intervention includes professional tissue debridement accompanied by rinsing. Although potentially uncomfortable, meticulous home care that includes brushing, flossing, and oral rinses is essential to alleviate the symptoms. Systemic effects often accompany NUG and include fever, malaise, and lymphadenopathy. Patients may seek treatment with the pediatrician before seeing the dentist; penicillin or metronidazole may be prescribed appropriately.[31] Necrotizing ulcerative gingivitis is thus an instance in which physicians and dentists are likely to interact on behalf of the adolescent patient.

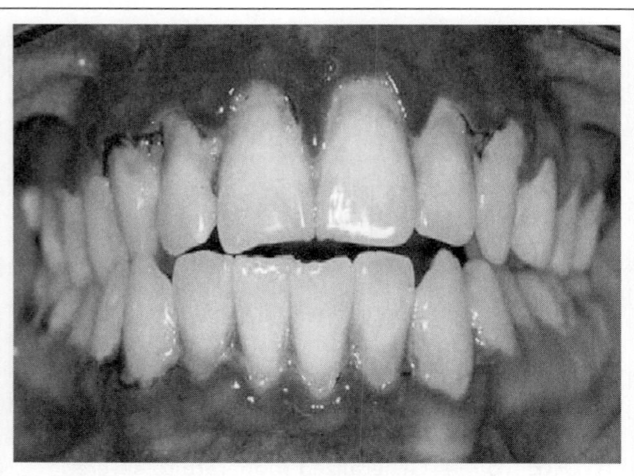

FIGURE 157-5 Acute phase of necrotizing ulcerative gingivitis demonstrating inflammation with tissue degradation. (See color insert.)

### HERPES SIMPLEX VIRUS

Another common periodontal disease in adolescent patients is associated with initial exposure to the herpes simplex virus (HSV). In addition, sexually active adolescents may present with sexually transmitted HSV-2 lesions in the oral cavity and perioral regions. According to a recent national survey, more than one-half of US teenagers have engaged in oral sex—including nearly one-quarter who have never experienced intercourse.[32] As a consequence, sexually transmitted diseases are spreading faster among adolescents than any other age group, with females more likely than their male counterparts to contract HSV-2 from a single act of unprotected sex.[33] Treatment is palliative and may include analgesics such as acetaminophen and antiviral medications such as acyclovir to alleviate symptoms. Recurrent herpes labialis may be treated with topical penciclovir cream for vesicular perioral lesions (Figure 157-6).[34] Thus, it is important for the pediatrician to address the adolescent's sexual activity history as a component of the overall medical history.

### PERICORONITIS

Another clinical situation in which the synergy between physicians and dentists is likely to occur relates to the development and eruption of the third molars—an event often anticipated by many teens as they transition from childhood into adulthood.

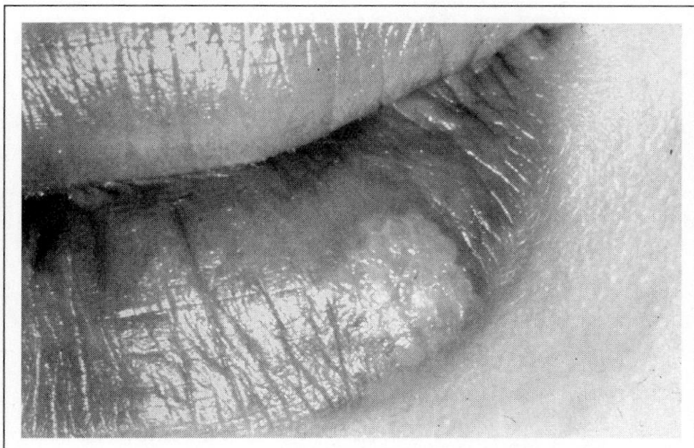

FIGURE 157-6 Vesicular lesion of recurrent herpes labialis on the lower lip. (See color insert.)

Active eruption of the third molars into the dental arch may be accompanied by irritation to the gingival tissues overlying the tooth. Bacterial ingress, particularly anaerobic bacteria, may cause formation of an inflammatory tissue operculum (pericoronitis) surrounding the crown of the erupting tooth (Figure 157-7), as well as systemic manifestations such as fever, malaise, and lymphadenopathy.[35] Unattended pericoronitis may result in alveolar bone loss and progression of periodontal disease to adjacent teeth.[36] Palliative treatment consists of determination of any periodontal pocketing, elimination of pathogens by debridement around/beneath the tissue operculum, irrigation with a solution of 0.2% chlorhexidine gluconate, and prescriptions for systemic antibiotics and pain medication as needed.

The full eruption of third molars frequently is inhibited by a tooth size-arch length discrepancy; the maxilla and/or the mandible are insufficient in length to accommodate the space needed for the third molars to erupt into occlusion. Definitive treatment consists of surgical removal of these teeth.

It is important to note that postoperative healing of third molar extraction sites may be compromised in some adolescents; for example, adolescent females on birth control pills and adolescent athletes on illicit anabolic steroids.[37,38] Further, susceptibility of mandibular gonial angle fractures may be increased in the presence of either an impacted mandibular third molar or a recently extracted mandibular third molar (Figure 157-8).

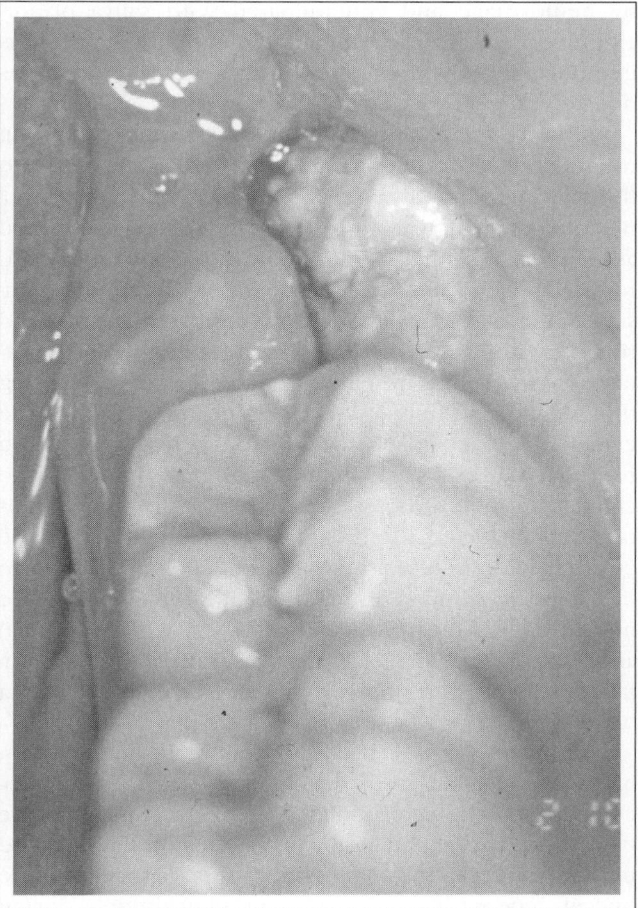

FIGURE 157-7 Pericoronitis surrounding the crown of an erupting mandibular permanent left third molar (Tooth #17). (See color insert.)

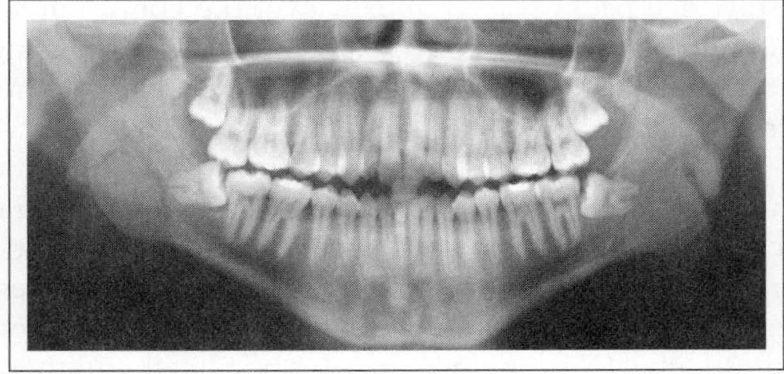

FIGURE 157-8 Panoramic radiograph of impacted third molars associated with bilateral mandibular fractures at the left and right gonial angles.

## SOFT TISSUE INJURIES

Injuries to the perioral and intraoral supporting soft tissues may occur separately from or in conjunction with dental injuries. Soft tissue trauma may result in a range of injuries from tissue abrasions, contusions, and lacerations to bite marks, puncture wounds, and tissue avulsions.[39] It should be emphasized that in cases of perioral and intraoral soft tissue injuries accompanied by hemorrhage and contaminated with saliva or foreign debris such as soil, the adolescent patient's tetanus immunization history should be reviewed and a tetanus booster administered as indicated.

Abrasions to the perioral tissues from scraping along rough surfaces often result in superficial damage to the skin, not usually deeper than the epidermal layer. Bleeding is generally minimal and treatment is directed at reducing healing time, preventing infection, and reducing the potential for scarring.[40] Treatment consists of cleansing the area with an antibacterial soap and rinsing with water to remove any debris. It is important to note that research contraindicates cleansing the wounds with hydrogen peroxide solution as the evidence has indicated that it is ineffective in reducing bacteria, causes tissue inflammation, and impedes the cellular healing process. Following appropriate, thorough cleansing of the area, the abrasion may then be covered with an antibiotic ointment such as Neosporin or bacitracin to prevent infection and to maintain tissue moisture. In adolescents with allergies to these topical antibiotics, petroleum jelly may be substituted to maintain tissue moisture. The wound may be dressed with a bandage.

Contusions are caused by traumatic forces from blunt objects that result in capillary damage and subcutaneous tissue ecchymosis. These hematomas may be painful and are readily visible as bruises on the face and perioral regions. Intraorally, they often appear on the buccal mucosa from inadvertent cheek-biting during mastication or on the hard and soft palate from oral sex. Cutaneous contusions progress through the various color changes from black and blue to greenish-yellow associated with the healing process over a 10- to 14-day period. Deeper firmness may take 1 to 2 months to resolve. Ice packs placed initially over the contusion for a 15-minute interval per hour are beneficial in reducing the posttraumatic edema, and analgesics may be prescribed as needed to alleviate pain.

Small lacerations to the lips, oral mucosa, and tongue often heal well without surgical intervention. Intraoral lacerations frequently are associated with traumatic forces against the teeth,[41] particularly in those adolescents wearing orthodontic appliances. Thus, it is important to check for mobile or chipped teeth in these patients. Control of bleeding for small lacerations consists of a sterile gauze compress and the application of an ice pack as needed. At home, salt water rinses should be recommended (Figure 157-9A, B, and C).

In adolescents with more extensive lacerations, in addition to hemorrhage and infection control, it is necessary to approximate the wound edges and place sutures that will promote a functional scar and an acceptable cosmetic result.[42] A local anesthetic with epinephrine

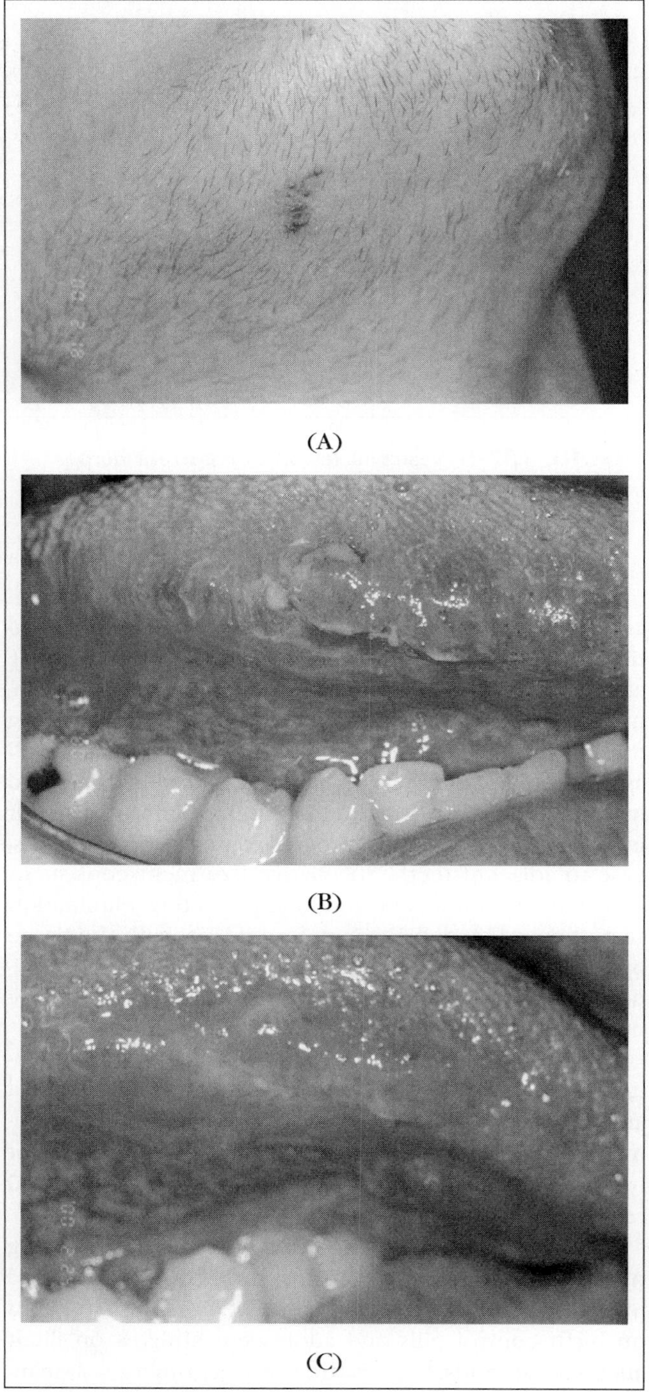


**FIGURE 157-9** (A) A 17-year-old white male wrestler received a blow to the mandible resulting in an abrasion with tissue edema; (B) The injury caused the patient to bite through the right lateral border of the tongue as demonstrated in the photo taken 2 days after the injury occurred; (C) Five days postinjury the tongue laceration healed spontaneously. (See color insert.)

may be infiltrated into the surrounding soft tissue to reduce pain and help control bleeding. The wound should be irrigated with saline and visualized to determine the presence of any foreign objects or tooth fragments within the laceration, which must be removed prior to suture placement. Suturing will depend on the length, depth, and location of the laceration. Deep lacerations extending into the underlying muscle tissue should be sutured in layers beginning in the deepest portion of the injury. For lacerations involving the buccal mucosa, the parotid duct and facial nerves should be evaluated. Postsuturing, an appropriate antibiotic, analgesic, and salt water home rinses may be prescribed. The patient should be placed on a soft diet and should avoid hot liquids for the first 4 to 6 hours and recalled in 48 hours for a follow-up evaluation.

As indicated in the section on contusions, patients may inadvertently bite the inside of their cheeks or may accidentally bite through the lateral borders of their tongue. Generally lacerations of the tongue heal quickly due to the rich blood supply and often do not require suturing. Another common site for self-inflicted bite wounds is the lower lip (Figure 157-10). Depending on the length and width of the laceration, sutures may be required. Long term, lip lacerations should be observed for the development of posttraumatic mucous retention cysts (mucocele). Habitual self-induced bite marks to other areas of the body may be indicative of a psychological disorder and require further questioning and referral as appropriate.

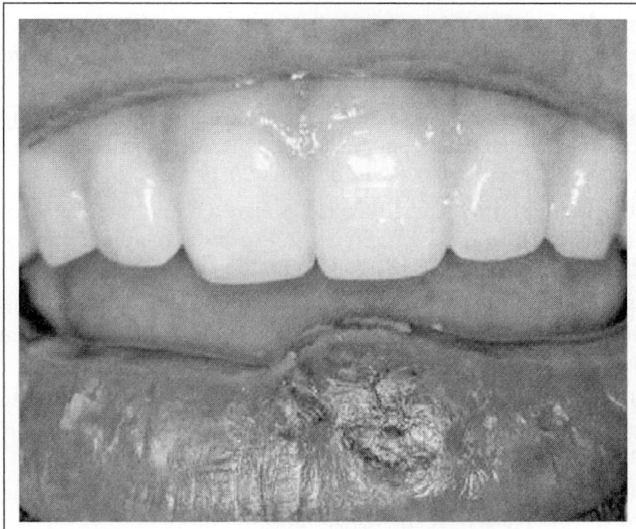

**FIGURE 157-10** Adolescent women's varsity basketball player with a self-inflicted bite wound to the lower lip that later developed into a mucocele. (See color insert.)

Bite marks inflicted on the adolescent by others may be the result of altercations, sexual activity, or abuse. Dentists are able to take impressions of the bite marks for forensic comparison to alleged perpetrators. In addition, the bite mark may be swabbed for DNA analysis. Human bite marks should trigger a cautionary note for potential infection. Bacterial inoculum from human bites is often more infectious than from animal bites.[39] Treatment consists of thoroughly cleansing the wound and prescribing antibiotics.

Animal bite marks have distinctive patterns different from human bite mark patterns. Human-pattern bite marks are elliptical or ovoid in shape with a central area of ecchymosis caused by tissue compression, whereas, dog or other carnivorous animal bites tear flesh and avulse tissue. Generally, an intercanine distance of greater than 3 centimeters is indicative of a suspected adult human bite mark.

Puncture wounds result from objects that penetrate the oral soft tissues, forcing a stream of bacteria into the injury. Management of accidental puncture wounds includes controlling bleeding, cleansing the wound, and administering antibiotics to prevent infection. Oral piercings are likely to be the most common type of puncture wounds seen among adolescents. The tongue and lips are the most frequent sites for piercings, and occasionally even the uvula. Often performed in less than ideal circumstances, a multiplicity of postpiercing complications has been reported in the scientific literature ranging from mild localized tissue reactions to life-threatening conditions (Figure 157-11). A listing of reported postpiercing sequelae is presented in Table 157-1. Health care providers should advise their adolescent patients

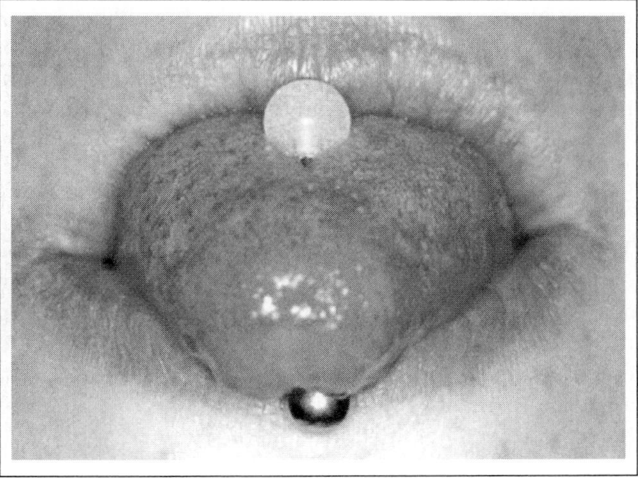

**FIGURE 157-11** Localized tissue reaction following tongue piercing and placement of jewelry. (See color insert.)

**Table 157-1**

**Reported Oral Piercing Complications**

| | |
|---|---|
| Airway obstruction | Mastication interference |
| Allergic reaction | Nerve damage |
| Aspirating jewelry | Numbness |
| Bleeding | Pain |
| Burning | Salivary flow increase |
| Cephalic tetanus | Scarring |
| Endocarditis | Septicemia |
| Fractured cusps | Speech interference |
| Fractured incisors | Swallowing interference |
| Gingival recession | Swallowing jewelry |
| Hepatitis | Swelling |
| HIV | Taste loss |
| Hypotensive collapse | Tissue overgrowth |
| Ludwig's angina | Toxic shock |

about these adverse consequences and discourage them from participating in the current fad. For those who do present with postpiercing complications, health care providers will be expected to manage the aftermath.

In addition to tissue avulsion as a result of carnivorous animal bites, such injuries may also occur from high-velocity sporting activities such as cycling and all-terrain vehicle accidents, or from gun shot wounds or hunting accidents. Basic life support should be instituted immediately and the patient referred for definitive care at an emergency department of a hospital.

Determination of the tetanus immunization status of the adolescent patient with soft tissue injuries is essential, with the administration of a booster as indicated.

## SUMMARY

The overarching theme of this chapter is to provide foundational dental information to pediatricians who treat adolescent patients in their practices. Understanding the fundamentals of adolescent dentistry is intended to enhance the physician's awareness of the role that good adolescent oral health contributes to the overall good health and well-being of adolescent patients.

## REFERENCES

1. American Academy of Pediatrics. Protecting all children's teeth (PACT): a pediatric oral health training program. American Academy of Pediatrics Web site. 2009. Available at: www.aap.org/oralhealth/pact.cfm. Accessed November 13, 2009

2. National Institute of Dental Research. Oral health of United States children. The national survey of dental caries in US schoolchildren, 1986-87. NIH Publication No. 80-2274, 1989

3. Majewski RF. Dental caries in adolescents associated with caffeinated carbonated beverages. *Pediatr Dent.* 2001;23(3):198-203

4. Bruzzese JM, Bonner S, Vincent EJ, et al. Asthma education: the adolescent experience. *Patient Educ Couns.* 2004;55(3):396-406

5. Adair SM. Dietary counseling—time for a nutritionist in the office? *Pediatr Dent.* 2004;26(5):389

6. Peldyak J, Makinen KK. Xylitol for caries prevention. *J Dent Hyg.* 2002;76(4):276-285

7. Beauchamp H, Caulfield PW, Crall JJ, et al. Evidence-based clinical recommendations for the use of pit-and-fissure sealants. A report of the American Dental Association Council on Scientific Affairs. *J Am Dent Assoc.* 2008;139(3):257-267

8. American Dental Association. Methamphetamine use (meth mouth). A-Z topics. American Dental Association Web site. 2009. Available at: www.ada.org/2711.aspx?currentTab=2. Accessed July 26, 2010

9. Klasser GD, Epstein JB. The methamphetamine epidemic and dentistry. *Gen Dent.* 2006;55(6):431-440

10. McGeary SP, Studen-Pavlovich D, Ranalli DN. Oral piercing in athletes: implications for general dentists. *Gen Dent.* 2002;50(2):168-172

11. Ranalli DN. Dental injuries in sports. *Curr Sports Med Reports.* 2005;4:12-17

12. Kelly JP, Rosenberg JH. Diagnosis and management of concussions in sports. *Neurology.* 1997;48(3):575-580

13. Flores MT, Andreasen JO, Bakland LK. Guidelines for the evaluation and management of traumatic dental injuries. *Dent Traumatol.* 2001;17:97-102

14. Andreasen JO, Andreasen FM, Mejàre I, Cvek M. Healing of 400 intra-alveolar root fractures. 1. Effect of preinjury and injury factors. *Dent Traumatol.* 2004;20:192-202

15. Andreasen JO, Andreasen FM, Mejàre I, Cvek M. Healing of 400 intra-alveolar root fractures. 2. Effect of treatment factors. *Dent Traumatol.* 2004;20:203-211

16. Nikoui M, Kenny DJ, Barrett EJ. Clinical outcomes of permanent incisor luxation in pediatric population. III: Lateral luxations. *Dent Traumatol.* 2003;19:280-285

17. Trope M. Clinical management of the avulsed tooth: present strategies and future directions. *Dent Traumatol.* 2002;18:1-11

18. Krasner P, Rankow HJ. New philosophy for the treatment of avulsed teeth. *Oral Surg, Oral Med, Oral Path.* 1995;79(5):616-623

19. Ranalli DN. Prevention of sports-related traumatic dental injuries. *Dent Clin North Am.* 2000;44:35-51

20. Vogel RI. Intrinsic and extrinsic discoloration of the dentition (a literature review). *J Oral Med.* 1975;30(4):99-104

21. Nathoo SA. The chemistry and mechanisms of extrinsic and intrinsic discoloration. *J Am Dent Assoc.* 1997;128(suppl): 6S-10S

22. Nelson R, Parker SR. Doxycycline-induced staining of adult teeth: the first reported case. *Arch Dermatol.* 2006;142(8): 1081-1082

23. Van Der Bijl P, Pitigoi-Aron G. Tetracyclines and calcified tissues. *Ann Dent.* 1995;54(1-2):69-72

24. Den Besten PK. Biological mechanisms of dental fluorosis relevant to the use of fluoride supplements. *Community Dent Oral Epidemiol.* 1999;27(1):41-47

25. Croll TP. Enamel microabrasion: observation after 10 years. *J Am Dent Assoc.* 1997;128(suppl):45S-50S

26. McGuire J, Szabo A, Jackson S, et al. Erosive tooth wear among children in the United States: relationship to race/ethnicity and obesity. *Int J Paediatr Dent.* 2009;19:91-98

27. Wagoner SN, Marshall TA, Qian F, Wefel JS. In vitro enamel erosion associated with commercially available original-flavor and sour versions of candies. *J Am Dent Assoc.* 2009;140(7): 906-913

28. Studen-Pavlovich D, Elliott MA. Eating disorders in women's oral health. *Dent Clin N Amer.* 2001;45(3):491-512

29. American Academy of Periodontology. Periodontal diseases of children and adolescents. *J Periodontol.* 2003;74(11): 1696-1704

30. Mombelli A, Rutar A, Lang NP. Correlation of the periodontal status 6 years after puberty with clinical and microbiological conditions during puberty. *J Clin Periodontol.* 1995;22:300-305

31. Johnson B, Engel D. Acute necrotizing gingivitis. A review of diagnosis, etiology, and treatment. *J Periodontol.* 1986;57: 141-150

32. US Department of Health and Human Services. Mosher WD, Chandra A, Jones JO. Sexual behavior and selected health measures: men and women 15-44 years of age, United States, 2002. (Released September 15, 2005.) Available at: www. cdc. gov/nchs/data/ad/ad362.pdf. Accessed November 13, 2009

33. Kaiser Family Foundation. *Emerging Issues in Reproductive Health.* Washington, DC: National Press Foundation; 1996

34. Emmert DH. Treatment of common cutaneous herpes simplex virus infections. *Am Fam Physician.* 2000;61:1697-1698

35. Khanuja A, Powers MP. Surgical management of impacted teeth. In: Fonseca RJ, ed. *Oral and Maxillofacial Surgery.* Vol 1. Philadelphia, PA: WB Saunders; 1999:245-280

36. White RP Jr. Third molar oral inflammation and systemic inflammation. *J Oral Maxillofac Surg.* 2005;62(suppl 8):5-6

37. Steinberg BJ. Women's oral health issues. *J Dent Educ.* 1999;63:271-275

38. Ranalli DN. Ergogenic substance abuse by adolescent athletes: perspectives for dental practitioners. *Northwest Dent.* 2007;86(5):396-400

39. Ranalli DN, Demas PN. Orofacial injuries from sport: preventive measures for sports medicine. *Sports Med.* 2002;32: 409-418

40. Basler RSW, Garcia MA, Gooding KS. Immediate steps for treating abrasions. *Physician Sports Med.* 2001;29(4):69-70

41. Pasini S, Bardellini E, Keller E, Conti G, Flocchini P, Majorana A. Surgical removal and immediate reattachment of coronal fragment embedded in lip. *Dental Traumatol.* 2006;22: 165-168

42. Silverstein LH, Kurtzman GM, Kurtzman D. Suturing for optimal soft tissue management. *Gen Dent.* 2007;55(2)95-100

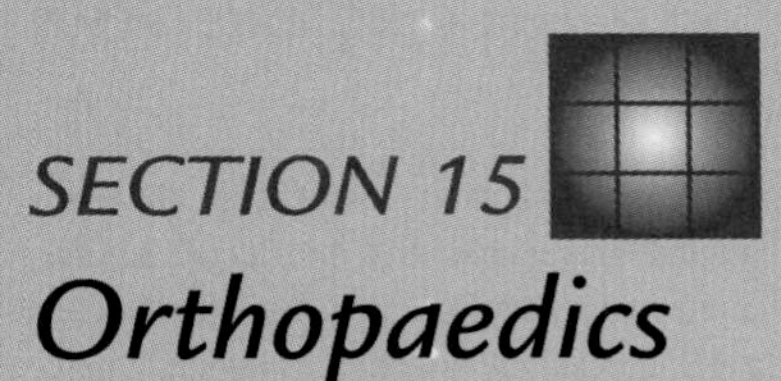

SECTION 15
# Orthopaedics

## CHAPTER 158

## Disorders of the Upper Extremities

JOSEPH N. CHORLEY, MD

In the pediatric athlete, about one-third of injuries will involve the upper extremity. Acute injuries are most often associated with contact collision sports (football, hockey, rugby) and falls, while chronic overuse injuries are more prevalent as pediatric athletes specialize earlier and train longer in sports like swimming, baseball, gymnastics, and volleyball.

### ANATOMY

The glenohumeral (GH) joint of the shoulder is generally an unstable joint, resulting in the major causes of shoulder pain in adolescents. The 3 bones of the shoulder are the clavicle, humerus, and scapula. A golf ball (humeral head) sitting on a golf tee (glenoid) is a useful analogy for understanding the GH joint. The glenoid is angled slightly forward, making the posterior rim more prominent (decreasing posterior humeral motion). The labrum is a rim of cartilage around the glenoid that increases the amount of joint congruity between the humeral head and the glenoid and is a buttress to protect the humeral head from subluxating (ball falling off the tee).

The muscles of the shoulder require coordination to work effectively. The function of the rotator cuff is to maintain the GH relationship (keeping the golf ball on the tee). The 4 muscles are the supraspinatus (humeral head depressor), infraspinatus and teres minor (external rotators), and subscapularis (internal rotator). The scapulothoracic muscles (serratus anterior, rhomboids, trapezius) provide a stable foundation for the shoulder and properly place the glenoid (so the rotator cuff does not overwork). The force generators of the shoulder (deltoids, latissimus dorsi, pectorals) contribute to instability primarily when there is asymmetric development that places stress on the shoulder. The rotator cuff interval is the space between the acromium and humeral head where the supraspinatus, subacromial bursa, and coracoacromial ligament are located. These structures are pinched by the humerus and acromium when the shoulder is forward flexed and internally rotated.

The elbow has 3 bones (humerus, radius, and ulna) and forms 3 interrelated joints. Flexion/extension of the elbow occurs at the ulnohumeral joint. Flexion is controlled by the biceps and extension by the triceps. Supination/pronation of the forearm occurs at the radiohumeral and proximal radioulnar joints under the control of the pronator teres and the supinator. At least 50° of pronation and supination and 30° of extension and 130° of flexion are necessary for the activities of daily living. The anterior band of the ulnar collateral ligament (UCL) provides stability to elbow valgus when the elbow is flexed.

The wrist consists of the articulations between the radius, ulna, and carpal bones. There are 8 carpal bones distributed in proximal (scaphoid, lunate, triquetrum, pisiform) and distal (trapezium, trapezoid, capitate, hamate) rows. Wrist flexion and extension (60°–80°) occurs at the radiocarpal (60%) and midcarpal joints (30%–40%). Between the distal ulna and the carpal bones is a meniscus-like shock-absorbing structure, the triangular fibrocartilage complex (TFCC). It is closely related to the distal radioulnar joint (DRUJ), which is the main point for forearm supination and pronation. The wrist is supported by a thin joint capsule, a thick complex of ligaments, and the fascia that binds the carpal bones and provides stability to the wrist. The palmar radiocarpal, scapholunate (SL), and lunotriquetral (LT) ligaments are the most important.

## ACUTE INJURIES

### TRAUMATIC BRACHIAL PLEXOPATHY

Traumatic brachial plexopathy results from a contralateral forced neck lateral flexion resulting in a stretch injury to the upper trunk of the brachial plexus. Direct trauma over Erb's point or neck hyperextension and lateral flexion toward the injury can cause a compression injury at the root level. These injuries are usually short-lived, with unilateral pain and altered sensation in the lateral arm and forearm and weakness in the deltoid and biceps muscles. With the risk of cervical spine injuries, patients with neck pain or altered mental status and neurological deficits must be immobilized and evaluated radiographically. Bilateral upper extremity symptoms are a red flag for spinal cord injury.

Plexus injuries are categorized based on the extent of damage to the nerve. **Neuropraxia** refers to altered axonal function with little sensory or autonomic dysfunction, no muscular atrophy, and no anatomic injury. Complete recovery usually occurs in less than 2 to 6 weeks. **Axonotemesis** refers to disruption of the axon and myelin with longer-lasting sensory, autonomic, and motor deficits. Healing requires Wallerian regeneration, so incomplete recovery may occur. **Neurotemesis** refers to disruption of the axon, myelin, and epineurium. Neurosurgical evaluation is required.

Electromyography and nerve conduction velocity (EMG/NCV) testing should be reserved for cases of continued nerve dysfunction that remains after 3 to 4 weeks postinjury. This testing can be helpful for localization of the level of injury and selection of the surgical approach. Decreasing fibrillations and denervation potentials will indicate healing even before motor function improves. A magnetic resonance imaging (MRI) study of the cervical spine can help show complicating congenital or acquired abnormalities.

Initial management starts with examination for other injuries and repeated examination every 10 minutes to monitor for changes. Return to play hinges on patients' ability to protect themselves from further injury; there should be no contact until there is a completely normal neurological examination and full, pain-free range of motion (active and resisted) of the neck and shoulder. Proper fitting shoulder pads, special neck rolls/collars, and addressing improper tackling are especially important in preventing recurrence and catastrophic neck injuries.

### SHOULDER SUBLUXATION/DISLOCATION

Shoulder subluxation/dislocation can occur at the GH joint anteriorly, inferiorly, and posteriorly. Each type of instability can be caused by a unique stress or properly placed tangential force that translocates the humerus. Anterior/inferior instability occurs with the shoulder abducted and externally rotated with a force that carries the arm posteriorly and further into external rotation (ie, fighting for a rebound or arm tackling). Throwing a punch can result in sufficient force forward to dislocate the shoulder anteriorly. Posterior instability can result from a fall on a forward-flexed, adducted arm or from extreme muscle contractions (seizures, electrocution).

The patient with a shoulder subluxation/dislocation will feel a pop and an uncomfortable shifting sensation and obvious pain. The deformity and arm position can help diagnose the type of instability (prominent acromium, swelling anteriorly, arm slightly abducted and externally rotated—anterior dislocation; more subtle prominence of the coracoid and flat anterior shoulder—posterior dislocation). Axillary nerve injury can occur in as many as one-third of anterior dislocations. During the anterior dislocation, the humeral head will injure the glenoid rim, GH ligament, and labrum (Bankart lesion—with or without glenoid rim fracture). When dislocated, the humeral head gets lodged on the anterior glenoid rim, resulting in a compression fracture of the posterior humeral head (referred to as a Hill-Sachs lesion).

Structural injuries can occur with dislocations and should be assessed with an examination, evaluation of clinical progression, and diagnostic imaging. Radiographic evaluation should include a routine trauma shoulder series and an axillary lateral West Point and Stryker-Notch view. The West Point view best visualizes fractures of the glenoid rim (boney Bankart lesion), which may occur in 45% of dislocations. The Stryker view optimizes the imaging of the Hill-Sachs lesion, which may occur in as many as 75% of anterior dislocations. Magnetic resonance imaging with intra-articular contrast has an increased sensitivity in identifying these lesions, chondral and ligament injuries, and labral tears. Magnetic resonance imaging is indicated in patients who have failed conservative management, or have recurrent instability.

The rate of recurrent dislocation, clinical instability, and an inability to return to preinjury levels of functioning have all been shown to be higher in young (20–30-year-old), active, athletes who have been managed conservatively when compared to those managed surgically. In general, however, studies have not looked at the younger, skeletally immature patient or those with multidirectionally unstable, atraumatic injuries and have not assessed for soft tissue injury prior to selection for conservative or surgical management. Surgical treatment may have advantages in older adolescent patients in high-demand sports, especially if the dislocation is associated with a soft tissue Bankart lesion. Those who fail conservative management or who have recurrence and then have a later repair do not have worse outcomes than those treated acutely.

### ACROMIOCLAVICULAR SEPARATION

Acromioclavicular (AC) separation occurs when the ligaments connecting the acromium to the distal clavicle are torn. The most common mechanism of injury occurs during contact/collision sports, when there is a direct blow to or a fall on the top of the shoulder (eg, tackling with the shoulder). The injuries are classified by the amount of displacement between the distal clavicle and the acromium (types 1-6). The physical examination demonstrates pain directly over the AC joint, and a palpable deformity in type 2 and above. Radiographs are indicated for types 4 to 6 and for a possible distal clavicle or coracoid process fracture.

Conservative management is recommended for types 1 to 3 and surgical referral is recommended for types 4 to 6. Conservative management includes providing protection from painful activities (temporarily using a sling to unload the AC joint); starting assisted pain-free range of motion; initiating isometric internal and external rotation and forward flexion exercises as pain allows; and progression to isotonic strengthening and range of motion. Return to full activity is allowed when the patient regains full, active range of motion and has sufficient strength to protect him or herself.

### GLENOID LABRAL TEARS

Glenoid labral tears are difficult to diagnose because they can mimic and coexist with other diagnoses. The mechanisms of acute injury can be an instability episode, a fall on an outstretched arm, a forceful biceps contraction (the long head of the biceps is anchored at the superior aspect of the labrum), or insidiously from repetitive overhead activity. The pain can be located discretely over the joint line or more diffusely throughout or "deep inside" the shoulder and may be accompanied by painful mechanical sensations.

Numerous physical examination techniques are used to investigate the labrum but most are not reliably sensitive or specific (O'Brien test, Hawkin, Jobe relocation test, crank test). These tests with joint line tenderness and history can raise the suspicion of a labral tear. An Magnetic resonance imaging with intra-articular contrast is the best way to confirm clinical suspicion and plan surgical management if needed. Although MRI is very good at diagnosing the most common type 2 lesions, it is less accurate with other types. The glenoid labrum has a number of normal variants that can mimic pathology (ie, sublabral recess or foramen or a Buford complex). The most common injuries in young athletes are type 1 (labral fraying) and 2 (tear of the labrum and bicep at its proximal glenoid insertion). Identified labral tears may not be the source of pain, and conservative treatment of other etiologies may improve the patient's symptoms and function. If symptoms continue, an experienced surgeon is necessary so that treatment by normal variants and pathology can be discerned intraoperatively. Postoperative rehabilitation will be needed to correct pathomechanics, regain range of motion, and improve rotator cuff and scapulothoracic function.

### ELBOW FRACTURE

Elbow fractures occur in the adolescent patient but not as often as in the younger patient. Although the usual pediatric type of fracture occurs in adolescents, as skeletal maturity approaches the more adult type of fracture pattern is seen. Plain radiographs should be obtained in 3 views: anterior–posterior (AP), lateral, and lateral oblique. It is extremely important to evaluate and monitor for neurovascular complications. Further evaluation and treatment is complicated and should be coordinated with a practitioner experienced in the management of elbow fractures.

### POSTERIOR ELBOW DISLOCATION

Posterior elbow dislocation occurs from a fall or a twisting elbow injury; its peak incidence is at 12 years of age. Fractures occur in 64% of cases. On examination, the olecranon is prominent posteriorly. Transient ulnar neuropathy occurs in 10% of cases, but more serious median nerve and brachial artery injuries can occur. Red flags for these injuries are severe pain not relieved by relocation, decreased skin temperature or pulse, and pallor distally. Unreduced, unwitnessed dislocations should be immobilized pending further evaluation. Uncomplicated injuries should be splint immobilized for 7 to 10 days, with early range-of-motion exercises. Long-term functional outcomes are excellent.

### SCAPHOID FRACTURE

Scaphoid fractures are the most common type of carpal fracture; they typically occur in young adults (15–30 years) after falling on an outstretched hand. Radial wrist pain is less severe than expected for a fracture, resulting in delayed presentation or the chief complaint of "wrist sprain not improving." Physical examination is significant for tenderness to palpation or with axial load of the thumb in the anatomic snuff box, decreased range of motion, and pain with radial deviation or extension of the wrist. On radiographs, fractures are best visualized in the AP view with 30° of ulnar deviation but may not be present acutely. If a scaphoid fracture is suspected, the wrist should be immobilized until follow-up examination (with radiographs) 10 to 14 days after the injury. Bone scan or MRI will be abnormal in the acute setting.

Management of scaphoid fractures continues to be debated. Most fractures will heal with cast immobilization with a thumb spica cast (distal pole, 4–6 weeks; waist, 10–12 weeks; proximal pole, 12–20 weeks). Indications for surgery include any displacement or rotation, associated SL injury, or nonunion after adequate immobilization. A nondisplaced wrist fracture treated with screw fixation will have a faster return to work and sports than those treated with cast immobilization. Complications of fractures (carpal instability, osteonecrosis, and nonunion) must be considered as possibly career threatening for athletes.

## TRIANGULOFIBROCARTILAGE COMPLEX TEAR

A triangulofibrocartilage complex tear can be the diagnosis in patients with either acute or chronic wrist pain. In acute injuries, the patient falls on an extended wrist or has sudden excessive pronation or supination. Insidious onset, particularly with mechanical sensations, can occur in patients who repetitively load with heavy lifting in ulnar deviation or ulnar loading of the wrist (eg, in racquet sports or golf). Physical examination will include tenderness in the hollow between the pisiform and the ulnar styloid and pain with the TFCC compression test. Associated radiographic abnormalities may include positive ulnar variance, fractures of the ulnar styloid, and DRUJ widening. Magnetic resonance imaging with intra-articular contrast demonstrates the TFCC, surrounding ligaments, DRUJ, and articular surfaces of the carpals and ulna. Acute TFCC tears (Palmar type I) are treated initially with immobilization in a sugar tong splint followed by a cast for 6 weeks. If patients are not improving, arthroscopy with either debridement or repair of the TFCC is indicated. Palmer type 2 TFCC tears usually are degenerative and do not occur in the adolescent patient.

## DISTAL RADIUS FRACTURE

Fractures of the distal radius are the most common fracture in children and adolescents. Distal radius fractures usually involve the metaphysis and occur most frequently during early adolescence, when a combination of increased body mass and decreased bone mineral density create the greatest risk. The mechanism of injury is usually a fall on a hyperextended wrist. Clinical findings of distal radius fractures include point tenderness, swelling, ecchymosis, and decreased grip strength. Associated injuries may include DRUJ injuries and TFCC tears. Fractures at the junction of the middle and distal one-third of the radius with associated dislocation of the DRUJ are known as Galeazzi fractures and require orthopedic consultation for reduction and stabilization.

Metaphyseal fractures are either torus or greenstick fractures. Torus fractures (also known as buckle fractures) do not require reduction and heal well with immobilization for the duration of pain. Greenstick fractures are incomplete fractures, usually of the palmar cortex of the radius, resulting in dorsal angulation. Angulation of more than 15° or displacement warrant closed reduction. Comminuted and intra-articular fractures require open reduction and internal fixation (ORIF).

The distal radial physis is susceptible to fracture during the adolescent growth spurt because of its rapid growth. The risk of this complication increases with the severity of the fracture based on the Salter Harris classification. Type III, IV, and V fractures are more severe than types I and II and sometimes require reduction and operative pin fixation. Growth arrest and resulting shortening of the radius can lead to ulnar impaction and TFCC tears.

## LIGAMENTOUS AND CAPSULAR INJURY

The complex anatomic relationship of the carpal bones and multiple ligamentous attachments helps stabilize the wrist while permitting considerable mobility. Ligamentous injuries encompass stretching (simple sprain) and partial or complete tears, which lead to instability and dislocation.

A simple sprain involves stretching of the supporting ligaments of the radiocarpal joint; the usual mechanism is a fall on an extended wrist. Simple sprains have mild pain or stiffness, normal range of motion, and normal radiographs. Most resolve within 2 weeks with conservative therapy (ice, immobilization, gentle stretching exercises). Carpal instability and dislocations may occur in adolescents, usually in association with a distal radius physeal injury. They are similar to simple sprains with the same mechanism of injury, but the pain and instability persist and often are made worse by physical therapy. Untreated injuries may result in chronic pain and functional deficits. Radiographs in patients with instability are usually normal but must be carefully reviewed for malalignment and frank dislocations. The early involvement of a hand specialist in the management of all carpal instability/dislocation is important to optimize long-term outcome of these injuries.

## GAMEKEEPER'S THUMB (SKIER'S THUMB)

Gamekeeper's thumb refers to a tear of the UCL of the thumb; it is the most common injury in downhill skiers and occurs when a valgus force occurs at the metacarpophalangeal (MCP) joint of the thumb (falling with a grip on the ski pole or a direct force on the thumb). When the UCL is torn, the injury may be associated with avulsion fractures. In the acute setting, a small pea-sized mass may be palpable over the medial MCP joint. This "Stener lesion" indicates that the ligament has been torn and is in a position that will not heal. There will be ulnar-sided MCP pain with swelling and/or ecchymosis and instability with prehension (holding a writing instrument). In the subacute setting, provocative testing should be done following radiographs to identify unstable fractures prior to stressing the fracture. Magnetic resonance imaging and ultrasound have been used for advanced anatomic study to distinguish between partial and complete tears and identification of Stener lesions. Conservative management is indicated for partial tears, nondisplaced fractures, pediatric fractures (usually up to a Salter Harris III—<2 mm of displacement), and late presentation (>6 weeks—with the realization that instability is likely). A short arm thumb spica or functional brace is used to prevent radial and ulnar deviation of the thumb for 4 to 8 weeks. Surgery is best performed early (<2 weeks) and is indicated for injuries with complete tears, Stener lesions, 3 mm or more of displacement of the proximal phalanx, avulsion fractures involving 30% or more of the joint space, fragment rotation or displacement.

### MALLET FINGER

A mallet finger results from forced flexion of the distal phalanx (ball trauma to the tip of the finger) in which the distal attachment of the terminal extensor tendon is avulsed from the dorsal aspect of the distal phalanx (with or without a fracture). The patient has pain with swelling and/or ecchymosis on the dorsum of the distal interphalangeal (DIP) joint and is unable to actively extend the joint. Plain radiographs for fracture identification are indicated, especially in the younger patient. Salter Harris II fractures in younger patients and III in older patients can mimic a mallet finger injury and, if displaced, may require ORIF. Surgery is warranted for extension lag following appropriate conservative management, volar subluxation of the distal phalanx, and fracture involving more than 30% of the articular surface. Conservative management is effective in most cases, utilizing extension splinting at neutral to 5° to 10° of hyperextension for 6 weeks, followed by 2 weeks of night splinting. The DIP cannot be flexed at all during splinting. Those who present with a chronic deformity from remote trauma, such as a swan neck deformity and early osteoarthritis of the joint, can be started on range-of-motion rehabilitation.

### JAMMED AND DISLOCATED FINGERS

This may represent a number of injuries including a collateral ligament injury, a tear of the central slip of the extensor mechanism, and a volar plate disruption. This type of injury most often occurs in basketball and football, from an axial or angular load on the finger. Signs and symptoms include pain with swelling and/or ecchymosis at the proximal interphalangeal (PIP) joint, as well as a dislocation deformity (lateral>dorsal>volar). If dislocated, the joint surface should be palpated for possible fracture. If none, steady axial distraction should easily reduce most dislocations. If not easy, there may be a fracture or soft tissue injury inhibiting the reduction. Loss of active extension indicates a central slip injury. Plain radiographs for fracture identification are important because epiphyseal fractures of the phalanx are the most common Salter Harris fractures. Surgery is indicated for inability to easily reduce a dislocation, central slip injuries, unstable fractures (with middle phalanx subluxation), or a dislocation that involves more than 30% of the articular surface.

## CHRONIC INJURIES

### SHOULDER

Shoulder rotator cuff tendonitis/subacromial bursitis/impingement syndromes are the most common source of insidious onset of shoulder pain associated with activity. Inadequate stability of the GH joint will result in impingement trauma to the subacromial bursa and rotator cuff. Etiologies of this excessive GH motion include the following:

- **Scapulothoracic dysfunction** occurs when the scapular stabilizing muscles either do not place the glenoid in the correct position or have inadequate strength to provide a stable foundation for energy transfer. An improper scapular position will cause inferior placement of the acromium, decreasing the rotator cuff interval and causing more impingement.
- **Hypermobility (innate or acquired).** If the capsule and ligaments are not controlling GH motion, the rotator cuff and scapulothoracic muscles will have to work harder.
- **Asymmetric muscular development and flexibility.** The forward flexed posture of adolescents, strength-training athletes, and swimmers will result in excessive anterior translation of the humeral head coupled with inadequate posterior muscle strength. Athletes who perform overhead activities can develop marked

posterior capsule tightness and weak external rotators, resulting in a posterior impingement syndrome in which the posterior glenoid and labrum and the supraspinatus and infraspinatus muscles pinch along the posterior joint line.

- **Inadequate core strength and proprioception to maintain posture and unrehabilitated injuries.** If an athlete is not able to maintain stability and translate force along the kinetic chain from the foot through the leg and hip up the spine and through the shoulder, the weakest link will be the first to get overloaded (ie, the shoulder and elbow). This can occur during the time of peak height velocity, when the adolescent's neuromuscular firing patterns are changing rapidly to accommodate the geometric body changes occurring. This can also occur in those with an unrehabilitated injury that causes a slight change in mechanics, which can then be magnified up the kinetic chain.
- **Overuse or improper mechanics with resulting muscular fatigue.** Excessive exercise that results in muscular fatigue can change the mechanics of any maneuver. If improper training continues, or if proper techniques were never learned, injury will occur.

In these situations, changing or modifying the etiology should prevent recurrence of the problem. Rotator cuff tendonitis is a self-perpetuating process whereby the injured supraspinatus cannot effectively act as a humeral head depressor, resulting in the humeral head being elevated, causing more impingement of the injured muscle.

The history usually has the insidious onset of pain related to overhead activity. It may be "deep in the shoulder" or referred over the deltoid tubercle. Nonpainful mechanical sensations and tenderness to palpation may occur over the anterior or posterior joint line; pain may be present, but painful mechanical sensations should increase suspicion that there may be labral pathology. Rotator cuff muscle testing will show weakness and pain. Provocative tests for anterior (Neer or Hawkin tests) and posterior impingement may reproduce the pain, and the relocation test (Fowler) will alleviate some of the symptoms. A subacromial bursa anesthetic injection can help distinguish between pain from the bursa versus other structures.

Radiographic evaluation is not usually required in the classic patient. Stress fractures and large unicameral bone cysts are not common but must be considered. Shoulder pain can also be the manifestation of neck, pulmonary, cardiac, or intra-abdominal pathology.

Treatment logically addresses the etiology of the shoulder pain and its consequences. Oral anti-inflammatory medications, taping, and injections can minimize the pain and allow patients to perform their rehabilitation more effectively. Rotator cuff and scapulothoracic strengthening and normalized firing patterns are important. Limitations on excessive participation may not be consistent with the expectations of the athlete or his or her parents, but may be necessary, especially during the time of peak height velocity.

"Little league shoulder" refers to proximal humeral epiphysiolysis, osteochondrosis of the proximal humeral epiphysis, and/or a stress fracture of the proximal humeral epiphyseal plate; it has been reported in throwers and tennis players. Physical examination findings are usually similar to those seen in rotator cuff tendonitis, but radiographs show the stress changes. Treatment requires complete restriction from provoking activities for a minimum of 4 to 6 weeks.

## LITTLE LEAGUE ELBOW

Little league elbow refers to a group of elbow problems related to the stress of throwing in young athletes. Throwing generates a valgus distraction force on the medial elbow and a compressive force on the lateral elbow. Microtrauma from overuse or improper throwing mechanics can cause injury. The skeletal maturity of the athlete affects the type of injury. The screening history and a physical examination of the ipsilateral shoulder will identify if there is pain or dysfunction causing a change in the throwing technique that increases stress on the elbow. Risk factors for elbow injuries requiring surgery are regularly pitching with arm fatigue, pitching more than 8 months per year, and averaging more than 80 pitches per appearance. Recommended measures to prevent these injuries include instruction in proper throwing techniques and education to facilitate early diagnosis and treatment.

Throwers with medial epicondyle apophysitis complain of medial elbow pain that progresses with continued throwing. Physical examination demonstrates pain to palpation of the medial epicondyle exacerbated by resisted wrist flexion and valgus testing of the elbow. Elbow extension may be limited. Radiographs demonstrate an open ossification center without separation. Treatment includes cessation of throwing for 4 to 6 weeks and symptomatic treatment.

Medial epicondyle avulsion fractures may coincide with a "pop" of the elbow during a throw, associated with pain. The physical examination is similar to that of epicondyle apophysitis. Radiographs demonstrate a separation of the medial epicondyle apophysis. Treatment of minimally displaced (<2 mm) medial epicondyle avulsion fractures involves brief immobilization for 1 to 2 weeks. Early range-of-motion exercises can be started once the athlete can perform them without pain. Referral for surgical intervention is advised if there is a >2 mm displacement or concomitant ulnar nerve findings.

Ulnar collateral ligament tears occur in the skeletally mature thrower from overuse and in athletes who sustain a traumatic valgus injury from a fall on an outstretched arm. On physical examination valgus stress at 30° of elbow flexion reproduces medial pain and instability. Ulnar collateral ligament tears may be seen on stress radiographs with the application of valgus force. Magnetic resonance imaging with contrast arthrography is sensitive for both partial and full thickness ligament injuries. Treatment includes conservative management for at least 6 months with no throwing activities. The associated strength and form deficits should be addressed through rehabilitation. If symptoms recur, surgical reconstruction may be necessary. The success rate of returning to the same throwing level has been reported to be 74% in adolescent patients.

For all of these injuries, once healing has occurred, correction of throwing mechanics is imperative. A progressive throwing program over 6 to 8 weeks will help the athlete return. A position change may help the player avoid reinjury.

### PANNER DISEASE

Panner disease is an osteochondrosis (developmental disorder of the epiphysis and secondary ossification centers) of the capitellum. Boys who pitch (ages 7–12 years) present with symptoms that include the sudden onset of lateral elbow tenderness, decreased elbow extension, and swelling. Fragmentation and sclerosis of the capitellum with an irregular joint surface may be seen on radiographs. Treatment is avoidance of elbow stress until radiographs and physical examination normalize (6–12 weeks). The capitellum has excellent potential for normal anatomic and functional healing in this injury.

### OSTEOCHONDRITIS DISSECANS

Osteochondritis dissecans (OCD) of the capitellum is an avascular necrosis of the articular cartilage and underlying subchondral bone that occurs in the capitellum. It occurs in athletes 13 to 15 years old, mostly in throwers and gymnasts. Symptoms include dull, poorly localized lateral elbow pain with decreased range of motion. Mechanical symptoms are usually late symptoms. Radiographs may show flattening of the capitellum with subchondral sclerosis, but may be normal initially. Computed tomography arthrography and MRI are helpful in early detection and staging of the lesion. Treatment is guided by the stage of the lesion. Long-term complications include radial head hypertrophy, early degenerative changes, and restricted motion. This may cause symptoms with activities of daily living in 50% of patients and is career threatening in athletes.

### DEQUERVAIN

DeQuervain is a tenosynovitis of the tendon sheath of the thumb at the radial wrist. It commonly occurs from overgripping and repetitive wrist motion in golf, fishing, and racquet sports. Treatment involves rest and splinting in a thumb spica splint, followed by stretching and strengthening exercises. Steroid injection into the tendon sheath has cure rates from 62% to 80%. If this conservative approach fails, surgical decompression should be considered.

### DISTAL RADIAL EPIPHYSIOLYSIS OF THE EPIPHYSIS

Distal radial epiphysiolysis of the epiphysis occurs with repetitive loading of the wrist; this is classically seen in female, competitive gymnasts who are 12 to 14 years old. Symptoms are reproduced with forced wrist extension; if caught early, radiographic changes will not be seen. If strength and range of motion normalize during 2 to 4 weeks of activity restriction, a progressive return to grip and tumbling exercises can begin. If the situation is more chronic, radiographic findings (including widening and irregularity of the epiphysis and volar spurring of the metaphysis) will be seen and a cast or splint immobilization for 4 to 8 weeks will be required. If radial shortening has occurred, restriction of activity is essential and surgical treatment of the ulnocarpal impingement may be needed.

## REFERENCES


1. Kaye A. Classification of nerve injuries. *Essential Neurosurgery*. Churchill Livingstone; 1991:333–334

2. Handoll HH, Al-Maiyah MA. Surgical versus non-surgical treatment for acute anterior shoulder dislocation. *Cochrane Database of Systematic Review.* Issue 4, 2008

3. Lawton RL, Choudhury S, Mansat P, et al. Pediatric shoulder instability: presentation, findings, treatment, and outcomes. *J Ped Ortho.* 22(1):52–61

4. Rockwood CA Jr, Green DP, Bucholz RW, et al. *Fractures in Adults.* 4th ed. Philadelphia, PA: Lippincott-Raven; 1996

5. Mikek M. Long-term shoulder function after type I and II AC joint disruption. *Am J Sports Med.* 2008;36:2147–2150

6. Jee WH, McCauley TR, Katz LD, et al. Superior labral anterior posterior (SLAP) lesions of the glenoid labrum. *Radiology.* 2001;218:127–132

7. Maffet M, Lowe W. Superior labral injuries. In Miller M, ed. *DeLee and Drez's Orthopeadic Sports Medicine: Principles and Practice*. 2 nd ed. Philadelphia, PA:WB Saunders; 2003

8. Rettig AC. Athletic injuries of the wrist and hand. Part I: traumatic injuries of the wrist. *Am J Sports Med.* 2003;31(6):1038–1048

9. Garcia-Elias M. Carpal instabilities and dislocations. *Green's Operative Hand Surgery*. New York, NY: Churchill Livingstone; 1999:865

10. Heyman P, Gelberman RH, Duncan K, et al. Injuries of the ulnar collateral ligament of the thumb metacarpophalangeal joint. *Clin Ortho & Rel Res.* 1993;292:165–171

11. Olsen SJ, Fleisig GS, Dun S, et al. Risk factors for shoulder and elbow injuries in adolescent baseball pitchers. *Am J Sports Med.* 2006:34:905–912

12. American Academy of Pediatrics Committee on Sports Medicine. Risk of injury from baseball and softball in children 5 to 14 years of age. *Pediatrics.* 1994;93:690

13. Plancher K, Peterson RK, Steichen JB. Compressive neuropathies and tendonopathies in the athletic elbow and wrist. *Clin Sports Med.* 1996:15(2):331–371

# CHAPTER 159

# Disorders of the Lower Extremities

ALBERT C. HERGENROEDER, MD

The prevalence of musculoskeletal complaints increases from childhood through adolescence. Reports have shown that up to one-third of adolescents had musculoskeletal complaints in a primary care setting over a 3-year period[1] and that 5% of adolescents experienced at least 1 sports-related injury that required medical attention over a 2-year period.[2] In 1 report, the annual incidence of all injuries in high school athletes was reported to be as high as 22%, with only 31% of these injuries having been seen by a physician.[3] Many physicians who care for adolescents lack training in the diagnosis and treatment of common musculoskeletal injuries.[4]

The goal of this chapter is to review the diagnosis and treatment of common acute and chronic overuse injuries to the lower extremities that occur during sports participation or exercise in adolescents. The lower extremity is the most common site of injury in male and female high school athletes.[5,6] The spectrum of injuries in the lower extremities includes the most serious, yet relatively infrequent, knee injuries to the more common, and less serious, chronic knee pain and ankle sprains. All of these injuries can have long-term sequelae if not diagnosed and treated properly. Demonstration of the physical examination tests referred to in this chapter are available in a teaching video referenced in the Internet Resources section at the end of this chapter.

## ACUTE INJURIES

### ACUTE KNEE INJURIES

#### Mechanisms of Injury, History, and Physical Examination Findings

For all of the acute knee injuries that will be discussed in this section, the patient is likely to report the sensations of pain, tearing or pulling, and swelling. The severity of pain and swelling after the injury often correlates with the severity of the injury; an initial inability to bear weight or a refusal to move the knee implies a serious injury. The adolescent who has just incurred a valgus injury (ie, the force is to the lateral knee, directed medially) resulting in tears of the medial collateral and anterior cruciate ligaments (ACL) along with a meniscal tear will have considerable disability, pain, and swelling. However, the severity of pain and swelling after the injury is not always predictive of injury severity. For example, in some cases the medial collateral ligament (MCL) can be completely torn, yet there can be relatively little swelling and pain soon after the injury. The adolescent may attempt to run or return to play unless he or she senses instability. The patient with a partial tear of the MCL, however, may have considerable pain with movement. A patient with a mild (ie, grade 1) MCL tear may have mild swelling the day of the injury, and if he/she does not elevate the leg or apply ice to the knee, may have a large effusion in the morning. Immediate hemarthrosis suggests an intra-articular fracture, ACL sprain, peripheral meniscal tear, or patellar dislocation. The absence of swelling does not necessarily imply a mild injury, as a large capsular tear can allow for leakage of fluid into soft tissue. The mechanisms, histories, and physical examination techniques for each injury are described, understanding that the mechanisms that result in injury are often multidirectional and more than one structure can be affected: One-half to two-thirds of acute ACL injuries are associated with meniscal tears; one-half are associated with collateral ligament tears; and 10% to 16% have associated chondral injuries or patellar dislocations.[7-8]

***Anterior Cruciate Ligament*** Anterior cruciate ligament injuries can result from a variety of mechanisms: Planting the foot to change direction, direct trauma (either a valgus force, applied to the outside of the knee directed medially; or a varus force, applied to the medial knee directed from the inside of the knee in a lateral direction), or landing in an off-balance position. Often the injury is a noncontact injury. The patient may report that the knee "shifted" or "went out" during a cutting or deceleration maneuver. The patient often points to the area of pain as being on both sides of the patellar tendon at the joint line. Hemarthrosis is often present. The Lachman, anterior drawer, and pivot shift tests are the physical examination tests used to diagnose ACL injuries. The latter is the most difficult to master. The anterior drawer is the easiest to perform and has a sensitivity and specificity of 62% and 67%, respectively, in adults.[9] If it is positive (ie, there is abnormal anterior translation of the tibia on the femur and no endpoint when pulling the tibia forward while the examiner is sitting on the patient's externally rotated foot), then other tests for ACL insufficiency can be deferred if the examiner is not comfortable with performing them. It would be important to master the anterior drawer test then to work on mastering the other examination techniques.

***Posterior Cruciate Ligament*** Posterior cruciate ligament (PCL) injuries can result from: (1) a direct posteriorly directed blow to the anterior aspect of the proximal tibia (eg, a kick during martial arts, a dashboard injury with the knee flexed, or falling from a bicycle); or (2) from a valgus or varus stress in which the MCL and lateral collateral ligament (LCL), respectively, are torn first, removing restraints to a PCL injury. In contrast to those with an ACL injury, patients with a PCL injury may try to return to play. A PCL tear will be indicated by a positive posterior drawer test or positive sag test. The posterior drawer test is the reverse of the anterior drawer test described previously under ACL injuries. A positive sag test is manifest when the tibia "sags" posteriorly, relative to the other leg, when the patient is in a supine position with the hips flexed to 45 degrees and the knees flexed to 90 degrees.

***Lateral Collateral Ligament*** The LCL can be injured via a varus force. Lateral collateral ligament injuries are manifest by tenderness to palpation along the course of the LCL and pain and laxity with varus testing at 30 degrees flexion. If the knee is markedly lax with varus testing at full extension, then consideration of an injury to the posterior lateral corner and PCL should be considered.

***Medial Collateral Ligament*** An MCL sprain tends to result from a valgus force. Physical examination evidence of the injury includes laxity with valgus testing and tenderness along the course of the MCL (from its origin at the distal, medial femoral condyle just anterior to the adductor tubercle to its insertion approximately 6 cm distal to the joint line under the insertion of the pes anserinus). In adolescents with open physes, the deep MCL fibers course from the distal femoral epiphysis to the proximal tibial epiphysis. If there is marked laxity of the MCL at full extension, then suspect an ACL injury in addition to a tear of the MCL. Laxity and pain along the course of the MCL, when tested with valgus stress at 30 degrees of knee flexion, support the diagnosis of a sprain of the MCL.

***Meniscal Injuries*** Meniscal injuries are rare under the age of 10 years, and when they occur in children the presence of a discoid meniscus should be considered. In contrast to adults in which medial meniscal tears are more frequent than lateral meniscal tears, medial and lateral meniscal tears occur with equal frequency in children. As the age/maturation of the patient increases, the pattern of meniscal tears should approach that of adult patients, with the exception of discoid menisci, which are more likely to involve the lateral meniscus and are more likely to be discovered in childhood/early adolescence. The mechanisms for meniscal injuries are similar to those for ACL injuries: twisting the knee while weight bearing. Mechanical symptoms may be more common than pain because only the periphery of the menisci contain nerve fibers. Mechanical symptoms include locking, popping, and catching. Joint line tenderness occurs in 50% to 75% of meniscal tears. Medial tenderness is present in up to 50% of lateral meniscal injuries in adults.[10] Positive McMurray, modified McMurray, and bounce home tests, along with joint line tenderness in a patient with an effusion who is unable to bear weight after an acute weight-bearing injury, suggest a meniscal tear.

***Fracture*** Fractures of the physes (growth plates) of the distal femur and proximal tibia are an important cause of knee pain in the young athlete. The physeal region is the weakest part of the child/adolescent's skeleton, compared to the periarticular ligaments and joint capsule; because of that, trauma is more likely to produce separation (ie, fracture) at the physis rather than dislocation and injury to ligaments. This situation is more likely to occur in high-energy accidents, such as motor vehicle or bicycle accidents. The MCL, ACL, and PCL all attach to the distal femoral and proximal tibial epiphyses. In a patient with open physes, the diagnosis of joint separation should prompt consideration of a physeal injury as well. In the knee, concomitant physeal and ligament injuries can occur, especially involving the ACL and MCL.[11] Pain and swelling will be present in such a case.

***Patellar Dislocation*** Patellar dislocation is usually a noncontact, weight-bearing injury, although it can be caused by midair maneuvers involving forceful quadriceps contraction (eg, in diving or gymnastics). It can also occur with valgus injuries. For the adolescent experiencing a first dislocation, with normal patellar mobility, the dislocation is audible and the swelling dramatic. Acute patellar dislocations can mimic ligamentous and meniscal injuries. The medial joint line can be tender yet there is usually diffuse medial knee tenderness and there can be pain with valgus testing, similar to findings with an MCL sprain. Palpation may indicate diffuse tenderness of the medial knee, and distinguishing between pain over the distal vastus medialis muscle, the MCL, and the medial retinaculum can be difficult. A positive apprehension test (marked tenderness or apprehension when the examiner tries to displace the patella laterally) can distinguish a patellar dislocation from an MCL injury.

### Diagnostic Evaluation

***Diagnostic Imaging*** Plain radiographs (anterior-posterior and lateral views) should be obtained if fractures are suspected. Sunrise views should be obtained after an acute patellar dislocation to look for condylar fractures. The Ottawa Knee Rules[12] indicate that the presence of any 1 of 4 criteria are an indication for a knee series. These are: (1) isolated tenderness of the patella; (2) inability to flex the knee to 90 degrees; (3) tenderness at the head of the fibula; and (4) inability to bear weight both immediately and in the emergency department for 4 steps (transferring weight back onto each limb twice, ie, 4 steps, regardless of limp). These rules are 100% sensitive and specific for detecting clinically significant fractures in adolescents.[13] The use of stress radiographs in patients with open physes, to rule out epiphyseal versus MCL injuries, is controversial. Valgus injuries to young adolescents can result in Salter fractures of the distal femur and proximal tibia and should be considered in the differential diagnosis. The author of this chapter does not routinely order stress radiographs in the initial evaluation.

Magnetic resonance imaging (MRI) is not necessary in patients with acute knee injuries if the diagnosis is established clinically. If the diagnosis is uncertain, then MRI should be ordered. Or if the patient is not progressing as expected, then an MRI should be considered. If there is marked laxity medially with valgus stress, especially with the knee extended, the integrity of the ACL should be questioned and an MRI done to evaluate the latter. If there is a suspicion of more than 1 structure being injured, for example, ligamentous and meniscal injuries, or more than 1 ligament injury, then an MRI is indicated. The MRI is approximately 90% accurate in identifying surgically confirmed ACL and meniscal injuries in adults and children.[14,15] However, it is no more accurate, and sometimes less accurate, than the physical examination of an experienced clinician.[16] For this reason, primary care physicians who are unskilled in the knee examination should consider referral of their patients with knee complaints to a sports medicine physician or orthopedic surgeon with training in sports medicine before making arrangements for an MRI. There are increased signal changes in the menisci of skeletally immature subjects compared to adults. Review of the findings with a radiologist trained in the musculoskeletal MRI, and familiarity with the differences between children and adults, will aid interpretation of findings.

***Arthrocentesis*** Joint aspiration is indicated if there is confusion about the etiology of the swelling, that is, if there is consideration of an infectious or immunologically mediated arthritis. However, given a presentation of acute hemarthrosis following trauma, the etiology is almost certainly traumatic, and arthrocentesis is not indicated unless the pain is unresponsive to analgesia, compression, and ice because of its size. In this case the arthrocentesis can be done therapeutically.

***Arthroscopy*** Arthroscopy is indicated only if the diagnosis cannot be established by history, physical examination and, if needed, MRI. The only absolute indication for arthroscopy is mechanical disruption of normal knee function.

### Initial Treatment of Acute Knee Injuries

***Indications for Immediate Referral*** Indications for immediate referral to an orthopedist following an acute knee injury include: penetrating wounds, neurovascular compromise, unreducible dislocation, and any fracture. These patients usually have gross deformity, inability to bear weight, or a rapidly expanding hemarthrosis. Neurovascular integrity is assessed by (1) palpating the dorsalis pedis and posterior tibialis pulses, and (2) testing sensation in the web space between the first and second toes (deep peroneal nerve), on plantarflexion (posterior tibial nerve), and on ankle eversion (peroneal nerve). Assuming these indications for immediate referral are not present, the patient with an acute hemarthrosis should be referred to an orthopedist or sports medicine physician within a few days in order to initiate physical therapy; the author of this chapter prefers that this take place within the first 72 hours.

***Routine Treatment*** The initial goal of therapy is to control pain and prevent further injury, and in doing the latter, to help assist with tissue healing. Initial treatment of acute knee hemarthrosis recommended by the author is represented by the pneumonic RICE: rest, ice, compression, and elevation.

- **Rest.** Crutches with nonweight bearing is indicated until the patient can start partial, pain-free weight bearing. If a brace is to be used, temporary immobilization in a hinged brace is appropriate. To prevent atrophy of the quadriceps muscles (especially the principal medial dynamic stabilizer of the patella, the vastus medialis obliquus) pain-free, isometric exercises, especially isometric extension of the knee, can start at once. These exercises consist of quadriceps setting ("quad set") and straight leg raising, performed by holding each contraction for 6 seconds, relaxing for 4 seconds, doing 10 repetitions at a time, and repeating that 10 times a day. In the first few days after the injury, the patient may have limited pain-free range of motion. Isotonic or isokinetic exercises can be started within the pain-free range of motion, under the direction of a physical therapist, in the interim between the initial evaluation and the sports medicine consultation. However, the physical therapist will be limited in the treatment program until a diagnosis is made. An attempt should be made to get the evaluation done within a few days of the injury. Unfortunately, insurance and other access barriers often delay definitive diagnosis and treatment, which, in turn, delays recovery.

- **Ice.** Apply ice for 20 minutes at a time, 3 to 4 times per day, with the ice in a plastic bag applied directly to the skin for as long as there is swelling. In practical terms, patients should ice at least once a day. Heat is not indicated with swelling.
- **Compression.** Applying an elastic bandage from mid-calf to mid-thigh during waking hours will prevent some swelling. Care should be taken to not wrap the elastic bandage so tightly that it will impede venous return from the lower leg and create the secondary problem of an ecchymosis distal to the injured knee.
- **Elevation.** Elevation promotes venous return and prevents further swelling. The patient should be advised to rest his or her foot on the edge of the couch or prop it up on a chair at school. He or she will need a physician's note to do so.

### Treatment after the Acute Period

After the treatment shown previously results in reduced swelling and decreased pain, a definitive diagnosis should be established. Referral to a physician trained in diagnosing and treating acute knee injuries is appropriate. The transition from acute care to rehabilitation, functional rehabilitation, and return to sports is discussed elsewhere.[17]

## ACUTE ANKLE INJURIES

### Mechanisms and Physical Examination Findings

Eighty-five percent of acute ankle injuries that present to an emergency department are the result of ankle inversion (foot turned under).[18] Eversion injuries, compared to inversion injuries, are associated with a higher rate of fractures. Physical examination of the injured ankle includes: (1) noting the presence of swelling and deformities, (2) evaluating neurovascular integrity, and (3) testing for active, passive, and resisted range of motion. (See link to video in references.) Palpation for point tenderness is performed to focus on possible fractured structures: the medial and lateral malleoli, base of the fifth metatarsal, navicular and talus (anterior joint line). In the absence of point tenderness over bone, the lateral ligaments (anterior talofibular, calcaneofibular, and posterior talofibular) will be tender, with the increasing number of ligaments torn reflecting the severity of injury. The sequence of ligaments torn is the same as that listed in the preceding sentence. In eversion injuries, the deltoid ligament (medially) is more likely to be injured. Because the mechanism of injury is not always known, palpation for all ligaments is indicated during the initial assessment. If the patient is able, weight bearing is assessed; if the patient is unable to bear weight, then a radiograph is indicated. If the ankle is diffusely swollen, palpation for crepitus is indicated; however, the discrimination of tenderness over discrete ligamentous structures will be poor. Neurovascular assessment is always indicated.

### Diagnostic Imaging

The Ottawa Rules[19,20] for ankle radiographs provide guidelines for obtaining anterior–posterior, lateral, and oblique ankle radiographs in the acute setting. The rules state that plain radiographs are indicated if there is pain in the area of the malleoli and 1 of the following: (1) inability to bear weight (taking 4 steps) both immediately and in the emergency department, or (2) bone tenderness at the posterior edge of the distal tibia or fibula.

### Initial Treatment of Ankle Injuries

As with acute knee injuries, the goal is to limit disability. Successful treatment is not defined by the absence of pain, but ultimately with the return to full range of motion, strength, and proprioception. As with knee injuries, the initial treatment is represented by the pneumonic RICE: rest, ice, compression, and elevation.

- **Rest.** Rest includes the use of crutches if the patient cannot bear weight pain free. Rest is facilitated by use of an air stirrup, which is easy to apply and remove, and allows for the use of an early mobilization program.[18] The air stirrup provides stability to inversion and eversion and also allows for active dorsiflexion and plantarflexion, which are important in rehabilitation. Patients can start rehabilitation exercises within days of the injury, as long as they are pain free. Casting is not indicated for ankle sprains unless they are complicated by a fracture or the patient is noncompliant with relative rest.[18] Casting should not be routine for ankle sprains as it actually worsens the outcome, specifically time to return to work.
- **Ice.** Applied as described previously for the acute treatment of knee injuries.
- **Compression.** If using an elastic wrap, always wrap distal to proximal from the base of the toes

to mid-calf. Advise the patient not to sleep with the elastic wrap still in place. As noted previously, compression and stability are best provided by an air stirrup, which should be used for all acute sprains not complicated by a fracture.

- **Elevation.** For the first 2 to 3 days, the ankle should be elevated as much as possible. Advise patients not to wait for definitive diagnosis and treatment of the injury (especially if discussing the injury by phone). Treatment should be instituted immediately to limit pain and disability and to promote the rehabilitative process. Waiting 1 to 2 weeks to see a sports medicine physician without ongoing RICE therapy will promote atrophy, and loss of strength, flexibility, and endurance and will only delay the patient's recovery. The author prefers to see patients with ankle sprains within days of the injury to make a diagnosis and initiate treatment.
- **Analgesia.** Nonsteroidal anti-inflammatory drugs (NSAIDs) can be used for pain relief and theoretically to control inflammation, but NSAIDs do not improve the time to recovery for ankle or knee injuries. Acetaminophen is another alternative.
- **Rehabilitation** starts on the first day of evaluation with the interventions described under the RICE pneumonic. (1) The relative rest can be extended to progressing off crutches as soon as the patient can bear weight pain free. Progression off crutches, from partial weight bearing to not using crutches, may take days. (2) Stretching, especially the soleus and gastrocnemius muscles by doing calf stretches is important to prevent a loss of dorsiflexion. The latter can result in reduced athletic performance. (3) Strengthening can be initiated with toe/heel walking for 2 minutes at a time. These can be done with the air stirrup on. Rubber bands can provide resistance exercises for all ankle motions, that is, plantar and dorsiflexion and inversion and eversion, and are indicated if the patient has those specific weaknesses identified on manual testing. All these exercises should be pain free and progressive. For example, the patient can start with 3 sets of 10 repetitions for several exercises, and then increase to 3 sets of 15, and then 20 using the same color band. Once 3 sets of 20 are achieved, the patient can transition to the next level of resistance with the bands, starting with 3 sets of 10 repetitions and progressing to 3 sets of 20 repetitions. (4) Proprioceptive retraining can occur with exercises such as raising on toes with little support (1 or 2 fingers on a chair) and eyes closed for 2 to 5 minutes a day. The patient can progress to standing on the injured leg while doing simple tasks such as brushing teeth or combing hair.
- **Functional rehabilitation.** The patient should not return directly to sports after an acute injury to the lower extremity, even with full strength, endurance, and flexibility restored in the clinic setting. To return too soon is to run the risk of reinjury. Functional progression of exercise toward returning to sports participation can take the form of a program such as: toe walking —> walking at a fast pace —> jogging —> jogging the curves of a quarter-mile track and sprinting along the straight part of the track —> sprinting in a 20-yard figure of 8 pattern —> to sprinting in a 10-yard figure of 8 pattern and if pain free at every stage, then can return to playing.[21] The air stirrup should be worn in competition for 6 months after the injury. The air stirrups are most comfortable with low-cut or three-quarters height shoes and provide excellent stability. Taping of the ankles does not prevent recurrent ankle sprains.

## OVERUSE INJURIES

### CHRONIC KNEE PAIN: PATELLOFEMORAL DYSFUNCTION, OSGOOD-SCHLATTER DISEASE, AND ILIOTIBIAL BAND TENDONITIS

Overuse injuries are caused by repetitive microtrauma that exceeds the body's rate of repair. Overuse injuries occur in patients of all ages. Puberty causes normal growth and development, including increased rates of height velocity. However, linear bone growth in puberty precedes attendant muscle-tendon growth, placing an intrinsic stress at tendon-bone and ligament-bone interfaces. Osgood-Schlatter disease (tibial tuberosity) and Sever disease (calcaneal apophysis) are examples of traction apophysitis that can occur as a result of this growth process when it is coupled with regular youth activities of daily living (ADL). When these normal forces are complicated by excessive, repetitive training in sports and exercise, especially as occurs in year-round sports with "travel" and "select" youth sports teams, an overuse injury may occur. The focus in this chapter is on lower extremity overuse injuries likely to result from running sports; however, overuse injuries have the potential to occur in any prolonged, repetitive training program, such as in weight training, cycling, gymnastics, pitching in baseball, practicing a string instrument, ballet, or swimming.

Several factors play a role in the development of overuse injuries in adolescents. These include the following:

### Training Error

Training error is the most frequently identified factor in overuse injuries. The training load (eg, pace, weekly mileage, and/or time spent running per week) and duration of the regimen create forces on the bone, muscle–tendon, and/or ligament that exceed the capacity of the bone or muscle–tendon unit to accommodate that training load. Examples are the runner who has not been training who tries out for the cross-country team and develops lower leg pain; the young cross-country runner who switches to basketball and develops knee pain; or the cheerleader who practices twice a week for her high school team, goes to a cheerleading camp and practices 8 hours a day for a week, and then develops back pain. Obtaining the exercise history (days/week, duration of sessions, numbers of repetitions and sets of exercises in each session, new exercises, and new techniques for doing existing exercises) and the pace of exercise or running is essential to try to identify the training error.

Often the pain is tolerable in the beginning of a new exercise program, occurring only after practice sessions. Over time, and with continuation or an increase in the training load, the pain may occur earlier in the exercise, and at the last phase occurs with routine ADL It is during these last 2 stages that the patient is often brought for evaluation, either because he/she is not performing well and it is a performance issue or because the pain is constant.

### Pressures to Compete

The implications for the roles of parents, coaches, and peer pressure in promoting the environment in which overtraining leads to injuries are obvious. It is not just the parents and coaches, however, as some youth are driven on their own to compete and to be "perfect" to maintain their self-esteem.

### Other Intrinsic Factors

Other intrinsic factors that put a youth at risk for overuse injuries include: (1) abnormal biomechanics that develop from specific physical characteristics of the individual; examples of this are leg length discrepancy, pes planus (flat feet), pes cavus (high arch), tarsal coalition (manifest as hyperpronation and recurrent ankle sprains), valgus heel, external tibial torsion, femoral anteversion, inability to control hip internal rotation because of weak hip external rotators and genu valgum ("knock knees"); (2) poor technique (eg, reduced external hip rotation causing poor turnout in a ballet dancer); (3) muscle imbalance or inflexibility (eg, quadriceps-hamstring imbalance, resulting from a previous acute injury that was not followed by proper rehabilitation; or overstrengthening the quadriceps with squats without increasing hamstring strengthening); and (4) medical conditions that lead to cardiovascular deconditioning (such as infectious mononucleosis requiring several weeks of bed rest).

### Extrinsic Factors

Extrinsic factors also play a role in overuse injuries. Athletes should be asked about their shoes, orthotics, or braces, running surfaces, and previous injuries and rehabilitation. When causative factors are identified, they can be addressed so that the athlete will be less likely to return to the same regimen and repeat the same mechanism of injury after rehabilitation is completed. The author prefers to address the intrinsic factors together with the shoe type. For example, a mild pronator is likely to benefit from wearing a stabilizing running shoe. However, in the absence of correcting the intrinsic factors, switching shoes is not likely to correct the problem.

### Differential Diagnosis

The presenting complaint of musculoskeletal pain can be the result of many processes, including traumatic, rheumatologic, infectious, hematologic, and oncologic processes. Symptoms such as fatigue, weight loss, rash, multiple joint complaints, fever, chronic or recent illness, or unexplained bleeding at another site suggest diagnoses other than an overuse injury. Incongruity between the patient's history and the physical examination findings require further evaluation. On the other hand, a normal review of systems with a history consistent with the physical examination findings suggests an overuse injury.

There are many overuse injuries of the lower extremity that can be discussed. The author has chosen 3 complaints/conditions that are common in his practice and in the literature of overuse injuries in youth: chronic knee pain, medial tibial stress syndrome (MTSS), and tibial stress fractures. As with acute lower extremity injuries discussed previously, mechanisms of injury, physical examination findings, diagnostic evaluation, and approaches to treatment are discussed.

## SPECIFIC INJURIES: PATELLOFEMORAL PAIN SYNDROME, OSGOOD-SCHLATTER DISEASE, AND ILIOTIBIAL BAND TENDONITIS

### Mechanism of Injury and Physical Examination Findings

Patellofemoral pain syndrome (PFPS), or patellofemoral dysfunction (PFD), is the most common cause of chronic anterior knee pain in adolescents. Typically it is worse going up stairs after sitting for prolonged periods (the "theater sign") or after squatting or running. It can follow a relatively rapid change in exercise and training, and there is usually not an acute injury causing the pain. However, it may be a result of an acute knee or ankle injury in which there was atrophy of the quadriceps while the patient was nonweight bearing and quadriceps-strengthening exercises were not done. The knee is usually stable; the patient will not describe "giving way" (manifest as falling to the ground, with the onset of swelling and pain), which would imply an unstable knee, as might occur with patellar dislocation or a meniscal or ligamentous tear as discussed previously. The "giving way" of PFPS is a transient inability to sustain a quadriceps contraction to decelerate or extend the knee, and feeling that insufficiency as "my knee felt like it was giving way," yet the patient does not fall suddenly or experience pain and swelling. Contributing mechanisms to PFPS include a relatively weak vastus medialis muscle, with relatively inflexible hamstring and quadriceps muscles, and abnormal biomechanics (as shown previously under "Other Intrinsic Factors"), which, if demonstrated on physical examination, provide evidence of factors contributing to PFPS. The diagnosis is confirmed with peripatellar tenderness.

Osgood-Schlatter disease is a traction apophysitis that should not be confused with PFPS, with the injury in the former occurring at the insertion of the patellar tendon on the tibial tuberosity. In contrast to PFPS, patients with Osgood-Schlatter disease should miss little if any time from sports.

Iliotibial band tendinitis is the most common cause of chronic lateral knee pain in adolescents. Generally it is not associated with swelling and instability. Tenderness should be elicited along the iliotibial band as it courses over the lateral femoral condyle, or at its insertion at Gerdy tubercle along the lateral tibial plateau, or with stretching the iliotibial band across the midline; tightness of the iliotibial band is also noted using a technique called the Ober test.

#### Diagnostic Imaging and Chronic Knee Pain

The Ottawa Knee Rules were discussed under acute knee injuries and apply here. If the knee pain that is the chief complaint can be reproduced on physical examination, the author does not routinely obtain radiographs in the diagnosis of PFPS, Osgood-Schlatter disease, or iliotibial band tendonitis.

#### Treatment of Patellofemoral Pain Syndrome

1. **Relative rest.** A cardinal rule in rehabilitation of overuse injuries is relative rest. The athlete can do whatever he or she wants as long as the injured structures do not hurt during or within 24 hours of the activity. Athletes who exceed this guideline will continue to reinjure tissue and not improve.
2. **Improving strength, flexibility, endurance.** The 3 overuse injuries described previously are characterized by the need to improve flexibility, strength, and endurance of the key structures involved. The treatment of PFPS includes quadriceps and hamstring stretching, and quadriceps strengthening ("quad sets" as discussed previously under the initial treatment of acute knee injuries). Correction of intrinsic factors will make it less likely that the PFPS will recur. For example, if the patient has weak hip external rotators, rehabilitating these along with the quadriceps and hamstrings will stabilize the patellofemoral joint. Likewise, if the patient has limited dorsiflexion and this is not corrected, this will likely cause continued medial stress on the knee during the push-off phase of gait and lead to recalcitrant PFPS even if the quadriceps and hamstrings are rehabilitated. If initial rehabilitative efforts fail to correct the problem, referral to a sports medicine specialist is indicated to address these biomechanical deficits.
3. **Icing,** as long as there is pain, is appropriate.
4. **Physical therapy.** A physical therapist is necessary to teach the patient the initial exercises to improve flexibility, strength, and endurance of all the muscles identified as contributing to the PFPS. For many patients, one physical therapy visit is adequate to teach proper performance of the exercises in the form of a home education program (HEP). In ordering the physical therapy prescription, for example, for the patient with mild PFPS the author would write "HEP for PFPS to address flexibility, strength deficits, one session." This is the most basic order. If a specific deficit is identified, such as unilateral hamstring inflexibility, then that should be highlighted in the prescription. The broadest order, and the one that physical therapists appreciate, is "Evaluate and Treat." This allows the physical therapist maximal latitude in doing a more thorough evaluation and initiating treatment of deficits. This latter order is appropriate if the physician does little musculoskeletal medicine. If the condition is longstanding, with significant strength or flexibility deficits or persistence in spite of initial physical therapy consultation, or if the patient has been through physical therapy and not improved, more thorough biomechanical evaluation and more hands-on physical therapy will be required. In that case, the physician should order an appropriate number of physical

therapy visits over weeks to months in dialogue with the physical therapist so that the appropriate number and type of physical therapy interventions can be ordered.

5. As pain inhibits full muscle contraction leading to deconditioning, continued pain will delay recovery. Therefore, analgesic medications have a role in the treatment of chronic knee pain. The author initiates medication if the patient reports pain with ADL The explanation for the use of analgesic medication, to break the pain-disuse-atrophy cycle and not allow the athlete to play with pain, is emphasized.
6. **Follow-up.** If there is no improvement in symptoms at one month, the patient has been following the relative rest guidelines, and has been compliant with the rehabilitation exercises, then the author will re-evaluate the gait looking for biomechanical problems such as those included in the "other intrinsic factors" mentioned previously.
7. **Functional rehabilitation.** Returning to sports and exercise following any overuse injury of the lower extremity requires a gradual resumption of walking, jogging, running, and then sprinting, as discussed under the functional rehabilitation of ankle sprains discussed previously. Once the intrinsic deficits are addressed, the author uses the walk–jog protocol used for 20 years in advising patients about returning to running sports. Once the patient is able to run pain free, then the author suggests a running program that includes the "10% rule": do not increase the training volume more than 10% per week. If the patient is unable to return to running pain free, then a reconsideration of the diagnosis, and a reappraisal of the biomechanics of the patient's gait, should be considered. The author advises patients to continue the strength and flexibility exercises they used during the rehabilitation period for another 4 to 6 weeks after resuming training.

### Treatment of Osgood-Schlatter Disease

Osgood-Schlatter disease is treated in a fashion similar to PFPS, with the addition of a protective Osgood-Schlatter pad, which protects the tibial tubercle from painful, direct trauma.

### Treatment of Iliotibial Band Tendonitis

Treatment principles follow those for patellofemoral syndrome, with the emphasis on improving strength, flexibility, and endurance of the iliotibial band, and the external hip rotators, as well as achieving improved dorsiflexion.

## SPECIFIC INJURIES: MEDIAL TIBIAL STRESS SYNDROME ("SHIN SPLINTS")

### Mechanism of Injury and History

The term medial tibial stress syndrome is the preferred term for chronic medial lower leg pain associated with weight-bearing activities. "Shin splints" is the term that exists in the athletic vernacular but should be replaced with MTSS in professional terminology. It appears that repetitive eccentric soleus contractions, especially in the individual who hyperpronates or has a varus heel, play a role in the etiology of MTSS.[22] The pain is usually of gradual onset, often occurring at the beginning of running and then improving during running, or occurring at the end of running, and the pain generally abates soon after running or other exercise is completed. If the level of exercise continues or increases, the duration of pain will extend for a greater portion of the exercise period, and if treatment is not instituted the pain will start to occur with ADL. The history should attempt to identify a problem in the training regimen, from an obvious change such as a teen with no running experience training with the cross-country team, to more subtle changes such as an established runner changing his/her shoes, running surface, or training regimen. Failure to identify the primary problem, that is, the training error or uncorrected intrinsic deficits, may result in solely treating the symptoms only to have the athlete return to the same training program and be reinjured.

### Physical Examination

The tenderness with MTSS is most often reproduced with palpation along the posteromedial border of the mid- to distal tibia, often for 10 to 15 cm. There may be mild swelling and some increased pain with resisted plantarflexion. If the tenderness is more discrete and over the bone, not at the posteromedial border of the tibia, then a stress fracture is suspected (see the following). Biomechanical analysis of the patient's gait is indicated, looking for such risk factors as discussed previously under "Chronic Knee Pain: Other Intrinsic Factors," such as heel or forefoot varus or valgus, hyperpronation, poor external hip strength, and limited dorsiflexion. Achilles tendon and hamstring flexibility should be noted and addressed in the treatment plan.

### Diagnostic Imaging

Plain radiographs are not mandatory with the history and physical examination findings described previously. The author does not routinely get plain radiographs on the initial visit if the diagnosis appears to be straightforward. However, if the patient is not improved at the first follow-up in 3 to 4 weeks and seems to be following the treatment plan, then radiologic evaluation should be considered. Plain radiographs are likely to be normal in most patients with MTSS; if abnormalities are present, they may include a periosteal reaction, which could be consistent with MTSS or a stress fracture. A triple-phase technetium scan will show diffuse uptake along the posteromedial border of the tibia with MTSS. An MRI will allow the identification of muscle inflammation consistent with MTSS but will also examine the bone for inflammation consistent with a stress fracture; in this regard, MRI is the preferred evaluation tool.

### Treatment of MTSS

There is no single established method for treating MTSS. What follows is a discussion of common interventions for MTSS.

***Relative Rest*** As with PFPS, the initial treatment of MTSS includes relative rest. Those who are having pain with ADL should not be running. If there is pain with just walking, a walking boot or crutches may be required temporarily. In the interim, patients may be able to cycle, swim, or water jog to maintain cardiovascular fitness.

***Flexibility, Strength, Endurance, and Proprioceptive Rehabilitation*** A physical therapy consult is indicated to improve lower extremity flexibility, especially dorsiflexion, and strength, endurance, and proprioception deficits where identified. The latter will include but may not be confined to improved flexibility of the Achilles tendon. It may require mobilization of the subtalar joint and strengthening of the dynamic support of the arch. This may require referral to a sports medicine specialist and/or a physical therapist with expertise in biomechanical evaluation. A 7-day course of analgesic medication is reasonable if there is pain with ADL.

***Functional Rehabilitation*** The functional rehabilitation of MTSS follows similar principles as for rehabilitation of PFPS with emphasis on correcting intrinsic factors and shoe type.

***Training Errors*** If the athlete returns to the same training regimen that led to the MTSS, then there is a great risk of reinjury. The author prescribes the amount of running that the athlete should be doing and encourages the athlete to give a copy of the training program to the coach and to call the physician if there are questions.

## SPECIFIC INJURIES: STRESS FRACTURES OF THE LOWER LEG

### Mechanism of Injury and History

The mechanism of injury and history are the same as for MTSS. The most common site of stress fractures in adolescent athletes is the medial tibia.[23] In inexperienced runners who start a running program, for instance soldiers in basic training, the metatarsals may also be a frequent site of injury. Metatarsal stress fractures are not discussed here.

The description of the pain of the medial tibial stress fracture overlaps with that of MTSS, although it is likely to last longer after the running is complete and to occur for a greater portion of the run.

### Physical Examination

The medial tibia is palpated for a discrete area of bone tenderness, ~ 2 to 5 cm in length, in contrast to MTSS, in which the tenderness is likely to be more diffuse and at the posteromedial border, along the bone–muscle interface. The same biomechanical analysis of gait, flexibility, and strength is indicated. Assessment for tenderness over the middle anterior tibia should be done, as the implications for treatment differ from that of the medial tibial stress fracture (see "Treatment," following).

### Diagnostic Imaging

Plain radiographs are normal in most cases of medial tibial stress fractures. Symptoms generally need to be present for at least 3 weeks before bone changes are evident on plain radiographs. If the tenderness is in the anterior portion of the tibia, plain radiographs are indicated to rule out a stress fracture complicated by the "dreaded black line"; see the following under "Treatment."

Technetium scans and MRI are both sensitive modalities for diagnosing stress reactions and fractures. Stress reactions are a milder form of bone injury characterized by marrow edema, whereas stress fractures are characterized by a greater extent of bone injury, from the endosteal to the periosteal surfaces.[24] The author has used both methods to confirm the clinical diagnosis of a stress reaction. However, if the athlete is willing to forgo running/weight-bearing sports, follow the relative rest guidelines in treatment and accept that the length of treatment will be ≥6 to 12 weeks before reinitiating training, then radiologic assessment at the first visit is not necessarily required. In the case of an elite athlete, however, in whom the decision about returning to sports has career and financial implications, an MRI may provide timely information in making that decision. Radiation exposure during the technetium scan has made the MRI the test of choice in the author's practice.

If in follow-up at 3 to 4 weeks the patient is following the relative rest guideline and has not improved, radiologic assessment should be reconsidered to confirm the diagnosis and suggest duration of treatment before returning to running. The technetium scan is not helpful in following the patient because once it is positive it is likely to remain so for up to 18 months.

### Treatment of Stress Fractures

The treatment strategy for medial tibial stress fractures is the same as for MTSS with the exception that the duration of time before returning to running is likely to be longer. The average length of time the patient has to rest for the treatment of a medial tibial stress fracture is 4 to 6 weeks. The average time to resuming full athletic competition is 3 months.[25] Once the patient is pain free for 10 consecutive days, defined as having no pain for any part of the day (including when the patient lays down at night), then a walk-jog program should be implemented as discussed under MTSS.

If the "dreaded black line" is seen, representing a cortical fracture on the tension side of the tibia, which has a high rate of nonunion, the patient should be made nonweight bearing and referral to a sports medicine specialist is indicated. This injury requires nonweight bearing for at least 6 weeks, and if not healing in that time may require surgery. In this setting the use of a bone stimulator is indicated for ~3 months. The average time lost to sports participation is 8 months.

Amenorrheic athletes, specifically runners and ballet dancers, are at risk for stress fractures when compared to their eumenorrheic counterparts. There is no evidence that stress fractures could be prevented using estrogen replacement with at-risk female athletes.

## INTERNET RESOURCES

- www.sportsmedkids.com: The author has created a teaching videotape of the physical examination techniques described in this chapter, as well as for the shoulder and back. The videos are also available on YouTube.com.

## REFERENCES


1. De Inocencio J. Epidemiology of musculoskeletal pain in primary care. *Arch Dis Child.* 2004;89:431–434

2. Cheng TL, Fields CB, Brenner RA, Wright JL, Lomax T, Scheldt PC. Sports injuries: an important cause of morbidity in urban youth. *Pediatr.* 2000;105(3):E32

3. McLain LG, Reynolds S. Sports injuries in a high school. *Pediatrics.* 1989;84:446–450

4. Stirling JM, Landry GL. Sports medicine training during pediatric residency. *Arch Pediatr Adolesc Med.* 1996;150:211–215

5. Garrick JG. The frequency of injury, mechanism of injury, and epidemiology of ankle sprains. *Am J Sports Med.* 1977;5:241–242

6. Beachy G, Akau CK, Martinson M, Olderr TF. High school sports injuries: a longitudinal study at Punahou School. *Am J Sports Med.* 1997;25:675–681

7. Bomberg BC. Acute hemarthrosis of the knee: indications for diagnostic arthroscopy. *Arthroscopy.* 1990;6(3):221–225

8. Zachazewski JE, Magee DJ, Quillen WS. *Athletic Injuries and Rehabilitation.* Philadelphia, PA: WB Saunders; 1996

9. Solomon DH, Simel DL, Bates DW, Katz JN, Schaffer JL. The rational clinical examination. Does this patient have a torn meniscus or ligament of the knee? Value of the physical examination. *JAMA.* 2001;286:1610–1620

10. Metcalf MH, Barrett GR. Prospective evaluation of 1485 meniscal tear patterns in patients with stable knees. *Am J Sports Med.* 2004;32(3):675–680

11. Bertin KC, Goble EM. Ligament injuries associated with physeal fractures about the knee. *Clin Orthop.* 1983;177:188–195

12. Stiell IG, Greenberg GH, Wells GA, et al. Prospective validation of a decision rule for the use of radiography in acute knee injuries. *JAMA.* 1996;275:611–615

13. Bulloch B, Neto G, Plint A, et al. Validation of the Ottawa knee rule in children: a multicenter study. *Ann Emerg Med.* 2003;42(1):48–55

14. Lee K, Siegel MJ, Lau DM, Hildebolt CF, Matava MJ. Anterior cruciate ligament tears: MR imaging-based diagnosis in a pediatric population. *Radiology.* 1999;213(3):697–704

15. Vincken PW, Ter Braak BP, Van Erkell AR, et al. Effectiveness of MR imaging in selection of patients for arthroscopy of the knee. *Radiology.* 2002;223:739–746

16. Stanitski CL. Correlation of arthroscopic and clinical examinations with magnetic resonance imaging findings of injured knees in children and adolescents. *Am J Sports Med.* 1998;26(1):2–6

17. Hergenroeder AC. Acute shoulder, knee, and ankle injuries. Part 2: rehabilitation. *Adolescent Health Update.* 1996;8: 1–8

18. Brostrom C. Sprained ankles. V. Treatment and prognosis in recent ligament ruptures. *Acta Chir Scand.* 1966;132:537–550

19. Steill IG, Greenberg GH, McKnight RD, Wells GA. The "real" Ottawa ankle rules. *Ann Emerg Med.* 1996;27(1):103–104

20. Leddy JJ, Smolinski RJ, Lawrence J, Snyder JL, Priore RL. Prospective evaluation of the Ottawa ankle rules in a university sports medicine center. *Am J Sports Med.* 1998;26(2):158–165

21. Garrick JG, Webb DR. *Sports Injuries: Diagnosis and Management.* Philadelphia, PA: WB Saunders Co; 1999

22. Michael RH, Holder LE. The soleus syndrome: a cause of medical tibial stress (shin splints). *Am J Sports Med.* 1985;13(2):87–94

23. Yngve DA. Stress fractures in the pediatric athlete. In: Sullivan JA, Grana WA, eds. *The Pediatric Athlete.* Park Ridge, IL: American Academy of Orthopedic Surgeons; 1988

24. Arendt EA, Griffiths JH. The use of MR imaging in the assessment and clinical management of stress reactions of none in high-performance athletes. *Clin Sports Med.* 1997;16:291–306

25. Orava S, Hulkko A. Stress fractures in athletes. *Int J Sports Med.* 1987;8:221–226

# CHAPTER 160

## Bone and Joint Infections

NATHAN LITMAN, MD

Osteomyelitis and septic arthritis are major infections of bones and joints almost always requiring hospitalization for initial diagnosis and management. Initial short-course parenteral antibiotic therapy can be followed by an extended course of oral therapy to achieve a successful elimination of infection and return to function.

## OSTEOMYELITIS

Osteomyelitis refers to infection of bone—usually by bacteria, less frequently by fungi or mycobacteria, and rarely by viruses, parasites, or other organisms. Despite the availability of improved diagnostic techniques, potent antibiotics, and effective surgical procedures, osteomyelitis continues to present problems in diagnosis and treatment. Optimal evaluation and management of the adolescent patient with osteomyelitis requires the collaboration of the primary care physician, orthopaedist, radiologist, and infectious diseases consultant.

### PATHOGENESIS

Osteomyelitis can develop from 1 of 3 mechanisms: hematogenous seeding of the bone, direct extension from a contiguous focus of infection, or direct inoculation of organisms into the bone by various forms of trauma. The vascular anatomy of the metaphysis provides the explanation for the pathogenesis of hematogenous osteomyelitis. Capillaries from the nutrient artery make sharp loops in the metaphysis near the growth plate, and these vessels have 3 characteristics that enhance the local susceptibility to infection: (1) nonanastomosing branches that allow for avascular necrosis following any vascular obstruction, (2) the absence of functional phagocytic cells, and (3) slow and turbulent flow.[1] There is a history of nonpenetrating trauma to the bone subsequently involved in almost half the patients with hematogenous osteomyelitis; this is presumed to provide an area of avascular necrosis that is a receptive environment for developing infection should there be a subsequent transient and asymptomatic bacteremia. Consistent with this theory is the male-to-female ratio of 2:1 to 3:1 in cases of hematogenous osteomyelitis, presumably due to the increased frequency of trauma in males; however, this form of infection is seen less often in adolescents than in younger children. The periosteum is relatively impenetrable to infection originating in the soft tissues; osteomyelitis secondary to a contiguous focus of infection is seen with decubitus or neuropathic ulcers, in which case the infection is usually indolent or is an extension from sinusitis or mastoiditis. Organisms can be directly introduced into bone with surgical procedures such as osteotomy or orthopedic pins, as a complication of an open fracture, or with a puncture wound from a nail through a sneaker.

### CLINICAL

Adolescents with acute hematogenous osteomyelitis present initially with localized pain in the end of a long bone that frequently is misdiagnosed as a sprain. Fever then develops over the next day or 2. The ends of the long tubular bones comprise the location of 85% of hematogenous osteomyelitis with the femur and tibia contributing at least half of all cases. Physical examination reveals erythema, indurative swelling, and warmth over the metaphysis of the involved bone, with tenderness out of proportion to what would be expected if this were a cellulitis. There is also not a break in the skin from an abrasion or insect bite to explain the inflammatory findings. If the lower extremity is involved, the patient ambulates with a limp or may refuse to put weight on the involved extremity. Percussion of the opposite end of the bone may also elicit pain. Unifocal bone involvement is the rule. The joint capsule of the hip and the shoulder extend onto the metaphysis; if the infection breaks through the cortex laterally, a secondary septic arthritis will develop; for other joints this results in only a soft tissue abscess. Unless there is a secondary septic arthritis, there is minimal discomfort with motion of the adjacent joint. Chills, malaise, anorexia, and toxicity tend to be less in the teenager than in the child.

Patients with sickle cell disease are more likely to have diaphyseal involvement and multifocal disease; differentiation from vaso-occlusive crisis may be difficult, but localized swelling is uncommon and the fever and pain of vaso-occlusive crises tend to respond promptly to intravenous hydration. Sickle cell patients with osteomyelitis have persistent fever and pain despite appropriate antibiotic therapy.

Patients with osteomyelitis secondary to a contiguous focus of infection or associated with penetrating trauma usually present in a more subacute fashion with complaints primarily of pain, swelling, tenderness, and discharge from the wound; they are often afebrile and nontoxic.

Brodie abscess is a subacute osteomyelitis in which patients present with localized bone pain and tenderness of weeks to months duration, usually without fever, swelling, or erythema of the area; the white blood cell count is usually normal. Plain films of the area reveal a well-circumscribed lytic lesion usually of the metaphysis.

Chronic osteomyelitis may develop after acute osteomyelitis, surgery, or penetrating trauma. Patients have chronic pain with or without drainage and occasional exacerbations associated with increased swelling, discharge, pain, and fever. Long-term complications include secondary amyloidosis and epidermoid carcinoma.

## LABORATORY AND RADIOLOGY

Leukocytosis with a left shift of the differential and elevated erythrocyte sedimentation rate (ESR) and C-reactive protein (CRP) are usually present in teens with hematogenous osteomyelitis. With an aggressive diagnostic approach, the etiologic agent should be identified in more than 80% of patients. Blood culture is positive in more than 50% of patients. Needle aspiration or surgical biopsy of bone will yield the infecting organism in most patients. In healthy adolescents, *Staphylococcus aureus* is the responsible organism in 75% to 80% of cases and *Streptococcus pyogenes* accounts for another 10%. In patients with sickle hemoglobinopathy, *Salmonella* species are the most frequent pathogens;[2] other enteric gram-negative bacilli are seen along with *S aureus*. Immunocompromised hosts, especially in certain geographic areas, may present with osteomyelitis due to endemic fungi such as *Coccidioides*, *Blastomyces*, or *Histoplasma*.

Patients with nail puncture wounds of the foot resulting in osteochondritis tend to have a normal white blood cell count and a modestly elevated ESR; *Pseudomonas aeruginosa* is the most common pathogen[3] isolated and has been demonstrated to originate in the inner layer of the sneaker sole. Infection following surgery is most often due to *Staphylococcus* species and/or resistant gram-negative bacilli. Osteomyelitis due to a contiguous focus of infection such as a decubitus ulcer or an open fracture is commonly polymicrobial, including gram-negative bacilli, *Staphylococci*, and anaerobes. Blood cultures are rarely positive in these conditions. Osteomyelitis due to *Mycobacterium tuberculosis* most commonly affects adjacent vertebrae causing persistent back pain, but usually without fever; a history of exposure, chest x-ray abnormalities, and/or a positive purified protein derivative test (PPD) should raise the index of suspicion; pathology and acid fast stain and culture of a biopsy specimen will confirm the diagnosis.

Initial radiographic studies consist of plain films of the involved extremity; unfortunately the earliest findings in patients with osteomyelitis consist of nonspecific soft tissue swelling, but the films do exclude other conditions that need to be considered such as fractures and tumors. Specific findings for osteomyelitis such as demineralization or lytic areas of the metaphysis and periosteal elevation require 10 to 14 days from the onset of illness to be appreciated; x-rays at clinical presentation may serve as a baseline for comparison with later studies. Radiographic improvement lags behind clinical resolution; plain films will show progressive changes at a time when clinical findings have resolved. Technetium 99 bone scans are positive in nearly all patients at the time of presentation; this radionuclide identifies areas of increased osteoblastic activity and will also be positive in many patients with tumor, trauma, and infarction. Focal uptake of technetium in the metaphysis at the time of the late (2-4 hour) scan is consistent with osteomyelitis. Indium-labeled white blood cell and gallium-67 scans have been advocated for diagnosis of osteomyelitis, but the gallium scan takes a minimum of 2 days to complete and involves more radiation exposure than the technetium scan, and the indium scan is not widely available. Magnetic resonance imaging with gadolinium has become the radiologic diagnostic study of choice for the diagnosis of osteomyelitis;[4] it is more sensitive than computed tomography (CT) scan (Figure 160-1). Medullary space edema and exudate appear as a low-signal intensity on T1-weighted images and as high-signal intensity on T2-weighted images; intravenous gadolinium reveals abscesses on the T1-weighted sequence with fat suppression. Ultrasound can detect subperiosteal abscesses and guide needle drainage.

## DIAGNOSIS

Diagnosis of osteomyelitis is based on the clinical, laboratory, and radiologic findings. The only unequivocal confirmation of osteomyelitis is the demonstration of organisms from a needle aspirate or surgical biopsy of bone. This is a markedly underused technique; not only is it a gold standard diagnostic test, but it will also be therapeutic if there is abscess formation and will provide the organism so that susceptibility testing can be performed to ensure that optimal antibiotic treatment is administered. The differential diagnosis includes cellulitis, necrotizing fasciitis, trauma, malignancy, infarction, SAPHO (synovitis, acne, palmoplantar pustulosis, hyperostosis, osteomyelitis), and infectious and noninfectious arthritis.

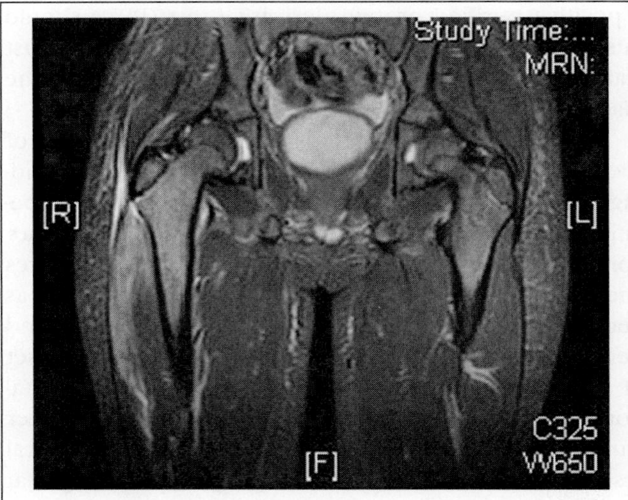


FIGURE 160-1 This adolescent male presented with fever, localized pain, and tenderness over the right greater trochanter. Blood cultures were positive for *S aureus*. Proximal femur demonstrates a high signal in the marrow on the inversion recovery sequence, compatible with marrow edema; edema is also noted in the overlying soft tissues. Marrow enhancement was seen after gadolinium contrast. These features are characteristic of osteomyelitis.

**TREATMENT**

After obtaining blood and bone specimens for culture, parenteral antibiotic therapy should be promptly started. Nafcillin or cefazolin can be the initial agent in healthy teens because of their excellent coverage of *S aureus* and *S pyogenes*. Unfortunately, in many areas of the country, community-associated methicillin-resistant *S aureus* (CA-MRSA) has become common,[5] and penicillins and cephalosporins are not effective against this organism. Vancomycin is the gold standard for treatment of MRSA; many but not all MRSA are susceptible to clindamycin. Discussion with your local microbiology laboratory staff will provide information about the percentage of CA-MRSA in your community and the susceptibility to clindamycin; keep in mind that if initial Kirby-Bauer disc susceptibility testing reveals an erythromycin-resistant, clindamycin-susceptible MRSA, a D-test must be performed to ensure that the MRSA does not have inducible clindamycin resistance, which could render the drug ineffective. Linezolid is active against almost all MRSA; it can be administered both intravenously and orally. Although it has not been Food and Drug Administration (FDA) approved for treatment of osteomyelitis, it has been used successfully for this indication in a compassionate use program.[6] Other drugs that might be useful for treating MRSA osteomyelitis include tetracyclines, trimethoprim-sulfamethoxazole, daptomycin, and quinupristin-dalfopristin, but there is insufficient evidence to recommend their routine use in this infection.

Parenteral antibiotic therapy should continue in the hospital until the patient has become afebrile and the local manifestations have improved. At that time, 1 of 2 options can be considered: continue parenteral antibiotic therapy as an outpatient or switch to an oral antibiotic regimen. A sequential parenteral-oral antibiotic regimen has been demonstrated to be equally effective as an all-parenteral regimen;[7] one must use well-absorbed antibiotics at high dose (cephalexin or dicloxacillin at 100 mg/kg/day, or clindamycin at 30 to 40 mg/kg/day) and ensure adherence with the regimen; this avoids the cost, inconvenience, and hazards of an intravenous line. If oral therapy is selected, many consultants recommend ensuring a peak serum cidal titer against the infecting organism of at least 1:8; this test can be performed if the etiologic agent has been isolated by sending to the lab a serum specimen obtained approximately 45 minutes after the dose of oral antibiotic is administered. Minimum duration of therapy is 3 weeks; shorter durations are associated with unacceptably high rates of failure.[8] Most experts advocate a 4- to 6-week course.

Surgical intervention is required if there is a subperiosteal or intraosseous abscess or if the patient fails to respond after a few days of therapy. Immobilization of the extremity by splinting may reduce pain in the first few days of therapy; nonweight bearing should be advocated for patients with extensive bone destruction involving a lower extremity bone until there is extensive healing to avoid the risk of a pathologic fracture.

Patients with sickle cell disease should have a third-generation cephalosporin such as ceftriaxone or cefotaxime included in their regimen initially to ensure coverage of *Salmonella* and other gram-negative bacilli; therapy can be tailored once the etiologic agent is known. Because of the impaired blood supply to the infected area due to the underlying hemoglobinopathy, many would continue a parenteral regimen for longer than the usual course.

Patients with foot puncture wound-associated osteochondritis should have therapy directed against *Pseudomonas* and *S aureus*; piperacillin-tazobactam provides that coverage, and ciprofloxacin is an alternative for the older adolescent; if debridement and curettage of the infected bone is carried out, antibiotic therapy can be completed a week after the surgery: otherwise a 4-week course of antibiotics is indicated.

Initial treatment of osteomyelitis secondary to adecubitus or neuropathic ulcer should cover the likely polymicrobial spectrum; agents such as cefoxitin or piperacillin-tazobactam are suitable choices while awaiting the results of culture from surgical debridement.

Most patients with osteomyelitis will recover without sequelae. Delayed diagnosis and/or therapy, short courses of antibiotics, or poor selection of drugs will increase the risk for chronic osteomyelitis. Treatment of chronic osteomyelitis requires surgical removal of devitalized bone and antibiotic therapy of 6 to 12 months.

Brodie abscess is managed with curettage and antibiotics directed against the infecting pathogen, usually *S aureus*. Isoniazid, rifampin, pyrazinamide, and ethambutol is the initial regimen for tuberculous bone infection; once susceptibility studies are known, 2 drugs active against the isolate can be continued to complete a 12-month course.

Antibiotic prophylaxis for elective orthopedic surgery should be administered intravenously starting 30 minutes prior to surgery and can be discontinued within 24 hours. Cefazolin is the drug of choice. Patients with open fractures should also receive one day of cefazolin if therapy can begin within 6 hours of the injury and operative repair will be prompt.[9]

## SEPTIC ARTHRITIS

Septic arthritis is a pyogenic infection of the joint usually caused by bacteria, less commonly by fungi or mycobacteria. In the adolescent, septic arthritis is less common than osteomyelitis. Similar to osteomyelitis, infection can be introduced into the joint by 3 different pathways: hematogenous seeding, contiguous spread from an adjacent osteomyelitis, or direct inoculation from penetrating trauma, surgery, or joint injection.

### CLINICAL

The lower extremities are involved more frequently than the upper extremities with the hips or knees being the site of involvement in two-thirds of patients. Males are affected twice as often as females in nongonococcal septic arthritis. The patient complains of pain and swelling of the joint accompanied by fever in most cases, and limp when the lower extremity is the site of infection. With hip involvement, the pain may be referred to the thigh or knee. Physical examination reveals erythema, warmth, and swelling of the joint; increased joint fluid is readily detected when the knee is involved. Active movement is restricted by pain and exquisite pain is elicited by passive movement.

Gonococcal joint involvement may present with the disseminated gonococcal arthritis/dermatitis syndrome,[10] and patients are usually asymptomatic at their primary mucosal site of infection. In the recent past, this was the most common cause of septic arthritis in the teenager, but the frequency has declined with the advent of AIDS and increased safe sex practices resulting in a decreased incidence of gonorrhea. The full-blown syndrome may be appreciated as a 2-phase illness, but only 1 or the other may be clinically recognized. The first phase is the bacteremic stage in which the patient may or may not have fever, toxicity, and leukocytosis. During this phase, painless skin lesions appear that start as erythematous macules, progress to papules, then pustules or hemorrhagic/necrotic lesions, and eventually scab and resolve. The lesions are generally less than 10 in number and present over the acral aspects of the extensor surfaces of the extremities such as the elbow, wrist, knuckle, knee, and ankle. Simultaneous with the skin lesions is a migratory polyarthritis and tenosynovitis. Patients will complain of joint pain, although on examination the swelling and tenderness is really a tenosynovitis. After 7 to 10 days of this bacteremic phase, the illness may entirely resolve or it may progress to the second stage recognized as the septic or suppurative stage. In this phase, fever, toxicity and leukocytosis are almost always present. The patient has a large joint (most common joints in decreasing order: knee, wrist, ankle, elbow) with swelling, erythema, warmth, and exquisite pain on motion; more than one joint may be affected. Up to 90% of patients with disseminated gonococcal infection are female and the illness often begins within a week after the onset of menses. Patients with congenital or acquired complement deficiencies are at increased risk for disseminated gonococcal infection.

### LABORATORY AND RADIOLOGY

Most patients with septic arthritis will have leukocytosis with a left shift and an elevated ESR and CRP. Plain films of the joint will usually reveal a joint effusion and serve to exclude other pathology such as fracture, osteomyelitis, or neoplasm. Ultrasound can be especially helpful in confirming increased joint fluid in the hip and guiding needle aspiration of the fluid. Arthrocentesis should be performed using a heparinized syringe to decrease clot formation; fluid should be sent for cell count and differential, culture and gram stain, and glucose and protein; the specimen for culture should be placed in a blood culture bottle for optimal yield of pathogens. In patients with nongonococcal septic arthritis or the suppurative phase of gonococcal septic arthritis, cell count of the joint fluid usually reveals >50,000 wbc/mm$^3$ with more than 75% polymorphonuclear leukocytes and synovial fluid glucose level more than 25 mg/dL less than the serum glucose level; bacteria will be seen on gram stain or grown in culture in only about 50% of the cases. In patients in the bacteremic phase of disseminated gonococcal infection syndrome, joint fluid is more typical of patients with noninfectious, inflammatory arthritis with

<20,000 wbc/mm$^3$, glucose within 25 mg/dL of the serum glucose level, and negative gram stain and culture for bacteria. Blood culture should always be obtained, but even with blood and synovial fluid cultures obtained before antibiotic administration, the yield of an etiologic agent in septic arthritis is only about 70%. Sexually active teenagers should have gonococcal cultures obtained from urethra or cervix, rectum, and pharynx; a positive culture from one of these sites in the clinical context of disseminated gonococcal syndrome confirms the diagnosis.

## DIAGNOSIS

The teenager with an acutely inflamed joint as manifested by swelling, erythema, warmth, tenderness, pain on movement, and fever should be assumed to have septic arthritis until proven otherwise because this entity requires immediate management to avoid destructive joint changes. Arthrocentesis is both diagnostic in terms of joint fluid cell count, chemistry, and culture as well as therapeutic in terms of relieving pressure within the joint and removing white cell enzymes and bacterial toxins damaging to cartilage. Differential diagnosis includes reactive arthritis, Reiter syndrome, viral infection, acute rheumatic fever, Henoch-Schonlein purpura, rheumatologic disorders, bursitis, trauma, cellulitis, crystal-induced arthritis, Lyme disease, serum sickness, malignancy, and adjacent osteomyelitis.

## TREATMENT

Antibiotic therapy directed against *S aureus* should be initiated immediately after cultures of blood and joint fluid have been obtained; nafcillin or cefazolin are excellent agents. As discussed previously in the treatment of osteomyelitis, in areas where MRSA is prevalent, vancomycin should be started pending susceptibility studies of the etiologic organism. Treatment can be switched to an oral agent active against the pathogen after several days if fever and local manifestations of inflammation have resolved; monitoring to ensure a peak serum cidal titer of 1:8 is recommended. The usual course of therapy is 3 to 4 weeks.

For sexually active teenagers, treatment for gonococcal infection should also be initiated; ceftriaxone 1 g every 24 hours is the first choice; cefotaxime or ceftizoxime 1 g every 8 hours, spectinomycin 2 g every 12 hours, or parenterally administered ciprofloxacin, ofloxacin, or levofloxacin are alternative regimens.[11] There is increasing resistance to quinolones, and susceptibility testing of isolates is mandatory. Particularly, patients with the bacteremic form of disseminated gonococcal infection will have dramatic responses to therapy within 24 to 48 hours. After improvement begins, therapy can be switched to cefixime 400 mg twice daily to complete a 7- to 14-day course of therapy; if quinolone susceptible, ciprofloxacin 500 mg twice daily, ofloxacin 400 mg twice daily, or levofloxacin 500 mg daily are alternative oral regimens. Patients treated for gonococcal infection should also be treated for *C trachomatis* unless infection has been excluded by appropriate tests. Sex partners of patients should be referred for evaluation and treatment.

Repeated needle aspiration of the joint is indicated if there is reaccumulation of synovial fluid after the initial tap. Open surgical drainage is required initially if the hip joint is involved or if fluid continues to reaccumulate after 3 to 5 days of antibiotic therapy and daily arthrocentesis. Antibiotic administration directly into the joint is not indicated.

Long-term sequelae such as decreased range of motion, chronic pain, and degenerative arthritis occur in approximately 25% of patients.

## REFERENCES

1. Waldvogel FA, Medoff G, Swartz MN. Osteomyelitis: a review of clinical features, therapeutic considerations, and unusual aspects. *N Engl J Med.* 1970;282:198–206, 260–266, 316–322

2. Burnett MW, Bass JW, Cook BA. Etiology of osteomyelitis complicating sickle cell disease. *Pediatrics.* 1998;101:296–297

3. Jacobs RF, McCarthy RE, Elser JM. Pseudomonas osteochondritis complicating puncture wounds of the foot in children: a 10-year evaluation. *J Infect Dis.* 1989;161:657–661

4. Pineda C, Vargas A, Rodriguez AV. Imaging of osteomyelitis: current concepts. *Infect Dis Clin N Am.* 2006;20:789–825

5. Kaplan SL, Hulten KG, Gonzalez BE, et al. Three-year surveillance of community-acquired Staphylococcus aureus infections in children. *Clin Infect Dis.* 2005;40:1785–1791

6. Rayner CR, Baddour LM, Birmingham MC, et al. Linezolid in the treatment of osteomyelitis: results of compassionate use experience. *Infection.* 2004;32:8–14

7. Tetzlaff TR, McCracken GH, Nelson JD. Oral antibiotic therapy for skeletal infections of children. *J Pediatr.* 1978;92:485–490

8. Dich VQ, Nelson JD, Haltalin KC. Osteomyelitis in infants and children. *Am J Dis Child.* 1975;129:1273–1278

9. Lew DP, Waldvogel FA. Osteomyelitis. *N Engl J Med.* 1997;336:999–1007

10. Rice PA. Gonococcal arthritis (disseminated gonococcal infection). *Infect Dis Clin N Am.* 2005;19:853–861

11. Centers for Disease Control and Prevention. Sexually transmitted diseases treatment guidelines, 2006. *MMWR.* 2006;55(No RR-11):46–47

# CHAPTER 161

## Bone Tumors

RICHARD GORLICK, MD

### INTRODUCTION

Although primary bone tumors are rare in adolescents and young adults, in this age group they are the third most frequent neoplasms, with only leukemias and lymphomas being more common. Malignant bone tumors occur in the United States at an annual rate of approximately 8.7 cases per million children and adolescents. Only half the bone tumors in childhood are malignant; of these, osteosarcoma is the most frequent, accounting for approximately 35% of all primary sarcomas of bone. Ewing sarcoma, the second most frequent primary bone cancer in adolescents, is more common than osteosarcoma in children younger than 10 years.[1] Many malignancies can metastasize to bone, but this is rarer than the incidence of discovering primary bone lesions, which is unique to adolescence. Lymphoma can metastasize as well as arise primarily in the bone and will be the subject of another chapter and therefore will not be discussed further here. Similarly, chondrosarcoma, which is the second most common bone tumor overall, is rare in those under age 21 and therefore will not be discussed further. The focus of this chapter is the 2 most common malignant bone tumors that afflict adolescents, which are Ewing sarcoma (including primitive neuroectodermal tumors) and osteosarcoma. It is important to recognize that a heterogeneous variety of benign bone tumors occur in adolescents as well, and these will be briefly presented in the following paragraphs.

Benign tumors can be categorized into lesions that produce osteoid, lesions that produce collagen, lesions that produce cartilage, and lesions of vascular or other etiologies. Bone-producing tumors include osteoid osteoma and osteoblastoma; collagen-producing lesions include non-ossifying fibroma and fibrous dysplasia; cartilage-producing lesions include osteochondroma, enchondroma, and chondroblastoma, and bone lesions of other or unknown origin include aneurysmal bone cysts, giant cell tumors, eosinophilic granuloma, and stress fractures.[2] Space precludes a discussion of each of these conditions. Many of these are included in the differential diagnosis of malignant tumors and can mimic their clinical presentation, radiographic or histologic appearance. These lesions, although capable of local recurrence, rarely metastasize, thus management is primarily surgical. As an example of the category of benign bone tumors, osteoid osteoma will be presented in additional detail, particularly given its peak incidence during adolescence.

Osteoid osteoma is a benign bone lesion clinically characterized by pain and sometimes swelling. The most common sites of osteoid osteoma are the femur and tibia, although they can occur anywhere in the skeleton. The radiographic appearance of an osteoid osteoma is characteristically a sclerotic lesion in the long bones with a lucent nidus. Pathologically the lesion comprises a peripheral area with less mature bone and prominent osteoblastic rimming, and a central part, which is commonly referred to as the nidus, comprising a denser, woven bone with less prominent osteoblastic rimming.[3] The clinical history of an osteoid osteoma involves the abrupt onset of pain in the area of the lesion, which classically awakens the patient at night. In many patients (75%), pain (the predominant clinical feature) is relieved by aspirin or nonsteroidal anti-inflammatory medications. Surgery is recommended for patients whose pain is not relieved with aspirin or other nonsteroidal medication. The only part of an osteoid osteoma that needs to be removed surgically is the nidus, with the nidus being the neoplastic portion of the tumor and the remainder of the tumor being reactive normal bone.[3]

### OSTEOSARCOMA

Although osteosarcoma and Ewing sarcoma have little in common beyond being malignant tumors arising in bone, it is useful to contrast the 2 entities to highlight the features specific to each entity (Table 161-1).[4] Osteosarcoma, the most common primary malignant bone tumor, is a highly aggressive disease in which dramatic progress has been made in treatment and outcome over the past several decades. Osteosarcoma is a disease primarily of adolescents and young adults.[5]

#### PRESENTATION

The most common clinical presentation of osteosarcoma is pain in the involved region, with or without an associated soft tissue mass. Pain is often attributed to trauma or vigorous physical exercise, both of which are common in the patient population. Trauma is not causally related

**Table 161-1**

**Comparison of Clinical Features of Ewing Sarcoma and Osteosarcoma**

| | *Ewing Sarcoma* | *Osteosarcoma* |
|---|---|---|
| Peak incidence/epidemiology | Peak incidence in second decade<br>Rare after age 30<br>No known causal factor | Peak incidence in second decade<br>Occurs in adults, particularly in Paget disease, radiation exposure, or genetically predisposed |
| Racial predilection | Uncommon in blacks and Asians | None |
| Genetics | A consistent chromosomal translocation is observed<br>Simple karyotype | Frequent genetic abnormalities at the p53 and retinoblastoma gene loci<br>Complex chromosomal derangements |
| Pathology | Small round blue cell tumor | Spindle cell sarcoma with osteoid |
| Skeletal location | Diaphyses | Metaphyses |
| Common sites of metastases | Lungs, bone, bone marrow | Lungs, bone |
| Treatment modalities | Surgery, radiation, chemotherapy | Surgery, chemotherapy |

to the development of osteosarcoma. Symptoms are usually present for several months before the diagnosis is made.[2-5] Occasionally patients can present more dramatically with a pathologic fracture. Osteosarcoma can occur in any bone of the body. Among young patients, the most common site is the metaphysis of a long bone. Approximately half of all osteosarcomas originate in the region around the knee. The most frequent primary site is the distal femur, followed by the proximal tibia. The proximal humerus is the third most common location. Involvement of the axial skeleton, most commonly the pelvis, occurs in fewer than 10% of cases in the adolescent age group (Figure 161-1).[3]

Osteosarcoma, which is typically high grade when it presents in adolescents, metastasizes very early in its evolution. Approximately 20% of patients present with radiographically detectable metastatic disease, but more than 80% of patients have subclinical, microscopic metastasis. The evidence for this comes from large clinical reports in which patients without clinically detectable metastatic disease were treated with surgical resection of the primary tumor alone.[6] The most frequent site for metastatic presentation is the lung. Much less frequently, metastases at initial diagnosis can occur in other bones. When osteosarcoma is widely metastatic, more frequently at recurrence than at the time of initial diagnosis, it can spread to the central nervous system or gastrointestinal tract. Death from osteosarcoma is almost always the result of progressive pulmonary metastasis. Bone lesions, although extremely painful, are usually not life threatening.[2-5]

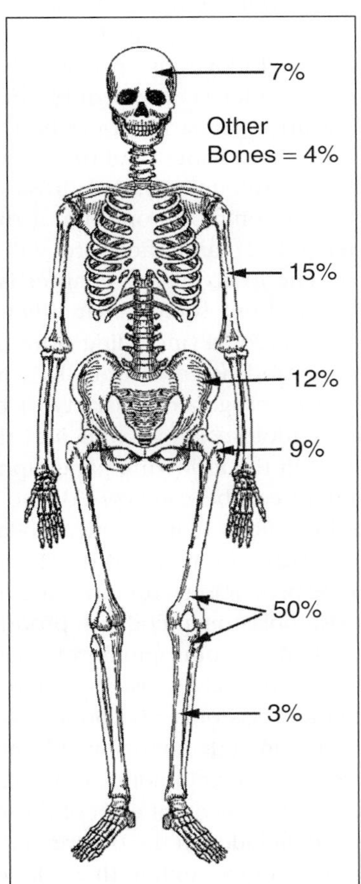


**FIGURE 161-1** Site of primary tumor in patients with osteosarcoma.

The evaluation of suspected osteosarcoma begins with history, physical examination, and plain radiographs. Pain at multiple sites does not rule out the possibility of osteosarcoma, as this may represent metastatic disease. Metastases in the lungs produce only respiratory symptoms with extensive involvement.[5] Systemic symptoms, such as fever and weight loss, occur rarely.[6] Physical examination is typically remarkable only for the soft tissue mass at the primary site, which is not invariably present. Laboratory evaluation is seldom revealing. Elevations of the serum alkaline phosphatase and lactate dehydrogenase are observed in a large proportion of patients but are not reliable. The differential diagnosis for pain at a bony site in this age group includes the malignant bone tumors, osteosarcoma, and Ewing sarcoma, as well as the benign bone tumors listed previously, and a variety of nonneoplastic conditions with osteomyelitis among the more common. In a patient with a suspected bone tumor, obtaining a plain radiograph of the site is most critical.[2-5]

The diagnosis of osteosarcoma is typically suspected by its radiographic appearance. Osteosarcoma can present as a lytic or sclerotic lesion or as a mixed lytic-sclerotic lesion. As with other malignant tumors in bone, plain films reveal permeative destruction with poorly defined zones of transition. Ossification in the soft tissue in a "sunburst" pattern is classic for osteosarcoma but is not a sensitive or specific feature. Periosteal new bone formation with lifting of the cortex leads to the appearance of a Codman triangle. Features such as the eccentric location of the tumor in the metaphyseal portion of the bone and the skeletal location help distinguish osteosarcoma and Ewing sarcoma, the second most frequent tumor in this age group.[2-5]

The diagnosis of osteosarcoma can be accurately predicted in two-thirds of cases based on radiographic location and appearance but should never be made from images alone. It is mandatory to obtain a biopsy for pathological confirmation of the diagnosis.[2-5] The biopsy must be performed by someone experienced in performing these procedures, as a poorly placed biopsy can necessitate a subsequent amputation or have other morbidities. The diagnosis of osteosarcoma is made by histologic examination of the biopsy. To determine the local and distant extent of disease at presentation various radiographic studies are indicated as part of the diagnostic evaluation. The extent of osteosarcoma in bone and soft tissue is best appreciated with cross-sectional imaging techniques such as computed tomography (CT) or magnetic resonance imaging (MRI).[2-5] A radionuclide bone scan with methylene diphosphonate labeled with technetium-99m defines the extent of the primary tumor and is useful in the detection of "skip lesions" within the same bone, as well as distant bone metastases.[7] An unusual presentation of osteosarcoma is multifocal osteosarcoma, a rare entity in which multiple synchronous skeletal tumors are present at diagnosis with each lesion resembling the primary tumor radiographically, suggesting a multicentric origin. It is unclear whether such sarcomas arise in multiple sites or if one of the lesions is the true primary that has metastasized rapidly to other skeletal sites in the absence of lung metastases.[2-5] Routine posteroanterior and lateral radiographs of the chest allow detection of metastases in most cases. Computed tomography of the chest is more sensitive in detecting pulmonary metastases and has become the imaging procedure of choice. However, there are false-positive results, particularly with smaller lesions.[2-5] Successful treatment of high-grade osteosarcoma requires the use of systemic chemotherapy. Many of the agents have acute and long-term toxicity; therefore, it is essential to obtain baseline studies before initiating chemotherapy so that toxicity can be monitored. Baseline evaluations are usually performed of renal function, cardiac function, and hearing. All young men past the age of puberty should be offered the opportunity for sperm banking.[2-5] Newer techniques for maintaining fertility of women have been developed, but their indications have not completely been established.

The most widely used staging system for bone tumors including osteosarcoma is the system developed by Enneking and associates.[8] This system categorizes localized malignant bone tumors by grade (low grade—stage I, or high grade—stage II) and by the local anatomic extent (intracompartmental—A, or extracompartmental—B). The compartmental status is determined by whether the tumor extends through the cortex. Patients with distant metastases are stage III. There are very few high-grade intramedullary lesions (ie, stage IIA) because most high-grade osteosarcomas break through the cortex early in their natural history. In the younger age groups most osteosarcomas are high-grade lesions, hence virtually all patients are stage IIB or III distinguished by the presence or absence of detectable metastatic disease.[2-5]

## EPIDEMIOLOGY AND PATHOGENESIS

Osteosarcoma has a bimodal age distribution with the first peak in adolescence and the second among older adults. In older patients osteosarcoma arises in abnormal bone, including those affected by longstanding Paget disease. The peak incidence occurs in the second decade of life during the adolescent growth spurt. The modal age of incidence is 16 years for girls and 18 for boys. It is estimated that approximately 400 children and adolescents younger than 20 years of age are diagnosed with osteosarcoma each year in the United States.[1] Boys are affected more frequently, and the incidence in black children is slightly higher than in whites.

There is limited understanding of the etiology of osteosarcoma. The peak age of incidence coincides with a period of rapid bone growth in young people, suggesting a correlation between rapid bone growth and the development of osteosarcoma.[2-5] Other evidence supporting this relationship includes the higher incidence of osteosarcoma in large dog breeds as compared with small breeds, and the earlier peak age in girls as compared with boys, corresponding to the earlier age of their growth spurt.[9] Some evidence suggests a higher incidence in tall people as compared with short people. At the same time, it is important to recognize that osteosarcoma arises in many patients both well before and long after the adolescent growth spurt. Radiation exposure is a well-documented etiologic factor but as the interval between irradiation and the appearance of osteosarcoma is typically long this is not relevant to most adolescent patients.[10] The incidence of osteosarcoma is dramatically increased among survivors of retinoblastoma. Most second malignancies are sarcomas, and almost 50% are osteosarcomas.[11] In the hereditary form of osteosarcoma, germline mutations of the retinoblastoma tumor suppressor gene are common. This is the probable basis of increased frequency of secondary cancers in this population, because the rate in survivors of unilateral sporadic retinoblastoma is much less.[12] Germline mutations in the p53 tumor suppressor gene can lead to a high risk of developing malignancies including osteosarcoma, which has been described as the Li-Fraumeni syndrome.[13] Loss of function of the p53 and retinoblastoma tumor suppressor genes are believed to have an important role in tumorigenesis in osteosarcoma, but numerous other oncogenes and tumor suppressor genes are found to be altered in osteosarcoma tumor cells. Although it is clear that alterations in tumor suppressor genes and oncogenes are necessary to produce osteosarcomas, it is not clear which of these events occurs first and why or how it occurs.[14] A viral etiology has been suggested by some based on several lines of evidence, but no convincing data have emerged that they are a major etiologic factor. Trauma often has been associated with the diagnosis of osteosarcoma, but little evidence exists to support a causal relationship.[2-5]

The diagnosis of osteosarcoma is based on histopathologic criteria and depends on the presence of malignant spindle cells associated with the production of tumor osteoid. Great variability exists in the histologic patterns seen in this tumor and in the degree of osteoid production, so that extensive review of the pathologic material may be required to demonstrate tumor osteoid. Osteosarcomas arise from mesenchymal tissue capable of differentiating toward fibrous tissue, cartilage, or bone; as such osteosarcoma can have chondroblastic, fibroblastic, and osteoblastic components.[3]

## TREATMENT

Almost all patients with osteosarcoma have microscopic metastatic disease at the time of diagnosis. The successful treatment requires systemic chemotherapy.[2-5] Prior to the early 1970s, the only therapy available for osteosarcoma was surgery. Despite the use of radical surgery, the outcome was poor. Approximately 85% to 90% of patients who presented with apparently localized disease and underwent radical surgery rendering them grossly free of disease had recurrences of disease.[6] In the 1970s, several investigators reported that chemotherapy had activity against relapsed or metastatic osteosarcoma. The agents that were reported to demonstrate activity included doxorubicin, cisplatin, high-dose methotrexate with leucovorin rescue, and ifosfamide.[15,16] When these agents were administered to patients with relapsed or metastatic osteosarcoma, tumor responses were observed. It must be noted that compared with other pediatric malignancies, the list of drugs effective against macroscopic disease is relatively short. It was recognized that in the absence of any clinically detectable or bulk disease, chemotherapy may be even more effective and may result in long-term disease-free survival. With this rationale, many investigators embarked on trials of adjuvant chemotherapy for the treatment of osteosarcoma. In the 1970s and early 1980s, all of these trials were single-arm, nonrandomized treatments employing adjuvant chemotherapy, comparing results against historical controls.[17] Every reported trial of adjuvant chemotherapy for osteosarcoma reported a disease-free survival superior to the historical rate of 20%.[2-5]

Not all investigators were convinced that chemotherapy is appropriate for all patients with osteosarcoma because the use of historical comparisons can be flawed. To clarify the issues surrounding the value of adjuvant chemotherapy, the Multi-Institution Osteosarcoma Study was initiated.[18] Patients were eligible for study entry after amputation or tumor resection if they did not have clinically detectable metastatic disease. The intent of the study was to randomize patients between observation and adjuvant multiagent chemotherapy. Patients who did not receive chemotherapy after surgery had a probability of disease-free survival of 11% as compared with 66% for those who received chemotherapy.[18] This study unequivocally demonstrated that adjuvant chemotherapy was of clear benefit, establishing chemotherapy as a clinical standard.

In the same era, Rosen et al[19] introduced the concept of giving chemotherapy before carrying out definitive surgery on the primary tumor. This treatment has been referred to as preoperative or neoadjuvant chemotherapy, or more recently, induction chemotherapy. The concept of induction chemotherapy arose from the need for time to make the custom endoprosthesis required for limb salvage procedures, creating an interval during which chemotherapy could be administered. In addition, theoretical advantages of induction chemotherapy included early treatment of micrometastatic disease and facilitation of the eventual surgical procedure because of tumor shrinkage and decreased vascularity. It also became possible to examine the histologic response of the tumor to induction chemotherapy to assess the effectiveness of therapy.[19] A strong correlation between the degree of necrosis and the probability of subsequent disease-free survival was observed. Given the advantages in facilitating limb salvage procedures and in assessing chemotherapeutic efficacy, the use of induction chemotherapy has become the standard treatment approach for osteosarcoma. Numerous trials have been conducted to clarify the role of the various chemotherapeutic agents in the treatment of osteosarcoma as well as their method of delivery.[20] Most adolescents treated for osteosarcoma receive treatment from pediatric oncologists at specialized centers. In North America most newly diagnosed patients are treated in phase III clinical trials led by a National Cancer Institute-funded cooperative clinical trials group, the Children's Oncology Group. It is the collective view of pediatric oncologists that only through clinical trials will prognosis be improved. The phase III trials generally compare an experimental arm, which is believed to be better with standard therapy. Standard therapy remains the chemotherapy agents, cisplatin, doxorubicin, high-dose methotrexate, ifosfamide, and etoposide, outlined previously both prior to and following definitive surgery typically for an approximately 32-week course.[20]

Despite the effectiveness of chemotherapy against microscopic disease it cannot control clinically detectable disease. The successful treatment of osteosarcoma requires local control and systemic chemotherapy. Osteosarcoma is considered resistant to radiation therapy, and the only effective tool for local control is surgery. Historically this surgery was amputation of the affected extremity, but at present most patients undergo a limb salvage procedure. The limb salvage procedure involves a wide excision of the entire affected region with replacement of the resected area by an autologous graft, allograft, or endoprosthesis. A wide range of surgical techniques and options for preservation of limbs and limb function are currently available.[2-5] For the successful treatment of osteosarcoma, all sites of radiographically visible metastatic disease need to be resected as well, including pulmonary metastases. This is usually accomplished through bilateral staged thoracotomies.[2-5]

### PROGNOSIS

The outcome of osteosarcoma patients depends on several factors, including how it is treated. The most consistent prognostic factor at diagnosis is the presence of clinically detectable metastatic disease, which confers an unfavorable prognosis. The site of the primary tumor has some prognostic significance, with axial lesions prognostically inferior to tumors of the appendicular skeleton. Both serum lactate dehydrogenase and the alkaline phosphatase can correlate with outcome; higher levels of either enzyme predict an inferior prognosis. These factors most likely influence outcome by reflecting its resectability. With currently available regimens, approximately 60% to 70% of patients with nonmetastatic osteosarcoma of the extremity will survive without evidence of recurrence. In nonextremity lesions particularly, prognosis is influenced by resectability because complete surgical resection is necessary for cure. In most large reported studies only 10% to 20% of patients who presented with clinically detectable metastatic disease were continuously free of disease 5 years from diagnosis.[2-5]

## EWING SARCOMA

The Ewing sarcoma family of tumors (ESFT) comprises 2 major entities, Ewing sarcoma and primitive neuroectodermal tumors, which although initially considered to be distinct are now believed to be a spectrum of the same entity.[2,3] Ewing sarcoma is a bone tumor first described by James Ewing in 1921.[21] In the early 1980s it was discovered that Ewing sarcoma and primitive neuroectodermal tumor have the same reciprocal translocation between chromosomes 11 and 22, t(11;22)(q24;q12).[22] It was the combination of the shared translocation and the similar clinical behavior that led these 2 tumors along with Askin tumor (a similar tumor specifically of the chest wall) to be described subsequently as the ESFT.[23]

### PRESENTATION

Patients with ESFT usually present with pain and a palpable mass. As compared with osteosarcoma there is a greater propensity to develop in the axial skeleton, although appendicular sites remain the most common site of presentation. Long bone lesions can present with a pathologic fracture. Back pain may indicate tumors in a paraspinal, retroperitoneal, or deep pelvic location and must be considered in the differential diagnosis of this symptom.[2-5] Systemic symptoms of fever and weight loss can occur and often indicate the presence of metastatic disease. Ewing sarcoma family of tumors can occur in virtually any location, even remote from bones rarely, so that careful examination of painful sites by inspection and palpation is critical. Because ESFT can present in close juxtaposition to vertebrae, tumors can result in neuropathic pain mimicking sciatica or producing nerve dysfunction. Thus, a comprehensive neurological exam is critical to evaluate asymmetric weakness or numbness, which should increase one's index of suspicion. Patients with lung metastases may present with asymmetric breath sounds, pleural signs, or rales. Unlike osteosarcoma, ESFT metastasizes to the bone marrow, and patients with significant disease in this site can present with petechiae or purpura from thrombocytopenia.[2-5]

The most frequent primary sites for ESFT include the pelvis (25%), femur (16%), ribs (12%), and spine (8%) (Figure 161-2). Approximately 25% of patients will present with metastatic disease at diagnosis.[24] Fewer than 40% of the patients who present with metastatic disease at diagnosis will have it confined to lung or pleura. Most with metastatic disease will have bone and/or bone marrow metastases either alone or in addition to pulmonary/pleural disease, which again contrasts with osteosarcoma.[24] A pelvic location of the tumor, high levels of lactate dehydrogenase, fever, an interval between onset of symptoms and diagnosis less than 3 months, and age older than 12 years tend to associate with having clinically evident metastatic disease at diagnosis.[25] There are no blood tests with which to diagnose ESFT. Serum lactate dehydrogenase level, if elevated, suggests malignancy but is neither sensitive nor specific. Anemia, neutropenia, and thrombocytopenia can suggest bone marrow infiltration but are also not specific for ESFT.

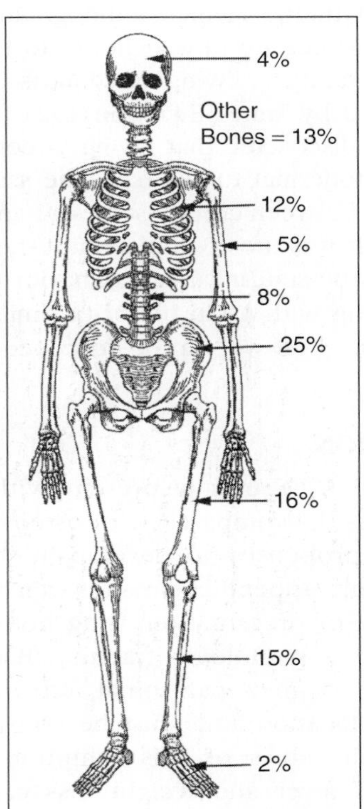


**FIGURE 161-2** Site of primary tumor in patients with Ewing sarcoma family tumors of the bone.

Ewing sarcoma family of tumors should be included in the differential diagnosis of any bone or soft tissue mass in patients from age 3 through the third decade of life. The differential diagnosis of a bone lesion should include other neoplasms both malignant and benign including osteosarcoma and other nonneoplastic entities such as osteomyelitis. If a mass is palpated or if persistent bone pain is reported, plain radiographs are indicated.[2-4,26] The classic radiological description of an ESFT is a lamellar (onion skin) lesion on plain film, which if it involves a long bone is typically in the diaphysis. Additional radiographic findings may include bone sclerosis, elevation of the periosteum with periosteal reaction (Codman triangle), and radial streaks of bone beyond the cortical walls. Once a bone tumor is suspected from a radiograph, a priority is to image the suspected primary lesion for biopsy planning purposes among other reasons.[2-4,26] Magnetic resonance imaging (MRI) of the region can help identify extent of disease and is generally more precise than CT scan. The CT scan, however, better delineates bone involvement. Tumors that are adjacent to critical neurologic structures require rapid MRI and consideration of emergency therapy to prevent neurologic deterioration. A metastatic evaluation includes a chest CT scan and radioisotope bone scans. Bone marrow aspiration and biopsy are required to exclude malignant infiltration as this is a potential site of metastases.[2-4,26] The definitive diagnosis for ESFT requires a biopsy specimen exactly analogous to the scenario in osteosarcoma. If a patient is suspected of having ESFT, consultation with a pediatric oncologist and/or pathologist prior to the biopsy may help ensure that the specimen is processed appropriately to permit molecular confirmation of the diagnosis, which will be discussed further subsequently. Biopsies need to be performed with consideration of further therapy, because all ESFT patients will require some form of definitive local management of their disease. Inappropriate biopsy or resection similar to the scenario in osteosarcoma can result in increased morbidity or mortality for the patient. Ewing sarcoma family of tumors are typically staged based on the radiographic findings and grade of the tumor (which is always high grade) using the Enneking staging system described previously. Prechemotherapy treatment evaluations should be performed as described for osteosarcoma.

## EPIDEMIOLOGY AND PATHOGENESIS

Based on SEER data, the incidence of ESFT from birth to 20 years is 2.9/1,0,000,00 per year. It has a slightly younger age distribution compared with osteosarcoma, being the most common malignant bone tumor in children younger than 10 years despite a lower overall incidence. Ewing sarcoma family of tumors is rare in those older than 30 years, whereas osteosarcoma is seen in adults.[1] It has a slight male preponderance with a peak incidence in the latter half of the second decade of life. Approximately 64% of ESFT are diagnosed during adolescence. The incidence in whites is much higher than in blacks or Asians, in contrast to osteosarcoma, which has a relatively equal race distribution. This racial predisposition does not vary geographically.[1]

All cases of ESFT are thought to be sporadic with no known genetic or environmental predisposing factors. Unlike osteosarcoma, growth parameters such as height and weight have not been linked to developing an ESFT.[2-4,26] Ewing sarcoma family of tumors is thought to derive from cells of primitive neuroectodermal origin, although the exact cell of origin of ESFT has yet to be identified. The translocation t(11;22)(q24;q12) or another in a series of related translocations occurs in more than 95% of ESFT.[27] The classic t(11;22)(q24;q12) translocation joins the *EWS* gene (Ewing sarcoma) located on chromosome 22 to an ets family gene, FLI1 (Friend leukemia insertion) located on chromosome 11. The EWS/FLI1 fusion creates a novel protein that acts as an aberrant transcription factor.[28] The translocation is believed to be central in the pathogenesis of ESFT, but the reason the translocation occurs and the primary mechanisms by which the fusion protein induces transformation remain poorly understood and are areas of active research.

To make the diagnosis of an ESFT, the biopsy material is typically evaluated by routine staining as well as by immunohistochemistry. On routine staining the ESFT appears as a small round blue cell tumor that is histologically similar to many other tumors that occur in adolescence including lymphoma and soft tissue sarcomas such as rhabdomyosarcoma. The Ewing sarcoma family of tumors can range from completely undifferentiated (Ewing sarcoma) to differentiated (primitive neuroectodermal tumor). Ewing sarcoma family of tumors is typically distinguished from other small round blue cell tumors by immunohistochemical staining. Immunohistochemical markers include membranous staining of CD99 (MIC2), which is present on more than 90% of ESFT.[2-4,26] Muscle, lymphoid, and adrenergic markers should be negative in ESFT. Immature tumors lack most immunohistochemical markers but contain abundant glycogen. More differentiated tumors express membrane and cytoplasmic markers including neuron specific enolase, S-100, neurofilaments, CD57, CD45, and synaptophysin. Differentiating tumors may contain pseudorosettes or have classical rosette formation.[2-5,20] The diagnosis can be confirmed by using cytogenetics, RT-PCR, and fluorescent in situ hybridization (FISH) to identify the t(11;22), or a related translocation as these are pathognomonic.[2-5,26] For the molecular studies it is helpful if a small piece of tumor is snap frozen in liquid nitrogen at the time of biopsy.

## TREATMENT

Survival of patients with ESFT prior to identification of chemotherapy was invariably poor, with studies reporting a 5-year survival of 10%.[2-5,26] The first chemotherapy agents with reported efficacy in ESFT were cyclophosphamide, actinomycin-D, and vincristine. Patients with ESFT began to be treated with these agents individually in the early 1960s and in combination by the late 1960s.[2-5,26] All of these studies demonstrated improvements in survival for patients presenting with localized disease. Unlike the scenario in osteosarcoma, a randomized study to prove the efficacy of chemotherapy was not undertaken, with the pediatric oncology community accepting the efficacy of chemotherapy based on the outcomes with chemotherapy as compared to historical controls. Chemotherapy treatment in ESFT has slowly evolved over the last several decades with information acquired through a series of clinical trials mounted in North America and in other countries that have generally resulted in consistent progress.[29] Space precludes describing these clinical trials, and therefore only the general principles of treatment at present will be covered.

In general for the treatment of ESFT the chemotherapy class of alkylating agents (cyclophosphamide, ifosfamide, melphalan, and busulfan), actinomycin-D, vincristine, and doxorubicin are active in the treatment of ESFT. Typical front-line chemotherapy regimens alternate noncross-resistant chemotherapy combinations. As an example, alternating cycles of cyclophosphamide/doxorubicin/vincristine and ifosfamide/etoposide.[29] The doses used in each cycle of therapy and the total duration of therapy have varied considerably over time, with clinical trials testing issues such as dose intensity and timing intensity in attempts to optimize the regimens. In addition to the agents listed previously, ESFT has been identified as responding to several other classes of chemotherapy more recently, most notably the camptothecins such as topotecan. Compared to osteosarcoma, many more chemotherapies have been demonstrated to have activity in ESFT. In contrast to osteosarcoma, not all of the active drugs are typically incorporated into routine front-line chemotherapy, as use of some would preclude the use of others. Approaches such as the use of high-dose chemotherapy with stem cell support have been applied by some to the treatment of high-risk patients, but the use of such approaches remains experimental.[2-5,26] Patients treated for ESFT are at high risk for the development of a second malignancy. Most second malignancies following successful treatment of ESFT are acute myeloid leukemia, myelodysplastic syndrome, and sarcomas in the radiation field. The overall likelihood of developing a second malignancy is approximately 2%.[30]

Ewing sarcoma family of tumors requires local and systemic therapy to achieve a cure. Similar to the scenario in osteosarcoma, chemotherapy alone cannot control clinically detectable disease. Local therapy needs to be directed to all sites of bulky tumor including the primary site and metastases. Unlike osteosarcoma, ESFT are radiation responsive. In ESFT options for local control therefore include radiation therapy and surgery. Which modality is utilized depends on a number of factors including resectability of the tumor, likely functional consequences of surgery, concern over late effects, and treating physician preferences.[2] To obtain local control, some tumors are treated with radiation and surgery.[2-5,26] In these cases radiation therapy can be administered as an external beam pre- or postoperatively, intraoperatively, or as radioactive implants.

### PROGNOSIS

Overall survival in patients with ESFT is 60%; however, for patients with localized disease it approaches 70%, whereas patients with metastatic disease have less than a 25% likelihood of surviving.[2-5,26] Metastatic disease at diagnosis is the most significant adverse prognostic factor in patients with ESFT despite aggressive chemotherapy. In early ESFT clinical trials, prognostic factors in patients who present with localized disease include tumor volume and site. In general, larger tumors (often pelvis) had a poorer prognosis. Aggressive, multiagent chemotherapy as well as effective local control have markedly reduced the prognostic value of these features.[2-5,26]

## CONCLUSIONS

Although rare, a number of benign and malignant bone tumors have their highest incidence during adolescence. Maintaining these entities in the differential diagnosis of musculoskeletal pain is necessary for the prompt recognition of these conditions, particularly the malignant bone tumors osteosarcoma and ESFT. The tumors are treated with complex treatment plans involving systemic chemotherapy and local control measures. The 2 diseases osteosarcoma and ESFT differ considerably in their epidemiology, pathology, and treatment. With aggressive treatment most patients who are diagnosed with localized osteosarcoma or ESFT will remain free of their disease. In the minority of patients who present with metastatic disease a cure is relatively rare. It is hoped clinical trials in patients with osteosarcoma and ESFT will lead to further improvements in their treatment.

## REFERENCES

1. Gurney JG, Swensen AR, Bulterys M. Malignant bone tumors. In: Ries LAG, Smith MA, Gurney JG, Linet M, Tamra T, Young JL, Bunin GR, eds. *Cancer Incidence and Survival among Children and Adolescents: United States SEER Program 1975-1995*. NIH Pub No 99-4649. Bethesda, MD: National Cancer Institute; 1999:99-110

2. Gorlick R, Bernstein ML, Toretsky JA, et al. Bone tumors. In: Holland J, Frei E, eds. *Cancer Medicine*. 7th ed. Hamilton, Ontario: BC Decker; 2006:2019-2027

3. Huvos A. *Bone Tumors: Diagnosis, Treatment, and Prognosis*. 2nd ed. Philadelphia, PA: WB Saunders; 1991

4. Meyers PA, Gorlick R. Osteosarcoma. *Ped Clin N Amer.* 1997;44:973-989

5. Link MP, Eilber E. Osteosarcoma. In: Pizzo PA, Poplack DG, eds. *Principles and Practice of Pediatric Oncology*. 3rd ed. Philadelphia, PA: Lippincott-Raven; 1997:889-920

6. Dahlin D, Coventry M. Osteogenic sarcoma: a study of six hundred cases. *J Bone Joint Surg.* 1967;49:101-110

7. McKillop J, Etcubanas E, Goris M. The indications for and limitations of bone scintigraphy in osteogenic sarcoma. A review of 55 patients. *Cancer.* 1981;48:1133-1138

8. Wolf RE, Enneking WF. The staging and surgery of musculoskeletal neoplasms. *Orthop Clin North Am.* 1996;27: 473-481

9. Tjalma RA. Canine bone sarcoma: estimation of relative risk as a function of body size. *J Natl Cancer Inst.* 1966;36:1137-1150

10. Newton WA, Meadows AT, Shimada H, et al. Bone sarcomas as second malignant neoplasms following childhood cancer. *Cancer.* 1991;67:193-201

11. Abramson D, Ellsworth R, Kitchin F, Tung G. Second nonocular tumors in retinoblastoma survivors. Are they radiation induced? *Ophthalmology.* 1984;91:1351-1355

12. Friend S, Bernards R, Rogelj S, et al. A human DNA segment with properties of the gene that predisposes to retinoblastoma and osteosarcoma. *Nature.* 1986;323:643-646

13. Toguchida J, Yamaguchi T, Dayton SH, et al. Prevalence and spectrum of germline mutations of the p53 gene among patients with sarcoma. *N Engl J Med.* 1992;326:1301-1308

14. Ladanyi M, Gorlick R. The molecular pathology and pharmacology of osteosarcoma. *Ped Pathol Molec Med.* 2000;19:391-413

15. Jaffe N, Frei E, Traggis D, Bishop Y. Adjuvant methotrexate and citrovorum-factor treatment of osteogenic sarcoma. *N Engl J Med.* 1974;291:994-997

16. Goorin A, Delorey M, Gelber R, et al. The Dana-Farber Cancer Institute/The Children's Hospital adjuvant chemotherapy trials for osteosarcoma: three sequential studies. *Cancer Treat Rep.* 1986;3:155-159

17. Sutow WW, Sullivan MP, Fernbach DJ, et al. Adjuvant chemotherapy in primary treatment of osteogenic sarcoma. A Southwest Oncology Group Study. *Cancer.* 1975;36:1598-1602

18. Link MP, Goorin AM, Miser AW, et al. The effect of adjuvant chemotherapy on relapse-free survival in patients with osteosarcoma of the extremity. *N Engl J Med.* 1986;314: 1600-1606

19. Rosen G, Marcove RC, Caparros B, et al. Primary osteogenic sarcoma. The rationale for preoperative chemotherapy and delayed surgery. *Cancer.* 1979;43:2163-2177

20. Meyers PA, Schwartz CL, Krailo M, et al. Osteosarcoma: a randomized, prospective trial of the addition of ifosfamide and/or muramyl tripeptide to cisplatin, doxorubicin, and high-dose methotrexate. *J Clin Oncol.* 2005;23:2004-2011

21. Ewing J. Diffuse endothelioma of bone. *Proc NY Path Soc.* 1921;21:17

22. Whang PJ, Triche TJ, Knutsen T, Miser J, Douglass EC, Israel MA. Chromosome translocation in peripheral neuroepithelioma. *N Engl J Med.* 1984;311:584-585

23. McKeon C, Thiele CJ, Ross RA, et al. Indistinguishable patterns of proto-oncogene expression in two distinct but closely related tumors: Ewing's sarcoma and neuroepithelioma. *Cancer Res.* 1988;48:4307-4311

24. Paulussen M, Ahrens S, Burdach S, et al. Primary metastatic (stage IV) Ewing tumor: survival analysis of 171 patients from the EICESS studies. European Intergroup Cooperative Ewing Sarcoma Studies. *Ann Oncol.* 1998;9:275-281

25. Ferrari S, Bertoni F, Mercuri M, Sottili S, Versari M, Bacci G. Ewing's sarcoma of bone: relation between clinical characteristics and staging. *Oncol Rep.* 2001;8:553-556

26. Horowitz ME, Malawer MM, Shiao YW, Woo SY, Hicks MJ. Ewing's sarcoma family of tumors: Ewing's sarcoma of bone and soft tissue and the peripheral primitive neuroectodermal tumors. In: Pizzo PA, Poplack DG, eds. *Principles and Practice of Pediatric Oncology*. 3rd ed. Philadelphia, PA: Lippincott-Raven; 1997:921-957

27. Delattre O, Zucman J, Melot T, et al. The Ewing family of tumors—a subgroup of small-round-cell tumors defined by specific chimeric transcripts. *N Engl J Med.* 1994;331:294-299

28. May WA, Lessnick SL, Braun BS, et al. The Ewing's sarcoma EWS/FLI-1 fusion gene encodes a more potent transcriptional activator and is a more powerful transforming gene than FLI-1. *Mol Cell Biol.* 1993;13:7393-7398

29. Grier H, Krailo M, Tarbell M. Adding ifosfamide and etoposide to vincristine, cyclophosphamide, adriamycin, and actinomycin improves outcome in non-metastatic Ewing's and PNET: update of CCG/POG study. *Med Pediatr Oncol.* 1996;32:O193

30. Dunst J, Ahrens S, Paulussen M, et al. Second malignancies after treatment for Ewing's sarcoma: a report of the CESS-studies. *Int J Radiat Oncol Biol Phys.* 1998;42:379-384

# CHAPTER 162

# Disorders of the Spine

PAUL T. RUBERY, MD

Adolescence is an important period of spinal growth and development. The increasing activities of the young adult can place the spine at risk for injury. These factors combine to accentuate the importance of spinal diagnosis and treatment in the care of adolescents. Adolescent patients typically present with complaints of either pain or deformity in the spine. An organized approach to the analysis and initial treatment of these complaints enhances efficiency and patient satisfaction and occasionally averts serious consequences.

## BACK PAIN

It is a misconception among physicians that children and adolescents are unlikely to have back pain. In fact, recent studies have shown that low back pain (LBP) in particular is quite common in these age groups. The reported 1-year prevalence of LBP among older children and adolescents is 17% to 26%.[1] One in 20 children is estimated to be experiencing back pain at any one time. The prevalence of LBP increases with age and seems to be higher among girls than boys. Interestingly, an increased prevalence of LBP is not correlated with either a sedentary lifestyle or extensive computer use. Efforts to establish a causal relationship between book bag weight and back pain have to date been unsuccessful. There is, however, a strong correlation between the presence of LBP and symptoms of depression.

Establishing a diagnosis for the adolescent with back pain can be challenging. Turner et al[2] analyzed referrals to a pediatric orthopaedic service at a large British children's hospital. Nearly 50% of patients were diagnosed as having nonspecific pathology, 13% had spondylolysis, 8% had infection, 6% had tumors, and 6% had a disc herniation. The differential diagnosis of back pain in the adolescent includes 7 categories (Table 162-1).

### MUSCULOSKELETAL STRAIN

Soft tissue injuries or "strains" of the back (especially the lumbar region) are perhaps the most common injury to the spine. Generally, these are self-limited and it is rare for patients to present to a physician for these injuries. Patients who present with pain or spasm in the back frequently report a history of lifting or twisting. Pain is the predominate finding on examination, and imaging is generally not indicated. Patients can expect resolution over 3 to 7 days.[3] Patients should be encouraged to use nonsteroidal anti-inflammatory drugs (NSAIDs) and limit bed rest to no more than 24 to 48 hours.[4–6] The spinal care community strongly discourages the use of narcotics, and opinion differs with regard to centrally acting antispasmodic medications. Muscular strain is unlikely to be the diagnosis in a patient whose back pain persist beyond 14 days.

### TRAUMA

Adolescent trauma can result from collisions involving sports, skateboards, bicycles snowboards, all-terrain vehicles, and trampolines. Such innocuous sounding situations can result in serious spinal injuries, and the clinician should have an extremely low threshold for ordering imaging and seeking subspecialty consultation.

Patient history should attempt to assess the magnitude of the energy the patient's body has absorbed and identify the presence of neurologic symptoms. In the author's experience, the frightened adolescent will often speak of a few seconds of numbness or tingling after a major incident; however, true neural injury is rarely so short-lived. Physical examination should focus on identifying the site of tenderness. The posterior ligaments of the spine (supraspinous and interspinous ligaments) form a continuous midline structure punctuated by the spinous processes. The most severe spinal injuries result in a disruption of this osteoligamentous structure, which will be exquisitely tender and may feel discontinuous. A neurologic examination including dermatomal sensation and myotomal strength assessment is important.

Adolescents who have suffered spinal trauma and have pain should undergo a plain radiographic examination. In cases where the initial x-rays are normal and the pain is substantial, a computed tomography (CT) scan of the spine without contrast enhancement will often reveal a fracture not seen on x-ray. Magnetic resonance imaging (MRI) is the imaging modality of choice for patients with neurologic signs or symptoms.

**Table 162-1**

**Differential Diagnosis of Adolescent Back Pain**

| *Diagnosis* | *Diagnostic Keys* |
|---|---|
| Musculoskeletal strain | Pain often begins after lifting or twisting. Unlikely to radiate to leg. Rarely symptomatic >14 days. |
| Trauma | History of injury. Physical examination of back and spinal nerve function and radiographic imaging of suspicious regions required. Higher energy events yield more significant injuries. |
| Spondylolysis and spondylolisthesis | Often insidious onset of back pain with "tight" hamstrings. Pain increases with extension of lumbar spine. Radiographic imaging may be normal. Bone scan with SPECT can be diagnostic. |
| Intervertebral disc disorders | "Typically atypical" in adolescence. Classic radiculopathy vs "pulled hamstring." MRI is imaging of choice. |
| Infection | Presentation differs as patients age from childhood through adulthood. Back pain, occasionally fever. See Table 162-2. |
| Neoplasm | Rare. Usually presents with back pain, especially pain that causes nighttime awakening. Radiographic imaging, bone scan, and MRI. Early referral to specialists for biopsy and treatment. |
| Spondyloarthropathy | An evolving area in adolescent medicine. Morning stiffness, which "works itself out." Physical examination maneuvers, particularly spinal mobility. Radiographic findings lag behind clinical symptoms. See Table 162-3. |

SPECT, single photon emission computed tomography; MRI, magnetic resonance imaging

Although a detailed discussion of all aspects of spine trauma is beyond the scope of this chapter, a brief review of the most common injuries is germane. Most spinal fractures in the adolescent occur in the thoracic or lumbar spine. These include fractures of the transverse processes, compression fractures of the vertebra, and bursting fractures of the vertebra (Figure 162-1).

The most commonly fractured transverse processes are those of the lumbar spine. Generally, this is a result of direct blunt trauma to the back and the injury does not result in spinal instability or neural injury. Renal contusions frequently occur in association with these fractures. No formal treatment or immobilization is required and clinical resolution occurs over 4 to 6 weeks. The fracture does not always unite radiographically, but nonunion is not usually symptomatic.[7]

Compression fractures result from axial loading of the spine and are, by definition, fractures of the anterior half of the vertebral body. These fractures usually are mechanically stable and do not result in neurologic symptoms. A small number of compression fractures are associated with disruption of the posterior ligaments, therapy rendering the spine unstable. These more dangerous injuries can be identified by extreme tenderness of the spine and the marked loss of height or angular deformity seen on x-ray. These rarer unstable fractures are treated surgically. However, most compression fractures are stable and can be managed with a prefabricated "extension orthosis" (brace). The brace is worn when the patient is out of bed, and works by shifting load from the anterior spine to the posterior spine, resulting in diminished pain. Bracing continues for 6 to 12 weeks and is often followed by physical therapy to recondition the abdominal and paraspinal muscles.[8]

Burst fractures also result from axial loading and involve the anterior and posterior halves of the vertebral body. These fractures are mechanically unstable and can result in neurologic deficit from bone being retropulsed against the neural elements. Patients with deficits or substantial fracture deformity are often treated surgically. Despite the mechanical "instability," most patients with bust fractures can be managed with orthoses. These braces tend to be more restrictive than those used for compression fractures, and many are custom made for the patient. The brace is often worn full-time to enhance stability of the spinal column. Typically bracing is for 10 to 12 weeks, and is followed by physical therapy.[9]

## SPONDYLOLYSIS AND SPONDYLOLISTHESIS

Spondylolysis and spondylolisthesis are common lumbar spine disorders in the adolescent. Spondylolysis is a defect of the pars. Spondylolisthesis is a forward translation of the one vertebra on the adjacent caudal neighbor. There are 5 different subclasses of spondylolisthesis, based on the pathoanatomy of the posterior vertebral elements. For practical purposes, the most clinically relevant types for adolescent care are *isthmic* and

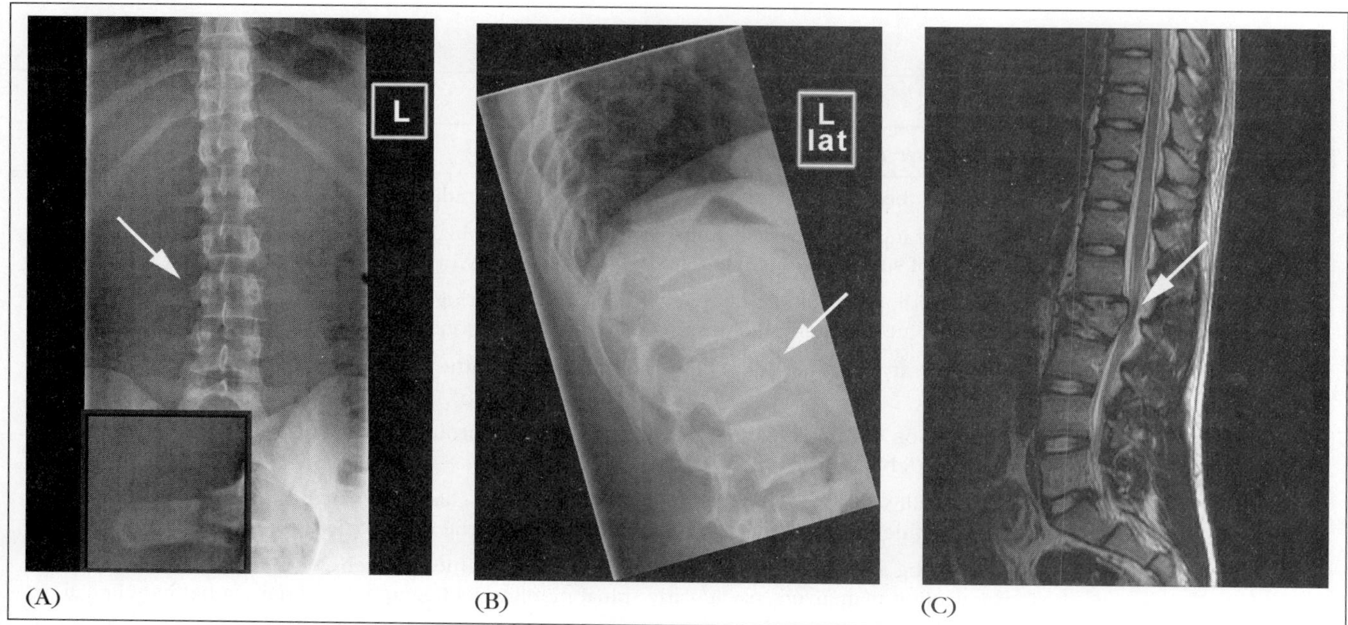


FIGURE 162-1 Anatomic differences between the 3 most common fractures of the vertebral body. (A) X-ray of a transverse process fracture. These processes are the site of origin of the psoas and do not contribute to spinal stability; (B) compression fracture in which the anterior half of the vertebra fails; (C) MRI of a bursting fracture in which the anterior and posterior halves of the vertebra fracture and there is retropulsion of fragments toward the neural elements.

*dysplastic spondylolisthesis*. Isthmic spondylolisthesis is characterized by a disruption in the pars and is present in approximately 5% of white males by age 9 years.[10] The pars is a thin bridge of cortical bone linking the superior and inferior articular facets. This bone is subject to substantial force concentration when humans stand upright. The cortical nature of this bone and its relatively poor vascularization predispose the pars to stress fractures and nonunion. The lesion can often be visualized on oblique radiographs (Figure 162-2). The appearance of

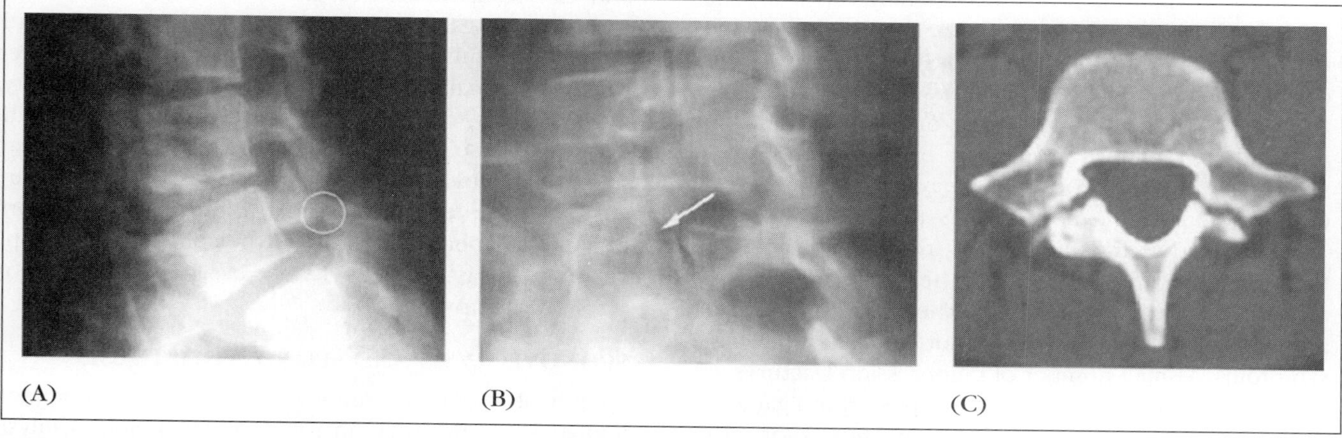

FIGURE 162-2 Disruption in the pars interarticularis of the fifth lumbar vertebra (A and B). Lateral views; (C) oblique view. The appearance on oblique views is that of a collar around the neck of a "Scotty dog" whose head is formed by the pedicle, superior facet, and transverse process, and whose body is formed by the lamina, inferior facet, and spinous process. CT scans can be useful in confirming the presence of the spondylolysis, which is not always easily seen on x-ray. (Reprinted with permission from Cavalier et al. Spondylolysis and spondylolisthesis: 1 diagnosis, natural history, and nonsurgical management. *J Am Acad Orthop Surg*. 2006;14:421. © 2006 American Academy of Orthopaedic Surgeons.)

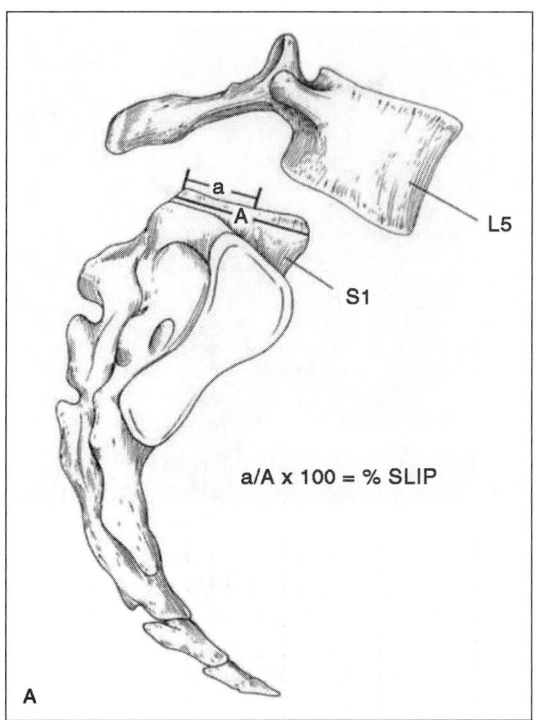


FIGURE 162-3 The method by which the percentage of slippage is calculated in spondylolisthesis. Increasing percentages are categorized as grades I through IV on the Meyerding grading scale. (Reprinted with permission from Elsevier from Herman MJ, Pizzutillo PD, Cavalier R. Spondylolysis and spondylolisthesis in the child and the adolescent athlete. *Orthop Clin North Am.* 2003;34:461–467 as appearing in the *Journal of the American Academy of Orthopaedic Surgeons* 2006;14(7):417-424.)

the posterior elements on an oblique radiograph is reminiscent of a "Scotty dog." The fracture appears as a collar on the dog's neck. When slippage or anterolisthesis is present, it is quantified using the Meyerding grading scale (Figure 162-3). The progression of the sliding vertebra's posterior cortex across the superior endplate below is measured and a percentage slip is calculated. This is then categorized into grade I (0% to 24%), II (25% to 49%), III (50% to 74%), or IV (75% to 100%). Complete anterior dislocation is called spondyloptosis, and is rare.[10]

Patients with symptomatic spondylolysis and spondylolisthesis complain of back pain. The classic patient with spondylolysis is an athlete involved in sports or activities that require substantial extension of the lumbar spine including gymnasts, football linemen, soccer "throw-in" specialists, divers, and cricket bowlers. Occasionally, patients will present with radicular complaints, and rarely with an isolated, painless neurologic deficit. The isthmic lysis is most commonly at L5, and nerve root symptoms are usually related to the L5 nerve root. In addition to the patient's symptoms, the amount of spinal growth remaining is an important consideration because patients with spondylolysis or spondylolisthesis may experience an increase in the grade of the slip with the adolescent growth spurt.[10]

The clinical examination can be deceptively benign in these patients. Common findings include increased LBP with passive extension of the lumbar spine, tight hamstrings, and occasionally mild weakness (often of the extensor hallucis longus). Radiographs are often diagnostic, but as many as 30% of patients with active spondylolysis may have normal lumbar x-rays.

Axial images by bone scan with single photon emission computed tomography (SPECT) are the preferred second level of testing if plain radiographs are unsatisfying.[11] Both CT, and increasingly MRI, can be used to identify disruptions in the pars interarticularis. An MRI is promising in its ability to identify physiologic stress in bone.

Treatment for most adolescents is aimed at decreasing their pain. For patients who are at the beginning of their adolescent growth spurt, monitoring and potentially treating, progressive vertebral slippage is a second critical goal. Key elements of initial treatment are activity modification, NSAID, and strengthening of the core stabilizing muscles. Physical therapy is a very important part of treating spondylolysis pain. Physicians should beware of writing overly simplistic referrals to physical therapy. Although traditional (adult) LBP is most effectively treated with therapy that focuses on lumbar extension exercises, these may exacerbate symptoms in spondylolysis. Rather, patients should pursue *flexion-based exercise*. Using NSAIDs are another cornerstone of conservative management, and patient acceptance is increased by explaining the role inflammation plays in the pain. The most difficult aspect of instituting treatment is getting active youngsters to decrease their sporting activities. When symptoms subside a gradual reintroduction of activity is prudent. If symptoms do not subside, institution of a flexion-molded brace to unload the pars interarticularis region is common. The author favors 3–6 months of concerted nonsurgical attempts to resolve symptomatic spondylolysis. Patients who remain symptomatic, and patients with either documented progressive spondylolisthesis or greater than grade II slips with significant growth remaining, are candidates for surgical treatment.[10]

## INTERVERTEBRAL DISC DISORDERS

It is generally assumed that disc pathology is rare among teens; however, prevalence studies are lacking (Figure 162-4). An intervertebral disc disorder generally implies herniation of the nucleus pulposus through the annulus fibrosus. In adolescence, however, it is also

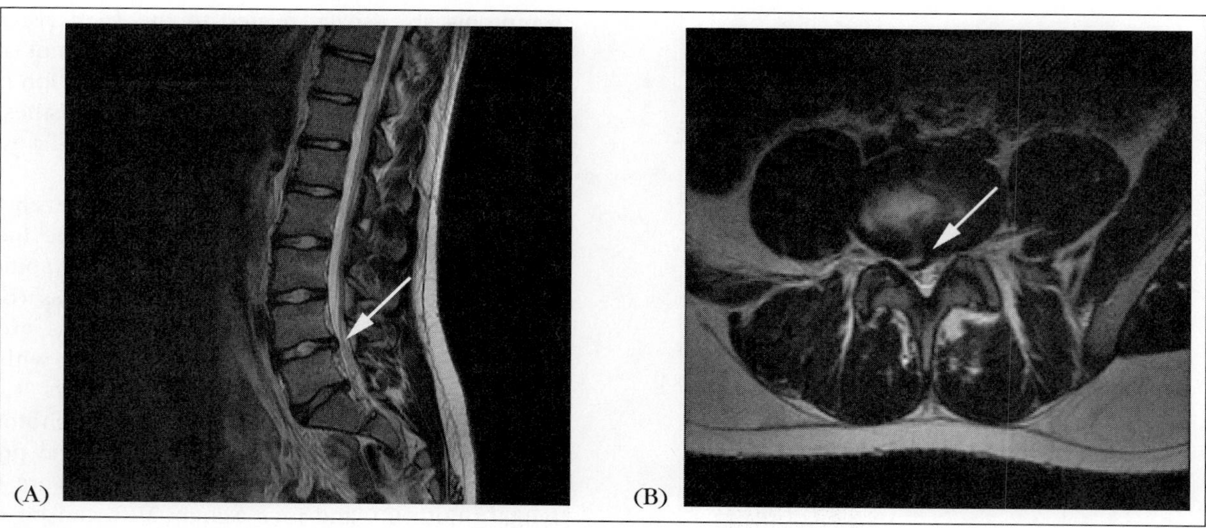


FIGURE 162-4 T2-weighted MRI images demonstrate a right-sided L4-L5 disc herniation. (A) Sagittal view; (B) axial view. This 15-year-old boy had radiculopathy including numbness on the dorsum of his foot, and a feeling like a "chronic hamstring pull."

possible to sustain a fracture through the ring apophysis of the vertebral body resulting in fragments of growth plate cartilage and bone lodging in the spinal canal. Spine care specialists associate disc herniations with lumbar nerve root irritation, radiculopathy, or sciatica more so than back pain. In adolescents, the clinical presentation of a lumbar disc herniation is "typically atypical" and may not involve the classic "sciatica" seen in the adult. Adolescent patients may present with odd complaints, such as a chronically "pulled hamstring" or a painless motor deficit. Physical findings may be nonspecific but will often include tight hamstrings and a straight leg raising sign. An MRI scan is the diagnostic test of choice, although plain x-rays may be used to eliminate the more common diagnosis of spondylolysis.[12]

Most patients with disc herniation (80% to 90%) get better on their own over 6 to 8 weeks. NSAIDs and brief courses of narcotics can ease the symptoms. In adult populations, epidural steroid injections and nerve root blocks have been successful in preventing surgery.[13] There is not good data on their use in adolescence. Surgery is reserved for those who fail conservative care and for those who present with clinical "red flags." The cardinal signs of lumbar disease include less than antigravity strength in a major muscle group (eg, "complete foot drop"), bowel and bladder compromise, and intractable pain.

## DISCITIS AND VERTEBRAL OSTEOMYELITIS

Spinal infection remains an important cause of pathology throughout the world. In developing countries these infections, particularly tuberculosis, are the most common cause of paralysis. In the developed world, pyogenic infections are more likely, although atypical mycobacterial and fungal infections are prevalent among immunocompromised patients.[14]

The unique vascular anatomy of the developing intervertebral disc in childhood and adolescence influences the clinical presentation of spinal infections in different age groups. During infancy and childhood, blood vessels traverse the disc. As the child approaches adulthood, these vascular channels are lost and the disc becomes relatively avascular. In adolescents and adults the blood supply of the disc arises from the vertebra, and "low flow" capillary loops supply the margins of the disc. Bacteria circulating in the bloodstream can be deposited at the junction of the vertebral endplate and the disc, and infection can take hold (Figure 162-5). The infection often grows rapidly within the low oxygen tension environment of the disc space and spreads to the adjacent bone, resulting in osteomyelitis. Further growth and suppuration leads to the development of abscess cavities. The abscess may drain into the spinal canal resulting in an epidural abscess and potential spinal cord compression.[15,16]

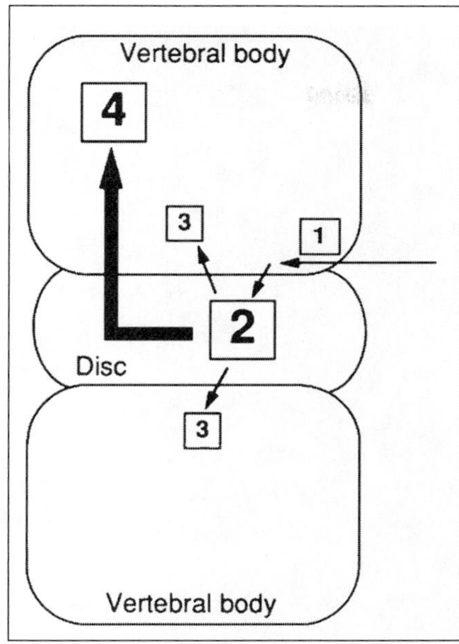


**FIGURE 162-5** Proposed sequence of intervertebral disc infection and progression to osteomyelitis: (1) Microabscess in metaphysis (adjacent to endplate). (2) Disc colonized and infected. (3) Reactive process (or low-grade infection of opposite endplate). (4) Diagnosis and treatment delayed—development of vertebral osteomyelitis. (Reprinted with permission from Wenger et al. Pyogenic infectious spondylitis. In Weinstein, ed. *The Pediatric Spine.* 2nd ed. Baltimore, MD: Lippincott Williams & Wilkins; 2001:622.)

**Table 162-2**

**Discitis and Vertebral Osteomyelitis Evaluation**

| | |
|---|---|
| Symptoms | Back pain, fever, occasional nerve deficits |
| Imaging | X-rays and MRI |
| Laboratory studies | White blood cell count, sedimentation rate, C-reactive protein, peripheral blood culture |
| Diagnostic testing | CT-guided needle aspiration |
| Treatment | Parenteral antibiotics, bracing, occasionally surgical debridement |

At one time, childhood discitis was considered a separate entity from the discitis and osteomyelitis of the adult. The child's discitis was marked by irritability and a refusal to walk. Tenderness and disc space narrowing on x-ray were hallmarks. Biopsy was avoided, the spine was often immobilized, and antibiotic treatment for presumptive gram-positive bacteria was debated by various authors. Clinical resolution and good results were the rule.[14] Current opinion is that the alterations in the disc's blood supply during development explain not only the differences in presentation but also guide the differing treatment for adolescent infection. As the disc takes on more adult vascular anatomy, the infections become more like vertebral and disc space infections in the adult.[15,16] Evaluation and treatment of infection is summarized in Table 162-2.

Adolescents with spinal infection complain of back pain. Fever is a common manifestation, but the absence of fever by no means precludes infection. Neurologic deficits can be present, although most adolescent patient's infections are neurologically intact. Laboratory testing is variable and nonspecific. The white blood cell (WBC) count may be normal or minimally elevated. The erythrocyte sedimentation rate (ESR) is also variable. In the early phases it may be normal.[16] The author particularly values the C-reactive protein (CRP), which is often elevated early in the course and which may begin to revert to normal within approximately 10 days of initiating treatment.[14] Peripheral blood cultures are often not diagnostic.

Clinical suspicion is the key to early diagnosis. Imaging can be very helpful. X-rays will often show narrowing of the disc space, and may show loss of the vertebral endplate contours. Bone scintigraphy (bone scan) is a sensitive test for bone pathology in the spine, but is not specific. Tagged WBC studies are unreliable in the presence of abscesses with necrosis. By far the most sensitive and specific, and thus most clinically useful, test is the MRI (Figure 162-6). Magnetic resonance scans will often show changes suggestive of disc space infection (especially a fluid signal within the disc space) well before there are x-ray abnormalities.[14-16]

The increasingly "adult character" of the adolescent spine infection argues for tissue biopsy to guide antibiotic choice. The use of presumptive antibiotics, broad spectrum antibiotics, and antibiotics based on a peripheral blood culture is discouraged in treating adult spinal infections. True tissue diagnosis, often obtained via CT-guided needle biopsy, is the standard for selecting treatments in adults and is increasingly so for adolescent patients, especially older adolescents. Infectious disease specialists are invaluable in helping to choose antibiotics and dosing. Antibiotics are usually administered parenterally and can be administered via home infusion programs. A custom-molded brace makes the

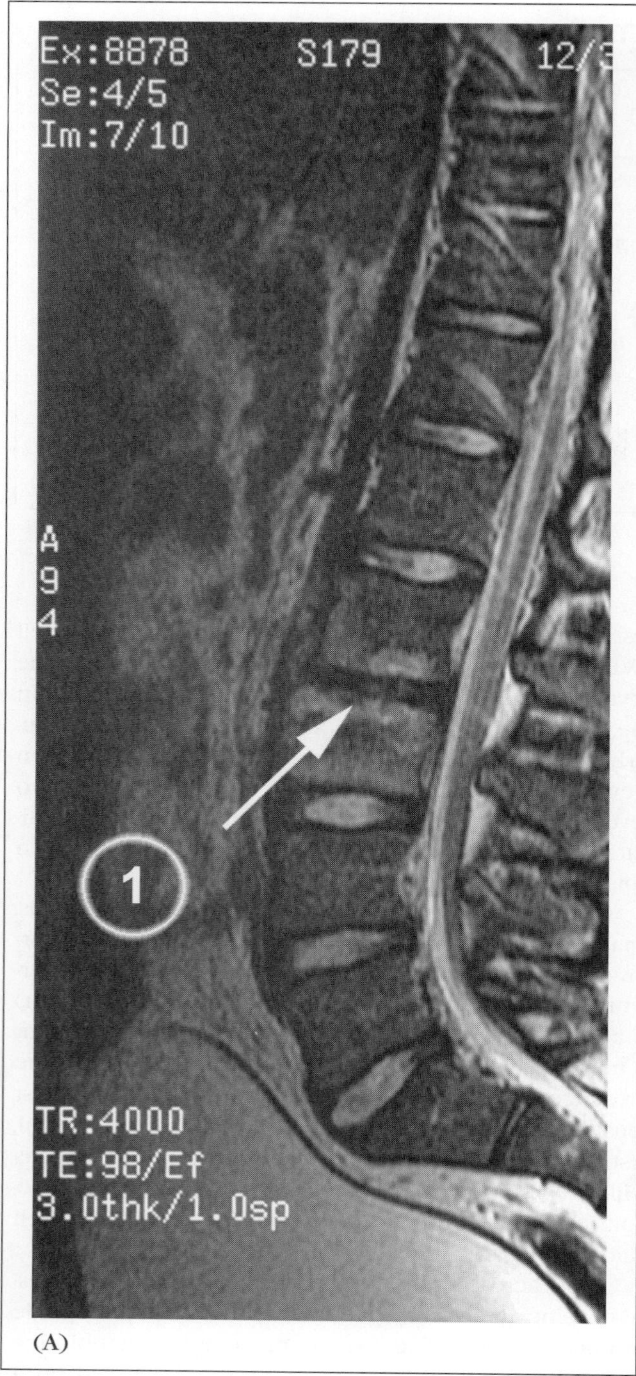


(A)

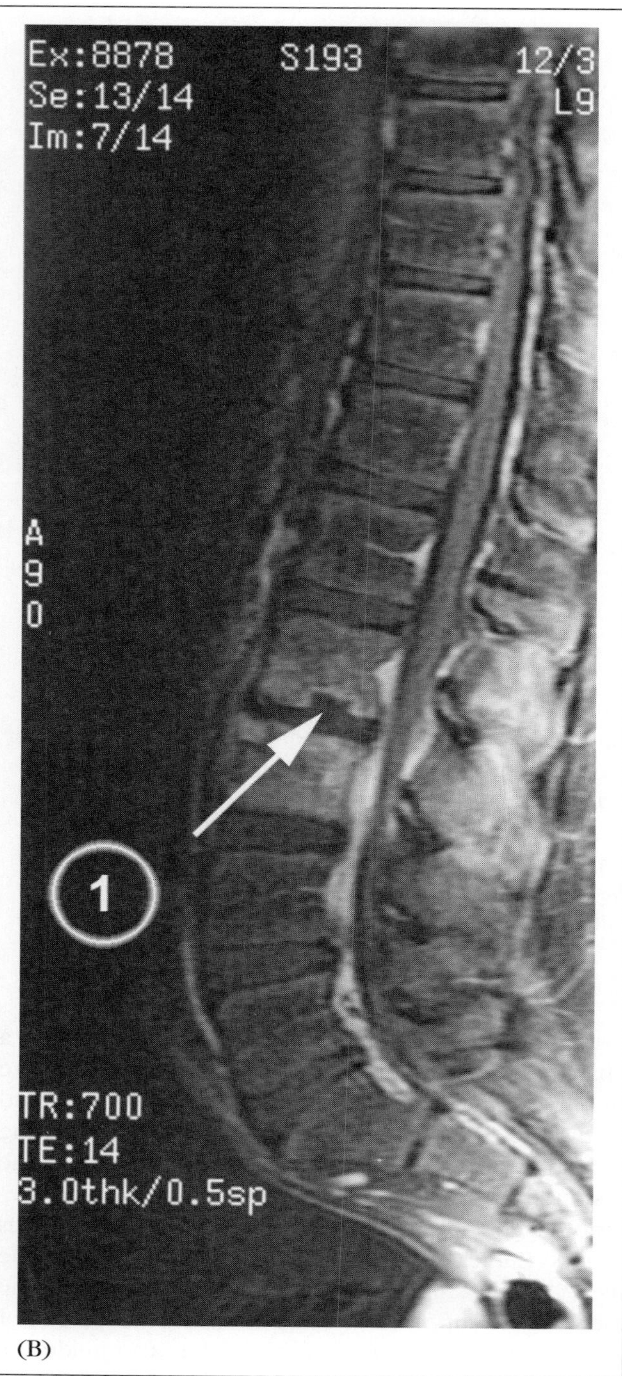


(B)

**FIGURE 162-6** (*Continued on the following page*)

patient more comfortable and may speed resolution. The clearing of infection is best tracked by the subjective reports of improvement from the patient and return of the ESR and CRP to normal values. Spontaneous fusion of the disc space is a common radiographic finding. Surgery to debride the infection and restore spinal stability is indicated in patients who present with a significant motor deficit, patients with systemic sepsis and abscess, patients in whom a tissue diagnosis cannot be made, patients with disease progression despite antibiotics, and those who develop a painful deformity after eradication of the infection.[17]

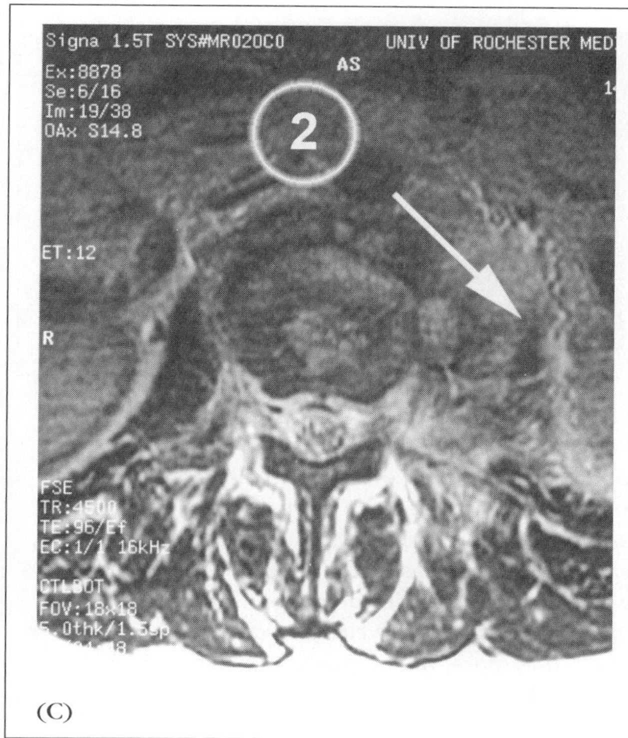


**FIGURE 162-6** MRI images demonstrate typical findings in vertebral osteomyelitis and discitis. (A and B) Note the signal change within the disc space with bone marrow signal change in the endplates adjacent to the infected disc (Arrow 1); (C) axial images will often show psoas muscle abscesses such as that seen in the left psoas of this 13-year-old boy with staphylococcal osteomyelitis of T12-L1 (Arrow 2).

## NEOPLASMS

There is understandable fear on the part of parents that the adolescent with back pain may have a tumor. The statistical likelihood of this is quite low; in the rare case of neoplasm, benign disease far outnumbers malignancy. As the primary care provider, the adolescent medicine specialist is called upon to decide when and how far to proceed with diagnostic testing. Back pain is the most common presenting symptom of spinal neoplasm. Pain that awakens the patient from sleep is classically considered to be more ominous than either activity-related back pain or pain at the end of an active day. It is rare for the child or adolescent to present with neurologic complaints.[18]

Initial imaging should be an x-ray. Second line imaging in patients with recalcitrant pain is bone scanning. The MRI provides the most detailed imaging, but expense makes this an inefficient screening test. The author obtains a complete blood count (CBC), an ESR, and a CRP. The combination of x-ray, bone scan, ESR, CBC, and CRP is said to identify more than 95% of occult neoplasms.[19]

Most spinal neoplasms in adolescents occur in the posterior elements (pedicles, facets, lamina, spinous process) and are benign. Common examples are osteoid osteoma and osteoblastoma. Lesions occurring in the vertebral body have greater statistical likelihood of being malignant. Although rare, osteosarcoma and Ewing sarcoma are the most common primary malignancies of the adolescent spine. Biopsy is a critical step in planning treatment. Musculoskeletal oncologists strongly believe that biopsy should be planned or performed by the surgeon ultimately responsible for treating the tumor. Thus, there is an emphasis on early referral to a subspecialist.[18]

## SPONDYLOARTHROPATHY

Juvenile spondyloarthropathy is a rare, important, and likely underdiagnosed cause of back pain in the adolescent age group. The annual incidence in Canada was recently estimated at 1.44 per 100,000 children.[20] Physicians have learned more about these disorders in the past 30 years, and the diagnostic criteria have become clearer. This greater understanding has increased the frequency with which these disorders are diagnosed and has created the impression that the prevalence of spondyloarthropathy is increasing.

Juvenile spondyloarthropathy is a group of disorders occurring in children younger than age 16 and associated with HLA-B27. Spondyloarthropathy is characterized by arthritis and enthesitis (inflammation of the insertions of tendons and ligaments).[21] Controversy exists regarding subclassification schemes that would aid both in further delineating diagnosis and in guiding therapy. There is agreement that the spondyloarthropathies can be divided into "differentiated" and "undifferentiated" types (Table 162-3). Importantly, many

**Table 162-3**

**Spondyloarthropathies**

| | |
|---|---|
| **Differentiated** | Ankylosing spondylitis |
| | Reactive arthritis (previously Reiter syndrome) |
| | Arthropathy associated with irritable bowel syndrome |
| | Arthropathy associated with psoriasis |
| **Undifferentiated** | Seronegative enthesopathy and arthropathy syndrome (SEA) |

pediatric rheumatologists believe that children present with undifferentiated spondyloarthropathy and progress gradually to differentiated forms over the years.[22]

The etiology of spondyloarthropathy remains poorly understood. There is clearly a strong association between juvenile spondyloarthropathy, especially ankylosing spondylitis, and HLA-B27. Sixty percent to 90% of patients with juvenile spondyloarthropathy will be HLA-B27 positive, often HLA-B27*05.[22] However, the presence of HLA-B27 is not necessary for diagnosis, and being HLA-B27 positive does not necessarily result in pathology. Ineffective clearance of bacterial DNA after infection has been suggested to influence the clinical expression of juvenile arthropathy. Infections that have been implicated include *Chlamydia, Salmonella, Campylobacter*, and *Mycobacterium tuberculosis*, although the exact pathophysiologic role of the bacterial DNA is not understood.[21] Recent research has focused on the role of tumor necrosis factor (TNF-α) in spondyloarthropathies. Although the exact role TNF plays is unclear, it appears that higher synovial fluid concentrations of this cytokine result in greater degrees of bone and cartilage destruction.[23]

The typical patient diagnosed with spondyloarthropathy is in his or her late teens or early 20s, and the major clinical complaint is chronic back pain. Many patients report 5 to 10 years of pain prior to diagnosis. This delay in treatment may have prognostic importance, as patients diagnosed with ankylosing spondylitis prior to age 16 are known to have poorer outcomes.[24] The pain is often a generalized soreness and is classically worst upon awakening in the morning, with a gradual "loosening up" during the day. The author finds careful history-taking to be particularly useful in identifying spondyloarthropathy in the adolescent. Helpful physical examination maneuvers include measuring chest expansion and Schober test. Chest expansion is measured at the nipple line with a tape measure between maximum expiration and inspiration. In the adolescent this value should be close to 5 cm, with values less than 2.5 cm in the adolescent bearing further investigation. The Schober test assesses lumbar spinal mobility. It is performed by placing 2 marks on the patient's skin over the spinous processes of the lumbar spine. They should be 15 cm apart. When the patient flexes forward, the distance between the marks should increase by 5 cm (Figure 162-7).

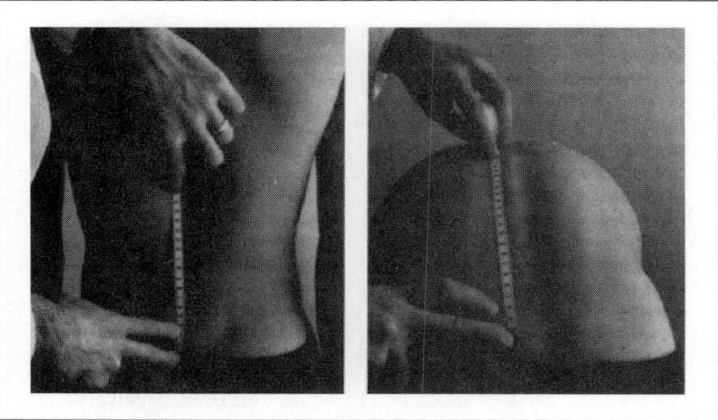

FIGURE 162-7 The Schober test, a measurement of lumbar spinal mobility, is useful in diagnosing spondyloarthropathy. Two lines are placed on the standing child's back; one 5 cm below and one 10 cm above the lumbosacral junction. With forward bending, there should be at least 5 cm of excursion between the lines. (Reprinted with permission from Moore M. Rheumatic diseases. In Weinstein, ed. *The Pediatric Spine*. 2nd ed. Baltimore, MD: Lippincott Williams & Wilkins; 2001:664.)

One of the factors that contributes to delays in diagnosis is that all the current diagnostic criteria require radiographic changes for diagnosis. Although changes may not appear for several years. The earliest x-ray finding is widening and erosion of the sacroiliac joint. Recent investigators have suggested that MRI of the sacroiliac joints may be a more sensitive test and may allow earlier diagnosis. To date, these recommendations have not been adopted.[25]

Treatment of spondyloarthropathy includes physical and pharmacologic treatment. Patients who are diagnosed with spondyloarthropathy should go through a course of physical therapy. This should include participation in a home exercise routine focusing on maintaining range of motion of the joints and proper spinal posture. Patients should be discouraged from using multiple pillows at night. Later in life, many patients with spondyloarthropathy go on to develop ankylosis of the spine, and can develop debilitating kyphotic deformities necessitating risky surgery. If the young patient can understand the natural history of the disease and is willing to take steps to ensure that the final spinal position is functional, future surgery can be avoided.

Until recently, pharmacologic management has been about symptom relief. Nonsteroidal anti-inflammatory drugs can decrease symptoms, but do not arrest disease progression. Gastropathy due to NSAIDs is a concern in patients taking these drugs for years. Standard disease-modifying antirheumatoid drugs (DMARDs) have some efficacy for the joint pain of spondyloarthropathy, but are less effective, or ineffective, for axial skeleton (spine) disease.[25] The recent introduction of anti-TNF drugs (infliximab and etanercept) has been an important advance. Both medications have been shown in randomized, prospective, placebo-controlled, double-blind trials to decrease disease activity in ankylosing spondylitis. Further developments in these therapies (which are discussed further in Chapter 121, Juvenile Idiopathic Arthritis) are likely in the near future.[23,24]

## SPINAL DEFORMITIES (SCOLIOSIS AND KYPHOSIS)

### ADOLESCENT IDIOPATHIC SCOLIOSIS

Rapid spinal growth can lead to progressive spinal deformity. The common spinal deformities encountered in the adolescent patient are scoliosis and kyphosis. Observant families and school screening programs refer a number of adolescent patients each year for evaluation of spinal deformity. At first exposure, the analysis and treatment of spinal deformity can seem hopelessly confusing. In fact, there are several themes that serve to organize this material into a relatively manageable form.

Scoliosis is a 3 plane deformation of the spine. Although lateral deviation of the spine from the midline in the coronal plane is the most easily recognized component, rotation of the spine in the axial plane and variations in the sagittal alignment also contribute to overall deformity. Angular deformation of the spine is measured on standing radiographs using the "Cobb angle." It is the angle created by the 2 intersecting lines drawn parallel to the endplates of the vertebra at the upper and lower limit of the curve. The Scoliosis Research Society has defined scoliosis as curvatures with a magnitude greater than 10 degrees. Kyphotic deformities are pathologic accentuations of the normal sagittal or lateral view alignment of the spine[26] (Figure 162-8).

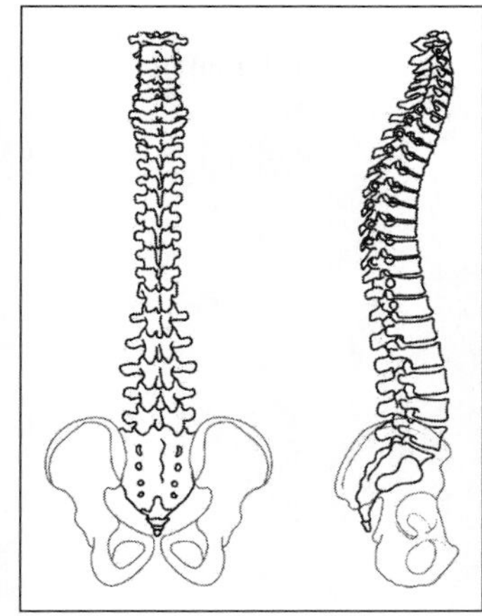

FIGURE 162-8 Normal coronal and sagittal alignment of the spine. Alterations in coronal alignment are scoliosis, abnormalities in the normal sagittal curvatures, or kyphosis. These may present in adolescence. (Reprinted with permission from Parent S, Newton PO, Wenger DR: Etiology, Anatomy, and Natural History, in Newton PO (ed): *Adolescent Idiopathic Scoliosis*. Rosemont, IL: American Academy of Orthopaedic Surgeons; 2004.)

Scoliosis can be subdivided by cause. Congenital curves arise due to abnormalities of vertebral shape. Neuromuscular curves arise from abnormalities of the neuroaxis (eg, cerebral palsy) or of the muscle/motor endplate (eg, Duchenne muscular dystrophy). By far, the most common type of scoliosis in adolescents is idiopathic scoliosis (Figure 162-9). Two percent to 3% of the population has scoliosis, and approximately 0.1% will require treatment.[27]

Adolescent idiopathic scoliosis (AIS) typically becomes clinically important during the adolescent growth spurt and is usually not a concern once skeletal maturity is reached. AIS affects mostly young women, with the male-to-female ratio among those requiring treatment being 1:10.[27] School screening programs, family concerns, and well child visits result in the greatest number of referrals, because most AIS patients are asymptomatic. Common physical clues to the diagnosis of scoliosis include shoulder asymmetry and rib rotational prominence on the Adam forward bending test (Figure 162-10). Other critical components of patient assessment include a brief neurologic examination, examination of the back for dimples or hair patches, which are possible indicators of underlying spinal cord abnormalities, and measurement of leg lengths (Figure 162-11). Leg length inequality is a common cause of mild nonstructural curves (curves lacking the rotation characteristic of true AIS).[28]

Many clinicians are familiar with the scoliometer. This device is a simple inclinometer used during the forward bending test to quantify the degree of rib rotational prominence (Figure 162-12). The scoliometer is calibrated in degrees (of incline). Large school screening studies suggest that a scoliometer reading of 7 degrees is the optimal value for referral for spine x-rays.[28] Interestingly, there is poor correlation between the scoliometer reading and the Cobb angle measured on x-ray. Measurement of the Cobb angle value is very important in determining treatment recommendations. Significant interobserver variability occurs on measurement of the Cobb angle and selection of end vertebrae.[27,28] Unfortunately, the author finds that his measurements often differ significantly from those provided to the primary care physician by radiologists, and consequently advises the reader to be very careful making treatment decisions based on radiology reports of the value of the Cobb angle.

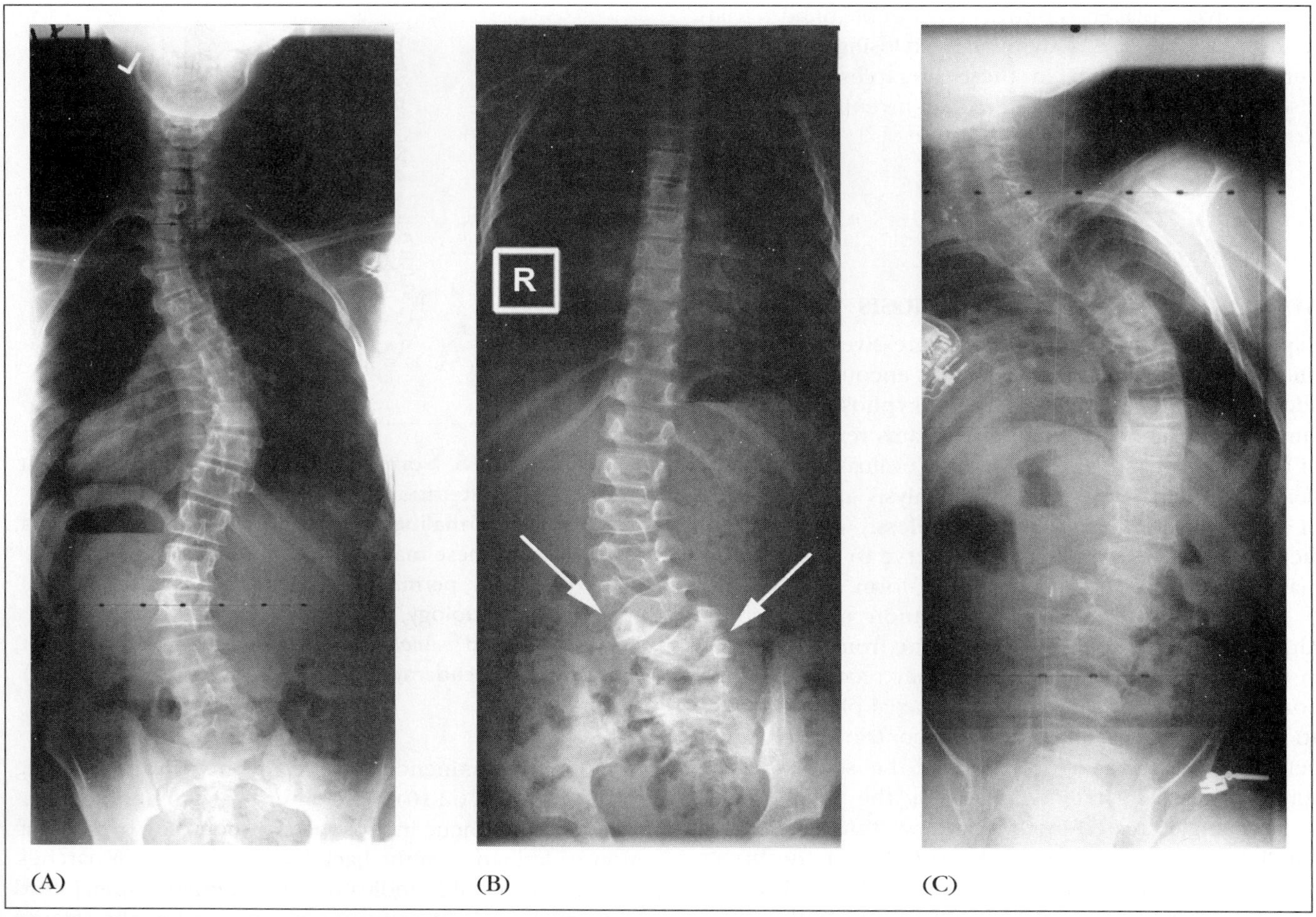

(A) (B) (C)

**FIGURE 162-9** Idiopathic, congenital, and neuromuscular scolioses. X-rays showing the essential differences in the types of curvature seen in various patient groups. (A) Idiopathic scoliosis typically seen during the adolescent growth spurt; (B) a congenital scoliosis arising due to a variation or abnormality in the formation of the vertebra embryologically. Arrows indicate hemivertebrae in the lumbar region; (C) a neuromuscular curvature seen in children with abnormalities of the central nervous system such as cerebral palsy or in the motor endplate such as Duchenne muscular dystrophy.

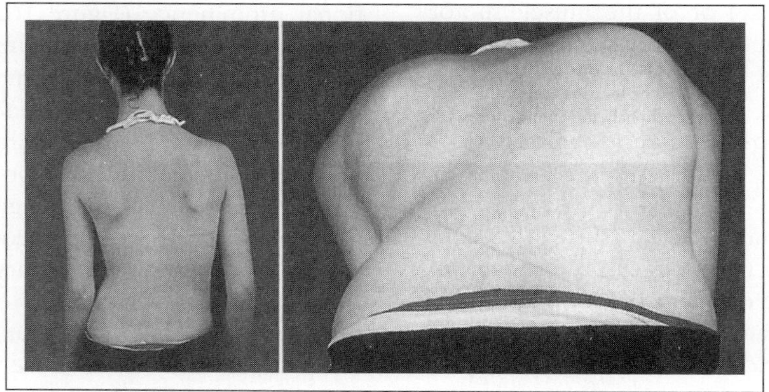

**FIGURE 162-10** The Adam forward bending test is used for scoliosis screening. Asymmetry of the scapulae, uneven shoulders or waistline, and rotational prominence of the rib cage on forward bending are clues to potential underlying scoliosis. (Reprinted from Dormans JP. *Core Knowledge in Orthopaedics: Pediatric Orthopaedics.* St Louis, MO: Mosby; 2005:267, with permission from Elsevier.)

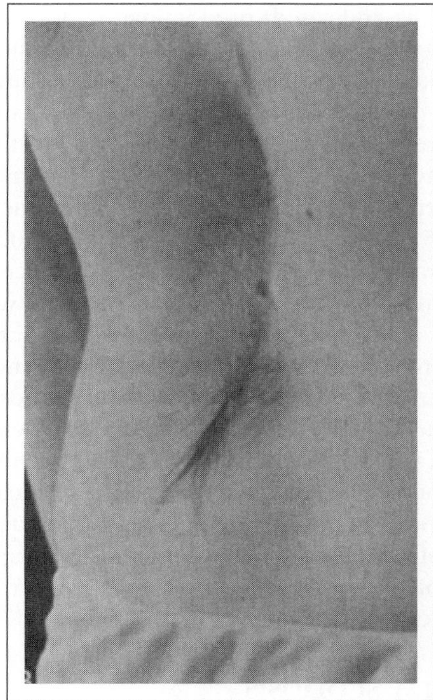

FIGURE 162-11 Visual inspection of the adolescent spine may reveal clues to underlying spinal dysraphism such as this midline hair patch. Other clues include dimples, fistulae, and birthmarks or nevi. (Reprinted from Lonstein JE, Bradford DS, Winter RB, Ogilvie JW (eds). *Moe's Textbook of Scoliosis and Other Spinal Deformities*. 3rd ed. Philadelphia, PA: WB Saunders; 1995:52, with permission from Elsevier.)

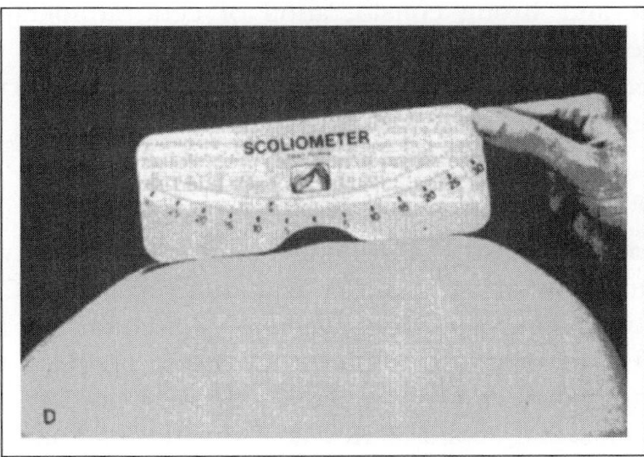


FIGURE 162-12 The scoliometer is an office tool for quantifying the slope or incline of the rib rotational prominence seen during the Adam test. Seven degrees of incline is considered to be an indication for referral for scoliosis x-rays. The scoliometer measurement does not correlate with the scoliosis or Cobb angle measured on x-rays. (Reprinted from Lonstein JE, Bradford DS, Winter RB, Ogilvie JW (eds). *Moe's Textbook of Scoliosis and Other Spinal Deformities*. 3rd ed. Philadelphia, PA: WB Saunders; 1995:49, with permission from Elsevier.)

Treatment of AIS is dependent on curve direction, the magnitude of the curve, and the degree of skeletal maturity. Curves can occur in the cervical, thoracic, or lumbar spine. There can be multiple curves, although typically one curve is the predominant or major curve and the others are compensatory or minor curves. The prototypical AIS patient is an adolescent girl with a thoracic curve. Most curves are convex to the right. Thoracic curves convex to the left receive special consideration. Although most patients with left thoracic curves are normal, there are a higher percentage of these patients who have underlying spinal cord anomalies. Patients with left thoracic curves should undergo MRI of the entire spine to assess for underlying abnormality of the neuroaxis.[26]

Pediatricians employ multiple measures to assess increasing physical maturity in their patients. In treating AIS, gauging the patient's proximity to the adolescent growth spurt, and more importantly to peak growth velocity, plays an important role. Much of the published data in the scoliosis literature deal with the progressive ossification of the iliac apophysis as a marker of increasing skeletal maturity. As seen on the anterior–posterior (AP) x-ray, the iliac apophysis begins its ossification laterally and progresses medially. Arbitrarily, spinal orthopedists refer to the degree of ossification as 1 of 5 "Risser" stages. Stage 0 shows no ossification, stage 1 is ossification of up to 25% of the apophysis, 2 is up to 50%, 3 up to 75%, and 4 is all the way across. Risser stages 0, 1, and 2 correspond with the period of most rapid spinal growth, and constitute the time of greatest risk for progression of curves[26] (Figure 162-13). When reviewing radiographs of patients with AIS, 2 analyses are germane:

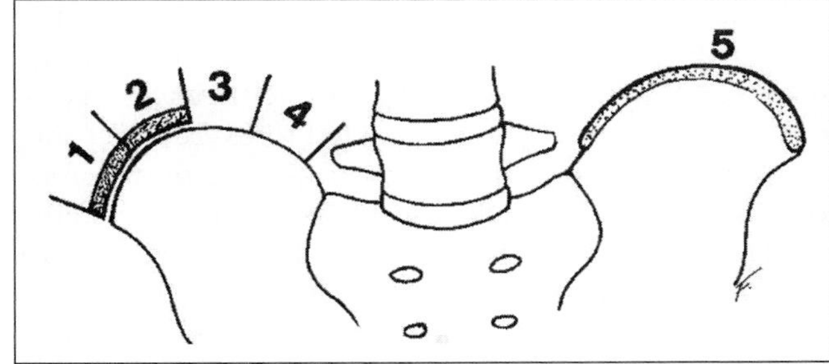


FIGURE 162-13 Progressive medial ossification of the iliac wing apophysis is referred to as the Risser sign. Measured on x-ray, it has been used by scoliosis specialists as a rough indicator of spinal maturity, and thus as a guide to the risk of curve progression. (Reprinted from Lonstein JE, Bradford DS, Winter RB, Ogilvie JW (eds). *Moe's Textbook of Scoliosis and Other Spinal Deformities*. 3rd ed. Philadelphia, PA: WB Saunders; 1995:76, with permission from Elsevier.)

**Table 162-4**

**Risser Stages and Prognosis of Scoliosis**

| *Risser Stage* | *Curve Magnitude <19°* | *Curve Magnitude 20–29°* |
|---|---|---|
| 0–1 | 22% incidence of progression | 68% incidence of progression |
| 2–4 | 1.6% incidence of progression | 23% incidence of progression |

1. What is the appropriate treatment at this point?
2. What is the risk of future progression in this patient?

The latter can be nicely summarized from the work of Lonstein and Carlson as reflected in Table 162-4.

Treatment should be individualized for each child. As a general rule, in children with significant growth remaining curves from 10 degrees up to 25 or 30 degrees are watched with intermittent x-ray, typically every 3 to 6 months. Curves of 25 degrees (in the very skeletally immature) or 30 degrees are braced. Curves of 40 to 45 degrees with growth remaining, or 55 degrees at maturity, typically are treated surgically with spinal instrumentation and fusion.[26-28]

Braces are custom-made for each child. *The purpose of a scoliosis brace is to prevent curve progression and avoid surgery. Scoliosis braces do not correct the curve or straighten the spine.* They are of 2 basic types. Thoracolumbar sacral orthoses (TLSO braces) are made with pads placed to make the brace functional enough to wear 23 hours a day. Patients are given extra time out of the brace for athletics. Nighttime bending braces are also TLSO braces but are molded to overcorrect the spine. They are worn at night, because the overcorrection makes ambulation in the brace exceedingly difficult. These braces are popular with patients. There has been considerable debate as to the efficacy of bracing as a treatment modality. There have been numerous papers and complex statistical analyses, showing that bracing does appear to influence the natural history of scoliosis for a percentage of patients but does not control all curves. Some adolescents who are carefully evaluated, treated early, and comply consistently with bracing will still progress to scoliosis surgery. The reasons are unclear. There are data to suggest that bracing may not be as effective for boys as it is for girls. At this point, the statistical evidence for 23-hour bracing is slightly more compelling than that for nighttime bracing.[27-29]

Surgery is indicated predominantly for failure of nonsurgical care, and for curves of such magnitude that they are likely to increase after skeletal maturity. Such curvatures can become painful in later life as the scoliosis progresses and as arthritis develops in the joints of the spine. As a rule, scoliosis does not significantly impair heart or lung functions unless the thoracic curve exceeds 95 degrees. Curves of less than 50 degrees in the thoracic spine and less than 30 degrees in the lumbar spine at maturity are not associated with progression in adulthood, nor with significant increases in back pain-related disability.[27] Surgical treatments are intended to correct the curve as much as possible by inserting metal rods attached with hooks or screws and then fusing the bones of the spine in the corrected position. Patients will generally have some residual curve. Differing approaches and implants have been developed for different scenarios. Most patients do not experience any functionally appreciable loss of motion from their fusion surgery[30,31] (Figure 162-14).

### CONGENITAL SCOLIOSIS

Congenital scoliosis arises during weeks 6 to 8 of embryogenesis. Thus, there are often important comorbidities. Twenty-five percent of these children will have spinal cord anomalies, 20% will have genito-urinary system anomalies, and 20% will have cardiac abnormalities, especially atrial septal defects. For these reasons, scoliosis specialists suggest that all children with congenital scoliosis have a spinal cord MRI, a renal ultrasound, and strong consideration of echocardiography. Congenital scoliosis requires careful monitoring by the subspecialist. Braces are ineffective, and early surgery is not unusual.[32]

### NEUROMUSCULAR SCOLIOSIS

Neuromuscular scoliosis encompasses a large variety of curvatures with vastly differing natural histories. Children with neuroaxis abnormalities (eg, cerebral palsy, spinal cord injury) and muscle or motor endplate disease (eg, Duchenne muscular dystrophy) can develop neuromuscular scoliosis. Key goals include treating the whole child, working to re-establish and preserve near normal sitting ability (ie, without complex wheelchair modifications), protecting skin and pulmonary function, and preventing progressive, painful deformity. Braces do not control these curves, although they are occasionally used to help position the patient upright until such time as surgery is advisable. Surgery is generally the rule, and the fusions often involve surgery on both the anterior and posterior spine, with spinal instrumentation extending all the way from the upper thoracic region to the pelvic bones.[33]

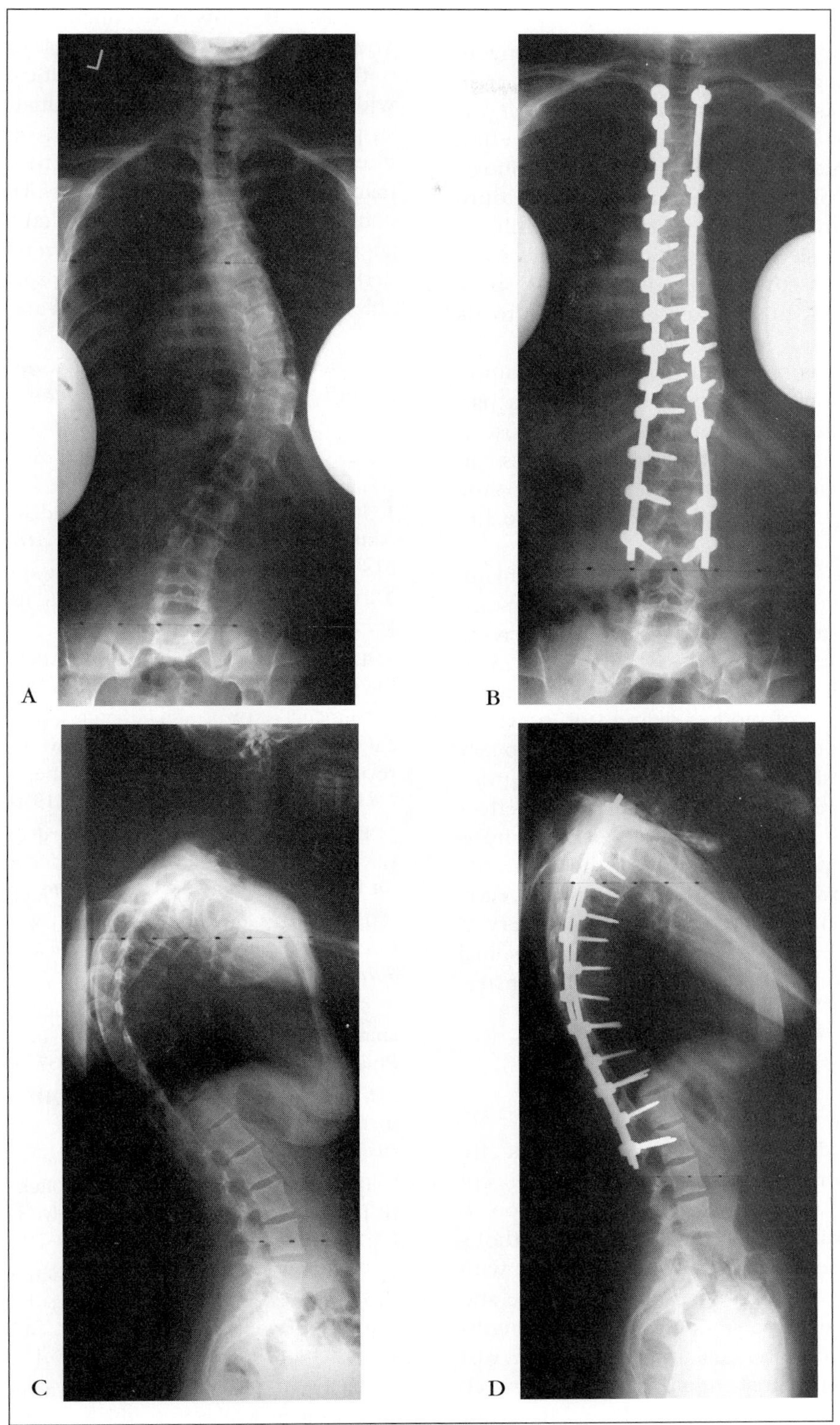


FIGURE 162-14 Surgical treatment of adolescent idiopathic scoliosis and Scheuermann kyphosis. These radiographs represent typical before and after x-rays in modern adolescent spinal deformity surgery. (A) and (B) are a 17-year-old woman with an approximately 50-degree right thoracic scoliosis treated with pedicle screw and rod instrumentation and spinal fusion. (C) and (D) are a 15-year-old woman with a 75-degree Scheuermann kyphosis treated with anterior spinal release and fusion followed by posterior pedicle screw instrumentation and fusion.

**KYPHOSIS**

Kyphoses can also be divided etiologically into congenital and developmental. The congenital kyphoses arise during embryogenesis due to *failures of vertebral formation and failures of segmentation* of the vertebral anlage. Like congenital scoliosis, congenital kyphosis has associated anomalies of the spinal cord, genitourinary system, and cardiovascular system.[34] Juvenile or developmental kyphosis is idiopathic; however, a differential vertebral growth rate in the anterior spine versus the posterior seems a likely contributor to its progression.

Congenital kyphosis can be a dangerous condition and can result in spinal cord dysfunction. This is particularly true of failures of formation. Although most of these deformities remain stable, those that progress can do so precipitously. Subspecialty evaluation at the time of diagnosis is wise, and some patients will require surgical stabilization.[34]

Juvenile kyphosis is also known as Scheuermann kyphosis It is often identified on the Adam forward bending test and is frequently found on school screenings. The normal thoracic kyphosis is a range of 25 to 45 degrees. Spinal deformity specialists disagree as to the clinical significance of modest degrees of increased kyphosis, but there is the possibility of cardiopulmonary difficulties at kyphosis angles more than 95 degrees. Patients often are particularly sensitive to the effect of kyphosis on body image. Unlike scoliosis, kyphosis braces may result in partial correction of the deformity if the patient has growth remaining. Consequently, early initiation of treatment can affect outcome. Surgery is occasionally required and often involves anterior spinal release and fusion followed by posterior spinal instrumentation and fusion.[35]

## SUMMARY

In conclusion, disorders of the back and neck are common maladies for patients of all ages. Adolescent medicine physicians will be frequently called upon to evaluate patients with a broad range of spinal pathologies. Consequently, they should develop familiarity with the anatomy of the spine, examination of the spine and spinal nerves, and an understanding of the strengths and weaknesses of common imaging studies. The vast majority of common spinal injuries are self-limited and usually not seen in the doctor's office. Physicians should suspect an identifiable source for pains that persist beyond 14 days, those which occur after trauma, or those that are associated with constitutional symptoms such as fever or night pain. Efficient use of imaging tests and timely consultation with specialists can speed accurate diagnosis and enhance recovery for patients. The rapid growth of the adolescent spine presents both challenges and opportunities for young patients with spinal deformity. Early evaluation of patients with suspected deformity may help to avoid major surgical interventions. "Back pain" is a frustrating condition for many adults and their physicians. Thankfully, the adolescent patient can often be provided with a more specific, accurate diagnosis, and thereby rendered more effective early treatment. The adolescent spine patient is usually able to be returned to a full and active life.

*The AAP thanks John F. Sarwark, MD, for his thoughtful review of this chapter.*

## REFERENCES

1. Jones GT, Macfarlane GJ. Epidemiology of low back pain in children and adolescents. *Arch Dis Child.* 2005;90: 312-316

2. Turner PG, Green JH, Galasko CS. Back pain in childhood. *Spine.* 1989;14:812-814

3. D'Hemecourt PA, Gerbino PG, Micheli LJ. Back injuries in the young athlete. *Clin Sports Med.* 2000;19(4):663-679

4. Van Tulder MW, Scholten RJP, Koes BW, Deyo RH. Nonsteroidal anti-inflammatory drugs for low back pain, a systematic review within the framework of the Cochrane collaboration back review group. *Spine.* 2000;25(19):2501-2513

5. Hagen KB, Gunvor H, Jamtvedt G, Winnem MF. The Cochrane review of advice to stay active as a single treatment for low back pain and sciatica. *Spine.* 2002;27:1736-1741

6. Hagen KB, Gunvor H, Jamtvedt G, Winnem MF. The updated Cochrane review of bed rest for low back pain and sciatica. *Spine.* 2005;30:542-546

7. Chambers HG, Akbarnia BA. Thoracic, lumbar, and sacral spine fractures and dislocations. In: *The Pediatric Spine.* Philadelphia, PA: Lippincott; 2001:567-583

8. Vaccaro AR, Kim DH, Brodke DS, et al. Diagnosis and management of thoracolumbar spine fractures. *AAOS Instructional Course Lectures.* 2004;53:359-373

9. Frederickson BE, Baker D, McHolick WJ, Yuan HA, Lubicky JP. The natural history of spondylolysis and spondylolisthesis. *J Bone Joint Surg Am.* 1984;66:699-707

10. Cavalier R, Herman MJ, Cheung EV, Pizzutillo PD. Spondylolysis and spondylolisthesis in children and adolescents: I. Diagnosis, natural history, and nonsurgical management. *J Am Acad Orthop Surg.* 2006;14:417-424

11. Bellah RD, Summerville DA, Treves ST, Micheli LJ. Low back pain in adolescent athletes: detection of stress injury to the pars interarticularis with SPECT. *Radiology.* 1991;180: 509-512

12. Parisini P, DiSilvestre M, Greggi T, Miglietta A, Paderni S. Lumbar disc excision in children and adolescents. *Spine.* 2001;26:1997-2000

13. Buttermann G. Treatment of lumbar disc herniation: epidural steroid injection compared with discectomy: a prospective, randomized study. *J Bone Joint Surg Am.* 2004;86:670–679

14. Early SD, Kay RM, Tolo VT. Childhood diskitis. *J Am Acad Orthop Surg.* 2003;11:413–420

15. Song KS, Ogden JA, Ganey T, Guidera KJ. Contiguous discitis and osteomyelitis in children. *J Pediatric Orthopedics.* 1997;17470–17477

16. Fernandez M, Carrol CL, Baker CJ. Discitis and vertebral osteomyelitis in children: an 18-year review. *Pediatrics.* 2000;105:1299–1304

17. Swanson AN, Pappoul P, Cammisa FP, Girardi FP. Chronic infections of the spine: surgical indications and treatments. *Clin Orthop Relat Res.* 2006;444:100–106

18. Garg S, Dormans JP. Tumors and tumor-like conditions of the spine in children. *J Am Acad Orthop Surg.* 2005;13:372–381

19. Joines JD, McNutt RA, Carey TS, Deyo RA, Rouhani R. Finding cancer in primary care outpatients with low back pain: a comparison of diagnostic strategies. *J Gen Intern Med.* 2001;16:14–23

20. Malleson PN, Fung MY, Rosenberg AM. The incidence of pediatric rheumatic diseases: results from the Canadian Pediatric Rheumatology Association Disease Registry. *J Rheumatol.* 1996;23(11):1834–1837

21. Tse SML, Laxer RM. Juvenile spondyloarthropathy. *Curr Opin Rheum.* 2003;15:374–379

22. Burgos-Vargas R. Juvenile onset spondyloarthropathy: therapeutic aspects. *Rheum Dis.* 2002;61:iii33–iii39

23. Tse SL, Burgos-Vargas R, Laxer RM. Anti-tumor necrosis factor alpha blockade in the treatment of juvenile spondyloarthropathy. *Arthritis Rheum.* 2005;52:2103–2108

24. Khan MA. Ankylosing spondylitis: introductory comments on its diagnosis and treatment. *Ann Rheum Dis.* 2002;61:iii3–iii7

25. Pepmueller PH, Moore TL. Juvenile spondyloarthropathies. *Curr Opin Rheum.* 2000;12:269–273

26. Reamy BV, Slakey JB. Adolescent idiopathic scoliosis: review and current concepts. *Am Fam Physician.* 2001;64:111–116

27. Lonstein JE. Scoliosis, surgical vs. nonsurgical treatment. *Clin Orthop Relat Res.* 2006;443:248–259

28. Roach JW. Adolescent idiopathic scoliosis. *Orthop Clin N Amer.* 1999;30:353–365

29. Dickson RA. Spinal deformity-adolescent idiopathic scoliosis, non-operative treatment. *Spine.* 1999;24:2601–2606

30. Bridwell KH. Surgical treatment of idiopathic adolescent scoliosis. *Spine.* 1999;24:2607–2616

31. Lenke LG, Betz RR, Harms J, et al. Adolescent idiopathic scoliosis: a new classification to determine extent of spinal arthrodesis. *J Bone Joint Surg Am.* 2001;83:1169–1181

32. Hedequist D, Emans J. Congenital scoliosis. *J Am Acad Orthop Surg.* 2004;12:266–275

33. McCarthy RE. Management of neuromuscular scoliosis. *Orthop Clin N Amer.* 1999;30:435–449

34. Lonstein JE. Congenital spine deformities: scoliosis, kyphosis, and lordosis. *Orthop Clin N Amer.* 1999;30:387–405

35. Tribus CB. Scheuermann's kyphosis in adolescents and adults: diagnosis and management. *J Am Aca Orthop Surg.* 1998;6:36–43

# CHAPTER 163

# Chest Wall Abnormalities

CHAD HAMNER, MD • DAVID H. ROTHSTEIN, MD • ANDREW R. HONG, MD

## PECTUS EXCAVATUM

### BACKGROUND

Pectus excavatum (PE), known archaically as funnel chest, is the most frequently occurring chest wall deformity, with an incidence of approximately 1:400 live births.[1] Males are more often affected than females (5:1) and there is a clear familial association; approximately 40% of patients have a family member with the condition.[2] However, longitudinal family studies have been unable to find a consistent inheritance pattern, and the relative risk for offspring or siblings of those with PE is not well established.[3] Other musculoskeletal abnormalities may be found in association with PE, including scoliosis (15%), kyphosis, Marfan syndrome, equinus varus, syndactyly, Ehlers-Danlos syndrome, osteogenesis imperfecta, Klippel-Feil syndrome, and congenital diaphragmatic hernia.[4,5] Rarely, these patients may have coexisting congenital cardiac defects (1.5%).[6] Although the association with multiple musculoskeletal abnormalities suggests that a connective tissue defect may play a role, the underlying etiology of PE remains uncertain. Multiple theories have been proposed, including poor development of the anterior diaphragm,[7,8] aberrant substernal ligamentous attachment,[9] and unbalanced costochondral growth,[10,11] but none is confirmed.

### PRESENTATION AND DIAGNOSIS

The presentation of PE is usually straightforward on physical examination by the classic appearance of a symmetrical depression of the middle and lower sternum, but the extent and severity of sternal involvement can vary. Infants and children often have a subtle, symmetric defect that may be accompanied by paradoxical inward motion of the sternum during inspiration, slumped shoulder posture, and a protuberant abdomen. Children with significant PE defects typically are brought for medical evaluation by age 3 years. Spontaneous regression is extremely rare, and physicians should not counsel parents that their child will "outgrow" the problem. For those whose defect is not particularly noticeable in childhood, rapid growth changes during adolescence cause the deformity to become prominent. At this stage, the deformity may still be symmetrical, but as many as 50% of patients will have an asymmetric appearance with the right side of the chest more significantly depressed than the left.[2]

Symptoms attributed to PE are unusual in children, but they often exhibit shy and reclusive personality traits, including reluctance to participate in swimming, sports, or other social events with their peers. Approximately half of PE patients report intermittent, vague, atypical chest pain at the lower anterior chest with exercise or, infrequently, with rest.[2] The pain may be relieved temporarily by nonsteroidal anti-inflammatory drugs (NSAIDs). As children and adolescents with PE become more active in sports, they will often experience easy tiredness, shortness of breath, wheezing, and decreased stamina and endurance. Older-age patients may note a fall off in their performance level or lose interest in physical activities. Many of these patients are diagnosed with exercise-induced asthma. However, pulmonary function testing in PE patients typically reveals a mild restrictive pattern with normal to low-normal lung capacities.[12,13] Response to bronchodilators is an indication of concomitant reactive airway disease. The reduction in pulmonary capacities and exercise-related symptoms roughly correlates with the severity of the deformity.[14] Overall, studies of exercise tolerance and pulmonary function have shown varied, often discrepant results, but it is believed that real exercise limitations exist in PE patients and that these may be more related to cardiac compression than to restrictive pulmonary mechanics.[15]

### EVALUATION

The evaluation of a patient with PE involves a thorough history and physical examination, pulmonary function and consultation with a pediatric cardiologist for echocardiography and possible exercise tolerance testing. Because the deformity is easily recognizable, the diagnosis is usually not difficult. However, a thorough history of exercise tolerance and respiratory status must be obtained to detail the severity of symptoms. The authors, and others, have utilized formal exercise tolerance testing as a way to document the presence of symptoms in certain cases. We evaluate pulmonary function in all patients to rule out reactive airway disease, which

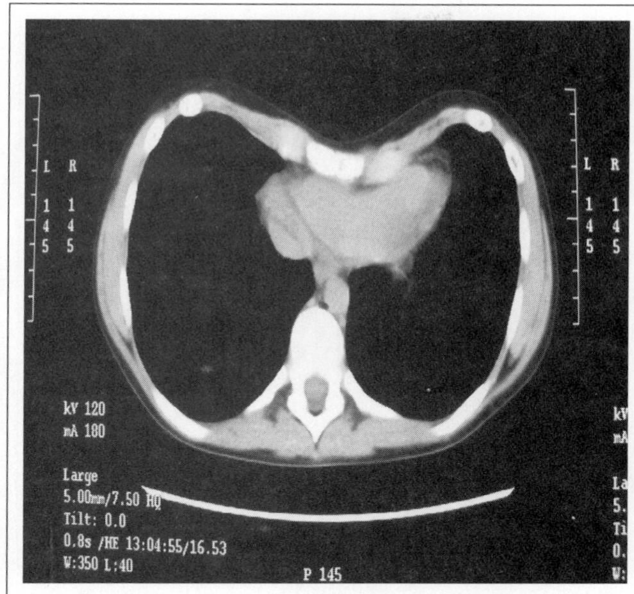


FIGURE 163-1 Noncontrast CT scan in typical PE patient showing significant cardiac compression.

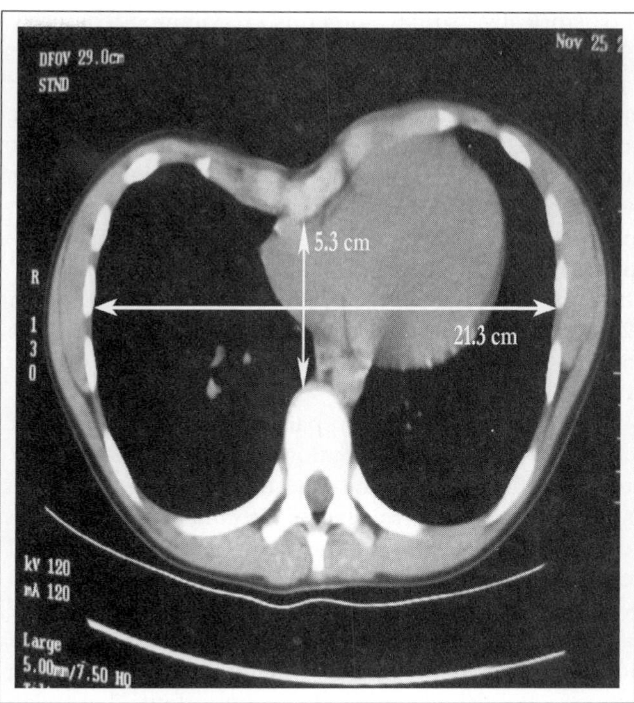


FIGURE 163-2 CT of chest with measurement of the AP and transverse diameters showing a Haller index of 4.0.

should be optimally treated before any surgical repair is attempted.

A limited, noncontrast computed tomography (CT) scan of the chest may demonstrate cardiac compression (Figure 163-1) and allows calculation of the Haller index, the ratio of the transverse chest diameter to the anterior–posterior diameter at the deepest depression of the sternum (Figure 163-2). The average index in normal individuals is 2.2; an index of more than 3.25 is considered indicative of a severe defect. The Haller index also may predict which patients will have significant symptomatic improvement following repair.[16] Other radiographic indices have been proposed, and controversy exists among pediatric surgeons regarding the utility of CT scans in the evaluation of PE due to the risk of radiation exposure. Individual surgical practice varies.

Cardiology evaluation is paramount to rule out occult congenital or acquired cardiac anomalies that may be responsible for a patient's symptoms. Approximately 15% of PE patients will have mitral valve prolapse (MVP), particularly those with Marfan syndrome. Although MVP is common, typically it is clinically insignificant in PE patients.[2] It is important, however, to refer those who fit the criteria for Marfan syndrome to an ophthalmologist and geneticist. Electrocardiograms are often abnormal, with right bundle block and right axis deviation, presumably due to cardiac displacement into the left hemithorax, and not intrinsic cardiac disease. An insignificant, functional systolic murmur may be present in 18% of patients due to compression of the right ventricular outflow tract.[2]

## THERAPEUTIC OPTIONS

Physical therapy and exercise programs are not effective in delaying the progression of a PE deformity, and are only mentioned here briefly as they remain in some treatment algorithms.[17] Surgical repair of PE has been the mainstay of treatment since Ravitch[18] first described his method of repair in 1949. Surgery is indicated in those patients with significant limitations in exercise tolerance or pulmonary mechanics and no other cause for symptoms. Although most patients voice great concern regarding their body image, insurance companies will rarely reimburse for the cost of surgical repair in asymptomatic patients. It is the authors' opinion that most adolescents will benefit psychologically from the repair and that the procedure allows these adolescents and young adults to go from having a distinctly abnormal body habitus to a relatively normal one. We view the procedure as a reconstructive one and not necessarily just cosmetic.

Historically, some surgeons recommended early repair in children between 2 and 5 years of age, as the repair was technically easier at that time. This practice has been abandoned in the last few decades, with most surgeons recommending repair in the late adolescent to early adult years. The rationale for this change is that most young children are physiologically asymptomatic, and the risk of either recurrence or acquired asphyxiating thoracic dystrophy is higher with early repair.[19,20] The optimum age to repair PE seems to be between 12 and 16 years of age, although good results in adult patients have been achieved as late as the fifth decade of life.[2]

For 50 years, the open repair has been used by most surgeons with minor variations on Ravitch's original procedure. Under general anesthesia, the sternum is exposed through a transverse inframammary or vertical incision placed over the point of maximal sternal depression; typically the transverse incision is preferred as it is more appealing cosmetically. Skin and muscle flaps are raised circumferentially, exposing the deformed cartilages, which are then resected bilaterally, leaving the perichondrium intact. It is important that bilateral resections are performed even if an asymmetric defect exists. After the anterior mediastinum and pleura are mobilized from the back of the sternum, a wedge-shaped, transverse osteotomy is made in the posterior table of the sternum above the superior aspect of the depression. Now the sternum and xyphoid are mobile and can be elevated and stabilized in the neutral position. Several methods to stabilize the sternum have been described, including a retrosternal steel bar,[21,22] a mesh sling "hammock,"[23] or a polytetrafluoroethylene (PTFE) strut.[24] This internal support provides several advantages to external support devices (abandoned in current practice) including improved pain control, respiratory mechanics, early ambulation, reduced hospitalization, and superior permanent repair.[2] Complications related to struts are few but include dislodgement and migration, and the steel bars must be removed at a second operation.

In 1998, Nuss and colleagues[17] described a new minimally invasive repair for PE (MIRPE), developed based on the concept of bracing for correction of skeletal deformities in children. This approach avoids any cartilage resection or sternal osteotomy. Under general anesthesia, a convex steel bar is passed under the sternum at the point of deepest depression through small bilateral incisions (Figure 163-3). The bar is positioned to force the sternum outward into a more neutral position and is secured to the chest wall with sutures or lateral stabilizers, as needed (Figure 163-4). Occasionally, a second bar is required for larger defects. Initially MIRPE was performed in a "blind" fashion, in which a large clamp was passed across the anterior mediastinum by palpation alone. However, reports of myocardial injury[25] prompted

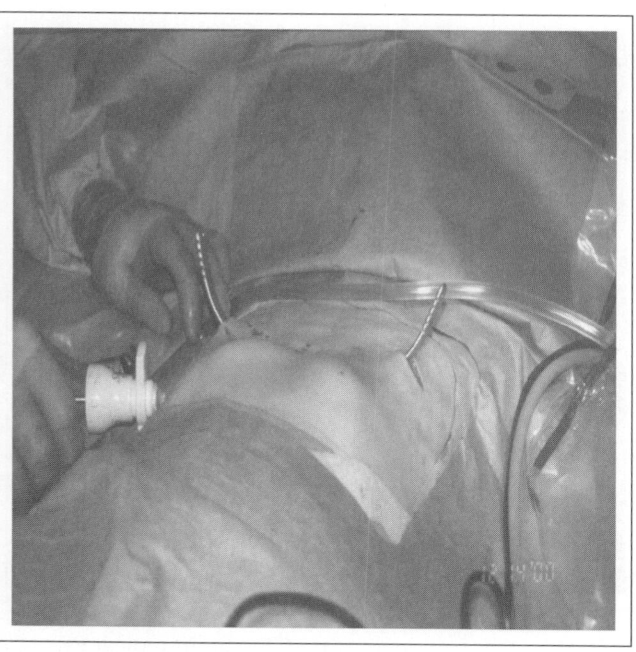

**FIGURE 163-3** Intraoperative photograph of VAPER showing convex bar in place before eversion of the sternum. (See color insert.)

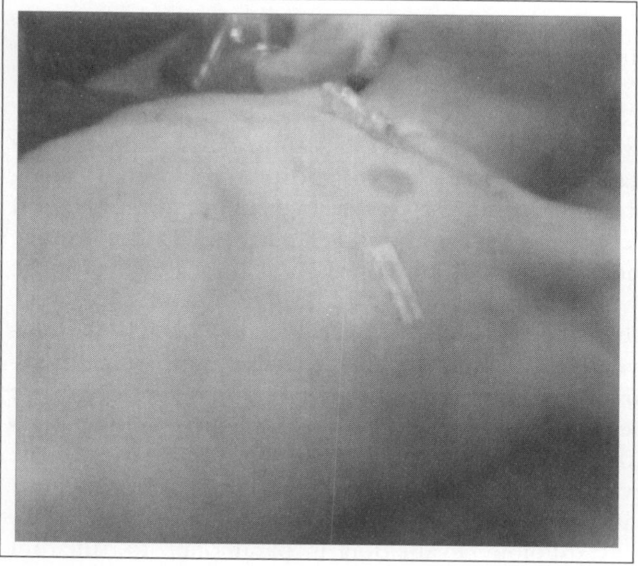

**FIGURE 163-4** Immediate postoperative photograph after eversion of sternum. (See color insert.)

many surgeons to abandon the "blind" technique in favor of videoscopic-assisted PE repair (VAPER).[26] This is the preferred method in the authors' institution. The VAPER technique modifies Nuss's approach by placing small trocars into one or both pleural spaces followed by carbon dioxide insufflation to assist lung collapse away from the chest wall. Thoracoscopy provides excellent visualization of the anterior mediastinum for careful dissection and controlled retrosternal strut positioning. The bar is left in place for 2 to 3 years to allow sufficient time for chest wall remodeling, at which time it is removed at a second outpatient procedure.

Postoperative care for any of the described procedures centers on stringent pain control to improve respiratory mechanics, minimize atelectasis, and prevent development of pneumonia from poor secretion clearance. In the authors' experience, epidural catheters placed at the time of surgery were initially used for postoperative pain control, but that method has been abandoned because of the temperamental nature of the delivery system. Instead, patient-controlled analgesia with intravenous narcotics and NSAIDs is now utilized in the immediate postoperative period, followed by a combination of oral NSAIDs, narcotics, and muscle relaxants for up to a month. Also added is a promotility agent to prevent constipation. Patients are encouraged to ambulate early, but activity restrictions are maintained for approximately 12 weeks to discourage strut dislodgement during the initial healing period. Hospitalization averages 3 to 6 days for either the open or minimally invasive repair, and blood loss is minimal.[15]

Mortality from either operation is exceedingly rare, and complications are few and easily managed, including seroma, infection, hemo/pneumothorax, pericarditis, and pneumonia. For minimally invasive repairs, bar dislodgement or flipping may occur in 3% to 11% of patients.[15,27-29] Satisfactory cosmetic results can be expected in 85% to 97% of patients regardless of technique (Figure 163-4).[2,25,27,30] Functional outcome assessments for the open and minimally invasive techniques have had variable results, but most patients experience moderate to marked improvement in exercise tolerance and stamina with much less dyspnea. Palpitations are frequently reduced and asthmatic patients often require less bronchodilator therapy for wheezing[2] (Figure 163-5).

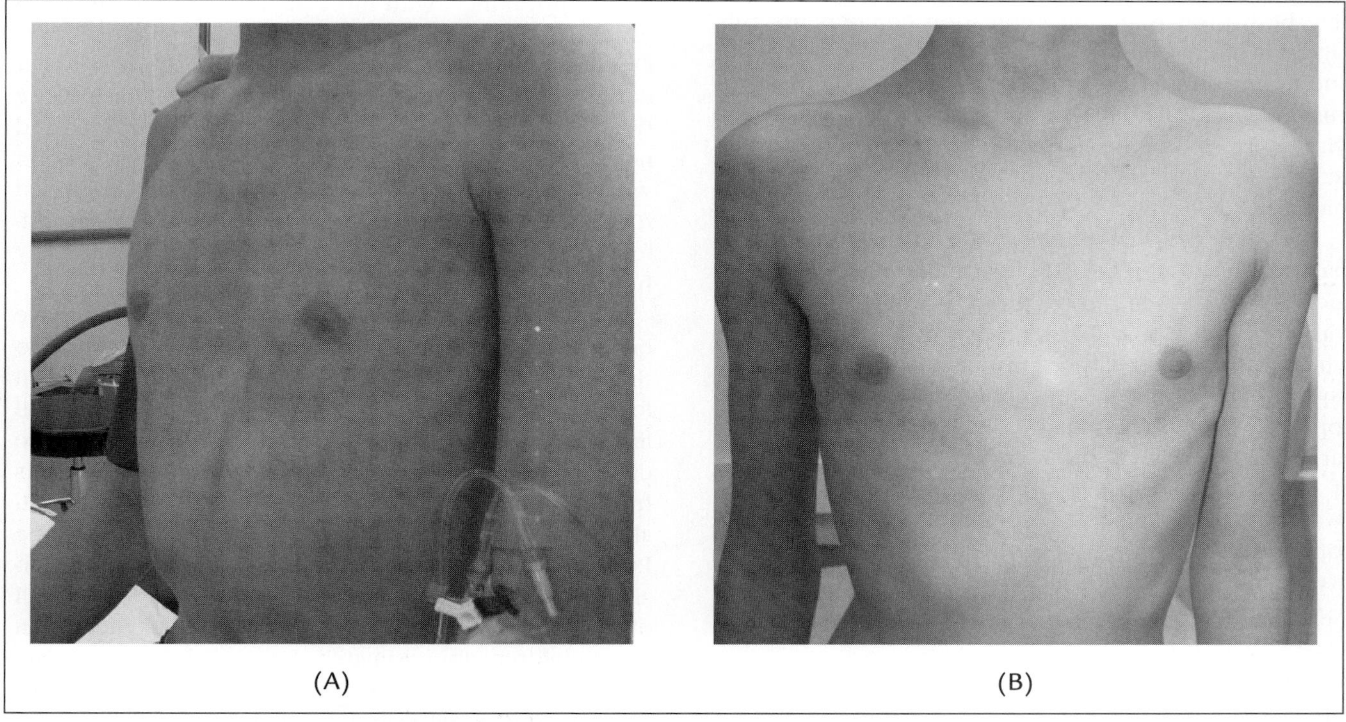


FIGURE 163-5 PE patient (A) before and (B) after VAPER. (See color insert.)

## PECTUS CARINATUM

### BACKGROUND

Pectus carinatum (PC), also known as pigeon breast, is 5 times less common than PE, occurring in approximately 1:2,000 children,[31,32] with males more often affected than females (4:1).[33] As many as 26% of patients will have a family history of some type of chest wall defect, but there is no known genetic abnormality predisposing to PC.[31] Although PC usually occurs in isolation, associated skeletal anomalies may be found, including scoliosis (15%), Marfan syndrome, Ehlers-Danlos syndrome, and myopathies.[34] Up to 10% of patients may have a congenital cardiac defect.[35] Similar to PE, no well-established cause is known, but abnormal growth of ribs or costal cartilages is thought to push the sternum outward in PC.[36]

### PRESENTATION AND DIAGNOSIS

Like PE, the characteristic appearance of PC makes the diagnosis relatively straightforward. Two major patterns are described: chondrogladiolar and chondromanubrial (1%).[37,38] Most children have a symmetric chondrogladiolar deformity with protrusion of the sternal body and costal cartilages. However, chondrogladiolar deformities may also be asymmetric, limited to one side of the sternum, producing a keel-like protrusion. Mixed chondrogladiolar deformities are described that combine both protrusion and depression components; this variant is often seen in patients with Poland syndrome.[38] Chondromanubrial deformities are characterized by protrusion of the manubrium and upper costal cartilages with depression of the sternal body.[38] Congenital cardiac defects are more commonly found with the chondromanubrial deformity.[39]

Most PC deformities are subtle in early childhood, masked by the normal childhood abdominal protuberance. Rapid growth during puberty worsens the chest wall appearance in adolescence, which is the point at which most patients present for medical evaluation. Psychosocial problems are common, arising from the appearance of the PC deformity, but other symptoms vary considerably. Atypical chest pain and symptoms of costochondritis are the most common complaints. Dyspnea and poor endurance during exercise are less common than in patients with PE.[40] Significant objective cardiopulmonary derangements are rare, except in very severe cases.[41]

### EVALUATION

The evaluation of the patient with PC comprises a careful history and physical examination, particularly aimed at uncovering associated musculoskeletal and cardiac abnormalities that may need to be addressed prior to definitive treatment. Computed tomography scanning may be helpful in operative planning, but it is less often necessary than with PE. In the absence of symptoms, pulmonary function tests and echocardiography are usually unnecessary.

### TREATMENT

The mainstay of treatment for more than 50 years has been surgical repair, as described by Ravitch[42] in 1952. Since his report, other approaches have been devised,[43,44] but modern surgical techniques continue to be modeled after Ravitch's original procedure (see previous discussion). Indications for repair remain the same as those for PE; however, because significant objective cardiorespiratory derangements are usually absent in PC, repair is generally undertaken for subjective symptoms or cosmesis. Optimal timing of correction is unclear; some surgeons advocate for repair after puberty to reduce the incidence of recurrence during the pubertal growth spurt,[45] whereas others propose that surgical repair be offered when the defect becomes obvious.[37] Unlike PE, development of asphyxiating thoracic dystrophy is usually not a concern with PC, because the deformity does not present until later in childhood.[15]

The success of PC repair is mostly related to cosmetic appearance, with most patients enjoying good to excellent appearance on long-term follow-up.[31,33,40,45] Operative mortality and morbidity are similar to that described previously for PE. Poor cosmetic results are typically due to incomplete operative resection, and not to recurrence, and usually can be improved upon with reoperation.[31,40] Few studies have addressed functional outcome, but most find minimal or no difference in quantifiable measures of cardiorespiratory function.[31,41]

Recently, form-fitting, adjustable orthotic braces have been developed that apply anteroposterior pressure to the sternum. Therapeutic regimens vary, but most call for a minimum duration of 2 years of therapy or until linear growth ceases. The duration of wear during the day diminishes as therapy progresses. Initial results from multiple institutions have been encouraging, with almost no complications. Significant improvement in the PC deformity and subjective appearance is reported in all patients completing therapy.[46-49] The main shortfall of bracing is adherence with the duration of therapy in older children; approximately 10% to 13% do not complete therapy.[48,49] However, those who fail nonoperative therapy do well with surgical repair.

It is our current practice to recommend bracing for all PC patients with symptoms. We have not found adherence to be a significant issue, and because a change in the appearance of the chest wall occurs relatively rapidly, most patients are willing to complete the course of therapy and avoid surgery.

## SKELETAL DISORDERS

There are several rare dysplastic syndromes that manifest a wide range of skeletal anomalies including chest wall defects. Only those disorders that have been long recognized and well documented are summarized: asphyxiating thoracic dystrophy (Jeune syndrome), spondylothoracic dysplasia (Jarcho-Levin syndrome), spodylocostal dystosis, and Poland syndrome.

### ASPHYXIATING THORACIC DYSTROPHY (JEUNE SYNDROME)

First described by Jeune and colleagues[50] in 1954, asphyxiating thoracic dystrophy is an autosomal recessive disease characterized by abnormalities of the thoracic cage, pelvis, and phalanges, accompanied by varying degrees of renal dysplasia.[51-53] Irregular costochondral junctions and horizontal, flattened ribs create a rigid, bell-shaped thorax, which markedly reduces thoracic dimensions[54] and restricts intercostal muscle excursion.[55]

The age of presentation and degree of pulmonary compromise vary greatly.[1,56,57] In severe cases, patients develop profound pulmonary hypertension, respiratory failure, and death in the newborn period. Children with milder forms develop recurrent pneumonia and progress to respiratory failure within the first year of life; ventilator dependence or death results without treatment.[55-57] Patients who survive childhood and are diagnosed late often maintain adequate respiratory capacity and may improve over time.[53,58] The only potentially correctable component of the disease is expansion of the chest cavity by expanding the sternum or lateral chest wall with either autologous bone grafts or prostheses.[58-61] Results vary and no consensus exists regarding which technique is superior.

### SPONDYLOTHORACIC DYSPLASIA AND SPONDYLOCOSTAL DYSTOSIS

Jarcho and Levin[62] first described a rare spectrum of skeletal anomalies, including abnormal vertebral and rib formation associated with short-trunk dwarfism, in 1938. Since that time, molecular, clinical, and radiologic studies have further characterized Jarcho-Levin syndrome, giving rise to a spectrum of disorders best classified into 2 distinct phenotypes, spondylothoracic dysplasia (STD) and spondylocostal dystosis (SCD).[63-69]

Spondylothoracic dysplasia is an autosomal recessive disorder recently linked to mutations on the long arm of chromosome 2.[70] In contrast, SCD mostly exhibits autosomal dominant inheritance, although recessive patterns have been described, with genetic mutations mapped to chromosome 19.[71,72] Both disorders typically display segmentation and formation defects throughout the spine in conjunction with variable rib anomalies leading to dwarfism. Symmetric, posterior fusion and anterior fanning of the ribs involving 60% to 90% of the thoracic cage is prominent in STD, whereas broadening, bifurcation, and asymmetric fusion of the ribs, frequently leading to progressive thoracic scoliosis, is more typical of SCD.[69] Other defects may be encountered with each disorder including inguinal and umbilical hernias, diaphragmatic hernia, urogenital tract defects, anal abnormalities, and congenital heart disease.[69]

Diagnosis is increasingly being made on prenatal screening, but regardless of timing, family genetic counseling should be offered once diagnosis is confirmed.[73] Poor pulmonary mechanics are more prominent in STD and seem to be secondary to reduced chest wall adherence and not necessarily intrinsic lung disease. However, long-term pulmonary insufficiency may develop related to bronchopulmonary dysplasia and recurrent pneumonia; thus, optimal management of pulmonary function and infection is paramount to prevent chronic lung disease.[69] Operative intervention for STD is rarely indicated, but favorable outcomes with chest wall reconstruction to improve adherence have been obtained in some SCD cases.[69,74,75] Spinal fusion often may be required in SCD patients to stabilize the development of progressive scoliosis.[75]

Prognosis varies with type and severity of disease. Although STD was once considered uniformly fatal in the neonatal period, recent studies[76] indicate survival may be expected in 56% of all cases and 100% of those living beyond infancy. Most SCD patients can expect a normal life expectancy.[69] Patients with either disease who survive into adulthood may achieve normal intelligence and a good independent quality of life.[69]

### POLAND SYNDROME

Poland syndrome is a rare congenital anomaly characterized by unilateral chest wall hypoplasia and ipsilateral hand abnormalities. The constellation of anomalies bears the namesake of Alfred Poland, who described a single anatomical case in the English literature in 1841 while just a medical student, but earlier reports exist in the foreign press dating to 1826.[77-79] Between 1 in 7,000 to 100,000 individuals are born annually with the defect, and males are more often affected than females (2 to 3:1).[80-83] Most cases are sporadic and the risk of familial transmission is less than 1%.[84] Congenital hypoplasia of the ipsilateral subclavian artery or one of its branches is thought to produce hypoperfusion and hypoplasia of the developing chest wall and arm.[85,86] The right chest wall appears affected more often in males (75%), whereas females have either side affected equally.[84]

Although clinical presentation varies, minimal diagnostic criteria include ipsilateral absence of the pectoralis major muscle and breast hypoplasia.[84] Involvement of one or more chest wall muscles with rib and cartilage hypoplasia (segments II to IV or III to V) is usually present, producing a sunken chest wall on the affected side. Furthermore, fusion of aplastic ribs may rotate the sternum toward the involved side, producing an asymmetric, contralateral PC defect. Breast abnormalities from unilateral aplasia to mild hypoplasia affect greater than a third of female patients. Hand abnormalities occur in 13% to 56% of patients, ranging from hypoplasia and webbing of the middle phalanges (mitten hand) to complete absence of the hand, but individuals without hand involvement are more common.[87-89] Poland syndrome may coexist with other abnormalities, including dextrocardia (6%),[86] Mobius syndrome,[90] Klippel-Feil syndrome,[86] and unilateral renal duplication or agenesis.[91] Those with renal abnormalities may develop hypertension; therefore, renal studies are recommended in all patients with pectoralis major aplasia.[92] Poland syndrome has also been associated with multiple malignancies including leukemia, non-Hodgkin lymphoma, leiomyosarcoma, and cancer of the lung, cervix, and breast.[93-95]

Most children are asymptomatic and can enjoy normal activities without treatment. However, in cases of severe rib aplasia, chest wall reconstruction may be done at an early age with muscle flaps, autologous bone grafts, or prosthetic implants to provide adequate protection of the heart and lung or to prevent paradoxical movement during respiration. Breast reconstruction with muscle flaps and breast implants may be undertaken for cosmesis and is best offered after puberty to optimize matching between the reconstructed and contralateral breast.[84,87,94]

## STERNAL DISORDERS

Sternal defects are very rare and arise from failure of midline fusion of embryonic mesoderm, independent of rib abnormalities.[96] These defects have been classified since 1818, but the earliest accounts may be found in ancient tablets comprising the Royal Library of Ninevah.[38] Multiple different classification schemes have been proposed, but current reports only recognize 4 different sternal defects based upon tissue coverage of the heart, severity, and associated anomalies: ectopia cordis (either thoracic, thoracoabdominal, or cervical) and sternal cleft.[97]

### ECTOPIA CORDIS

In ectopia cordis, classically the heart is exposed with no overlying somatic structures. Three variants of ectopia cordis are now recognized: thoracic, thoracoabdominal, and cervical, which differ in severity of the sternal defect, cardiac position, and associated anomalies. Thoracic ectopia cordis (Figure 163-6) is the most common anomaly, with a severe lack of midline tissues producing a small thoracic cavity with either a total or central sternal defect; occasionally the manubrium remains intact. The heart is displaced anteriorly and superiorly and often has intrinsic anomalies. Upper abdominal wall defects are common, including omphalocoele, diastasis recti, and eventration of abdominal viscera.[97] In contrast, patients with thoracoabdominal ectopia cordis always have abdominal wall defects that include omphalocoele, diastasis recti, and ventral hernia, along with variable anterior diaphragmatic and pericardial defects. However, the heart is covered by a thin membrane of pigmented skin and lacks the severe anterior displacement seen in the thoracic variant. Cardiac position may vary, either lying within the thoracic cavity, with only the diaphragmatic and pericardial defect below it, or entirely in the abdominal cavity. Intrinsic cardiac defects and diverticula of the left ventricle are common.[38,97] Cantrell and Ravitch[98] described this complex of intrinsic cardiac defects with thoracoabdominal ectopia cordis in 1958; it archaically had been referred to as Cantrell pentalogy. Cervical ectopia cordis, the rarest of the group, differs from other variants by the severity of superior displacement of the cardiac apex, which is often fused with the mouth.[99] Severe craniofacial defects also are frequently associated with the cervical variant.[38]

Treatment options for all types of ectopia cordis are few, and most patients eventually succumb from

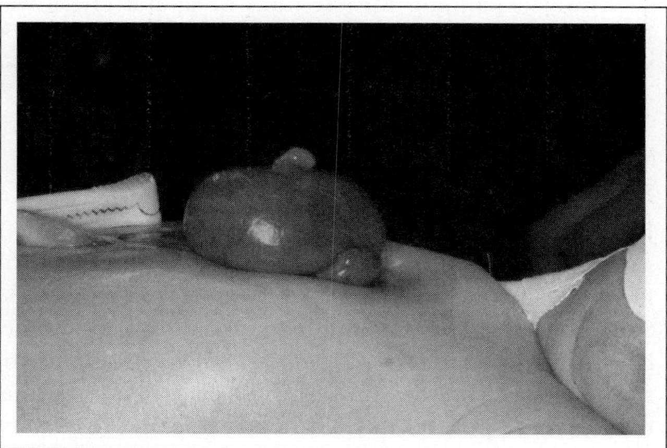

FIGURE 163-6 Thoracic ectopia cordis. (See color insert.)

complications of intrinsic cardiac anomalies. However, long-term survival has been reported following chest wall reconstruction and correction of cardiac anomalies and is most successful for the thoracoabdominal variant. No survivors of cervical ectopia cordis have been reported. Despite the once grim prognosis of ectopia cordis, advances in pediatric cardiac surgery support an aggressive approach to this anomaly.[38,97]

### CLEFT (BIFID) STERNUM

Cleft, or bifid, sternum is the least severe of sternal anomalies. Unlike ectopia cordis, the heart is usually structurally normal, positioned within a normal-sized thoracic cavity, and covered by normal skin and pericardium.[38] Most cases involve primarily the upper sternum; the lower third of the sternal body and xyphoid remain intact. Other associated anomalies are rare, but cervicofacial hemangiomas and band-like scars extending from the defect inferiorly to the umbilicus or superiorly to the mandible have been reported.[100,101] Most infants and children are asymptomatic, but occasionally paradoxical chest wall motion may compromise pulmonary mechanics.[38] Sternal reconstruction is usually indicated to provide protective covering for the heart. Reconstruction is ideally performed in infancy when chest wall adherence provides the best opportunity for primary closure.[97,102] Successful repair may be achieved in older children as well, but often requires more complicated techniques, including autologous bone or cartilage transfers or prosthetic grafts.[97] Sternal cleft defects are rarely lethal.

## REFERENCES


1. Fonkalsrud EW, DeUgarte D, Choi E. Repair of pectus excavatum and carinatum deformities in 116 adults. *Ann Surg.* 2002;236(3):304–312

2. Fonkalsrud EW. Current management of pectus excavatum. *World J Surg.* 2003;27(5):502–508

3. Creswick H, Stacey MW, Kelly RE, et al. Family study of the inheritance of pectus excavatum. *J Ped Surg.* 2006;41:1699–1703

4. Williams AM, Crabbe DC. Pectus deformities of the anterior chest wall. *Paediatr Respir Rev.* 2003;4:237–242

5. Shamberger RC, Welch KJ. Surgical repair of pectus excavatum. *J Pediatr Surg.* 1988;23:615–622

6. Shamberger RC, Welch KJ, Castaneda AR, Keane JF, Fyler DC. Anterior chest wall deformities and congenital heart disease. *J Thorac Cardiovasc Surg.* 1988;96:427–432

7. Brodkin HA. Congenital anterior chest wall deformities of diaphragmatic origin. *Dis Chest.* 1953;24(3):259–277

8. Chin EF, Adler RH. The surgical treatment of pectus excavatum (funnel chest). *BMJ.* 1954;4870:1064–1066

9. Brown AL. Pectus excavatum (funnel chest): anatomic basis, surgical treatment of the incipient stage in infancy, and correction of the deformity in the fully developed stage. *J Thorac Surg.* 1939;9:164–184

10. Davis WC, Berley FV. Pectus excavatum and pectus carinatum: report on the surgical treatment of eleven patients. *Am J Surg.* 1956;91:770–776

11. Ravitch MM. Operative treatment of congenital deformities of the chest. *Am J Surg.* 1961;101:588–597

12. Castile RG, Staats BA, Westbrook PR. Symptomatic pectus deformities of the chest. *Am Rev Respir Dis.* 1982;126: 564–568

13. Quigley PM, Haller JA, Jelus KL, et al. Cardiorespiratory function before and after corrective surgery in pectus excavatum. *J Pediatr.* 1996;128:638–643

14. Malek MH, Fonkalsrud EW, Cooper CB. Ventilatory and cardiovascular responses to exercise in patients with pectus excavatum. *Chest.* 2003;124:870–872

15. McQuigan RM, Azarow KS. Congenital chest wall defects. *Surg Clin N Am.* 2006;86:353–370

16. Haller JA, Kramer SS, Lietman SA. Use of CT scans in selection of patients for pectus excavatum surgery: a preliminary report. *J Pediatr Surg.* 1987;22:904–906

17. Nuss D, Kelly RE, Croitoru DP, et al. A 10-year review of a minimally invasive technique for the correction of pectus excavatum. *J Pediatr Surg.* 1998;33:545–552

18. Ravitch M. The operative treatment of pectus excavatum. *Ann Surg.* 1949;129:429–444

19. Haller JA, Colombani P, Humphries C, et al. Chest wall constriction after too extensive and too early operations for pectus excavatum. *Ann Thorac Surg.* 1996;61:1618–1625

20. Martinez D, Juame J, Stein T, et al. The effect of costal cartilage resection on chest wall development. *Pediatr Surg Int.* 1990;5:170–173

21. Rehbein F, Wernick HH. The operative treatment of the funnel chest. *Arch Dis Child.* 1957;32:5–8

22. Adkins PC, Blades B. A stainless steel strut for correction of pectus excavatum. *Suvr Med.* 1961;113:111–113

23. Robicsek F, Fokin A. Surgical correction of pectus excavatum and carinatum. *J Cardiovasc Surg.* 1999;40: 725–731

24. Gene A, Mutaf O. Polytertafluoroethylene bars in stabilizing the reconstructed sternum for pectus excavatum operations in children. *Plast Reconstr Surg.* 2002;110: 54–57

25. Moss RL, Albanese CT, Reynolds M. Major complications after minimally invasive repair of pectus excavatum: case reports. *J Pediatr Surg.* 2001;36:155–158

26. Hebra A. Minimally invasive pectus surgery. *Chest Surg Clin N Am.* 2000;10:329–339

27. Croitoru DP, Kelly RE, Goretsky MJ, et al. Experience and modification update for the minimally invasive Nuss technique for pectus excavatum repair in 303 patients. *J Pediatr Surg.* 2002;37:437–445

28. Molik KA, Engum SA, Rescorla FJ, et al. Pectus excavatum repair: experience with standard and minimally invasive techniques. *J Pediatr Surg.* 2001;36:324-328

29. Wu PC, Knauer EM, McGowan GE, et al. Repair of pectus excavatum deformities in children: a new perspective of treatment using minimal access surgical technique. *Arch Surg.* 2001;136:419-424

30. Lacquet LK, Morshius WJ, Folgering HT. Long-term results after correction of anterior chest wall deformities. *J Cardiovasc Surg.* 1998;39:683-688

31. Shamberger RC, Welch KJ. Surgical correction of pectus carinatum. *J Pediatr Surg.* 1987;22:48-53

32. Fonkalsrud EW, Beanes S. Surgical management of pectus carinatum: 30 years' experience. *Worl J Surg.* 2001;25: 898-903

33. Fonkalsrud EW, Anselmo DM. Less extensive techniques for repair of pectus carinatum: the undertreated chest deformity. *J Am Coll Surg.* 2004;198:898-905

34. Golladay ES. Pectus carinatum and other deformities of the chest wall. In: Ziegler MM, Azizkhan RG, Weber TR, eds. *Operative Pediatric Surgery*. New York, NY: McGraw-Hill; 2003:269-277

35. Lees RF, Caldicott JH. Sternal anomalies and congenital heart disease. *AMA J Roentgenol Radium Ther Nucl Med.* 1975;124:423-427

36. Pena A, Perez L, Nurko S, et al. Pectus carinatum and pectus excavatum: are they the same disease? *Am Surg.* 1981;47: 215-218

37. Shamberger RC, Welch KJ. Surgical correction of chondromanubrial deformity (Currarino Silverman syndrome). *J Pediatr Surg.* 1988;23:319-322

38. Shamberger RC. Congenital chest wall deformities. In: Grosfeld JL, O'Neil JA, Fonkalsrud EW, Coran AG, eds. *Pediatric Surgery*. 6th ed. Philadelphia, PA: Mosby-Elsevier; 2006: 894-921

39. Curriarino G, Silverman FN. Premature obliteration of the sternal sutures and pigeon-breast deformity. *Radiology.* 1958;70:532-540

40. Robicsek F, Cook JW, Daugherty HK, et al. Pectus carinatum. *J Thorac Cardiovasc Surg.* 1979;78:52-61

41. Cahill JL, Lees GM, Robertson HT. A summary of preoperative and postoperative cardiorespiratory performance in patients undergoing pectus excavatum and carinatum repair. *J Pediatr Surg.* 1984;19:430-433

42. Ravitch MM. Unusual sternal deformity with cardiac symptoms operative correction. *J Thorac Surg.* 1952;23:138-144

43. Lester CW. Pigeon breast (pectus carinatum) and other protrusion deformities of the chest of developmental origin. *Ann Surg.* 1953;137:482-489

44. Brodkin HA. Pigeon breast, congenital chondrosternal prominence, etiology, and surgical treatment by xiphosternopexy. *AMA Arch Surg.* 1958;77:261-270

45. Pickard LR, Tepas JJ, Shermeta DW, et al. Pectus carinatum: results of surgical therapy. *J Pediatr Surg.* 1979;14: 228-230

46. Haje SA, Bowen JR. Preliminary results of orthotic treatment of pectus deformities in children and adolescents. *J Pediatr Orthop.* 1992;12:795-800

47. Egan JC, DuBois JJ, Morphy M, et al. Compressive orthotics in the treatment of asymmetric pectus carinatum: a preliminary report with an objective radiologic marker. *J Pediatr Surg.* 2000;35:1183-1186

48. Frey AS, Garcia VF, Brown RL, et al. Nonoperative management of pectus carinatum. *J Pediatr Surg.* 2006;41:40-45

49. Kravarusic D, Dicken BJ, Dewar R, et al. The Calgary protocol for bracing of pectus carinatum: a preliminary report. *J Pediatr Surg.* 2006;41:923-926

50. Jeune M, Carron R, Beraud C, et al. Polychondrodystrophie avec Blcage Thoracique d' Evolution fatale. *Pediatrie.* 1954;9:390-392

51. Langer LO. Thoracic pelvic phalangeal dystrophy: asphyxiating thoracic dystrophy of the newborn, infantile thoracic dystrophy. *Radiology.* 1968;91:447-456

52. Herdman RC, Langer LO. The thoracic asphyxiant dystrophy and renal disease. *Am J Dis Child.* 1977;52:192-201

53. Oberklaid F, Danks DM, Mayne V, et al. Asphyxiating thoracic dysplasia. *Arch Dis Child.* 1977;52:758-765

54. Ravitch MM. *Congenital Deformities of the Chest Wall and Their Operative Correction.* Philadelphia, PA: WB Saunders; 1977:273-284

55. Borland LM. Anesthesia for children with Jeune's syndrome (asphyxiating thoracic dystrophy). *Anesthesiology.* 1987;66:86-88

56. Tahernia AC, Stamps P. Jeune's syndrome (asphyxiating thoracic dystrophy). *Clin Pediatr.* 1977;16:903-907

57. Schmidt R, Pajewski M, Mundel G. Unusual features in familial asphyxiating thoracic dystrophy (Jeune's disease). *Clin Genet.* 1972;3:90-98

58. Weber TR, Kurkchubasche AG. Operative management of asphyxiating thoracic dystrophy after pectus repair. *J Pediatr Surg.* 1998;33:262-265

59. Barnes ND, Hull D, Milner AD, et al. Chest reconstruction in thoracic dystrophy. *Arch Dis Child.* 1971;46:833-837

60. Todd DW, Tinguely SJ, Norberg WJ. A thoracic expansion technique for Jeune's asphyxiating thoracic dystrophy. *J Pediatr Surg.* 1986;21:161-163

61. Davis JT, Heisten JB, Castile RG, et al. Lateral thoracic expansion for Jeune's syndrome: midterm results. *Ann Thorac Surg.* 2001;72:872-878

62. Jarcho S, Levin P. Hereditary malformation of the vertebral bodies. *Bull John Hopkins Hosp.* 1938;62:216-226

63. Lavy NW, Palmer CG, Merritt AD. A syndrome of bizarre vertebral anomalies. *J Pediatr.* 1966;69:1121-1125

64. Rimoin DL, Fletcher BD, McKusick V. Spondylocostal dysplasia: a dominantly inherited form of short-trunked dwarfism. *Am J Med.* 1968;45:948-953

65. Moseley JE, Bonforte RJ. Spondylothoracic dysplasia, a syndrome of congenital anomalies. *Am J Roentgenol.* 1969;106:166-169

66. Perez-Comas A, Garcia-Castro JM. Occipito-facial-cervicothoracic-abdomino-digital dysplasia; Jarcho-Levin syndrome of vertebral anomalies. *J Pediatr.* 1974;85:388-391

67. Solomon L, Bosch-Jinemez R, Reiner L. Spondylothoracic dystosis. *Arch Pathol Lab Med.* 1978;102:201-205

68. Mortier GR, Lachman RS, Bocian M, et al. Multiple vertebral segmentation defects: analysis of 26 new patients and review of the literature. *Am J Med Genet.* 1996;61:310-319

69. Cornier AS, Ramirez N, Carlo S, et al. Controversies surrounding Jarcho-Levin syndrome. *Curr Opin Pediatr.* 2003;15: 614-620

70. Santiago-Cornier A, Ramirez N, Franceschini V, et al. Mapping of spondylothoracic dysplasia (Jarcho-Levin syndrome) to chromosome 2q32.1 in Puerto Rican population. *Am J Hum Genet.* 2001;69-S:514

71. Turnpenny PD, Whittock N, Duncan J, et al. Novel mutations in DLL3, a somitogenesis gene encoding a ligand for Notch signaling pathway, cause a consistent pattern of abnormal vertebral segmentation in spondylocostal dystosis. *J Med Genet.* 2003;40:333-339

72. Dunwoodie SL, Clements M, Duncan S, et al. Axial skeletal defects caused by mutation in the spondylocostal dysplasia/pudgy gene DLL3 are associated with disruption of the segmentation clock within the presomitic mesoderm. *Development.* 2002;129:1795-1806

73. Kauffman E, Roman H, Barau G, et al. Case report: a prenatal case of Jarcho-Levin syndrome diagnosed during the first trimester of pregnancy. *Prenat Diagn.* 2003;23:163-165

74. Mooney JF, Emans JB. Progressive kyphosis and neurologic compromise complicating spondylothoracic dysplasia in infancy (Jarcho-Levin syndrome). *Spine.* 1995;20:1938-1942

75. Teli M, Hosalkar H, Gill I, et al. Spondylocostal dysostosis: thirteen new cases treated by conservative and surgical means. *Spine.* 2004;29:1447-1451

76. Cornier AS, Ramírez N, Arroyo S, et al. Phenotype characterization and natural history of spondylothoracic dysplasia syndrome: a series of 27 new cases. *Am J Med Genet A.* 2004;128:120-126

77. Poland A. Deficiency of the pectoralis muscles. *Guy's Hospital Reports.* 1841;6:191-193

78. Lallemand LM. Absence de trios cotes simulant un enfoncement accidental. *Ephemerides Medicales de Montpelier.* 1826;1:144-147

79. Froriep R. Beobachtung eines Falles von Mangel der Brustdruse. *Notizen aus dem Gebiete der Natururnd Heilkinde.* 1839;10:9-14

80. Freire-Maia N, Chautard EA, Opitz JM, et al. The Poland syndrome - clinical and genealogical data, dermatoglyphic analysis, and incidence. *Human Heredity.* 1973;23:97-104

81. McGillivray BC, Lowry RB. Poland syndrome in British Columbia: incidence and reproductive experience of affected persons. *Am J Med Genet.* 1977;1:65-74

82. Merlob P, Schonfeld A, Ovadia Y, et al. Real-time echo-Doppler Duplex Scanner in the evaluation of patients with Poland sequence. *Eur J Obstet Gynecol Reprod Biol.* 1989;32: 103-108

83. Azner JM, Urbano J, Laborda EG, et al. Breast and pectoralis muscle hypoplasia. A mil degree of Poland's syndrome. *Acta Radiologica.* 1996;37:759-762

84. Fokin AA, Robicsek F. Poland's syndrome revisited. *Ann Thorac Surg.* 2002;74:2218-2225

85. Bouvet JP, Leveque D, Bernetieres F, et al. Vascular origin of Poland syndrome. *Eur J Pediatr.* 1978;128:17-26

86. Bavinck JN, Weaver DD. Subclavian artery supply disruption sequence: hypothesis of a vascular etiology for Poland, Klippeil-Feil, and Mobius anomalies. *Am J Med Genet.* 1986;23: 903-918

87. Shamberger RC, Welch KJ, Upton J. Surgical treatment of thoracic deformity in Poland's syndrome. 1989;24:760-765; discussion 766

88. Ireland DC, Takayama N, Flatt AE. Poland's syndrome. *J Bone Joint Surg.* 1976;58:52-58

89. Al-Quattan MM. Classification of hand anomalies in Poland's syndrome. *Br J Plast Surg.* 2001;54:132-136

90. Kuklik M. Poland-Mobius syndrome and disruption spectrum affecting the face and extremities: a review paper and presentation of five cases. *Acta Chir Plast.* 2000;42:95-103

91. Hedge HR, Leung AK. Aplasia of pectoralis major muscle and renal anomalies. *Am J Med Genet.* 1989;32:109-111

92. Pranava VM, Rao PS, Neelachalam A, et al. Poland's syndrome with renal hypertension. *JAPI.* 2000;48:452-453

93. Ahn MI, Park SH, Park YH. Poland's syndrome with lung cancer. A case report. *Acta Radiologica.* 2000;41:432-434

94. Ravitch MM. Poland's syndrome. In: Wada J, Yokoyama M, eds. *Chest Wall Deformities and Their Operative Treatment.* Tokyo: AD Printing Inc; 1990:197-208

95. Fukushima T, Otake T, Yashima R, et al. A case report. Breast cancer in two patients with Poland's syndrome. *Breast Cancer.* 1998;6:127-130

96. Ravitch MM. Congenital deformities of the chest wall. In: Welch KS, Randolph GJ, Ravitch MM, O'Neal JA, Rowel M, eds. *Pediatric Surgery.* Vol I. 4th ed. Chicago: Year Book Medical Publishers Inc; 1986:563-568

97. Shamberger R, Welch KJ. Sternal defects. *Pediatr Surg Unt.* 1990;5:156-164

98. Cantrell HJ, Ravitch MM. A syndrome of congenital defects involving the abdominal wall, sternum, diaphragm, pericardium, and heart. *Surg Gynecol Obstet.* 1958;107:602-614

99. Shao-tsu L. Ectopia cordis congenital. *Thoraxchirurgie.* 1957;5:197-212

100. Fisher H. Fissura sterno congenital mit partieller Bauchspalte. *Disch Z Chir.* 1879;12:367-369

101. Ingelrans P, Debeugny P. [Case of bifidity of the sternum associated with tracheal angiomatosis]. *Ann Chir Infant.* 1965;6:123-128

102. Maier HC, Bortone F. Complete failure of sternal fusion with herniation of pericardium. *J Thorac Surg.* 1949;18: 851-859

SECTION 16

Sports Medicine

# CHAPTER 164

## Preparticipation Evaluation

ERIC SMALL, MD

More than 6 million high school students participate in sports each year. With this many participants, the preparticipation physical evaluation (PPE) is one of the most commonly performed examinations by medical providers. In the past, consistent guidelines for performing the sports physical were lacking. However, the PPE has evolved to allow physicians nationwide to provide quality examinations. In the early 1990s, the American Academy of Family Physicians (AAFP), the American Academy of Pediatrics (AAP), the American Medical Society for Sports Medicine (AMSSM), the American Orthopaedic Society for Sports Medicine (ASSM), and the American Osteopathic Academy of Sports Medicine (AOASM) formed the Preparticipation Examination Task Force to standardize the conduct and content of these examinations. In 1992, the Task Force published recommendations for the PPE based on the consensus of the current literature. These guidelines were updated in 1997, 2002, 2004, and 2010, and serve as the basis for the current PPE.[1]

### GOALS OF THE PPE

The purpose of the PPE is not to disqualify athletes; fewer than 2% are actually disqualified based on the results of the evaluation. Rather, the primary goals of the PPE are to detect conditions that might predispose the athlete to injury, to detect conditions that might be life threatening or disabling, and to meet legal or insurance requirements. The secondary goals are to determine general health, to counsel athletes on health-related issues, and to assess fitness level.[1]

Identifying athletes who may need further diagnostic testing, counseling, and/or rehabilitation is the primary goal of the PPE, but there are a number of other expectations. Sometimes, parents expect the PPE to be a comprehensive evaluation of the athlete's health, including areas that may be considered unrelated to sports participation, such as teenage sexuality, substance abuse, immunizations, behavioral counseling, and others. Parents frequently use the PPE as the only medical evaluation for their child or adolescent, expecting it to be comprehensive.[2] In contrast, many physicians view the PPE as a cursory examination, intended only to detect conditions that might limit or impair athletic endeavors. Because parents and physicians view the evaluation differently, it is critical that parents be clearly advised about the intent of the PPE to clarify its scope and purpose. The most recent PPE manual as well as members of the PPE task force suggest creating and re-establishing a medical home for all athletes.

### METHODS OF CONDUCTING THE PPE

The PPE is typically conducted in 1 of 3 ways: the locker room method, the station method, and the office-based method.[1]

In the locker room method, athletes traditionally are lined up single file while the physician examines each athlete individually. One benefit of this method is that it requires few personnel and can be done with little preparation. However, it affords little privacy for the athlete, is usually noisy so that the physician has a difficult time auscultating the heart and lungs, and is often too brief.

The station method divides the examination into several components with physicians, nurses, athletic trainers, and coaches, each assigned one task. This method is ideally suited for screening large numbers of athletes. Two benefits of this method are its relative efficiency and its high yield in identifying abnormalities. However, this method affords less rapport with athletes and a lack of privacy. Athletes have limited or no opportunity to ask questions of the physicians regarding their own health or other medical or personal issues.

The individual office-based method has the advantages of an established physician–patient relationship in which the past medical history is known and continuity of care is fostered. The disadvantages can include a lack of consistency among physicians, potential unfamiliarity with the sport and disqualifying conditions by the physician, and the lack of cost-effectiveness.

## TIMING

Ideally, the PPE is performed early enough in the preseason to ensure that athletes who have medical problems can be thoroughly evaluated and treated, but not so early that intervening injuries are likely to occur. Most sources recommend that the evaluation take place at least 4 to 6 weeks before the first scheduled practice.

The AAP recommends yearly health supervisions for adolescents. In the *Preparticipation Physical Evaluation*, 4/e, PPE is recommended every year.[1] Most sources recommend that the PPE be conducted before the beginning of each new level of competition (ie, middle school or junior high, high school, and college) with annual updates of the history and targeted physical examinations for areas of concern. Most state high school athletic associations require annual evaluations. A recent survey of all 50 states and the District of Columbia found that 65% of states require annual examination of all athletes competing in high school sports.

## HISTORY

As with any health evaluation, the history identifies most potential problems for young athletes.[2–4] The key to identifying these problems is the questionnaire that systematically screens for conditions that frequently cause problems in athletes or that could lead to sudden death during athletic activity. Table 164-1 lists some of the most important questions to ask in the examination. Note that the PPE forms provided by state high school athletic associations do not incorporate all of the screening questions recommended by the Preparticipation Examination Task Force. It is recommended that the Task Force form be used, it is available on the AAP Web site at www.aap.org.

Most experts agree that despite the best screening of athletes for sudden death, illness in only a few who die could have been detected through the screening history and physical examination. However, cardiovascular screening questions are increasingly being considered an important part of the PPE.

Athletes typically complete their history forms without input from their parents. One study showed that only 40% of PPE forms matched when filled out independently by parent and child. It is essential that both the athlete and the parents complete the form together, so that a thorough and accurate history is obtained. Adolescent privacy about certain topics, such as sexuality and substance abuse, should be respected.

## PHYSICAL EXAMINATION

Two key components of the physical examination identify most athletes who warrant further evaluation or disqualification. The musculoskeletal history and physical examination detects most of the problems noted on the evaluation and should be the focus of any preparticipation screening. The medical evaluation form recommended by the Preparticipation Examination Task Force is shown in Figure 164-1.

## CARDIOVASCULAR EXAMINATION

The cardiovascular examination should include evaluation of peripheral pulses, murmurs, and blood pressure. Table 164-2 summarizes important aspects of the screening cardiovascular examination. Note that all diastolic murmurs and grade 3/6 systolic murmurs warrant further evaluation. Hypertrophic cardiomyopathy (HCM) may produce a systolic murmur that cannot be distinguished from an innocent murmur. The murmur of HCM increases in intensity with a Valsalva maneuver (decreased ventricular filling, increased obstruction) and decreases with squatting (increased ventricular filling, decreased obstruction). Note that it will also increase in intensity when the athlete moves from a squatting to standing position.

Blood pressures obtained during the PPE are often elevated; sometimes, this is due to the use of a blood pressure cuff that is too small, particularly in large adolescents. However, at times, the athlete's blood pressure is truly elevated, given that a table with age-based norms is used. Hypertension is rarely severe enough to disqualify an athlete from participation, but it needs to be identified and followed by the athlete's primary care

**Table 164-1**

**Medical History Questions**

| *Question* | *Reason* |
|---|---|
| 1. Injury or illness since last checkup? | Targets potential physical examination concerns |
| 2. Chronic illnesses, hospitalizations, or surgeries? | Identifies potential counseling or rehabilitation issues |
| 3. Any medications or supplements of any type? | Identifies drugs that may inhibit or interfere with sports participation |
| 4. Allergies to medications, insects, food? | Alerts physicians and trainers for potential allergic reactions |
| 5. Dizziness, passed out, chest pain with exercise; history of sudden death in a close relative <50 years old? | Identifies potential causes of sudden death due to cardiovascular problems |
| 6. History of hypertension or murmur? | Targets cardiovascular concerns |
| 7. Ever been restricted from sports by physician? | Identifies potential disqualifying problems |
| 8. Any skin problems? | Identifies potential transmittable disease during contact |
| 9. Concussion, "knocked out," unconsciousness, or memory loss, seizure, or severe/frequent headache? | Targets neurologic concerns |
| 10. Stinger, burner, pinched nerve, numbness/tingling in extremities? | Targets neurologic concerns |
| 11. Problems while exercising in the heat? | Targets heat illness concerns |
| 12. Asthma, allergies, wheezing, difficulty breathing, chest pain? | Identifies potential for exercise-induced asthma |
| 13. Special equipment or devices not usually used in your sport? | Identifies potential concerns for physician follow-up |
| 14. Glasses, contacts, or vision or eye problems? | Identifies ophthalmologic concerns |
| 15. Strain, sprain, fracture, joint pain, or swelling? | Identifies potential musculoskeletal problems |
| 16. Concerns about weight, do you lose weight regularly for your sport? | Identifies potential disordered eating |
| 17. Feel stressed out? | Clue to ask follow-up questions regarding drug use, eating problems, sexuality, home/school problems |
| 18. Recent immunizations (tetanus, measles, hepatitis B, chickenpox) | Health maintenance issues |
| 19. Female only: menstrual history | Identifies oligomenorrhea and amenorrhea and potential risk for poor nutrition, stress fractures |

physician. Recent cardiovascular research performed in Italy shows that screening may prevent sudden death due to cardiomyopathy.[5]

At this time, there is no role for screening electrocardiogram and echocardiogram.[1]

## MUSCULOSKELETAL EXAMINATION

The musculoskeletal examination is of particular importance because it typically accounts for 50% of the abnormal physical findings identified on the PPE. The examination should focus on areas previously injured or on areas that are symptomatic. Ninety-two percent of orthopaedic injuries are detected on the basis of the history alone.[6] The 2-minute orthopaedic screening examination is a quick screening for detecting musculoskeletal problems in asymptomatic individuals. Box 164-1 lists the components of this examination.

Some authorities recommend a sport-specific approach to the physical examination.[7] This method emphasizes those areas that are most commonly injured or diseased in each specific sport (Box 164-2). For example, a swimmer's examination would focus on the shoulders and ears (otitis externa), whereas a football player's exam should focus on concussions (neurologic status) and shoulder injuries.

PREPARTICIPATION PHYSICAL EVALUATION

# PHYSICAL EXAMINATION FORM

Name ______________________________ Date of birth ______________

PHYSICIAN REMINDERS

1. Consider additional questions on more sensitive issues
   - Do you feel stressed out or under a lot of pressure?
   - Do you ever feel sad, hopeless, depressed, or anxious?
   - Do you feel safe at your home or residence?
   - Have you ever tried cigarettes, chewing tobacco, snuff, or dip?
   - During the past 30 days, did you use chewing tobacco, snuff, or dip?
   - Do you drink alcohol or use any other drugs?
   - Have you ever taken anabolic steroids or used any other performance supplement?
   - Have you ever taken any supplements to help you gain or lose weight or improve your performance?
   - Do you wear a seat belt, use a helmet, and use condoms?
2. Consider reviewing questions on cardiovascular symptoms (questions 5–14).

| EXAMINATION | | |
|---|---|---|
| Height Weight | ☐ Male ☐ Female | |
| BP / ( / ) Pulse | Vision R 20/ L 20/ | Corrected ☐ Y ☐ N |
| **MEDICAL** | **NORMAL** | **ABNORMAL FINDINGS** |
| Appearance<br>• Marfan stigmata (kyphoscoliosis, high-arched palate, pectus excavatum, arachnodactyly, arm span > height, hyperlaxity, myopia, MVP, aortic insufficiency) | | |
| Eyes/ears/nose/throat<br>• Pupils equal<br>• Hearing | | |
| Lymph nodes | | |
| Heart[a]<br>• Murmurs (auscultation standing, supine, +/- Valsalva)<br>• Location of point of maximal impulse (PMI) | | |
| Pulses<br>• Simultaneous femoral and radial pulses | | |
| Lungs | | |
| Abdomen | | |
| Genitourinary (males only)[b] | | |
| Skin<br>• HSV, lesions suggestive of MRSA, tinea corporis | | |
| Neurologic[c] | | |
| **MUSCULOSKELETAL** | | |
| Neck | | |
| Back | | |
| Shoulder/arm | | |
| Elbow/forearm | | |
| Wrist/hand/fingers | | |
| Hip/thigh | | |
| Knee | | |
| Leg/ankle | | |
| Foot/toes | | |
| Functional<br>• Duck-walk, single leg hop | | |

[a]Consider ECG, echocardiogram, and referral to cardiology for abnormal cardiac history or exam.
[b]Consider GU exam if in private setting. Having third party present is recommended.
[c]Consider cognitive evaluation or baseline neuropsychiatric testing if a history of significant concussion.

☐ Cleared for all sports without restriction

☐ Cleared for all sports without restriction with recommendations for further evaluation or treatment for ______________________________

☐ Not cleared

- ☐ Pending further evaluation
- ☐ For any sports
- ☐ For certain sports ______________________________

Reason ______________________________

Recommendations ______________________________

**I have examined the above-named student and completed the preparticipation physical evaluation. The athlete does not present apparent clinical contraindications to practice and participate in the sport(s) as outlined above. A copy of the physical exam is on record in my office and can be made available to the school at the request of the parents. If conditions arise after the athlete has been cleared for participation, the physician may rescind the clearance until the problem is resolved and the potential consequences are completely explained to the athlete (and parents/guardians).**

Name of physician (print/type) ______________________________ Date ______________

Address ______________________________ Phone ______________

Signature of physician ______________________________, MD or DO



FIGURE 164-1 Medical evaluation form: physical examination.

**Table 164-2**

**Cardiovascular Screening in Athletes**

| *Condition* | *Cardiovascular Examination* | *Abnormality* |
|---|---|---|
| Hypertension | Blood pressure | Varies with age—See Chapter 118, Hypertension |
| Coarctation of aorta | Femoral pulses | Decreased intensity of pulse |
| Hypertrophic cardiomyopathy | Auscultation with provocative maneuvers (standing, supine, Valsalva) | Systolic ejection murmur that intensifies with standing or Valsalva maneuver |
| Marfan syndrome | Auscultation | Aortic (decrescendo diastolic murmur) or mitral insufficiency (holosystolic murmur) |

Based on Maron BJ, Thompson PO, Puffer JC. Cardiovascular preparticipation screening of competitive athletes: A Statement from the Sudden Death Committee [clinical cardiology] and Congenital Cardiac Defects Committee [cardiovascular disease in the young] American Heart Association. *Circulation* 1996;94:850–856.

**Box 164-1**

***The General Musculoskeletal Screening Examination***

1. Inspection, athlete standing, facing toward examiner (symmetry of trunk, upper extremities);
2. Forward flexion, extension, rotation, lateral flexion of neck (range of motion, cervical spine);
3. Resisted shoulder shrug (strength, trapezius);
4. Resisted shoulder abduction (strength, deltoid);
5. Internal and external rotation of shoulder (range of motion, glenohumeral joint);
6. Extension and flexion of elbow (range of motion, elbow);
7. Pronation and supination of elbow (range of motion, elbow and wrist);
8. Clench fist, then spread fingers (range of motion, hand and fingers);
9. "Duck walk" 4 steps (motion of hip, knee, and ankle; strength; balance);
10. Inspection, athlete facing away from examiner (symmetry of trunk, upper extremities);
11. Back extension, knees straight (spondylolysis/ spondylolisthesis);
12. Back flexion with knees straight, facing toward and away from examiner (range of motion, thoracic and lumbosacral spine; spine curvature; hamstring flexibility);
13. Inspection of lower extremities, contraction of quadriceps muscles (alignment, symmetry);
14. Standing on toes, then on heels (symmetry, calf; strength; balance).

**Box 164-2**

***Special Considerations for the Examination of Injured or Symptomatic Joints***

- Inspect for visual deformity, muscle mass, asymmetry, and swelling
- Palpate for localized areas of tenderness, warmth, and effusion
- Assess range of motion (eg, an athlete with hip pain should be tested for loss of internal rotation and abduction, which can be seen in slipped capital femoral epiphysis and Legg-Calvé-Perthes disease)
- Test neurovascular status by evaluating muscle strength, sensation, reflexes, and pulses of the involved limb (eg, an athlete with a history of burners should undergo complete neurovascular testing of the neck and upper extremities)
- Test joint stability (eg, an athlete with knee pain should undergo tests for valgus and varus stress, the Lachman test, and the posterior drawer test)

## LABORATORY STUDIES

Laboratory studies have not been shown to be cost-effective or warranted in young athletes who are asymptomatic. Obtaining a routine urinalysis and hematocrit on all athletes has been largely abandoned, as these tests do not identify athletes who require disqualification and have a high rate of false-positive results. Similarly, electrocardiogram, echocardiogram, and stress testing are not recommended as screening tests for asymptomatic individuals because of the high rate of false-positive tests and their high costs.

## SPORTS CLASSIFICATION

Sports are classified based on the likelihood of collision injury and on the strenuousness of exercise. These classifications are used to guide physicians on the risk of injury and the degree of cardiopulmonary fitness required. The AAP has established classification guidelines that can be found in Table 164-3 and Table 164-4.

## CLEARANCE TO PLAY

Few athletes are disqualified from activity based on conditions identified during the PPE. Table 164-5 lists the most current recommendations regarding medical conditions and contraindications to participation. This table is designed to be understood by medical and nonmedical personnel. In the "Explanation" section, "needs evaluation" means that a physician with appropriate knowledge and experience should assess the safety of a given sport for an athlete with the listed medical condition. Unless otherwise noted, this is because of the variability of the severity of the disease or of the risk of injury among the specific sports, or both. It is important to work with athletes to find safe, enjoyable sports in which they can participate and not eliminate all sports participation, depending on the condition that is detected. For specific cardiac conditions, refer to the proceedings of the 26th Bethesda Conference on cardiovascular abnormalities and participation in sports.[8] Figure 164-2 is a sample Clearance to Return to Play form.

Occasionally, an athlete or parent will disagree with a physician's recommendation for restricting participation

**Table 164-3**

**Sport Classification by Contact**

| *Contact/Collision* | *Limited Contact* | *Noncontact* |
|---|---|---|
| Basketball | Baseball | Archery |
| Boxing | Bicycling | Badminton |
| Diving | Cheerleading | Body building |
| Field hockey | Canoeing/kayaking (white water) | Canoeing/kayaking (flat water) |
| Football (flag, tackle) | Fencing | Crew/rowing |
| Ice hockey | Field (high jump, pole vault) | Curling |
| Lacrosse | Floor hockey | Dancing |
| Martial arts | Gymnastics | Field events (discus, javelin, shot put) |
| Rodeo | Handball | Golf |
| Rugby | Horseback riding | Orienteering |
| Ski jumping | Racquetball | Power lifting |
| Soccer | Skating (ice, in-line, roller) | Race walking |
| Team handball | Skiing (downhill, water) | Riflery |
| Water polo | Softball | Rope jumping |
| Wrestling | Squash | Running |
| | Ultimate frisbee | Sailing |
| | Volleyball | Scuba diving |
| | Windsurfing/surfing | Strength training |
| | | Swimming |
| | | Table tennis |
| | | Tennis |
| | | Track |
| | | Weightlifting |

Adapted from American Academy of Pediatrics Committee on Sports Medicine and Fitness. Medical conditions affecting sports participation. *Pediatrics*. 1994;94:757-760.

**Table 164-4**

**Sports Classification by Intensity**

| *High to Moderate Dynamic and Static Intensity* | *High to Moderate Dynamic and Low Static Intensity* | *High to Moderate Static and Low Dynamic Intensity* | *Low Dynamic and Low Intensity* |
|---|---|---|---|
| Boxing | Badminton | Archery | Bowling |
| Crew/rowing | Baseball | Auto racing | Cricket |
| Cross-country skiing | Basketball | Diving | Curling |
| Cycling | Field hockey | Equestrian | Golf |
| Downhill skiing | Lacrosse | Field events (jumping) | Riflery |
| Fencing | Orienteering | Field events (throwing) | |
| Football | Ping-pong | Gymnastics | |
| Ice hockey | Race walking | Karate or judo | |
| Rugby | Racquetball | Motorcycling | |
| Running (sprint) | Soccer | Rodeoing | |
| Speed skating | Squash | Sailing | |
| Water polo | Swimming | Ski jumping | |
| Wrestling | Tennis | Water skiing | |
| | Volleyball | Weightlifting | |

Adapted from American Academy of Pediatrics Committee on Sports Medicine and Fitness: Medical conditions affecting sports participation. *Pediatrics*. 1994;94:757–760.

**Table 164-5**

**Medical Conditions and Sports Participation**

| *Condition* | *Participate?* | *Explanation* |
|---|---|---|
| Atlantoaxial instability (instability of the joint between cervical vertebrae 1 and 2) | Qualified yes | Athlete needs evaluation to assess risk of spinal cord injury during sports participation. |
| Bleeding disorder | Qualified yes | Athlete needs evaluation. |
| Cardiovacular diseases | | |
| • Carditis (inflammation of the heart) | No | Carditis may result in sudden death with exertion. |
| • Hypertension (high blood pressure) | Qualified yes | Those with significant essential (unexplained) hypertension should avoid weight and power lifting, body building, and strength training. Those with secondary hypertension (hypertension caused by a previously identified disease), or severe essential hypertension, need evaluation. |
| • Congenital heart disease (structural heart defects present at birth) | Qualified yes | Those with mild forms may participate fully; those with moderate or severe forms, or who have undergone surgery, need evaluation. |
| • Dysrhythmia (irregular heart rhythm) | Qualified yes | Athlete needs evaluation because some types require therapy or make certain sports dangerous, or both. |

*(Continued)*

**Table 164-5 (Continued)**

| *Condition* | *Participate?* | *Explanation* |
|---|---|---|
| • Mitral valve prolapse (abnormal heart valve) | Qualified yes | Those with symptoms (chest pain, symptoms of possible dysrhythmia), or evidence of mitral regurgitation (leaking) on physical examination need evaluation. All others may participate fully. |
| • Heart murmur | Qualified yes | If the murmur is innocent (does not indicate heart disease), full participation is permitted. Otherwise the athlete needs evaluation (see "Congenital heart disease" and "Mitral valve prolapse" previously). |
| Cerebral palsy | Qualified yes | Athlete needs evaluation. |
| Diabetes mellitus | Yes | All sports can be played with proper attention to diet, hydration, and insulin therapy. Particular attention is needed for activities that last 30 minutes or more. |
| Diarrhea | Qualified no | Unless disease is mild, no participation is permitted, because diarrhea may increase the risk of dehydration and heat illness. See "Fever" below. |
| Eating disorders<br>• Anorexia nervosa<br>• Bulimia nervosa | Qualified yes | These patients need both medical and psychiatric assessment before participation. |
| Eyes<br>• Functionally 1-eyed athlete<br>• Loss of an eye<br>• Detached retina<br>• Previous eye surgery or serious eye injury | Qualified yes | A functionally 1-eyed athlete has a best corrected visual acuity of <20/40 in the worse eye. These athletes would suffer significant disability if the better eye was seriously injured as would those with loss of an eye. Some athletes who have previously undergone eye surgery or had a serious eye injury may have an increased risk of injury because of weakened eye tissue. Availability of eye guards approved by the American Society of Testing Materials (ASTM) and other protective equipment may allow participation in most sports, but this must be judged on an individual basis. |
| Fever | No | Fever can increase cardiopulmonary effort, reduce maximum exercise capacity, make heat illness more likely, and increase orthostatic hypotension during exercise. Fever may rarely accompany myocarditis or other infections that may make exercise dangerous. |
| Heat illness, history of | Qualified yes | Because of the increased likelihood of recurrence, the athlete needs individual assessment to determine the presence of predisposing conditions and to arrange a prevention strategy. |
| HIV infection | Yes | Because of the apparent minimal risk to others, all sports may be played that the state of health allows. In all athletes, skin lesions should be properly covered, and athletic personnel should use universal precautions when handling blood or body fluids with visible blood. |
| Kidney: absence of 1 | Qualified yes | Athlete needs individual assessment for contact/collision and limited contact sports. |
| Liver: enlarged | Qualified yes | If the liver is acutely enlarged, participation should be avoided because of risk of rupture. If the liver is chronically enlarged, individual assessment is needed before collision/contact or limited contact sports are played. |
| Malignancy | Qualified yes | Athlete needs individual assessment. |

*(Continued)*

**Table 164-5 (Continued)**

| *Condition* | *Participate?* | *Explanation* |
|---|---|---|
| Musculoskeletal disorders | Qualified yes | Athlete needs individual assessment. |
| Neurologic | | |
| History of serious head or spine trauma, severe or repeated, concussions, or craniotomy | Qualified yes | Athlete needs individual assessment for collision/contact or limited contact sports, and also for noncontact sports if there are deficits in judgment or cognition. Recent research supports a conservative approach to management of concussions. Risk of convulsion during participation is minimal. |
| Convulsive disorder, well controlled | Yes | |
| Convulsive disorder, poorly controlled | Qualified yes | Athlete needs individual assessment for collision/contact or limited contact sports. Avoid the following noncontact sports: archery, riflery, swimming, weight or power lifting, strength training, or sports involving heights. In these sports, occurrence of a convulsion may be a risk to self or others. |
| Obesity | Qualified yes | Because of the risk of heat illness, obese persons need careful acclimatization and hydration. |
| Organ transplant recipient | Qualified yes | Athlete needs individual assessment. |
| Ovary: absence | | Risk of severe injury to the remaining ovary is minimal. |
| Respiratory | | |
| • Pulmonary compromise including cystic fibrosis | | Athlete needs individual assessment, but generally all sports may be played if oxygenation remains satisfactory during a graded exercise test. Patients with cystic fibrosis need acclimatization and good hydration to reduce the risk of heat illness. |
| • Asthma | Yes | With proper medication and education, only athletes with the most severe asthma will have to modify their participation. |
| • Acute upper respiratory infection | Qualified yes | Upper respiratory obstruction may affect pulmonary function. Athlete needs individual assessment for all but mild diseases. See "Fever" previously. |
| Sickle cell disease | Qualified yes | Athlete needs individual assessment. In general if status of the illness permits, all but high exertion, collision/contact sports may be played. Overheating, dehydration, and chilling must be avoided. |
| Sickle cell trait | Yes | It is unlikely that individuals with sickle cell trait (AS) have an increased risk of sudden death or other medical problems during athletic participation except under the most extreme condition of heat, humidity, and possibly increased altitude. These individuals, like all athletes, should be carefully conditioned, acclimatized, and hydrated to reduce any possible risk. |
| Skin: boils, herpes simplex, impetigo, scabies, molluscum contagiosum | Qualified yes | While the patient is contagious, participation in gymnastics with mats, martial arts, wrestling, or other collision/contact or limited contact sports is not allowed. Herpes simplex virus probably is not transmitted via mats. |
| Spleen, enlarged | Qualified yes | Patients with acutely enlarged spleens should avoid all sports because of risk of rupture. Those with chronically enlarged spleens need individual assessment before playing collision/contact or limited contact sports. |
| Testicle: absent or undescended | Yes | Certain sports may require a protective cup. |

Adapted from American Academy of Pediatrics Committee on Sports Medicine and Fitness. Medical conditions affecting sports participation. *Pediatrics*. 1994;94:757-760.

PREPARTICIPATION PHYSICAL EVALUATION

**CLEARANCE FORM**

Name ______________________ Sex ☐ M ☐ F Age __________ Date of birth __________

☐ Cleared for all sports without restriction

☐ Cleared for all sports without restriction with recommendations for further evaluation or treatment for ______________________

☐ Not cleared

☐ Pending further evaluation

☐ For any sports

☐ For certain sports ______________________

Reason ______________________

Recommendations ______________________

**I have examined the above-named student and completed the preparticipation physical evaluation. The athlete does not present apparent clinical contraindications to practice and participate in the sport(s) as outlined above. A copy of the physical exam is on record in my office and can be made available to the school at the request of the parents. If conditions arise after the athlete has been cleared for participation, the physician may rescind the clearance until the problem is resolved and the potential consequences are completely explained to the athlete (and parents/guardians).**

Name of physician (print/type) ______________________ Date __________

Address ______________________ Phone __________

Signature of physician ______________________, MD or DO

**EMERGENCY INFORMATION**

Allergies ______________________

Other information ______________________



**FIGURE 164-2** Sample Clearance to Return to Play form.

in a particular sport. In these cases, it is important to fully explain the reasons for the recommendation and consider having the athlete and parent sign a document acknowledging that this discussion occurred and that they were informed of the risks. Athletes who request a second opinion should be encouraged to do so. Ultimately, the team physician is responsible for ensuring that athletes are able to participate safely and without undue risk of injury.

## SPECIAL CONSIDERATIONS

### NUTRITIONAL SUPPLEMENTS

Sports supplements have become a billion-dollar industry. Athletes as young as 11 are taking performance-enhancing supplements. Sports supplements contain impurities and, when taken inappropriately, may lead to adverse side effects ranging from muscle cramps, dehydration, abdominal bloating, tachycardia, arrhythmia, and even death. Supplement use should be discouraged. If a young athlete is taking them, advice should be given as to ill effects such as muscle cramping, dehydration, and palpitations. The PPE is an ideal time to briefly question about supplement use.

### OBESITY

Childhood obesity has reached epidemic proportions. Up to 30% of children are obese; many of these youngsters are seeking to participate in sports. Obesity is not a contraindication to sports participation unless there is a comorbid finding such as severe hypertension. Sports participation should be encouraged for the obese adolescent.

### CONCUSSION

A history of concussions should be addressed during the PPE. As a result of recent research, consensus about classifying concussions has been revised and the system of using 3 grades of severity is no longer being used by many practitioners. The classification system now includes 2 classifications: simple and complicated.[9] Complicated includes amnesia, loss of consciousness, seizure, or prolonged symptoms. With repeated concussion or a complicated concussion, neuropsychological testing is recommended. Patients must meet 3 criteria to return to play: asymptomatic at rest, aymptomatic with exercise, and no neurocognitive deficits (memory loss, concentration problems, fatigue, "fogginess," or confusion). Concussion management is also discussed in Chapter 130, Central Nervous System Trauma.

### THE MEDICAL HOME

Adolescents are an underserved population in terms of comprehensive primary care. Often, the only contact with the medical system is the PPE. It is important to refer all young athletes to a primary care provider for routine care and for follow-up of any ongoing medical conditions. If the primary care provider is performing the PPE, a more comprehesive psychosocial assessment should be performed as part of the medical history.

## KEY SUMMARY POINTS

1. The PPE is performed to prevent injury and assess medical conditions; it is not performed to disqualify an athlete.
2. The PPE should be done by one provider even if there is a mass screening.
3. Sudden cardiac death in young athletes is a rare event, but a history of syncope, chest pain with exercise, or family history of sudden death under age 50 should be evaluated.
4. The musculoskeletal history and physical examination provide the highest yield on finding problems.
5. Concussion, heat injury, and nutritional supplement use are topics that need to be discussed and emphasized during the PPE. Box 164-3 lists answers to questions parents may have.

### Box 164-3

#### *Partnering with Parents*

***My son had a preparticipation physical examination for participating in football last year. Does he still need to see his physician this year?***
While the PPE is often quite comprehensive, it was never designed to take the place of a regular physician visit. The setting or time allocation for the PPE is often not conducive to discussions of health issues that are of primary importance during the adolescent years, such as drug and alcohol use, smoking, sexual activity education, safety issues, and diagnosis of depression.

***When should my child have a PPE, relative to the beginning of an athletic season?***
The best time for the PPE is about 4 to 6 weeks before the beginning of the athletic season. This allows enough time for thorough evaluations, consultations, and rehabilitation of any identified musculoskeletal injuries.

***Do I need to attend the PPE with my child?***
Although you may not be asked to attend the PPE with your child, it is very important that you review the accuracy and completeness of the past medical history and family history that is given. Your child may not know or remember some of the history. Most of the important information obtained in the PPE is obtained from the history.

***How often will my son or daughter need a PPE?***
The frequency of required evaluations varies by state. Most commonly, a physical evaluation is required every year. To determine the requirements of your state, check with the school district or the state high school athletic association.

***Will my child need to undergo any laboratory or radiographic studies at the PPE?***
Routine laboratory studies and radiographs are not generally indicated. Based on information obtained during the history and physical examination, however, further studies may be indicated.

## REFERENCES

1. American Academy of Family Physicians, American Academy of Pediatrics, American College of Sports Medicine, American Medical Society for Sports Medicine, American Orthopaedic Society for Sports Medicine, American Osteopathic Academy

of Sports Medicine. *The Preparticipation Physical Evaluation*. 4th ed. Elk Grove Village, IL: American Academy of Pediatrics; 2010

2. Krowchuk DP, Krowchuk HV, Hunter M, et al. Parents' knowledge of the purposes and content of the preparticipation physical examination. *Arch Pediatr Adolesc Med.* 1995;149(6):L653–L657

3. Corrado D, Basso C, Pavei A, Michieli P, Schiavon M, Thiene G. Trends in sudden cardiovascular death in young competitive athletes after implementation of a preparticipation screening program. *JAMA.* 2006;296(13):1593–1601

4. Koester MC, Amundson Cl. Preparticipation screening of high school athletes: are recommendations enough? *Phys Sportsmed*. 2003;31(3):35–38

5. Corrado D, Basso C, Pavei A, Michieli P, Schiavon M, Thiene G. Trends in sudden cardiovascular death in young competitive athletes after implementation of a preparticipation screening program. *JAMA.* 2006;296(13):1593–1601

6. High Blood Pressure Education Working Group on Hypertension Control in Children and Adolescents. Update on the 1987 task force report on high blood pressure in children and adolescents: a working group report on the National High Blood Pressure Education Program. *Pediatrics.* 1996;98 (4 pt 1):649–658

7. Smith J, Laskowski ER. The preparticipation physical examination: Mayo Clinic experience with 2,739 examinations. *Mayo Clinic Proc.* 1998;73(5):419–429

8. 26th Bethesda Conference: recommendations for determining eligibility for competition in athletes with cardiovascular abnormalities. *Med Sci Sports Exerc.* 1994;26(10 suppl):S223–S283

9. McCrory P, Johnston K, Meeuwisse W, et al. Summary and agreement statement report of the 2nd International Conference on Concussion in Sport, Prague 2004. *Br J Sports Med.* 2005;39:196–204

# CHAPTER 165

# Rehabilitation and Strength Training

GREGORY J. MULFORD, MD • MICHAL E. EISENBERG, MD

## BASIC PRINCIPLES OF REHABILITATION FOR ADOLESCENTS

There are 5 phases of rehabilitation that provide a rational and sequential approach to assessing the progress of an athlete with an acute injury and that assist in determining when an athlete can return to play. These are summarized in Box 165-1[1] and discussed in the section that follows. The rehabilitation program should be based on physiological healing of tissues and restoration of function, as presented in Table 165-1.[2]

### DECREASE PAIN AND CONTROL INFLAMMATION

The initial phase of treatment is to control tissue damage and minimize the inflammatory reaction and associated pain that occur following an acute musculoskeletal injury. The PRICE (Protection, Relative rest, Ice, Compression, Elevation) approach, a variation of the familiar RICE (Rest, Ice, Compression, Elevation) paradigm for the initial management of acute musculoskeletal injuries, is used in this phase.[1]

Immediately following an acute musculoskeletal injury, the affected area should be protected by splinting, bracing, wrapping, or taping. Most ligamentous or musculoskeletal injuries do not require rigid, nonremovable casting, which is usually avoided to minimize the negative effects of immobilization. The period of muscle-tendon immobilization should usually be less than a week in order to limit the extent of undesirable connective tissue proliferation at the site of the injury.[2] Crutch ambulation (usually weight bearing as tolerated) for lower extremity injuries is helpful until a normal, pain-free gait pattern is possible. Bracing should stabilize and protect the specific area involved while allowing normal motion of other joints and body areas. The same brace that is used to facilitate early protective motion can often also serve to facilitate return to functional activities later in the rehabilitation process.

> **Box 165-1**
>
> ***Phases of Sports Rehabilitation***
>
> - Resolving pain and inflammation
> - Restoring range of motion
> - Strengthening
> - Proprioceptive training
> - Sports/task-specific activities

Rest should be prescribed carefully in order to prevent or minimize deconditioning and the numerous negative effects of bed rest and immobility. Relative rest serves to protect and facilitate the healing process of injured structures while preventing deconditioning during recovery and the rehabilitation process. Deconditioning leads to fatigue, resulting in decreased neuromuscular functioning and joint control, thereby placing a greater load on the static stabilizers (ie, the ligaments and joint capsules), thus increasing the risk for further injury. Cardiovascular conditioning can be safely and effectively accomplished by utilizing exercises that protect the injured area while achieving aerobic and anaerobic intensities, durations, and frequencies similar to those the athlete had been training at prior to the acute injury.

Ice is a cooling modality that helps reduce pain, swelling, inflammation, and muscle spasm when applied immediately following an injury. Cooling of tissues results in vasoconstriction, reduction of edema, decreased release of vasoactive and pain-sensitizing chemicals (eg, bradykinins, leukotrienes), and decreased conduction of nerve fibers. Ice applied intermittently at 10-minute intervals several times per day has been shown to provide effective cooling of tissues.[3]

Compression also serves to limit swelling and edema in the injured area. Wrapping with an elastic bandage or use of various compressive braces, sleeves, stockings, or garments is useful in providing proper compression to injured tissues. Care must be taken to avoid excessive pressure over bony prominences, superficial nerves, or blood vessels to minimize potential adverse events.[4] Devices that combine icing with compression are very useful and effective in the postinjury and postoperative rehabilitation of musculoskeletal injuries.[1]

Elevation is another means to control postinjury swelling. The injured limb should be elevated above the level of the heart to optimally assist with venous and lymphatic drainage and control of edema. The injured body part should not be kept in a dependent position

**Table 165-1**

**Guidelines for Rehabilitation Program Based on Stages of Healing**

| *Time* | *Stages of Healing* | *Rehabilitation Program* | *Therapeutic Goals* |
|---|---|---|---|
| **Phase 1**<br>Days 1-3 | Acute inflammation | Modified activities, ice, compression, elevation; crutches, braces, supportive devices as needed | **1. Control pain and inflammation.**<br>Provide acute management. Protect affected area (protective weight bearing in lower extremity injuries). Reduce swelling and inflammation. |
| Days 4-7 | Repair/substrate/ inflammation | Isometric exercise<br>Gentle "pain-free" active ROM | Minimize hypoxic damage. Gradually increase "pain-free" ROM. |
| **Phase 2**<br>Days 7-21 | Proliferation | Restore active full ROM<br>Gentle progressive resistive exercises | **2. Promote healing.**<br>Decrease protected status as indicated and tolerated.<br>Reduce muscle atrophy. Improve ROM, flexibility, and strength. |
| **Phase 3**<br>Weeks 3-6 | Healing and maturation | Functional activities as tolerated<br>More complex movements<br>Progressive loading (ie, cycling, light weights) as tolerated | **3. Restore function.**<br>Continue to restore ROM and strength.<br>Restore proper muscle activation and biomechanics.<br>Improve proprioception and endurance. |
| **Phases 4 and 5**<br>Week 6-6 months | Tissue remodeling | Sport-specific training<br>Simulate demands of sport/activity<br>Coordination and balance exercises<br>Eccentric loading exercises | **4. Return to activities and sports.**<br>Restore form and function.<br>Improve conditioning.<br>Return to play/sport.<br>**5. Prevent future injury.**<br>Use protective equipment. Practice injury prevention exercises/programs. |

ROM, range of motion.

Adapted from Jarvinen TAH, Jarvinen TLN, Kaariainen M, et al. Muscle injuries: biology and treatment. *Am J Sports Med*. 2005;33(5): 745-764, reprinted by permission of SAGE Publications

in order to limit the pooling of edema and inflammatory and post-traumatic products.

Short duration use of nonsteroidal anti-inflammatory medications (NSAIDs), if not contraindicated for other reasons, can also assist in reducing inflammation and pain. However, NSAIDs may interfere with normal tissue healing, and prolonged or excessive use can lead to gastrointestinal, renal, and hepatic problems. Long-term use of NSAIDs is not indicated for children or adolescents, and use in order to enable an athlete to compete should be discouraged.[5]

## RESTORE NORMAL/SYMMETRIC RANGE OF MOTION

Pain and swelling can inhibit motion or produce altered movement patterns. In the early stages of rehabilitation, pain-free movement of a joint and gentle stretching and mobilization of joints and soft tissues are encouraged. Active or active-assisted range of motion (ROM) and non–weight-bearing movements can be done with gravity eliminated or in water at first if pain is severe. As pain and inflammation subside, more aggressive stretching, joint mobilization, and ROM continue until motion and movement patterns are symmetric with the unaffected side.

## RESTORE NORMAL/SYMMETRIC STRENGTH

Strengthening a painful, inflamed limb that lacks normal ROM can delay recovery. In the early postinjury phases, pain-free isometric contractions are encouraged in an effort to minimize muscular atrophy. Isometric contractions involve muscle contractions without any joint or limb movements and should be performed several times throughout the day as tolerated. A simple isometric protocol is to recommend that the athlete perform 10-second contractions, with 10 repetitions, 10 times per day. As the injured area recovers and normal ROM is restored, isotonic strengthening can begin. Isokinetic strengthening has fallen out of favor as a routine method of strength training during the rehabilitation process due to limited functional carry-over and a high potential for injury. Sport-specific strengthening and conditioning programs are important to ensure that the athlete addresses all muscle groups that are integral to performance of his or her sport.

### NEUROMUSCULAR CONTROL (PROPRIOCEPTIVE) RETRAINING

In addition to restoring normal ROM, strength, stability, and aerobic conditioning, dynamic motor control is an important component of a comprehensive rehabilitation program. An injured joint must be stabilized by synchronous and coordinated activation of appropriate muscle groups so that larger, more powerful muscles may safely produce the forces necessary in sporting activities. Many musculoskeletal injuries result in a loss of pro-prioception that may predispose an athlete to recurrent injury. The proprioceptive system needs to be progressively challenged in order for function and performance to improve. Simple proprioceptive training progresses to higher-level activities as tolerated. Proprioceptive training requires a great deal of one-on-one work with a therapist or trainer, and creativity is important to simulate sport-specific movement patterns. Core muscles, which include the abdominals, spine extensors and rotators, and other large proximal muscle groups, are critical in maintaining optimal alignment of the trunk and pelvis; strengthening and stabilizing these core muscle groups is important in rehabilitation and performance enhancement.[5]

### RETURN TO SPORT ACTIVITIES

As the athlete progresses through the phases of the rehabilitation process, the therapist or trainer facilitates the transition to return to sport. As the athlete successfully meets the challenges of the previous, less challenging phases of functional progression, he or she is put through sequentially more challenging activities that simulate the demands of the particular sport. For example, an athlete will be given various drills that include running, cutting, and jumping (and landing), using optimal form and biomechanics. Once the athlete demonstrates the ability to successfully complete the different drills under controlled situations, he or she can advance to more challenging and less controlled competitive situations. This concept is often referred to as functional progressions. Any significant increase in pain, swelling, instability, or loss of function that occurs when an athlete progresses to a higher level of activity during these functional progressions results in having the athlete reduce the level of activity to a lower level that previously did not precipitate such symptoms. When performed properly with adequate supervision, these functional progressions facilitate earlier return to play while avoiding returning athletes to competition prematurely. Return to play criteria include full and pain-free ROM, appropriate aerobic conditioning, normal strength, and a demonstrated ability to perform sports-related skills without pain.[6]

## STRENGTH TRAINING FOR ADOLESCENTS

Strength training is an important component of the rehabilitation process and is one of the most popular and rapidly growing means of enhancing athletic performance. There is continued debate on the proper role of strength training for children and adolescents, but its effectiveness, risks, and methods are well established for adults.[7]

Strength training can be defined as the use of progressive resistance methods to increase the ability to exert or resist force. It is controlled and progressive, using various modalities, such as individual body weight, hydraulics, free weights, weight machines, elastic bands, or other equipment, to generate the resistance needed for increases in strength to occur.

Common questions that arise for parents, pediatricians, coaches, and others caring for children and adolescents include whether young athletes can increase strength with strength training programs; whether strength training is safe for adolescents; and whether strength training will improve athletic performance.

Terms that may be used synonymously with strength training include "weight training" or "resistance training," but these terms should be distinguished from "weight lifting," "power lifting," and "bodybuilding." In contrast to strength training, weight lifting and power lifting include techniques of training at high intensities with the goal of lifting maximal amounts of weight, often competitively. The competitive sport of weight lifting involves 2 lifts, the clean-and-jerk and the snatch, whereas power lifting includes 3 lifts, the squat, bench press, and dead lift. Bodybuilding does not involve competitive lifts. It is an aesthetic sport that relies largely on weight training/resistance exercise to achieve the desired degree of muscular development, size, and symmetry on which success is based.

### SAFETY

The safety of strength training in adolescents is now well documented.[8] Unlike strength training, the sports of weight lifting, power lifting, and bodybuilding are to be avoided by children and young adolescents until Tanner stage 5. These recommendations have been established by the American Academy of Pediatrics (AAP) and the American Orthopaedic Society for Sports Medicine due to an increased risk of musculoskeletal injuries and a risk of acute medical events in young athletes with these competitive activities.[9] Some studies have demonstrated the safety of weight lifting for children and adolescents, noting that proper technique and qualified supervision can provide safe practices for this activity.[10]

Any effective regimen for strength training must be individualized and should include progression of intensity to achieve strength gain beyond that which would be associated with normal growth and development.

Various national leading medical and sports organizations have established position statements on strength training in youth. The AAP originally published a statement by its Committee on Sports Medicine and Fitness in 2001, establishing its support for strength training, as well as recommendations for safety and guidelines[11]; the committee updated the policy statement in 2008.[12] The National Strength and Conditioning Association has published a position statement supporting the concept that children can safely increase strength with an appropriate and supervised strength training program.[13] An evidence-based review of youth experimental resistance training protocols found the training to be "relatively safe."[14] Youth resistance training was also endorsed by the President's Council on Physical Fitness and Sports in 2003.[15]

## BENEFITS

It is clear that adolescents are able to increase muscle strength; a meta-analysis of studies of strength training in children has shown the achievement of increased strength. Preadolescents have been shown to achieve strength gains with strength training, without muscle hypertrophy. Some studies show that increased strength correlates with improved motor skills and sports performance; these have been demonstrated in studies involving the long jump, the vertical jump, and sprint speed. Other studies have shown increased strength, but no improvement in motor performance skills.[8]

Advantages of youth strength training include cardiovascular fitness, improved body composition, stimulus for bone mineralization and increased bone density, improved lipids, and improved psychosocial measures that include increased self-efficacy and general self-esteem. Strength training offers similar benefits as team sports for children and adolescents in the areas of socialization and mental discipline. With an increase in childhood obesity, strength training has the potential to decrease obesity and help reduce the risks of non-insulin-dependent diabetes mellitus and cardiovascular disease.

It was previously believed that early sports-specific specialization was the best method to increase sports performance. However, it now appears that greater sports performance can be achieved by participating in a variety of activities with the development of different skills. Furthermore, strength training itself can help eliminate an emphasis on competitive sports activities, which may discriminate against those youth with poorer motor skills. The American College of Sports Medicine estimates that 50% of overuse injuries in young athletes could be prevented if more emphasis was placed on fundamental fitness and skills rather than sports-specific training.[16]

As children and adolescents spend more time watching television and less time in unstructured physical activity, young athletes are less physically prepared for sports and competition. This has been especially noted in young female athletes, who are particularly susceptible to knee injuries. It has been shown that adolescent athletes who participate in strength training programs have lower injury rates and less rehabilitation time compared with teammates who do not participate in strength training.[17] Furthermore, preseason strength training in adolescents has been shown to reduce sports-related injuries overall and to decrease the number and severity of knee injuries in high school football players.[18]

Recent and ongoing studies continue to investigate the benefits of strength training in adolescents. A study of 12- to 15-year-olds, comparing soccer training alone versus soccer training with strength training, showed that the strength training group had significantly improved strength.[19]

## MISCONCEPTIONS

Various misconceptions about strength training have previously discouraged the athletic community from recommending strength training for adolescents, and some of these misperceptions still persist among parents, coaches, physicians, and athletes. Studies have shown that strength training is relatively safe compared to sports and other regular adolescent activities.[20] One possible source for the commonly held misconception that weight training will stunt growth may be due to the history of children subjected to heavy labor, but there is no evidence that strength training contributes to decreased stature. Another perceived danger is that too much exercise leads to bone loss and increased susceptibility to fracture, but this is refuted in the literature with studies showing increased bone density with proper strength training.[21]

The presumed high risk for injury in adolescent strength training have been based on data from the National Electronic Injury Surveillance System (NEISS).[22] The NEISS reports make nationwide estimates of injuries incurred due to exercise and equipment, and is based on hospital emergency department data. The most commonly reported exercise-related injuries are sprains and strains. These reports, however, do not distinguish between injuries that occur during properly designed and supervised programs versus those involving unsupervised activities or improper use of equipment. The NEISS reports also do not distinguish between injuries due to strength training versus those due to the competitive sports of powerlifting or weightlifting.

The concern for epiphyseal (growth) plate or cartilage damage due to strength training may be related to reports from weight lifting because improper lifting techniques and heavy overhead lifts have resulted in injury to the epiphyseal plate. Strength training programs do not appear to negatively affect linear growth or to have any negative effects on cardiovascular health.[23]

It was previously believed that prepubescent athletes could not derive any benefit from strength training due to insufficient circulating androgens. This early perception of strength training was noted in the AAP position paper of 1983, stating that "prepubertal boys do not significantly improve strength or increase muscle mass in a weight training program because of insufficient circulating androgens."[24] This belief has been disproven, however, and it has been shown that young athletes do gain strength with proper strength training programs. The flawed conclusions of the earlier studies were most likely due to an inadequate intensity and duration of training used in those studies.[25]

Strength training was once believed to contribute to reduced ROM and loss of flexibility, which are important components of optimal performance. However, studies have shown that athletes demonstrate increased flexibility when flexibility training is incorporated into a strength training program.[24]

Currently, 2 main concerns should be considered when embarking on a strength training program. First, unethical coaching and excessive pressure can have a negative influence.[26] Second, the awareness of the potential risk for overuse soft tissue injury seems to be the greatest concern in adolescent strength training.[8] Proper supervision and attention to safety, technique, and training principles can ensure a safe and successful experience.

## GUIDELINES

The 2008 revised statement of the AAP states that strength training can improve sports performance, rehabilitate injuries, prevent injuries, and enhance long-term health (Box 165-2). The recommendation also notes that strength training in the preadolescent and adolescent population can be safe and effective if proper techniques and safety measures are followed.[12] The statement further recommends a medical evaluation before initiating a formal strength training program. The medical evaluation should evaluate for risk factors for injury and review training goals, techniques, and expectations.

**Box 165-2**

***American Academy of Pediatrics 2008 Recommendations for Strength Training***

- Before beginning a formal strength training program, undergo a medical evaluation by a pediatrician and, if indicated, a sports medicine physician.
- Combine aerobic conditioning with resistance training if the goal of the program is general health.
- Strength training programs should include warm-up and cool-down periods.
- Exercises should be learned initially with no load, and then gradually have load added once the skill is learned.
- Before increasing weight or resistance, 8–15 repetitions showing good form should be mastered.
- All muscle groups and full joint range of motion should be incorporated into the exercise program.
- Specific exercises should be stopped until further evaluation if any sign of injury or illness develops.
- Three sets of 15 repetitions of a given exercise maintained over 3 training sessions should be mastered before adding weight.

Adapted from American Academy of Pedatrics Council on Sports Medicine and Fitness. Strength training by children and adolescents. *Pediatrics*. 2008;121(4):835–840.

Strength training programs should begin with low-resistance exercises until correct technique is mastered. Twenty to 30 minutes of exercise are needed to achieve strength gains, 2–3 times per week. Adding weight or increasing the number of repetitions should be continued as strength develops.[11] A glossary of definitions used in strength training is provided in Box 165-3.

## ADVICE ON CHOOSING A STRENGTH TRAINING PROGRAM

Key factors to consider when deciding to initiate a strength training program for young athletes are the psychological and physical preparedness of the individual,

## Box 165-3

### *Common Terms Used in Strength Training*

**Strength training.** The use of resistance methods to increase one's ability to exert or resist force. The training may use free weights, the individual's own body weight, machines, and/or other resistance devices to attain this goal.

**Set.** A group of repetitions separated by scheduled rest periods (eg, 3 sets of 20 reps).

**Reps.** Abbreviation for repetitions.

**One rep max (1RM).** The maximum amount of weight that can be displaced in a single repetition.

**Concentric contraction.** The muscle shortens during contraction (eg, arm curl, leg press).

**Eccentric contraction.** The muscle lengthens during contraction (eg, lowering a weight).

**Isometric contraction.** The muscle length is unchanged during contraction (eg, wall sits).

**Progressive resistive exercises.** An exercise regimen in which the athlete progressively increases the amount of weight lifted and/or the number of repetitions. The more repetitions, the greater the work performed and the greater the endurance development. The more weight lifted, the greater the strength development.

**Weight lifting.** A competitive sport that involves maximum lifting ability. Olympic weight lifting includes the "snatch" and the "clean and jerk."

**Power lifting.** A competitive sport that also involves maximum lifting ability. Power lifting includes the "dead lift," the "squat," and the "bench press."

**Bodybuilding.** A competition in which muscle size, symmetry, and definition are judged.

Reprinted from American Academy of Pediatrics Committee on Sports Medicine and Fitness. Strength training by children and adolescents. *Pediatrics*. 2001;107(6):1470–1472.

such as preparticipation evaluation and minimizing pressure and stress to perform. The young athlete needs to understand that the goals of a strength training program should be to gain strength and thereby increase performance rather than to achieve maximal lifts or increase visible muscle size. Education prior to initiating a strength training program must include an emphasis on safety. Finally, the training program should be tailored to the individual needs and goals of the young athlete.[24]

Strength training programs should be evaluated on the basis of the following features:[25]

- Safety factors are determined by the degree of proper adult supervision. No more than 10 participants should be allocated to a single adult supervisor.
- The training facility should be clean and equipped with weight equipment suitable for young athletes (ie, sized for children or adolescents and with weights in 1- to 5-pound increments). Proper clothing and footwear should be another requirement.
- Initial exercises should begin with simple movements and progress to more complex movements as the athlete masters the simpler tasks. The use of body weight, elastic tubing, and medicine balls should precede and prepare the adolescent for the use of weights and higher-intensity training.
- Each exercise should generally involve sets of 10 to 15 repetitions. A weight is too heavy and should be reduced if the adolescent is unable to do 10 repetitions per set for a given weight while maintaining proper form.
- Strength training programs should meet no more frequently than 3 days per week, with at least 1 day of rest after each session.

**SUMMARY**

Strength training is currently accepted by the medical and sports communities as an important, safe, and effective component of physical training for young athletes. Current guidelines and recommendations support integrating strength training into physical activity and rehabilitation programs for children and adolescents, provided that adequate adult supervision and proper techniques, training, and safety are maintained. The advantages of strength training in adolescents significantly outweigh the potential dangers, especially given the high level of sports participation and physical demands placed on many of today's young athletes. Previous misconceptions and fears about strength training have been clarified, and strength training is considered a safe and advantageous physical activity

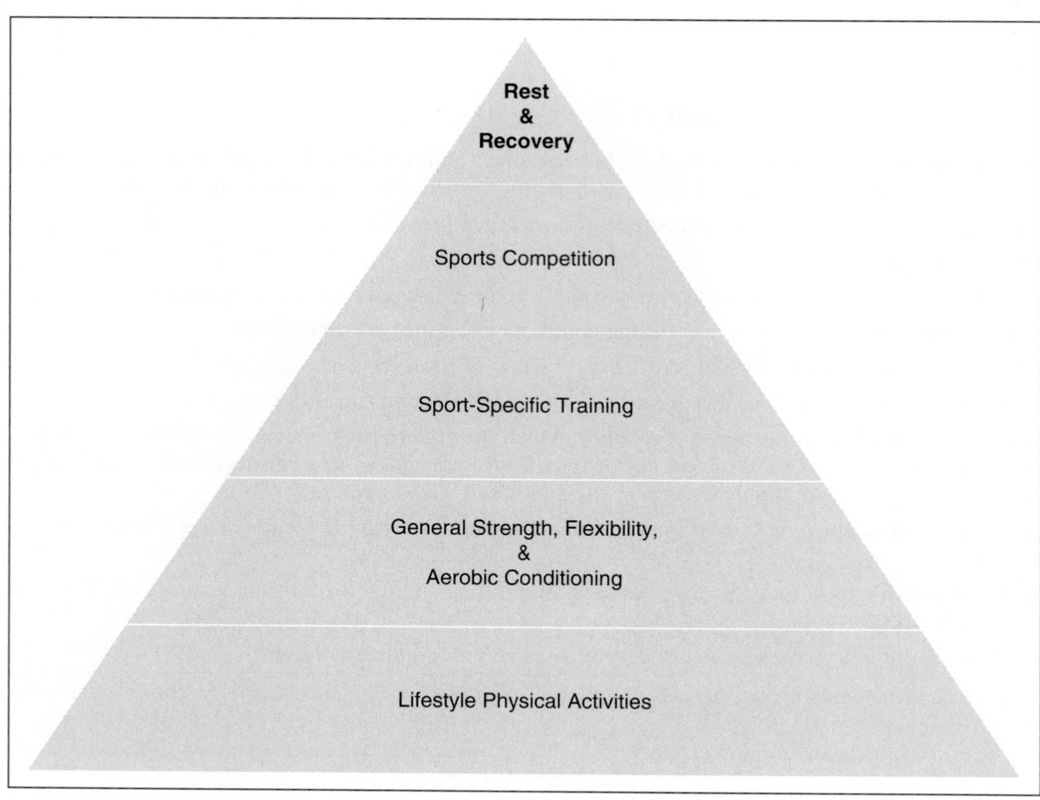


**FIGURE 165-1** Physical activity recommendations for children and adolescents.

for youth and an important component of a comprehensive rehabilitation program. A general concept of physical activity recommendations for children and adolescents, including these principles, is presented in Figure 165-1.

## REFERENCES

1. Malanga GA. Sports medicine. In: DeLisa JA, Gans BM, Walsh NE, Bockenek WL, Frontera WR, eds. *Physical Medicine and Rehabilitation: Principles and Practice.* Philadelphia: Lippincott Williams & Wilkins; 2009

2. Jarvinen TAH, Jarvinen TLN, Kaariainen M, et al. Muscle injuries: biology and treatment. *Am J Sports Med.* 2005;33(5):745-764

3. Bleakley GA, McDonough S, MacAuley D. The use of ice in the treatment of acute soft tissue injury: a systematic review of randomized trials. *Am J Sports Med.* 2004;32:251-261

4. Kaul MP, Herring SA. Superficial heat and cold: how to maximize the benefits. *Phys Sports Med.* 1994;22(12):65-74

5. Cassella MC, Richards K. Principles of rehabilitation. In: Micheli L, Purcell L, eds. *The Adolescent Athlete.* New York: Springer Science+Business Media; 2007:25

6. Herring SA, Kibler WB. A framework for rehabilitation. In: Kibler WB, Herring SA, Press JM, et al, eds. *Functional Rehabilitation of Sports and Musculoskeletal Injuries.* Gaithersburg, MD: Aspen; 1998:1-8

7. Guy JA, Micheli LJ. Strength training for children and adolescents. *J Am Acad Orthop Surg.* 2001;9(1):29-36

8. Faigenbaum A. Strength training for children and adolescents. *Clin Sports Med.* 2000;19(4):593-619

9. American Academy of Pediatrics Committee on Sports Medicine. Strength training, weight and power lifting, and body building by children and adolescents. *Pediatrics.* 1990;86(5):801-803

10. Faigenbaum AD, Polakowski C. Olympic-style weightlifting, kid style. *J Strength Cond Res.* 1999;21(3):73-76

11. American Academy of Pediatrics Committee on Sports Medicine and Fitness. Strength training by children and adolescents. *Pediatrics.* 2001;107 (6):1470-1472

12. American Academy of Pediatrics Council on Sports Medicine and Fitness. Strength training by children and adolescents. *Pediatrics.* 2008;121(4):835-840

13. National Strength and Conditioning Association *(NSCA). Position Statement: Youth Resistance Training*. Colorado Springs, CO: NSCA; 2001. Available at: www.nsca-lift.org/Publications/YouthforWeb.pdf. Accessed April 25, 2010

14. Malina RM. Weight training in youth—growth, maturation, and safety: an evidence-based review. *Clin J Sport Med.* 2006;16(6):478-487

15. Faigenbaum AD. Youth resistance training. President's Council on Physical Fitness and Sports. *Res Digest.* 2003;4(3): 1-8

16. Smith A, Andrish J, Micheli L. The prevention of sports injuries of children and adolescents. *Med Sci Sports Exerc.* 1993;25(suppl 8):1-7

17. Hejna W, Rosenberg A, Buturusis D, et al. The prevention of sports injuries in high school students through strength training. *Natl Strength Coaches Assoc J* 1982;4:28-31

18. Cahill B, Griffith E. Effect of preseason conditioning on the incidence and severity of high school football knee injuries. *Am J Sports Med.* 1978;6:180-184

19. Christou M, Smilios I, Sotiropoulos K, et al. Effects of resistance training on the physical capacities of adolescent soccer players. *J Strength Cond Res.* 2006;20(4):783-791

20. Hamill B. Relative safety of weight lifting and weight resistance training. *J Strength Cond Res.* 1994;8:53-57

21. Morris F, Naughton G, Gibbs J, et al. Prospective ten-month exercise intervention in premenarcheal girls: positive effects on bone and lean mass. *J Bone Miner Res.* 1997; 12:1453-1462

22. US Consumer Product Safety Commission. National Electronic Injury Surveillance System (NEISS) On-line [database]. Available at: www.cpsc.gov/library/neiss.html. Accessed April 25, 2010

23. American Academy of Pediatrics Committee on Sports Medicine and Fitness. Strength training by children and adolescents. *Pediatrics.* 2001;107(6):1470-1472

24. Guy JA, Micheli LJ. Strength training for children and adolescents. *J Am Acad Orthop Surg.* 2001;9(1): 29-36

25. Benjamin HJ, Glow KM. Strength training for children and adolescents. *Phys Sports Med.* 2003;31(9):19-28

26. Gould D. Intensive sport participation and the prepubescent athlete: competitive stress and burnout. In: Cahill B, Pearl A, eds. *Intensive Participation in Children's Sports.* Champaign, IL: Human Kinetics;1993:19-38

# CHAPTER 166

# Exertional Heat-Related Illnesses

DILIP R. PATEL, MD

One of the most important factors affecting the sports performance and well-being of an athlete is environmental heat stress and the athlete's physiologic ability to effectively dissipate heat generated during exercise. Heat-related illnesses (or heat illnesses) are common; however, many go unreported because of minor symptoms. This chapter provides an overview of temperature regulation mechanisms, clinical aspects of exertional heat-related disorders, and prevention measures. The terms sport, physical activity, and exercise, although used interchangeably in the present discussion, have somewhat different connotations.[1] The term *physical fitness* refers to a set of attributes that individuals have or achieve that relates to the ability to perform physical activity. *Physical activity* is defined as bodily movement produced by the contraction of skeletal muscle that increases energy metabolism above basal metabolic rate. *Exercise* (or exercise training) is a type of physical activity that is planned, structured, repetitive, and done to improve or maintain one or more components of physical fitness. *Sport* is also a type of physical activity that has a distinct psychosocial dimension.

## EPIDEMIOLOGY

The exact incidence of different heat-related illnesses occurring in adolescents while they participate in sports or various physical activities is not known. Exertional heat-related illnesses are most common in adolescents participating in sports that require strenuous and prolonged physical activity in hot and humid weather. Sports that have a relatively higher incidence of exertional heat-related illnesses include tennis, long-distance running, long-distance cycle races, and (American) football.[2-7] Deaths due to exertional heat stroke in (American) football players are reported to be most common when the ambient temperature is more than 78°F (26°C) and relative humidity is more than 50%.[7] Between 1995 and 2001 there were 21 deaths among young football players from heat stroke, and it is the third-leading cause of mortality among high school athletes.[3,8] The incidence of nonfatal heat stroke in adolescents is not known.

Exertional heat exhaustion is the most common heat-related illness at all ages, although its exact incidence in adolescents participating in sports is not known. The estimated incidence varies depending on the particular physical activity and its intensity and duration; examples include 14 per 10,000 participants per day in a 14-km road race and 85 per 10,000 participants in a 6-day youth soccer tournament.[7] The incidence of other exertional heat-related illnesses, such as exercise-associated muscle cramps, heat edema, and heat syncope is not known. Factors that contribute to an increased risk for heat-related illness in adolescent athletes are listed in Box 166-1.[4,5,7-15]

## THERMOREGULATION

Maintenance of body temperature homeostasis depends on a number of physiologic processes (Box 166-2). Human beings are homeothermic; they must maintain a constant core body temperature between 96.8°F and 99.5°F (36°C-37.5°C).[16-18] Heat is continuously generated by basal metabolic activity at a rate of 1 kcal/kg/hour.[16] A significantly increased amount of heat is generated by muscular activity during exercise and sports. During physical exercise, contractions of muscles can generate heat 20 times the basal metabolic rate.[16,18] Increases in temperature of the blood reaching the hypothalamus, along with input from skin thermoreceptors, trigger the heat regulatory mechanisms.[16] A number of environmental and intrinsic factors that influence the dissipation of heat are listed in Box 166-3.[5,7,9-11,16]

Generally heat is lost from the body via radiation, convection, or conduction. However, the tremendous amount of heat generated during sports activity is largely dissipated by evaporation of sweat. Evaporation of 1 liter of sweat can lead to a loss of 600 to 700 kcal of heat, and trained athletes can produce up to 3 liters of sweat per hour.[16] Evaporation of sweat cools the skin and can take place at any ambient temperature.[5,7,16] Thus, effective production and evaporation of sweat become critical factors for the athlete to maintain body temperature.

**Box 166-1**

***Factors that Predispose to Exertional Heat Illness***

**A. Nonenvironmental**

1. Individual characteristics
   a. Genetic predisposition
   b. High body mass index
   c. Past history of heat-related illness
   d. Very young and very old age
2. Medical conditions
   a. Acute
      i. Gastroenteritis
      ii. Acute febrile illness
      iii. Sunburn
      iv. Malignant hyperthermia
   b. Chronic
      i. Diabetes mellitus
      ii. Diabetes insipidus
      iii. Myelomeningocele
      iv. Cystic fibrosis
      v. Hyperthyroidism
      vi. Anorexia nervosa
      vii. Scleroderma
      viii. Sickle cell disease
   c. Drugs
      i. Anticholinergic drugs
      ii. Antiepileptic drugs
      iii. Antihistamine drugs
      iv. Phenothiazines
      v. Tricyclic antidepressants
      vi. Amphetamines
      vii. Ephedra and ephedrine
      viii. Diuretics
      ix. Beta blockers
      x. Thyroid hormones
      xi. Alcohol
3. Other factors
   a. Lack of acclimation/acclimatization
   b. Poor conditioning
   c. Excessive clothing
   d. Sport equipment (eg, helmet, padding)
   e. Sleep deprivation
   f. Prolonged strenuous physical exertion

**B. Environmental factors**

1. High ambient temperature
2. High relative humidity
3. High radiant heat
4. Low air velocity

**Box 166-2**

***Mechanisms of Body Heat Gain and Loss***

**Heat Gain**

- High basal metabolic rate
- Sustained muscular contractions
- Thermic effects of food
- High environmental heat
- Hormonal action

**Heat Loss**

- Conduction
- Convection
- Radiation
- Evaporation (both respiratory and sweat)

**Box 166-3**

***Factors that Influence Heat Dissipation***

**Extrinsic**

- Ambient temperature
- Relative humidity
- Air current or wind velocity
- Radiant heat from sun
- Clothing

**Intrinsic**

- Hydration status
- Acclimation and acclimatization
- Rate and amount of sweating
- Rate of evaporation of sweat
- Menstrual cycle phase (heat dissipation is reduced in the luteal phase because of an elevated hypothalamic temperature set point)

Adequate hydration before, during, and after exercise is important to maintain the circulating blood volume and to also allow for the production of large amounts of sweat.[9] Thus, dehydration can adversely affect the dissipation of heat. Dehydration in the range of even 1% to 3% has been shown to impair heat regulatory mechanisms and sports performance.

Relative humidity of the environment is an important factor affecting heat loss from the body; higher environmental humidity allows for less efficient evaporation of sweat. Environmental temperature is obviously also a critical determinant for body temperature and dissipation of heat generated during physical activity. When the environmental temperature exceeds that of the skin, the ability of the body to lose heat is significantly impaired.[16,18] Higher radiant heat from the sun, low wind velocity, and clothing covering the skin all tend to decrease the ability of the body to dissipate heat via evaporation of sweat.[16]

Sweat is generally hypotonic; in otherwise healthy adolescents there is relatively more water loss and very little loss of electrolytes during exercise.[7,16,19] The body tends to conserve sodium efficiently during intense endurance sports activities. Lack of acclimation or acclimatization, prolonged repeated exercise in heat, and ultra-endurance activity (eg, a triathlon) may potentially predispose the athlete to increased sodium loss. Potassium loss is not clinically significant, and plasma concentrations are maintained within normal limits during exercise in otherwise healthy individuals. Electrolyte disturbances may be a consideration in certain disease states such as cystic fibrosis.

### ACCLIMATION AND ACCLIMATIZATION

The body adapts to heat stress either by acclimation or acclimatization.[7,10,12,16] Although the terms acclimation and acclimatization are often used interchangeably, in the present discussion of exertional heat-related illnesses, acclimation is the preferred term and is used in the discussion that follows. Physiologic adaptation occurs naturally in acclimatization and following repeated exposures in acclimation.[10] In acclimatization, long-term exposure to a hot climate leads to physiologic and metabolic adaptations. On the other hand, acclimation results from repeatedly exercising in a hot climate and occurs over a period of several weeks.[20]

In order to achieve acclimation, the physical exertion should be of an intensity that elevates both the skin and core temperatures and is accompanied by profuse sweating.[16,20] Typically the exercise sessions should last 1.5 to 2 hours per day and the intensity should be at about 50% to 70% of maximum effort.[5,7,12,20] The effects of acclimation typically persist from 1 to 4 weeks after returning to a cooler environment. Physiologic adaptations that occur as a result of acclimation to heat stress are listed in Box 166-4.[12,16,20]

**Box 166-4**

***Physiologic Adaptations to Acclimation***

- Increased blood flow to the skin
- Increased rate of sweat production
- Increased evaporation of sweat
- Earlier onset of sweating relative to body temperature
- Increase in plasma volume
- Decreased rate of carbohydrate utilization
- Increased efficiency of conserving electrolytes
- Decreased core temperature
- Lower heart rate relative to intensity of exercise
- Decreased fatigue
- Increased total extracellular volume
- Increased plasma volume
- Increased aldosterone secretion and urinary sodium excretion

### ASPECTS UNIQUE TO ADOLESCENTS

There are several differences in the physiologic responses to heat stress in children, adolescents, and adults. In general, prepubescent children take longer to acclimatize, have a lower sweat rate and lower ability to enhance the sweating mechanism, and tend to have greater adverse effects due to dehydration. In children, the onset of sweating occurs at a higher body temperature, they produce more metabolic heat at a given level of activity compared to adults, and they have a lower cardiac output.[10] The changes that take place during the adolescent years that have effects on thermoregulation and are listed in Table 166-1.[10]

## SPECTRUM OF CLINICAL SYNDROMES

A wide clinical spectrum of exertional heat-related illnesses have been described in athletes. These range in order from minor to life threatening: heat edema, heat cramps, heat exhaustion, heat syncope, and heat stroke.[5,7,13,18,21,22] In the discussion that follows, body temperature refers to rectal temperature, which in practice provides the closest approximation to actual core body temperature.[23] Actual core temperature in research is measured by using an esophageal probe and thermister.[23] In the present discussion, all of the heat-related illnesses refer to those that occur within the context of physical exertion in a hot climate.

### HEAT EDEMA

#### Definition

Heat edema is characterized by transient edema noted in the extremities following sustained physical exertion.

#### Pathophysiology

Exercise leads to increased heat production and vasodilatation in the exercising muscles. The heat is dissipated by an increased rate of sweating and there is thus

**Table 166-1**

**Changes Occurring during Puberty that Might Influence Thermoregulation**

| *Change* | *Effect on Thermoregulation* |
|---|---|
| Decrease in body surface area to mass ratio | Decrease in heat gain in a hot environment |
| | Decrease in heat loss in a cold environment |
| Increase in body density among boys (not consistent in all studies) | Increase in the specific heat of the body |
| Decrease in body density among girls | Decrease in the specific heat of the body |
| Decrease in oxygen cost of walking or running | Decrease in metabolic heat production per kilogram body mass |
| Increase in maximal cardiac output | Enhancement of peripheral perfusion and, therefore, convective heat loss |
| Increase in blood volume per body surface area | Decrease in the proportion of blood volume necessary for adequate peripheral perfusion and, therefore, enhanced perfusion of muscles |
| Increase in sweat gland size | Increase in sweat gland output |
| Increase in sweat gland sensitivity | Decrease in sweat threshold and time to sweat onset. Increase in sweating rate |
| Increase in sweat gland anaerobic metabolism | Increase in sweating rate |
| Change in hormonal status | Change in sweat electrolyte composition |

Reprinted with permission from Falk B. Physiologic and health aspects of exercise in hot and cold climates. In: Bar-Or O, ed. *The Child and Adolescent Athlete*. London: Blackwell Science; 1996:331.

a relative loss of plasma volume; this may trigger an increased secretion of aldosterone resulting in sodium and water retention and edema.[5,20]

### Clinical Presentation

The clinical picture is characterized by puffiness and edema, mainly noted in the distal lower extremities and to a lesser extent the upper extremities. Facial edema is very rare.

### Treatment

The edema is transient and the athlete is advised to elevate the legs while resting. The tendency to develop heat edema decreases (or disappears) within a few days of proper conditioning and acclimation in heat.

## EXERCISE-ASSOCIATED MUSCLE CRAMPS

### Definition

Exercise-associated muscle cramps (or EAMC) are characterized by the sudden onset of painful skeletal muscle spasms during or after prolonged and strenuous physical exertion; these occur mostly in hot climates (hence they are commonly known as "heat cramps").[7,24]

### Pathophysiology

The pathophysiology of EAMC has not been clearly elucidated. Most research suggests that the muscle cramps are due mainly to continued muscle activity resulting in fatigue and altered neural impulses.[5,7,22] Thus, muscle cramps can occur at any temperature, although they are certainly more common when exercising in the heat. Exercise-induced muscle fatigue, along with water and sodium losses in the sweat, are believed to be the main contributory factors for EAMC.

### Clinical Presentation

The leg and thigh muscles are most commonly affected, with the abdominal muscles sometimes also affected. Exercise-associated muscle cramps are most often reported in football players, tennis players, and long-distance runners.[7,22] Heat cramps are typically seen in well-conditioned athletes after several hours of physical exertion. The athlete experiences sudden and sustained acute muscle spasm and pain in the affected muscle. The acute pain can be severe and the muscle spasm usually lasts between 1 to 3 minutes. In some athletes, intermittent acute painful spasms can continue for up to 4 to 8 hours.[7]

### Treatment

Treatment involves stopping the activity, starting oral hydration, and initiating muscle stretching and massage; there is generally rapid resolution in most athletes. Adequate sodium and fluid intake before and during physical activity can effectively prevent EAMC in most cases. Suggested guidelines for ensuring adequate sodium intake include consumption of sports drinks or fluids with added salt: about 1/8 to 1/4 teaspoonful of table salt or 1 to 2 salt tablets to 300 to 500 ml of sport drinks or fluids.[7] In very rare instances of sustained muscle spasms with excruciating pain, intravenous normal saline has been reported to be effective in relieving the spasm. The athlete can usually return to play soon after the pain and spasm have resolved.[7,24]

> **Box 166-5**
>
> ***Differential Diagnosis of the Collapsed Athlete***
>
> Heat exhaustion
> Heat syncope
> Heat stroke
> Hypoglycemia
> Cardiac arrhythmia
> Hypertrophic cardiomyopathy
> Anomalous origin of coronary artery
> Noncontact cerebral concussion

## HEAT EXHAUSTION

### Definition

Heat exhaustion is characterized by an inability to continue or sustain exercise (at any ambient temperature) because of muscle fatigue and a normal to elevated core temperature (between 100°F [38°C] and 104°F [40°C]).[5,7]

### Pathophysiology

Neural mechanisms have been implicated in the pathogenesis of heat exhaustion.[7,14,16] It is postulated that strenuous and prolonged physical activity induces central fatigue and triggers peripheral vasodilatation with consequent tachycardia, high cardiac output, and collapse, effectively leading to cessation of further physical exertion, thus potentially preventing further complications (the so-called safety brake effect).[7] Because of peripheral vasodilatation, the blood is pooled in the peripheral muscles and the transport of heat from the core to the periphery is impaired. A high body mass index and dehydration have been shown to increase the risk for heat exhaustion.

### Clinical Presentation

Clinical symptoms and signs of heat exhaustion include nausea, vomiting, intestinal cramps, urge to defecate, irritability, headaches, weakness, confusion, dizziness or fainting, profuse sweating, chills, goose bumps, muscle fatigue, myalgias, rapid breathing, rapid pulse, and decreased blood pressure.[5,7] Heat exhaustion tends to occur relatively early in the course of an exercise session and is likely to be more common in athletes who are dehydrated.

Making a clinical distinction between heat exhaustion and incipient heat stroke is often difficult, and onset of heat exhaustion symptoms should prompt initiation of aggressive treatment. A temperature not exceeding 102.2°F (39°C) and absence of neurological signs favor the diagnosis of heat exhaustion. The athlete with exertional heat exhaustion may collapse during exercise, and other conditions should be carefully considered in the differential diagnosis (Box 166-5).[25-28] It is especially important to consider exercise-associated hyponatremia (EAH) (see the following), which warrants different treatment considerations. Although the differentiation between hyponatremic (salt depleting) and hypernatremic (water depleting) types of heat exhaustion is difficult to make clinically, because of nonspecific symptoms, most cases are a mixed type.

### Treatment

The primary goal of treatment of heat exhaustion is to restore the intravascular volume. Treatment includes removal from the sport or exercise activity, rest under shade in a cool environment, removal of excessive clothing, immediate oral rehydration with an electrolyte and carbohydrate solution and, rarely, intravenous rehydration with a normal saline and 5% dextrose solution.[5,7,8,14] One to 2 liters of fluid over 2 to 4 hours may be needed. Ice bags may be applied to the neck, axillae and groin areas. Fanning will greatly enhance the evaporation of sweat. The rectal temperature must be monitored closely (every 5 minutes), and a continued or rapid increase is a sign of impending heat stroke. Also, the onset of confusion and altered sensorium may indicate progression to heat stroke. In these circumstances the athlete must be transported to a hospital emergency department to receive aggressive and intensive treatment. The athlete may return to sports 24 to 48 hours after a full clinical recovery.[7,24]

## HEAT SYNCOPE

### Definition

Heat syncope is characterized by sudden fainting and transient loss of consciousness in an athlete upon cessation of or at the end of the physical activity or exercise.[5,7]

### Pathophysiology

During sustained exercise there is a steady increase in heat production and core temperature that triggers cutaneous vasodilatation to facilitate dissipation of the heat. At the same time there is vasodilatation of the exercising muscles and an increased intravascular space. Continued muscle contractions tend to compensate for the relative decrease in intravascular volume. When the athlete stops physical activity (and thereby muscle contractions) there is a sudden decrease in venous return to the heart and decreased cardiac output that results in postural or orthostatic hypotension, decreased cerebral blood flow, and syncope.

### Clinical Presentation

The athlete collapses and has a transient loss of consciousness on cessation of relatively sustained activity in a hot climate. Heat syncope occurs most commonly during the initial 5 days of sports participation in the heat. The core temperature is usually normal to only slightly elevated. The athlete should always be examined carefully for any injury, especially to the head and neck, as a result of the fall, and consideration should be given to other conditions in the differential diagnosis of the collapsed athlete (Box 166-5).[24,25] Sudden collapse during exercise should prompt investigation of a cardiac cause.[25,27]

### Treatment

The athlete should be moved to a cool place and the rectal temperature should be measured. The athlete typically recovers spontaneously and is fully alert, awake, and oriented. The athlete should consume electrolyte/carbohydrate drinks. Appropriate acclimation and conditioning can effectively prevent the likelihood of heat syncope. After full clinical resolution and hydration the athlete may resume sports participation.[5,24]

## EXERTIONAL HEAT STROKE

### Definition

Exertional heat stroke is characterized by elevation of the core body temperature to 104°F (40°C) or more and central nervous system signs and symptoms in athletes engaged in prolonged strenuous physical activity, most commonly in a hot and humid climate.[21]

### Pathophysiology

The pathogenesis of heat stress leading to heat stoke is depicted in Figure 166-1.[21,29-31]

### Clinical Presentation

Exertional heat stroke is a life-threatening illness with mortality ranging from 50% to 70%.[18] The greatest risk of exertional heat stroke has been reported to be with

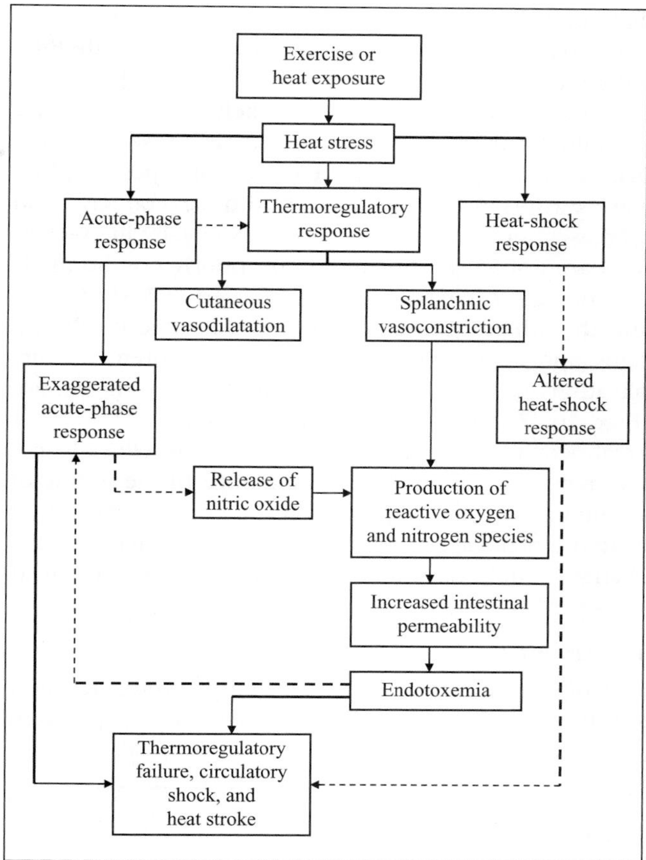


**FIGURE 166-1** The sequence of events in the progression of heat stress to heat stroke. Heat stress induces thermoregulatory, acute-phase, and heat-shock responses. Thermoregulatory failure, exaggeration of the acute-phase response, and alteration in the expression of heat-shock proteins, individually or collectively, may contribute to the development of heat stroke. Active cutaneous vasodilatation and splanchnic vasoconstriction permit the shift of heated blood from the central organs to the periphery, from which heat is then dissipated to the environment. This change may also lead to splanchnic hypoperfusion and ischemia, resulting in increased production of reactive oxygen and nitrogen species, which may in turn induce intestinal mucosal injury and hyperpermeability. Endotoxins may then leak into the circulation and enhance the acute-phase response, leading to increased production of pyrogenic cytokines and nitric oxide. Both cytokines and nitric oxide can interfere with thermoregulation and precipitate hyperthermia, hypotension, and heat stroke. The solid arrows indicate pathways for which there is clinical or experimental evidence, and the broken arrows indicate putative pathways. (From Bouchama A, Knochel JP. Heat stroke. *New Engl J Med.* 2002;346:1982, with permission.)

high intensity (at 75% or more $Vo_{2max}$) exercise in a hot climate 82.4°F [28°C] or more) that typically lasts longer than one hour.[7,18] Similar to the risk of heat exhaustion, heat stroke is most likely to occur during the initial 5 days of activity, such as in preseason football practice.[7] The cumulative effects of repeated physical exertion in heat over a period of several days also increases the risk for heat stroke, especially in athletes who are not yet acclimated or are poorly conditioned.

The rectal temperature may exceed 105.8°F (41°C) and the athlete presents with a wide range of clinical signs and symptoms (Box 166-6) and potential complications as a result of multiorgan system failure (Box 166-7) with irreversible sequealae.[5,7,15,16,21,29-31] Treatment must be initiated based on the clinical findings regardless of the core temperature. In the setting of strenuous and prolonged physical activity, especially in heat, the presence of confusion and other mental status changes should be sufficient indications to suspect heat stroke.[7,14,21]

### Treatment

The higher the degree of core temperature elevation and the longer the duration that the core temperature remains elevated, the worse the prognosis.[5,7,21] Therefore rapid external cooling must be initiated as soon as heat stroke is suspected based on signs and symptoms.[7,21,31]

Rapid external cooling is best initiated by the removal of clothes and ice water immersion.[7,32-35] The athlete's core temperature should be checked every 5 minutes and ice water immersion continued until the temperature reaches 102°F (38.8°C); it should then be discontinued to prevent hypothermia. Further cooling should be continued with bags of crushed ice placed over the neck, axillae, and groin, along with fanning, to enhance evaporative heat loss. Body massage during external cooling is recommended to reduce cutaneous vasoconstriction associated with cooling.[7]

Emergency medical services (EMS) should be called, intravenous normal saline should be started, and the athlete should be transported to the emergency department. Further treatment is best accomplished in the hospital intensive care setting by critical care specialists.[18,21]

The athlete should rest and refrain from returning to all sports activities for at least a week after complete clinical recovery.[5,7,24] A follow-up clinical and laboratory evaluation is recommended at that time before allowing

## Box 166-6

### *Signs and Symptoms of Exertional Heat Stroke*

**General (nonspecific)**
Dehydration
Diarrhea
Dry or wet hot skin
Elevated core body temperature of 40° C or more
Hyperventilation
Hypotension
Tachycardia
Vomiting
Weakness and fatigue

**Central Nervous System**
Apathy
Aggressiveness
Confusion
Coma
Delirium
Disorientation
Drowsiness
Emotional instability
Irritability
Irrational behaviors
Loss of consciousness
Seizures
Staggered gait

## Box 166-7

### *Systemic Complications of Exertional Heat Stroke*

**Multiorgan System Dysfunction**
Hypovolemic shock
Encephalopathy
Rhabdomyolysis
Acute renal failure
Acute respiratory distress syndrome
Myocardial irritability and cellular injury
Hepatocellular damage
Gastrointestinal tract injury
Disseminated intravascular coagulation
Thrombocytopenia

**Metabolic Disturbances**
*Early phase*
Respiratory alkalosis
Lactic acidosis
Hypophosphatemia
Hypocalcemia
Hypokalemia

*Late phase*
Hyperphosphatemia
Hypercalcemia
Hyperkalemia

the athlete to return to sports. The athlete should resume gradually increasing levels of physical activities, should acclimatize herself or himself slowly, and then return to regular sport participation in about 4 weeks following recovery.

### EXERCISE-ASSOCIATED HYPONATREMIA AND COLLAPSE

#### Definition

Exercise-associated hyponatremia is characterized by hyponatremia (serum sodium concentration below normal for the laboratory, generally below 135 mmol/L), mostly seen in endurance athletes participating in events lasting 4 or more hours.[19]

#### Pathophysiology

Exercise-associated hyponatremia is the sudden onset of dilutional hyponatremia secondary to an increased volume of total body water relative to the amount of total serum sodium.[19,26] Consumption during exercise of sports drinks and water (hypotonic liquids) in excess of total body water loss (respiratory, gastrointestinal, sweat, and urine) is the primary mechanism for the increase in total body water relative to the amount of serum sodium.[19,26] Some evidence implicates inappropriate secretion of antidiuretic hormone during sustained endurance activity as a contributing factor in the development of EAH.[19]

#### Clinical Presentation

Mild cases are generally asymptomatic. Although there is considerable individual variability, the development of clinical signs and symptoms generally correlates with the serum levels of sodium. Athletes with a serum sodium level in the range of 130 to 134 mmol/L are generally asymptomatic, whereas those with a serum sodium level less than 130 mmol/L are generally symptomatic. The initial symptoms are nonspecific and include malaise, fatigue, nausea, vomiting, headache, bloating, and puffiness. With a further drop in the serum sodium level, signs and symptoms of cerebral edema develop; these include confusion, disorientation, and agitation. Severe cases can result in seizures, respiratory distress, collapse (see differential diagnosis, Box 166-5), coma, and death.

Early detection is imperative to prevent progressive worsening and life-threatening complications. The on-site or on-field capability of measuring serum sodium for events involving prolonged endurance activities is critical.

#### Treatment

Asymptomatic and mildly symptomatic cases generally resolve with fluid restriction until the onset of diuresis. Intravenous normal saline can exacerbate the dilutional hyponatremia and is contraindicated.

Athletes who are moderately symptomatic need urgent emergency care and should be transported to an emergency department for further treatment. Administration of intravenous 3% sodium chloride, with close clinical and laboratory monitoring, is the mainstay of treatment in severe cases.[19,26,36]

Exercise-associated hyponatremia can be effectively prevented by drinking fluids (with adequate sodium and carbohydrates) to replace losses during exercise. A general guideline is not to consume more than 500 to 1,000 ml of fluid per hour of physical activity.[19,36] The athlete can estimate his or her own typical fluid loss by weighing himself or herself before and after the exercise session and customize his or her fluid intake during exercise accordingly.[9,19,36]

## RISK REDUCTION AND PREVENTION

Prevention of heat-related illnesses must be a priority for all of those involved in the care and training of young athletes. Various preventive measures are outlined in Box 166-8.[5,11,15,37–40]

### ENVIRONMENTAL HEAT STRESS

Sports activities should be appropriately modified based on the environmental risk for heat illnesses as indicated by measurement of the heat index. Actual temperature and relative humidity measurements on the field or court are needed to accurately assess the degree of environmental heat stress. Environmental heat stress can be determined using various methods.[11,15,16]

#### Heat Index Thermometer

The Wet Bulb Globe Temperature (WBGT) index is a measure of temperature, relative humidity, and solar radiation. The WBGT index is calculated using the formula: WBGT = 0.7 wet bulb temperature + 0.2 black globe temperature + 0.1 shaded dry bulb temperature. Measurement of wet bulb temperature, black bulb temperature, and dry bulb temperature is somewhat complex and requires setting up equipment on the site.

#### Sling Psychrometer

A simpler way to determine the WBGT is the use of a sling psychrometer, which is available commercially. The sling psychrometer (Figure 166-2) allows for the measurement of dry bulb and wet bulb temperatures on the field, from which WBGT can be approximated using a standard formula: WBGT = (dry bulb temperature + wet bulb temperature) / 2. A sling psychrometer device is comprised of a dry bulb and a wet bulb thermometer.

**Box 166-8**

***Preventive Measures***

**Event Planning**

- Advance planning for treatment of heat-related illnesses
- On-field availability for external cooling
- Availability of adequate fluid and electrolyte beverages
- Ability to measure core temperature
- Ability to measure serum sodium
- Prearrangement with emergency medical services
- Assessment of environmental conditions
- Implementation of participation guidelines

**Preparticipation Evaluation**

- Identify predisposing factors
- Review drugs, supplements, nutrition, and hydration status
- Educate regarding early signs and symptoms of heat illness

**Individual Considerations by Athletes**

- Acclimation
- Proper conditioning
- Avoid "heroic" exertion in the heat
- Ensure proper food and fluid intake
- Routine pre- and postexercise weight to estimate personal water loss in sweat
- Rest and sleep well
- Appropriate clothing and use of equipment

The globe of the wet bulb thermometer is covered with a wetted cotton sleeve. The sling psychrometer is rotated or swung overhead, which allows evaporative cooling and measurement of the wet bulb temperature. The dry bulb thermometer measures the air temperature in a shaded area. Digital devices are now commercially available that directly display the calculated WBGT.

Guidelines for modification of activity using the WBGT index are listed in Table 166-2.

### Heat Index Chart

A practical way to assess environmental heat stress based on the air temperature and relative humidity is the use of the heat index chart shown in Figure 166-3. Local temperature, relative humidity, and wind velocity can be easily obtained from regional sources or the National Weather Service.

## GUIDELINES FOR HYDRATION

Proper hydration must be maintained throughout all activities. For short-duration activities generally lasting less than an hour, cool water is adequate fluid; for activities lasting longer than an hour, sports drinks containing electrolytes and carbohydrates are recommended.[5,7,11] The carbohydrate content (mixed sugars—glucose, sucrose, fructose, maltodextrin) of the sports drink should not exceed 6%; the sodium content should be 30 to 40 mEq per liter and the potassium content should not exceed 5 mEq per liter.[5,7,9,36,41] Sports drinks are generally more palatable than plain water, and studies suggest that athletes are more likely to consume them.

The sweat rate during exercise can range from 0.5 to 2 liters per hour, resulting in large amounts of water and electrolyte losses; exact amounts vary significantly between individual athletes and types of physical activities.[7,16] The sweat rate is influenced by many factors including genetic predisposition, body mass index, acclimation status, metabolic efficiency, clothing and equipment, ambient temperature, relative humidity, and intensity of the physical activity. Thus, a wide range of individual variability in the amount of fluid loss and sweat rates precludes the ability to offer a universal recommendation for replacement of fluids and electrolytes during exercise.[5,7,36,42,43] The athlete should regularly weigh himself or herself before and after practice or exercise to determine individual fluid loss to develop a customized or individualized plan for fluid replacement.

The American College of Sports Medicine Position Stand[9] on exercise and fluid replacement (2007) provides the following set of guidelines for fluid replacement before, during, and following exercise:

### Before Exercise

Generally, consumption of regular meals and beverages with adequate salt over several hours prior to exercise is sufficient to maintain a state of euhydration before exercise. If the athlete is not in a state of euhydration before exercise, hydration is achieved slowly over a period of 4 hours before exercise by drinking approximately 5 to 7 ml of fluid/electrolyte drinks per kilogram of body weight. In the absence of adequate urinary output the athlete should drink approximately 3 to 5 ml of fluid/electrolyte drink per kilogram of body weight about 2 hours prior to exercise.

### During Exercise

Fluid intake during exercise or sports should be individualized based on the estimated fluid losses for the athlete calculated using previous monitoring of weight loss relative to the type of physical activity the athlete

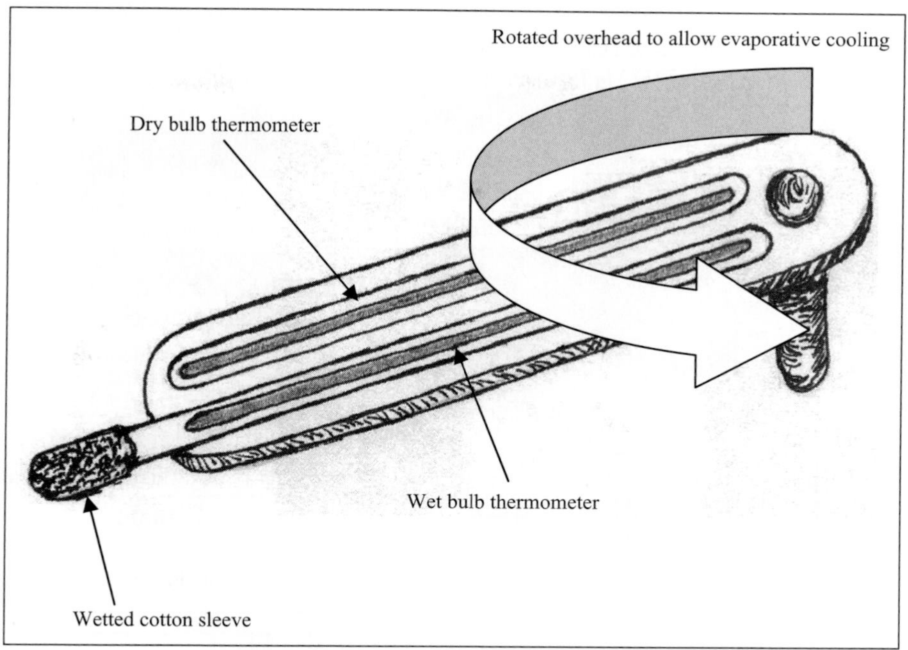


FIGURE 166-2 Sling psychrometer schematic drawing

**Table 166-2**

**Restraints on Activities at Different Levels of Heat Stress**

| *WGBT* | | *Restraints on Activities* |
|---|---|---|
| °*C* | °*F* | |
| <24 | <75 | All activities allowed, but be alert for prodromes of heat-related illness in prolonged events |
| 24.0–25.9 | 75.0–78.6 | Longer rest periods in the shade; enforce drinking every 15 minutes |
| 26–29 | 79–84 | Stop activity of unacclimatized persons and other persons with high risk; limit activities of all others (disallow long-distance races, cut down further duration of other activities) |
| >29 | >85 | Cancel all athletic activities |

From American Academy of Pediatrics Committee on Sports Medicine and Fitness. Climatic heat stress and the exercising child and adolescent. *Pediatrics*. 2000;106:158-159.

is engaged in. The athlete should drink periodically during exercise to replace ongoing fluid losses. The athlete may need to consume between 0.4 and 0.8 liters per hour of fluid. The American Academy of Pediatrics recommends that adolescent athletes consume about 250 ml (9 oz) of fluid every 20 minutes during exercise.[11]

### After Exercise

Adequate consumption of regular meals and beverages over several hours following exercise is generally sufficient to restore fluid and electrolyte homeostasis. For rapid rehydration, the athlete should drink about 1.5 liters of fluid per kilogram of body weight lost over a period of a few hours.

## SUMMARY

For the clinician who is caring for adolescents that participate in sports activities, the following "take away" points from this chapter are useful to remember in the prevention and management of heat-related illnesses:

- Exertional heat exhaustion is the most common heat-related illness at any age.
- Effective production and evaporation of sweat are the most critical factors for dissipation of heat.

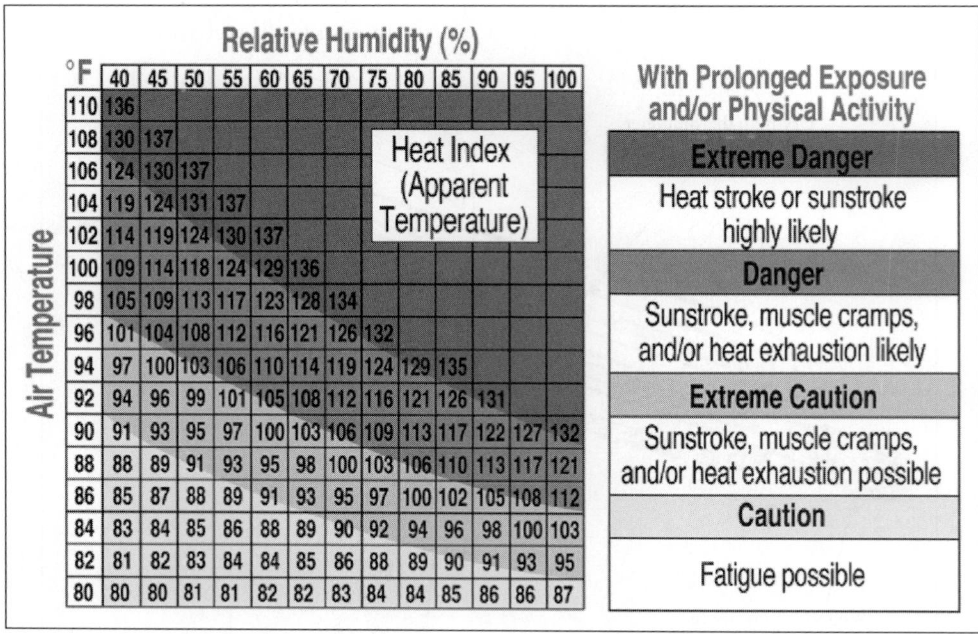

Relative Humidity (%)

| °F (Air Temperature) | 40 | 45 | 50 | 55 | 60 | 65 | 70 | 75 | 80 | 85 | 90 | 95 | 100 |
|---|---|---|---|---|---|---|---|---|---|---|---|---|---|
| 110 | 136 | | | | | | | | | | | | |
| 108 | 130 | 137 | | | | | | | | | | | |
| 106 | 124 | 130 | 137 | | | | | | | | | | |
| 104 | 119 | 124 | 131 | 137 | | | | | | | | | |
| 102 | 114 | 119 | 124 | 130 | 137 | | | | | | | | |
| 100 | 109 | 114 | 118 | 124 | 129 | 136 | | | | | | | |
| 98 | 105 | 109 | 113 | 117 | 123 | 128 | 134 | | | | | | |
| 96 | 101 | 104 | 108 | 112 | 116 | 121 | 126 | 132 | | | | | |
| 94 | 97 | 100 | 103 | 106 | 110 | 114 | 119 | 124 | 129 | 135 | | | |
| 92 | 94 | 96 | 99 | 101 | 105 | 108 | 112 | 116 | 121 | 126 | 131 | | |
| 90 | 91 | 93 | 95 | 97 | 100 | 103 | 106 | 109 | 113 | 117 | 122 | 127 | 132 |
| 88 | 88 | 89 | 91 | 93 | 95 | 98 | 100 | 103 | 106 | 110 | 113 | 117 | 121 |
| 86 | 85 | 87 | 88 | 89 | 91 | 93 | 95 | 97 | 100 | 102 | 105 | 108 | 112 |
| 84 | 83 | 84 | 85 | 86 | 88 | 89 | 90 | 92 | 94 | 96 | 98 | 100 | 103 |
| 82 | 81 | 82 | 83 | 84 | 84 | 85 | 86 | 88 | 89 | 90 | 91 | 93 | 95 |
| 80 | 80 | 80 | 81 | 81 | 82 | 82 | 83 | 84 | 84 | 85 | 86 | 86 | 87 |

Heat Index (Apparent Temperature)

| With Prolonged Exposure and/or Physical Activity |
|---|
| Extreme Danger |
| Heat stroke or sunstroke highly likely |
| Danger |
| Sunstroke, muscle cramps, and/or heat exhaustion likely |
| Extreme Caution |
| Sunstroke, muscle cramps, and/or heat exhaustion possible |
| Caution |
| Fatigue possible |

**FIGURE 166-3** Heat Stress Index (Reprinted from www.wrh.noaa.gov).

- Sweat is generally hypotonic, and in otherwise healthy adolescents during exercise there is relatively more water loss in sweat than sodium loss.
- Acclimation is best achieved over a period of 2 to several weeks by repeated exercise for about 1.5 to 2 hours per day in a hot climate at 50% to 70% of maximum effort.
- Changes of puberty uniquely affect thermoregulation.
- In practice, the rectal temperature provides the closest approximation to the core body temperature.
- Onset of confusion and altered mental status herald progression to heat stroke and indicate prompt initiation of treatment.
- Treatment for heat stroke should be initiated based on clinical signs and symptoms.
- Rapid external cooling is best achieved by ice water immersion.
- Ad lib consumption of hypotonic fluids during prolonged physical activity may lead to exercise-associated dilutional hyponatremia and collapse.
- To prevent heat-related illnesses, sports activities should be modified based on environmental heat stress.
- A wide range of individual variability in sweat rates and fluid loss during exercise precludes universal fluid and electrolyte replacement recommendations; fluid and electrolyte replacement should be individualized accordingly.

*Acknowledgments: The author thanks Ms Laurie Grimm for her assistance in preparing the manuscript.*

## REFERENCES


1. US Department of Health and Human Services. *Physical Activity and Health:A Report of the Surgeon General.* Atlanta, GA: US Department of Health and Human Services, Centers for Disease Control and Prevention, National Center for Chronic Disease Prevention and Health Promotion, 1996
2. Bugbee S, Knopp WD. Medical coverage of tennis events. *Curr Sports Med Rep.* 2006;5(3):131–134
3. Bergerson MF, McKeag DB, Casa PM, et al. Youth football: heat stress and injury risk. *Med Sci Sports Exerc.* 2005;37(8): 1421–1430
4. Bytomski JR, Squire DL. Heat illness in children. *Curr Sports Med Rep.* 2003;2(6):320–324
5. Binkley HM, Beckett J, Casa DJ, Kleiner DM, Plummer PE. National Athletic Trainers' Association Position Statement: exertional heat illnesses. *J Athl Training.* 2002;37(3):329–343
6. Cooper ER, Ferrara MS, Broglio SP. Exertional heat illness and environmental conditions during a single football season in the southeast. *J Athl Train.* 2006;41(3):332–336
7. American College of Sports Medicine. Position Stand: exertional heat illness during training and competition. *Med Sci Sports Exerc.* 2007;39(3): 556–572

8. Coris EE, Ramirez AM, Van Durme DJ. Heat illness in athletes: the dangerous combination of heat, humidity, and exercise. *Sports Med.* 2004;34(1):9-16

9. American College of Sports Medicine. Position Stand: exercise and fluid replacement. *Med Sci Sports Exerc.* 2007;39(2): 377-390

10. Falk B. Physiological and health aspects of exercise in hot and cold climate. In: Bar-Or O, ed. *The Child and Adolescent Athlete*. London: Blackwell Science; 1996:326-352

11. American Academy of Pediatrics Committee on Sports Medicine and Fitness. Climatic heat stress and the exercising child and adolescent. *Pediatrics.* 2000;106(1):158-159

12. Maughan RJ, Shirreffs SM. Preparing athletes for competition in the heat: developing an effective acclimatization strategy. *Sports Science Exchange*. 1997;10(2)

13. Bytomski JR, Squire DL. Heat illness in children. *Curr Sport Med Rep.* 2003;2:320-324

14. Seto CK, Way D, O'Connor N. Environmental illness in athletes. *Clin Sports Med.* 2005;24(3):695-718

15. Jardine DS. Heat illness and heat stroke. *Pediatrics in Review.* 2007;28(7):249-258

16. McArdle WD, Katch FI, Katch VL. *Exercise Physiology: Energy, Nutrition, and Human Performance*. 6th ed. Baltimore, MD: Williams & Wilkins; 2006

17. Byrne C, Lee JK, Chew SA, Lim CL, Tan EY. Continuous thermoregulatory responses to mass-participation distance running in heat. *Med Sci Sports Exerc.* 2006;38(5):803-810

18. Khosla R, Guntupalli K. Heat-related illnesses. *Crit Care Clin*. 1999;15:251

19. Hew-Butler T, Almond C, Ayus JC, et al. Consensus statement of the 1*st* International Exercise-Associated Hyponatremia Consensus Development Conference, Cape Town, South Africa 2005. *Clin J Sport Med.* 2005;15(4): 206-211

20. Carter R, Cheuvront SN, Sawka MN. Heat-related illnesses. *Sports Science Exchange.* 2006;19(3):1-6

21. Bouchana A, Knochel JP. Heat stroke. *N Engl J Med.* 2002;346:1978-1988

22. Bergeron MF. Heat cramps: fluid and electrolyte challenges during tennis in the heat. *J Sci Med Sport.* 2003;6(1):19-27

23. Moran DS, Mendal L. Core temperature measurement: methods and current insights. *Sports Med.* 2002;32(14): 879-885

24. Inter-Association Task Force on Exertional Heat Illnesses Consensus Statement. Available at: www.naspem.org/LinkClick.aspx?fileticket=yRFeKM7Y9nw%3D&tabid=64. Accessed June 22, 2010

25. Blue JG, Pecci MA. The collapsed athlete. *Orthop Clin North Am.* 2002;33(3):471-478

26. Noakes T. Hyponatremia in distance runners: fluid and sodium balance during exercise. *Curr Sports Med Rep.* 2002;4: 197-207

27. Drezner JA, Courson RW, Roberts WO, Mosesso VN Jr, Link MS, Maron BJ. Inter-association task force recommendations on emergency preparedness and management of sudden cardiac arrest in high school and college athletic programs: a consensus statement. *Heart Rhythm.* 2007;4(4): 549-565

28. Holtzhausen LM, Noakes TD. Collapsed ultraendurance athlete: proposed mechanisms and an approach to management. *Clin J Sport Med.* 1997;7(4):292-301

29. Heled Y, Deuster PA. Severe heat stroke with multiple organ dysfunction. *Crit Care.* 2006;10(2):406.

30. Lambert GP. Role of gastrointestinal permeability in exertional heatstroke. *Exercise Sport Sci Rev.* 2004;32(4): 185-190

31. Casa DJ, Armstrong LE, Ganio MS, Yeargin SW. Exertional heat stroke in competitive athletes. *Curr Sports Med Rep.* 2005;4:309-317

32. Webborn N, Price MJ, Castle PC, Goosey-Tolfrey VL. Effects of 2 cooling strategies on thermoregulatory responses of tetraplegic athletes during repeated intermittent exercise in the heat. *J Appl Physiol.* 2005;98(6):2101-2107

33. Coris EE, Walz SM, Duncanson R, Ramirez AM, Roetzheim RG. Heat illness symptom index (HISI): a novel instrument for the assessment of heat illness in athletes. *South Med J.* 2006;99(4):340-345

34. Smith JE. Cooling methods used in the treatment of exertional heat illness. *Br J Sports Med.* 2005;39:503-507

35. Hadad E, Moran DS, Epstein Y. Cooling heat stroke patients by available field measures. *Intensive Care Med.* 2004;2:338.

36. Noakes T. Fluid replacement during marathon running. *Clin J Sport Med.* 2003;13(5):309-318

37. Brotherhood JR. Guidelines for the prevention of heat illness in community-based sports participants and officials. *J Sci Med Sport.* 2007;10(3):191-192. Epub 2007 Mar 27

38. Wexler R. Preventing heat illness in athletes. *South Med J.* 2006;99(4):334

39. Dallam GM, Jonas S, Miller TK. Medical considerations in triathlon competition: recommendations for triathlon organizers, competitors, and coaches. *Sports Med.* 2005;35(2): 143-161

40. Larsen T, Kumar S, Grimmer K, Potter A, Farquharson T, Sharpe P. A systematic review of guidelines for the prevention of heat illness in community-based sports participants and officials. *J Sci Med Sport.* 2007;10(1):11-26

41. Burns JH, Berning JR. Sports beverages. In: Driskell JA, Wolinsky I, eds. *Macroelements, Water, and Electrolytes in Sports Nutrition*. New York, NY: CRC Press; 1999:211-240

42. Ganio MS, Casa DJ, Armstrong LE, Maresh CM. Evidence-based approach to lingering hydration questions. *Clin Sport Med.* 2007;26:1-16

43. Maughan RJ, Leiper JB. Limitations to fluid replacement during exercise. *Can J Appl Physiol.* 1999;24(2):173-187

# CHAPTER 167

## Sport Psychology

GLORIA BALAGUE, PhD

Adolescence is by definition a phase of change, of transition, moving from childhood to adulthood. Many demands are placed on the adolescent to start firming up his or her goals, academic skills, interests, personality style, and values. The importance of adult influence progressively decreases during this time and the role of peers becomes more central. Why focus on sport? Because sport offers more possibilities than most in terms of affect on the adolescent: Peer status, social acceptance, and integration are linked to physical skills and abilities. Many boys and girls younger than 15 years of age answer 'good at sports' when asked "Would you rather be good at sports or good at school?" Being physically skilled is a valued quality in childhood and adolescence, which then affects the development of self-image and contributes to self-esteem.[1]

Some researchers have demonstrated that youth engaged in competitive sports get better grades and choose more challenging coursework than their nonathletic counterparts.[2] Others have shown that positive youth development is associated with continued and intense sport involvement.[3] It is therefore helpful, to the degrees possible and reasonable, to encourage youth to be engaged in sports activities.

### SPORTS ACTIVITIES AND YOUTH DEVELOPMENT

How does sport contribute to youth development? We hear a lot about the positive things sport can do. It teaches self-discipline, teamwork, responsibility, healthy lifestyles, and leadership. We also see many examples of young people learning entitlement, aggressive behavior, and self-centeredness in sports. And we know that many of the values in sports are conveyed by adults, especially parents and coaches, in the ways they organize and conduct formal sports activities. In the upcoming section of this chapter we focus on a few main areas of emphasis in psychological development, and the effects of parents and coaches, for young adolescents who participate in sports activities. These concepts were reviewed in a book by Ginsburg, Durant, and Baltzell[4] published in 2006.

### CONFIDENCE, RELATIONSHIPS, JUDGMENT, EMOTIONAL CONTROL

#### Confidence

A central skill to develop during the adolescent's search for identity is confidence. The discovery of one's strengths and weaknesses is important, and although failures, errors, and mistakes can be a great source of challenges and steps to improvement, they can also demoralize a young person, particularly if they are not balanced with the knowledge of one's improvements, successes, and positive qualities.

If coaches and parents define success as "winning" or "being better than others," the young athlete is asked to do something he or she cannot fully control, because the outcome depends to a great degree on the other people who are competing. In particular, care must be taken with young adolescents, especially those who mature later and are therefore physically behind some of their peers. If young athletes think their inability to "win" means they are a failure, then they will lose confidence in their skills and abilities and likely withdraw from sports before reaching maturity.

Many well-meaning parents and coaches believe that the best way to improve the young athlete's performance is by pointing out what should be done better, so they criticize often, and when they praise they use the dreadful "yes, but." The message heard by the athlete is "you are never good enough," which lowers confidence and destroys motivation. Encouraging, emphasizing improvement, and comparing the young athlete to his or her previous performance are the best tools for helping to build confident athletes.[5]

Almost as damaging is an opposite behavior on the rise, which is when parents think that any negative feedback or any information that can be seen as negative (such as not starting) is unacceptable, because it will damage their child's confidence or self-esteem. As such, they want to protect their child from any disappointment and unpleasant emotions. But sports and physical activity are an effective way to learn that we do not have everything we want, that skills and talents are not distributed equally, and that being good at 1 activity does not make one good at all activities, nor does it make one a better person. That is an insight that needs to be taught. How can a smaller teen engage in sports with bigger peers and still learn to be confident? Not by being spared the reality that some are better than him or her "right now," but instead by setting personally controllable goals that will allow for success. *Improvement* is one such goal, and *effort* should be the primary means to achieve it. Everyone can improve if they work hard, but not everyone can be number 1, regardless of how much they try. If the adults go to great lengths to protect the teen from disappointment, they not only miss a great teaching opportunity, they convey a very damaging message: "You are so fragile that you cannot handle any negative information or a disappointing outcome." If that message gets integrated into the newly forming identity, the consequences can be more severe than just learning that one is not very good at a particular sport.

If we agree that one of the roles of youth sports is to keep adolescents engaged in their sports activities, then we should make sure that as many young athletes as possible become confident in their capacity to improve. They would learn to compare their current performances to their past performances, not just to the performances of others (which they cannot control), and that would allow them to feel competent and remain engaged in the activity. Even for more highly competitive athletes in the later adolescent years, where successful outcomes in themselves are emphasized, focusing on improvement and on controllable aspects of performance are better strategies to achieve success than focusing on winning.

### Relationships

Sports can provide an ideal medium for expanding relationship knowledge. Friendships within the team, cross-age friendships with older or younger players, and relationships with coaches are all integral parts of sports.[6] Some coaches believe they should generate rivalries within the team to maintain a "competitive spirit." Some parents end up disliking their children's strongest competitors because they see them as obstacles in their child's path to success, so they try to prevent friendships from developing. That is not helpful and does not work. It is recommended that parents leave their adolescents alone to navigate the complex world of interpersonal relationships, with all of the issues of jealousy, loyalty, conflict, and team spirit. It should be the teenager's world, not the parents'.

When possible, parents should look for a team where personal respect is emphasized and no one is ridiculed or ostracized. Parents also need to model the behaviors they want their sons and daughters to learn, so the behavior of parents during games and competitions is very important. Blaming coaches, referees, or other competitors for the young athlete's results teaches entitlement and lack of responsibility. Disrespecting the other team, the referees, and the coaches is also contrary to what should be taught to young adolescents in sport. So from a developmental perspective for the young athlete, it is important that the values of the coaches and the team are positive and clear, accepted by the other parents, and modeled by all.

### Judgment and Emotional Control

Sport can teach young athletes to make good decisions, but in order to do that they have to be allowed the responsibility to make some choices. They will need support and guidance, although progressively less, as they learn to anticipate the consequences of their choices and learn from them.[7] A coach who never allows for input, or parents who control every single aspect of the training and competition regimen (such as parents who "pack the sports bag" of 14- or 15-year-olds because "otherwise he or she forgets important stuff"), are teaching neither good judgment nor emotional control.

Adolescence is a time of emotional intensity, with peaks and valleys. In sport, one's performance is publicly displayed, and this may result in a strong positive or negative emotional reaction. For that reason it also provides an unusually good stage for learning to win and lose with composure. However, these values have to be taught and to be seen as desirable goals by the adults and reinforced as such.

## THE ROLES OF SUCCESSFUL COACHES AND PROGRAMS

### COACHES WHO SUCCEED

Gould and Carson[2] describe the characteristics of successful coaches who have a positive affect on their athletes. These coaches are motivated to win, but see personal development as a priority, they set clear expectations and rules regarding player behavior and team expectations, and they provide feedback that enhances competence. These positive coaches ultimately have less attrition among their players. Smith and Smoll[8] found that providing youth coaches with training in positive reinforcement, and decreasing punishment and control, resulted in a more positive atmosphere, with increased enjoyment and decreased attrition of athletes. Coaches who place an emphasis exclusively on winning are likely to exploit their athletes for their own success, eventually resulting in burnout and increased dropout.

## CHARACTERISTICS OF PROGRAMS THAT PROMOTE POSITIVE YOUTH DEVELOPMENT

Research by the National Research Council and the Institute of Medicine[9] highlights features that should be present in sports programs for youth if they are to promote positive development:

- *Physical and psychological safety:* An environment of respect that encourages safe practices and interactions.
- *Appropriate structure:* The presence of clear and consistent expectations, rules, and limits.
- *Supportive relationships:* Coaches and administrators who promote positive communication and connectedness.
- *Opportunities to belong:* Programs that make sure that everyone has a role and promote team unity and cohesion.
- *Positive social norms*: Emphasis on cooperation, responsibility, fair play, and self-control.
- *Support for efficacy and mattering*: Providing opportunities for taking responsibility, emphasizing intrinsic motivations for involvement, and empowering youth's decision-making capabilities.
- *Opportunities for skill building*: Providing learning experiences for everyone, with organized, deliberate practices.
- *Integration of family, school, and community efforts:* Programs that integrate parents and are community based tend to increase persistence and a commitment to achievement of goals.
- *Time*: Changing activities over time to adjust to the developmental stages of the young athlete.

## CHOOSING APPROPRIATE PROGRAMS

When it comes time to choose specific programs, Ginsburg et al[4] offer 3 simple rules: (1) Know your child, (2) know yourself, and (3) know your child's sports environment. Some young athletes are better suited to individual rather than team sports, or to noncontact rather than contact sports. Parents who were themselves serious competitors in a sport should be aware that it may be hard for them to abstain from "coaching" or providing comparisons and expectations, and if so, their child may be much happier participating in a different sport. Finally, parents should be familiar with the specific sports environment in which their child is placed to make sure basic requirements for a positive experience are met. Box 167-1 lists do's and don'ts for parents of adolescent athletes, and Box 167-2 lists do's and don'ts for coaches.

### Box 167-1

### *Do's and Don'ts for Parents of Adolescent Athletes*

**Do**

- Set clear expectations for behavior and effort (attendance, work, improvement)
- Ask about how practice or competition went
- Ask the coach directly if needed
- Provide praise: Be specific, not just a generic "that was nice"
- Give responsibility
- Conduct yourself with composure
- After a competition, ask, "How did you play? Did you work/play hard?"

**Don't**

- Set outcome expectations (winning, being a starter)
- Coach or criticize the coach
- Show conditional love (given with good results, withheld with poor performances)
- Get overly involved or make it "your activity"
- Attack/blame others (your child, opponents, referees, other team)
- Make "Did you win?" your first question

### Box 167-2

### *Do's and Don'ts for Coaches*

**Do**

- Set clear rules and expectations for behavior, effort, sportsmanship
- Reinforce the right behavior, provide feedback on what to do
- Respect the developmental level of your athletes. Treat fairly, not equally
- Reward effort, define success as improvement
- Show respect for the athletes, other teams, referees, parents
- Keep parents informed, set expectations for parents

**Don't**

- Compare players to others but to their previous performance
- Ridicule, use too much criticism, or punish
- Overcontrol or reward only for outcome (just winning or losing)
- Lose your composure
- Encourage cheating, disrespect

## STRESS AND NEGATIVE CONSEQUENCES IN YOUTH SPORT

We have seen that sports can contribute positive aspects to the physical, psychological, and social development of the adolescent. There are also numerous examples of physical and psychological stressors in youth sports: from the "entrapped" athletes who feel they "have to" participate to satisfy their parents, coaches, etc, to the athletes who feel they have to succeed all of the time to keep their parents' love and approval. Often these athletes show classic stress reactions, including decreased school performance and a variety of injuries, and they may eventually drop out of sports. Parents are often not aware of their role in these situations, but many outside observers can see what is happening. Teachers, trainers, coaches, and physicians may be the first to observe the syndrome and should look for ways to help the adolescent and his or her family.

The issue of sports dropouts seems to peak during adolescence, in part because of the emergence of competing interests, but often because of the undue pressure young athletes experience from negative coaches or overly involved parents. For female athletes, the subtle message of the contradiction between the characteristics of sports, strength, competitiveness and persistence, and the traditional "feminine" values of softness, passivity, and empathy, often results in abandoning athletics. The specific issues of body image and eating disorders found disproportionally among young female athletes is addressed in other chapters of this book (see Chapter 76, Anorexia Nervosa, Chapter 77, Bulimia Nervosa, and Chapter 78, The Female Athlete Triad.).

Finally, the issue of premature specialization is becoming a major stressor in youth sports. The professional model of sports has been applied to the domain of youth sport with negative consequences. Early specialization has been linked to dropout in elite-level hockey players,[10] and Barynina and Vaitsekhovskii[11] found that national team members of the Russian swim team who specialized earlier arrived later to the national team, retired earlier, and did not stay as long. Evidence of overtraining, injury, burnout, and depression abound when looking at early specialization. A great resource for what sport could look like at different levels is provided by Côté's Developmental Model of Sport Participation.[10]

## DEALING WITH TALENTED YOUNG ATHLETES

Bloom[12] studied the pathways of successful people in a variety of areas, including sports. His findings provide a road map for helping talented youngsters reach their potential.

### THE EARLY YEARS

Development at that level is characterized by supportive, enthusiastic parents who model a good work ethic and reward "trying hard and doing your best." The teachers/coaches at that point make initial learning pleasant, fun, and rewarding. These teachers are described as "being rarely critical, using positive reinforcement, and setting standards for improvement." According to Bloom, during this phase, motivation and effort count more than specific qualities. A small percentage of these successful and talented individuals (<10%) are identified as gifted at ages 11 to 13 years, indicating that being good at 1 developmental phase does not necessarily imply being good at all phases.

### THE MIDDLE YEARS

These are the years when commitment is established. The role of the parents changes now to providing emotional and financial support, and the athlete becomes more responsible for his or her activity as the motivation becomes more intrinsic. Seeing improvement and reaching desired goals become the main motivations. The coach, at this stage, is now more of an expert, focusing on precision, endurance, and setting specific goals.

### THE LATER YEARS

Perfecting the craft is now the task. Reaching the highest levels possible requires that the athletes become increasingly responsible for their own motivation. Elite athletes have to be committed to the activity, and cannot diffuse their energies in a variety of domains. As the demand increases, so do the sacrifices required of the family. The family must now allocate more financial and emotional resources toward the young athlete, and at times the whole family is affected because it may have to reschedule vacations or miss family events due to the competitive schedule and demands of the elite athlete. The main authority for planning training and competition schedules is the master coach, and the parents' role becomes almost exclusively a supportive one.

Clearly, no one can be "pushed" to greatness. Stress and difficulties arise when the parents want athletic success more than the young athlete.

## PSYCHOLOGICAL SKILLS FOR YOUNG ATHLETES

Adolescence is the time to learn and train psychological skills. To succeed in competitive sports one must train and improve physical skills, technical skills, and psychological skills. A number of athletes drop out because excessive competition anxiety makes participation unbearable, or they have negative experiences with coaches or teammates. Finally, some athletes are so self-critical that they undermine their own confidence and cannot handle close competitions.

Learning to regulate one's level of arousal, relaxing if tension is too high or activating if the level is too low, is a basic trainable skill. Identifying effective self-talk and focus of attention (what Vealey[13] calls productive thinking) is also trainable. Goal setting is a major tool, useful to keep motivation on track during training and during competitions. Emotional self-regulation allows the young athlete to identify emotional states and regulate expression. All of these are extremely helpful life skills, and should be taught and practiced during the training sessions. They help the learning process and improve the overall experience of the athletes, helping them to be better prepared for the competition of life, which ultimately is what really matters.

## REFERENCES

1. Duda JL. *A Cross-Cultural Analysis of Achievement Motivation in Sport and the Classroom.* Champaign, IL: University of Illinois; 1981

2. Gould D, Carson S. Personal development through sport. In: Bar-Or O, ed. *The Encyclopedia of Sports Medicine—The Child and Adolescent Athlete*. Oxford: Blackwell Science; 2005

3. Zarrett N. *The Dynamic Relation between Out-of-School Activities and Adolescent Development.* Ann Arbor: University of Michigan; 2006

4. Ginsburg R, Durant S, Baltzell A. *Whose Game Is It Anyway?* New York, NY: Houghton Mifflin Company; 2006

5. Thompson J. *The Double-Goal Coach.* New York, NY: HarperCollins Books; 2003

6. Weiss MR, Smith AL. Friendship quality in youth sport: relationship to age, gender, and motivation variables. Sport friendship quality scale. *J Sport Exercise Psychol.* 2002;24(4):420-437

7. Hamilton SF, Hamilton A, Pittman K. Principles for youth development. In: Hamilton SF, Hamilton MA, eds. *The Youth Development Handbook*. Thousand Oaks, CA: Sage Publications; 2004

8. Smith R, Smoll F. *Way to Go Coach.* Portola Valley, CA: Warde Publishers; 2001

9. National Research Council and Institute of Medicine. *Community Programs to Promote Youth Development*. Washington, DC: National Academy Press; 2002

10. Wall M, Cote J. Developmental activities that lead to drop out and investment in sport. *Physical Education and Sport Pedagogy.* 2007;12:77-87

11. Barynina I, Vaitsekhovskii SM. The aftermath of early sports specialization for highly qualified swimmers. *Fitness and Sport Review International.* 1992;27:132-133

12. Bloom BS, ed. *Developing Talent in Young People*. New York, NY: Ballantine Books; 1985

13. Vealey RS. *Coaching for the Inner Edge.* Morgantown, WV: Fitness Information Technology; 2005

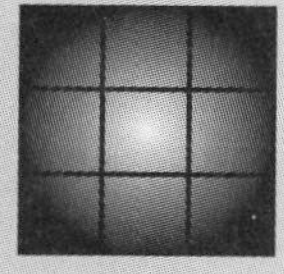

# Part 4

# Psychosocial Issues

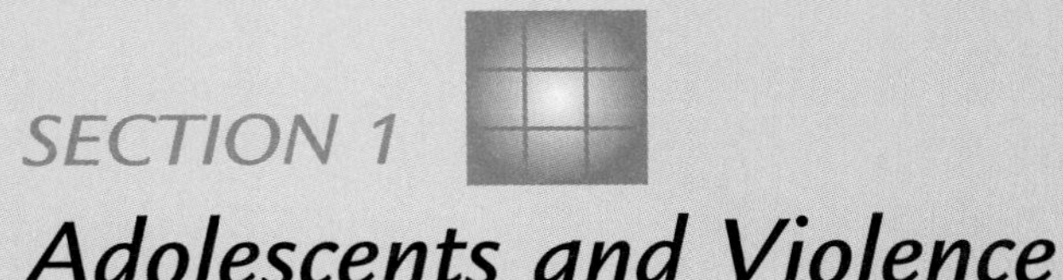

SECTION 1

# Adolescents and Violence

## CHAPTER 168

## Physical Abuse

MOLLY CURTIN BERKOFF, MD, MPH • ADAM J. ZOLOTOR, MD • DESMOND K. RUNYAN, MD, DrPH

There are serious health risks associated with adolescent physical abuse, including significant mental health sequelae, as psychological abuse frequently occurs with physical abuse and the 2 forms of maltreatment are tightly intertwined. Where health care providers are aware of the extent and seriousness of the problem, it is important to facilitate primary prevention, identification, and treatment.

### DIFFERENTIATING PHYSICAL ABUSE FROM CORPORAL PUNISHMENT

Parents are permitted to use corporal punishment on minor children in their care. The permission usually takes the form of an exemption from the crime of physical assault. This exemption gives parents the right to use "reasonable force" for purposes of discipline and control. However, the specific acts considered to be reasonable force are not identified by the law. Thus, the boundary between "reasonable force" and "physical abuse" is left to the judgment of the law enforcement and judicial systems. The definition of physical abuse has therefore reflected cultural norms concerning what exceeds reasonable force. Perhaps the most important criterion embedded in Western cultural norms concerns injury. Essentially, parents are permitted to use force that does not result in a recognizable injury (such as a bruise) or does not involve an extremely high risk of injury. Therefore, parents are not proscribed from hitting with objects such as belts and wooden paddles, as long as there are no obvious resulting injuries.

There is an inherent tension between the criterion of injury that defines abuse on the basis of demonstrated injury and the criterion of abuse as constituting acts that entail a high risk of injury, such as kicking or punching an adolescent, even though in most cases no injury occurs. This is in contrast to laws addressing the physical assault of adults and the sexual abuse of children, defined on the basis of the act occurring rather than whether it resulted in an injury. From 1962 to 1970, every state passed legislation to define, prevent, and treat child abuse. These statutes make the presence of injury the primary criterion but allow for determining presence of abuse on the basis of a high risk of injury. Although the inclusion of risk for injury would seem to expand the definition to include severe assaults by parents that do not result in an injury, in practice it is rare for physical abuse to be confirmed unless it results in injury requiring medical attention and treatment. Instead, this legislation had the ironic effect of codifying the right of parents to hit adolescents by declaring that the law was not intended to prohibit corporal punishment. In effect, the criminal justice system, child protective system, and informal cultural norms are in agreement that if an assault by a parent on an adolescent results in an injury requiring medical care, it is physical abuse, but if no injury results, as long as it is not considered "excessive" or "unlawful," in many states it is considered an acceptable means of discipline. This principle is supported by a New Hampshire Supreme Court[1] ruling that a mother had not committed physical abuse by hitting her child with a leather belt because the child did not suffer an injury that required medical care. Although the child abuse legislation has not clarified the boundary between corporal punishment and physical abuse, it may have laid the basis for long-term change in what is accepted as corporal punishment and what is considered abusive.

## CORPORAL PUNISHMENT OF ADOLESCENTS AS A FORM OF ABUSE

There are important reasons to include corporal punishment in a consideration of physical abuse of adolescents. One reason is the evidence that most cases of physical abuse occur when corporal punishment escalates out of control. In addition, as shown in the following, ordinary corporal punishment of adolescents is associated with an increased risk of many serious social and mental health problems.

Although the law continues to give parents the right to hit adolescents, the cultural norms are changing. The American Academy of Pediatrics[2] suggests encouraging and assisting parents to develop methods other than spanking for managing undesired behaviors. Types of physical punishment other than spanking are considered unacceptable and are reported to be possibly dangerous to the health and well-being of the child.

## PREVALENCE STUDIES

Two main types of data have been used to compute rates of physical abuse of adolescents: (1) reports of abuse to state child protection agencies, and (2) interviews with parents and/or adolescents in household epidemiologic surveys.

### REPORTS TO CHILD PROTECTION AGENCIES

#### Child Protective Services

The most widely used rates come from the National Child Abuse and Neglect Data System (NCANDS) based upon citizen reports to state Child Protective Service (CPS) agencies under the mandatory reporting acts (hereafter called CPS data).[3] Approximately 16% of all confirmed cases are for physical abuse. Applied to adolescents, that means a rate of physical abuse of about 1.6 per 1,000 children aged 12 to 15 years, and about 1.0 per 1,000 children aged 16 to 17 years.

In 1999 the Children's Bureau funded the National Survey of Child and Adolescent Well-Being (NSCAW).[4] This study included detailed interviews of children and families referred to CPS for concerns of child abuse and/or neglect, not just cases of substantiated abuse and/or neglect. Almost a third of adolescents reported experiencing physical abuse.

The National Survey of Child and Adolescent Well-Being also contained interviews of adolescents and their parents who had come to the attention of social service agencies to determine the level of agreement in the lifetime prevalence of physical assault for the child. Sixty percent of adolescents reported a lifetime prevalence of physical assault whereas 73% of parents reported a history of physically assaulting their child. Adolescents reported a 21% lifetime prevalence of severe physical assault by their parent (eg, choking, or being burned on purpose), whereas parents reported only a 3% lifetime prevalence.

Child Protective Services data are limited; the data only reflect cases reported to authorities. Because many cases are unknown and there is therefore no report or investigation, CPS data underestimate the prevalence of abuse. The decrease with age in the NCANDS data may reflect age differences in reporting rather than a lesser underlying prevalence.

#### National Incidence Studies

Another source of data for estimating physical abuse of adolescents are the National Incidence Studies (NIS),[5,6,7] conducted in 1980, 1986, and 1995. Data from the fourth NIS are being collected and tabulated. In its earlier iterations, the NIS interviewed a variety of human service professionals in a randomly selected nationally stratified sample of 29 counties. The respondents were asked for information on all instances of children who had suffered demonstrable harm from maltreatment in the previous 12 months. The NIS data include only cases known to service providers. Consequently, the NIS data, like the CPS data, result in a measure closer to an intervention rate than to a prevalence rate. A key difference, however, is that the service providers were asked about all cases, regardless of whether they had been reported to CPS. The inclusion of cases that were not officially reported explains why the 1995 NIS rate (6 per 1,000 for children aged 12 to 14 years) is almost 4 times higher than the estimate from CPS reports. The NIS findings on adolescents also differ from the CPS rates in demonstrating a greater prevalence of physical abuse of adolescents than that of younger children. This, too, could be the result of including cases that are known but not officially reported because these did not involve an injury that required medical attention.

### HOUSEHOLD EPIDEMIOLOGIC SURVEYS

#### Patient Surveys

***National Family Violence Surveys (NFVS)*** These surveys, conducted in 1976, 1985, and 1995, interviewed one parent from each household in large and nationally representative samples. The NFVS measured physical abuse by means of the Conflict Tactics Scales (CTS). The CTS ask parents about how often they engaged in each of a list of acts during the previous 12 months when they had trouble with a randomly selected child. These acts are used to compute 4 scales: nonviolent discipline (eg, explaining), psychologic aggression (eg, calling the child a name), corporal punishment (eg, slapping or spanking), and physical abuse (eg, kicking or punching).

The physical abuse rate for children 12 to 17 years old in the NFVS was about 25 per 1,000 in all 3 surveys, which is 15 times greater than the CPS rate and 4 times greater than the NIS rate.[8] Moreover, these are lower bound estimates because it can be assumed that some of the parents interviewed did not disclose instances of abuse. In addition, only one parent was interviewed in each household. If the rate of 25 per 1,000 applies to the 24 million US adolescents, it means that a minimum of 600,000 adolescents were severely assaulted by 1 of their parents during the survey year. Fortunately, this does not mean 600,000 adolescents required medical care. The NFVS did not measure injuries requiring medical attention.

***CarolinaSAFE*** Conducted in 2002, CarolinaSAFE (Carolinas Survey of Abuse in the Family Environment) used random-digit dialing and targeted sampling of 1,435 mothers in 2 states (North and South Carolina) with anonymous telephone interviews regarding child-rearing and discipline practices.[9] Interviews were conducted in English and Spanish. Questions regarding harsh physical discipline were assessed using the Parent-Child CTS. The measure for harsh physical discipline included whether a parent had beaten, kicked, burned, or hit their child with an object somewhere other than the buttocks. Among 13- to 17-year-olds, mothers reported rates of harsh physical discipline to be 39 per 1,000.

### Adolescent Surveys

***Youth Risk Behavior Surveys*** Beginning in 1990, the Youth Risk Behavior Surveys (YRBS), a survey of adolescents in grades 9 to 12, has been sponsored by the Centers for Disease Control and Prevention.[10] The YRBS includes national samples, state samples, and some smaller local samples and is administered every 2 years. The 1993 Oregon survey included 3 questions about physical abuse. The survey asked whether the person had ever been physically abused (hit, kicked, or struck with an object) when not involved in a fight. It also asked when was the last time this occurred and whether the adolescent tried to talk with someone about the abuse. This survey was administered to 3,211 students in 25 high schools in Oregon, using a stratified cluster design. A total of 32% of the adolescents reported that they had ever been abused. For some the abuse was quite recent; 3.7% reported having been abused in the past week, and 16.3% reported that the most recent occurrence was in the last year.

***Developmental Victimization Study*** In 2002, the Developmental Victimization Study[11] completed interviews of 2,030 parents and children aged 2 to 17 years using questions from the Juvenile Victimization Questionnaire. The main telephone interview was completed with the child if the child was older than 10 years. The adolescent was asked if any adult in his or her life had hit, kicked, or physically abused him or her in any way. Physical abuse was determined to be highest among children older than 13 years of age, with rates of 67 per 1,000 reporting physical abuse.

## SUMMARY

The CPS data indicate lower rates of adolescent physical abuse than survey data from either parents or teens themselves. CPS data are limited as they only include reported physical abuse. Not all physical abuse events are reported to CPS as they may not require medical attention or involvement with law enforcement.

When interviewed, one-third of adolescents involved with CPS report a history of physical abuse by their parents, with 1 in 5 reporting a lifetime prevalence of severe physical abuse. The true rate of adolescent physical abuse is likely high as non-CPS data show rates ranging from 2.5% to 6.7% of teens each year.

## SUBSEQUENT TRENDS

Until the mid-1990s, reports of abuse to CPS increased steadily since these data began to be compiled in 1976. The 1988 NIS also found a substantially higher rate than the first NIS found in 1980. Child maltreatment rates based on CPS and NIS reports roughly doubled from 1980 to 1990. However, for adolescents the rates were the same in all 3 NFVS. These seemingly contradictory trends are consistent if it is recognized that the CPS and NIS data measure interventions to treat and prevent child abuse, and that the focus of these interventions has been on infants and young children. To the extent that these interventions are effective, it should result in a decrease in the incidence rates for young children, but not for adolescents, and that is exactly what the NFVS have found. This should not be taken to mean that treatment and prevention efforts are the only, or even the main, reason for the decrease in prevalence of physical abuse found by the NFVS. Many other changes in American society have lowered the risk of child maltreatment, including a decrease in the prevalence of alcoholism, later marriage, more egalitarian marriages, and fewer children per couple. These have probably outweighed other changes that increase the risk of child abuse, such as a growing underclass, the crack cocaine epidemic, and a greater proportion of children in 1-parent households.

## CLINICAL CHARACTERISTICS

Survey data from parents and teens suggest that significant amounts of physical and sexual abuse are occurring and that the rates of physical abuse among adolescents are not much lower than for younger children. Child Protective Services data, in contrast, find much higher rates for younger children. The higher rate for younger children in the CPS reports likely occurs because younger children are more likely to be injured and thus be confirmed as cases of physical abuse.

## ETIOLOGY OF ADOLESCENT ABUSE

### ONSET DURING ADOLESCENCE

Little is known about the extent to which abuse of adolescents begins during the adolescent years as opposed to cases that are a continuation of a longstanding pattern. This information could be helpful in determining prevention and treatment because the dynamics of adolescent-onset abuse might be different from those of early-onset abuse. National Survey of Child and Adolescent Well-Being data show the majority of adolescent abuse beginning in adolescence (86%).[4] Libbey and Bybee[12] found that in nearly half their 24 cases of abuse began in adolescence and that these cases were less often characterized by major disorganization and parental inadequacy than early-onset cases. This is consistent with the report of Moran and Eckenrode,[13] who found that adolescent onset is associated with a lower risk of psychologic injury to the child. It is also consistent with the theory that much adolescent abuse occurs as a response by previously nonabusive parents to delinquency and rebelliousness emerging during adolescence. If this is correct, treatment and primary prevention of such cases must include work with the adolescent as well as the parents.

### ETIOLOGIC THEORIES

Libbey and Bybee[12] argue that understanding abuse of adolescents requires considering not only the characteristics of the parents but also the characteristics of the adolescent, and the social circumstances of the family such as stress, poverty, and social isolation. They identify theories that emphasize 1 or the other of these 3 types of etiologic factors, starting with what might be called "developmental vulnerability" theories. These theories postulate that the developmental tasks of separation and control during adolescence make the adolescent vulnerable. What they perceive to be the typical case involves parents who have not previously abused but who, in responding to adolescent misbehavior, may "go too far."

A second theoretical approach involves parental "inadequacy theories." Researchers who advocate this perspective focus on characteristics of the parents that put them at risk of abusing an adolescent, such as psychopathology, alcoholism, disorganized and dysfunctional family patterns, and rigid and controlling discipline.

The third theoretical approach is "sociologic." These theories focus on socially generated stresses such as social isolation, unemployment, and poverty.

As useful as it is to identify the predominant focus of these 3 theories, Libbey and Bybee[12] emphasize that "all of these models include the relation parent + child + crises = abuse." In addition, although they do not identify it as a theory, these authors put forward what can be called an escalation from corporal punishment theory. They report that 22 of the 24 most recent abusive incidents were immediately preceded by "typical adolescent-parent conflicts." They also found that most of the abusing parents believed they were disciplining the youth.

## PSYCHOSOCIAL HEALTH RISKS ASSOCIATED WITH PHYSICAL ABUSE

Physically abused adolescents experience a greater risk of a wide variety of psychosocial and behavioral problems than other adolescents. Adolescents who report physical abuse have higher rates of drug use, partner violence, and commission of crimes in adolescence and adulthood as compared to adolescents who do not report being victims of physical abuse.[14,15] The YRBS[10] found a strong association between a history of abuse and a variety of serious outcomes. When adolescents who were physically abused were compared with those who were not, the odds for a poor self-image were 6:1; the odds for having seriously considered suicide in the past year, 2:1; the odds for alcohol, cigarettes, and marijuana use, each approximately 7:1; and the odds for more than 3 sex partners in a lifetime and for involvement in a pregnancy, 9:1. Aggressive behaviors in physically abused adolescents also increased. The odds of fighting in the previous year were increased to 2:2, and the odds for carrying a weapon in the past 30 days were 9:1. These findings are all consistent with previously reported associations.

As mentioned previously, in addition to physical abuse, more than half of American adolescents experience less severe assaults by parents in the form of corporal punishment, such as a slap in the face.[16] This widely occurring practice is associated with an increased risk of such problems as depression, delinquency, and impaired school performance in the adolescent.

## PREVENTION AND TREATMENT

### SCREENING FOR PHYSICAL ABUSE

An evidence-based screen for adolescent physical abuse does not exist. In 2004, the US Preventive Services Task Force[17] concluded that there was insufficient evidence to recommend for or against routine screening of physical abuse in a primary care setting. Most guidelines and professional groups suggest asking adolescents open-ended questions during well-child visits to assess whether they are victims of physical abuse. The American Academy of Pediatrics[2] suggests discussing discipline practices with parents during well-child visits when the child is young to help parents establish reasonable control.

### PRIMARY PREVENTION

Because more than 90% of parents spank and slap toddlers, and just more than 50% use corporal punishment on adolescents, it is possible that a large percentage of adolescent physical abuse represents escalation of a pattern that began with slapping the hand of an infant. This suggests that the most important step for primary prevention of adolescent abuse is the same as the most important primary prevention step to prevent physical abuse of young children: total avoidance of corporal punishment as a means of discipline. A prevention approach that begins with avoiding corporal punishment of toddlers is also likely to apply to parents who gradually reduce the amount of corporal punishment as the child grows older. For these parents, the onset of adolescence, with attendant difficulties in monitoring and directing the child's behavior, can lead some to revert to corporal punishment. During adolescence, a slap in the face for "mouthing off" or staying out late carries a greater risk of escalation into physical abuse because the adolescent may retaliate verbally or physically. The furious parent may use physical force in retaliation.

### TREATMENT

Treatment and secondary prevention is more difficult because it often involves addressing the combination of an entrenched pattern of harsh but inconsistent discipline, including corporal punishment, and the acting out of rebellious youth. The combination manifests itself as a vicious circle of coercion, abuse, and acting out. To end this pattern, parents can be helped (1) to understand that corporal punishment, especially at this age, is counterproductive; and (2) to learn and practice more effective disciplinary methods.

Mandatory reporting laws require the reporting of abuse of adolescents to CPS agencies in all 50 states. The process of recognizing and reporting adolescent abuse can serve to begin a discussion directed at helping the family and the adolescent. Treatment begins at the point of recognition of the problem through the responses of the observing professional. It may first be necessary to deal with concerns related to making the mandatory report. Protective service agency involvement connotes both treatment and punishment. In most states the protective service agency must share all confirmed reports with police authorities. However, CPS agencies have a mandate to protect the child and preserve the family. The risk of foster home placement and/or criminal prosecution is low. Adolescents whose physical abuse is substantiated by protective service agencies are less likely to be put into foster care than either adolescents associated with sexual abuse allegations or younger children. This may result from the increased difficulty in finding placements for adolescents, or from a perception by CPS workers that physical abuse of adolescents is less serious.

Successful treatment of adolescent abuse is likely to involve multiple agencies and disciplines working with families. In addition to working with parents, treatment may involve agencies that deal with the adolescent's behaviors. The schools, courts, police, and protective service agencies all play an important role in supporting the adolescent and the family engaged in treatment. Treatment must be directed at the child and parents as individuals and at the family unit. The behaviors and responses of abusing parents and their children have developed over a long time. Consequently, treatment is not likely to be brief.

The more effective treatments are based on the discipline already practiced by almost all parents, but not consistently enough. These include providing clear standards and expectations, recognizing and praising good behavior, and the sparing use of nonviolent punishments. The behavior of acting-out or rebellious youth must also be addressed. Just as parents need to understand that corporal punishment is counterproductive and dangerous, adolescents should recognize that defiance and delinquency are also counterproductive. The methods of resolving conflicts with peers being taught in school-based violence prevention programs are also effective in preventing conflicts with parents. Mediation is an element of these programs applicable to parent-child conflict. In some states, such as New Hampshire, parent–child mediation is currently the largest single category of cases among members of the mediators association.

Adolescents experience a high rate of severe physical violence by parents. In addition, just more than half of early teenagers experience less dangerous forms of violence by parents, such as a slap. Although the less serious violence rarely results in a physical injury requiring treatment, it puts the child at increased risk of serious social and mental health problems, resulting in reduced school performance, violence, delinquency, and depression.

*This material is part of a research program on family violence at the Family Research Laboratory, University of New Hampshire, Durham, NH 03824. A publications list will be sent on request. It is a pleasure to express appreciation to Nancy Asdigian for assistance with the literature review and statistical analysis. The work has been supported by grants from several organizations, including National Institute of Mental Health grants T32MH15161.*

## REFERENCES

1. NH vs Johnson. No 90-533 (Supreme Court, Hillsborough. June 25, 1992); 1992

2. Stein MT, Perrin EL. Guidance for effective discipline. American Academy of Pediatrics Committee on Psychosocial Aspects of Child and Family Health. *Pediatrics.* 1998;101(4 Pt 1):723–728

3. United States Department of Health and Human Services. Child maltreatment annual reports. Available at: www.acf.hhs.gov/programs/cb/stats_research/index.htm#can. Accessed May 11, 2010

4. United States Department of Health and Human Services. National Survey of Child and Adolescent Well-Being. Available at: www.acf.hhs.gov/programs/opre/abuse_neglect/nscaw/index.html. Accessed May 11, 2010

5. National Center on Child Abuse and Neglect (DHHS). *National Study of Incidence and Severity of Child Abuse and Neglect: Executive Summary*. Rockville, MD; 1981

6. National Center on Child Abuse and Neglect (DHHS). *Study Findings. Study of National Incidence and Prevalence of Child Abuse and Neglect: 1988.* Westat, Inc.; 1988

7. Sedlak AJ, Broadhurst DD. Third National Incidence Study of Child Abuse and Neglect. Available at: www.childwelfare.gov/pubs/statsinfo/nis3.cfm. Accessed May 11, 2010

8. Straus M. *Trends in Physical Abuse by Parents from 1975 to 1992: A Comparison of Three National Surveys.* Boston, MA: American Society of Criminology; 1995

9. Theodore AD, Chang JJ, Runyan DK, Hunter VM, Bangdiwala SI, Agans R. Epidemiologic features of the physical and sexual maltreatment of children in the Carolinas. *Pediatrics.* 2005;115(3):e331–e337

10. Centers for Disease Control. Youth Risk Behavior Surveillance System. Available at: www. cdc.gov/HealthyYouth/yrbs/index.htm. Accessed May 11, 2010

11. Finkelhor D, Ormond R, Turner H, Hamby SL. The victimization of children and youth: a comprehensive, national survey. *Child Maltreat.* 2005;10(1):5–25

12. Libbey P, Bybee R. The physical abuse of adolescents. *J Soc Issues.* 1979;35:101–126

13. Moran P, Eckenrode J. Protective personality characteristics among adolescent victims of maltreatment. *Child Abuse Negl.* 1992;16:743–754

14. Fagan A. The relationship between adolescent physical abuse and criminal offending: support for an enduring and generalized cycle of violence. *J Fam Violence.* 2005;20(5):279–289

15. Kaplan SJ, Pelcovitz D, Salzinger S, et al. Adolescent physical abuse: risk for adolescent psychiatric disorders. *Am J Psychiatry.* 1998;155(7):954–959

16. Straus MA. *Beating the Devil Out of Them: Corporal Punishment in American Families.* San Francisco, CA: Jossey-Bass/Lexington Books; 1994

17. United States Preventive Services Task Force. Screening for family and intimate partner violence. Available at: www.uspreventiveservicestaskforce.org/uspstf/uspsfamv.htm. Accessed November 26, 2010

# CHAPTER 169

## Sexual Abuse and Assault

MARTIN A. FINKEL, DO • MARITA E. LIND, MD

### OVERVIEW

Sexual victimization of adolescents is a common occurrence for which primary care providers need to possess special knowledge and skill to appropriately address concerns in an empathetic and protective manner. Although recent literature suggests the prevalence of sexual victimization of children and youth is declining, it continues to be a common adverse experience.[1-5] Frequently cited prevalence rates indicate that approximately 1 in 4 girls, and 1 in 7 boys experience some form of unwanted sexual experience.[6-9]

There is ample research to demonstrate that inappropriate sexual experiences have the potential for long-term medical and mental health consequences for children and adolescents, and that early intervention has the greatest potential for mitigating future damage.[10] Children and adolescents who experience sexual abuse are at significantly higher risk for depression, cigarette smoking, marijuana use, regular alcohol use and binge drinking, obesity, engaging in violent behaviors, and fair/poor overall health.[11] Adolescent girls and boys with a history of sexual abuse are also more likely to report sexual risk-taking than nonabused adolescents.[12,13] Primary care physicians should routinely screen adolescents for a history of sexual abuse both to address previously undisclosed abuse and to provide anticipatory guidance regarding how to respond to inappropriate sexual encounters that might occur in the future. For example, adolescents presenting with depression, eating disorders, high-risk behaviors, and/or self-mutilation should be queried regarding a history of sexual abuse. Using empathetic nonstigmatizing and nonjudgmental questioning, adolescents may for the first time disclose a history of sexual abuse. This disclosure provides an opportunity for the physician to begin the process of addressing the potential underpinnings of emotional difficulties and to provide recommendations for mental health evaluation and treatment.

### CLINICAL RELEVANCE OF THE DYNAMICS OF SEXUAL VICTIMIZATION

As is true of other clinical situations in adolescent health care, the diagnosis of sexual abuse involves integration of the medical history, physical examination findings, and laboratory or other testing. Among the challenges in applying the traditional medical model to the diagnosis of sexual abuse are the emotionally charged nature of the issue, its intersection with the legal system, and the often limited training of clinicians regarding the dynamics of sexual victimization. As is also true in other cases of medical diagnosis, the "chief complaint" and medical history are often the most readily available sources of "evidence." However, in cases of sexual abuse the link between the chief complaint and an underlying dynamic of sexual victimization may not be obvious, and the disclosure of the abuse itself may not come to light for months or years, if ever. Therefore, it is crucial for the clinician to understand the dynamics of sexual victimization and disclosure.[14]

#### ENGAGEMENT/SEXUAL INTERACTION

Most perpetrators who engage adolescents in sexual activities are known and trusted by the adolescent. Perpetrators also have easy access to the adolescent or create opportunities for such. Sexual abuse often begins at an age inappropriate for either noncontact or contact sexual interaction. Unlike sexual assault, most perpetrators of sexual abuse intend to engage the adolescent in sexual activities repeatedly and in an increasingly more intrusive manner over time. The medical history should seek the details of early contact, progression of sexual activities over time, and the rewards or intimidating threats used to assure secrecy.[15,16]

#### SECRECY

Secrecy is an essential dynamic of sexual victimization. Once an adolescent experiences a sexually inappropriate interaction, the primary goal of the perpetrator is to engage and maintain secrecy. From the perpetrator's perspective, secrecy removes accountability and sets the stage for repeating the abusive acts. Secrecy may be accomplished by: (1) targeting adolescents who are nonverbal or with limited communication skills; (2) making direct statements to the victims such as bribery with money, gifts, or other favors, or a variety of threats or intimidating remarks directed at the adolescent, the family, or friends; (3) encouraging shame, embarrassment, or guilt on the part of the adolescent; or (4) some combination of the previous.

### DISCLOSURE

Adolescents frequently fail to disclose their victimization or disclose long after the event. When adolescents experience sexually inappropriate interactions they may find it difficult to disclose for a variety of reasons, including stigmatization, embarrassment, fear of threats, fear of not being believed, and feelings of culpability for their experience. Males may find it particularly difficult to disclose due to fear that they may be labeled homosexual.[9] The relationship of the perpetrator to the adolescent is also a significant factor in whether disclosure occurs. When the perpetrator is not a caretaker, family member, or significant other of a parent, adolescents are more likely to be comfortable disclosing and more likely to be believed.

Disclosures generally can be categorized as planned, accidental, or elicited. Accidental disclosures occur under circumstances that are unanticipated, such as a parent finding a diary describing inappropriate sexual interactions. Planned disclosures are the result of a conscious decision to tell someone about the abuse. Even when adolescents make a decision to disclose, their disclosure may be limited and incomplete. When an adolescent makes a conscious decision to tell, ask him/her why s/he decided to tell and what she or he wants to happen after the disclosure. Asking the adolescent why it was difficult to tell either in a delayed disclosure or accidental circumstance provides insight into the fears and anxieties that will need to be addressed. Elicited disclosures are the result of questioning the adolescent when a behavior or statement warrants suspicion.

### RECANTATION

When adolescents disclose abuse they do so primarily because they want the abuse to stop, but generally they do not have an understanding of the cascade of events that might be precipitated by the disclosure. Adolescents frequently feel responsible for what happened to them, even when the interactions were clearly not consensual. This sense of culpability increases as the number of sexual interactions, or the duration of the abuse prior to disclosure, increases. If the adolescent is not believed or supported following disclosure, or if the unanticipated consequences of the disclosure, such as prosecution of a family member, result in the adolescent feeling guilt, the adolescent may recant the initial disclosure.

## HISTORY OF CHIEF COMPLAINT

It is better to rely on a physician-obtained history rather than reviewing a videotaped law enforcement interview or a summary from child protection or law enforcement. Adolescents may share information with a physician that they have not otherwise shared with anyone else based on their trusting relationship with their doctor.

The physician should meet independently with the adolescent and in an unhurried manner obtain a history of the sequence of events concerning the circumstances that led up to the first incident and the details up to and following disclosure. The history should elicit details of the possible dynamics of victimization listed in the previous section. When obtaining the medical history, it is important to ask questions in a nonjudgmental, empathetic, and open-ended manner without leading questions. The medical record should accurately reflect the history obtained, using exact quotations when appropriate, and not be simply a summary or synthesis of the adolescent's history.

When obtaining a history of sexual victimization it is best to obtain the chronology of events from the time of initial engagement until disclosure and determine the relationship of the perpetrator to the victim. An assessment of how the activities were represented (coercive, deceptive, playful, or threatening) should also be documented. The age differential between the adolescent and the alleged perpetrator can be relevant; generally, if the age differential is more than 5 years, there is an imbalance of power and the autonomy of the younger adolescent is compromised. Additionally, the age difference between the victim and the perpetrator may have varied legal implications as age of consent laws differ from state to state.

It is also important to obtain any history of possible signs and symptoms of sexual abuse.[17] Did the child report experiencing physical discomfort during or after the abuse? Did she/he observe anything that made them know she/he was hurt? Attempt to ask open-ended questions that obtain idiosyncratic descriptions of experiences that an adolescent may not otherwise identify unless she/he had personal knowledge. It is also important to determine whether she/he has any worries or concerns about his/her body as a result of the experience. Common concerns include questions about physical "intactness," whether people can tell something happened, the ability to have children as adults and the possibility of sexually transmitted infection (STI). Reassure them that the physical examination will provide an opportunity to address all of these concerns.

## MEDICAL HISTORY

The medical history is the cornerstone of understanding the adolescent's experience and is obtained in the context of a complete assessment that should include a medical history and detailed review of systems focused on genitourinary and gastrointestinal systems, obtained from the caretaker and the adolescent separately. The caretaker should be queried independently about his/her understanding of what the adolescent experienced along with any observations and concerns.

Questions regarding prior consensual sexual activities and signs and symptoms associated with such are important to obtain. Parents may be unaware of consensual sexual activities. This information should be kept confidential until such time that the adolescent can share this information with her/his parent. However, the physician should be aware that prior consensual activities may have forensic value and therefore may not remain confidential.

## PHYSICAL EXAMINATION

A disclosure of sexual abuse almost always precipitates a crisis, and the need for a parent, guardian, or caretaker "to know" has resulted in many adolescents unnecessarily being taken to a hospital emergency department (ED) for an examination. Therefore, the interval between the last inappropriate sexual contact and clinical presentation influences decisions regarding therapeutic or investigative interventions. If the primary care physician is contacted following a disclosure of abuse, the physician should determine the timing of the most recent incident. If the last sexual contact occurred within the last 5 days and was of a type to result in foreign DNA being deposited on the adolescent's body, then an evaluation is necessary both to examine the adolescent and to collect forensic evidence. In addition, emergency contraception should be offered if there was intercourse within the last 5 days. The longer the interval between the abuse and the examination, the less likely forensic evidence will be retrievable. In cases where the perpetrator is unknown to the adolescent, DNA evidence can play a role in the confirmation and identification of the perpetrator. Although most cases of sexual abuse involve the identity of the perpetrator being known, DNA evidence can confirm that sexual contact took place. Non-DNA types of evidence may be used to confirm other aspects of the adolescent's history. Additionally, if the patient has any ano-genital complaints, physical examination is required to determine the need for further evaluation or treatment. Adolescents who experience physical discomfort and/or observe bleeding following the contact are more likely to demonstrate findings on examination.

A guiding principle in clinical decision making is to assure that the adolescent undergoes only one examination at a facility where knowledgeable and skilled physicians can identify acute and healed trauma, collect and preserve forensic evidence, and initiate treatment for STIs or pregnancy prevention. Some communities have facilities outside of hospitals specifically designed to address the needs of children and adolescents who are abused physically or sexually. These facilities provide a safe and secure setting in which professionals who are experts in the assessment and treatment of sexual abuse work together as a team. At such facilities, adolescents who experience sexual assault may be examined by sexual assault nurse examiners (SANEs) or be responded to by sexual assault response teams (SARTs) whose clinical response is to identify injuries and collect forensic evidence. Depending upon the clinical situation of the adolescent and the scope of licensure of the facility and the SANE/SART nurses, it may be possible for the adolescent to have comprehensive diagnosis, treatment, and follow-up, including interaction with legal authorities, and social service and mental health providers. Because hospital EDs are often busy, crowded, somewhat impersonal, and often intimidating for adolescents, if available, such community-based centers devoted specifically to handling sexual abuse are often preferred by patients, parents, and legal authorities. Regardless of where the adolescent patient is evaluated, when there is an opportunity to identify and preserve physical evidence, a "rape kit" is used. This provides both the instructions and materials necessary to collect physical evidence. The completed rape kit must be handled in a manner that preserves a chain of custody prior to being handed to law enforcement.[18]

All adolescents deserve an opportunity for a complete, comprehensive physical examination, even when considerable time has elapsed since the last contact. The examination is conducted to address possible medical consequences of the contact such as extragenital, genital, and/or anal trauma and STIs. Equally important is conducting the examination even when the likelihood of identifying acute trauma is remote for the purpose of assuring "normality." The examination is best conducted by a provider who has experience evaluating children and adolescents who are suspected of being sexually abused. In most communities there are physicians available to either conduct or assist the primary care doctor in providing care for the patient. The physical examination should focus not only on the health consequences of suspected sexual abuse but also on the identification and collection of evidence. Evidence such as seminal products is most frequently collected from either the patient's clothing and/or bedding rather than during the physical examination.[19] For the purpose of this chapter the focus will be on the identification of acute and healed genital, anal, and extragenital trauma.

The presence of injury is increased under circumstances where force and restraint are used to complete the sexual acts. When the alleged perpetrator is a family member or person with caretaking responsibilities for the adolescent, the potential for injury is reduced. Most perpetrating caretakers do not intend to harm the adolescent because of the common intention, as noted previously, to engage the adolescent in repeated activities over time.

Most injuries incurred as part of sexual abuse are superficial and heal without consequences.[20,21] Variables related to the extent of physical findings—from none to readily visible—following vaginal and/or anal penetration include the (1) degree of force used, (2) "cooperativeness" of the victim, (3) use of lubrication, and (4) size and type of object used for penetration. A common myth is that the hymen is impenetrable until first vaginal penetration, so that first penetration is always associated with bleeding. Once the hymen is estrogenized, the tissue that forms the hymen becomes very elastic. It is this distensibility that allows the hymenal orifice to admit objects such as a penis without any sign or symptoms of injury. In a study of college girls' first intercourse experiences, 44% had no bleeding and 35% had only slight bleeding.[22] In a study of 36 pregnant adolescents only 2 had hymenal findings that were diagnostic of prior penetration.[23] Diagnostic findings following anal penetration are uncommon as well due to the ability of the anal sphincter to dilate to accommodate the passage of large bowel movements. Because of the highly vascular nature of the vaginal and perianal tissues, injuries often heal quickly and usually without diagnostic findings.

Less frequently, sexual abuse results in more severe injuries. Extragenital trauma may be observed in the form of ligature marks, bite marks, or residual to a struggle and/or physical altercation. Acute abrasions, contusions, or healed trauma to the labia majora, minora, fossa navicularis, posterior fourchette, hymenal membrane, or internal vaginal structures may be present. Anal trauma may be evident as abrasions, lacerations of the anal verge and, depending upon the degree of penetration and the object utilized, trauma to the rectosigmoid. In extreme cases there may be either vaginal or anal perforation into the peritoneal cavity. Acute signs of genital trauma may also be accompanied by symptoms such as genital pain with or without dysuria.

Although there are few genital or anal findings that are diagnostic of sexual abuse on their own, genital injuries can result in recognizable lacerations/transections of the genital/anal tissues and the formation of scar tissue.[24] Occasionally scar tissue may also be noted in the fossa, fourchette, or on the perineum. Genital trauma may be evident as a complete or partial transection of the hymenal membrane edge. An acute or healed transection when located between the 4 and 7 o'clock position supine that extends to the base of the hymenal attachment is diagnostic of blunt force penetrating trauma. There may be acute bruising of the anal verge tissue, mucosal lacerations, perineal trauma, and with extreme force, complete transections of the sphincter. The history should include the object that resulted in such injuries.

The genital examination of the adolescent female will generally entail the use of a vaginal speculum, if tolerated. The pelvic examination also provides an opportunity to collect seminal products from the endocervix and posterior fornix, obtain cultures, and perform a Pap smear, if needed. The examination may be enhanced with the use of colposcopy, which affords an excellent light source and magnification capabilities that are particularly helpful in identifying mucosal abrasions. Another advantage of colposcopy is that when fitted with either a video or digital camera, a permanent record of observed injuries can be documented. With a history of acute anal penetration, anoscopy may be used to examine the rectosigmoid for signs of trauma and to collect cultures and seminal products as well. When either acute or healed diagnostic findings are observed the examiner should make every attempt to photograph the injuries accompanied by a detailed description in the medical record.

## ADOLESCENT CONCERNS REGARDING SEXUALLY TRANSMITTED INFECTIONS AND PREGNANCY

Some of the most commonly expressed concerns of the adolescent patient are whether they may have contracted an STI or could be pregnant. Sexually transmitted infections are more commonly seen in adolescent victims of sexual abuse than in prepubertal victims, but they remain relatively uncommon.[25] The medical interview should explore what the adolescent experienced and the reasons for his/her concern. Rather than accepting at face value statements such as "we had sex," clarifying questions may help regarding concerns about STIs and/or pregnancy, such as the presence of symptoms or anxiety about complications of the sexual contact. This interchange also provides an opportunity to answer questions and educate about sexuality.

**SEXUALLY TRANSMITTED INFECTIONS**

In cases where there is a history of contact between mucous membranes of the adolescent and the bodily fluids and/or mucous membranes of a perpetrator of sexual abuse, testing for STIs is necessary.[26] Both the Centers for Disease Control and Prevention (CDC)[27] and *Red Book of Infectious Diseases,* published by the American Academy of Pediatrics, provide guidelines for testing, treatment, and follow-up of STIs. When cultures are obtained they should be sent directly to the laboratory for processing rather than being submitted with the same kit used to collect forensic evidence.

Testing for STIs should be based on the previously mentioned guidelines and the history provided. Screening for STIs in adolescents following an acute sexual assault may have mixed forensic value due to the possibility of pre-existing infections. However, such testing is medically indicated especially if the adolescent refuses antibiotic prophylaxis. Cultures for chlamydia and gonorrhea from the endocervix are the standard for the evaluation of adolescent females; other forms of testing may have false-positive results. A wet mount for trichomoniasis and bacterial vaginosis should be performed if clinically indicated. In males, urethral swabs may be indicated if signs and symptoms indicate this is necessary. In both males and females, the history may indicate that swabs from the rectum and oropharynx are needed. During the physical examination of the adolescent, lesions suggestive of herpes or syphilis may be identified. Although herpes is often a clinical diagnosis, the physician should culture ulcerative lesions to confirm the diagnosis. Typing of the herpes virus can be considered but may be of limited forensic value. Serologic testing for HIV, hepatitis B and C, and syphilis should also be completed.

Treatment decisions regarding STIs are best guided by the history. In cases where the sexual contact has been ongoing or is not recent, it is appropriate to let STI test results guide the treatment plan. In cases of acute (less than 72 hours) sexual contact with mucous membrane exposure to bodily fluids, prophylactic treatment for gonorrhea and chlamydia should be provided. After an acute assault, follow-up STI testing and re-examination should be performed in 2 weeks. Counseling regarding STIs and other health risks can be provided at that time to adolescent patients.

Communication with local infectious disease specialists can help guide decisions regarding the cost and benefit of prophylactic HIV treatment in the setting of an acute sexual assault. In addition, the clinician should recommend that the family request HIV testing of the perpetrator because this may provide important information for the care of the adolescent.

To successfully provide acute and ongoing care of adolescents who have experienced sexual abuse, policies and protocols with reference laboratories and area emergency departments must be developed. Good communication regarding the testing that is required and how the results of the tests will be communicated will enable the clinician to more effectively treat and reassure families regarding STIs promptly.

**PREGNANCY**

A pregnancy test is indicated in all female adolescents being evaluated for possible sexual abuse. A history of prior or current pregnancy in a young adolescent may indicate previous or ongoing sexual abuse. In cases of acute sexual assault, counseling regarding pregnancy prophylaxis should be provided.[25]

Adolescents who are being evaluated for sexual abuse may have never received reproductive health care. The care they receive after reporting sexual abuse should include appropriate anticipatory guidance as well as appropriate testing and treatment for health risks identified by the history provided. If the adolescent is not emotionally able to have a physical examination in the acute setting, a follow-up examination should be scheduled. In this instance, a urine pregnancy test as well as testing for STIs by urine nucleic acid amplification and serologic testing, can provide useful clinical information.

## FORMULATING AND DOCUMENTING A DIAGNOSIS

When formulating a diagnosis of sexual abuse the clinician must consider and incorporate salient aspects of each of the following:

1. Historical details and/or behavioral indicators that reflect suspected inappropriate sexual contact
2. Symptoms that can be directly associated with the contact
3. Acute and healed genital/anal injuries
4. Extragenital injuries
5. STIs
6. Other forensic evidence

The following common clinical scenarios reflect the potential combinations of the previously noted considerations, each of which may have a varying degree of importance when formulating a diagnostic assessment. It is important to keep in mind that a complete understanding of what a child experienced may be apparent only when the collaborative insights of other disciplines are considered. Case scenario presentation examples are as follows:

1. An adolescent offers a history of inappropriate sexual contact and/or there is suspicion of inappropriate sexual contact due to the adolescent's behavior, but there are no diagnostic findings on examination.
2. Diagnostic findings are present that indicate inappropriate sexual contact, such as trauma, STI, and/or seminal products, but there has been no disclosure of inappropriate contact.
3. Diagnostic findings are present that indicate inappropriate sexual contact, such as trauma, STI, and/or seminal products and these findings support the adolescent's disclosure.
4. Inappropriate sexual contact can be confirmed without medical findings, such as contact witnessed by a third party or documented and preserved in pornographic materials.
5. There are insufficient historical or behavioral details to support a concern of inappropriate sexual contact and the physical examination is not diagnostic of sexual abuse.

The medical record is the key element of the medical evaluation. The medical record will potentially undergo legal scrutiny and must provide an accurate reflection of the historical details obtained to form the basis of the diagnosis.[28] Because the most available form of "evidence" in cases of child and adolescent sexual abuse is the patient's report, it is essential that the historical details from the medical history be accurately preserved in the record along with the specific questions asked to elicit the information. In a legal setting, it is possible that the medical history will be analyzed regarding how leading and/or suggestible the questions are. Familiarity with the continuum of leading and suggestible questions will serve the historian well when framing questions in a developmentally appropriate manner.[29,30] Where physical evidence exists to support the diagnosis, this should be documented via photographs or through digital or videocolposcopy.[31] Visual documentation is important and has the potential to reduce the chance of an adolescent being subjected to a second opinion re-examination when the initial examining physician's opinion is challenged. The diagnosis must be formulated in a manner that is clear, balanced, and defensible.

The diagnostic formulation section of the medical record should also document: (1) discrepancies between an adolescent's perception of his or her experience and what actually happened; (2) clear histories of injuries as a result of the contact that may not have diagnostic residual; (3) symptoms secondary to trauma anticipated when an adolescent experiences genital fondling, genital-to-genital contact, or anal trauma.

## MENTAL HEALTH TREATMENT RECOMMENDATIONS

Overall, the most significant impact of sexual abuse is related to the mental health and psychological sequelae. Without appropriate treatment these patients have the potential of long-term consequences that can involve sexual acting out, substance abuse, depression, self-injurious behavior, and engagement in high-risk activities.[32-34]

In any adolescent in which the diagnostic assessment concludes that he or she experienced inappropriate sexual contact, the patient should be referred for a comprehensive psychological assessment to determine the type of mental health treatment required. The mental health treatment of choice for most patients is trauma-focused cognitive behavioral therapy.[35,36] Successful treatment models provide group role-playing opportunities, individual therapy, and active engagement of the nonoffending parent in the treatment. Effective therapy can be relatively short-term with the trauma-focused cognitive behavioral therapy approach for most patients.

## SUMMARY

The primary care physician can play a significant role in caring for the adolescent patient who discloses sexual abuse. An understanding of the dynamics of sexual victimization can make it possible to sensitively elicit a medical history and examine adolescents who have been sexually abused. Even though caring for a patient who has been sexually abused can be emotionally challenging, substantiating suspected sexual abuse is the first step to protecting the patient and securing the critically important services necessary for the adolescent's treatment and recovery.

## REFERENCES


1. Dube SR, Anda RF, Whitfield CL, et al. Long-term consequences of childhood sexual abuse by gender of victim. *Am J Prev Med.* 2005;28(5):430–438

2. Dube SR, Miller JW, Brown DW, et al. Adverse childhood experiences and the association with ever using alcohol and initiating alcohol use during adolescence. *J Adolesc Health.* 2006;38(4):444 e1–e10

3. Finkelhor D, Hotaling G, Lewis IA, Smith C. Sexual abuse in a national survey of adult men and women: prevalence, characteristics, and risk factors. *Child Abuse Negl.* 1990;14(1):19–28

4. Finkelhor D, Ormrod R, Turner H, Hamby SL. The victimization of children and youth: a comprehensive, national survey. [erratum appears in *Child Maltreat.* 2005;10(2):207]. *Child Maltreat.* 2005;10(1):5–25

5. Jones LM, Finkelhor D, Kopiec K. Why is sexual abuse declining? A survey of state child protection administrators. [see comment]. *Child Abuse Negl.* 2001;25(9):1139-1158

6. Finkelhor D, Dziuba-Leatherman J. Children as victims of violence: a national survey. *Pediatrics.* 1994;94(4 Pt 1):413-420

7. Helweg-Larsen K, Boving Larsen H. The prevalence of unwanted and unlawful sexual experiences reported by Danish adolescents: results from a national youth survey in 2002. *Acta Paediatrica.* 2006;95(10):1270-1276

8. Trocme NM, Tourigny M, MacLaurin B, Fallon B. Major findings from the Canadian incidence study of reported child abuse and neglect. *Child Abuse Negl.* 2003;27(12):1427-1439

9. Watkins B, Bentovim A. The sexual abuse of male children and adolescents: a review of current research. *J Child Psychol Psych Allied Disc.* 1992;33(1):197-248

10. Edwards VJ, Holden GW, Felitti VJ, Anda RF. Relationship between multiple forms of childhood maltreatment and adult mental health in community respondents: results from the adverse childhood experiences study. *Am J Psych.* 2003;160(8):1453-1460

11. Hussey JM, Chang JJ, Kotch JB. Child maltreatment in the United States: prevalence, risk factors, and adolescent health consequences. *Pediatrics.* 2006;118(3):933-942

12. Champion HL, Foley KL, DuRant RH, Hensberry R, Altman D, Wolfson M. Adolescent sexual victimization, use of alcohol and other substances, and other health risk behaviors. *J Adolesc Health.* 2004;35(4):321-328

13. Raj A, Silverman JG, Amaro H. The relationship between sexual abuse and sexual risk among high school students: findings from the 1997 Massachusetts Youth Risk Behavior Survey. *Maternal and Child Health Journal.* 2000;4(2):125-134

14. Finkelhor D. The victimization of children: a developmental perspective. *Am J Orthopsych.* 1995;65(2):177-193

15. Finkelhor D, Browne A. The traumatic impact of child sexual abuse: a conceptualization. *Am J Orthopsych.* 1985;55(4):530-541

16. Summit RC. The child sexual abuse accommodation syndrome. *Child Abuse Negl.* 1983;7(2):177-193

17. DeLago C, Deblinger ED, Schroeder C, Finkel MA. Girls who disclose sexual abuse: urogenital symptoms and signs following sexual contact. *Pediatrics.* 2008;122(8):e221-e226

18. US Department of Justice. *A National Protocol for Sexual Assault Medical Forensic Examination Adults/Adolescents: President's DNA Initiative.* In: Women of VA, ed; 2004

19. Christian CW, Lavelle JM, De Jong AR, Loiselle J, Brenner L, Joffe M. Forensic evidence findings in prepubertal victims of sexual assault. *Pediatrics.* 2000;106(1 Pt 1):100-104

20. Finkel MA. Anogenital trauma in sexually abused children. *Pediatrics.* 1989;84(2):317-322

21. Heger A, Ticson L, Velasquez O, Bernier R. Children referred for possible sexual abuse: medical findings in 2,384 children. *Child Abuse Negl.* 2002;26(6-7):645-659

22. Whitley N. The first coital experience of one hundred women. *JOGN Nursing.* 1978;7(4):41-45

23. Kellogg ND, Menard SW, Santos A. Genital anatomy in pregnant adolescents: "normal" does not mean "nothing happened." *Pediatrics.* 2004;113(1 Pt 1):e67-e69

24. Adams JA, Harper K, Knudson S, Revilla J. Examination findings in legally confirmed child sexual abuse: it's normal to be normal [see comment]. *Pediatrics.* 1994;94(3):310-317

25. Kellogg N, American Academy of Pediatrics Committee on Child Abuse and Neglect. The evaluation of sexual abuse in children. *Pediatrics.* 2005;116(2):506-512

26. Siegel RM, Schubert CJ, Myers PA, Shapiro RA. The prevalence of sexually transmitted diseases in children and adolescents evaluated for sexual abuse in Cincinnati: rationale for limited STD testing in prepubertal girls. *Pediatrics.* 1995;96(6):1090-1094

27. Centers for Disease Control. Sexual Assault or Abuse of Children. Sexually Transmitted Diseases Treatment Guidelines 2006. Available at: www.cdc.gov/std/treatment/2006/sexual-assault.htm. Accessed August 3, 2010

28. Finkel MA, Giardino AP. *Medical Evaluation of Child Sexual Abuse: A Practical Guide*. 3rd ed. Elk Grove Village, IL: American Academy of Pediatrics; 2009

29. Myers JE. Role of physician in preserving verbal evidence of child abuse. *J Pediatr.* 1986;109(3):409-411

30. Myers JEB. Investigative interviewing regarding child maltreatment. *Legal Issues in Child Abuse and Neglect Practice*. 2nd ed. Thousand Oaks, CA: Sage; 1998:102-152

31. Finkel MA, Ricci LR. Documentation and preservation of visual evidence in child abuse. *Child Maltreatment.* 1997;2(4):322-330

32. Turner HA, Finkelhor D, Ormrod R. The effect of lifetime victimization on the mental health of children and adolescents. *Soc Sci Med.* 2006;62(1):13-27

33. Widom CS, Kuhns JB. Childhood victimization and subsequent risk for promiscuity, prostitution, and teenage pregnancy: a prospective study. *Am J Pub Health.* 1996;86(11):1607-1612

34. Widom CS, Weiler BL, Cottler LB. Childhood victimization and drug abuse: a comparison of prospective and retrospective findings. *J Consult Clin Psych.* 1999;67(6):867-880

35. Deblinger E, Mannarino AP, Cohen JA, Steer RA. A follow-up study of a multisite, randomized, controlled trial for children with sexual abuse-related PTSD symptoms. *J Am Acad Child and Adolesc Psych.* 2006;45(12):1474-1484

36. Deblinger E, Steer RA, Lippmann J. Two-year follow-up study of cognitive behavioral therapy for sexually abused children suffering post-traumatic stress symptoms. *Child Abuse Negl.* 1999;23(12):1371-1378

# CHAPTER 170

## Prostitution and Sex Trafficking

CURREN WARE, MD, MS Ed

### INTRODUCTION

Common pathways of adolescent sexual development are described in Chapters 7, Sexual Development, and 49, Adolescent Sexual Behaviors. For some young people there are significant obstacles in the path toward healthy sexual development. Responding to the demands of survival when homeless or in other desperate conditions, exploitation by adults, enmeshment in drug abuse, or in the expression of early childhood trauma, sex may come to be exchanged for needs or material desires. The psychological and physical risks incurred by individuals engaged in survival sex are among the most severe faced by young people. These risks include contracting HIV and other sexually transmitted infections (STIs), becoming enmeshed in drug use, being the victim of sexual or physical assault (including homicide), mental health problems, and suicide. In a 1999 study,[1] female prostitutes in London had a mortality rate 12 times that of noninvolved women of similar age. This chapter reviews health care issues related to prostitution and sex trafficking and offers suggestions for interventions by health care professionals for adolescents and young adults involved in these activities.

### DEFINITION OF TERMS

Because of the stigmatization associated with the term prostitution, and because it tends to imply a moral judgment about the individual rather than a description of context or behavior, alternative terms have emerged to describe behavior in which sexual activity is offered in exchange for needs and desires. Among adolescents, this behavior generally is linked to obtaining necessities of life, so the term "survival sex" is often used. Survival sex is the exchange of sex for food, drugs, money, and/or a place to stay.

Youth in more stable environments may also engage in sexually related activities as employment or as a means to meet material needs and desires. These include pornography, strip (or exotic) dancing, erotic massage, and others. Though there are clearly sexually exploitative aspects to these activities, and some overlap of these behaviors with prostitution, they are not usually considered forms of survival sex by themselves. There are other forms of sexual exploitation of youth, such as familial sexual abuse, but these are not the focus of the current chapter (see Chapter 168, Sexual Abuse and Assault), although many young people who become involved in survival sex have a history of familial sexual abuse.[2]

### PREVALENCE OF SURVIVAL SEX

There are few data regarding the prevalence of adolescent involvement in survival sex. However, studies of specified high-risk populations indicate that certain groups are likely to engage in survival sex. For example, among homeless youth in Hollywood, California, surveyed in 1994, 43% of the sample (46% of males and 32% of females) disclosed having ever engaged in survival sex; a survey[3] in 2008 found that 15% of females and 22% of males disclosed having engaged in survival sex. The reasons for engaging in survival sex included making money (82%), obtaining food or a place to stay (48%), or drugs (22%).[3] Other studies of homeless youth estimate involvement in survival sex ranging from 10% to 50%. Much of the variability is related to differing definitions of what constitutes survival sex. For example, it may be limited in definition to the exchange of sex for money, or more broadly defined as the exchange of sex for other necessities and desires. A multi-city study[4] found a prevalence of involvement in survival sex among youth on the streets to be 27.5%. Among homeless youth staying in shelters, only 9.5% reported survival sex.

### CONTEXTS OF SURVIVAL SEX

Survival sex can take place almost anywhere, indoors or outdoors, in cars, alleys, abandoned buildings, where drugs are sold, apartments, or houses. In most large cities there are areas and streets known for prostitution. These areas may shift as police conduct surveillance and arrests, and neighborhoods change. Adolescents may solicit or be contacted in diverse areas including shopping malls or secondary schools. With the widespread availability of cell phones and pagers, much sexual solicitation has been removed from the streets. There are many cases of young immigrants being subjected to sexual exploitation in households where they work, in transient brothels located in apartment buildings, near migrant worker camps, or other areas. Various types of coercion such as threats of making a report to police or deportation may be used to enforce adolescent involvement in prostitution under these circumstances.

## PROCESS OF INVOLVEMENT IN SURVIVAL SEX

### ADULT MODELING

As with other youth behavior, adult modeling can have a significant influence on involvement in survival sex. It is not uncommon for adolescents, particularly girls who are involved in the exchange of sex for money, to have contact with adult women, sometimes in their own family—such as sisters, aunts, even mothers—who act as adult models. These individuals may deliberately, or by example, normalize involvement in prostitution. Among runaways, youth may encounter seemingly supportive and understanding adults on the streets who guide them into providing sexual favors for survival needs.

### PEER INVOLVEMENT

Many teen girls involved in survival sex are homeless runaways who had left an abusive or conflictual home environment, or "throwaways" who are forced out of home by caregivers because of conflict. They frequently encounter girls in similar situations on the streets. Some of these young people have been in and out of juvenile detention, psychiatric hospitals, or both, and have made contacts with peers who have been engaged in similar behavior. These relationships may be very close. Initially sex for money may seem exciting and provide access to seemingly easy money and drugs. In addition, though survival sex remains a behavior predominately of young people with a paucity of alternative means of self-support, there are also girls and boys who engage in the exchange of sex for commodities or money who are not homeless to satisfy perceived needs for fashionable clothing, drugs, or other desires.

Because of the vulnerability of many adolescents to the influence of peers, particularly if they feel estranged from adult society, clinicians need to be aware of potential unintended consequences of cohorting adolescents involved in high-risk behaviors together, such as in juvenile justice facilities. The idea of commercial sex involvement can be reinforced among vulnerable young people, with relationships formed in group settings frequently continuing after release. When there have been inadequate preparations for housing and stabilization for youth released from juvenile detention, they may become homeless and be faced with the same survival imperatives that led them to the attention of the authorities in the first place.

### IMPACT OF CHILD SEXUAL ABUSE

Correlational or cross-sectional studies have had conflicting findings regarding associations between child abuse, including child sexual abuse, with later sexual behaviors such as prostitution, promiscuity, and early childbearing; because of limitations due to study design conclusions about causal relationships cannot be made. Factors other than child abuse, such as parental alcoholism, drug problems, family violence, and unemployment can have a significant effect on the experiences of young children and behaviors of adolescents and frequently underlie running away and homelessness. One longitudinal cohort study[5] found no significant relationship between sexual abuse and promiscuity or early pregnancy, but it did find a relationship between sexual abuse, physical abuse, and neglect and prostitution in females. The only prospective cohort study[6] of homeless youth evaluating precursors for survival sex found no direct connection between sexual abuse and later involvement in prostitution. A cross-sectional study[7] of homeless girls in Hollywood did not find an increased rate of childhood sexual abuse among girls who had been involved in survival sex. It is likely that the connection between sexual abuse and involvement in prostitution exists principally for youth who run away, become homeless, and develop significant drug abuse.[8]

### RUNAWAY BEHAVIOR AND HOMELESSNESS

Adolescents who run away from home are faced with the challenges of survival without job skills, a poor education, and lack of family support. These individuals often live furtive lives, avoiding contact with agencies that they believe may return them to an unacceptable home situation or otherwise "institutionalize" them. On their own at a young age, they are generally destitute. They resort to extraordinary means to survive, including eating discarded food from restaurant dumpsters and sleeping in outdoor areas. Their self-care is compromised through neglect of dental hygiene and extended periods without access to bathing. The options for meeting survival needs are limited and include utilization of available youth services, panhandling or begging, taking odd jobs, or becoming involved in drug sales. The exchange of sex for survival needs may come to seem increasingly acceptable, and given the lack of alternatives it can seem to offer easy money, excitement, and, even if illusory, a sense of control over one's life. It is estimated that runaway and homeless youth make up about 75% of all juveniles involved in prostitution.[9] In a review of characteristics of 1,180 homeless and runaway adolescents and young adults 12 to 24 years old living in Hollywood and surrounding communities, 46% disclosed a history of involvement in survival sex.[10] Youth require a surprisingly brief period to acculturate to street life, as little as 2 weeks. Predictors of involvement in survival sex among homeless/runaway youth include: age younger than 16 years at first homelessness; recent and frequent use of cocaine or heroin; and use of injection drugs before age 16.[6]

### DRUG USE

In several studies,[11] drug dependence was highly correlated with involvement in survival sex; the exchange of sex for drugs was the most prevalent form of exchange. Historically, adolescents have been disproportionately represented among those engaged in the exchange of sex for drugs in the crack cocaine trade, which is prevalent in urban areas characterized by economic and physical decay, high unemployment, and high levels of poverty. These environments may be particularly risky and degrading, with girls coerced to perform sex publicly with multiple partners.[12] Young people on the streets engaged in survival sex commonly become immersed in the use of methamphetamine, which further complicates their situation by contributing to significant mental health and personality changes, including thought disorders and psychosis.

## SEXUAL BEHAVIORS, SEXUAL ORIENTATION, AND GENDER IDENTITY

The media usually portray females as survival sex workers, but males are also involved in survival sex, often providing sexual services for much older adult males. The boys engaged in this behavior may identify as either heterosexual or homosexual, or may be confused about their own sexual orientation. Some identify themselves as transgender, usually biologic males that identify as having female gender identity.

Heterosexual males who engage in survival sex with other males usually do so out of desperation to meet survival needs. Sometimes the behavior is a component of a criminal plan to rob or assault the customer. Individuals engaged in these criminal activities may be able to avoid apprehension and continue for some time because of the embarrassment and shame of their client/victims that prevents them from contacting the police.

A disproportionate number of gay youth experience homelessness after running away from, or being thrown out of, their homes. They commonly have experienced a family environment that is unable to accept them, and may encounter a family member who makes life intolerable. Many of these boys find themselves in urban centers, naïve and continuing to attempt to define their sexual orientation. Faced with immediate survival needs, some of these youth become involved in survival sex. Many of them encounter a "sugar daddy" who provides food, clothing, and a place to stay in exchange for sexual favors over a period of time. These youth encounter significant danger, such as contracting HIV or other STIs, being assaulted, or being arrested. Tragically, homeless gay youth are disproportionately represented among completed suicides. Most homeless male youth do not engage in survival sex. Homeless males who do engage in survival sex are distinguished by a longer period of homelessness (>6 months), a history of sexual abuse, and a higher risk of alcohol abuse and injection drug use.[13]

## INFLUENCE OF SOCIAL AND ECONOMIC ENVIRONMENTAL FACTORS

Many factors influence adolescents to become engaged in survival sex, almost all beyond their control. Poverty, poor education, familial substance abuse, and child abuse contribute to an adolescent's engagement in survival sex. Youth who grow up in stable home environments where they are valued and loved and who have educational and recreational opportunities rarely become engaged in prostitution. Community environments with a high prevalence of poverty, poorly functioning schools, lack of productive opportunities for youth, substance abuse, and gangs are fertile areas for young people to become engaged in survival sex.

Particularly in the Southwest, unaccompanied immigrant youth who have left their family of origin, usually because of poverty, travel to the United States in an attempt to find work, and often encounter insurmountable challenges. Some of these adolescents are forced to survive through various types of exchange of sexual favors for money or other necessities.

## HEALTH RISKS

There is an obvious risk to male and female adolescents engaged in survival sex of acquiring HIV and other STIs. This risk can be significantly reduced by the use of condoms, as demonstrated by an English study[14] of 402 adult women working in the sex trade. With an average of 250 clients per year, most of whom wore condoms, there were no new cases of HIV infection attributable to sexual contact with a client. Unfortunately, it is not uncommon for clients of young people engaged in survival sex to pay more if the youth agrees not to use a condom, increasing the probability of the transmission of HIV and other STIs.

When survival sex is combined with substance abuse, particularly in the exchange of sex for drugs, the health risks escalate dramatically. In a study[15] of male and female sex workers in San Francisco, Miami, and New York City who were engaged in the exchange of crack cocaine for sex, with a median age of initiation of 19 for girls and 18 for boys, 25% of females and 39% of males were HIV positive, and 40% of females and 25% of males had syphilis.

Other health risks of involvement in the sex trade include the consequences of sexual and physical assault. Among sex workers studied in New York City, more than 50% had experienced violence from commercial clients and 73% from intimate partners.[16] A 2008 survey[7] of homeless youth in Hollywood found that 36% had been physically assaulted and 39% sexually assaulted while engaged in survival sex.

## PREGNANCY AND CHILDBEARING

Homeless and runaway youth's circumstances create perhaps the most difficult environments in which to care for an infant or child. Nonetheless, the perception that having a baby will offer a solution to problems can be compelling to adolescents in these situations. For a teen whose future is difficult to envision, who has failed in school, and who is estranged from her family, the belief that a baby will offer hope and a future can be extraordinarily powerful. The adolescent may believe that a baby will provide someone to love, and who will love her, increase her social status as a mother, provide a compelling reason to stop using drugs, and improve the bond with her boyfriend. These perceptions are rarely grounded in reality, however. A girl who remains on the streets with a baby will almost invariably have him or her removed by child protective services. The emotional turmoil resulting from the loss of an infant under these circumstances can contribute to a spiraling deterioration in substance use, depression, and other mental health problems, and pursuit of another pregnancy.

## SEXUAL TRAFFICKING

Trafficking in humans for prostitution is a worldwide phenomenon and a significant human rights issue akin to modern-day slavery.[17] The extent of trafficking in adolescents is not known, but annually about 45,000 women and children in the United States are estimated to be trafficked, of whom 30,000 are from Southeast Asia and an additional 10,000 from Latin America.[18] The Immigration and Naturalization Service has identified more than 250 brothels in 26 American cities. These brothels are usually located in apartment complexes; however, sexual trafficking also occurs in secured warehouses where trafficked girls are isolated by their foreign language and culture, and fear of arrest, deportation, or violence. They may be controlled through threats against loved ones in their home country. The hidden nature of the phenomenon, the isolation from mainstream society, the language barriers, and the difficulty apprehending, prosecuting, and convicting the trafficker all create almost insurmountable challenges to preventing its occurrence. Trafficking adolescent females as a sexual commodity is a distinct phenomenon from prostitution. They are victims who do not receive pay and are generally kept captive through powerlessness, threats, fear, and isolation.[19]

Trafficking of immigrant adolescent females, regardless of national origin, takes place mainly across the United States–Mexico border. Trafficked children have been found in many American cities, in particular Miami, New York City, Chicago, Los Angeles, and San Diego.[20] Young women and teens are lured with promises of jobs as waitresses, nannies, or factory workers, and are sometimes kidnapped *en route*. The abduction, transport, and utilization of young women as sexual commodities frequently involves organized crime originating in other countries. They may be subjected to sexual exploitation in temporary shelters on the outskirts of migrant labor camps.

In addition to adolescent females being brought to the United States for the commercial sex industry, men are known to travel to Mexico, Thailand, or the Philippines for sex with underage girls. It is a federal crime, with a sentence of up to 30 years per offense, for any person to enter the United States or to travel abroad for the purpose of sex tourism involving underage individuals.[19,21]

In addition to the obvious human rights violations inherent in human trafficking, there are many serious health and medical problems. These include STI, HIV, hepatitis C, substance abuse, and injuries incurred by assault. Physicians and others who may interface with this population have a special responsibility, beyond the treatment of acute infections and injuries, to follow state law in reporting child sexual abuse and exploitation to child protective services and/or law enforcement.

## INTERNATIONAL PERSPECTIVES

The United Nations International Children's Fund (UNICEF) characterizes child prostitution as "one of the gravest infringements of rights that children can endure."[22] Under the United Nations Convention on the Rights of the Child, signed by every country (except Somalia and the United States), children have the right to be protected from prostitution. Worldwide, some 9 million girls and 1 million boys are estimated to be prostituted annually, resulting in at least 300,000 cases of HIV, more than 1.2 million induced abortions, and more than 360,000 abortion-related complications.[23] Prostitution of teenage girls and young women, particularly of street youth, has emerged as a significant factor in the spread of HIV and other STI in the developing world. The World Health Organization found that "sexual abuse and family and economic pressures to engage in prostitution present adverse environments for adolescent health, including exposure to sexually transmitted diseases."[24] HIV infection risk is attracting men to increasingly younger sexual partners.[24] About 75% of the 40 million refugees in the world are women and children. When family and social ties break down, prostitution represents a way for them to earn money in exchange for food. Thus, prostitution often becomes established around refugee camps.[25] In addition to refugees, prostitution involving adolescents is prevalent around military bases, migrant worker camps, and along trucking routes. In every respect, the prostitution of adolescents and its attendant risks are created by conditions that result from poverty or lack of adult protection, not of adolescent misconduct.

## PREVENTION AND INTERVENTION

For youth who are on the streets and have not been engaged in survival sex, it is important to appreciate that they are at significant risk of becoming engaged in this activity to meet basic needs, particularly if they are using drugs. Although there have been no longitudinal studies evaluating the efficacy of prevention strategies, there are some promising approaches, including:

- Developing a culture that does not tolerate physical or sexual abuse, or severe neglect, of children or adolescents, and reframing adolescents involved in survival sex as victims of poverty, child abuse, and social rejection, rather than seductive aggressors.
- Building a culture of acceptance of sexual minority youth, including homosexual and transgender youth (see Chapter 51) that overcomes biases and rejection and encourages young people to stay at home through adolescence, or provides an alternative, accepting, safe environment for nonheterosexual adolescents whose families cannot accept them.
- Prosecuting adult perpetrators who act as pimps for adolescents involved in survival sex or who are involved in human trafficking.
- Providing appropriate, mandated substance abuse and mental health treatment for youth who are incarcerated or on probation, and avoiding the cohorting in social service or detention facilities of adolescents involved with survival sex and those who have not been involved. In addition, incarcerated minors must be segregated from adults, as required by federal law. The "Standards for Health Services in Juvenile Detention and Confinement Facilities" by the National Commission on Correctional Health Care[26] also should be adhered to.
- Providing easy availability of condoms for sexually active youth.

## INCARCERATED YOUTH

Young people who are engaged in survival sex are frequently apprehended by the police, and if younger than 18 years of age, they are placed under juvenile judicial custody. The environment during detention or incarceration may further complicate the problem. Juvenile females are typically cohorted with other females who have had similar experiences, potentially contributing to a sense of normalization of the behavior. Other girls may be initiated into prostitution for "easy money." Males engaged in survival sex on the street sometimes continue the behavior after they have been incarcerated. Adolescents and young adults who have a history of engaging in survival sex often have concomitant substance abuse and mental health problems, in addition to poor education and lack of job skills. Many juvenile judicial facilities are poorly equipped to provide substance abuse or mental health treatment for adolescents who are incarcerated. Some innovative urban centers provide alternative courts for youth with nonviolent drug-related offenses (teen drug court) and for youth with mental illness (family court).

Adolescents who are arrested for survival sex frequently have a childhood characterized by emotional, sexual, or physical abuse, or severe neglect. They often have been wards of the state through child protective or family court action before arrest. In addition, they may be homeless after running away from placement. Therefore, involvement in survival sex should be interpreted as a warning signal for child abuse and neglect.

## HEALTH INSURANCE AND HEALTH CARE ACCESS

Child protective services generally enrolls adolescents in its custody in Medicaid, and some states have extended the age of eligibility of youth in foster care for health services to age 21, or even 24. Unfortunately, adolescents in the delinquency system, though their background and problems are similar, usually do not receive these benefits after release. Extending Medicaid benefits to youth leaving juvenile delinquency custody would avoid the gap in health insurance coverage that occurs when adolescents transition out of the system. In addition, the incarceration of adolescents and young adults provides a unique opportunity to address educational gaps, provide job training, and include substance abuse and mental health treatment so that there may be an alternative to survival sex after leaving child protective custody.

## SPECIFIC ISSUES FOR PHYSICIANS AND OTHER HEALTH CARE PROVIDERS

In developing services appropriate for young people who have been engaged in stigmatized behaviors, it is essential to approach them nonjudgmentally and with a positive demeanor that communicates respect, acceptance, interest, and caring. Critical to working with adolescents engaged in highly stigmatized or illegal activities, such as prostitution or child pornography, is the assurance of privacy and confidentiality. In addition, clinical expertise includes the ability to balance the pursuit of interview questions with the recognition of when to not force sensitive issues that may be emotionally upsetting. It is also important to let the adolescent know the limits of confidentiality that require health care providers to protect youth by disclosing to other helping individuals or agencies any plans the adolescent may have to harm herself or himself or others (including retaliating for a perceived wrong), as well as any history of maltreatment of himself or herself (if a minor), or the endangerment of another minor. It is essential for the health professional interviewer to know the availability of community resources to whom young people can be referred and the specific state laws governing minor consent and confidentiality.

Young people who are involved in survival sex frequently experience significant negative events in their own lives and in the lives of friends. These include physical or sexual assault, serious illness, HIV and other STI (or the fear of them), and drug overdose. Because of their living situations, various infestations such as pubic and hair lice and scabies are also common. In addition, living on the street or involvement in survival sex for many young people takes a cumulative toll that may eventually cause them to consider giving up this behavior. Thus, one must always maintain hope for improvement.

Health care services for youth involved in prostitution or child pornography should be connected to available mental health and substance abuse treatment resources in the community. Commonly, the adolescent's presenting medical complaint may be relatively minor, but it may act as a bridge to mental health and social services if the clinician is alert and is familiar with the appropriate referral sources. Many urban child protective service agencies have specific teams that are skilled in addressing the unique challenges of homeless and runaway youth. Many of the young people engaged in survival sex respond to individual case management, which in addition to providing access to resources may provide a responsible young adult case worker who can act as a role model and guide.

Young people with a history of survival sex are vulnerable to multiple infections, complications of substance abuse (in particular injection drug use), injuries from accidents and assaults, other acute biomedical problems, and mental health disorders. They need reproductive health care, including provision of condoms and contraception, with pregnancy termination or prenatal care as indicated.

There are several health care-related concerns for youth who have been involved in survival sex:

- They should be screened for chlamydia and gonorrhea, syphilis, HIV, hepatitis C, and hepatitis BsAg.
- Those engaged in oral or anal sex should receive a pharyngeal or anal swab for gonorrhea as indicated (these should be direct cultures rather than DNA amplification tests).
- Positive diagnoses of gonorrhea, chlamydia, syphilis, and other reportable diseases should be reported to the public health department.
- Individuals who present within 72 hours of a sexual assault should be referred to an emergency department or other facility capable of conducting a forensic examination, if he or she is willing to do so. Police reports should be made in compliance with local regulations, or the youth should at least be given the option of making a report to police.
- Injection drug users commonly develop abscesses related to methicillin-resistant *Staphylococcal aureus*. They should be referred for access to clean needles and instructed on practical

methods of needle sterilization using bleach as appropriate. They should be strongly advised against sharing needles.

## IMPORTANT AREAS FOR FUTURE RESEARCH

Continued monitoring of the prevalence of survival sex behaviors among urban youth is essential to understanding the scope of the problem and targeting interventions. In addition, little is known about survival sex behaviors outside of major metropolitan areas in the United States. There are few academic studies of the phenomenon of human trafficking of adolescents for the sex trade in the United States. Circumstances related to entry into survival sex and continued participation have not been studied. Understanding these factors may help the design of programs that prevent youth from high-risk environments and backgrounds from entering into survival sex practices.

There are no evaluations of intervention models for youth engaged in survival sex, limiting the development of evidence-based approaches. Though experience-based programs, particularly with homeless and runaway youth, have been designed and implemented, more rigorous longitudinal evaluations are needed.

## SUMMARY

Although the emotional and behavioral manifestations of normal development can take a variety of pathways, some contemporary adolescents are forced into an unhealthy direction in which sexual activity is exchanged for things having nothing to do with the meaningful relationships in which healthy adolescent sexual development occurs. Whether an adolescent is forced into sexual activity through human trafficking, survival sex, or forced into exchanging sex for material goods, the potential risks to health and development are significant. Health care providers who see adolescents engaged in various forms of prostitution need to be aware of the complex interplay of factors that lead to such behavior, but also to approach the adolescent in a supportive and nonjudgmental manner, engaging the help of professionals from other disciplines.

## REFERENCES

1. Ward H, Day S, Weber J. Risky business: health and safety in the sex industry over a 9-year period. *Sex Transm Infect.* 1999;75:1406–1409

2. Widom C, Kuhns JB. Childhood victimization and subsequent risk for promiscuity, prostitution, and teenage pregnancy: a prospective study. *Am J Public Health.* 1996;86(11):1607–1612

3. Kipke M, O'Conner S, Palmer R, MacKenzie R. Street youth in Los Angeles profile of a group at high risk for human immunodeficiency virus infection. *Arch Pediatr Adolesc Med.* 1995;149:513–519

4. Greene JM, Enett ST, Ringwalt C. Prevalence and correlates of survival sex among runaway and homeless youth. *Am J Public Health.* 1999;89(9):1406–1409

5. Widom C, Kuhns J. Childhood victimization and subsequent risk for promiscuity, prostitution, and teenage pregnancy: a prospective study. *Am J Public Health.* 1996;86(11):1607–1612

6. Weber AE, Boivin J, Blais L, Haley N, Roy E. Predictors of initiation into prostitution among female street youths bulletin. NY Academy of Medicine. *J Urban Health.* 2004;81(4):584–595

7. Warf C, Desai M, Clark LF. *Early Involvement in Survival Sex among Homeless Girls; a Comparative Study*. APHA Conference, San Diego (Nov 2008)

8. Seng MJ. Child sexual abuse and adolescent prostitution: a comparative analysis. *Adolescence.* 1989;24:664–675

9. Cohen M. *Identifying and Combating Juvenile Prostitution*. Washington, DC: National Association of Counties Research;1987

10. Runaway/Homeless Youth Network Summary, July 2000–June 2001, Division of Adolescent Medicine, Children's Hospital Los Angeles, unpublished data

11. Jones D, Irwin K, Inciardi J, et al. The high risk of sexual practices of crack-smoking sex workers recruited from the streets of three American cities. *Sexually Transmitted Dis.* 1998;25(4):187–193

12. Inciardi J. Crack, crack house sex, and HIV risk. *Arch Sex Behav.* 1995;24:249–269

13. Haley N, Roy E, Leclerc P, Boudreau J-F, Boivin J-F. HIV risk profile of male street youth involved in survival sex. *Sex Transm Infect.* 2004;80:526–530

14. Ward H, Day S, Weber J. Risky business: health and safety in the sex industry over a 9-year period. *Sex Transm Infect.* 1999;75(5):340–343

15. Jones D, Irwin K, Inciardi J, et al. The high risk sexual practices of crack-smoking sex workers recruited from the streets of three American cities. *Sex Transm Dis.* 1998; 25(4):187–193

16. El-Bassel N, Witte S, Wada T, Gilbert L, Wallace J. Correlates of partner violence among female street-based sex workers: substance abuse, history of childhood abuse, and HIV risks. *AIDS Patient Care and STDs.* 2001;15(1):41–51

17. US Department of State. Trafficking in persons report, June 2008. Available at: www.state.gov/g/tip/rls/tiprpt/2008/. Accessed March 16, 2010

18. Richard AO. International trafficking in women to the United States: a contemporary manifestation of slavery and organized crime. DCI Report. US Department of State. Available at: www.cia.gov/library/center-for-the-study-of-intelligence/csi-publications/books-and-monographs/trafficking.pdf. Accessed March 16, 2010

19. Ugarte MB, Zarate L, Farley M. Prostitution and trafficking of women and children from Mexico to the United States. In: Farley M, ed. *Prostitution, Trafficking, and Traumatic Stress.* London: The Haworth Press; 2004:147-165, 2330

20. Estes RJ, Weiner NA. The Commercial Exploitation of Children in the US, Canada and Mexico. University of Pennsylvania School of Social Work, Center for the Study of Youth Policy, September 10, 2001

21. Landesman P. The girls next door. *The New York Times.* January 25, 2004

22. UNICEF. The progress of nations. *Child Rights—the Ultimate Abuse*. New York, NY: UNICEF;1995

23. Willis B, Levy B. Child prostitution: global health burden, research needs, and interventions. *Lancet.* 2002;359:1417-1422

24. World Health Organization. *Women's Health: Across Age and Frontier*. Geneva: WHO;1992:35

25. Refugees and AIDS, UNAIDS Point of View, April 1997. Available at: data.unaids.org/publications/IRC-pub04/refugpov_en.pdf. Accessed March 16, 2010

26. Standards for Health Services in Juvenile Detention and Confinement Facilities; National Commission on Correctional Health Care, 2nd Printing, June 2000

# CHAPTER 171

## Adolescents in Gangs

CURREN WARE, MD, MS Ed • MICHAEL J. FALK, MD

### OVERVIEW

Gangs have been a part of large urban centers in America for at least 200 years. Over the last 20 years, there have been significant changes in the number and nature of gangs, as well as the extent to which their activities have lethal outcomes. This chapter provides a brief history and description of the social context of gangs, describes risk factors for involvement and the effect on youth, and discusses clinical prevention and evaluation approaches. The focus of this chapter is youth gangs. Other types of gangs, such as motorcycle gangs, criminal or drug gangs, prison gangs, and hate-based gangs, will not be discussed.

### HISTORY OF GANGS IN AMERICA

During the latter part of the 19th century, gangs were reported in Boston, New York, Philadelphia, Chicago, and many other urban settings.[1] In Chicago alone in the 1920s there were about 1,300 separate gangs.[2] In the early 20th century, gangs arose within economically disadvantaged communities and reflected the process of industrialization and the deterioration of specific parts of these metropolitan centers. Gang members in these areas were overwhelmingly of European descent, being largely comprised of the children of recent immigrants from countries including Germany, Ireland, Italy, and Poland. On the West Coast, gangs such as White Fence developed within the Hispanic communities of the barrios and shanty towns during the early part of the 20th century. Other gangs, such as the 18th Street Gang, with a reputed membership today of 20,000—thought to be the largest in Los Angeles—began in the 1960s. The ethnic makeup of gangs has varied over the years, frequently reflecting disproportionately the groups who are displaced and marginalized. Early in American history, the children of Irish immigrants made up the majority of gang members in Eastern cities. In the latter part of the 19th century, Jewish youth made up a significant proportion of gangs in New York City. Thus, the current ethnic makeup of gangs is likely related to the extent to which these racial and ethnic groups are marginalized within modern American society.[3]

Other gangs mirror international events and immigration patterns. *Mara Salvatrucha*, a predominantly Salvadoran gang in Los Angeles, now considered 1 of the most violent gangs, began in the 1980s initially as a self-protection organization against existing gangs, but soon took in people fleeing the wars in Central America, including unaccompanied immigrant youth, soldiers, and even death-squad members. Some members have been deported to El Salvador, with the consequence that the same gang has taken root in that country.[4]

### DEFINING GANGS

There is no consensus regarding what constitutes a gang.[3,5] However, most definitions include the following 5 features:

1. Involvement in delinquent or criminal activity distinguishes a "gang" from other peer groups
2. Control of a specific territory, structure, or enterprise
3. Use of "inside" symbols or specific slang language to communicate
4. Coming together through common or shared interests
5. Self-identification as a gang/group

Adolescent and young adult gangs tend to specialize either in violence or entrepreneurial activities.[5,6] The violent turf gang is organized around the defense of the gang's home "turf" and often has territorial conflicts with other gangs. Entrepreneurial gangs exist to make money from criminal activity such as drug sales, extortion, or robbery. They tend to use violence only to further their goal of making money or in the defense of territory. Unfortunately, most youth gangs in America today are violent turf gangs.[3,5]

Although youth may affiliate with larger gangs dominated by adults, many youth gangs are small and formed spontaneously in communities. Younger teens may affiliate with or aspire to join a gang, and may participate in marking territory through graffiti or other means, acting as lookouts, or performing other ancillary activities. Additionally, an individual who is in the company of a known gang member who is arrested by the police may be entered into a database as a gang member, even though he/she does not have an ongoing affiliation with a gang. He/she may even be subject to severe gang enhancement sentencing guidelines. For example, the state of California maintains a gang database that lists every person who is *thought* to be a gang member. Once entered on that database, it is very difficult for an individual's name to be removed.

## PREVALENCE OF GANGS IN AMERICA

The National Youth Gang Survey[7] for 2006 estimated that there were 26,500 gangs with 785,000 members in the United States. Gangs can be found in every large urban center with a population of at least 250,000, as well as 40% of suburban counties and 12% of rural counties.[6] Although more than 80% of rural counties with gang activity reported 6 or fewer gangs, 61% of large urban centers reported 30 or more gangs. Urban centers account for 85% of all gang members. Specific cities have long been identified as having a significant and chronic gang problem. For example, in 2003, Los Angeles had an estimated 50,000 gang members in more than 400 gangs. Chicago had more than 130 gangs with an estimated 30,000 to 50,000 gang members. Thus, urban areas remain the centers of gang activity in America.

Most national data collection occurs through the Office of Juvenile Justice and Delinquency Prevention of the United States Department of Justice (OJJDP; ojjdp.ncjrs.org). The OJJDP conducts the National Youth Gang Survey annually, surveying law enforcement officials in urban, suburban, and rural settings regarding the number of gangs, gang members, their activities, and criminal involvement. In addition, many state departments of corrections or justice, and municipal agencies ranging from police departments to school districts, collect data independently.

Because these different sources use different definitions for a gang, gang member, or gang-related activity, their data should be interpreted with caution. For example, the National Youth Gang Center[8] defines a gang as "a group of youths or young adults in your jurisdiction that you or other responsible persons in your agency or community are willing to identify as a 'gang.'" Definitions for gang-related crimes also vary by jurisdiction. For example, Chicago employs a highly restrictive definition for a gang-related crime: the crime must have been committed for specific reasons that are thought to benefit the gang. In Los Angeles, on the other hand, the police and sheriff's office only require that the crime be committed by a "known" gang member for it to be counted as gang-related. Clearly, these definitions result in highly variable rates of gang-related crime.[9] Finally, "troublesome" youth groups are more likely to be labeled gangs if the community believes them to be a problem.[10]

Media attention and public perception suggest that gangs are related to specific ethnic or racial populations. Black and Hispanic youth are more commonly identified as being gang affiliated. Nationally, the OJJDP reports that 94% are male and 49% and 37% of identified gang members are Hispanic and black, respectively.[11] Hispanic and black youth in the United States each represent less than 20% of the population overall.

However, when youth themselves are surveyed regarding their own gang affiliation, the proportion of minority youth and the gender of youth who report gang involvement changes significantly. In a study of public school eighth graders, of those who reported gang involvement 38% were female and 25% were identified as white. One study comparing 3 groups of criminally active youth in different neighborhoods of New York City found that early involvement in illegal activities were similar across groups.[12] However, youth from white working-class areas aged out of crime faster than their black or Hispanic peers living in neighborhoods characterized by racial and ethnic segregation, concentrated poverty, adult joblessness, and single-parent households.

An appreciation of the immigrant experience is critical to understanding the current disproportionate involvement of Hispanic youth in gangs. First-generation immigrants typically come to America with ambitions to take advantage of employment and educational opportunities and thereby advance their economic situation. Through low wages, job instability, and discrimination, some families experience a collapse of family structure and resources, as well as extreme poverty from which they do not recover. For many adolescents growing up in these highly stressed families, difficulties are compounded by poor schools and education, ongoing discrimination, and poor prospects for employment. They experience marginalization and alienation from dominant social values. The disadvantaged families from which many young gang members emerge contrast sharply with the traditional Latino family that generally includes extended family members, is close-knit, and provides a protective environment for children and youth along with elders, who are viewed with respect.[4]

Adolescents in some black communities face similar challenges. Gangs became prominent in the 1980s in the black communities of Los Angeles, when unemployment rates exceeded 40% for young black men. Schools in these communities were poorly funded and administered, with dropout rates that typically exceeded 50%.

Decades of discrimination in housing, employment, and education ensured that many blacks were unable to escape chronic unemployment, social marginalization, and poverty. In addition, relationships with legal authorities were extremely negative, particularly for young men, characterized by harassment, arrests, and beatings. This led to many young people gravitating toward gangs that offered emotional support, protection, and friendship. Unfortunately, in some parts of Los Angeles, conditions are not qualitatively different today.

Other ethnic groups, too, have their own gangs, including Vietnamese, Filipinos, Chinese, and Armenians. Although these "ethnic gangs" have distinct characteristics, their members share a sense of marginalization and exclusion from dominant society and a perceived need for self-protection.[4]

### GIRLS IN GANGS

Historically, teenage girls in gangs functioned as "auxiliaries" to male gang members, acting as lookouts, drivers, supporters, and girlfriends. In some gangs they may also be sexually exploited. However, there is evidence that female youth gang members have been increasingly involved in criminal activities, including violent crimes. Gang-involved females are much more likely to engage in serious delinquency than females who are not gang-involved.[13,14] In a study of Los Angeles Latino gangs, whereas boys were found to come from conventional working-class families in which "being out on the streets" was more acceptable, girls in gangs were more likely to come from abusive homes in which the adolescent and the family were stigmatized by the community. Though only one-third of boys had run away from home, three-quarters of the girls had done so.[15] Girls who joined gangs were more likely than boys to be labeled as bad and deviant.

Girls in gangs frequently become pregnant, and the responsibilities of childrearing fall primarily on them rather than on the father of the baby. This increased responsibility enables many young women to leave the gang. For this and other reasons, the gang experience of most females is restricted to adolescence. Girls who may have had a reputation as "loose" may reinvent themselves socially by becoming "good mothers." These girls typically stay single mothers.[16]

## ADOLESCENT DEVELOPMENT AND GANGS

The key to successful navigation of the transition from childhood to adulthood is the development of competency to maintain employment and to develop moral and ethical values that allow one to live with others in society. This process is shaped by relationships with peers, older youth, and adults who provide direct guidance, as well as modeling appropriate behavior. Gang-involved youth, who typically have poor educational backgrounds, similarly disadvantaged peers, and adult role models themselves involved in antisocial activities, have little opportunity to develop the competencies and moral and ethical grounding to enable them to survive, much less prosper, in mainstream society.

In communities where there are few opportunities for young people, where gangs are well established, where there is significant pressure to conform with peer norms to participate in gang activities, or where refusal to do so may be dangerous, joining a gang may seem a reasonable option. In many ways, the vulnerability of many young people to gang involvement is a reflection of the failure of our society, communities, schools, and families to provide youth with the healthy environment they need to grow and thrive. Many youth come to realize this and do not stay in gangs for long. For most youth, gang involvement represents a temporary period of their adolescence. As they mature cognitively and emotionally, and are faced with adult responsibilities, they commonly join the work force as they leave gangs behind. Most youth who join gangs leave them in less than a year.

## WHY YOUTH JOIN GANGS

Although the duration of gang membership may be relatively short for many adolescents, a significant number of teenagers will join a gang at some point during adolescence. A survey of eighth graders in 11 cities found that 9% were current gang members and 17% had never belonged to a gang. Other surveys have reported that gang members represent 4% to 14% of youth in cities that have been identified as having a gang problem.[3] Outside of the United States, a survey of Canadian youth in high school in Toronto found that 6% described themselves as current gang members and another 5% identified as having been gang-involved at some time.[17]

To date, 3 long-term studies in Rochester, Pittsburgh, and Seattle have examined youth delinquency and gang involvement, and have identified 5 major categories of risk factors for joining a gang. These have been summarized in a document by the OJJDP.[3,18]

### INDIVIDUAL CHARACTERISTICS

Individual characteristics of youth that are strongly predictive of gang involvement include:

- Having negative life experiences
- Delinquent or violent behavior
- Low self-esteem/poor sense of self

- Drug use, especially before age 12
- Mental health diagnoses such as depression, post-traumatic stress disorder (PTSD), or conduct disorder
- Externalizing behaviors

**FAMILY CHARACTERISTICS**

A number of family characteristics are also associated with gang involvement. These include:

- Family disorganization or poverty
- Poor parent–child bonding or parenting skills
- Parental violence or lack of education
- Lack of adult role models
- Single-parent households
- Parental alcohol or substance use
- Family poverty
- Family member who is involved in a gang

**EDUCATIONAL AND SCHOOL FACTORS**

Research has shown that youth who perform poorly in the educational system are at higher risk than other youth for gang involvement. A number of factors in this domain predict gang involvement, including:

- Academic failure
- Negative labeling by teachers
- Having a learning disorder
- Frequent troubles at school
- Low familial or personal expectations

For members of immigrant ethnic groups who had extensive kinship networks in their communities of origin, the transition to school and the care of nonfamily members can be especially stressful, particularly in circumstances where the parents are preoccupied with working multiple low-wage jobs. These immigrant children may have negative and damaging experiences in schools that are segregated, underfunded, and academically inferior, where they encounter cultural insensitivity and ethnic bias.[4] Dropping out of school, though obviously damaging in the long run, may seem to be of short-term benefit.

Gang activity can take place inside or outside of schools. Among the students 12 to 18 years of age who were surveyed in the School Crime Supplement to the National Crime Victimization Survey, 20% reported that gangs had been present on their school campus in the past 6 months. The number was much higher for Hispanic students; 42% reported gangs being on their campuses. However, campus fatalities related to gang activity are extraordinarily rare; schools remain among the safest environments for young people.

**PEER FACTORS**

In contrast to classmates and schools, which are often experienced negatively, peers on the streets may offer a sense of belonging, affection, protection, friendship, and acceptance. These peers fill a void left by poorly funded schools and highly stressed families, leading to a romanticized perception of gang life. Peer factors that are strongly associated with gang involvement include a commitment to delinquent peers and a high degree of street socialization and having friends who are gang members.

**NEIGHBORHOOD CHARACTERISTICS**

A number of studies have shown that gangs tend to cluster in communities with high levels of violence and crime, which are socially disorganized, have high degrees of endemic poverty, and where barriers to social and economic opportunity exist. In gang-prone neighborhoods, there are also substantial subsidized or community housing ("projects") and readily available illegal drugs. Gangs arise in communities that are overwhelmed by the features mentioned previously and where young people experience a significant degree of alienation and isolation from mainstream society.

Because many youth in America have one or more of the risk factors noted previously, the reliable prediction of gang membership is difficult. To address this, Thornberry and colleagues[18] conducted a variable-based analysis of these multiple risk factors to determine the antecedents of and cumulative risk for future gang membership. More than 40 variables associated with future gang involvement were studied. Only 0.7% of males younger than 11 years old who had less than 11 risk factors became gang members. For males in that age group with 11 to 15 risk factors, 13% became gang involved. Of those preadolescent boys with 16 to 20 risk factors, 23.4% became gang involved. This proportion almost doubled to 43.5% for those who had more than 20 risk factors. Therefore, even a moderate reduction in risk factors might have a significant effect on preventing gang involvement.

**CULTURAL REFLECTIONS**

Despite the negative reputation that gangs have with law enforcement and much of the public, residents of the communities where gangs operate may be ambivalent about gangs. Youth in gangs are composed of community residents and have productive roles in the community besides gang affiliation. Affiliation with a gang may commonly be viewed as a youthful rite of passage, and there are usually expectations that gang members will ultimately join the work force and raise families. Community residents, including many adults and parents, have had difficult relationships with the legal system and may have family members or friends who have experienced lengthy incarceration. Many parents of youth gang members may have had an affiliation with gangs themselves as teenagers. For these reasons and others, the relationship of the gang members to their community is complex.

Ethnographic studies of Hispanic gangs in Los Angeles found that they tend to be based in a specific neighborhood, are characterized by fighting, and provide a sense of "family" for adolescents who are alienated from their native and adopted cultures.[4] Ties to the neighborhood link them to the larger culture. Much of the violence is perceived as a defense of the neighborhood turf. These characteristics are neither unique to Los Angeles nor to Hispanic gangs.

## CONCEPTUAL FRAMEWORK

Data regarding gangs should be considered within a conceptual framework that takes into account how youth interact and are influenced by these and other societal influences. In *A Rainbow of Gangs*, Vigil[4] developed a theoretical framework called "Multiple Marginality" that examines the influences on young people's lives within the micro and macro environments they inhabit (Figure 171-1). This framework envisions the exertion of social control at different levels. For a young person, this starts at home and continues within the environments of school and the neighborhood as a whole. In this context, general codes of conduct for society are introduced and accepted. For a young person who does not accept these codes, a variety of factors (personal, familial, peer, academic, and societal) operate to leave youth open to "street socialization." Once adolescents become "street socialized" they enter into a different social network and adopt a new set of social codes and rules of behavior. When this pathway is complete, these adolescents become the next generation of "street-culture carriers" that can influence other young people to accept or reject either traditional or gang codes of behavior.

## CONSEQUENCES OF GANG MEMBERSHIP

Gangs have a significant affect on the lives of the young men and women who join them. Many youth who join gangs report that the gang fills many needs.[4,9] For youth who have little parental involvement, or for young men who have no positive male role models, the "OGs" (original gangsters or older members) often serve as father figures or role models. Frequently youth

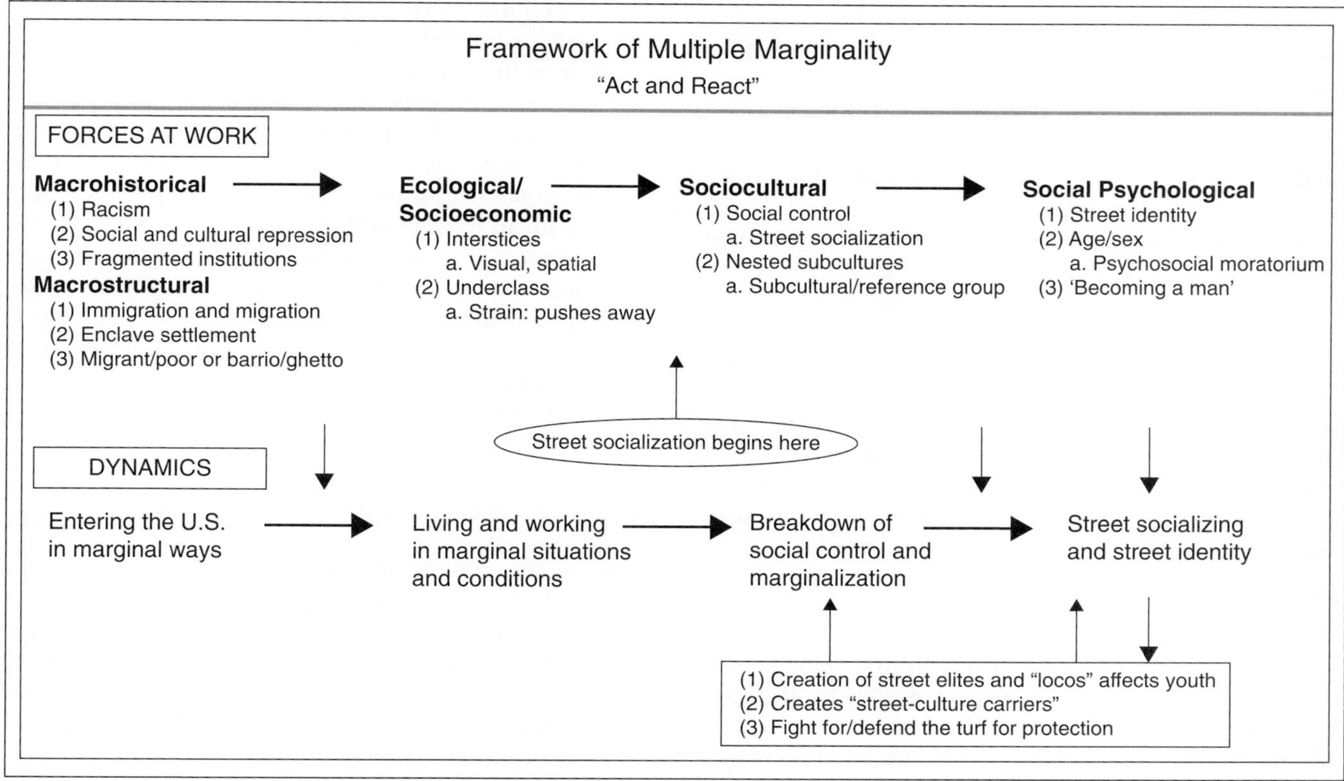


FIGURE 171-1 Framework of multiple marginality (From *A Rainbow of Gangs: Street Cultures in the Mega-City* by James Diego Vigil. Copyright (c) 2002, by permission of the University of Texas Press.)

report feeling that they have found a "place where they belong" and a sense of kinship or identity that was missing from their lives in these relationships. Finally, many youth who join gangs acquire a feeling of safety or protection. Although they are definitely less safe, many youth who live in unsafe communities feel less endangered knowing that they have a group of friends who will always "have their back" and who will offer them protection from others.

### Social Networking

Gangs can also serve a social function. Gang members spend most of their time involved in relatively normal social activities such as hanging out, partying, playing sports, and other common adolescent behaviors.[19] One-third of all gang members in a Toronto survey of high school youth reported belonging to a "social gang." They were no more likely to engage in criminal behavior than other high school youth.[17]

### Violence

Although some "gangs" are engaged in relatively prosocial behavior, most modern youth gangs are characterized by violence and delinquent behavior. For many youth gangs the initiation rites involve being assaulted by multiple other members, called "jumping-in." The goal is for the new recruit to demonstrate his or her toughness in the face of serious adversity, and the recruit often sustains injuries in the process. Furthermore, gangs are often in conflict with each other, with serious consequences. One study found that most homicides of youth 14 to 24 years of age living in California were gang-related. These fatalities accounted for 80% of all gang-related homicides in the state between 1990 and 1999.[20]

Over the past 25 years, the total amount of violence within and between gangs has increased. Miller's[10] research demonstrated that gang-related violence had risen because of a significant increase in the level of conflict related to defending personal or gang honor, local turf or facilities, as well as monetary gain and crime-related activities. Block's[6] research in Chicago showed that the increase in the amount of violence between gangs and spikes in gang-related homicides and violent crime were directly related to gang conflicts between rival or neighboring gangs.

### Firearm Possession and Use

There has also been a significant increase in the use of firearms among gang members.[5] Of the gang-related homicides in California, 85% were caused by handguns.[20] Gang members are much more likely to carry a firearm and report being willing to use it than gang members of previous generations. Because of the increased use of firearms by gang members in a fight, gang fight, robbery, or other criminal activity, injuries and death are much more likely. In addition, the types of guns used have changed significantly. Gang members in Chicago and Los Angeles are more likely to use a handgun to commit an assault, homicide, or drive-by shooting than any other type of firearm, including assault weapons. This is significant because the types of handguns used today are much larger caliber, have a larger clip capacity, use more powerful ammunition, and are more likely to be semiautomatic or fully automatic than they were previously.[21] Research has clearly shown that these newer types of handguns are associated with much higher rates of morbidity and mortality than the old "Saturday night specials," which had been the handgun of choice in the last quarter of the 20th century.[21] Thus, advances in firearm technology have led to an increase in the amount of violence, and the likelihood a gang encounter will result in serious injury or death.

## JUVENILE AND CRIMINAL JUSTICE SYSTEMS

In the United States, youth who are involved in gangs are frequently incarcerated. Consequently, youth who are not gang involved but who are incarcerated for some other reason commonly come in contact with representatives of gangs during their incarceration. Adolescents in juvenile detention may feel the need for protection and safety, which can compel them to affiliate with a gang. Gangs have been widely reported within most juvenile correctional facilities. In fact, one survey noted that 40% of juveniles in a juvenile justice facility self-identified as gang members.[3] Some of the largest and most influential gangs got their start among incarcerated youth. For example, the Vice Lords, a Chicago youth gang, originated in the Illinois State Training School for Boys.[22] Thus, the juvenile justice system may inadvertently contribute to the increase in gang membership. Confinement in juvenile corrections is one of the strongest predictors of adult prison gang membership.[23]

## PREVENTING GANG INVOLVEMENT

Due to the complexity of the phenomenon of gangs, prevention strategies are complex and multidimensional. Preventive strategies must target children and youth at different developmental stages and differing levels of risk, as well as parents and families, schools, and communities that have the previously described risk factors. Because most intervention models are beyond the scope of medical clinics, health care providers who encounter young people at risk for gang involvement need to utilize external community agencies. No controlled longitudinal studies exist for gang prevention. However, there are models for prevention based on diminishing known risk factors and reinforcing assets and resiliency factors, and these have shown promising results.

School is the central prosocial community agency for most adolescents. Preventing school dropout and maintaining student engagement are powerful factors in preventing gang involvement. Thus, the early identification of learning disabilities and appropriate educational interventions to keep adolescents interested in continuing their schooling, the referral to counseling or other mental health services as needed, and the availability of activities such as vocational training, sports, and artistic activities in which at-risk youth can succeed, all can play an important role in diverting young people from gangs. In communities with prominent gang activity, programs targeting at-risk youth can be successful in providing alternative activities to gang involvement. Examples of preventive activities at a community level include identifying and acknowledging personal assets and strengths in a youth development approach, providing shared activities and therapy to strengthen families, and facilitating relationships with positive adult mentors.[24]

In addition, unsupervised after-school time is the main portion of the day for youth to engage in troublesome behaviors, including antisocial behavior. After-school programs in athletics, music, art, employment, and recreation have demonstrated roles in providing a safe environment for adolescents and in helping them to develop relationships with responsible adults while engaging in constructive activities. The creation and maintenance of community- and school-based gang prevention efforts depends on adequate funding and supportive social policy. Limitations on funding to schools, parks and recreation, and other social agencies that serve adolescents, especially those living in impoverished communities, create a climate of deprivation that significantly enhances the attractions gangs may hold.

As noted earlier, the more risk factors that adolescents accumulate, the greater the likelihood of becoming involved in a gang. In addition, a study of young people in the Orange County, California, juvenile justice system showed that only 8% of incarcerated adolescents were likely to become adult offenders and that these youth could be identified by age 12.[25] Therefore, early identification and intervention to identify and address risk factors, such as school failure, learning disorders, family conflict, lack of role models, and lack of prosocial activities, can play an important part in diverting children from gangs. Screening for these risk factors should be included in the annual visit by any health care provider who works with children or teens.

Many opportunities exist in the emergency department and hospital settings to have a positive influence on the lives of gang-involved youth. For many of these adolescents, their most frequent contact with the medical system will be as a victim of a violent injury when they require medical or surgical care. This is a vulnerable moment and excellent time for them to consider the consequences of their behavior. It is important to assess the adolescent's risk for further injury after discharge, as well as his or her intent to retaliate for the injury. It is advisable to involve hospital social workers to assist in identifying resources for referral. The management of an adolescent who has sustained a significant injury from a gang conflict requires a multidisciplinary approach with mental health, social work, and medical care providers. Becker and colleagues[26] describe an exciting and effective model of a hospital-based, peer-intervention, violence prevention program directed at injured youth.

## INTERVIEWING GANG-INVOLVED YOUTH

When in a clinical setting and interviewing an adolescent who might be involved in a gang, it is important to assess the environmental (family, school, peers) factors that might be related to gang activity and to determine the level of danger that the patient may be in. As is true of adolescent history-taking and interviewing in general, it is important for the adolescent and the health care provider to know the purpose of the interview, and the information that needs (and does not need) to be collected. In addition, both need to be aware of the health care provider's responsibility to maintain confidentiality and the limits of confidentiality. It is important to acknowledge that young people do not have an obligation to disclose the details of their lives. However, the patient needs to be made aware of the clinician's responsibility to report child maltreatment, suicidal intent, or intent to harm others. This should be presented as concern for the safety and well-being of the patient and others in the patient's life. In asking about violence and gang-related issues, it is important to remain neutral and nonjudgmental in tone, without presumption. The clinician interviewing the potentially gang-involved adolescent is not a criminal investigator and has a role distinct from that played by members of the judicial system and/or law enforcement.

The interview that is appropriate in the setting of a private community clinic may be very different from what is appropriate when providing health services in a detention facility or jail. It is usually not appropriate to ask youth in detention settings the reasons for their incarceration or to inquire about the circumstances surrounding events in which they were involved. If this information is considered necessary, it should be available from the staff at the facility.

As with most youth, the Home, Education, Activities, Drugs, Sex, Suicide (HEADSS)[27] interviewing approach addresses the main areas for psychosocial assessment in a reasonably time-efficient, focused manner. Many gang-involved youth have problems in multiple areas such as strained relationships with adults and families, truancy, dropout or poor school performance, substance use, and unsafe sexual practices. Frequently these issues underlie the strong attraction to and involvement with gangs. When possible, it is important to make appropriate referrals to community agencies for individual and/or family therapy. Youth who are interviewed in a hospital setting following an injury should be evaluated for risk of further harm or intent of retaliation after discharge.

## CONCLUSION

Gangs are found in all major urban centers in the United States. They have a strong attraction for young people, providing a sense of belonging and protection, in communities characterized by poverty, poor schools, lack of recreational activity, and highly stressed families. Though most adolescents who affiliate with a gang leave within a year and ultimately join the work force, those who are involved are at significant risk for sustaining serious injury, in particular a firearm injury, or developing a criminal record. Identifying youth at risk and providing access to alternative activities can play a significant role in diminishing the attraction of gangs to young people.

## REFERENCES


1. Asbury H. *The Gangs of New York.* New York, NY: Thunder's Mouth Press; 1927

2. Thrasher FM. *The Gang*. Chicago, IL: University of Chicago Press; 1927

3. Howell JC. *Youth Gangs: An Overview*. Juvenile Justice Bulletin. Washington, DC: Office of Juvenile Justice and Delinquency Prevention; August 1998

4. Vigil JD. *A Rainbow of Gangs*. Austin, TX: University of Texas Press; 2002:142

5. Klein MW. *The American Street Gang: It's Nature, Prevalence, and Control.* New York, NY: Oxford University Press; 1995

6. Block CR, Christakos A, Jacob A, Przybylski R. *Street Gangs and Crime: Patterns and Trends in Chicago*. Research Bulletin. Chicago, IL: Criminal Justice Information Authority; 1996

7. Egley A, O'Donnell C. Highlights of the 2006 National Youth Gang Survey, OJJDP Factsheet. Washington, DC: US Department of Justice, Office of Juvenile Justice and Delinquency Prevention; July 2008. Available at: www.ncjrs.gov/pdffiles1/ojjdp/fs200805.pdf. Accessed March 16, 2010

8. Egley A, Ritz C. *Office of Juvenile Justice and Delinquency Prevention (OJJDP) Highlights of the 2004 National Youth Gang Survey*. OJJDP Fact Sheet; April 2006

9. Klein MW, Maxson CL. *Defining Gang Homicide in Gangs in America*. Huff RC, ed. 2nd ed. Thousand Oaks, CA: Sage; 1996

10. Miller WB. *Crime by Youth Gangs and Groups in the United States*. Washington, DC: Office of Juvenile Justice and Delinquency Prevention, Department of Justice; 1992

11. Snyder HS, Sickmund M. Office of Juvenile Justice and Delinquency Prevention (OJJDP), Juvenile Offenders and Victims: 2006 National Report. Washington, DC: Department of Justice; 2006. Available at: ojjdp.ncjrs.org/ojstatbb/nr2006/downloads/chapter3.pdf. Accessed March 16, 2010

12. Sullivan M. *Getting Paid: Youth Crime and Employment in the Inner City*. Ithaca, NY: Cornell University Press, quoted in Juvenile Crime, Juvenile Justice, National Research Council, Institute of Medicine, National Academy Press; 2001:95

13. Fagan JE. Social process of delinquency and drug use among urban gangs. In: Huff CR, ed. *Gangs in America*. Newbury Park, CA: Sage; 1990:183–219

14. Bjerregaard B, Smith C. Gender differences in gang participation, delinquency, and substance use. *J Quant Criminol.* 1993;9:329–355

15. Moore JW. The chola life course: chica heroin users and the barrio gang. *Int J Addictions.* 1994;29(9):1115–1126

16. Horowitz R. *Honor and the American Dream: Culture and Identity in a Chicano Community.* New Brunswick, NJ: Rutgers University Press, referenced by Joan W. Moore and John M. Hagedorn in Peterson RD. *What Happens to Girls in the Gang, Understanding Contemporary Gangs in America, an Interdisciplinary Approach.* San Antonio, TX: Prentice Hall; 2004

17. Wortley S, Tanner J. Immigration, social disadvantage, and urban youth gangs. *Can J Urban Res.* 2006;15:2S

18. Thornberry TP, Krohn MD, Lizotte AJ, Smith CA, Tobin K. *The Antecedents of Gang Membership in The Modern Gang Reader.* Egley A et al, eds. Los Angeles, CA: Roxbury; 2006

19. Decker SH, Van Winkle B. *Life in the Gang: Family, Friends, and Violence.* New York, NY: Cambridge University Press; 1996

20. Falk M, Chan LS, MacKenzie RG. *Gang-Involved Homicides among Californian Youth from 1990 to 1999: An Analysis of Demographic Differences.* Washington, DC: Society for Pediatric Research; 2005

21. Wintemute GJ. The relationship between firearm design and firearm violence: handguns in the 1990s. *JAMA.* 1996;275(22):1035

22. Dawley D. 1992. *A Nation of Lords: The Autobiography of the Vice Lords.* 2nd ed. Prospect Heights, IL: Waveland, referenced in Youth Gangs: An Overview, OJJDP, US Department of Justice; August 1998

23. Ralph P, Hunter RJ, Marquart JW, Cuvelier SJ, Merianos D. Exploring the differences between gang and non-gang prisoners. In: Huff CR, ed. *Gangs in America.* 2nd ed. Thousand Oaks, CA: Sage: 1996;241-256

24. *Best Practices of Youth Violence Prevention, a Sourcebook for Community Action.* Washington, DC: Department of Health and Human Resources, CDC; 2002

25. Schumacher M, Kurz GA. *The 8% Solution: Preventing Serious, Repeat Juvenile Crime.* Thousand Oaks, CA: Sage; 2000

26. Becker MG, Hall JS, Ursic CM, Jain S, Calhoun D. Caught in the crossfire: the effects of peer-based intervention program for violently injured youth. *J Adol Health.* 2004;34(3): 177-183

27. Goldenring JM, Rosen DS. Getting into adolescent heads: An essential update. *Contemp Pediatr.* 2004;21:64-90

SECTION 2

# Substance Abuse

## CHAPTER 172

## Overview: Substance Abuse

JOHN KULIG, MD, MPH

Adolescent substance abuse may be the most commonly overlooked medical disorder in primary care practice. Despite the high prevalence of alcohol, tobacco, and other drug (ATOD) use among adolescents, clinicians may be unaware of common presentations of substance use, uncertain about how to screen or assess for problem use, and unacquainted with the variety of treatment resources available in their communities.[1-3]

### EPIDEMIOLOGY

Although alcohol and tobacco use remains prevalent, use of specific illicit drugs varies over time and location. In a phenomenon described as "generational forgetting" each new generation of youth discovers a drug for seemingly the first time. Initial use is associated with few reports of adverse reactions; therefore use soon becomes widespread, then eventually declines as adverse reactions become apparent. This pattern was noted with cocaine in the 1980s and Ecstasy (MDMA [methylenedioxymethamphetamine]) in the late 1990s. Geographic variation in use may vary regionally or even within the neighborhoods of a city. In the United States, widespread abuse of methamphetamine ("crystal meth") spread from the West Coast in the early 1990s to the Midwest, then to the East Coast by 2002, while sparing the northeast states. Heroin and synthetic opioid abuse moved from isolated urban areas into the suburbs in the past decade.

Principles of illicit drug use are summarized in Box 172-1.

**Box 172-1**

***Principles of Illicit Drug Use (NIDA)[a]***

- Drug abuse patterns not only change over time but vary by area and by populations within areas.
- Although a particular drug or drugs may dominate in a given area, most drug abusers use multiple drugs, including alcohol.
- Drugs are administered in different ways, resulting in different effects and different health consequences.
- Illicit drugs are sold in different forms and at different purity levels, factors that have immediate and long-term health consequences.

[a]National Institute on Drug Abuse

In the United States, patterns of alcohol, tobacco, and illicit drug use are assessed by 3 prominent national surveys. The *Monitoring the Future Study*,[4] initiated in 1975 at the University of Michigan, is an annual anonymous, cross-sectional survey of approximately 50,000 representative 8th-, 10th-, and 12th-grade students across the country. Findings are valid, reproducible, and consistent with the biannual *Youth Risk Behavior Survey* (YRBS) conducted by the Centers for Disease Control and Prevention (CDC), and the *National Survey on Drug Use and Health* (NSDUH), formerly called the *National Household Survey on Drug Abuse* (NHSDA). It is important to note that surveys of students attending school miss home-schooled youth as well as school dropouts.

Figure 172-1 illustrates the pattern of illicit drug use over time, from 1975 to 2006. After peaking in the late 1970s, illicit use fell dramatically through the 1980s, rose again in the 1990s, then reached a plateau, with small subsequent annual declines. This largely reflects marijuana use, the most widely available illicit drug. Figure 172-2 demonstrates that binge drinking

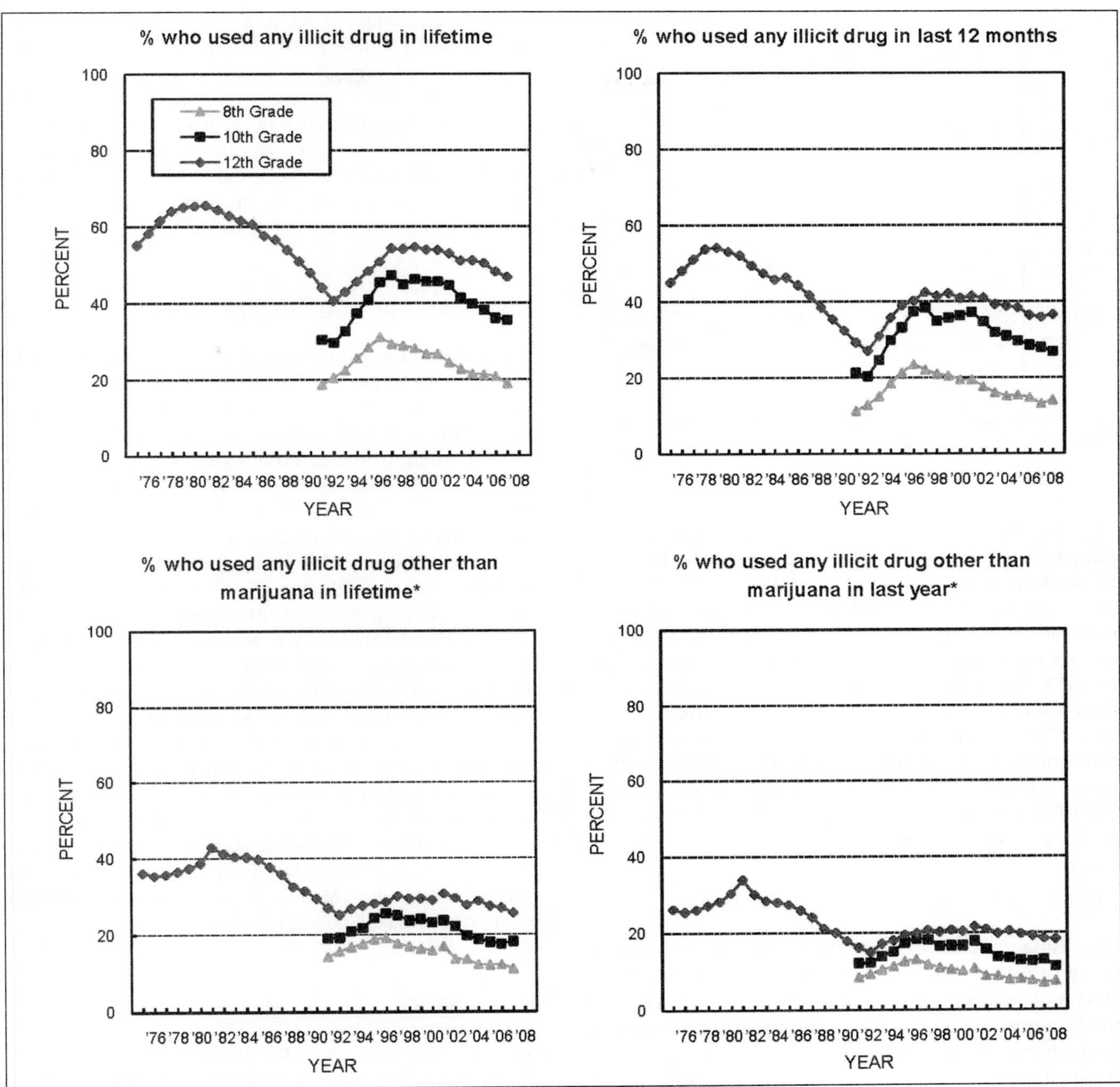


**FIGURE 172-1** Trends in annual prevalence of an illicit drug use 8th-, 10th-, and 12th-graders. *Beginning in 2001, revised sets of questions on other hallucinogen and tranquilizer use were introduced. Data for "any illicit drug other than marijuana" were affected by these changes. (Source: Johnston LD, O'Malley PM, Bachman JG, Schulenberg JE. Monitoring the Future national results on adolescent drug use: Overview of key findings, 2008. [NIH Publication No. 07-7401]. Bethesda, MD: National Institute on Drug Abuse; 2009.)

of alcohol by 8th-, 10th-, and 12th-graders has changed little from 1990 through 2008. Trends in use of any substance by adolescents closely parallel availability in a positive manner and perception of risk and peer disapproval in a negative manner. Figure 172-3 demonstrates this phenomenon for tobacco use.[4] The inverse relationship between use and risk perception is even more striking for marijuana.

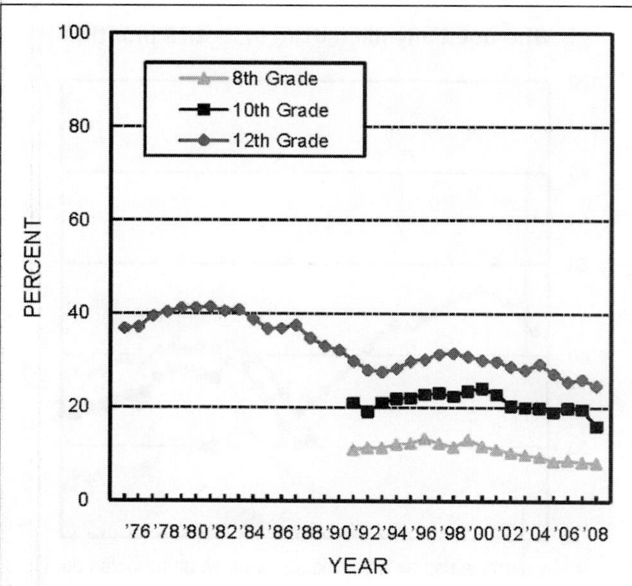


FIGURE 172-2 Alcohol: trends in binge drinking—8th-, 10th-, 12th-graders. Use: percentage who had 5+ drinks in a row in previous 2 weeks. For 8th- and 10th-graders only: The 1991–2007 estimates for 5 or more drinks in a row differ slightly from some previous reports due to an error in the data-editing process prior to 2008. The revised estimates average about 2% lower than previous estimates. These have been corrected here. (Source: Johnston LD, O'Malley PM, Bachman JG, Schulenberg JE. Monitoring the Future national results on adolescent drug use: Overview of key findings, 2008. [NIH Publication No. 07-7401]. Bethesda, MD: National Institute on Drug Abuse;2009.)

## CATEGORIES OF SUBSTANCE ABUSE

Increasing concern has recently focused on the misuse of prescription drugs, such as opioid analgesics, stimulants, and benzodiazepines, and abuse of over-the-counter medications, such as cough suppressants containing dextromethorphan. Inhalants are readily accessible at minimal cost, and toxicity can affect every organ system. Anabolic steroids remain a concern among adolescent males in particular, because they are used in high doses in hopes of enhancing athletic performance or simply for body sculpting. (Subsequent chapters will address specific categories of drugs.)

## MORBIDITY AND MORTALITY

Analysis of actual causes of death in the United States population in total reveals that tobacco use is first, alcohol consumption is second, and illicit drug use is ninth, accounting for 537,000 deaths, or 22.3% of the total annually (Table 172-1).[5] Each of these behaviors is most likely adopted during adolescence.

Among adolescents and young adults ages 15 to 24 years, unintentional injury, homicide, and suicide are the top 3 causes of mortality, accounting for 26,135 deaths or 75% of the total each year (Table 172-2). Alcohol, marijuana, and other illicit and prescription drugs may be involved in as many as half of these deaths.

## RISK AND PROTECTIVE FACTORS

Substance abuse is increasingly recognized as a disorder of the brain rather than a failure of will or a defect in character. Multiple risk and protective factors interact in several domains to determine outcome (Table 172-3).[6]

According to the gateway hypothesis, progression to abuse of illicit drugs is the outcome of a predictable temporal sequence that begins with beer or wine, progresses to hard liquor or tobacco, then marijuana, and results ultimately in the use of "hard drugs." Although this may be a common pattern, high rates of nonconformance with this sequence have been noted among males. Cocaine, heroin, stimulant, and LSD use may actually begin first and precede marijuana use, often in the setting of availability in the neighborhood environment and low parental supervision.[7] Predictions that rising rates of marijuana use among youth born in the 1970s would lead to dramatic increases in progression to use of hard drugs in the 1990s proved to be incorrect.[8] Progression is not inevitable, and substance use commonly declines in young adult life.

The stages of adolescent substance use outlined in Table 172-4 also do not imply an inevitable progression through the stages. Many adolescents remain abstinent or do not progress beyond experimentation.[9]

## SCREENING

Clinical preventive services guidelines advocate annual screening and assessment for adolescent substance abuse, yet adherence by clinicians is brief and superficial at best. A recent study identified "6 Ts" as barriers to screening for adolescent substance abuse in a primary care setting. In rank order, the barriers cited were: (1) Insufficient **T**ime, (2) Lack of **T**raining to manage positive screen, (3) Need to **T**riage competing medical problems, (4) Lack of **T**reatment resources, (5) **T**enacious parents (won't leave room), and (6) Unfamiliarity with screening **T**ools.[10]

Informative questioning for substance use works best when yes/no questions are avoided. The clinician may share general information about social norms in the community, assure conditional confidentiality, and solicit

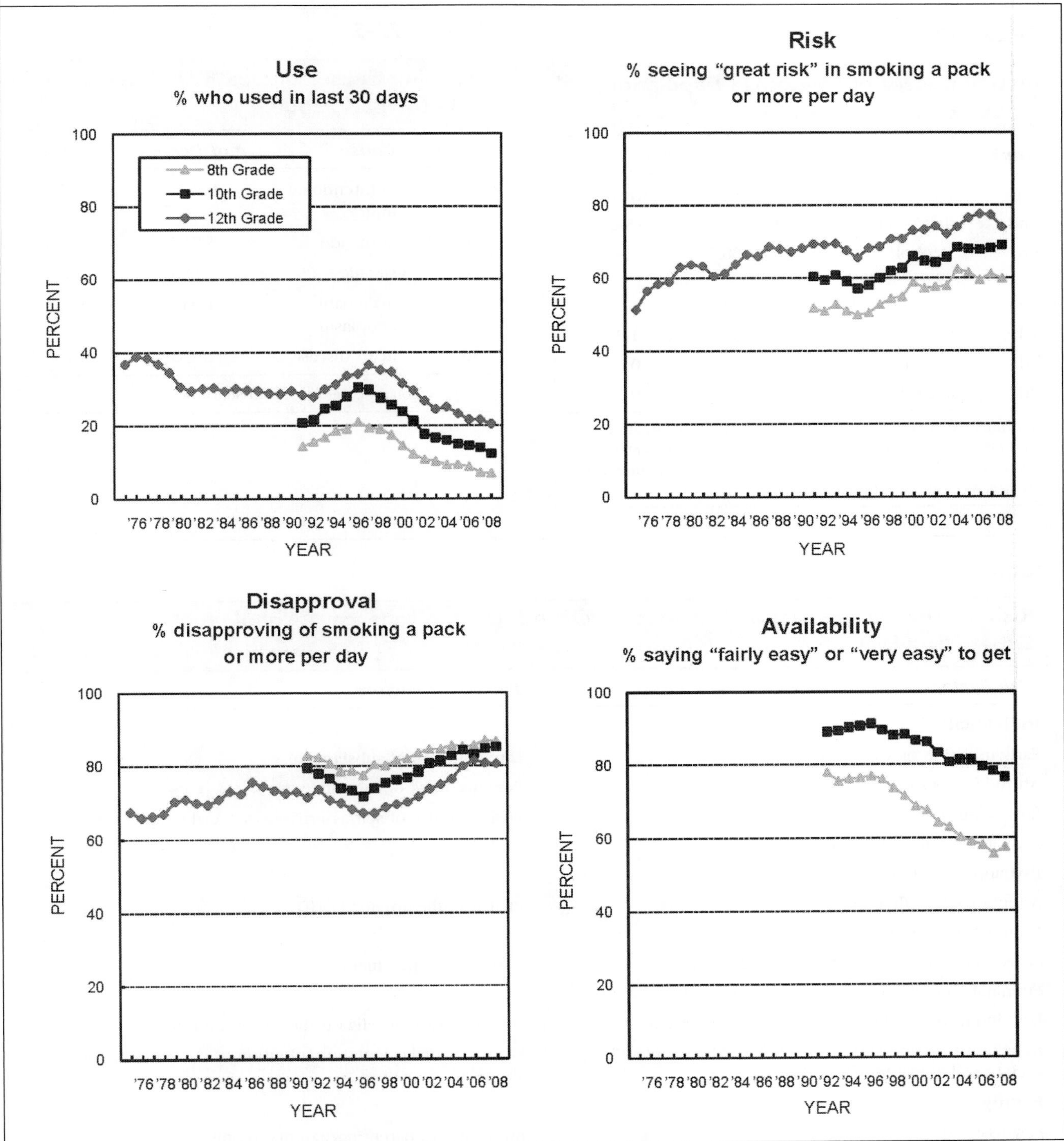


**FIGURE 172-3** Cigarettes: trends in 30-day use, risk, disapproval, and availability 8th-, 10th-, and 12th-graders. (Source: Johnston LD, O'Malley PM, Bachman JG, Schulenberg JE. Monitoring the Future national results on adolescent drug use: Overview of key findings, 2008 [NIH Publication No. 09-7401]. Bethesda, MD: National Institute on Drug Abuse; 2009.)

**Table 172-1**

**Actual Causes of Death: US Population, Total, 2000**

| *Rank* | *Cause* | *# of Deaths* | *% of Total* |
|---|---|---|---|
| 1st | tobacco | 435,000 | 18.1 |
| 2nd | diet/inactivity | 365,000 | 15.2 |
| 3rd | alcohol consumption | 85,000 | 3.5 |
| 6th | motor vehicles | 43,000 | 1.8 |
| 7th | firearms | 29,000 | 1.2 |
| 8th | sexual behavior | 20,000 | 0.8 |
| 9th | illicit drug use | 17,000 | 0.7 |

Reprinted with permission from Mokdad AH, Marks JS, Stroup DF, Gerberding JL. Actual causes of death in the United States, 2000. *JAMA*. 2004;291:1238–1245. 

**Table 172-2**

**Leading Causes of Death US Population, 15–24 Years, 2006**

| *Rank* | *Cause* | *# of Deaths* | *% of Total* |
|---|---|---|---|
| 1st | unintentional injury | 16,229 | 46.5% |
| 2nd | homicide | 5,717 | 16.4% |
| 3rd | suicide | 4,189 | 12.0% |
| 4th | malignant neoplasm | 1,644 | 4.7% |
| 5th | heart disease | 1,076 | 3.1% |

CDC. National Center for Health Statistics

**Table 172-3**

**Risk and Protective Factors Associated with Adolescent Tobacco, Alcohol, and Other Drug Use**

| *Risk Factors* | *Protective Factors* |
|---|---|
| **Individual** | |
| Early initiation of substance use | Late initiation of substance use |
| Attitude favorable to substance use | Perceived risk of substance use |
| Low self-esteem/poor coping skills | Positive sense of self/assertiveness/social competence |
| Early antisocial or delinquent behavior | |
| Psychopathology, particularly depression | |
| Attention-deficit/hyperactivity disorder (ADHD) | Pharmacotherapy for ADHD |
| Conduct disorder/aggressive behavior | |
| Sensation seeking/impulsivity/distractibility | Resilient temperament |
| Perinatal complications or brain injury | |
| Low intensity of religious beliefs and observance | High intensity of religious beliefs and observance |
| Rebelliousness and alienation from the dominant values of society and conventional norms | Positive social orientation/adoption of conventional norms about substance use |
| **Family** | |
| Permissive or authoritarian parenting | Authoritative parenting/parental monitoring of activities |
| Parental and older sibling use of alcohol, tobacco, or other drugs | Clearly communicated parental expectation of nonuse/clear rules of conduct, consistently enforced |
| Family history of alcoholism | |
| High levels of family conflict | Positive, supportive relationships with family |
| Parental divorce during adolescence | Open communication with parents |
| Child abuse and neglect/sexual abuse | Supportive relationships with prosocial adults |

(*Continued*)

**Table 172-3 (Continued)**

| *Risk Factors* | *Protective Factors* |
|---|---|
| **Peers** | |
| Friends who drink, smoke, or use other drugs | Friends not engaged in substance use |
| Perceived peer drug use | Peer disapproval of substance use |
| **School** | |
| Poor academic achievement and school failure | High academic achievement and school success |
| Low interest in school and achievement | High academic aspirations |
| **Community** | |
| Disorganization in the community/neighborhood | Lower acculturation and higher ethnic identification |
| Availability of tobacco and alcohol | Increased legal smoking and drinking ages |
| Marketing of tobacco and alcohol | Increased excise taxes on tobacco and alcohol |
| Availability of licit and illicit drugs | Strict law enforcement |
| **Sociocultural** | |
| Media portrayal of substance use | Media literacy |
| Advertising licit substances | Formal antidrug education programs |

From Kulig JW and the Committee on Substance Abuse. Tobacco, alcohol, and other drugs. The role of the pediatrician in prevention, identification, and management of substance abuse. *Pediatrics*. 2005;115:816–821.

**Table 172-4**

**Stages of Adolescent Substance Abuse**

| *Stage* | *Description* |
|---|---|
| 1 | **Potential for abuse** |
| | Decreased impulse control |
| | Need for immediate gratification |
| | Availability of tobacco, drugs, alcohol, inhalants |
| | Need for peer acceptance |
| 2 | **Experimentation: learning the euphoria** |
| | Use of tobacco, marijuana, inhalants, and alcohol with friends |
| | Few, if any, consequences |
| | Possible increase to regular weekend use |
| | Little change in behavior |
| 3 | **Regular use: seeking the euphoria** |
| | Use of other drugs, eg, cocaine, club drugs, opioids |
| | Behavioral changes and some consequences |
| | Increased frequency of use; use alone |
| | Buying or stealing drugs |
| 4 | **Regular use: preoccupation with the "high"** |
| | Daily use of drugs |
| | Loss of control |
| | Multiple consequences and risk-taking |
| | Estrangement from family and "clean" friends |
| 5 | **Addiction: use of drugs to feel normal** |
| | Use of multiple substances; cross-addiction |
| | Guilt, withdrawal, shame, remorse, depression |
| | Physical and mental deterioration |
| | Increased risk-taking, self-destructive or suicidal behavior |

Reprinted with permission from Comerci GD. Recognizing the 5 stages of substance abuse. *Contemp Pediatr.* 1985;2:57–68

information about school climate and peer behavior before inquiring about the individual patient's behavior. As with any psychosocial assessment of an adolescent, the clinician should explore function at home, in school, at work, and with peers.[11-13] Conditional confidentiality can be maintained, but clinicians should be guided by applicable state consent laws when treating minors.[14] Substance abuse that places the adolescent patient or others at life-threatening risk requires the involvement of parents, and potentially school officials or law enforcement authorities. Patients should be notified when disclosure will occur and be offered a chance to join the conversation.[15]

A structured approach to screening is recommended as clinical impressions of adolescents' alcohol and drug involvement have been shown to underestimate substance-related pathology.[16]

The CRAFFT screen is a questionnaire that can be applied in a primary care setting. Two "yes" answers indicate the need for further assessment and intervention.[17] See Chapter 181, Office Management and Laboratory Testing, for more detail on the CRAFFT screening questions. Alternate screening instruments include the 159-item Drug Use Screening Inventory—Adolescents (DUSI-A), which documents level of involvement and quantifies consequences of drug use, and the 139-item Problem-Oriented Screening Instrument for Teenagers (POSIT),[18] which identifies problems in 10 functional areas, including substance use. When an adolescent patient screens positive, the clinician's response may range from brief office interventions to referral for addiction treatment, depending upon severity at presentation.

## CLINICAL PRESENTATION

Adolescents with substance abuse problems may present with behavioral, mental health, or medical complaints. Parents may note declining school performance, a new peer group, or discover drugs or related paraphernalia. They may note obvious signs of intoxication or secondary findings such as the smell of marijuana smoke. Mental health presentations include disorders comorbid with substance use, when the illicit drug may be used to self-medicate a mood disorder or may trigger a psychotic disorder. Medical presentations may include fatigue, malaise, and headaches following a weekend of alcohol and drug use, as well as specific adverse effects such as gastritis, hepatitis, and pancreatitis. Findings on examination suggestive of substance abuse are listed in Box 172-2.[19] Substance abuse during pregnancy is associated with increased risk of preterm delivery, low birthweight, and sudden infant death syndrome (SIDS). Infants may require prolonged hospitalization after birth for treatment of neonatal abstinence syndrome (NAS).

### Box 172-2

### *Examination Findings Suggestive of Addiction or Its Complications*

**General**

- Odor of alcohol on breath
- Odor of marijuana on clothing
- Odor of nicotine or smoke on breath or clothing
- Poor nutritional status
- Poor personal hygiene

**Behavior**

- Intoxicated behavior during examination
- Slurred speech
- Staggering gait
- Scratching

**Skin**

- Signs of physical injury
- Bruises
- Lacerations
- Scratches
- Burns
- Needle marks
- Skin abscesses
- Cellulitis
- Jaundice
- Palmar erythema
- Hair loss
- Diaphoresis
- Rash
- Puffy hands

**Head, Eyes, Ears, Nose, Throat (HEENT)**

- Conjunctival irritation or injection
- Inflamed nasal mucosa
- Perforated nasal septum
- Blanched nasal septum
- Sinus tenderness
- Gum disease, gingivitis
- Gingival ulceration
- Rhinitis
- Sinusitis
- Pale mucosa
- Burns in oral cavity

**Gastrointestinal**

- Hepatomegaly
- Liver tenderness
- Positive stool hemoccult

**Immune**

- Lymphadenopathy

*(Continued)*

**Box 172-2 (continued)**

**Cardiovascular**
- Hypertension
- Tachycardia
- Cardiac arrhythmia
- Heart murmurs, clicks
- Edema
- Swelling

**Pulmonary**
- Wheezing, rales, rhonchi
- Cough
- Respiratory depression

**Female Reproductive/Endocrine**
- Pelvic tenderness
- Vaginal discharge

**Male Reproductive/Endocrine**
- Testicular atrophy
- Penile discharge
- Gynecomastia

**Neurologic**
- Sensory impairment
- Memory impairment
- Motor impairment
- Ophthalmoplegia
- Myopathy
- Neuropathy
- Tremor
- Cognitive defects
- Ataxia
- Pupillary dilation or constriction

Center for Substance Abuse Treatment. *Clinical Guidelines for the Use of Buprenorphine in the Treatment of Opioid Addiction.* Treatment Improvement Protocol (TIP) Series 40. DHHS Publication No (SMA) 04-3939. Rockville, MD: Substance Abuse and Mental Health Services Administration; 2004.

**Box 172-3**

***Drug Class and Urine Detection Period***

- Alcohol: 6–10 hours
- Amphetamines: 1–2 days
- Anabolic steroids: 3 weeks–3 months
- Barbiturates: 2–10 days
- Benzodiazepines: 1–6 weeks
- Cannabinoids: 2–8 days short-term and 14–42 days long-term
- Cocaine: 2–4 days short-term and up to 8 days long-term
- LSD: 8 hours
- Opiates: 1–2 days
- Phencyclidine: 2–8 days
- Psilocybin (mushrooms): 2–8 days

www.nida.nih.gov

**Box 172-4**

***Urine Drug Testing: "The NIDA 5"***

- Cannabinoids (marijuana, hashish)
- Cocaine (cocaine, benzoylecgonine, cocaethylene)
- Amphetamines (amphetamine, methamphetamine)
- Opiates (heroin, opium, codeine, morphine)
- Phencyclidine (PCP)

www.nida.nih.gov

## DRUG TESTING

The use of routine drug testing as a screening tool for adolescent substance abuse is of limited value. Many drugs of abuse are not included in routine testing, and most remain detectable in the urine for a relatively brief period of time, often only 1 to 2 days (Box 172-3). The "NIDA 5" is a standard panel that includes the drugs listed in Box 172-4. Drug testing is most useful as part of a drug treatment program or in an emergency department when evaluating an unresponsive patient. Patient consent for testing should be obtained whenever possible.[20]

## ASSESSMENT AND MANAGEMENT

The American Academy of Pediatrics recommends that clinicians: (1) become familiar with DSM-IV and DSM-PC criteria for distinguishing experimental from problem drug use (Box 172-5 and Box 172-6), (2) recognize the limitations of drug testing, (3) recognize psychiatric comorbidity (dual diagnosis) and refer for psychiatric consultation, (4) develop a close working relationship with local community resources, and (5) advocate for quality substance abuse and mental health services under managed care.[21,22]

As part of anticipatory guidance, patients and their families should be advised that even casual use of ATOD by adolescents, regardless of amount or frequency, is illegal and has potential adverse health consequences.[6]

### Box 172-5

## *Criteria for Substance Abuse [305.90]*

A maladaptive pattern of substance use leading to clinically significant impairment or distress, as manifested by 1 (or more) of the following, occurring within a 12-month period:

- Recurrent substance use resulting in a failure to fulfill major role obligations at work, school, or home (eg, repeated absences or poor work performance related to substance use; substance-related absences, suspensions, or expulsions from school; neglect of children or household
- Recurrent substance use in situations in which it is physically hazardous (eg, driving an automobile or operating a machine when impaired by substance use)
- Recurrent substance-related legal problems (eg, arrests for substance-related disorderly conduct)
- Continued substance use despite having persistent or recurrent social or interpersonal problems caused or exacerbated by the effects of the substance (eg, arguments with spouse about consequence of intoxication, physical fights)

The symptoms have never met the criteria for substance dependence for this class of substance.

Reprinted with permission from American Psychiatric Association. *Diagnostic and Statistical Manual of Mental Disorders,* 4th ed., Text Revision. Washington, DC: American Psychiatric Association; 2000: 199.

### Box 172-6

## *Criteria for Substance Dependence [304.90]*

A maladaptive pattern of substance use, leading to clinically significant impairment or distress, as manifested by 3 (or more) of the following, occurring at any time in the same 12-month period:

- Tolerance, as defined by either of the following:
    - A need for markedly increased amounts of the substance to achieve intoxication or desired effect

  -or-

    - Markedly diminished effect with continued use of the same amount of the substance
- Withdrawal, as manifested by either of the following:
    - The characteristic withdrawal syndrome for the substance

  -or-

    - The same (or a closely related) substance is taken to relieve or avoid withdrawal symptoms
- The substance is often taken in larger amounts or over a longer period than was intended
- There is a persistent desire or unsuccessful efforts to cut down or control substance use
- A great deal of time is spent on activities necessary to obtain the substance (eg, visiting multiple doctors or driving long distances), use the substance (eg, chain-smoking), or recover from its effects
- Important social, occupational, or recreational activities are given up or reduced because of substance use
- The substance use is continued despite knowledge of having a persistent physical or psychological problem that is likely to have been caused or exacerbated by the substance (eg, current cocaine use despite recognition of cocaine-induced depression, or continued drinking despite recognition that an ulcer was made worse by alcohol consumption)

Specify if:

- With physiological dependence: Evidence of tolerance or withdrawal (ie, either item 1 or 2 is present)
- Without physiological dependence: No evidence of tolerance or withdrawal (ie, neither item 1 nor 2 is present)

Reprinted with permission from American Psychiatric Association: *Diagnostic and Statistical Manual of Mental Disorders*, 4th ed., Text Revision. American Psychiatric Association; 2000: 279.

Brief office-based interventions should be based upon the level of risk and the patient's progression through the stages of behavioral change. Studies of tobacco cessation in adults have shown that even 10 minutes of counseling by a physician more than doubles the likelihood of success when compared with no counseling. An adolescent who reports abstinence from substance use deserves strong encouragement, support, and anticipatory guidance. A patient who reports experimental substance use should be provided with risk reduction guidance and refusal skills. Parental involvement and protective strategies may be required if a patient is engaging in life-threatening behavior such as driving while impaired. A signed parent–teen contract may prove useful to guarantee a safe ride home. Dysfunctional behavior and comorbid mental health disorders (dual diagnosis) require referral for assessment and treatment beyond the primary care office setting.[23]

A work group of the American Academy of Child and Adolescent Psychiatry[18] has published a practice parameter for the assessment and treatment of children and adolescents with substance use disorders. The document highlights impairment in psychosocial and academic functioning as hallmarks of substance use disorder in adolescents and provides clinical guidance with 15 specific recommendations.

Principles of effective drug addiction treatment are listed in Box 172-7. Clinicians should be aware of community services for evaluation, referral, and treatment of substance-abuse disorders and be available to provide aftercare for adolescent patients completing substance-abuse treatment programs. They should also be able to assist with reintegration into the community.

Finally, prevention and treatment of adolescent substance abuse cannot be solely addressed in a clinical setting. The Healthy People goals for 2010[24] (Table 172-5) emphasize the need for including health education, law enforcement, and changing social norms. Substance abuse prevention programs are difficult to evaluate, and initial efficacy trial findings may not be replicated in effectiveness trials, suggesting that program assessments must be ongoing.

## Box 172-7

### *Principles of Effective Drug Addiction Treatment*

1. No single treatment is appropriate for all individuals.
2. Treatment needs to be readily available.
3. Effective treatment attends to multiple needs of the individual, not just drug use.
4. Treatment needs to be flexible.
5. Remaining in treatment for an adequate period of time is critical for treatment effectiveness.
6. Individual and/or group counseling and other behavioral therapies are critical components of effective treatment for addiction.
7. Medications are an important element of treatment for many patients.
8. Addicted or individuals who abuse drugs and have coexisting mental disorders should have an integrated treatment plan.
9. Medical detoxification is only the first stage of addiction treatment and by itself does little to change long-term drug use.
10. Treatment does not need to be voluntary to be effective.
11. Possible drug use during treatment must be monitored continuously.
12. Treatment programs should provide assessment for HIV/AIDS, hepatitis B and C, tuberculosis, and other infectious diseases.
13. Recovery from addiction can be a long-term process.

National Institute on Drug Abuse. *Principles of Drug Addiction Treatment: A Research-Based Guide*, 2nd ed. NIH Publication No. 09-4180. Bethesda, MD: National Institute on Drug Abuse; 2009.

## Table 172-5

### Healthy People 2010: Child- and Adolescent-Specific Goals for Substance Use

| *Goal Number* | *Description* |
|---|---|
| 7-2 | Increase the proportion of middle, junior high, and senior high schools that provide school health education to prevent health problems in the following areas: unintentional injury; violence; suicide; tobacco use and addiction; alcohol and other drug use; unintended pregnancy, HIV/AIDS, and STD infection; unhealthy dietary patterns; inadequate physical activity; and environmental health |
| 16-18 | Reduce the occurrence of fetal alcohol syndrome (FAS) |
| 26-1 | Reduce deaths and injuries caused by alcohol- and drug-related motor vehicle crashes |
| 26-6 | Reduce the proportion of adolescents who report that they rode, during the previous 30 days, with a driver who had been drinking alcohol |
| 26-9 | Increase the age and proportion of adolescents who remain alcohol and drug free |
| 26-10 | Reduce past-month use of illicit substances. |
| 26-11 | Reduce the proportion of persons engaging in binge drinking of alcoholic beverages |
| 26-14 | Reduce steroid use among adolescents |
| 26-15 | Reduce the proportion of adolescents who use inhalants |
| 26-16 | Increase the proportion of adolescents who disapprove of substance abuse |
| 26-17 | Increase the proportion of adolescents who perceive great risk associated with substance abuse |
| 27-2 | Reduce tobacco use by adolescents |
| 27-3 | Reduce the initiation of tobacco use among children and adolescents |
| 27-4 | Increase the average age of first use of tobacco products by adolescents and young adults. |
| 27-7 | Increase tobacco use cessation attempts by adolescent smokers |
| 27-9 | Reduce the proportion of children who are regularly exposed to tobacco smoke at home |
| 27-14 | Reduce the illegal buy rate among minors through enforcement of laws prohibiting the sale of tobacco products to minors |
| 27-16 | Eliminate tobacco advertising and promotions that influence adolescents and young adults |
| 27-17 | Increase adolescents' disapproval of smoking |

US Department of Health and Human Services. *Healthy People 2010. Understanding and Improving Health and Objectives for Improving Health*. Vols I and II. 2nd ed. Washington, DC: US Government Printing Office; 2000.

## INTERNET RESOURCES

### GOVERNMENT AGENCY WEB SITES

- NIDA: www.drugabuse.gov/
- NIAAA: www.niaaa.nih.gov/
- SAMHSA: www.samhsa.gov/

### NATIONAL SURVEY WEB SITES

- MTF: www.monitoringthefuture.org
- YRBSS: www.cdc.gov/nccdphp/dash/yrbs/
- NSDUH: oas.samhsa.gov/nsduh.htm

### STREET DRUG NAME WEB SITES

- Government: www.whitehousedrugpolicy.gov/streetterms/default.asp
- Private: www.drug-rehabs.org/slang-names.htm

## REFERENCES

1. Schydlower M, ed. *Substance Abuse: A Guide for Health Professionals.* 2nd ed. Elk Grove Village, IL: American Academy of Pediatrics; 2002

2. Rogers PD, Heyman RB, eds. Addiction medicine: adolescent substance abuse. *Pediatr Clinics North Am.* 2002;49:1-496

3. Schydlower M, Arredondo RM, eds. Substance abuse among adolescents. *Adolesc Med Clinics.* 2006;17:1-504

4. Johnston LD, O'Malley PM, Bachman JG, et al. *Monitoring the Future: National Results on Adolescent Drug Use: Overview of Key Findings, 2006.* (NIH Publication No. 07-6202). Bethesda, MD: National Institute on Drug Abuse; 2007

5. Mokdad AH, Marks JS, Stroup DF, et al. Actual causes of death in the United States, 2000. *JAMA.* 2005;293:293-294

6. Kulig JW and the Committee on Substance Abuse. Tobacco, alcohol, and other drugs: the role of the pediatrician in prevention, identification, and management of substance abuse. *Pediatrics.* 2005;115:816-821

7. Tarter RE, Vanykov M, Kirisci L, et al. Predictors of marijuana use in adolescents before and after licit drug use: examination of the gateway hypothesis. *Am J Psychiatry.* 2006;163:2134-2140

8. Golub A, Johnson BD. Variation in youthful risks of progression from alcohol and tobacco to marijuana and hard drugs across generations. *Am J Public Health.* 2001;91:225-232

9. American Academy of Pediatrics Committee on Substance Abuse. Indications for management and referral of patients involved in substance abuse. *Pediatrics.* 2000;106:143-148

10. Van Hook S, Harris SK, Brooks T, et al. "The Six Ts": barriers to screening teens for substance abuse in primary care. *J Adolesc Health.* 2007;40:456-461

11. American Academy of Pediatrics. Office management of substance abuse. *Adolescent Health Update.* 2003;15:1-8

12. American Academy of Pediatrics Committee on Substance Abuse. Tobacco's toll: implications for the pediatrician. *Pediatrics.* 2001;107:794-798

13. American Academy of Pediatrics Committee on Substance Abuse. Alcohol use and abuse: a pediatric concern. *Pediatrics.* 2001;108:185-189

14. English A, Kenney KE. *State Minor Consent Laws: A Summary.* 2nd ed. Chapel Hill, NC: Center for Adolescent Health & the Law; 2003

15. Joffe A. Confidentiality in dealing with adolescents. In: Graham AW, Schultz TK, Mayo-Smith MF, et al, eds. *Principles of Addiction Medicine.* 3rd ed. Chevy Chase, MD: American Society of Addiction Medicine; 2003:1555-1557

16. Wilson CR, Sherritt L, Gates E, et al. Are clinical impressions of adolescent substance abuse accurate? *Pediatrics.* 2004;114:e536-e540

17. Knight JR, Sherritt L, Shrier LA, Harris SK, Chang G. Validity of the CRAFFT substance abuse screening test among adolescent clinic patients. *Arch Pediatr Adolesc Med.* 2002;156:607-614

18. Bukstein OG, Bernet W, Arnold V, et al. Work Group on Quality Issues. Practice parameter for the assessment and treatment of children and adolescents with substance use disorders. *J Am Acad Child Adolesc Psychiatry.* 2005;44:609-621

19. Center for Substance Abuse Treatment. *Clinical Guidelines for the Use of Buprenorphine in the Treatment of Opioid Addiction.* Treatment Improvement Protocol (TIP) Series 40. DHHS Publication No (SMA) 04-3939. Rockville, MD: Substance Abuse and Mental Health Services Administration; 2004

20. Casavant MJ. Urine drug screening in adolescents. *Pediatr Clin N Am.* 2002;49:317-327

21. American Academy of Pediatrics. Insurance coverage of mental health and substance abuse services for children and adolescents: a consensus statement. *Pediatrics.* 2000;106:860-862

22. American Academy of Pediatrics Committee on Child Health Financing and Committee on Substance Abuse. Improving substance abuse prevention, assessment, and treatment financing for children and adolescents. *Pediatrics.* 2001;108:1025-1029

23. Fournier ME, Levy S. Recent trends in adolescent substance use, primary care screening, and updates in treatment options. *Curr Opin Pediatrics.* 2006;18:352-358

24. Hallfors D, Cho H, Sanchez V, et al. Efficacy vs effectiveness trial results of an indicated "model" substance abuse program: implications for public health. *Am J Public Health.* 2006;96:2254-2259

# CHAPTER 173

# Tobacco

SETH D. AMMERMAN, MD

*"If current trends hold, tobacco will kill a billion people this century, 10 times more than in the 20th century."*

WORLD HEALTH ORGANIZATION[1]

## INTRODUCTION

Although progress has been made in smoking prevention and cessation efforts in the United States, use of tobacco still kills almost 450,000 people each year in this country.[2-8] Compared to other public health problems of high concern such as illegal drugs, alcohol, homicide, suicide, acquired immunodeficiency syndrome, and motor vehicle accidents, tobacco use results in two-thirds more deaths each year than all of the others combined. Not only do users of all tobacco products suffer high rates of morbidity and mortality, but so do those exposed to secondhand (ie, the smoking of others) and thirdhand (ie, smoking residue in walls, clothes, hair, skin) tobacco smoke.[9] Use of any tobacco products can negatively effect virtually every organ system in the body (Box 173-1).

One area of special concern is tobacco use by pregnant women, as the mother and developing fetus and baby can be adversely affected. Problems can include an increased risk of ectopic pregnancy and spontaneous abortion; prematurity, lower birth weights, and small for gestational age; and an increase in stillborn and early neonatal deaths, including sudden infant death syndrome (SIDS).

Approximately 20% of health care dollars spent in the United States is due to tobacco-related illnesses. Additionally, fires started by cigarettes cause thousands of deaths and injuries each year.[10] Worldwide, 20% of 13- to 15-year-old students use tobacco, evenly split between cigarettes and all other tobacco products.[11] Many youth smokers report a desire to quit smoking, but once addicted, find it very difficult to do.[12] At the same time, a significant number of middle and high school students who have never smoked cigarettes state that they might try smoking in the next year. *Healthy People 2010*, a US national health promotion and disease prevention initiative, had a primary tobacco use objective of reducing smoking prevalence to 16% or less in youth by 2010; this is unfortunately not being met.

Besides direct use of tobacco products by a patient, exposure to environmental tobacco smoke (ETS or secondhand smoke) is a serious problem. More than 50% of youth are exposed to ETS each week, with a third exposed to >3 hours of ETS. A report on ETS released by the United States Surgeon General in 2006, "The Health Consequences of Involuntary Exposure to Tobacco Smoke,"[8] had 4 key findings, which are listed in Box 173-2. Because most tobacco use starts in the adolescent age group, with almost 90% of all cigarette smokers starting before the age of 18, clinicians who provide health care to adolescents have an important role to play in tobacco use prevention and cessation.

### Box 173-1

### *Negative Systemic Effects of Cigarette Use*

Negative effects may include:

- Heart and lung disease—ischemic heart disease, cerebrovascular and peripheral vascular disease
- Cancers—lung, head, and neck, esophageal, gastric, colorectal, bladder, renal, prostate, and cervical tumors
- Diminished bone density
- Pulmonary—chronic obstructive pulmonary disease and small airway disease
- Gastrointestinal—gastroesophageal reflux and peptic ulcer disease
- Cataracts
- Premature wrinkling of the skin
- Potential adverse effects on immune system
- Pregnancy-related problems including low-birth-weight babies and higher rates of spontaneous abortions
- Erectile dysfunction (impotence)

Smokeless tobacco users may also suffer from:

- Higher rates of various cancers, including oral, prostate, pancreas, and cervical
- Dental, periodontal, and oral soft tissue problems, including gingival recession, periodontal attachment loss, tooth staining, halitosis, and leukoplakia
- Inflammatory bowel disease

**Box 173-2**

***The Health Consequences of Involuntary Exposure to Environmental Tobacco Smoke (ETS)***

- ETS exposure causes disease and premature death in children and adults who do not smoke
- ETS exposure leads to an increased risk of sudden infant death syndrome
- ETS exposure in adults has immediate negative effects on the cardiovascular system and causes coronary heart disease and lung cancer
- There is no safe level of exposure to ETS

## PREVALENCE

Cigarette use by adolescents remains a serious problem. Each day approximately 6,000 American youth under the age of 18 start smoking for the first time, and 2,000 youth become established daily smokers.[13] Although cigarette use rates for youth under age 18 had declined 40% in the last decade, recent data reveal that the percentage of high school students reporting that they have smoked cigarettes in the past month (defined as current smokers) has recently increased (Table 173-1 and Table 173-2).

Cigarettes are the most commonly used tobacco product by adolescents, followed by cigars, smokeless tobacco, pipes, bidis, and kreteks. Bidis and kreteks are hand-rolled cigarettes, often flavored, that typically contain a mixture consisting of tobacco, cloves, and other additives. Clove cigarettes are similar to bidis and kreteks. Adolescents may mistakenly believe that these formulations are safer than conventional cigarettes; however, in reality, they may actually deliver more nicotine, carbon monoxide, and tar than regular cigarettes. Menthol cigarettes are as dangerous as regular cigarettes, and those who smoke menthol brands may have a harder time quitting. Black smokers are more than twice as likely to smoke menthol cigarettes as white smokers. Tobacco products labeled "light" or "low" are equally harmful as products not labeled as such and should not be proposed as a safer alternative.[14]

Smokeless tobacco use, mainly chewing tobacco and snuff, is also a serious problem. Chewing tobacco comes in loose leaf, plug, or twist forms. Snuff is finely ground tobacco that comes in dry, moist, or sachet (pouch)

(continued on p. 1741)

**Table 173-1**

**Percentage of High School Students who Reported Lifetime Cigarette Use,[a] Current Cigarette Use,[b] and Current Frequent Cigarette Use[c]—Youth Risk Behavior Survey, United States, 1991–2007[d]**

| *Category* | *1991 (95% CI[e])* | *1993 (95% CI)* | *1995 (95% CI)* | *1997 (95% CI)* | *1999 (95% CI)* | *2001 (95% CI)* | *2003 (95% CI)* | *2005 (95% CI)* | *2007 (95% CI)* |
|---|---|---|---|---|---|---|---|---|---|
| Lifetime[f] | 70.1 (67.8–72.3) | 69.5 (68.1–70.8) | 71.3 (69.5–73.0) | 70.2 (68.2–72.1) | 70.4 (67.3–73.3) | 63.9 (61.6–66.0) | 58.4 (55.1–61.6) | 54.3 (51.2–57.3) | 50.3 (47.2–53.5) |
| Current[g] | 27.5 (24.8–30.3) | 30.5 (28.6–32.4) | 34.8 (32.5–37.2) | 36.4 (34.1–38.7) | 34.8 (32.3–37.4) | 28.5 (26.4–30.6) | 21.9 (19.8–24.2) | 23.0 (20.7–25.5) | 20.0 (17.6–22.5) |
| Current frequent[f] | 12.7 (10.6–15.5) | 13.8 (12.1–15.5) | 16.1 (13.6–19.1) | 16.7 (14.8–18.7) | 16.8 (14.3–19.6) | 13.8 (12.3–15.5) | 9.7 (8.3–11.3) | 9.4 (7.9–11.0) | 8.1 (6.7–9.8) |

[a]Ever smoked cigarettes, even 1 or 2 puffs.

[b]Smoked cigarettes on at least 1 day during the 30 days before the survey.

[c]Smoked cigarettes on 20 or more days during the 30 days before the survey.

[d]Linear, quadratic, and cubic trend analyses were conducted using a logistic regression model controlling for sex, race/ethnicity, and grade. These prevalence estimates are not standardized by demographic variables.

[e]Confidence interval.

[f]Significant linear and quadratic effects only ($p<0.05$).

[g]Significant linear, quadratic, and cubic effects ($p<0.05$).

CDC. Cigarette use among high school students–1991-2007. *MMWR*, June 27, 2008/57(25);689-691.

**Table 173-2**

**Percentage of High School Students who Reported Current Cigarette Use,[a] by Sex, Race/Ethnicity, and Grade—Youth Risk Behavior Survey, United States, 1991–2007[b]**

| *Characteristic* | *1991 (95% CI[c])* | *1993 (95% CI)* | *1995 (95% CI)* | *1997 (95% CI)* | *1999 (95% CI)* | *2001 (95% CI)* | *2003 (95% CI)* | *2005 (95% CI)* | *2007 (95% CI)* |
|---|---|---|---|---|---|---|---|---|---|
| Sex | | | | | | | | | |
| Female[d] | 27.3 (23.9–31.0) | 31.2 (29.1–33.4) | 34.3 (31.0–37.7) | 34.7 (31.8–37.6) | 34.9 (32.3–37.7) | 27.7 (25.6–30.0) | 21.9 (19.2–24.9) | 23.0 (20.4–25.8) | 18.7 (16.5–21.1) |
| Male[d] | 27.6 (24.6–30.9) | 29.8 (27.4–32.3) | 35.4 (32.9–37.9) | 37.7 (35.0–40.6) | 34.7 (31.8–37.7) | 29.2 (36.7–32.0) | 21.8 (19.8–24.1) | 22.9 (20.7–25.3) | 21.3 (18.3–24.6) |
| Race/Ethnicity[e] | | | | | | | | | |
| White, non-Hispanic[d] | 30.9 (27.6–34.5) | 33.7 (31.4–36.0) | 38.3 (35.6–41.1) | 39.7 (37.3–42.2) | 38.6 (35.5–41.9) | 31.9 (29.6–34.4) | 24.9 (22.4–27.5) | 25.9 (22.9–29.2) | 23.2 (20.4–26.2) |
| Female[d] | 31.7 (27.1–36.7) | 35.3 (32.6–38.0) | 39.8 (36.3–43.5) | 39.9 (36.6–43.2) | 39.1 (35.4–42.9) | 31.2 (28.7–33.7) | 26.6 (22.9–30.5) | 27.0 (23.4–31.0) | 22.5 (19.6–25.7) |
| Male[d] | 30.2 (26.5–34.3) | 32.2 (29.4–35.0) | 37.0 (33.7–40.5) | 39.6 (35.8–43.5) | 38.2 (34.6–41.8) | 32.7 (29.7–35.9) | 23.3 (20.7–26.0) | 24.9 (22.2–27.7) | 23.8 (20.2–27.8) |
| Black, non-Hispanic[f] | 12.6 (10.2–15.5) | 15.4 (12.9–18.2) | 19.1 (16.1–22.6) | 22.7 (19.0–26.8) | 19.7 (15.8–24.3) | 14.7 (12.0–17.9) | 15.1 (12.4–18.2) | 12.9 (11.1–14.8) | 11.6 (9.5–14.1) |
| Female[g] | 11.3 (9.2–13.9) | 14.4 (11.9–17.4) | 12.2 (9.3–15.7) | 17.4 (13.8–21.7) | 17.7 (14.4–21.7) | 13.3 (10.1–17.2) | 10.8 (8.2–14.2) | 11.9 (10.2–13.8) | 8.4 (6.6–10.6) |
| Male[f] | 14.1 (10.1–19.4) | 16.3 (12.4–21.1) | 27.8 (22.5–33.9) | 28.2 (23.0–34.1) | 21.8 (15.4–29.9) | 16.3 (13.2–19.8) | 19.3 (15.8–23.5) | 14.0 (11.5–16.9) | 14.9 (11.7–18.8) |

*(Continued)*

**Table 173-2 (Continued)**

| *Characteristic* | *1991 (95% CI[c])* | *1993 (95% CI)* | *1995 (95% CI)* | *1997 (95% CI)* | *1999 (95% CI)* | *2001 (95% CI)* | *2003 (95% CI)* | *2005 (95% CI)* | *2007 (95% CI)* |
|---|---|---|---|---|---|---|---|---|---|
| Hispanic[d] | 25.3 (22.5–28.2) | 28.7 (25.8–31.8) | 34.0 (28.7–39.6) | 34.0 (31.3–36.9) | 32.7 (29.0–36.6) | 26.6 (22.4–31.2) | 18.4 (16.1–20.9) | 22.0 (18.7–25.8) | 16.7 (13.5–20.4) |
| Female[d] | 22.9 (19.2–27.1) | 27.3 (23.5–31.5) | 32.9 (27.4–39.0) | 32.3 (28.6–36.2) | 31.5 (26.8–36.5) | 26.0 (22.3–30.0) | 17.7 (15.6–19.9) | 19.2 (16.4–22.5) | 14.6 (11.3–18.8) |
| Male[d] | 27.8 (24.3–31.8) | 30.2 (26.7–33.8) | 34.9 (26.6–44.3) | 35.5 (31.9–39.2) | 34.0 (29.7–38.7) | 27.2 (20.6–35.0) | 19.1 (15.8–23.0) | 24.8 (20.0–30.4) | 18.7 (15.0–23.2) |
| Grade | | | | | | | | | |
| 9th[d] | 23.2 (19.5–27.4) | 27.8 (25.4–30.3) | 31.2 (29.5–32.9) | 33.4 (28.4–38.9) | 27.6 (24.0–31.6) | 23.9 (21.1–27.0) | 17.4 (15.0–20.1) | 19.7 (17.5–22.1) | 14.3 (11.9–17.1) |
| 10th[d] | 25.2 (22.5–28.1) | 28.0 (24.7–31.6) | 33.1 (29.3–37.1) | 35.3 (31.2–39.7) | 34.7 (32.2–37.2) | 26.9 (23.8–30.3) | 21.8 (19.0–24.9) | 21.4 (18.4–24.8) | 19.6 (16.7–22.8) |
| 11th[d] | 31.6 (27.8–35.7) | 31.1 (27.9–34.4) | 35.9 (32.0–39.9) | 36.6 (32.9–40.4) | 36.0 (33.1–39.1) | 29.8 (26.1–33.7) | 23.6 (20.5–27.0) | 24.3 (21.2–27.7) | 21.6 (18.4–25.2) |
| 12th[d] | 30.1 (25.7–34.8) | 34.5 (30.7–38.5) | 38.2 (34.6–41.9) | 39.6 (34.7–44.6) | 42.8 (37.2–48.5) | 35.2 (31.1–39.5) | 26.2 (23.4–29.3) | 27.6 (24.0–31.5) | 26.5 (22.5–30.8) |

[a]Smoked cigarettes on at least 1 day during the 30 days before the survey.

[b]Linear, quadratic, and cubic trend analyses were conducted using a logistic regression model controlling for sex, race/ethnicity, and grade. These prevalence estimates shown here were not standardized by demographic variables.

[c]Confidence interval.

[d]Significant linear, quadratic, and cubic effects ($p<0.05$).

[e]Numbers for other racial/ethnic groups were too small for meaningful analysis.

[f]Significant quadratic and cubic effects only ($p<0.05$).

[g]Significant linear and quadratic effects only ($p<0.05$).

CDC. Cigarette use among high school students–1991-2007. *MMWR,* June 27, 2008/57(25);689–691.

forms. Usually, smokeless tobacco is placed in the cheek or put between the gum and the cheek. The tobacco is sucked on and the juices spit out. Gutka (betel quid with tobacco) is a form of flavored or spiced smokeless tobacco primarily from India, Pakistan, and Bangladesh that is becoming more popular among youth in the United States.

Smokeless tobacco contains a number of cancer-causing agents, and smokeless tobacco is addictive. In addition, use of smokeless tobacco may also lead to use of cigarettes. Smokeless tobacco rates are higher among young white males, American Indian and Alaskan natives, in the south and north-central United States, and among those who are unemployed or in blue-collar or service/laborer jobs. Seven percent of high school students are current users of smokeless tobacco. Use of smokeless tobacco products is not an effective harm reduction strategy for cigarette users.

Tobacco use also remains a serious problem for college students and young adults.[15] In 2004, 36% of college students reported having used a tobacco product. For young adults ages 18 to 24, 26.3% of men and 21.5% of women are current smokers. Additionally, use rates by young adults (ages 18–24) have only shown minimal declines. The tobacco industry spends more than $1 million a day in the United States sponsoring events and giveaways targeting college students.

There are several reasons being proposed for the recent increases in smoking among adolescents and young adults that have followed several years of decreases in these age groups. These include the findings that taxes on cigarettes are too low to discourage smoking in many states;[16] that there is less media education on tobacco in many states than there should be;[17,18] that there has been a substantial increase in the amount of money that the tobacco industry spends on tobacco advertising and promotions, from $5.7 billion in 1997 to $15.2 billion in 2003; and that there has been a substantial increase in smoking portrayed in the movies (see the following concerning the Smoke-Free Movies campaign).[19–23]

The tobacco industry continues to target youth, as a source of new users and as a replacement for those who have quit using or died. Adolescents are exposed to significant amounts of tobacco advertising on the Internet, and more importantly, to tobacco use in movies. Lack of adherence with status laws (ie, asking for proof of age before selling cigarettes to those <18 years of age) also leads to increased youth smoking. Additionally, there are reports that the tobacco companies raised the levels of nicotine in cigarettes by 10% between 1998 and 2004, making smoking more addictive for young smokers and making it harder for older smokers to quit.[24]

## FACTORS ASSOCIATED WITH TOBACCO USE

Psychosocial and biological addiction issues are important in adolescent tobacco use.[25–28] Adolescents are more likely to use tobacco if their parents, siblings, or friends do. Thus a tobacco-free environment at home and with friends is to be encouraged (see Box 173-3). Other psychosocial factors include smoking by teen girls as a method of weight control and maintenance of a thin appearance, and smoking by teen boys as a way of risk-taking. Low self-esteem and depression in adolescents are also associated with tobacco use. Gay, lesbian, or bisexual teens smoke at rates more than 50% higher than those of their straight counterparts and are 4 times more likely to use smokeless tobacco products.[29] Preteens and early adolescents may not understand the addictive nature of cigarettes and may believe there are positive attributes to smoking.

As time goes on, tobacco use becomes more of a biological addiction problem, which can be addressed in part by providing patients with nicotine replacement therapies and/or nonnicotine medication treatments (see the following for details). Thus, for adolescent tobacco users, helping patients deal with the psychosocial and addiction aspects of tobacco use will be most helpful. Research

### Box 173-3

#### *Tobacco as the "5th" Vital Sign*

Adolescents may not come in at regular intervals for office visits. Therefore, it is important to raise the tobacco use issue at every visit, regardless of chief complaint.

**For the Adolescent**

P _____ R _____ T _____ BP _____ Height _____ Weight _____

"We now ask teens about tobacco use at each visit. This is confidential. Do you ever use any tobacco products? Are you around tobacco smoke at home or with friends?"

Teen tobacco use? Yes _____ No _____ Advice given _____

Teen tobacco exposure? Yes _____ No _____ Advice given_____

**For the Parent**

P _____ R _____ T _____ BP _____ Height _____ Weight _____

"We now ask parents about their child's exposure to tobacco at each visit. Is your child ever exposed to tobacco smoke? Does your child/teen use tobacco?"

Teen tobacco exposure? Yes _____ No _____ Advice given _____

Teen tobacco use? Yes _____ No _____ Advice given_____

has shown that for addicted adolescent patients, a combination of psychosocial support and pharmacotherapy has a better outcome than either approach alone.

### ADVERTISING

The advertising of tobacco products is primarily geared toward adolescents and plays an important role in recruiting adolescent users.[30–32] The tobacco industry, as noted previously, spends more than $13 billion a year in the United States alone. Tobacco industry advertising virtually ignores all health concerns and uses themes that appeal to adolescents. Advertising tobacco in the context of other businesses and services (eg, household detergents, movies, clothing) helps legitimize tobacco use. Multiple media are utilized to promote tobacco use; these include neighborhood-based, bus-stop shelter illuminated billboards, magazines with a youth or young-adult focus, the Internet, and movies. Smoking portrayed in the movies is a particularly potent inducement to use tobacco. The Smoke Free Movies campaign has proposed 4 measures to make sure that the United States film industry does not act as a marketing arm for the tobacco industry (Box 173-4); this campaign has been endorsed by numerous health organizations, including the American Academy of Pediatrics, the Society for Adolescent Medicine, the World Health Organization, the American Heart Association and the American Medical Association. Additionally, promotional offerings and contests, as well as offers of free items (eg, hats, jackets) that usually are redeemable after mailing in a specified number of empty cigarette packs are also offered as inducements to youth to smoke.

## NICOTINE PATHOPHYSIOLOGY, ADDICTION, TOXINS, SECOND- AND THIRDHAND SMOKE

Pathophysiologically, nicotine can cause vasoconstriction of blood vessels throughout the body, leading to abnormal blood flow to tissues and tissue compromise.[33] Nicotine primarily affects dopamine and similar neurotransmitters, which are involved in pleasure and reward dependence and addiction. Nicotine is a highly addictive drug. There are likely genetic factors involved in the susceptibility to tobacco addiction, for example, the genes of the dopamine receptor. Initial symptoms of nicotine dependence occur in some adolescents within days to weeks after the onset of use. When trying to quit using tobacco, most users experience a variety of withdrawal symptoms including anxiety, irritability, and difficulty concentrating. Cravings are also common. Relapse rates are high without psychosocial and/or pharmacotherapeutic support; reports indicate that only 5% of adult smokers remain tobacco free for longer than one year after a quit attempt.

Besides nicotine, cigarettes contain tar, which is also a toxic compound. Cigarettes usually contain literally thousands of other chemicals, many poisonous and cancer causing, including ammonia, cadmium, carbon monoxide, cyanide, formaldehyde, nitrosamines, and polynuclear aromatic hydrocarbons. Toxins in tobacco products, and in second- and thirdhand smoke, can lead to ongoing destruction of cells and abnormal cell function, including the development of cancer.

More than 126 million Americans are exposed to ETS (secondhand smoke), causing an estimated 3,400 lung cancer deaths per year among nonsmokers. Secondhand smoke is a mixture of the smoke given off by the burning end of tobacco products (sidestream smoke) and the smoke exhaled by smokers (mainstream smoke). Sidestream and mainstream smoke contain many chemicals (including formaldehyde, cyanide, carbon monoxide, and ammonia), some of which are known carcinogens. Environmental tobacco smoke has numerous serious adverse health effects. Children exposed to ETS may have development and/or worsening of asthma, higher rates of lower respiratory tract infections (eg, bronchitis, pneumonia), and higher rates of otitis media. Heart disease, lung cancer, and nasal sinus cancer are also more common with exposure to ETS, as are pulmonary hypertension of the newborn, SIDS, and postanesthesia pulmonary complications.

Another danger from cigarettes may be that of "thirdhand smoke," toxic particles and gases from cigarette smoke residue that remain in walls, clothes, hair, and skin. Cigarette smoke residue may linger for months, depending on the level of contamination and ventilation of the affected area. Thirdhand smoke may be a particular problem in enclosed areas in which smoking is allowed, such as bars, hotel rooms, and casinos.

## PREVENTION AND TREATMENT

### SCHOOL- AND COMMUNITY-BASED PREVENTION

School-based tobacco prevention programs, often partnering with community-based tobacco control programs, are commonly utilized with adolescent patients. These prevention programs usually focus on improving knowledge, increasing helpful social skills, and emphasizing positive youth development. The effectiveness of these programs has been mixed, with reported results of a 0% to 40% decrease in smoking onset among adolescents receiving these prevention programs.[34–36] Higher success rates have been associated with programs that are adequately funded, comprehensive in nature, and presented over the course of a semester, through a number of years of school grades, using developmentally appropriate material. Schools typically welcome clinician involvement in an advisory capacity for these programs to help ensure that sound, practical, and up-to-date medical advice is included in the classes. Interested pediatricians can contact their local schools and talk with the "TUPE" ("Tobacco Use Prevention Education") coordinator.

### BRIEF INTERVENTIONS BY PHYSICIANS

Just 3-minute discussions of tobacco use *(brief interventions)* with patients and parents can have a significant effect on smoking prevention or smoking cessation.[37-39] Using progress notes with "tobacco as the 5th vital sign" (Box 173-3) is a simple and effective way to bring up the tobacco use issue. Of note, if an adolescent is using tobacco, it is common for she or he to be involved in other risk behaviors. These other behaviors may include alcohol and other drug use, and sexual activity without using condoms or hormonal contraception. Thus the pediatrician should inquire about other risk behaviors in a confidential manner. As with tobacco use, adolescents should be praised for not engaging in other risk behaviors or encouraged to stop if they are engaging in other risk behaviors.

> **Box 173-4**
>
> ***Smoke-Free Movies Campaign Platform***
>
> 1. Certify no payoffs. Every new smoking movie should run the following affidavit in the closing credits: "No person or entity involved in this motion picture accepted anything from any tobacco company, its agents, or fronts."
> 2. Require antismoking ads. Exhibitors should run effective antitobacco spots before all feature films. Spots should also be added to newly released videos and DVDs of smoking films, regardless of rating; many teens view R-rated movies through those media.
> 3. Stop displaying brands. Use of specific brands gives the appearance of violating agreements against brand placement.
> 4. Rate new smoking movies "R." All new movies with smoking and tobacco should receive an R rating from the Motion Picture Association of America (MPAA). Doing so will reduce the amount of smoking in the movies teens see by more than 60%. Because the effects of smoking in the movies depend on the "dose" kids get, an R rating will prevent 535 kids from starting to smoke every day.
>
> For more information: www.smokefreemovies.ucsf.edu; www.who.int/tobacco/smoke_free_movies/en/index.html.

Brief interventions should include praising nontobacco users and encouraging users to stop. Setting a formal quit date for users has been shown to be particularly effective in helping users quit. More intensive interventions and treatments including nicotine replacement therapy (patch, gum, lozenge, inhaler, and nasal spray), nonnicotine medications (bupropion and varenicline),[40] telephone quit-lines, and counseling can all be effective with patients, and combining counseling with pharmacotherapy can be more effective than either one alone. In adults, using effective tobacco cessation interventions can double or triple quit rates. However, there are only a handful of studies published that have specifically looked at success rates utilizing pharmacotherapy in adolescent smokers, and the results are modest at best. Typically reported cessation rates for adolescents at 6 months postintervention average ~12%.[41-45] Factors related to successful quitting may include shorter history of cigarette use, fewer cigarettes smoked per day, fewer cravings and withdrawal symptoms when attempting to quit, and provision of psychosocial support to life skills training. Significantly decreasing cigarette use rather than complete cessation may be a reasonable outcome for adolescents. For information on currently available nicotine replacement therapies and non-nicotine therapies, including prescribing information, see Table 173-3. Note that in prescribing these therapies, even if one doesn't work, another one may, so trying more than one, if needed, is indicated. Nicotine replacement treatment and non-nicotine treatment can be used together if they don't work alone. And, more than one nicotine replacement therapy can be used alternately if a patient feels it will be helpful, for example, chewing gum in one situation and using the inhaler in another situation may be better than just using one therapy at a time.

Clinical practice guidelines have been developed for helping patients quit smoking.[46,47] Using *the five "A's"*:

1. Ask about tobacco use at every visit;
2. Advise patients to quit smoking;
3. Assess the patient's willingness to quit;
4. Assist patients in quitting; and
5. Arrange follow-up

is an easy and brief method to help patients remain tobacco-free or decrease or quit using tobacco (Box 173-5). There are 3 parts to quitting. Part 1 is consciously preparing ahead of the quit date. Part 2 is taking the step to be tobacco-free on the quit date. Part 3 is maintaining a tobacco-free life. A brief patient guide to quitting can be found in Box 173-6. During a quit attempt, depression

**Table 173-3**

**Pharmacotherapy for Tobacco Use Cessation**

| *NRT* | *Indications* | *Warnings* | *Adverse Effects* | *Dosage* | *Rx or OTC* | *Prescribing Instructions* |
|---|---|---|---|---|---|---|
| Gum | Patients who prefer oral method | Not studied in pregnant women; cardiac symptoms | Mouth soreness, hiccups, dyspepsia, and aching jaw | 2 and 4 mg<br>Use 4 mg for >25 cigarettes/day; use 2 mg for <25 cigarettes/ day; Preferable to chew at least 1 piece every 1–2 hours; may chew up to 30 pieces of 2 mg or 20 pieces of 4 mg gum per day; usually used for 2–3 months | OTC | Don't smoke while using the gum<br>Chew gum slowly until it tastes minty, peppery, or orange, then park it between the cheek and gum to enhance nicotine absorption<br>Chew slowly and park intermittently for about 30 minutes<br>Reduce number of pieces chewed gradually over time |
| Lozenge | Same as gum | Same | Same as gum | 2 and 4 mg<br>Use 4 mg if first cigarette of day is within a half-hour of awakening; otherwise, use 2 mg; usually used for 2–3 months | OTC | Don't chew or swallow the lozenge<br>Allow lozenge to slowly dissolve over 20 or 30 minutes<br>There may be a warm or tingly sensation in the mouth<br>Intermittently shift the lozenge around in the mouth<br>Reduce number of lozenges used gradually over time |
| Patch | Patients who prefer 24-hour method | Same | Skin rash | 21 mg for >10 cigarettes/day; otherwise start with 14 mg × 6 weeks, then 7 mg × 2 weeks; worn 24 hours/day; usually used for 2–3 months | OTC | Start first patch on awakening on quit day<br>Don't smoke while using the patch; if you must smoke, take off the patch<br>Each morning, place a new patch on a relatively hairless spot between the neck and waist<br>Use a different spot each day to reduce skin irritation |
| Inhaler | Patients who prefer hand and mouth activities | Same | May cause wheezing in asthmatics | Up to 20 cartridges per day, up to 6 months | Rx | Insert cartridge into mouthpiece; cartridge lasts about 20 minutes of inhaling time<br>Lack of a distinct taste means cartridge is empty |
| Nasal spray | For highly addicted patients | Same | Nasal irritation | 1–2 sprays in each nostril per hour, at least 8 times per day, to a maximum of 80 sprays per day; use no more than 3 months | Rx | Use as frequently as needed to counter withdrawal symptoms for about 8 weeks, then reduce use over the next 4–6 weeks |

(*Continued*)

## Table 173-3 (Continued)

| *Non-nicotine medications* | *Indications* | *Warnings* | *Adverse Effects* | *Dosage* | *Rx or OTC* | *Prescribing Instructions* |
|---|---|---|---|---|---|---|
| Bupropion (Zyban) | For patients who have failed to quit using nicotine medications alone, or who prefer a pill or non-NRT medication | Should not be used in patients already on bupropion, or in patients with anorexia nervosa, bulimia nervosa, or seizure disorders (it lowers the seizure threshold especially in those who are vomiting) | Dry mouth, insomnia, headache, rhinitis | 150 mg qd or bid for up to 6 months | Rx | Start with 150 mg qod for 3 days, increase as needed to a maximum of 300 mg/day<br>Initiate 1 week qod before quit date to allow time for blood levels to build up<br>May use in conjunction with nicotine replacement products |
| Varenicline (Chantix) | Same as bupropion | No studies in patients under age 18 or pregnant women | Nausea, sleep disturbance, constipation, flatulence, vomiting | 0.5 mg on days 1–3; 0.5 mg bid on days 4–7; 1.0 mg bid from day 8 to end of treatment; for up to 6 months | Rx | Initiate 1 week before quit date, to allow time for blood levels to build up |

bid, twice a day; OTC, over-the-counter; NRT, nicotine replacement therapy; qd, once a day; qod, every other day

Addiction is usually defined as smoking half a pack of cigarettes or more per day, smoking the first cigarette of the day within 1 hour after awakening, or having had withdrawal symptoms during a previous quit attempt.

## Box 173-5

### *Brief Interventions for the Busy Practitioner: The 5 A's*

1. ***Ask*** about tobacco use at each visit. Use "TVS," tobacco as the fifth vital sign, to ask about tobacco use (See Box 173-3).
2. ***Advise*** all smokers to quit. Praise nontobacco users for being tobacco-free.
3. ***Assess*** patient willingness to make a quit attempt. Ask the patient 2 questions using a 1–10 scale: (1) How much confidence do you have in being able to successfully quit? (2) How important is it for you to quit? Patients who state high self-confidence and high importance are more likely to do well, whereas patients who state low self-confidence and low importance will likely do poorly. It is usual for patients to be somewhere in the middle on both scales, so the patient and clinician can strategize about doing better on both.
4. ***Assist*** the patient in stopping smoking. Setting a quit date is important and effective. Deadlines are helpful in achieving goals, even if patients don't meet them right away. The quit date is an actual calendar date. A quit date should be selected that is within a realistic time frame (within a few months is best), so that the patient can prepare to become a nontobacco user. Support from family and friends has been shown to lead to more successful quit attempts. The clinician or designated office staff should call the patient on the quit date. If the patient forgot about the quit date, or wasn't able to quit on that day, another quit date can be set and successful quitting next time can be encouraged. Pharmacotherapy can be prescribed to help addicted tobacco users better deal with cravings and withdrawal symptoms (see Table 173-3). Distraction and relaxation techniques (eg, writing in a journal, deep breathing) should be encouraged to help patients deal with withdrawal and craving symptoms.

*(Continued)*

## Box 173-5 (Continued)

5. ***Arrange*** follow-up. Cessation rates have been shown to significantly improve with regular follow-up. Following up in person or by phone every 1 or 2 weeks during the first 3 months of the quit attempt can make a big difference, as this is the time of greatest relapse. It is rare for a patient to relapse after remaining tobacco-free for an entire year. Remind patients that:
   - Tobacco is an addictive drug and that the cessation process is usually difficult.
   - They should not get discouraged if the first few quit attempts are unsuccessful.
   - They should view unsuccessful quit attempts as learning experiences.
   - The average number of quit attempts before successful cessation is about 7!

## Box 173-6

### *Patient Guide to Quitting Smoking*

Quitting smoking isn't easy, but millions of people have done it and so can you. These tips will help:

**Getting ready to quit**

- Set a quit date on the calendar. Let your family and friends know that you are trying to quit; they can help you through the harder times and give you ongoing encouragement.
- Write down your "triggers"—the situations when you feel like smoking or times that you do smoke. Think of ways other than smoking to deal with the triggers.
- Designate 1 place to smoke—outside—and don't smoke anywhere else.
- When you get a craving for a cigarette, try to wait a few minutes before you light up. Try a cigarette substitute during these few minutes—like slow deep breaths, chewing gum, drinking a glass of water, or eating sunflower seeds. Often the urge will go away after a few minutes.
- Ask your doctor about medications that help decrease withdrawal symptoms and cravings.

**Quit day**

- Get rid of all your tobacco products.
- Think of yourself as a nonsmoker.
- When you have a craving, do something else instead.
- Have small items to chew or suck on, such as chewing gum, hard candy, or toothpicks.

**Making it work**

- Symptoms of nicotine withdrawal and cravings may come and go; they are common and will go away.
- Physical activity helps. Do something you enjoy—walking, dancing, sports.
- Remember why you want to quit smoking and write it down. Look at the reasons every day.
- Plan ahead when you are about to be in a trigger situation—use the alternatives you came up with to deal with triggers.
- Save up the money you would have spent on tobacco products. Treat yourself with the money you've saved up.
- Tell your friends and family how you're doing. They can help you through the tough and the good times.
- If you do smoke a cigarette, don't get discouraged. Most former smokers tried to quit a number of times before successfully quitting. Start over and congratulate yourself for keeping at it.

Ammerman S. Helping kids kick butts. *Contemp Pediatr.* 1998;15:71.

can occur, so it is helpful to assess a patient's mood prior to and during the quitting process. If depression does occur, brief counseling can be helpful, and patients can be reassured that the depression will usually be transient.

Pediatricians should also provide tobacco cessation referrals for parents who use tobacco, explaining that use of pharmacotherapy, and referral for more extensive psychosocial and behavioral counseling as needed, can be very helpful. Providing a handout of available

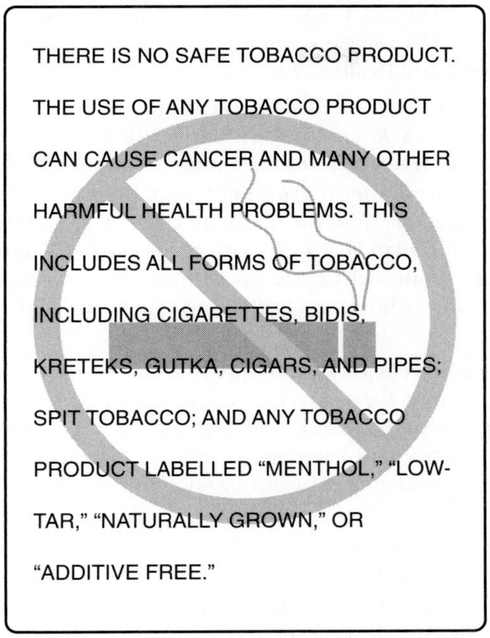

THERE IS NO SAFE TOBACCO PRODUCT.

THE USE OF ANY TOBACCO PRODUCT CAN CAUSE CANCER AND MANY OTHER HARMFUL HEALTH PROBLEMS. THIS INCLUDES ALL FORMS OF TOBACCO, INCLUDING CIGARETTES, BIDIS, KRETEKS, GUTKA, CIGARS, AND PIPES; SPIT TOBACCO; AND ANY TOBACCO PRODUCT LABELLED "MENTHOL," "LOW-TAR," "NATURALLY GROWN," OR "ADDITIVE FREE."

**FIGURE 173-1** Sample office poster.

doctors and community resources (eg, smoking cessation classes sponsored by the American Lung Association) is useful. Pediatricians should also explicitly encourage parents to maintain smoke-free homes, not only because of second- and thirdhand smoke exposure, but also because parents are role models for their children's behaviors.

Promoting a tobacco-free culture includes making tobacco-free office and clinic space environments. Toward this end try the following: make sure no office staff use tobacco products in front of any patients while on break; post "No Smoking" signs and posters (Figure 173-1) in all office areas; prominently display cessation materials and information in the waiting and examination rooms; eliminate all tobacco advertising from magazines in the waiting room; and take advantage of high-profile events such as the "Great American Smoke-Out," which is always the Thursday before Thanksgiving, and "World No-Tobacco Day," which is always May 31.

## ADVOCACY ISSUES

Advocacy efforts can significantly reduce the morbidity, mortality, and health care costs associated with tobacco use. There are a variety of efforts that have been shown to be effective. These include (1) increasing taxes on tobacco products; youth are particularly sensitive to the pricing of tobacco products, with an increase in the price of cigarettes by 10% leading to a 4% decrease in youth smoking; (2) banning advertising of tobacco products in all youth-oriented media (see Box 173-4, concerning the Smoke-Free Movies Campaign) and youth-frequented activities such as sporting events; (3) enforcing status laws (requiring identification) and banning cigarette vending machines; and (4) promoting adoption of clean indoor air laws and smoke-free facilities in such venues as schools, day care centers, office buildings, hotels, apartment buildings, casinos, restaurants, and bars. Additionally, the Food and Drug Administration now has regulatory oversight of nicotine as a drug; this will likely lead to changes in levels of nicotine allowed in tobacco products, as well as eliminating misleading advertising using words such as "light" or "low tar." On an international level, the WHO has sponsored a treaty on tobacco control, the International Framework Convention on Tobacco Control (www.who.int/fctc/en/). More than 90 countries have ratified the treaty, although the United States is not one of them. Advocating for the United States to join this international tobacco control effort would have worldwide significance.

## SUMMARY

Tobacco use remains a serious health problem among youth. Prevention and cessation efforts can have a significant impact on decreasing morbidity and mortality from tobacco use. Praising adolescents for nonuse of tobacco, and providing psychosocial support and pharmacotherapy as needed for tobacco users to aid in quitting can be helpful. It is important to educate patients that all tobacco products can cause serious disease, addiction, and death, and that there is no safe tobacco product. Advocacy efforts including higher tobacco taxes, smoke-free movies, clean indoor air laws, and smoke-free zones in youth-frequented areas, also play an important role in decreasing tobacco use.

## INTERNET RESOURCES

- Americans for Nonsmokers' Rights: www.no-smoke.org
- Campaign for Tobacco-Free Kids: www.tobaccofreekids.org (also with youth focus at tobaccofreekids.org/youthaction
- Action on Smoking and Health: www.ash.org

- The American Legacy Foundation: www.legacyforhealth.org (also with youth focus at www.thetruth.com)
- Smokefree.net: www.smokefree.net
- Centers for Disease Control and Prevention: www. cdc.gov/tobacco (also with youth focus at www. cdc.gov/tobacco/youth.htm)
- American Academy of Pediatrics: www.aap.org
- World Health Organization: tobacco.who.int
- American Cancer Society: www.cancer.org
- American Lung Association: www.lungusa.org/stop-smoking
- List of magazines that do not accept tobacco advertising: www.tobacco.org/Misc/tob_ad_mags.html
- Free pamphlets for download about ETS (English and Spanish): California Office of Environmental Health Hazard Assessment: www.oehha.ca.gov/air/environmental_tobacco/pdf/smoke2final.pdf (brochure in English); www.oehha.ca.gov/air/environmental_tobacco/pdf/smoke2final_span.pdf (brochure in Spanish)
- ETS Science Summary: California Environmental Protection Agency, Air Resources Board: "Proposed Identification of Environmental Tobacco Smoke as a Toxic Air Contaminant." www.arb.ca.gov/toxics/ets/finalreport/finalreport.htm
- Tobacco Free Initiative: WHO calls for enforceable policies to restrict smoking in movies: www.who.int/tobacco/smoke_free_movies/en/

## REFERENCES

1. WHO. Framework Convention on Tobacco Control. Available at: www.who.int/fctc/en/ Accessed May 30, 2009

2. US Department of Health and Human Services. *The Health Consequences of Smoking: Nicotine Addiction: A Report of the Surgeon General.* Atlanta, GA: US Department of Health and Human Services, Centers for Disease Control and Prevention, National Center for Chronic Disease Prevention and Health Promotion, Office on Smoking and Health; 1988

3. US Department of Health and Human Services. *Reducing the Health Consequences of Smoking: 25 Years of Progress. A Report of the Surgeon General.* US Department of Health and Human Services, Centers for Disease Control and Prevention, National Center for Chronic Disease Prevention and Health Promotion, Office on Smoking and Health. DHHS Publication No (CDC) 89-8411; 1989

4. US Department of Health and Human Services. *Youth and Tobacco: Preventing Tobacco Use among Young People.* Atlanta, GA: US Department of Health and Human Services, Centers for Disease Control and Prevention, National Center for Chronic Disease Prevention and Health Promotion, Office on Smoking and Health; 1994

5. US Department of Health and Human Services. *Tobacco Use among US Racial /Ethnic Minority Groups—African Americans, American Indians and Alaska Natives, Asian Americans and Pacific Islanders, and Hispanics: A Report of the Surgeon General.* Atlanta, GA: US Department of Health and Human Services, Centers for Disease Control and Prevention, National Center for Chronic Disease Prevention and Health Promotion, Office on Smoking and Health; 1998

6. US Department of Health and Human Services. *Reducing Tobacco Use: A Report of the Surgeon General.* Atlanta, GA: US Department of Health and Human Services, Centers for Disease Control and Prevention, National Center for Chronic Disease Prevention and Health Promotion, Office on Smoking and Health; 2000

7. US Department of Health and Human Services. *The Health Consequences of Smoking: A Report of the Surgeon General.* Atlanta, GA: US Department of Health and Human Services, Centers for Disease Control and Prevention, National Center for Chronic Disease Prevention and Health Promotion, Office on Smoking and Health; 2004

8. US Department of Health and Human Services. *The Health Consequences of Involuntary Exposure to Tobacco Smoke: A Report of the Surgeon General.* Atlanta, GA: US Department of Health and Human Services, Centers for Disease Control and Prevention, National Center for Chronic Disease Prevention and Health Promotion, Office on Smoking and Health; 2006

9. Matt GE, Quintana PJ, Hovell MF, et al. Households contaminated by environmental tobacco smoke: sources of infant exposures. *Tob Control.* 2004;13(1):29–37

10. Leistikow BN, Martin DC, Milano CE. Fire injuries, disasters, and costs from cigarettes and cigarette lights: a global overview. *Prev Med.* 2000;31:91

11. Centers for Disease Control and Prevention. Use of cigarettes and other tobacco products among students aged 13–15 years—worldwide, 1999–2005. *Morb Mortal Wkly Rep.* 2005;55:553

12. Centers for Disease Control and Prevention. High school students who tried to quit smoking cigarettes—United States, 2007. *Morb Mortal Wkly Rep.* 2009;58(16):428–431

13. Centers for Disease Control and Prevention. Youth Risk Behavior Surveillance—United States, 2007. *Morb Mortal Wkly Rep.* 2008;57(SS04):1–31

14. US Department of Health and Human Services. Risks associated with smoking cigarettes with low machine-measured yields of tar and nicotine. *Smoking and Tobacco Control Monograph 13.* Bethesda, MD: National Cancer Institute; 2001

15. American Lung Association. Tobacco policy project monograph: big tobacco on campus: ending the addiction. Available

at: www.lungusa.org/stop-smoking/tobacco-control-advocacy/reports-resources/tobacco-policy-trend-reports/college-report.pdf. Accessed May 28, 2009

16. Farrelly MC, Davis KC, Haviland ML, et al. Evidence of a dose-response relationship between "truth" antismoking ads and youth smoking prevalence. *Am J Pub Health.* 2005;95(3):425

17. Centers for Disease Control and Prevention. Strategies for reducing exposure to environmental tobacco smoke, increasing tobacco use cessation, and reducing initiation in communities and health care systems: a report on the recommendations of the Task Force on Community Preventive Services. *Morb Mortal Wkly Rep.* 2000;47(suppl):RR-12

18. Pizacani BA, Dent CW, Maher JE, et al. Smoking patterns in Oregon youth: effects of funding and defunding of a comprehensive state tobacco control program. *J Adolesc Health.* 2009;44(3)229–236

19. Dalton DA, Sargent JD, Beach ML, et al. Effect of viewing smoking in movies on adolescent smoking initiation: a cohort study. *Lancet.* 2003;362(9380):281

20. Glantz G, Kacirk K, McCulloch C. Back to the future: smoking in movies in 2002 compared with 1950 levels. *Am J Pub Health.* 2004;94(2):261

21. Sargent JD, Stoolmiller M, Worth KA, et al. Exposure to smoking depictions in movies: its association with established adolescent smoking. *Arch Pediatr Adolesc Med.* 2007;161(9):849–856

22. Sargent JD, Gibson J, Heatherton TF. Comparing the effects of entertainment media and tobacco marketing on youth smoking. *Tob Control.* 2009

23. Titus K, Polansky JR, Glantz S. Smoking presentation trends in US movies, 1991–2008. Center for Tobacco Control Research and Education. Tobacco Control Policy Making: United States. *Paper Movies* 2008. San Francisco: University of California, 2009. Available at: repositories.cdlib.org/ctcre/tcpmus/Movies2008. Accessed May 30, 2009

24. Massachusetts Department of Public Health. Change in nicotine yields 1998–2004. Available at: www.mass.gov/Eeohhs2/docs/dph/tobacco_control/nicotine_yields_1998_2004_report.pdf. Accessed June 22, 2009

25. Becklake MR, Ghezzo H, Ernst P. Childhood predictors of smoking in adolescence: a follow-up study of Montreal children. *CMAJ.* 2005;173(4):377

26. Bush T. Preteen attitudes about smoking and parental factors associated with favorable attitudes. *Am J Health Prom.* 2005;19:410

27. DiFranza JR, Savageau JA, Rigotta NA, et al. Development of symptoms of tobacco dependence in youths: 30-month follow-up data from the DANDY study. *Tob Control.* 2002;11:228

28. Killen J, Ammerman S, Rojas N, et al. Do adolescent smokers experience withdrawal when deprived of nicotine? *Exp Clin Psychopharmacol.* 2001;9(2):176

29. Remafedi G, Carol H. Preventing tobacco use among lesbian, gay, bisexual, and transgender youth. *Nicotine Tob Res.* 2005;7(2):249

30. Ammerman SD, Nolden M. Neighborhood-based tobacco advertising targeting adolescents. *West J Med.* 1995;162:514

31. DiFranza JR, Wellman RJ, Sargent D, et al. Tobacco promotion and the initiation of tobacco use: assessing the evidence for casualty. *Pediatrics.* 2006;117(6):e1237

32. Centers for Disease Control and Prevention. Cigarette brand preferences among middle and high school students who are established smokers, 2004 and 2006. *Morb Mortal Wkly Rep.* 2009;58(5):112–115

33. Pletcher MJ, Hulley BJ, Houston T, Kiefe CI, Benowitz N, Sidney S. Menthol cigarettes, smoking cessation, atherosclerosis, and pulmonary function: the coronary artery risk development in young adults (CARDIA) study. *Arch Intern Med.* 2006;166:1915–1922

34. Flay BR. School-based smoking prevention programs with the promise of long-term effects. *Tob Induc Dis.* 2009;5(1):6

35. Flay BR. The promise of long-term effectiveness of school-based smoking prevention programs: a critical review of reviews. *Tob Induc Dis.* 2009;5(1):7

36. Wiehe SE, Garrison MM, Christakis DA, Ebel BE, Rivara FP. A systematic review of school-based smoking prevention trials with long-term follow-up. *J Adolesc Health.* 2005;36(3):162–169

37. Ammerman SD. Helping kids kick butts. *Contemp Pediatr.* 1998;15(2):64

38. Colby SM, Monti PM, O'Leary TT, et al. Brief motivational intervention for adolescents in medical settings. *Addict Behav.* 2005;30(5):865

39. Grimshaw GM, Stanton A. Tobacco cessation interventions for young people. *Cochrane Database Syst Rev.* Oct 18, 2006;(4):CD003289

40. Nides M, Oncken C, Gonzales D, et al. Smoking cessation with varenicline, a selective alpha4beta2 nicotinic receptor partial agonist: results from a 7-week, randomized, placebo- and bupropion-controlled trial with 1-year follow-up. *Arch Intern Med.* 2006;166(15):1561

41. Hurt RD, Croghan GA, Beede SD, et al. Nicotine patch therapy in 101 adolescent smokers: efficacy, withdrawal symptom relief, and carbon monoxide and plasma cotinine levels. *Arch Pediatr Adolesc Med.* 2000;154:31

42. Killen JD, Robinson TN, Ammerman S, et al. Randomized clinical trial of the efficacy of bupropion combined with nicotine patch in the treatment of the adolescent smokers. *J Consult Clin Psychol.* 2004;72(4):729

43. Killen JD, Robinson TN, Ammerman S, et al. Major depression among adolescent smokers undergoing treatment for nicotine dependence. *Addict Beh.* 2004;29:1517

44. Rojas N, Killen JD, Haydel KF, et al. Nicotine dependence and withdrawal symptoms in adolescent smokers. *Arch Pediatr Adolesc Med.* 1998;152:151

45. Smith TA, House RF, Croghan IT, et al. Nicotine patch therapy in adolescent smokers. *Pediatrics.* 1996;98:659

46. Milton MH, Maule CO, Yee SI, et al. Youth tobacco cessation: a guide for making informed decision. Washington, DC: US Department of Health and Human Services, Centers for Disease Control and Prevention; 2004

47. Fiore MC, Jaen CR, Bailey TB, et al. A clinical practice guideline for treating tobacco use and dependence: 2008 update. A US public health service report. *Am J Prev Med.* 2008;35(2):158–176

# CHAPTER 174

## Alcohol

MEGAN A. MORENO, MD, MS Ed, MPH • PATRICIA K. KOKOTAILO, MD

### INTRODUCTION

Among adolescents in the United States, alcohol use is common and is not without consequences. The use of alcohol at an early age is associated with myriad of health risk behaviors, social problems, and future alcohol misuse.[1-3] The circumstances that contribute to adolescent alcohol use are complex and include psychosocial, environmental, genetic, and neurobiological factors.[4] Recent research has demonstrated that brain development continues into early adulthood and that alcohol consumption during adolescence can negatively affect this development. These findings highlight the importance of adolescent alcohol use as a serious health concern.[5,6] Adolescent providers should be comfortable with available screening tools and treatment strategies for adolescents regarding alcohol use.

### EPIDEMIOLOGY

Data on trends and current use of alcohol among US teenagers can be found in the annual Monitoring the Future Study, which is sponsored by the National Institute on Drug Abuse and implemented by the University of Michigan.[7] This study has consistently reported that alcohol is the drug most commonly used by youth, exceeding tobacco and all illicit drugs. The lifetime prevalence of alcohol use in 2008 is reported as 71.9% for students in 12th grade, 58.3% for those in 10th grade, and 38.9% for those in 8th grade. This means that by the middle of high school, most adolescents have tried alcohol. In addition, 54.7% of those in 12th grade reported "having been drunk," compared with 37.2% of those in 10th grade and 18% of those in 8th grade. For 12th graders, 43.1% reported having consumed alcohol in the past month, and 27.6% reported having been drunk in the past month. It is not surprising, therefore, that only 10% of 12th graders indicated that they considered having 1 or 2 drinks of an alcoholic beverage as an activity involving "great risk." Recent binge drinking, defined as the consumption of 5 or more drinks in a row on at least 1 occasion in the previous 2 weeks, was reported by 24.6% of 12th graders, 16.0% of 10th graders, and 8.1% of 8th graders. Binge drinking is a particular concern in the adolescent population given its association with risk behaviors and negative consequences, as described later in this chapter.

### DEFINITIONS

Adolescent alcohol use represents a spectrum from primary abstinence to alcohol dependence. Because the diagnostic criteria were developed and evaluated in adult populations, there are limitations when applying the definitions to adolescents.[8]

*DSM-IV* criteria for "alcohol misuse" may be a more useful concept applied to the adolescent population. This term encompasses alcohol use and dependence, as well as earlier stages of problem alcohol use that do not meet the other criteria. It may be a more useful concept clinically in pediatrics and when developing alcohol use prevention programs for youth.[8]

### RISK FACTORS

Risk factors for problem use of alcohol by adolescents are multifactorial. These include individual factors, such as genetics, neurobiology, development and related comorbidities; and environmental and social factors, such as family, peers, and media.

#### INDIVIDUAL FACTORS

Genetic influences on use and abuse of alcohol have been illustrated via twin studies. One study found that for adolescents, the magnitude of genetic influences was higher than environmental influences for problem alcohol or drug use.[9]

Adolescent brain development also plays a role in susceptibility to alcohol misuse. Studies have shown that brain development, particularly frontal lobe maturation via myelination, continues throughout adolescence into early adulthood.[10] The frontal lobes play a major role in functions such as response inhibition, emotional regulation, planning, and organization. The effects of alcohol on the developing adolescent brain are probably multiple. Given that brain processes surrounding inhibition, planning, and organization are not fully developed in adolescents, they may be more at risk for engaging in alcohol use at risky levels due to lack of inhibition or planning. Furthermore, the immaturity of the adolescent brain likely confers greater vulnerability to both the toxic and/or addictive actions of drugs, and drug use itself may directly affect brain development.[11]

Other individual-level risk factors for substance abuse include poor school performance, untreated attention-deficit/hyperactivity disorder (ADHD), and conduct disorder.[12] Psychiatric conditions most likely to co-occur with alcohol use disorders include mood disorders, anxiety disorders, ADHD, conduct disorders, bulimia nervosa, and schizophrenia.[13-16] Alcohol use disorders are also a risk factor for suicide attempts.[17]

### ENVIRONMENTAL AND SOCIAL FACTORS

Families play a critical role in the development of alcohol problems in youth by providing the primary environment in which norms and attitudes toward alcohol are developed. Parental drug use and permissive attitudes toward drug use predict greater risk of drugs and alcohol use in youth.[12]

Given the well-known influence of peers on adolescent behavior, it is not surprising that one of the strongest predictors of adolescent substance use is having peers who use alcohol or drugs. The community environment, including community socioeconomic status and racial composition, also contributes to variations in alcohol use among teens, even after controlling for individual factors.[18]

The media are another strong influence on adolescent norms, attitudes, and behaviors toward alcohol use. Research has consistently shown that adolescents are exposed to alcohol messages in a variety of media formats, including magazines, television, movies, music, and the Internet. These messages typically highlight social benefits of alcohol use and tend to underplay any risks or negative consequences. Studies have shown that media messages affect adolescents' attitudes toward alcohol use as favorable and can affect their intention to drink alcohol.[19,20]

## PHARMACOLOGY

Alcohol, like other drugs of abuse, increases the firing of ventral tegmental area dopamine neurons and subsequent dopamine release. Other ion channels and receptor systems within the brain have also been shown to be sensitive to alcohol. The challenge remains to identify which sites are important for specific electrophysiological and behavioral actions of alcohol.[4]

Acute effects of alcohol depend on the time course of drinking. During the initial period of up to 30 minutes after ingesting even small amounts of alcohol, there is typically mood elevation, followed by sedative and anxiolytic effects with increasing amounts of alcohol.[4]

## COMPLICATIONS OF ALCOHOL USE

### ACUTE EFFECTS

The acute complications most often seen in adolescents are consequences of how they use alcohol and the related risk behaviors they engage in while under the influence of alcohol.[4] When compared with use by adults, alcohol use by adolescents is much more likely to be episodic ("binge") and heavy, making their alcohol use particularly dangerous. Alcohol use is the primary contributor to the leading causes of adolescent mortality (ie, motor vehicle crashes, homicide, suicide) in the United States.[21] The research literature consistently reports the association of alcohol use or abuse with other risk-taking behaviors and morbidity in this population, including assault, sexual risk-taking, and other drug use.[13,22]

Physical complications following the acute consumption of large amounts of alcohol can include profound respiratory depression followed by coma and death. Although there can be wide variability between individuals, based on such factors as metabolism and body weight, a blood alcohol level of 0.2% to 0.3% will generally lead to stupor, 0.3% to 0.4% to coma, and 0.4% to 0.5% and above to death.

### ONGOING OR CHRONIC EFFECTS

Alcohol use in the early teenage years may have long-term consequences. Recent research supports the view that early adolescence is a potential "critical period" during which the direction of biopsychosocial development can be altered. Alcohol misuse and alcohol use disorders in adolescents are associated with long-term physical and mental health disorders.

The best known health complication of alcohol disorders is liver disease, but this is a late-stage complication not usually seen in teens. However, it is important to note that use of alcohol at an early age increases the risks of future alcohol use problems.[23] Evidence has shown that those who reported having their first alcoholic drink before age 14 or their first drug use before age 15 were 3 times more likely to develop alcohol or drug dependence, compared with those whose first use of these substances was at age 15 or older.[24] Associated physical health problems include sequelae of trauma, sleep disturbances, elevated serum liver enzyme levels, and dental and other oral abnormalities.[14]

Research on ways in which alcohol alters adolescent brain development suggests that adolescents with an alcohol use disorder use fewer learning strategies and have reduced memory skills, and that these continue to decline with ongoing alcohol use. Neuroimaging studies of patients with adolescent-onset alcohol use disorders have documented reduced hippocampal volumes and subtle white matter abnormalities.[25]

Social problems linked to teenage alcohol use may also continue beyond adolescence. By young adulthood, early alcohol use is associated with employment problems, other substance abuse, aggression, and criminal behavior.[26]

## ASSESSMENT

Adolescent health providers should help prevent, identify, and treat alcohol and other substance use by youth. Pursuing an effective treatment initially requires a recognition that the individual is in need of treatment.

### SCREENING

The American Academy of Pediatrics guidelines for the health care of children and adolescents recommend that pediatricians and adolescent providers discuss substance use as part of anticipatory guidance and preventive care for children and adolescents.[27] The American Medical Association Guidelines for Adolescent Preventive Services[28] and the Bright Futures guidelines[29] recommend that health care providers who work with adolescents conduct routine annual substance abuse screening of all adolescents and offer brief interventions as appropriate. It is also recommended that providers be familiar with community resources and be able to refer for the treatment of substance abuse.

Despite these recommendations and strong research to support them, many providers find universal screening of adolescents for substance use problems a challenging task. Health providers at all levels identify barriers to screening for adolescent substance abuse in primary care. These barriers include insufficient Time, lack of Training to manage a positive screen, the need to Triage other medical problems, lack of Treatment resources, a Tenacious parent who won't leave the examination room, and unfamiliarity with screening Tools ("the 6 Ts").[30]

Several screening surveys for adolescent substance use are available. Among these, the CRAFFT has emerged as a brief, validated, and easy-to-use verbal screening tool that has good discriminative properties for determining the presence of substance abuse disorders in this age group.[31] See Chapter 181, Office Management and Laboratory Testing, for more detail on the CRAFFT screening questions.

### CONFIDENTIALITY

When discussing substance use with adolescents, it is important to conduct discussions in a way that ensures patient confidentiality. An essential first step is to conduct discussions with the teen patient alone, asking any accompanying parent, friend, or partner to step out of the room. Informing the teen about the confidentiality of the information that he or she may share, as well as the limits to confidentiality, are essential steps prior to beginning any discussion of substance use. Knowledge of one's state laws regarding confidentiality and adolescent substance use assessment and treatment for adolescents is important.

## TREATMENT

### ACUTE

Adult treatment guidelines for acute alcohol overdose include use of flumazenil (a benzodiazepine antagonist) to reverse alcohol-related respiratory suppression.[4] Typically, this is administered in a highly supervised hospital setting. Severe withdrawal is unusual in adolescents and requires hospitalization.

### ONGOING OR CHRONIC CARE

Early treatments for adolescent alcohol misuse used adult treatments and applied them to teens without developmental modifications. Fortunately, progress has been made in treating adolescent alcohol use disorders with evidence-based modalities developed for the adolescent population. The current challenge lies in replication and wider implementation of these programs. These treatments can include interventions at the individual, family, and community level.

Treatments tailored to the individual adolescent include behavioral therapy, motivational interviewing (MI), and harm reduction. Behavioral therapy targets substance use in the context of the individual's environment. Approaches are based on classic and operant conditioning. These therapies focus on the identification of behaviors that promote substance use and teach skills to avoid or disrupt these behaviors. Essential elements of this approach include functional analysis, skills training, and relapse prevention. Cognitive behavioral therapy (CBT) extends behavioral therapy by integrating the impact of cognitive elements in addressing substance use.

Motivational interviewing is a technique used to enhance an individual's motivation to make changes regarding substance use and the life situations that may trigger or sustain substance use. This approach is often appealing to adolescent providers because adolescents are a population that is not typically seeking treatment, so teens may need to be motivated to engage in treatment. Primary tenets of the MI approach include empathetic nonjudgmental stance, reflective listening, developing discrepancy, rolling with resistance and avoiding arguments, and supporting self-efficacy for change. Research has shown that MI as a counseling style has been effective in decreasing alcohol use in both younger and older adolescents. A recent Cochrane Systematic Review of primary prevention for alcohol misuse in young people noted the poor quality of much research investigating the effectiveness of alcohol interventions, but remarked on the potential value of MI.[32]

A harm reduction strategy is often employed in drug education and treatment. This strategy recognizes the frequent chronic and relapsing nature of substance abuse and focuses on minimizing the potential hazards associated with use rather than the use itself. Harm reduction messages can often be considered as a stepped framework tailored to populations of increasing risk. For example, the messages of harm reduction may include warnings about the dangers of binge drinking to those at lowest risk and warnings about drinking while driving to those at higher risk.[33]

Family-based intervention remains the most investigated psychosocial treatment modality. Its approach is grounded in family systems theory, which posits that an individual's behavior is integrally related to his or her primary relational context, the family. In this approach, alcohol use is assessed and treated in the context of how a teen functions in the family, including communication patterns within the family and relationships to extended family and social systems.

Ongoing treatment can also involve helping an adolescent find a new environment and community that does not involve alcohol-using peers and lifestyle. This may involve tackling obstacles such as homelessness, educational exclusion, incarceration, and handling a negative home situation. Tailoring services to meet an adolescent's needs may include flexible meeting arrangements, home visits, text messages, telephone calls, and transportation assistance. Given the long-term effort involved in ongoing engagement of adolescents in treatment programs, a final key strategy is to work with other networks designed to assist in the longer-term strain. These may include education, social work, criminal justice, nongovernmental organizations, and health and mental health agencies.

## RECOMMENDATIONS FOR PROVIDERS

Many opportunities exist for health providers to be effective in the prevention, assessment, and treatment of adolescent alcohol use. The following list includes strategies to employ at the patient, family, community, and individual provider levels. We encourage providers to adopt as many of these as are feasible to help improve the care of adolescents regarding alcohol use.

### INDIVIDUAL PATIENTS

- Provide information regarding the dangers of alcohol and other substance use with patients and families during clinic/office visits, including but not limited to health maintenance visits.
- Recognize risk factors for alcohol and other substance use among youth and be aware of coexisting health problems, such as depression, that may occur in teens.
- Regularly screen for adolescent substance use, using nonjudgmental validated screening methods and appropriate attention to confidentiality.
- Offer brief intervention and referral to treatment as appropriate.
- Continue to support patients with substance use disorders both during and following their treatment.

### FAMILIES

- Obtain a complete family medical and social history to explore potential genetic and family influences regarding alcohol and other substance use.
- Encourage parents to be good role models for healthy life choices and discourage parents from allowing any underage drinking in their home or on their property.

### COMMUNITY

- Know appropriate guidelines regarding adolescent confidentiality in your state.
- Know appropriate referring agencies for adolescent substance use in your community.
- Participate in school and other community alcohol abuse prevention programs.
- Participate in advocacy efforts to promote appropriate media modeling of alcohol.
- Participate in advocacy efforts to promote legislation; examples include but are not limited to

- Graduated driver's licensing that reduces alcohol-related morbidity and mortality.
- Treatment parity from third-party payers.
- Legal ramifications for parents sponsoring teen drinking.

- Support further research into prevention, evidence-based screening and identification, brief intervention, management, and treatment of alcohol and other substance use by adolescents.

**PROVIDER**

- Complete substance abuse training during residency or via continuing medical education.

## INTERNET RESOURCES

- Al-Anon/Alateen: For adolescents with problem alcohol use and those who have parents with problem alcohol use: www.al-anon.alateen.org
- US Department of Health and Human Services and SAMHSA's National Clearinghouse for Alcohol and Drug Information: ncadi.samhsa.gov
- National Institute on Alcohol Abuse and Alcoholism: Resources for parents, clinicians, and researchers: www.niaaa.nih.gov
- American Academy of Pediatrics Children's Health Topics: Substance Abuse: Parents page regarding substance use: www.aap.org/health-topics/subabuse.cfm
- Erowid: Although not affiliated with an official medical group, this site is frequently referenced by patients and families: www.erowid.org

## REFERENCES

1. Grant BF, Stinson FS, Harford TC. Age at onset of alcohol use and DSM-IV alcohol abuse and dependence: a 12-year follow-up. *J Subst Abuse.* 2001;13(4):493–504

2. DeWit DJ, Adlaf EM, Offord DR, Ogborne AC. Age at first alcohol use: a risk factor for the development of alcohol disorders. *Am J Psychiatry.* 2000;157(5):745–750

3. Stueve A, O'Donnell LN. Early alcohol initiation and subsequent sexual and alcohol risk behaviors among urban youths. *Am J Public Health.* 2005;95(5):887–893

4. Ruiz P, Strain EC, Langrod JG. *The Substance Abuse Handbook*. Philadelphia: Lippincott Williams & Wilkins; 2007

5. Chambers RA, Taylor JR, Potenza MN. Developmental neurocircuitry of motivation in adolescence: a critical period of addiction vulnerability. *Am J Psychiatry.* 2003;160(6):1041–1052

6. Giedd JN. The teen brain: insights from neuroimaging. *J Adolesc Health.* 2008;42(4):335–343

7. Johnston LD, O'Malley PM, Bachman JG, Schulenberg JE. 2009. *Monitoring the Future national results on adolescent drug use: Overview of key findings, 2008* (NIH Publication No. 09-7401). Bethesda, MD: National Institute on Drug Abuse

8. American Academy of Pediatrics, Committee on Substance Abuse. Policy statement: Alcohol use by youth and adolescents: A pediatric concern. *Pediatrics*. 2010;125:1078-1087

9. Rhee SH, et al. Genetic and environmental influences on substance initiation, use, and problem use in adolescents. *Arch Gen Psychiatry.* 2003;60(12):1256–1264

10. Sowell ER, et al. In vivo evidence for post-adolescent brain maturation in frontal and striatal regions. *Nat Neurosci.* 1999;2(10):859–861

11. Casey BJ, Jones RM, Hare TA. The adolescent brain. *Ann NY Acad Sci.* 2008;1124:111–126

12. Hawkins JD. Risk and protective factors and their implications for preventive interventions for the health care professional. In: American Academy of Pediatrics, ed. *Substance Abuse: A Guide for Health Professionals*. Elk Grove Village, IL: American Academy of Pediatrics; 2001

13. Simkin D. Adolescent substance use disorders and comorbidity. In: Rogers PD, Heyman RB, eds. *Addiction Medicine: Adolescent Substance Use.* 2002:463–477

14. Clark DB, et al. Health problems in adolescents with alcohol use disorders: self-report, liver injury, and physical examination findings and correlates. *Alcohol Clin Exp Res.* 2001;25(9):1350–1359

15. Arria AM, et al. Self-reported health problems and physical symptomatology in adolescent alcohol abusers. *J Adolesc Health.* 1995;16(3):226–231

16. Vitale S, van deMheen D. Illicit drug use and injuries: a review of emergency room studies. *Drug Alcohol Depend.* 2006;82(1):1–9

17. Windle M. Suicidal behaviors and alcohol use among adolescents: a developmental psychopathology perspective. *Alcohol Clin Exp Res.* 2004;28(5 suppl):29S–37S

18. Song EY, et al. Selected community characteristics and underage drinking. *Subst Use Misuse.* 2009;44(2):179–194

19. American Academy of Pediatrics, Committee on Communications. Policy statement: Children, adolescents, and advertising. *Pediatrics.* 2006;118(6):2563–2569

20. Robinson TN, Chen HL, Killen JD. Television and music video exposure and risk of adolescent alcohol use. *Pediatrics.* 1998;102(5):E54

21. National Institute on Alcohol Abuse and Alcoholism (NIAAA). Underage drinking: a major public health challenge. *Alcohol Alert.* 2003;59. Available at: pubs.niaaa.nih.gov/publications/aa59.htm. Accessed April 25, 2010

22. Clark DB. The natural history of adolescent alcohol use disorders. *Addiction.* 2004;99(Suppl 2):5–22

23. Grant BF, Dawson DA. Age at onset of alcohol use and its association with DSM-IV alcohol abuse and dependence: results from the National Longitudinal Alcohol Epidemiologic Survey. *J Subst Abuse.* 1997;9:103–110

24. Hingson RW, Heeren T, Winter MR. Age at drinking onset and alcohol dependence: age at onset, duration, and severity. *Arch Pediatr Adolesc Med.* 2006;160(7):739–746

25. Brown SA, Tapert SF. Adolescence and the trajectory of alcohol use: basic to clinical studies. *Ann NY Acad Sci.* 2004; 1021:234–244

26. Ellickson PL, Tucker JS, Klein DJ. Ten-year prospective study of public health problems associated with early drinking. *Pediatrics.* 2003;111(5 pt 1):949–955

27. Kulig JW. Tobacco, alcohol, and other drugs: the role of the pediatrician in prevention, identification, and management of substance abuse. *Pediatrics.* 2005;115(3): 816–821

28. Elster A, Kuznets N. *AMA Guidelines for Adolescent Preventive Services (GAPS).* Baltimore, MD: Williams & Wilkins; 1994

29. Hagan JF, Shaw JS, Duncan P. *Bright Futures: Guidelines for Health Supervision of Infants, Children, and Adolescents.* 3rd ed. Elk Grove Village, IL: American Academy of Pediatrics; 2007

30. Van Hook S, et al. The "six T's": barriers to screening teens for substance abuse in primary care. *J Adolesc Health.* 2007; 40(5):456–461

31. Knight JR, et al. A new brief screen for adolescent substance abuse. *Arch Pediatr Adolesc Med.* 1999;153(6):591–596

32. Foxcroft DR, et al. Longer-term primary prevention for alcohol misuse in young people: a systematic review. *Cochrane Database Syst Rev.* 2002

33. Bonomo YA, Bowes G. Putting harm reduction into an adolescent context. *J Paediatr Child Health.* 2001;37(1): 5–8

# CHAPTER 175

# Marijuana

ALAIN JOFFE, MD, MPH

## EPIDEMIOLOGY AND PHARMACOLOGY

Use of marijuana by adolescents has declined steadily over the last decade; still, it is the illicit drug most often used by this age group. In the 2008 Monitoring the Future Survey,[1] 10.9% of 8th graders, 23.9% of 10th graders, and 32.4% of 12th graders reported using marijuana or hashish in the past year, and 5.8%, 13.8%, and 19.4% of 8th, 10th, and 12th graders, respectively, reported use in the last 30 days.[1] Previous research has shown that marijuana use among adolescents is most strongly linked to their perception of the risk associated with its use and not to its perceived availability (Figure 175-1).[2] As perception of risk increases, prevalence of use falls, only to rise again if perception of risk decreases. Advances in our understanding of the ongoing development of the adolescent brain and how marijuana affects the brain, coupled with new data derived from longitudinal studies of marijuana users, have helped to better define the risks associated with use of this illicit substance.

Marijuana is obtained from the dried flowering tops and leaves of the hemp plant, with Δ-9 tetrahydrocannabinol (THC) being its most psychoactive molecule (Figure 175-2). The concentration of THC varies according to the part of the plant that is used, ranging from 0.5% to 5% in leaves and stems to 7% to 14% in

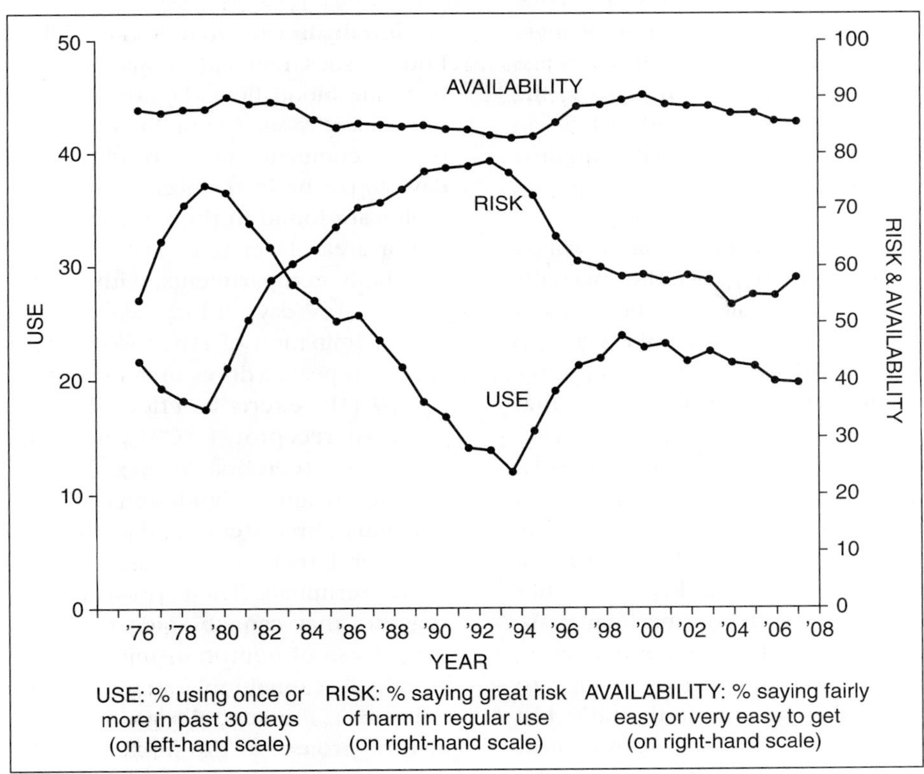


**FIGURE 175-1** Marijuana: Trends in perceived availability, perceived risk of regular use, and prevalence of use in past 30 days for 12th graders. (From Johnston LD, O'Malley PM, Bachman JG, Schulenberg JE (2009). *Monitoring the Future National Survey Results on Drug Use, 1975–2008: Volume 1, Secondary School Students* (NIH Publication No. 09-7402). Bethesda, MD: National Institute on Drug Abuse, 382. The Monitoring the Future Study, the University of Michigan.)

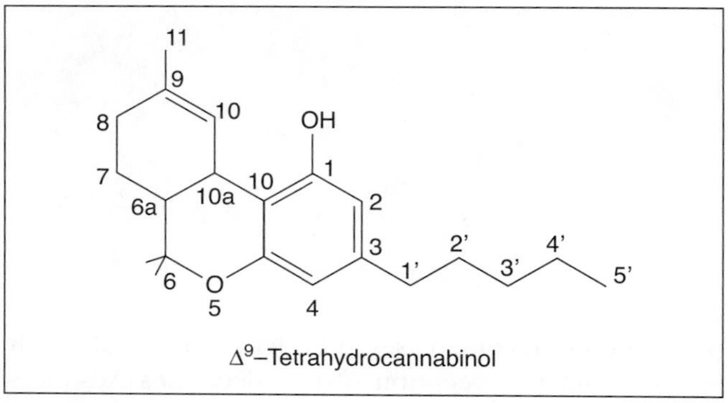

$\Delta^9$–Tetrahydrocannabinol

**FIGURE 175-2** Δ-9 THC, the active product in marijuana. (Reprinted with permission from Ameri A. The effects of cannabinoids on the brain. *Prog Neurobiol* 1999;58:315–348.)

the flowering tops of unfertilized female plants.[3] Resin secreted by the female plant or mixed with compressed flowers (hashish) has a THC concentration of 2% to 8%; if an organic solvent is used further to extract THC from hashish, the resulting hashish oil can reach THC concentrations of 15% to 50%. There is disagreement about whether selective breeding of plants and improved growing methods have increased the potency of marijuana available today compared with 20 to 30 years ago (THC concentrations from confiscated marijuana in the United States did increase from 2% in 1980 to 8.5% in 2006), in part because there is no consistent sampling method and trends in THC concentrations vary among countries.[4,5]

Most marijuana is smoked, either as joints (rolled in cigarette papers) or as blunts (cigars either partially or completely hollowed out). It can also be smoked in pipes or in devices that filter the smoke through water (bongs). Because THC is not water soluble, using bongs does not decrease the THC content that reaches the lungs; in fact, the amount of THC being absorbed may be increased as the amount of side-stream smoke is decreased and the cooled smoke can be held longer in the lungs, allowing greater absorption. Approximately one-half of the THC is absorbed when the user inhales deeply and holds his or her breath. With smoking, the effects of marijuana are noticeable in seconds, with the full effects occurring in 15 to 30 minutes and then tapering off over 2 to 3 hours. Marijuana can also be ingested orally but first pass metabolism through the liver delays onset of action (with blood concentrations being only one-third of those achieved through smoking); however, the resulting slow, sustained absorption prolongs the effects on the user. Concomitant alcohol use enhances the absorption of THC.

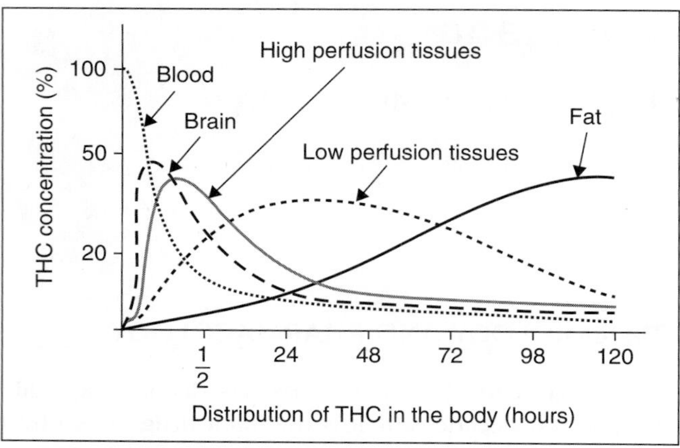


**FIGURE 175-3** Distribution of THC in the body. The distribution of THC after a single administration in plasma and body tissues. Note the "biphasic" disappearance in plasma. The rapid phase (in minutes) indicates a rapid uptake of the drug by fat-containing tissues. The slow phase (in days) shows the release of THC by these tissues (Nahas, 1975). THC, tetrahydrocannabinol. (Reprinted with permission from Ashton CH. Pharmacology and effects of cannabis: a brief review. *Br J Psych* 2001;175:104.)

Tetrahydrocannabinol is rapidly distributed to all body tissues; concentrations are generally proportional to tissue blood flow (Figure 175-3).[4] The major exception is fatty tissue (including the brain): THC is lipophilic so it accumulates in fat, reaching peak levels in 4 to 5 days. In the brain, the greatest concentrations of cannabinoids are found in the neocortical, limbic, sensory, and motor areas. Over time, THC is gradually released back into body compartments, with the tissue half-life being about 5 to 7 days. It may take almost a month for complete elimination of THC following a single dose. Exposure to repeated doses increases tissue concentrations.

Δ-9 THC exerts its effects by interacting with cannabinoid receptor 1 (CB1) in peripheral nerves and the brain (cerebral cortex, limbic area [including the hippocampus and amygdala], the basal ganglia, thalamus, brainstem, and cerebellum). Cannabinoid receptor 1 receptors are located mainly on axons and nerve terminals. Their presynaptic location strongly suggests that cannabinoids play a role in controlling the release of neurotransmitters from axon terminals.[6] Tetrahydrocannabinol stimulates dopamine-releasing neurons in the ventral tegmental area of the brain that in turn project to the nucleus accumbens. This effect is blocked by naloxone.[7,8] Characterization of the CB1 receptors led to the discovery of the endogenous cannabinoids, including anandamide (arachidonoyl ethanolamide) and 2-arachidonoyl glycerol (Figure 175-4). Tetrahydrocannabinol also reacts with cannabinoid

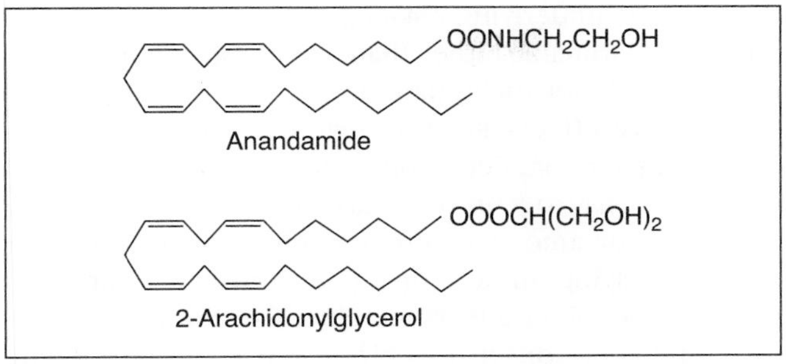

$OONHCH_2CH_2OH$

Anandamide

$OOOCH(CH_2OH)_2$

2-Arachidonylglycerol

**FIGURE 175-4** The endogenous cannabinoids, anandamide, and 2-arachidonylglycerol. (Reprinted with permission from Ameri A. The effects of cannabinoids on the brain. *Prog Neurobiol* 1999;58:315–348.)

receptor 2 (CB2) in splenic macrophages and other immune system cells. Endogenous cannabinoids bind to CB receptors for a shorter period of time and are less potent than Δ-9 THC.

Animal studies have shown that THC acts at the same μ1 G protein coupled receptors as do other drugs of abuse such as opioids (heroin), cocaine, amphetamines, hallucinogens, and phencyclidine.[9] Stimulation of these receptors releases dopamine from the prefrontal cortex and the shell of the nucleus accumbens and by retrograde messenger in the ventral tegmental area. These latter 2 areas are part of the brain's "reward system" involved in the reinforcing properties associated with use of these drugs. Cocaine, nicotine, and amphetamine also produce their reinforcing effects through increasing dopamine levels in the shell of this area. Marijuana use during adolescence may induce permanent changes in these receptors and neurons. In a rat model, dopaminergic neurons of adolescent, but not adult, rats exposed to marijuana developed a cross-tolerance to morphine, cocaine, and amphetamine.[10]

SR141716 A, a synthetic CB1 receptor antagonist, blocks the action of THC in mice and can be used to precipitate withdrawal symptoms (Figure 175-5). In contrast, WIN55,212-2, a CB1 agonist, can be used to mimic the effects of THC (Figure 175-6). Studies in rats demonstrate that chronic exposure to Δ-9 THC produces time-dependent downregulation and desensitization of cannabinoid receptors in the brain. This phenomenon would help provide a physiologic basis for "tolerance," the observation that experienced smokers need to smoke more marijuana to achieve the same effects.[11]

## ACUTE EFFECTS

The acute effects of marijuana are generally pleasurable. Users describe feeling euphoric or "high" as well as feeling less anxious and less depressed; there is

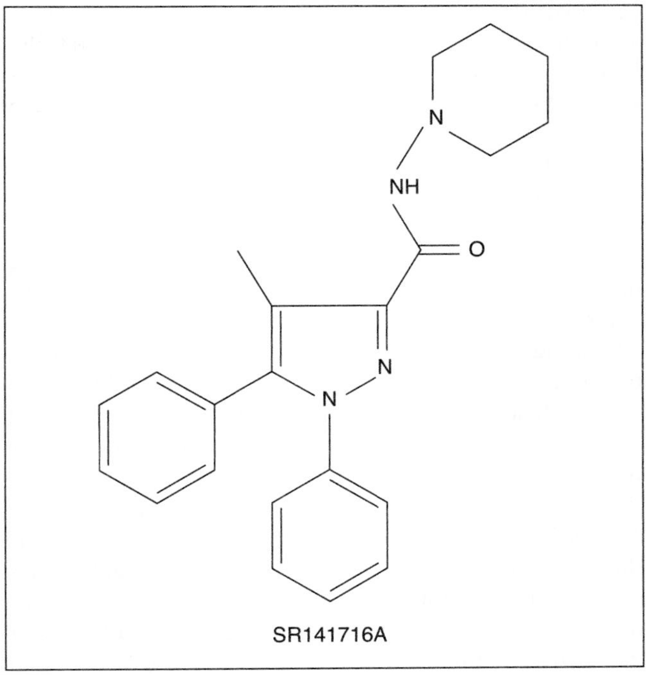

N

NH

O

N

N

SR141716A

**FIGURE 175-5** The potent synthetic CB1 receptor antagonist, SR14176 A. (Reprinted with permission from Ameri A. The effects of cannabinoids on the brain. *Prog Neurobiol* 1999;58:315–348.)

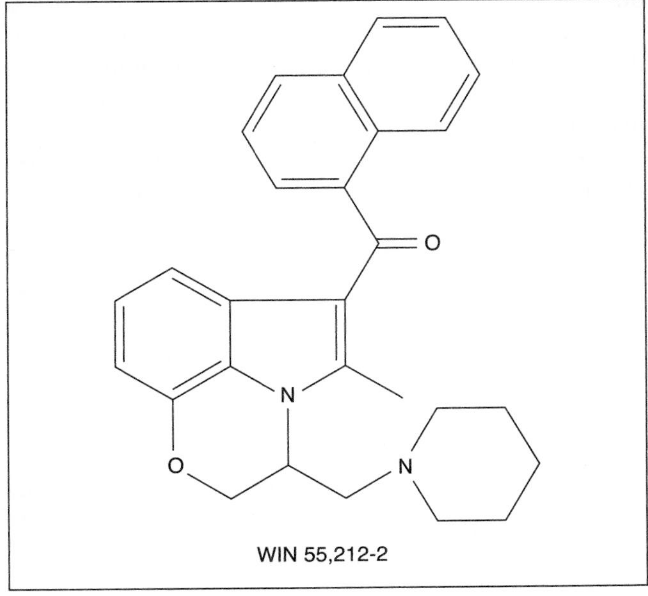


**FIGURE 175-6** The synthetic CB1 agonist WIN 55,212-2. (Reprinted with permission from Ameri A. The effects of cannabinoids on the brain. *Prog Neurobiol* 1999;58:315–348.)

some overlap with the "tipsy" feeling one experiences after drinking alcohol. As does alcohol, marijuana also increases feelings of sociability. Users claim that music sounds better and that colors are brighter, more visually appealing, and more vivid; time also seems to pass more quickly. Physiologically, heart rate and cardiac output are increased and blood pressure goes up. Initially, bronchoconstriction occurs but is soon followed by bronchodilation; there is also conjunctival injection and a feeling of dry mouth. Users also report increased appetite (the "munchies").

Marijuana also acutely affects cognitive and psychomotor performance. Short-term memory, the ability to sustain or divide one's attention, complex decision making, and the ability to concentrate are all reduced, even at relatively low doses. Reaction time and motor coordination are both negatively affected. These negative effects are particularly worrisome when considered within the context of adolescent driving. Several studies have shown that smoking marijuana affects driving performance to a degree comparable to that seen with alcohol use. However, unlike alcohol, marijuana's negative effects on driving performance can be objectively measured for up to 24 hours, even though the adolescent may feel completely normal. Used together, alcohol and marijuana cause far more impairment than either used alone.[12,13]

In many countries, marijuana is the second most commonly detected drug after alcohol in drivers involved in fatal car crashes; however, many jurisdictions do not test for marijuana routinely. Many of these drivers either do not have alcohol in their bloodstream or have blood alcohol concentrations below the legal limit for impaired driving. Although the known psychomotor impairments associated with marijuana use and the detection of marijuana in the blood of many drivers involved in fatal car crashes suggests a direct link between marijuana use and motor vehicle accidents,[14,15] one study[16] suggests that it is the underlying risk-taking tendencies of drivers who use marijuana, rather than the marijuana itself, that is responsible for the apparent relationship.

Negative effects, such as severe anxiety or feelings of panic, paranoia, depersonalization, derealization, and dysphoria, may occur with casual use; typically, these effects occur among first-time users or among people with underlying anxiety or among those who are otherwise psychologically vulnerable. Psychotic reactions, including acute onset of schizophrenia, can also occur; true hallucinations may occur at high doses.

## DEPENDENCE AND WITHDRAWAL

Overall, about 8% to 9% of adolescents who ever use marijuana will meet criteria for dependence within 10 years of first use; most cases occur in youth between 15 and 25 years of age.[17] Approximately one-fifth of adolescents who use marijuana more than 5 times will become daily users and another 10% to 20% will use almost every day. One-third of those who use almost every day or daily meet diagnostic criteria for dependence. Marijuana is the primary substance of abuse for adolescents who are admitted to drug treatment facilities (Figure 175-7),[18] and the prevalence of marijuana use disorders in the United States increased by 25% over the decade from 1991–1992 to 2001–2002.[19] The higher potency of today's marijuana may also increase the risk for development of dependence. Adolescents can develop dependence while using marijuana at lower doses and less frequently compared with adults.[7]

Because THC stored in fatty tissues gradually escapes into the bloodstream as an individual ceases smoking marijuana, demonstration of withdrawal has been difficult. However, a marijuana withdrawal syndrome has been clearly demonstrated in humans, with typical

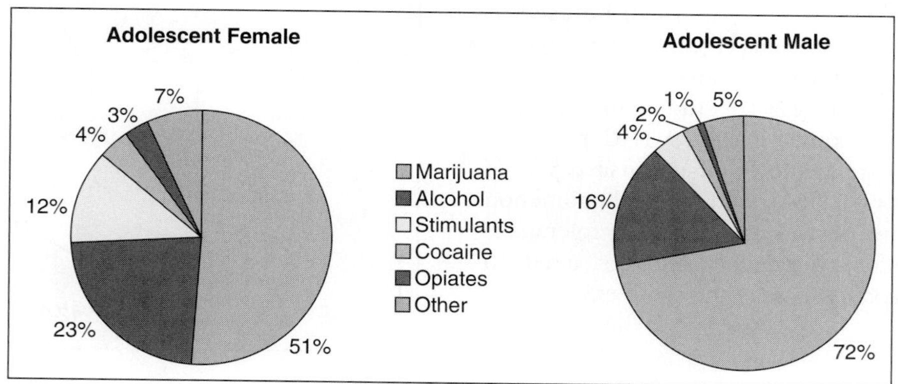


**FIGURE 175-7** Adolescent treatment admissions by gender: 2005. (From: Office of Applied Studies, Substance Abuse and Mental Health Services Administration. The DASIS Report. 2007. Available at: www.oas.samhsa.gov/2k7/youthTX/youthTX.pdf. Accessed November 1, 2009. 2005 SAMHSA Treatment Episode Data Set.)

symptoms including insomnia, irritability, depression, decreased appetite, tremor, and physical tension.[20] Withdrawal symptoms generally appear after about 24 hours of nonuse, peak at 3 days, and disappear by 7 to 10 days. In mice, administration of the cannabinoid receptor antagonist SR141716 A produces an acute withdrawal syndrome. These mice also display elevated levels of corticotropin-releasing factor; peak levels of this stress hormone correlate with peak withdrawal symptoms. A similar hormonal response is viewed during withdrawal from other drugs.[21]

## LONG-TERM EFFECTS

### MENTAL HEALTH PROBLEMS

Two retrospective cohort studies have demonstrated that cannabis users report more psychotic symptoms and have higher rates of diagnosed psychosis (including schizophrenia) than those who have never used marijuana. In a 15-year follow-up of almost 50,000 Swedish army conscripts, the risk of developing schizophrenia was 6 times greater among those who had used at least 50 times in their lives compared to nonusers. The results persisted even after controlling for other psychiatric illnesses and social background.[22] A more comprehensive reanalysis of these data, combined with a longer follow-up period, confirmed these findings. The reanalysis showed a dose–response relationship, even after controlling for other drug use and excluding subjects who developed schizophrenia within 5 years of conscription (prodromal cases).[23]

Numerous longitudinal studies highlight the association between cannabis use and subsequent development of mental health problems among adolescents. In general, the risk is directly proportional to frequency of use and is highest for adolescents who begin using before age 16 (even after controlling for frequency of use). Analysis of data from the Dunedin multidisciplinary health and development study (1,057 individuals followed from birth to age 26) showed that those who used cannabis by age 15 were significantly more likely to display schizophrenia symptoms than control subjects (those who never used or used only once or twice), even after controlling for psychotic symptoms at age 11 and other drug use at age 15 to 18.[24] A longitudinal study of Australian students showed that female (but not male) teenagers who ever used marijuana at least weekly were more likely to report depression or anxiety 7 years later than those who used less than weekly, even after controlling for such variables as prior depression or anxiety and alcohol use.[25] In a birth cohort of 1,265 New Zealand children followed for 21 years, cannabis use was related to depression, suicidal ideation, suicide attempts, and participation in violent crimes. These effects held true for both males and females, with the effect being greatest for those using marijuana by age 14 to 15.[26] Even though these studies attempt to control for a wide variety of potential confounders and use sophisticated statistical analyses, there remains the concern that associations between cannabis use and adverse psychological outcomes are due to some unmeasured construct related to both (residual confounding). The interested reader is directed to 2 recent review articles that address this issue.[27,28]

### SCHOOL DROPOUT

Two longitudinal studies, 1 in the United States and 1 in Australia, explored the effect of marijuana use on school dropout. In the US study of almost 1,400 students, ever users of marijuana were twice as likely to leave school as were never users, controlling for race, gender, parental education, number of parents in the home, youth report of grades, and other drug use.[29] In an Australian study, 1,600 students were followed from age 15 to age 21. Students who used marijuana weekly at age 14 to 15 were more than 5 times as likely to drop out of school than students who used marijuana less often; marijuana use after age 15 was not related to school dropout. Again, the study controlled for such important baseline characteristics as place of birth, parental separation or divorce, parental education, students' alcohol and tobacco use, antisocial behavior, and psychiatric morbidity.[30]

### MARIJUANA AND OTHER DRUG USE

A longitudinal study in New Zealand, controlling for a broad range of potential confounders (including markers of deviant behavior), found a significant dose–response relationship between frequency of marijuana use and other drug use. Compared to never users, those who used 1 to 2 times were almost 3 times as likely to use other drugs. Those who used between 12 and 49 times were 21 times as likely to use other drugs, and those who used 50 times or more were almost 60 times as likely to use other drugs. Additional work from this study showed that use at 14 to 15 years of age was critical, with those using less than monthly at 14 to 15 years of age being 6 times as likely and those using at least monthly at 14 to 15 years of age being 38 times as likely to use other drugs compared to never users.[31]

Marijuana users may be more likely to use other drugs compared to nonusers because they are both more likely to have the opportunity to try other drugs and to use them if offered. A study of more than 26,000 12- to 18-year-olds showed a clear progression in drug use. Alcohol and tobacco users (compared to nonusers) were significantly more likely to have an opportunity to try marijuana and were significantly more likely to start using marijuana if offered. In turn, marijuana users were more likely to have an opportunity to try cocaine than nonusers and were also more likely to try cocaine than nonusers if offered. These associations held true even if one excluded individuals who started using a drug within a year of having the opportunity to do so.[32]

## ORGAN SYSTEM EFFECTS

### ENDOCRINE

Δ-9 THC acts either directly or indirectly at the hypothalamus, mediated by CB1 receptors located there. Secretion of gonadotropins from the pituitary gland is inhibited. It may also act at CB1 receptors located in the testes and ovaries. Δ-9 THC inhibits binding of dihydrotestosterone to androgen receptors, and a noncannabinoid component of Δ-9 THC may bind to estrogen receptors. Chronic marijuana use disrupts the hypothalamic-pituitary-gonadal axis but the effect weakens with time, likely due to downregulation of the CB1 receptors. In men, chronic marijuana use causes a dose-related but reversible drop in sperm count and an increase in abnormal sperm forms; in women, chronic use may lead to anovulatory cycles and a shortened luteal phase. Marijuana use may also impair cortisol and growth hormone secretion, but the clinical implication of these findings is unknown.[33]

### HUMAN COGNITION AND NEUROTOXIC EFFECTS

Almost all studies show that adult chronic marijuana users display deficits in memory, attention, and cognition for periods of up to 28 days after cessation of marijuana use.[34,35] However, beyond that period, virtually no differences can be found between long-term users and controls.[36,37] Results from studies of adolescents are only now beginning to emerge; although the overall pattern of deficits following periods of abstinence is similar to that observed in adults, noted deficits may persist longer in adolescents; age of first use is an important variable.[38]

The study of the effect of marijuana use on adolescent brain structure, development, and function is still in its infancy. A variety of structural changes have been noted in the brains of marijuana users compared to controls, but long-term studies are needed to determine which abnormalities predated onset of use, which are due to marijuana use alone (versus other factors such as depression or concomitant use of other drugs), and which changes persist after a period of abstinence. Similarly, use of functional magnetic resonance imaging has demonstrated abnormalities in brain function in adolescent cannabis users after a month of abstinence. Whether these alterations persist after longer periods of abstinence and into adulthood requires long-term longitudinal studies.[38]

### PULMONARY

Marijuana's long-term effects are clearest in the pulmonary system; smoking the drug is associated with significant airway inflammation. Numerous studies show that marijuana smokers (2–3 joints per day), compared with tobacco smokers (20–30 cigarettes per day), have the same amount of cough, wheeze, and sputum production, and the same degree of airway erythema, inflammation, edema, and goblet cell hyperplasia. Marijuana smokers have been shown to have mild airflow obstruction, acute and chronic bronchitis, altered expression of nuclear and cytoplasmic proteins involved in the pathogenesis of bronchogenic carcinoma, and disturbances of alveolar macrophage function. Biopsies of individuals who smoke marijuana but not tobacco demonstrate premalignant changes. These findings are not surprising, given that the tar phase of marijuana smoke contains increased concentrations of carcinogenic polycyclic aromatic hydrocarbons and that there is a fourfold greater deposition of tar while smoking marijuana than cigarettes. The long-term epidemiologic significance of these findings is uncertain because the number of chronic marijuana users who do not also smoke cigarettes is small.[39,40] Marijuana smoking does not seem to lead to development of chronic obstructive pulmonary disease in adulthood.[41]

### MALIGNANCIES

In the laboratory, THC has tumor-promoting and antitumor properties. It enhances the transcription of P4501A1, an enzyme that converts polycyclic aromatic hydrocarbons into carcinogens. In contrast, other laboratory studies show that THC causes apoptosis in human prostate cancer cells and the regression of malignant gliomas in rats.[42] Not surprisingly, data regarding the link between marijuana smoking and cancer risk in humans are conflicting, although the bulk of the evidence does not support a link.[43,44] One study showed a dose–response relationship between marijuana smoking (both frequency and duration) and the development of head and neck cancers, but more recent studies did not confirm this association.[45] Two studies of marijuana use and lung cancer, both conducted in Africa, suggest a relationship between smoking marijuana and lung cancer, but it is not clear that the studies adequately controlled for tobacco and snuff use. A recent epidemiologic review points out the difficulties in this kind of research: collecting in-depth information about use of an illegal drug, identifying enough cases and controls to maximize statistical power, and adequately controlling for alcohol and tobacco use, both of which have been linked to a variety of cancers.[43]

## CONCLUSION

Marijuana shares many neuropharmacologic properties with other drugs of abuse. Although residual confounding remains a concern regarding its long-term effects, marijuana use appears to be related to a number of adverse psychosocial outcomes for youth. The effect is strongest for adolescents who begin using marijuana by age 15 years.

## REFERENCES


1. Johnston LD, O'Malley PM, Bachman JG, Schulenberg JE. *Monitoring the Future National Results on Adolescent Drug Use: Overview of Key Findings 2008.* Bethesda, MD: National Institute on Drug Abuse; 2009. NIH Publication No. 09-7401

2. Johnston LD, O'Malley PM, Bachman JG, Schulenberg JE. *Monitoring the Future National Survey Results on Drug Use, 1975-2008: Volume 1: Secondary School Students*. Bethesda, MD: National Institute on Drug Abuse; 2009. NIH Publication No. 09-7402

3. Welch SP, Martin BR. The pharmacology of marijuana. In: Graham AW, Schultz TK, Mayo-Smith MF, Ries RK, Wilford BB, eds. *Principles of Addiction Medicine*. 3rd ed. Chevy Chase, MD: American Society of Addiction Medicine; 2003: 249-270

4. Ashton CH. Pharmacology and effects of cannabis: a brief review. *Br J Psychiatry.* 2001;178:101-106

5. McLaren J, Swift W, Dillon P, Allsop S. Cannabis potency and contamination: a review of the literature. *Addiction.* 2008;103:1100-1109

6. Iversen L. Cannabis and the brain. *Brain.* 2003;126: 1252-1270

7. Gruber AJ, Pope Jr HG. Marijuana use among adolescents. *Pediatr Clin N Am.* 2002;49:389-413

8. Tanda G, Pontieri FE, Di Chiara G. Cannabinoid and heroin activation of mesolimbic dopamine transmission by a common μ1 opioid receptor mechanism. *Science.* 1997;276:2048-2050

9. Camí J, Farré M. Drug addiction. *N Engl J Med.* 2003;349: 975-986

10. Pistis M, Perra S, Pillolla G, et al. Adolescent exposure to cannabinoids induces long-lasting changes in the response to drugs of abuse of rat midbrain dopamine neurons. *Biol Psychiatry.* 2004;56:86-94

11. Breivogel CS, Childers SR, Deadwyler SA, et al. Chronic Δ-9 tetrahydrocannabinol treatment produces a time-dependent loss of cannabinoid receptors and cannabinoid receptor-activated G proteins in rat brain. *J Neurochem.* 1999;73:2447-2459

12. Hall W, Solowij N. Adverse effects of cannabis. *Lancet.* 1998;352:1611-1616

13. Ameri A. The effects of cannabinoids on the brain. *Progress Neurobiol.* 1999;58:315-348

14. Richer I, Bergeron J. Driving under the influence of cannabis: links with dangerous driving, psychological predictors, and accident involvement. *Accid Anal Prev.* 2009;41:299-307

15. Hall W, Degenhardt L. Adverse health effects of non-medical cannabis use. *Lancet.* 2009;374:1383-1391

16. Fergusson DM, Horwood LJ. Cannabis use and traffic accidents in a birth cohort of young adults. *Accid Anal Prev.* 2001;33:703-711

17. Wagner FA, Anthony JC. From drug use to drug dependence: developmental periods of risk for dependence upon marijuana, cocaine, and alcohol. *Neuropsychopharm.* 2002;26: 479-488

18. Office of Applied Studies, Substance Abuse and Mental Health Services Administration. The DASIS Report. Adolescent Treatment Admissions by Gender. 2005. Available at: www.oas.samhsa.gov/2k7/youthTX/youthTX.pdf. Accessed November 1, 2009

19. Compton WM, Grant BF, Colliver JD, Glantz MD, Stinson FS. Prevalence of marijuana use disorders in the United States: 1991-1992 and 2001-2002. *JAMA.* 2004;291:2114-2121

20. Budney AJ, Moore BA. Development and consequences of cannabis dependence. *J Clin Pharmacol.* 2002;42:28S-33S

21. Rodriguez de Fonseca F, Carrera MRA, Navarro M, Koob GF, Weiss F. Activation of corticotropin-releasing factor in the limbic system during cannabinoid withdrawal. *Science.* 1997;276:2050-2054

22. Andreasson S, Allebeck P, Engstrom A, Rydberg U. Cannabis and schizophrenia. A longitudinal study of Swedish conscripts. *Lancet.* 1987;8574:1483-1486

23. Zammit S, Allebeck P, Andreasson S, Lundberg I, Lewis G. Self-reported cannabis use as a risk factor for schizophrenia in Swedish conscripts of 1969: historical cohort study. *BMJ.* 2002;325:1199-1203

24. Arseneault L, Cannon M, Poulton R, et al. Cannabis use in adolescence and risk for adult psychosis: longitudinal prospective study. *BMJ.* 2002;325:1212-1213

25. Patton GC, Coffey C, Cardin JB, et al. Cannabis use and mental health in young people: cohort study. *BMJ.* 2002;325: 1195-1198

26. Fergusson DM, Horwood LJ, Swain-Campbell N. Cannabis use and psychosocial adjustment in adolescence and young adulthood. *Addiction.* 2002;97:1123-1135

27. Macleod J, Oakes R, Copello A, et al. Psychological and social sequelae of cannabis and other illicit drug use by young people: a systematic review of longitudinal, general population studies. *Lancet.* 2004;363:1579-1588

28. Degenhardt L, Hall W. Is cannabis use a contributory cause of psychosis? *Can J Psychiatry.* 2006;51:556-565

29. Bray JW, Zarkin GA, Ringwalt C, Qi J. The relationship between marijuana initiation and dropping out of school. *Health Econ.* 2000;9:9-18

30. Lynskey MT, Coffey C, Degenhardt L, Carlin JB, Patton G. A longitudinal study of the effects of adolescent cannabis use on high school completion. *Addiction.* 2003;98:685-692

31. Fergusson DM, Horwood LJ. Does cannabis use encourage other forms of illicit drug use? *Addiction.* 2000;95:505-520

32. Wagner FA, Anthony JC. Into the world of illegal drug use: exposure opportunity and other mechanisms linking the use of alcohol, tobacco, marijuana, and cocaine. *Am J Epidemiol.* 2002;155:918-925

33. Brown T, Dobs AS. Endocrine effects of marijuana. *J Clin Pharmacol.* 2002;42: 90S-96S

34. Solowij N, Stephens RS, Roffman RA, et al. Cognitive functioning of long-term heavy cannabis users seeking treatment. *JAMA.* 2002;287:1123-1131

35. Pope HG, Gruber AJ, Hudson JI, Huestis MA, Yurgelun-Todd D. Cognitive measures in long-term cannabis users. *J Clin Pharmacol.* 2002;42:41S-47S

36. Gonzalez R, Carey C, Grant I. Nonacute (residual) neuropsychological effects of cannabis use: a qualitative analysis and systematic review. *J Clin Pharmacol.* 2002;42:48S-57S

37. Pope HG. Cannabis, cognition, and residual confounding. *JAMA.* 2002;287:1172-1174

38. Jacobus J, Bava S, Cohen-Zion M, Mahmood O, Tapert SF. Functional consequences of marijuana use in adolescents. *Pharmacol Biochem Behav.* 2009;92:559-565

39. Roth MD, Arora A, Barsky SH, et al. Airway inflammation in young marijuana and tobacco smokers. *Am J Respir Crit Care Med.* 1998;157:928-937

40. Tashkin DP, Baldwin GC, Sarafian T, Dubinett S, Roth MD. Respiratory and immunologic consequences of marijuana smoking. *J Clin Pharmacol.* 2002;42:71S-81S

41. Tan WC, Lo C, Jong A, et al, for the Vancouver Burden of Obstructive Lung Disease (BOLD) Research Group. Marijuana and chronic obstructive lung disease: a population-based study. *CMAJ.* 2009;180:814-820

42. Hashibe M, Ford DE, Zhang Z-F. Marijuana smoking and head and neck cancer. *J Clin Pharmacol.* 2002;42:103S-107S

43. Hashibe M, Straif K, Tashkin DP,et al. Epidemiologic review of marijuana use and cancer risk. *Alcohol.* 2005;35: 265-275

44. Hashibe M, Morgenstern H, Cui Y,et al. Marijuana use and the risk of ling and upper aerodigestive tract cancers: results of a population-based case-control study. *Cancer Epidemiol Biomarkers Prev.* 2006;15:1829-1834

45. Berthiller J, Lee YC, Boffetta P, et al. Marijuana smoking and the risk of head and neck cancer: pooled analysis in the INHANCE consortium. *Cancer Epidemiol Biomarkers Prev.* 2009;18:1544-1551

# CHAPTER 176

## Stimulants

MELISSA WEDDLE, MD, MPH • PATRICIA K. KOKOTAILO, MD, MPH

Stimulants are compounds that have direct neurologic effects, including heightened alertness, increased energy with decreased sense of fatigue, appetite suppression, mood elevation, and sometimes euphoria (Table 176-1). Amphetamine, methylphenidate, and methamphetamine are used clinically, primarily for the treatment of attention-deficit hyperactivity disorder (ADHD) and narcolepsy. Cocaine has limited medical use as a mucosal anesthetic, but is more commonly produced and used illegally. Other illegal stimulants include methcathinone, 3,4-methylenedioxyamphetamine (MDA), and 3,4-methylenedioxymethamphetamine (MDMA, ecstasy).

Stimulants closely resemble the chemical structures of the catecholamine neurotransmitters norepinephrine, epinephrine, and dopamine. It is not, then, surprising that these drugs have autonomic nervous system activity, including sympathomimetic and mood-altering effects. Amphetamines and closely related drugs can activate receptors that normally bind catecholamines and serotonin, cause the release of these neurotransmitters from nerve endings, and prevent their reuptake. Neuropsychological effects of catecholamine receptor activation may include increased alertness, insomnia, euphoria, decreased appetite, and, at higher doses, psychosis. Peripheral effects include vasoconstriction with resulting hypertension, mydriasis, and tachycardia. These compounds have a wide range of affinities to catecholamine and serotonin receptors. For each given stimulant, the pattern of receptor binding is unique and contributes to the distinctive behavioral effects of a given compound.[1]

### AMPHETAMINE AND METHYLPHENIDATE

#### BACKGROUND

Amphetamines were first clinically used in the early 1920s (as Benzedrine) to treat asthma and, in the 1950s, were used more widely to treat obesity, mild depression, and fatigue.[2,3] During the 1950s, methylphenidate was developed, and along with amphetamine, was found to be effective in treatment of ADHD. Both amphetamine (Adderall) and methylphenidate (Ritalin, Metadate, Concerta) are US Food and Drug Administration approved to treat attention-deficit hyperactivity disorder and narcolepsy. Because of their high potential for abuse, these medications are controlled by the Drug Enforcement Agency as schedule II drugs. Chapter 199, ADHD, contains an in-depth discussion of ADHD and medical treatment with stimulants.

**Table 176-1**

**Common Stimulants**

| *Compound* | *Trade or Common Name* | *Schedule* |
|---|---|---|
| Amphetamine | Adderall, Dexedrine | C-II |
| Methylphenidate | Ritalin, Concerta, Metadate | C-II |
| Methamphetamine | Desoxyn, ice, crystal meth, speed | C-II |
| Cocaine (methylbenzoylecgonine) | Coke, crack | C-II |
| 3,4-Methylenedioxyamphetamine | MDA, love drug | C-I |
| 3,4-Methylenedioxymethamphetamine | MDMA, ecstasy | C-I |

### EPIDEMIOLOGY

The 2008 Monitoring the Future Survey shows annual prevalence rates of illicit amphetamine use at 4.5% for 8th graders, 6.4% for 10th graders, and 6.8% for 12th graders. From 1996 to 2008, nonmedical amphetamine use decreased for all 3 groups. For Ritalin, 1.6% of 8th graders, 2.9% of 10th graders, and 3.4% of 12th graders reported use in the previous year.[4] Because of a change in survey questions about Ritalin use that occurred in 2001, it is difficult to assess the trend prior to that time.[5]

In the 2007 Monitoring the Future Survey, 3.7% of college students reported use of Ritalin, and 6.9% reported use of amphetamine in the previous year; these rates are similar to use rates for same-aged young adults not attending college.[5] Although it is likely that many college students use prescription stimulants as a method to stay awake while studying or to increase test performance, one study[6] showed that more than 50% of college students using nonmedical stimulants reported using them to "get high."

Prescription of stimulants has steadily increased over the past 20 years. Using data from a 2003 to 2004 US survey, an estimated 2.5 million children aged 4 to 17 years were receiving medication to treat ADHD.[7] It would be expected that along with increases in prescribing frequency, the potential for abuse of these medications has increased. One study found that out of children and adolescents who had been prescribed methylphenidate, nearly 1 in 5 had been asked to sell, give, or trade their medication at least once in the preceding 5 years.[8]

### PHARMACOLOGY

The central nervous system (CNS) effects of amphetamine and methylphenidate are mediated primarily through the block of dopamine and norepinephrine reuptake.[9] Central nervous system effects include heightened alertness, decreased sense of fatigue, increased ability to concentrate, mood elevation, euphoria, and increase in motor and speech activity. These medications may cause appetite suppression and have been used in treatment of obesity. Peripheral adrenergic effects can include increased blood pressure and slowing of heart rate.[10]

The acute toxic effects of these drugs include restlessness, dizziness, tremor, hyperactive reflexes, irritability, weakness, insomnia, fever, and sometimes euphoria. Confusion, anxiety, delirium, paranoia, hallucinations, panic, or convulsions may develop. Cardiovascular effects can include pallor or flushing, palpitation, cardiac arrhythmias, hypertension or hypotension, and circulatory collapse.[11]

Both amphetamine and methylphenidate are available in immediate-release and sustained-release preparations. On oral dosing, both medications are rapidly and completely absorbed from the gastrointestinal tract, with peak concentrations occurring 1 to 2 hours after dose administration and a half-life of 2 to 8 hours. In addition to being used orally, methylphenidate may be taken intravenously or intranasally.[12] Amphetamine may also be smoked or injected. Amphetamines can be detected in the urine for up to 2 days following recreational use. Newer-generation assays react with MDA, MDMA, and methamphetamine.[13] Methylphenidate is usually not detected in urine drug screens.

### ABUSE POTENTIAL

When methylphenidate is used intranasally, effects are immediate and similar to those of cocaine. When the drug is used intranasally and intravenously, it may be addictive.[12] Although the pharmacologic effects of methylphenidate are similar to those of cocaine, methylphenidate seems to have lower abuse potential, possibly due to different pharmacokinetics within the brain.[14] With amphetamine, both tolerance and physical dependence occur with regular heavy use. Symptoms of amphetamine withdrawal can include depression, intense dreaming, insomnia or hypersomnia, increased appetite, and depression.

### OVERDOSE

Amphetamines and methylphenidate have similar overdose effects, which include restlessness, confusion, irritability, insomnia, tremor, hyperreflexia, diaphoresis, mydriasis, flushing, palpitations, tachycardia, and elevated blood pressure. More severe toxic effects can include delirium, hypertension, dysrhythmias, hyperthermia, delusions, hallucinations, seizures, coma, cardiovascular collapse, and death.

## COCAINE

### BACKGROUND

Cocaine is an alkaloid found in the plant *Erythroxylon coca,* grown primarily in the Andes Mountains in South America. The leaves are harvested, dried, and converted into a cocaine paste, eventually used to produce cocaine hydrochloride (HCl). Illicit cocaine is typically available as the HCl salt and crack. The salt form varies considerably in purity, and may be diluted with other agents such as mannitol, lactose, and sucrose. Other stimulants such as caffeine, phenylpropanolamine, and ephedrine, and local anesthetics such as lidocaine, procaine, and benzocaine, may be added to simulate the actual drug. Adding baking soda to aqueous cocaine HCl and heating it to remove the water transforms it into its smokable form, known as "freebase" or "crack." As it cools, the freebase cocaine precipitates into small pellets, or "rocks."[15] Cocaine is a schedule II drug, with its only medical indication as a topical local anesthetic.

### EPIDEMIOLOGY

Data from the 2008 Monitoring the Future Survey show that over the preceding decade, annual prevalence use of both cocaine and crack use has decreased among 8th, 10th, and 12th graders. The annual prevalence use for powder cocaine is 1.8% for 8th graders, 3.0% for 10th graders, and 4.4% for 12th graders, whereas the annual prevalence use for crack cocaine is 1.1% for 8th graders, 1.3% for 10th graders, and 1.6% for 12th graders.[4] Cocaine and crack use has increased among college students and young adults.[5]

### PHARMACOLOGY

Cocaine powder is readily absorbed through the nasal mucosa and is most commonly used intranasally, by "snorting." Because it is water soluble, cocaine powder can be injected intravenously. When converted to freebase or crack, cocaine is smokable. Cocaine has a very rapid onset of action, less than 1 minute when smoked, 0.5 to 2 minutes when used intravenously, and 2 to 30 minutes when snorted. Duration of effect is from 4 to 15 minutes when smoked, 12 to 30 minutes when used intravenously, and 30 to 60 minutes when snorted.[16] Cocaine can be detected in urine up to 2 to 3 days after use.[17]

When used intermittently, cocaine blocks reuptake of norepinephrine and dopamine. Adrenergic effects include mydriasis, vasoconstriction, hypertension, tachycardia, and tachypnea. The behavioral effects appear to be mediated by its dopaminergic effects, and include euphoria, heightened sexual excitement, and mood elevation. Undesirable effects of the drug may include paranoia, hallucinations, and dysphoria. The central stimulatory effects (the "rush") are followed by depression ("crash").

### ABUSE POTENTIAL

The intense high with cocaine is short-lived, leading to a pattern of repeated use at short intervals. The feelings of euphoria, energy, and confidence may be particularly appealing to adolescents as a way to overcome shyness, inhibitions, or low self-esteem.[2] The physical effects of cocaine withdrawal are negatively reinforcing, another factor that makes it difficult for an individual to stop cocaine use. Repeated use of cocaine has been shown to result in tolerance and dependence.

As with other addictive drugs, dependence on cocaine is obvious by lack of control over use, urges and cravings for the drug, and continued use despite adverse consequences. Although there is usually no dramatic physical withdrawal syndrome associated with abrupt discontinuation of the drug, cocaine is considered to be physically addictive because of the cravings and urges that propel compulsive drug-taking behavior.

Symptoms of chronic use are typically related to the mode of administration. Those who use intranasally may experience rhinitis, nasal bleeding, and nasal septum perforation, whereas those who smoke crack cocaine may develop shortness of breath or sore throat. Chronic cocaine users may develop mood swings, irritability, erratic sleep patterns, difficulty concentrating, and social withdrawal.

### OVERDOSE

Acute cocaine toxicity may result in profound CNS stimulation with psychosis and repeated grand mal convulsions, ventricular arrhythmias and respiratory dysfunction, mydriasis, hypertension leading to hypotension and small muscle twitching, and extreme hyperthermia. Acute myocardial infarction may occur.

## METHAMPHETAMINE

### BACKGROUND

Methamphetamine, an amphetamine derivative, was a common drug of abuse in the 1960s, and was recognized for its potential for tolerance and physical dependence. Use of methamphetamine, commonly known as "crystal meth," "ice," "crank," "crystal," or "speed," has undergone a resurgence, particularly in the western and midwestern regions of the United States. Although available as a schedule II pharmaceutical preparation (Desoxyn), methamphetamine is most commonly used in an illicit preparation. "Super labs" in California and Mexico produce most of the methamphetamine used in the United States, although ease of production and readily available ingredients have facilitated rapid growth of "do-it-yourself" labs throughout the country, primary in rural areas.[18] The term "ice" refers to extremely pure d-methamphetamine that has the appearance of a chunk of quartz crystal.

### PHARMACOLOGY

Methamphetamine can be ingested orally, smoked, used intranasally, or injected intravenously. With adolescents, intranasal use is the most common route of administration. Unlike cocaine, methamphetamine does not have to be converted to a "freebase" form to be smoked. Effects of methamphetamine are almost instantaneous when smoked or injected, and occur within 20 minutes after oral ingestion. Methamphetamine effects last longer than cocaine, typically 8 to 13 hours.[19] Methamphetamine can be detected in the urine for up to 2 days.[13]

The N-methyl group that differentiates amphetamine from methamphetamine decreases polarity and allows better penetration of the blood–brain barrier. It is a white, odorless, bitter, crystalline powder that is soluble in water and alcohol. Like the other stimulants, methamphetamine effects are mediated by dopamine and norepinephrine, although methamphetamine has significantly higher CNS stimulant activity and less peripheral nervous system and cardiovascular stimulation compared with amphetamine.[20] Continued use of methamphetamine leads to depletion of stores, and a clinical binge–crash cycle occurs.

The desirable effects of methamphetamine are euphoria, increased alertness, concentration, and hypersexuality. Other CNS effects include increased motor and speech activity, repetitive or stereotypic behaviors, and insomnia. Peripheral effects include increased blood pressure, increased respiratory rate, diaphoresis, increased gastrointestinal motility, and tachycardia. Negative side effects can include hyperthermia, stroke, cardiac arrhythmia, increased anxiety, aggression, paranoia, and hallucinations.[21] The hallucinations of chronic methamphetamine use are typically visual or tactile in contrast to the usual auditory hallucinations of schizophrenia.[20]

### EPIDEMIOLOGY

The 2008 Monitoring the Future Survey reflects annual prevalence rates for methamphetamine use at 1.2%, 1.5%, and 1.2% for 8th, 10th, and 12th graders, respectively. These levels are down from 1999, the first year students were asked about use.[4] Methamphetamine use has been highest in the West and lowest in the Northeast.[5] Extensive evidence indicates that in many western US cities, methamphetamine is used extensively by gay males and is associated with high-risk sexual behavior, a significant factor in transmission of HIV.[22] Annual prevalence use for college students is 0.4%, less than the 1.9% prevalence use for similarly aged respondents not attending college.[5]

### ABUSE POTENTIAL

Methamphetamine is a highly addictive drug, cheaper and longer acting than cocaine. After a binge and before the "crash," users may develop restless anxiety, irritability, fatigue, and dysphoria, including paranoia and hallucinations, termed "tweaking." Further use of methamphetamine temporarily improves the symptoms and further reinforces the addiction. After days of sleeplessness, users may "crash" into a nonrestful sleep.[18] Skin ulcers, repetitive behaviors, and hallucinations (primarily tactile and visual) may be signs of chronic methamphetamine use.

### OVERDOSE

Because methamphetamine has fewer peripheral side effects than the other stimulants, methamphetamine toxicity is typically manifested by CNS effects, primarily anxiety, paranoia, violent behavior, acute psychosis, and hallucinations. Peripheral sympathetic effects are similar to those of the other stimulants.

## TREATMENT OF STIMULANT OVERDOSE

Stimulant overdose may be severe and life threatening, requiring respiratory assistance and a life support system. Treatment for complications may include fluid resuscitation, cooling measures, airway management, benzodiazepines for agitation or seizures, defibrillation, or cardioversion. If the drug has been taken orally, activated charcoal and a cathartic should be given. Patients without life-threatening signs or symptoms typically are treated with sedation and observation in a quiet and calm environment. Short-acting betablockers may be used to treat hypertension. Neuroleptic agents may be used to treat the delusions or psychosis seen with methamphetamine use, and benzodiazepines for milder anxiety.[23]

## TREATMENT OF STIMULANT ADDICTION

Treatment of cocaine, amphetamine, and methamphetamine addiction is similar and should be conducted in a specialized chemical dependency program. The matrix model is a psychosocial approach that has been effective in treating adults with methamphetamine addiction, but it has not been studied in adolescents.[24] Withdrawal syndrome is not life threatening and usually does not require hospitalization. Close monitoring with frequent urine testing may be needed as an adjunct to relapse prevention.[2]

## REFERENCES

1. Foley KF. Mechanism of action and therapeutic uses of psychostimulants. *Clin Lab Sci.* 2003;18(2):107–118

2. Coupey SM. Specific drugs. In: Schydlower M, ed. *Substance Abuse: A Guide for Health Professional.* Elk Grove Village, IL: American Academy of Pediatrics; 2002:191–276

3. Wilens TE, Spencer TJ. The stimulants revisited. *Child Adolesc Psychiatr Clin N Am.* 2000;9(3):573–603

4. Johnston LD, O'Malley PM, Bachman JG, Schulenberg JE. Various stimulant drugs show continuing gradual declines among teens in 2008, most illicit drugs hold steady. December 11, 2008. Press release. University of Michigan News Service. Available at: monitoringthefuture.org/pressreleases/08drugpr.pdf. Accessed September 21, 2009

5. Johnston LD, O'Malley PM, Bachman JG, Schulenberg JE. *Monitoring the Future National Survey Results on Drug Use, 1975-2007.* Bethesda, MD: National Institute on Drug Abuse; 2008. NIH publication 08-6418A, 08-6413B

6. McCabe SE, Knight JR, Teter CJ, Wechsler H. Non medical use of prescription stimulants among US college students: prevalence and correlates from a national survey. *Addiction.* 2005;99:96-106

7. Visser SN, Lesesne CA. Mental health in the United States: prevalence of diagnosis and medication treatment for attention-deficit/hyperactivity disorder—United States, 2003. *MMWR Morb Mortal Wkly Rep.* 2005;54(34):842-847

8. Musser CJ, Ahmann PA, Mundt P, et al. Stimulant use and the potential for abuse in Wisconsin as reported by school administrators and longitudinally followed children. *Dev Behav Pediatr.* 1998;19(3):187-192

9. Greenhill LL. The science of stimulant abuse. *Pediatr Ann.* 2006;35(8):552-556

10. Brunton LL, Lazo JS, Parker KL. *Goodman & Gilman's The Pharmacological Basis of Therapeutics.* 11th ed. New York: McGraw-Hill; 2006

11. Klein-Schwartz W. Abuse and toxicity of methylphenidate. *Curr Opin Pediatr.* 2002;14:219-223

12. Morton WA, Stockton GG. Methylphenidate abuse and psychiatric side effects. *Prim Care Companion J Clin Psychiatry.* 2000;2(5):159-164

13. Ford M, Delaney KA, Ling L, Erickson T. *Clinical Toxicology.* Philadelphia: WB Saunders; 2001

14. Volkow ND, Ding YS, Fowler JS, et al. Is methylphenidate like cocaine? *Arch Gen Psychiatry.* 1995;52:456-463

15. Isenschmid DS. Cocaine—effects of human performance and behavior. *Forensic Sci Rev.* 2002;14(1-2):62-100

16. Substance abuse. In: Strasburger VC, Brown RT, Braverman PK, Rogers PD, Holland-Hall C, Coupey SM. *Adolescent Medicine: A Handbook for Primary Care.* Philadelphia: Lippincott Williams & Wilkins; 2006:147-171

17. Rosenfeld W, Wingert WE. Scientific issues in drug testing and use of the laboratory. *Substance Abuse: A Guide for Health Professionals.* Elk Grove Village, IL: American Academy of Pediatrics; 2002:105-121

18. Lineberry TW, Bostwick M. Methamphetamine abuse: a perfect storm of complications. *Mayo Clin Proc.* 2006;81(1): 77-84

19. Nordahl TE, Salo R, Leamon M. Neuropsychological effects of chronic methamphetamine use on neurotransmitters and cognition: a review. *J Neuropsychiatry Clin Neurosci.* 2003;15:317-325

20. MacKenzie RG, Heischober B. Methamphetamine. *Pediatr Rev.* 1997;18(9):305-309

21. Rawson RA, Gonzales R, Brethen P. Treatment of methamphetamine use disorders: an update. *J Subst Abuse Treat.* 2002;23:145-150

22. Shoptaw S, Reback CJ, Freese TE. Patient characteristics, HIV serostatus, and risk behaviors among gay and bisexual males seeking treatment for methamphetamine abuse and dependence in Los Angeles. *J Addict Dis.* 2002;21(1):91-105

23. Gawin FH, Ellinwood EH. Cocaine and other stimulants. *N Engl J Med.* 1988;318(18):1173-1182

24. Rawson RA, Marinelli-Casey P, Anglin MD, et al. A multi-site comparison of psychosocial approaches for the treatment of methamphetamine dependence. *Addiction.* 2004;99:708-717

# CHAPTER 177

# Opiates

JOHN KULIG, MD, MPH

Opiates, derived from *Papaver somniferum*, the opium poppy, include opium, morphine, codeine, and heroin. Raw opium contains 10% morphine by weight, and heroin is synthesized by diacetylating morphine. Heroin is 2 to 3 times more potent than morphine and penetrates the blood-brain barrier more readily. Intravenous administration produces rapid onset of euphoria and peak intensity in less than 1 minute, while smoking or snorting heroin produces a peak effect in 10 to 15 minutes. The drug is typically administered 3 times a day. Tolerance and addiction develop with any method of heroin use. Heroin is also used in combination with other illicit drugs, including cocaine, methamphetamine, psilocybin, LSD, phencyclidine, marijuana, and even other opioids such as fentanyl. Codeine can be extracted from opium or synthesized from morphine as methylmorphine. Multiple semisynthetic and synthetic opioids are listed in Table 177-1. These drugs can be ingested orally ("eating"), inhaled nasally ("snorting" or "sniffing"), smoked, and injected (intravenous, intramuscular, or subcutaneous).[1]

**Table 177-1**

**Opiates versus Opioids Classification**

| *Classification* | *Examples* |
|---|---|
| Opiates | Opium<br>Morphine<br>Codeine<br>Heroin |
| Semisynthetic/synthetic opioids | Buprenorphine<br>Butorphanol<br>Dihydrocodeine<br>Fentanyl<br>Hydrocodone<br>Hydromorphone<br>Levorphanol<br>Meperidine<br>Methadone<br>Nalbuphine<br>Nicomorphine<br>Oxycodone<br>Oxymorphone<br>Pentazocine<br>Propoxyphene |

## EPIDEMIOLOGY

Heroin use has fallen dramatically from its peak in the 1960s and 1970s, but recent trends suggest a rise in abuse of synthetic opioids, diverted from legitimate prescribed use as potent analgesics. Among US 12th graders in 2009, reported lifetime prevalence was 1.3% for heroin use, but 13.2% for use of "other narcotics." Annual prevalence of reported OxyContin use in 2009 was 2.0% for 8th graders, 3.6% for 10th graders, and 4.7% for 12th graders. Annual prevalence of reported Vicodin use in 2009 was 2.9% for 8th graders, 6.7% for 10th graders, and 9.7% for 12th graders. Trends in use of heroin and other narcotics are demonstrated in Figures 177-1 and 177-2. The apparent rise beginning in 2002 is attributed to the introduction of a revised set of questions on "other narcotics" use, in which Talwin, laudanum, and paregoric were replaced with Vicodin, OxyContin, and Percocet.[2]

## PATTERNS OF USE

A typical pattern leading to opioid addiction in adolescence involves early use of synthetic opioids such as Percocet, Vicodin, or OxyContin by mouth or by snorting, as early as age 14 or 15 years. Heroin use follows due to the increasing cost of synthetic opioids as dosing increases to achieve the desired effect due to the development of tolerance. At a street cost of $1 per mg, a typical user of 3 or 4 OxyContin 80-mg tablets daily must raise $240 to $320 a day or $1,680 to $2,240 a week. Heroin is considerably less costly and may initially be snorted or "sniffed" in the mistaken belief that this route will be less addictive. Use by injection soon follows because the nasal membranes cannot tolerate ever-increasing doses. Even with needle exchange programs and bleaching syringes, intravenous drug injection is associated with skin abscesses; bacterial endocarditis; and risk of hepatitis B, hepatitis C, and HIV infection. Dependence may develop in as few as 3 or 4 weeks

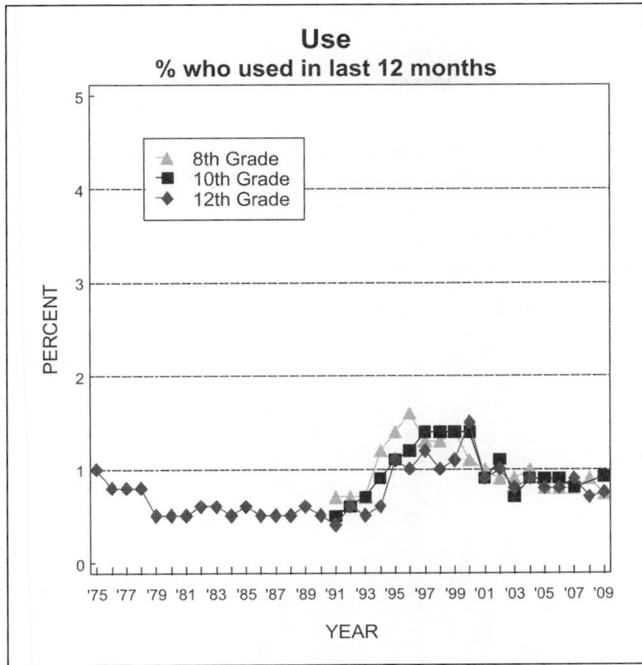


**FIGURE 177-1** Trends in annual use of heroin in grades 8, 10, and 12 (percent who used in last 12 months). (Johnston LD, O'Malley PM, Bachman JG, Schulenberg JE. *Monitoring the Future national results on adolescent drug use: Overview of key findings, 2009* (NIH Publication No. 10-7583). Bethesda, MD: National Institute on Drug Abuse; 2010.)

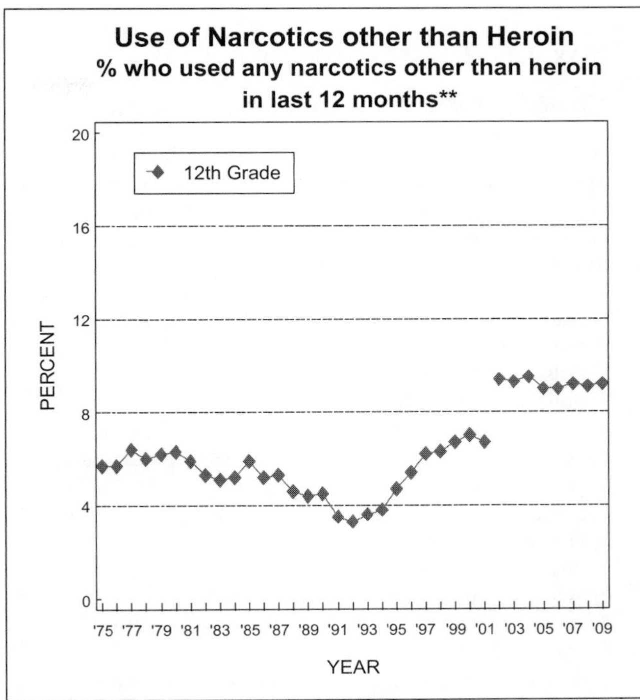


**FIGURE 177-2** Trends in annual use of narcotics other than heroin (percent who used in last 12 months, 12th grade). (Johnston LD, O'Malley PM, Bachman JG, Schulenberg JE. *Monitoring the Future national results on adolescent drug use: Overview of key findings, 2009* (NIH Publication No. 10-7583). Bethesda, MD: National Institute on Drug Abuse; 2010.)

of regular use of opiates such as heroin or morphine. Death by overdose can result because the purity and concentration of heroin, as well as the amount ingested, may vary considerably.

## MORBIDITY AND MORTALITY

The mortality rate in persons who regularly inject heroin has been estimated at 2% annually.[3] In 2006, 167,568 (33%) of the 741,425 emergency department (ED) visits involving nonmedical use of pharmaceuticals were attributed to hydrocodone, oxycodone, and methadone.[4] Data on drug abuse–related deaths from the 28 metropolitan areas included in the Drug Abuse Warning Network indicated a 97% increase from 1997 to 2002 in reported opioid analgesic deaths. Deaths reported with oxycodone increased 728%, and by 2002, deaths from opioid analgesics were more frequent than heroin or cocaine.[5]

## CLINICAL PRESENTATIONS

A high index of suspicion or a positive CRAFFT screen (Chapter 181, Office Management and Laboratory Testing) may lead to a frank discussion of opioid use. By late adolescence, youth may voluntarily seek treatment. Opioid-dependent youth, as a group, tend to avoid alcohol, but commonly use tobacco and marijuana, and occasionally cocaine. Examination findings suggestive of addiction or its complications are reported in Chapter 172 (Box 172-2), along with DSM-IV-TR criteria for substance abuse (Box 172-5) and substance dependence (Box 172-6). Clinical manifestations of opiate withdrawal can be quantified by using the Clinical Opiate Withdrawal Scale (Box 177-1).

## OVERDOSE

An acute overdose with heroin or opioids may present with life-threatening respiratory depression, along with depressed sensorium, mioisis, and signs of recent inhalation or injection. Diagnostic criteria include altered

## Box 177-1

### *Clinical Opiate Withdrawal Scale*

For each item, circle the number that best describes the patient's signs or symptoms. Rate just on the apparent relationship to opiate withdrawal. For example, if heart rate is increased because the patient was jogging just prior to assessment, the increased pulse rate would not add to the score.

**Patient Name:** ______________________ **Date:** __________ **Time:** ______

**Reason for this assessment:** ______________________________________

**1. Resting pulse rate:** _____ **beats/minute.**

***Measured after the patient is sitting or lying for 1 minute***

0 Pulse rate 80 or below
1 Pulse rate 81–100
2 Pulse rate 101–120
4 Pulse rate greater than 120

**2. Sweating:** ***over past half hour not accounted for by room temperature or patient activity***

0 No reports of chills or flushing
1 Subjective reports of chills or flushing
2 Flushed or observable moisture on face
3 Beads of sweat on brow or face
4 Sweat streaming off face

**3. Restlessness:** ***observation during assessment***

0 Able to sit still
1 Reports difficulty sitting still, but is able to do so
3 Frequent shifting or extraneous movements of legs/arms
5 Unable to sit still for more than a few seconds

**4. Pupil size**

0 Pupils pinned or normal size for room light
1 Pupils possibly larger than normal for room light
2 Pupils moderately dilated
5 Pupils so dilated that only the rim of the iris is visible

**5. Bone or joint aches:** ***if patient was having pain previously, only the additional component attributed to opiate withdrawal is scored***

0 Not present
1 Mild diffuse discomfort
2 Patient reports severe diffuse aching of joints/muscles
4 Patient is rubbing joints or muscles and is unable to sit still because of discomfort

**6. Runny nose or tearing:** ***not accounted for by cold symptoms or allergies***

0 Not present
1 Nasal stuffiness or unusually moist eyes
2 Nose running or tearing
4 Nose constantly running or tears streaming down cheeks

**7. GI upset:** ***over last half hour***

0 No GI symptoms
1 Stomach cramps
2 Nausea or loose stool
3 Vomiting or diarrhea
5 Multiple episodes of diarrhea or vomiting

**8. Tremor:** ***observation of outstretched hands***

0 No tremor
1 Tremor can be felt, but not observed
2 Slight tremor observable
4 Gross tremor or muscle twitching

**9. Yawning:** ***observation during assessment***

0 No yawning
1 Yawning once or twice during assessment
2 Yawning three or more times during assessment

(*Continued*)

**Box 177-1 (Continued)**

***Clinical Opiate Withdrawal Scale***

4 Yawning several times/minute

**10. Anxiety or irritability**

0 None

1 Patient reports increasing irritability or anxiousness

2 Patient obviously irritable, anxious

4 Patient so irritable or anxious that participation in the assessment is difficult

**11. Gooseflesh skin**

0 Skin is smooth

3 Piloerection of skin can be felt or hairs standing up on arms

5 Prominent piloerection

**Total Score:__________**

**[The total score is the sum of all 11 items.]**

**Signature of person completing assessment:______________________________**

**Score: 5–12=Mild; 13–24=Moderate; 25–36=Moderately severe; >36=Severe withdrawal**

*Source:* Center for Substance Abuse Treatment. *Clinical Guidelines for the Use of Buprenorphine in the Treatment of Opioid Addiction.* Treatment Improvement Protocol (TIP) Series 40. Rockville, MD: Substance Abuse and Mental Health Services Administration; 2004. DHHS publication no. (SMA) 04-3939.

level of consciousness plus one of the following: (1) respiratory rate <12 breaths/minute, (2) miotic pupils, and (3) circumstantial evidence or history of heroin use. Polydrug abuse and hypoglycemia should be ruled out, the airway should be assessed, and respiration should be supported by bag and mask ventilation or endotracheal intubation, as needed. Naloxone (Narcan), a narcotic antagonist, should be administered in an initial dose of 0.2 to 0.4 mg intravenously, subcutaneously, or intramuscularly, and repeated in doses up to 2 mg after 5 to 7 minutes. Onset of action is approximately 2 minutes. In patients who respond to naloxone, an ED stay of 2 to 3 hours is warranted to observe for complications.[3,6] Special consideration should be given to the possibility of "body packing," when an ingested heroin packet bursts in the gastrointestinal tract, leading to a massive unintentional overdose. Hospitalization for medical complications is otherwise uncommon, but transfer for inpatient detoxification should be considered.

## LIMITATIONS OF DRUG TESTING

Urine drug testing is most useful for monitoring abstinence while undergoing treatment for opioid addiction, or in the ED for evaluating an unresponsive patient. Initial urine screening is done by immunoassay (enzyme-linked immunosorbent assay). Positive results are confirmed by gas chromatography-mass spectrometry. Basic urine screening for drugs of abuse (the NIDA 5) includes opiates such as heroin and morphine, but does not include synthetic opioids such as hydrocodone and oxycodone. Testing for semisynthetic and synthetic opioids must be specifically requested. Procedures must be in place to avoid sample substitution, dilution, and adulteration, and chain of custody must be preserved for the specimen. Interpretation of results is important in that the detection period for opiates in the urine is only 1 to 2 days, and false positives may occur with ingestion of poppy seeds in baked goods.[7]

## ASSESSMENT AND MANAGEMENT

The advent of office-based treatment with buprenorphine has expanded pharmacologic management of opiate addiction beyond methadone clinics.[8,9] Primary care clinicians with 8 hours of accredited training are licensed by the US Food and Drug Administration to prescribe buprenorphine for outpatient management of opiate/opioid addiction. A Substance Abuse and Mental Health Services Administration–sponsored educational resource for clinicians treating patients with opioid dependence is available at www.pcssmentor.org (Box 177-2). Most clinicians use the combination of buprenorphine-naloxone (Suboxone), available in 8.0/2.0 mg and 2.0/0.5 mg sublingual tablets. Buprenorphine-naloxone tablets must be allowed to dissolve sublingually for a minimum of 4 minutes. Swallowing the tablets inactivates the drug, and if the

**Box 177-2**

***Physician Clinical Support System***

Includes clinical guidance on

1. Patient assessment
   a. Selection for office-based opioid treatment
   b. Considerations of appropriateness for opioid maintenance
   c. Considerations of appropriateness for opioid withdrawal
   d. The use of DSM-IV checklists and opioid withdrawal scales
   e. Pharmacologic withdrawal follow-up procedures
2. Induction
   a. Induction methods
   b. Physician or nurse availability during induction and early stabilization
3. Dosing and patient monitoring
   a. Buprenorphine dosing
   b. Appropriate use of ancillary medications
   c. Frequency of monitoring
   d. Complications and treatment of complications
   e. Timing and processes of referrals to higher levels of care
4. Treatment of poly substance dependence or comorbid conditions, including
   a. Psychiatric conditions
   b. Medical conditions, especially hepatitis C
5. Issues related to treatment of special populations
   a. Adolescents
   b. Pregnant patients
   c. Elderly
   d. HIV/AIDS, including HIV and HCV screening, counseling, and referrals
   e. Pain
6. Development of support and referral networks
   a. Involvement of nurse, nonphysician health professionals, pharmacists, and certified alcohol and other drug abuse counselors
   b. Collaboration with opioid treatment programs
   c. Integrating counseling and urine toxicology testing into treatment regimen
   d. Involvement of family members and significant others
   e. Patient and family education for appropriate expectations on symptom decrease and treatment outcomes
7. Use of nonpharmacologic strategies
   a. Motivational counseling
   b. Limit setting
   c. Appropriate use of contingencies
   d. Use of 12-step and other self-help programs
8. Patient tracking
   a. Tracking procedures
   b. Recommended visit schedules
9. Office logistics
   a. Staff education
   b. Paper work
   c. Screening and initial and follow-up visit forms
   d. Coding with proper CPT codes and billing

*Source:* Physician Clinical Support System. PCSS-Methadone, PCSS-Buprenorphine. Available at www.pcssmentor.org.

crushed tablets are injected, naloxone will induce withdrawal. Following an induction process, most young patients can be managed with buprenorphine in a daily dose of 16 mg, with weekly or biweekly follow-up. Buprenorphine is not approved for use during pregnancy, so use of effective contraception should be encouraged. Although buprenorphine can also be used for rapid detoxification, relapse rates are high without maintenance therapy. With the recent increase in availability of "street Suboxone," patients may self-medicate and present for maintenance treatment having already initiated therapy.[10] As with all addiction treatment, behavioral therapy with participation in individual or group counseling is an essential component of treatment. A daily exercise regimen may also assist in recovery through the release of endorphins in the brain.

Optimal duration of buprenorphine maintenance therapy for adolescents is unknown, but patients may be offered an opportunity to taper or discontinue the drug after 12 months of abstinence. Another alternative under study is transitioning from daily sublingual buprenorphine to monthly injectable depot naltrexone.[11] The primary reason for treatment failure in adolescents is continued association with peers and family members who use. Long-term placement in residential programs for up to 12 months or more can be successful, but dropouts and relapse rates remain high. Many residential programs also prohibit or limit maintenance pharmacotherapy.

Additional pharmacologic options for treatment of opiate addiction include full agonist therapy with methadone and full antagonist therapy with oral or injectable naltrexone. Methadone has been used for short-term detoxification of adolescents, but has not been widely used in maintenance because adherence to the required frequent follow-up visits has been poor. A 28-day outpatient treatment regimen for 36 adolescents aged 13 to 18 years who met DSM-IV criteria for opioid dependence compared buprenorphine with clonidine for detoxification in combination with thrice weekly behavioral counseling and incentives. Treatment with buprenorphine was associated with 72% treatment retention and 61% initiating ongoing treatment with naltrexone, whereas treatment with clonidine was associated with 39% treatment retention and 5% initiating treatment with naltrexone.[12] Further study is needed to determine the optimal combination of behavioral counseling and pharmacotherapy to maintain remission in youth with opioid dependence.

## REFERENCES

1. Schydlower M, ed. *Substance Abuse: A Guide for Health Professionals*. 2nd ed. Elk Grove Village, IL: American Academy of Pediatrics; 2002

2. Johnston LD, O'Malley PM, Bachman JG, et al. *Monitoring the Future: National Results on Adolescent Drug Use: Overview of Key Findings, 2008*. Bethesda, MD: National Institute on Drug Abuse; 2009. NIH publication no. 09-7401

3. Sporer KA. Acute heroin overdose. *Ann Intern Med*. 1999;130:584–590

4. Substance Abuse and Mental Health Services Administration, Office of Applied Studies. *Drug Abuse Warning Network, 2006: National Estimates of Drug-Related Emergency Department Visits*. DAWN Series D-30. Rockville, MD: 2008. DHHS publication no. (SMA) 08-4339

5. Paulozzi LJ. Opioid analgesic involvement in drug abuse deaths in American metropolitan areas. *Am J Public Health*. 2006;96:1755–1757

6. O'Connor PG, Kosten TR, Stine SM. Management of opioid intoxication and withdrawal. In: Graham AW, Schultz TK, Mayo-Smith MF, et al, eds. *Principles of Addiction Medicine*. 3rd ed. Chevy Chase, MD: American Society of Addiction Medicine; 2003:651–663

7. Eskridge KD, Guthrie SK. Clinical issues associated with urine testing of substances of abuse. *Pharmacotherapy*. 1997;17:497–510

8. Johnson RE, Strain EC, Amass L. Buprenorphine: how to use it right. *Drug Alcohol Depend*. 2003;70:S59–S77

9. Fiellin DA, Pantalon MV, Chawarski MC, et al. Counseling plus buprenorphine-naloxone maintenance therapy for opioid dependence. *N Engl J Med*. 2006;355:365–374

10. Fiellin DA. The first three years of buprenorphine in the United States: experience to date and future directions. *J Addict Med*. 2007;1:62–67

11. Stine SM, Greenwald MK, Kosten TR. Pharmacologic interventions for opioid addiction. In: Graham AW, Schultz TK, Mayo-Smith MF, et al, eds. *Principles of Addiction Medicine*. 3rd ed. Chevy Chase, MD: American Society of Addiction Medicine; 2003:735–744

12. Marsch LA, Bickel WK, Badger G, et al. Comparison of pharmacological treatments for opioid-dependent adolescents: a randomized controlled trial. *Arch Gen Psychiatry*. 2005;62:1157–1164

# CHAPTER 178

# Hallucinogens, Club Drugs, Inhalants, and Other Substances of Abuse

PIERRE-PAUL TELLIER, MD

As providers of adolescent health care, we are faced with parents, adolescents, and others asking questions about drugs and the risks involved. The most common substances of abuse by adolescents are alcohol and marijuana. However, there are other drugs such as hallucinogens, club drugs, inhalants, and stimulants that teenagers may use or experiment with, and it is important that we know about them. Data on the less commonly used substances are often missing, and the available information is confusing. An approach is to understand the general principles of drug use and then become familiar with individual substances and their potential short- and long-term effects.

## GENERAL PRINCIPLES

Adolescents use a variety of substances in an attempt to get "high." These may include illicit drugs such as marijuana, hallucinogens, stimulants, or new "designer drugs," such as 3,4-methylene dioxy-N-methylamphetamine (MDMA, or Ecstasy), or legal substances such as alcohol, prescription, and over-the-counter OTC medications, or household products used as inhalants.[1] A more in-depth discussion of many of these substances of abuse may be found in other chapters in this section of the textbook. Some of these drugs are synthetic products, whereas others are derivatives of plants.[2] Some are new compounds whereas others are older products that have regained popularity. Therefore, when trying to determine if a patient is using drugs, it is important to inquire not only about "drug use," but also about the abuse of medications that have been prescribed for the patient, the patient's friends or family, and the use of over-the-counter (OTC) pharmaceuticals and herbal products.

The prevalence of use of these products is difficult to assess. Large cross-sectional surveys provide us with information about trends of use in the population at large, whereas smaller studies may give us data relevant to certain subpopulations. From these smaller studies we know that prevalence of use and risk of use is higher in such groups as gay, lesbian, bisexual and transgender youth, rave attendees, and youth who are incarcerated.

"Monitoring the Future" is a long-term, school-based survey supported by grants from the National Institute of Drug Abuse. It reports on substance use among junior high school, high school, and college students. The use of almost all known illicit drugs, alcohol, cigarettes, and inhalants, as well as nonprescribed uses of prescription drugs, is monitored and the results are published annually. Relevant information from this survey is that the lifetime use of illicit drugs peaked in 1996 for all grades and has been decreasing since then, especially for eighth graders.[3] The most commonly used drugs in the past year by eighth-grade students after alcohol are marijuana, inhalants, amphetamines, OTC cough/cold medicines, and Vicodin, in that order.[3] For 10th- and 12th-grade students inhalants drop out of the top 5 and tranquilizers are added to the list as the fifth most commonly used substance by these age groups.[3] A striking phenomenon in the past decade has been the marked decrease of Ecstasy for all age groups as one of the most frequent drugs of use.

The Substance Abuse and Mental Health Services Administration sponsors the "National Survey on Drug Use and Health."[4] Findings from this survey demonstrate that drug use increases with age in adolescents, with a peak in the 18 to 20 year-old group. More boys than girls use drugs; boys use more marijuana, and girls abuse more psychotherapeutics such as tranquilizers.[4] American Indians/Alaska natives have the greatest prevalence of use of illicit drugs, followed by persons who report being 2 or more races, blacks, whites, Hispanics, and Asians.[4] Individuals living in larger metropolitan areas are the most likely to use illicit drugs, whereas those living in rural areas are the least likely.[4]

Patterns of use in those adolescents who use drugs vary. Youth may use drugs at home, at house parties, at raves, or at larger venues such as concerts. Most adolescents who use drugs have 1 or 2 drugs of choice that they use on a regular basis alone or with friends.

In special circumstances such as raves or large parties, they may choose to use other drugs. In these environments, polydrug use is frequent and drugs may be taken simultaneously or sequentially. The nature of these combinations is not based on any credible or reliable data. A dangerous method of combining drugs consists of taking a handful of pills of an unknown nature and consuming them at one time with or without alcohol; this is called a "trail mix." When taken this way, the effect of a specific drug is difficult to assess, and the observed reactions by the adolescent to the combination of drugs often result in unexpected interactions and side effects.

The composition of most substances bought illegally is unreliable. Analyses of these substances reveal that many of the pills or powders, even if they resemble actual products sold legally, often are adulterated and may not even contain the substance they are purported to be.[1] In illegal laboratories, contaminants may be purposely or inadvertently added, and each time a drug is transferred from one person to another it is often "cut" with other products. Therefore, when a patient claims to have consumed a given compound he may be right, but more often than not he is mistaken and the reaction being experienced or observed by a third party is a mystery to all.

The identification and study of various receptors in the brain using modern technology such as positron emission tomography (PET) scan have led to a better understanding of the neuropharmacology of many of these products. Serotonin receptors have been associated with Ecstasy, dopamine receptors with methamphetamine, cannabinoid receptors with marijuana, and various opiod receptors with narcotics.[1,5] Large twin studies being performed in Europe and Australia are also providing us with more information on the genetic aspects of substance use.[6] This research will hopefully lead to a better understanding of substance use and its impact on humans.

Harm to the user also varies according to the mode of ingestion. Illegal drugs may be ingested orally, nasally, by inhalation, by injection, anally, or vaginally. The risks related to oral use include nausea, heartburn, and erosion of the wall of the stomach. Nasal or oral inhalation of fumes, powder, or vapors can irritate the nasal mucosa, sometimes leading to ulceration, infection, and perforation of the nasal mucosa, sinuses, and lungs. Intravenous drug use has multiple risks depending on the site of injection and on whether needles are shared. These risks are thrombophlebitis, emboli, arteriovenous fistula, and infections with HIV, syphilis, hepatitis B and C, mycotic emboli, and abscesses.[7] Anal and vaginal use can lead to erosion of mucous membranes. An assessment of risk must include a history on the mode of ingestion.

It is very difficult to predict the reaction a patient may have after the ingestion of a specific drug. Reactions are idiosyncratic and depend on gender, genetics, premorbid personality, the physical and emotional health of the person, and coingestion of other chemicals that may affect the rate of metabolism. Despite the confusion that may exist, being familiar with the expected reaction is helpful in treating and counseling patients. See Table 178-1 for detailed information.

## SPECIFIC SUBSTANCES

### HALLUCINOGENS

The hallucinogens are a broad variety of naturally occurring and synthetic compounds. They are one of the more popular drugs used by adolescents of all ages.[3] They have been defined as "any agent that causes alterations in perception, cognition, and mood as its primary psychological actions in the presence of an other wise clear sensorium."[8] These include 3 different groups of compounds based on their chemical structure: (1) ergolines (eg, LSD), (2) simple indoleamine hallucinogens (eg, psilocybin), (3) ring-substituted phenethyamine hallucinogens (eg, mescaline, Ecstasy).[9] Other compounds used by adolescents have hallucinogenic effects: piperidines (eg, phencyclidine or ketamine) and cannabinoids (marijuana), and have been included in this category by other authors.[10] The major concern related to the use of these drugs is psychiatric complications, mainly psychosis.

### CLUB DRUGS

Club drugs are a disparate group that have the common characteristic of frequently being used during dance events or in the club environment. They include amphetamine and its many derivatives, ketamine, and other hallucinogens such as psilocybin and LSD, gamma hydroxybutyrate (GHB) and its precursors, marijuana, and pharmaceutical compounds such as benzodiazepines and medications used to treat erectile dysfunction. As amphetamine and methamphetamine, MDMA (or Ecstasy), Ketamine, and GHB are the most commonly used, they will be discussed in the following.

Amphetamine, a stimulant, is available in various formulations and is used commonly by adolescents. Amphetamines were first synthesized in the early 20th century and first entered medical use in the 1930s.[1] They are often synthesized in illegal laboratories, although one of their most common formulations is dextroamphetamine used in the treatment of attention-deficit disorder.[11] The rate of absorption varies depending on the compound and the mode of ingestion. The duration of the effect also varies, from 8 hours for amphetamine to up to 24 hours for methamphetamine. The high is usually followed by a marked depression 2 to 3 days later. Ecstasy (MDMA) is an analogue of amphetamine. Ecstasy comes as a crystallized powder pressed into tablets with fashionable logos imprinted on the surface. Its popularity as a club drug has been decreasing in the last 10 years.[3]

**Table 178-1**

**Characteristics of Substances of Abuse**

| *Categories/Names* | *Ingestion/ Metabolism/ Excretion* | *Desired Effects* | *Toxic Effects* | *Long-Term Effects* | *Withdrawal* |
|---|---|---|---|---|---|
| ***I—Stimulants*** | | | | | |
| **Amphetamines** speed, whiz, billy, wake up, peach, uppers, pep pills, jolly beans, truck drivers, copilots, eye-openers, footballs, dexies, bennies, dexedrine, adderall, benzedrine | Ingestion: oral, intranasal, intravenous, vaginally, anally, dabbing on gums<br>Site of action: catecholamine, dopamine, and serotonin transmitters<br>Metabolism: liver<br>Excretion: urine; detected for 2–3 days; crosses placental fetal blood barrier, excreted in human milk<br>Duration of effect: up to 8 hours | Euphoria; increased energy, physical activity, and self-esteem; emotional disinhibition | Psychosis; paranoia; anxiety; vomiting; increase in blood pressure, arterial pulse, and body temperature; arrhythmias; seizures; CVA; rhabdomyolysis, erectile dysfunction | Neurotoxic, possibly related to early onset of Parkinson like symptoms, psychosis, paranoia, insomnia, irritability<br>Dependence | Depression, fatigue, lethargy |
| **Methamphetamine** ice, crystal, tweak, crank, glass, tina | Ingestion: as per amphetamines; inhaling of vapors produced when heated<br>Site of action: as per amphetamines<br>Metabolism: as per amphetamines<br>Excretion: urine<br>Duration of effect: up to 24 hours | As per amphetamines | As per amphetamines | As per amphetamines<br>Associated with an increase in STIs and HIV<br>Damage to dopamine receptors<br>Dependence | As per amphetamines |
| **Ecstasy** MDMA, X, E, XTC, Adam | Ingestions: pills orally or crushed and inhaled nasally<br>Site of action: serotonin and dopamine receptors<br>Metabolism: liver, P450 system, rate dependent on amount ingested and genetics<br>Excretion: urine<br>Duration: 6 hours | Stimulation but not as marked with amphetamines; perception of time acceleration; increased feeling of wellness, self-esteem, better communication | Similar to amphetamines but not as marked, trismus, hyperthermia, renal insufficiency, cerebral hemorrhage, serotonin syndrome, erectile dysfunction, decreased vaginal lubrication | Neurotoxic to serotonin receptors, clinical manifestation of memory loss<br>Dependence less frequent than with amphetamines | As per amphetamines |

*(Continued)*

**Table 178-1 (Continued)**

| *Categories/Names* | *Ingestion/ Metabolism/ Excretion* | *Desired Effects* | *Toxic Effects* | *Long-Term Effects* | *Withdrawal* |
|---|---|---|---|---|---|
| **Cocaine** Coke, Charlie, snow, powder, nose candy, crack, white lady, toot | Ingestion: oral, intranasal, rectal, intravenous, smoked Site of action: norepinephrine, dopamine, and serotonin receptors Metabolism: liver or plasma esterases Excretion: urine 2–3 days and up to 8 days for chronic users, hair for weeks or months, blood assay can also be performed Duration: a half-hour intranasal, 10 minutes when smoked as "crack" | Intense euphoria and excitation, increased self-confidence and sexuality, indifference to worries and cares | As per other stimulants Increased risk of MI | Dependence | Despair, depression, fatigue |
| **Ephedrine, pseudoephedrine, ephedra, Ma Hwang** | Ingestion: oral, nasal, or brewed in tea Duration: up to 8 hours | Increased awareness, physical arousal | Anxiety, hypertension, seizures, agitation, muscular spasms, palpitations, dry mouth, MI | | |
| **Ritalin, methylphenidate** | Ingestion: oral, nasal, intravenous | Increased physical arousal and wakefulness | As per stimulants | Dependence | Depression |
| **Caffeine, guarana** | Ingestion: oral as pills or liquid | Increased physical arousal and wakefulness | Nervousness; anxiety; increased pulse rate, blood pressure, and body temperature; nausea; vomiting; headaches; insomnia; seizures | Dependence | Depression, headaches |
| **Methcathinone** Cat, Khat, Dqat | Ingestion: chewing of herb (catha edulis) | Increased physical arousal and wakefulness | As per amphetamines | | |

*(Continued)*

**Table 178-1 (Continued)**

| *Categories/Names* | *Ingestion/ Metabolism/ Excretion* | *Desired Effects* | *Toxic Effects* | *Long-Term Effects* | *Withdrawal* |
|---|---|---|---|---|---|
| ***II—Hallucinogens*** | | | | | |
| **Amphetamine derivatives**<br>MDMA = Ecstasy<br>MDA = Love Pill<br>MDE = Eve<br>2-CB = Nexus | As per Ecstasy and other stimulants | Hallucinogen effect increases with progression down the list | As per stimulants | As per stimulants | As per stimulants |
| **Ketamine** | See sedatives | See sedatives | See sedatives | See sedatives | See sedatives |
| **Marijuana** | See sedatives | See sedatives | See sedatives | See sedatives | See sedatives |
| **Dextromethorphan**<br>DMX, Robo, DM, Robitussin DM | Ingestion: orally as a pill or syrup<br>Metabolism: liver, some individuals lack P450-2D6, which may lead to toxicity<br>Excretion: urine may give a positive PCP test result | Euphoria and hallucinations | Lethargy, dizziness, perspiration, ataxia, tachycardia, hypertension, hyperthermia, seizures<br>Several side effects from other products included in the pill or syrup | Depression; psychosis; suicidal tendencies; decreased language capacity, motor function, and memory | |
| **Lysergic acid**<br>LSD, acid, blotter, candy, sugar cube, A, microdots, 25+, pink jesus, purple wedges | Ingestion: orally on blotting paper, sugar cubes, or gelatin leaves<br>Duration: up to 12 hours | Auditory and visual hallucinations, euphoria | Depression; panic; increased body temperature, heart rate, and blood pressure; insomnia | | |
| **Phencyclidine**<br>PCP, angel dust, mess, PeaCe pill, rocket fuel, magic dust, DOA, elephant tranquilizer, wack | Ingestion: orally by capsules or pills, occasionally intravenously, intranasally, and smoked<br>Site of action: inhibition of dopamine, norepinephrine, serotonin, and GABA receptors<br>Metabolism: liver<br>Excretion: urine for 7–14 days | Hallucinations and euphoria | Low dose: disinhibition; dysphoria; myosis with nystagmus; shallow, quick breathing; increased pulse and arterial pressure; numbness<br>Large dose: psychosis; agitation; catatonia; decreased pulse, arterial pressure, and respiratory rate; nausea; vomiting; seizures; hypoglycemia; death | Psychosis, which may last days or weeks; flashbacks | |

*(Continued)*

**Table 178-1 (Continued)**

| *Categories/Names* | *Ingestion/ Metabolism/ Excretion* | *Desired Effects* | *Toxic Effects* | *Long-Term Effects* | *Withdrawal* |
|---|---|---|---|---|---|
| **Psilocybin** magic mushroom, mushroom, mush, shrooms, liberty caps | Ingestion: orally whole, or stewed into a liquid that is ingested<br>Metabolism: liver<br>Excretion: urine | Auditory and visual hallucinations | Dysphoria, paranoia | | |
| **Derivatives of tryptamine dimethyltryptamine (DMT)** happy pill, love pill | Ingestion: orally as a capsule | Euphoria, hallucinations | Aggressiveness, agitation, twitching, decreased blood pressure | | |
| **Nutmeg** | Ingestion: orally 2–3 nuts at a time<br>Duration: up to 24 hours | Hallucinations | Nausea, vomiting, dry mouth, abdominal pain, palpitations, weak pulse, and shallow breathing | | |
| **Hallucinogenic plants** peyote, San Pedro cactus, salvia, morning glory, Hawaiian baby woodrose, jimson weed | Ingestion: orally or in a tea<br>Source of mescaline | Hallucinations | Nausea, vomiting, abdominal pain, death since jimson weed is poisonous | | |
| ***III—Sedatives*** | | | | | |
| **Gamma hydroxybutyrate** GHB, liquid Ecstasy, cherry meth, G, Easy Lay, grievous bodily harm, gook, gamma 10, liquid G | Ingestion: orally in a capsule, as a powder, or dissolved in a liquid<br>Metabolism: in the liver to $CO_2$<br>Excretion: lungs<br>Duration: 1-3 hours | Euphoria, disinhibition, sexual interest; like alcohol but without a hangover | Mydriasis or myosis, nightmare, myoclonic movement, agitation, bradycardia, hypotension, nausea, vomiting, respiratory distress, amnesia, comatose state, respiratory arrest when mixed with alcohol | Dependence | Tremors, confusion, insomnia, nightmares, seizures, severe delirium with hallucinations |
| **Gamma butyrolactone** Blue nitro, Gamma-G, renewtrient, GHR<br>**1,4 butanediol** Thunder nectar, serenity | Ingestion: orally<br>Metabolism: in liver to GHB | As per GHB but onset takes longer because must be metabolized by liver first | As per GHB | As per GHB | As per GHB |

*(Continued)*

## Table 178-1 (Continued)

| *Categories/Names* | *Ingestion/ Metabolism/ Excretion* | *Desired Effects* | *Toxic Effects* | *Long-Term Effects* | *Withdrawal* |
|---|---|---|---|---|---|
| **Ketamine**<br>Special K, vitamin K, Ketalar, Ketaject, new Ecstasy | Ingestion: as a liquid orally or injected; as a powder orally, nasally, smoked<br>Excretion: urine may give a positive PCP test result<br>Duration: 2–3 hours with some effects lasting up to 24 hours | Relaxation<br>Hallucinations and visual distortions (K-land) | Dissociation, loss of time perception and identity, depression, flashbacks, delirium, amnesia, decreased motor function, hypertension, increased cardiac output, nausea, vomiting, decreased pain sensation and potential for increased injury, comatose state (K-hole) | Dependence<br>Still controversial as to neurological damage | Nervousness |
| **Marijuana**<br>pot, hash, weed, boom, Mary Jane, reefer, grass, roaches, dope, spiff, herb<br>**Hashish**<br>**Hash oil** | Ingestion: smoked in cigarettes (joints), pipe, cigar (blunt), eaten or drunk as a tea<br>Site of action: dopamine pathways, cannabinoid receptors<br>Metabolized: in liver by cytochrome P450<br>Stored in fatty tissue, brain, and testis<br>Excretion: 60% in feces; rest in urine; urine, 1–7 days for light use and up to 1 month with chronic use; blood assay can give quantitative levels | Euphoria, relaxation, mild hallucinations | Loss of coordination, slowed reaction time, anxiety, panic attacks, paranoia, injected conjunctiva, increased pulse rate | Memory loss, lung damage, decreased sperm count, gynecomastia | Anxiety |
| **Temazepam**<br>Jellies, wobbly eggs | Ingestion: orally as a capsule or pill, or dissolved and injected | Muscle relaxation, somnolence | | | |
| **Flunitrazepam**<br>Rohypnol, roofies, roach, Roche, Mexican valium<br>**Other benzodiazepines**<br>Pumpkin seeds | Ingestion: orally as a pill or dissolved in liquid<br>Site of action: GABA receptors (alpha subsite)<br>Excretion: urine<br>Duration: 6–8 hours | Relaxation, somnolence | Deep sedation, coordination problems, amnesia, respiratory distress | Dependence | Anxiety |

(*Continued*)

## Table 178-1 (Continued)

| *Categories/Names* | *Ingestion/ Metabolism/ Excretion* | *Desired Effects* | *Toxic Effects* | *Long-Term Effects* | *Withdrawal* |
|---|---|---|---|---|---|
| **Barbiturates**<br>Amobarbital (Amytal), pentobarbital (Nembutal), secobarbital (Seconal), phenobarbital (Fiorinal), barbs, goof balls, red devils, downers, block busters, pinks, reds and blues, yellow jackets, downers, Ace | Ingestion: orally<br>Site of action: GABA-A receptors suppressing serotonin, norepinephrine, and dopamine receptors<br>Metabolism: liver<br>Excretion: urine | Relaxation, somnolence | Hypothermia, myosis, nystagmus, hypoventilation, somnolence, paranoia, coma | Dependence | Seizures; unstable arterial pressure, cardiac rate, and temperature |
| **Opioids**<br>Heroin<br>Propoxiphene = lily<br>Methadone = orange<br>Fentanyls = STP, six pack<br>Codeine<br>Meperidine<br>Oxycodone<br>Hydrocodone<br>China cat, skag | Ingestion: oral; rectal; intranasal; injected subcutaneously, intradermally, intravenously<br>Site of action: mu, kappa, and delta opioid receptors<br>Excretion: urine, 1–3 days | Euphoria, relaxation, somnolence | Decreased body temperature, myosis, nausea, vomiting, tearing, rhinorrhea, pulmonary edema, cardiac arrhythmia | Dependence | Seizures, muscular pain, anxiety, insomnia, constipation |
| ***IV—Inhalants*** | | | | | |
| **Nitrites; amyl-, alkyl-, and iso-butyl**<br>Poppers, rush, locker room | Ingestion: orally | Euphoria, smooth muscle relaxation | Headaches, fainting, nausea, myocardial infarct, sinusitis | Neurological damage<br>Methemoglobinemia<br>Associated with the transmission of HIV | |
| **Solvents, anesthetic agents, and hydrocarbons**<br>Ether, toluene, benzene, chloroform, gasoline, glue, paint, and paint thinners | Ingestion: inhalation, sniffing, snorting, bagging (from a bag), huffing (saturating a bag and placing the rag in the mouth), spraying in the mouth<br>Metabolism: liver<br>Excretion: lungs | Disinhibition, euphoria, hallucinations | Confusion, hallucinations, ataxia, aggressivity, arrhythmias, coma<br>Freezing of larynx from spray<br>Dependence | Hepatotoxicity, sensitization of myocardium to endogenous catecholamines, cerebral atrophy (toluene), distal renal tubular acidosis (toluene), peripheral neuropathy (n-hexane), aplastic anemia (benzene), leukemia (benzene) | |
| **Nitrous oxide**<br>Whippets | Ingestion: nasally or orally | Mild dissociative experience | Freezing of larynx leading to vagal reflex causing arrhythmias, hypoxia, nausea | Peripheral neuropathy | |

CVA, cerebrovascular accident; MI, myocardial infarction; STIs, sexually transmitted infections

Methamphetamine is another derivative of amphetamine causing concern due to its high addictive potential and its relationship to unsafe sexual practices leading to a higher incidence of sexually transmitted infections (STIs) including HIV in users. It is a powerful central nervous system stimulant that is cheaply synthesized in illegal or clandestine home labs with easily available ingredients. "Meth," "speed," "crystal," and "ice" are names used to refer to this substance. The crystalline form can be smoked in a pipe like "crack," but other formulations can be ingested orally, nasally, rectally, and injected. Methamphetamine is lipophilic, readily crosses the blood–brain barrier, and has a long half-life ranging from 10 to 20 hours. There is solid evidence that chronic use of this drug leads to cerebral damage.

Two anesthetics used in the club environment are ketamine (special K, K, or vitamin K) and GHB, or G. Ketamine was developed in 1962 and is currently used as an anesthetic in veterinary medicine, pediatrics, and in the management of chronic pain.[12-14] It is taken for its hallucinogenic potential. Gamma hydroxy butyrate and its precursors butyrolactone and 1,4 butanediol are usually sold as a liquid and taken in their concentrated form from small vials or diluted in water or other liquids.[13] It was developed as an adjunct to anesthesia in the early 1950s and is now used primarily in the treatment of narcolepsy. Both of these substances, as well as rohypnol, have been used as "date rape drugs." For this purpose, they are usually added to a drink of some sort that has been left unattended by the victim. However, it is important to remember that the substance most often implicated in nonconsensual sex is alcohol.

Pharmaceuticals used by adolescents may include barbiturates, benzodiazepines, and opioids. All of these can create dependence, with withdrawal from barbiturates potentially life threatening. Opioids are of concern because they are commonly used intravenously, which may lead to several serious medical complications. The prevalence of use of 2 narcotics, Vicodin and OxyContin, has been increasing since the early 1990s.[3]

### INHALANTS

Inhalants are the second most commonly used drugs by eighth-grade students after marijuana, excluding alcohol and nicotine.[3] This group includes numerous compounds normally found around the home and easily accessible to most adolescents. They are defined as being volatile at room temperature, not included in a pharmacologically distinct class, and used by sniffing, snorting, bagging, huffing, or spraying in the mouth.[15] They can be divided into 3 main groups: volatile solvents, nitrous oxide, and nitrites.[15] The solvents are the most commonly used. These include household or industrial products, such as glues, shoe polish, Liquid Paper, lighter fluid, gasoline, paint thinner, and spray paints. They usually contain several compounds including such products as toluene, n-hexane, chlorohydrocarbons, or benzene.[15-17] Nitrous oxide or "laughing gas" may be used by adolescents at home or in the rave environment. It is inhaled from balloons, or from "whippets," which are small gas-filled containers used to make whipped cream in restaurants. The sudden release of nitrous oxide from these "whippets" may lead to cooling or freezing of the larynx, causing a reflex vagal inhibition leading to arrhythmias and sudden death.[17] Nitrites include amyl, butyl, and isobutyl nitrites. They are used most commonly by an older age group and are more closely associated with the gay community.[18] They are known as "poppers" and are used to induce euphoria and to enhance sexual experience. They produce a relaxation of smooth muscle, making anal penetration easier.[18]

## CONCLUSION

Despite what parents like to believe, experimenting with substances both legal and illegal is a common occurrence during adolescence. Most adolescents will use them a few times and nothing will come of it; however, others will get into trouble. Some problems will occur because of the potential effects these substances may have on physical and mental health, others because of the legal complications that may result from the possession, distribution, and consumption of these products. Finally, a number of adolescents will become habitual users. The risk factors related to potential substance use may be individual, family, and peer-related as outlined in Table 178-2. It is therefore important to identify young people at risk and to provide them with appropriate and timely counseling.

As previously mentioned, the substances most frequently used by adolescents are alcohol, marijuana, and cocaine. This chapter deals with other drugs less commonly used by the teenage population. However, it is important to be familiar with these products, because they are the drugs of choice used in specific situations by some subgroups of adolescents. Although you are provided with current information on many of these substances, remember this is a continuously evolving field, and you should keep yourself updated using a variety of sources including scientific literature, the popular media, your local law enforcement officer, and most importantly, your patients.

**Table 178-2**

**Risk Factors for Substance Abuse**

| *Category of Risk* | *Description* |
|---|---|
| Individual | Male sex |
| | Biogenetic influences |
| | Low socioeconomic factors in childhood |
| | Adverse life events |
| | Beginning to use harmful substances at an early age |
| | Poor self-esteem |
| | Personality and temperamental problems |
| | Sensation seeking |
| | Comorbid mental health problems |
| Family | Lack of family connectedness |
| | Dysfunctional parenting traits |
| | Substance use by family members |
| | Physical or sexual abuse |
| Peers | Peers who use substances |
| | Peers who engage in risky behavior |
| | Lack of group identity |

## REFERENCES

1. Tellier P-P. The adolescent and substance use, an approach to office management. *Prim Care.* 2006;33:517–530

2. Tellier P-P. Club drugs: is it all ecstasy? *Pediatr Ann.* 2002;31(9):550–556

3. Johnston LD, O'Malley PM, Bachman JG, Schulenberg JE. *Monitoring the Future National Results on Adolescent Drug Use: Overview of Key Findings, 2008.* NIH Publication No. 09-7401. Bethesda, MD: National Institute of Drug Abuse; 2006

4. Substance Abuse and Mental Health Administration, Office of Applied Studies. *Results from the 2007 National Survey on Drug Use and Health: National Findings.* Rockville, MD: Office of Applied Studies, NSDUH Series H-34, DHHS Publication No SMA 08-4343; 2008

5. Obrocki J, Schmoldt A, Buchert R, Andresen B, Petersen K, Thomasius R. Specific neurotoxicity of chronic use of ecstasy. *Toxicology Lett.* 2002;127(1-3):285–297

6. Lynskey MT, Grant JD, Nelson EC, et al. Duration of cannabis use—a novel phenotype? *Addict Behav.* 2006;31(6):984–994

7. Stein MD. Medical consequences of substance abuse. *Psychiatr Clin North Am.* 1999;22(2):351–370

8. Abraham HD, Aldridge AM, Gogia P. The psychopharmacology of hallucinogens. *Neuropsychopharmacology.* 1996; 14(4):285–298

9. Marek GJ, Aghajanian GK. Indoleamine and the phenethylamine hallucinogens: mechanisms of psychotomimetic action. *Drug Alcohol Depend.* 1998;51(1-2):189–198

10. Salomone JA. III. Toxicity, hallucinogen. eMedicine. Available at: www.emedicine.com/emerg/topic223.htm. Accessed July 23, 2009

11. Derlet R, Albertson T. Toxicity, methamphetamine. eMedicine. Available emedicine.medscape.com/article/820918-overview. Accessed July 27, 2010

12. Dotson JW, Ackerman DL, West LJ. Ketamine abuse. *J Drug Issues.* 1995;25(4):751–757

13. Nicholson KL, Balster RL. GHB: a new and novel drug of abuse. *Drug Alcohol Depend.* 2001;63(1):1–22

14. Jansen KLR. A review of nonmedical use of ketamine: use, users, and consequences. *J Psychoactive Drugs.* 2000; 32(4):419–433

15. Brouette T, Anton R. Clinical review of inhalants. *Am J Addict.* 2001;10(1):79–94

16. Kurtzman TL, Otsuka KN, Wahl RA. Inhalant abuse by adolescents. *J Adolesc Health.* 2001;28(3):170–180

17. Lorenc JD. Inhalant abuse in the pediatric population: a persistent challenge. *Curr Opin Pediatr.* 2003;15(2):204–209

18. Haverkos HW, Kopstein AN, Wilson H, Drotman P. Nitrite inhalants: history, epidemiology, and possible links to AIDS. *Environ Health Perspect.* 1994;102(10):858–861

# CHAPTER 179

# Abuse of Prescription Drugs

SUSAN R. BRILL, MD

## INTRODUCTION

Clinicians who take care of adolescents are aware of the increasing misuse of prescription drugs. The growing recreational use of prescription medications such as stimulants, narcotics, and tranquilizers has caught the attention of medical researchers and lay people alike. The Partnership for a Drug-Free America has referred to today's teenagers as "Generation Rx."[1] An article in *Reader's Digest* entitled "The Dangerous New High" detailed several cases of such substance abuse.[2] Although prescription drugs have been abused in the past, the increased variety and prescriptions of narcotics and stimulants, in particular, have led to more availability for young people. In addition, many adolescents have misperceived the pills as "safer" than street drugs because they have observed their parents and family members using these drugs appropriately; and the ease of acquisition is no more difficult than looking in the family medicine cabinet.

The spectrum of prescription drug use and misuse is important to define. A patient who is taking a prescribed stimulant drug for attention-deficit/hyperactivity disorder (ADHD) in appropriate doses is following a doctor's direction. However, particular patterns of use can engender greater risk of harm than benefit. Escalating use of a drug without discussion with a physician, use of the substance for effects beyond the medical condition for which it is prescribed (using to "get high"), or continued use despite negative consequences all connote inappropriate medication use.[3]

## EPIDEMIOLOGY

Increasing nonmedical use of prescription drugs has been noted since the 1990s. Data obtained from the National Household Survey on Drug Abuse noted an increase of 452% in emergency department visits related to the use of oxycodone hydrochloride (Oxycodone) from 1994 to 2001. This survey is now known as the National Survey on Drug Use and Health (NSDUH). It is a telephone survey that collects data for both teenagers and adults. Respondents ages 12 and older are asked questions related to their drug and alcohol use. One category queried is the nonmedical use of "psychotherapeutic prescription drugs." This includes pain relievers, tranquilizers, stimulants, and sedatives.

When the adolescent data from NSDUH are analyzed, several trends emerge. Among children ages 12 to 17, lifetime use of any psychotherapeutic prescription drug was reported as 13.5% in 2004 and had decreased to 11.9% by 2005. Most of the drugs used were pain relievers. Interestingly, females ages 12 to 17 reported 12.7% lifetime use of prescription drugs in 2005, whereas 12- to 17-year-old males reported 11.1%. However, among young adults ages 18 to 20, the nonmedical use of these drugs increased from 27.7% in 2004 to 28.1% lifetime use in 2005. There was a greater frequency of use among these young people; in fact, 6.7% reported use in the past month.

There are also data on mean age of first use among past year initiates of substances. Among those questioned by NSDUH who had used before age 21, 16.3 years was the mean age of first use of psychotherapeutics. Those who started before 18 years of age used their first psychotherapeutic at age 15.1 years. The same individuals in both groups also began using marijuana at the same relative ages. Therefore, it may be inferred that nonmedical use of prescription drugs begins at the same time as marijuana use; often both can be considered "gateway" drugs. The NSDUH data also support the notion that teens who use any substance early, such as tobacco and alcohol, often use "harder" drugs earlier as well. Finally, teenagers ages 12 to 17 were asked the source of the drugs they obtained. Almost 50% of them responded "friend or relative for free." Young adults also obtained the pills in this manner, but a substantial percentage reported getting them from a doctor or more than one doctor.[4]

Another yearly study that focuses only on teenagers is the Monitoring the Future study sponsored by the National Institute on Drug Abuse, which is designed and conducted by researchers at the University of Michigan. The study annually surveys a representative sample of approximately 50,000 students in 400 public and private secondary schools in the United States. Although widely referenced, this study does have a limitation in that it does not survey youth not enrolled in school, who are presumed to be at higher risk of substance use and abuse.

The Monitoring the Future study analyzes current data and tracks use over the past 3 decades. The survey included more than 46,000 students for 2008. In this survey year, tables that combined data among 8th, 10th, and 12th graders were introduced that allow for analysis of overall trends. For all students surveyed, there has been continued decline in lifetime illicit drug use, reported as 32.6% in 2008, since the peak of 43.3% in 1997. However, there were continued high rates of nonmedical use of prescription medications, especially opioid painkillers. In 2008, lifetime nonmedical use by 12th graders of Percocet, Vicodin, and Oxycontin was 13.2%, not much change from 13.5% in 2004, but representing a huge increase from the 2001 report of 9.9%. Past year use was broken out by drug: Oxycontin was used by 2.1% of 8th graders, 3.6% of 10th graders, and 4.7% of 12th graders, and Vicodin was used by 2.9% of 8th graders, 6.7% of 10th graders, and 9.7% of 12th-grade students within the past year. From these data, the age of first use of these agents is in early to mid-adolescence. Overall trends that compare prescription drug use to other frequently abused drugs are illustrated in Figure 179-1.[5]

Stimulant use was queried by asking about amphetamines or Ritalin (not prescribed by a doctor). The annual prevalence in 2008 for amphetamine use was 4.5% for 8th graders, 6.4% for 10th graders, and 6.8% for 12th graders; the Ritalin prevalence data were 1.6%, 2.9%, and 3.4%, respectively. These are relatively static numbers and, in fact, represent a decreasing trend over the past decade. Finally, sedatives (barbiturates) were tried by 5.8% of 12th graders (a significant decrease from 7.2% in 2005), and tranquilizers (Xanax) were used by 6.2% of senior students.[5]

Subjects are also asked about perceived availability of drugs. When asked about the availability of "other narcotic drugs" (which includes Vicodin, Oxycontin, and Percocet), a full 35% of youth in 12th grade reported they were "fairly easy" or "very easy" to get. Availability of amphetamines was reported as "fairly easy" or "very easy" to get by almost 50% of 12th graders, and even by 21% of 8th graders. Because this category includes several prescription drugs prescribed for ADHD, drug diversion from legitimate prescriptions remains a significant source of nonmedical use of these stimulants.

## SPECIFIC PRESCRIPTION DRUGS COMMONLY ABUSED

Clinicians should be aware of effects of commonly used prescription drugs.[6] Recognition of these symptoms are especially important when adolescents present with altered levels of consciousness. Table 179-1 provides a summary of the physiological effects and signs of opioid, amphetamine, and sedative overdose.

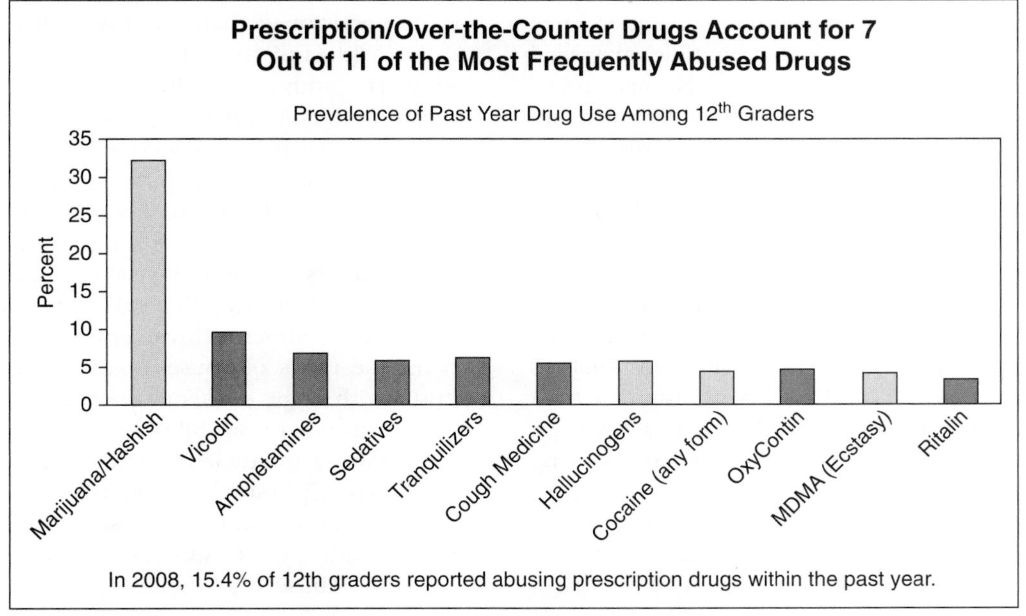


**FIGURE 179-1** Past year use of prescription drugs and commonly abused illicit drugs. (Johnston LD, O'Malley PM, Bachman JG, Schulenberg JE. *Monitoring the Future national results on adolescent drug use: Overview of key findings, 2008* (NIH Publication No. 09-7401). Bethesda, MD: National Institute on Drug Abuse; 2009.)

**Table 179-1**

**Effects of Commonly Abused Prescription Drugs**

| *Prescription Drug Class* | *Common Drugs Abused* | *Physiological Effects* | *Overdose Effects* | *Treatment of Overdosage* | *Withdrawal Symptoms* |
|---|---|---|---|---|---|
| Opioid | Vicodin<br>Lortab<br>Dilaudid<br>Oxycontin | Pain relief<br>Euphoria<br>Drowsiness<br>Constipation | Respiratory depression<br>Miosis<br>Hypotension | Monitored setting<br>Naloxone | Insomnia<br>Rhinorrhea<br>Diarrhea<br>Hypertension<br>Tachycardia |
| Stimulants | Ritalin<br>Dexedrine<br>Adderall<br>Concerta | Increased alertness<br>Increased attention and concentration | Restlessness<br>Insomnia<br>Arrhythmias<br>Seizures<br>Psychosis | Activated charcoal<br>Supportive care | Depression<br>Drug craving |
| Sedatives/ tranquilizers | Valium<br>Xanax<br>Klonopin | Sleepiness<br>Relaxation | Nystagmus<br>Respiratory<br>Depression<br>Ataxia, Confusion | Monitored setting<br>Supportive care | Anxiety<br>Hallucinations<br>Seizures |

**OPIOIDS**

Oxycodone, hydrocodone (Vicodin, Lortab), hydromorphone (Dilaudid), and morphine (MS Contin) are considered opioids. Common street names include "killers," OC, Oxy, and Oxycotton. These medicines are prescribed for acute or chronic pain relief, or relief of cough or diarrhea. They work by attaching to opioid receptors in the brain and spinal cord, such as mu ($\mu$), kappa ($\kappa$), and delta ($\delta$) receptors, that are mediators of analgesia. They also activate reward pathways that in time may lead to addiction. In the short term, they cause pain relief, drowsiness, and decreased contractility of the small and large intestine, leading to constipation. Overdose may cause respiratory depression, particularly if combined with other respiratory depressants such as alcohol. In addition, miosis and central nervous system depression are seen. Management should be done in a monitored setting because pulmonary edema may develop. Naloxone may be administered as an antagonist to make the diagnosis, as well as to reverse symptoms such as respiratory depression. Withdrawal symptoms such as restlessness, insomnia, rhinorrhea, diarrhea, tachycardia, and hypertension can usually be managed by offering supportive care.

Sung et al[7] provided a large-scale analysis of data from the NSDUH over the past 30 years to identify trends and correlates of prescription opioid use. The first wave of increasing misuse was in the early 1970s, when use increased from less than 0.5% to 2.1% lifetime use. The prevalence decreased during the 1980s, but a second youth epidemic was identified starting in the early 1990s, with an increase in the prevalence rate of 618% by 2002. After analysis of several demographic and social variables was conducted, the authors found that females, older adolescents, whites, and individuals from low-income families constituted the higher-risk groups for past year misuse. The prevalence rates were higher among those who had a history of delinquent activities or recent mental health problems. Rates of misuse were higher among users of alcohol and tobacco and "nearly endemic" among users of illicit drugs or those that misused other prescription drugs. The authors conclude that the current trend of prescription opioid misuse "looks remarkably like an epidemic...which has coincided with the increase in medical use of newer opioids for pain management."[7]

One group of adolescents especially vulnerable to abuse of opioids are those with chronic illness. Often these patients are medically savvy with regard to brand and dose of drugs that they have experienced for legitimate pain treatment. However, they can be vulnerable to unique types of abuse. Box 179-1 describes a case report with tragic consequences.

The growing availability of these drugs creates new opportunities for their illegal diversion, trafficking, and abuse. When physicians prescribe drugs, they may not always ask about previous substance abuse history. Data from a study by the National Center on Addiction and Substance Abuse of Columbia University reported that 43% did not ask about prescription drug abuse when taking a patient's history, and one-third did not regularly call or obtain records from previous physicians before prescribing potentially addictive drugs.[9]

## Box 179-1

### *Case Report*

Smith et al[8] reported an unusual case of an adolescent with cystic fibrosis (CF) who presented with declining pulmonary function and worsening disease. The patient had a 6-month history of recurring episodes of cough, exercise intolerance, and declining pulmonary function tests. She was treated aggressively with antibiotics and supportive care but continued to do poorly. Her chest CT showed clustered micronodular opacities. On lung biopsy, these were identified as crystalline material resembling calcium oxalate. One day after her hospital discharge, she unfortunately had an acute onset of chest pain and shortness of breath, and expired while at home. On autopsy, the lung was analyzed and found to have material identified as crospovidone, an insoluble polymer used as a disintegrant in pharmaceutical tablets. Prescription records showed that the patient had filled 4 prescriptions for Vicodin during the previous 16 months, the most recent of which was filled the day before her death. Because the patient had an indwelling central venous catheter, the clinicians surmised that the patient was crushing the Vicodin and injecting it into the port on a regular basis. The authors concluded that adolescent and young adult patients with chronic illness such as CF, sickle cell disease, and malignancy may be at higher risk for intravenous abuse of prescription drugs.[8] Clinicians need to be aware of untoward reactions and unexplained clinical deterioration, as well as social and emotional deterioration commonly seen with advanced abuse of these drugs.

## STIMULANTS

The commonly prescribed stimulants include dextroamphetamine (Dexedrine and Adderall) and methylphenidate (Ritalin, Concerta). Slang names for Ritalin, in particular, include "kibbles and bits" and "pineapple." Stimulants are usually prescribed for ADHD, or occasionally for narcolepsy. They act on dopaminergic receptors to increase alertness, attention, and energy. In the short term, they cause dilated pupils, blood pressure and heart rate elevation, sleep interference, and appetite suppression. In the long term, there is potential for physical dependence and addiction to stimulants. Risks of stimulant overdose include arrhythmias, seizures, or heart failure. Paranoia is also reported with high doses. Drug-induced psychosis is also possible, which includes both visual and auditory hallucinations. Overdose can be treated with activated charcoal and cathartics for recent ingestions, and supportive care for hypertension and tachycardia. Withdrawal symptoms, which are possible with continued use of high doses of the drug, include severe mood swings, exhaustion, and increased appetite.

Many researchers have noted an increase in college students engaging in nonmedical use of stimulants. A study from a small US college surveyed 150 psychology students via anonymous questionnaires. Low et al[10] reported that approximately one-third (35.3%) of these students used amphetamine-dextroamphetamine, methylphenidate, or dextroamphetamine without a prescription. Of these users, 10% used them monthly, and about 8% weekly. Motivations for use included "to improve intellectual performance" and "to be more efficient on academic assignments." Some students commented that the stimulants enabled them to "party longer and drink more." Correlates of past year nonmedical use of prescription stimulants include previous mental health treatment utilization and use of marijuana and other illegal drugs. Adolescents who reported high family conflict and sensation seeking were also more likely to use these drugs.[11]

It is important for primary care providers to recognize adolescents who may be at high risk for nonmedical use and/or abuse of prescription stimulants. The precollege physical is an ideal time to educate adolescents about the ubiquitous nature of these drugs on college campuses, and a discussion of risk factors and warning signs would be appropriate in this setting.

## SEDATIVES/TRANQUILIZERS

Prescription medications included in this category include drugs such as pentobarbital (Nembutal) and benzodiazepines, such as diazepam (Valium), alprazolam (Xanax), and clonazepam (Klonopin). These drugs are usually prescribed for anxiety disorders, panic attacks, or sleep disorders. Sedatives act on the gamma amino butyric acid (GABA) system and slow brain activity. Sedatives are classified by duration of action. Ultra short-acting barbiturates, such as thiopental, act within 30 minutes and are used for anesthesia induction. Short-acting agents, such as pentobarbital and secobarbital, take 3 to 8 hours to demonstrate their effects, which are sedative and hypnotic. They are the most likely to be misused by teenagers. The shorter-acting agents that are more lipid soluble and protein bound are metabolized almost entirely in the liver to inactive products via the P450 microsomal enzyme.[11] Long-acting phenobarbital takes 1 to 2 days for clinical effect and is rarely abused. Short-term clinical effects result in users feeling sleepy and uncoordinated. There is a marked tolerance to these drugs, and a physical dependence and addiction may develop. If sedatives are stopped abruptly, seizures may result. If combined with alcohol, respiratory depression can ensue. Toxic effects of sedatives include nystagmus, ataxia, and mental confusion. Barbiturate withdrawal, which can be severe, may include anxiety, nausea and vomiting, hallucinations, delirium, and seizures.

In the Monitoring the Future survey, sedative use has demonstrated a decade-long rise in use from 1993 to 2003. Since then, the lifetime, past year, and past month use has declined somewhat. The combined 8th-, 10th-, and 12th-grade data from 2008 reported a lifetime prevalance of tranquilizers of 6.3%, a decrease from 7.9% noted in the earlier part of this decade.[5] Availability data indicate that 40% of 12th graders reported that sedatives are "fairly easy" to get, and 22% reported it was "fairly to very easy" to get tranquilizers. This is actually a significant decrease from the 1970s and 1980s.

## SPECIAL CONCERNS

Medical providers are the source of prescription drugs that teenagers abuse. Therefore, clinicians are responsible for how and to whom they prescribe psychoactive substances. To avoid diversion of drugs, clinicians need to be cognizant of common tactics patients would use to obtain prescription drugs with a high potential for abuse. A student may come in with vague concerns about attention problems in order to obtain stimulant medication, for example. Unclear pain syndromes or seeing multiple physicians for such problems are also a common modality to obtain narcotics with continued refills. In general, if the patient seems more concerned about getting medication than the problem itself, claims to have lost prescriptions, and seems sophisticated about various drug effects, these would be red flags for drug-seeking behavior. Clinicians should also be aware that parents may be the "index patient" as well. Prescription medication for another family member may be abused by the adolescent.[3]

Adolescents have been creative about obtaining drugs and resourceful in seeking information about them. The Internet may provide a source of the drugs and also a ready supply of information about the effects of various drugs they may find at home. The Internet contains several Web sites devoted to the use and effects of a variety of psychoactive substance. One study conducted a cross-sectional survey of patients being treated for substance abuse. Out of the 12 patients surveyed, 100% of them reported that information found on the Internet affected the ways in which they had used psychoactive substances. They reported changes in the uses of over-the-counter and prescription pharmaceuticals, such as dextromethorphan, Oxycontin, and Ritalin. One such online drug encyclopedia cited was Erowid (www.erowid.org). This Web site contains 20,000 documents that detail practical aspects of drug use, such as dosage, administration, and effects, covering more than 200 psychoactive substances. The site receives 6 million visits annually. Government Web sites that may more accurately detail the risks of these drugs are less accessible on search engines and may be less accepted by adolescents in general. The authors conclude that as adolescents become "experts" in a particular drug's effects, they can then disseminate that knowledge to peers to proliferate or increase the popularity of a particular pill or even brand name.[12] Clinicians may consider discussing such Web sites with their patients who are experimenting with prescription drugs to achieve a meaningful dialog about the benefits and risks of information on the Internet.

It is important to recognize that adolescents are in some sense surrounded by prescription drugs. As more teens are treated with psychoactive drugs to regulate mood, attention, and sleep, it is not surprising that they are becoming savvy consumers regarding the effects and variety of these drugs. They are also able to obtain them easily from friends, parents of friends, and the Internet. The perception of safety also blurs the line between legitimate prescriptions and misuse of the drugs. One director of a college psychiatry service observed that it is "nearly impossible to open a newspaper, turn on the television, or search the Internet without encountering an advertisement for a prescription medication... direct-to-consumer advertising...increased to $4.2 billion in 2004. One effect has been to foster an image of prescription drugs as an integral and routine aspect of everyday life." He urges that physicians should assess their patients for substance abuse and psychiatric illness before prescribing psychoactive drugs, and that they should be discussing the risk of diverted medications with their adult patients who have teenage children at home.[13]

## REFERENCES

1. The Partnership for a Drug-Free America. Generation Rx: National Study Reveals New Category of Substance Abuse Emerging: Teens Abusing Rx and OTC Medications Intentionally to Get High [news release]. November 16, 2005. Available at: www.westlakeparentconnection.com/DrugFacts/GenRxAbuseOTCDrugs.htm. Accessed November 30, 2010

2. Kaufman J. The dangerous new high. *Reader's Digest.* November 2006

3. Isaacson JH, Hopper JA, Alford DP, Parran T. Prescription drug use and abuse: risk factors, red flags, and prevention strategies. *Postgrad Med.* 2005;118(1):19–26

4. Substance Abuse and Mental Health Services Administration (SAMHSA), Office of Applied Studies. The National Survey on Drug Use and Health. 2006;(22). Available at: www.oas.samhsa.gov. Accessed November 3, 2006

5. Johnston LD, O'Malley PM, Bachman JG, Schulenberg JE. Monitoring the Future national results on adolescent drug use: Overview of key findings, 2008 (NIH Publication No. 09-7401). Bethesda, MD: National Institute on Drug Abuse; 2009

6. Schydlower M, ed. *Substance Abuse: A Guide for Health Professionals.* 2nd ed. Elk Grove Village, IL: American Academy of Pediatrics; 2002

7. Sung HE, Richter L, Vaughan R, Johnson P, Thom B. Nonmedical use of prescription opioids among teenagers in the United States: trends and correlates. *J Adolesc Health.* 2005;37(1):44-51

8. Smith K, Epidemic O, Dishop M, Eldin K, Tatevian N, Moore R. Intravenous injection of pharmaceutical tablets presenting as multiple pulmonary nodules and declining pulmonary function in an adolescent with cystic fibrosis. *Pediatrics.* 2006;118(3):e924-e928

9. Doe J. *Under the Counter: The Diversion and Abuse of Controlled Prescription Drugs in the U.S.* New York: National Center on Addiction and Substance Abuse, Columbia University; 2005

10. Low KG, Gendaszek AE. Illicit use of psychostimulants among college students: a preliminary study. *Psychol Health Med.* 2002;7(3):283-287

11. Herman-Stahl MA, Krebs CP, Kroutil LA, Heller DC. Risk and protective factors for nonmedical use of prescription stimulants and methamphetamine among adolescents. *J Adolesc Health.* 2006;39(3):374-380. Epub 2006 July 10

12. Boyer E, Shannon M, Hibberd P. The Internet and psychoactive substance use among innovative drug users. *Pediatrics.* 2005;115(2):302-305

13. Friedman R. The changing face of teenage drug abuse—the trend toward prescription drugs. *N Engl J Med.* 2006;354(14):1448-1450

# CHAPTER 180

# Overdose of Prescription Drugs

MICHELE J. FAGAN, MD • YOUNG-JIN SUE, MD

## INTRODUCTION

Toxic exposures in the pediatric population occur in a bimodal distribution. The first peak consists of newly mobile toddlers who, exploring their surroundings, find themselves momentarily undersupervised. Typically these accidental exposures, which involve a single agent in small quantities, are often of low medical consequence. In contrast, toxic exposures involving adolescents are typically intentional. Whether suicidal or recreational, adolescent exposures more often involve multiple substances in greater quantities. Although toxic exposures occur predominantly in young children, adolescents suffer disproportionately from clinical consequences and death.

The *2004 Annual Report of the American Association of Poison Control Centers Toxic Exposure Surveillance System* reported 51% of total exposures occurred in children younger than age 6. Most (74%) of the 27 fatalities were classified as accidental. In contrast, children aged 13 to 19 years totalled only 7% of total exposures. Yet in this group there were 90 fatalities, of which 79 (88%) were due to intentional causes.[1]

A myriad of physiologic and psychosocial changes an adolescent endures conspires to place the teen in a unique position of risk with respect to toxic exposures. Developing independence, the experience of sexual maturation, and increasing pressures of middle school social dynamics cultivate opportunities ripe for experimentation with both legally available and illicit psychoactive substances. Social isolation, conflict with parents and teachers, and nascent abstract thinking unchecked by underdeveloped coping skills contribute to feelings of hopelessness and thoughts of suicide. Adolescents who are dating may fall prey to drug-assisted sexual assault. Competitive athletes may feel pressure to pharmacologically enhance their performance potential. Dissatisfaction with body image contributes to anorexia nervosa and bulimia with abuse of emetics and cathartics for weight loss.[2] Chronic medical conditions such as diabetes are perceived as especially burdensome by adolescents. Some adolescents enter the job market where their lack of experience and risk-taking behavior place them at added risk for occupational hazards.[3] Pregnant adolescents suffer consequences of toxic exposures not only to themselves but also to their developing fetuses.[4,5]

## GENERAL APPROACH

In adolescent toxic exposures, the identity of the toxic substance is often unknown. The adolescent may be unwilling, unaware, or too symptomatic to share vital information. In addition to the identity of the substance, treating the poisoning requires knowledge of the quantity of substance, the route of exposure (eg, ingestion, inhalation, dermal, parenteral), and time of exposure. Contributory medical history and knowledge of medications and allergies are required for expeditious management of the exposure.

Three questions are central to the management of toxic exposures in adolescents:

1. Will there be adverse medical consequences?
2. What can be done to avoid those consequences?
3. How much time is available to decide on and institute intervention?

It is true that the dose makes the poison. As occurs with most toddler toxic exposures, there may be little or no medical consequences if the dose is small. In these cases, overzealous or inappropriate intervention may be more harmful than the exposure. Many substances are harmful if exposure occurs above the toxic threshold. This is true for therapeutic compounds that are acceptable in recommended doses but toxic in overdose. Some substances are considered poisonous in any amount—medications with narrow therapeutic windows and naturally occurring highly toxic substances, cyanide and arsenic, for example.

Once a toxic exposure is deemed medically consequential, information is required concerning the substances' unique toxicities, decontamination options, specific therapies and, for the critically ill patient, resuscitation measures. The physician should access the local poison information hotline for help in identifying the substance and managing the exposure.

If the patient is in extremis, resuscitative measures are initiated simultaneously with information gathering.

Fortunately, diagnostic and therapeutic decisions may more often be made less emergently. The pharmacodynamic and toxicokinetic features of a given substance determine whether the anticipated medical consequences will occur within minutes or days.

## EMERGENCY MANAGEMENT

The goals of emergency management are to stabilize, evaluate, diagnose, treat, and monitor. In the adolescent with altered level of consciousness, there must be efforts to ascertain effective ventilation and perfusion. Standard advanced pediatric life support protocols are often but not always appropriate in the setting of toxic exposures. Care should be taken to limit ongoing exposure to patient and providers by removing contaminated clothing and using personal protective barriers such as masks, gowns, and gloves.

## HISTORY

Evaluation begins with a toxin-focused history and physical examination. Eliciting an accurate history often requires persistent detective work. The adolescent may not be candid when the goal is to evade legal or parental consequences. The truly suicidal will be reticent to share information that may thwart the attempt. When a poisoning occurs from malicious action perpetrated by one teen against another, the victims are unaware of the substances to which they have been exposed. Sometimes, the adolescent is impaired or even unconscious. The examiner needs to doggedly pursue the substance's identity by repeatedly interviewing the patient, friends, significant others, bystanders, parents, and siblings. Identification is aided by knowledge of current substances favored by the local adolescent population and by the contents of the patient's home and medicine cabinet. A history of depression, past suicide attempt, or a story that doesn't make sense should raise suspicion of toxic exposure.

## PHYSICAL EXAMINATION AND TOXIDROMES

All adolescent patients whose physical presentation is inconsistent with the story should be considered to have had a possible toxic exposure. Abnormal vital signs, specific neurologic findings, odors, and toxidromes, (groups of signs and symptoms that characterize a specific class of compounds) all hold clues to the identity of the toxic exposure. Classes of agents reliably produce alterations of specific vital signs. Sympathomimetic agents such as pseudoephedrine or cocaine produce tachycardia, hypertension, and agitation. Overdose of opioid agents leads to hypotension, bradycardia, hypothermia, and hypoventilation. Calcium channel blocker overdose results in refractory hypotension and bradycardia. Overdose of phenylpropanolamine, an agent with nearly pure alpha-receptor agonism, results in hypertension and reflex beta-receptor-mediated bradycardia. Hyperthermia is seen in cocaine and salicylate overdose. Salicylates cause hyperventilation following overdose via a centrally mediated stimulation of respiratory drive.

### Box 180-1

#### *Altered Mental Status Toxicological Differential Diagnosis*

| ***Primary CNS Depression*** | ***Secondary CNS Depression*** |
|---|---|
| Benzodiazepines | Simple asphyxiants displace oxygen, eg, carbon dioxide |
| Opioids | Chemical asphyxiants impair oxygen-carrying capacity, eg, carbon monoxide |
| Barbiturates | Hypoglycemic agents |
| Alcohol | Hypotensive agents |
| Clonidine | |
| Antidepressants | |
| Antipsychotics | |
| Anticonvulsants | |
| Antihistamines | |
| Anticholinergics | |

Note that this is a general, not exhaustive list

CNS, central nervous system.

Numerous classes of compounds cause sedation in overdose (Box 180-1). Many compounds have primary sedative properties. Other compounds cause sedation by producing hypoglycemia, hypoxia, hypotension, or hypothermia. Many drugs have proconvulsant activity. Isoniazid (INH) in overdose produces seizures by causing a functional depletion of gamma-aminobutyric acid (GABA), a major inhibitory neurotransmitter. Pupillary changes occur with autonomically active drugs. Sympathetic and anticholinergic agents produce mydriasis, whereas parasympathetic agents cause miosis. Several compounds emit characteristic odors that aid in diagnosis. Toxidromes are sets of physical findings shared by a given class of compounds (Box 180-2).

## DIAGNOSTIC STRATEGIES

A number of therapeutic agents help diagnose toxic exposures. Clinical improvement upon administration of oxygen uncovers hypoxia and implicates substances

**Box 180-2**
***Toxidromes***

| *Toxidrome* | *Signs and Symptoms* |
|---|---|
| **Opioids** | Altered level of consciousness<br>Respiratory depression<br>Miosis |
| **Sympathomimetics** | Excitation, agitation<br>Tachycardia<br>Hypertension<br>Mydriasis<br>Diaphoresis<br>Seizures |
| **Parasympathomimetics**<br>Muscarinic stimulation<br>"DUMBBELS" | Diarrhea<br>Urination<br>Miosis<br>Bronchorrhea<br>Bradycardia<br>Emesis<br>Lacrimation<br>Salivation |
| **Parasympathomimetic**<br>Nicotinic stimulation | Fasciculations<br>Weakness<br>Paralysis<br>Hypertension/Hypotension<br>Tachycardia/Bradycardia |
| **Opioid withdrawal** | Nausea, vomiting, diarrhea<br>Tachycardia<br>Yawning<br>Piloerection<br>Rhinorrhea<br>Diaphoresis<br>Myalgia<br>Anxiety, drug craving |
| **Anticholinergic** | Altered level of consciousness<br>Tachycardia<br>Mydriasis<br>Hyperthermia<br>Dry mucous membranes<br>Urinary retention<br>Seizures |

that impair ventilation. Resolution of lethargy after intravenous glucose points to drugs that cause hypoglycemia. Naloxone is a pure opioid antagonist that reverses the sedation and respiratory depression caused by naturally occurring and synthetic opioids.

A variety of laboratory abnormalities result from toxic exposures. Sympathomimetic agents may cause leukocytosis. Many agents cause metabolic acidosis associated with an increased anion gap. Blood chemistries and blood gas analysis help manage acid base disturbances and diagnose ventilatory distress. Co-oximetry is required to measure carbon monoxide and methemoglobin. Toxic alcohols contribute to unmeasured osmoles not accounted for by glucose, blood urea nitrogen, and serum sodium. Superwarfarins in rodenticides cause coagulopathies manifested by deranged clotting studies.

Some compounds may be visible on plain radiographs. These include heavy metals, sustained-release medications, and foreign bodies such as heroin packets and crack vials. Radiographs reveal aspiration pneumonitis, which may occur with hydrocarbon ingestions, and gastrointestinal (GI) perforation, a consequence of severe caustic ingestions. Comprehensive toxicology screens are not only unfeasible but cost ineffective. Specific assays should be selected based upon the patient's history and presentation. Limited qualitative urine drug screens may be used when drug abuse is suspected. Quantitative drug levels help guide management of drugs whose levels correlate with clinical toxicity or drugs for which accepted treatment nomograms exist. Adolescent toxic exposures should be considered unknown exposures. An electrocardiogram (ECG) and acetaminophen level should always be obtained. Many psychoactive substances may manifest subtle electrocardiogram changes before frank toxicity develops. Acetaminophen is a ubiquitous drug that causes few early symptoms and irreversible hepatic failure in later stages. Moreover, an antidote is available that is completely effective if administered early.

## THERAPY

The goals of therapy are to limit exposure, enhance elimination, and treat consequences. Skin and mucous membranes should be irrigated and fresh air provided for respiratory exposures. Medical personnel should protect themselves from secondary exposure with barriers and ventilatory precautions. For ingestions, GI decontamination comprises 3 therapeutic efforts: gastric emptying, administration of a sorbent, and use of a cathartic. Gastric emptying is achieved by 2 methods: induction of emesis with syrup of ipecac or gastric lavage via a large bore orogastric tube. Activated charcoal adsorbs a wide variety of substances to prevent absorption in the GI tract. Its adsorbent capacity is optimum when present in tenfold excess of toxin, but gastric capacity more often limits the dose to 1 gram per kilogram body weight or 50 grams for adults. Commonly used cathartics are sorbitol and magnesium citrate. Although shown to decrease GI transit time, cathartics have not proven to improve other therapeutic parameters such as survival or length of hospitalization. Nevertheless, as long as they are administered judiciously with careful monitoring of fluid and electrolyte balance, they may be useful, particularly for substances not well adsorbed to activated charcoal.

The first consideration in the treatment of toxic exposures is determining that treatment is indeed necessary. The physician must weigh the anticipated therapeutic gains against the risks inherent to therapy. This is true in particular with respect to gastric emptying. Gastric emptying is an intuitively attractive intervention, as removal of toxin from the stomach would reasonably be expected to lessen its consequences. However, whether accomplished by emesis or gastric lavage, its significant risks limit its utility.

Time of onset to vomiting after administration of ipecac is variable among individuals. Delayed or persistent vomiting may hamper other possibly more effective modes of GI decontamination. Until recently, syrup of ipecac was prescribed for home administration by parents of toddlers for selected ingestions. Although emesis may have a limited role in ingestions for which no therapeutic alternatives exist or when medical care is remote and no antidote is available, it is no longer routinely recommended because its use would rarely be considered sufficient intervention to supplant subsequent physician evaluation.[6]

The foremost risk of gastric emptying is aspiration of gastric contents due to impaired airway protective response. This is especially true for patients who are obtunded or seizing, or for patients who have ingested low-viscosity hydrocarbons. Increased intraluminal pressure from forceful emesis or trauma from large orogastric tubes may extend partial thickness burns from caustic ingestions to frank perforation. Possible benefit of gastric emptying was demonstrated only when it was employed within 1 hour following ingestion. A greater interval may apply for substances that delay gastric emptying or tend to form insoluble masses in the stomach.[7,8] Due to its risks and lack of clear evidence of improved clinical outcome, gastric lavage has fallen out of favor as routine therapy for acutely poisoned patients. Gastric lavage should be considered for critically ill intubated patients with massive ingestions for which there are inadequate alternative treatments.[9]

Toxin load may be decreased by augmenting postabsorptive elimination. Methods include hemodialysis, hemoperfusion, exchange transfusion, alkaline diuresis, and multiple dose-activated charcoal. Toxic alcohols and lithium are removed by hemodialysis. Salicylates are removed most efficiently by hemoperfusion, but hemodialysis has the added advantage of correcting electrolyte abnormalities. Exchange transfusion removes drugs that cause hemolysis and replaces hemolysed blood with intact cells. Alkaline diuresis maximizes renal excretion of salicylates when hepatic mechanisms are overwhelmed. Multiple dose-activated charcoal enhances elimination of drugs that back diffuse across mesenteric vessels into the gut (GI dialysis) and drugs excreted into bile (enterohepatic recirculation).

Antidotes work in numerous ways to treat specific poisonings (Box 180-3). Careful monitoring must be maintained beyond the initial evaluation and treatment phase, as poisonings are a dynamic process. Fine adjustment of ongoing management is guided by periodic assessment of vital signs, physical examination, and laboratory analyses.

**Box 180-3**
***Antidotes***

| *Antidote* | *Drug* | *Mechanism of Rescue* |
|---|---|---|
| Deferroxamine | Iron | Chelation |
| Vitamin K | Coumadin | Cofactor |
| Naloxone | Morphine | Receptor antagonist |
| Ethanol | Methanol | Inhibition of toxic conversion |
| Digibind | Digoxin | Immunoneutralization |

## SPECIFIC SUBSTANCES

In-depth discussion of specific poisonings is beyond the scope of this text. However, several substances deserve brief directive comments.

### OVER-THE-COUNTER MEDICATIONS

#### Acetaminophen

Acetaminophen is ubiquitous in over-the-counter analgesics, alone and in combination with other compounds and as regular and extended release formulations. Acetaminophen toxicity is readily treated if diagnosed early. The treatment nomogram is based on the assumption that absorption of regular acetaminophen, even in overdose, is rapid and complete.[10,11] In therapeutic doses, acetaminophen is metabolized in the liver by glucuronidation and sulfation. A small fraction undergoes oxidation by the P450 mixed-function oxidase system to form the hepatotoxic compound, N-acetyl-p-benzoquinoneimine (NAPQI), which is quickly detoxified by glutathione (GSH).

Following overdose, normal detoxification reactions are overwhelmed, and NAPQI accumulates, leading to centrilobular hepatic necrosis.

Early symptoms of acetaminophen overdose are few and nonspecific. Therefore, a high index of suspicion for acetaminophen overdose must be maintained for all adolescents who present with a possible overdose of any substance. Although 150 mg/kg is generally accepted as the threshold toxic dose, any adolescent acetaminophen ingestion should be considered potentially toxic, and an acetaminophen level should be obtained at 4 hours or greater following ingestion. Standard GI decontamination efforts are appropriate until the need for an antidote can be determined. As with all adolescent poisonings, coingestants must be considered. At 24 to 48 hours following a toxic ingestion, transaminase levels begin to rise even as the patient continues to feel well. A progressive rise in transaminase levels, bilirubin, and prothrombin time occurs over 3 to 4 days, accompanied by the clinical symptoms of encephalopathy, bleeding, and coma. Patients may recover over the ensuing weeks with complete hepatic recovery by 3 to 4 months or succumb to hepatic failure. The mortality rate of untreated acetaminophen overdose is low (<5%), but a poor prognosis is predicted by an arterial pH <7.30, peak prothrombin time >100 seconds, and creatinine >300 mmols/L in patients with grade III or IV encephalopathy.[12] Cerebral edema, renal failure, hypotension, and hemorrhage are late indicators of poor prognosis.

The antidote for acetaminophen overdose is N-acetylcysteine (NAC), which is thought to prevent acetaminophen toxicity by both serving as a GSH precursor and as a GSH analog. The optimum window for administration of NAC is 8 hours, the interval from ingestion and formation of NAPQI to onset of irreversible hepatotoxicity. N-acetylcysteine is maximally effective throughout this interval with decremental efficacy thereafter. Although the efficacy of NAC in preventing hepatotoxicity does not extend beyond 24 hours following an acute ingestion, nonspecific benefits to organ function have been demonstrated even following hepatic failure.[13] N-acetylcysteine is indicated if a single acetaminophen level at 4 hours following ingestion is at or above 150 ug/mL or at any point above the potential toxicity line of the treatment nomogram (line connecting 150 ug/mL at 4 hours and 37.5 ug/mL at 12 hours).[14] For an overdose of the extended release product, a second level should be obtained 4 to 6 hours after the first.[15] Treatment should be initiated if either level is above the potential toxicity line. In addition to NAC, fluids, dextrose, vitamin K, and hemodialysis may be beneficial.

N-acetylcysteine had been administered orally as a 140 mg/kg loading dose of a 5% solution followed by 17 doses of 70 mg/kg at 4-hour intervals. However, due to its emetogenic sulfuric odor, the intravenous preparation is preferred. Available as a 20% solution, it is dosed at 300 mg/kg over 21 hours according to the following schedule: 150 mg/kg over the first hour followed by 50 mg/kg over 4 hours followed by 100 mg/kg over 16 hours.[16]

### Salicylates

Salicylates are irreversible nonspecific inhibitors of cyclo-oxygenase (COX). Therapeutic effects are analgesic, antipyretic, and anti-inflammatory. In overdose, salicylates uncouple oxidative phosphorylation, leading to increased metabolic rate, hyperthermia, dehydration, and multiple metabolic derangements. Early on, salicylates centrally stimulate medullary respiratory drive manifesting primary respiratory alkalosis. Both local gastric mucosal irritation and central stimulation of the chemotrigger zone contribute to nausea, vomiting, and GI distress. Inner ear toxicity causes tinnitus. Central nervous system (CNS) manifestations include irritability, lethargy, and seizures. Direct myocardial toxicity and metabolic disturbances may contribute to development of dysrhythmias.[17] In severe salicylate poisoning, elevated anion-gap metabolic acidosis with primary and compensatory respiratory alkalosis evolve to deepening lethargy with loss of respiratory drive and worsening metabolic acidosis.[18]

Although frequently associated with acetaminophen, it differs from the latter in important ways. Symptoms of salicylate overdose develop early in poisoning. Unlike acetaminophen, which is rapidly absorbed, large quantities of salicylates may form poorly soluble gastric masses, resulting in prolonged absorption and delayed peak levels. A single early salicylate level might underestimate the severity of the overdose.[19] Conversely, ingestion of methylsalicylate, a highly concentrated liquid form of salicylate (1.4 grams salicylate per mL), could lead to rapid attainment of consequential levels.

Salicylates are well adsorbed to activated charcoal. Multiple doses should be administered to prevent ongoing absorption of gastric masses.[20] Salicylate levels correlate poorly with toxicity. Chronic salicylate toxicity manifests greater severity at lower serum levels likely due to higher tissue levels. Serial salicylate assays confirm effective decontamination and falling levels. Salicylate levels should be obtained early in methylsalicylate overdose, as absorption is rapid. Dehydration and electrolyte abnormalities should be identified and treated. Urine alkalinization with intravenous sodium bicarbonate enhances renal elimination of unchanged salicylates. As weak acids, salicylates acquire a charge in alkaline medium and become trapped in renal collecting ducts. Urine alkalinization should be considered for patients with salicylate levels greater than 30 mg/dL. Ion trapping is achieved at a urine pH of 7.5 to 8.0. Hypokalemia needs to be corrected for successful alkalinization of urine. A bolus of 1 to 2 meq/kg of sodium bicarbonate followed by infusion of D51/3 NS with 2 amps of NaHCO3/L and 40 meg/L of KCl at twice the maintenance rate is effective to achieve urine alkalinization, repletion of potassium, and replacement of fluid deficits.

Extracorporeal methods of elimination are effective for the removal of salicylates from blood. Although hemoperfusion effects greater clearance of the drug, hemodialysis is preferred as it produces the added benefit of treating fluid and electrolyte abnormalities.[21] Hemodialysis is indicated for progressive clinical deterioration, renal failure, or an acute salicylate level of 100 mg/dL or greater. Hemodialysis should be considered at lower levels for ill patients with chronic exposure to salicylates.

### *NSAIDS*

Nonsteroidal anti-inflammatory agents (NSAIDS) are compounds that decrease prostaglandin, prostacycline, and thromboxane synthesis by inhibiting COX. Prostaglandins are a heterogenous group of compounds that produce vasodilatation, GI cytoprotection, pain, fever, and inflammation. Prostacyclines cause vasodilatation and platelet antagonism. Thromboxanes produce vasoconstriction and platelet aggregation. COX inhibition produces increased substrate for lipooxygenase, leading to increased production of leukotrienes. Desired effects of NSAIDs are analgesia, antipyresis, and anti-inflammatory activity. Adverse effects include GI toxicity, renal vascular toxicity, platelet dysfunction, and leukotriene-mediated bronchospasm in susceptible individuals.

There are 2 isoforms of COX: COX-1 catalyzes the formation of the cytoprotective prostaglandins; COX-2 catalyzes the production of prostaglandins that mediate pain and inflammation. COX-2 selective inhibitors were developed to reduce adverse effects of COX-1 inhibition, namely dose-limiting GI toxicity.

Nonspecific COX inhibitors include salicylates (discussed earlier), ibuprofen, naproxen, indomethacin, and ketorolac. COX-2 selective inhibitors include celecoxib and rofecoxib. Rofecoxib was withdrawn from the market for increased incidence of cardiovascular events during clinical trials.[22] The pathophysiology underlying cardiovascular events with COX inhibitors is not well understood, although cardiovascular risk from nonselective NSAIDS is felt to be small.[23] COX inhibitors disturb the balance of thromboxanes and prostacyclines. Decreased thromboxane production leads to increased bleeding, whereas decreased prostacyclines would have thrombotic effects.[24] The US Food and Drug Administration (FDA) has called for a boxed warning on all NSAIDS to emphasize this cardiovascular risk.[25]

Acute NSAID overdose is generally mild with a predominance of GI symptoms. Severe overdose may be accompanied by altered mental status or metabolic acidosis. Chronic use of NSAIDS can lead to interstitial nephritis and papillary necrosis. NSAIDS are well adsorbed to activated charcoal, so gastric emptying is unnecessary as spontaneous emesis is usually present. Care must be taken to exclude other causes of lethargy and anion-gap metabolic acidosis. As always, toxic acetaminophen ingestion must be excluded. Electrolytes, arterial blood gas determination, blood urea nitrogen, and creatinine help guide fluid management and assess renal function.

### Iron

Iron is a heavy metal available over the counter in multivitamins and prenatal supplements. Serious toddler ingestions have decreased in frequency since the adoption of blister packaging of individual tablets, but fatal overdose still occurs among determined adolescents and adults. Iron is a nutritional requirement for the synthesis of heme, the iron-carrying core of hemoglobin. In overdose, it is a mitochondrial toxin, leading to production of free radicals, lipid peroxidation, and disruption of cellular aerobic metabolism. In addition to its metabolic consequences, it is directly corrosive to the GI tract. Clinical manifestations of iron overdose occur in stages. The initial stage, occurring within 6 hours of ingestion consists of nausea, abdominal pain, vomiting, and diarrhea, often bloody. Vomiting, although nonspecific, is a *sine qua non* of serious iron poisoning. The second "latent" stage is described as 1 of relative quiescence as the initial GI symptoms subside from 6 to 24 hours postingestion. Seriously poisoned patients are not completely asymptomatic, however, usually displaying some degree of tachycardia. The systemic stage occurring from 4 to 40 hours describes the onset of cardiovascular instability, lethargy, and coagulopathy. During the ensuing 2 to 4 days, patients may progress to hepatic and renal failure. Recovery over 2 to 8 weeks may be complicated by GI strictures and scarring.

Heavy metals as a class are not well adsorbed to activated charcoal. Spontaneous emesis renders the controversy of gastric emptying moot. Whole bowel irrigation with polyethylene glycol may be useful in helping eliminate residual GI iron tablets as demonstrated on abdominal radiographs.

Mild toxicity occurs with doses as low as 10 to 20 mg/kg.[26] Moderate toxicity occurs at doses greater than 20 mg/kg. Any ingestion in excess of 20 mg/kg and any intentional iron overdose should be treated as potentially consequential. Iron intoxication is diagnosed clinically. Persistent vomiting and lethargy should alert the physician to the likelihood of serious poisoning. Iron levels should be determined at 4 to 6 hours following ingestion, although follow-up levels should confirm that levels have peaked. Levels between 300 and 500 ug/dL are associated with serious toxicity. Levels greater than 500 ug/dL should be managed as potentially life threatening. Elevated white blood cell count and blood glucose level are nonspecific indicators of iron intoxication. Excess total iron binding capacity (TIBC) is an unreliable method for determining serious iron toxicity. The increase in TIBC in iron poisoning is a laboratory aberration and should not be considered a protective effect.[27]

Blood chemistries, complete blood count, and arterial blood gas are useful for identifying and managing acidosis, fluid and electrolyte disturbances, and blood loss. Radiographs may help identify persistence of GI iron and guide whole bowel irrigation, but a normal film does not exclude ingestion. Deferroxamine (DFO) is indicated for serious iron poisoning as manifested by metabolic acidosis, hemodynamic instability, or iron level >500 ug/dL. Achievement of the "vin rose" hue of urine following intramuscular administration of "test dose" of DFO is an unreliable method for assessing need for further chelation. The recommended dose is empiric and limited by the toxicity of DFO. The immediate rate-limiting adverse effect is hypotension. Adult respiratory distress syndrome can occur with prolonged infusion at high doses.[28] Based on these factors, an accepted regimen is 15 mg/kg/hr for 24 hours. If hemodynamic instability, continued metabolic acidosis, or evidence of ongoing renal excretion of iron persists beyond 24 hours, additional DFO should be administered with care at decreased doses. Iron and DFO do not cross the placenta.[29] The fetus is at far greater risk from the hemodynamic effects of iron upon the mother than any risk demonstrated with the antidote. Deferroxamine should not be withheld in seriously poisoned pregnant women.

### Anticholinergic Agents

Diphenhydramine (DPH) is a compound widely available in over-the-counter preparations to treat allergy, upper respiratory symptoms, and insomnia. It blocks the H subtype of histamine receptor. Adverse effects of DPH include sedation and anticholinergic symptoms of tachycardia, hyperthermia, urinary retention, mydriasis, flushed skin, dry mucous membranes, and seizures. Two early second-generation H blockers, the long-acting terfenadine and astemizole, were withdrawn for their association with torsades de pointes.[30] Newer second-generation H blockers were developed to minimize affinity for CNS and cholinergic receptors.

Diagnosis of DPH toxicity is made by history and characteristic symptoms of anticholinergic overactivity. Physostigmine, the reversible inhibitor of cholinesterase, alleviates both central and peripheral antagonism of cholinergic receptors. Its use may obviate the need for other diagnostic measures, for example CNS imaging or lumbar puncture, in the seizing or obtunded patient with DPH toxicity. Its use is appropriate for known ingestions of DPH alone. The dose of physostigmine is 0.5 to 2 mg in adults and 0.02 mg/kg up to 0.5 mg/dose in children by slow intravenous push, monitoring carefully for signs of cholinergic excess. The use of physostigmine is relatively contraindicated in mixed or unknown overdose and contraindicated in patients who manifest symptoms of epileptogens or membrane stabilizers such as Class 1A and 1C antiarrhythmic agents. Additional therapies include benzodiazepines, support, and sodium bicarbonate for ECG changes.

## PSYCHOACTIVE MEDICATIONS

### Anxiolytic Drugs

Anxiolytics are prescription drugs to treat and prevent anxiety disorders. Benzodiazepines are the drugs most often prescribed to manage anxiety. In 2004, the 2 most commonly prescribed anxiolytics were the drugs lorazepam (Ativan) and alprazolam (Xanax).[31] Benzodiazepine anxiolytics enhance the actions of GABA, an inhibitory neurotransmitter. Increased central neuroinhibition is postulated to alleviate symptoms of anxiety. Similar in activity to the older barbiturate anxiolytics, benzodiazepines have a much wider margin of safety.

In addition to sedation, benzodiazepine anxiolytics produce confusion, poor concentration, ataxia, dysarthria, motor incoordination, diplopia, muscle weakness, and vertigo. These effects are more pronounced at the beginning of therapy and after dosage increases. Paradoxical disinhibition may occur in some individuals manifested as increased excitement, irritability, aggression, hostility, and impulsivity. When anxiolytics are used in high doses or taken with other depressant drugs such as alcohol or barbiturates, respiratory depression results. Due to the potential for abuse, the Drug Enforcement Administration classifies benzodiazepine anxiolytics as controlled substances. Physical dependence develops when these medications are used at high doses or for prolonged periods of time. When discontinued abruptly, withdrawal symptoms occur: return of anxiety, tachycardia, hypertension, tremors, diaphoresis, seizures, and delirium tremens.

Benzodiazepine overdose should be suspected in obtunded patients with relatively preserved vital signs. Consideration should be given to GI decontamination and the possibility of coingestants. Hemodynamic monitoring and respiratory support are the mainstays of treatment.

Flumazenil is a competitive benzodiazepine antagonist that rapidly reverses sedative effects. Its use is contraindicated in mixed or unknown overdose. Reversal of benzodiazepine depressant activity may lead to withdrawal in habituated patients or seizures or dysrhythmias in patients who have also ingested epileptogenic or dysrhythmogenic agents such as tricyclic antidepressants.

### Antidepressants

Antidepressants treat or alleviate the symptoms of clinical depression. The newer antidepressants have an improved side effect profile and are safer in overdose. The first medications used as antidepressants were the monoamine oxidase inhibitors (MAOIs), originally an antituberculosis drug. Tricyclic antidepressants (TCAs) followed MAOIs in the treatment of depression. Currently, the most widely prescribed antidepressants are selective serotonin reuptake inhibitors (SSRIs).

Nonselective MAOIs irreversibly block presynaptic breakdown of monoamines resulting in their increased neuronal release. Present as 2 subtypes, monoamine oxidase A (MAO-A) is found in the GI tract and breaks down epinephrine, norepinephrine, tyramine, and serotonin. Monoamine oxidase B (MAO-B) functions predominantly in the brain, its principal substrate being dopamine. Nonspecific MAOIs produce severe hypertension if taken with foods that contain high levels of tyramine, for example, certain cheeses and wine. Following overdose, initial symptoms of sympathetic overactivity may be delayed for greater than 24 hours. Severe hypertension, tachycardia, and excitation evolve toward a state of catecholamine depletion resulting in cardiovascular collapse. Treatment is aimed at decontamination, cardiovascular support, and avoidance of harmful drug interactions. The newer reversible inhibitors of monoamine oxidase A (RIMA) have a much greater safety profile.

Tricyclic antidepressants (TCAs) prevent the reuptake of neurotransmitters at central presynaptic terminals, increasing synaptic catecholamines. In addition, they produce anticholinergic symptoms, hypotension from peripheral alpha adrenergic blockade, and quinidine-like membrane stabilization. Earliest signs of TCA overdose consist of sedation and tachycardia. The quinidine-like effect, inhibition of fast sodium channels, manifests electrocardiographically as right axis deviation of the terminal 40 msecs of the QRS complex, which generalizes to widening of the entire QRS complex. In 1 series of patients, seizures were associated with QRS duration of 100 msec or longer. Ventricular dysrhythmias were seen with QRS duration of 160 msec or longer.[32,33]

Gastrointestinal decontamination efforts must be aggressive and ongoing. Reports of late decompensation following initial stabilization presumably resulted from ongoing absorption of TCAs from anticholinergically slowed gut.[34] QRS widening on the ECG responds to sodium bicarbonate, administered intravenously as a bolus of 1–2 mEq/kg.[35] Physostigmine for treatment of anticholinergic symptoms is contraindicated as its use in this setting has been associated with asystole.[36] Although largely supplanted by the safer SSRIs for use in depression, TCAs are still prescribed for treatment of enuresis, obsessive-compulsive disorder, attention-deficit/hyperactivity disorder, and chronic pain.

As their name suggests, SSRIs increase synaptic serotonin levels by preventing reuptake of serotonin. Overdose of SSRIs results in nausea, vomiting, dizziness, blurred vision, and, less commonly, CNS depression and sinus tachycardia. One SSRI, citalopram, has been associated with QTc prolongation on the ECG and seizures.

Although reasonably safe as single agents, serious adverse effects occur when SSRIs are used in conjunction with other drugs with serotonergic activity. Serotonin syndrome describes the altered mental status, agitation, hyperthermia, hyperreflexia, myoclonus, and seizures associated with the coadministration of meperidine and phenelzine or other drugs with like serotonin activity.[37] Benzodiazepines, hydration, and aggressive correction of hyperthermia are essential for the treatment of serotonin syndrome.

Suicidal ideation is relatively common during the initial phases of antidepressant treatment. Although not definitive, there is some evidence that antidepressants may worsen depression and increase suicidality in teenagers.[38]

### Antipsychotics

Antipsychotic drugs are prescribed for a variety of psychiatric and medical disorders including bipolar disease, pervasive developmental delay and autism, conduct disorders, anxiety, tics, schizophrenia, and eating disorders.

There are several classes of antipsychotic medications that are structurally distinct. Their therapeutic effect has been attributed to antagonism of central dopamine and serotonin receptors. The older antipsychotic agents, for example chlorpromazine and haloperidol, seem to alleviate the "positive" symptoms of schizophrenia (hallucinations, delusions, paranoia, disorganized thought). Newer or "atypical" antipsychotics such as clozapine and risperidone have greater affinity for serotonin receptors and seem to better alleviate negative symptoms of schizophrenia (blunted affect, social withdrawal, apathy). Adverse effects include antagonism of muscarinic, histamine, and alpha-adrenergic receptors resulting in anticholinergic symptoms, sedation, and orthostatic hypotension. Thioridazine and mesoridazine are 2 older agents with sodium channel-blocking activity and consequent cardiotoxicity.

Although the antipsychotic agents possess a wide therapeutic index, extrapyramidal and anticholinergic symptoms range from the uncomfortable to the life threatening. Dystonia, akathisia, parkinsonism, and neuroleptic malignant syndrome (NMS) may complicate recently initiated therapy, whereas the risk for tardive dyskinesia, as the name implies, increases with duration of treatment. Newer atypical antipsychotic agents have been developed with fewer extrapyramidal and anticholinergic adverse effects and have largely replaced the traditional drugs. The adverse event of greatest concern is consisting of altered mental state, muscular rigidity, hyperthermia, and dysautonomia. The syndrome may persist for as long as a week following discontinuation of the offending drug. In addition to decontamination and meticulous supportive care, benzodiazepines treat agitation, and bromocriptine, a centrally acting dopamine agonist, has been associated with clinical improvement.

### STIMULANTS

Therapeutic uses of amphetamines include treatment of attention-deficit/hyperactivity disorder, short-term weight loss, and narcolepsy. Amphetamines cause the release of neurotransmitters, dopamine, and norepinephrine from presynaptic terminals, as well as prevent the breakdown of these neurotransmitters. The clinical picture that results from overdose is one of sympathetic overdrive. Signs and symptoms include hypertension, anxiety, aggression, hallucinations, tachycardia, mydriasis, diaphoresis, and hyperthermia. Life-threatening events include severe hyperthermia, dysrhythmia, cerebrovascular events, and myocardial hypoperfusion.

Qualitative urine immunoassay confirms the presence of amphetamines, but diagnosis is more quickly made by recognition of the toxidrome. Management of amphetamine overdose centers on aggressive external cooling and treatment wtih benzodiazepines.

### ISONIAZID

Isoniazid is an antibiotic widely used for both the prophylaxis and treatment of tuberculosis. Important adverse effects are hepatitis in therapeutic use and seizures with overdose. Isoniazid blocks conversion of pyridoxine to its active state. Pyridoxine is a necessary cofactor in the production of GABA, the major inhibitory neurotransmitter in the CNS. What results is a state of functional GABA depletion, CNS disinhibition, and seizures.

The risk for hepatitis increases with chronic overdose, advanced age, and concomitant use of other hepatotoxic antituberculous agents. There are genetic variations in the ability to metabolize INH. In general, a greater number of Asians are fast acetylators when compared with persons of white or African derivation.[39] Hepatitis is thought to be caused by a hepatotoxic intermediate produced between 2 acetylation steps. Although fast acetylators might be at decreased risk of seizures following INH overdose, their risk for hepatitis is less clear. The hepatotoxic intermediate, although formed more rapidly, would dissipate quickly as well. Clinical hepatitis occurred in 0.1%[40] and death in 0.001%[41] in 2 series of patients. Significant liver function abnormalities should prompt immediate discontinuation of INH. Monitoring and support should accompany timely referral for liver transplant in patients with fulminant hepatitis. Seizures induced by INH are treated with benzodiazepines and pyridoxine. The latter is dosed gram per gram of INH overdosed or empirically at 70 mg/kg up to 5 grams.[42]

## CONCLUSIONS

Adolescents suffer disproportionate risk from drug overdose when compared with younger children. Intentionality, greater quantities, numbers of agents, and reticence all contribute to greater morbidity seen in this population. When treating drug overdose in adolescents, the clinician must be aware of the patient's past medical history, medications, and potential interactions. Adolescent overdoses should all be managed as potentially unknown ingestions, particularly in the suicidal adolescent. Acetominophen level, ECG, screening labs, and knowledge of toxidromes guide management.

## REFERENCES

1. Watson WA, Litovitz TL, Rodgers Jr GC, et al. 2004 Annual Report of the American Association of Poison Control Centers Toxic Exposure Surveillance System. Available at: www.poison.org/prevent/documents/TESS%20Annual%20Report%202004.pdf. Accessed November 30, 2010

2. Woolf AD. Acute poisonings among adolescents and young adults with anorexia nervosa. *Am J Dis Child.* 1990;144(7):785–788

3. Bearer C. Specific unique susceptibilities of the fetus, infant, and adolescent. *Neurotoxicology.* 2000;21(1–2):240

4. Murray L. Drug therapy during pregnancy and lactation. *Emerg Med Clin North Am.* 1994;12(1):129–149

5. Briggs GG, Freeman RK, Yaffe SJ. *Drugs in Pregnancy and Lactation, Sixth Edition*. Philadelphia, PA: Lippincott Williams Wilkins; 2002

6. American Academy of Pediatrics Committee on Injury, Violence, and Poison Prevention. Poison treatment in the home. *Pediatrics.* 2003;112:1182–1185

7. Kulig K, Bar-Or D, Cantrill S, et al. Management of acutely poisoned patients without gastric emptying. *Ann Emerg Med.* 1985;14:562-567

8. Pond SM, Lewis-Driver DJ, Williams GM, et al. Gastric emptying in acute overdose: a prospective randomized controlled trial. *Med J Aust.* 1995;163:345-349

9. Bond GR. The role of activated charcoal and gastric emptying in gastrointestinal decontamination. *Ann Emerg Med.* 2002;39:273-286

10. Rumack BH, Matthew HM. Acetaminophen poisoning and toxicity. *Pediatrics.* 1975;55:871-876

11. Smilkstein MJ, Knapp GL, Kulig KW, Rumack BH. Efficacy of oral N-acetylcysteine in the treatment of acetaminophen overdose. *N Eng J Med.* 1988;319:1557-1562

12. O'Grady JG, Alexander GJ, Hayllar KM, Williams R. Early indicators of prognosis in fulminant hepatic failure. *Gastroenterology.* 1989;97:439-445

13. Harrison PM, Wendon JA, Gimson AE, Alexander GJ, Williams R. Improvement by acetylcysteine of hemodynamics and oxygen transport in fulminant hepatic failure. *N Eng J Med.* 1991;324:1852-1857

14. Smilkstein MJ, Bronstein AC, Linden C, Augenstein WL, Kulig KW, Rumack BH. Acetaminophen overdose: a 48-hour intravenous N-acetylcysteine treatment protocol. *Ann Emerg Med.* 1991;20:1058-1063

15. Cetaruk EW. Tylenol Extended Relief overdose. *Ann Emerg Med.* 1997;30(1):104-108

16. Acetadote prescribing information. Cumberland Pharmaceuticals Web site. Available at: www.acetadote.net/AcetadotePI_rDec08.pdf Accessed May 13, 2010

17. Mukerji V, Alpert MA, Flaker GC, Beach CL, Weber RD. Cardiac conduction abnormalities and atrial arrhythmias associated with salicylate toxicity. *Pharmacotherapy.* 1986;6:41-43

18. Hill JB. Salicylate intoxication. *N Eng J Med.* 1973;288:1110-1113

19. Wortzman DJ, Grunfeld A. Delayed absorption following enteric-coated aspirin overdose. *Ann Emerg Med.* 1987;16:434-436

20. Barone JA, Raia JJ, Huang YC. Evaluation of the effects of multiple-dose activated charcoal on the absorption of orally administered salicylate in a simulated toxic ingestion model. *Ann Emerg Med.* 1988;17:34-37

21. Borkan SC. Extracorporeal therapies for acute intoxications. *Crit Care Clin.* 2002;18(2):393-420, vii

22. Sibbald B. Rofecoxib (Vioxx) voluntarily withdrawn from market. *CMAJ.* 2004;171(9):1027-1028

23. Salpeter SR. Meta-analysis: cardiovascular events associated with nonsteroidal anti-inflammatory drugs. *Am J Med.* 2006;119(7):552-559

24. Weir MR. Selective COX-2 inhibition and cardiovascular effects: a review of the rofecoxib development program. *Am Heart J.* 2003;146(4):591-604

25. COX-2 selective (includes Bextra, Celebrex, and Vioxx) and non selective non steroidal anti-inflammatory drugs (NSAIDs). 2005. Available at: www.fda.gov/cder/drug/infopage/cox2/ Accessed August 17, 2006

26. Ling LJ, Hornfeldt CS, Winter JP. Absorption of iron after experimental overdose of chewable vitamins. *Am J Emerg Med.* 1991;9:24-26

27. Tenenbein M, Yatscoff RW. The total iron-binding capacity in iron poisoning—is it useful? *AJDC.* 1991;145:437-439

28. Tenenbein M. Pulmonary toxic effects of continuous desferrioxamine administration in acute iron poisoning. *Lancet.* 1992;339(8795):699-701

29. McElhatton PR, Roberts JC, Sullivan FM. The consequences of iron overdose and its treatment with desferrioxamine in pregnancy. *Hum Exp Toxicol.* 1991;10(4):251-259

30. Kao LW. Drug-induced Q-T prolongation. *Med Clin North Am.* 2005;89(6):1125-1144

31. The top 300 prescriptions for 2005 by number of US prescriptions dispensed. The Internet Drug Index. 2005. Available at: www.rxlist.com/script/main/hp.asp. Accessed May 13, 2010

32. Wolfe TR, Caravati EM, Rollins DE. Terminal 40-ms frontal plane QRS axis as a marker for tricyclic antidepressant overdose. *Ann Emerg Med.* 1989;18(4):348-351

33. Boehnert MT, Lovejoy FH. Value of the QRS duration versus the serum drug level in predicting seizures and ventricular arrhythmias after an acute overdose of tricyclic antidepressants. *N Eng J Med.* 1985;313:474-479

34. McAlpine SB, Calabro JJ, Robinson MD, Burkle FM Jr. Late death in tricyclic antidepressant overdose revisited. *Ann Emerg Med.* 1986;15:1349-1352

35. Pentel P, Benowitz N. Efficacy and mechanism of action of sodium bicarbonate in the treatment of desipramine toxicity in rats. *J Pharmacol Exp Ther.* 1984;230:12-19

36. Pentel P, Peterson CD. Asystole complicating physostigmine treatment of tricyclic overdose. *Ann Emerg Med.* 1980;9:588-590

37. Gnanadesigan N, Espinoza RT, Smith RL. The serotonin syndrome. *N Engl J Med.* 2005;352(23):2454-2456

38. Bostic JQ, Rubin DH, Prince J, Schlozman S. Treatment of depression in children and adolescents. *J Psychiatr Pract.* 2005;11(3):141-154

39. Ellard GA. The potential clinical significance of the isoniazid acetylator phenotype in the treatment of pulmonary tuberculosis. *Tubercle.* 1984;65(3):211-227

40. Nolan CM, Goldberg SV, Buskin SE. Hepatotoxicity associated with isoniazid preventive therapy: a 7-year survey from a public health tuberculosis clinic. *JAMA.* 1999;281(11):1014-1018

41. Salpeter SR. Fatal isoniazid-induced hepatitis. Its risk during chemoprophylaxis. *West J Med.* 1993;15(5):560-564

42. Sievers ML, Herrier RN. Treatment of acute isoniazid toxicity. *Am J Hosp Pharm.* 1975;32:202-206

# CHAPTER 181

# Office Management and Laboratory Testing

SHARON J. LEVY, MD • JOHN R. KNIGHT, MD

## INTRODUCTION

Use of alcohol and drugs by American teenagers is a major public health problem. According to the Monitoring the Future Survey, in 2008, 72% of high school seniors had tried alcohol, and 50.4% had tried an illicit drug in their lifetime.[1] Use of psychoactive substances puts teenagers at risk of significant morbidity and mortality from accidents, violence, unwanted sex, and overdose. Furthermore, the 2008 National Household Survey on Drug Abuse found that 7.6% of teenagers (aged 12–17 years) and 20.8% of young adults (aged 18–25 years) met diagnostic criteria for drug or alcohol abuse or dependence, putting them at risk of developing chronic health, psychological, and social problems.[2] Primary health care providers can play an important role by screening all adolescent patients for drug and alcohol use, giving brief advice to low-risk teens and referring high-risk teens for additional assessment and treatment.

## SCREENING

### ASKING ABOUT DRUG AND ALCOHOL USE

The American Academy of Pediatrics,[3] the American Medical Association,[4] and the Bureau of Maternal Child Health[5] recommend that every adolescent be screened for alcohol and drug use at every yearly health maintenance visit. Screening should begin when the preteen or young adolescent is old enough to be interviewed alone and should always be done privately, after reviewing the rules of confidentiality. Adolescents should be afforded confidentiality if they are not in acute danger of harming themselves or others. Determining what constitutes "acute danger" is a matter of clinical judgment. Generally, a report of intermittent use of alcohol and marijuana can be kept confidential, although confidentiality may need to be breached if a teen is reporting use in high-risk situations (eg, while driving). Past use of other drugs (eg, cocaine, amphetamines, opiates) can also usually be kept confidential; however, ongoing use may need to be reported to parents. Diagnoses of a substance use disorder should be ultimately shared with parents whenever possible. In many cases, parents are already aware of their child's substance use, and the adolescent may give permission to discuss the plan together. If parents are unaware, informing them should be a goal of treatment. Physicians should consider breaking confidentiality if an adolescent has a diagnosis of substance dependence (addiction) and is unwilling to enter treatment.

After explaining confidentiality, the clinician should ask about alcohol and drug use. Questions should be simple, direct, and unambiguous, such as, "During the past 12 months, did you drink any alcohol (more than a few sips?); Smoke any marijuana or hashish? Use anything else to get high?" Some clinicians prefer to introduce the topic by asking about drug use by peers, classmates, and friends first; others prefer to ask directly. The screen should be considered negative if a teen reports consuming sips of alcohol under a parent's supervision, such as at a wedding or religious ceremony.

### BRIEF SCREENING TOOLS

All teens who report a history of alcohol or drug use should be screened with a structured questionnaire to determine whether they are low or high risk for a substance use disorder. Recent research has shown that when relying on clinical impressions alone, even experienced clinicians frequently miss serious substance use disorders.[6] A number of screening tools have been validated with adolescents, including written instruments such as the AUDIT,[7] which screens for alcohol problems, and the POSIT,[8] which screens for a variety of mental health disorders, and the orally administered CRAFFT,[9] which screens for drug and alcohol disorders simultaneously. CRAFFT is a mnemonic for a key word in each of the tool's 6 questions (Figure 181-1).

Each affirmative answer is scored 1 point, and a score of 2 or more is considered a positive screen, indicating that the adolescent is at high risk of a substance use disorder and in need of further assessment.

The CAGE is an orally administered tool designed to detect alcohol disorders and has been validated with adults. However, it has poor psychometric properties when used with adolescents and is thus not recommended with this age group.[10]

# The CRAFFT Screening Questionnaire

Please answer all questions honestly; your answers will be kept confidential.

### *Part A*

**During the PAST 12 MONTHS, did you:**

| | No | | Yes | |
|---|---|---|---|---|
| **1.** Drink any alcohol (more than a few sips)? | ☐ | If you answered NO to ALL (A1, A2, A3) answer **only B1** below, then STOP. | ☐ | If you answered YES to ANY (A1, A2, A3), answer **B1 to B6** below. |
| **2.** Smoke any marijuana or hashish? | ☐ | | ☐ | |
| **3.** Use anything else to get high? ("anything else" includes illegal drugs, over-the-counter and prescription drugs, and things that you sniff or "huff") | ☐ | | ☐ | |

### *Part B*

| | No | Yes |
|---|---|---|
| **1.** Have you ever ridden in a **CAR** driven by someone (including yourself) who was "high" or had been using alcohol or drugs? | ☐ | ☐ |
| **2.** Do you ever use alcohol or drugs to **RELAX**, feel better about yourself, or fit in? | ☐ | ☐ |
| **3.** Do you ever use alcohol or drugs while you are by yourself, or **ALONE**? | ☐ | ☐ |
| **4.** Do you ever **FORGET** things you did while using alcohol or drugs? | ☐ | ☐ |
| **5.** Do your **FAMILY** or **FRIENDS** ever tell you that you should cut down on your drinking or drug use? | ☐ | ☐ |
| **6.** Have you ever gotten into **TROUBLE** while you were using alcohol or drugs? | ☐ | ☐ |

**NOTICE TO CLINIC STAFF AND MEDICAL RECORDS:**
The information on this page may be protected by special federal confidentiality rules (42 CFR Part 2), which prohibit disclosure of this information unless authorized by specific written consent. A general authorization for release of medical information is NOT sufficient.



**FIGURE 181-1** CRAFFT screening questionnaire.

## ASSESSMENT

### SUBSTANCE HISTORY

Every adolescent who screens positive for high-risk alcohol or drug use should be assessed further. In some instances, a return visit will be required so that adequate time can be devoted. When the clinician has determined that another appointment is needed, but confidentiality is to be protected, the parents should honestly be told that more time is needed to cover the issues important to their child's health.

An assessment should begin with a substance use history. The clinician should use open-ended questions and a nonjudgmental style to explore the current pattern of drug use, how the pattern has evolved over time, and any associated problems for any drug that has been used on a regular basis (Box 181-1). The clinician should also review the list of drugs commonly used by adolescents to determine whether the adolescent has used other substances (Box 181-2). A well-conducted history can have therapeutic value by encouraging the teenager to consider the problems that have resulted, either directly or indirectly, from his or her drug use.

### COLLATERAL HISTORY

A collateral history is particularly important if a parent, teacher, coach, or other adult presents concerns about drug use or deterioration in functioning. The clinician should determine the nature of the parents' concerns. Excessive fatigue or moodiness, new onset or worsening academic problems, loss of interest in hobbies, change in friends, lying, stealing, and possession of drug paraphernalia can all be nonspecific signs of drug use. General concerns such as living in a bad neighborhood, family history of drug problems, or personal history of attention deficit-hyperactivity disorder can be met with reassurance if an adolescent's screen is negative.

**Box 181-1**

***Substance Use History***

- How old were you when you started using?
- What was your pattern of use at first?
- What is your pattern of use like now?
- Have you ever tried to cut down or quit? If so, why?
- Have you had problems associated with use of drugs or alcohol (eg, accidents, injuries, interpersonal difficulties, school problems, legal problems)?

**Box 181-2**

***List of Psychoactive Substances Commonly Used by Adolescents***

- Alcohol
- Marijuana
- Cocaine
- 3,4-Methylenedioxymethamphetamine (MDMA, Ecstasy)
- Amphetamines or stimulants (ie, methylphenidate [Ritalin, Concerta], dextroamphetamine [Adderall], amphetamine [Adderall], methamphetamine)
- Opioids or pain killers (eg, OxyContin ["OCs"], Percocet ["percs"], Vicodin ["vics"], heroin)
- Benzodiazepines or tranquilizers (eg, Klonopin ["K-pins"], Ativan, Valium)
- Hallucinogens (eg, mushrooms, LSD ["acid"], PCP ["angel dust"], Salvia)
- Cold medications (eg, dextromethorphan ["DXM"], Coricidin ["triple C"], Robitussin)
- Inhalants (eg, whipped cream aerosol cans, gasoline)
- "Club drugs" (eg, ketamine, gamma hydroxybutyrate ["GHB"], Rohypnol ["roofies"])
- Other (eg, caffeine pills, diet pills, antidepressants, antihistamines)

### PHYSICAL EXAMINATION

A physical examination should always be part of a complete assessment for a substance use disorder. Signs of acute intoxication include drowsiness or hyperalert state, slowed or rapid speech, pupil changes, conjunctivitis, and irregular heart beat. Signs of chronic drug use are uncommon in adolescents, but include phlebitis, cellulitis, and nasal septum irritation or erosion. Thought disorders and mood disorders may also be associated with drug use; symptoms should be noted if present.

### DRUG TESTING

Laboratory testing for substances of abuse may be a useful part of an assessment if parents present valid concerns, but the adolescent denies drug use. Parents and clinicians, however, should be aware of the significant limitations of this procedure. A drug test will be negative in the context of ongoing drug use if the adolescent has used a drug not detected by a routine panel; the window of detection (48–72 hours for most substances) has been missed; or the adolescent has substituted, adulterated, or diluted the specimen. A drug test may be positive even though a teen has not used illicit drugs if a prescription or over-the-counter medication or food substance has cross-reacted with the screening panel. To avoid these errors, physicians should use recommended testing procedures (Box 181-3). A negative drug test may support a history of no recent drug use, but should be repeated at random intervals over the course of several weeks if the suspicion of drug use is high. A positive drug test is neither necessary nor sufficient to make a diagnosis of a substance use disorder, but may provide an opportunity for a more honest history. Drug testing should be voluntary. Surreptititious drug testing should never be performed on a competent adolescent without his or her knowledge.

**Box 181-3**

***Recommended Drug Testing Procedures***

- All urine specimens should be collected either using the federal collection protocol[a] or *directly* observed.
- A urine creatinine level and specific gravity should be obtained for every specimen. Urine specimens with a creatinine level 25–50 mg/dL are considered moderately dilute and should be repeated. Specimens with a creatinine level <25 mg/dL and a specific gravity <1.005 should be considered too dilute for proper interpretation.
- All positive screens must be confirmed by a more specific testing procedure, such as gas chromatography/mass spectrometry (GC/MS), to rule out substances cross-reacting with a screen to cause a false positive.
- Ensure that all substances of concern are included in the testing panel. In general, multiscreen panels include marijuana, cocaine, amphetamines, opiates (morphine and codeine), and phencyclidine (PCP) to meet the requirements of federal drug testing programs. Many laboratories use screens that can detect additional substances as well; however, alcohol, opioids (eg, oxycodone, hydrocodone), 3,4-methylenedioxymethamphetamine ("Ecstasy"), and many of the benzodiazepines may not be reliably detected. These substances can be detected via more specific tests, which must be ordered separately.

[a]This protocol requires positive photographic identification, removal of outer garments and pocket contents, and hand washing. The bathroom must have all sources of running water shut off, and standing water should be stained blue. A temperature check must be completed immediately after the specimen has been produced, and the specimen should be discarded if the temperature does not fall within the specified range. Many commercial laboratories offer this service.

## BRIEF ADVICE IN PRIMARY CARE PRACTICE

### POSITIVE REINFORCEMENT

Positive reinforcement is the best technique for modifying or encouraging many different behaviors, including abstinence from substance use. All adolescents who have never used drugs or alcohol should be given positive reinforcement in the form of a brief statement such as, "It sounds like you have made some good decisions about drugs and alcohol, and I am proud of you." It is important that the adolescent is comfortable enough to return to you with questions and to report an honest history. Adding an invitation to ask questions about drugs in the future, such as "Please let me know if you ever have questions about drugs, if you are tempted to use them, or even if you try them," can indicate your willingness to discuss drug use openly.

### ADVICE TO STOP

All adolescents who are using drugs and alcohol should be given clear advice to stop. Even if an adolescent is not willing to discontinue drug use entirely, he or she should understand that the medical advice from their clinician is to stop. Teens who have reported problems associated with drug use, even minor ones, should be asked how they intend to address these problems in the future. For example, "You don't think that drinking is a problem for you, but your parents have said that you are not allowed to drive at all unless you can commit to stop. What do you want to do about it?"

Adolescents who are willing to stop using alcohol and other drugs should be challenged to make a time-limited commitment—usually 3 to 6 months—because it can be difficult for teens to make long-term or lifetime commitments. A written contract may be useful. Patients who sign such a contract should be seen at the end of the time period to determine how well they achieved their goals, what changed for the worse and what changed for the better when they were not using, and what are their long-range plans. Many adolescents who are successful in maintaining abstinence for a period of 3 to 6 months note positive changes in their lives, including better relationships with parents and improved school and sports performance.

### CONTRACT FOR LIFE

Although most adolescents understand that drinking and driving is dangerous, some may be tempted to drive after drinking, believing that they can "handle their alcohol" or "know their limits." Many adolescents think that they concentrate better and therefore drive better after using marijuana. However, research has shown that driving after marijuana use is associated with an increase in accidents.[11,12] All adolescents should be advised to avoid driving or riding with a driver who has used drugs or alcohol or drugs that day. The Contract for Life is a tool developed by Students Against Destructive Decisions (SADD) that asks adolescents to commit not to drive or ride with an intoxicated driver and parents to commit to providing transportation home if a teenager has no access to a safe form of transportation.[13] Parents also agree not to ask questions on the day of the incident.

### HELPING PARENTS SET LIMITS

Parental limits are an extremely important determinant of adolescent behavior. Parents should be advised to maintain a clear "no alcohol or other drugs" policy in their home and establish consequences for use, such as suspending driving privileges and limiting social activities until the teenager is willing to commit to behavior change. Parents whose children have drug problems should also monitor or limit access to resources that allow teenagers to obtain drugs, such as money, credit cards, cell phone, and Internet access. If parents are unable to control their child's drug use, a "Child in Need of Supervision (CHINS)" or similar order may be filed with the police department. These orders help support parents by providing a probation officer and other services to teens with drug problems. The primary care clinician can support parents in the decision to file an order and report transgressions to their probation officer when this is in the best interest of the adolescent.

### MAKING A REFERRAL

Teens who meet criteria for abuse of more than one substance, who have a diagnosis of alcohol or drug dependence (see Chapter 172, Overview: Substance Abuse for the diagnostic criteria), or who have a significant comorbid mental health disorder should be referred to an addiction specialist or a mental health provider with experience in working with adolescents with drug problems. A variety of counseling styles and services, reviewed more thoroughly in Chapter 182, Treatment Options, may be useful to them. Patients may be more likely to accept a referral after a thorough evaluation by their primary care clinician. As with other disorders, clinicians who refer patients for more intensive services for drug and alcohol problems should continue to see them for follow-up visits in order to help monitor their progress and demonstrate their ongoing commitment to the individual patient.

## SUMMARY

Alcohol and drug use is common among adolescents. Primary care clinicians can have a major effect on reducing alcohol- and drug-related morbidity and mortality to adolescents by using a standardized approach. All adolescents should be asked about drug and alcohol use at every yearly health visit; those who have used substances should be screened with a structured screening tool to determine their risk level. Most adolescents are at low risk for developing chronic substance use disorders; these teens should be given brief advice in the office. Adolescents who are at high risk of developing chronic alcohol or drug problems should be referred for more intensive services. All adolescents should be followed over time; low-risk adolescents should be rescreened yearly, and high-risk teens should be seen intermittently to monitor their progress in treatment.

## REFERENCES

1. Johnston L, O'Malley P, Bachman J, Schulenbert J. *Monitoring the Future National Survey Results on Adolescent Drug Use: Overview of Key Findings.* NIH Publication No. 09-7401. Bethesda, MD: National Institute on Drug Abuse; 2009

2. U. S. Department of Health and Human Services, Substance Abuse and Mental Health Services Administration, Office of Applied Studies. *Results from the 2008 National Survey on Drug Use and Health: National Findings.* NSDUH Series H-36, HHS Publication No. SMA 09-4434. September 10, 2009. Available at: www.oas.samhsa.gov/nsduh/2k8nsduh/2k8Results.cfm. Accessed March 9, 2010

3. American Academy of Pediatrics Committee on Substance Abuse. Tobacco, alcohol, and other drugs: the role of the pediatrician in prevention and management of substance abuse. *Pediatrics.* 1998;101:125-128

4. American Medical Association. *Guidelines for Adolescent Preventive Services (GAPS).* Chicago: American Medical Association; 1997

5. National Center for Education in Maternal and Child Health. *Bright Futures: Guidelines for Health Supervision of Infants, Children, and Adolescents.* 2nd ed. rev. Washington, DC: Georgetown University; 2002

6. Wilson CR, Sherritt L, Gates E, Knight JR. Are clinical impressions of adolescent substance use accurate? *Pediatrics.* 2004;114:e536-e540

7. Reinert D, Allen J. The Alcohol Use Disorders Identification Test (AUDIT): a review of recent research. *Alcohol Clin Exp Res.* 2002;26(2):272-279

8. *Problem Oriented Screening Instrument for Teenagers (POSIT), Version 2.* [computer program]. Landover, MD: PowerTrain; 1998

9. Knight J, Shrier L, Bravender T, Farrell M, VanderBilt J, Shaffer H. A new brief screen for adolescent substance abuse. *Arch Pediatr Adolesc Med.* 1999;153:591-596

10. Knight JR, Sherritt L, Harris SK, Gates EC, Chang G. Validity of brief alcohol screening tests among adolescents: a

comparison of the AUDIT, POSIT, CAGE, and CRAFFT. *Alcohol Clin Exp Res.* 2002;27:67-73

11. National Institute on Drug Abuse (NIDA). *NIDA InfoFacts: Drugged Driving.* October 2009. Available at: www.drugabuse.gov/Infofacts/driving.html. Accessed March 9, 2010

12. Ehrlich P, Brown J, Drongowski R. Characterization of the drug-positive adolescent trauma population: should we, do we, and does it make a difference if we test? *J Pediatr Surg.* 2006;41(5):927-930

13. SADD. *Contract for Life.* Available at: www.sadd.org/contract.htm#cfl. Accessed March 9, 2010

# CHAPTER 182

## Treatment Options

SHARON LEVY, MD, MPH • JOHN R. KNIGHT, MD

### INTRODUCTION

Many adolescents who have used alcohol or other drugs can be treated within a primary care setting. However, patients who are diagnosed with abuse of more than 1 substance, or who are dependent on 1 or more drugs, are more likely to benefit from referral to more intensive ongoing addiction treatment. No single treatment is appropriate for all individuals; the primary care physician can play a key role in developing a treatment plan and assisting patients in finding appropriate resources. Treatment for adolescents should be developmentally appropriate, family oriented, and based on the latest scientific research. Younger adolescents who use substances may have a more rapid progression from casual use to dependence[1] and are more likely to have problems associated with their drug use[2] than older patients. This chapter describes the therapeutic modalities, formats and treatment settings used to treat substance use disorders in adolescents.

### OUTPATIENT TREATMENTS

Among the various treatment methods for adolescents with substance use disorders, outpatient counseling is a mainstay. Individual therapy methods shown to be effective include motivational interviewing (MI) and cognitive behavioral therapy (CBT).[3,4] Research has demonstrated that even brief interventions, comprised of a small number of short sessions, can significantly impact drug and alcohol use.

Group therapies may be process oriented, such as the traditional 12-step model, or based on a psychoeducational curriculum. Effective family therapies include multisystemic therapy (MST) and multidimensional family therapy (MDFT).[5–8] Many patients benefit from a simultaneous combination of therapeutic modalities.

#### BRIEF INTERVENTIONS

Within the substance abuse treatment literature, brief interventions are generally defined as a limited number of counseling sessions (eg, 1–12) administered over a relatively brief period of time (eg, 1–6 months). These interventions are primarily aimed at moving patients along the stages of change continuum described by Prochaska and DiClemente[9] (Figure 182-1). Thus, an intervention that results in an adolescent moving from precontemplation to contemplation should be

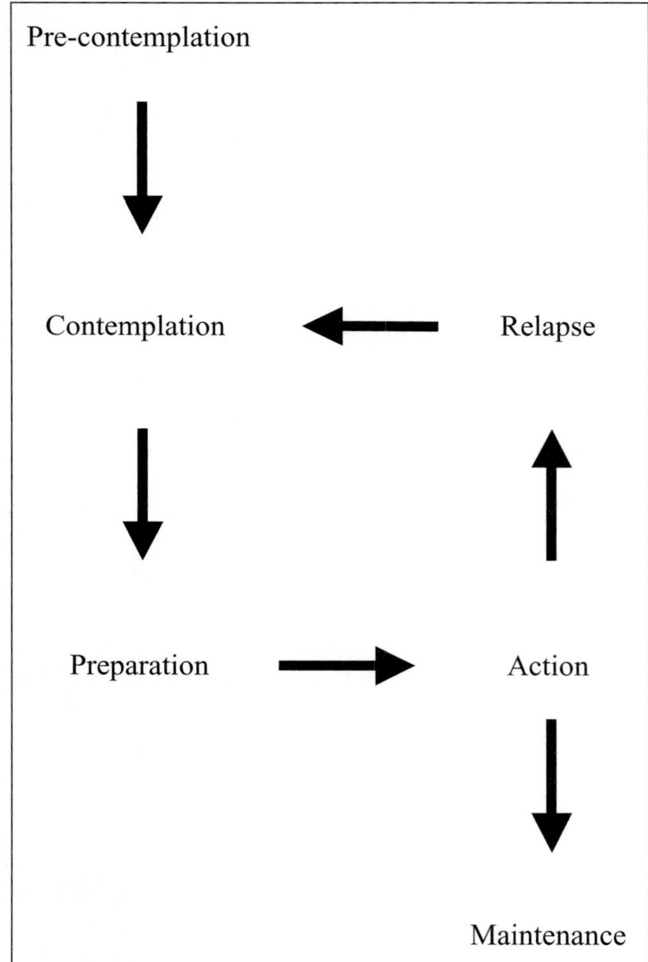


FIGURE 182-1 Stages of change model. (Reprinted from Feldman HM, Coleman WL, Carey WB, Crocker AC, Elias ER, eds. *Developmental-Behavioral Pediatrics*. 4th ed. Philadelphia: Saunders; 2009, with permission from Elsevier.)

considered a success, even though no observed behavior change will be noted at that time. Motivational interviewing and CBT approaches are well suited for brief interventions and form a core set of treatment strategies from which many brief interventions are designed.

### Motivational Interviewing

Motivational interviewing is an empathetic, patient-focused, directive counseling style that aims at creating conditions necessary for behavior change.[10] It is based on 2 core assumptions: (1) motivation is a product of interpersonal interaction, not an innate character trait; and (2) ambivalence toward changing behavior and breaking habits is normal and acceptable.

According to this view, adolescents who use alcohol and drugs are in constant conflict, simultaneously experiencing positive and negative feelings about their use. Their "decisional balance" can be viewed as an old-fashioned pan scale, with the pros and cons of substance use represented by the relative weights on the 2 sides.

What the counselor does or says in counseling sessions can either help or hinder a patient in changing his or her behavior. Confrontation leads to polarization and resistance, with the patient arguing the case for drug use as an ego defense.

Exploration of the negative consequences (the cons) of drug use with empathy and understanding leads to motivation toward positive behavior change. In this model, the counselor elicits "change talk" by encouraging the adolescent to consider all aspects of drug and alcohol use, including negative consequences that have already occurred and those that may occur in the future if the current pattern of use remains the same. By exploring alcohol and drug use in this way, the adolescent presents the arguments for change. The counselor facilitates the discussion by asking thought-provoking, open-ended questions; listening carefully for the ambivalence in the patient's own words; and repeating and reinforcing the negative aspects of drug use and positive aspects of change. He or she also looks for opportunities to support self-efficacy by pointing out strengths and previous successes, regardless of how small. For example, a counselor might support self-efficacy by reframing a single use of marijuana as a success ("You used only one time this month, which is much less than before") for an adolescent attempting abstinence who has a "slip." Acknowledging the difficulties of making behavioral change helps create a supportive atmosphere for the adolescent. The counselor avoids resistance by refraining from lecturing or arguing with the patient.

### Cognitive Behavioral Therapy

Cognitive behavioral therapy is a structured, goal-oriented counseling style that has been effective for patients with substance abuse disorders.[11] Substance use is regarded as a learned behavioral response to environmental stimuli. The counselor shows patients how thoughts affect behavior and then teaches them to identify the thoughts and feelings that precede drug use. Once patients can recognize the precursors of drug use, they learn to avoid situations that trigger their use, or to substitute new behavioral responses instead of drug use. Cognitive behavioral therapy is most effective when patients are motivated to stop using and are willing and able to practice newly acquired skills.

## GROUP THERAPY

Group therapy for adolescents with substance use disorders offers several treatment advantages. Many teens can benefit from support from peers, and congregating with peers is a developmentally normal preference of adolescents. Group therapy offers adolescents the opportunity to meet other young people who are working on similar goals and may diminish the sense of isolation, or feeling of being singled out for drug treatment. In addition, group therapy may be cost effective and maximize the number of treatment opportunities available. Group composition must be carefully planned, and groups should be closely supervised because teens may also put peers at risk by encouraging drug use, providing information, or even supplying drugs outside the group meetings. Adolescents with co-occurring conduct disorders may be particularly disruptive, diminishing the ability of sessions to help others.[12] Thus, precautions are necessary when recommending group treatment.

### Twelve-Step Model

Twelve-step facilitation (TSF) therapy describes the process-oriented model developed by Alcoholics Anonymous (AA) and Narcotics Anonymous (NA).[13] In addition to being an effective treatment for adults with alcohol or drug problems,[14] the TSF method has shown promise with adolescents.[15] There is no prescribed curriculum, and each meeting is unique. Participants meet in small groups to share their drug and alcohol "stories," and provide support for each other. Other groups consider "working the 12 steps," a core group of spiritual principles that includes acknowledgment of powerlessness, developing belief in a "higher power," performing a critical self-inventory of one's character, making amends to those one has harmed, and helping other alcoholics achieve sobriety.[16] Many patients who are successful in recovering from drug and alcohol disorders using TSF continue to attend meetings for years after they have achieved abstinence. The TSF fellowship thus becomes an important social structure and provides the opportunity to meet others in recovery, and, ultimately, to provide service to the community in the form of mentoring.

Alcoholics Anonymous and NA have specially designated "young people's" meetings. These meetings are usually attended by young adults and may also be appropriate for adolescents. Adolescents who are referred to AA or NA meetings should be accompanied by a sponsor, such as an adult relative or family friend. This will allow the adolescent to process the content after the meeting has concluded, and also may serve to protect the adolescent from anyone who is still actively using drugs or alcohol who may be in attendance or near the premises of the meeting. Attendance at AA meetings has been shown to be a correlate of positive outcomes among adolescents in substance abuse treatment.[17]

### Psychoeducational Groups

In many communities, curriculum-based, psychoeducational groups are available for adolescents with substance use disorders. Many of these groups use the CBT modality. Cognitive behavioral therapy groups focus on skills training, problem solving, and role-playing. Participants also learn relaxation, stress reduction, and anger management techniques, because many adolescents with substance use disorders have had limited opportunities to develop skills in these areas.[18] For these groups to be successful, group composition must be carefully planned. Generally, adolescents should be in groups with peers who are close in age and who have had similar experiences. It may be best to avoid having adolescents who know each other from the community in the same group because attending a meeting together with "old friends" may trigger old behavior patterns. Adolescents with co-occurring disorders such as depression or anxiety should be treated and stable before beginning group therapy.

## FAMILY THERAPY

Parents and guardians play an important role in the treatment and recovery of adolescents with substance use disorders. Family therapies teach parents and guardians to monitor the behavior of their adolescent child, promote appropriate behavior with positive reinforcement, and provide negative consequences for inappropriate behavior. These therapies have reduced drug abuse and thus are practical and useful outpatient treatment options.[19]

### Functional Family Therapy

Functional family therapy (FFT) strives to alter dysfunctional family patterns that have influenced an individual's substance use. The work in FFT occurs in phases. In the first phase, counselors work to develop alliances with and between family members, improve communication, decrease polarization, and reduce negativity and hopelessness. In the next phase, individualized plans for change are developed and implemented, and in the final phase, changes are generalized and maintained to prevent relapse.[20]

### Multidimensional Family Therapy

Multidimensional family therapy is intended to treat adolescents with substance abuse and behavioral problems. It is a family-directed therapy that focuses on identifying and addressing the interaction patterns among the adolescent, parents, and other family members that contribute to problem behaviors. Therapy includes individual meetings with the adolescent, separate meetings with the parents, and family sessions. Frequent meetings and interim phone contact are a hallmark of this modality. This treatment has been manualized to ensure accurate replication.[21]

### Multisystemic Therapy

Multisystemic therapy attempts to address the adolescent's entire social network, including family, friends, and school. Treatment goals are developed on an individualized basis and in collaboration with family members. Parents are taught to set firm limits, recognize and reinforce positive behaviors, and use appropriate discipline for negative behaviors. Academic problems are assessed and addressed, and adolescents are assisted in breaking ties with drug-using peers. MST services are delivered at home. Counselors have only a few active patients at once, allowing them to provide intensive time-limited service to each family.[22,23]

## PHARMACOTHERAPY

Pharmacotherapy is a useful adjunct to psychotherapy for patients addicted to certain drugs. Opioid replacement therapy has a long history of safety and efficacy.[24,25] Several medications have also become available to treat patients with alcohol addictions. Newer medications for the treatment of cocaine addictions are currently being investigated. However, few medication trials have been conducted with adolescents.

### Opioids

Opioid replacement therapy has been a mainstay of the treatment of opioid-addicted patients for more than 4 decades. Methadone, a long-acting opioid agonist, has a long history of safety and efficacy for adult patients, although certain features make this option less attractive for adolescents. Because of legal restrictions, methadone can only be prescribed as opioid replacement therapy from specific methadone clinics, many of which do not accept adolescent patients. Attending methadone programs may also put adolescents at risk of exposure to drug-using patients in the vicinity of the clinic. Buprenorphine is a new synthetic partial opioid agonist that has several advantages over methadone, including lower abuse potential and a stronger safety profile. Buprenorphine is a partial agonist of the μ-opioid receptor that is as effective in treating opioid dependence as high-dose methadone[25] and can be prescribed by primary care physicians, thus providing better access for adolescents and reducing stigma. Buprenorphine is commonly prescribed in a combination sublingual tablet that includes naloxone, a μ-opioid antagonist with a higher affinity for the receptor than buprenorphine, to prevent patients from injecting their medication in an attempt to get high.

### Alcohol

Three medications have been approved by the US Food and Drug Administration to treat alcohol addiction: naltrexone, disulfiram, and acamprosate. None of these medications are specifically approved for use with adolescents, although they may be helpful in some cases. Each adolescent should be carefully evaluated before deciding whether a particular medication would be appropriate for that individual.

Naltrexone is an opioid-receptor antagonist that blocks μ-opioid receptors, leading to decreased feelings of intoxication and decreased drug cravings. Adherence may be an issue because of a side effect of nausea. A long-acting injected formulation, developed to improve treatment adherence, is available and has been used in adults with alcohol dependence.

Disulfiram inhibits acetaldehyde dehydrogenase, causing a highly unpleasant reaction to ingestion of even small amounts of alcohol while taking this medication. Disulfiram has been used for the treatment of alcohol dependence for the past 40 years, although patient adherence is generally poor, limiting its efficacy.[26] Because adolescents are relatively more impulsive compared to adults, disulfiram may be contraindicated. Acamprosate is used to reduce alcohol cravings in dependent patients. Acamprosate blocks glutaminergic N-methyl-D-aspartate receptors and activates gamma-aminobutyric acid type A receptors, although the exact neural mechanism involved in alcoholic craving is unknown. It has been shown to be helpful in reducing relapse rates, especially when combined with psychosocial treatments.

## INPATIENT TREATMENTS

Substance abuse treatment should be provided in the least restrictive setting possible.[27,28] Some adolescents need a greater level of supervision than can be provided by outpatient visits, because of safety issues, patient or family motivation, or medical or psychiatric complications. Adolescents who fail to improve significantly in an outpatient setting may need more intensive treatment. Adolescents with severe behavioral or psychiatric symptoms may require inpatient psychiatric hospitalization or acute residential treatment (ART) for stabilization in a safe, structured setting. Inpatient treatment programs form a spectrum from brief detoxification to long-term residential programs.

### DETOXIFICATION

Adolescents who are at risk of withdrawing from alcohol or sedatives should be monitored in a medically supervised setting because withdrawal symptoms may be life threatening. Adolescents withdrawing from opioids or stimulants may also benefit from a detoxification program to relieve the symptoms of withdrawal, although these symptoms are not generally life threatening in otherwise healthy young people. Detoxification is an essential first step in recovery, but is not adequate treatment for long-term recovery.

### PARTIAL HOSPITALIZATION PROGRAMS

Partial hospitalization, or day treatment, is an option for patients who require more intensive therapy than outpatient treatment can provide, yet do not need inpatient care. Adolescents spend several hours per day attending groups and individual counseling, and return home in the evening. A benefit of participating in a partial hospitalization program is that patients are given the opportunity to practice newly acquired skills in their daily lives at home and in their interactions with parents and friends. Most partial hospitalization programs use a combination of individual, family, and group therapy, and many provide skill development sessions and self-help groups, along with recreation, creative therapy techniques, and schooling. Little research has been done on these programs; existing studies have found participants to have similar rates of completion and reductions in substance use as those in residential programs.

### ACUTE RESIDENTIAL TREATMENT

Acute residential treatment typically lasts 1 to 4 weeks and can be useful for accomplishing the earliest phases of drug treatment in an intensive, highly structured setting. Acute residential treatment programs intervene with adolescents and families in crisis. For many adolescents, the first few weeks of abstinence can be the most challenging, and ART programs allow patients to establish new behaviors away from the environment in which their drug use behaviors may be entrenched. More specific psychiatric assessment and treatment are also initiated when indicated. After achieving stabilization in an ART program, adolescents may return home or enter a long-term residential treatment program for more intensive therapy.

**LONG-TERM RESIDENTIAL TREATMENT/ THERAPEUTIC SCHOOLS**

Residential programs offer 24-hour care for adolescents with substance use disorders. These programs provide therapy via a variety of modalities (individual counseling, group programs, family meetings, schooling and structured recreational activities). Adolescents with significant disruption in multiple aspects of their lives benefit from the intensive treatment provided, particularly if they are unable to function at school and at home, or if they present a risk to themselves or others. Therapeutic schools are residential educational institutions that also offer substance abuse and mental health treatment. These settings provide a supervised educational milieu that supports the adolescent's emotional, behavioral, social, and academic growth. Long-term residential programs and therapeutic schools may grant either high school diplomas or credits that can be transferred to another school.

**OTHER: WILDERNESS THERAPY PROGRAMS**

Other treatment approaches have not been scientifically evaluated, but may be an option for adolescents who have failed at other forms of treatment. Wilderness therapy programs take advantage of adolescents' physical abilities, a natural strength during this phase of life, in an attempt to promote personal growth through a strenuous physical curriculum. Traditional wilderness therapy programs encourage independence and promote self-esteem by teaching problem-solving skills.[29] Adolescents learn to take responsibility for their actions and improve decision making by assessing consequences. Many wilderness programs include daily individual and group therapy. Wilderness therapy programs treat adolescents with a variety of behavioral problems. Although not specifically designed as a treatment for substance use disorders, many of the adolescents in these programs have drug problems, and drug use is often addressed in the various curricula. Wilderness therapy programs vary greatly, and parents should be cautioned to consider only those programs that are licensed by their host state.

## AFTER-CARE

All adolescents who have successfully completed treatment for a substance use disorder will need after-care for monitoring, relapse prevention, and to help them reestablish functioning in school, at home, and in other aspects of their lives. All adolescents should be followed by their primary care physician to demonstrate ongoing support and caring, and to reduce the stigma associated with substance abuse treatment. Adolescents who successfully complete brief interventions with good results can be referred back to their primary care physician for ongoing monitoring. Adolescents who have completed more intensive programs may benefit from subsequent participation in a less intensive setting, such as individual treatment or after-care groups.

**RECOVERY HIGH SCHOOLS**

Many adolescents who complete an intensive substance abuse treatment program are placed at risk of relapse by returning to the settings, such as their school, where they used drugs or spent time with drug-using peers. Recovery high schools integrate educational, therapeutic, and mentoring services for adolescents who have completed substance abuse treatment and pledged to stay sober. These schools reinforce positive, drug-free behavior and allow adolescents to be in a milieu of peers with similar experiences and goals. There are currently 30 recovery high schools nationwide, and new programs are being developed rapidly.[30]

## SUMMARY

Adolescents with substance use disorders need specific, targeted interventions to help them replace and maintain drug use behaviors with healthy behavior patterns. Treatment can take various forms and can be given in a variety of modalities and settings. The primary care physician can be instrumental in helping design an individualized treatment program based on the severity of the substance use disorder, presence of co-occurring disorders, patient and family preferences, and availability of resources. Primary care physician should always follow up with patients after they have completed their treatment to determine whether treatment was effective, whether additional resources or treatments would be beneficial, and to provide ongoing monitoring and support for patients and families.

## REFERENCES

1. Hingson R, Heeren T, Winter M. Age at drinking onset and alcohol dependence. *Arch Pediatr Adolesc Med*. 2006;160:739-746

2. Boys A, Marsden J. Perceived functions predict intensity of use and problems in young polysubstance users. *Addiction*. 2003;98:951-963

3. Tevyaw T, Monti P. Motivational enhancement and other brief interventions for adolescent substance abuse: foundations, applications, and evaluations. *Addiction*. 2004;99(suppl 2): 63-75

4. Waldron H, Kaminer Y. On the learning curve: the emerging evidence supporting cognitive-behavioral therapies for adolescent substance abuse. *Addiction*. 2004;99(suppl 2):93-105

5. Randall J, Cunningham P. Multisystemic therapy: a treatment for violent substance-abusing and substance dependent juvenile offenders. *Addict Behav*. 2003;28(9):1737–1739

6. Liddle H, Dakof G, Parker K, Diamond G, Barrett K, Tejeda M. Multidimensional family therapy for adolescent drug abuse: results of a randomized clinical trial. *Am J Drug Alcohol Abuse*. 2001;27(4):651–688

7. Henggeler S, Pickrel S, Brondino M. Multisystemic treatment of substance-abusing and dependent delinquents: outcomes, treatment fidelity, and transportability. *Ment Health Serv Res*. 1999;1(3):171–184

8. Liddle H. Family-based therapies for adolescent alcohol and drug use: research contributions and future research needs. *Addiction*. 2004;99(suppl 2):76–92

9. Prochaska JO, DiClemente CC. Stages of change in the modification of problem behaviors. *Prog Behav Modif*. 1992;28: 183–218

10. Miller W, Rollnick S, eds. *Motivational Interviewing: Preparing People to Change Addictive Behavior*. New York: Guilford Press; 1991

11. Kadden R, Carroll K, Donovan D, et al. *Cognitive-Behavioral Coping Skills Therapy Manual: A Clinical Research Guide for Therapists Treating Individuals with Alcohol Abuse and Dependence*. Rockville, MD: National Institute on Alcohol Abuse and Alcoholism; 1994

12. Dishion T, Poulin F, Burraston B. Peer group dynamics associated with iatrogenic effects in group interventions with high-risk young adolescents. In: Nangle D, Erdley C, eds. *The Role of Friendship in Psychological Adjustment: New Directions for Child and Adolescent Development*. No. 91. San Francisco: Jossey-Bass; 2001:79

13. Nowinski J, Baker S, Carroll KM. *Twelve-Step Facilitation Therapy Manual: A Clinical Research Guide for Therapists Treating Individuals with Alcohol Abuse and Dependence*. Rockville, MD: National Institute on Alcohol Abuse and Alcoholism; 1994

14. Vaillant G. Alcoholics Anonymous: cult or cure? *Aust N Z J Psychiatry*. 2005;39:431–436

15. Alford G, Koehler R, Leonard J. Alcoholics Anonymous-Narcotics Anonymous model inpatient treatment of chemically dependent adolescents: a 2-year outcome study. *J Stud Alcohol*. 1991;52(2):118–126

16. Alcoholics Anonymous. *Twelve Steps and Twelve Traditions*. New York: Alcoholics Anonymous World Services; 1995

17. Kelly JF, Myers MG, Brown SA. Do adolescents affiliate with 12-step groups? A multivariate process model of effects. *J Stud Alcohol*. 2002;63(3):293–304

18. Carroll KM. *Therapy Manuals for Drug Addiction. Manual 1—A Cognitive-Behavioral Approach: Treating Cocaine Addiction*. Rockville, MD: National Institute on Drug Abuse; 1998. NIDA publication 98-4308

19. Deas D, Thomas S. An overview of controlled studies of adolescent substance abuse treatment. *Am J Addict*. 2001;10 (2):178–189

20. Sexton T, Alexander J. *Functional Family Therapy*. Washington, DC: Office of Justice Programs; 2000.

21. Liddle H. *Multidimensional Family Therapy for Adolescent Cannabis Users*. Rockville, MD: Center for Substance Abuse Treatment, Substance Abuse and Mental Health Services Administration, US Department of Health and Human Services; 2002

22. Henggeler S, Schoenwald S, Borduin C, Rowland M, Cunningham P. *Multisystemic Treatment of Antisocial Behavior in Children and Adolescents*. New York: Guilford Press; 1998

23. Henggeler S, Clingempeel W, Brondino M, Pickrel S. Four-year follow-up of multisystemic therapy with substance-abusing and substance-dependent juvenile offenders. *J Am Acad Child Adolesc Psychiatry*. 2002;41(7):868–874

24. Sees K, Delucchi K, Masson C, et al. Methadone maintenance vs 180-day psychosocially enriched detoxification for treatment of opioid dependence: a randomized controlled trial. *JAMA*. 2000;283(10):1303–1310

25. Fudala P, Bridge T, Herbert S, et al. Office-based treatment of opiate addiction with a sublingual-tablet formulation of buprenorphine and naloxone. *N Eng J Med*. 2003;349 (10):949–958

26. O'Farrell T, Allen J, Litten R. Disulfram (Antabuse) contracts in treatment of alcoholism. *NIDA Res Monogr*. 1995;150:65–91

27. American Academy of Child and Adolescent Psychiatry. Practice parameter for the assessment and treatment of children and adolescents with substance use disorders. *J Am Acad Child Adolesc Psychiatry*. 2005;44(6):609

28. American Society of Addiction Medicine (ASAM). *ASAM Patient Placement Criteria for the Treatment of Substance-Related Disorders*. Chevy Chase, MD; American Society of Addiction Medicine; 2001

29. Russell KC, Hendee JC, Phillips-Miller D. How wilderness therapy works: an examination of the wilderness therapy process to treat adolescents with behavioral problems and addictions. In: Cole DN, McCool SF, eds. *Proceedings: Wilderness Science in a Time of Change*. Proc. Ogden, UT: US Department of Agriculture, Forest Service, Rocky Mountain Research Station; 2000. Proc. RMRS-P-000

30. Association of Recovery Schools. Schools, associates, and foundational members. 2006. Available at: www.recoveryschools.org/schools.html. Accessed on September 21, 2009

## SECTION 3

# Psychiatric, Behavioral, and Developmental Health Problems

## CHAPTER 183

# Somatoform Disorders in Adolescents

RICHARD E. KREIPE, MD

*Partially supported by HRSA/MCHB Grant 5 T71MC00012-09-00.*

## INTRODUCTION

Somatoform disorders in adolescents include a variety of conditions in which somatic symptoms are not adequately explained by a physical condition but are associated with significant functional impairment. The approaches to adolescents with somatoform symptoms that are often used by clinicians can hinder acceptance by the patient and the family of the diagnosis and effective treatment. In contrast, a biopsychosocial approach that uses a "systems" model that considers all levels of impairment (from the molecular, to the patient, to the family, and beyond) in interactive dynamics allows for the development of therapeutic partnerships in which the adolescent and the family are active agents in symptom improvement (Figure 183-1).

This chapter addresses the practical application of the biopsychosocial approach to somatoform disorders in either primary or specialty care for adolescents. Existing classification and diagnostic criteria, as well as potential pitfalls in diagnosing somatoform disorders using the suggested algorithm in the *Diagnostic and Statistical Manual-IV-TR Fourth Edition, Text Revision (DSM-IV-TR)*, are addressed first. This is followed by a discussion of practical strategies, skills, and techniques for providers to use in evaluating, treating, and referring adolescents with somatoform disorder.

## CLASSIFICATION OF SOMATOFORM DISORDERS IN *DSM-IV-TR*

Somatoform disorders comprise 6 distinct diagnoses: somatization disorder, conversion disorder, pain disorder, hypochondriasis, body dysmorphic disorder, and undifferentiated or not-otherwise-specified somatoform disorder. All of these share 2 features in common: (1) physical (somatic) symptoms that suggest a medical condition but are not fully explained by a medical or mental disorder or the direct effects of a substance, and (2) symptoms that "must cause clinically significant distress or impairment in social, occupational, or other areas of functioning."[1]

Because the symptoms are physical, patients with somatoform disorders generally present to a primary care provider or medical specialist rather than to a mental health provider. Although patients with factitious disorder and malingering can present with similar symptoms and are often considered in the differential diagnosis, they each are placed in separate categories in the *DSM-IV-TR*.[1] They will be discussed here, however, because of the similarities of these disorders with classic somatoform disorders and because they are included in the *DSM-IV-TR* somatoform diagnostic algorithm.

### SOMATIZATION DISORDER

Adolescents with somatization disorder (Box 183-1) display a pattern of multiple, recurring, somatic symptoms that are not fully explained by a general medical condition nor by the direct effects of a substance and that result in medical or surgical treatment(s) because of significant impairment in social, occupational, or other important areas of functioning. Although the *DSM-IV-TR* criteria require the onset of symptoms before 30 years of age, most affected individuals have their onset in the teenage years. Because the pattern of multiple symptoms may not be recognized in primary care during adolescence,

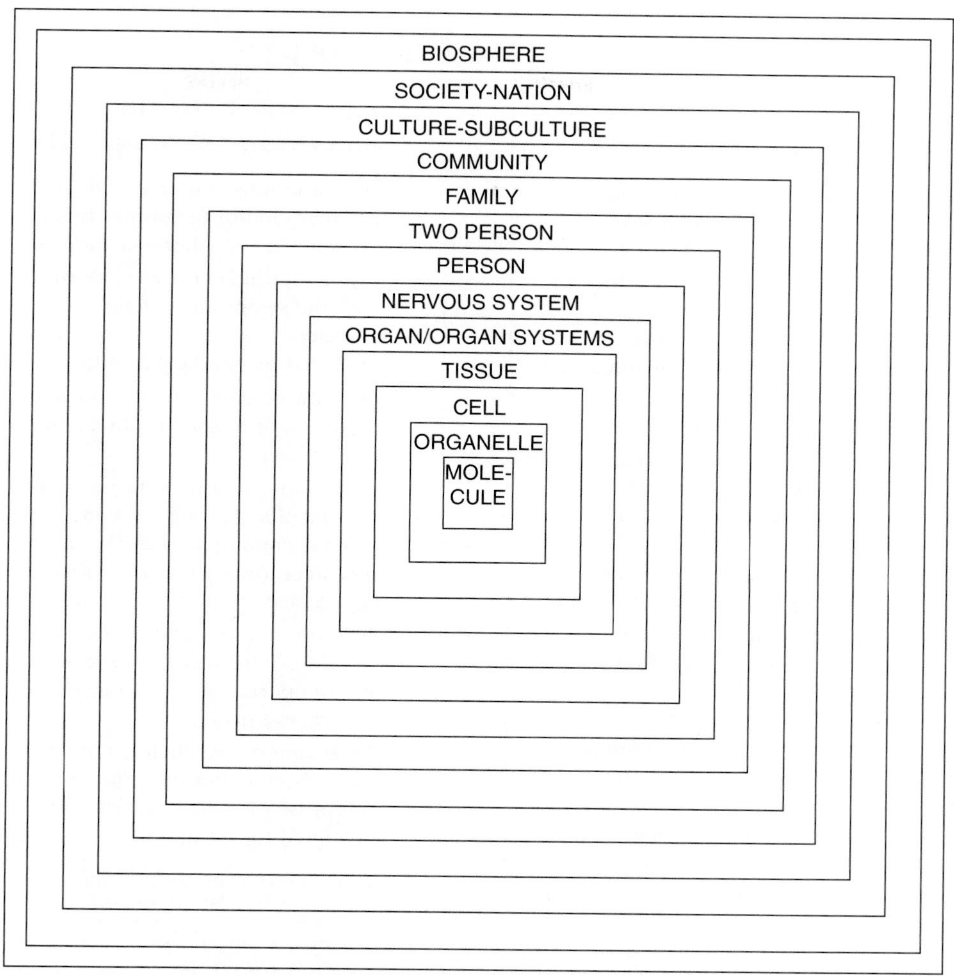


**FIGURE 183-1** Biopsychosocial model of systems-level interactions. (Reprinted with permission from Engel GL. The clinical application of the biopsychosocial model. *Amer J of Psychiatry*. 1980;137:537.)

affected individuals often are treated as if they have a series of unrelated health problems. This can make treatment in adulthood more difficult because of longstanding impairments in educational, social, and work domains.

Somatization disorder in adolescents may be associated with an underlying anxiety disorder or depression.[2] Although the disorder is classified as a psychiatric condition, adolescents with somatization disorder benefit from regular contact with their primary care provider, with brief, scheduled visits to avoid prolonged, urgent visits as new symptoms arise.[3] Psychiatric consultation in somatization disorder has been shown to reduce hospitalization and the overall cost of care.[4]

## CONVERSION DISORDER

The core feature of conversion disorder (Box 183-2) is the presence of symptoms affecting motor or sensory function for which no underlying medical condition is found, but psychological factors are thought to be related. Common neurologic findings include motor symptoms that are incongruous with known neuroanatomy or neurologic function, impaired coordination or balance (eg, wide-based "astasia-abasia" gait), paralysis or localized weakness, dysphonia, dysphagia, or convulsions, and sensory symptoms that include loss of touch or pain sensation, double vision, blindness, or deafness.

The diagnosis of conversion disorder should be preceded by a thorough history and comprehensive physical examination.[5] These are required not only to establish that the history and physical examination are not consistent with any known medical condition, but also to provide positive evidence regarding the underlying psychological issues.[6] Once the diagnosis is made, close medical follow-up is needed because medical etiologies are later found in up to half of individuals originally diagnosed with conversion symptoms.

## Box 183-1

### *Diagnostic Criteria for 300.81, Somatization Disorder* (DSM-IV-TR)

A. History of many physical complaints beginning before age 30 that occur over a period of several years and result in treatment being sought or significant impairment in social, occupational, or other important areas of functioning.

B. Each of the following criteria must have been met, with individual symptoms occurring at any time during the course of the disturbance:

1. *four pain symptoms:* a history of pain related to at least 4 different sites or functions (eg, head, abdomen, back, joints, extremities, chest, rectum, during menstruation, during sexual intercourse, or during urination)
2. *two gastrointestinal symptoms:* a history of at least 2 gastrointestinal symptoms other than pain (eg, nausea, bloating, vomiting other than during pregnancy, diarrhea, or intolerance of several different foods)
3. *one sexual symptom:* a history of at least 1 sexual or reproductive symptom other than pain (eg, sexual indifference, erectile or ejaculatory dysfunction, irregular menses, excessive menstrual bleeding, vomiting throughout pregnancy)
4. *one pseudoneurological symptom:* a history of at least 1 symptom or deficit suggesting a neurological condition not limited to pain (conversion symptoms such as impaired coordination or balance, paralysis or localized weakness, difficulty swallowing or lump in throat, aphonia, urinary retention, hallucinations, loss of touch or pain sensation, double vision, blindness, deafness, seizures; dissociative symptoms such as amnesia; or loss of consciousness other than fainting)

C. Either (1) or (2):

1. after appropriate investigation, each of the symptoms in criterion B cannot be fully explained by a known general medical condition or the direct effects of a substance (eg, a drug of abuse, a medication)
2. when there is a related general medical condition, the physical complaints or resulting social or occupational impairment are in excess of what would be expected from the history, physical examination, or laboratory findings

D. The symptoms are not intentionally produced or feigned (as in factitious disorder or malingering).

---

Reprinted with permission from American Psychiatric Association. *Diagnostic and Statistical Manual of Mental Disorders.* 4th ed. Text Revision. Washington, DC: American Psychiatric Association; 2000: 490.

## Box 183-2

### *Diagnostic Criteria for 300.11, Conversion Disorder* (DSM-IV-TR)

A. One or more symptoms or deficits affecting voluntary motor or sensory function that suggest a neurological or other general medical condition.

B. Psychological factors are judged to be associated with the symptom or deficit because the initiation or exacerbation of the symptom or deficit is preceded by conflicts or other stressors.

C. The symptom or deficit is not intentionally produced or feigned (as in factitious disorder or malingering).

D. The symptom or deficit cannot, after appropriate investigation, be fully explained by a general medical condition, or by the direct effects of a substance, or as a culturally sanctioned behavior or experience.

E. The symptom or deficit causes clinically significant distress or impairment in social, occupational, or other important areas of functioning or warrants medical evaluation.

F. The symptom or deficit is not limited to pain or sexual dysfunction, does not occur exclusively during the course of somatization disorder, and is not better accounted for by another mental disorder.

---

*Specify* type of symptom or deficit: motor; sensory; seizures or convulsions; mixed.

---

Reprinted with permission from American Psychiatric Association. *Diagnostic and Statistical Manual of Mental Disorders.* 4th ed. Text Revision. Washington, DC: American Psychiatric Association; 2000: 498.

## PAIN DISORDER

The diagnostic features of pain disorder (Box 183-3) are parallel to those for conversion disorder, except the symptom that brings the adolescent to the attention of the clinician is pain rather than a neurologic or general medical disorder. The dynamics of an underlying psychological problem and treatment approach are also similar to conversion disorder, although often more complicated in pain disorder because of the availability of powerful analgesics, many of which have addictive potential. The diagnosis is sometimes not considered until the realization that the adolescent has sought pain medications from several different providers.

Emerging evidence demonstrates that stressors and proinflammatory cytokines play an important role in somatic amplification of a number of "illness" symptoms seen in somatoform disorders, especially pain.[7] Functional magnetic resonance imaging (*f*MRI) of the

**Box 183-3**

### *Diagnostic Criteria for Pain Disorder* (DSM-IV-TR)

A. Pain in 1 or more anatomical sites is the predominant focus of the clinical presentation and is of sufficient severity to warrant clinical attention.

B. The pain causes clinically significant distress or impairment in social, occupational, or other important areas of functioning.

C. Psychological factors are judged to have an important role in the onset, severity, exacerbation, or maintenance of the pain.

D. The symptom or deficit is not intentionally produced or feigned (as in factitious disorder or malingering).

E. The pain is not better accounted for by a mood, anxiety, or psychotic disorder and does not meet criteria for dyspareunia.

*Code* as follows:

**307.80 Pain Disorder Associated with Psychological Factors:** Psychological factors are judged to have the major role in the onset, severity, exacerbation, or maintenance of the pain. (If a general medical condition is present, it does not have a major role in the onset, severity, exacerbation, or maintenance of the pain.) This type of pain disorder is not diagnosed if criteria are also met for somatization disorder.

*Specify:* Acute if duration <6 months; chronic if duration ≥6 months.

**307.89 Pain Disorder Associated with Both Psychological Factors and a General Medical Condition:** Both psychological factors and a general medical condition are judged to have important roles in the onset, severity, exacerbation, or maintenance of the pain. The associated general medical condition or anatomical site of the pain (see the following) is coded on Axis III.

*Specify:* Acute if duration <6 months; chronic if duration ≥6 months.

Reprinted with permission from American Psychiatric Association. *Diagnostic and Statistical Manual of Mental Disorders.* 4th ed. Text Revision. Washington, DC: American Psychiatric Association; 2000: 503.

brain shows common neural response patterns to both actual and hypnotically suggested painful stimuli.[8] Additionally, *f*MRI studies have been performed in subjects dichotomized into low and high pain sensitivity groups who received identical painful stimuli. These studies have shown that the high pain sensitivity subjects, when compared to the low sensitivity subjects, demonstrated increased activation of the anterior cingulate, somatosensory, and prefrontal cortex.[9]

## HYPOCHONDRIASIS

Hypochondriasis (Box 183-4) is uncommon among adolescents, but is included under the umbrella of somatoform disorders because of the prominent role of concern about bodily symptoms resulting in psychosocial morbidity. Although a criterion for the diagnosis is the persistence of preoccupation with symptoms despite appropriate medical evaluation and reassurance,[1] it is important for the evaluation to address all of the concerns of the adolescent or young adult and not only what the clinician deems appropriate. This is especially important if the patient has anxiety because of a heightened concern about body symptoms with anxiety.

## BODY DYSMORPHIC DISORDER

Symptoms of body dysmorphic disorder (Box 183-5) may at times appear to mimic anorexia nervosa, but the focus is an imagined or exaggerated physical defect. It occurs as commonly in males as in females, and is often associated with obsessive-compulsive symptoms, but

**Box 183-4**

### *Diagnostic Criteria for 300.7 Hypochondriasis* (DSM-IV-TR)

A. Preoccupation with fears of having, or the idea that one has, a serious disease based on the person's misinterpretation of bodily symptoms.

B. The preoccupation persists despite appropriate medical evaluation and reassurance.

C. The belief in criterion A is not of delusional intensity (as in delusional disorder, somatic type) and is not restricted to a circumscribed concern about appearance (as in body dysmorphic disorder).

D. The preoccupation causes clinically significant distress or impairment in social, occupational, or other important areas of functioning.

E. The duration of the disturbance is at least 6 months.

F. The preoccupation is not better accounted for by generalized anxiety disorder, obsessive-compulsive disorder, panic disorder, a major depressive episode, separation anxiety, or another somatoform disorder.

*Specify:* With poor insight if for most of the time during the current episode, the person does not recognize that the concern about having a serious illness is excessive or unreasonable.

Reprinted with permission from American Psychiatric Association. *Diagnostic and Statistical Manual of Mental Disorders.* 4th ed. Text Revision. Washington, DC: American Psychiatric Association; 2000: 507.

**Box 183-5**

***Diagnostic Criteria for 300.7 Body Dysmorphic Disorder* (DSM-IV-TR)**

A. Preoccupation with an imagined defect in appearance. If a slight physical anomaly is present, the person's concern is markedly excessive.
B. The preoccupation causes clinically significant distress or impairment in social, occupational, or other important areas of functioning.
C. The preoccupation is not better accounted for by another mental disorder (eg, dissatisfaction with body shape and size in anorexia nervosa).

Reprinted with permission from American Psychiatric Association. *Diagnostic and Statistical Manual of Mental Disorders.* 4th ed. Text Revision. Washington, DC: American Psychiatric Association; 2000: 510.

can take on strongly delusional qualities.[10] In men, body dysmorphia is often related to small size generally or to inadequately large or developed musculature; in women it may be the presence of a small facial mole or the absence of adequate breast tissue.

### UNDIFFERENTIATED AND NOT-OTHERWISE-SPECIFIED SOMATOFORM DISORDERS

As is true of many conditions in the *DSM-IV-TR*, most patients with somatoform symptoms do not reach the level of a full syndrome, but fall into an undifferentiated or not-otherwise-specified category. For *undifferentiated*, symptoms are fewer in number but are present for at least 6 months (Box 183-6); for *not otherwise specified*, all that is required is that the adolescent's condition does not meet the criteria for a specific somatoform disorder (Box 183-7). The symptoms may be as vague as fatigue or weakness of fewer than 6 months duration. Although over time both undifferentiated and not-otherwise-specified somatoform disorders may develop into full syndromes, health care providers presented with symptoms suggestive of a somatoform disorder should not delay the identification and early intervention for these conditions.

### CONDITIONS WITH "VOLUNTARY" SOMATIC SYMPTOMS

All of the somatic symptoms in the diagnoses listed previously are not considered to be under voluntary control. Two diagnostic categories that may mimic somatoform disorders, but are thought to be under voluntary control, are malingering and factitious disorders.

**Box 183-6**

***Diagnostic Criteria for 300.82 Undifferentiated Somatoform Disorder* (DSM-IV-TR)**

A. One or more physical complaints (eg, fatigue, loss of appetite, gastrointestinal, or urinary complaints).
B. Either (1) or (2):
   1. after appropriate investigation, the symptoms cannot be fully explained by a known general medical condition or the direct effects of a substance (eg, a drug of abuse, a medication).
   2. when there is a related general medical condition, the physical complaints or resulting social or occupational impairment is in excess of what would be expected from the history, physical examination, or laboratory findings.
C. The symptoms cause clinically significant distress or impairment in social, occupational, or other important areas of functioning.
D. The duration of the disturbance is at least 6 months.
E. The disturbance is not better accounted for by another mental disorder (eg, another somatoform disorder, sexual dysfunction, mood disorder, anxiety disorder, sleep disorder, or psychotic disorder).
F. The symptom is not intentionally produced or feigned (as in factitious disorder or malingering).

Reprinted with permission from American Psychiatric Association. *Diagnostic and Statistical Manual of Mental Disorders.* 4th ed. Text Revision. Washington, DC: American Psychiatric Association; 2000: 492.

#### Malingering

Malingering is characterized by the intentional production of nonexistent or grossly exaggerated physical or psychological symptoms that is motivated by external incentives, such as not going to school, avoiding work, obtaining financial compensation in litigation for an injury, or obtaining narcotic analgesics (Box 183-8). It can be adaptive, depending on the circumstances. In clinical situations, however, consideration of the diagnosis of malingering tends to raise a barrier between the adolescent and the health care provider because the patient often complains about not being believed and the clinician often feels that he or she is being lied to or manipulated. As discussed later, the determination of symptoms being intentionally produced for some external gain is challenging and clinically counterproductive.

**Box 183-7**

***300.81 Somatoform Disorder Not Otherwise Specified* (DSM-IV-TR)**

This category includes disorders with somatoform symptoms that do not meet the criteria for any specific somatoform disorder. Examples include:

1. Pseudocyesis: a false belief of being pregnant that is associated with objective signs of pregnancy, which may include abdominal enlargement (although the umbilicus does not become everted), reduced menstrual flow, amenorrhea, subjective sensation of fetal movement, nausea, breast engorgement and secretions, and labor pains at the expected date of delivery. Endocrine changes may be present, but the syndrome cannot be explained by a general medical condition that causes endocrine changes (eg, a hormone-secreting tumor).
2. A disorder involving nonpsychotic hypochondriacal symptoms of less than 6 months duration.
3. A disorder involving unexplained physical complaints (eg, fatigue or body weakness) of less than 6 months duration that are not due to another mental disorder.

Reprinted with permission from American Psychiatric Association. *Diagnostic and Statistical Manual of Mental Disorders.* 4th ed. Text Revision. Washington, DC: American Psychiatric Association; 2000: 511.

**Box 183-8**

***V65.2 Malingering* (DSM-IV-TR)**

The essential feature of malingering is the intentional production of false or grossly exaggerated physical or psychological symptoms, motivated by external incentives such as avoiding military duty, avoiding work, obtaining financial compensation, evading criminal prosecution, or obtaining drugs. Under some circumstances, malingering may represent adaptive behavior—for example, feigning illness while a captive of the enemy during wartime. Malingering should be strongly suspected if any combination of the following is noted:

1. Medicolegal context of presentation (eg, the person is referred by an attorney to the clinician for examination)
2. Marked discrepancy between the person's claimed stress or disability and the objective findings
3. Lack of cooperation during the diagnostic evaluation and in complying with the prescribed treatment regimen
4. The presence of antisocial personality disorder

Reprinted with permission from American Psychiatric Association. *Diagnostic and Statistical Manual of Mental Disorders.* 4th ed. Text Revision. Washington, DC: American Psychiatric Association; 2000: 739.

### Factitious Disorder

Factitious disorders are characterized by physical or psychological symptoms that are intentionally produced or feigned, without a recognizable external incentive as is found in malingering (Box 183-9). The presumed goal is to assume the sick role, in which the adolescent may be relieved of certain responsibilities or able to avoid conflict because of being "sick." Unlike malingering, which can be adaptive, the diagnosis of factitious disorder always implies psychopathology. In simple factitious disorder, the adolescent has psychopathology; in factitious disorder by proxy, the psychopathology is in a proxy agent.

Because of the difficulties associated with diagnosing factitious disorder, as well as with presenting the diagnosis to adolescents and families, the clinician needs concrete evidence by direct observation (eg, surveillance video) and/or by tests that cannot be manipulated. Disclosure of the presumptive diagnosis should be done with psychiatric consultation, especially in cases by proxy, because of the aforementioned psychopathology that may emerge acutely when the defense has been breached.

**Box 183-9**

***Diagnostic Criteria for Factitious Disorder* (DSM-IV-TR)**

A. Intentional production or feigning of physical or psychological signs or symptoms.

B. The motivation for the behavior is to assume the sick role.

C. External incentives for the behavior (such as economic gain, avoiding legal responsibility, or improving physical well-being, as in malingering) are absent.

*Code* based on type:

300.16 With predominantly *psychological* signs and symptoms: if psychological signs and symptoms predominate in the clinical presentation.

300.19 With predominantly *physical* signs and symptoms: if physical signs and symptoms predominate in the clinical presentation.

300.19 With *combined* psychological and physical signs and symptoms: if both psychological and physical signs and symptoms are present but neither predominates in the clinical presentation.

Reprinted with permission from American Psychiatric Association. *Diagnostic and Statistical Manual of Mental Disorders*. 4th ed. Text Revision. Washington, DC: American Psychiatric Association; 2000: 517.

## CHALLENGES USING THE *DSM-IV-TR* DIAGNOSTIC SCHEME WITH ADOLESCENTS

In clinical practice, mental health symptoms associated with somatoform disorders tend to be considered the *result* of a physical illness by adolescent patients and their parents. Health care providers, however, often interpret underlying psychiatric problems as the *cause* of the symptoms. Medical care providers who dichotomize somatic symptoms into mutually exclusive, linear "organic" or "psychologic" categories often use an approach that leads to conflict and dissatisfaction for everyone (adolescents, parents, *and* health care providers), as discussed later in this chapter.

### LIMITATIONS OF THE *DSM-IV-TR* DIAGNOSTIC ALGORITHM

There are at least 3 dilemmas facing clinicians using the *DSM-IV-TR* diagnostic algorithm for somatoform disorders. First, the need to rule out an underlying medical condition; second, the requirement to differentiate between voluntary and involuntary symptoms; and third, the need to identify any underlying conflict or stressor. Problems that arise as a result of these elements are detailed in the following.

#### Ruling Out Underlying Medical Conditions

"Ruling out" underlying medical conditions in the patient with somatoform disorders involves diagnostic testing that may include: (1) analysis of blood, urine, stool, or spinal fluid; (2) indirect imaging by ultrasound, x-rays, computed tomography (CT), or magnetic resonance imaging (MRI); (3) direct imaging of internal organs by endoscopy or laparoscopy; and (4) procedures related to the function of the heart (eg, echocardiogram), lungs (eg, pulmonary function test), brain (eg, electroencephalogram; EEG), metabolism (eg, breath hydrogen test), or other targets suggested by the symptoms. When presented with symptoms not accounted for by the history or physical examination, physicians may perform a battery of tests, some of which will be neither informative nor necessary, but are performed for the sake of completeness or in response to pressures by the patient and/or parents to "figure out what is causing the problem." However, few diagnostic tests have 100% sensitivity in detecting pathology. Also, the more tests that are performed the greater the likelihood that some abnormal results will appear due to random error rather than pathology.

Although such an unfocused strategy may lead a clinician to conclude that a medical condition has been excluded, a series of negative or normal test results often trigger requests or demands for additional tests from the adolescent and/or parent(s). A major source of misinformation leading to such requests is the Internet. Sometimes the requests are for unusual tests, such as to detect "dysbiosis" related to "yeast overgrowth," diagnosed by the presence of antibodies of unknown significance. Thus, in practice, diagnostic testing to either rule out or determine the cause of symptoms often confuses rather than clarifies the source of the symptoms. Just as the absence of proof does not constitute proof of absence of a medical condition, the presence of abnormal findings, such as gallstones, does not necessarily account for symptoms of abdominal pain. The presence of a medical diagnosis may distract from the recognition of an underlying psychiatric condition.

A physician who reports normal diagnostic test findings to a somatic adolescent may not be reassuring because of the possible interpretation of "there is nothing wrong with you." If mention of normal diagnostic tests is followed by questions about underlying stress or emotional problems, the patient may conclude that the physician assumes that "the doctor thinks that this is all in my head." Therefore, adolescents and/or their parents may be *disappointed* when told of normal test results. When diagnostic tests are obtained with a belief that the tests will identify the cause of the symptoms, there is hope that the test(s) will result in a diagnosis. Normal test results are not reassuring if the diagnosis remains unknown and the prognosis remains uncertain; the logical next step is often to obtain more tests. "Negative" test results are also distressing because adolescents may believe that without a positive test, no treatment will be offered and the symptoms could continue indefinitely. This exacerbates the suffering already being caused by the symptoms.

If the physician notes that no further studies are indicated because testing has been normal so far, the adolescent and parents may be resentful that the severity of the symptoms is not being fully appreciated. Likewise, there may be a sense of abandonment when the patient is told "there's nothing more I can do for you," "you'll just have to learn to live with it," or "you need to see a psychiatrist, because I can't find anything wrong with you physically." Obtaining more tests may temporarily give the patient and family hope, but more negative test results fuel a vicious cycle with unacceptable outcomes.

Some health care providers believe that to perform too many tests only reinforces the belief that a medical condition exists, sometimes termed "feeding into the illness." However, *not* performing tests may suggest to the patient that the symptoms are not being taken seriously, often leading to families consulting with a series of specialists. The medical care of adolescents with somatoform disorders requires a balance of art and science that can help to avoid some of these pitfalls. A detailed and comprehensive history and physical examination, performed with the explicit intention of looking for clues that will lead to the diagnosis, raises these essential elements of medical care to the level of importance of diagnostic testing in the perception of patients and parents.

Furthermore, caution regarding the difficulty of "ruling out" an underlying medical condition is based on emerging evidence from psychoneuroimmunology and other fields. A variety of studies suggest the presence of important biological substrates that modulate symptoms but cannot be determined by the history, physical examination, or laboratory testing.[11] For example, rats exposed to inescapable tailshock became sensitized to the innate immune response to a dose of bacterial endotoxin and later had an enhanced induction of proinflammatory cytokines compared to controls.[12] Moreover, there is strong evidence that the brain recognizes cytokines as molecular signals of sickness.[13] Although our understanding of how the brain processes information generated by the innate immune system has been accompanied by an improved understanding of the cellular and molecular components of the intricate system that mediates cytokine-induced sickness behavior, much remains to be clarified.

### Involuntary vs Voluntary (Intentional) Symptoms

The purpose of distinguishing if somatic symptoms are involuntary or intentionally produced is to differentiate somatoform disorders from malingering and factitious disorders, in which symptoms are under voluntary control. Although somatoform disorders are characterized by symptoms *not* under voluntary control, attempting to determine if symptoms *are* intentionally produced tends to be counterproductive in clinical practice. Adolescents who *are not* intentionally producing symptoms are offended and suffer further because they are not believed; adolescents who *are* intentionally producing symptoms may become indignant or escalate or modify their symptoms.

If the diagnosis of factitious disorder is being considered, data from numerous sources should be obtained prior to any direct confrontation of the adolescent or parent with the diagnosis. The production of signs or symptoms to assume the sick role in factitious disorder, whether by the adolescent or by a proxy, can be associated with significant harm, including death, because of the associated major psychiatric illness. Ultimately, the patient and/or proxy must be approached cautiously, with appropriate input from psychiatry, but not avoided.

### Symptoms Caused by Unresolved Conflict or Stress

The third step in the *DSM-IV-TR* somatoform diagnostic algorithm is the determination if unconscious, unresolved conflict or stress is related to the symptom pattern. In conversion disorder, stress or unresolved conflict that cannot be dealt with on a conscious level submerges below the level of awareness, but is "converted" into somatic, often neurologic, symptoms. The symptom often has symbolic meaning and reflects symptoms in a "model."[5] Apparent indifference to the symptoms (*la belle indifference*) is not common in adolescents and is difficult to operationalize.[2] In classic conversion disorder, there are primary and secondary gains that can be identified, representing something that the adolescent is avoiding and is approaching, respectively. The avoidance-approach dynamic is not unique to conversion disorder but provides homeostatic balance by allowing the adolescent to avoid the source of stress or unresolved conflict (primary) and also approach something desirable, such as attention (secondary). As is true of the other elements of the *DSM-IV-TR* algorithm, this criterion is difficult to apply clinically because it is not clear how a clinician determines if psychological factors *are* etiologically related to the somatic symptoms.

Similar to the dilemma of determining if symptoms are intentionally produced, there is little advantage for the clinician to definitively link cause–effect emotional distress and physical symptoms to patients or parents. If the symptoms are due to stress or a conflict that *could not be dealt with* on a conscious level, it is clinically useless and potentially countertherapeutic to bring these issues to conscious awareness during symptom assessment. Merely making explicit the proposed link between somatic symptoms and emotional distress does not help affected adolescents deal with underlying problems, and in the case of conversion disorder may cause symptoms to worsen. Also, the presence of significant stress or unresolved conflict does not necessarily mean that the symptoms are causally related. Treatment is directed at helping adolescents learn how problems might make their bodies not function properly, how they can resolve the conflict, and how they can develop alternative coping skills.

## CLINICAL ISSUES RELATED TO ADOLESCENT SOMATOFORM DISORDERS

Faced with all of the problems noted previously, it is understandable that many clinicians are "baffled" by the onslaught of symptoms, become annoyed by the time consumed in caring for patients who are "not really sick," or feel frustrated by the "never-ending, recurrent complaints."[6] The traditional biomedical paradigm reduces the patient's subjective distress and impairment to a diagnosed, objective disease, whereas pathophysiological processes are understood only in terms of biophysical or chemical processes.[14]

Persistent somatic complaints are common in primary care,[14–18] with recurrent abdominal pain accounting for up to 5% of pediatric office visits, and headaches, nausea, chest pain, or fatigue reported by 10% of adolescents.[6] Furthermore, some somatizing adolescents have coexisting psychopathology, family conflict, school absenteeism, and increased use of health and mental health services,[15] as well as emotional problems[16–18] and persistent physical symptoms later in adulthood.[19–21] Thus, a primary care approach that addresses both the diagnosis and treatment of these challenging conditions, such as the biopsychosocial model, is needed.

## THE BIOPSYCHOSOCIAL APPROACH TO SOMATOFORM DISORDERS

First described in 1977, the biopsychosocial approach[22] incorporates existing as well as emerging scientific areas such as psychoneuroimmunology that explain the cause and treatment of somatic symptoms in adolescents.[7] It thereby supplements and enriches the discoveries of biomedicine, rather than undermining them.[23] Central to the biopsychosocial model is a continuum of interactive hierarchical systems that affect an adolescent's experience of somatic symptoms.[11] In practice, all aspects of care from diagnosis to treatment require an understanding of both linear and nonlinear processes associated with disease and illness.[24,25]

Although often considered distinct and separate, *subjective domains*, such as patient- or parent-reported history and symptoms, and *objective domains*, such as physical examination or laboratory findings, are equally important and iterative. Regardless of the diagnosis or underlying emotional issues, it has been noted that patients do not have the option, nor the interest, of being objective about their own illness.[26] Although the diagnostic process begins with the history, a history is unavoidably and actually an *exchange* of information.[26]

As noted in the chapter on psychopharmacology (Chapter 190, Adolescent Psychopharmacology), medication can be a useful tool in the treatment of adolescents with psychiatric symptoms, but its optimal effect is realized when it is used as a component of a multipronged therapeutic approach. In somatoform disorders, this includes the active involvement of a primary care provider or adolescent medicine specialist who can address physical symptoms in the context of the adolescent's personal life and environment. Cassell emphasizes that"suffering is experienced by persons, not merely by bodies, and has its source in challenges that threaten the intactness of the person as a complex social and psychological entity."[27] Cassell also notes that "physicians are less skilled at what were once thought to be the basic skills of doctors—discovering the history of an illness through questioning and physical examination, and working toward healing the whole person."[28] The role of the history and physical examination in this context is discussed in detail in the next section.

### Dysmenorrhea: Scientific Knowledge Changes Diagnostic Assumptions

Dysmenorrhea provides an excellent example of how our understanding of adolescent somatic symptoms and their relationship to psychological issues changes with new knowledge. Almost 40 years ago, primary dysmenorrhea was defined in a pediatric quarterly publication as "the presence of painful menstruation in the absence of any somatic or pelvic lesion. The term intrinsic…was derived from the belief, sometimes still held, that the etiology for the pain lay in the uterus itself."[29] Based on this primitive understanding of the pathophysiology of menstrual pain, the conclusion was that "the cause… that can account for the vast number of cases is and remains psychogenic. As stated, this is almost 100% true in the patient in her teens or younger."[29] With the lack of scientific information available at the time, this formulation would have placed an adolescent experiencing dysmenorrhea in 1 of 2 *DSM-IV-TR* categories: conversion disorder, or pain disorder associated with psychological factors.

Ten years later (about 30 years ago), primary dysmenorrhea was defined in the same publication as "painful menstruation without *significant* pelvic pathology."[30] Citing scientific findings over the previous 5 years based on microtransducer techniques, studies of pain receptor physiology, and new information on a variety of prostaglandins and their metabolites, the authors concluded that the "common denominator in women with primary dysmenorrhea is excess myometrial activity…and the importance of psychological factors in dysmenorrhea is dubious."[30] This formulation would not fit into any *DSM-IV-TR* category.

A more balanced, biopsychosocial approach than either of these dualistic conceptualizations was offered in the same publication about 20 years ago, using a synthesis of knowledge about both the physiology and psychology of dysmenorrhea; at this point, the authors of the article on dysmenorrhea concluded that adolescents may have disability out of proportion to the severity of the pain, and that occasionally an underlying psychosocial, personal, or family problem "may be contributing to the decreased pain tolerance and heightened anxiety centered around the menses…."[31] This formulation considers pain in the context of the adolescent female experiencing it, as well as the various external domains that may affect it. In this formulation, the symptom of dysmenorrhea might not fit into any *DSM-IV-TR* category or may fit into the category Pain Disorder Associated with Both Psychological Factors and a General Medical Condition (307.89). Furthermore, as scientific knowledge regarding the pathophysiology of symptoms and conditions continues to emerge, the number of diagnoses attributable to "nonorganic" causes will undoubtedly diminish.

## APPLIED PRINCIPLES OF THE BIOPSYCHOSOCIAL APPROACH IN ADOLESCENT SOMATOFORM DISORDERS

There is not a large evidence base regarding the treatment of somatoform disorders in adolescents.[2,6,9,32] Rather than address the specific diagnoses separately, as occurs in the *DSM-IV-TR*, the approach used by family physicians and internists[3,33] is more applicable in the primary care of adolescents.[34] In this approach, the diagnosis is based on a thorough history and physical examination, but with the physician displaying emotional empathy and a concerned attitude emanating from acknowledgment of the adolescent's suffering, regardless of the presumed diagnosis. The successful approach to treatment relies on giving an acceptable, physiologically based explanation of the symptoms to the patient and family, avoiding unwarranted testing and procedures, establishing reasonable treatment goals, and arranging for brief but regular and frequent office visits to provide the patient with ongoing medical attention that is independent of symptom development.[2,3,6,35] Antidepressant medications and/or cognitive psychotherapy may be of benefit for willing participants.[36,37]

### Agreeing on the Diagnostic and Therapeutic Approach

A first step in the process of exchanging information (mistakenly labeled as "taking" a history) in somatoform disorders is to have all parties (clinician, adolescent, and parent) agree that physical symptoms *are* physical, but that these may be due to *pathological* and/or *functional* processes. Pathological processes, such as inflammation, infection, or cancer, cause cellular disruption, tissue damage, or anatomical distortions that can be detected by a variety of tests or imaging procedures or direct visualization with endoscopy. Other pathological conditions, such as epilepsy, cardiac conduction defects, or lactose intolerance, are detected through procedures such as an electroencephalogram (EEG), electrocardiogram (ECG), or breath hydrogen measurement. Pathological processes may require medication, surgery, or both, but may also benefit from supportive treatments that are prescribed with functional disorders. Thus, a daily routine including a healthy diet and good sleep hygiene, physical activity, social supports and skills to deal with stress can be helpful if there are problems with nutrition, sleep, activity, or social interactions related to the symptoms.[34]

Functional processes can result in symptoms that are just as debilitating as pathological ones, but are related to disruption of normal physiologic function to a degree that might not be detected by "testing." Thus, the history and physical examination become essential elements in diagnosis. The example of a muscle spasm in the calf ("charley horse") can help patients and parents understand what is meant by a functional disorder.[34] Functional disorders are generally diagnosed by history and physical examination; testing is performed to exclude conditions that might represent a threat to health or may require different treatments.

### Detailed History Focused on the Presenting Symptoms

When somatoform disorders are in the differential diagnosis, some practitioners focus on psychosocial issues in an effort to avoid reinforcing any notion that something is physically wrong. Experience suggests that it is better to focus meticulously on symptoms. This is the adolescent's "ticket of admission"; paying attention to it does not reinforce illness; instead, it sends the message that the symptoms are being taken seriously and prepares the patient for *talking about* symptoms rather than *testing for* symptoms.[34] The timing, location, radiation, quality, severity, precipitants, and relievers of target symptoms, as well as any associated symptoms, should be explored. With respect to neurological symptoms, even if not in keeping with recognized neuroanatomy (eg, stocking-glove anesthesia) or function (eg, unable to bend at the waist from standing but able to sit up from supine), the *story of the symptoms* should be obtained in detail.[34]

Although the history should focus on the details of symptoms, medical and psychosocial issues should be examined together, rather than in sequence, because the assessment lays the groundwork for treatment. Thus, when an adolescent reports that her body "hurts all over," asking "What does that hurt stop you from doing ?" puts the symptoms in the context of relevant psychosocial issues. Even if a patient has a serious medical or surgical condition, it is important to know something about how an adolescent patient might cope with such a condition. With a "horizontal" assessment, medical symptoms and psychosocial factors are addressed side-by-side; psychosocial issues are considered not only as a context to understand medical diagnoses, but also because they reveal strengths and vulnerabilities of the adolescent and family.[34] This increases the likelihood of making a positive somatoform diagnosis, rather than by exclusion.

### History Between Visits Essential to Establish Patterns

A written daily journal of symptoms kept by the adolescent helps to establish patterns of what makes symptoms worse or better. An emphasis on the latter will be useful in the treatment phase, because somatizing patients often report that "nothing makes it better." If an adolescent is asked to keep a journal, it is important to review the log each visit; if a parent completes the symptom journal for an adolescent, this can be interpreted as the suffering being extended to the rest of the family.[34] Eventually the journal becomes less important as the adolescent is able to discuss not only physical symptoms, but also psychosocial issues.

### Physical Examination Focused on Symptoms

Regardless of how unlikely it may seem that any abnormalities will be detected based on the history, a targeted physical examination to determine the cause of functional symptoms should be performed on the initial, as well as subsequent, visits. Patients with neurological symptoms should have a neurologic examination, using as many techniques employing "laying on of hands" as possible; the examination should include indirect ophthalmoscopy, deep tendon reflex testing, cranial nerve evaluation, and evaluation of cerebellar function. On follow-up visits, this can be done quickly; the interval history can be obtained and feedback regarding findings given during the examination.

Performance of the physical examination for adolescents with suspected somatoform disorders will (1) reinforce for the physician the diagnosis of a somatic condition, (2) identify any changes that might occur over time, acknowledging that a positive diagnosis of a somatoform disorder is never 100% certain, and (3) demonstrate to the adolescent and parent(s) that the illness will be closely monitored, even though this may not include diagnostic testing.

### Laboratory and Imaging Studies

Laboratory and imaging studies in suspected somatoform disorders should be selected on the basis of the history and physical examination. Somatizing adolescents and/or their parent(s) may ask for specific tests to be performed, such as an MRI for a headache or an upper gastrointestinal series for abdominal pain. Such requests need to be interpreted with care; they may be generated by (mis)information obtained from television, the Internet, friends, or family members. Rather than rejecting a request for testing outright, a clinician might respond, "We could get that test, but it only would tell us about anatomy. Based on your story, I suspect that muscle spasms are causing your headaches and they will not show up on an MRI, or any other test."[34]

If the symptoms and physical examination cause diagnostic uncertainty, the least invasive test that will still provide necessary information should be obtained. For example, an ultrasound of the abdomen can provide a great deal of detailed information for an adolescent with abdominal pain. Before actually performing diagnostic procedures, however, it is worthwhile to prepare the adolescent and parent(s) for the expected results, including a positive framing on "negative" studies, and using charts or illustrations to explain the normal anatomy and physiology of the affected system, as well as to provide insight into the dysfunction causing the symptom(s). When tests are "normal," it is useful to review with the adolescent and parent(s) the details of the study, both in visual form—the actual study—as well as the written report. Similar to the detailed history and physical examination, this transmits the fact that the diagnostic process is being conducted carefully to identify any pathological processes.

### Applied Physiology in Diagnosis and the Development of Intervention Strategies

Without an explanatory model for the symptoms, negative findings provide little reassurance to the patient and family.[38] Once a somatoform disorder is being considered, the clinician should present the diagnostic impression clearly, frankly, and directly, but this should be done in a manner that will build a foundation for intervention.[2] Three physiologic explanations can be used to provide an understanding of the likely cause of symptoms, alone or in combination.[34]

***1. Conditioned responses*** Conditioned responses are well-recognized patterns based on normal physiology, in which a repeated stimulus causes a repeated response, with the result that the response can occur in the absence of the original conditioning stimulus, especially if it is linked with another stimulus. With operant conditioning, symptoms become self-perpetuating after the inciting factor (such as an injury or virus) has passed, possibly related to cytokines induced by a preceding medical illness. In this way, the symptoms take on a life of their own. Most adolescents and parents are familiar with the concepts of conditioned response in the context of training desired animal behaviors. Using this paradigm, symptoms are viewed as *undesired* conditioned responses, and *operant deconditioning* can be included as an element of treatment. To avoid the impression that this treatment is being *done to* the adolescent, one should include the adolescent in the development of the deconditioning strategies employed for symptom reduction.[34]

Patients and parents may find it helpful to learn that coexisting symptoms, such as depression, can also be explained on a biological basis. For instance, infections cause the peripheral release of the proinflammatory cytokines interleukin-1 (IL-1) and tumor necrosis factor-α (TNF-α) in the brain via rapid transmission of primary afferent nerves innervating the affected site(s).[39] Thus, there is a biological substrate for depression associated with viral infections such as infectious mononucleosis.[40] Reciprocally, IL-1 from a previous infection is known to sensitize the pituitary–adrenal response to inescapable shock in rats.[12]

***2. Multiple triggers and precipitants*** Because mind-body disconnections often lead to polarized viewpoints about the causes of symptoms, patients often interpret any psychologic interpretation as "you think it's all in my head." To avoid this conflict, one can discuss with the adolescent how the body has a limited number of ways to respond to various triggers. That is, the muscles of the digestive track can either contract or relax, and bowel wall spasm or distension are each painful. However, there are many different things that can trigger a "final common pathway."[34] Bowel wall spasm causes pain, whether it is related to irritable bowel syndrome or to lymphoma. Included in the list of triggers discussed should be factors mediated through the central nervous system, and therefore made worse by anxiety or depression.[41]

Citing multiple potential causes for symptoms prepares the adolescent with abdominal pain to work on psychological issues, *in addition to* diet (including fiber), physical activity, bowel habits, antispasmodic medications, and relaxation techniques. One can avoid dichotomization with the question, "If working on psychological issues can help your symptoms improve by 10%, wouldn't that be worth it? I believe that you can improve a lot more than that, but there is no single thing that is going to provide you full relief."

***3. Reflexes*** Because adolescents with somatoform disorders are often sensitive to implications that their symptoms are voluntary, purposeful, or intentional, it often helps to emphasize to the patient that there are numerous automatic, involuntary, subcortical "reflexes" at work causing symptoms.[34] Function in the autonomic nervous system is based on the balance of sympathetic and parasympathetic tone. Insufficient or excessive activity, or an imbalance between the 2, can result in symptoms. The vagus nerve, carrying autonomic efferents from the brain to the heart, lungs, stomach, and intestines, has numerous outputs that can result in symptoms. Most adolescents are familiar with feeling "butterflies" in their stomach when nervous, and all parents are familiar with the gastro-colic reflex of infants.

### Prescribe Face-Saving Interventions

The biopsychosocial approach is highly interactive, involving a therapeutic partnership with the adolescent patient. Depending on the nature of the symptom(s), the somatic interventions prescribed may relate to the daily structure of eating and sleep; physical, occupational or speech therapy; and/or various integrative therapies, such as biofeedback, yoga, massage, or acupuncture.

Including the family can be critical in this phase of symptom management, because the family (especially grandparents) may have beneficial folk remedies that could be suggested.[34] If physical, occupational, or speech therapy are prescribed, or any integrative therapies pursued, there should be a clear explanation regarding expected outcomes and delineation of how family members will be able to support these modalities.

Return to school is also important. Symptoms may make it difficult to attend school, and not attending school may cause the adolescent to fall behind academically, which makes return to school a source of anxiety. After a prolonged school absence, it is useful for the adolescent to have a prescribed, time-limited period of tutoring, based on the tutor's assessment, to ensure that the patient is caught up with classwork prior to returning to school. Some schools allow in-school tutoring, providing a gradual re-entry into school in which the adolescent is physically in the school building, but without the pressure of performing in the classroom. The resultant socialization often facilitates a return to the classroom. Returning to school for half-days initially can smooth the re-entry process for adolescents who have missed a great deal of school because of somatic symptoms.[34] Whatever plan is developed for school return, it should be previewed with the school nurse and guidance counselor to ensure that it is feasible and that someone will be able to monitor progress. Because of the dynamics of parental protectiveness that sometimes arises with somatoform disorders, a parent may actually impede return to school. When such collusion is suspected, it may help to contact the other parent directly to engage his or her help in carrying out the plan.

### Inclusion of Mental Health Services

Underlying mood disturbance, anxiety, stress, or unresolved conflict need to be addressed as an integral part of treatment. However, because the presentation is somatic, the treatment must include some kind of somatic interventions, as described previously, in combination with a variety of cognitive behavioral interventions (Chapter 191). Family therapy can also be helpful,[42] especially if the symptoms are disruptive to family functioning. Mental health treatment may be more readily accepted if the health care provider emphasizes that this is part of the treatment plan for all such cases and that the purpose of mental health intervention is to prevent the symptoms from causing secondary problems that might perpetuate symptoms. Framing the therapist as a professional who will help the clinician manage the overall care of the adolescent's symptoms is generally received more positively than "you need to see a psychiatrist." It should also be made clear that the primary care or specialty provider will continue to monitor the adolescent's symptoms in partnership with the mental health therapist.

### EVIDENCE FOR TREATMENTS FOR SOMATOFORM DISORDERS

A recent synthesis of the literature regarding effective psychiatric treatments of somatoform disorders[43] found that cognitive behavioral therapy is consistently effective across a spectrum of somatoform disorders.[44] A psychiatric consultation letter to the primary care physician regarding strategies for managing symptoms was found to improve physical functioning and reduce costs. Finally, preliminary evidence indicates that antidepressants, especially the selective serotonin reuptake inhibitors (SSRIs), are effective across a range of somatoform disorders, although it is not known whether the benefits are due to reduced depression, anxiety, or somatic symptoms.

Because there is no clear evidence-based strategy for primary care providers to address somatoform disorders, especially with respect to adolescents, clinicians often turn to the advice of those who have experience with these issues.[38] A recent article by an internist proposes that primary care providers consider the following advice: (1) Patience: a long-term perspective is required because symptoms can be deeply rooted, resistant to change, and often embedded in a mutually suspicious relationship with physicians; (2) Selective referral: select subjective psychological distress as the target for referral for mental health services, rather than physician-perceived excessive somatic concerns; (3) A psychiatric consultation letter to the primary care provider: to legitimize physical symptoms, avoid excessive examinations and unnecessary tests, give appointments at regular intervals, perform brief physical examinations, provide reassurance, and invite the patient to talk about personal issues; (4) Consider depression: excessive somatic concerns frequently occur with depression; (5) Consider antidepressant medication: SSRIs and tricyclic antidepressants can be effective, even for patients who are not depressed and at doses lower than used to treat depression; and, (6) Make common cause with your patient: although patients with somatoform disorders can be antagonistic, a collaborative relationship results in improved therapeutic results.[45]

Because psychological factors play a role in the development and treatment of somatoform disorders, primary care physicians need a strategy to refer patients to mental health providers in a manner that will facilitate acceptance of these referrals. As noted previously, patients and families tend to consider mental health symptoms associated with somatoform disorders the result of a physical illness. Thus, the primary care provider should take this viewpoint in referring a patient for psychiatric services and make the referral because of stress, worry, or other target symptoms. In addition, rather than referring the patient "out" for psychological treatment, it may be advantageous to bring the mental health provider "in" to the treatment team. That is, the primary care provider continues as the central health professional, whereby the referral is framed as, "In order for me to treat all of your symptoms, I want to bring in Dr. Brown. She is a psychiatrist (or psychologist, or social worker) who helps my patients with their worries and stress that come from having symptoms like yours." It should be emphasized that the primary care provider will continue to see the adolescent for regular check-up visits. This reinforces the concept that recovery benefits most from the adolescent forming a therapeutic alliance with both the primary care and mental health providers.

## SUMMARY

The challenges in primary and specialty care presented by adolescents with somatoform symptoms can be minimized by an awareness of the diagnostic features of the 6 disorders in this category. This awareness prepares the clinician to obtain a detailed history and physical examination and to minimize testing or procedures that may distract from the underlying dynamics. The interaction of the psyche and the soma is central in the etiology of these disorders, with a dualistic conceptualization of somatic symptoms as either organic or psychiatric being counterproductive. The biopsychosocial approach offers a practical means of working toward symptom relief in a way that is developmentally growth promoting and benefits not only the adolescent and the family but also provides the clinician with a sense of functioning as a healer.

## REFERENCES

1. American Psychiatric Association. *Diagnostic and Statistical Manual of Mental Disorders*. 4th ed. Text Revision. Washington, DC: American Psychiatric Association; 2000

2. Campo JV, Fritz G. A management model for somatization. *Psychosomatics.* 2001;42:467-476

3. Epstein RM, Quill TE, McWhinney IR. Somatization reconsidered: incorporating the patient's experience of illness. *Arch Intern Med.* 1999;159(3):215-222

4. Smith GR Jr, Monson RA, Ray DC. Psychiatric consultation in somatization disorder. a randomized controlled study. *N Engl J Med.* 1986;314:1407-1413

5. Gold MA, Friedman SB. Conversion reactions in adolescents. *Pediatr Ann.* 1995;24:296-306

6. Silber TJ, Pao M. Somatization disorders in children and adolescents. *Pediatr Rev.* 2003;24(8):255-264

7. Dimsdale J, Dantzer R. A biological substrate for somatoform disorders: importance of pathophysiology. In: Dimsdale JE, Xin Y, Kleinman A, Patel V, Narrow WE, Sirovatka PJ, Regier DA, eds. Somatic Presentations of Mental Disorders: Refining the Research Agenda for DSM-V. Arlington, VA: American Psychiatric Association; 2009;63-73

8. Raij TT, Numminem J, Narvanen S, Hiltunen J, Han R. Brain correlates of subjective reality of physically and psychologically induced pain. *Proc Natl Acad Sci.* 2005;102:2147-2151

9. Coghill RC, McHaffie JG, Yen YF. Neural correlates of interindividual differences in the subjective experience of pain. *Proc Natl Acad Sci.* 2003;100:8538-8542

10. Castle DJ, Rossell SL. An update on body dysmorphic disorder. *Current Opinion Psychiatry.* 2006;19:74-78

11. Engel CC. Explanatory and pragmatic perspectives regarding idiopathic physical symptoms and related syndromes. *CNS Spectr.* 2006;11:225-232

12. Johnson JD, O'Connor KA, Deak T, Stark M, Watkins LR, Maier SF. Prior stressor exposure sensitizes LPS-induced cytokine production. *Brain Behav Immun.* 2002;16:461-476

13. Konsman JP, Parnet P, Dantzer R. Cytokine-induced sickness behaviour: mechanisms and implications. *Trends Neurosci.* 2002;25:154-159

14. Fabrega H. The concept of somatization as a cultural and historical product of Western medicine. *Psychosom Med.* 1990;52:653-672

15. Fritz GK, Fritsch S, Hagino O. Somatoform disorders in children and adolescents: a review of the past 10 years. *J Am Acad Child Adolesc Psychiatry.* 1997;36:1329-1338

16. Alfven G. Preliminary findings on increased muscle tension and tenderness, and recurrent abdominal pain in children. A clinical study. *Acta Pediatrica.* 1993;82:400-403

17. Garber J, Walker LS, Zeman J. Somatization symptoms in a community sample of children and adolescents: further validation of the children's somatization inventory. *Psychol Assess.* 1991;3:588-595

18. Walker LS, Guite JW, Duke M, et al. Recurrent abdominal pain: a potential precursor of irritable bowel syndrome in adolescents and young adults. *J Pediatr.* 1998;132:1010-1015

19. Campo JV, McWilliams L, Comer D, et al. Somatization in pediatric primary care: association with psychopathology, functional impairment, and use of services. *J Am Acad Child Adolesc Psychiatry.* 1999;38:1093-1101

20. Campo JV, DiLorenzo C, Chiappetta L, et al. Adult outcomes of pediatric recurrent abdominal pain: do they "just grow out of it"? *Pediatrics.* 2001;108:e1-e7

21. Hotopf M, Carr S, Mayou R, et al. Why do children have chronic abdominal pain, and what happens to them when they grow up? Population based cohort study. *BMJ.* 1998;316:1196-1200

22. Engel GL. The need for a new medical model: a challenge for biomedicine. *Science.* 1977;196:129-136

23. Frankel RM, Quill RE, McDaniel SH. The future of the biopsychosocial approach. In: Frankel RM, Quill TE, McDaniel SH, eds. *The Biopsychosocial Approach: Past, Present, Future.* Rochester, NY: The University of Rochester Press; 2003

24. Engel GL. The application of the biopsychosocial model. In: Frankel RM, Quill TE, McDaniel SH, eds. *The Biopsychosocial Approach: Past, Present, Future.* Rochester, NY: The University of Rochester Press; 2003

25. Frankel RM, Quill RE, McDaniel SH. Introduction to the biopsychosocial approach. In: Frankel RM, Quill TE, McDaniel SH, eds. *The Biopsychosocial Approach: Past, Present, Future.* Rochester, NY: The University of Rochester Press; 2003

26. Cassell EJ. *Talking with Patients.* Cambridge, MA: MIT Press; 1985

27. Cassell EJ. The nature of suffering and the goals of medicine. *NEJM.* 1982;306:639-645

28. Cassell EJ. *The Nature of Suffering and the Goals of Medicine.* 2nd ed. Oxford, UK: Oxford University Press; 2003

29. Sloan D. Pelvic pain and dysmenorrhea. *Pediatr Clin North Am.* 1972;19:669-680

30. Gantt PA, McDonough PG. Adolescent dysmenorrhea. *Pediatr Clin North Am.* 1981;28:389-395

31. Coupey SM, Ahlstrom P. Common menstrual disorders. *Pediatr Clin North Am.* 1989;36:551-571

32. Lieb R, Pfister H, Masraler M, Wittchen HU. Somatoform syndromes and disorders in a representative population sample of adolescents and young adults: prevalence, comorbidity, and impairments. *Acta Psychiatr Scand.* 2000;101:194-208

33. Servan-Schreiber D, Kolb NR, Tabas G. Somatizing patients: part I. Practical diagnosis. *Am Fam Physician.* 2000;61:1073-1078

34. Kreipe RE. The biopsychosocial approach to adolescents with somatoform disorders. *Adolesc Med Clin.* 2006;17:1-24

35. Servan-Schreiber D, Kolb NR, Tabas G. Somatizing patients: part II. Practical management. *Am Fam Physician.* 2000;61:1423-1428

36. O'Malley PG, Jackson JL, Sanroro J, Tomkins G, Balden E, Kroenke K. Antidepressant therapy for unexplained medical symptoms and syndromes. *J Fam Pract.* 1999;48:980-990

37. Price J. Review: antidepressants are effective for clinical unexplained symptoms and syndromes. *Evid Based Ment Health.* 2000;3:84

38. Barsky AJ, Borus JF. Functional somatic syndromes. *Ann Intern Med.* 1999;130:910-921

39. Dantzer R. Cytokine-induced sickness behavior: where do we stand? *Brn Behav Immun.* 2001;15:7-24

40. Raison CL, Capuron L, Miller AH. Cytokines sing the blues: inflammation and the pathogenesis of depression. *Trends Immunol.* 2006;27:24–31

41. Lieb R, Meinlschmidt G, Araya R. Epidemiology of the association between somatoform disorders and anxiety and depressive disorders: an update. In: Dimsdale JE, Xin Y, Kleinman A, Patel V, Narrow WE, Sirovatka PJ, and Regier DA, eds. *Somatic Presentations of Mental Disorders: Refining the Research Agenda for DSM-V.* Arlington, VA: American Psychiatric Association; 2009;1–7

42. Sanders MR, Shepherd RW, Cleghorn G, et al. The treatment of recurrent abdominal pain in children: a controlled comparison of cognitive-behavioral family intervention and standard pediatric care. *J Consult Clin Psychol.* 1994;62:306–314

43. Kroenke K. Efficacy of treatment for somatoform disorders. In: Dimsdale JE, Xin Y, Kleinman A, Patel V, Narrow WE, Sirovatka PJ, Regier DA, eds. *Somatic Presentations of Mental Disorders: Refining the Research Agenda for DSM-V.* Arlington, VA: American Psychiatric Association; 2009;143–163

44. Kroenke K, Swindle R. Cognitive-behavioral therapy for somatization and symptom syndromes: a critical review of controlled clinical trials. *Psychother Psychosom.* 2000;69:205–215

45. Levenstein S. The evidence for treatments for somatoform disorders: a view from the trenches. In: Dimsdale JE, Xin Y, Kleinman A, Patel V, Narrow WE, Sirovatka PJ, Regier DA. *Somatic Presentations of Mental Disorders: Refining the Research Agenda for DSM-V.* Arlington, VA: American Psychiatric Association; 2009;165–169

# CHAPTER 184

# Mood Disorders in Adolescents

PETER J. SIMON, MPH • CYNTHIA P. RICKERT, PhD • DAWN NERO, PsyD • VAUGHN I. RICKERT, PsyD

## INTRODUCTION

Mood disorders are characterized by their ability to influence the affective experience of the adolescent. These disorders can significantly impair the health and life trajectories of adolescents through their effects on energy level, motivation, sociability, feelings of self-worth, and perceptions of agency and control.[1] Mood disorders are divided into 4 major groups: depressive disorders, bipolar disorders, mood disorders due to a general medical condition, and substance-induced mood disorders.[2]

### EPIDEMIOLOGY

Depression is one of the most common mood disorders among adolescents, present in 5% of this population at any given time.[3] If all subtypes of depression are included in the estimate, the prevalence roughly doubles.[4] The prevalence of depression rapidly increases after the initiation of puberty and by late adolescence reaches a level comparable to the 5% to 8% rate found in adults.[5,6]Although community samples of adolescents show a 3% to 5% prevalence for major depressive disorder (MDD), the prevalence rises to 14% among urban adolescents presenting for health care,[7] with lifetime occurrence of depression as high as 30%.[6]

Bipolar disorder is much rarer, having an estimated lifetime prevalence between 0.4% and 1.6%.[8,9] The period of peak onset, however, is between 15 and 25 years of age.[10] Moreover, approximately 10% to 15% of adolescents with recurrent MDD will subsequently develop bipolar disorder.[10] These facts highlight the importance of not only being vigilant for symptoms of bipolar disorder in adolescents but also of identifying those adolescents at increased risk of developing bipolar disorder in the future.

### RISK FACTORS

Research has identified a number of risk factors associated with depression.Whereas boys and girls are at equal risk prior to puberty, after puberty the rate of depression is about twice as high in girls.[3,4] Having a parent with a history of depression increases an adolescent's risk of a depressive episode two- to fourfold.[3] An individual adolescent who has previously had a depressive episode is at increased risk for subsequent episodes.[4] Finally, chronic illness increases the risk for depressive symptoms.[4]

In the case of bipolar disorders, evidence suggests that there is a genetic basis to the disorder. Bipolar disorders occur more frequently among biological relatives; having first-degree relatives with the disorder has been associated with increased risk.[9,11] In addition, among adolescents presenting with MDD, those who respond negatively to antidepressants with manic or hypomanic symptoms, or who have a rapid onset of depressive symptoms, are more likely to eventually develop bipolar disorder.[12] For those reasons, adolescents who have a rapid progression of initial depressive symptoms or a family history of bipolar disorder should be prescribed antidepressants with caution.[12] Finally, adolescents whose depressive symptoms are accompanied by psychotic symptoms are at increased risk to develop bipolar disorder.There is little gender difference in the incidence of bipolar disorders.[12]

### SCREENING

If left untreated, depression can seriously influence an adolescent's functioning.[1,4] Thus, reliable and valid screening tools are an effective first step in identifying depression symptoms.[4] Table 184-1 provides a summary of some existing screening tools available to clinicians. Evidence suggests that self-report is an unreliable measure, as an adolescent may be unaware of changes in affect.[4]

## DIAGNOSIS OF DEPRESSION

In the United States, mood disorders are diagnosed using criteria detailed in the *Diagnostic and Statistical Manual of Mental Disorders, Fourth Edition, Text Revision (DSM-IV-TR)*.[2] The *DSM-IV-TR* provides criteria for identifying various *mood episodes*. Mood episodes are constellations of specific symptoms that co-occur for specified durations, which are then used to diagnose

**Table 184-1**

**Screening Measures for Depression in Children and Adolescents**

| *Measure* | *Age* | *Reading Level* | *Spanish Version Available* | *# of Items* | *Time Needed to Complete (Minutes)* | *Psychometrics/Cutoff* |
|---|---|---|---|---|---|---|
| Children's Depression Inventory (CDI) | 7-17 | 1 | Yes | 27 | 10-15 | Alpha: 0.81; test-retest: 0.60/above 19 |
| Center for Epidemiological Studies-Depression Scale (CES-D) | 14 and older | 6 | No | 20 | 5-10 | Sensitivity: 84% Specificity: 75%/above 15 |
| Reynolds Adolescent Depression Scale | 13-18 | 3 | No | 30 | 10-15 | Alpha: 0.87-0.91; test-retest: 0.80-0.93/refer to manual |
| Beck Depression Inventory | 14 and older | 6 | Yes | 21 | 5-10 | Sensitivity: 84% Specificity: 81%/above 15 |
| Kutcher Adolescent Depression 6-Item Scale (KADS-6) | 12-18 | NA | NA | 6 | 5 | Sensitivity: 92% Specificity: 71%/above 6 |

Adapted with permission from Sharp LK, Lipsky MS. Screening for depression across the lifespan: a review of measures for use in primary care settings. *Am Fam Physician*. 2002;66:1001-1008.

mood disorders. Mood disorders are defined and diagnosed by the presence or absence of specific mood episodes.

## THE ROLE OF LABORATORY STUDIES IN DIAGNOSING MOOD DISORDERS

Although some laboratory findings among individuals with depressive or bipolar disorders have been found to differ from those in healthy individuals, these findings are unreliable and inconclusive. There is no diagnostic laboratory study for mood disorders, except for organic conditions related to depression and treated. The important exception to this rule is the use of laboratory studies for diagnosing or ruling out the 2 etiology-based mood disorders.

## ETIOLOGY-BASED DISORDERS

Mood disorders due to a general medical condition and substance-induced mood disorders are categories of conditions in which symptoms contain some or all of the symptoms of specific mood disorders.[2] However, the underlying cause is due to a medical condition or reaction to a drug or pharmacologic treatment. Taking a detailed medical and drug history and obtaining appropriate laboratory studies (if indicated) is essential. Hypothyroidism, hypoadrenalism, and beta-blocker medications are examples of medical conditions and substances that can be associated with depression.[3]

## DEPRESSIVE DISORDERS

There are 3 diagnostic categories of depressive disorders: *major depressive disorder, dysthymic disorder*, and *depressive disorder, not otherwise specified* (DD NOS).[2]

### Major Depressive Disorder

The diagnosis of MDD requires the presence of one or more major depressive episodes (MDE) in the absence of any manic episodes.[2] The identification of an MDE requires the presence of 5 symptoms from the following list experienced for most of the day, nearly every day, for at least a 2-week period, and significantly affecting normal function.[3] One of the 5 symptoms must be (a) or (b).

(a) Depressed or irritable mood (reported or observed)

(b) Diminished pleasure or interest in activities (reported or observed)

(c) Weight loss of more than 5% in 1 month or failure to make expected weight gains

(d) Insomnia or hypersomnia

(e) Psychomotor agitation or retardation (observed only)

(f) Fatigue or loss of energy
(g) Feelings of worthlessness or excessive guilt
(h) Diminished ability to think or concentrate or indecisiveness (reported or observed)
(i) Thoughts of death, suicidal ideation, or suicide attempt[2]

Symptoms of bereavement are excluded if the duration is less than 6 months.[2] However, if the symptoms include marked functional impairment, feelings of worthlessness, suicidal ideation, psychotic symptoms, or psychomotor retardation, treatment is warranted.

### Dysthymic Disorder (Dysthymia)

Dysthymia represents a milder but more protracted depressive disorder than MDD and requires the presence of depressed or irritable mood for most of the day for most days for at least 1 year AND 2 or more of the following (without any symptom-free periods lasting longer than 2 months):

- Poor appetite or overeating
- Insomnia or hypersomnia
- Low energy level or fatigue
- Low self-esteem
- Poor concentration or difficulty making decisions
- Feelings of hopelessness[2]

Adolescents with dysthymic disorder present with low self-esteem, feelings of inadequacy or guilt, poor social skills, and are pessimistic, irritable, and excessively angry.[4,12]

### Depressive Disorder Not Otherwise Specified

The diagnosis of DD NOS is reserved for adolescents who present with depressive symptoms that fail to meet the criteria for any other depressive disorder.[2] Consensus surrounding this disorder category is less complete, and some practitioners have suggested that medical intervention is not justified for adolescents under this classification.

## TREATMENT OF DEPRESSION

Recent advances with respect to talking therapies and medications have brought the treatment of milder depressive symptoms and depression in adolescents into the realm of primary adolescent health care. Chapters 193 and 194 describe in-depth the important elements of psychopharmacology and mental health treatment modalities for adolescents, respectively.

### PSYCHOTHERAPEUTIC TREATMENT

Cognitive behavioral therapy (CBT), developed by Beck and colleagues, and interpersonal therapy (IPT), developed by Klerman and Weissman, have been shown to have therapeutic efficacy when compared to other forms of psychotherapy. Cognitive behavioral therapy is more widely used and focuses on the cognitive distortions that lead to negative moods and behaviors associated with depression.[13] Effective CBT for adolescents is facilitated by the provider working collaboratively with the patient to ensure that the between-visit "take-home exercises" are completed and the overall cognitive development is taken into account.[13] Motivational interviewing techniques can facilitate engagement in CBT. Interpersonal therapy focuses on the decreased pleasure derived from, or decreased motivation to engage in, social interactions.[14] Mufson and colleagues[15] have adapted IPT for adolescents, and preliminary findings indicate that it is effective in reducing depressive symptoms. Individual or family psychotherapy for the adolescent may also be appropriate to help address continuing difficulties the adolescent may be having in interactions with friends and family.

### PHARMACOLOGIC TREATMENT

Despite US Food and Drug Administration (FDA) "Black Box" labeling, selective serotonin reuptake inhibitors (SSRIs) remain the most commonly used medication for adolescent depression. Placebo-controlled trials of fluoxetine,[16] citalopram,[17] sertraline,[18] and paroxetine[19] with a response of approximately 60% (with placebo response rates of 30% to 40%) and favorable side effect profiles underlie their accepted efficacy.

The recommended prescribing practice for children and adolescents with depression is to begin with half the usual therapeutic dose of an SSRI (10 mg of fluoxetine, citalopram, or paroxetine per day) for 1 week to help the patient adjust to side effects, and to then increase the dose to the equivalent of 20 mg of fluoxetine for another 3 weeks.[3] The dose can be increased at intervals of no less than 4 weeks, as it takes at least 4 weeks at steady state to determine whether a given dose will be helpful. Because adolescents metabolize SSRIs more rapidly than adults, they may often require doses above the equivalent of 20 mg of fluoxetine to attain a clinical response for depression.[3] Once an adequate clinical response has been achieved, treatment should be continued for at least 6 months to 1 year to reduce the risk of relapse (see Chapter 190, Adolescent Psychopharmacology, for more detailed coverage of SSRI side effects and usage).

It is important for providers to remember that tricyclic antidepressants are no longer considered first line agents. Controlled trials have found them to be no better than placebo, and the risk of fatal overdose with tricyclic antidepressants is much greater than the risk with SSRIs.[3]

Areas of uncertainty in the management of adolescents with depression include identifying the specific indications for using antidepressant medication and psychotherapy, determining whether to use one alone or both in combination, and establishing the optimal duration of maintenance treatment.[20] It should be noted that although some studies have shown that a combination of psychotherapy and medication is the most effective treatment regimen, one study showed that medication alone offered almost as much benefit as the combined regimen.[20] Adolescents with chronic depression lasting longer than 12 months should receive medication and psychotherapy.[21]

One of the most serious potential consequences of depression among adolescents is suicide, and managing the increased risk of suicide in depressed adolescents is an important part of treating this population.[4] The clinician should determine past suicidal behavior or ideation, identify any family history of suicide, and advise parents to take the preventive measure of removing firearms from the home. Providers who are treating suicidal teens *should not* rely solely on "safety contracts" with the adolescent. Parents and other caretakers of suicidal adolescents should be educated to monitor the adolescent in their care for changing suicidal thoughts and associated behaviors. Suicide risk is often highest at the beginning of depressive episodes, suggesting that expeditious treatment or referral is crucial.[22]

Lastly, adolescents with depressive symptoms are at increased risk for substance and alcohol abuse and dependence.[4] These issues should be addressed and monitored throughout treatment.

## BIPOLAR DISORDERS

Bipolar disorders are characterized by fluctuation of mood between low, depressed states and elevated, highly active states.[11,23,24] The clinical features of depression are the same as those listed previously, but the distinguishing feature is the presence of behaviors in the manic spectrum.[11,12,23,24] They are being increasingly recognized in adolescents as awareness of the spectrum of manifestations is more widespread.

### DIAGNOSIS OF BIPOLAR DISORDERS

There are 4 diagnostic categories of bipolar disorders: type I bipolar disorder, type II bipolar disorder, cyclothymic disorder, and bipolar disorder, not otherwise specified.[2,24]

#### Type I Bipolar Disorder

Representing the "classic" form of bipolar disorder, also known as manic-depressive disorder or manic-depressive illness, type I bipolar disorder presents with an episode of mania that may occur without a preceding MDE, or with a mixed picture of both mania and depressed mood.[24] Generally, however, adolescents have experienced at least one MDE prior to the first manic episode. Adolescents with type I bipolar disorder experience recurrent, debilitating episodes of mania and depression. Type I bipolar disorder must be differentiated from substance-induced mood disorder, or mood disorder due to a general medical condition, as well as from schizoaffective disorder, schizophrenia, schizophreniform disorder, delusional disorder, or psychotic disorder not otherwise specified.[2,24]

***Mania and Hypomania*** Mania and hypomania are characterized by a distinct period of persistently elevated, expansive, or irritable mood and require the presence of at least 3 of the following symptoms:

- Inflated self-esteem or grandiosity (reaching delusional levels in mania)
- Decreased need for sleep
- Flight of ideas or racing thoughts
- Rapid and pressured speech that rapidly moves from one idea to the next
- Easy distractibility
- Increase in goal-directed activity (increased creativity in hypomania) or psychomotor agitation
- Excessive involvement in pleasurable activities with high potential for harmful consequences (eg, spending sprees, speeding when driving)[2,24]

Manic and hypomanic episodes are distinguished from each other by the duration and degree of the impairment that these symptoms produce. "Full-blown" manic episodes are characterized by serious symptomatic behaviors that persist for at least one week and can lead to hospitalization because of symptoms of psychosis such as hallucinations, or can cause significant impairment in social and occupational functioning.[2,11,23,24] Episodes of mania and depression in adolescents are often not clearly demarcated and are more likely to present as chronic mood dysregulation or irregularity, with minor remission of symptoms between episodes. Moreover, manic episodes in adolescents may sometimes (but not always) present as irritability or extreme anger, rather than euphoria.[10,24]

### Type II Bipolar Disorder

Occuring 5 to 10 times more commonly than type I, type II bipolar disorder is characterized by 1 or more MDE accompanied by at least 1 hypomanic, but no manic, episodes; the presence of mania automatically places the patient in the type I category.[2,11,24] Hypomanic behavior is milder than that seen in mania and is characterized by optimism, pressure of speech and activity, and the decreased need for sleep. This combination of features often causes the affected adolescent to feel good and to appear happy and productive.[11,24] Other adolescents with hypomania may demonstrate poor judgment and irritability. Delusions and hallucinations, however, do not occur in hypomania, but may occur in mania. Hypomania may be difficult to recognize because the individual may appear to have unusually high levels of energy and creativity, and the symptoms are ego-syntonic and associated with an inflated sense of abilities. Objectively, hypomanic episodes represent a clear, marked change from usual function observable by others and last at least 4 days.[2,24] Peers, family, and others who are in contact with the adolescent often perceive hypomanic behaviors as erratic or problematic.

Attention-deficit/hyperactivity disorder (ADHD) may be confused with manic or hypomanic episodes because of the shared symptoms of distractibility, increased speech amount and pressure, hyperactivity, and impulsive behavior.[2] ADHD, however, can be distinguished from bipolar disorders by its early onset (usually before 7 years), chronic rather than episodic nature, and absence of elevated or expansive mood or psychotic features.[2]

### Cyclothymic Disorder (Cyclothymia)

Cyclothymia is characterized by chronic, fluctuating mood disturbances involving numerous periods of hypomanic symptoms and numerous periods of depressive symptoms, neither of which are sufficient in number, intensity, or duration to meet the criteria for either a major depressive or a manic episode.[2] These symptoms must cause clinically significant impairment in normal functioning, and must persist for 1 year with no single symptom-free period lasting longer than 2 months.[2]

### Bipolar Disorder, Not Otherwise Specified (BP NOS)

This disorder category is reserved for adolescents having disorders with bipolar features that do not meet criteria for any specific bipolar disorder. Many adolescents with disorders with bipolar features receive this diagnosis before their disorder takes on more easily classifiable features that fit into either type I or type II categories.[2]

## TREATMENT OF BIPOLAR DISORDERS

Bipolar disorder, especially type I, can be devastating to an adolescent's development, but effective treatments are available.[10,11,23,24]

### Psychotherapeutic Treatment

Adolescents with bipolar disorders often exhibit poor social skills and, as a result, have few friends and exhibit higher levels of conflict with their families and peers when compared to healthy adolescents.[10] Psychotherapeutic treatment is recommended to help with family and peer relationships.[10] Four treatment modalities have been investigated and found to improve adolescents' social functioning or to reduce some disordered mood symptoms. These include: (1) family psychoeducation, (2) family-focused therapy, (3) interpersonal social rhythm therapy (IPSRT), and (4) CBT.[10] These therapies seek to provide education to the adolescent and family, teach conflict resolution skills, and provide social, interpersonal behavior-change skills training, respectively. Rarely does treatment focus on only one of these elements, because optimal functioning requires competence in all of these domains. Psychotherapeutic treatment has been shown to be an effective adjunct to drug therapy in the treatment of bipolar disorders.[23,24]

### Pharmacologic Treatment

The FDA has recently recommended 3 atypical antipsychotics, Seroquel, Geodon, and Zyprexa, for the treatment of bipolar disorder in adolescents.[25] Prior evidence of clinical trials and professional experience strongly supported the use of "mood stabilizers," lithium or anticonvulsants (eg, valproic acid, carbamazepine, or lamotrigine), and atypical antipsychotics (eg, olanzepine, aripiprazole, or risperidone) as the best option for the acute stabilization of manic symptoms and symptom remission.[23,24] Research on combination therapy is limited, but studies suggest that combination therapy may be more effective for adolescent patients who remain symptomatic while on drug monotherapy.[23] Treatment is recommended for 12 to 24 months after acute manic symptoms have stabilized. It should be noted that all of these medications carry risks of significant side effects, and the use of these compounds in adolescents who do not meet strict *DSM-IV-TR* diagnostic criteria is not encouraged.[24] See Chapter 190, Adolescent Psychopharmacology, for more detailed description of the use of these medications.

Special attention should be paid to adolescents with bipolar disorders where depressive symptoms are being managed with antidepressants. In these cases, antidepressant monotherapy has been shown to cause depressed adolescents who are predisposed to develop bipolar disorder (eg, who have a family history of bipolar illness) to have a manic episode, often very abruptly.[10,24] Therefore, antidepressants should be used with caution in this population, and if used, should only serve as an adjunct to mood stabilizers.

**Special Treatment Considerations**

Because treatment and predicted long-term outcome differ dramatically in adolescents with depressive disorders from those with bipolar disorders, early identification is of paramount importance.[24] Adolescents with bipolar disorders who are not identified and treated early may go on to suffer from increasingly severe episodes of depression as well as potentially to face an increased risk of physical and psychosocial trauma related to the risk-taking, impulsivity, and aggression that accompanies manic episodes.[11,23,24]

## MANAGEMENT

### DIAGNOSTIC CONSIDERATIONS

Diagnosing mood disorders in adolescents is challenging, as symptoms often mimic what is thought to be normal adolescent development. Adolescence is characterized by wide changes in mood, which challenges providers to distinguish between a mental health disorder and troubling but essentially normal behavior. For example, an adolescent who says he feels "totally depressed" may not really be depressed at all, but is instead expressing frustration with a given situation. A teen who stops answering phone calls from friends for a few days, eats less, or who makes comments about "wanting to die" similarly sends mixed messages to a provider. Although these behaviors may, indeed, be indicators of an underlying psychiatric concern, they may also simply represent expressions of the enhanced emotionality of the adolescent years. Proper assessment and diagnosis may require more than one session and information-sharing with parents or teachers to better understand and frame the teen's *normal* range of behaviors.

At the same time, special attention is required when interviewing adolescents to ensure that mood symptoms are properly elicited.[24] Adolescents, for example, are less likely than adults to disclose depressive symptoms if they are not asked directly about them.[3] Specific depression screening tools, such as those listed in Table 184-1, as well as more general adolescent health screening instruments such as the Guidelines for Adolescent Preventive Services (GAPS) forms (see Chapter 13, Screening, and Chapter 15, Anticipatory Guidance) alert the provider for the need for more in-depth exploration of diagnostic criteria. In addition to the presence or absence of symptoms, the duration of symptoms and the amount of time each day experiencing symptoms should be explored. Symptoms related to impairments in thinking or concentration may not be reported directly even when asked, but might be suggested by a sudden decrease in school performance.

Clinicians should rely on the adolescent's report to gain knowledge about internal processes and experiences, and rely on the parents' reports to gain information about observed behaviors or attitudes, of which the adolescent may not be aware or may not disclose. However, relying on parents' reports is not without its risks. In the case of reported sleep, for example, parents may look in on the adolescent and report that the adolescent went to bed early and appeared to be sleeping soundly. The adolescent, in turn, may more accurately report that he or she was experiencing difficulties falling asleep.

It is important for clinicians not to confuse the feelings adolescents experience following negative life experiences with clinical depression.[12] Typically, depressive disorders do not have a sudden onset; instead, their onset is usually slow and insidious.[12] Breaking up with a boyfriend or girlfriend, performing in school below expectations, relocating to a new house, neighborhood, city, or state, or having difficulties with social or familial relations all may fall within the scope of an adolescent's normal experience and may produce emotional distress. A diagnosis of clinical depression requires the presence of a specific set of symptoms for a specific duration.[3,4,12] Failure to recover from these transitory events is more appropriately understood as an adjustment disorder with depressive symptoms.[2]

### PATIENT EDUCATION

Once the diagnosis of a mood disorder is made, it is valuable to provide education to the adolescent and the family about the disorder and to allow them to ask questions and express their fears and concerns.[12] This is especially important with respect to their experience with family members who may share a diagnosis of depression or bipolar illness with the adolescent. This situation may result in stereotyping, with the adolescent and/or parents assuming that the treatment and course of illness will follow that of the affected family member. For example, if an uncle has type I bipolar disorder and has required repeated psychiatric hospitalizations associated with suicide attempts and frequent motor vehicle crashes, there may be an unspoken belief that the adolescent is destined to the same outcome because of having the same diagnostic label. If the other affected individual is a first-degree relative with whom the adolescent lives on a daily basis, such concerns tend to be especially prominent. For example, an adolescent who has a parent who is severely disabled by MDD, and is resistant to multiple medications and intensive therapy, may resist taking medications or engaging in CBT because they are assumed to be ineffective. Prepared protocols, worksheets, and Web pages can be helpful sources of information. Specific resources that may be useful to parents and adolescents are listed at the end of this chapter. Talking to an adolescent's school guidance counselor may be indicated if the disorder has a serious effect on the adolescent's behavior in the classroom or academic performance.

### MONITORING

Monitoring is an essential component of managing the adolescent patient with mood disorders, useful in the context of continued care and in those cases when the adolescent is later referred to another practitioner.[12,23,24] Thorough monitoring consists of taking a baseline measure, as well as continued measures of mood symptom severity, functional impairment, and somatic symptoms. Rigorous monitoring is essential in measuring treatment efficacy, in distinguishing symptoms that are part of the underlying disorder from those that emerge as treatment side effects, and in noting important changes in symptom severity such as signs of mania or increases in suicidal ideation in response to antidepressant therapy.[12]

Symptom severity is best measured using a tool that incorporates the rating of symptoms by an observer. One such tool useful with adolescents is the 12-item Clinical Assessment of Adolescent Depression, or CAAD (www.cprf.ca/education/Openmind2006/CAAD.pdf).[12] This instrument can be used to establish a baseline and to continuously monitor symptoms over the course of the treatment to measure response. Functional impairment related to depression should be monitored along 5 domains important in adolescent development: family function, school function, work function, peer interactions, and recreational functioning. In addition, safety should be assessed. It is not unusual for adolescents to show marked impairment in some domains while showing only mild to moderate impairment in others. In these cases, therapeutic attention should be placed on those domains with the greatest impairment. Progress in each of these 5 domains can be monitored by making sure to ask about and assess functioning in each domain during clinical visits. A scale of 0–3 can be used (0 for no problems in the given domain, 1 for some problems, 2 for significant problems, and 3 for severe problems). Three of the 12 items in the CAAD[12] relate to somatic symptoms; somatic complaints are often the presenting symptom in depressed adolescents. Monitoring somatic symptoms from baseline and then over time will provide important information that may help identify which somatic symptoms are somatic manifestations of the mood disorder and which are side effects of attempted treatments.

### REFERRAL

Perhaps the most important aspect of managing an adolescent with a mood disorder is having the knowledge and skill to refer the patient to another professional at the right time and to the appropriate person. This decision depends on the training, experience, expertise, and degree of comfort treating adolescents with these disorders. However, the presence of manic episodes or risk factors associated with an increased risk of bipolar disorders indicates that the management of the adolescent will be considerably more complex.[11,12,24] Immediate referral in the case of mania, and expedited referral in the case of hypomania, to a more experienced practitioner is appropriate. Similarly, adolescents presenting with psychotic features deserve immediate attention and require careful management best handled by experienced psychiatric providers. Finally, the importance of being vigilant for and managing suicidality in adolescents with mood disorders cannot be overemphasized, and despite an absence of evidence on the efficacy of such a practice, adolescents presenting with suicidal intent or action should still be hospitalized for their protection and further evaluation.[22]

## SUMMARY

Patients with depressive symptoms, whether alone or in association with manic or hypomanic behaviors, are fairly common in adolescent health care. Recognizing common signs, symptoms, and predisposing risk factors will aid in the early recognition and diagnosis of the entire range of conditions from mild dysthymia to severe manic-depressive episodes. Although treatment for the more disabling conditions in this category of psychiatric disturbance may require hospitalization and/or psychoactive medications under the supervision of a psychiatrist, professionals providing health care to adolescents should be familiar with the concepts presented in this chapter.

## INTERNET RESOURCES

- American Academy of Child and Adolescent Psychiatry. Information on depression and bipolar disorder: www.aacap.org/cs/root/facts_for_families/facts_for_families
- National Mental Health Association. Fact sheet and other information on adolescent depression: www.nmha.org/go/information/get-info/depression/depression-in-teens

- National Library of Medicine. Information regarding adolescent depression: www.nlm.nih.gov/medlineplus/ency/article/001518.htm
- National Institutes of Mental Health. Information on bipolar disorder: www.nimh.nih.gov/health/publications/bipolar-disorder/complete-index.shtml
- National Institutes of Mental Health. *Bipolar Disorder in Children and Teens: A Parent's Guide:* www.nimh.nih.gov/health/publications/bipolar-disorder-in-children-and-teens-a-parents-guide/nimh_bipolar_children_parents_guide.pdf

## REFERENCES

1. National Academy of Sciences. *Report Brief for Researchers. Preventing Mental, Emotional, and Behavioral Disorders among Young People: Progress and Possibilities.* Washington, DC: The National Academies; March 2009

2. American Psychiatric Association. Diagnostic and Statistical Manual of Mental Disorders, 4th ed, Text Revision. Washington, DC: American Psychiatric Association; 2000

3. Brent DA, Birmaher B. Adolescent depression. *N Engl J Med.* 2000;347:667–671

4. Birmaher B, Brent D, AACAP Work Group on Quality Issues, et al. Practice parameter for the assessment and treatment of children and adolescents with depressive disorders. *J Am Acad Child Adolesc Psychiatry.* 2007;46:1502–1526

5. Pratt LA, Brody DJ. *National Center for Health Statistics Data Brief.* Sept 2008, Number 7: 1–7. CDC/NCHS. Available at: www. cdc.gov/nchs/data/databriefs/db07.htm. Accessed July 2, 2009

6. Winter LB, Steer RA, Jones-Hicks L, Beck AT. Screening for major depression disorders in adolescent medical outpatients with the Beck depression inventory for primary care. *J Adolesc Health.* 1999;24:389–394

7. Asarnow JR, Jaycox LH, Anderson M. Depression among youth in primary care models for delivering health services. *Child Adolesc Psychiatr Clin N Am.* 2002;11:477–497

8. Lewisohn PM, Klein DN, Seeley JR. Bipolar disorder during adolescence and young adulthood in a community sample. *Bipolar Disord.* 2000;2:281–293

9. Birmaher B, Axelson D, Monk K, et al. Lifetime psychiatric disorders in school-aged offspring of parents with bipolar disorder. *Arch Gen Psychiatry.* 2009;66:287–296

10. Birmaher B, Axelson D. Course and outcome of bipolar spectrum disorder in children and adolescents: a review of the existing literature. *Dev Psychopathol.* 2006;18(4):1023–1035

11. Townsend LD, Demeter CA, Wilson M, Findling RL. Update on pediatric bipolar disorder. *Curr Psychiatry Rep.* 2007;9(6):529–534

12. Kutcher S, Chehil S. Adolescent depression and anxiety disorders. In: Neinstein LS, Gordon C, Katzman D, Woods ER, Rosen D, eds. *Adolescent Healthcare: A Practical Guide.* 5th ed. Philadelphia, PA: Lippincott, Williams, and Wilkins; 2007:994–1017

13. Beck AT. The current state of cognitive therapy. *Arch Gen Psychiatry.* 2005;62:953–959

14. Weissman MM. Interpersonal therapy: current status. *Keio J Med.* 1997;46:105–1101

15. Mufson L, Weissman MM, Moreau D, Garfinkel R. Efficacy of interpersonal psychotherapy for depressed adolescents. *Arch Gen Psychiatry.* 1999;56:573–579

16. Emslie GJ, Rush AJ, Weinberg WA, et al. A double-blind, randomized, placebo-controlled trial of fluoxetine in children and adolescents with depression. *Arch Gen Psychiatry.* 1997;54(11):1031–1037

17. von Knorring AL, Olsson GI, Thomsen PH, Lemming OM, Hultén A. A randomized, double-blind, placebo-controlled study of citalopram in adolescents with major depressive disorder. *J Clin Psychopharmacol.* 2006;25:311–315

18. Wagner KD, Ambrosini P, Rynn M, et al. Efficacy of sertraline in the treatment of children and adolescents with major depressive disorder: two randomized controlled trials. *JAMA.* 2003;290:1033–1041

19. Berard R, Fong R, Carpenter DJ, Thomason C, Wilkinson C. An international, multi-center, placebo-controlled trial of paroxetine in adolescents with major depressive disorder. *J Clin Adolesc Psychopharmacol.* 2006;16:59–75

20. Brent DA, Maalouf FT. Pediatric depression: is there evidence to improve evidence-based treatments? *J Clin Psychol Psychiatry.* 2009;50:143–152

21. Keller MB, McCullough JP, Klein DN, et al. A comparison of nefazodone, the cognitive behavioral-analysis system of psychotherapy, and their combination for the treatment of chronic depression. *N Engl J Med.* 2000;342:1462–1470

22. Zametkin AJ, Alter MR, Yemini T. Suicide in teenagers: assessment, management, and prevention. *JAMA.* 2001;286:3120–3125

23. Findling RL, Steiner H, Weller EB. Use of antipsychotics in children and adolescents. *J Clin Psychiatry.* 2005;66(suppl 7):29–40

24. Kowatch RA, Del Bellow MP. Pediatric bipolar disorder: emerging diagnostic and treatment approaches. *Child Adolesc Psychiatric Clinic N Am.* 2006;15:73–108

25. Psych Central News Editor. FDA panel recommends approval of Seroquel, Geodon, and Zyprexa for children, teens. Psych Central. Available at: psychcentral.com/news/2009/06/10/fda-panel-recommends-approval-of-seroquel-geodon-and-zyprexa-for-children-teens/6457.html. Accessed July 6, 2009

# CHAPTER 185

# Disorders of Anxiety in Adolescents

MARGERY R. JOHNSON, MD • POONAM JHA, MD

## INTRODUCTION

Anxiety disorders constitute one of the most common categories of psychiatric disorders affecting adolescents, with a prevalence of 6% to 20%.[1] Although anxiety disorders can greatly impair emotional, cognitive, and social development, early detection and treatment of adolescents with anxiety have been shown to mitigate these possible sequelae.[1] Seven anxiety disorders will be discussed in this chapter: separation anxiety disorder, specific phobia, social anxiety disorder, generalized anxiety disorder, panic disorder, obsessive–compulsive disorder (OCD), and post-traumatic stress disorder (PTSD). Age of onset and course vary among the different anxiety disorders. Although many disorders may remit with or without treatment, it is generally believed that pediatric anxiety disorders increase the risk of future psychopathology and adult functional impairment. Poor prognostic factors include early onset, chronic course of active symptoms, greater severity of symptoms, greater functional impairment, family psychopathology, and lack of treatment.[1] This chapter addresses the etiology, evaluation, classification, treatment, and prognosis for anxiety disorders of adolescents, with an emphasis on practical information in routine adolescent health care rather than on psychiatric care.

## ETIOLOGY

The etiology of anxiety disorders is multidimensional. Biological contributors include genetic predisposition (as evidenced by twin studies and familial aggregation), neurobiological abnormalities (neuroendocrine abnormalities and variant neurocircuitry), and immunologic abnormalities. A type of temperament called "behavioral inhibition" associated with increased physiologic reactivity and behavioral withdrawal to novel stimuli or challenging situations is commonly seen in adolescents with anxiety. Parenting styles, such as overprotectiveness or low nurturing, may increase the likelihood of particular anxiety disorders. Exposure to an anxious parent may lead to modeling of anxious behavior in addition to the genetic contribution of one (or both) parent(s) who have an anxiety disorder. Lastly, adverse life events, such as the death of a loved one, personal or familial illness, or abuse, may lead to the development of an anxiety disorder in adolescents.[2]

## EVALUATION

Evaluation of anxiety disorders relies on the clinical interview of the adolescent and of the parent or primary caregiver. Older children and adolescents are better able to recognize and report symptoms related to anxiety. Because some adolescents may have difficulty describing their internal experience due to a developmental inability to describe abstract concepts such as feelings associated with anxiety, parents may not be aware of their son's or daughter's anxiety. However, parents may be more accurate reporters of an adolescent's functioning (eg, behavior, social activities, and academics). Self-report questionnaires may augment the clinical interview, because an adolescent may be better able to endorse or decline the presence of a list of symptoms than to describe them directly. Examples include the Screen for Child Related Anxiety Disorders (SCARED, for patients older than age 8)[3] or the Multidimensional Anxiety Scale for Children (MASC, for patients 8–19 years of age).[4] There are also scales for specific disorders, such as the Children's Yale Brown Obsessive-Compulsive Scale (C-YBOCS for patients 8–14 years of age, or the YBOCS for adolescents older than 14),[5] which measures symptoms of OCD. School functioning may be assessed using teacher rating scales.

Because anxiety, like depression, may present with somatic symptoms, a comprehensive medical evaluation (history, physical examination, and laboratory screening) of an adolescent presenting with anxiety is indicated. The history should include the taking of medications and illegal drugs, such as amphetamines or marijuana. Panic disorder, generalized anxiety disorder, and separation anxiety disorder are likely to present with physical symptoms, including abdominal pain, headache, difficulty breathing, or dizziness, which should be evaluated on physical examination. Because the abrupt onset of generalized anxiety with obsessive–compulsive symptoms may follow a Group A beta-hemolytic streptococcal infection; a throat culture and streptococcal antibody titer may be indicated. Other biologic conditions that may be associated with anxiety in adolescents include (1) hyperthyroidism, (2) excessive caffeine intake, (3) migraine headaches, (4) asthma, (5) seizure disorders, and (6) lead intoxication. Less common conditions that can present with anxiety are hypoglycemia, pheochromocytoma, brain tumors, delirium, and cardiac arrhythmias. Many medications can produce anxiety as a side effect, including (1) beta agonist bronchodilators, (2) sympathomimetics, (3) corticosteroids, (4) selective serotonin reuptake inhibitors (SSRIs), (5) antipsychotics, (6) diet pills, and (7) antihistamines.[1]

## CLASSIFICATION OF ANXIETY DISORDERS IN ADOLESCENTS

Anxiety disorders in adolescents are classified into 7 categories, as described in the following. The common features across anxiety disorders include situational fear and avoidance, autonomic arousal, and anticipatory worry. The categories fall into 3 groups, characterized by worry/distress, fear, or obsessive/compulsive features.[6]

### SEPARATION ANXIETY DISORDER

Separation anxiety disorder is characterized by developmentally inappropriate and excessive anxiety following thoughts of, or actual, separation from a primary attachment figure. Box 185-1 lists the *Diagnostic and Statistical Manual of Mental Disorders*, 4th Edition, Text Revision (*DSM-IV-TR*) diagnostic criteria for separation anxiety disorder. Prevalence ranges from 2% to 5%, with peak age of onset between 7 to 9 years of age, continuing into adolescence. Gender ratio differs among studies.[7] The symptoms are manifested in cognitive, affective, somatic, and behavioral domains. School avoidance, sometimes mislabeled school phobia, is seen in approximately 75% of affected individuals.[8] The reason for not attending school in these cases is the presence of physical symptoms, commonly a combination of headaches and abdominal pain. The somatic manifestations dominate the clinical presentation to the point that reaction to the separation from an attachment figure

**Box 185-1**

***DSM-IV-TR Diagnostic Criteria for Separation Anxiety Disorder (309.21)***

Diagnostic criteria for separation anxiety in adolescents

A. Developmentally inappropriate and excessive anxiety concerning separation from home or from those to whom the individual is attached, as evidenced by 3 (or more) of the following:
   1. Recurrent excessive distress when separation from home or major attachment figures occurs or is anticipated
   2. Persistent and excessive worry about losing, or about possible harm befalling, major attachment figures
   3. Persistent and excessive worry that an event will lead to separation from a major attachment figure (eg, getting lost or being kidnapped)
   4. Persistent reluctance or refusal to go to school or elsewhere because of fear of separation
   5. Persistent and excessive fear or reluctance to be alone or without major attachment figures at home or without significant adults in other settings
   6. Persistent reluctance or refusal to go to sleep without being near a major attachment figure or to sleep away from home
   7. Repeated nightmares involving the theme of separation
   8. Repeated complaints of physical symptoms (such as headaches, abdominal pain, nausea, or vomiting) when separation from major attachment figures occurs or is anticipated

B. Duration of the disturbance is at least 4 weeks.

C. Onset is before age 18 years.

D. The disturbance causes clinically significant distress or impairment in social, academic (occupational), or other important areas of functioning.

E. The disturbance does not occur exclusively during the course of a pervasive developmental disorder, schizophrenia, or other psychotic disorder and, in adolescents and adults, is not better accounted for by panic disorder with agoraphobia.

Specify: Early Onset: if onset occurs before age 6 years

Modified with permission from American Psychiatric Association. *Diagnostic and Statistical Manual of Mental Disorders*, 4th ed., Text Revision. Washington, DC: American Psychiatric Association; 2000: 125.

is easily missed. In fact, when a clinician asks about avoiding (or being "phobic" about) school, the patient and the parent (usually the mother) express a very strong desire for school attendance, but it is impossible because of the physical symptoms. Separation anxiety disorder usually is recurrent, with acute exacerbations seen at the beginning of school, after school holidays, after starting a new school, after a family move, after parental separation, or after the death of a loved one. Comorbidity of separation anxiety disorder exists with other anxiety disorders, depression, attention-deficit/hyperactivity disorder (ADHD), and oppositional defiant disorder (ODD). Many affected children do not receive treatment, and in most cases the condition will improve with or without treatment, although distress may be reduced with treatment.[8]

## SPECIFIC PHOBIA

In specific phobias, an adolescent experiences a persistent fear in response to a specific stimulus that triggers anxiety, so that the individual attempts to avoid the stimulus or risks exposure to it, with resultant increased anxiety. The avoidant behaviors can become elaborate and may not be easily recognized by either the patient or others as related to stimulus avoidance. Box 185-2 lists the *DSM-IV-TR* diagnostic criteria for specific phobia, formerly known as simple phobia. Specific phobia should be distinguished from developmentally normal fears. Phobias are excessive, cannot be reasoned away, are beyond voluntary control, lead to avoidance of the feared stimulus, persist over time, and are maladaptive. Common stimuli for specific phobias in adolescents include heights, small animals, injections, darkness, loud noises, and storms. Prevalence of specific phobia is estimated at 1.7% to 16%. Generally females are more often and severely affected by phobias than males. Comorbidity is high with other anxiety disorders, depression, somatoform disorders, and substance abuse. Specific phobias tend to persist into adulthood, although intensity of distress and impairment appears to lessen.[9]

## SOCIAL PHOBIA (SOCIAL ANXIETY DISORDER)

Social phobia, also known as social anxiety disorder, is defined as excessive fear of social or performance situations in which the adolescent is exposed to scrutiny or possible humiliation by other people. Box 185-3 lists the *DSM-IV-TR* diagnostic criteria for social phobia. Commonly feared situations are public speaking, social gatherings, public artistic or athletic performances, speaking with strangers, and dealing with authority figures. Prevalence is estimated at 2% to 4% in adolescence. Age of onset may be 2 to 4 years with an insidious, subthreshold presentation progressing to more impairment seen in

### Box 185-2

### *DSM-IV-TR Diagnostic Criteria for Specific Phobia (300.20)*

Diagnostic criteria for specific phobia in adolescents

A. Marked and persistent fear that is excessive or unreasonable, cued by the presence or anticipation of a specific object or situation (eg, flying, heights, animals, receiving an injection, seeing blood).
B. Exposure to the phobic stimulus almost invariably provokes an immediate anxiety response, which may take the form of a situationally bound or situationally predisposed panic attack.
C. The person recognizes that the fear is excessive or unreasonable.
D. The phobic situation(s) is avoided or else is endured with intense anxiety or distress.
E. The avoidance, anxious anticipation, or distress in the feared situation(s) interferes significantly with the person's normal routine, occupational (or academic) functioning, or social activities or relationships, or there is marked distress about having the phobia.
F. In individuals under age 18 years, the duration is at least 6 months.
G. The anxiety, panic attacks, or phobic avoidance associated with the specific object or situation are not better accounted for by another mental disorder, such as obsessive–compulsive disorder (eg, fear of dirt in someone with an obsession about contamination), post-traumatic stress disorder (eg, avoidance of stimuli associated with a severe stressor), separation anxiety disorder (eg, avoidance of school), social phobia (eg, avoidance of social situations because of fear of embarrassment), panic disorder with agoraphobia, or agoraphobia without history of panic disorder.

Specify: type: 1) Animal Type; 2) Natural Environment Type (eg, heights, storms, water); 3) Blood-Injection-Injury Type; 4) Situational Type (eg, airplanes, elevators, enclosed places), or 5) Other Type (eg, fear of choking, vomiting, or contracting an illness)

Modified with permission from American Psychiatric Association. *Diagnostic and Statistical Manual of Mental Disorders*, 4th ed., Text Revision. Washington, DC: American Psychiatric Association; 2000: 449.

**Box 185-3**

***DSM-IV-TR* Diagnostic Criteria for Social Phobia (300.23)**

Diagnostic criteria for social phobia (social anxiety disorder) in adolescents

A. Marked and persistent fear of 1 or more social or performance situations in which the person is exposed to unfamiliar people or to possible scrutiny by others. The adolescent fears that he or she will act in a way (or show anxiety symptoms) that will be humiliating or embarrassing.

B. Exposure to the feared social situations provokes anxiety, which may take the form of a situationally bound or situationally predisposed panic attack.

C. The adolescent recognizes that the fear is excessive or unreasonable. Note: In children, this feature may be absent.

D. The feared social or performance situations are avoided or else are endured with intense anxiety or distress.

E. The avoidance, anxious anticipation, or distress in the feared social or performance situation(s) interferes significantly with the person's normal routine, occupational (academic) functioning, or social activities or relationships, or there is marked distress about having the phobia.

F. In individuals under age 18 years, the duration is at least 6 months.

G. The fear or avoidance is not due to the direct physiological effects of a substance (eg, a drug of abuse, a medication) or a general medical condition and is not better accounted for by another mental disorder (eg, panic disorder with or without agoraphobia, separation anxiety disorder, body dysmorphic disorder, a pervasive developmental disorder, or schizoid personality disorder).

H. If a general medical condition or another mental disorder is present, the fear in Criterion A is unrelated to it, eg, the fear is not of stuttering, trembling in Parkinson's disease, or exhibiting abnormal eating behavior in anorexia nervosa or bulimia nervosa.

Specify: Generalized: if the fears include most social situations (also consider the additional diagnosis of avoidant personality disorder)

Modified with permission from American Psychiatric Association. *Diagnostic and Statistical Manual of Mental Disorders,* 4th ed., Text Revision. Washington, DC: American Psychiatric Association; 2000: 456.

adolescence. Comorbidity is seen with depression, substance use disorders, and other anxiety disorders. Social anxiety disorder may have significant negative effects in adulthood such as educational/occupational underachievement, social isolation/loneliness, depression, and substance abuse.[10]

## GENERALIZED ANXIETY DISORDER

Generalized anxiety disorder is characterized by marked anxiety and worry that is difficult to control. Box 185-4 lists the *DSM-IV-TR* diagnostic criteria for generalized anxiety disorder. Affected individuals are often described as "worry warts," overly conscientious, self-doubting, pessimistic, pseudomature, or perfectionistic. They often have nervous habits such as nail biting, hair pulling, or thumb sucking. Anxiety commonly manifests by somatic symptoms such as headaches, stomach aches, and excessive fatigue. Common themes are worry about future events, peer relations, social acceptance, competency, and pleasing others. Prevalence rates are 2% to 4%, with a greater proportion of affected individuals being adolescents. Prevalence is higher in girls. Comorbidity is high with depression, anorexia nervosa, ADHD, and substance abuse disorders. Generalized anxiety disorder may have significant negative sequelae on academic achievement, self-esteem, and peer relationships.[11]

## PANIC DISORDER

Panic disorder is characterized by the presence of recurrent, unexpected panic attacks followed by persistent worry about future attacks or the behavioral or affective implications of the attack. Box 185-5 lists the *DSM-IV-TR* diagnostic criteria for panic disorder and Box 185-6 includes the criteria for the requisite panic attack. Prevalence of full panic disorder is estimated to be 1% in community samples and as high as 10% in clinic-based populations.[12] Panic attacks are common, with 1 study reporting 20% lifetime prevalence. The mean age of onset is mid-adolescence to mid-20s. Females and males are equally affected. Comorbidity is high with anxiety disorders, depressive disorders, ADHD, OCD, and agoraphobia; the absence or presence of agoraphobia results in 2 different diagnoses. The course of the disorder is chronic with periods marked by acute exacerbations.[13]

Panic attacks are an essential feature of panic disorder, but they are considered a symptom, rather than a

## Box 185-4

### *DSM-IV-TR Diagnostic Criteria for Generalized Anxiety Disorder (300.02)*

Diagnostic criteria for generalized anxiety disorder in adolescents

A. Excessive anxiety and worry about a number of events or activities (such as work or school performance), occurring on most days for at least 6 months.

B. The adolescent finds it difficult to control the worry.

C. The anxiety and worry are associated with 3 (or more) of the following 6 symptoms (with at least some symptoms present for more days than not for the past 6 months).

1. Restlessness or feeling keyed up or on edge
2. Being easily fatigued
3. Difficulty concentrating or mind going blank
4. Irritability
5. Muscle tension
6. Sleep disturbance (difficulty falling or staying asleep, or restless unsatisfying sleep)

D. The focus of the anxiety and worry is not confined to features of an Axis I disorder, eg, the anxiety or worry is not about having a panic attack (as in panic disorder), being embarrassed in public (as in social phobia), being contaminated (as in obsessive–compulsive disorder), being away from home or close relatives (as in separation anxiety disorder), gaining weight (as in anorexia nervosa), having multiple physical complaints (as in somatization disorder), or having a serious illness (as in hypochondriasis), and the anxiety and worry do not occur exclusively during post-traumatic stress disorder.

E. The anxiety, worry, or physical symptoms cause clinically significant distress or impairment in social, occupational, or other important areas of functioning.

F. The disturbance is not due to the direct physiological effects of a substance (eg, a drug of abuse, a medication) or a general medical condition (eg, hyperthyroidism) and does not occur exclusively during a mood disorder, a psychotic disorder, or a pervasive developmental disorder.

Modified with permission from American Psychiatric Association. *Diagnostic and Statistical Manual of Mental Disorders*, 4th ed., Text Revision. Washington, DC: American Psychiatric Association; 2000: 476.

## Box 185-5

### *DSM-IV-TR Diagnostic Criteria for Panic Disorder*

Diagnostic criteria for panic disorder in adolescents

A. Both (1) and (2):

1. Recurrent, unexpected panic attacks
2. At least 1 of the attacks has been followed by at least 1 month (or more) of 1 (or more) of the following:
    (a) Persistent concern about having additional attacks
    (b) Worry about the implications of the attack or its consequences (eg, losing control, having a heart attack, "going crazy")
    (c) A significant change in behavior related to the attacks

B. Agoraphobia absent (DSM-IV-TR code 300.01) OR present (DSM-IV-TR code 300.21, see Criteria for Agoraphobia).

C. The panic attacks are not due to the direct physiological effects of a substance (eg, a drug of abuse, a medication) or a general medical condition (eg, hyperthyroidism).

D. The panic attacks are not better accounted for by another mental disorder, such as social phobia (eg, occurring on exposure to feared social situations), specific phobia (eg, on exposure to a specific phobic situation), obsessive–compulsive disorder (eg, on exposure to dirt in someone with an obsession about contamination), post-traumatic stress disorder (eg, in response to stimuli associated with a severe stressor), or separation anxiety disorder (eg, in response to being away from home or close relatives).

Modified with permission from American Psychiatric Association. *Diagnostic and Statistical Manual of Mental Disorders*, 4th ed., Text Revision. Washington, DC: American Psychiatric Association; 2000: 440.

## Box 185-6

### *DSM-IV-TR Criteria for Panic Attack*

A discrete period of intense fear or discomfort, in which at least 4 of the following symptoms develop abruptly and reach a peak within 10 minutes:

1. Palpitations, pounding heart, or accelerated heart rate
2. Sweating
3. Trembling or shaking
4. Sensations of shortness of breath or smothering
5. Feeling of choking
6. Chest pain or discomfort
7. Nausea or abdominal distress
8. Feeling dizzy, unsteady, light-headed, or faint
9. Derealization (feelings of unreality) or depersonalization (being detached from oneself)
10. Fear of losing control or going crazy
11. Fear of dying
12. Paresthesias (numbness or tingling sensations)
13. Chills or hot flushes

Modified with permission from American Psychiatric Association. *Diagnostic and Statistical Manual of Mental Disorders*, 4th ed., Text Revision. Washington, DC: American Psychiatric Association; 2000: 432.

separate illness, and do not have a separate code in the *DSM-IV* schema. As noted previously, they are several-fold more common than full-blown panic disorder in adolescents in which there is also associated emotional and/or behavioral morbidity. Even without panic disorder, panic attacks are significantly distressing, but discrete and time limited events that include overwhelming emotional and physical symptoms associated with an impending sense of doom or danger during an attack. The features of a panic attack are listed in Box 185-6.

Because panic disorder is often associated with agoraphobia, the absence or presence of this feature should be determined when considering the diagnosis of panic disorder. As is true with panic attacks, agoraphobia is a symptom and not a codable disorder in *DSM-IV.* The essential feature of agoraphobia is anxiety about being "trapped" in places or situations from which escape might be difficult or embarrassing, or in which aid may not be available in the event of having a panic attack or symptoms. The characteristics of agoraphobia are listed in Box 185-7.

## Box 185-7

### *DSM-IV-TR Criteria for Agoraphobia*

A. Anxiety about being in places or situations from which escape might be difficult or embarrassing, or in which help may not be available in the event of having an unexpected or situationally predisposed panic attack or panic-like symptoms. Agoraphobic fears typically involve characteristic clusters of situations that include being outside the home alone; being in a crowd or standing in a line; being on a bridge; or traveling in a bus, train, or automobile. Of note, if the avoidance is limited to 1 or only a few specific situations, or is limited to social situations, the diagnosis of specific phobia or social phobia, respectively, should be considered.

B. The situations are avoided (eg, travel is restricted) or else are endured with marked distress or with anxiety about having a panic attack or panic-like symptoms, or require the presence of a companion.

C. The anxiety or phobic avoidance is not better accounted for by another mental disorder, such as social phobia (eg, avoidance limited to social situations because of fear of embarrassment), specific phobia (eg, avoidance limited to a single situation like elevators), obsessive–compulsive disorder (eg, avoidance of dirt in someone with an obsession about contamination), post-traumatic stress disorder (eg, avoidance of stimuli associated with a severe stressor), or separation anxiety disorder (eg, avoidance of leaving home or relatives).

Modified with permission from American Psychiatric Association. *Diagnostic and Statistical Manual of Mental Disorders*, 4th ed., Text Revision. Washington, DC: American Psychiatric Association; 2000: 433.

## OBSESSIVE–COMPULSIVE DISORDER

Obsessive–compulsive disorder (OCD) is characterized by recurrent obsessions and compulsions that are distressful or interfere in functioning. Box 185-8 lists the *DSM-IV-TR* diagnostic criteria for obsessive–compulsive disorder. Obsessions are persistent thoughts, images, or impulses that are intrusive, unwanted, and distressing. Compulsions are repetitive, purposeful, and intentional behaviors that are performed in response to an obsession or rule; they are done to decrease anxiety or prevent a dreaded event. Common themes of obsessions are contamination fears, harm fears, scrupulosity, intrusive sexual thoughts, and need for order. The resultant compulsive behaviors include repetitive hand washing, frequent showering, checking, hoarding, counting, and/or touching things. Prevalence ranges from 0.3% to 4%. Post-pubescent-onset OCD is seen equally in boys and girls. Association of OCD and neurobiological abnormality is supported by the association with pediatric autoimmune neuropsychiatric disorders

## Box 185-8

### *DSM-IV-TR Criteria for Obsessive–Compulsive Disorder (300.3)*

Diagnostic criteria for obsessive-compulsive disorder in adolescents

A. Either obsessions or compulsions:
- Obsessions are defined by all 4 of the following:
  1. Recurrent and persistent thoughts, impulses, or images that are experienced, at some time as intrusive and inappropriate and that cause marked anxiety or distress, and
  2. The thoughts, impulses, or images are not simply excessive worries about real-life problems, and
  3. The adolescent attempts to ignore or suppress such thoughts, impulses, or images, or to neutralize them with some other thought or action, and
  4. The adolescent recognizes that the obsessional thoughts, impulses, or images are a product of his or her own mind (not imposed from without as in thought insertion).
- Compulsions as defined by both of the following:
  1. Repetitive behaviors (eg, hand washing, ordering, checking) or mental acts (eg, praying, counting, repeating words silently) that the adolescent feels driven to perform in response to an obsession, or according to rules that must be applied rigidly, and
  2. The behaviors or mental acts are aimed at preventing or reducing distress or preventing some dreaded event or situation; however, these behaviors or mental acts either are not connected in a realistic way with what they are designed to neutralize or prevent or are clearly excessive.

B. At some point during the course of the disorder, the adolescent has recognized that the obsessions or compulsions are excessive or unreasonable.

C. The obsessions or compulsions cause marked distress, are time-consuming (take more than 1 hour a day), or significantly interfere with the adolescent's normal routine, occupational (or academic) functioning, or usual social activities or relationships.

D. If another Axis I disorder is present, the content of the obsessions or compulsions is not restricted to it (eg, preoccupation with food in the presence of an eating disorder; hair pulling in the presence of trichotillomania; concern with appearance in the presence of body dysmorphic disorder; preoccupation with drugs in the presence of a substance use disorder; preoccupation with having a serious illness in the presence of hypochondriasis; preoccupation with sexual urges or fantasies in the presence of a paraphilia; or guilty ruminations in the presence of major depressive disorder).

E. The disturbance is not due to the direct physiological effects of a substance (eg, a drug of abuse, a medication) or a general medical condition.

Specify: With poor insight: if, for most of the time during the current episode, the person does not recognize that the obsessions and compulsions are excessive or unreasonable

Modified with permission from American Psychiatric Association. *Diagnostic and Statistical Manual of Mental Disorders*, 4th ed., Text Revision. Washington, DC: American Psychiatric Association; 2000: 462.

associated with streptococcal infection (PANDAS) in which an abrupt onset of OCD symptoms occurs after an infection with group A beta-hemolytic streptococcus. Comorbidity is seen with mood disorders, other anxiety disorders, tic disorders, ADHD, and ODD. Obsessive-compulsive disorder is a chronic, waxing/waning disorder. It may have a significant effect on school performance, peer relationships, and physical manifestations (eg, dermatological problems from repetitive hand washing).[14]

### POST-TRAUMATIC STRESS DISORDER

Post-traumatic stress disorder (PTSD) is characterized by the experience of an extreme traumatic event in which the person felt or experienced actual or threatened death, serious injury, or physical integrity of self or others and anxiety, fear, or horror after the event. Box 185-9 lists the *DSM-IV-TR* diagnostic criteria for PTSD. After the trauma, the individual endures intrusive re-experiencing of the traumatic event, has persistent avoidance of stimuli associated with the trauma, and has persistent physiological arousal. Traumatic events may include an isolated event (eg, accident, natural disaster) or may be chronic (eg, recurrent abuse, warfare). Prevalence of PTSD varies depending on the type of trauma. Overall, the rate is estimated to be 1% to 14%. Comorbidity with depressive disorders is most common; symptoms consistent with ADHD and ODD may present after the trauma.[15]

**Box 185-9**

***DSM-IV Criteria for Post-traumatic Stress Disorder (309.81)***

Diagnostic criteria for post-traumatic stress disorder in adolescents

A. The adolescent has been exposed to a traumatic event in which both of the following were present:
  1. The adolescent experienced, witnessed, or was confronted with an event or events that involved actual or threatened death or serious injury, or a threat to the physical integrity of self or others
  2. The adolescent's response involved intense fear, helplessness, or horror

B. The traumatic event is persistently re-experienced in 1 (or more) of the following ways:
  1. Recurrent and intrusive distressing recollections of the event, including images, thoughts, or perceptions
  2. Recurrent distressing dreams of the event
  3. Acting or feeling as if the traumatic event were recurring (includes a sense of reliving the experience, illusions, hallucinations, and dissociative flashback episodes, including those that occur on awakening or when intoxicated)
  4. Intense psychological distress at exposure to internal or external cues that symbolize or resemble an aspect of the traumatic event
  5. Physiological reactivity on exposure to internal or external cues that symbolize or resemble an aspect of the traumatic event

C. Persistent avoidance of stimuli associated with the trauma and numbing of general responsiveness (not present before the trauma), as indicated by 3 (or more) of the following:
  1. Efforts to avoid thoughts, feelings, or conversations associated with the trauma
  2. Efforts to avoid activities, places, or people that arouse recollections of the trauma
  3. Inability to recall an important aspect of the trauma
  4. Markedly diminished interest or participation in significant activities
  5. Feeling of detachment or estrangement from others
  6. Restricted range of affect (eg, unable to have loving feelings)
  7. Sense of a foreshortened future (eg, does not expect to have a career, marriage, children, or a normal life span)

D. Persistent symptoms of increased arousal (not present before the trauma), as indicated by 2 (or more) of the following:
  1. Difficulty falling or staying asleep
  2. Irritability or outbursts of anger
  3. Difficulty concentrating
  4. Hypervigilance
  5. Exaggerated startle response

E. Duration of the disturbance (symptoms in Criteria B, C, and D) is more than 1 month

F. The disturbance causes clinically significant distress or impairment in social, occupational, or other important areas of functioning

Specify: *Acute*: if duration of symptoms is less than 3 months; *Chronic*: if duration of symptoms is 3 months or more

Specify: *With delayed onset*: if onset of symptoms is at least 6 months after the stressor

Modified with permission from American Psychiatric Association. *Diagnostic and Statistical Manual of Mental Disorders*, 4th ed., Text Revision. Washington, DC: American Psychiatric Association; 2000: 467–468.

## TREATMENT OF ANXIETY DISORDERS IN ADOLESCENTS

Because early diagnosis and treatment of anxiety disorders can greatly improve academic and social functioning in affected adolescents, the primary care provider is in a position to directly intervene with the patient and the family, as well as make a referral to a mental health professional for more specific modalities of treatment. A general principle in the treatment of anxiety is that the anxiety must be faced in order to be overcome.[16] Allowing avoidance and withdrawal, and even well-meaning, overly sympathetic support allows the anxiety to persist or grow. The adolescent with separation anxiety that precludes school attendance must return to school as soon as possible; the teen with social anxiety needs to have more contact with peers; and the traumatized patient needs to tolerate reminders of the trauma. Although a positive, empathic, and supportive relationship with a primary care or mental health professional is important, there are also an increasing number of psychotherapeutic and psychopharmacologic evidence-based treatments specific for anxiety disorders. A multimodal treatment program is often necessary, taking into consideration such factors as impairment in the school setting (which may require involvement of school personnel), the overall severity of the anxiety, and the preferences of the adolescent and his or her family.[17]

## PSYCHOTHERAPY

A number of psychotherapeutic methods are effective in the treatment of anxiety disorders. The following section describes the methods (see Chapter 181) framed in the context of the conditions for which they are most commonly applied.

### Cognitive Behavioral Therapy

Cognitive behavioral therapy (CBT) actively addresses the faulty thinking and the avoidant behaviors seen in anxiety disorders.[18] There is a growing body of evidence for the effectiveness of this treatment, and the primary care providers can also use CBT principles in working with an anxious adolescent and his or her family. The patient is taught to identify unrealistic fears and develop active coping skills that will help him or her master situations associated with fear or anxiety. The basic idea is to face fears, beginning with the least severe, and move slowly to more challenging situations. The therapist's task is to help the adolescent move steadily forward without becoming overwhelmed and regressing.

There are a number of components of CBT in a successful treatment plan. Psychoeducation for the adolescent and the parents is a necessary first step, helping them understand what anxiety is, when it becomes a disorder, and how it must be confronted and overcome. In cognitive restructuring, the adolescent examines and challenges negative thought patterns that create and perpetuate anxiety, and with the therapist's assistance, replaces them with positive thoughts and self-talk. Exposure, both in imagination and in real life, to the feared situations works to gradually desensitize the adolescent. As exposure produces an initial increase in anxiety, it is often done in conjunction with a reward or positive reinforcement program, to increase motivation for what can be a difficult treatment process, and methods such as relaxation or controlled breathing exercises to reduce the somatic manifestations of anxiety.

### Obsessive–Compulsive Disorder

Exposure and response prevention (ERP) is a specific and effective treatment for OCD.[19] The adolescent and therapist first develop a hierarchy of feared objects or situations and, beginning with the easiest situation, develop a treatment plan in which the patient, often with the help and support of a parent, purposefully and repeatedly exposes herself or himself to the feared situation, but avoids the usual ritual response behavior. For example, a teenager who has to wash his hands if he touches a toy belonging to his baby sister, is encouraged to "practice" touching one of his sister's toys and is kept from washing for a specified amount of time. An adolescent prevented from performing a ritual initially experiences an increase in anxiety but, with repeated practice, the anxiety eventually decreases until it is extinguished, at which time he can proceed to the next more difficult item on the list.

### Post-traumatic Stress Disorder

Treatment of PTSD is an excellent example of how the key to overcoming anxiety is to confront it. Adolescents with PTSD almost always want to avoid anything that reminds them of the traumatic incident. The more the patient avoids people, places, and things, the more various benign situations are perceived as threatening, and the more the adolescent's life becomes restricted by the fears. The goal for the therapist, the parent, or the adolescent health care professional is to help the adolescent to tolerate remembering, but also to move on with his or her life. In formal therapy, the therapist guides the adolescent through graded exposure to feared stimuli. This exposure may be in the real world (*in vivo*) or in the imagination (imaginal exposure); both are generally used in therapy. This sort of treatment is easiest with situations that are common and benign; most trips in a car do not result in an accident, and most days at the beach do not involve a near-drowning. The treatment approach is different, however, for situations in which the traumatic incident involved a dangerous situation or abuse by an adult, when exposure could retraumatize the adolescent. In such situations, the therapy focuses on helping the adolescent correct cognitive distortions about the trauma; the therapist helps the patient realize that she or he was not responsible for the abuse, did not provoke it, and need not be abused again. It may also be important for the adolescent to regain a sense of control by being involved in the legal process if the perpetrator of the abuse is facing criminal charges.

### Separation Anxiety Disorder

The therapy of separation anxiety disorder inevitably involves treating the adolescent and the parents, because a parent often is the attachment object. The teen needs to work toward tolerating more autonomy, which the parents need to support, despite any ambivalence by any member of the family. In some cases the parents do not agree between themselves on this issue.

As noted in the classification section of this chapter, about 75% of adolescents with separation anxiety do not attend school regularly, generally because of physical symptoms but without clear symptoms of anxiety. This may be associated with one parent, often the father, being excluded from the management of the presenting somatic symptoms. The inclusion of the father in management can be critical to success in shifting the focus from continued search for "organic" causes of the symptoms to a more balanced approach focused on healthy adolescent and family development. This can allow the parents to examine how one or both of them are reinforcing their adolescent's anxiety and to explore reasons why that might be occurring and ways to support autonomy. While increasing insight proceeds, the adolescent and the parents have to push forward to develop an age-appropriate degree of autonomy. This includes return to school, if school absence due to physical symptoms has occurred.

Separation anxiety that manifests itself as difficulty attending school because of physical symptoms often occurs after a vacation break, or after an absence due to illness. In such cases, the underlying anxiety increases each day the student misses school (heralded by an increase in symptoms), as he or she gets progressively further behind in school and homework assignments. For the teen who has been ill, the anxiety may result in lingering physical symptoms that may cause further school absence. In such cases, it is best not to challenge the validity of the physical symptoms, but rather help the patient function at school despite feeling unwell, perhaps with support from the school nurse. The opportunity to return to school gradually should be offered for an adolescent who has been out of school for a substantial amount of time. As long as he or she spends more time at school each day compared with the previous day, it should be considered acceptable progress. Making a plan for the teen to catch up on school work, either by dropping a course, going to summer school, or having a scheduled plan of remediation in place is appropriate, often with the inclusion of a medical excuse, to facilitate a return to normalcy. Consistency, clarity, and agreement on the plan of action by all relevant parties can help the patient get past feeling hopelessly burdened and overwhelmed.

### Panic Disorder

Treatment of panic disorder includes strategies to address the acute panic symptoms and the accompanying anticipatory anxiety and avoidant behaviors. The affected adolescent experiences somatic symptoms and subjective fears during an attack. Techniques such as deep breathing, relaxation, or various maneuvers to focus on autonomic tranquility and calming helps to distract the adolescent from symptoms such as shortness of breath or tachycardia. Cognitive techniques help reorient thinking about the panic experience; an explanation of the autonomic and other physiologic processes causing the symptoms increases an appreciation that the symptoms are not "all in my head."

Patients may fear dying of a heart attack in a panic attack, for example, because of the associated tachycardia and palpitations due to sympathetic discharge. Simple cardiac auscultation can be used to reassure the patient that his or her heart is normal, and that the rapid pulse and sensation of pounding in the chest is due to epinephrine released from the adrenal gland during an attack. It is less helpful to just provide reassurance that "everything is fine," because this may be perceived as minimizing the ominous feeling of a panic attack. Many also fear embarrassment if a panic attack were to happen in public, which often leads to anticipatory anxiety. As the adolescent becomes anxious about being anxious, avoiding public places or situations in which a panic attack has occurred can escalate. In such cases, the first step is to explore what the patient thinks would be the worst thing that could happen, and then help him or her develop strategies to deal with those feared outcomes. Imagining the worst-case scenario and figuring out what to do usually helps the patient realize that she could, in fact, survive the "worst."

### Social Phobia

In treating social phobia, social skills training as well as cognitive behavioral techniques are used. The first step is to explore what the teen's fears are about social interaction. Is there a specific fear, is there a distortion in body image or a particular source of self-consciousness, or is there a general sense of people being rejecting or judgmental? The therapist attempts to identify distortions that can be addressed and hopefully modified while also identifying real challenges that need to be overcome. The behavioral component of treating social phobia is to help the patient take small steps toward the cause of anxiety, proceeding up a hierarchy of fears from the easiest situation to the most intimidating. A therapist or primary care provider can encourage an adolescent to find his or her social niche in the complex multiple cultures of a high school. A small group of friends with a shared sense of purpose can reduce social anxiety; membership in a group, such as a computer interest group or a choral group, can help alleviate social phobia.

### Specific Phobias

The therapeutic approach to specific phobias is behavioral. Many patients and parents want to understand *why* the child has a specific phobia. The search for answers may not be fruitful, and discovering the cause does not make the phobia go away. Desensitization by exposure to the phobic object, either imaginal or *in vivo*, is necessary. The cognitive component of the therapy involves a rational discussion of the actual danger, or lack thereof, of the phobic object. Recognizing that few people die in elevator accidents or are bitten by spiders does not, alone, help an adolescent overcome these phobias. Most affected adolescents realize that their phobias are irrational; merely pointing that out often makes them feel worse. Exposure and desensitization are also required. Specific relaxation exercises are often used, either alone or in conjunction with CBT and exposure techniques.

## ADJUNCTIVE TREATMENT METHODS

Progressive muscle relaxation is helpful for generalized anxiety and for anxiety-related insomnia. Controlled breathing exercises are especially helpful for panic disorder, specific phobias, and separation anxiety, but may be applied to any other anxiety disorders as well. Relaxation exercises may be done in association with techniques, such as exposure, that cause a transient increase in anxiety. By using these techniques, the adolescent can gain a sense of mastery by learning to calm down on his or her own. Parental involvement in psychotherapy is essential, especially for the younger adolescent.[20] Parents need to examine how they are contributing to the development or perpetuation of the adolescent's anxiety and they need to be actively involved in the behavioral treatments, to provide encouragement, support, and positive reinforcement.

## PHARMACOTHERAPY

The decision to treat anxiety with medication is a complex and difficult one for many patients and parents (see Chapter 190, Adolescent Psychopharmacology). They often have preconceived ideas, true and false, about the use of medication. Given the familial clustering of anxiety, these ideas may be influenced by the response, or lack thereof, to medications for anxiety by family members. Ambivalence about pharmacotherapy is common. Often, patients and parents want to start with psychotherapy, then add medication if there is not sufficient progress; this is often a very reasonable approach. However, in cases where the anxiety is so severe as to prevent participation in psychotherapy, or when the appropriate psychotherapy is not readily available, medication as the first step is reasonable. Medication treatment, however, even when effective, does not eliminate the need for the patient and parents to deal with confronting anxiety-provoking situations.

The SSRIs are the current first line of pharmacological treatment for most anxiety disorders.[21] Essentially all of the SSRIs, as well as the combined serotonin and norepinephrine reuptake inhibitor venlafaxine, are used to treat anxiety disorders. Not surprisingly, many parents and patients with anxiety disorders are apprehensive about using medications, and patients whose anxiety manifests itself with somatic symptoms are often exquisitely sensitive to medication side effects. The old maxim "start low and go slow" is an effective strategy to avoid side effects such as gastrointestinal upset, insomnia, or agitation that may feel like an exacerbation of the anxiety disorder and decrease the likelihood that the adolescent will discontinue the medication prematurely. Dose reduction or a switch to another SSRI may resolve side effects. Many adolescents with anxiety respond to very low doses, but some, especially those with OCD, require much higher doses for optimal effect. Frequent monitoring of the patient for response and adverse effects is essential. Serotonin reuptake inhibitors are generally safe, and especially the absence of cardiovascular side effects, or lethality in overdose, makes these the most acceptable medication for anxious patients. Despite the US Food and Drug Administration (FDA) "Black Box Warning," there is currently no evidence of increased or emergent suicidality in any of the clinical trials of Serotonin reuptake inhibitors in the treatment of anxiety disorders.

Tricyclic antidepressants are older antidepressant/antianxiety medications and are less commonly used, primarily because of side effects. Anticholinergic effects, cardiovascular side effects, and lethality in overdose are major deterrents to their use. They do, however, have a place in treatment of patients with anxiety who either have intolerable side effects, especially activation or disinhibition, or who have not responded to an SSRI. Clomipramine is a unique medication, as it is almost purely serotonergic, which makes it an alternative for a patient with OCD who has not responded to an SSRI.

Buspirone is also an option for treating generalized or background anxiety, but it is not effective for panic, OCD, or other acute types of anxiety. It has the advantages of having few side effects and not being habituating, which makes it an acceptable alternative for patients or parents who are concerned about addiction or side effects.

Benzodiazepines are occasionally used for severe anxiety, to augment an SSRI, or to provide immediate relief to a very anxious patient whose SSRI treatment has not yet taken effect. They can be used regularly but can also be used as needed, which may provide an extra "safety net" for a patient who fears an attack of panic or anxiety.

Low doses of the second generation, or atypical, antipsychotics are occasionally used to augment SSRI treatment in severe anxiety, especially in OCD. Risperidone and quetiapine are most commonly used, as side effects are generally rare at low doses, but this is usually a relatively short-term intervention because of concern about side effects such as weight gain and sedation.

Beta blockers are used primarily for acute, short-term anxiety such as performance anxiety, which manifests itself with prominent physiological symptoms such as shaking, sweating, and dry mouth. The medication is taken approximately a half-hour before the performance or other predictable source of anxiety, and the patient is usually advised to make a "dry run," to be sure he or she can tolerate the medication prior to using it before a performance.

How long do you treat with medication? There are some general concepts to consider when advising a specific patient. Anxiety disorders may be a response to acute stress but may also be chronic problems, with a remitting and relapsing course. For example, OCD, which is generally longterm, and which has usually gone untreated for quite a while, often requires long-term treatment. In general, most patients who have responded to medication for anxiety should continue treatment for about a year. After that, the decision to discontinue medication is most often based on the patient's preference. Some adolescents are eager to discontinue medication as soon as possible; whereas others are so relieved to be feeling better that they are reluctant to make any changes. If a patient has been successfully involved in psychotherapy and has achieved a sense of mastery and ability to cope with stress, it is more likely that medication can be discontinued without relapse. In any case, the patient who is discontinuing medication treatment should do so at a time of relatively low stress, should be helped to identify signs of relapse, and should be encouraged to resume treatment promptly should that happen.

## PROGNOSIS

A propensity toward anxiety disorders is often a lifelong vulnerability that manifests itself differently at different life stages. Critical points such as leaving the relatively sheltered setting of elementary school for the chaos of high school, leaving home for college, a first really serious romantic involvement, or becoming pregnant may trigger anxiety. Chronic, unremitting anxiety can have a devastating effect on quality of life and may result in hopelessness and suicidal tendencies. It is also a risk factor for alcohol or drug abuse, as the patient tries to self-medicate. Vulnerability to anxiety is often lifelong, but treatment and self-awareness can make the difference between someone who is profoundly anxious, or even suicidal, and someone who copes, overcomes, and has a successful life in spite of a tendency to anxiety.

## SUMMARY

Anxiety disorders in adolescents encompass a number of different specific disorders that fall into a variety of diagnoses. Symptoms can range from mild to incapacitating. The constellation of symptoms span physical, psychological, and emotional domains. In some cases, such as adolescents who are unable to attend school because of severe headaches and abdominal pain (separation anxiety or "school phobia"), traditional emotional features of anxiety may not be apparent or are overshadowed by incapacitating physical symptoms, effectively masking the underlying anxious component. Primary care clinicians who have a working knowledge of the panoply of manifestations of anxiety disorders and an awareness of the effective treatment methods described in this chapter can provide adolescents and their families with significant relief of symptoms and return to health.

## INTERNET RESOURCES

- US Department of Health and Human Services, Substance Abuse and Mental Health Services Administration, National Mental Health Information Center. Children and Adolescents with Anxiety Disorders. www.mentalhealth.samhsa.gov/publications/allpubs/ca-0007/default.asp. Accessed May 30, 2009.
- American Academy of Child and Adolescent Psychiatry. Anxiety Disorders Resource Center. www.aacap.org/cs/Anxiety Disorders. ResourceCenter. Accessed May 30, 2009.
- National Alliance on Mental Illness. Anxiety Disorders in Children and Adolescents. www.nami.org/Content/ContentGroups/Helpline1/Anxiety_Disorders_in_Children_and_Adolescents.htm Accessed May 30, 2009.

## REFERENCES

1. Connolly S, Bernstein GA, Work Group on Quality Issues. Practice parameter for the assessment and treatment of children and adolescents with anxiety disorders. *J Am Acad Child Adolesc Psychiatry.* 2007;46(2):267–283

2. Merikangas KR. Vulnerability factors for anxiety disorders in children and adolescents. *Child Adolesc Psychiatr Clin N Am.* 2005;14(4):649–679

3. Birmaher B, Brent DA, Chiappetta L, Bridge J, Monga S, Baugher M. Psychometric properties of the Screen for Child Anxiety Related Emotional Disorders Scale (SCARED): a replication study. *J Am Acad Child Adolesc Psychiatry.* 1999;38(10):1230–1236

4. March JS, Parker JD, Sullivan K, Stallings P, Conners CK. The Multidimensional Anxiety Scale for Children (MASC): factor structure, reliability, and validity. *J Am Acad Child Adolesc Psychiatry.* 1997;36:554–565

5. Scahill L, Riddle MA, McSwiggin-Harden M, et al. Children's Yale-Brown Obsessive-Compulsive Scale: reliability and validity. *J Am Acad Child Adolesc Psychiatry.* 1997;36:844–852

6. Watson D. Rethinking the mood and anxiety disorders: a quantitative hierarchical model for DSM-V. *J Abnorm Psychol.* 2005;114:522–536

7. Suveg C, Aschenbrand SG, Kendall PC. Separation anxiety disorder, panic disorder, and school refusal. *Child Adolesc Psychiatr Clin N Am.* 2005;14(4):773–795

8. Dulcan MK, Martini DR, Lake MB. *Concise Guide to Child and Adolescent Psychiatry*, 3rd ed. Washington, DC: American Psychiatric Publishing; 2003

9. Silverman WK, Moreno J. Specific phobia. *Child Adolesc Psychiatr Clin N Am.* 2005;14(4):819–843

10. Chavira DA, Stein MB. Childhood social anxiety disorders: from understanding to treatment. *Child Adolesc Psychiatr Clin N Am.* 2005;14(4):797–818

11. Dulcan MK, Wiener JM. *Essentials of Child and Adolescent Psychiatry.* Washington, DC: American Psychiatric Publishing; 2004

12. Essau C, Conradt J, Petermann F. Frequency, comorbidity, and psychosocial impairment of anxiety disorders in German adolescents. *J Anxiety Disord.* 2000;14(3):263–279

13. Suveg C, Aschenbrand SG, Kendall PC. Separation anxiety disorder, panic disorder, and school refusal. *Child Adolesc Psychiatr Clin N Am.* 2005;14(4):773–795

14. Leonard HL, Ale CM, Freeman JB, Garcia AM, Ng JS. Obsessive-compulsive disorder. *Child Adolesc Psychiatr Clin N Am.* 2005;14(4):727-743

15. De Bellis MD, Van Dillen T. Childhood post-traumatic stress disorder: an overview. *Child Adolesc Psychiatr Clin N Am.* 2005;14(4):745–772

16. Evans DL, Foa ED, Gur RE et al, eds. Treatment of anxiety disorders. In: *Treating and Preventing Adolescent Mental Health Disorders: What We Know and What We Don't Know.* New York: Oxford University Press; 2005:184–220

17. March JS. Combining medication and psychosocial treatments: an evidence-based medicine approach. *Int Rev Psychiatry.* 2002;14:155–163

18. Compton SN, March JS, Brent D, Albano AM, Weersing VR, Curry J. Cognitive-behavioral psychotherapy for anxiety and depressive disorders in children and adolescents: an evidence-based medicine review. *J Am Acad Child Adolesc Psychiatry.* 2004;43:930–959

19. Freeman JB, Garcia AM, Swedo SE. Obsessive-compulsive disorder. In: Dulcan MK, Wiener JM, eds. *Essentials of Child and Adolescent Psychiatry.* Washington, DC: American Psychiatric Publishing; 2006:441–453

20. Bogels SM, Siqueland L. Family cognitive behavioral therapy for children and adolescents with clinical anxiety disorders. *J Am Acad Child Adolesc Psychiatry.* 2006;45:134–141

21. Birmaher B, Yelovich K, Renaud J. Pharmacologic treatment for children and adolescents with anxiety disorders. *Pediatr Clin North Am.*1998;45:1187–1204

# CHAPTER 186

# Disorders of Behavior

NIRANJAN S. KARNIK, MD, PhD • ARASH ANOSHIRAVANI, MD, MPH •
DR MED UNIV HANS STEINER

## OVERVIEW

As noted throughout this textbook, adolescence is a dynamic period in which growth and maturation occur at variable paces in multiple domains. In addition to the obvious physical changes associated with puberty are a variety of behaviors typically considered "being an adolescent." These features include demonstrating independence, risk-taking, thrill-seeking, limit-testing, challenging rules, and questioning authority. Although research has shown that significant disruptive behavior is not displayed by most adolescents (see Chapter 6, Psychosocial Development and Behavior), disruptive behaviors sometimes are considered normative as adolescents develop a sense of autonomy and identity in their families, their peer group, their school, and other environments in the process of "growing up." However, when these behaviors develop into patterns, they can be dangerous to the adolescent or to others and become repetitive, fixed, or show evidence of a maladaptive trajectory. Then, they often require attention by medical and mental health professionals.[1]

Increasingly, research has shown that disruptive behaviors are the final common pathway with multiple etiologies and trajectories. Biologically, there is growing evidence that some adolescents may be predisposed to aggressive behaviors and conduct disorders, based on particular neurochemical and neuroanatomical variations.[2-5] These biological variables likely interact with individual psychological factors and the social environment. It is clear that the development of personality and attitudinal variables both play significant roles in the evolution of disruptive patterns. Finally, the influences of social and family factors can modulate and ameliorate underlying predispositions to some extent. An ecological view—in which the adolescent influences the environment and the environment influences the adolescent—is essential to understanding adolescent development and the role disruptive behaviors play in this process.[6] This chapter focuses on the diagnostic features of disruptive behaviors in adolescents. The clinical features of disruptive behaviors are discussed and treatment options are detailed.

## BASIC CONCEPTS AND TRENDS

The basic social patterns and behavioral norms that define the boundaries of disruptive behaviors emerge from social consensus about acceptable and unacceptable behavior. These boundaries are widely understood and are based on both cultural definitions handed down from one generation to the next and on legal definitions in the juvenile justice system. Neither of these forces is fixed or constant. What is socially inappropriate or illegal in one circumstance may be considered understandable or even acceptable in another situation. For example, an adolescent living in the midst of a civil war who kills an armed warrior who invades his home would generally be considered to have done what was needed to protect himself and his family. He would probably even be considered a hero. Another adolescent living in an impoverished inner city as a gang member who kills another adolescent to protect his "turf" would generally be seen as profoundly antisocial and could serve a prolonged sentence in jail. Similarly, an affluent teenage girl who steals food from a supermarket for friends on a dare would be considered a shoplifter, but a poor teenage girl who steals food from a supermarket for her family would be perceived as trying to survive and would be considered for social services rather than legal action. Context defines behaviors and how we understand them, and hence the importance of taking an ecological and systemic approach to understanding disruptive behaviors in adolescents.

The *Diagnostic and Statistical Manual of Mental Disorders,* 4th Edition, Text Revision (*DSM-IV-TR*),[7] defines a series of syndromes characterized by disruptive behaviors, aggression, and criminality. Often called "externalizing disorders" because the behavior is directed externally toward others, they include oppositional defiant disorder (ODD), conduct disorder (CD), antisocial personality disorder (ASPD), and disruptive behavior disorder, not otherwise specified. These diagnoses generally follow a trajectory that begins with oppositional behaviors at younger ages that evolves into CD and its associated police and legal interventions, and ultimately developing into a personality-driven pattern in ASPD. Such a trajectory is not fixed, however, because interventions are possible at each stage to avert continued progression down a maladaptive pathway (see Chapter 187 for discussion of personality disorders).

Disruptive disorders show significant gender differences. Adolescent males exhibit externalizing and aggressive patterns of behavior at 4 to 5 times the rate of females. Despite this difference, recent studies have noted that girls are one of the fastest-growing segments in the juvenile justice system. Research has shown that girls tend to use social aggression and ostracism as a means of violence rather than the physical aggression that is more typical of boys. It also appears that aggression by girls can be linked to early physical maturity, which predisposes them at several levels to greater degrees of aggression.[8]

Comorbid trauma histories are especially important in the development of disruptive behaviors. Retrospective studies of adolescents in the juvenile justice system have shown extremely high levels of traumatic experiences.[9-12] These experiences result in a high degree of dissociative symptoms and can make these adolescents have significant mental health morbidities.[13,14] Early screening and intervention can help these adolescents avoid further exacerbation of their symptoms, leading to potential maladaptive patterns.

## OPPOSITIONAL DEFIANT DISORDER

Oppositional defiant disorder generally presents in preadolescents with a pattern of intentional and persistent antagonism and blame toward others. See Box 186-1 for clinical features of ODD.

Youth with ODD often have tantrum and rage outbursts that are disproportionate to initiating stressors. As a syndromic diagnosis, it tends to present between 6 and 10 years of age, and often shows an escalating pattern. Treatment for ODD focuses on behavioral therapy for the child combined with parent management training for the caregivers. Medications have generally not been shown to have significant benefit, unless there are marked comorbid conditions, such as attention-deficit/hyperactivity disorder (ADHD).[2,3]

### Box 186-1

### *Clinical Features of Oppositional Defiant Disorder*

**Criteria**

- Argumentative
- Intentionally irritates people
- Struggles to comply with rules made by adults
- Absence of psychosis or mood disorders
- Exhibits behavior in excess of what is typical for developmental age

**Symptoms**

- Blames others for own misdeeds or when things go wrong
- Irritable
- Easily angered
- Spiteful
- Resentful of attempts by others to control behavior
- Loses temper readily

**Other Factors**

- Persistence of disruptive behavior for > 6 months
- Impairment in multiple functional domains: home, school, work, peers
- Age at onset
- Level of severity

Reprinted with permission from American Psychiatric Association. *Diagnostic and Statistical Manual of Mental Disorders*, 4th Edition, Text Revision. Washington, DC: American Psychiatric Association; 2000:102–103.

## CONDUCT DISORDER

While ODD is quintessentially the disruptive disorder of childhood, CD can be considered the disruptive behavior of adolescence. Conduct disorder is characterized by a repeated pattern of violating the rights of others. The pattern involves a combination of physical aggression that causes harm or threatens others, nonaggressive behaviors that include vandalism, theft, and lying; and rule violations, such as truancy and breaking normal social rules set by adults and authorities. Two types of CD are identified in the *DSM-IV-TR*. Childhood-onset CD begins before age 10. Adolescent-onset begins between 10 and 17 years of age. The childhood-onset variant generally has a worse prognosis, with 30% to 50% of these youth progressing to ASPD in adulthood and greater risk of developing adult substance abuse and dependence as well as other psychiatric conditions.[7,15] See Box 186-2 for the clinical features of CD.

Recent research supports treatment of youth with CD that focuses on the nature of the aggressive acts that these adolescents commit. Multiple lines of evidence have led to an understanding that there are 2 major subtypes of aggression in CD:

- Reactive/Affective/Defensive/Impulsive (RADI) or "hot" aggression, in which the aggression is largely unplanned and often overt. The anticipated outcome of the aggression from the perspective of the aggressor is negative emotional affect. Associated emotions in this subtype of aggression include anger, frustration, irritability, and fear.

**Box 186-2**

***Diagnostic Criteria for Conduct Disorder***

A. A repetitive and persistent pattern of behavior in which the basic rights of others or major age-appropriate societal norms or rules are violated, as manifested by the presence of 3 (or more) of the following 15 criteria in the past 12 months, with at least 1 criterion present in the past 6 months:

**Aggression to people and animals**

(1) Often bullies, threatens, or intimidates others
(2) Often initiates physical fights
(3) Has used a weapon that can cause serious physical harm to others
(4) Has been physically cruel to people
(5) Has been physically cruel to animals
(6) Has stolen while confronting a victim
(7) Has forced someone into sexual activity

**Destruction of property**

(8) Has deliberately engaged in fire setting with the intention of causing serious damage
(9) Has deliberately destroyed others' property (other than by fire setting)

**Deceitfulness or theft**

(10) Has broken into someone else's house, building, or car
(11) Often lies to obtain goods or favors or to avoid obligations; "cons" others
(12) Has stolen items of nontrivial value without confronting a victim

**Serious violations of rules**

(13) Often stays out at night despite parental prohibitions, beginning before age 13 years
(14) Has run away from home overnight at least twice while living in parental or parental surrogate home (or once without returning for a lengthy period)
(15) Is often truant from school, beginning before age 13 years

B. The disturbance in behavior causes clinically significant impairment in social, academic, or occupational functioning.

C. If the individual is age 18 years or older, criteria are not met for ASPD.

Specify type based on age at onset:

Childhood-onset type: onset of at least one criterion characteristic of conduct disorder prior to 10 years of age

Adolescent-onset type: absence of any criteria characteristic of conduct disorder prior to 10 years of age

Adapted from American Psychiatric Association. *Diagnostic and Statistical Manual of Mental Disorders*, 4th Edition, Text Revision. Washington, DC: American Psychiatric Association; 2000: 98–99.

- Proactive/Instrumental/Planned (PIP) or "cold" aggression, in which there is a planned execution of aggression. This type of aggression is often covert and the anticipated outcome from the perspective of the aggressor is positive emotional affect. Associated emotions in this subtype of aggression include interest and happiness about the act or outcome, or feelings of disgust or contempt directed toward the object of the aggression.

Individuals with hot and cold aggression begin with a maladaptive form of aggression. If a pattern continues these individuals develop psychiatric diagnosis(es). If the pattern worsens despite efforts at intervention, individuals may diverge into acute or chronic forms of aggression. For individuals who are on the "PIP pathway" there are early signs of maladaptive "cold" aggression that is planned, covert, and without remorse or bad feelings, other than blaming others for it. If this pattern persists into adolescence, the diagnosis would become CD and subsequently ASPD if it persists into adulthood. Individuals with acute onset of aggressive behaviors, rather than a persistent pattern, are more likely to be diagnosed with psychopathy.

Reactive/Affective/Defensive/Impulsive aggression begins with a maladaptive type of reactive or emotional aggression that has a primarily negative affect. If the pattern persists in childhood, the psychiatric diagnosis becomes ODD. Should the pattern of aggression continue into adulthood, the diagnosis would be irritable personality disorder if a chronic and fixed pattern is demonstrated, or intermittent explosive disorder if marked by discrete episodes of extremely violent behavior.

These 2 major new taxa for aggression lead to markedly different approaches to the treatment of these disorders.[16] The RADI subtype may be more responsive to psychopharmacological[17] and psychotherapeutic interventions, whereas the PIP subtype may require more structured environments that include methods of behavioral modification as well as psychotherapy. The PIP form may not be as pharmacologically responsive as the RADI subtype.

## MEDICAL COMORBIDITIES AND DISRUPTIVE PATTERNS

Adolescents with chronic medical illnesses may be at risk for the development of behavioral problems but follow patterns of behavior and development that fall well outside of those described for youth with ODD and CD. The Ontario Child Health Study[18] found that children and adolescents with chronic illness and significant disability are 3 times as likely to have psychiatric morbidity and social problems, and those without disability were twice as likely to have psychiatric illnesses, but without social dysfunction. Siblings of youth with chronic illnesses are at risk for higher rates of internalizing disorders (ie, depression and anxiety) as well as poorer peer relationships, but do not appear to have increased risks of CD, ADHD, or somatization.[19]

Nonadherence to treatment recommendations is one of the most common presentations of disruptive behavior,[20] and more commonly occurs with family problems, affective problems, and possible substance abuse. This behavior may be related to the stress that chronic illness exerts on adolescents. Nonadherence has been well documented in the areas of transplantation,[21-23] asthma,[24-26] and rheumatic disease.[27] Empirical interventions have been developed for pediatric nonadherence asthma, juvenile rheumatoid arthritis, and diabetes.[28]

## TREATMENT

Although physicians and other primary care providers might not provide direct interventions for disruptive patterns among adolescents, it is important for these providers to be familiar with available therapies so that appropriate referrals can be made. Most available research data suggest that ODD is best treated with individual and family therapy. Under this rubric many different modalities can be used, but the common theme should be to educate parents about behavioral management techniques and parenting approaches. Adolescents can benefit significantly from interpersonal and cognitive behavioral psychotherapy. These approaches can help them to understand their own behaviors and their responses to situations from a new vantage point, and the effects of their behaviors on others. The length of therapy cannot easily be predicted and will vary by the specific psychotherapeutic modality and the approach of the clinician. Kazdin and colleagues[29,30] have been studying the variety of psychotherapeutic approaches present to address youth with CD. In their research they find 3 therapeutic models that have proven efficacy.

- Parent management training (PMT) focuses on changing the parent–adolescent dynamics so that coercive techniques are minimized in favor of longer-lasting teaching modalities.
- Problem-solving skills training (PSST) is related to CBT modalities and attempts to address the cognitions and social underpinnings that create CD and ODD. This modality will likely work for adolescents who are more cognizant and reflective about themselves.
- Multisystemic therapy (MST) attempts to address the adolescent, the family, and the nonfamily influences on behavior in an attempt to make rules and normative patterns more consistent across time and space.

Another intervention that is re-emerging in the treatment of disruptive behavior is "sociotherapy." This modality, popularized in community-based mental health and centers, applies social and community interventions to help facilitate behavioral changes. In the case of ODD, structured after-school programs and weekend activities can significantly help adolescents learn social behaviors and boundaries. Adolescents with CD may require more intensive sociotherapy, including attempts to intervene at the group or gang level. Some rehabilitation programs focus on the peer group as the unit of intervention, because focusing on the individual neglects group dynamics and peer pressure.

Conduct disorder is among the most difficult of adolescent psychiatric conditions to treat. All of the approaches outlined previously are applicable. In the context of an acute episode, time may not permit psychotherapeutic or sociotherapeutic modalities to reach their full potential. At these times it may be appropriate to consider medication intervention.[17] The first line of therapy for CD is mood stabilizers or anticonvulsants. Among the best-studied medications are valproic acid and its derivatives, as well as lithium. Extended release formulations of these medications facilitate dosing and adherence. Clinicians should take a careful medical history before starting these medications and regularly monitor relevant laboratory studies (see Chapter 190 for a detailed discussion of adolescent psychopharmacology). Should mood stabilizers fail to produce an adequate effect, an atypical antipsychotic can be added. This class of medications is being widely used for multiple off-label uses and can benefit mood stabilization when used in low doses. Attention needs to be paid to possible extrapyramidal and akathisic side effects, and careful monitoring should be done when prescribing any antipsychotic.

Should outpatient interventions fail, hospitalization can be used as an intervention of last resort or in the context of acute behavioral decompensation where the safety of the adolescent or individuals around the adolescent is at risk. Hospitalization should focus on rapid interventions to de-escalate the crisis, build a safety network around the adolescent, and change the direction of care. Careful follow-up and consideration of a partial hospitalization or other specialized treatment program need to be part of discharge planning. Primary care physicians can play an essential role in helping to coordinate care at all levels and enabling consistency over the course of treatment.

## CONCLUSIONS

Disruptive behaviors among adolescents should be expected, as they are normative aspects of development and often emerge in the transition from childhood to adulthood. When these patterns become fixed and maladaptive, they then deserve more focused and concerted therapeutic attention. Disruptive behaviors rarely emerge *de novo*, and can be linked to other factors such as family, peer, social, environmental, and academic stressors. These behavioral patterns can also emerge in the context of a chronic illness that exerts a significant stressor in a child's life. Providers who work with adolescents should be attentive to multiple comorbidities that can characterize disruptive behaviors including ADHD. In addition, screening for past trauma and abuse as well as current substance abuse is essential along with trying to understand the social and family situation the adolescent lives within. Referrals and comanagement with experienced mental health professionals are warranted when the fixed patterns of behavior are evident.

## REFERENCES


1. Karnik NS, McMullin MA, Steiner H. Disruptive behaviors: conduct and oppositional disorders in adolescents. *Adolesc Med Clin.* 2006;17(1):97-114

2. Nada-Raja S, Langley JD, McGee R, Williams SM, Begg DJ, Reeder AI. Inattentive and hyperactive behaviors and driving offenses in adolescence.*J Am Acad Child Adolesc Psychiatry.* 1997;36(4):515-522

3. Newcorn JH, Halperin JM, Jensen PS, et al. Symptom profiles in children with ADHD: effects of comorbidity and gender. *J Am Acad Child Adolesc Psychiatry.* 2001;40(2): 137-146

4. Blair RJ. Neurobiological basis of psychopathy. *Br J Psychiatry.* 2003;182:5-7

5. Blair RJ, Coccaro EF, Connor DF, et al. Juvenile maladaptive aggression: a review of the neuroscientific data. *Biol Psychiatry. Under review*

6. Karnik NS. The social environment. In: Steiner H, ed. *Handbook of Mental Health Interventions in Children and Adolescents: An Integrated Developmental Perspective.* San Francisco, CA: Jossey-Bass; 2004

7. American Psychiatric Association. Task Force on DSM-IV. *Diagnostic and Statistical Manual of Mental Disorders:* DSM-IV-TR. 4th ed. Text Revision. Washington, DC: American Psychiatric Association; 2000

8. Celio M, Karnik NS, Steiner H. Early maturation as a risk factor for aggression and delinquency in adolescent girls: a review. *Int J Clin Pract.* 2006;60(10):1254-1262. Epub 2006 Aug 22

9. Cauffman E, Feldman SS, Waterman J, Steiner H. Posttraumatic stress disorder among female juvenile offenders. *J Am Acad Child Adolesc Psychiatry.* 1998;37(11):1209-1216

10. Ruchkin VV, Schwab-Stone M, Koposov R, Vermeiren R, Steiner H. Violence exposure, posttraumatic stress, and personality in juvenile delinquents. *J Am Acad Child Adolesc Psychiatry.* 2002;41(3):322-329

11. Steiner H, Garcia IG, Matthews Z. Posttraumatic stress disorder in incarcerated juvenile delinquents. *J Am Acad Child Adolesc Psychiatry.* 1997;36(3):357-365

12. Vermeiren R, De Clippele A, Deboutte D. A descriptive survey of Flemish delinquent adolescents. *J Adolesc.* 2000;23(3): 277-285

13. Plattner B, Silvermann MA, Redlich AD, et al. Pathways to dissociation: intrafamilial versus extrafamilial trauma in juvenile delinquents. *J Nerv Ment Dis.* 2003;191(12):781-788

14. Steiner H, Carrion V, Plattner B, Koopman C. Dissociative symptoms in posttraumatic stress disorder: diagnosis and treatment. *Child Adolesc Psychiatr Clin N Am.* 2003;12(2):231-249, viii

15. Loeber R. Antisocial behavior: more enduring than changeable? *J Am Acad Child Adolesc Psychiatry.* 1991;30(3):393-397

16. Connor DF, Carlson GA, Chang KD, et al. Juvenile maladaptive aggression: a review of prevention, treatment, and service configuration and a proposed research agenda. *J Clin Psychiatry.* 2006;67(5):808-820

17. Soller MV, Karnik NS, Steiner H. Psychopharmacologic treatment in juvenile offenders. *Child Adolesc Psychiatr Clin N Am.* 2006;15(2):477-499, x

18. Cadman D, Boyle M, Szatmari P, Offord DR. Chronic illness, disability, and mental and social well-being: findings of the Ontario Child Health Study. *Pediatrics.* 1987;79(5):805-813

19. Cadman D, Boyle M, Offord DR. The Ontario Child Health Study: social adjustment and mental health of siblings of children with chronic health problems. *J Dev Behav Pediatr.* 1988;9(3):117-121

20. Smith BA, Shuchman M. Problem of nonadherence in chronically ill adolescents: strategies for assessment and intervention. *Curr Opin Pediatr.* 2005;17(5):613-618

21. Hsu DT. Biological and psychological differences in the child and adolescent transplant recipient. *Pediatr Transplant.* 2005;9(3):416-421

22. Shaw RJ, Palmer L, Blasey C, Sarwal M. A typology of non-adherence in pediatric renal transplant recipients. *Pediatr Transplant.* 2003;7(6):489-493

23. Griffin KJ, Elkin TD. Non-adherence in pediatric transplantation: a review of the existing literature. *Pediatr Transplant.* 2001;5(4):246-249

24. Bender BG. Risk taking, depression, adherence, and symptom control in adolescents and young adults with asthma. *Am J Respir Crit Care Med.* 2006;173(9):953-977

25. Adams CD, Dreyer ML, Dinakar C, Portnoy JM. Pediatric asthma: a look at adherence from the patient and family perspective. *Curr Allergy Asthma Rep.* 2004;4(6):425-432

26. McQuaid EL, Kopel SJ, Klein RB, Fritz GK. Medication adherence in pediatric asthma: reasoning, responsibility, and behavior. *J Pediatr Psychol.* 2003;28(5):323-333

27. Rapoff MA. Management of adherence and chronic rheumatic disease in children and adolescents. *Best Pract Res Clin Rheumatol.* 2006;20(2):301-314

28. Lemanek KL, Kamps J, Chung NB. Empirically supported treatments in pediatric psychology: regimen adherence. *J Pediatr Psychol.* 2001;26(5):253-275

29. Kazdin AE. Treatments for aggressive and antisocial children. *Child Adolesc Psychiatr Clin N Am.* 2000;9(4):841-858

30. Kazdin AE. Family and parenting interventions for conduct disorder and delinquency: a meta-analysis of randomized controlled trials. *J Pediatr.* 2002;141(5):738

# CHAPTER 187

# Personality Disorders in Adolescents

NISHKA R. VIJAY, MD • JOHN LANGLEY, MD • PAUL S. LINKS, MD, MSc

## INTRODUCTION

Adolescent personality disorders, sometimes termed *character pathology*, include pervasive, inflexible, and maladaptive constellations of symptoms that manifest themselves across all domains of interpersonal interactions and relationships, and often are assumed to be immutable and a barrier to positive interactions in health care settings. Because personality development continues into adulthood, the younger the adolescent, the more difficult it is to make a definitive diagnosis of a personality disorder. The determinants and risk factors include biological, psychological, social, and environmental factors that appear to interact in complex ways in the origin and maintenance of personality disorders. In addition, the diagnosis of a personality disorder in an adolescent can be confusing because there are 10 different personality disorders grouped into 3 different clusters.[1] Within the diagnostic classification system in the American Psychiatric Association's *Diagnostic and Statistical Manual of Mental Disorders*, 4th Edition, Text Revision (DSM-IV-TR), personality disorders are placed on Axis II; the more common mental health conditions encountered in adolescents (with which they may coexist), such as depression, anxiety, or schizophrenia, are placed on Axis I. Furthermore, compared to other psychiatric conditions, personality disorders have not been studied extensively in adolescents, and much remains to be learned about these poorly understood but challenging conditions.

Nonetheless, a discussion of personality disorder is appropriate in this textbook for several reasons: (1) the symptoms associated with a personality disorder in young adulthood can be traced back to adolescence and even childhood, (2) the behavioral patterns associated with certain personality disorders put the adolescent at risk for a number of different health problems, such as suicide and substance abuse, and (3) adolescent health care providers may be one of the few sources of continuity for adolescents during the transition to young adulthood, which is characteristically a difficult time for individuals with a personality disorder. The interpersonal style, emotional lability, and impulsivity exhibited in some personality disorders can threaten therapeutic relationships with health care providers and disrupt the health care team unless common pitfalls are avoided. In addition, clinicians who are aware that the behavioral patterns found in certain personality disorders are often associated with somatoform disorders can recognize these symptoms more readily and initiate proper treatment while minimizing iatrogenic complications. This chapter emphasizes two personality disorders most likely to present challenges in adolescent health care: borderline personality disorder (BPD) and antisocial personality disorder (ASPD). It also touches on diagnoses frequently associated with ASPD, such as oppositional defiant disorder (ODD) and externalizing disorders, which are discussed in greater detail in Chapter 186, Disorders of Behavior.

## DEFINITIONS

Personality disorders are enduring patterns of inner experience and behavior that deviate markedly from the expectation of an individual's culture and that are consistently exhibited in a variety of settings. They have their onset in adolescence or early adulthood, becoming pronounced during young and middle adulthood. Being pervasive and relatively stable in patients between ages 15 and 25 years, personality disorders lead to impairment of the day-to-day functioning of affected individuals in the second and third decades of life.[2] Such impairment is often associated with a variety of behaviors that bring the adolescent to the attention of health care providers. Although affected individuals experience emotional distress due to their behavior, personality disorders are remarkable for their ability to elicit a variety of responses, almost all of them negatively reinforcing, from individuals and groups in the patient's environment. There are 10 distinct patterns of behaviors that are grouped into 3 clusters based on whether the behavior patterns are oddly eccentric, dramatically emotional, or anxiously fearful, as outlined in Box 187-1.

The behavior patterns listed in Box 187-1 indicate that adolescents with personality disorders have

## Box 187-1

### *Personality Disorders Grouped into 3 Clusters by Patterns of Behavior*

**Cluster A (oddly eccentric)**

*Paranoid personality disorder*: Pervasive distrust and suspiciousness, with the following beliefs commonly held: (1) others are exploiting or deceiving the person, (2) friends and associates are untrustworthy, (3) information confided to others will be used maliciously, (4) there is hidden meaning in remarks or events others perceive as benign, (5) the spouse or partner is unfaithful.

*Schizoid personality disorder*: Marked detachment from others, with little desire for close relationships, resulting in little pleasure in activities, indifference to praise or criticism, and seeming cold or aloof due to lack of interest in interpersonal interaction or emotional connections.

*Schizotypal personality disorder*: Marked eccentricities of thought, perception, and behavior, exhibited by (1) ideas of reference; (2) odd beliefs or magical thinking; (3) vague, circumstantial, or stereotyped speech; (4) social anxiety that does not diminish with familiarity; (5) idiosyncratic perceptual experiences or bodily illusions.

**Cluster B (dramatically emotional)**

*Antisocial personality disorder* (ASPD): See Box 187-2.

*Borderline personality disorder* (BPD): Unstable and intense interpersonal relationships, self-perception, and moods with marked impulse control impairment with at least 5 of the following 9 criteria: (1) frantic efforts to avoid expected abandonment; (2) unstable and intense interpersonal relationships; (3) marked, persistently unstable self-image; (4) impulsivity in at least 2 areas that are potentially self-damaging (eg, sex, substance abuse, reckless driving); (5) recurrent suicidal behaviors or threats of self-mutilation; (6) marked affective instability; (7) chronic feelings of emptiness; (8) intense and inappropriate anger; (9) transient paranoia or dissociation.

*Histrionic personality disorder*: Excessively emotional and emotionally labile, with dramatic, often sexually provocative, attention-seeking behavior.

*Narcissistic personality disorder*: Grandiose and requiring admiration from others, with the following features: (1) exaggeration of their own talents or accomplishments; (2) a sense of entitlement; (3) exploitation of others; (4) lack of empathy; (5) envy of others; (6) arrogant, haughty attitude.

**Cluster C (anxiously fearful)**

*Avoidant personality disorder*: Extreme shyness resulting in social inhibition and isolation. Despite feelings of inadequacy and heightened sensitivity to rejection, maintains a desire to have relationships with others but is unable to do so because of fear and sensitivity.

*Dependent personality disorder*: Excessive need to be taken care of that results in submissive and clinging behavior, regardless of the consequences, exhibited as at least 5 of the following 8 criteria: (1) difficulty making decisions without guidance and reassurance, (2) need for others to assume responsibility for major areas of the person's life, (3) difficulty expressing disagreement with others, (4) difficulty initiating activities because of lack of confidence, (5) excessive measures to obtain nurturance and support, (6) discomfort or helplessness when alone, (7) urgent seeking for another relationship after one has ended, (8) unrealistic preoccupation with fears of being left to fend for self.

*Obsessive-compulsive personality disorder*: Markedly preoccupied with orderliness, perfectionism, and control, while lacking flexibility or openness. Despite being highly task oriented, their preoccupying thoughts and compulsive behaviors interfere with their efficiency at completing tasks. Strong willed and often scrupulous.

Adapted from American Psychiatric Association. *Diagnostic and Statistical Manual of Mental Disorders*, 4th Edition, Text Revision. Washington, DC: American Psychiatric Association; 2000.

symptoms in least 2 of the following areas: (1) *thoughts*, reflected in the way that an individual views self and others; (2) *interpersonal functioning and skills*, reflected in relationships with others; (3) *emotions*, reflected in the range, intensity, and appropriateness of their expression; and (4) *impulse control*, reflected in the external expression of internally experienced emotional states. Recognizing these patterns when they exist will assist the practitioner in diagnosing the condition, understanding the patient's needs, facilitating appropriate treatment, and avoiding potential pitfalls in patient care.

## BORDERLINE PERSONALITY DISORDER

### DIAGNOSTIC ISSUES

The DSM-IV-TR defines BPD as a pervasive pattern of instability in interpersonal relationships, self-image, affect, and marked impulsivity. In addition, it notes that personality disorder categories may be applied to children and adolescents, in which the individual's particular maladaptive personality traits appear to be pervasive, persistent, and, unlikely to be limited to a particular developmental stage or episode of an Axis 1 disorder.[1] It also stipulates that because traits for a personality disorder that appear in childhood may be transient, to diagnose a personality disorder in an individual younger than 18 years, the features must have been present for at least 1 year.[1] Although making the diagnosis of BPD early may seem unjustified, failing to recognize the behavior patterns as dysfunctional may prevent the affected adolescent from gaining insight or receiving appropriate treatment.

There are few studies of BPD focused exclusively on adolescents. Longitudinal and epidemiological research suggests that, similar to adult samples, about 15% of adolescents living in the community meet criteria for BPD, and the diagnosis remains stable over time.[3] In a 2-year prospective study of adolescents, those with a personality disorder were more likely to abuse drugs and to require inpatient treatment. Hospitalized adolescents have had BPD rates comparable to those reported in adults but with different symptoms. Compared with adults, adolescents are more likely to have uncontrolled anger and affective instability;[4] however, there seems to be a more variable range of psychopathology and diminished internal consistency of the BPD criteria among adolescents. For these reasons, clinicians are cautioned that "borderline pathology of childhood should not be thought of as an earlier version of the adult category."[5]

There is a diverse array of early presentations, including irritability, anger and defiance, affective instability, dissociative symptoms, psychotic symptoms, and even neuropsychological abnormalities, that encompass the "soft signs" of organicity. Adolescent manifestations of BPD are more plastic than in adults and may evolve over time. For example, bipolar illness is often preceded by depression; 20% of adolescents and 32% of children younger than 11 years who present with depression eventually develop bipolar disorder.[6] In addition to the lack of symptom uniformity, children with borderline pathology do not necessarily become adults with BPD.[7]

### RISK FACTORS AND COMORBIDITIES

There are a variety of risk factors for the development of BPD, including (1) trauma and abuse, (2) neglect, (3) early separations, (4) unpredictable environments, (5) childhood conduct problems, (6) severe family dysfunction, and (7) family history.[8-12] However, much of the research identifying these risk factors is retrospective and limited by recall bias. Adults with BPD tend to remember more childhood difficulties than those without BPD. No single risk factor is uniformly associated with the diagnosis.[13] In addition, risk factors are difficult to separate from early presentations of the illness. For example, an adolescent exhibiting problem behaviors at home (eg, acting out) may be triggered by stressors (eg, parental conflict, separation, divorce). Likewise, the behavior may be the first manifestation of underlying traits that will eventually be exhibited across multiple other domains.

Any Axis I disorder can co-occur with borderline pathology, and adolescents with mood disorders have an elevated risk of demonstrating borderline traits.[14] Furthermore, over the course of the disorder, adolescents with BPD may have significant comorbidities, such as major depressive disorder (MDD), post-traumatic stress disorder, or both. Some evidence suggests that comorbidities may be related to gender and that there may be a "specialization effect," with males who have borderline traits tending to develop a substance use disorder, whereas females are more likely to develop an eating disorder, particularly bulimia nervosa.[15] This same evidence indicates that a lifetime pattern of complex comorbidity itself is strongly predictive of BPD.[15]

Some of the most unclear distinctions, however, appear between the affective spectrum illnesses and BPD. Major depressive disorder and BPD share features of anergia, irritability, and dependence. Overlap is even more significant between BPD and bipolar II disorder; shared characteristics include impulsivity, affective instability, inappropriate anger, recurrent suicidality, and unstable relationships.[16] Therefore, efforts to distinguish whether behavioral symptoms reflect Axis I or Axis II pathology or early borderline traits requires a careful longitudinal history and close follow-up to determine how behaviors change over time.

### CLINICAL IMPLICATIONS

Opinions regarding the advantages and disadvantages of making an early diagnosis vary. An argument against early diagnosis is the need to avoid the stigma associated with the label of BPD and the belief that BPD is nothing more than "an adjective in search of a noun."[17] In favor of early diagnosis is the belief in the ability to optimize preventive care and treatment, possibly reducing the heightened risk of chronic physical conditions, poor health-related lifestyle choices, costly forms of medical services,[18] and extensive use of mental health resources.[19] Borderline personality disorder is associated with significantly more impairment at work, in social relationships, and at leisure than is seen in MDD.[19] Adolescents with personality disorders are more than twice as likely to have anxiety, disruptive, mood, and substance use disorders during early childhood. They are also at risk for Axis I disorders in young adulthood.[20]

Although morbidities associated with BPD are significant, the most alarming data regarding BPD relates to mortality. The risk of completed suicide is estimated to approach 10% over time, with adolescents and young adults at the highest risk for death by suicide.[21] This alone could justify making the diagnosis early in life, so that appropriate treatment may be instituted, with the goal of preventing suicide. This argument is bolstered by limited but positive adolescent treatment studies. In one 12-week clinical trial comparing an adaptation of dialectical behavior therapy (DBT) to usual treatment, the adolescents in the DBT group had fewer hospitalizations, less suicidal ideation, and reduced general symptoms.[22] In a 1-year follow-up study comparing adolescents admitted to an inpatient unit who engaged in DBT to those who had usual treatment, both were doing well at the time of the study, but the DBT group had fewer behavioral incidents while in the hospital.[23] A 6-year prospective naturalistic study recently showed high remission rates in adults, suggesting that treatment is possible and perhaps prognosis is better than previously recognized.[24] This is consistent with other studies that have shown DBT to be effective in decreasing suicidal behavior in adults. In many respects, the diagnosis of BPD itself is less harmful than the psychosocial fallout and iatrogenic consequences of being "labeled" with this diagnosis. Health care professionals tend to consider patients with BPD to be more in control of their negative behavior than those with a label of depression, and the attribution of the ability to control behavior was associated with less sympathy toward these patients than those with other mental health conditions.[25] Rather than perceiving the diagnosis of BPD as a "label," it should be seen as a severe and persistent but treatable mental illness.

In summary, although the clinician is faced with the challenging task of diagnosing BPD in an adolescent, emerging treatment studies are encouraging. More research is needed to understand the phenotypic variability of adolescent presentations and the impact of comorbidities on primary Axis II pathology, and to develop more effective treatments. Primary care providers should take a lead in the management of this disorder and should continue to combat against the tendencies toward countertransference and stigmatization that negatively affects these patients and their families. The National Association for Personality Disorder's Treatment and Research Advancements (TARA) offers valuable resources online.[26]

## ANTISOCIAL PERSONALITY DISORDER

### DIAGNOSIS

The DSM-IV-TR defines ASPD as a pervasive pattern of disregard for and violation of the rights of others occurring since age 15 years. At least 3 of 7 of the behavioral criteria listed in Box 187-2 need to be present to diagnose ASPD. An adolescent must have also met criteria earlier for conduct disorder (CD) (see Chapter 186, Disorders of Behavior, for the diagnostic criteria for CD). Thus, the diagnosis of ASPD in adulthood places an enormous weight on history in adolescence. Antisocial personality disorder is the only diagnosis on Axis II that requires an earlier analogous diagnosis of preceding condition. A chronic condition, ASPD is associated with multiple medical and social concerns, including substance use, violence, self-harm, and crime, and is found in up to 60% of male prisoners.[27] Because of the constellation of symptoms, adolescents with ASPD are frequently treated in hospital emergency departments and inpatient units.

#### Box 187-2

#### *Diagnostic Features of Antisocial Personality Disorder*

A. Pervasive pattern of disregard for and violation of the rights of others, occurring since age 15 years, as indicated by three (or more) of the following:
   (1) Failure to conform to social norms with respect to lawful behaviors, as indicated by repeatedly performing acts that are grounds for arrest
   (2) Deceitfulness, as indicated by repeated lying, use of aliases, or conning others for personal profit or pleasure
   (3) Impulsivity or failure to plan ahead
   (4) Irritability and aggressiveness, as indicated by repeated physical fights or assaults
   (5) Reckless disregard for safety of self or others
   (6) Consistent irresponsibility, as indicated by repeated failure to sustain consistent work behavior or honor financial obligations
   (7) Lack of remorse, as indicated by being indifferent to or able to rationalize having hurt, mistreated, or stolen from another
B. At least 18 years old
C. Evidence of conduct disorder with onset before age 15 years
D. Occurrence of antisocial behavior is not exclusively during the course of schizophrenia or a manic episode

Adapted from American Psychiatric Association. *Diagnostic and Statistical Manual of Mental Disorders*, 4th ed, Text Revision. Washington, DC: American Psychiatric Association; 2000: 706.

## COURSE OVER TIME

Most of what is known about the natural history of ASPD is based on the seminal work of Robins in the late 1960s on "sociopathic personality disorder," the forerunner to ASPD.[28] This research established that adult antisocial behavior basically requires antisocial behavior during adolescence because 95% of males with at least 4 symptoms of ASPD in adulthood had at least 1 symptom of the disorder in childhood or adolescence.[29] However, it is important to emphasize that most antisocial children with ODD or CD do not go on to develop ASPD as adults. For example, the prevalence of CD is about 5% in children and more than 10% in adolescents,[30] but the prevalence then drops to far less than 10% in adults. No single antisocial behavior in childhood predicts adult psychopathology. Childhood conduct problems, however, are a stronger predictor of adult antisocial behavior than either family background or social class.[27]

There is good evidence that a number of antisocial personality traits and behaviors emerge early in life, and retrospective studies have traced the onset of severely antisocial symptoms back to children as young as 6 years old. However, fewer than 50% of severely conduct-disordered children go on to become antisocial adults. A recent study indicated that of 483 psychiatrists given vignettes depicting adolescent antisocial behaviors in various social settings revealed that when identical hypothetical behaviors were posed as occurring in different environments and settings, psychiatrists made different judgments about the predicted course, etiology, and treatment responsiveness of adolescents who had identical behaviors being demonstrated in different social contexts.[31] Because behaviors demonstrated by adolescents are judged to be antisocial relative to the social context in which they occur, an argument could be made for focusing on the contextual psychosocial factors as much as the behaviors themselves.

## TEMPERAMENT AND OTHER DIAGNOSTIC ISSUES

Until recently, discussion about characteristics and behaviors related to personality disorders were considered independent of temperament. Difficulties with emotional regulation are common in the temperamental style of adolescents who are at risk for ASPD.[32] This is typically characterized by a tendency to display negative affect. Although external processes such as harsh environmental influences and poor parental modeling can affect emotional regulation, behavioral difficulties arise from deficits in internal processes, involving experiencing, modulating, and at times suppressing emotions.[33] For example, an adolescent who by temperament cannot regulate strong, angry, and hostile emotions may demonstrate a tendency to act aggressively and without concern for the potential consequences to him- or herself or others. This may lead to punitive or even sadistic external behaviors that further reinforce the intensity of the anger, and reinforce and further entrench the pathology. Over time, he becomes desensitized to the negative consequences of behavior and develops a callous disregard for others. Thus, one observes the transformation of a temperamental predisposition into a set of pervasive personality characteristics and behaviors.

Other adolescents may not be prone to negative affect or direct confrontation but have innate callousness or lack of emotionality. Their behavior problems are "covert."[34] The lack of emotional response, if associated with a lack of "fearful inhibition," is particularly problematic because the development of "conscience" depends on an adolescent's fear of certain situations, which results in inhibition of aggressive behaviors. Without normative fearful inhibition, an adolescent may exhibit a tendency to be remorseless or exploitative. These callous and unemotional traits confer a high risk of antisocial behavior, as has been demonstrated in studies of adult prisoners possessing these traits.[35]

A critical diagnostic challenge in adolescents is the differentiation between normative behavior and the more pervasive and fixed patterns of behavior seen in ODD and CD. This distinction is largely based on the degree of academic, social, and functional impairment. Also complicating this diagnostic process are associated comorbidities. For ASPD, associated comorbidities include attention-deficit/hyperactivity disorder (ADHD), ODD, substance use disorders, and MDD, and thus include the other externalizing disorders. Depression is particularly important in this regard because suicide is a complication of CD with comorbid depression. This is particularly true in young adults, although suicidality may be related to both impulsivity and depression. Behavior problems occur in more than half of children with ADHD and may be difficult to differentiate from CD.[36] To disentangle the 2 diagnoses, one needs to determine whether the behaviors arise out of a temperamental domain. Behaviors related to temperament suggest CD, whereas those not related to temperament suggest ADHD.

Antisocial personality disorder is closely associated with substance use disorders and conduct disorders, which may exacerbate each other. The severity of substance abuse relates directly to the severity of CD. Chronic substance abuse not only impairs cognitive function, but also impairs impulse control, which further exacerbates the behavior problems. Adolescents who present as hostile, negativistic, and defiant, without violating the basic rights of others, are often mislabeled as suffering from CD when they actually have ODD (see Chapter 186, Disorders of Behavior, for the diagnostic criteria for ODD). This distinction is important to make because ODD does not usually persist beyond adolescence and has a more favorable prognosis. The differential diagnosis for ODD, however, is similar to CD and includes the other externalizing disorders, mood disorders, substance use disorders, and learning disabilities. Given that the psychological health of an adolescent may be exquisitely sensitive to numerous factors and that the diagnostic issues can be subtle and intricate, a low threshold to arrange a mental health referral is warranted.

### TREATMENT

Usual psychiatric interventions are not successful in the treatment of ASPD. In settings such as in the military or in prison, some affected individuals may demonstrate some change in behavior when confronted by consistent structure and peers. Additionally, long-term studies indicate that individuals with ASPD can gain insight and learn from experiences and alter their dysfunctional behavior.

If used, medications should target specific symptoms such as aggression or impulsivity, rather than ASPD *per se*. For details about medication management, see Chapter 190, Adolescent Psychopharmacology. Psychosocially, a number of options exist, including parent training, clinic-based treatments with a focus on short-term therapies such as cognitive behavioral therapy, and community-based interventions with an emphasis on risk reduction and prevention programs. Therapy can be frustrating at times. However, the ramifications of neglecting this condition are too great to ignore. Conduct disorder and ASPD both pose great costs to society, in terms of direct and indirect expenditures, although the exact amount is unknown. Unfortunately, most estimates are confined to the costs of imprisonment. The juvenile court system often plays a significant role in the lives of this population and may insist on their participation in community programs or their commitment to therapy. In general, more treatment studies are needed to examine a variety of interventions, and more longitudinal data would be helpful to better understand the course and outcome of this disorder.

## SUMMARY

Although there are 10 different personality disorders divided into 3 clusters, BPD and ASPD are the 2 most likely to include behaviors that bring an affected adolescent to a health care setting and interact with a variety of health care professionals. Early careful diagnosis and management can diminish the long-term morbidity of these illnesses, and offer the hope of a better outcome. Traditionally, personality disorders were thought to define a person and to be immutable. However, recognition of the patterns of behavior and awareness of their associated morbidities empowers a clinician to address elements of behavior that threaten the health of the adolescent and the successful transition to adulthood.

## REFERENCES

1. American Psychiatric Association. *Diagnostic and Statistical Manual of Mental Disorders*. 4th ed. Text revision. Washington, DC: American Psychiatric Association; 2000: 710

2. Skodol AE, Gunderson JG, McGlashan TH, et al. Functional impairment in patients with schizotypal, borderline, avoidant or obsessive compulsive personality disorder. *Am J Psychiatry.* 2002;159(2):276–283

3. Bernstein DP, Cohen P, Velez CN, Schwab-Stone M, Siever LJ, Shinsato L. Prevalence and stability of the DSM-III-R disorders in a community-based survey of adolescents. *Am J Psychiatry.* 1993;150:1237–1243

4. Becker DF, Grilo CM, Edell WS, McGlashan TH. Diagnostic efficiency of borderline personality disorder criteria in hospitalized adolescents: comparison with hospitalized adults. *Am J Psychiatry.* 2002;159 (12):2042–2047

5. Paris J. *Personality Disorders Over Time: Precursors, Course, and Outcome.* Arlington, VA: American Psychiatric Publishing; 2003

6. Geller B, Todd RD, Luby J, Botteron KN. Treatment resistant depression in children and adolescents. *Psychiatr Clin North Am.* 1996;19(2):253–267

7. Lofgren DP, Bemporad J, King J, Lindem K, O'Driscoll G. A prospective follow-up study of so-called borderline children. *Am J Psychiatry.* 1991;148(11):1541–1547

8. Links PS, Heslegrave R, van Reekum R. Prospective follow-up study of borderline personality disorder: prognosis, prediction of outcome, and axis II co-morbidity. *Can J Psychiatry.* 1998;43(3):265–270

9. Herman JL, Perry JC, Van Der Kolk BA. Childhood trauma in borderline personality disorder. *Am J Psychiatry*. 1989;146:490–495

10. Zanarini MC, Gunderson JG, Marino MF, Schwartz EO, Frankenburg FR. Childhood experiences of borderline patients. *Compr Psychiatry.* 1989;30:18–25

11. Paris J. Personality disorders over time: precursors, course, and outcome. *J Personal Disord.* 2003;17 (6):479–488

12. Paris J. Antisocial and borderline personality disorders: 2 separate diagnoses or 2 aspects of the same psychopathology? *Compr Psychiatry.* 1997;38(4):237–242

13. Reich DB, Zanarini MC. Developmental aspects of borderline personality disorder. *Harv Rev Psychiatry.* 2001;9(6): 294–301

14. Oldham JM, Skodol AE, Kellman HD, et al. Comorbidity of axis I and axis II disorders. *Am J Psychiatry.* 1995;152: 571–578

15. Zanarini MC, Frankenburg FR, Dubo ED, et al. Axis I comorbidity of borderline personality disorder. *Am J Psychiatry.* 1998;155(12):1733–1739

16. Gunderson JG. *Borderline Personality Disorder: A Clinical Guide.* Washington, DC: American Psychiatric Publishing, Inc; 2001

17. Akiskal HS, Chen SE, Davis GC, Puzantian VR, Kashgarian M, Bolinger JM. Borderline: an adjective in search of a noun. *J Clin Psychiatry.* 1985;46(2):41–48

18. Frankenburg FR, Zanarini MC. The association between borderline personality disorder and chronic medical illnesses, poor health-related lifestyle choices, and costly forms of health care utilization. *J Clin Psychiatry.* 2004;65:1660–1665

19. Bender DS, Dolan RT, Skodol AE, et al. Treatment utilization by patients with borderline personality disorder. *Am J Psychiatry.* 2001;158(2):295–302

20. Johnson JG, Cohen P, Skodol AE, Oldham JM, Kasen S, Brook JS. Personality disorders in adolescence and risk of major mental disorders and suicidality during adulthood. *Arch Gen Psychiatry.* 1999;56(9):805–811

21. Paris J, Zweig-Frank H. A 27-year follow-up of patients with borderline personality disorder. *Compr Psychiatry.* 2001;42:482–487

22. Rathus JH, Miller AL. Dialectical behaviour therapy adapted for suicidal adolescents. *Suicide Life Threat Behav.* 2002;32 (2):146–157

23. Katz LY, Cox BJ, Gunasekara S, Miller AL. Feasibility of dialectical behaviour therapy for suicidal adolescent inpatients. *J Am Acad Child Adolesc Psychiatry.* 2004;43 (3):276–282

24. Zanarini MC, Frankenburg FC, Hennen J, Silk KR. The longitudinal course of borderline psychopathology: 6-year prospective follow-up of the phenomenology of borderline personality disorder. *Am J Psychiatry.* 2003;160(2):274–283

25. Markham D, Trower P. The effects of the psychiatric label "borderline personality disorder" on nursing staff's perceptions and causal attributions for challenging behaviours. *Br J Clin Psychol.* 2003;42(pt 3):242–256

26. National Association for Personality Disorder Treatment and Research Advancements (TARA) Web site. Available at: www.tara4bpd.org/tara.html. Accessed July 28, 2009

27. Moran P. The epidemiology of antisocial personality disorder. *Soc Psychiatry Psychiatr Epidemiol.* 1999;34:231–242

28. Robins LN. *Deviant Children Grown Up.* Baltimore, MD: Williams & Wilkins; 1966

29. Robins LN. Antisocial personality. In: Robins LN, Regier DN eds. *Psychiatric Disorders in America: The Epidemiologic Catchment Area Study.* New York: MacMillan Free Press; 1991:255–280

30. Anderson CA, Hinshaw SP, Simmel C. Mother–child interactions in ADHD and comparison boys: relations with onset and covert externalizing behaviour. *J Abnorm Child Psychol.* 1994;22(2):247–265

31. Hsieh DK, Kirt SA. The effect of social context on psychiatrists' judgments of adolescent antisocial behaviour. *J Child Psychol Psychiatry.* 2003;44(6):877–887

32. Krueger RF, Caspi A, Moffitt TE, White J, Stouthamer-Loeber M. Delay of gratification, psychopathology, and personality: is low self-control specific to externalizing problems? *J Pers.* 1996;64:107–129

33. Frick PJ, Morris AS. Temperament and developmental pathways to conduct problems. *J Clin Child Adolesc Psychol.* 2004;33(1):54–68

34. Frick PJ, Lahey BB, Loeber R, et al. Oppositional defiant disorder and conduct disorder: a meta-analytic review of factor analyses and cross-validation in a clinical sample. *Clin Psychol Rev.* 1993;13:319–340

35. Lykken DT. *The Antisocial Personalities.* Hillsdale, NJ: Lawrence Erlbaum Associates, Inc; 1995

36. Biederman J, Newcorn J, Sprich S. Comorbidity of attention deficit hyperactivity disorder with conduct, depressive, anxiety, and other disorders. *Am J Psychiatry.* 1991;148:564–577

# CHAPTER 188

# Psychotic Disorders in Adolescents

CHRISTOPHER H. HODGMAN, MD

## OVERVIEW

Adolescents with psychosis display grossly impaired reality testing, including delusions, hallucinations, incoherent speech, and disorganized, often agitated, behavior. The term *psychosis* also refers to significant psychological dysfunction that renders an affected adolescent unable to meet everyday life demands.[1] Adolescents with a psychotic illness may not be readily recognizable as such because they may not actually be psychotic when they are seen in the office, clinic, or other settings. Psychotic illnesses include schizophrenia and its associated conditions, the affective disorders (psychotic depression, bipolar disorder), and delirium and substance use. Uncommon psychotic presentations without an apparent organic cause must also be considered, such as shared (conversion) psychosis, delusional disorder, and psychotic malingering. Early or prodromal presentations may be puzzling. In every case, it is essential to recognize that psychosis may be present and then to respond quickly for effective treatment and for the safety of the patient and those nearby. All of these conditions are generally first recognized in adolescence. This chapter addresses the initial assessment of psychosis in adolescents using the mental status examination, then describes the clinical presentations of various psychotic illnesses, and concludes with the management of patients with acute or chronic psychosis.

## INITIAL ASSESSMENT: THE ADOLESCENT MENTAL STATUS EXAMINATION

Although psychotic behaviors nearly always have organic components, these are not usually detectable in everyday adolescent health care practice. Accordingly, a mental status examination remains critical. Much of the mental status is revealed in the course of the complete interview and history-taking, but it begins with encountering the adolescent. The clinician may become aware of personally feeling anxious, puzzled, depressed, elated, or in some way different when interacting with a psychotic adolescent. Family members accompanying the patient should be present, at least for the start of the interview, to determine how the adolescent relates to them as well as to the health care provider. The general rules for the visit can then be clarified with everyone present, including an understanding of the purpose of the interview, as well as issues of confidentiality and acknowledging limits when safety is in question. The ease with which the patient separates from the family, and the family from the adolescent, can then be assessed. All of these elements help to define the mental status, which should include an assessment of the following:

1. **Appearance**—dress, grooming, posture, eye contact, overall comfort or discomfort. Note any dysmorphic features, scars, or bruises.
2. **Behavior**—motor activity (heightened or slowed), repetitive or stereotyped gestures or movements, degree of self-control.
3. **Relatedness**—ability to maintain eye contact, establish rapport, engage in appropriate conversation, with attention to how the clinician feels in this context.
4. **Communication**—quality of speech (monotonous, histrionic), volume, rate.
5. **Mood and affect**—both as displayed and in response to direct questions, range of responses, changes in mood or affect during the course of the interview.
6. **Thought**—both the process of thinking as expressed by the adolescent spontaneously and in response to questions, as well as its content (appropriate vs bizarre), including fantasies. Reality testing as assessed by the context of discussion and in response to questions including perceptual disturbances, such as hallucinations or delusions.
7. **Cognitive examination**—usually by content of interview, size and appropriateness of vocabulary, and accuracy of history as related by the patient.

## KEY FEATURES OF PSYCHOSIS

Certain elements are required for a formal diagnosis of psychosis. These include delusions, hallucinations, disorders of thought, and behavior. Each are detailed in the following.

**Delusions** are beliefs that strike the interviewer as false, odd, or unusual, without cultural or social support. Younger adolescents' delusions are often less detailed or fixed than those of older patients. Direct, supportive inquiry can be helpful. Delusions may be grandiose (unusual powers or skills); persecutory (being pursued, ridiculed, spied upon, or tricked); delusions of reference (eg, when gestures or comments on television are seen as directed specifically at the patient); religious (as distinguished from cultural beliefs); or somatic (bizarre physical complaints, often linked to other delusional features).

**Hallucinations** are sensory perceptions without objective environmental origin. They may be *auditory, visual, tactile, olfactory*, or *gustatory*. These can be explored with a question like, "Do your eyes or ears ever play tricks on you?" Hallucinating adolescents often appear preoccupied, with involuntary movements, especially of the eyes. Hallucinations are disconcerting and often frightening; patients are often reluctant to acknowledge them, and adolescents who readily refer to hallucinations are often dissimulating. Chronically psychotic adolescents and young adults often learn that concealing hallucinations is desirable.

**Thought disorder** can result in incoherent, illogical thinking, often disconcerting or puzzling to the interviewer. Adolescent thought disorder is often less fixed or explicable than in adults, particularly in younger patients.

**Behavior** may be agitated, disorganized, or inappropriate. If the interviewer is puzzled by behaviors apparently unrelated to circumstances or situation, the possibility of psychosis should be considered. Sympathetic, direct inquiry may reveal an underlying psychotic explanation.

## PSYCHOTIC ILLNESSES IN ADOLESCENTS

The adolescent psychotic illnesses include schizophrenia, bipolar disorder, major depressive disorder with psychotic features, psychotic disorders due to a general medical condition or induced by substances, and other psychotic presentations. These are discussed in detail in the following.

### SCHIZOPHRENIA

Schizophrenia is the most common cause of chronic psychosis in adolescents. The epidemiology and symptom presentation in the various subtypes of schizophrenia are important to recognize.

#### Epidemiology

Although the worldwide incidence of schizophrenia is about 1%, in developed countries, acute episodes seem to be seen less commonly than in the past, probably from early use of medication. Genetic factors are revealed by a higher concordance rate in monozygotic twins than in dizygotic twins,[2] but no single gene is apparently responsible.[3] Obstetrical factors[4] and maternal infection[5] also increase the incidence of psychosis in adolescents.[6] Social and psychological circumstances may alter the presentation.

Onset is often earlier in males (18–25 years of age) than in females, where estrogen seems to ameliorate symptoms.[7] Academic function often begins to decline months before the onset of overt symptoms, so school history may be significant. Social behavior often may have been less effective than that of the patient's siblings for years.

Brain pathology in schizophrenia includes gray matter loss even before treatment, as well as diminished prefrontal and thalamic blood flow on positive emission tomography (PET) scanning.[8] Such findings, for example as evidence of accelerated gray matter loss in early onset schizophrenia, confirm that schizophrenia is a brain disorder,[9–11] albeit often set off and shaped by psychological forces (Figure 188-1).

#### Symptoms

Symptoms of schizophrenia are dichotomized into positive and negative. Positive symptoms include delusions, hallucinations, disorganized speech (loosened associations, acceleration or slowing) and behavior (agitation, inappropriateness). Negative symptoms include flat or inappropriate affect, isolation, apathy, anhedonia (loss of pleasure), and lack of insight. Cognitive deterioration (precocious dementia, "dementia praecox") has long been identified and is increasingly viewed as central to the schizophrenias.[12] It may account for the academic decline often noted before overt symptoms. Features of the principal subtypes of schizophrenia with psychotic symptoms are listed in Table 188-1. Schizotypal, paranoid, and schizoid personality disorders do not present with psychosis.

### BIPOLAR DISORDER

Most bipolar disorder behavior is not psychotic, but severe (eg, classically paranoid) presentations may be indistinguishable from schizophrenia. More common, but less severe, psychotic episodes often include acceleration, euphoria, and irritability. The long-term treatment of bipolar disorders differs from that of schizophrenia.

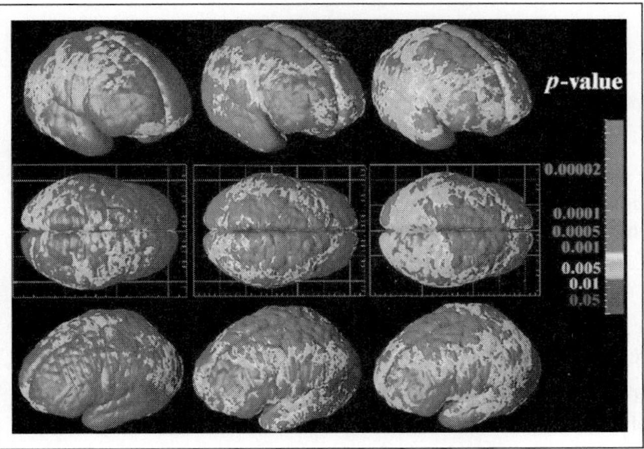


FIGURE 188-1 Compared to gray matter loss pattern in normal adolescents (left), adolescents with schizophrenia (right) experience progressive gray matter loss in the parietal, motor, supplementary motor, and superior frontal cortices, with broad regions of the temporal cortex, including the superior temporal gyrus most severely affected. (Reprinted with permission from Thompson PM, Vidal C, Giedd JN, et al. Mapping adolescent brain change reveals dynamic wave of accelerated gray matter loss in very early-onset schizophrenia. *Proc Nat Acad Sci USA*. 2001;98(20):11652. Copyright 2001 National Academy of Sciences, U.S.A.) (See color insert.)

**Table 188-1**

**Major Features of the Schizophrenias**

| *Type* | *Speech* | *Thinking* | *Actions* | *Cognition* | *Prognosis* |
|---|---|---|---|---|---|
| Paranoid | Clear, often forceful | Hallucinations (mostly auditory; delusional [paranoid]) | Sometimes violent, suicide-prone | Often largely preserved | Better than most other schizophrenias |
| Catatonic | Usually slurred, minimal; echolalia, echopraxia (parroting speech or actions) | Same, but less clear | Usually slowed, even rigid; uncommonly frenzied | Varies with motoric state | Highly variable |
| Disorganized (formerly "hebephrenic") | Quite fragmented, even silly | Same, but tangential ("poverty of thinking") | Erratic, impulsive | Most decline | Poor |
| Undifferentiated | Tangential | Delusions, hallucinations, often unclear | Erratic, sometimes violent | Varies with duration | Uncertain |
| Schizophreniform | Resembles paranoid | Resembles paranoid, but less fixed | Resembles paranoid | Brief, less severe | By definition, <6 months |
| Schizoaffective | Varies with mood; resembles bipolar disorder (see Table 188-2) | Varies with mood, paranoid features | Varies with mood, resembles bipolar disorder | Less decline | Better than schizophrenia, worse than bipolar disorder |
| Brief psychotic disorder | Fragmented | Fragmented | Erratic, ungoverned | Often drug effect | Brief (<30 days) |

American Psychiatric Association. *Diagnostic and Statistical Manual of Mental Disorders*, 4th ed, Text Revision. Washington, DC: American Psychiatric Association; 2000:297–298.

**Table 188-2**

**Major Features of Affective and Organic Psychoses**

| *Type* | *Speech* | *Thinking* | *Action* | *Other* |
|---|---|---|---|---|
| Bipolar manic | Accelerated, loud (can mimic schizophrenia) | Accelerated, "flight of ideas" (can mimic schizophrenia) | Impulsive, spendthrift, can be suicidal | Often depressed before, after, or mixed |
| Depressed | Low volume, slowed | Slowed, self-depreciative to a psychotic degree | Serious risk of suicide | Usually precedes first manic episode |
| Psychosis due to general medical condition | Variable, sometimes unpredictable | Hallucinations (often visual, tactile, olfactory, even gustatory); often delusional | Erratic; risk of suicide | Duration depends on medical condition |
| Substance-induced psychosis | Variable, sometimes unpredictable | (See general medical condition) | Erratic, risk of suicide | Usually briefer than brief psychotic disorder |

American Psychiatric Association. *Diagnostic and Statistical Manual of Mental Disorders*, 4th ed, Text Revision. Washington, DC: American Psychiatric Association; 2000:297–298.

Bipolar disorder generally shows less cognitive deterioration, but both conditions pose serious risks of suicidal behavior.

A family history of bipolar disorder is common and should always be diligently sought. It is often overlooked because all psychotic symptoms in the past tended to be called "schizophrenic"; thus an older relative's symptoms may be more revealing than the formal diagnosis. In bipolar disorder, premorbid cognitive and especially social functions tend to be less impaired than in schizophrenia. Onset of classical bipolar disorder can be seen prepubertally, but it is most common in late adolescence and early adulthood.

Biological findings in bipolar disorder occur in the ventral prefrontal cortex and its subcortical connection to the amygdala, striatum, and thalamus. Abnormalities in subcortical areas may be seen in early adolescence, but such ventral prefrontal cortex changes are often not detectable until late adolescence or early adulthood. This may explain the timing of onset of symptoms.[13,14] The common findings and differential features on mental status examination in bipolar and other psychoses are listed in Table 188-2.

## MAJOR DEPRESSIVE DISORDER WITH PSYCHOTIC FEATURES

Major depression in adolescents uncommonly presents with the psychotic symptoms characteristic of classical melancholia; even serious adolescent depression generally lacks these classical symptoms. Only rarely does the full panoply of melancholic grandiose self-abasement, motor retardation, weight loss, and early-morning awakening occur. Depression in adolescents often has atypical physical symptoms such as weight gain and excessive sleep. Psychotic symptoms are seen in up to 10% of adolescents hospitalized for depression.[15]

## PSYCHOTIC DISORDER DUE TO A GENERAL MEDICAL CONDITION

Psychosis related to a medical condition may be transient, but it does occur in adolescents and uncommonly may linger. The distinctive hallucinations are noted in Table 188-2. The presence of visual, tactile, olfactory, or gustatory hallucinations warrants careful assessment for biological causes, such as intoxication or trauma. The general medical conditions that can be associated with psychosis in adolescents are noted in Box 188-1.

## PSYCHOTIC DISORDERS INDUCED BY SUBSTANCES

Psychosis, whether affective or schizophrenic, is significantly comorbid with substance abuse.[16] Tobacco use is impressively frequent and intense in adolescents with schizophrenia, some of whose cognitive functions are altered by nicotine.[17] Psychotic youth often find cannabis and other compounds socially adaptive and normalizing. Psychosis may begin before substance use, or substances may be sought during the prodromal period

**Box 188-1**

***General Medical Conditions Causing Psychosis in Adolescents***

- Brain trauma, particularly left/frontal
- Neurologic disorders
  - Epilepsy, especially from temporal lobe sites, rarely as atypical status epilepticus
  - Central nervous system infections, both acute and in their sequelae
  - Neoplasms of many types, especially cortical
  - Multiple sclerosis (especially depressive manic psychoses)
  - Early-onset Huntington disease
  - Wilson disease (psychosis may precede choreoathetosis)
- Endocrine disorders
  - Thyroid (hypothyroid "myxedema madness," hyperthyroid toxicosis)
  - Adrenal (Addison, Cushing diseases)
  - Acute intermittent porphyria
  - Autoimmune disorders (eg, systemic lupus erythematosis)

before active psychotic symptoms emerge. Both the use of, and withdrawal from substances can precipitate psychotic episodes in adolescents. Accordingly, the care provider should always inquire about psychotic symptoms among adolescent substance users, and about substance use by schizophrenic and bipolar adolescents in whom substance use is too often overlooked.

Substance-induced psychosis, like other medical conditions, is more likely than schizophrenia to involve visual hallucinations, as well as a family history of substance use. Psychotic symptoms have been reported to occur in as many as 15% of marijuana users,[18] but are probably less frequent in casual use. The source and purity of the intoxicant may also be significant. Negative symptoms of schizophrenia and the "amotivational symptoms" of the chronic cannabis user may be difficult to differentiate; affective psychosis may be distinguishable from negative symptoms by the communicated mood.[19] Amphetamines, ecstasy (MDMA), and cocaine can elicit paranoid states and visual and tactile hallucinations.[20,21] Ephedrine psychosis has been reported[22] but should be seen less frequently with its recently restricted availability. In all cases, exclusion of the comorbidity of drug use and underlying psychosis can be difficult over the short term, but several days' stay in a safe, ordered environment, such as an adolescent psychiatric unit, generally clarifies the diagnosis.

In addition to illicit drugs, a variety of prescribed medications can induce psychosis. These include diuretics, anticholinergics, antihistamines, antibiotics (especially quinolones),[23] chemotherapeutic agents, and corticosteroids.[24] Inhalants and other toxic agents can also cause psychosis.[25] Most such episodes are of limited duration (see Table 188-2).

#### OTHER PSYCHOTIC PRESENTATIONS

Other conditions that may present with psychotic features include shared psychosis, delusional disorders, delirium, and psychotic malingering. Although uncommon, they may be seen in adolescent patients.

**Shared psychosis** (*folie à deux*, even *folie à famille*) is an uncommon condition in which a passive, dependent person, often younger, shares a delusional system with a dominant psychotic patient, often a parent, in the case of adolescents. Separation of the 2 often results in improvement in the dependent patient, in whom the psychosis can be seen as a form of conversion disorder.[26]

**Delusional disorder** in adolescents is most commonly seen as body dysmorphic disorder, in which minor, even invisible, "defects" become the focus of utter preoccupation.[27] Anorexia nervosa involves eating behaviors and distortions of body image, often to a psychotic degree. In both conditions, patients often cannot be convinced of the inappropriateness of their perceptions.

**Delirium** may induce agitation delusions, hallucinations, and speech disturbance, frequently accompanied by significant cognitive impairment. Abnormalities in the brain of people with delirium are often revealed on electroencephalogram, which is not the case for most psychosis. Other physical findings and history usually are diagnostic.

**Psychotic malingering** is uncommon, except in the occasional youth who feigns hallucinosis in hopes of hospitalization in lieu of some other less desirable placement.[28] As noted previously, the truly psychotic patient mentions hallucinations uncommonly, because they are quite disconcerting and disquieting.

### MANAGEMENT OF ADOLESCENTS WITH PSYCHOSIS IN PRIMARY CARE SETTINGS

Different management strategies are employed in acute, compared to chronic, psychotic conditions in adolescents. The highlights of each are discussed in the following.

#### ACUTE PSYCHOSIS

Acutely psychotic behavior constitutes an emergency (see Chapter 189, Psychiatric Emergencies in Adolescents).

Safety for the patient and for those in the environment, including health care providers, is the first priority. It is desirable and often essential to:

- Ensure that there are enough staff in a secure setting. Treating a disturbed or violent adolescent may heighten the anxiety of everyone if professional personnel do not feel calm and safe. Most acutely psychotic patients are quite aware that they are in difficulty. An unfamiliar setting and insufficient help are likely to make them feel all the more vulnerable and upset.
- Remove the acutely upset patient from a disruptive environment, if necessary by ambulance, to prevent running away and to ensure safety.
- Provide staff of both genders to allay potential sexual panic.
- Ensure that appropriate pharmaceuticals are always readily available for emergencies in the pediatric office or clinic (see Chapter 190, Adolescent Psychopharmacology).
- Restrain by medication, rather than physically, if possible. Physical restraints can provoke fear and vulnerability, but if medication does not suffice, physical restraints can be calming and reassuring if accompanied by a clear explanation and instructions to the patient.
- Limit the number of staff involved once violent behavior is controlled, to minimize disorientation and consequent anxiety. To prevent elopement, both 1-to-1 staffing and a locked door may be essential.
- Clarify the etiology of the acute episode as the immediate distress is allayed. A careful history often reveals difficulties long before the crisis, and detailed family history may be of immediate value. Ideally, continuity between acute management and ongoing care can improve the ultimate outcome.

## CHRONIC PSYCHOSIS

Chronic conditions can be conveniently divided into prodromal, subacute, and truly chronic psychotic illnesses. Prodromal states are of increasing interest because it is still unclear whether early identification and treatment can prevent decompensation.

**Prodromal schizophrenia** has been identified retrospectively in young children by reviewing childhood family movies, but clinically it often becomes apparent from 2 to 6 years before obvious psychosis.[29] Symptoms include diminished attention and concentration, with resultant academic difficulties; social ineffectiveness and withdrawal; and anxiety, depression, irritability, and sleep problems. Engaging patients and parents at this time can be daunting, but early evaluation and intervention may forestall and possibly prevent deterioration.[30] Early treatment is more likely if the adolescent and family have sufficient confidence in the primary care provider. Also, timely intervention may lessen the academic, familial, and social stressors often implicated in the decompensation of acute schizophrenia. There is evidence that atypical antipsychotics can diminish or prevent loss of gray matter volume over time.[31] This could favor early use of antipsychotics in prodromal patients.

**Prodromal bipolar disorder** is less well studied. It has long been known that bipolar patients often realize that they have had affective swings for years before bipolar illness declares itself. There seems to be some, but less, cognitive deterioration and social damage from incipient bipolar disorder than from prodromal schizophrenia, but studies are only preliminary.

**Subacute psychosis**, whether of schizophrenic or bipolar origin, dictates immediate treatment in hopes of preventing serious decompensation. Psychotropic medications (atypical antipsychotics for probable schizophrenia or mood stabilizers for potential bipolar illness), as well as evaluation of stressors in the adolescent, the family, and the environment, may be useful in subacute psychosis. At this stage, uncovering potential problems may be easier than after decompensation occurs.

**Chronic psychosis** in adolescents may go untreated because the environment has not, for some reason, identified the problem. Usually hospitalization is not required. Such conditions may only emerge in the course of treatment for a serious medical or surgical condition. In such cases it is best, if possible, to manage such patients on the medical or surgical service with appropriate psychiatric support because they can usually accept illness as a physical reality. Psychotropic medications may be indicated, and effective ongoing care of the psychosis can thus be initiated.

## SUBTLE PSYCHOTIC STATES

Alert observers may note subtle disturbances suggestive of psychosis that should not be dismissed as normal adolescent behavior. These may constitute prodromal illness, or may stem from one of the personality disorders, or may be examples of pervasive developmental disorder in the autism spectrum. Usually any psychotic content is minor or sequestered. If academic and social functions are not seriously compromised, "watchful waiting" may suffice. Psychological testing may be valuable if school performance is diminished, with possible academic interventions as suggested by the testing; and socialization techniques, particularly through group activities, may be helpful. Occasionally, psychotropic medication is useful because patients can identify diminished stress when taking them. Because these are likely to be lifelong conditions, however, the desirability of introducing long-term medication must be weighed carefully.

## SUMMARY

Psychotic behavior in adolescence is uncommon, but it is likely to emerge in any busy pediatric practice. Precise diagnosis is less important initially than assuring safety and early treatment, with referral to an experienced mental health specialist once that has occurred. The primary care provider should offer active, continued support after such referral to ensure effective adherence and to maintain continuity of care.

## REFERENCES

1. American Psychiatric Association. *Diagnostic and Statistical Manual of Mental Disorders,* 4th ed, Text Revision. Washington, DC: American Psychiatric Association; 2000:297–298

2. Sullivan PH, Kendler K, Neale MC. Schizophrenia as a complex trait: evidence from a meta-analysis of twin studies. *Arch Gen Psychiatry.* 2003;60(12):1187–1192

3. McClellan JM, Susser E, King MC. Schizophrenia: a common disease caused by multiple rare alleles. *Brit J Psychiatry.* 2007;190(3):194–199

4. Ballon AS, Dean KA. Obstetrical complications in people at risk for developing schizophrenia. *Schizophrenia Research.* 2008;98(1-3):307–311

5. Brown AS, Begg MD, Gravenstein S, et al. Serological evidence of prenatal influenza in the etiology of schizophrenia. *Arch Gen Psychiatry.* 2004;61(8):774–780

6. Brown AS, Schaefer CA, Quesenberry CF, Liu L, Babulus VP, Susser ES. Maternal exposure to toxoplasmosis and risk of schizophrenia in adult offspring. *Amer J Psychiatry.* 2005;162(4):767–773

7. Rao ML, Kolsch H. Effects of estrogen on brain development and neuroprotection—implications for negative symptoms in schizophrenia. *Psychoneuroendocrinology.* 2003;28(S2): 83–96

8. Lehrer DS, Christian BT, Mantil J, et al. Thalamic and prefrontal FDG uptake in never-medicated patients with schizophrenia. *Amer J Psychiatry.* 2005;162(5):931–938

9. Thompson TM, Vidaal C, Giedd JN, et al. Mapping adolescent brain change reveals dynamic wave of accelerated gray matter loss in very early-onset schizophrenia. *Proc Nat Acad Sci USA.* 2001;98(20):11652

10. Ho BC, Alicata D, Ward J, et al. Untreated initial psychosis: relation to cognitive deficits and brain morphology in first-episode schizophrenia. *Amer J Psychiatry.* 2003;160(1):14214–14218

11. Arango C, Moreno C, Martinez S, et al. Longitudinal brain changes in early-onset psychosis. *Schizophrenia Bulletin.* 2008;34(2):341–353

12. Heinrichs RW. The primacy of cognition in schizophrenia. *Amer Psychologist.* 2005;60(3):229–242

13. Blumberg HP, Kaufman J, Martin A, Charney DS, Krystal JH, Peterson BS. Significance of adolescent neurodevelopment for the neural circuitry of bipolar disorder. *Ann NY Acad Sciences.* 2004;1021:376–383

14. Doty TJ, Payne ME, Steffens DC, Bever JL, Krishnan KR, LaBar KS. Age-dependent reduction of amygdala volume in bipolar disorder. *Psychiatry Res.* 2008;163(1):84–94

15. Quinlan PE, King CA, Hanna GL, Ghaziuddin N. Psychotic versus nonpsychotic depression in hospitalized adolescents. *Depression and Anxiety.* 1997;6(1):40–42

16. Cayton CL, Drake RE, Hasin DS, et al. Differences between early-phase primary psychotic disorders with substance abuse and substance-induced psychosis. *Arch Gen Psychiatry.* 2005;62(2):137–145

17. Sacco KA, Termine A, Segal A, et al. Effect of cigarette smoking on spatial working memory and attentional deficits in schizophrenia: involvement of nicotine receptor mechanisms. *Arch Gen Psychiatry.* 2005;62(6):649–659

18. Miettunen J, Tormanen S, Murray GK, et al. Association of cannabis use with prodromal symptoms of psychosis in adolescence. *Brit J Psychiatry.* 2008;192(6):470–471

19. Rey JM, Martin A, Krabman P. Is the party over? Cannabis and juvenile psychiatric disorder: the past 10 years. *J Amer Child and Adol Psychiatry.* 2004;43(10):1194–1205

20. Chen CK, Lin SK, Sham PC, et al. Premorbid characteristics and co-morbidity of methamphetamine users with and without psychosis. *Psychological Med.* 2003;33(8):1407–1414

21. Williamson S, Gossop M, Powis B, Griffiths P, Fountain J, Strang J. Adverse effects of stimulant drugs in a community sample of drug users. *Drug Alcohol Depend.* 1997;44(2–3): 87–94

22. Maglione M, Miotto K, Iguchi M, Jungvig L, Morton SC, Shekelle PG. Psychiatric effects of ephedrine use: an analysis of food and drug administration reports of adverse events. *Amer J Psychiatry.* 2005;162(1):189–191

23. Mulhall JP, Bergman LS. Ciprofloxacin-induced acute psychosis. *Urology.* 1995;46(1):102–103

24. Stuart FA, Segal TY, Keady S. Adverse psychological effects of corticosteroids in children and adolescents. *Arch Dis Childhood.* 2005;90(5):500–506

25. Wu L-T, Pilowsky DJ, Schlenger WE. Inhalant abuse and dependence among adolescents in the United States. *J Amer Acad Child Adol Psychiatry.* 2004;43(10):1206–1214

26. Wehmeier PM, Barth IV, Remschmidt H. Induced delusional disorder: a review of the concept and an unusual case of folie à famille. *Psychopathology.* 2003;36(1):37–45

27. Philips KA. Psychosis in body dysmorphic disorder. *J Psychiatric Research.* 2004;38(1):63–72

28. Penn JV, Thomas C. Practice parameter for the assessment and treatment of youth in juvenile detention and correctional facilities. *J Amer Acad Child Adol Psychiatry.* 2005; 44(10):1085-1098

29. Hafner H, Loeffler W, Maurer K, Hambrecht M, an der Heiden W. Depression, negative symptoms, social stagnation, and social decline in the early course of schizophrenia. *Acta Psychiatrica Scandinavia.* 1999;100(2):105-118

30. McGorry PD, Young AF, Phillips LJ, et al. Randomized controlled trial of interventions designed to reduce the progression to first-episode psychosis in a clinical sample with sub-threshold symptoms. *Arch Gen Psych*iatry. 2002;59(10):921-928

31. Lieberman JA, Tollefson GD, Charles C, et al. Antipsychotic drug effects on brain morphology in first-episode psychosis. *Arch Gen Psy*chiatry. 2005;62(4): 361-370

# CHAPTER 189

## Psychiatric Emergencies in Adolescents

GAIL A. EDELSOHN, MD, MSPH • JOHN-PAUL GOMEZ, MD

### INTRODUCTION

Only 1 in 5 of the 10% of adolescents having a mental illness associated with functional impairment receive the mental health treatment that they need.[1] The dearth of child and adolescent psychiatrists available in the United States (fewer than 7,000) means that a significant proportion of even the most severely ill adolescents will not have access to a trained specialist.[2] Therefore, medical triage is needed to obtain a rapid assessment of the condition of the patient to prioritize treatment to the most ill before meeting the needs of patients who are more stable.

Because of the high proportion of affected youth who receive no mental health services, increasing demands are being placed on primary care physicians and hospital emergency departments (EDs) to manage a variety of urgent and nonurgent pediatric mental health problems. Page[3] noted a 59% increase in pediatric psychiatric visits to a children's hospital ED between 1995 and 1999. At a national level, a study of the National Hospital Ambulatory Medical Care Survey examining pediatric mental health visits to the ED from 1993 to 1996 found an annual average rate of 326.8 visits/10,000 youth.[4] Mental health visits accounted for 1.6% of all ED visits for those younger than 18 years of age. Of note, 71% of mental health visits were for adolescents; 67.2% of the visits were classified as "urgent." Almost 20% of these visits resulted in admission to a hospital, with nearly 9% being admitted from the ED directly to an intensive care unit.

However, the increase in ED mental health visits during those 4 years cannot be attributed to suicide attempts or psychosis, as the rates of those conditions were unchanged. The data suggest that the overall increase in ED visits reflect non life-threatening problems, which in turn may be related to inadequate access to primary mental health care services that might otherwise avert such crises. Identifying a psychiatric emergency is based not only on the behavior itself, but also on the resources and demands of the family and the local human services available.

One study conducted in a busy urban psychiatric emergency service found that 40% of the visits were for nonurgent reasons.[5] The authors developed a tool to quickly classify adolescent psychiatric emergencies based on Rosenn's[6] 4 part classification of urgency: (1) potentially life-threatening emergencies; (2) urgent but not life-threatening disturbances; (3) serious situations requiring prompt but not immediate intervention; and (4) nonurgent situations deemed by someone as an emergency. An adolescent with new onset psychosis accompanied by command hallucinations telling him or her to jump out of a window would fall into Class I, whereas an adolescent with a history of schizophrenia who has been stable and ran out of medication because of failure to keep appointments would be in Class 4.

Application of such a triage framework can mitigate the frustration of treating nonurgent cases in the ED. The triage tool developed by Edelsohn[7] can be used to efficiently prioritize patients and quickly identify when case management services are needed. Based on the categorization, a medical or mental health provider in the ED may request psychiatric consultation only for adolescents falling into Classes I or II, whereas those falling into Class III or IV may be referred for linkage with and follow-up by a nurse practitioner, social worker, or other appropriate provider.

This chapter presents a practical review of the epidemiology, risk/protective factors, issues in assessment, and treatment options of common emergencies in the 4 classes of urgency. It is not designed to be an exhaustive review of the complexities of psychiatric diagnosis and treatment; rather, it may serve as guide for the physician caring for an adolescent in a psychiatric emergency, either in a hospital ED or other community setting. Essential legal considerations in conducting emergency evaluations are discussed at the end of the chapter.

### CLASS I: POTENTIALLY LIFE-THREATENING, WITH IMMEDIATE RISK TO THE ADOLESCENT

#### 1. SUICIDALITY

Suicide is a major public health concern in adolescents. In 2004, it was the third-leading cause of death in 10- to 24-year-olds and accounted for 4,559 deaths.[8] In some suburban populations where homicide is less common, it is often the second-leading cause of death. Although suicidal ideation is common, risk assessment for suicide is imperfect and predicting repeat attempts is difficult. In the United States, more than 70% of deaths among 10- to 24-year-olds are attributable to 4 causes: motor vehicle crashes (32.3%), homicide (15.1%), suicide (11.7%), and unintentional injuries (11.7%).[9] In the United States, roughly 2,000 adolescents die of suicide each year.[10] Suicidal teens may be labeled as "attention-getters" or "acting-out" by parents, foster parents, or child protective workers, and clinical staff may have negative attitudes toward suicidal patients.[11] Nonetheless, "suicidal gestures" by teens who may not appreciate their true risk, or who may view themselves as invincible, can prove fatal. Decisions regarding hospital admission or discharge must be tempered by the high rate of missed outpatient appointments by suicidal adolescents.[12,13]

Assessment of the suicidal adolescent requires that both the adolescent and his or her guardian be interviewed separately. In addition, multiple informants should be sought that may include school personnel, individuals close to the patient, and current mental health providers. For suicidal ideation, the physician must, at a minimum, explore the following: (1) frequency (how often do you think of hurting yourself?), (2) intensity (how strong are these thoughts? What makes them better? What makes them worse?), (3) duration (When did you first start to have these thoughts?), and (4) specificity of suicidal plan (How and when would you do it?). This is similar to the evaluation of physical pain, now considered an essential "fifth vital sign" in outpatient encounters, only the domain is emotional, rather than somatic, pain.

### History

For those who have attempted suicide, a detailed history of the events preceding and following the suicidal behavior is critical.[13] Information gathered reflects the previously noted risk factors, including symptoms of mood disorder (depression and bipolar disorder, with special emphasis on mania or hypomania), substance abuse, impulsive behavior, a wish to die or influence others, and the presence of contagion. Coping skills and family supports should be evaluated. Lethality is not synonymous with intention. Lethality refers to a measure of how likely death might occur, based on the relevant details of the event, such as method, location, and likelihood of being discovered. Adolescents are known to both overestimate and underestimate the lethality of the attempt. Suicidal intention, on the other hand, refers to the adolescent's expected outcome of the attempt. Questions related to: (1) expected outcome (Did you expect to die after the overdose?), (2) reversibility (Could you do something to undo the attempt?), and (3) ambivalence about living (Do the reasons for living outweigh the reasons for dying? Did you care whether you lived or died after the attempt?) can probe intent. The adolescent's intention is important, because it is related to the belief of repeat attempters that death will be a likely, or desired, outcome, regardless of medical lethality.

### Mental Status Examination

The mental status examination of the suicidal adolescent should address: (1) depression and feelings of hopelessness or helplessness, (2) perceptions that the adolescent would be better off dead, (3) disappointment regarding being found or rescued before death, (4) any wish to join a dead relative or friend, (5) any suicidal "pact" that might have been made with a friend, (6) belief that death might be transient or pleasant, (7) psychosis, (8) presence of intoxication at the time of the incident or the evaluation, and (9) willingness to notify some responsible adult if suicidal urges return. The clinical interview must be tailored to the individual adolescent and his or her environment. When determining disposition for a suicidal adolescent and whether to hospitalize the patient or not, safety is always the first consideration. The mental status examination, the details surrounding the suicide attempt, and the environment (stressors and supports), along with history of individual risk factors guide the decision when to hospitalize.

### Hospitalization

Several factors should be taken into account when considering hospitalization for a suicidal adolescent: (1) medical or surgical necessity to treat complications of the attempt, (2) abnormal mental state (acute depression or acute psychosis), (3) persistent wish to die, (4) highly lethal, unusual, or painful method, (5) family history of suicide, (6) male gender, (7) prior suicide attempts, (8) active substance or alcohol abuse, and (9) inadequate supervision at home or unresponsive family to suicidal behavior. The presence of any 1 of the first 4 factors is an indication for inpatient treatment. Although no single other factor is an indicator for hospitalization, as more factors accumulate, hospitalization is increasingly justified. Despite the clinical rationale for hospitalization, there are no controlled studies demonstrating that hospitalization is effective in preventing subsequent attempted or completed suicide.[11,13]

### Follow-Up

Adolescents are at risk of another suicide attempt in the days and weeks after discharge from the ED following suicidal behavior. There are limited follow-up studies, with rates of subsequent attempts about 10% at 3 months, and between 6% and 14% a year after discharge. If the decision is made not to hospitalize a suicidal teen, the following 3 conditions should be met: (1) an outpatient follow-up visit is scheduled with a provider within a few days (ideally with a mental health provider, but possibly with the primary care provider), (2) the residence where the adolescent will be living is "sanitized" (remove or lock firearms securely, with ammunition stored and locked separately, and keys for both kept in a secure hiding place; lock away any potentially lethal medications; and lock away knives or other potential weapons), and (3) contract for safety is agreed on (patient promises to contact a trusted adult who can help if she or he begins to think about hurting her or himself). Although there is no evidence that a safety contract prevents subsequent suicide, it remains a standard of practice because clinical experience suggests that it opens discussion about how the patient might respond in the future ("What would you do differently?") and provides teens and caretakers a way of having their concerns heard.[10] Some clinicians would reconsider a decision to discharge if the adolescent cannot contract for safety. A disturbing finding following discharge from the ED is the high rate of not having any mental health follow-up treatment. Between 16% and 59% of suicidal adolescent inpatients receive no aftercare, similar to that for suicidal outpatients discharged from the ED (18%–42%).[11] Enhancing outpatient follow-up is improved if the adolescent is given a specific time, location, and name of a provider for the appointment, and if there is follow-up contact after discharge but before the initial outpatient visit.

## 2. SELF-DESTRUCTIVE ACTS

Self-destrutive acts include failure to take necessary medications (such as insulin for adolescents with diabetes, or bronchodilators for asthma) or self-induced starvation for those with anorexia nervosa. Adolescent patients who seriously jeopardize their physical well-being by nonadherence with medical interventions may require acute hospitalization on a pediatric unit with consultation from child and adolescent psychiatry. Anorexia nervosa and bulimia nervosa have been estimated to occur in approximately 1% and 3% of adolescent females, respectively, and the prevalence in men has been estimated to be only one-tenth of that in women.[14]

Patients with anorexia nervosa tend to deny that their behaviors are self-destructive despite significant symptoms. This denial is central to the maintenance of the disorder, but also may be related to the abnormal metabolic and cognitive states associated with weight loss. In this case, the capacity of the patient to consent to or refuse treatment may need to be considered. Most adolescents with bulimia freely admit that their compulsive behaviors are self-destructive and ego-dystonic, but feel powerless to control the binge eating, vomiting, and laxative abuse.[15] Another self-destructive behavior exhibited by adolescents with bulimia nervosa is cutting or other self-injurious behaviors. These may be performed to inflict punishment, to feel pain rather than emotional numbness, or to dissociate from emotional "flooding" commonly associated with posttraumatic stress disorder (PTSD). It is important to evaluate the intent of the self-destructive act in the context of the presence of other psychiatric disorders that may increase the risk for suicide, their judgment, and availability/adequacy of adult supervision.

Adolescents with an eating disorder may present to the ED needing medical clearance for admission to an eating disorder unit, or with a variety of acute medical symptoms. Regardless of their reason for presentation, they should be evaluated for comorbid psychiatric conditions such as anxiety disorders, mood disorders (major depression and bipolar disorder), substance abuse disorder, and cognitive deficits. Admission to an inpatient medical unit should be considered if the patient has a weight of less than 75% of average for sex, age, and height; periods of hypoglycemia; syncope; severe dehydration or electrolyte abnormalities; cardiac dysrhythmias or hypotension; or small bowel obstruction due to superior mesenteric artery syndrome.[16] If a patient with an eating disorder is hospitalized, it should be for a specific, achievable indication, preferably on a unit where the staff is familiar with the inpatient treatment of eating disorders.

## 3. PHYSICAL ABUSE OR SEVERE NEGLECT

In 2006, there were 753,357 reported cases of child abuse in the United States. Abused 12- to 17-year-olds have a fatality rate of 6%.[17] Signs and symptoms of physical abuse that should elicit further exploration include an adolescent with: unexplained burns, bites, bruises, broken bones, or black eyes; lesions at different stages of healing; fading marks after an absence from school; unexplained fear of a guardian; resistance to return home; or a report of injury by a caregiver. Signs of neglect include frequent school absences, begging or stealing food or money, lack of routine medical care, chronically dirty, inappropriate dress for the weather, drug or alcohol abuse, and adolescent complaints of no adult caretaker at home. Emotional abuse frequently goes unrecognized. Combinations of physical, sexual, emotional abuse, and neglect are common. The goal of evaluating an adolescent with suspected abuse is to ensure safety and prevent repeated abuse. Physically traumatized patients may require hospitalization, but if safety cannot be ensured, psychiatric admission may be indicated. If the youth is psychiatrically stable, alternative placement such as with relatives or placement through child protective services (CPS) should be arranged.

## 4. DELIRIUM AND OTHER ACUTE CONFUSIONAL STATES

The fourth Class I group of adolescents includes those who experience an acute state of confusion, with a change in mental status, delirium, acute intoxication, or acute psychosis with inability to maintain safety. Younger patients may be especially vulnerable to toxins, and to metabolic, infectious, and traumatic effects on their central nervous system (CNS), and developmental difficulties in communication and cognition may place the younger patient at a higher risk of having his or her altered mental status unrecognized. However, most data regarding delirium are derived from adults.

Delirium is a neuropsychiatric disorder characterized by global cortical dysfunction that is attributable to a variety of medical or surgical causes. Delirium includes 4 features: (1) disturbance in consciousness with reduced clarity of awareness of the environment and reduced ability to focus, sustain, or shift attention, (2) change in cognition, such as memory deficit, disorientation, language disturbance, or the development of a perceptual disturbance that is not better accounted for by a pre-existing, established, or evolving dementia, (3) the disturbance develops over hours to days and fluctuates during the course of the day, and (4) the disturbance being caused by the direct physiologic consequences of a general medical condition.[15]

The first step in recognizing delirium is to suspect it from history. Diagnosing delirium can be challenging because youth may present with either a hypoactive or hyperactive state, further complicated by fluctuating periods of confusion and lucidity. In addition to fluctuating awareness, there frequently are associated changes in anxiety or activity (sleepiness) that may include attempts to pull out an IV or a catheter or to become combative. Multiple examinations are needed to observe these changes over time. A thorough history, including recent medication changes, should be carefully scrutinized for potential causes of delirium.[18]

### Mental Status Examination in Adolescents Experiencing Acute Confusional States

The mental status examination should assess the appearance, level of consciousness, activity, attitude, thought process and content, speech, attention, orientation, memory, and mood. If the patient has impaired consciousness, the adolescent requires a thorough neurologic examination including (1) pupil reactivity; (2) extraocular movements; (3) nuchal rigidity; (4) muscle tone, strength, coordination, and gait (if possible); (5) deep tendon reflexes, Babinski reflexes, asterixis, and (6) temperature and vibratory, and position senses. Frontal release signs include snout, grasp, glabelar, and palmomental reflexes. If the patient is awake and responsive, test the patient's attention with digit span forward and backward (5-7 is normal), identifying the letters of the alphabet that rhyme with "tree," or listing the months of the year backward. The ability to write is a sensitive indicator of impaired consciousness.[19] Drawing a clock face is another commonly used task that can be helpful in assessing the adolescent's executive function.

### Laboratory Tests, Imaging, and Electroencephalography in the Diagnosis of Adolescents Experiencing Acute Confusional States

Laboratory blood tests commonly ordered for acute changes in mental status include: (1) electrolytes, (2) glucose, (3) blood urea nitrogen and creatinine, (4) calcium and magnesium, (5) complete blood count, (6) urinalysis and urine toxicology screen, (7) alcohol and prescription drug levels, and (8) liver function tests. Other lab tests that may aid in the diagnosis based on findings from the history and physical examination might include: thyroid function tests, blood lead, ammonia, or ceruloplasmin levels, arterial blood gas, blood and urine cultures, lumbar puncture, syphilis screening tests, erythrocyte sedimentation rate, antinuclear antibody test, cortisol, vitamin $B_{12}$/folate, and heavy metal and HIV screening. Computed tomography (CT) scans of the brain are commonly ordered to rule out a mass lesion, subdural hematoma, intracerebral hemorrhage, and hydrocephalus. The electroencephalogram (EEG) in delirium is commonly abnormal and can be useful in the diagnosis of certain metabolic encephalopathies as well as seizure disorders. A normal EEG does not completely rule out seizure as a cause because the deeper limbic structures may not be captured on a surface EEG.

### Toxidromes Associated with Acute Confusional States in Adolescents

Younger patients may be less able to report hallucinations and delusions.[20] There are several toxidromes—syndromes associated with medication-induced delirium—that deserve mention. *Anticholinergic* delirium classically presents with confusion, hallucinations, dry and red skin, tachycardia, mydriasis, inactive bowel sounds, and urinary retention ("red as a beet, dry as a bone, blind as a bat, and mad as a hatter"). *Cholinergic* excess presents with excessive salivation, lacrimation, urination, defecation, gastrointestinal activity and emesis (resulting in the mnemonic SLUDGEing). *Adrenergic* excess is marked by hyperthermia, diaphoresis, and tachycardia. *Opioid* intoxication presents with CNS depression, pinpoint pupils, bradypnea, and possible hypotension. *Extrapyramidal* presentations include cogwheel rigidity, torticollis, bradykinesia, oculogyric crisis, opisthotonos, trismus, dysphonia, akathesia, and laryngospasm. Cassem and colleagues[21] hypothesize that the increased release of endogenous dopamine during surgery and the decrease in endogenous acetylcholine may be responsible for the clinical manifestations of delirium.

### Treatment of Delirium

The treatment of delirium begins with the removal, supplementation, or correction of the offending agent or state. Educating the family and staff about the diagnosis and implementing procedures to limit stimulation, provide frequent reorientation, and limit disruptions of sleep can be helpful in lessening the intensity of the confusional state. Haloperidol is considered the treatment of choice for the acute management of delirium that is not caused by alcohol withdrawal or seizure (for which a benzodiazepine is more effective). It has minimal effects on blood pressure, pulmonary artery pressure, heart rate, and respiration and does not have clinically significant anticholinergic properties. The goal is to have the adolescent remain calm, but arousable. The starting dose of haloperidol is 1 to 2 mg by mouth or 0.5 to 1.0 mg IV, but should be titrated based on clinical response. One should routinely check for extrapyramidal side effects, which can be treated with benztropine mesylate, and also follow the magnesium, potassium, and corrected QT interval when using haloperidol. Physostigmine has been used to correct anticholinergic delirium and is usually given in doses of 0.5 mg to 2 mg IV. It should be used cautiously because it can cause profound bradycardia and hypotension.

### 5. RUNAWAY BEHAVIOR

Chronic runaway behavior in the face of longstanding behavioral problems is excluded as Class I and may be more appropriately considered as Class III or IV depending on the specifics leading to the presentation. However, runaway behavior becomes as Class I emergency with threats of, or actual abuse, or when the patient is very young, immature, or has developmental delay. A cause of adolescent females running away is sexual abuse; likewise, runaway males and females are at increased risk of sexual misuse when living on the streets.

## CLASS I: POTENTIALLY LIFE-THREATENING WITH IMMEDIATE RISK TO OTHERS

The fundamentals of emergency psychiatric interventions include: (1) ensuring safety of the patient, family, and staff, (2) excluding medical and substance-related conditions before making a psychiatric diagnosis, (3) stabilizing the presenting condition, and (4) facilitating the appropriate disposition for the necessary level of continued care. The first step of the assessment is to decide if the adolescent is out of control. Clinicians are encouraged to trust their intuition and clinical judgment and consider the circumstances of the adolescent's presentation (eg, victim of violence, pervasive developmental disorder, availability of a family member). Inquiring about pain or offering something to eat or drink may transform a situation from confrontational to therapeutic. This can be especially important when treating a trauma victim who requires restraints, because the administration of intramuscular medications may retraumatize the patient. The ED may be an adolescent's first interaction with mental health services; steps to reassure and assist in coping may improve adherence to future treatment recommendations.

When a patient with a profound developmental disorder presents with agitation, a thorough search for physical causes, such as a tooth abscess or otitis media, is indicated because physical discomfort commonly leads to agitation in this population. A family member can often assist the patient in calming down. The Treatment Recommendations for the use of Antipsychotics for Aggressive Youth (TRAAY) includes adding an orally disintegrating atypical antipsychotic (eg, risperidone or olanzapine, 0.5 to 1.0 mg or 2.5 to 5 mg, respectively).[22] If the patient is agitated or out of control, medications should be used to keep everyone, including the adolescent patient and staff, safe. Depending on the size of the patient, haloperidol 2.5 to 5 mg IM with 1 to 2 mg of lorazepam IM can be given to ensure the safety of the adolescent and those in the immediate environment. This combination regimen should be followed by close monitoring both to assess the therapeutic response and to recognize the emergence of extrapyramidal side effects. Benztropine 1 to 2 mg IM or diphenhydramine 25 to 50 mg IV or IM may be used to treat extrapyramidal side effects. The atypical antipsychotics ziprasidone and olanzapine have recently become available in IM formulations and have been used in open trials with small numbers of patients. The atypical antipsychotics have a lower incidence of extrapyramidal side effects and may become more widely used with adolescent patients.

A clinician should approach the agitated patient cautiously and have assistance available. The door of the examination room should be kept open and the clinician should be positioned between the patient and the door, close enough to it to allow for a quick exit, if needed. Lights and sounds should be kept low, sometimes a difficult challenge in a busy ED or clinic. Such caution should not preclude demonstration of a respectful, calm, and confident attitude, however, toward the adolescent. Prolonged direct eye contact with an agitated adolescent may be interpreted as threatening and should be avoided. Speech should be slow and include an explanation of the clinician's role in helping the patient feel better and describe all actions that will occur. Once the patient is more in control, the assessment can be completed, including history and review of symptoms, vital signs, physical examination, urine drug screen, and if the patient is a female of child-bearing age, a urine pregnancy test. Measurement of levels of blood alcohol, prescription drugs, and glucose are performed depending on the patient's presentation. As is true of Class I situations in which the adolescent is at risk of self-harm, the history should focus on the onset, severity, frequency, associated manifestations, and exacerbating or mitigating factors of symptoms. Information from a collateral source (parent, foster parent, therapist, teacher, and previous presentations) may clarify the answer to "Why now?" A thorough physical and neurologic examination, review of symptoms, laboratory and other diagnostic tests, and medication regimen changes often point to a likely cause. The neurologic examination is the most neglected part of the physical examination of psychiatric patients in the ED, but is critical to diagnosis and in guiding treatment.[23]

### 1. VIOLENCE

The assessment of the violent adolescent includes an evaluation of the precipitant, the presence of any underlying conditions, and risk factors for future violence. Behaviors that may contribute to future violence include: (1) a history of violence, (2) expressing a direct threat toward another, (3) access to, or carrying, a weapon, (4) physical fighting, (5) history of being victimized, (6) history of head trauma, epilepsy, neurologic impairment, or substance abuse, (7) persecutory or jealous delusions, (8) command hallucinations, and (9) inability of the family to control the patient.

The treatment of the violent patient should be focused on maintaining the safety of the patient and others, treating acute agitation with antipsychotic medication, diagnosing and initiating treatment of accompanying psychiatric conditions that may be contributing to violence (substance dependence, attention-deficit/hyperactivity disorder [ADHD], psychotic disorders, and affective disorders). If an adolescent has made a specific threat against an individual, the physician should consider local laws and consult hospital counsel regarding the duty to warn.

### 2. PSYCHOSIS

Psychotic adolescents are out of touch with reality and may demonstrate hallucinations, delusions, disorganized speech (loosening of associations), disorganized behavior, and negative symptoms (blunted affect, decreased speech, or avolition), and may present to the ED due to these factors. The differential diagnosis of psychosis in adolescents includes: anxiety disorders, mood disorders (depression and manic depression), PTSD, externalizing disorders (ADHD, oppositional defiant disorder [ODD], conduct disorders), delirium, borderline personality traits, factitious disorder, and malingering. As noted in Chapter 188 (Psychotic Disorders in Adolescents), adolescents presenting with psychotic symptoms should have a thorough work-up to exclude medical and substance-related causes as described in the section on delirium.[24] Acutely psychotic patients are at risk for aggression and violence and should be treated with antipsychotic medications if they become agitated (see section on treatment of agitation). Adolescents with command hallucinations, paranoid/persecutory delusions, or both should be admitted to an acute inpatient psychiatry unit for further treatment and diagnostic clarification once medical causes have been excluded.

### 3. SEVERE UNTREATED HYPERACTIVITY

Adolescents with ADHD left untreated or undertreated can present in the ED with significant risk of self-harm and injury to others due to impulsivity and failure to consider the consequences of their behaviors. In a study of a high-volume urban psychiatric emergency service, the authors[5] found that 48% of children and adolescents with ADHD were classified as urgent, either Class I or II. These youth should be treated in the ED as described in the section on the aggressive patient and may require hospitalization to be stabilized.

### 4. FIRE-SETTING

Half of all arrested arsonists in the United States are juveniles. Roughly 300 people die and $300 million worth of property is destroyed by juvenile fire-setters.[25] Given the serious consequences of their behavior, adolescent fire-setters may be brought to the ED even though their mental health problems are likely to include disruptive behaviors that preceded the fire-setting. A distinction needs to be made between fire play and fire-setting. Fire play is characterized by curiosity and fascination and does not imply malice, with a low level to harm. Fire-setting involves a higher level of malicious intent and may be associated with aggression, social skills deficits, and other social deviance (lying, truancy, vandalism). In the ED setting, the evaluation should cover the type of fire behavior (play or setting), the extent of the incident, previous history of fire-setting, the family's capacity for supervision, and other psychiatric disorders that might affect the adolescent or his or her parents.[26] The disposition to an inpatient or outpatient treatment setting depends on the level of danger. Given the multiple origins of fire-setting, a multisystem approach involving the family, school, local fire departments and law-enforcement agencies is recommended. Fire departments can provide fire safety and prevention education programs.

## CLASS II: URGENT, BUT NOT LIFE-THREATENING DISTURBANCES

Adolescents falling into the Class II category require urgent intervention because they include: (1) being a victim of rape or sexual abuse (especially immediately following disclosure of incest), (2) witnessing trauma, (3) experiencing the death of a parent, sibling, or close friend, (4) suffering from a severe anxiety attack or hyperventilation, (5) presenting with somatoform or conversion symptoms, (6) recent diagnosis or disclosure of unplanned pregnancy.

### VICTIM OF RAPE, SEXUAL ABUSE

Adolescents who have been sexually abused or raped by a stranger, rather than by a family member or friend, are more likely to present to an ED. Victims of both genders, but especially males, may be reluctant to discuss the event and often experience significant shame. Medical care, including evidence gathering, psychiatric consultation, and CPS for sexually misused adolescents should interact collaboratively in evaluation and treatment (see Chapters 168, Physical Abuse, and 169, Sexual Abuse and Assault).

### SEVERE ANXIETY/PANIC ATTACKS

A panic attack is an acute episode of intense fear or discomfort that usually peaks within 10 minutes and typically includes at least 4 of the following symptoms: palpitations, sweating, trembling, shortness of breath, feeling of choking, chest pain, nausea, dizziness, derealization or depersonalization, fear of losing control, and a fear of dying (see Chapter 185, Disorders of Anxiety). Panic attacks can occur with all anxiety disorders. The history and circumstances associated with the onset of symptoms are important factors in making a diagnosis. Routine medical work-up for panic attacks may include vital signs, inquiring about the amount of caffeine and nicotine intake, an electrocardiogram (ECG), thyroid screen, and a urine drug screen. The acute treatment includes ruling out medical causes and administering a low dose of a benzodiazepine. Anxiety and panic attacks generally do not require inpatient hospitalization, but create a great deal of distress, and more in-depth outpatient evaluation and treatment may be facilitated by the patient's primary care physician.

### SOMATOFORM DISORDERS

Adolescents may present in an urgent manner with various kinds of somatic complaints (see Chapter 183, Somatoform Disorders) that generally do not meet full criteria for the somatoform disorders (somatization disorder, conversion disorder, pain disorder, and hypochondriasis).[15] Because of its striking symptom complex, conversion disorder is the most likely somatoform disorder to present acutely to the ED. Physicians evaluating patients with conversion symptoms need to recognize that (1) these are serious conditions that require treatment, even though "organic" illness may be confidently ruled out, (2) emphasis on their "psychological" nature should be downplayed, as this is usually interpreted as a belief that the symptoms are "all in the head" and often leads to requests for "more tests," (3) talking about the effects of "stress" on the body is better received, and (4) comprehensive treatment should include not only referral for mental health services but also a recommendation for scheduled close follow-up with the primary care physician to continue to monitor and evaluate the presenting physical symptoms.

### PREGNANCY

Pregnancy may be discovered in the medical evaluation of an adolescent female with other physical or emotional symptoms. Any adolescent with secondary amenorrhea presenting to an ED requires a urine pregnancy test, even if her chief complaint is a physical symptom unrelated to pregnancy. The reaction to the pregnancy, identification of available supports, and an assessment of danger to self or others must be determined. The ED physician serves a critical role in the timely referral for medical and obstetric care, along with mental health, and social services.

## CLASS III: PROMPT BUT NOT IMMEDIATE INTERVENTION

Class III conditions are those that are serious enough to need prompt, but not immediate, intervention. "Emergency" conditions that fall into this category include (1) school refusal, (2) crises in caretakers' lives, (3) major impending stressor, such as hospitalization or surgery, or disruption in home life, and (4) verbal threats of suicide or violence, where the adolescent is unmanageable, but not dangerous.

Presenting problems that fall into Class III can be referred to an outpatient setting for more comprehensive assessment. It is important to acknowledge the concern of the caregiver and make a prompt and appropriate referral to either a partial hospital program, school-based services, in-home services including wrap-around services (therapeutic support staff, mobile therapist, and a behavioral specialist), and family-based interventions.

### SCHOOL REFUSAL

Adolescents who refuse to attend school or are chronically absent may have separation anxiety, lax or inconsistent parental limits, fears of being bullied, and other psychiatric conditions. School absences due to truancy may be associated with conduct disorder. Truant adolescents may appear to leave for school but either do not arrive, or leave school property without permission so that they can socialize with peers, who may also have conduct disorder. Adolescents who do not attend school because of physical symptoms may, in fact, have significant separation anxiety (sometimes mislabeled as "school phobia," see Chapter 185, Disorders of Anxiety in Adolescents). Thus, when the issue of returning to school is raised, both the mother and adolescent typically respond that there is a desire to go to school, but the symptoms prevent that from occurring. The symptom complex frequently consists of headaches and abdominal pain resulting in chronic school absence and often begins in childhood. Separation anxiety that begins in or persists into adolescence is more ominous and often more difficult to treat than the childhood variety. Because the physical symptoms are so incapacitating, the underlying dynamic of separation anxiety, most commonly related to maternal attachment, may go undetected. The dynamic is more related to staying at home than avoiding school. The immediate goal is for the adolescent to return to school as soon as possible, because the longer she or he remains out of school, the more resistance there is to return to school and to treatment.[27]

## CLASS IV: NONURGENT SITUATIONS

Class IV situations require an intervention, but are not medically urgent, even though someone in the adolescent's life believes that an emergency exists that must be addressed immediately. This often occurs in the context of an overburdened family, school, or other system that can no longer deal with the problems raised by the adolescent.

Examples of Class IV presentations include (1) lack of awareness of proper mental health channels, (2) parents who wish to punish or "teach the teenager a lesson" for misbehavior, (3) consumer frustration with overburdened mental health system (eg, long wait for appointments, ran out of medication), (4) "school says he ***has*** to be seen," (5) interagency struggle, and (6) chronic antisocial behavior requiring placement outside the home. These reasons illustrate the broad concept of urgency, underscoring the notion that a situation becomes an emergency when the typical systems in the community cannot handle it. These situations typically reflect system failures of access, of quality, and of engagement with youth and family.

## LEGAL ISSUES

In an emergency situation, consent to treatment is not needed if the delay in treatment caused by attempting to secure consent before beginning treatment would increase risk to the adolescent's life or health. However, in the pressured environment of the ED, the most relevant legal issues may get lost. In true emergencies involving adolescents, which Class IV conditions are not, the standard practice is to have a physician begin taking the history and performing the physical examination while an associate, such as a social worker, attempts to contact a parent or guardian. In cases that fall into Class IV, the history and physical examination can be performed, but administering medications or performing laboratory tests would not be justified until issues related to legal consent for treatment, guardianship, rights of minors to consent, involuntary commitment, and disclosure of information are all clarified.

At the time of triage, it is important to quickly identify who has legal custody of the minor, not just physical custody. It may be incorrectly assumed that if a youth is in CPS or in the delinquency (juvenile justice) system, that CPS or the court or the state has legal custody. It is also critical, however, to be aware of state laws regarding the legal rights of minors to consent for their own care, based on a variety of factors, including the condition for which they are seeking care, such as reproductive health care or mental illness (see Chapter 11, Legal and Ethical Framework). Although initiating care related to mental illness in minor adolescents without parental consent can be justified legally, it rarely would continue without parental involvement. Typically foster parents, agency workers, juvenile probation officers, relatives, or those providing kinship care do not have legal custody for treatment matters. Documents designating the legal custodian should be requested. Child protective services generally can provide consent for routine medical and dental care, but not for mental health treatment for adolescents in their custody. If parents are unavailable or unwilling to give consent, court-ordered psychiatric treatment may be needed. Although parents, CPS, and other agencies may be needed to be involved in decision making regarding emergency mental health services, adolescents may have the right to consent for themselves. Being placed outside of the home does not result in the loss of any rights that adolescents would otherwise have. Physicians should be familiar with their state's involuntary commitment regulations.

## SUMMARY

The burden of providing mental health treatment for adolescents has been shifted to primary care and ED due to a large need and a scarcity of child and adolescent psychiatrists. Using a triage approach may assist in determining the level of severity of presentations and prioritizing the level of care based on urgency. Understanding the range of urgency can minimize frustration, enhance the clinician's ability to accurately assess complex situations, and make a tremendous difference in the patient's receipt of future mental health services. Adolescent health care providers need to be familiar with the conditions discussed in this chapter, because many may present in primary care settings such as physician's offices, and outpatient or school-based clinics, as well as in EDs.

## REFERENCES

1. US Department of Health and Human Services. *Mental Health: A Report of the Surgeon General.* Bethesda, MD: US Department of Health and Human Services, Substance Abuse and Mental Health Services Administration Center for Mental Health, National Institutes of Health; 1999

2. Kim WJ. Child and adolescent psychiatry workforce: a critical shortage and national challenge. *Acad Psychiatry.* 2003;23(4):278–282

3. Page D. Pediatric psychiatry: more blues in ED? *Hosp Health Netw.* 2000;74:24

4. Sills ME, Bland SD. Summary statistics for pediatric psychiatric visits to US emergency departments, 1993–1999. *Pediatrics.* 2002;110:e40 [40-DOI: 10.1542]. Available at: www.pediatrics.org/cgi/content/full/110/4/e40. Accessed November 12, 2005

5. Edelsohn GA, Braitman LE, Rabinovich H, et al. Predictors of urgency in a pediatric psychiatric emergency service. *J Am Acad Child Adolesc Psychiatr.* 2003;42:1197–1202

6. Rosenn DW. Psychiatric emergencies in children and adolescents. In: Bassuk EL, Birk AW, eds. *Emergency Psychiatry: Concepts, Methods, and Practices.* New York, NY: Plenum; 1984:303–349

7. Edelsohn GA. Urgency counts: the why behind pediatric psychiatric emergency visits. *Clin Ped Emerg Med.* 2004;5:146–153

8. National Center for Health Statistics. *Multiple Cause of-Death Public-Use Data Files, 1990 through 2004.* Hyattsville, MD: US Department of Health and Human Services, CDC, National Center for Health Statistics; 2007

9. Grunbaum JA, Kann L, Kinchen S, et al. Youth risk behavior surveillance—United States, 2003. *MMWR.* 2004; 53(SS-2):1–96

10. Dulcan MK, Martini DR, Lake M. *Concise Guide to Child and Adolescent Psychiatry.* 3rd ed. Washington, DC: APPI; 2003:209–257

11. Stewart SE, Manion IG, Davidson S. Emergency management of the adolescent suicide attempter. *J Adolesc Health.* 2002;30:312–325

12. Piacentini J, Rotheram-Borus MJ, Gillis JR, et al. Demographic predictors of treatment attendance among adolescent suicide attempters. *J Cons Clin Psychol.* 1995;63:469–473

13. Spirito A, Lewander WJ, Levy S, et al. Emergency department assessment of adolescent suicide attempters: factors related to short-term follow-up outcome. *Pediatr Emerg Care.* 1994;10:6–12

14. Hoek HW, Van Hoeken D. Review of the prevalence and incidence of eating disorders. *Int J Eat Disord.* 2003;34:383–396

15. American Psychiatric Association. *Diagnostic and Statistical Manual of Mental Disorders* 4th ed. Text Revision. Washington, DC: American Psychiatric Association; 2000:143, 486–498, 583–595

16. Robb AS. Master of disguise: eating disorders in the emergency department. *Clinical Pediatric Emergency Medicine* 2004;5:161–186

17. National Clearinghouse on Child Abuse and Neglect Information. Child maltreat 2003: summary of key findings. Available at: ncfm.org/libraryfiles/Children/Abuse/canstats.pdf. Accessed December 1, 2010

18. The Medical Letter. *Drugs That Cause Psychiatric Symptoms.* 35 (901): 65–69. New Rochelle, NY: The Medical Letter, Inc; 1993

19. Chedu F, Geschwind N. Writing disturbances in acute confusional states. *Neuropsychologia* 1972;10:343–353

20. Turkel SB, Braslow K, Tavare CJ, Trzepacz PT. The Delirium Rating Scale in Children and Adolescents. *Psychosomatics* 2003;44:126–129

21. Cassem NH, Murray GB, Lafayette JM, Stern TA. *Massachusetts General Hospital Handbook of General Hospital Psychiatry.* 5th ed. St. Louis, MO: Mosby; 2004:119–134

22. Pappadopulos E, MacIntyreII JC, Crimson ML, et al. Treatment recommendations for the use of antipsychotics for aggressive youth (TRAAY). Part II. *J Am Acad Child Adolesc Psychiatr.* 2003;42:145-161

23. Tintinalli JE, Peacock IV FW, Wright MA. Emergency medical evaluation of psychiatric patients. *Ann Emerg Med.* 1994;23:859-862

24. Sosland MD, Edelsohn GA. Hallucinations in children and adolescents. *Curr Psychiatry Rep.* 2005;7:180-188

25. Office of Juvenile Justice and Delinquency Prevention. Juvenile firesetting: a research overview. Juvenile Justice Bulletin May 2005. Available at: www.ojp.usdoj.gov/ojjdp. Accessed August 28, 2005

26. Slavkin ML. What every clinician needs to know about juvenile firesetters. *Psychiatr Serv.* 2002;53(10):1237-1238

27. Dulcan MK, Martini DR, Lake M. *Concise Guide to Child and Adolescent Psychiatry.* 3rd ed. Washington, DC: APPI; 2003:68-69

# CHAPTER 190

# Adolescent Psychopharmacology

MICHAEL A. SCHARF, MD • THOMAS WILLIAMS, MD, PhD

## OVERVIEW

The treatment of an adolescent with a mental health disorder or multiple mental health problems, especially with respect to using medications, should proceed only after a thorough understanding of the individual patient has been achieved through a comprehensive assessment that includes individual and family history, with information ideally obtained from multiple sources. A complete physical examination and possibly laboratory studies should also precede definitive treatment that might include the use of medications. Adolescent health care providers who employ psychopharmaceutical agents as a tool to treat mental health conditions should not fit the patient to available medications based on labels or presenting complaints. Instead, when prescribed, medications should be used based on the adolescent's unique needs. To do so, clinicians need to understand normative expectations, to define quantitative and qualitative differences in several developmental lines, and use judgment in interpreting feelings and behaviors in all of their contexts. This chapter addresses biological, psychological, and social contexts that need to be understood in the assessment phases. The initiation of treatment is discussed, followed by a description of how to assess the response to treatment. Finally, pharmacologic treatment of adolescents for specific syndromes, including disorders of mood and emotion, disorders of thought, and disruptive behaviors are discussed. Based on this information, adolescent health care providers will be enabled to make judicious decisions about the use of medications in the treatment of mental health disorders in adolescents.

## ASSESSMENT

Assessment should always precede intervention, especially when considering the use of psychopharmacologic agents. Psychiatric assessment can be complicated and time intensive. Because mental health conditions continue to be negatively stigmatized by many individuals and groups, adolescents may be reluctant to undergo assessment because of concerns about being labeled "crazy." Likewise, because mental health diagnoses in adolescents are often associated with a family history of similar diagnoses, there may be resistance on the part of the parent(s) to undergo a psychiatric assessment. This is more likely if family members have had a negative experience in receiving mental health services. Family members who have benefited from mental health treatment, including medications, can, conversely, facilitate acceptance of such an assessment. Given the many constraints that may be encountered, a clinician may feel pressure to make the evaluation compact and efficient. This is more likely when there is a specific request for medication to help with an emotional or behavioral problem. However, such pressure should not deter clinicians from being thorough. Consultation with a mental health provider may be necessary to complete an adequate assessment.

A distinction between diagnosis and formulation needs to be made. A diagnosis is a label. In the most commonly used current diagnostic scheme, the *Diagnostic and Statistical Manual of Mental Disorders Fourth edition, Text Revision (DSM IV-TR),* diagnoses are based on a categorical approach to classification. A diagnosis is confirmed or refuted based on the use of checklists of reportable phenomena.[1] An underlying biologic or genetic basis is not currently considered an element of diagnosis. However, a biologic basis is inferred when a psychopharmacologic intervention is chosen.

Formulation is an attempt at more complete understanding. A careful review of family history and biologic determinants, the adolescent's perceptions and interpretations of experiences, as well as the context in which they live, provides the basis for such understanding. The biopsychosocial model, as proposed by Engel,[2] is one method of organizing a formulation. Although a synthetic, integrated formulation for any case is the goal, separate consideration of the biological, psychological, and social factors may be useful. When considering psychopharmacologic intervention, it may be tempting to exclusively consider biologic factors, but such a limited approach is a disservice to the patient. What follows is an elaboration on biological, psychological, and social factors that influence diagnostic formulation generally and pharmacotherapy specifically.

## BIOLOGICAL FACTORS

Genetic factors, identified or implied by family history, central nervous system (CNS) development, physiology, pharmacology, developmental history, history of illness, injury, trauma, current medications, other substance use, and prior responses to medications, in the patient and family members, are all biologic factors to be considered for a proper formulation.

Genetic factors play a critical role in the biological vulnerability and developmental progress of an adolescent. Family history of mental health conditions, both of the biological parents and across multiple generations, is useful in considering diagnostic alternatives, and in recognizing risks and pitfalls. Asking about family history of specific symptoms or behaviors is generally more useful than asking about specific diagnoses. Many diagnosable psychiatric conditions in families never come to the attention of a professional, but can be surmised from characteristic patterns of behavior.[3]

To obtain a personal view of the familial basis of an adolescent's symptoms, one can ask the patient and the parent(s) their perspectives. For example, one could ask the adolescent: "Who are you most like in your family?"; "How are you like that person?"; "In what ways are you like your mother and your father?" The parent(s) could be asked: "How is your child like you?, like your spouse/ex?"; "How is your daughter's/son's adolescence alike or different from yours?"; "Is there a relative who your daughter/son reminds you of?"; "Who else in the family has (describe adolescent's symptoms) like your daughter/son?" These questions help to identify potential subtle genetic relationships and may also provide a window into family dynamics, as well as parental and adolescent perspectives.

Individual differences in biological development result in a wide range of sensitivities and expression along many developmental lines, as well as variable responses to medications.[4] Hepatic capacity to clear medications and their metabolites typically decreases, relative to body mass, from childhood to adulthood. Therefore compared with older adolescents, younger adolescents of the same body size may need more frequent dosing and higher doses of medication. Likewise, older adolescents may need more frequent and higher doses than adults to achieve similar effects. Varying volumes of distribution and body composition, such as body fat content, lead to shorter effective half-lives and possible need for more frequent dosing to achieve a steady state.[5]

Psychotropic medications are believed to have their therapeutic actions by affecting neurotransmitters, though suggesting that psychopharmacology is merely a matter of leveling a "chemical imbalance" is an oversimplification. Individual genetic variations affect psychotropic medication action at the neurotransmitter level, as well as medication metabolism. This variability has potential treatment implications that are being studied.[6] Neurotransmitter systems change during puberty and continue to change throughout life,[4,7] so that distinct effects of psychotropic medications can be seen at different ages.[8–10]

Puberty affects CNS development, which has cognitive, emotional, and behavioral implications. Sex hormones have evident neuroactivity, but without a specific correlation to particular diagnoses. Increases in emotional reactivity are popularly described as being related to "hormonal imbalance," but cannot be specifically tied to changes in sex hormone levels. Testosterone has been repeatedly linked to aggression. However, a causal relationship has not been clarified. Emotional symptoms related to the menstrual cycle have been a target of pharmacotherapy, with selective serotonin reuptake inhibitors (SSRIs) and certain oral contraceptive formulations, each apparently helpful with some patients. However, none has been found effective for all, highlighting the complexity of such issues.[11]

## PSYCHOLOGICAL FACTORS

The psychological development of adolescents entails their unique personality; their perceptions, interpretations, and patterned and creative responses; and interactions with the world. Various exposures to trauma, maltreatment, abandonment, bullying, hardship, and subtler caregiver manipulations can result in a wide variety of styles of understanding the world and interacting with others. The very nature of adolescence, as a time of great change, adds another layer of variability. Adolescents may seek conformity with peers, affecting how they present themselves in different settings. One of the greatest challenges of caregivers for adolescents is to empathically recognize their internal struggle for emotional stability and rational understanding as their body, identity, and environmental contexts are rapidly evolving.

Risk-taking behaviors, a subjective sense of invulnerability, and intense emotional states are common to adolescence and have implications for diagnostic assessment[12] and treatment adherence. Complicated regimens, medications with potential withdrawal symptoms, abuse potential, or which may interact with common drugs of abuse, should be used with caution in adolescents.

Piaget[13] described the shift in cognitive processing that begins during late childhood to early adolescence as a move from concrete to formal operational thinking, with increasing capacity to use metaphor, to think about thinking, and to consider situational rather than black-white decision making. This cognitive advance, which does not occur in all adolescents, represents a major shift in how well the adolescent may understand and be autonomously involved in the diagnostic and treatment process. This cognitive process also affects the ability of the adolescent to enjoin with treatment and self-monitor and report over time.

As an adolescent is confronted with issues of identity, independence, and autonomy, these intrinsic drives can create conflict with parents, requiring finesse in understanding the relative role of the adolescent and the parent(s) in decisions about treatment. Clinicians should make every attempt to include adolescents and parents in decision making regarding psychotropic medications, recognizing the variations in adolescents' capacities and in the ability of adolescents and parents to work collaboratively. It is always necessary to discuss the limits of confidentiality as early in treatment as possible, clarifying safety issues that require informing parents, including thoughts about harming self or others.[14]

Adolescents may view the prescription of psychoactive medication as an accusation or implication that something is wrong with them.[15] This may trigger feelings of being controlled, resulting in poor adherence. However, confronting the adolescent about poor adherence may cause alienation and further resistance to treatment. To avoid this, a nonjudgmental approach with open-ended questions is preferable: "What is it like for you when a dose is missed?" If the individual adolescent's awareness, expectations, and goals for treatment are not addressed, then medications that might otherwise be initially effective may lose their effectiveness, with the adolescent's perception as being immune, allergic, or tolerant to the medicine ("it stopped working"). In fact, the adolescent may feel the need to resist external expectations, and it may be that the adolescent and/or family cannot, or will not, tolerate change.

Unconscious mental processes are potentially critical to the presentation of emotional and behavioral symptoms and responses to medications.[16] Deeply rooted memories, perceptions, development of defensive coping mechanisms, internalized conflicts, emotional experiences and expressions, and personality development warrant consideration and require careful listening over time.

### SOCIAL FACTORS

Social contexts generally determine the presentation of symptoms and influence treatment options. For the adolescent, the contexts that profoundly affect self-awareness, self-esteem, role identification, symptom expression, coping, expectations and goals, and adherence are the family (immediate, extended, and step/other); peers; school; and community. The relationship of an adolescent to parents, peers, other adults, and mentors affects the presentation of the adolescent and investment in treatment.

The relationship of the caregiver with the adolescent and family can elicit patient and parent investment in positive change. The adolescent and family need to be involved in exploring treatment options. Parents and many adolescents *want* to be involved in decision making and are most invested when enlisted in decisions about medication trials. It is recommended to encourage questions about, and discussion of, the variety of information available from peers, organizations, and media (including the Internet), as adolescents and their families will be exposed to such ideas and information whether discussed openly or not.

## INITIATING TREATMENT

Once the assessment is complete, a biopsychosocial treatment plan to match the biopsychosocial formulation should be considered and pursued. Psychopharmacologic intervention may be 1 part of such a comprehensive treatment plan. Psychotherapy is sometimes the most critical component, and usually is provided by a different clinician. Communication between therapist and medical provider are essential for effective care.[17]

When used, medications are directed toward target symptoms of the designated disorder or dysfunction, rather than a diagnostic label. In adolescents, the evidence basis for use of psychopharmacologic interventions is severely lacking, especially considering the increasing use of these medications. Therefore, much of our prescribing is off-label, or not US Food and Drug Administration (FDA) approved for the condition for which it is prescribed. Our best option is to extrapolate information from available reports, including those in adults, and to consider our own anecdotal experiences. Thus, every medication trial is a *trial*, an opportunity to consider the benefits, side effects, and risks inherent in this intervention and treatment continuation. A linear approach that implies "you have this diagnosis and you need this treatment" has minimal support in the literature. Nonetheless, linear and directed pharmacologic treatment occurs frequently. An adolescent-centered approach, in which the primary consideration is the adolescent as a unique individual, is recommended. An algorithm summarizing this approach is presented in Box 190-1.

**Box 190-1**

***Algorithm for Adolescent Psychopharmacology***

**Assessment**

1. Clarify the presenting symptoms.
2. Determine the dysfunction, distress, and effect of symptoms for the adolescent and family.
3. Establish a differential diagnosis.
   a Consider environmental stresses—family, social, abuse.
   b Rule out medical causes.
   c Determine psychiatric diagnoses and rule-outs.
4. Determine comorbid diagnoses.
5. Determine biophysical formulation, including family history and response to treatment.
6. Determine severity of symptoms and urgency of treatment.

**Treatment**

1. Consider a trial of psychotherapeutic intervention by an experienced clinician.
2. Use pharmacotherapy for moderate to severe suffering alone or as an adjunct to psychotherapy.

*If symptoms persist or respond only minimally*

1. Assess for nonresponse vs partial response to interventions.
2. Reconsider diagnoses or comorbidity; consider referral to an experienced mental health clinician for further assessment, if necessary.
3. Reconsider trial of psychotherapeutic intervention if not part of care plan.
4. Consider alternate medications (nonresponse) or combinations (partial response) as indicated.
5. Consultation with or referral to a child and adolescent psychiatrist for complex psychopharmacologic management.

Reprinted from Scharf MA, Williams TP. Psychopharmacology in adolescent medicine. *Adolesc Med Clin*. 2006;17(1):165-181, with permission from Elsevier.

Individualize the plan by establishing the hoped for goals that the adolescent and family have for the medication. Unrealistic expectations need to be identified and adapted to the limitations of the medications. Alternatives and choices are presented, with recommendations and support of the decision-making process over time. It is important to introduce ideas, establish dialogue, promote autonomy by supporting self-awareness, and education to engender appropriate medication trials. The pace of the treatment plan should be flexible to adapt to the adolescent's changes over time. A partnership with the involved decision makers will minimize mixed and ambivalent expectations and optimize a positive direction for continued development and growth of the individual.

**Table 190-1**

**Levels of Recommendation for Psychopharmacologic Intervention**

| *Level* | *Description* |
|---|---|
| 0 | Medication has no role in this case or situation at this time. |
| 1 | Medicine exists that some people use and find relief with and I'd be happy to discuss it with you if you're interested. |
| 2 | Medicine exists that will probably help your suffering, and is 1 of many appropriate options. |
| 3 | I believe your condition warrants treatment with medication and you should strongly consider taking it. |
| 4 | Medication is an essential part of the appropriate management of your condition and it is not acceptable to me, as your physician, to participate in your care without it. |

A useful way to enhance autonomy for the adolescent patient and facilitate appropriate discussion is to present medication recommendations with a weight or level of recommendation. The suggested scale of 0 to 4 and each number's meaning is presented in Table 190-1. Assigning a specific level to medication recommendations is based on anticipated benefit versus risk of side effects. When using this approach, the clinician should explain the "levels" and what each one means in general before presenting the specific medication recommendation for any given patient. For example, in a case of initial presentation for treatment of generalized anxiety, after explaining the levels one might say, "Using an SSRI to treat your anxiety symptoms would be a 2 on this scale."

Any enlistment of the placebo response is by definition helpful, and pre-existing positive ideas about a medication seem to have a positive effect on treatment adherence and outcome.[18] Statements such as "This medication saved my life," or "That medicine nearly killed his sister" by patients or family members should be listened for and may help guide specific medication choices within a class for more than just the potential biologic implications. Clinicians, however, should stop short of misleading or withholding full informed consent from patients and families.

The legal capacity of adolescents to seek and consent to mental health care varies geographically, and clinicians need to be aware of state laws[19] and financial implications[20] of care.

## DOSING

Suggested initial target doses for psychopharmacologic agents are listed in Table 190-2. It may be necessary to exceed these target doses to achieve full therapeutic effect. Metabolic issues, body mass index (BMI), and concurrent medications must also be considered when choosing a specific medication and dose.

Alternative formulations are also included in Table 190-2. These may be useful in situations where swallowing pills is a problem or there is concern about treatment adherence. If there are concerns about adherence, medication administration should be observed by an adult; liquids and orally dissolving tablets are more difficult to hide in the mouth than solid pills or capsules. Some medications are available in "sustained release" (SR, XR, XL, ER, or CR) formulations, which enables less frequent, typically daily, dosing than regular formulations. Almost no oral formulations make dosing less frequent than once per day; the lone exception being the sustained release form of fluoxetine, dosed once weekly (Prozac Weekly). Depot injections are available for risperidone and some first-generation antipsychotics, such as haloperidol and fluphenazine; these may be helpful for treatment adherence when chronic antipsychotic treatment is necessary.

**Table 190-2**

**Dosing Suggestions and Alternative Formulations**

| *Medication* | *Start* | *Maintenance* | *Alternative Formulations SR = Sustained Release ODT = Orally Dissolving Tablet* |
|---|---|---|---|
| **Antidepressants** | | | |
| Fluoxetine | 10 mg | 20–40 mg | Liquid, weekly dosed tablet |
| Sertraline | 25–50 mg | 150–200 mg | Liquid |
| Fluvoxamine | 25–50 mg | 150–300 mg | |
| Paroxetine | 10–20 mg | 20–40 mg | Liquid, SR (CR) |
| Citalopram | 10–20 mg | 20–40 mg | Liquid |
| Escitalopram | 5–10 mg | 10–20 mg | Liquid |
| Venlafaxine | 37.5–75 mg | 150–300 mg | SR (XR) |
| Bupropion | 75–100 mg | 150–300 mg | SR (SR, XL) |
| **Antianxiety**[a] | | | |
| Buspirone | 10–20 mg | 40 mg | |
| Propranolol | 20–40 mg | 400–600 mg | Liquid, SR (LA, XL) |
| *Benzodiazepines* | | | |
| Long-acting | | | |
| Clonazepam | 0.5 mg | 1–2 mg | ODT (wafers) |
| Diazepam | 1–2 mg | 5–10 mg | Liquid, IM, IV |
| Short-acting | | | |
| Lorazepam | 0.5 mg | 1–2 mg | Liquid, IM, IV |
| Alprazolam | 0.25 mg | 0.5–2 mg | Liquid, ODT (Niravam), SR (XR) |

*(Continued)*

**Table 190-2 (Continued)**

| *Medication* | *Start* | *Maintenance* | *Alternative Formulations SR = Sustained Release ODT = Orally Dissolving Tablet* |
|---|---|---|---|
| **Antipsychotics** | | | |
| Risperidone | 0.5–1 mg | 2–4 mg | Liquid, ODT (M-tab), long-acting IM (Consta) |
| Olanzapine | 2.5–5 mg | 10–20 mg | ODT (Zydis), IM |
| **Mood Stabilizers** | | | |
| Lithium | 150–300 mg | Serum level = 0.6–1.2 meq/L | SR (Lithobid, CR) |
| Divalproex | 250–500 mg | Serum level = 50–100 mcg/mL | SR (ER), sprinkles, liquid (valproic acid), IV (valproate sodium) |
| Gabapentin | 200–400 mg | 2,400 mg | Liquid |
| **Miscellaneous** | | | |
| Clonidine | 0.1–0.2 mg | 0.2–0.5 mg | Transdermal patch (TDS) |

[a]SSRIs are first line medications for chronic anxiety.

IM, intramuscular; IV, intravenous

Reprinted from Scharf MA, Williams TP. Psychopharmacology in adolescent medicine. *Adolesc Med Clin*. 2006;17(1):165–181, with permission from Elsevier.

## ASSESSING RESPONSE TO TREATMENT

A clear list of target symptoms, documented in the patient's record, should be followed over time. Side effects should be inquired about directly at regular intervals. Patients and families should be encouraged to bring up any concerns as they arise. Adolescent patients should not be the sole source of data regarding response, because they may have responses clearly manifested to others (such as parents) that are not readily apparent to themselves. Evaluating treatment response often requires balancing achieved desired therapeutic effects with undesired side effects. Drawing conclusions and decisions for next steps should be in the adolescent's purview, to the extent possible.

Treatment "failure" refers to a lack of any desired effect from a given medication, as opposed to intolerability of side effects, sensitivity, allergy, or other adverse reaction, or treatment nonadherence that prevents an adequate trial. Treatment failure requires reconsideration of diagnosis and formulation and consideration of another trial with a different medication or psychotherapy.

"Partial response" refers to achieving some desired effect without complete resolution of target symptoms. Next steps may be to either increase the dose, add psychotherapy, or augment pharmacotherapy by adding a second medication, typically with a different mechanism of action. One example of augmentation is adding a second-generation antipsychotic (SGA) to augment the therapeutic effects of an anticonvulsant in treating emotional dysregulation. Augmentation is distinguished from other medications to treat or prevent unwanted side effects, such as using anticholinergic medications for extrapyramidal symptoms associated with antipsychotics.

Treatment "success" refers to sufficient improvement in symptoms to be acceptable to the adolescent and other concerned persons. Decisions about continuation of treatment need to balance the desire to stop medication with the risk of recurrence of symptoms. Consideration of decreasing the dose or discontinuation of a successful medication once a year is recommended.

## PHARMACOLOGIC TREATMENTS FOR SPECIFIC SYNDROMES

As previously noted, medication choices are not directed by diagnoses, but target the symptoms of these conditions. Medications specifically affect the underlying predisposing biologic factors of any particular mental illness. Mental processes affected by medications are more specifically related to emotion and emotional regulation; thought processes; and biological determinates of disruptive behavior (rather than the specific behavior itself).

## DISORDERS OF EMOTIONS AND EMOTIONAL REGULATION

Disorders of emotions and emotional regulation conceptually refers to specific mood or "feeling" states that cause suffering and dysfunction or emotional sensitivity or reactivity to environmental stimuli that is extreme and not consistent with developmental expectations.

### Depressive Disorders

Having a deliberate and careful approach to deciding whether to medicate depressive disorders is critical. This is especially true given the consistently high placebo rates and less than overwhelming treatment effect of antidepressants in adolescents demonstrated in many published studies,[21] as well as recent controversy about their safety.

Although antidepressant medications may be considered for any persistent depressive symptoms or syndromes, actual treatment choice will be guided by formulation and accurate diagnosis. A depressed adolescent with known bipolar disorder should be treated with a "mood stabilizer" before considering antidepressant medication to avoid triggering mania. If psychotic features, such as disordered thought processes, delusions, or hallucinations are present, antipsychotic medications, in addition to antidepressant medication, may be necessary for successful treatment outcome.[22] For depressive symptoms that present in the context of trauma or a loss, psychotherapy alone may be the preferred treatment.

Concern regarding possible risks of suicidality associated with antidepressants has resulted in much attention and discussion. An analysis conducted for the FDA[23] suggested a 1.7% greater risk of "suicidal ideations or behavior"—but no completed suicides—in pediatric patients who received antidepressant medications compared to placebo. Two more recent meta-analyses, conducted by the FDA found that this risk may continue into young adulthood, up to age 24.[24] The finding of increased risk of suicidal ideations or behaviors is controversial; some other analyses have not found such increased risk[24,25] or found that benefits exceeded risks from suicidal ideation and attempt.[26] In an attempt to examine the relationship of antidepressant medications with actual suicide risk, Gibbons and colleagues[27] compared the rates of antidepressant prescriptions with rates of adolescent suicides in counties in the United States and found higher rates of antidepressant prescription associated with *lower* rates of completed suicide. In practice, the potential risk for increased suicidal ideations needs to be balanced against the risks associated with not treating or undertreating major depressive and other disorders, recognizing that major depressive disorder has a lifetime suicide rate of up to 15%.[28] Clinicians should acknowledge this potential risk when discussing antidepressant medications as a treatment option with patients and parents. Information to facilitate such discussions is available through the American Academy of Child and Adolescent Psychiatry, including information for parents and practical prescribing information for physicians.[29]

For depression in adolescents, SSRIs (fluoxetine [Prozac, Serafem], sertraline [Zoloft], citalopram [Celexa], escitalopram [Lexapro], paroxetine [Paxil, Pexeva], and fluvoxamine [Luvox]) are considered first line.[22] Monoamine oxidase inhibitors (MAOIs) are also effective, but are rarely used in adolescents due to necessary dietary restrictions and the risk of hypertensive crisis or serotonin syndrome.

Tricyclic antidepressants (TCAs) are not effective for depression in children and adolescents[8] but may still have other uses in clinical practice, including for chronic pain, nocturnal enuresis, anxiety,[30] or attention-deficit/hyperactivity disorder (ADHD).[31] Other antidepressants, such as venlafaxine (Effexor), bupropion (Wellbutrin), mirtazapine (Remeron), and duloxetine (Cymbalta) have minimal evidence to establish their safety or efficacy among adolescents, but may be considered second line or third line. The active stereoisomer of venlafaxine, desvenlafaxine (Pristiq), is currently being marketed, but there is no information about its use in children or adolescents at this time. Many clinicians prefer a second SSRI trial as a second-line medication. Some of these agents are also used for augmentation of SSRIs. Augmentation should not properly be considered an evidence-based practice in adolescents, given the lack of available data. FDA-approved augmentation strategies, which do have supporting evidence of efficacy in adults, include adding lithium, liothyronine (Cytomel), or aripiperazole (Abilify) to antidepressant medications.[32]

## BIPOLAR DISORDERS

The prevalence and presentation of bipolar disorders in adolescence is controversial.[33,34] The *DSM-IV-TR*[1] recognizes 2 defined subtypes of bipolar disorder and reserves the "not otherwise specified" category for persons with clinically significant symptoms not better classified elsewhere. Youth diagnosed with a bipolar disorder often present in a different manner than adults, with rapidly changing mood states and behaviors rather than discrete episodes of mania and depression. Despite the controversy, it is generally agreed that a diagnosis of bipolar disorder warrants treatment with medication.[34]

The term "mood stabilizer" is frequently used. However, this is not 1 pharmacologic class or category, and it can be misleading. The term implies efficacy in treating bipolar disorders, but many agents included in the common vernacular, such as "mood stabilizers," have only demonstrated efficacy as antimanic agents, if there is evidence to support their use at all.[34] A true "mood stabilizer" should be effective in treating the acute phases of mania and possibly depression, and should also be effective in preventing or decreasing the frequency or severity of discrete episodes or symptoms associated with bipolar disorders. Most clinicians use the "mood stabilizer" label to refer to lithium and anticonvulsants with efficacy in treating bipolar disorders. Antipsychotic medications could be included under this umbrella label, given the nonspecific nature of the term, but many clinicians refer to those medications separately. Reliance on a nonspecific label or terminology for selection of therapeutic agent is not advised.

Until recently, lithium was the only medication with an FDA indication for the treatment of pediatric bipolar disorder. More recently, risperidone (Risperdal) and aripiperazole (Abilify) have received indications for treating acute manic and mixed episodes of bipolar disorder type I in patients 10 to 17 years old.[32] The FDA was in the process of reviewing further indications for other "atypical" or "second-generation" antipsychotics at the time this book was published.[30]

In practice, clinicians use agents with established efficacy to treat bipolar disorder symptoms in adults in all phases of illness,[34] including: lithium, valproic acid (Depakote), carbamazepine (Tegretol), lamotrigine (Lamictal), and SGA medications such as risperidone (Risperdal), olanzapine (Zyprexa), quetiapine (Seroquel), ziprasidone (Geodon), aripiperazole (Abilify), and clozapine (Clozaril). Honest discussion with careful attention to potential benefits and risks or side effects is necessary before initiating trials of these medications.

Anticonvulsants without demonstrated efficacy to treat bipolar disorder in any age group, for example gabapentin (Neurontin), topiramate (Topamax), and oxcarbazepine (Trileptal) have been used as "mood stabilizers" due to favorable side effect profiles. Consideration of such agents on a case-by-case basis may be warranted in certain situations, but needs a careful discussion and informed consent process given the lack of clear evidence to support their efficacy.

### OTHER AFFECTIVE DYSREGULATION

Adolescents may have affective dysregulation, which is clinically significant but does not meet diagnostic criteria for any bipolar disorder. These cases can be difficult to manage and highlight once again the importance of adequate diagnostic evaluation and a thoughtful formulation. A target symptom-based approach to treatment may lead one to consider medications used as "mood stabilizers," which may be helpful but should be pursued cautiously and with careful informed consent given the paucity of evidence to support such interventions.

### ANXIETY DISORDERS

Treatment of anxiety disorders should always include behavioral or psychotherapeutic interventions, and psychopharmacologic intervention should only be considered in adjunct with these.[35] Benzodiazepines may be used for brief treatment of acute anxiety; these are generally well tolerated and effective, but are considered short-term interventions due to their abuse and addiction potential.[35] Antihistamines such as hydroxyzine may also be used and are sometimes effective in acute anxiety. For acute panic and performance anxiety, beta blockers have been shown to be effective.

Selective serotonin reuptake inhibitors are considered the first-line medication choice for chronic anxiety.[35] Tricyclic antidepressants are also effective for anxiety in adolescents but are not first-line agents, due to less preferable tolerability/side effect profiles compared with SSRIs. Some clinicians will consider prescribing a short-term course of a benzodiazepine or an antihistamine at the same time as an SSRI, anticipating discontinuing the short-term medication in a few weeks after the estimated time necessary to see efficacy from the SSRI. When contemplating antidepressant medications in the treatment of anxiety disorders, one must remember and include in the informed consent, potential suicidality risk as discussed earlier in this chapter.

## DISORDERS OF THOUGHT

The capacity to self-reflect, understand meaning and the role of emotion and behavior, consider alternatives, generalize coping, and be flexible are critical to improvement in mentally ill individuals. The construct of disorders based on deficits of thought or cognition assists us in targeting critical underlying determinants of presentation of psychiatric diagnoses. Cognitive processes including capacity (IQ), perceptions, interpretations, reality testing, order, organization, and coherence are representative of or associated with several psychiatric conditions. These dysfunctional elements represent specific targets of several medications.

### PSYCHOTIC DISORDERS

Psychotic symptoms need to be interpreted in terms of the context in which they develop. For example, severe trauma can lead to re-experiencing symptoms or dissociation, either of which may be mistaken for psychosis if not explored and understood. In addition, psychosis can be the initial manifestation of a variety of medical conditions, such as systemic lupus erythematosus. For confirmed psychotic disorders and psychotic symptoms associated with other conditions, treatment with antipsychotic medications is indicated.[36] Antipsychotic medications are also used to treat symptoms other than psychosis and mania, including aggression, perseverations, and tics.

Although there are multiple classes of antipsychotic medications, each with some differences in mechanisms of action and side effects, the most significant distinction currently is between "first-generation antipsychotics" such as haloperidol (Haldol) and chlorpromazine (Thorazine) and SGAs such as risperidone and olanzapine. Second-generation antipsychotics are generally considered to have similar efficacy, but preferable side effect profiles to older antipsychotic medications. As a result, most clinicians pursue an exhaustive trial of the newer antipsychotics before prescribing a first-generation antipsychotic.

The SGAs are considered less likely to cause neurologic side effects such as tardive dyskinesia or extrapyramidal side effects,[37] although some instances of tardive dyskinesia, extrapyramidal side effects, and neuroleptic malignant syndrome have been reported with each of these newer agents. Weight gain, dyslipidemia, and hyperglycemia are commonly associated with SGAs. Acute diabetic ketoacidosis and increased rates of diabetes mellitus have also been reported.[38] Evaluating weight, body mass index fasting lipid profile, and fasting glucose prior to initiating treatment and at regular intervals is necessary when prescribing these agents.[39]

### EATING DISORDERS

Psychopharmacologic intervention is not an essential part of the treatment of anorexia nervosa (AN). Selective serotonin reuptake inhibitors may be helpful during the weight maintenance phase of treatment.[40] Comorbid psychiatric conditions may exist with AN, and it would be appropriate to treat those with medications as indicated, but caution is advised in assessment; symptoms that have their onset during an acute malnourished state may be secondary to the starvation and may resolve with nutritional stabilization.

Serotonergic antidepressants are effective in reducing the symptoms of binge eating and vomiting associated with bulimia nervosa (BN).[40] Fluoxetine is the only SSRI with FDA approval for the treatment of BN. The dose of fluoxetine required to treat BN is higher than that for depression, often 60 mg or more.

### AUTISTIC SPECTRUM DISORDERS

Psychotropic medications may be helpful in targeting certain symptoms or behaviors associated with autism or other pervasive developmental disorders,[31] but there is no medication designed or indicated for these diagnoses. Antipsychotic medications are often used for aggression and may also be helpful with perseverations. Antidepressants may be effective in treating anxiety and obsessive-compulsive symptoms.

## DISRUPTIVE BEHAVIOR DISORDERS

Behaviors are not specifically targeted by medications, and the statement "it's just behavioral" highly misrepresents the individual and underlying mental and emotional processes leading to behaviors. Factors such as impulse control, coping styles, learned and reinforced patterns of stimulus-response, capacity to predict outcome and generalize expectations, self and other awareness, and capacity for empathy can strongly effect behavioral choices and are more specifically targeted by medications. Behaviors also occur in the context of other mental illnesses, which must be addressed. Attention deficit/hyperactivity disorder (ADHD) presentation has been theorized as a "final common pathway" for several psychiatric conditions, which must be considered, especially in nonresponsive adolescents.

### ATTENTION DEFICIT/HYPERACTIVITY DISORDER

Psychostimulants are long established and well researched as the treatment of choice for symptoms of ADHD, with reported response rates as high as 96%.[41] There are 2 basic agents, each available in multiple formulations: methylphenidate (Ritalin, Concerta, Metadate, Methylin, and Focalin) and amphetamine (Dexedrine, Adderall). Recently lisdexamfetamine (Vyvanse) was introduced as the first "prodrug" in this class, being metabolized to the active amphetamine in the gastrointestinal system. Different formulations are designed to vary in time of onset and duration of action. Some patients report variable therapeutic responses and side effects to different formulations.

Intolerable side effects, a history of abuse or addiction to stimulants, multiple failed trials, or a desire to use alternative medications with stimulants to enhance efficacy or combat side effects are reasons to consider medications outside the stimulant class. Options include atomoxetine (Straterra), bupropion, TCAs, and α-adrenergic agents such as guanfacine (Tenex) or clonidine (Catapres). These medications are generally less effective than the stimulants but may have some benefits.[41]

### OPPOSITIONAL DEFIANT DISORDER AND CONDUCT DISORDER

Diagnosis of these behavior clusters as medical conditions is controversial, and there is no medication indicated for their treatment. When medication is considered, the target symptom is typically aggression. Reassessing diagnosis and considering behavioral approaches to managing the aggression is warranted before initiating medication. If comorbid conditions are present, they should be treated before using medication to sedate or suppress aggressive behaviors.

In clinical practice, antipsychotic medications, α-adrenergic medications, and all agents used as mood stabilizers have been used to treat aggression, with varying levels of success and no significant evidence base to distinguish their efficacy in adolescents.[42] If medications are to be used, those with the least potential for harm (side effects) should generally be considered first. Safety issues may make the most sedating or "potent" agents desirable, which leads to increased use of antipsychotics in clinical practice.

### PSYCHIATRIC EMERGENCIES

In situations where a patient's acute agitation or safety risk requires immediate medication intervention, antipsychotic (tranquilizing) medications and benzodiazepines are used, alone or in combination. Oral medication should always be offered prior to using involuntary, intramuscular (IM) options. When IM medications are required, SGAs with immediate-acting IM formulations (ziprasidone, olanzapine, and aripiprazole) are preferred for severe agitation, alone or with benzodiazepines (typically, lorazepam), due to the decreased likelihood of serious neurologic side effects compared to first-generation antipsychotics. Clinicians should familiarize themselves with what is actually on hand in whatever settings they work, as waiting for a delivery from the pharmacy may not be feasible, depending on the situation.

## CONCLUSIONS

Following the biopsychosocial model, psychopharmacologic agents will rarely be used as the sole means to treat adolescents. Pharmacologic agents have their main effect in the biological domain, but psychological and social factors must also be addressed for treatment to be successful.

## REFERENCES

1. American Psychiatric Association. *Diagnostic and Statistical Manual of Mental Disorders*. 4th ed. Text Revision. Washington, DC: American Psychiatric Association; 2000

2. Engel GL. The need for a new medical model: a challenge for biomedicine. *Science.* 1977;196(4286):129–136

3. Gray GV, Brody DS, Hart MT. Primary care and the de facto mental health care system: improving care where it counts. *Managed Care Interface.* 2000;13(3):62–65

4. Tosyali MC, Greenhill LL. Child and adolescent psychopharmacology. Important developmental issues. *Ped Clin North Am.* 1998;45(5):1021–1035

5. Scharf MA, Williams TP. Psychopharmacology in adolescent medicine. *Adolesc Med Clin.* 2006;17(1):165–181

6. Mrazek D. Psychiatric pharmacogenomics. *Focus.* 2006; 4:339–343

7. Ziegler MG, Lake CR, Kopin IJ. Plasma norepinephrine increases with age. *Nature.* 1976;261:333–335

8. Ryan ND. Pharmacotherapy of adolescent major depression: beyond TCAs. *Psychopharmacol Bull.* 1990;26:75–79

9. Keepers GA, Casey DE. Prediction of neuroleptic-induced dystonia. *J Clin Psychopharm.* 1987;7:342–345

10. US Food and Drug Administration. Psychopharmacologic Drugs Advisory Committee Meeting (transcript). Rockville, MD: Food and Drug Administration; 2006. Available at: www.fda.gov/ohrms/dockets/ac/cder06.html#Psychopharmacologic. Accessed March 16, 2010

11. Rapkin A. A review of treatment of premenstrual syndrome and premenstrual dysphoric disorder. *Psychoneuroendocrinology.* 2003;28(suppl 3):39–53

12. Golombek H, Kutcher S. Feeling states during adolescence. *Psych Clin North Am.* 1990;13(3):443–454

13. Flavell JH. *The Developmental Psychology of Jean Piaget.* New York, NY: Van Nostrand; 1963

14. Judge B, Billick SB. Suicidality in adolescence: review and legal considerations. *Behav Sci Law.* 2004;22(5):681–695

15. Corrigan PW, Lurie BD, Goldman HH, Slopen N, Medasani K, Phelan S. How adolescents perceive the stigma of mental illness and alcohol abuse. *Psychiatr Serv.* 2005;56(5):544–550

16. Goetzmann L, Holzapfel M, Toygar A. Psychotropic agents in psychotherapy: the subjective meaning of medication in different levels of self/object differentiation (neurosis, borderline, psychosis). *Int J Psychotherapy.* 2003;8(3):213–222

17. Lazarus JA. Ethics in split treatment. *Psychiatr Ann.* 2001;31(10):611–614

18. Krell HV, Leuchter AF, Morgan M, Cook IA, Abrams M. Subject expectations of treatment effectiveness and outcome of treatment with an experimental antidepressant. *J Clin Psychiatry.* 2004;65(9):1174–1179

19. Vukadinovich DM. Minors' rights to consent to treatment: navigating the complexity of state laws. *J Health Law.* 2004;37(4):667–691

20. English A. Treating adolescents. Legal and ethical considerations. *Med Clin North Am.* 1990;74(5):1097–1112

21. Moncrieff J, Wessely S, Hardy R. Active placebos versus antidepressants for depression. *Cochrane Database of Systematic Reviews.* 2004;(1):CD003012

22. Birmaher B, Brent DA, Benson RS. Summary of the practice parameters for the assessment and treatment of children and adolescents with depressive disorders. American Academy of Child and Adolescent Psychiatry. *J Am Acad Child Adolesc Psychiatry.* 1998;37(11):1234–1238

23. Brent DA. Antidepressants and pediatric depression—the risk of doing nothing. *N Eng J Med.* 2004;351(16):1598–1601

24. Valuck RJ, Libby AM, Sills MR, Giese AA, Allen RR. Antidepressant treatment and risk of suicide attempt by adolescents with major depressive disorder: a propensity-adjusted retrospective cohort study. *CNS Drugs.* 2004;18(15):1119–1132

25. Jick H, Kaye JA, Jick SS. Antidepressants and the risk of suicidal behaviors. *JAMA.* 2004;292(3):338–343

26. Bridge JA, Iyengar S, Salary CB, et al. Clinical response and risk for reported suicidal ideation and suicide attempts in pediatric antidepressant treatment: a meta-analysis of randomized controlled trials. *JAMA.* 2007;297(15):1683–1696

27. Gibbons RD, Hur K, Bhaumik DK, Mann JJ. The relationship between antidepressant prescription and rate of early adolescent suicide. *Am J Psychiatry.* 2006;163(11):1898–1904

28. Angst J. Major depression in 1998: are we providing optimal therapy? *J Clin Psychiatry.* 1999;60(suppl 6):5–9

29. The American Psychiatric Association and American Academy of Child and Adolescent Psychiatry. *Parent's Medical Guide: Parents Medication Guide*. Available at: www.parentsmedguide.org. Accessed March 16, 2010

30. Department of Health and Human Services, Food and Drug Administration. Psychopharmacologic Drugs Advisory Committee Notice of Meeting. Available at: www.fda.gov/AdvisoryCommittees/Calendar/ucm221386.htm. Accessed September 2, 2010

31. Volkmar F, Cook EH Jr, Pomeroy J, Realmuto G, Tanguay P. Practice parameters for the assessment and treatment of children, adolescents, and adults with autism and other pervasive developmental disorders. American Academy of Child and Adolescent Psychiatry Working Group on Quality Issues. *J Am Acad Child Adolesc Psychiatry.* 1999;38(12 suppl):32S–54S

32. *Physician's Desk Reference.* 63rd ed. Thomson Healthcare; 2009

33. Carlson GA. Early onset bipolar disorder: clinical and research considerations. *J Clin Child and Adolesc Psych.* 2005;34(2):333–343

34. McClellan J, Kowatch R, Findling RL. Practice parameters for the assessment and treatment of children and adolescents with bipolar disorder. American Academy of Child and Adolescent Psychiatry. *J Am Acad Child and Adolesc Psychiatry.* 2007;46(1):107–125

35. Bernstein GA, Shaw K. Practice parameters for the assessment and treatment of children and adolescents with anxiety disorders. American Academy of Child and Adolescent Psychiatry. *J Am Acad Child and Adolesc Psychiatry.* 1997;36(10 suppl):69S–84S

36. McClellan J, Werry J. Practice parameter for the assessment and treatment of children and adolescents with schizophrenia. American Academy of Child and Adolescent Psychiatry. *J Am Acad Child and Adolesc Psychiatry.* 2001; 40(7 suppl):4S–23S

37. Correll CU, Leucht S, Kane JM. Lower risk for tardive dyskinesia associated with second-generation antipsychotics: a systematic review of 1-year studies. *Am J Psychiatry.* 2004;161(3):414–425

38. Newcomer JW. Second-generation (atypical) antipsychotics and metabolic effects: a comprehensive literature review. *CNS Drugs.* 2005;19(suppl 1):1–93

39. American Diabetes Association. American Psychiatric Association. American Association of Clinical Endocrinologists. North American Association for the Study of Obesity. Consensus development conference on antipsychotic drugs and obesity and diabetes. *Diabetes Care.* 2004;27(2):596–601

40. American Psychiatric Association. Practice guideline for the treatment of patients with eating disorders (revision). American Psychiatric Association Work Group on Eating Disorders. *Am J Psychiatry.* 2000;157(1 suppl):1–39

41. Dulcan M. Practice parameters for the assessment and treatment of children, adolescents, and adults with attention-deficit/hyperactivity disorder. American Academy of Child and Adolescent Psychiatry. *J Am Acad Child Adolesc Psychiatry.* 1997;36(10 suppl):85S–121S

42. Steiner H. Practice parameters for the assessment and treatment of children and adolescents with conduct disorder. American Academy of Child and Adolescent Psychiatry. *J Am Acad Child Adolesc Psychiatry.* 1997;36(10 suppl):122S–139S

# CHAPTER 191

# Mental Health Treatment Modalities for Adolescents

PIETER LE ROUX, D LITT ET PHIL • CHRISTINA M. MCCANN, PhD

## OVERVIEW

This chapter focuses on the most prevalent modalities of psychotherapeutic treatment for adolescents and several theoretical orientations that guide treatment. These modalities include individual, family, and group psychotherapies, and are typically used when treating a variety of conditions. Some conditions responsive to the treatment modalities discussed in this chapter include: (1) common mental health disorders, such as mood and anxiety disorders; (2) developmental problems, including autism spectrum disorders, developmental delays, and learning problems accompanied by behavioral problems, and (3) adjustment disorders related to various life changes including divorce, grief, and loss, or transitions that adolescents experience. Treatment is discussed within the context of new developments in neuroscience, while the specific role of the primary care provider is outlined.

## THE CHANGING LANDSCAPE IN ADOLESCENT MENTAL HEALTH TREATMENT

Treatment for adolescent mental health problems has gone through continuous changes over the past century. From the initial work of Anna Freud and Melanie Klein, the psychotherapeutic approaches used with young children and adolescents have been influenced by a broad range of theoretical perspectives and scientific developments.[1] Adolescents are now benefiting from improved diagnostics that can result in earlier intervention. In addition, there is a better understanding of how to use combination therapies, such as pharmacology, in conjunction with outpatient psychotherapy (see Chapter 190, Adolescent Psychopharmacology).

Adolescents face different stressors and information overload based on the rapid progress in the field of technology and the ever-expanding role of the media. These trends parallel the increasing need for mental health and therapeutic services, given the growing pattern of earlier age of problem onset, greater problem severity, and increasing comorbidities in psychiatric and emotional disorders during childhood and adolescence. The prevalence of psychopathology in adolescents has been reported at 15%.[2] Specific issues that arise during adolescence can further affect mental health, such as male homosexual teenagers being at greater risk for attempted suicide.[3]

## RECENT CONTRIBUTIONS IN NEUROSCIENCE RELATED TO MENTAL HEALTH

Advances in brain imaging technology have facilitated a better understanding of specific neuronal growth patterns (see Chapter 5, Adolescent Brain and Cognitive Development). Magnetic resonance imaging (MRI) now allows for research on the structure of healthy developing brains, and functional MRI (*f*MRI) similarly poses no risk of radiation but assesses brain functioning using oxygenated versus nonoxygenated hemoglobin, which have different magnetic properties.[4] These technologies have helped define 2 critical periods of neuronal development after birth: infancy through 3 years, and the period approximately between 10 to 13 years of age.[5] These stages of development offer windows of opportunity for addressing genetic predisposition and environmental factors on mental health.

The principle "use it or lose it" applies during the adolescent phase of growth and development, when there is a significant increase in the brain's gray matter. The gray matter goes through a "pruning" stage[4,6] during this period. Giedd[4] notes there is a specific pattern to the pruning that starts caudally and progresses rostrally toward the frontal lobes, the last parts of the brain to mature.[4] The frontal cortex controls executive functioning, which affects the teenager's ability to make decisions, think about "thinking," and engage in planning or other higher-order processing.[4] Awareness of this critical period of brain growth throughout adolescence guides mental health treatment providers as they formulate diagnostic impressions and determine the best treatment plan.

The surge of brain growth during adolescence suggests that adolescents have increased opportunity to form and strengthen neural connections based on the activities in which they engage. The primary care provider can help guide the adolescent and family during this time to make the best choices for the future, especially because some adolescents are not yet equipped with long-term thinking aptitudes. For example, the adolescent who mainly plays video games and watches television during free time will enhance neural connections involved with these activities. Playing sports, learning a musical instrument, and engaging in positive and supportive relationships will affect other neural pathways that can help build skills used in adulthood and enhance self-esteem.

## MENTAL HEALTH TREATMENT AND THE ROLE OF PRIMARY CARE

Amid all of the neurological changes, adolescents are faced with matters requiring complex decision making, social and identity issues, and different environmental stressors.[7] Depending upon genetic predisposition, some adolescents are more vulnerable to development of mental health disorders, particularly when confronted with more stressful environments. The diathesis stress hypothesis proposes that individuals born with a higher predisposition to develop mental health problems would be more likely to develop these disorders even with less environmental stressors than individuals who do not have the genetic loading for mental health problems.[8] This highlights the need for primary care providers to be aware of potential life stressors during this life stage and to screen for mental health issues in adolescents as needed. It is not surprising that primary care providers are often confronted, and even challenged by overwhelming surges of problems that can arise in their patients during this period.

As discussed earlier, there is a window of opportunity in early adolescence during which this formative, transitional phase of development can be affected. Cognitive behavioral, interpersonal, family, and psychoeducational therapies have been shown to be effective in helping adolescents and their families through these difficult developmental periods, particularly when mental health problems arise.[9] Given the complexity of the psychoneurological development, together with the intricate needs of the adolescent and family, the most appropriate treatments for adolescents often are multimodal approaches, which can incorporate a combination of individual, family, and/or group therapies. Primary care providers can play a large role in assessing the need for mental health treatment, facilitating referral, and following up with patients to ensure their needs are being met.

## PSYCHOTHERAPEUTIC TREATMENT WITH ADOLESCENTS

The unique developmental trajectories of adolescents are important factors in understanding the key elements in adolescent psychotherapy. Successful treatment of adolescents therefore depends on multiple factors specific to the developmental needs and contextual factors surrounding the individual adolescent. Psychotherapy is not "one thing" or a single process. The American Psychological Association Task Force on Evidence-Based Practice defines evidence-based practice in psychology as "the integration of the best available research with clinical expertise in the context of patient characteristics, culture, and preferences."[10] The American Academy of Child and Adolescent Psychiatry Psychotherapy Task Force describes 3 essential elements of psychotherapy: (1) a clearly defined therapist/patient relationship, (2) specific relational context, such as an individual, group, or family therapy framework, and (3) conducted by a professional psychotherapist according to a theoretical model within specific frameworks for understanding psychopathology.[11] Adolescents can benefit from psychotherapy not only for treatment of major mental health disorders, but also to help address the array of developmental and transitional needs that they and their families face during this sometimes turbulent period.

A comprehensive intake process will help determine the best psychotherapeutic treatment plan. When collecting family history, the genogram or family tree is a useful tool that provides a structure for gathering relevant information, such as mental and physical health history, facts and perceptions about relationships, and knowledge about recent events, such as marriage, divorce, deaths, or other significant life events, in an easy-to-read format.[12] It often takes 2 or more sessions to complete the assessment, allowing for time alone with the adolescent and time with the adolescent and her or his parents.

A standard protocol used by clinicians during the intake process typically includes several key elements. The history of the presenting problem provides the focus of treatment. A mental status exam identifies thought and behavior patterns, as well as emotional strengths and vulnerabilities. The developmental and medical history is needed to uncover any predisposing conditions that might affect therapy. An educational and social history provides the 2 important contexts in which the adolescent is developing. The family history, including psychiatric and medical problems, is critical to identifying conditions that affect the presentation of adolescents with mental health problems. The family assessment should also include an exploration of important cultural and ethnic factors, as well as any stressors that the adolescent and/or family may have encountered over the past year. Taken together, this information will enable the goals for treatment to be established.[13]

## TREATMENT OUTCOMES

Treatment outcomes for mental health treatments for adolescents are influenced by several different factors. Developmental changes, the therapeutic alliance, and environmental and social influences are important factors that can affect successful change, as discussed in the following. Of note, the quality of the therapeutic relationship itself forms an important part of the therapeutic effectiveness.[14] Often, the parents' level of motivation for change is higher than that of the adolescent. Therefore, positive reinforcement, which can include verbal praise, privileges, and monetary rewards, can increase the adolescent's motivation level, thereby improving treatment outcome.

### DEVELOPMENTAL CHANGES

When working with adolescents, treatment providers should pay attention to developmental needs and changes. Some adolescents will present with additional challenges, such as verbal learning disabilities, which could affect talk therapy and how it is conducted. Even without any problems, several normative developmental changes of adolescence should be noted:

- Shifts in thinking include a move from preformal to formal operational thinking.[15] For example, adolescents begin to develop the capacity for abstract thought, even though they may still show impulsivity during decision making.
- Identity is not yet established and the personality is still developing, which can lead to a more egocentric view of the world.
- Self-concept is changing, so it can be confusing to identify and define the self. "What are my own feelings and thoughts? Who am I?"
- Sexuality issues and heightened emotional states are prominent. The therapist should be aware of any sexualized ways that the adolescent relates to others and help adolescents identify the emotions that they feel, which can lead to better understanding of what they are thinking. Adolescents often prefer same-sex therapists.
- Adolescents may lack good judgment on a developmental basis. There is a significant disconnect between their world and the real world, which puts them at risk to be exploited by peers and adults, especially with the continuing growth of "cyberspace."

### THERAPEUTIC ALLIANCE

It is especially important to establish a good therapeutic alliance with adolescents in treatment. Often times, adolescents are "dragged into treatment" by their parents and are sensitive and resistant to the idea that they need help. Key components of establishing a therapeutic relationship in preparation for effective mental health treatment with adolescents include:

- Establishing a collaborative, rather than a hierarchical or authoritarian, relationship with adolescent patients. The therapist should help the adolescent effectively communicate with parents and authority figures but be careful not to align too closely with either side.
- Establishing a good working relationship with the parents. The parents of adolescents are often equally challenged by the intensity of the developmental shifts displayed by their teenager.
- Demonstrating good listening skills, building trust and showing empathy, and being congruent.[14] When these factors are in place, adolescents will be more likely to disclose important issues they may not otherwise share.
- Approaching adolescents in psychotherapy with proactive, directive, and empathic interactions that include collaboration with immediate support systems, such as parents and families.[14]

### ENVIRONMENTAL AND SOCIAL FACTORS

Environmental and social influences strongly affect teenagers, and the inclusion of people involved in their social circle, such as family members, school personnel, other providers, or friends, can help address issues more effectively. To successfully address these factors the therapist can:

- Comment on emotional shifts during sessions to help the adolescent communicate what he or she is thinking and feeling;
- Avoid blaming the adolescent by externalizing the problem, rather than by indicating that the problem is caused by something inherently wrong with the patient;
- Explore issues further by showing curiosity and interest in the adolescent, not just the presenting problem or "chief complaint," which will also prevent misunderstanding on the part of the therapist;
- Model skills while doing therapy so the patient can learn by example and through experiencing new ways of relating with adults.

## BASIC PRINCIPLES OF INDIVIDUAL, FAMILY, AND GROUP PSYCHOTHERAPIES

Therapeutic interventions, such as individual, family, or group therapy can complement one another and be used alone or in combination, depending on the needs of the patient. Each of the modalities has a specific treatment focus for adolescents: **individual therapy** has an important role in helping adolescents develop a sense of identity; **family therapy** can help adolescents and their parents relate in new ways as the adolescent approaches adulthood, but sometimes can still slip back into the child role; **group therapy** can help validate adolescents' common experiences, particularly when they are facing a similar adversity such as a major mental health disorder, substance abuse, divorce of parents, or surviving sexual abuse. Adolescents often benefit from a combination of individual therapy that alternates with family therapy.

Regardless of modality and theoretical orientation, the therapeutic alliance is fundamentally important to successful outcomes. If the adolescent, adolescent's family member(s), or others closely involved with the adolescent are not comfortable with the therapist, this will likely have a detrimental effect on treatment outcome. Treatment techniques vary according to modality, although there can be some overlap, such as in the use of homework tasks and in-session activities including expressing feelings and learning about emotion regulation.

## INDIVIDUAL PSYCHOTHERAPY

Individual psychotherapy is based on the configuration of the therapist meeting alone with the patient. In the traditional sense of the word, it is a relationship based on confidentiality that excludes other people. However, for adolescents it is often useful to meet with the adolescent and the parent(s) together at times. The therapist can, for example, meet with the adolescent for a series of sessions alone, and then include a parent after the series of meetings. Alternatively, sessions including the parent can alternate with sessions involving the adolescent alone with the therapist. A session can also be split in half, meeting with the adolescent alone for part of the session and with both the parent and the adolescent for the rest of the session.

The task of the therapist is to elicit goals from the parent(s) and the adolescent. The adolescent may not initially have any goals, especially if he or she does not agree that treatment is needed in the first place. The therapist assists the adolescent in identifying treatment goals and creatively thinking about these goals. For example, establishing a goal such as "how to get your parents to leave you alone" could be a useful treatment goal to build communication skills: "Why don't you call your parent(s) when you will be late, so they will not need to call you." The therapist typically draws on a broad range of therapeutic techniques such as journaling, validating emotions, role-playing, and creative arts to help the adolescent achieve specified therapeutic goals. Individual therapy provides a protected space for the adolescent to define a sense of self and increase feelings of responsibility and accountability.

## FAMILY THERAPY

Family therapy is often indicated when treating adolescents. A family can be defined as "any group of people related either biologically, emotionally, or legally."[12] This broader definition of family reflects changes in family configurations in recent years and the importance of secure attachment to significant care providers during different stages of the developmental cycle for children as well as adolescents. Family therapy can include various combinations of people to meet treatment needs, ranging from parent–child; sibling–sibling; all or some immediate family members; extended family members; and people who are involved and important in the adolescent's life such as primary care providers, close friends, clergy members, school personnel, and other professionals or mentors.

Family therapy sessions typically last for 45 to 50 minutes, and duration of treatment depends on the specific needs of the family. Typical presenting problems include chaos in the family caused by poor boundaries and lack of parental control and limit setting, or when the family is experiencing a life transition, such as death, marriage, birth, or relocation. In family therapy, emphasis is placed on how external and relational factors among family members affect one another. The role of the therapist is to build rapport and engage all family members with goal-focused, strength-based communication to help them address the presenting problem. Homework tasks and in-session activities, such as mapping the family tree, focusing on specific family communication patterns, and strengthening the parental role to help with unclear boundaries, are designed to facilitate an active therapeutic approach that involves all family members, instead of focusing on the adolescent.

## GROUP PSYCHOTHERAPY

Adolescents relate strongly to their peers as they are pursuing autonomy and identity development, making group treatment particularly relevant. Group therapy is often more efficient for adolescents, helping several adolescents during one session. Groups tend to have 6 to 8 members, and sessions are typically 90 minutes with a predetermined duration of treatment, such as 12 weeks. The group therapist first facilitates group cohesion, which will allow group members to work effectively together in a safe environment.[16]

Based on the nature of the group and specific goals, the rules of communication, participation, and confidentiality are established. The group therapist relies heavily on "here and now" activities during group sessions, designed to facilitate skills building and to process emotion by utilizing interpersonal relationships within the group. Thus, group treatment can be especially helpful for adolescents when they are learning new skills (social skills, communication, anger management) or coping with a similar physiological or psychological adversity, such as cancer, sexual abuse, eating disorders, or substance abuse.

## THEORETICAL ORIENTATIONS OF INDIVIDUAL, FAMILY, AND GROUP PSYCHOTHERAPIES

Another dimension of mental health treatment for adolescents is the theoretical orientation and associated treatment modalities that emerge from those theories. Therefore, the format of each session can include the adolescent as an individual, as a member of a family, or as a member of a group. The process of therapy in each of these sessions, however, is directed by certain assumptions about how to best effect change during treatment. Cognitive behavioral therapy (CBT) is based on the assumption that an adolescent's emotions are the result of thoughts and behaviors. Interpersonal psychotherapy (IPT) focuses on an adolescent's behaviors in the context of relationships with others. Psychodynamic therapy is based on assumptions about the influence of past events in shaping internalized psychological processes. Systems theory makes assumptions about the way individuals in a family, which represents a system, can upset homeostasis and how treatment can re-establish balance in the family. Each of these treatment modalities will be explored in the following section.

### COGNITIVE BEHAVIORAL THERAPY

Cognitive behavioral therapy (CBT) utilizes a theoretical framework that focuses on how the patient perceives, thinks about, and interprets various situations, which leads to emotional and behavioral responses.[17] The way through which meaning is ascribed can trigger automatic thoughts or distorted thinking, resulting in problematic symptoms. For example, the teen who has a pimple on her cheek may notice that the cashier at the store smiles at her. She assumes the cashier is laughing because of her appearance, and she then treats the cashier in a rude manner. In reality, the cashier could have smiled because there was a baby in the shopping cart behind the teen.

Treatment using CBT is typically short term, with up to 20 sessions to successfully treat symptoms. The therapist structures the session with direct questions to find out the adolescent's unique interpretation of events. Questioning should be more casual and conversational in nature to help prevent the adolescent from feeling as if he or she is being interrogated.[18] It can be helpful to offer the adolescent "multiple choice answers" to question(s) asked if he or she cannot come up with an answer on his or her own or often states "I don't know." Some adolescents, especially younger ones, are not as verbal as others, so assigning journaling or brief writing assignments, or playing a game while talking, can help them express themselves further. Cognitive behavioral therapy is solution-focused and problem-solving oriented, with an emphasis on the "here and now." Specific techniques used in CBT include:[18]

- Thought stopping: prior to an exam at school, the adolescent imagines a "stop" sign every time she or he starts to think she or he is going to fail;
- Imagery: to improve self-image, the adolescent imagines walking down a school corridor, greeting peers with smiles and feeling confident;
- Relaxation training: the adolescent practices abdominal/deep breathing techniques that can be used with imagery to reduce anxiety and gain a sense of calm;
- Identifying and challenging distorted thoughts: the adolescent who says "I have no friends" (but parents can list several friends, and the patient has good social skills) can be challenged to provide proof to back up the distortion. When the evidence does not support that thought, alternative thoughts can be considered.

### INTERPERSONAL PSYCHOTHERAPY

Interpersonal psychotherapy is a short-term, goal-directed approach used to treat interpersonal difficulties related to conflict, disputes, role transitions, and loss.[19] Unlike CBT, IPT relies less on techniques to cope with symptoms and emphasizes how the adolescent relates to others. It focuses on the interpersonal domain by assessing how patterns of behavior relate to significant people in the adolescent's life. The therapist and adolescent enter into treatment together based on their formulation of a therapeutic contract that specifies the conditions for treatment, length of treatment, and goals. An important feature of IPT is that treatment ends when the contract specifies, instead of continuing.[19]

Treatment starts with developing a thorough interpersonal inventory designed to develop specific goals for therapy.[19] Central interpersonal systems for adolescents, including sources of significant relationships such as key family members, peers, and the school environment, are listed in the interpersonal inventory. One way to gather information for the inventory is to use the "closeness circle" approach, which involves a series of concentric circles that represent important relationships in the adolescent's life. The distance of the other person's circle from the adolescent's circle (center circle) represents the closeness of that relationship. Once the inventory has been completed, each relationship is discussed in more detail by assessing: (a) each person's interactions with the adolescent, (b) expectations for that relationship, (c) positive and negative features to the relationship, (d) changes that the adolescent would like to make in the relationship, and (e) how the presenting problem affects the relationship.[19]

During the middle phase of treatment, problem areas are explored in more detail and specific interpersonal problem-solving skills are built. The adolescent learns how to put these skills to use to reach the goals set in the contract. In the last phase of therapy, the adolescent and therapist review how the contract goals have been met and how to sustain positive changes. There are 4 areas where IPT is known to be effective:[19]

- Grief and loss (death of a loved one, rejection by a parent, diagnosis of a chronic illness);
- Interpersonal role disputes (parent sets limits for the adolescent, who fights against this, not wanting parent to set limits that restrict his or her freedom);
- Interpersonal role transitions (difficulty going away to college and leaving home);
- Interpersonal deficits (inability to express self to others, difficulty initiating contact with others, inability to share emotions).

## PSYCHODYNAMIC PSYCHOTHERAPY

Psychodynamic psychotherapy is rooted in the psychoanalytic theory of Sigmund Freud. The theory follows the concept that symptomatic behavior is learned in the past and maintained in the present by the patient's reaction to unconscious and internalized psychological processes. The therapist focuses on uncovering resistances that oppose self-knowledge and growth, and attempts to uncover repressed impulses by using interpretation of the interpersonal dynamics in the therapeutic relationship, as well as the patient's representation of behavior outside of therapy sessions.[20]

An essential part of psychodynamic treatment is the understanding of transference and countertransference. Transference refers to the adolescent projecting feelings toward the therapist that are meant for another person, and it can be helpful in treatment.[20] This allows the patient to work out issues with another person even if that person is not involved in treatment. Countertransference is a process that could interfere with the therapeutic relationship. Countertransference occurs when the therapist experiences emotional reactions toward the patient that originate from other interpersonal relationships in the therapist's life. It is important for the therapist to recognize countertransference and to seek consultation if needed.[20]

Theorists who base their work on Freud's initial ideas have acknowledged the importance of developmental crises, environmental factors, relationships with parents (attachment), and the influence of the family. Today, the principles of psychodynamic therapy can be found across the modalities of individual, family, and group therapy. Time-limited approaches, in contrast to the long-term approach followed by earlier psychodynamic therapists, have been developed in recent years.[21]

Psychodynamic treatment can be used with older adolescents who have repressed feelings and unresolved emotions caused by problems such as trauma, abuse, loss of a loved one, or internal conflict about sexual, race, or gender identity. For example, an adolescent girl might have recently lost her father in an automobile accident. He was having an affair with a woman who died in the car with him. The adolescent's mother is angry about the affair while also grieving her husband's death. The adolescent, who recently experienced her first sexual intercourse with her boyfriend, is now presenting with medically unexplained pelvic pain and is refusing further sexual relations with her boyfriend. There is no medical explanation for the pelvic pain, and the presence of major mental health disorders has been ruled out. Therefore, treatment would involve helping the adolescent work through her feelings, such as anger, guilt, sadness, and protectiveness toward her father. She also eventually expresses fears about trusting males. As she is able to identify and express these feelings, the pelvic pain resolves.

## SYSTEMS THEORY

Systems theory is based on the principle that "the whole is more than the sum of the parts." Systems maintain themselves through a process of homeostasis in which the behavior of one part affects the behavior of the others in the system to sustain continuity and predictability.[22] The family is considered an organic system that adapts to internal or external changes over time. Therefore, systems theory has been applied to the family to help create positive change. Systems theory can be used when working either with the family or just an individual in the family. Therapeutic approaches to family therapy vary in technique and focus of treatment.

As discussed earlier, adolescents are in the midst of identity development and are therefore focused on themselves and typically less tuned in to the needs of their family. Teenagers are often conflicted because they want to be independent, yet they also are not ready to sever ties with their families and live on their own. Parents can have a difficult time when their adolescent seeks independence, often feeling rejected by their "child" who used to look up to them. The principles of systems theory are well suited to help the adolescent and family through these developmental transitions. Interdependency among family members can be addressed specifically, as one person's behavior in the family affects all other family members. Family involvement in treatment helps sustain changes for each member of the family.

## CONCLUSION

The major psychotherapeutic modalities used for treatment with adolescents include individual, family, and group therapy. Various theoretical orientations help guide therapists as they work with adolescents and their families and offer specialized methods to help effect change and enhance problem solving. Different psychotherapies can work well in combination, such as individual and family therapy. A current trend in mental health treatment for adolescents includes multimodal and multisystemic approaches to severe problems such as ongoing juvenile delinquency, physical aggression, or chronic substance abuse, and outcome data for these approaches are promising.[23] In addition, treatment modalities are used in a variety of community contexts to better address specific needs, such as school-based and partial hospitalization programs. Neuroscience continues to shed new light on adolescent behavior by helping explain why adolescents have difficulty with planning and other higher-order processing and by identifying an additional period of neuronal growth during adolescence that can be used to help promote mental health. The primary care provider plays a pivotal role in screening for mental health problems and therefore needs to understand the treatment options available. The provider also recommends appropriate referrals while collaborating with those involved in the care of the adolescent.

## REFERENCES


1. Bernstein A. The psychoanalytic technique. In: Wolman BB, ed. *Handbook of Clinical Psychology*. New York, NY: McGraw-Hill; 1965:1168–1199

2. Staller JA. Diagnostic profiles in outpatient child psychiatry. *Amer J Orthopsychiatry.* 2006;76(1):98–102

3. Gutgesell ME, Payne N. Issues of adolescent psychological development in the 21st century. *Ped Review.* 2004;25(3): 79–85

4. Giedd JN. Structural magnetic resonance imaging of the adolescent brain. *Ann NY Acad Sci.* 2004;1021:77–85

5. Thompson PM, Giedd JN, Woods RP, MacDonald D, Evans A, Toga AW. Growth patterns in the developing brain detected by using continuum mechanical tensor maps. *Nature.* 2000;404(6774):190–193

6. Powell K. How does the teenage brain work? *Nature.* 2006;442:865–867

7. Siegel DJ. *The Developing Mind: Toward a Neurobiology of Interpersonal Experience*. New York, NY: Guilford Press; 1999

8. Butcher JN, Mineka S, Hooley JM. *Abnormal Psychology.* 12th ed. Boston, MA: Pearson Education, Inc; 2004

9. Chang K, Gallelli K, Howe M. Early identification and prevention of early-onset bipolar disorder. In: Romer D, Walker EF, eds. *Adolescent Psychopathology and the Developing Brain*. New York, NY: Oxford University Press, Inc; 2007:315–346

10. APA Presidential Task Force on Evidence-Based Practice. Evidence-based practice in psychology. *Amer Psychologist.* 2006;61(4):271–285

11. Ritvo R, Al-Mateen C, Ascherman L, et al. Report of the psychotherapy task force of the American Academy of Child and Adolescent Psychiatry. *J Psychother Pract Res.* 1999;8:93–102

12. McDaniel SH, Campbell TL, Hepworth J, Lorenz A. *Family-oriented Primary Care.* 2nd ed. New York, NY: Springer; 2005

13. McCann CM, le Roux P. Individual, family, and group therapy for adolescents. *Adolesc Med.* 2006;17:217–231

14. Oetzel KB, Bolton K, Scherer D. Therapeutic engagement with adolescents in psychotherapy. *Psychotherapy: Theory, Research, Practice, Training.* 2003;40(3):215–225

15. Piaget J. *The Growth of Logical Thinking from Childhood to Adolescence*. New York, NY: Basic Books; 1958

16. Yalom ID. *The Theory and Practice of Group Psychotherapy.* 5th ed. New York, NY: Basic Books; 2005

17. Beck JS. *Cognitive Therapy; Basics and Beyond*. New York, NY: Guilford Press; 1995

18. Wilkes TR, Belsher G, Rush AJ, Frank E. *Cognitive Therapy for Depressed Adolescents*. New York, NY: Guilford Press; 1994

19. Mufson L, Dorta KP, Moreau D, Weissman MM. *Interpersonal Psychotherapy for Depressed Adolescents.* New York, NY: Guilford Press; 2004

20. Meissner WW. The psychotherapies: individual, family, and group. In: Nicholi AM, ed. *The New Harvard Guide to Psychiatry*. Cambridge, MA: The Belknap Press of Harvard University Press; 1988:449–480

21. Levenson H. Time-limited dynamic psychotherapy: an integrationist perspective. *J Psychother Integrat.* 2003;13(324): 300–333

22. von Bertalanffy L. General system theory and psychiatry. In: *American Handbook of Psychiatry.* 2nd ed. (The foundations of psychiatry, vol. 1). New York, NY: Basic Books; 1974:1095–1117

23. Hogue A, Dauber S, Samuolis J, Liddle H. Treatment techniques and outcomes in multidimensional family therapy for adolescent behavioral problems. *J Family Psychol.* 2006; 20(4):535–543

# CHAPTER 192

# Neuropsychologic Testing of Adolescents

HEATHER R. ADAMS, PhD

## INTRODUCTION

Psychological assessment encompasses a range of methods and tools for evaluating cognitive, behavioral, mental health, and personality function. Any psychological assessment tool should optimally meet empirical standards of reliability and validity. Such assessment can be useful for establishing baseline functioning, informing treatment planning, and evaluating change in psychological or cognitive functions within the context of disease and its treatment. For example, psychological screening tools can serve as an efficient method to screen for mental health or behavioral concerns that present during a routine exam and to evaluate response to treatment. This chapter will review the indications for neuropsychological testing and then the process itself, with attention to the most common approaches to the assessment of adolescents with a suspected neuropsychiatric condition, including neuropsychological testing (NPT) and the assessment of behavior or personality disorders.

## NEUROPSYCHOLOGICAL TESTING

A primary goal of NPT is to describe an adolescent's pattern of cognitive strengths and weaknesses, and the relationship between cognitive test performance and underlying brain processes or pathology. Neuropsychological testing involves in-depth evaluation of attention, memory, language, visuomotor and visuoperceptual skills, and other cognitive functions. Neuropsychological testing can often identify subtle cognitive difficulties that may not be evident on a general assessment of intellectual ability or academic achievement. This is particularly true for adolescents with neurodevelopmental or neurological disorders, or injuries that may not be well understood in the school setting. Neuropsychological testing can also help determine if specific and potentially subtle cognitive profiles are consistent with underlying neuropathology. Within that context, recommendations can be made for cognitive rehabilitation and prognostic guides for expected recovery or for change in function over time.

### INDICATIONS FOR NEUROPSYCHOLOGICAL TESTING

Adolescents for whom NPT may be indicated include those with: (1) traumatic brain injury, (2) epilepsy, (3) spina bifida and hydrocephalus, (4) inherited and congenital neurodevelopmental conditions, (5) metabolic disorders such as phenylketonuria, (6) infections with central nervous system impact (such as meningitis or HIV), (7) neurotoxic exposures (eg, *in utero* drug exposure, lead, carbon monoxide poisoning, or extensive cancer treatment), (8) a history of prematurity or low birth weight. For example, adolescents with a history of being born at <33 weeks gestation and/or at very low birth weight have been found to have deficient performances on neuropsychological tests of abstract reasoning, learning, visuomotor integration, processing speed, and executive function.[1-4]

A school-based evaluation may identify global cognitive or achievement delays but fail to recognize other aspects of this cognitive pattern that could inform diagnosis, treatment, and monitoring. Neuropsychological impairments may also be found among adolescents with attention-deficit/hyperactivity disorder (ADHD), seizure disorders, and autism spectrum disorders. In these latter groups, NPT is not required for diagnostic purposes but can be useful to clarify individual patterns of cognitive strength and weakness that may help guide educational and treatment planning, and to monitor treatment response (eg, improved attentional performances in adolescents treated for ADHD with stimulant medication), as well as potential cognitive side effects of medical intervention (eg, antiepileptic drugs, surgical interventions).

Likewise, most school-based academic evaluations can establish the fundamental diagnosis and functional defects of a learning disability, but NPT can further elucidate neurocognitive processes affecting successful learning in a student with a learning disability. Neuropsychological testing may be warranted for adolescents for whom school-based evaluations and interventions have not resulted in satisfactory or expected improvement in learning difficulties, or the nature of the learning disability is not well understood.

## NEUROPSYCHOLOGICAL TESTING PROCESS

The role of the primary care physician is often the individual in the best position to initiate the referral of an adolescent for neuropsychological assessment to rule out organic brain disorder secondary to a neurodevelopmental or neurological condition. Although NPT can be quite useful in many instances, it may be contraindicated or not diagnostically necessary for teenagers with primary psychiatric diagnoses. These adolescents should first receive appropriate pharmacotherapy and psychotherapy to stabilize psychiatric symptoms before determining if NPT is indicated.

Many neuropsychologists who evaluate adolescents prefer to review any prior evaluations completed by the school. These evaluations can inform a deeper understanding of any school testing within the context of the neuropsychological evaluation results. Table 192-1 lists and describes some common neuropsychological

**Table 192-1**

**Some Common Neuropsychological Measures for Assessment of Adolescents**

| *Test Name* | *Domains Assessed* |
|---|---|
| **Fixed or flexible "omnibus" neuropsychological test batteries for adolescents** | |
| Halstead Reitan Neuropsychological Test Battery for Adults[5] | Attention, sensory functions (visual, auditory, tactual), language, spatial organization, executive function, memory, motor strength/dexterity |
| Luria-Nebraska Neuropsychological Battery[6] | Sensory functions, motor function, expressive and receptive language, reading, arithmetic, memory |
| NEPSY-II[7] | Attention, memory, expressive and receptive language, motor dexterity and speed, visuospatial function, executive function |
| Halstead Reitan Neuropsychological Test Battery for Children[8] | Attention, sensory functions (visual, auditory, tactual), language, visuospatial function, executive function, memory, motor strength/dexterity |
| **Tests of attention** | |
| Test of Everyday Attention for Children (TEA-Ch)[9] | Sustained, selective, divided attention, attentional switching, response inhibition |
| Trail-making tasks[5] | Visual attention and processing speed |
| Cancellation tasks[5] | Visual selective attention and processing speed |
| Digit span tasks (eg, WISC-IV; WAIS-III; WMS-III)[5] | Auditory attention and working memory |
| Visual span tasks (eg, Wechsler tests spatial span; WRAML Finger Windows)[5] | Visual attention and working memory |
| Children's Paced Auditory Serial Addition Task (CHIPASAT)[10] | Auditory selective attention, working memory, cognitive flexibility, math calculation |
| Continuous Performance Tasks: Test of Variables of Attention; Conners' Continuous Performance Test[5] | Computerized tests of visual and/or auditory selective and sustained attention, response inhibition, and reaction time |
| **Tests of memory and learning** | |
| Test of Memory and Learning-2 Edition (TOMAL-2)[11] | Verbal and nonverbal learning and memory; rote learning; contextual learning; associative learning sequential memory; immediate vs delayed recall; attention |
| Children's Memory Scale (CMS)[12] | Verbal and nonverbal learning and memory; rote learning, contextual learning, immediate vs delayed recall; attention and working memory |
| Verbal learning tests (eg, Hopkins, Rey Auditory Verbal Learning Test; California Verbal Learning Test; CVLT-Children's Version, Wide Range Assessment of Memory & Learning, etc)[5] | Rote verbal learning. Target word list is presented multiple times with recall tested after each presentation. Measures of immediate and delayed recall, cued and free recall, recognition |

*(Continued)*

**Table 192-1 (Continued)**

| *Test Name* | *Domains Assessed* |
|---|---|
| Complex Figure Tests (recall trials)[5] | Nonverbal/visual recall |
| Benton Visual Retention Test[13] | Nonverbal/visual recall |
| **Tests of executive function** | |
| Card sorting tests[5] | Concept formation, flexible thinking |
| Category tests[5] | Concept formation, flexible thinking |
| Contingency Naming Test; Stroop Color-Word Test[5] | Flexible thinking, rapid processing, response inhibition |
| Tower tests (eg, Tower of London; NEPSY Tower test)[5] | Planning |
| Delis Kaplan Executive Function System (DKEFS)[14] | Concept formation, flexible thinking, response inhibition, processing speed, fluency, abstract thinking |
| Verbal Fluency; Design Fluency tasks[5] | Verbal/visual processing speed, fluency, cognitive flexibility |
| Mazes tasks[5] | Visual reasoning, planning |
| Behavior Rating Inventory of Executive Function (BRIEF)[15] | Parent, teacher, and self-informant ratings of executive function domains: planning, working memory, organization, behavioral inhibition, emotional regulation, self-monitoring |
| **Tests of expressive and receptive language** | |
| Peabody Picture Vocabulary Test-Fourth Edition (PPVT-IV)[16] | Single word recognition |
| Boston Naming Test[17] | Single word naming |
| Expressive One Word Picture Vocabulary Test (EOWPVT)[18] | Single word naming |
| Token Test for Children (versions reviewed in Baron, 2004)[19] | Comprehension of multistep verbal instructions |
| SSPT[19,20] | Attention, auditory perception/discrimination |
| Clinical Evaluation of Language Fundamentals (CELF-4)[21] | Expressive and receptive language |
| **Tests of visuospatial processing** | |
| Rey-Osterrieth Complex Figure (ROCF)[5] | Visuomotor integration; reproduction of complex geometric design |
| Beery VMI[22] | Visuomotor integration of 2-dimensional designs |
| Judgment of Line Orientation test (JLO)[23] | Nonmotor visuospatial/visuoperceptual function |
| Hooper Visual Organization Test (VOT)[24] | Nonmotor visual integration |
| **Motor function** | |
| Pegboard tests (eg, Grooved Pegboard test; Purdue Pegboard test)[5] | Bilateral dexterity and motor speed |
| Grip Strength[5] | Bilateral hand grip strength |
| Finger Tapping[5] | Bilateral dexterity and speed |
| Reitan-Kløve Sensory Perceptual Examination[25] | Sensation and perception (visual, tactile, auditory) |
| **Further reading in neuropsychology** | |
| Lezak et al (2004). Neuropsychological Assessment, 4th Edition | |
| Baron IS (2004). Neuropsychological Evaluation of the Child | |
| Strauss et al (2006). A Compendium of Neuropsychological Tests, 3rd Edition | |
| Spreen et al (1995). Developmental Neuropsychology | |
| Reynolds CR, Fletcher-Janzen E (2008). Handbook of Clinical Child Neuropsychology | |

measures used with adolescents. Comprehensive reviews of many more neuropsychological tests, including discussions of clinical applications, reliability, and validity, are available.[19,26,27] Evaluation of adolescents typically involves a "flexible" testing approach in which a core set of neuropsychological tests are used for all adolescents being assessed for standardized evaluation of key cognitive processes, such as attention and memory, with additional tests included as dictated by the clinical questions and practical constraints, such as time limits and the adolescent's own tolerance of the evaluation.

In some cases, a "fixed" battery of invariant tests is administered to all patients. For adolescents, options for a fixed test battery include the Halstead Neuropsychological Test Battery (9–14 years) or the Halstead Reitan Neuropsychological Test Battery (age ≥15).[8] Another fixed test battery for adolescents (ages ≥12) is the Luria-Nebraska test.[28] Within the constraints of this fixed test battery there is room for clinical interpretation of individual test performances.

Intrinsic and extrinsic factors can affect the reliability and validity of NPT. Mood and mental state, effort and motivation, and energy and physical health on the day of the evaluation can influence performance. Generalized anxiety or test performance anxiety can interfere with attentional focus, processing speed, and recall of information. Extrinsic factors such as noisy or disruptive test setting or an unqualified examiner can also affect the validity of testing results. When possible, acute medical and psychiatric problems should be stabilized before undertaking NPT.

## BEHAVIOR, MOOD, AND PERSONALITY ASSESSMENT IN ADOLESCENTS

In providing health care to adolescents, behavioral assessments and related screening tools are among the most widely used measures by clinicians. Assessment of adolescent behavioral problems, mood, and personality may be critical to assist with screening, diagnosis, and treatment management of common presenting problems including ADHD, depression, anxiety, and oppositional-defiant or conduct disorders. Multi-informant rating scales that collate information from parents, teachers, and self-ratings of problem behaviors are useful for describing a broad range of mood and behavior problems across multiple settings and perspectives. For evaluation of externalizing problems, such as ADHD or conduct problems, adult ratings by parents and teachers are useful as adolescents with externalizing behaviors may minimize or not be fully aware of the impact of their negative behaviors upon others. For internalizing problems, such as anxiety or depression, self-ratings by the adolescent provide insight into mood experiences that may not be well understood by outside observers.

### BEHAVIOR AND MOOD ASSESSMENT

Among the most commonly used and most extensively validated scales are the Achenbach System of Empirically Based Assessment (ASEBA).[29-32] The ASEBA forms include self, parent, and teacher-rating scales for individuals from preschool age through adulthood. Problem behavior items on the ASEBA forms are organized in empirically derived factors defining various symptom clusters or syndromes: (1) anxiety, (2) depressed mood, (3) physical complaints, (4) social problems, (5) thought problems, (6) inattention, and (7) noncompliance/defiance. These syndrome scales include age- and sex-based normative comparisons. Thus, parental ratings of depressive symptoms in an adolescent girl can be compared to those of her same-age peers to assess their clinical significance and severity.

The Child Behavior Check List (CBCL) is a key Achenbach tool that is hierarchically organized; groups of lower-order syndrome scales combine to define intermediate composite factors of internalizing (anxious and depressed mood, somatic complaints) and externalizing (rule-breaking and aggression) problems. When combined with other syndrome scales, the CBCL defines an overarching "Total Problems" factor. Finally, there are *DSM-IV-TR* oriented scales containing CBCL items that are keyed to the *Diagnostic and Statistical Manual of Mental Disorders, Fourth Edition, Text Revision* (*DSM-IV-TR*) symptom criteria for various adolescent mental health concerns, including anxiety, depression, ADHD, conduct disorder, and oppositional-defiant disorder. Although these *DSM-IV-TR*-based CBCL scales cannot be used in isolation to establish diagnoses of adolescent behavior/mood disorders, elevations on these scales can serve as "red flags" for further assessment.

Other well-validated multi-informant tests include the recently revised Conners' Comprehensive Behavior Rating Scales[33] and the second edition of the Behavioral Assessment System for Children (BASC-2).[34] These form sets and the CBCL are available in Spanish and various other languages, and each have been used to evaluate behavioral problems in a range of medical and psychiatric disorders, in addition to unselected adolescent groups. There are also rating scales that target specific problem areas when further information is desired for an already-identified area of concern. For example, the Children's Depression Inventory (CDI)[35] normed for adolescents up to 18 years of age consists of 27 multiple-choice items. Easily completed within 15 minutes, the CDI provides details on affective, cognitive, and physiologic symptoms of depression, such as sad mood,

**Table 192-2**

**Tools to Assess Behavioral, Emotional, and Personality Problems in Adolescents**

| *Test Name* | *Informants* |
|---|---|
| **Omnibus assessment measures of behavioral/emotional function in adolescents** | |
| Achenbach System of Empirically Based Assessment (ASEBA)[29,31] | Parent, teacher, self-rating forms |
| Conners' Rating Scales[36] | Parent, teacher, self-rating forms |
| Behavior Assessment System for Children—Second Edition (BASC-2)[34] | Parent, teacher, self-rating forms |
| NIMH Diagnostic Interview Schedule for Children (DISC)[37] | Parent, self-report |
| Schedule for Affective Disorders and Schizophrenia for School-Age Children—Present and Lifetime Version (K-SADS-PL)[38] | Parent, self-report |
| Revised Version of the Diagnostic Interview for Children and Adolescents (DICA-R)[39] | Parent, self-report |
| **Depression** | |
| Children's Depression Inventory (CDI)[40] | Parent, teacher, self-rating forms |
| Beck Depression Inventory (BDI)[41] | Self-report |
| Reynolds Adolescent Depression Scale (RADS)[42] | Self-report |
| **Anxiety** | |
| Revised Children's Manifest Anxiety Scale —Second Edition (RCMAS-2)[43] | Self-report |
| Multidimensional Anxiety Scale for Children (MASC)[44] | Self-report |
| Anxiety Disorders Interview Schedule for Children —Child & Parent Versions[45] | Parent, self-report |
| **Further reading** | |
| Silverman WK Ollendick TH. Evidence-based assessment of anxiety and its disorders in children and adolescents. *J Clin Child Adolesc Psychol.* 2005;34(3):380–411. | |
| **Attention-deficit/hyperactivity disorder (ADHD)** | |
| DuPaul ADHD Rating Scale[46] | Adult informant |
| Vanderbilt ADHD Rating Scales[47–49] | Parent, teacher |
| Brown Attention-Deficit Disorder Scales for Adolescents and Adults[50] | Parent, teacher, self-report |
| **Further reading** | |
| Pelham WE Jr et al. Evidence-based assessment of attention deficit hyperactivity disorder in children and adolescents. *J Clin Child Adolesc Psychol.* 2005; 34(3):449–476. | |
| **Personality** | |
| Minnesota Multiphasic Personality Inventory for Adolescents (MMPI-A)[51] | Self-report |
| Personality Assessment Inventory—Adolescents[52] | Self-report |
| Millon Adolescent Personality Inventory (MAPI)[53] | Self-report |

negative thoughts, and sleep and appetite problems, respectively. Comprehensive guidelines for assessment and treatment of adolescent disorders were published recently in *Pediatrics*.[54,55] A list of various common omnibus rating scales and problem-specific rating forms are summarized in Table 192-2.

In addition to diagnostic screening, rating forms can be helpful for monitoring treatment progress over time. For example, in adolescents with ADHD, serial assessment with the 18-item ADHD Rating Scale[56,57] can monitor therapeutic response during dose titration of a stimulant medication. In a primary adolescent health care practice, broad-based, multi-informant measures can ensure that "no stone is left unturned" during comprehensive screening of most common behavioral and emotional disorders. On the other hand, the symptom- or syndrome-specific measures are useful for more detailed evaluation and monitoring of treatment response. Whenever there are concerns for clinically significant problems based on rating scale results, an in-depth psychological and/or psychiatric evaluation may be warranted.

**PERSONALITY ASSESSMENT**

There are several common personality assessment measures for adolescents including the Minnesota Multiphasic Personality Assessment for Adolescents (MMPI-A), the Personality Inventory for Children (PIC; ages 6–19), and the Personality Assessment Inventory for Adolescents (PAI-A; ages 12–18). Each is a well-validated omnibus measure of adolescent personality and is used for in-depth evaluation of adolescent psychopathology. These measures are also used in empirical research of personality characteristics associated with adolescent substance abuse, criminal behavior, eating disorders, emergent adult personality disorders, sexual abuse, and various psychiatric disorders. However, their length (may involve 200–300 questions and at least 1 hour to administer) and the complexity of interpretation generally precludes their use in a general office, clinic, or school-based adolescent health care practice.

**PROJECTIVE TESTS**

On occasion, a health care provider may be asked to review the results of projective psychological testing. Projective evaluation methods, used in tests such as the Rorschach Inkblot test or the Thematic Apperception Test (TAT), are based upon the assumption that an adolescent's responses to ambiguous stimuli may provide insight into underlying personality characteristics and psychological states. Projective testing can be lengthy and should be done only by psychologists or psychiatrists fully trained in projective assessment methods. Projective assessment of adolescents and adults remains controversial. In summarizing research and controversies on the Rorschach test, it has been recommended that "clinicians choosing the Rorschach should be able to articulate a rationale explaining why it is likely to be valuable with a particular patient who presents a distinctive set of referral questions to be addressed."[58] This advice would also seem applicable to other projective methods and more generally to psychological assessment overall.

## SUMMARY

Psychological assessment of the adolescent serves a broad range of purposes including evaluation of general intellectual ability and a range of specific cognitive processes, identification and monitoring of learning disabilities, determination of academic and vocational placements, screening for behavioral and mental health concerns, and evaluating treatment response. The relevant clinical highlights related to the assessment of behavior, mood, and personality have been detailed. The clinician needs to keep in mind that in conducting any form of psychological assessment, emphasis should be placed upon the use of reliable and valid assessment methods and measures, and a clear understanding of the reason for the evaluation and the type of information to be gained.

## REFERENCES

1. Nosarti C, Giouroukou E, Micali N, Rifkin L, Morris RG, Murray RM. Impaired executive functioning in young adults born very preterm. *J Int Neuropsychol Soc.* 2007;13(4):571–581

2. D'Angio C, Sinkin RA, Stevens TP, et al. Longitudinal, 15-year follow-up of children born at less than 29 weeks' gestation after introduction of surfactant therapy into a region: neurologic, cognitive, and educational outcomes. *Pediatrics.* 2002;110(6):1094–1102

3. Allin M, Salaria S, Nosarti C, Wyatt J, Rifkin L, Murray RM. Vermis and lateral lobes of the cerebellum in adolescents born very preterm. *NeuroReport.* 2005;16(16):1821–1824

4. Parker J, Mitchell A, Kalpakidou A, et al. Cerebellar growth and behavioural and neuropsychological outcome in preterm adolescents. *Brain.* 2008;131(5):1344–1351

5. Lezak M, Howieson D, Loring D, Hannay J, Fischer J. *Neuropsychological Assessment-4th Edition.* New York, NY: Oxford University Press; 2004

6. Golden C, Hammeke T, Purisch A. *A Manual for the Administration and Interpretation of the Luria-Nebraska Neuropsychological Battery.* Los Angeles, CA: Western Psychological Services; 1980

7. Korkman M, Kirk U, Kemp S. *NEPSY®-Second Edition (NEPSY®-II).* San Antonio, TX: Psychological Corporation; 2007

8. Reitan R. *The Halstead Reitan Neuropsychological Test Battery: Theory and Clinical Interpretation.* Tucson, AZ: Neuropsychology Press; 1993

9. Manly T, Robertson I, Anderson A, Nimmo-Smith I. *The Test of Everyday Attention for Children (TEA-Ch).* Bury St Edmunds, Suffolk, England: Thames Valley Test Company; 1999

10. Johnson D, Roethig-Johnston K, Middleton J. *Children's Paced Auditory Serial Addition Test (Chi-PASAT)*; 1988

11. Reynolds C, Voress J. *Test of Memory and Learning-2nd Edition (TOMAL-2).* Austin, TX: Pro-Ed; 2007

12. Cohen M. *Children's Memory Scale.* San Antonio, TX: The Psychological Corporation; 1997

13. Benton Sivan A. *Benton Visual Retention Test-5th Edition.* San Antonio, TX: The Psychological Corporation; 1991

14. Delis D, Kaplan E, Kramer J. *Delis Kaplan Executive Function System (DKEFS).* San Antonio, TX: The Psychological Corporation; 2001

15. Gioia G, Isquith P, Guy S, Kenworthy L. *Behavior Rating Inventory of Executive Function (BRIEF)*. Odessa, FL: PAR, Inc; 2000

16. Dunn L, Dunn L. *Peabody Picture Vocabulary Test–Third Edition (PPVT-III)*. Circle Pines, MN: American Guidance Service, Inc; 1997

17. Kaplan E, Goodglass H, Weintraub S. *Boston Naming Test (revised 60-item version)*. Philadelphia, PA: Lea & Febiger; 1983

18. Gardner M. *Expressive One-Word Picture Vocabulary Test–2000 Edition*. Novato, CA: Academic Therapy Publications; 2000

19. Baron I. *Neuropsychological Evaluation of the Child*. New York, NY: Oxford University Press; 2004

20. Reitan R. Manual for Administration of Neuropsychological Test Batteries for Adults and Children. Unpublished manuscript; 1969

21. Semel E, Wiig E, Secord W. *Clinical Evaluation of Language Fundamentals, 4th Edition (CELF-4)*. San Antonio, TX: The Psychological Corporation; 2003

22. Beery K, Beery N. *Beery VMI (The Beery-Buktenica Developmental Test of Visual-Motor Integration, 5th Edition)*. San Antonio, TX: Pearson; 2004

23. Benton A, Varney N, Hamsher K. Visuospatial judgment: a clinical test. *Archives of Neurology.* 1978;35:364–367

24. Hooper H. *Hooper Visual Organization Test.* Los Angeles, CA: Western Psychological Services; 1983

25. Reitan R. *Aphasia and Sensory-Perceptual Deficits in Children*. Tucson, AZ: Neuropsychology Press; 1984

26. Lezak M, Howieson D, Loring D, Hannay H, Fischer J. *Neuropsychological Assessment*. New York, NY: Oxford University Press; 2004

27. Strauss E, Sherman E, Spreen O. *A Compendium of Neuropsychological Tests: Administration, Norms, and Commentary*. 3rd ed. New York, NY: Oxford University Press; 2006

28. Golden C, Purisch A, Hammeke T. *The Luria-Nebraska Neuropsychological Battery: A Manual for Clinical and Experimental Uses*. Lincoln, NE: University of Nebraska Press; 1979

29. Achenbach T, Rescorla L. *Manual for the ASEBA School-Age Forms and Profiles*. Burlington, VT: University of Vermont, Research Center for Children, Youth, & Families; 2001

30. Achenbach TM. *Child Behavior Checklist/1 1/2–5*. TM Achenbach; 2002

31. Achenbach TM. *Child Behavior Checklist/6–18*. TM Achenbach; 2002

32. Achenbach TM, Rescorla LA. *Manual for ASEBA Adult Forms and Profiles*. Burlington, VT: Research Center for Children, Youth, & Families; 2003

33. Conners K. *Conners' Comprehensive Behavior Rating System*. North Tonawanda, NY: Multi-Health Systems; 2008

34. Reynolds C, Kamphaus RW. *Behavior Assessment System for Children–2 nd Edition (BASC-2)*. Bloomington, MN: Pearson Assessments; 2004

35. Kovacs M. *Children's Depression Inventory*. North Tonawanda, NY: Multi-Health Systems; 1992

36. Conners C. Conners' *Rating Scales – Revised*. North Tonawanda, NY: Multi-Health Systems, Inc; 2001

37. Schaffer D, Fisher P, Lucas C, Comer J. *Scoring Manual: Diagnostic Interview Schedule for Children (DISC-IV)*. New York, NY: Columbia University; 2003

38. Kaufman J, Birmaher B, Brent D, et al. Schedule for affective disorders and schizophrenia for school-age children—present and lifetime version (K-SADS-PL): initial reliability and validity data. *J Am Acad Child Adolesc Psychiatry.* 1997;36:980–988

39. Reich W, Welner Z. *Revised Version of the Diagnostic Interview for Children and Adolescents (DICA-R)*. St Louis, MO: Department of Psychiatry, Washington University School of Medicine; 1988

40. Kovacs M. *Children's Depression Inventory. Technical Manual Update.* North Tonawanda, NY: Multi-Health Systems, Inc; 2003

41. Beck A, Steer R, Brown G. *Beck Depression Inventory®-II (BDI®-II)*. Bloomington, MN; Pearson Assessments; 1996

42. Reynolds W. *Reynolds Adolescent Depression Scale–2nd Ed (RADS-2).* Lutz, FL: PAR, Inc; 1988

43. Reynolds C, Richmond B. *Revised Children's Manifest Anxiety Scale: Second Edition (RCMAS-2).* Los Angeles, CA: Western Psychological Services; 2008

44. March J. *Multidimensional Anxiety Scale for Children (MASC)*. North Tonawanda, NY: Multi-Health Systems, Inc; 1997

45. Silverman WK, Nelles WB. The anxiety disorders interview schedule for children. *J Am Acad Child Adolesc Psychol*. 1988;27:772–778

46. DuPaul G, Power T, Anastopoulos A, Reid R. *ADHD Rating Scale-IV. Checklists, Norms, and Clinical Interpretation* New York, NY: The Guilford Press; 1998

47. Wolraich M, Feurer I, Hannah J, Baumgaertel A, Pinnock T. Obtaining systematic teacher reports of disruptive behavior disorders utilizing DSM-IV. *J Abnorm Child Psychol.* 1998;26(2):141–152

48. Wolraich M, Hannah J, Baumgaertel A, Feurer I. Examination of DSM-IV criteria for ADHD in a county-wide sample. *J Dev Behav Pediatrics.* 1998;19:162–168

49. Wolraich M, Lambert W, Doffing M, Bickman L, Simmons T, Worley K. Psychometric properties of the Vanderbilt ADHD Diagnostic Parent Rating Scale. *J Pediatr Psychol.* 2004;28:559–568

50. Brown T. *Brown ADD Scales for Children and Adolescents*. San Antonio, TX: Psychological Corp; 2001

51. Butcher J, Williams C, Graham J, et al. *Minnesota Multiphasic Personality Inventory-Adolescent*. Bloomington, MN: Pearson Assessments; 2006

52. Morey LC. *Personality Assessment Inventory-Adolescent*. Lutz, FL: PAR, Inc; 2005. Available at: www4.parinc.com/products/product.aspx?Productid=PAI-A. Accessed June 21, 2009

53. Millon T, Green C, Meagher Jr R. *Millon Adolescent Personality Inventory*. Bloomington, IN: Pearson Education Assessments; 2008. Available at: www.pearsonassessments.com/mapi.aspx. Accessed June 21, 2009

54. Cheung A, Zuckerbrot R, Jensen P, et al. Guidelines for adolescent depression in primary care (GLAD-PC): II. Treatment and ongoing management. *Pediatrics*. 2007;120(5):e1313–e1326

55. Zuckerbrot R, Cheung A, Jensen P, Stein R, Laraque D, and the GLAD-PC Steering Group. Guidelines for adolescent depression in primary care (GLAD-PC): I. Identification, assessment, and initial management. *Pediatrics*. 2007;120(5):e1299–e1312

56. DuPaul G. Parent and teacher ratings of ADHD symptoms: psychometric properties in a community-based sample. *J Clin Child Psychol*. 1981;20:245–253

57. DuPaul G. *ADHD Rating Scale-IV: Checklists, Norms, and Clinical Interpretation*. New York, NY: The Guilford Press; 1998

58. Meyer G, Archer R. The hard science of Rorschach research: what do we know and where do we go? *Psychological Assessment*. 2001;13(4):486–502

SECTION 4

# Educational Issues

# CHAPTER 193

## Academic Overachievement and Underachievement

STEVEN E. TOBIAS, PsyD • NANETTE C. SUDLER, PhD

### DEFINITIONS

Overachievement (OA) and underachievement (UA) are significant discrepancies between ability and performance that cause emotional distress. Both are matters of degree and there are no universally accepted specific criteria for determining OA or UA, either in terms of academic performance or emotional impairment. In addition, a formal judgment of OA or UA requires that the problem behaviors be habitual; however, inconsistencies may be seen in school performance, either within subjects or between subjects. Frequently, parents experience emotional distress and, in fact, it is often the parent who will express concern rather than the adolescent. It is common for adolescents who underachieve or overachieve to deny the problem and the emotional difficulty and state that it is the reporting parent or teacher with the problem.

Overachievement and UA can be seen as variations of the "fight or flight" response to stress during the adolescent years, when OA and UA are most common. The stress may be due to normal adolescent issues such as a search for individual identity, conflicted relations with parents, or concerns related to independence, responsibility, and self-reliance. Other more severe causal or comorbid impairments can exist. These include obsessive–compulsive disorder (OCD), drug use, parent–child problems, anxiety, or depression. To complicate this further, disabilities such as attention-deficit/hyperactivity disorder (ADHD) and learning disabilities, if undiagnosed, may present similarly to UA or be exacerbated by UA. Adolescents may have various combinations of these disorders, such as an individual with UA, ADHD, a learning disability, depression, and parent–child conflict, all of which may lead the adolescent to engage in risk-taking behaviors.

With OA, the response to stress is to "fight" or accelerate one's effort. Although this may be seen as a positive reaction and some have noted better adjustment in students who perform above their innate intelligence, others have found negative consequences such as anxiety, depression, or social withdrawal.[1] Overachievement, as defined, is accompanied by significant emotional distress. It may be an attempt to compensate for feelings of inadequacy related to fear of failure, or an attempt to be "perfect" to please a parent. Ironically, the attempt to excel can ultimately inhibit career achievement. Just because one has achieved at a high level in school does not ensure that one will succeed in the workplace where different skills, especially in the social–emotional area, are necessary. An additional concern regarding OA is the potential for "burnout," where an individual literally pushes so hard that he or she is left exhausted with little emotional resources remaining to persevere, leaving him or her in despair.

Underachievement can be seen as a "flight" response to stress, an avoidance of the academic stressor. By definition UA cannot be due primarily to a learning disability, which also is a discrepancy between potential and achievement. The distinction is that students with learning disabilities have processing deficits that inhibit learning whereas motivation is the primary impediment to learning for the UA students. Interestingly, a primary group of underachievers is gifted students and it has been estimated that 15% to 40% of gifted students potentially are underachieving.[2] Most supplemental educational programs address low-achieving students rather than the gifted. For example, the "No Child Left Behind Act" addresses the needs of students who are functioning below grade level rather than those who are not meeting their potential, thus perhaps underrecognizing and underserving the needs of this population.

## ETIOLOGY

Societal factors potentially are escalating the incidence of OA and UA. Academic demands are intensifying in schools at all levels. A generation ago, the focus of kindergarten was socialization, now it is academic achievement. The more academic stress placed on some students and the less time they are allowed to mature and develop social and emotional skills, the more they will either internalize the expectation and overachieve, or reject it and underachieve.

Another societal factor is ubiquitous entertainment technology. One symptom of UA is distraction from schoolwork. From video games to text messaging, there are abundant opportunities for students to do something other than their work. Ironically, UA students do not end up enjoying their leisure time when they are procrastinating from their work.[3]

An additional societal factor is the nature of family involvement. If parents and extended family are not physically and/or psychologically present to monitor and guide adolescents, achievement difficulties can arise. Similarly, the opposite parenting extreme of overinvolvement creates children who are insecure and overly dependent on their parents, adversely affecting achievement and emotional well-being. Although cultural factors may contribute to OA and UA, this aspect is beyond the scope of this chapter and, regardless, students must be viewed as individuals, each with unique circumstances and motivations.

Depression can be associated with OA and UA. In each case, there is a lack of emotional meaning in work. Work is not enjoyed, nor is pride taken in achievement. It is either a necessity that must be done, or a burden to avoid. Overachievement may be an attempt to ward off feelings of inadequacy and low self-esteem. Underachievement may be due to the inability to exert mental energy toward a goal. Some students may be afraid of growing up and accepting adult responsibility due to their feelings of inadequacy; UA successfully maintains their dependency.

Anxiety often accompanies OA and UA. Students with OA may use work to overcompensate for feelings of inadequacy. In addition, the stress of maintaining a high level of performance may cause undue anxiety. Perfectionism and other traits of OCD can be related to OA. The student with UA may be responding to the same stresses but have the opposite reaction. They worry they are not "good enough" and therefore do not try. They avoid doing schoolwork so they have an external reason for failure, which is a defense against internal feelings of inadequacy. For example, their cognitions may be, "I could do it if I tried, I just don't want to." Procrastination, although commonly perceived as laziness, is usually an indication of underlying anxiety and work avoidance.

Underachievement is more readily noted as a problem, and, therefore, more thoroughly researched. Underachieving students tend to be bright but do not put forth the effort necessary to consistently achieve grades commensurate with their ability. This becomes increasingly apparent as the student progresses in school. In elementary school, these students rely on their innate intelligence. An early warning sign is good grades despite difficulty with homework, mundane tasks, studying, and completing long-term assignments. By middle and high school, these students' grades begin to decline as the work becomes increasingly complex and substantial, especially if enrolled in academically advanced classes. At this point it is likely that the students with UA have failed to establish the work-study habits needed to achieve at higher academic levels. An important note is that most students who underachieve will verbalize motivation to do well. They do care about their grades and are ashamed of their poor performance. Underachievement is a chronic problem, which is not likely to be outgrown unless treated. Some adolescents eventually are able to overcome their UA independently, but many grow into underachieving adults. As employability becomes progressively more related to education, nonacademic avenues to success will be increasingly limited.

Students with UA are not a homogeneous group[4] but do share several characteristics. They lack self-discipline, which basically is the ability to do what you do not feel like doing at the moment. Difficulty delaying gratification makes them focus on immediate pleasures rather than on future goals. Ordinary, mundane tasks as well as challenging tasks are avoided. Some students with UA escape into socializing, video games, or even reading. They fail to accept responsibility for themselves because they fear personal responsibility. Thus, this avoidance results in students externalizing blame for their UA (eg, "It is the teacher's fault" or "It was a dumb assignment"). Some students with UA pathologize themselves and blame a learning disability, ADHD, or some other diagnosed excuse for failure (although they may indeed also have these disabilities). Believing that they cannot succeed results in feelings of low self-efficacy. Their success or failure is perceived to be beyond their own control. Consequently, they do not set goals for themselves or set unrealistic goals and engage in magical thinking that things will "just happen" for them. Generally, they have negative feelings about work and careers, which inadvertently may have been modeled by parents.

Students with UA are dependent in their work. They fail to regulate their own behavior and require close monitoring to complete tasks. They may do well on tests due to their innate intelligence but have difficulty with homework and long-term assignments. Their grades are inconsistent and may depend on their relationship with the teacher. A lack of self-awareness creates the capacity to lie to themselves. Thus, they can truly be unaware of their feelings, goals, actions, and consequences.

There are a variety of potential causes of UA. As previously mentioned, parents may be over- or under-involved with their children. Overinvolved parents can cause the student to underachieve as a means of rebelling and establishing a separate identity. Underinvolved parents do not teach students to value education or work and do not provide necessary limit-setting and guidance. Early health problems or tragic experiences can put children at risk for UA in that they are perceived as fragile, resulting in few demands and expectations placed on them. Having a high-achieving older sibling is another risk factor because the younger child may feel like he or she cannot compete with the older sibling, or he or she develops a separate identity by not achieving. Children who have been labeled by parents as "lazy" or "not a student" can fulfill these expectations. Family stress is another potential cause, such as divorce, illness, or death; in these cases, the child's emotional needs may be unmet and he or she then lacks the emotional resources to cope with the additional challenges of schoolwork. Peer influences can contribute to UA. Often, students' grades correlate with the grades of their friends; adolescents are particularly peer group oriented, and students will rise or fall according to the norms of their group. Finally, giftedness is one of the leading causes of UA noted in the literature. These students may underachieve due to a lack of appropriate challenges in school, little experience coping with academic frustration, or underdeveloped work-study habits.

Schools have been blamed for causing UA.[2] Factors such as teacher expectations, student boredom, inadequate academic programming, and the teacher–student relationship have been noted. However, when working with adolescents, it is important to focus on their contribution to their UA and the need for them to do something about it rather than reinforcing their tendency to externalize blame and avoid responsibility.

Prior to a discussion of potentially effective interventions, it is equally important to be cognizant of what does not work. By the time a parent is confronted with OA or UA, the usual array of interventions has probably been tried. Adult-delivered logic, lectures, and power struggles do not work for this and most other adolescent problems. External rewards and punishments do not motivate UA students, whether these are social (praise and acceptance from adults) or material. Reasoning does not work with OA students. Tutoring is ineffective for UA students because they usually have the necessary academic skills; it is motivation and independence they lack. Finally, suffering the consequences of their OA or UA behavior does not work; OA and UA are maladaptive responses that tend to maintain themselves.

## ASSESSMENT

Diagnosis of OA and UA can be difficult because they are conditions observed on a continuum of behavior where specific criteria do not exist and also because the accompanying emotional distress may be denied. Objective measures of both ability and performance need to be obtained along with clinical interviews of the parents and adolescent.

### OBJECTIVE MEASURES

Standardized intelligence tests should be administered such as the *Wechsler Intelligence Scale for Children*[5] or *Stanford-Binet Intelligence Scales*,[6] as well as academic achievement tests such as the *Woodcock-Johnson Psycho-Educational Battery*.[7] The results from these tests should be analyzed, specifically examining if there is a statistically significant discrepancy between an adolescent's potential and achievement. Typically, at least 1 standard deviation (15 points) needs to exist to be considered a significant discrepancy. In addition to these standardized tests, objective data from the school should be collected and reviewed. For example, level of academic achievement can be ascertained from report cards and other results from class tests. Objective behavioral data also are critical to collect. This gives the evaluator an idea of the amount of effort adolescents are putting into school achievement and how that is balanced with other aspects of their lives. For example, it would be important to know how many hours they are working on homework, how much time is spent doing other things, what activities they are engaged in, and what is their daily as well as weekly schedule for work and leisure activities.

### CLINICAL INTERVIEWS

Besides objective measures, clinical interviews can provide crucial information not obtained by the objective measures. This can give the evaluator a much better overall picture of the individual adolescent. Clinical interviews with the parents (preferably both) and adolescent should be conducted together and separately to obtain the most valid information. First, physical, mental, or emotional problems that could be the cause for the OA or UA need to be ruled out through a medical history (eg, sleep, nutrition, drug use, etc). Other areas that should be assessed include

(1) the adolescent's desire to change, without which no change can occur, (2) emotional stress about school performance, (3) academic self-concept (eg, smart, lazy, failure) and self-efficacy, (4) attitude toward school and their future, (5) underlying cognitions (eg, "I'm not good enough." "I have to be perfect"), (6) balance in life (eg, too many or too few extracurricular activities), (7) parental involvement (eg, pushing or neglecting), (8) long- and short-term goals (eg, are they realistic and obtainable?), (9) friendships (eg, who are their friends and how are they doing in school?), (10) positive and negative coping skills, and (11) strengths and weaknesses, academic and extracurricular. When evaluating OA, assess possible indicators that have been chronic (lasting more than a year), including (1) social withdrawal, (2) fear of failure, (3) feelings of inadequacy, (4) significant distress, (5) feelings of being "burned out," (6) lack of recreational activities or overscheduling, (7) depression and low self-esteem, and (8) anxiety and/or features of OCD. Underachievement evaluations should include possible indicators that have been chronic (lasting more than a year), including (1) poor organizational skills (eg, "forgetting" homework) and lack of time management (starting homework late in the evening), (2) low frustration tolerance and avoidance of challenges, lack of persistence despite motivation, (3) feelings of shame or embarrassment about poor performance, although he/she may deny this, (4) engagement in more than 2 hours of electronics (eg, TV, video games, computer), (5) lack of independence in schoolwork, (6) lack of self-discipline, commitment, the ability to delay gratification, and future goal orientation, (7) social withdrawal or social aggression, (8) inconsistent academic performance determined by social-emotional factors, (9) depression and low self-esteem, and (10) anxiety and avoidance.

## TREATMENT SUGGESTIONS

If OA or UA seem related to significant emotional difficulty, either as cause or effect, a referral should be made to an appropriate mental health professional. If a learning disability has not been ruled out, refer for psychoeducational evaluation to rule out a processing deficit that could inhibit learning. Although UA and OA should be viewed as the adolescent's problem, treatment should involve the adolescent and the parents.

**Parent training** should focus on how parents can (a) support schoolwork without over- or underinvolvement, (b) empathize and validate the student's feelings, (c) communicate effectively with their teenager, and (d) model positive attitudes about work. Parents should not make excuses for the adolescent; the adolescent must accept responsibility. Clinicians can facilitate this process by clearly outlining the following principles and suggestions:

- Parents need to work together to solve the problem. When differences of opinion exist, they should first come to an agreement on their position regarding their child. They also need to set the values by example and frequent communication. Parents should strive toward having a positive, supportive parent–child relationship and not a critical, rejecting one. Simultaneously, parents need to set and enforce limits that teach the concept of balance between work and play.
- Fostering independence and responsibility in the child with OA or UA is critical. One concrete way for parents to do this is to develop a list of household chores for the child.
- Parents can request the implementation of weekly reports from the school so that the student and the parents can monitor the student's work.

Although clinicians can do some of the **adolescent training** directly, parents will find most of these suggestions extremely useful:

- Focus on a student's strengths, not weaknesses. Further develop the strengths while working on improving the weaknesses if necessary.
- Have the student set realistic goals and plans. Try to anticipate potential obstacles and create ways to effectively overcome any problems that may arise.
- Work on improving coping skills especially when dealing with frustration and disappointment, rather than the maladaptive fight–flight response.
- Increase self-awareness. Students may have difficulty self-monitoring and being self-aware. "I don't know" may actually be a true statement when asked what their goals are or what's going on with school.
- For UA, work on developing simple organizational skills (eg, self-monitoring, breaking down tasks into manageable parts, and devoting the same block of time to schoolwork everyday, regardless of the amount of work, and then work to fill the time). For OA, have them set reasonable limits on the time they spend on schoolwork.
- Use a Socratic approach, questioning adolescents so that they come up with answers that have the potential to change their outlook and awareness of their current situation.

- Work on creating balance in the adolescent's life (school, activities, family, friends, and fun).

Although all of the aforementioned suggestions can be used by clinicians and parents, the severity of the problem, parental limitations, or other factors may require additional interventions. Cognitive behavioral therapy tends to be effective in these circumstances and one should become familiar with community resources where this specific treatment is available. Overachievement and UA are complex issues with no one or simple answer. They require careful evaluation and multiple intervention strategies involving home, school, and the individual student.

## REFERENCES

1. Parsons A, Frydenberg E, Poole C. Overachievement and coping strategies in adolescent males. *Br J Edu Psychology.* 1996;66:109–114

2. Baker JA, Bridger R, Evans K. Models of underachievement among gifted preadolescents: the role of personal, family, and school factors. *Gifted Child Quarterly.* 1998;42(1):5–15

3. Gustafson SB. Female underachievement and overachievement: parental contributions and long-term consequences. *Int J Beh Dev.* 1994;17(3):469–484

4. McCoach DB, Siegle D. Factors that differentiate underachieving gifted students from high-achieving gifted students. *Gifted Child Quarterly.* 2003;47(2):144–154

5. Wechsler D. *Wechsler Intelligence Scale for Children*. 4th ed. San Antonio, TX: The Psychological Corporation; 2003

6. Roid GH. *Stanford-Binet Intelligence Scales*. 5th ed. Itasca, IL: Riverside Publishing; 2003

7. Woodcock RW, Johnson MB. *Woodcock-Johnson Psycho-Educational Battery—Revised.* Itasca, IL: Riverside Publishing; 1989, 1990

# CHAPTER 194

## Psychoeducational Assessment of Adolescents

HEATHER R. ADAMS, PhD

## INTRODUCTION

Adolescents who have difficulty in educational settings frequently benefit from formal assessment of psychoeducational status with standardized measures. As noted in the previous chapter, optimal tools used for this purpose need to meet empirical standards of reliability and validity. Psychoeducational testing can be used to establish a function baseline, identify strengths and vulnerabilities in various domains of learning, inform treatment planning, and evaluate change in function within the context of education and learning in response to various interventions. This chapter addresses psychological assessment related to intelligence (IQ) testing and achievement testing in adolescents.

## INTELLIGENCE TESTS FOR ADOLESCENTS

Intelligence quotient (IQ) tests provide an estimate of an adolescent's cognitive function and potential. An IQ test score is a statistically reliable estimate of overall intellectual ability within a certain range of scores, the confidence interval. Most IQ tests in use today are hierarchically organized with the highest-order factor reflecting global cognitive abilities, with selected lower-order factors defining constructs such as verbal and nonverbal reasoning, perceptual/spatial abilities, attention, processing speed, and other cognitive processes.

The Wechsler tests[1,2] including the Wechsler Intelligence Scale for Children (WISC-IV) and Wechsler Adult Intelligence Scale (WAIS-III) are among the most common IQ measures in use. Each provides a global Full Scale IQ (FSIQ) score, a Verbal IQ (VIQ) score reflecting verbal knowledge and verbal reasoning skills, and a Performance IQ (PIQ) score reflecting nonverbal and visual reasoning skills. Wechsler scales also evaluate auditory attention (Working Memory Index) and speeded visual processing (Processing Speed Index). In addition to the Wechsler scales there are a number of other well-validated, psychometrically sound IQ tests appropriate for evaluating adolescents and young adults. Table 194-1 summarizes common IQ tests used for adolescents.

Intelligence quotient scores are standardized to indicate performance in relation to an age-normative distribution of scores. Most IQ tests today use Deviation IQ scores, which generally have an average standard score of 100 and a standard deviation of 15. Thus, an adolescent with an IQ score of 100 would be considered to have average intellectual function, in comparison to his or her same-age peers. Lower scores reflect lower cognitive ability. Adolescents obtaining IQ test scores below approximately 70 may qualify for a clinical diagnosis of "mental retardation" (see Table 194-2), but only when cognitive deficit is paired with significant impairment in the performance of age-expected functional skills such as activities of daily living.[3] Functional abilities can be systematically evaluated in relation to same-age peers using measures such as the second edition of the Vineland Adaptive Behavior Scales (VABS-II)[4] or the Scales of Independent Behavior, Revised (SIB-R).[5]

Whether adolescents are newly diagnosed as meeting criteria for mental retardation or were identified in childhood, the family, school, and health care team should begin planning, during the middle and early high school years, for their transition to adult living.[6] Adolescents with mental retardation or borderline IQ test scores may benefit from an educational curriculum focused on functional academics, activities of daily living, and vocational training; these students may also require considerable lead time in their curriculum to master these skills. The "Arc" (originally known as The National Association for Retarded Children) is a national organization that provides support for families of individuals with intellectual disability, including a Web site (www.thearc.org) that includes state chapters and state-specific family resource guides that include a directory of transitional services for adolescents.

### "SHORT-FORM" IQ TESTS

Short-form IQ tests are either constructed as stand-alone measures that are independently validated and normed or that use statistical algorithms to generate IQ estimates based on selected subtests of a full-length test battery or selected items from subtests. Examples of the stand-alone measures include the Kaufman Brief Intelligence Test-2 (KBIT-2)[7] or the Wechsler Abbreviated Scales of

**Table 194-1**

**Some Common Tests of Intelligence for Assessment of Adolescents**

| *Test Name* | *Domains Assessed* | *Approximate Time* |
|---|---|---|
| Wechsler Intelligence Scale for Children, Fourth Edition (WISC-IV)[1] | Full Scale IQ (FSIQ)<br>• Verbal comprehension<br>• Perceptual reasoning<br>• Working memory<br>• Processing speed | 60–90 minutes |
| Wechsler Adult Intelligence Scale, Third Edition (WAIS-III)[2] | Full Scale IQ (FSIQ)<br>• Verbal comprehension<br>• Perceptual reasoning<br>• Working memory<br>• Processing speed | 60–90 minutes |
| Differential Abilities Scale, Second Edition (DAS-II), School-Age Cognitive Battery[8] | General conceptual ability (GCA)<br>• Verbal<br>• Nonverbal reasoning<br>• Spatial<br>Special nonverbal composite (SNC)<br>• *Nonverbal reasoning + spatial*<br>Diagnostic battery<br>• Processing speed<br>• Working memory<br>• Selected subtests (auditory attention, visual learning/recall, phonological processing) | Core battery: 45–60 minutes<br>Diagnostic battery: 30 minutes |
| Woodcock-Johnson III Normative Update Test of Cognitive Abilities (WJ-III-NU:COG)[9] | General intellectual ability (GIA)<br>• Verbal ability<br>• Thinking ability<br>• Cognitive efficiency | 45–60 minutes |
| Stanford-Binet[10] | Full Scale IQ<br>• Verbal IQ<br>• Nonverbal IQ<br>Factors:<br>• Fluid reasoning<br>• Knowledge<br>• Quantitative reasoning<br>• Visual-spatial processing<br>• Working memory | |
| Test of Nonverbal Intelligence, Third Edition (TONI-3)[11] | Brief assessment of nonverbal abilities; minimal demand for motor responses; reduced culture biases | 20 minutes |

Intelligence (WASI).[12] Short-form IQ tests offer a considerable time benefit, with completion time in as little as 20 to 30 minutes. However, these brief measures are often less reliable and informative than full tests,[13,14] and the tests with the greatest time-saving may sacrifice the most in terms of precision. Therefore, a number of psychometric standards have been proposed for short-form IQ measures to be clinically useful,[15] although it

**Table 194-2**

**IQ Score Classifications and Diagnostic Criteria for Mental Retardation[1,3]**

| *Deviation IQ Standard Score M = 100, SD = 15* | *Clinical Classification* |
|---|---|
| IQ ≥ 130 | Very superior |
| IQ = 120–129 | Superior |
| IQ = 110–119 | High average |
| IQ = 90–109 | Average |
| IQ = 80–89 | Low average |
| IQ = 70–79 | Below average |
| IQ = 50–55 to about 70 | Mild mental retardation[a] |
| IQ = 35–40 to 50–55 | Moderate mental retardation[a] |
| IQ = 20–25 to 35–40 | Severe mental retardation[a] |
| IQ < 20–25 | Profound mental retardation[a] |

[a]Note: Diagnosis of mental retardation requires dual criteria met: deficient IQ score (IQ ≤ approx 70) and impairment in at least 2 domains of adaptive living skills. The diagnosis must be made based on the presence of dual impairments within a developmental framework, for example, before age 18.

is unlikely that any single short form will fit all clinical purposes.[16] It has been proposed that algorithm-based short forms should not be used to classify an adolescent for clinical or psychoeducational purposes, or for programming decisions.[13] This guideline is reasonable for the stand-alone brief IQ tests as well.

Collectively, the utility of most brief and short-form IQ tests is limited mainly to screening for cognitive difficulty to indicate whether subsequent in-depth evaluation is necessary, and for monitoring specific cognitive abilities over time. The Test of Nonverbal Intelligence, Third Edition (TONI-3)[17] provides a brief (approximately 20 minutes), language-free assessment of nonverbal/perceptual abilities. It may be useful to screen adolescents who are unable to communicate verbally, have limited or no exposure to the English or Spanish languages (the most common formats for IQ tests), or where cultural aspects of English or Spanish language-based tasks may lead to a biased assessment of abilities.

## LEARNING DISABILITIES IN ADOLESCENTS

A primary reason for referring an adolescent for academic skills testing is for the diagnosis and monitoring of a learning disability (LD). The Individuals with Disabilities Education Improvement Act (IDE-IA), which reauthorized and revised federal education laws in 2004, defines an LD as:

"A disorder in 1 or more of the basic psychological processes involved in understanding or in using language, spoken or written, which disorder may manifest itself in the imperfect ability to listen, think, speak, read, write, spell, or do mathematical calculations.... [including] such conditions as perceptual disabilities, brain injury, minimal brain dysfunction, dyslexia, and developmental aphasia...[but not including] a learning problem that is primarily the result of visual, hearing, or motor disabilities, of mental retardation, of emotional disturbance, or of environmental, cultural, or economic disadvantage."[18] [Part A, Sec. 602(30)(A),(B)]

### ACHIEVEMENT TESTS IN ADOLESCENTS

Achievement testing is performed to assess an adolescent's current academic level, to identify specific areas of academic skills and deficits, and to aid in the diagnosis and monitoring of LDs. The second edition of the Wechsler Individual Achievement Test (WIAT-II)[19] and the third edition of the Woodcock-Johnson Achievement Test (WJ-III)[20] are common omnibus measures of academic achievement in adolescents. The WIAT-II and WJ-III each assess: (1) reading in the areas of phonemic awareness, word recognition, and reading comprehension, (2) math domains of numeracy, calculation, and math reasoning, (3) writing with respect to spelling and written expression, and (4) listening comprehension. The WIAT-II and WJ-III contain tasks that evaluate speeded performance in which the presentation of a stimulus is brief and the reaction time is considered. As with IQ tests, achievement tests provide age-normalized scores in the form of standard scores and percentile ranks.

Many achievement tests also report grade equivalent (GE) or age equivalent (AE) scores to describe performance in relation to grade- or age-based curriculum standards. For example, a GE = 10.5 reflects academic skill at the level expected of a student in the fifth month of the Grade 10 school year, not the fifth calendar month. Grade equivalent and AE scores can be difficult to interpret because their metrics are not standardized across the many different achievement tests. Thus, GE scores on one reading measure may not be comparable to GE scores on another reading measure and may not be referenced against the adolescent's actual curriculum within the respective grade. In general, age-normalized scores are recommended for interpreting achievement tests.

In certain cases, GE and AE scores are useful. For example, GE scores may best describe the achievement level of adolescents with significant interruptions in schooling due to illness, geographic instability, or truancy. Age-equivalent scores can provide a developmental benchmark for academic skills in developmentally delayed individuals. Early developing adolescents with cognitive and academic limitations may have unreasonably high demands placed on them because of mature physical size and appearance. Understanding the GE and AE level of such adolescents can help adults adjust their expectations accordingly and target interventions at an appropriate level.

## IDENTIFYING LEARNING DISABILITIES IN ADOLESCENTS

Learning disabilities have historically been diagnosed on the basis of a significant discrepancy between lower achievement relative to the capacity for higher intellectual function. Considerable research, however, shows that differentiating learners on the basis of a discrepancy model has limited sensitivity or prognostic value. IQ-discrepant and nondiscrepant low-achievers exhibit similar kinds of deficits in achievement and core processes; the developmental course of their achievement performance is not significantly different,[21–23] and neither the low-achievement nor discrepancy-based definitions of LD adequately predict academic outcomes.[24] Additionally, relying on a discrepancy model delays identification of and intervention for LD until larger numerical score differences emerge, essentially creating a "wait to fail" scenario. Based on revisions in the 2004 IDE-IA legislation, schools are not required to employ the discrepancy model and may choose to consider whether a student fails to progress despite reasonable, evidence-based interventions.

With the advent of a "response to intervention" standard, there may be more emphasis on early identification and dynamic, serial monitoring of children and adolescents at risk for academic problems without the requirement for a formal diagnostic label. The integration of research findings on prevention, diagnosis, and remediation of LDs, a "hybrid" model, has been proposed in which a multistep assessment swiftly intervenes once lagging achievement is noted.[25]

In this approach, formal achievement testing and diagnosis may be deferred pending implementation of evidence-based intervention based on observations of an adolescent's academic difficulties. Serial assessment of an adolescent's response to intervention can then be utilized to determine if achievement has been normalized or warrants further evaluation. Effective interventions for LDs include combining bottom-up training and drilling on an adolescent's deficient academic skills with top-down strategies of instruction to expand the student's academic problem-solving repertoire.[26] The Learning Disabilities Association (LDA) has local chapters in each of the 50 states and provides online information and resources at its Web site (www.ldanatl.org/) including materials for parents, teachers, and health care professionals.

Adolescents with LDs have higher rates of academic failure, school dropout, and behavioral and adjustment problems in comparison with their non-LD peers,[27] and only half as many students labeled as having an LD go on to postsecondary education in comparison with general education students (30.5% vs 68.3%).[28,29] Furthermore, although young adults with LDs attain employment rates comparable to their non-LD peers,[28] their earning potential and job status appear to be lower.[30] In the practice of adolescent medicine, a physician can serve as a primary advocate for school evaluation and intervention when patients: (1) have chronic academic problems but have not yet been formally evaluated for an LD, (2) are receiving suboptimal interventions for an already-identified learning problem, or (3) encounter new challenges as academic demands increase.

Identification and intervention for teens with LDs should also consider social and psychological factors potentially affecting academic achievement, such as a family history of learning problems, and highly associated comorbidities, such as attention-deficit/hyperactivity disorder, that may require adjunctive treatment to maximize success of academic interventions. Adolescents with significant LDs that preclude a rigorous academic program may benefit from exposure to vocational training as a component of their transition to independent adult living.

## DYSLEXIA IN ADOLESCENTS

Dyslexia, or specific reading disability, is estimated to occur in 5% to 15% of the population and is the single most prevalent LD.[31,32] Dyslexia is defined simply as "an unexpected difficulty in reading,"[33] in contrast to a persisting, but inaccurate, lay perception that individuals with dyslexia "see letters and words backwards." Dyslexia involves core deficits in phonemic processing, sound recognition, and mapping sounds to the written code of letters and letter groups.[34–37] Neurobiologic studies demonstrate morphological[38] differences detected on functional magnetic resonance imaging (*f*MRI), particularly underactivation and disrupted activation and functional connectivity of the posterior regions in the left temporo-parieto-occipital regions,[39–41] in dysfluent readers compared to fluent readers (Figure 194-1).

Scientific studies of individuals with dyslexia have elucidated the phenomenology of dyslexia, associated risk factors, clinical course, and longitudinal reading outcomes.[42] Dyslexia is heritable, and candidate genes are being identified.[43] Although an adolescent with an affected parent is at risk of up to 60% for developing reading problems, the development of reading skills can be moderated, in part by an enriched home and school environment and to a lesser extent by socioeconomic status.[44] In addition, brain activation patterns in individuals with dyslexia can be normalized following successful reading interventions.[45,46]

Effective, early remediation of dyslexia consists of training that combines bottom-up skills of decoding and phonemics with top-down skills, such as analysis of context cues and classroom/instructional accommodations, that enable students to keep pace with academic content, despite reading problems. However, even teens with early diagnosis and intervention for reading disabilities may have difficulties with phonemic decoding, fluency, and reading comprehension.[40] These students may have reasonably accurate but inefficient and laborious reading and can become overwhelmed with the dual burdens of the technical aspects of reading recognition and the analytic components of reading comprehension. Reading efficiency or "fluency" can also be improved but must be incorporated explicitly as 1 component of remediation for dyslexia. In addition, anxiety disorders and lowered self-esteem may develop as comorbidities among adolescents with dyslexia.[47,48] Therefore, reassessment of teenage students with dyslexia, including screening for mood problems, can be helpful to identify persisting deficits and develop more advanced interventions.

## SUMMARY

Psychological assessment of the adolescent serves a broad range of purposes including evaluating general intellectual ability and a range of specific cognitive processes, identifying and monitoring of LDs, determining academic and vocational placements, screening for behavioral and mental health concerns, and evaluating treatment response. When conducting any form of psychological assessment, emphasis should be placed on the use of reliable and valid assessment methods and measures, and a clear understanding of the reason for the evaluation and the type of information to be gained.

This chapter provides primary care providers with the information they need to identify adolescents along the entire range of intelligence levels. In addition, the most commonly encountered LD, dyslexia, is now known to be heritable and have recognizable changes on *f*MRI. Nonetheless, there are now robust data that indicate that dyslexia is remediable with specific reading-focused interventions.

## REFERENCES


1. Wechsler D. *Wechsler Intelligence Scale for Children (WISC-IV)*. 4th ed. San Antonio, TX: The Psychological Corporation; 2003
2. Wechsler D. *Wechsler Adult Intelligence Test (WAIS-III)*. 3rd ed. San Antonio,TX:The Psychological Corporation; 1997
3. American Psychiatric Association. *Diagnostic and Statistical Manual of Mental Disorders,* Fourth Edition, Text Revision. Washington, DC: American Psychiatric Association; 2000
4. Sparrow S, Ciccetti D, Balla D. *Vineland Adaptive Behavior Scales (Vineland II)*. 2nd ed. Bloomington, MN: American Guidance Services Publishing; 2005
5. Bruininks R, Woodcock R, Weatherman R, Hill B. *Scales of Independent Behavior—Revised*. Chicago, IL: Riverside Publishing; 1996
6. Smith T, Puccini I. *Position statement: secondary curricula and policy issues for students with mental retardation. Education & Training in Mental Retardation & Developmental Disabilities.* 1995;30:275–282
7. Kaufman A, Kaufman N. *Kaufman Brief Intelligence Test (KBIT-2)*. 2nd ed. Minneapolis, MN: Pearson Assessments; 1997
8. Elliott C. *Differential Ability Scales*. San Antonio, TX: The Psychological Corporation; 1990
9. Woodcock R, McGrew K, Schrank F, Mather N. *Woodcock-Johnson-III Normative Update*. Rolling Meadows, IL: Riverside Publishing; 2001, 2007
10. Roid G. *Stanford-Binet Intelligence Scales (SB5)*. 5th ed. Itasca, IL: Riverside Publishing; 2003
11. Hammill D, Pearson N, Wiederholt J. *Comprehensive Test of Nonverbal Intelligence (CTONI)*. Austin, TX: Pro-Ed; 1997
12. The Psychological Corporation. *Wechsler Abbreviated Scale of Intelligence (WASI)*. San Antonio,TX:The Psychological Corporation; 1999
13. Axelrod B. Validity of the Wechsler Abbreviated Scale of Intelligence and other very short forms of estimating intellectual functioning. *Assessment.* 2002;9:17–23
14. Sattler J, Dumont R. *Assessment of Children: WISC-IV and WPPSI-III Supplement*. San Diego, CA: Jerome M. Sattler, Inc; 2004
15. Silverstein A. Short forms of individual intelligence tests. *J Consult Clin Psychol.* 1990;2:3–11
16. Donders J, Axelrod B. Two-subtest estimations of WAIS-III factor index scores. *Psychol Assess.* 2002;14: 360–364
17. Brown L, Sherbenou R, Johnsen S. *Test of Nonverbal Intellilgence (TONI-3)*. 3rd ed. Austin, TX: Pro-Ed; 1997
18. Individuals with Disabilities Education Improvement Act (IDEA 2004), in 20 U.S.C. §1401 [30]; 2004
19. Wechsler D. *Wechsler Individual Achievement Test (WIAT-II)*. 2nd ed. San Antonio, TX: The Psychological Corporation; 2002

20. Woodcock R, McGrew K, Mather N. *Woodcock Johnson III Tests of Achievement*. Rolling Meadows, IL: Riverside Publishing; 2001

21. Steubing, K, Fletcher, J, LaDoux, et al. Validity of IQ-discrepancy classifications of reading disabilities: a meta-analysis. *Am Educa Res J.* 2002;39:469–518

22. Hoskyn M, Swanson H. Cognitive processing of low achievers and children with reading disabilities: a selective meta-analytic review of the published literature. *Sch Psychol Rev.* 2000;29:102–119

23. Shaywitz BA, Fletcher JM, Holahan JM, Shaywitz SE. Discrepancy compared to low achievement definitions of reading disability: results from the Connecticut Longitudinal Study. *J Learn Disabil.* 1992;25:639–648

24. Francis DJ, Fletcher JM, Stuebing KK, Lyon GR, Shaywitz BA, Shaywitz SE. Psychometric approaches to the identification of LD: IQ and achievement scores are not sufficient. *J Learn Disabil.* 2005;38:98–108

25. Fletcher JM, Francis DJ, Morris RD, Lyon GR. Evidence-based assessment of learning disabilities in children and adolescents. *J Clin Child Adolesc Psychol.* 2005;34: 506–522

26. Swanson HL, Hoskyn M, Lee C. *Interventions for Students with Learning Disabilities: A Meta-Analysis of Treatment Outcomes*. New York, NY: The Guilford Press; 1999

27. Swanson H, Deshler D. Instructing adolescents with learning disabilities: converting a meta-analysis to practice. *J Learn Disabil.* 2003;36:124

28. Wagner M, Blackorby J. Transition from high school to work or college: how special education students fare. *The Future of Children: Special Education for Students with Disabilities.* 1996;6(1)

29. Sitlington P, Frank A. Are adolescents with learning disabilities successfully crossing the bridge into adult life? *Learn Disabil Q.* 1990;13

30. Blackorby J, Wagner M. Longitudinal postschool outcomes of youth with disabilities: findings from the National Longitudinal Transition Study. *Except Child.* 1996;62:399–413

31. Interagency Committee on Learning Disabilities. *Learning Disabilities: A Report to the US Congress*. Washington, DC: Government Printing Office; 1987

32. Shaywitz SE, Fletcher JM, Shaywitz BA. Issues in the definition and classification of attention deficit disorder. *Top Lang Disord.* 1994;14:1–25

33. Shaywitz S, Shaywitz B. Dyslexia (specific reading disability). *Biol Psychiatry.* 2005;57:1301–1309

34. Bradley L, Bryant P. Categorizing sounds and learning to read: a causal connection. *Nature.* 1983;301:419–421

35. Stanovich K, Siegel L. Phenotypic performance of children with reading disabilities: a regression-based test of the phonological-core variable-difference model. *J Educ Psychol.* 1994;86:24–53

36. Wagner R, Torgesen J. The nature of phonological processing and its causal role in the acquisition of reading skills. *Psychol Bull.* 1987;101:192–212

37. Bradley L, Bryant P. Difficulties in auditory organization as a possible cause of reading backwardness. *Nature.* 1978;271:746–747

38. Phinney E, Pennington BF, Olson RK, Filley, CM, Filipek PA. Brain structure correlates of component reading processes: implications for reading disability. *Cortex.* 2008;43:777–791

39. Horwitz B, Rumsey J, Donohue B. Functional connectivity of the angular gyrus in normal reading and dyslexia. *Proc Natl Acad Sci USA.* 1998;95:8939–8944

40. Pugh K, Mencl W, Shaywitz B, et al. The angular gyrus in developmental dyslexia: task-specific differences in functional connectivity within posterior cortex. *Science.* 2000;11:51–56

41. Shaywitz BA, Shaywitz SE, Pugh KR, et al. Disruption of posterior brain systems for reading in children with developmental dyslexia. *Biol Psychiatry.* 2002;52:101–110

42. Shaywitz S, Morris R, Shaywitz B. The education of dyslexic children from childhood to young adulthood. *Ann Rev Psychol.* 2008;59:451–475

43. Schumacher J, Hoffmann P, Schmal C, Schulte-Korn G, Nothen MM. Genetics of dyslexia: the evolving landscape. *J Med Genet.* 2007;44:289–297

44. Molfese F, Modglin A, Molfese D. The role of environment in the development of readings skills: a longitudinal study of preschool and school-age measures. *J Learn Disabil.* 2007;36:59–67

45. Simos PG, Fletcher JM, Bergman E, et al. Dyslexia-specific brain activation profile becomes normal following successful remedial training. *Neurology.* 2002;58:1203–1213

46. Simos PG, Fletcher JM, Sarkari S, Billingsley RL, Denton C, Papanicolaou AC. Altering the brain circuits for reading through intervention: a magnetic source imaging study. *Neuropsychology.* 2007;21:485–496

47. Goldston D, et al. Reading problems, psychiatric disorders, and functional impairment from mid- to late adolescence. *J Am Acad Child Adolesc Psychiatry.* 2008;46:25–32

48. McNulty M. Dyslexia and the life course. *J Learn Disabil.* 2003;36:363–381

# CHAPTER 195

# Gifted Adolescents

NANETTE C. SUDLER, PhD • STEVEN E. TOBIAS, PsyD

## DEFINITIONS

There are no established standardized criteria for giftedness, although an intelligence quotient (IQ) of 130 or above is commonly used. An IQ of 130, with a standard deviation of 15, represents approximately the 97.72 nd percentile; this criterion is often used in schools to qualify for a gifted program, although other criteria, such as teacher recommendations and/or grades, are used as well. Instruments used to assess IQ and giftedness during adolescence are the Wechsler Intelligence Scale for Children (ages 6–16),[1] the Wechsler Adult Intelligence Scale (ages 16–adult),[2] and the Stanford-Binet Intelligence Scale, Fourth Edition (ages 2–23).[3] Individually administered tests, such as those noted previously, are more valid and reliable than tests administered in a group setting.

Other definitions of giftedness encompass academic aptitude, creative thinking, artistic ability, leadership, and sometimes athletic ability.[4] The concept of giftedness is sometimes broadened as "gifted and talented" to accommodate a wider segment of the population. For the purpose of this chapter, the definition of giftedness is limited to intellectual ability as represented by an IQ of 130 or above. Adolescents who meet this criterion require some form of special attention by parents and educators. The level of academic achievement is not being included in the definition because it may not correlate with intellectual potential. Some gifted students underachieve (see Chapter 193, Academic Overachievement and Underachievement) whereas other gifted students may be considered "twice-exceptional." This latter group encompasses students who are gifted intellectually and have one or more deficits in learning, attention, physical/sensory functioning, and/or emotional functioning that impede their academic achievement.

## CHALLENGES

Generally, the more gifted the student, the more challenging it is for their academic and social needs to be met. Typically, there are a number of gifted students in the 130 to 140 range in a school district and their academic and social needs can usually be met with some special programming. It has been argued that adolescents with IQs in the 140 to 160 range (99.62%-99.99%) require significant modification of the entire school curriculum (which may include skipping grades), and for those rare students with IQs above 160, regular school resources will be unable to provide for their needs and an individualized program needs to be developed.[5] Although the needs of gifted students can vary significantly, schools often do not make distinctions in degrees of giftedness, which is done for those with disabilities; therefore, it is common for all gifted students to be categorized under the same label.

In addition, the national No Child Left Behind Act has placed an emphasis on students passing state tests that establish minimum standards. Public school curricula and programming are therefore geared toward meeting minimum standards rather than establishing educational programming that seeks to have all children reach their potential. In fact, it has been suggested that gifted adolescents are a group that has remained invisible on the national agenda[6] and at best are viewed as a low priority by educational administrations.[4] Specifically, gifted adolescents are even less recognized than their younger counterparts. Unfortunately, much of the research in the field has focused on younger children, and many school districts consider gifted education to end in middle school because once students are in high school, advanced placement and honors classes are often considered sufficient.[7] This ignores special qualities possessed by gifted students as well as how giftedness interacts with identity formation and the need for social connections in adolescence.

Overall, the literature on giftedness indicates that when gifted students are identified and their academic and social needs are met, there are no differences in their emotional or social adjustment and they are not more vulnerable than their more average peers. Gifted adolescents do not have greater suicidal ideation than their peers[8] and, in fact, are under-represented in the delinquent population.[9] However, because of their different profile (which may include asynchronous development, perfectionism, social isolation, and sensitivity) and needs, there may be greater stress on gifted students,[9] and they may have more difficulty coping with typical adolescent issues.[7] It is important to note that there is not a direct relationship between IQ and emotional intelligence (EQ).[10] In fact, IQ and EQ rarely keep pace with each other.[4] With gifted students, EQ is often beyond chronological age, but not commensurate with the expectation based on intellectual age.[9]

One of the greatest sources of stress for adolescents emanates from teen culture and its social implications, which emphasize belonging and conformity. Being different in any way can be a challenge. Affiliation and achievement conflict when adolescents perceive that their peer group does not validate achievement goals. The need to belong can affect achievement and self-concept.[11] Many adolescents perceive their giftedness as having negative social consequences. Interestingly, in the early grades social status can be obtained by being smart, but this is less so in adolescence.[12] To cope with this, females are likely to use denial of their abilities as a defense mechanism, whereas males tend to use humor as their social coping strategy. Low-income students may be particularly vulnerable to denying their ability because it causes dissonance with their culture and identity.[11] To complicate this further, giftedness is not evenly spread across all activities and interests. Therefore, it becomes necessary for the gifted adolescent to have many different kinds of peers. For example, a friend who may be well matched intellectually may not have similar physical or emotional skills.[4]

If available educational programs do not sufficiently address students' giftedness, then the school experience can become unpleasant and unmotivating. Giving gifted students boring busywork can add additional stress. Research has found that gifted students tend to have higher intrinsic academic motivation,[13-16] but this does not always generalize to classroom skills and performance.[17,18] Younger gifted students who have not been appropriately challenged may feel schoolwork is too easy. However, by the time they are older and schoolwork becomes more difficult, they may have not developed the sufficient study skills and frustration tolerance to maintain a high level of achievement. This can also create a high level of stress, which can exacerbate tendencies toward anxiety and/or depression. In addition, a lack of academic stimulation can cause attentional, behavioral, and emotional problems.

"Twice-exceptional" students are gifted and have deficits in learning, attention, physical/sensory functioning, and/or emotional functioning that impede their academic achievement; these include dyslexia, developmental delays (in speech, language, and/or motor coordination), disruptive behaviors (such as conduct disorder or oppositional defiant disorder), hearing/visual/perceptual impairments, anxieties, eating disorders, attentional issues (such as attention-deficit/hyperactivity disorder), learning disorders, and Asperger syndrome. Due to the fact that being twice-exceptional is so complex and convoluted many students can be misdiagnosed or underdiagnosed. A comprehensive evaluation utilizing multiple testing methods and integrating various sources of information is necessary (eg, subtest patterns on IQ tests, classroom performance, time and support needed to complete assignments, and specific assessment of talent areas may be used). Many twice-exceptional students are not accurately identified until adolescence or even adulthood because their abilities and disabilities may mask each other. Schools frequently do not identify these students because they may not be falling below grade level; they are able to use their giftedness to compensate for their disabilities. Furthermore, once these students are identified, educational settings tend to focus on the areas of weakness for twice-exceptional students. This can have a negative effect on motivation and self-concept and can further frustrate these students by ignoring their intellectual, social, and emotional needs. This places them at greater risk for underachievement, and they are a particularly challenging and at-risk population.[7]

Healthy emotional adjustment in life requires positive work experiences and supportive relationships with others. These are important needs of gifted students as well but are often the ones that are hardest to meet. When gifted students have problems, it is often because of a lack of academic stimulation and/or lack of peer connections. It is perplexing that more attention, services, and resources are not specifically designated for the gifted population. It is these students who could best serve as future leaders and pioneers in various fields if given proper programming and guidance. Thus, society and the human condition would ultimately benefit from their accomplishments.

## OPPORTUNITIES

The primary need of gifted students is to have opportunities for accelerated instruction with their intellectual peers. Some research has correlated opportunities for academic acceleration with self-esteem, life satisfaction, and career achievement even when the gifted students have been placed with older peers.[19] Academic challenges not only teach advanced learning, but also work-study habits such as perseverance, frustration tolerance, self-discipline, organization, and time-management skills, all of which are critical for life success. Hard work also gives a feeling of accomplishment and enhances self-esteem. These opportunities need to be individualized but, unfortunately, are sometimes based on what is available rather than what is best. "Best" tends to be a homogeneous grouping with a compacted curriculum, an instructional pace based on mastery and opportunities for experiential learning. However, being placed with older students in a mainstream setting can also be "good" for these students. The general rule is for the student to be taught with his or her intellectual peers.[20] In addition, providing students with meaningful and challenging opportunities for personal growth[21] and talent development are helpful (eg, special classes, internships and mentorships, college classes, competitions, clubs, and activities).[22,23]

Gifted students need to develop positive coping strategies when confronted with the achievement–affiliation conflict. They should have opportunities to share their experiences and feelings as well as problem solve with other similar students and caring adults. In contrast, not having strategies to cope with social and self-identity issues can have deleterious effects.

Gifted students need a mentor or role model, even if it is a literary or historical character. This is important for guidance, motivation, and inspiration. They need to feel support from someone else and have someone with whom they can identify. Similarly, family support and understanding are critical. Parents who set high and clear expectations, have strong extended family support, and use an authoritative rather than authoritarian parenting style will have a more positive affect on achievement. In contrast, permissive parents, although emotionally supportive, tend to set few goals and limits, which discourages achievement. Adults need to be careful with praise and recognition; it is important to focus on effort rather than innate ability or specific achievement, which may have been accomplished effortlessly.

Gifted students benefit from early career exploration because of their advanced pace of learning and achievement. They may have to choose a college major when most students are choosing high school activities. This is especially important for those with strengths in multiple areas because it can be harder for them to choose an area within which to specialize.

When difficulties do arise, it is important to seek professional assistance as early as possible. It has been found that psychologists have been identified as most influential in gifted education.[24] Many gifted adolescents can benefit from instruction in stress management, as they can be at higher risk due to self-imposed expectations, expectations of others, being different, or a lack of academic challenge. Also, nurturing a positive explanatory style has been associated with optimism,[25,26] which can help minimize the negative effects of anxiety and depression. Optimists tend to attribute the causes of negative events to local, temporary, and changeable factors, whereas pessimists tend to see them as stable and global. In addition, proactive instruction in social and emotional learning can avoid potential difficulties.[9] Professionals can also serve as a clearinghouse for information about gifted programs.

The effect of technology on gifted students is an unexplored area but is likely a heightened parallel to the affect it can have on all children in terms of how it can help and hurt. Obviously, the computer can allow gifted adolescents to have access to their true peer group, especially in less populated areas, which helps foster a positive identity and sense of belonging. It also allows students to have access to college-level courses and independent research. However, it can be harmful by fostering social isolation, inhibiting the practice of social skills, and limiting the experiences of gratifying emotional interactions. Text lacks the nonverbal aspects of communication, which is how most emotions get expressed and how empathy is experienced and shared. This can exacerbate any pre-existing imbalance between the cognitive and social–emotional skills of gifted teens.

When interacting with gifted adolescents, it is important to view them as adolescents first and gifted second. It is likely that their social–emotional skills are more commensurate with their chronological age and it is necessary to take this into consideration in terms of maturity, degree of independence, and judgment. It can be easy to assume social–emotional skills consistent with their reasoning skills; however, adolescents can be unreasonable at times because they are often driven by social–emotional impulses rather than cognitive thoughts. As with all adolescents, a balance among schoolwork, friends, family, nonacademic interests (hobbies, sports, music), and downtime should be encouraged. It is helpful to keep in mind the individual nature of gifted teens when offering support in the development of their gifts and maintenance of their positive peer relationships. Finally, when a program for gifted adolescents is being developed to address their academic and social needs, it is essential to include adolescents in the process by asking for their insights, opinions, goals, and desires. Once implemented, the gifted adolescent's feedback should be included in the program evaluation and assessment of its effectiveness.

## REFERENCES

1. Wechsler D. *Wechsler Intelligence Scale for Children.* 4th ed. San Antonio, TX: The Psychological Corporation; 2003

2. Wechsler D. *Wechsler Adult Intelligence Scale.* 3rd ed. San Antonio, TX: The Psychological Corporation; 1997

3. Roid GH. *Stanford Binet Intelligence Scales,* 5th ed. Itasca, IL: Riverside Publishing; 2003

4. Webb JT, Meckstroth EA, Tolan SS. *Guiding the Gifted Child: A Practical Source for Parents and Teachers.* Scottsdale, AZ: Gifted Psychology Press; 1994

5. Delisle JR. *Parenting Gifted Kids.* Waco, TX: Prufrock Press Inc; 2006

6. Colangelo N, Assouline SG, Gross MUM. *A Nation Deceived: How Schools Hold Back America's Brightest Students.* Vols 1 and 2. Iowa City: The University of Iowa, The Connie Belin and Jacqueline N. Black International Center for Gifted Education and Talent Development; 2004

7. Dixon FA, Moon SM, eds. *The Handbook of Secondary Gifted Education.* Waco, TX: Prufrock Press Inc; 2006

8. Cross TL, Cassady JC, Miller KA. Suicide ideation and personality characteristics among gifted adolescents. *Gifted Child Quarterly.* 2006;50(4):295–309

9. Neihart M, Reis SM, Robinson NM, Moon SM, eds. *The Social and Emotional Development of Gifted Children: What Do We Know?* Waco, TX: Prufrock Press, Inc; 2002

10. Lee SY, Olszewski-Kubilius P. The emotional intelligence, moral judgment, and leadership of academically gifted adolescents. *J Educ Gifted.* 2006;30(1): 29–67

11. Neihart M. Dimensions of underachievement, difficult contexts, and perceptions of self: achievement/affiliation conflicts in gifted adolescents. *Roeper Review.* 2006;28(4): 196–203

12. Rimm SB, Rimm-Kaufman S, Rimm L. *See Jane Win: The Rimm Report on How 1,000 Girls Became Successful Women.* New York, NY: Crown Publishing Group; 1999

13. Davis HB, Connell JP. The effect of aptitude and achievement status on the self-system. *Gifted Child Quarterly.* 1985;29: 131–135

14. Gottfried AE, Gottfried AW. A longitudinal study of academic intrinsic motivation in intellectually gifted children: childhood through early adolescence. *Gifted Child Quarterly.* 1996;40:179–184

15. Li AKF. Self-perception and motivational orientation in gifted children. *Roeper Review.* 1988;10:175–180

16. Vallerand RJ, Gagne F, Senecal C, Pelletier LG. A comparison of the school intrinsic motivation and perceived competence of gifted and regular students. *Gifted Child Quarterly.* 1994;38:172–175

17. Janos PM, Robinson NM. Psychosocial development in intellectually gifted children. In: Horowitz FD, O'Brien M, eds. *The Gifted and Talented: Developmental Perspectives.* Washington, DC: American Psychological Association; 1985:149–195

18. Robinson NM, Noble KD. Social-emotional development and adjustment of gifted children. In: Wang MG, Reynolds MC, Walberg HJ, eds. *Handbook of Special Education: Research and Practice.* Vol 4. New York, NY: Pergamon Press; 1991: 57–76

19. Gross MUM. Exceptionally gifted children: long-term outcomes of academic acceleration and nonacceleration. *Journal for the Education of the Gifted.* 2006;29(4):404–432

20. Cross TL. *The Social and Emotional Lives of Gifted Kids: Understanding and Guiding Their Development.* Waco, TX: Prufrock Press Inc; 2005

21. Hoekman K, McCormick J, Barnett K. The important role of optimism in a motivational investigation of the education of gifted adolescents. *Gifted Child Quarterly.* 2005;49(2): 99–110

22. Olenchek FR, Reis SM. Gifted students with learning disabilities. In: Neihart M, Reis S, Robinson N, Moon S, eds. *The Social & Emotional Needs of Gifted Students: What Do We Know?* Waco, TX: Prufrock; 2002:177–192

23. Weinfeld R, Barnes-Robinson L, Jeweler S, Shevitz B. Academic programs for gifted and talented/learning disabled students. *Roeper Review.* 2002;24:226–233

24. Karnes FA, Nugent SA. Influential people in gifted education. *Gifted Child Today.* 2002;25(4):60–63

25. Seligman MEP. *Learned Optimism.* New York, NY: Knopf; 1991

26. Seligman MEP. *Authentic Happiness: Using the New Positive Psychology to Realize Your Potential for Lasting Fulfillment.* New York, NY: The Free Press; 2002

# CHAPTER 196

# ADHD in Adolescents

ARTHUR L. ROBIN, PhD • ANJU SAWNI, MD

Attention-deficit/hyperactivity disorder (ADHD) is a relatively common neurobiological disorder, with most US epidemiological studies estimating ADHD prevalence rates at between 4% and 8%.[1] Classically, the core symptoms of ADHD have been regarded as inattention, impulsivity, and hyperactivity, although in recent years these symptoms have been recast as deficits in executive functions and behavioral inhibition. Prospective follow-up studies have found that approximately 78% of children with ADHD continue to display the full clinical syndrome as adolescents.[2] Inattention and impulsivity persist more than overt physical hyperactivity, which transforms into mental restlessness. Many adolescents with ADHD also have at least one comorbid psychiatric condition: 59% to 65% with oppositional defiant disorder (ODD), 22% to 43% with conduct disorder (CD), 29% with major depressive disorder, 11% with bipolar disorder, and 27% with multiple anxiety disorders.[2] Even when they do not have comorbid psychiatric disorders, adolescents with ADHD may do poorly in school, become embroiled in frequent conflicts with their parents, experience peer relationship problems, suffer from low self-esteem, and make poor drivers of motor vehicles.

## COMMON PRESENTATIONS

Here are 3 common initial presentations of adolescents diagnosed as having ADHD:

Fifteen-year-old Sarah presented as depressed during an office visit. She was failing 3 classes in the 10th grade, argued with her parents about school, and was "grounded" until her grades improved. Sarah was an A student who had a positive relationship with her parents until seventh grade, when her world "collapsed."

Thirteen-year-old Bill defies every request from his parents, refuses to do chores, homework, or participate in family activities, and talks to his parents in disrespectful language. Failing most of his eighth-grade classes, Bill devotes all of his time to playing violent video games. When his parents attempt to turn off the video games, he flies into a rage, pushing and shoving them and punching holes in the wall until they back off. Although he was always stubborn and hyperactive, Bill did not reach this level of defiance until he entered middle school and became obsessed with the video games. His parents seek advice for dealing with his "video game addiction."

Intellectually gifted 18-year-old Joan coasted through middle and high school with As and Bs, doing very little work, and then enrolled in a large public university. By the end of her first year at college, Joan was on academic probation for failing most of her classes. She devoted her time to socializing and dating instead of studying. Now she was back home and depressed about her situation, asking for help.

Sarah, Bill, and Joan illustrate the heterogeneity of clinical presentations in adolescents with ADHD. Sarah and Joan both presented for depression; neither had ever displayed hyperactivity. Both excelled in school early in their education but eventually "hit a brick wall" of failure when the demands of more independent learning overwhelmed their executive functions. Because of her giftedness, Joan did not hit a brick wall until college. By contrast, Bill had always been stubborn and hyperactive. When he entered puberty these characteristics intensified and he hyperfocused on video games, avoiding school work. Like many adolescents with ADHD, the high-stimulation environment of video games took on addictive properties.

The *Diagnostic and Statistical Manual*, Fourth Edition, Text Revision (*DSM-IV-TR*)[3] criteria for ADHD do not adequately capture the heterogeneity inherent in these examples of adolescent ADHD. The astute clinician needs to filter these criteria through the lens of adolescent development when conducting an evaluation.

## EVALUATION AND DIAGNOSIS

A thorough clinical interview, rating scales, and psychological tests remain the "gold standards" for evaluating an adolescent for possible ADHD. The parents and the adolescent should be interviewed, both individually and together. The interviews should include a careful review of the 18 *DSM-IV-TR* symptoms for ADHD, developmental, school, and medical histories, and a review of common medical or psychiatric disorders that may either be comorbid with ADHD or in the differential diagnoses for ADHD. The clinician should also assess

**Box 196-1**

***ADHD Interview Questions for Adolescents***

- Does your mind often drift when you try to pay attention in class?
- Do you lose track of your place when reading a textbook for school?
- Do you "space out" during conversations?
- Does every little noise distract you from doing school work or homework?
- Do you forget things at school (planner, book, paper, etc)?
- Do you put off doing chores or homework until the last minute?
- Do you have trouble finishing tests by the end of the class period?
- Do you have a short fuse and blow up easily?
- Do you get frustrated easily?
- Do you have to say things so impatiently that you interrupt others?
- Do you make careless mistakes in math or writing?
- Do you misunderstand the directions for assignments?
- Do you get restless during class lectures?

family functioning and peer relationships. A specific, abbreviated ADHD symptom and comorbidity interview should be conducted with the adolescent. Box 196-1 illustrates questions to ask the adolescent that might elicit useful information about ADHD symptoms.

Parent, teacher, and adolescent rating scales should supplement the clinical interviews. Common parent rating scales include the DSM-IV ADHD Rating Scale,[2] the Vanderbilt Assessment Scale,[4] the Conners 3 Parent Rating Scale,[5] the Child Behavior Checklist,[2] and the Behavior Assessment System for Children (BASC).[2] There are also teacher versions of these parent rating scales; brief teacher rating scales, such as the Child Attention Profile and Classroom Performance Survey,[2] are useful because multiple copies from each of the adolescent's teachers can easily be scored. Adolescent self-report instruments include the Brown Adolescent ADD Scale[2] and the Conners 3 Self-Report Form.[5] The parent–adolescent relationship can also be assessed through comprehensive questionnaires such as the Parent Adolescent Relationship Questionnaire,[6] which is independently completed by each parent and the adolescent.

Although a clinical diagnosis of ADHD can be made through the use of interviews and rating scales without psychological tests, such tests are essential to explore the possibility that the adolescent has a learning disability requiring specific educational intervention (see Chapter 193 for details of psychoeducational testing). A licensed clinical or school psychologist should administer a standardized IQ test (Wechsler Intelligence Scale for Children-IV Edition)[7] and a standardized achievement test (Wechsler Individual Achievement Test, nd Edition).[8] The psychologist compares intellectual ability and achievement, looking for possible discrepancies indicative of learning disabilities. Continuous performance tests and neuropsychological tests of executive function may also provide useful information but are not essential for diagnostic purposes.

All of the data are integrated to answer these questions: (1) Does the adolescent currently meet the *DSM-IV-TR* criteria for ADHD? (2) Do comorbid psychiatric disorders also apply to the adolescent? (3) Does the adolescent have a learning disability requiring special education services? (4) What family and peer relationship problems are occurring that might require behavioral/psychological interventions?

## INTERVENTION: OVERVIEW

Because there is currently no "cure" for ADHD, a comprehensive intervention provides the adolescent and family with the appropriate tools for coping adequately with ADHD. These tools include (1) psychoeducation, (2) medication, (3) school/educational interventions, (4) family interventions, (5) individual cognitive behavioral therapy (CBT), and (6) complementary and alternative medicine (CAM) interventions.

### PSYCHOEDUCATION

As described in various chapters in this textbook, the developing adolescent individuates from his/her parents and develops an identity. To accomplish these goals, teenagers may rebel against their parents and other authority figures; this includes health care professionals asking the adolescent to take medication or participate in therapy for ADHD. This individuation process is particularly intense from 12 to 15 years of age. The clinician presenting the ADHD diagnosis and interventions to the patient and family must consider the context of adolescent development. This means fitting the interventions to the developing adolescent rather than forcing the adolescent to fit into the professional's preconceived notions about interventions. The clinician needs to involve the adolescent in all decisions regarding the management of ADHD, discuss rather than lecture, listen and respond to the adolescent's concerns, and relate to the adolescent in an informal, authoritative but nonauthoritarian manner. Keeping these principles in mind, the clinician should give a brief definition of ADHD to the adolescent and then address the common concerns in Table 196-1. It is also helpful to connect an adolescent with peers successfully coping with ADHD. Educating parents about ADHD usually involves giving them a "crash course" in adolescent development, providing reading material on ADHD, and answering questions about it. Parents might also be referred to national support organizations for individuals with ADHD such as Children and Adults with Attention Deficit Disorder (CHADD: see www.chadd.org and www.help4adhd.org for details).

**MEDICATION**

For most adolescents with ADHD, medication is a necessary but not sufficient intervention for coping with ADHD. They need the "biological edge" provided by medication to pull their lives together at school, at home, and in the community. Because of the adolescent development issues noted previously, teenagers with ADHD often resist taking medication. Instead of trying to force medication on an adolescent, the skillful clinician should explain how medication provides chemicals needed by the brain for improved concentration and impulse control, describe its advantages and disadvantages, and offer the adolescent the choice to try medication. The physician should make it clear that the adolescent will be involved in every decision about medication. The adolescent should be encouraged to voice concerns about medication, which should be met with clear-cut information. If a teenager still refuses to try medication, this decision should be respected, but the physician should develop a written "performance contract" whereby the adolescent is asked to achieve goals for change in school and at home without medication over a few months, and if these goals are not achieved, to revisit the question of medication.

Stimulant medications remain first line agents to prescribe for adolescents with ADHD, followed by the nonstimulant atomoxetine as the second line agent. Because responses to each medication cannot be predicted reliably and vary from adolescent to adolescent, the decision regarding specific medication and dosing needs to be individualized following certain principles that universally apply. ADHD is a 24-hour disorder. Most adolescents with ADHD need the biological edge on self-control provided by medication 7 days per week, most of their waking hours. A combination of short- and long-acting stimulant medications are typically needed to achieve this goal. For such a medication regimen to be palatable, unpleasant side effects need to be kept to a

**Table 196-1**

**Adolescent Concerns about ADHD and Clinician Responses**

| *Adolescent Concern or Myth about ADHD* | *Clinician Responses* |
|---|---|
| I must be crazy if I have ADHD. | ADHD is not a mental illness. It is the way your brain is wired—it makes self-control over the mind and body difficult. |
| I will outgrow ADHD pretty soon. | ADHD changes as you grow but does not usually go away. |
| ADHD only has to do with school. | ADHD affects more than school—it also affects getting along with people, sports, health, driving. |
| Well, Doc, if ADHD is inherited and I have bad genes, then I don't have to do homework or chores. | ADHD is a challenge, not an excuse. |
| I must be stupid if I have ADHD. | ADHD has nothing to do with IQ. Some of the smartest people have ADHD. |
| I will lose my friends. They will think I'm a nerd. | If they really are your friends, they will stick by you. |
| I'll be forced to take medicine and become a "zombie." | No one can force you to take medicine. If you choose to take medicine, it will sharpen your focus, not make you a "zombie." |
| This ADHD thing is just one more way for my parents to control me. | The issue is not whether your parents are controlling you, but whether you can control yourself. |
| I will never have any fun because I will spend all my time seeing doctors, therapists, and tutors. | Doctors, therapists, and tutors usually take about 2 hours per week, only 1% of the hours in a week. |

minimum. Thus, the clinician needs to listen carefully to the adolescent's concerns about side effects and make adjustments to doses or changes in medication to minimize them.

Table 196-2[9] lists the commonly available stimulant medications and their lengths of action.

The positive and negative side effects of all these forms of stimulant medication are similar. They all increase concentration, reduce distractibility, enhance executive functions, increase impulse control, and decrease physical and mental restlessness. Side effects include appetite suppression, delayed sleep onset, headaches, and stomachaches. There have been concerns about stimulant medications promoting substance abuse, but research is now clear that treatment of ADHD with stimulant medication does not cause substance abuse. There is some evidence that long-term use of stimulant medication can slightly slow physical growth, so careful monitoring of growth is essential for adolescents treated with stimulants.

The adolescent should be started on a relatively low dose of a long-acting stimulant, and the dose should be increased every 3 days until the adolescent has tried 3 to 4 different doses of the medicine and can select the best dose. In the case of extended-release mixed salts of amphetamine, for example, the dose schedule might be 10, 15, 20, and 25 mg once a day for 3 days at each dose. Having tried different doses, the adolescent is in the best position to indicate which dose worked best. The rapid titration schedule is recommended because impatient adolescents lose interest in medication if they are kept on initial, ineffective doses for too long.

Clinicians should titrate stimulant medication based on feedback from the adolescent and parents, with some input from the teachers. Teenagers should be prompted to select "medication target behaviors" and monitor the performance of these behaviors on various doses of the selected stimulant. Reading a boring textbook, listening to a teacher, and remaining focused during homework time exemplify such medication target behaviors.

Atomoxetine (Strattera) is the primary nonstimulant medication indicated for ADHD. A selective norepinephrine uptake inhibitor, it has the potential advantages of 24-hour action and is dosed once per day. It takes several weeks to obtain an optimal effect, a disadvantage with adolescents who need a more immediate response in school or at home. Stomach upset and drowsiness are the 2 primary side effects of atomoxetine, but these can be minimized by taking it in the evening with food. Other nonstimulants sometimes used to treat adolescents with ADHD include bupropion (Wellbutrin), clonidine (Catepres), and guanfacine, now available as a short- and long-acting preparation. For specific dosing information and more details about using these medications with adolescents who have ADHD and/or comorbid conditions, the reader should consult the

**Table 196-2**

**Common Stimulant Formulations and Durations of Action**

| *Medication, generic description* | *Examples of commercial formulations* | *Approximate duration of action in hours* |
|---|---|---|
| Methylphenidate | Ritalin, Methylin, Metadate | 3–4 |
| Methylphenidate | Ritalin SR, Methylin ER, Metadate ER | 6–8 |
| Methylphenidate | Ritalin LA, Metadate CD | 8–9 |
| Methylphenidate | Concerta | 12 |
| Methylphenidate patch | Daytrana | 12+ |
| Dextromethylphenidate | Focalin | 4 |
| Dextromethylphenidate | Focalin XR | 8–12 |
| Dextroamphetamine | Dexedrine, Dextrostat | 4–6 |
| Mixed amphetamine salts | Adderall | 4–6 |
| Mixed amphetamine salts | Adderall XR | 8–12 |
| Lisdexamphetamine | Vyvanse | 12+ |

Reproduced with permission from Soileau EJ. Medication for adolescents with attention-deficit/hyperactivity disorder. *Adolescent Medicine: State of the Art Reviews.* 2008;19:254–267.

current literature, such as the monograph published by the American Academy of Pediatrics Section on Adolescent Health.[9]

### SCHOOL-RELATED INTERVENTIONS

Adolescents with ADHD commonly present with one or more of the following school difficulties: (1) failure to complete homework; (2) poor test preparation and test-taking skills; (3) poor organizational skills; (4) poor understanding of material; (5) poor classroom participation and failure to ask teachers for needed help; (6) disruptive behavior in the classroom; and/or (7) truancy. Many adolescents with ADHD also have associated learning disabilities in reading, written expression, or mathematics. As a result of these problems, they receive low grades on report cards and tests, get in trouble with teachers, and have seemingly endless conflicts over school with their parents.

Effective interventions for these school difficulties occur at multiple levels: (1) the adolescent medicine physician can make selected recommendations in an anticipatory guidance mode; (2) a psychologist or other therapist can help the family develop home-based interventions for homework, study, and related problems as well as help parents and adolescents advocate for school-based interventions; (3) school personnel can use behavioral and academic interventions in regular and special education classrooms to enhance academic success and improve social behavior for an individual adolescent; and (4) innovative school-wide programs can promote academic and social success for all youngsters with ADHD in a middle or high school. Most adolescents with ADHD need all 4 levels of intervention. An example of each level of intervention follows.

**Box 196-2**

***Advice to Parents Regarding Homework Completion***

- Prompt the adolescent to use a student planner regularly to record all assignments.
- Arrange for teachers to initial the planner daily.
- Periodically check the accuracy of the planner through contacts with teachers.
- Decide upon a regular time and quiet place to do homework.
- Prompt the adolescent once to start homework at the designated time.
- Check up on whether the adolescent is completing homework (every 15–20 minutes.)
- Break assignments into small chunks, permitting brief rests between chunks.
- Coach the adolescent to use a calendar to plan completion of projects and long-term assignments.
- Make sure medication is in effect during homework time.
- Coach the adolescent to put all completed assignments in the backpack in an organized fashion.
- Make a back-up of the files for any assignments done on a computer.
- Provide positive incentives for carrying out all of these steps.
- Arrange with the teachers to obtain a weekly report of the status of homework, preferably by e-mail.
- Ask for a second set of textbooks at home.

The adolescent medicine practitioner can provide the type of advice concerning homework contained in Box 196-2 during an office or clinic visit. A therapist can help the family implement homework strategies, deal with conflict around school issues, obtain a weekly home and school report of the status of the adolescent's assignments, and teach the adolescent study and organizational skills. School personnel can certify an adolescent as eligible either for an Individual Educational Plan under the Individuals with Disabilities Education Act or for accommodations under Section 504 of the Rehabilitation of the Handicapped Law. The student who has learning problems associated with ADHD can then access resource rooms, individual tutoring services, adjustments such as extended time for testing and note-taking assistance, or a variety of other helpful strategies. School personnel can also create programs that benefit all youngsters with ADHD in a middle or high school. The Challenging Horizons Program (CHP)[10] exemplifies an after-school program designed to foster academic success for all middle school youngsters with ADHD in a given middle school. Two to 3 days per week, each student participates after school in a homework management group, a study skills group, a social problem-solving group, and recreation. Each student also has an individual counselor who tailors these interventions to the student's needs and meets with the parents monthly. A series of studies with the CHP system demonstrated that it resulted in increased grades and improved social behavior.

### FAMILY INTERVENTIONS

Family interventions are designed to teach parents effective skills for parenting the adolescent with ADHD, improve the parent–adolescent relationship, reduce conflict, and ameliorate oppositional/defiant behavior. Such interventions are essential for adolescents who have ODD or CD in addition to ADHD. Behavior management training (BMT) for parents and problem-solving communication training (PSCT) for families are the 2 primary family interventions used to achieve these goals. Behavior management training involves teaching parents the systematic use of reinforcement and punishment contingencies to modify problem behaviors of their children. Problem-solving communication training involves teaching parents and adolescents to replace negative with positive communication behaviors and to negotiate mutually acceptable solutions to disagreements through the use of problem-solving steps. Two studies have demonstrated the effectiveness of these interventions in reducing parent–adolescent conflict for families with adolescents diagnosed with ADHD and ODD and suggested that a combination of BMT and PSCT works best.[11] The combined 18-session intervention, known as "the defiant teen approach," has been described in detail in 2 books[11,12] and is summarized next.

During the first portion of the "defiant teen" program, parents attend sessions without their adolescent. After a session focused on understanding the nature of coercive interchanges between parents and adolescents, the therapist first teaches the parents to conduct "one-on-one" time with their adolescent. Designed to restore positiveness in the parent–adolescent relationship, one-on-one time involves engaging the adolescent in an activity of his/her choice for 15 to 20 minutes, 5 to 6 times per week; the parent refrains from ordering, commanding, directing, or giving any negative feedback, instead simply enjoying time with the adolescent. Second, the therapist teaches the parents how to "catch the adolescent being good" and frequently praise appropriate behaviors while ignoring minor negative behaviors. Third, as the parents use one-on-one time and contingent praise regularly, they are taught to give short, clear, effective commands. Fourth, the therapist spends several sessions helping parents successfully implement positive incentives in the form of point systems and behavior "contracts" to encourage the adolescent to comply with instructions, complete chores, homework, and self-care tasks. Only when positive incentive systems have taken hold does the therapist introduce the fifth step, punishment systems such as taking away privileges and groundings.

During the second portion of the intervention the parents and the adolescent attend all of the sessions together. A distinction is made between nonnegotiable issues (bottom line rules for living in civilized society such as no violence, no drugs, no alcohol, attend school) and negotiable issues (everything else). Parents are coached to rely upon behavior management to handle nonnegotiable issues. The therapist uses instructions, modeling, behavior rehearsal, and feedback to teach the family the 4 steps of problem solving to resolve negotiable issues: (1) *define the problem:* each person makes a short, clear nonaccusatory statement of the problem; (2) *generate the solutions*: the adolescent starts, and then each person takes a turn brainstorming creative ideas to solve the problem; (3) *evaluate the solutions and reach an agreement:* again starting with the adolescent, each person rates each solution "plus" or "minus," and then the family reaches an agreement on those solutions endorsed by everyone; and (4) *plan to implement the solution:* the family discusses what has to be done to carry out the agreed-upon solution(s). After the family has learned problem solving, the therapist switches the emphasis to communication training. Common negative communication patterns such as accusations, criticisms, interrupting, poor eye contact, and lecturing are identified, and the therapist prompts the family to practice replacing them with more positive, alternative responses.

### OTHER INTERVENTIONS

Adolescents who have anxiety or depression in addition to ADHD need additional interventions. Cognitive behavioral therapy is the psychological treatment of choice for anxiety or depression. Pharmacological interventions with antidepressant medication may also be indicated.

The use of CAM for the treatment of ADHD has increased by parents and health care providers in recent years. Even though there are limited data and research on many of these CAM therapies as sole treatments for ADHD, some of these therapies are considered safe, with potential for few side effects, and they may be effective as adjunctive therapies.[13] Complementary and alternative medicine therapies that might be useful adjuncts include: mind-body therapies such as yoga/meditation, biofeedback, hypnotherapy, and massage; some nutritional supplements, such as omega 3-essential fatty acids; and certain herbs such as chamomile, melatonin, valerian, and St John's wort. Asking about CAM use needs to be a part of the ADHD evaluation.

## CONCLUSIONS

The adolescent medicine practitioner is often on the front line when it comes to identifying and treating ADHD. It is important to become familiar with the many different ways in which ADHD may present and to screen for it as needed. Interviews, rating scales, and psychological tests are the 3 methods used to evaluate adolescents for ADHD. After diagnosing ADHD, the clinician should educate the patient and the parents about it, and if the patient is willing to try medication, prescribe a rapidly increasing titration schedule of a long-acting stimulant. The adolescent should be referred to the school for educational interventions and to a psychologist or other mental health professional for individual and family interventions. Psychological interventions are especially important for addressing the many comorbid conditions that accompany ADHD. Complementary and alternative medicine may also be suggested as an adjunctive intervention.

## REFERENCES

1. Faraone SV, Sergeant J, Gillberg C, Biederman J. The worldwide prevalence of ADHD: is it an American condition? *World Psychiatry.* 2003;2(2):104–113

2. Robin AL. *ADHD in Adolescents: Diagnosis and Treatment.* New York, NY: Guilford Press; 1998

3. American Psychiatric Association. *Diagnostic and Statistical Manual of Mental Disorders.* 4th ed. Text Revision. Washington, DC: American Psychiatric Association; 2000

4. Wolraich ML, Lambert W, Doffing MA, Bickman L. Psychometric properties of the Vanderbilt ADHD diagnostic parent rating scale in a referred population. *J Ped Psych.* 2003;28(8):559–568

5. Conners CK. *Conners Manual.* 3rd ed. Toronto, Ontario: Multi-Health Systems; 2008

6. Robin AL, Koepke T, Moye A. *Parent Adolescent Relationship Questionnaire.* Lutz, FL: Psychological Assessment Resources; 2009

7. Wechsler D. *Wechsler Intelligence Scale for Children.* 4th ed. San Antonio, TX: The Psychological Corporation; 2003

8. Wechsler D. *Wechsler Individual Achievement Test.* 2nd ed. San Antonio, TX: The Psychological Corporation; 2002

9. Soileau EJ. Medications for adolescents with attention- deficit/hyperactivity disorder. *AM:STARs.* 2008;19:254–267

10. DuPaul GJ, Evans SW. School-based interventions for adolescents with attention-deficit/hyperactivity disorder. *AM:STARs.* 2008;19:300–312

11. Barkley RA, Edwards G, Robin AL. *Defiant Teens: A Clinician's Manual for Family Assessment and Intervention.* New York, NY: Guilford Press; 1999

12. Barkley RA, Robin AL, Benton C. *Your Defiant Teen.* New York, NY: Guilford Press; 2008

13. Sawni A. Attention-deficit/hyperactivity disorder and complementary/alternative medicine. *AM:STARs.* 2008;19: 313–326

# Index

## C

## E

## F

## G

## J

## K



## L

## Q



## R

## W

## X



## Y



## Z